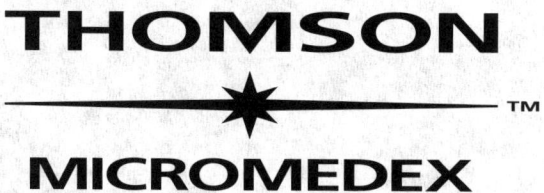

THOMSON

MICROMEDEX

Volume II

Advice
for the Patient®
Drug
Information in
Lay Language

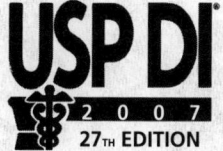

USP DI®

2007

27TH EDITION

NOTICE AND WARNING

Read the "To the Reader" section before consulting individual monographs.

The inclusion in *USP Dispensing Information (USP DI®)* of a monograph on any drug in respect to which patent or trademark rights may exist shall not be deemed, and is not intended as, a grant of, or authority to exercise, any rights or privilege protected by such patent or trademark. All such rights and privileges are vested in the patent or trademark owner, and no other person may exercise the same without express permission, authority, or license secured from such patent or trademark owner.

The listing of selected brand names is intended only for ease of reference. The inclusion of a brand name does not mean the authors have any particular knowledge that the brand listed has properties different from other brands of the same drug, nor should it be interpreted as an endorsement. Similarly, the fact that a particular brand has not been included does not indicate that the product has been judged to be unsatisfactory or unacceptable.

Attention is called to the fact that all volumes of *USP Dispensing Information* are fully copyrighted: Volume I *—Drug Information for the Health Care Professional;* Volume II—*Advice for the Patient®;* Volume III—*Approved Drug Products and Legal Requirements.*

For permission to copy or utilize limited excerpts of this text, address inquiries to *USP DI* Reprint Requests, Thomson Micromedex, 6200 S. Syracuse Way, Suite 300, Greenwood Village, CO 80111.

Physicians, pharmacists, nurses, and other health practitioners are hereby given permission to reproduce a limited number of one or more pages of advice from the *Advice for the Patient* volume of *USP DI* but only when for direct distribution, without charge, to their patients or clients receiving the prescribed drug, provided that such reproduction shall include the copyright notice appearing on the pages from which it was copied.

Library of Congress Catalog Card Number 81-640842
ISBN 1-56363-575-5
ISSN 0740-4174

Printed by Quebecor World, Versailles, Kentucky 40383.
Published & distributed by Thomson Micromedex, 6200 S. Syracuse Way, Suite 300, Greenwood Village, CO 80111.

PIMECROLIMUS (Topical route) - pim-e-KROE-li-mus

Black Box Warning

Long-term safety of topical calcineurin inhibitors has not been established. Although a causal relationship has not been established, rare cases of malignancy (e.g., skin and lymphoma) have been reported in patients treated with topical calcineurin inhibitors, including pimecrolimus cream. Therefore:

Continuous long-term use of topical calcineurin inhibitors, including pimecrolimus cream, in any age group should be avoided, and application limited to areas of involvement with atopic dermatitis. Pimecrolimus cream is not indicated for use in children less than 2 years of age.

Commonly used brand name(s)

In the U.S.—
Elidel

Available Dosage Forms:
• Cream

Therapeutic Class: Dermatological Agent

Uses For This Medicine

Pimecrolimus cream is used for mild to moderate atopic dermatitis. This is a skin condition where there is itching, redness and inflammation, much like an allergic reaction. Pimecrolimus helps to suppress these symptoms which are a reaction caused by the body's immune system. It can be used for short-term or long-term periodic treatment (not beyond one year). It is often used when other types of treatment are either not working or when you cannot tolerate other types of treatment.

Pimecrolimus is available only with your doctor's prescription.

Once a medicine has been approved for marketing for a certain use, experience may show that it is also useful for other medical problems. Although this use is not included in product labeling, pimecrolimus is used in certain patients with the following medical condition:

• Atopic dermatitis in children less than 2 years of age

Before Using This Medicine

In deciding to use a medicine, the risks of taking the medicine must be weighed against the good it will do. This is a decision you and your doctor will make. For this medicine, the following should be considered:

Allergies—Tell your doctor if you have ever had any unusual or allergic reaction to this medicine or any other medicines. Also tell your health care professional if you have any other types of allergies, such as to foods, dyes, preservatives, or animals. For non-prescription products, read the label or package ingredients carefully.

Pediatric—This medicine is not known to cause different types of side effects or problems in children over the age of two, than it does in adults, although some side effects may occur more often than they do in adult patients. This medicine has not been tested and should not be used in children under 2 years of age.

Geriatric—There is no specific information comparing the use of pimecrolimus in the elderly with the use in other age groups. Pimecrolimus is not expected to cause different side effects or problems in older people than it does in younger adults.

Pregnancy—

	Pregnancy Category	Explanation
All Trimesters	C	Animal studies have shown an adverse effect and there are no adequate studies in pregnant women OR no animal studies have been conducted and there are no adequate studies in pregnant women.

Breast Feeding—There are no adequate studies in women for determining infant risk when using this medication during breastfeeding. Weigh the potential benefits against the potential risks before taking this medication while breastfeeding.

Other medicines—Although certain medicines should not be used together at all, in other cases two different medicines may be used together even if an interaction might occur. In these cases, your doctor may want to change the dose, or other precautions may be necessary. Tell your healthcare professional if you are taking any other prescription or non-prescription (over-the-counter [OTC]) medicine.

Interactions with Food/Tobacco/Alcohol—Certain medicines should not be used at or around the time of eating food or eating certain types of food since interactions may occur. Using alcohol or tobacco with certain medicines may also cause interactions to occur. Discuss with your healthcare professional the use of your medicine with food, alcohol, or tobacco.

Other medical problems—The presence of other medical problems may affect the use of this medicine. Make sure you tell your doctor if you have any other medical problems, especially:

• Eczema herpeticum (Kaposi's varicelliform eruption), or
• Herpes simplex virus infection or
• Varicella zoster virus infection (chicken pox or shingles) — Increases the risk of skin infections
• Erythroderma (exfoliative dermatitis [ED]) — The safety of this medicine is not known for patients who have this condition.
• Immunocompromised patients (weakened immune system) — The safety of these patients using pimecrolimus cream has not been established.
• Lymphadenopathy or
• Mononucleosis, acute infectious — May cause enlargement of lymph nodes
• Netherton's syndrome — May cause too much of the pimecrolimus cream to be absorbed into the body
• Precancerous condition of the skin or
• Skin cancer — You should not use this medicine.
• Skin infections — Safety of using pimecrolimus cream for some skin infections is unknown.
• Skin papilloma or
• Warts — May worsen condition

Proper Use of This Medicine

Dosing—The dose of this medicine will be different for different patients. Follow your doctor's orders or the directions on the label. The following information includes only the average doses of this medicine. If your dose is different, do not change it unless your doctor tells you to do so.

The amount of medicine that you take depends on the strength of the medicine. Also, the number of doses you take each day, the time allowed between doses, and the length of time you take the medicine depend on the medical problem for which you are using the medicine.

Infections in the affected areas should be treated before starting treatment with pimecrolimus cream.

Apply a thin layer of pimecrolimus cream and rub it in well to cover the affected areas.

Do not use this medicine in the eyes and do not swallow it.

Wash hands thoroughly after applying pimecrolimus cream, unless your hands are part of the area for treatment.

Use of this medicine may cause reactions at the site of application such as a mild to moderate feeling of warmth and/or sensation of burning. You should contact your doctor if this reaction is severe or persists for more than 1 week.

While using pimecrolimus, if symptoms of your skin condition go away, consult your doctor.

If after your doctor tells you to stop using pimecrolimus, your skin condition reoccurs, consult your doctor.

Do not use any occlusive dressings (a dressing that seals the area that is being treated such as a plastic exercise suit or plastic wraps used to store foods).

Do not bathe, shower or swim right after applying this medicine. This could wash off the cream.

• For cream dosage form
  ○ For atopic dermatitis
    • Adults — Gently apply cream to skin that is clean and dry two times a day. Stop using when the signs and symptoms of eczema, such as itching, rash, and redness go away, as directed by your doctor.
    • Children over 2 years old — Gently apply cream to skin that is clean and dry two times a day. Stop using when the signs and symptoms of eczema, such as itching, rash, and redness go away, as directed by your doctor.
    • Children under 2 years of age — Use and dose must be determined by your doctor.

Storage—Store the medicine in a closed container at room temperature, away from heat, moisture, and direct light. Keep from freezing.

Keep out of the reach of children.

Do not keep outdated medicine or medicine no longer needed.

Ask your healthcare professional how you should dispose of any medicine you do not use.

Precautions While Using This Medicine

It is very important that your doctor check your progress at regular visits. Your doctor will want to make sure the pimecrolimus cream is working properly and to check for unwanted

effects. If your condition has not improved after 6 weeks, your doctor will want to reexamine you.

Report any adverse reactions or side effects to your doctor or if your skin condition seems to be getting worse.

Use this medicine only for the condition for which it was prescribed by your doctor.

You should not use this medicine beyond a year.

Exposure to natural or artificial sunlight should be minimized or avoided.

• Stay out of direct sunlight, especially between the hours of 10:00 a.m. and 3:00 p.m., if possible.
• Wear protective clothing, including a hat. Also, wear sunglasses.
• Apply a sun block product that has a skin protection factor (SPF) of at least 15. Some people may require a product with a higher SPF number, especially if they have a fair complexion. If you have any questions about this, check with your health care professional.
• Apply a sun block lipstick that has an SPF of at least 15 to protect your lips.
• Do not use a sunlamp or tanning bed or booth.

Side Effects of This Medicine

Along with its needed effects, a medicine may cause some unwanted effects. Although not all of these side effects may occur, if they do occur they may need medical attention.

Check with your doctor as soon as possible if any of the following side effects occur:

More common
  Abdominal or stomach pain; body aches or pain; burning, itching, redness, skin rash, swelling, or soreness at site; change in hearing; chills; cold or flu-like symptoms; congestion, ear or nasal; cough producing mucus; diarrhea; difficulty breathing or shortness of breath; dryness or soreness of throat; earache or pain in ear, ear drainage; fever; general feeling of discomfort or illness; headache; hoarseness; itching; joint pain; loss of appetite; loss of voice; muscle aches and pains; nausea; pain; redness; runny nose; shivering; sneezing; sore throat; sweating; swelling; tenderness; tender, swollen glands in neck; tightness in chest, wheezing; trouble in swallowing; trouble sleeping; unusual tiredness or weakness; voice changes; vomiting; warmth on skin

Less common
  Blistering, crusting, irritation, itching, or reddening of skin; blurred vision or other change in vision; eye pain; fast heartbeat; hives; hives or welts, itching, redness of skin; hoarseness; itching; itchy, raised, round, smooth, skin-colored bumps found on just one area of the body that are oozing, thick, white fluid; irritation; joint pain, stiffness or swelling; rash; redness of eye; redness of skin; sensitivity of eye to light; shortness of breath; skin rash on face, scalp, or stomach; swelling of eyelids, face, lips, hands, or feet; tearing; tightness in chest; troubled breathing or swallowing; wheezing

Incidence not known
  Black, tarry stools; change in size, shape or color of existing mole; cough; dizziness; itching, puffiness or swelling of the eyelids or around the eyes, face, lips or tongue; large, hive-like swelling on face; mole that

How to use Volume II

This book provides information about prescription and over-the-counter medicines. It is written in everyday language, making it a valuable reference guide for consumers.

On this page, you'll find general information about how to use this book. An illustration showing how the listings are organized appears on the back of this page.

About the entries

The drug entries are arranged alphabetically like an encyclopedia. **If you already know which entry the drug belongs to,** you can turn directly to it.

If you know only the drug's generic or brand name, the best way to find your information is to use the index at the front of this book. It will tell you which entry includes that drug and the page number on which the entry starts.

For more information

For general guidelines about medicines, see *To the Reader* (page v), which also discusses this book's content in-depth. In addition to the entries, this book contains general information about the use of medicines, a glossary with over 400 medical terms plus a four-color medicine chart and the following supplemental appendixes:

▶ *Excluded Monograph Listing*

▶ *Poison Control Center Listing*

▶ *Pregnancy Precaution Listing*

▶ *Breast-feeding Precaution Listing*

See illustration on the back of this page.

Contents

USP DI–Volume II
Advice for the Patient

To The Reader

When purchasing a medicine, whether over-the-counter (nonprescription) or with a doctor's prescription, you may have questions about its usefulness to you, the best way to take it, possible side effects, and precautions to take to avoid complications. For instance, some medicines should be taken with meals, others between meals. Some may make you drowsy while others may tend to keep you awake. Alcoholic or other beverages, other medicines, certain foods, or smoking may affect the way your medicine works. As for side effects, some are merely bothersome and may go away while others may require medical attention.

Advice for the Patient contains information that may provide general answers to some of your questions as well as suggestions for the correct use of your medicine. *It is important to remember, however, that the human body is very complex and medicines may act differently on different people—and even in the same person at different times. If you want additional information about your medicine or its possible side effects, ask your doctor, nurse, pharmacist, or other health care provider. They are there to help you.*

Notice:

The information about the drugs contained herein is general in nature and is intended to be used in consultation with your health care providers. It is not intended to replace specific instructions or directions or warnings given to you by your physician or other prescriber or accompanying a particular product. The information is selective and it is not claimed that it includes all known precautions, contraindications, effects, or interactions possibly related to the use of a drug. The information may differ from that contained in the product labeling which is required by law. The information is not sufficient to make an evaluation as to the risks and benefits of taking a particular drug in a particular case and is not medical advice for individual problems and should not alone be relied upon for these purposes. Since the inclusion or exclusion of particular information about a drug is judgmental in nature and since opinion as to drug usage may differ, you may wish to consult additional sources. Should you desire additional information or if you have any questions as to how this information may relate to you in particular, ask your doctor, nurse, pharmacist, or other health care provider.

Since new drugs are constantly being marketed and since previously unreported side effects, newly recognized precautions, or other new information for any given drug may come to light at any time, continuously updated drug information sources should be consulted as necessary.

There are many brands of drugs on the market. The listing of selected brand names is intended only for ease of reference. The inclusion of a brand name does not mean the authors have any particular knowledge that the brand listed has properties different from other brands of the same drug, nor should it be interpreted as an endorsement. Similarly, the fact that a brand name has not been included does not indicate that that particular brand has been judged to be unsatisfactory or unacceptable.

If any of the information in this book causes you special concern, do not decide against taking any medicine prescribed for you without first checking with your doctor.

How To Use This Book

Advice for the Patient contains a section of general information about the appropriate use of any medicine, as well as individual discussions of a wide variety of commonly and not so commonly used medicines. *You should read both the general information and the information specific to the medicine you are taking.* See page G-1 for this general information.

Each medicine has a generic name that all manufacturers who make that medicine must use. Some manufacturers also create a brand name to put on the label and to use in advertising. *Look in the index* for the generic name or the brand name of the medicine about which you have questions. We have put the generic names and common brand names in the same index, so you do not have to know whether the name you have is a generic name or a brand name. However, it is a good idea for you to learn both the generic and the brand names of the medicines you are using and to write them down and keep them for future use.

Although the informational entries generally appear in alphabetical order by generic name, there are numerous occasions when closely related medicines are grouped under a family name. Therefore, the surest way to quickly find the page number of the information about each medicine is to *look in the index first.*

The information for each medicine is presented according to the route of administration (i.e., how the medicine is taken or used). As a general rule, dosing, precautionary, and side effect information may not be the same as for other types of use. For example, if you take tetracycline capsules by mouth to treat an infection, the information will not be the same as for tetracycline ointment which is applied directly to the skin. And both of these will be different from the information for tetracyclines used in the eye. The common routes used in this publication are:

- *BUCCAL MUCOSA*—For systemic (e.g., general effects throughout the body) when a medicine is placed in the cheek pocket, allowed to dissolve, and slowly absorbed.
- *DENTAL*—For local effects when applied to the teeth or gums.
- *INHALATION*—For local, and in some cases systemic, effects when inhaled into the lungs.
- *INJECTION*—For general effects throughout the body when a medicine is injected in the skin (given as a shot).
- *INTRACAVERNOSAL*—For local effects in the penis when a medicine is given by injection.

- *LINGUAL*—For general effects throughout the body when a medicine is absorbed through the lining of the mouth
- *MUCOUS MEMBRANE*—For local effects when applied directly to mucous membranes (for example, the inside of the mouth)
- *NASAL*—For local effects when used in the nose
- *OPHTHALMIC*—For local effects when applied directly to the eyes.
- *ORAL*—For general effects throughout the body when a medicine is taken by mouth.
- *OTIC*—For local effects when used in the ear..
- *RECTAL*—For local, and in some cases systemic, effects when used in the rectum.
- *SUBLINGUAL*—For general effects throughout the body when a medicine is placed under the tongue, allowed to dissolve, and slowly absorbed.
- *TOPICAL*—For local effects when applied directly to the skin.
- *VAGINAL*—For local, and in some cases systemic, effects when used in the vagina.

About *USP DI*

USP DI was first published in 1980 by the Untied States Pharmacopeia. In September of 1998, the USP Board of Trustees entered into agreements with MICROMEDEX for the sale of the USP DI Volume I and Volume II databases and licensing of the USP DI trademarks. At that time, USP continued to have editorial involvement in the creation of the drug monographs. As of May 2004, MICROMEDEX and USP modified their relationship. MICROMEDEX now has sole editorial responsibility for this content. USP DI is continuously reviewed and revised by a staff of distinguished physicians, pharmacists, nurses, toxicologists and other healthcare specialists ensuring the most current and accurate data is presented.

Advice for the Patient® is Volume II of *USP DI*. Volume I contains drug use information in technical language for the physician, dentist, pharmacist, nurse, or other health care provider, and Volume II is its lay language counterpart for use by consumers. Volume III provides information on approved drug products and legal requirements. Together, the volumes form the foundation of a coordinated approach to drug-use education.

About MICROMEDEX

Since 1974, MICROMEDEX, headquartered in Greenwood Village, Colorado, has been the leading provider of clinical information and decision support tools within the healthcare community. Today, in over 9,000 facilities and more than 90 countries, MICROMEDEX knowledge bases are relied upon to provide current, comprehensive information on drugs, diseases, toxicology, alternative medicine, and patient education.

For further information about *USP DI* or to comment on how the information published in this volume might better meet your information needs, please contact: MICROMEDEX, 6200 S. Syracuse Way, Suite 300, Greenwood Village, CO 80111; telephone (303) 486-6400; telefax (303) 486-6464; or access support via the web at http://www.micromedex.com/support/request/. There are drugs for which monographs are not included in this published version of the *USP DI* database due to space constraints. Copies of the monographs are available on the MICROMEDEX website. See the inside front cover of this book for details on how to access the site.

Index Guide

Index

The following excerpts are examples of the information included in the Index:

Brand name – manufacturer brand name is identified by *italics*.

    Lanoxin — 556

Combination Listing – Includes a series of ingredients that act together.

    Propoxyphene, Aspirin, and Caffeine —1069

Drug Effect/Route – Identifies the drug's effect on the body and/or administration. It is identified by parenthesis (e.g., topical route, oral route, otic, nasal route, systemic). A systemic effect would affect the entire body, topical route- the skin, otic route - the ears, nasal route- the nose, ophthalmic route- the eyes, etc.

    Mometasone (Nasal)

Family Monograph Title – Groups multiple drugs into a common grouping. A reference to a family monograph typically appears in bold.

    Calcium Channel Blocking Agents (Systemic), 3265

Generic or common name – Identified by bold.

    Fexofenadine (oral route), 697

Page number - Identifies the location of the drug entry in the first page of a drug entry.

    Relafen —171

Pound sign – Identifies a drug not published in the printed version of the *USP DI*. Exclusions can be accessed on the *USP DI* Updates Online website. See the front cover of book for details on accessing the site.

    Talc (Intrapleural-route), **#**

Single Entry Title - Includes one drug; each drug may have multiple brand names and common names but only one generic name.

    Celecoxib (oral route), 358

Index

Brand names are in *italics*. There are many brands of drugs and the listing of selected American and Canadian brand names in this index are intended only for ease of reference. There are additional brands that have not been included in the book. The inclusion of a brand name does not mean the authors have any particular knowledge that the brand listed has properties different from other brands of the same drug, nor should it be interpreted as an endorsement. Similarly, the fact that a particular brand has not been included does not indicate that the product has been judged to be unsatisfactory or unacceptable.

\# — Drugs for which monographs are not included in this published version of the *USP DI* database due to space constraints. Copies of the monographs are available on the MICROMEDEX *USP DI* Updates Online website. See the front cover of this book for details on how to access the site.

Apidra, 911
Aplicare One Tincture Of Iodine, #
Aplisol, 1609
Apo-Acetazolamide, 344
Apo-Alpraz, 237
Apo-Amitriptyline, 120
Apo-Amoxi Sugar-Free, 1280
Apo-Amoxi, 1280
Apo-Asa, 1442
Apo-ASEN, 1442
Apo-Benztropine, 126
Apo-Bisacodyl, 973
Apo-Bisacodyl, 979
Apo-Cal, 323
Apo-Cefaclor, 361
Apo-Chlordiazepoxide, 237
Apo-Chlorthalidone, 589
Apo-Cimetidine, 853
Apo-Clonazepam, 237
Apo-Clorazepate, 237
Apo-Cloxi, 1280
Apo-Cyclosporine, 500
Apo-Diazepam, 237
Apo-Diclo, 164
Apo-Diflunisal, 164
Apo-Diltiaz, 318
Apo-Dimenhydrinate, 141
Apo-Doxy, 1543
Apo-Doxy-Tabs, 1543
Apo-Erythro E-C, 669
Apo-Erythro, 669
Apo-Erythro-ES, 669
Apo-Erythro-S, 669
Apo-Famotidine, 853
Apo-Ferrous Gluconate, 937
Apo-Ferrous Sulfate, 937
Apo-Fluphenazine, 1302
Apo-Flurazepam, 237
Apo-Flurbiprofen, 164
Apo-Gain, 1102
Apo-Haloperidol, 839
Apo-Hydro, 589
Apo-Hydroxyzine, 141
Apo-Ibuprofen, 164
Apo-Imipramine, 120
Apo-Indomethacin, 164
Apo-ISDN, 1194
Apo-ISDN, 1196
Apo-K, 1334
Apo-Keto, 164
Apo-Keto-E, 164
Apo-Lorazepam, 237
Apo-Megestrol, 1363
Apo-Minocycline, 1543
Apomorphine (Injection Route), 181
Apo-Napro-Na DS, 164
Apo-Napro-Na, 164
Apo-Naproxen, 164
Apo-Nifed, 318
Apo-Oxazepam, 237
Apo-Oxtriphylline, 290
Apo-Pen-Vk, 1280
Apo-Perphenazine, 1302
Apo-Phenylbutazone, 164
Apo-Piroxicam, 164
Apo-Prednisone, 461
Apo-Salvent, 278
Apo-Sulfamethoxazole, 1494
Apo-Sulfatrim DS, 1498
Apo-Sulfatrim, 1498
Apo-Sulfisoxazole, 1494
Apo-Sulin, 164

Apo-Temazepam, 237
Apo-Tenoxicam, 164
Apo-Tetra, 1543
Apo-Theo LA, 290
Apo-Thioridazine, 1302
Apo-Timop, #
Apo-Tobramycin, 1571
Apo-Triazide, 586
Apo-Triazo, 237
Apo-Trifluoperazine, 1302
Apo-Trihex, 126
Apo-Trimip, 120
Apo-Verap, 318
Appearex, #
Appetite Suppressants, Sympathomimetic (Systemic), 182
Apra, 12
Apraclonidine (Ophthalmic Route), 186
Aprepitant (Oral Route), 188
Apresoline, 860
Aprobarbital, 223
Aqua Gem-E, 1644
Aquachloral Supprettes, #
AquaMEPHYTON, 1646
Aquasol A, 1636
Aquasol E, 1644
Aquatensen, 589
Aralast, #
Aralen Phosphate, 382
Aranesp, 524
Arava, 981
Arcet, 300
Arco Pain Tablet, 1442
Ardeparin (Subcutaneous Route), #
Aredia, 1257
Aricept, 600
Arimidex, 77
Aripiprazole (Oral Route), 189
Aristocort A, 468
Aristocort C, 468
Aristocort D, 468
Aristocort Forte, 461
Aristocort Intralesional, 461
Aristocort R, 468
Aristocort, 468
Aristocort, 461
Aristopak, 461
Aristospan, 461
Arixtra, 780
Arm-a-Med Isoetharine, 278
Arm-a-Med Metaproterenol, 278
Armour Thyroid, 1554
Aromasin, 717
Aromatic Ammonia Spirit (Inhalation, Oral/Nebulization Route), #
Arsenic Trioxide (Intravenous Route), #
Artane Sequels, 126
Artane, 126
Arthricare For Women, 333
Arthrisin, 1442
Arthritis Pain Ascriptin, 1442
Arthritis Pain Formula, 1442
Arthritis Strength Bufferin, 1442
Arthropan, 1442
Arthrotec, 552
Articaine, #
Articulose-50, 461
Articulose-L.A., 461
Artria S.R, 1442
Asacol 800, 1056
Asacol, 1056
Ascarel, #

Ascocid, 191
Ascomp with Codeine No.3, 229
Ascorbic Acid (Oral Route), 191
Asendin, 120
Asmalix, 290
Asmanex Twist, 1117
Asparaginase (Injection Route), 194
A-Spas S/L, 102
Aspergum, 1442
Aspirin and Caffeine, 1442
Aspirin and Codeine, 1146
Aspirin And Dipyridamole (Oral Route), 196
Aspirin Caplets, 1442
Aspirin Children's Tablets, 1442
Aspirin Plus Stomach Guard Extra Strength, 1442
Aspirin Plus Stomach Guard Regular Strength, 1442
Aspirin Regimen Bayer Adult Low Dose, 1442
Aspirin Regimen Bayer Regular Strength Caplets, 1442
Aspirin Tablets, 1442
Aspirin, 1442
Aspirin, Caffeine, and Dihydrocodeine, 1146
Aspirin, Coated, 1442
Aspirin, Codeine, and Caffeine, 1146
Aspirin, Codeine, and Caffeine, Buffered, 1146
Aspirin, Sodium Bicarbonate, And Citric Acid (Oral Route), 198
Aspir-Low, 1442
Aspirtab, 1442
Aspirtab-Max, 1442
Assure Sore Throat, #
Astelin Ready-Spray, 212
Astelin, 212
Asthmahaler Mist, 278
AsthmaNefrin, 278
Astone, 1442
Astracaine 4% Forte, #
Astracaine 4%, #
Astramorph PF, 1133
Astramorph PF, 1140
Astramorph, 1140
Astrin, 1442
Atacand HCT, #
Atacand, 327
Atarax, 141
Atasol, 12
Atasol-15, 1142
Atasol-30, 1142
Atasol-8, 1142
Atazanavir Sulfate (Oral Route), 201
Atenolol and Chlorthalidone, #
Athlete's Foot Gel, #
Ativan, 237
Atomoxetine (Oral Route), 202
Atorvastatin (Oral Route), 204
Atovaquone (Oral Route), #
Atovaquone And Chloroguanide (Oral Route), #
Atridox, #
Atrohist Pediatric Suspension Dye Free, 147
Atrohist Pediatric, 147
Atropair, #
Atropine and Phenobarbital, #
Atropine Care, #
Atropine Sulfate S.O.P., #

Atropine, 102
Atropine, #
Atropine, Homatropine, and Scopolamine (Ophthalmic), #
Atropine, Hyoscyamine, Methenamine, Methylene Blue, Phenyl Salicylate, And Benzoic Acid (Oral Route), #
Atropine, Hyoscyamine, Scopolamine, and Phenobarbital, #
Atropisol, #
Atrosulf, #
Atrovent, 930
Atrovent, 927
Attapulgite (Oral Route), #
Attenuvax, 1029
Augmentin, 1286
Auranofin, #
Aureomycin, #
Aurodex, 177
Aurothioglucose, #
Auroto, 177
Avage, 1522
Avandamet, 1436
Avandia, 1433
Avapro, 932
Avastin, 260
AVC, 1496
Aveeno Anti-Itch, #
Avelox I.V., 752
Avelox, 752
Aventyl, 120
AVINZA, 1133
Avita, 1598
Avodart, 625
Avonex, 917
Avosil, #
Axert, #
Axid Ar, 853
Axid Pulvules, 853
Axid, 853
Axotal, 303
Axsain, 333
Aygestin, 1363
Azacitidine (Subcutaneous Route), 207
Azactam, 217
Azasan, 208
Azatadine and Pseudoephedrine, 147
Azatadine, 141
Azathioprine (Oral Route, Intravenous Route), 208
Azelaic Acid (Topical Route), 211
Azelastine (Nasal Route), 212
Azelastine (Ophthalmic Route), 214
Azelex, 211
Azilect, 1389
Azithromycin (Intravenous Route), 215
Azmacort, 452
Azo Gantanol, #
Azo Gantrisin, #
Azo-Gesic, 1300
Azopt 1%, #
Azopt, #
Azo-Septic, 1300
Azo-Standard, 1300
Azo-Sulfamethoxazole, #
Azo-Sulfisoxazole, #
Azo-Truxazole, #
Aztreonam (Intravenous Route, Injection Route), 217
Azulfidine Entabs, 1491
Azulfidine, 1491

B

Babee Cof Syrup, 547
Baby Gasz, 1466
Bacillus Of Calmette And Guerin Vaccine, Live (Intradermal Route), #
Bacillus Of Calmette And Guerin Vaccine, Live (Intravesical Route), #
Bacitracin-Neomycin-Polymyxin, 1168
Bacitracin-Neomycin-Polymyxin, 1169
Backache Caplets, 1442
Baclofen (Intrathecal Route), 218
Baclofen (Oral Route), 220
Bactine, 466
Bactocill, 1280
Bactrim DS, 1498
Bactrim I.V., 1498
Bactrim Pediatric, 1498
Bactrim, 1498
Bactroban, #
Bactroban, 1122
Baldex, #
Balsalazide (Oral Route), 222
Bancap, 300
Bancap-HC, 1142
Banophen Caplets, 141
Banophen, 141
Banthine, 102
Baraclude, 648
Barbidonna No. 2, #
Barbidonna, #
Barbita, 223
Barbiturates (Systemic), 223
Barbiturates, Aspirin, and Codeine (Systemic), 229
Baridium, 1300
Barium Sulfate (Oral Route, Rectal Route), 233
Baro-Cat, 233
Barophen, #
Barosperse Enema, 233
Barriere-HC, 466
Bar-Test, 233
Basaljel, 93
Basaljel, 93
Basiliximab (Intravenous Route), #
Bayer Children's Aspirin, 1442
Bayer Select Ibuprofen Pain Relief Formula Caplets, 164
Bayer Select Maximum Strength Backache Pain Relief Formula, 1442
Baygam, 888
Bayhep B, 850
Bayrab, #
Bayrho-D, #
Baytet, 1541
Baza Antifungal, 1091
BCG Vaccine Freeze Dried, #
BCG Vaccine, #
Beben, 468
Bebulin Vh, #
Becaplermin (Topical Route), 234
Because, 1482
Beclodisk, 452
Becloforte, 452
Beclomethasone, 452
Beclomethasone, 457
Beclomethasone, 468
Beclovent Rotacaps, 452
Beclovent, 452
Beconase AQ, 457
Beconase, 457

Bedoz, #
Belcomp-PB, 842
Belladonna Alkaloids and Barbiturates (Systemic), #
Belladonna and Butabarbital, #
Belladonna, 102
Bellalphen, #
Benadryl Allergy Decongestant Liquid Medication, 147
Benadryl Allergy, 141
Benadryl Allergy/Sinus Headache Caplets, 151
Benadryl, 141
Benadryl, #
Benazepril and Hydrochlorothiazide, #
Bendroflumethiazide, 589
Benefix, #
Benemid, 1348
Benicar HCT, 1215
Benicar, 1217
Bentiromide (Oral Route), #
Bentoquatam (Topical Route), 236
Bentyl, 102
Bentylol, 102
Benylin 4 Flu, 471
Benylin DM-D for Children, 471
Benylin DM-D, 471
Benylin DM-D-E Extra Strength, 471
Benylin DM-D-E, 471
Benylin DM-E Extra Strength, 471
Benylin DM-E, 471
Benylin E Extra Strength Chest Congestion, 835
Benylin Expectorant, 471
Benylin Pediatric Formula, 547
Benylin-E, 835
Benzac Ac, 246
Benzac W, 246
Benzacot, #
Benzagel Wash, 246
Benzagel-10, 246
Benzagel-5, 246
10 Benzagel Acne Gel, 246
2.5 Benzagel Acne Gel, 246
5 Benzagel Acne Gel, 246
2.5 Benzagel Acne Lotion, 246
5 Benzagel Acne Lotion, 246
5 Benzagel Acne Wash, 246
Benzalkonium Chloride, 1482
Benzashave, 246
Benzocaine and Menthol, #
Benzocaine and Menthol, 89
Benzocaine and Phenol, #
Benzocaine, #
Benzocaine, 87
Benzocaine, 89
Benzodent, #
Benzodiazepines (Systemic), 237
Benzonatate (Oral Route), 244
Benzoyl Peroxide (Topical Route), 246
Benzphetamine, 182
Benztropine, 126
Benzyl Benzoate (Topical Route), 248
Bepridil, 318
Berotec, 278
17 beta-estradiol and norgestimate, 697
Beta Carotene (Oral Route), 249
Beta Med, #
Beta-2, 278
Beta-Adrenergic Blocker (Oral Route, Injection Route, Intravenous Route), 251

C

C.E.S., 682
C2 Buffered with Codeine, 1146
C2 Buffered, 1442
C2 with Codeine, 1146
C2, 1442
C-500, 191
Cabergoline (Oral Route), 314
Caduet, 63
Cafcit, 315
Cafergot, 842
Caffedrine Caplets, 315
Caffeine (Systemic), 315
Caffeine and Sodium Benzoate, 315
Caffeine, 315
Calamine (Topical Route), #
Calamine Lotion, #
Calan SR, 318
Calan, 318
Calcarb 600, 323
Calcibind, #
Calci-Chew, 323
Calciday 667, 323
Calcifediol, 1639
Calciferol Drops, 1639
Calciferol, 1639
Calciject, 323
Calcijex, 1639
Calcilac, 323
Calci-Mix, 323
Calcionate, 323
Calcipotriene (Topical Route), #
Calcite 500, 323
Calcitonin (Salmon) (Nasal Route), #
Calcitriol, 1639
Calcium 600, 323
Calcium Acetate (Oral Route), #
Calcium Acetate, 323
Calcium and Magnesium Carbonates, 93
Calcium Carbonate and Magnesia, 93
Calcium Carbonate and Simethicone, 93
Calcium Carbonate, 93
Calcium Carbonate, 323
Calcium Carbonate, Magnesia, and Simethicone, 93
Calcium Channel Blocking Agents (Systemic), 318
Calcium Chloride, 323
Calcium Citrate, 323
Calcium Glubionate, 323
Calcium Gluceptate and Calcium Gluconate, 323
Calcium Gluceptate, 323
Calcium Gluconate, 323
Calcium Glycerophosphate and Calcium Lactate, 323
Calcium Lactate, 323
Calcium Lactate-Gluconate and Calcium Carbonate, 323
Calcium Stanley, 323
Calcium Supplements (Systemic), 323
Calcium-Sandoz Forte, 323
Calcium-Sandoz, 323
CaldeCORT Anti-Itch, 466
CaldeCORT Light, 466
Calderol, 1639
Caldesene, #
Calglycine, 93
Calglycine, 323

Calm X, 141
Calmine, 1442
Calmydone, 471
Calmylin #2, 471
Calmylin #3, 471
Calmylin #4, 471
Calmylin Cough and Flu, 471
Calmylin DM-D-E Extra Strength, 471
Calmylin Original with Codeine, 471
Calmylin Pediatric, 471
Calphosan, 323
Cal-Plus, 323
Calsan, 323
Caltrate 600, 323
Caltrate Jr, 323
Cama Arthritis Pain Reliever, 1442
Campath, #
Campral, 8
Camptosar, 934
Canasa, #
Cancidas, 354
Candesartan And Hydrochlorothiazide (Oral Route), #
Candesartan Cilexetil (Oral Route), 327
Canesten 1-Day Cream Combi-Pak, 135
Canesten 1-Day Therapy, 135
Canesten 3-Day Therapy, 135
Canesten 6-Day Therapy, 135
Canesten Combi-Pak 1-Day Therapy, 135
Canesten Combi-Pak 3-Day Therapy, 135
Canesten, 435
Cantil, 102
Capastat Sulfate, 332
Capecitabine (Oral Route), 329
Capital with Codeine, 1142
Capitrol, 384
Capoten, #
Capozide, #
Capreomycin (Injection Route), 332
Capsagel, 333
Capsagesic-HP Arthritis Relief, 333
Capsaicin (Topical Route), 333
Capsaicin HP, 333
Capsaicin, 333
Capsin, 333
Captopril and Hydrochlorothiazide, #
Carac, 759
Carafate, 1488
Carbachol (Ophthalmic Route), 335
Carbamazepine (Oral Route), 336
Carbatrol, 336
Carbetocin (Intravenous Route), #
Carbidopa, Entacapone, And Levodopa (Oral Route), 340
Carbinoxamine and Pseudoephedrine, 147
Carbinoxamine Compound-Drops, 471
Carbinoxamine, Pseudoephedrine, and Dextromethorphan, 471
Carbocaine with Neo-Cobefrin, #
Carbocaine, #
Carbocaine, #
Carbohydrates and Electrolytes (Systemic), 342
Carbol-Fuchsin Solution (Topical Route), #
Carbonic Anhydrase Inhibitors (Systemic), 344
Carboplatin (Intravenous Route), 347
Carboprost (Intramuscular Route), #
Cardec DM, 471
Cardene, 318
Cardioquin, 1378

Cardizem CD, 318
Cardizem LA, 318
Cardizem SR, 318
Cardizem, 318
Cardura Xl, 607
Cardura, 607
Carimune Nf, 888
Carimune, 888
Carisoprodol, 1470
Cari-Tab, 1648
Carmol-HC, 466
Carmustine (Implantation Route), #
Carmustine (Intravenous Route), 349
Carnitine, #
Carnitor, #
Carrington Antifungal, 1091
Carteolol, #
Carter's Little Pills, 973
Carticel, #
Cartrol, 251
Carvedilol (Oral Route), 351
Casanthranol and Docusate, 973
Casanthranol, 973
Cascara Sagrada and Aloe, 973
Cascara Sagrada and Bisacodyl, 973
Cascara Sagrada, 973
Casodex, 99
Caspofungin (Intravenous Route), 354
Castor Oil, 973
Cataflam, 164
Catapres, 427
Catapres-Tts-1, 427
Catapres-Tts-2, 427
Catapres-Tts-3, 427
Caverject, 48
Cavirinse, 1472
Ceclor, 361
Cecon, 191
Cedax, 361
Cedocard-SR, 1194
Ceenu, #
Cefaclor, 361
Cefditoren Pivoxil (Oral Route), 355
Cefizox, 361
Cefobid, 361
Cefotan, 361
Cefotaxime, 361
Ceftin, 361
Cefuroxime (Injection Route, Intravenous Route), 357
Cefuroxime, 361
Cefzil, 361
Celebrex, 358
Celecoxib (Oral Route), 358
Celestoderm-V, 468
Celestoderm-V/2, 468
Celestone Phosphate, 461
Celestone Soluspan, 461
Celestone, 461
Celexa, 402
Cellcept, 1123
Celontin, 115
Cemill 1000, 191
Cemill 500, 191
Cenafed, 1370
Cena-K, 1334
Centany, 1122
Ceo-Two, 979
Cepacol Maximum Strength, #
Cephalosporin (Oral Route, Injection Route, Intravenous Route, Intramuscular Route), 361
Ceptaz, 361

Fexofenadine And Pseudoephedrine (Oral Route), 738
Fexofenadine, 141
Fiberall, 973
Fibercon Caplets, 973
Fiber-Lax, 973
FiberNorm, 973
Finacea, 211
Finasteride (Oral Route), 740
Fiorgen, 303
Fioricet, 300
Fiorinal with Codeine No.3, 229
Fiorinal, 303
Fiorinal-C ¼, 229
Fiorinal-C ½, 229
Fiormor, 303
Flagyl Er, 1082
Flagyl I.V. Rtu, 1082
Flagyl I.V., 1082
Flagyl, 1085
Flagyl, 1082
Flamazine, 1464
Flarex, #
Flavocoxid (Oral Route), 741
Flavoxate (Oral Route), 742
Flecainide (Oral Route), 743
Fleet Babylax, 979
Fleet Bisacodyl, 979
Fleet Enema for Children, 979
Fleet Enema Mineral Oil, 979
Fleet Enema, 979
Fleet Glycerin Laxative, 979
Fleet Laxative, 973
Fleet Laxative, 979
Fleet Mineral Oil, 973
Fleet Pediatric Enema, 979
Fleet Phospho-Soda, 973
Fleet Relief, 87
Fleet Soflax Gelcaps, 973
Fleet Soflax Overnight Gelcaps, 973
Fletcher's Castoria, 973
Fletcher's Castoria, 973
Flexeril, 491
Floctafenine, 164
Flolan, #
Flomax, 1521
Flonase, 457
Flonase, #
Florinef Acetate, 750
Florone E, 468
Florone, 468
Flovent Hfa, 764
Flovent Rotadisk, 764
Flovent, 764
Floxin, 1211
Floxin, 752
Floxuridine (Injection Route), 745
Fluanxol Depot, #
Fluanxol, #
Fluarix, 897
Fluconazole, 130
Flucytosine (Oral Route), 747
Fludarabine (Oral Route), 748
Fludeoxyglucose F 18, #
Fludrocortisone (Oral Route), 750
Flumadine, 1415
Flumethasone, 466
Flumist, 897
Flunarizine, 318
Flunisolide, 452
Flunisolide, 457
Fluocet, 468
Fluocin, 468

Fluocinolone, 468
Fluocinonide, 468
Fluoderm, 468
Fluolar, 468
Fluonid, 468
Fluonide, 468
Fluorabon, 1472
Fluor-A-Day, 1472
Fluorigard, 1472
Fluorinse, 1472
Fluorometholone, #
Fluor-Op, #
Fluoroplex, 759
Fluoroquinolone (Oral Route, Injection Route, Intravenous Route), 752
Fluorosol, 1472
Fluorouracil (Intravenous Route, Injection Route), 757
Fluorouracil (Topical Route), 759
Fluothane, #
Fluoxetine (Oral Route), 761
Fluoxymesterone, 79
Flupenthixol, #
Fluphenazine, 1302
Flura-Drops, 1472
Flura-Loz, 1472
Flurandrenolide, 468
Flurandrenolide, 466
Flurazepam, 237
Flurbiprofen, #
Flurbiprofen, 164
Flurosyn, 468
Flutamide, 99
Flutex, 468
Fluticasone (Inhalation, Oral/Nebulization Route), 764
Fluticasone (Nasal Route), #
Fluticasone And Salmeterol (Inhalation, Oral/Nebulization Route), 767
Fluticasone, 457
Fluticasone, 468
Fluvirin, 897
Fluvoxamine (Oral Route), 770
Fluzone Pediatric, 897
Fluzone, 897
FML Forte, #
FML Liquifilm, #
FML S.O.P., #
Foamicon, 93
Focalin Xr, 544
Focalin, 544
FoilleCort, 466
Folacin-800, 772
Folic Acid (Oral Route, Injection Route), 772
Follicle Stimulating Hormone And Luteinizing Hormone (Intramuscular Route, Subcutaneous Route), 774
Follistim Aq, 778
Follistim, 778
Follitropin Alfa (Subcutaneous Route), 776
Follitropin Beta (Subcutaneous Route), 778
Fomivirsen (Intraocular Route), #
Fondaparinux (Subcutaneous Route), 780
Foradil Aerolizer, 782
Foradil, 278
Forane, #
Formoterol (Inhalation, Oral/Nebulization Route), 782
Formoterol, 278

Formula E 400, 1644
Formulex, 102
Fortabs, 303
Fortamet, 1058
Fortaz, 361
Forteo, #
Fortical, #
Fortovase, 1450
Fosamax, 42
Fosamprenavir (Oral Route), 784
Foscarnet (Intravenous Route), 786
Foscavir, 786
Fosfomycin (Oral Route), 788
Fosphenytoin, 111
Fosrenol, 969
Fototar, 439
Fragmin, 512
Framycetin (Ophthalmic Route), #
Freezone - One Step Callus Remover Pad, #
Freezone - One Step Corn Remover Pad, #
Freezone, #
Frigiderm, #
Frisium, 237
Froben SR, 164
Froben, 164
Frova, 789
Frovatriptan (Oral Route), 789
Fructose, Dextrose, And Phosphoric Acid (Oral Route), #
Fucidin Suspension, #
Fudr, 745
Fulvestrant (Intramuscular Route), 791
Fulvicin P/G, 830
Fulvicin-U/F, 830
Fumasorb, 937
Fumerin, 937
Fungi-Guard, #
Fungi-Nail, #
Fungizone, #
Fung-O, #
Fungoid, 1091
Furacin, #
Furadantin, 1201
Furazolidone (Oral Route), #
Furocot, 580
Furomide M.D., 580
Fusidic Acid (Oral Route, Injection Route), #
Fuzeon, 642

G

Gabapentin (Oral Route), 793
Gabarone, 793
Gabitril, 1557
Gadodiamide, #
Gadopentetate, #
Gadoteridol, #
Gadoversetamide, #
Galantamine (Oral Route), 795
Gallium Citrate Ga 67, #
Gallium Nitrate (Intravenous Route), #
Galsulfase (Injection Route), 797
Gamimmune N 10 %, 888
Gamma E Plus, 1644
Gamma E-Gems, 1644
Gammagard S/D, 888
Gammar-P I.V., 888
Gamunex, 888
Ganciclovir (Intraocular Route), 798

Ganciclovir (Oral Route, Intravenous Route), 799
Ganirelix (Subcutaneous Route), 801
Ganite, #
Gantanol, 1494
Gantrisin, #
Gantrisin, 1494
Garamycin, 57
Garamycin, #
Garamycin, 813
Gas Aid Maximum Strength, 1466
Gasmas, 93
Gastrocrom, 488
Gastrolyte, 342
Gastrosed, 102
Gastrozepin, 102
Gas-X, 1466
Gatifloxacin (Ophthalmic Route), 803
Gaviscon Acid Plus Gas Relief, 93
Gaviscon Acid Relief, 93
Gaviscon Extra Strength Acid Relief, 93
Gaviscon Extra Strength Relief Formula, 93
Gaviscon Heartburn Relief Extra Strength, 93
Gaviscon Heartburn Relief, 93
Gaviscon, 93
Gaviscon-2, 93
Gebauer's Ethyl Chloride, #
Gefitinib (Oral Route), 804
Gelpirin, 14
Gelusil Extra Strength, 93
Gelusil, 93
Gelusil, 93
Gemcitabine (Intravenous Route), 805
Gemfibrozil (Oral Route), 807
Gemifloxacin (Oral Route), 809
Gemonil, 223
Gemtuzumab Ozogamicin (Intravenous Route), 811
Gemzar, 805
Genahist, 141
Gen-Allerate, 141
Gen-Alprazolam, 237
Gen-Amoxicillin, 1280
Genapap, 12
Genaphed, 1370
Genarc, #
Genasal, 1245
Genasoft Plus Softgels, 973
Genasyme, 1466
Genaton Extra Strength, 93
Genaton, 93
Genatuss DM, 471
Gen-Bromazepam, 237
Gencalc 600, 323
Gen-Cefaclor, 361
Gen-Clonazepam, 237
Gengraf, 500
Gen-K, 1334
Gen-Medroxy, 1363
Gen-Minocycline, 1543
Gen-Minoxidol, 1102
Genoptic S.O.P., 813
Genoptic, 813
Genora 0.5/35, 691
Genora 1/35, 691
Genora 1/50, 691
Genotropin Miniquick, 832
Genotropin, 832
Genpril Caplets, 164
Genpril, 164
Gen-Salbutamol Sterinebs P.F., 278

Gensan, 1442
Gentacidin, 813
Gentafair, 813
Gentak, 813
Gentamicin (Ophthalmic Route), 813
Gentamicin (Otic Route), 814
Gentamicin (Topical Route), #
Gentamicin, 57
Gentasol, 813
Genteal Mild, 871
Genteal, 871
Gentian Violet (Topical Route), #
Gentian Violet (Vaginal Route), #
Gentle Laxative, 973
Gent-L-Tip, 979
Gen-Triazolam, 237
Genuine Bayer Aspirin Caplets, 1442
Genuine Bayer Aspirin Tablets, 1442
Geocillin, 1280
Geodon, 1663
Geref Diagnostic, #
Geref, #
Gesterol 50, 1363
Gesterol LA 250, 1363
Gets-It Corn/Callus Remover, #
Gin Pain Pills, 1442
Glatiramer Acetate (Subcutaneous Route), #
Glaucon, #
Gleevec, 882
Gliadel, #
Glipizide And Metformin (Oral Route), 816
Glucagen Diagnostic Kit, 818
Glucagen, 818
Glucagon (Injection Route), 818
Glucagon Diagnostic Kit, 818
Glucagon Emergency Kit, 818
Glucagon, 818
Glucophage Xr, 1058
Glucophage, 1058
Glucotrol Xl, 1502
Glucotrol, 1502
Glucovance, 822
Glu-K, 1334
Glutamine (Oral Route), 821
Glyburide And Metformin (Oral Route), 822
Glycerin (Oral Route), #
Glycerin, 979
Glycerin, #
Glycopyrrolate, 102
Gly-Cort, 466
Glycron, 1502
Glynase Pres-Tab, 1502
Glysennid, 973
Glyset, 1095
G-Mycin, 57
Gold Compounds (Systemic), #
Gold Sodium Thiomalate, #
Golytely, 1332
Gonadorelin (Intravenous Route, Injection Route), 825
Gonak, 871
Gonal-F Rff, 776
Gonal-F Rff, 778
Gonal-F, 776
Goniosoft, 871
Goody's Fast Pain Relief, 14
Goody's Headache Powders, 14
Gordofilm, #
Goserelin (Subcutaneous Route), 827
GP-500, 471

Gramcal, 323
Granisetron (Oral Route, Intravenous Route), 829
Gravergol, 842
Gravol Filmkote (Junior Strength), 141
Gravol Filmkote, 141
Gravol I/M, 141
Gravol I/V, 141
Gravol L/A, 141
Gravol Liquid, 141
Gravol, 141
Grifulvin V, 830
Griseofulvin (Oral Route), 830
Gris-Peg, 830
Growth Hormone (Systemic), 832
Guaifed, 471
Guaifenesin (Oral Route), 835
Guaifenex G, 835
Guaifenex La, 835
Guaifenex PSE 120, 471
Guaifenex PSE 60, 471
GuaiMAX-D, 471
Guai-Vent/PSE, 471
Guanabenz (Oral Route), #
Guanadrel (Oral Route), #
Guanethidine (Oral Route), #
Guanfacine (Oral Route), #
Guiatuss A.C., 471
Guiatuss CF, 471
Guiatuss DAC, 471
Guiatuss PE, 471
Gyne Cure, 1566
Gynecort 10, 466
Gynecort, 466
GyneCure Ovules, 135
GyneCure Vaginal Ointment Tandempak, 135
GyneCure Vaginal Ovules Tandempak, 135
GyneCure, 135
Gyne-Lotrimin Combination Pack, 135
Gyne-Lotrimin, 135
Gyne-Lotrimin3 Combination Pack, 135
Gyne-Lotrimin3, 135
Gynol II Extra Strength Contraceptive Jelly, 1482
Gynol II Original Formula Contraceptive Jelly, 1482

H

Habitrol, 1186
Haemophilus b Conjugate Vaccine (HbOC—Diphtheria CRM 197 Protein Conjugate), 836
Haemophilus b Conjugate Vaccine (PRP-D—Diphtheria Toxoid Conjugate), 836
Haemophilus b Conjugate Vaccine (PRP-OMP—Meningococcal Protein Conjugate), 836
Haemophilus b Conjugate Vaccine (PRP-T—Tetanus Protein Conjugate), 836
Haemophilus b Conjugate Vaccine (Systemic), 836
Haemophilus B Polysaccharide Vaccine (Intramuscular Route, Injection Route), 838
Hair Regrowth Treatment, 1102
Hairgro, 1102
Halazepam, 237

Halcinonide, 468
Halcion, 237
Haldol Decanoate, 839
Haldol, 839
Haley's M-O, 973
Halfprin, 1442
Halobetasol, 468
Halofantrine (Oral Route), #
Halog, 468
Halog-E, 468
Haloperidol (Oral Route, Intramuscular Route, Injection Route), 839
Halotestin, 79
Halothane, #
Haltran, 164
Harmonyl, #
Havrix Pediatric, 849
Havrix, 849
Hayfebrol, 147
Headache Medicines, Ergot Derivative-Containing (Systemic), 842
Headache Tablet, 1442
Healthprin Adult Low Strength, 1442
Healthprin Full Strength, 1442
Healthprin Half-Dose, 1442
Heartburn Relief, 853
Hectorol, 1639
Helidac, 266
Helixate Fs, #
Hemabate, #
Hemocyte, 937
Hemofil-M, #
Hemorrhoidal HC, #
Hemril-HC Uniserts, #
Hepagam B, 850
Heparin (Intravenous Route, Injection Route), #
Hepatitis A Vaccine Inactivated And Hepatitis B Vaccine Recombinant (Intramuscular Route), 847
Hepatitis A Vaccine, Inactivated (Intramuscular Route), 849
Hepatitis B Immune Globulin (Intramuscular Route), 850
Hepatitis B Vaccine Recombinant (Intramuscular Route), 852
Hepflush-10, #
Hep-Lock U/P, #
Hep-Lock, #
Hepsera, 34
Heptovir, 959
Herbal Laxative, 973
Herbal Laxative, 973
Herbopyrine, 1442
Herceptin, #
Herplex, 877
Hexadrol Phosphate, 461
Hexalen, 52
Hibtiter, 836
Hi-Cor 1.0, 466
Hi-Cor 2.5, 466
Hiprex, #
Histamine (Injection Route), #
Histamine H2 Antagonist (Oral Route, Injection Route, Intravenous Route), 853
Histantil, 159
Histatab Plus, 147
Histenol, 471
Histinex HC, 471
Histinex PV, 471
Histrelin (Implantation Route), #
Hivid, 1654

Hmg-Coa Reductase Inhibitor (Oral Route), 858
HMS Liquifilm, #
Homapin, 102
Homatropine, 102
Homatropine, #
12 Hour Cold Maximum Strength, 1370
Humalog, 913
Humatrope, 832
Humira, 30
Humorsol, 138
Humulin 10/90, 899
Humulin 20/80, 899
Humulin 30/70, 899
Humulin 40/60, 899
Humulin 50/50, 899
Humulin 70/30 Pen, 899
Humulin 70/30, 899
Humulin L, 899
Humulin N Pen, 899
Humulin N, 899
Humulin R, 899
Humulin R, Regular U-500 (Concentrated), 899
Humulin U, 899
Humulin-L, 899
Humulin-N, 899
Humulin-R, 899
Humulin-U, 899
Hurricane, #
Hy/Gestrone, 1363
Hyaluronate Sodium (Injection Route), #
Hyaluronidase (Subcutaneous Route, Injection Route), #
Hyate:C, #
Hybolin Decanoate, 71
Hybolin-Improved, 71
Hycamtin, 1579
Hycodan, 471
Hycodan, 1133
Hycomed, 1142
Hycomine Compound, 471
Hycomine, 471
Hyco-Pap, 1142
Hycort, #
Hydergine, 656
Hyderm, 466
Hydralazine (Oral Route, Injection Route, Intravenous Route), 860
Hydralazine And Hydrochlorothiazide (Oral Route), #
Hydrate, 141
Hydrea, 869
Hydrisalic, #
Hydrobexan, #
Hydrocet, 1142
Hydro-chlor, 589
Hydrochlorothiazide, 589
Hydrocil Instant, 973
Hydro-Cobex, #
Hydrocodone and Acetaminophen, 1142
Hydrocodone and Aspirin, 1146
Hydrocodone and Guaifenesin, 471
Hydrocodone and Homatropine, 471
Hydrocodone And Ibuprofen (Oral Route), 862
Hydrocodone and Potassium Guaiacol-sulfonate, 471
Hydrocodone, 1133
Hydrocortisone acetate, 466

Hydrocortisone acetate, #
Hydrocortisone And Acetic Acid (Otic Route), 864
Hydrocortisone butyrate, 468
Hydrocortisone or hydrocortisone acetate, 466
Hydrocortisone probutate, 468
Hydrocortisone valerate, 468
Hydrocortisone, #
Hydrocortisone, #
Hydrocortisone, 461
Hydrocortisone, 466
Hydrocortisone, #
Hydrocortone Acetate, 461
Hydrocortone Phosphate, 461
Hydrocortone, 461
Hydro-Crysti-12, #
Hydro-D, 589
HydroDIURIL, 589
Hydroflumethiazide, 589
Hydrogesic, 1142
Hydromorphone, 1133
Hydromox, 589
Hydropane, 471
Hydropres-50, #
Hydrostat IR, 1133
Hydro-Tex, 466
Hydroxocobalamin, #
Hydroxyamphetamine And Tropicamide (Ophthalmic Route), #
Hydroxychloroquine (Oral Route), 866
Hydroxy-Cobal, #
Hydroxyprogesterone, 1363
Hydroxypropyl Cellulose (Ophthalmic Route), 868
Hydroxyurea (Oral Route), 869
Hydroxyzine, 141
Hygroton, 589
Hylan Polymers A And B (Injection Route), #
Hylenex, #
Hylorel, #
Hylutin, 1363
Hyoscyamine, 102
Hyosophen, #
Hyperhep B, 850
Hyperrab S/D, #
Hyperrho S/D, #
HY-PHEN, 1142
Hypromellose (Intraocular Route), #
Hypromellose (Ophthalmic Route), 871
Hyrexin, 141
Hytakerol, 1639
Hytinic, 937
Hytone, 466
Hytrin, 1535
Hyzaar, #
Hyzine-50, 141

I

Ibandronate (Oral Route, Injection Route), 873
Ibifon 600 Caplets, 164
Ibren, 164
Ibritumomab Tiuxetan (Intravenous Route), #
Ibu, 164
Ibu-200, 164
Ibu-4, 164
Ibu-6, 164
Ibu-8, 164

M2 Potassium, #
Maalox Antacid Caplets, 93
Maalox Antacid Caplets, 323
Maalox Anti-Gas, 1466
Maalox Heartburn Relief Formula, 93
Maalox HRF, 93
Maalox Plus, 93
Maalox Plus, Extra Strength, 93
Maalox TC, 93
Maalox, 93
Macrodantin, 1201
Mafenide (Topical Route), 1025
Mag 2, #
Mag-200, #
Magaldrate and Simethicone, 93
Magaldrate, 93
Magan, 1442
Mag-L-100, #
Maglucate, #
Magnalox Plus, 93
Magnalox, 93
Magnaprin, 1442
Magnesium Carbonate and Sodium Bi-carbonate, 93
Magnesium Chloride, #
Magnesium Citrate, 973
Magnesium Citrate, #
Magnesium Gluceptate, #
Magnesium Gluconate, #
Magnesium Hydroxide, 93
Magnesium Hydroxide, 973
Magnesium Hydroxide, #
Magnesium Lactate, #
Magnesium Oxide, 93
Magnesium Oxide, 973
Magnesium Oxide, #
Magnesium Pidolate, #
Magnesium Salicylate, 1442
Magnesium Sulfate, 973
Magnesium Sulfate, #
Magnesium Supplements (Systemic), #
Magnesium-Rougier, #
Magnetic Resonance Imaging Contrast Agents (Diagnostic), #
Magnetic Resonance Imaging Contrast Agents, Iron-containing (Diagnostic), #
Magnolax, 973
Magonate, #
Mag-Ox 400, 93
Mag-Ox 400, 973
Mag-Ox 400, #
Mag-Tab SR, #
Magtrate, #
Majeptil, 1302
Malarone Pediatric, #
Malarone, #
Malatal, #
Malathion (Topical Route), #
Mallamint, 93
Mallamint, 323
Malogen in Oil, 79
Malt Soup Extract and Psyllium, 973
Malt Soup Extract, 973
Maltsupex, 973
Mandelamine, #
Mandol, 361
Mangafodipir (Intravenous Route), #
Manganese Chloride, #
Manganese Sulfate, #
Manganese Supplements (Systemic), #
Maolate, 1470
Maox 420, 93

Maox, #
Mapap Cold Formula, 471
Maprotiline (Oral Route), 1027
Marblen, 93
Marcaine Hcl, #
Marcaine Spinal, #
Marcaine With Epinephrine, #
Marcaine, #
Marcof Expectorant, 471
Margesic #3, 1142
Margesic-H, 1142
Marinol, 616
Marnal, 303
Marplan, 117
Marthritic, 1442
Marvelon, 691
Matulane, 1356
Mavik, #
Maxair Autohaler, 278
Maxair, 278
Maxalt, 1430
Maxalt-Mlt, 1430
Maxaquin, 752
Maxidex, #
Maxiflor, 468
Maximum Strength Arthritis Foundation Safety Coated Aspirin, 1442
Maximum Strength Ascriptin, 1442
Maximum Strength Cortaid, 466
Maximum Strength Doan's Analgesic Caplets, 1442
Maximum Strength SnapBack Stimulant Powders, 315
Maxipime, 361
Maxivate, 468
Maxzide, 586
May be available in other countries., #
Mazanor, 182
Mazindol, 182
Mb-Tab, #
Me-500, #
Measles And Rubella Virus Vaccine Live (Intramuscular Route, Injection Route), #
Measles Virus Vaccine, Live (Subcutaneous Route), 1029
Measles, Mumps, And Rubella Virus Vaccine Live (Subcutaneous Route, Intramuscular Route), 1030
Mebaral, 223
Mebendazole (Oral Route), 1032
Mecamylamine (Oral Route), #
Mecasermin (Subcutaneous Route), 1034
Mechlorethamine (Intravenous Route), 1036
Mechlorethamine (Topical Route), #
Meclan, #
Meclocycline, #
Meclofenamate, 164
Meclomen, 164
Med Amoxicillin, 1280
Med Minoxidil, 1102
Med Valproic, 1616
Medigesic, 300
Medihaler-Iso, 278
Medi-Lice Maximum Strength, 1372
Mediplast, #
Medipren Caplets, 164
Medipren, 164
Medotar, 439
Medrogestone, 1363
Medrol, 461

Medroxyprogesterone, 1359
Medroxyprogesterone, 1363
Medrysone, #
Mefenamic Acid, 164
Mefloquine (Oral Route), 1038
Mefoxin, 361
Mega-C, 191
Megace OS, 1363
Megace, 1363
Megestrol, 1363
Meglumine Antimoniate (Intravenous Route, Injection Route), #
Melate, #
Melfiat, 182
Mellaril Concentrate, 1302
Mellaril, 1302
Mellaril-S, 1302
Meloxicam (Oral Route), 1040
Melphalan (Oral Route, Intravenous Route), 1043
Memantine (Oral Route), 1045
Menactra, 1048
Menadiol, 1646
Menest, 682
Meningococcal Polysaccharide Vaccine (Subcutaneous Route), 1047
Meningococcal Vaccine, Diphtheria Conjugate (Intramuscular Route), 1048
Menomune-A/C/Y/W-135, 1047
Menopur, 774
Mentax, 310
Mepenzolate, 102
Meperidine, 1133
Meperidine, 1140
Mephenytoin, 111
Mephobarbital, 223
Mephyton, 1646
Mepivacaine, #
Meprobamate (Oral Route), #
Meprobamate And Aspirin (Oral Route), 1050
Meprolone, 461
Mepron, #
Mequinol And Tretinoin (Topical Route), 1053
Mercaptopurine (Oral Route), 1054
Meribin, #
Meridia, 1460
Meropenem (Intravenous Route), #
Merrem Iv, #
Mersyndol with Codeine, 471
Meruvax Ii, #
Mesalamine (Oral Route), 1056
Mesalamine (Rectal Route), #
Mesantoin, 111
Mesasal, #
Mescolor, 156
M-Eslon, 1133
Mesna (Intravenous Route), #
Mesnex, #
Mesoridazine, 1302
Mestinon Timespans, 175
Mestinon, 175
Mestinon-SR, 175
Metadate Cd, 1076
Metadate Er, 1076
Metaderm Mild, 468
Metaderm Regular, 468
Metaglip, 816
Metahydrin, 589
Metamucil Apple Crisp Fiber Wafers, 973
Metamucil Cinnamon Spice Fiber Wafers, 973

8-Mop, 1070
Moricizine (Oral Route), #
Morphine Extra-Forte, 1133
Morphine Forte, 1133
Morphine H.P., 1133
Morphine, 1133
Morphine, 1140
Morphitec, 1133
Mosco Corn & Callus Remover, #
Motofen, #
Motrin Chewables, 164
Motrin IB Sinus Caplets, 529
Motrin IB Sinus, 529
Motrin, 164
Motrin, Children's Oral Drops, 164
Motrin, Children's, 164
Motrin, Junior Strength Caplets, 164
Motrin-IB Caplets, 164
Motrin-IB, 164
Moxifloxacin (Ophthalmic Route), 1121
MS IR, 1133
MS/L Concentrate, 1133
MS/L, 1133
MS/S, 1133
MSIR, 1133
Mucinex, 835
Mucomyst, 19
Multipax, 141
Multiple Vitamins and Fluoride, 1648
Mulvidren-F, 1648
Mumps Virus Vaccine, Live (Subcuta-
  neous Route), #
Mumpsvax, #
Mupirocin (Nasal Route), #
Mupirocin (Topical Route), 1122
Muro-128, #
Muromonab-Cd3 (Intravenous Route),
  #
Muse Micro, 48
Muse, 48
Mustargen, 1036
Mutamycin, 1108
Myambutol, 704
Mycamine, #
Mycelex Troche, 433
Mycelex Twin Pack, 135
Mycelex, 435
Mycelex-7, 135
Mycelex-G, 135
Myclo-Derm, 435
Myclo-Gyne, 135
Mycobutin, 1402
Mycolog-II, #
Mycophenolate Mofetil (Oral Route, In-
  travenous Route), 1123
MyCort, 466
Mycostatin Cream, 1206
Mycostatin Ointment, 1206
Mycostatin Powder, 1206
Mycostatin Suspension, 1204
Mycostatin Vaginal Cream, 1207
Mycostatin, 1207
Mycostatin, 1206
Mydfrin, #
Mydral, #
Mydriacyl, #
My-E, 669
Mygel II, 93
Mygel, 93
Mykrox, 589
Mylanta Double Strength Plain, 93
Mylanta Double Strength, 93
Mylanta Double Strength, 93

Mylanta Extra Strength, 93
Mylanta Gas, 1466
Mylanta Gelcaps, 93
Mylanta Natural Fiber Supplement, 973
Mylanta Sugar Free Natural Fiber Supple-
  ment, 973
Mylanta, 93
Mylanta, 93
Mylicon, 1466
Mylotarg, 811
Myobloc, #
Myochrysine, #
Mysoline, 1347
Mytab Gas, 1466
Mytelase Caplets, 175
Mytrex, #
MZM, 344

N

N.E.E. 1/35, 691
N.E.E. 1/50, 691
Nabi-Hb Novaplus, 850
Nabi-Hb, 850
Nabilone (Oral Route), #
Nabumetone, 164
Nadolol and Bendroflumethiazide, #
Nadopen V 200, 1280
Nadopen V 400, 1280
Nadostine Sucrose-Free, 1204
Nadostine, 1207
Nadostine, 1206
Nadostine, 1204
Nadroparin (Subcutaneous Route),
  1125
Nafarelin (Nasal Route), 1127
Nafcil, 1280
Naftifine (Topical Route), #
Naftin, #
Naftin-Mp, #
Nail-Ex, #
Nalbuphine, 1133
Nalbuphine, 1140
Nalex DH, 471
Nalex-A, 147
Nalfon 200, 164
Nalfon, 164
Nalidixic Acid (Oral Route), #
Naltrexone (Oral Route), #
Namenda, 1045
Nandrolone, 71
Naphazoline (Ophthalmic Route), 1130
Naphcon, 1130
Naprelan, 164
Naprosyn, 164
Naprosyn-E, 164
Naprosyn-SR, 164
Naproxen, 164
Naqua, 589
Naratriptan (Oral Route), 1131
Narcotic Analgesics (Systemic), 1133
Narcotic Analgesics (Systemic), 1140
Narcotic Analgesics and Acetamino-
  phen (Systemic), 1142
Narcotic Analgesics and Aspirin
  (Systemic), 1146
Nardil, 117
Naropin, #
Naropin, #
Nasacon, 1245
Nasacort AQ, 457
Nasacort, 457

Nasahist B, 141
Nasalcrom, 485
Nasalide, 457
Nasarel, 457
Nascobal, #
Nasin, 1245
Nasonex, 457
Nasonex, #
Natacyn, #
Natalizumab (Intravenous Route), 1151
Natamycin (Ophthalmic Route), #
Nateglinide (Oral Route), 1153
Natrecor, 1175
Natural Source Fibre Laxative, 973
Natural Vitamin Blend E-400iu, 1644
Naturalyte, 342
Nature's Blend Folic Acid, 772
Nature's Remedy, 973
Nature's Tears, 871
Naturetin, 589
Navane, #
Navelbine, 1634
Naxen, 164
ND Clear T.D., 147
ND-Gesic, 151
Nebcin, 57
Nebupent, 1289
Necon 0.5/35, 691
Necon 1/35, 691
Necon 1/50, 691
Necon 10/11, 691
Nedocromil (Inhalation, Oral/Nebuliza-
  tion Route), 1155
Nedocromil (Ophthalmic Route), 1158
Nefazodone (Oral Route), 1159
Neggram, #
Nelfinavir (Oral Route), 1162
Nelova 0.5/35E, 691
Nelova 1/35E, 691
Nelova 1/50M, 691
Nelova 10/11, 691
Nembutal, 223
Neo Citran A, 147
Neo Citran Extra Strength Colds and Flu,
  151
Neo Citran Extra Strength Sinus, 529
Neo Citran Nutrasweet, 151
Neo-Calglucon, 323
NeoCitran DM Coughs and Colds, 471
Neo-Codema, 589
Neocontrast, #
Neo-Estrone, 682
Neo-Fer, 937
Neo-Fradin, 1163
Neofrin, #
Neo-K, 1334
Neoloid, 973
Neo-Metric, 1085
Neomycin (Ophthalmic Route), #
Neomycin (Oral Route), 1163
Neomycin (Topical Route), 1165
Neomycin And Polymyxin B (Topical
  Route), 1166
Neomycin, 57
Neomycin, Polymyxin B, And Bacitra-
  cin (Ophthalmic Route), 1168
Neomycin, Polymyxin B, And Bacitra-
  cin (Topical Route), 1169
Neomycin, Polymyxin B, And Gramici-
  din (Ophthalmic Route), 1170
Neomycin, Polymyxin B, And Hydro-
  cortisone (Ophthalmic Route), 1171
Neomycin, Polymyxin B, And Hydro-
  cortisone (Otic Route), 1173

Novolin ge 30/70 Penfill, 899
Novolin ge 30/70, 899
Novolin ge 40/60 Penfill, 899
Novolin ge 50/50 Penfill, 899
Novolin ge Lente, 899
Novolin ge NPH Penfill, 899
Novolin ge NPH, 899
Novolin ge Toronto Penfill, 899
Novolin ge Toronto, 899
Novolin ge Ultralente, 899
Novolin L, 899
Novolin N PenFill, 899
Novolin N Prefilled, 899
Novolin N, 899
Novolin R PenFill, 899
Novolin R Prefilled, 899
Novolin R, 899
Novolog Flexpen, 905
Novolog, 905
Novo-Lorazem, 237
Novo-Medrone, 1363
Novo-Methacin, 164
Novo-Miconazole Vaginal Ovules, 135
Novo-Minocycline, 1543
Novo-Naprox Sodium DS, 164
Novo-Naprox Sodium, 164
Novo-Naprox, 164
Novo-Niacin, 1180
Novo-Nifedin, 318
Nov-Onxol, 1250
Novopentobarb, 223
Novo-Peridol, 839
Novo-Pheniram, 141
Novo-Pirocam, 164
Novo-Poxide, 237
Novopramine, 120
Novo-Profen, 164
Novoreserpine, #
Novo-Ridazine, 1302
Novo-rythro Encap, 669
Novo-rythro, 669
Novo-rythro, 669
Novo-Salmol, 278
Novosecobarb, 223
Novoseven, #
Novo-Soxazole, 1494
Novospiroton, 583
Novo-Spirozine, 586
Novo-Sundac, 164
Novo-Temazepam, 237
Novo-Tenoxicam, 164
Novo-Tetra, 1543
Novo-Thalidone, 589
Novo-Timol, #
Novo-Tolmetin, 164
Novo-Triamzide, 586
Novo-Trifluzine, 1302
Novo-Trimel D.S., 1498
Novo-Trimel, 1498
Novo-Triolam, 237
Novo-Tripramine, 120
Novotriptyn, 120
Novo-Valproic, 1616
Novo-Veramil, 318
Novoxapam, 237
Nozinan Liquid, 1302
Nozinan Oral Drops, 1302
Nozinan, 1302
NPH Iletin II, 899
NPH Iletin, 899
NPH Purified Insulin, 899
Nrs-Nasal Relief, 1245
Nu-Alpraz, 237

Nubain, 1133
Nubain, 1140
Nu-Cal, 323
Nu-Cefaclor, 361
Nucofed Expectorant, 471
Nucofed Pediatric Expectorant, 471
Nu-Cotrimox DS, 1498
Nu-Cotrimox, 1498
Nucotuss Expectorant, 471
Nucotuss Pediatric Expectorant, 471
Nu-Diclo, 164
Nu-Diltiaz, 318
Nu-Doxycycline, 1543
Nu-Flurbiprofen, 164
Nu-Ibuprofen, 164
Nu-Indo, 164
Nu-Iron 150, 937
Nu-Iron, 937
Nujol, 973
Nu-Loraz, 237
Numorphan, 1133
Numzident, #
Num-Zit Gel, #
Num-Zit Lotion, #
Nu-Naprox, 164
Nu-Nifed, 318
Nupercainal Cream, 89
Nupercainal Ointment, 89
Nupercainal, 87
Nupercainal, #
Nu-Pirox, 164
Nuprin Caplets, 164
Nuprin, 164
Nu-Prochlor, 1302
Nu-Tetra, 1543
Nutracort, 466
Nutr-E-Sol, 1644
Nutropin AQ, 832
Nutropin, 832
Nu-Valproic, 1616
Nuvaring, 705
Nu-Verap, 318
Nyaderm Cream, 1206
Nyaderm Ointment, 1206
Nyaderm Vaginal Cream, 1207
Nyaderm, 1204
Nycoff, 547
Nydrazid, 943
Nylidrin (Oral Route), #
Nystatin (Oral Route), 1204
Nystatin (Topical Route), 1206
Nystatin (Vaginal Route), 1207
Nystatin And Triamcinolone (Topical Route), #
Nystop, 1206
Nytcold Medicine, 471
Nytime Cold Medicine Liquid, 471
Nytol QuickCaps, 141
Nytol QuickGels, 141

O

Obenix, 182
Obezine, 182
Occlusal-Hp, #
Occulocort, 468
Octagam, 888
Octocaine, #
Octocaine-100, #
Octocaine-50, #
Octoxynol 9, 1482

Octreotide (Injection Route, Intramuscular Route), 1208
Ocu-Carpine, 1317
Ocu-Chlor, 375
Ocuclear, 1247
Ocu-Dex, #
Ocufen, #
Ocuflox, 1210
Ocuflox, 752
Ocu-Mycin, 813
Ocu-Pentolate, 493
Ocu-Phrin, #
Ocu-Pred Forte, #
Ocu-Pred, #
Ocu-Pred-A, #
Ocupress, #
Ocusert Pilo, 1317
Ocu-Spor-G, 1170
Ocu-Sul-10, #
Ocu-Sul-15, #
Ocu-Sul-30, #
Ocusulf-10, #
Ocu-Tropic, #
Ocu-Tropine, #
Ocu-Zoline, 1130
Oestrilin, 688
Off-Ezy, #
Ofloxacin (Ophthalmic Route), 1210
Ofloxacin (Otic Route), 1211
Ofloxacin, 1210
Ogen .625, 682
Ogen 1.25, 682
Ogen 2.5, 682
Ogen, 682
Olanzapine (Intramuscular Route), 1213
Olmesartan And Hydrochlorothiazide (Oral Route), 1215
Olmesartan Medoxomil (Oral Route), 1217
Olopatadine (Ophthalmic Route), 1219
Olsalazine (Oral Route), 1221
Olux, 468
Omacor, 1223
Omalizumab (Subcutaneous Route), 1222
Omega-3-Acid Ethyl Esters (Oral Route), 1223
Omeprazole (Oral Route), 1225
Omnicef, 361
OMNIhist L.A., 156
OMS Concentrate, 1133
Oncaspar, 1267
Oncet, 1142
Oncovin, 1633
Ondansetron (Oral Route, Injection Route, Intravenous Route), 1227
One-Alpha, 1639
One-Gram C, 191
Ontak, 537
Onxol, 1250
Ophthacet, #
Ophthaine, #
Ophthetic, #
Ophtho-Bunolol, #
Ophtho-Chloram, 375
Ophtho-Flox, 1210
Ophtho-Tate, #
Opium Injection, 1133
Opium Preparations (Systemic), #
Opium Tincture, #
Oprelvekin (Subcutaneous Route), #
Optimine, 141

The Medicine Chart

The Medicine Chart presents sample photographs of prescribed medicines in the United States. In general, commonly used brand name products and a representative sampling of generic products have been included. The pictorial listing is not intended to be inclusive and does not represent all products on the market. The inclusion of a product does not mean the authors have any particular knowledge that the product included has properties different from other products, nor should it be interpreted as an endorsement. Similarly, the fact that a particular product has not been included does not indicate that the product has been judged to be unsatisfactory or unacceptable.

The drug products in *The Medicine Chart* are listed alphabetically by generic name of active ingredient(s). In some instances, not all dosage forms and sizes are pictured. If others are available, a † symbol proceeds the products name. Letters or numbers representing the manufacturer's identification code are followed by an asterisk.

The size and color of the products shown are intended to match the actual product as closely as possible; however, there may be some differences due to variations caused by the photographic process. Also, manufacturers may occasionally change the color, imprinting, or shape of their products, and for a period of time both the "old" and the newly changed dosage forms may be on the market. Such changes may not occur uniformly throughout the different dosages of the product. When applicable these types of changes will be incorporated in the subsequent versions of *The Medicine Chart* as they are brought to our attention.

Use of this chart is limited to serving as an initial guide in identifying drug products. The identity of a product should be verified further before any action is taken.

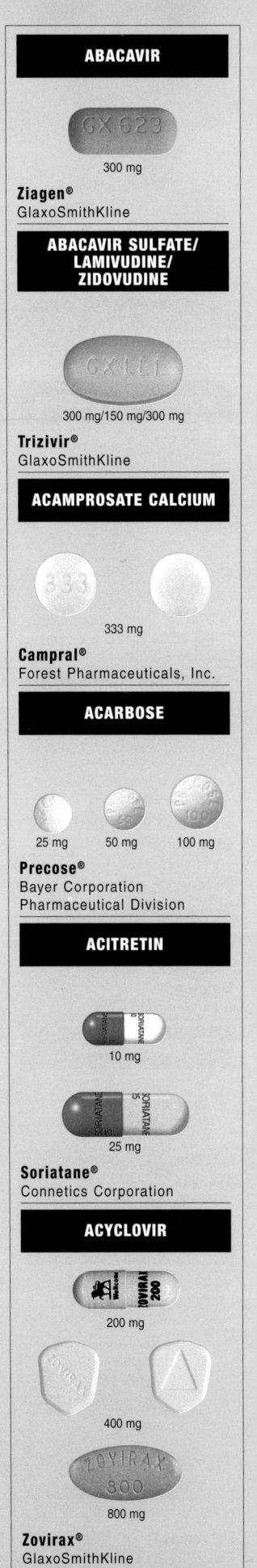

ABACAVIR

GX 623
300 mg

Ziagen®
GlaxoSmithKline

ABACAVIR SULFATE/ LAMIVUDINE/ ZIDOVUDINE

GX LL1
300 mg/150 mg/300 mg

Trizivir®
GlaxoSmithKline

ACAMPROSATE CALCIUM

333
333 mg

Campral®
Forest Pharmaceuticals, Inc.

ACARBOSE

25 mg   50 mg   100 mg

Precose®
Bayer Corporation
Pharmaceutical Division

ACITRETIN

10 mg

25 mg

Soriatane®
Connetics Corporation

ACYCLOVIR

ZOVIRAX 200
200 mg

400 mg

ZOVIRAX 800
800 mg

Zovirax®
GlaxoSmithKline

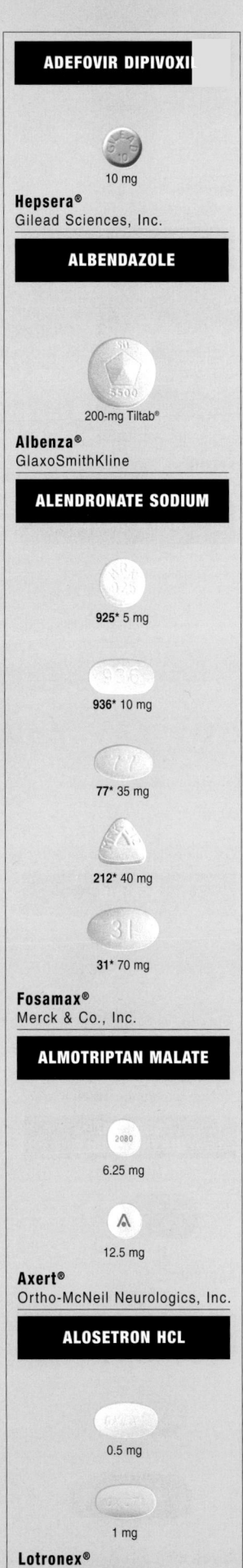

ADEFOVIR DIPIVOXIL

GILEAD 10
10 mg

Hepsera®
Gilead Sciences, Inc.

ALBENDAZOLE

5500
200-mg Tiltab®

Albenza®
GlaxoSmithKline

ALENDRONATE SODIUM

925* 5 mg

936* 10 mg

77* 35 mg

212* 40 mg

31* 70 mg

Fosamax®
Merck & Co., Inc.

ALMOTRIPTAN MALATE

2080
6.25 mg

A
12.5 mg

Axert®
Ortho-McNeil Neurologics, Inc.

ALOSETRON HCL

0.5 mg

1 mg

Lotronex®
GlaxoSmithKline

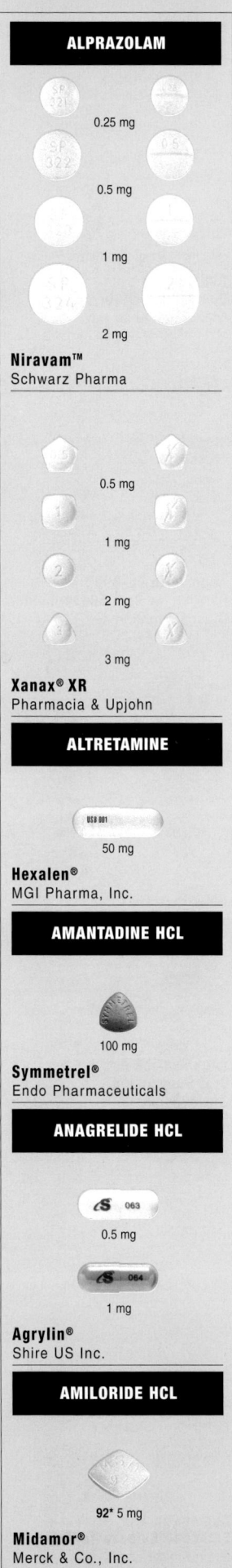

ALPRAZOLAM

0.25 mg

0.5 mg

1 mg

2 mg

Niravam™
Schwarz Pharma

0.5 mg

1 mg

2 mg

3 mg

Xanax® XR
Pharmacia & Upjohn

ALTRETAMINE

USB 001
50 mg

Hexalen®
MGI Pharma, Inc.

AMANTADINE HCL

100 mg

Symmetrel®
Endo Pharmaceuticals

ANAGRELIDE HCL

S 063
0.5 mg

S 064
1 mg

Agrylin®
Shire US Inc.

AMILORIDE HCL

92* 5 mg

Midamor®
Merck & Co., Inc.

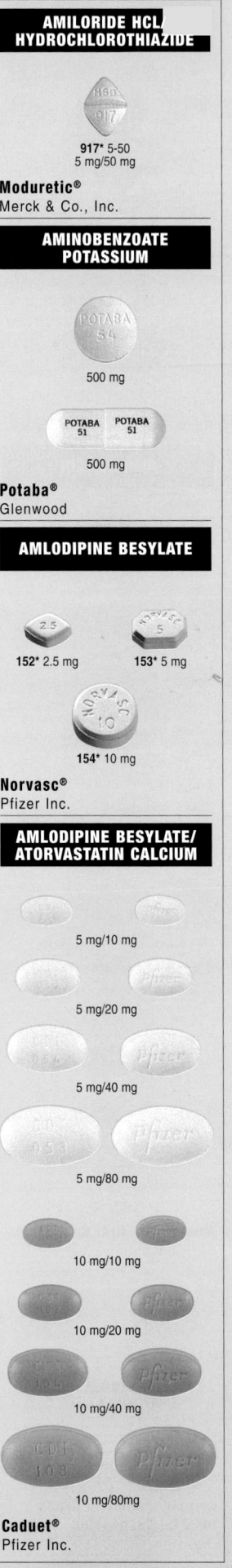

AMILORIDE HCL/ HYDROCHLOROTHIAZIDE

MSD 917
917* 5-50
5 mg/50 mg

Moduretic®
Merck & Co., Inc.

AMINOBENZOATE POTASSIUM

POTABA 54
500 mg

POTABA 51   POTABA 51
500 mg

Potaba®
Glenwood

AMLODIPINE BESYLATE

2.5
152* 2.5 mg

NORVASC 5
153* 5 mg

NORVASC 10
154* 10 mg

Norvasc®
Pfizer Inc.

AMLODIPINE BESYLATE/ ATORVASTATIN CALCIUM

5 mg/10 mg

5 mg/20 mg

5 mg/40 mg

5 mg/80 mg

10 mg/10 mg

10 mg/20 mg

10 mg/40 mg

10 mg/80mg

Caduet®
Pfizer Inc.

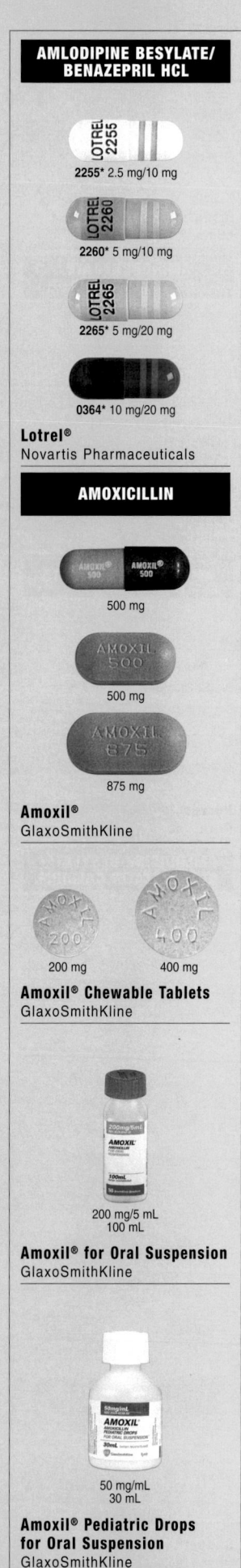

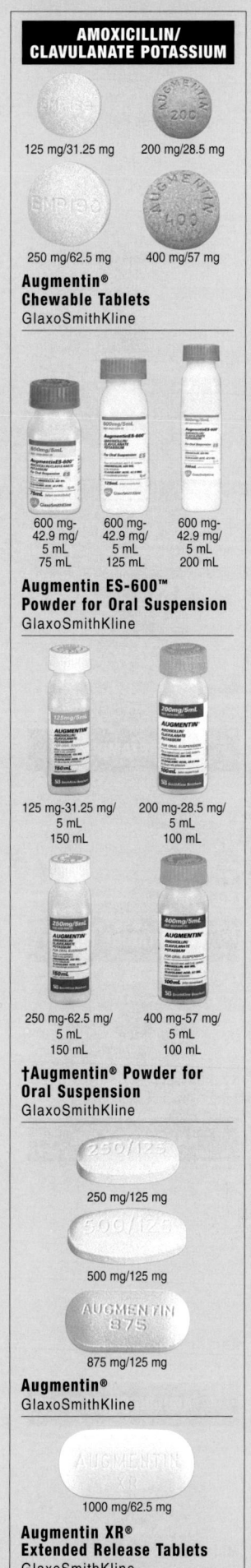

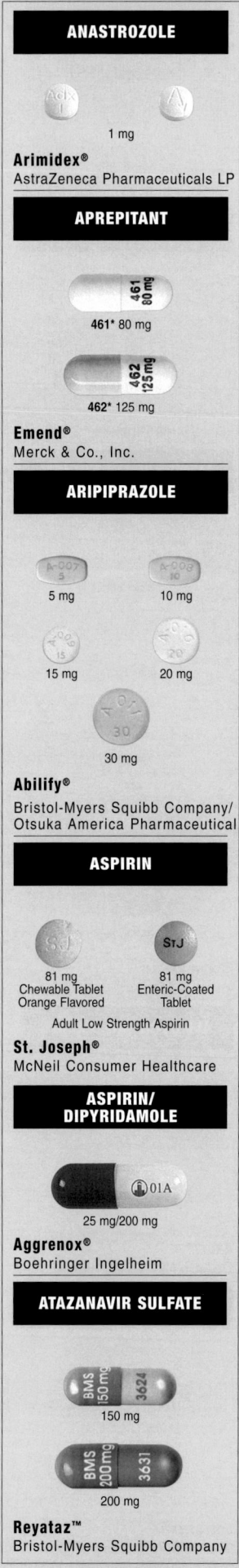

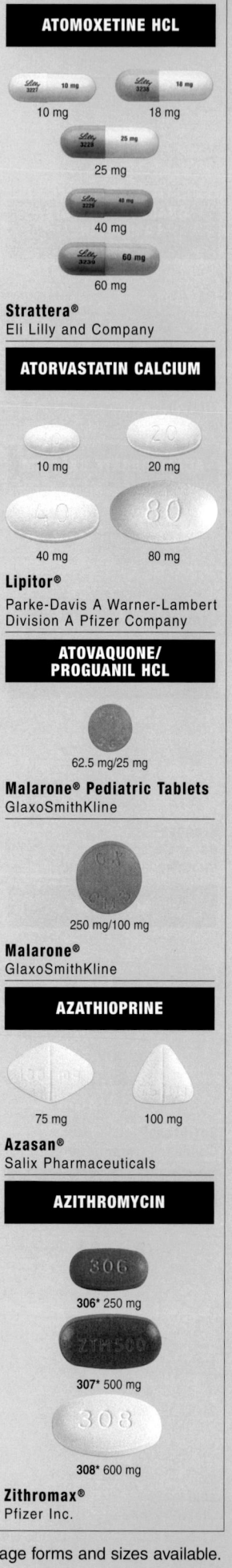

AMLODIPINE BESYLATE/ BENAZEPRIL HCL

2255* 2.5 mg/10 mg

2260* 5 mg/10 mg

2265* 5 mg/20 mg

0364* 10 mg/20 mg

Lotrel®
Novartis Pharmaceuticals

AMOXICILLIN

500 mg

500 mg

875 mg

Amoxil®
GlaxoSmithKline

200 mg   400 mg

Amoxil® Chewable Tablets
GlaxoSmithKline

200 mg/5 mL
100 mL

Amoxil® for Oral Suspension
GlaxoSmithKline

50 mg/mL
30 mL

**Amoxil® Pediatric Drops
for Oral Suspension**
GlaxoSmithKline

AMOXICILLIN/ CLAVULANATE POTASSIUM

125 mg/31.25 mg   200 mg/28.5 mg

250 mg/62.5 mg   400 mg/57 mg

**Augmentin®
Chewable Tablets**
GlaxoSmithKline

600 mg-   600 mg-   600 mg-
42.9 mg/   42.9 mg/   42.9 mg/
5 mL   5 mL   5 mL
75 mL   125 mL   200 mL

**Augmentin ES-600™
Powder for Oral Suspension**
GlaxoSmithKline

125 mg-31.25 mg/   200 mg-28.5 mg/
5 mL   5 mL
150 mL   100 mL

250 mg-62.5 mg/   400 mg-57 mg/
5 mL   5 mL
150 mL   100 mL

**†Augmentin® Powder for
Oral Suspension**
GlaxoSmithKline

250 mg/125 mg

500 mg/125 mg

875 mg/125 mg

Augmentin®
GlaxoSmithKline

1000 mg/62.5 mg

**Augmentin XR®
Extended Release Tablets**
GlaxoSmithKline

ANASTROZOLE

1 mg

Arimidex®
AstraZeneca Pharmaceuticals LP

APREPITANT

461* 80 mg

462* 125 mg

Emend®
Merck & Co., Inc.

ARIPIPRAZOLE

5 mg   10 mg

15 mg   20 mg

30 mg

Abilify®
Bristol-Myers Squibb Company/
Otsuka America Pharmaceutical

ASPIRIN

81 mg   81 mg
Chewable Tablet   Enteric-Coated
Orange Flavored   Tablet
Adult Low Strength Aspirin

St. Joseph®
McNeil Consumer Healthcare

ASPIRIN/ DIPYRIDAMOLE

25 mg/200 mg

Aggrenox®
Boehringer Ingelheim

ATAZANAVIR SULFATE

150 mg

200 mg

Reyataz™
Bristol-Myers Squibb Company

ATOMOXETINE HCL

10 mg   18 mg

25 mg

40 mg

60 mg

Strattera®
Eli Lilly and Company

ATORVASTATIN CALCIUM

10 mg   20 mg

40 mg   80 mg

Lipitor®
Parke-Davis A Warner-Lambert
Division A Pfizer Company

ATOVAQUONE/ PROGUANIL HCL

62.5 mg/25 mg

Malarone® Pediatric Tablets
GlaxoSmithKline

250 mg/100 mg

Malarone®
GlaxoSmithKline

AZATHIOPRINE

75 mg   100 mg

Azasan®
Salix Pharmaceuticals

AZITHROMYCIN

306* 250 mg

307* 500 mg

308* 600 mg

Zithromax®
Pfizer Inc.

* Manufacturer's Identification Code   † Additional dosage forms and sizes available.

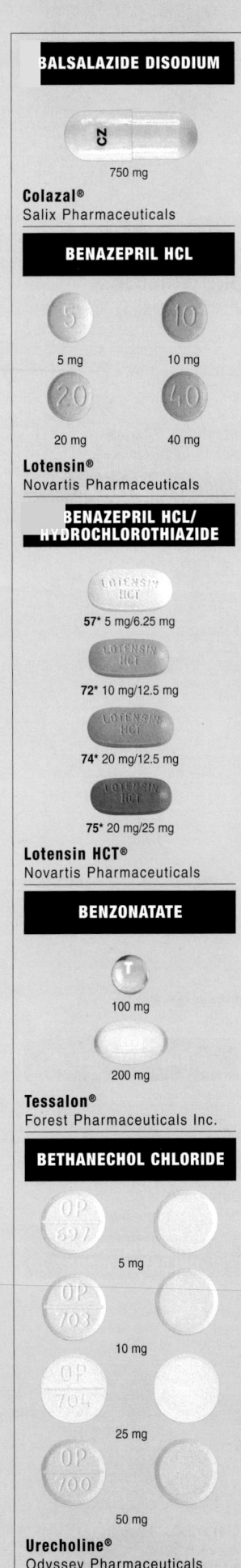

BALSALAZIDE DISODIUM

CZ
750 mg

Colazal®
Salix Pharmaceuticals

BENAZEPRIL HCL

5
5 mg

10
10 mg

20
20 mg

40
40 mg

Lotensin®
Novartis Pharmaceuticals

BENAZEPRIL HCL/ HYDROCHLOROTHIAZIDE

LOTENSIN HCT
57* 5 mg/6.25 mg

LOTENSIN HCT
72* 10 mg/12.5 mg

LOTENSIN HCT
74* 20 mg/12.5 mg

LOTENSIN HCT
75* 20 mg/25 mg

Lotensin HCT®
Novartis Pharmaceuticals

BENZONATATE

T
100 mg

200 mg

Tessalon®
Forest Pharmaceuticals Inc.

BETHANECHOL CHLORIDE

OP 697
5 mg

OP 703
10 mg

OP 704
25 mg

OP 700
50 mg

Urecholine®
Odyssey Pharmaceuticals

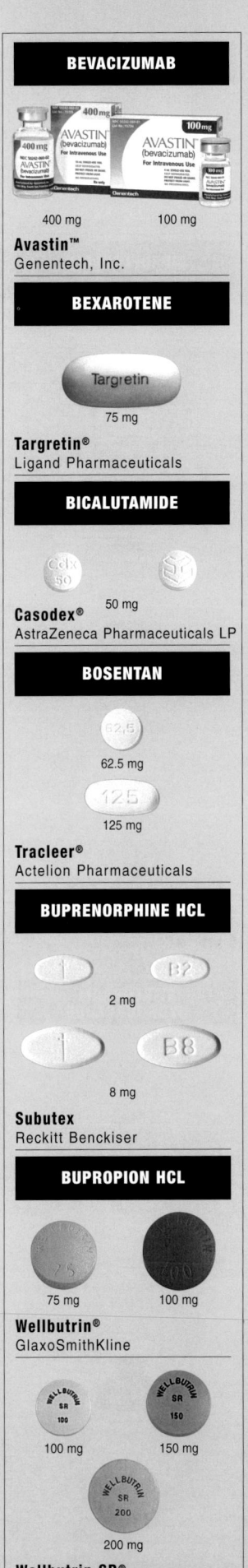

BEVACIZUMAB

400 mg

100 mg

Avastin™
Genentech, Inc.

BEXAROTENE

Targretin
75 mg

Targretin®
Ligand Pharmaceuticals

BICALUTAMIDE

Cdx 50

50 mg

Casodex®
AstraZeneca Pharmaceuticals LP

BOSENTAN

62.5
62.5 mg

125
125 mg

Tracleer®
Actelion Pharmaceuticals

BUPRENORPHINE HCL

B2
2 mg

B8
8 mg

Subutex
Reckitt Benckiser

BUPROPION HCL

25
75 mg

100
100 mg

Wellbutrin®
GlaxoSmithKline

WELLBUTRIN SR 100
100 mg

WELLBUTRIN SR 150
150 mg

WELLBUTRIN SR 200
200 mg

Wellbutrin SR®
GlaxoSmithKline

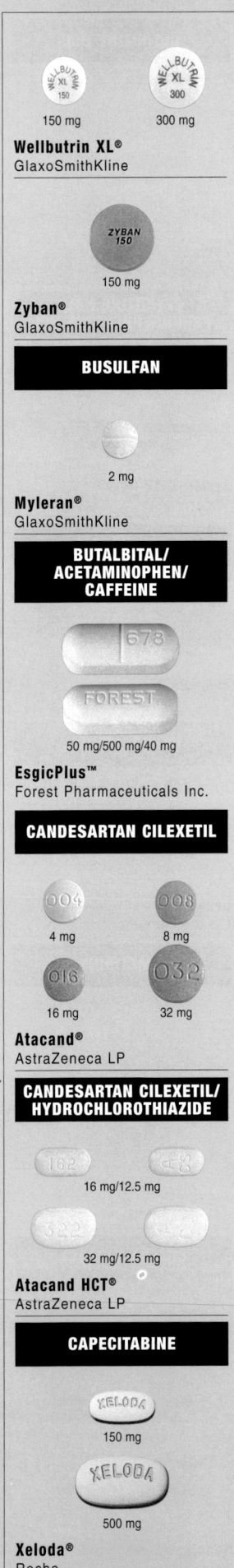

WELLBUTRIN XL 150
150 mg

WELLBUTRIN XL 300
300 mg

Wellbutrin XL®
GlaxoSmithKline

ZYBAN 150
150 mg

Zyban®
GlaxoSmithKline

BUSULFAN

2 mg

Myleran®
GlaxoSmithKline

BUTALBITAL/ ACETAMINOPHEN/ CAFFEINE

678

FOREST

50 mg/500 mg/40 mg

EsgicPlus™
Forest Pharmaceuticals Inc.

CANDESARTAN CILEXETIL

004
4 mg

008
8 mg

016
16 mg

032
32 mg

Atacand®
AstraZeneca LP

CANDESARTAN CILEXETIL/ HYDROCHLOROTHIAZIDE

162

16 mg/12.5 mg

322

32 mg/12.5 mg

Atacand HCT®
AstraZeneca LP

CAPECITABINE

XELODA
150 mg

XELODA
500 mg

Xeloda®
Roche

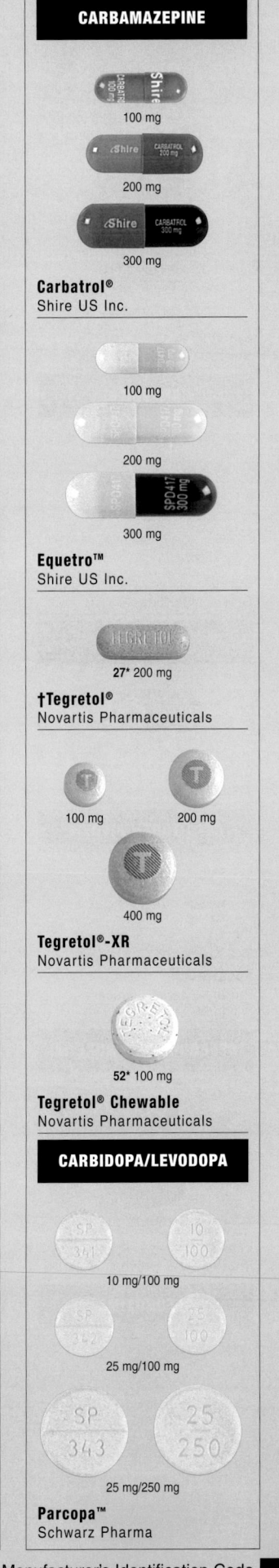

CARBAMAZEPINE

100 mg

200 mg

300 mg

Carbatrol®
Shire US Inc.

100 mg

200 mg

SPD417 300 mg
300 mg

Equetro™
Shire US Inc.

TEGRETOL
27* 200 mg

†Tegretol®
Novartis Pharmaceuticals

T
100 mg

T
200 mg

T
400 mg

Tegretol®-XR
Novartis Pharmaceuticals

TEGRETOL
52* 100 mg

Tegretol® Chewable
Novartis Pharmaceuticals

CARBIDOPA/LEVODOPA

SP 341

10 100

10 mg/100 mg

SP 342

25 100

25 mg/100 mg

SP 343

25 250

25 mg/250 mg

Parcopa™
Schwarz Pharma

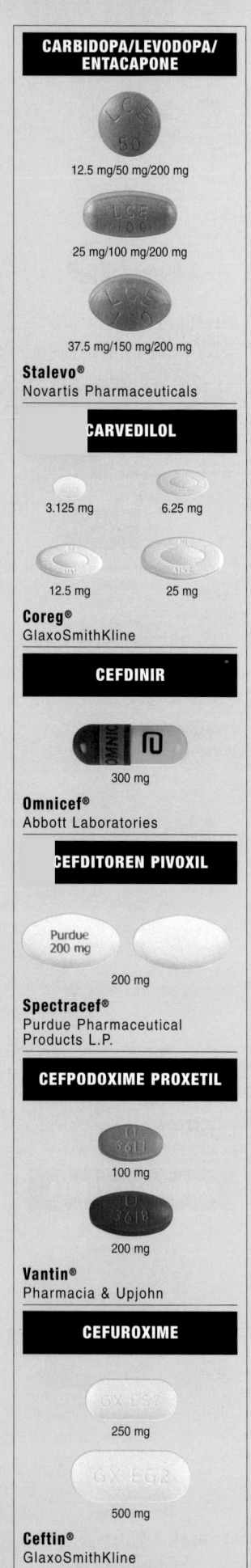

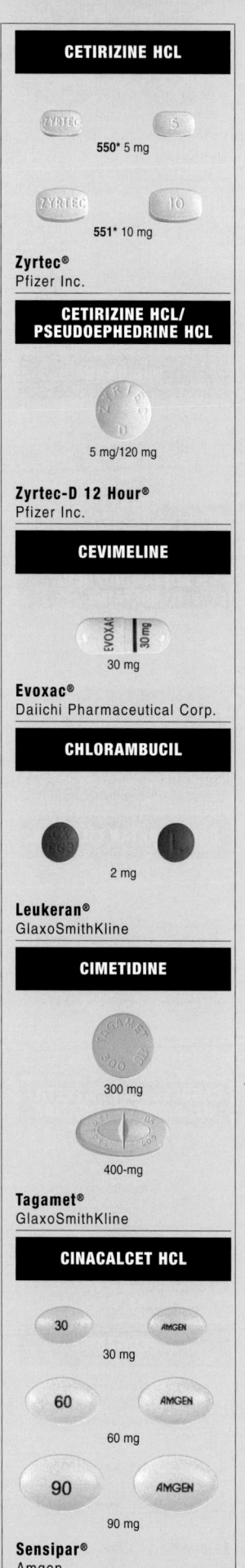

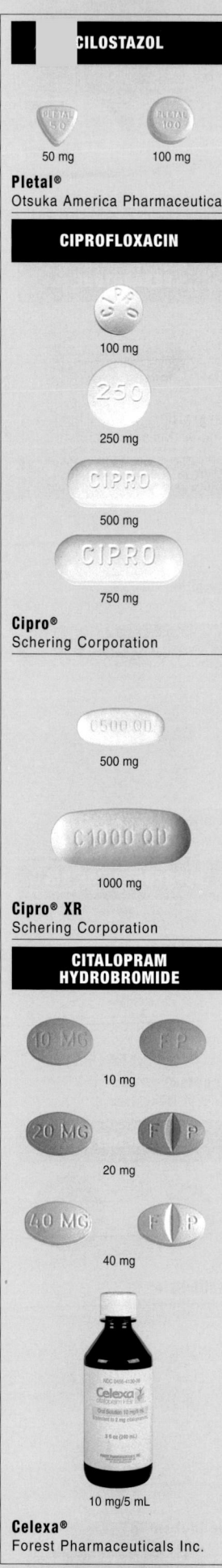

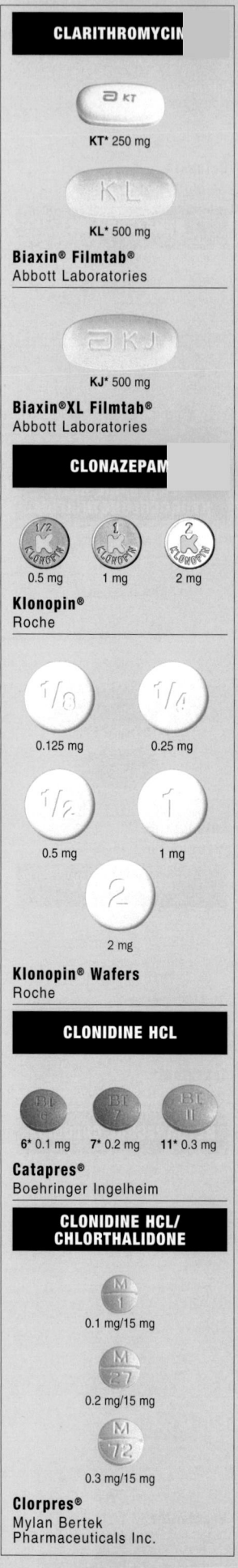

CARBIDOPA/LEVODOPA/ENTACAPONE

12.5 mg/50 mg/200 mg

25 mg/100 mg/200 mg

37.5 mg/150 mg/200 mg

Stalevo®
Novartis Pharmaceuticals

CARVEDILOL

3.125 mg   6.25 mg

12.5 mg   25 mg

Coreg®
GlaxoSmithKline

CEFDINIR

300 mg

Omnicef®
Abbott Laboratories

CEFDITOREN PIVOXIL

Purdue 200 mg

200 mg

Spectracef®
Purdue Pharmaceutical
Products L.P.

CEFPODOXIME PROXETIL

100 mg

200 mg

Vantin®
Pharmacia & Upjohn

CEFUROXIME

250 mg

500 mg

Ceftin®
GlaxoSmithKline

CETIRIZINE HCL

550* 5 mg   5

551* 10 mg   10

Zyrtec®
Pfizer Inc.

CETIRIZINE HCL/PSEUDOEPHEDRINE HCL

5 mg/120 mg

Zyrtec-D 12 Hour®
Pfizer Inc.

CEVIMELINE

30 mg

Evoxac®
Daiichi Pharmaceutical Corp.

CHLORAMBUCIL

2 mg

Leukeran®
GlaxoSmithKline

CIMETIDINE

300 mg

400-mg

Tagamet®
GlaxoSmithKline

CINACALCET HCL

30   AMGEN
30 mg

60   AMGEN
60 mg

90   AMGEN
90 mg

Sensipar®
Amgen

CILOSTAZOL

50 mg   100 mg

Pletal®
Otsuka America Pharmaceutical

CIPROFLOXACIN

100 mg

250 mg

500 mg

750 mg

Cipro®
Schering Corporation

500 mg

1000 mg

Cipro® XR
Schering Corporation

CITALOPRAM HYDROBROMIDE

10 MG   F P
10 mg

20 MG   F P
20 mg

40 MG   F P
40 mg

10 mg/5 mL

Celexa®
Forest Pharmaceuticals Inc.

CLARITHROMYCIN

KT* 250 mg

KL* 500 mg

Biaxin® Filmtab®
Abbott Laboratories

KJ* 500 mg

Biaxin®XL Filmtab®
Abbott Laboratories

CLONAZEPAM

0.5 mg   1 mg   2 mg

Klonopin®
Roche

0.125 mg   0.25 mg

0.5 mg   1 mg

2 mg

Klonopin® Wafers
Roche

CLONIDINE HCL

6* 0.1 mg   7* 0.2 mg   11* 0.3 mg

Catapres®
Boehringer Ingelheim

CLONIDINE HCL/CHLORTHALIDONE

0.1 mg/15 mg

0.2 mg/15 mg

0.3 mg/15 mg

Clorpres®
Mylan Bertek
Pharmaceuticals Inc.

* Manufacturer's Identification Code   † Additional dosage forms and sizes available.

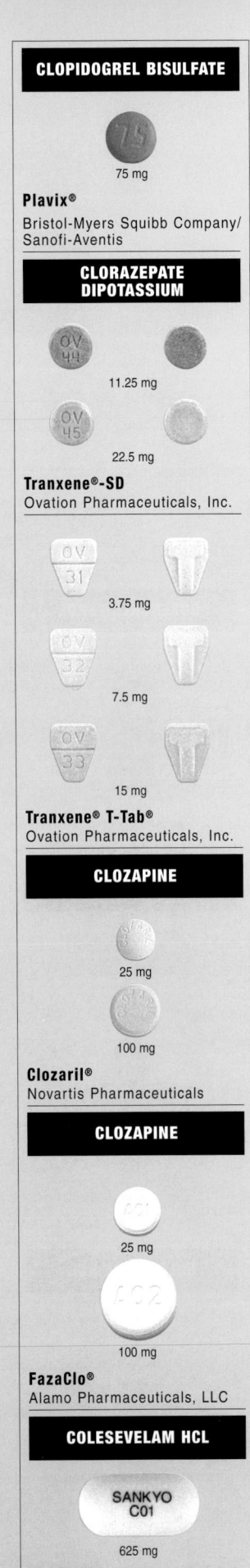

CLOPIDOGREL BISULFATE

75 mg

Plavix®
Bristol-Myers Squibb Company/
Sanofi-Aventis

CLORAZEPATE DIPOTASSIUM

11.25 mg

22.5 mg

Tranxene®-SD
Ovation Pharmaceuticals, Inc.

3.75 mg

7.5 mg

15 mg

Tranxene® T-Tab®
Ovation Pharmaceuticals, Inc.

CLOZAPINE

25 mg

100 mg

Clozaril®
Novartis Pharmaceuticals

CLOZAPINE

25 mg

100 mg

FazaClo®
Alamo Pharmaceuticals, LLC

COLESEVELAM HCL

SANKYO
C01

625 mg

WelChol®
Sankyo Pharma Inc.

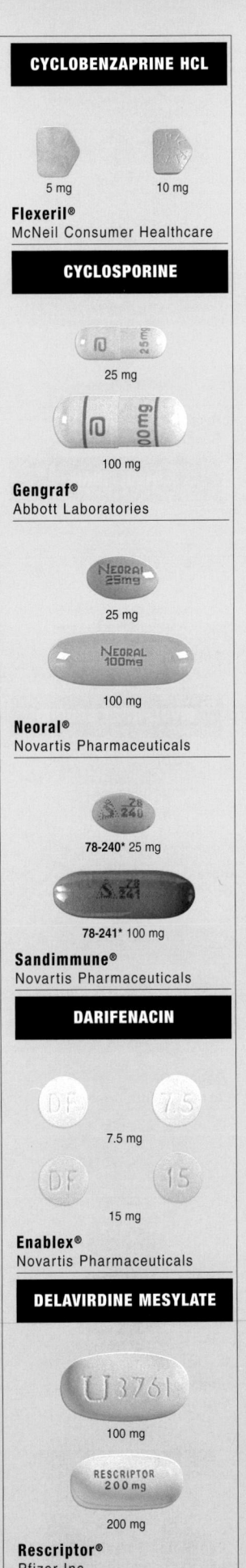

CYCLOBENZAPRINE HCL

5 mg   10 mg

Flexeril®
McNeil Consumer Healthcare

CYCLOSPORINE

25 mg

100 mg

Gengraf®
Abbott Laboratories

25 mg

100 mg

Neoral®
Novartis Pharmaceuticals

78-240* 25 mg

78-241* 100 mg

Sandimmune®
Novartis Pharmaceuticals

DARIFENACIN

7.5 mg

15 mg

Enablex®
Novartis Pharmaceuticals

DELAVIRDINE MESYLATE

U 3761

100 mg

RESCRIPTOR
200 mg

200 mg

Rescriptor®
Pfizer Inc.

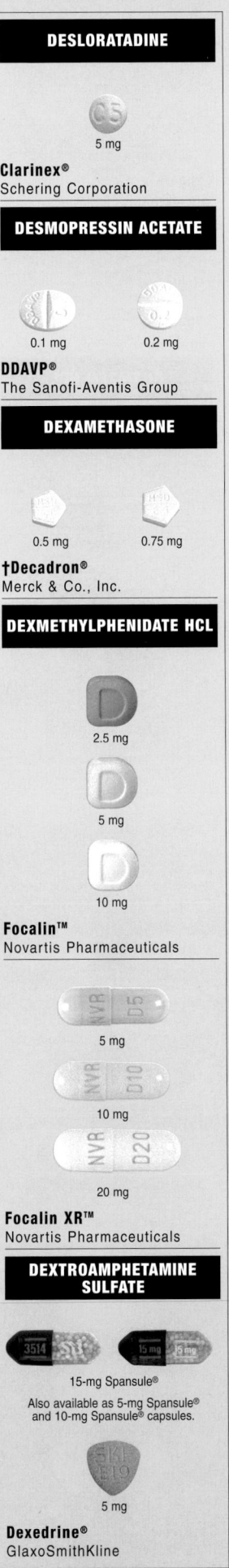

DESLORATADINE

5 mg

Clarinex®
Schering Corporation

DESMOPRESSIN ACETATE

0.1 mg   0.2 mg

DDAVP®
The Sanofi-Aventis Group

DEXAMETHASONE

0.5 mg   0.75 mg

†Decadron®
Merck & Co., Inc.

DEXMETHYLPHENIDATE HCL

2.5 mg

5 mg

10 mg

Focalin™
Novartis Pharmaceuticals

5 mg

10 mg

20 mg

Focalin XR™
Novartis Pharmaceuticals

DEXTROAMPHETAMINE SULFATE

15-mg Spansule®

Also available as 5-mg Spansule®
and 10-mg Spansule® capsules.

5 mg

Dexedrine®
GlaxoSmithKline

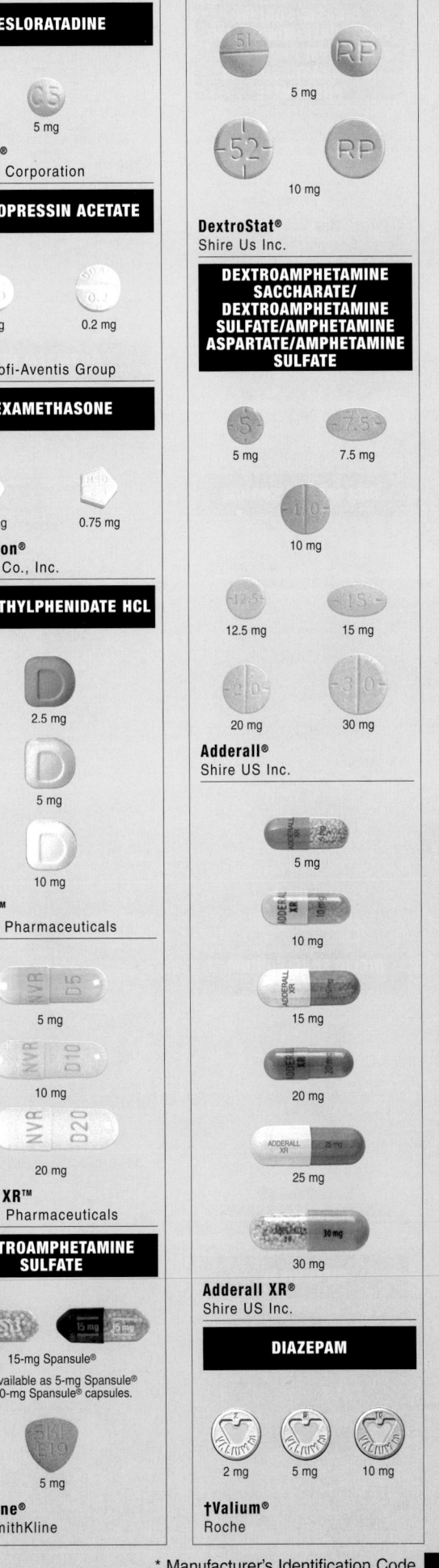

5 mg

10 mg

DextroStat®
Shire US Inc.

DEXTROAMPHETAMINE SACCHARATE/ DEXTROAMPHETAMINE SULFATE/AMPHETAMINE ASPARTATE/AMPHETAMINE SULFATE

5 mg   7.5 mg

10 mg

12.5 mg   15 mg

20 mg   30 mg

Adderall®
Shire US Inc.

5 mg

10 mg

15 mg

20 mg

25 mg

30 mg

Adderall XR®
Shire US Inc.

DIAZEPAM

2 mg   5 mg   10 mg

†Valium®
Roche

---

† Additional dosage forms and sizes available.

* Manufacturer's Identification Code   **MC 5**

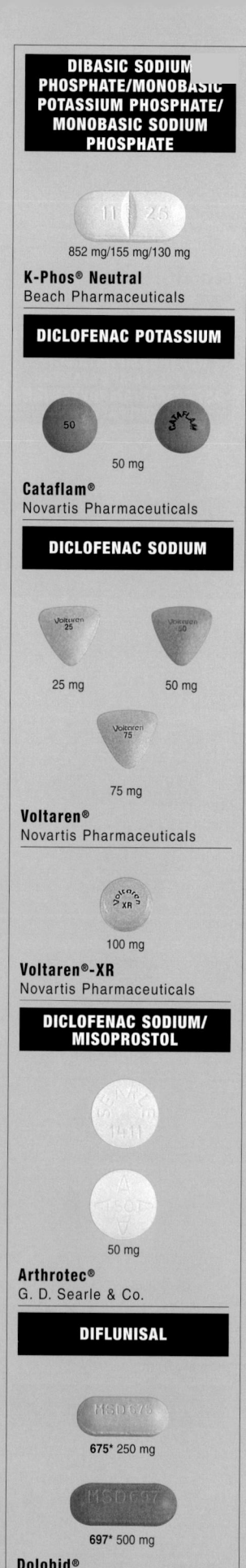

DIBASIC SODIUM PHOSPHATE/MONOBASIC POTASSIUM PHOSPHATE/MONOBASIC SODIUM PHOSPHATE

852 mg/155 mg/130 mg

K-Phos® Neutral
Beach Pharmaceuticals

DICLOFENAC POTASSIUM

50 mg

Cataflam®
Novartis Pharmaceuticals

DICLOFENAC SODIUM

25 mg   50 mg

75 mg

Voltaren®
Novartis Pharmaceuticals

100 mg

Voltaren®-XR
Novartis Pharmaceuticals

DICLOFENAC SODIUM/ MISOPROSTOL

50 mg

Arthrotec®
G. D. Searle & Co.

DIFLUNISAL

675* 250 mg

697* 500 mg

Dolobid®
Merck & Co., Inc.

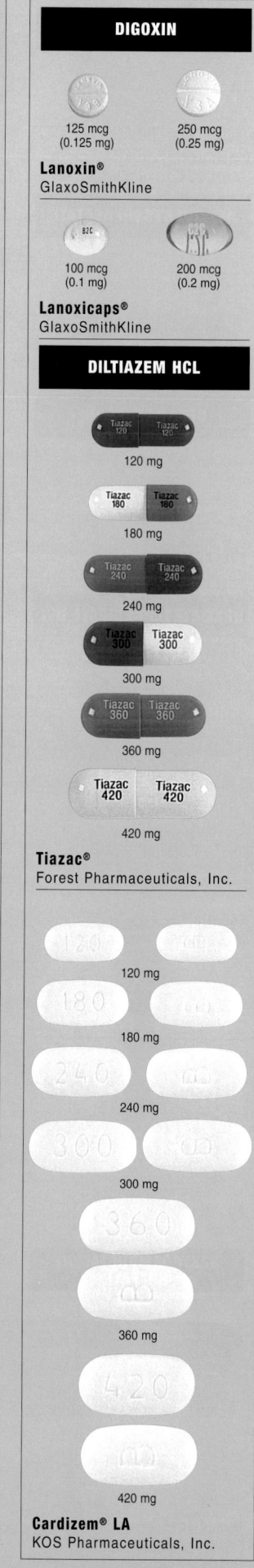

DIGOXIN

125 mcg (0.125 mg)   250 mcg (0.25 mg)

Lanoxin®
GlaxoSmithKline

100 mcg (0.1 mg)   200 mcg (0.2 mg)

Lanoxicaps®
GlaxoSmithKline

DILTIAZEM HCL

120 mg

180 mg

240 mg

300 mg

360 mg

420 mg

Tiazac®
Forest Pharmaceuticals, Inc.

120 mg

180 mg

240 mg

300 mg

360 mg

420 mg

Cardizem® LA
KOS Pharmaceuticals, Inc.

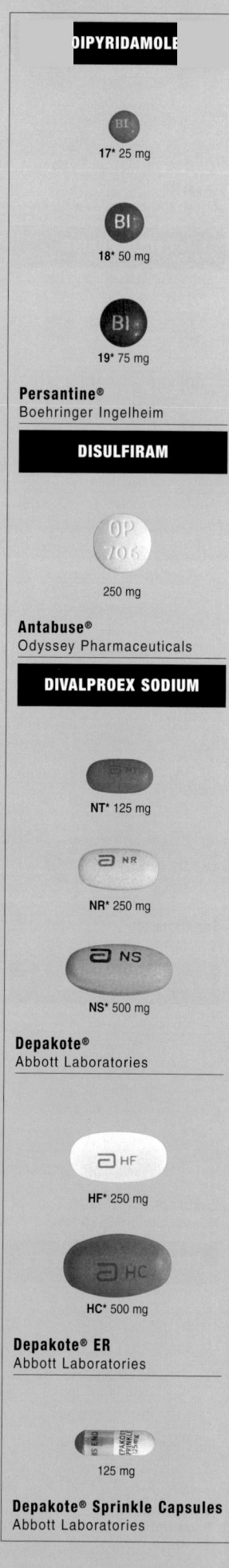

DIPYRIDAMOLE

17* 25 mg

18* 50 mg

19* 75 mg

Persantine®
Boehringer Ingelheim

DISULFIRAM

250 mg

Antabuse®
Odyssey Pharmaceuticals

DIVALPROEX SODIUM

NT* 125 mg

NR* 250 mg

NS* 500 mg

Depakote®
Abbott Laboratories

HF* 250 mg

HC* 500 mg

Depakote® ER
Abbott Laboratories

125 mg

Depakote® Sprinkle Capsules
Abbott Laboratories

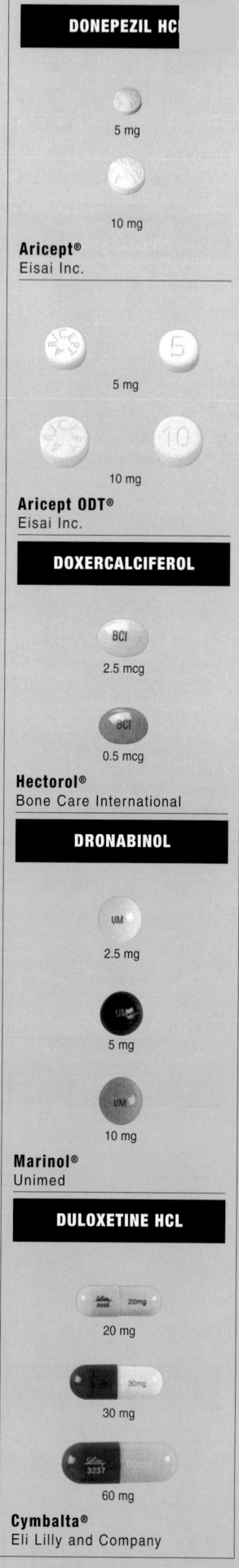

DONEPEZIL HCL

5 mg

10 mg

Aricept®
Eisai Inc.

5 mg

10 mg

Aricept ODT®
Eisai Inc.

DOXERCALCIFEROL

2.5 mcg

0.5 mcg

Hectorol®
Bone Care International

DRONABINOL

2.5 mg

5 mg

10 mg

Marinol®
Unimed

DULOXETINE HCL

20 mg

30 mg

60 mg

Cymbalta®
Eli Lilly and Company

* Manufacturer's Identification Code

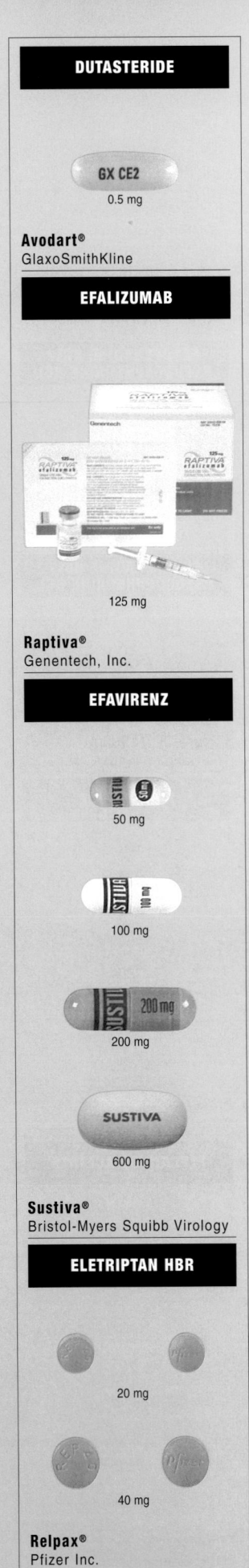

DUTASTERIDE

GX CE2
0.5 mg

Avodart®
GlaxoSmithKline

EFALIZUMAB

125 mg

Raptiva®
Genentech, Inc.

EFAVIRENZ

50 mg

100 mg

200 mg

SUSTIVA
600 mg

Sustiva®
Bristol-Myers Squibb Virology

ELETRIPTAN HBR

20 mg

40 mg

Relpax®
Pfizer Inc.

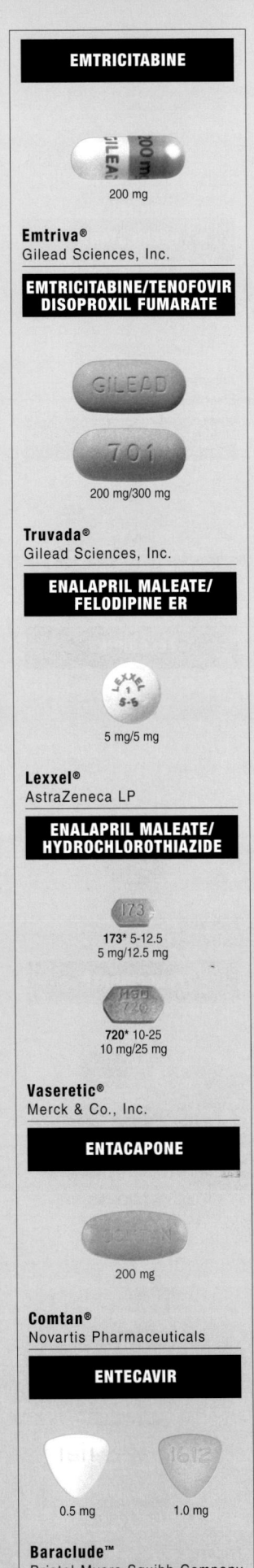

EMTRICITABINE

200 mg

Emtriva®
Gilead Sciences, Inc.

**EMTRICITABINE/TENOFOVIR
DISOPROXIL FUMARATE**

GILEAD

701

200 mg/300 mg

Truvada®
Gilead Sciences, Inc.

**ENALAPRIL MALEATE/
FELODIPINE ER**

LEXXEL
1
5-5

5 mg/5 mg

Lexxel®
AstraZeneca LP

**ENALAPRIL MALEATE/
HYDROCHLOROTHIAZIDE**

173
173* 5-12.5
5 mg/12.5 mg

720
720* 10-25
10 mg/25 mg

Vaseretic®
Merck & Co., Inc.

ENTACAPONE

200 mg

Comtan®
Novartis Pharmaceuticals

ENTECAVIR

0.5 mg   1.0 mg

Baraclude™
Bristol-Myers Squibb Company

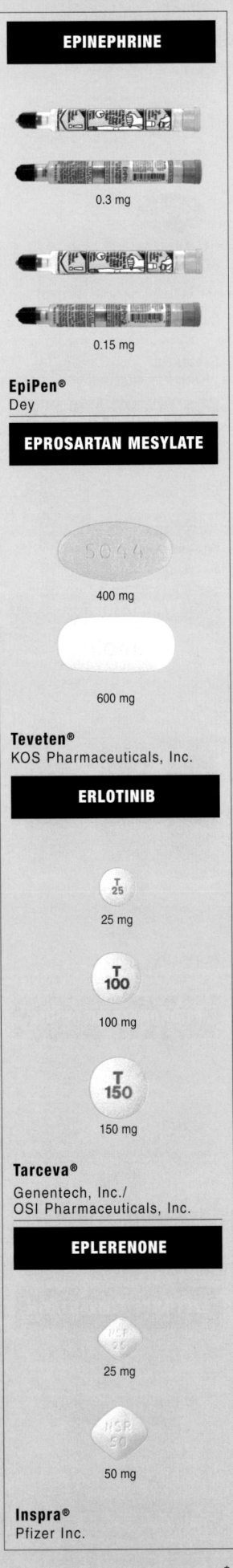

EPINEPHRINE

0.3 mg

0.15 mg

EpiPen®
Dey

EPROSARTAN MESYLATE

5044

400 mg

600 mg

Teveten®
KOS Pharmaceuticals, Inc.

ERLOTINIB

T
25
25 mg

T
100
100 mg

T
150
150 mg

Tarceva®
Genentech, Inc./
OSI Pharmaceuticals, Inc.

EPLERENONE

25 mg

50 mg

Inspra®
Pfizer Inc.

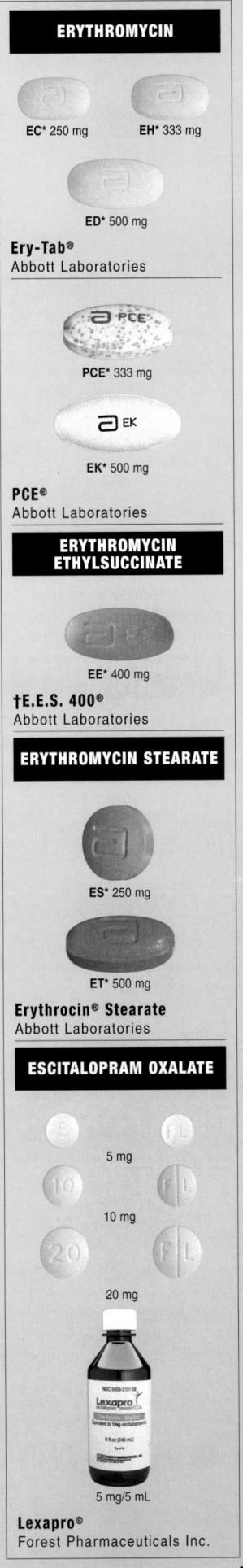

ERYTHROMYCIN

EC* 250 mg   EH* 333 mg

ED* 500 mg

Ery-Tab®
Abbott Laboratories

PCE
PCE* 333 mg

EK
EK* 500 mg

PCE®
Abbott Laboratories

**ERYTHROMYCIN
ETHYLSUCCINATE**

EE* 400 mg

†E.E.S. 400®
Abbott Laboratories

ERYTHROMYCIN STEARATE

ES* 250 mg

ET* 500 mg

Erythrocin® Stearate
Abbott Laboratories

ESCITALOPRAM OXALATE

5 mg

10 mg

20 mg

Lexapro
5 mg/5 mL

Lexapro®
Forest Pharmaceuticals Inc.

† Additional dosage forms and sizes available.

* Manufacturer's Identification Code

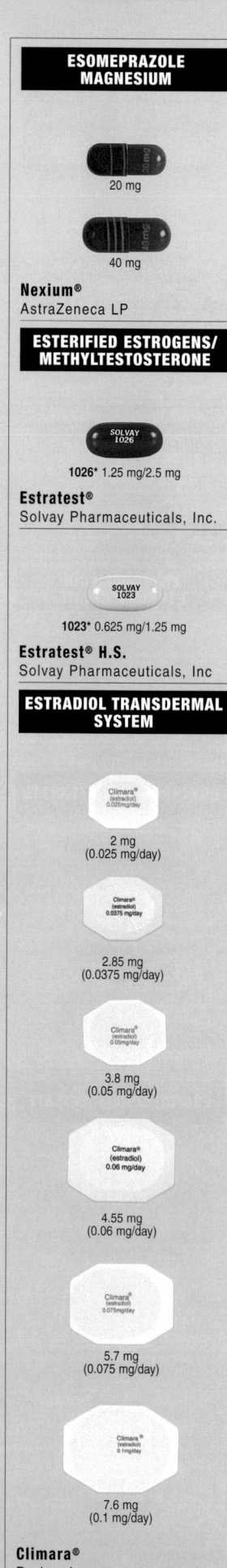

ESOMEPRAZOLE MAGNESIUM

20 mg

40 mg

Nexium®
AstraZeneca LP

ESTERIFIED ESTROGENS/ METHYLTESTOSTERONE

SOLVAY 1026
1026* 1.25 mg/2.5 mg

Estratest®
Solvay Pharmaceuticals, Inc.

SOLVAY 1023
1023* 0.625 mg/1.25 mg

Estratest® H.S.
Solvay Pharmaceuticals, Inc

ESTRADIOL TRANSDERMAL SYSTEM

Climara® (estradiol) 0.025 mg/day
2 mg (0.025 mg/day)

Climara® (estradiol) 0.0375 mg/day
2.85 mg (0.0375 mg/day)

Climara® (estradiol) 0.05 mg/day
3.8 mg (0.05 mg/day)

Climara® (estradiol) 0.06 mg/day
4.55 mg (0.06 mg/day)

Climara® (estradiol) 0.075mg/day
5.7 mg (0.075 mg/day)

Climara® (estradiol) 0.1mg/day
7.6 mg (0.1 mg/day)

Climara®
Berlex, Inc.

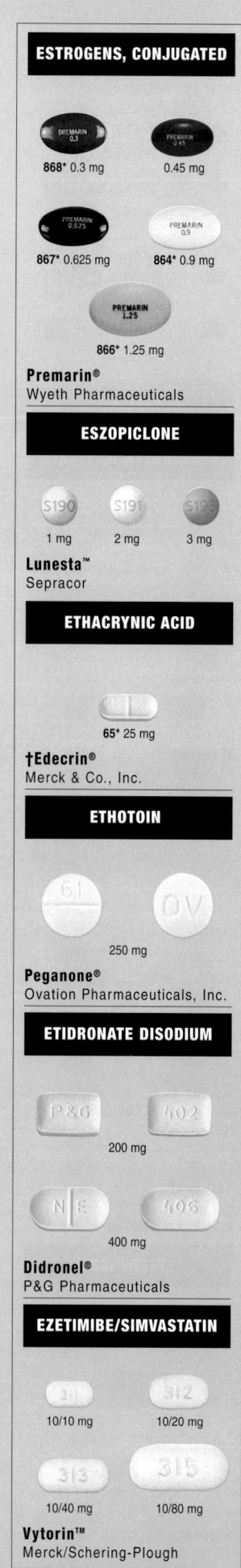

ESTROGENS, CONJUGATED

PREMARIN 0.3
868* 0.3 mg

PREMARIN 0.45
0.45 mg

PREMARIN 0.625
867* 0.625 mg

PREMARIN 0.9
864* 0.9 mg

PREMARIN 1.25
866* 1.25 mg

Premarin®
Wyeth Pharmaceuticals

ESZOPICLONE

S190
1 mg

S191
2 mg

S193
3 mg

Lunesta™
Sepracor

ETHACRYNIC ACID

166
65* 25 mg

†Edecrin®
Merck & Co., Inc.

ETHOTOIN

61

OV

250 mg

Peganone®
Ovation Pharmaceuticals, Inc.

ETIDRONATE DISODIUM

P&G

402

200 mg

N E

406

400 mg

Didronel®
P&G Pharmaceuticals

EZETIMIBE/SIMVASTATIN

311
10/10 mg

312
10/20 mg

313
10/40 mg

315
10/80 mg

Vytorin™
Merck/Schering-Plough

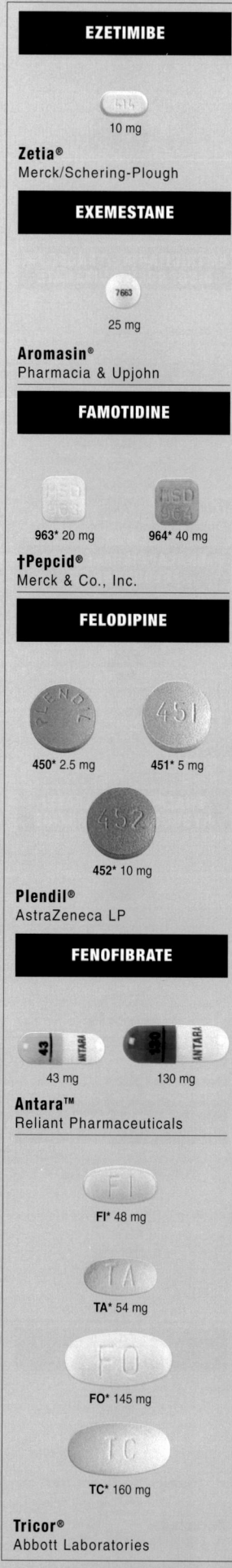

EZETIMIBE

414
10 mg

Zetia®
Merck/Schering-Plough

EXEMESTANE

7663
25 mg

Aromasin®
Pharmacia & Upjohn

FAMOTIDINE

MSD 963
963* 20 mg

MSD 964
964* 40 mg

†Pepcid®
Merck & Co., Inc.

FELODIPINE

PLENDIL
450* 2.5 mg

451
451* 5 mg

452
452* 10 mg

Plendil®
AstraZeneca LP

FENOFIBRATE

43 ANTARA
43 mg

130 ANTARA
130 mg

Antara™
Reliant Pharmaceuticals

FI
FI* 48 mg

TA
TA* 54 mg

FO
FO* 145 mg

TC
TC* 160 mg

Tricor®
Abbott Laboratories

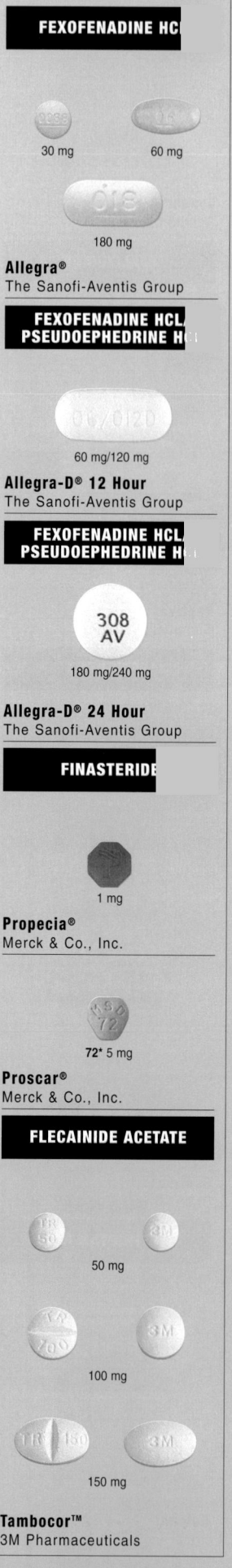

FEXOFENADINE HCl

0938
30 mg

016
60 mg

018
180 mg

Allegra®
The Sanofi-Aventis Group

FEXOFENADINE HCL/ PSEUDOEPHEDRINE HCl

06/012D
60 mg/120 mg

Allegra-D® 12 Hour
The Sanofi-Aventis Group

FEXOFENADINE HCL/ PSEUDOEPHEDRINE HCl

308 AV
180 mg/240 mg

Allegra-D® 24 Hour
The Sanofi-Aventis Group

FINASTERIDE

1 mg

Propecia®
Merck & Co., Inc.

MSD 72
72* 5 mg

Proscar®
Merck & Co., Inc.

FLECAINIDE ACETATE

TR 50
3M
50 mg

TR 100
3M
100 mg

TR 150
3M
150 mg

Tambocor™
3M Pharmaceuticals

* Manufacturer's Identification Code

† Additional dosage forms and sizes available.

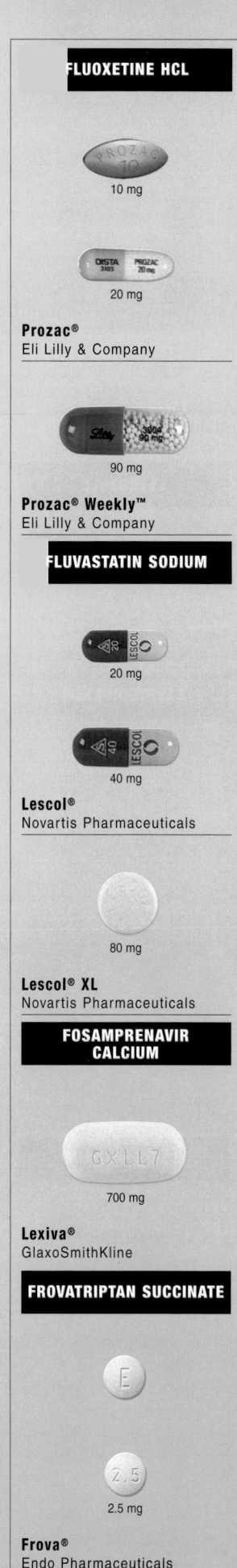

FLUOXETINE HCL

PROZAC 10
10 mg

DISTA 3105 PROZAC 20 mg
20 mg

Prozac®
Eli Lilly & Company

Lilly 3004 90 mg
90 mg

Prozac® Weekly™
Eli Lilly & Company

FLUVASTATIN SODIUM

20
20 mg

40
40 mg

Lescol®
Novartis Pharmaceuticals

80 mg

Lescol® XL
Novartis Pharmaceuticals

FOSAMPRENAVIR CALCIUM

GXLL7
700 mg

Lexiva®
GlaxoSmithKline

FROVATRIPTAN SUCCINATE

E

2.5
2.5 mg

Frova®
Endo Pharmaceuticals

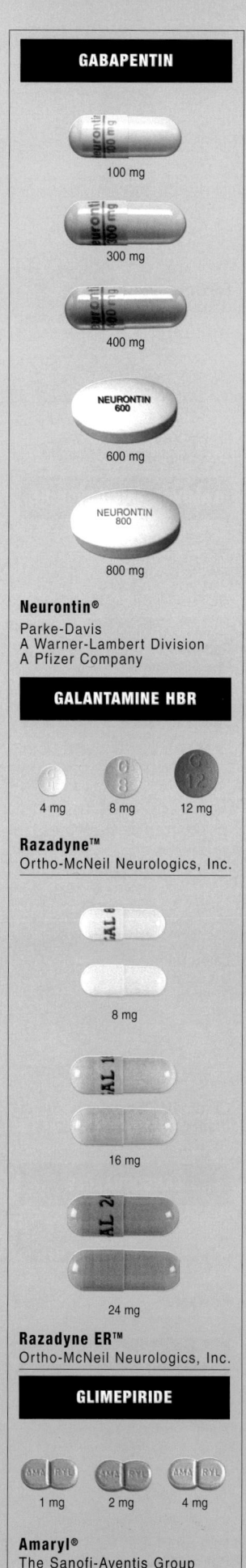

GABAPENTIN

Neurontin 100 mg
100 mg

Neurontin 300 mg
300 mg

Neurontin 400 mg
400 mg

NEURONTIN 600
600 mg

NEURONTIN 800
800 mg

Neurontin®
Parke-Davis
A Warner-Lambert Division
A Pfizer Company

GALANTAMINE HBR

4 mg   8 mg   12 mg

Razadyne™
Ortho-McNeil Neurologics, Inc.

8 mg

16 mg

24 mg

Razadyne ER™
Ortho-McNeil Neurologics, Inc.

GLIMEPIRIDE

AMA RYL   AMA RYL   AMA RYL
1 mg   2 mg   4 mg

Amaryl®
The Sanofi-Aventis Group

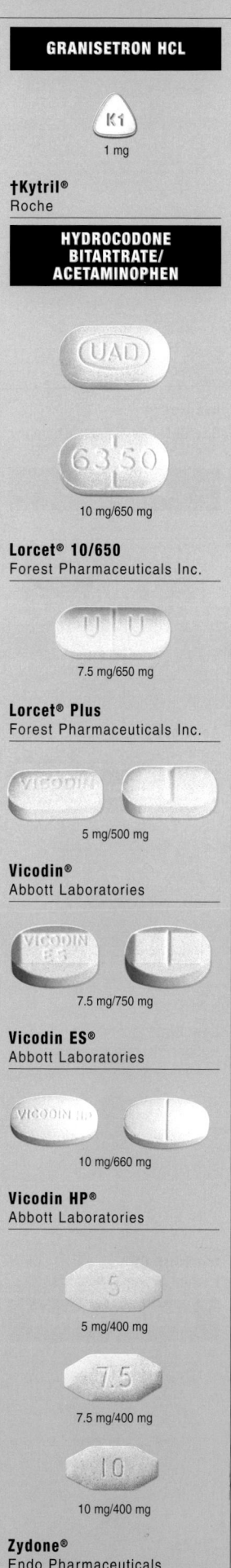

GRANISETRON HCL

K1
1 mg

†Kytril®
Roche

HYDROCODONE BITARTRATE/ ACETAMINOPHEN

UAD

63 50
10 mg/650 mg

Lorcet® 10/650
Forest Pharmaceuticals Inc.

U U
7.5 mg/650 mg

Lorcet® Plus
Forest Pharmaceuticals Inc.

VICODIN
5 mg/500 mg

Vicodin®
Abbott Laboratories

VICODIN ES
7.5 mg/750 mg

Vicodin ES®
Abbott Laboratories

VICODIN HP
10 mg/660 mg

Vicodin HP®
Abbott Laboratories

5
5 mg/400 mg

7.5
7.5 mg/400 mg

10
10 mg/400 mg

Zydone®
Endo Pharmaceuticals

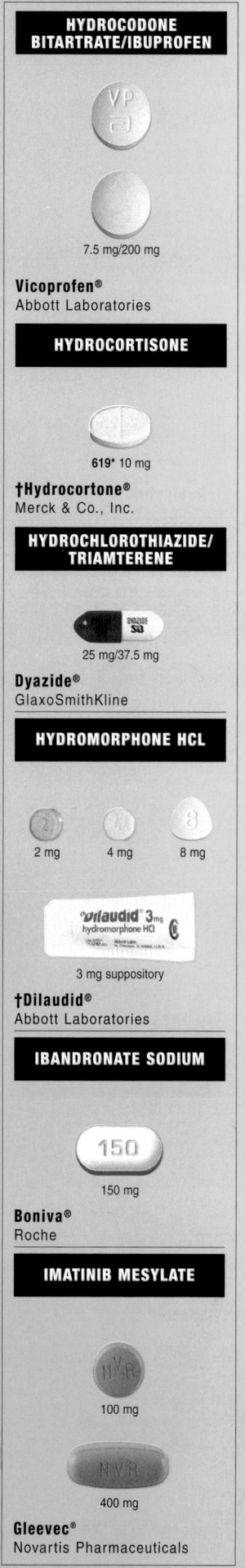

HYDROCODONE BITARTRATE/IBUPROFEN

VP a

7.5 mg/200 mg

Vicoprofen®
Abbott Laboratories

HYDROCORTISONE

619* 10 mg

†Hydrocortone®
Merck & Co., Inc.

HYDROCHLOROTHIAZIDE/ TRIAMTERENE

DN2101 SQ
25 mg/37.5 mg

Dyazide®
GlaxoSmithKline

HYDROMORPHONE HCL

2   4   8
2 mg   4 mg   8 mg

Dilaudid 3 mg
hydromorphone HCl
3 mg suppository

†Dilaudid®
Abbott Laboratories

IBANDRONATE SODIUM

150
150 mg

Boniva®
Roche

IMATINIB MESYLATE

NVR
100 mg

NVR
400 mg

Gleevec®
Novartis Pharmaceuticals

† Additional dosage forms and sizes available.

* Manufacturer's Identification Code

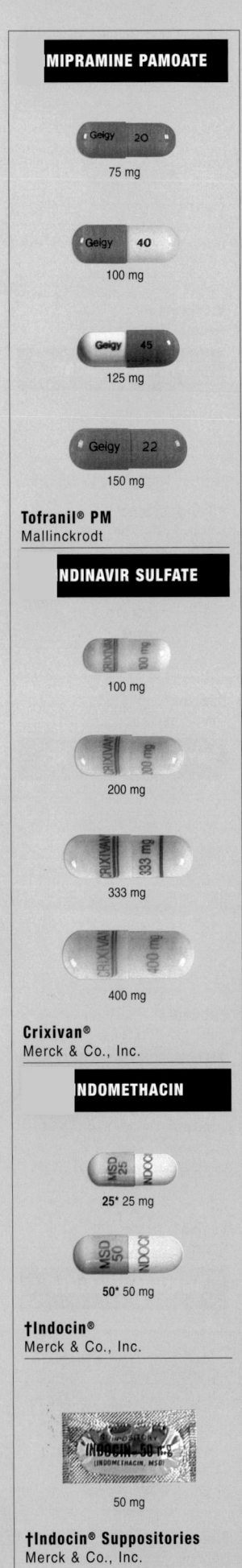

IMIPRAMINE PAMOATE

Geigy 20
75 mg

Geigy 40
100 mg

Geigy 45
125 mg

Geigy 22
150 mg

Tofranil® PM
Mallinckrodt

INDINAVIR SULFATE

CRIXIVAN 100 mg
100 mg

CRIXIVAN 200 mg
200 mg

CRIXIVAN 333 mg
333 mg

CRIXIVAN 400 mg
400 mg

Crixivan®
Merck & Co., Inc.

INDOMETHACIN

MSD 25 INDOCIN
25* 25 mg

MSD 50 INDOCIN
50* 50 mg

†Indocin®
Merck & Co., Inc.

INDOCIN-50 R-S
(INDOMETHACIN, MSD)
50 mg

†Indocin® Suppositories
Merck & Co., Inc.

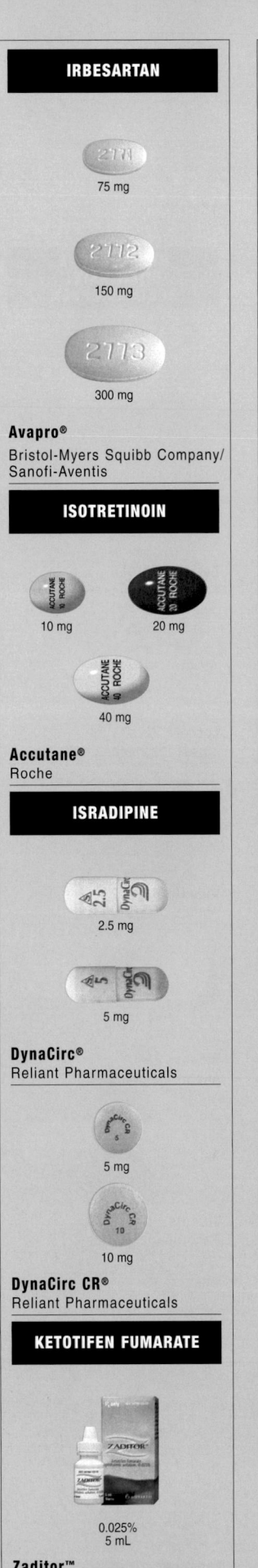

IRBESARTAN

2771
75 mg

2772
150 mg

2773
300 mg

Avapro®
Bristol-Myers Squibb Company/
Sanofi-Aventis

ISOTRETINOIN

ACCUTANE 10 ROCHE
10 mg

ACCUTANE 20 ROCHE
20 mg

ACCUTANE 40 ROCHE
40 mg

Accutane®
Roche

ISRADIPINE

2.5 DynaCirc
2.5 mg

5 DynaCirc
5 mg

DynaCirc®
Reliant Pharmaceuticals

DynaCirc CR 5
5 mg

DynaCirc CR 10
10 mg

DynaCirc CR®
Reliant Pharmaceuticals

KETOTIFEN FUMARATE

ZADITOR

0.025%
5 mL

Zaditor™
Novartis Ophthalmics

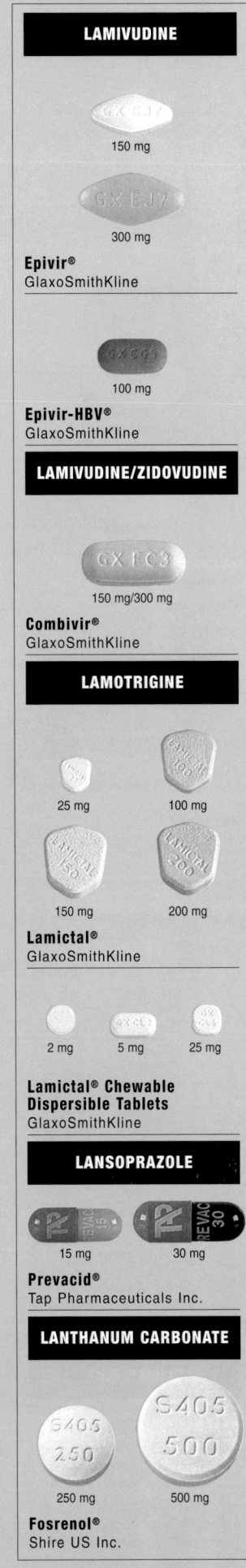

LAMIVUDINE

GX CJ7
150 mg

GX EJ7
300 mg

Epivir®
GlaxoSmithKline

GX CG5
100 mg

Epivir-HBV®
GlaxoSmithKline

LAMIVUDINE/ZIDOVUDINE

GX FC3
150 mg/300 mg

Combivir®
GlaxoSmithKline

LAMOTRIGINE

25 mg

100 mg

LAMICTAL 150
150 mg

LAMICTAL 200
200 mg

Lamictal®
GlaxoSmithKline

2 mg

GX CL2
5 mg

GX CL5
25 mg

**Lamictal® Chewable
Dispersible Tablets**
GlaxoSmithKline

LANSOPRAZOLE

TAP PREVAC 15
15 mg

TAP PREVAC 30
30 mg

Prevacid®
Tap Pharmaceuticals Inc.

LANTHANUM CARBONATE

S405 250
250 mg

S405 500
500 mg

Fosrenol®
Shire US Inc.

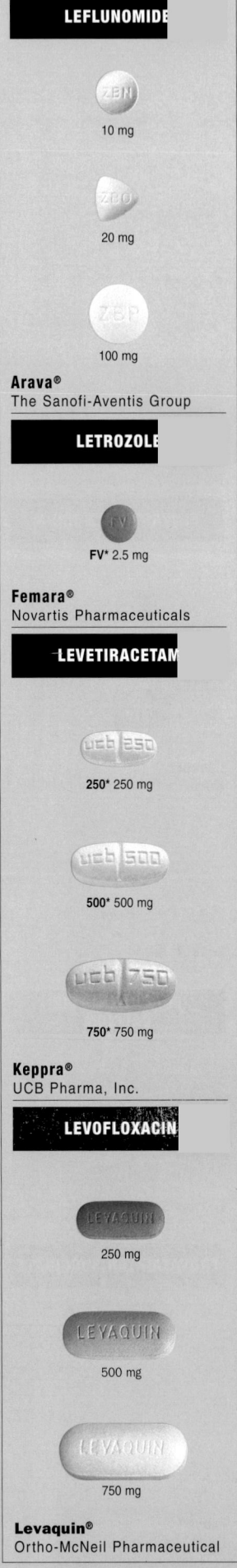

LEFLUNOMIDE

ZBN
10 mg

ZBO
20 mg

ZBP
100 mg

Arava®
The Sanofi-Aventis Group

LETROZOLE

FV
FV* 2.5 mg

Femara®
Novartis Pharmaceuticals

LEVETIRACETAM

ucb 250
250* 250 mg

ucb 500
500* 500 mg

ucb 750
750* 750 mg

Keppra®
UCB Pharma, Inc.

LEVOFLOXACIN

LEVAQUIN
250 mg

LEVAQUIN
500 mg

LEVAQUIN
750 mg

Levaquin®
Ortho-McNeil Pharmaceutical

* Manufacturer's Identification Code   † Additional dosage forms and sizes available.

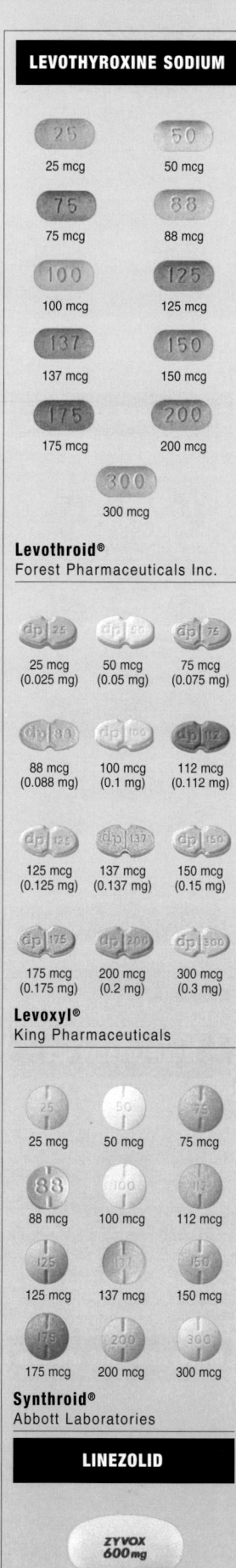

LEVOTHYROXINE SODIUM

25 — 25 mcg	50 — 50 mcg
75 — 75 mcg	88 — 88 mcg
100 — 100 mcg	125 — 125 mcg
137 — 137 mcg	150 — 150 mcg
175 — 175 mcg	200 — 200 mcg
300 — 300 mcg	

Levothroid®
Forest Pharmaceuticals Inc.

dp 25 — 25 mcg (0.025 mg)	dp 50 — 50 mcg (0.05 mg)	dp 75 — 75 mcg (0.075 mg)
dp 88 — 88 mcg (0.088 mg)	dp 100 — 100 mcg (0.1 mg)	dp 112 — 112 mcg (0.112 mg)
dp 125 — 125 mcg (0.125 mg)	dp 137 — 137 mcg (0.137 mg)	dp 150 — 150 mcg (0.15 mg)
dp 175 — 175 mcg (0.175 mg)	dp 200 — 200 mcg (0.2 mg)	dp 300 — 300 mcg (0.3 mg)

Levoxyl®
King Pharmaceuticals

25 — 25 mcg	50 — 50 mcg	75 — 75 mcg
88 — 88 mcg	100 — 100 mcg	112 — 112 mcg
125 — 125 mcg	137 — 137 mcg	150 — 150 mcg
175 — 175 mcg	200 — 200 mcg	300 — 300 mcg

Synthroid®
Abbott Laboratories

LINEZOLID

ZYVOX 600mg — 600 mg

Zyvox®
Pharmacia & Upjohn

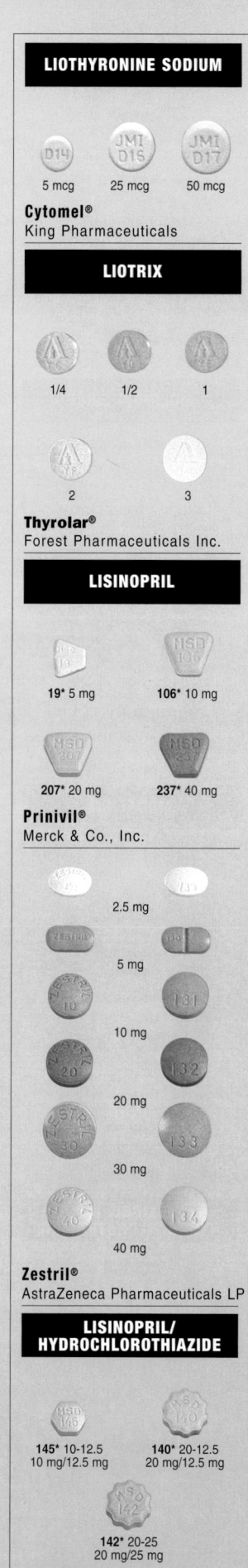

LIOTHYRONINE SODIUM

D14 — 5 mcg	JMI D15 — 25 mcg	JMI D17 — 50 mcg

Cytomel®
King Pharmaceuticals

LIOTRIX

1/4	1/2	1
2	3	

Thyrolar®
Forest Pharmaceuticals Inc.

LISINOPRIL

19* 5 mg	106* 10 mg
207* 20 mg	237* 40 mg

Prinivil®
Merck & Co., Inc.

	2.5 mg
ZESTRIL	5 mg
ZESTRIL 10 — 10 mg	131
ZESTRIL 20 — 20 mg	132
ZESTRIL 30 — 30 mg	133
ZESTRIL 40 — 40 mg	134

Zestril®
AstraZeneca Pharmaceuticals LP

LISINOPRIL/ HYDROCHLOROTHIAZIDE

145* 10-12.5 10 mg/12.5 mg	140* 20-12.5 20 mg/12.5 mg
142* 20-25 20 mg/25 mg	

Prinzide®
Merck & Co., Inc.

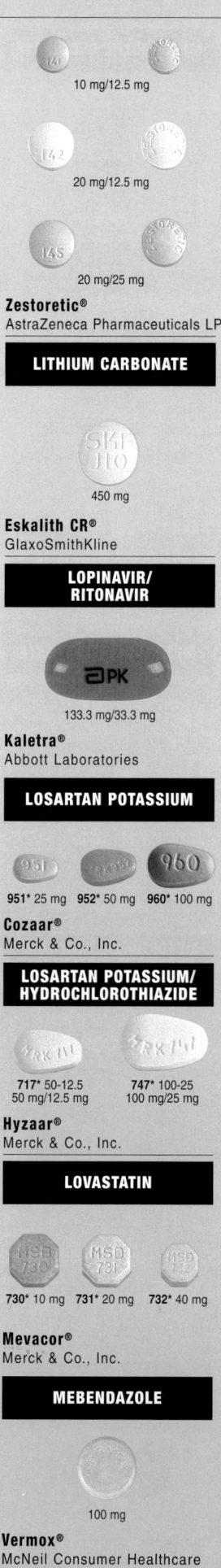

141 — 10 mg/12.5 mg
142 — 20 mg/12.5 mg
145 — 20 mg/25 mg

Zestoretic®
AstraZeneca Pharmaceuticals LP

LITHIUM CARBONATE

SKF J10 — 450 mg

Eskalith CR®
GlaxoSmithKline

LOPINAVIR/ RITONAVIR

PK — 133.3 mg/33.3 mg

Kaletra®
Abbott Laboratories

LOSARTAN POTASSIUM

951* 25 mg	952* 50 mg	960* 100 mg

Cozaar®
Merck & Co., Inc.

LOSARTAN POTASSIUM/ HYDROCHLOROTHIAZIDE

717* 50-12.5 50 mg/12.5 mg	747* 100-25 100 mg/25 mg

Hyzaar®
Merck & Co., Inc.

LOVASTATIN

MSD 730 — 730* 10 mg	MSD 731 — 731* 20 mg	MSD 732 — 732* 40 mg

Mevacor®
Merck & Co., Inc.

MEBENDAZOLE

100 mg

Vermox®
McNeil Consumer Healthcare

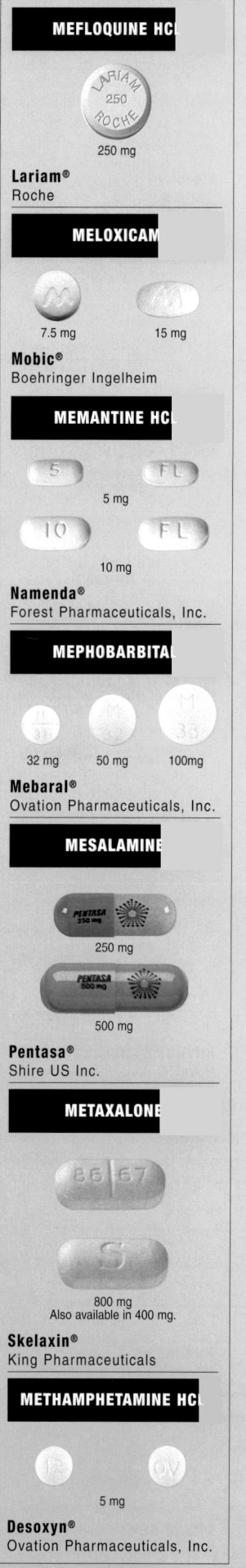

MEFLOQUINE HCl

LARIAM 250 ROCHE — 250 mg

Lariam®
Roche

MELOXICAM

M — 7.5 mg	M — 15 mg

Mobic®
Boehringer Ingelheim

MEMANTINE HCl

5 — 5 mg	FL
10 — 10 mg	FL

Namenda®
Forest Pharmaceuticals, Inc.

MEPHOBARBITAL

M 31 — 32 mg	M 32 — 50 mg	M 33 — 100mg

Mebaral®
Ovation Pharmaceuticals, Inc.

MESALAMINE

PENTASA 250 mg — 250 mg

PENTASA 500 mg — 500 mg

Pentasa®
Shire US Inc.

METAXALONE

86 67 — 800 mg

S

800 mg
Also available in 400 mg.

Skelaxin®
King Pharmaceuticals

METHAMPHETAMINE HCl

12	OV
5 mg	

Desoxyn®
Ovation Pharmaceuticals, Inc.

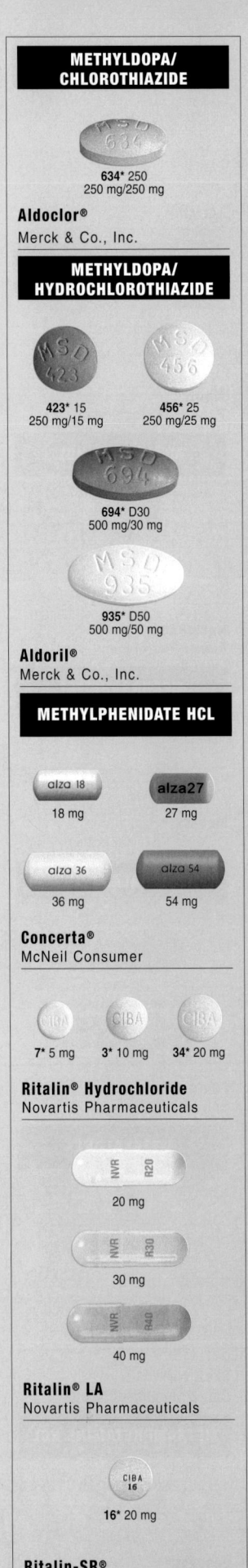

METHYLDOPA/ CHLOROTHIAZIDE

634* 250
250 mg/250 mg

Aldoclor®
Merck & Co., Inc.

METHYLDOPA/ HYDROCHLOROTHIAZIDE

423* 15
250 mg/15 mg

456* 25
250 mg/25 mg

694* D30
500 mg/30 mg

935* D50
500 mg/50 mg

Aldoril®
Merck & Co., Inc.

METHYLPHENIDATE HCL

18 mg   27 mg

36 mg   54 mg

Concerta®
McNeil Consumer

7* 5 mg   **3*** 10 mg   **34*** 20 mg

Ritalin® Hydrochloride
Novartis Pharmaceuticals

20 mg

30 mg

40 mg

Ritalin® LA
Novartis Pharmaceuticals

16* 20 mg

Ritalin-SR®
Novartis Pharmaceuticals

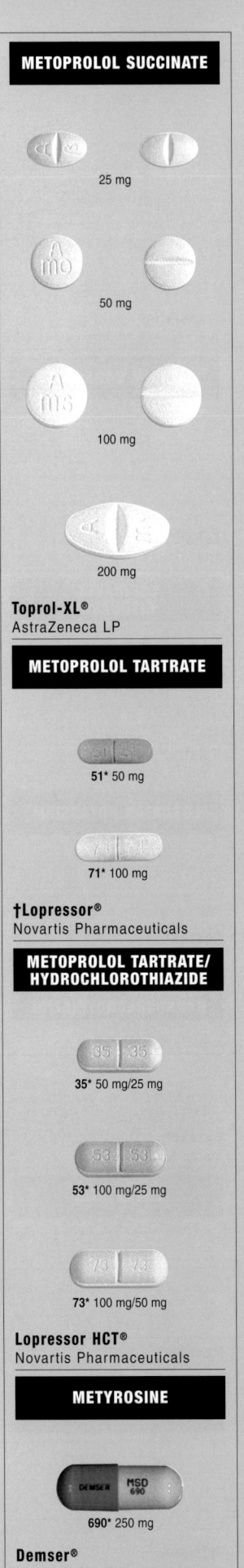

METOPROLOL SUCCINATE

25 mg

50 mg

100 mg

200 mg

Toprol-XL®
AstraZeneca LP

METOPROLOL TARTRATE

51* 50 mg

71* 100 mg

†Lopressor®
Novartis Pharmaceuticals

METOPROLOL TARTRATE/ HYDROCHLOROTHIAZIDE

35* 50 mg/25 mg

53* 100 mg/25 mg

73* 100 mg/50 mg

Lopressor HCT®
Novartis Pharmaceuticals

METYROSINE

690* 250 mg

Demser®
Merck & Co., Inc.

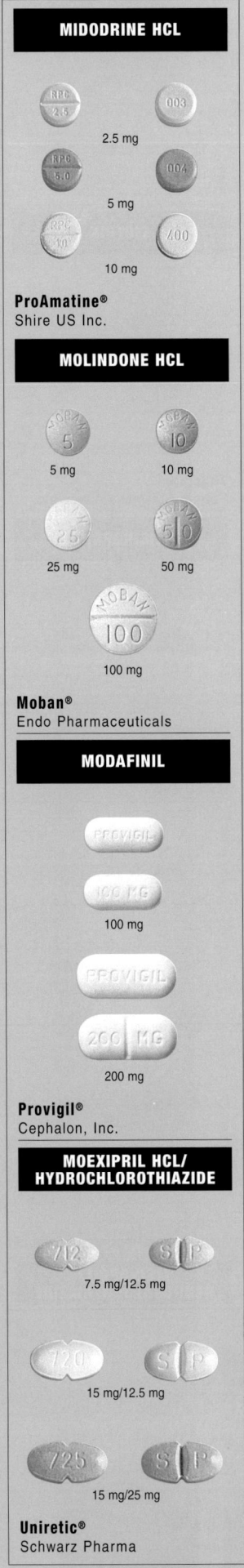

MIDODRINE HCL

2.5 mg

5 mg

10 mg

ProAmatine®
Shire US Inc.

MOLINDONE HCL

5 mg   10 mg

25 mg   50 mg

100 mg

Moban®
Endo Pharmaceuticals

MODAFINIL

100 mg

200 mg

Provigil®
Cephalon, Inc.

MOEXIPRIL HCL/ HYDROCHLOROTHIAZIDE

7.5 mg/12.5 mg

15 mg/12.5 mg

15 mg/25 mg

Uniretic®
Schwarz Pharma

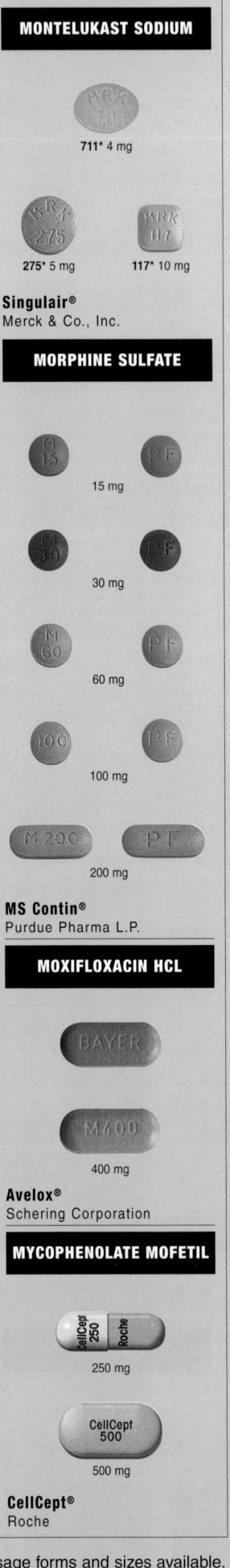

MONTELUKAST SODIUM

711* 4 mg

275* 5 mg   **117*** 10 mg

Singulair®
Merck & Co., Inc.

MORPHINE SULFATE

15 mg

30 mg

60 mg

100 mg

200 mg

MS Contin®
Purdue Pharma L.P.

MOXIFLOXACIN HCL

400 mg

Avelox®
Schering Corporation

MYCOPHENOLATE MOFETIL

250 mg

500 mg

CellCept®
Roche

* Manufacturer's Identification Code   † Additional dosage forms and sizes available.

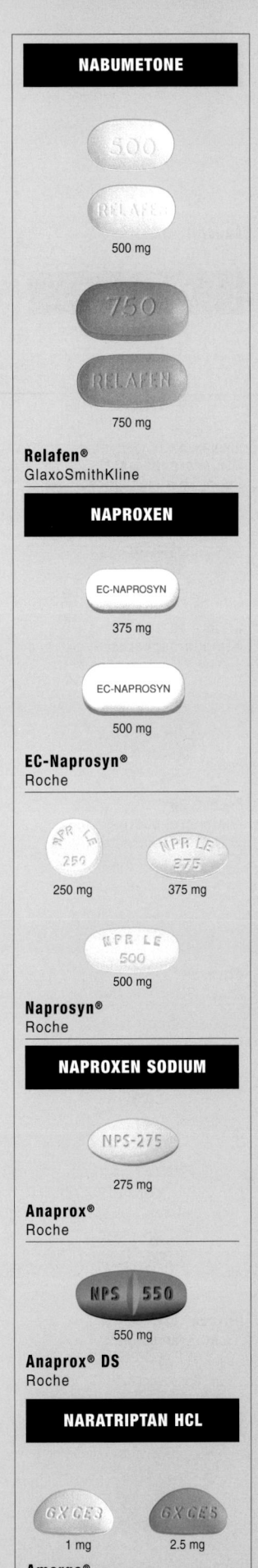

NABUMETONE

500 mg

750 mg

Relafen®
GlaxoSmithKline

NAPROXEN

EC-NAPROSYN
375 mg

EC-NAPROSYN
500 mg

EC-Naprosyn®
Roche

NPR LE 250
250 mg

NPR LE 375
375 mg

NPR LE 500
500 mg

Naprosyn®
Roche

NAPROXEN SODIUM

NPS-275
275 mg

Anaprox®
Roche

NPS 550
550 mg

Anaprox® DS
Roche

NARATRIPTAN HCL

GX CE3
1 mg

GX CE5
2.5 mg

Amerge®
GlaxoSmithKline

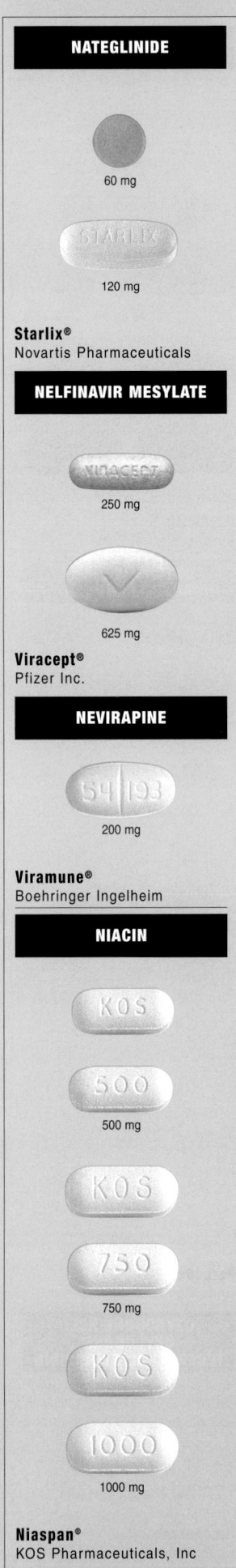

NATEGLINIDE

60 mg

STARLIX
120 mg

Starlix®
Novartis Pharmaceuticals

NELFINAVIR MESYLATE

VIRACEPT
250 mg

V
625 mg

Viracept®
Pfizer Inc.

NEVIRAPINE

54 193
200 mg

Viramune®
Boehringer Ingelheim

NIACIN

KOS

500
500 mg

KOS

750
750 mg

KOS

1000
1000 mg

Niaspan®
KOS Pharmaceuticals, Inc

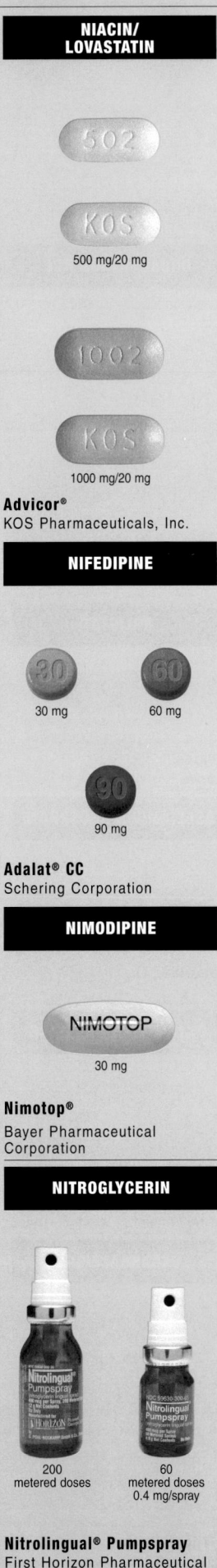

NIACIN/LOVASTATIN

502

KOS
500 mg/20 mg

1002

KOS
1000 mg/20 mg

Advicor®
KOS Pharmaceuticals, Inc.

NIFEDIPINE

30 mg   60 mg

90
90 mg

Adalat® CC
Schering Corporation

NIMODIPINE

NIMOTOP
30 mg

Nimotop®
Bayer Pharmaceutical
Corporation

NITROGLYCERIN

200
metered doses

60
metered doses
0.4 mg/spray

Nitrolingual® Pumpspray
First Horizon Pharmaceutical

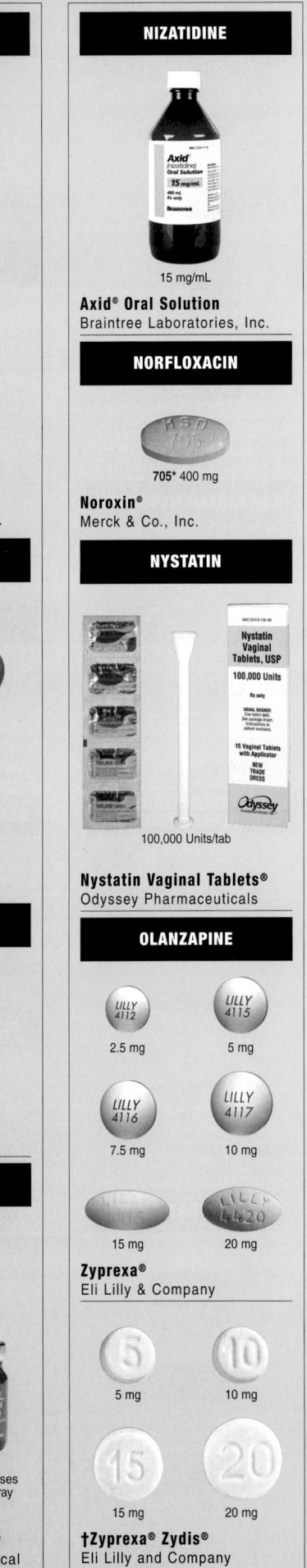

NIZATIDINE

15 mg/mL

Axid® Oral Solution
Braintree Laboratories, Inc.

NORFLOXACIN

MSD
705
705* 400 mg

Noroxin®
Merck & Co., Inc.

NYSTATIN

100,000 Units/tab

Nystatin Vaginal Tablets®
Odyssey Pharmaceuticals

OLANZAPINE

LILLY 4112
2.5 mg

LILLY 4115
5 mg

LILLY 4116
7.5 mg

LILLY 4117
10 mg

15 mg

LILLY 4420
20 mg

Zyprexa®
Eli Lilly & Company

5 mg   10 mg

15 mg   20 mg

†Zyprexa® Zydis®
Eli Lilly and Company

---

† Additional dosage forms and sizes available.

* Manufacturer's Identification Code **MC 13**

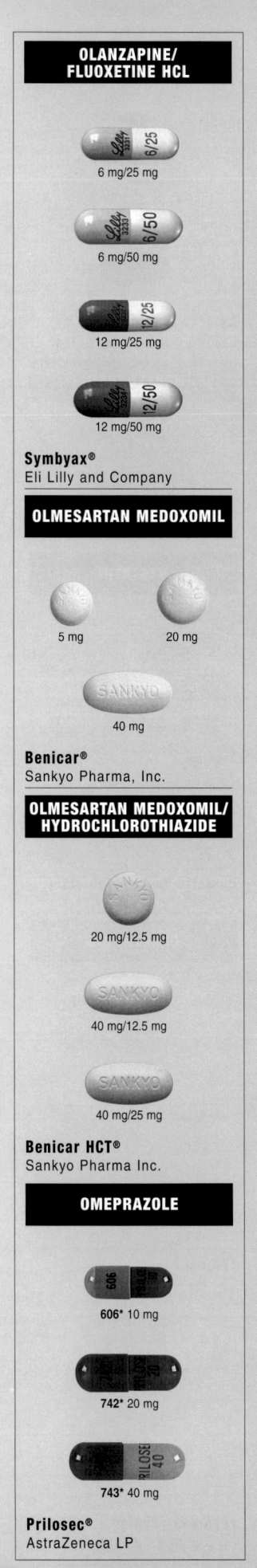
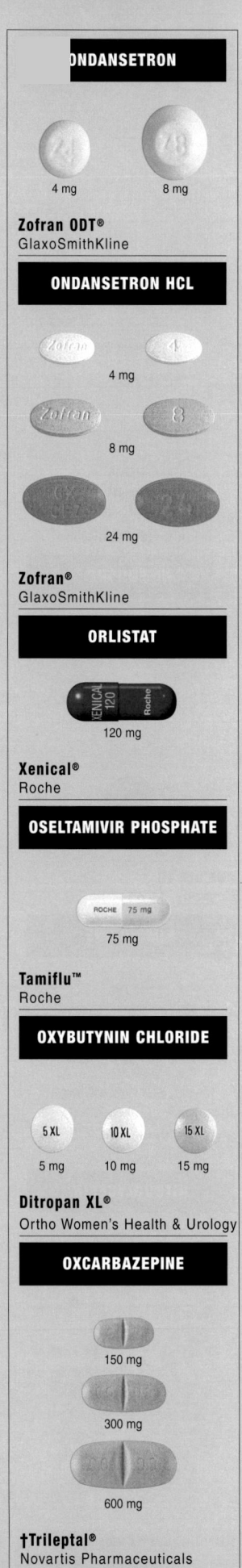
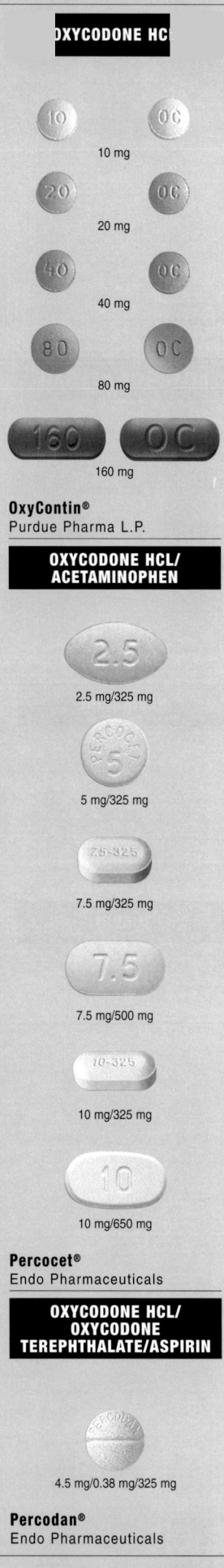
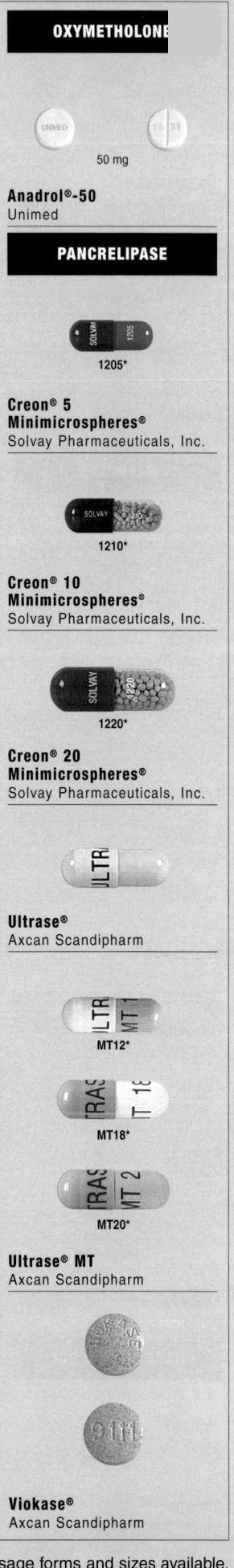

OLANZAPINE/ FLUOXETINE HCL

6 mg/25 mg

6 mg/50 mg

12 mg/25 mg

12 mg/50 mg

Symbyax®
Eli Lilly and Company

OLMESARTAN MEDOXOMIL

5 mg   20 mg

40 mg

Benicar®
Sankyo Pharma, Inc.

OLMESARTAN MEDOXOMIL/ HYDROCHLOROTHIAZIDE

20 mg/12.5 mg

40 mg/12.5 mg

40 mg/25 mg

Benicar HCT®
Sankyo Pharma Inc.

OMEPRAZOLE

606* 10 mg

742* 20 mg

743* 40 mg

Prilosec®
AstraZeneca LP

ONDANSETRON

4 mg   8 mg

Zofran ODT®
GlaxoSmithKline

ONDANSETRON HCL

4 mg

8 mg

24 mg

Zofran®
GlaxoSmithKline

ORLISTAT

120 mg

Xenical®
Roche

OSELTAMIVIR PHOSPHATE

75 mg

Tamiflu™
Roche

OXYBUTYNIN CHLORIDE

5 mg   10 mg   15 mg

Ditropan XL®
Ortho Women's Health & Urology

OXCARBAZEPINE

150 mg

300 mg

600 mg

†Trileptal®
Novartis Pharmaceuticals

OXYCODONE HCL

10 mg

20 mg

40 mg

80 mg

160 mg

OxyContin®
Purdue Pharma L.P.

OXYCODONE HCL/ ACETAMINOPHEN

2.5 mg/325 mg

5 mg/325 mg

7.5 mg/325 mg

7.5 mg/500 mg

10 mg/325 mg

10 mg/650 mg

Percocet®
Endo Pharmaceuticals

OXYCODONE HCL/ OXYCODONE TEREPHTHALATE/ASPIRIN

4.5 mg/0.38 mg/325 mg

Percodan®
Endo Pharmaceuticals

OXYMETHOLONE

50 mg

Anadrol®-50
Unimed

PANCRELIPASE

1205*

Creon® 5 Minimicrospheres®
Solvay Pharmaceuticals, Inc.

1210*

Creon® 10 Minimicrospheres®
Solvay Pharmaceuticals, Inc.

1220*

Creon® 20 Minimicrospheres®
Solvay Pharmaceuticals, Inc.

Ultrase®
Axcan Scandipharm

MT12*

MT18*

MT20*

Ultrase® MT
Axcan Scandipharm

Viokase®
Axcan Scandipharm

* Manufacturer's Identification Code   † Additional dosage forms and sizes available.

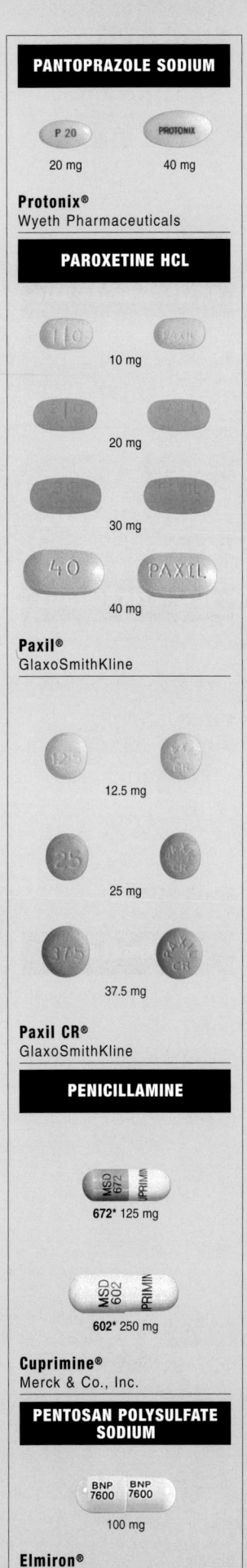

PANTOPRAZOLE SODIUM

P 20 — 20 mg
PROTONIX — 40 mg

Protonix®
Wyeth Pharmaceuticals

PAROXETINE HCL

10 mg
20 mg
30 mg
40 mg

Paxil®
GlaxoSmithKline

12.5 mg
25 mg
37.5 mg

Paxil CR®
GlaxoSmithKline

PENICILLAMINE

672* 125 mg
602* 250 mg

Cuprimine®
Merck & Co., Inc.

PENTOSAN POLYSULFATE SODIUM

BNP 7600 BNP 7600
100 mg

Elmiron®
Ortho Women's Health & Urology

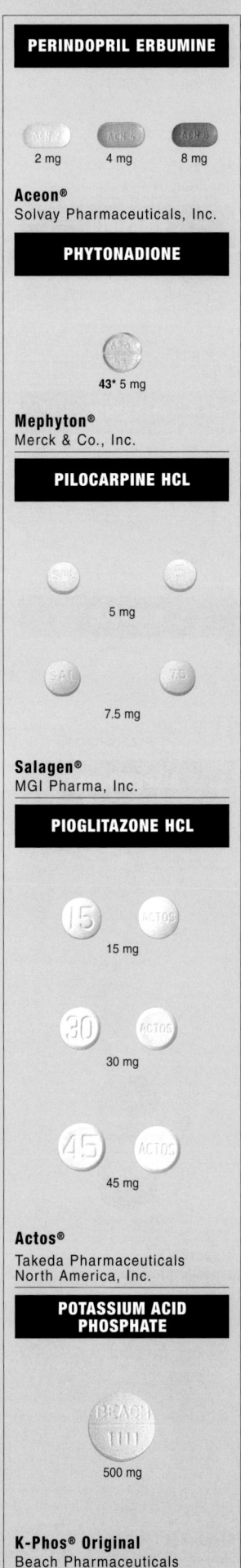

PERINDOPRIL ERBUMINE

2 mg
4 mg
8 mg

Aceon®
Solvay Pharmaceuticals, Inc.

PHYTONADIONE

43* 5 mg

Mephyton®
Merck & Co., Inc.

PILOCARPINE HCL

5 mg
7.5 mg

Salagen®
MGI Pharma, Inc.

PIOGLITAZONE HCL

15 mg
30 mg
45 mg

Actos®
Takeda Pharmaceuticals
North America, Inc.

POTASSIUM ACID PHOSPHATE

BEACH 1111
500 mg

K-Phos® Original
Beach Pharmaceuticals

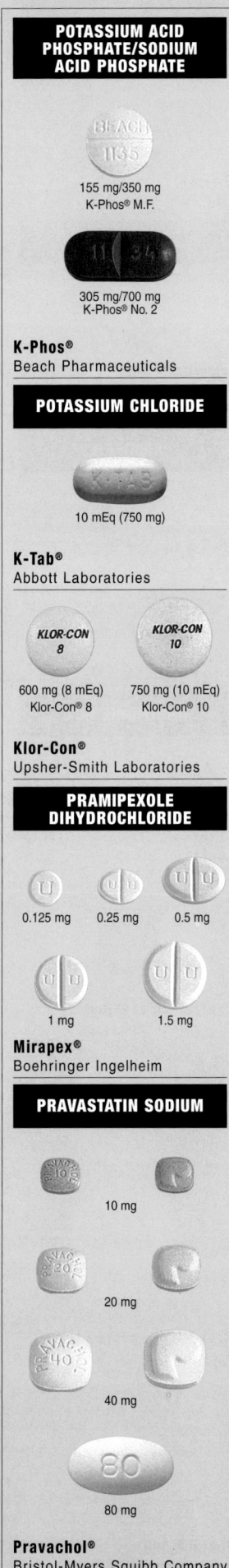

POTASSIUM ACID PHOSPHATE/SODIUM ACID PHOSPHATE

BEACH 1135
155 mg/350 mg
K-Phos® M.F.

11 34
305 mg/700 mg
K-Phos® No. 2

K-Phos®
Beach Pharmaceuticals

POTASSIUM CHLORIDE

K-TAB
10 mEq (750 mg)

K-Tab®
Abbott Laboratories

KLOR-CON 8 — 600 mg (8 mEq) Klor-Con® 8
KLOR-CON 10 — 750 mg (10 mEq) Klor-Con® 10

Klor-Con®
Upsher-Smith Laboratories

PRAMIPEXOLE DIHYDROCHLORIDE

0.125 mg
0.25 mg
0.5 mg
1 mg
1.5 mg

Mirapex®
Boehringer Ingelheim

PRAVASTATIN SODIUM

10 mg
20 mg
40 mg
80 mg

Pravachol®
Bristol-Myers Squibb Company

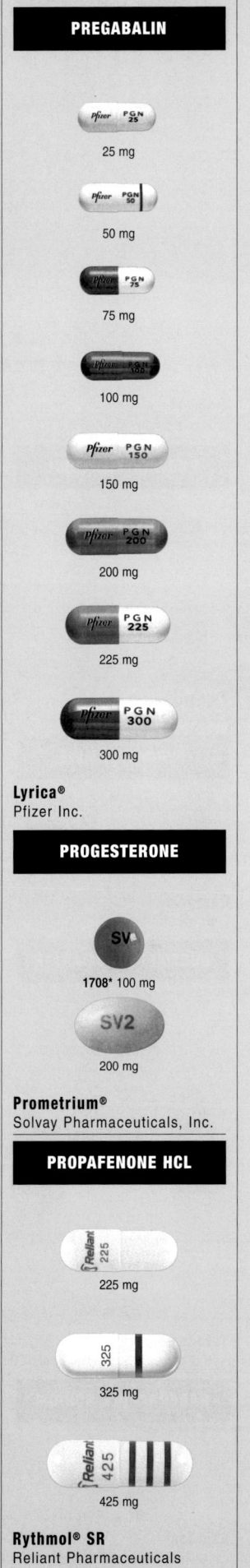

PREGABALIN

Pfizer PGN 25 — 25 mg
Pfizer PGN 50 — 50 mg
Pfizer PGN 75 — 75 mg
Pfizer PGN 100 — 100 mg
Pfizer PGN 150 — 150 mg
Pfizer PGN 200 — 200 mg
Pfizer PGN 225 — 225 mg
Pfizer PGN 300 — 300 mg

Lyrica®
Pfizer Inc.

PROGESTERONE

SV — 1708* 100 mg
SV2 — 200 mg

Prometrium®
Solvay Pharmaceuticals, Inc.

PROPAFENONE HCL

Reliant 225 — 225 mg
325 — 325 mg
Reliant 425 — 425 mg

Rythmol® SR
Reliant Pharmaceuticals

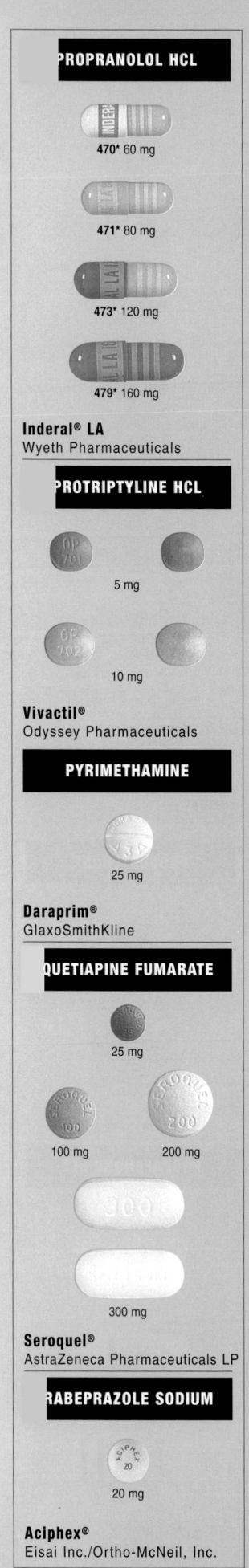

PROPRANOLOL HCL

470* 60 mg

471* 80 mg

473* 120 mg

479* 160 mg

Inderal® LA
Wyeth Pharmaceuticals

PROTRIPTYLINE HCL

5 mg

10 mg

Vivactil®
Odyssey Pharmaceuticals

PYRIMETHAMINE

25 mg

Daraprim®
GlaxoSmithKline

QUETIAPINE FUMARATE

25 mg

100 mg   200 mg

300 mg

Seroquel®
AstraZeneca Pharmaceuticals LP

RABEPRAZOLE SODIUM

20 mg

Aciphex®
Eisai Inc./Ortho-McNeil, Inc.

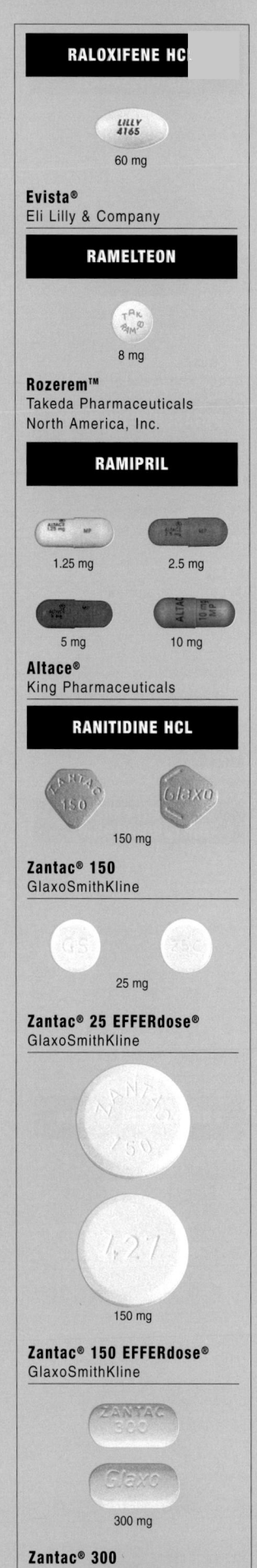

RALOXIFENE HCL

60 mg

Evista®
Eli Lilly & Company

RAMELTEON

8 mg

Rozerem™
Takeda Pharmaceuticals
North America, Inc.

RAMIPRIL

1.25 mg   2.5 mg

5 mg   10 mg

Altace®
King Pharmaceuticals

RANITIDINE HCL

150 mg

Zantac® 150
GlaxoSmithKline

25 mg

Zantac® 25 EFFERdose®
GlaxoSmithKline

150 mg

Zantac® 150 EFFERdose®
GlaxoSmithKline

300 mg

Zantac® 300
GlaxoSmithKline

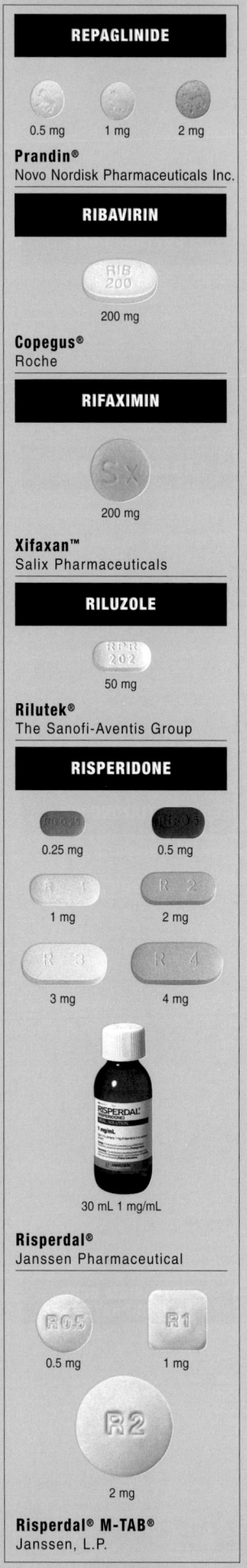

REPAGLINIDE

0.5 mg   1 mg   2 mg

Prandin®
Novo Nordisk Pharmaceuticals Inc.

RIBAVIRIN

200 mg

Copegus®
Roche

RIFAXIMIN

200 mg

Xifaxan™
Salix Pharmaceuticals

RILUZOLE

50 mg

Rilutek®
The Sanofi-Aventis Group

RISPERIDONE

0.25 mg   0.5 mg

1 mg   2 mg

3 mg   4 mg

30 mL 1 mg/mL

Risperdal®
Janssen Pharmaceutical

0.5 mg   1 mg

2 mg

Risperdal® M-TAB®
Janssen, L.P.

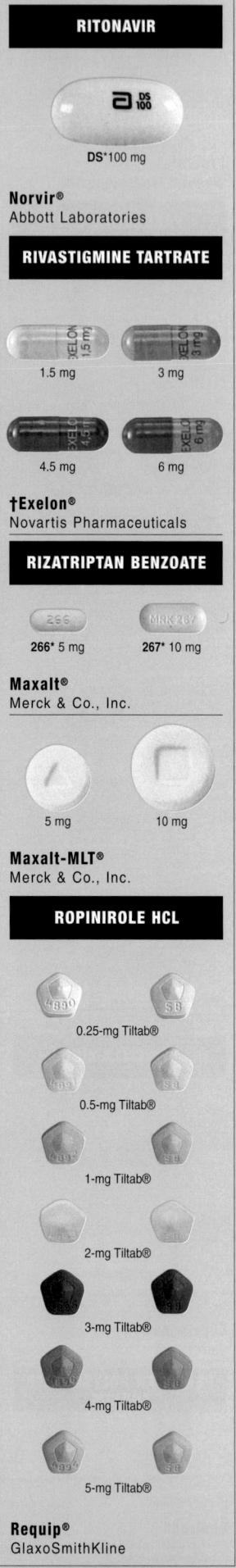

RITONAVIR

DS*100 mg

Norvir®
Abbott Laboratories

RIVASTIGMINE TARTRATE

1.5 mg   3 mg

4.5 mg   6 mg

†Exelon®
Novartis Pharmaceuticals

RIZATRIPTAN BENZOATE

266* 5 mg   **267*** 10 mg

Maxalt®
Merck & Co., Inc.

5 mg   10 mg

Maxalt-MLT®
Merck & Co., Inc.

ROPINIROLE HCL

0.25-mg Tiltab®

0.5-mg Tiltab®

1-mg Tiltab®

2-mg Tiltab®

3-mg Tiltab®

4-mg Tiltab®

5-mg Tiltab®

Requip®
GlaxoSmithKline

* Manufacturer's Identification Code   † Additional dosage forms and sizes available.

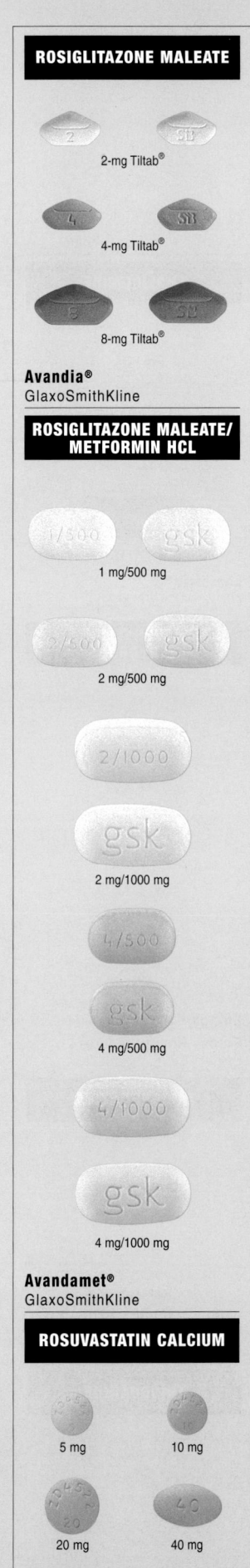

ROSIGLITAZONE MALEATE

2-mg Tiltab®

4-mg Tiltab®

8-mg Tiltab®

Avandia®
GlaxoSmithKline

ROSIGLITAZONE MALEATE/ METFORMIN HCL

1 mg/500 mg

2 mg/500 mg

2 mg/1000 mg

4 mg/500 mg

4 mg/1000 mg

Avandamet®
GlaxoSmithKline

ROSUVASTATIN CALCIUM

5 mg

10 mg

20 mg

40 mg

Crestor®
Astrazeneca Pharmaceuticals LP

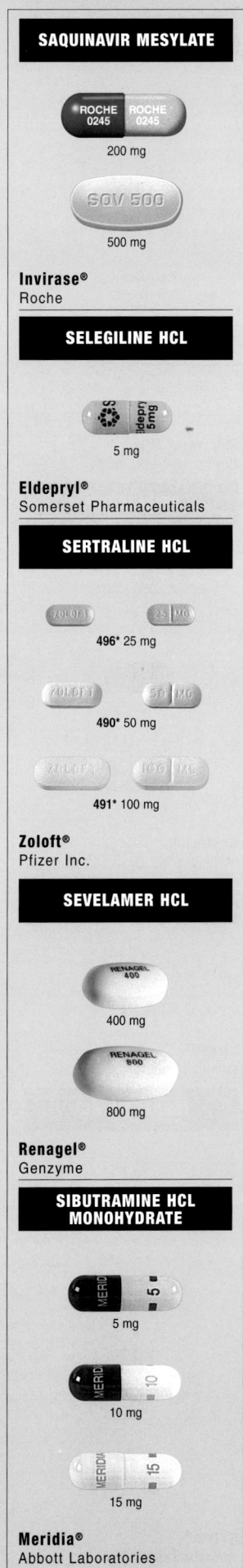

SAQUINAVIR MESYLATE

200 mg

SQV 500

500 mg

Invirase®
Roche

SELEGILINE HCL

5 mg

Eldepryl®
Somerset Pharmaceuticals

SERTRALINE HCL

496* 25 mg

490* 50 mg

491* 100 mg

Zoloft®
Pfizer Inc.

SEVELAMER HCL

RENAGEL 400

400 mg

RENAGEL 800

800 mg

Renagel®
Genzyme

SIBUTRAMINE HCL MONOHYDRATE

5 mg

10 mg

15 mg

Meridia®
Abbott Laboratories

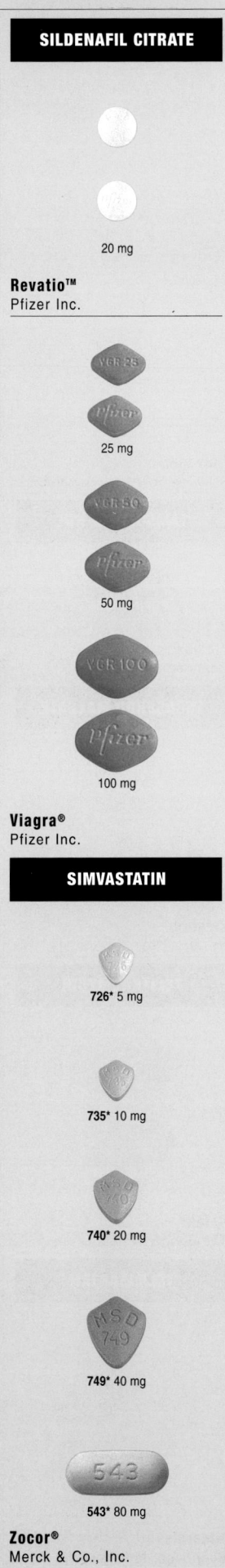

SILDENAFIL CITRATE

20 mg

Revatio™
Pfizer Inc.

VGR 25

25 mg

50 mg

VGR 100

100 mg

Viagra®
Pfizer Inc.

SIMVASTATIN

726* 5 mg

735* 10 mg

740* 20 mg

MSD 749

749* 40 mg

543

543* 80 mg

Zocor®
Merck & Co., Inc.

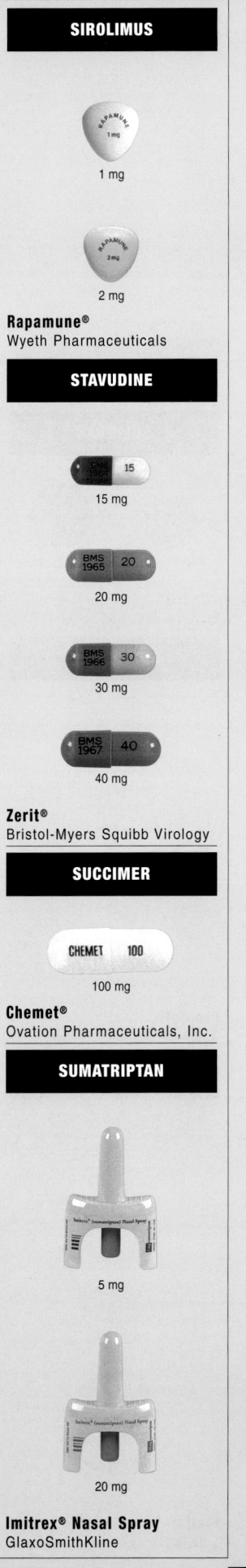

SIROLIMUS

1 mg

2 mg

Rapamune®
Wyeth Pharmaceuticals

STAVUDINE

15

15 mg

BMS 1965 20

20 mg

BMS 1966 30

30 mg

BMS 1967 40

40 mg

Zerit®
Bristol-Myers Squibb Virology

SUCCIMER

CHEMET 100

100 mg

Chemet®
Ovation Pharmaceuticals, Inc.

SUMATRIPTAN

5 mg

20 mg

Imitrex® Nasal Spray
GlaxoSmithKline

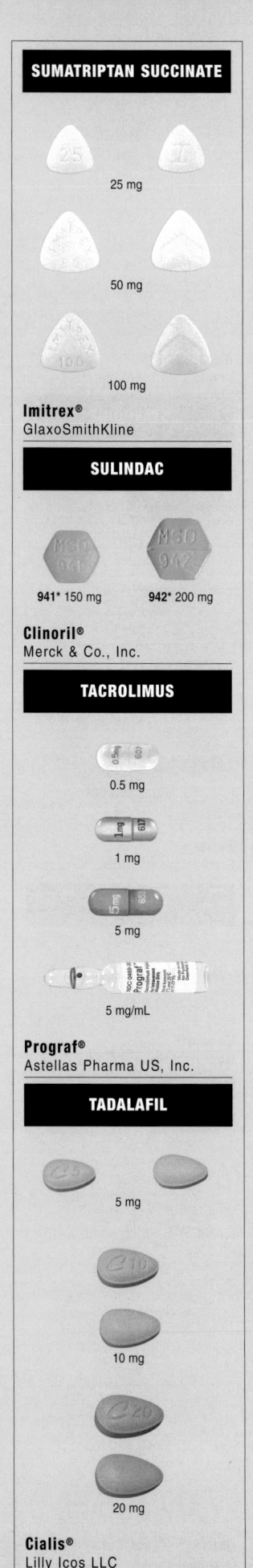

SUMATRIPTAN SUCCINATE

25 mg

50 mg

100 mg

Imitrex®
GlaxoSmithKline

SULINDAC

941* 150 mg   942* 200 mg

Clinoril®
Merck & Co., Inc.

TACROLIMUS

0.5 mg

1 mg

5 mg

5 mg/mL

Prograf®
Astellas Pharma US, Inc.

TADALAFIL

5 mg

10 mg

20 mg

Cialis®
Lilly Icos LLC

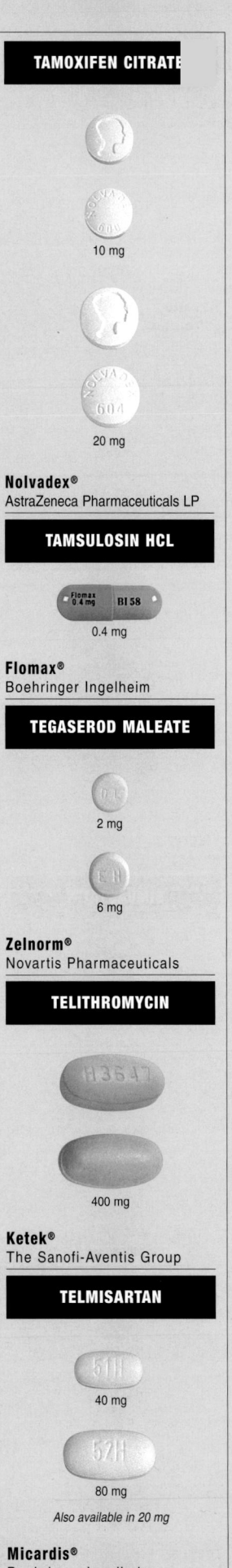

TAMOXIFEN CITRATE

10 mg

20 mg

Nolvadex®
AstraZeneca Pharmaceuticals LP

TAMSULOSIN HCL

0.4 mg

Flomax®
Boehringer Ingelheim

TEGASEROD MALEATE

2 mg

6 mg

Zelnorm®
Novartis Pharmaceuticals

TELITHROMYCIN

400 mg

Ketek®
The Sanofi-Aventis Group

TELMISARTAN

40 mg

80 mg

Also available in 20 mg

Micardis®
Boehringer Ingelheim

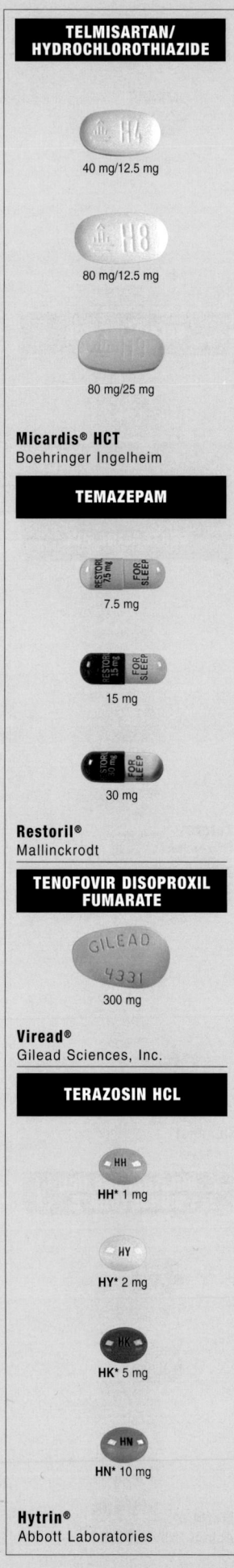

TELMISARTAN/ HYDROCHLOROTHIAZIDE

40 mg/12.5 mg

80 mg/12.5 mg

80 mg/25 mg

Micardis® HCT
Boehringer Ingelheim

TEMAZEPAM

7.5 mg

15 mg

30 mg

Restoril®
Mallinckrodt

TENOFOVIR DISOPROXIL FUMARATE

300 mg

Viread®
Gilead Sciences, Inc.

TERAZOSIN HCL

HH* 1 mg

HY* 2 mg

HK* 5 mg

HN* 10 mg

Hytrin®
Abbott Laboratories

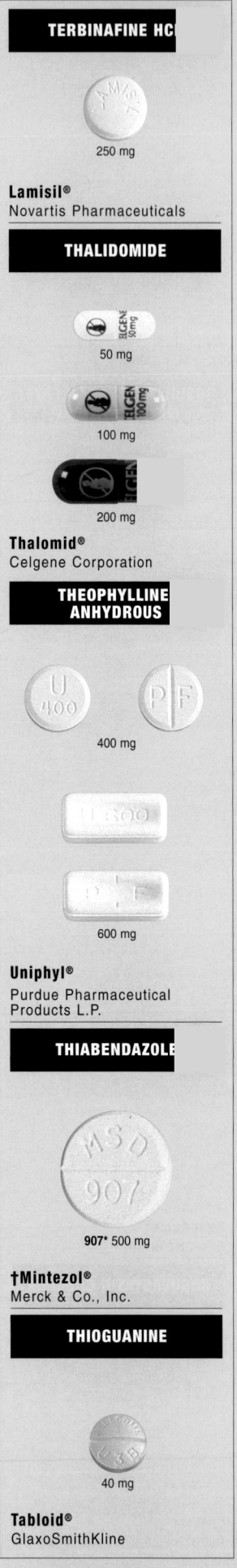

TERBINAFINE HCL

250 mg

Lamisil®
Novartis Pharmaceuticals

THALIDOMIDE

50 mg

100 mg

200 mg

Thalomid®
Celgene Corporation

THEOPHYLLINE ANHYDROUS

400 mg

600 mg

Uniphyl®
Purdue Pharmaceutical Products L.P.

THIABENDAZOLE

907* 500 mg

†Mintezol®
Merck & Co., Inc.

THIOGUANINE

40 mg

Tabloid®
GlaxoSmithKline

* Manufacturer's Identification Code   † Additional dosage forms and sizes available.

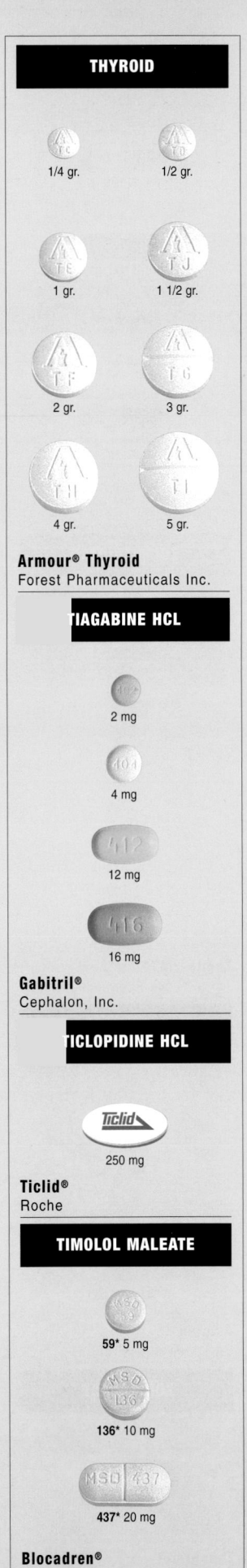

THYROID

1/4 gr.   1/2 gr.

1 gr.   1 1/2 gr.

2 gr.   3 gr.

4 gr.   5 gr.

Armour® Thyroid
Forest Pharmaceuticals Inc.

TIAGABINE HCL

2 mg

4 mg

12 mg

16 mg

Gabitril®
Cephalon, Inc.

TICLOPIDINE HCL

250 mg

Ticlid®
Roche

TIMOLOL MALEATE

59* 5 mg

136* 10 mg

437* 20 mg

Blocadren®
Merck & Co., Inc.

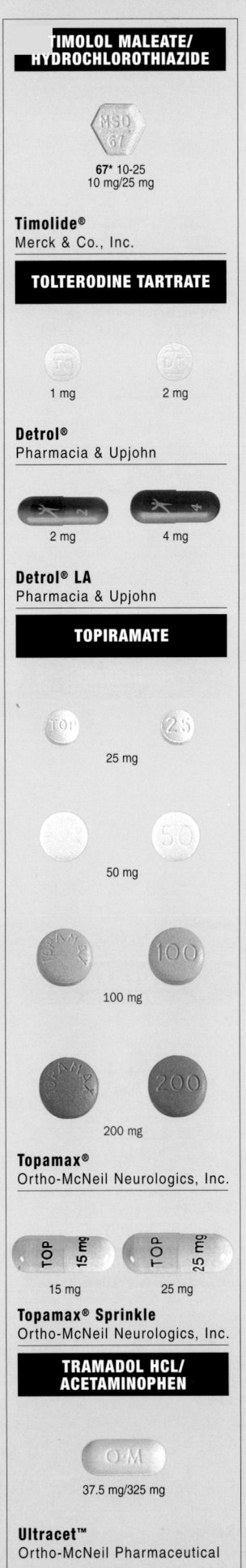

TIMOLOL MALEATE/ HYDROCHLOROTHIAZIDE

67* 10-25
10 mg/25 mg

Timolide®
Merck & Co., Inc.

TOLTERODINE TARTRATE

1 mg   2 mg

Detrol®
Pharmacia & Upjohn

2 mg   4 mg

Detrol® LA
Pharmacia & Upjohn

TOPIRAMATE

25 mg

50 mg

100 mg

200 mg

Topamax®
Ortho-McNeil Neurologics, Inc.

15 mg   25 mg

Topamax® Sprinkle
Ortho-McNeil Neurologics, Inc.

TRAMADOL HCL/ ACETAMINOPHEN

37.5 mg/325 mg

Ultracet™
Ortho-McNeil Pharmaceutical

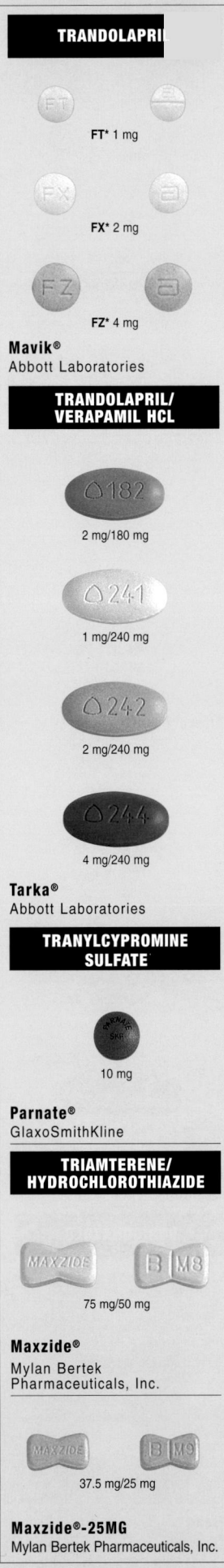

TRANDOLAPRIL

FT* 1 mg

FX* 2 mg

FZ* 4 mg

Mavik®
Abbott Laboratories

TRANDOLAPRIL/ VERAPAMIL HCL

2 mg/180 mg

1 mg/240 mg

2 mg/240 mg

4 mg/240 mg

Tarka®
Abbott Laboratories

TRANYLCYPROMINE SULFATE

10 mg

Parnate®
GlaxoSmithKline

TRIAMTERENE/ HYDROCHLOROTHIAZIDE

75 mg/50 mg

Maxzide®
Mylan Bertek
Pharmaceuticals, Inc.

37.5 mg/25 mg

Maxzide®-25MG
Mylan Bertek Pharmaceuticals, Inc.

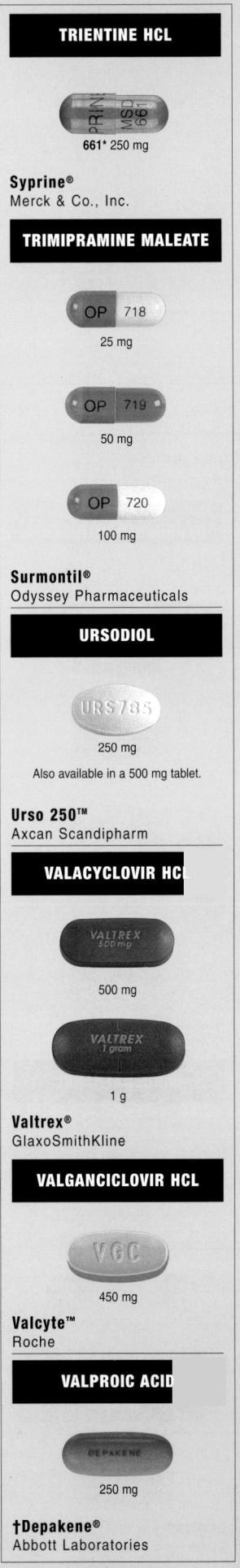

TRIENTINE HCL

661* 250 mg

Syprine®
Merck & Co., Inc.

TRIMIPRAMINE MALEATE

OP 718
25 mg

OP 719
50 mg

OP 720
100 mg

Surmontil®
Odyssey Pharmaceuticals

URSODIOL

URS785
250 mg

Also available in a 500 mg tablet.

Urso 250™
Axcan Scandipharm

VALACYCLOVIR HCL

500 mg

1 g

Valtrex®
GlaxoSmithKline

VALGANCICLOVIR HCL

450 mg

Valcyte™
Roche

VALPROIC ACID

250 mg

†Depakene®
Abbott Laboratories

---

† Additional dosage forms and sizes available.

* Manufacturer's Identification Code

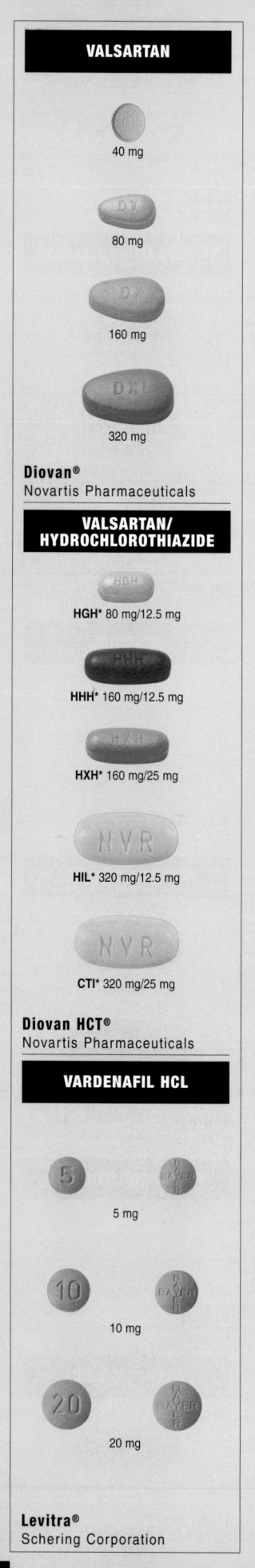
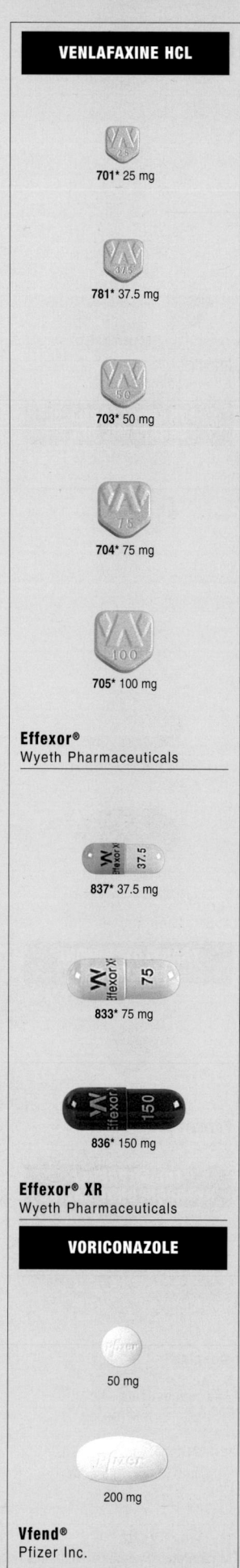
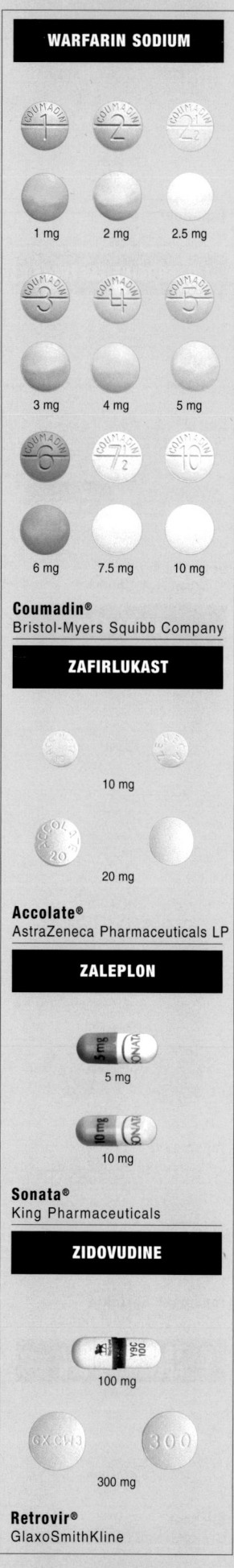
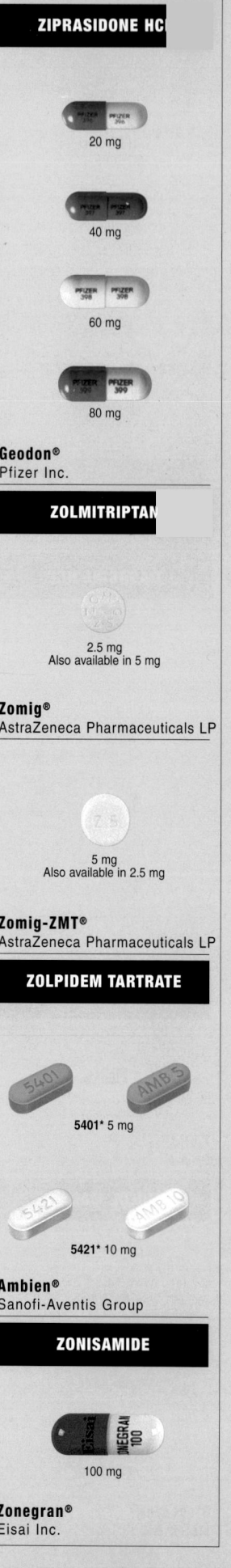

VALSARTAN

40 mg

80 mg

160 mg

320 mg

Diovan®
Novartis Pharmaceuticals

VALSARTAN/ HYDROCHLOROTHIAZIDE

HGH* 80 mg/12.5 mg

HHH* 160 mg/12.5 mg

HXH* 160 mg/25 mg

HIL* 320 mg/12.5 mg

CTI* 320 mg/25 mg

Diovan HCT®
Novartis Pharmaceuticals

VARDENAFIL HCL

5 mg

10 mg

20 mg

Levitra®
Schering Corporation

VENLAFAXINE HCL

701* 25 mg

781* 37.5 mg

703* 50 mg

704* 75 mg

705* 100 mg

Effexor®
Wyeth Pharmaceuticals

837* 37.5 mg

833* 75 mg

836* 150 mg

Effexor® XR
Wyeth Pharmaceuticals

VORICONAZOLE

50 mg

200 mg

Vfend®
Pfizer Inc.

WARFARIN SODIUM

1 mg   2 mg   2.5 mg

3 mg   4 mg   5 mg

6 mg   7.5 mg   10 mg

Coumadin®
Bristol-Myers Squibb Company

ZAFIRLUKAST

10 mg

20 mg

Accolate®
AstraZeneca Pharmaceuticals LP

ZALEPLON

5 mg

10 mg

Sonata®
King Pharmaceuticals

ZIDOVUDINE

100 mg

300 mg

Retrovir®
GlaxoSmithKline

ZIPRASIDONE HCL

20 mg

40 mg

60 mg

80 mg

Geodon®
Pfizer Inc.

ZOLMITRIPTAN

2.5 mg
Also available in 5 mg

Zomig®
AstraZeneca Pharmaceuticals LP

5 mg
Also available in 2.5 mg

Zomig-ZMT®
AstraZeneca Pharmaceuticals LP

ZOLPIDEM TARTRATE

5401* 5 mg

5421* 10 mg

Ambien®
Sanofi-Aventis Group

ZONISAMIDE

100 mg

Zonegran®
Eisai Inc.

* Manufacturer's Identification Code

General Information

GENERAL INFORMATION ABOUT USE OF MEDICINES

There are two kinds of information about the proper use of medicines. One type applies to a certain medicine or group of medicines only. The other type is more general and applies to the use of any medicine.

The information that follows is general in nature. For your own safety, health, and well being, however, it is important that you learn about the proper use of your specific medicines as well. You can get this information from your health care professional, or find it in the individual listings of this book.

Black Box Warning

Before you use any medicine with a black box warning, tell your health care professional if you have any conditions or concerns related to this warning. A black box warning provides information that alerts the healthcare professional and consumer to any serious side effect or other important safety information.

Before Using Your Medicine

Before you use any medicine, tell your health care professional:

—if you have ever had an allergic or unusual reaction to any medicine, food, or other substance, such as yellow dye or sulfites.

—if you are on a low-salt, low-sugar, or any other special diet. Most medicines contain more than their active ingredient, and many liquid medicines contain alcohol.

—*if you are pregnant or if you plan to become pregnant.* Certain medicines may cause birth defects or other problems in the unborn child. For other medicines, safe use during pregnancy has not been established. *The use of any medicine during pregnancy must be carefully considered* and should be discussed with a health care professional.

—*if you are breast-feeding.* Some medicines may pass into the breast milk and cause unwanted effects in the baby.

—*if you are now taking or have taken any medicines or dietary supplements in the recent past.* Do not forget over-the-counter (nonprescription) medicines such as pain relievers, laxatives, antacids or dietary supplements.

—*if you use alcohol or tobacco.* Using alcohol or tobacco while you are taking certain medicines could cause unwanted effects and should be discussed with a health care professional.

—*if you have any medical problems* other than the one(s) for which your medicine was prescribed.

—*if you have difficulty remembering things or reading labels.*

Storage of Your Medicine

It is important to store your medicines properly. Guidelines for proper storage include:

Keep out of the reach of children.
- Keep medicines in their original containers.
- Store away from heat and direct light.
- Do not store capsules or tablets in the bathroom, near the kitchen sink, or in other damp places. Heat or moisture may cause the medicine to break down. Also, do not leave the cotton plug in a medicine container that has been opened, since it may draw moisture into the container.
- Keep liquid medicines from freezing.
- Do not store medicines in the refrigerator unless directed to do so.
- Do not leave your medicines in an automobile for long periods of time.
- Do not keep outdated medicine or medicine that is no longer needed. Be sure that any discarded medicine is out of the reach of children.

Proper Use of Your Medicine

Take medicine only as directed, at the right time, and for the full length of your prescribed treatment. If you are using an over-the-counter (nonprescription) medicine, follow the directions on the label unless otherwise directed by your health care professional. If you feel that your medicine is not working for you, check with your health care professional.

Unless your pharmacist has packaged different medicines together in a "bubble-pack," different medicines should never be mixed in one container. It is best to keep your medicines tightly capped in their original containers when not in use. Do not remove the label since directions for use and other important information may appear on it.

To avoid mistakes, do not take medicine in the dark. Always read the label before taking, especially noting the expiration date and any directions for use.

For oral (by mouth) medicines:
- In general, it is best to take oral medicines with a full glass of water. However, follow your health care professional's directions. Some medicines should be taken with food, while others should be taken on an empty stomach.
- When taking most long-acting forms of a medicine, each dose should be swallowed whole. Do not break, crush, or chew before swallowing unless you have been specifically told that it is all right to do so.
- If you are taking liquid medicines, you should use a specially marked measuring spoon or other device to measure each dose accurately. Ask your pharmacist about these devices. The average household teaspoon may not hold the right amount of medicine.
- Oral medicine may come in a number of different dos-

age forms, such as tablets, capsules, and liquids. If you have trouble swallowing the dosage form prescribed for you, check with your health care professional. Another dosage form that you can swallow more easily may be available.

- Child-resistant caps on medicine containers have decreased greatly the number of accidental poisonings that occur each year. Use of these caps is required by law. However, if you find it hard to open such caps, you may ask your pharmacist for a regular, easier-to-open cap. He or she can provide you with a regular cap if you request it. However, you must make this request each time you get a prescription filled.

For skin patches:

- Apply the patch to a clean, dry skin area that has little or no hair and is free of scars, cuts, or irritation. Remove the previous patch before applying a new one.
- Apply a new patch if the first one becomes loose or falls off.
- Apply each patch to a different area of skin to prevent skin irritation or other problems.
- Do not try to trim or cut the adhesive patch to adjust the dosage. Check with your health care professional if you think the medicine is not working as it should.

For inhalers:

- Medicines that come in inhalers usually come with patient directions. Read the directions carefully before using the medicine. If you do not understand the directions, or if you are not sure how to use the inhaler, check with your health care professional.
- Since different types of inhalers may be used in different ways, it is very important to follow carefully the directions given to you.

For ophthalmic (eye) drops:

- To prevent contamination, do not let the tip of the eye drop applicator touch any surface (including the eye) and keep the container tightly closed.
- The bottle may not be full; this is to provide proper drop control.
- How to apply: First, wash your hands. Tilt your head back and, with the index finger, pull the lower eyelid away from the eye to form a pouch. Drop the medicine into the pouch and gently close your eyes. Do not blink. Keep your eyes closed for 1 to 2 minutes.
- If your medicine is for glaucoma or inflammation of the eye: Follow the directions for application that are listed above. However, immediately after placing the drops in your eye, apply pressure to the inside corner of the eye with your middle finger. Continue to apply pressure for 1 to 2 minutes after the medicine has been placed in the eye. This will help prevent the medicine from being absorbed into the body and causing side effects.
- After applying the eye drops, wash your hands to remove any medicine.

For ophthalmic (eye) ointments:

- To prevent contamination of the eye ointment, do not let the tip of the applicator touch any surface (including the eye). After using, wipe the tip of the ointment tube with a clean tissue and keep the tube tightly closed.
- How to apply: First, wash your hands. Pull the lower eyelid away from the eye to form a pouch. Squeeze a thin strip of ointment into the pouch. A 1-cm (approximately 1/3-inch) strip of ointment is usually enough unless otherwise directed. Gently close your eyes and keep them closed for 1 to 2 minutes.
- After applying the eye ointment, wash your hands to remove any medicine.

For nasal (nose) drops:

- How to use: Blow your nose gently. Tilt your head back while standing or sitting up, or lie down on your back on a bed and hang your head over the side. Place the drops into each nostril and keep your head tilted back for a few minutes to allow the medicine to spread throughout the nose.
- Rinse the dropper with hot water and dry with a clean tissue. Replace the cap right after use. To avoid the spread of infection, do not use the container for more than one person.

For nasal (nose) spray:

- How to use: Blow your nose gently. With your head upright, spray the medicine into each nostril. Sniff briskly while squeezing the bottle quickly and firmly.
- Rinse the tip of the spray bottle with hot water, taking care not to suck water into the bottle, and dry with a clean tissue. Replace the cap right after cleaning. To avoid the spread of infection, do not use the container for more than one person.

For otic (ear) drops:

- To prevent contamination of the ear drops, do not touch the applicator tip to any surface (including the ear).
- The bottle may not be full; this is to provide proper drop control.
- How to apply: Lie down or tilt the head so the ear needing treatment faces up. For adults, gently pull the earlobe up and back (pull down and back for children). Drop the medicine into the ear canal. Keep the ear facing up for about 5 minutes so the medicine can run to the bottom of the ear canal (For young children and other patients who cannot stay still for 5 minutes, try to keep the ear facing up for at least 1 or 2 minutes.)
- Do not rinse the dropper after use. Wipe the tip of the dropper with a clean tissue and keep the container tightly closed.

For rectal suppositories:

- How to insert suppository: First, wash your hands. Remove the foil wrapper and moisten the suppository with water. Lie down on your side. Push the suppository well up into the rectum with your finger. If the suppository is too soft to insert, chill it in the refrigerator for 30 minutes or run cold water over it before removing the foil wrapper.
- Wash your hands after you have inserted the suppository.

For rectal cream or ointment:

- Clean and dry the rectal area. Apply a small amount of cream or ointment and rub it in gently.
- If your health care professional wants you to insert the medicine into the rectum: First, attach the plastic

applicator tip onto the opened tube. Insert the applicator tip into the rectum and gently squeeze the tube to deliver the cream. Remove the applicator tip from the tube and wash with hot, soapy water. Replace the cap of the tube after use.
- Wash your hands after you have inserted the medicine.

For vaginal medicines:
- How to insert the medicine: First, wash your hands. Use the special applicator. Follow any special directions that are provided by the manufacturer. If you are pregnant, however, check with your health care professional before using the applicator to insert the medicine.
- Lie on your back, with your knees drawn up. Using the applicator, insert the medicine into the vagina as far as you can without using force or causing discomfort. Release the medicine by pushing on the plunger. Wait several minutes before getting up.
- Wash the applicator and your hands with soap and warm water.

Precautions While Using Your Medicine

Never give your medicine to anyone else. It has been prescribed for your personal medical problem or condition and may be harmful to another person.

Many medicines should not be taken with other medicines or with alcoholic beverages. Follow your health care professional's directions to help avoid problems.

Before having any kind of surgery (including dental surgery) or emergency treatment, tell the physician or dentist about any medicine you are taking.

If you think you have taken an overdose of any medicine or if a child has taken a medicine by accident: Call your poison control center or your health care professional at once. Keep those telephone numbers handy. Also, keep a bottle of Ipecac Syrup safely stored in your home in case you are told to cause vomiting. Read the directions on the label of Ipecac Syrup before using.

Side Effects of Your Medicine

Along with its intended effects, a medicine may cause some unwanted effects. Some of these side effects may need medical attention, while others may not. It is important for you to know what side effects may occur and what you should do if you notice signs of them. Check with your health care professional about the possible side effects of the medicines you are taking, or if you notice any unusual reactions or side effects.

Other Information

It is a good idea for you to learn both the generic and brand names of your medicine and even to write them down for future use.

Many prescriptions may not be refilled until your pharmacist checks with your health care professional. *To save time, do not wait until you have run out of medicine before requesting a refill.* This is especially important if you must take your medicine every day.

When traveling:
- Carry your medicine with you rather than putting it in your checked luggage. Checked luggage may get lost or stored in very cold or very hot areas.
- Make sure a source of medicine is available where you are traveling, or take a large enough supply to last during your visit. It is also a good idea to take a copy of your written prescription with you.

If you want more information about your medicines, ask your health care professional. *Do not be embarrassed to ask questions* about any medicine you are taking. To help you remember, it may be useful to write down any questions and bring them with you on your next visit to your health care professional.

AVOIDING MEDICINE MISHAPS

Tips Against Tampering

Over-the-counter (OTC) or nonprescription medicines are now packaged so that it will be easier to notice signs of tampering. A tamper-evident package is required either to be unique so that it cannot be copied easily, or to have a barrier or indicator (with an identifying characteristic, such as a pattern, picture, or logo) that will be easily noticed if broken. For two-piece, unsealed, hard gelatin capsules, two tamper-evident features are required. Improved packaging also includes using special wrappers, seals, or caps on the outer and/or inner containers, or sealing each dose in its own pouch.

Even with such packaging, however, no system is completely safe. It is important that you do your part by checking for signs of tampering whenever you buy or use a medicine.

The following information may help you detect possible signs of tampering.

Protecting yourself

General common sense suggestions include the following:
- When buying a drug product, *consider* the dosage form (for example, capsules, tablets, syrup), the type of packaging, and the tamper-evident features. Ask yourself: Would it be easy for someone to tamper with this product? Will I be able to determine whether or not this product has been tampered with?
- *Look very carefully* at the outer packaging of the drug product before you buy it. After you buy it, also check the inner packaging as soon as possible.
- If the medicine has a protective packaging feature, it should be described in the labeling. This description is required to be placed so that it will not be affected if the feature is broken or missing. If the feature is broken or missing, *do not buy or use* the product. If you have already purchased the product, return it to the store.

Always be sure to tell someone in charge about any problems.

- *Do not take* medicines that show even the slightest signs of tampering or do not seem quite right.
- Never take medicines in the dark or in poor lighting. *Read* the label and check each dose of medicine before you take it.

What to look for

Packaging

- Are there breaks, cracks, or holes in the outer or inner wrapping or protective cover or seal?
- Does the outer or inner covering appear to have been disturbed, unwrapped, or replaced?
- Does a plastic or other shrink band (tight-fitting wrap) around the top of the bottle appear distorted or stretched, as though it had been rolled down and then put back into place? Is the band missing? Has the band been slit and retaped?
- Is the bottom of the container intact?
- Does the container appear to be too full or not full enough?
- Is the cap on tight?
- Are there bits of paper or glue stuck on the rim of the container (does it seem like the container once had a bottle seal)?
- Is the cotton plug or filler in the bottle torn, sticky, or stained, or does it appear to have been taken out and put back?
- Do eye drops have a protective seal? All eye drops must be sealed when they are made, in order to keep them germ-free. Do not use if there is any sign of a broken or removed seal.
- Check the bottom as well as the top of a tube. Is the tube properly sealed? Metal tubes crimped up from the bottom like a tube of toothpaste should be firmly sealed.
- Are the expiration date, lot number, and other information the same on both the container and its outer wrapping or box?

Liquids

- Is the medicine the usual color? Thickness?
- Is a normally clear liquid cloudy or colored?
- Are there particles (small pieces) in the bottom of the bottle or floating in the solution? For some liquids, called suspensions, floating particles are normal.
- Does the medicine have a strange or different taste or odor (for example, bleach, acid, gasoline-like, or other pungent or sharp odor)? Do not taste the medicine if it has a strange odor.

Tablets

- Do the tablets look different than they usually do? Do they have unusual spots or markings? If they normally are shiny and smooth, are some dull or rough? Is there anything unusual about the color?
- Are the tablets all the same size and thickness?
- If there is printing on the tablets, do they all have the same imprint? Is the imprint missing from any?
- Do the tablets have a strange or different odor or taste?
- Are any of the tablets broken?

Capsules

- Do the capsules look different than they usually do? Are any cracked or dented? Are they all the same size and color?
- Do they have their normal shiny appearance or are some dull? Do some have fingerprints on them as though they have been handled?
- Are the capsules all the same length?
- If there is printing on the capsules, do they all have the same imprint? Is the imprint missing from any? Do the imprints all line up the same way?
- Do the capsules have an unexpected or unusual odor or taste?

Tubes and jars (ointments, creams, pastes, etc.)

- Does the product or container look different than usual?
- Are ointments and creams smooth and non-gritty? Have they separated?

Be a wise consumer. Look for signs of tampering before you buy a medicine and again each time you take a dose. Also, pay attention to the daily news in order to learn about any reported tampering.

It is important to understand that a change in the appearance or condition of a product may not mean that the package has been tampered with. The manufacturer may have changed the color of a medicine or its packaging. Also, the product may be breaking down with age or it may have had rough or unusual handling in shipping. In addition, some minor product variations may be normal.

Whenever you suspect that something is unusual about a medicine or its packaging, take it to your pharmacist. He or she is familiar with most products and their packaging. If there are serious concerns or problems, your pharmacist should report them to the FDA MedWatch Program at 1-800-FDA-1088.

Unintentional Poisoning

According to information provided by the American Association of Poison Control Centers, over one million children 6 years of age and under were unintentionally poisoned in 2001.

Adults also may be unintentionally poisoned. This happens most often through carelessness or lack of information. For example, people can be poisoned by taking medicines in the dark and getting the wrong one, or taking medicine prescribed for a friend to treat "the same symptoms."

Drug poisoning from an unintentional overdose is one type of accidental poisoning contributing to these figures. Other causes include household chemical poisoning from unintentional ingestion or contact, and inhaled poisoning—for example, carbon monoxide from a car.

Children are ready victims

The natural curiosity of children makes them ready victims of poisoning. Children explore everywhere and investigate their environment. What they find frequently goes into their mouths. They do not understand the danger and possibly cannot read warning labels.

Accidental poisoning from medicine is especially dangerous in small children because a medicine's strength is usually based on its use in adults. Even a small quantity of an adult dose can sometimes poison a child.

Preventing poisoning from medicines

- Store medicines out of the sight and reach of children, preferably in a locked cabinet—not in the bathroom medicine cabinet or in a food cabinet. Always store your medicines in a secure place.
- If you have children living with you or as occasional guests, you should have child-resistant caps on your medicine containers. These will help ensure that an accidental poisoning does not occur in your home. (Adults who have difficulty opening child-resistant closures may request traditional, easy-to-open packaging for their medicines.)
- If you are called to the telephone or to answer the door while you are taking a medicine, take the container with you or put the medicine out of the reach of small children. Children act quickly—usually when no one is watching.
- Always replace lids and return medicines to their storage place after use, even if you will be using them again soon.
- Date medicines when purchased and clean out your medicines periodically. Discard prescription medicines that are past their expiration or "beyond use" date. As medicines grow old, the chemicals in them may change. In general, medicines that do not have an expiration date should not be kept for more than 1 year. Carefully dis- card any medicines so children cannot get them. Rinse containers well before discarding in the trash.
- Take only those medicines prescribed for you and give medicines only to those for whom they are prescribed. A medicine that worked well for one person may harm another.
- It is best to keep all medicines in their original containers with their labels intact. The label contains valuable information for taking the medicine properly. Also, in case of accidental poisoning, it is important to know the ingredients in a drug product and any emergency instructions from the manufacturer. While prescription medicines usually do not list ingredients, information on the label makes it possible for your pharmacist to identify the contents.
- Ask your pharmacist to include on the label the number of tablets or capsules that he or she put in the container. In case of poisoning, it may be important to know roughly how many tablets or capsules were taken.
- Do not trust your memory—read the label before using the medicine, and take it as directed.
- If a medicine container has no label or the label has been defaced so you are not absolutely sure what it says, do not use it.
- Turn on a light when taking or giving medicines at night or in a dark room.
- Label medicine containers with poison symbols, especially if you have children, individuals with poor vision, or other persons in your home who cannot read well.
- Teach children that medicine is not candy by calling each medicine by its proper name.
- Do not take medicines in front of children. They may wish to imitate you.
- Communicate these safety rules to any babysitters you have and remember them if you babysit or are visiting a house with children. Children are naturally curious and can get into a pocketbook, briefcase, or overnight bag that contains medicines.

What to do if a poisoning happens

Remember:

- There may be no immediate, significant symptoms or warning signs, particularly in a child.
- Nothing you can give will work equally well in all cases of poisoning. In fact, one "antidote" may counteract the effects of another.
- Many poisons act quickly, leaving little time for treatment.

Therefore:

- If you think someone has swallowed medicine or a household product, and the person is unconscious, having seizures (convulsions), or is not breathing, immediately call for an ambulance. Otherwise, do not wait to see what effect the poison will have or if symptoms of overdose develop; immediately call a poison control center (listed in the white pages of your telephone book under "Poison Control" or inside the front cover with other emergency numbers). These numbers should be posted beside every telephone in the house, as should those of your pharmacist, the police, the fire department, and ambulance services. (Some poison control centers have TTY capability for the deaf. Check with your local center if you or someone in your family requires this service.)
- Have the container with you when you call so you can read the label on the product for ingredients.
- Describe what, when, and how much was taken and the age and condition of the person poisoned—for example, if the person is vomiting, choking, drowsy, shows a change in color or temperature of skin, is conscious or unconscious, or is convulsing.
- *Do not induce vomiting* unless instructed by medical personnel. *Do not induce vomiting or force liquids* into a person who is convulsing, unconscious, or very drowsy.
- Stay calm and in control of the situation.

Keep a bottle of Ipecac Syrup stored in a secure place in your home for emergency use. It is available at pharmacies in 1 ounce bottles without prescription. Ipecac Syrup is often recommended to induce vomiting in cases of poisoning.

Activated Charcoal also is sometimes recommended in certain types of poisoning and you may wish to add a supply to your emergency medicines. It is available without a prescription. Before using this medicine for poisoning, however, call a poison control center for advice.

Getting the Most Out of Your Medicines

To get the most out of your medicines, there are certain things that you must do. Your health care professionals will be working with you, but you also have a responsibility for your own health.

Communicating With Your Health Care Provider

Communication between you and your health care professional is central to good medical care. Your health care professional needs to know about you, your medical history, and your current problems. In turn, you need to understand the recommendations he or she is making and what you will need to do to follow the treatment. You will have to ask questions—and answer some too. Communication is a two-way process.

Giving information

Your health care professional needs to know some details about your past and present medical history. In discussing these details, you should always be completely open and honest. Your health professional's diagnosis and treatment will be based in part on the information that you provide. A complete list of the details that should be included in a full medical history is provided below.

"Medical history" checklist

A "medical history" checklist covers the following information:

- All the serious illnesses you have ever had and the approximate dates.
- Your current symptoms, if any.
- **All** the medicines and dietary supplements you are tak-ing or have taken in the recent past. This includes pre-scription and nonprescription medicines (such as pain relievers, antacids, laxatives, and cold medicines, etc.) and herbal medicines and home remedies. This is especially important if you are seeing more than one health care professional; if you are having surgery, including dental or emergency treatment; or if you get your medicines from more than one source.
- **Any** allergies or sensitivities to medicines, foods, or other substances.
- Your smoking, drinking, and exercise habits.
- Any recent changes in your lifestyle or personal habits. New job? Retired? Change of residence? Death in family? Married? Divorced? Other?
- Any special diet you are on—low-sugar, low-sodium, low-fat, or a diet to lose or gain weight.
- If you are pregnant, plan to become pregnant, or if you are breast-feeding.
- All the vaccinations and vaccination boosters you have had, with dates if possible.
- Any operations you have had, including dental and those performed on an outpatient basis, and any accidents that have required hospitalization.
- Illnesses or conditions that run in your family.
- Cause of death of closest relatives.

Remember, be sure to tell your health care professional at each visit if there have been any changes since your last visit.

Medical history forms

Many health care professionals have a standard "medical history" form they will ask you to fill out when they see you for the first time. Some may ask the questions and write down the answers for you. If you will be visiting a health care professional for the first time, prepare yourself before you go by thinking about the questions that might be asked and jotting down the answers—including dates—so that you will not forget an important detail. Once your "medical history" is in the files, subsequent visits will take less time.

You will have to supply each health care provider you see—every time you see one—with complete information about what happened since your last visit. It is important that your records are updated so he or she can make sound recommendations for your continued treatment, or treatment of any new problems.

Medical history file

It will simplify things if you develop a "medical history" file at home for yourself and each family member for whom you are responsible. Setting up the file will take time. However, once it is established, you need only to keep it up-to-date and remember to take it with you when you see a health care professional. This will be easier than having to repeat the information each time and running the risk of confusing or forgetting details.

It is also a good idea to carry in your wallet a card that summarizes your chronic medical conditions, the medicines you are taking, and your allergies and drug sensitivities. You should keep this card as up-to-date as possible. Many pharmacists provide these cards as a service.

Getting information

In order to benefit from your health care professional's advice you must understand completely everything that he or she tells you. Do not be embarrassed to ask questions, or to ask him or her to explain again any instruction or detail that you do not understand. Then it is up to you to carry out those instructions precisely. If there is a failure in any part of this system, you will pay an even higher price—physically and financially—for your health care.

Your health care professional may provide instructions to you in written form. If he or she does not, you may want to write them down or ask the health care professional to write them down for you. If you do not have time to jot down everything while you are still with your health care professional, sit down in the waiting room before you leave and write down the information while it is still fresh in your mind and you can still ask questions. If you have been given a prescription, ask for written information about the drug and how to take it. Your pharmacist can also answer questions when you have your prescription filled.

What you need to know about your medicines

There are a number of things that you should know about each medicine you are taking. These include:

- The medicine's generic and brand name.
- How the medicine will help you and the expected results. How it makes you feel. How long it takes to begin working.
- How much to take at one time.
- How often to take the medicine.
- How long it will be necessary to take the medicine.
- When to take it. Before, during, after meals? At bedtime? At any other special times?
- How to take it. With water? With fruit juice? With food?
- What to do if you forget to take it (miss a dose).
- Foods, drinks, or other medicines that you should not take while taking the medicine.
- Restrictions on activities while taking the medicine, such as driving a car or operating other motor vehicles.
- Possible side effects. What to do if they appear. How to minimize the side effects. How soon they will go away.
- When to seek help if there are problems.
- How long to wait before reporting no change in your symptoms.
- How to store the medicine.
- The expiration date.
- The cost of the medicine.
- How to have your prescription refilled, if necessary.

Other information

Following are some other issues and information that you may want to consider:

- Ask your health care professional about the ingredients in the medicines (both prescription and over-the-counter [OTC]) you are taking and whether there may be a conflict with other medicines. Your health care professional can help you avoid dangerous combinations or drug products that contain ingredients to which you are allergic or sensitive.
- Ask your health care professional for help in developing a system for taking your medicines properly, particularly if you are taking a number of them on a daily basis. When you are a patient in a hospital, ask for instructions before you are discharged. Do not hesitate or be embarrassed to ask questions or ask for help.
- If you are over 60 years of age, ask your health care professional if the dose of the medicine is right for you. Some medicines should be given in lower doses to certain older individuals.
- If you are taking several different medicines, ask your health care professional if all of them are necessary for you. You should take only those medicines that you need.
- Medicines should be kept in the container they came

in. If this is not possible when you are at work or away from home, ask your pharmacist to provide or recommend a container to transport your medicines safely. The use of "pill boxes" can also cause some problems, such as broken or chipped tablets, mistaking one medicine for another, and even interactions between the medicine and the metal of these boxes.

- Some people have trouble taking tablets or capsules. Your health care professional will know if another dosage form is available, and if tablet or capsule contents can be taken in a liquid. If this is an ongoing problem, ask your prescriber to write the prescription for the dosage form you can take most comfortably.
- To protect children from accidental poisoning, child-resistant caps are required by law on most oral prescription medicines. These containers are designed so children will have difficulty opening them. Since many adults also find these containers hard to open, the law allows consumers to request traditional, easy-to-open packaging for their drugs. If you do not use child-resistant packaging, make sure that your medicines are stored where small children cannot see or reach them. If you use child-resistant containers, ask your pharmacist to show you how to open them.

Consumer education is one of your health care professional's most important responsibilities. To supplement what you learn during your visit, ask if there is any written information about your medicines that you can take home with you. Your health care professional may also have available various reference books or computerized drug information that you can consult for details about precautions, side effects, and proper use of your medicines.

Your Health Care Team

Your health care team will be made up of several different health care professionals. Each of these individuals will play an important part in the overall provision of your health care. It is important that you understand the roles of each of these providers and what you should be able to expect from each of them.

Your dentist

In addition to providing care and maintenance of your mouth, teeth, and gums, your dentist is also an essential member of your overall health care team since your oral health and general health often affect one another.

In providing dental treatment, your dentist should base his or her decisions upon an extensive knowledge of your current condition and past medical and dental history. Because the dentist is a prescriber of medications, it is very important that he or she is aware of your **full** medical and dental history. A complete medical and dental history should include the information that is listed in the "Medical history checklist" section above. Even if you do not consider this information important, you should inform your dentist as fully as possible.

In the treatment of any dental/oral problem your dentist should make every effort to inform you as fully as possible about the nature of the problem. He or she should explain why this problem has occurred, the advantages and disadvantages of available treatments (including no treatment), and what types of preventive measures can be employed to avoid future problems. These measures may include periodic visits to the dentist, and a general awareness of the manner in which dental and overall health may affect one another. In any type of treatment, your dentist should always allow you to ask questions, and should be willing to answer them to your satisfaction.In selecting a dentist, it is important to keep in mind the role of the dentist as a member of the health care team, and the extent of the information that he or she should be asking for and providing. There are also several practical issues that you should consider, such as:

- Is the dentist a specialist or general practitioner?
- What are the office hours?
- Is the dentist or his/her associates available after office hours by phone? In emergencies, will you be able to contact a dentist?
- What is the office policy on cancellations?
- What types of payment are accepted at the office?
- What is the office policy on x-ray procedures?
- Is the dentist willing to work with other medical and/or dental specialists that you may be seeing?

Your dentist should be an integral part of your health care team. In treating problems and providing general maintenance of your oral health, your dentist should base decisions upon a full dental and medical history. He or she should also be willing to answer any questions that you have regarding your oral health, any medications prescribed, and preventive measures to avoid future problems.

Your nurse

Depending upon the setting, type of therapy being administered, and state regulations, the role of the nurse in your health care team may vary. Registered nurses practice in diverse health care settings, such as hospitals, outpatient clinics or physicians' offices, schools, workplaces, homes, and long-term care facilities like nursing homes and retirement centers. Some nurses, including certified nurse practitioners and midwives, hold a master's degree in nursing and may assume the role of primary health care professional, either in practice by themselves or in joint practices with physicians. In most states, nurse practitioners may prescribe selected medications. Clinical nurse specialists also have a master's degree in nursing and specialize in a particular area of health care. In some hospitals, long-term care facilities, and out-patient care settings, licensed practical nurses (LPNs) have certain responsibilities in administering medication to patients. LPNs usually work under the supervision of a RN or physician. Nursing aides assist RNs and LPNs with different kinds of patient care activities. In most places where people receive health care, RNs may be the primary source of information for drug therapies and other medical treatments. It is important that you be aware of the roles and responsibilities of the nurses participating in your health care.

Professional nurses participate with other health professionals to ensure that your medication therapy is safe and effective and to monitor any effects (both desired and negative) from the medication. You may be admitted to the hospital so that nurses can administer medications and monitor your response to therapy. In hospitals or long-term care facilities, nurses are responsible for administering your medications in their proper dosage form and dose, and at correct time intervals, as well as monitoring your response to these medications. At home or in outpatient settings, nurses should ensure that you have the proper information and support of others, if needed, to get the medication and take it as prescribed. When nurses administer medication, they should explain why you are receiving this medication, how it works, any possible side effects, special precautions or actions that you must take while using the medication, and any potential interactions with other medications.

If you experience any side effects or symptoms from a medication, you should always tell your health care provider. It is important that these reactions be detected before they become serious or permanent. You can seek advice about possible ways to minimize these side effects from your nurse. Your health care professional should also be made aware of any additional medical problems or conditions (such as pregnancy) that you may have, since these can also affect the safety and effectiveness of a medication.

The professional nurse is someone who can help to clarify drug information. In most health care settings, nurses are accessible and can answer your questions or direct you to others who can assist you. Professional nurses are skilled in the process of patient teaching. To make sure that patients learn important information about their health problem and its treatment, RNs often use a combination of teaching methods, such as verbal instruction, written materials, demonstration, and audio-visual instructions. Above all, professional nurses should teach at a pace and level that are appropriate for you. RNs can also help you design a medication schedule that fits your lifestyle and may be less likely to cause unwanted side effects.

Your pharmacist

Your pharmacist is an important member of your health care team. In addition to performing traditional services, such as dispensing medications, your pharmacist can help you understand your medications and how to take them safely and effectively. By keeping accurate and up-to-date records and monitoring your use of medications, your pharmacist can help to protect you from improper medication therapy, unwanted side effects, and dangerous drug interactions. Because your pharmacist can play a vital role in protecting and improving your health, you should seek a pharmacist who will provide these services.

To provide you with the best possible care, your pharmacist should be informed about your current condition and medication history. Your personal medication history should include the information that is listed in the "Medical history checklist" section above. Your pharmacist should also be aware of any special packaging needs that you may have (such as child-resistant or easy-to-open containers). Your pharmacist should keep accurate and up-to-date records that contain this information. If you visit a new pharmacy that does not have access to your medication records, it is important that you inform that pharmacist as fully as possible about your medical history or provide him or her with a copy of your medication records from your previous pharmacy. In general, in order to get the most out of your pharmacy services, it is best to get all of your medications (including OTCs) from the same pharmacy. Your pharmacist should be a knowledgeable and approachable source of information about your medications. Some of the information that your pharmacist should explain is listed in the "What you need to know about your medicines" section above. Ideally, this information should also be provided in written form, so that you may refer to it later if you have any questions or problems. The pharmacist should always be willing to answer any questions that you have regarding your medications, and should also be willing to contact your physician or other health care professionals (dentist, nurses, etc.) on your behalf if necessary.

Your pharmacist can also help you with information on the costs of your medicines. Many medicines are available from more than one company. They may have equal effects but different costs. Your insurance company, HMO, or other third-party payment group may reimburse you for only some of these medications or only for part of their costs. Your pharmacist will be able to tell you which of these medications are covered by your payment plan or which cost less.

In selecting a pharmacist, it is important that you understand the role of the pharmacist as a member of your health care team and the extent of information that he or she should be asking for and providing. Because pharmacies can offer different types of services and have different policies regarding patient information, some of the issues that you should consider in selecting a pharmacist also relate to the pharmacy where that person practices. There are several issues regarding the pharmacist and pharmacy that you should consider, such as:

- Does the pharmacy offer written information that you can take home? Home delivery?
- Are you able to talk to your pharmacist without other people hearing you?
- Can the pharmacist be reached easily by phone? In an emergency, is a pharmacist available twenty-four hours (including weekends and holidays) by phone?
- What types of payment are accepted in the pharmacy?
- Does the pharmacy accept your HMO or third-party payment plan?
- Does the pharmacy offer any specialized services, such as diabetes education?

You should select your pharmacist and pharmacy as carefully as you select your physician, and stay with the same pharmacy so that all of your medication records are in the same place. This will help to ensure that your records are accurate and up-to-date and will allow you to develop a beneficial relationship with your pharmacist.

Your physician

One of the most important health care decisions that you will make is your choice of a personal physician. The physician is central to your health care team, and is responsible for helping you maintain your overall health. In addition to detecting and treating ailments or adverse conditions, your physician and his or her coworkers should also serve as primary sources of health care information. Because the physician plays such an important role in your overall health care, it is important that you understand the full range of the physician's role as health care and information provider.

In providing any type of treatment or counseling, your physician should base his or her decisions upon an extensive knowledge of your current condition and past medical history. A complete medical history should include the information that is listed in the "Medical history checklist" section above. Your physician should keep accurate and comprehensive medical records containing this information. Because your treatment (and your health) is dependent upon a full disclosure of your medical history, as well as any factors that may currently be affecting your health (i.e., stress, smoking, drug use, etc.), it is important that you inform your physician as fully as possible, even if you might not consider this information important.

It is important that you inform your personal physician of any other physicians (such as specialists or subspecialists), dentists, or other health care professionals that you are seeing. You should also inform your physician of the pharmacy that you use or intend to use, so that he or she can contact the pharmacist if necessary.

In treating any health problem, your physician should make every effort to help you understand completely the nature of the problem and its treatment. He or she should take the time to explain the problem, why it may have occurred, and what preventive measures (if any) can be taken to avoid it in the future. Your physician should explain fully the reasons for any prescribed treatment. He or she should also be willing to discuss alternative therapies, especially if you are uncomfortable with the one that has been prescribed. Your physician should always be willing to answer all of your questions to your satisfaction.

In selecting a physician, you should look for one who will provide a full range of services. You may also want to consider your physician's medical credentials. Your local medical society should be able to provide specific facts about your physician's traning, experience, and membership in professional societies.

Cost and payment are two of the most important issues in contemporary health care. Your physician should be sensitive to the costs of your treatment and the manner in which you intend to pay for this and related medications. If you belong to an HMO or third-party payment plan, be sure that your physician is aware of your involvement in the plan. You should also be aware of the different types of payment that are accepted at the physician's office.

In prescribing medications, your physician should take

into account the manner in which you intend to pay for your drugs, and should be aware of any specific concerns regarding the costs of your treatment and medication. He or she should also explain why brand or generic medication may be preferable in certain situations.

In selecting a physician, there are also several practical issues and matters of convenience that you should consider, such as:

- Is the office convenient to your home or work?
- What are the office hours?
- Is your physician or his/her associates or partners available (twenty-four hours) by phone? In emergencies, will you be able to contact a physician?
- Are you able to arrange appointments to fit your schedule? What is the office policy on cancellations?
- Is the physician well regarded in the community? Does he or she have a reputation for listening to patients and answering questions?
- Does the physician have admitting privileges at a hospital of your preference?
- Does he/she participate in your health plan?

In addition to the considerations already mentioned, your physician should be sensitive to the special concerns of treating the elderly. Older patients can present disease processes differently from younger adults, can react differently to certain drugs and dosages, and may have preexisting conditions that require special treatments to be prescribed.

There are also several special issues to consider in your selection of a pediatrician or family physician. If your child is not old enough to understand all instructions and information, it is important that your child's physician explain to you any information about a problem and all instructions for treatment. When your child is of school age, the physician should speak directly to the child as well, asking and answering questions, and providing information about cause and prevention of medical problems and the use of medications. He or she should choose a dosage form and dose that is appropriate for your child's age and explain what to do if the child has certain symptoms, such as fever, vomiting, etc. (including the amount and type of medicine to give, if any, and when to call him or her for advice).

Your physician should be a primary source of information about your health and any medications that you are taking. In providing treatment for medical problems or conditions, the physician should base decisions on a full medical history and be willing to answer any questions that you have regarding your health, treatment, and medications.

Managing Your Medicines

To get the full benefit and reduce risks in taking your medicines, it is important to follow instructions exactly. This means taking the right medicine and dose, at correct time intervals, for the length of time prescribed. Bad effects can result from taking too much or too little of a medicine, or taking it too often or not often enough.

Establishing a system

Whether you are taking one or several medicines, you should develop a system for taking them. It can be just as difficult to remember whether you took your once-a-day medicine as it can be to keep track of a number of medicines that need to be taken several times a day. Many medicines also have special instructions that can further complicate proper use.

Establish a way of knowing whether you took your medicines properly, then make that a part of your daily routine. If you take one or two medicines a day, you may only need to take them at the same time that you perform some other regular task, such as brushing your teeth or getting dressed.

For most people, a check-off record can also be a handy way of managing multiple medicines. Keep your medicine record in a handy, visible place next to where you take your medicines. Check off each dose as you take it. If you miss a dose, make a note about what happened and what you did on the back of the record or the bottom of the sheet.

Be sure to note any unwanted effects or anything unusual that you think may be connected with your medicines. Also note if a medicine does not do what you expect, but remember that some medicines take a while before having a noticeable effect.

If you keep a check-off record faithfully, you will know for sure whether or not you took your medicine. You will also have a complete record for your health care professionals to review when you visit them again. This information can help them determine if the medicine is working properly or causing unwanted side effects, or whether adjustments should be made in your medicines and/or doses.

If your medicines or the instructions for taking them are changed, correct your record or make a new one. Keep the old record until you are sure this information is no longer needed.

You might want to color code your medicine containers to help tell them apart. If you are having trouble reading labels or if you are color-blind, codes that can be recognized by touch (rubber bands, a cotton ball, or a piece of emery board, for instance) can be attached to the container. If you code your medicines, be sure these identifications are included on any medicine record you use. If necessary, ask your pharmacist to type medicine labels in large letters for easier reading.

A check-off list is not the only method for recording medicine use. If this system does not work for you, ask your health care professional for help in developing an alternative. Be sure he or she knows all the medicines prescribed for you and any nonprescription medicines you take regularly, the hours you usually eat your meals, and any special diet you are following.

Informed management

Your medicines have been prescribed for you and your condition. Ask your health care professional what benefits to expect, what side effects may occur, and when to report any side effects. If your symptoms go away, do not decide you are well and stop taking your medicine. If you stop too soon, the symptoms may come back. Finish all of the medicine if you have been told to do so. However, if you develop diarrhea or other unpleasant side effects, do not continue with the medicine; call your health care professional and report these effects. A change in dose or in the kind of medicine you are taking may be necessary.

When you are given a prescription for a medicine, ask the person who wrote it to explain it to you. For example, does "four times a day" mean one in the morning, one at noon, one in the evening, and one at bedtime; or does it mean every six hours around the clock? When a prescription says "take as needed," ask how close together the doses can be taken and what the maximum number of doses you can take in one day should be. Does "take with liquids" mean with water, milk, or something else? Are there some liquids that should avoided? What does "take with food" mean? At every mealtime (some people must eat six meals a day), or with a snack? Do not trust your memory—have the instructions written down. You must understand exactly what the prescriber wants you to do in order to "take as directed."

When the pharmacist dispenses your medicine, you have another opportunity to clarify information or to ask other questions. Before you leave, check the label on your medicine to be sure it matches the prescription and your understanding of what you are to do. If it does not, ask more questions.

The key to getting the most from your prescribed treatments is following instructions accurately and intelligently. If you have questions or doubts about the prescribed treatment, do not decide to stop taking the medicine or fail to follow the prescribed regimen. Discuss your questions and doubts with your health care professional.

The time and effort put into setting up a system to manage your medicines and establishing a routine for taking them will pay off by relieving anxiety and helping you get the most from your prescribed treatment.

Taking Your Medicine

To take medicines safely and get the greatest benefit from them, it is important to establish regular habits so you are less likely to make mistakes.

Before taking any medicine, read the label and any accompanying information. You can also consult books to learn more about the medicine. If you have unanswered questions, check with your health care professional.

The label on the container of a prescription medicine should bear your first and last name; the name of the prescriber; the pharmacy address and telephone number; the prescription number; the date of dispensing; and directions for use. Some states or provinces may have additional requirements. If the name of the drug product is not on the label, ask the pharmacist to include the brand (if any) and generic names. An expiration date may also appear. All of this information is important in identifying your medicines and using them properly. The labels on containers should never be removed and all medicines should be kept in their original containers.

Some tips for taking medicines safely and accurately include the following:

- Read the label of each medicine container three times:
  —before you remove it from its storage place,
  —before you take the lid off the container to remove the dose, and
  —before you replace the container in its storage place.
- Never take medicines in the dark, even if you think you know exactly where to find them.
- Use standard measuring devices to take your medicines (household teaspoons, cups, or glasses vary widely in the amount they hold). Ask your pharmacist for help with measuring.
- Set bottles and boxes of medicines on a clear area, well back from the edge of the surface to prevent containers and/or caps from being knocked to the floor.
- When pouring liquid medicines, pick up the container with the label against the palm of your hand to protect it from being stained by dripping medicine.
- Wipe off the top and neck of bottles of liquid medicines to keep labels from being obscured, and to make it less likely that the lid will stick.
- Shake all liquid suspensions of drug products before pouring so that ingredients are mixed thoroughly.
- If you are taking medicine with water, use a full, 8 ounce glassful, not just enough to get it down. Too little liquid with some medicines can prevent the medicine from working properly, and can cause throat irritation if the medicine does not get completely to the stomach.
- To avoid accidental confusion of lids, labels, and medicines, replace the lid on one container before opening another.
- When you are interrupted while taking your medicine, take the container with you or put the medicine out of the reach of small children. It only takes a second for them to take an overdose. When you return, check the label of the medicine to be sure you have the right one.
- Crush tablets or open capsules to take with food or beverages if your health care professional has told you that this will not affect the way the medicine works. If you have difficulty swallowing a tablet or capsule, check with your health care professional about the availability of a different dosage form.
- Follow any diet instructions or other treatment measures prescribed by your health care professional.
- If at any point you realize you have taken the wrong medicine or the wrong amount, call your health care professional immediately. In an emergency, call your local emergency number.

When you have finished taking your medicines, mark it down immediately on your medication calendar to avoid "double dosing." Also make note of any unusual changes in your body, including change in weight, color or amount of urine, perspiration, or coughed-up matter; as well as your pulse, temperature, or any other items you may have been instructed to observe for your condition or your medicine.

Try to take your medicines on time, but a half-hour early or late will usually not upset your schedule. If you are more than several hours late and are getting close to your next scheduled dose, check any instructions that were given to you by your health care professional. If you did not receive instructions about missed doses, check with your health care professional. You may also find missed dose information in the entries included in this book.

When your medicines are being managed by someone else (for example, when you are a patient in a hospital or nursing home), question what is happening to you and communicate what you know about your previous drug therapy or any other treatments. If you know you always take one, not two, of a certain tablet, say so and ask that your record be checked before you take the medicine. If you think you are receiving the wrong treatment or medication, do not hesitate to say so. You should always remain involved in your own therapy.

Many hospitals and nursing homes now offer counseling in medicine management as part of their discharge planning for patients. If you or a family member are getting ready to come home, ask your health care professional if you can be part of such instruction.

The "Expiration Date" on Medicine Labels

To assure that a drug product meets applicable standards of identity, strength, quality, and purity at the time of use, an "expiration date" is added by the manufacturer to the label of most prescription and nonprescription drug products.

The expiration date on a drug product is valid only as long as the product is stored in the original, unopened container under the storage conditions specified by the manufacturer. Among other things, humidity, temperature, light, and even air can effect drugs. A medicine taken after the expiration date may have changed in potency or may have formed harmful material as it deteriorates. Contamination with germs can also occur. The safest rule is not to use any medicine beyond the expiration date.

Preventing deterioration

A drug begins to deteriorate the minute it is made. The manufacturer in calculating the expiration date factors in this rate of deterioration. Keeping the drug product in the container supplied by the pharmacist helps slow down deterioration. Storing the drug in a proper manner—for example, in a light-resistant container or in a cool, dry place (not the bathroom medicine cabinet)—also helps. The need for medicines to be kept in their containers and stored properly cannot be overstressed.

Patients sometimes ask their health care professionals to prescribe a large quantity of a particular medicine in order to "economize." Although this may be all right in some cases, this practice may backfire. If you have a large supply of your medicine and it deteriorates before you can use it all, or if your doctor changes your medicine, you may lose out.

Sometimes deterioration can be recognized by physical changes in the drug, such as a change in odor or appearance. For example, aspirin tablets develop a vinegar odor when they break down. These changes are not true of all drugs, however, and the absence of physical changes should not be assumed to mean that no deterioration has occurred.

Some liquid medicines mixed at the pharmacy will have a "beyond use" date on the label. This is an expiration date that is calculated from the date of preparation in the pharmacy. This is a definite date, after which you should throw away any remaining medicine.

If your prescription medicines do not bear an "expiration" or "beyond use" date, your dispensing pharmacist is the best person to advise you about how long they can be safely used.

ABOUT THE MEDICINES YOU ARE TAKING

New Drugs—From Idea to Marketplace

To be sold legitimately in the United States, new drugs must pass through a rigorous system of approval specified in the Food, Drug, and Cosmetic Act and supervised by the Food and Drug Administration (FDA). Except for certain drugs subject to other regulatory provisions, no new drug for human use may be marketed in this country unless FDA has approved a "New Drug Application" (NDA) for it.

The idea

The creation of a new drug usually starts with an idea. Most likely that idea results from the study of a disease or group of symptoms. Ideas can also come from observations of clinical research. This may involve many years of study, or the idea may occur from an accidental discovery in a research laboratory. Some may be coincidental discoveries, as in the case of penicillin.

Idea development takes place most often in the laboratory of a pharmaceutical company, but may also happen in laboratories at research institutions like the National Institutes of Health, at medical centers and universities, or in the laboratory of a chemical company.

Animal testing

A new drug is first tested on animals to help determine how toxic the substance may be. Most drugs interfere in some way with normal body functions. These animal studies are designed to discover the degree of that interference and the extent of the toxic effects.

After successful animal testing, perhaps over several years, the sponsors of the new drug apply to the FDA for an Investigational New Drug (IND) application. This status allows the drug to be tested in humans. As part of their request, the sponsoring manufacturer must submit the results of the animal studies, plus a detailed outline of the proposed human testing and information about the researchers that will be involved.

Human testing

Drug testing in humans usually consists of three consecutive phases. "Informed consent" must be secured from all volunteers participating in this testing.

Phase I testing is most often done on young, healthy adults. This testing is done on a relatively small number of subjects, generally between 20 and 80. Its purpose is to learn more about the biochemistry of the drug: how it acts on the body and how the body reacts to it. The procedure differs for some drugs, however. For example, Phase I testing of cancer drugs involves actual cancer patients from the beginning of testing.

During Phase II, small controlled clinical studies are designed to test the effectiveness and relative safety of the drug. These are done on closely monitored patients who have the disease for which the drug is being tested. Their numbers seldom go beyond 100 to 200 patients. Some volunteers for Phase II testing who have severely complicated conditions may be excluded.

A "control" group of people of comparable physical and disease types is used in double-blind, controlled experiments for most drugs. These experiments are conducted by medical investigators thoroughly familiar with the disease and this type of research. In a double-blind experiment, the patient, the health professional, and other personnel do not know whether the patient is receiving the drug being tested, another active drug, or no medicine at all (a placebo or "sugar pill"). This helps eliminate bias and assures the accuracy of results. The findings of these tests are statistically analyzed to determine whether they are "significant" or due to chance alone.

Phase III consists of larger studies. This testing is performed after effectiveness of the drug has been established and is intended to gather additional evidence of effectiveness for specific uses of the drug. These studies also help discover adverse drug reactions that may occur with the drug. Phase III studies involve a few hundred to several thousand patients who have the disease the drug is intended to treat.

Patients with additional diseases or those receiving other therapy may be included in later Phase II and Phase III studies. They would be expected to be representative of certain segments of the population who would receive the drug following approval for marketing.

Final approval

When a sponsor believes the investigational studies on a drug have shown it to be safe and effective in treating specific conditions, a New Drug Application (NDA) is submitted to FDA. This application is accompanied by all the documentation from the company's research, including complete records of all the animal and human testing. This documentation can run to many thousands of pages.

The NDA and its documentation must then be reviewed by FDA physicians, pharmacologists, chemists, statisticians, and other professionals experienced in evaluating new drugs. Proposed labeling information for the physician and pharmacist is also screened for accuracy, completeness, and conformity to FDA-approved wording.

Regulations call for the FDA to review an NDA within 180 days. This period may be extended if additional data is required and, in some cases, may take several years. When all research phases are considered, the actual time it takes from idea to marketplace may be 8 to 10 years or even longer. However, for drugs representing major therapeutic advances, FDA may "fast-track" the approval process to try to get those drugs to patients who need them as soon as possible.

After approval

After a drug is marketed, the manufacturer must inform the FDA of any unexpected side effects or toxicity that comes to its attention. Consumers and health care professionals have an important role in helping to identify any previously unreported effects. If new evidence indicates that the drug may present an "imminent hazard," the FDA can withdraw approval for marketing or add new information to the drug's labeling at any time.

Generic drugs

After a new drug is approved for marketing, a patent will generally protect the financial interests of the drug's developer for a number of years. The traditional protection period is for 17 years. In reality, however, the period is much less due to the extended period of time needed to gain approval before marketing can begin. Recognizing that a considerable part of a drug's patent life may be tied up in the approval process, in 1984 the U.S. Congress passed a law providing patent extension for drugs whose commercial sale may have been unduly delayed by the approval process.

Any manufacturer can apply for permission to produce and market a drug after the patent for the drug has expired. Following a procedure called an Abbreviated New Drug Application (ANDA), the applicant must show that its product has a comparable potency and effect to the original product. Although the extensive clinical testing completed by the originator during the drug's development does not have to be repeated, comparative testing between the products must be done.

Drug Names

Every drug must have a nonproprietary name, a name that is available for each manufacturer to use. These names are commonly called generic names.

The FDA requires the generic name of a drug product to be placed on its labeling. However, manufacturers often use brand names in promoting their products. In general, brand names are shorter and easier to use than the corresponding generic name. The manufacturer then emphasizes its brand name (which cannot be used by anyone else) in advertising and other promotions. Often, the consumer may not realize that a brand name drug is also available under other brand names or by generic name. Ask your pharmacist if you have any questions about the names of your medicines.

Drug Quality

After an NDA or an ANDA has been approved for a product, the manufacturer must then meet all requirements relating to production. These include the FDA's current Good Manufacturing Practice regulations and any applicable standards relating to strength, quality, purity, packaging, and labeling that are established by the United States Pharmacopeia (USP).

Routine product testing by the manufacturer is required by the Good Manufacturing Practice regulations of the FDA (the FDA itself does not routinely test all products, except in cases where there is a suspicion that something may be wrong). In addition to governmental requirements, drug products must meet public standards of strength, quality, and purity that are developed by USP. In order to market their products, all manufacturers in the United States must meet USP-established standards unless they specifically choose not to meet the standards for a particular product. In this case, that product's label must state that it is "not USP" and how it differs from USP standards (this occurs very rarely).

Differences in Drug Products

Although standards to ensure strength, quality, purity, and bioequivalence (comparable potency and effect) exist, the standards allow for variations in certain factors that may produce other differences from product to product. These product variations may be important to some patients, since not all patients are "equivalent." For example, the size, shape, and coating may vary and, therefore, be harder or easier for some patients to swallow; an oral liquid will taste good to some patients and bad to others; one manufacturer may use lactose as an inactive ingredient in its product, while another product may contain a different inactive ingredient; one product may contain sugar or alcohol while another product does not.

In deciding to use one therapeutically equivalent product over another, consumers should keep the following in mind:

- Consider convenience factors of drug products (for example, ease of taking a particular dosage form).
- Don't overlook the convenience of the package. The package must protect the drug in accordance with USP requirements, but packages can be quite different in their ease of carrying, storing, opening, and measuring.
- If you have an allergy or any type of dietary restriction, you need to be aware of the "inactive" ingredients that may be present in different medicines. These inactive ingredients may vary from product to product.

- Price is always a consideration. The price difference between products (e.g., different brands, or brands versus generics) may be a major factor in the overall price of a prescription. Talk to your pharmacist about price considerations. Some states require that the pharmacist dispense exactly what is prescribed. However, other states allow the pharmacist to dispense less expensive medicines when appropriate.

Aside from differences in the drug product, there are many other factors that may influence the effectiveness of a medicine. For example, your diet, body chemistry, medical conditions, or other drugs you are taking may affect how much of a dose of a particular medicine gets into the body.

For the majority of drugs, slight differences in the amount of drug made available to the body will not make any therapeutic difference. For other drugs, the precise amount that gets into the body is more critical. For example, some heart or epilepsy medicines may create problems for the patient if the dose delivered to the body varies for some reason.

For those drugs in the critical category, it is a good idea to stay on the specific product you started on. Changes should only be made after a consultation with the health care professional who prescribed the medicine. If you feel that a certain batch of your medicine is more potent or does not work as well as other batches, or if you have other questions, check with your health care professional.

ABACAVIR (Oral route) - a-BAK-a-veer

Black Box Warning

Hypersensitivity reactions: Serious and sometimes fatal hypersensitivity reactions have been associated with abacavir sulfate. Hypersensitivity to abacavir is a multi-organ clinical syndrome usually characterized by a sign or symptom in 2 or more of the following groups: 1) fever, 2) rash, 3) gastrointestinal (including nausea, vomiting, diarrhea, or abdominal pain), 4) constitutional (including generalized malaise, fatigue, or achiness), and 5) respiratory (including dyspnea, cough, or pharyngitis). Discontinue abacavir sulfate as soon as a hypersensitivity reaction is suspected. Permanently discontinue abacavir sulfate if hypersensitivity cannot be ruled out, even when other diagnoses are possible.

Following a hypersensitivity reaction to abacavir, NEVER restart abacavir sulfate or any other abacavir-containing product because more severe symptoms can occur within hours and may include life-threatening hypotension and death.

Reintroduction of abacavir sulfate or any other abacavir-containing product, even in patients who have no identified history or recognized symptoms of hypersensitivity to abacavir therapy, can result in serious or fatal hypersensitivity reactions. Such reactions can occur within hours.

Lactic acidosis and severe hepatomegaly: Lactic acidosis and severe hepatomegaly with steatosis, including fatal cases, have been reported with the use of nucleoside analogues alone or in combination, including abacavir sulfate and other antiretrovirals.

Commonly used brand name(s)

In the U.S.—
Ziagen

Available Dosage Forms:
- Tablet
- Solution

Therapeutic Class: Antiretroviral Agent
Pharmacologic Class: Nucleoside Reverse Transcriptase Inhibitor

Uses For This Medicine

Abacavir is used, in combination with other medicines, in the treatment of the infection caused by the human immunodeficiency virus (HIV). HIV is the virus that causes acquired immunodeficiency syndrome (AIDS).

Abacavir will not cure or prevent HIV infection or AIDS; however, it helps keep HIV from reproducing and appears to slow down the destruction of the immune system. This may help delay the development of problems usually related to AIDS or HIV disease. Abacavir will not keep you from spreading HIV to other people. People who receive this medicine may continue to have other problems usually related to AIDS or HIV disease.

This medicine is available only with your doctor's prescription.

Before Using This Medicine

In deciding to use a medicine, the risks of taking the medicine must be weighed against the good it will do. This is a decision you and your doctor will make. For this medicine, the following should be considered:

Allergies—Tell your doctor if you have ever had any unusual or allergic reaction to this medicine or any other medicines. Also tell your health care professional if you have any other types of allergies, such as to foods, dyes, preservatives, or animals. For non-prescription products, read the label or package ingredients carefully.

Pediatric—This medicine has been tested in children 3 months of age and older and, in effective doses, has not been shown to cause different side effects or problems than it does in adults.

Geriatric—Many medicines have not been studied specifically in older people. Therefore, it may not be known whether they work exactly the same way they do in younger adults or if they cause different side effects or problems in older people. There is no specific information comparing use of abacavir in the elderly with use in other age groups.

Pregnancy—

	Pregnancy Category	Explanation
All Trimesters	C	Animal studies have shown an adverse effect and there are no adequate studies in pregnant women OR no animal studies have been conducted and there are no adequate studies in pregnant women.

Breast Feeding—There are no adequate studies in women for determining infant risk when using this medication during breastfeeding. Weigh the potential benefits against the potential risks before taking this medication while breastfeeding.

Other medicines—

Using this medicine with any of the following medicines is usually not recommended, but may be required in some cases. If both medicines are prescribed together, your doctor may change the dose or how often you use one or both of the medicines.

Ribavirin

Interactions with Food/Tobacco/Alcohol—Certain medicines should not be used at or around the time of eating food or eating certain types of food since interactions may occur. Using alcohol or tobacco with certain medicines may also cause interactions to occur. Discuss with your healthcare professional the use of your medicine with food, alcohol, or tobacco.

Other medical problems—The presence of other medical problems may affect the use of this medicine. Make sure you tell your doctor if you have any other medical problems, especially:
- Allergy to abacavir or any ingredients in the medicine— You should tell your doctor immediately if you have signs of an allergic reaction. If you have ever taken abacavir in the past, you should tell your doctor right away.
- Liver problems, moderate or severe—Abacavir has not been studied in patient with liver problems, so it should not be used.
- Risk factors for liver disease such as:

- Being overweight or
- Taking other HIV medicines for long periods of time—Serious side effects could occur; caution should be used

Proper Use of This Medicine

Take this medicine exactly as directed by your doctor. Do not take it more often, and do not take it for a longer time than your doctor ordered.

Dosing—The dose of this medicine will be different for different patients. Follow your doctor's orders or the directions on the label. The following information includes only the average doses of this medicine. If your dose is different, do not change it unless your doctor tells you to do so.

The amount of medicine that you take depends on the strength of the medicine. Also, the number of doses you take each day, the time allowed between doses, and the length of time you take the medicine depend on the medical problem for which you are using the medicine.

- For oral dosage form (oral solution or tablets):
  - For HIV infection:
    - Adults and adolescents 16 years of age and older—300 milligrams (mg) two times a day or 600 mg once a day. This medicine can be taken with or without food.
    - Children 3 months to 16 years of age—Dose is based on body weight and must be determined by your doctor. The usual dose is 8 mg per kilogram (kg) (3.6 mg per pound) of body weight two times a day.

Missed dose—If you miss a dose of this medicine, take it as soon as possible. However, if it is almost time for your next dose, skip the missed dose and go back to your regular dosing schedule. Do not double doses.

Storage—Store the medicine in a closed container at room temperature, away from heat, moisture, and direct light. Keep from freezing.

Keep the bottle closed when you are not using it. Store it at room temperature, away from light and heat. Do not freeze.

Keep out of the reach of children.

Do not keep outdated medicine or medicine no longer needed.

Precautions While Using This Medicine

This medicine may cause a severe allergic reaction in some patients. This reaction usually occurs within 6 weeks after the medicine is started but may occur at any time. If untreated, it can lead to severe low blood pressure and even death. Stop taking this medicine and check with your doctor immediately if you notice sudden fever, skin rash, diarrhea, nausea, stomach pain, vomiting, or a feeling of unusual tiredness or illness, cough, shortness of breath, or sore throat.

When you begin taking this medicine, you will be given a warning card which describes symptoms of severe allergic reactions that may be caused by abacavir. The warning card also provides information about how to treat these allergic reactions. For your safety, you should carry the warning card with you at all times.

Side Effects of This Medicine

Along with its needed effects, a medicine may cause some unwanted effects. Although not all of these side effects may occur, if they do occur they may need medical attention.

Stop taking this medicine and get emergency help immediately if any of the following effects occur:

Less common

Abdominal or stomach pain; cough; diarrhea; difficult or labored breathing; fever; headache; joint or muscle pain; nausea; numbness or tingling of hands, feet, or face; redness and soreness of eyes; shortness of breath; skin rash; sore throat; sores in mouth; swelling of feet or lower legs; vomiting; unusual feeling of discomfort or illness; unusual tiredness

Incidence not known— occurred during clinical practice

Blistering, peeling, loosening of skin; chills; dark urine; itching; light-colored stools; red, irritated eyes; red skin lesions, often with a purple center; sores, ulcers or white spots in mouth or on lips; unusual weakness; upper right abdominal pain; yellow eyes and skin

Check with your doctor as soon as possible if any of the following side effects occur:

Rare

Abdominal swelling; decreased appetite; fast, shallow breathing; sleepiness

Some side effects may occur that usually do not need medical attention. These side effects may go away during treatment as your body adjusts to the medicine. Also, your health care professional may be able to tell you about ways to prevent or reduce some of these side effects. Check with your health care professional if any of the following side effects continue or are bothersome or if you have any questions about them:

More common

Headache

Less common

Trouble in sleeping

Incidence not known— occurred during clinical practice

Breast enlargement; buffalo hump; central obesity; facial wasting; peripheral wasting

Other side effects not listed may also occur in some patients. If you notice any other effects, check with your healthcare professional.

ABACAVIR AND LAMIVUDINE (Oral route) - a-BAK-a-veer, la-MI-vyoo-deen

Black Box Warning

Abacavir sulfate/lamivudine contains 2 nucleoside analogues (abacavir sulfate and lamivudine) and is intended only for patients whose regimen would otherwise include these 2 components.

Hypersensitivity Reactions: Serious and sometimes fatal hypersensitivity reactions have been associated with abacavir sulfate, a component of abacavir sulfate/lamivudine. Hypersensitivity to abacavir is a multi-organ clinical syndrome usually characterized by a sign or symptom in 2 or more of the following groups: fever, rash, gastrointestinal (including nausea, vomiting, diarrhea, or abdominal pain), constitutional (including generalized malaise, fatigue, or achiness) and respiratory (including dyspnea, cough, or pharyngitis). Discontinue abacavir sulfate/lamivudine as soon as a hypersensitivity reaction is suspected. Permanently discontinue abacavir sulfate/lamivudine if hypersensitivity cannot be ruled out, even when other diagnoses are possible.

Following a hypersensitivity reaction to abacavir, never restart abacavir sulfate/lamivudine or any other-abacavir containing product because more severe symptoms can occur within hours and may include life-threatening hypotension and death.

Reintroduction of abacavir sulfate/lamivudine or any other-abacavir containing product, even in patients who have no identified history or unrecognized symptoms of hypersensitivity to abacavir therapy, can result in serious or fatal hypersensitivity reactions. Such reactions can occur within hours.

Lactic Acidosis and Severe Hepatomegaly: Lactic acidosis and severe hepatomegaly with steatosis, including fatal cases, have been reported with the use of nucleoside analogues alone or in combination, including abacavir, lamivudine, and other antiretrovirals.

Exacerbations of Hepatitis B: Severe acute exacerbations of hepatitis B have been reported in patients who are co-infected with hepatitis B virus (HBV) and human immunodeficiency virus (HIV) and have discontinued lamivudine, which is one component of abacavir sulfate/lamivudine. Hepatic function should be monitored closely with both clinical and laboratory follow-up for at least several months in patients who discontinue abacavir sulfate/lamivudine and are co-infected with HIV and HBV. If appropriate, initiation of anti-hepatitis B therapy may be warranted.

Commonly used brand name(s)

In the U.S.—
   Epzicom

Available Dosage Forms:
- Tablet

Therapeutic Class: Antiretroviral Agent
Pharmacologic Class: Abacavir

Uses For This Medicine

Abacavir and lamivudine combination is used in the treatment of human immunodeficiency virus (HIV) infection. HIV is the virus that causes acquired immune deficiency syndrome (AIDS).

Abacavir, and lamivudine combination will not cure or prevent HIV infection or the symptoms of AIDS; however, it helps keep HIV from reproducing, and appears to slow down the destruction of the immune system. This may help delay the development of serious health problems usually related to AIDS or HIV infection. Abacavir and lamivudine combination will not keep you from spreading HIV to other people. People who receive this medicine may continue to have other problems usually related to AIDS or HIV infection.

This medicine is available only with your doctor's prescription.

Before Using This Medicine

In deciding to use a medicine, the risks of taking the medicine must be weighed against the good it will do. This is a decision you and your doctor will make. For this medicine, the following should be considered:

Allergies—Tell your doctor if you have ever had any unusual or allergic reaction to this medicine or any other medicines. Also tell your health care professional if you have any other types of allergies, such as to foods, dyes, preservatives, or animals. For non-prescription products, read the label or package ingredients carefully.

Pediatric—Studies on this medicine have been done only in adult patients, and there is no specific information comparing use of abacavir and lamivudine in children with the use in other age groups.

Geriatric—Many medicines have not been studied specifically in older people. Therefore, it may not be known whether they work exactly the same way they do in younger adults or if they cause different side effects or problems in older people. There is no specific information comparing use of abacavir in the elderly with use in other age groups.

Other medicines—

Using this medicine with any of the following medicines is usually not recommended, but may be required in some cases. If both medicines are prescribed together, your doctor may change the dose or how often you use one or both of the medicines.

Interferon Alfa, Ribavirin, Zalcitabine

Interactions with Food/Tobacco/Alcohol—Certain medicines should not be used at or around the time of eating food or eating certain types of food since interactions may occur. Using alcohol or tobacco with certain medicines may also cause interactions to occur. Discuss with your healthcare professional the use of your medicine with food, alcohol, or tobacco.

Other medical problems—The presence of other medical problems may affect the use of this medicine. Make sure you tell your doctor if you have any other medical problems, especially:
- Allergy to abacavir—You should tell your doctor immediately if you have signs of an allergic reaction. If you have ever taken abacavir in the past, you should tell your doctor right away.
- Kidney disease or
- Liver problems—Patients with kidney or liver disease may have more side effects
- Risk factors for liver disease such as:
- Being overweight or
- Taking other HIV medicines for long periods of time—Serious side effects could occur; caution should be used

---

Proper Use of This Medicine

Take this medicine exactly as directed by your doctor. Do not take it more often, and do not take it for a longer time than your doctor ordered.

Do not stop taking abacavir and lamivudine combination without checking with your doctor first.

Dosing—The dose of this medicine will be different for different patients. Follow your doctor's orders or the directions on the label. The following information includes only the average doses of this medicine. If your dose is different, do not change it unless your doctor tells you to do so.

The amount of medicine that you take depends on the strength of the medicine. Also, the number of doses you take each day, the time allowed between doses, and the length of time you take the medicine depend on the medical problem for which you are using the medicine.

This medicine works best when there is a constant amount in the blood. To help keep the amount constant, do not miss any doses. If you need help in planning the best times to take your medicine, check with your health care professional.

Only take medicine your doctor has prescribed for you. Do not share your medicine with others.

Abacavir and lamivudine combination contains a fixed amount of each medicine.

- For oral dosage form (tablets):
  - For HIV infection:
    - Adults—600 milligrams (mg) of abacavir, and 300 mg of lamivudine (equal to one tablet) once a day. This medicine can be taken with or without food.
    - Children—Use and dose must be determined by your doctor

Missed dose—If you miss a dose of this medicine, take it as soon as possible. However, if it is almost time for your next dose, skip the missed dose and go back to your regular dosing schedule. Do not double doses.

Storage—Store the medicine in a closed container at room temperature, away from heat, moisture, and direct light. Keep from freezing.

Keep out of the reach of children.

Do not keep outdated medicine or medicine no longer needed.

Precautions While Using This Medicine

It is very important that your doctor check your progress at regular visits. Abacavir and lamivudine combination may cause blood problems, and your doctor will want to test your blood regularly.

This medicine may cause a severe allergic reaction in some patients. This reaction usually occurs within 6 weeks after the medicine is started but may occur at any time. If untreated, it can lead to severe low blood pressure and even death. Stop taking this medicine and check with your doctor immediately if you notice sudden fever, skin rash, diarrhea, nausea, stomach pain, vomiting, or a feeling of unusual tiredness or illness, cough, shortness of breath, or sore throat.

When you begin taking this medicine, you will be given a warning card which describes symptoms of severe allergic reactions that may be caused by abacavir and lamivudine combination. The warning card also provides information about how to treat these allergic reactions. For your safety, you should carry the warning card with you at all times.

Side Effects of This Medicine

Along with its needed effects, a medicine may cause some unwanted effects. Although not all of these side effects may occur, if they do occur they may need medical attention.

Check with your doctor immediately if any of the following side effects occur:
  More common
  Hypersensitivity reaction, including abdominal or stomach pain; cough; diarrhea; fever; headache; nausea; numbness or tingling of face, feet, or hands; pain in joints; pain in muscles; shortness of breath; skin rash; sore throat; swelling of feet or lower legs; unusual feeling of discomfort or illness; unusual tiredness or weakness; or vomiting
  Incidence not known— occurred during clinical practice
  Blistering, peeling, loosening of skin; bloating; burning, numbness, tingling, or painful sensations; chest pain; chills; constipation; convulsions; dark urine; decreased appetite; diarrhea; difficulty swallowing; dizziness; fast heartbeat; fast, shallow breathing; feeling of fullness; general feeling of discomfort; hives or welts; indigestion; itching; light-colored stools; loss of appetite; loss of bladder control; muscle cramping; muscle spasm or jerking of all extremities; pains in stomach, side, or abdomen, possibly radiating to the back; pale skin; puffiness or swelling of the eyelids or around the eyes, face, lips or tongue; red irritated eyes; redness of skin; red skin lesions, often with a purple center; sleepiness; sores, ulcers, or white spots on lips or in mouth; sudden loss of consciousness; swollen, painful, or tender lymph glands in neck, armpit, or groin; tightness in chest; troubled breathing with exertion; unsteadiness or awkwardness; unusual bleeding or bruising; upper right abdominal pain; weakness in arms, hands, legs, or feet; wheezing; yellow eyes and skin

Some side effects may occur that usually do not need medical attention. These side effects may go away during treatment as your body adjusts to the medicine. Also, your health care professional may be able to tell you about ways to prevent or reduce some of these side effects. Check with your health care professional if any of the following side effects continue or are bothersome or if you have any questions about them:
  More common
  Abnormal dreams; burning feeling in chest or stomach; fear; feeling of constant movement of self or surroundings; lightheadedness; nervousness; sensation of spinning; severe and throbbing headache; sleeplessness; stomach upset; tenderness in stomach area; trouble sleeping; unable to sleep
  Incidence not known—occurred during clinical practice
  Abnormal breathing sounds; blurred vision; burning, crawling, itching, numbness, prickling, "pins and needles", or tingling feelings; dry mouth; dry skin; fruit-like breath odor; flushed; hair loss; increased hunger; increased thirst; increased urination; muscle weakness; redistribution/accumulation of body fat; sweating; swelling or inflammation of the mouth; thinning of hair; unexplained weight loss

Other side effects not listed may also occur in some patients. If you notice any other effects, check with your healthcare professional.

ABACAVIR, LAMIVUDINE, AND ZIDOVUDINE (Oral route) - a-BAK-a-veer, la-MI-vyoo-deen, zye-DOE-vyoo-deen

Black Box Warning

The three nucleoside analogues (abacavir sulfate/lamivudine/zidovudine) are intended only for patients whose regimen would otherwise include these 3 components.

Hypersensitivity reactions: Serious and sometimes fatal hypersensitivity reactions have been associated with abacavir sulfate. Hypersensitivity to abacavir is a multi-organ clinical syndrome usually characterized by a sign or symptom in 2 or more of the following groups: fever, rash, gastrointestinal (including nausea, vomiting, diarrhea, or abdominal pain), constitutional (including generalized malaise, fatigue, or achiness), and respiratory (including dyspnea, cough, or pharyngitis). Discontinue abacavir sulfate/lamivudine/zidovudine as soon as a hypersensitivity reaction is suspected. Permanently discontinue abacavir sulfate/lamivudine/zidovudine if hypersensitivity cannot be ruled out, even when other diagnoses are possible.

Following a hypersensitivity reaction to abacavir, never restart abacavir sulfate/lamivudine/zidovudine or any other abacavir-containing product because more severe symptoms can occur within hours and may include life-threatening hypotension and death.

Reintroduction of abacavir sulfate/lamivudine/zidovudine or any other abacavir-containing product, even in patients who have no identified history or unrecognized symptoms of hypersensitivity to abacavir therapy, can result in serious or fatal hypersensitivity reactions. Such reactions can occur within hours.

Hematologic toxicity: Zidovudine has been associated with hematologic toxicity including neutropenia and severe anemia, particularly in patients with advanced Human Immunodeficiency Virus (HIV) disease. Prolonged use of zidovudine has been associated with symptomatic myopathy.

Lactic acidosis and severe hepatomegaly: Lactic acidosis and severe hepatomegaly with steatosis, including fatal cases, have been reported with the use of nucleoside analogues alone or in combination, including abacavir, lamivudine, zidovudine, and other antiretrovirals.

Exacerbations of hepatitis B: Severe acute exacerbations of hepatitis B have been reported in patients who are co-infected with hepatitis B virus (HBV) and human immunodeficiency virus (HIV) and have discontinued lamivudine, which is one component of abacavir sulfate/lamivudine/zidovudine. Hepatic function should be monitored closely with both clinical and laboratory follow-up for at least several months in patients who discontinue abacavir sulfate/lamivudine/zidovudine and are co-infected with HIV and HBV. If appropriate, initiation of anti-hepatitis B therapy may be warranted.

Commonly used brand name(s)

In the U.S.—
Trizivir

Available Dosage Forms:
• Tablet

Therapeutic Class: Antiretroviral Agent
Pharmacologic Class: Abacavir

Uses For This Medicine

Abacavir, lamivudine, and zidovudine combination is used in the treatment of human immunodeficiency virus (HIV) infection. HIV is the virus that causes acquired immune deficiency syndrome (AIDS).

Abacavir, lamivudine, and zidovudine combination will not cure or prevent HIV infection or the symptoms of AIDS; however, it helps keep HIV from reproducing, and appears to slow down the destruction of the immune system. This may help delay the development of serious health problems usually related to AIDS or HIV infection. Abacavir, lamivudine, and zidovudine combination will not keep you from spreading HIV to other people. People who receive this medicine may continue to have other problems usually related to AIDS or HIV infection.

This medicine is available only with your doctor's prescription.

Before Using This Medicine

In deciding to use a medicine, the risks of taking the medicine must be weighed against the good it will do. This is a decision you and your doctor will make. For this medicine, the following should be considered:

Allergies—Tell your doctor if you have ever had any unusual or allergic reaction to this medicine or any other medicines. Also tell your health care professional if you have any other types of allergies, such as to foods, dyes, preservatives, or animals. For non-prescription products, read the label or package ingredients carefully.

Pediatric—Abacavir, lamivudine, and zidovudine combination contains a fixed amount of each medicine that cannot be decreased. Therefore, this medicine is not recommended for patients who weigh less than 40 kilograms (88 pounds) because the amounts of abacavir, lamivudine, and zidovudine in this product cannot be adjusted for smaller body sizes.

Geriatric—Many medicines have not been studied specifically in older people. Therefore, it may not be known whether they work exactly the same way they do in younger adults or if they cause different side effects or problems in older people. There is no specific information comparing use of abacavir, lamivudine, and zidovudine combination in the elderly with use in other age groups.

Other medicines—

Using this medicine with any of the following medicines is usually not recommended, but may be required in some cases. If both medicines are prescribed together, your doctor may change the dose or how often you use one or both of the medicines.

Dapsone, Doxorubicin Hydrochloride, Flucytosine, Ganciclovir, Interferon Alfa, Pyrazinamide, Pyrimethamine, Ribavirin, Stavudine, Vinblastine, Vincristine, Vincristine Liposome, Zalcitabine

Interactions with Food/Tobacco/Alcohol—Certain medicines should not be used at or around the time of eating food or eating certain types of food since interactions may occur. Using alcohol or tobacco with certain medicines may also cause interactions to occur. Discuss with your healthcare

professional the use of your medicine with food, alcohol, or tobacco.

Other medical problems—The presence of other medical problems may affect the use of this medicine. Make sure you tell your doctor if you have any other medical problems, especially:

- Blood problems, including anemia and decreased bone marrow production—Abacavir, lamivudine, and zidovudine combination may make these conditions worse

- Kidney disease or

- Liver disease—Patients with kidney or liver disease may have more side effects

Proper Use of This Medicine

Take this medicine exactly as directed by your doctor. Do not take more of it, do not take it more often, and do not take it for a longer time than your doctor ordered. Also, do not stop taking abacavir, lamivudine, and zidovudine combination without checking with your doctor first.

This medicine works best when there is a constant amount in the blood. To help keep the amount constant, do not miss any doses. If you need help in planning the best times to take your medicine, check with your health care professional.

Only take medicine that your doctor has prescribed specifically for you. Do not share your medicine with others.

Dosing—The dose of this medicine will be different for different patients. Follow your doctor's orders or the directions on the label. The following information includes only the average doses of this medicine. If your dose is different, do not change it unless your doctor tells you to do so.

The amount of medicine that you take depends on the strength of the medicine. Also, the number of doses you take each day, the time allowed between doses, and the length of time you take the medicine depend on the medical problem for which you are using the medicine.

Abacavir, lamivudine, and zidovudine combination contains a fixed amount of each medicine.

- For oral dosage form (tablets):

- For human immunodeficiency virus (HIV) infection:

- Adults, teenagers, and children who weigh more than 40 kilograms (kg) (88 pounds)—300 milligrams (mg) of abacavir, 150 mg of lamivudine, and 300 mg of zidovudine (equal to one tablet) two times a day.

- Adults, teenagers, and children who weigh 40 kg (88 pounds) or less—Use is not recommended.

Missed dose—If you miss a dose of this medicine, take it as soon as possible. However, if it is almost time for your next dose, skip the missed dose and go back to your regular dosing schedule. Do not double doses.

Storage—Store the medicine in a closed container at room temperature, away from heat, moisture, and direct light. Keep from freezing.

Keep out of the reach of children.

Do not keep outdated medicine or medicine no longer needed.

Precautions While Using This Medicine

It is very important that your doctor check your progress at regular visits. Abacavir, lamivudine, and zidovudine combination may cause blood problems, and your doctor will want to test your blood regularly.

This medicine may cause a severe allergic reaction in some patients. This reaction usually occurs within 6 weeks after the medicine is started but may occur at any time. If untreated, it can lead to severe low blood pressure and even death. Stop taking this medicine and check with your doctor immediately if you notice abdominal or stomach pain; cough; diarrhea; fever; headache; nausea; numbness or tingling of face, feet, or hands; pain in joints; pain in muscles; shortness of breath; skin rash; sore throat; swelling of feet or lower legs; unusual feeling of discomfort or illness; unusual tiredness or weakness; or vomiting.

When you begin taking this medicine, you will be given a warning card which describes symptoms of severe allergic reactions that may be caused by abacavir, lamivudine, and zidovudine combination. The warning card also provides information about how to treat these allergic reactions. For your safety, you should carry the warning card with you at all times.

Side Effects of This Medicine

Along with its needed effects, a medicine may cause some unwanted effects. Although not all of these side effects may occur, if they do occur they may need medical attention.

Stop taking this medicine and get emergency help immediately if any of the following effects occur:

Less common
Hypersensitivity reaction, including abdominal or stomach pain; cough; diarrhea; fever; headache; nausea; numbness or tingling of face, feet, or hands; pain in joints; pain in muscles; shortness of breath; skin rash; sore throat; swelling of feet or lower legs; unusual feeling of discomfort or illness; unusual tiredness or weakness; or vomiting

Check with your doctor as soon as possible if any of the following side effects occur:

More common
Chills

Less common
Muscle weakness; pale skin; yellow eyes or skin

Rare
Black tarry stools; blood in urine or stools; pinpoint red spots on skin; unusual bleeding or bruising

Some side effects may occur that usually do not need medical attention. These side effects may go away during treatment as your body adjusts to the medicine. Also, your health care professional may be able to tell you about ways to prevent or reduce some of these side effects. Check with your health care professional if any of the following side effects continue or are bothersome or if you have any questions about them:

More common
Bone pain; loss of appetite; sleeplessness; trouble sleeping

Other side effects not listed may also occur in some patients. If you notice any other effects, check with your healthcare professional.

ABARELIX (Intramuscular route) - a-ba-REL-iks

Black Box Warning

Immediate-onset systemic allergic reactions, some resulting in hypotension and syncope, have occurred after administration of abarelix. These immediate-onset reactions have been reported to occur following any administration of abarelix, including after the initial dose. The cumulative risk of such a reaction increases with the duration of treatment. Following each injection of abarelix, patients should be observed for at least 30 minutes in the office and in the event of an allergic reaction, managed appropriately.

Abarelix is indicated for the palliative treatment of men with advanced symptomatic prostate cancer, in whom LHRH agonist therapy is not appropriate and who refuse surgical castration, and have one or more of the following: (1) risk of neurological compromise due to metastases, (2) ureteral or bladder outlet obstruction due to local encroachment or metastatic disease, or (3) severe bone pain from skeletal metastases persisting on narcotic analgesia.

The effectiveness of abarelix in suppressing serum testosterone to castrate levels decreases with continued dosing in some patients. Effectiveness beyond 12 months has not been established. Treatment failure can be detected by measuring serum total testosterone concentrations just prior to administration on Day 29 and every 8 weeks thereafter.

- PLENAXIS®
  - Only physicians who have enrolled in the Plenaxis® PLUS Program (Plenaxis® User Safety Program), based on their attestation of qualifications and acceptance of prescribing responsibilities, may prescribe Plenaxis®.

Commonly used brand name(s)

In the U.S.—
Plenaxis

Available Dosage Forms:

- Powder for Suspension

Therapeutic Class: Antineoplastic Agent
Pharmacologic Class: Luteinizing Hormone Releasing Hormone Antagonist

Uses For This Medicine

Abarelix is a type of medicine called a gonadotropin-releasing hormone (GnRH) antagonist that lowers the male hormone testosterone in your blood. Testosterone makes most prostate cancers grow. Other ways to treat your prostate cancer are taking other hormone medicines to lower testosterone or surgery to remove your testicles. Abarelix is used when these other ways to treat prostate cancer cannot be used or are refused.

Abarelix is to be given only under the supervision of your doctor. It is to be injected into your buttocks.

Before Using This Medicine

In deciding to use a medicine, the risks of taking the medicine must be weighed against the good it will do. This is a decision you and your doctor will make. For this medicine, the following should be considered:

It is very important that you read the Patient Information for abarelix before you start getting injections. You will need to sign the last page if you agree with treatment with abarelix. If you have any questions about this ask your doctor.

Allergies—Tell your doctor if you have ever had any unusual or allergic reaction to this medicine or any other medicines. Also tell your health care professional if you have any other types of allergies, such as to foods, dyes, preservatives, or animals. For non-prescription products, read the label or package ingredients carefully.

Pediatric—Studies on this medicine have only been done in adult patients, and there is no specific information comparing the use of abarelix in children with other age groups. Abarelix is not for use in children.

Geriatric—This medicine has been tested and has not been shown to cause different side effects or problems in older people than it does in younger adults.

Pregnancy—

	Pregnancy Category	Explanation
All Trimesters	X	Studies in animals or pregnant women have demonstrated positive evidence of fetal abnormalities. This drug should not be used in women who are or may become pregnant because the risk clearly outweighs any possible benefit.

Breast Feeding—There are no adequate studies in women for determining infant risk when using this medication during breastfeeding. Weigh the potential benefits against the potential risks before taking this medication while breastfeeding.

Other medicines—

Using this medicine with any of the following medicines may cause an increased risk of certain side effects, but using both drugs may be the best treatment for you. If both medicines are prescribed together, your doctor may change the dose or how often you use one or both of the medicines.

Amiodarone, Quinidine, Sotalol

Interactions with Food/Tobacco/Alcohol—Certain medicines should not be used at or around the time of eating food or eating certain types of food since interactions may occur. Using alcohol or tobacco with certain medicines may also cause interactions to occur. Discuss with your healthcare professional the use of your medicine with food, alcohol, or tobacco.

Other medical problems—The presence of other medical problems may affect the use of this medicine. Make sure you tell your doctor if you have any other medical problems, especially:

- Osteoporosis—May be worsened by this medicine.
- QT prolongation (rare heart condition)—May be worsened by abarelix

Proper Use of This Medicine

Abarelix is only prescribed by doctors who are part of Plenaxis PLUS Program (Plenaxis User Safety Program) that is run by the pharmaceutical (drug) company that makes the medicine.

Abarelix is given as an injection (shot) in your buttocks. Your doctor or nurse will give you the injection. It is important that you keep your appointment with your doctor's office when your injection is due. If you are unable to keep your appointment, contact your doctor's office to be rescheduled as soon as possible. It is very important that you follow the schedule that your doctor planned for your treatment.

You must always wait in your doctor's office for at least 30 minutes after getting each abarelix injection (shot). If a serious or life-threatening allergic reaction happens it is usually soon after getting an abarelix injection. Tell your doctor right away if you feel warm, faint or lightheaded or if you have chest tightness, shortness of breath, redness of your skin, or swelling of your face, eyelids, tongue, or throat. These could be signs of an allergic reaction.

Abarelix is only used for treating advanced symptomatic prostate cancer when a patient cannot have or refuses other treatments for prostate cancer

Dosing—The dose of this medicine will be different for different patients. Follow your doctor's orders or the directions on the label. The following information includes only the average doses of this medicine. If your dose is different, do not change it unless your doctor tells you to do so.

The amount of medicine that you take depends on the strength of the medicine. Also, the number of doses you take each day, the time allowed between doses, and the length of time you take the medicine depend on the medical problem for which you are using the medicine.

- For parenteral dosage form (injection):
  - For advanced prostate cancer:
    - Adults—100 milligrams (mg) in the muscle (buttock) on Day 1, 15, 29 (week 4) and every 4 weeks thereafter.

Precautions While Using This Medicine

It is very important that your doctor check you at regular visits. Your doctor will also want to do regular blood tests about every 8 weeks to check your testosterone level to see if abarelix is working for you. If you weigh more than 225 pounds there may be a greater chance that abarelix may stop working. Your doctor may also want to do blood tests to check your liver function before and during treatment with abarelix.

This medicine may cause loss in bone mineral density with extended treatment. Loss in bone mineral density can lead to the thinning of bones (osteoporosis). If you have any questions about this ask your doctor.

This medicine can cause a change in heart rhythm called prolongation of the QTc interval. This condition may change the way your heart beats and can cause fainting and serious side effects in some patients. Contact your doctor right away if you have any of these symptoms or any questions about this.

Side Effects of This Medicine

Along with its needed effects, a medicine may cause some unwanted effects. Although not all of these side effects may occur, if they do occur they may need medical attention.

Check with your doctor immediately if any of the following side effects occur:
> *Less common*
>> Fainting or loss of consciousness; fast or irregular breathing; itching; skin rash; swelling of eyes or eyelids; tightness in chest and/or wheezing; trouble in breathing

Some side effects may occur that usually do not need medical attention. These side effects may go away during treatment as your body adjusts to the medicine. Also, your health care professional may be able to tell you about ways to prevent or reduce some of these side effects. Check with your health care professional if any of the following side effects continue or are bothersome or if you have any questions about them:
> *More common*
>> Back pain; bladder pain; breast enlargement; breast pain; bloating or swelling of face, arms, hands, lower legs, or feet; bloody or cloudy urine; body aches or pain; burning while urinating; chills; cough; decrease in frequency of urination; decrease in urine volume; diarrhea; difficult, burning, or painful urination; difficulty having a bowel movement (stool); difficulty in passing urine [dribbling]; dizziness; ear congestion; feeling of warmth; fever; frequent urge to urinate; headache; loss of voice; lower back or side pain; nasal congestion; nausea; pain; rapid weight gain; nipple enlargement; redness of the face, neck, arms and occasionally upper chest; runny nose; sneezing; sore throat; sweating; tingling of hands or feet; trouble in holding or releasing urine; trouble in sleeping; unusual tiredness or weakness; unusual weight gain or loss

Other side effects not listed may also occur in some patients. If you notice any other effects, check with your healthcare professional.

ACAMPROSATE   (Oral route) - a-kam-PRO-sate

Commonly used brand name(s)

In the U.S.—
Campral

Available Dosage Forms:
- Tablet, Enteric Coated

Therapeutic Class: Ethanol Dependency

Uses For This Medicine

Acamprosate is used to help overcome your drinking problem. It is not a cure for alcoholism, but rather will help you maintain abstinence.

This medicine is available only with your doctor's prescription.

Before Using This Medicine

In deciding to use a medicine, the risks of taking the medicine must be weighed against the good it will do. This is a decision

you and your doctor will make. For this medicine, the following should be considered:

Allergies—Tell your doctor if you have ever had any unusual or allergic reaction to this medicine or any other medicines. Also tell your health care professional if you have any other types of allergies, such as to foods, dyes, preservatives, or animals. For non-prescription products, read the label or package ingredients carefully.

Pediatric—Safety and efficacy in pediatric patients have not been established.

Geriatric—This medicine has been tested and has not been shown to cause different side effects or problems in older people than it does in younger adults.

Pregnancy—

	Pregnancy Category	Explanation
All Trimesters	C	Animal studies have shown an adverse effect and there are no adequate studies in pregnant women OR no animal studies have been conducted and there are no adequate studies in pregnant women.

Breast Feeding—There are no adequate studies in women for determining infant risk when using this medication during breastfeeding. Weigh the potential benefits against the potential risks before taking this medication while breastfeeding.

Other medicines—Although certain medicines should not be used together at all, in other cases two different medicines may be used together even if an interaction might occur. In these cases, your doctor may want to change the dose, or other precautions may be necessary. Tell your healthcare professional if you are taking any other prescription or non-prescription (over-the-counter [OTC]) medicine.

Interactions with Food/Tobacco/Alcohol—Certain medicines should not be used at or around the time of eating food or eating certain types of food since interactions may occur. Using alcohol or tobacco with certain medicines may also cause interactions to occur. Discuss with your healthcare professional the use of your medicine with food, alcohol, or tobacco.

Other medical problems—The presence of other medical problems may affect the use of this medicine. Make sure you tell your doctor if you have any other medical problems, especially:

- Kidney disease (severe)—Acamprosate is not recommended; serious side effects could occur
- Depression or
- Suicidal thinking—Acamprosate may make the condition worse

Proper Use of This Medicine

Beginning treatment as soon as possible after the period of alcohol withdrawal, and after you have achieved abstinence.

Using acamprosate as part of a treatment program that includes counseling and support.

Continuing acamprosate therapy, even in the event of a relapse.

In addition to beverages, alcohol is found in many other products. Reading the list of ingredients on foods and other products before using them will help you to avoid alcohol. Do not use alcohol-containing foods such as sauces and vinegars.

Dosing—The dose of this medicine will be different for different patients. Follow your doctor's orders or the directions on the label. The following information includes only the average doses of this medicine. If your dose is different, do not change it unless your doctor tells you to do so.

The amount of medicine that you take depends on the strength of the medicine. Also, the number of doses you take each day, the time allowed between doses, and the length of time you take the medicine depend on the medical problem for which you are using the medicine.

- For oral dosage form (tablets):
  - To help overcome drinking problems:
    - Adults—Two tablets (666 mg per dose) taken three times daily.
    - Children—Use and dose must be determined by your doctor.

Missed dose—If you miss a dose of this medicine, take it as soon as possible. However, if it is almost time for your next dose, skip the missed dose and go back to your regular dosing schedule. Do not double doses.

Storage—Store the medicine in a closed container at room temperature, away from heat, moisture, and direct light. Keep from freezing.

Keep out of the reach of children.

Do not keep outdated medicine or medicine no longer needed.

Precautions While Using This Medicine

If you will be taking this medicine for a long time, it is very important that your doctor check you at regular visits

This medicine may cause some people to become drowsy, dizzy, or less alert than they are normally. Make sure you know how you react to this medicine before you drive, use machines, or do anything else that could be dangerous if you are dizzy or are not alert.

Side Effects of This Medicine

Along with its needed effects, a medicine may cause some unwanted effects. Although not all of these side effects may occur, if they do occur they may need medical attention.

Check with your doctor immediately if any of the following side effects occur:

More common

Agitation; coma; confusion; decreased urine output; depression; dizziness; headache; hostility; irritability; lethargy; muscle twitching; nausea; rapid weight gain; seizures; stupor; swelling of face, ankles, or hands; unusual tiredness or weakness

Symptoms of overdose

Get emergency help immediately if any of the following symptoms of overdose occur:

Abdominal pain; confusion; constipation; depression; diarrhea; dry mouth; headache; incoherent speech; increased urination; loss of appetite; metallic taste; muscle weakness; nausea; thirst; unusual tiredness; vomiting; weight loss

Some side effects may occur that usually do not need medical attention. These side effects may go away during treatment as your body adjusts to the medicine. Also, your health care professional may be able to tell you about ways to prevent or reduce some of these side effects. Check with your health care professional if any of the following side effects continue or are bothersome or if you have any questions about them:

More common

Discouragement; feeling sad or empty; irritability; lack of appetite; loss of interest or pleasure; tiredness; trouble concentrating; trouble sleeping; diarrhea; sleeplessness; trouble sleeping; unable to sleep

Less common

Accidental injury; pain; loss of appetite; weight loss; fear; nervousness; dry mouth; bloated full feeling; excess air or gas in stomach or intestines; passing gas; burning, crawling, itching, numbness, prickling, "pins and needles", or tingling feelings; itching skin; sweating

Other side effects not listed may also occur in some patients. If you notice any other effects, check with your healthcare professional.

ACARBOSE   (Oral route) - AY-kar-bose

Commonly used brand name(s)

In the U.S.—
    Precose

Available Dosage Forms:
  • Tablet

Therapeutic Class: Antidiabetic
Pharmacologic Class: Alpha-Glucosidase Inhibitor

Uses For This Medicine

Acarbose is used to treat type 2 diabetes. Normally, your pancreas releases insulin into the blood stream after you eat. Insulin is used by all the cells in your body to help turn the food you eat into energy. This is done by using glucose (sugar) in the blood as quick energy. When you have type 2 diabetes, insulin is still produced by your pancreas, but the amount of insulin produced may not be enough or your body may not be using it properly and you may still need more. Because of this, the insulin is not able to lower your blood sugar properly and you will have too much sugar in your blood. Acarbose lowers your blood sugar by preventing the breakdown of starch into sugar. It may be used alone or in combination with another type of oral diabetes medicine called a sulfonylurea.

This medicine is available only with your doctor's prescription.

Before Using This Medicine

In deciding to use a medicine, the risks of taking the medicine must be weighed against the good it will do. This is a decision you and your doctor will make. For this medicine, the following should be considered:

Allergies—Tell your doctor if you have ever had any unusual or allergic reaction to this medicine or any other medicines. Also tell your health care professional if you have any other types of allergies, such as to foods, dyes, preservatives, or animals. For non-prescription products, read the label or package ingredients carefully.

Pediatric—Studies on this medicine have been done only in adult patients, and there is no specific information comparing use of acarbose in children with use in other age groups.

Geriatric—This medicine has been tested in a limited number of elderly people and has not been shown to cause different side effects or problems in older people than it does in younger adults.

Pregnancy—

	Pregnancy Category	Explanation
All Trimesters	B	Animal studies have revealed no evidence of harm to the fetus, however, there are no adequate studies in pregnant women OR animal studies have shown an adverse effect, but adequate studies in pregnant women have failed to demonstrate a risk to the fetus.

Breast Feeding—There are no adequate studies in women for determining infant risk when using this medication during breastfeeding. Weigh the potential benefits against the potential risks before taking this medication while breastfeeding.

Other medicines—

Using this medicine with any of the following medicines is usually not recommended, but may be required in some cases. If both medicines are prescribed together, your doctor may change the dose or how often you use one or both of the medicines.

Acetohexamide, Alatrofloxacin, Balofloxacin, Chlorpropamide, Ciprofloxacin, Clinafloxacin, Enoxacin, Fleroxacin, Flumequine, Gatifloxacin, Gemifloxacin, Gliclazide, Glipizide, Glyburide, Grepafloxacin, Levofloxacin, Lomefloxacin, Moxifloxacin, Norfloxacin, Ofloxacin, Pefloxacin, Pruliflaxacin, Rufloxacin, Sparfloxacin, Temafloxacin, Tolazamide, Tolbutamide, Tosufloxacin, Trovafloxacin Mesylate

Interactions with Food/Tobacco/Alcohol—Certain medicines should not be used at or around the time of eating food or eating certain types of food since interactions may occur. Using alcohol or tobacco with certain medicines may also cause interactions to occur. Discuss with your healthcare professional the use of your medicine with food, alcohol, or tobacco.

Other medical problems—The presence of other medical problems may affect the use of this medicine. Make sure you tell your doctor if you have any other medical problems, especially:

  • Diabetic ketoacidosis or

  • Fever or

  • Infection or

- Surgery or
- Trauma—Insulin is needed to control these conditions
- Digestion problems or
- Inflammatory bowel disease or
- Intestinal blockage or
- Other intestinal problems—Acarbose should not be used
- Kidney disease (severe)—Higher blood levels of acarbose may occur; acarbose should not be used
- Liver disease—Acarbose may make this condition worse

Proper Use of This Medicine

Follow carefully the special meal plan your doctor gave you. This is the most important part of controlling your condition, and is necessary if the medicine is to work properly. Also, exercise regularly and test for sugar in your blood or urine as directed.

For this medicine to work properly it must be taken at the beginning of each main meal.

Dosing—The dose of this medicine will be different for different patients. Follow your doctor's orders or the directions on the label. The following information includes only the average doses of this medicine. If your dose is different, do not change it unless your doctor tells you to do so.

The amount of medicine that you take depends on the strength of the medicine. Also, the number of doses you take each day, the time allowed between doses, and the length of time you take the medicine depend on the medical problem for which you are using the medicine.

- For oral dosage form (tablets):
  - For type 2 diabetes:
    - Adults—At first the dose is 25 milligrams (mg) three times a day, at the start of each main meal. Your dose may then be adjusted by your doctor.
    - Children—Use and dose must be determined by your doctor.

Missed dose—If you miss a dose of this medicine, skip the missed dose and go back to your regular dosing schedule. Do not double doses.

If you finish a meal and you have forgotten to take the medicine, do not take the missed dose. Instead, take the next dose at the beginning of your next meal, as scheduled.

Storage—Store the medicine in a closed container at room temperature, away from heat, moisture, and direct light. Keep from freezing.

Keep out of the reach of children.

Do not keep outdated medicine or medicine no longer needed.

Precautions While Using This Medicine

Your doctor will want to check your progress at regular visits, especially during the first few weeks you take this medicine.

It is very important to follow carefully any instructions from your health care team about:
- Alcohol—Drinking alcohol may cause severe low blood sugar. Discuss this with your health care team.

- Other medicines—Do not take other medicines during the time you are taking acarbose unless they have been discussed with your doctor. This especially includes non-prescription medicines such as aspirin, and medicines for appetite control, asthma, colds, cough, hay fever, or sinus problems.
- Counseling—Other family members need to learn how to prevent side effects or help with side effects if they occur. Also, patients with diabetes may need special counseling about diabetes medicine dosing changes that might occur because of lifestyle changes, such as changes in exercise and diet. Furthermore, counseling on contraception and pregnancy may be needed because of the problems that can occur in patients with diabetes during pregnancy.
- Travel—Keep a recent prescription and your medical history with you. Be prepared for an emergency as you would normally. Make allowances for changing time zones and keep your meal times as close as possible to your usual meal times.

In case of emergency—There may be a time when you need emergency help for a problem caused by your diabetes. You need to be prepared for these emergencies. It is a good idea to wear a medical identification (ID) bracelet or neck chain at all times. Also, carry an ID card in your wallet or purse that says that you have diabetes and a list of all of your medicines.

Acarbose does not cause hypoglycemia (low blood sugar). However, low blood sugar can occur if you take acarbose with another type of diabetes medicine, delay or miss a meal or snack, exercise more than usual, drink alcohol, or cannot eat because of nausea or vomiting. Symptoms of low blood sugar must be treated before they lead to unconsciousness (passing out). Different people may feel different symptoms of low blood sugar. It is important that you learn which symptoms of low blood sugar you usually have so that you can treat it quickly.

Symptoms of low blood sugar include anxiety; behavior change similar to being drunk; blurred vision; cold sweats; confusion; cool, pale skin; difficulty in thinking; drowsiness; excessive hunger; fast heartbeat; headache (continuing); nausea; nervousness; nightmares; restless sleep; shakiness; slurred speech; or unusual tiredness or weakness.

If symptoms of low blood sugar occur, eat glucose tablets or gel or honey, or drink fruit juice to relieve the symptoms. Table sugar (sucrose) or regular (nondiet) soft drinks will not work. Also, check your blood for low blood sugar. Glucagon is used in emergency situations when severe symptoms such as seizures (convulsions) or unconsciousness occur. Have a glucagon kit available, along with a syringe and needle, and know how to use it. Members of your household also should know how to use it.

Hyperglycemia (high blood sugar) may occur if you do not take enough or skip a dose of your antidiabetic medicine, overeat or do not follow your meal plan, have a fever or infection, or do not exercise as much as usual.

Symptoms of high blood sugar include blurred vision; drowsiness; dry mouth; flushed, dry skin; fruit-like breath odor; increased urination; ketones in urine; loss of appetite; stomachache, nausea, or vomiting; tiredness; troubled breathing (rapid and deep); unconsciousness; or unusual thirst.

If symptoms of high blood sugar occur, check your blood sugar level and then call your doctor for instructions.

Side Effects of This Medicine

Along with its needed effects, a medicine may cause some unwanted effects. Although not all of these side effects may occur, if they do occur they may need medical attention.

Check with your doctor as soon as possible if any of the following side effects occur:

Rare

Yellow eyes or skin

Some side effects may occur that usually do not need medical attention. These side effects may go away during treatment as your body adjusts to the medicine. Also, your health care professional may be able to tell you about ways to prevent or reduce some of these side effects. Check with your health care professional if any of the following side effects continue or are bothersome or if you have any questions about them:

More common

Abdominal or stomach pain; bloated feeling or passing of gas; diarrhea

Other side effects not listed may also occur in some patients. If you notice any other effects, check with your healthcare professional.

ACETAMINOPHEN (Oral route, Rectal route) - a-seet-a-MIN-oh-fen

Commonly used brand name(s)

In the U.S.—

Actamin Maximum Strength	Children's Nortemp
Altenol	Comtrex Sore Throat Relief
Aminofen	Dolono
Anacin Aspirin Free	Feverall
Apra	Genapap
Cetafen	Tylenol

In Canada—

Abenol	Children's Acetaminophen
Acetaminophen	Grape Flavor
Actimol Children's	Children's Acetaminophen
Actimol Infant	Suspension Bubble Gum
Atasol	Flavor - Ages 2 To 11
Children's Acetaminophen	Children's Acetaminophen
Children's Acetaminophen	Suspension Cherry Flavor
Bubble Gum Flavor	Children's Acetaminophen
Children's Acetaminophen	Suspension Grape Flavor -
Cherry Flavor	Ages 2 To 11

Available Dosage Forms:

- Tablet, Chewable
- Suppository
- Liquid
- Capsule
- Syrup
- Tablet, Extended Release
- Solution
- Tablet
- Suspension
- Elixir
- Powder for Solution

Therapeutic Class: Analgesic

Uses For This Medicine

Acetaminophen is used to relieve pain and reduce fever. Unlike aspirin, it does not relieve the redness, stiffness, or swelling caused by rheumatoid arthritis. However, it may relieve the pain caused by mild forms of arthritis.

This medicine is available without a prescription.

Before Using This Medicine

In deciding to use a medicine, the risks of taking the medicine must be weighed against the good it will do. This is a decision you and your doctor will make. For this medicine, the following should be considered:

Allergies—Tell your doctor if you have ever had any unusual or allergic reaction to this medicine or any other medicines. Also tell your health care professional if you have any other types of allergies, such as to foods, dyes, preservatives, or animals. For non-prescription products, read the label or package ingredients carefully.

Pediatric—This medicine has been tested in children and has not been shown to cause different side effects or problems than it does in adults. However, some children's products containing acetaminophen also contain aspartame, which may be dangerous if it is given to children with phenylketonuria.

Geriatric—Acetaminophen has been tested and has not been shown to cause different side effects or problems in older people than it does in younger adults.

Breast Feeding—There are no adequate studies in women for determining infant risk when using this medication during breastfeeding. Weigh the potential benefits against the potential risks before taking this medication while breastfeeding.

Other medicines—

Using this medicine with any of the following medicines may cause an increased risk of certain side effects, but using both drugs may be the best treatment for you. If both medicines are prescribed together, your doctor may change the dose or how often you use one or both of the medicines.

Acenocoumarol, Carbamazepine, Isoniazid, Phenytoin, Warfarin, Zidovudine

Interactions with Food/Tobacco/Alcohol—Certain medicines should not be used at or around the time of eating food or eating certain types of food since interactions may occur. Using alcohol or tobacco with certain medicines may also cause interactions to occur. The following interactions have been selected on the basis of their potential significance and are not necessarily all-inclusive.

Using this medicine with any of the following is usually not recommended, but may be unavoidable in some cases. If used together, your doctor may change the dose or how often you use this medicine, or give you special instructions about the use of food, alcohol, or tobacco.

Ethanol

Using this medicine with any of the following may cause an increased risk of certain side effects but may be unavoidable in some cases. If used together, your doctor may change the dose or how often you use this medicine, or give you special instructions about the use of food, alcohol, or tobacco.

Cabbage

Other medical problems—The presence of other medical problems may affect the use of this medicine. Make sure you tell your doctor if you have any other medical problems, especially:

- Alcohol abuse or
- Kidney disease (severe) or
- Hepatitis or other liver disease—The chance of serious side effects may be increased
- Phenylketonuria—Some brands of acetaminophen contain aspartame, which can make your condition worse

Proper Use of This Medicine

Unless otherwise directed by your medical doctor or dentist:

- Do not take more of this medicine than is recommended on the package label. If too much is taken, liver and kidney damage may occur.
- Children up to 12 years of age should not take this medicine more than 5 times a day.

To use acetaminophen oral granules (e.g., Snaplets-FR):

- Just before the medicine is to be taken, open the number of packets needed for one dose. Mix the granules inside of the packets with a small amount of soft food, such as applesauce, ice cream, or jam. Eat the acetaminophen granules along with the food.

To use acetaminophen oral powders (e.g., Feverall Sprinkle Caps [Children's or Junior Strength]):

- These capsules are not intended to be swallowed whole. Instead, just before the medicine is to be taken, open the number of capsules needed for one dose. Empty the powder from each capsule into 1 teaspoonful of water or other liquid. Drink the medicine along with the liquid. You may drink more liquid after taking the medicine. You may also mix the powder with a small amount of soft food, such as applesauce, ice cream, or jam. Eat the acetaminophen powder along with the food.

For patients using acetaminophen suppositories:

- If the suppository is too soft to insert, chill it in the refrigerator for 30 minutes or run cold water over it before removing the foil wrapper.
- To insert the suppository:
  - First remove the foil wrapper and moisten the suppository with cold water. Lie down on your side and use your finger to push the suppository well up into the rectum.

Dosing—The dose of this medicine will be different for different patients. Follow your doctor's orders or the directions on the label. The following information includes only the average doses of this medicine. If your dose is different, do not change it unless your doctor tells you to do so.

The amount of medicine that you take depends on the strength of the medicine. Also, the number of doses you take each day, the time allowed between doses, and the length of time you take the medicine depend on the medical problem for which you are using the medicine.

- For oral dosage forms (capsules, granules, powders, solution, suspension, or tablets) and rectal dosage forms (suppositories):
  - For pain or fever:
    - Adults and teenagers—325 or 500 milligrams (mg) every three or four hours, 650 mg every four to six hours, or 1000 mg every six hours as needed. The total dose should not be more than 4000 mg (for example, eight 500-mg tablets) a day.
  - Children—Acetaminophen dose is based on the child's age.
    - Infants up to 3 months of age: 40 mg every four hours as needed.
    - Infants 4 to 12 months of age: 80 mg every four hours as needed.
    - Children 1 to 2 years of age: 120 mg every four hours as needed.
    - Children 2 to 4 years of age: 160 mg every four hours as needed.
    - Children 4 to 6 years of age: 240 mg every four hours as needed.
    - Children 6 to 9 years of age: 320 mg every four hours as needed.
    - Children 9 to 11 years of age: 320 to 400 mg every four hours as needed.
    - Children 11 to 12 years of age: 320 to 480 mg every four hours as needed.

Storage—Store the medicine in a closed container at room temperature, away from heat, moisture, and direct light. Keep from freezing.

Keep the bottle closed when you are not using it. Store it at room temperature, away from light and heat. Do not freeze.

You may store the suppositories in the refrigerator, but do not freeze them.

Keep out of the reach of children.

Do not keep outdated medicine or medicine no longer needed.

Precautions While Using This Medicine

Check with your medical doctor or dentist:

- If you are taking this medicine to relieve pain, including arthritis pain, and the pain lasts for more than 10 days for adults or 5 days for children or if the pain gets worse, new symptoms occur, or the painful area is red or swollen. These could be signs of a serious condition that needs medical or dental treatment.
- If you are taking this medicine to bring down a fever, and the fever lasts for more than 3 days or returns, the fever gets worse, new symptoms occur, or redness or swelling is present. These could be signs of a serious condition that needs treatment.
- If you are taking this medicine for a sore throat, and the sore throat is very painful, lasts for more than 2 days, or occurs together with or is followed by fever, headache, skin rash, nausea, or vomiting.

Check the labels of all prescription and nonprescription (over-the-counter [OTC]) medicines you now take. If any contain acetaminophen, check with your health care professional. Taking them together with this medicine may cause an overdose.

If you will be taking more than an occasional 1 or 2 doses of acetaminophen, do not drink alcoholic beverages. To do so may increase the chance of liver damage, especially if you drink large amounts of alcoholic beverages regularly, if you take more acetaminophen than is recommended on the package label, or if you take it regularly for a long time.

Taking certain other medicines together with acetaminophen may increase the chance of unwanted effects. The risk will depend on how much of each medicine you take every day, and on how long you take the medicines together. If your medical doctor or dentist directs you to take these medicines together on a regular basis, follow his or her directions carefully. However, do not take any of the following medicines together with acetaminophen for more than a few days unless your doctor has directed you to do so and is following your progress:

- Aspirin or other salicylates
- Diclofenac (e.g., Voltaren)
- Diflunisal (e.g., Dolobid)
- Etodolac (e.g., Lodine)
- Fenoprofen (e.g., Nalfon)
- Floctafenine (e.g., Idarac)
- Flurbiprofen, oral (e.g., Ansaid)
- Ibuprofen (e.g., Motrin)
- Indomethacin (e.g., Indocin)
- Ketoprofen (e.g., Orudis)
- Ketorolac (e.g., Toradol)
- Meclofenamate (e.g., Meclomen)
- Mefenamic acid (e.g., Ponstel)
- Nabumetone (e.g., Relafen)
- Naproxen (e.g., Naprosyn)
- Oxaprozin (e.g., Daypro)
- Phenylbutazone (e.g., Butazolidin)
- Piroxicam (e.g., Feldene)
- Sulindac (e.g., Clinoril)
- Tenoxicam (e.g., Apo-Tenoxicam)
- Tiaprofenic acid (e.g., Surgam)
- Tolmetin (e.g., Tolectin)

Acetaminophen may interfere with the results of some medical tests. Before you have any medical tests, tell the person in charge if you have taken acetaminophen within the past 3 or 4 days. If possible, it is best to call the laboratory where the test will be done about 4 days ahead of time, to find out whether this medicine may be taken during the 3 or 4 days before the test.

For diabetic patients:

- Acetaminophen may cause false results with some blood glucose (sugar) tests. If you notice any change in your test results, or if you have any questions about this possible problem, check with your health care professional. This is especially important if your diabetes is not well-controlled.

For patients taking one of the products that contain caffeine in addition to acetaminophen:

- Caffeine may interfere with the results of a test that uses adenosine (e.g., Adenocard) or dipyridamole (e.g., Persantine) to help find out how well your blood is flowing through certain blood vessels. Therefore, you should not have any caffeine for 8 to 12 hours before the test.

If you think that you or anyone else may have taken an overdose of acetaminophen, get emergency help at once, even if there are no signs of poisoning. Signs of severe poisoning may not appear for 2 to 4 days after the overdose is taken, but treatment to prevent liver damage or death must be started as soon as possible. Treatment started more than 24 hours after the overdose is taken may not be effective.

Side Effects of This Medicine

Along with its needed effects, a medicine may cause some unwanted effects. Although not all of these side effects may occur, if they do occur they may need medical attention.

Check with your doctor immediately if any of the following side effects occur:

Rare
   Yellow eyes or skin

Symptoms of overdose
   Diarrhea; increased sweating; loss of appetite; nausea or vomiting; stomach cramps or pain; swelling, pain, or tenderness in the upper abdomen or stomach area

Check with your doctor as soon as possible if any of the following side effects occur:

Rare
   Bloody or black, tarry stools; bloody or cloudy urine; fever with or without chills (not present before treatment and not caused by the condition being treated); pain in lower back and/or side (severe and/or sharp); pinpoint red spots on skin; skin rash, hives, or itching; sores, ulcers, or white spots on lips or in mouth; sore throat (not present before treatment and not caused by the condition being treated); sudden decrease in amount of urine; unusual bleeding or bruising; unusual tiredness or weakness

Other side effects not listed may also occur in some patients. If you notice any other effects, check with your healthcare professional.

ACETAMINOPHEN AND SALICYLATES (Systemic)

Some commonly used brand names are:

In the U.S.—

Excedrin Extra-Strength Caplets (1)	Goody's Headache Powders (1)
Excedrin Extra-Strength Tablets (1)	Rid-A-Pain Compound (4)
Excedrin Migraine (1)	Saleto (3)
Gelpirin (2)	Supac (2)
Goody's Fast Pain Relief (1)	Vanquish Caplets (2)

This information applies to the following medicines:

1. Acetaminophen, Aspirin, and Caffeine (a-seat-a-MIN-oh-fen AS-pir-in and kaf-EEN)
2. Acetaminophen, Aspirin, and Caffeine, Buffered (a-seat-a-MIN-oh-fen AS-pir-in and kaf-EEN, BUF-fered)
3. Acetaminophen, Aspirin, Salicylamide, and Caffeine (a-seat-a-MIN-oh-fen AS-pir-in sal-i-SILL-a-mide and kaf-EEN)
4. Acetaminophen, Salicylamide, and Caffeine (a-seat-a-MIN-oh-fen sal-i-SILL-a-mide and kaf-EEN)

Category

- **Analgesic**—Acetaminophen, Aspirin, and Caffeine; Acetaminophen, Aspirin, and Caffeine, Buffered; Acetaminophen, Aspirin, Salicylamide, and Caffeine; Acetaminophen, Salicylamide, and Caffeine

- **Antipyretic**—Acetaminophen, Aspirin, and Caffeine; Acetaminophen, Aspirin, and Caffeine, Buffered; Acetaminophen, Aspirin, Salicylamide, and Caffeine; Acetaminophen, Salicylamide, and Caffeine
- **Antimigraine**—Acetaminophen, Aspirin, and Caffeine

Description

Acetaminophen and salicylate combination medicines relieve pain and reduce fever. They may be used to relieve occasional pain caused by mild inflammation or arthritis (rheumatism). The acetaminophen, aspirin, and caffeine combination also may be used to relieve pain associated with migraine headaches.

Neither acetaminophen nor salicylamide is as effective as aspirin for treating chronic or severe pain, or other symptoms, caused by inflammation or arthritis. Some of these combination medicines do not contain any aspirin. Even those that do contain aspirin may not contain enough to be effective in treating these conditions.

A few reports have suggested that acetaminophen and salicylates used together may cause kidney damage or cancer of the kidney or urinary bladder. This may occur if large amounts of both medicines are taken together for a very long time. However, taking usual amounts of these combination medicines for a short time has not been shown to cause these unwanted effects. Also, these effects are not likely to occur with either acetaminophen or a salicylate used alone, even if large amounts have been taken for a long time. Therefore, for long-term use, it may be best to use either acetaminophen or a salicylate, but not both, unless you are under a doctor's care.

Before giving any of these combination medicines to a child, check the package label very carefully. Some of these medicines are too strong for use in children. If you are not certain whether a specific product can be given to a child, or if you have any questions about the amount to give, check with your health care professional.

These medicines are available without a prescription. However, your doctor may have special instructions on the proper dose of these medicines for your medical condition.

These medicines are available in the following dosage forms:

Oral
- Acetaminophen, Aspirin, and Caffeine
  - Oral powders
  - Tablets
- Acetaminophen, Aspirin, and Caffeine, Buffered
  - Tablets
- Acetaminophen, Aspirin, Salicylamide, and Caffeine
  - Tablets
- Acetaminophen, Salicylamide, and Caffeine
  - Capsules

Before Using This Medicine

If you are taking this medicine without a prescription, carefully read and follow any precautions on the label. For acetaminophen and salicylate combinations, the following should be considered:

Allergies—Tell your doctor if you have ever had any unusual or allergic reaction to acetaminophen, aspirin or other salicylates including methyl salicylate (oil of wintergreen), or to any of the following medicines:
- Diclofenac (e.g., Voltaren)
- Diflunisal (e.g., Dolobid)
- Etodolac (e.g., Lodine)
- Fenoprofen (e.g., Nalfon)
- Floctafenine (e.g., Idarac)
- Flurbiprofen, oral (e.g., Ansaid)
- Ibuprofen (e.g., Motrin)
- Indomethacin (e.g., Indocin)
- Ketoprofen (e.g., Orudis)
- Ketorolac (e.g., Toradol)
- Meclofenamate (e.g., Meclomen)
- Mefenamic acid (e.g., Ponstel)
- Nabumetone (e.g., Relafen)
- Naproxen (e.g., Naprosyn)
- Oxaprozin (e.g., Daypro)
- Phenylbutazone (e.g., Butazolidin)
- Piroxicam (e.g., Feldene)
- Sulindac (e.g., Clinoril)
- Tenoxicam (e.g., Mobiflex)
- Tiaprofenic acid (e.g., Surgam)
- Tolmetin (e.g., Tolectin)

Also tell your health care professional if you are allergic to any other substances, such as foods, preservatives, or dyes.

Pregnancy—
- *For acetaminophen:* Studies on birth defects have not been done in humans. However, acetaminophen has not been reported to cause birth defects or other problems.
- *For aspirin:* Studies in humans have not shown that aspirin causes birth defects. However, aspirin has been shown to cause birth defects in animals. *Do not take aspirin during the last 3 months of pregnancy unless it has been ordered by your doctor.* Some reports have suggested that too much use of aspirin late in pregnancy may cause a decrease in the newborn's weight and possible death of the fetus or newborn infant. However, the mothers in these reports had been taking much larger amounts of aspirin than are usually recommended. Studies of mothers taking aspirin in the doses that are usually recommended did not show these unwanted effects. However, there is a chance that regular use of aspirin late in pregnancy may cause unwanted effects on the heart or blood flow in the fetus or newborn infant. Use of aspirin during the last 2 weeks of pregnancy may cause bleeding problems in the fetus before or during delivery, or in the newborn infant. Also, too much use of aspirin during the last 3 months of pregnancy may increase the length of pregnancy, prolong labor, cause other problems during delivery, or cause severe bleeding in the mother before, during, or after delivery.
- *For salicylamide:* Studies on birth defects have not been done in humans.
- *For caffeine:* Studies in humans have not shown that caffeine causes birth defects. However, use of large amounts of caffeine by the mother during pregnancy

may cause problems with the heart rhythm of the fetus and may affect the growth of the fetus. Studies in animals have shown that caffeine causes birth defects when given in very large doses (amounts equal to the amount of caffeine in 12 to 24 cups of coffee a day).

Breast-feeding—

- *For acetaminophen and for aspirin:* Acetaminophen and aspirin pass into breast milk; however, they have not been reported to cause problems in nursing babies.

- *For caffeine:* Caffeine (contained in some of these combination medicines) passes into breast milk in small amounts. Taking caffeine in the amounts present in these medicines has not been reported to cause problems in nursing babies. However, studies have shown that babies may appear jittery and have trouble in sleeping when their mothers drink large amounts of caffeine-containing beverages. Therefore, breast-feeding mothers who use these medicines probably should limit the amount of caffeine they take in from other medicines or from beverages.

Children—

- *For acetaminophen:* Acetaminophen has been tested in children and, in effective doses, has not been shown to cause different side effects or problems than it does in adults.

- *For aspirin and for salicylamide: Do not give a medicine containing aspirin or salicylamide to a child with symptoms of a virus infection, especially flu or chickenpox, without first discussing its use with your child's doctor.* This is very important because aspirin may cause a serious illness called Reye's syndrome in children with fever caused by a virus infection, especially flu or chickenpox. Children who do not have a virus infection may also be more sensitive to the effects of aspirin, especially if they have a fever or have lost large amounts of body fluid because of vomiting, diarrhea, or sweating. This may increase the chance of side effects during treatment.

- *For caffeine:* There is no specific information comparing use of caffeine in children younger than 12 years of age with use in other age groups. However, caffeine is not expected to cause different side effects or problems in children than it does in adults.

Older adults—Elderly people may be more likely than younger adults to develop serious kidney problems if they take large amounts of these combination medicines for a long time. Therefore, it is best that elderly people not take this medicine for more than 5 days in a row unless they are under a doctor's care.

- *For acetaminophen:* Acetaminophen has been tested and, in effective doses, has not been shown to cause different side effects or problems in older people than it does in younger adults.

- *For aspirin:* People 60 years of age and older are especially sensitive to the effects of aspirin. This may increase the chance of side effects during treatment.

- *For caffeine:* Many medicines have not been studied specifically in older people. Therefore, it may not be known whether they work exactly the same way they do in younger adults or if they cause different side effects or problems in older people. There is no specific information comparing use of caffeine in the elderly with use in other age groups.

Other medicines—Although certain medicines should not be used together at all, in other cases two different medicines may be used together even if an interaction might occur. In these cases, your doctor may want to change the dose, or other precautions may be necessary. When you are taking an acetaminophen and salicylate combination, it is especially important that your health care professional know if you are taking any of the following:

- Anticoagulants (blood thinners) or
- Carbenicillin by injection (e.g., Geopen) or
- Cefamandole (e.g., Mandol) or
- Cefoperazone (e.g., Cefobid) or
- Cefotetan (e.g., Cefotan) or
- Dipyridamole (e.g., Persantine) or
- Divalproex (e.g., Depakote) or
- Heparin or
- Inflammation or pain medicine, except narcotics, or
- Pentoxifylline (e.g., Trental) or
- Plicamycin (e.g., Mithracin) or
- Ticarcillin (e.g., Ticar) or
- Valproic acid (e.g., Depakene)—Taking these medicines together with aspirin (present in some of these combination medicines) may increase the chance of serious bleeding
- Antidiabetics, oral (diabetes medicine you take by mouth)—Aspirin (present in some of these combination medicines) may increase the effects of the antidiabetic medicine; a change in dose may be needed if aspirin is taken regularly
- Ciprofloxacin (e.g., Cipro) or
- Enoxacin (e.g., Penetrex) or
- Itraconazole (e.g., Sporanox) or
- Ketoconazole (e.g., Nizoral) or
- Lomefloxacin (e.g., Maxaquin) or
- Norfloxacin (e.g., Noroxin) or
- Ofloxacin (e.g., Floxin) or
- Tetracyclines (medicine for infection), taken by mouth—Antacids (present in buffered forms of acetaminophen and salicylate combination medicines) can keep these other medicines from working properly if the medicines are taken too closely together
- Methotrexate (e.g., Mexate)—Taking aspirin (present in some of these combination medicines) together with methotrexate may increase the chance of serious side effects
- Probenecid (e.g., Benemid)—Aspirin (present in some of these combination medicines) can keep probenecid from working properly for treating gout
- Sulfinpyrazone (e.g., Anturane)—Aspirin (present in some of these combination medicines) can keep sulfinpyrazone from working properly for treating gout; also, taking aspirin together with sulfinpyrazone may increase the chance of bleeding
- Urinary alkalizers (medicine that makes the urine less acid, such as acetazolamide [e.g., Diamox], calcium- and/or magnesium-containing antacids, dichlorphenamide [e.g., Daranide], methazolamide [e.g., Neptazane], potassium or sodium citrate and/or citric acid, so-

dium bicarbonate [baking soda])—These medicines may make aspirin (present in some of these combination medicines) less effective by causing it to be removed from the body more quickly

Other medical problems—The presence of other medical problems may affect the use of acetaminophen and salicylate combinations. Make sure you tell your doctor if you have any other medical problems, especially:

- Alcohol abuse or
- Asthma, allergies, and nasal polyps (history of) or
- Hepatitis or other liver disease or
- Kidney disease—The chance of serious side effects may be increased
- Anemia or
- Stomach ulcer or other stomach problems—Aspirin (present in some of these combination medicines) may make these conditions worse
- Gout—Aspirin (present in some of these combination medicines) can make this condition worse and can also lessen the effects of some medicines used to treat gout
- Heart disease—Caffeine (present in some of these combination medicines) can make your condition worse
- Hemophilia or other bleeding problems—Aspirin (present in some of these combination medicines) increases the chance of serious bleeding

Proper Use of This Medicine

Take this medicine with food or a full glass (8 ounces) of water to lessen the chance of stomach upset.

Unless otherwise directed by your doctor:

- *Do not take more of this medicine than directed on the package label.* Taking too much acetaminophen may cause liver damage or lead to other medical problems because of an overdose. Also, taking too much aspirin can cause stomach problems or lead to other medical problems because of an overdose.
- *Children up to 12 years of age should not take this medicine more often than five times a day.*

Check with your doctor before taking one of these combination medicines to treat severe or chronic inflammation or arthritis (rheumatism). These combination medicines may not relieve the severe pain, redness, swelling, or stiffness caused by these conditions unless very large amounts are taken for a long time. *It is best not to take acetaminophen and salicylate combination medicines in large amounts for a long time* unless you are under a doctor's care.

If a combination medicine containing aspirin has a strong vinegar-like odor, do not use it. This odor means the medicine is breaking down. If you have any questions about this, check with your pharmacist.

Dosing—The dose of acetaminophen and salicylate combination medicines will be different for different patients. *Follow your doctor's orders or the directions on the label.* The following information includes only the average doses of these combination medicines. *If your dose is different, do not change it* unless your doctor tells you to do so.

The number of capsules, tablets (including caplets), or packets of oral powders that you take depends on the total amount of acetaminophen and salicylate (aspirin and/or salicylamide) in one capsule, tablet, or packet of oral powder. Also, the number of doses you take each day and the time allowed between doses depend on the strength of the medicine.

- For *oral (capsules or tablets [including caplets])* dosage forms:
  - For pain, fever, or mild arthritis symptoms:
    - Adults and teenagers—The usual dose is 1 or 2 capsules or tablets every three, four, or six hours, depending on the strength of the product. Do not take any of these combination medicines for more than ten days, unless otherwise directed by your doctor.
    - Children—Use and dose must be determined by your doctor.
  - For migraine headaches:
    - Adults and teenagers—The usual dose is 2 tablets (250 mg acetaminophen, and 250 mg of aspirin, and 65 mg of caffeine in combination) every six hours as necessary for relief from migraine headaches. Do not take for relief of migraine headache for more than two days, unless otherwise directed by your doctor.
    - Children—Use and dose must be determined by your doctor.
- For *oral (powder)* dosage form:
  - For pain, fever, or mild arthritis symptoms:
    - Adults and teenagers—This medicine is very strong. Each packet of powder contains 260 mg of acetaminophen and 520 mg of aspirin (a total of 780 mg of both medicines). The usual dose is one packet of powder every four to six hours. Do not take this medicine for more than ten days, unless otherwise directed by your doctor.
    - Children—The oral powder dosage form is too strong to use in children 12 years of age or younger.

Storage—To store this medicine:

- Keep out of the reach of children. Overdose of the salicylates in these combination medicines is very dangerous in young children.
- Store away from heat and direct light.
- Do not store tablets (including caplets), capsules, or powders in the bathroom, near the kitchen sink, or in other damp places. Heat or moisture may cause the medicine to break down.
- Do not keep outdated medicine or medicine no longer needed. Be sure that any discarded medicine is out of the reach of children.

Precautions While Using This Medicine

If you will be taking this medicine for a long time, or in high doses, *your doctor should check your progress at regular visits.* This is especially important for elderly people, who may be more likely than younger adults to develop serious kidney problems if they take large amounts of this medicine for a long time.

Check with your doctor:

- If you are taking this medicine to relieve pain and the pain lasts for more than 10 days (5 days for children), if the pain gets worse, if new symptoms occur, or if the painful area is red or swollen. These could be signs of a serious condition that needs treatment.

- If you are taking this medicine to bring down a fever, and the fever lasts for more than 3 days or returns, if your fever gets worse, if new symptoms occur, or if redness or swelling is present. These could be signs of a serious condition that needs treatment.
- If you are taking this medicine for a sore throat, and the sore throat is very painful, lasts for more than 2 days, or occurs together with or is followed by fever, headache, skin rash, nausea, or vomiting.

Do not take any of the combination medicines containing aspirin for 5 days before any surgery, including dental surgery, unless otherwise directed by your medical doctor or dentist. Taking aspirin during this time may cause bleeding problems.

Check the label of all over-the-counter (OTC), nonprescription, and prescription medicines you now take. If any of them contain acetaminophen, aspirin, other salicylates such as bismuth subsalicylate (e.g., Pepto Bismol) or magnesium salicylate (e.g., Nuprin Backache Caplets), or salicylic acid (present in some shampoos and skin products), *check with your health care professional. Using any of them together with this medicine may cause an overdose.*

Stomach problems may be more likely to occur if you drink three or more alcoholic beverages while you are taking aspirin. Also, liver damage may be more likely to occur if you drink three or more alcoholic beverages while you are taking acetaminophen.

Taking certain other medicines together with acetaminophen and salicylates may increase the chance of unwanted effects. The risk will depend on how much of each medicine you take every day, and on how long you take the medicines together. If your medical doctor or dentist directs you to take these medicines together on a regular basis, follow his or her directions carefully. However, *do not take any of the following medicines together with any of these combination medicines for more than a few days unless your doctor has directed you to do so and is following your progress:*

- Diclofenac (e.g., Voltaren)
- Diflunisal (e.g., Dolobid)
- Etodolac (e.g., Lodine)
- Fenoprofen (e.g., Nalfon)
- Floctafenine (e.g., Idarac)
- Flurbiprofen, oral (e.g., Ansaid)
- Ibuprofen (e.g., Motrin)
- Indomethacin (e.g., Indocin)
- Ketoprofen (e.g., Orudis)
- Ketorolac (e.g., Toradol)
- Meclofenamate (e.g., Meclomen)
- Mefenamic acid (e.g., Ponstel)
- Nabumetone (e.g., Relafen)
- Naproxen (e.g., Naprosyn)
- Oxaprozin (e.g., Daypro)
- Phenylbutazone (e.g., Butazolidin)
- Piroxicam (e.g., Feldene)
- Sulindac (e.g., Clinoril)
- Tenoxicam (e.g., Mobiflex)
- Tiaprofenic acid (e.g., Surgam)
- Tolmetin (e.g., Tolectin)

The antacid present in buffered forms of these combination medicines can keep other medicines from working properly. If you need to take a buffered form of this medicine, and you are also taking one of the following medicines, *be sure to take the buffered acetaminophen and salicylate combination medicine:*

- *At least 6 hours before or 2 hours after taking ciprofloxacin (e.g., Cipro) or lomefloxacin (e.g., Maxaquin).*
- *At least 8 hours before or 2 hours after taking enoxacin (e.g., Penetrex).*
- *At least 2 hours after taking itraconazole (e.g., Sporanox).*
- *At least 3 hours before or after taking ketoconazole (e.g., Nizoral).*
- *At least 2 hours before or after taking norfloxacin (e.g., Noroxin) or ofloxacin (e.g., Floxin).*
- *At least 3 or 4 hours before or after taking a tetracycline antibiotic by mouth.*
- *At least 1 or 2 hours before or after taking any other medicine by mouth.*

If you are taking a laxative containing cellulose, do not take it within 2 hours of taking this medicine. Taking the laxative and this medicine close together may make this medicine less effective by preventing the salicylate in it from being absorbed by your body.

Acetaminophen and salicylate combinations may interfere with the results of some medical tests. Before you have any medical tests, tell the person in charge if you have taken any of these combination medicines within the past 3 or 4 days. If possible, it is best to call the laboratory where the test will be done about 4 days ahead of time to find out whether the medicine may be taken during the 3 or 4 days before the test.

For patients with diabetes:

- Acetaminophen and salicylate combinations may cause false results with some blood and urine glucose (sugar) tests. If you notice any change in your test results, or if you have any questions about this possible problem, check with your health care professional. This is especially important if your diabetes is not well-controlled.

For patients taking one of the products that contain *caffeine:*

- Caffeine may interfere with the results of a test that uses adenosine (e.g., Adenocard) or dipyridamole (e.g., Persantine) to help find out how well your blood is flowing through certain blood vessels. Therefore, you should not have any caffeine for 8 to 12 hours before the test.

If you think that you or anyone else may have taken an overdose of this medicine, get emergency help at once. Taking an overdose of a salicylate may cause unconsciousness or death. The first symptom of an aspirin overdose may be ringing or buzzing in the ears. Other signs include convulsions (seizures), hearing loss, confusion, severe drowsiness or tiredness, severe excitement or nervousness, and unusually fast or deep breathing. Signs of severe acetaminophen overdose may not appear until 2 to 4 days after the overdose is taken, but treatment to prevent liver damage or death must be started within 24 hours or less after the overdose is taken.

Side Effects of This Medicine

Along with its needed effects, a medicine may cause some unwanted effects. Although not all of these side effects may occur, if they do occur they may need medical attention.

Check with your doctor immediately if any of the following side effects occur:
Less common or rare
Coughing; difficulty in swallowing; dizziness, lightheadedness, or feeling faint (severe); flushing, redness, or other change in skin color; shortness of breath, troubled breathing, tightness in chest, or wheezing; sudden decrease in amount of urine; swelling of eyelids, face, or lips

Signs and symptoms of overdose
Agitation, anxiety, excitement, irritability, nervousness, or restlessness; any loss of hearing; bloody urine; confusion or delirium; convulsions (seizures); diarrhea (severe or continuing); dizziness or lightheadedness; drowsiness (severe); fast or deep breathing; fast or irregular heartbeat (for medicines containing caffeine); fever; frequent urination (for medicines containing caffeine); hallucinations (seeing, hearing, or feeling things that are not there); headache (severe or continuing); increased sensitivity to touch or pain (for medicines containing caffeine); increased sweating; increased thirst; loss of appetite; muscle trembling or twitching (for medicines containing caffeine); nausea or vomiting (continuing, sometimes with blood); ringing or buzzing in ears (continuing); seeing flashes of "zig-zag" lights (for medicines containing caffeine); stomach cramps or pain (severe or continuing); swelling, pain, or tenderness in the upper abdomen or stomach area; trouble in sleeping (for medicines containing caffeine); uncontrollable flapping movements of the hands, especially in elderly patients; unexplained fever; vision problems

Signs of overdose in children
Changes in behavior; drowsiness or tiredness (severe); fast or deep breathing

Also, check with your doctor as soon as possible if any of the following side effects occur:
Less common or rare
Bloody or black, tarry stools; bloody or cloudy urine; fever with or without chills (not present before treatment and not caused by the condition being treated); pain in lower back and/or side (severe and/or sharp); pinpoint red spots on skin; skin rash, hives, or itching; sores, ulcers, or white spots on lips or in mouth; sore throat (not present before treatment and not caused by the condition being treated); stuffy nose; swelling of face, fingers, feet, or lower legs; unusual bleeding or bruising; unusual tiredness or weakness; vomiting of blood or material that looks like coffee grounds; weight gain; yellow eyes or skin

Other side effects may occur that usually do not need medical attention. These side effects may go away during treatment as your body adjusts to the medicine. However, check with your doctor if any of the following side effects continue or are bothersome:
More common
Heartburn or indigestion (for medicines containing aspirin); nausea, vomiting, or stomach pain (for medicines containing aspirin)

Less common
Drowsiness (for medicines containing salicylamide); trouble in sleeping, nervousness, or jitters (for medicines containing caffeine)

Some side effects may occur after you have stopped taking these combination medicines, especially if you have taken large amounts of them for a long time. *Check with your doctor immediately* if any of these side effects occur after you have stopped taking these medicines:
Rare
Bloody or cloudy urine; decreased urination; swelling of face, fingers, feet, or lower legs; weight gain

Other side effects not listed above may also occur in some patients. If you notice any other effects, check with your doctor.

ACETYLCYSTEINE   (Inhalation, oral/nebulization route) - a-se-teel-SIS-teen

Commonly used brand name(s)
In the U.S.—
Mucomyst

Available Dosage Forms:
• Solution

Therapeutic Class: Mucolytic

Uses For This Medicine

Acetylcysteine is a mucolytic (medicine that destroys or dissolves mucus). It is usually given by inhalation but may be given in other ways in a hospital.

Acetylcysteine is used for certain lung conditions when increased amounts of mucus make breathing difficult. Acetylcysteine liquefies (thins) or dissolves mucus so that it may be coughed up. Sometimes the mucus may have to be removed by suction.

This medicine is available only with your doctor's prescription.

Before Using This Medicine

In deciding to use a medicine, the risks of taking the medicine must be weighed against the good it will do. This is a decision you and your doctor will make. For this medicine, the following should be considered:

Allergies—Tell your doctor if you have ever had any unusual or allergic reaction to this medicine or any other medicines. Also tell your health care professional if you have any other types of allergies, such as to foods, dyes, preservatives, or animals. For non-prescription products, read the label or package ingredients carefully.

Pediatric—Although there is no specific information comparing use of acetylcysteine in children with use in other age groups, this medicine is not expected to cause different side effects or problems in children than it does in adults.

Geriatric—Many medicines have not been studied specifically in older people. Therefore, it may not be known whether they work exactly the same way they do in younger adults or if they cause different side effects or problems in older people. There is no specific information comparing use of acetylcysteine in the elderly with use in other age groups.

Pregnancy—

	Pregnancy Category	Explanation
All Trimesters	B	Animal studies have revealed no evidence of harm to the fetus, however, there are no adequate studies in pregnant women OR animal studies have shown an adverse effect, but adequate studies in pregnant women have failed to demonstrate a risk to the fetus.

Breast Feeding—There are no adequate studies in women for determining infant risk when using this medication during breastfeeding. Weigh the potential benefits against the potential risks before taking this medication while breastfeeding.

Other medicines—

Using this medicine with any of the following medicines may cause an increased risk of certain side effects, but using both drugs may be the best treatment for you. If both medicines are prescribed together, your doctor may change the dose or how often you use one or both of the medicines.

Carbamazepine, Nitroglycerin

Interactions with Food/Tobacco/Alcohol—Certain medicines should not be used at or around the time of eating food or eating certain types of food since interactions may occur. Using alcohol or tobacco with certain medicines may also cause interactions to occur. Discuss with your healthcare professional the use of your medicine with food, alcohol, or tobacco.

Other medical problems—The presence of other medical problems may affect the use of this medicine. Make sure you tell your doctor if you have any other medical problems, especially:

- Asthma—Acetylcysteine may make the condition worse
- Decreased ability to cough—The mucus may have to be removed by suctioning

Proper Use of This Medicine

Use acetylcysteine only as directed. Do not use more of it and do not use it more often than your doctor ordered. To do so may increase the chance of side effects.

If you are using this medicine at home, make sure you understand exactly how to use it. If you have any questions about this, check with your doctor.

After using acetylcysteine, try to cough up the loosened or thinned mucus. If this does not work, it may have to be suctioned out. This will prevent too much mucus from building up in the lungs. If you have any questions about this, check with your doctor.

Dosing—The dose of this medicine will be different for different patients. Follow your doctor's orders or the directions on the label. The following information includes only the average doses of this medicine. If your dose is different, do not change it unless your doctor tells you to do so.

The amount of medicine that you take depends on the strength of the medicine. Also, the number of doses you take each day, the time allowed between doses, and the length of time you take the medicine depend on the medical problem for which you are using the medicine.

- For inhalation dosage form (solution):
  - To thin or dissolve mucus in lung diseases:
    - Adults and children—
      - 3 to 5 milliliters (mL) of a 20% solution or 6 to 10 mL of a 10% solution used in a nebulizer three or four times a day. The medicine is inhaled through a face mask, mouthpiece, or tracheostomy.
      - The 10 or 20% solution may be used for inhalation as a heavy mist in a tent or croupette.
      - Sometimes the 10 or 20% solution is placed directly into the trachea or through a catheter into the trachea for certain conditions.
  - For use in tests to diagnose lung problems:
    - Adults and children—1 to 2 mL of a 20% solution or 2 to 4 mL of a 10% solution used for inhalation or placed directly into the trachea two or three times before the test.

Missed dose—If you miss a dose of this medicine, take it as soon as possible. However, if it is almost time for your next dose, skip the missed dose and go back to your regular dosing schedule. Do not double doses.

Storage—Store in the refrigerator. Do not freeze.

Keep out of the reach of children.

Do not keep outdated medicine or medicine no longer needed.

Store unopened vials of this medicine in the refrigerator. Do not freeze. An open vial of medicine must be used right away.

The opened container should be discarded after 4 days.

Precautions While Using This Medicine

If your condition does not improve or if it becomes worse, check with your doctor.

Side Effects of This Medicine

Along with its needed effects, a medicine may cause some unwanted effects. Although not all of these side effects may occur, if they do occur they may need medical attention.

Check with your doctor as soon as possible if any of the following side effects occur:

Less common
Wheezing, tightness in chest, or difficulty in breathing (especially in asthma patients)

Rare
Skin rash or other irritation

Some side effects may occur that usually do not need medical attention. These side effects may go away during treatment as your body adjusts to the medicine. Also, your health care professional may be able to tell you about ways to prevent or reduce some of these side effects. Check with your health care professional if any of the following side effects continue or are bothersome or if you have any questions about them:

Less common
Clammy skin; fever; increase in amount of mucus in lungs; irritation or soreness of mouth, throat, or lungs; nausea or vomiting; runny nose

For patients using a face mask for inhalation of acetylcysteine: the mask may leave a stickiness on your face. This can be removed with water.

When you use acetylcysteine, you may notice that the medicine has an unpleasant odor at first. However, this smell will go away soon after you use the medicine.

Other side effects not listed may also occur in some patients. If you notice any other effects, check with your healthcare professional.

ACITRETIN   (Oral route) - a-si-TRE-tin

Black Box Warning

- Contraindications and Warnings:
  - Acitretin must not be used by females who are pregnant, or who intend to become pregnant during therapy or at any time for at least 3 years following discontinuation of therapy. acitretin also must not be used by females who may not use reliable contraception while undergoing treatment and for at least 3 years following discontinuation of treatment. Acitretin is a metabolite of etretinate, and major human fetal abnormalities have been reported with the administration of acitretin and etretinate. Potentially, any fetus exposed can be affected.
  - Clinical evidence has shown that concurrent ingestion of acitretin and ethanol has been associated with the formation of etretinate, which has a significantly longer elimination half-life than acitretin. Because the longer elimination half-life of etretinate would increase the duration of teratogenic potential for female patients, ethanol must not be ingested by female patients either during treatment with acitretin or for 2 months after cessation of therapy. This allows for elimination of acitretin, thus removing the substrate for transesterification to etretinate. The mechanism of the metabolic process for conversion of acitretin to etretinate has not been fully defined. It is not known whether substances other than ethanol are associated with transesterification.
  - Acitretin has been shown to be embryotoxic and/or teratogenic in rabbits, mice, and rats at oral doses of 0.6, 3 and 15 mg/kg, respectively. These doses are approximately 0.2, 0.3 and 3 times the maximum recommended therapeutic dose, respectively, based on a mg/m(2) comparison.
  - Major human fetal abnormalities associated with acitretin and/or etretinate administration have been reported including meningomyelocele, meningoencephalocele, multiple synostoses, facial dysmorphia, syndactyly, absence of terminal phalanges, malformations of hip, ankle and forearm, low-set ears, high palate, decreased cranial volume, cardiovascular malformation and alterations of the skull and cervical vertebrae.
  - Acitretin should be prescribed only by those who have special competence in the diagnosis and treatment of severe psoriasis, are experienced in the use of systemic retinoids, and understand the risk of teratogenicity.

- Important Information for Women of Childbearing Potential:
  - Acitretin should be considered only for women with severe psoriasis unresponsive to other therapies or whose clinical condition contraindicates the use of other treatments.
  - Females of reproductive potential must not be given a prescription for acitretin until pregnancy is excluded. acitretin is contraindicated in females of reproductive potential unless the patient meets all of the following conditions:
    - Must have had 2 negative urine or serum pregnancy tests with a sensitivity of at least 25 mIU/mL before receiving the initial acitretin prescription. The first test (a screening test) is obtained by the prescriber when the decision is made to pursue acitretin therapy. The second pregnancy test (a confirmation test) should be done during the first 5 days of the menstrual period immediately preceding the beginning of acitretin therapy. For patients with amenorrhea, the second test should be done at least 11 days after the last act of unprotected sexual intercourse (without using 2 effective forms of contraception [birth control] simultaneously). Timing of pregnancy testing throughout the treatment course should be monthly or individualized based on the prescriber's clinical judgment.
    - Must have selected and have committed to use 2 effective forms of contraception (birth control) simultaneously, at least 1 of which must be a primary form, unless absolute abstinence is the chosen method, or the patient has undergone a hysterectomy or is clearly postmenopausal.
    - Patients must use 2 effective forms of contraception (birth control) simultaneously for at least 1 month prior to initiation of acitretin therapy, during acitretin therapy, and for at least 3 years after discontinuing acitretin therapy. A acitretin Patient Referral Form is available so that patients can receive an initial free contraceptive counseling session and pregnancy testing. Counseling about contraception and behaviors associated with an increased risk of pregnancy must be repeated on a regular basis by the prescriber. To encourage compliance with this recommendation, a limited supply of the drug should be prescribed.
    - Effective forms of contraception include both primary and secondary forms of contraception. Primary forms of contraception include: tubal ligation, partner's vasectomy, intrauterine devices, birth control pills, and injectable/implantable/insertable/topical hormonal birth control products. Secondary forms of contraception include diaphragms, latex condoms, and cervical caps; each secondary form must be used with a spermicide.
    - Any birth control method can fail. Therefore, it is critically important that women of childbearing potential use 2 effective forms of contraception (birth control) simultaneously. It has not been established if there is a pharmacokinetic interaction between acitretin and combined oral contraceptives. However, it has been established that acitretin interferes with the contraceptive effect of microdosed progestin preparations. Microdosed "minipill" progestin preparations are not recommended

for use with acitretin. It is not known whether other progestational contraceptives, such as implants and injectables, are adequate methods of contraception during acitretin therapy.

- Prescribers are advised to consult the package insert of any medication administered concomitantly with hormonal contraceptives, since some medications may decrease the effectiveness of these birth control products. Patients should be prospectively cautioned not to self-medicate with the herbal supplement St. John's Wort because a possible interaction has been suggested with hormonal contraceptives based on reports of breakthrough bleeding on oral contraceptives shortly after starting St. John's Wort. Pregnancies have been reported by users of combined hormonal contraceptives who also used some form of St. John's Wort.

- Must have signed a Patient Agreement/Informed Consent for Female Patients that contains warnings about the risk of potential birth defects if the fetus is exposed to acitretin, about contraceptive failure, and about the fact that they must not ingest beverages or products containing ethanol while taking acitretin and for 2 months after acitretin treatment has been discontinued.

- If pregnancy does occur during acitretin therapy or at any time for at least 3 years following discontinuation of acitretin therapy, the prescriber and patient should discuss the possible effects on the pregnancy. The available information is as follows:
  - Acitretin, the active metabolite of etretinate, is teratogenic and is contraindicated during pregnancy. The risk of severe fetal malformations is well established when systemic retinoids are taken during pregnancy. Pregnancy must also be prevented after stopping acitretin therapy, while the drug is being eliminated to below a threshold blood concentration that would be associated with an increased incidence of birth defects. Because this threshold has not been established for acitretin in humans and because elimination rates vary among patients, the duration of posttherapy contraception to achieve adequate elimination cannot be calculated precisely. It is strongly recommended that contraception be continued for at least 3 years after stopping treatment with acitretin, based on the following considerations:
    - In the absence of transesterification to form etretinate, greater than 98% of the acitretin would be eliminated within 2 months, assuming a mean elimination half-life of 49 hours.
    - In cases where etretinate is formed, as has been demonstrated with concomitant administration of acitretin and ethanol,
      - greater than 98% of the etretinate formed would be eliminated in 2 years, assuming a mean elimination half-life of 120 days.
      - greater than 98% of the etretinate formed would be eliminated in 3 years, based on the longest demonstrated elimination half-life of 168 days.
      - However, etretinate was found in plasma and subcutaneous fat in one patient reported to have had sporadic alcohol intake, 52 months after she stopped acitretin therapy.

- Severe birth defects have been reported where conception occurred during the time interval when the patient was being treated with acitretin and/or etretinate. In addition, severe birth defects have also been reported when conception occurred after the mother completed therapy. These cases have been reported both prospectively (before the outcome was known) and retrospectively (after the outcome was known). The events below are listed without distinction as to whether the reported birth defects are consistent with retinoid-induced embryopathy or not.
  - There have been 318 prospectively reported cases involving pregnancies and the use of etretinate, acitretin or both. In 238 of these cases, the conception occurred after the last dose of etretinate (103 cases), acitretin (126) or both (9). Fetal outcome remained unknown in approximately one-half of these cases, of which 62 were terminated and 14 were spontaneous abortions. Fetal outcome is known for the other 118 cases and 15 of the outcomes were abnormal (including cases of absent hand/wrist, clubfoot, GI malformation, hypocalcemia, hypotonia, limb malformation, neonatal apnea/anemia, neonatal ichthyosis, placental disorder/death, undescended testicle and 5 cases of premature birth). In the 126 prospectively reported cases where conception occurred after the last dose of acitretin only, 43 cases involved conception at least 1 year but less than 2 years after the last dose. There were 3 reports of abnormal outcomes out of these 43 cases (involving limb malformation, GI tract malformations and premature birth). There were only 4 cases where conception occurred at least 2 years after the last dose but there were no reports of birth defects in these cases.
  - There is also a total of 35 retrospectively reported cases where conception occurred at least one year after the last dose of etretinate, acitretin or both. From these cases there are 3 reports of birth defects when the conception occurred at least 1 year but less than 2 years after the last dose of acitretin (including heart malformations, Turner's Syndrome, and unspecified congenital malformations) and 4 reports of birth defects when conception occurred 2 or more years after the last dose of acitretin (including foot malformation, cardiac malformations [2 cases] and unspecified neonatal and infancy disorder). There were 3 additional abnormal outcomes in cases where conception occurred 2 or more years after the last dose of etretinate (including chromosome disorder, forearm aplasia, and stillbirth).
  - Females who have taken Tegison (etretinate) must continue to follow the contraceptive recommendations for Tegison. Tegison is no longer marketed in the US; for information, call Connetics at 1–888–500–DERM (3376).
  - Patients should not donate blood during and for at least 3 years following the completion

of acitretin therapy because women of child-bearing potential must not receive blood from patients being treated with acitretin.

- Important Information For Males Taking acitretin:
  - Patients should not donate blood during and for at least 3 years following acitretin therapy because women of childbearing potential must not receive blood from patients being treated with acitretin.
  - Samples of seminal fluid from 3 male patients treated with acitretin and 6 male patients treated with etretinate have been assayed for the presence of acitretin. The maximum concentration of acitretin observed in the seminal fluid of these men was 12.5 ng/mL. Assuming an ejaculate volume of 10 mL, the amount of drug transferred in semen would be 125 ng, which is 1/200,000 of a single 25 mg capsule. Thus, although it appears that residual acitretin in seminal fluid poses little, if any, risk to a fetus while a male patient is taking the drug or after it is discontinued, the no-effect limit for teratogenicity is unknown and there is no registry for birth defects associated with acitretin. The available data are as follows:
    - There have been 25 cases of reported conception when the male partner was taking acitretin. The pregnancy outcome is known in 13 of these 25 cases. Of these, 9 reports were retrospective and 4 were prospective (meaning the pregnancy was reported prior to knowledge of the outcome). When the paternal acitretin treatment occurred at the time of conception, there were 5 healthy neonates delivered (4 of 5 cases were prospective), 5 spontaneous abortions, and 1 induced abortion. When the paternal acitretin treatment was discontinued 4 weeks prior to conception, there was 1 induced abortion with malformation pattern not typical of retinoid embryopathy (bilateral cystic hygromas of neck, hypoplasia of lungs bilateral, pulmonary atresia, VSD with overriding truncus arteriosus). When the paternal acitretin treatment was discontinued 6 to 8 months prior to conception, there was 1 spontaneous abortion.
  - For All Patients: An acitretin medication guide must be given to the patient each time acitretin is dispensed, as required by law

Commonly used brand name(s)

In the U.S.—
Soriatane

Available Dosage Forms:
- Capsule

Therapeutic Class: Antipsoriatic

Uses For This Medicine

Acitretin is used to help relieve and control severe skin disorders, such as severe psoriasis. It works by allowing normal growth and development of the skin. Acitretin may continue to work after you stop taking it, but usually after a time, the skin condition returns and you may need to begin taking it again.

Acitretin must not be used to treat women who are able to bear children unless other forms of treatment have been tried first and failed. Acitretin must not be taken during pregnancy because it causes birth defects in humans. If you are able to bear children, it is very important that you read, understand, and follow the pregnancy warnings for acitretin.

You must take important precautions while taking acitretin and continue with them for a period of time after you stop taking the medicine. The precautions are:

- Women should not become pregnant and should use two methods of very effective birth control. The birth control methods should begin 1 month before starting the medicine and continue for at least 2 or 3 years after discontinuing the medicine or as directed by your doctor.
- Men and women should not donate blood for transfusion purposes during treatment and for 2 or 3 years after discontinuing the medicine or as directed by your doctor.
- Men and women should not drink alcohol during treatment and for 2 months after discontinuing the medicine.

If you do not think these precautions are reasonable, you should discuss this with your doctor before starting to take this medicine.

This medicine is available only with your doctor's prescription.

Before Using This Medicine

In deciding to use a medicine, the risks of taking the medicine must be weighed against the good it will do. This is a decision you and your doctor will make. For this medicine, the following should be considered:

Allergies—Tell your doctor if you have ever had any unusual or allergic reaction to this medicine or any other medicines. Also tell your health care professional if you have any other types of allergies, such as to foods, dyes, preservatives, or animals. For non-prescription products, read the label or package ingredients carefully.

Pediatric—This medicine has been tested in some children and has been shown not to cause different side effects or problems in children than it does in adults. However, children may be more sensitive to some of the medicine's effect on bones, which may prevent normal bone growth during puberty. This can cause them to grow up to be shorter adults than expected. Therefore, it is especially important that you discuss with the child's doctor the good that this medicine may do as well as the risks of using it.

Geriatric—This medicine has been tested and has not been shown to cause different side effects or problems in older people than it does in younger adults. However, some older patients may have higher levels of the medicine in the blood stream as compared to younger adults, and they may be more sensitive to its effects. This may increase their chance of developing side effects during treatment.

Pregnancy—

	Pregnancy Category	Explanation
All Trimesters	X	Studies in animals or pregnant women have demonstrated positive evidence of fetal abnormalities. This drug should not be used in women who are or may become pregnant because the risk clearly outweighs any possible benefit.

Breast Feeding—There are no adequate studies in women for determining infant risk when using this medication during

breastfeeding. Weigh the potential benefits against the potential risks before taking this medication while breastfeeding.

Other medicines—

Using this medicine with any of the following medicines is not recommended. Your doctor may decide not to treat you with this medication or change some of the other medicines you take.

Chlortetracycline, Demeclocycline, Doxycycline, Methacycline, Minocycline, Oxytetracycline, Rolitetracycline, Tetracycline

Interactions with Food/Tobacco/Alcohol—Certain medicines should not be used at or around the time of eating food or eating certain types of food since interactions may occur. Using alcohol or tobacco with certain medicines may also cause interactions to occur. The following interactions have been selected on the basis of their potential significance and are not necessarily all-inclusive.

Using this medicine with any of the following is usually not recommended, but may be unavoidable in some cases. If used together, your doctor may change the dose or how often you use this medicine, or give you special instructions about the use of food, alcohol, or tobacco.

Ethanol

Other medical problems—The presence of other medical problems may affect the use of this medicine. Make sure you tell your doctor if you have any other medical problems, especially:

- Diabetes mellitus (sugar diabetes) or
- High cholesterol or triglycerides, uncontrollable (or history of) or
- Inflammation of pancreas (or history of)—Acitretin may make these conditions worse or increase cholesterol or triglyceride problems
- Hypervitaminosis A (or history of)—If you have past or current problems with toxic symptoms from vitamin A, acitretin may increase the chance that they will occur again
- Kidney disease, severe or
- Liver disease, severe—May cause acitretin to stay in the body for a longer period of time and increase the chance of side effects

Proper Use of This Medicine

Make certain your health care provider knows if you are on any special diet, such as a low-sodium, low-cholesterol, or low-sugar diet. Discuss with your doctor how often you drink alcohol, even if it is only an occasional drink.

Patient information is usually provided with acitretin. Read it carefully before using this medicine.

Take acitretin with a main meal or with a glass of milk.

For women—This medicine may cause birth defects. To make sure you are not pregnant before beginning treatment, your doctor will ask you to:

- Use two effective forms of birth control (contraception) for at least 1 month before beginning treatment.
- Report when your menstrual periods are normal.
- Take a pregnancy test within 1 week before beginning the treatment to make sure you are not pregnant.
- Begin your acitretin treatment on Day 2 or Day 3 of your next menstrual period.

- Sign a paper to show that you understand the importance of not becoming pregnant for at least 2 to 3 years after you stop taking this medicine, according to the advice of your doctor.

Using two effective forms of birth control for at least 2 or 3 years after you stop taking acitretin, according to the advice of your doctor, is very important to help prevent an unplanned pregnancy. If you do not think this is reasonable, you should discuss this with your doctor before you start taking this medicine.

Dosing—The dose of this medicine will be different for different patients. Follow your doctor's orders or the directions on the label. The following information includes only the average doses of this medicine. If your dose is different, do not change it unless your doctor tells you to do so.

The amount of medicine that you take depends on the strength of the medicine. Also, the number of doses you take each day, the time allowed between doses, and the length of time you take the medicine depend on the medical problem for which you are using the medicine.

Take acitretin with food. Taking with food is important for getting the right amount of medicine out of your stomach.

It is important that you do not share this medicine with anyone else because of the risk of birth defects and other serious side effects.

- For oral dosage form (tablets):
  - For severe psoriasis:
    - Adults—25 to 50 milligrams (mg) a day as a single dose. After four weeks, your doctor may increase your dose depending on how well this medicine is working for you
    - Children—Use and dose must be determined by your doctor.
  - For other severe skin disorders (such as bullous or nonbullous erythroderma, lamellar ichthyoses, and keratosis follicularis):
    - Adults—25 milligrams (mg) a day. After four weeks, a dose of 10 to 75 mg a day is used.
    - Children—Use and dose must be determined by your doctor.

Missed dose—If you miss a dose of this medicine, take it as soon as possible. However, if it is almost time for your next dose, skip the missed dose and go back to your regular dosing schedule. Do not double doses.

Storage—Store the medicine in a closed container at room temperature, away from heat, moisture, and direct light. Keep from freezing.

Keep out of the reach of children.

Do not keep outdated medicine or medicine no longer needed.

Precautions While Using This Medicine

It is important that your doctor check your progress at regular visits while you are taking this medicine. If your condition has improved and you are no longer taking acitretin, your progress must still be checked. This is especially important for children or elderly patients, who may be more sensitive to the effects of this medicine, and for women who want to become pregnant after they stop taking the medicine.

It is important that you check with your doctor before taking any medicines including vitamins, herbal products or over-the-counter (OTC) medicines. Some of these medicines or nutritional supplements (e.g., St. John's wort) may make your birth control pills not work.

Your skin condition may improve or get worse during the first 3 weeks of treatment and you also may notice some skin irritation from the medicine. With continued use, the expected skin irritation will lessen after a few weeks. Check with your health care professional any time skin irritation becomes severe or if your skin condition does not improve within 8 to 12 weeks.

Do not drink alcohol while taking this medicine or for at least 2 months after discontinuing treatment.

- Drinking alcohol can change the medicine in the body to a product that stays in your body for an extended period of time. This can increase your chance of developing side effects for a longer period of time than if you hadn't consumed alcohol.
- If a woman consumes alcohol during acitretin treatment, she should consider delaying a pregnancy for longer than 2 or 3 years or as directed by her doctor.

Do not donate blood during treatment with acitretin, for 2 or 3 years following treatment, or as otherwise directed by your doctor. Although problems resulting from a blood transfusion are not likely, this precaution prevents the possibility that your blood would be used in pregnant women.

Acitretin can cause dryness of the eyes, blur your vision, or cause other vision problems. Be aware that while using acitretin you may see a sudden decrease in your night vision (ability to see before the sun rises or after the sun goes down). Also, acitretin may cause your eyes to be more sensitive to light, including sunlight, than they are normally. These effects can make certain activities dangerous, such as driving or operating machines.

Check with your doctor if you experience any vision or eye problem. Wearing contact lenses may become uncomfortable. Your doctor may suggest using artificial tears to keep your eyes from getting too dry.

Acitretin may cause dryness of the mouth, nose, and throat. For temporary relief of mouth dryness, use sugarless candy or gum, melt bits of ice in your mouth, or use a saliva substitute. However, if your mouth continues to feel dry for more than 2 weeks, check with your medical doctor or dentist. Continuing dryness of the mouth may increase the chance of developing dental disease, including tooth decay, gum disease, and fungus infections.

Avoid overexposing your skin to wind, cold weather, and sunlight, even on cloudy days. Your skin will be more prone to sunburn, dryness, or irritation, especially during the first 2 or 3 weeks. However, you should not stop taking this medicine, unless the skin irritation becomes too severe. For best results:

- Wear sunglasses that can block ultraviolet (UV) light. Ordinary sunglasses may not protect your eyes.
- Regularly use sunscreen or sunblocking lotions with a sun protection factor (SPF) of at least 15.
- Wear protective clothing and hats and stay out of direct sunlight, especially between the hours of 10 a.m. and 3 p.m.
- Apply creams, lotions, or moisturizers often. Your health care professional can help you choose the right skin products for you to reduce skin dryness and irritation.
- Do not use an artificial light, such as a sunlamp, unless directed otherwise by your doctor.

Unless your doctor tells you otherwise, it is especially important to avoid using the following skin products:

- Any topical acne product or skin product containing a peeling agent (such as benzoyl peroxide, resorcinol, salicylic acid, or sulfur).
- Hair products that are irritating, such as permanents or hair removal products.
- Skin products that cause sensitivity to the sun, such as those containing spices or limes.
- Skin products containing a large amount of alcohol, such as astringents, shaving creams, or after-shave lotions.
- Skin products that are too drying or abrasive, such as some cosmetics, soaps, or skin cleansers.

Using these products when taking acitretin may cause mild to severe irritation of the skin.

Do not take doses of vitamin A or any vitamin supplement containing vitamin A that exceeds the minimum recommended allowance (RDA) while you are taking this medicine. To do so may increase the chance of developing side effects.

Side Effects of This Medicine

Along with its needed effects, a medicine may cause some unwanted effects. Although not all of these side effects may occur, if they do occur they may need medical attention.

Check with your doctor immediately if any of the following side effects occur:
 More common
　Headache (severe and continuing); nausea or vomiting (severe and continuing)
 Less common
　Blurred vision; eye pain
 Rare
　Abdominal or stomach pain; bleeding gums; bleeding time increased; chest pain; coughing up blood; diarrhea; difficulty in breathing or swallowing; double vision or other problems in seeing, including decreased night vision after sunset and before sunrise; darkened urine; increased menstrual flow; or vaginal bleeding; light-colored stools; nosebleeds; pale or cold hands or feet; paralysis; prolonged bleeding from cuts; red or dark brown urine; shortness of breath; unpleasant breath odor; unusual tiredness or weakness; vomiting of blood; yellowing of the skin or eyes
 Incidence not known
　Assault; attack; burning, numbness, tingling, or painful sensations; chest pain or discomfort; confusion; difficulty breathing; difficulty in speaking; doing things to injure oneself; force; inability to move arms, legs, or facial muscles; inability to speak; pain in chest, groin, or legs, especially calves; pain or discomfort in arms, jaw, back or neck; shortness of breath; slurred speech; slow speech; sudden loss of coordination; sudden, severe weakness or numbness in arm or leg; sudden, unexplained shortness of breath; sweating; thoughts of killing oneself; unsteadiness or awkwardness; vision changes; weakness in arms, hands, legs, or feet

Check with your doctor as soon as possible if any of the following side effects occur:
 More common
　Back pain; bad, unusual or unpleasant (after)taste; bone or joint pain; change in taste; continuing ringing

or buzzing or other unexplained noise in ears; degenerative disease of the joint; difficulty in moving or walking; excessive muscle tone; feeling of warmth redness of the face, neck, arms and occasionally, upper chest; headache; hearing loss; increased sensitivity to pain; increased sensitivity to touch; muscle stiffness; muscle tension or tightness; redness of skin; sleeplessness; stiff, painful muscles; thinning of skin with easy bruising; tingling in the hands and feet; tongue irritation; trouble sleeping; unable to sleep

Less common

Acid or sour stomach; belching; breast pain; eye problems, such as loss of eyebrows or eyelashes, redness or swelling of the eyelid, redness of the eyes, sensitivity of eyes to light, or watery eyes; general feeling of discomfort or illness; heartburn; increased hair growth on forehead, back, arms, and legs; indigestion; itching of the vagina or genital area; loosening of the fingernails; pain during sexual intercourse; redness or soreness around fingernails; sore mouth or tongue; thick, white vaginal discharge with no odor or with a mild odor; white patches in mouth and/or on tongue

Rare

Coughing, hoarseness, trouble in speaking, or influenza-like symptoms; itchy or painful ears; skin problems, such as abnormal sensation of burning or stinging of skin, cracking of skin, redness of skin, skin irritation or rash (including a rash that looks like psoriasis), skin infection, skin ulcers, skin odor (unusual), or small red spots in skin; sore on the edge of the eyelid (stye); thick, white, curd-like vaginal discharge; vaginal itching or irritation

Symptoms of overdose

Dizziness or lightheadedness; feeling of constant movement of self or surroundings; headache; sensation of spinning; vomiting

Some side effects may occur that usually do not need medical attention. These side effects may go away during treatment as your body adjusts to the medicine. Also, your health care professional may be able to tell you about ways to prevent or reduce some of these side effects. Check with your health care professional if any of the following side effects continue or are bothersome or if you have any questions about them:

More common

Chapped, red, or swollen lips; difficulty in wearing contact lenses; dryness of eyes; dry or runny nose; increased ability to sunburn; increased amount of ear wax (unusual); itchy skin; nosebleeds; irritation in mouth or swollen gums; loss of hair (usually reversible); scaling and peeling of eyelids, fingertips, palms, and soles of feet; sticky skin; unusual thirst

Less common

Constipation; diarrhea; fatigue; increased sweating

Incidence not known

Cracking fingernails or fingernails break easily; muscular pain, tenderness, wasting or weakness

Other side effects not listed may also occur in some patients. If you notice any other effects, check with your healthcare professional.

ACYCLOVIR   (Oral route, Intravenous route) - ay-SYE-kloe-veer

Commonly used brand name(s)

In the U.S.—
Zovirax

In Canada—
Acyclovir

Available Dosage Forms:

- Tablet
- Capsule
- Suspension
- Solution
- Powder for Solution

Therapeutic Class: Antiviral
Pharmacologic Class: Viral DNA Polymerase Inhibitor

Uses For This Medicine

Acyclovir belongs to the family of medicines called antivirals, which are used to treat infections caused by viruses. Usually these medicines work for only one kind or group of virus infections.

Acyclovir is used to treat the symptoms of chickenpox, shingles, herpes virus infections of the genitals (sex organs), the skin, the brain, and mucous membranes (lips and mouth), and widespread herpes virus infections in newborns. Acyclovir is also used to prevent recurrent genital herpes infections. Although acyclovir will not cure herpes, it does help relieve the pain and discomfort and helps the sores (if any) heal faster.

Acyclovir may also be used for other virus infections as determined by your doctor. However, it does not work in treating certain virus infections, such as the common cold.

Acyclovir is available only with your doctor's prescription.

Once a medicine has been approved for marketing for a certain use, experience may show that it is also useful for other medical problems. Although not specifically included in product labeling, acyclovir by injection is used in certain patients with the following medical conditions:

- Herpes simplex (for prevention of repeated infections) in people with a weak immune system
- Herpes zoster infections of the eye
- Shingles (for prevention of repeated infections) in people with a weak immune system

Before Using This Medicine

In deciding to use a medicine, the risks of taking the medicine must be weighed against the good it will do. This is a decision you and your doctor will make. For this medicine, the following should be considered:

Allergies—Tell your doctor if you have ever had any unusual or allergic reaction to this medicine or any other medicines. Also tell your health care professional if you have any other types of allergies, such as to foods, dyes, preservatives, or animals. For non-prescription products, read the label or package ingredients carefully.

Pediatric—A limited number of studies have been done using oral acyclovir in children, and it has not caused different effects or problems in children than it does in adults.

Geriatric—Agitation, confusion, dizziness, and drowsiness may be especially likely to occur in elderly patients who are usually more sensitive than younger adults to the central nervous system effects of acyclovir.

Pregnancy—

	Pregnancy Category	Explanation
All Trimesters	B	Animal studies have revealed no evidence of harm to the fetus, however, there are no adequate studies in pregnant women OR animal studies have shown an adverse effect, but adequate studies in pregnant women have failed to demonstrate a risk to the fetus.

Breast Feeding—Studies in women suggest that this medication poses minimal risk to the infant when used during breastfeeding.

Other medicines—

Using this medicine with any of the following medicines is usually not recommended, but may be required in some cases. If both medicines are prescribed together, your doctor may change the dose or how often you use one or both of the medicines.

Varicella Virus Vaccine

Interactions with Food/Tobacco/Alcohol—Certain medicines should not be used at or around the time of eating food or eating certain types of food since interactions may occur. Using alcohol or tobacco with certain medicines may also cause interactions to occur. Discuss with your healthcare professional the use of your medicine with food, alcohol, or tobacco.

Other medical problems—The presence of other medical problems may affect the use of this medicine. Make sure you tell your doctor if you have any other medical problems, especially:

- Dehydration or
- Kidney disease—Dehydration or kidney disease may increase blood levels of acyclovir, increasing the chance of side effects.
- Nervous system problems—Acyclovir may make these problems worse.

Proper Use of This Medicine

Patient information about the treatment of herpes, chickenpox, or shingles is available with this medicine. Read it carefully before using this medicine.

Acyclovir is best used as soon as possible after the symptoms of herpes infection or shingles (for example, pain, burning, blisters) *begin to appear*.

If you are taking acyclovir for the *treatment of chickenpox*, it is best to *start taking acyclovir as soon as possible after the first sign of the chickenpox rash*, usually within one day.

Acyclovir capsules, tablets, and oral suspension may be taken with meals or on an empty stomach.

Acyclovir is best taken with a full glass (8 ounces) of water.

If you are using *acyclovir oral suspension*, use a specially marked measuring spoon or other device to measure each dose accurately. The average household teaspoon may not hold the right amount of liquid.

To help clear up your herpes infection, chickenpox, or shingles, *keep taking acyclovir for the full time of treatment*, even if your symptoms begin to clear up after a few days. *Do not miss any doses*. However, *do not use this medicine more often or for a longer time than your doctor ordered*.

If you are taking acyclovir capsules, tablets, or oral suspension, you should drink plenty of water to avoid becoming dehydrated.

Dosing—The dose of this medicine will be different for different patients. Follow your doctor's orders or the directions on the label. The following information includes only the average doses of this medicine. If your dose is different, do not change it unless your doctor tells you to do so.

The amount of medicine that you take depends on the strength of the medicine. Also, the number of doses you take each day, the time allowed between doses, and the length of time you take the medicine depend on the medical problem for which you are using the medicine.

- For oral dosage forms (capsules, oral suspension, or tablets):
  - For treatment of genital herpes:
    - Adults and children 12 years of age and older—200 milligrams (mg) five times a day for ten days.
    - Children up to 12 years of age—Use and dose must be determined by the doctor.
  - For prevention of recurrent outbreaks of genital herpes infections:
    - Adults and children 12 years of age and older—200 to 400 mg two to five times a day for five days or up to twelve months, depending on how often your outbreaks of infection occur.
    - Children up to 12 years of age—Use and dose must be determined by the doctor.
  - For treatment of chickenpox:
    - Adults and children who weigh over 88 pounds (40 kilograms)—800 mg four times a day for five days.
    - Children 2 years of age and older and weighing 88 pounds (40 kilograms) or less—Dose is based on body weight and must be determined by the doctor. The usual dose is 20 mg per kilogram (kg) of body weight, up to 800 mg, four times a day for five days.
    - Children up to 2 years of age—Use and dose must be determined by the doctor.
  - For treatment of shingles:
    - Adults and children 12 years of age and older—800 mg five times a day for seven to ten days.
    - Children up to 12 years of age—Use and dose must be determined by the doctor.
- For injection dosage form:
  - For treatment of herpes of the brain, genitals, or mucous membranes, or for the treatment of shingles:
    - Adults and children 12 years of age and older—Dose is based on body weight and must be determined by the doctor. The usual dose is 5 to 10 mg of acyclovir per kg (2.3 to 4.5 mg per pound) of body weight, injected slowly into a vein over at least a one-hour period, and repeated every eight hours for five to ten days.
    - Children up to 12 years of age—Dose is based on body weight and must be determined by the

doctor. The usual dose is 10 mg to 20 mg of acyclovir per kg (4.5 mg to 9.1 mg per pound) of body weight, injected slowly into a vein over at least a one-hour period and repeated every eight hours for seven to ten days.

- ○ For treatment of widespread herpes virus infection in newborns:
    - ▪ Infants from birth to 3 months of age—Dose is based on body weight and must be determined by the doctor. The usual dose is 10 mg of acyclovir per kg (4.5 mg per pound) of body weight, injected slowly into a vein over at least a one-hour period and repeated every eight hours for ten days.

Missed dose—If you miss a dose of this medicine, take it as soon as possible. However, if it is almost time for your next dose, skip the missed dose and go back to your regular dosing schedule. Do not double doses.

Storage—Store the medicine in a closed container at room temperature, away from heat, moisture, and direct light. Keep from freezing.

Keep out of the reach of children.

Do not keep outdated medicine or medicine no longer needed.

Precautions While Using This Medicine

If your symptoms do not improve within a few days, or if they become worse, check with your doctor.

The areas affected by herpes, chickenpox, or shingles should be kept as clean and dry as possible. Also, wear loose-fitting clothing to avoid irritating the sores (blisters).

It is important to remember that acyclovir will not keep you from spreading herpes to others.

Herpes infection of the genitals can be caught from or spread to your partner during any sexual activity. Even though you may get herpes if your partner has no symptoms, the infection is more likely to be spread if sores are present. This is true until the sores are completely healed and the scabs have fallen off. *Therefore, it is best to avoid any sexual activity if either you or your sexual partner has any symptoms of herpes.* The use of a latex condom ("rubber") may help prevent the spread of herpes. However, spermicidal (sperm-killing) jelly or a diaphragm will probably not help.

Side Effects of This Medicine

Along with its needed effects, a medicine may cause some unwanted effects. Although not all of these side effects may occur, if they do occur they may need medical attention.

Check with your doctor immediately if any of the following side effects occur:

More common—For acyclovir injection only
    Pain, swelling, or redness at place of injection

Less common
    Abdominal or stomach pain; decreased frequency of urination or amount of urine; increased thirst; loss of appetite; nausea or vomiting; unusual tiredness or weakness

Rare
    Black, tarry stools; blood in urine or stools; chills, fever, or sore throat; confusion; convulsions (seizures); hallucinations (seeing, hearing, or feeling things that are

not there); hives; pinpoint red spots on skin; trembling; unusual bleeding or bruising

Frequency not determined
    Bleeding or oozing from puncture sites or mucous membranes (bowel, mouth, nose, or urinary bladder), continuing; blistering, peeling, or loosening of skin; bluish coloring, especially of the hands and feet; blurred vision; bruising at the place of injection; changes in facial skin color; changes in vision; clumsiness; coughing; decreased consciousness; difficulty in breathing or swallowing; dizziness or feeling faint, severe; fast heartbeat; irritability; itching or skin rash; large hive-like swelling on face, eyelids, lips, tongue, throat, hands, legs, feet, sex organs; mood or mental changes; muscle cramps, pain, or weakness; pale skin; red or irritated eyes; sense of agitation or uneasiness; shakiness and unsteady walk; sores, ulcers, or white spots in mouth or on lips; swelling of eyelids, face, feet, hands, lower legs or lips; swollen, painful, or tender lymph nodes (glands) in neck, armpit, or groin; unsteadiness or other problems with muscle control or coordination; yellow eyes or skin

Some side effects may occur that usually do not need medical attention. These side effects may go away during treatment as your body adjusts to the medicine. Also, your health care professional may be able to tell you about ways to prevent or reduce some of these side effects. Check with your health care professional if any of the following side effects continue or are bothersome or if you have any questions about them:

More common—Especially seen with high doses
    General feeling of discomfort or illness

Less common—Especially seen with long-term use or high doses
    Diarrhea; headache

Frequency not determined
    Burning, prickling, or tingling sensations; drowsiness; loss of hair

Other side effects not listed may also occur in some patients. If you notice any other effects, check with your healthcare professional.

ACYCLOVIR (Topical route) - ay-SYE-kloe-veer

Commonly used brand name(s)
In the U.S.—
    Zovirax

In Canada—
    Acyclovir

Available Dosage Forms:
- Cream
- Ointment

Therapeutic Class: Antiviral
Pharmacologic Class: Viral DNA Polymerase Inhibitor

Uses For This Medicine

Acyclovir belongs to the family of medicines called antivirals. Antivirals are used to treat infections caused by viruses. Usually they work for only one kind or group of virus infections.

Topical acyclovir is used to treat the symptoms of herpes simplex virus infections of the skin, mucous membranes, and genitals (sex organs). Although topical acyclovir will not cure herpes simplex, it may help relieve the pain and discomfort and may help the sores (if any) heal faster. Topical acyclovir may also be used for other conditions as determined by your doctor.

Acyclovir is available only with your doctor's prescription.

Before Using This Medicine

In deciding to use a medicine, the risks of taking the medicine must be weighed against the good it will do. This is a decision you and your doctor will make. For this medicine, the following should be considered:

Allergies—Tell your doctor if you have ever had any unusual or allergic reaction to this medicine or any other medicines. Also tell your health care professional if you have any other types of allergies, such as to foods, dyes, preservatives, or animals. For non-prescription products, read the label or package ingredients carefully.

Pediatric—Studies on this medicine have been done only in adult patients, and there is no specific information comparing use of topical acyclovir in children with use in other age groups.

Geriatric—Many medicines have not been studied specifically in older people. Therefore, it may not be known whether they work exactly the same way they do in younger adults. Although there is no specific information comparing the use of topical acyclovir in the elderly with use in other age groups, this medicine is not expected to cause different side effects or problems in older people than it does in younger adults.

Pregnancy—

	Pregnancy Category	Explanation
All Trimesters	B	Animal studies have revealed no evidence of harm to the fetus, however, there are no adequate studies in pregnant women OR animal studies have shown an adverse effect, but adequate studies in pregnant women have failed to demonstrate a risk to the fetus.

Breast Feeding—Studies in women suggest that this medication poses minimal risk to the infant when used during breastfeeding.

Other medicines—

Using this medicine with any of the following medicines is usually not recommended, but may be required in some cases. If both medicines are prescribed together, your doctor may change the dose or how often you use one or both of the medicines.

Varicella Virus Vaccine

Interactions with Food/Tobacco/Alcohol—Certain medicines should not be used at or around the time of eating food or eating certain types of food since interactions may occur. Using alcohol or tobacco with certain medicines may also cause interactions to occur. Discuss with your healthcare professional the use of your medicine with food, alcohol, or tobacco.

Other medical problems—Tell your doctor if your herpes simplex infection keeps coming back while you are using acyclovir.

Proper Use of This Medicine

Acyclovir may come with patient information about herpes simplex infections. Read this information carefully. If you have any questions, check with your health care professional.

Do not use this medicine in the eyes.

Acyclovir is best used as soon as possible after the signs and symptoms of herpes infection (for example, pain, burning, or blisters) begin to appear.

Use a finger cot or rubber glove when applying this medicine. This will help keep you from spreading the infection to other areas of your body and will prevent the transmission of the infection to other persons. Apply enough medicine to completely cover all the sores (blisters). A 1.25–centimeter (approximately ½-inch) strip of ointment applied to each area of the affected skin measuring 5 × 5 centimeters (approximately 2 × 2 inches) is usually enough, unless otherwise directed by your doctor.

To help clear up your herpes infection, continue using acyclovir for the full time of treatment, even if your symptoms begin to clear up after a few days. Do not miss any doses. However, do not use this medicine more often or for a longer time than your doctor ordered.

Dosing—The dose of this medicine will be different for different patients. Follow your doctor's orders or the directions on the label. The following information includes only the average doses of this medicine. If your dose is different, do not change it unless your doctor tells you to do so.

The amount of medicine that you take depends on the strength of the medicine. Also, the number of doses you take each day, the time allowed between doses, and the length of time you take the medicine depend on the medical problem for which you are using the medicine.

- For topical dosage form (cream):
  - For herpes simplex infection:
    - Adults—Apply to the affected area(s), four to six times a day, for up to ten days.
    - Children—Use and dose must be determined by your doctor.
- For topical dosage form (ointment):
  - For herpes simplex infection:

    In the U.S.
    - Adults—Apply to the affected area(s), every three hours, for a total of six times a day, for seven days.
    - Children—Use and dose must be determined by your doctor.

    In Canada
    - Adults—Apply to the affected area(s), four to six times a day, for up to ten days.

• Children—Use and dose must be determined by your doctor.

Missed dose—If you miss a dose of this medicine, apply it as soon as possible. However, if it is almost time for your next dose, skip the missed dose and go back to your regular dosing schedule.

Storage—Store the medicine in a closed container at room temperature, away from heat, moisture, and direct light. Keep from freezing.

Keep out of the reach of children.

Do not keep outdated medicine or medicine no longer needed.

Precautions While Using This Medicine

Women with genital herpes may be more likely to get cancer of the cervix (opening to the womb). Therefore, it is very important that Pap tests be taken at least once a year to check for cancer. Cervical cancer can be cured if found and treated early.

If your symptoms do not improve within 1 week, or if they become worse, check with your doctor.

Consider the possibility of viral resistance to acyclovir if little or no improvement in symptoms during therapy.

The areas affected by herpes should be kept as clean and dry as possible. Also, wear loose-fitting clothing to avoid irritating the sores (blisters).

Herpes infection of the genitals can be caught from or spread to your partner during any sexual activity. Although you may get herpes even though your sexual partner has no symptoms, the infection is more likely to be spread if sores are present. This is true until the sores are completely healed and the scabs have fallen off. The use of a condom (prophylactic) may help prevent the spread of herpes. However, spermicidal (sperm-killing) jelly or a diaphragm will not help prevent the spread of herpes. Therefore, it is best to avoid any sexual activity if either you or your partner has any symptoms of herpes. It is also important to remember that acyclovir will not keep you from spreading herpes to others.

Side Effects of This Medicine

Along with its needed effects, a medicine may cause some unwanted effects. Although not all of these side effects may occur, if they do occur they may need medical attention.

Some side effects may occur that usually do not need medical attention. These side effects may go away during treatment as your body adjusts to the medicine. Also, your health care professional may be able to tell you about ways to prevent or reduce some of these side effects. Check with your health care professional if any of the following side effects continue or are bothersome or if you have any questions about them:

More common
Mild pain, burning, or stinging

Less common
Itching

Rare
Itching, stinging, or redness of the genital area; skin rash

Other side effects not listed may also occur in some patients. If you notice any other effects, check with your healthcare professional.

ADALIMUMAB (Subcutaneous route) -
ay-da-LIM-yoo-mab

Black Box Warning

Risk of infections: Tuberculosis (frequently disseminated or extrapulmonary at clinical presentation), invasive fungal infections, and other opportunistic infections, have been observed in patients receiving adalimumab. Some of these infections have been fatal. Anti-tuberculosis treatment of patients with latent tuberculosis infection reduces the risk of reactivation in patients receiving treatment with adalimumab. However, active tuberculosis has developed in patients receiving adalimumab whose screening for latent tuberculosis infection was negative.

Patients should be evaluated for latent tuberculosis infection with a tuberculin skin test. Treatment of latent tuberculosis infection should be initiated prior to therapy with adalimumab. Physicians should monitor patients receiving adalimumab for signs and symptoms of active tuberculosis, including patients who are tuberculin skin test negative.

Commonly used brand name(s)

In the U.S.—
Humira

Available Dosage Forms:

• Solution

Therapeutic Class: Antirheumatic
Pharmacologic Class: Monoclonal Antibody

Uses For This Medicine

Adalimumab is used to decrease signs, symptoms, and progression of moderately to severely active rheumatoid arthritis and ankylosing spondylitis. It is also used to treat psoriatic arthritis which is a type of arthritis that causes pain and swelling of the joints and patches of scaly skin on some areas of the body. Psoriatic arthritis is related to the skin condition, psoriasis. Adalimumab can be used in combination with methotrexate or other Disease Modifying Antirheumatic Drugs (DMARDs)

This medicine is available only with your doctor's prescription.

Before Using This Medicine

In deciding to use a medicine, the risks of taking the medicine must be weighed against the good it will do. This is a decision you and your doctor will make. For this medicine, the following should be considered:

Allergies—Tell your doctor if you have ever had any unusual or allergic reaction to this medicine or any other medicines. Also tell your health care professional if you have any other types of allergies, such as to foods, dyes, preservatives, or animals. For non-prescription products, read the label or package ingredients carefully.

Pediatric—Studies on adalimumab have been done only in adult patients, and there is no specific information comparing the use adalimumab in children with use in other age groups.

Geriatric—Elderly people are especially sensitive to the effects of certain drugs. Specific side effects may be especially likely to occur in elderly patients, who are usually more sensitive than younger adults to the effects of adalimumab. Adalimumab causes more serious infections and malignancies in the elderly.

Pregnancy—

	Pregnancy Category	Explanation
All Trimesters	B	Animal studies have revealed no evidence of harm to the fetus, however, there are no adequate studies in pregnant women OR animal studies have shown an adverse effect, but adequate studies in pregnant women have failed to demonstrate a risk to the fetus.

Breast Feeding—There are no adequate studies in women for determining infant risk when using this medication during breastfeeding. Weigh the potential benefits against the potential risks before taking this medication while breastfeeding.

Other medicines—

Using this medicine with any of the following medicines is usually not recommended, but may be required in some cases. If both medicines are prescribed together, your doctor may change the dose or how often you use one or both of the medicines.

Abatacept, Anakinra

Interactions with Food/Tobacco/Alcohol—Certain medicines should not be used at or around the time of eating food or eating certain types of food since interactions may occur. Using alcohol or tobacco with certain medicines may also cause interactions to occur. Discuss with your healthcare professional the use of your medicine with food, alcohol, or tobacco.

Other medical problems—The presence of other medical problems may affect the use of this medicine. Make sure you tell your doctor if you have any other medical problems, especially:

- Heart failure—This medicine may cause heart failure to become worse or for new heart failure symptoms and adverse effects to occur. Caution should be used and your doctor should monitor you carefully.
- Infections—This medicine should not be started in patients who have active infections of any type. It may also cause reactivation of previous infections such as hepatitis B. This medicine may need to be stopped if you develop an infection.
- Tuberculosis or
- Demyelinating disorders—This medicine may make these medical problems worse.

Proper Use of This Medicine

Dosing—The dose of this medicine will be different for different patients. Follow your doctor's orders or the directions on the label. The following information includes only the average doses of this medicine. If your dose is different, do not change it unless your doctor tells you to do so.

The amount of medicine that you take depends on the strength of the medicine. Also, the number of doses you take each day, the time allowed between doses, and the length of time you take the medicine depend on the medical problem for which you are using the medicine.

- For injection dosage form:
  - For psoriatic arthritis, rheumatoid arthritis, or ankylosing spondylitis:
    - Adults—40 milligrams (mg) given under the skin by injection every other week alone or in combination with methotrexate, glucocorticoids, aspirin, non-steroidal anti-inflammatories (NSAIDS), analgesics, or other disease modifying antirheumatic drugs (DMARDS); or 40 mg given under the skin by injection every week for patients with rheumatoid arthritis who are not taking methotrexate.
    - Children—Use and dose must be determined by your doctor.

Missed dose—If you miss a dose of this medicine, take it as soon as possible. However, if it is almost time for your next dose, skip the missed dose and go back to your regular dosing schedule. Do not double doses.

Storage—Store in the refrigerator. Do not freeze.

Keep out of the reach of children.

Do not keep outdated medicine or medicine no longer needed.

Throw away used needles in a hard, closed container that the needles cannot poke through. Keep this container away from children and pets.

Precautions While Using This Medicine

If you will be taking this medicine for a long time, it is very important that your doctor check you at regular visits. This will allow your doctor to see if the medicine is working properly. Your doctor can then decide if you should continue to take it.

You will need to have a skin test for tuberculosis before you start using this medicine. Tell your doctor if you or anyone in your home has ever had a positive reaction to a tuberculosis test.

Call your doctor right away if you start to have persistent cough, weight loss, night sweats, fever, chills, or flu-like symptoms such as runny or stuffy nose, headache, feeling generally ill, unusual bleeding, bruising or paling of the skin. This may be signs that you are already having an infection.

Do not take other medicines unless they have been discussed with your doctor. Your doctor will discuss with you any changes in your medicine. Ask your doctor if you have any questions.

Make sure you know how you react to this medicine before you drive, use machines, or do anything else that could be dangerous if you are dizzy or are not alert.

This medicine may cause other unwanted effects that may not occur until months or years after this medicine is used. A small number of people who have used this medicine have developed lymphoma or skin cancer. Discuss these possible effects with your doctor.

Side Effects of This Medicine

Along with its needed effects, a medicine may cause some unwanted effects. Although not all of these side effects may occur, if they do occur they may need medical attention.

Check with your doctor immediately if any of the following side effects occur:

More common

Abdominal fullness; body aches or pain; cough or hoarseness; ear congestion; gaseous abdominal pain;

infection; lightheadedness; loss of voice; lower back or side pain; muscle aches and pains; nasal congestion; pain or tenderness around eyes or cheekbones; rapid sometimes shallow breathing; runny nose; shivering; stuffy nose; sunken eyes; thirst; trouble sleeping; warmth on skin; wrinkled skin

Less common

Abdominal pain; abnormal vaginal bleeding or discharge; agitation; anxiety; arm, back, or jaw pain; a sore on the skin of the breast that doesn't heal; back pain; black, tarry stools; bleeding from gums or nose; blindness; bloating or swelling of face, arms, hands, lower legs, or feet; blood in stool or change in bowel habits; bloody or cloudy urine; blurred vision; broken bones; change in size, shape, or color of an existing mole; change in skin color; chest tightness or heaviness; chest pain; chills; clear or bloody discharge from nipple; cold hands and feet; confusion; constipation; cough; coughing or spitting up blood; decreased urination; decreased vision; depression; difficulty, burning, or painful urination; difficult or frequent urination; difficulty breathing; dimpling of breast skin; dizziness; drowsiness; eye pain; fainting; fast, slow or irregular heartbeat; fever; forgetfulness; frequent urge to urinate; general feeling of illness; hair loss; hallucinations; headache; increased thirst; inverted nipple; irregular breathing; irregular pulse; irritability; itching; light colored stools; loss of appetite; lump in breast or under your arm; lump or swelling in the abdomen; mole that leaks fluid or bleeds; mood or mental changes; muscle cramps or spasms; nausea; new mole; night sweats; no blood pressure or pulse; noisy breathing; numbness or tingling in your arms, legs, or face; pain, redness, or swelling in arms or legs without any injury present; pale skin; persistent non-healing sore on your skin; pink growth; puffiness or swelling of the eyelids or around the eyes, face, lips or tongue; raised, firm, bright red patch; rash; redness or swelling of the breast; seizures; sharp back pain just below your ribs; shiny bump on your skin; shortness of breath; skin rash; slurred speech or problems swallowing; sneezing; sore throat; sores, ulcers, or white spots on lips or mouth; spitting up blood; stiff neck; stopping of the heart; sudden high fever or low grade fever for months; sweating; swelling of the face, fingers, feet, or lower legs; swollen glands; swollen neck veins; tightness in chest; tiredness; trouble breathing with activity; trouble thinking; unconsciousness; unexplained bruising or bleeding; unpleasant breath odor; unusual tiredness or weakness; unusual weight gain or loss; visual disturbances; vomiting; vomiting of blood or material that looks like coffee grounds; yellow skin or eyes; wheezing

Frequency not determined—occurred during clinical practice; frequency not known

Pinpoint red spots on skin; unusual bleeding or bruising

Some side effects may occur that usually do not need medical attention. These side effects may go away during treatment as your body adjusts to the medicine. Also, your health care professional may be able to tell you about ways to prevent or reduce some of these side effects. Check with your health care professional if any of the following side effects continue or are bothersome or if you have any questions about them:

More common

Bladder pain; bleeding; blistering; burning; coldness; discoloration of skin; feeling of pressure; general feeling of discomfort or illness; hives; infection; inflam-

mation; joint pain; large amount of cholesterol in your blood; large amount of fat in your blood; lumps; numbness; pounding in the ears; redness; scarring; soreness; stinging; swelling; tenderness; tingling; ulceration; warmth

Less common

Abnormal healing; decrease in height; difficulty in moving; difficulty in walking; difficulty swallowing; dry mouth; heartburn; indigestion; loss of hearing; loss of strength or energy; menstrual changes; muscle or joint stiffness, tightness, or rigidity; muscle pain or stiffness; muscle pain or weakness; pain in back, ribs, arms, or legs; pain or burning in throat; passing of gas; shakiness in legs, arms, hands, and feet; sores; stomach pain, fullness, or discomfort; swelling or redness in joints; weakness

Other side effects not listed may also occur in some patients. If you notice any other effects, check with your healthcare professional.

ADAPALENE (Topical route) - a-DAP-a-leen

Commonly used brand name(s)

In the U.S.—
  Differin

Available Dosage Forms:

- Solution
- Gel/Jelly
- Cream
- Swab

Therapeutic Class: Antiacne

Uses For This Medicine

Adapalene is used to treat acne. It works partly by keeping skin pores clear.

Adapalene is available only with your doctor's prescription.

Before Using This Medicine

In deciding to use a medicine, the risks of taking the medicine must be weighed against the good it will do. This is a decision you and your doctor will make. For this medicine, the following should be considered:

Allergies—Tell your doctor if you have ever had any unusual or allergic reaction to this medicine or any other medicines. Also tell your health care professional if you have any other types of allergies, such as to foods, dyes, preservatives, or animals. For non-prescription products, read the label or package ingredients carefully.

Pediatric—Studies of this medicine have been done only in adult patients, and there is no specific information comparing use of adapalene in children up to 12 years of age with use in other age groups. In teenagers, adapalene is not expected to cause different side effects or problems than it does in adults.

Geriatric—Many medicines have not been studied specifically in older people. Therefore, it may not be known whether they work exactly the same way they do in younger adults or if they cause different side effects or problems in older people. There is no specific information comparing use of adapalene in the elderly with use in other age groups. Older adults are not likely to develop acne.

Pregnancy—

	Pregnancy Category	Explanation
All Trimesters	C	Animal studies have shown an adverse effect and there are no adequate studies in pregnant women OR no animal studies have been conducted and there are no adequate studies in pregnant women.

Breast Feeding—There are no adequate studies in women for determining infant risk when using this medication during breastfeeding. Weigh the potential benefits against the potential risks before taking this medication while breastfeeding.

Other medicines—Although certain medicines should not be used together at all, in other cases two different medicines may be used together even if an interaction might occur. In these cases, your doctor may want to change the dose, or other precautions may be necessary. Tell your healthcare professional if you are taking any other prescription or non-prescription (over-the-counter [OTC]) medicine.

Interactions with Food/Tobacco/Alcohol—Certain medicines should not be used at or around the time of eating food or eating certain types of food since interactions may occur. Using alcohol or tobacco with certain medicines may also cause interactions to occur. Discuss with your healthcare professional the use of your medicine with food, alcohol, or tobacco.

Other medical problems—The presence of other medical problems may affect the use of this medicine. Make sure you tell your doctor if you have any other medical problems, especially:

- Eczema or
- Seborrheic dermatitis—Use of this medicine may cause or increase the irritation associated with eczema or seborrheic dermatitis

Proper Use of This Medicine

It is very important that you use this medicine only as directed. Do not use more of it, do not use it more often, and do not use it for a longer time than your doctor ordered. To do so may cause irritation of the skin.

Do not apply this medicine to windburned or sunburned skin or on open wounds.

Do not use this medicine in or around the eyes, lips, or inside of the nose. Spread the medicine away from these areas when applying. If the medicine accidently gets on these areas, wash with water at once.

Apply the medicine to clean, dry areas of the skin affected by acne. Rub in gently and well. Wash your hands afterwards to remove any medicine that may remain on them.

To help clear up your acne completely, it is very important that you keep using this medicine for the full time of treatment, even if your symptoms begin to clear up after a short time. If you stop using this medicine too soon, your acne may return or get worse.

Dosing—The dose of this medicine will be different for different patients. Follow your doctor's orders or the directions on the label. The following information includes only the average doses of this medicine. If your dose is different, do not change it unless your doctor tells you to do so.

The amount of medicine that you take depends on the strength of the medicine. Also, the number of doses you take each day, the time allowed between doses, and the length of time you take the medicine depend on the medical problem for which you are using the medicine.

- For topical dosage form (gel):
  - For acne:
    - Adults and teenagers—Apply a small amount as a thin film once a day, at least one hour before bedtime. Apply the medicine to dry, clean areas affected by acne. Rub in gently and well.
    - Children—Use and dose must be determined by your doctor.

Missed dose—If you miss a dose of this medicine, skip the missed dose and go back to your regular dosing schedule. Do not double doses.

Storage—Store the medicine in a closed container at room temperature, away from heat, moisture, and direct light. Keep from freezing.

Keep out of the reach of children.

Do not keep outdated medicine or medicine no longer needed.

Precautions While Using This Medicine

During the first 3 weeks you are using adapalene, your acne may seem to get worse before it gets better. Full improvement should be seen within 12 weeks, especially if you use the medicine every day. You should not stop using adapalene if your acne seems worse at first, unless irritation or other symptoms become severe. Check with your doctor if your acne does not improve within 8 to 12 weeks.

Do not apply any topical product to the same area where you are using adapalene, unless otherwise directed by your doctor. If applied to the same area treated with adapalene, the following products may cause mild to severe irritation of the skin:

- Hair products that irritate the skin, such as permanents or hair removal products
- Skin products for acne (such as clindamycin or erythromycin) or other skin products containing a peeling agent (such as benzoyl peroxide, resorcinol, salicylic acid, or sulfur)
- Skin products that cause one to be more sensitive to the sun, such as those containing spices or lime
- Skin products that are too drying or that contain a large amount of alcohol, such as astringents, cosmetics, shaving creams, or after-shave lotions
- Skin products that are abrasive, such as some soaps or skin cleansers

Your doctor may ask you to use other topical products, such as benzoyl peroxide, clindamycin, or erythromycin, during your treatment with adapalene. Applying the products at different times of the day will lessen the chance of causing skin irritation.

If your skin becomes too dry or red at any time, discuss with your doctor whether you should continue using adapalene. Applying creams, lotions, or moisturizers as needed helps lessen these skin problems.

During treatment with this medicine, avoid getting too much sun on treated areas and do not use sunlamps. Since your skin may be more prone to sunburn or skin irritation, use sunscreen or sunblocking lotions regularly with a sun protection factor (SPF) of 15 or more. Wear protective clothing against sun, wind, and cold weather.

Side Effects of This Medicine

Along with its needed effects, a medicine may cause some unwanted effects. Although not all of these side effects may occur, if they do occur they may need medical attention.

Check with your doctor as soon as possible if any of the following side effects occur:

More common—especially during the first month of use
Burning sensation or stinging of skin; dryness and peeling of skin; itching of skin; redness of skin

Some side effects may occur that usually do not need medical attention. These side effects may go away during treatment as your body adjusts to the medicine. Also, your health care professional may be able to tell you about ways to prevent or reduce some of these side effects. Check with your health care professional if any of the following side effects continue or are bothersome or if you have any questions about them:

Rare—more common during the first month of use
Worsening of acne

Other side effects not listed may also occur in some patients. If you notice any other effects, check with your healthcare professional.

ADEFOVIR DIPIVOXIL   (Oral route)

Black Box Warning

Severe acute exacerbations of hepatitis have been reported in patients who have discontinued anti-hepatitis B therapy including adefovir dipivoxil. Hepatic function should be monitored closely with both clinical and laboratory follow-up for at least several months in patients who discontinue anti-hepatitis B therapy. If appropriate, resumption of anti-hepatitis B therapy may be warranted.

In patients at risk of or having underlying renal dysfunction, chronic administration of adefovir dipivoxil may result in nephrotoxicity. These patients should be monitored closely for renal function and may require dose adjustment.

HIV resistance may emerge in chronic hepatitis B patients with unrecognized or untreated Human Immunodeficiency Virus (HIV) infection treated with anti-hepatitis B therapies, such as therapy with adefovir dipivoxil, that may have activity against HIV.

Lactic acidosis and severe hepatomegaly with steatosis, including fatal cases, have been reported with the use of nucleoside analogs alone or in combination with other antiretrovirals.

Commonly used brand name(s)

In the U.S.—
Hepsera

Available Dosage Forms:
• Tablet

Therapeutic Class: Antiviral
Pharmacologic Class: Nucleotide Reverse Transcriptase Inhibitor

Uses For This Medicine

Adefovir is used to treat adults with chronic infections of active hepatitis B. Adefovir is not a cure for the hepatitis B virus, but it may lower the amount of hepatitis B virus in your body. It may also lower the ability of the virus to multiply in your body.

This medicine is available only with your doctor's prescription.

Before Using This Medicine

In deciding to use a medicine, the risks of taking the medicine must be weighed against the good it will do. This is a decision you and your doctor will make. For this medicine, the following should be considered:

Allergies—Tell your doctor if you have ever had any unusual or allergic reaction to this medicine or any other medicines. Also tell your health care professional if you have any other types of allergies, such as to foods, dyes, preservatives, or animals. For non-prescription products, read the label or package ingredients carefully.

Pediatric—Studies on adefovir have been done only in adult patients, and there is no specific information comparing the use of adefovir in children with use in other age groups.

Geriatric—Many medicines have not been studied specifically in older people. Therefore, it may not be known whether they work exactly the same way they do in younger adults. Older patients should use this medicine with caution. Elderly people can be especially sensitive to the effects of medicines.

Pregnancy—

	Pregnancy Category	Explanation
All Trimesters	C	Animal studies have shown an adverse effect and there are no adequate studies in pregnant women OR no animal studies have been conducted and there are no adequate studies in pregnant women.

Breast Feeding—There are no adequate studies in women for determining infant risk when using this medication during breastfeeding. Weigh the potential benefits against the potential risks before taking this medication while breastfeeding.

Other medicines—Although certain medicines should not be used together at all, in other cases two different medicines may be used together even if an interaction might occur. In these cases, your doctor may want to change the dose, or other precautions may be necessary. Tell your healthcare professional if you are taking any other prescription or nonprescription (over-the-counter [OTC]) medicine.

Interactions   with   Food/Tobacco/Alcohol—Certain medicines should not be used at or around the time of eating food or eating certain types of food since interactions may occur. Using alcohol or tobacco with certain medicines may also cause interactions to occur. Discuss with your healthcare professional the use of your medicine with food, alcohol, or tobacco.

Other medical problems—The presence of other medical problems may affect the use of this medicine. Make sure you tell your doctor if you have any other medical problems, especially:
• Human immunodeficiency virus (HIV)—It is important to talk to your doctor about the HIV virus before starting this medicine. Adefovir can make this condition worse.

• Kidney problems—Adefovir can cause kidney problems and your doctor may want to change your dose.

Proper Use of This Medicine

Dosing—The dose of this medicine will be different for different patients. Follow your doctor's orders or the directions on the label. The following information includes only the average doses of this medicine. If your dose is different, do not change it unless your doctor tells you to do so.

The amount of medicine that you take depends on the strength of the medicine. Also, the number of doses you take each day, the time allowed between doses, and the length of time you take the medicine depend on the medical problem for which you are using the medicine.

• For oral dosage form (tablets):
  ○ For treatment of hepatitis B infection:
    ▪ Adults: 10 milligrams (mg) once daily. May take with or without food.
    ▪ Children—Use and dose must be determined by your doctor.

Missed dose—If you miss a dose of this medicine, take it as soon as possible. However, if it is almost time for your next dose, skip the missed dose and go back to your regular dosing schedule. Do not double doses.

Storage—Store the medicine in a closed container at room temperature, away from heat, moisture, and direct light. Do not refrigerate. Keep from freezing.

Keep out of the reach of children.

Do not keep outdated medicine or medicine no longer needed.

Precautions While Using This Medicine

It is very important that your doctor check your progress and kidney function at regular visits. This will allow your doctor to see if the medicine is working properly.

Notify your doctor immediately if you think that you may be pregnant or plan to become pregnant. Certain medications may cause birth defects or other problems in the baby if taken during pregnancy.

Notify your doctor immediately if there is a chance you were exposed to HIV.

Be sure to follow up with your doctor after you stop this medicine so that your doctor can watch your liver function

Be sure that you notify your doctor immediately or get immediate medical attention if you notice abdominal discomfort or cramping, diarrhea, decreased appetite, discomfort, muscle cramping or pain, or unusual tiredness or weakness. These may be symptoms of a serious condition called lactic acidosis.

Side Effects of This Medicine

Along with its needed effects, a medicine may cause some unwanted effects. Although not all of these side effects may occur, if they do occur they may need medical attention.

Check with your doctor immediately if any of the following side effects occur:
  More common
    Blood in your urine
  Less common
    Sugar in your urine

Some side effects may occur that usually do not need medical attention. These side effects may go away during treatment as your body adjusts to the medicine. Also, your health care professional may be able to tell you about ways to prevent or reduce some of these side effects. Check with your health care professional if any of the following side effects continue or are bothersome or if you have any questions about them:
  More common
    Abdominal pain; headache; lack or loss of strength
  Less common
    Acid or sour stomach; belching; bloated or full feeling; diarrhea; excess air or gas in stomach or intestines; heartburn or indigestion; nausea; passing gas; stomach discomfort, upset, or pain

Other side effects not listed may also occur in some patients. If you notice any other effects, check with your healthcare professional.

ALBENDAZOLE   (Oral route) - al-BEN-da-zole

Commonly used brand name(s)
In the U.S.—
  Albenza

Available Dosage Forms:
• Tablet

Therapeutic Class: Anthelmintic

Uses For This Medicine

Albendazole is used to treat infections caused by worms. Albendazole works by keeping the worm from absorbing sugar (glucose), so that the worm loses energy and dies.

Albendazole is used to treat:
• Hydatid disease (echinococcosis);
• Infection of the nervous system caused by pork tapeworms (neurocysticercosis).

Albendazole is available only with your doctor's prescription.

Once a medicine has been approved for marketing for a certain use, experience may show that it is also useful for other medical problems. Although these uses are not included in product labeling in the U.S., albendazole is used in certain patients with the following infections:
• Capillariasis;
• Cutaneous larva migrans;
• Common roundworms (ascariasis);
• Hookworms (ancylostomiasis and necatoriasis);
• Pinworms (enterobiasis or oxyuriasis);
• Strongyloidiasis;
• Tapeworms (taeniasis);
• Trichostrongyliasis;
• Whipworms (trichuriasis).

For patients taking albendazole for hookworms:
• In hookworm infections, anemia may occur. Therefore, your doctor may want you to take iron supplements. If so, it is important to take iron every day while you are being treated for hookworm infection. Do not miss any doses. Your doctor may also want you to keep taking

iron supplements for at least 3 to 6 months after you stop taking albendazole. If you have any questions about this, check with your doctor.

For patients taking albendazole for pinworms:

- In some patients, pinworms may return after treatment with albendazole. Wear pajamas and underwear to sleep, take a bath every day, and wash (not shake) all bedding and nightclothes (pajamas) after treatment to help prevent reinfection. Treatment may be repeated after 3 weeks.
- Pinworms may be easily passed from one person to another, especially among persons in the same household. Therefore, all household members may have to be treated at the same time to prevent their infection or reinfection.

Before Using This Medicine

In deciding to use a medicine, the risks of taking the medicine must be weighed against the good it will do. This is a decision you and your doctor will make. For this medicine, the following should be considered:

Allergies—Tell your doctor if you have ever had any unusual or allergic reaction to this medicine or any other medicines. Also tell your health care professional if you have any other types of allergies, such as to foods, dyes, preservatives, or animals. For non-prescription products, read the label or package ingredients carefully.

Pediatric—Although there is very little specific information comparing use of albendazole in children with use in other age groups, this medicine is not expected to cause different side effects or problems in children than it does in adults.

Geriatric—Many medicines have not been studied specifically in older people. Therefore, it may not be known whether they work exactly the same way they do in younger adults or if they cause different side effects or problems in older people. There is no specific information comparing use of albendazole in the elderly with use in other age groups.

Pregnancy—

	Pregnancy Category	Explanation
All Trimesters	C	Animal studies have shown an adverse effect and there are no adequate studies in pregnant women OR no animal studies have been conducted and there are no adequate studies in pregnant women.

Breast Feeding—There are no adequate studies in women for determining infant risk when using this medication during breastfeeding. Weigh the potential benefits against the potential risks before taking this medication while breastfeeding.

Other medicines—Although certain medicines should not be used together at all, in other cases two different medicines may be used together even if an interaction might occur. In these cases, your doctor may want to change the dose, or other precautions may be necessary. Tell your healthcare professional if you are taking any other prescription or nonprescription (over-the-counter [OTC]) medicine.

Interactions with Food/Tobacco/Alcohol—Certain medicines should not be used at or around the time of eating food or eating certain types of food since interactions may occur. Using alcohol or tobacco with certain medicines may also cause interactions to occur. The following interactions have been selected on the basis of their potential significance and are not necessarily all-inclusive.

Using this medicine with any of the following may cause an increased risk of certain side effects but may be unavoidable in some cases. If used together, your doctor may change the dose or how often you use this medicine, or give you special instructions about the use of food, alcohol, or tobacco.

Grapefruit Juice

Other medical problems—The presence of other medical problems may affect the use of this medicine. Make sure you tell your doctor if you have any other medical problems, especially:

- Cysticercosis involving the eye—Patients who are being treated with albendazole for pork tapeworms of the nervous system (neurocysticercosis) should be examined for lesions in the eye; use of albendazole may increase the chance of side effects involving the eye

- Liver disease—Patients with liver disease may have an increased chance of side effects

Proper Use of This Medicine

No special preparations (fasting, laxatives, or enemas) or other steps are necessary before, during, or immediately after treatment with albendazole.

Albendazole is best taken with meals, especially with food containing fat, to help your body absorb the medicine better.

For patients taking the tablet form of albendazole:

- Tablets should be swallowed whole with a small amount of liquid.

To help clear up your infection completely, take this medicine exactly as directed by your doctor for the full time of treatment. In some infections, additional treatments with this medicine may be needed at 2–week intervals to clear up the infection completely. Do not miss any doses.

Dosing—The dose of this medicine will be different for different patients. Follow your doctor's orders or the directions on the label. The following information includes only the average doses of this medicine. If your dose is different, do not change it unless your doctor tells you to do so.

The amount of medicine that you take depends on the strength of the medicine. Also, the number of doses you take each day, the time allowed between doses, and the length of time you take the medicine depend on the medical problem for which you are using the medicine.

- For oral dosage form (tablets):
  - For hydatid disease:
    - Adults, teenagers, and children weighing 60 kilograms (132 pounds) and over—400 milligrams (mg) two times a day for twenty-eight days. Treatment may need to be repeated in fourteen days.

- Adults, teenagers, and children weighing less than 60 kilograms (132 pounds)—15 mg per kilogram (6.8 milligrams per pound) of body weight per day divided into two doses and taken for twenty-eight days. Treatment may need to be repeated in fourteen days.
  - For infections of the nervous system caused by pork tapeworm (neurocysticercosis):
    - Adults, teenagers, and children weighing 60 kilograms (132 pounds) and over—400 milligrams (mg) two times a day for eight to thirty days.
    - For adults, teenagers, and children weighing less than 60 kilograms (132 pounds)—15 mg per kilogram (6.8 mg per pound) of body weight per day divided into two doses and taken for eight to thirty days.

Missed dose—If you miss a dose of this medicine, take it as soon as possible. However, if it is almost time for your next dose, skip the missed dose and go back to your regular dosing schedule. Do not double doses.

Storage—Store the medicine in a closed container at room temperature, away from heat, moisture, and direct light. Keep from freezing.

Keep the bottle closed when you are not using it. Keep it in the refrigerator. Do not freeze.

Keep out of the reach of children.

Do not keep outdated medicine or medicine no longer needed.

Precautions While Using This Medicine

It is important that your doctor check your progress after treatment. This is to make sure that the infection is cleared up completely, and to allow your doctor to check for any unwanted effects.

If your symptoms do not improve after you have taken this medicine for the full course of treatment, or if they become worse, check with your doctor.

For women of childbearing age, it is important that you use birth control while taking albendazole since this medicine can cause birth defects or other problems.

Side Effects of This Medicine

Along with its needed effects, a medicine may cause some unwanted effects. Although not all of these side effects may occur, if they do occur they may need medical attention.

Check with your doctor as soon as possible if any of the following side effects occur:
  Rare
    Fever; skin rash or itching; sore throat; unusual tiredness and weakness

Some side effects may occur that usually do not need medical attention. These side effects may go away during treatment as your body adjusts to the medicine. Also, your health care professional may be able to tell you about ways to prevent or reduce some of these side effects. Check with your health care professional if any of the following side effects continue or are bothersome or if you have any questions about them:

Less common
    Abdominal pain; diarrhea; dizziness; headache; nausea; vomiting
Rare
    Thinning or loss of hair

Other side effects not listed may also occur in some patients. If you notice any other effects, check with your healthcare professional.

ALBUTEROL AND IPRATROPIUM
(Inhalation, oral/nebulization route) - al-BYOO-ter-ol, i-pra-TROE-pee-um

Commonly used brand name(s)
In the U.S.—
    Combivent
    Duoneb

Available Dosage Forms:
- Solution
- Aerosol Powder
- Aerosol Liquid

Therapeutic Class: Bronchodilator
Pharmacologic Class: Ipratropium

Uses For This Medicine

Albuterol and ipratropium combination is a bronchodilator (medicine that opens up narrowed breathing passages). It is taken by inhalation to help control the symptoms of lung diseases, such as asthma, chronic bronchitis, and emphysema.

Albuterol in combination with ipratropium helps decrease coughing, wheezing, shortness of breath, and troubled breathing by increasing the flow of air into the lungs.

This medicine is available only with your doctor's prescription.

Before Using This Medicine

In deciding to use a medicine, the risks of taking the medicine must be weighed against the good it will do. This is a decision you and your doctor will make. For this medicine, the following should be considered:

Allergies—Tell your doctor if you have ever had any unusual or allergic reaction to this medicine or any other medicines. Also tell your health care professional if you have any other types of allergies, such as to foods, dyes, preservatives, or animals. For non-prescription products, read the label or package ingredients carefully.

Pediatric—Studies comparing the effects of the inhalation aerosol dosage form of ipratropium and albuterol in children with those in other age groups have not been done.

Geriatric—Albuterol and ipratropium combination has been tested in elderly patients and has not been found to cause different side effects or problems in older people than it does in younger adults.

Other medicines—

Using this medicine with any of the following medicines is usually not recommended, but may be required in some cases. If both medicines are prescribed together, your doctor

may change the dose or how often you use one or both of the medicines.

Atomoxetine, Clorgyline, Iproniazid, Isocarboxazid, Moclobemide, Nialamide, Pargyline, Phenelzine, Procarbazine, Selegiline, Toloxatone, Tranylcypromine

Interactions with Food/Tobacco/Alcohol—Certain medicines should not be used at or around the time of eating food or eating certain types of food since interactions may occur. Using alcohol or tobacco with certain medicines may also cause interactions to occur. Discuss with your healthcare professional the use of your medicine with food, alcohol, or tobacco.

Other medical problems—The presence of other medical problems may affect the use of this medicine. Make sure you tell your doctor if you have any other medical problems, especially:

- Difficult urination—This medicine may make the condition worse
- Glaucoma—This medicine may make the condition worse if it gets into the eyes
- Heart rhythm problems or
- High blood pressure (hypertension) or
- Problems with blood circulation to the heart—The albuterol contained in this combination medicine can cause unwanted effects on the heart in some patients

Proper Use of This Medicine

This medicine usually comes with patient directions. Read them carefully before using this medicine. If you do not understand the directions or you are not sure how to use the inhaler or nebulizer, ask your doctor, nurse, or pharmacist to show you how to use it.

When you use the inhaler for the first time, or if you have not used it for more than 24 hours, the inhaler may not give the right amount of medicine with the first puff. Therefore, before using the inhaler, prime it by spraying the medicine into the air three times. The inhaler will now be ready to give the right amount of medicine when you use it.

When you use the inhalation solution, make sure you use a jet nebulizer that is connected to an air compressor with a good air flow. Use a face mask or mouthpiece to inhale the medicine.

Keep the spray away from the eyes because this medicine may cause irritation or blurred vision. This is especially important for people with glaucoma. Closing your eyes while you are inhaling this medicine may help keep it out of your eyes.

It is very important that you use albuterol and ipratropium combination only as directed. Do not use more of it and do not use it more often than directed. To do so may increase the chance of serious side effects.

Dosing—The dose of this medicine will be different for different patients. Follow your doctor's orders or the directions on the label. The following information includes only the average doses of this medicine. If your dose is different, do not change it unless your doctor tells you to do so.

The amount of medicine that you take depends on the strength of the medicine. Also, the number of doses you take each day, the time allowed between doses, and the length of time you take the medicine depend on the medical problem for which you are using the medicine.

- For inhalation aerosol dosage form:
  - For symptoms of chronic obstructive pulmonary disease:
    - Adults—2 puffs four times a day and as needed. No more than a total of 12 puffs should be used in any twenty-four-hour period.
    - Children—Use and dose must be determined by your doctor.
- For inhalation solution dosage form (used with a nebulizer):
  - For symptoms of chronic obstructive pulmonary disease:
    - Adults—Use one 3 mL (milliliter) vial in the nebulizer 4 times a day. You may have 2 additional treatments per day if needed.
    - Children—Use and dose must be determined by your doctor.

Missed dose—If you miss a dose of this medicine, take it as soon as possible. However, if it is almost time for your next dose, skip the missed dose and go back to your regular dosing schedule. Do not double doses.

Storage—Store the medicine in a closed container at room temperature, away from heat, moisture, and direct light. Keep from freezing.

Keep the medicine in the foil pouch until you are ready to use it. Store at room temperature, away from heat and direct light. Do not freeze.

Keep out of the reach of children.

Do not keep outdated medicine or medicine no longer needed.

Precautions While Using This Medicine

Check with your doctor at once if difficulty in breathing continues after using a dose of this medicine or if your condition gets worse.

Side Effects of This Medicine

Along with its needed effects, a medicine may cause some unwanted effects. Although not all of these side effects may occur, if they do occur they may need medical attention.

Check with your doctor as soon as possible if any of the following side effects occur:
  Rare
    Chest discomfort or pain; fast or irregular heartbeat; shortness of breath or wheezing; skin rash or hives; swelling of the face, lips, eyelids, mouth, or throat

Some side effects may occur that usually do not need medical attention. These side effects may go away during treatment as your body adjusts to the medicine. Also, your health care professional may be able to tell you about ways to prevent or reduce some of these side effects. Check with your health care professional if any of the following side effects continue or are bothersome or if you have any questions about them:
  Less common or rare
    Change in sense of taste; coughing; dizziness; dryness of mouth; headache; nausea; nervousness; tremor

Other side effects not listed may also occur in some patients. If you notice any other effects, check with your healthcare professional.

ALDESLEUKIN (Intravenous route) -
al-des-LOO-kin

Black Box Warning

Therapy with aldesleukin for injection should be restricted to patients with normal cardiac and pulmonary functions as defined by thallium stress testing and formal pulmonary function testing. Extreme caution should be used in patients with a normal thallium stress test and a normal pulmonary function test who have a history of cardiac or pulmonary disease.

Aldesleukin should be administered in a hospital setting under the supervision of a qualified physician experienced in the use of anticancer agents. An intensive care facility and specialists skilled in cardiopulmonary or intensive care medicine must be available.

Aldesleukin administration has been associated with capillary leak syndrome (CLS) which is characterized by a loss of vascular tone and extravasation of plasma proteins and fluid into the extravascular space. CLS results in hypotension and reduced organ perfusion which may be severe and can result in death. CLS may be associated with cardiac arrhythmias (supraventricular and ventricular), angina, myocardial infarction, respiratory insufficiency requiring intubation, gastrointestinal bleeding or infarction, renal insufficiency, edema, and mental status changes.

Aldesleukin treatment is associated with impaired neutrophil function (reduced chemotaxis) and with an increased risk of disseminated infection, including sepsis and bacterial endocarditis. Consequently, preexisting bacterial infections should be adequately treated prior to initiation of aldesleukin therapy. Patients with indwelling central lines are particularly at risk for infection with gram positive microorganisms. Antibiotic prophylaxis with oxacillin, nafcillin, ciprofloxacin, or vancomycin has been associated with a reduced incidence of staphylococcal infections.

Aldesleukin administration should be withheld in patients developing moderate to severe lethargy or somnolence; continued administration may result in coma.

Commonly used brand name(s)

In the U.S.—
  Proleukin

Available Dosage Forms:
  • Powder for Solution

Therapeutic Class: Antineoplastic Agent
Pharmacologic Class: Interleukin

Uses For This Medicine

Aldesleukin is a synthetic (man-made) version of a substance called interleukin-2. Interleukins are produced naturally by cells in the body to help white blood cells work. Aldesleukin is used to treat cancer of the kidney and skin cancer that has spread to other parts of the body.

Aldesleukin causes some other very serious effects in addition to its helpful effects. Some effects can be fatal. For that reason, aldesleukin is given only in the hospital. If severe side effects occur, which is common, treatment in an intensive care unit (ICU) may be necessary. Other effects may not be serious but may cause concern. Before you begin treatment with aldesleukin, you and your doctor should talk about the good this medicine will do as well as the risks of using it.

Aldesleukin is to be administered only by or under the immediate supervision of your doctor.

Before Using This Medicine

In deciding to use a medicine, the risks of taking the medicine must be weighed against the good it will do. This is a decision you and your doctor will make. For this medicine, the following should be considered:

Allergies—Tell your doctor if you have ever had any unusual or allergic reaction to this medicine or any other medicines. Also tell your health care professional if you have any other types of allergies, such as to foods, dyes, preservatives, or animals. For non-prescription products, read the label or package ingredients carefully.

Pediatric—There is no specific information comparing use of aldesleukin in children with use in other age groups.

Geriatric—Many medicines have not been studied specifically in older people. Therefore, it may not be known whether they work exactly the same way they do in younger adults. There is no specific information comparing use of aldesleukin in the elderly with use in other age groups.

Pregnancy—

	Pregnancy Category	Explanation
All Trimesters	C	Animal studies have shown an adverse effect and there are no adequate studies in pregnant women OR no animal studies have been conducted and there are no adequate studies in pregnant women.

Breast Feeding—There are no adequate studies in women for determining infant risk when using this medication during breastfeeding. Weigh the potential benefits against the potential risks before taking this medication while breastfeeding.

Other medicines—

Using this medicine with any of the following medicines is not recommended. Your doctor may decide not to treat you with this medication or change some of the other medicines you take.

Rotavirus Vaccine, Live

Interactions with Food/Tobacco/Alcohol—Certain medicines should not be used at or around the time of eating food or eating certain types of food since interactions may occur. Using alcohol or tobacco with certain medicines may also cause interactions to occur. Discuss with your healthcare professional the use of your medicine with food, alcohol, or tobacco.

Other medical problems—The presence of other medical problems may affect the use of this medicine. Make sure you tell your doctor if you have any other medical problems, especially:

- Chickenpox (including recent exposure) or
- Herpes zoster (shingles)—Risk of severe disease affecting other parts of the body
- Heart disease or
- Immune system problems or
- Liver disease or
- Lung disease or
- Psoriasis or
- Underactive thyroid—May be worsened by aldesleukin
- Infection—Aldesleukin may decrease your body's ability to fight infection
- Kidney disease—Effects of aldesleukin may be increased because of slower removal from the body
- Mental problems—Aldesleukin may make them worse
- Seizures (history of)—Aldesleukin can cause seizures

Proper Use of This Medicine

Dosing—The dose of this medicine will be different for different patients. Follow your doctor's orders or the directions on the label. The following information includes only the average doses of this medicine. If your dose is different, do not change it unless your doctor tells you to do so.

The amount of medicine that you take depends on the strength of the medicine. Also, the number of doses you take each day, the time allowed between doses, and the length of time you take the medicine depend on the medical problem for which you are using the medicine.

Precautions While Using This Medicine

Aldesleukin can temporarily affect the white blood cells in your blood, increasing the chance of getting an infection. It can also lower the number of platelets, which are necessary for proper blood clotting. If this occurs, there are certain precautions you can take, especially when your blood count is low, to reduce the risk of infection or bleeding:

- If you can, avoid people with infections. Check with your doctor immediately if you think you are getting an infection or if you get a fever or chills, cough or hoarseness, lower back or side pain, or painful or difficult urination.
- Check with your doctor immediately if you notice any unusual bleeding or bruising; black, tarry stools; blood in urine or stools; or pinpoint red spots on your skin.
- Be careful when using a regular toothbrush, dental floss, or toothpick. Your medical doctor, dentist, or nurse may recommend other ways to clean your teeth and gums. Check with your medical doctor before having any dental work done.
- Do not touch your eyes or the inside of your nose unless you have just washed your hands and have not touched anything else in the meantime.
- Be careful not to cut yourself when you are using sharp objects such as a safety razor or fingernail or toenail cutters.
- Avoid contact sports or other situations where bruising or injury could occur.

Side Effects of This Medicine

Along with its needed effects, a medicine may cause some unwanted effects. Some side effects will have signs or symptoms that you can see or feel. Your doctor may watch for others by doing certain tests.

Check with your doctor immediately if any of the following side effects occur:
  More common
    Fever or chills; shortness of breath

  Less common
    Black, tarry stools; blisters on skin; blood in urine; bloody vomit; chest pain; cough or hoarseness; lower back or side pain; painful or difficult urination; pinpoint red spots on skin; stomach pain (severe); unusual bleeding or bruising

Check with your doctor as soon as possible if any of the following side effects occur:
  More common
    Agitation; confusion; diarrhea; dizziness; drowsiness; mental depression; nausea and vomiting; sores in mouth and on lips; tingling of hands or feet; unusual decrease in urination; unusual tiredness; weight gain of 5 to 10 pounds or more

  Less common
    Bloating and stomach pain; blurred or double vision; faintness; fast or irregular heartbeat; loss of taste; rapid breathing; redness, swelling, and soreness of tongue; trouble in speaking; yellow eyes and skin

  Rare
    Changes in menstrual periods; clumsiness; coldness; convulsions (seizures); listlessness; muscle aches; pain or redness at site of injection; sudden inability to move; swelling in the front of the neck; swelling of feet or lower legs; weakness

This medicine may also cause the following side effects that your doctor will watch for:
  More common
    Anemia; heart problems; kidney problems; liver problems; low blood pressure; low platelet counts in blood; low white blood cell counts; other blood problems; underactive thyroid

Some side effects may occur that usually do not need medical attention. These side effects may go away during treatment as your body adjusts to the medicine. Also, your health care professional may be able to tell you about ways to prevent or reduce some of these side effects. Check with your health care professional if any of the following side effects continue or are bothersome or if you have any questions about them:
  More common
    Dry skin; loss of appetite; skin rash or redness with burning or itching, followed by peeling; unusual feeling of discomfort or illness

  Less common
    Constipation; headache; joint pain; muscle pain

Other side effects not listed may also occur in some patients. If you notice any other effects, check with your healthcare professional.

ALEFACEPT (Intravenous route, Intramuscular route) - a-LE-fa-sept

Commonly used brand name(s)

In the U.S.—
Amevive

Available Dosage Forms:
- Powder for Solution

Therapeutic Class: Immune Suppressant

Uses For This Medicine

Alefacept is used in adult patients to treat moderate to severe psoriasis. This medicine is for patients who have used other medicines that have not worked for their psoriasis.

This medicine is available only with your doctor's prescription.

Before Using This Medicine

In deciding to use a medicine, the risks of taking the medicine must be weighed against the good it will do. This is a decision you and your doctor will make. For this medicine, the following should be considered:

Allergies—Tell your doctor if you have ever had any unusual or allergic reaction to this medicine or any other medicines. Also tell your health care professional if you have any other types of allergies, such as to foods, dyes, preservatives, or animals. For non-prescription products, read the label or package ingredients carefully.

Pediatric—Studies on this medicine have been done only in adult patients, and there is no specific information comparing the use of alefacept in children with use in other age groups.

Geriatric—Many medicines have not been studied specifically in older people and it may not be known if they work the same way they do in younger adults. Elderly people may have more age related problems than younger people and may need less of this medicine.

Pregnancy—

	Pregnancy Category	Explanation
All Trimesters	B	Animal studies have revealed no evidence of harm to the fetus, however, there are no adequate studies in pregnant women OR animal studies have shown an adverse effect, but adequate studies in pregnant women have failed to demonstrate a risk to the fetus.

Breast Feeding—There are no adequate studies in women for determining infant risk when using this medication during breastfeeding. Weigh the potential benefits against the potential risks before taking this medication while breastfeeding.

Other medicines—Although certain medicines should not be used together at all, in other cases two different medicines may be used together even if an interaction might occur. In these cases, your doctor may want to change the dose, or other precautions may be necessary. Tell your healthcare professional if you are taking any other prescription or non-prescription (over-the-counter [OTC]) medicine.

Interactions with Food/Tobacco/Alcohol—Certain medicines should not be used at or around the time of eating food or eating certain types of food since interactions may occur. Using alcohol or tobacco with certain medicines may also cause interactions to occur. Discuss with your healthcare professional the use of your medicine with food, alcohol, or tobacco.

Other medical problems—The presence of other medical problems may affect the use of this medicine. Make sure you tell your doctor if you have any other medical problems, especially:
- Human immunodeficiency virus (HIV) infection—This medicine should not be used in patients who have HIV infection.
- Infection, moderate to severe—Alefacept could make your infections worse; your doctor may want to stop this medicine if you get an infection.
- Lymphopenia (small amount of white blood cells)—This medicine could make this condition worse; your doctor may want to stop this medicine if your white blood cell counts are too low.
- Cancer, history of—This medicine should not be used in patients with a history of cancer and it should be used with caution in patients at risk for cancer.

Proper Use of This Medicine

Dosing—The dose of this medicine will be different for different patients. Follow your doctor's orders or the directions on the label. The following information includes only the average doses of this medicine. If your dose is different, do not change it unless your doctor tells you to do so.

The amount of medicine that you take depends on the strength of the medicine. Also, the number of doses you take each day, the time allowed between doses, and the length of time you take the medicine depend on the medical problem for which you are using the medicine.
- For parenteral dosage form
  - Psoriasis
    - Adults—15 milligrams (mg) injected into a muscle once a week for 12 weeks OR 7.5 milligrams (mg) injected into a vein once a week for 12 weeks
    - Children—Use and dose must be determined by your doctor.

Missed dose—If you miss a dose of this medicine, take it as soon as possible. However, if it is almost time for your next dose, skip the missed dose and go back to your regular dosing schedule. Do not double doses.

Storage—Store the medicine in a closed container at room temperature, away from heat, moisture, and direct light. Keep from freezing.

Keep out of the reach of children.

Do not keep outdated medicine or medicine no longer needed.

Ask your healthcare professional how you should dispose of any medicine you do not use.

Precautions While Using This Medicine

It is very important that your doctor check you at regular visits for any blood problems or any other side effects that may be caused by this medicine.

It is important to check with your doctor if you have any symptoms of an infection such as fever or chills, cough or hoarseness, lower back or side pain, painful or difficult urination. If your symptoms do not improve within a few days or if they become worse, check with your doctor.

You should contact your doctor right away if you develop persistent nausea, anorexia, fatigue, vomiting, abdominal pain, jaundice (yellow eyes and/or skin), easy bruising, dark urine, or pale stools.

It is important to tell your doctor if you become pregnant. Your doctor may want you join a pregnancy registry for patients taking this medicine.

Side Effects of This Medicine

Along with its needed effects, a medicine may cause some unwanted effects. Although not all of these side effects may occur, if they do occur they may need medical attention.

Check with your doctor immediately if any of the following side effects occur:

More common
    Chills; cough; fever; hoarseness; lower back or side pain; painful or difficult urination

Less common
    Body aches or pain; congestion; dryness or soreness of throat; infections, serious; runny nose; tender, swollen glands in neck; trouble in swallowing; voice changes

Rare
    Arm, back or jaw pain; cardiovascular events; chest pain or discomfort; chest tightness or heaviness; fast or irregular heartbeat; nausea; pain or discomfort in arms, jaw, back or neck; shortness of breath; sweating; vomiting

Some side effects may occur that usually do not need medical attention. These side effects may go away during treatment as your body adjusts to the medicine. Also, your health care professional may be able to tell you about ways to prevent or reduce some of these side effects. Check with your health care professional if any of the following side effects continue or are bothersome or if you have any questions about them:

More common
    Injection site reactions, including pain, swelling, bleeding, skin rash or lumps

Less common
    Difficulty in moving; dizziness; itching skin; joint pain; muscle aching or cramping; muscle pains or stiffness; swollen joints

Rare
    Headache

Other side effects not listed may also occur in some patients. If you notice any other effects, check with your healthcare professional.

ALENDRONATE (Oral route) - a-LEN-droe-nate

Commonly used brand name(s)

In the U.S.—
    Fosamax

Available Dosage Forms:
  • Tablet
  • Solution

Therapeutic Class: Calcium Regulator

Uses For This Medicine

Alendronate is used to prevent or treat osteoporosis (thinning of the bone) in women after menopause and to treat osteoporosis in men. It may also be used to treat Paget's disease of bone and osteoporosis (thinning of the bone) caused by glucocorticoid treatment.

Alendronate is available only with your doctor's prescription.

Before Using This Medicine

In deciding to use a medicine, the risks of taking the medicine must be weighed against the good it will do. This is a decision you and your doctor will make. For this medicine, the following should be considered:

Allergies—Tell your doctor if you have ever had any unusual or allergic reaction to this medicine or any other medicines. Also tell your health care professional if you have any other types of allergies, such as to foods, dyes, preservatives, or animals. For non-prescription products, read the label or package ingredients carefully.

Pediatric—Studies on this medicine have been done only in adult patients and there is no specific information comparing use of alendronate in children with use in other age groups.

Geriatric—This medicine has been tested and has not been shown to cause different side effects or problems in older people than it does in younger adults.

Pregnancy—

	Pregnancy Category	Explanation
All Trimesters	C	Animal studies have shown an adverse effect and there are no adequate studies in pregnant women OR no animal studies have been conducted and there are no adequate studies in pregnant women.

Breast Feeding—There are no adequate studies in women for determining infant risk when using this medication during breastfeeding. Weigh the potential benefits against the potential risks before taking this medication while breastfeeding.

Other medicines—Although certain medicines should not be used together at all, in other cases two different medicines may be used together even if an interaction might occur. In these cases, your doctor may want to change the dose, or other precautions may be necessary. Tell your healthcare

professional if you are taking any other prescription or non-prescription (over-the-counter [OTC]) medicine.

Interactions with Food/Tobacco/Alcohol—Certain medicines should not be used at or around the time of eating food or eating certain types of food since interactions may occur. Using alcohol or tobacco with certain medicines may also cause interactions to occur. The following interactions have been selected on the basis of their potential significance and are not necessarily all-inclusive.

Using this medicine with any of the following may cause an increased risk of certain side effects but may be unavoidable in some cases. If used together, your doctor may change the dose or how often you use this medicine, or give you special instructions about the use of food, alcohol, or tobacco.

Dairy Food

Other medical problems—The presence of other medical problems may affect the use of this medicine. Make sure you tell your doctor if you have any other medical problems, especially:

- Digestion problems—Taking alendronate may be harmful to the esophagus, intestine, or stomach
- Esophagus problems or
- Intestine problems or
- Stomach problems—Alendronate may make these conditions worse
- Kidney problems—The effects of alendronate may be increased

Proper Use of This Medicine

Make certain your health care professional knows if you are on any special diet, such as a low-sodium or low-sugar diet. Your doctor may recommend that you eat a balanced diet with an adequate amount of calcium and vitamin D (found in milk or other dairy products).

Take alendronate with a full glass (6 to 8 ounces) of plain water on an empty stomach. It should be taken in the morning at least 30 minutes before any food, beverage, or other medicines. Food and beverages, such as mineral water, coffee, tea, or juice, will decrease the amount of alendronate absorbed by the body. Waiting longer than 30 minutes will allow more of the drug to be absorbed. Medicines such as antacids or calcium or vitamin supplements will also decrease the absorption of alendronate.

Do not lie down for 30 minutes after taking alendronate. This will help alendronate reach your stomach faster. It will also help prevent irritation to your esophagus.

Your doctor may recommend that you eat a balanced diet with an adequate amount of calcium and vitamin D (found in milk or other dairy products). However, do not take any food, beverages, or calcium or vitamin supplements within 30 minutes of taking alendronate. To do so may keep this medicine from working properly.Waiting longer than 30 minutes will allow more of the drug to be absorbed.

Dosing—The dose of this medicine will be different for different patients. Follow your doctor's orders or the directions on the label. The following information includes only the average doses of this medicine. If your dose is different, do not change it unless your doctor tells you to do so.

The amount of medicine that you take depends on the strength of the medicine. Also, the number of doses you take each day, the time allowed between doses, and the length of time you take the medicine depend on the medical problem for which you are using the medicine.

- For treatment of Paget's disease of bone:
  - Adults—40 milligrams (mg) once a day in the morning, taken at least thirty minutes before the first food, beverage, or medication. You should take alendronate with six to eight ounces of plain water. Your treatment may continue for six months. Your doctor may repeat the treatment.
  - Children—Use and dose must be determined by your doctor.
- For treatment of osteoporosis in men (thinning of bone):
  - Adults—10 mg once a day in the morning, taken at least thirty minutes before the first food, beverage, or medication. You should take alendronate with six to eight ounces of plain water.
- For treatment of postmenopausal osteoporosis (thinning of bone):
  - Adults—10 mg once a day in the morning or 70 mg once a week, taken at least thirty minutes before the first food, beverage, or medication. You should take alendronate with six to eight ounces of plain water.
- For prevention of postmenopausal osteoporosis (thinning of bone):
  - Adults—5 mg once a day in the morning or 35 mg once a week, taken at least thirty minutes before the first food, beverage, or medication. You should take alendronate with six to eight ounces of plain water.
- For treatment of osteoporosis (thinning of bone) caused by glucocorticoid treatment:
  - Adults—5 mg once a day in the morning, taken at least thirty minutes before the first food, beverage, or medication. In postmenopausal women not receiving estrogen, the dose is 10 mg once a day in the morning, taken at least thirty minutes before the first food, beverage, or medication. You should take alendronate with six to eight ounces of plain water.

Missed dose—If you miss a dose of this medicine, skip the missed dose and go back to your regular dosing schedule. Do not double doses.

Storage—Store the medicine in a closed container at room temperature, away from heat, moisture, and direct light. Do not refrigerate. Keep from freezing.

Keep out of the reach of children.

Do not keep outdated medicine or medicine no longer needed.

Side Effects of This Medicine

Along with its needed effects, a medicine may cause some unwanted effects. Although not all of these side effects may occur, if they do occur they may need medical attention.

Check with your doctor as soon as possible if any of the following side effects occur:

More common
 Abdominal pain
Less common
 Difficulty in swallowing; heartburn; irritation or pain of the esophagus; muscle pain

Rare
    Skin rash

Some side effects may occur that usually do not need medical attention. These side effects may go away during treatment as your body adjusts to the medicine. Also, your health care professional may be able to tell you about ways to prevent or reduce some of these side effects. Check with your health care professional if any of the following side effects continue or are bothersome or if you have any questions about them:
Less common
    Constipation; diarrhea; full or bloated feeling; gas; headache; nausea

Other side effects not listed may also occur in some patients. If you notice any other effects, check with your healthcare professional.

ALFUZOSIN (Oral route) - al-FYOO-zoe-sin

Commonly used brand name(s)
In the U.S.—
    Uroxatral

Available Dosage Forms:
• Tablet, Extended Release

Therapeutic Class: Benign Prostatic Hypertrophy Agent
Pharmacologic Class: Alpha-1 Adrenergic Blocker

Uses For This Medicine

Alfuzosin is used to treat the signs and symptoms of benign enlargement of the prostate (benign prostatic hyperplasia or BPH). Benign enlargement of the prostate is a problem that can occur in men as they get older. The prostate gland is located below the bladder. As the prostate gland enlarges, certain muscles in the gland may become tight and get in the way of the tube that drains urine from the bladder. This can cause problems in urinating, such as a need to urinate often, a weak stream when urinating, or a feeling of not being able to empty the bladder completely. Alfuzosin helps relax the muscles in the prostate and the opening of the bladder. This may help increase the flow of urine and/or decrease the symptoms.

This medicine is available only with your doctor's prescription.

Before Using This Medicine

In deciding to use a medicine, the risks of taking the medicine must be weighed against the good it will do. This is a decision you and your doctor will make. For this medicine, the following should be considered:

Allergies—Tell your doctor if you have ever had any unusual or allergic reaction to this medicine or any other medicines. Also tell your health care professional if you have any other types of allergies, such as to foods, dyes, preservatives, or animals. For non-prescription products, read the label or package ingredients carefully.

Pregnancy—

	Pregnancy Category	Explanation
All Trimesters	B	Animal studies have revealed no evidence of harm to the fetus, however, there are no adequate studies in pregnant women OR animal studies have shown an adverse effect, but adequate studies in pregnant women have failed to demonstrate a risk to the fetus.

Breast Feeding—There are no adequate studies in women for determining infant risk when using this medication during breastfeeding. Weigh the potential benefits against the potential risks before taking this medication while breastfeeding.

Other medicines—

Using this medicine with any of the following medicines is not recommended. Your doctor may decide not to treat you with this medication or change some of the other medicines you take.

Itraconazole, Ketoconazole, Ritonavir

Interactions with Food/Tobacco/Alcohol—Certain medicines should not be used at or around the time of eating food or eating certain types of food since interactions may occur. Using alcohol or tobacco with certain medicines may also cause interactions to occur. The following interactions have been selected on the basis of their potential significance and are not necessarily all-inclusive.

Using this medicine with any of the following may cause an increased risk of certain side effects but may be unavoidable in some cases. If used together, your doctor may change the dose or how often you use this medicine, or give you special instructions about the use of food, alcohol, or tobacco.

Grapefruit Juice

Other medical problems—The presence of other medical problems may affect the use of this medicine. Make sure you tell your doctor if you have any other medical problems, especially:
• Prostatic carcinoma (cancer of the prostate)—This medical condition may have the same symptoms as your medical condition. Your doctor will want to know because different treatment is need for prostatic carcinoma.
• Liver disease, moderate or severe—Patients with this condition should not use alfuzosin.

Proper Use of This Medicine

This medicine should be taken with food and with the same meal every day.

It is very important to not chew or crush the tablets.

Dosing—The dose of this medicine will be different for different patients. Follow your doctor's orders or the directions on the label. The following information includes only the average doses of this medicine. If your dose is different, do not change it unless your doctor tells you to do so.

The amount of medicine that you take depends on the strength of the medicine. Also, the number of doses you take each day, the time allowed between doses, and the length of time you take the medicine depend on the medical problem for which you are using the medicine.
• For oral dosage form (tablets):
    ◦ Adults—10 milligrams (mg) once a day taken after the same meal each day, tablets should be swallowed whole. Not for use in women.
    ◦ Children—Not for use in children

Missed dose—If you miss a dose of this medicine, take it as soon as possible. However, if it is almost time for your next dose, skip the missed dose and go back to your regular dosing schedule. Do not double doses.

Storage—Store the medicine in a closed container at room temperature, away from heat, moisture, and direct light. Keep from freezing.

Keep out of the reach of children.

Do not keep outdated medicine or medicine no longer needed.

Ask your healthcare professional how you should dispose of any medicine you do not use.

Precautions While Using This Medicine

This medicine may cause some people to become drowsy, dizzy, or less alert than they are normally. Make sure you know how you react to this medicine before you drive, use machines, or do anything else that could be dangerous if you are dizzy or are not alert.

Side Effects of This Medicine

Along with its needed effects, a medicine may cause some unwanted effects. Although not all of these side effects may occur, if they do occur they may need medical attention.

Check with your doctor immediately if any of the following side effects occur:
> *Rare*
>> Chest pain; fast, pounding, or irregular heartbeat or pulse; painful or prolonged erection of the penis

Some side effects may occur that usually do not need medical attention. These side effects may go away during treatment as your body adjusts to the medicine. Also, your health care professional may be able to tell you about ways to prevent or reduce some of these side effects. Check with your health care professional if any of the following side effects continue or are bothersome or if you have any questions about them:
> *More common*
>> Dizziness
>
> *Less common*
>> Abdominal pain; acid or sour stomach; belching; body aches or pain; chills; congestion; cough; cough producing mucus; decreased interest in sexual intercourse; difficulty breathing; difficulty having a bowel movement (stool); dryness or soreness of throat; ear congestion; fever; headache; heartburn; hoarseness; inability to have or keep an erection; indigestion; loss in sexual ability, desire, drive, or performance; loss of voice; nasal congestion; nausea; pain; pain or tenderness around eyes and cheekbones; runny nose; shortness of breath; sneezing; sore throat; stomach discomfort, upset, or pain; stuffy or runny nose; tender, swollen glands in neck; tightness in chest; trouble in swallowing; unusual tiredness or weakness; wheezing; voice changes
>
> *Rare*
>> Rash

Other side effects not listed may also occur in some patients. If you notice any other effects, check with your healthcare professional.

ALITRETINOIN (Topical route) - a-li-TRET-i-noyn

Commonly used brand name(s)

In the U.S.—
> Panretin

Available Dosage Forms:
- Gel/Jelly

Therapeutic Class: Dermatological Agent

Uses For This Medicine

Alitretinoin is used as a topical treatment for cutaneous AIDS-related Kaposi's sarcoma in cases when there is no need for oral or intravenous medication.

This medicine is available only with your doctor's prescription.

Before Using This Medicine

In deciding to use a medicine, the risks of taking the medicine must be weighed against the good it will do. This is a decision you and your doctor will make. For this medicine, the following should be considered:

Allergies—Tell your doctor if you have ever had any unusual or allergic reaction to this medicine or any other medicines. Also tell your health care professional if you have any other types of allergies, such as to foods, dyes, preservatives, or animals. For non-prescription products, read the label or package ingredients carefully.

Pediatric—Studies of this medicine have been done only in adult patients, and there is no specific information comparing the use of alitretinoin in children with use in other age groups.

Geriatric—Many medicines have not been studied specifically in older people. Therefore, it may not be known whether they work exactly the same way they do in younger adults or if they cause different side effects or problems in older people. There is no specific information comparing the use of alitretinoin in the elderly with use in other age groups.

Other medicines—Although certain medicines should not be used together at all, in other cases two different medicines may be used together even if an interaction might occur. In these cases, your doctor may want to change the dose, or other precautions may be necessary. Tell your healthcare professional if you are taking any other prescription or non-prescription (over-the-counter [OTC]) medicine.

Interactions with Food/Tobacco/Alcohol—Certain medicines should not be used at or around the time of eating food or eating certain types of food since interactions may occur. Using alcohol or tobacco with certain medicines may also cause interactions to occur. Discuss with your healthcare professional the use of your medicine with food, alcohol, or tobacco.

Other medical problems—The presence of other medical problems may affect the use of this medicine. Make sure you tell your doctor if you have any other medical problems, especially:
- Cutaneous T-cell lymphoma—May be more likely to experience side effects of alitretinoin gel.

Proper Use of This Medicine

Avoid the use of occlusive dressings

Dosing—The dose of this medicine will be different for different patients. Follow your doctor's orders or the directions on the label. The following information includes only the average doses of this medicine. If your dose is different, do not change it unless your doctor tells you to do so.

The amount of medicine that you take depends on the strength of the medicine. Also, the number of doses you take each day, the time allowed between doses, and the length of time you take the medicine depend on the medical problem for which you are using the medicine.

- For topical dosage form (gel):
  - For cutaneous Kaposi's sarcoma:
    - Adults—Apply a generous amount to the affected area of the skin two times day, or as directed by your doctor, and allow to dry for three to five minutes before covering with clothing.
    - Children—Use and dose must be determined by your doctor.

Missed dose—If you miss a dose of this medicine, take it as soon as possible. However, if it is almost time for your next dose, skip the missed dose and go back to your regular dosing schedule. Do not double doses.

Storage—Store the medicine in a closed container at room temperature, away from heat, moisture, and direct light. Keep from freezing.

Keep out of the reach of children.

Do not keep outdated medicine or medicine no longer needed.

Precautions While Using This Medicine

It is very important that your doctor check your progress at regular visits to make sure that this medicine is working properly and to check for unwanted effects.

This medicine increases the sensitivity of the treated areas of your skin to sunlight or sun lamps. Therefore, exposure to the sun, even through window glass or on a cloudy day, could cause a serious burn.

Avoid application of the gel to normal skin surrounding the lesions or to mucous membranes

Side Effects of This Medicine

Along with its needed effects, a medicine may cause some unwanted effects. Although not all of these side effects may occur, if they do occur they may need medical attention.

Check with your doctor as soon as possible if any of the following side effects occur:

More common
Abrasion of skin; blisters on skin; burning pain; cracking, crusting, drainage, or oozing of the skin; groove in the skin; peeling of skin; severe rash; skin redness; sloughing of skin; swelling at the site of application

Less common
Stinging or tingling of skin

Some side effects may occur that usually do not need medical attention. These side effects may go away during treatment as your body adjusts to the medicine. Also, your health care professional may be able to tell you about ways to prevent or reduce some of these side effects. Check with your health care professional if any of the following side effects continue or are bothersome or if you have any questions about them:

More common
Itching; rash

Less common
Increased sensitivity to the sun

Other side effects not listed may also occur in some patients. If you notice any other effects, check with your healthcare professional.

ALOSETRON (Oral route) - a-LOE-se-tron

Black Box Warning

Infrequent but serious gastrointestinal adverse events have been reported with the use of alosetron hydrochloride. These events, including ischemic colitis and serious complications of constipation, have resulted in hospitalization, and rarely, blood transfusion, surgery, and death.

The Prescribing Program for LOTRONEX® was implemented to help reduce risks of serious gastrointestinal adverse events. Only physicians who have enrolled in GlaxoSmith-Kline's Prescribing Program for LOTRONEX®, based on their understanding of the benefits and risks, should prescribe Lotronex®

Alosetron hydrochloride is indicated only for women with severe diarrhea-predominant irritable bowel syndrome (IBS) who have not responded adequately to conventional therapy. Before receiving the initial prescription for alosetron hydrochloride, the patient must read and sign the Patient-Physician Agreement for alosetron hydrochloride.

Alosetron hydrochloride should be discontinued immediately in patients who develop constipation or symptoms of ischemic colitis. Patients should immediately report constipation or symptoms of ischemic colitis to their physician. Alosetron hydrochloride should not be resumed in patients who develop ischemic colitis. Patients who have constipation should immediately contact their physician if the constipation does not resolve after alosetron hydrochloride is discontinued. Patients with resolved constipation should resume alosetron hydrochloride only on the advice of their treating physician.

Commonly used brand name(s)

In the U.S.—
Lotronex

Available Dosage Forms:
- Tablet

Therapeutic Class: Antidiarrheal
Pharmacologic Class: Serotonin Receptor Antagonist, 5–HT3

Uses For This Medicine

Alosetron is a medicine used to treat irritable bowel syndrome (IBS) in women who have diarrhea as their main symptom. IBS has been called by many names, including irritable colon and spastic colon. IBS is a medical condition causing cramping abdominal pain, abdominal discomfort, urgency (a sudden need to have a bowel movement), and irregular bowel habits, such as diarrhea and constipation. It is not clear why some people develop IBS. It may be caused by your body's overreaction to a body chemical called serotonin. This overreaction may cause your intestinal system to be overactive. Alosetron works by blocking the action of serotonin on the intestinal system. This reduces the cramping abdominal pain, abdominal discomfort, urgency, and diarrhea caused by IBS. Alosetron does not cure IBS and it may not help every person who takes it.

Alosetron is available through a restricted marketing program. The restricted marketing program is because of serious bowel side effects seen with the use of this medication. Only doctors enrolled in the prescribing program for alosetron can write a prescription.

Before Using This Medicine

In deciding to use a medicine, the risks of taking the medicine must be weighed against the good it will do. This is a decision you and your doctor will make. For this medicine, the following should be considered:

Allergies—Tell your doctor if you have ever had any unusual or allergic reaction to this medicine or any other medicines. Also tell your health care professional if you have any other types of allergies, such as to foods, dyes, preservatives, or animals. For non-prescription products, read the label or package ingredients carefully.

Pediatric—Studies on this medicine have been done only in adult patients, and there is no specific information comparing use of alosetron in children with use in other age groups.

Geriatric—Older adults or adults weak from an illness may be especially sensitive to the effects of alosetron. This may increase the chance of serious constipation problems.

Pregnancy—

	Pregnancy Category	Explanation
All Trimesters	B	Animal studies have revealed no evidence of harm to the fetus, however, there are no adequate studies in pregnant women OR animal studies have shown an adverse effect, but adequate studies in pregnant women have failed to demonstrate a risk to the fetus.

Breast Feeding—There are no adequate studies in women for determining infant risk when using this medication during breastfeeding. Weigh the potential benefits against the potential risks before taking this medication while breastfeeding.

Other medicines—

Using this medicine with any of the following medicines is not recommended. Your doctor may decide not to treat you with this medication or change some of the other medicines you take.

Apomorphine, Fluvoxamine

Interactions with Food/Tobacco/Alcohol—Certain medicines should not be used at or around the time of eating food or eating certain types of food since interactions may occur. Using alcohol or tobacco with certain medicines may also cause interactions to occur. Discuss with your healthcare professional the use of your medicine with food, alcohol, or tobacco.

Other medical problems—The presence of other medical problems may affect the use of this medicine. Make sure you tell your doctor if you have any other medical problems, especially:

- Constipation or
- Crohn's disease (inflammatory bowel disease) or
- Diverticulitis (abnormal pouches in the colon that become inflamed) or
- Excessive blood clotting problems or
- Intestinal blood circulation problems or
- Intestinal adhesions, obstructions, perforations, or strictures (colon blockage) or
- Ischemic colitis (poor blood flow to your colon) or
- Severe liver problems or
- Thrombophlebitis or
- Toxic megacolon or
- Ulcerative colitis—This medicine should not be taken if you have any of these conditions. Check with your doctor if you have any of these conditions before you take this medicine.
- Mild or moderate liver problems—May have an increased risk of serious side effects

Proper Use of This Medicine

Read the Medication Guide before starting alosetron for the first time and each time you refill your alosetron prescription.

Your doctor will ask you to sign a Patient-Physician Agreement after you have read the Medication Guide for the first time. Signing the agreement means that you understand the risks and benefits of alosetron therapy and that you have read and understand the Medication Guide.

Do not start taking alosetron if you are constipated.

This medicine may be taken with or without food.

If constipation develops while your are taking alosetron, stop taking alosetron and check with your doctor.

Dosing—The dose of this medicine will be different for different patients. Follow your doctor's orders or the directions on the label. The following information includes only the average doses of this medicine. If your dose is different, do not change it unless your doctor tells you to do so.

The amount of medicine that you take depends on the strength of the medicine. Also, the number of doses you take each day, the time allowed between doses, and the length of time you take the medicine depend on the medical problem for which you are using the medicine.

- For oral dosage form (tablets):
  - For irritable bowel syndrome associated with diarrhea:
    - Adults—0.5 milligram (mg) twice daily for 4 weeks to see how alosetron affects you. Your doctor will decide if you should continue to take alosetron and how much you should take.
    - Children—Use and dose must be determined by your doctor.

Missed dose—If you miss a dose of this medicine, skip the missed dose and go back to your regular dosing schedule. Do not double doses.

Storage—Store the medicine in a closed container at room temperature, away from heat, moisture, and direct light. Keep from freezing.

Keep out of the reach of children.

Do not keep outdated medicine or medicine no longer needed.

Ask your healthcare professional how you should dispose of any medicine you do not use.

Precautions While Using This Medicine

It is very important that your doctor check you at regular visits.

Stop taking alosetron and check with your doctor right away if you become constipated or have symptoms of poor blood flow to your intestines (ischemic colitis), such as new or worsening abdominal pain, bloody diarrhea, or blood in the stool.

Check with your doctor again if the constipation does not resolve after stopping alosetron.

Do not start taking alosetron again unless your doctor tells you to do so.

Stop taking alosetron and check with your doctor if alosetron does not adequately control irritable bowel syndrome (IBS) symptoms after 4 weeks of taking alosetron.

Side Effects of This Medicine

Along with its needed effects, a medicine may cause some unwanted effects. Although not all of these side effects may occur, if they do occur they may need medical attention.

Check with your doctor immediately if any of the following side effects occur:
> *More common*
>> Constipation
> *Rare*
>> Bloody diarrhea; new or worsening stomach pain or discomfort; rectal bleeding
> *Frequency not determined*
>> Abdominal or stomach pain, cramping, or burning; black, tarry stools; diarrhea; fever; heartburn; indigestion; nausea; vomiting with or without blood or material that looks like coffee grounds

Get emergency help immediately if any of the following symptoms of overdose occur:
> *Symptoms of overdose*
>> Clumsiness, unsteadiness, trembling, or other problems with muscle control or coordination; convulsions (seizures); difficulty breathing; shakiness and unsteady walk; withdrawn or socially detached behavior

Some side effects may occur that usually do not need medical attention. These side effects may go away during treatment as your body adjusts to the medicine. Also, your health care professional may be able to tell you about ways to prevent or reduce some of these side effects. Check with your health care professional if any of the following side effects continue or are bothersome or if you have any questions about them:
> *Less common or rare*
>> Bleeding after defecation; full or bloated feeling; pressure in the stomach; swelling of abdominal or stomach area; uncomfortable swelling around anus
> *Frequency not determined*
>> Headache; skin rash

Other side effects not listed may also occur in some patients. If you notice any other effects, check with your healthcare professional.

ALPROSTADIL   (Intraurethral route, Intravenous route, Intracavernosal route)
- al-PROS-ta-dil

Black Box Warning

Apnea is experienced by about 10% to 12% of neonates with congenital heart defects treated with alprostadil injection. Apnea is most often seen in neonates weighing less than 2 kg at birth and usually appears during the first hour of drug infusion. Therefore, respiratory status should be monitored through out treatment, and alprostadil injection should be used where ventilatory assistance is immediately available.

Commonly used brand name(s)
In the U.S.—
> Caverject
> Edex

> Muse
> Prostin VR Pediatric

In Canada—
> Muse Micro

Available Dosage Forms:
> • Powder for Solution
> • Solution

> • Suppository
> • Kit

Therapeutic Class: Erectile Dysfunction Agent
Pharmacologic Class: Prostaglandin

Uses For This Medicine

Alprostadil belongs to a group of medicines called vasodilators that can increase blood flow by expanding blood vessels. Alprostadil is used to produce erections in some men who need treatment for erectile dysfunction (sexual impotence). This medicine causes an erection because it increases the blood flow to the penis.

Alprostadil injection should not be used as a sexual aid by men who do not have erectile dysfunction. If the medicine is not used properly, permanent damage to the penis and loss of the ability to have erections could result.

Alprostadil is used alone or with medical tests to help diagnose erectile dysfunction that may be caused by nerve or blood vessel problems in the penis.

Alprostadil is available only with your doctor's prescription.

Before Using This Medicine

In deciding to use a medicine, the risks of taking the medicine must be weighed against the good it will do. This is a decision you and your doctor will make. For this medicine, the following should be considered:

Allergies—Tell your doctor if you have ever had any unusual or allergic reaction to this medicine or any other medicines. Also tell your health care professional if you have any other types of allergies, such as to foods, dyes, preservatives, or animals. For non-prescription products, read the label or package ingredients carefully.

Geriatric—This medicine has been tested and has not been shown to cause different side effects or problems in older people than it does in younger adults.

Pregnancy—

	Pregnancy Category	Explanation
All Trimesters	C	Animal studies have shown an adverse effect and there are no adequate studies in pregnant women OR no animal studies have been conducted and there are no adequate studies in pregnant women.

Breast Feeding—There are no adequate studies in women for determining infant risk when using this medication during breastfeeding. Weigh the potential benefits against the potential risks before taking this medication while breastfeeding.

Other medicines—

Using this medicine with any of the following medicines is usually not recommended, but may be required in some cases. If both medicines are prescribed together, your doctor may change the dose or how often you use one or both of the medicines.

Heparin

Interactions with Food/Tobacco/Alcohol—Certain medicines should not be used at or around the time of eating food or eating certain types of food since interactions may occur. Using alcohol or tobacco with certain medicines may also cause interactions to occur. Discuss with your healthcare professional the use of your medicine with food, alcohol, or tobacco.

Other medical problems—The presence of other medical problems may affect the use of this medicine. Make sure you tell your doctor if you have any other medical problems, especially:

- Abnormal penis, including curved penis and birth defects of the penis—Chance of problems occurring may be increased
- Bleeding problems—Chance of bleeding at the place of injection may be increased
- Infection of penis or
- Red or itchy (inflamed) penis—Conditions may worsen with the use of alprostadil suppositories. Also, local skin problems and minor bleeding from inserting the suppository may occur
- Conditions causing thickened blood or slower blood flow, including leukemia; multiple myeloma (tumors of the bone marrow); polycythemia, sickle cell disease, or thrombocythemia (blood problems) or
- Priapism (history of)—Patients with these conditions have an increased risk of priapism (erection lasting longer than 6 hours) while using alprostadil

Proper Use of This Medicine

Special patient directions come with the suppositories and some of the injection medicines. *Read the directions carefully before using the medicine.*

For the injections—There are several alprostadil products that can be injected. Although the injection method is the same, the mixing procedures are different. *Be sure you know which of these products you will be using and the proper way to mix the injection.*

- One product called Alprostadil for Injection (brand names Caverject and Edex) is available as a powder in an injection bottle (vial). Caverject must be mixed with a solution called Bacteriostatic Water for Injection USP. Edex must be mixed with a solution called Sodium Chloride Injection USP. The solution for mixing comes with your product and may be already loaded into a syringe or contained in another injection bottle (vial).
- Another product is called Alprostadil Injection (brand names Prostin VR Pediatric and Prostin VR). Although the medicine is already in solution, it is much too strong to be injected into the penis. The solution must be mixed (diluted) with another liquid that is sold as a separate prescription, called 0.9% Sodium Chloride Injection USP. In most cases, a pharmacist will make this solution for you, giving you the proper strength that you need. Check with your doctor or pharmacist to make sure the solution has been diluted before using it.

It is important to follow several steps to prepare your alprostadil injection correctly. Before drawing up the medicine into the syringe:

- Wash your hands with soap and water.
- Set the bottles on a clean surface. Wipe the top of the injection bottles with an alcohol swab. Do not wipe the needle. Throw away the alcohol swab.
- You may need to attach the needle to the syringe. Do not take the cap off yet.

How to mix Caverject:

- If the syringe already contains the Bacteriostatic Water for Injection USP, then you need only add the plunger to the syringe. To do this:
  ○ Pick up the rod-like plunger and place it within the barrel of the syringe until it touches the rubber piece. Gently screw the plunger into the rubber piece until it seems secure. Do not use a lot of force.
  ○ Hold the syringe by the barrel (not the plunger) and take the cap off the needle.
  ○ You are now ready to mix the water and the powder. Skip to the directions under the title, "To mix the water and powder."
- If the syringe does not already contain the Bacteriostatic Water for Injection USP, you must withdraw 1 milliliter (mL) of it from the bottle provided. To do this:
  ○ Pick up the syringe and take the cap off the needle. Pull the plunger back to the 1–mL mark on the syringe. This pulls air into the syringe. Insert the needle into rubber top of the bottle while it is upright and inject the 1 mL of air into the bottle.
  ○ Turn the bottle upside down using one hand. Be sure the tip of the needle is covered by solution.
  ○ With your other hand, pull the plunger back slowly to withdraw 1 mL of solution into the syringe. Remove the needle and skip to the directions under the title, "To mix the water and powder."
- To mix the water and powder:
  ○ Insert the needle into the bottle of alprostadil and inject 1 milliliter of Bacteriostatic Water for Injection USP from your syringe into the bottle of alprostadil.
  ○ Remove the needle from the bottle, holding the barrel of the syringe.

- Gently swirl the bottle to mix the powder into the solution, turning it upside down to wet all the powder in the bottle.
- Follow the directions below, "How to draw your dose into the syringe."

How to mix Edex:

- The syringe already contains the Sodium Chloride Injection USP. You need only attach the needle to the syringe and add the plunger. To do this:
  - Remove the needle from its package. Do not remove the needle cap. Gently screw the needle into place on the syringe tip.
  - Pick up the rod-like plunger and place it within the barrel of the syringe until it touches the rubber piece. Gently screw the plunger into the rubber piece until it seems secure. Do not use a lot of force.
  - Hold the syringe by the barrel (not the plunger) and take the cap off the needle.
  - You are now ready to mix the Sodium Chloride Injection USP and the powder.
  - Insert the needle into the bottle of alprostadil and inject 1.2 milliliters of the Sodium Chloride Injection USP from your syringe into the bottle of alprostadil.
  - Remove the needle from the bottle, holding the barrel of the syringe.
  - Gently swirl the bottle to mix the powder into the solution, turning it upside down to wet all the powder in the bottle.
  - Follow the directions below, "How to draw your dose into the syringe."

How to mix Prostin VR or Prostin VR Pediatric:

- You will need to get exact mixing instructions from your doctor or pharmacist if you are given two solutions to be mixed. Follow them carefully, asking the pharmacist or doctor any questions that you might have before injecting the medicine.
- After you or the pharmacist has mixed these solutions, follow the directions below, "How to draw your dose into the syringe."

How to draw your dose into the syringe (for all injection products):

- Check the solution to make sure it is clear. Do not use the mixture if you can see anything solid in the solution or if the solution is cloudy or colored.
- After the alprostadil solution is mixed and the needle is inserted into the alprostadil bottle, turn the bottle with the syringe as a unit upside down in one hand. Be sure the tip of the needle is covered by the solution. With your other hand, pull the plunger back slowly to draw the correct dose of the medicine into the syringe.
- Hold the syringe with the measuring scale at eye level to see that the proper dose is withdrawn and to check for air bubbles. To remove air bubbles, tap gently on the measuring scale of the syringe to move any bubbles to the top of the syringe near the needle.
- If your dose measures too low in the syringe, withdraw more solution from the bottle. If there is too much medicine in the syringe, put some back into the bottle. Then check your dose again.
- Remove the needle from the bottle, holding the barrel of the syringe, not the plunger.

- Place the cover back on the needle. You are now ready to inject your dose. Follow the directions below, "How to give the alprostadil injection."

How to give the alprostadil injection:

- Choose a spot on your penis as directed by your doctor where you will give the injection.
- Clean the injection site with alcohol. Sitting upright or slightly reclined, hold your penis against the side of your thigh so that it cannot move.
- Remove the cover from the needle and hold the needle at a 90–degree angle to the place of injection.
- Insert the needle until almost all of the metal part of the needle is inserted into the penis.
- Do not inject the medicine just under the surface of the skin, at the top or head of the penis, or at the base of the penis near the scrotum or testes. Avoid injecting the medicine into blood vessels that you can see.
- Press the plunger down slowly, taking 5 to 10 seconds to release the dose into the penis.
- The injection is usually not painful. If the injection is very painful or if you notice bruising or swelling at the place of injection, that means you are injecting the medicine under the skin. Stop, withdraw the needle, and reposition it properly before continuing with the injection.
- Remove the needle and recap it.
- After you have completed the injection, put pressure on the place of injection for about 5 minutes or until any bleeding stops. This will prevent bruising. Then massage your penis as instructed by your doctor. This helps the medicine spread to all parts of the penis, so that the medicine will work better.

Choose a different place of injection each time you use the medicine to prevent skin problems. This includes switching the place of injection from the right side of the penis for one injection to the left side for the next injection.

After a single-use injection is mixed, the medicine must be used immediately. Throw away any unused mixture in the syringe. It cannot be stored for a later injection.

Do not reuse your needles.

How to throw away the syringes and bottles safely:

Dispose of your materials properly. *Caverject* comes in a plastic case that can be permanently locked with the red locking device that is included with the packaging. When the case label is removed, you can see a hole in the center of the case. The red locking device can be inserted and, by firmly pressing it down with your thumb, you will permanently lock the case. The locked case is safe to be thrown away.

If you do not have the plastic case or are using *Prostin VR* or *Prostin VR Pediatric* injection, unscrew the needle from the barrel of the syringe. Then bend, break, or cut the needle into two pieces with wire cutters. The pieces can be placed in a heavy plastic container, such as a bleach container, and thrown away. Or you may give them to a health care professional to throw away. If you have any questions about disposing of the syringe and needles, ask your health care professional.

For suppositories—*Before inserting the suppository, you should urinate.* The small amount of urine normally left in your urethra will help dissolve the suppository after it is inserted.

How to insert suppositories:

- Remove the delivery device containing the suppository from the foil. Remove the cap from the applicator stem.
- Stretch your penis upward to extend its length, pressing your penis top and bottom. Gently insert the delivery stem up to its collar into your urethra (located at the top of the penis). If you have pain or a pulling feeling in the penis, withdraw the device and start again.
- Press the button down slowly as far as it will go. This releases the suppository into the urethra. After holding the delivery device within your penis still for 5 seconds, carefully rock the penis and delivery device as a unit from side to side. This helps remove the suppository from the device.
- Remove the delivery device while your penis is upright. Look at the device to make sure that the suppository was completely released.
- Repeat the process if a part of the suppository remains in the device.
- After the suppository is completely released, roll your penis between your hands for 10 seconds. This helps to dissolve the suppository. If you feel any stinging, continue this motion to help stop it.
- Sitting, standing, or walking for 10 minutes while an erection is developing helps increase the blood flow to your penis to gain a proper erection.

How to throw away the suppository delivery device safely:

- Replace the cap on the delivery device. After storing it in the foil, fold and throw away.

For injections or suppositories—This medicine usually begins to work in about 5 to 10 minutes. You should attempt intercourse within 10 to 30 minutes after using the medicine. An erection may continue after ejaculation.

Dosing—The dose of this medicine will be different for different patients. Follow your doctor's orders or the directions on the label. The following information includes only the average doses of this medicine. If your dose is different, do not change it unless your doctor tells you to do so.

The amount of medicine that you take depends on the strength of the medicine. Also, the number of doses you take each day, the time allowed between doses, and the length of time you take the medicine depend on the medical problem for which you are using the medicine.

- For the treatment of erectile dysfunction:
  - For injection dosage form:
    - Adults—1.25 to 60 micrograms (mcg) as a single dose once a day. Your exact dose will be determined by your doctor. Inject this medicine very slowly into your penis as shown to you by your doctor ten to thirty minutes before intercourse. Allow five to ten seconds to completely inject the dose. Do not inject more than one dose within twenty-four hours. Also, do not use this medicine for more than two days in a row or more than three times a week.
  - For suppository dosage form:
    - Adults—125, 250, 500, or 1000 mcg as a single dose once a day. Your exact dose will be determined by your doctor. Insert this medicine into the urethra of your penis as shown to you by your doctor ten to thirty minutes before intercourse. Do

not insert more than two doses within twenty-four hours.

Storage—Store in the refrigerator. Do not freeze.

You may store the suppositories in the refrigerator, but do not freeze them.

Keep out of the reach of children.

Do not keep outdated medicine or medicine no longer needed.

Alprostadil for Injection while in the powder form can be stored at room temperature (between 15 and 25 °C or 59 and 77 °F) for 3 months. After it is mixed, the solution must be used immediately. Suppositories may be stored at room temperature

---

Precautions While Using This Medicine

Do not use alprostadil if you have a penile implant unless advised by doctor.

If using the alprostadil suppository, use a condom when having sexual intercourse with a pregnant female. Although harm to the fetus is unlikely, using a condom will protect the fetus from exposure to this medicine. If a woman can become pregnant, use of contraceptive methods is recommended because the effects of this medicine on early pregnancy are not known.

Use alprostadil exactly as directed by your doctor. Do not use more of it and do not use it more often than your doctor ordered. If too much is used, the erection lasts too long and does not reverse when it should. This condition is called priapism. If the erection is not reversed, the blood supply to the penis may be cut off and permanent damage may occur.

Contact your doctor immediately if the erection lasts longer than 4 hours or if it becomes painful. This may be a sign of priapism and must be treated right away to prevent permanent damage.

If you notice bleeding at the place where you injected the medicine, put pressure on the spot until the bleeding stops. If it doesn't stop within 10 minutes, check with your doctor.

Side Effects of This Medicine

Along with its needed effects, a medicine may cause some unwanted effects. Although not all of these side effects may occur, if they do occur they may need medical attention.

Check with your doctor immediately if any of the following side effects occur:
Rare
  Curving of penis with pain during erection; erection continuing for 4 to 6 hours; erection continuing longer than 6 hours with severe and continuing pain of the penis; swelling in or pain of the testes

Symptoms of too much medicine being absorbed into the body
  Dizziness; faintness; pelvic pain; flu-like symptoms

Some side effects may occur that usually do not need medical attention. These side effects may go away during treatment as your body adjusts to the medicine. Also, your health care professional may be able to tell you about ways to prevent or reduce some of these side effects. Check with your health care professional if any of the following side effects

continue or are bothersome or if you have any questions about them:

More common

Bleeding at place of injection, short-term; mild bleeding or spotting from urethra (suppository only); pain at place of injection; painful erection; stinging of urethra (suppository only)

Rare

Bruising or clotted blood in penis at place of injection, usually caused by an incorrect injection

Female partners may experience itching or stinging of vagina when you first begin using the alprostadil suppository. These side effects may not be caused from the medicine but may result if female partner has not had frequent or recent sexual intercourse.

Other side effects not listed may also occur in some patients. If you notice any other effects, check with your healthcare professional.

ALTRETAMINE   (Oral route) - al-TRET-a-meen

Black Box Warning

Altretamine should only be given under the supervision of a physician experienced in the use of antineoplastic agents.

Peripheral blood counts should be monitored at least monthly, prior to the initiation of each course of altretamine, and as clinically indicated.

Because of the possibility altretamine-related neurotoxicity, neurologic examination should be performed regularly during altretamine administration.

Commonly used brand name(s)

In the U.S.—

Hexalen

Available Dosage Forms:

• Capsule

Therapeutic Class: Antineoplastic Agent

Uses For This Medicine

Altretamine belongs to the group of medicines called antineoplastics. It is used to treat cancer of the ovaries. It may also be used to treat other kinds of cancer, as determined by your doctor.

Altretamine interferes with the growth of cancer cells, which are eventually destroyed. Since the growth of normal body cells may also be affected by altretamine, other effects will also occur. Some of these may be serious and must be reported to your doctor. Other effects may not be serious but may cause concern. Some effects may not occur for months or years after the medicine is used.

Before you begin treatment with altretamine, you and your doctor should talk about the good this medicine will do as well as the risks of using it.

Altretamine is available only with your doctor's prescription.

Once a medicine has been approved for marketing for a certain use, experience may show that it is also useful for other medical problems. Although this use is not included in product labeling, altretamine is used in certain patients with the following medical condition:

• Cancer of the lung

Before Using This Medicine

In deciding to use a medicine, the risks of taking the medicine must be weighed against the good it will do. This is a decision you and your doctor will make. For this medicine, the following should be considered:

Allergies—Tell your doctor if you have ever had any unusual or allergic reaction to this medicine or any other medicines. Also tell your health care professional if you have any other types of allergies, such as to foods, dyes, preservatives, or animals. For non-prescription products, read the label or package ingredients carefully.

Pediatric—There is no specific information comparing use of altretamine in children with use in other age groups.

Geriatric—Many medicines have not been studied specifically in older people. Therefore, it may not be known whether they work exactly the same way they do in younger adults. Although there is no specific information comparing use of altretamine in the elderly with use in other age groups, this medicine is not expected to cause different side effects or problems in older people than it does in younger adults.

Pregnancy—

	Pregnancy Category	Explanation
All Trimesters	D	Studies in pregnant women have demonstrated a risk to the fetus. However, the benefits of therapy in a life threatening situation or a serious disease, may outweigh the potential risk.

Breast Feeding—There are no adequate studies in women for determining infant risk when using this medication during breastfeeding. Weigh the potential benefits against the potential risks before taking this medication while breastfeeding.

Other medicines—

Using this medicine with any of the following medicines is not recommended. Your doctor may decide not to treat you with this medication or change some of the other medicines you take.

Rotavirus Vaccine, Live

Interactions with Food/Tobacco/Alcohol—Certain medicines should not be used at or around the time of eating food or eating certain types of food since interactions may occur. Using alcohol or tobacco with certain medicines may also cause interactions to occur. Discuss with your healthcare professional the use of your medicine with food, alcohol, or tobacco.

Other medical problems—The presence of other medical problems may affect the use of this medicine. Make sure you tell your doctor if you have any other medical problems, especially:

• Chickenpox (including recent exposure) or

• Herpes zoster (shingles)—Risk of severe disease affecting other parts of the body

- Nervous system problems—May be worsened by altretamine
- Infection—Altretamine may decrease your body's ability to fight infection
- Kidney disease—Effects of altretamine may be increased because of slower removal from the body
- Liver disease—Effects may be changed because altretamine is activated and cleared from the body by the liver

Proper Use of This Medicine

This medicine often causes nausea and vomiting. However, it is very important that you continue to receive the medicine even if you begin to feel ill. Taking this medicine after meals will lessen stomach upset. Ask your health care professional for other ways to lessen these effects.

Dosing—The dose of this medicine will be different for different patients. Follow your doctor's orders or the directions on the label. The following information includes only the average doses of this medicine. If your dose is different, do not change it unless your doctor tells you to do so.

The amount of medicine that you take depends on the strength of the medicine. Also, the number of doses you take each day, the time allowed between doses, and the length of time you take the medicine depend on the medical problem for which you are using the medicine.

Missed dose—If you miss a dose of this medicine, take it as soon as possible. However, if it is almost time for your next dose, skip the missed dose and go back to your regular dosing schedule. Do not double doses.

Storage—Store the medicine in a closed container at room temperature, away from heat, moisture, and direct light. Keep from freezing.

Keep out of the reach of children.

Do not keep outdated medicine or medicine no longer needed.

Precautions While Using This Medicine

It is very important that your doctor check your progress at regular visits to make sure that this medicine is working properly and to check for unwanted effects.

While you are being treated with altretamine, and after you stop treatment with it, do not have any immunizations (vaccinations) without your doctor's approval. Altretamine may lower your body's resistance and there is a chance you might get the infection the immunization is meant to prevent. In addition, other persons living in your household should not take oral polio vaccine since there is a chance they could pass the polio virus on to you. Also, avoid persons who have taken oral polio vaccine within the last several months. Do not get close to them and do not stay in the same room with them for very long. If you cannot take these precautions, you should consider wearing a protective face mask that covers the nose and mouth.

Altretamine can temporarily lower the number of white blood cells in your blood, increasing the chance of getting an infection. It can also lower the number of platelets, which are necessary for proper blood clotting. If this occurs, there are certain precautions you can take, especially when your blood count is low, to reduce the risk of infection or bleeding:

- If you can, avoid people with infections. Check with your doctor immediately if you think you are getting an infection or if you get a fever or chills, cough or hoarseness, lower back or side pain, or painful or difficult urination.
- Check with your doctor immediately if you notice any unusual bleeding or bruising; black, tarry stools; blood in urine or stools; or pinpoint red spots on your skin.
- Be careful when using a regular toothbrush, dental floss, or toothpick. Your medical doctor, dentist, or nurse may recommend other ways to clean your teeth and gums. Check with your medical doctor before having any dental work done.
- Do not touch your eyes or the inside of your nose unless you have just washed your hands and have not touched anything else in the meantime.
- Be careful not to cut yourself when you are using sharp objects such as a safety razor or fingernail or toenail cutters.
- Avoid contact sports or other situations where bruising or injury could occur.

Side Effects of This Medicine

Along with its needed effects, a medicine may cause some unwanted effects. Although not all of these side effects may occur, if they do occur they may need medical attention.

Also, because of the way these medicines act on the body, there is a chance that they might cause other unwanted effects that may not occur until months or years after the medicine is used. These delayed effects may include certain types of cancer, such as leukemia. Discuss these possible effects with your doctor.

Check with your doctor immediately if any of the following side effects occur:
> *Less common or rare*
>> Black, tarry stools; blood in urine or stools; cough or hoarseness, accompanied by fever or chills; fever or chills; lower back or side pain, accompanied by fever or chills; painful or difficult urination, accompanied by fever or chills; pinpoint red spots on skin; unusual bleeding or bruising; unusual tiredness

Check with your doctor as soon as possible if any of the following side effects occur:
> *More common*
>> Anxiety; clumsiness; confusion; convulsions (seizures); dizziness; mental depression; numbness in arms or legs; weakness
>
> *Rare*
>> Skin rash or itching

Some side effects may occur that usually do not need medical attention. These side effects may go away during treatment as your body adjusts to the medicine. Also, your health care professional may be able to tell you about ways to prevent or reduce some of these side effects. Check with your health care professional if any of the following side effects continue or are bothersome or if you have any questions about them:
> *More common*
>> Nausea and vomiting
>
> *Less common*
>> Diarrhea; loss of appetite; stomach cramps

Other side effects not listed may also occur in some patients. If you notice any other effects, check with your healthcare professional.

AMANTADINE   (Oral route) - a-MAN-ta-deen

Commonly used brand name(s)

In the U.S.—
  Symmetrel

Available Dosage Forms:
  • Capsule, Liquid Filled
  • Syrup
  • Tablet

Therapeutic Class: Antiparkinsonian
Pharmacologic Class: Anticholinergic

Uses For This Medicine

Amantadine is an antiviral. It is used to prevent or treat certain influenza (flu) infections (type A). It may be given alone or along with flu shots. Amantadine will not work for colds, other types of flu, or other virus infections.

Amantadine also is an antidyskinetic. It is used to treat Parkinson's disease, sometimes called paralysis agitans or shaking palsy. It may be given alone or with other medicines for Parkinson's disease. By improving muscle control and reducing stiffness, this medicine allows more normal movements of the body as the disease symptoms are reduced. Amantadine is also used to treat stiffness and shaking caused by certain medicines used to treat nervous, mental, and emotional conditions.

Amantadine may be used for other conditions as determined by your doctor.

Amantadine is available only with your doctor's prescription.

Once a medicine has been approved for marketing for a certain use, experience may show that it is also useful for other medical problems. Although this use is not included in product labeling, amantadine is used in certain patients with the following medical condition:
  • Unusual tiredness or weakness associated with multiple sclerosis

Before Using This Medicine

In deciding to use a medicine, the risks of taking the medicine must be weighed against the good it will do. This is a decision you and your doctor will make. For this medicine, the following should be considered:

Allergies—Tell your doctor if you have ever had any unusual or allergic reaction to this medicine or any other medicines. Also tell your health care professional if you have any other types of allergies, such as to foods, dyes, preservatives, or animals. For non-prescription products, read the label or package ingredients carefully.

Pediatric—This medicine has been tested in children over 1 year of age and has not been shown to cause different side effects or problems in these children than it does in adults. There is no specific information comparing the use of amantadine in children under 1 year of age with use in other age groups.

Geriatric—Elderly people are especially sensitive to the effects of amantadine. Confusion, difficult urination, blurred vision, constipation, and dry mouth, nose, and throat may be especially likely to occur.

Pregnancy—

	Pregnancy Category	Explanation
All Trimesters	C	Animal studies have shown an adverse effect and there are no adequate studies in pregnant women OR no animal studies have been conducted and there are no adequate studies in pregnant women.

Breast Feeding—There are no adequate studies in women for determining infant risk when using this medication during breastfeeding. Weigh the potential benefits against the potential risks before taking this medication while breastfeeding.

Other medicines—

Using this medicine with any of the following medicines may cause an increased risk of certain side effects, but using both drugs may be the best treatment for you. If both medicines are prescribed together, your doctor may change the dose or how often you use one or both of the medicines.

Betel Nut, Bromperidol, Bupropion, Triamterene

Interactions   with   Food/Tobacco/Alcohol—Certain medicines should not be used at or around the time of eating food or eating certain types of food since interactions may occur. Using alcohol or tobacco with certain medicines may also cause interactions to occur. Discuss with your healthcare professional the use of your medicine with food, alcohol, or tobacco.

Other medical problems—The presence of other medical problems may affect the use of this medicine. Make sure you tell your doctor if you have any other medical problems, especially:
  • Eczema (recurring)—Amantadine may cause or worsen eczema
  • Epilepsy or other seizure disorder (history of)—Amantadine may increase the frequency of convulsions (seizures) in patients with a seizure disorder
  • Heart disease or other circulation problems or
  • Swelling of feet and ankles—Amantadine may increase the chance of swelling of the feet and ankles, and may worsen heart disease or circulation problems
  • Kidney disease—Amantadine is removed from the body by the kidneys; patients with kidney disease will need to receive a lower dose of amantadine
  • Mental or emotional illness—Higher doses of amantadine may cause confusion, hallucinations, and nightmares
  • Substance abuse (drug or alcohol abuse), history of—The chance of side effects from this medicine may be increased

Proper Use of This Medicine

For patients taking amantadine to prevent or treat flu infections:
  • Talk to your doctor about the possibility of getting a flu shot if you have not had one yet.

- This medicine is best taken before exposure, or as soon as possible after exposure, to people who have the flu.
- To help keep yourself from getting the flu, keep taking this medicine for the full time of treatment. Or if you already have the flu, continue taking this medicine for the full time of treatment even if you begin to feel better after a few days. This will help to clear up your infection completely. If you stop taking this medicine too soon, your symptoms may return. This medicine should be taken for at least 2 days after all your flu symptoms have disappeared.
- This medicine works best when there is a constant amount in the blood. To help keep the amount constant, do not miss any doses. Also, it is best to take the doses at evenly spaced times day and night. For example, if you are to take two doses a day, the doses should be spaced about 12 hours apart. If this interferes with your sleep or other daily activities, or if you need help in planning the best times to take your medicine, check with your health care professional.
- If you are using the oral liquid form of amantadine, use a specially marked measuring spoon or other device to measure each dose accurately. The average household teaspoon may not hold the right amount of liquid.

For patients taking amantadine for Parkinson's disease or movement problems caused by certain medicines used to treat nervous, mental, and emotional conditions:

- Take this medicine exactly as directed by your doctor. Do not miss any doses and do not take more medicine than your doctor ordered.
- Improvement in the symptoms of Parkinson's disease usually occurs in about 2 days. However, in some patients this medicine must be taken for up to 2 weeks before full benefit is seen.

Dosing—The dose of this medicine will be different for different patients. Follow your doctor's orders or the directions on the label. The following information includes only the average doses of this medicine. If your dose is different, do not change it unless your doctor tells you to do so.

The amount of medicine that you take depends on the strength of the medicine. Also, the number of doses you take each day, the time allowed between doses, and the length of time you take the medicine depend on the medical problem for which you are using the medicine.

- For oral dosage forms (capsules, syrup, and tablets):
  - For the treatment or prevention of flu:
    - Older adults—100 milligrams once a day.
    - Adults and children 12 years of age and older—200 milligrams once a day, or 100 milligrams two times a day.
    - Children 9 to 12 years of age—100 milligrams two times a day.
    - Children 1 to 9 years of age—Dose is based on body weight and must be determined by the doctor.
    - Children up to 1 year of age—Use and dose must be determined by your doctor
  - For the treatment of Parkinson's disease or movement problems:
    - Older adults—100 milligrams once a day to start. The dose may be increased slowly over time, if needed.

- Adults—100 milligrams one or two times a day. Your doctor may increase this dose, if needed.
- Children—Dose has not been determined.

Missed dose—If you miss a dose of this medicine, take it as soon as possible. However, if it is almost time for your next dose, skip the missed dose and go back to your regular dosing schedule. Do not double doses.

Storage—Store the medicine in a closed container at room temperature, away from heat, moisture, and direct light. Keep from freezing.

Keep the bottle closed when you are not using it. Keep it in the refrigerator. Do not freeze.

Keep out of the reach of children.

Do not keep outdated medicine or medicine no longer needed.

Precautions While Using This Medicine

Drinking alcoholic beverages while taking this medicine may cause increased side effects such as circulation problems, dizziness, lightheadedness, fainting, or confusion. Therefore, do not drink alcoholic beverages while you are taking this medicine.

This medicine may cause some people to become dizzy, confused, or lightheaded, or to have blurred vision or trouble concentrating. Make sure you know how you react to this medicine before you drive, use machines, or do anything else that could be dangerous if you are dizzy or are not alert or able to see well. If these reactions are especially bothersome, check with your doctor.

Getting up suddenly from a lying or sitting position also may be a problem because of the dizziness, lightheadedness, or fainting that may be caused by this medicine. Getting up slowly may help. If this problem continues or gets worse, check with your doctor.

If amantadine causes you to feel very depressed or to have thoughts of suicide, check with your doctor immediately.

Amantadine may cause dryness of the mouth, nose, and throat. For temporary relief of mouth dryness, use sugarless candy or gum, melt bits of ice in your mouth, or use a saliva substitute. However, if your mouth continues to feel dry for more than 2 weeks, check with your doctor or dentist. Continuing dryness of the mouth may increase the chance of dental disease, including tooth decay, gum disease, and fungus infections.

This medicine may cause purplish red, net-like, blotchy spots on the skin. This problem occurs more often in females and usually occurs on the legs and/or feet after this medicine has been taken regularly for a month or more. Although the blotchy spots may remain as long as you are taking this medicine, they usually go away gradually within 2 to 12 weeks after you stop taking the medicine. If you have any questions about this, check with your doctor.

For patients taking amantadine to prevent or treat flu infections:

- If your symptoms do not improve within a few days, if they become worse, or you develop new symptoms, check with your doctor.

For patients taking amantadine for Parkinson's disease or movement problems caused by certain medicines used to treat nervous, mental, and emotional conditions:

- Patients with Parkinson's disease must be careful not to overdo physical activities as their condition improves and body movements become easier since injuries resulting from falls may occur. Such activities must be gradually increased to give your body time to adjust to changing balance, circulation, and coordination.
- Some patients may notice that this medicine gradually loses its effect while they are taking it regularly for a few months. If you notice this, check with your doctor. Your doctor may want to adjust the dose or stop the medicine for a while and then restart it to restore its effect.
- Do not suddenly stop taking this medicine without first checking with your doctor since your Parkinson's disease may get worse very quickly. Your doctor may want you to reduce your dose gradually before stopping the medicine completely.

Side Effects of This Medicine

Along with its needed effects, a medicine may cause some unwanted effects. Although not all of these side effects may occur, if they do occur they may need medical attention.

Check with your doctor immediately if any of the following side effects occur:

Less common
Blurred vision; confusion (especially in elderly patients); difficult urination (especially in elderly patients); fainting; hallucinations (seeing, hearing, or feeling things that are not there); swelling of hands, feet, or lower legs

Rare
Convulsions (seizures); decreased vision or any change in vision; difficulty in coordination; fever, chills, or sore throat; increased blood pressure; increase in body movements; irritation and swelling of the eye; loss of memory; mental depression; severe mood or mental changes; skin rash; slurred speech; thoughts of suicide or attempts at suicide; unexplained shortness of breath

Some side effects may occur that usually do not need medical attention. These side effects may go away during treatment as your body adjusts to the medicine. Also, your health care professional may be able to tell you about ways to prevent or reduce some of these side effects. Check with your health care professional if any of the following side effects continue or are bothersome or if you have any questions about them:

More common
Agitation, anxiety, or nervousness; difficulty concentrating; dizziness or lightheadedness; headache; irritability; loss of appetite; nausea; purplish red, net-like, blotchy spots on skin; trouble in sleeping or nightmares

Less common or rare
Constipation; decrease in sexual desire; diarrhea; drowsiness; dryness of the mouth, nose, and throat; false sense of well-being; headache; vomiting; unusual tiredness or weakness

Other side effects not listed may also occur in some patients. If you notice any other effects, check with your healthcare professional.

AMIFOSTINE (Intravenous route) - am-i-FOS-teen

Commonly used brand name(s)
In the U.S.—
Ethyol

Available Dosage Forms:
- Powder for Solution

Therapeutic Class: Cytoprotective Agent

Uses For This Medicine

Amifostine is used to help prevent or lessen some side effects caused by other medicines or radiation therapy that are used to treat cancer.

This medicine is available only with your doctor's prescription.

Once a medicine has been approved for marketing for a certain use, experience may show that it is also useful for other medical problems. Although this use is not included in the product labeling, amifostine is used in certain patients with the following medical conditions:
- Mucositis in patients receiving radiation therapy or radiation combined with chemotherapy
- Myelodysplastic syndromes

Before Using This Medicine

In deciding to use a medicine, the risks of taking the medicine must be weighed against the good it will do. This is a decision you and your doctor will make. For this medicine, the following should be considered:

Allergies—Tell your doctor if you have ever had any unusual or allergic reaction to this medicine or any other medicines. Also tell your health care professional if you have any other types of allergies, such as to foods, dyes, preservatives, or animals. For non-prescription products, read the label or package ingredients carefully.

Pediatric—Although this medicine has been given to a limited number of children, there is no specific information comparing use of amifostine in children with use in other age groups.

Geriatric—Many medicines have not been studied specifically in older people. Therefore, it may not be known whether they work exactly the same way they do in younger adults or if they cause different side effects or problems in older people. Although amifostine has been given to a limited number of elderly people, there is no specific information comparing use of amifostine in the elderly with use in other age groups.

Pregnancy—

	Pregnancy Category	Explanation
All Trimesters	C	Animal studies have shown an adverse effect and there are no adequate studies in pregnant women OR no animal studies have been conducted and there are no adequate studies in pregnant women.

Breast Feeding—There are no adequate studies in women for determining infant risk when using this medication during

breastfeeding. Weigh the potential benefits against the potential risks before taking this medication while breastfeeding.

Other medicines—Although certain medicines should not be used together at all, in other cases two different medicines may be used together even if an interaction might occur. In these cases, your doctor may want to change the dose, or other precautions may be necessary. Tell your healthcare professional if you are taking any other prescription or non-prescription (over-the-counter [OTC]) medicine.

Interactions with Food/Tobacco/Alcohol—Certain medicines should not be used at or around the time of eating food or eating certain types of food since interactions may occur. Using alcohol or tobacco with certain medicines may also cause interactions to occur. Discuss with your healthcare professional the use of your medicine with food, alcohol, or tobacco.

Other medical problems—The presence of other medical problems may affect the use of this medicine. Make sure you tell your doctor if you have any other medical problems, especially:

- Dehydration or
- Heart or blood vessel disease or
- Low blood pressure or
- Nausea, history of, or
- Vomiting, history of, or
- Stroke (history of) or
- Transient ischemic attacks (sometimes called TIAs or "ministrokes"), history of—Some of amifostine's side effects can cause harm to patients with these conditions
- Kidney disease—The chance of low blood calcium may be increased in people with some forms of kidney disease

Proper Use of This Medicine

Dosing—The dose of this medicine will be different for different patients. Follow your doctor's orders or the directions on the label. The following information includes only the average doses of this medicine. If your dose is different, do not change it unless your doctor tells you to do so.

The amount of medicine that you take depends on the strength of the medicine. Also, the number of doses you take each day, the time allowed between doses, and the length of time you take the medicine depend on the medical problem for which you are using the medicine.

- For parenteral dosage form (injection):
  ○ For preventing or lessening side effects caused by medicines used to treat cancer:
    ▪ Adults—910 milligrams (mg) for each square meter of body surface area, injected into a vein starting 30 minutes before the cancer medicine.
    ▪ Children—Use and dose will have to be determined by the doctor.
  ○ For preventing or lessening side effects caused by radiation therapy used to treat cancer:
    ▪ Adults—200 milligrams (mg) for each square meter of body surface area, injected into a vein starting 15 to 30 minutes before the radiation treatment.
    ▪ Children—Use and dose will have to be determined by the doctor.

Side Effects of This Medicine

Along with its needed effects, a medicine may cause some unwanted effects. Although not all of these side effects may occur, if they do occur they may need medical attention.

Check with your doctor immediately if any of the following side effects occur:
More common
Blurred vision; confusion; dizziness, faintness, or lightheadedness when getting up from a lying or sitting position suddenly; fainting or loss of consciousness; fast or irregular breathing; itching; nausea and vomiting; red, scaly, swollen, or peeling areas of skin; swelling of eyes or eyelids; trouble in breathing; tightness in chest; wheezing; skin rash; sweating; unusual tiredness or weakness
Rare
Burning or tingling sensation; convulsions; fast, slow or irregular heartbeat or pulse; loss of bladder control; muscle cramps; muscle spasm or jerking of all extremities; palpitations

Some side effects may occur that usually do not need medical attention. These side effects may go away during treatment as your body adjusts to the medicine. Also, your health care professional may be able to tell you about ways to prevent or reduce some of these side effects. Check with your health care professional if any of the following side effects continue or are bothersome or if you have any questions about them:
Less common or rare
fever; headache; nervousness; pounding in the ears; sleepiness (severe)

Other side effects that sometimes occur are harmless and will go away without treatment. These are:
Less common or rare
Feeling unusually warm or cold; flushing or redness of face or neck; hiccups

Other side effects not listed may also occur in some patients. If you notice any other effects, check with your healthcare professional.

AMINOGLYCOSIDES (Systemic)

Some commonly used brand names are:

In the U.S.—

Amikin (1)	Kantrex (3)
Garamycin (2)	Nebcin (7)
G-Mycin (2)	Netromycin (5)
Jenamicin (2)	

In Canada—

Amikin (1)	Nebcin (7)
Garamycin (2)	Netromycin (5)

The information applies to the following medicines:

1. Amikacin (am-i-KAY-sin)
2. Gentamicin (jen-ta-MYE-sin)
3. Kanamycin (kan-a-MYE-sin)
4. Neomycin (nee-oh-MYE-sin)
5. Netilmicin (ne-til-MYE-sin)
6. Streptomycin (strep-toe-MYE-sin)
7. Tobramycin (toe-bra-MYE-sin)

Category

- **Antibacterial, antimycobacterial**—Streptomycin
- **Antibacterial, systemic**—Amikacin; Gentamicin; Kanamycin; Netilmicin; Streptomycin; Tobramycin

Description

Aminoglycosides (a-mee-noe-GLYE-koe-sides) are used to treat serious bacterial infections. They work by killing bacteria or preventing their growth.

Aminoglycosides are given by injection to treat serious bacterial infections in many different parts of the body. In addition, some aminoglycosides may be given by irrigation (applying a solution of the medicine to the skin or mucous membranes or washing out a body cavity) or by inhalation into the lungs. Streptomycin may also be given for tuberculosis (TB). These medicines may be given with 1 or more other medicines for bacterial infections, or they may be given alone. Aminoglycosides may also be used for other conditions as determined by your doctor. However, aminoglycosides will not work for colds, flu, or other virus infections.

Aminoglycosides given by injection are usually used for serious bacterial infections for which other medicines may not work. However, aminoglycosides may also cause some serious side effects, including damage to your hearing, sense of balance, and kidneys. These side effects may be more likely to occur in elderly patients and newborn infants. *You and your doctor should talk about the good these medicines may do as well as the risks of receiving them.*

Aminoglycosides are to be administered only by or under the immediate supervision of your doctor. They are available in the following dosage forms:

Inhalation
- Amikacin
  - Inhalation solution
- Gentamicin
  - Inhalation solution
- Kanamycin
  - Inhalation solution
- Tobramycin
  - Inhalation solution

Irrigation
- Kanamycin
  - Irrigation solution

Parenteral
- Amikacin
  - Injection
- Gentamicin
  - Injection
- Kanamycin
  - Injection
- Neomycin
  - Injection
- Netilmicin
  - Injection
- Streptomycin
  - Injection
- Tobramycin
  - Injection

Before Receiving This Medicine

In deciding to use a medicine, the risks of taking the medicine must be weighed against the good it will do. This is a decision you and your doctor will make. For aminoglycosides, the following should be considered:

Allergies—Tell your doctor if you have ever had any unusual or allergic reaction to any of the aminoglycosides. Also tell your health care professional if you are allergic to any other substances, such as foods, sulfites, or other preservatives.

Pregnancy—Studies on most of the aminoglycosides have not been done in pregnant women. Some reports have shown that aminoglycosides, especially streptomycin and tobramycin, may cause damage to the infant's hearing, sense of balance, and kidneys if the mother was receiving the medicine during pregnancy. However, this medicine may be needed in serious diseases or other situations that threaten the mother's life. Be sure you have discussed this with your doctor.

Breast-feeding—Aminoglycosides pass into breast milk in small amounts. However, they are not absorbed very much when taken by mouth. To date, aminoglycosides have not been reported to cause problems in nursing babies.

Children—Children are especially sensitive to the effects of aminoglycosides. Damage to hearing, sense of balance, and kidneys is more likely to occur in premature infants and neonates.

Older adults—Elderly people are especially sensitive to the effects of aminoglycosides. Serious side effects, such as damage to hearing, sense of balance, and kidneys may occur in elderly patients.

Other medicines—Although certain medicines should not be used together at all, in other cases two different medicines may be used together even if an interaction might occur. In these cases, your doctor may want to change the dose, or other precautions may be necessary. When you are receiving aminoglycosides it is especially important that your health care professional knows if you are taking any of the following:

- Aminoglycosides, used on the skin or mucous membranes and by injection at the same time; or more than one aminoglycoside at a time or
- Anti-infectives by mouth or by injection (medicine for infection) or
- Capreomycin (e.g., Capastat) or
- Carmustine (e.g., BiCNU) or
- Chloroquine (e.g., Aralen) or
- Cisplatin (e.g., Platinol) or
- Combination pain medicine containing acetaminophen and aspirin (e.g., Excedrin) or other salicylates (with large amounts taken regularly) or
- Cyclosporine (e.g., Sandimmune) or
- Deferoxamine (e.g., Desferal) (with long-term use) or
- Gold salts (medicine for arthritis) or
- Hydroxychloroquine (e.g., Plaquenil) or
- Inflammation or pain medicine, except narcotics, or
- Lithium (e.g., Lithane) or

- Methotrexate (e.g., Mexate) or
- Penicillamine (e.g., Cuprimine) or
- Plicamycin (e.g., Mithracin) or
- Quinine (e.g., Quinamm) or
- Streptozocin (e.g., Zanosar) or
- Tiopronin (e.g., Thiola)—Use of any of these medicines with aminoglycosides may increase the chance of hearing, balance, or kidney side effects.

Other medical problems—The presence of other medical problems may affect the use of the aminoglycosides. Make sure you tell your doctor if you have any other medical problems, especially:

- Kidney disease—Patients with kidney disease may have increased aminoglycoside blood levels and increased chance of side effects
- Loss of hearing and/or balance (eighth-cranial-nerve disease)—High aminoglycoside blood levels may cause hearing loss or balance disturbances
- Myasthenia gravis or
- Parkinson's disease—Aminoglycosides may cause muscular problems, resulting in further muscle weakness

Proper Use of This Medicine

To help clear up your infection completely, *aminoglycosides must be given for the full time of treatment,* even if you begin to feel better after a few days. Also, this medicine works best when there is a certain amount in the blood or urine. To help keep the correct level, aminoglycosides must be given on a regular schedule.

Dosing—The dose of aminoglycosides will be different for different patients. *Follow your doctor's orders or the directions on the label.* The following information includes only the average doses of aminoglycosides. Your dose may be different if you have kidney disease. *If your dose is different, do not change it* unless your doctor tells you to do so.

The dose of most aminoglycosides is based on body weight and must be determined by your doctor. The medicine is injected into a muscle or vein. Depending on the aminoglycoside prescribed, doses are given at different times and for different lengths of time. These times are as follows:

For amikacin
- For *all* dosage forms:
  ○ Adults and children: The dose is given every eight or twelve hours for seven to ten days.
  ○ Newborn babies: The dose is given every twelve hours for seven to ten days.
  ○ Premature babies: The dose is given every eighteen to twenty-four hours for seven to ten days.

For gentamicin
- For *all* dosage forms:
  ○ Adults and children: The dose is given every eight hours for seven to ten days or more.
  ○ Infants: The dose is given every eight to sixteen hours for seven to ten days or more.
  ○ Premature and full-term newborn babies: The dose is given every twelve to twenty-four hours for seven to ten days or more.

For kanamicin
- For *all* dosage forms:
  ○ Adults and children: The dose is given every eight or twelve hours for seven to ten days.

For netilmicin
- For *all* dosage forms:
  ○ Adults and children: The dose is given every eight or twelve hours for seven to fourteen days.

For streptomycin
- For *all* dosage forms—The dose of streptomycin is often not based on body weight and the amount given depends on the disease being treated.
  ○ *Treatment of tuberculosis (TB):*
    ▪ Adults: Dose is based on body weight and must be determined by your doctor. This dose is injected into a muscle. The dosing schedule will also be determined by your doctor, usually once daily or twice weekly or three times-a-week. This medicine must be given with other medicines for tuberculosis (TB).
    ▪ Children and adolescents: Dose is based on body weight and must be determined by your doctor. This dose is injected into a muscle. The dosing schedule will also be determined by your doctor, usually once daily or twice weekly or three times-a-week. This medicine must be given with other medicines for tuberculosis (TB).
  ○ *Treatment of bacterial infections:*
    ▪ Adults: 250 to 500 milligrams of streptomycin is injected into a muscle every six hours; or 500 milligrams to 1 gram of streptomycin is injected into a muscle every twelve hours.
    ▪ Children and adolescents: Dose is based on body weight and must be determined by your doctor. This dose is injected into a muscle every six to twelve hours.

For tobramycin
- For *all* dosage forms:
  ○ Adults and adolescents: The dose is given every six to eight hours for seven to ten days or more.
  ○ Older infants and children: The dose is given every six to sixteen hours.
  ○ Premature and full-term newborn babies: The dose is given every twelve to twenty-four hours.

Side Effects

Along with its needed effects, a medicine may cause some unwanted effects. Although not all of these side effects may occur, if they do occur they may need medical attention.

Check with your health care professional immediately if any of the following side effects occur:

More common
   Any loss of hearing; clumsiness or unsteadiness; dizziness; greatly increased or decreased frequency of urination or amount of urine; increased thirst; loss of appetite; nausea or vomiting; numbness, tingling, or burning of face or mouth (streptomycin only); muscle twitching, or convulsions (seizures); ringing or buzzing or a feeling of fullness in the ears

Less common
   Any loss of vision (streptomycin only); skin rash, itching, redness, or swelling

Rare—Once-daily or "high dose" gentamicin only-
   Shaking; chills; fever

All aminoglycosides—In addition, leg cramps, skin rash,
   fever, and convulsions (seizures) may occur when gentamicin is given by injection into the muscle or a vein, and
   into the spinal fluid.

   Difficulty in breathing; drowsiness; weakness

For up to several weeks after you stop receiving this medicine, it may still cause some side effects that need medical
attention. Check with your doctor if you notice any of the following side effects or if they get worse:

   Any loss of hearing; clumsiness or unsteadiness; dizziness; greatly increased or decreased frequency of urination or amount of urine; increased thirst; loss of appetite;
   nausea or vomiting; ringing or buzzing or a feeling of fullness in the ears

Other side effects not listed above may also occur in some
patients. If you notice any other effects, check with your
doctor.

AMINOLEVULINIC ACID (Topical route) - a-MEE-noh-lev-yoo-lin-ik AS-id

Commonly used brand name(s)

In the U.S.—
   Levulan Kerastick

Available Dosage Forms:
- Kit
- Stick

Therapeutic Class: Photosensitizing Agent

Uses For This Medicine

Aminolevulinic acid application followed by exposure to a certain type of light (blue light using the BLU–U Blue Light Photodynamic Therapy Illuminator) treats the skin condition
called actinic keratoses.

This medicine is available only with your doctor's prescription.

Before Using This Medicine

In deciding to use a medicine, the risks of taking the medicine
must be weighed against the good it will do. This is a decision
you and your doctor will make. For this medicine, the following
should be considered:

Allergies—Tell your doctor if you have ever had any unusual or allergic reaction to this medicine or any other medicines. Also tell your health care professional if you have any
other types of allergies, such as to foods, dyes, preservatives,
or animals. For non-prescription products, read the label or
package ingredients carefully.

Pediatric—Studies on this medicine have been done only
in adult patients, and there is no specific information comparing use of aminolevulinic acid in children with use in other
age groups.

Geriatric—Many medicines have not been studied specifically in older people. Therefore, it may not be known whether
they work exactly the same way they do in younger adults or
if they cause different side effects or problems in older people.
There is no specific information comparing use of aminolevulinic acid in the elderly with use in other age groups.

Pregnancy—

	Pregnancy Category	Explanation
All Trimesters	C	Animal studies have shown an adverse effect and there are no adequate studies in pregnant women OR no animal studies have been conducted and there are no adequate studies in pregnant women.

Breast Feeding—There are no adequate studies in
women for determining infant risk when using this medication during breastfeeding. Weigh the potential benefits
against the potential risks before taking this medication
while breastfeeding.

Other medicines—Although certain medicines should not
be used together at all, in other cases two different medicines
may be used together even if an interaction might occur. In
these cases, your doctor may want to change the dose, or
other precautions may be necessary. Tell your healthcare
professional if you are taking any other prescription or non-
prescription (over-the-counter [OTC]) medicine.

Interactions with Food/Tobacco/Alcohol—Certain
medicines should not be used at or around the time of eating
food or eating certain types of food since interactions may
occur. Using alcohol or tobacco with certain medicines may
also cause interactions to occur. Discuss with your healthcare
professional the use of your medicine with food, alcohol, or
tobacco.

Other medical problems—The presence of other medical
problems may affect the use of this medicine. Make sure you
tell your doctor if you have any other medical problems, especially:
- Skin sensitivity to light or
- Porphyria—May be worsened by aminolevulinic acid

Proper Use of This Medicine

Dosing—The dose of this medicine will be different for different patients. Follow your doctor's orders or the directions
on the label. The following information includes only the average doses of this medicine. If your dose is different, do not
change it unless your doctor tells you to do so.

The amount of medicine that you take depends on the
strength of the medicine. Also, the number of doses you take
each day, the time allowed between doses, and the length of
time you take the medicine depend on the medical problem
for which you are using the medicine.

Aminolevulinic acid is applied to your skin in your doctor's
office. Blue light illumination treatment must be followed with
BLU–U Blue Light Photodynamic Therapy Illuminator in your
doctor's office 14 to 18 hours after the application. The blue
light treatment lasts approximately 17 minutes. Your doctor
may want to re-treat you after 8 weeks if your skin condition
did not completely resolve.

Call your doctor if you cannot return for the blue light illumination treatment after the aminolevulinic acid application. You should then protect the treated skin from sunlight and prolonged or intense light for at least 40 hours.

Precautions While Using This Medicine

After aminolevulinic acid application you should avoid exposure to sunlight or bright indoor light (e.g., from examination lamps, operating room lamps, tanning beds, or being close to lights) up until the time of the blue light treatment. Wide-brimmed hats or similar head covering can help protect you from sunlight or sources of light.

Sunscreens will not protect you from sunlight or sources of light.

Reduce your exposure to light if you experience stinging or burning on the treated areas before blue light treatment.

Do not wash the treated areas before the blue light treatment.

You and the doctor will wear eye protection during the blue light treatment.

During the blue light treatment you will experience sensations of tingling, stinging, prickling or burning of the treated skin. These feelings of discomfort should improve at the end of the light treatment.

Following treatment, the actinic keratoses and possibly the surrounding skin will redden and swelling and scaling may also occur. These changes are temporary and should completely resolve by 4 weeks after treatment.

Side Effects of This Medicine

Along with its needed effects, a medicine may cause some unwanted effects. Although not all of these side effects may occur, if they do occur they may need medical attention.

Check with your doctor immediately if any of the following side effects occur:
> *Less common*
> Bleeding

Some side effects may occur that usually do not need medical attention. These side effects may go away during treatment as your body adjusts to the medicine. Also, your health care professional may be able to tell you about ways to prevent or reduce some of these side effects. Check with your health care professional if any of the following side effects continue or are bothersome or if you have any questions about them:
> *More common*
> Burning, crawling, itching, numbness, prickling, "pins and needles," stinging, or tingling feelings; darkening of treated skin; lightening of treated skin; scaling or crusting; skin sore; small red raised itchy bumps; swelling of skin
> *Less common*
> Blister; oozing; open sore on skin; pain; pus filled blister or pimple; raw skin; scabbing; tenderness.

Other side effects not listed may also occur in some patients. If you notice any other effects, check with your healthcare professional.

AMLODIPINE (Oral route) - am-LOE-di-peen

Commonly used brand name(s)
In the U.S.—
> Norvasc

Available Dosage Forms:
- Tablet

Therapeutic Class: Cardiovascular Agent
Pharmacologic Class: Calcium Channel Blocker

Uses For This Medicine

Amlodipine is a calcium channel blocker used to treat angina (chest pain) and high blood pressure. Amlodipine affects the movement of calcium into the cells of the heart and blood vessels. As a result, amlodipine relaxes blood vessels and increases the supply of blood and oxygen to the heart while reducing its workload.

High blood pressure adds to the workload of the heart and arteries. If it continues for a long time, the heart and arteries may not function properly. This can damage the blood vessels of the brain, heart, and kidneys, resulting in a stroke, heart failure, or kidney failure. High blood pressure may also increase the risk of heart attacks. These problems may be less likely to occur if blood pressure is controlled.

This medicine is available only with your doctor's prescription.

Before Using This Medicine

In deciding to use a medicine, the risks of taking the medicine must be weighed against the good it will do. This is a decision you and your doctor will make. For this medicine, the following should be considered:

Allergies—Tell your doctor if you have ever had any unusual or allergic reaction to this medicine or any other medicines. Also tell your health care professional if you have any other types of allergies, such as to foods, dyes, preservatives, or animals. For non-prescription products, read the label or package ingredients carefully.

Pediatric—Studies on this medicine have been done only in adult patients, and there is no specific information comparing use of amlodipine in children with use in other age groups.

Geriatric—Elderly people may be especially sensitive to the effects of amlodipine. This may increase the chance of side effects during treatment.

Pregnancy—

	Pregnancy Category	Explanation
All Trimesters	C	Animal studies have shown an adverse effect and there are no adequate studies in pregnant women OR no animal studies have been conducted and there are no adequate studies in pregnant women.

Breast Feeding—There are no adequate studies in women for determining infant risk when using this medication during

breastfeeding. Weigh the potential benefits against the potential risks before taking this medication while breastfeeding.

Other medicines—

Using this medicine with any of the following medicines is usually not recommended, but may be required in some cases. If both medicines are prescribed together, your doctor may change the dose or how often you use one or both of the medicines.

Amiodarone, Atazanavir, Droperidol, Fentanyl

Interactions with Food/Tobacco/Alcohol—Certain medicines should not be used at or around the time of eating food or eating certain types of food since interactions may occur. Using alcohol or tobacco with certain medicines may also cause interactions to occur. Discuss with your healthcare professional the use of your medicine with food, alcohol, or tobacco.

Other medical problems—The presence of other medical problems may affect the use of this medicine. Make sure you tell your doctor if you have any other medical problems, especially:

- Congestive heart failure—There is a small chance that amlodipine may make this condition worse
- Liver disease—Higher blood levels of amlodipine may result and a smaller dose may be needed
- Very low blood pressure—Amlodipine may make this condition worse

Proper Use of This Medicine

Take this medicine exactly as directed even if you feel well and do not notice any chest pain. Do not take more of this medicine and do not take it more often than your doctor ordered. Do not miss any doses.

For patients taking this medicine for high blood pressure:

- In addition to the use of the medicine your doctor has prescribed, treatment for your high blood pressure may include weight control and care in the types of food you eat, especially foods high in sodium (salt). Your doctor will tell you which of these are most important for you. You should check with your doctor before changing your diet.
- Many patients who have high blood pressure will not notice any signs of the problem. In fact, many may feel normal. It is very important that you take your medicine exactly as directed and that you keep your appointments with your doctor even if you feel well.
- Remember that this medicine will not cure your high blood pressure but it does help control it. Therefore, you must continue to take it as directed if you expect to lower your blood pressure and keep it down. You may have to take high blood pressure medicine for the rest of your life. If high blood pressure is not treated, it can cause serious problems such as heart failure, blood vessel disease, stroke, or kidney disease.

Dosing—The dose of this medicine will be different for different patients. Follow your doctor's orders or the directions on the label. The following information includes only the average doses of this medicine. If your dose is different, do not change it unless your doctor tells you to do so.

The amount of medicine that you take depends on the strength of the medicine. Also, the number of doses you take each day, the time allowed between doses, and the length of time you take the medicine depend on the medical problem for which you are using the medicine.

- For oral dosage form (tablets):
  - For angina (chest pain):
    - Adults—5 to 10 milligrams (mg) once a day.
    - Children—Use must be determined by your doctor.
  - For high blood pressure:
    - Adults—2.5 to 10 mg once a day.
    - Children 6 years of age and older—2.5 to 5 mg once a day.
    - Children younger than 6 years of age—Use must be determined by your doctor.

Missed dose—If you miss a dose of this medicine, take it as soon as possible. However, if it is almost time for your next dose, skip the missed dose and go back to your regular dosing schedule. Do not double doses.

Storage—Store the medicine in a closed container at room temperature, away from heat, moisture, and direct light. Do not refrigerate. Keep from freezing.

Keep out of the reach of children.

Do not keep outdated medicine or medicine no longer needed.

Precautions While Using This Medicine

It is important that your doctor check your progress at regular visits. This will allow your doctor to make sure the medicine is working properly and to change the dosage if needed.

If you have been using this medicine regularly for several weeks, do not suddenly stop using it. Stopping suddenly may cause your chest pain or high blood pressure to come back or get worse. Check with your doctor for the best way to reduce gradually the amount you are taking before stopping completely.

Chest pain resulting from exercise or physical exertion usually is reduced or prevented by this medicine. This may tempt you to be too active. Make sure you discuss with your doctor a safe amount of exercise for your medical problem.

After taking a dose of this medicine you may get a headache that lasts for a short time. This should become less noticeable after you have taken this medicine for a while. If this effect continues, or if the headaches are severe, check with your doctor.

In some patients, tenderness, swelling, or bleeding of the gums may appear soon after treatment with this medicine is started. Brushing and flossing your teeth carefully and regularly and massaging your gums may help prevent this. See your dentist regularly to have your teeth cleaned. Check with your medical doctor or dentist if you have any questions about how to take care of your teeth and gums, or if you notice any tenderness, swelling, or bleeding of your gums.

For patients taking this medicine for high blood pressure:

- Do not take other medicines unless they have been discussed with your doctor. This especially includes over-the-counter (nonprescription) medicines for appetite control, asthma, colds, cough, hay fever, or sinus problems, since they may tend to increase your blood pressure.

Side Effects of This Medicine

Along with its needed effects, a medicine may cause some unwanted effects. Although not all of these side effects may occur, if they do occur they may need medical attention.

Check with your doctor as soon as possible if any of the following side effects occur:

More common
Swelling of ankles or feet

Less common
Dizziness; pounding heartbeat

Rare
Chest pain; dark yellow urine; dizziness or lightheadedness when getting up from a lying or sitting position; slow heartbeat; yellow eyes or skin

Some side effects may occur that usually do not need medical attention. These side effects may go away during treatment as your body adjusts to the medicine. Also, your health care professional may be able to tell you about ways to prevent or reduce some of these side effects. Check with your health care professional if any of the following side effects continue or are bothersome or if you have any questions about them:

More common
Abdominal pain; flushing; headache; sleepiness or unusual drowsiness

Less common
Nausea; unusual tiredness or weakness

Other side effects not listed may also occur in some patients. If you notice any other effects, check with your healthcare professional.

AMLODIPINE AND ATORVASTATIN
(Oral route) - am-LOE-di-peen, a-TORE-va-sta-tin

Commonly used brand name(s)

In the U.S.—
Caduet

Available Dosage Forms:
• Tablet

Therapeutic Class: Calcium Channel Blocker/HMG-COA Reductase Inhibitor Combination
Pharmacologic Class: Amlodipine

Uses For This Medicine

Amlodipine and atorvastatin is a combination of a calcium channel blocker and HMG-CoA reductase inhibitor. Amlodipine is used to treat angina (chest pain) or high blood pressure. Atorvastatin is used to lower cholesterol and triglyceride (fat-like substances) levels in the blood.

High blood pressure adds to the workload of the heart and arteries. If it continues for a long time, the heart and arteries may not function properly. This can damage the blood vessels of the brain, heart, and kidneys, resulting in a stroke, heart failure, or kidney failure. High blood pressure may also increase the risk of heart attacks. These problems may be less likely to occur if blood pressure is controlled.

The exact way in which this medicine works is not known. Amlodipine is a type of medicine known as a calcium channel blocker. Calcium channel blocking agents affect the movement of calcium into the cells of the heart and blood vessels. Atorvastatin is used to lower cholesterol and triglyceride (fat-like substances) levels in the blood. The action of both medicines together is to relax blood vessels, lower blood pressure, and decrease the amount of cholesterol in the blood.

Amlodipine and atorvastatin is available only with your doctor's prescription.

Importance of Diet—Before prescribing the atorvastatin and amlodipine combination for your condition, your doctor will probably try to control your condition by prescribing a personal diet for you. Such a diet may be low in fats, sugars, and/or cholesterol. Many people are able to control their condition by carefully following their doctor's orders for proper diet and exercise. Medicine is prescribed only when additional help is needed and is effective only when a schedule of diet and exercise is properly followed.

Also, this medicine is less effective if you are greatly overweight. It may be very important for you to go on a weight-reducing diet. However, check with your doctor before going on any diet.

Before Using This Medicine

In deciding to use a medicine, the risks of taking the medicine must be weighed against the good it will do. This is a decision you and your doctor will make. For this medicine, the following should be considered:

Allergies—Tell your doctor if you have ever had any unusual or allergic reaction to this medicine or any other medicines. Also tell your health care professional if you have any other types of allergies, such as to foods, dyes, preservatives, or animals. For non-prescription products, read the label or package ingredients carefully.

Pediatric—Studies on this combination medicine have been done only in adult patients, and there is no specific information comparing use of amlodipine and atorvastatin in children with use in other age groups.

Atorvastatin alone is safe to use in boys and some girls 10 to 17 years of age for treating certain types of high cholesterol.

Adolescent girls taking atorvastatin should be counseled on appropriate contraceptive methods.

Geriatric—Many medicines have not been studied specifically in older people. Therefore, it may not be known whether they work exactly the same way they do in younger adults or if they cause different side effects or problems in older people. However, elderly people may be especially sensitive to the effects of amlodipine which may increase the chance of side effects during treatment.

Other medicines—

Using this medicine with any of the following medicines is usually not recommended, but may be required in some cases. If both medicines are prescribed together, your doctor may change the dose or how often you use one or both of the medicines.

Amiodarone, Atazanavir, Bezafibrate, Ciprofibrate, Clarithromycin, Clofibrate, Cyclosporine, Dalfopristin, Diltiazem, Droperidol, Erythromycin, Fenofibrate, Fentanyl, Fluconazole, Fosamprenavir, Fusidic Acid, Gemfibrozil, Indinavir, Itraconazole, Ketoconazole, Lopinavir, Mibefradil, Nefazodone, Nelfinavir, Niacin, Quinupristin, Saquinavir, Telithromycin, Tipranavir, Troleandomycin, Verapamil

Interactions with Food/Tobacco/Alcohol—Certain medicines should not be used at or around the time of eating food or eating certain types of food since interactions may occur. Using alcohol or tobacco with certain medicines may also cause interactions to occur. The following interactions have been selected on the basis of their potential significance and are not necessarily all-inclusive.

Using this medicine with any of the following may cause an increased risk of certain side effects but may be unavoidable in some cases. If used together, your doctor may change the dose or how often you use this medicine, or give you special instructions about the use of food, alcohol, or tobacco.

Grapefruit Juice

Other medical problems—The presence of other medical problems may affect the use of this medicine. Make sure you tell your doctor if you have any other medical problems, especially:

- Alcohol abuse (or history of) or
- Liver disease (or history of) or
- Liver enzymes, persistently high levels—Use of this medicine may make liver problems worse
- Aortic stenosis, severe (abnormally narrow aorta)—Use of this medicine may increase the chance of low blood pressure
- Congestive heart failure—There is a small chance that amlodipine may make this condition worse
- Convulsions (seizures), not well-controlled, or
- Electrolyte or metabolic enzyme deficiencies or disorders or
- Infection, severe or
- Low blood pressure or
- Major surgery or trauma, recent or
- Myopathy (a disorder of muscle tissue or muscles)—Patients with these conditions may be at risk of developing muscle problems (causing the release of muscle pigment into the urine) that may lead to kidney failure
- Coronary artery disease, severe, obstructive—Use of this medicine may result in other heart problems

Proper Use of This Medicine

Use this medicine only as directed by your doctor. Do not use more or less of it, and do not use it more often or for a longer time than your doctor ordered. Also, this medicine works best if there is a constant amount in the blood. To help keep this amount constant, do not miss any doses and take the medicine at the same time each day.

Before prescribing the atorvastatin and amlodipine combination for your condition, your doctor will probably try to control your condition by prescribing a personal diet for you. *Follow carefully the special diet your doctor gave you.* Such a diet may be low in fats, sugars, and/or cholesterol. Many people are able to control their condition by carefully following their doctor's orders for proper diet and exercise. *Medicine is prescribed only when additional help is*

needed and is effective only when a schedule of diet and exercise is properly followed.

Also, this medicine is less effective if you are greatly overweight. It may be very important for you to go on a weight-reducing diet. However, check with your doctor before going on any diet.

Dosing—The dose of this medicine will be different for different patients. Follow your doctor's orders or the directions on the label. The following information includes only the average doses of this medicine. If your dose is different, do not change it unless your doctor tells you to do so.

The amount of medicine that you take depends on the strength of the medicine. Also, the number of doses you take each day, the time allowed between doses, and the length of time you take the medicine depend on the medical problem for which you are using the medicine.

- For oral dosage form (tablets):
  - Adults—1 tablet a day, tablet strength is determined by your doctor.
  - Children—Use and dose must be determined by your doctor.

Missed dose—If you miss a dose of this medicine, take it as soon as possible. However, if it is almost time for your next dose, skip the missed dose and go back to your regular dosing schedule. Do not double doses.

Storage—Store the medicine in a closed container at room temperature, away from heat, moisture, and direct light. Keep from freezing.

Keep out of the reach of children.

Do not keep outdated medicine or medicine no longer needed.

Precautions While Using This Medicine

It is important that your doctor check your progress at regular visits. This will allow your doctor to make sure the medicine is working properly and to change the dosage if needed.

Check with your doctor immediately if you think that you may be pregnant. HMG-CoA reductase inhibitors may cause birth defects or other problems in the baby if taken during pregnancy.

Before having any kind of surgery (including dental surgery) or emergency treatment, tell the medical doctor or dentist in charge that you are taking this medicine.

Do not take over-the-counter (OTC) niacin preparations without consulting your doctor. Niacin may increase atorvastatin's adverse effects on muscle, which can lead to serious kidney problems.

Do not use excessive amounts of alcohol while taking atorvastatin because it can worsen the adverse effects of this medicine on the liver.

Check with your doctor immediately if you experience unexplained muscle pain, tenderness, or weakness, especially if it is accompanied by unusual tiredness or fever, because the medicine's adverse effects on muscle can lead to serious kidney problems.

Checking with physician before discontinuing medication because a gradual reduction in dose may be necessary

Side Effects of This Medicine

Along with its needed effects, a medicine may cause some unwanted effects. Although not all of these side effects may occur, if they do occur they may need medical attention.

Check with your doctor immediately if any of the following side effects occur:

More common-Atorvastatin
Cough; difficulty swallowing; dizziness; fast heartbeat; hives; itching; puffiness or swelling of the eyelids or around the eyes, face, lips or tongue; shortness of breath; skin rash; tightness in chest; unusual tiredness or weakness; wheezing

Rare-Amlodipine
Chest pain or discomfort; dilated neck veins; extra heartbeats; extreme fatigue; irregular breathing; irregular heartbeat; pulse irregularity; shortness of breath; swelling of face, fingers, feet, or lower legs; weight gain

Observed post-marketing frequency unknown-Atorvastatin
Blistering, peeling, loosening of skin; chills; dark-colored urine; diarrhea; fever; itching; joint or muscle pain; muscle cramps or spasms; muscle pain or stiffness; red irritated eyes; red skin lesions, often with a purple center; sore throat; sores, ulcers, or white spots in mouth or on lips

Symptoms of overdose

Get emergency help immediately if any of the following symptoms of overdose occur:

Blurred vision; confusion; dizziness, faintness, or lightheadedness when getting up from a lying or sitting position suddenly; flushing; sweating; unusual tiredness or weakness

Some side effects may occur that usually do not need medical attention. These side effects may go away during treatment as your body adjusts to the medicine. Also, your health care professional may be able to tell you about ways to prevent or reduce some of these side effects. Check with your health care professional if any of the following side effects continue or are bothersome or if you have any questions about them:

More common-Amlodipine
Headache

More common-Atorvastatin
Body aches or pain; congestion; difficulty in moving; dryness or soreness of throat; fever or chills; hoarseness; lower back or side pain; muscle pain or stiffness; pain in joints; pain or tenderness around eyes and cheekbones; painful or difficult urination; runny nose; stuffy nose; tender, swollen glands in neck; voice changes

Less common-Amlodipine
Feeling of warmth; nausea; redness of the face, neck, arms and occasionally, upper chest; sleepiness or unusual drowsiness; stomach pain

Less common-Atorvastatin
Accidental injury; acid or sour stomach; belching; bloated full feeling; diarrhea; difficulty having a bowel movement (stool); excess air or gas in stomach or intestines; general feeling of discomfort or illness; heartburn; indigestion; lack or loss of strength; loss of appetite; nausea; passing gas; rash; shivering; stomach discomfort upset or pain; sweating; trouble sleeping; vomiting

Rare-Amlodipine
Anxiety; bad unusual or unpleasant (after) taste; blistering, crusting, irritation, itching, or reddening of skin; burning feeling in chest or stomach; burning while urinating; change in near or distance vision; change in taste; change in color of skin; cold and clammy skin; cracked, dry, scaly skin; difficult or painful urination; difficulty in focusing eyes; dry mouth; dryness of eyes; excessive muscle tone; frequent urination; hair loss, thinning of hair; hives or welts; hyperventilation; increased appetite; increased volume of pale, dilute urine; irritability; lack of feeling or emotion; loose stools; loss of memory; muscle tension or tightness; muscle weakness; nervousness; problems with memory; restlessness; severe and throbbing headache; shakiness and unsteady walk; sneezing; tenderness in stomach area; transient, mild, pleasant aromatic odor; trembling, or other problems with muscle control or coordination; trouble sleeping; twitching; uncaring; unsteadiness

Other side effects not listed may also occur in some patients. If you notice any other effects, check with your healthcare professional.

AMLODIPINE AND BENAZEPRIL
(Oral route) - am-LOE-di-peen, ben-AY-ze-pril

Black Box Warning

When used in pregnancy during the second and third trimesters, ACE inhibitors can cause injury and even death to the developing fetus. When pregnancy is detected, amlodipine besylate/benazepril hydrochloride should be discontinued as soon as possible.

Commonly used brand name(s)

In the U.S.—
Lotrel

Available Dosage Forms:
• Capsule

Therapeutic Class: ACE Inhibitor/Calcium Channel Blocker Combination
Pharmacologic Class: Amlodipine

Uses For This Medicine

Amlodipine and benazepril combination belongs to the class of medicines called high blood pressure medicines (antihypertensives). It is used to treat high blood pressure (hypertension).

High blood pressure adds to the workload of the heart and arteries. If it continues for a long time, the heart and arteries may not function properly. This can damage the blood vessels of the brain, heart, and kidneys, resulting in a stroke, heart failure, or kidney failure. High blood pressure may also increase the risk of heart attacks. These problems may be less likely to occur if blood pressure is controlled.

The exact way in which this medicine works is not known. Amlodipine is a type of medicine known as a calcium channel blocker. Calcium channel blocking agents affect the movement of calcium into the cells of the heart and blood vessels. Benazepril is a type of medicine known as an angiotensin-converting enzyme (ACE) inhibitor. It blocks an enzyme in the body that is necessary in producing a substance that causes blood vessels to tighten. The action of both medicines together is to relax blood vessels, lower blood pressure, and increase the supply of blood and oxygen to the heart.

This medicine is available only with your doctor's prescription.

Before Using This Medicine

In deciding to use a medicine, the risks of taking the medicine must be weighed against the good it will do. This is a decision you and your doctor will make. For this medicine, the following should be considered:

Allergies—Tell your doctor if you have ever had any unusual or allergic reaction to this medicine or any other medicines. Also tell your health care professional if you have any other types of allergies, such as to foods, dyes, preservatives, or animals. For non-prescription products, read the label or package ingredients carefully.

Pediatric—Studies on this medicine have been done only in adult patients, and there is no specific information comparing use of amlodipine and benazepril combination in children with use in other age groups.

Geriatric—This medicine has been tested in patients 65 years of age or older and has not been shown to cause different side effects or problems in older people than it does in younger adults. However, blood levels of amlodipine may be increased in the elderly and elderly people may be more sensitive to the effects of this medicine.

Other medicines—

Using this medicine with any of the following medicines is usually not recommended, but may be required in some cases. If both medicines are prescribed together, your doctor may change the dose or how often you use one or both of the medicines.

Allopurinol, Amiloride, Amiodarone, Atazanavir, Azathioprine, Canrenoate, Droperidol, Fentanyl, Potassium, Spironolactone, Triamterene

Interactions with Food/Tobacco/Alcohol—Certain medicines should not be used at or around the time of eating food or eating certain types of food since interactions may occur. Using alcohol or tobacco with certain medicines may also cause interactions to occur. Discuss with your healthcare professional the use of your medicine with food, alcohol, or tobacco.

Other medical problems—The presence of other medical problems may affect the use of this medicine. Make sure you tell your doctor if you have any other medical problems, especially:

- Bee-sting allergy treatments or
- Dialysis—Increased risk of serious allergic reaction occurring
- Dehydration—Lowering effects on blood pressure may be increased

- Diabetes mellitus (sugar diabetes)—Increased risk of potassium levels in the body becoming too high
- Heart or blood vessel disease—Lowering blood pressure may make problems resulting from these conditions worse
- Kidney disease or
- Liver disease—Effects may be increased because of slower removal of this medicine from the body
- Scleroderma or
- Systemic lupus erythematosus (SLE) (or history of)—Increased risk of blood problems caused by ACE inhibitors

Proper Use of This Medicine

Take this medicine exactly as directed by your doctor, at the same time each day. Do not take more of it and do not take it more often than directed.

Dosing—The dose of this medicine will be different for different patients. Follow your doctor's orders or the directions on the label. The following information includes only the average doses of this medicine. If your dose is different, do not change it unless your doctor tells you to do so.

The amount of medicine that you take depends on the strength of the medicine. Also, the number of doses you take each day, the time allowed between doses, and the length of time you take the medicine depend on the medical problem for which you are using the medicine.

- For oral dosage form (capsules):
    - For high blood pressure:
        - Adults—1 capsule a day. Your doctor may increase your dose if needed.
        - Children—Use and dose must be determined by your doctor.

Missed dose—If you miss a dose of this medicine, take it as soon as possible. However, if it is almost time for your next dose, skip the missed dose and go back to your regular dosing schedule. Do not double doses.

Storage—Store the medicine in a closed container at room temperature, away from heat, moisture, and direct light. Keep from freezing.

Keep out of the reach of children.

Do not keep outdated medicine or medicine no longer needed.

Precautions While Using This Medicine

It is very important that your doctor check your progress at regular visits. This will allow your doctor to make sure the medicine is working properly, to check for unwanted effects, and to change the dosage if needed.

If you think that you may have become pregnant, check with your doctor immediately. Use of this medicine, especially during the second and third trimesters (after the first 3 months) of pregnancy, may cause serious injury or even death to the unborn child.

Do not take any other medicines, especially potassium supplements, or salt substitutes that contain potassium unless approved or prescribed by your doctor.

Dizziness, lightheadedness, or fainting may occur after the first dose, especially if you have been taking a diuretic (water pill). Make sure you know how you react to the medicine before you drive, use machines, or do other things that could be dangerous if you experience these effects.

Check with your doctor if you notice any signs of fever, sore throat, or chills. These could be symptoms of an infection resulting from low white blood cell counts.

Check with your doctor if you notice difficult breathing or swelling of the face, arms, or legs. These could be symptoms of a serious allergic reaction.

Check with your doctor if you become sick while taking this medicine, especially with severe or continuing vomiting or diarrhea. These conditions may cause you to lose too much water, possibly resulting in low blood pressure.

Check with your doctor if you have strong stomach pain. This could be a symptom of a condition called intestinal angioedema. Your doctor may have to use a CT scan or an ultrasound to diagnose this condition.

Dizziness, lightheadedness, or fainting may also occur if you exercise or if the weather is hot. Heavy sweating can cause loss of too much water and result in low blood pressure. Use extra care during exercise or hot weather.

In some patients, tenderness, swelling, or bleeding of the gums may appear soon after treatment with this medicine is started. Brushing and flossing your teeth carefully and regularly and massaging your gums may help prevent this. See your dentist regularly to have your teeth cleaned. Check with your medical doctor or dentist if you have any questions about how to take care of your teeth and gums, or if you notice any tenderness, swelling, or bleeding of your gums.

Before having any kind of surgery (including dental surgery) or emergency treatment, tell the medical doctor or dentist in charge that you are taking this medicine.

Black patients may be less sensitive to the blood pressure-lowering effects of this medicine. In addition, the risk of a serious allergic reaction involving swelling of the face, mouth, hands, or feet may be increased.

Side Effects of This Medicine

Along with its needed effects, a medicine may cause some unwanted effects. Although not all of these side effects may occur, if they do occur they may need medical attention.

Check with your doctor immediately if any of the following side effects occur:

Rare
  Swelling of face, mouth, hands, or feet; trouble in swallowing or breathing (sudden) and/or hoarseness

Incidence not determined
  Chest pain; difficulty in swallowing; heartburn; pain or burning in throat; vomiting; sores, ulcers, or white spots on lips or tongue or inside the mouth; stomach pain

Check with your doctor as soon as possible if any of the following side effects occur:

Less common
  Dizziness, lightheadedness, or fainting; swelling of ankles, feet, or lower legs

Signs and symptoms of too much potassium in the body
  Confusion; irregular heartbeat; nervousness; numbness or tingling in hands, feet, or lips; shortness of breath; weakness or heaviness of legs

Rare
  Bleeding gums, fatigue, nosebleeds, and/or pale skin; blisters in mouth spreading to trunk, scalp, or other

areas; chills, fever, or sore throat; nausea or vomiting; sores in mouth, or on arms, feet, hands, legs, or lips (sudden); stomach pain or bloating with fever, nausea, or vomiting; unusual bleeding or bruising; yellow eyes or skin

Some side effects may occur that usually do not need medical attention. These side effects may go away during treatment as your body adjusts to the medicine. Also, your health care professional may be able to tell you about ways to prevent or reduce some of these side effects. Check with your health care professional if any of the following side effects continue or are bothersome or if you have any questions about them:

Less common
  Awareness of heartbeat; cough (dry, continuing); feeling of warmth; redness of the face, neck, arms and occasionally upper chest; sleepiness

Incidence not determined
  acid or sour stomach; belching; blistering, crusting, irritation, itching, or reddening of skin; body aches or pain; congestion; cracked, dry, scaly skin; decreased interest in sexual intercourse; difficulty having a bowel movement (stool); dryness or soreness of throat; fear; fever; frequent urination; hoarseness; inability to have or keep an erection; increased volume of pale, dilute urine; indigestion; lack or loss of strength; loss in sexual ability, desire, drive, or performance; muscle or bone pain; nervousness; runny nose; shakiness in legs, arms, hands, feet; sleeplessness; small lump under the skin; sudden sweating; swelling; stomach discomfort or upset; tender, swollen glands in neck; trembling or shaking of hands or feet; trouble in swallowing; trouble sleeping; unable to sleep; unusual tiredness or weakness; voice changes

Other side effects not listed may also occur in some patients. If you notice any other effects, check with your healthcare professional.

AMPHETAMINES (Systemic)

Some commonly used brand names are:

In the U.S.—

Adderall (3)	Dexedrine (2)
Adderall XR	Dexedrine Spansule (2)
Desoxyn (4)	DextroStat (2)
Desoxyn Gradumet (4)	

In Canada—
  Dexedrine (2)
  Dexedrine Spansule (2)

This information applies to the following medicines:

1. Amphetamine (am-FET-a-meen)
2. Dextroamphetamine (dex-troe-am-FET-a-meen)
3. Dextroamphetamine and amphetamine (dex-troe-am-FET-a-meen and am-FET-a-meen)
4. Methamphetamine (meth-am-FET-a-meen)

Category

- **Stimulant, central nervous system**—Amphetamine; Dextroamphetamine; Methamphetamine

Description

Amphetamines (am-FET-a-meens) belong to the group of medicines called central nervous system (CNS) stimulants. They are used to treat attention-deficit hyperactivity disorder (ADHD). Amphetamines increase attention and decrease restlessness in patients who are overactive, unable to concentrate for very long or are easily distracted, and have unstable emotions. These medicines are used as part of a total treatment program that also includes social, educational, and psychological treatment.

Amphetamine and dextroamphetamine are also used in the treatment of narcolepsy (uncontrollable desire for sleep or sudden attacks of deep sleep).

Amphetamines should not be used for weight loss or weight control or to combat unusual tiredness or weakness or replace rest. When used for these purposes, they may be dangerous to your health.

Amphetamines may also be used for other conditions as determined by your doctor.

These medicines are available only with a doctor's prescription. Prescriptions cannot be refilled. A new prescription must be obtained from your doctor each time you or your child needs this medicine.

Amphetamines are available in the following dosage forms:

Oral
- Amphetamine
  - Tablets
- Amphetamine and dextroamphetamine
  - Tablets
  - Extended-release capsules
- Dextroamphetamine
  - Extended-release capsules
  - Tablets
- Methamphetamine
  - Tablets
  - Extended-release tablets

Before Using This Medicine

In deciding to use a medicine, the risks of taking the medicine must be weighed against the good it will do. This is a decision you and your doctor will make. For amphetamines, the following should be considered:

Allergies—Tell your doctor if you have ever had any unusual or allergic reaction to amphetamine, dextroamphetamine, ephedrine, epinephrine, isoproterenol, metaproterenol, methamphetamine, norepinephrine, phenylephrine, phenylpropanolamine, pseudoephedrine, or terbutaline. Also tell your health care professional if you are allergic to any other substances, such as foods, preservatives, or dyes.

Pregnancy—Studies have not been done in humans. However, animal studies have shown that amphetamines may increase the chance of birth defects if taken during the early months of pregnancy. Before taking this medicine, make sure your doctor knows if you are pregnant of if you may become pregnant.

In addition, overuse of amphetamines during pregnancy may increase the chances of a premature delivery and of having a baby with a low birth weight. Also, the baby may become dependent on amphetamines and experience withdrawal effects such as agitation and drowsiness.

Breast-feeding—Amphetamines pass into breast milk. Although this medicine has not been reported to cause problems in nursing babies, it is best not to breast-feed while you are taking an amphetamine. Be sure you have discussed this with your doctor.

Children—When amphetamines are used for long periods of time in children, they may cause unwanted effects on behavior and growth. Before these medicines are given to a child, you should discuss their use with your child's doctor.

Older adults—Many medicines have not been studied specifically in older people. Therefore, it may not be known whether they work exactly the same way they do in younger adults or if they cause different side effects or problems in older people. There is no specific information comparing use of amphetamines in the elderly with use in other age groups.

Other medicines—Although certain medicines should not be used together at all, in many cases two different medicines may be used together even if an interaction might occur. In these cases, changes in dose or other precautions may be necessary. When you are taking amphetamines, it is especially important that your health care professional know if you are taking any of the following:
- Amantadine (e.g., Symmetrel) or
- Caffeine (e.g., NoDoz) or
- Chlophedianol (e.g., Ulone) or
- Methylphenidate (e.g., Ritalin) or
- Nabilone (e.g., Cesamet) or
- Pemoline (e.g., Cylert)—Use of these medicines may increase the CNS stimulation effects of amphetamines and cause unwanted effects such as nervousness, irritability, trouble in sleeping, and possibly convulsions (seizures)
- Appetite suppressants (diet pills) or
- Medicine for asthma or other breathing problems or
- Medicine for colds, sinus problems, or hay fever or other allergies (including nose drops or sprays)—Use of these medicines may increase the CNS stimulation effects of amphetamines and cause unwanted effects such as nervousness, irritability, trouble in sleeping, or convulsions (seizures), as well as unwanted effects on the heart and blood vessels
- Beta-adrenergic blocking agents (acebutolol [e.g., Sectral], atenolol [e.g., Tenormin], betaxolol [e.g., Kerlone], carteolol [e.g., Cartrol], labetalol [e.g., Normodyne], metoprolol [e.g., Lopressor], nadolol [e.g., Corgard], oxprenolol [e.g., Trasicor], penbutolol [e.g., Levatol], pindolol [e.g., Visken], propranolol [e.g., Inderal], sotalol [e.g., Sotacor], timolol [e.g., Blocadren])—Use of amphetamines with beta-blocking agents may increase the chance of high blood pressure and heart problems
- Cocaine—Use by persons taking amphetamines may cause a severe increase in blood pressure and other unwanted effects, including nervousness, irritability, trouble in sleeping, or convulsions (seizures)
- Digitalis glycosides (heart medicine)—Amphetamines may cause additive effects, resulting in irregular heartbeat

- Meperidine—Use of meperidine by persons taking amphetamines is not recommended because the chance of serious side effects (such as high fever, convulsions, or coma) may be increased

- Monoamine oxidase (MAO) inhibitor activity—(isocarboxazid [e.g., Marplan], phenelzine [e.g., Nardil], procarbazine [e.g., Matulane], selegiline [e.g., Eldepryl], tranylcypromine [e.g., Parnate])—Taking amphetamines while you are taking or within 2 weeks of taking monoamine oxidase (MAO) inhibitors may increase the chance of serious side effects such as sudden and severe high blood pressure or fever

- Thyroid hormones—The effects of either these medicines or amphetamines may be increased; unwanted effects may occur in patients with heart or blood vessel disease

- Tricyclic antidepressants (amitriptyline [e.g., Elavil], amoxapine [e.g., Asendin], clomipramine [e.g., Anafranil], desipramine [e.g., Pertofrane], doxepin [e.g., Sinequan], imipramine [e.g., Tofranil], nortriptyline [e.g., Aventyl], protriptyline [e.g., Vivactil], trimipramine [e.g., Surmontil])—Although tricyclic antidepressants may be used with amphetamines to help make them work better, using the two medicines together may increase the chance of fast or irregular heartbeat, severe high blood pressure, or high fever

Other medical problems—The presence of other medical problems may affect the use of amphetamines. Make sure you tell your doctor if you have any other medical problems, especially:

- Anxiety or tension (severe) or

- Drug abuse or dependence (history of) or

- Glaucoma or

- Heart or blood vessel disease or

- High blood pressure, severe or moderate or

- Mental illness (severe), especially in children, or

- Overactive thyroid—This medicine should not be used if any of these conditions exist. Serious unwanted effects could occur.

- Heart abnormalities or birth defects—*This medicine should not be used in children or adults with this condition.* Severe unwanted heart problems including death have been reported.

- Mild high blood pressure—Caution should be used. May make condition worse.

- Tourette's syndrome (history of) or other tics—Children and their families should be checked by their doctor for this condition before taking this medicine.

Proper Use of This Medicine

Take this medicine only as directed by your doctor. Do not take more or less of it, do not take it more often, and do not take it for a longer time than your doctor ordered. If too much is taken, it may become habit-forming (causing mental or physical dependence).

If you think this medicine is not working properly after you have taken it for several weeks, *do not increase the dose.* Instead, check with your doctor.

For patients taking *the short-acting form* of this medicine:

- Take the last dose for each day at least 6 hours before bedtime to help prevent trouble in sleeping.

For patients taking *the long-acting form* of this medicine:

- Take the daily dose when you wake up to help prevent trouble in sleeping.

- These capsules or tablets should be swallowed whole. Do not break, crush, or chew them before swallowing.

Amphetamines may be taken with or without food or on a full or empty stomach. However, if your doctor tells you to take the medicine a certain way, take it exactly as directed.

Dosing—The dose of amphetamines will be different for different patients. *Follow your doctor's orders or the directions on the label.* The following information includes only the average doses of amphetamines. *If your dose is different, do not change it* unless your doctor tells you to do so.

The number of capsules or tablets that you take depends on the strength of the medicine. Also, *the number of doses you take each day, the time allowed between doses, and the length of time you take the medicine depend on the medical problem for which you are taking amphetamines.*

For amphetamine
- For *oral* dosage form (tablets):
  - For attention-deficit hyperactivity disorder:
    - Adults—At first, 5 milligrams (mg) one to three times a day. Your doctor may increase your dose if needed.
    - Children 6 years of age and older—At first, 5 mg one or two times a day. Your doctor may increase your dose if needed.
    - Children 3 to 6 years of age—At first, 2.5 mg once a day. Your doctor may increase your dose if needed.
    - Children younger than 3 years of age—Use is not recommended.
  - For narcolepsy:
    - Adults—At first, 5 mg one to three times a day. Your doctor may increase your dose if needed.
    - Children 12 years of age and older—At first, 5 mg two times a day. Your doctor may increase your dose if needed.
    - Children 6 to 12 years of age—At first, 2.5 mg two times a day. Your doctor may increase your dose if needed.
    - Children younger than 6 years of age—Dose must be determined by your doctor.

For amphetamine and dextroamphetamine
- For *oral extended-release* dosage form (capsules):
  - For attention-deficit hyperactivity disorder:
    - Adults—20 mg one time a day in the morning.
    - Children 6 years of age and older—At first, 10 mg one time a day in the morning. Your doctor may increase your child's dose as needed.
    - Children less than 6 years of age—Use is not recommended.

- For *oral* dosage form (tablets):
  - For attention-deficit hyperactivity disorder:
    - Children 6 years of age and older—At first, 5 milligrams (mg) one or two times a day. Your doctor may increase your dose if needed.

- Children 3 to 6 years of age—At first, 2.5 mg once a day. Your doctor may increase your dose if needed.
- Children younger than 3 years of age—Use is not recommended.
  - For narcolepsy:
    - Adults—Usually 5 to 60 mg a day, divided into two or three smaller doses.
    - Children 12 years of age and older—At first, 10 mg a day. Your doctor may increase your dose if needed.
    - Children 6 to 12 years of age—At first, 5 mg a day. Your doctor may increase your dose if needed.
    - Children younger than 6 years of age—Dose must be determined by your doctor.

For dextroamphetamine
- For *oral extended-release capsule* dosage form:
  - For attention-deficit hyperactivity disorder:
    - Adults—5 to 60 milligrams (mg) a day.
    - Children 6 years of age and older—At first, 5 mg one or two times a day. Your doctor may increase your dose if needed.
    - Children 3 to 6 years of age—At first, 2.5 mg a day. Your doctor may increase your dose if needed.
    - Children younger than 3 years of age—Use is not recommended.
  - For narcolepsy:
    - Adults—5 to 60 mg a day.
    - Children 12 years of age and older—At first, 10 mg a day. Your doctor may increase your dose if needed.
    - Children 6 to 12 years of age—At first, 5 mg a day. Your doctor may increase your dose if needed.
    - Children 3 to 6 years of age—Dose must be determined by your doctor.
    - Children younger than 3 years of age—Use is not recommended.
- For *oral tablet* dosage form:
  - For attention-deficit hyperactivity disorder:
    - Adults—5 to 60 mg a day.
    - Children 6 years of age and older—At first, 5 mg one or two times a day. Your doctor may increase your dose if needed.
    - Children 3 to 6 years of age—At first, 2.5 mg a day. Your doctor may increase your dose if needed.
    - Children younger than 3 years of age—Use is not recommended.
  - For narcolepsy:
    - Adults—5 to 60 mg a day.
    - Children 12 years of age and older—At first, 10 mg a day. Your doctor may increase your dose if needed.
    - Children 6 to 12 years of age—At first, 5 mg a day. Your doctor may increase your dose if needed.
    - Children younger than 6 years of age—Dose must be determined by your doctor.

For methamphetamine
- For *oral tablet* dosage form:
  - For attention-deficit hyperactivity disorder:
    - Children 6 years of age and older—At first, 5 milligrams (mg) one or two times a day. Your doctor may increase your dose if needed.

- Children younger than 6 years of age—Use is not recommended.
- For *oral extended-release tablet* dosage form:
  - For attention-deficit hyperactivity disorder:
    - Children 6 years of age and older—20 to 25 mg a day.
    - Children younger than 6 years of age—Use is not recommended.

Missed dose—If you miss a dose of this medicine and your dosing schedule is:

- One dose a day—Take the missed dose as soon as possible, but not later than stated above, to prevent trouble in sleeping. However, if you do not remember the missed dose until the next day, skip it and go back to your regular dosing schedule. Do not double doses.
- Two or three doses a day—If you remember within an hour or so of the missed dose, take the dose right away. However, if you do not remember until later, skip it and go back to your regular dosing schedule. Do not double doses.

Storage—To store this medicine:

- Keep out of the reach of children.
- Store away from heat and direct light.
- Do not store the capsule or tablet form of this medicine in the bathroom, near the kitchen sink, or in other damp places. Heat or moisture may cause the medicine to break down.
- Do not keep outdated medicine or medicine no longer needed. Be sure that any discarded medicine is out of the reach of children.

Precautions While Using This Medicine

Your doctor should check your progress at regular visits to make sure that this medicine does not cause unwanted effects.

If you will be taking this medicine in large doses for a long time, *do not stop taking it without first checking with your doctor*. Your doctor may want you to reduce gradually the amount you are taking before stopping completely.

Do not take amphetamines within 14 days of taking an MAO inhibitor.

This medicine may cause some people to feel a false sense of well-being or to become dizzy, lightheaded, or less alert than they are normally. *Make sure you know how you react to this medicine before you drive, use machines, or do anything else that could be dangerous if you are dizzy or are not alert.*

Amphetamines may cause your skin to be more sensitive to sunlight than it is normally. Exposure to sunlight, even for brief periods of time, may cause a skin rash, itching, redness or other discoloration of the skin, or a severe sunburn. When you begin taking this medicine:

- Stay out of direct sunlight, especially between the hours of 10:00 a.m. and 3:00 p.m., if possible.
- Wear protective clothing, including a hat. Also, wear sunglasses.
- Apply a sun block product that has a skin protection factor (SPF) of at least 15. Some patients may require a product with a higher SOF number, especially if they

have a fair complexion. If you have any questions about this, check with your health care professional.

- Apply a sun block lipstick that has an SPF of at least 15 to protect your lips.
- Do not use a sunlamp or tanning bed or booth.

If you have a severe reaction from the sun, check with your doctor.

Before you have any medical tests, tell the medical doctor in charge that you are taking this medicine. The results of the metyrapone test may be affected by this medicine.

If you have been using this medicine for a long time and you think you may have become mentally or physically dependent on it, check with your doctor. Some signs of dependence on amphetamines are:

- A strong desire or need to continue taking the medicine.
- A need to increase the dose to receive the effects of the medicine.
- Withdrawal effects (for example, mental depression, nausea or vomiting, stomach cramps or pain, trembling, unusual tiredness or weakness) occurring after the medicine is stopped.

Side Effects of This Medicine

Along with its needed effects, a medicine may cause some unwanted effects. Although not all of these side effects may occur, if they do occur they may need medical attention.

Check with your doctor as soon as possible if any of the following side effects occur:

More common
Anxiety; crying; depersonalization; dry mouth; dysphoria; euphoria; fast, pounding, or irregular heartbeat or pulse; hyperventilation; irritability; mental depression; nervousness; paranoia; quick to react or overreact emotionally; rapidly changing moods; restlessness; shaking; shortness of breath; trouble sleeping

Less common
Chills; cold flu-like symptoms; cough or hoarseness; difficult or labored breathing; lower back or side pain; painful or difficult urination; tightness in chest; wheezing

Rare
Chest pain; fever, unusually high; skin rash or hives; uncontrolled movements of head, neck, arms, and legs

With long-term use or high doses
Difficulty in breathing; dizziness or feeling faint; increased blood pressure; mood or mental changes; pounding heartbeat; unusual tiredness or weakness

Other side effects may occur that usually do not need medical attention. These side effects may go away during treatment as your body adjusts to the medicine. However, check with your doctor if any of the following side effects continue or are bothersome:

More common
False sense of well-being; irritability; nervousness; restlessness; trouble in sleeping

Less common
Accidental injury; bladder pain; bloody or cloudy urine; blurred vision; changes in sexual desire or decreased sexual ability; constipation; cramps; diarrhea; difficult, burning, or painful urination; difficulty in speaking; diz-

ziness or lightheadedness; dryness of mouth or unpleasant taste; fast or pounding heartbeat; frequent urge to urinate; headache; heavy bleeding with menstrual period; inability to have or keep an erection; increased sensitivity of skin to sunlight; increased sweating; itching, redness or other discoloration of skin; loss of appetite; lower back or side pain; nausea or vomiting; pain; severe sunburn; sleepiness or unusual drowsiness; stomach cramps or pain; tooth disorder; twitching; weight loss

After you stop using this medicine, your body may need time to adjust. The length of time this takes depends on the amount of medicine you were using and how long you used it. During this period of time check with your doctor if you notice any of the following side effects:

Mental depression; nausea or vomiting; stomach cramps or pain; trembling; unusual tiredness or weakness

Other side effects not listed above may occur also in some patients. If you notice any other effects check with your doctor.

ANABOLIC STEROIDS (Systemic)

Some commonly used brand names are:

In the U.S.—

Anadrol-50 (3)	Hybolin-Improved (1)
Deca-Durabolin (1)	Kabolin (1)
Durabolin (1)	Oxandrin (2)
Durabolin-50 (1)	Winstrol (4)
Hybolin Decanoate (1)	

In Canada—

Anapolon 50 (3)
Deca-Durabolin (1)

This information applies to the following medicines:
1. Nandrolone (NAN-droe-lone)
2. Oxandrolone (ox-AN-droe-lone)
3. Oxymetholone (ox-i-METH-oh-lone)
4. Stanozolol (stan-OH-zoe-lole)

Category

- **Anabolic steroid**—Nandrolone; Oxandrolone; Oxymetholone; Stanozolol
- **Antianemic**—Nandrolone; Oxymetholone; Stanozolol
- **Antiangioedema, hereditary, agent**—Oxymetholone; Stanozolol
- **Antineoplastic**—Nandrolone

Description

This medicine belongs to the group of medicines known as anabolic (an-a-BOL-ik) steroids. They are related to testosterone, a male sex hormone. Anabolic steroids help to rebuild tissues that have become weak because of serious injury or illness. A diet high in proteins and calories is necessary with anabolic steroid treatment.

Anabolic steroids are used for several reasons:
- to help patients gain weight after a severe illness, injury, or continuing infection. They also are used when patients

fail to gain or maintain normal weight because of unexplained medical reasons.
- to treat certain types of anemia.
- to treat certain kinds of breast cancer in some women.
- to treat hereditary angioedema, which causes swelling of the face, arms, legs, throat, windpipe, bowels, or sexual organs.

Anabolic steroids may also be used for other conditions as determined by your doctor.

Anabolic steroids are available only with your doctor's prescription, in the following dosage forms:

Oral
- Oxandrolone
  - Tablets
- Oxymetholone
  - Tablets
- Stanozolol
  - Tablets

Parenteral
- Nandrolone
  - Injection

Before Using This Medicine

In deciding to use a medicine, the risks of taking the medicine must be weighed against the good it will do. This is a decision you and your doctor will make. For anabolic steroids, the following should be considered:

Allergies—Tell your doctor if you have ever had any unusual or allergic reaction to anabolic steroids or androgens (male sex hormones). Also tell your health care professional if you are allergic to any other substances, such as foods, preservatives, or dyes.

Pregnancy—Anabolic steroids should not be used during pregnancy. They may cause the development of male features in the female fetus and premature growth and development of male features in the male fetus. Be sure you have discussed this with your doctor.

Breast-feeding—It is not known whether anabolic steroids pass into breast milk.

Children—Anabolic steroids should be used with caution in pediatric patients. This medicine may cause children to stop growing or their bone growth to slow down. In addition, they may make male children develop too fast sexually and may cause male-like changes in female children.

Older adults—When elderly male patients are treated with anabolic steroids, they may have an increased risk of enlarged prostate or cancer of the prostate.

Other medicines—Although certain medicines should not be used together at all, in other cases two different medicines may be used together even if an interaction might occur. In these cases, your doctor may want to change the dose, or other precautions may be necessary. When you are taking anabolic steroids, it is especially important that your health care professional know if you are taking any of the following:

- Acetaminophen (e.g., Tylenol) (with long-term, high-dose use) or
- Amiodarone (e.g., Cordarone) or
- Androgens (male hormones) or

- Anti-infectives by mouth or by injection (medicine for infection) or
- Antithyroid agents (medicine for overactive thyroid) or
- Carbamazepine (e.g., Tegretol) or
- Carmustine (e.g., BiCNU) or
- Chloroquine (e.g., Aralen) or
- Dantrolene (e.g., Dantrium) or
- Daunorubicin (e.g., Cerubidine) or
- Disulfiram (e.g., Antabuse) or
- Divalproex (e.g., Depakote) or
- Estrogens (female hormones) or
- Etretinate (e.g., Tegison) or
- Gold salts (medicine for arthritis) or
- Hydroxychloroquine (e.g., Plaquenil) or
- Mercaptopurine (e.g., Purinethol) or
- Methotrexate (e.g., Mexate) or
- Methyldopa (e.g., Aldomet) or
- Naltrexone (e.g., Trexan) (with long-term, high-dose use) or
- Oral contraceptives (birth control pills) containing estrogen or
- Phenothiazines (acetophenazine [e.g., Tindal], chlorpromazine [e.g., Thorazine], fluphenazine [e.g., Prolixin], mesoridazine [e.g., Serentil], perphenazine [e.g., Trilafon], prochlorperazine [e.g., Compazine], promazine [e.g., Sparine], promethazine [e.g., Phenergan], thioridazine [e.g., Mellaril], trifluoperazine [e.g., Stelazine], triflupromazine [e.g., Vesprin], trimeprazine [e.g., Temaril]) or
- Phenytoin (e.g., Dilantin) or
- Plicamycin (e.g., Mithracin) or
- Valproic acid (e.g., Depakene)—Taking anabolic steroids with any of these medicines may increase the chances of liver damage. Your doctor may want you to have extra blood tests to check for this if you must take both medicines
- Anticoagulants, oral (blood thinners you take by mouth)—Anabolic steroids can increase the effect of these medicines and possibly cause excessive bleeding

Other medical problems—The presence of other medical problems may affect the use of anabolic steroids. Make sure you tell your doctor if you have any other medical problems, especially:
- Breast cancer (in males and some females)
- Diabetes mellitus (sugar diabetes)—Anabolic steroids can decrease blood sugar levels
- Enlarged prostate or
- Prostate cancer—Anabolic steroids may make these conditions worse by causing more enlargement of the prostate or more growth of a tumor
- Heart or blood vessel disease—Anabolic steroids can worsen these conditions by increasing blood cholesterol levels
- Kidney disease
- Liver disease

- Too much calcium in the blood (or history of) (in females)—Anabolic steroids may worsen this condition by raising the amount of calcium in the blood even more

Proper Use of This Medicine

Take this medicine only as directed. Do not take more of it and do not take it more often than your doctor ordered. To do so may increase the chance of side effects.

In order for this medicine to work properly, it is important that you follow a diet high in proteins and calories. If you have any questions about this, check with your health care professional.

Dosing—The dose of these medicines will be different for different patients. *Follow your doctor's orders or the directions on the label.* The following information includes only the average doses of these medicines. *If your dose is different, do not change it* unless your doctor tells you to do so.

The number of tablets that you take depends on the strength of the medicine. Also, *the number of doses you take each day, the time allowed between doses, and the length of time you take the medicine depend on the medical problem for which you are taking the anabolic steroid.*

For nandrolone decanoate
- For *injection* dosage form:
  - For treatment of certain types of anemia:
    - Women and girls 14 years of age and older—50 to 100 milligrams (mg) injected into a muscle every one to four weeks.
    - Men and boys 14 years of age and older—50 to 200 mg injected into a muscle every one to four weeks.Your doctor may want to continue treatment for up to twelve weeks. After a four-week rest period without receiving this medicine, your doctor may want you to repeat the cycle.
    - Children up to 2 years of age—Dose must be determined by your doctor.
    - Children 2 to 13 years of age—25 to 50 mg injected into a muscle every three to four weeks.

For nandrolone phenpropionate
- For *injection* dosage form:
  - For treatment of certain breast cancers in women:
    - Adults—25 to 100 milligrams (mg) injected into a muscle once a week for up to twelve weeks. After a four-week rest period without receiving this medicine, your doctor may want you to repeat the cycle.
    - Children—Dose must be determined by your doctor.

For oxandrolone
- For *oral* dosage form (tablets):
  - For treatment in rebuilding tissue after a serious illness or injury:
    - Adults and teenagers—2.5 milligrams (mg) two to four times a day for up to four weeks. Your doctor may increase your dose up to 20 mg a day.
    - Children—Dose is based on body weight and must be determined by your doctor. The usual dose is 0.25 mg per kilogram (kg) (0.11 mg per pound) of body weight a day.

For oxymetholone
- For *oral* dosage form (tablets):
  - For treatment of certain types of anemia:
    - Adults, teenagers, children, and older infants—Dose is based on body weight and must be determined by your doctor. The usual dose is 1 to 5 milligrams (mg) per kilogram (kg) (0.45 to 2.3 mg per pound) of body weight a day.
    - Premature and newborn infants—Dose is based on body weight or size and must be determined by your doctor. The usual dose is 0.175 mg per kg (0.08 mg per pound) of body weight once a day.

For stanozolol
- For *oral* dosage form (tablets):
  - To prevent hereditary angioedema, which causes swelling of the face, arms, legs, throat, windpipe, bowels, or sexual organs:
    - Adults and teenagers—At first, 2 milligrams (mg) three times a day to 4 mg four times a day for five days. Then, your doctor may slowly lower the dose to 2 mg once a day or once every other day.

Missed dose—If you miss a dose of this medicine and your dosing schedule is:

- One dose a day—Take the missed dose as soon as possible. However, if you do not remember it until the next day, skip the missed dose and go back to your regular dosing schedule. Do not double doses.
- More than one dose a day—Take the missed dose as soon as possible. However, if it is almost time for your next dose, skip the missed dose and go back to your regular dosing schedule. Do not double doses.

If you have any questions about this, check with your doctor.

Storage—To store this medicine:
- Keep out of the reach of children.
- Store away from heat and direct light.
- Do not store the tablet form of this medicine in the bathroom, near the kitchen sink, or in other damp places. Heat or moisture may cause the medicine to break down.
- Keep the liquid form of this medicine from freezing.
- Do not keep outdated medicine or medicine no longer needed. Be sure that any discarded medicine is out of the reach of children.

Precautions While Using This Medicine

Your doctor should check your progress at regular visits to make sure that this medicine does not cause unwanted effects.

If your child or teenager is taking this medicine, it is important that the doctor take x-rays every 6 months to check your child for bone growth and height. Anabolic steroids may interfere with normal bone growth.

For diabetic patients:
- This medicine may affect blood sugar levels. If you notice a change in the results of your blood or urine sugar tests or if you have any questions, check with your doctor.

Side Effects of This Medicine

Tumors of the liver, liver cancer, or peliosis hepatis, a form of liver disease, have occurred during long-term, high-dose therapy with anabolic steroids. Although these effects are rare, they can be very serious and may cause death. Discuss these possible effects with your doctor.

Along with its needed effects, a medicine may cause some unwanted effects. Although not all of these side effects may occur, if they do occur they may need medical attention.

Check with your doctor immediately if any of the following side effects occur:

  For both females and males
    Less common
      Yellow eyes or skin
    Rare (with long-term use)
      Black, tarry, or light-colored stools; dark-colored urine; purple- or red-colored spots on body or inside the mouth or nose; sore throat and/or fever; vomiting of blood

Also, check with your doctor as soon as possible if any of the following side effects occur:

  For both females and males
    Less common
      Bone pain; nausea or vomiting; sore tongue; swelling of feet or lower legs; unusual bleeding; unusual weight gain
    Rare (with long-term use)
      Abdominal or stomach pain; feeling of discomfort (continuing); headache (continuing); hives; loss of appetite (continuing); unexplained weight loss; unpleasant breath odor (continuing)
    Incidence not known
      Lack or slowing of normal bone growth
  For females only
    More common
      Acne or oily skin; enlarging clitoris; hoarseness or deepening of voice; irregular menstrual periods; unnatural hair growth; unusual hair loss
    Less common
      Mental depression; unusual tiredness
  For young males (boys) only
    More common
      Acne; enlarging penis; increased frequency of erections; unnatural hair growth
    Less common
      Unexplained darkening of skin
  For sexually mature males only
    More common
      Enlargement of breasts or breast soreness; frequent or continuing erections; frequent urge to urinate
  For elderly males only
    Less common
      Difficult or frequent urination

Other side effects may occur that usually do not need medical attention. These side effects may go away during treatment as your body adjusts to the medicine. However, check with your doctor if any of the following side effects continue or are bothersome:

  For both females and males
    Less common
      Chills; diarrhea; feeling of abdominal or stomach fullness; muscle cramps; trouble in sleeping; unusual decrease or increase in sexual desire
  For males only
    More common
      Acne

  Less common
      Decreased sexual ability

Other side effects not listed above may also occur in some patients. If you notice any other effects, check with your doctor.

Additional Information

Once a medicine has been approved for marketing for a certain use, experience may show that it is also useful for other medical problems. Although these uses are not included in product labeling, anabolic steroids may be used in certain patients with the following medical conditions:

- Certain blood clotting diseases
- Growth failure
- Turner's syndrome

Other than the above information, there is no additional information relating to proper use, precautions, or side effects for these uses.

ANAGRELIDE (Oral route) - an-AG-re-lide

Commonly used brand name(s)

In the U.S.—
  Agrylin

Available Dosage Forms:

- Capsule

Therapeutic Class: Platelet Reducing Agent

Uses For This Medicine

Anagrelide is used to decrease the risk of blood clots in patients who have too many platelet cells in their blood.

This medicine is available only with your doctor's prescription.

Before Using This Medicine

In deciding to use a medicine, the risks of taking the medicine must be weighed against the good it will do. This is a decision you and your doctor will make. For this medicine, the following should be considered:

Allergies—Tell your doctor if you have ever had any unusual or allergic reaction to this medicine or any other medicines. Also tell your health care professional if you have any other types of allergies, such as to foods, dyes, preservatives, or animals. For non-prescription products, read the label or package ingredients carefully.

Pediatric—This medicine has been tested in children and, in effective doses, has not been shown to cause different side effects or problems than it does in adults.

Pregnancy—

	Pregnancy Category	Explanation
All Trimesters	C	Animal studies have shown an adverse effect and there are no adequate studies in pregnant women OR no animal studies have been conducted and there are no adequate studies in pregnant women.

Breast Feeding—There are no adequate studies in women for determining infant risk when using this medication during breastfeeding. Weigh the potential benefits against the potential risks before taking this medication while breastfeeding.

Other medicines—

Using this medicine with any of the following medicines is usually not recommended, but may be required in some cases. If both medicines are prescribed together, your doctor may change the dose or how often you use one or both of the medicines.

Ginkgo

Interactions with Food/Tobacco/Alcohol—Certain medicines should not be used at or around the time of eating food or eating certain types of food since interactions may occur. Using alcohol or tobacco with certain medicines may also cause interactions to occur. Discuss with your healthcare professional the use of your medicine with food, alcohol, or tobacco.

Other medical problems—The presence of other medical problems may affect the use of this medicine. Make sure you tell your doctor if you have any other medical problems, especially:

- Heart disease (known or suspected)—Anagrelide can cause unwanted effects on the heart
- Kidney disease—Anagrelide rarely causes unwanted effects on the kidney
- Liver disease—Blood levels of anagrelide may be increased, possibly increasing the chance of side effects. Also, this medicine sometimes causes unwanted effects on the liver

Proper Use of This Medicine

Dosing—The dose of this medicine will be different for different patients. Follow your doctor's orders or the directions on the label. The following information includes only the average doses of this medicine. If your dose is different, do not change it unless your doctor tells you to do so.

The amount of medicine that you take depends on the strength of the medicine. Also, the number of doses you take each day, the time allowed between doses, and the length of time you take the medicine depend on the medical problem for which you are using the medicine.

- For oral dosage form (capsules):
  - For too many platelets in the blood:
    - Adults—0.5 milligrams (mg) four times a day, or 1 mg two times a day, for at least one week. After that, the dose is adjusted to the dose that keeps the number of platelets normal.
    - Children—0.5 mg one time per day, for at least one week. After that, the dose is adjusted to the dose that keeps the number of platelets normal.

Storage—Store the medicine in a closed container at room temperature, away from heat, moisture, and direct light. Keep from freezing.

Keep out of the reach of children.

Do not keep outdated medicine or medicine no longer needed.

Precautions While Using This Medicine

It is very important that your doctor check your progress at regular visits to make sure that this medicine is working properly and to check for unwanted effects.

Anagrelide can cause unwanted effects on the heart, including a heart attack. Check with your doctor and/or get emergency help immediately if you experience any signs or symptoms of a heart attack.

Side Effects of This Medicine

Along with its needed effects, a medicine may cause some unwanted effects. Although not all of these side effects may occur, if they do occur they may need medical attention.

Check with your doctor immediately if any of the following side effects occur:
  Less common
    Sudden severe headache or weakness; symptoms of a heart attack, which may include anxiety, cold sweating, increased heart rate, nausea or vomiting, severe pain or pressure in the chest and/or the jaw, neck, back, or arms, and shortness of breath

Check with your doctor as soon as possible if any of the following side effects occur:
  More common
    Abdominal or stomach pain; dizziness; irregular heartbeat; weakness
  Less common
    Blood in urine; blurred or double vision; difficulty in breathing; faintness; flushing; numbness or tingling in hands or feet; painful or difficult urination; swelling of feet or lower legs; unusual bleeding or bruising; unusual tiredness

Some side effects may occur that usually do not need medical attention. These side effects may go away during treatment as your body adjusts to the medicine. Also, your health care professional may be able to tell you about ways to prevent or reduce some of these side effects. Check with your health care professional if any of the following side effects continue or are bothersome or if you have any questions about them:
  More common
    Diarrhea; gas or bloating of stomach; headache; heartburn; pain
  Less common or rare
    Back pain; canker sore; confusion; constipation; fever or chills; general feeling of discomfort or illness; joint pain; leg cramps; loss of appetite; mental depression; muscle pain; nervousness; ringing in the ears; skin rash or itching; sleepiness; stuffy or runny nose; trouble in sleeping; unusual sensitivity to light

Anagrelide may cause a temporary loss of hair in some people.

Other side effects not listed may also occur in some patients. If you notice any other effects, check with your healthcare professional.

ANAKINRA (Subcutaneous route) - an-a-KIN-ra

Commonly used brand name(s)

In the U.S.—
Kineret

Available Dosage Forms:
* Solution

Therapeutic Class: Immune Stimulant
Pharmacologic Class: Interleukin-1 Inhibitor

Uses For This Medicine

Anakinra is used to treat moderate to severe symptoms of rheumatoid arthritis. It may relieve redness, pain, tenderness, and warmth in hands, feet, wrists, shoulders, elbows, and ankles. This medicine is used in patients 18 years of age or older. Anakinra will not cure the disease, but will help with the symptoms as long as you continue to take it.

This medicine is available only with your doctor's prescription.

Before Using This Medicine

In deciding to use a medicine, the risks of taking the medicine must be weighed against the good it will do. This is a decision you and your doctor will make. For this medicine, the following should be considered:

Allergies—Tell your doctor if you have ever had any unusual or allergic reaction to this medicine or any other medicines. Also tell your health care professional if you have any other types of allergies, such as to foods, dyes, preservatives, or animals. For non-prescription products, read the label or package ingredients carefully.

Pediatric—Studies on this medicine have been done only in adult patients, and there is no specific information comparing use of anakinra in children with use in other age groups.

Geriatric—This medicine has been tested and has not been shown to cause different side effects or problems in older people than it does in younger adults.

Pregnancy—

	Pregnancy Category	Explanation
All Trimesters	B	Animal studies have revealed no evidence of harm to the fetus, however, there are no adequate studies in pregnant women OR animal studies have shown an adverse effect, but adequate studies in pregnant women have failed to demonstrate a risk to the fetus.

Breast Feeding—There are no adequate studies in women for determining infant risk when using this medication during breastfeeding. Weigh the potential benefits against the potential risks before taking this medication while breastfeeding.

Other medicines—

Using this medicine with any of the following medicines is usually not recommended, but may be required in some cases. If both medicines are prescribed together, your doctor may change the dose or how often you use one or both of the medicines.

Abatacept, Adalimumab, Etanercept, Infliximab

Interactions with Food/Tobacco/Alcohol—Certain medicines should not be used at or around the time of eating food or eating certain types of food since interactions may occur. Using alcohol or tobacco with certain medicines may also cause interactions to occur. Discuss with your healthcare professional the use of your medicine with food, alcohol, or tobacco.

Other medical problems—The presence of other medical problems may affect the use of this medicine. Make sure you tell your doctor if you have any other medical problems, especially:

* Active infections—May be worsened by anakinra
* Asthma—Patients with asthma may be at higher risk of getting a serious infection when taking anakinra.
* Immunosuppression—Anakinra has not been studied in patients who have immune system problems. The effects of the medicine in these patients is not known
* Kidney disease—Higher blood levels of anakinra may occur

Proper Use of This Medicine

Your health care professional will teach you or your caregiver how to give the injection. You must demonstrate the procedure so that your health care professional knows you understand. Before taking the injection, check the medicine to make sure it is clear and doesn't have any particles in it. If it looks cloudy or discolored, or has any particles floating in it, you should throw it away. Do not shake the syringe. Give the entire dose and then throw away the syringe. Your health care professional will tell you how to dispose of your syringes. Do not reuse syringes. Do not keep part of a dose for later use. Take the medicine at the same time each day. If you have questions or problems with the procedure, call your health care professional.

Dosing—The dose of this medicine will be different for different patients. Follow your doctor's orders or the directions on the label. The following information includes only the average doses of this medicine. If your dose is different, do not change it unless your doctor tells you to do so.

The amount of medicine that you take depends on the strength of the medicine. Also, the number of doses you take each day, the time allowed between doses, and the length of time you take the medicine depend on the medical problem for which you are using the medicine.

* For injection dosage form
  * For rheumatoid arthritis:
    * Adults—100 milligrams (mg) a day injected under the skin.

- Children—Use and dose must be determined by your doctor. Anakinra is not usually recommended for use in children.

Missed dose—If you miss a dose of this medicine, take it as soon as possible. However, if it is almost time for your next dose, skip the missed dose and go back to your regular dosing schedule. Do not double doses.

Storage—Store in the refrigerator. Do not freeze.

Keep out of the reach of children.

Do not keep outdated medicine or medicine no longer needed.

Precautions While Using This Medicine

It is important that your doctor check your progress at regular visits to make sure that this medicine is working properly and to check for unwanted effects.

Your body's ability to fight infection may be reduced while you are being treated with anakinra, it is very important that you call your doctor at the first signs of any infection (for example, if you get a fever or chills).

While you are being treated with anakinra, do not have any immunizations (vaccinations) without your doctor's approval.

Side Effects of This Medicine

Along with its needed effects, a medicine may cause some unwanted effects. Although not all of these side effects may occur, if they do occur they may need medical attention.

Check with your doctor immediately if any of the following side effects occur:

More common
Chest pain; cough; diarrhea; fever or chills; general feeling of discomfort or illness; headache; itching, pain, redness, swelling, tenderness or warmth on skin; joint pain; loss of appetite; muscle aches and pains; nausea; pain or tenderness around eyes and cheekbones; redness, bruising pain at the injection site; runny nose; shivering; shortness of breath; sneezing; sore throat; sweating; tightness in chest; trouble sleeping; unusual tiredness or weakness; vomiting; wheezing

Less common or rare
Black, sticky stools; difficulty in swallowing; itching; lower back pain or side pain; painful or difficult urination; pale skin; rash; hives; swelling of face or lips; ulcers, sores or white spots in mouth; unusual bruising or bleeding

Some side effects may occur that usually do not need medical attention. These side effects may go away during treatment as your body adjusts to the medicine. Also, your health care professional may be able to tell you about ways to prevent or reduce some of these side effects. Check with your health care professional if any of the following side effects continue or are bothersome or if you have any questions about them:

More common
Abdominal or stomach pain

Other side effects not listed may also occur in some patients. If you notice any other effects, check with your healthcare professional.

ANASTROZOLE (Oral route) - an-AS-troe-zole

Commonly used brand name(s)

In the U.S.—
Arimidex

Available Dosage Forms:
- Tablet

Therapeutic Class: Antineoplastic Agent
Pharmacologic Class: Aromatase Inhibitor

Uses For This Medicine

Anastrozole is a medicine that is used to treat breast cancer.

Many breast cancer tumors grow in response to estrogen. This medicine interferes with the production of estrogen in the body. As a result, the amount of estrogen that the tumor is exposed to is reduced, limiting the growth of the tumor.

This medicine is available only with your doctor's prescription.

Once a medicine has been approved for marketing for a certain use, experience may show that it is also useful for other medical problems. Although these uses are not included in product labeling, anastrozole is used in certain patients with the following medical conditions:
- Breast cancer, neoadjuvant treatment for hormone receptor-positive, operable or potentially operable, locally advanced disease in postmenopausal women (treatment for advanced breast cancer that may be operable in women who have already gone through menopause)

Before Using This Medicine

In deciding to use a medicine, the risks of taking the medicine must be weighed against the good it will do. This is a decision you and your doctor will make. For this medicine, the following should be considered:

Allergies—Tell your doctor if you have ever had any unusual or allergic reaction to this medicine or any other medicines. Also tell your health care professional if you have any other types of allergies, such as to foods, dyes, preservatives, or animals. For non-prescription products, read the label or package ingredients carefully.

Pediatric—Studies on this medicine have been done only in adult patients, and there is no specific information comparing use of anastrozole in children with use in other age groups.

Geriatric—This medicine has been tested in a limited number of patients 65 years of age or older and has not been shown to cause different side effects or problems in older people than it does in younger adults.

Pregnancy—

	Pregnancy Category	Explanation
All Trimesters	D	Studies in pregnant women have demonstrated a risk to the fetus. However, the benefits of therapy in a life threatening situation or a serious disease, may outweigh the potential risk.

Breast Feeding—There are no adequate studies in women for determining infant risk when using this medication during breastfeeding. Weigh the potential benefits against the potential risks before taking this medication while breastfeeding.

Other medicines—

Using this medicine with any of the following medicines may cause an increased risk of certain side effects, but using both drugs may be the best treatment for you. If both medicines are prescribed together, your doctor may change the dose or how often you use one or both of the medicines.

Tamoxifen

Interactions with Food/Tobacco/Alcohol—Certain medicines should not be used at or around the time of eating food or eating certain types of food since interactions may occur. Using alcohol or tobacco with certain medicines may also cause interactions to occur. Discuss with your healthcare professional the use of your medicine with food, alcohol, or tobacco.

Other medical problems—The presence of other medical problems may affect the use of anastrozole. Make sure you tell your doctor if you have any other medical problems.

Proper Use of This Medicine

Take this medicine only as directed by your doctor. Do not use more or less of it, and do not use it more often than your doctor ordered.

Anastrozole sometimes causes nausea, vomiting, and diarrhea. However, it is very important that you continue to use the medicine, even if you begin to feel ill. Ask your doctor, nurse, or pharmacist for ways to lessen these effects.

Dosing—The dose of this medicine will be different for different patients. Follow your doctor's orders or the directions on the label. The following information includes only the average doses of this medicine. If your dose is different, do not change it unless your doctor tells you to do so.

The amount of medicine that you take depends on the strength of the medicine. Also, the number of doses you take each day, the time allowed between doses, and the length of time you take the medicine depend on the medical problem for which you are using the medicine.

- For oral dosage form (tablets):
  - For breast cancer:
    - Adults—1 mg once a day. Your doctor will determine how long you need to take this medicine.
    - Children—Use and dose must be determined by your doctor.

Missed dose—If you miss a dose of this medicine, skip the missed dose and go back to your regular dosing schedule. Do not double doses.

Storage—Store the medicine in a closed container at room temperature, away from heat, moisture, and direct light. Do not refrigerate. Keep from freezing.

Keep out of the reach of children.

Do not keep outdated medicine or medicine no longer needed.

Precautions While Using This Medicine

It is important that your doctor check your progress at regular visits to make sure this medicine is working properly and to check for unwanted effects.

Side Effects of This Medicine

Along with its needed effects, a medicine may cause some unwanted effects. Although not all of these side effects may occur, if they do occur they may need medical attention.

Check with your doctor immediately if any of the following side effects occur:

More common
> Chest pain; shortness of breath; swelling of feet or lower legs

Check with your doctor as soon as possible if any of the following side effects occur:

Less common
> Cough or hoarseness; difficult or painful urination; dizziness, severe; fever or chills; headache, continuing; increased blood pressure; lower back or side pain; pain, tenderness, bluish color, or swelling of foot or leg; sore throat; sudden shortness of breath; unusual tiredness or weakness; vaginal bleeding (unexpected and heavy)

Frequency not known—occurred during clinical practice; number of times side effect occurred is not known
> Blistering, peeling, loosening of skin; Fast heartbeat; hives; itching, puffiness or swelling of the eyelids or around the eyes, face, lips or tongue; large, hive-like swelling on face, eyelids, lips, tongue, throat, hands, legs, feet, sex organs; red skin lesions, often with a purple center; sores, ulcers, or white spots in mouth or on lips; welts

Some side effects may occur that usually do not need medical attention. These side effects may go away during treatment as your body adjusts to the medicine. Also, your health care professional may be able to tell you about ways to prevent or reduce some of these side effects. Check with your health care professional if any of the following side effects continue or are bothersome or if you have any questions about them:

More common
> Back pain; body aches or pain; bone pain; congestion; constipation; cough; diarrhea; dizziness; dry mouth; dryness or soreness of throat; feeling of warmth; fever; flushing or redness of skin, especially on face and neck; headache; hoarseness; hot flashes; increased appetite; loss of appetite and weight loss; mood or mental changes; nausea or vomiting; pain, general; pelvic pain; runny nose; skin rash; stomach pain; sweating; tender, swollen glands in neck; trouble in swallowing; voice changes; weakness

Less common
> Anxiety and confusion; breast pain; chills; cough or a cough producing mucus; diarrhea; difficulty breathing; dryness of the vagina; fever; general feeling of discomfort or illness; headache; itching of skin; joint pain and stiffness; loss of appetite; loss of hair; muscle pain; nausea; nervousness; numbness or tingling of hands or feet; shivering; shortness of breath; sleepiness or unusual drowsiness; sore throat; stuffy or runny nose; sweating; tightness in chest; trouble sleeping or sleeplessness; unusual tiredness or weakness; vaginal dryness; vomiting; weight gain; wheezing

Other side effects not listed may also occur in some patients. If you notice any other effects, check with your healthcare professional.

ANDROGENS (Systemic)

Some commonly used brand names are:

In the U.S.—

Androderm (3)	ORETON Methyl (2)
AndroGel (3)	T-Cypionate (3)
Android (2)	Testamone 100 (3)
Android-F (1)	Testaqua (3)
Andro L.A. 200 (3)	Testex (3)
Andronate 100 (3)	Testoderm (3)
Andronate 200 (3)	Testoderm with Adhesives (3)
Andropository 200 (3)	Testoderm TTS (3)
Andryl 200 (3)	Testopel Pellets (3)
Delatest (3)	Testred (2)
Delatestryl (3)	Testred Cypionate 200 (3)
Depotest (3)	Testrin-P.A. (3)
Depo-Testosterone (3)	Virilon (2)
Everone 200 (3)	Virilon IM (3)
Halotestin (1)	

In Canada—

Andriol (3)	Halotestin (1)
Delatestryl (3)	Malogen in Oil (3)
Depo-Testosterone	Metandren (2)
Cypionate (3)	Scheinpharm Testone-Cyp (3)

This information applies to the following medicines

1. Fluoxymesterone (floo-ox-i-MES-te-rone)
2. Methyltestosterone (meth-il-tes-TOS-te-rone)
3. Testosterone (tes-TOS-te-rone)

Category

- **Androgen**—Fluoxymesterone; Methyltestosterone; Testosterone
- **Antianemic**—Fluoxymesterone; Testosterone
- **Antineoplastic**—Fluoxymesterone; Methyltestosterone; Testosterone

Description

Androgens (AN-droe-jens) are male hormones. Some androgens are naturally produced in the body and are necessary for the normal sexual development of males.

Androgens are used for several reasons, such as:
- to replace the hormone when the body is unable to produce enough on its own.
- to stimulate the beginning of puberty in certain boys who are late starting puberty naturally.
- to treat certain types of breast cancer in females.

In addition, some of these medicines may be used for other conditions as determined by your doctor.

Androgens are available only with your doctor's prescription, in the following dosage forms:

Oral
- Fluoxymesterone
  - Tablets
- Methyltestosterone
  - Capsules
  - Tablets
- Testosterone
  - Capsules

Parenteral
- Testosterone
  - Injection

Subcutaneous
- Testosterone
  - Implants (Pellets)

Topical
- Testosterone
  - Gel
  - Ointment
  - Transdermal systems (skin patches)

Before Using This Medicine

In deciding to use a medicine, the risks of taking the medicine must be weighed against the good it will do. This is a decision you and your doctor will make. For androgens, the following should be considered:

Allergies—Tell your doctor if you have ever had any unusual or allergic reaction to androgens. Also tell your health care professional if you are allergic to any other substances, such as foods, preservatives, or dyes.

Pregnancy—Androgens are not recommended during pregnancy. When given to pregnant women, the medicine has caused male features to develop in female babies.

Breast-feeding—Use is not recommended in nursing mothers, since androgens may pass into the breast milk and may cause unwanted effects in the nursing baby, such as premature (too early) sexual development in males and development of male features in female babies.

Children—Androgens may cause children to stop growing. In addition, androgens may make male children develop too fast sexually and may cause male-like changes in female children.

Older adults—When older male patients are treated with androgens, they may have an increased risk of enlarged prostate (a male gland) or their existing prostate cancer may get worse. For these reasons, a prostate examination and a blood test to check for prostate cancer is often done before androgens are prescribed for men over 50 years of age. These examinations may be repeated during treatment.

Other medicines—Although certain medicines should not be used together at all, in other cases two different medicines may be used together even if an interaction might occur. In these cases, your doctor may want to change the dose, or other precautions may be necessary. When you are taking androgens, it is especially important that your health care professional know if you are taking any of the following:
- Acetaminophen (e.g., Tylenol) (with long-term, high-dose use) or
- Amiodarone (e.g., Cordarone) or
- Anabolic steroids (nandrolone [e.g., Anabolin], oxandrolone [e.g., Anavar], oxymetholone [e.g., Anadrol], stanozolol [e.g., Winstrol]) or
- Anti-infectives by mouth or by injection (medicines for infection) or
- Antithyroid agents (medicines for overactive thyroid) or
- Carbamazepine (e.g., Tegretol) or
- Carmustine (e.g., BiCNU) or
- Chloroquine (e.g., Aralen) or
- Dantrolene (e.g., Dantrium) or
- Daunorubicin (e.g., Cerubidine) or
- Disulfiram (e.g., Antabuse) or
- Divalproex (e.g., Depakote) or

- Estrogens (female hormones) or
- Etretinate (e.g., Tegison) or
- Gold salts (medicines for arthritis) or
- Hydroxychloroquine (e.g., Plaquenil) or
- Mercaptopurine (e.g., Purinethol) or
- Methotrexate (e.g., Mexate) or
- Methyldopa (e.g., Aldomet) or
- Naltrexone (e.g., Trexan) (with long-term, high-dose use) or
- Oral contraceptives (birth control pills) containing estrogen or
- Phenothiazines (acetophenazine [e.g., Tindal], chlorpromazine [e.g., Thorazine], fluphenazine [e.g., Prolixin], mesoridazine [e.g., Serentil], perphenazine [e.g., Trilafon], prochlorperazine [e.g., Compazine], promazine [e.g., Sparine], promethazine [e.g., Phenergan], thioridazine [e.g., Mellaril], trifluoperazine [e.g., Stelazine], triflupromazine [e.g., Vesprin], trimeprazine [e.g., Temaril]) or
- Phenytoin (e.g., Dilantin) or
- Plicamycin (e.g., Mithracin) or
- Valproic acid (e.g., Depakene)—Use of these medicines with androgens may increase the chance of liver problems. Your doctor may want you to have extra blood tests that check your liver while you are taking any of these medicines with an androgen
- Anticoagulants (blood thinners)—Androgens can increase the effect of these medicines and possibly cause excessive bleeding

Other medical problems—The presence of other medical problems may affect the use of androgens. Make sure you tell your doctor if you have any other medical problems, especially:

- Breast cancer (in males) or
- Prostate cancer—Androgens can cause growth of these tumors
- Breast cancer (in females)—Androgens may cause high calcium levels in the blood to become worse
- Diabetes mellitus (sugar diabetes)—Androgens can increase or decrease blood sugar levels. Careful monitoring of blood glucose should be done
- Edema (swelling of face, hands, feet, or lower legs) or
- Kidney disease or
- Liver disease—These conditions can be worsened by the fluid retention (keeping too much water in the body) that can be caused by androgens. Also, liver disease can prevent the body from removing the medicine from the bloodstream as fast as it normally would. This could increase the chance of side effects occurring
- Enlarged prostate—Androgens can cause further enlargement of the prostate
- Heart or blood vessel disease—Androgens can make these conditions worse because androgens may increase blood cholesterol levels. Also, androgens can cause fluid retention (keeping too much water in the body), which also can worsen heart or blood vessel disease

Proper Use of This Medicine

Take this medicine only as directed. Do not take more of it and do not take it more often than your doctor ordered. Doing so may increase the chance of side effects.

There are two types of testosterone skin patches. The matrix-type is applied to skin of the scrotum. The reservoir-type is never applied to the skin of the scrotum. It is applied to other parts of the body. Be sure you know which type you are using so that you will apply it properly. These skin patches come with patient directions. Read them carefully before using the patch.

For patients taking *fluoxymesterone* or *methyltestosterone:*

- Take this medicine with food to lessen possible stomach upset, unless otherwise directed by your doctor.

For patients using the *matrix-type skin patch of testosterone (Testoderm or Testoderm with Adhesives):*

- You must apply the patch to the scrotum because the medicine easily passes into your body at this area. Other areas of your skin are too thick for the medicine to work properly.
- Wash and dry your hands thoroughly before and after handling the patch.
  - Before applying the patch:
    - Clean and dry your scrotum.
    - You should also dry-shave this area once a week by using a shaver only (no soap or water). To dry-shave, stretch the skin of your scrotum with your fingers. Use short gentle strokes with no pressure on the razor to remove the hair. Do not use shaving cream or hair-removing creams (e.g., Nair).
    - You may sit with your legs apart or stand while applying the patch.
  - To apply the patch:
    - Open the wrapper containing the patch at the point shown on the package.
    - Carefully remove the patch from its protective plastic liner by peeling the patch from the liner starting at the corner.
    - Warm your scrotum for a few seconds before applying the patch to achieve the best results. Stretch the skin of your scrotum gently to remove the folds by pulling the penis up and to the side. Another way is to pull your scrotum down. Use your first and middle fingers to stretch the skin of your scrotum.
    - Place the shiny side of the patch onto the warm stretched skin of your scrotum.
    - Press the shiny side of the patch firmly in place with the palm of your hand for about 10 seconds. Make sure there is good contact, especially around the edges. The patch should stick to your scrotum and show the natural wrinkles of your scrotum.
    - Put on comfortable, close-fitting briefs (underwear) after applying the patch.
    - If a patch becomes loose or falls off, you may reapply it or discard it and apply a new patch.

- To remove the skin patch:
  - Gently peel the patch from the skin.
  - You may reuse the patch after removing it for swimming, bathing, showering, or sexual activity. First, remove the patch and place the shiny (sticky) side up on a counter. Before you reapply the patch, be sure the skin on your scrotum is dry. Then, follow the directions to reapply the patch.
  - When the wearing period is over, fold the patch in half with the sticky sides together. Place the folded, used patch in its protective pouch or in aluminum foil. Be sure to throw it away out of the reach of children and pets.

For patients using the *reservoir-type skin patch of testosterone (Androderm or Testoderm TTS):*

- Apply the patch called *Androderm* to the abdomen, back, thighs, or arms. Apply the patch called *Testoderm TTS* to the back, arms, or upper buttocks. *Do not apply these patches to the scrotum.*

- Do not apply the patch to areas of the body that seem bony, such as the top of the shoulders or near the elbows, or to areas that may have to support your body while sleeping or sitting, such as the hips or shoulder blades. Apply each new patch to a different place. Do not reapply a patch to the same area of skin for 7 days.

- Wash and dry your hands thoroughly before and after handling the patch.
  - Before applying the patch, clean and dry the application site.
  - To apply the patch:
    - Open the wrapper containing the patch at the point shown on the package.
    - Carefully remove the patch from its protective plastic liner by peeling the patch from the liner, starting at the corner.
    - Place the shiny side of the patch onto the skin.
    - Press the shiny side of the patch firmly in place with the palm of your hand for about 10 seconds. Be sure there is good contact, especially around the edges.
    - If a patch becomes loose or falls off, you may reapply it or discard it and apply a new patch.
  - To remove the skin patch:
    - Gently peel the patch from the skin.
    - You do not need to remove this patch for swimming, bathing, showering, or sexual activity.
    - When the wearing period is over, fold the patch in half with the sticky sides together. Place the folded, used patch in its protective pouch or in aluminum foil. Be sure to throw it away out of the reach of children and pets.

Dosing—The dose of these medicines will be different for different patients. *Follow your doctor's orders or the directions on the label.* The following information includes only the average doses of these medicines. *If your dose is different, do not change it* unless your doctor tells you to do so.

The number of capsules or tablets that you take depends on the strength of the medicine. Also, *the number of doses you take each day, the time between doses, and the length of time you take the medicine depend on the medical problem for which you are taking the androgen.*

For fluoxymesterone
- For *oral* dosage form (tablets):
  - For androgen hormone replacement in men:
    - Adults—5 milligrams (mg) one to four times a day.
  - For treatment of breast cancer in women:
    - Adults—10 to 40 mg a day in divided doses.
  - For treatment of delayed sexual development in boys:
    - Children—2.5 to 10 mg a day for four to six months.

For methyltestosterone
- For *oral* dosage forms (capsules or tablets):
  - For androgen hormone replacement in men:
    - Adults—10 to 50 milligrams (mg) a day.
  - For treatment of breast cancer in women:
    - Adults—50 mg one to four times a day. Your doctor may decrease your dose to 50 mg two times a day after two to four weeks.
  - For treatment of delayed sexual development in boys:
    - Children—5 to 25 mg a day for four to six months.

For testosterone
- For *injection* dosage form:
  - For androgen hormone replacement in men:
    - Adults—25 to 50 milligrams (mg) injected into a muscle two or three times a week.
  - For treatment of breast cancer in women:
    - Adults—50 to 100 mg injected into a muscle three times a week.
  - For treatment of delayed sexual development in boys:
    - Children—Up to 100 mg injected into a muscle once a month for four to six months.

- For *subcutaneous* dosage form (implants):
  - For androgen hormone replacement in men:
    - Adults—150 to 450 milligram (mg) (two to six implants) inserted into the skin every three to six months.

  - For treatment of delayed sexual development in boys:
    - Children—Use and dose must be determined by your doctor.

- For *topical* dosage forms:
  - For androgen hormone replacement in men:

  When using the brand name AndroGel 1% testosterone gel
    - Adults—The recommended starting dose is 5 grams applied once daily (preferably in the morning) to clean, dry, intact skin of the shoulders and upper arms and/or abdomen. Allow the application sites to dry prior to dressing and wash hands with soap and water after application.
    - Children—Use and dose must be determined by your doctor.

  When using the brand name Testoderm or Testoderm with Adhesives patches (matrix-type)
    - Adults—4 or 6 mg (one patch) applied to your scrotum once a day at about 8 a.m. The patch should be worn at least twenty-two of the twenty-four hours in a day.

- Children—Use and dose must be determined by your doctor.

When using the brand name Androderm patches (reservoir-type)
- Adults and teenagers 15 years of age and older—2.5 to 7.5 mg (one to three patches) applied to the abdomen, back, thighs, or upper arms once a day at about 10 p.m. The patch(es) should be worn for twenty-four hours a day.
- Children up to 15 years of age—Use and dose must be determined by your doctor.

When using the brand name Testoderm TTS patches (reservoir-type)
- Adults—5 mg (one patch) applied to the back, arms, or upper buttocks once a day at about 8 a.m. Your doctor may increase your dose if necessary. The patch should be worn at least twenty-two of the twenty-four hours in a day.
- Children up to 18 years of age—Use and dose must be determined by your doctor.

For testosterone cypionate or testosterone enanthate
- For *injection* dosage form:
  - For androgen hormone replacement in men:
    - Adults—50 to 400 milligrams (mg) injected into a muscle every two to four weeks.
  - For treatment of breast cancer in women:
    - Adults—200 to 400 mg injected into a muscle every two to four weeks.
  - For treatment of delayed sexual development in boys:
    - Children—Up to 100 mg injected into a muscle once a month for four to six months.

For testosterone propionate
- For *injection* dosage form:
  - For androgen hormone replacement in men:
    - Adults—25 to 50 milligrams (mg) injected into a muscle two or three times a week.
  - For treatment of breast cancer in women:
    - Adults—50 to 100 mg injected into a muscle three times a week.
  - For treatment of delayed sexual development in boys:
    - Children—Up to 100 milligrams injected into a muscle once a month for four to six months.

For testosterone undecanoate
- For *oral* dosage form (capsules):
  - For androgen hormone replacement in men:
    - Adults—120 to 160 milligrams (mg) divided into two doses a day taken with meals for two to three weeks. Then dose is reduced to 40 to 120 mg a day, taken with meals, and divided into 2 doses a day when possible.

Missed dose—For oral dosage forms: If you miss a dose of this medicine and your dosing schedule is:
- One dose a day—Take, use, or apply the missed dose as soon as possible. However, if you do not remember it until the next day, skip the missed dose and go back to your regular dosing schedule. Do not double doses.
- More than one dose a day—Take or use the missed dose as soon as possible. However, if it is almost time for your next dose, skip the missed dose and go back to your regular dosing schedule. Do not double doses.

For topical dosage forms (patches): If you miss a dose of this medicine or your patch falls off within 12 hours after applying it and cannot be reapplied, skip the rest of the dose and go back to your regular dosing schedule. Do not double doses.

If you have any questions about this, check with your doctor.

Storage—To store this medicine:
- Keep out of the reach of children.
- Store away from heat and direct light.
- Do not store in the bathroom, near the kitchen sink, or in other damp places. Heat or moisture may cause the medicine to break down.
- Keep the injection form of this medicine from freezing.
- Do not keep outdated medicine or medicine no longer needed. Be sure that any discarded medicine is out of the reach of children.

Precautions While Using This Medicine

Your doctor should check your progress at regular visits to make sure this medicine does not cause unwanted effects.

For patients with diabetes mellitus (sugar diabetes):
- This medicine may affect blood sugar levels. If you notice a change in the results of your blood or urine sugar tests or if you have any questions, check with your doctor.

For patients using the brand name Testoderm patches (matrix-type):
- In some cases, this medicine can pass from you to your sexual partner. Tell your doctor if your female sex partner has a great increase in acne. Also, tell your doctor if her hair begins to grow in odd places like her upper lip, chest, or back. This will not occur if you are using the reservoir-type skin patch because it is not applied to the scrotum and because it has a protective liner.

For patients using the brand name Androgel
- Wait 5 or 6 hours after applying the gel before showering or swimming.
- Gel contains alcohol which is flammable- avoid fire, flame or smoking until the gel is dried.

Side Effects of This Medicine

Discuss these possible effects with your doctor:
- Tumors of the liver, liver cancer, or peliosis hepatis (a form of liver disease) have occurred during long-term, high-dose therapy with androgens. Although these effects are rare, they can be very serious and may cause death.
- Androgens can stimulate existing prostate cancer in men who already have it but have not yet been diagnosed. Also, the prostate (a male gland) may become enlarged. Enlargement of the prostate does not mean that cancer will develop. If enlargement occurs and you have difficulty in urinating, it is a good idea to be checked by your doctor.
- When androgens are used in women, especially in high doses, male-like changes may occur, such as hoarseness or deepening of the voice, unnatural hair growth, or unusual hair loss. Most of these changes will go away if the medicine is stopped as soon as the changes are

noticed. However, some changes, such as voice changes or enlarged clitoris, may not go away.

- When androgens are used in high doses in males, they interfere with the production of sperm. This effect is usually temporary and only happens during the time you are taking the medicine. However, discuss this possible effect with your doctor if you are planning on having children.

Along with its needed effects, a medicine may cause some unwanted effects. Although not all of these side effects appear very often, when they do occur they may require medical attention. Check with your doctor as soon as possible if any of the following side effects occur:

More common
For females only
Acne or oily skin; decreased breast size; irregular menstrual cycles; hoarseness or deepening of voice; increase in size of female genitals; increase in unnatural hair growth or male pattern baldness

For males only
Blistering of skin under patch (especially when the nonscrotal patch is applied to bony areas of the skin); breast soreness or enlargement; frequent or continuing erection of penis lasting up to 4 hours or painful penile erections lasting longer than 4 hours; frequent urge to urinate; itching or redness of skin under patch (less likely with nonscrotal patch) or at site of implants, mild to severe

For prepubertal boys only
Acne; early growth of pubic hair; enlargement of penis; frequent or continuing erections

Less common
For males or females
Dizziness; frequent or continuing headache; lack or loss of strength; nausea; overall body flushing, redness, or itching of skin; rapid weight gain; rapidly changing moods, such as depersonalization, dysphoria, euphoria, depression, paranoia, and quick to react or overreact emotionally; swelling of feet or lower legs; unusual bleeding; unusual tiredness; vomiting; yellow skin or eyes (occurring with fluoxymesterone or methyltestosterone more often than with testosterone)

For females with breast cancer or bedridden males or females— in addition to the side effects listed above
Confusion or mental depression; constipation; increased thirst; increased urge to urinate or increased amount of urine

For males only
Black, tarry stools; burning sensation or hardening or thickening of skin under patch; chills; continuing pain at site of implants; difficulty in urinating; itching, skin redness, or rash under patch, severe (less likely with nonscrotal patch); pain in scrotum or groin; vomiting of blood or material that looks like coffee grounds

Rare
For males or females— more likely with oral androgens or long-term or high doses of androgens
Abdominal or stomach pain, continuing; bad breath odor, continuing; black, tarry or light-colored stools or dark urine; fever; hives; loss of appetite, continuing; mood or mental changes; purple or red spots on body or inside the mouth or nose; sore throat; swelling, pain, or tenderness of abdomen; vomiting of blood

Other side effects may occur that usually do not need medical attention. These side effects may go away during treatment as your body adjusts to the medicine. However, check with your doctor if any of the following side effects continue or are bothersome:

Less common
For males and females
Acne, mild; diarrhea; hair loss or thinning of hair; increase in pubic hair growth; infection, pain, redness, or other irritation at site of injection; decrease or increase in sexual desire or drive; nervousness; stomach pain; trouble in sleeping

For males only
Decrease in testicle size; infection, pain, redness, swelling, sores, or other skin irritation underneath patch

Other side effects not listed above may also occur in some patients. If you notice any other effects, check with your doctor.

Additional Information

Once a medicine has been approved for marketing for a certain use, experience may show that it is also useful for other medical problems. Although these uses are not included in product labeling, androgens are used in certain patients with the following medical conditions:

- Anemias (blood problems)
- Delayed growth spurt
- Development of male features in transsexuals
- Microphallus (underdevelopment of the penis)
- Lichen sclerosus (a skin problem of the vulva)

Other than the above information, there is no additional information relating to proper use, precautions, or side effects for these uses.

ANDROGENS AND ESTROGENS (Systemic)

Some commonly used brand names are:

In the U.S.—
Depo-Testadiol (2)   Estratest H.S. (1)
Estratest (1)   Valertest No. 1 (2)

In Canada—
Climacteron (2)

This information applies to the following medicines:

1. Estrogens, Esterified, and Methyltestosterone (ESS-troe-jenz, ess-TAIR-i-fyed, and meth-il-tes-TOSS-ter-one)
2. Testosterone and Estradiol (tess-TOSS-ter-own and ess-tra-DYE-ole)

Category

- **Androgen-estrogen—**
- **This monograph includes information on the following:**—Estrogens, Esterified, and Methyltestosterone; Testosterone and Estradiol

Description

Androgens and estrogens (AN-droe-jens and ESS-troe-jens) are hormones. Estrogens are produced by the body in greater amounts in females. They are necessary for normal sexual development of the female and for regulation of the menstrual cycle during the childbearing years. Androgens are produced by the body in greater amounts in males. However, androgens are also present in females in small amounts.

The ovaries and adrenal glands begin to produce less of these hormones after menopause. This combination product is prescribed to make up for this lower production of hormones. This may relieve signs of menopause, such as hot flashes and unusual sweating, chills, faintness, or dizziness.

Androgens and estrogens may also be used for other conditions as determined by your doctor.

There is no medical evidence to support the belief that the use of estrogens (contained in this combination medicine) will keep the patient feeling young, keep the skin soft, or delay the appearance of wrinkles. Nor has it been proven that the use of estrogens during the menopause will relieve emotional and nervous symptoms, unless these symptoms are caused by other menopausal symptoms, such as hot flashes.

A paper called "Information for the Patient" should be given to you with your prescription. Read this carefully. Also, before you use an androgen and estrogen product, you and your doctor should discuss the good that it will do as well as the risks of using it.

This medicine is available only with your doctor's prescription, in the following dosage forms:

Oral
- Estrogens, Esterified, and Methyltestosterone
  - Tablets

Parenteral
- Testosterone and Estradiol
  - Injection

Before Using This Medicine

In deciding to use a medicine, the risks of taking the medicine must be weighed against the good it will do. This is a decision you and your doctor will make. For androgen and estrogen combination products, the following should be considered:

Allergies—Tell your doctor if you have ever had any unusual or allergic reaction to androgens, anabolic steroids, or estrogens. Also tell your health care professional if you are allergic to any other substances, such as foods, preservatives, or dyes.

Pregnancy—Estrogens (contained in this combination medicine) are not recommended for use during pregnancy, since some estrogens have been shown to cause serious birth defects in humans. Some daughters of women who took diethylstilbestrol (DES) during pregnancy have developed reproductive (genital) tract problems and, rarely, cancer of the vagina and/or uterine cervix when they reached childbearing age. Some sons of women who took DES during pregnancy have developed urinary-genital tract problems.

Androgens (contained in this combination medicine) should not be used during pregnancy because they may cause male-like changes in a female baby.

Breast-feeding—Use of this medicine is not recommended in nursing mothers. Estrogens pass into the breast milk and their possible effect on the baby is not known. It is not known if androgens pass into breast milk. However, androgens may cause unwanted effects in nursing babies such as too early sexual development in males or male-like changes in females.

Older adults—This medicine has been tested and has not been shown to cause different side effects or problems in older women than it does in younger females.

Other medicines—Although certain medicines should not be used together at all, in other cases two different medicines may be used together even if an interaction might occur. In these cases, your doctor may want to change the dose, or other precautions may be necessary. When you are taking an androgen and estrogen combination product, it is especially important that your health care professional know if you are taking any of the following:

- Acetaminophen (e.g., Tylenol) (with long-term, high-dose use) or
- Amiodarone (e.g., Cordarone) or
- Anabolic steroids (nandrolone [e.g., Anabolin], oxandrolone [e.g., Anavar], oxymetholone [e.g., Anadrol], stanozolol [e.g., Winstrol]) or
- Anti-infectives by mouth or by injection (medicine for infection) or
- Antithyroid agents (medicine for overactive thyroid) or
- Carbamazepine (e.g., Tegretol) or
- Carmustine (e.g., BiCNU) or
- Chloroquine (e.g., Aralen) or
- Dantrolene (e.g., Dantrium) or
- Daunorubicin (e.g., Cerubidine) or
- Disulfiram (e.g., Antabuse) or
- Divalproex (e.g., Depakote) or
- Etretinate (e.g., Tegison) or
- Gold salts (medicine for arthritis) or
- Hydroxychloroquine (e.g., Plaquenil) or
- Mercaptopurine (e.g., Purinethol) or
- Methotrexate (e.g., Mexate) or
- Methyldopa (e.g., Aldomet) or
- Naltrexone (e.g., Trexan) (with long-term, high-dose use) or
- Phenothiazines (acetophenazine [e.g., Tindal], chlorpromazine [e.g., Thorazine], fluphenazine [e.g., Prolixin], mesoridazine [e.g., Serentil], perphenazine [e.g., Trilafon], prochlorperazine [e.g., Compazine], promazine [e.g., Sparine], promethazine [e.g., Phenergan], thioridazine [e.g., Mellaril], trifluoperazine [e.g., Stelazine], triflupromazine [e.g., Vesprin], trimeprazine [e.g., Temaril]) or
- Phenytoin (e.g., Dilantin) or
- Plicamycin (e.g., Mithracin) or
- Valproic acid (e.g., Depakene)—Androgens, estrogens, and all of these medicines can cause liver damage. Your doctor may want you to have extra blood tests that tell about your liver, while you are taking any of these medicines with an androgen and estrogen combination product.

- Anticoagulants (blood thinners)—Androgens can cause an increased effect of blood thinners, which could lead to uncontrolled or excessive bleeding
- Cyclosporine (e.g., Sandimmune)—Estrogens can increase the chances of toxic effects to the kidney or liver from cyclosporine because estrogens can interfere with the body's ability to get the cyclosporine out of the bloodstream as it normally would

Other medical problems—The presence of other medical problems may affect the use of androgen and estrogen combination products. Make sure you tell your doctor if you have any other medical problems, especially:

- Blood clots (or history of during previous estrogen therapy)—Estrogens may worsen blood clots or cause new clots to form
- Breast cancer (active or suspected)—Estrogens may cause growth of the tumor
- Changes in vaginal bleeding of unknown causes—Some irregular vaginal bleeding is a sign that the lining of the uterus is growing too much or is a sign of cancer of the uterus lining; estrogens may make these conditions worse
- Diabetes mellitus (sugar diabetes)—Androgens can decrease blood sugar levels
- Edema (swelling of feet or lower legs caused by retaining [keeping] too much body water) or
- Heart or circulation disease or
- Kidney disease or
- Liver disease—Androgens can worsen these conditions because androgens cause the body to retain extra fluid (keep too much body water). Also, heart or circulation disease can be worsened by androgens because androgens may increase blood cholesterol levels
- Endometriosis—Estrogens may worsen endometriosis by causing growth of endometriosis implants
- Fibroid tumors of the uterus—Estrogens may cause fibroid tumors to increase in size
- Gallbladder disease or gallstones (or history of)—There is no clear evidence as to whether estrogens increase the risk of gallbladder disease or gallstones
- Jaundice (or history of during pregnancy)—Estrogens use may worsen or cause jaundice in these patients
- Liver disease—Toxic drug effects may occur in patients with liver disease because the body is not able to get this medicine out of the bloodstream as it normally would
- Porphyria—Estrogens can worsen porphyria

Proper Use of This Medicine

For patients taking any of the androgen and estrogen products by mouth:

- *Take this medicine only as directed by your doctor. Do not take more of it and do not take it for a longer time than your doctor ordered.*
- Try to take the medicine at the same time each day to reduce the possibility of side effects and to allow it to work better.
- Nausea may occur during the first few weeks after you start taking estrogens. This effect usually disappears with continued use. If the nausea is bothersome, it can usually be prevented or reduced by taking each dose with food or immediately after food.

Dosing—The dose of these medicines will be different for different patients. *Follow your doctor's orders or the directions on the label.* The following information includes only the average doses of these medicines. *If your dose is different, do not change it* unless your doctor tells you to do so.

The number of tablets that you take depends on the strength of the medicine. Also, *the number of doses you take each day, the time allowed between doses, and the length of time you take the medicine depend on the medical problem for which you are taking combinations of androgen and estrogen.*

For esterified estrogens and methyltestosterone
- For *oral* dosage form (tablets):
  - For treatment of certain signs of menopause, such as hot flashes and unusual sweating, chills, faintness, or dizziness:
    - Adults—0.625 to 2.5 mg of esterified estrogens and 1.25 to 5 mg of methyltestosterone once a day for twenty-one days. Stop the medicine for seven days, then repeat the twenty-one day cycle.

For testosterone cypionate and estradiol cypionate
- For *injection* dosage form:
  - For treatment of certain signs of menopause, such as hot flashes and unusual sweating, chills, faintness, or dizziness:
    - Adults—50 milligrams (mg) of testosterone cypionate and 2 mg of estradiol cypionate injected into a muscle once every four weeks.

For testosterone enanthate and estradiol valerate
- For *injection* dosage form:
  - For treatment of certain signs of menopause, such as hot flashes and unusual sweating, chills, faintness, or dizziness:
    - Adults—90 milligrams (mg) of testosterone enanthate and 4 mg of estradiol valerate injected into a muscle once every four weeks.

For testosterone enanthate benzilic acid hydrazone, estradiol dienanthate, and estradiol benzoate
- For *injection* dosage form:
  - For treatment of bone loss (osteoporosis) or certain signs of menopause, such as hot flashes and unusual sweating, chills, faintness, or dizziness:
    - Adults—150 milligrams (mg) of testosterone enanthate benzilic acid hydrazone, 7.5 mg of estradiol dienanthate, and 1 mg of estradiol benzoate injected into a muscle once every four to eight weeks or less.

Missed dose—If you miss a dose of this medicine and your dosing schedule is:

- One dose a day—Take the missed dose as soon as possible. However, if you do not remember it until the next day, skip the missed dose and go back to your regular dosing schedule. Do not double doses.
- More than one dose a day—Take the missed dose as soon as possible. However, if it is almost time for your next dose, skip the missed dose and go back to your regular dosing schedule. Do not double doses.

If you have any questions about this, check with your doctor.

Storage—To store this medicine:

- Keep out of the reach of children.
- Store away from heat and direct light.
- Do not store in the bathroom medicine cabinet because the heat or moisture may cause the medicine to break down.
- Keep the injectable form of this medicine from freezing.
- Do not keep outdated medicine or medicine no longer needed. Be sure that any discarded medicine is out of the reach of children.

Precautions While Using This Medicine

It is very important that your doctor check your progress at regular visits to make sure this medicine does not cause unwanted effects. These visits will usually be every 6 to 12 months, but many doctors require them more often.

It is not yet known whether the use of estrogen increases the risk of breast cancer in women. Therefore, it is very important that you regularly check your breasts for any unusual lumps or discharge. You should also have a mammogram (x-ray picture of the breasts) done if your doctor recommends it.

In some patients using estrogens, tenderness, swelling, or bleeding of the gums may occur. Brushing and flossing your teeth carefully and regularly and massaging your gums may help prevent this. See your dentist regularly to have your teeth cleaned. Check with your medical doctor or dentist if you have any questions about how to take care of your teeth and gums, or if you notice any tenderness, swelling, or bleeding of your gums.

For diabetic patients:

- This medicine may affect blood sugar levels. If you notice a change in the results of your blood or urine sugar tests or if you have any questions, check with your doctor.

If you think that you may have become pregnant, check with your doctor immediately. Continued use of this medicine during pregnancy may cause birth defects or future health problems in the child.

In studies with oral contraceptives (birth control pills) containing estrogens, cigarette smoking during the use of estrogens was shown to cause an increased risk of serious side effects affecting the heart or blood circulation, such as dangerous blood clots, heart attack, or stroke. The risk increased as the amount of smoking and the age of the smoker increased. Women aged 35 and over were at greatest risk when they smoked while using oral contraceptives containing estrogens. It is not known if this risk exists with the use of androgens and estrogens for symptoms of menopause. However, smoking may make estrogens less effective.

Do not give this medicine to anyone else. Your doctor has prescribed it specifically for you after studying your health record and the results of your physical examination. Androgens and estrogens may be dangerous for some people because of differences in their health and body chemistry.

Side Effects

Discuss these possible effects with your doctor:

- Tumors of the liver, liver cancer, and peliosis hepatis (a form of liver disease) have occurred during long-term, high-dose therapy with androgens. Although these ef-

fects are rare, they can be very serious and may cause death.

- When androgens are used in women, especially in high doses, male-like changes may occur, such as hoarseness or deepening of the voice, unnatural hair growth, or unusual hair loss. Most of these changes will go away if the medicine is stopped as soon as the changes are noticed. However, some changes, such as voice changes, may not go away.
- The prolonged use of estrogens has been reported to increase the risk of endometrial cancer (cancer of the uterus lining) in women after menopause. The risk seems to increase as the dose and the length of use increase. When estrogens are used in low doses for less than one year, there is less risk. The risk is also reduced if a progestin (another female hormone) is added to, or replaces part of, your estrogen dose. If the uterus has been removed by surgery (total hysterectomy), there is no risk of endometrial cancer.
- It is not yet known whether the use of estrogens increases the risk of breast cancer in women. Although some large studies show an increased risk, most studies and information gathered to date do not support this idea.

Along with its needed effects, a medicine may cause some unwanted effects. Although not all of these side effects may occur, if they do occur they may need medical attention.

Check with your doctor immediately if any of the following side effects occur:

Less common
Yellow eyes or skin

Rare
Uncontrolled jerky muscle movements; vomiting of blood (with long-term use or high doses)

Also, check with your doctor as soon as possible if any of the following side effects occur:

More common
Acne or oily skin (severe); breast pain or tenderness; changes in vaginal bleeding (spotting, breakthrough bleeding, prolonged or heavier bleeding, or complete stoppage of bleeding); enlarged clitoris; enlargement or decrease in size of breasts; hoarseness or deepening of voice; swelling of feet or lower legs; unnatural hair growth; unusual hair loss; weight gain (rapid)

Less common or rare
Confusion; dizziness; flushing or redness of skin; headaches (frequent or continuing); hives (especially at place of injection); shortness of breath (unexplained); skin rash, hives, or itching; unusual bleeding; unusual tiredness or drowsiness

With long-term use or high doses
Black, tarry, or light-colored stools; dark-colored urine; general feeling of discomfort or illness (continuing); hives (frequent or continuing); loss of appetite (continuing); lump in, or discharge from breast; nausea (severe); pain, swelling, or tenderness in stomach or upper abdomen (continuing); purple- or red-colored spots on body or inside the mouth or nose; sore throat or fever (continuing); unpleasant breath odor (continuing); vomiting (severe)

Other side effects may occur that usually do not need medical attention. These side effects may go away during treatment

as your body adjusts to the medicine. However, check with your doctor if any of the following side effects continue or are bothersome:

More common

Bloating of abdomen or stomach; cramps of abdomen or stomach; loss of appetite (temporary); nausea (mild); stomach pain (mild); unusual increase in sexual desire; vomiting (mild)

Less common

Constipation; diarrhea (mild); dizziness (mild); headaches (mild); infection, redness, pain, or other irritation at place of injection; migraine headaches; problems in wearing contact lenses; trouble in sleeping

Also, many women who are taking a progestin (another type of female hormone) with this medicine will begin to have monthly vaginal bleeding again, similar to menstrual periods. This effect will continue for as long as this medicine is used. However, monthly bleeding will not occur in women who have had the uterus removed by surgery (total hysterectomy).

Other side effects not listed above may also occur in some patients. If you notice any other effects, check with your doctor.

ANESTHETICS (Rectal)

Some commonly used brand names are:

In the U.S.—

Americaine Hemorrhoidal (1)   Pontocaine Ointment (5)
Nupercainal (2)   ProctoFoam/non-steroid (3)
Fleet Relief (3)   Tronolane (3)
Pontocaine Cream (4)   Tronothane (3)

In Canada—

Nupercainal (2)
Tronothane (3)

This information applies to the following medicines:

1. Benzocaine (BEN-zoe-kane)
2. Dibucaine (DYE-byoo-kane)
3. Pramoxine (pra-MOX-een)
4. Tetracaine (TET-ra-kane)
5. Tetracaine and Menthol (TET-ra-kane and MEN-thol)

Category

- **Anesthetic (mucosal-local)**—Benzocaine; Dibucaine; Pramoxine; Tetracaine; Tetracaine and Menthol

Description

Rectal anesthetics (an-ess-THET-iks) are used to relieve the pain and itching of hemorrhoids (piles) and other problems in the rectal area. However, if you have hemorrhoids that bleed, especially after a bowel movement, check with your doctor before using this medicine. Bleeding may mean that you have a condition that needs other treatment.

These medicines are available without a prescription; however, your doctor may have special instructions on the proper use and dose for your medical problem.

These medicines are available in the following dosage forms:

Rectal

- Benzocaine
  - Ointment
- Dibucaine
  - Ointment
- Pramoxine
  - Aerosol foam
  - Cream
  - Ointment
- Tetracaine
  - Cream
- Tetracaine and Menthol
  - Ointment

Before Using This Medicine

If you are using this medicine without a prescription, carefully read and follow any precautions on the label. For rectal anesthetics, the following should be considered:

Allergies—Tell your doctor if you have ever had any unusual or allergic reaction to a local anesthetic, especially one that was applied to any part of the body as a liquid, cream, ointment, or spray. Also tell your health care professional if you are allergic to any other substances, such as foods, preservatives, or dyes.

Pregnancy—Rectal anesthetics have not been reported to cause birth defects or other problems in humans.

Breast-feeding—Rectal anesthetics have not been reported to cause problems in nursing babies.

Children—Children may be especially sensitive to the effects of local anesthetics. This may increase the chance of side effects during treatment.

Older adults—Elderly people are especially sensitive to the effects of local anesthetics. This may increase the chance of side effects during treatment.

Other medicines—Although certain medicines should not be used together at all, in other cases two different medicines may be used together even if an interaction might occur. In these cases, your doctor may want to change the dose, or other precautions may be necessary. Before you use a rectal anesthetic, check with your health care professional if you are taking any other prescription or nonprescription (over-the-counter [OTC]) medicine.

Other medical problems—The presence of other medical problems may affect the use of rectal anesthetics. Make sure you tell your doctor if you have any other medical problems, especially:

- Infection at or near place of treatment or
- Large sores, broken skin, or severe injury at or near place of treatment—The chance of unwanted effects may be increased

---

Proper Use of This Medicine

For safe and effective use of this medicine:

- Rectal anesthetics usually come with patient directions. Read them carefully before using the medicine, even if it was prescribed by your doctor. Check with your pharmacist if you have any questions about how to use the product.

- Follow your doctor's instructions if this medicine was prescribed.
- Follow the manufacturer's package directions if you are treating yourself.
- *Do not use more of this medicine, do not use it more often, and do not use it for a longer time than directed*. To do so may increase the chance of absorption into the body and the chance of unwanted effects.

This medicine should be used only for conditions being treated by your doctor or for problems listed on the package label. *Do not use it for other problems without first checking with your doctor*. This medicine should not be used if certain kinds of infections are present.

For *applying a rectal anesthetic to the area around the rectum:*

- First, clean the area, using mild soap and water or a cleansing wipe. Rinse the area carefully and dry it gently with a soft towel or toilet paper.
- Apply a small amount of medicine to the sore area, using a piece of gauze, a tissue, or a "finger cot."

For *inserting a rectal cream or ointment inside the rectum:*

- Use only products that come packaged in pre-filled applicators or that come packaged with a special inserter called a rectal tube.
- If you are using a product that has an inserter (rectal tube) packaged separately from the tube of cream or ointment:
  - Remove the cap from the tube of cream or ointment. Attach the inserter to the top of the tube. Squeeze the tube until a little cream or ointment comes out on the inserter. Then spread the cream or ointment over the inserter.
  - Place the inserter into your rectum and squeeze the tube until a small amount of medicine comes out. Then remove the inserter from your body.
  - Remove the inserter from the tube and replace the cap. Then wash the applicator carefully.
- If you are using the product that comes in pre-filled applicators:
  - Follow the manufacturer's directions for using the applicator and inserting the medicine. Each applicator is meant to be used only once. Throw the applicator away after using it.

For *inserting the rectal aerosol foam (e.g., Proctofoam/ nonsteroid) into the rectum:*

- Do not insert the container itself into your rectum. Use the applicator provided.
- To fill the container—First, shake the container hard for several seconds. Then, holding the container upright, insert it into the applicator. Press the cap of the container until the foam reaches the fill line of the applicator. Remove the applicator from the container.
- To use the medicine—Place a small amount of foam on the tip of the applicator. Insert the applicator into your rectum, then push the plunger as far as possible. Remove the applicator. Then take it apart and wash it carefully.

Dosing—The dose of rectal anesthetics will be different for different patients. *Follow your doctor's orders or the di-*

rections on the label. The following information includes only the average doses of these medicines. *If your dose is different, do not change it* unless your doctor tells you to do so.

For *benzocaine*

- For pain and itching of hemorrhoids or other problems in the rectal area:
  - For *rectal ointment* dosage form:
    - Adults—Apply a small amount of ointment to the area around the rectum up to six times a day.
    - Children—Use and dose must be determined by the doctor.

For *dibucaine*

- For pain and itching of hemorrhoids or other problems in the rectal area:
  - For *rectal ointment* dosage form:
    - Adults—Insert a small amount of ointment into the rectum three or four times a day, in the morning, in the evening, and after bowel movements. Or, apply a small amount of ointment to the area around the rectum three or four times a day.
    - Children—Use and dose must be determined by the doctor.

For *pramoxine*

- For pain and itching of hemorrhoids or other problems in the rectal area:
  - For *rectal cream* dosage form:
    - Adults—Apply a small amount to the area around the rectum up to five times a day, in the morning, in the evening, and after bowel movements.
    - Children—Use and dose must be determined by the doctor.
  - For *rectal ointment* dosage form:
    - Adults—Insert a small amount of ointment into the rectum up to five times a day, in the morning, in the evening, and after bowel movements. Or, apply a small amount to the area around the rectum up to five times a day, in the morning, in the evening, and after bowel movements.
  - For the *rectal aerosol foam* dosage form:
    - Adults—Insert 1 applicatorful into the rectum two or three times a day. Or, apply a small amount to the area around the rectum two or three times a day.
    - Children—Use and dose must be determined by the doctor.

For *tetracaine and for tetracaine and menthol*

- For pain and itching of hemorrhoids or other problems in the rectal area:
  - For the *rectal cream* or *rectal ointment* dosage form:
    - Adults—Insert a small amount into the rectum up to six times a day. Or, apply a small amount to the area around the rectum up to six times a day.
    - Children—Use and dose must be determined by the doctor.

Missed dose—If your doctor has directed you to use this medicine on a regular schedule and you miss a dose, use it as soon as possible. However, if it is almost time for your next dose, skip the missed dose and go back to your regular dosing schedule.

Storage—To store this medicine:

- Keep out of the reach of children.
- Store away from heat and direct light.

- Keep the medicine from freezing.
- Do not puncture, break, or burn the pramoxine aerosol foam container, even after it is empty.
- Do not keep outdated medicine or medicine no longer needed. Be sure that any discarded medicine is out of the reach of children.

Precautions While Using This Medicine

Check with your doctor:
- If your condition does not improve after you have been using this medicine regularly for 7 days, or if it becomes worse.
- If any bleeding from the rectum occurs.
- If you notice any rash, redness, or irritation that was not present before you started using this medicine.

False test results may occur if benzocaine or tetracaine is present in your body when a certain laboratory test is done. This test uses a medicine called bentiromide (e.g., Chymex) to show how well your pancreas is working. You should not use any products containing benzocaine or tetracaine for about 72 hours (3 days) before this test is done.

Side Effects

Along with its needed effects, a medicine may cause some unwanted effects. Although not all of these side effects may occur, if they do occur they may need medical attention.

Stop using this medicine and check with your doctor immediately if any of the following side effects occur:
Signs and symptoms of too much medicine being absorbed by the body
Blurred or double vision; confusion; convulsions (seizures); dizziness or lightheadedness; drowsiness; feeling hot, cold, or numb; increased sweating; ringing or buzzing in ears; shivering or trembling; slow or irregular heartbeat; unusual anxiety, excitement, nervousness, or restlessness; unusual paleness

Also, check with your doctor as soon as possible if any of the following side effects occur:
Less common
Burning, stinging, swelling, or tenderness not present before treatment; skin rash, redness, itching, or hives at or near place of application

Other side effects not listed above may also occur in some patients. If you notice any other effects, check with your doctor.

ANESTHETICS (Topical)

Some commonly used brand names are:

In the U.S.—

Almay Anti-itch Lotion (7)
Americaine Topical Anesthetic First Aid Ointment (1)
Americaine Topical Anesthetic Spray (1)
Butesin Picrate (3)
DermaFlex (5)
Dermoplast (2)
Lagol (1)
Nupercainal Cream (4)
Nupercainal Ointment (4)
Pontocaine Cream (8)
Pontocaine Ointment (9)
Pramegel (7)
Prax (6)
Tronothane (6)
Xylocaine (5)

In Canada—

After Burn Double Strength Gel (5)
After Burn Double Strength Spray (5)
After Burn Gel (5)
After Burn Spray (5)
Alphacaine (5)
Dermoplast (2)
Endocaine (1)
Norwood Sunburn Spray (5)
Nupercainal Ointment (4)
Pramegel (7)
Shield Burnasept Spray (1)
Tronothane (6)
Xylocaine (5)

This information applies to the following medicines:

1. Benzocaine (BEN-zoe-kane)
2. Benzocaine and Menthol (BEN-zoe-kane and MEN-thol)
3. Butamben (byoo-TAM-ben)
4. Dibucaine (DYE-byoo-kane)
5. Lidocaine (LYE-doe-kane)
6. Pramoxine (pra-MOX-een)
7. Pramoxine and Menthol (pra-MOX-een and MEN-thol)
8. Tetracaine (TET-ra-kane)
9. Tetracaine and Menthol (TET-ra-kane and MEN-thol)

Category

- **Anesthetic, local—**Benzocaine; Benzocaine and Menthol; Butamben; Dibucaine; Lidocaine; Pramoxine; Pramoxine and Menthol; Tetracaine; Tetracaine and Menthol

Description

This medicine belongs to a group of medicines known as topical local anesthetics (an-ess-THET-iks). Topical anesthetics are used to relieve pain and itching caused by conditions such as sunburn or other minor burns, insect bites or stings, poison ivy, poison oak, poison sumac, and minor cuts and scratches.

Topical anesthetics deaden the nerve endings in the skin. They do not cause unconsciousness as do general anesthetics used for surgery.

Most topical anesthetics are available without a prescription; however, your doctor may have special instructions on the proper use and dose for your medical problem.

These medicines are available in the following dosage forms:

Topical
- Benzocaine
  - Cream
  - Ointment
  - Topical aerosol
  - Topical spray solution
- Benzocaine and Menthol
  - Lotion
  - Topical aerosol solution
- Butamben
  - Ointment
- Dibucaine
  - Cream
  - Ointment
- Lidocaine
  - Film-forming gel
  - Jelly
  - Ointment

- ◦ Topical aerosol
- ◦ Topical spray solution
- • Pramoxine
  - ◦ Cream
  - ◦ Lotion
- • Pramoxine and Menthol
  - ◦ Gel
  - ◦ Lotion
- • Tetracaine
  - ◦ Cream
- • Tetracaine and Menthol
  - ◦ Ointment

Before Using This Medicine

If you are using this medicine without a prescription, carefully read and follow any precautions on the label. For topical anesthetics, the following should be considered:

Allergies—Tell your doctor if you have ever had any unusual or allergic reaction to a local anesthetic, especially when applied to the skin or other areas of the body. Also tell your health care professional if you are allergic to any other substances, such as foods, preservatives, or dyes, especially aminobenzoic acid (also called para-aminobenzoic acid [PABA]), to parabens (preservatives in many foods and medicines), or to paraphenylenediamine (a hair dye).

Pregnancy—Although studies on effects in pregnancy have not been done in humans, topical anesthetics have not been reported to cause problems in humans. Lidocaine has not been shown to cause birth defects or other problems in animal studies. Other topical anesthetics have not been studied in animals.

Breast-feeding—Topical anesthetics have not been reported to cause problems in nursing babies.

Children—Benzocaine may be absorbed through the skin of young children and cause unwanted effects. There is no specific information comparing use of other topical anesthetics in children with use in other age groups, but it is possible that they may also cause unwanted effects in young children. Check with your doctor before using any product that contains a topical anesthetic for a child younger than 2 years of age.

Older adults—Many medicines have not been studied specifically in older people. Therefore, it may not be known whether they work exactly the same way they do in younger adults or if they cause different side effects or problems in older people. There is no specific information comparing use of topical anesthetics in the elderly with use in other age groups.

Other medicines—Although certain medicines should not be used together at all, in other cases two different medicines may be used together even if an interaction might occur. In these cases, your doctor may want to change the dose, or other precautions may be necessary. Tell your health care professional if you are taking any other prescription or nonprescription (over-the-counter [OTC]) medicine.

Other medical problems—The presence of other medical problems may affect the use of topical anesthetics. Before using a topical anesthetic, check with your health care professional if you have any other medical problems, especially:

- • Infection at or near the place of application or

- • Large sores, broken skin, or severe injury at the area of application—The chance of side effects may be increased

Proper Use of This Medicine

For safe and effective use of this medicine:

- • Follow your doctor's instructions if this medicine was prescribed.
- • Follow the manufacturer's package directions if you are treating yourself.
- • Unless otherwise directed by your doctor, *do not use this medicine on large areas, especially if the skin is broken or scraped. Also, do not use it more often than directed on the package label, or for more than a few days at a time.* To do so may increase the chance of absorption through the skin and the chance of unwanted effects. This is especially important when benzocaine is used for children younger than 2 years of age.

This medicine should be used only for problems being treated by your doctor or conditions listed in the package directions. *Check with your doctor before using it for other problems, especially if you think that an infection may be present.* This medicine should not be used to treat certain kinds of skin infections or serious problems, such as severe burns.

Read the package label very carefully to see if the product contains any alcohol. Alcohol is flammable and can catch on fire. *Do not use any product containing alcohol near a fire or open flame, or while smoking. Also, do not smoke after applying one of these products until it has completely dried.*

If you are using this medicine on your face, *be very careful not to get it in your eyes, mouth, or nose.* If you are using an aerosol or spray form of this medicine, do not spray it directly on your face. Instead, use your hand or an applicator (for example, a sterile gauze pad or a cotton swab) to apply the medicine.

For patients using *butamben:*

- • Butamben may stain clothing and discolor hair. It may not be possible to remove the stains. To avoid this, do not touch your clothing or your hair while applying the medicine. Also, cover the treated area with a loose bandage after applying butamben, to protect your clothes.

To use *lidocaine film-forming gel* (e.g., DermaFlex):

- • First dry the area with a clean cloth or a piece of gauze. Then apply the medicine. The medicine should dry, forming a clear film, after about 1 minute.

Dosing—The dose of a topical anesthetic will be different for different patients. *Follow your doctor's orders or the directions on the label.* The following information includes only the average doses of these medicines. *If your dose is different, do not change it* unless your doctor tells you to do so.

For benzocaine and for benzocaine and menthol combination

- • For *topical* dosage forms (aerosol solution, cream, lotion, ointment, and spray solution):
  - ◦ For pain and itching caused by minor skin conditions:
    - ▪ Adults and children 2 years of age and older—Apply to the affected area three or four times a day as needed.

- Children younger than 2 years of age—Dose must be determined by your doctor.

For *butamben*
- For *topical* dosage form (ointment):
  - For pain and itching caused by minor skin conditions:
    - Adults—Apply to the affected area three or four times a day as needed.
    - Children—Dose must be determined by your doctor.

For *dibucaine*
- For *topical cream* dosage form:
  - For pain and itching caused by minor skin conditions:
    - Adults and children 2 years of age and older—Apply to the affected area three or four times a day as needed.
    - Children up to 2 years of age—Dose must be determined by your doctor.
- For *topical ointment* dosage form:
  - For pain and itching caused by minor skin conditions:

    - Adults—Apply to the affected area three or four times a day as needed. The largest amount that may be used in a twenty-four-hour period is 30 grams, but much smaller amounts are usually enough.
    - Children 2 years of age and older—Apply to the affected area three or four times a day as needed. Do not use more than 7.5 grams in a twenty-four-hour period.
    - Children up to 2 years of age—Dose must be determined by your doctor.

For *lidocaine*
- For *topical* dosage forms (aerosol solution, film-forming gel, jelly, ointment, and spray solution):
  - For pain and itching caused by minor skin conditions:
    - Adults—Apply to the affected area three or four times a day as needed.
    - Children—Dose must be determined by your doctor.

For *pramoxine and for pramoxine and menthol combination*
- For *topical* dosage forms (cream, gel, and lotion):
  - For pain and itching caused by minor skin conditions:
    - Adults and children 2 years of age and older—Apply to the affected area three or four times a day as needed.
    - Children younger than 2 years of age—Dose must be determined by your doctor.

For *tetracaine and for tetracaine and menthol combination*
- For *topical* dosage forms (cream and ointment):
  - For pain and itching caused by minor skin conditions:
    - Adults and teenagers—Apply to the affected area three or four times a day as needed. The largest amount that may be used in a twenty-four-hour period is 30 grams (a whole tube of the medicine), but much smaller amounts are usually enough.
    - Children 2 years of age and older—Apply to the affected area three or four times a day as needed. Do not use more than 7 grams (about one-fourth of a tube of the medicine) in a twenty-four-hour period.
    - Children younger than 2 years of age—Dose must be determined by your doctor.

Missed dose—If your doctor has ordered you to use this medicine according to a regular schedule and you miss a dose, use it as soon as possible. However, if it is almost time for your next dose, skip the missed dose and use your next dose at the regularly scheduled time.

Storage—To store this medicine:
- Keep out of the reach of children.
- Store away from heat and direct light.
- Keep the medicine from freezing.
- Do not puncture, break, or burn aerosol containers, even when they are empty.
- Do not keep outdated medicine or medicine no longer needed. Be sure that any discarded medicine is out of the reach of children.

Precautions While Using This Medicine

After applying this medicine to the skin of a child, *watch the child carefully to make sure that he or she does not get any of the medicine into his or her mouth.* Topical anesthetics can cause serious side effects, especially in children, if any of the medicine gets into the mouth or is swallowed.

Stop using this medicine and check with your doctor:
- *If your condition does not improve within 7 days, or if it gets worse.*
- *If the area you are treating becomes infected.*
- *If you notice a skin rash, burning, stinging, swelling, or any other sign of irritation that was not present when you began using this medicine.*
- *If you swallow any of the medicine.*

Side Effects

Along with its needed effects, a medicine may cause some unwanted effects. Although not all of these side effects may occur, if they do occur they may need medical attention.

Check with your doctor immediately if any of the following side effects occur:
Less common
   Large swellings that look like hives on the skin or in the mouth or throat
Symptoms of too much medicine being absorbed by the body—very rare
   Blurred or double vision; confusion; convulsions (seizures); dizziness or lightheadedness; drowsiness; feeling hot, cold, or numb; headache; increased sweating; ringing or buzzing in the ears; shivering or trembling; slow or irregular heartbeat; troubled breathing; unusual anxiety, excitement, nervousness, or restlessness; unusual paleness; unusual tiredness or weakness

Also, check with your doctor as soon as possible if any of the following side effects occur:
   Burning, stinging, or tenderness not present before treatment; skin rash, redness, itching, or hives

Other side effects not listed above may also occur in some patients. If you notice any other effects, check with your doctor.

ANIDULAFUNGIN   (Intravenous route)
- ay-nid-yoo-la-FUN-jin

Commonly used brand name(s)
In the U.S.—
  Eraxis

Available Dosage Forms:
  • Powder for Solution

Therapeutic Class: Antifungal
Pharmacologic Class: Glucan Synthesis Inhibitor

Uses For This Medicine

Anidulafungin is an antifungal. It is used to help the body overcome serious fungus infections. This medicine is available only with your doctor's prescription.

Before Using This Medicine

In deciding to use a medicine, the risks of taking the medicine must be weighed against the good it will do. This is a decision you and your doctor will make. For this medicine, the following should be considered:

Allergies—Tell your doctor if you have ever had any unusual or allergic reaction to this medicine or any other medicines. Also tell your health care professional if you have any other types of allergies, such as to foods, dyes, preservatives, or animals. For non-prescription products, read the label or package ingredients carefully.

Pediatric—Studies on this medicine have been done only in adult patients, and there is no specific information comparing the use of anidulafungin in children with use in other age groups.

Geriatric—This medicine has been tested and has not been shown to cause different side effects or problems in older people than it does in younger adults.

Pregnancy—

	Pregnancy Category	Explanation
All Trimesters	C	Animal studies have shown an adverse effect and there are no adequate studies in pregnant women OR no animal studies have been conducted and there are no adequate studies in pregnant women.

Breast Feeding—There are no adequate studies in women for determining infant risk when using this medication during breastfeeding. Weigh the potential benefits against the potential risks before taking this medication while breastfeeding.

Other medicines—Although certain medicines should not be used together at all, in other cases two different medicines may be used together even if an interaction might occur. In these cases, your doctor may want to change the dose, or other precautions may be necessary. Tell your healthcare professional if you are taking any other prescription or non-prescription (over-the-counter [OTC]) medicine.

Interactions with Food/Tobacco/Alcohol—Certain medicines should not be used at or around the time of eating food or eating certain types of food since interactions may occur. Using alcohol or tobacco with certain medicines may also cause interactions to occur. Discuss with your healthcare professional the use of your medicine with food, alcohol, or tobacco.

Other medical problems—The presence of other medical problems may affect the use of this medicine. Make sure you tell your doctor if you have any other medical problems, especially:

  • Allergies to other echinocandin antifungal drugs (Caspofungin [e.g., Cancidas], Micafungin [e.g., Mycamine])—You should not use anidulafungin.
  • Liver problems—This medicine may cause liver problems to become worse.

Proper Use of This Medicine

Dosing—The dose of this medicine will be different for different patients. Follow your doctor's orders or the directions on the label. The following information includes only the average doses of this medicine. If your dose is different, do not change it unless your doctor tells you to do so.

The amount of medicine that you take depends on the strength of the medicine. Also, the number of doses you take each day, the time allowed between doses, and the length of time you take the medicine depend on the medical problem for which you are using the medicine.

  • For injection dosage form:
    ○ Adults—At first, the dose is 200 milligrams (mg) injected into a vein. After that, the dose is 100 mg a day injected into a vein. For a fungal infection of the esophagus, the first dose is 100 mg and after that the dose is 50 mg a day.
    ○ Children—Use and dose must be determined by your doctor.

Precautions While Using This Medicine

It is important that you adhere to your doctor's treatment plan for you.

Side Effects of This Medicine

Along with its needed effects, a medicine may cause some unwanted effects. Although not all of these side effects may occur, if they do occur they may need medical attention.

Check with your doctor immediately if any of the following side effects occur:
  Less common
    Black, tarry stools; chills; cough; decreased urine; dry mouth; fever; increased thirst; irregular heartbeat; loss of appetite; lower back or side pain; mood or mental changes; muscle pain or cramps; nausea or vomiting; numbness or tingling in hands, feet or lips; painful or difficult urination; pale skin; seizures; shortness of breath; sore throat; sores, ulcers, or white spots on lips or in mouth; unusual bleeding or bruising; unusual tiredness or weakness
  Rare
    Abdominal or stomach pain; back pain; bleeding gums; blood in urine or stools; bloody stools; bluish color of skin; blurred or loss of vision; changes in skin color; chest pain; chest tightness; clay-colored stools; confusion; constipation; dark urine; depression; diarrhea; dizziness; dizziness, faintness, or lightheadedness

when getting up from a lying or sitting position suddenly; drowsiness; extra heartbeats; fainting; fast heartbeat; fatigue; flushed, dry skin; flushing; fruit-like breath odor; headache; high blood pressure; hives or welts; incoherent speech; increased hunger; increased urination; infection of blood; irregular fast heartbeat; irritability; itching; large, hive-like swelling on face, eyelids, lips, tongue, throat, hands, legs, feet, sex organs; light-colored stools; metallic taste; muscle spasms (tetany) or twitching; muscle weakness; nervousness; pain, redness or swelling in arm or leg; pain, tenderness, and swelling of foot or leg; palpitations; pinpoint red spots on skin; pounding in the ears; redness of skin; restlessness; skin rash; slow heartbeat; sore mouth or tongue; sweating; swelling of feet or lower legs; swollen glands; trembling; trouble breathing; unexplained weight loss; unpleasant breath odor; unusually warm skin; vomiting of blood; weakness; weight loss; white patches in the mouth or throat or on the tongue; white patches with diaper rash; yellow eyes or skin

Some side effects may occur that usually do not need medical attention. These side effects may go away during treatment as your body adjusts to the medicine. Also, your health care professional may be able to tell you about ways to prevent or reduce some of these side effects. Check with your health care professional if any of the following side effects continue or are bothersome or if you have any questions about them:

Rare

Acid or sour stomach; belching; bloating or swelling of face, arms, hands, lower legs, or feet; disturbed color perception; double vision; eye pain; feeling of warmth; feeling unusually cold; halos around light; hot flushes; indigestion; loss of bowel control; night blindness; over bright appearance of lights; rapid weight gain; redness of the face, neck, arms and occasionally, upper chest; shivering; stomach discomfort, upset, or pain; tingling of hands or feet; tunnel vision; unusual weight gain or loss; upper stomach pain

Other side effects not listed may also occur in some patients. If you notice any other effects, check with your healthcare professional.

ANTACIDS (Oral)

Some commonly used brand names are:

In the U.S.—

Advanced Formula Di-Gel (29)	Aludrox (9)
Alamag (2)	Alu-Tab (25)
Alamag Plus (9)	Amitone (27)
Alenic Alka (15)	Amphojel (25)
Alenic Alka Extra Strength (18)	Antacid Gelcaps (31)
	Antacid Liquid (9)
Alka-Mints (27)	Antacid Liquid Double Strength (9)
Alkets (27)	
Alkets Extra Strength (27)	Basaljel (23)
Almacone (9)	Calglycine (27)
Almacone II (9)	Chooz (27)
AlternaGEL (21)	Dicarbosil (27)
Alu-Cap (25)	Di-Gel (29)
	Equilet (27)

Foamicon (19)	Mygel (9)
Gaviscon (15)	Mygel II (9)
Gaviscon-2 (20)	Mylanta (11)
Gaviscon Extra Strength Relief Formula (17)	Mylanta Double Strength (12)
	Mylanta Gelcaps (28)
Gelusil (9)	Nephrox (25)
Genaton (15)	Phillips' (35)
Genaton Extra Strength (18)	Phillips' Chewable (35)
Kudrox Double Strength (9)	Phillips' Concentrated Double Strength (35)
Losopan (32)	
Losopan Plus (33)	Riopan (32)
Lowsium Plus (33)	Riopan Plus (33)
Maalox (2)	Riopan Plus Double Strength (33)
Maalox Antacid Caplets (31)	
Maalox Heartburn Relief Formula (14)	Rolaids (28)
	Rulox (2)
Maalox Plus (9)	Rulox No. 1 (2)
Maalox Plus, Extra Strength (9)	Rulox No. 2 (2)
	Rulox Plus (9)
Maalox TC (2)	Simaal Gel (9)
Magnalox (9)	Simaal 2 Gel (9)
Magnalox Plus (9)	Tempo (4)
Mag-Ox 400 (36)	Titralac (27)
Mallamint (27)	Titralac Extra Strength (27)
Maox 420 (36)	Titralac Plus (30)
Marblen (31)	Tums (27)
Mi-Acid (10)	Tums Anti-gas/Antacid (30)
Mi-Acid Double Strength (9)	Tums E-X (27)
Mintox (2)	Tums Ultra (27)
Mintox Extra Strength (9)	Uro-Mag (36)

In Canada—

Almagel 200 (2)	Maalox HRF (13)
Alugel (25)	Maalox Plus (9)
Alu-Tab (25)	Maalox Plus, Extra Strength (9)
Amphojel (25)	
Amphojel 500 (2)	Maalox TC (2)
Amphojel Plus (8)	Mylanta (9)
Basaljel (25)	Mylanta Double Strength (9)
Diovol (6)	Mylanta Double Strength Plain (2)
Diovol Caplets (2)	
Diovol Ex (2)	Mylanta Extra Strength (9)
Diovol Plus (8)	Neutralca-S (2)
Diovol Plus AF (29)	Phillips' (35)
Gasmas (7)	PMS Alumina, Magnesia, and Simethicone (9)
Gaviscon Acid Plus Gas Relief (29)	
	Rafton (3)
Gaviscon Acid Relief (28)	Riopan (32)
Gaviscon Extra Strength Acid Relief (28)	Riopan Extra Strength (32)
	Riopan Plus (33)
Gaviscon Heartburn Relief (13)	Riopan Plus Extra Strength (33)
Gaviscon Heartburn Relief Extra Strength (13)	Rolaids (28)
	Rolaids Extra Strength (28)
Gelusil (2)	Trial (27)
Gelusil Extra Strength (2)	Tums (27)
Life Antacid (2)	Tums Extra Strength (27)
Life Antacid Plus (9)	Tums Ultra (27)
Maalox (2)	Univol (2)
Maalox Antacid Caplets (31)	

This information applies to the following medicines:

1. Alumina, Calcium Carbonate, and Sodium Bicarbonate (a-LOO-mi-na, KAL-see-um KAR-bon-ate, and SOE-dee-um bi-KAR-bon-ate)
2. Alumina and Magnesia (a-LOO-mi-na and mag-NEE-zha)
3. Alumina, Calcium Carbonate, and Sodium Bicarbonate or Alumina, Magnesium Trisilicate, and Sodium Bicarbonate (a-LOO-mi-na, KAL-see-um KAR-bon-ate, and SOE-dee-um bi-KAR-bon-ate or a-LOO-mi-na, mag-NEE-zhum trye-SILL-i-kate, and SOE-dee-um bi-KAR-bon-ate)
4. Alumina, Magnesia, Calcium Carbonate, and Simethicone (a-LOO-mi-na, mag-NEE-zha, KAL-see-um KAR-bon-ate, and Si-METH-i-kone)

5. Alumina, Magnesia, and Magnesium Carbonate (a-LOO-mi-na, mag-NEE-zha, and mag-NEE-zhum KAR-bon-ate)
6. Alumina, Magnesia, and Magnesium Carbonate or Alumina, Magnesia, and Simethicone (a-LOO-mi-na, mag-NEE-zha, and mag-NEE-zhum KAR-bon-ate or a-LOO-mi-na, mag-NEE-zha, and Si-METH-i-kone)
7. Alumina, Magnesia, Magnesium Carbonate, and Simethicone (a-LOO-mi-na, mag-NEE-zha, mag-NEE-zhum KAR-bon-ate, and Si-METH-i-kone)
8. Alumina, Magnesia, Magnesium Carbonate, and Simethicone or Alumina, Magnesia, and Simethicone (a-LOO-mi-na, mag-NEE-zha, mag-NEE-zhum KAR-bon-ate, and Si-METH-i-kone or a-LOO-mi-na, mag-NEE-zha, and Si-METH-i-kone)
9. Alumina, Magnesia, and Simethicone (a-LOO-mi-na, mag-NEE-zha, and Si-METH-i-kone)
10. Alumina, Magnesia, and Simethicone or Calcium and Magnesium Carbonates (a-LOO-mi-na, mag-NEE-zha, and Si-METH-i-kone or KAL-see-um and mag-NEE-zhum KAR-bon-ates)
11. Alumina, Magnesia, and Simethicone or Calcium Carbonate or Calcium Carbonate and Magnesia (a-LOO-mi-na, mag-NEE-zha, and Si-METH-i-kone or KAL-see-um KAR-bon-ate or KAL-see-um KAR-bon-ate and mag-NEE-zha,)
12. Alumina, Magnesia, and Simethicone or Calcium Carbonate and Magnesia (a-LOO-mi-na, mag-NEE-zha, and Si-METH-i-kone or KAL-see-um KAR-bon-ate and mag-NEE-zha,)
13. Alumina, Magnesium Alginate, and Magnesium Carbonate (a-LOO-mi-na, mag-NEE-zhum al-JI-nate, and mag-NEE-zhum KAR-bon-ate)
14. Alumina and Magnesium Carbonate (a-LOO-mi-na and mag-NEE-zhum KAR-bon-ate)
15. Alumina and Magnesium Carbonate or Alumina, Magnesium Trisilicate, and Sodium Bicarbonate (a-LOO-mi-na and mag-NEE-zhum KAR-bon-ate or a-LOO-mi-na, mag-NEE-zhum trye-SILL-i-kate, and SOE-dee-um bi-KAR-bon-ate)
16. Alumina, Magnesium Carbonate, and Simethicone (a-LOO-mi-na, mag-NEE-zhum KAR-bon-ate, and Si-METH-i-kone)
17. Alumina, Magnesium Carbonate, and Simethicone or Alumina, Magnesium Carbonate, and Sodium Bicarbonate (a-LOO-mi-na, mag-NEE-zhum KAR-bon-ate, and Si-METH-i-kone or a-LOO-mi-na, mag-NEE-zhum KAR-bon-ate, and SOE-dee-um bi-KAR-bon-ate)
18. Alumina, Magnesium Carbonate, and Sodium Bicarbonate (a-LOO-mi-na, mag-NEE-zhum KAR-bon-ate, and SOE-dee-um bi-KAR-bon-ate)
19. Alumina and Magnesium Trisilicate (a-LOO-mi-na and mag-NEE-zhum trye-SILL-i-kate)
20. Alumina, Magnesium Trisilicate, and Sodium Bicarbonate (a-LOO-mi-na, mag-NEE-zhum trye-SILL-i-kate, and SOE-dee-um bi-KAR-bon-ate)
21. Alumina and Simethicone (a-LOO-mi-na and Si-METH-i-kone)
22. Alumina and Sodium Bicarbonate (a-LOO-mi-na and SOE-dee-um bi-KAR-bon-ate)
23. Aluminum Carbonate, Basic (a-LOO-mi-num KAR-bon-ate, BA-sic)
24. Aluminum Carbonate, Basic, and Simethicone (a-LOO-mi-num KAR-bon-ate, BA-sic, and Si-METH-i-kone)
25. Aluminum Hydroxide (a-LOO-mi-num hye-DROX-ide)
26. Aluminum Hydroxide, Magnesium Carbonate, and Sodium Bicarbonate (a-LOO-mi-num hye-DROX-ide, mag-NEE-zhum KAR-bon-ate, and SOE-dee-um bi-KAR-bon-ate)
27. Calcium Carbonate (KAL-see-um KAR-bon-ate)
28. Calcium Carbonate and Magnesia (KAL-see-um KAR-bon-ate and mag-NEE-zha,)
29. Calcium Carbonate, Magnesia, and Simethicone (KAL-see-um KAR-bon-ate, mag-NEE-zha, and Si-METH-i-kone)
30. Calcium Carbonate and Simethicone (KAL-see-um KAR-bon-ate and Si-METH-i-kone)
31. Calcium and Magnesium Carbonates (KAL-see-um and mag-NEE-zhum KAR-bon-ates)
32. Magaldrate (MAG-al-drate)
33. Magaldrate and Simethicone (MAG-al-drate and Si-METH-i-kone)

34. Magnesium Carbonate and Sodium Bicarbonate (mag-NEE-zhum KAR-bon-ate and SOE-dee-um bi-KAR-bon-ate)
35. Magnesium Hydroxide (mag-NEE-zhum hye-DROX-ide)
36. Magnesium Oxide (mag-NEE-zhum OX-ide)

Category

- **Antacid**—Alumina, Calcium Carbonate, and Sodium Bicarbonate; Alumina and Magnesia; Alumina, Magnesia, Calcium Carbonate, and Simethicone; Alumina, Magnesia, and Magnesium Carbonate; Alumina, Magnesia, Magnesium Carbonate, and Simethicone; Alumina, Magnesia, and Simethicone; Alumina, Magnesium Alginate, and Magnesium Carbonate; Alumina and Magnesium Carbonate; Alumina, Magnesium Carbonate, and Simethicone; Alumina, Magnesium Carbonate, and Sodium Bicarbonate; Alumina and Magnesium Trisilicate; Alumina, Magnesium Trisilicate, and Sodium Bicarbonate; Alumina and Simethicone; Alumina and Sodium Bicarbonate; Aluminum Carbonate, Basic; Aluminum Carbonate, Basic, and Simethicone; Aluminum Hydroxide; Calcium Carbonate; Calcium Carbonate and Magnesia; Calcium Carbonate, Magnesia, and Simethicone; Calcium Carbonate and Simethicone; Calcium and Magnesium Carbonates; Magaldrate; Magaldrate and Simethicone; Magnesium Carbonate and Sodium Bicarbonate; Magnesium Hydroxide; Magnesium Oxide
- **Antiurolithic (phosphate calculi)**—Aluminum Carbonate, Basic; Aluminum Hydroxide
- **Laxative, hyperosmotic, saline**—Magnesium Hydroxide; Magnesium Oxide
- **Antihyperphosphatemic**—Aluminum Carbonate, Basic; Aluminum Hydroxide; Calcium Carbonate
- **Antihypocalcemic**—Calcium Carbonate
- **Antiurolithic (calcium calculi)**—Magnesium Hydroxide

Description

Antacids are taken by mouth to relieve heartburn, sour stomach, or acid indigestion. They work by neutralizing excess stomach acid. Some antacid combinations also contain simethicone, which may relieve the symptoms of excess gas. Antacids alone or in combination with simethicone may also be used to treat the symptoms of stomach or duodenal ulcers.

With larger doses than those used for the antacid effect, magnesium hydroxide (magnesia) and magnesium oxide antacids produce a laxative effect. The information that follows applies only to their use as an antacid.

Some antacids, like aluminum carbonate and aluminum hydroxide, may be prescribed with a low-phosphate diet to treat hyperphosphatemia (too much phosphate in the blood). Aluminum carbonate and aluminum hydroxide may also be used with a low-phosphate diet to prevent the formation of some kinds of kidney stones. Aluminum hydroxide may also be used for other conditions as determined by your doctor.

These medicines are available without a prescription. However, your doctor may have special instructions on the proper use and dose of these medicines for your medical problem. They are available in the following dosage forms:

Oral
- Alumina, Calcium Carbonate, and Sodium Bicarbonate
  - Oral suspension

- Alumina and Magnesia
  - Oral suspension
  - Tablets
  - Chewable tablets
- Alumina, Magnesia, Calcium Carbonate, and Simethicone
  - Chewable tablets
- Alumina, Magnesia, and Magnesium Carbonate
  - Chewable tablets
- Alumina, Magnesia, Magnesium Carbonate, and Simethicone
  - Chewable tablets
- Alumina, Magnesia, and Simethicone
  - Oral suspension
  - Chewable tablets
- Alumina, Magnesium Alginate, and Magnesium Carbonate
  - Oral suspension
  - Chewable tablets
- Alumina and Magnesium Carbonate
  - Oral suspension
  - Chewable tablets
- Alumina, Magnesium Carbonate, and Simethicone
  - Oral suspension
- Alumina, Magnesium Carbonate, and Sodium Bicarbonate
  - Chewable tablets
- Alumina and Magnesium Trisilicate
  - Chewable tablets
- Alumina, Magnesium Trisilicate, and Sodium Bicarbonate
  - Chewable tablets
- Alumina and Simethicone
  - Gel
- Alumina and Sodium Bicarbonate
  - Chewable tablets
- Aluminum Carbonate, Basic
  - Capsules
  - Tablets
- Aluminum Carbonate, Basic, and Simethicone
  - Oral suspension
- Aluminum Hydroxide
  - Capsules
  - Oral suspension
  - Gel
  - Tablets
  - Chewable tablets
- Calcium Carbonate
  - Chewing gum
  - Lozenges
  - Oral suspension
  - Tablets
  - Chewable tablets
- Calcium Carbonate and Magnesia
  - Oral suspension
  - Tablets
  - Chewable tablets
- Calcium Carbonate, Magnesia, and Simethicone
  - Oral suspension
  - Chewable tablets
- Calcium Carbonate and Simethicone
  - Oral suspension
  - Chewable tablets

- Calcium and Magnesium Carbonates
  - Oral suspension
  - Tablets
- Magaldrate
  - Oral suspension
  - Chewable tablets
- Magaldrate and Simethicone
  - Oral suspension
  - Chewable tablets
- Magnesium Carbonate and Sodium Bicarbonate
  - Chewable tablets
- Magnesium Hydroxide
  - Milk of magnesia
  - Chewable tablets
- Magnesium Oxide
  - Capsules
  - Tablets

Before Using This Medicine

If you are taking this medicine without a prescription, carefully read and follow any precautions on the label. For antacids, the following should be considered:

Allergies—Tell your health care professional if you have ever had any unusual or allergic reaction to aluminum-, calcium-, magnesium-, simethicone-, or sodium bicarbonate-containing medicines. Also, tell your health care professional if you are allergic to any other substances, such as foods, preservatives, or dyes.

Diet—Make certain your health care professional knows if you are on a low-sodium diet. Some antacids contain large amounts of sodium.

Pregnancy—Studies on effects in pregnancy have not been done in either humans or animals. However, there have been reports of antacids causing side effects in •babies whose mothers took antacids for a long time, especially in high doses during pregnancy. Also, sodium-containing medicines should be avoided if you tend to retain (keep) body water.

Breast-feeding—Some aluminum-, calcium-, or magnesium-containing antacids may pass into breast milk. However, these medicines have not been reported to cause problems in nursing babies.

Children—Antacids should not be given to young children (under 6 years of age) unless ordered by their doctor. Since children cannot usually describe their symptoms very well, a doctor should first check the child. The child may have a condition that needs other treatment. If so, antacids will not help and may even cause unwanted effects or make the condition worse. In addition, aluminum- or magnesium-containing medicines should not be given to premature or very young children because they may cause serious side effects, especially when given to children who have kidney disease or who are dehydrated.

Older adults—Aluminum-containing antacids should not be used by elderly persons with bone problems or with Alzheimer's disease. The aluminum may cause their condition to get worse.

Other medicines—Although certain medicines should not be used together at all, in other cases two different medicines may be used together even if an interaction might occur. In these cases, your doctor may want to change the dose, or other precautions may be necessary. When you are taking antacids, it is especially important that your health care professional know if you are taking any of the following:

- Cellulose sodium phosphate (e.g., Calcibind)—Calcium-containing antacids may decrease the effects of cellulose sodium phosphate; use with magnesium-containing antacids may prevent either medicine from working properly; antacids should not be taken within 1 hour of cellulose sodium phosphate

- Fluoroquinolones (medicine for infection)—Antacids may decrease the effects of these medicines

- Isoniazid taken by mouth (e.g., INH)—Aluminum-containing antacids may decrease the effects of isoniazid; isoniazid should be taken at least 1 hour before or after the antacid

- Ketoconazole (e.g., Nizoral) or

- Methenamine (e.g., Mandelamine)—Antacids may decrease the effects of ketoconazole or methenamine; these medicines should be taken 3 hours before the antacid

- Mecamylamine (e.g., Inversine)—Antacids may increase the effects and possibly the side effects of mecamylamine

- Sodium polystyrene sulfonate resin (SPSR) (e.g., Kayexalate)—This medicine may decrease the effects of antacids

- Tetracyclines (medicine for infection) taken by mouth—Use with antacids may decrease the effects of both medicines; antacids should not be taken within 3 to 4 hours of tetracyclines

Other medical problems—The presence of other medical problems may affect the use of antacids. Make sure you tell your doctor if you have any other medical problems, especially:

- Alzheimer's disease (for aluminum-containing antacids only) or

- Appendicitis (or signs of) or

- Bone fractures or

- Colitis or

- Constipation (severe and continuing) or

- Hemorrhoids or

- Intestinal blockage or

- Intestinal or rectal bleeding—Antacids may make these conditions worse

- Colostomy or

- Ileostomy or

- Inflamed bowel—Use of antacids may cause the body to retain (keep) water and electrolytes such as sodium and/or potassium

- Diarrhea (continuing)—Aluminum-containing antacids may cause the body to lose too much phosphorus; magnesium-containing antacids may make diarrhea worse

- Edema (swelling of feet or lower legs) or

- Heart disease or

- Liver disease or

- Toxemia of pregnancy—Use of sodium-containing antacids may cause the body to retain (keep) water

- Kidney disease—Antacids may cause higher blood levels of aluminum, calcium, or magnesium, which may increase the risk of serious side effects

- Sarcoidosis—Use of calcium-containing antacids may cause kidney problems or too much calcium in the blood

- Underactive parathyroid glands—Use with calcium-containing antacids may cause too much calcium in the blood

Proper Use of This Medicine

For patients taking the *chewable tablet form* of this medicine:

- Chew the tablets well before swallowing. This is to allow the medicine to work faster and be more effective.

For patients taking this medicine for a *stomach or duodenal ulcer:*

- *Take it exactly as directed and for the full time of treatment as ordered by your doctor*, to obtain maximum relief of your symptoms.

- Take it 1 and 3 hours after meals and at bedtime for best results, unless otherwise directed by your doctor.

For patients taking *aluminum carbonate* or *aluminum hydroxide* to *prevent kidney stones:*

- Drink plenty of fluids for best results, unless otherwise directed by your doctor.

For patients taking *aluminum carbonate* or *aluminum hydroxide* for *hyperphosphatemia* (too much phosphate in the blood):

- Your doctor may want you to follow a low-phosphate diet. If you have any questions about this, check with your doctor.

Dosing—The dose of an antacid will be different for different patients. *Follow your doctor's orders or the directions on the label.*

Missed dose—If your doctor has told you to take this medicine on a regular schedule and you miss a dose, take it as soon as possible. However, if it is almost time for your next dose, skip the missed dose and go back to your regular dosing schedule. Do not double doses.

Storage—To store this medicine:

- Keep out of the reach of children.

- Store away from heat and direct light.

- Do not store the capsule, tablet, or lozenge form of this medicine in the bathroom, near the kitchen sink, or in other damp places. Heat or moisture may cause the medicine to break down.

- Keep the liquid or gel form of this medicine from freezing.

- Do not keep outdated medicine or medicine no longer needed. Be sure that any discarded medicine is out of the reach of children.

Precautions While Using This Medicine

If this medicine has been ordered by your doctor and you will be taking it in large doses, or for a long time, your doctor should check your progress at regular visits. This is to make sure the medicine does not cause unwanted effects.

Some tests may be affected by this medicine. Tell the doctor in charge that you are taking this medicine before you have any tests to determine how much acid your stomach produces.

Do not take this medicine:
- *if you have any signs of appendicitis or inflamed bowel* (such as stomach or lower abdominal pain, cramping, bloating, soreness, nausea, or vomiting). Instead, check with your doctor as soon as possible.
- *within 1 to 2 hours or more of taking other medicine by mouth.* To do so may keep the other medicine from working properly.

For patients on a *sodium-restricted diet:*
- Some antacids (especially those containing sodium bicarbonate) contain a large amount of sodium. If you have any questions about this, check with your health care professional.

For patients taking this medicine for increased stomach acid:
- *Do not take it for more than 2 weeks unless otherwise directed by your doctor.* Antacids should be used only for occasional relief.
- If your stomach problem is not helped by the antacid or if it keeps coming back, check with your doctor.
- Using magnesium- or sodium bicarbonate-containing antacids too often, or in high doses, may produce a laxative effect. This happens fairly often and depends on the individual's sensitivity to the medicine.

For patients taking *aluminum-containing antacids* (including magaldrate):
- Before you have any test in which a radiopharmaceutical will be used, tell the doctor in charge that you are taking this medicine. The results of the test may be affected by aluminum-containing antacids.

For patients taking *calcium—*or *sodium bicarbonate-containing antacids:*
- *Do not take the antacid with large amounts of milk or milk products.* To do so may increase the chance of side effects.

Side Effects

Along with its needed effects, a medicine may cause some unwanted effects. Although the following side effects occur very rarely when this medicine is taken as recommended, they may be more likely to occur if:
- too much medicine is taken
- it is taken in large doses
- it is taken for a long time
- it is taken by patients with kidney disease

Check with your doctor as soon as possible if any of the following side effects (which may be signs of overdose) occur:
For aluminum-containing antacids (including magaldrate)
   Bone pain; constipation (severe and continuing); feeling of discomfort (continuing); loss of appetite (continuing); mood or mental changes; muscle weakness; swelling of wrists or ankles; weight loss (unusual)
For calcium-containing antacids
   Constipation (severe and continuing); difficult or painful urination; frequent urge to urinate; headache (contin-

uing); loss of appetite (continuing); mood or mental changes; muscle pain or twitching; nausea or vomiting; nervousness or restlessness; slow breathing; unpleasant taste; unusual tiredness or weakness
For magnesium-containing antacids (including magaldrate)
   Difficult or painful urination (with magnesium trisilicate); dizziness or lightheadedness; feeling of discomfort (continuing); irregular heartbeat; loss of appetite (continuing); mood or mental changes; muscle weakness; unusual tiredness or weakness; weight loss (unusual)
For sodium bicarbonate-containing antacids
   Frequent urge to urinate; headache (continuing); loss of appetite (continuing); mood or mental changes; muscle pain or twitching; nausea or vomiting; nervousness or restlessness; slow breathing; swelling of feet or lower legs; unpleasant taste; unusual tiredness or weakness

Other side effects may occur that usually do not need medical attention. These side effects may go away during treatment as your body adjusts to the medicine. However, check with your doctor if any of the following side effects continue or are bothersome:
More common
   Chalky taste
Less common
   Constipation (mild); diarrhea or laxative effect; increased thirst; speckling or whitish discoloration of stools; stomach cramps

Other side effects not listed above may also occur in some patients. If you notice any other effects, check with your doctor.

ANTHRALIN (Topical route) - AN-thra-lin

Commonly used brand name(s)

In the U.S.—
   Drithocreme
   Dritho-Scalp
   Psoriatec

In Canada—
   Anthraforte 2%
   Anthraforte 3%
   Anthrascalp

Available Dosage Forms:
- Paste
- Ointment
- Cream

Therapeutic Class: Antipsoriatic

Uses For This Medicine

Anthralin is used to treat psoriasis. It may also be used to treat other skin conditions as determined by your doctor.

In the U.S., this medicine is available only with your doctor's prescription.

Once a medicine has been approved for marketing for a certain use, experience may show that it is also useful for other medical problems. Although this use is not included in product labeling, anthralin is used in certain patients with the following medical condition:

- Alopecia areata (patchy hair loss)

Before Using This Medicine

In deciding to use a medicine, the risks of taking the medicine must be weighed against the good it will do. This is a decision you and your doctor will make. For this medicine, the following should be considered:

Allergies—Tell your doctor if you have ever had any unusual or allergic reaction to this medicine or any other medicines. Also tell your health care professional if you have any other types of allergies, such as to foods, dyes, preservatives, or animals. For non-prescription products, read the label or package ingredients carefully.

Pediatric—Studies on this medicine have been done only in adult patients, and there is no specific information comparing use of anthralin in children with use in other age groups.

Geriatric—Many medicines have not been studied specifically in older people. Therefore, it may not be known whether they work exactly the same way they do in younger adults or if they cause different side effects or problems in older people. There is no specific information comparing use of anthralin in the elderly with use in other age groups.

Pregnancy—

	Pregnancy Category	Explanation
All Trimesters	C	Animal studies have shown an adverse effect and there are no adequate studies in pregnant women OR no animal studies have been conducted and there are no adequate studies in pregnant women.

Breast Feeding—There are no adequate studies in women for determining infant risk when using this medication during breastfeeding. Weigh the potential benefits against the potential risks before taking this medication while breastfeeding.

Other medicines—Although certain medicines should not be used together at all, in other cases two different medicines may be used together even if an interaction might occur. In these cases, your doctor may want to change the dose, or other precautions may be necessary. Tell your healthcare professional if you are taking any other prescription or non-prescription (over-the-counter [OTC]) medicine.

Interactions with Food/Tobacco/Alcohol—Certain medicines should not be used at or around the time of eating food or eating certain types of food since interactions may occur. Using alcohol or tobacco with certain medicines may also cause interactions to occur. Discuss with your healthcare professional the use of your medicine with food, alcohol, or tobacco.

Other medical problems—The presence of other medical problems may affect the use of this medicine. Make sure you tell your doctor if you have any other medical problems, especially:

- Skin diseases or problems (other)—Anthralin may make the condition worse

Proper Use of This Medicine

Keep this medicine away from the eyes and mucous membranes, such as the mouth and the inside of the nose.

Do not apply this medicine to blistered, raw, or oozing areas of the skin or scalp.

Do not use this medicine on your face or sex organs or in the folds and creases of your skin. If you have any questions about this, check with your doctor.

Use this medicine only as directed. Do not use more of it, do not use it more often, and do not use it for a longer time than your doctor ordered. To do so may increase the chance of side effects.

Anthralin may be used in different ways. In some cases, it is applied at night and allowed to remain on the affected areas overnight, then washed off the next morning or before the next application. In other cases, it may be applied and allowed to remain on the affected areas for a short period of time (usually 10 to 30 minutes), then washed off. (This is called short contact treatment.) Make sure you understand exactly how you are to use this medicine. If you have any questions about this, check with your doctor.

Anthralin may cause irritation of normal skin. If it does, petrolatum may be applied to the skin or scalp around the affected areas for protection.

Apply a thin layer of anthralin to only the affected area of the skin or scalp and rub in gently and well.

Immediately after applying this medicine, wash your hands to remove any medicine that may be on them.

For patients using anthralin for short contact (usually 10 to 30 minutes) treatment:

- After applying anthralin, allow the medicine to remain on the affected area for 10 to 30 minutes or as directed by your doctor. Then remove the medicine by bathing, if the anthralin was applied to the skin, or by shampooing, if it was applied to the scalp.

For patients using the cream form of anthralin for overnight treatment:

- If anthralin cream is applied to the skin, any medicine remaining on the affected areas the next morning should be removed by bathing.
- If anthralin cream is applied to the scalp, shampoo to remove the scales and any medicine remaining on the affected areas from the previous application. Dry the hair and, after parting, rub the cream into the affected areas. Check with your doctor to see when the cream should be removed.

For patients using the ointment form of anthralin for overnight treatment:

- If anthralin ointment is applied to the skin at night, any ointment remaining on the affected areas the next morning should be removed with warm liquid petrolatum followed by bathing.
- If anthralin ointment is applied to the scalp at night, shampoo the next morning to clean the scalp.

Dosing—The dose of this medicine will be different for different patients. Follow your doctor's orders or the directions on the label. The following information includes only the average doses of this medicine. If your dose is different, do not change it unless your doctor tells you to do so.

The amount of medicine that you take depends on the strength of the medicine. Also, the number of doses you take each day, the time allowed between doses, and the length of time you take the medicine depend on the medical problem for which you are using the medicine.

- For psoriasis:
  - For cream dosage form:
    - Adults—Apply to the dry, affected area(s) of the skin once a day, preferably at night, or as directed by your doctor. Wash medicine off skin at the proper time.
    - Children—Use and dose must be determined by your doctor.
  - For ointment dosage form:
    - Adults—Apply to the dry, affected area(s) of the skin once a day or as directed by your doctor. Wash medicine off skin at the proper time.
    - Children—Use and dose must be determined by your doctor.

Missed dose—If you miss a dose of this medicine, apply it as soon as possible. However, if it is almost time for your next dose, skip the missed dose and go back to your regular dosing schedule.

Storage—Store the medicine in a closed container at room temperature, away from heat, moisture, and direct light. Keep from freezing.

Keep out of the reach of children.

Do not keep outdated medicine or medicine no longer needed.

Precautions While Using This Medicine

Anthralin may stain the skin, hair, fingernails, clothing, bed linens, or bathtub or shower. The stain on the skin or hair will wear off in several weeks after you stop using this medicine. Some ways to prevent or lessen anthralin staining include:
- Wear plastic gloves when you apply this medicine.
- Avoid getting the medicine on your clothing or on bed linens. Ask your doctor if you can wear a plastic cap while sleeping if you apply your medicine to your scalp at bedtime.
- Remove any medicine on the surface of the bathtub or shower stall by immediately rinsing it with hot water after bathing or showering. Afterwards wash the bathtub or shower stall with a household cleanser to remove any remaining deposits.

Side Effects of This Medicine

Anthralin has been shown to cause tumors in animals. However, there have been no reports of anthralin causing tumors in humans.

Along with its needed effects, a medicine may cause some unwanted effects. Although not all of these side effects may occur, if they do occur they may need medical attention.

Check with your doctor as soon as possible if any of the following side effects occur:
More common
Redness or other skin irritation of treated or uninvolved skin not present before use of this medicine
Rare
Skin rash

Other side effects not listed may also occur in some patients. If you notice any other effects, check with your healthcare professional.

ANTIANDROGENS, NONSTEROIDAL   (Systemic)

Some commonly used brand names are:

In the U.S.—
Casodex (1)
Eulexin (2)
Nilandron (3)

In Canada—
Anandron (3)
Casodex (1)
Euflex (2)

This information applies to the following medicines:
1. Bicalutamide (bye-ka-LOO-ta-mide)
2. Flutamide (FLOO-ta-mide)
3. Nilutamide (nye-LOO-ta-mide)

Category

- **Antineoplastic**—Bicalutamide; Flutamide; Nilutamide

Description

Nonsteroidal antiandrogens are used to treat cancer of the prostate gland. The prostate gland is present only in males; therefore, females do not get prostate cancer.

Nonsteroidal antiandrogens block the effect of the male hormone testosterone in the body. Giving a nonsteroidal antiandrogen together with another treatment that decreases the amount of testosterone produced in the body is one way of treating this type of cancer.

These medicines are available only with your doctor's prescription, in the following dosage form(s):
Oral
- Bicalutamide
  - Tablets
- Flutamide
  - Capsules
  - Tablets
- Nilutamide
  - Tablets

Before Using This Medicine

In deciding to use a medicine, the risks of taking the medicine must be weighed against the good it will do. This is a decision you and your doctor will make. For the nonsteroidal antiandrogens, the following should be considered:

Allergies—Tell your doctor if you have ever had any unusual or allergic reaction to any of the nonsteroidal antiandrogens. Also tell your health care professional if you are allergic to any other substances, such as foods, preservatives, or dyes.

Fertility—Nonsteroidal antiandrogens, and other treatments for prostate cancer that are used together with these medicines, may cause low sperm counts or otherwise decrease a man's ability to father a child. In some cases, these effects may be permanent. Men who wish to have children should discuss this with their doctors before starting treatment.

Pregnancy—Nonsteroidal antiandrogens are usually given to men. However, if one of these medicines is needed by a woman, it is very important that an effective method of avoiding pregnancy be used during treatment. Because these medicines block the effect of the male hormone, testosterone, they may interfere with the normal development of a male fetus.

Breast-feeding—Nonsteroidal antiandrogens are usually given to men, and it is not known whether any of these medicines passes into breast milk. However, nonsteroidal antiandrogens can cause serious side effects. Therefore, if a woman needs one of these medicines, she should not breast-feed during treatment.

Children—Studies with the nonsteroidal antiandrogens have been done only in adults, and there is no specific information comparing the use of these medicines in children with use in other age groups. There is a chance that a nonsteroidal antiandrogen could interfere with the development of boys. However, cancer of the prostate gland usually occurs in middle-aged or older men, so it is very unlikely that a child would need these medicines.

Older adults—Nonsteroidal antiandrogens have been tested in elderly people and have not been shown to cause different side effects or problems than they do in younger adults.

Race—A serious side effect of nilutamide that affects the lungs may be more likely to occur in Asian patients than in Caucasian patients.

Other medicines—Although certain medicines should not be used together at all, in other cases two different medicines may be used together even if an interaction might occur. In these cases, your doctor may want to change the dose, or other precautions may be necessary. When you are taking a nonsteroidal antiandrogen, it is especially important that your health care professional know if you are taking any of the following:

- Anticoagulants such as warfarin (e.g., Coumadin)—Bicalutamide, flutamide, or nilutamide may increase the effects of the anticoagulant. Your doctor may recommend having your blood tested more often so that the dose of anticoagulant can be changed if necessary.

- Phenytoin (e.g., Dilantin) or

- Theophylline (e.g., Theo-Dur; Theolair)—Nilutamide may increase the blood levels of these medicines in your body, which can increase the risk of serious side effects.

Also tell your doctor if you smoke tobacco. Tobacco smoking may increase the risk of a rare side effect of flutamide.

Other medical problems—The presence of other medical problems may affect the use of nonsteroidal antiandrogens. Make sure you tell your doctor if you have any other medical problems, especially:

- Certain blood deficiencies or disorders or

- Tobacco smoking—Increased risk of anemia, other blood disorders, and jaundice

- Liver disease—The chance of serious side effects may be increased.

- Lung disease or other breathing problems—One side effect of nilutamide can make your condition worse; your doctor may want to select a different antiandrogen.

Proper Use of This Medicine

Take this medicine exactly as directed by your doctor. Do not take more or less of it, and do not take it more often than your doctor ordered. The exact amount of medicine you need has been carefully worked out. Taking too much may increase the chance of side effects, while taking too little may not improve your condition.

It is best to take this medicine at the same time each day. If you have been directed to take the medicine once a day, you may take it either in the morning or in the evening.

Bicalutamide and nilutamide may be taken with food or on an empty stomach.

A nonsteroidal antiandrogen is often used together with another medicine, which is given by injection. *It is very important that the two medicines be used as directed. Follow your doctor's instructions very carefully about when to use these medicines.*

Unwanted effects, including hot flashes and decreased sexual ability, may occur during treatment for prostate cancer. Also, symptoms that often occur in men with prostate cancer, including difficult or painful urination, bloody urine, and urinary tract infections, may occur or continue to occur for a while, until your condition starts to improve. *It is very important that you continue to take the medicine, even if it causes side effects or if you start to feel better. Do not stop taking this medicine without first checking with your doctor.*

If you vomit shortly after taking a dose of this medicine, check with your doctor. You will be told whether to take the dose again or to wait until the next scheduled dose.

Dosing—The doses of these medicines will be different for different patients. *Follow your doctor's orders or the directions on the label.* The following information includes only the average doses of these medicines. *If your dose is different, do not change it* unless your doctor tells you to do so.

The number of capsules or tablets that you take depends on the strength of the medicine. Also, *the number of doses you take each day, the time allowed between doses, and the length of time you take the medicine depend on which of these medicines you are taking.*

For bicalutamide
- For the *oral* dosage form (tablets):
  - For prostate cancer:
    - Adults—50 milligrams (mg) (one tablet) once a day.
    - Children—It is unlikely that bicalutamide would be needed to treat cancer of the prostate in a child. If a child needs this medicine, the dose would have to be determined by the doctor.

For flutamide
- For *oral* dosage forms (capsules or tablets):
  - For prostate cancer:
    - Adults—250 milligrams (mg) (two 125–mg capsules or one 250–mg tablet) every eight hours.
    - Children—It is unlikely that flutamide would be needed to treat cancer of the prostate in a child. If a child needs this medicine, the dose would have to be determined by the doctor.

For nilutamide
- For the *oral* dosage form (tablets):
  ○ For prostate cancer:
    ▪ Adults—300 milligrams (mg) (six 50–mg tablets) once a day for the first thirty days, then 150 mg (three 50–mg tablets) once a day.
    ▪ Children—It is unlikely that nilutamide would be needed to treat cancer of the prostate in a child. If a child needs this medicine, the dose would have to be determined by the doctor.

Missed dose—If you miss a dose of this medicine, take it as soon as possible.

For bicalutamide or nilutamide: If you do not remember your missed dose until the next day, skip the missed dose and go back to your regular dosing schedule. Do not double doses.

For flutamide: If it is almost time for your next dose, skip the missed dose and go back to your regular dosing schedule. Do not double doses.

Storage—To store this medicine:
- Keep out of the reach of children.
- Store away from heat and direct light.
- Do not store in the bathroom, near the kitchen sink, or in other damp places. Heat or moisture may cause the medicine to break down.
- Do not keep outdated medicine or medicine no longer needed. Be sure that any discarded medicine is out of the reach of children.

Precautions While Using This Medicine

It is very important that your doctor check your progress at regular visits to make sure that this medicine is working properly and to check for unwanted effects.

Nonsteroidal antiandrogens rarely cause liver problems during treatment. The most important signs of this side effect are pain or tenderness in the upper right side of the abdomen (stomach) and yellow eyes or skin. *Check with your doctor immediately if either of these occurs. Also, check with your doctor as soon as possible* if itching occurs or your urine appears unusually dark. Other possible symptoms, such as loss of appetite, nausea or vomiting, and "flu-like" symptoms (headache, muscle or joint pain, or tiredness), can occur during treatment even if you are not having any liver problems. These symptoms usually do not need medical attention. However, if two or more of them occur at the same time, and they last for more than a few days, check with your doctor even if you do not have any of the other symptoms mentioned earlier.

For patients taking *nilutamide:*
- *Check with your doctor right away* if shortness of breath or difficult breathing occurs or gets worse during treatment.
- *Be very careful while driving, especially when you drive into or out of tunnels.* Nilutamide can temporarily change the way your eyes react to light. You may not be able to see as well as usual for up to several minutes after going from bright light to darkness or from dark to lighted areas. Also, nilutamide can cause your eyes to be more sensitive to light than they are normally. Wearing eyeglasses with tinted lenses or sunglasses may help reduce these effects.

- Drinking alcoholic beverages while taking nilutamide may cause unwanted effects in some people. Possible effects include feeling dizzy, lightheaded, or faint; flushing of the face; or a general feeling of illness. *If you notice any of these effects, do not drink any more alcoholic beverages while you are being treated with this medicine.*

Side Effects of This Medicine

Along with its needed effects, a medicine may cause some unwanted effects. Although not all of these side effects may occur, if they do occur they may need medical attention.

Check with your doctor immediately if any of the following side effects occur:
  Less common
    Chest pain; shortness of breath or difficult or troubled breathing
  Rare
    Pain or tenderness in the upper right side of the abdomen (stomach); yellow eyes or skin

Also, check with your doctor as soon as possible if any of the following side effects occur:
  More common
    Cough or hoarseness; fever; runny nose; sneezing; sore throat; tightness in chest or wheezing
  Less common
    Bloody or black, tarry stools; chills (flutamide only); itching; lower back or side pain (flutamide only); mental depression; numbness, tingling, pain, or muscle weakness in hands, arms, feet, or legs; skin rash; swelling of face, fingers, feet, or lower legs; unusual tiredness or weakness
  Rare
    Bluish-colored lips, fingernails, or palms of hands (flutamide only); dark urine; dizziness (severe) or fainting (flutamide only); feeling of severe pressure in head (flutamide only); pinpoint red spots on skin; unusual bleeding or bruising

Other side effects may occur that usually do not need medical attention. These side effects may go away during treatment as your body adjusts to the medicine. However, check with your doctor if any of the following side effects continue or are bothersome:
  More common
    Constipation; decrease in or loss of appetite; diarrhea; dizziness; headache; impotence or decrease in sexual desire; nausea; swelling of breasts with pain or tenderness; trouble in sleeping
  Less common
    Bloated feeling, gas, or indigestion; change in color vision (nilutamide only); confusion; drowsiness; dryness of mouth; "flu-like" symptoms, such as headache, muscle or joint pain, or tiredness (occurring together); nervousness; vomiting

Although not all of the side effects listed above have been reported for all of these medicines, they have been reported for at least one of them. However, because all nonsteroidal antiandrogens are very similar, it is possible that any of the above side effects may occur with any of these medicines.

In addition to the effects listed above, hot flashes (flushing, sudden sweating, and feeling of warmth) often occur during treatment with these medicines. Also, flutamide may cause your urine to have an amber or a yellow-green color. These effects are harmless and do not need medical attention.

Other side effects not listed above may also occur in some patients. If you notice any other effects, check with your doctor.

ANTICHOLINERGICS/ ANTISPASMODICS (Systemic)

Some commonly used brand names are:

In the U.S.—

Anaspaz (8)	Levbid (8)
A-Spas S/L (8)	Levsin (8)
Banthine (10)	Levsinex Timecaps (8)
Bentyl (5)	Levsin/SL (8)
Cantil (9)	Pro-Banthine (13)
Cystospaz (8)	Quarzan (4)
Cystospaz-M (8)	Robinul (6)
Donnamar (8)	Robinul Forte (6)
ED-SPAZ (8)	Symax SL (8)
Gastrosed (8)	Transderm-Scō p (14)
Homapin (7)	

In Canada—

Bentylol (5)	Propanthel (13)
Buscopan (14)	Robinul (6)
Formulex (5)	Robinul Forte (6)
Gastrozepin (12)	Spasmoban (5)
Levsin (8)	Transderm-V (14)
Pro-Banthine (13)	

This information applies to the following medicines:

1. Anisotropine (an-iss-oh-TROE-peen)
2. Atropine (A-troe-peen)
3. Belladonna (bell-a-DON-a)
4. Clidinium (kli-DI-nee-um)
5. Dicyclomine (dye-SYE-kloe-meen)
6. Glycopyrrolate (glye-koe-PYE-roe-late)
7. Homatropine (hoe-MA-troe-peen)
8. Hyoscyamine (hye-oh-SYE-a-meen)
9. Mepenzolate (me-PEN-zoe-late)
10. Methantheline (meth-AN-tha-leen)
11. Methscopolamine (meth-skoe-POL-a-meen)
12. Pirenzepine (peer-EN-ze-peen)
13. Propantheline (proe-PAN-the-leen)
14. Scopolamine (scoe-POL-a-meen)

Category

- **Anesthesia adjunct**—Scopolamine
- **Antiarrhythmic**—Atropine; Glycopyrrolate; Hyoscyamine; Scopolamine
- **Anticholinergic**—Anisotropine; Atropine; Belladonna; Clidinium; Dicyclomine; Glycopyrrolate; Homatropine; Hyoscyamine; Mepenzolate; Methantheline; Methscopolamine; Pirenzepine; Propantheline; Scopolamine
- **Antidiarrheal**—Glycopyrrolate
- **Antidote, to cholinesterase inhibitors**—Atropine; Hyoscyamine
- **Antidote, to muscarine**—Atropine; Hyoscyamine
- **Antidote, to organophosphate pesticides**—Atropine
- **Antidysmenorrheal**—Belladonna; Scopolamine
- **Antiemetic**—Scopolamine

- **Antispasmodic, gastrointestinal**—Dicyclomine; Scopolamine
- **Antispasmodic, urinary tract**—Atropine; Scopolamine
- **Antivertigo agent**—Belladonna; Scopolamine
- **Cholinergic adjunct, curariform block**—Atropine; Glycopyrrolate; Hyoscyamine

Description

The anticholinergics/antispasmodics are a group of medicines that include the natural belladonna alkaloids (atropine, belladonna, hyoscyamine, and scopolamine) and related products.

The anticholinergics/antispasmodics are used to relieve cramps or spasms of the stomach, intestines, and bladder. Some are used together with antacids or other medicine in the treatment of peptic ulcer. Others are used to prevent nausea, vomiting, and motion sickness.

Anticholinergics/antispasmodics are also used in certain surgical and emergency procedures. In surgery, some are given by injection before anesthesia to help relax you and to decrease secretions, such as saliva. During anesthesia and surgery, atropine, glycopyrrolate, hyoscyamine, and scopolamine are used to help keep the heartbeat normal. Scopolamine is also used to prevent nausea and vomiting after anesthesia and surgery. Atropine is also given by injection to help relax the stomach and intestines for certain types of examinations. Some anticholinergics are also used to treat poisoning caused by medicines such as neostigmine and physostigmine, certain types of mushrooms, and poisoning by "nerve'" gases or organic phosphorous pesticides (for example, demeton [Systox], diazinon, malathion, parathion, and ronnel [Trolene]). Also, anticholinergics can be used for painful menstruation, runny nose, and to prevent urination during sleep.

These medicines may also be used for other conditions as determined by your doctor.

The anticholinergics/antispasmodics are available only with your doctor's prescription in the following dosage forms:

Oral
- Anisotropine
  - Tablets
- Atropine
  - Tablets
  - Soluble tablets
- Belladonna
  - Tincture
- Clidinium
  - Capsules
- Dicyclomine
  - Capsules
  - Syrup
  - Tablets
- Glycopyrrolate
  - Tablets
- Homatropine
  - Tablets
- Hyoscyamine
  - Extended-release capsules
  - Extended-release tablets
  - Elixir
  - Oral solution
  - Tablets

- Mepenzolate
  - Tablets
- Methantheline
  - Tablets
- Methscopolamine
- Pirenzepine
  - Tablets
- Propantheline
  - Tablets
- Scopolamine
  - Tablets

Parenteral
- Atropine
  - Injection
- Dicyclomine
  - Injection (U.S.)
- Glycopyrrolate
  - Injection
- Hyoscyamine
  - Injection (U.S.)
- Scopolamine
  - Injection

Rectal
- Scopolamine
  - Suppositories

Transdermal
- Scopolamine
  - Transdermal disk

Before Using This Medicine

In deciding to use a medicine, the risks of taking the medicine must be weighed against the good it will do. This is a decision you and your doctor will make. For anticholinergics/antispasmodics the following should be considered:

Allergies—Tell your doctor if you have ever had any unusual or allergic reaction to any of the natural belladonna alkaloids (atropine, belladonna, hyoscyamine, and scopolamine), or any related products. Also, tell your health care professional if you are allergic to any other substances, such as foods, preservatives, or dyes.

Pregnancy—If you are pregnant or if you may become pregnant, make sure your doctor knows if your medicine contains any of the following:

- *Atropine*—Atropine has not been shown to cause birth defects or other problems in animals. However, when injected into humans during pregnancy, atropine has been reported to increase the heartbeat of the fetus.
- *Belladonna*—Studies on effects in pregnancy have not been done in either humans or animals.
- *Clidinium*—Clidinium has not been studied in pregnant women. However, clidinium has not been shown to cause birth defects or other problems in animal studies.
- *Dicyclomine*—Dicyclomine has been associated with a few cases of human birth defects but dicyclomine has not been confirmed as the cause.
- *Glycopyrrolate*—Glycopyrrolate has not been studied in pregnant women. However, glycopyrrolate did not cause birth defects in animal studies, but did decrease the chance of becoming pregnant and the newborn's chance of surviving after weaning.

- *Hyoscyamine*—Studies on effects in pregnancy have not been done in either humans or animals. However, when injected into humans during pregnancy, hyoscyamine has been reported to increase the heartbeat of the fetus.
- *Mepenzolate*—Mepenzolate has not been studied in pregnant women. However, studies in animals have not shown that mepenzolate causes birth defects or other problems.
- *Propantheline*—Studies on effects in pregnancy have not been done in either humans or animals.
- *Scopolamine*—Studies on effects in pregnancy have not been done in either humans or animals.

Breast-feeding—Although these medicines may pass into the breast milk, they have not been reported to cause problems in nursing babies. However, the flow of breast milk may be reduced in some patients. The use of dicyclomine in nursing mothers has been reported to cause breathing problems in infants.

Children—Unusual excitement, nervousness, restlessness, or irritability and unusual warmth, dryness, and flushing of skin are more likely to occur in children, who are usually more sensitive to the effects of anticholinergics. Also, when anticholinergics are given to children during hot weather, a rapid increase in body temperature may occur. In infants and children, especially those with spastic paralysis or brain damage, this medicine may be more likely to cause severe side effects. Shortness of breath or difficulty in breathing has occurred in children taking dicyclomine.

Older adults—Confusion or memory loss; constipation; difficult urination; drowsiness; dryness of mouth, nose, throat, or skin; and unusual excitement, nervousness, restlessness, or irritability may be more likely to occur in the elderly, who are usually more sensitive than younger adults to the effects of anticholinergics. Also, eye pain may occur, which may be a sign of glaucoma.

Other medicines—Although certain medicines should not be used together at all, in other cases two different medicines may be used together even if an interaction might occur. In these cases, your doctor may want to change the dose, or other precautions may be necessary. When you are taking anticholinergics/antispasmodics, it is especially important that your health care professional know if you are taking any of the following:

- Antacids or
- Diarrhea medicine containing kaolin or attapulgite or
- Ketoconazole (e.g., Nizoral)—Using these medicines with an anticholinergic may lessen the effects of the anticholinergic
- Central nervous system (CNS) depressants (medicines that cause drowsiness)—Taking scopolamine with CNS depressants may increase the effects of either medicine
- Other anticholinergics (medicine for abdominal or stomach spasms or cramps) or
- Tricyclic antidepressants (amitriptyline [e.g., Elavil], amoxapine [e.g., Asendin], clomipramine [e.g., Anafranil], desipramine [e.g., Pertofrane], doxepin [e.g., Sinequan], imipramine [e.g., Tofranil], nortriptyline [e.g., Aventyl], protriptyline [e.g., Vivactil], trimipramine [e.g., Surmontil])—Taking anticholinergics with tricyclic antidepressants or other anticholinergics may cause an increase in the effects of the anticholinergic

- Potassium chloride (e.g., Kay Ciel)—Using this medicine with an anticholinergic may make gastrointestinal problems caused by potassium worse

Other medical problems—The presence of other medical problems may affect the use of anticholinergics/antispasmodics. Make sure you tell your doctor if you have any other medical problems, especially:

- Bleeding problems (severe)—These medicines may increase heart rate, which would make bleeding problems worse
- Brain damage (in children)—May increase the CNS effects of this medicine
- Colitis (severe) or
- Dryness of mouth (severe and continuing) or
- Enlarged prostate or
- Fever or
- Glaucoma or
- Heart disease or
- Hernia (hiatal) or
- High blood pressure (hypertension) or
- Intestinal blockage or other intestinal problems or
- Lung disease (chronic) or
- Myasthenia gravis or
- Toxemia of pregnancy or
- Urinary tract blockage or difficult urination—These medicines may make these conditions worse
- Down's syndrome—These medicines may cause an increase in pupil dilation and heart rate
- Kidney disease or
- Liver disease—Higher blood levels may occur and cause an increase in side effects
- Overactive thyroid—These medicines may further increase heart rate
- Spastic paralysis (in children)—This condition may increase the effects of the anticholinergic

---

Proper Use of This Medicine

Take this medicine only as directed. Do not take more of it, do not take it more often, and do not take it for a longer time than your doctor ordered. To do so may increase the chance of side effects.

Dosing—The dose of the anticholinergic/antispasmodic will be different for different patients. *Follow your doctor's orders or the directions on the label.* The following information includes only the average doses of your medicine. *If your dose is different, do not change it* unless your doctor tells you to do so.

The number of capsules or tablets or teaspoonfuls of solution or syrup that you take depends on the strength of the medicine. Also, *the number of doses you take each day, the time allowed between doses, and the length of time you take the medicine depends on the medical problem for which you are taking this medicine.*

For anisotropine
- For *oral* dosage forms (tablets):
  - To treat duodenal or stomach ulcers:

- Older adults, adults, and teenagers—50 milligrams (mg) three times a day. Your doctor may change the dose if needed.
- Children—Dose must be determined by your doctor.

For atropine
- For *oral* dosage form (tablets):
  - To treat duodenal or stomach ulcers, intestine problems, or urinary problems:
    - Older adults, adults, and teenagers—300 to 1200 micrograms (mcg) every four to six hours.
    - Children—Dose is based on body weight. The usual dose is 10 mcg per kilogram (kg) (4.5 mcg per pound) of body weight every four to six hours. However, the dose will not be more than 400 mcg every four to six hours.
- For *injectable* dosage form:
  - To treat duodenal or stomach ulcers or intestine problems:
    - Older adults, adults, and teenagers—400 to 600 mcg injected into a muscle, vein, or under the skin every four to six hours.
    - Children—The dose is based on body weight. The usual dose is 10 mcg per kilogram (kg) (4.5 mcg per pound) of body weight injected under the skin every four to six hours. However, the dose will not be more than 400 mcg every four to six hours.
  - To treat heart problems:
    - Older adults, adults, and teenagers—400 to 1000 mcg injected into a vein every one to two hours as needed. The total dose will not be more than 2 mg.
    - Children—The dose is based on body weight. The usual dose is 10 to 30 mcg per kilogram (kg) (4.5 to 13.6 mcg per pound) of body weight injected under the skin.

For belladonna
- For *oral* dosage form (oral solution):
  - To treat duodenal or stomach ulcers or intestine problems:
    - Older adults, adults, and teenagers—180 to 300 micrograms (mcg) three or four times a day. The dose should be taken 30 to 60 minutes before meals and at bedtime. Your doctor may change the dose if needed.
    - Children—The dose is based on body weight. The usual dose is 9 mcg per kilogram (kg) (4 mcg per pound) of body weight three or four times a day.

For clidinium
- For *oral* dosage form (capsules):
  - To treat duodenal or stomach ulcers:
    - Older adults, adults, and teenagers—2.5 to 5 milligrams (mg) three or four times a day. The dose should be taken before meals and at bedtime. Your doctor may change the dose if needed.
    - Children—Dose must be determined by your doctor.

For dicyclomine
- For *oral* dosage forms (capsules, extended-release tablets, syrup, tablets):
  - To treat intestine problems:
    - Older adults, adults, and teenagers—10 to 20 milligrams (mg) three or four times a day. Some

people may take 30 mg two times a day. Your doctor may change the dose if needed. Your dose will not be more than 160 mg a day.

- Children 2 years of age and older—5 to 10 mg three or four times a day. Your doctor may change the dose if needed.
- Children 6 months to 2 years of age—5 to 10 mg of the syrup three or four times a day. Your doctor may change the dose if needed.
- Children up to 6 months of age—Use is not recommended.

- For *injectable* dosage form:
  - To treat intestine problems:
    - Older adults, adults, and teenagers—20 mg injected into a muscle every four to six hours. Your doctor may change the dose if needed.
    - Children—Dose must be determined by your doctor.

For glycopyrrolate
- For *oral* dosage form (tablets):
  - To treat duodenal or stomach ulcers:
    - Older adults, adults, and teenagers—To start, 1 to 2 milligrams (mg) two or three times a day. Some people may also take 2 mg at bedtime. Your doctor may change the dose if needed. However, your dose will not be more than 8 mg a day.
    - Children—Dose must be determined by your doctor.
- For *injectable* dosage form:
  - To treat duodenal or stomach ulcers:
    - Older adults, adults, and teenagers—100 to 200 micrograms (mcg) injected into a muscle or vein. The dose may be repeated every four hours up to four times a day.
    - Children—Dose must be determined by your doctor.

For homatropine
- For *oral* dosage form:
  - To treat duodenal or stomach ulcers:
    - Older adults, adults, and teenagers—5 to 10 milligrams (mg) three or four times a day. Your doctor may change the dose if needed.
    - Children—Dose must be determined by your doctor.

For hyoscyamine
- For *oral* dosage forms (capsules, elixir, oral solution, tablets):
  - To treat duodenal or stomach ulcers, intestine problems, or urinary problems:
    - Older adults, adults, and teenagers—125 to 500 micrograms (mcg) four to six times a day. Some people may take 375 mcg two times a day. The tablets should be taken 30 to 60 minutes before meals. Your doctor may change the dose if needed.
    - Children—Dose is based on body weight. The usual dose is 12.5 to 187 mcg every four hours if needed.
- For *injectable* dosage form:
  - To treat duodenal or stomach ulcers or intestine problems:
    - Older adults, adults, and teenagers—250 to 500 mcg injected into a muscle, vein, or under the skin every four to six hours.

- Children—Dose must be determined by your doctor.

For mepenzolate
- For *oral* dosage form (tablets):
  - To treat duodenal or stomach ulcers or intestine problems:
    - Older adults, adults, and teenagers—25 to 50 milligrams (mg) four times a day, with meals and at bedtime. Your doctor may change the dose if needed.
    - Children—Dose must be determined by your doctor.

For methantheline
- For *oral* dosage form (tablets):
  - To treat intestine or stomach ulcers, intestine problems, or urinary problems:
    - Older adults, adults, and teenagers—50 to 100 milligrams (mg) every six hours. Your doctor may change the dose if needed.
    - Children 1 year of age and older—12.5 to 50 mg four times a day. Your doctor may change the dose if needed.
    - Children 1 month to 1 year of age—12.5 mg four times a day. Your doctor may change the dose if needed.
    - Children up to 1 month of age—12.5 mg two times a day. Your doctor may change the dose if needed.

For methscopolamine
- For *oral* dosage form (tablets):
  - To treat duodenal or stomach ulcers or intestine problems:
    - Older adults, adults, and teenagers—2.5 to 5 milligrams (mg) four times a day, one-half hour before meals and at bedtime. Your doctor may change the dose if needed.
    - Children—Dose is based on body weight. The usual dose is 200 micrograms (mcg) per kilogram (kg) (90.9 mcg per pound) of body weight four times a day. The dose should be taken before meals and at bedtime.

For pirenzepine
- For *oral* dosage form (tablets):
  - To treat duodenal or stomach ulcers or intestine problems:
    - Older adults, adults, and teenagers—50 milligrams (mg) two times a day, in the morning and at bedtime. Your doctor may change the dose if needed.
    - Children—Dose must be determined by your doctor.

For propantheline
- For *oral* dosage form (tablets):
  - To treat duodenal or stomach ulcers:
    - Older adults, adults, and teenagers—7.5 to 15 milligrams (mg) three times a day, one-half hour before meals, and 30 mg at bedtime. Your doctor may change the dose if needed.
    - Children—Dose is based on body weight. The usual dose is 375 micrograms (mcg) per kilogram (kg) (170 mcg per pound) of body weight four times a day. Your doctor may change the dose if needed.

For scopolamine
- For *oral* dosage form (tablets):
  - To treat urinary problems or intestine problems or painful menstruation:
    - Older adults, adults, and teenagers—10 to 20 milligrams (mg) three or four times a day. Your doctor may change the dose if needed.
    - Children—Dose must be determined by your doctor.
- For *injectable* dosage form:
  - To treat urinary problems or intestine problems:
    - Older adults, adults, and teenagers—10 to 20 mg three or four times a day. Your doctor may change the dose if needed.
    - Children—Dose must be determined by your doctor.
- For *rectal* dosage form (suppository):
  - To treat urinary problems or intestine problems or painful menstruation:
    - Older adults, adults, and teenagers—Insert one 10 mg suppository rectally three or four times a day. Your doctor may change the dose if needed.
    - Children—Dose must be determined by your doctor.
- For *transdermal* dosage form (patch):
  - To treat motion sickness:
    - Older adults, adults, and teenagers—Apply one 1.0 milligram (mg) patch behind ear at least four hours before antinausea effect is needed.
    - Children—Use is not recommended.
  - To treat nausea and vomiting after surgery
    - Older adults, adults and teenagers—Apply one 1.0 mg patch behind the ear the evening before surgery to prevent nausea and vomiting after surgery
    - Children—Use is not recommended.

Missed dose—If you miss a dose of this medicine, take it as soon as possible. However, if it is almost time for your next dose, skip the missed dose and go back to your regular dosing schedule. Do not double doses.

For patients *taking any of these medicines by mouth:*
- Take this medicine 30 minutes to 1 hour before meals unless otherwise directed by your doctor.

To use the *rectal suppository* form of *scopolamine:*
- If the suppository is too soft to insert, chill it in the refrigerator for 30 minutes or run cold water over it before removing the foil wrapper.
- To insert the suppository: First remove the foil wrapper and moisten the suppository with cold water. Lie down on your side and use your finger to push the suppository well up into the rectum.

To use the *transdermal disk* form of *scopolamine:*
- This medicine usually comes with patient directions. Read them carefully before using this medicine.
- Wash and dry your hands thoroughly before and after handling.
- Apply the disk to the hairless area of skin behind the ear. Do not place over any cuts or irritations.

Storage—To store this medicine:
- Keep out of the reach of children. Overdose is especially dangerous in young children.

- Store away from heat and direct light.
- Do not store the capsule or tablet form of this medicine in the bathroom, near the kitchen sink, or in other damp places. Heat or moisture may cause the medicine to break down.
- Keep the liquid form of this medicine tightly closed and keep it from freezing. Do not refrigerate the syrup form of this medicine.
- Do not keep outdated medicine or medicine no longer needed. Be sure that any discarded medicine is out of the reach of children.

Precautions While Using This Medicine

If you think you or someone else may have taken an overdose, get emergency help at once. Taking an overdose of any of the belladonna alkaloids or taking scopolamine with alcohol or other CNS depressants may lead to unconsciousness and possibly death. Some signs of overdose are clumsiness or unsteadiness; dizziness; severe drowsiness; fever; hallucinations (seeing, hearing, or feeling things that are not there); confusion; shortness of breath or troubled breathing; slurred speech; unusual excitement, nervousness, restlessness, or irritability; fast heartbeat; and unusual warmth, dryness, and flushing of skin.

These medicines may make you sweat less, causing your body temperature to increase. *Use extra care not to become overheated during exercise or hot weather while you are taking this medicine,* since overheating may result in heat stroke. Also, hot baths or saunas may make you dizzy or faint while you are taking this medicine.

Check with your doctor before you stop using this medicine. Your doctor may want you to reduce gradually the amount you are using before stopping completely. Stopping this medicine may cause withdrawal side effects such as vomiting, sweating, and dizziness.

Anticholinergics may cause some people to have blurred vision. *Make sure your vision is clear before you drive or do anything else that could be dangerous if you are not able to see well.* These medicines may also cause your eyes to become more sensitive to light than they are normally. Wearing sunglasses may help lessen the discomfort from bright light.

These medicines, especially in high doses, may cause some people to become dizzy or drowsy. *Make sure you know how you react to this medicine before you drive, use machines, or do anything else that could be dangerous if you are dizzy or are not alert.*

Dizziness, lightheadedness, or fainting may occur, especially when you get up from a lying or sitting position. Getting up slowly may help lessen this problem.

These medicines may cause dryness of the mouth, nose, and throat. For temporary relief of mouth dryness, use sugarless candy or gum, melt bits of ice in your mouth, or use a saliva substitute. However, if your mouth continues to feel dry for more than 2 weeks, check with your medical doctor or dentist. Continuing dryness of the mouth may increase the chance of dental disease, including tooth decay, gum disease, and fungus infections.

For patients taking *scopolamine:*
- This medicine will add to the effects of alcohol and other CNS depressants (medicines that slow down the nervous system, possibly causing drowsiness). Some ex-

amples of CNS depressants are antihistamines or medicine for hay fever, other allergies, or colds; sedatives, tranquilizers, or sleeping medicine; prescription pain medicine or narcotics; barbiturates; medicine for seizures; muscle relaxants; or anesthetics, including some dental anesthetics. *Check with your doctor before taking any of the above while you are using this medicine.*

For patients *taking any of these medicines by mouth:*
- Do not take this medicine within 2 or 3 hours of taking antacids or medicine for diarrhea. Taking antacids or antidiarrhea medicines and this medicine too close together may prevent this medicine from working properly.

Side Effects of This Medicine

Along with its needed effects, a medicine may cause some unwanted effects. Although not all of these side effects may occur, if they do occur they may need medical attention.

Check with your doctor as soon as possible if any of the following side effects occur:

Rare
Confusion (especially in the elderly); dizziness, lightheadedness (continuing), or fainting; eye pain; skin rash or hives

Incidence not known
Cough; difficulty swallowing; fast irregular, pounding, or racing heartbeat or pulse; fever; hives or welts; hoarseness; irritation; itching skin; joint pain, stiffness, or swelling; puffiness or swelling of the eyelids or around the eyes, face, lips, or tongue; redness of skin; shortness of breath; skin rash; tightness in chest; troubled breathing or swallowing; wheezing

Symptoms of overdose
Blurred vision (continuing) or changes in near vision; clumsiness or unsteadiness; confusion; convulsions (seizures); difficulty in breathing, muscle weakness (severe), or tiredness (severe); dizziness; drowsiness (severe); dryness of mouth, nose, or throat (severe); fast heartbeat; fever; hallucinations (seeing, hearing, or feeling things that are not there); slurred speech; unusual excitement, nervousness, restlessness, or irritability; unusual warmth, dryness, and flushing of skin

Other side effects may occur that usually do not need medical attention. These side effects may go away during treatment as your body adjusts to the medicine. However, check with your doctor if any of the following side effects continue or are bothersome:

More common
Constipation (less common with hyoscyamine); decreased sweating; dryness of mouth, nose, throat, or skin

Less common or rare
Bloated feeling; blurred vision; decreased flow of breast milk; difficult urination; difficulty in swallowing; drowsiness (more common with high doses of any of these medicines and with usual doses of scopolamine when given by mouth or by injection); false sense of wellbeing (for scopolamine only); headache; increased sensitivity of eyes to light; lightheadedness (with injection); loss of memory; nausea or vomiting; redness or

other signs of irritation at place of injection; trouble in sleeping (for scopolamine only); unusual tiredness or weakness

Incidence not known
Decreased interest in sexual intercourse; inability to have or keep an erection; loss in sexual ability, desire, drive, or performance; loss of taste

For patients using *scopolamine:*
- After you stop using scopolamine, your body may need time to adjust. The length of time this takes depends on the amount of scopolamine you were using and how long you used it. During this period of time check with your doctor if you notice any of the following side effects: Anxiety; irritability; nightmares; trouble in sleeping

For patients using the *transdermal disk* of *scopolamine:*
- While using the disk or even after removing it, your eyes may become more sensitive to light than usual. You may also notice the pupil in one eye is larger than the other. Check with your doctor if this side effect continues or is bothersome

Other side effects not listed above may also occur in some patients. If you notice any other effects, check with your doctor.

Additional Information

Once a medicine has been approved for marketing for a certain use, experience may show that it is also useful for other medical problems. Although these uses are not included in product labeling, anticholinergics/antispasmodics are used in certain patients with the following medical conditions:

- Diarrhea
- Excessive watering of mouth
- Asthma treatment (atropine)

Other than the above information, there is no additional information relating to proper use, precautions, or side effects for these uses.

ANTICOAGULANTS (Systemic)

Some commonly used brand names are:

In the U.S.—
Coumadin (4)
Miradon (2)

In Canada—
Coumadin (4)
Sintrom (1)
Warfilone (4)

This information applies to the following medicines:
1. Acenocoumarol (a-see-no-COOM-a-rol)
2. Anisindione (an-iss-in-DYE-one)
3. Dicumarol (dye-KOO-ma-role)
4. Warfarin (WAR-far-in)

Category

- **Anticoagulant**—Acenocoumarol; Anisindione; Dicumarol; Warfarin

Description

Anticoagulants decrease the clotting ability of the blood and therefore help to prevent harmful clots from forming in the blood vessels. These medicines are sometimes called blood thinners, although they do not actually thin the blood. They also will not dissolve clots that already have formed, but they may prevent the clots from becoming larger and causing more serious problems. They are often used as treatment for certain blood vessel, heart, and lung conditions.

In order for an anticoagulant to help you without causing serious bleeding, it must be used properly and all of the precautions concerning its use must be followed exactly. Be sure that you have discussed the use of this medicine with your doctor. It is very important that you understand all of your doctor's orders and that you are willing and able to follow them exactly.

Anticoagulants are available only with your doctor's prescription, in the following dosage forms:

Oral
- Acenocoumarol
  ◦ Tablets
- Anisindione
  ◦ Tablets
- Dicumarol
  ◦ Tablets
- Warfarin
  ◦ Tablets

Parenteral
- Warfarin
  ◦ Injection

Before Using This Medicine

In deciding to use a medicine, the risks of taking the medicine must be weighed against the good it will do. This is a decision you and your doctor will make. For anticoagulants, the following should be considered:

Allergies—Tell your doctor if you have ever had any unusual or allergic reaction to an anticoagulant. Also tell your health care professional if you are allergic to any other substances, such as foods, preservatives, or dyes.

Pregnancy—Anticoagulants may cause birth defects. They may also cause other problems affecting the physical or mental growth of the fetus or newborn baby. In addition, use of this medicine during the last 6 months of pregnancy may increase the chance of severe, possibly fatal, bleeding in the fetus. If taken during the last few weeks of pregnancy, anticoagulants may cause severe bleeding in both the fetus and the mother before or during delivery and in the newborn infant.

Do not begin taking this medicine during pregnancy, and do not become pregnant while taking it, unless you have first discussed the possible effects of this medicine with your doctor. Also, if you suspect that you may be pregnant and you are already taking an anticoagulant, check with your doctor at once. Your doctor may suggest that you take a different anticoagulant that is less likely to harm the fetus or the newborn infant during all or part of your pregnancy. Anticoagulants may also cause severe bleeding in the mother if taken soon after the baby is born.

Breast-feeding—Warfarin is not likely to cause problems in nursing babies. Other anticoagulants may pass into the breast milk. A blood test can be done to see if unwanted effects are occurring in the nursing baby. If necessary, another medicine that will overcome any unwanted effects of the anticoagulant can be given to the baby.

Children—Very young babies may be especially sensitive to the effects of anticoagulants. This may increase the chance of bleeding during treatment.

Older adults—Elderly people are especially sensitive to the effects of anticoagulants. This may increase the chance of bleeding during treatment.

Other medicines—Although certain medicines should not be used together at all, in other cases two different medicines may be used together even if an interaction might occur. In these cases, your doctor may want to change the dose, or other precautions may be necessary. *Many different medicines can affect the way anticoagulants work in your body.* Therefore, it is very important that your health care professional knows if you are taking *any* other prescription or nonprescription (over-the-counter [OTC]) medicine, especially:

- Amiodarone (e.g., Cordarone) or
- Cimetidine (e.g., Tagamet) or
- Metronidazole (e.g., Flagyl) or
- Omeprazole (e.g., Prilosec) or
- Zafirlukast (e.g., Accolate)—Effects of anticoagulants may be increased because of slower removal from the body
- Anabolic steroids (nandrolone [e.g., Anabolin], oxandrolone [e.g., Anavar], oxymetholone [e.g., Anadrol], stanozolol [e.g., Winstrol]) or
- Androgens (male hormones) or
- Antifungals, azole (e.g., Diflucan) or
- Antithyroid agents (medicine for overactive thyroid) or
- Aspirin or other salicylates, including bismuth subsalicylate (e.g., Pepto-Bismol) or
- Cephalosporins (medicine for infection) or
- Cinchophen or
- Clofibrate (e.g., Abitrate, Atromid-S) or
- Danazol (e.g., Danocrine) or
- Dextrothyroxine or
- Diflunisal or
- Disulfiram (e.g., Antabuse) or
- Fluvoxamine (e.g., Luvox) or
- Inflammation or pain medicine (except narcotics) or
- Lepirudin (e.g., Refludan) or
- Medications causing low platelet count or
- Paroxetine (e.g., Paxil) or
- Propafenone (e.g., Rythmol) or
- Quinidine (e.g., Quinidex) or
- Sertraline (e.g., Zoloft) or
- Sulfapyridine or
- Sulfasalazine (e.g., Azulfidine) or
- Thyroid hormones or

- Ticlopidine (e.g., Ticlid) or
- Zileuton (e.g., Zyflo)—These medications may increase the effects of anticoagulants and may increase the chance of bleeding
- Carbenicillin by injection (e.g., Geopen) or
- Dipyridamole (e.g., Persantine) or
- Divalproex (e.g., Depakote) or
- Moxalactam (e.g., Moxam) or
- Pentoxifylline (e.g., Trantal) or
- Plicamycin (e.g., Mithracin) or
- Sulfinpyrazone (e.g., Anturane) or
- Thrombolytic agents (medicine for blood clots) or
- Ticarcillin (e.g., Ticar) or
- Valproic acid (e.g., Depakene)—Using any of these medicines together with anticoagulants may increase the chance of bleeding
- Alcohol (with chronic use) or
- Barbiturates or
- Carbamazepine (e.g., Tegretol) or
- Corticosteroids (cortisone-like medicine) or
- Glutethimide (e.g., Doriden) or
- Griseofulvin (e.g., Fulvicin) or
- Phenylbutazone (e.g., Butazolidin) or
- Phenytoin (e.g., Dilantin) or
- Primidone (e.g., Mysoline) or
- Rifampin (e.g., Rifadin)—Effects of anticoagulants may be decreased because of faster removal from the body
- Vitamin K (e.g., AquaMEPHYTON)—Vitamin K helps produce some important blood clotting factors and may decrease the effects of anticoagulants if used at the same time

Other medical problems—The presence of other medical problems may affect the use of anticoagulants. *Many medical problems and treatments will affect the way your body responds to this medicine.* Make sure you tell your doctor if you have *any* other medical problems, or if you have recently had any of the following conditions or medical procedures, especially:

- Aneurysm (swelling in a blood vessel) especially in the head or chest or
- Bleeding in the brain or
- Blood disorders or diseases, especially thrombocytopenia (low platelet count), polycythemia (high red blood cell count), or leukemia or
- Bruising, excessive or
- Cancer of the internal organs, especially of the abdomen or
- Childbirth, recent or
- Diabetes mellitus (sugar diabetes) or
- Diverticulitis or
- Falls or blows to the body or head or
- Heart infection or
- Hemophilia or other bleeding problems or
- Hypertension (high blood pressure) or

- Inflammation of blood vessels or
- Intestinal problems, especially conditions that may affect the absorption of food or vitamins or
- Liver disease or
- Pregnancy, terminated or
- Spinal anesthetics or spinal puncture or
- Surgery, major, especially of the head or eye, or dental surgery or
- Toxemia of pregnancy or
- Ulcers, active, of the stomach, lung, or urinary tract or
- Vitamin K deficiency or
- Wounds, open, surgical or from an ulcer—These conditions may increase the chance of bleeding

In addition, it is important that you tell your doctor if you are now being treated by any other medical doctor or dentist.

Proper Use of This Medicine

Take this medicine only as directed by your doctor. Do not take more or less of it, do not take it more often, and do not take it for a longer time than your doctor ordered. This is especially important for elderly patients, who are especially sensitive to the effects of anticoagulants. Also, it is best if you take this medicine at the same time each day.

Your doctor or health care professional should check your progress at regular visits. A blood test must be taken regularly to see how fast your blood is clotting. This will help your doctor decide on the proper amount of anticoagulant you should be taking each day. Some patients may be able to test their blood at home; discuss with your doctor whether or not this is possible for you.

Dosing—The dose of these medicines will be different for different patients. *Follow your doctor's orders or the directions on the label.* The following information includes only the average doses of these medicines. *If your dose is different, do not change it* unless your doctor tells you to do so.

For acenocoumarol
- For *oral* dosage form (tablets):
  - For preventing or treating harmful blood clots:
    - Adults—The usual dose is 1 to 10 milligrams (mg) per day, adjusted according to blood tests.
    - Children—Dose must be determined by your doctor.

For anisindione
- For *oral* dosage form (tablets):
  - For preventing or treating harmful blood clots:
    - Adults—The usual dose is 25 to 250 milligrams (mg) per day, adjusted according to blood tests.
    - Children—Dose must be determined by your doctor.

For dicumarol
- For *oral* dosage form (tablets):
  - For preventing or treating harmful blood clots:
    - Adults—The usual dose is 25 to 200 milligrams (mg) per day, adjusted according to blood tests.
    - Children—Dose must be determined by your doctor.

For warfarin
- For *oral* dosage form (tablets):
  - For preventing or treating harmful blood clots:
    - Adults—The starting dose is usually 2 to 5 milligrams (mg) per day for two to four days. Then, your dose may be adjusted, depending on your condition and results of routine blood tests.
    - Children—Dose must be determined by your doctor.

- For *injection* dosage form:
  - For preventing or treating harmful blood clots:
    - Adults—The starting dose is usually 2 to 5 milligrams (mg) per day for two to four days. Then, your dose may be adjusted, depending on your condition and results of routine blood tests.
    - Children—Dose must be determined by your doctor.

Missed dose—If you miss a dose of this medicine, take it as soon as possible. Then go back to your regular dosing schedule. If you do not remember until the next day, do not take the missed dose at all and do not double the next one. *Doubling the dose may cause bleeding.* Instead, go back to your regular dosing schedule. It is recommended that you keep a record of each dose as you take it to avoid mistakes. Also, be sure to give your doctor a record of any doses you miss. If you have any questions about this, check with your doctor.

Storage—To store this medicine:
- Keep out of the reach of children.
- Store away from heat and direct light.
- Do not store this medicine in the bathroom, near the kitchen sink, or in other damp places. Heat or moisture may cause the medicine to break down.
- Do not keep outdated medicine or medicine no longer needed. Be sure that any discarded medicine is out of the reach of children.

Precautions While Using This Medicine

Tell all medical doctors, dentists, and pharmacists you go to that you are taking this medicine.

Check with your doctor right away if you notice any unusual bleeding or bruising.

Check with your health care professional before you start or stop taking any other medicine, or change the amount you are taking. This includes any nonprescription (over-the-counter [OTC]) medicine, even aspirin or acetaminophen. Many medicines change the way this medicine affects your body. You may not be able to take the other medicine, or the dose of your anticoagulant may need to be changed.

It is important that you carry identification stating that you are using this medicine. If you have any questions about what kind of identification to carry, check with your health care professional.

While you are taking this medicine, it is very important that you avoid sports and activities that may cause you to be injured. Report to your doctor any falls, blows to the body or head, or other injuries, since serious internal bleeding may occur without your knowing about it.

Be careful to avoid cutting yourself. This includes taking special care in brushing your teeth and in shaving. Use a soft toothbrush and floss gently. Also, it is best to use an electric shaver rather than a blade.

Drinking too much alcohol may change the way this anticoagulant affects your body. You should not drink regularly on a daily basis or take more than 1 or 2 drinks at any time. If you have any questions about this, check with your doctor.

The foods that you eat may also affect the way this medicine affects your body. Eat a normal, balanced diet while you are taking this medicine. *Do not go on a reducing diet, make other changes in your eating habits, start taking vitamins, or begin using other nutrition supplements unless you have first checked with your health care professional.* Also, check with your doctor if you are unable to eat for several days or if you have continuing stomach upset, diarrhea, or fever. These precautions are important because the effects of the anticoagulant depend on the amount of vitamin K in your body. Therefore, it is best to have the same amount of vitamin K in your body every day. Some multiple vitamins and some nutrition supplements contain vitamin K. Vitamin K is also present in green, leafy vegetables (such as broccoli, cabbage, collard greens, kale, lettuce, and spinach) and some vegetable oils. It is especially important that you do not make large changes in the amounts of these foods that you eat every day while you are taking an anticoagulant.

Check with your doctor if you are unable to eat for several days or if you have continuing stomach upset, diarrhea, or fever. This could decrease the amount of vitamin K that gets into your body and could affect this medicine.

Be careful if the weather is very hot for several days. This could increase the effects of the medicine.

After you stop taking this medicine, your body will need time to recover before your blood clotting ability returns to normal. Your health care professional can tell you how long this will take depending on which anticoagulant you were taking. *Use the same caution during this period of time as you did while you were taking the anticoagulant.*

Side Effects

Along with its needed effects, a medicine may cause some unwanted effects. Although not all of these side effects may occur, if they do occur they may need medical attention.

Since many things can affect the way your body reacts to this medicine, you should always watch for signs of unusual bleeding. Unusual bleeding may mean that your body is getting more medicine than it needs. *Check with your doctor immediately if any of the following signs of bleeding or overdose occur:*
Signs and symptoms of bleeding inside the body—dose-related

Abdominal or stomach pain or swelling; back pain or backaches; black, tarry stools; bleeding in eye; blood in stools; blood in vomit or vomit that looks like coffee grounds; blood in urine; blurred vision; chest pain; confusion; constipation; coughing up blood; diarrhea (sudden and severe); dizziness or fainting; headache (continuing or severe); joint pain, stiffness, or swelling; loss of appetite; nausea and vomiting (severe); nervousness; numbness or tingling of hands, feet, or face; paralysis; shortness of breath; weakness (sudden); Bleeding from gums when brushing teeth; blood in urine; nosebleeds; pinpoint red spots on skin; unusual bleeding or bruising; unusually heavy bleeding or oozing from cuts or wounds; unusually heavy or un-expected menstrual bleeding

Also, check with your doctor as soon as possible if any of the following side effects occur:

Less common
> Cough or hoarseness; fever or chills; lower back or side pain; painful or difficult urination; skin rash, hives, or itching

Rare
> Blisters or itching on skin; blue or purple toes; dark urine; pain in toes; painful red sores on skin, especially on thighs, breasts, penis, or buttocks; sores, ulcers, or white spots in mouth or throat; sudden increase or de-crease in amount of urine; swelling of face, feet, and/or lower legs; trouble in breathing; yellow eyes or skin

Other side effects may occur that usually do not need medical attention. These side effects may go away during treatment as your body adjusts to the medicine. However, check with your doctor if any of the following side effects continue or are bothersome:

Less common or rare
> Bloated stomach or gas (with dicumarol); cold intoler-ance; diarrhea (more common with dicumarol); loss of appetite; nausea or vomiting (more common with di-cumarol); stomach cramps or pain

These medicines sometimes cause temporary loss of hair on the scalp.

Depending on your diet, *anisindione* may cause your urine to turn orange. Since it may be hard to tell the difference between blood in the urine and this normal color change, check with your doctor if you notice any color change in your urine.

Other side effects not listed above may also occur in some patients. If you notice any other effects, check with your doctor.

ANTICONVULSANTS, HYDANTOIN (Systemic)

Some commonly used brand names are:

In the U.S.—

Cerebyx (2)	Dilantin Kapseals (4)
Dilantin (4)	Mesantoin (3)
Dilantin-125 (4)	Peganone (1)
Dilantin Infatabs (4)	Phenytek (4)

In Canada—

Cerebyx (2)	Dilantin-125 (4)
Dilantin (4)	Dilantin Infatabs (4)
Dilantin-30 (4)	

This information applies to the following medicines:

1. Ethotoin (ETH-oh-toyn)
2. Fosphenytoin (fos-FEN-i-toyn)
3. Mephenytoin (me-FEN-i-toyn)
4. Phenytoin (FEN-i-toyn)

Category

- **Antiarrhythmic**—Phenytoin
- **Anticonvulsant**—Ethotoin; Fosphenytoin; Mepheny-toin; Phenytoin

- **Antineuralgic, trigeminal neuralgia**—Phenytoin
- **Skeletal muscle relaxant**—Phenytoin

Description

Hydantoin anticonvulsants (hye-DAN-toyn an-tye-kon-VUL-sants) are used most often to control certain convulsions or seizures in the treatment of epilepsy. Phenytoin also may be used for other conditions as determined by your doctor.

In seizure disorders, these medicines act on the central ner-vous system (CNS) to reduce the number and severity of sei-zures. Hydantoin anticonvulsants may also produce some unwanted effects. These depend on the patient's individual condition, the amount of medicine taken, and how long it has been taken. It is important that you know what the side effects are and when to call your doctor if they occur.

Hydantoin anticonvulsants are available only with your doctor's prescription, in the following dosage forms:

Oral
- Ethotoin
  - Tablets
- Mephenytoin
  - Tablets
- Phenytoin
  - Extended capsules
  - Prompt capsules
  - Oral suspension
  - Chewable tablets

Parenteral
- Fosphenytoin
  - Injection
- Phenytoin
  - Injection

Because fosphenytoin is converted to phenytoin in your body, it has the same effects as those listed for phenytoin in the following sections.

Before Using This Medicine

In deciding to use a medicine, the risks of taking the medicine must be weighed against the good it will do. This is a decision you and your doctor will make. For hydantoin anticonvulsants, the following should be considered:

Allergies—Tell your doctor if you have ever had any un-usual or allergic reaction to any hydantoin anticonvulsant medicine. Also tell your health care professional if you are allergic to any other substance, such as foods, preservatives, or dyes.

Pregnancy—Although most mothers who take medicine for seizure control deliver normal babies, there have been re-ports of increased birth defects when these medicines were used during pregnancy. It is not definitely known if any of these medicines are the cause of such problems.

Also, pregnancy may cause a change in the way hydantoin anticonvulsants are absorbed in your body. You may have more seizures, even though you are taking your medicine regularly. Your doctor may need to increase the anticonvul-sant dose during your pregnancy.

In addition, when taken during pregnancy, this medicine may cause a bleeding problem in the mother during delivery and in the newborn. This may be prevented by giving vitamin K to the mother during delivery, and to the baby immediately after birth.

Breast-feeding—Ethotoin and phenytoin pass into the breast milk in small amounts. It is not known whether mephenytoin passes into breast milk. Be sure you have discussed the risks and benefits of the medicine with your doctor.

Children—Some side effects, especially bleeding, tender, or enlarged gums and enlarged facial features, are more likely to occur in children and young adults. Also, unusual and excessive hair growth may occur, which is more noticeable in young girls. In addition, some children may not do as well in school after using high doses of this medicine for a long time.

Older adults—Some medicines may affect older patients differently than they do younger patients. Overdose is more likely to occur in elderly patients and in patients with liver disease.

Other medicines—Although certain medicines should not be used together at all, in other cases two different medicines may be used together even if an interaction might occur. In these cases, your doctor may want to change the dose, or other precautions may be necessary. When you are taking or receiving hydantoin anticonvulsants, it is especially important that your health care professional know if you are taking any of the following:

- Alcohol or
- Central nervous system (CNS) depressants (medicine that causes drowsiness)—Long-term use of alcohol may decrease the blood levels of hydantoin anticonvulsants, resulting in decreased effects; use of hydantoin anticonvulsants in cases where a large amount of alcohol is consumed may increase the blood levels of the hydantoin, resulting in an increased risk of side effects
- Amiodarone (e.g., Cordarone)—Use with phenytoin and possibly with other hydantoin anticonvulsants may increase blood levels of the hydantoin, resulting in an increase in serious side effects
- Antacids or
- Medicine containing calcium—Use of antacids or calcium supplements may decrease the absorption of phenytoin; doses of antacids and phenytoin or calcium supplements and phenytoin should be taken 2 to 3 hours apart
- Anticoagulants (blood thinners) or
- Chloramphenicol (e.g., Chloromycetin) or
- Cimetidine (e.g., Tagamet) or
- Disulfiram (e.g., Antabuse) (medicine for alcoholism) or
- Isoniazid (INH) (e.g., Nydrazid) or
- Fluconazole (e.g., Diflucan) or
- Fluoxetine (e.g., Prozac) or
- Itraconazole (e.g., Sporanox) or
- Ketoconazole (e.g., Nizoral) or
- Miconazole (e.g., Monistat) or
- Phenylbutazone (e.g., Butazolidin) or
- Sulfonamides (sulfa drugs)—Blood levels of hydantoin anticonvulsants may be increased, increasing the risk of serious side effects; hydantoin anticonvulsants may increase the effects of the anticoagulants at first, but with continued use may decrease the effects of these medicines

- Corticosteroids (cortisone-like medicines) or
- Estrogens (female hormones) or
- Oral contraceptives (birth-control pills) containing estrogens or progestins or
- Progestin injection contraceptives (e.g., Depo-Provera) or
- Progestin implant contraceptives (e.g., Norplant)—Hydantoin anticonvulsants may decrease the effects of these medicines; use of hydantoin anticonvulsants with estrogen- or progestin-containing contraceptives may result in breakthrough bleeding and contraceptive failure; additional birth control measures may be needed to decrease the risk of pregnancy
- Diazoxide (e.g., Proglycem)—Use with hydantoin anticonvulsants may decrease the effects of both medicines; therefore, these medicines should not be taken together
- Felbamate (e.g., Felbatrol)—Blood levels of hydantoin anticonvulsants may be increased, and blood levels of felbamate may be decreased. Your doctor may need to adjust your dosage
- Lidocaine—Risk of slow heartbeat may be increased. Other effects of lidocaine may be decreased because hydantoin anticonvulsants may cause it to be removed from the body more quickly
- Methadone (e.g., Dolophine, Methadose)—Long-term use of phenytoin may bring on withdrawal symptoms in patients being treated for drug dependence
- Phenacemide (e.g., Phenurone)—Use with hydantoin anticonvulsants may increase the risk of serious side effects
- Rifampin (e.g., Rifadin)—Use with phenytoin may decrease the effects of phenytoin; your doctor may need to adjust your dosage
- Streptozocin (e.g., Zanosar)—Phenytoin may decrease the effects of streptozocin; therefore, these medicines should not be used together
- Sucralfate (e.g., Carafate)—Use of sucralfate may decrease the absorption of hydantoin anticonvulsants
- Theophylline (e.g., Theo-Dur)—Hydantoin anticonvulsants may make this medicine less effective
- Valproic acid (e.g., Depakene, Depakote)—Use with phenytoin, and possibly other hydantoin anticonvulsants, may increase seizure frequency and increase the risk of serious side effects affecting the liver, especially in infants

Other medical problems—The presence of other medical problems may affect the use of hydantoin anticonvulsants. Make sure you tell your doctor if you have any other medical problems, especially:

- Alcohol abuse—Blood levels of phenytoin may be decreased, decreasing its effects
- Blood disease—Risk of serious infections rarely may be increased by hydantoin anticonvulsants
- Diabetes mellitus (sugar diabetes) or
- Porphyria or
- Systemic lupus erythematosus—Hydantoin anticonvulsants may make the condition worse

- Fever above 101 °F for longer than 24 hours—Blood levels of hydantoin anticonvulsants may be decreased, decreasing the medicine's effects
- Heart disease—Administration of phenytoin by injection may change the rhythm of the heart
- Kidney disease or
- Liver disease—Blood levels of hydantoin anticonvulsants may be increased, leading to an increase in serious side effects
- Thyroid disease—Blood levels of thyroid hormones may be decreased

Proper Use of This Medicine

For patients taking the *liquid form* of this medicine:

- Shake the bottle well before using.
- Use a specially marked measuring spoon, a plastic syringe, or a small measuring cup to measure each dose accurately. The average household teaspoon may not hold the right amount of liquid.

For patients taking the *chewable tablet form* of this medicine:

- Tablets may be chewed or crushed before they are swallowed, or may be swallowed whole.

For patients taking the *capsule form* of this medicine:

- Swallow the capsule whole.

If this medicine upsets your stomach, take it with food, unless otherwise directed by your doctor. The medicine should always be taken at the same time in relation to meals to make sure that it is absorbed in the same way.

To control your medical problem, *take this medicine every day* exactly as ordered by your doctor. Do not take more or less of it than your doctor ordered. To help you remember to take the medicine at the correct times, try to get into the habit of taking it at the same time each day.

Dosing—The dose of hydantoin anticonvulsants will be different for different patients. *Follow your doctor's orders or the directions on the label.* The following information includes only the average doses of ethotoin, fosphenytoin, mephenytoin, and phenytoin. *If your dose is different, do not change it* unless your doctor tells you to do so.

The number of capsules or tablets or teaspoonfuls of suspension that you take or the number of injections you receive depends on the strength of the medicine. Also, *the number of doses you take each day, the time allowed between doses, and the length of time you take the medicine depend on the medical problem for which you are using a hydantoin anticonvulsant.*

For ethotoin
- For *oral* dosage form (tablets):
  - As an anticonvulsant:
    - Adults and teenagers—To start, 125 to 250 milligrams (mg) four to six times a day. Your doctor may increase your dose gradually over several days if needed. However, the dose is usually not more than 3000 mg a day.
    - Children—To start, up to 750 mg a day, based on the age and weight of the child. The doctor may increase the dose gradually if needed.

For fosphenytoin
- For *injection* dosage form:
  - As an anticonvulsant:
    - Adults and children—Dose is based on the illness being treated, and the body weight or size of the patient. The medicine is injected into a vein or muscle.

For mephenytoin
- For *oral* dosage form (tablets):
  - As an anticonvulsant:
    - Adults and teenagers—To start, 50 to 100 milligrams (mg) once a day. Your doctor may increase your dose by 50 to 100 mg a day at weekly intervals if needed. However, the dose is usually not more than 1200 mg a day.
    - Children—To start, 25 to 50 mg once a day. The doctor may increase the dose by 25 to 50 mg a day at weekly intervals if needed. However, the dose is usually not more than 400 mg a day.

For phenytoin
- For *oral* dosage forms (capsules, chewable tablets, or suspension):
  - As an anticonvulsant:
    - Adults and teenagers—To start, 100 to 125 milligrams (mg) three times a day. Your doctor may adjust your dose at intervals of seven to ten days if needed.
    - Children—Dose is based on body weight or body surface area. The usual dose is 5 mg of phenytoin per kilogram (kg) (2.3 mg per pound) of body weight to start. The doctor may adjust the dose if needed.
    - Older adults—Dose is based on body weight. The usual dose is 3 mg per kg (1.4 mg per pound) of body weight. The doctor may need to adjust the dose based on your response to the medicine.
- For *injection* dosage form:
  - As an anticonvulsant:
    - Adults and children—Dose is based on the illness being treated, and the body weight or size of the patient. The medicine is usually injected into a vein.

Missed dose—*If you miss a dose of this medicine* and your dosing schedule is:

- One dose a day—Take the missed dose as soon as possible. However, if you do not remember the missed dose until the next day, skip it and go back to your regular dosing schedule. Do not double doses.
- More than one dose a day—Take the missed dose as soon as possible. However, if it is within 4 hours of your next dose, skip the missed dose and go back to your regular dosing schedule. Do not double doses.

If you miss doses for 2 or more days in a row, check with your doctor.

Storage—To store this medicine:

- Keep out of the reach of children.
- Store away from heat and direct light.
- Do not store in the bathroom, near the kitchen sink, or in other damp places. Heat or moisture may cause the medicine to break down.

- Keep the liquid form of this medicine from freezing. Do not refrigerate.
- Do not keep outdated medicine or medicine no longer needed. Be sure any discarded medicine is out of the reach of children.

Precautions While Using This Medicine

Your doctor should check your progress at regular visits, especially during the first few months of treatment with this medicine. During this time the amount of medicine you are taking may have to be changed often to meet your individual needs.

Do not start or stop taking any other medicine without your doctor's advice. Other medicines may affect the way this medicine works.

This medicine will add to the effects of alcohol and other CNS depressants (medicines that may make you drowsy or less alert). Some examples of CNS depressants are antihistamines or medicine for hay fever, other allergies, or colds; sedatives, tranquilizers, or sleeping medicine; prescription pain medicine or narcotics; barbiturates; other medicine for seizures; muscle relaxants; or anesthetics, including some dental anesthetics. *Check with your doctor before taking any of the above while you are using this medicine.*

Do not take this medicine within 2 to 3 hours of taking antacids or medicine for diarrhea. Taking these medicines and hydantoin anticonvulsants too close together may make the hydantoins less effective.

Do not change brands or dosage forms of phenytoin without first checking with your doctor. Different products may not work the same way. If you refill your medicine and it looks different, check with your pharmacist.

If you have been taking this medicine regularly for several weeks or more, do not suddenly stop taking it. Your doctor may want you to reduce gradually the amount you are taking before stopping completely.

Your doctor may want you to carry a medical identification card or bracelet stating that you are taking this medicine.

For diabetic patients:
- This medicine may affect blood sugar levels. If you notice a change in the results of your blood or urine sugar tests or if you have any questions, check with your doctor.

Before you have any medical tests, tell the doctor in charge that you are taking this medicine. The results of some tests (including the dexamethasone, metyrapone, or Schilling tests, and certain thyroid function tests) may be affected by this medicine.

Before having any kind of surgery, dental treatment, or emergency treatment, tell the medical doctor or dentist in charge that you are taking this medicine. Taking hydantoin anticonvulsants together with medicines that are used during surgery or dental or emergency treatments may cause increased side effects.

This medicine may cause some people to become dizzy, lightheaded, drowsy, or less alert than they are normally. After you have taken this medicine for a while, this effect may not be so bothersome. However, *make sure you know how you react to this medicine before you drive, use machines, or do anything else that could be dangerous if you are dizzy or are not alert.*

Oral contraceptives (birth control pills) containing estrogen or progestin, contraceptive progestin injections (e.g., Depo-Provera), and implant contraceptive forms of progestin (e.g., Norplant) may not work properly if you take them while you are taking hydantoin anticonvulsants. Unplanned pregnancies may occur. You should use a different or additional means of birth control while you are taking hydantoin anticonvulsants. If you have any questions about this, check with your health care professional.

For patients taking *phenytoin* or *mephenytoin:*
- In some patients (usually younger patients), tenderness, swelling, or bleeding of the gums (gingival hyperplasia) may appear soon after phenytoin or mephenytoin treatment is started. To help prevent this, brush and floss your teeth carefully and regularly and massage your gums. Also, *see your dentist every 3 months to have your teeth cleaned. If you have any questions about how to take care of your teeth and gums, or if you notice any tenderness, swelling, or bleeding of your gums, check with your doctor or dentist.*

Side Effects

Along with its needed effects, a medicine may cause some unwanted effects. Although not all of these side effects may occur, if they do occur they may need medical attention.

Check with your doctor as soon as possible if any of the following side effects or signs of overdose occur:
More common
Bleeding, tender, or enlarged gums (rare with ethotoin); burning, tingling, pain, or itching, especially in the groin— following fosphenytoin injection; clumsiness or unsteadiness; confusion; continuous, uncontrolled back-and-forth and/or rolling eye movements— may be sign of overdose; swollen glands in neck or underarms; fever; muscle pain; skin rash or itching; slurred speech or stuttering— may be sign of overdose; sore throat; trembling— may be sign of overdose; unusual excitement, nervousness, or irritability

Rare
Bone malformations; burning pain at place of injection; chest discomfort; chills and fever; dark urine; dizziness; frequent breaking of bones; headache; joint pain; learning difficulties— in children taking high doses for a long time; light gray– colored stools; loss of appetite; nausea or vomiting; pain of penis on erection; restlessness or agitation; slowed growth; stomach pain (severe); troubled or quick, shallow breathing; uncontrolled jerking or twisting movements of hands, arms, or legs; uncontrolled movements of lips, tongue, or cheeks; unusual bleeding (such as nosebleeds) or bruising; unusual tiredness or weakness; weight loss (unusual); yellow eyes or skin

Rare (with long-term use of phenytoin)
Numbness, tingling, or pain in hands or feet

Symptoms of overdose
Blurred or double vision; clumsiness or unsteadiness (severe); confusion (severe); dizziness or drowsiness (severe); seizures; staggering walk; stuttering or slurred speech

Other side effects may occur that usually do not need medical attention. These side effects may go away during treatment

as your body adjusts to the medicine. However, check with your doctor if any of the following side effects continue or are bothersome:

More common
Constipation; dizziness (mild); drowsiness (mild)

Less common
Diarrhea (with ethotoin); enlargement of jaw; muscle twitching; swelling of breasts—in males; thickening of lips; trouble in sleeping; unusual and excessive hair growth on body and face (more common with phenytoin); widening of nose tip

Other side effects not listed above may also occur in some patients. If you notice any other effects, check with your doctor.

Additional Information

Once a medicine has been approved for marketing for a certain use, experience may show that it is also useful for other medical problems. Although these uses are not included in product labeling, phenytoin is used in certain patients with the following medical conditions:

- Cardiac arrhythmias (changes in your heart rhythm) caused by digitalis medicine
- Myotonia congenita or
- Myotonic muscular dystrophy or
- Neuromyotonia (certain muscle disorders)
- Paroxysmal choreoathetosis (certain movement disorders)
- Tricyclic antidepressant poisoning
- Trigeminal neuralgia (tic douloureux)

Other than the above information, there is no additional information relating to proper use, precautions, or side effects for these uses.

ANTICONVULSANTS, SUCCINIMIDE (Systemic)

Some commonly used brand names are:

In the U.S.—
Celontin (2)
Zarontin (1)

In Canada—
Celontin (2)
Zarontin (1)

This information applies to the following medicines:

1. Ethosuximide (eth-oh-SUX-i-mide)
2. Methsuximide (meth-SUX-i-mide)

Category

- **Anticonvulsant**—Ethosuximide; Methsuximide

Description

Succinimide anticonvulsants are used to control certain seizures in the treatment of epilepsy. These medicines act on the central nervous system (CNS) to reduce the number and severity of seizures.

This medicine is available only with your doctor's prescription, in the following dosage forms:

Oral
- Ethosuximide
  - Capsules
  - Syrup
- Methsuximide
  - Capsules

Before Using This Medicine

In deciding to use a medicine, the risks of taking the medicine must be weighed against the good it will do. This is a decision you and your doctor will make. For succinimide anticonvulsants, the following should be considered:

Allergies—Tell your doctor if you have ever had any unusual or allergic reaction to anticonvulsant medicines. Also tell your health care professional if you are allergic to any other substances, such as foods, preservatives, or dyes.

Pregnancy—Although succinimide anticonvulsants have not been shown to cause problems in humans, there have been unproven reports of increased birth defects associated with the use of other anticonvulsant medicines.

Breast-feeding—Ethosuximide passes into breast milk. It is not known whether methsuximide passes into breast milk. However, these medicines have not been reported to cause problems in nursing babies.

Children—Succinimide anticonvulsants are not expected to cause different side effects or problems in children than they do in adults.

Older adults—Many medicines have not been studied specifically in older people. Therefore, it may not be known whether they work exactly the same way they do in younger adults. Although there is no specific information comparing use of succinimide anticonvulsants in the elderly to use in other age groups, they are not expected to cause different side effects or problems in older people than they do in younger adults.

Other medicines—Although certain medicines should not be used together at all, in other cases two different medicines may be used together even if an interaction might occur. In these cases, your doctor may want to change the dose, or other precautions may be necessary. When you are taking succinimide anticonvulsants, it is especially important that your health care professional know if you are taking any of the following:

- Central nervous system (CNS) depressants (medicines that cause drowsiness)—Using these medicines together may increase CNS depressant effects
- Haloperidol (e.g., Haldol)—A change in the pattern and/ or the frequency of seizures may occur; the dose of either medicine may need to be changed

Other medical problems—The presence of other medical problems may affect the use of succinimide anticonvulsants. Make sure you tell your doctor if you have any other medical problems, especially:

- Blood disease or
- Intermittent porphyria or
- Kidney disease (severe) or

• Liver disease—Succinimide anticonvulsants may make the condition worse

Proper Use of This Medicine

This medicine must be taken every day in regularly spaced doses as ordered by your doctor. Do not take more or less of it than your doctor ordered.

If this medicine upsets your stomach, take it with food or milk unless otherwise directed by your doctor.

Dosing—The dose of succinimide anticonvulsants will be different for different patients. *Follow your doctor's orders or the directions on the label.* The following information includes only the average doses of ethosuximide and methsuximide. *If your dose is different, do not change it* unless your doctor tells you to do so.

The number of capsules or teaspoonfuls of syrup that you take depends on the strength of the medicine. Also, *the number of doses you take each day, the time allowed between doses, and the length of time you take the medicine depend on the medical problem for which you are taking a succinimide anticonvulsant.*

For ethosuximide
• For *oral* dosage form (capsules or syrup):
  ○ As an anticonvulsant:
    ▪ Adults and children 6 years of age and over—To start, 250 milligrams (mg) twice a day. Your doctor may increase your dose gradually if needed. However, the dose is usually not more than 1500 mg a day.
    ▪ Children up to 6 years of age—To start, 250 mg once a day. Your doctor may increase your dose gradually if needed. However, the dose is usually not more than 1000 mg a day.

For methsuximide
• For *oral* dosage form (capsules):
  ○ As an anticonvulsant:
    ▪ Adults, teenagers, and children—To start, 300 milligrams (mg) once a day. Your doctor may increase your dose gradually if needed. However, the dose is usually not more than 1200 mg a day.

Missed dose—If you miss a dose of this medicine, take it as soon as possible. However, if it is within 4 hours of your next dose, skip the missed dose and go back to your regular dosing schedule. Do not double doses.

Storage—To store this medicine:
• Keep out of the reach of children.
• Store away from heat and direct light.
• Do not store the capsule form of this medicine in the bathroom, near the kitchen sink, or in other damp places. Heat or moisture may cause the medicine to break down.
• Keep the liquid form of this medicine from freezing. Do not refrigerate.
• Do not keep outdated medicine or medicine that is no longer needed. Be sure any discarded medicine is out of the reach of children.

Precautions While Using This Medicine

Your doctor should check your progress at regular visits, especially during the first few months of treatment with this medicine. During this time the amount of medicine you are taking may have to be changed often to meet your individual needs.

If you have been taking a succinimide anticonvulsant regularly, do not stop taking it without first checking with your doctor. Your doctor may want you to reduce gradually the amount you are taking before stopping completely. Stopping this medicine suddenly may cause seizures.

Do not start or stop taking any other medicine without your doctor's advice. Other medicines may affect the way this medicine works.

This medicine will add to the effects of alcohol and other CNS depressants (medicines that slow down the nervous system, possibly causing drowsiness). Some examples of CNS depressants are antihistamines or medicine for hay fever, other allergies, or colds; sedatives, tranquilizers, or sleeping medicine; prescription pain medicine or narcotics; barbiturates; medicine for seizures; muscle relaxants; or anesthetics, including some dental anesthetics. *Check with your doctor before taking any of the above while you are using this medicine.*

This medicine may cause some people to become drowsy or less alert than they are normally. *Make sure you know how you react to this medicine before you drive, use machines, or do anything else that could be dangerous if you are not alert.* After you have taken this medicine for a while, this effect may lessen.

Before having any kind of surgery, dental treatment, or emergency treatment, tell the medical doctor or dentist in charge that you are taking this medicine. Taking succinimide anticonvulsants together with medicines that are used during surgery or dental or emergency treatments may increase the CNS depressant effects.

Your doctor may want you to carry a medical identification card or bracelet stating that you are taking this medicine.

For patients taking *methsuximide:*
• Do not use capsules that are not full or in which the contents have melted, because they may not work properly.

Side Effects

Along with its needed effects, a medicine may cause some unwanted effects. Although not all of these side effects may occur, if they do occur they may need medical attention.

Check with your doctor as soon as possible if any of the following side effects occur:
More common
  Muscle pain; skin rash and itching; swollen glands; sore throat and fever
Less common
  Aggressiveness; difficulty in concentration; mental depression; nightmares
Rare
  Chills; increased chance of certain types of seizures; mood or mental changes; nosebleeds or other unusual bleeding or bruising; shortness of breath; sores, ulcers, or white spots on lips or in mouth; unusual tiredness or weakness; wheezing, tightness in chest, or troubled breathing

Symptoms of overdose
Drowsiness (severe); nausea and vomiting (severe); troubled breathing

Other side effects may occur that usually do not need medical attention. These side effects may go away during treatment as your body adjusts to the medicine. However, check with your doctor if any of the following side effects continue or are bothersome:

More common
Clumsiness or unsteadiness; dizziness; drowsiness; headache; hiccups; loss of appetite; nausea or vomiting; stomach cramps

Less common
Irritability

Other side effects not listed above may also occur in some patients. If you notice any other effects, check with your doctor.

ANTIDEPRESSANTS, MONOAMINE OXIDASE INHIBITOR (MAO) (Systemic)

Some commonly used brand names are:

In the U.S.—
Nardil (2)
Parnate (3)
Marplan (1)

In Canada—
Nardil (2)
Parnate (3)

This information applies to the following medicines:

1. Isocarboxazid (eye-so-car-BOX-a-zid)
2. Phenelzine (FEN-el-zeen)
3. Tranylcypromine (tran-ill-SIP-roe-meen)

Category

- **Antidepressant**—Isocarboxazid; Phenelzine; Tranylcypromine
- **Antipanic agent**—Phenelzine; Tranylcypromine
- **Headache, tension, prophylactic**—Phenelzine; Tranylcypromine
- **Vascular headache prophylactic**—Phenelzine; Tranylcypromine

---

Description

Monoamine oxidase (MAO) inhibitors are used to relieve certain types of mental depression. They work by blocking the action of a chemical substance known as monoamine oxidase (MAO) in the nervous system.

Although these medicines are very effective for certain patients, they may also cause some unwanted reactions if not taken in the right way. It is very important to avoid certain foods, beverages, and medicines while you are being treated with an MAO inhibitor. Your health care professional will help you obtain a list to carry in your wallet or purse as a reminder of which products you should avoid.

MAO inhibitors are available only with your doctor's prescription, in the following dosage forms:

Oral
- Isocarboxazid
  - Tablets
- Phenelzine
  - Tablets
- Tranylcypromine
  - Tablets

Before Using This Medicine

In deciding to use a medicine, the risks of taking the medicine must be weighed against the good it will do. This is a decision you and your doctor will make. For monoamine oxidase (MAO) inhibitors, the following should be considered:

Allergies—Tell your doctor if you have ever had any unusual or allergic reaction to any MAO inhibitor. Also tell your health care professional if you are allergic to any other substances, such as foods, preservatives, or dyes.

Diet—Dangerous reactions such as sudden high blood pressure may result when MAO inhibitors are taken with certain foods or drinks. The following foods should be avoided:

- Foods that have a high tyramine content (most common in foods that are aged or fermented to increase their flavor), such as cheeses; fava or broad bean pods; yeast or meat extracts; smoked or pickled meat, poultry, or fish; fermented sausage (bologna, pepperoni, salami, summer sausage) or other fermented meat; sauerkraut; or any overripe fruit. If a list of these foods and beverages is not given to you, ask your health care professional to provide one.
- Alcoholic beverages or alcohol-free or reduced-alcohol beer and wine.
- Large amounts of caffeine-containing food or beverages such as coffee, tea, cola, or chocolate.

Pregnancy—A limited study in pregnant women showed an increased risk of birth defects when these medicines were taken during the first 3 months of pregnancy. In animal studies, MAO inhibitors caused a slowing of growth and increased excitability in the newborn when very large doses were given to the mother during pregnancy.

Breast-feeding—Tranylcypromine passes into the breast milk; it is not known whether isocarboxazid or phenelzine passes into breast milk. Problems in nursing babies have not been reported.

Children—Antidepressants must be used with caution in children with depression. Studies have shown occurrences of children thinking about suicide or attempting suicide in clinical trials for this medicine. More study is needed to be sure antidepressants are safe and effective in children

Animal studies have shown that these medicines may slow growth in the young. Therefore, be sure to discuss with your doctor the use of these medicines in children.

Older adults—Dizziness or lightheadedness may be especially likely to occur in elderly patients, who are usually more sensitive than younger adults to these effects of MAO inhibitors.

Other medicines—Although certain medicines should not be used together at all, in other cases two different medicines may be used together even if an interaction might occur. In these cases, your doctor may want to change the dose, or other precautions may be necessary. When you are taking MAO inhibitors, it is especially important that your health care professional know if you are taking any of the following:

- Amphetamines or
- Antihypertensives (high blood pressure medicine) or
- Appetite suppressants (diet pills) or
- Cyclobenzaprine (e.g., Flexeril) or
- Fluoxetine (e.g., Prozac) or
- Levodopa (e.g., Dopar, Larodopa) or
- Maprotiline (e.g., Ludiomil) or
- Medicine for asthma or other breathing problems or
- Medicines for colds, sinus problems, or hay fever or other allergies (including nose drops or sprays) or
- Meperidine (e.g., Demerol) or
- Methylphenidate (e.g., Ritalin) or
- Monoamine oxidase (MAO) inhibitors, other, including furazolidone (e.g., Furoxone), procarbazine (e.g., Matulane), or selegiline (e.g., Eldepryl), or
- Paroxetine (e.g., Paxil), or
- Sertraline (e.g., Zoloft), or
- Tricyclic antidepressants (amitriptyline [e.g., Elavil], amoxapine [e.g., Asendin], clomipramine [e.g., Anafranil], desipramine [e.g., Pertofrane], doxepin [e.g., Sinequan], imipramine [e.g., Tofranil], nortriptyline [e.g., Aventyl], protriptyline [e.g., Vivactil], trimipramine [e.g., Surmontil])—Using these medicines while you are taking or within 2 weeks of taking MAO inhibitors may cause serious side effects such as sudden rise in body temperature, extremely high blood pressure, severe convulsions, and death; however, sometimes certain of these medicines may be used with MAO inhibitors under close supervision by your doctor
- Antidiabetics, oral (diabetes medicine you take by mouth) or
- Insulin—MAO inhibitors may change the amount of antidiabetic medicine you need to take
- Bupropion (e.g., Wellbutrin)—Using bupropion while you are taking or within 2 weeks of taking MAO inhibitors may cause serious side effects such as seizures
- Buspirone (e.g., BuSpar)—Use with MAO inhibitors may cause high blood pressure
- Carbamazepine (e.g., Tegretol)—Use with MAO inhibitors may increase seizures
- Central nervous system (CNS) depressants (medicines that cause drowsiness)—Using these medicines with MAO inhibitors may increase the CNS and other depressant effects
- Cocaine—Cocaine use by persons taking MAO inhibitors, including furazolidone and procarbazine, may cause a severe increase in blood pressure
- Dextromethorphan—Use with MAO inhibitors may cause excitement, high blood pressure, and fever
- Trazodone or
- Tryptophan used as a food supplement or a sleep aid— Use of these medicines by persons taking MAO inhibitors, including furazolidone and procarbazine, may

cause mental confusion, excitement, shivering, trouble in breathing, or fever

Other medical problems—The presence of other medical problems may affect the use of MAO inhibitors. Make sure you tell your doctor if you have any other medical problems, especially:

- Alcohol abuse—Drinking alcohol while you are taking an MAO inhibitor may cause serious side effects
- Angina (chest pain) or
- Headaches (severe or frequent)—These conditions may interfere with warning signs of serious side effects of MAO inhibitors
- Asthma or bronchitis—Some medicines used to treat these conditions may cause serious side effects when used while you are taking an MAO inhibitor
- Diabetes mellitus (sugar diabetes)—These medicines may change the amount of insulin or oral antidiabetic medication that you need
- Epilepsy—Seizures may occur more often
- Heart or blood vessel disease or
- Liver disease or
- Mental illness (or history of) or
- Parkinson's disease or
- Recent heart attack or stroke—MAO inhibitors may make the condition worse
- High blood pressure—Condition may be affected by these medicines
- Kidney disease—Higher blood levels of MAO inhibitors may occur, which increases the chance of side effects
- Overactive thyroid or
- Pheochromocytoma (PCC)—Serious side effects may occur

Proper Use of This Medicine

Sometimes this medicine must be taken for several weeks before you begin to feel better. Your doctor should check your progress at regular visits, especially during the first few months of treatment, to make sure that this medicine is working properly and to check for unwanted effects.

Take this medicine only as directed by your doctor. Do not take more of it, do not take it more often, and do not take it for a longer time than your doctor ordered.

MAO inhibitors may be taken with or without food or on a full or empty stomach. However, if your doctor tells you to take the medicine a certain way, take it exactly as directed.

Dosing—The dose of MAO inhibitors will be different for different patients. *Follow your doctor's orders or the directions on the label.* The following information includes only the average doses of phenelzine and tranylcypromine. *If your dose is different, do not change it* unless your doctor tells you to do so.

The number of tablets that you take depends on the strength of the medicine. Also, *the number of doses you take each day, the time allowed between doses, and the length of time you take the medicine depend on the medical problem for which you are using an MAO inhibitor.*

For isocarboxazid
- For *oral* dosage form (tablets):
  - For treatment of depression:
    - Adults—To start, 10 milligrams (mg) twice a day. Your doctor may increase your dose gradually as needed. However, the dose usually is not more than 60 mg a day.
    - Children younger than 16 years of age—Use and dose must be determined by the doctor.

For phenelzine
- For *oral* dosage form (tablets):
  - For treatment of depression:
    - Adults—Dose is based on your body weight. To start, the usual dose is 1 milligram (mg) per kilogram (kg) of body weight (0.45 mg per pound) a day. Your doctor may decrease or increase your dose as needed. However, the dose usually is not more than 90 mg a day.
    - Children younger than 16 years of age—Use and dose must be determined by the doctor.
    - Older adults—To start, 15 mg in the morning. Your doctor may increase your dose gradually as needed. However, the dose usually is not more than 60 mg a day.

For tranylcypromine
- For *oral* dosage form (tablets):
  - For treatment of depression:
    - Adults—To start, 30 milligrams (mg) a day. Your doctor may increase your dose gradually as needed. However, the dose usually is not more than 60 mg a day.
    - Children younger than 16 years of age—Use and dose must be determined by the doctor.
    - Older adults—To start, 2.5 to 5 mg a day. The doctor may increase your dose as needed. However, the dose usually is not more than 45 mg a day.

Missed dose—If you miss a dose of this medicine, take it as soon as possible. However, if it is within 2 hours of your next dose, skip the missed dose and go back to your regular dosing schedule. Do not double doses.

Storage—To store this medicine:
- Keep out of the reach of children.
- Store away from heat and direct light.
- Do not store in the bathroom, near the kitchen sink, or in other damp places. Heat or moisture may cause the medicine to break down.
- Do not keep outdated medicine or medicine no longer needed. Be sure that any discarded medicine is out of the reach of children.

Precautions While Using This Medicine

When taken with certain foods, drinks, or other medicines, MAO inhibitors can cause very dangerous reactions such as sudden high blood pressure (also called hypertensive crisis). To avoid such reactions, *obey the following rules of caution:*
- Do not eat foods that have a high tyramine content (most common in foods that are aged or fermented to increase their flavor), such as cheeses; fava or broad bean pods; yeast or meat extracts; smoked or pickled meat, poultry, or fish; fermented sausage (bologna, pepperoni, salami, and summer sausage) or other fermented meat; sauerkraut; or any overripe fruit. If a list of these foods is not given to you, ask your health care professional to provide one.
- Do not drink alcoholic beverages or alcohol-free or reduced-alcohol beer and wine.
- Do not eat or drink large amounts of caffeine-containing food or beverages such as coffee, tea, cola, or chocolate.
- Do not take any other medicine unless approved or prescribed by your doctor. This especially includes nonprescription (over-the-counter [OTC]) medicine, such as that for colds (including nose drops or sprays), cough, asthma, hay fever, and appetite control; "keep awake" products; or products that make you sleepy.

This medicine will add to the effects of alcohol and other CNS depressants (medicines that slow down the nervous system, possibly causing drowsiness). Some examples of CNS depressants are antihistamines or medicine for hay fever, other allergies, or colds; sedatives, tranquilizers, or sleeping medicine; prescription pain medicine or narcotics; barbiturates; medicine for seizures; muscle relaxants; or anesthetics, including some dental anesthetics. *Check with your doctor before taking any of the above while you are using this medicine.*

Check with your doctor or hospital emergency room immediately if severe headache, stiff neck, chest pains, fast heartbeat, or nausea and vomiting occur while you are taking this medicine. These may be symptoms of a serious side effect that should have a doctor's attention.

Do not stop taking this medicine without first checking with your doctor. Your doctor may want you to reduce gradually the amount you are using before stopping completely.

Dizziness, lightheadedness, or fainting may occur, especially when you get up from a lying or sitting position. *Getting up slowly may help.* When you get up from lying down, sit on the edge of the bed with your feet dangling for 1 or 2 minutes. Then stand up slowly. If the problem continues or gets worse, check with your doctor.

This medicine may cause blurred vision or make some people drowsy or less alert than they are normally. *Make sure you know how you react to this medicine before you drive, use machines, or do anything else that could be dangerous if you are unable to see well or are not alert.*

Antidepressants may cause some people to be agitated, irritable or display other abnormal behaviors. It may also cause some people to have suicidal thoughts and tendencies or to become more depressed. If you or your caregiver notice any of these adverse effects, tell your doctor right away.

Before having any kind of surgery, dental treatment, or emergency treatment, tell the medical doctor or dentist in charge that you are using this medicine or have used it within the past 2 weeks. Taking MAO inhibitors together with medicines that are used during surgery or dental or emergency treatments may increase the risk of serious side effects.

Your doctor may want you to carry an identification card stating that you are using this medicine.

For patients with *angina* (chest pain):
- This medicine may cause you to have an unusual feeling of good health and energy. However, *do not suddenly increase the amount of exercise you get without discussing it with your doctor.* Too much activity could bring on an attack of angina.

For *diabetic* patients:
- This medicine may affect blood sugar levels. While you are using this medicine, be especially careful in testing for sugar in your blood or urine. If you have any questions about this, check with your doctor.

After you stop using this medicine, you must continue to obey the rules of caution for at least 2 weeks concerning food, drink, and other medicine, since these things may continue to react with MAO inhibitors.

Side Effects of This Medicine

Along with its needed effects, a medicine may cause some unwanted effects. Although not all of these side effects may occur, if they do occur they may need medical attention.

Stop taking this medicine and get emergency help immediately if any of the following side effects occur:

Symptoms of unusually high blood pressure (hypertensive crisis)
Chest pain (severe); enlarged pupils; fast or slow heartbeat; headache (severe); increased sensitivity of eyes to light; increased sweating (possibly with fever or cold, clammy skin); nausea and vomiting; stiff or sore neck

Check with your doctor as soon as possible if any of the following side effects occur:

More common
Dizziness or lightheadedness (severe), especially when getting up from a lying or sitting position

Less common
Diarrhea; fast or pounding heartbeat; swelling of feet or lower legs; unusual excitement or nervousness

Rare
Dark urine; fever; skin rash; slurred speech; sore throat; staggering walk; yellow eyes or skin

Symptoms of overdose
Anxiety (severe); confusion; convulsions (seizures); cool, clammy skin; dizziness (severe); drowsiness (severe); fast and irregular pulse; fever; hallucinations (seeing, hearing, or feeling things that are not there); headache (severe); high or low blood pressure; muscle stiffness; sweating; troubled breathing; trouble in sleeping (severe); unusual irritability

Other side effects may occur that usually do not need medical attention. These side effects may go away during treatment as your body adjusts to the medicine. However, check with your doctor if any of the following side effects continue or are bothersome:

More common
Blurred vision; decreased amount of urine; decreased sexual ability; dizziness or lightheadedness (mild), especially when getting up from a lying or sitting position; drowsiness; headache (mild); increased appetite (especially for sweets) or weight gain; increased sweating; muscle twitching during sleep; nausea; restlessness; shakiness or trembling; tiredness and weakness; trouble in sleeping

Less common or rare
Chills; constipation; decreased appetite; dryness of mouth

Other side effects not listed above may also occur in some patients. If you notice any other effects, check with your doctor.

Additional Information

Once a medicine has been approved for marketing for a certain use, experience may show that it is also useful for other medical problems. Although these uses are not included in product labeling, phenelzine and tranylcypromine are used in certain patients with the following medical conditions:

- Headache
- Panic disorder

Other than the above information, there is no additional information relating to proper use, precautions, or side effects for these uses.

ANTIDEPRESSANTS, TRICYCLIC (Systemic)

Some commonly used brand names are:

In the U.S.—

Anafranil (3)	Pamelor (7)
Asendin (2)	Sinequan (5)
Aventyl (7)	Surmontil (9)
Elavil (1)	Tipramine (6)
Endep (1)	Tofranil (6)
Norfranil (6)	Tofranil-PM (6)
Norpramin (4)	Vivactil (8)

In Canada—

Anafranil (3)	Novopramine (6)
Apo-Amitriptyline (1)	Novo-Tripramine (9)
Apo-Imipramine (6)	Novotriptyn (1)
Apo-Trimip (9)	Pertofrane (4)
Asendin (2)	Rhotrimine (9)
Aventyl (7)	Sinequan (5)
Elavil (1)	Surmontil (9)
Impril (6)	Tofranil (6)
Levate (1)	Triadapin (5)
Norpramin (4)	Triptil (8)
Novo-Doxepin (5)	

This information applies to the following medicines:

1. Amitriptyline (a-mee-TRIP-ti-leen)
2. Amoxapine (a-MOX-a-peen)
3. Clomipramine (cloe-MIP-ra-meen)
4. Desipramine (dess-IP-ra-meen)
5. Doxepin (DOX-e-pin)
6. Imipramine (im-IP-ra-meen)
7. Nortriptyline (nor-TRIP-ti-leen)
8. Protriptyline (proe-TRIP-ti-leen)
9. Trimipramine (trye-MIP-ra-meen)

Category

- **Antibulimic**—Amitriptyline; Clomipramine; Desipramine; Imipramine
- **Anticataplectic**—Clomipramine; Desipramine; Imipramine; Protriptyline

- **Antidepressant**—Amitriptyline; Amoxapine; Clomipramine; Desipramine; Doxepin; Imipramine; Nortriptyline; Protriptyline; Trimipramine
- **Antienuretic**—Amitriptyline; Imipramine Hydrochloride
- **Antinarcolepsy adjunct**—Imipramine; Protriptyline
- **Antineuralgic**—Amitriptyline; Clomipramine; Desipramine; Doxepin; Imipramine; Nortriptyline; Trimipramine
- **Antiobsessive-compulsive agent**—Clomipramine
- **Antipanic agent**—Clomipramine; Desipramine; Doxepin; Imipramine; Nortriptyline
- **Antipruritic**—Doxepin
- **Antiulcer agent**—Amitriptyline; Doxepin; Trimipramine

Description

Tricyclic antidepressants are used to relieve mental depression.

One form of this medicine (imipramine) is also used to treat enuresis (bedwetting) in children. Another form (clomipramine) is used to treat obsessive-compulsive disorders. Tricyclic antidepressants may be used for other conditions as determined by your doctor.

These medicines are available only with your doctor's prescription, in the following dosage forms:

Oral
- Amitriptyline
  - Syrup
  - Tablets
- Amoxapine
  - Tablets
- Clomipramine
  - Capsules
  - Tablets
- Desipramine
  - Tablets
- Doxepin
  - Capsules
  - Oral solution
- Imipramine
  - Capsules
  - Tablets
- Nortriptyline
  - Capsules
  - Oral solution
- Protriptyline
  - Tablets
- Trimipramine
  - Capsules
  - Tablets

Parenteral
- Amitriptyline
  - Injection
- Imipramine
  - Injection

Before Using This Medicine

In deciding to use a medicine, the risks of taking the medicine must be weighed against the good it will do. This is a decision you and your doctor will make. For tricyclic antidepressants, the following should be considered:

Allergies—Tell your doctor if you have ever had any unusual or allergic reaction to any tricyclic antidepressant or to carbamazepine, maprotiline, or trazodone. Also tell your health care professional if you are allergic to any other substances, such as foods, preservatives, or dyes.

Pregnancy—Studies have not been done in pregnant women. However, there have been reports of newborns suffering from muscle spasms and heart, breathing, and urinary problems when their mothers had taken tricyclic antidepressants immediately before delivery. Also, studies in animals have shown that some tricyclic antidepressants may cause unwanted effects in the fetus.

Breast-feeding—Tricyclic antidepressants pass into the breast milk. Doxepin has been reported to cause drowsiness in the nursing baby.

Children—Children are especially sensitive to the effects of this medicine. This may increase the chance of side effects during treatment. However, side effects in children taking this medicine for bedwetting usually disappear upon continued use. The most common of these are nervousness, sleeping problems, tiredness, and mild stomach upset. If these side effects continue or are bothersome, check with your doctor.

Antidepressants must be used with caution in children with depression. Studies have shown occurrences of children thinking about suicide or attempting suicide in clinical trials for this medicine. More study is needed to be sure antidepressants are safe and effective in children

Older adults—Drowsiness, dizziness, confusion, vision problems, dryness of mouth, constipation, and problems in urinating are more likely to occur in elderly patients, who are usually more sensitive than younger adults to the effects of tricyclic antidepressants.

Other medicines—Although certain medicines should not be used together at all, in other cases 2 different medicines may be used together even if an interaction might occur. In these cases, your doctor may want to change the dose, or other precautions may be necessary. When you are taking a tricyclic antidepressant, it is especially important that your health care professional know if you are taking any of the following:
- Amphetamines or
- Appetite suppressants (diet pills) or
- Ephedrine or
- Epinephrine (e.g., Adrenalin) or
- Isoproterenol (e.g., Isuprel) or
- Medicine for asthma or other breathing problems or
- Medicine for colds, sinus problems, or hay fever or other allergies or
- Phenylephrine (e.g., Neo-Synephrine)—Using these medicines with tricyclic antidepressants may increase the risk of serious effects on the heart
- Antipsychotics (medicine for mental illness) or
- Clonidine (e.g., Catapres)—Using these medicines with tricyclic antidepressants may increase the CNS depressant effects and increase the chance of serious side effects
- Antithyroid agents (medicine for overactive thyroid) or

- Cimetidine (e.g., Tagamet)—Using these medicines with tricyclic antidepressants may increase the chance of serious side effects
- Central nervous system (CNS) depressants (medicine that causes drowsiness)—Using these medicines with tricyclic antidepressants may increase the CNS depressant effects
- Guanadrel (e.g., Hylorel) or
- Guanethidine (e.g., Ismelin)—Tricyclic antidepressants may keep these medicines from working as well
- Methyldopa (e.g., Aldomet) or
- Metoclopramide (e.g., Reglan) or
- Metyrosine (e.g., Demser) or
- Pemoline (e.g., Cylert) or
- Pimozide (e.g., Orap) or
- Promethazine (e.g., Phenergan) or
- Rauwolfia alkaloids (alseroxylon [e.g., Rauwiloid], deserpidine [e.g., Harmonyl], rauwolfia serpentina [e.g., Raudixin], reserpine [e.g., Serpasil]) or
- Trimeprazine (e.g., Temaril)—Tricyclic antidepressants may cause certain side effects to be more severe and occur more often
- Metrizamide—The risk of seizures may be increased
- Monoamine oxidase (MAO) inhibitor activity (isocarboxazid [e.g., Marplan], isocarboxazid [e.g., Marplan], phenelzine [e.g., Nardil], procarbazine [e.g., Matulane], selegiline [e.g., Eldepryl], tranylcypromine [e.g., Parnate])—Taking tricyclic antidepressants while you are taking or within 2 weeks of taking MAO inhibitors may cause sudden high body temperature, extremely high blood pressure, severe convulsions, and death; however, sometimes certain of these medicines may be used together under close supervision by your doctor

Other medical problems—The presence of other medical problems may affect the use of tricyclic antidepressants. Make sure you tell your doctor if you have any other medical problems, especially:

- Alcohol abuse (or history of)—Drinking alcohol may cause increased CNS depressant effects
- Asthma or
- Bipolar disorder (manic-depressive illness) or
- Blood disorders or
- Convulsions (seizures) or
- Difficult urination or
- Enlarged prostate or
- Glaucoma or increased eye pressure or
- Heart disease or
- High blood pressure (hypertension) or
- Schizophrenia—Tricyclic antidepressants may make the condition worse
- Kidney disease or
- Liver disease—Higher blood levels of tricyclic antidepressants may result, increasing the chance of side effects
- Overactive thyroid or

- Stomach or intestinal problems—Tricyclic antidepressants may cause an increased chance of serious side effects

---

Proper Use of This Medicine

To lessen stomach upset, take this medicine with food, even for a daily bedtime dose, unless your doctor has told you to take it on an empty stomach.

Take this medicine only as directed by your doctor, to benefit your condition as much as possible. Do not take more of it, do not take it more often, and do not take it for a longer time than your doctor ordered.

Sometimes this medicine must be taken for several weeks before you begin to feel better. Your doctor should check your progress at regular visits.

To use *doxepin oral solution:*

- This medicine is to be taken by mouth even though it comes in a dropper bottle. The amount you should take should be measured with the dropper provided with your prescription and diluted just before you take each dose. Dilute each dose with about one-half glass (4 ounces) of water, milk, citrus fruit juice, tomato juice, or prune juice. Do not mix this medicine with grape juice or carbonated beverages since these may decrease the medicine's effectiveness.
- Doxepin oral solution must be mixed immediately before you take it. Do not prepare it ahead of time.

Dosing—The dose of tricyclic antidepressants will be different for different patients. *Follow your doctor's orders or the directions on the label.* The following information includes only the average doses of tricyclic antidepressants. *If your dose is different, do not change it* unless your doctor tells you to do so.

The number of capsules or tablets, or the amount of solution or syrup that you take depends on the strength of the medicine. Also, *the number of doses you take each day, the time allowed between doses, and the length of time you take the medicine depend on the medical problem for which you are taking tricyclic antidepressants.*

For amitriptyline
- For *tablet* dosage form:
  - For depression:
    - Adults—At first, 25 milligrams (mg) two to four times a day. Your doctor may increase your dose gradually as needed. However, the dose is usually not more than 150 mg a day, unless you are in the hospital. Some hospitalized patients may need higher doses.
    - Teenagers—At first, 10 mg three times a day, and 20 mg at bedtime. Your doctor may increase your dose gradually as needed. However, the dose is usually not more than 100 mg a day.
    - Children 6 to 12 years of age—10 to 30 mg a day.
    - Children up to 6 years of age—Use and dose must be determined by your doctor.
    - Older adults—At first, 25 mg at bedtime. Your doctor may increase your dose gradually as needed. However, the dose is usually not more than 100 mg a day.

- For *syrup* dosage form:
  - For depression:
    - Adults—At first, 25 mg two to four times a day. Your doctor may increase your dose gradually as needed.
    - Teenagers—At first, 10 mg three times a day, and 20 mg at bedtime. Your doctor may increase your dose gradually as needed. However, the dose is usually not more than 100 mg a day.
    - Children 6 to 12 years of age—10 to 30 mg a day.
    - Children up to 6 years of age—Use and dose must be determined by your doctor.
    - Older adults—At first, 10 mg three times a day, and 20 mg at bedtime. Your doctor may increase your dose gradually as needed. However, the dose is usually not more than 100 mg a day.
- For *injection* dosage form:
  - For depression:
    - Adults—20 to 30 mg four times a day, injected into a muscle.
    - Children up to 12 years of age—Use and dose must be determined by your doctor.

For amoxapine
- For *tablet* dosage form:
  - For depression:
    - Adults—At first, 50 milligrams (mg) two to three times a day. Your doctor may increase your dose gradually as needed.
    - Children up to 16 years of age—Use and dose must be determined by your doctor.
    - Older adults—At first, 25 mg two to three times a day. Your doctor may increase your dose gradually as needed.

For clomipramine
- For *capsule or tablet* dosage forms:
  - For obsessive-compulsive disorders:
    - Adults—At first, 25 milligrams (mg) once a day. Your doctor may increase your dose gradually as needed. However, the dose is usually not more than 250 mg a day, unless you are in the hospital. Some hospitalized patients may need higher doses.
    - Teenagers and children 10 years of age and over—At first, 25 mg once a day. Your doctor may increase your dose gradually as needed. However, the dose is usually not more than 200 mg a day.
    - Children up to 10 years of age—Use and dose must be determined by your doctor.
    - Older adults—At first, 20 to 30 mg a day. Your doctor may increase your dose gradually as needed.

For desipramine
- For *tablet* dosage form:
  - For depression:
    - Adults—100 to 200 milligrams (mg) a day. Your doctor may increase your dose gradually as needed. However, the dose is usually not more than 300 mg a day.
    - Teenagers—25 to 50 mg a day. Your doctor may increase your dose gradually as needed. However, the dose is usually not more than 100 mg a day.
    - Children 6 to 12 years of age—10 to 30 mg a day.

- Older adults—25 to 50 mg a day. Your doctor may increase your dose gradually as needed. However, the dose is usually not more than 150 mg a day.

For doxepin
- For *capsule or solution* dosage forms:
  - For depression:
    - Adults—At first, 25 milligrams (mg) three times a day. Your doctor may increase your dose gradually as needed. However, the dose is usually not more than 150 mg a day, unless you are in the hospital. Some hospitalized patients may need higher doses.
    - Children up to 12 years of age—Use and dose must be determined by your doctor.
    - Older adults—At first, 25 to 50 mg a day. Your doctor may increase your dose gradually as needed.

For imipramine
- For *tablet* dosage form:
  - For depression:
    - Adults—25 to 50 milligrams (mg) three to four times a day. Your doctor may increase your dose gradually as needed. However, the dose is usually not more than 200 mg a day, unless you are in the hospital. Some hospitalized patients may need higher doses.
    - Adolescents—25 to 50 mg a day. Your doctor may increase your dose gradually as needed. However, the dose is usually not more than 100 mg a day.
    - Children 6 to 12 years of age—10 to 30 mg a day.
    - Children up to 6 years of age—Use and dose must be determined by your doctor.
    - Older adults—At first, 25 mg at bedtime. Your doctor may increase your dose gradually as needed. However, the dose is usually not more than 100 mg a day.
  - For bedwetting:
    - Children—25 mg once a day, taken one hour before bedtime. Your doctor may increase the dose as needed, based on the child's age.
- For *capsule* dosage form:
  - For depression:
    - Adults—At first, 75 mg a day taken at bedtime. Your doctor may increase your dose gradually as needed. However, the dose is usually not more than 200 mg a day, unless you are in the hospital. Some hospitalized patients may need higher doses.
    - Children up to 12 years of age—Use and dose must be determined by your doctor.
- For *injection* dosage form:
  - For depression:
    - Adults—Dose must be determined by your doctor. It is injected into a muscle. The dose is usually not more than 300 mg a day.
    - Children up to 12 years of age—Use and dose must be determined by your doctor.

For nortriptyline
- For *capsule or solution* dosage forms:
  - For depression:
    - Adults—25 milligrams (mg) three to four times a day. Your doctor may increase your dose gradu-

ally as needed. However, the dose is usually not more than 150 mg a day.

- Teenagers—25 to 50 mg a day. Your doctor may increase your dose gradually as needed.
- Children 6 to 12 years of age—10 to 20 mg a day.
- Older adults—30 to 50 mg a day. Your doctor may increase your dose gradually as needed.

For protriptyline
- For *tablet* dosage form:
  ○ For depression:
    - Adults—At first, 5 to 10 milligrams (mg) three to four times a day. Your doctor may increase your dose gradually as needed. However, the dose is usually not more than 60 mg a day.
    - Teenagers—At first, 5 mg three times a day. Your doctor may increase your dose gradually as needed.
    - Children up to 12 years of age—Use and dose must be determined by your doctor.
    - Older adults—At first, 5 mg three times a day. Your doctor may increase your dose gradually as needed.

For trimipramine
- For *capsule or tablet* dosage forms:
  ○ For depression:
    - Adults—At first, 75 milligrams (mg) a day. Your doctor may increase your dose as needed. However, the dose is usually not more than 200 mg a day, unless you are hospitalized. Some hospitalized patients may need higher doses.
    - Teenagers—At first, 50 mg a day. Your doctor may increase your dose gradually as needed. However, the dose is usually not more than 100 mg a day.
    - Children up to 12 years of age—Use and dose must be determined by your doctor.
    - Older adults—At first, 50 mg a day. Your doctor may increase your dose gradually as needed. However, the dose is usually not more than 100 mg a day.

Missed dose—If you miss a dose of this medicine and your dosing schedule is:

- One dose a day at bedtime—Do not take the missed dose in the morning since it may cause disturbing side effects during waking hours. Instead, check with your doctor.
- More than one dose a day—Take the missed dose as soon as possible. However, if it is almost time for your next dose, skip the missed dose, and go back to your regular dosing schedule. Do not double doses.

If you have any questions about this, check with your doctor.

Storage—To store this medicine:

- Keep out of the reach of children. Overdose of this medicine is very dangerous in young children.
- Store away from heat and direct light.
- Do not store the tablet or capsule form of this medicine in the bathroom, near the kitchen sink, or in other damp places. Heat or moisture may cause the medicine to break down.
- Keep the liquid form of this medicine from freezing.

- Do not keep outdated medicine or medicine no longer needed. Be sure that any discarded medicine is out of the reach of children.

Precautions While Using This Medicine

It is very important that your doctor check your progress at regular visits to allow dosage adjustments and to help reduce side effects.

This medicine will add to the effects of alcohol and other CNS depressants (medicines that make you drowsy or less alert). Some examples of CNS depressants are antihistamines or medicine for hay fever, other allergies, or colds; sedatives, tranquilizers, or sleeping medicine; prescription pain medicine or narcotics; barbiturates; medicine for seizures; muscle relaxants; or anesthetics, including some dental anesthetics. *Check with your medical doctor or dentist before taking any of the above while you are taking this medicine.*

Antidepressants may cause some people to be agitated, irritable or display other abnormal behaviors. It may also cause some people to have suicidal thoughts and tendencies or to become more depressed. If you or your caregiver notice any of these adverse effects, tell your doctor right away.

This medicine may cause some people to become drowsy. *If this occurs, do not drive, use machines, or do anything else that could be dangerous if you are not alert.*

Dizziness, lightheadedness, or fainting may occur, especially when you get up from a lying or sitting position. Getting up slowly may help. If this problem continues or gets worse, check with your doctor.

This medicine may cause dryness of the mouth. For temporary relief, use sugarless gum or candy, melt bits of ice in your mouth, or use a saliva substitute. However, if your mouth continues to feel dry for more than 2 weeks, check with your medical doctor or dentist. Continuing dryness of the mouth may increase the chance of dental disease, including tooth decay, gum disease, and fungus infections.

Tricyclic antidepressants may cause your skin to be more sensitive to sunlight than it is normally. Exposure to sunlight, even for brief periods of time, may cause a skin rash, itching, redness or other discoloration of the skin, or a severe sunburn. When you begin taking this medicine:

- Stay out of direct sunlight, especially between the hours of 10:00 a.m. and 3:00 p.m., if possible.
- Wear protective clothing, including a hat. Also, wear sunglasses.
- Apply a sun block product that has a skin protection factor (SPF) of at least 15. Some patients may require a product with a higher SPF number, especially if they have a fair complexion. If you have any questions about this, check with your health care professional.
- Apply a sun block lipstick that has an SPF of at least 15 to protect your lips.
- Do not use a sunlamp or tanning bed or booth.

If you have a severe reaction from the sun, check with your doctor.

Before you have any medical tests, tell the medical doctor in charge that you are taking this medicine. The results of the metyrapone test may be affected by this medicine.

Before having any kind of surgery, dental treatment, or emergency treatment, tell the medical doctor or dentist in charge that you are using this medicine. Taking tricyclic antidepressants together with medicines used during surgery or dental or emergency treatments may increase the risk of side effects.

For diabetic patients:
- This medicine may affect blood sugar levels. If you notice a change in the results of your blood or urine sugar tests or if you have any questions, check with your doctor.

Do not stop taking this medicine without first checking with your doctor. Your doctor may want you to reduce gradually the amount you are using before stopping completely. This may help prevent a possible worsening of your condition and reduce the possibility of withdrawal symptoms such as headache, nausea, and/or an overall feeling of discomfort.

The effects of this medicine may last for 3 to 7 days after you have stopped taking it. Therefore, all the precautions stated here must be observed during this time.

For patients taking protriptyline:
- If taken late in the day, protriptyline may interfere with nighttime sleep.

Side Effects

Along with its needed effects, a medicine may cause some unwanted effects. Although not all of these side effects may occur, if they do occur they may need medical attention.

Stop taking this medicine and get emergency help immediately if any of the following side effects occur:
Reported for amoxapine only—rare
Convulsions (seizures); difficult or fast breathing; fever with increased sweating; high or low (irregular) blood pressure; loss of bladder control; muscle stiffness (severe); pale skin; unusual tiredness or weakness

Check with your doctor as soon as possible if any of the following side effects occur:
Less common
Blurred vision; confusion or delirium; constipation (especially in the elderly); decreased sexual ability (more common with amoxapine and clomipramine); difficulty in speaking or swallowing; eye pain; fainting; fast or irregular heartbeat (pounding, racing, skipping); hallucinations; loss of balance control; mask-like face; nervousness or restlessness; problems in urinating; shakiness or trembling; shuffling walk; slowed movements; stiffness of arms and legs

Reported for amoxapine only (in addition to the above)—less common
Lip smacking or puckering; puffing of cheeks; rapid or worm-like movements of tongue; uncontrolled chewing movements; uncontrolled movements of hands, arms, or legs

Rare
Anxiety; breast enlargement in both males and females; hair loss; inappropriate secretion of milk— in females; increased sensitivity to sunlight; irritability; muscle twitching; red or brownish spots on skin; ringing, buzzing, or other unexplained sounds in the ears; seizures (more common with clomipramine); skin rash and itching; sore throat and fever; swelling of face and tongue; swelling of testicles (more common with amoxapine); trouble with teeth or gums (more common with clomipramine); weakness; yellow eyes or skin

Symptoms of acute overdose
Confusion; convulsions (seizures); disturbed concentration; drowsiness (severe); enlarged pupils; fast, slow, or irregular heartbeat; fever; hallucinations (seeing, hearing, or feeling things that are not there); restlessness and agitation; shortness of breath or troubled breathing; unusual tiredness or weakness (severe); vomiting

Other side effects may occur that usually do not need medical attention. These side effects may go away during treatment as your body adjusts to the medicine. However, check with your doctor if any of the following side effects continue or are bothersome:
More common
Dizziness; drowsiness; dryness of mouth; headache; increased appetite (may include craving for sweets); nausea; tiredness or weakness (mild); unpleasant taste; weight gain
Less common
Diarrhea; heartburn; increased sweating; trouble in sleeping (more common with protriptyline, especially when taken late in the day); vomiting

Certain side effects of this medicine may occur after you have stopped taking it. Check with your doctor if you notice any of the following effects:
Headache; irritability; nausea, vomiting, or diarrhea; restlessness; trouble in sleeping, with vivid dreams; unusual excitement
Reported for amoxapine only (in addition to the above)
Lip smacking or puckering; puffing of cheeks; rapid or worm-like movements of the tongue; uncontrolled chewing movements; uncontrolled movements of arms or legs

Other side effects not listed above also may occur in some patients. If you notice any other effects, check with your doctor.

Additional Information

Once a medicine has been approved for marketing for a certain use, experience may show that it is also useful for other medical problems. Although these uses are not included in product labeling, tricyclic antidepressants are used in certain patients with the following medical conditions:

- Attention deficit hyperactivity disorder (hyperactivity in children) (desipramine, imipramine, and protriptyline)
- Bulimia (uncontrolled eating, followed by vomiting) (amitriptyline, clomipramine, desipramine, and imipramine)
- Cocaine withdrawal (desipramine and imipramine)
- Headache prevention (for certain types of frequent or continuing headaches) (most tricyclic antidepressants)
- Itching with hives due to cold temperature exposure (doxepin)
- Narcolepsy (extreme tendency to fall asleep suddenly) (clomipramine, desipramine, imipramine, and protriptyline)
- Neurogenic pain (a type of continuing pain) (amitriptyline, clomipramine, desipramine, doxepin, imipramine, nortriptyline, and trimipramine)
- Nicotine dependence (as an aid to other smoking cessationn therapy) (nortriptyline)
- Panic disorder (clomipramine, desipramine, doxepin, nortriptyline, and trimipramine)

- Stomach ulcer (amitriptyline, doxepin, and trimipramine)
- Urinary incontinence (imipramine)

Other than the above information, there is no additional information relating to proper use, precautions, or side effects for these uses.

ANTIDYSKINETICS (Systemic)

Some commonly used brand names are:

In the U.S.—

Akineton (2)	Kemadrin (4)
Artane (5)	Parsidol (3)
Artane Sequels (5)	Trihexane (5)
Cogentin (1)	Trihexy (5)

In Canada—

Akineton (2)	Kemadrin (4)
Apo-Benztropine (1)	Parsitan (3)
Apo-Trihex (5)	PMS Benztropine (1)
Artane (5)	PMS Procyclidine (4)
Artane Sequels (5)	PMS Trihexyphenidyl (5)
Cogentin (1)	Procyclid (4)

This information applies to the following medicines:

1. Benztropine (BENZ-troe-peen)
2. Biperiden (bye-PER-i-den)
3. Ethopropazine (eth-oh-PROE-pa-zeen)
4. Procyclidine (proe-SYE-kli-deen)
5. Trihexyphenidyl (trye-hex-ee-FEN-i-dill)

Category

- **Antidyskinetic**—Benztropine; Biperiden; Ethopropazine; Procyclidine; Trihexyphenidyl

Description

Antidyskinetics are used to treat Parkinson's disease, sometimes referred to as "shaking palsy." By improving muscle control and reducing stiffness, this medicine allows more normal movements of the body as the disease symptoms are reduced. It is also used to control severe reactions to certain medicines such as reserpine (e.g., Serpasil) (medicine to control high blood pressure) or phenothiazines, chlorprothixene (e.g., Taractan), thiothixene (e.g., Navane), loxapine (e.g., Loxitane), and haloperidol (e.g., Haldol) (medicines for nervous, mental, and emotional conditions).

Antidyskinetics may also be used for other conditions as determined by your doctor.

These medicines are available only with your doctor's prescription in the following dosage forms:

Oral
- Benztropine
  - Tablets
- Biperiden
  - Tablets
- Ethopropazine
  - Tablets
- Procyclidine
  - Elixir
  - Tablets

- Trihexyphenidyl
  - Extended-release capsules
  - Elixir
  - Tablets

Parenteral
- Benztropine
  - Injection
- Biperiden
  - Injection

Before Using This Medicine

In deciding to use a medicine, the risks of taking the medicine must be weighed against the good it will do. This is a decision you and your doctor will make. For antidyskinetics, the following should be considered:

Allergies—Tell your doctor if you have ever had any unusual or allergic reaction to antidyskinetics. Also tell your health care professional if you are allergic to any other substances, such as foods, preservatives, or dyes.

Pregnancy—Studies on effects in pregnancy have not been done in either humans or animals. However, antidyskinetics have not been shown to cause problems in humans.

Breast-feeding—It is not known if antidyskinetics pass into breast milk. Although most medicines pass into breast milk in small amounts, many of them may be used safely while breast-feeding. Mothers who are taking these medicines and who wish to breast-feed should discuss this with their doctor.

Since antidyskinetics tend to decrease the secretions of the body, it is possible that the flow of breast milk may be reduced in some patients.

Children—Children may be especially sensitive to the effects of antidyskinetics. This may increase the chance of side effects during treatment.

Older adults—Agitation, confusion, disorientation, hallucinations, memory loss, and mental changes are more likely to occur in elderly patients, who are usually more sensitive to the effects of antidyskinetics.

Other medicines—Although certain medicines should not be used together at all, in other cases 2 different medicines may be used together even if an interaction might occur. In these cases, your doctor may want to change the dose, or other precautions may be necessary. When you are taking an antidyskinetic, it is especially important that your health care professional know if you are taking any of the following:

- Anticholinergics (medicine for abdominal or stomach spasms or cramps) or
- Central nervous system (CNS) depressants (medicine that causes drowsiness) or
- Tricyclic antidepressants (medicine for depression)—Using these medicines together with antidyskinetics may result in additive effects, increasing the chance of unwanted effects

Other medical problems—The presence of other medical problems may affect the use of antidyskinetics. Make sure you tell your doctor if you have any other medical problems, especially:

- Difficult urination or
- Enlarged prostate or
- Glaucoma or

- Heart or blood vessel disease or
- High blood pressure or
- Intestinal blockage or
- Myasthenia gravis or
- Uncontrolled movements of hands, mouth, or tongue—Antidyskinetics may make the condition worse
- Kidney disease or
- Liver disease—Higher blood levels of the antidyskinetics may result, increasing the chance of side effects

Proper Use of This Medicine

Take this medicine only as directed by your doctor. Do not take more of it, do not take it more often, and do not take it for a longer period of time than your doctor ordered. To do so may increase the chance of side effects.

To lessen stomach upset, take this medicine with meals or immediately after meals, unless otherwise directed by your doctor.

Dosing—The dose of antidyskinetics will be different for different patients. *Follow your doctor's orders or the directions on the label.* The following information includes only the average doses of benztropine, biperiden, ethopropazine, procyclidine, and trihexyphenidyl. *If your dose is different, do not change it* unless your doctor tells you to do so.

The number of capsules, tablets, or teaspoonfuls of elixir that you take depends on the strength of the medicine. Also, *the number of doses you take each day, the time allowed between doses, and the length of time you take the medicine depend on the medical problem for which you are taking antidyskinetics.*

For benztropine
- For *oral* dosage forms (tablets):
  - For Parkinson's disease or certain severe side effects caused by some other medicines:
    - Adults—To start, 0.5 to 4 milligrams (mg) a day, depending on your condition. Your doctor will adjust your dose as needed; however, the dose is usually not more than 6 mg a day.
    - Children—Use and dose must be determined by your doctor.
- For *injection* dosage form:
  - For Parkinson's disease or certain severe side effects caused by some other medicines:
    - Adults—1 to 4 mg a day, depending on your condition. Your doctor will adjust your dose as needed; however, the dose is usually not more than 6 mg a day.
    - Children—Use and dose must be determined by your doctor.

For biperiden
- For *oral* dosage forms (tablets):
  - For Parkinson's disease or certain severe side effects caused by some other medicines:
    - Adults—2 mg up to four times a day. Your doctor will adjust your dose, depending on your condition; however, the dose is usually not more than 16 mg a day.
    - Children—Use and dose must be determined by your doctor.
- For *injection* dosage form:
  - For Parkinson's disease or certain severe side effects caused by some other medicines:

- Adults—2 mg, injected into a muscle or vein. The dose may be repeated if needed; however, the dose is usually not given more than four times a day.
- Children—Use and dose is based on body weight and must be determined by your doctor.

For ethopropazine
- For *oral* dosage forms (tablets):
  - For Parkinson's disease or certain severe side effects caused by some other medicines:
    - Adults—50 mg one or two times a day. Your doctor will adjust your dose as needed; however, the dose is usually not more than 600 mg a day.
    - Children—Use and dose must be determined by your doctor.

For procyclidine
- For *oral* dosage forms (elixir or tablets):
  - For Parkinson's disease or certain severe side effects caused by some other medicines:
    - Adults—To start, 2.5 mg three times a day after meals. Your doctor may need to adjust your dose, depending on your condition.
    - Children—Use and dose must be determined by your doctor.

For trihexyphenidyl
- For *extended-release oral* dosage forms (extended-release capsules):
  - For Parkinson's disease or certain severe side effects caused by some other medicines:
    - Adults—5 mg after breakfast. Your doctor may add another 5 mg dose to be taken twelve hours later, depending on your condition.
    - Children: Use and dose must be determined by your doctor.
- For other *oral* dosage forms (elixir or tablets):
  - For Parkinson's disease or certain severe side effects caused by some other medicines:
    - Adults—To start, 1 to 2 mg a day. Your doctor may adjust your dose as needed; however, the dose is usually not more than 15 mg a day.
    - Children—Use and dose must be determined by your doctor.

Missed dose—If you miss a dose of this medicine, take it as soon as possible. However, if it is within 2 hours of your next dose, skip the missed dose and go back to your regular dosing schedule. Do not double doses.

Storage—To store this medicine:
- Keep out of the reach of children.
- Store away from heat and direct light.
- Do not store the capsule or tablet form of this medicine in the bathroom, near the kitchen sink, or in other damp places. Heat or moisture may cause the medicine to break down.
- Keep the liquid form of this medicine from freezing.
- Do not keep outdated medicine or medicine no longer needed. Be sure that any discarded medicine is out of the reach of children.

Precautions While Using This Medicine

Your doctor should check your progress at regular visits, especially for the first few months you take this medicine. This will allow your dosage to be changed as necessary to meet your needs.

Your doctor may want you to have your eyes examined by an ophthalmologist (eye doctor) before and also sometime later during treatment.

Do not stop taking this medicine without first checking with your doctor. Your doctor may want you to reduce gradually the amount you are taking before stopping completely, to prevent side effects or the worsening of your condition.

This medicine will add to the effects of alcohol and other CNS depressants (medicines that slow down the nervous system, possibly causing drowsiness). Some examples of CNS depressants are antihistamines or medicine for hay fever, other allergies, or colds; sedatives, tranquilizers, or sleeping medicine; prescription pain medicine or narcotics; barbiturates; medicine for seizures; muscle relaxants; or anesthetics, including some dental anesthetics. *Check with your doctor before taking any of the above while you are using this medicine.*

Do not take this medicine within 1 hour of taking medicine for diarrhea. Taking these medicines too close together will make this medicine less effective.

If you think you or anyone else has taken an overdose of this medicine, get emergency help at once. Taking an overdose of this medicine may lead to unconsciousness. Some signs of an overdose are clumsiness or unsteadiness; seizures; severe drowsiness; severe dryness of mouth, nose and throat; fast heartbeat; hallucinations (seeing, hearing, or feeling things that are not there); mood or mental changes; shortness of breath or troubled breathing; trouble in sleeping; and unusual warmth, dryness, and flushing of skin.

This medicine may cause your eyes to become more sensitive to light than they are normally. Wearing sunglasses and avoiding too much exposure to bright light may help lessen the discomfort.

This medicine may cause some people to have blurred vision or to become drowsy, dizzy, or less alert than they are normally. *Make sure you know how you react to this medicine before you drive, use machines, or do anything else that could be dangerous if you are dizzy or are not alert or able to see well.*

Dizziness, lightheadedness, or fainting may occur, especially when you get up from lying or sitting. Getting up slowly may help. If the problem continues or gets worse, check with your doctor.

This medicine may make you sweat less, causing your body temperature to increase. *Use extra care to avoid becoming overheated during exercise or hot weather while you are taking this medicine, since overheating may result in heat stroke.* Also, hot baths or saunas may make you feel dizzy or faint while you are taking this medicine.

This medicine may cause dryness of the mouth. For temporary relief, use sugarless candy or gum, melt bits of ice in your mouth, or use a saliva substitute. However, if your mouth continues to feel dry for more than 2 weeks, check with your medical doctor or dentist. Continuing dryness of the mouth may increase the chance of dental disease, including tooth decay, gum disease, and fungus infections.

Side Effects

Along with its needed effects, a medicine may cause some unwanted effects. Although not all of these side effects may occur, if they do occur they may need medical attention.

Check with your doctor as soon as possible if any of the following side effects occur:

Rare

Confusion (more common in the elderly or with high doses); eye pain; skin rash

Symptoms of overdose

Clumsiness or unsteadiness; drowsiness (severe); dryness of mouth, nose, or throat (severe); fast heartbeat; hallucinations (seeing, hearing, or feeling things that are not there); mood or mental changes; seizures; shortness of breath or troubled breathing; trouble in sleeping; warmth, dryness, and flushing of skin

Other side effects may occur that usually do not need medical attention. These side effects may go away during treatment as your body adjusts to the medicine. However, check with your doctor if any of the following side effects continue or are bothersome:

More common

Blurred vision; constipation; decreased sweating; difficult or painful urination (especially in older men); drowsiness; dryness of mouth, nose, or throat; increased sensitivity of eyes to light; nausea or vomiting

Less common or rare

Dizziness or lightheadedness when getting up from a lying or sitting position; false sense of well-being (especially in the elderly or with high doses); headache; loss of memory (especially in the elderly); muscle cramps; nervousness; numbness or weakness in hands or feet; soreness of mouth and tongue; stomach upset or pain; unusual excitement (more common with large doses of trihexyphenidyl)

After you stop using this medicine, your body may need time to adjust. The length of time this takes depends on the amount of medicine you were using and how long you used it. During this period of time check with your doctor if you notice any of the following side effects:

Anxiety; difficulty in speaking or swallowing; dizziness or lightheadedness when getting up from a lying or sitting position; fast heartbeat; loss of balance control; mask-like face; muscle spasms, especially of face, neck, and back; restlessness or desire to keep moving; shuffling walk; stiffness of arms or legs; trembling and shaking of hands and fingers; trouble in sleeping; twisting movements of body

Other side effects not listed above may also occur in some patients. If you notice any other effects, check with your doctor.

ANTIFIBRINOLYTIC AGENTS (Systemic)

Some commonly used brand names are:

In the U.S.—

Amicar (1)
Cyklokapron (2)

In Canada—

Amicar (1)
Cyklokapron (2)

This information applies to the following medicines:

1. Aminocaproic Acid (a-mee-noe-ka-PROE-ik ASS-id)
2. Tranexamic Acid (tran-ex-AM-ik ASS-id)

Category

- **Antifibrinolytic—**
- **Antihemorrhagic—**Aminocaproic Acid; Tranexamic Acid

Description

Antifibrinolytic (an-tee-fye-bri-noh-LIT-ik) agents are used to treat serious bleeding, especially when the bleeding occurs after dental surgery (particularly in patients with hemophilia) or certain other kinds of surgery. These medicines are also sometimes given before an operation to prevent serious bleeding in patients with medical problems that increase the chance of serious bleeding.

Antifibrinolytic agents may also be used for other conditions as determined by your doctor.

Antifibrinolytic agents are available only with your doctor's prescription, in the following dosage forms:

Oral
- Aminocaproic acid
  - Syrup
  - Tablets
- Tranexamic acid
  - Tablets

Parenteral
- Aminocaproic acid
  - Injection
- Tranexamic acid
  - Injection

Before Using This Medicine

In deciding to use a medicine, the risks of taking the medicine must be weighed against the good it will do. This is a decision you and your doctor will make. For antifibrinolytic agents, the following should be considered:

Allergies—Tell your doctor if you have ever had any unusual or allergic reaction to aminocaproic acid or tranexamic acid. Also tell your health care professional if you are allergic to any other substances, such as foods, preservatives, or dyes.

Pregnancy—Studies on birth defects have not been done in humans. However, these medicines have been given to pregnant women without causing birth defects or other problems.

Studies on effects of aminocaproic acid in pregnancy have not been done in animals. Tranexamic acid has not been shown to cause birth defects or other problems in animal studies.

Before taking this medicine, make sure your doctor knows if you are pregnant or if you may become pregnant.

Breast-feeding—These medicines have not been reported to cause problems in nursing babies. However, small amounts of tranexamic acid pass into the breast milk. Mothers who are taking this medicine and who wish to breast-feed should discuss this with their doctor.

Children—Although there is no specific information comparing use of aminocaproic acid or tranexamic acid in children with use in other age groups, these medicines are not expected to cause different side effects or problems in children than they do in adults.

Aminocaproic acid injection *should not* be given to newborns. It contains a preservative called benzyl alcohol that can cause a condition called "gasping syndrome" with very serious unwanted effects.

Older adults—
- *For aminocaproic acid:* Although there is no specific information comparing use of aminocaproic acid in the elderly with use in other age groups, this medicine is not expected to cause different side effects or problems in older people than it does in younger adults.
- *For tranexamic acid:* Tranexamic acid has been tested and has not been shown to cause different side effects or problems in older people than it does in younger adults.

Other medicines—Although certain medicines should not be used together at all, in other cases two different medicines may be used together even if an interaction might occur. In these cases, your doctor may want to change the dose, or other precautions may be necessary. Tell your health care professional if you are taking any other prescription or nonprescription (over-the-counter [OTC]) medicine.

Other medical problems—The presence of other medical problems may affect the use of antifibrinolytic agents. Make sure you tell your doctor if you have any other medical problems, especially:
- Blood clots or a history of medical problems caused by blood clots or
- Blood in the urine or
- Color vision problems or
- Heart disease or
- Kidney disease or
- Liver disease—The chance of side effects may be increased

Proper Use of This Medicine

Take this medicine only as directed by your doctor. Do not take more or less of it, do not take it more often, and do not take it for a longer time than your doctor ordered. To do so may increase the chance of unwanted effects.

Dosing—The dose of these medicines will be different for different patients. *Follow your doctor's orders or the directions on the label.* The following information includes only the average doses of these medicines. *If your dose is different, do not change it* unless your doctor tells you to do so.

For aminocaproic acid
- To prevent or treat serious bleeding:
  - For *oral* dosage forms (syrup or tablets):
    - Adults—For the first hour, the dose is 5 grams. Then the dose is 1 or 1.25 grams per hour for eight hours.
    - Children—Dose is based on body weight or size and must be determined by your doctor. For the first hour, the dose is usually 100 milligrams (mg) per kilogram (kg) (45.4 mg per pound) of body weight. Then the dose is 33.3 mg per kg (15.1 mg per pound) of body weight per hour.
  - For *injection* dosage form:
    - Adults—At first, the dose is 4 to 5 grams injected into a vein, over a period of one hour. Then the

dose is 1 gram per hour, injected into a vein over a period of eight hours.

- Children—Dose is based on body weight or size and must be determined by your doctor. At first, the dose is usually 100 mg per kg (45.4 mg per pound) of body weight, injected into a vein over a period of one hour. Then the dose is 33.3 mg per kg (15.1 mg per pound) of body weight per hour, injected into a vein.

For tranexamic acid
- To prevent or treat serious bleeding after dental surgery:
  ○ For *oral* dosage form (tablets):
    - Adults and children—Dose is based on body weight and must be determined by your doctor. The dose is usually 25 milligrams (mg) per kilogram (kg) (11.4 mg per pound) of body weight every six to eight hours, beginning one day before surgery. After surgery, the dose is usually 25 mg per kg (11.4 mg per pound) of body weight every six to eight hours for two to eight days.
  ○ For *injection* dosage form:
    - Adults and children—Dose is based on body weight and must be determined by your doctor. The dose is usually 10 mg per kg (4.5 mg per pound) of body weight, injected into a vein just before surgery. After surgery, the dose is usually 10 mg per kg (4.5 mg per pound) of body weight, injected into a vein every six to eight hours for seven to ten days.

Missed dose—
- *For aminocaproic acid* (e.g., Amicar): If you miss a dose, take it as soon as possible. However, if you do not remember until it is almost time for your next dose, double the next dose. Then go back to your regular dosing schedule.
- *For tranexamic acid* (e.g., Cyklokapron): If you miss a dose, take it as soon as possible. Then take any remaining doses for the day at regularly spaced times. Do not double doses. If you have any questions about this, check with your doctor.

Storage—To store this medicine:
- Keep out of the reach of children.
- Store away from heat and direct light.
- Do not store the tablet form of this medicine in the bathroom, near the kitchen sink, or in other damp places. Heat or moisture may cause the medicine to break down.
- Do not keep outdated medicine or medicine no longer needed. Be sure that any discarded medicine is out of the reach of children.

Precautions While Using This Medicine

If you will be taking tranexamic acid for longer than several days, your doctor may want you to have your eyes checked regularly by an ophthalmologist (eye doctor). This will allow your doctor to check for unwanted effects that may be caused by this medicine.

If you are using aminocaproic acid syrup as a mouth rinse to control oral bleeding, and you are in the first or second trimester of pregnancy, you should spit out the syrup after rinsing without swallowing it.

Side Effects

Along with its needed effects, a medicine may cause some unwanted effects. Although not all of these side effects may occur, if they do occur they may need medical attention.

The same effect that makes aminocaproic acid or tranexamic acid help prevent or stop bleeding also may cause blood clots that could be dangerous. Check with your doctor immediately if any of the following possible signs and symptoms of blood clots occur:

Less common or rare
Headache (severe and sudden); loss of coordination (sudden); pains in chest, groin, or legs, especially the calves; shortness of breath (sudden); slurred speech (sudden); vision changes (sudden); weakness or numbness in arm or leg

Also, check with your doctor as soon as possible if any of the following side effects occur:

Less common or rare
For aminocaproic acid
Dizziness; headache; muscle pain or weakness (severe and continuing); ringing or buzzing in ears; skin rash; slow or irregular heartbeat— with the injection only; stomach cramps or pain; stuffy nose; sudden decrease in amount of urine; swelling of face, feet, or lower legs; unusual tiredness or weakness; weight gain (rapid)

For tranexamic acid
Blurred vision or other changes in vision; dizziness or lightheadedness; unusual tiredness or weakness

Other side effects may occur that usually do not need medical attention. These side effects may go away during treatment as your body adjusts to the medicine. However, check with your doctor if any of the following side effects continue or are bothersome:

Diarrhea; dry ejaculation; nausea or vomiting; unusual menstrual discomfort; watery eyes

Other side effects not listed above may also occur in some patients. If you notice any other effects, check with your doctor.

ANTIFUNGALS, AZOLE (Systemic)

Some commonly used brand names are:

In the U.S.—
Diflucan (1)
Nizoral (3)
Sporanox (2)

In Canada—
Diflucan (1)   Nizoral (3)
Diflucan-150 (1)   Sporanox (2)

This information applies to the following medicines:

1. Fluconazole (floo-KOE-na-zole)
2. Itraconazole (i-tra-KOE-na-zole)
3. Ketoconazole (kee-toe-ko-NA-zole)

Category

- **Antiadrenal**—Ketoconazole
- **Antifungal, systemic**—Fluconazole; Itraconazole; Ketoconazole
- **Antineoplastic**—Ketoconazole

Description

Azole antifungals are used to treat serious fungus infections that may occur in different parts of the body. These medicines may also be used for other problems as determined by your doctor.

Azole antifungals are available only with your doctor's prescription, in the following dosage forms:

Oral
- Fluconazole
  - Capsules
  - Oral suspension
  - Tablets
- Itraconazole
  - Capsules
  - Oral solution
- Ketoconazole
  - Oral suspension
  - Tablets

Parenteral
- Fluconazole
  - Injection
- Itraconazole
  - Injection

Before Using This Medicine

In deciding to use a medicine, the risks of taking the medicine must be weighed against the good it will do. This is a decision you and your doctor will make. For the azole antifungals, the following should be considered:

Allergies—Tell your doctor if you have ever had any unusual or allergic reaction to any of the azole antifungals. Also tell your health care professional if you are allergic to any other substances, such as foods, preservatives, or dyes.

Pregnancy—Studies have not been done in pregnant women. However, studies in some animals have shown that azole antifungals, taken in high doses, may cause harm to the mother and the fetus. They have caused birth defects in animals. During clinical practice of itraconazole, cases of birth defects including skeletal, GI tract, heart, and eye malformations and genetic malformations have been reported. Itraconazole should not be given to pregnant women or women who may become pregnant for the treatment of onychomycosis. Women who could become pregnant should use birth control while taking itraconazole and for 2 months after itraconazole treatment is stopped. Before taking these medicines, make sure your doctor knows if you are pregnant or if you may become pregnant.

Breast-feeding—Azole antifungals pass into breast milk. Mothers who are taking these medicines and who wish to breast-feed should discuss this with their doctors.

Children—A small number of children have been safely treated with azole antifungals. Be sure to discuss with your child's doctor the use of these medicines in children.

Older adults—Many medicines have not been studied specifically in older people. Therefore, it may not be known whether they work exactly the same way they do in younger adults or if they cause different side effects or problems in older people. There is no specific information comparing use of azole antifungals in the elderly with use in other age groups.

Other medicines—Although certain medicines should not be used together at all, in other cases two different medicines may be used together even if an interaction might occur. In these cases, your doctor may want to change the dose, or other precautions may be necessary. When you are taking azole antifungals, it is especially important that your health care professional know if you are taking any of the following:
- Acetaminophen (e.g., Tylenol) (with long-term, high-dose use) or
- Amiodarone (e.g., Cordarone) or
- Anabolic steroids (nandrolone [e.g., Anabolin], oxandrolone [e.g., Anavar], oxymetholone [e.g., Anadrol], stanozolol [e.g., Winstrol]) or
- Androgens (male hormones) or
- Antithyroid agents (medicine for overactive thyroid) or
- Carmustine (e.g., BiCNU) or
- Chloroquine (e.g., Aralen) or
- Dantrolene (e.g., Dantrium) or
- Daunorubicin (e.g., Cerubidine) or
- Disulfiram (e.g., Antabuse) or
- Divalproex (e.g., Depakote) or
- Estrogens (female hormones) or
- Etretinate (e.g., Tegison) or
- Gold salts (medicine for arthritis) or
- Hydroxychloroquine (e.g., Plaquenil) or
- Mercaptopurine (e.g., Purinethol) or
- Methotrexate (e.g., Mexate) or
- Methyldopa (e.g., Aldomet) or
- Naltrexone (e.g., Trexan) (with long-term, high-dose use) or
- Oral contraceptives (birth control pills) containing estrogen or
- Other anti-infectives by mouth or by injection (medicine for infection) or
- Phenothiazines (acetophenazine [e.g., Tindal], chlorpromazine [e.g., Thorazine], fluphenazine [e.g., Prolixin], mesoridazine [e.g., Serentil], perphenazine [e.g., Trilafon], prochlorperazine [e.g., Compazine], promazine [e.g., Sparine], promethazine [e.g., Phenergan], thioridazine [e.g., Mellaril], trifluoperazine [e.g., Stelazine], triflupromazine [e.g., Vesprin], trimeprazine [e.g., Temaril]) or
- Plicamycin (e.g., Mithracin) or
- Valproic acid (e.g., Depakene)—Use of these medicines with azole antifungals may increase the chance of side effects affecting the liver
- Alprazolam (e.g., Xanax) or
- Diazepam (e.g., Valium) or
- Midazolam (e.g., Versed) or

- Triazolam (e.g., Halcion)—Sedative effects are increased when taken with fluconazole, itraconazole or ketoconazole. These medicines should not be taken together with itraconazole.
- Amantadine (e.g., Symmetrel) or
- Anticholinergics (medicine for abdominal or stomach spasms or cramps) or
- Antidepressants (medicine for depression) or
- Antidyskinetics (medicine for Parkinson's disease or other conditions affecting control of muscles) or
- Antihistamines or
- Antipsychotics (medicine for mental illness) or
- Buclizine (e.g., Bucladin) or
- Cyclizine (e.g., Marezine) or
- Cyclobenzaprine (e.g., Flexeril) or
- Disopyramide (e.g., Norpace) or
- Flavoxate (e.g., Urispas) or
- Ipratropium (e.g., Atrovent) or
- Meclizine (e.g., Antivert) or
- Methylphenidate (e.g., Ritalin) or
- Orphenadrine (e.g., Norflex) or
- Oxybutynin (e.g., Ditropan) or
- Procainamide (e.g., Pronestyl) or
- Promethazine (e.g., Phenergan) or
- Quinidine (e.g., Quinidex) or
- Trimeprazine (e.g., Temaril)—Use of these medicines may decrease the effects of itraconazole and ketoconazole; these medicines should be taken at least 2 hours after itraconazole or ketoconazole
- Antidiabetic agents, oral (chlorpropamide [e.g., Diabinese], glipizide [e.g., Glucotrol], glyburide [e.g., DiaBeta, Micronase], tolbutamide [e.g., Orinase])—May cause hypoglycemia (low blood sugar). Your doctor may need to adjust your dose.
- Antacids or
- Histamine H_2-receptor antagonists (cimetidine [e.g., Tagamet], famotidine [e.g., Pepcid], nizatidine [e.g., Axid], ranitidine [e.g., Zantac]) or
- Proton pump inhibitors (esomeprazole [e.g., Nexium], omeprazole [e.g., Losec]) or
- Sucralfate (e.g., Carafate)—These medicines may decrease itraconazole concentrations. They should be taken at least 1 hour before or 2 hours after you take itraconazole. Itraconazole should be taken with a cola beverage if you are taking any of these medicines.
- Astemizole (e.g., Hismanal) or
- Terfenadine (e.g., Seldane)—These medicines should not be taken with fluconazole, itraconazole, or ketoconazole; these azole antifungals may increase the chance of serious side effects of astemizole or terfenadine
- Atorvastatin (e.g., Lipitor) or
- Cerivastatin (e.g., Baycol) or
- Lovastatin (e.g., Mevacor) or
- Simvastatin (e.g., Zocor)—Use of these drugs with itraconazole or ketoconazole since increased levels of these drugs can cause serious muscular disorders. Lo-

vastatin and simvastatin should not be used together with itraconazole.
- Busulfan (e.g., Myleran) or
- Docetaxel (e.g., Taxotere) or
- Vinblastine (e.g., Velban) or
- Vincristine (e.g., Oncovin)—Metabolism of these drugs may be delayed by itraconazole.
- Felodipine (e.g., Plendil) or
- Nifedipine (e.g., Procardia) or
- Verapamil (e.g., Isoptin, Covera)—Concurrent use can cause water retention or slow the heart rate.
- Carbamazepine (e.g., Tegretol) or
- Phenobarbital (e.g., Luminal) or
- Phenytoin (e.g., Dilantin)—Concurrent use with itraconazole may decrease itraconazole concentrations. Carbamazepine and phenytoin concentrations may be increased.
- Cisapride (e.g., Propulsid)—Cisapride should not be taken with fluconazole, itraconazole or oral ketoconazole; these azole antifungals may increase the chance of serious side effects of cisapride.
- Cyclosporine (e.g., Sandimmune, Neoral) or
- Sirolimus (e.g., Rapamune) or
- Tacrolimus (e.g., Prograf)—Concomitant use may cause increased concentrations of these drugs, resulting in toxicity.
- Didanosine (e.g., ddI, Videx)—Use of didanosine with itraconazole or ketoconazole may decrease the effects of itraconazole or ketoconazole, as well as of didanosine. Itraconazole and ketoconazole should be taken at least 2 hours before or 2 hours after didanosine is given
- Digoxin (e.g., Lanoxin)—Digoxin concentrations may be increased, resulting in toxicity.
- Dofetilide (e.g., Tikosyn) or
- Pimozide (e.g., Orap) or
- Quinidine (e.g., Quinaglute, Cardioquin, Quinidex)—Pimozide, dofetilide and quinidine should not be taken with itraconazole; itraconazole may increase the chance of serious side effects of pimozide, dofetilide and quinidine.
- Ergot alkaloids (dihydroergotamine [e.g., Migranal], ergonovine [e.g., Ergotrate], ergotamine [e.g., Ergomar, Ergostat], methylergonovine [e.g., Methergine])—These medicines should not be taken with itraconazole; itraconazole may increase risk of serious side effects.
- Erythromycin (e.g., Ery-Tab)—Should not be used together with azole antifungals; severe heart problems may result.
- Indinavir (e.g., Crixivan) or
- Ritonavir (e.g., Norvir) or
- Saquinavir (e.g., Invirase)—Use of these drugs with itraconazole or ketoconazole may increase your risk of side effects from these medicines.
- Isoniazid or
- Rifampin (e.g., Rifadin)—These medicines may decrease the effects of azole antifungals
- Clarithromycin (e.g., Biaxin)—Plasma concentrations of itraconazole may be increased.

- Levomethadyl (e.g., Orlaam)—Itraconazole should not be used with levomethadyl; serious heart problems could result.
- Nevirapine (e.g., Viramune)—Plasma concentrations of itraconazole or ketoconazole may be decreased.
- Warfarin (e.g., Coumadin)—Anticoagulant effects may be increased.

Other medical problems—The presence of other medical problems may affect the use of azole antifungals. Make sure you tell your doctor if you have any other medical problems, especially:

- Congestive heart failure or
- Other heart problems—Itraconazole may make these conditions worse.
- Achlorhydria (absence of stomach acid) or
- Hypochlorhydria (decreased amount of stomach acid)—Itraconazole and ketoconazole may not be absorbed from the stomach as well in patients who have low levels of or no stomach acid
- Alcohol abuse (or history of) or
- Liver disease—Alcohol abuse or liver disease may increase the chance of side effects caused by azole antifungals
- Kidney disease—The effects of fluconazole may be increased in patients with kidney disease

Proper Use of This Medicine

Ketoconazole and the *capsule form of itraconazole* should be taken with a full meal. The *oral solution form of itraconazole* should be taken on an empty stomach. If you have any questions about the antifungal medicine you are taking, check with your health care professional.

For patients taking the *oral liquid form of fluconazole, itraconazole, or ketoconazole:*

- Use a specially marked measuring spoon or other device to measure each dose accurately. The average household teaspoon may not hold the right amount of liquid.

If you have achlorhydria (absence of stomach acid) or hypochlorhydria (decreased amount of stomach acid), and you are taking itraconazole or ketoconazole, your doctor may want you to take your medicine with an acidic drink. You may dissolve your medicine in cola or seltzer water and drink the solution, or your may take your medicine with a glass of cola or seltzer water. Your doctor may suggest that you dissolve each capsule or tablet in a teaspoonful of weak hydrochloric acid solution to help you absorb the medicine better. Your health care professional can prepare the solution for you. After you dissolve the tablet in the acid solution, add this mixture to a small amount (1 or 2 teaspoonfuls) of water in a glass. Drink the mixture through a plastic or glass drinking straw. Place the straw behind your teeth, as far back in your mouth as you can. This will keep the acid from harming your teeth. Be sure to drink all the liquid to get the full dose of medicine. Next, swish around in your mouth about one-half glass of water and then swallow it. This will help wash away any acid that may remain in your mouth or on your teeth.

To help clear up your infection completely, *it is very important that you keep taking this medicine for the full time of treatment,* even if your symptoms begin to clear up or you begin to feel better after a few days. Since fungus infections may be very slow to clear up, you may have to continue taking this medicine every day for as long as 6 months to a year or more. Some fungus infections never clear up completely and require continuous treatment. If you stop taking this medicine too soon, your symptoms may return.

This medicine works best when there is a constant amount in the blood. *To help keep the amount constant, do not miss any doses. Also, it is best to take each dose at the same time every day.* If you need help in planning the best time to take your medicine, check with your health care professional.

Dosing—The dose of azole antifungals may be different for different patients. *Follow your doctor's orders or the directions on the label.* The following information includes only the average doses of azole antifungals. Your dose of fluconazole may be different if you have kidney disease. *If your dose is different, do not change it* unless your doctor tells you to do so.

The number of capsules or tablets, or the amount of oral suspension or injection that you take depends on the strength of the medicine. Also, *the number of doses you take each day, the time allowed between doses, and the length of time you take the medicine depend on the medical problem for which you are taking azole antifungals.*

For fluconazole
- For fungus infections:
  - For *capsule* dosage form:
    - Adults—150 milligrams (mg) as a single dose to treat vaginal yeast infections.
    - Children up to 18 years of age—Dose must be determined by your doctor.
  - For *oral suspension* and *tablet* dosage forms:
    - Adults and teenagers—200 to 400 mg on the first day, then 100 to 400 mg once a day for weeks or months, depending on the medical problem being treated. A vaginal yeast infection is treated with a single dose of 150 mg.
    - Children 6 months of age and older—6 to 12 mg per kilogram (mg/kg) (2.7 to 5.4 mg per pound) of body weight on the first day, then 3 to 12 mg/kg (1.35 to 5.4 mg per pound) of body weight once a day for weeks or months, depending on the medical problem being treated.
    - Infants and children up to 6 months of age—Dose must be determined by your doctor.
  - For *injection* dosage form:
    - Adults and teenagers—200 to 400 mg on the first day, then 100 to 400 mg once a day, injected into a vein, for weeks or months, depending on the medical problem being treated.
    - Children 6 months of age and older—6 to 12 mg per kilogram (mg/kg) (2.7 to 5.4 mg per pound) of body weight on the first day, then 3 to 12 mg/kg (1.35 to 5.4 mg per pound) of body weight once a day, injected into a vein, for weeks or months, depending on the medical problem being treated.
    - Infants and children up to 6 months of age—Dose must be determined by your doctor.

For itraconazole
- For fungus infections:
  - For *capsule* dosage form:
    - Adults and teenagers—200 milligrams (mg) once a day, which may be increased up to 400 mg once a day for weeks or months, depending on the medical problem being treated. Fingernail and toenail

infections are treated with 200 mg one or two times a day for weeks or months.
- Children up to 16 years of age—Dose must be determined by your doctor.
  - ° For *injection* dosage form:
    - Adults—200 milligrams (mg) twice a day for 4 doses, then 200 mg once a day.
    - Children—Dose must be determined by your doctor.
  - ° For *oral solution* dosage form:
    - Adults and teenagers—100 to 200 mg once a day for days or weeks, depending on the medical problem being treated.
    - Children up to 12 years of age—Dose must be determined by your doctor.
- For febrile neutropenia (low white blood cell count with a fever):
  - ° For *oral solution* dosage form:
    - Adults and teenagers—200 milligrams (mg) twice a day until your doctor tells you to stop taking this medicine. Your doctor will have you use itraconazole for injection before being switched to oral solution.
    - Children up to 16 years of age—Dose must be determined by your doctor.
  - ° For *injection* dosage form:
    - Adults—200 milligrams (mg) twice a day for 4 doses, then 200 mg once a day for up to 14 days. Your doctor will have you start taking oral solution after you have completed your treatment with this injection dosage form.
    - Children—Dose must be determined by your doctor.

For ketoconazole
- For fungus infections:
  - ° For *oral* dosage form (oral suspension and tablets):
    - Adults and teenagers—200 to 400 milligrams (mg) once a day for days or weeks, depending on the medical problem being treated.
    - Children over 2 years of age—3.3 to 6.6 mg per kilogram (1.5 to 3 mg per pound) of body weight once a day for days or weeks, depending on the medical problem being treated.
    - Infants and children up to 2 years of age—Dose must be determined by your doctor.

Missed dose—If you miss a dose of this medicine, take it as soon as possible. This will help to keep a constant amount of medicine in the blood. However, if it is almost time for your next dose, skip the missed dose and go back to your regular dosing schedule. Do not double doses.

Storage—To store this medicine:
- Keep out of the reach of children.
- Store away from heat and direct light.
- Do not store the capsule or tablet form of this medicine in the bathroom, near the kitchen sink, or in other damp places. Heat or moisture may cause the medicine to break down.
- Keep the oral liquid form of this medicine from freezing.
- Do not keep outdated medicine or medicine no longer needed. Be sure that any discarded medicine is out of the reach of children.

Precautions While Using This Medicine

It is important that your doctor check your progress at regular visits. This will allow your doctor to check for any unwanted effects.

If your symptoms do not improve within a few weeks (or months for some infections), or if they become worse, check with your doctor.

These medicines should not be taken with astemizole (e.g., Hismanal), cisapride (e.g., Propulsid), dofetilide (e.g., Tikosyn) or terfenadine (e.g., Seldane). Doing so may increase the risk of serious side effects affecting the heart.

Liver problems may be more likely to occur if you drink alcoholic beverages while you are taking ketoconazole. Alcoholic beverages may also cause stomach pain, nausea, vomiting, headache, or flushing or redness of the face. Other alcohol-containing preparations (for example, elixirs, cough syrups, tonics) may also cause problems. These problems may occur for at least a day after you stop taking ketoconazole. Therefore, *you should not drink alcoholic beverages or use alcohol-containing preparations while you are taking this medicine and for at least a day after you stop taking it.*

If you are taking antacids, cimetidine (e.g., Tagamet), famotidine (e.g., Pepcid), nizatidine (e.g., Axid), omeprazole (e.g., Prilosec), or ranitidine (e.g., Zantac) while you are taking itraconazole or ketoconazole, take the other medicine at least 2 hours after you take itraconazole or ketoconazole. If you take these medicines at the same time that you take itraconazole or ketoconazole, they will keep your antifungal medicine from working properly.

Ketoconazole may cause your eyes to become more sensitive to light than they are normally. Wearing sunglasses and avoiding too much exposure to bright light may help lessen the discomfort.

Side Effects of This Medicine

Along with its needed effects, a medicine may cause some unwanted effects. Although not all of these effects may occur, if they do occur they may need medical attention.

Check with your doctor immediately if any of the following side effects occur:
> *Less common*
>> Fever and chills; skin rash or itching
> *Rare*
>> Dark or amber urine; fever and sore throat; loss of appetite; pale stools; reddening, blistering, peeling, or loosening of skin and mucous membranes; stomach pain; unusual bleeding or bruising; unusual tiredness or weakness; yellow eyes or skin
> *Incidence not known—Itraconazole—*occurred during clinical practice for itraconazole
>> Abdominal pain; black, tarry stools; blistering, peeling or loosening of skin; bloating or swelling of face, arms, hands, lower legs, or feet; blue lips and fingernails; blurred vision; burning, numbness, tingling, or painful sensations; chest pain; chills; continuing vomiting; convulsions; cough; coughing that sometimes produces a pink frothy sputum; decreased urine output; difficult, fast, noisy breathing, sometimes with wheezing; difficulty swallowing; dilated neck veins; dry mouth; extreme fatigue; fast heartbeat; fatigue; flushed, dry skin;

fruit-like breath odor; general feeling of tiredness or weakness; hives or welts; increased hunger; increased sweating; increased thirst; increased urination; irregular breathing; irregular heartbeat; itching skin; joint or muscle pain; large amount of triglyceride in the blood; large, hive-like swelling on face, eyelids, lips, tongue, throat, hands, legs, feet, sex organs; light-colored stools; lower back or side pain; mood changes; muscle pain or cramps; numbness or tingling in hands, feet, or lips; painful or difficult urination; pale skin; pale stools; puffiness; rapid weight gain; red skin lesions, often with a purple center; red, irritated eyes; redness of skin; shortness of breath; skin rash or itching; sores, ulcers, or white spots in mouth or on lips; sweating; swelling in legs and ankles; swelling of face, fingers, feet, or lower legs; swelling of the eyelids or around the eyes, face, lips, or tongue; tightness in chest; tingling of hands or feet; troubled breathing; unexplained weight loss; unsteadiness or awkwardness; unusual weight gain or loss; upper right abdominal pain; weakness in arms, hands, legs, or feet; weight gain; wheezing

Incidence not known—Fluconazole—occurred during clinical practice for fluconazole

black, tarry, stools; chest pain or discomfort; convulsions; cough; decreased urine; diarrhea; dry mouth; fainting; increased thirst; irregular or slow heartbeat; joint or muscle pain; large amount of cholesterol in the blood; large amount of triglyceride in the blood; large, hive-like swelling on face, eyelids, lips, tongue, throat, hands, legs, feet, sex organs; loss of bladder control; lower back or side pain; mood changes; muscle pain or cramps; muscle spasm or jerking of all extremities; nausea or vomiting; numbness or tingling in hands, feet, or lips; painful or difficult urination; pale skin; red irritated eyes; red skin lesions, often with a purple center; shortness of breath; sore throat; sores, ulcers, or white spots in mouth or on lips; sudden loss of consciousness

Other side effects may occur that usually do not need medical attention. These side effects may go away during treatment as your body adjusts to the medicine. However, check with your doctor if any of the following side effects continue or are bothersome:

Less common

Constipation; diarrhea; dizziness; drowsiness; headache; nausea; vomiting

Rare—for ketoconazole

Decreased sexual ability in males; enlargement of the breasts in males; increased sensitivity of the eyes to light; menstrual irregularities

Incidence not known—Fluconazole—occurred during clinical practice for fluconazole

acid or sour stomach; bad unusual or unpleasant taste in mouth; belching; change in taste; hair loss; heartburn; indigestion; stomach discomfort, upset or pain; swelling of face; thinning of hair

Other side effects not listed above may also occur in some patients. If you notice any other effects, check with your doctor.

Additional Information

Once a medicine has been approved for marketing for a certain use, experience may show that it is also useful for other medical problems. Although these uses are not included in

product labeling, azole antifungals are used in certain patients with the following medical conditions:

- Cryptococcosis
- Cushing's syndrome
- Fungus infections in newborns
- Hirsutism
- Histoplasmosis
- Paronychia (infection of the tissue surrounding the nail)
- Penicillium marneffei infection
- Pneumonia caused by fungus
- Prostate cancer
- Ringworm of the beard, hand, or scalp
- Septicemia (infection of the blood) caused by fungus
- Skin infection (including leishmaniasis and sporotrichosis)

Other than the above information, there is no additional information relating to proper use, precautions, or side effects for these uses.

ANTIFUNGALS, AZOLE (Vaginal)

Some commonly used brand names are:

In the U.S.—

FemCare (2)	Monistat 3 (4)
Femizol-M (4)	Monistat 3 Combination Pack
Femstat 3 (1)	(4)
Gyne-Lotrimin (2)	Monistat 5 Tampon (4)
Gyne-Lotrimin Combination	Monistat 7 (4)
Pack (2)	Monistat 7 Combination Pack
Gyne-Lotrimin3 (2)	(4)
Gyne-Lotrimin3 Combination	Mycelex-7 (2)
Pack (2)	Mycelex-G (2)
Miconazole-7 (4)	Mycelex Twin Pack (2)
Monistat 1 (6)	Terazol 3 (5)
Monistat 1 Combination Pack	Terazol 7 (5)
(4)	Vagistat-1 (6)

In Canada—

Canesten Combi-Pak 1–Day	Micozole (4)
Therapy (2)	Monazole 7 (4)
Canesten Combi-Pak 3–Day	Monistat 3 Dual-Pak (4)
Therapy (2)	Monistat 3 Vaginal Ovules (4)
Canesten 1–Day Cream	Monistat 7 (4)
Combi-Pak (2)	Monistat 7 Dual-Pak (4)
Canesten 1–Day Therapy (2)	Monistat 7 Vaginal
Canesten 3–Day Therapy (2)	Suppositories (4)
Canesten 6–Day Therapy (2)	Myclo-Gyne (2)
Clotrimaderm (2)	Novo-Miconazole Vaginal
Ecostatin Vaginal Ovules (3)	Ovules (4)
GyneCure (6)	Terazol 3 (5)
GyneCure Ovules (6)	Terazol 3 Dual Pak (5)
GyneCure Vaginal Ointment	Terazol 3 Vaginal Ovules (5)
Tandempak (6)	Terazol 7 (5)
GyneCure Vaginal Ovules	
Tandempak (6)	

This information applies to the following medicines

1. Butoconazole (byoo-toe-KON-a-zole)
2. Clotrimazole (kloe-TRIM-a-zole)
3. Econazole (e-KON-a-zole)
4. Miconazole (mi-KON-a-zole)
5. Terconazole (ter-KON-a-zole)
6. Tioconazole (tye-oh-KON-a-zole)

Category

- **Antifungal, vaginal**—Butoconazole; Clotrimazole; Econazole; Miconazole; Terconazole; Tioconazole

Description

Vaginal azoles (A-zoles) are used to treat yeast (fungus) infections of the vagina.

For first-time users, make sure your doctor has checked and confirmed that you have a vaginal yeast infection before you use the vaginal azole antifungal medicines that do not require a prescription. Vaginal yeast infections can reoccur over time and, when the same symptoms occur again, self-treating with these medicines is recommended. However, you should see your doctor if the symptoms occur again within 2 months.

Some vaginal azoles are available only with your doctor's prescription. Most are available without a prescription; however, your doctor may have special instructions on the proper use of this medicine.

Vaginal azoles are available in the following dosage forms:

Vaginal
- Butoconazole
  - Cream
- Clotrimazole
  - Cream
  - Tablets
- Econazole
  - Suppositories
- Miconazole
  - Cream
  - Suppositories
  - Tampons (U.S.—California only)
- Terconazole
  - Cream
  - Suppositories
- Tioconazole
  - Ointment
  - Suppositories

Before Using This Medicine

In deciding to use a medicine, the risks of using the medicine must be weighed against the good it will do. This is a decision you and your doctor will make. For vaginal azoles, the following should be considered:

Allergies—Tell your doctor if you have ever had any unusual or allergic reaction to any of the azoles. Also tell your health care professional if you are allergic to any other substances, such as foods, preservatives, or dyes.

Pregnancy—Studies have not been done in humans for use of all azole antifungals during the first trimester of pregnancy. These medicines are safe and effective when used for at least 7 days during the second and third trimesters of pregnancy. However, check with your doctor before using this medicine during the first trimester of pregnancy. Also, use of 1– and 3–day treatments may not be effective during pregnancy.

Breast-feeding—It is not known whether vaginal azoles pass into the breast milk. However, these medicines have not been shown to cause problems in nursing babies.

Children—Studies on these medicines have been done only in adult patients, and there is no specific information comparing use of vaginal azoles in children with use in other age groups. It is recommended that these medicines not be used in children up to 12 years of age.

Older adults—Many medicines have not been studied specifically in older people. Therefore, it may not be known whether they work exactly the same way they do in younger adults. Although there is no specific information comparing use of vaginal azoles in the elderly with use in other age groups, they are not expected to cause different side effects or problems in older people than they do in younger adults.

Other medicines—Although certain medicines should not be used together at all, in other cases two different medicines may be used together even if an interaction might occur. In these cases, your doctor may want to change the dose, or other precautions may be necessary. Tell your health care professional if you are using any other vaginal prescription or nonprescription (over-the-counter [OTC]) medicine. When you are taking miconazole, it is especially important that your health care professional know if you are taking any of the following:

- Warfarin (e.g., Coumadin; Warfilone)—Using with warfarin may cause bleeding and/or bruising

Proper Use of This Medicine

Vaginal azoles usually come with patient directions. Read them carefully before using this medicine.

Use this medicine at bedtime, unless otherwise directed by your doctor. The vaginal tampon form of miconazole should be left in the vagina overnight and removed the next morning.

This medicine is usually inserted into the vagina with an applicator. However, if you are pregnant, check with your doctor before using the applicator.

Some of the vaginal suppositories or tablets come packaged with a small tube of cream. This cream can be applied outside of the vagina in the genital area to treat itching. The packages are called combination, dual, or twin packs.

To help clear up your infection completely, *it is very important that you keep using this medicine for the full time of treatment*, even if your symptoms begin to clear up after a few days. If you stop using this medicine too soon, your symptoms may return. *Do not miss any doses. Also, do not stop using this medicine if your menstrual period starts during the time of treatment.*

Dosing—The dose of these medicines will be different for different patients. *Follow your doctor's orders or the directions on the label.* The following information includes only the average doses of these medicines. *If your dose is different, do not change it* unless your doctor tells you to do so.

For butoconazole
- For yeast infection:
  - For *vaginal cream* dosage form:
    - Adults and teenagers:
      — Women who are not pregnant: 100 milligrams (mg) (one full applicator) of 2% cream inserted into the vagina at bedtime for three nights in a row.
      — Pregnant women, after the third month: 100 mg (one full applicator) of 2% cream inserted into the vagina at bedtime for six nights in a row.
    - Children up to 12 years of age—Use and dose must be determined by your doctor.

- For *vaginal suppository* dosage form:
  - Adults and teenagers:
    - Women who are not pregnant: 100 mg (one suppository) inserted into the vagina at bedtime for three nights in a row.
    - Children up to 12 years of age—Use and dose must be determined by your doctor.

For clotrimazole
- For yeast infection:
  - For *vaginal cream* dosage form:
    - Adults and teenagers—The dose depends on the strength of the cream.
      - 1% cream: 50 milligrams (mg) (one full applicator) inserted into the vagina at bedtime for six to fourteen nights in a row.
      - 2% cream: 100 mg (one full applicator) inserted into the vagina at bedtime for three nights in a row.
      - 10% cream: 500 mg (one full applicator) inserted into the vagina at bedtime for one night only.
    - Children up to 12 years of age—Use and dose must be determined by your doctor.
  - For *vaginal tablet* dosage form:
    - Adults and teenagers—The dose depends on the strength of the vaginal tablet.
      - Women who are not pregnant:
        - 100–mg tablet: Insert one tablet into the vagina at bedtime for six or seven nights in a row.
        - 200–mg tablet: Insert one tablet into the vagina at bedtime for three nights in a row.
        - 500–mg tablet: Insert one tablet into the vagina at bedtime for one night only.
      - Pregnant women: 100 mg (one vaginal tablet) inserted into the vagina at bedtime for seven nights in a row.
    - Children up to 12 years of age—Use and dose must be determined by your doctor.

For econazole
- For yeast infection:
  - For *vaginal suppository* dosage form:
    - Adults and teenagers—150 milligrams (mg) (one vaginal suppository) inserted into the vagina at bedtime for three nights in a row.
    - Children up to 12 years of age—Use and dose must be determined by your doctor.

For miconazole
- For yeast infection:
  - For *vaginal cream* dosage form:
    - Adults and teenagers—20 milligrams (one full applicator) inserted into the vagina at bedtime for seven nights in a row. Treatment may be repeated if needed.
    - Children up to 12 years of age—Use and dose must be determined by your doctor.
  - For *vaginal suppository* dosage form:
    - Adults and teenagers—The dose depends on the strength of the suppository.
      - 100–milligram (mg) suppository: Insert one vaginal suppository into the vagina at bedtime for seven nights in a row. Treatment may be repeated if needed.
      - 200–mg suppository or

- 400–mg suppository: Insert one vaginal suppository into the vagina at bedtime for three nights in a row. Treatment may be repeated if needed.
      - 1200–mg suppository: Insert one vaginal suppository into the vagina at bedtime for one night.
    - Children up to 12 years of age—Use and dose must be determined by your doctor.
  - For *tampon* dosage form:
    - Adults and teenagers—100 mg (one tampon) inserted into the vagina at bedtime and then removed the next morning. This is repeated every night for five nights in a row.
    - Children up to 12 years of age—Use and dose must be determined by your doctor.

For terconazole
- For yeast infection:
  - For *vaginal cream* dosage form:
    - Adults and teenagers—The dose depends on the strength of the cream.
      - 0.4% cream: 20 milligrams (mg) (one full applicator) inserted into the vagina at bedtime for seven nights in a row.
      - 0.8% cream: 40 mg (one full applicator) inserted into the vagina at bedtime for three nights in a row.
    - Children up to 12 years of age—Use and dose must be determined by your doctor.
  - For *vaginal suppository* dosage form:
    - Adults and teenagers—80 mg (one vaginal suppository) inserted into the vagina at bedtime for three nights in a row.
    - Children up to 12 years of age—Use and dose must be determined by your doctor.

For tioconazole
- For yeast infection:
  - For *vaginal ointment* dosage form:
    - Adults and teenagers—300 milligrams (mg) (one full applicator) of 6.5% ointment inserted into the vagina at bedtime for one night only.
    - Children up to 12 years of age—Use and dose must be determined by your doctor.
  - For *vaginal suppository* dosage form:
    - Adults and teenagers—300 mg (one vaginal suppository) inserted into the vagina at bedtime for one night only.
    - Children up to 12 years of age—Use and dose must be determined by your doctor.

Missed dose—If you miss a dose of this medicine, insert it as soon as possible. However, if it is almost time for your next dose, skip the missed dose and go back to your regular dosing schedule.

Storage—To store this medicine:
- Keep out of the reach of children.
- Store away from heat and direct light.
- Do not store the vaginal suppository or vaginal tablet form of this medicine in the bathroom, near the kitchen sink, or in other damp places. Heat or moisture may cause the medicine to break down.
- Keep the vaginal cream, ointment, and suppository forms of this medicine from freezing.

• Do not keep outdated medicine or medicine no longer needed. Be sure that any discarded medicine is out of the reach of children.

Precautions While Using This Medicine

If your symptoms do not improve within 3 days or have not disappeared in 7 days, or if they become worse, check with your doctor. The 1– or 3–day treatments may take up to 7 days to completely clear up your infection. However, not all vaginal infections are caused by yeast. If symptoms occur again within 2 months, check with your doctor.

Vaginal medicines usually will come out of the vagina during treatment. To keep the medicine from getting on your clothing, wear a minipad or sanitary napkin. The use of non-medicated tampons (like those used for menstrual periods) is not recommended since they may soak up the medicine.

To help clear up your infection completely and to help make sure it does not return, good health habits are also required.

• Wear cotton panties (or panties or pantyhose with cotton crotches) instead of synthetic (for example, nylon or rayon) panties.

• Wear only clean panties.

If you have any questions about this, check with your health care professional.

Vaginal yeast infections are not usually spread by having sex and your sex partner does not need to be treated. However, if the sex partner has symptoms of local itching or skin irritation of the penis, he may benefit by being treated also.

If you use latex or rubber birth control devices (condoms, diaphragms, or cervical caps), you should wait 3 days after treatment with azole antifungal agents before using them again. Many brands of vaginal azoles contain oils in the product that can weaken these devices. This increases the chances of a condom breaking during sexual intercourse. The rubber in cervical caps or diaphragms may break down faster and wear out sooner. Check with your health care professional to make sure the vaginal azole product you are using can be used with latex rubber birth control devices.

Check with your doctor before douching to obtain advice about whether you may douche and, if allowed, the proper method.

Side Effects

Along with its needed effects, a medicine may cause some unwanted effects. Although not all of these side effects may occur, if they do occur they may need medical attention.

Check with your doctor as soon as possible if any of the following side effects occur:

Less common
Vaginal burning, itching, discharge, or other irritation not present before use of this medicine

Rare
Skin rash or hives

Other side effects may occur that usually do not need medical attention. These side effects may go away during treatment as your body adjusts to the medicine. However, check with your doctor if any of the following side effects continue or are bothersome:

Less common or rare
Abdominal or stomach cramps or pain; burning or irritation of penis of sexual partner; headache

Other side effects not listed above may also occur in some patients. If you notice any other effects, check with your doctor.

ANTIGLAUCOMA AGENTS, CHOLINERGIC, LONG-ACTING (Ophthalmic)

Some commonly used brand names are:

In the U.S.—
Humorsol (1)
Phospholine Iodide (2)

In Canada—
Phospholine Iodide (2)

This information applies to the following medicines:

1. Demecarium (dem-e-KARE-ee-um)
2. Echothiophate (ek-oh-THYE-oh-fate)
3. Isoflurophate (eye-soe-FLURE-oh-fate)

Category

• **Antiglaucoma agent, ophthalmic**—Demecarium; Echothiophate; Isoflurophate

• **Cyclostimulant, accommodative esotropia**—Demecarium; Echothiophate; Isoflurophate

• **Diagnostic aid, accommodative esotropia**—Demecarium; Echothiophate; Isoflurophate

Description

Demecarium, echothiophate, and isoflurophate are used in the eye to treat certain types of glaucoma and other eye conditions, such as accommodative esotropia. They may also be used in the diagnosis of certain eye conditions, such as accommodative esotropia.

These medicines are available only with your doctor's prescription, in the following dosage forms:

Ophthalmic
• Demecarium
  ◦ Ophthalmic solution (eye drops)
• Echothiophate
  ◦ Ophthalmic solution (eye drops)
• Isoflurophate
  ◦ Ophthalmic ointment (eye ointment) (France)

Before Using This Medicine

In deciding to use a medicine, the risks of using the medicine must be weighed against the good it will do. This is a decision you and your doctor will make. For demecarium, echothiophate, or isoflurophate, the following should be considered:

Allergies—Tell your doctor if you have ever had any unusual or allergic reaction to demecarium, echothiophate, or isoflurophate. Also tell your health care professional if you are allergic to any other substances, such as preservatives.

Pregnancy—Because of the toxicity of these medicines in general, demecarium, echothiophate, and isoflurophate are not recommended during pregnancy.

Breast-feeding—Demecarium, echothiophate, and isoflurophate may be absorbed into the body. These medicines are not recommended during breast-feeding, because they may cause unwanted effects in nursing babies. It may be necessary for you to use another medicine or to stop breast-feeding during treatment. Be sure you have discussed the risks and benefits of the medicine with your doctor.

Children—Demecarium, echothiophate, or isoflurophate can cause serious side effects in any patient. When this medicine is used for a long time, eye cysts may occur. These eye cysts occur more often in children than in adults. Therefore, it is especially important that you discuss with the child's doctor the good that this medicine may do as well as the risks of using it.

Older adults—Many medicines have not been studied specifically in older people. Therefore, it may not be known whether they work exactly the same way they do in younger adults or if they cause different side effects or problems in older people. There is no specific information comparing use of these medicines in the elderly with use in other age groups. However, demecarium, echothiophate, or isoflurophate can cause serious side effects in any patient.

Other medicines—Although certain medicines should not be used together at all, in other cases two different medicines may be used together even if an interaction might occur. In these cases, your doctor may want to change the dose, or other precautions may be necessary. When you are taking demecarium, echothiophate, or isoflurophate, it is especially important that your health care professional know if you are taking any of the following:

- Amantadine (e.g., Symmetrel) or
- Anticholinergics (medicine for abdominal or stomach spasms or cramps) or
- Antidepressants (medicine for depression) or
- Antidyskinetics (medicine for Parkinson's disease or other conditions affecting control of muscles) or
- Antihistamines or
- Antimyasthenics (ambenonium [e.g., Mytelase], neostigmine [e.g., Prostigmin], pyridostigmine [e.g., Mestinon]) or
- Antipsychotics (medicine for mental illness) or
- Buclizine (e.g., Bucladin) or
- Carbamazepine (e.g., Tegretol) or
- Cyclizine (e.g., Marezine) or
- Cyclobenzaprine (e.g., Flexeril) or
- Disopyramide (e.g., Norpace) or
- Flavoxate (e.g., Urispas) or
- Ipratropium (e.g., Atrovent) or
- Meclizine (e.g., Antivert) or
- Methylphenidate (e.g., Ritalin) or
- Orphenadrine (e.g., Norflex) or
- Oxybutynin (e.g., Ditropen) or
- Procainamide (e.g., Pronestyl) or
- Promethazine (e.g., Phenergan) or
- Quinidine (e.g., Quinidex) or
- Trimeprazine (e.g., Temaril)—May increase the possibility of side effects or toxic effects; use of these medicines with demecarium, echothiophate, or isoflurophate is not recommended except under close supervision by your doctor

- Malathion (topical) (e.g., Prioderm)—May increase the possibility of side effects or toxic effects, especially if large amounts of malathion are used

Pesticides or insecticides—Make sure you tell your doctor if you have been exposed recently to pesticides or insecticides.

Other medical problems—The presence of other medical problems may affect the use of demecarium, echothiophate, or isoflurophate. Make sure you tell your doctor if you have any other medical problems, especially:

- Asthma or
- Epilepsy or
- Heart disease or
- High or low blood pressure (severe) or
- Myasthenia gravis or
- Overactive thyroid or
- Parkinsonism or
- Stomach ulcer or other stomach problems or
- Urinary tract blockage—If this medicine is absorbed into the body, it may make the condition worse
- Down's syndrome (mongolism)—This medicine may cause these children to become hyperactive
- Eye disease or problems (other)—May increase absorption of this medicine into the body or this medicine may make the condition worse

Proper Use of This Medicine

To use the *ophthalmic solution (eye drops) form* of this medicine:

- First, wash your hands. Tilt the head back and, pressing your finger gently on the skin just beneath the lower eyelid, pull the lower eyelid away from the eye to make a space. Drop the medicine into this space. Let go of the eyelid and gently close the eyes. Do not blink. Keep the eyes closed and apply pressure to the inner corner of the eye with your finger for 1 or 2 minutes to allow the medicine to be absorbed by the eye.
- Remove any excess solution around the eye with a clean tissue, being careful not to touch the eye.
- Immediately after using the eye drops, wash your hands to remove any medicine that may be on them.
- To keep the medicine as germ-free as possible, do not touch the applicator tip to any surface (including the eye). Also, keep the container tightly closed.
- The preservative in the eye drops containing the medicine, demecarium, may be absorbed by soft contact lenses. If you wear soft contact lenses, and your doctor has informed you that you can wear them while taking this medication, you should wait at least 15 minutes after applying the eye drops before inserting your lenses.

To use the *ophthalmic ointment (eye ointment) form* of this medicine:

- First, wash your hands. Tilt the head back and, pressing your finger gently on the skin just beneath the lower eyelid, pull the lower eyelid away from the eye to make a space. Squeeze a thin strip of ointment into this space. A ½-cm (approximately ¼-inch) strip of ointment is usually enough, unless you have been told by your doctor to use a different amount. Let go of the eyelid and gently close the eyes. Keep the eyes closed for 1 to 2 minutes to allow the medicine to be absorbed by the eye.

- Immediately after using the eye ointment, wash your hands to remove any medicine that may be on them.
- Since isoflurophate loses its effectiveness when exposed to moisture, do not wash the tip of the ointment tube or allow it to touch any moist surface (including the eye).
- To keep the medicine as germ-free as possible, do not touch the applicator tip to any surface (including the eye). After using this eye ointment, wipe the tip of the ointment tube with a clean tissue and keep the tube tightly closed.

It is very important that you use this medicine only as directed. Do not use more of it and do not use it more often than your doctor ordered. To do so may increase the chance of too much medicine being absorbed into the body and the chance of side effects.

If the applicator tip touches any surface (including the eye), it may become contaminated with bacteria, which may increase the chance of developing an eye infection. If you think the applicator has become contaminated, notify your doctor immediately.

Eye ointment usually causes blurred vision for a short time after you use it, and eye drops containing these medicines may affect your vision for several hours after you use them. Therefore, ask your doctor if the dose (or one of the doses if you use more than 1 dose a day) can be used at bedtime.

Dosing—The doses of these medicines will be different for different patients. *Follow your doctor's orders or the directions on the label.* The following information includes only the average doses of these medicines. *If your dose is different, do not change it* unless your doctor tells you to do so.

For demecarium
- For *ophthalmic solution (eye drops)* dosage form:
  ○ For glaucoma:
    ▪ Adults and older children—Use one drop in the eye one or two times a day.
    ▪ Infants and young children—Use and dose must be determined by your doctor.
  ○ For treatment of accommodative esotropia:
    ▪ Adults and older children—Use one drop in the eye once a day for two to three weeks, then one drop in the eye once every two days for three to four weeks, then use as determined by the doctor.
    ▪ Infants and young children—Use and dose must be determined by your doctor.
  ○ For diagnosis of accommodative esotropia:
    ▪ Adults and older children—Use one drop in the eye once a day for two weeks, then one drop in the eye once every two days for two to three weeks.
    ▪ Infants and young children—Use and dose must be determined by your doctor.

For echothiophate
- For *ophthalmic solution (eye drops)* dosage form:
  ○ For glaucoma:
    ▪ Adults and older children—Use one drop in the eye one or two times a day.
    ▪ Infants and younger children—Use and dose must be determined by your doctor.
  ○ For treatment of accommodative esotropia:
    ▪ Adults and older children—Use one drop in the eye once a day or one drop in the eye once every two days.

- Infants and young children—Use and dose must be determined by your doctor.
  ○ For diagnosis of accommodative esotropia:
    ▪ Adults and older children—Use one drop in the eye once a day at bedtime for two to three weeks.
    ▪ Infants and young children—Use and dose must be determined by your doctor.

For isoflurophate
- For *ophthalmic ointment* dosage form:
  ○ For glaucoma:
    ▪ Adults and older children—Use the ointment in the eyes once every three days or as often as three times a day as directed by the doctor.
    ▪ Infants and young children—Use and dose must be determined by your doctor.
  ○ For treatment of accommodative esotropia:
    ▪ Adults and older children—Use the ointment in the eyes once a day at bedtime for two weeks, then once a week or as often as once every two days as directed by the doctor.
    ▪ Infants and young children—Use and dose must be determined by your doctor.
  ○ For diagnosis of accommodative esotropia:
    ▪ Adults and older children—Use the ointment in the eyes once a day at bedtime for two weeks.
    ▪ Infants and young children—Use and dose must be determined by your doctor.

Missed dose—If you miss a dose of this medicine and your dosing schedule is:

- One dose every other day—Use the missed dose as soon as possible if you remember it on the day it should be used. However, if you do not remember the missed dose until the next day, use it at that time. Then skip a day and start your dosing schedule again. Do not double doses.

- One dose a day—Use the missed dose as soon as possible. However, if you do not remember the missed dose until the next day, skip the missed dose and go back to your regular dosing schedule. Do not double doses.

- More than one dose a day—Use the missed dose as soon as possible. However, if it is almost time for your next dose, skip the missed dose and go back to your regular dosing schedule. Do not double doses.

If your dosing schedule is different from all of the above and you miss a dose of this medicine, or if you have any questions about this, check with your doctor.

Storage—To store this medicine:

- Keep out of the reach of children. Overdose of demecarium, echothiophate, or isoflurophate is very dangerous in young children.
- Store away from heat and direct light.
- Keep this medicine from freezing.
- Do not keep outdated medicine or medicine no longer needed. Be sure that any discarded medicine is out of the reach of children.

Precautions While Using This Medicine

If you are using this medicine for glaucoma, your doctor should check your eye pressure at regular visits to make sure the medicine is working.

If you will be using this medicine for a long time, your doctor should examine your eyes at regular visits to make sure this medicine does not cause unwanted effects.

Before you have any kind of surgery (including eye surgery), dental treatment, or emergency treatment, tell the medical doctor or dentist in charge and the anesthesiologist or anesthetist (the person who puts you to sleep) that you are using this medicine or have used it within the past month.

These medicines should not be used if an eye infection is present, or if the eye is wounded or injured. If redness, pain, or discharge develops, or if a foreign object becomes lodged in one or both eyes, or if you suffer a blow to the eye or eye area, notify your doctor immediately.

Avoid breathing in even small amounts of carbamate- or organophosphate-type insecticides or pesticides (for example, carbaryl [Sevin], demeton [Systox], diazinon, malathion, parathion, ronnel [Trolene], or TEPP). They may add to the effects of this medicine. Farmers, gardeners, residents of communities undergoing insecticide or pesticide spraying or dusting, workers in plants manufacturing such products, or other persons exposed to such poisons should protect themselves by wearing a mask over the nose and mouth, changing clothes frequently, and washing hands often.

Make sure your vision is clear before you drive, use machines, or do anything else that could be dangerous if you are not able to see well. This is because:
- After you apply this medicine to your eyes, your pupils may become unusually small. This may cause you to see less well at night or in dim light.
- After you begin using this medicine, your vision may be blurred or there may be a change in your near or distance vision.
- The eye ointment form of this medicine usually causes blurred vision for a short time after you apply it.

Side Effects

Along with its needed effects, a medicine may cause some unwanted effects. Although not all of these side effects may occur, if they do occur they may need medical attention.

Check with your doctor immediately if any of the following side effects occur:

Rare
Burning, redness, stinging, or other eye irritation; eye pain; veil or curtain appearing across part of vision

Symptoms of too much medicine being absorbed into the body
Increased sweating; loss of bladder control; muscle weakness; nausea, vomiting, diarrhea, or stomach cramps or pain; shortness of breath, tightness in chest, or wheezing; slow or irregular heartbeat; unusual tiredness or weakness; watering of mouth

Other side effects may occur that usually do not need medical attention. These side effects may go away during treatment as your body adjusts to the medicine. However, check with your doctor if any of the following side effects continue or are bothersome:
Blurred vision or change in near or distance vision; difficulty in seeing at night or in dim light; headache or browache; twitching of eyelids; watering of eyes

Other side effects not listed above may also occur in some patients. If you notice any other effects, check with your doctor.

ANTIHISTAMINES (Systemic)

Some commonly used brand names are:

In the U.S.—

Alavert (14)	Genahist (10)
Allegra (12)	Gen-Allerate (4)
Aller-Chlor (4)	Hydrate (9)
AllerMax Caplets (10)	Hyrexin (10)
Aller-med (10)	Hyzine-50 (13)
Atarax (13)	Nasahist B (2)
Banophen (10)	Nervine Nighttime Sleep-Aid
Banophen Caplets (10)	(10)
Benadryl (10)	Nolahist (15)
Benadryl Allergy (10)	Nytol QuickCaps (10)
Bromphen (2)	Nytol QuickGels (10)
Calm X (9)	Optimine (1)
Chlo-Amine (4)	PediaCare Allergy Formula (4)
Chlorate (4)	Periactin (6)
Chlor-Trimeton (4)	Phenetron (4)
Chlor-Trimeton Allergy (4)	Polaramine (8)
Chlor-Trimeton Repetabs	Polaramine Repetabs (8)
(4)	Siladryl (10)
Clarinex (7)	Sleep-Eze D (10)
Claritin (14)	Sleep-Eze D Extra Strength
Claritin Reditabs (14)	(10)
Compoz (10)	Sominex (10)
Contac 12 Hour Allergy (5)	Tavist (5)
Cophene-B (2)	Tavist-1 (5)
Dexchlor (8)	Telachlor (4)
Dimetapp Allergy Liqui-Gels	Teldrin (4)
(2)	Triptone Caplets (9)
Dinate (9)	Twilite Caplets (10)
Diphen Cough (10)	Unisom Nighttime Sleep Aid
Diphenhist (10)	(11)
Diphenhist Captabs (10)	Unisom SleepGels Maximum
Dormarex 2 (10)	Strength (10)
Dramamine (9)	Vistaril (13)
Dramanate (9)	Zyrtec (3)

In Canada—

Aerius (7)	Gravol L/A (9)
Allegra (12)	Gravol Liquid (9)
Allerdryl (10)	Multipax (13)
Apo-Dimenhydrinate (9)	Novo-Hydroxyzin (13)
Apo-Hydroxyzine (13)	Novo-Pheniram (4)
Atarax (13)	Optimine (1)
Benadryl (10)	Periactin (6)
Chlor-Tripolon (4)	PMS-Cyproheptadine (6)
Claritin (14)	PMS-Dimenhydrinate (9)
Dimetane (2)	Polaramine (8)
Gravol (9)	Polaramine Repetabs (8)
Gravol Filmkote (9)	Reactine (3)
Gravol Filmkote (Junior	Tavist (5)
Strength) (9)	Traveltabs (9)
Gravol I/M (9)	Zyrtec (3)
Gravol I/V (9)	

This information applies to the following medicines:

1. Azatadine (a-ZA-ta-deen)
2. Brompheniramine (brome-fen-EER-a-meen)
3. Cetirizine (se-TI-ra-zeen)
4. Chlorpheniramine (klor-fen-EER-a-meen)
5. Clemastine (KLEM-as-teen)
6. Cyproheptadine (si-proe-HEP-ta-deen)
7. Desloratadine (des-LOR-at-a-deen)
8. Dexchlorpheniramine (dex-klor-fen-EER-a-meen)
9. Dimenhydrinate (dye-men-HYE-dri-nate)
10. Diphenhydramine (dye-fen-HYE-dra-meen)
11. Doxylamine (dox-ILL-a-meen)
12. Fexofenadine (fex-o-FEN-a-deen)
13. Hydroxyzine (hye-DROX-i-zeen)
14. Loratadine (lor-AT-a-deen)
15. Phenindamine (fen-IN-da-meen)

Category

- **Antianxiety agent**—Hydroxyzine
- **Antiasthmatic**—Cetirizine; Loratadine
- **Antidyskinetic**—Diphenhydramine
- **Antiemetic**—Dimenhydrinate; Diphenhydramine; Hydroxyzine (parenteral)
- **Antihistaminic, H₁-receptor**—Azatadine; Brompheniramine; Cetirizine; Chlorpheniramine; Clemastine; Cyproheptadine; Desloratadine; Dexchlorpheniramine; Dimenhydrinate; Diphenhydramine; Doxylamine; Fexofenadine; Hydroxyzine; Loratadine; Phenindamine
- **Antitussive**—Diphenhydramine Syrup
- **Antivertigo agent**—Dimenhydrinate; Diphenhydramine
- **Appetite stimulant**—Cyproheptadine
- **Sedative-hypnotic**—Diphenhydramine; Doxylamine; Hydroxyzine
- **Vascular headache suppressant**—Cyproheptadine

Description

Antihistamines are used to relieve or prevent the symptoms of hay fever and other types of allergy. They work by preventing the effects of a substance called histamine, which is produced by the body. Histamine can cause itching, sneezing, runny nose, and watery eyes. Also, in some persons histamine can close up the bronchial tubes (air passages of the lungs) and make breathing difficult.

Some of the antihistamines are also used to prevent motion sickness, nausea, vomiting, and dizziness. In patients with Parkinson's disease, diphenhydramine may be used to decrease stiffness and tremors. Also, the syrup form of diphenhydramine is used to relieve the cough due to colds or hay fever. In addition, since antihistamines may cause drowsiness as a side effect, some of them may be used to help people go to sleep.

Hydroxyzine is used in the treatment of nervous and emotional conditions to help control anxiety. It can also be used to help control anxiety and produce sleep before surgery.

Some antihistamines are used in the treatment of chronic urticaria, which is a persistent hive-like rash.

Antihistamines may also be used for other conditions as determined by your doctor.

Some antihistamine preparations are available only with your doctor's prescription. Others are available without a prescription. However, your doctor may have special instructions on the proper dose of the medicine for your medical condition.

These medicines are available in the following dosage forms:

Oral
- Azatadine
  - Tablets
- Brompheniramine
  - Capsules
  - Elixir
  - Tablets
- Cetirizine
  - Syrup
  - Tablets
- Chlorpheniramine
  - Extended-release capsules
  - Syrup
  - Tablets
  - Chewable tablets
  - Extended-release tablets
- Clemastine
  - Syrup
  - Tablets
- Cyproheptadine
  - Syrup
  - Tablets
- Desloratadine
  - Tablets
- Dexchlorpheniramine
  - Syrup
  - Tablets
  - Extended-release tablets
- Dimenhydrinate
  - Extended-release capsules
  - Oral Solution
  - Syrup
  - Tablets
  - Chewable tablets
- Diphenhydramine
  - Capsules
  - Elixir
  - Tablets
- Doxylamine
  - Tablets
- Fexofenadine
  - Tablets
  - Capsules (U.S.)
- Hydroxyzine
  - Capsules
  - Oral suspension
  - Syrup
  - Tablets
- Loratadine
  - Syrup
  - Tablets
- Phenindamine
  - Tablets

Parenteral
- Brompheniramine
  - Injection
- Chlorpheniramine
  - Injection
- Dimenhydrinate
  - Injection
- Diphenhydramine
  - Injection
- Hydroxyzine
  - Injection

Rectal
- Dimenhydrinate
  - Suppositories

Before Using This Medicine

In deciding to use a medicine, the risks of taking the medicine must be weighed against the good it will do. This is a decision

you and your doctor will make. For antihistamines, the following should be considered:

Allergies—Tell your doctor if you have ever had any unusual or allergic reaction to antihistamines. Also tell your health care professional if you are allergic to any other substances, such as foods, preservatives, or dyes.

Diet—Make certain your health care professional knows if you are on a low-sodium, low-sugar, or any other special diet. Most medicines contain more than their active ingredient, and many liquid medicines contain alcohol.

Pregnancy—Hydroxyzine is not recommended for use in the first months of pregnancy since it has been shown to cause birth defects in animal studies when given in doses many times higher than the usual human dose. Be sure you have discussed this with your doctor.

Desloratadine and fexofenadine have not been studied in pregnant women. However, studies in animals have shown that these medicines cause birth defects or other problems when given in doses higher than the usual human dose. Before taking this medicine, make sure your doctor knows if you are pregnant or if you may become pregnant.

Azatadine, brompheniramine, cetirizine, chlorpheniramine, clemastine, cyproheptadine, dexchlorpheniramine, dimenhydrinate, diphenhydramine, doxylamine, and loratadine have not been studied in pregnant women. However, these medicines have not been shown to cause birth defects or other problems in animal studies.

Breast-feeding—Small amounts of antihistamines pass into the breast milk. Use is not recommended since babies are more susceptible to the side effects of antihistamines, such as unusual excitement or irritability. Also, since these medicines tend to decrease the secretions of the body, it is possible that the flow of breast milk may be reduced in some patients. It is not known yet whether cetirizine, desloratadine, or loratadine cause these same side effects.

Children—Serious side effects, such as convulsions (seizures), are more likely to occur in younger patients and would be of greater risk to infants than to older children or adults. In general, children are more sensitive to the effects of antihistamines. Also, nightmares or unusual excitement, nervousness, restlessness, or irritability may be more likely to occur in children.

Older adults—Elderly patients are usually more sensitive to the effects of antihistamines. Confusion; difficult or painful urination; dizziness; drowsiness; feeling faint; or dryness of mouth, nose, or throat may be more likely to occur in elderly patients. Also, nightmares or unusual excitement, nervousness, restlessness, or irritability may be more likely to occur in elderly patients.

Other medicines—Although certain medicines should not be used together at all, in other cases different medicines may be used together even if an interaction might occur. In these cases, your doctor may want to change the dose, or other precautions may be necessary. When you are taking antihistamines it is especially important that your health care professional knows if you are taking any of the following:

- Anticholinergics (medicine for abdominal or stomach spasms or cramps)—Side effects, such as dryness of mouth, of antihistamines or anticholinergics may be more likely to occur
- Erythromycin (e.g., E-Mycin) or

- Ketoconazole (e.g., Nizoral)—Use of these medicines with fexofenadine may cause an increased amount of fexofenadine in the blood.
- Central nervous system (CNS) depressants (medicines that cause drowsiness)—Effects, such as drowsiness, of CNS depressants or antihistamines may be worsened; also, taking maprotiline or tricyclic antidepressants may cause some side effects of either of these medicines, such as dryness of mouth, to become more severe
- Monoamine oxidase (MAO) inhibitor activity (isocarboxazid [e.g., Marplan], isocarboxazid [e.g., Marplan], phenelzine [e.g., Nardil], procarbazine [e.g., Matulane], selegiline [e.g., Eldepryl], tranylcypromine [e.g., Parnate])—If you are now taking, or have taken within the past 2 weeks, any of the MAO inhibitors, the side effects of the antihistamines, such as drowsiness and dryness of mouth, may become more severe; these medicines should not be used together

Other medical problems—The presence of other medical problems may affect the use of antihistamines. Make sure you tell your doctor if you have any other medical problems, especially:
- Enlarged prostate or
- Urinary tract blockage or difficult urination—Antihistamines may make urinary problems worse
- Glaucoma—These medicines may cause a slight increase in inner eye pressure that may make the condition worse
- Intestinal obstruction or
- Stomach ulcer—Use of cyproheptadine may make these conditions worse.
- Liver disease or
- Kidney disease—Effects of desloratadine may be increased because of slower removal from the body.

Proper Use of This Medicine

Antihistamines are used to relieve or prevent the symptoms of your medical problem. Take them only as directed. Do not take more of them and do not take them more often than recommended on the label, unless otherwise directed by your doctor. To do so may increase the chance of side effects.

Dosing—The dose of an antihistamine will be different for different patients. *Follow your doctor's orders or the directions on the label.* The following information includes only the average doses of antihistamines. *If your dose is different, do not change it* unless your doctor tells you to do so.

The number of capsules or tablets or teaspoonfuls of liquid that you take or the number of suppositories you use depends on the strength of the medicine. Also, *the number of doses you take each day and the time between doses depends on whether you are taking a short-acting or long-acting form of antihistamine.*

- For use as an antihistamine:
  - *For azatadine*
    - For *oral* dosage form (tablets):
      — Adults: 1 to 2 milligrams (mg) every eight to twelve hours as needed.

— Children younger than 12 years of age: Use and dose must be determined by your doctor.
— Children 12 years of age and older: 0.5 mg to 1 mg two times a day as needed.

○ *For brompheniramine*
  ▪ For *regular (short-acting) oral* dosage forms (capsules, tablets, or liquid):
    — Adults and teenagers: 4 milligrams (mg) every four to six hours as needed.
    — Children 2 to 6 years of age: 1 mg every four to six hours as needed.
    — Children 6 to 12 years of age: 2 mg every four to six hours as needed.
  ▪ For *injection* dosage form:
    — Adults and teenagers: 10 milligrams (mg) injected into a muscle, under the skin, or into a vein every eight to twelve hours.
    — Children younger than 12 years of age: 0.125 mg per kilogram (0.06 mg per pound) of body weight injected into a muscle, under the skin, or into a vein three or four times a day as needed.

○ *For cetirizine*
  ▪ For *oral* dosage forms (syrup and tablets):
    — Adults: 5 to 10 milligrams (mg) once a day.
    — Children younger than 2 years of age: Use and dose must be determined by your doctor.
    — Children 2 to 6 years of age: 2.5 mg once a day, up to a maximum of 5 mg once a day or 2.5 mg twice a day.
    — Children 6 years of age and older: 5 to 10 mg once a day.

○ *For chlorpheniramine*
  ▪ For *regular (short-acting) oral* dosage forms (tablets or liquid):
    — Adults and teenagers: 4 milligrams (mg) every four to six hours as needed.
    — Children younger than 6 years of age: Use and dose must be determined by your doctor.
    — Children 6 to 12 years of age: 2 mg three or four times a day as needed.
  ▪ For *long-acting oral* dosage forms (capsules or tablets):
    — Adults: 8 or 12 milligrams (mg) every eight to twelve hours as needed.
    — Children younger than 12 years of age: Use and dose must be determined by your doctor.
    — Children 12 years of age and older: 8 mg every twelve hours as needed.
  ▪ For *injection* dosage form:
    — Adults: 5 to 40 milligrams (mg) injected into a muscle, into a vein, or under the skin.
    — Children: 0.0875 mg per kilogram (0.04 mg per pound) of body weight injected under the skin every six hours as needed.

○ *For clemastine*
  ▪ For *oral* dosage forms (tablets or liquid):
    — Adults and teenagers: 1.34 milligrams (mg) two times a day or 2.68 mg one to three times a day as needed.
    — Children younger than 6 years of age: Use and dose must be determined by your doctor.
    — Children 6 to 12 years of age: 0.67 to 1.34 mg two times a day.

○ *For cyproheptadine*
  ▪ For *oral* dosage forms (tablets or liquid):
    — Adults and children 14 years of age and older: 4 milligrams (mg) every eight hours. The doctor may increase the dose if needed.
    — Children 2 to 6 years of age: 2 mg every eight to twelve hours as needed.
    — Children 6 to 14 years of age: 4 mg every eight to twelve hours as needed.

○ *For desloratadine*
  ▪ For *oral* dosage form (tablets):
    — Adults and children 12 years of age and older: 5 milligrams (mg) once a day.
    — Children younger than 12 years of age: Use and dose must be determined by your doctor.

○ *For dexchlorpheniramine*
  ▪ For *regular (short-acting) oral* dosage forms (tablets or liquid):
    — Adults and teenagers: 2 milligrams (mg) every four to six hours as needed.
    — Children 2 to 5 years of age: 0.5 mg every four to six hours as needed.
    — Children 5 to 12 years of age: 1 mg every four to six hours as needed.
  ▪ For *long-acting oral* dosage form (tablets):
    — Adults: 4 or 6 milligrams (mg) every eight to twelve hours as needed.
    — Children: Use and dose must be determined by your doctor.

○ *For diphenhydramine*
  ▪ For *oral* dosage forms (capsules, tablets, or liquid):
    — Adults and teenagers: 25 to 50 milligrams (mg) every four to six hours as needed.
    — Children younger than 6 years of age: 6.25 to 12.5 mg every four to six hours.
    — Children 6 to 12 years of age: 12.5 to 25 mg every four to six hours.
  ▪ For *injection* dosage form:
    — Adults: 10 to 50 milligrams (mg) injected into a muscle or into a vein.
    — Children: 1.25 mg per kg (0.6 mg per pound) of body weight injected into a muscle four times a day.

○ *For doxylamine*
  ▪ For *oral* dosage form (tablets):
    — Adults and teenagers: 12.5 to 25 milligrams (mg) every four to six hours as needed.
    — Children younger than 6 years of age: Use and dose must be determined by your doctor.
    — Children 6 to 12 years of age: 6.25 to 12.5 mg every four to six hours as needed.

○ *For fexofenadine*
  ▪ For *oral* dosage forms (capsules):
    — Adults and teenagers: 60 milligrams (mg) two times a day as needed or 180 mg once a day
    — Children 6 to 11 years of age: 30 mg twice a day as needed.
    — Children under 6 years of age: Use and dose must be determined by your doctor.

○ *For loratadine*
  ▪ For *oral* dosage forms (tablets or liquid):
    — Adults and children 6 years of age and older: 10 milligrams (mg) once a day.

— Children 2 to 5 years of age: 5 mg once a day.

○ *For phenindamine*
- For *oral* dosage form (tablets):
  — Adults and teenagers: 25 milligrams (mg) every four to six hours as needed.
  — Children younger than 6 years of age: Use and dose must be determined by your doctor.
  — Children 6 to 12 years of age: 12.5 mg every four to six hours as needed.

• For nausea, vomiting, and vertigo (only dimenhydrinate and diphenhydramine are used for vertigo):
  ○ *For dimenhydrinate*
  - For *regular (short-acting) oral* dosage forms (tablets or liquid):
    — Adults and teenagers: 50 to 100 milligrams (mg) every four to six hours as needed.
    — Children 2 to 6 years of age: 12.5 to 25 mg every six to eight hours as needed.
    — Children 6 to 12 years of age: 25 to 50 mg every six to eight hours as needed.
  - For *long-acting oral* dosage form (capsules):
    — Adults: 1 capsule (contains 25 milligrams [mg] for immediate action and 50 mg for long action) every twelve hours.
    — Children: Use and dose must be determined by your doctor.
  - For *injection* dosage form:
    — Adults: 50 milligrams (mg) injected into a muscle or into a vein every four hours as needed.
    — Children: 1.25 mg per kg (0.6 mg per pound) of body weight injected into a muscle or into a vein every six hours as needed.
  - For *suppository* dosage form:
    — Adults: 50 to 100 milligrams (mg) inserted into the rectum every six to eight hours as needed.
    — Children younger than 6 years of age: Use and dose must be determined by your doctor.
    — Children 6 to 8 years of age: 12.5 to 25 mg inserted into the rectum every eight to twelve hours as needed.
    — Children 8 to 12 years of age: 25 to 50 mg inserted into the rectum every eight to twelve hours as needed.
    — Children 12 years of age and older: 50 mg inserted into the rectum every eight to twelve hours as needed.

  ○ *For diphenhydramine*
  - For *oral* dosage forms (capsules, tablets, or liquid):
    — Adults: 25 to 50 milligrams (mg) every four to six hours as needed.
    — Children: 1 to 1.5 mg per kg (0.45 to 0.7 mg per pound) of body weight every four to six hours as needed.
  - For *injection* dosage form:
    — Adults: 10 milligrams (mg) injected into a muscle or into a vein. Dose may be increased to 25 to 50 mg every two to three hours.
    — Children: 1 to 1.5 mg per kg (0.45 to 0.68 mg per pound) of body weight injected into a muscle every six hours.

○ *For hydroxyzine*
- For *oral* dosage forms (capsules, tablets, or liquid):
  — Adults: 25 to 100 milligrams (mg) three or four times a day as needed.
  — Children younger than 6 years of age: 12.5 mg every six hours as needed.
  — Children 6 years of age and older: 12.5 to 25 mg every six hours as needed.

For *injection* dosage form:
  — Adults: 25 to 100 milligrams (mg) injected into a muscle.
  — Children: 1 mg per kg (0.45 mg per pound) of body weight injected into a muscle.

• For Parkinson's disease:
  ○ *For diphenhydramine*
  - For *oral* dosage forms (capsules, tablets, or liquid):
    — Adults: 25 milligrams (mg) three times a day when starting treatment. Your doctor may increase the dose gradually later if needed.
  - For *injection* dosage form:
    — Adults: 10 to 50 milligrams (mg) injected into a muscle or into a vein.
    — Children: 1.25 mg per kg (0.6 mg per pound) of body weight four times a day injected into a muscle.

• For use as a sedative (to help sleep):
  ○ *For diphenhydramine*
  - For *oral* dosage forms (capsules, tablets, or liquid):
    — Adults: 50 milligrams (mg) twenty to thirty minutes before bedtime if needed.
  ○ *For doxylamine*
  - For *oral* dosage form (tablets):
    — Adults: 25 milligrams (mg) thirty minutes before bedtime if needed.
    — Children: Use and dose must be determined by your doctor.
  ○ *For hydroxyzine*
  - For *oral* dosage forms (capsules, tablets, or liquid):
    — Adults: 50 to 100 milligrams (mg).
    — Children: 0.6 mg per kg (0.3 mg per pound) of body weight.
  - For *injection* dosage form:
    — Adults: 50 milligrams (mg) injected into a muscle.

• For anxiety:
  ○ *For hydroxyzine*
  - For *oral* dosage forms (capsules, tablets, or liquid):
    — Adults: 50 to 100 milligrams (mg).
    — Children: 0.6 mg per kilogram (0.3 mg per pound) of body weight.
  - For *injection* dosage form:
    — Adults: 50 to 100 milligrams (mg) injected into a muscle every four to six hours as needed.
    — Children: 1 mg per kilogram (0.45 mg per pound) of body weight injected into a muscle.

Missed dose—If you are taking this medicine regularly and you miss a dose, take it as soon as possible. However, if it is almost time for your next dose, skip the missed dose and go back to your regular dosing schedule. Do not double doses.

For patients *taking this medicine by mouth:*

- Antihistamines can be taken with food or a glass of water or milk to lessen stomach irritation if necessary.
- If you are taking the extended-release tablet form of this medicine, swallow the tablets whole. Do not break, crush, or chew before swallowing.

For patients taking *dimenhydrinate or diphenhydramine for motion sickness:*

- Take this medicine at least 30 minutes or, even better, 1 to 2 hours before you begin to travel.

For patients using the *suppository form of this medicine:*

- To insert suppository: First remove the foil wrapper and moisten the suppository with cold water. Lie down on your side and use your finger to push the suppository well up into the rectum. If the suppository is too soft to insert, chill the suppository in the refrigerator for 30 minutes or run cold water over it before removing the foil wrapper.

For patients using the *injection form of this medicine:*

- If you will be giving yourself the injections, make sure you understand exactly how to give them. If you have any questions about this, check with your health care professional.

Storage—To store this medicine:

- Keep out of the reach of children, since overdose may be very dangerous in children.
- Store away from heat and direct light.
- Do not store the capsule or tablet form of this medicine in the bathroom medicine cabinet, near the kitchen sink, or in other damp places. Heat or moisture may cause the medicine to break down.
- Keep the liquid form of this medicine from freezing.
- Do not keep outdated medicine or medicine no longer needed. Be sure that any discarded medicine is out of the reach of children.

Precautions While Using This Medicine

Before you have any skin tests for allergies, tell the doctor in charge that you are taking this medicine. The results of the test may be affected by this medicine.

When taking antihistamines on a regular basis, make sure your doctor knows if you are taking large amounts of aspirin at the same time (as for arthritis or rheumatism). Effects of too much aspirin, such as ringing in the ears, may be covered up by the antihistamine.

Antihistamines will add to the effects of alcohol and other CNS depressants (medicines that slow down the nervous system, possibly causing drowsiness). Some examples of CNS depressants are sedatives, tranquilizers, or sleeping medicine; prescription pain medicine or narcotics; barbiturates; medicine for seizures; muscle relaxants; or anesthetics, including some dental anesthetics. *Check with your doctor before taking any of the above while you are using this medicine.*

This medicine may cause some people to become drowsy or less alert than they are normally. Even if taken at bedtime, it may cause some people to feel drowsy or less alert on arising. Some antihistamines are more likely to cause drows-

iness than others. Drowsiness is less likely with cetirizine, and rare with desloratadine and loratadine. *Make sure you know how you react to the antihistamine you are taking before you drive, use machines, or do anything else that could be dangerous if you are not alert.*

Antihistamines may cause dryness of the mouth, nose, and throat. Some antihistamines are more likely to cause dryness of the mouth than others. For temporary relief of mouth dryness, use sugarless candy or gum, melt bits of ice in your mouth, or use a saliva substitute. However, if your mouth continues to feel dry for more than 2 weeks, check with your medical doctor or dentist. Continuing dryness of the mouth may increase the chance of dental disease, including tooth decay, gum disease, and fungus infections.

For patients using *dimenhydrinate, diphenhydramine, or hydroxyzine:*

- This medicine controls nausea and vomiting. For this reason, it may cover up the signs of overdose caused by other medicines or the symptoms of appendicitis. This will make it difficult for your doctor to diagnose these conditions. Make sure your doctor knows that you are taking this medicine if you have other symptoms of appendicitis such as stomach or lower abdominal pain, cramping, or soreness. Also, if you think you may have taken an overdose of any medicine, tell your doctor that you are taking this medicine.

For patients using *diphenhydramine or doxylamine as a sleeping aid:*

- If you are already taking a sedative or tranquilizer, do not take this medicine without consulting your doctor first.

Side Effects

Along with its needed effects, a medicine may cause some unwanted effects. Although not all of these side effects may occur, if they do occur they may need medical attention.

Check with your doctor immediately if the following side effect occurs:

Less common or rare
Fast or irregular heartbeat; fever; abdominal or stomach pain; burning; chills; clay-colored stools or dark urine; cough; diarrhea; difficulty swallowing; dizziness; fast heartbeat; fever; headache; hives; itching; prickly sensations; puffiness or swelling of the eyelids or around the eyes, face, lips or tongue; redness of skin; seizures; shortness of breath; skin rash; swelling; tightness in chest; tingling; unusual tiredness or weakness; wheezing

Also, check with your doctor as soon as possible if any of the following side effects occur:

Less common or rare
Sore throat; unusual bleeding or bruising; unusual tiredness or weakness

Symptoms of overdose
Clumsiness or unsteadiness; convulsions (seizures); drowsiness (severe); dryness of mouth, nose, or throat (severe); feeling faint; flushing or redness of face; hallucinations (seeing, hearing, or feeling things that are not there); shortness of breath or troubled breathing; trouble in sleeping

Other side effects may occur that usually do not need medical attention. These side effects may go away during treatment as your body adjusts to the medicine. However, check with your health care professional if any of the following side effects continue or are bothersome:

More common

Drowsiness; dry mouth, nose, or throat; gastrointestinal upset, stomach pain, or nausea; headache; increased appetite and weight gain; thickening of mucus

Less common or rare

Acid or sour stomach; belching; blurred vision or any change in vision; clumsiness or unsteadiness; body aches or pain; confusion (not with diphenhydramine); congestion; constipation; cough; diarrhea; difficult or painful urination; difficulty in moving; difficult or painful menstruation; dizziness (not with brompheniramine or hydroxyzine; drowsiness (with high doses of desloratadine and loratadine); dryness of mouth, nose, or throat; early menstruation; fast heartbeat; fatigue; fever; gastrointestinal upset, stomach pain or nausea; heartburn; hoarseness; increased appetite and weight gain; increased sensitivity of skin to sun; increased sweating; indigestion; loss of appetite; joint pain; muscle aching or cramping; muscle pains or stiffness; nausea; nightmares (not with azatadine, chlorpheniramine, cyproheptadine, desloratadine, hydroxyzine, or loratadine); ringing or buzzing in ears; runny nose; skin rash; swollen joints; stomach discomfort, upset or pain; tender swollen glands in neck; thickening of mucus; tremor; unusual excitement, nervousness, restlessness, or irritability; vomiting

Other side effects not listed above may also occur in some patients. If you notice any other effects, check with your health care professional.

Additional Information

Once a medicine has been approved for marketing for a certain use, experience may show that it is also useful for other medical problems. Although this use is not included in product labeling, cetirizine and loratadine are used in certain patients with asthma together with asthma medicines. The antihistamine is used before and during exposure to substances that cause reactions, to prevent or reduce bronchospasm (wheezing or difficulty in breathing).

Cyproheptadine is used as an appetite stimulant, in adults and children

Cyproheptadine is used for treatment of vascular headaches.

Other than the above information, there is no additional information relating to proper use, precautions, or side effects for this use.

ANTIHISTAMINES AND DECONGESTANTS (Systemic)

Some commonly used brand names are:

In the U.S.—

Allerest Maximum Strength (7)	Benadryl Allergy
Allerphed (14)	Decongestant Liquid
Atrohist Pediatric (7)	Medication (10)
Atrohist Pediatric Suspension	Brofed Liquid (3)
Dye Free (8)	Bromadrine TR (3)

Bromfed (3)	Lodrane Liquid (3)
Bromfed-PD (3)	Mooredec (4)
Bromfenex (3)	Nalex-A (6)
Bromfenex PD (3)	ND Clear T.D. (7)
Chlordrine S.R. (7)	Novafed A (7)
Chlorfed A (7)	PediaCare Cold Formula (7)
Chlor-Trimeton 4 Hour Relief (7)	Poly Hist Forte (8)
	Promethazine VC (13)
Chlor-Trimeton 12 Hour Relief (7)	Prometh VC Plain (13)
	Pseudo-Chlor (7)
Chlor-Trimeton Allergy-D 12 Hour (7)	Rescon (7)
	Rescon-ED (7)
Claritin-D 12 Hour (11)	Rescon JR (7)
Claritin-D 24 Hour (11)	Respahist (3)
Colfed-A (7)	Rhinosyn (7)
Comhist (6)	Rhinosyn-PD (7)
CP Oral (4)	Rinade B.I.D. (7)
Dallergy Jr (3)	Rondamine (4)
Deconamine (7)	Rondec (4)
Deconamine SR (7)	Rondec Chewable (3)
Deconomed SR (7)	Rondec Drops (4)
Dexaphen SA (9)	Rondec-TR (4)
Disobrom (9)	R-Tannamine (8)
Disophrol Chronotabs (9)	R-Tannamine Pediatric (8)
Drixomed (9)	R-Tannate (8)
Drixoral Cold and Allergy (9)	Semprex-D (1)
Ed A-Hist (5)	Silafed (14)
Hayfebrol (7)	Tanafed (7)
Histatab Plus (5)	Trinalin Repetabs (2)
Iofed (3)	Triotann (8)
Iofed PD (3)	Triotann Pediatric (8)
Kronofed-A Jr. Kronocaps (7)	Triotann-S Pediatric (8)
	Tri-Tannate (8)
Kronofed-A Kronocaps (7)	ULTRAbrom (3)
Lodrane LD (3)	ULTRAbrom PD (3)

In Canada—

Claritin Extra (11)	Neo Citran A (12)
Drixoral (9)	Trinalin Repetabs (2)
Drixoral Night (9)	Vasofrinic (7)
Drixtab (9)	

This information applies to the following medicines:

1. Acrivastine and Pseudoephedrine (AK-ri-vas-teen and soo-doe-e-FED-rin)
2. Azatadine and Pseudoephedrine (a-ZA-ta-deen and soo-doe-e-FED-rin)
3. Brompheniramine and Pseudoephedrine (brome-fen-EER-a-meen and soo-doe-e-FED-rin)
4. Carbinoxamine and Pseudoephedrine (kar-bi-NOX-a-meen and soo-doe-e-FED-rin)
5. Chlorpheniramine and Phenylephrine (klor-fen-EER-a-meen and fen-ill-EF-rin)
6. Chlorpheniramine, Phenyltoloxamine, and Phenylephrine (klor-fen-EER-a-meen fen-ill-toe-LOX-a-meen and fen-ill-EF-rin)
7. Chlorpheniramine and Pseudoephedrine (klor-fen-EER-a-meen and soo-doe-e-FED-rin)
8. Chlorpheniramine, Pyrilamine, and Phenylephrine (klor-fen-EER-a-meen peer-ILL-a-meen and fen-ill-EF-rin)
9. Dexbrompheniramine and Pseudoephedrine (dex-brom-fen-EER-a-meen and soo-doe-e-FED-rin)
10. Diphenhydramine and Pseudoephedrine (dye-fen-HYE-dra-meen and soo-doe-e-FED-rin)
11. Loratadine and Pseudoephedrine (lor-AT-a-deen and soo-doe-e-FED-rin)
12. Pheniramine and Phenylephrine (fen-EER-a-meen and fen-ill-EF-rin)
13. Promethazine and Phenylephrine (proe-METH-a-zeen and fen-ill-EF-rin)
14. Triprolidine and Pseudoephedrine (trye-PROE-li-deen and soo-doe-e-FED-rin)
15. Cetirizine and Pseudoephedrine (trye-PROE-li-deen and soo-doe-e-FED-rin)

Category

- **Antihistaminic (H₁-receptor)-decongestant**—Acrivastine and Pseudoephedrine; Azatadine and Pseudoephedrine; Brompheniramine and Pseudoephedrine; Carbinoxamine and Pseudoephedrine; Cetirizine and Pseudoephedrine; Chlorpheniramine and Phenylephrine; Chlorpheniramine and Pseudoephedrine; Chlorpheniramine, Phenyltoloxamine, and Phenylephrine; Chlorpheniramine, Pyrilamine, and Phenylephrine; Dexbrompheniramine and Pseudoephedrine; Diphenhydramine and Pseudoephedrine; Loratadine and Pseudoephedrine; Pheniramine and Phenylephrine; Promethazine and Phenylephrine; Triprolidine and Pseudoephedrine

Description

Antihistamine and decongestant combinations are used to treat the nasal congestion (stuffy nose), sneezing, and runny nose caused by colds and hay fever.

Antihistamines work by preventing the effects of a substance called histamine, which is produced by the body. Histamine can cause itching, sneezing, runny nose, and watery eyes. Antihistamines contained in these combinations are:

acrivastine, azatadine, brompheniramine, carbinoxamine, chlorpheniramine, clemastine, dexbrompheniramine, diphenhydramine, loratadine, pheniramine, phenyltoloxamine, promethazine, pyrilamine, and triprolidine.

The decongestants, such as phenylephrine, and pseudoephedrine, produce a narrowing of blood vessels. This leads to clearing of nasal congestion, but it may also cause an increase in blood pressure in patients who have high blood pressure.

Some of these combinations are available only with your doctor's prescription. Others are available without a prescription; however, your doctor may have special instructions on the proper dose of the medicine for your medical condition. They are available in the following dosage forms:

Oral

- Acrivastine and Pseudoephedrine
  - Capsules
- Azatadine and Pseudoephedrine
  - Extended-release tablets
- Brompheniramine and Pseudoephedrine
  - Extended-release capsules
  - Oral solution
  - Syrup
  - Tablets
  - Chewable tablets
- Carbinoxamine and Pseudoephedrine
  - Oral solution
  - Syrup
  - Tablets
  - Extended-release tablets
- Cetirizine and Pseudoephedrine
  - Extended-release tablets
- Chlorpheniramine and Phenylephrine
  - Elixir
  - Oral solution
  - Oral suspension
  - Syrup
  - Tablets
  - Extended-release tablets
- Chlorpheniramine, Phenyltoloxamine, and Phenylephrine
  - Extended-release capsules
  - Tablets
  - Extended-release tablets
- Chlorpheniramine and Pseudoephedrine
  - Capsules
  - Extended-release capsules
  - Oral solution
  - Oral suspension
  - Syrup
  - Tablets
  - Chewable tablets
  - Extended-release tablets
- Chlorpheniramine, Pyrilamine, and Phenylephrine
  - Oral suspension
  - Tablets
- Dexbrompheniramine and Pseudoephedrine
  - Tablets
  - Extended-release tablets
- Diphenhydramine and Pseudoephedrine
  - Capsules
  - Oral solution
  - Tablets
- Loratadine and Pseudoephedrine
  - Extended-release tablets
- Pheniramine and Phenylephrine
  - for Oral solution
- Promethazine and Phenylephrine
  - Syrup
- Triprolidine and Pseudoephedrine
  - Syrup
  - Tablets

Before Using This Medicine

If you are taking this medicine without a prescription, carefully read and follow any precautions on the label. For antihistamine and decongestant combinations, the following should be considered:

Allergies—Tell your doctor if you have ever had any unusual or allergic reaction to antihistamines or to amphetamine, dextroamphetamine (e.g., Dexedrine), ephedrine (e.g., Ephed II), epinephrine (e.g., Adrenalin), isoproterenol (e.g., Isuprel), metaproterenol (e.g., Alupent), methamphetamine (e.g., Desoxyn), norepinephrine (e.g., Levophed), phenylephrine (e.g., Neo-Synephrine), pseudoephedrine (e.g., Sudafed), PPA (e.g., Dexatrim), or terbutaline (e.g., Brethine).

Pregnancy—The occasional use of antihistamine and decongestant combinations is not likely to cause problems in the fetus or in the newborn baby. However, when these medicines are used at higher doses and/or for a long time, the chance that problems might occur may increase. For the individual ingredients of these combinations, the following apply:

- *Alcohol*—Some of these combination medicines contain alcohol. Too much use of alcohol during pregnancy may cause birth defects.

- *Antihistamines*—Antihistamines have not been shown to cause problems in humans.

- *Phenylephrine*—Studies on birth defects have not been done in either humans or animals with phenylephrine.

- *Promethazine*—Phenothiazines, such as promethazine (contained in some of these combination medicines [e.g., Phenergan-D]), have been shown to cause jaundice and muscle tremors in a few newborn infants whose mothers received phenothiazines during pregnancy. Also, the newborn baby may have blood clotting problems if promethazine is taken by the mother within 2 weeks before delivery.

- *Pseudoephedrine*—Studies on birth defects with pseudoephedrine have not been done in humans. In animal studies pseudoephedrine did not cause birth defects but did cause a decrease in average weight, length, and rate of bone formation in the animal fetus when administered in high doses.

Breast-feeding—Small amounts of antihistamines and decongestants pass into the breast milk. Use is not recommended since the chances are greater for this medicine to cause side effects, such as unusual excitement or irritability, in the nursing baby. Also, since antihistamines tend to decrease the secretions of the body, it is possible that the flow of breast milk may be reduced in some patients. It is not known yet whether loratadine causes these same side effects.

Children—Very young children are usually more sensitive to the effects of this medicine. Increases in blood pressure, nightmares or unusual excitement, nervousness, restlessness, or irritability may be more likely to occur in children. *Before giving any of these combination medicines to a child, check the package label very carefully. Some of these medicines are too strong for use in children.* If you are not certain whether a specific product can be given to a child, or if you have any questions about the amount to give, check with your health care professional.

Older adults—Confusion, difficult and painful urination, dizziness, drowsiness, dryness of mouth, or convulsions (seizures) may be more likely to occur in the elderly, who are usually more sensitive to the effects of this medicine. Also, nightmares or unusual excitement, nervousness, restlessness, or irritability may be more likely to occur in elderly patients.

Other medicines—Although certain medicines should not be used together at all, in other cases different medicines may be used together even if an interaction might occur. In these cases, your doctor may want to change the dose, or other precautions may be necessary. When you are taking antihistamines it is especially important that your health care professional know if you are taking any of the following:

- Alcohol—Effects such as drowsiness may be worsened.

- Anticholinergics (medicine for abdominal or stomach spasms or cramps)—Side effects, such as dryness of mouth, of antihistamines or anticholinergics may be more likely to occur

- Central nervous system (CNS) depressants—Effects, such as drowsiness, of CNS depressants or antihistamines may be worsened

- Digitalis glycosides (e.g., Digoxin)—Use of this medicine may affect heartbeats.

- Maprotiline (e.g., Ludiomil) or

- Tricyclic antidepressants (amitriptyline [e.g., Elavil], amoxapine [e.g., Asendin], clomipramine [e.g., Anafranil], desipramine [e.g., Pertofrane], doxepin [e.g., Sinequan], imipramine [e.g., Tofranil], nortriptyline [e.g., Aventyl], protriptyline [e.g., Vivactil], trimipramine [e.g.,

Surmontil])—Effects, such as drowsiness, of CNS depressants or antihistamines may be worsened; also, taking these medicines together may cause some of their side effects, such as dryness of mouth, to become more severe

- Monoamine oxidase (MAO) inhibitor activity (isocarboxazid [e.g., Marplan], phenelzine [e.g., Nardil], procarbazine [e.g., Matulane], selegiline [e.g., Eldepryl], tranylcypromine [e.g., Parnate])—If you are now taking, or have taken within the past 2 weeks, any of the MAO inhibitors, the side effects of the antihistamines may become more severe; these medicines should not be used together

- Rauwolfia alkaloids (alseroxylon [e.g., Rauwiloid], deserpidine [e.g., Harmonyl], rauwolfia serpentina [e.g., Raudixin], reserpine [e.g., Serpasil])—These medicines may increase or decrease the effect of the decongestant

Also, if you are taking one of the combinations containing pseudoephedrine and are also taking:

- Amantadine (e.g., Symmetrel) or

- Amphetamines or

- Appetite suppressants (diet pills), except fenfluramine (e.g., Pondimin) or

- Caffeine (e.g., NoDoz) or

- Chlophedianol (e.g., Ulone) or

- Medicine for asthma or other breathing problems or

- Medicine for colds, sinus problems, or hay fever or other allergies (including nose drops or sprays) or

- Methylphenidate (e.g., Ritalin) or

- Nabilone (e.g., Cesamet) or

- Pemoline (e.g., Cylert)—Using any of these medicines together with an antihistamine and decongestant combination may cause excessive stimulant side effects, such as difficulty in sleeping, heart rate problems, nervousness, and irritability

- Beta-adrenergic blocking agents (acebutolol [e.g., Sectral], atenolol [e.g., Tenormin], betaxolol [e.g., Kerlone], bisoprolol [e.g., Zebeta], carteolol [e.g., Cartrol], labetalol [e.g., Normodyne], metoprolol [e.g., Lopressor], nadolol [e.g., Corgard], oxprenolol [e.g., Trasicor], penbutolol [e.g., Levatol], pindolol [e.g., Visken], propanolol [e.g., Inderal], sotalol [e.g., Sotacor], timolol [e.g., Blocadren])—Using any of these medicines together with an antihistamine and decongestant combination may cause high blood pressure and heart problems (e.g., unusually slow heartbeat)

Other medical problems—The presence of other medical problems may affect the use of antihistamine and decongestant combinations. Make sure you tell your doctor if you have any other medical problems, especially:

- Diabetes mellitus (sugar diabetes)—The decongestant in this medicine may put diabetic patients at a greater risk of having heart or blood vessel disease

- Enlarged prostate or

- Urinary tract blockage or difficult urination—Some of the effects of antihistamines may make urinary problems worse

- Glaucoma—A slight increase in inner eye pressure may occur

- Heart or blood vessel disease or

- High blood pressure—The decongestant in this medicine may cause the blood pressure to increase and may also speed up the heart rate

- Kidney disease—Higher blood levels of loratadine may result, which may increase the chance of side effects. The dosage of loratadine-containing combination may need to be reduced

- Liver disease—Higher blood levels of loratadine may result, which may increase the chance of side effects

- Overactive thyroid—If the overactive thyroid has caused a fast heart rate, the decongestant in this medicine may cause the heart rate to speed up further

- Urinary retention—Condition may be worsened with use of pseudoephedrine

Proper Use of This Medicine

Take this medicine only as directed. Do not take more of it and do not take it more often than recommended on the label, unless otherwise directed by your doctor. To do so may increase the chance of side effects.

If this medicine irritates your stomach, you may take it with food or a glass of water or milk, to lessen the irritation.

For patients *taking the extended-release capsule or tablet form of this medicine:*

- Swallow it whole.

- Do not crush, break, or chew before swallowing.

- If the capsule is too large to swallow, you may mix the contents of the capsule with applesauce, jelly, honey, or syrup and swallow without chewing.

Dosing—There is a large variety of antihistamine and decongestant combination products on the market. Some products are for use in adults only, while others may be used in children. If you have any questions about this, check with your health care professional.

The dose of antihistamines and decongestants will be different for different products. The number of capsules or tablets or teaspoonfuls of liquid or granules that you take depends on the strengths of the medicines. Also, *the number of doses you take each day and the time between doses depend on whether you are taking a short-acting or long-acting form of antihistamine and decongestant. Follow your doctor's orders if this medicine was prescribed. Or, follow the directions on the box if you are buying this medicine without a prescription.*

Missed dose—If you are taking this medicine regularly and you miss a dose, take it as soon as possible. However, if it is almost time for your next dose, skip the missed dose and go back to your regular dosing schedule. Do not double doses.

Storage—To store this medicine:

- Keep out of the reach of children.

- Store away from heat and direct light.

- Do not store in the bathroom, near the kitchen sink, or in other damp places. Heat or moisture may cause the medicine to break down.

- Keep the liquid form of this medicine from freezing.

- Do not keep outdated medicine or medicine no longer needed. Be sure that any discarded medicine is out of the reach of children.

Precautions While Using This Medicine

Before you have any skin tests for allergies, tell the doctor in charge that you are taking this medicine. The results of the test may be affected by the antihistamine in this medicine.

When taking antihistamines (contained in this combination medicine) on a regular basis, make sure your doctor knows if you are taking large amounts of aspirin at the same time (as for arthritis or rheumatism). Effects of too much aspirin, such as ringing in the ears, may be covered up by the antihistamine.

The antihistamine in this medicine will add to the effects of alcohol and other CNS depressants (medicines that slow down the nervous system, possibly causing drowsiness). Some examples of CNS depressants are other antihistamines or medicine for hay fever, other allergies, or colds; sedatives, tranquilizers, or sleeping medicine; prescription pain medicine or narcotics; barbiturates; medicine for seizures; muscle relaxants; or anesthetics, including some dental anesthetics. *Check with your doctor before taking any of the above while you are taking this medicine.*

The antihistamine in this medicine may cause some people to become drowsy, dizzy, or less alert than they are normally. *Some antihistamines are more likely to cause drowsiness than others (loratadine, for example, rarely produces this effect). Make sure you know how you react before you drive, use machines, or do anything else that could be dangerous if you are dizzy or are not alert.*

The decongestant in this medicine may add to the central nervous system (CNS) stimulant and other effects of diet aids. *Do not use medicines for diet or appetite control while taking this medicine unless you have checked with your doctor.*

The decongestant in this medicine may cause some people to be nervous or restless or to have trouble in sleeping. If you have trouble in sleeping, *take the last dose of this medicine for each day a few hours before bedtime.* If you have any questions about this, check with your doctor.

Antihistamines may cause dryness of the mouth, nose, and throat. Some antihistamines are more likely to cause dryness of the mouth than others (loratadine, for example, rarely produces this effect). For temporary relief, use sugarless candy or gum, melt bits of ice in your mouth, or use a saliva substitute. However, if your mouth continues to feel dry for more than 2 weeks, check with your dentist. Continuing dryness of the mouth may increase the chance of dental disease, including tooth decay, gum disease, and fungus infections.

For patients *using promethazine-containing medicine:*

- This medicine controls nausea and vomiting. For this reason, it may cover up the signs of overdose caused by other medicines or the symptoms of intestinal blockage. This will make it difficult for your doctor to diagnose these conditions. Make sure your doctor knows that you are taking this medicine if you have other symptoms such as stomach or lower abdominal pain, cramping, or soreness. Also, if you think you may have taken an overdose of any medicine, tell your doctor that you are taking this medicine.

Side Effects

Along with its needed effects, a medicine may cause some unwanted effects. Although serious side effects occur rarely when this medicine is taken as recommended, they may be more likely to occur if:

- too much medicine is taken
- it is taken in large doses
- it is taken for a long period of time

Get emergency help immediately if any of the following symptoms of overdose occur:

> *For promethazine only*
> Muscle spasms (especially of neck and back); restlessness; shuffling walk; tic-like (jerky) movements of head and face; trembling and shaking of hands
> Clumsiness or unsteadiness; convulsions (seizures); drowsiness (severe); dryness of mouth, nose, or throat (severe); flushing or redness of face; hallucinations (seeing, hearing, or feeling things that are not there); headache (continuing); shortness of breath or troubled breathing; slow, fast, or irregular heartbeat; trouble in sleeping

Also, check with your doctor as soon as possible if any of the following side effects occur:

> *Rare*
> Back, leg or stomach pain; black, sticky stools; bleeding gums; blood, cloudy or dark urine, or sudden decrease in amount of urine; blood pressure increased; blurred vision; chest pain; confusion; diarrhea; dizziness; faintness, or lightheadedness when getting up from a lying or sitting position; fever or chills; light-colored stools; mood or mental changes; nosebleeds; sore throat and fever; skin rash or hives; stillbirth; swollen mouth, throat, face, fingers, feet, glands or lower legs; sweating suddenly; tightness in chest; troubled breathing; twitching, twisting, or uncontrolled repetitive movements of face; unusual bleeding or bruising; unusual tiredness or weakness; vomiting of blood; weight gain suddenly; yellow or pale eyes or skin

Other side effects may occur that usually do not need medical attention. These side effects may go away during treatment as your body adjusts to the medicine. However, check with your health care professional if any of the following side effects continue or are bothersome:

> *More common*—rare with loratadine-containing combination
> Drowsiness; thickening of the bronchial secretions
> *Less common*—more common with high doses
> Blurred vision; confusion; difficult or painful urination; dizziness; dryness of mouth, nose, or throat; headache; loss of appetite; nightmares; pounding heartbeat; ringing or buzzing in ears; skin rash; stomach upset or pain (more common with pyrilamine); unusual excitement, nervousness, restlessness, or irritability; unusual sleepiness, weakness or drowsiness, extreme tiredness

Other side effects not listed above may also occur in some patients. If you notice any other effects, check with your doctor.

ANTIHISTAMINES, DECONGESTANTS, AND ANALGESICS (Systemic)

Some commonly used brand names are:

In the U.S.—

Actifed Cold & Sinus Caplets (3)	Singlet for Adults (3)
Alka-Seltzer Plus Cold Medicine Liqui-Gels (3)	TheraFlu/Flu and Cold Medicine (3)
Benadryl Allergy/Sinus Headache Caplets (6)	TheraFlu/Flu and Cold Medicine for Sore Throat (3)
Children's Tylenol Cold Multi-Symptom (3)	Tylenol Allergy Sinus Medication Maximum Strength Caplets (3)
Comtrex Allergy-Sinus (3)	
Comtrex Allergy-Sinus Caplets (3)	Tylenol Allergy Sinus Medication Maximum Strength Gelcaps (3)
Contac Allergy/Sinus Night Caplets (6)	Tylenol Allergy Sinus Medication Maximum Strength Geltabs (3)
Dimetapp Cold & Fever Suspension (1)	
Dristan Cold Multi-Symptom Formula (2)	Tylenol Allergy Sinus Night Time Medicine Maximum Strength Caplets (6)
Drixoral Allergy-Sinus (5)	
Drixoral Cold and Flu (5)	Tylenol Flu NightTime Hot Medication Maximum Strength (6)
Kolephrin Caplets (3)	
ND-Gesic (4)	
Scot-Tussin Original 5–Action Cold Formula (8)	Tylenol Flu NightTime Medication Maximum Strength Gelcaps (6)
Sinarest (3)	
Sine-Off Sinus Medicine Caplets (3)	

In Canada—

Actifed Plus Extra Strength Caplets (10)	Sinutab Regular Caplets (3)
Dristan (2)	Tylenol Allergy Sinus Medication Extra Strength Caplets (3)
Dristan Extra Strength Caplets (2)	
Neo Citran Nutrasweet (7)	Tylenol Cold Medication Children's (3)
Neo Citran Extra Strength Colds and Flu (7)	Tylenol Flu NightTimeMedication Extra Strength Gelcaps (6)
Sinutab Extra Strength Caplets (3)	

This information applies to the following medicines:

1. Brompheniramine, Pseudoephedrine, and Acetaminophen (brome-fen-IR-a-meen soo-doe-e-FED-rin and a-set-a-MIN-oh-fen)
2. Chlorpheniramine, Phenylephrine, and Acetaminophen (klor-fen-EER-a-meen fen-il-EF-rin and a-set-a-MIN-oh-fen)
3. Chlorpheniramine, Pseudoephedrine, and Acetaminophen (klor-fen-EER-a-meen soo-doe-e-FED-rin and a-set-a-MIN-oh-fen)
4. Chlorpheniramine, Pyrilamine, Phenylephrine, and Acetaminophen (klor-fen-EER-a-meen peer-ILL-a-meen fen-il-EF-rin and a-set-a-MIN-oh-fen)
5. Dexbrompheniramine, Pseudoephedrine, and Acetaminophen (dex-brome-fen-EER-a-meen soo-doe-e-FED-rin and a-set-a-MIN-oh-fen)
6. Diphenhydramine, Pseudoephedrine, and Acetaminophen (dye-fen-HYE-dra-meen soo-doe-e-FED-rin and a-set-a-MIN-oh-fen)
7. Pheniramine, Phenylephrine, and Acetaminophen (fen-EER-a-meen fen-il-EF-rin and a-set-a-MIN-oh-fen)
8. Pheniramine, Phenylephrine, Sodium Salicylate, and Caffeine (fen-EER-a-meen fen-il-EF-rin SOE-dee-um sa-LI-si-late and kaf-EEN)
9. Pyrilamine, Phenylephrine, Aspirin, and Caffeine (peer-ILL-a-meen fen-il-EF-rin AS-pir-in and kaf-EEN)
10. Triprolidine, Pseudoephedrine, and Acetaminophen (trye-PROE-li-deen soo-doe-e-FED-rin and a-set-a-MIN-oh-fen)

Category

- **Antihistaminic (H₁-receptor)-decongestant-analgesic**—Brompheniramine, Pseudoephedrine, and Acetaminophen; Chlorpheniramine, Phenylephrine, and Acetaminophen; Chlorpheniramine, Pseudoephedrine, and Acetaminophen; Chlorpheniramine, Pyrilamine, Phenylephrine, and Acetaminophen; Dexbrompheniramine, Pseudoephedrine, and Acetaminophen; Diphenhydramine, Pseudoephedrine, and Acetaminophen; Pheniramine, Phenylephrine, and Acetaminophen; Pheniramine, Phenylephrine, Sodium Salicylate, and Caffeine; Pyrilamine, Phenylephrine, Aspirin, and Caffeine; Triprolidine, Pseudoephedrine, and Acetaminophen

Description

Antihistamine, decongestant, and analgesic combinations are taken by mouth to relieve the sneezing, runny nose, sinus and nasal congestion (stuffy nose), fever, headache, and aches and pain of colds, influenza, and hay fever. These combinations do not contain any ingredient to relieve coughs.

Antihistamines are used to relieve or prevent the symptoms of hay fever and other types of allergy. They may also help relieve some symptoms of the common cold, such as sneezing and runny nose. They work by preventing the effects of a substance called histamine, which is produced by the body. Antihistamines contained in these combinations are:

brompheniramine, chlorpheniramine, dexbrompheniramine, diphenhydramine, pheniramine, phenyltoloxamine, pyrilamine, and triprolidine.

Decongestants, such as phenylephrine, and pseudoephedrine, produce a narrowing of blood vessels. This leads to clearing of nasal congestion, but it may also cause an increase in blood pressure in patients who have high blood pressure.

Analgesics, such as acetaminophen and salicylates (e.g., aspirin, sodium salicylate), are used in these combination medicines to help relieve fever, headache, aches, and pain.

Some of these medicines are available without a prescription. However, your doctor may have special instructions on the proper dose of these medicines for your medical condition. These medicines are available in the following dosage forms:

Oral
- Brompheniramine, Pseudoephedrine, and Acetaminophen
  - Oral suspension
  - Tablets
- Chlorpheniramine, Phenylephrine, and Acetaminophen
  - Capsules
  - Tablets
  - Extended-release tablets
- Chlorpheniramine, Pseudoephedrine, and Acetaminophen
  - Capsules
  - For oral solution
  - Oral solution
  - Tablets
  - Chewable tablets
- Chlorpheniramine, Pyrilamine, Phenylephrine, and Acetaminophen
  - Tablets
- Dexbrompheniramine, Pseudoephedrine, and Acetaminophen
  - Extended-release tablets
- Diphenhydramine, Pseudoephedrine, and Acetaminophen
  - For oral solution
  - Tablets
- Pheniramine, Phenylephrine, and Acetaminophen
  - For oral solution
- Pheniramine, Phenylephrine, Sodium Salicylate, and Caffeine
  - Oral solution
- Pyrilamine, Phenylephrine, Aspirin, and Caffeine
  - Tablets
- Triprolidine, Pseudoephedrine, and Acetaminophen
  - Tablets

Before Using This Medicine

If you are taking this medicine without a prescription, carefully read and follow any precautions on the label. For antihistamine, decongestant, and analgesic combinations, the following should be considered:

Allergies—Tell your doctor if you have ever had any unusual or allergic reaction to any of the ingredients contained in this medicine. If this medicine contains *aspirin* or *another salicylate*, before taking it, check with your doctor if you have ever had any unusual or allergic reaction to any of the following medicines:

- Diclofenac (e.g., Voltaren)
- Diflunisal (e.g., Dolobid)
- Etodolac (e.g., Lodine)
- Fenoprofen (e.g., Nalfon)
- Floctafenine
- Flurbiprofen, by mouth (e.g., Ansaid)
- Ibuprofen (e.g., Motrin)
- Indomethacin (e.g., Indocin)
- Ketoprofen (e.g., Orudis)
- Meclofenamate (e.g., Meclomen)
- Mefenamic acid (e.g., Ponstel)
- Methyl salicylate (oil of wintergreen)
- Nabumetone (e.g., Relafen)
- Naproxen (e.g., Naprosyn)
- Oxaprozin (e.g., Daypro)
- Oxyphenbutazone (e.g., Tandearil)
- Phenylbutazone (e.g., Butazolidin)
- Piroxicam (e.g., Feldene)
- Sulindac (e.g., Clinoril)
- Suprofen (e.g., Suprol)
- Tenoxicam (e.g., Mobiflex)
- Tiaprofenic acid (e.g., Surgam)
- Tolmetin (e.g., Tolectin)
- Zomepirac (e.g., Zomax)

Also tell your health care professional if you are allergic to any other substances, such as foods, preservatives, or dyes.

Pregnancy—The occasional use of antihistamine, decongestant, and analgesic combinations is not likely to cause problems in the fetus or in the newborn baby. However, when these medicines are used at higher doses and/or for a long time, the chance that problems might occur may increase. For the individual ingredients of these combinations, the following apply:

- *Acetaminophen*—Acetaminophen has not been shown to cause birth defects or other problems in humans. However, studies on birth defects have not been done in humans.

- *Alcohol*—Some of these combination medicines contain large amounts of alcohol. Too much use of alcohol during pregnancy may cause birth defects.

- *Antihistamines*—Antihistamines have not been shown to cause problems in humans.

- *Caffeine*—Studies in humans have not shown that caffeine causes birth defects. However, studies in animals have shown that caffeine causes birth defects when given in very large doses (amounts equal to the amount of caffeine contained in 12 to 24 cups of coffee a day).

- *Phenylephrine*—Studies on birth defects have not been done in either humans or animals with phenylephrine.

- *Pseudoephedrine*—Studies on birth defects with pseudoephedrine have not been done in humans. In animal studies pseudoephedrine did not cause birth defects but did cause a decrease in average weight, length, and rate of bone formation in the animal fetus when administered in high doses.

- *Salicylates (e.g., aspirin)*—Salicylates have not been shown to cause birth defects in humans. Studies on birth defects in humans have been done with aspirin. However, salicylates have been shown to cause birth defects in animals. Regular use of salicylates late in pregnancy may cause unwanted effects on the heart or blood flow in the fetus or newborn baby. Use of salicylates during the last 2 weeks of pregnancy may cause bleeding problems in the fetus before or during delivery, or in the newborn baby. Also, too much use of salicylates during the last 3 months of pregnancy may increase the length of pregnancy, prolong labor, cause other problems during delivery, or cause severe bleeding in the mother before, during, or after delivery. *Do not take aspirin during the last 3 months of pregnancy unless it has been ordered by your doctor.*

Breast-feeding—If you are breast-feeding the chance that problems might occur depends on the ingredients of the combination. For the individual ingredients of these combinations, the following apply:

- *Acetaminophen*—Acetaminophen passes into the breast milk. However, it has not been shown to cause problems in nursing babies.

- *Alcohol*—Alcohol passes into the breast milk. However, the amount of alcohol in recommended doses of this medicine does not usually cause problems in nursing babies.

- *Antihistamines*—Use is not recommended since the chances are greater for this medicine to cause side effects, such as unusual excitement or irritability, in the nursing baby. Also, since antihistamines tend to de-

crease the secretions of the body, it is possible that the flow of breast milk may be reduced in some women.

- *Caffeine*—Small amounts of caffeine pass into the breast milk and may build up in the nursing baby. However, the amount of caffeine in recommended doses of this medicine does not usually cause problems in nursing babies.

- *Decongestants (e.g., phenylephrine, pseudoephedrine)*—Decongestants may pass into the breast milk and may cause unwanted effects in nursing babies of mothers taking this medicine.

- *Salicylates (e.g., aspirin, sodium salicylate)*—Salicylates pass into the breast milk. Although salicylates have not been reported to cause problems in nursing babies, it is possible that problems may occur if large amounts are taken regularly.

Children—Very young children are usually more sensitive to the effects of this medicine. Increases in blood pressure, nightmares, unusual excitement, nervousness, restlessness, or irritability may be more likely to occur in children. Also, mental changes may be more likely to occur in young children taking these combination medicines.

Before giving any of these combination medicines to a child, check the package label very carefully. Some of these medicines are too strong for use in children. If you are not certain whether a specific product can be given to a child, or if you have any questions about the amount to give, check with your health care professional.

Do not give aspirin or other salicylates to a child with a fever or other symptoms of a virus infection, especially flu or chickenpox, without first discussing their use with your child's doctor. This is very important because salicylates may cause a serious illness called Reye's syndrome in children with fever caused by a virus infection, especially flu or chickenpox. Also, children may be more sensitive to the aspirin or other salicylates contained in some of these medicines, especially if they have a fever or have lost large amounts of body fluid because of vomiting, diarrhea, or sweating.

Teenagers—*Do not give aspirin or other salicylates to a teenager with a fever or other symptoms of a virus infection, especially flu or chickenpox, without first discussing their use with your child's doctor.* This is very important because salicylates may cause a serious illness called Reye's syndrome in teenagers with fever caused by a virus infection, especially flu or chickenpox.

Older adults—The elderly are usually more sensitive to the effects of this medicine. Confusion, difficult or painful urination, dizziness, drowsiness, feeling faint, or dryness of mouth, nose, or throat may be more likely to occur in elderly patients. Also, nightmares or unusual excitement, nervousness, restlessness, or irritability may be more likely to occur in the elderly.

Other medicines—Although certain medicines should not be used together at all, in other cases two different medicines may be used together even if an interaction might occur. In these cases, your doctor may want to change the dose, or other precautions may be necessary. When you are taking antihistamine, decongestant, and analgesic combinations it is especially important that your health care professional know if you are taking *any* other prescription or nonprescription (over-the-counter [OTC]) medicine, for example, aspirin or other medicine for allergies. Some medicines may change the way this medicine affects your body. Also, the effect of other medicines may be increased or reduced by some of the ingredients in this medicine.

Other medical problems—The presence of other medical problems may affect the use of antihistamine, decongestant, and analgesic combinations. Make sure you tell your doctor if you have any other medical problems, especially:

- Alcohol abuse—Acetaminophen-containing medicines increase the chance of liver damage
- Anemia—Taking a salicylate-containing medicine may make the anemia worse
- Asthma, allergies, and nasal polyps, history of, or
- Asthma attacks—Taking a salicylate-containing medicine may cause an allergic reaction in which breathing becomes difficult; also, although antihistamines open tightened bronchial passages, other effects of the antihistamines may cause secretions to become thick so that during an asthma attack it might be difficult to cough them up
- Diabetes mellitus (sugar diabetes)—The decongestant in this medicine may put the patient with diabetes at a greater risk of having heart or blood vessel disease
- Enlarged prostate or
- Urinary tract blockage or difficult urination—Some of the effects of antihistamines may cause urinary problems to get worse
- Glaucoma—A slight increase in inner eye pressure may occur
- Gout—Aspirin- or sodium salicylate-containing medicine may make the gout worse and reduce the benefit of the medicines used for gout
- Hemophilia or other bleeding problems—Aspirin- or sodium salicylate-containing medicine increases the chance of bleeding
- Hepatitis or other liver disease—There is a greater chance of side effects because the medicine is not broken down and may build up in the body; also, if liver disease is severe there is a greater chance that aspirin-containing medicine may cause bleeding
- Heart or blood vessel disease or
- High blood pressure—The decongestant in this medicine may cause the blood pressure to increase and may also speed up the heart rate; also, caffeine-containing medicine, if taken in large amounts, may have a similar effect on the heart
- Kidney disease (severe)—The kidneys may be affected, especially if too much of this medicine is taken for a long time
- Overactive thyroid—If the overactive thyroid has caused a fast heart rate, the decongestant in this medicine may cause the heart rate to speed up further
- Stomach ulcer or other stomach problems—Salicylate-containing medicine may make the ulcer worse or cause bleeding of the stomach

Proper Use of This Medicine

Take this medicine only as directed. Do not take more of it and do not take it more often than recommended on the label,

unless otherwise directed by your doctor. To do so may increase the chance of side effects.

If this medicine irritates your stomach, you may take it with food or a glass of water or milk, to lessen the irritation.

For patients taking the extended-release tablet form of this medicine:

- Swallow the tablets whole.
- Do not crush, break, or chew before swallowing.

If a combination medicine containing aspirin has a strong vinegar-like odor, do not use it. This odor means the medicine is breaking down. If you have any questions about this, check with your pharmacist.

Dosing—The dose of these combination medicines will be different for different products. *Follow the directions on the box if you are taking this medicine without a prescription. Or, follow your doctor's orders if this medicine was prescribed.* The following information includes only the average doses for these combinations.

The number of capsules or tablets or teaspoonfuls of liquid that you take depends on the strength of the medicine.

There is a large variety of antihistamine, decongestant, and analgesic combination products on the market. Some products are for use in adults only, while others may be used in children. If you have any questions about this, check with your health care professional.

For cold symptoms and sinus pain and congestion:

- For *regular (short-acting) oral* dosage forms (chewable tablets, capsules, liquid, or tablets):
  - Adults and children 12 years of age and older: Usually the dose is 1 to 2 capsules or tablets, or 1 teaspoonful of liquid, every four to six hours.
  - Children 6 to 12 years of age: Usually the dose is 1 tablet, 4 chewable tablets, or 1 to 2 teaspoonfuls of liquid every four hours.
  - Children up to 6 years of age: Use and dose must be determined by your doctor.
- For *oral* dosage forms that *must be dissolved* (effervescent tablets or powder):
  - Adults and children 12 years of age and older: Usually the dose is 2 effervescent tablets or the contents of 1 packet of powder dissolved as directed on the package.
  - Children up to 12 years of age: Use and dose must be determined by your doctor.
- For *long-acting oral* dosage form (tablets):
  - Adults and children 12 years of age and older: Usually the dose is 1 to 2 tablets every 12 hours.
  - Children up to 12 years of age: Use and dose must be determined by your doctor.

Missed dose—If you must take this medicine regularly and you miss a dose, take it as soon as possible. However, if it is almost time for your next dose, skip the missed dose and go back to your regular dosing schedule. Do not double doses.

Storage—To store this medicine:

- Keep this medicine out of the reach of children. Overdose is very dangerous in young children.
- Store away from heat and direct light.
- Do not store the capsule or tablet form of this medicine in the bathroom, near the kitchen sink, or in other damp

places. Heat or moisture may cause the medicine to break down.

- Keep the liquid form of this medicine from freezing.

- Do not keep outdated medicine or medicine no longer needed. Be sure that any discarded medicine is out of the reach of children.

Precautions While Using This Medicine

Before you have any skin tests for allergies, tell the doctor in charge that you are taking this medicine. The results of the test may be affected by the antihistamine in this medicine.

Check with your doctor if your symptoms do not improve or become worse, or if you have a high fever.

The antihistamine in this medicine will add to the effects of alcohol and other central nervous system (CNS) depressants (medicines that slow down the nervous system, possibly causing drowsiness). Some examples of CNS depressants are other antihistamines or medicine for hay fever, other allergies, or colds; sedatives, tranquilizers, or sleeping medicine; prescription pain medicine or narcotics; barbiturates; medicine for seizures; muscle relaxants; or anesthetics, including some dental anesthetics. *Check with your doctor before taking any of the above while you are taking this medicine.*

Also, stomach problems may be more likely to occur if you drink alcoholic beverages while taking a medicine that contains aspirin. In addition, drinking large amounts of alcoholic beverages while taking a medicine that contains acetaminophen may cause liver damage.

The antihistamine in this medicine may cause some people to become drowsy, dizzy, or less alert than they are normally. *Make sure you know how you react to this medicine before you drive, use machines, or do anything else that could be dangerous if you are dizzy or are not alert.*

The decongestant in this medicine may cause some people to become nervous or restless or to have trouble in sleeping. If you have trouble in sleeping, *take the last dose of this medicine for each day a few hours before bedtime.* If you have any questions about this, check with your doctor.

Also, this medicine may add to the CNS stimulant and other effects of diet aids. *Do not use medicines for diet or appetite control while taking this medicine unless you have checked with your doctor.*

Before having any kind of surgery (including dental surgery) or emergency treatment, tell the medical doctor or dentist in charge that you are taking this medicine.

Antihistamines may cause dryness of the mouth, nose, and throat. For temporary relief of mouth dryness, use sugarless candy or gum, melt bits of ice in your mouth, or use a saliva substitute. However, if your mouth continues to feel dry for more than 2 weeks, check with your dentist. Continuing dryness of the mouth may increase the chance of dental disease, including tooth decay, gum disease, and fungus infections.

Check the label of all over-the-counter (OTC), nonprescription, and prescription medicines you now take. If any contain acetaminophen or aspirin or other salicylates, including diflunisal or bismuth subsalicylate (e.g., Pepto-Bismol), be especially careful. This combination medicine contains acetaminophen and/or a salicylate. Therefore, taking it while taking any other medicine that contains these

drugs may lead to overdose. If you have any questions about this, check with your health care professional.

For patients taking *aspirin-containing medicine:*
- Do not take aspirin-containing medicine within 5 days before any surgery, including dental surgery, unless otherwise directed by your medical doctor or dentist. Taking aspirin during this time may cause bleeding problems.

For diabetic patients taking *salicylate-containing medicine,* false urine sugar test results may occur:
- If you take 8 or more 325–mg (5–grain) doses of aspirin every day for several days in a row.
- If you take 8 or more 325–mg (5–grain), or 4 or more 500–mg (10–grain), doses of sodium salicylate a day.

Smaller doses or occasional use usually will not affect urine sugar tests. If you have any questions about this, check with your health care professional, especially if your diabetes is not well controlled.

Side Effects

Along with its needed effects, a medicine may cause some unwanted effects. Although serious side effects occur rarely when this medicine is taken as recommended, they may be more likely to occur if:
- too much medicine is taken
- it is taken in large doses
- it is taken for a long time

Get emergency help immediately if any of the following symptoms of overdose occur:
  For all combinations
    Clumsiness or unsteadiness; convulsions (seizures); drowsiness (severe); dryness of mouth, nose, or throat (severe); fast heartbeat; flushing or redness of face; hallucinations (seeing, hearing, or feeling things that are not there); headache (continuing and/or severe); increased sweating; nausea or vomiting (severe or continuing); shortness of breath or troubled breathing; stomach cramps or pain (severe or continuing); trouble in sleeping

  For acetaminophen-containing only
    Diarrhea; loss of appetite; swelling or tenderness in the upper abdomen or stomach area

  For salicylate-containing only
    Any loss of hearing; bloody urine; changes in behavior (in children); confusion; diarrhea (severe or continuing); drowsiness or tiredness (severe, especially in children); fast or deep breathing (especially in children); fever; ringing or buzzing in ears (continuing); uncontrollable flapping movements of the hands (especially in elderly patients); unusual thirst; vision problems

Also, check with your doctor as soon as possible if any of the following side effects occur:
  More common
    Nausea or vomiting; stomach pain (mild)

  Less common or rare
    Bloody or black tarry stools; changes in urine or problems with urination; skin rash, hives, or itching; sore throat and fever; swelling of face, feet, or lower legs; tightness in chest; unusual bleeding or bruising; unusual tiredness or weakness; vomiting of blood or ma-

terial that looks like coffee grounds; weight gain (unusual); yellow eyes or skin

Other side effects may occur that usually do not need medical attention. These side effects may go away during treatment as your body adjusts to the medicine. However, check with your doctor if any of the following side effects continue or are bothersome:

More common
Drowsiness; heartburn or indigestion (for salicylate-containing medicines); thickening of mucus

Less common—more common with high doses
Blurred vision; confusion; difficult or painful urination; dizziness; dryness of mouth, nose, or throat; headache; loss of appetite; nightmares; pounding heartbeat; ringing or buzzing in ears; skin rash; stomach upset or stomach pain; unusual excitement, nervousness, restlessness, or irritability

Not all of the side effects listed above have been reported for each of these medicines, but they have been reported for at least one of them. There are some similarities among these combination medicines, so many of the above side effects may occur with any of these medicines.

Other side effects not listed above may also occur in some patients. If you notice any other effects, check with your doctor.

ANTIHISTAMINES, DECONGESTANTS, AND ANTICHOLINERGICS (Systemic)

Some commonly used brand names are:

In the U.S.—

AH-chew (1)	Extendryl JR (1)
D.A. Chewable (1)	Extendryl SR (1)
Dallergy (1)	Mescolor (2)
Dura-Vent/DA (1)	OMNIhist L.A. (1)
Extendryl (1)	Stahist (3)

This information applies to the following medicines:

1. Chlorpheniramine, Phenylephrine, and Methscopolamine (klor-fen-EER-a-meen fen-ill-EF-rin and meth-skoe-POL-a-meen)
2. Chlorpheniramine, Pseudoephedrine, and Methscopolamine (klor-fen-EER-a-meen soo-doe-e-FED-rin and meth-skoe-POla-meen)
3. Chlorpheniramine, Phenylephrine, Pseudoephedrine, Atropine, Hyoscyamine, and Scopolamine (soo-doe-e-FED-rin fen-ill-EF-rin klor-fen-EER-a-meen hye-oh-SYE-a-meen scoe-POL-a-meen and A-troe-peen)

Category

- **Antihistaminic (H$_1$-receptor)-decongestant-anticholinergic**—Chlorpheniramine, Phenylephrine, and Methscopolamine

Description

Antihistamine, decongestant, and anticholinergic combinations are used to treat the nasal congestion (stuffy nose) and runny nose caused by allergies and/or the common cold.

Antihistamines work by preventing the effects of a substance called histamine, which is produced by the body. Histamine can cause itching, sneezing, runny nose, and watery eyes.

The antihistamine contained in these combinations is chlorpheniramine.

The decongestants in these combinations, phenylephrine, and pseudoephedrine produce a narrowing of blood vessels. This leads to clearing of nasal congestion, but it may also cause an increase in blood pressure in patients who have high blood pressure.

Anticholinergics, such as atropine, hyoscyamine, methscopolamine, and scopolamine may help produce a drying effect in the nose and chest.

These combinations are available only with your doctor's prescription in the following dosage forms:
- Chlorpheniramine, Phenylephrine, and Methscopolamine
  - Extended-release capsules
  - Syrup
  - Tablets
  - Chewable tablets
  - Extended-release tablets
- Chlorpheniramine, Pseudoephedrine, and Methscopolamine
  - Extended-release tablets

Before Using This Medicine

In deciding to use a medicine, the risks of taking the medicine must be weighed against the good it will do. This is a decision you and your doctor will make. For antihistamine, decongestant, and anticholinergic combinations, the following should be considered:

Allergies—Tell your doctor if you have ever had any unusual or allergic reactions to antihistamines or anticholinergics, or to amphetamine, dextroamphetamine (e.g., Dexedrine), ephedrine (e.g., Ephed II), epinephrine (e.g., Adrenalin), isoproterenol (e.g., Isuprel), metaproterenol (e.g., Alupent), methamphetamine (e.g., Desoxyn), norepinephrine (e.g., Levophed), phenylephrine (e.g., Neo-Synephrine), pseudoephedrine (e.g., Sudafed), or terbutaline (e.g., Brethine). Also, tell your health care professional if you are allergic to any other substances, such as foods, preservatives, or dyes.

Pregnancy—For the individual ingredients of these combinations, the following apply:
- *Antihistamines*—Antihistamines have not been shown to cause problems in humans.
- *Atropine*—Studies on effects in pregnancy have not been done in humans. Atropine has not been shown to cause birth defects or other problems in animals.
- *Hyoscyamine*—Studies on effects in pregnancy have not been done in either humans or animals.
- *Methscopolamine*—Studies on effects in pregnancy have not been done in either humans or animals.
- *Phenylephrine*—Studies on birth defects have not been done in either humans or animals.
- *Pseudoephedrine*—Studies on birth defects have not been done in humans. Pseudoephedrine has not been shown to cause birth defects in animal studies. However, studies in animals have shown that pseudoephedrine causes a reduction in average weight, length, and rate of bone formation in the animal fetus.
- *Scopolamine*—Studies on effects in pregnancy have not been done in pregnant women. However, studies in animals at doses many times the human dose have

shown that scopolamine causes a small increase in the number of fetal deaths.

Breast-feeding—Small amounts of antihistamines, decongestants, and anticholinergics may pass into the breast milk. Use is not recommended since this medicine may cause side effects, such as unusual excitement or irritability, in the nursing baby. Also, since this medicine tends to decrease the secretions of the body, it is possible that the flow of breast milk may be reduced in some women.

Children—Very young children are usually more sensitive than adults to the effects of this medicine. Increases in blood pressure, nightmares or unusual excitement, nervousness, restlessness, or irritability may be more likely to occur in children. Also, when anticholinergics are given to children during hot weather, a rapid increase in body temperature may occur, which may lead to heat stroke. In infants and children, especially those with spastic paralysis or brain damage, this medicine may be especially likely to cause severe side effects.

Older adults—Confusion or memory loss, difficult and painful urination, dizziness, drowsiness, dryness of mouth, or convulsions (seizures) may be more likely to occur in the elderly, who are usually more sensitive than younger adults to the effects of this medicine. Also, nightmares or unusual excitement, nervousness, restlessness, or irritability may be more likely to occur in elderly patients. In addition, eye pain may occur, which may be a sign of glaucoma.

Other medicines—Although certain medicines should not be used together at all, in other cases different medicines may be used together even if an interaction might occur. In these cases, your doctor may want to change the dose, or other precautions may be necessary. When you are taking this medicine it is especially important that your health care professional know if you are taking any of the following:

- Amantadine (e.g., Symmetrel) or
- Amphetamines or
- Appetite suppressants (diet pills), except fenfluramine (e.g., Pondimin), or
- Beta-adrenergic blocking agents (acebutolol [e.g., Sectral], atenolol [e.g., Tenormin], betaxolol [e.g., Kerlone], bisoprolol [e.g., Zebeta], carteolol [e.g., Cartrol], labetalol [e.g., Normodyne], metoprolol [e.g., Lopressor], nadolol [e.g., Corgard], oxprenolol [e.g., Trasicor], penbutolol [e.g., Levatol], pindolol [e.g., Visken], propranolol [e.g., Inderal], sotalol [e.g., Sotacor], timolol [e.g., Blocadren]) or
- Caffeine (e.g., NoDoz) or
- Chlophedianol (e.g., Ulone) or
- Cocaine or
- Digitalis medicine (heart medicine) or
- Medicine for asthma or other breathing problems or
- Medicine for colds, sinus problems, or hay fever or other allergies (including nose drops or sprays) or
- Methylphenidate (e.g., Ritalin) or
- Nabilone (e.g., Cesamet) or
- Pemoline (e.g., Cylert)—Using any of these medicines together with a decongestant-containing combination may cause excessive stimulant side effects, such as difficulty in sleeping, heart rate problems, nervousness, and irritability

- Central nervous system (CNS) depressants—Using these combinations with CNS depressants may worsen the effects (e.g., drowsiness) of CNS depressants or antihistamines
- Monoamine oxidase (MAO) inhibitors (furazolidone [e.g., Furoxone], isocarboxazid [e.g., Marplan], phenelzine [e.g., Nardil], procarbazine [e.g., Matulane], selegiline [e.g., Eldepryl], tranylcypromine [e.g., Parnate])—Taking an antihistamine, decongestant, and anticholinergic combination while you are taking or within 2 weeks of taking MAO inhibitors, may make the side effects of the antihistamines, decongestants, and anticholinergics more severe; these medicines should not be used together
- Other anticholinergics (medicine for abdominal or stomach spasms or cramps)—Side effects of antihistamines or anticholinergics, such as dryness of mouth, may be more likely to occur
- Potassium chloride (e.g., Kay Ciel)—Using this medicine with an anticholinergic-containing medicine may make gastrointestinal problems caused by potassium worse
- Rauwolfia alkaloids (alseroxylon [e.g., Rauwiloid], deserpidine [e.g., Harmonyl], rauwolfia serpentina [e.g., Raudixin], reserpine [e.g., Serpasil])—These medicines may increase or decrease the effect of the decongestant in this medicine
- Tricyclic antidepressants (amitriptyline [e.g., Elavil], amoxapine [e.g., Asendin], clomipramine [e.g., Anafranil], desipramine [e.g., Pertofrane], doxepin [e.g., Sinequan], imipramine [e.g., Tofranil], nortriptyline [e.g., Aventyl], protriptyline [e.g., Vivactil], trimipramine [e.g., Surmontil])—Effects, such as drowsiness, may be worsened; also, taking these medicines together may make some of the anticholinergic side effects, such as dryness of mouth, more severe

Other medical problems—The presence of other medical problems may affect the use of antihistamine, decongestant, and anticholinergic combinations. Make sure you tell your doctor if you have any other medical problems, especially:
- Brain damage in children or
- Down syndrome or
- Dryness of mouth (severe and continuing) or
- Enlarged prostate or
- Fever or
- Glaucoma or
- Intestinal blockage or other intestinal problems or
- Kidney disease or
- Liver disease or
- Lung disease or
- Mental or emotional problems or
- Myasthenia gravis or
- Toxemia of pregnancy or
- Urinary tract blockage or difficult urination—These medicines may make these conditions worse
- Diabetes mellitus (sugar diabetes)—The decongestant in this medicine may put diabetic patients at greater risk of having heart or blood vessel disease
- Heart or blood vessel disease or

- High blood pressure—The decongestant and anticholinergic in this medicine may cause the blood pressure to increase and may also speed up the heart rate
- Overactive thyroid—If the overactive thyroid has caused a fast heartbeat, the decongestant and anticholinergic in this medicine may cause the heart rate to speed up further

Proper Use of This Medicine

Take this medicine only as directed. Do not take more of it and do not take it more often than recommended on the label, unless otherwise directed by your doctor. To do so may increase the chance of side effects.

If this medicine irritates your stomach, you may take it with food or a glass of water or milk, to lessen the irritation.

For patients *taking the extended-release capsule or extended-release tablet form of this medicine:*

- Swallow the capsule or tablet whole.
- Do not crush, break, or chew before swallowing.
- If the capsule is too large to swallow, you may mix the contents of the capsule with applesauce, jelly, honey, or syrup and swallow without chewing.

Dosing—The dose of these combination medicines will be different for different patients. *Follow your doctor's orders or the directions on the label.* The following information includes only the average doses for these combinations. *If your dose is different, do not change it* unless your doctor tells you to do so.

The number of capsules or tablets or teaspoonfuls of syrup that you take depends on the strength of the medicine. Also, the number of doses you take each day and the time between doses depend on whether you are taking a short-acting or a long-acting form of this medicine.

- For *regular (short-acting)* dosage forms (syrup, tablets, or chewable tablets):
  - For allergy and cold symptoms:
    - Adults and children 12 years of age and older— 1 or 2 tablets or chewable tablets, or 1 to 2 teaspoonfuls of syrup every four to six hours.
    - Children up to 6 years of age—Use and dose must be determined by your doctor.
    - Children 6 to 12 years of age—1 chewable tablet or 1 teaspoonful of syrup every four hours.
- For *long-acting* dosage forms (extended-release capsules or tablets):
  - For allergy and cold symptoms:
    - Adults and children 12 years of age and older— 1 capsule or tablet every twelve hours.
    - Children up to 12 years of age—Use and dose must be determined by your doctor.

Missed dose—If you miss a dose of this medicine, take it as soon as possible. However, if it is almost time for your next dose, skip the missed dose and go back to your regular dosing schedule. Do not double doses.

Storage—To store this medicine:

- Keep out of the reach of children.
- Store away from heat and direct light.
- Do not store in the bathroom, near the kitchen sink, or in other damp places. Heat or moisture may cause the medicine to break down.
- Keep the liquid form of this medicine from freezing.

- Do not keep outdated medicine or medicine no longer needed. Be sure that any discarded medicine is out of the reach of children.

Precautions While Using This Medicine

Check with your doctor if your symptoms do not improve or become worse, or if you have a high fever.

Before you have any skin tests for allergies, tell the doctor in charge that you are taking this medicine. The results of the test may be affected by the antihistamine in this medicine.

These medicines may make you sweat less, causing your body temperature to increase. *Use extra care not to become overheated during exercise or hot weather while you are taking this medicine,* since overheating may result in heat stroke. Also hot baths or saunas may make you dizzy or faint while you are taking this medicine.

The anticholinergic contained in this medicine may cause some people to have blurred vision. *Make sure your vision is clear before you drive or do anything else that could be dangerous if you are not able to see well.* These medicines may also cause your eyes to become more sensitive to light than they are normally. Wearing sunglasses may help lessen the discomfort from bright light.

These medicines may cause some people to become dizzy or drowsy. *Make sure you know how you react to this medicine before you drive, use machines, or do anything else that could be dangerous if you are dizzy or are not alert.*

The decongestant in this medicine may cause some people to be nervous or restless or to have trouble in sleeping. If you have trouble in sleeping, *take the last dose of this medicine for each day a few hours before bedtime.* If you have any questions about this, check with your doctor.

Before having any kind of surgery (including dental surgery) or emergency treatment, tell the medical doctor or dentist in charge that you are taking this medicine.

This medicine may cause dryness of the mouth, nose, and throat. For temporary relief, use sugarless candy or gum, melt bits of ice in your mouth, or use a saliva substitute. However, if your mouth continues to feel dry for more than 2 weeks, check with your dentist. Continuing dryness of the mouth may increase the chance of dental disease, including tooth decay, gum disease, and fungus infections.

If you think you or someone else may have taken an overdose, get emergency help at once. Taking an overdose of this medicine or taking this medicine with alcohol or other CNS depressants may lead to unconsciousness and possibly death.

Side Effects

Along with its needed effects, a medicine may cause some unwanted effects. Although not all of these side effects may occur, if they do occur they may need medical attention.

Get emergency help immediately if any of the following symptoms of overdose occur:

Clumsiness or unsteadiness; convulsions (seizures); drowsiness (severe); dryness of mouth, nose, or throat (severe); fast heartbeat; flushing or redness of face; hallucinations (seeing, hearing, or feeling things that are not there); headache (continuing); shortness of breath or troubled breathing; trouble in sleeping

For pseudoephedrine only
    Unusual nervousness, restlessness, or excitement
Also, check with your doctor as soon as possible if any of the following side effects occur:
Rare
    Irregular or slow heartbeat; mood or mental changes; skin rash, hives, or itching; sore throat and fever; tightness in chest; unusual bleeding or bruising; unusual tiredness or weakness

Other side effects may occur that usually do not need medical attention. These side effects may go away during treatment as your body adjusts to the medicine. However, check with your health care professional if any of the following side effects continue or are bothersome:
More common
    Drowsiness; nervousness; restlessness; thickening of mucus; trouble in sleeping
Less common—more common with high doses
    Blurred vision; confusion; difficult or painful urination; dizziness; dryness of mouth, nose, or throat; fast or pounding heartbeat; headache; increased sweating; loss of appetite; nausea or vomiting; nightmares; ringing or buzzing in ears; trembling; unusual excitement, nervousness, restlessness, or irritability; unusual paleness; weakness

Other side effects not listed above may also occur in some patients. If you notice any other effects, check with your doctor.

ANTIHISTAMINES, PHENOTHIAZINE-DERIVATIVE (Systemic)

Some commonly used brand names are:

In the U.S.—

Anergan 25 (2)	Pro-50 (2)
Anergan 50 (2)	Promacot (2)
Antinaus 50 (2)	Pro-Med 50 (2)
Pentazine (2)	Promet (2)
Phenazine 25 (2)	Prorex-25 (2)
Phenazine 50 (2)	Prorex-50 (2)
Phencen-50 (2)	Prothazine (2)
Phenergan (2)	Prothazine Plain (2)
Phenergan Fortis (2)	Shogan (2)
Phenergan Plain (2)	Tacaryl (1)
Phenerzine (2)	V-Gan-25 (2)
Phenoject-50 (2)	V-Gan-50 (2)

In Canada—

Histantil (2)	Phenergan (2)
Panectyl (3)	

This information applies to the following medicines:

1. Methdilazine (meth-DILL-a-zeen)
2. Promethazine (proe-METH-a-zeen)
3. Trimeprazine (trye-MEP-ra-zeen)

Category

- **Antiemetic**—Promethazine
- **Antihistaminic, H₁-receptor**—Methdilazine; Promethazine; Trimeprazine
- **Antivertigo agent**—Promethazine
- **Sedative-hypnotic**—Promethazine; Trimeprazine

Description

Phenothiazine (FEE-noe-THYE-a-zeen)-derivative antihistamines are used to relieve or prevent the symptoms of hay fever and other types of allergy. They work by preventing the effects of a substance called histamine, which is produced by the body. Histamine can cause itching, sneezing, runny nose, and watery eyes. Also, in some persons histamine can close up the bronchial tubes (air passages of the lungs) and make breathing difficult.

Some of these antihistamines are also used to prevent motion sickness, nausea, vomiting, and dizziness. In addition, some of them may be used to help people go to sleep and control their anxiety before or after surgery.

Phenothiazine-derivative antihistamines may also be used for other conditions as determined by your doctor.

In the U.S. these antihistamines are available only with your doctor's prescription. In Canada some are available without a prescription. However, your doctor may have special instructions on the proper dose of the medicine for your medical condition.

These medicines are available in the following dosage forms:

Oral
- Methdilazine
    - Syrup
    - Tablets
    - Chewable tablets
- Promethazine
    - Syrup
    - Tablets
- Trimeprazine
    - Extended-release capsules
    - Syrup
    - Tablets

Parenteral
- Promethazine
    - Injection

Rectal
- Promethazine
    - Suppositories

Before Using This Medicine

In deciding to use a medicine, the risks of taking the medicine must be weighed against the good it will do. This is a decision you and your doctor will make. For phenothiazine-derivative antihistamines, the following should be considered:

Allergies—Tell your doctor if you have ever had any unusual or allergic reaction to these medicines or to phenothiazines. Also tell your health care professional if you are allergic to any other substances, such as foods, preservatives, or dyes.

Pregnancy—Methdilazine, promethazine, and trimeprazine have not been studied in pregnant women. In animal studies, promethazine has not been shown to cause birth defects. However, other phenothiazine medicines caused jaundice and muscle tremors in a few newborn babies whose mothers received these medicines during pregnancy. Also, the newborn baby may have blood clotting problems if promethazine is taken by the mother within 2 weeks before delivery. Before taking this medicine, make sure your doctor knows if you are pregnant or if you may become pregnant.

Breast-feeding—Small amounts of antihistamines pass into the breast milk. Use by nursing mothers is not recommended since babies are more sensitive to the side effects of antihistamines, such as unusual excitement or irritability. Also, with the use of phenothiazine-derivative antihistamines there is the chance that the nursing baby may be more at risk of having difficulty in breathing while sleeping or of the sudden infant death syndrome (SIDS). However, more studies are needed to confirm this.

In addition, since these medicines tend to decrease the secretions of the body, it is possible that the flow of breast milk may be reduced in some patients.

Children—Serious side effects, such as convulsions (seizures), are more likely to occur in younger patients and would be of greater risk to infants than to older children or adults. In general, children are more sensitive to the effects of antihistamines. Also, nightmares or unusual excitement, nervousness, restlessness, or irritability may be more likely to occur in children. *The use of phenothiazine-derivative antihistamines is not recommended in children who have a history of difficulty in breathing while sleeping, or a family history of sudden infant death syndrome (SIDS).*

Children younger than 2 years of age **should not** take promethazine because it may cause severe and sometimes fatal breathing and lung problems. *Check with your doctor or pharmacist right away if you are unsure about whether or not your child or infant should be taking promethazine.*

Children who show signs of Reye's syndrome should not be given phenothiazine-derivative antihistamines, especially by injection. Uncontrolled movements that may occur with phenothiazine-derivative antihistamines may be mistakenly confused with symptoms of Reye's syndrome.

Teenagers—Adolescents who show signs of Reye's syndrome should not be given phenothiazine-derivative antihistamines, especially by injection. Uncontrolled movements that may occur with phenothiazine-derivative antihistamines may be mistakenly confused with symptoms of Reye's syndrome.

Older adults—Elderly patients are especially sensitive to the effects of antihistamines. Confusion; difficult or painful urination; dizziness; drowsiness; feeling faint; or dryness of the mouth, nose, or throat may be more likely to occur in elderly patients. Also, nightmares or unusual excitement, nervousness, restlessness, or irritability may be more likely to occur in elderly patients. In addition, uncontrolled movements may be more likely to occur in elderly patients taking phenothiazine-derivative antihistamines.

Other medicines—Although certain medicines should not be used together at all, in other cases two different medicines may be used together even if an interaction might occur. In these cases, your doctor may want to change the dose, or other precautions may be necessary. When taking phenothiazine-derivative antihistamines, it is especially important that your health care professional know if you are taking/receiving any of the following:

- Amoxapine (e.g., Asendin) or
- Antipsychotics (medicine for mental illness) or
- Methyldopa (e.g., Aldomet) or
- Metoclopramide (e.g., Reglan) or
- Metyrosine (e.g., Demser) or
- Pemoline (e.g., Cylert) or
- Pimozide (e.g., Orap) or

- Rauwolfia alkaloids (alseroxylon [e.g., Rauwiloid], deserpidine [e.g., Harmonyl], rauwolfia serpentina [e.g., Raudixin], reserpine [e.g., Serpasil])—Side effects of these medicines, such as uncontrolled body movements, may become more severe and frequent if they are used together with phenothiazine-derivative antihistamines
- Anticholinergics (medicine for abdominal or stomach spasms or cramps)—Side effects of phenothiazine-derivative antihistamines or anticholinergics, such as dryness of mouth, may be more likely to occur
- Central nervous system (CNS) depressants (medicines that cause drowsiness) or
- Maprotiline or
- Tricyclic antidepressants (medicine for depression)—Effects of CNS depressants or antihistamines, such as drowsiness, may become more severe; also, taking maprotiline or tricyclic antidepressants may cause some side effects of antihistamines, such as dryness of mouth, to become more severe; taking promethazine with these medicines may make very serious lung problems worse
- Contrast agent, injected into spinal canal—If you are having an x-ray test of the head, spinal canal, or nervous system for which you are going to receive an injection into the spinal canal, phenothiazine-derivative antihistamines may increase the chance of seizures; stop taking any phenothiazine-derivative antihistamine 48 hours before the test and do not start taking it until 24 hours after the test
- Levodopa—When used together with phenothiazine-derivative antihistamines, the levodopa may not work as it should
- Monoamine oxidase (MAO) inhibitor activity (isocarboxazid [e.g., Marplan], isocarboxazid [e.g., Marplan], phenelzine [e.g., Nardil], procarbazine [e.g., Matulane], selegiline [e.g., Eldepryl], tranylcypromine [e.g., Parnate])—If you are now taking or have taken within the past 2 weeks any of the MAO inhibitors, the side effects of the phenothiazine-derivative antihistamines may become more severe; these medicines should not be used together

Other medical problems—The presence of other medical problems may affect the use of antihistamines. Make sure you tell your doctor if you have any other medical problems, especially:

- Blood disease or
- Heart or blood vessel disease—These medicines may cause more serious conditions to develop
- Airway blockage or
- Breathing/lung problems or
- Sleep apnea (stop breathing while asleep)—Promethazine should not be used; may make condition much worse
- Comatose state (unconscious)—These medicines should not be given to patients who are in a coma.
- Encephalopathy (brain disease) or
- Reye's syndrome—Phenothiazine-derivative antihistamines, especially promethazine, may increase the chance of uncontrolled movements. Promethazine use should be avoided in children with these conditions.
- Enlarged prostate or

- Urinary tract blockage or difficult urination—Phenothiazine-derivative antihistamines may cause urinary problems to become worse

- Epilepsy or

- Seizure disorders—Phenothiazine-derivative antihistamines, especially promethazine, may increase the chance of seizures

- Glaucoma—These medicines may cause a slight increase in inner eye pressure that may worsen the condition

- Intestinal tract obstruction or

- Stomach ulcer—Phenothiazine-derivative antihistamines should be used with caution. They may make the condition worse.

- Jaundice—Phenothiazine-derivative antihistamines may make the condition worse

- Liver disease—Phenothiazine-derivative antihistamines may build up in the body, which may increase the chance of side effects such as muscle spasms

Proper Use of This Medicine

Antihistamines are used to relieve or prevent the symptoms of your medical problem. Take them only as directed. Do not take more of them and do not take them more often than recommended on the label, unless otherwise directed by your doctor. To do so may increase the chance of side effects.

For patients *taking this medicine by mouth:*

- Antihistamines can be taken with food or a glass of water or milk to lessen stomach irritation if necessary.

- If you are taking the *extended-release capsule* form of this medicine, swallow it whole. Do not break, crush, or chew before swallowing.

For patients taking *promethazine for motion sickness:*

- Take this medicine 30 minutes to 1 hour before you begin to travel.

For patients using the *suppository form of this medicine:*

- To insert suppository: First remove the foil wrapper and moisten the suppository with cold water. Lie down on your side and use your finger to push the suppository well up into the rectum. If the suppository is too soft to insert, chill the suppository in the refrigerator for 30 minutes or run cold water over it before removing the foil wrapper.

For patients using the *injection form of this medicine:*

- If you will be giving yourself the injections, make sure you understand exactly how to give them. If you have any questions about this, check with your health care professional.

Dosing—The dose of an antihistamine will be different for different patients. *Follow your doctor's orders or the directions on the label.* The following information includes only the average doses of antihistamines. *If your dose is different, do not change it* unless your doctor tells you to do so.

The number of capsules or tablets or teaspoonfuls of liquid that you take depends on the strength of the medicine. Also, *the number of doses you take each day and the time be-* tween doses depends on whether you are taking a short-acting or long-acting form of antihistamine.

For methdilazine
- For *regular (short-acting) oral* dosage forms (tablets or liquid):
  - For allergy symptoms:
    - Adults and teenagers—8 milligrams (mg) every six to twelve hours as needed.
    - Children younger than 3 years of age—Use and dose must be determined by your doctor.
    - Children 3 to 12 years of age—4 mg every six to twelve hours as needed.

For promethazine
- For *regular (short-acting) oral* dosage forms (tablets or liquid):
  - For allergy symptoms:
    - Adults and teenagers—10 to 12.5 mg four times a day before meals and at bedtime; or 25 mg at bedtime as needed.
    - Children younger than 2 years of age—Should not be used
    - Children 2 years of age and older—Your doctor will determine dose based on the weight and/or size of the child. Children usually are given 5 to 12.5 mg three times a day or 25 mg at bedtime as needed.
  - For nausea and vomiting:
    - Adults and teenagers—25 mg for the first dose, then 10 to 25 mg every four to six hours if needed.
    - Children younger than 2 years of age—Should not be used
    - Children 2 years of age and older—Your doctor will determine dose based on the weight and/or size of the child. Children usually are given 10 to 25 mg every four to six hours as needed.
  - For prevention of motion sickness:
    - Adults and teenagers—25 mg taken one-half to one hour before traveling. The dose may be repeated eight to twelve hours later if needed.
    - Children younger than 2 years of age—Should not be used
    - Children 2 years of age and older—Your doctor will determine dose based on the weight and/or size of the child. Children usually are given 10 to 25 mg one-half to one hour before traveling. The dose may be repeated eight to twelve hours later if needed.
  - For vertigo (dizziness):
    - Adults and teenagers—25 mg two times a day as needed.
    - Children younger than 2 years of age—Should not be used
    - Children 2 years of age and older—Your doctor will determine dose based on the weight and/or size of the child. Children usually are given 10 to 25 mg two times a day as needed.
  - For use as a sedative:
    - Adults and teenagers—25 to 50 mg.
    - Children younger than 2 years of age—Should not be used
    - Children 2 years of age and older—Your doctor will determine dose based on the weight and/or size of the child. Children usually are given 10 to 25 mg.

- For *injection* dosage form:
  - For allergy symptoms:
    - Adults and teenagers—25 mg injected into a muscle or into a vein.
    - Children younger than 2 years of age—Use and dose must be determined by your doctor.
    - Children 2 years of age and older—Your doctor will determine dose based on the weight and/or size of the child. Children usually are given 6.25 to 12.5 mg injected into a muscle three times a day or 25 mg at bedtime as needed.
  - For nausea and vomiting:
    - Adults and teenagers—12.5 to 25 mg injected into a muscle or into a vein every four hours as needed.
    - Children younger than 2 years of age—Use and dose must be determined by your doctor.
    - Children 2 years of age and older—Your doctor will determine dose based on the weight and/or size of the child. Children usually are given 12.5 to 25 mg injected into a muscle every four to six hours as needed.
  - For use as a sedative:
    - Adults and teenagers—25 to 50 mg injected into a muscle or into a vein.
    - Children younger than 2 years of age—Use and dose must be determined by your doctor.
    - Children 2 years of age and older—Your doctor will determine dose based on the weight and/or size of the child. Children usually are given 12.5 to 25 mg injected into a muscle.
- For *suppository* dosage form:
  - For allergy symptoms:
    - Adults and teenagers—25 mg inserted in rectum. Another 25-mg suppository may be inserted two hours later if needed.
    - Children younger than 2 years of age—Should not be used
    - Children 2 years of age and older—Your doctor will determine dose based on the weight and/or size of the child. Children usually are given 6.25 to 12.5 mg inserted into the rectum three times a day or 25 mg at bedtime as needed.
  - For nausea and vomiting:
    - Adults and teenagers—25 mg inserted into the rectum for the first dose, then 12.5 to 25 mg every four to six hours if needed.
    - Children younger than 2 years of age—Should not be used
    - Children 2 years of age and older—Your doctor will determine dose based on the weight and/or size of the child. Children usually are given 12.5 to 25 mg inserted into the rectum every four to six hours as needed.
  - For vertigo (dizziness):
    - Adults and teenagers—25 mg inserted into the rectum, two times a day as needed.
    - Children younger than 2 years of age—Should not be used
    - Children 2 years of age and older—Your doctor will determine dose based on the weight and/or size of the child. Children usually are given 12.5 to 25 mg inserted into the rectum two times a day as needed.

- For use as a sedative:
  - Adults and teenagers—25 to 50 mg inserted into the rectum.
  - Children younger than 2 years of age—Should not be used
  - Children 2 years of age and older—Your doctor will determine dose based on the weight and/or size of the child. Children usually are given 12.5 to 25 mg inserted into the rectum.

For trimeprazine
- For *regular (short-acting) oral* dosage forms (tablets or liquid):
  - For allergy symptoms:
    - Adults and teenagers—2.5 mg four times a day as needed.
    - Children younger than 2 years of age—Use and dose must be determined by your doctor.
    - Children 2 to 3 years of age—1.25 mg at bedtime or three times a day as needed.
    - Children 3 to 12 years of age—2.5 mg at bedtime or three times a day as needed.
- For *long-acting oral* dosage forms (extended-release capsules):
  - For allergy symptoms:
    - Adults and teenagers—5 mg every twelve hours as needed.
    - Children younger than 6 years of age—Use and dose must be determined by your doctor.
    - Children 6 to 12 years of age—5 mg once a day as needed.

Missed dose—If you are taking this medicine regularly and you miss a dose, take it as soon as possible. However, if it is almost time for your next dose, skip the missed dose and go back to your regular dosing schedule. Do not double doses.

Storage—To store this medicine:
- Keep out of the reach of children, since overdose may be very dangerous in children.
- Store away from heat and direct light.
- Do not store the capsule or tablet form of this medicine in the bathroom medicine cabinet, near the kitchen sink, or in other damp places. Heat or moisture may cause the medicine to break down.
- Keep the liquid form of this medicine from freezing.
- Do not keep outdated medicine or medicine no longer needed. Be sure that any discarded medicine is out of the reach of children.

Precautions While Using This Medicine

Tell the doctor in charge that you are taking this medicine before you have any skin tests for allergies. The results of the tests may be affected by this medicine.

When taking phenothiazine-derivative antihistamines on a regular basis, make sure your doctor knows if you are taking large amounts of aspirin at the same time (as for arthritis or rheumatism). Effects of too much aspirin, such as ringing in the ears, may be covered up by the antihistamine.

Phenothiazine-derivative antihistamines will add to the effects of alcohol and other CNS depressants (medicines that slow down the nervous system, possibly causing drowsiness). Some examples of CNS depressants are sedatives, tranquilizers, or sleeping medicine; prescription pain medicine or narcotics; barbiturates; medicine for seizures; muscle relaxants; or anesthetics, including some dental anesthetics. *Check with your doctor before taking any of the above while you are using this medicine.*

Check with your doctor right away if you have symptoms of pale or blue lips, fingernails, or skin, difficult or troubled breathing, irregular, fast, slow or shallow breathing or shortness of breath. These could be signs of a condition called respiratory depression.

Check with your doctor right away and stop taking your medicine (if directed by your doctor) if you have muscle rigidity, fever, difficult or fast breathing, seizures, fast heartbeat, increased sweating, loss of bladder control, unusually pale skin, or tiredness or weakness. These may be symptoms of a serious condition called neuroleptic malignant syndrome.

This medicine may cause some people to become drowsy or less alert than they are normally. Even if taken at bedtime, it may cause some people to feel drowsy or less alert on arising. *Make sure you know how you react to the phenothiazine-derivative antihistamine you are taking before you drive, use machines, or do anything else that could be dangerous if you are not alert.*

Phenothiazine-derivative antihistamines may cause dryness of the mouth, nose, and throat. For temporary relief of mouth dryness, use sugarless candy or gum, melt bits of ice in your mouth, or use a saliva substitute. However, if your mouth continues to feel dry for more than 2 weeks, check with your medical doctor or dentist. Continuing dryness of the mouth may increase the chance of dental disease, including tooth decay, gum disease, and fungus infections.

This medicine controls nausea and vomiting. For this reason, it may cover up some of the signs of overdose caused by other medicines or the symptoms of appendicitis. This will make it difficult for your doctor to diagnose these conditions. Make sure your doctor knows that you are taking this medicine if you have other symptoms of appendicitis such as stomach or lower abdominal pain, cramping, or soreness. Also, if you think you may have taken an overdose of any medicine, tell your doctor that you are taking this medicine.

Side Effects of This Medicine

Along with its needed effects, a medicine may cause some unwanted effects. Although not all of these side effects may occur, if they do occur they may need medical attention.

Check with your doctor as soon as possible if any of the following side effects occur:

Less common or rare
Sore throat and fever; unusual bleeding or bruising; unusual tiredness or weakness

Incidence not known
Abdominal or stomach pain; area rash; black, tarry stools; bleeding gums; blood in urine or stools; bloody nose; bluish skin or lips; chest pain or discomfort; chills; clay-colored stools; confusion about identity, place, and time; continuing ringing or buzzing or other unexplained noise in ears; convulsions; cough or hoarseness; dark urine; decreased awareness or responsiveness; difficult or troubled breathing; difficulty in speaking; drooling; fainting; fever with or without chills; fixed position of eye; general feeling of tiredness or weakness; headache; hearing loss; heavier menstrual periods; high fever; high or low blood pressure; hives or welts; hysteria; irregular,

fast, slow, or shallow breathing; itching; large, hive-like swelling on face, eyelids, lips, tongue, throat, hands, legs, feet, sex organs; lightheadedness; loss of balance control; loss of bladder control; loss of strength or energy; lower back or side pain; menstrual periods; mimicry of speech or movements; muscle pain or weakness; muscle spasm or jerking of all extremities; muscle trembling, jerking or stiffness; mutism; nausea; negativism; not breathing; painful or difficult urination; pale or blue lips, fingernails, or skin; peculiar postures or movements, mannerisms, or grimacing; pinpoint red spots on skin; redness of skin; restlessness; seeing, hearing, or feeling things that are not there; severe muscle stiffness; severe muscle stiffness; severe sleepiness; shortness of breath; shuffling walk; slow or irregular heartbeat; sore throat; sores, ulcers, or white spots on lips or in mouth; sticking out of tongue; stiffness of limbs; sudden loss of consciousness; swollen glands; tiredness; trouble thinking, speaking, or walking; twisting movements of body; uncontrolled movements, especially of face, neck, and back; uncontrolled twisting movements of neck; unpleasant breath odor; unusual bleeding or bruising; unusual tiredness or weakness; unusual weak feeling; unusually pale skin; vomiting of blood; weakness, numbness or tingling in arms or legs; yellow eyes or skin

Symptoms of overdose
Clumsiness or unsteadiness; convulsions (seizures); drowsiness (severe); dryness of mouth, nose, or throat (severe); feeling faint; flushing or redness of face; hallucinations (seeing, hearing, or feeling things that are not there); muscle spasms (especially of neck and back); restlessness; shortness of breath or troubled breathing; shuffling walk; tic-like (jerky) movements of head and face; trembling and shaking of hands; trouble in sleeping

Other side effects may occur that usually do not need medical attention. These side effects may go away during treatment as your body adjusts to the medicine. However, check with your health care professional if any of the following side effects continue or are bothersome:

More common
Drowsiness (less common with methdilazine); thickening of mucus

Less common or rare
Blurred vision or any change in vision; burning or stinging of rectum (with rectal suppository); confusion; difficult or painful urination; dizziness; dryness of mouth, nose, or throat; fast heartbeat; feeling faint; increased sensitivity of skin to sun; increased sweating; loss of appetite; nightmares; ringing or buzzing in ears; skin rash; unusual excitement, nervousness, restlessness, or irritability

Incidence not known
blistering, crusting, irritation, itching, or reddening of skin; cracked, dry, scaly skin; double vision; false or unusual sense of well being; lack of coordination; nasal stuffiness; nervousness; noisy breathing; relaxed and calm; seeing double; sleepiness or unusual drowsiness; sleeplessness; swelling; tightness in chest; trouble sleeping; unable to sleep; vomiting; wheezing

Other side effects not listed above may also occur in some patients. If you notice any other effects, check with your health care professional.

ANTI-INFLAMMATORY DRUGS, NONSTEROIDAL (Systemic)

Some commonly used brand names are:

In the U.S.—

Actron (9)	Indocin SR (8)
Advil (7)	Lodine (3)
Advil Caplets (7)	Lodine XL (3)
Advil, Children's (7)	Meclomen (10)
Aleve (14)	Medipren (7)
Anaprox (14)	Medipren Caplets (7)
Anaprox DS (14)	Midol IB (7)
Ansaid (6)	Mobic (12)
Bayer Select Ibuprofen Pain	Motrin (7)
Relief Formula Caplets (7)	Motrin Chewables (7)
Cataflam (1)	Motrin, Children's (7)
Clinoril (18)	Motrin, Children's Oral Drops
Cotylbutazone (16)	(7)
Cramp End (7)	Motrin-IB (7)
Daypro (15)	Motrin-IB Caplets (7)
Dolgesic (7)	Motrin, Junior Strength
Dolobid (2)	Caplets (7)
EC-Naprosyn (14)	Nalfon (4)
Excedrin IB (7)	Nalfon 200 (4)
Excedrin IB Caplets (7)	Naprelan (14)
Feldene (17)	Naprosyn (14)
Genpril (7)	Nuprin (7)
Genpril Caplets (7)	Nuprin Caplets (7)
Haltran (7)	Orudis (9)
Ibifon 600 Caplets (7)	Orudis KT (9)
Ibren (7)	Oruvail (9)
Ibu (7)	Pamprin-IB (7)
Ibu-200 (7)	Ponstel (11)
Ibu-4 (7)	Q-Profen (7)
Ibu-6 (7)	Relafen (13)
Ibu-8 (7)	Rufen (7)
Ibuprin (7)	Tolectin 200 (21)
Ibuprohm (7)	Tolectin 600 (21)
Ibuprohm Caplets (7)	Tolectin DS (21)
Ibu-Tab (7)	Trendar (7)
Indocin (8)	Voltaren (1)

In Canada—

Actiprofen Caplets (7)	Froben SR (6)
Advil (7)	Idarac (5)
Advil Caplets (7)	Indocid (8)
Albert Tiafen (20)	Indocid SR (8)
Alka Butazolidin (16)	Medipren Caplets (7)
Anaprox (14)	Mobiflex (19)
Anaprox DS (14)	Motrin (7)
Ansaid (6)	Motrin-IB (7)
Apo-Diclo (1)	Nalfon (4)
Apo-Diflunisal (2)	Naprosyn (14)
Apo-Flurbiprofen (6)	Naprosyn-E (14)
Apo-Ibuprofen (7)	Naprosyn-SR (14)
Apo-Indomethacin (8)	Naxen (14)
Apo-Keto (9)	Novo-Difenac (1)
Apo-Keto-E (9)	Novo-Difenac SR (1)
Apo-Napro-Na (14)	Novo-Diflunisal (2)
Apo-Napro-Na DS (14)	Novo-Flurprofen (6)
Apo-Naproxen (14)	Novo-Keto-EC (9)
Apo-Phenylbutazone (16)	Novo-Methacin (8)
Apo-Piroxicam (17)	Novo-Naprox (14)
Apo-Sulin (18)	Novo-Naprox Sodium (14)
Apo-Tenoxicam (19)	Novo-Naprox Sodium DS (14)
Butazolidin (16)	Novo-Pirocam (17)
Clinoril (18)	Novo-Profen (7)
Daypro (15)	Novo-Sundac (18)
Dolobid (2)	Novo-Tenoxicam (19)
Feldene (17)	Novo-Tolmetin (21)
Froben (6)	Nu-Diclo (1)

Nu-Flurbiprofen (6)	Rhodis (9)
Nu-Ibuprofen (7)	Rhodis-EC (9)
Nu-Indo (8)	Surgam (20)
Nu-Naprox (14)	Surgam SR (20)
Nu-Pirox (17)	Synflex (14)
Orudis (9)	Synflex DS (14)
Orudis-E (9)	Tolectin 200 (21)
Orudis-SR (9)	Tolectin 400 (21)
Oruvail (9)	Tolectin 600 (21)
PMS-Piroxicam (17)	Voltaren (1)
Ponstan (11)	Voltaren Rapide (1)
Relafen (13)	Voltaren SR (1)

This information applies to the following medicines:

1. Diclofenac (dye-KLOE-fen-ak)
2. Diflunisal (dye-FLOO-ni-sal)
3. Etodolac (ee-TOE-doe-lak)
4. Fenoprofen (fen-oh-PROE-fen)
5. Floctafenine (flok-ta-FEN-een)
6. Flurbiprofen (flure-BI-proe-fen)
7. Ibuprofen (eye-byoo-PROE-fen)
8. Indomethacin (in-doe-METH-a-sin)
9. Ketoprofen (kee-toe-PROE-fen)
10. Meclofenamate (me-kloe-FEN-am-ate)
11. Mefenamic Acid (me-fe-NAM-ik)
12. (mel-OX-i-cam)
13. Nabumetone (na-BYOO-me-tone)
14. Naproxen (na-PROX-en)
15. Oxaprozin (ox-a-PROE-zin)
16. Phenylbutazone (fen-ill-BYOO-ta-zone)
17. Piroxicam (peer-OX-i-kam)
18. Sulindac (sul-IN-dak)
19. Tenoxicam (ten-OX-i-kam)
20. Tiaprofenic Acid (tie-a-pro-FEN-ik)
21. Tolmetin (TOLE-met-in)

Category

- **Analgesic**—Diclofenac; Diflunisal; Etodolac; Fenoprofen; Floctafenine; Ibuprofen; Ketoprofen; Meclofenamate; Mefenamic Acid; Naproxen

- **Anti-inflammatory, nonsteroidal**—Flurbiprofen; Indomethacin; Naproxen; Sulindac; Tenoxicam

- **Antidysmenorrheal**—Diclofenac; Flurbiprofen; Ibuprofen; Indomethacin; Ketoprofen; Meclofenamate; Mefenamic Acid; Naproxen; Piroxicam

- **Antigout agent**—Diclofenac; Diflunisal; Etodolac; Fenoprofen; Floctafenine; Ibuprofen; Indomethacin; Ketoprofen; Naproxen; Phenylbutazone; Piroxicam; Sulindac

- **Antipyretic**—Ibuprofen; Indomethacin; Naproxen

- **Antirheumatic, nonsteroidal anti-inflammatory**—Diclofenac; Diflunisal; Etodolac; Fenoprofen; Flurbiprofen; Ibuprofen; Indomethacin; Ketoprofen; Meclofenamate; Nabumetone; Naproxen; Oxaprozin; Phenylbutazone; Piroxicam; Sulindac; Tenoxicam; Tiaprofenic Acid; Tolmetin

- **Prostaglandin synthesis inhibitor, renal, Bartter's syndrome**—Indomethacin

- **Vascular headache prophylactic**—Fenoprofen; Ibuprofen; Indomethacin; Mefenamic Acid; Naproxen

- **Vascular headache suppressant**—Diclofenac; Diflunisal; Etodolac; Fenoprofen; Floctafenine; Ibuprofen; Indomethacin; Ketoprofen; Meclofenamate; Mefenamic Acid; Naproxen

Description

Nonsteroidal anti-inflammatory drugs (also called NSAIDs) are used to relieve some symptoms caused by arthritis (rheumatism), such as inflammation, swelling, stiffness, and joint pain. However, this medicine does not cure arthritis and will help you only as long as you continue to take it.

Some of these medicines are also used to relieve other kinds of pain or to treat other painful conditions, such as:

- gout attacks;
- bursitis;
- tendinitis;
- sprains, strains, or other injuries; or
- menstrual cramps.

Ibuprofen and naproxen are also used to reduce fever.

Meclofenamate is also used to reduce the amount of bleeding in some women who have very heavy menstrual periods.

Nonsteroidal anti-inflammatory drugs may also be used to treat other conditions as determined by your doctor.

Any nonsteroidal anti-inflammatory drug can cause side effects, especially when it is used for a long time or in large doses. Some of the side effects are painful or uncomfortable. Others can be more serious, resulting in the need for medical care and sometimes even death. If you will be taking this medicine for more than one or two months or in large amounts, you should discuss with your doctor the good that it can do as well as the risks of taking it. Also, it is a good idea to ask your doctor about other forms of treatment that might help to reduce the amount of this medicine that you take and/or the length of treatment.

One of the nonsteroidal anti-inflammatory drugs, phenylbutazone, is especially likely to cause very serious side effects. These serious side effects are more likely to occur in patients 40 years of age or older than in younger adults, and the risk becomes greater as the patient's age increases. Before you take phenylbutazone, be sure that you have discussed its use with your doctor. *Also, do not use phenylbutazone to treat any painful condition other than the one for which it was prescribed by your doctor.*

Although ibuprofen and naproxen may be used instead of aspirin to treat many of the same medical problems, they must not be used by people who are allergic to aspirin.

The 200–mg strength of ibuprofen and the 220–mg strength of naproxen are available without a prescription. However, your health care professional may have special instructions on the proper dose of these medicines for your medical condition.

Other nonsteroidal anti-inflammatory drugs and other strengths of ibuprofen and naproxen are available only with your medical doctor's or dentist's prescription. These medicines are available in the following dosage forms:

Oral
- Diclofenac
  - Tablets
  - Delayed-release tablets
  - Extended-release tablets
- Diflunisal
  - Tablets
- Etodolac
  - Capsules
  - Tablets
  - Extended-release tablets
- Fenoprofen
  - Capsules
  - Tablets
- Floctafenine
  - Tablets
- Flurbiprofen
  - Extended-release capsules
  - Tablets
- Ibuprofen
  - Oral suspension
  - Tablets
  - Chewable tablets
- Indomethacin
  - Capsules
  - Extended-release capsules
  - Oral suspension
- Ketoprofen
  - Capsules
  - Extended-release capsules
  - Tablets
  - Delayed-release tablets
  - Extended-release tablets
- Meclofenamate
  - Capsules
- Mefenamic Acid
  - Capsules
- Meloxicam
  - Tablets
- Nabumetone
  - Tablets
- Naproxen
  - Oral suspension
  - Tablets
  - Delayed-release tablets
  - Extended-release tablets
- Oxaprozin
  - Tablets
- Phenylbutazone
  - Capsules
  - Tablets
  - Buffered tablets
- Piroxicam
  - Capsules
- Sulindac
  - Tablets
- Tenoxicam
  - Tablets
- Tiaprofenic Acid
  - Extended-release capsules
  - Tablets
- Tolmetin
  - Capsules
  - Tablets

Rectal
- Diclofenac
  - Suppositories
- Indomethacin
  - Suppositories
- Ketoprofen
  - Suppositories
- Naproxen
  - Suppositories
- Piroxicam
  - Suppositories

Before Using This Medicine

In deciding to use a medicine, the risks of taking the medicine must be weighed against the good it will do. This is a decision you and your health care professional will make. For the nonsteroidal anti-inflammatory drugs, the following should be considered:

Allergies—Tell your health care professional if you have ever had any unusual or allergic reaction to any of the nonsteroidal anti-inflammatory drugs, or to any of the following medicines:

- Aspirin or other salicylates
- Ketorolac (e.g., Toradol)
- Oxyphenbutazone (e.g., Oxalid, Tandearil)
- Suprofen (e.g., Suprol)
- Zomepirac (e.g., Zomax)

Also tell your health care professional if you are allergic to any other substances, such as foods, preservatives, or dyes.

Diet—Make certain your health care professional knows if you are on any special diet, such as a low-sodium or low-sugar diet. Some of these medicines contain sodium or sugar.

Pregnancy—Studies on birth defects with these medicines have not been done in humans. However, there is a chance that these medicines may cause unwanted effects on the heart or blood flow of the fetus or newborn baby if they are taken regularly during the last few months of pregnancy. Also, studies in animals have shown that these medicines, if taken late in pregnancy, may increase the length of pregnancy, prolong labor, or cause other problems during delivery. If you are pregnant, do not take any of these medicines, including nonprescription (over-the-counter [OTC]) ibuprofen or naproxen, without first discussing its use with your doctor.

Studies in animals have not shown that fenoprofen, floctafenine, flurbiprofen, ibuprofen, ketoprofen, nabumetone, phenylbutazone, piroxicam, tiaprofenic acid, or tolmetin causes birth defects. Diflunisal caused birth defects of the spine and ribs in rabbits, but not in mice or rats. Diclofenac and meclofenamate caused unwanted effects on the formation of bones in animals. Etodolac and oxaprozin caused birth defects in animals. Indomethacin caused slower development of bones and damage to nerves in animals. In some animal studies, sulindac caused unwanted effects on the development of bones and organs. Studies on birth defects with mefenamic acid have not been done in animals.

Even though most of these medicines did not cause birth defects in animals, many of them did cause other harmful or toxic effects on the fetus, usually when they were given in such large amounts that the pregnant animals became sick.

For naproxen: Before taking this medicine, make sure your doctor knows if you are pregnant or if you may become pregnant.

Breast-feeding—Although other anti-inflammatory analgesics have not been reported to cause problems in nursing babies, diclofenac, diflunisal, fenoprofen, flurbiprofen, meclofenamate, mefenamic acid, naproxen, piroxicam, and tolmetin pass into the breast milk. It is not known whether etodolac, floctafenine, ibuprofen, ketoprofen, nabumetone, oxaprozin, sulindac, or tiaprofenic acid passes into human breast milk.

- *For indomethacin:* Indomethacin passes into the breast milk and has been reported to cause unwanted effects in nursing babies.

- *For meclofenamate:* Use of meclofenamate by nursing mothers is not recommended, because in animal studies it caused unwanted effects on the newborn's development.

- *For nabumetone:* Use of nabumetone is not recommended because it may cause unwanted effects in nursing babies

- *For naproxen:* Use of naproxen is not recommended because it may cause unwanted effects in nursing babies

- *For phenylbutazone:* Phenylbutazone passes into the breast milk and may cause unwanted effects, such as blood problems, in nursing babies.

- *For piroxicam:* Studies in animals have shown that piroxicam may decrease the amount of milk.

Although other anti-inflammatory analgesics have not been reported to cause problems in nursing babies, diclofenac, diflunisal, fenoprofen, flurbiprofen, meclofenamate, mefenamic acid, naproxen, piroxicam, and tolmetin pass into the breast milk. It is not known whether etodolac, floctafenine, ibuprofen, ketoprofen, nabumetone, oxaprozin, sulindac, or tiaprofenic acid passes into human breast milk.

Children—Most of these medicines, especially indomethacin and phenylbutazone, can cause serious side effects in any patient. Therefore, it is especially important that you discuss with the child's doctor the good that this medicine may do as well as the risks of using it.

- *For ibuprofen:* Ibuprofen has been tested in children 6 months of age and older. It has not been shown to cause different side effects or problems than it does in adults.

- *For indomethacin and for tolmetin:* Indomethacin and tolmetin have been tested in children 2 years of age and older and have not been shown to cause different side effects or problems than they do in adults.

- *For naproxen:* Studies with naproxen in children 2 years of age and older have shown that skin rash may be more likely to occur.

- *For oxaprozin:* Oxaprozin has been used in children with arthritis. However, there is no specific information comparing use of this medicine in children with use in other age groups.

- *For phenylbutazone:* Use of phenylbutazone in children up to 15 years of age is not recommended.

- *For other anti-inflammatory analgesics:* There is no specific information on the use of other anti-inflammatory analgesics in children.

Most of these medicines, especially indomethacin and phenylbutazone, can cause serious side effects in any patient. Therefore, it is especially important that you discuss with the child's doctor the good that this medicine may do as well as the risks of using it.

Older adults—Certain side effects, such as confusion, swelling of the face, feet, or lower legs, or sudden decrease in the amount of urine, may be especially likely to occur in elderly patients, who are usually more sensitive than younger adults to the effects of nonsteroidal anti-inflammatory drugs. Also, elderly people are more likely than younger adults to get very sick if these medicines cause stomach problems. With phenylbutazone, blood problems may also be more likely to occur in the elderly.

Other medicines—Although certain medicines should not be used together at all, in other cases two different medicines may be used together even if an interaction might occur. In these cases, your doctor may want to change the dose, or other precautions may be necessary. When you are taking a nonsteroidal anti-inflammatory drug, it is especially important that your health care professional know if you are taking any of the following:

- Alcohol or
- Corticosteroids taken orally (cortisone-like medicine) or
- Corticotropin (e.g., HP Acthar) or
- Potassium supplements (e.g., K-Dur, Slow-K)—May increase the risk of serious stomach problems such as ulcers and bleeding
- Anticoagulants (blood thinners) or
- Cefamandole (e.g., Mandol) or
- Cefoperazone (e.g., Cefobid) or
- Cefotetan (e.g., Cefotan) or
- Heparin or
- Plicamycin (e.g., Mithracin) or
- Valproic acid—The chance of bleeding may be increased
- Aspirin—The chance of serious side effects may be increased if aspirin is used together with a nonsteroidal anti-inflammatory drug on a regular basis
- Ciprofloxacin (e.g., Cipro) or
- Enoxacin (e.g., Penetrex) or
- Itraconazole (e.g., Sporanox) or
- Ketoconazole (e.g., Nizoral) or
- Lomefloxacin (e.g., Maxaquin) or
- Norfloxacin (e.g., Noroxin) or
- Ofloxacin (e.g., Floxin) or
- Tetracyclines, oral—The buffered form of phenylbutazone (e.g., Alka Butazolidin) may keep these medicines from working properly if the 2 medicines are taken too close together
- Cyclosporine (e.g., Sandimmune) or
- Digitalis glycosides (heart medicine) or
- Lithium (e.g., Lithane) or
- Methotrexate (e.g., Mexate) or
- Phenytoin (e.g., Dilantin)—Higher blood levels of these medicines and an increased chance of side effects may occur
- Penicillamine (e.g., Cuprimine)—The chance of serious side effects may be increased, especially with phenylbutazone (e.g., Cotylbutazone)
- Probenecid (e.g., Benemid)—Higher blood levels of the nonsteroidal anti-inflammatory drug and an increased chance of side effects may occur
- Triamterene (e.g., Dyrenium)—The chance of kidney problems may be increased, especially with indomethacin
- Zidovudine (e.g., AZT, Retrovir)—The chance of serious side effects may be increased, especially with indomethacin

Other medical problems—The presence of other medical problems may affect the use of nonsteroidal anti-inflammatory drugs. Make sure you tell your doctor if you have any other medical problems, especially:

- Alcohol abuse or
- Bleeding problems or
- Colitis, Crohn's disease, diverticulitis, stomach ulcer, or other stomach or intestinal problems or
- Diabetes mellitus (sugar diabetes) or
- Hemorrhoids or
- Hepatitis or other liver disease or
- Kidney disease (or history of) or
- Rectal irritation or bleeding, recent, or
- Stomach or colon irritation or bleeding, recent, or
- Systemic lupus erythematosus (SLE) or
- Tobacco use (or recent history of)—The chance of side effects may be increased
- Anemia or
- Asthma or
- Epilepsy or
- Fluid retention (swelling of feet or lower legs) or
- Heart disease or
- High blood pressure or
- Kidney stones (or history of) or
- Low platelet count or
- Low white blood cell count or
- Mental illness or
- Parkinson's disease or
- Polymyalgia rheumatica or
- Porphyria or
- Temporal arteritis—Some nonsteroidal anti-inflammatory drugs may make these conditions worse
- Ulcers, sores, or white spots in mouth—Ulcers, sores, or white spots in the mouth sometimes mean that the medicine is causing serious side effects; if these sores or spots are already present before you start taking the medicine, it will be harder for you and your doctor to recognize that these side effects might be occurring

Proper Use of This Medicine

For patients taking *a capsule, tablet (including caplet), or liquid form* of this medicine:

- *Take tablet or capsule forms of these medicines with a full glass (8 ounces) of water*. Also, do not lie down for about 15 to 30 minutes after taking the medicine. This helps to prevent irritation that may lead to trouble in swallowing.
- To lessen stomach upset, these medicines should be taken with food or an antacid. This is especially important when you are taking indomethacin, mefenamic acid, phenylbutazone, or piroxicam, which should always be taken with food or an antacid. Taking the extended-release tablet dosage form of flurbiprofen or naproxen and taking nabumetone with food may also help the medicine be absorbed into your body more quickly. However, your doctor may want you to take the first 1 or 2 doses of other nonsteroidal anti-inflammatory drugs 30 minutes before meals or 2 hours after meals. This helps the medicine start working a little faster when you first begin to

take it. However, after the first few doses, take the medicine with food or an antacid.

- It is not necessary to take delayed-release (enteric-coated) tablets with food or an antacid, because the enteric coating helps protect your stomach from the irritating effects of the medicine. Also, it is not necessary to take ketoprofen extended-release capsules (e.g., Oruvail) with food or an antacid, because the medicine inside the capsules is enteric coated.

- If you will be taking your medicine together with an antacid, one that contains magnesium and aluminum hydroxides (e.g., Maalox) may be the best kind of antacid to use, unless your doctor has directed you to use another antacid. However, do not mix the liquid form of ibuprofen, indomethacin, or naproxen together with an antacid, or any other liquid, before taking it. To do so may cause the medicine to break down. If stomach upset (indigestion, nausea, vomiting, stomach pain, or diarrhea) continues or if you have any questions about how you should be taking this medicine, check with your health care professional.

- Some of these medicines must be swallowed whole. Tablets should not be crushed, chewed, or broken, and capsules should not be emptied out, before you take the medicine. These include delayed-release (enteric-coated) or extended-release tablets or capsules, diflunisal tablets (e.g., Dolobid), and phenylbutazone tablets (e.g., Butazolidin). If you are not sure whether you are taking a delayed-release or extended-release form of your medicine, check with your pharmacist.

For patients using *a suppository form* of this medicine:

- If the suppository is too soft to insert, chill it in the refrigerator for 30 minutes or run cold water over it before removing the foil wrapper.

- To insert the suppository: First remove the foil wrapper and moisten the suppository with cold water. Lie down on your side and use your finger to push the suppository well up into the rectum.

- Indomethacin suppositories should be kept inside the rectum for at least one hour so that all of the medicine can be absorbed by your body. This helps the medicine work better.

For patients taking *nonprescription (over-the-counter [OTC]) ibuprofen or naproxen:*

- This medicine comes with a patient information sheet. Read it carefully. If you have any questions about this information, check with your health care professional.

For safe and effective use of this medicine, do not take more of it, do not take it more often, and do not take it for a longer time than ordered by your health care professional or directed on the nonprescription (over-the-counter [OTC]) package label. Taking too much of any of these medicines may increase the chance of unwanted effects, especially in elderly patients.

When used for severe or continuing arthritis, a nonsteroidal anti-inflammatory drug must be taken regularly as ordered by your doctor in order for it to help you. These medicines usually begin to work within one week, but in severe cases up to two weeks or even longer may pass before you begin to feel better. Also, several weeks may pass before you feel the full effects of the medicine.

For patients taking *mefenamic acid:*

- *Always take mefenamic acid with food or antacids.*

- *Do not take mefenamic acid for more than 7 days at a time* unless otherwise directed by your doctor. To do so may increase the chance of side effects, especially in elderly patients.

For patients taking *phenylbutazone:*

- Phenylbutazone is intended to treat your current medical problem only. *Do not take it for any other aches or pains.* Also, phenylbutazone should be used for the shortest time possible because of the chance of serious side effects, especially in patients who are 40 years of age or older.

Dosing—The dose of these medicines will be different for different patients. *Follow your doctor's orders or the directions on the label.* The following information includes only the average doses of these medicines. *If your dose is different, do not change it* unless your doctor tells you to do so.

The number of capsules or tablets or teaspoonfuls of suspension that you take, or the number of suppositories that you use, depends on the strength of the medicine. Also, *the number of doses you take each day, the time allowed between doses, and the length of time you take the medicine depend on the medical problem for which you are taking the medicine.*

People with arthritis usually need to take more of a nonsteroidal anti-inflammatory drug during a flare-up than they do between flare-ups of arthritis symptoms. Therefore, your dose may need to be increased or decreased as your condition changes.

For diclofenac
- For *tablet* dosage form:
  - For relieving pain or menstrual cramps:
    - Adults—50 milligrams (mg) three times a day as needed. Your doctor may direct you to take 100 mg for the first dose only.
    - Children—Use and dose must be determined by your doctor.
  - For rheumatoid arthritis:
    - Adults—At first, 50 mg three or four times a day. Your doctor may increase the dose, if necessary, up to a total of 225 mg a day. After your condition improves your doctor may direct you to take a lower dose.
    - Children—Use and dose must be determined by your doctor.
  - For osteoarthritis:
    - Adults—At first, 50 mg two or three times a day. Usually, no more than a total of 150 mg a day should be taken. After your condition improves your doctor may direct you to take a lower dose.
    - Children—Use and dose must be determined by your doctor.
  - For spondylitis (lower back pain):
    - Adults—At first, 25 mg four or five times a day. After your condition improves your doctor may direct you to take a lower dose.
    - Children—Use and dose must be determined by your doctor.
- For *delayed-release tablet* dosage form:
  - For rheumatoid arthritis:
    - Adults—At first, 50 mg three or four times a day. Your doctor may increase the dose, if necessary,

up to a total of 225 mg a day. After your condition improves your doctor may direct you to take a lower dose.
- Children—Use and dose must be determined by your doctor.
  - For osteoarthritis:
    - Adults—At first, 50 mg two or three times a day. Usually, no more than a total of 150 mg a day should be taken. After your condition improves your doctor may direct you to take a lower dose.
    - Children—Use and dose must be determined by your doctor.
  - For spondylitis (lower back pain):
    - Adults—At first, 25 mg four or five times a day. After your condition improves your doctor may direct you to take a lower dose.
    - Children—Use and dose must be determined by your doctor.
- For *extended-release tablet* dosage form:
  - For rheumatoid arthritis, osteoarthritis, or spondylitis:
    - Adults—Usually 75 or 100 mg once a day, in the morning or evening. Some people may need 75 mg twice a day, in the morning and evening. Take the medicine at the same time every day.
    - Children—Use and dose must be determined by your doctor.
- For *rectal* dosage form (suppositories):
  - For rheumatoid arthritis, osteoarthritis, or spondylitis:
    - Adults—One 50–mg or 100–mg suppository, inserted into the rectum. The suppository is usually used only at night by people who take tablets during the day. Usually, no more than a total of 150 mg of diclofenac should be used in a day from all dosage forms combined.
    - Children—Use and dose must be determined by your doctor.

For *diflunisal*
- For *oral* dosage form (tablets):
  - For pain:
    - Adults—1000 milligrams (mg) for the first dose, then 500 mg every eight to twelve hours as needed. Some people may need only 500 mg for the first dose, then 250 mg every eight to twelve hours as needed. Usually, no more than a total of 1500 mg a day should be taken.
    - Children—Dose must be determined by your doctor.
  - For rheumatoid arthritis or osteoarthritis:
    - Adults—At first, 250 or 500 mg twice a day. Your doctor may increase the dose, if necessary, up to a total of 1500 mg a day. After your condition improves your doctor may direct you to take a lower dose.
    - Children—Dose must be determined by your doctor.

For *etodolac*
- For *oral* dosage forms (capsules or tablets):
  - For pain:
    - Adults—400 milligrams (mg) for the first dose, then 200 to 400 mg every six to eight hours as needed. Usually, no more than a total of 1200 mg a day should be taken.
    - Children—Use and dose must be determined by your doctor.

- For osteoarthritis:
  - Adults—At first, 400 mg two or three times a day or 300 mg three or four times a day. Usually, no more than a total of 1200 mg a day should be taken. After your condition improves your doctor may direct you to take a lower dose.
  - Children—Use and dose must be determined by your doctor.
- For *extended-release tablet* dosage form:
  - For rheumatoid arthritis, osteoarthritis, or spondylitis:
    - Adults—Usually 400 to 1000 mg once a day. Take the medicine at the same time every day.
    - Children—Use and dose must be determined by your doctor.

For *fenoprofen*
- For *oral* dosage forms (capsules or tablets):
  - For pain:
    - Adults—200 milligrams (mg) every four to six hours as needed.
    - Children—Use and dose must be determined by your doctor.
  - For arthritis:
    - Adults—At first, 300 to 600 mg three or four times a day. Your doctor may increase the dose, if necessary, up to a total of 3200 mg a day. After your condition improves your doctor may direct you to take a lower dose.
    - Children—Use and dose must be determined by your doctor.

For *floctafenine*
- For *oral* dosage form (tablets):
  - For pain:
    - Adults—200 to 400 milligrams (mg) every six to eight hours, as needed. Usually, no more than 1200 mg a day should be taken.
    - Children—Use is not recommended.

For *flurbiprofen*
- For *oral tablet* dosage form:
  - For menstrual cramps:
    - Adults—50 milligrams (mg) four times a day.
    - Children—Use and dose must be determined by your doctor.
  - For bursitis, tendinitis, or athletic injuries:
    - Adults—50 mg every four to six hours as needed.
    - Children—Use and dose must be determined by your doctor.
  - For rheumatoid arthritis or osteoarthritis:
    - Adults—At first, 200 to 300 mg a day, divided into smaller amounts that are taken two to four times a day. Usually, no more than a total of 300 mg a day should be taken. After your condition improves your doctor may direct you to take a lower dose.
    - Children—Use and dose must be determined by your doctor.
  - For spondylitis (lower back pain):
    - Adults—At first, 50 mg four times a day. Your doctor may increase the dose, if necessary, up to a total of 300 mg a day. After your condition improves your doctor may direct you to take a lower dose.
    - Children—Use and dose must be determined by your doctor.

- For *extended-release capsule* dosage form:
  - For arthritis:
    - Adults—200 mg once a day, in the evening. Take the medicine at the same time every day.
    - Children—Use and dose must be determined by your doctor.

For ibuprofen

- For *oral* dosage forms (oral suspension, tablets, chewable tablets):
  - For pain or menstrual cramps:
    - Adults and teenagers—200 to 400 milligrams (mg) every four to six hours as needed. If you are taking the medicine without a prescription from your health care professional, do not take more than a total of 1200 mg (six 200–mg tablets) a day.
    - Children up to 12 years of age—Use and dose must be determined by your doctor.
  - For fever:
    - Adults and teenagers—200 to 400 mg every four to six hours as needed. If you are taking the medicine without a prescription from your health care professional, do not take more than a total of 1200 mg (six 200–mg tablets) a day.
    - Children 6 months to 12 years of age—The medicine should be used only with a prescription from your doctor. The dose is based on body weight and on the body temperature. For fevers lower than 102.5 °F (39.2 °C) the dose is 5 mg per kilogram (kg) (about 2.2 mg per pound) of body weight. For higher fevers the dose is 10 mg per kg (about 4.5 mg per pound) of body weight.
    - Infants younger than 6 months of age—Use and dose must be determined by your doctor.
  - For arthritis:
    - Adults and teenagers—At first, a total of 1200 to 3200 mg a day, divided into smaller amounts that are taken three or four times a day. After your condition improves your doctor may direct you to take a lower dose.
    - Children 6 months to 12 years of age—The dose is based on body weight. At first, a total of 30 to 40 mg per kg (about 13.6 to 18 mg per pound) of body weight a day, divided into smaller amounts that are taken three or four times a day. Your doctor may increase the dose, if necessary, up to a total of 50 mg per kg (about 21 mg per pound) of body weight a day. After your condition improves your doctor may direct you to take a lower dose.
    - Infants younger than 6 months of age—Use and dose must be determined by your doctor.

For indomethacin

- For *capsule or oral suspension* dosage forms:
  - For arthritis:
    - Adults—At first, 25 or 50 milligrams (mg) two to four times a day. Your doctor may increase the dose, if necessary, up to a total of 200 mg a day. After your condition improves your doctor may direct you to take a lower dose.
    - Children—The dose is based on body weight. At first, 1.5 to 2.5 mg per kilogram (kg) (about 0.7 to 1.1 mg per pound) of body weight a day, divided into smaller amounts that are taken three or four times a day. Your doctor may increase the dose, if necessary, up to a total of 4 mg per kg (about 1.8 mg per pound) of body weight or 200 mg a

day, whichever is less. After your condition improves your doctor may direct you to take a lower dose.

  - For gout:
    - Adults—100 mg for the first dose, then 50 mg three times a day. After the pain is relieved, your doctor may direct you to take a lower dose for a while before stopping treatment completely.
    - Children—Use and dose must be determined by your doctor.
  - For bursitis or tendinitis:
    - Adults—25 mg three or four times a day or 50 mg three times a day.
    - Children—Use and dose must be determined by your doctor.
- For *extended-release capsule* dosage form:
  - For arthritis:
    - Adults—75 mg once a day, in the morning or evening. Some people may need to take 75 mg twice a day, in the morning and evening. Take the medicine at the same time each day.
    - Children—Dose must be determined by your doctor.
- For *rectal suppository* dosage form:
  - For arthritis, bursitis, tendinitis, or gout:
    - Adults—One 50–mg suppository, inserted into the rectum up to four times a day.
    - Children—One 50–mg suppository, inserted into the rectum up to four times a day. The suppository dosage form is too strong for small children. However, the suppositories may be used for large or heavy children if they need doses as large as 50 mg.

For ketoprofen

- For *capsule, tablet, or delayed-release tablet* dosage forms:
  - For pain or menstrual cramps:
    - Adults—25 to 50 milligrams (mg) every six to eight hours as needed. Some people may need to take as much as 75 mg every six to eight hours. Doses larger than 75 mg are not likely to give better relief.
    - Over-the-counter medication—12.5 mg every 4 to 6 hours.
    - Children—Use and dose must be determined by your doctor.
  - For arthritis:
    - Adults—At first, 50 mg four times a day or 75 mg three times a day. Your doctor may increase the dose, if necessary, up to a total of 300 mg a day. After your condition improves your doctor may direct you to take a lower dose.
    - Children—Use and dose must be determined by your doctor.
- For *extended-release capsule or extended-release tablet* dosage forms:
  - For arthritis:
    - Adults—150 or 200 mg once a day, in the morning or evening. Take the medicine at the same time every day.
    - Children—Use and dose must be determined by your doctor.
- For *rectal suppository* dosage form:
  - For arthritis:
    - Adults—50 or 100 mg twice a day, inserted into the rectum, in the morning and evening. Sometimes, the suppository is used only at night by

people who take an oral dosage form (capsules or delayed-release tablets) during the day. Usually, no more than a total of 300 mg of ketoprofen should be used in a day from all dosage forms combined.

- Children—Use and dose must be determined by your doctor.

For meclofenamate
- For *oral* dosage form (capsules):
  - For arthritis:
    - Adults and teenagers 14 years of age and older—At first, 50 milligrams (mg) four times a day. Your doctor may increase the dose, if necessary, up to a total of 400 mg a day. After your condition improves your doctor may direct you to take a lower dose.
    - Children up to 14 years of age—Use and dose must be determined by your doctor.
  - For pain:
    - Adults and teenagers 14 years of age and older—50 mg every four to six hours. Some people may need as much as 100 mg every four to six hours.
    - Children up to 14 years of age—Use and dose must be determined by your doctor.
  - For menstrual cramps and heavy menstrual bleeding:
    - Adults and teenagers 14 years of age and older—100 mg three times a day for up to six days.
    - Children up to 14 years of age—Use and dose must be determined by your doctor.

For mefenamic acid
- For *oral* dosage form (capsules):
  - For pain and for menstrual cramps:
    - Adults and teenagers 14 years of age and older—500 milligrams (mg) for the first dose, then 250 mg every six hours as needed for up to seven days.
    - Children up to 14 years of age—Use and dose must be determined by your doctor.

For meloxicam
- For *oral* dosage form (tablets):
  - For osteoarthritis:
    - Adults—7.5 milligrams (mg) daily in a single dose.

For nabumetone
- For *oral* dosage form (tablets):
  - For arthritis:
    - Adults—At first, 1000 milligrams (mg) once a day, in the morning or evening, or 500 mg twice a day, in the morning and evening. Your doctor may increase the dose, if necessary, up to a total of 2000 mg a day. After your condition improves your doctor may direct you to take a lower dose.
    - Children—Use and dose must be determined by your doctor.

For naproxen
- For *naproxen (e.g., Naprosyn) tablet and oral suspension* dosage forms:
  - For rheumatoid arthritis, osteoarthritis, and spondylitis (lower back pain):
    - Adults—At first, 250, 375, or 500 milligrams (mg) two times a day, in the morning and evening. Your doctor may increase the dose, if necessary, up to a total of 1500 mg a day. After your condition improves your doctor may direct you to take a lower dose.

- Children—The dose is based on body weight. At first, 5 mg per kilogram (kg) (about 2.25 mg per pound) of body weight twice a day. After your condition improves your doctor may direct you to take a lower dose.
  - For bursitis, tendinitis, menstrual cramps, and other kinds of pain:
    - Adults—500 mg for the first dose, then 250 mg every six to eight hours as needed.
    - Children—Use and dose must be determined by your doctor.
  - For gout:
    - Adults—750 mg for the first dose, then 250 mg every eight hours until the attack is relieved.
    - Children—Use and dose must be determined by your doctor.

- For *naproxen delayed-release tablet (e.g., EC-Naprosyn)* dosage form:
  - For rheumatoid arthritis, osteoarthritis, and spondylitis (lower back pain):
    - Adults—At first, 375 or 500 milligrams (mg) two times a day, in the morning and evening. Your doctor may increase the dose, if necessary, up to a total of 1500 mg a day. After your condition improves your doctor may direct you to take a lower dose.
    - Children—The delayed-release tablets are too strong for use in children.

- For *naproxen extended-release tablet (e.g., Naprelan)* dosage form:
  - For arthritis and pain:
    - Adults—750 to 1000 mg once a day, in the morning or evening.
    - Children—The extended-release tablets are too strong for use in children.

- For *naproxen (e.g., Naprosyn) rectal suppository* dosage form:
  - For arthritis:
    - Adults—One 500-mg suppository, inserted into the rectum at bedtime. The suppository is usually used only at night by people who take an oral dosage form (tablets, oral suspension, or delayed-release tablets) during the day. Usually, no more than a total of 1500 mg of naproxen should be used in a day from all dosage forms combined.
    - Children—The suppositories are too strong for use in children.

- For *naproxen sodium (e.g., Aleve, Anaprox) tablet* dosage form:
  - For arthritis:
    - Adults—At first, 275 or 550 mg two times a day, in the morning and evening, or 275 mg in the morning and 550 mg in the evening. Your doctor may increase the dose, if necessary, up to a total of 1650 mg a day. After your condition improves your doctor may direct you to take a lower dose.
    - Children—Naproxen sodium tablets are too strong for most children. Naproxen (e.g., Naprosyn) tablets or oral suspension are usually used for children.
  - For bursitis and tendinitis:
    - Adults—550 mg for the first dose, then 275 mg every six to eight hours as needed.
    - Children—Use and dose must be determined by your doctor. Naproxen sodium tablets are too strong for most children.

○ For gout:
  ▪ Adults—825 mg for the first dose, then 275 mg every eight hours until the attack is relieved.
  ▪ Children—Use and dose must be determined by your doctor. Naproxen sodium tablets are too strong for most children.
○ For pain, fever, and menstrual cramps:
  ▪ Adults and children 12 years of age or older—For nonprescription (over-the-counter [OTC]) use: 220 mg (one tablet) every eight to twelve hours as needed. Some people may get better relief if they take 440 mg (two tablets) for the first dose, then 220 mg twelve hours later on the first day only. If you are taking this medicine without a prescription from your health care professional, do not take more than three 220–mg tablets a day. If you are older than 65 years of age, do not take more than two 220–mg tablets a day. Your health care professional may direct you to take larger doses.
  ▪ Children up to 12 years of age—Use and dose must be determined by your doctor.

For oxaprozin
• For *oral* dosage form (tablets):
  ○ For arthritis:
    ▪ Adults—At first, 600 milligrams (mg) once or twice a day, or 1200 mg once a day. Some people may need a larger amount for the first dose only. Your doctor may increase the dose, if necessary, up to 1800 mg a day. This large dose should always be divided into smaller amounts that are taken two or three times a day. After your condition improves your doctor may direct you to take a lower dose.
    ▪ Children—Use and dose must be determined by your doctor.

For phenylbutazone
• For *oral* dosage forms (capsules, tablets, and buffered tablets):
  ○ For severe arthritis:
    ▪ Adults and teenagers 15 years of age and older—At first, 100 milligrams (mg) three or four times a day. Some people may need a higher dose of 200 mg three times a day. After your condition improves your doctor may direct you to take a lower dose for a while before stopping treatment completely. This medicine should not be taken for longer than a few weeks.
    ▪ Children up to 15 years of age—Use is not recommended.
  ○ For gout:
    ▪ Adults—400 mg for the first dose, then 100 mg every four hours for one week or less.
    ▪ Children up to 15 years of age—Use is not recommended.

For piroxicam
• For *oral* dosage form (capsules):
  ○ For arthritis:
    ▪ Adults—20 milligrams (mg) once a day or 10 mg twice a day.
    ▪ Children—Dose must be determined by your doctor.
  ○ For menstrual cramps:
    ▪ Adults—40 mg once a day for one day only, then 20 mg once a day if needed.
    ▪ Children—Dose must be determined by your doctor.

• For *rectal* dosage form (suppositories):
  ○ For arthritis:
    ▪ Adults—20 mg once a day or 10 mg twice a day.
    ▪ Children—Dose must be determined by your doctor.

For sulindac
• For *oral* dosage form (tablets):
  ○ For arthritis:
    ▪ Adults—At first, 150 or 200 milligrams (mg) twice a day. After your condition improves, your doctor may direct you to take a lower dose.
    ▪ Children—Use and dose must be determined by your doctor.
  ○ For gout, bursitis, or tendinitis:
    ▪ Adults—At first, 200 mg twice a day. After the pain is relieved, your doctor may direct you to take a lower dose for a while before treatment is stopped completely.
    ▪ Children—Use and dose must be determined by your doctor.

For tenoxicam
• For *oral* dosage form (tablets):
  ○ For arthritis:
    ▪ Adults and teenagers 16 years of age and older—At first, 20 milligrams (mg) once a day, at the same time each day. For some people, a smaller dose of 10 mg (one-half tablet) a day may be enough.
    ▪ Children and teenagers up to 16 years of age—Dose must be determined by your doctor.

For tiaprofenic acid
• For *oral tablet* dosage form:
  ○ For arthritis:
    ▪ Adults—At first, 200 milligrams (mg) three times a day or 300 mg twice a day. After your condition improves, your doctor may direct you to take a lower dose.
    ▪ Children—Use and dose must be determined by your doctor.
• For *extended-release capsule* dosage form:
  ○ For arthritis:
    ▪ Adults—600 mg (two capsules) once a day, at the same time each day.
    ▪ Children—Use and dose must be determined by your doctor.

For tolmetin
• For *oral* dosage forms (capsules or tablets):
  ○ For arthritis:
    ▪ Adults—At first, 400 milligrams (mg) three times a day. Your doctor may increase the dose, if necessary, up to a total of 1800 mg a day. After your condition improves, your doctor may direct you to take a lower dose.
    ▪ Children 2 years of age and older—The dose is based on body weight. At first, 20 mg per kilogram (kg) (about 9 mg per pound) of body weight a day, divided into smaller amounts that are taken three or four times a day. Your doctor may increase the dose, if necessary, up to 30 mg per kg (about 13.5 mg per pound) of body weight a day. After your condition improves, your doctor may direct you to take a lower dose.
    ▪ Children up to 2 years of age—Dose must be determined by your doctor.

Missed dose—If your health care professional has ordered you to take this medicine according to a regular schedule, and you miss a dose, take it as soon as you remember. However, if it is almost time for your next dose, skip the missed dose and go back to your regular dosing schedule. (For long-acting medicines or extended-release dosage forms that are only taken once or twice a day, take the missed dose only if you remember within an hour or two after the dose should have been taken. If you do not remember until later, skip the missed dose and go back to your regular dosing schedule.) Do not double doses.

Storage—To store this medicine:

- Keep out of the reach of children.
- Store away from heat and direct light.
- Do not store tablets or capsules in the bathroom, near the kitchen sink, or in other damp places. Heat or moisture may cause the medicine to break down.
- Keep liquid and suppository forms of this medicine from freezing.
- Do not keep outdated medicine or medicine no longer needed. Be sure that any discarded medicine is out of the reach of children.

Precautions While Using This Medicine

If you will be taking this medicine for a long time, as for arthritis (rheumatism), your doctor should check your progress at regular visits. Your doctor may want to do certain tests to find out if unwanted effects are occurring, especially if you are taking phenylbutazone. The tests are very important because serious side effects, including ulcers, bleeding, or blood problems, can occur without any warning.

Stomach problems may be more likely to occur if you drink alcoholic beverages while being treated with this medicine. Also, alcohol may add to the depressant side effects of phenylbutazone.

If you consume 3 or more alcoholic beverages per day, check with your doctor before taking this medicine.

Taking two or more of the nonsteroidal anti-inflammatory drugs together on a regular basis may increase the chance of unwanted effects. Also, taking acetaminophen, aspirin or other salicylates, or ketorolac (e.g., Toradol) regularly while you are taking a nonsteroidal anti-inflammatory drug may increase the chance of unwanted effects. The risk will depend on how much of each medicine you take every day, and on how long you take the medicines together. If your health care professional directs you to take these medicines together on a regular basis, follow his or her directions carefully. However, *do not take acetaminophen or aspirin or other salicylates together with this medicine for more than a few days, and do not take any ketorolac (e.g., Toradol) while you are taking this medicine, unless your doctor has directed you to do so and is following your progress.*

Serious side effects can occur during treatment with this medicine. Sometimes serious side effects can occur without any warning. However, possible warning signs often occur, including swelling of the face, fingers, feet, and/or lower legs; severe stomach pain, black, tarry stools, and/or vomiting of blood or material that looks like coffee grounds; unusual weight gain; and/or skin rash. Also, signs of serious heart problems could occur such as chest pain, tightness in chest, fast or irregular heartbeat, or unusual flushing or warmth of skin. *Stop taking this medicine and check with your doctor immediately if you notice any of these warning signs.*

Before having any kind of surgery (including dental surgery), tell the medical doctor or dentist in charge that you are taking this medicine. If possible, this should be done when your surgery is first being planned. Some of the nonsteroidal anti-inflammatory drugs can increase the chance of bleeding during and after surgery. It may be necessary for you to stop treatment for a while, or to change to a different nonsteroidal anti-inflammatory drug that is less likely to cause bleeding.

This medicine may cause some people to become confused, drowsy, dizzy, lightheaded, or less alert than they are normally. It may also cause blurred vision or other vision problems in some people. *Make sure you know how you react to this medicine before you drive, use machines, or do anything else that could be dangerous if you are confused, dizzy, or drowsy, or if you are not alert and able to see well.* If these reactions are especially bothersome, check with your doctor.

For patients taking *the buffered form of phenylbutazone (e.g., Alka-Butazolidin):*

- This medicine contains antacids that can keep other medicines from working properly if the 2 medicines are taken too close together. *Always take this medicine:*
  - *At least 6 hours before or 2 hours after taking ciprofloxacin (e.g., Cipro) or lomefloxacin (e.g., Maxaquin).*
  - *At least 8 hours before or 2 hours after taking enoxacin (e.g., Penetrex).*
  - *At least 2 hours after taking itraconazole (e.g., Sporanox).*
  - *At least 3 hours before or after taking ketoconazole (e.g., Nizoral).*
  - *At least 2 hours before or after taking norfloxacin (e.g., Noroxin) or ofloxacin (e.g., Floxin).*
  - *At least 1 to 3 hours before or after taking a tetracycline antibiotic by mouth.*
  - *At least 1 or 2 hours before or after taking any other medicine by mouth.*

For patients taking *mefenamic acid:*

- If diarrhea occurs while you are using this medicine, *stop taking it and check with your doctor immediately. Do not take it again without first checking with your doctor,* because severe diarrhea may occur each time you take it.

Some people who take nonsteroidal anti-inflammatory drugs may become more sensitive to sunlight than they are normally. Exposure to sunlight, even for brief periods of time, may cause severe sunburn; blisters on the skin; skin rash, redness, itching, or discoloration; or vision changes. When you begin taking this medicine:

- Stay out of direct sunlight, especially between the hours of 10:00 a.m. and 3:00 p.m., if possible.
- Wear protective clothing, including a hat and sunglasses.
- Apply a sun block product that has a skin protection factor (SPF) of at least 15. Some patients may require a product with a higher SPF number, especially if they have a fair complexion. If you have any questions about this, check with your health care professional.
- Do not use a sunlamp or tanning bed or booth.

If you have a severe reaction from the sun, check with your doctor.

Serious side effects, including ulcers or bleeding, can occur during treatment with this medicine. Sometimes serious side effects can occur without any warning. However, possible warning signs often occur, including severe abdominal or stomach cramps, pain, or burning; black, tarry stools; severe, continuing nausea, heartburn, or indigestion; and/or vomiting of blood or material that looks like coffee grounds. *Stop taking this medicine and check with your doctor immediately if you notice any of these warning signs.*

Check with your doctor immediately if chills, fever, muscle aches or pains, or other influenza-like symptoms occur, especially if they occur shortly before, or together with, a skin rash. Very rarely, these effects may be the first signs of a serious reaction to this medicine.

Nonsteroidal anti-inflammatory drugs may cause a serious type of allergic reaction called anaphylaxis. Although this is rare, it may occur more often in patients who are allergic to aspirin or to any of the nonsteroidal anti-inflammatory drugs. *Anaphylaxis requires immediate medical attention.* The most serious signs of this reaction are very fast or irregular breathing, gasping for breath, wheezing, or fainting. Other signs may include changes in color of the skin of the face; very fast but irregular heartbeat or pulse; hive-like swellings on the skin; and puffiness or swellings of the eyelids or around the eyes. If these effects occur, get emergency help at once. Ask someone to drive you to the nearest hospital emergency room. If this is not possible, do not try to drive yourself. Call an ambulance, lie down, cover yourself to keep warm, and prop your feet higher than your head. Stay in that position until help arrives.

For patients taking *ibuprofen* or *naproxen* without a prescription:
- Check with your medical doctor or dentist:
  ◦ if your symptoms do not improve or if they get worse.
  ◦ if you are using this medicine to bring down a fever and the fever lasts more than 3 days or returns.
  ◦ if the painful area is red or swollen.

Side Effects of This Medicine

Along with its needed effects, a medicine may cause some unwanted effects. Although not all of these side effects may occur, if they do occur they may need medical attention.

Stop taking this medicine and get emergency help right away if any of the following side effects occur:
Rare—For all nonsteroidal anti-inflammatory drugs
Fainting; fast or irregular breathing; fast, irregular heartbeat or pulse; hive-like swellings (large) on face, eyelids, mouth, lips, or tongue; puffiness or swelling of the eyelids or around the eyes; shortness of breath, troubled breathing, wheezing, or tightness in chest

Also, stop taking this medicine and check with your doctor immediately if any of the following side effects occur:

More common—for mefenamic acid only
Diarrhea
More common—for phenylbutazone only
Swelling of face, hands, feet, or lower legs; weight gain (rapid)
Symptoms of phenylbutazone overdose
Bluish color of fingernails, lips, or skin; headache (severe and continuing)

Rare—for all nonsteroidal anti-inflammatory drugs
Abdominal or stomach pain, cramping, or burning (severe); bloody or black, tarry stools; chest pain; convulsions (seizures); fever with or without chills; nausea, heartburn, and/or indigestion (severe and continuing); pinpoint red spots on skin; sores, ulcers, or white spots on lips or in mouth; spitting up blood; unexplained nosebleeds; unusual bleeding or bruising; vomiting of blood or material that looks like coffee grounds

Also, check with your doctor as soon as possible if any of the following side effects occur:
More common
Bleeding from rectum (with suppositories); headache (severe), especially in the morning (for indomethacin only); skin rash
Less common or rare
Bladder pain; bleeding from cuts or scratches that lasts longer than usual; bleeding or crusting sores on lips; bloody or cloudy urine or any problem with urination, such as difficult, burning, or painful urination; change in urine color or odor; frequent urge to urinate; sudden, large increase or decrease in the amount of urine; or loss of bladder control; blurred vision or any change in vision; burning feeling in throat, chest, or stomach; confusion, forgetfulness, mental depression, or other mood or mental changes; cough or hoarseness; decreased hearing, any other change in hearing, or ringing or buzzing in ears; difficulty in swallowing; eye pain, irritation, dryness, redness, and/or swelling; hallucinations (seeing, hearing, or feeling things that are not there); headache (severe), throbbing, or with stiff neck or back; hives, itching of skin, or any other skin problem, such as blisters, redness or other color change, tenderness, burning, peeling, thickening, or scaliness; increased blood pressure; irritated tongue; light-colored stools; loosening or splitting of fingernails; muscle cramps, pain, or weakness; numbness, tingling, pain, or weakness in hands or feet; pain in lower back and/or side (severe); swelling and/or tenderness in upper abdominal or stomach area; swelling of face, feet, or lower legs (if taking phenylbutazone, stop taking it and check with your doctor immediately); swelling of lips or tongue; swollen and/or painful glands (especially in the neck or throat area); thirst (continuing); trouble in speaking; unexplained runny nose or sneezing; unexplained, unexpected, or unusually heavy vaginal bleeding; unusual tiredness or weakness; weight gain (rapid) (if taking phenylbutazone, stop taking it and check with your doctor immediately); yellow eyes or skin

Other side effects may occur that usually do not need medical attention. These side effects may go away during treatment as your body adjusts to the medicine. However, check with your doctor if any of the following side effects continue or are bothersome:
More common
Abdominal or stomach cramps, pain, or discomfort (mild to moderate); diarrhea (if taking mefenamic acid, stop taking it and check with your doctor immediately); dizziness, drowsiness, or lightheadedness; headache (mild to moderate); heartburn, indigestion, nausea, or vomiting
Less common or rare
Bitter taste or other taste change; bloated feeling, gas, or constipation; decreased appetite or loss of appetite;

fast or pounding heartbeat; flushing or hot flashes; general feeling of discomfort or illness; increased sensitivity of eyes to light; increased sensitivity of skin to sunlight; increased sweating; irritation, dryness, or soreness of mouth; nervousness, anxiety, irritability, trembling, or twitching; rectal irritation (with suppositories); trouble in sleeping; unexplained weight loss; unusual tiredness or weakness without any other symptoms

Although not all of the side effects listed above have been reported for all of these medicines, they have been reported for at least one of them. However, since all anti-inflammatory analgesics are very similar, it is possible that any of the above side effects may occur with any of these medicines.

Some side effects may occur many days or weeks after you have stopped using phenylbutazone. During this time *check with your doctor immediately* if you notice any of the following side effects:

Sore throat and fever; ulcers, sores, or white spots in mouth; unusual bleeding or bruising; unusual tiredness or weakness

Other side effects not listed above may also occur in some patients. If you notice any other effects, check with your doctor.

ANTIMYASTHENICS (Systemic)

Some commonly used brand names are:

In the U.S.—

Mestinon (3)	Prostigmin (2)
Mestinon Timespans (3)	Regonol (3)
Mytelase Caplets (1)	

In Canada—

Mestinon (3)	Prostigmin (2)
Mestinon-SR (3)	Regonol (3)

This information applies to the following medicines:

1. Ambenonium (am-be-NOE-nee-um)
2. Neostigmine (nee-oh-STIG-meen)
3. Pyridostigmine (peer-id-oh-STIG-meen)

Category

- **Antidote, to nondepolarizing neuromuscular block**—Neostigmine; Pyridostigmine

- **Antimyasthenic**—Ambenonium; Neostigmine; Pyridostigmine

- **Cholinergic, cholinesterase inhibitor**—Ambenonium; Neostigmine; Pyridostigmine

- **Diagnostic aid, myasthenia gravis**—Neostigmine

Description

Antimyasthenics are given by mouth or by injection to treat myasthenia gravis. Neostigmine may also be given by injection as a test for myasthenia gravis. Sometimes neostigmine is given by injection to prevent or treat certain urinary tract or intestinal disorders. In addition, neostigmine or pyridostig-

mine may be given by injection as an antidote to certain types of muscle relaxants used in surgery.

These medicines are available only with your doctor's prescription in the following dosage forms:

Oral
- Ambenonium
  - Tablets
- Neostigmine
  - Tablets
- Pyridostigmine
  - Syrup
  - Tablets
  - Extended-release tablets

Parenteral
- Neostigmine
  - Injection
- Pyridostigmine
  - Injection

Before Using This Medicine

In deciding to use a medicine, the risks of taking the medicine must be weighed against the good it will do. This is a decision you and your doctor will make. For the antimyasthenics, the following should be considered:

Allergies—Tell your doctor if you have ever had any unusual or allergic reaction to ambenonium, bromides, neostigmine, or pyridostigmine. Also tell your health care professional if you are allergic to any other substances, such as foods, preservatives, or dyes.

Pregnancy—Antimyasthenics have not been reported to cause birth defects; however, muscle weakness has occurred temporarily in some newborn babies whose mothers took antimyasthenics during pregnancy.

Breast-feeding—Antimyasthenics have not been reported to cause problems in nursing babies.

Children—Although there is no specific information comparing use of antimyasthenics in children with use in other age groups, these medicines are not expected to cause different side effects or problems in children than they do in adults.

Older adults—Many medicines have not been studied specifically in older people. Therefore, it may not be known whether they work exactly the same way they do in younger adults. Although there is not much information comparing use of antimyasthenics in the elderly with use in other age groups, these medicines are not expected to cause different side effects or problems in older people than they do in younger adults.

Other medicines—Although certain medicines should not be used together at all, in other cases 2 different medicines may be used together even if an interaction might occur. In these cases, your doctor may want to change the dose, or other precautions may be necessary. When you are taking an antimyasthenic, it is especially important that your health care professional knows if you are using any of the following:

- Demecarium (e.g., Humorsol) or
- Echothiophate (e.g., Phospholine Iodide) or
- Isoflurophate (e.g., Floropryl) or
- Malathion (e.g., Prioderm)—Using these medicines with antimyasthenics may result in serious side effects

- Guanadrel (e.g., Hylorel) or
- Guanethidine (e.g., Ismelin) or
- Mecamylamine (e.g., Inversine) or
- Procainamide (e.g., Pronestyl) or
- Trimethaphan (e.g., Arfonad)—The effects of these medicines may interfere with the actions of the antimyasthenics

Other medical problems—The presence of other medical problems may affect the use of the antimyasthenics. Make sure you tell your doctor if you have any other medical problems, especially:

- Intestinal blockage or
- Urinary tract blockage or
- Urinary tract infection—These medicines may make the condition worse

---

Proper Use of This Medicine

Your doctor may want you to take this medicine with food or milk to help lessen the chance of side effects. If you have any questions about how you should be taking this medicine, check with your doctor.

Take this medicine only as directed. Do not take more of it, do not take it more often, and do not take it for a longer time than your doctor ordered. To do so may increase the chance of side effects.

If you are taking this medicine *for myasthenia gravis:*

- When you first begin taking this medicine, your doctor may want you to keep a daily record of:
  ○ the time you take each dose.
  ○ how long you feel better after taking each dose.
  ○ how long you feel worse.
  ○ any side effects that occur.

This is to help your doctor decide whether the dose of this medicine should be increased or decreased and how often the medicine should be taken in order for it to be most effective in your condition.

Dosing—The dose of these medicines will be different for different patients. *Follow your doctor's orders or the directions on the label.* The following information includes only the average doses of these medicines. *If your dose is different, do not change it* unless your doctor tells you to do so.

The number of tablets or teaspoonfuls of syrup that you take depends on the strength of the medicine. Also, *the number of doses you take each day, the time allowed between doses, and the length of time you take the medicine depend on the medical problem for which you are taking these medicines.*

For ambenonium
- For *oral* dosage form (tablets):
  ○ For myasthenia gravis:
    ▪ Adults and teenagers—At first, the dose is 5 milligrams (mg) three or four times per day. Then, if needed, the dose will be adjusted by your doctor.
    ▪ Children—The dose is based on body weight or size and must be determined by your doctor. The total daily dose is usually 300 micrograms (mcg) per kilogram (kg) (136 mcg per pound) of body weight or 10 mg per square meter of body surface area. This dose may be divided into three or four smaller doses. If needed, the total daily dose will be increased to 1.5 mg per kg (0.68 mg per pound) of body weight or 50 mg per square meter of body surface area. This dose may be divided into three or four smaller doses.

For neostigmine
- For *oral* dosage form (tablets):
  ○ For myasthenia gravis:
    ▪ Adults and teenagers—At first, the dose is 15 milligrams (mg) every three or four hours. Then, the dose is 150 mg taken over a twenty-four-hour period.
    ▪ Children—The dose is based on body weight or size and must be determined by your doctor. The total daily dose is usually 2 mg per kilogram (kg) (0.91 mg per pound) of body weight or 60 mg per square meter of body surface area. This dose may be divided into six to eight smaller doses.
- For *injection* dosage form:
  ○ For myasthenia gravis:
    ▪ Adults and teenagers—The usual dose is 500 micrograms (mcg) injected into a muscle or under the skin.
    ▪ Children—The dose is based on body weight and must be determined by your doctor. It is usually 10 to 40 mcg per kg (4.5 to 18.2 mcg per pound) of body weight, injected into a muscle or under the skin, every two or three hours.
  ○ For urinary tract or intestinal disorders:
    ▪ Adults and teenagers—The usual dose is 250 to 500 mcg, injected into a muscle or under the skin, as needed.
    ▪ Children—Use and dose must be determined by your doctor.

For pyridostigmine
- For *oral* dosage forms (syrup and tablets):
  ○ For myasthenia gravis:
    ▪ Adults and teenagers—At first, the dose is 30 to 60 milligrams (mg) every three or four hours. Then, the dose is 60 mg to 1.5 grams (usually 600 mg) per day.
    ▪ Children—The dose is based on body weight or size and must be determined by your doctor. The total daily dose is usually 7 mg per kilogram (kg) (3.2 mg per pound) of body weight or 200 mg per square meter of body surface area. This dose may be divided into five or six smaller doses.
- For *long-acting oral* dosage form (extended-release tablets):
  ○ For myasthenia gravis:
    ▪ Adults and teenagers—The usual dose is 180 to 540 mg one or two times per day.
    ▪ Children—Dose must be determined by your doctor.
- For *injection* dosage form:
  ○ For myasthenia gravis:
    ▪ Adults and teenagers—The usual dose is 2 mg, injected into a muscle or vein, every two or three hours.

• Children—The dose is based on body weight and must be determined by your doctor. It is usually 50 to 150 micrograms (mcg) per kg (22.7 to 68.1 mcg per pound) of body weight, injected into a muscle every four to six hours.

Missed dose—If you miss a dose of this medicine, take it as soon as you remember. However, if it is almost time for your next dose, skip the missed dose and go back to your regular dosing schedule. Do not double doses.

Storage—To store this medicine:

- Keep out of the reach of children.
- Store away from heat and direct light.
- Do not store the tablet form of this medicine in the bathroom, near the kitchen sink, or in other damp places. Heat or moisture may cause the medicine to break down.
- Keep the syrup form of pyridostigmine from freezing.
- Do not keep outdated medicine or medicine no longer needed. Be sure that any discarded medicine is out of the reach of children.

Side Effects

Along with its needed effects, a medicine may cause some unwanted effects. Although not all of these side effects may occur, if they do occur they may need medical attention.

Check with your doctor immediately if any of the following side effects occur:

Symptoms of overdose

Blurred vision; clumsiness or unsteadiness; confusion; convulsions (seizures); diarrhea (severe); increase in bronchial secretions or watering of mouth (excessive); increasing muscle weakness (especially in the arms, neck, shoulders, and tongue); muscle cramps or twitching; nausea or vomiting (severe); shortness of breath, troubled breathing, wheezing, or tightness in chest; slow heartbeat; slurred speech; stomach cramps or pain (severe); unusual irritability, nervousness, restlessness, or fear; unusual tiredness or weakness

Also, check with your doctor as soon as possible if any of the following side effects occur:

Rare

Redness, swelling, or pain at place of injection (for pyridostigmine injection only); skin rash (does not apply to ambenonium)

Other side effects may occur that usually do not need medical attention. These side effects may go away during treatment as your body adjusts to the medicine. However, check with your doctor if any of the following side effects continue or are bothersome:

More common

Diarrhea; increased sweating; increased watering of mouth; nausea or vomiting; stomach cramps or pain

Less common

Frequent urge to urinate; increase in bronchial secretions; unusually small pupils; unusual watering of eyes

Other side effects not listed above may also occur in some patients. If you notice any other effects, check with your doctor.

ANTIPYRINE AND BENZOCAINE
(Otic route) - an-tee-PYE-reen, BEN-zoe-kane

Commonly used brand name(s)

In the U.S.—

A/B Otic	Benzotic
Aurodex	Dec-Agesic A.B.
Auroto	Dolotic

Available Dosage Forms:

• Solution

Therapeutic Class: Anesthetic Combination
Pharmacologic Class: NSAID

Uses For This Medicine

Antipyrine and benzocaine combination is used in the ear to help relieve the pain, swelling, and congestion of some ear infections. It will not cure the infection itself. An antibiotic will be needed to treat the infection. This medicine is also used to soften earwax so that the earwax can be washed away more easily.

In the U.S., this medicine is available only with your doctor's prescription.

Before Using This Medicine

In deciding to use a medicine, the risks of taking the medicine must be weighed against the good it will do. This is a decision you and your doctor will make. For this medicine, the following should be considered:

Allergies—Tell your doctor if you have ever had any unusual or allergic reaction to this medicine or any other medicines. Also tell your health care professional if you have any other types of allergies, such as to foods, dyes, preservatives, or animals. For non-prescription products, read the label or package ingredients carefully.

Pediatric—Infants, especially infants up to 3 months of age, may be especially sensitive to the effects of the benzocaine in this combination medicine. This may increase the chance of side effects. However, this medicine is not expected to cause different side effects or problems in older children than it does in adults.

Geriatric—Many medicines have not been studied specifically in older people. Therefore, it may not be known whether they work exactly the same way they do in younger adults. Although there is no specific information comparing use of antipyrine and benzocaine in the elderly with use in other age groups, this medicine is not expected to cause different side effects or problems in older people than it does in younger adults.

Other medicines—Although certain medicines should not be used together at all, in other cases two different medicines may be used together even if an interaction might occur. In these cases, your doctor may want to change the dose, or other precautions may be necessary. Tell your healthcare professional if you are taking any other prescription or non-prescription (over-the-counter [OTC]) medicine.

Interactions with Food/Tobacco/Alcohol—Certain medicines should not be used at or around the time of eating

food or eating certain types of food since interactions may occur. Using alcohol or tobacco with certain medicines may also cause interactions to occur. Discuss with your healthcare professional the use of your medicine with food, alcohol, or tobacco.

Other medical problems—The presence of other medical problems may affect the use of this medicine. Make sure you tell your doctor if you have any other medical problems, especially:

- Your ear is draining—The chance of unwanted effects may be increased

---

Proper Use of This Medicine

You may warm the ear drops to body temperature (37 °C or 98.6 °F) by holding the bottle in your hand for a few minutes before applying the drops.

To use:

- Lie down or tilt the head so that the affected ear faces up. Gently pull the earlobe up and back for adults (down and back for children) to straighten the ear canal. Drop the medicine into the ear canal. Keep the ear facing up for about 5 minutes to allow the medicine to coat the ear canal. (For young children and other patients who cannot stay still for 5 minutes, try to keep the ear facing up for at least 1 or 2 minutes.) A sterile cotton plug may be moistened with a few drops of this medicine and gently placed at the ear opening for no longer than 5 to 10 minutes to help keep the medicine from leaking out. If you have any questions about this, check with your doctor.

- To keep the medicine as germ-free as possible, do not touch the dropper to any surface (including the ear).

- Do not rinse the dropper after use. Wipe the tip of the dropper with a clean tissue and keep the container tightly closed.

If you are using this medicine to help remove earwax, the ear should be flushed with warm water after you have used this medicine for 2 or 3 days. This is usually done by your doctor. If you have been directed to flush the ear out yourself, make sure that you have learned how to do it correctly. Follow the instructions carefully.

Dosing—The dose of this medicine will be different for different patients. Follow your doctor's orders or the directions on the label. The following information includes only the average doses of this medicine. If your dose is different, do not change it unless your doctor tells you to do so.

The amount of medicine that you take depends on the strength of the medicine. Also, the number of doses you take each day, the time allowed between doses, and the length of time you take the medicine depend on the medical problem for which you are using the medicine.

- For otic dosage form (ear drops):
  - Adults and children:
    - For ear pain caused by an infection—Use enough medicine to fill the entire ear canal every one or two hours until the pain is relieved.
    - For softening earwax before removal—Use enough medicine to fill the entire ear canal three times a day for two or three days.

Missed dose—If you miss a dose of this medicine, take it as soon as possible. However, if it is almost time for your next dose, skip the missed dose and go back to your regular dosing schedule. Do not double doses.

Storage—Store the medicine in a closed container at room temperature, away from heat, moisture, and direct light. Keep from freezing.

Keep out of the reach of children.

Do not keep outdated medicine or medicine no longer needed.

Side Effects of This Medicine

Along with its needed effects, a medicine may cause some unwanted effects. The following side effects may mean that you are having an allergic reaction to the medicine.

Stop using the medicine right away if any of them occur. Check with your doctor if any of the following effects continue or are bothersome:

Itching, burning, redness, or oozing sores in the ear

Other side effects not listed may also occur in some patients. If you notice any other effects, check with your healthcare professional.

ANTITHYROID AGENTS   (Systemic)

Some commonly used brand names are:

In the U.S.—
Tapazole (1)

In Canada—
Propyl-Thyracil (2)
Tapazole (1)

This information applies to the following medicines:

1. Methimazole (meth-IM-a-zole)
2. Propylthiouracil (proe-pill-thye-oh-YOOR-a-sill)

Category

- **Antihyperthyroid agent**—Methimazole; Propylthiouracil

Description

Methimazole and propylthiouracil are used to treat conditions in which the thyroid gland produces too much thyroid hormone.

These medicines work by making it harder for the body to use iodine to make thyroid hormone. They do not block the effects of thyroid hormone that was made by the body before their use was begun.

Methimazole and propylthiouracil are available only with your doctor's prescription, in the following dosage forms:

Oral
- Methimazole
  - Tablets
- Propylthiouracil
  - Tablets

Before Using This Medicine

In deciding to use a medicine, the risks of taking the medicine must be weighed against the good it will do. This is a decision you and your doctor will make. For antithyroid agents, the following should be considered:

Allergies—Tell your doctor if you have ever had any unusual or allergic reaction to methimazole or propylthiouracil. Also tell your health care professional if you are allergic to any other substances, such as foods, preservatives, or dyes.

Pregnancy—Use of too large a dose during pregnancy may cause problems in the fetus. However, use of the proper dose, with careful monitoring by the doctor, is not likely to cause problems.

Breast-feeding—These medicines pass into breast milk. (Methimazole passes into breast milk more freely and in higher amounts than propylthiouracil.) However, your doctor may allow you to continue to breast-feed, if your dose is low and the infant gets frequent check-ups. If you are taking a large dose, it may be necessary for you to stop breast-feeding during treatment.

Children—This medicine has been used in children and, in effective doses, has not been shown to cause different side effects or problems in children than it does in adults.

Teenagers—This medicine has been used in teenagers and, in effective doses, has not been shown to cause different side effects or problems in teenagers than it does in adults.

Older adults—Elderly people may have an increased chance of certain side effects during treatment. Your doctor may need to take special precautions while you are taking this medicine.

Other medicines—Although certain medicines should not be used together at all, in other cases two different medicines may be used together even if an interaction might occur. In these cases, your doctor may want to change the dose, or other precautions may be necessary. When you are taking antithyroid agents, it is especially important that your health care professional know if you are taking any of the following:

- Amiodarone or
- Iodinated glycerol or
- Potassium iodide (e.g., Pima)—The use of these medicines may change the effect of antithyroid agents
- Anticoagulants (blood thinners)—The use of antithyroid agents may affect the way anticoagulants work in your body
- Beta-adrenergic blocking agents (e.g., Inderal, Metoprolol, Sotalol)—The use of antithyroid agents may change the amount of beta-blockers you need to take.
- Digitalis glycosides—The use of antithyroid agents may affect the amount of digitalis glycosides in the bloodstream

Other medical problems—The presence of other medical problems may affect the use of antithyroid agents. Make sure you tell your doctor if you have any other medical problems, especially:

- Liver disease—The body may not get this medicine out of the bloodstream at the usual rate, which may increase the chance of side effects

Proper Use of This Medicine

Use this medicine only as directed by your doctor. Do not use more or less of it and do not use it more often or for a longer time than your doctor ordered. To do so may increase the chance of side effects.

This medicine works best when there is a constant amount in the blood. *To help keep the amount constant, do not miss any doses. Also, if you are taking more than one dose a day, it is best to take the doses at evenly spaced times day and night.* For example, if you are to take 3 doses a day, the doses should be spaced about 8 hours apart. If this interferes with your sleep or other daily activities, or if you need help in planning the best times to take your medicine, check with your health care professional.

Food in your stomach may change the amount of methimazole that is able to enter the bloodstream. To make sure that you always get the same effects, try to take methimazole at the same time in relation to meals every day. That is, always take it with meals or always take it on an empty stomach.

Dosing—The dose of these medicines will be different for different patients. *Follow your doctor's orders or the directions on the label.* The following information includes only the average doses of these medicines. *If your dose is different, do not change it* unless your doctor tells you to do so.

The number of tablets that you take or the number of suppositories that you use depends on the strength of the medicine. Also, *the number of doses you take each day, the time allowed between doses, and the length of time you take the medicine depend on the medical problem for which you are taking antithyroid agents.*

For methimazole
- For *oral* dosage form (tablets):
  - For treatment of hyperthyroidism (overactive thyroid):
    - Adults and teenagers—At first, 15 to 60 milligrams (mg) a day for up to six to eight weeks. Later, your doctor may want to lower your dose to 5 to 30 mg a day. This may be taken once a day or it may be divided into two doses a day.
    - Children—Dose is based on body weight and must be determined by your doctor. The usual dose is 0.4 mg per kilogram (kg) (0.18 mg per pound) of body weight a day. Later, your doctor may want to lower the dose to 0.2 mg per kg (0.09 mg per pound) of body weight a day. The dose may be taken once a day or it may be divided into two doses a day.
  - For treatment of thyrotoxicosis (a thyroid emergency):
    - Adults and teenagers—15 to 20 mg every four hours.
- For *rectal* dosage form (suppositories):
  - For treatment of thyrotoxicosis (a thyroid emergency):
    - Adults and teenagers—15 to 20 mg inserted into the rectum every four hours. Your doctor may change your dose as needed.
    - Children—The dose is based on body weight and must be determined by your doctor. The usual dose is 0.4 mg per kg (0.18 mg per pound) of body weight inserted into the rectum a day. This may be

used as a single dose or it may be divided into two doses a day.

For propylthiouracil
- For *oral* dosage form (tablets):
  - For treatment of hyperthyroidism (overactive thyroid):
    - Adults and teenagers—At first, 300 to 900 milligrams (mg) a day. Some people may need up to 1200 mg a day. This may be taken as a single dose or it may be divided into two to four doses in a day. Later, your doctor may lower your dose to 50 to 600 mg a day.
    - Children 6 to 10 years of age—At first, 50 to 150 mg a day. This may be taken as a single dose or it may be divided into two to four doses in a day. Later, your doctor may change your dose as needed.
    - Children 10 years of age and older—At first, 50 to 300 mg a day. This may be taken as a single dose or it may be divided into two to four doses in a day. Then, your doctor may change your dose as needed.
  - For treatment of thyrotoxicosis (a thyroid emergency):
    - Adults and teenagers—200 to 400 mg every four hours. Your doctor will lower your dose as needed.
    - Newborn infants—Dose is based on body weight and must be determined by your doctor. The usual dose is 10 mg per kilogram (kg) (4.5 mg per pound) of body weight a day. This is usually divided into more than one dose a day.
- For *rectal* dosage forms (enemas or suppositories):
  - For treatment of thyrotoxicosis (a thyroid emergency):
    - Adults and teenagers—200 to 400 mg inserted into the rectum every four hours. Your doctor may change your dose as needed.
    - Children 6 to 10 years of age—50 to 150 mg inserted into the rectum a day. This dose may be used as a single dose or it may be divided into two to four doses in a day. Your doctor may change your dose as needed.
    - Children 10 years of age and older—50 to 300 mg inserted into the rectum a day. This dose may be used as a single dose or it may be divided into two to four doses in a day. Your doctor may change your dose as needed.
    - Newborn infants—Dose is based on body weight and must be determined by your doctor. The usual dose is 10 mg per kg (4.5 mg per pound) of body weight inserted into the rectum. This is usually divided into more than one dose a day. Your doctor may change your dose as needed.

Missed dose—If you miss a dose of this medicine, take it as soon as possible. If it is almost time for your next dose, take both doses together. Then go back to your regular dosing schedule. If you miss more than one dose or if you have any questions about this, check with your doctor.

Storage—To store this medicine:
- Keep out of the reach of children.
- Store away from heat and direct light.
- Do not store in the bathroom, near the kitchen sink, or in other high-moisture areas. Heat or moisture may cause the medicine to break down.

- Do not keep outdated medicine or medicine no longer needed. Be sure that any discarded medicine is out of the reach of children.

Precautions While Using This Medicine

It is very important that your doctor check your progress at regular visits to make sure that this medicine is working properly and to check for unwanted effects.

It may take several days or weeks for this medicine to work. However, *do not stop taking this medicine without first checking with your doctor*. Some medical problems may require several years of continuous treatment.

Before having any kind of surgery (including dental surgery) or emergency treatment, *tell the medical doctor or dentist in charge that you are taking this medicine.*

Check with your doctor right away if you get an injury, infection, or illness of any kind. Your doctor may want you to stop taking this medicine or change the amount you are taking.

While you are being treated with antithyroid agents, and after you stop treatment with it, *do not have any immunizations (vaccinations) without your doctor's approval.* Antithyroid agents may lower your body's resistance and there is a chance you might get the infection the immunization is meant to prevent. In addition, other persons living in your household should not take or have recently taken oral polio vaccine since there is a chance they could pass the polio virus on to you. Also, avoid other persons who have taken oral polio vaccine. Do not get close to them, and do not stay in the same room with them for very long. If you cannot take these precautions, you should consider wearing a protective face mask that covers the nose and mouth.

Before you have any medical tests, tell the doctor in charge that you are taking this medicine. The results of some tests may be affected by this medicine.

Side Effects of This Medicine

Along with its needed effects, a medicine may cause some unwanted effects. Although not all of these side effects may occur, if they do occur they may need medical attention.

Check with your doctor immediately if any of the following side effects occur:
  Less common
      Cough; fever or chills (continuing or severe); general feeling of discomfort, illness or weakness; hoarseness; mouth sores; pain, swelling, or redness in joints; throat infection
  Rare
      Yellow eyes or skin
Check with your doctor as soon as possible if any of the following side effects occur:
  More common
      Fever (mild and temporary); skin rash or itching
  Rare
      Backache; black, tarry stools; blood in urine or stools; shortness of breath; increase in bleeding or bruising; increase or decrease in urination; numbness or tingling of fingers, toes, or face; pinpoint red spots on skin; swelling of feet or lower legs; swollen lymph nodes; swollen salivary glands

Symptoms of overdose

Changes in menstrual periods; coldness; constipation; dry, puffy skin; headache; listlessness or sleepiness; muscle aches; swelling in the front of the neck; unusual tiredness or weakness; weight gain (unusual)

Other side effects may occur that usually do not need medical attention. These side effects may go away during treatment as your body adjusts to the medicine. However, check with your doctor if any of the following side effects continue or are bothersome:

Less common

Dizziness; loss of taste (for methimazole); nausea; stomach pain; vomiting

Other side effects not listed above may also occur in some patients. If you notice any other effects, check with your doctor.

APOMORPHINE (Injection route) - a-poe-MOR-feen

Uses For This Medicine

Apomorphine is used to treat Parkinson's disease, sometimes referred to as "shaking palsy." By improving muscle control and reducing stiffness, this medicine allows more normal movements of the body as the disease symptoms are reduced.

This medicine is available only with your doctor's prescription.

Before Using This Medicine

In deciding to use a medicine, the risks of taking the medicine must be weighed against the good it will do. This is a decision you and your doctor will make. For this medicine, the following should be considered:

Allergies—Tell your doctor if you have ever had any unusual or allergic reaction to this medicine or any other medicines. Also tell your health care professional if you have any other types of allergies, such as to foods, dyes, preservatives, or animals. For non-prescription products, read the label or package ingredients carefully.

Pediatric—Studies on this medicine have been done only in adult patients, and there is no specific information comparing use of apomorphine in children with use in other age groups.

Geriatric—Confusion, hallucinations, falls causing bone and joint injuries, heart, lung, or stomach problems may be especially likely to occur in elderly patients, who are usually more sensitive than younger adults to the effects of apomorphine.

Pregnancy—

	Pregnancy Category	Explanation
All Trimesters	C	Animal studies have shown an adverse effect and there are no adequate studies in pregnant women OR no animal studies have been conducted and there are no adequate studies in pregnant women.

Breast Feeding—There are no adequate studies in women for determining infant risk when using this medication during breastfeeding. Weigh the potential benefits against the potential risks before taking this medication while breastfeeding.

Other medicines—

Using this medicine with any of the following medicines is not recommended. Your doctor may decide not to treat you with this medication or change some of the other medicines you take.

Alosetron, Dolasetron, Granisetron, Ondansetron, Palonosetron

Interactions with Food/Tobacco/Alcohol—Certain medicines should not be used at or around the time of eating food or eating certain types of food since interactions may occur. Using alcohol or tobacco with certain medicines may also cause interactions to occur. Discuss with your healthcare professional the use of your medicine with food, alcohol, or tobacco.

Other medical problems—The presence of other medical problems may affect the use of this medicine. Make sure you tell your doctor if you have any other medical problems, especially:

- Dyskinesia (difficulty performing voluntary movements without tics and spasms)—May be worsened by apomorphine.
- Heart disease or problems or
- Hypokalemia (abnormally low potassium in the blood) or
- Hypomagnesemia (abnormally low magnesium in the blood) or
- Stroke—Extra caution should be used because heart problems have been reported with apomorphine use.
- Kidney problems—The starting dose of apomorphine will need to be reduced.
- Liver problems—Caution should be used because the amount of apomorphine in the blood may be increased.
- Psychotic disorder—The doctor needs to know if the patient is being treated with an antipsychotic medicine to decide whether or not to use this medicine.
- Sleeping disorder—This medicine could increase the risk of being drowsy or sleepy during daily activities.

Proper Use of This Medicine

Some medicines given by injection may sometimes be given at home to patients who do not need to be in the hospital. If you are using this medicine at home, make sure you clearly understand and carefully follow your doctor's instructions.

Use this medicine only as directed by your doctor. Do not use more or less of it, do not use it more often, and do not use it for a longer time than your doctor ordered. To do so may increase the chance of side effects.

This medicine should be injected just under the skin (i.e., subcutaneously), and not into a vein (i.e., intravenously).

Your doctor will also prescribe another medicine called an antiemetic to take when you are using apomorphine. Antiemetic medicines help reduce the nausea and vomiting that can occur with apomorphine use.

Dosing—The dose of this medicine will be different for different patients. Follow your doctor's orders or the directions on the label. The following information includes only the average doses of this medicine. If your dose is different, do not change it unless your doctor tells you to do so.

The amount of medicine that you take depends on the strength of the medicine. Also, the number of doses you take each day, the time allowed between doses, and the length of time you take the medicine depend on the medical problem for which you are using the medicine.

- For parenteral dosage form (injection):
  - For treatment of Parkinson's disease:
    - Adults—Your doctor will use a test dose of 0.2 mL and base your starting dose on how your body responds to the test dose.
    - Children—Use and dose must be determined by your doctor.

Missed dose—Call your doctor or pharmacist for instructions.

Storage—Keep out of the reach of children.

Store the medicine in a closed container at room temperature, away from heat, moisture, and direct light. Keep from freezing.

Ask your healthcare professional how you should dispose of any medicine you do not use.

Precautions While Using This Medicine

When you are using apomorphine, you should avoid drinking alcohol.

Do not take medicines that cause sleepiness while taking apomorphine.

Do not take other medicines unless they have been discussed with your doctor.

If you take too much apomorphine, you may experience more side effects or they may be stronger than usual. *You should contact your doctor or have someone take you to an emergency room right away.*

Tell your doctor if you are having trouble with drowsiness and sleepiness during the day.

This medicine may cause some people to become drowsy, dizzy, or less alert than they are normally. *Make sure you know how you react to this medicine before you drive, use machines, or do anything else that could be dangerous if you are dizzy or not alert.*

Do not get up too quickly from a lying or sitting position. This could cause dizziness and faintness to occur.

Side Effects of This Medicine

Along with its needed effects, a medicine may cause some unwanted effects. Although not all of these side effects may occur, if they do occur they may need medical attention.

Check with your doctor immediately if any of the following side effects occur:

More common
   Chest pain, discomfort, or pressure; chills; cold sweats; confusion; dizziness, faintness, or light-headedness when getting up from lying or sitting position; falling asleep during activity; mood or mental changes; seeing, hearing, or feeling things that are not there; swelling; twitching, twisting, uncontrolled repetitive movements of tongue, lips, face, arms, or legs

Less common
   Arm, back, neck or jaw pain or discomfort; chest tightness or heaviness; fainting; fast or irregular heartbeat; low blood pressure or pulse; nausea; shortness of breath; sweating; unconsciousness; vomiting

Rare
   Irregular heartbeat; recurrent fainting

Some side effects may occur that usually do not need medical attention. These side effects may go away during treatment as your body adjusts to the medicine. Also, your health care professional may be able to tell you about ways to prevent or reduce some of these side effects. Check with your health care professional if any of the following side effects continue or are bothersome or if you have any questions about them:

More common
   Bleeding, blistering, burning, coldness, discoloration of skin, feeling of pressure, hives, infection, inflammation, itching, lumps, numbness, pain, rash, redness, scarring, soreness, stinging, swelling, tenderness, tingling, ulceration, or warmth at injection site; blurred vision; dizziness; drowsiness; runny nose; sleepiness; yawning

Rare
   Painful or prolonged erection of the penis

Other side effects not listed may also occur in some patients. If you notice any other effects, check with your healthcare professional.

APPETITE SUPPRESSANTS, SYMPATHOMIMETIC (Systemic)

Some commonly used brand names are:

In the U.S.—

Adipex-P (5)	Phentercot (5)
Adipost (4)	Phentride (5)
Bontril PDM (4)	Plegine (5)
Bontril Slow-Release (4)	Prelu-2 (4)
Didrex (1)	Pro-Fast (5)
Fastin (5)	PT 105 (4)
Ionamin (5)	Sanorex (3)
Mazanor (3)	Tenuate (2)
Melfiat (4)	Tenuate Dospan (2)
Obenix (5)	Tepanil Ten-Tab (2)
Obezine (4)	Teramine (5)
Phendiet (4)	Zantryl (5)
Phendiet-105 (4)	

In Canada—

Ionamin (5)	Tenuate (2)
Sanorex (3)	Tenuate Dospan (2)

This information applies to the following medicines:

1. Benzphetamine (benz-FET-a-meen)
2. Diethylpropion (dye-eth-il-PROE-pee-on)
3. Mazindol (MAY-zin-dole)
4. Phendimetrazine (fen-dye-MET-ra-zeen)
5. Phentermine (FEN-ter-meen)

Category

- **Appetite suppressant**—Benzphetamine; Diethylpropion; Mazindol; Phendimetrazine; Phentermine

Description

Sympathomimetic appetite suppressants are used in the short-term treatment of obesity. Their appetite-reducing effect tends to decrease after a few weeks. Because of this, these medicines are useful only during the first few weeks of a weight-loss program. The sympathomimetic appetite suppressants can help you to lose weight while you are learning new ways to eat and to exercise. Changes in eating habits and activity level must be developed and continued long-term in order for you to continue losing weight and to keep the lost weight from returning.

These medicines are available only with your doctor's prescription, in the following dosage forms:

Oral
- Benzphetamine
  - Tablets
- Diethylpropion
  - Tablets
  - Extended-release tablets
- Mazindol
  - Tablets
- Phendimetrazine
  - Extended-release capsules
  - Tablets
- Phentermine
  - Capsules
  - Resin capsules
  - Tablets

Before Using This Medicine

In deciding to use a medicine, the risks of taking the medicine must be weighed against the good it may do. This is a decision you and your doctor will make. For sympathomimetic appetite suppressants, the following should be considered:

Allergies—Tell your doctor if you have ever had any unusual or allergic reaction to this medicine or amphetamine, dextroamphetamine, ephedrine, epinephrine, isoproterenol, metaproterenol, methamphetamine, norepinephrine, phenylephrine, phenylpropanolamine, pseudoephedrine, terbutaline, or other appetite suppressants. Also tell your health care professional if you are allergic to any other substances, such as foods, preservatives, or dyes.

Diet—You must follow a reduced-calorie diet while using an appetite suppressant in order to lose weight. Also, in order to keep the lost weight from returning, changes in diet and exercise must be continued after the weight has been lost.

Pregnancy—If a pregnant woman takes this medicine in high doses or more often than the doctor has directed, it may cause withdrawal symptoms in the newborn baby. Also, medicines similar to sympathomimetic appetite suppressants can cause birth defects in the newborn baby if a pregnant woman takes them in high doses. Before taking this medicine, make sure your doctor knows if you are pregnant or if you may become pregnant.

Breast-feeding—Diethylpropion and benzphetamine pass into breast milk. It is not known if other sympathomimetic appetite suppressants pass into breast milk. However, use of sympathomimetic appetite suppressants during breast-feeding is not recommended, because it may cause unwanted effects in nursing babies.

Children—Studies on these medicines have been done only in adult patients, and there is no specific information comparing use of sympathomimetic appetite suppressants in children with use in other age groups. The use of these medicines by children younger than 16 years of age is not recommended.

Older adults—Many medicines have not been studied specifically in older people. Therefore, it may not be known whether they work exactly the same way they do in younger adults or if they cause different side effects or problems in older people. There is no specific information comparing use of appetite suppressants in the elderly with use in other age groups.

Other medicines—Although certain medicines should not be used together at all, in other cases two different medicines may be used together even if an interaction might occur. In these cases, your doctor may want to change the dose, or other precautions may be necessary. When you are taking appetite suppressants, it is especially important that your health care professional know if you are taking any of the following:

- Amantadine (e.g., Symmetrel) or
- Amphetamines or
- Caffeine (e.g., NoDoz) or
- Chlophedianol (e.g., Ulone) or
- Cocaine or
- Medicine for asthma or other breathing problems or
- Medicine for colds, sinus problems, or hay fever or other allergies (including nose drops or sprays) or
- Methylphenidate (e.g., Ritalin) or
- Nabilone (e.g., Cesamet) or
- Pemoline (e.g., Cylert)—Using these medicines with sympathomimetic appetite suppressants may increase the central nervous system (CNS) stimulant effects, such as irritability, nervousness, trembling or shaking, or trouble in sleeping
- Appetite suppressants (diet pills), other or
- Selective serotonin reuptake inhibitors (citalopram [e.g., Celexa], fluoxetine [e.g., Prozac], fluvoxamine [e.g., Luvox], paroxetine [e.g., Paxil], sertraline [e.g., Zoloft])—It is not known whether using two different appetite suppressants together or using a sympathomimetic appetite suppressant with a selective serotonin reuptake inhibitor is safe and effective. There have been some serious unwanted effects on the hearts of people who used two different appetite suppressants together
- Monoamine oxidase (MAO) inhibitor activity (isocarboxazid [e.g., Marplan], isocarboxazid [e.g., Marplan], phenelzine [e.g., Nardil], procarbazine [e.g., Matulane], selegiline [e.g., Eldepryl], tranylcypromine [e.g., Parnate])—*Do not take an appetite suppressant while you are taking or less than 14 days after taking a monoamine oxidase (MAO) inhibitor*. If you do, you may develop sudden extremely high blood pressure
- Tricyclic antidepressants (amitriptyline [e.g., Elavil], amoxapine [e.g., Asendin], clomipramine [e.g., Anafranil], desipramine [e.g., Pertofrane], doxepin [e.g., Sinequan], imipramine [e.g., Tofranil], nortriptyline [e.g., Aventyl], protriptyline [e.g., Vivactil], trimipramine [e.g., Surmontil])—Using these medicines with sympathomimetic appetite suppressants may cause high blood pressure or irregular heartbeat

Other medical problems—The presence of other medical problems may affect the use of appetite suppressants. Make sure you tell your doctor if you have any other medical problems, especially:
- Alcohol abuse (or history of) or
- Drug abuse or dependence (or history of)—Dependence on appetite suppressants may be more likely to develop

- Diabetes mellitus (sugar diabetes)—The amount of insulin or oral antidiabetic medicine that you need to take may change
- Epilepsy—Diethylpropion may increase the risk of having seizures
- Family history of mental illness—Mental depression or other mental illness may be more likely to occur
- Glaucoma or
- Heart or blood vessel disease or
- High blood pressure or
- Mental illness or
- Overactive thyroid—Appetite suppressants may make the condition worse
- Kidney disease—Higher blood levels of the appetite suppressant may occur, increasing the chance of serious side effects

Proper Use of This Medicine

In order to prevent trouble in sleeping, if you are taking:

- One dose of this medicine a day, take it about 10 to 14 hours before bedtime.
- More than one dose of this medicine a day, take the last dose of the day about 4 to 6 hours before bedtime.

For patients taking a *long-acting form* of this medicine:

- Swallow these capsules or tablets whole. Do not break, crush, or chew before swallowing.

For patients taking *mazindol:*

- This medicine may be taken with food, if needed, to prevent stomach upset.

Take this medicine only as directed by your doctor. Do not take more of it, do not take it more often, and do not take it for a longer time than your doctor ordered. If too much is taken, it may cause unwanted effects or become habit-forming.

If you think this medicine is not working properly after you have taken it for a few weeks, *do not increase the dose.* Instead, check with your doctor.

Dosing—The dose of appetite suppressants will be different for different patients. *Follow your doctor's orders or the directions on the label.* The following information includes only the average doses of appetite suppressants. *If your dose is different, do not change it* unless your doctor tells you to do so.

For benzphetamine
- For *oral* dosage form (tablets):
  - For appetite suppression:
    - Adults—At first, 25 to 50 milligrams (mg) once a day, taken in midmorning or midafternoon. Your doctor may need to adjust your dose.
    - Children up to 16 years of age—Use is not recommended.

For diethylpropion
- For *oral* dosage form (tablets):
  - For appetite suppression:
    - Adults—25 milligrams (mg) three times a day, taken one hour before meals.
    - Children up to 16 years of age—Use is not recommended.

- For *long-acting oral* dosage form (extended-release tablets):
  - For appetite suppression:
    - Adults—75 mg once a day, taken in midmorning.
    - Children up to 16 years of age—Use is not recommended.

For mazindol
- For *oral* dosage form (tablets):
  - For appetite suppression:
    - Adults—At first, 1 milligram (mg) once a day. Your doctor may need to adjust your dose.
    - Children up to 16 years of age—Use is not recommended.

For phendimetrazine
- For *long-acting oral* dosage form (extended-release capsules):
  - For appetite suppression:
    - Adults—105 mg once a day, taken thirty to sixty minutes before the morning meal.
    - Children up to 16 years of age—Use is not recommended.
- For *oral* dosage form (tablets):
  - For appetite suppression:
    - Adults—17.5 to 35 mg two or three times a day, taken one hour before meals.
    - Children up to 16 years of age—Use is not recommended.

For phentermine
- For *oral* dosage form (capsules):
  - For appetite suppression:
    - Adults—15 to 37.5 milligrams (mg) once a day, taken before breakfast or one to two hours after breakfast.
    - Children up to 16 years of age—Use is not recommended.
- For *oral* dosage form (tablets):
  - For appetite suppression:
    - Adults—15 to 37.5 mg once a day, taken before breakfast or one to two hours after breakfast. Instead of taking it once a day, your doctor may tell you to take smaller doses thirty minutes before meals.
    - Children up to 16 years of age—Use is not recommended.
- For *oral resin* dosage form (capsules):
  - For appetite suppression:
    - Adults—15 to 30 mg once a day, taken before breakfast.
    - Children up to 16 years of age—Use is not recommended.

Missed dose—If you miss a dose of this medicine, skip the missed dose and continue with your regular dosing schedule. Do not double doses.

Storage—To store this medicine:

- Keep out of the reach of children.
- Store away from heat and direct light.
- Do not store in the bathroom, near the kitchen sink, or in other damp places. Heat or moisture may cause the medicine to break down.
- Do not keep outdated medicine or medicine no longer needed. Be sure that any discarded medicine is out of the reach of children.

Precautions While Using This Medicine

Your doctor should check your progress at regular visits to make sure that this medicine does not cause unwanted effects.

If you think this medicine is not working properly after you have taken it for a few weeks, *do not increase the dose.* Instead, check with your doctor.

Do not take an appetite suppressant with or less than 14 days after taking a monoamine oxidase (MAO) inhibitor. If you do, you may very suddenly develop extremely high blood pressure.

Taking a sympathomimetic appetite suppressant may cause a positive result in urine screening tests for amphetamines.

Sympathomimetic appetite suppressants may cause dryness of the mouth. For temporary relief, use sugarless candy or gum, melt bits of ice in your mouth, or use a saliva substitute. However, if your mouth continues to feel dry for more than 2 weeks, check with your medical doctor or dentist. Continuing dryness of the mouth may increase the chance of developing dental disease, including tooth decay, gum disease, and fungus infections.

This medicine may cause some people to feel a false sense of well-being or to become dizzy, lightheaded, drowsy, or less alert than they are normally. *Make sure you know how you react to this medicine before you drive, use machines, or do anything else that could be dangerous if you are dizzy or are not alert.*

Before having any kind of surgery, dental treatment, or emergency treatment, tell the medical doctor or dentist in charge that you are using this medicine. Taking appetite suppressants together with medicines that are used during surgery or dental or emergency treatments may cause serious side effects.

Check with your doctor immediately if you notice a decrease in your ability to exercise, if you faint, or if you have chest pain, swelling of your feet or lower legs, or trouble in breathing. These may be symptoms of very serious heart or lung problems.

If you have been taking this medicine for a long time or in large doses and *you think you may have become mentally or physically dependent on it, check with your doctor.*
- Some signs of dependence on appetite suppressants are:
  - a strong desire or need to continue taking the medicine.
  - a need to increase the dose to receive the effects of the medicine.
  - withdrawal side effects (for example, mental depression, nausea or vomiting, stomach cramps or pain, trembling, unusual tiredness or weakness) when you stop taking the medicine.

For *patients with diabetes:*
- This medicine may affect blood sugar levels. If you notice a change in the results of your urine or blood sugar test or if you have any questions, check with your doctor.

If you have been taking this medicine in large doses or for a long time, *do not stop taking it without first checking with your doctor.* Your doctor may want you to reduce gradually the amount you are taking before stopping completely. This will help prevent withdrawal side effects.

Side Effects

Appetite suppressants may cause some serious side effects, including heart and lung problems. *You and your doctor should discuss the good this medicine may do as well as the risks of taking it.*

Along with its needed effects, a medicine may cause some unwanted effects. Although not all of these side effects may occur, if they do occur they may need medical attention.

Check with your doctor immediately if any of the following side effects occur:
Rare
    Chest pain; decreased ability to exercise; fainting; swelling of feet or lower legs; trouble in breathing

Check with your doctor as soon as possible if any of the following side effects occur:
More common
    Increased blood pressure
Less common or rare
    Difficult or painful urination; fast or irregular heartbeat; feeling that others can hear your thoughts; feeling that others are watching you or controlling your behavior; hallucinations (feeling, seeing, or hearing things that are not there); headache (severe); mental depression; numbness, especially on one side of the face or body; skin rash or hives; sore throat and fever (with diethylpropion); talking, feeling, and acting with excitement and activity you cannot control; unusual bleeding or bruising (with diethylpropion)
Symptoms of overdose
    Abdominal or stomach cramps; coma; confusion; convulsions (seizures); diarrhea (severe); dizziness, lightheadedness, or fainting; fast breathing; feeling of panic; fever; hallucinations (seeing, hearing or feeling things that are not there); high or low blood pressure; hostility with urge to attack; irregular heartbeat; nausea or vomiting (severe); overactive reflexes; restlessness; trembling or shaking; tiredness, weakness, and mental depression following effects of excitement

Abuse of a sympathomimetic appetite suppressant (taking the medicine in larger doses or taking it more frequently or for a longer time than the doctor ordered) can cause the following side effects:
    Changes in personality; excessive, excited activity; irritability (severe); mental illness (severe), similar to schizophrenia; skin disease; trouble in sleeping (severe)

Other side effects may occur that usually do not need medical attention. These side effects may go away during treatment as your body adjusts to the medicine. However, check with your doctor if any of the following side effects continue or are bothersome:
More common
    Constipation; dizziness or lightheadedness; dryness of mouth; false sense of well-being; headache; irritability; nausea or vomiting; nervousness or restlessness; stomach cramps or pain; trembling or shaking; trouble in sleeping
Less common or rare
    Blurred vision; changes in sexual desire or decreased sexual ability; diarrhea; drowsiness; frequent urge to urinate or increased urination; increased sweating; unpleasant taste

Although not all of the side effects listed above have been reported for all of these medicines, they have been reported for at least one of them. However, since all of the sympathomimetic appetite suppressants are similar, any of the above side effects may occur with any of these medicines.

After you stop using this medicine, your body may need time to adjust. The length of time this takes depends on the amount of medicine you were using and how long you used it. During this time check with your doctor if you notice any of the following side effects:

Extreme tiredness or weakness; mental depression; nausea or vomiting; stomach cramps or pain; trembling; trouble in sleeping or nightmares

Other side effects not listed above may also occur in some patients. If you notice any other effects, check with your doctor.

APRACLONIDINE (Ophthalmic route)
- a-pra-KLOE-ni-deen

Commonly used brand name(s)

In the U.S.—
Iopidine

Available Dosage Forms:
• Solution

Therapeutic Class: Antiglaucoma
Pharmacologic Class: Alpha-2 Adrenergic Agonist

Uses For This Medicine

Apraclonidine 0.5% is used to treat glaucoma when the medications you have been using for glaucoma do not reduce your eye pressure enough.

Apraclonidine 1% is used just before and after certain types of eye surgery (argon laser trabeculoplasty, argon laser iridotomy, and Nd:YAG laser posterior capsulotomy). The medicine is used to control or prevent a rise in pressure within the eye (ocular hypertension) that can occur after this type of surgery.

Apraclonidine 0.5% is available only with your doctor's prescription.

Before Using This Medicine

In deciding to use a medicine, the risks of taking the medicine must be weighed against the good it will do. This is a decision you and your doctor will make. For this medicine, the following should be considered:

Allergies—Tell your doctor if you have ever had any unusual or allergic reaction to this medicine or any other medicines. Also tell your health care professional if you have any other types of allergies, such as to foods, dyes, preservatives, or animals. For non-prescription products, read the label or package ingredients carefully.

Pediatric—Studies on this medicine have been done only in adult patients, and there is no specific information comparing use of apraclonidine in children with use in other age groups.

Geriatric—Many medicines have not been studied specifically in older people. Therefore, it may not be known whether they work exactly the same way they do in younger adults or if they cause different side effects or problems in older people. There is no specific information comparing use of apraclonidine in the elderly with use in other age groups.

Pregnancy—

	Pregnancy Category	Explanation
All Trimesters	C	Animal studies have shown an adverse effect and there are no adequate studies in pregnant women OR no animal studies have been conducted and there are no adequate studies in pregnant women.

Breast Feeding—There are no adequate studies in women for determining infant risk when using this medication during breastfeeding. Weigh the potential benefits against the potential risks before taking this medication while breastfeeding.

Other medicines—Although certain medicines should not be used together at all, in other cases two different medicines may be used together even if an interaction might occur. In these cases, your doctor may want to change the dose, or other precautions may be necessary. Tell your healthcare professional if you are taking any other prescription or non-prescription (over-the-counter [OTC]) medicine.

Interactions   with   Food/Tobacco/Alcohol—Certain medicines should not be used at or around the time of eating food or eating certain types of food since interactions may occur. Using alcohol or tobacco with certain medicines may also cause interactions to occur. Discuss with your healthcare professional the use of your medicine with food, alcohol, or tobacco.

Other medical problems—The presence of other medical problems may affect the use of this medicine. Make sure you tell your doctor if you have any other medical problems, especially:

• Depression or

• Heart or blood vessel disease or

• High blood pressure—Apraclonidine may make the condition worse

• Kidney disease or

• Liver disease—Higher blood levels of apraclonidine may result, which may lead to increased side effects

• Unusual reaction to a medicine that reduces the pressure within the eye—Apraclonidine is a strong reducer of eye pressure and could also cause this reaction

• Vasovagal attack (history of)—The signs and symptoms are paleness, nausea, sweating, slow heartbeat, sudden and severe tiredness or weakness, and possibly fainting, usually brought on by emotional stress caused by fear or pain. Apraclonidine may cause this reaction to happen again

Proper Use of This Medicine

If your doctor ordered two different eye drops to be used together, wait at least 10 minutes between the times you apply the medicines. This will help to keep the second medicine from" washing out" the first one.

To use the eye drops:

- First, wash your hands. Tilt the head back and, pressing your finger gently on the skin just beneath the lower eyelid, pull the lower eyelid away from the eye to make a space. Drop the medicine into this space. Let go of the eyelid and gently close the eyes. Do not blink. Keep the eyes closed and apply pressure to the inner corner of the eye with your finger for 1 or 2 minutes to allow the medicine to be absorbed by the eye.
- If you think you did not get the drop of medicine into your eye properly, use another drop.
- To keep the medicine as germ-free as possible, do not touch the applicator tip to any surface (including the eye). Also, keep the container tightly closed.

Use this medicine only as directed. Do not use more of it and do not use it more often than your doctor ordered. To do so may increase the chance of too much medicine being absorbed into the body and the chance of side effects.

It is important that your doctor check your progress at regular visits. This is to make sure the medicine is working properly.

Dosing—The dose of this medicine will be different for different patients. Follow your doctor's orders or the directions on the label. The following information includes only the average doses of this medicine. If your dose is different, do not change it unless your doctor tells you to do so.

The amount of medicine that you take depends on the strength of the medicine. Also, the number of doses you take each day, the time allowed between doses, and the length of time you take the medicine depend on the medical problem for which you are using the medicine.

- For ophthalmic solution (eye drops) dosage form:
  - For glaucoma (0.5% apraclonidine):
    - Adults—Use one drop in each eye two or three times a day.
    - Children—Use and dose must be determined by your doctor.
  - For preventing ocular hypertension before and after eye surgery (1% apraclonidine):
    - Adults—One drop is placed in the affected eye one hour before surgery, then one drop in the same eye immediately after surgery.
    - Children—Use and dose must be determined by your doctor.

Missed dose—If you miss a dose of this medicine, take it as soon as possible. However, if it is almost time for your next dose, skip the missed dose and go back to your regular dosing schedule. Do not double doses.

Storage—Store the medicine in a closed container at room temperature, away from heat, moisture, and direct light. Keep from freezing.

Keep out of the reach of children.

Do not keep outdated medicine or medicine no longer needed.

The 0.5% eye drops may be stored in the refrigerator.

Precautions While Using This Medicine

This medicine may cause some people to become dizzy, drowsy, or less alert than they are normally. Make sure you know how you react to this medicine before you drive, use machines, or do anything else that could be dangerous if you are not alert.

Apraclonidine may cause your eyes to become more sensitive to light than they are normally. Wearing sunglasses and avoiding too much exposure to bright light may help lessen the discomfort.

Side Effects of This Medicine

Along with its needed effects, a medicine may cause some unwanted effects. Although not all of these side effects may occur, if they do occur they may need medical attention.

Check with your doctor as soon as possible if any of the following side effects occur:

For 0.5% apraclonidine
  More common
    Allergic reaction (redness, itching, tearing of eye)

  Less common or rare
    Blurred vision or change in vision; chest pain; clumsiness or unsteadiness; depression; dizziness; eye discharge, irritation, or pain; irregular heartbeat; numbness or tingling in fingers or toes; raising of upper eyelid; rash around eyes; redness of eyelid, or inner lining of eyelid; swelling of eye, eyelid, or inner lining of eyelid; swelling of face, hands, or feet; wheezing or troubled breathing

For 1% apraclonidine
  Less common or rare
    Allergic reaction (redness of eye or inner lining of eyelid, swelling of eyelid, watering of eye); irregular heartbeat

Some side effects may occur that usually do not need medical attention. These side effects may go away during treatment as your body adjusts to the medicine. Also, your health care professional may be able to tell you about ways to prevent or reduce some of these side effects. Check with your health care professional if any of the following side effects continue or are bothersome or if you have any questions about them:

For 0.5% apraclonidine
  More common
    Dryness of mouth; eye discomfort

  Less common or rare
    Change in taste or smell; constipation; crusting or scales on eyelid or corner of eye; discoloration of white part of eyes; drowsiness or sleepiness; dry nose or eyes; general feeling of discomfort or illness; headache; increased sensitivity of eyes to light; muscle aches; nausea; nervousness; paleness of eye or inner lining of eyelid; runny nose; sore throat; tiredness or weakness; trouble in sleeping

For 1% apraclonidine
  More common
    Increase in size of pupil of eye; paleness of eye or inner lining of eyelid; raising of upper eyelid

  Less common or rare
    Runny nose

Other side effects not listed may also occur in some patients. If you notice any other effects, check with your healthcare professional.

APREPITANT (Oral route) - ap-RE-pi-tant

Commonly used brand name(s)
In the U.S.—
  Emend

Available Dosage Forms:
  • Capsule

Therapeutic Class: Antiemetic
Pharmacologic Class: Neurokinin-1 Receptor Antagonist

Uses For This Medicine

Aprepitant is used in combination with other antiemetics to prevent acute and delayed nausea and vomiting associated with cancer chemotherapy.

This medicine is available only with your doctor's prescription.

Before Using This Medicine

In deciding to use a medicine, the risks of taking the medicine must be weighed against the good it will do. This is a decision you and your doctor will make. For this medicine, the following should be considered:

Allergies—Tell your doctor if you have ever had any unusual or allergic reaction to this medicine or any other medicines. Also tell your health care professional if you have any other types of allergies, such as to foods, dyes, preservatives, or animals. For non-prescription products, read the label or package ingredients carefully.

Pediatric—Studies on this medicine have been done only in adult patients, and there is no specific information comparing use of aprepitant in children with use in other age groups.

Geriatric—This medicine has been studied in the elderly and has not been shown to cause different side effects or problems in older people than it does in younger adults. However, elderly people may be more sensitive to the adverse effects of aprepitant which may require caution.

Pregnancy—

	Pregnancy Category	Explanation
All Trimesters	B	Animal studies have revealed no evidence of harm to the fetus, however, there are no adequate studies in pregnant women OR animal studies have shown an adverse effect, but adequate studies in pregnant women have failed to demonstrate a risk to the fetus.

Breast Feeding—There are no adequate studies in women for determining infant risk when using this medication during breastfeeding. Weigh the potential benefits against the potential risks before taking this medication while breastfeeding.

Other medicines—
Using this medicine with any of the following medicines is not recommended. Your doctor may decide not to treat you with this medication or change some of the other medicines you take.

Astemizole, Cisapride, Pimozide, Terfenadine

Interactions with Food/Tobacco/Alcohol—Certain medicines should not be used at or around the time of eating food or eating certain types of food since interactions may occur. Using alcohol or tobacco with certain medicines may also cause interactions to occur. Discuss with your healthcare professional the use of your medicine with food, alcohol, or tobacco.

Other medical problems—The presence of other medical problems may affect the use of this medicine. Make sure you tell your doctor if you have any other medical problems, especially:
  • Severe liver problems—Aprepitant has not been studied in patients with severe liver problems.

Proper Use of This Medicine

Read the patient information provided with your medicine before starting therapy with aprepitant and each time you refill your aprepitant prescription.

Do not start taking aprepitant if you already have nausea and vomiting. Contact your doctor about what to do.

Dosing—The dose of this medicine will be different for different patients. Follow your doctor's orders or the directions on the label. The following information includes only the average doses of this medicine. If your dose is different, do not change it unless your doctor tells you to do so.

The amount of medicine that you take depends on the strength of the medicine. Also, the number of doses you take each day, the time allowed between doses, and the length of time you take the medicine depend on the medical problem for which you are using the medicine.

You may take aprepitant with or without food.
  • For oral dosage form (capsules):
    ○ For chemotherapy induced nausea and vomiting:
      ▪ Adults—125 milligrams (mg) one hour before chemotherapy treatment (Day 1) and 80 mg once a day in the morning on Days 2 and 3.
      ▪ Children—Use and dose must be determined by your doctor.

Missed dose—If you miss a dose of this medicine, take it as soon as possible. However, if it is almost time for your next dose, skip the missed dose and go back to your regular dosing schedule. Do not double doses.

Storage—Store the medicine in a closed container at room temperature, away from heat, moisture, and direct light. Keep from freezing.

Keep out of the reach of children.

Do not keep outdated medicine or medicine no longer needed.

Precautions While Using This Medicine

It is very important that your doctor check your progress at regular visits to make sure that this medicine is working properly and to check for unwanted effects.

Oral contraceptives (birth control pills) may not work properly if you take them while you are taking aprepitant. Unplanned pregnancies may occur. You should use a different or additional means os birth control while you are taking aprepitant. If you have any questions about this, check with your health care professional.

If your symptoms do not improve or if they become worse, check with your doctor.

Do not take other medicines unless they have been discussed with your doctor.

Side Effects of This Medicine

Along with its needed effects, a medicine may cause some unwanted effects. Although not all of these side effects may occur, if they do occur they may need medical attention.

Check with your doctor immediately if any of the following side effects occur:

Less common
Black or tarry stools; chills; cough; fever; lower back or side pain; painful or difficult urination; pale skin; shortness of breath; sore throat; ulcers, sores, or white spots in mouth; unusual bleeding or bruising; unusual tiredness or weakness

Some side effects may occur that usually do not need medical attention. These side effects may go away during treatment as your body adjusts to the medicine. Also, your health care professional may be able to tell you about ways to prevent or reduce some of these side effects. Check with your health care professional if any of the following side effects continue or are bothersome or if you have any questions about them:

Incidence unknown
Blistering, peeling, loosening of skin; diarrhea; itching; joint or muscle pain; large, hive-like swelling on face, eyelids, lips, tongue, throat, hands, legs, feet, sex organs; red irritated eyes; redness of skin; red skin lesions, often with a purple center; skin rash; slow or irregular heartbeat

Some side effects may occur that usually do not need medical attention. These side effects may go away during treatment as your body adjusts to the medicine. Also, your health care professional may be able to tell you about ways to prevent or reduce some of these side effects. Check with your health care professional if any of the following side effects continue or are bothersome or if you have any questions about them:

More common
Acid or sour stomach; belching; confusion; decreased urination; dizziness; dry mouth; fainting; heartburn; hiccups; increase in heart rate; indigestion; lack or loss of strength; lightheadedness; loss of appetite; nausea; rapid breathing; stomach discomfort upset or pain; swelling or inflammation of the mouth; sunken eyes; thirst; weight loss; wrinkled skin

Less common
Burning feeling in chest or stomach; hot flashes; indigestion; pain or discomfort in chest, upper stomach, or throat; tenderness in stomach area

Incidence unknown
Confusion about identity, place, and time

Other side effects not listed may also occur in some patients. If you notice any other effects, check with your healthcare professional.

ARIPIPRAZOLE (Oral route) - ay-ri-PIP-ray-zole

Black Box Warning

Elderly patients with dementia-related psychosis treated with atypical antipsychotic drugs are at an increased risk of death compared to placebo. Analyses of seventeen placebo-controlled trials (modal duration of 10 weeks) in these patients revealed a risk of death in the drug-treated patients of between 1.6 times to 1.7 times that seen in placebo-treated patients. Over the course of a typical 10–week controlled trial, the rate of death in drug-treated patients was about 4.5%, compared to a rate of about 2.6% in the placebo group. Although the causes of death were varied, most of the deaths appeared to be either cardiovascular (eg, heart failure, sudden death) or infectious (eg, pneumonia) in nature. Aripiprazole is not approved for the treatment of patients with dementia-related psychosis.

Commonly used brand name(s)

In the U.S.—
Abilify
Abilify Discmelt

Available Dosage Forms:
- Tablet
- Tablet, Disintegrating
- Solution

Therapeutic Class: Antipsychotic
Pharmacologic Class: Dopamine Antagonist

Uses For This Medicine

Aripiprazole is used to treat schizophrenia, which is a mental disorder. It is also used to treat the mania phase of bipolar disorder (manic-depressive illness). This medicine should NOT be used to treat behavioral problems in older adult patients who have dementia.

This medicine is available only with your healthcare professional's prescription.

Before Using This Medicine

In deciding to use a medicine, the risks of taking the medicine must be weighed against the good it will do. This is a decision you and your doctor will make. For this medicine, the following should be considered:

Allergies—Tell your doctor if you have ever had any unusual or allergic reaction to this medicine or any other medicines. Also tell your health care professional if you have any other types of allergies, such as to foods, dyes, preservatives, or animals. For non-prescription products, read the label or package ingredients carefully.

Pediatric—Studies on this medicine have only been done in adult patients, and there is no specific information comparing the use of aripiprazole in children with use in other age groups.

Geriatric—Many medicines have not been studied specifically in older people. Therefore, it may not be known whether they work exactly the same way they do in younger adults or if they cause different side effects or problems in older people. There is no specific information comparing the use of aripiprazole in the elderly with use in other age groups. Older patients who take this medicine for psychosis (mental disturbances) related to their dementia may be at risk for serious side effects and their doctor will need to use extra caution. This medicine should NOT be used to treat behavioral problems in older adult patients who have dementia.

Pregnancy—

	Pregnancy Category	Explanation
All Trimesters	C	Animal studies have shown an adverse effect and there are no adequate studies in pregnant women OR no animal studies have been conducted and there are no adequate studies in pregnant women.

Breast Feeding—

There are no adequate studies in women for determining infant risk when using this medication during breastfeeding. Weigh the potential benefits against the potential risks before taking this medication while breastfeeding.

Other medicines—

Using this medicine with any of the following medicines is not recommended. Your doctor may decide not to treat you with this medication or change some of the other medicines you take.

Ranolazine

Interactions with Food/Tobacco/Alcohol—

Certain medicines should not be used at or around the time of eating food or eating certain types of food since interactions may occur. Using alcohol or tobacco with certain medicines may also cause interactions to occur. Discuss with your healthcare professional the use of your medicine with food, alcohol, or tobacco.

Other medical problems—

The presence of other medical problems may affect the use of this medicine. Make sure you tell your doctor if you have any other medical problems, especially:

- Alcohol or drug abuse or dependence, history of—This medicine may make these conditions worse
- Alzheimer's disease—Risk of seizures, aspiration pneumonia, accidental injury, difficulty swallowing, or excessive drowsiness may be increased
- Conditions that lower the seizure threshold or
- Seizures, history of—Seizures may increase
- Aspiration pneumonia, risk or history of—May increase risk of adverse events
- Blood vessel disease or
- Conduction abnormalities (abnormalities of the heart's electrical impulses) or
- Dehydration or
- Heart disease or
- Heart failure or
- Hypovolemia (decrease in the volume of blood) or
- Ischemic heart disease, history of or
- Myocardial infarction (heart attack), history of—Risk of hypotension (abnormally low blood pressure) is increased

- Diabetes or family history of diabetes—May make condition worse and cause serious side effects
- Drug abuse or dependence, history of—May be more likely to develop dependence on this medicine
- Exposure to extreme heat or
- Strenuous exercise—Increased risk of heat stroke because aripiprazole effects the body's ability to cool itself
- Neuroleptic Malignant Syndrome (NMS), history of—May cause condition to worsen

Proper Use of This Medicine

Dosing—The dose of this medicine will be different for different patients. Follow your doctor's orders or the directions on the label. The following information includes only the average doses of this medicine. If your dose is different, do not change it unless your doctor tells you to do so.

The amount of medicine that you take depends on the strength of the medicine. Also, the number of doses you take each day, the time allowed between doses, and the length of time you take the medicine depend on the medical problem for which you are using the medicine.

Aripiprazole may be taken with or without food, on a full or an empty stomach. If your doctor tells you to take it a certain way, follow your doctor's instructions.

- For oral dosage form (solution):
  - For schizophrenia:
    - Adults—Oral, 10 to 15 milligrams (mg) a day, once a day, without regard to food. Dose increases should not be made before 2 weeks.
  - For bipolar mania:
    - Adults—Oral, 25 mg a day, once a day, without regard to food.
- For oral dosage form (tablets):
  - For schizophrenia:
    - Adults—Oral, 10 to 15 milligrams (mg) a day, once a day, without regard to food. Dose increases should not be made before 2 weeks.
  - For bipolar mania:
    - Adults—Oral, 30 mg a day, once a day, without regard to food.

Missed dose—If you miss a dose of this medicine, take it as soon as possible. However, if it is almost time for your next dose, skip the missed dose and go back to your regular dosing schedule. Do not double doses.

Storage—Store the medicine in a closed container at room temperature, away from heat, moisture, and direct light. Keep from freezing.

Keep out of the reach of children.

Do not keep outdated medicine or medicine no longer needed.

Ask your healthcare professional how you should dispose of any medicine you do not use.

Precautions While Using This Medicine

It is very important that your healthcare professional check you at regular visits to allow for changes in your dose and help reduce any unwanted effects.

This medicine may add to the effects of alcohol and other central nervous system (CNS) depressants (medicines that make you drowsy or less alert). Some examples of CNS depressants are antihistamines or medicine for hay fever, other allergies, or colds; sedatives, tranquilizers, or sleeping medicine; prescription pain medicine or narcotics; barbiturates; medicine for seizures; muscle relaxants; or anesthetics, including some dental anesthetics. Check with your doctor before taking any CNS depressants while you are taking this medicine.

Aripiprazole may cause drowsiness, trouble in thinking, or trouble in controlling movements. Make sure you know how you react to this medicine before you drive, use machines, or do other jobs that require you to be alert, well-coordinated, or able to think well.

If you experience difficulty swallowing or extreme sleepiness (especially if you are an older adult taking this medicine for psychosis [mental disturbances] related to dementia), contact your doctor immediately. It could increase your risk for serious unwanted effects.

This medicine may make it more difficult for your body to cool itself down. Use care not to become overheated during exercise or hot weather since overheating may result in heat stroke.

For diabetic patients: This medicine may affect blood sugar levels. Also, the oral solution contains sugar.

Side Effects of This Medicine

Along with its needed effects, a medicine may cause some unwanted effects. Although not all of these side effects may occur, if they do occur they may need medical attention.

Check with your doctor immediately if any of the following side effects occur:

More common
Difficulty speaking; drooling; loss of balance control; muscle trembling, jerking, or stiffness; restlessness; shuffling walk; stiffness of limbs; twisting movements of body; uncontrolled movements, especially of face, neck, and back

Less common
Blurred vision; dizziness; headache; nervousness; pounding in the ears; slow or fast heartbeat

Rare
Convulsions; difficulty in breathing; fast heartbeat; high fever; high or low blood pressure; increased sweating; lip smacking or puckering; loss of bladder control; muscle spasm or jerking of all extremities; puffing of cheeks; rapid or worm-like movements of tongue; severe muscle stiffness; sudden loss of consciousness; tiredness; uncontrolled chewing movements; uncontrolled movements of arms and legs; unusually pale skin

Incidence not known
Difficulty swallowing; hives or welts; itching, puffiness or swelling of the eyelids or around the eyes, face, lips, or tongue; itching skin; large, hive-like swelling on face, eyelids, lips, tongue, throat, hands, legs, feet, sex organs; redness of skin; shortness of breath; skin rash; tightness in chest; trouble in breathing; unusual tiredness or weakness; wheezing

Symptoms of overdose
Get emergency help immediately if any of the following symptoms of overdose occur:
Diarrhea; difficulty in speaking; drooling; fast, pounding, or irregular heartbeat or pulse; lack or loss of strength; loss of balance control; loss of consciousness; muscle trembling, jerking, or stiffness; nausea; restlessness; shuffling walk; stiffness of limbs; sleepiness or unusual drowsiness; twisting movements of body; uncontrolled movements, especially of face, neck, and back; vomiting

Some side effects may occur that usually do not need medical attention. These side effects may go away during treatment as your body adjusts to the medicine. Also, your health care professional may be able to tell you about ways to prevent or reduce some of these side effects. Check with your health care professional if any of the following side effects continue or are bothersome or if you have any questions about them:

More common
Acid or sour stomach; anxiety; belching; difficulty having a bowel movement (stool); dry mouth; fear; headache; heartburn; hyperventilation; inability to sit still; indigestion; irregular heartbeats; irritability; lack or loss of strength; lightheadedness; nausea; need to keep moving; nervousness; rash; restlessness; shaking; sleepiness or unusual drowsiness; sleeplessness; stomach discomfort, upset, or pain; trouble sleeping; unable to sleep; vomiting; weight gain

Less common
Accidental injury; bloating or swelling of face, arms, hands, lower legs, or feet; blurred vision; body aches or pain; congestion; coughing; difficulty in moving; dryness or soreness of throat; fever; hoarseness; increased salivation; joint pain; muscle aching or cramping; muscle pains or stiffness; rapid weight gain; runny nose; stuffy nose; sneezing; swollen joints; tender, swollen glands in neck; tingling of hands or feet; tremor; trouble in swallowing; unusual weight gain or loss; voice changes

Other side effects not listed may also occur in some patients. If you notice any other effects, check with your healthcare professional.

ASCORBIC ACID (Oral route) - a-SKOR-bik AS-id

Commonly used brand name(s)
In the U.S.—

Ascocid	C-Time w/Rose Hips
C-500	Mega-C
Cecon	One-Gram C
Cemill 1000	Protexin
Cemill 500	Sunkist Vitamin C
Cevi-Bid	

In Canada—

Ce-Vi-Sol	Vitamin C Powder
Revitalose-C-1000	
Revitonus C-1000 Yellow Ampule	

Available Dosage Forms:

- Tablet
- Tablet, Chewable
- Tablet, Extended Release
- Solution
- Liquid
- Granule
- Powder for Suspension
- Powder
- Capsule, Liquid Filled
- Syrup
- Lozenge/Troche
- Capsule
- Capsule, Extended Release

Therapeutic Class: Nutritive Agent
Pharmacologic Class: Vitamin C

Uses For This Dietary Supplement

Vitamins are compounds that you must have for growth and health. They are needed in small amounts only and are usually available in the foods that you eat. Ascorbic acid, also known as vitamin C, is necessary for wound healing. It is needed for many functions in the body, including helping the body use carbohydrates, fats, and protein. Vitamin C also strengthens blood vessel walls.

Lack of vitamin C can lead to a condition called scurvy, which causes muscle weakness, swollen and bleeding gums, loss of teeth, and bleeding under the skin, as well as tiredness and depression. Wounds also do not heal easily. Your health care professional may treat scurvy by prescribing vitamin C for you.

Some conditions may increase your need for vitamin C. These include:

- AIDS (acquired immune deficiency syndrome)
- Alcoholism
- Burns
- Cancer
- Diarrhea (prolonged)
- Fever (prolonged)
- Infection (prolonged)
- Intestinal diseases
- Overactive thyroid (hyperthyroidism)
- Stomach ulcer
- Stress (continuing)
- Surgical removal of stomach
- Tuberculosis

Also, the following groups of people may have a deficiency of vitamin C:

- Infants receiving unfortified formulas
- Smokers
- Patients using an artificial kidney (on hemodialysis)
- Patients who undergo surgery
- Individuals who are exposed to long periods of cold temperatures

Increased need for vitamin C should be determined by your health care professional.

Vitamin C may be used for other conditions as determined by your health care professional.

Claims that vitamin C is effective for preventing senility and the common cold, and for treating asthma, some mental problems, cancer, hardening of the arteries, allergies, eye ulcers, blood clots, gum disease, and pressure sores have not been proven. Although vitamin C is being used to reduce the risk of cardiovascular disease and certain types of cancer, there is not enough information to show that these uses are effective.

Injectable vitamin C is given by or under the supervision of a health care professional. Other forms of vitamin C are available without a prescription.

Once a medicine or dietary supplement has been approved for marketing for a certain use, experience may show that it is also useful for other medical problems. Although these uses are not included in product labeling, vitamin C is used in certain patients with the following medical conditions:

- Overdose of iron (to help another drug in decreasing iron levels in the body)
- Methemoglobinemia (a blood disease)

Importance of Diet—For good health, it is important that you eat a balanced and varied diet. Follow carefully any diet program your health care professional may recommend. For your specific dietary vitamin and/or mineral needs, ask your health care professional for a list of appropriate foods. If you think that you are not getting enough vitamins and/or minerals in your diet, you may choose to take a dietary supplement.

Vitamin C is found in various foods, including citrus fruits (oranges, lemons, grapefruit), green vegetables (peppers, broccoli, cabbage), tomatoes, and potatoes. It is best to eat fresh fruits and vegetables whenever possible since they contain the most vitamins. Food processing may destroy some of the vitamins. For example, exposure to air, drying, salting, or cooking (especially in copper pots), mincing of fresh vegetables, or mashing potatoes may reduce the amount of vitamin C in foods. Freezing does not usually cause loss of vitamin C unless foods are stored for a very long time.

Vitamins alone will not take the place of a good diet and will not provide energy. Your body also needs other substances found in food such as protein, minerals, carbohydrates, and fat. Vitamins themselves often cannot work without the presence of other foods.

The daily amount of vitamin C needed is defined in several different ways.

For U.S.—

- Recommended Dietary Allowances (RDAs) are the amount of vitamins and minerals needed to provide for adequate nutrition in most healthy persons. RDAs for a given nutrient may vary depending on a person's age, sex, and physical condition (e.g., pregnancy).
- Daily Values (DVs) are used on food and dietary supplement labels to indicate the percent of the recommended daily amount of each nutrient that a serving provides. DV replaces the previous designation of United States Recommended Daily Allowances (USRDAs).

For Canada—

- Recommended Nutrient Intakes (RNIs) are used to determine the amounts of vitamins, minerals, and protein needed to provide adequate nutrition and lessen the risk of chronic disease.

Normal daily recommended intakes for vitamin C are generally defined as follows:

Persons	U.S. (mg)	Canada (mg)
Infants and children		
Birth to 3 years of age	30–40	20
4 to 6 years of age	45	25
7 to 10 years of age	45	25
Adolescent and adult males	50–60	25–40
Adolescent and adult females	50–60	25–30
Pregnant females	70	30–40
Breast-feeding females	90–95	55
Smokers	100	45–60

Before Using This Dietary Supplement

If you are taking this dietary supplement without a prescription, carefully read and follow any precautions on the label. For this supplement, the following should be considered:

Allergies—Tell your doctor if you have ever had any unusual or allergic reaction to this medicine or any other medicines. Also tell your health care professional if you have any other types of allergies, such as to foods, dyes, preservatives, or animals. For non-prescription products, read the label or package ingredients carefully.

Pediatric—Problems in children have not been reported with intake of normal daily recommended amounts.

Geriatric—Problems in older adults have not been reported with intake of normal daily recommended amounts.

Pregnancy—

	Pregnancy Category	Explanation
All Trimesters	C	Animal studies have shown an adverse effect and there are no adequate studies in pregnant women OR no animal studies have been conducted and there are no adequate studies in pregnant women.

Breast Feeding—There are no adequate studies in women for determining infant risk when using this medication during breastfeeding. Weigh the potential benefits against the potential risks before taking this medication while breastfeeding.

Other medicines—

Using this dietary supplement with any of the following medicines is usually not recommended, but may be required in some cases. If both medicines are prescribed together, your doctor may change the dose or how often you use one or both of the medicines.

Amygdalin

Interactions with Food/Tobacco/Alcohol—Certain medicines should not be used at or around the time of eating food or eating certain types of food since interactions may occur. Using alcohol or tobacco with certain medicines may also cause interactions to occur. Discuss with your healthcare professional the use of your medicine with food, alcohol, or tobacco.

Other medical problems—The presence of other medical problems may affect the use of this dietary supplement. Make sure you tell your doctor if you have any other medical problems, especially:

- Blood problems—High doses of vitamin C may cause certain blood problems
- Type 2 diabetes mellitus—Very high doses of vitamin C may interfere with tests for sugar in the urine
- Glucose-6–phosphate dehydrogenase (G6PD) deficiency—High doses of vitamin C may cause hemolytic anemia
- Kidney stones (history of)—High doses of vitamin C may increase risk of kidney stones in the urinary tract

Proper Use of This Dietary Supplement

Dosing—The dose of this medicine will be different for different patients. Follow your doctor's orders or the directions on the label. The following information includes only the average doses of this medicine. If your dose is different, do not change it unless your doctor tells you to do so.

The amount of medicine that you take depends on the strength of the medicine. Also, the number of doses you take each day, the time allowed between doses, and the length of time you take the medicine depend on the medical problem for which you are using the medicine.

- For oral dosage form (capsules, tablets, oral solution, syrup):
  - To prevent deficiency, the amount taken by mouth is based on normal daily recommended intakes:

    For the U.S.
    - Adult and teenage males—50 to 60 milligrams (mg) per day.
    - Adult and teenage females—50 to 60 mg per day.
    - Pregnant females—70 mg per day.
    - Breast-feeding females—90 to 95 mg per day.
    - Smokers—100 mg per day.
    - Children 4 to 10 years of age—45 mg per day.
    - Children birth to 3 years of age—30 to 40 mg per day.

    For Canada
    - Adult and teenage males—25 to 40 mg per day.
    - Adult and teenage females—25 to 30 mg per day.
    - Pregnant females—30 to 40 mg per day.
    - Breast-feeding females—55 mg per day.
    - Smokers—45 to 60 mg per day.
    - Children 4 to 10 years of age—25 mg per day.
    - Children birth to 3 years of age—20 mg per day.
  - To treat deficiency:
    - Adults and teenagers—Treatment dose is determined by prescriber for each individual based on the severity of deficiency. The following dose has been determined for scurvy: 500 mg a day for at least 2 weeks.
    - Children—Treatment dose is determined by prescriber for each individual based on the severity of deficiency. The following dose has been determined for scurvy: 100 to 300 mg a day for at least 2 weeks.

For those individuals taking the oral liquid form of vitamin C:

- This preparation is to be taken by mouth even though it comes in a dropper bottle.

- This dietary supplement may be dropped directly into the mouth or mixed with cereal, fruit juice, or other food.

Missed dose—If you miss a dose of this medicine, take it as soon as possible. However, if it is almost time for your next dose, skip the missed dose and go back to your regular dosing schedule. Do not double doses.

If you miss taking a vitamin for one or more days there is no cause for concern, since it takes some time for your body to become seriously low in vitamins.

Storage—Store the dietary supplement in a closed container at room temperature, away from heat, moisture, and direct light. Keep from freezing.

Keep out of the reach of children.

Do not keep outdated medicine or medicine no longer needed.

Precautions While Using This Dietary Supplement

Vitamin C is not stored in the body. If you take more than you need, the extra vitamin C will pass into your urine. Very large doses may also interfere with tests for sugar in diabetics and with tests for blood in the stool.

Side Effects of This Dietary Supplement

Along with its needed effects, a medicine may cause some unwanted effects. Although not all of these side effects may occur, if they do occur they may need medical attention.

Check with your doctor as soon as possible if any of the following side effects occur:
Less common or rare—with high doses
　Side or lower back pain

Some side effects may occur that usually do not need medical attention. These side effects may go away during treatment as your body adjusts to the medicine. Also, your health care professional may be able to tell you about ways to prevent or reduce some of these side effects. Check with your health care professional if any of the following side effects continue or are bothersome or if you have any questions about them:
Less common or rare—with high doses
　Diarrhea; dizziness or faintness (with the injection only); flushing or redness of skin; headache; increase in urination (mild); nausea or vomiting; stomach cramps

Other side effects not listed may also occur in some patients. If you notice any other effects, check with your healthcare professional.

ASPARAGINASE　(Injection route) - a-SPARE-a-ji-nase

Black Box Warning

It is recommended that asparaginase be administered to patients only in a hospital setting under the supervision of a physician who is qualified by training and experience to administer cancer chemotherapeutic agents, because of the possibility of severe reactions, including anaphylaxis and sudden death. The physician must be prepared to treat anaphylaxis at each administration of the drug. In the treatment of each patient the physician must weigh carefully the possibility of achieving therapeutic benefit versus the risk of toxicity.

Special handling procedures should be followed.

Commonly used brand name(s)

In the U.S.—
　Elspar

Available Dosage Forms:
- Powder for Solution

Therapeutic Class: Antineoplastic Agent
Pharmacologic Class: Asparaginase (class)

Uses For This Medicine

Asparaginase belongs to the group of medicines known as enzymes. It is used to treat some kinds of cancer of the blood. It may also be used to treat other kinds of cancer, as determined by your doctor.

All cells need a chemical called asparagine to stay alive. Normal cells can make this chemical for themselves, while cancer cells cannot. Asparaginase breaks down asparagine in the body. Since the cancer cells cannot make more asparagine, they die.

Before you begin treatment with asparaginase, you and your doctor should talk about the good this medicine will do as well as the risks of using it.

Asparaginase is to be administered only by or under the supervision of your doctor.

Once a medicine has been approved for marketing for a certain use, experience may show that it is also useful for other medical problems. Although these uses are not included in product labeling, asparaginase is used in certain patients with the following condition:
- Cancer of the lymph system (certain types)

Before Using This Medicine

In deciding to use a medicine, the risks of taking the medicine must be weighed against the good it will do. This is a decision you and your doctor will make. For this medicine, the following should be considered:

Allergies—Tell your doctor if you have ever had any unusual or allergic reaction to this medicine or any other medicines. Also tell your health care professional if you have any other types of allergies, such as to foods, dyes, preservatives, or animals. For non-prescription products, read the label or package ingredients carefully.

Pediatric—This medicine has been tested in children and has not been shown to cause different side effects or problems than it does in adults. In fact, the side effects of this medicine seem to be less severe in children than in adults.

Geriatric—Many medicines have not been studied specifically in older people. Therefore, it may not be known whether they work exactly the same way they do in younger adults or if they cause different side effects or problems in older people. There is no specific information comparing use of asparaginase in the elderly with use in other age groups.

Pregnancy—

	Pregnancy Category	Explanation
All Trimesters	C	Animal studies have shown an adverse effect and there are no adequate studies in pregnant women OR no animal studies have been conducted and there are no adequate studies in pregnant women.

Breast Feeding—There are no adequate studies in women for determining infant risk when using this medication during breastfeeding. Weigh the potential benefits against the potential risks before taking this medication while breastfeeding.

Other medicines—

Using this medicine with any of the following medicines is not recommended. Your doctor may decide not to treat you with this medication or change some of the other medicines you take.

Rotavirus Vaccine, Live

Interactions with Food/Tobacco/Alcohol—Certain medicines should not be used at or around the time of eating food or eating certain types of food since interactions may occur. Using alcohol or tobacco with certain medicines may also cause interactions to occur. Discuss with your healthcare professional the use of your medicine with food, alcohol, or tobacco.

Other medical problems—The presence of other medical problems may affect the use of this medicine. Make sure you tell your doctor if you have any other medical problems, especially:

- Chickenpox (including recent exposure) or
- Herpes zoster (shingles)—Risk of severe disease affecting other parts of the body
- Type 2 diabetes mellitus—Asparaginase may increase glucose (sugar) in the blood
- Gout or
- Kidney stones—Asparaginase may increase levels of uric acid in the body, which can cause gout or kidney stones
- Infection—Asparaginase can reduce your body's ability to fight infection
- Liver disease—Asparaginase may worsen the condition
- Pancreatitis (inflammation of the pancreas)—Asparaginase may cause pancreatitis

Proper Use of This Medicine

This medicine is usually given together with certain other medicines. If you are using a combination of medicines, it is important that you receive each one at the proper time. If you are taking some of these medicines by mouth, ask your health care professional to help you plan a way to remember to take them at the right times.

While you are using this medicine, your doctor may want you to drink extra fluids so that you will pass more urine. This will help prevent kidney problems and keep your kidneys working well.

This medicine often causes nausea, vomiting, and loss of appetite. However, it is very important that you continue to re-

ceive the medicine, even if you begin to feel ill. After several doses, your stomach upset should lessen. Ask your health care professional for ways to lessen these effects.

Dosing—The dose of this medicine will be different for different patients. Follow your doctor's orders or the directions on the label. The following information includes only the average doses of this medicine. If your dose is different, do not change it unless your doctor tells you to do so.

The amount of medicine that you take depends on the strength of the medicine. Also, the number of doses you take each day, the time allowed between doses, and the length of time you take the medicine depend on the medical problem for which you are using the medicine.

Precautions While Using This Medicine

It is very important that your doctor check your progress at regular visits to make sure that this medicine is working properly and to check for unwanted effects.

While you are being treated with asparaginase, and after you stop treatment with it, do not have any immunizations (vaccinations) without your doctor's approval. Asparaginase may lower your body's resistance and there is a chance you might get the infection the immunization is meant to prevent. In addition, other persons living in your household should not take oral polio vaccine since there is a chance they could pass the polio virus on to you. Also, avoid persons who have taken oral polio vaccine within the last several months. Do not get close to them, and do not stay in the same room with them for very long. If you cannot take these precautions, you should consider wearing a protective face mask that covers the nose and mouth.

Before you have any medical tests, tell the medical doctor in charge that you are receiving this medicine. The results of thyroid tests may be affected by this medicine.

Side Effects of This Medicine

Along with its needed effects, a medicine may cause some unwanted effects. Some side effects will have signs or symptoms that you can see or feel. Your doctor may watch for others by doing certain tests. Some of the unwanted effects that may be caused by asparaginase are listed below. Although not all of these effects may occur, if they do occur, they may need medical attention.

Also, because of the way these medicines act on the body, there is a chance that they might cause other unwanted effects that may not occur until months or years after the medicine is used. These delayed effects may include certain types of cancer, such as leukemia. Discuss these possible effects with your doctor.

Check with your doctor immediately if any of the following side effects occur:
More common
  Joint pain; puffy face; skin rash or itching; stomach pain (severe) with nausea and vomiting; trouble in breathing
Less common
  Frequent urination; swelling of feet or lower legs; unusual thirst
Rare
  Fever or chills; headache (severe); inability to move arm or leg; infection; pain in lower legs; unusual bleeding or bruising

Check with your doctor as soon as possible if any of the following side effects occur:

Less common

Confusion; drowsiness; hallucinations (seeing, hearing, or feeling things that are not there); lower back or side pain; mental depression; nervousness; sores in mouth or on lips; unusual tiredness

This medicine may also cause the following side effect that your doctor will watch for:

More common

Bleeding problems; liver problems

Some side effects may occur that usually do not need medical attention. These side effects may go away during treatment as your body adjusts to the medicine. Also, your health care professional may be able to tell you about ways to prevent or reduce some of these side effects. Check with your health care professional if any of the following side effects continue or are bothersome or if you have any questions about them:

More common

Headache (mild); loss of appetite; nausea or vomiting; stomach cramps; weight loss

After you stop using this medicine, it may still produce some side effects that need attention. During this period of time, *check with your doctor immediately* if you notice the following side effects:

Headache (severe); inability to move arm or leg; stomach pain (severe) with nausea and vomiting

Other side effects not listed may also occur in some patients. If you notice any other effects, check with your healthcare professional.

ASPIRIN AND DIPYRIDAMOLE
(Oral route) - AS-pir-in, dye-peer-ID-a-mole

Commonly used brand name(s)

In the U.S.—
Aggrenox

Available Dosage Forms:

• Capsule, Extended Release

• Capsule

Therapeutic Class: Platelet Aggregation Inhibitor, Phosphodiesterase Inhibitor/Salicylate, Aspirin Combination

Pharmacologic Class: NSAID

Uses For This Medicine

Dipyridamole and aspirin is used to lessen the chance of stroke that may occur when a blood vessel in the brain is blocked by blood clots. It is given only when there is a larger-than-usual chance that these problems may occur. For example, it is given to people who have had a stroke, because dangerous blood clots are especially likely to occur in these patients. Dipyridamole and aspirin work by helping to prevent dangerous blood clots from forming.

This medicine is available only with your doctor's prescription.

Before Using This Medicine

In deciding to use a medicine, the risks of taking the medicine must be weighed against the good it will do. This is a decision you and your doctor will make. For this medicine, the following should be considered:

Allergies—Tell your doctor if you have ever had any unusual or allergic reaction to this medicine or any other medicines. Also tell your health care professional if you have any other types of allergies, such as to foods, dyes, preservatives, or animals. For non-prescription products, read the label or package ingredients carefully.

Pediatric—

• Dipyridamole—There is no specific information comparing use of dipyridamole in children with use in other age groups.

• Aspirin—Do not give aspirin to a child or a teenager with a fever or other symptoms of a virus infection, especially flu or chickenpox, without first discussing its use with your child's doctor. This is very important because salicylates may cause a serious illness called Reye's syndrome in children and teenagers caused by a virus infection, especially flu or chickenpox.

Geriatric—

• Dipyridamole—Dipyridamole has not been studied specifically in older people taking the medicine regularly to prevent blood clots from forming. Although there is no specific information comparing this use of dipyridamole in the elderly with use in other age groups, it is not expected to cause different side effects or problems in older people than it does in younger adults.

• Aspirin—Elderly people are especially sensitive to the effects of aspirin. However, this is not expected to limit the usefulness of this drug.

Other medicines—

Using this medicine with any of the following medicines is not recommended. Your doctor may decide not to treat you with this medication or change some of the other medicines you take.

Ketorolac

Interactions with Food/Tobacco/Alcohol—Certain medicines should not be used at or around the time of eating food or eating certain types of food since interactions may occur. Using alcohol or tobacco with certain medicines may also cause interactions to occur. The following interactions have been selected on the basis of their potential significance and are not necessarily all-inclusive.

Using this medicine with any of the following may cause an increased risk of certain side effects but may be unavoidable in some cases. If used together, your doctor may change the dose or how often you use this medicine, or give you special instructions about the use of food, alcohol, or tobacco.

Other medical problems—The presence of other medical problems may affect the use of this medicine. Make sure you tell your doctor if you have any other medical problems, especially:

• Alcohol use, chronic or

• Vitamin K deficiency or other bleeding problems—The chance of bleeding may be increased

• Asthma, allergies, and nasal polyps (history of) or

• Heart disease or

- Liver disease or
- Low blood pressure—The side effects may be increased
- Glucose–6– phosphate dehydrogenase enzyme deficiency—This condition may worsen, increasing risk of anemia
- Gout—The medicine used to treat this condition may not work properly
- Kidney disease—This condition may be made worse
- Stomach inflammation or ulcer—These conditions may worsen, increasing the risk of bleeding

Proper Use of This Medicine

The capsules must be swallowed whole. Do not chew them, crush them or break them up before taking.

Dosing—The dose of this medicine will be different for different patients. Follow your doctor's orders or the directions on the label. The following information includes only the average doses of this medicine. If your dose is different, do not change it unless your doctor tells you to do so.

The amount of medicine that you take depends on the strength of the medicine. Also, the number of doses you take each day, the time allowed between doses, and the length of time you take the medicine depend on the medical problem for which you are using the medicine.

- For preventing stroke:
  - For oral dosage form (capsules):
    - Adults—The usual dose is one capsule twice a day, one in the morning and one in the evening.
    - Children—Use is not recommended.

Missed dose—If you miss a dose of this medicine, take it as soon as possible. However, if it is almost time for your next dose, skip the missed dose and go back to your regular dosing schedule. Do not double doses.

Storage—Store the medicine in a closed container at room temperature, away from heat, moisture, and direct light. Keep from freezing.

Keep out of the reach of children.

Do not keep outdated medicine or medicine no longer needed.

Ask your healthcare professional how you should dispose of any medicine you do not use.

Precautions While Using This Medicine

Dipyridamole and aspirin combination provide better protection against the formation of blood clots than either of the medicines used alone. However, the risk of bleeding may also be increased. To reduce the risk of bleeding:

- Do not take aspirin, or any combination medicine containing aspirin in addition to this medicine unless the same doctor who directed you to take dipyridamole and aspirin also directs you to take aspirin.
- If you need a medicine to relieve pain or a fever, your doctor may not want you to take extra aspirin. It is a good idea to discuss this with your doctor, so that you will know ahead of time what medicine to take.
- Your doctor should check your progress at regular visits.

Tell all medical doctors and dentists you go to that you are taking dipyridamole and aspirin.

Dizziness, lightheadedness, or fainting may occur, especially when you get up from a lying or sitting position. Getting up slowly may help. If this problem continues or gets worse, check with your doctor.

Do not stop taking this medicine for any reason without first checking with the doctor who directed you to take it.

Side Effects of This Medicine

Along with its needed effects, a medicine may cause some unwanted effects. Although not all of these side effects may occur, if they do occur they may need medical attention.

Check with your doctor immediately if any of the following side effects occur:

   Confusion, difficulty in speaking, slow speech, inability to speak, inability to move arms, legs, or facial muscles, or double vision; difficulty breathing, tightness in chest, or wheezing
Symptoms of overdose

   Get emergency help immediately if any of the following symptoms of overdose occur:

   Blurred vision; Continuing ringing or buzzing or other unexplained noise in ears, or hearing loss; dizziness, faintness, or lightheadedness when getting up from a lying or sitting position sudden, sweating, or unusual tiredness or weakness; fast or irregular heartbeat; restlessness; warm feeling, flushes

Check with your doctor as soon as possible if any of the following side effects occur:
More common
   Stomach or abdomen pain; vomiting

Less common
   Bloody or black, tarry stools, blood or coffee ground materials in the vomit, or bleeding from the rectum; convulsions (seizures); memory loss; pale skin, troubled breathing, exertional, unusual bleeding or bruising; purple or red spots on skin

Rare
   Abdominal fullness, gaseous abdominal pain, recurrent fever, chills, clay-colored stools, loss of appetite, nausea, yellow eyes or skin; blood in the urine; collection of blood under skin, deep, dark purple bruise; cough; noisy breathing; shortness of breath; itching, pain, redness, or swelling of eye or eyelid watering of eyes, or severe skin rash or hives

Some side effects may occur that usually do not need medical attention. These side effects may go away during treatment as your body adjusts to the medicine. Also, your health care professional may be able to tell you about ways to prevent or reduce some of these side effects. Check with your health care professional if any of the following side effects continue or are bothersome or if you have any questions about them:
More common
   Diarrhea; headache; pain, swelling, or redness in joints, muscle pain or stiffness, or difficulty in moving; stomach discomfort upset or pain, heartburn, belching, acid or sour stomach, or indigestion

Less common or rare
   Back pain; bloody mucous, or unexplained nosebleeds; burning feeling in chest or stomach tenderness in stomach area stomach upset indigestion; loss of

strength or energy; rectal pain or swelling; sleepiness or unusual drowsiness; taste loss

Other side effects not listed may also occur in some patients. If you notice any other effects, check with your healthcare professional.

ASPIRIN, SODIUM BICARBONATE, AND CITRIC ACID (Oral route) - AS-pir-in, SOE-dee-um bye-KARB-oh-nate, SI-trik AS-id

Available Dosage Forms:
- Tablet
- Tablet, Effervescent

Therapeutic Class: Salicylate, Aspirin Combination
Pharmacologic Class: NSAID

Uses For This Medicine

Aspirin, sodium bicarbonate, and citric acid combination is used to relieve pain occurring together with heartburn, sour stomach, or acid indigestion.

The aspirin in this combination is the pain reliever. Aspirin belongs to the group of medicines known as salicylates and to the group of medicines known as anti-inflammatory analgesics. The sodium bicarbonate in this medicine is an antacid. It neutralizes stomach acid by combining with it to form a new substance that is not an acid.

Aspirin, sodium bicarbonate, and citric acid combination may also be used to lessen the chance of heart attack, stroke, or other problems that may occur when a blood vessel is blocked by blood clots. The aspirin in this medicine helps prevent dangerous blood clots from forming. However, this effect of aspirin may increase the chance of serious bleeding in some people. Therefore, aspirin should be used for this purpose only when your doctor decides, after studying your medical condition and history, that the danger of blood clots is greater than the risk of bleeding. Do not take aspirin to prevent blood clots or a heart attack unless it has been ordered by your doctor.

This combination medicine is available without a prescription.

Before Using This Medicine

In deciding to use a medicine, the risks of taking the medicine must be weighed against the good it will do. This is a decision you and your doctor will make. For this medicine, the following should be considered:

Allergies—Tell your doctor if you have ever had any unusual or allergic reaction to this medicine or any other medicines. Also tell your health care professional if you have any other types of allergies, such as to foods, dyes, preservatives, or animals. For non-prescription products, read the label or package ingredients carefully.

Pediatric—Do not give any medicine containing aspirin to a child with fever or other symptoms of a virus infection, especially flu or chickenpox, without first discussing its use with your child's doctor. This is very important because aspirin may cause a serious illness called Reye's syndrome in children with fever caused by a virus infection, especially flu or chickenpox. Children who do not have a virus infection may also be more sensitive to the effects of aspirin, especially if they have a fever or have lost large amounts of body fluid because of vomiting, diarrhea, or sweating. This may increase the chance of side effects during treatment.

Geriatric—People 60 years of age and older are especially sensitive to the effects of aspirin. This may increase the chance of side effects during treatment. Also, the sodium in this combination medicine can be harmful to some elderly people, especially if large amounts of the medicine are taken regularly. Therefore, it is best that older people not use this medicine for more than 5 days in a row, unless otherwise directed by their doctor.

Pregnancy—

	Pregnancy Category	Explanation
All Trimesters	D	Studies in pregnant women have demonstrated a risk to the fetus. However, the benefits of therapy in a life threatening situation or a serious disease, may outweigh the potential risk.

Breast Feeding—There are no adequate studies in women for determining infant risk when using this medication during breastfeeding. Weigh the potential benefits against the potential risks before taking this medication while breastfeeding.

Other medicines—

Using this medicine with any of the following medicines is not recommended. Your doctor may decide not to treat you with this medication or change some of the other medicines you take.

Ketorolac

Interactions with Food/Tobacco/Alcohol—Certain medicines should not be used at or around the time of eating food or eating certain types of food since interactions may occur. Using alcohol or tobacco with certain medicines may also cause interactions to occur. The following interactions have been selected on the basis of their potential significance and are not necessarily all-inclusive.

Using this medicine with any of the following may cause an increased risk of certain side effects but may be unavoidable in some cases. If used together, your doctor may change the dose or how often you use this medicine, or give you special instructions about the use of food, alcohol, or tobacco.

Ethanol

Other medical problems—The presence of other medical problems may affect the use of this medicine. Make sure you tell your doctor if you have any other medical problems, especially:
- Anemia or
- Stomach ulcer or other stomach problems—Aspirin can make these conditions worse
- Appendicitis (symptoms of, such as stomach or lower abdominal pain, cramping, bloating, soreness, nausea, or vomiting)—Sodium bicarbonate can make your con-

dition worse; also, people who may have appendicitis need medical attention and should not try to treat themselves

- Asthma, allergies, and nasal polyps (history of) or
- Kidney disease or
- Liver disease—The chance of serious side effects may be increased
- Edema (swelling of face, fingers, feet, or lower legs caused by too much water in the body) or
- Heart disease or
- High blood pressure or
- Toxemia of pregnancy—The sodium in this combination medicine can make these conditions worse
- Gout—Aspirin can make this condition worse and can also keep some medicines used to treat gout from working properly
- Hemophilia or other bleeding problems—Aspirin increases the chance of serious bleeding

Proper Use of This Medicine

Make certain your health care professional knows if you are on any special diet, such as a low-sodium or low-sugar diet. This medicine contains a large amount of sodium (more than 500 mg in each tablet).

Unless otherwise directed by your doctor, do not take more of this medicine than is recommended on the package label. If too much is taken, serious side effects may occur.

Do not take this medicine if it has a strong vinegar-like odor. This odor means the aspirin in it is breaking down. If you have any questions about this, check with your health care professional.

To use this medicine:

- The tablets must be dissolved in water before taking. Do not swallow the tablets or any pieces of the tablets.
- Place the number of tablets needed for one dose (1 or 2 tablets) into a glass. Then add ½ glass (4 ounces) of cool water.
- Check to be sure that the tablets have disappeared completely. This shows that all of the medicine is in the liquid. Then drink all of the liquid. You may drink the liquid while it is still fizzing or after the fizzing stops.
- Add a little more water to the glass and drink that, to make sure that you get the full amount of the medicine.

Dosing—The dose of this medicine will be different for different patients. Follow your doctor's orders or the directions on the label. The following information includes only the average doses of this medicine. If your dose is different, do not change it unless your doctor tells you to do so.

The amount of medicine that you take depends on the strength of the medicine. Also, the number of doses you take each day, the time allowed between doses, and the length of time you take the medicine depend on the medical problem for which you are using the medicine.

- For oral dosage forms (effervescent tablets):
  - For pain and upset stomach:
    - Adults and teenagers—One or two regular-strength (325–milligram [mg]) tablets every four to six hours as needed, one extra-strength (500–mg) tablet every four to six hours as needed, or two extra-strength (500–mg) tablets every six hours as

needed, dissolved in water. Elderly people should not take more than four regular-strength or extra-strength tablets a day. Other adults and teenagers should not take more than 6 regular-strength flavored tablets, 8 regular-strength unflavored tablets, or 7 extra-strength tablets a day.
    - Children—The dose depends on the child's age.
      — Children younger than 3 years of age: Use and dose must be determined by your doctor.
      — Children 3 to 5 years of age: One-half of a regular-strength (325–mg) tablet, dissolved in water, every four to six hours as needed.
      — Children 6 to 12 years of age: One regular-strength (325–mg) tablet, dissolved in water, every four to six hours as needed.
  - For reducing the chance of heart attack, stroke, or other problems that may occur when a blood vessel is blocked by blood clots:
    - Adults—One regular-strength (325–mg) tablet a day, dissolved in water.
    - Children and teenagers—Use and dose must be determined by your doctor.

Missed dose—If you miss a dose of this medicine, take it as soon as possible. However, if it is almost time for your next dose, skip the missed dose and go back to your regular dosing schedule. Do not double doses.

Storage—Store the medicine in a closed container at room temperature, away from heat, moisture, and direct light. Keep from freezing.

Keep out of the reach of children.

Do not keep outdated medicine or medicine no longer needed.

Precautions While Using This Medicine

If you will be taking this medicine for a long time (more than 5 days in a row for children or 10 days in a row for adults), your doctor should check your progress at regular visits.

Check with your doctor if your pain and/or upset stomach last for more than 10 days for adults or 5 days for children or if they get worse, if new symptoms occur, or if the painful area is red or swollen. These could be signs of a serious condition that needs medical treatment.

The sodium bicarbonate in this combination medicine can keep other medicines from working properly if the 2 medicines are taken too close together. Always take this medicine:

- At least 6 hours before or 2 hours after taking ciprofloxacin (e.g., Cipro) or lomefloxacin (e.g., Maxaquin).
- At least 8 hours before or 2 hours after taking enoxacin (e.g., Penetrex).
- At least 2 hours after taking itraconazole (e.g., Sporanox).
- At least 3 hours before or after taking ketoconazole (e.g., Nizoral).
- At least 2 hours before or after taking norfloxacin (e.g., Noroxin) or ofloxacin (e.g., Floxin).
- At least 3 or 4 hours before or after taking a tetracycline antibiotic by mouth.
- At least 1 or 2 hours before or after taking any other medicine by mouth.

If you are also taking a laxative that contains cellulose, take this combination medicine at least 2 hours before or after you take the laxative. Taking the medicines too close together may lessen the effects of aspirin.

Check the labels of all nonprescription (over-the-counter [OTC]) and prescription medicines you now take. If any contain aspirin or other salicylates, including bismuth subsalicylate (e.g., Pepto-Bismol), magnesium salicylate (e.g., Nuprin Backache Caplets), or salsalate (e.g., Disalcid); if any contain salicylic acid (present in some shampoos or medicines for your skin); or if any contain sodium, check with your health care professional. Taking other salicylate-containing or other sodium-containing products together with this medicine may cause an overdose.

Do not take aspirin for 5 days before any surgery, including dental surgery, unless otherwise directed by your medical doctor or dentist. Taking aspirin during this time may cause bleeding problems.

For patients taking this medicine to lessen the chance of a heart attack, stroke, or other problems caused by blood clots:

- Take only the amount of aspirin ordered by your doctor. If you need a medicine to relieve pain, a fever, or arthritis, your doctor may not want you to take extra aspirin. It is a good idea to discuss this with your doctor, so that you will know ahead of time what medicine to take.

- Do not stop taking this medicine for any reason without first checking with the doctor who directed you to take it.

Taking certain other medicines together with a salicylate may increase the chance of unwanted effects. The risk will depend on how much of each medicine you take every day, and on how long you take the medicines together. If your doctor directs you to take these medicines together on a regular basis, follow his or her directions carefully. However, do not take any of the following medicines together with a salicylate for more than a few days, unless your doctor has directed you to do so and is following your progress:

- Acetaminophen (e.g., Tylenol)
- Diclofenac (e.g., Voltaren)
- Diflunisal (e.g., Dolobid)
- Etodolac (e.g., Lodine)
- Fenoprofen (e.g., Nalfon)
- Floctafenine (e.g., Idarac)
- Flurbiprofen, oral (e.g., Ansaid)
- Ibuprofen (e.g., Motrin)
- Indomethacin (e.g., Indocin)
- Ketoprofen (e.g., Orudis)
- Ketorolac (e.g., Toradol)
- Meclofenamate (e.g., Meclomen)
- Mefenamic acid (e.g., Ponstel)
- Nabumetone (e.g., Relafen)
- Naproxen (e.g., Naprosyn)
- Oxaprozin (e.g., Daypro)
- Phenylbutazone (e.g., Butazolidin)
- Piroxicam (e.g., Feldene)
- Sulindac (e.g., Clinoril)
- Tenoxicam (e.g., Mobiflex)
- Tiaprofenic acid (e.g., Surgam)
- Tolmetin (e.g., Tolectin)

If you will be taking more than an occasional 1 or 2 doses of this medicine:

- Do not drink alcoholic beverages. Drinking alcoholic beverages while you are taking aspirin, especially if you take aspirin regularly or in large amounts, may increase the chance of stomach problems.

- Do not drink a lot of milk or eat a lot of milk products. To do so may increase the chance of side effects.

- To prevent side effects caused by too much sodium in the body, you may need to limit the amount of sodium in the foods you eat. Some foods that contain large amounts of sodium are canned soup, canned vegetables, pickles, ketchup, green and ripe (black) olives, relish, frankfurters and other sausage-type meats, soy sauce, and carbonated beverages. If you have any questions about this, check with your health care professional.

Before you have any medical tests, tell the person in charge that you are taking this medicine. The results of some tests may be affected by the aspirin in this combination medicine.

For diabetic patients:

- Aspirin can cause false urine glucose (sugar) test results if you regularly take 8 or more 324–mg, or 4 or more 500–mg (extra-strength), tablets a day. Smaller amounts or occasional use of aspirin usually will not affect the test results. However, check with your health care professional if you notice any change in your urine glucose test results. This is especially important if your diabetes is not well-controlled.

If you think that you or anyone else may have taken an overdose, get emergency help at once. Taking an overdose of aspirin may cause unconsciousness or death, especially in young children. Signs of overdose include convulsions (seizures), hearing loss, confusion, ringing or buzzing in the ears, severe drowsiness or tiredness, severe excitement or nervousness, and fast or deep breathing.

Side Effects of This Medicine

Along with its needed effects, a medicine may cause some unwanted effects. Although the following side effects occur very rarely when 1 or 2 doses of this combination medicine is taken occasionally, they may be more likely to occur if: too much medicine is taken, the medicine is taken several times a day, or the medicine is taken for more than a few days in a row.

Check with your doctor immediately if any of the following side effects occur:

Any loss of hearing; bloody urine; confusion; convulsions (seizures); diarrhea (severe or continuing); difficulty in swallowing; dizziness, lightheadedness, or feeling faint (severe); drowsiness (severe); excitement or nervousness (severe); fast or deep breathing; flushing, redness, or other change in skin color; hallucinations (seeing, hearing, or feeling things that are not there); nausea or vomiting (severe or continuing); shortness of breath, troubled breathing, tightness in chest, or wheezing; stomach pain (severe or continuing); swelling of eyelids, face, or lips; unexplained fever; uncontrollable flapping movements of the hands (especially in elderly patients); vision problems

Signs of overdose in children

Changes in behavior; drowsiness or tiredness (severe); fast or deep breathing

Check with your doctor as soon as possible if any of the following side effects occur:

Less common or rare

Bloody or black, tarry stools; frequent urge to urinate; headache (severe or continuing); increased blood pressure; loss of appetite (continuing); mood or mental changes; muscle pain or twitching; ringing or buzzing in ears (continuing); skin rash, hives, or itching; slow breathing; swelling of face, fingers, ankles, feet, or lower legs; unpleasant taste; unusual tiredness or weakness; vomiting of blood or material that looks like coffee grounds; weight gain (unusual)

Some side effects may occur that usually do not need medical attention. These side effects may go away during treatment as your body adjusts to the medicine. Also, your health care professional may be able to tell you about ways to prevent or reduce some of these side effects. Check with your health care professional if any of the following side effects continue or are bothersome or if you have any questions about them:

Heartburn or indigestion; increased thirst; nausea or vomiting; stomach pain (mild)

Other side effects not listed may also occur in some patients. If you notice any other effects, check with your healthcare professional.

ATAZANAVIR SULFATE (Oral route)
- at-a-za-NA-veer SUL-fate

Commonly used brand name(s)

In the U.S.—
Reyataz

Available Dosage Forms:
- Capsule

Therapeutic Class: Antiretroviral Agent
Pharmacologic Class: Atazanavir

Uses For This Medicine

Atazanavir is used with other medicines, in the treatment of the infection caused by the human immunodeficiency virus (HIV). HIV is the virus that causes acquired immune deficiency syndrome (AIDS).

Atazanavir will not cure or prevent HIV infection or AIDS; however, it helps keep HIV from reproducing and appears to slow down the destruction of the immune system. This may help delay the development of problems usually related to AIDS or HIV disease. Atazanavir will not keep you from spreading HIV to other people. People who receive this medicine may continue to have other problems usually related to AIDS or HIV disease.

This medicine is available only with your doctor's prescription.

Before Using This Medicine

In deciding to use a medicine, the risks of taking the medicine must be weighed against the good it will do. This is a decision you and your doctor will make. For this medicine, the following should be considered:

Allergies—Tell your doctor if you have ever had any unusual or allergic reaction to this medicine or any other medicines. Also tell your health care professional if you have any other types of allergies, such as to foods, dyes, preservatives, or animals. For non-prescription products, read the label or package ingredients carefully.

Pediatric—Studies on this medicine have been done only in adult patients, and there is limited recommendations comparing the use of atazanavir in children with use in other age groups. Atazanavir should not be administered to children under the age of 3 months.

Geriatric—Many medicines have not been studied specifically in older people. Therefore, it may not be known whether they work exactly the same way they do in younger adults. There is no specific information comparing use of atazanavir in the elderly with use in other age groups.

Pregnancy—

	Pregnancy Category	Explanation
All Trimesters	B	Animal studies have revealed no evidence of harm to the fetus, however, there are no adequate studies in pregnant women OR animal studies have shown an adverse effect, but adequate studies in pregnant women have failed to demonstrate a risk to the fetus.

Breast Feeding—There are no adequate studies in women for determining infant risk when using this medication during breastfeeding. Weigh the potential benefits against the potential risks before taking this medication while breastfeeding.

Other medicines—

Using this medicine with any of the following medicines is not recommended. Your doctor may decide not to treat you with this medication or change some of the other medicines you take.

Alprazolam, Cisapride, Clonazepam, Diazepam, Dihydroergotamine, Ergoloid Mesylates, Ergonovine, Ergotamine, Methylergonovine, Methysergide, Midazolam, Pimozide, Ranolazine, St John's Wort, Triazolam

Interactions with Food/Tobacco/Alcohol—Certain medicines should not be used at or around the time of eating food or eating certain types of food since interactions may occur. Using alcohol or tobacco with certain medicines may also cause interactions to occur. Discuss with your healthcare professional the use of your medicine with food, alcohol, or tobacco.

Other medical problems—The presence of other medical problems may affect the use of this medicine. Make sure you tell your doctor if you have any other medical problems, especially:
- Diabetes mellitus (sugar diabetes) or
- Hyperglycemia—Atazanavir may increase or decrease the amount of sugar in your blood, dose adjustments of insulin or other medicines for diabetes may be needed. Talk to your doctor about this.

- Heart conduction problems, preexisting—Atazanavir may change the way your heart beats and increase your chance of getting side effects.
- Hemophilia, type A and B—Use of atazanavir may increase your chance of having serious bleeding problems.
- Hepatitis, or
- Transaminase, elevated—Use of atazanavir may make these problems worse.
- Liver disease—May increase your chance of getting side effects.

Proper Use of This Medicine

It is important that atazanavir be taken with food.

Dosing—The dose of this medicine will be different for different patients. Follow your doctor's orders or the directions on the label. The following information includes only the average doses of this medicine. If your dose is different, do not change it unless your doctor tells you to do so.

The amount of medicine that you take depends on the strength of the medicine. Also, the number of doses you take each day, the time allowed between doses, and the length of time you take the medicine depend on the medical problem for which you are using the medicine.

- For oral dosage form (capsules):
  - For treatment of HIV infection:
    - Adults—300 to 400 mg once daily with food
    - Children (3 months and older)—Use and dose must be determined by your doctor.

Note: This medicine may be taken in combination with other medicines that are used to treat HIV infection. Check with your health care professional for information and dose amounts.

Missed dose—If you miss a dose of this medicine, take it as soon as possible. However, if it is almost time for your next dose, skip the missed dose and go back to your regular dosing schedule. Do not double doses.

Storage—Store the medicine in a closed container at room temperature, away from heat, moisture, and direct light. Keep from freezing.

Keep out of the reach of children.

Do not keep outdated medicine or medicine no longer needed.

Ask your healthcare professional how you should dispose of any medicine you do not use.

Precautions While Using This Medicine

Do not take any other medicines without checking with your doctor first. To do so may increase the chance of side effects from atazanavir.

It is very important that your doctor check your progress at regular visits to make sure this medicine is working properly and to check for unwanted effects.

Side Effects of This Medicine

Along with its needed effects, a medicine may cause some unwanted effects. Although not all of these side effects may occur, if they do occur they may need medical attention.

Check with your doctor immediately if any of the following side effects occur:
  Incidence not determined
  Abdominal discomfort; blurred vision; chills; decreased appetite; diarrhea; dizziness or lightheadedness; dry mouth; fast, shallow breathing; fatigue; fever; flushed, dry skin; fruit-like breath odor; general feeling of discomfort; hives; increased hunger; increased thirst; increased urination; itching; loss of consciousness; muscle pain or cramping; nausea; shortness of breath; skin rash; sleepiness; stomachache; sweating; tightness in chest; trouble in breathing; unexplained weight loss; unusual tiredness or weakness; vomiting; wheezing; yellow eyes or skin
  Symptoms of overdose
  Get emergency help immediately if any of the following symptoms of overdose occur:
  Abdominal or stomach pain; area rash; chills; clay-colored stools; dark urine; dizziness; dizziness or lightheadedness; fever; headache; itching; loss of appetite; nausea; unpleasant breath odor; unusual tiredness or weakness; vomiting of blood; yellow eyes or skin

Some side effects may occur that usually do not need medical attention. These side effects may go away during treatment as your body adjusts to the medicine. Also, your health care professional may be able to tell you about ways to prevent or reduce some of these side effects. Check with your health care professional if any of the following side effects continue or are bothersome or if you have any questions about them:
  More common
  Back pain; cough, increased; discouragement; feeling sad or empty; headache; irritability; lack of appetite; loss of interest or pleasure; redistribution or accumulation of body fat; trouble concentrating; trouble sleeping
  Less common
  Burning, numbness, tingling, or painful sensations; difficulty in moving; muscle stiffness; pain; pain in joints; sleeplessness; unable to sleep; unsteadiness or awkwardness; weakness in arms, hands, legs, or feet

Other side effects not listed may also occur in some patients. If you notice any other effects, check with your healthcare professional.

ATOMOXETINE (Oral route) - AT-oh-mox-e-teen

Black Box Warning

Suicidal ideation in children and adolescents: atomoxetine increased the risk of suicidal ideation in short-term studies in children or adolescents with Attention-Deficit/Hyperactivity Disorder (ADHD). Anyone considering the use of atomoxetine in a child or adolescent must balance this risk with the clinical need. Patients who are started on therapy should be monitored closely for suicidality (suicidal thinking and behavior), clinical worsening, or unusual changes in behavior. Families and caregivers should be advised of the need for close observation and communication with the prescriber. Atomoxetine is approved for ADHD in pediatric and adult patients. Atomoxetine is not approved for major depressive disorder.

Pooled analyses of short-term (6 to 18 weeks) placebo-controlled trials of atomoxetine in children and adolescents (a total of 12 trials involving over 2200 patients, including 11 trials in ADHD and 1 trial in enuresis) have revealed a greater risk of suicidal ideation early during treatment in those receiving atomoxetine compared to placebo. The average risk of suicidal ideation in patients receiving atomoxetine was 0.4% (5/1357 patients), compared to none in placebo-treated patients (851 patients). No suicides occurred in these trials

Commonly used brand name(s)

In the U.S.—
  Strattera

Available Dosage Forms:
  • Capsule

Therapeutic Class: Central Nervous System Agent
Pharmacologic Class: Norepinephrine Reuptake Inhibitor

Uses For This Medicine

Atomoxetine belongs to the group of medicines called selective norepinephrine reuptake inhibitor. It is used to treat children, adolescents, and adults with attention-deficit hyperactivity disorder (ADHD).

Atomoxetine increases attention and decreases restlessness in people who are overactive, cannot concentrate for very long or are easily distracted, and are emotionally unstable. This medicine is used as part of a total treatment program that also includes social, educational, and psychological treatment.

This medicine is available only with your doctor's prescription.

Before Using This Medicine

In deciding to use a medicine, the risks of taking the medicine must be weighed against the good it will do. This is a decision you and your doctor will make. For this medicine, the following should be considered:

Allergies—Tell your doctor if you have ever had any unusual or allergic reaction to this medicine or any other medicines. Also tell your health care professional if you have any other types of allergies, such as to foods, dyes, preservatives, or animals. For non-prescription products, read the label or package ingredients carefully.

Pediatric—Safety and effectiveness has not been established in pediatric patients less than 6 years of age; increases chance of suicidal thinking in children and adolescents with ADHD.

Geriatric—Atomoxetine has not been studied specifically in older people. Therefore, it is not known whether it causes different side effects or problems in the elderly than it does in younger adults.

Pregnancy—

	Pregnancy Category	Explanation
All Trimesters	C	Animal studies have shown an adverse effect and there are no adequate studies in pregnant women OR no animal studies have been conducted and there are no adequate studies in pregnant women.

Breast Feeding—There are no adequate studies in women for determining infant risk when using this medication during breastfeeding. Weigh the potential benefits against the potential risks before taking this medication while breastfeeding.

Other medicines—

Using this medicine with any of the following medicines is not recommended. Your doctor may decide not to treat you with this medication or change some of the other medicines you take.

Clorgyline, Isocarboxazid, Lazabemide, Moclobemide, Phenelzine, Selegiline, Tranylcypromine

Interactions with Food/Tobacco/Alcohol—Certain medicines should not be used at or around the time of eating food or eating certain types of food since interactions may occur. Using alcohol or tobacco with certain medicines may also cause interactions to occur. Discuss with your healthcare professional the use of your medicine with food, alcohol, or tobacco.

Other medical problems—The presence of other medical problems may affect the use of this medicine. Make sure you tell your doctor if you have any other medical problems, especially:

• Blood disorder or
• Dehydration—May make hypotension (decreased blood pressure) caused by this medicine worse
• Blood vessel problems or
• Heart disease or
• Hypertension (high blood pressure) or
• Tachycardia (rapid heart rate)—Atomoxetine may make these conditions worse.
• Glaucoma, narrow angle (eye disease)—Atomoxetine may make this condition worse.
• Liver disease—The dose of atomoxetine may need to be adjusted

Proper Use of This Medicine

Dosing—The dose of this medicine will be different for different patients. Follow your doctor's orders or the directions on the label. The following information includes only the average doses of this medicine. If your dose is different, do not change it unless your doctor tells you to do so.

The amount of medicine that you take depends on the strength of the medicine. Also, the number of doses you take each day, the time allowed between doses, and the length of time you take the medicine depend on the medical problem for which you are using the medicine.

• For oral dosage form (capsules):
  ○ Attention deficit hyperactivity disorder [ADHD]
    ▪ Adults—Oral, 40 milligrams (mg) once a day; your doctor may want to increase or decrease your dose and change the number of times a day you take your medicine.
    ▪ Children (6 years of age and older)—Oral, to start 0.5 milligram per kilogram (mg per kg) of body weight once daily; your doctor may want to increase or decrease your dose and change the number of times a day you take your medicine.
    ▪ Children (less than 6 years of age)—Use and dose must be determined by your doctor.

Missed dose—If you miss a dose of this medicine, take it as soon as possible. However, if it is almost time for your next

dose, skip the missed dose and go back to your regular dosing schedule. Do not double doses.

Storage—Store the medicine in a closed container at room temperature, away from heat, moisture, and direct light. Keep from freezing.

Keep out of the reach of children.

Do not keep outdated medicine or medicine no longer needed.

Ask your healthcare professional how you should dispose of any medicine you do not use.

Precautions While Using This Medicine

It is very important that your doctor check you at regular visits.

This medicine may cause some people to become drowsy, dizzy, or less alert than they are normally. Make sure you know how you react to this medicine before you drive, use machines, or do anything else that could be dangerous if you are dizzy or are not alert.

Tell your doctor about all the medicines you take or plan to take, including prescription and nonprescription medicines, dietary supplements, and herbal remedies.

Tell your doctor if you are nursing, pregnant, or thinking of becoming pregnant.

Call your doctor right away if you get swelling, hives, or if you develop any symptoms that concern you.

Tell your doctor right away if you get a skin rash, dark urine, persistent loss of appetite, yellow eyes or skin, flu-like symptoms or right upper quadrant tenderness. These could be symptoms of a serious liver problem.

Do not give atomoxetine to other people, even if they have the same symptoms as you have.

Tell your doctor right away if you or your family notices any unusual changes in behavior such as an increase in aggression, hostility, agitation, irritability, or suicidal thinking or behaviors.

Atomoxetine may be taken with or without food.

Atomoxetine may cause your mouth to feel dry. You may use sugarless candy or gum, ice or saliva substitute for relief. Tell you doctor or dentist if dry mouth continues for more than 2 weeks.

Side Effects of This Medicine

Along with its needed effects, a medicine may cause some unwanted effects. Although not all of these side effects may occur, if they do occur they may need medical attention.

Check with your doctor immediately if any of the following side effects occur:

Less common or rare
Hives or welts; irregular heartbeat; itching; large, hive-like swelling on face, eyelids, lips, tongue, throat, hands, legs, feet, or sex organs; redness of skin; skin rash

Incidence not known
Dark urine; flu-like symptoms; persistent anorexia; pruritus; right upper quadrant tenderness; yellow eyes or skin

Some side effects may occur that usually do not need medical attention. These side effects may go away during treatment as your body adjusts to the medicine. Also, your health care

professional may be able to tell you about ways to prevent or reduce some of these side effects. Check with your health care professional if any of the following side effects continue or are bothersome or if you have any questions about them:

More common
Acid or sour stomach; belching; bleeding between periods; change in amount of bleeding during periods; change in pattern of monthly periods; cough; decreased appetite; decreased interest in sexual intercourse; decrease in frequency of urination; decrease in urine volume; difficulty having a bowel movement (stool); difficulty in passing urine [dribbling] dizziness; dry mouth; fever; headache; heartburn; heavy bleeding; inability to have or keep an erection; indigestion; irritability; loss in sexual ability, desire, drive, or performance; nausea; painful urination; pain or tenderness around eyes and cheekbones; shortness of breath or troubled breathing; sleepiness or unusual drowsiness; sleeplessness; stomach discomfort, upset, cramps, or pain; stuffy or runny nose; tightness of chest or wheezing; trouble sleeping; unable to sleep; unusual drowsiness, dullness, tiredness, weakness or feeling of sluggishness; unusual stopping of menstrual bleeding; unusual tiredness or weakness; vomiting

Less common
Abnormal dreams; abnormal orgasm; back pain; blistering, crusting, irritation, itching, or reddening of skin; bloated, full feeling; burning, crawling, itching, numbness, prickling, "pins and needles" or tingling feelings; change in hearing; change or problem with discharge of semen; chills; cold sweats; confusion; cough; cracked, dry, scaly skin; crying; decreased weight; diarrhea; difficulty in moving; dizziness, faintness, or lightheadedness when getting up from lying or sitting position; ear drainage; earache or pain in ear; excess air or gas in stomach or intestines; feeling of warmth redness of the face, neck, arms and occasionally, upper chest; feeling unusually cold; frequent urination; general feeling of discomfort or illness; groin pain; increased or sudden sweating; joint pain; loss of appetite; mood swings; muscle aches, cramping, pains, or stiffness; pain or burning with urination; passing gas; shivering; sinus headache; sleep disorder; swelling of skin; swollen joints; swollen, tender prostate

Other side effects not listed may also occur in some patients. If you notice any other effects, check with your healthcare professional.

ATORVASTATIN (Oral route) - a-TORE-va-sta-tin

Commonly used brand name(s)

In the U.S.—
Lipitor

Available Dosage Forms:
• Tablet

Therapeutic Class: Antihyperlipidemic
Pharmacologic Class: HMG-COA Reductase Inhibitor

Uses For This Medicine

Atorvastatin is used to lower cholesterol and triglyceride (fat-like substances) levels in the blood. Using this medicine may help prevent medical problems caused by such substances clogging the blood vessels. This medicine may also be used to prevent certain types of heart problems in adults with risk factors for heart problems.

Atorvastatin belongs to the group of medicines called 3–hydroxy-3–methylglutaryl coenzyme A (HMG-CoA) reductase inhibitors. It works by blocking an enzyme that is needed by the body to make cholesterol, thereby reducing the amount of cholesterol in the blood.

Atorvastatin is available only with your doctor's prescription.

Before Using This Medicine

In deciding to use a medicine, the risks of taking the medicine must be weighed against the good it will do. This is a decision you and your doctor will make. For this medicine, the following should be considered:

In addition to its helpful effects in treating your medical problem, this type of medicine may have some harmful effects.

Allergies—Tell your doctor if you have ever had any unusual or allergic reaction to this medicine or any other medicines. Also tell your health care professional if you have any other types of allergies, such as to foods, dyes, preservatives, or animals. For non-prescription products, read the label or package ingredients carefully.

Pediatric—This medicine is safe to use in boys and some girls 10 to 17 years of age for treating certain types of high cholesterol.

Geriatric—This medicine has been tested in a limited number of patients 65 years of age or older and has not been shown to cause different problems in older people than it does in younger adults. However, blood levels of atorvastatin tend to be higher in older people than they do in younger adults.

Pregnancy—

	Pregnancy Category	Explanation
All Trimesters	X	Studies in animals or pregnant women have demonstrated positive evidence of fetal abnormalities. This drug should not be used in women who are or may become pregnant because the risk clearly outweighs any possible benefit.

Breast Feeding—There are no adequate studies in women for determining infant risk when using this medication during breastfeeding. Weigh the potential benefits against the potential risks before taking this medication while breastfeeding.

Other medicines—

Using this medicine with any of the following medicines is usually not recommended, but may be required in some cases. If both medicines are prescribed together, your doctor may change the dose or how often you use one or both of the medicines.

Atazanavir, Bezafibrate, Ciprofibrate, Clarithromycin, Clofibrate, Cyclosporine, Dalfopristin, Diltiazem, Erythromycin, Fenofibrate, Fluconazole, Fosamprenavir, Fusidic Acid, Gemfibrozil, Indinavir, Itraconazole, Ketoconazole, Lopinavir, Mibefradil, Nefazodone, Nelfinavir, Niacin, Quinupristin, Saquinavir, Telithromycin, Tipranavir, Troleandomycin, Verapamil

Interactions with Food/Tobacco/Alcohol—Certain medicines should not be used at or around the time of eating food or eating certain types of food since interactions may occur. Using alcohol or tobacco with certain medicines may also cause interactions to occur. The following interactions have been selected on the basis of their potential significance and are not necessarily all-inclusive.

Using this medicine with any of the following may cause an increased risk of certain side effects but may be unavoidable in some cases. If used together, your doctor may change the dose or how often you use this medicine, or give you special instructions about the use of food, alcohol, or tobacco.

Grapefruit Juice

Other medical problems—The presence of other medical problems may affect the use of this medicine. Make sure you tell your doctor if you have any other medical problems, especially:

- Alcohol abuse (or history of) or
- Liver disease (or history of) or
- Liver enzymes, persistently high levels—Use of this medicine may make liver problems worse
- Convulsions (seizures), not well-controlled, or
- Electrolyte or metabolic enzyme deficiencies or disorders or
- Infection, severe or
- Low blood pressure or
- Major surgery or trauma, recent—Patients with these conditions may be at risk of developing muscle problems (causing the release of muscle pigment into the urine) that may lead to kidney failure

Proper Use of This Medicine

Before prescribing medicine for your condition, your doctor will probably try to control your condition by prescribing a personal diet for you. Such a diet may be low in fats, sugars, and/or cholesterol. Many people are able to control their condition by carefully following their doctor's orders for proper diet and exercise. Medicine is prescribed only when additional help is needed and is effective only when a schedule of diet and exercise is properly followed.

Also, this medicine is less effective if you are greatly overweight. It may be very important for you to go on a weight-reducing diet. However, check with your doctor before going on any diet.

Use this medicine only as directed by your doctor. Do not use more or less of it, and do not use it more often or for a longer time than your doctor ordered. Also, this medicine works best if there is a constant amount in the blood. To help keep this amount constant, do not miss any doses and take the medicine at the same time each day.

Remember that this medicine will not cure your condition but it does help control it. Therefore, you must continue to take it as directed if you expect to keep your cholesterol levels down.

Follow carefully the special diet your doctor gave you. This is the most important part of controlling your condition and is necessary if the medicine is to work properly.

Atorvastatin should not be taken with large amounts of grapefruit juice or other grapefruit products because these may increase the concentrations of atorvastatin in the body

Dosing—The dose of this medicine will be different for different patients. Follow your doctor's orders or the directions on the label. The following information includes only the average doses of this medicine. If your dose is different, do not change it unless your doctor tells you to do so.

The amount of medicine that you take depends on the strength of the medicine. Also, the number of doses you take each day, the time allowed between doses, and the length of time you take the medicine depend on the medical problem for which you are using the medicine.

- For oral dosage form (tablets):
  - Adults: 10 milligrams (mg) once daily. Your doctor may increase your dose if needed.
  - Children (10 to 17 years of age): 10 milligrams (mg) once daily. Your doctor may increase your dose if needed.
  - Children (less than 10 years of age): Use and dose must be determined by your doctor.

Missed dose—If you miss a dose of this medicine, take it as soon as possible. However, if it is almost time for your next dose, skip the missed dose and go back to your regular dosing schedule. Do not double doses.

Storage—Store the medicine in a closed container at room temperature, away from heat, moisture, and direct light. Keep from freezing.

Keep out of the reach of children.

Do not keep outdated medicine or medicine no longer needed.

Precautions While Using This Medicine

It is very important that your doctor check your progress at regular visits. This will allow your doctor to see if the medicine is working properly to lower your cholesterol and triglyceride levels and to decide if you should continue to take it.

Check with your doctor immediately if you think that you may be pregnant. HMG-CoA reductase inhibitors may cause birth defects or other problems in the baby if taken during pregnancy.

Before having any kind of surgery (including dental surgery) or emergency treatment, tell the medical doctor or dentist in charge that you are taking this medicine.

Do not take over-the-counter (OTC) niacin preparations without consulting your doctor. Niacin may increase atorvastatin's adverse effects on muscle, which can lead to serious kidney problems.

Do not use excessive amounts of alcohol while taking atorvastatin because it can worsen the adverse effects of this medicine on the liver.

Check with your doctor immediately if you experience unexplained muscle pain, tenderness, or weakness, especially if it is accompanied by unusual tiredness or fever, because the medicine's adverse effects on muscle can lead to serious kidney problems.

Side Effects of This Medicine

Along with its needed effects, a medicine may cause some unwanted effects. Although not all of these side effects may occur, if they do occur they may need medical attention.

Check with your doctor immediately if any of the following side effects occur:
Less common or rare
Cough; difficulty swallowing; dizziness; fast heartbeat; hives; itching; muscle cramps, pain, stiffness, swelling, or weakness, especially if accompanied by unusual tiredness or fever; persistent elevation of liver function tests; puffiness or swelling of the eyelids or around the eyes, face, lips or tongue; shortness of breath; skin rash; tightness in chest; unusual tiredness or weakness; wheezing

Frequency not determined
Blistering, peeling, loosening of skin; chills; dark-colored urine; diarrhea; fever; itching; joint pain; large, hive-like swelling on face, eyelids, lips, tongue, throat, hands, legs, feet, sex organs; red irritated eyes; redness, tenderness, itching, burning, or peeling of skin; red skin lesions, often with a purple center sore; sore throat; sores, ulcers, or white spots in mouth or on lips

Some side effects may occur that usually do not need medical attention. These side effects may go away during treatment as your body adjusts to the medicine. Also, your health care professional may be able to tell you about ways to prevent or reduce some of these side effects. Check with your health care professional if any of the following side effects continue or are bothersome or if you have any questions about them:
More common
Headache; hoarseness; lower back or side pain; painful or difficult urination; pain or tenderness around eyes and cheekbones; stuffy or runny nose

Less common
Abdominal pain; accidental injury; back pain; belching or excessive gas; constipation; general feeling of discomfort or illness; heartburn, indigestion, or stomach discomfort; lack or loss of strength; loss of appetite; nausea; shivering; sweating; trouble sleeping; vomiting

Frequency not determined
Appetite increased; black tarry stools; blindness; bloody nose; bloody or cloudy urine; bluish color changes in skin; blurred vision; bruising, large, flat, blue patches on the skin; chapped, red, or swollen lips; continuing ringing or buzzing or other unexplained noise in ears; depersonalization; difficult, burning or painful urination; difficulty seeing at night; dysphoria; euphoria; excessive muscle tone or tension; frequent urge to urinate or defecate; fruit-like breath odor; groin or scrotum pain; inability to have or keep an erection; increased body movements; increased sensitivity of eyes to light; increased sensitivity to touch or pain; increased thirst; increased urination; loss of bladder control; loss of sexual ability, drive, or desire; lumps in breasts; mental depression; nervousness; nightmares; normal menstrual bleeding occurring earlier or lasting longer; pale skin; paranoia; pinpoint red spots on skin; slurred speech; swollen or tender lymph glands in neck, armpit or groin; transient, mild, pleasant aromatic odor; unable to move or feel face; unusual bleeding or bruising; weight loss; yellow skin or eyes

Other side effects not listed may also occur in some patients. If you notice any other effects, check with your healthcare professional.

AZACITIDINE (Subcutaneous route) -
ay-za-SYE-ti-deen

Commonly used brand name(s)

In the U.S.—
Vidaza

Available Dosage Forms:
• Powder for Suspension

Therapeutic Class: Antineoplastic Agent

Uses For This Medicine

Azacitidine belongs to the group of medicines known as antimetabolites. It is used to treat some kinds of cancer.

Azacitidine interferes with the growth of cancer cells, which are eventually destroyed. Since the growth of normal body cells may also be affected by azacitidine, other effects will also occur. Some of these may be serious and must be reported to your doctor. Some effects may not occur for months or years after the medicine is used.

This medicine is available only with your doctor's prescription.

Before Using This Medicine

In deciding to use a medicine, the risks of taking the medicine must be weighed against the good it will do. This is a decision you and your doctor will make. For this medicine, the following should be considered:

Allergies—Tell your doctor if you have ever had any unusual or allergic reaction to this medicine or any other medicines. Also tell your health care professional if you have any other types of allergies, such as to foods, dyes, preservatives, or animals. For non-prescription products, read the label or package ingredients carefully.

Pediatric—There is no specific information comparing use of azacitidine in children with use in other age groups.

Geriatric—Azacitidine has been tested in elderly patients and has not been shown to cause different side effects or problems in older people than it does in younger adults. However, older patients are more likely to have age-related kidney problems which may require monitoring

Pregnancy—

	Pregnancy Category	Explanation
All Trimesters	D	Studies in pregnant women have demonstrated a risk to the fetus. However, the benefits of therapy in a life threatening situation or a serious disease, may outweigh the potential risk.

Breast Feeding—There are no adequate studies in women for determining infant risk when using this medication during breastfeeding. Weigh the potential benefits against the potential risks before taking this medication while breastfeeding.

Other medicines—
Using this medicine with any of the following medicines is not recommended. Your doctor may decide not to treat you with this medication or change some of the other medicines you take.

Rotavirus Vaccine, Live

Interactions with Food/Tobacco/Alcohol—Certain medicines should not be used at or around the time of eating food or eating certain types of food since interactions may occur. Using alcohol or tobacco with certain medicines may also cause interactions to occur. Discuss with your healthcare professional the use of your medicine with food, alcohol, or tobacco.

Other medical problems—The presence of other medical problems may affect the use of this medicine. Make sure you tell your doctor if you have any other medical problems, especially:
• Cancerous liver tumors—The risk of side effects that affect the liver may be increased. Azacitidine should not be used in patients with cancerous liver tumors.
• Kidney disease or
• Liver disease—These conditions sometimes increase the effects of medicines by causing them to be removed from the body more slowly.

Proper Use of This Medicine

Azacitidine sometimes causes nausea and vomiting. Tell your doctor if this occurs, especially if you have stomach pain

Dosing—The dose of this medicine will be different for different patients. Follow your doctor's orders or the directions on the label. The following information includes only the average doses of this medicine. If your dose is different, do not change it unless your doctor tells you to do so.

The amount of medicine that you take depends on the strength of the medicine. Also, the number of doses you take each day, the time allowed between doses, and the length of time you take the medicine depend on the medical problem for which you are using the medicine.

Missed dose—Call your doctor or pharmacist for instructions.

Precautions While Using This Medicine

It is very important that your doctor check your progress at regular visits to make sure that this medicine is working properly. Blood tests will be needed to check for unwanted effects.

Side Effects of This Medicine

Along with its needed effects, a medicine may cause some unwanted effects. Although not all of these side effects may occur, if they do occur they may need medical attention.

Also, because of the way these medicines act on the body, there is a chance that they might cause other unwanted effects that may not occur until months or years after the medicine is used. These may include certain types of cancer, such as leukemia or bladder cancer. Discuss these possible effects with your doctor.

Check with your doctor immediately if any of the following side effects occur:

More common

Black, tarry stools; bladder pain; bleeding gums; blood in urine or stools; cloudy urine; body aches or pain; burning or stinging of skin; chest pain; chills; congestion; cough; difficult breathing; difficulty swallowing; dizziness; ear congestion; fast heartbeat; fever; frequent urge to urinate; headache; hives; hoarseness; itching; loss of voice; lower back or side pain; muscle aches; nasal congestion; nausea; pain or tenderness around eyes and cheekbones; painful cold sores or blisters on lips, nose, eyes, or genitals; painful or difficult urination; pain, redness, swelling, tenderness, warmth on skin; pale skin; pinpoint red spots on skin; puffiness or swelling of the eyelids or around the eyes, face, lips or tongue; rapid heartbeat; runny nose; shortness of breath; skin rash; sneezing; sore throat; sores, ulcers, or white spots on lips or in mouth; stuffy nose; swollen glands; tender, swollen glands in neck; tightness in chest; troubled breathing with exertion; unusual bleeding or bruising; unusual tiredness or weakness; voice changes; vomiting; wheezing

Less common

Change in consciousness; convulsions; decreased urine; drowsiness; dry mouth; increased blood creatinine; increased blood pressure; increased thirst; irregular heartbeat; loss of appetite; mood changes; muscle pain or cramps; numbness or tingling in hands, feet, or lips; loss of consciousness

Symptoms of overdose

Get emergency help immediately if any of the following symptoms of overdose occur:

Diarrhea; nausea; vomiting

Some side effects may occur that usually do not need medical attention. These side effects may go away during treatment as your body adjusts to the medicine. Also, your health care professional may be able to tell you about ways to prevent or reduce some of these side effects. Check with your health care professional if any of the following side effects continue or are bothersome or if you have any questions about them:

More common

Acid or sour stomach; appetite decreased; belching; bleeding after defecation; bloody nose; blurred vision; bruise; bumps on skin; burning, crawling, itching, numbness, prickling, "pins and needles'; or tingling feelings; burning while urinating; confusion; diarrhea; difficulty having a bowel movement (stool); difficulty in moving; discouragement; dizziness, faintness, or lightheadedness when getting up from a lying or sitting position suddenly; dry skin; fainting; fear; feeling of discomfort or illness; feeling of sluggishness; feeling sad or empty; feeling unusually cold; flushing; full or bloated feeling or pressure in the stomach; heartburn; heart murmur; indigestion; inflamed tissue from infection at the site of injection; injection site bruising; irritability; itching at injection site; joint pain; lack of appetite; large, flat, blue or purplish patches in the skin; loss of interest or pleasure; mouth hemorrhage; muscle stiffness; nervousness; night sweats; pain in joints; postnasal drip; post procedural hemorrhage; redness of skin; shivering; sleeplessness; small clicking, bubbling, or rattling sounds in the lung when listening with a stethoscope;

small lumps under the skin; small red or purple spots in mouth; soreness or discomfort to touch or pressure on stomach; stomach discomfort upset or pain; sweating; swelling of abdominal or stomach area; swelling of hands, ankles, feet, or lower legs; swelling or inflammation of the mouth; swelling with pits or depressions visible on skin; swollen joints; tongue ulceration; trouble concentrating; trouble sleeping; uncomfortable swelling around anus; unusual drowsiness; unusually warm skin; upper abdominal pain; weight loss

Other side effects not listed may also occur in some patients. If you notice any other effects, check with your healthcare professional.

AZATHIOPRINE (Oral route, Intravenous route) - ay-za-THYE-oh-preen

Black Box Warning

Chronic immunosuppression with this purine antimetabolite increases risk of neoplasia in humans. Physicians using this drug should be very familiar with this risk as well as with the mutagenic potential to both men and women and with possible hematologic toxicities.

Commonly used brand name(s)

In the U.S.—
Azasan
Imuran

Available Dosage Forms:

- Tablet
- Powder for Solution

Therapeutic Class: Antirheumatic, Cytotoxic
Pharmacologic Class: Antimetabolite

Uses For This Medicine

Azathioprine belongs to the group of medicines known as immunosuppressive agents. It is used to reduce the body's natural immunity in patients who receive organ transplants. It is also used to treat rheumatoid arthritis. Azathioprine may also be used for other conditions as determined by your doctor.

Azathioprine is a very strong medicine. You and your doctor should talk about the need for this medicine and its risks. Even though azathioprine may cause side effects that could be very serious, remember that it may be required to treat your medical problem.

Azathioprine is available only with your doctor's prescription.

Once a medicine has been approved for marketing for a certain use, experience may show that it is also useful for other medical problems. Although these uses are not included in product labeling, azathioprine is used in certain patients with the following medical conditions:

- Bowel disease, inflammatory
- Cirrhosis, biliary
- Dermatomyositis, systemic
- Glomerulonephritis
- Hepatitis, chronic active

- Lupus erythematosus, systemic
- Myasthenia gravis
- Myopathy, inflammatory
- Nephrotic syndrome
- Pemphigoid
- Pemphigus

Before Using This Medicine

In deciding to use a medicine, the risks of taking the medicine must be weighed against the good it will do. This is a decision you and your doctor will make. For this medicine, the following should be considered:

Allergies—Tell your doctor if you have ever had any unusual or allergic reaction to this medicine or any other medicines. Also tell your health care professional if you have any other types of allergies, such as to foods, dyes, preservatives, or animals. For non-prescription products, read the label or package ingredients carefully.

Pediatric—This medicine has been tested in children and, in effective doses, has not been shown to cause different side effects or problems than it does in adults.

Geriatric—Many medicines have not been studied specifically in older people. Therefore, it may not be known whether they work exactly the same way they do in younger adults. Although there is no specific information comparing use of azathioprine in the elderly with use in other age groups, this medicine is not expected to cause different side effects or problems in older people than it does in younger adults.

Pregnancy—

	Pregnancy Category	Explanation
All Trimesters	D	Studies in pregnant women have demonstrated a risk to the fetus. However, the benefits of therapy in a life threatening situation or a serious disease, may outweigh the potential risk.

Breast Feeding—There are no adequate studies in women for determining infant risk when using this medication during breastfeeding. Weigh the potential benefits against the potential risks before taking this medication while breastfeeding.

Other medicines—

Using this medicine with any of the following medicines is usually not recommended, but may be required in some cases. If both medicines are prescribed together, your doctor may change the dose or how often you use one or both of the medicines.

Alacepril, Alfalfa, Allopurinol, Bacillus of Calmette and Guerin Vaccine, Live, Benazepril, Black Cohosh, Captopril, Cilazapril, Enalaprilat, Enalapril Maleate, Fosinopril, Lisinopril, Measles Virus Vaccine, Live, Mercaptopurine, Moexipril, Mumps Virus Vaccine, Live, Pentopril, Perindopril, Poliovirus Vaccine, Live, Quinapril, Ramipril, Rotavirus Vaccine, Live, Rubella Virus Vaccine, Live, Smallpox Vaccine, Spirapril, Trandolapril, Typhoid Vaccine, Varicella Virus Vaccine, Yellow Fever Vaccine, Zofenopril

Interactions with Food/Tobacco/Alcohol—Certain medicines should not be used at or around the time of eating food or eating certain types of food since interactions may occur. Using alcohol or tobacco with certain medicines may also cause interactions to occur. Discuss with your healthcare professional the use of your medicine with food, alcohol, or tobacco.

Other medical problems—The presence of other medical problems may affect the use of this medicine. Make sure you tell your doctor if you have any other medical problems, especially:

- Chickenpox (including recent exposure) or
- Herpes zoster (shingles)—Risk of severe disease affecting other parts of the body
- Gout—Allopurinol (used to treat gout) may increase wanted and unwanted effects of azathioprine
- Infection—Azathioprine decreases your body's ability to fight infection
- Kidney disease or
- Liver disease—Effects of azathioprine may be increased because of slower removal from the body
- Pancreatitis (inflammation of the pancreas)—Azathioprine can cause pancreatitis

Proper Use of This Medicine

Use this medicine only as directed by your doctor. Do not use more or less of it, and do not use it more often than your doctor ordered. The exact amount of medicine you need has been carefully worked out. Taking too much may increase the chance of side effects, while taking too little may not properly treat your condition.

This medicine is sometimes given together with certain other medicines. If you are using a combination of medicines, make sure that you take each one at the proper time and do not mix them up. Ask your health care professional to help you plan a way to remember to take your medicines at the right times.

Do not stop taking this medicine without first checking with your doctor.

Azathioprine sometimes causes nausea or vomiting. Taking this medicine after meals or at bedtime may lessen stomach upset. Ask your health care professional for other ways to lessen these effects.

If you vomit shortly after taking a dose of azathioprine, check with your doctor. You will be told whether to take the dose again or to wait until the next scheduled dose.

Dosing—The dose of this medicine will be different for different patients. Follow your doctor's orders or the directions on the label. The following information includes only the average doses of this medicine. If your dose is different, do not change it unless your doctor tells you to do so.

The amount of medicine that you take depends on the strength of the medicine. Also, the number of doses you take each day, the time allowed between doses, and the length of time you take the medicine depend on the medical problem for which you are using the medicine.

- For oral dosage form (tablets):
  - For transplant rejection:
    - Adults, teenagers, and children: Dose is based on body weight or size. The usual beginning dose is 3 to 5 milligrams (mg) per kilogram (kg) (1.5 to 2 mg per pound) of body weight a day. As time

goes on, your doctor may lower your dose to 1 to 3 mg per kg (0.5 to 1.5 mg per pound) of body weight a day.

- For rheumatoid arthritis:
  - Adults, teenagers, and children: Dose is based on body weight or size. The usual beginning dose is 1 mg per kg (0.5 mg per pound) of body weight a day. Your doctor will increase this dose as needed. The highest dose is usually not more than 2.5 mg per kg (1 mg per pound) of body weight a day. Your doctor may then lower your dose as needed.
- For injection dosage form:
  - For transplant rejection:
    - Adults, teenagers, and children: Dose is based on body weight or size. The usual beginning dose is 3 to 5 milligrams (mg) per kilogram (kg) (1.5 to 2 mg per pound) of body weight a day. As time goes on, your doctor may lower your dose to 1 to 3 mg per kg (0.5 to 1.5 mg per pound) of body weight a day.

Missed dose—If you miss a dose of this medicine, skip the missed dose and go back to your regular dosing schedule. Do not double doses.

If you are taking more than one dose a day, take the missed dose as soon as you remember it. If it is time for your next dose, take both doses together, then go back to your regular dosing schedule. If you miss more than one dose, check with your doctor.

Storage—Store the medicine in a closed container at room temperature, away from heat, moisture, and direct light. Keep from freezing.

Keep out of the reach of children.

Do not keep outdated medicine or medicine no longer needed.

Precautions While Using This Medicine

It is very important that your doctor check your progress at regular visits to make sure that this medicine is working properly and to check for unwanted effects.

While you are being treated with azathioprine, and after you stop treatment with it, it is important to see your doctor about the immunizations (vaccinations) you should receive. Do not get any immunizations without your doctor's approval. Azathioprine lowers your body's resistance to infections. For some immunizations, there is a chance you might get the infection the immunization is meant to prevent. For other immunizations, it may be especially important to receive the immunization to prevent a disease. In addition, other persons living in your household should not take oral polio vaccine since there is a chance they could pass the polio virus on to you. Also, avoid persons who have recently taken oral polio vaccine. Do not get close to them, and do not stay in the same room with them for very long. If you cannot take these precautions, you should consider wearing a protective face mask that covers the nose and mouth.

Azathioprine can temporarily lower the number of white blood cells in your blood, increasing the chance of getting an infection. It can also lower the number of platelets, which are necessary for proper blood clotting. If this occurs, there are certain precautions you can take, especially when your blood count is low, to reduce the risk of infection or bleeding:

- If you can, avoid people with infections. Check with your doctor as soon as possible if you think you are getting an infection or if you get a fever or chills, cough or hoarseness, lower back or side pain, or painful or difficult urination.
- Check with your doctor as soon as possible if you notice any unusual bleeding or bruising; black, tarry stools; blood in urine or stools; or pinpoint red spots on your skin.
- Be careful when using a regular toothbrush, dental floss, or toothpick. Your medical doctor, dentist, or nurse may recommend other ways to clean your teeth and gums. Check with your health care professional before having any dental work done.
- Do not touch your eyes or the inside of your nose unless you have just washed your hands and have not touched anything else in the meantime.
- Be careful not to cut yourself when you are using sharp objects such as a safety razor or fingernail or toenail cutters.
- Avoid contact sports or other situations where bruising or injury could occur.

The effects of azathioprine may cause increased infections and delayed healing. Dental work, whenever possible, should be completed prior to beginning this medicine.

Side Effects of This Medicine

Along with its needed effects, a medicine may cause some unwanted effects. Some side effects will have signs or symptoms that you can see or feel. Your doctor will watch for others by doing certain tests.

Also, because of the way this medicine acts on the body, there is a chance that it might cause other unwanted effects that may not occur until months or years after the medicine is used. These delayed effects may include certain types of cancer, such as leukemia, lymphoma, or skin cancer. However, the risk of cancer seems to be lower in people taking azathioprine for arthritis. Discuss these possible effects with your doctor.

Check with your doctor as soon as possible if any of the following side effects occur:

More common
  Cough or hoarseness; fever or chills; lower back or side pain; painful or difficult urination; unusual tiredness or weakness

Less common
  Black, tarry stools; blood in urine or stools; pinpoint red spots on skin; unusual bleeding or bruising

Rare
  Fast heartbeat; fever (sudden); muscle or joint pain; nausea, vomiting, and diarrhea (severe); redness or blisters on skin; shortness of breath; sores in mouth and on lips; stomach pain; swelling of feet or lower legs; unusual feeling of discomfort or illness (sudden)

This medicine may also cause the following side effect that your doctor will watch for:

Less common
  Liver problems

For patients taking this medicine for rheumatoid arthritis:

Signs and symptoms of blood problems (black, tarry stools; blood in urine or stools; cough or hoarseness; fever or chills; lower back or side pain; painful or difficult urination; pinpoint red spots on skin; unusual tiredness or weakness; or unusual bleeding or bruising) are less likely to occur in patients taking azathioprine for rheumatoid arthritis than in patients taking azathioprine for transplant rejection. This is because lower doses are often used.

Some side effects may occur that usually do not need medical attention. These side effects may go away during treatment as your body adjusts to the medicine. Also, your health care professional may be able to tell you about ways to prevent or reduce some of these side effects. Check with your health care professional if any of the following side effects continue or are bothersome or if you have any questions about them:

More common
    Loss of appetite; nausea or vomiting

Less common
    Skin rash

After you stop using this medicine, it may still produce some side effects that need attention. During this period of time, *check with your doctor immediately* if you notice the following side effects:

    Black, tarry stools; blood in urine; cough or hoarseness; fever or chills; lower back or side pain; painful or difficult urination; pinpoint red spots on skin; unusual bleeding or bruising

Other side effects not listed may also occur in some patients. If you notice any other effects, check with your healthcare professional.

AZELAIC ACID (Topical route) - ay-ze-LAY-ik AS-id

Commonly used brand name(s)

In the U.S.—
    Azelex
    Finacea

Available Dosage Forms:
- Cream
- Gel/Jelly

Therapeutic Class: Antiacne Antibacterial

Uses For This Medicine

Azelaic acid is used to treat mild to moderate acne. It works in part by stopping the growth of skin bacteria that can help cause acne. Azelaic acid also helps to lessen acne by keeping skin pores (tiny openings on the skin's surface) clear.

It may also be used to treat other conditions as determined by your doctor.

Azelaic acid is available only with your doctor's prescription.

Once a medicine has been approved for marketing for a certain use, experience may show that it is also useful for other medical problems. Although this use is not included in product labeling, azelaic acid is used in certain patients with the following medical condition:
- Melasma

Before Using This Medicine

In deciding to use a medicine, the risks of taking the medicine must be weighed against the good it will do. This is a decision you and your doctor will make. For this medicine, the following should be considered:

Allergies—Tell your doctor if you have ever had any unusual or allergic reaction to this medicine or any other medicines. Also tell your health care professional if you have any other types of allergies, such as to foods, dyes, preservatives, or animals. For non-prescription products, read the label or package ingredients carefully.

Pediatric—Studies of this medicine have been done only in adult patients, and there is no specific information comparing use of azelaic acid in children with use in other age groups.

Geriatric—Many medicines have not been studied specifically in older people. Therefore, it may not be known whether they work exactly the same way they do in younger adults or if they cause different side effects or problems in older people. There is no specific information comparing use of azelaic acid in the elderly with use in other age groups.

Pregnancy—

	Pregnancy Category	Explanation
All Trimesters	B	Animal studies have revealed no evidence of harm to the fetus, however, there are no adequate studies in pregnant women OR animal studies have shown an adverse effect, but adequate studies in pregnant women have failed to demonstrate a risk to the fetus.

Breast Feeding—There are no adequate studies in women for determining infant risk when using this medication during breastfeeding. Weigh the potential benefits against the potential risks before taking this medication while breastfeeding.

Other medicines—Although certain medicines should not be used together at all, in other cases two different medicines may be used together even if an interaction might occur. In these cases, your doctor may want to change the dose, or other precautions may be necessary. Tell your healthcare professional if you are taking any other prescription or non-prescription (over-the-counter [OTC]) medicine.

Interactions with Food/Tobacco/Alcohol—Certain medicines should not be used at or around the time of eating food or eating certain types of food since interactions may occur. Using alcohol or tobacco with certain medicines may also cause interactions to occur. Discuss with your healthcare professional the use of your medicine with food, alcohol, or tobacco.

Proper Use of This Medicine

When applying the cream, use only a small amount of medicine and apply a thin film to clean, dry skin that is affected by acne. It is important to rub it in gently but well.

After applying azelaic acid cream, wash your hands well to remove any medicine that may remain on them.

Keep this medicine away from the eyes, other mucous membranes, such as the mouth, lips, and inside of the nose, and sensitive areas of the neck. If the medicine accidently gets on these areas, wash with water at once.

To help clear up your acne completely, it is very important that you keep using this medicine for the full time of treatment, even if your symptoms begin to clear up after a short time. If you stop using this medicine too soon, your acne may return or get worse.

Dosing—The dose of this medicine will be different for different patients. Follow your doctor's orders or the directions on the label. The following information includes only the average doses of this medicine. If your dose is different, do not change it unless your doctor tells you to do so.

The amount of medicine that you take depends on the strength of the medicine. Also, the number of doses you take each day, the time allowed between doses, and the length of time you take the medicine depend on the medical problem for which you are using the medicine.

- For topical dosage form (cream):
  - For acne:
    - Adults and teenagers—Apply a small amount two times a day, usually in the morning and the evening, to areas affected by acne. Rub in gently but well. When you are just beginning to use the medicine, your doctor may want you to apply the medicine only one time a day for a few days, to reduce the chance of skin irritation.
    - Children—Use and dose must be determined by your doctor.

Missed dose—If you miss a dose of this medicine, take it as soon as possible. However, if it is almost time for your next dose, skip the missed dose and go back to your regular dosing schedule. Do not double doses.

Storage—Store the medicine in a closed container at room temperature, away from heat, moisture, and direct light. Keep from freezing.

Keep out of the reach of children.

Do not keep outdated medicine or medicine no longer needed.

Precautions While Using This Medicine

If your acne does not improve within 4 weeks, or if it becomes worse, check with your health care professional. However, it may take longer than 4 weeks before you notice full improvement in your acne even if you use the medicine every day.

If this medicine causes too much redness, peeling, or dryness of your skin, check with your doctor. It may be necessary for you to reduce the number of times a day that you use the medicine or to stop using the medicine for a short time until your skin is less irritated.

If your doctor has ordered another medicine to be applied to the skin along with this medicine, it is best to apply them at different times. This may help keep your skin from becoming too irritated. Also, if the medicines are used at or near the same time, they may not work properly.

You may continue to use cosmetics (make-up) while you are using this medicine for acne. However, it is best to use only water-base cosmetics. Also, it is best not to use cosmetics too heavily or too often. They may make your acne worse. If you have any questions about this, check with your doctor.

Side Effects of This Medicine

Along with its needed effects, a medicine may cause some unwanted effects. Although not all of these side effects may occur, if they do occur they may need medical attention.

Check with your doctor as soon as possible if any of the following side effects occur:

Rare

White spots or lightening of treated areas of dark skin—in patients with dark complexions, although usually not lightened beyond normal skin color

Some side effects may occur that usually do not need medical attention. These side effects may go away during treatment as your body adjusts to the medicine. Also, your health care professional may be able to tell you about ways to prevent or reduce some of these side effects. Check with your health care professional if any of the following side effects continue or are bothersome or if you have any questions about them:

More common

Burning, stinging, or tingling of skin, mild; dryness of skin; itching of skin; peeling of skin; redness of skin

Other side effects not listed may also occur in some patients. If you notice any other effects, check with your healthcare professional.

AZELASTINE   (Nasal route) - a-ZEL-as-teen

Commonly used brand name(s)

In the U.S.—
   Astelin
   Astelin Ready-Spray

Available Dosage Forms:
- Spray

Therapeutic Class: Nasal Agent
Pharmacologic Class: Antihistamine

Uses For This Medicine

Azelastine nasal solution is used to help treat the symptoms (runny nose, sneezing, itching) of seasonal (short-term) allergic rhinitis and vasomotor rhinitis.

This medicine works by blocking the effect of histamine on certain cells.

This medicine is available only with your doctor's prescription.

Before Using This Medicine

In deciding to use a medicine, the risks of taking the medicine must be weighed against the good it will do. This is a decision you and your doctor will make. For this medicine, the following should be considered:

Allergies—Tell your doctor if you have ever had any unusual or allergic reaction to this medicine or any other medicines. Also tell your health care professional if you have any other types of allergies, such as to foods, dyes, preservatives, or animals. For non-prescription products, read the label or package ingredients carefully.

Pediatric—This medicine has been tested in children and, in effective doses, has not been shown to cause different side effects or problems in children, older than 5 years of age, than it does in adults.

Geriatric—Many medicines have not been studied specifically in older people. Therefore, it may not be known whether they work exactly the same way they do in younger adults. Although there is no specific information comparing use of nasal azelastine in the elderly with use in other age groups, this medicine has been used in a small number of older patients and is not expected to cause different side effects or problems in older people than it does in younger adults.

Pregnancy—

	Pregnancy Category	Explanation
All Trimesters	C	Animal studies have shown an adverse effect and there are no adequate studies in pregnant women OR no animal studies have been conducted and there are no adequate studies in pregnant women.

Breast Feeding—There are no adequate studies in women for determining infant risk when using this medication during breastfeeding. Weigh the potential benefits against the potential risks before taking this medication while breastfeeding.

Other medicines—

Using this medicine with any of the following medicines may cause an increased risk of certain side effects, but using both drugs may be the best treatment for you. If both medicines are prescribed together, your doctor may change the dose or how often you use one or both of the medicines.

Cimetidine

Interactions with Food/Tobacco/Alcohol—Certain medicines should not be used at or around the time of eating food or eating certain types of food since interactions may occur. Using alcohol or tobacco with certain medicines may also cause interactions to occur. Discuss with your healthcare professional the use of your medicine with food, alcohol, or tobacco.

Other medical problems—The presence of other medical problems may affect the use of this medicine. Make sure you tell your doctor if you have any other medical problems, especially:
- Kidney disease—Blood levels of azelastine may be increased, leading to increased effects

---

Proper Use of This Medicine

This medicine usually comes with patient directions. Read them carefully before using the medicine.

Before using this medicine, clear the nasal passages by blowing your nose.

To prepare this medicine:
- Before you use a new bottle of azelastine spray, the spray pump will need to be primed (started). If your pharmacist assembled the unit for you, check to see if it has already been primed by pumping the unit once. If a full spray comes out, the unit has already been primed; if not you must prime the pump.
- To prime a new bottle, hold the bottle upright and away from you, then pump it four times or until you see a fine spray.
- If you have not used the spray for 3 or more days, pump it two times or until you see a fine spray.

To keep the applicator clean, wipe the nosepiece with a clean tissue and replace the dust cap after each use.

Use this medicine only as directed. Do not use more of it and do not use it more often than your doctor ordered. To do so may increase the chance of side effects.

Dosing—The dose of this medicine will be different for different patients. Follow your doctor's orders or the directions on the label. The following information includes only the average doses of this medicine. If your dose is different, do not change it unless your doctor tells you to do so.

The amount of medicine that you take depends on the strength of the medicine. Also, the number of doses you take each day, the time allowed between doses, and the length of time you take the medicine depend on the medical problem for which you are using the medicine.
- For nasal dosage form (nose spray):
  - For treatment of seasonal allergic rhinitis:
    - Adults and teenagers—Use 1 or 2 sprays in each nostril two times a day.
    - Children 5 to 11 years of age—Use 1 spray in each nostril two times a day.
    - Children younger than 5 years of age—Use and dose must be determined by your doctor.
  - For treatment of vasomotor rhinitis:
    - Adults and teenagers—Use 2 sprays in each nostril two times a day.
    - Children younger than 12 years of age—Use and dose must be determined by your doctor.

Missed dose—If you miss a dose of this medicine, take it as soon as possible. However, if it is almost time for your next dose, skip the missed dose and go back to your regular dosing schedule. Do not double doses.

Storage—Store the medicine in a closed container at room temperature, away from heat, moisture, and direct light. Keep from freezing.

Keep out of the reach of children.

Do not keep outdated medicine or medicine no longer needed.

Store the bottle upright with the pump tightly closed.

Precautions While Using This Medicine

This medicine will add to the effects of alcohol and other CNS depressants (medicines that slow down the nervous system, possibly causing drowsiness). Some examples of CNS depressants are antihistamines or medicine for hay fever, other allergies, or colds; sedatives, tranquilizers, or sleeping medicine; prescription pain medicine or narcotics; medicine for seizures; muscle relaxants; or anesthetics, including some dental anesthetics. Check with your doctor before taking any of the above while you are using this medicine.

This medicine may cause some people to become dizzy, drowsy, or less alert than they are normally. Even if used at bedtime, it may cause some people to feel drowsy or less alert on arising. Make sure you know how you react to this medicine before you drive, use machines, or do anything else that could be dangerous if you are not alert.

Keep the spray away from the eyes because this medicine may cause irritation or blurred vision. Closing your eyes while you are using this medicine may help keep it out of your eyes.

Side Effects of This Medicine

Along with its needed effects, a medicine may cause some unwanted effects. Although not all of these side effects may occur, if they do occur they may need medical attention.

Check with your doctor as soon as possible if any of the following side effects occur:

Rare

Blood in urine; cough; eye pain, eye redness, blurred vision or other change in vision; rapid heartbeat; shortness of breath, tightness in chest, troubled breathing, or wheezing; skin rash, hives, or itching; sores in mouth or on lips

Some side effects may occur that usually do not need medical attention. These side effects may go away during treatment as your body adjusts to the medicine. Also, your health care professional may be able to tell you about ways to prevent or reduce some of these side effects. Check with your health care professional if any of the following side effects continue or are bothersome or if you have any questions about them:

More common

Bitter taste in mouth; drowsiness or sleepiness

Less common

Bloody mucus or unexplained nosebleeds; burning inside the nose; dizziness; dryness of mouth; headache; muscle aches or pain; nausea; sore throat; sudden outbursts of sneezing; unusual tiredness or weakness; weight gain

Other side effects not listed may also occur in some patients. If you notice any other effects, check with your healthcare professional.

AZELASTINE (Ophthalmic route) - a-ZEL-as-teen

Commonly used brand name(s)

In the U.S.—
Optivar

Available Dosage Forms:

• Solution

Therapeutic Class: Ophthalmologic Agent
Pharmacologic Class: Antihistamine

Uses For This Medicine

Azelastine ophthalmic (eye) solution is used to treat itching of the eye caused by a condition known as allergic conjunctivitis. It works by preventing the effects of certain inflammatory substances, which are produced by cells in your eyes and sometimes cause allergic reactions.

This medicine is available only with your doctor's prescription.

Before Using This Medicine

In deciding to use a medicine, the risks of taking the medicine must be weighed against the good it will do. This is a decision you and your doctor will make. For this medicine, the following should be considered:

Allergies—Tell your doctor if you have ever had any unusual or allergic reaction to this medicine or any other medicines. Also tell your health care professional if you have any other types of allergies, such as to foods, dyes, preservatives, or animals. For non-prescription products, read the label or package ingredients carefully.

Pediatric—Studies on this medicine have been done only in adult patients, and there is no specific information comparing use of azelastine in children under the age of 3 years with use in other age groups.

Geriatric—This medicine has been tested and has not been shown to cause different side effects or problems in older people than it does in younger adults.

Pregnancy—

	Pregnancy Category	Explanation
All Trimesters	C	Animal studies have shown an adverse effect and there are no adequate studies in pregnant women OR no animal studies have been conducted and there are no adequate studies in pregnant women.

Breast Feeding—There are no adequate studies in women for determining infant risk when using this medication during breastfeeding. Weigh the potential benefits against the potential risks before taking this medication while breastfeeding.

Other medicines—

Using this medicine with any of the following medicines may cause an increased risk of certain side effects, but using both drugs may be the best treatment for you. If both medicines are prescribed together, your doctor may change the dose or how often you use one or both of the medicines.

Cimetidine

Interactions with Food/Tobacco/Alcohol—Certain medicines should not be used at or around the time of eating food or eating certain types of food since interactions may occur. Using alcohol or tobacco with certain medicines may also cause interactions to occur. Discuss with your healthcare professional the use of your medicine with food, alcohol, or tobacco.

Proper Use of This Medicine

Do not wear contact lenses if your eyes are red. If your eyes are not red, contact lenses should be removed before you use this medicine. Also, you should wait at least 10 minutes after using this medicine before putting the contact lenses back in.

To use:

• The bottle is only partially full to provide proper drop control.
• First, wash your hands. Tilt the head back and, pressing your finger gently on the skin just beneath the lower

eyelid, pull the lower eyelid away from the eye to make a space. Drop the medicine into this space. Let go of the eyelid and gently close the eyes. Do not blink. Keep the eyes closed for 1 to 2 minutes to allow the medicine to be absorbed by the eye.

- If you think you did not get the drop of medicine into your eye properly, use another drop.
- Immediately after using the eye drops, wash your hands to remove any medicine that may be on them.

To keep the medicine as germ-free as possible, do not touch the applicator tip to any surface (including the eye). Also, keep the container tightly closed. Serious damage to the eye and possible loss of vision may result from using contaminated eye drops.

Dosing—The dose of this medicine will be different for different patients. Follow your doctor's orders or the directions on the label. The following information includes only the average doses of this medicine. If your dose is different, do not change it unless your doctor tells you to do so.

The amount of medicine that you take depends on the strength of the medicine. Also, the number of doses you take each day, the time allowed between doses, and the length of time you take the medicine depend on the medical problem for which you are using the medicine.

- For ophthalmic dosage form (eye drops):
  ○ For eye allergy:
    ▪ Adults and children 3 years of age and older— Use one drop in the affected eye twice a day.
    ▪ Children younger than 3 years of age—Use and dose must be determined by your doctor.

Missed dose—If you miss a dose of this medicine, take it as soon as possible. However, if it is almost time for your next dose, skip the missed dose and go back to your regular dosing schedule. Do not double doses.

Storage—Store the medicine in a closed container at room temperature, away from heat, moisture, and direct light. Keep from freezing.

Keep out of the reach of children.

Do not keep outdated medicine or medicine no longer needed.

Ask your healthcare professional how you should dispose of any medicine you do not use.

Keep bottle in an upright position.

Precautions While Using This Medicine

If your symptoms do not improve within a few days or if they become worse, check with your doctor.

Side Effects of This Medicine

Along with its needed effects, a medicine may cause some unwanted effects. Although not all of these side effects may occur, if they do occur they may need medical attention.

Check with your doctor immediately if any of the following side effects occur:

Less common
Cough; difficulty breathing; noisy breathing; shortness of breath; tightness in chest; wheezing

Some side effects may occur that usually do not need medical attention. These side effects may go away during treatment as your body adjusts to the medicine. Also, your health care professional may be able to tell you about ways to prevent or reduce some of these side effects. Check with your health care professional if any of the following side effects continue or are bothersome or if you have any questions about them:

More common
Bitter taste in mouth; headaches; temporary eye burning or stinging

Less common
Burning, dry or itching eyes; blurred vision, temporary; chills; diarrhea; eye discharge or excessive tearing; fever; general feeling of discomfort or illness; hoarseness or other voice changes; itching skin; joint pain; loss of appetite; muscle aches and pains; nausea; redness, pain, swelling of eye, eyelid, or inner lining of eyelid; runny nose; shivering; sneezing; sore throat; stuffy nose; sweating; tender, swollen glands in neck; trouble in swallowing; trouble sleeping; unusual tiredness or weakness; vomiting

Other side effects not listed may also occur in some patients. If you notice any other effects, check with your healthcare professional.

AZITHROMYCIN   (Intravenous route) - az-ith-roe-MYE-sin

Commonly used brand name(s)

In the U.S.—
Zithromax

Available Dosage Forms:
- Powder for Solution

Therapeutic Class: Antibiotic

Uses For This Medicine

Azithromycin is used to treat bacterial infections in many different parts of the body. It is also used to prevent Mycobacterium avium complex (MAC) disease in patients infected with the human immunodeficiency virus (HIV). It works by killing bacteria or preventing their growth. However, this medicine will not work for colds, flu, or other viral infections. Azithromycin may be used for other problems as determined by your doctor.

Azithromycin is available only with your doctor's prescription.

Once a medicine has been approved for marketing for a certain use, experience may show that it is also useful for other medical problems. Although these uses are not included in product labeling, azithromycin is used in certain patients with the following medical condition:

- Trachoma (treatment)

Before Using This Medicine

In deciding to use a medicine, the risks of taking the medicine must be weighed against the good it will do. This is a decision

you and your doctor will make. For this medicine, the following should be considered:

Allergies—Tell your doctor if you have ever had any unusual or allergic reaction to this medicine or any other medicines. Also tell your health care professional if you have any other types of allergies, such as to foods, dyes, preservatives, or animals. For non-prescription products, read the label or package ingredients carefully.

Pediatric—This medicine has been tested in a limited number of children up to the age of 16. In effective doses, the medicine has not been shown to cause different side effects or problems than it does in adults.

Geriatric—This medicine has been tested in a limited number of elderly patients and has not been shown to cause different side effects or problems in older people than it does in younger adults.

Pregnancy—

	Pregnancy Category	Explanation
All Trimesters	B	Animal studies have revealed no evidence of harm to the fetus, however, there are no adequate studies in pregnant women OR animal studies have shown an adverse effect, but adequate studies in pregnant women have failed to demonstrate a risk to the fetus.

Breast Feeding—Studies in women suggest that this medication poses minimal risk to the infant when used during breastfeeding.

Other medicines—

Using this medicine with any of the following medicines is not recommended. Your doctor may decide not to treat you with this medication or change some of the other medicines you take.

Dihydroergotamine, Ergoloid Mesylates, Ergonovine, Ergotamine, Methylergonovine, Methysergide, Pimozide

Interactions with Food/Tobacco/Alcohol—Certain medicines should not be used at or around the time of eating food or eating certain types of food since interactions may occur. Using alcohol or tobacco with certain medicines may also cause interactions to occur. Discuss with your healthcare professional the use of your medicine with food, alcohol, or tobacco.

Other medical problems—The presence of other medical problems may affect the use of this medicine. Make sure you tell your doctor if you have any other medical problems, especially:

- Liver disease—Patients with severe liver disease may have an increased chance of side effects

Proper Use of This Medicine

Azithromycin capsules and pediatric oral suspension should be taken at least 1 hour before or at least 2 hours after meals. Azithromycin tablets and adult single dose oral suspension may be taken with or without food.

To help clear up your infection completely, keep taking azithromycin for the full time of treatment, even if you begin to feel better after a few days. If you stop taking this medicine too soon, your symptoms may return.

Dosing—The dose of this medicine will be different for different patients. Follow your doctor's orders or the directions on the label. The following information includes only the average doses of this medicine. If your dose is different, do not change it unless your doctor tells you to do so.

The amount of medicine that you take depends on the strength of the medicine. Also, the number of doses you take each day, the time allowed between doses, and the length of time you take the medicine depend on the medical problem for which you are using the medicine.

- For the oral suspension dosage form:
  - For chancroid in men and chlamydia infections:
    - Adults and adolescents—1 gram taken once as a single dose.
    - Children 6 months to 12 years of age—Use and dose must be determined by your doctor.
  - For gonococcal infections:
    - Adults and adolescents—2 grams taken once as a single dose.
    - Children 6 months to 12 years of age—Use and dose must be determined by your doctor.
  - For otitis media and pneumonia:
    - Children 6 months to 12 years of age—10 milligrams (mg) per kilogram (kg) (4.5 mg per pound) of body weight once a day on the first day, then 5 mg per kg (2.2 mg per pound) of body weight once a day on days two through five.
  - For strep throat:
    - Adults and adolescents—The oral suspension is usually not used. Refer to azithromycin capsules or tablets.
    - Children 2 to 12 years of age—12 mg per kg (5.4 mg per pound) of body weight once a day for five days.
    - Children up to 2 years of age—Use and dose must be determined by your doctor.

- For the tablet dosage form:
  - For bronchitis, strep throat, pneumonia, and skin infections:
    - Adults and adolescents 16 years of age and older—500 milligrams (mg) on the first day, then 250 mg once a day on days two through five.
    - Children up to 16 years of age—Use and dose must be determined by your doctor.
  - For chlamydia infections:
    - Adults and adolescents 16 years of age and older—1000 mg taken once as a single dose.
    - Children up to 16 years of age—Use and dose must be determined by your doctor.
  - For prevention of Mycobacterium avium complex (MAC) disease:
    - Adults and adolescents 16 years of age and older—1200 mg once a week.
    - Children up to 16 years of age—Use and dose must be determined by your doctor.
  - For sinusitis:
    - Adults and adolescents—500 mg a day for 3 days
    - Children up to 16 years of age—Use and dose must be determined by your doctor.

- For injection dosage form:
  - For pelvic inflammatory disease:
    - Adults and adolescents 16 years of age and older—500 milligrams (mg) once a day for one or two days, injected into a vein.
    - Children up to 16 years of age—Use and dose must be determined by your doctor.
  - For pneumonia:
    - Adults and adolescents 16 years of age and older—500 mg once a day for at least two days, injected into a vein.
    - Children up to 16 years of age—Use and dose must be determined by your doctor.

Missed dose—If you miss a dose of this medicine, take it as soon as possible. However, if it is almost time for your next dose, skip the missed dose and go back to your regular dosing schedule. Do not double doses.

Storage—Store the medicine in a closed container at room temperature, away from heat, moisture, and direct light. Keep from freezing.

Keep out of the reach of children.

Do not keep outdated medicine or medicine no longer needed.

Store the pediatric suspension form in the refrigerator.

Precautions While Using This Medicine

If your symptoms do not improve within a few days, or if they become worse, check with your doctor.

Side Effects of This Medicine

Along with its needed effects, a medicine may cause some unwanted effects. Although not all of these side effects may occur, if they do occur they may need medical attention.

Stop taking this medicine and get emergency help immediately if any of the following effects occur:
  More common (for injection form only)
    Pain, redness, and swelling at site of injection
  Rare
    Abdominal or stomach cramps or pain (severe); abdominal tenderness; diarrhea (watery and severe, which may be bloody); difficulty in breathing; fever; joint pain; skin rash; swelling of face, mouth, neck, hands, and feet

Some side effects may occur that usually do not need medical attention. These side effects may go away during treatment as your body adjusts to the medicine. Also, your health care professional may be able to tell you about ways to prevent or reduce some of these side effects. Check with your health care professional if any of the following side effects continue or are bothersome or if you have any questions about them:
  Less common
    Diarrhea (mild); nausea; stomach pain or discomfort
  Rare
    Dizziness; headache

Other side effects not listed may also occur in some patients. If you notice any other effects, check with your healthcare professional.

AZTREONAM (Intravenous route, Injection route) - AZ-tree-oh-nam

Commonly used brand name(s)

In the U.S.—
    Azactam

Available Dosage Forms:
- Powder for Solution
- Solution

Therapeutic Class: Antibiotic

Uses For This Medicine

Aztreonam is an antibiotic that is used to treat infections caused by bacteria. It works by killing bacteria or preventing their growth.

Aztreonam is used to treat bacterial infections in many different parts of the body. It is sometimes given with other antibiotics. This medicine will not work for colds, flu, or other viral infections.

This medicine is available only with your doctor's prescription.

Before Receiving This Medicine

In deciding to use a medicine, the risks of taking the medicine must be weighed against the good it will do. This is a decision you and your doctor will make. For this medicine, the following should be considered:

Allergies—Tell your doctor if you have ever had any unusual or allergic reaction to this medicine or any other medicines. Also tell your health care professional if you have any other types of allergies, such as to foods, dyes, preservatives, or animals. For non-prescription products, read the label or package ingredients carefully.

Pediatric—Studies have been done in children and have shown that aztreonam is effective in treating certain bacterial infections and that side effects in children are similar to those experienced by adults. Elevations of liver enzymes and reductions in white blood cell counts were seen in children who were given high doses of this medicine or who had more serious infections.

Geriatric—Aztreonam has been tested in a limited number of patients 65 years of age or older and has not been shown to cause different side effects or problems in older people than it does in younger adults.

Pregnancy—

	Pregnancy Category	Explanation
All Trimesters	B	Animal studies have revealed no evidence of harm to the fetus, however, there are no adequate studies in pregnant women OR animal studies have shown an adverse effect, but adequate studies in pregnant women have failed to demonstrate a risk to the fetus.

Breast Feeding—Studies in women suggest that this medication poses minimal risk to the infant when used during breastfeeding.

Other medicines—Although certain medicines should not be used together at all, in other cases two different medicines may be used together even if an interaction might occur. In these cases, your doctor may want to change the dose, or other precautions may be necessary. Tell your healthcare professional if you are taking any other prescription or non-prescription (over-the-counter [OTC]) medicine.

Interactions with Food/Tobacco/Alcohol—Certain medicines should not be used at or around the time of eating food or eating certain types of food since interactions may occur. Using alcohol or tobacco with certain medicines may also cause interactions to occur. Discuss with your healthcare professional the use of your medicine with food, alcohol, or tobacco.

Other medical problems—The presence of other medical problems may affect the use of this medicine. Make sure you tell your doctor if you have any other medical problems, especially:

- Liver disease—Patients receiving high doses of aztreonam for a long time, who also have severe liver disease, may have an increased chance of side effects

- Kidney disease—Patients with kidney disease may have an increased chance of side effects

Proper Use of This Medicine

To help clear up your infection completely, aztreonam must be given for the full time of treatment, even if you begin to feel better after a few days. Also, this medicine works best when there is a constant amount in the blood or urine. To help keep the amount constant, aztreonam must be given on a regular schedule.

Dosing—The dose of this medicine will be different for different patients. Follow your doctor's orders or the directions on the label. The following information includes only the average doses of this medicine. If your dose is different, do not change it unless your doctor tells you to do so.

The amount of medicine that you take depends on the strength of the medicine. Also, the number of doses you take each day, the time allowed between doses, and the length of time you take the medicine depend on the medical problem for which you are using the medicine.

- For injection dosage form:
  ○ Adults and children 16 years of age and older: 1 to 2 grams injected slowly into a vein over a twenty- to sixty-minute period. This is repeated every six to twelve hours.
  ○ Children up to 16 years of age: Dosage is based on body weight and must be determined by your doctor.

Side Effects of This Medicine

Along with its needed effects, a medicine may cause some unwanted effects. Although not all of these side effects may occur, if they do occur they may need medical attention.

Check with your doctor immediately if any of the following side effects occur:

Less common or rare

Black, tarry stools; blood in urine or stools; burning or itching of vagina; chest pain; chills; confusion; convulsions (seizures); cough; dark urine; diarrhea; difficulty in breathing; discharge from vagina; discomfort, inflammation, or swelling at the injection site; dizziness; eye pain; fever; flu-like symptoms; general feeling of illness; headache; hives; light gray-colored stools; loss of appetite; numbness of tongue; pinpoint red spots on skin; seeing double; skin rash, redness, or itching; sore throat; unusual bleeding or bruising; unusual tiredness or weakness; yellow skin or eyes

Some side effects may occur that usually do not need medical attention. These side effects may go away during treatment as your body adjusts to the medicine. Also, your health care professional may be able to tell you about ways to prevent or reduce some of these side effects. Check with your health care professional if any of the following side effects continue or are bothersome or if you have any questions about them:

Less common or rare

Abdominal or stomach cramps; altered sense of taste; bad breath; breast tenderness; burning or prickling feeling of skin; flushing; increased sweating; mouth ulcers; muscular aches; nasal congestion; nausea or vomiting; ringing, buzzing, or noise in ear; small, non-raised, round, purplish or red spots on skin; sneezing; trouble in sleeping

Other side effects not listed may also occur in some patients. If you notice any other effects, check with your healthcare professional.

BACLOFEN (Intrathecal route) - BAK-loe-fen

Black Box Warning

Abrupt discontinuation of intrathecal baclofen, regardless of the cause, has resulted in sequelae that include high fever, altered mental status, exaggerated rebound spasticity, and muscle rigidity, that in rare cases has advanced to rhabdomyolysis, multiple organ-system failure and death.

Prevention of abrupt discontinuation of intrathecal baclofen requires careful attention to programming and monitoring of the infusion system, refill scheduling and procedures, and pump alarms. Patients and caregivers should be advised of the importance of keeping scheduled refill visits and should be educated on the early symptoms of baclofen withdrawal. Special attention should be given to patients at apparent risk (eg, spinal cord injuries at T-6 or above, communication difficulties, history of withdrawal symptoms from oral or intrathecal baclofen). Consult the technical manual of the implantable infusion system for additional postimplant clinician and patient information.

Commonly used brand name(s)

In the U.S.—
Lioresal

Available Dosage Forms:
- Solution
- Kit

Therapeutic Class: Skeletal Muscle Relaxant, Centrally Acting

Uses For This Medicine

Intrathecal baclofen is used to help relax certain muscles in your body. It relieves the spasms, cramping, and tightness of muscles caused by medical problems such as multiple sclerosis, cerebral palsy, or certain injuries to the spine. Intrathecal baclofen does not cure these problems, but it may allow other treatment, such as physical therapy, to be more helpful in improving your condition.

Intrathecal baclofen acts on the central nervous system (CNS) to produce its muscle relaxant effects. Its actions on the CNS may also cause some of the medicine's side effects.

This medicine is delivered by a drug pump directly into the spinal fluid of your back. A doctor will surgically place the pump and monitor the dose of the medication that is delivered by the pump. The dose of intrathecal baclofen will be different for different patients and will depend on the type of muscle tightness that you have.

Intrathecal baclofen is given only by or under the direct supervision of a doctor.

Before Using This Medicine

In deciding to use a medicine, the risks of taking the medicine must be weighed against the good it will do. This is a decision you and your doctor will make. For this medicine, the following should be considered:

Allergies—Tell your doctor if you have ever had any unusual or allergic reaction to this medicine or any other medicines. Also tell your health care professional if you have any other types of allergies, such as to foods, dyes, preservatives, or animals. For non-prescription products, read the label or package ingredients carefully.

Pediatric—This medicine has been tested in children 4 years of age and older. Effective doses have not been shown to cause different side effects or problems in children than it does in adults. However, this medicine may not be safe for children younger than 4 years of age.

Geriatric—Side effects such as hallucinations, confusion or mental depression, other mood or mental changes, and severe drowsiness may be especially likely to occur in elderly patients, who may be more sensitive than younger adults to the effects of intrathecal baclofen.

Pregnancy—

	Pregnancy Category	Explanation
All Trimesters	C	Animal studies have shown an adverse effect and there are no adequate studies in pregnant women OR no animal studies have been conducted and there are no adequate studies in pregnant women.

Breast Feeding—There are no adequate studies in women for determining infant risk when using this medication during breastfeeding. Weigh the potential benefits against the potential risks before taking this medication while breastfeeding.

Other medicines—Although certain medicines should not be used together at all, in other cases two different medicines may be used together even if an interaction might occur. In these cases, your doctor may want to change the dose, or other precautions may be necessary. Tell your healthcare professional if you are taking any other prescription or non-prescription (over-the-counter [OTC]) medicine.

Interactions with Food/Tobacco/Alcohol—Certain medicines should not be used at or around the time of eating food or eating certain types of food since interactions may occur. Using alcohol or tobacco with certain medicines may also cause interactions to occur. Discuss with your healthcare professional the use of your medicine with food, alcohol, or tobacco.

Other medical problems—The presence of other medical problems may affect the use of this medicine. Make sure you tell your doctor if you have any other medical problems, especially:

- Breathing difficulties or
- Stroke or other brain disease—Baclofen may make these conditions worse
- Communication difficulties or
- Spinal cord injuries, at or above T−6 or
- Withdrawal symptoms, history of—These conditions may increase your risk for side effects of baclofen
- Epilepsy or
- Kidney disease or
- Mental or emotional problems or
- Spinal lesions—The chance of side effects may be increased
- Parkinson's disease—Baclofen may make this condition worse

Proper Use of This Medicine

Dosing—The dose of this medicine will be different for different patients. Follow your doctor's orders or the directions on the label. The following information includes only the average doses of this medicine. If your dose is different, do not change it unless your doctor tells you to do so.

The amount of medicine that you take depends on the strength of the medicine. Also, the number of doses you take each day, the time allowed between doses, and the length of time you take the medicine depend on the medical problem for which you are using the medicine.

Precautions While Using This Medicine

Your doctor should check your progress at regular visits, especially during the first few weeks of treatment with this medicine. During this time, the amount of medicine you are using may have to be changed often to meet your individual needs.

Make sure to keep all appointments to refill the pump. If the pump is not refilled on time, you may experience return of your muscle tightness and early withdrawal symptoms which might include:

- itching of the skin
- decreased blood pressure
  - blurred vision
  - confusion
  - dizziness, faintness, or lightheadedness when getting up from a lying or sitting position suddenly
  - sweating
  - unusual tiredness or weakness

- burning, crawling, itching, numbness, prickling, "pins and needles", or tingling feelings
- seizures

Intrathecal baclofen will add to the effects of alcohol and other CNS depressants (medicines that may make you drowsy or less alert). Some examples of CNS depressants are antihistamines or medicine for hay fever, other allergies, or colds; sedatives, tranquilizers, or sleeping medicine; prescription pain medicine or narcotics; barbiturates; medicine for seizures; other muscle relaxants; and anesthetics, including some dental anesthetics. Check with your doctor before taking any of the above while you are using intrathecal baclofen.

Intrathecal baclofen may cause dizziness, drowsiness, false sense of well-being, lightheadedness, vision problems, or clumsiness or unsteadiness in some people. Make sure you know how you react to this medicine before you drive, use machines, or do anything else that could be dangerous if you are not alert, well-coordinated, and able to see well.

Intrathecal baclofen may cause dryness of the mouth. For temporary relief, use sugarless candy or gum, melt bits of ice in your mouth, or use a saliva substitute. However, if dry mouth continues for more than 2 weeks, check with your medical doctor or dentist. Continuing dryness of the mouth may increase the chance of dental disease, including tooth decay, gum disease, and fungus infections.

Dizziness, lightheadedness, or fainting may occur when you get up suddenly from a lying or sitting position. Getting up slowly may help lessen this problem.

Side Effects of This Medicine

Along with its needed effects, a medicine may cause some unwanted effects. Although not all of these side effects may occur, if they do occur they may need medical attention.

Check with your doctor as soon as possible if any of the following side effects occur:

More common
Convulsions (seizures)

Less common or rare
Blurred vision or double vision; fainting; mental depression; muscle weakness; ringing or buzzing in ears; seeing, hearing, or feeling things that are not there; shortness of breath or troubled breathing

Symptoms of overdose
Convulsions (seizures); dizziness, drowsiness, or lightheadedness; increased watering of the mouth; mental confusion; muscle weakness; nausea and/or vomiting; shortness of breath or troubled breathing

Some side effects may occur that usually do not need medical attention. These side effects may go away during treatment as your body adjusts to the medicine. Also, your health care professional may be able to tell you about ways to prevent or reduce some of these side effects. Check with your health care professional if any of the following side effects continue or are bothersome or if you have any questions about them:

More common
Constipation; difficult urination; dizziness; headache; nausea and/or vomiting; numbness or tingling in hands or feet; sleepiness

Less common
Clumsiness, unsteadiness, trembling, or other problems with muscle control; diarrhea; difficulty sleeping;

dizziness or lightheadedness, especially when getting up from a lying or sitting position; dry mouth; frequent urge to urinate; irritation of the skin at the site where the pump is located; itching of the skin; sexual problems; slurred speech or other speech problems; swelling of ankles, feet, or lower legs; trembling or shaking

After you stop using this medicine, it may still produce some side effects that need attention. During this period of time, *check with your doctor immediately* if you notice the following side effects:

Convulsions (seizures); facial flushing, headache, increased sweating, or slow heartbeat; increased muscle spasms; seeing, hearing, or feeling things that are not there

Other side effects not listed may also occur in some patients. If you notice any other effects, check with your healthcare professional.

BACLOFEN (Oral route) - BAK-loe-fen

Commonly used brand name(s)

In Canada—
Lioresal
Lioresal Double Strength

Available Dosage Forms:
- Tablet

Therapeutic Class: Skeletal Muscle Relaxant, Centrally Acting

Uses For This Medicine

Baclofen is used to help relax certain muscles in your body. It relieves the spasms, cramping, and tightness of muscles caused by medical problems such as multiple sclerosis or certain injuries to the spine. Baclofen does not cure these problems, but it may allow other treatment, such as physical therapy, to be more helpful in improving your condition.

Baclofen acts on the central nervous system (CNS) to produce its muscle relaxant effects. Its actions on the CNS may also cause some of the medicine's side effects. Baclofen may also be used to relieve other conditions as determined by your doctor.

This medicine is available only with your doctor's prescription.

Once a medicine has been approved for marketing for a certain use, experience may show that it is also useful for other medical problems. Although this use is not included in product labeling, baclofen is used in certain patients with trigeminal neuralgia (severe burning or stabbing pain along the nerves in the face); also called "tic douloureux."

Before Using This Medicine

In deciding to use a medicine, the risks of taking the medicine must be weighed against the good it will do. This is a decision you and your doctor will make. For this medicine, the following should be considered:

Allergies—Tell your doctor if you have ever had any unusual or allergic reaction to this medicine or any other medicines. Also tell your health care professional if you have any

other types of allergies, such as to foods, dyes, preservatives, or animals. For non-prescription products, read the label or package ingredients carefully.

Pediatric—Studies on this medicine have been done only in adult patients, and there is no specific information comparing use of baclofen in children with use in other age groups.

Geriatric—Side effects such as hallucinations, confusion or mental depression, other mood or mental changes, and severe drowsiness may be especially likely to occur in elderly patients, who are usually more sensitive than younger adults to the effects of baclofen.

Pregnancy—

	Pregnancy Category	Explanation
All Trimesters	C	Animal studies have shown an adverse effect and there are no adequate studies in pregnant women OR no animal studies have been conducted and there are no adequate studies in pregnant women.

Breast Feeding—There are no adequate studies in women for determining infant risk when using this medication during breastfeeding. Weigh the potential benefits against the potential risks before taking this medication while breastfeeding.

Other medicines—Although certain medicines should not be used together at all, in other cases two different medicines may be used together even if an interaction might occur. In these cases, your doctor may want to change the dose, or other precautions may be necessary. Tell your healthcare professional if you are taking any other prescription or nonprescription (over-the-counter [OTC]) medicine.

Interactions with Food/Tobacco/Alcohol—Certain medicines should not be used at or around the time of eating food or eating certain types of food since interactions may occur. Using alcohol or tobacco with certain medicines may also cause interactions to occur. Discuss with your healthcare professional the use of your medicine with food, alcohol, or tobacco.

Other medical problems—The presence of other medical problems may affect the use of this medicine. Make sure you tell your doctor if you have any other medical problems, especially:
- Type 2 diabetes mellitus—Baclofen may raise blood sugar levels
- Epilepsy or
- Kidney disease or
- Mental or emotional problems or
- Stroke or other brain disease—The chance of side effects may be increased

Proper Use of This Medicine

Dosing—The dose of this medicine will be different for different patients. Follow your doctor's orders or the directions on the label. The following information includes only the average doses of this medicine. If your dose is different, do not change it unless your doctor tells you to do so.

The amount of medicine that you take depends on the strength of the medicine. Also, the number of doses you take

each day, the time allowed between doses, and the length of time you take the medicine depend on the medical problem for which you are using the medicine.
- For oral dosage form (tablets):
  - For muscle relaxation:
    - Adults and teenagers—At first, the dose is 5 milligrams (mg) three times a day. Then, each dose may be increased by 5 mg every three days until the desired response is reached. No more than 80 mg should be taken within a twenty-four-hour period.
    - Children—Use and dose must be determined by your doctor.

Missed dose—If you miss a dose of this medicine, take it as soon as possible. However, if it is almost time for your next dose, skip the missed dose and go back to your regular dosing schedule. Do not double doses.

Storage—Store the medicine in a closed container at room temperature, away from heat, moisture, and direct light. Keep from freezing.

Keep out of the reach of children.

Do not keep outdated medicine or medicine no longer needed.

Precautions While Using This Medicine

Do not suddenly stop taking this medicine. Unwanted effects may occur if the medicine is stopped suddenly. Check with your doctor for the best way to reduce gradually the amount you are taking before stopping completely.

This medicine will add to the effects of alcohol and other CNS depressants (medicines that slow down the nervous system, possibly causing drowsiness). Some examples of CNS depressants are antihistamines or medicine for hay fever, other allergies, or colds; sedatives, tranquilizers, or sleeping medicine; prescription pain medicine or narcotics; barbiturates; medicine for seizures; other muscle relaxants; or anesthetics, including some dental anesthetics. Check with your doctor before taking any of the above while you are using baclofen.

This medicine may cause drowsiness, dizziness, vision problems, or clumsiness or unsteadiness in some people. Make sure you know how you react to this medicine before you drive, use machines, or do anything else that could be dangerous if you are not alert, well-coordinated, and able to see well.

For diabetic patients:
- This medicine may cause your blood sugar levels to rise. If you notice a change in the results of your blood or urine sugar test or if you have any questions about this, check with your doctor.

Side Effects of This Medicine

Along with its needed effects, a medicine may cause some unwanted effects. Although not all of these side effects may occur, if they do occur they may need medical attention.

Check with your doctor as soon as possible if any of the following side effects occur:
Less common or rare
Bloody or dark urine; chest pain; fainting; hallucinations (seeing or hearing things that are not there); mental depression or other mood changes; ringing or buzzing in the ears; skin rash or itching

Symptoms of overdose

Blurred or double vision; convulsions (seizures); muscle weakness (severe); shortness of breath or unusually slow or troubled breathing; vomiting

Some side effects may occur that usually do not need medical attention. These side effects may go away during treatment as your body adjusts to the medicine. Also, your health care professional may be able to tell you about ways to prevent or reduce some of these side effects. Check with your health care professional if any of the following side effects continue or are bothersome or if you have any questions about them:

More common

Confusion; dizziness or lightheadedness; drowsiness; nausea; unusual weakness, especially muscle weakness

Less common or rare

Abdominal or stomach pain or discomfort; clumsiness, unsteadiness, trembling, or other problems with muscle control; constipation; diarrhea; difficult or painful urination or decrease in amount of urine; false sense of well-being; frequent urge to urinate or uncontrolled urination; headache; loss of appetite; low blood pressure; muscle or joint pain; numbness or tingling in hands or feet; pounding heartbeat; sexual problems in males; slurred speech or other speech problems; stuffy nose; swelling of ankles; trouble in sleeping; unexplained muscle stiffness; unusual excitement; unusual tiredness; weight gain

After you stop using this medicine, it may still produce some side effects that need attention. During this period of time, *check with your doctor immediately* if you notice the following side effects:

Convulsions (seizures); hallucinations (seeing or hearing things that are not there); increase in muscle spasm, cramping, or tightness; mood or mental changes; unusual nervousness or restlessness

Other side effects not listed may also occur in some patients. If you notice any other effects, check with your healthcare professional.

BALSALAZIDE   (Oral route) - bal-SAL-a-zide

Commonly used brand name(s)

In the U.S.—

Colazal

Available Dosage Forms:

• Capsule

Therapeutic Class: Gastrointestinal Agent

Uses For This Medicine

Balsalazide helps to decrease inflammation in the colon by blocking the production of certain chemicals that cause the bowel to become overactive.

This medicine is available only with your doctor's prescription.

Before Using This Medicine

In deciding to use a medicine, the risks of taking the medicine must be weighed against the good it will do. This is a decision you and your doctor will make. For this medicine, the following should be considered:

Allergies—Tell your doctor if you have ever had any unusual or allergic reaction to this medicine or any other medicines. Also tell your health care professional if you have any other types of allergies, such as to foods, dyes, preservatives, or animals. For non-prescription products, read the label or package ingredients carefully.

Pediatric—Studies on this medicine have been done only in adult patients, and there is no specific information comparing the use of balsalazide in children with use in other age groups.

Geriatric—Many medicines have not been studied specifically in older people. Therefore, it may not be known whether they work exactly the same way they do in younger adults or if they cause different side effects or problems in older people. There is no specific information comparing the use of balsalazide in the elderly with use in other age groups.

Pregnancy—

	Pregnancy Category	Explanation
All Trimesters	B	Animal studies have revealed no evidence of harm to the fetus, however, there are no adequate studies in pregnant women OR animal studies have shown an adverse effect, but adequate studies in pregnant women have failed to demonstrate a risk to the fetus.

Breast Feeding—Studies in women breastfeeding have demonstrated harmful infant effects. An alternative to this medication should be prescribed or you should stop breastfeeding while using this medicine.

Other medicines—

Using this medicine with any of the following medicines may cause an increased risk of certain side effects, but using both drugs may be the best treatment for you. If both medicines are prescribed together, your doctor may change the dose or how often you use one or both of the medicines.

Tamarind

Interactions with Food/Tobacco/Alcohol—Certain medicines should not be used at or around the time of eating food or eating certain types of food since interactions may occur. Using alcohol or tobacco with certain medicines may also cause interactions to occur. Discuss with your healthcare professional the use of your medicine with food, alcohol, or tobacco.

Other medical problems—The presence of other medical problems may affect the use of this medicine. Make sure you tell your doctor if you have any other medical problems, especially:

• Pyloric stenosis—Balsalazide capsules may take longer to reach the colon.

• Kidney problems—Balsalazide should be used with caution.

Proper Use of This Medicine

Dosing—The dose of this medicine will be different for different patients. Follow your doctor's orders or the directions on the label. The following information includes only the average doses of this medicine. If your dose is different, do not change it unless your doctor tells you to do so.

The amount of medicine that you take depends on the strength of the medicine. Also, the number of doses you take each day, the time allowed between doses, and the length of time you take the medicine depend on the medical problem for which you are using the medicine.

- For oral dosage form (capsules):
  ○ For treatment of ulcerative colitis
    ▪ Adults—Three 750–milligram (mg) balsalazide capsules three times a day for a total daily dose of 6.75 grams for eight weeks. You may need to take the medicine for up to twelve weeks as ordered by your doctor.
    ▪ Children—Use and dosage must be determined by your doctor.

Missed dose—If you miss a dose of this medicine, take it as soon as possible. However, if it is almost time for your next dose, skip the missed dose and go back to your regular dosing schedule. Do not double doses.

Storage—Store the medicine in a closed container at room temperature, away from heat, moisture, and direct light. Keep from freezing.

Keep out of the reach of children.

Do not keep outdated medicine or medicine no longer needed.

Ask your healthcare professional how you should dispose of any medicine you do not use.

Precautions While Using This Medicine

It is important that your doctor check your progress at regular visits. This will allow your doctor to check for any unwanted effects.

If your symptoms become worse, check with your doctor.

Side Effects of This Medicine

Some side effects may occur that usually do not need medical attention. These side effects may go away during treatment as your body adjusts to the medicine. Also, your health care professional may be able to tell you about ways to prevent or reduce some of these side effects. Check with your health care professional if any of the following side effects continue or are bothersome or if you have any questions about them:

More common
Diarrhea; stomach pain

Less common
Blood in urine; constipation; coughing; cramps; dry mouth; fever; flu-like symptoms; passing of gas; heart burn or upset stomach; joint pain; loss of appetite; lower back pain; muscle pain; pain or burning while urinating; stuffy nose; trouble sleeping or getting to sleep; unusual tiredness or weakness; yellowish skin

Other side effects not listed may also occur in some patients. If you notice any other effects, check with your healthcare professional.

BARBITURATES   (Systemic)

Some commonly used brand names are:

In the U.S.—

Alurate (2)	Mebaral (4)
Amytal (1)	Nembutal (6)
Barbita (7)	Sarisol No. 2 (3)
Busodium (3)	Seconal (8)
Butalan (3)	Solfoton (7)
Butisol (3)	Tuinal (9)
Luminal (7)	

In Canada—

Amytal (1)	Nova Rectal (6)
Ancalixir (7)	Novopentobarb (6)
Butisol (3)	Novosecobarb (8)
Mebaral (4)	Seconal (8)
Nembutal (6)	Tuinal (9)

This information applies to the following medicines:

1. Amobarbital (am-oh-BAR-bi-tal)
2. Aprobarbital (a-proe-BAR-bi-tal)
3. Butabarbital (byoo-ta-BAR-bi-tal)
4. Mephobarbital (me-foe-BAR-bi-tal)
5. Metharbital (meth-AR-bi-tal)
6. Pentobarbital (pen-toe-BAR-bi-tal)
7. Phenobarbital (fee-noe-BAR-bi-tal)
8. Secobarbital (see-koe-BAR-bi-tal)
9. Secobarbital and Amobarbital (see-koe-BAR-bi-tal and am-oh-BAR-bi-tal)

Category

- **Anticonvulsant**—Amobarbital (parenteral only); Mephobarbital; Metharbital; Pentobarbital (parenteral only); Phenobarbital; Secobarbital (parenteral only)
- **Antihyperbilirubinemic**—Phenobarbital
- **Sedative-hypnotic**—Amobarbital; Aprobarbital; Butabarbital; Pentobarbital; Phenobarbital (parenteral only); Secobarbital

Description

Barbiturates (bar-BI-tyoo-rates) belong to the group of medicines called central nervous system (CNS) depressants (medicines that cause drowsiness). They act on the brain and CNS to produce effects that may be helpful or harmful. This depends on the individual patient's condition and response and the amount of medicine taken.

Some of the barbiturates may be used before surgery to relieve anxiety or tension. In addition, some of the barbiturates are used as anticonvulsants to help control seizures in certain disorders or diseases, such as epilepsy. Barbiturates may also be used for other conditions as determined by your doctor.

The barbiturates have been used to treat insomnia (trouble in sleeping); but if they are used regularly (for example, every day) for insomnia, they are usually not effective for longer than 2 weeks. The barbiturates have also been used to re-

page _224_ _Barbiturates_ _(Systemic)_

lieve nervousness or restlessness during the daytime. However, the barbiturates have generally been replaced by safer medicines for the treatment of insomnia and daytime nervousness or tension.

If too much of a barbiturate is used, it may become habit-forming.

Barbiturates should not be used for anxiety or tension caused by the stress of everyday life.

These medicines are available only with your doctor's prescription, in the following dosage forms:

Oral
- Amobarbital
  - Capsules
  - Tablets
- Aprobarbital
  - Elixir
- Butabarbital
  - Capsules
  - Elixir
  - Tablets
- Mephobarbital
  - Tablets
- Metharbital
  - Tablets (Other countries)
- Pentobarbital
  - Capsules
  - Elixir
- Phenobarbital
  - Capsules
  - Elixir
  - Tablets
- Secobarbital
  - Capsules
- Secobarbital and Amobarbital
  - Capsules

Parenteral
- Amobarbital
  - Injection
- Pentobarbital
  - Injection
- Phenobarbital
  - Injection
- Secobarbital
  - Injection

Rectal
- Pentobarbital
  - Suppositories

Before Using This Medicine

In deciding to use a medicine, the risks of taking the medicine must be weighed against the good it will do. This is a decision you and your doctor will make. For barbiturates, the following should be considered:

Allergies—Tell your doctor if you have ever had any unusual or allergic reaction to barbiturates. Also tell your health care professional if you are allergic to any other substances, such as foods, preservatives, or dyes.

Pregnancy—Barbiturates have been shown to increase the chance of birth defects in humans. However, this medicine may be needed in serious diseases or other situations that threaten the mother's life. Be sure you have discussed this and the following information with your doctor:
- Taking barbiturates regularly during pregnancy may cause bleeding problems in the newborn infant. In addition, taking barbiturates regularly during the last 3 months of pregnancy may cause the baby to become dependent on the medicine. This may lead to withdrawal side effects in the baby after birth.
- One study in humans has suggested that barbiturates taken during pregnancy may increase the chance of brain tumors in the baby.
- Barbiturates taken for anesthesia during labor and delivery may reduce the force and frequency of contractions of the uterus; this may prolong labor and delay delivery.
- Use of barbiturates during labor may cause breathing problems in the newborn infant.

Breast-feeding—Barbiturates pass into the breast milk and may cause drowsiness, slow heartbeat, shortness of breath, or troubled breathing in babies of nursing mothers taking this medicine.

Children—Unusual excitement may be more likely to occur in children, who are usually more sensitive than adults to the effects of barbiturates.

Older adults—Confusion, mental depression, and unusual excitement may be more likely to occur in the elderly, who are usually more sensitive than younger adults to the effects of barbiturates.

Other medicines—Although certain medicines should not be used together at all, in other cases 2 different medicines may be used together even if an interaction might occur. In these cases, your doctor may want to change the dose, or other precautions may be necessary. When you are taking a barbiturate, it is especially important that your health care professional know if you are taking any of the following:
- Adrenocorticoids (cortisone-like medicine) or
- Anticoagulants (blood thinners) or
- Carbamazepine or
- Corticotropin (ACTH)—Barbiturates may decrease the effects of these medicines
- Central nervous system (CNS) depressants (medicines that cause drowsiness)—Using these medicines with barbiturates may result in increased CNS depressant effects
- Divalproex sodium or
- Valproic acid—Using these medicines with barbiturates may change the amount of either medicine that you need to take
- Oral contraceptives (birth control pills) containing estrogens—Barbiturates may decrease the effectiveness of these oral contraceptives, and you may need to change to a different type of birth control

Other medical problems—The presence of other medical problems may affect the use of barbiturates. Make sure you tell your doctor if you have any other medical problems, especially:
- Alcohol abuse (or history of) or
- Drug abuse or dependence (or history of)—Dependence on barbiturates may develop

© 2007 Thomson Micromedex All rights reserved.

- Anemia (severe) or
- Asthma (history of), emphysema, or other chronic lung disease or
- Diabetes mellitus (sugar diabetes) or
- Hyperactivity (in children) or
- Mental depression or
- Overactive thyroid or
- Porphyria (or history of)—Barbiturates may make the condition worse
- Kidney disease or
- Liver disease—Higher blood levels of barbiturates may result, increasing the chance of side effects
- Pain—Barbiturates may cause unexpected excitement or mask important symptoms of more serious problems
- Underactive adrenal gland—Barbiturates may interfere with the effects of other medicines needed for this condition

Proper Use of This Medicine

For patients taking the *extended-release capsule or tablet form* of this medicine:

- These capsules or tablets are to be swallowed whole. Do not break, crush, or chew before swallowing.

For patients using the *rectal suppository form* of this medicine:

- To insert the suppository: First remove the foil wrapper and moisten the suppository with cold water. Lie down on your side and use your finger to push the suppository well up into the rectum.
- Wash your hands with soap and water.

Use this medicine only as directed by your doctor. Do not use more of it, do not use it more often, and do not use it for a longer time than your doctor ordered. If too much is used, it may become habit-forming (causing mental or physical dependence).

If you think this medicine is not working properly after you have taken it for a few weeks, *do not increase the dose*. To do so may increase the chance of your becoming dependent on the medicine. Instead, check with your doctor.

If you are taking this medicine for epilepsy, it must be taken every day in regularly spaced doses as ordered by your doctor in order for it to control your seizures. This is necessary to keep a constant amount of medicine in the blood. To help keep the amount constant, do not miss any doses.

Dosing—The dose of barbiturates will be different for different patients. *Follow your doctor's orders or the directions on the label.* The following information includes only the average doses of barbiturates. *If your dose is different, do not change it* unless your doctor tells you to do so.

The number of capsules, tablets, or teaspoonfuls of elixir that you take, the number of suppositories you use, or the number of injections you receive depends on the strength of the medicine. Also, *the number of doses you take each day, the time allowed between doses, and the length of time you*

take the medicine depend on the medical problem for which you are taking barbiturates.

For amobarbital
- For *oral* dosage form (tablets or capsules):
  - For trouble in sleeping:
    - Adults—65 to 200 milligrams (mg) at bedtime.
    - Children—Dose must be determined by your doctor.
  - For daytime sedation:
    - Adults—50 to 300 mg, taken in smaller doses during the day.
    - Children—Dose is based on body weight or size and must be determined by your doctor. The usual dose is 2 mg per kilogram (kg) (0.9 mg per pound) of body weight taken three times a day.
  - For sedation before surgery:
    - Adults—200 mg taken one to two hours before surgery.
    - Children—Dose is based on body weight and must be determined by your doctor. The usual dose is 2 to 6 mg per kg (0.9 to 2.7 mg per pound) of body weight, taken before surgery. However, the dose is usually not more than 100 mg.
  - For sedation during labor:
    - Adults—200 to 400 mg every one to three hours if needed. However, the total dose is usually not more than 1000 mg.
- For *injection* dosage form:
  - For trouble in sleeping:
    - Adults—65 to 200 mg, injected into a muscle or vein.
    - Children up to 6 years of age—Dose is based on body weight and must be determined by your doctor. The usual dose is 2 to 3 mg per kg (0.9 to 1.4 mg per pound) of body weight, injected into a muscle.
    - Children 6 years of age and over—Dose is based on body weight and must be determined by your doctor. The usual dose is 2 to 3 mg per kg (0.9 to 1.4 mg per pound) of body weight, injected into a muscle, or 65 to 500 mg injected into a vein.
  - For daytime sedation:
    - Adults—30 to 50 mg two or three times a day, injected into a muscle or vein.
  - For sedation before surgery:
    - Children—Dose is based on body weight and must be determined by your doctor. The usual dose is 3 to 5 mg per kg (1.4 to 2.3 mg per pound) of body weight or 65 to 500 mg per dose, injected into a vein.
  - For control of seizures:
    - Adults and children 6 years of age and over—65 to 500 mg per dose, injected into a vein.
    - Children up to 6 years of age—Dose is based on body weight or size and must be determined by your doctor. The usual dose is 3 to 5 mg per kg (1.4 to 2.3 mg per pound) of body weight, injected into a muscle or vein.

For aprobarbital
- For *oral* dosage form (elixir):
  - For trouble in sleeping:
    - Adults—40 to 160 milligrams (mg) at bedtime.
    - Children—Dose must be determined by your doctor.

◦ For daytime sedation:
- Adults—40 mg three times a day.
- Children—Dose must be determined by your doctor.

For butabarbital
- For *oral* dosage form (elixir or tablets):
  ◦ For trouble in sleeping:
  - Adults—50 to 100 milligrams (mg) at bedtime.
  - Children—Dose must be determined by your doctor.
  ◦ For daytime sedation:
  - Adults—15 to 30 mg three or four times a day.
  - Children—Dose is based on body weight or size and must be determined by your doctor. The usual dose is 2 mg per kilogram (kg) (0.9 mg per pound) of body weight three times a day.
  ◦ For sedation before surgery:
  - Adults—50 to 100 mg sixty to ninety minutes before surgery.
  - Children—Dose is based on body weight and must be determined by your doctor. The usual dose is 2 to 6 mg per kg (0.9 to 2.7 mg per pound) of body weight. However, the dose is usually not more than 100 mg.

For mephobarbital
- For *oral* dosage form (tablets):
  ◦ For daytime sedation:
  - Adults—32 to 100 milligrams (mg) three or four times a day.
  - Children—16 to 32 mg three or four times a day.
  ◦ For control of seizures:
  - Adults—200 to 600 mg a day, taken in smaller doses during the day.
  - Children up to 5 years of age—16 to 32 mg three or four times a day.
  - Children 5 years of age and over—32 to 64 mg three or four times a day.

For metharbital
- For *oral* dosage form (tablets):
  ◦ For control of seizures:
  - Adults—At first, 100 milligrams (mg) one to three times a day. Your doctor may increase your dose if needed. However, the dose is usually not more than 800 mg a day.
  - Children—50 mg one to three times a day.

For pentobarbital
- For *oral* dosage form (elixir or capsules):
  ◦ For trouble in sleeping:
  - Adults—100 milligrams (mg) at bedtime.
  - Children—Dose must be determined by your doctor.
  ◦ For daytime sedation:
  - Adults—20 mg three or four times a day.
  - Children—Dose is based on body weight and must be determined by your doctor. The usual dose is 2 to 6 mg per kilogram (kg) (0.9 to 2.7 mg per pound) of body weight per day.
  ◦ For sedation before surgery:
  - Adults—100 mg before surgery.
  - Children—Dose is based on body weight and must be determined by your doctor. The usual dose is 2 to 6 mg per kilogram (0.9 to 2.7 mg per pound) of body weight, taken before surgery. However, the dose is usually not more than 100 mg.

- For *injection* dosage form:
  ◦ For trouble in sleeping:
  - Adults—150 to 200 mg, injected into a muscle. Or, 100 mg injected into a vein, with additional small doses given if needed. However, the dose is usually not more than 500 mg.
  - Children—Dose is based on body weight and must be determined by your doctor. The usual dose is 2 to 6 mg per kg (0.9 to 2.7 mg per pound) of body weight, injected into a muscle. Or, 50 mg injected into a vein, with additional small doses given if needed.
  ◦ For sedation before surgery:
  - Adults—150 to 200 mg, injected into a muscle.
  - Children—Dose is based on body weight and must be determined by your doctor. The usual dose is 2 to 6 mg per kg (0.9 to 2.7 mg per pound) of body weight, injected into a muscle. However, the dose is usually not more than 100 mg.
  ◦ For control of seizures:
  - Adults—At first, 100 mg injected into a vein. Additional small doses may be given if needed. However, the dose is usually not more than 500 mg.
  - Children—At first, 50 mg injected into a muscle or vein. Additional small doses may be given if needed.

- For *rectal* dosage form (suppositories):
  ◦ For trouble in sleeping:
  - Adults—120 to 200 mg inserted into the rectum at bedtime.
  - Children up to 2 months of age—Dose must be determined by your doctor.
  - Children 2 months to 1 year of age—30 mg inserted into the rectum at bedtime.
  - Children 1 to 4 years of age—30 or 60 mg inserted into the rectum at bedtime.
  - Children 5 to 12 years of age—60 mg inserted into the rectum at bedtime.
  - Children 12 to 14 years of age—60 or 120 mg inserted into the rectum at bedtime.
  ◦ For daytime sedation:
  - Adults—30 mg inserted into the rectum two to four times a day.
  - Children—Dose is based on body weight or size and must be determined by your doctor. The usual dose is 2 mg per kg (0.9 mg per pound) of body weight, inserted into the rectum three times a day.
  ◦ For sedation before surgery:
  - Children up to 2 months of age—Dose must be determined by your doctor.
  - Children 2 months to 1 year of age—30 mg inserted into the rectum.
  - Children 1 to 4 years of age—30 or 60 mg inserted into the rectum.
  - Children 5 to 12 years of age—60 mg inserted into the rectum.
  - Children 12 to 14 years of age—60 or 120 mg inserted into the rectum.

For phenobarbital
- For *oral* dosage form (elixir, capsules, or tablets):
  ◦ For trouble in sleeping:
  - Adults—100 to 320 milligrams (mg) at bedtime.
  - Children—Dose must be determined by your doctor.

- For daytime sedation:
  - Adults—30 to 120 mg a day, taken in smaller doses two or three times during the day.
  - Children—Dose is based on body weight or size and must be determined by your doctor. The usual dose is 2 mg per kilogram (kg) (0.9 mg per pound) of body weight three times a day.
- For sedation before surgery:
  - Children—Dose is based on body weight and must be determined by your doctor. The usual dose is 1 to 3 mg per kg (0.45 to 1.4 mg per pound) of body weight.
- For control of seizures:
  - Adults—60 to 250 mg a day.
  - Children—Dose is based on body weight and must be determined by your doctor. The usual dose is 1 to 6 mg per kg (0.45 to 2.7 mg per pound) of body weight a day.
- For *injection* dosage form:
  - For trouble in sleeping:
    - Adults—100 to 325 mg, injected into a muscle or vein, or under the skin.
    - Children—Dose must be determined by your doctor.
  - For daytime sedation:
    - Adults—30 to 120 mg a day, injected into a muscle or a vein, or under the skin, in smaller doses two or three times during the day,
    - Children—Dose must be determined by your doctor.
  - For sedation before surgery:
    - Adults—130 to 200 mg, injected into a muscle sixty to ninety minutes before surgery.
    - Children—Dose is based on body weight and must be determined by your doctor. The usual dose is 1 to 3 mg per kg (0.45 to 1.4 mg per pound) of body weight, injected into a muscle or vein sixty to ninety minutes before surgery.
  - For control of seizures:
    - Adults—100 to 320 mg injected into a vein. The dose may be repeated if needed, but is usually not more than 600 mg a day. However, higher doses may be needed for certain types of continuing seizures.
    - Children—Dose is based on body weight and must be determined by your doctor. At first, the usual dose is 10 to 20 mg per kg (4.5 to 9 mg per pound) of body weight, injected into a vein. Later, 1 to 6 mg per kg (0.45 to 2.7 mg per pound) of body weight a day, injected into a vein. Higher doses may be needed for certain types of continuing seizures.

For secobarbital
- For *oral* dosage form (capsules):
  - For trouble in sleeping:
    - Adults—100 milligrams (mg) at bedtime.
    - Children—Dose must be determined by your doctor.
  - For daytime sedation:
    - Adults—30 to 50 mg three or four times a day.
    - Children—Dose is based on body weight or size and must be determined by your doctor. The usual dose is 2 mg per kilogram (kg) (0.9 mg per pound) of body weight three times a day.

- For sedation before surgery:
  - Adults—200 to 300 mg one or two hours before surgery.
  - Children—Dose is based on body weight and must be determined by your doctor. The usual dose is 2 to 6 mg per kg (0.9 to 2.7 mg per pound) of body weight one or two hours before surgery. However, the dose is usually not more than 100 mg.
- For *injection* dosage form:
  - For trouble in sleeping:
    - Adults—100 to 200 mg injected into a muscle, or 50 to 250 mg injected into a vein.
    - Children—Dose is based on body weight or size and must be determined by your doctor. The usual dose is 3 to 5 mg per kg (1.4 to 2.3 mg per pound) of body weight, injected into a muscle. However, the dose is usually not more than 100 mg.
  - For sedation before dental procedures:
    - Adults—Dose is based on body weight and must be determined by your doctor. The usual dose is 1.1 to 2.2 mg per kg (0.5 to 1 mg per pound) of body weight, injected into a muscle ten to fifteen minutes before the procedure.
    - Children—Dose must be determined by your dentist.
  - For sedation before a nerve block:
    - Adults—100 to 150 mg, injected into a vein.
  - For sedation before surgery:
    - Children—Dose is based on body weight and must be determined by your doctor. The usual dose is 4 to 5 mg per kg (1.8 to 2.3 mg per pound) of body weight, injected into a muscle.
  - For seizures from tetanus:
    - Adults—Dose is based on body weight and must be determined by your doctor. The usual dose is 5.5 mg per kg (2.5 mg per pound) of body weight, injected into a muscle or vein. Dose may be repeated every three to four hours if needed.
    - Children—Dose is based on body weight and must be determined by your doctor. The usual dose is 3 to 5 mg per kg (1.4 to 2.3 mg per pound) of body weight, injected into a muscle or vein.

For secobarbital and amobarbital combination
- For *oral* dosage form (capsules):
  - For trouble in sleeping:
    - Adults—1 capsule at bedtime.
    - Children—Dose must be determined by your doctor.
  - For sedation before surgery:
    - Adults—1 capsule taken one hour before surgery.
    - Children—Dose must be determined by your doctor.

Missed dose—If you are taking this medicine regularly (for example, every day as in epilepsy) and you do miss a dose, take it as soon as possible. However, if it is almost time for your next dose, skip the missed dose and go back to your regular dosing schedule. Do not double doses.

Storage—To store this medicine:
- Keep out of the reach of children since overdose is especially dangerous in children.
- Store away from heat and direct light.

- Do not store the capsule or tablet form of this medicine in the bathroom, near the kitchen sink, or in other damp places. Heat or moisture may cause the medicine to break down.
- Keep the liquid form of this medicine from freezing.
- Store the suppository form of this medicine in the refrigerator.
- Do not keep outdated medicine or medicine no longer needed. Be sure that any discarded medicine is out of the reach of children.

Precautions While Using This Medicine

If you will be using this medicine regularly for a long time:
- Your doctor should check your progress at regular visits.
- Do not stop using it without first checking with your doctor. Your doctor may want you to reduce gradually the amount you are using before stopping completely.

This medicine will add to the effects of alcohol and other CNS depressants (medicines that slow down the nervous system, possibly causing drowsiness). Some examples of CNS depressants are antihistamines or medicine for hay fever, other allergies, or colds; sedatives, tranquilizers, or sleeping medicine; prescription pain medicine or narcotics; medicine for seizures; muscle relaxants; or anesthetics, including some dental anesthetics. *Check with your doctor before taking any of the above while you are using this medicine.*

Before you have any medical tests, tell the medical doctor in charge that you are taking this medicine. The results of the metyrapone test may be affected by this medicine.

If you have been using this medicine for a long time and you think that you may have become mentally or physically dependent on it, check with your doctor. Some signs of mental or physical dependence on barbiturates are:
- a strong desire or need to continue taking the medicine.
- a need to increase the dose to receive the effects of the medicine.
- withdrawal side effects (for example, anxiety or restlessness, convulsions [seizures], feeling faint, nausea or vomiting, trembling of hands, trouble in sleeping) occurring after the medicine is stopped.

If you think you or someone else may have taken an overdose of this medicine, get emergency help at once. Taking an overdose of a barbiturate or taking alcohol or other CNS depressants with the barbiturate may lead to unconsciousness and possibly death. Some signs of an overdose are severe drowsiness, severe confusion, severe weakness, shortness of breath or slow or troubled breathing, slurred speech, staggering, and slow heartbeat.

This medicine may cause some people to become dizzy, lightheaded, drowsy, or less alert than they are normally. Even if taken at bedtime, it may cause some people to feel drowsy or less alert on arising. *Make sure you know how you react to this medicine before you drive, use machines, or do anything else that could be dangerous if you are dizzy or are not alert.*

Oral contraceptives (birth control pills) containing estrogen may not work properly if you take them while you are taking barbiturates. Unplanned pregnancies may occur. You should use a different or additional means of birth control while you are taking barbiturates. If you have any questions about this, check with your health care professional.

Side Effects

Along with its needed effects, a medicine may cause some unwanted effects. Although not all of these side effects may occur, if they do occur they may need medical attention.

Check with your doctor immediately if any of the following side effects occur:
> *Rare*
>> Bleeding sores on lips; chest pain; fever; muscle or joint pain; red, thickened, or scaly skin; skin rash or hives; sores, ulcers, or white spots in mouth (painful); sore throat and/or fever; swelling of eyelids, face, or lips; wheezing or tightness in chest

Also, check with your doctor as soon as possible if any of the following side effects occur:
> *Less common*
>> Confusion; mental depression; unusual excitement
> *Rare*
>> Hallucinations (seeing, hearing, or feeling things that are not there); unusual bleeding or bruising; unusual tiredness or weakness
> *With long-term or chronic use*
>> Bone pain, tenderness, or aching; loss of appetite; muscle weakness; weight loss (unusual); yellow eyes or skin
> *Symptoms of overdose*
>> Confusion (severe); decrease in or loss of reflexes; drowsiness (severe); fever; irritability (continuing); low body temperature; poor judgment; shortness of breath or slow or troubled breathing; slow heartbeat; slurred speech; staggering; trouble in sleeping; unusual movements of the eyes; weakness (severe)

Other side effects may occur that usually do not need medical attention. These side effects may go away during treatment as your body adjusts to the medicine. However, check with your doctor if any of the following side effects continue or are bothersome:
> *More common*
>> Clumsiness or unsteadiness; dizziness or lightheadedness; drowsiness; "hangover" effect
> *Less common*
>> Anxiety or nervousness; constipation; feeling faint; headache; irritability; nausea or vomiting; nightmares or trouble in sleeping

For very ill patients:
- Confusion, mental depression, and unusual excitement may be more likely to occur in very ill patients

After you stop using this medicine, your body may need time to adjust. If you took this medicine in high doses or for a long time, this may take up to about 15 days. During this period of time check with your doctor if any of the following side effects occur (usually occur within 8 to 16 hours after medicine is stopped):
> Anxiety or restlessness; convulsions (seizures); dizziness or lightheadedness; feeling faint; hallucinations (seeing, hearing, or feeling things that are not there); muscle twitching; nausea or vomiting; trembling of hands; trouble in sleeping, increased dreaming, or nightmares; vision problems; weakness

Other side effects not listed above may also occur in some patients. If you notice any other effects, check with your doctor.

Additional Information

Once a medicine has been approved for marketing for a certain use, experience may show that it is also useful for other medical problems. Although this use is not included in product labeling, phenobarbital is used in certain patients with the following medical condition:

- Hyperbilirubinemia (high amount of bile pigments in the blood that may lead to jaundice)

Other than the above information, there is no additional information relating to proper use, precautions, or side effects for these uses.

BARBITURATES, ASPIRIN, AND CODEINE (Systemic)

Some commonly used brand names are:

In the U.S.—
Ascomp with Codeine No.3 (1)
Butalbital Compound with Codeine (1)

Butinal with Codeine No.3 (1)
Fiorinal with Codeine No.3 (1)
Idenal with Codeine (1)
Isollyl with Codeine (1)

In Canada—
Fiorinal-C ¼ (1)
Fiorinal-C ½ (1)
Phenaphen with Codeine No.3 (2)

Tecnal-C ¼ (1)
Tecnal-C ½ (1)

This information applies to the following medicines:

1. Butalbital, Aspirin, and Codeine (byoo-TAL-bi-tal AS-pir-in and KOE-deen)
2. Phenobarbital, Aspirin, and Codeine (fee-noe-BAR-bi-tal AS-pir-in and KOE-deen)

Category

- **Analgesic**—Butalbital, Aspirin, Caffeine, and Codeine; Phenobarbital, Aspirin, and Codeine

Description

Barbiturate (bar-BI-tyoo-rate), aspirin, and codeine combinations are used to relieve headaches and other kinds of pain. These combination medicines may provide better pain relief than either aspirin or codeine used alone. In some cases, relief of pain may come at lower doses of each medicine.

Codeine is a narcotic analgesic (nar-KOT-ik an-al-JEE-zik) that acts in the central nervous system (CNS) to relieve pain. Many of its side effects are also caused by actions in the CNS. Butalbital and phenobarbital belong to the group of medicines called barbiturates. Barbiturates also act in the CNS to produce their effects.

When you use a barbiturate or codeine for a long time, your body may get used to the medicine so that larger amounts are needed to produce the same effects. This is called tolerance to the medicine. Also, barbiturates and codeine may become habit-forming (causing mental or physical dependence) when they are used for a long time or in large doses. Physical dependence may lead to withdrawal symptoms when you stop taking the medicine. In patients who get headaches, the first symptom of withdrawal may be new (rebound) headaches.

The butalbital, aspirin, and codeine combination also contains caffeine (kaf-EEN). Caffeine may help to relieve headaches. However, caffeine can also cause physical dependence when it is used for a long time. This may lead to withdrawal (rebound) headaches when you stop taking it.

Aspirin is not a narcotic and does not cause physical dependence. However, it may cause other unwanted effects if too much is taken.

These combination medicines are available only with your doctor's prescription, in the following dosage forms:

Oral
- Butalbital, Aspirin, Caffeine, and Codeine
  - Capsules
  - Tablets
- Phenobarbital, Aspirin, and Codeine
  - Capsules

Before Using This Medicine

In deciding to use a medicine, the risks of taking the medicine must be weighed against the good it will do. This is a decision you and your doctor will make. For barbiturate, aspirin, and codeine combinations, the following should be considered:

Allergies—Tell your doctor if you have ever had any unusual or allergic reaction to aspirin or other salicylates including methyl salicylate (oil of wintergreen); butalbital, phenobarbital, or other barbiturates; caffeine; codeine; or any of the following medicines:
- Diclofenac (e.g., Voltaren)
- Diflunisal (e.g., Dolobid)
- Etodolac (e.g., Lodine)
- Fenoprofen (e.g., Nalfon)
- Floctafenine (e.g., Idarac)
- Flurbiprofen, oral (e.g., Ansaid)
- Ibuprofen (e.g., Motrin)
- Indomethacin (e.g., Indocin)
- Ketoprofen (e.g., Orudis)
- Ketorolac (e.g., Toradol)
- Meclofenamate (e.g., Meclomen)
- Mefenamic acid (e.g., Ponstel)
- Nabumetone (e.g., Relafen)
- Naproxen (e.g., Naprosyn)
- Oxaprozin (e.g., Daypro)
- Oxyphenbutazone (e.g., Tandearil)
- Phenylbutazone (e.g., Butazolidin)
- Piroxicam (e.g., Feldene)
- Sulindac (e.g., Clinoril)
- Suprofen (e.g., Suprol)
- Tenoxicam (e.g., Mobiflex)
- Tiaprofenic acid (e.g., Surgam)
- Tolmetin (e.g., Tolectin)
- Zomepirac (e.g., Zomax)

Also tell your health care professional if you are allergic to any other substances, such as foods, preservatives, or dyes.

Pregnancy—

- *For butalbital or phenobarbital:* Barbiturates have been shown to increase the chance of birth defects in humans. Also, one study in humans has suggested that barbiturates taken during pregnancy may increase the chance of brain tumors in the baby. Barbiturates may cause breathing problems in the newborn baby if taken just before or during delivery.

- *For aspirin:* Although studies in humans have not shown that aspirin causes birth defects, aspirin has caused birth defects in animal studies. *Do not take aspirin during the last 3 months of pregnancy unless it has been ordered by your doctor.* Some reports have suggested that use of aspirin late in pregnancy may cause a decrease in the newborn's weight and possible death of the fetus or newborn baby. However, the mothers in these reports had been taking much larger amounts of aspirin than are usually recommended. Studies of mothers taking aspirin in the doses that are usually recommended did not show these unwanted effects. There is a chance that regular use of aspirin late in pregnancy may cause unwanted effects on the heart or blood flow in the fetus or in the newborn baby. Also, use of aspirin during the last 2 weeks of pregnancy may cause bleeding problems in the fetus before or during delivery or in the newborn baby. In addition, too much use of aspirin during the last 3 months of pregnancy may increase the length of pregnancy, prolong labor, cause other problems during delivery, or cause severe bleeding in the mother before, during, or after delivery.

- *For codeine:* Although studies on birth defects with codeine have not been done in pregnant women, it has not been reported to cause birth defects. However, it may cause breathing problems in the newborn baby if taken just before or during delivery. Codeine did not cause birth defects in animal studies, but it caused slower development of bones and other harmful effects in the fetus.

- *For caffeine:* Studies in humans have not shown that caffeine causes birth defects. However, use of large amounts of caffeine during pregnancy may cause problems with the heart rhythm and the growth of the fetus. Also, studies in animals have shown that caffeine causes birth defects when given in very large doses (amounts equal to those in 12 to 24 cups of coffee a day).

Breast-feeding—Although this combination medicine has not been reported to cause problems, the chance always exists, especially if the medicine is taken for a long time or in large amounts.

- *For butalbital or phenobarbital:* Barbiturates pass into the breast milk and may cause drowsiness, unusually slow heartbeat, shortness of breath, or troubled breathing in nursing babies.

- *For aspirin:* Aspirin passes into the breast milk. However, taking aspirin in the amount present in these combination medicines has not been reported to cause problems in nursing babies.

- *For codeine:* Codeine passes into the breast milk in small amounts. However, it has not been reported to cause problems in nursing babies.

- *For caffeine:* The caffeine in the butalbital, aspirin, and codeine combination medicine passes into the breast milk in small amounts. Taking caffeine in the amounts present in this combination medicine has not been reported to cause problems in nursing babies. However, studies have shown that nursing babies may appear jittery when their mothers drink large amounts of caffeine-containing beverages. Therefore, breast-feeding mothers who use caffeine-containing medicines should probably limit the amount of caffeine they take in from other medicines or from beverages.

Children—

- *For butalbital or phenobarbital:* Although barbiturates often cause drowsiness, some children become excited after taking them.

- *For aspirin: Do not give a medicine containing aspirin to a child with fever or other symptoms of a virus infection, especially flu or chickenpox, without first discussing its use with your child's doctor.* This is very important because aspirin may cause a serious illness called Reye's syndrome in children with fever caused by a virus infection, especially flu or chickenpox. Children who do not have a virus infection may also be more sensitive to the effects of aspirin, especially if they have a fever or have lost large amounts of body fluid because of vomiting, diarrhea, or sweating. This may increase the chance of side effects during treatment.

- *For caffeine:* There is no specific information comparing use of caffeine in children up to 12 years of age with use in other age groups. However, caffeine is not expected to cause different side effects or problems in children than it does in adults.

Older adults—

- *For butalbital or phenobarbital:* Confusion, depression, or excitement may be especially likely to occur in elderly patients, who are usually more sensitive than younger adults to the effects of barbiturates.

- *For aspirin:* Elderly patients are more sensitive than younger adults to the effects of aspirin. This may increase the chance of side effects during treatment.

- *For codeine:* Breathing problems may be especially likely to occur in elderly patients, who are usually more sensitive than younger adults to the effects of codeine.

- *For caffeine:* Many medicines have not been studied specifically in older people. Therefore, it may not be known whether they work exactly the same way they do in younger adults or if they cause different side effects or problems in older people. There is no specific information comparing use of caffeine in the elderly with use in other age groups.

Other medicines—Although certain medicines should not be used together at all, in other cases two different medicines may be used together even if an interaction might occur. In these cases, your doctor may want to change the dose, or other precautions may be necessary. When you are taking this combination medicine, it is especially important that your health care professional know if you are taking any of the following:

- Antacids, large amounts taken regularly, especially calcium- and/or magnesium-containing antacids or sodium bicarbonate (baking soda), or

- Urinary alkalizers (medicine that makes the urine less acid, such as acetazolamide [e.g., Diamox], dichlorphenamide [e.g., Daranide], methazolamide [e.g., Neptazane], potassium or sodium citrate and/or citric acid)—These medicines may cause aspirin to be removed from the body faster than usual, which may shorten the length of time that aspirin is effective; acetazolamide, dichlorphenamide, and methazolamide may also increase the chance of side effects when taken together with aspirin

- Anticoagulants (blood thinners) or
- Heparin—Use of these medicines together with aspirin may increase the chance of bleeding; also, barbiturates, especially phenobarbital, may decrease the effects of anticoagulants
- Antidepressants, tricyclic (amitriptyline [e.g., Elavil], amoxapine [e.g., Asendin], clomipramine [e.g., Anafranil], desipramine [e.g., Pertofrane], doxepin [e.g., Sinequan], imipramine [e.g., Tofranil], nortriptyline [e.g., Aventyl], protriptyline [e.g., Vivactil], trimipramine [e.g., Surmontil]) or
- Central nervous system (CNS) depressants (medicines that often cause drowsiness)—These medicines may add to the effects of barbiturates and codeine and increase the chance of drowsiness or other side effects
- Carbamazepine or
- Contraceptives, oral (birth control pills) containing estrogens or
- Corticosteroids (cortisone-like medicines) or
- Corticotropin (ACTH)—Barbiturates, especially phenobarbital, may make these medicines less effective
- Divalproex (e.g., Depakote) or
- Methotrexate (e.g., Mexate) or
- Valproic acid (e.g., Depakene) or
- Vancomycin (e.g., Vancocin)—The chance of serious side effects may be increased
- Naltrexone (e.g., Trexan)—Naltrexone blocks the pain-relieving effect of codeine
- Probenecid (e.g., Benemid) or
- Sulfinpyrazone (e.g., Anturane)—Aspirin can keep these medicines from working properly for treating gout

Other medical problems—The presence of other medical problems may affect the use of butalbital, aspirin, and codeine combination. Make sure you tell your doctor if you have any other medical problems, especially:
- Alcohol abuse (or history of) or
- Drug abuse or dependence (or history of)—Dependence on barbiturates and/or codeine may develop
- Asthma, especially if occurring together with other allergies and nasal polyps (history of), or
- Brain disease or head injury or
- Colitis or
- Convulsions (seizures) (history of) or
- Emphysema or other chronic lung disease or
- Enlarged prostate or problems with urination or
- Gallbladder disease or gallstones or
- Hyperactivity (in children) or
- Kidney disease or
- Liver disease—The chance of serious side effects may be increased

- Diabetes mellitus (sugar diabetes) or
- Mental depression or
- Overactive thyroid or
- Porphyria (or history of)—Barbiturates can make these conditions worse
- Gout—Aspirin can make this condition worse and can also lessen the effects of some medicines used to treat gout
- Heart disease (severe)—The caffeine in the butalbital, aspirin, and codeine combination can make some kinds of heart disease worse
- Hemophilia or other bleeding problems or
- Vitamin K deficiency—Aspirin increases the chance of serious bleeding
- Stomach ulcer, especially with a history of bleeding, or other stomach problems—Aspirin can make your condition worse

Proper Use of This Medicine

Take this medicine with food or a full glass (8 ounces) of water to lessen stomach irritation.

Do not take this medicine if it has a strong vinegar-like odor. This odor means the aspirin in it is breaking down. If you have any questions about this, check with your health care professional.

Take this medicine only as directed by your doctor. Do not take more of it, do not take it more often, and do not take it for a longer time than your doctor ordered. If a barbiturate or codeine is taken regularly (for example, every day), it may become habit-forming (causing mental or physical dependence). Regular use of caffeine can also cause physical dependence. Dependence is especially likely to occur in people who take these medicines to relieve frequent headaches. Also, taking too much of this combination medicine may cause stomach problems or other medical problems.

This medicine will relieve a headache best if you *take it as soon as the headache begins*. If you get warning signs of a migraine, take this medicine as soon as you are sure that the migraine is coming. This may even stop the headache pain from occurring. *Lying down in a quiet, dark room for a while after taking the medicine also helps to relieve headaches.*

People who get a lot of headaches may need to take a different medicine to help prevent headaches. *It is important that you follow your doctor's directions about taking the other medicine, even if your headaches continue to occur.* Headache-preventing medicines may take several weeks to start working. Even after they do start working, your headaches may not go away completely. However, your headaches should occur less often, and they should be less severe and easier to relieve than before. This will reduce the amount of headache relievers that you need. If you do not notice any improvement after several weeks of headache-preventing treatment, check with your doctor.

Dosing—The dose of these medicines will be different for different patients. *Follow your doctor's orders or the directions on the label.* The following information includes only the average doses of these medicines. *If your dose is different, do not change it* unless your doctor tells you to do so.

The number of capsules or tablets that you take depends on the strength of the medicine.

For Butalbital, Aspirin, and Codeine combination
- For *oral* dosage forms (capsules and tablets):
  - For relieving pain:
    - Adults—One or 2 capsules or tablets every four hours as needed. You should not take more than six capsules or tablets a day.
    - Children—Dose must be determined by your doctor.

For Phenobarbital, Aspirin, and Codeine combination
- For *oral* dosage form (capsules):
  - For relieving pain:
    - Adults—One or 2 capsules every three or four hours as needed.
    - Children—Dose must be determined by your doctor.

Missed dose—If your doctor has ordered you to take this medicine according to a regular schedule and you miss a dose, take it as soon as you remember. However, if it is almost time for your next dose, skip the missed dose and go back to your regular dosing schedule. Do not double doses.

Storage—To store this medicine:
- Keep out of the reach of children. Overdose is especially dangerous in young children.
- Store away from heat and direct light.
- Do not store this medicine in the bathroom, near the kitchen sink, or in other damp places. Heat or moisture may cause the medicine to break down.
- Do not keep outdated medicine or medicine no longer needed. Be sure that any discarded medicine is out of the reach of children.

Precautions While Using This Medicine

Check with your doctor:
- If the medicine stops working as well as it did when you first started using it. This may mean that you are in danger of becoming dependent on the medicine. *Do not try to get better pain relief by increasing the dose.*
- *If you are having headaches more often than you did before you started using this medicine.* This is especially important if a new headache occurs within 1 day after you took your last dose of headache medicine, headaches begin to occur every day, or a headache continues for several days in a row. This may mean that you are dependent on the headache medicine. *Continuing to take this medicine will cause even more headaches later on.* Your doctor can give you advice on how to relieve the headaches.

Check the labels of all nonprescription (over-the-counter [OTC]) and prescription medicines you now take. If any contain a narcotic, a barbiturate, aspirin, or other salicylates, including diflunisal, check with your doctor or pharmacist. Taking them together with this medicine may cause an overdose.

The barbiturate and the codeine in this medicine will add to the effects of alcohol and other CNS depressants (medicines that slow down the nervous system, possibly causing drowsiness). Some examples of CNS depressants are antihistamines or medicine for hay fever, other allergies, or colds; sedatives, tranquilizers, or sleeping medicine; other prescription pain medicine or narcotics; other barbiturates; medicine for seizures; muscle relaxants; or anesthetics, including some dental anesthetics. Also, stomach problems may be more likely to occur if you drink alcoholic beverages while you are taking aspirin. Therefore, *do not drink alcoholic beverages, and check with your doctor before taking any of the medicines listed above, while you are using this medicine.*

This medicine may cause some people to become drowsy, dizzy, or lightheaded, or to feel a false sense of well-being. *Make sure you know how you react to this medicine before you drive, use machines, or do anything else that could be dangerous if you are dizzy or are not alert and clearheaded.*

Dizziness, lightheadedness, or fainting may occur, especially when you get up suddenly from a lying or sitting position. Getting up slowly may help lessen this problem. Lying down for a while may relieve these effects.

Nausea or vomiting may occur, especially after the first couple of doses. This effect may go away if you lie down for a while. However, if nausea or vomiting continues, check with your doctor.

Before having any kind of surgery (including dental surgery) or emergency treatment, tell the medical doctor or dentist in charge that you are taking this medicine. Serious side effects can occur if your medical doctor or dentist gives you certain medicines without knowing that you have taken a barbiturate or codeine.

Do not take this medicine for 5 days before any planned surgery, including dental surgery, unless otherwise directed by your medical doctor or dentist. Taking aspirin during this time may cause bleeding problems.

Before you have any medical tests, tell the person in charge that you are taking this medicine. The caffeine in the butalbital, aspirin, and codeine combination interferes with the results of certain tests that use dipyridamole (e.g., Persantine) to help show how well blood is flowing to your heart. Caffeine should not be taken for 8 to 12 hours before the test. The results of some other tests may also be affected by this medicine.

If you have been taking large amounts of this medicine, or if you have been taking it regularly for several weeks or more, *do not suddenly stop using it without first checking with your doctor*. Your doctor may want you to reduce gradually the amount you are taking before stopping completely, to lessen the chance of withdrawal side effects.

If you think you or anyone else may have taken an overdose of this medicine, get emergency help at once. Taking an overdose of this medicine or taking alcohol or CNS depressants with this medicine may lead to unconsciousness or death. Signs of overdose of this medicine include convulsions (seizures); hearing loss; confusion; ringing or buzzing in the ears; severe excitement, nervousness, or restlessness; severe dizziness; severe drowsiness; unusually slow or troubled breathing; and severe weakness.

Side Effects

Along with its needed effects, a medicine may cause some unwanted effects. Although not all of these side effects may occur, if they do occur they may need medical attention.

The following side effects may mean that a serious allergic reaction is occurring. Check with your doctor or get emergency help immediately if they occur, especially if several of them occur at the same time.

> *Less common or rare*
>> Bluish discoloration or flushing or redness of skin (occurring together with other effects listed in this section); coughing, shortness of breath, troubled breathing, tightness in chest, or wheezing; difficulty in swallowing; dizziness or feeling faint (severe); hive-like swellings (large) on eyelids, face, lips, or tongue; skin rash, itching, or hives; stuffy nose (occurring together with other effects listed in this section)

Also check with your doctor immediately if any of the following side effects occur, especially if several of them occur together:

> *Rare*
>> Bleeding or crusting sores on lips; chest pain; fever with or without chills; red, thickened, or scaly skin; sores, ulcers, or white spots in mouth (painful); sore throat (unexplained); tenderness, burning, or peeling of skin

> *Symptoms of overdose*
>> Anxiety, confusion, excitement, irritability, nervousness, restlessness, or trouble in sleeping (severe, especially with products containing caffeine); cold, clammy skin; convulsions (seizures); diarrhea (severe or continuing); dizziness, lightheadedness, drowsiness, or weakness (severe); frequent urination (for products containing caffeine); hallucinations (seeing, hearing, or feeling things that are not there); increased sensitivity to touch or pain (for products containing caffeine); increased thirst; low blood pressure; muscle trembling or twitching (for products containing caffeine); nausea or vomiting (severe or continuing), sometimes with blood; pinpoint pupils of eyes; ringing or buzzing in ears (continuing) or hearing loss; seeing flashes of "zig-zag" lights (for products containing caffeine); slow, fast, or irregular heartbeat; slow, fast, irregular, or troubled breathing; slurred speech; staggering; stomach pain (severe); uncontrollable flapping movements of the hands (especially in elderly patients); unusual movements of the eyes; vision problems

Also, check with your doctor as soon as possible if any of the following side effects occur:

> *Less common or rare*
>> Bloody or black, tarry stools; bloody urine; confusion or mental depression; pinpoint red spots on skin; skin rash, hives, or itching (without other signs of an allergic reaction to aspirin listed above); sore throat and fever; stomach pain (severe); swollen or painful glands; trembling or uncontrolled muscle movements; unusual bleeding or bruising; unusual excitement (mild); unusual tiredness or weakness (mild)

Other side effects may occur that usually do not need medical attention. These side effects may go away during treatment as your body adjusts to the medicine. However, check with your doctor if any of the following side effects continue or are bothersome:

> *More common*
>> Bloated or "gassy" feeling; dizziness, lightheadedness, or drowsiness (mild); heartburn or indigestion; nausea, vomiting, or stomach pain (occurring without other symptoms of overdose)

Other side effects not listed above may also occur in some patients. If you notice any other effects, check with your doctor.

BARIUM SULFATE (Oral route, Rectal route) - BA-ree-um SUL-fate

Commonly used brand name(s)

In the U.S.—
Bar-Test
E-Z-Disk

In Canada—

Acb	Esopho-Cat Esophageal
Baro-Cat	Cream
Barosperse Enema	E-Z-Cat
Colobar-100	E-Z-Hd
Epi-C	E-Z-Jug
Epi-Stat	E-Z-Paque
Esobar	

Available Dosage Forms:

- Paste
- Kit
- Suspension
- Powder for Suspension
- Enema
- Tablet
- Liquid

Therapeutic Class: Diagnostic Agent, Radiological Contrast Media

Uses For This Test

Barium sulfate is a radiopaque agent. Radiopaque agents are used to help diagnose certain medical problems. Since radiopaque agents are opaque to (block) x-rays, the areas of the body in which they are localized will appear white on the x-ray film. This creates the needed distinction, or contrast, between one organ and other tissues. The contrast will help the doctor see any special conditions that may exist in that organ or part of the body.

Barium sulfate is taken by mouth or given rectally by enema. If taken by mouth, it makes the esophagus, the stomach, and/or the small intestine opaque to the x-rays so that they can be "photographed'. If it is given by enema, the colon and/or the small intestine can be seen and photographed by x-rays.

The dose of barium sulfate will be different for different patients and depends on the type of test. The strength of the suspension and tablet is determined by how much barium they contain. Different tests will require a different strength and amount of suspension (some may require the tablet form), depending on the age of the patient, the contrast needed, and the x-ray equipment used.

Barium sulfate is to be used only by or under the direct supervision of a doctor.

Before Having This Test

In deciding to use a diagnostic test, any risks of the test must be weighed against the good it will do. This is a decision you and your doctor will make. Also, other things may affect test results. For this test, the following should be considered:

In deciding to use a diagnostic test, any risks of the test must be weighed against the good it will do. This is a decision you and your doctor will make. Also, test results may be affected by other things. For barium sulfate, the following should be considered:

Allergies—Tell your doctor if you have ever had any unusual or allergic reaction to this medicine or any other medicines. Also tell your health care professional if you have any other types of allergies, such as to foods, dyes, preservatives,

or animals. For non-prescription products, read the label or package ingredients carefully.

Pediatric—Although there is no specific information comparing use of barium sulfate in children with use in other age groups, this agent is not expected to cause different side effects or problems in children than it does in adults.

Geriatric—This contrast agent has been used in older people and has not been shown to cause different side effects or problems in them than it does in younger adults.

Other medicines—Although certain medicines should not be used together at all, in other cases two different medicines may be used together even if an interaction might occur. In these cases, your doctor may want to change the dose, or other precautions may be necessary. Tell your healthcare professional if you are taking any other prescription or non-prescription (over-the-counter [OTC]) medicine.

Interactions with Food/Tobacco/Alcohol—Certain medicines should not be used at or around the time of eating food or eating certain types of food since interactions may occur. Using alcohol or tobacco with certain medicines may also cause interactions to occur. Discuss with your healthcare professional the use of your medicine with food, alcohol, or tobacco.

Other medical problems—The presence of other medical problems may affect the use of this diagnostic test. Make sure you tell your doctor if you have any other medical problems, especially:

- Asthma, hay fever, or other allergies (history of)—If you have a history of these conditions, the risk of having a reaction, such as an allergic reaction to the additives in the barium sulfate preparation, is greater
- Cystic fibrosis—The risk of blockage in the small bowel is greater
- Dehydration—Barium sulfate may cause severe constipation
- Intestinal blockage or perforation—Barium sulfate may make this condition worse

Proper Use of This Test

Dosing—The dose of this medicine will be different for different patients. Follow your doctor's orders or the directions on the label. The following information includes only the average doses of this medicine. If your dose is different, do not change it unless your doctor tells you to do so.

The amount of medicine that you take depends on the strength of the medicine. Also, the number of doses you take each day, the time allowed between doses, and the length of time you take the medicine depend on the medical problem for which you are using the medicine.

Precautions When Having This Test

Make sure to drink plenty of liquids after the test. Otherwise, barium sulfate may cause severe constipation.

Side Effects of This Test

Along with its needed effects, a medicine may cause some unwanted effects. Although not all of these side effects may occur, if they do occur they may need medical attention.

Check with your doctor immediately if any of the following side effects occur:

Rare

Bloating; constipation (severe, continuing); cramping (severe); nausea or vomiting; stomach or lower abdominal pain; tightness in chest or troubled breathing; wheezing

Some side effects may occur that usually do not need medical attention. These side effects may go away during treatment as your body adjusts to the medicine. Also, your health care professional may be able to tell you about ways to prevent or reduce some of these side effects. Check with your health care professional if any of the following side effects continue or are bothersome or if you have any questions about them:

More common

Constipation or diarrhea; cramping

Other side effects not listed may also occur in some patients. If you notice any other effects, check with your healthcare professional.

BECAPLERMIN (Topical route) - be-KAP-ler-min

Commonly used brand name(s)

In the U.S.—

Regranex

Available Dosage Forms:

- Gel/Jelly

Therapeutic Class: Wound Care Agent
Pharmacologic Class: Platelet Derived Growth Factor

Uses For This Medicine

Becaplermin is used to treat skin ulcers, usually on the lower leg, in patients with type 2 diabetes mellitus. It works by locally stimulating the wound to heal. It is important to use other methods for good skin ulcer care when using becaplermin.

Becaplermin is available only with your doctor's prescription.

Before Using This Medicine

In deciding to use a medicine, the risks of taking the medicine must be weighed against the good it will do. This is a decision you and your doctor will make. For this medicine, the following should be considered:

Allergies—Tell your doctor if you have ever had any unusual or allergic reaction to this medicine or any other medicines. Also tell your health care professional if you have any other types of allergies, such as to foods, dyes, preservatives, or animals. For non-prescription products, read the label or package ingredients carefully.

Pediatric—Although there is no specific information comparing use of becaplermin in children 16 years of age or older with use in other age groups, this medicine is not expected to cause different side effects or problems in children than it does in adults. This medicine has not been studied in children up to 16 years of age.

Geriatric—Many medicines have not been studied specifically in older people. Therefore, it may not be known whether they work exactly the same way they do in younger adults or if they cause different side effects or problems in older people. There is no specific information comparing use of becaplermin in the elderly with use in other age groups.

Other medicines—Although certain medicines should not be used together at all, in other cases two different medicines may be used together even if an interaction might occur. In these cases, your doctor may want to change the dose, or other precautions may be necessary. Tell your healthcare professional if you are taking any other prescription or non-prescription (over-the-counter [OTC]) medicine.

Interactions with Food/Tobacco/Alcohol—Certain medicines should not be used at or around the time of eating food or eating certain types of food since interactions may occur. Using alcohol or tobacco with certain medicines may also cause interactions to occur. Discuss with your healthcare professional the use of your medicine with food, alcohol, or tobacco.

Other medical problems—The presence of other medical problems may affect the use of this medicine. Make sure you tell your doctor if you have any other medical problems, especially:

- Skin cancer or tumors at the site of the ulcer—Use of becaplermin is not recommended because its effect on these conditions is not known

- Wounds that show exposed joints, tendons, ligaments, or bone—Use of becaplermin is not recommended because it is not known if it would work for these conditions

- Wounds that are closed manually by your health care professional—Use of becaplermin is not recommended because these wounds require a sterile product

Proper Use of This Medicine

To make using becaplermin as safe and reliable as possible, you should understand how and when to use this medicine and what effects may be expected. A paper with information for the patient will be given to you with your filled prescription and will provide many details concerning the use of becaplermin. Read this paper carefully and ask your health care professional for any additional information or explanation.

It is important to prevent the tip of the tube from touching the skin ulcer or any other object to keep the medicine from becoming impure and a possible source of infection.

There are several important steps that will help you apply your medicine properly.

- Wash your hands before preparing your dose.

- The proper amount to measure depends on the size of the tube you are using and the size of the skin ulcer. You should expect the dose to change each week or every other week, depending on the rate your skin ulcer changes in size.

- Measure the proper amount carefully onto a clean surface such as wax paper. Then, transfer the medicine to your skin ulcer by using an applicator aid, such as a cotton swab or tongue depressor.

- Spread the medicine on your skin ulcer as a thin (about 1/16th of an inch), even, continuous film.

- After wetting a gauze pad with 0.9% Sodium Chloride Irrigation USP, apply it on top of your medicated skin ulcer.

- After 12 hours, remove the medicine left on the skin ulcer with 0.9% Sodium Chloride Irrigation USP or water.

- Keep the ulcer from becoming too dry. When changing the dressing, the existing bandage may need to be wetted with 0.9% Sodium Chloride Irrigation USP to help remove the bandage and prevent injury to the healing ulcer.

- Wet a new gauze pad with 0.9% Sodium Chloride Irrigation USP. Apply it on top of your skin ulcer that no longer has the medicine on it and wait 12 hours before applying the medicine again. Therefore, the medicine is reapplied every 24 hours, with a change in the wound dressing in between applications.

Dosing—The dose of this medicine will be different for different patients. Follow your doctor's orders or the directions on the label. The following information includes only the average doses of this medicine. If your dose is different, do not change it unless your doctor tells you to do so.

The amount of medicine that you take depends on the strength of the medicine. Also, the number of doses you take each day, the time allowed between doses, and the length of time you take the medicine depend on the medical problem for which you are using the medicine.

- For topical dosage form (gel):
  - For skin ulcers caused by type 2 diabetes mellitus:
    - Adults and children 16 years of age and over—Apply an amount of gel once a day and leave it on for twelve hours. The amount applied will change each week or every other week, depending on the changing size of the skin ulcer.
    - Children up to 16 years of age—Use and dose must be determined by the doctor.

Missed dose—If you miss a dose of this medicine, take it as soon as possible. However, if it is almost time for your next dose, skip the missed dose and go back to your regular dosing schedule. Do not double doses.

Storage—Store in the refrigerator. Do not freeze.

Keep out of the reach of children.

Do not keep outdated medicine or medicine no longer needed.

Precautions While Using This Medicine

Your doctor should check your progress at regular visits to make sure that this medicine does not cause unwanted effects. As your skin ulcer changes in size, your doctor may change your dose weekly or every other week.

Becaplermin works best when used with other methods for good skin ulcer care, such as not bearing weight on the leg that has the skin ulcer. Your doctor will discuss these methods with you.

Discuss with your doctor whether you should continue the medicine if your skin ulcer is not reduced by 30% in 10 weeks or your skin ulcer does not improve after 20 weeks. If your skin ulcer does improve, your doctor may keep you on the medicine until your skin ulcer is completely healed.

It is important to use the proper amount and not to use more than prescribed.

Check the expiration date before using becaplermin and do not use it if it is out of date. The expiration date is located stamped on the crimped portion at the bottom of the tube.

Side Effects of This Medicine

Along with its needed effects, a medicine may cause some unwanted effects. Although not all of these side effects may occur, if they do occur they may need medical attention.

Check with your doctor as soon as possible if any of the following side effects occur:

Less common
> Reddened skin near ulcer; skin rash near ulcer

Other side effects not listed may also occur in some patients. If you notice any other effects, check with your healthcare professional.

BENTOQUATAM   (Topical route) -
BEN-toe-kwa-tam

Commonly used brand name(s)

In the U.S.—
> Ivy Block

Available Dosage Forms:
- Suspension

Therapeutic Class: Protectant, Dermatological

Uses For This Medicine

Bentoquatam protects the skin like a shield against poison ivy, poison oak, and poison sumac by physically blocking skin contact with their resin. The best protection against getting these conditions is to avoid contact with these plants. This medicine does not dry oozing and weeping caused by the rash of poison ivy, poison oak, or poison sumac.

Bentoquatam is available without prescription.

Before Using This Medicine

In deciding to use a medicine, the risks of taking the medicine must be weighed against the good it will do. This is a decision you and your doctor will make. For this medicine, the following should be considered:

Allergies—Tell your doctor if you have ever had any unusual or allergic reaction to this medicine or any other medicines. Also tell your health care professional if you have any other types of allergies, such as to foods, dyes, preservatives, or animals. For non-prescription products, read the label or package ingredients carefully.

Pediatric—Although there is no specific information comparing use of bentoquatam in children 6 years of age or older with use in other age groups, this medicine is not expected to cause different side effects or problems in these children than it does in adults. Use is not recommended for children up to 6 years of age.

Geriatric—Many medicines have not been studied specifically in older people. Therefore, it may not be known whether they work exactly the same way they do in younger adults.

Although there is no specific information comparing use of bentoquatam in the elderly with use in other age groups, this medicine is not expected to cause different side effects or problems in older people than it does in younger adults.

Other medicines—Although certain medicines should not be used together at all, in other cases two different medicines may be used together even if an interaction might occur. In these cases, your doctor may want to change the dose, or other precautions may be necessary. Tell your healthcare professional if you are taking any other prescription or non-prescription (over-the-counter [OTC]) medicine.

Interactions   with   Food/Tobacco/Alcohol—Certain medicines should not be used at or around the time of eating food or eating certain types of food since interactions may occur. Using alcohol or tobacco with certain medicines may also cause interactions to occur. Discuss with your healthcare professional the use of your medicine with food, alcohol, or tobacco.

Other medical problems—The presence of other medical problems may affect the use of this medicine. Make sure you tell your doctor if you have any other medical problems, especially:
- Contact dermatitis, allergic, due to poison ivy, poison oak, or poison sumac—Bentoquatam should not be applied to the rash of poison ivy, poison oak, or poison sumac and should be discontinued if such a rash develops

Proper Use of This Medicine

Although this medicine provides some protection, avoiding contact with poison ivy, poison oak, or poison sumac is best.

Do not use this medicine in or near the eyes. If this medicine does get into your eyes, wash them out immediately for 20 minutes with large amounts of cool tap water. If your eyes still burn or are painful, check with your doctor.

To use bentoquatam lotion:
- Shake the lotion well before using.
- Rub on enough lotion to leave a smooth wet film on skin.
- Allow the medicine to dry on the skin at least 15 minutes before being exposed to poison ivy, poison oak, or poison sumac.
- Maximum protection lasts for 4 hours but lotion must be reapplied whenever the dried film on the skin cannot be seen.
- Remove medicine with soap and water when it is no longer needed.

Dosing—The dose of this medicine will be different for different patients. Follow your doctor's orders or the directions on the label. The following information includes only the average doses of this medicine. If your dose is different, do not change it unless your doctor tells you to do so.

The amount of medicine that you take depends on the strength of the medicine. Also, the number of doses you take each day, the time allowed between doses, and the length of time you take the medicine depend on the medical problem for which you are using the medicine.
- For prevention of skin irritation from poison ivy, poison oak, or poison sumac (allergic contact dermatitis):
  - For topical dosage form (lotion):
    - Adults and children six years of age and older— Apply to the area(s) of skin that may be affected

at least fifteen minutes before exposure. Reapply whenever dry film is not seen or every four hours as needed.

- Children up to six years of age—Use must be determined by the doctor.

Storage—Store the medicine in a closed container at room temperature, away from heat, moisture, and direct light. Keep from freezing.

Keep out of the reach of children.

Do not keep outdated medicine or medicine no longer needed.

Precautions While Using This Medicine

If a rash or irritation occurs, stop using bentoquatam and check with your health care professional.

Side Effects of This Medicine

Along with its needed effects, a medicine may cause some unwanted effects. Although not all of these side effects may occur, if they do occur they may need medical attention.

Check with your doctor as soon as possible if any of the following side effects occur:
Rare
  Mild redness of skin

Other side effects not listed may also occur in some patients. If you notice any other effects, check with your healthcare professional.

BENZODIAZEPINES (Systemic)

Some commonly used brand names are:

In the U.S.—

Alprazolam Intensol (1)	Niravam (1)
Ativan (12)	Paxipam (10)
Dalmane (9)	ProSom (8)
Diastat (7)	Restoril (17)
Diazepam Intensol (7)	Serax (14)
Dizac (7)	Tranxene-SD (6)
Doral (16)	Tranxene-SD Half Strength
Halcion (18)	(6)
Klonopin (5)	Tranxene T-Tab (6)
Librium (3)	Valium (7)
Lorazepam Intensol (12)	Xanax (1)

In Canada—

Alti-Alprazolam (1)	Ativan (12)
Alti-Bromazepam (2)	Clonapam (5)
Alti-Clonazepam (5)	Dalmane (9)
Alti-Triazolam (18)	Diazemuls (7)
Apo-Alpraz (1)	Frisium (4)
Apo-Chlordiazepoxide (3)	Gen-Alprazolam (1)
Apo-Clonazepam (5)	Gen-Bromazepam (2)
Apo-Clorazepate (6)	Gen-Clonazepam (5)
Apo-Diazepam (7)	Gen-Triazolam (18)
Apo-Flurazepam (9)	Halcion (18)
Apo-Lorazepam (12)	Lectopam (2)
Apo-Oxazepam (14)	Mogadon (13)
Apo-Temazepam (17)	Novo-Alprazol (1)
Apo-Triazo (18)	Novo-Clopate (6)

Novo-Dipam (7)	PMS-Diazepam (7)
Novo-Flupam (9)	Restoril (17)
Novo-Lorazem (12)	Rivotril (5)
Novo-Poxide (3)	Serax (14)
Novo-Temazepam (17)	Somnol (9)
Novo-Triolam (18)	Tranxene (6)
Novoxapam (14)	Valium (7)
Nu-Alpraz (1)	Vivol (7)
Nu-Loraz (12)	Xanax (1)
PMS-Clonazepam (5)	Xanax TS (1)

This information applies to the following medicines:

1. Alprazolam (al-PRAZ-oh-lam)
2. Bromazepam (broe-MA-ze-pam)
3. Chlordiazepoxide (klor-dye-az-e-POX-ide)
4. Clobazam (KLOE-ba-zam)
5. Clonazepam (kloe-NA-ze-pam)
6. Clorazepate (klor-AZ-e-pate)
7. Diazepam (dye-AZ-e-pam)
8. Estazolam (ess-TA-zoe-lam)
9. Flurazepam (flure-AZ-e-pam)
10. Halazepam (hal-AZ-e-pam)
11. Ketazolam (kee-TAY-zoe-lam)
12. Lorazepam (lor-AZ-e-pam)
13. Nitrazepam (nye-TRA-ze-pam)
14. Oxazepam (ox-AZ-e-pam)
15. Prazepam (PRAZ-e-pam)
16. Quazepam (KWA-ze-pam)
17. Temazepam (tem-AZ-e-pam)
18. Triazolam (trye-AY-zoe-lam)

Category

- **Amnestic**—Diazepam (parenteral only); Lorazepam (parenteral only)
- **Antianxiety agent**—Alprazolam; Bromazepam; Chlordiazepoxide; Clorazepate; Diazepam; Halazepam; Ketazolam; Lorazepam; Oxazepam; Prazepam
- **Anticonvulsant**—Clobazam; Clonazepam; Clorazepate; Diazepam; Lorazepam (parenteral only); Nitrazepam
- **Antiemetic, in cancer chemotherapy**—Lorazepam (parenteral only)
- **Antipanic agent**—Alprazolam; Chlordiazepoxide (parenteral only); Clonazepam; Diazepam; Lorazepam
- **Antitremor agent**—Alprazolam; Chlordiazepoxide (oral only); Diazepam (oral only); Lorazepam (oral only)
- **Sedative-hypnotic**—Alprazolam; Bromazepam; Chlordiazepoxide; Clonazepam; Clorazepate; Diazepam; Estazolam; Flurazepam; Halazepam; Ketazolam; Lorazepam; Nitrazepam; Oxazepam; Prazepam; Quazepam; Temazepam; Triazolam
- **Skeletal muscle relaxant adjunct**—Diazepam; Lorazepam

Description

Benzodiazepines (ben-zoe-dye-AZ-e-peens) belong to the group of medicines called central nervous system (CNS) depressants (medicines that slow down the nervous system).

Some benzodiazepines are used to relieve anxiety. However, benzodiazepines should not be used to relieve nervousness or tension caused by the stress of everyday life.

Some benzodiazepines are used to treat insomnia (trouble in sleeping). However, if used regularly (for example, every day) for insomnia, they usually are not effective for more than a few weeks.

Many of the benzodiazepines are used in the treatment of other conditions, also. Diazepam is used to help relax muscles or relieve muscle spasm. Diazepam injection is used before some medical procedures to relieve anxiety and to reduce memory of the procedure. Chlordiazepoxide, clorazepate, diazepam, and oxazepam are used to treat the symptoms of alcohol withdrawal. Alprazolam and clonazepam are used in the treatment of panic disorder. Clobazam, clonazepam, clorazepate, diazepam, and lorazepam are used in the treatment of certain convulsive (seizure) disorders, such as epilepsy. The benzodiazepines may also be used for other conditions as determined by your doctor.

Benzodiazepines may be habit-forming (causing mental or physical dependence), especially when taken for a long time or in high doses.

These medicines are available only with your doctor's prescription, in the following dosage forms:

Oral
- Alprazolam
  - Oral disintegrating tablets
  - Oral solution
  - Tablets
- Bromazepam
  - Tablets
- Chlordiazepoxide
  - Capsules
- Clobazam
  - Tablets
- Clonazepam
  - Tablets
- Clorazepate
  - Capsules
  - Tablets
  - Extended-release tablets
- Diazepam
  - Oral solution
  - Tablets
- Estazolam
  - Tablets
- Flurazepam
  - Capsules
  - Tablets
- Halazepam
  - Tablets
- Lorazepam
  - Oral concentrate
  - Tablets
  - Sublingual tablets
- Nitrazepam
  - Tablets
- Oxazepam
  - Capsules
  - Tablets
- Quazepam
  - Tablets
- Temazepam
  - Capsules
- Triazolam
  - Tablets

Parenteral
- Chlordiazepoxide
  - Injection
- Diazepam
  - Injection
- Lorazepam
  - Injection

Rectal
- Diazepam
  - For rectal solution (may be prepared in U.S. and Canada from diazepam injection)
  - Rectal gel

Before Using This Medicine

In deciding to use a medicine, the risks of taking the medicine must be weighed against the good it will do. This is a decision you and your doctor will make. For benzodiazepines, the following should be considered:

Allergies—Tell your doctor if you have ever had any unusual or allergic reaction to benzodiazepines. Also tell your health care professional if you are allergic to any other substances, such as foods, preservatives, or dyes. Certain benzodiazepine products may contain lactose, parabens, or soybean oil.

Pregnancy—Chlordiazepoxide and diazepam have been reported to increase the chance of birth defects when used during the first 3 months of pregnancy. Although similar problems have not been reported with the other benzodiazepines, the chance always exists since all of the benzodiazepines are related.

Studies in animals have shown that clonazepam, lorazepam, and temazepam cause birth defects or other problems, including death of the animal fetus.

Too much use of a benzodiazepine during pregnancy may cause the baby to become dependent on the medicine. This may lead to withdrawal side effects after birth. Also, use of benzodiazepines during pregnancy, especially during the last weeks, may cause body temperature problems, breathing problems, difficulty in feeding, drowsiness, or muscle weakness in the newborn infant.

Benzodiazepines given just before or during labor may cause weakness in the newborn infant. When diazepam is given in high doses (especially by injection) within 15 hours before delivery, it may cause breathing problems, muscle weakness, difficulty in feeding, and body temperature problems in the newborn infant.

Breast-feeding—Benzodiazepines may pass into the breast milk and cause drowsiness, difficulty in feeding, and weight loss in nursing babies of mothers taking these medicines.

Children—Most of the side effects of these medicines are more likely to occur in children, especially the very young. These patients are usually more sensitive than adults to the effects of benzodiazepines.

It is possible that using clonazepam for long periods of time may cause unwanted effects on physical and mental growth in children. If such effects do occur, they may not be noticed until many years later. Before this medicine is given to children for long periods of time, you should discuss its use with your child's doctor.

Older adults—Most of the side effects of these medicines are more likely to occur in the elderly, who are usually more sensitive to the effects of benzodiazepines.

Taking benzodiazepines for trouble in sleeping may cause more daytime drowsiness in elderly patients than in younger adults. In addition, falls and related injuries are more likely to occur in elderly patients taking benzodiazepines.

Other medicines—Although certain medicines should not be used together at all, in other cases two different medicines may be used together even if an interaction might occur. In these cases, your doctor may want to change the dose, or other precautions may be necessary. When you are taking or receiving benzodiazepines it is especially important that your health care professional know if you are taking any of the following:

- Central nervous system (CNS) depressants (medicines that cause drowsiness)—The CNS depressant effects of either these medicines or benzodiazepines may be increased; your doctor may want to change the dose of either or both medicines
- Fluvoxamine (e.g., Luvox) or
- Nefazodone (e.g., Serzone)—Higher blood levels of benzodiazepines may occur, increasing the chance that side effects will occur; your doctor may want to change the dose of either or both medicines, or give you a different medicine
- Itraconazole (e.g., Sporanox) or
- Ketoconazole (e.g., Nizoral)—These medicines should NOT be used if you are taking a benzodiazepine.

Other medical problems—The presence of other medical problems may affect the use of benzodiazepines. Make sure you tell your doctor if you have any other medical problems, especially:

- Alcohol abuse (or history of) or
- Drug abuse or dependence (or history of)—Dependence on benzodiazepines may be more likely to develop
- Brain disease—CNS depression and other side effects of benzodiazepines may be more likely to occur
- Difficulty in swallowing (in children) or
- Emphysema, asthma, bronchitis, or other chronic lung disease or
- Hyperactivity or
- Mental depression or
- Mental illness (severe) or
- Myasthenia gravis or
- Porphyria or
- Sleep apnea (temporary stopping of breathing during sleep)—Benzodiazepines may make these conditions worse
- Epilepsy or history of seizures—Although some benzodiazepines are used in treating epilepsy, starting or suddenly stopping treatment with these medicines may increase seizures
- Glaucoma, acute narrow angle—Benzodiazepines should NOT be used if you have this condition.
- Glaucoma, open angle—Benzodiazepines can be used but your doctor should be monitoring your condition carefully.

- Kidney or liver disease—Higher blood levels of benzodiazepines may result, increasing the chance that side effects will occur

Proper Use of This Medicine

For caregivers administering *diazepam rectal gel:*

- Discuss with the patient's medical doctor exactly when and how to use diazepam rectal gel.
- Discuss with the patient's medical doctor when you should call for emergency help.
- Read the instructions that you received with the medicine before you need to use it.
- Stay with the patient after administering diazepam rectal gel to check his or her condition as instructed by the doctor.

For patients taking *clorazepate extended-release tablets:*

- Swallow tablets whole.
- Do not crush, break, or chew before swallowing.

For patients taking *alprazolam, diazepam, or lorazepam concentrated oral solution:*

- Measure each dose carefully using the dropper provided with the medicine.
- It is recommended that each dose be mixed with water, soda or soda-like beverages, or semisolid food such as applesauce or pudding, just before it is taken.
- Take the entire mixture right away. It should not be saved to be used later.

For patients taking *lorazepam sublingual tablets:*

- Do not chew or swallow the tablet. This medicine is meant to be absorbed through the lining of the mouth. Place the tablet under your tongue (sublingual) and let it slowly dissolve there. Do not swallow for at least 2 minutes.

For patients taking *alprazolam oral disintegrating tablets:*

- Make sure your hands are dry. Just prior to taking the tablet, remove the tablet from the bottle. Immediately place the tablet on top of the tongue. The tablet will dissolve in seconds, and you may swallow it with your saliva. You do not need to drink water or other liquid to swallow the tablet. If you have split apart a tablet and only taken one half of the tablet, you should throw away the unused part of the tablet right away because it may not remain stable.

Take this medicine only as directed by your doctor. Do not take more of it, do not take it more often, and do not take it for a longer time than your doctor ordered. If too much is taken, it may become habit-forming (causing mental or physical dependence).

If you think this medicine is not working properly after you have taken it for a few weeks, *do not increase the dose.* Instead, check with your doctor.

For patients taking this medicine on a regular schedule *for epilepsy or other seizure disorder:*

- *In order for this medicine to control your seizures, it must be taken every day in regularly spaced doses as ordered by your doctor.* This is necessary to keep a constant amount of the medicine in the blood. To help keep the amount constant, do not miss any doses.

For patients taking this medicine *for insomnia:*

- *Do not take this medicine when your schedule does not permit you to get a full night's sleep (7 to 8 hours).* If you must wake up before this, you may continue to feel drowsy and may experience memory problems, because the effects of the medicine have not had time to wear off.

For patients taking *flurazepam:*

- *When you begin to take this medicine, your sleeping problem will improve somewhat the first night. However, 2 or 3 nights may pass before you receive the full effects of this medicine.*

Dosing—The dose of benzodiazepines will be different for different patients. *Follow your doctor's orders or the directions on the label.* The following information includes only the average doses of benzodiazepines. *If your dose is different, do not change it* unless your doctor tells you to do so.

The number of capsules or tablets, or the amount of solution that you take, or the number of injections you receive, depends on the strength of the medicine. Also, *the number of doses you take each day, the time allowed between doses, and the length of time you take the medicine depend on the medical problem for which you are taking benzodiazepines.*

For alprazolam
- For *oral* dosage form (solution or tablets):
  - For anxiety:
    - Adults—At first, 0.25 to 0.5 milligram (mg) three times a day. Your doctor may increase your dose if needed. However, the dose usually is not more than 4 mg a day.
    - Children younger than 18 years of age—Use and dose must be determined by your doctor.
    - Older adults—At first, 0.25 mg two or three times a day. Your doctor may increase your dose if needed.
  - For panic disorder:
    - Adults—At first, 0.5 mg three times a day. Your doctor may increase your dose if needed. However, the dose usually is not more than 10 mg a day.
    - Children younger than 18 years of age—Use and dose must be determined by your doctor.

For bromazepam
- For *oral* dosage form (tablets):
  - For anxiety:
    - Adults—6 to 30 milligrams (mg) a day, taken in smaller doses during the day.
    - Children younger than 18 years of age—Use and dose must be determined by your doctor.
    - Older adults—At first, up to 3 mg a day. Your doctor may change your dose if needed.

For chlordiazepoxide
- For *oral* dosage form (capsules):
  - For anxiety:
    - Adults—5 to 25 milligrams (mg) three or four times a day.
    - Children 6 years of age and older—5 mg two to four times a day. Your doctor may increase your dose if needed.
    - Children younger than 6 years of age—Use and dose must be determined by your doctor.
    - Older adults—At first, 5 mg two to four times a day. Your doctor may increase your dose if needed.
  - For sedation during withdrawal from alcohol:
    - Adults—At first, 50 to 100 mg, repeated if needed. However, the dose usually is not more than 400 mg a day.
    - Children—Use and dose must be determined by your doctor.
- For *injection* dosage form:
  - For anxiety:
    - Adults—At first, 50 to 100 mg, injected into a muscle or vein. Then, if needed, 25 to 50 mg three or four times a day.
    - Teenagers—25 to 50 mg, injected into a muscle or vein.
    - Children younger than 12 years of age—Use and dose must be determined by your doctor.
    - Older adults—25 to 50 mg, injected into a muscle or vein.
  - For sedation during withdrawal from alcohol:
    - Adults—At first, 50 to 100 mg, injected into a muscle or vein. If needed, the dose may be repeated in two to four hours.
    - Children—Use and dose must be determined by your doctor.

For clobazam
- For *oral* dosage form (tablets):
  - For control of seizures:
    - Adults—At first, 5 to 15 milligrams (mg) a day. Your doctor may increase your dose if needed. However, the dose usually is not more than 80 mg a day.
    - Children 2 to 16 years of age—At first, 5 mg a day. Your doctor may increase your dose if needed. However, the dose usually is not more than 40 mg a day.
    - Children younger than 2 years of age—Dose is based on body weight and must be determined by your doctor.

For clonazepam
- For *oral* dosage form (tablets):
  - For control of seizures:
    - Adults—At first, 0.5 milligram (mg) three times a day. Your doctor may increase your dose if needed. However, the dose usually is not more than 20 mg a day.
    - Infants and children younger than 10 years of age—Dose is based on body weight and must be determined by your doctor.
  - For panic disorder:
    - Adults—At first, 0.25 mg two times a day. Your doctor may increase your dose if needed. However, the dose usually is not more than 4 mg a day.
    - Children—Use and dose must be determined by your doctor.

For clorazepate
- For *oral* dosage form (capsules or tablets):
  - For anxiety:
    - Adults and teenagers—7.5 to 15 mg two to four times a day. Or your doctor may want you to start by taking 15 mg at bedtime.
    - Children younger than 12 years of age—Use and dose must be determined by your doctor.

- Older adults—At first, 3.75 to 15 mg a day. Your doctor may increase your dose if needed.
  ○ For sedation during withdrawal from alcohol:
    - Adults and teenagers—At first, 30 mg. Your doctor will set up a schedule that will gradually reduce your dose.
    - Children younger than 12 years of age—Use and dose must be determined by your doctor.
  ○ For control of seizures:
    - Adults and teenagers—At first, up to 7.5 mg taken three times a day. Your doctor may increase your dose if needed. However, the dose usually is not more than 90 mg a day.
    - Children 9 to 12 years of age—At first, up to 7.5 mg two times a day. Your doctor may increase your dose if needed. However, the dose usually is not more than 60 mg a day.
    - Children younger than 9 years of age—Use and dose must be determined by your doctor.

- For *oral* dosage form (extended-release tablets):
  ○ For anxiety:
    - Adults and teenagers—Your doctor may change your dosage form to the extended-release tablet if you are already taking 3.75 or 7.5 milligrams (mg) of clorazepate three times a day. The extended-release tablet is taken one time each day.
    - Children younger than 12 years of age—Use and dose must be determined by your doctor.
  ○ For control of seizures:
    - Adults, teenagers, and children 9 to 12 years of age—Your doctor may change your dosage form to the extended-release tablet if you are already taking 3.75 or 7.5 milligrams (mg) of clorazepate three times a day. The extended-release tablet is taken one time each day.
    - Children younger than 9 years of age—Use and dose must be determined by your doctor.

For diazepam
- For *oral* dosage form (solution or tablets):
  ○ For anxiety:
    - Adults—2 to 10 mg two to four times a day.
    - Children 6 months of age and older—Dose is based on body weight or size and must be determined by your doctor.
    - Children younger than 6 months of age—Use is not recommended.
    - Older adults—2 to 2.5 mg one or two times a day. Your doctor may increase your dose if needed.
  ○ For sedation during withdrawal from alcohol:
    - Adults—At first, 10 mg three or four times a day. Your doctor will set up a schedule that will gradually decrease your dose.
    - Children—Use and dose must be determined by your doctor.
  ○ For control of seizures:
    - Adults—2 to 10 mg two to four times a day.
    - Children 6 months of age and older—Dose is based on body weight or size and must be determined by your doctor.
    - Children younger than 6 months of age—Use is not recommended.
    - Older adults—2 to 2.5 mg one or two times a day. Your doctor may increase your dose if needed.

  ○ For relaxing muscles:
    - Adults—2 to 10 mg three or four times a day.
    - Children 6 months of age and older—Dose is based on body weight or size and must be determined by your doctor.
    - Children younger than 6 months of age—Use is not recommended.
    - Older adults—2 to 2.5 mg one or two times a day. Your doctor may increase your dose if needed.

- For *injection* dosage form:
  ○ For anxiety:
    - Adults—2 to 10 mg, injected into a muscle or vein.
    - Children—Use and dose must be determined by your doctor.
    - For older adults—2 to 5 mg, injected into a muscle or vein.
  ○ For sedation during withdrawal from alcohol:
    - Adults—At first, 10 mg injected into a muscle or vein. If needed, 5 to 10 mg may be given three or four hours later.
    - Children—Use and dose must be determined by your doctor.
  ○ For sedation before surgery or other procedures:
    - Adults—5 to 20 mg, injected into a muscle or vein.
    - Children—Use and dose must be determined by your doctor.
    - Older adults—2 to 5 mg, injected into a muscle or vein.
  ○ For control of seizures:
    - Adults—At first, 5 to 10 mg, usually injected into a vein every ten to fifteen minutes, stopping if the total dose reaches 30 mg. If needed, this treatment may be repeated in two to four hours.
    - Children 5 years of age and older—At first, 1 mg, usually injected into a vein every two to five minutes, stopping if the total dose reaches 10 mg. This treatment may be repeated in two to four hours.
    - Infants older than 30 days of age and children younger than 5 years of age—At first, 0.2 to 0.5 mg, usually injected into a vein every two to five minutes, stopping if the total dose reaches 5 mg. This treatment may be repeated in two to four hours.
    - Newborns and infants 30 days of age and younger—Use and dose must be determined by your doctor.
    - Older adults—2 to 5 mg, injected into a muscle or vein.
  ○ For relaxing muscle spasms:
    - Adults—At first, 5 to 10 mg injected into a muscle or vein. The dose may be repeated in three or four hours.
    - Children—Use and dose must be determined by your doctor.
    - Older adults—2 to 5 mg, injected into a muscle or vein.
  ○ For relaxing muscles in tetanus:
    - Adults—At first, 5 to 10 mg injected into a muscle or vein. Your doctor may increase your dose if needed.
    - Children 5 years of age and older—5 to 10 mg, injected into a muscle or vein. The dose may be repeated every three to four hours if needed.

- Infants older than 30 days of age and children younger than 5 years of age—1 to 2 mg, injected into a muscle or vein. The dose may be repeated every three to four hours if needed.
- Newborns and infants 30 days of age and younger—Use and dose must be determined by your doctor.
- For *rectal* dosage form (gel or solution):
  - For control of seizures:
    - Adults and teenagers—Dose is based on body weight and must be determined by your doctor.
    - Children—Dose is based on body weight and must be determined by your doctor.

For estazolam
- For *oral* dosage form (tablets):
  - For trouble in sleeping:
    - Adults—1 milligram (mg) at bedtime. Your doctor may increase your dose if needed. However, the dose usually is not more than 2 mg.
    - Children younger than 18 years of age—Use and dose must be determined by your doctor.

For flurazepam
- For *oral* dosage form (capsules or tablets):
  - For trouble in sleeping:
    - Adults—15 or 30 milligrams (mg) at bedtime.
    - Children younger than 15 years of age—Use and dose must be determined by your doctor.
    - Older adults—At first, 15 mg at bedtime. Your doctor may increase your dose if needed.

For halazepam
- For *oral* dosage form (tablets):
  - For anxiety:
    - Adults—20 to 40 milligrams (mg) three or four times a day.
    - Children younger than 18 years of age—Use and dose must be determined by your doctor.
    - Older adults—20 mg one or two times a day.

For lorazepam
- For *oral* dosage form (concentrate or tablets):
  - For anxiety:
    - Adults and teenagers—1 to 3 milligrams (mg) two or three times a day.
    - Children younger than 12 years of age—Use and dose must be determined by your doctor.
    - Older adults—0.5 to 2 mg a day, taken in smaller doses during the day.
  - For trouble in sleeping:
    - Adults and teenagers—2 to 4 mg taken at bedtime.
    - Children younger than 12 years of age—Use and dose must be determined by your doctor.
- For *sublingual tablet* dosage form:
  - For anxiety:
    - Adults—2 to 3 mg a day, in smaller doses placed under the tongue during the day. Your doctor may increase your dose if needed. However, the dose usually is not more than 6 mg a day.
    - Children younger than 18 years of age—Use and dose must be determined by your doctor.
    - Older adults—At first, 0.5 mg a day. Your doctor may increase your dose if needed.

- For sedation before surgery:
  - Adults—Dose is based on body weight and will be determined by your doctor. However, the dose usually is not more than 4 mg, placed under the tongue, one to two hours before surgery.
  - Children—Use and dose must be determined by your doctor.
- For *injection* dosage form:
  - For sedation before surgery or other procedures:
    - Adults—Dose is based on body weight and will be determined by your doctor. However, the dose usually is not more than 4 mg, injected into a muscle or vein.
    - Children younger than 18 years of age—Use and dose must be determined by your doctor.
  - For control of seizures:
    - Adults—At first, 4 mg slowly injected into a vein. The dose may be repeated after ten to fifteen minutes if needed.
    - Children younger than 18 years of age—Use and dose must be determined by your doctor.

For nitrazepam
- For *oral* dosage form (tablets):
  - For trouble in sleeping:
    - Adults—5 to 10 milligrams (mg) at bedtime.
    - Children—Use and dose must be determined by your doctor.
    - Older adults—At first, 2.5 mg taken at bedtime. Your doctor may increase your dose if needed.
  - For control of seizures:
    - Children less than 30 kilograms (66 pounds) of body weight—Dose is based on body weight and will be determined by your doctor.

For oxazepam
- For *oral* dosage form (capsules or tablets):
  - For anxiety:
    - Adults—10 to 30 milligrams (mg) three or four times a day.
    - Children younger than 12 years of age—Use and dose must be determined by your doctor.
    - Older adults—At first, 5 mg one or two times a day or 10 mg three times a day. Your doctor may increase your dose if needed. However, the dose usually is not more than 15 mg four times a day.
  - For sedation during withdrawal from alcohol:
    - Adults—15 to 30 mg three or four times a day.
    - Children younger than 12 years of age—Use and dose must be determined by your doctor.

For quazepam
- For *oral* dosage form (tablets):
  - For trouble in sleeping:
    - Adults—7.5 to 15 milligrams (mg) at bedtime.
    - Children younger than 18 years of age—Use and dose must be determined by your doctor.

For temazepam
- For *oral* dosage form (capsules):
  - For trouble in sleeping:
    - Adults—15 milligrams (mg) at bedtime. Your doctor may change your dose if needed.
    - Children younger than 18 years of age—Use and dose must be determined by your doctor.
    - Older adults—At first, 7.5 mg at bedtime. Your doctor may increase your dose if needed.

For triazolam
- For *oral* dosage form (tablets):
  - For trouble in sleeping:
    - Adults—0.125 to 0.25 milligram (mg) at bedtime.
    - Children younger than 18 years of age—Use and dose must be determined by your doctor.
    - Older adults—At first, 0.125 mg at bedtime. Your doctor may increase your dose if needed.

Missed dose—If you are taking this medicine regularly (for example, every day as for epilepsy) and you miss a dose, take it right away if you remember within an hour or so of the missed dose. However, if you do not remember until later, skip the missed dose and go back to your regular dosing schedule. Do not double doses.

Storage—To store this medicine:
- Keep out of the reach of children. Overdose of benzodiazepines may be especially dangerous in children.
- Store away from heat and direct light.
- Do not store the capsule or tablet form of this medicine in the bathroom, near the kitchen sink, or in other damp places. Heat or moisture may cause the medicine to break down.
- Keep the liquid form of this medicine from freezing.
- Keep the oral disintegrating tablet form of this medicine in a tightly sealed bottle and discard any cotton that was included in the bottle
- Do not keep outdated medicine or medicine no longer needed. Be sure that any discarded medicine is out of the reach of children.

Precautions While Using This Medicine

If you will be *taking a benzodiazepine regularly for a long time:*
- Your doctor should check your progress at regular visits to make sure that this medicine does not cause unwanted effects. If you are taking a benzodiazepine for convulsions (seizures), this is also important during the first few months of treatment.
- Check with your doctor at regular visits to see if you need to continue taking this medicine.

If you are taking a benzodiazepine for *epilepsy or another seizure disorder:*
- Your doctor may want you to carry a medical identification card or bracelet stating that you are taking this medicine.

If you are taking a benzodiazepine for *insomnia* (trouble in sleeping):
- If you think you need this medicine for more than 7 to 10 days, be sure to discuss it with your doctor. Insomnia that lasts longer than this may be a sign of another medical problem.
- You may have difficulty sleeping (rebound insomnia) for the first few nights after you stop taking this medicine.

Benzodiazepines may be habit-forming (causing mental or physical dependence), especially when taken for a long time or in high doses. Some signs of dependence on benzodiazepines are:
- A strong desire or need to continue taking the medicine.
- A need to increase the dose to receive the effects of the medicine.

- Withdrawal effects (for example, irritability, nervousness, trouble in sleeping, abdominal or stomach cramps, trembling or shaking) occurring after the medicine is stopped.

If you think you may have become mentally or physically dependent on this medicine, check with your doctor. Do not stop taking it suddenly.

If you have been taking this medicine in large doses or for a long time, do not stop taking it without first checking with your doctor. Your doctor may want you to reduce gradually the amount you are taking before stopping completely. Stopping this medicine suddenly may cause withdrawal side effects, including seizures. Stopping this medicine suddenly is most likely to cause seizures if you have been taking it for epilepsy or another seizure disorder.

This medicine will add to the effects of alcohol and other central nervous system (CNS) depressants (medicines that slow down the nervous system, possibly causing drowsiness). Some examples of CNS depressants are antihistamines or medicine for hay fever, other allergies, or colds; sedatives, tranquilizers, or sleeping medicine; prescription pain medicine or narcotics; barbiturates; medicine for seizures; muscle relaxants; or anesthetics, including some dental anesthetics. This effect may last for a few days after you stop taking this medicine. *Check with your doctor before taking any of the above while you are taking this medicine.*

If you think you or someone else may have taken an overdose of this medicine, get emergency help at once. Taking an overdose of a benzodiazepine or taking alcohol or other CNS depressants with the benzodiazepine may lead to unconsciousness and possibly death. Some signs of an overdose are continuing slurred speech or confusion, severe drowsiness, severe weakness, and staggering.

Before you have any medical tests, tell the medical doctor in charge that you are taking this medicine. The results of the metyrapone test may be affected by chlordiazepoxide.

If you develop any unusual and strange thoughts or behavior while you are taking this medicine, be sure to discuss it with your doctor. Some changes that have occurred in people taking this medicine are like those seen in people who drink alcohol and then act in a manner that is not normal. Other changes may be more unusual and extreme, such as confusion, agitation, and hallucinations (seeing, hearing, or feeling things that are not there).

This medicine may cause some people, especially older persons, to become drowsy, dizzy, lightheaded, clumsy or unsteady, or less alert than they are normally. Even if taken at bedtime, it may cause some people to feel drowsy or less alert on arising. *Make sure you know how you react to this medicine before you drive, use machines, or do anything else that could be dangerous if you are dizzy or are not alert.*

Side Effects of This Medicine

Along with its needed effects, a medicine may cause some unwanted effects. Although not all of these side effects may occur, if they do occur they may need medical attention.

Check with your doctor as soon as possible if any of the following side effects occur:
Less common
  Anxiety; confusion (may be more common in the elderly); fast, pounding, or irregular heartbeat; lack of

memory of events taking place after benzodiazepine is taken (may be more common with triazolam); mental depression

Rare

Abnormal thinking, including disorientation, delusions (holding false beliefs that cannot be changed by facts), or loss of sense of reality; agitation; behavior changes, including aggressive behavior, bizarre behavior, decreased inhibition, or outbursts of anger; convulsions (seizures); hallucinations (seeing, hearing, or feeling things that are not there); hypotension (low blood pressure); muscle weakness; skin rash or itching; sore throat, fever, and chills; trouble in sleeping; ulcers or sores in mouth or throat (continuing); uncontrolled movements of body, including the eyes; unusual bleeding or bruising; unusual excitement, nervousness, or irritability; unusual tiredness or weakness (severe); yellow eyes or skin

Symptoms of overdose

Confusion (continuing); convulsions (seizures); drowsiness (severe) or coma; shakiness; slow heartbeat; slow reflexes; slurred speech (continuing); staggering; troubled breathing; weakness (severe)

For patients having *chlordiazepoxide, diazepam, or lorazepam injected:*

- Check with your doctor if there is redness, swelling, or pain at the place of injection.

Other side effects may occur that usually do not need medical attention. These side effects may go away during treatment as your body adjusts to the medicine. However, check with your doctor if any of the following side effects continue or are bothersome:

More common

Clumsiness or unsteadiness; dizziness or lightheadedness; drowsiness; slurred speech

Less common or rare

Abdominal or stomach cramps or pain; blurred vision or other changes in vision; changes in sexual desire or ability; constipation; diarrhea; dryness of mouth or increased thirst; false sense of well-being; headache; increased bronchial secretions or watering of mouth; muscle spasm; nausea or vomiting; problems with urination; trembling or shaking; unusual tiredness or weakness

Not all of the side effects listed above have been reported for each of these medicines, but they have been reported for at least one of them. All of the benzodiazepines are similar, so any of the above side effects may occur with any of these medicines.

After you stop using this medicine, your body may need time to adjust. During this time, check with your doctor if you notice any of the following side effects:

More common

Irritability; nervousness; trouble in sleeping

Less common

Abdominal or stomach cramps; confusion; fast or pounding heartbeat; increased sense of hearing; increased sensitivity to touch and pain; increased sweating; loss of sense of reality; mental depression; muscle cramps; nausea or vomiting; sensitivity of eyes to light; tingling, burning, or prickly sensations; trembling or shaking

Rare

Confusion as to time, place, or person; convulsions (seizures); feelings of suspicion or distrust; hallucinations (seeing, hearing, or feeling things that are not there)

Other side effects not listed above may also occur in some patients. If you notice any other effects, check with your doctor.

Additional Information

Once a medicine has been approved for marketing for a certain use, experience may show that it is also useful for other medical problems. Although these uses are not included in product labeling, some of the benzodiazepines are used in certain patients with the following medical conditions:

- Nausea and vomiting caused by cancer chemotherapy
- Tension headache
- Tremors

Other than the above information, there is no additional information relating to proper use, precautions, or side effects for these uses.

BENZONATATE (Oral route) - ben-ZOE-na-tate

Commonly used brand name(s)

In the U.S.—
Tessalon Perles

Available Dosage Forms:

- Capsule, Liquid Filled
- Capsule

Therapeutic Class: Antitussive

Uses For This Medicine

Benzonatate is used to relieve coughs due to colds or influenza (flu). It is not to be used for chronic cough that occurs with smoking, asthma, or emphysema or when there is an unusually large amount of mucus or phlegm (pronounced flem) with the cough.

Benzonatate relieves cough by acting directly on the lungs and the breathing passages. It may also act on the cough center in the brain.

This medicine is available only with your doctor's prescription.

Before Using This Medicine

In deciding to use a medicine, the risks of taking the medicine must be weighed against the good it will do. This is a decision you and your doctor will make. For this medicine, the following should be considered:

Allergies—Tell your doctor if you have ever had any unusual or allergic reaction to this medicine or any other medicines. Also tell your health care professional if you have any other types of allergies, such as to foods, dyes, preservatives, or animals. For non-prescription products, read the label or package ingredients carefully.

Pediatric—It is very important that children do not chew or suck on the capsule before swallowing it. If the benzonatate contained in the capsules comes in contact with the mouth, it may cause the mouth and throat to become numb (loss of feeling) and choking may occur.

Geriatric—Many medicines have not been studied specifically in older people. Therefore, it may not be known whether they work exactly the same way they do in younger adults or if they cause different side effects or problems in older people. There is no specific information comparing use of benzonatate in the elderly with use in other age groups.

Pregnancy—

	Pregnancy Category	Explanation
All Trimesters	C	Animal studies have shown an adverse effect and there are no adequate studies in pregnant women OR no animal studies have been conducted and there are no adequate studies in pregnant women.

Breast Feeding—There are no adequate studies in women for determining infant risk when using this medication during breastfeeding. Weigh the potential benefits against the potential risks before taking this medication while breastfeeding.

Other medicines—Although certain medicines should not be used together at all, in other cases two different medicines may be used together even if an interaction might occur. In these cases, your doctor may want to change the dose, or other precautions may be necessary. Tell your healthcare professional if you are taking any other prescription or non-prescription (over-the-counter [OTC]) medicine.

Interactions with Food/Tobacco/Alcohol—Certain medicines should not be used at or around the time of eating food or eating certain types of food since interactions may occur. Using alcohol or tobacco with certain medicines may also cause interactions to occur. Discuss with your healthcare professional the use of your medicine with food, alcohol, or tobacco.

Other medical problems—The presence of other medical problems may affect the use of this medicine. Make sure you tell your doctor if you have any other medical problems, especially:

- Mucus or phlegm with cough—Since benzonatate decreases coughing, it makes it difficult to get rid of the mucus that may collect in the lungs and airways with some diseases

Proper Use of This Medicine

It is very important that you do not chew or suck on the capsule before swallowing it. If the benzonatate contained in the capsules comes in contact with the mouth, it may cause the mouth and throat to become numb (loss of feeling) and choking may occur.

Dosing—The dose of this medicine will be different for different patients. Follow your doctor's orders or the directions on the label. The following information includes only the average doses of this medicine. If your dose is different, do not change it unless your doctor tells you to do so.

The amount of medicine that you take depends on the strength of the medicine. Also, the number of doses you take each day, the time allowed between doses, and the length of time you take the medicine depend on the medical problem for which you are using the medicine.

- For oral dosage form (capsules):
  - For cough:
    - Adults—100 milligrams (mg) three times a day as needed.
    - Children—
      — Up to 10 years of age: Use and dose must be determined by your doctor.
      — 10 years of age and older: 100 mg three times a day as needed.

Missed dose—If you miss a dose of this medicine, take it as soon as possible. However, if it is almost time for your next dose, skip the missed dose and go back to your regular dosing schedule. Do not double doses.

Storage—Store the medicine in a closed container at room temperature, away from heat, moisture, and direct light. Keep from freezing.

Keep out of the reach of children.

Do not keep outdated medicine or medicine no longer needed.

Precautions While Using This Medicine

If your cough has not become better after 7 days or if you have a high fever, skin rash, or continuing headache with the cough, check with your doctor. These signs may mean that you have other medical problems.

Side Effects of This Medicine

Along with its needed effects, a medicine may cause some unwanted effects. Although not all of these side effects may occur, if they do occur they may need medical attention.

Check with your doctor as soon as possible if any of the following side effects occur:
Rare
Confusion; signs of hypersensitivity reactions, such as bronchospasm (shortness of breath, difficulty in breathing, tightness in chest, and/or wheezing) or laryngospasm (difficulty in speaking or breathing); visual hallucinations (seeing things that are not there)

Symptoms of overdose
Convulsions (seizures); restlessness; trembling

Some side effects may occur that usually do not need medical attention. These side effects may go away during treatment as your body adjusts to the medicine. Also, your health care professional may be able to tell you about ways to prevent or reduce some of these side effects. Check with your health care professional if any of the following side effects continue or are bothersome or if you have any questions about them:
Less common or rare
Burning sensation in the eyes; constipation; dizziness (mild); drowsiness (mild); headache; itching; nausea or vomiting; skin rash; stuffy nose

Other side effects not listed may also occur in some patients. If you notice any other effects, check with your healthcare professional.

BENZOYL PEROXIDE (Topical route)
- BEN-zoe-ill per-OX-ide

Commonly used brand name(s)

In the U.S.—

Benzac AC	Brevoxyl-4
Benzac W	Brevoxyl-8
Benzagel-10	Del-Aqua-10
Benzagel-5	Del-Aqua-5
Benzagel Wash	Desquam-E
Benzashave	Triaz

In Canada—

10 Benzagel Acne Gel	Acetoxyl 10
2.5 Benzagel Acne Gel	Acetoxyl 2.5
2.5 Benzagel Acne Lotion	Acetoxyl 20
5 Benzagel Acne Gel	Acetoxyl 5
5 Benzagel Acne Lotion	Acnomel Bp 5
5 Benzagel Acne Wash	Alquam-X Acne Therapy Gel

Available Dosage Forms:

- Pad
- Cream
- Gel/Jelly
- Liquid
- Soap
- Lotion
- Solution

Therapeutic Class: Antiacne Antibacterial

Uses For This Medicine

Benzoyl peroxide is used to treat acne.

It may also be used for other conditions as determined by your doctor.

Some of these preparations are available only with your doctor's prescription.

Once a medicine has been approved for marketing for a certain use, experience may show that it is also useful for other medical problems. Although these uses are not included in product labeling, benzoyl peroxide is used in certain patients with the following medical conditions:

- Decubital ulcer (bed sores)
- Stasis ulcer (a certain type of ulcer)

Before Using This Medicine

In deciding to use a medicine, the risks of taking the medicine must be weighed against the good it will do. This is a decision you and your doctor will make. For this medicine, the following should be considered:

Allergies—Tell your doctor if you have ever had any unusual or allergic reaction to this medicine or any other medicines. Also tell your health care professional if you have any other types of allergies, such as to foods, dyes, preservatives, or animals. For non-prescription products, read the label or package ingredients carefully.

Pediatric—For children up to 12 years of age: Studies on this medicine have been done only in adult patients, and there is no specific information comparing use of benzoyl peroxide with use in other age groups. For children 12 years of age and older: Although there is no specific information comparing use of benzoyl peroxide in children with use in other age groups, this medicine is not expected to cause different side effects or problems in children 12 years of age and older than it does in adults.

Geriatric—Many medicines have not been studied specifically in older people. Therefore, it may not be known whether they work exactly the same way they do in younger adults. Although there is no specific information comparing use of benzoyl peroxide in the elderly with use in other age groups, this medicine is not expected to cause different side effects or problems in older people than it does in younger adults.

Other medicines—Although certain medicines should not be used together at all, in other cases two different medicines may be used together even if an interaction might occur. In these cases, your doctor may want to change the dose, or other precautions may be necessary. Tell your healthcare professional if you are taking any other prescription or nonprescription (over-the-counter [OTC]) medicine.

Interactions with Food/Tobacco/Alcohol—Certain medicines should not be used at or around the time of eating food or eating certain types of food since interactions may occur. Using alcohol or tobacco with certain medicines may also cause interactions to occur. Discuss with your healthcare professional the use of your medicine with food, alcohol, or tobacco.

Other medical problems—The presence of other medical problems may affect the use of this medicine. Make sure you tell your doctor if you have any other medical problems, especially:

- Dermatitis, seborrheic or
- Eczema or
- Red or raw skin, including sunburned skin—Irritation will occur if benzoyl peroxide is used with these conditions

Proper Use of This Medicine

It is very important that you use this medicine only as directed. Do not use more of it and do not use it more often than recommended on the label, unless otherwise directed by your doctor. To do so may cause irritation of the skin.

Do not use this medicine in or around the eyes or lips, or inside the nose, or on sensitive areas of the neck. Spread the medicine away from these areas when applying. If the medicine gets on these areas, wash with water at once.

Do not apply this medicine to windburned or sunburned skin or on open wounds, unless otherwise directed by your doctor.

This medicine usually comes with patient directions. Read them carefully before using the medicine.

To use the cream, gel, lotion, or stick form of benzoyl peroxide:

- Before applying, wash the affected area with nonmedicated soap and water or with a mild cleanser and then gently pat dry with a towel.
- Apply enough medicine to cover the affected areas, and rub in gently.

To use the shave cream form of benzoyl peroxide:

- Wet the area to be shaved.
- Apply a small amount of the shave cream and gently rub over entire area.
- Shave.
- Rinse the area and pat dry.
- After-shave lotions or other drying face products should not be used without checking with your doctor first.

To use the cleansing bar, cleansing lotion, or soap form of benzoyl peroxide:

- Use to wash the affected areas as directed.

To use the facial mask form of benzoyl peroxide:

- Before applying, wash the affected area with a nonmedicated cleanser. Then rinse and pat dry.
- Using a circular motion, apply a thin layer of the mask evenly over the affected area.
- Allow the mask to dry for 15 to 25 minutes.
- Then rinse thoroughly with warm water and pat dry.

After applying the medicine, wash your hands to remove any medicine that might remain on them.

Dosing—The dose of this medicine will be different for different patients. Follow your doctor's orders or the directions on the label. The following information includes only the average doses of this medicine. If your dose is different, do not change it unless your doctor tells you to do so.

The amount of medicine that you take depends on the strength of the medicine. Also, the number of doses you take each day, the time allowed between doses, and the length of time you take the medicine depend on the medical problem for which you are using the medicine.

- For acne:
  - For cleansing bar dosage form:
    - Adults and children 12 years of age and over— Use two or three times a day, or as directed by your doctor.
    - Children up to 12 years of age—Use and dose must be determined by your doctor.
  - For cleansing lotion, cream, or gel dosage forms:
    - Adults and children 12 years of age and over— Use on the affected area(s) of the skin one or two times a day.
    - Children up to 12 years of age—Use and dose must be determined by your doctor.
  - For lotion dosage form:
    - Adults and children 12 years of age and over— Use on the affected area(s) of the skin one to four times a day.
    - Children up to 12 years of age—Use and dose must be determined by your doctor.
  - For facial mask dosage form:
    - Adults and children 12 years of age and over— Use one time a week or as directed by your doctor.
    - Children up to 12 years of age—Use and dose must be determined by your doctor.
  - For stick dosage form:
    - Adults and children 12 years of age and over— Use on the affected area(s) of the skin one to three times a day.
    - Children up to 12 years of age—Use and dose must be determined by your doctor.

Missed dose—If you miss a dose of this medicine, apply it as soon as possible. However, if it is almost time for your next dose, skip the missed dose and go back to your regular dosing schedule.

Storage—Store the medicine in a closed container at room temperature, away from heat, moisture, and direct light. Keep from freezing.

Keep out of the reach of children.

Do not keep outdated medicine or medicine no longer needed.

Precautions While Using This Medicine

During the first 3 weeks you are using benzoyl peroxide, your skin may become irritated. Also, your acne may seem to get worse before it gets better. If your skin problem has not improved within 4 to 6 weeks, check with your health care professional.

You should not wash the areas of the skin treated with benzoyl peroxide for at least 1 hour after application.

Avoid using any other topical medicine on the same area within 1 hour before or after using benzoyl peroxide. Otherwise, benzoyl peroxide may not work properly.

Unless your doctor tells you otherwise, it is especially important to avoid using the following skin products on the same area as benzoyl peroxide:

- Any other topical acne product or skin product containing a peeling agent (such as resorcinol, salicylic acid, sulfur, or tretinoin);
- Hair products that are irritating, such as permanents or hair removal products;
- Skin products that cause sensitivity to the sun, such as those containing lime or spices;
- Skin products containing a large amount of alcohol, such as astringents, shaving creams, or after-shave lotions; or
- Skin products that are too drying or abrasive, such as some cosmetics, soaps, or skin cleansers.

Using these products along with benzoyl peroxide may cause mild to severe irritation of the skin. Although skin irritation can occur, some doctors sometimes allow benzoyl peroxide to be used with tretinoin to treat acne. Usually tretinoin is applied at night so that it doesn't cause a problem with any other topical products that you might use during the day. Check with your doctor before using any other topical medicines with benzoyl peroxide.

This medicine may bleach hair or colored fabrics.

Check with your doctor at any time your skin becomes too dry or irritated. Your health care professional can help you choose the right skin products for you to reduce skin dryness and irritation.

Side Effects of This Medicine

Along with its needed effects, a medicine may cause some unwanted effects. Although not all of these side effects may occur, if they do occur they may need medical attention.

Check with your doctor as soon as possible if any of the following side effects occur:

Less common or rare
　Painful irritation of skin, including burning, blistering, crusting, itching, severe redness, or swelling; skin rash

Symptoms of overdose
　Burning, itching, scaling, redness, or swelling of skin (severe)

Some side effects may occur that usually do not need medical attention. These side effects may go away during treatment as your body adjusts to the medicine. Also, your health care professional may be able to tell you about ways to prevent or reduce some of these side effects. Check with your health care professional if any of the following side effects continue or are bothersome or if you have any questions about them:

Less common

Dryness or peeling of skin (may occur after a few days); feeling of warmth, mild stinging, and redness of skin

Other side effects not listed may also occur in some patients. If you notice any other effects, check with your healthcare professional.

BENZYL BENZOATE (Topical route)

Uses For This Medicine

Benzyl benzoate is used to treat lice and scabies infestations. This medicine is believed to be absorbed by the lice and mites and to destroy them by acting on their nervous system.

This medicine is available without a prescription.

Before Using This Medicine

In deciding to use a medicine, the risks of taking the medicine must be weighed against the good it will do. This is a decision you and your doctor will make. For this medicine, the following should be considered:

Allergies—Tell your doctor if you have ever had any unusual or allergic reaction to this medicine or any other medicines. Also tell your health care professional if you have any other types of allergies, such as to foods, dyes, preservatives, or animals. For non-prescription products, read the label or package ingredients carefully.

Pediatric—Although there is no specific information comparing use of benzyl benzoate in children with use in other age groups, this medicine is not expected to cause different side effects or problems in children than it does in adults.

Geriatric—Many medicines have not been studied specifically in older people. Therefore, it may not be known whether they work exactly the same way they do in younger adults or if they cause different side effects or problems in older people. There is no specific information comparing use of benzyl benzoate in the elderly with use in other age groups. However, older people may have dry skin and the medicine may make the condition worse.

Other medicines—Although certain medicines should not be used together at all, in other cases two different medicines may be used together even if an interaction might occur. In these cases, your doctor may want to change the dose, or other precautions may be necessary. Tell your healthcare professional if you are taking any other prescription or non-prescription (over-the-counter [OTC]) medicine.

Interactions   with   Food/Tobacco/Alcohol—Certain medicines should not be used at or around the time of eating food or eating certain types of food since interactions may occur. Using alcohol or tobacco with certain medicines may also cause interactions to occur. Discuss with your healthcare professional the use of your medicine with food, alcohol, or tobacco.

Other medical problems—The presence of other medical problems may affect the use of this medicine. Make sure you tell your doctor if you have any other medical problems, especially:

- Inflammation of the skin (severe)—Use of benzyl benzoate may make the condition worse

Proper Use of This Medicine

Benzyl benzoate usually comes with patient directions. Read them carefully before using this medicine.

Use this medicine only as directed. Do not use more of it and do not use it more often than recommended on the label. To do so may increase the chance of absorption through the skin and the chance of side effects.

Keep this medicine away from the eyes and other mucous membranes, such as the inside of the nose, because it may cause irritation. If you accidentally get some in your eyes, flush them thoroughly with water at once.

Do not use benzyl benzoate on open wounds, such as cuts or sores on the skin or scalp. To do so may increase the amount of absorption, which may increase the chance of side effects.

Your sexual partner or partners, especially, and all members of your household may need to be treated also, since the infestation may spread to persons in close contact. If these persons have not been examined for infestation or if you have any questions about this, check with your doctor.

To use this medicine for lice:

- If your hair has any cream, lotion, ointment, or oil-based product on it, shampoo, rinse, and dry your hair and scalp well before applying benzyl benzoate.
- Apply enough medicine to thoroughly wet the dry hair and scalp or skin.
- Allow the medicine to remain on the affected areas for 24 hours.
- Then, thoroughly wash the affected areas with warm water and soap or regular shampoo.
- Rinse thoroughly and dry with a clean towel.
- After rinsing and drying, use a fine-toothed comb (less than 0.3 mm between the teeth) to remove any remaining nits (eggs) or nit shells from your hair, or, if you have fine hair, you may use a tweezer or your fingernails to pick nits out.

To use this medicine for scabies:

- If your skin has any cream, lotion, ointment, or oil on it, wash, rinse, and dry your skin well before applying benzyl benzoate.
- If you take a bath or shower before using benzyl benzoate, dry the skin well before applying the medicine.
- Apply enough medicine to cover the entire skin surface from the neck down, including the soles of your feet, and rub in well.
- Allow the medicine to remain on the body for 24 hours.
- Then, thoroughly wash the body with warm water and soap.
- Rinse thoroughly and dry with a clean towel.

Immediately after using benzyl benzoate, wash your hands to remove any medicine that may be on them.

Treatment may need to be repeated for severe infestation.

Dosing—The dose of this medicine will be different for different patients. Follow your doctor's orders or the directions

on the label. The following information includes only the average doses of this medicine. If your dose is different, do not change it unless your doctor tells you to do so.

The amount of medicine that you take depends on the strength of the medicine. Also, the number of doses you take each day, the time allowed between doses, and the length of time you take the medicine depend on the medical problem for which you are using the medicine.

- For topical dosage form (emulsion):
  - For lice infestation:
    - Adults—Use just one time. For severe cases, treatment may be repeated two or three times after twenty-four hours.
    - Children—
      — For infants: Use mixed with three parts of water, just one time.
      — For older children: Use mixed with an equal quantity of water, just one time.
  - For scabies infestation:
    - Adults—Use just one time. For severe cases, treatment may be repeated after twenty-four hours one time anytime within five days.
    - Children—
      — For infants: Use mixed with three parts of water, just one time.
      — For older children: Use mixed with an equal quantity of water, just one time.

Storage—Store the medicine in a closed container at room temperature, away from heat, moisture, and direct light. Keep from freezing.

Keep out of the reach of children.

Do not keep outdated medicine or medicine no longer needed.

Precautions While Using This Medicine

To prevent reinfection or spreading of the infection to other people, good health habits are required. These include the following:

- For lice infestation:
  - Disinfecting or washing combs, curlers, and brushes in very hot water (65 °C or 150 °F) for about 10 minutes immediately after using.
  - Washing in very hot water all recently worn clothing and used bed linens and towels, and drying them in a hot dryer for at least 20 minutes. Articles that cannot be washed may be dry-cleaned, pressed with a hot iron, or just placed in a hot dryer.
  - Sealing stuffed toys and other non-washable articles in a plastic bag for 2 weeks, or placing these items in the freezer (in sealed plastic bags) for 12 to 24 hours.
  - Vacuuming all rugs, mattresses, pillows, furniture, and car seats to get rid of fallen hairs with lice.
- For scabies infestation: Washing all recently worn clothing such as underwear and pajamas, and used sheets, pillowcases, and towels in very hot water or dry-cleaning.

Side Effects of This Medicine

Along with its needed effects, a medicine may cause some unwanted effects. Although not all of these side effects may occur, if they do occur they may need medical attention.

Check with your doctor as soon as possible if any of the following side effects occur:

Symptoms of overdose

Blister formation, crusting, itching, oozing, reddening, or scaling of skin; difficulty in urinating (dribbling); jerking movements; sudden loss of consciousness

Some side effects may occur that usually do not need medical attention. These side effects may go away during treatment as your body adjusts to the medicine. Also, your health care professional may be able to tell you about ways to prevent or reduce some of these side effects. Check with your health care professional if any of the following side effects continue or are bothersome or if you have any questions about them:

Less common or rare

Burning or itching of skin

Other side effects not listed may also occur in some patients. If you notice any other effects, check with your healthcare professional.

BETA CAROTENE (Oral route) - bay-ta KARE-oh-teen

Commonly used brand name(s)

In the U.S.—
A-Caro-25
Lumitene

Available Dosage Forms:
- Capsule, Liquid Filled
- Tablet
- Liquid
- Capsule

Therapeutic Class: Nutritive Agent
Pharmacologic Class: Vitamin A (class)

Uses For This Dietary Supplement

Vitamins are compounds that you must have for growth and health. They are needed in small amounts only and are usually available in the foods that you eat. Beta-carotene is converted in the body to vitamin A, which is necessary for healthy eyes and skin.

A lack of vitamin A may cause a rare condition called night blindness (problems seeing in the dark). It may also cause dry eyes, eye infections, skin problems, and slowed growth. Your health care professional may treat these problems by prescribing either beta-carotene, which your body can change into vitamin A, or vitamin A for you.

Some conditions may increase your need for vitamin A. These include:
- Cystic fibrosis
- Diarrhea, continuing
- Illness, long-term
- Injury, serious
- Liver disease
- Malabsorption problems
- Pancreas disease

Increased need for vitamin A should be determined by your health care professional.

Claims that beta-carotene is effective as a sunscreen have not been proven. Although beta-carotene supplements are being studied for their ability to reduce the risk of certain types of cancer and possibly heart disease, there is not enough information to show that this is effective.

Beta-carotene may be used to treat other conditions as determined by your doctor.

Beta-carotene is available without a prescription.

Once a product has been approved for marketing for a certain use, experience may show that it is also useful for other medical problems. Although this use is not included in product labeling, beta-carotene is used in certain patients with the following medical conditions:

- Polymorphous light eruption (a type of reaction to sun)
- Erythropoietic protoporphyria photosensitivity reaction (a type of reaction to sun)

Other than the above information, there is no additional information relating to proper use, precautions, or side effects for these uses.

Importance of Diet—For good health, it is important that you eat a balanced and varied diet. Follow carefully any diet program your health care professional may recommend. For your specific dietary vitamin and/or mineral needs, ask your health care professional for a list of appropriate foods. If you think that you are not getting enough vitamins and/or minerals in your diet, you may choose to take a dietary supplement.

It is documented that people who consume diets high in fruits and vegetables have a reduced risk of heart disease and certain cancers. Fruits and vegetables are rich in beta-carotene and other nutrients that may be beneficial.

Beta-carotene is found in carrots; dark-green leafy vegetables, such as spinach and green leaf lettuce; sweet potatoes; broccoli; cantaloupe; and winter squash. The body converts beta-carotene into vitamin A. Ordinary cooking does not destroy beta-carotene.

Vitamins alone will not take the place of a good diet and will not provide energy. Your body needs other substances found in food, such as protein, minerals, carbohydrates, and fat. Vitamins themselves often cannot work without the presence of other foods. For example, some fat is needed so that beta-carotene can be absorbed into the body.

Before Using This Dietary Supplement

If you are taking this dietary supplement without a prescription, carefully read and follow any precautions on the label. For this supplement, the following should be considered:

Allergies—Tell your doctor if you have ever had any unusual or allergic reaction to this medicine or any other medicines. Also tell your health care professional if you have any other types of allergies, such as to foods, dyes, preservatives, or animals. For non-prescription products, read the label or package ingredients carefully.

Pediatric—Problems in children have not been documented with intake of normal daily recommended amounts.

Geriatric—Problems in older adults have not been documented with intake of normal daily recommended amounts.

Breast Feeding—There are no adequate studies in women for determining infant risk when using this medication during breastfeeding. Weigh the potential benefits against the potential risks before taking this medication while breastfeeding.

Other medicines—Although certain medicines should not be used together at all, in other cases two different medicines may be used together even if an interaction might occur. In these cases, your doctor may want to change the dose, or other precautions may be necessary. Tell your healthcare professional if you are taking any other prescription or non-prescription (over-the-counter [OTC]) medicine.

Interactions with Food/Tobacco/Alcohol—Certain medicines should not be used at or around the time of eating food or eating certain types of food since interactions may occur. Using alcohol or tobacco with certain medicines may also cause interactions to occur. Discuss with your healthcare professional the use of your medicine with food, alcohol, or tobacco.

Other medical problems—The presence of other medical problems may affect the use of this dietary supplement. Make sure you tell your doctor if you have any other medical problems, especially:

- Eating disorders or
- Kidney disease or
- Liver disease—These conditions may cause high blood levels of beta-carotene, which may increase the chance of side effects

---

Proper Use of This Dietary Supplement

Dosing—The dose of this medicine will be different for different patients. Follow your doctor's orders or the directions on the label. The following information includes only the average doses of this medicine. If your dose is different, do not change it unless your doctor tells you to do so.

The amount of medicine that you take depends on the strength of the medicine. Also, the number of doses you take each day, the time allowed between doses, and the length of time you take the medicine depend on the medical problem for which you are using the medicine.

For use as a dietary supplement:

- For oral dosage forms (capsules or chewable tablets):
  - Adults and teenagers: 6 to 15 milligrams (mg) of beta-carotene (the equivalent of 10,000 to 25,000 Units of vitamin A activity) per day.
  - Children: 3 to 6 mg of beta-carotene (the equivalent of 5,000 to 10,000 Units of vitamin A activity) per day.

For other uses:

- For oral dosage forms (capsules or tablets):
  - To treat or prevent a reaction to sun in patients with erythropoietic protoporphyria:
    - Adults and teenagers—30 to 300 milligrams (mg) of beta-carotene (the equivalent of 50,000 to 500,000 Units of vitamin A activity) a day.
    - Children—30 to 150 mg of beta-carotene (the equivalent of 50,000 to 250,000 Units of vitamin A activity) a day.
  - To treat or prevent a reaction to sun in patients with polymorphous light eruption:
    - Adults and teenagers—75 to 180 mg of beta-carotene (the equivalent of 125,000 to 300,000 Units of vitamin A activity) a day.
    - Children—30 to 150 mg of beta-carotene (the equivalent of 50,000 to 250,000 Units of vitamin A activity) a day.

If you have high blood levels of vitamin A, your body will convert less beta-carotene to vitamin A.

Missed dose—If you miss a dose of this medicine, take it as soon as possible. However, if it is almost time for your next dose, skip the missed dose and go back to your regular dosing schedule. Do not double doses.

If you miss taking a vitamin for one or more days there is no cause for concern, since it takes some time for your body to become seriously low in vitamins. However, if your health care professional has recommended that you take this vitamin, try to remember to take it as directed every day.

If you miss a dose and you are using it as medicine, take it as soon as possible. However, if it is almost time for your next dose, skip the missed dose and go back to your regular dosing schedule. Do not double doses.

Storage—Store the medicine in a closed container at room temperature, away from heat, moisture, and direct light. Do not refrigerate. Keep from freezing.

Store the dietary supplement in a closed container at room temperature, away from heat, moisture, and direct light. Keep from freezing.

Keep out of the reach of children.

Do not keep outdated medicine or medicine no longer needed.

Precautions While Using This Dietary Supplement

Use of beta-carotene has been associated with an increased risk of lung cancer in people who smoke or who have been exposed to asbestos. One study of 29,000 male smokers found an 18% increase in lung cancer in the group receiving 20 mg of beta-carotene a day for 5 to 8 years. Another study of 18,000 people found 28% more lung cancers in people with a history of smoking and/or asbestos exposure. These people took 30 mg of beta-carotene in addition to 25,000 Units of retinol (a form of vitamin A) a day for 4 years. However, one study of 22,000 male physicians, some of them smokers or former smokers, found no increase in lung cancer. These people took 50 mg of beta-carotene every other day for 12 years. If you smoke or have a history of smoking or asbestos exposure, you should not take large amounts of beta-carotene supplements for long periods of time. However, foods that are rich in beta-carotene are considered safe and appear to lower the risk of some types of cancer and possibly heart disease.

Side Effects of This Dietary Supplement

Along with its needed effects, a medicine may cause some unwanted effects. Although not all of these side effects may occur, if they do occur they may need medical attention.

Some side effects may occur that usually do not need medical attention. These side effects may go away during treatment as your body adjusts to the medicine. Also, your health care professional may be able to tell you about ways to prevent or reduce some of these side effects. Check with your health care professional if any of the following side effects continue or are bothersome or if you have any questions about them:

More common
Yellowing of palms, hands, or soles of feet, and to a lesser extent the face (this may be a sign that your dose of beta-carotene as a nutritional supplement is too high)

Rare
Diarrhea; dizziness; joint pain; unusual bleeding or bruising

Other side effects not listed may also occur in some patients. If you notice any other effects, check with your healthcare professional.

BETA-ADRENERGIC BLOCKER
(Oral route, Injection route, Intravenous route)

Commonly used brand name(s)
In the U.S.—

Betagan	Lopressor
Betapace	Normodyne
Betimol	Optipranolol
Betoptic S	Sectral
Brevibloc	Tenormin
Cartrol	Timoptic Ocudose
Coreg	Toprol XL
Corgard	Visken
Inderal	Zebeta
Levatol	

In Canada—

Alti-Nadolol	Alti-Sotalol
Alti-Pindolol	

Available Dosage Forms:

• Tablet	• Tablet, Extended Release
• Solution	• Injectable
• Capsule	• Capsule, Extended Release

Uses For This Medicine

This group of medicines is known as beta-adrenergic blocking agents, beta-blocking agents, or, more commonly, beta-blockers. Beta-blockers are used in the treatment of high blood pressure (hypertension). Some beta-blockers are also used to relieve angina (chest pain) and in heart attack patients to help prevent additional heart attacks. Beta-blockers are also used to correct irregular heartbeat, prevent migraine headaches, and treat tremors. They may also be used for other conditions as determined by your doctor.

Beta-blockers work by affecting the response to some nerve impulses in certain parts of the body. As a result, they decrease the heart's need for blood and oxygen by reducing its workload. They also help the heart to beat more regularly.

Once a medicine has been approved for marketing for a certain use, experience may show that it is also useful for other medical problems. Although these uses are not included in product labeling, some beta-blockers are used in certain patients with the following medical conditions:
• Glaucoma
• Neuroleptic-induced akathisia (restlessness or the need to keep moving caused by some medicines used to treat nervousness or mental and emotional disorders)

Before Using This Medicine

Allergies—Tell your doctor if you have ever had any unusual or allergic reaction to medicines in this group or any other medicines. Also tell your health care professional if you have any other types of allergies, such as to foods dyes, preservatives, or animals. For non-prescription products, read the label or package ingredients carefully.

Pediatric—Some of these medicines have been used in children and, in effective doses, have not been shown to cause different side effects or problems in children than they do in adults.

Geriatric—Some side effects are more likely to occur in the elderly, who are usually more sensitive to the effects of beta-blockers. Also, beta-blockers may reduce tolerance to cold temperatures in elderly patients.

Pregnancy—Use of some beta-blockers during pregnancy has been associated with low blood sugar, breathing problems, a lower heart rate, and low blood pressure in the newborn infant. Other reports have not shown unwanted effects on the newborn infant. Animal studies have shown some beta-blockers to cause problems in pregnancy when used in doses many times the usual human dose. Before taking any of these medicines, make sure your doctor knows if you are pregnant or if you may become pregnant.

Breast Feeding—It is not known whether bisoprolol, carvedilol, carteolol, or penbutolol passes into breast milk. All other beta-blockers pass into breast milk. Problems such as slow heartbeat, low blood pressure, and trouble in breathing have been reported in nursing babies. Mothers who are taking beta-blockers and who wish to breast-feed should discuss this with their doctor.

Other medicines—

Using medicines in this class with any of the following medicines is not recommended. Your doctor may decide not to treat you with a medication in this class or change some of the other medicines you take.

Bepridil, Cisapride, Grepafloxacin, Levomethadyl, Mesoridazine, Pimozide, Ranolazine, Sparfloxacin, Terfenadine, Thioridazine, Ziprasidone

Using medicines in this class with any of the following medicines is usually not recommended, but may be required in some cases. If both medicines are prescribed together, your doctor may change the dose or how often you use one or both of the medicines.

Acecainide, Acetazolamide, Ajmaline, Amiloride, Amiodarone, Amisulpride, Amitriptyline, Amoxapine, Aprindine, Arsenic Trioxide, Astemizole, Azimilide, Azosemide, Bemetizide, Bendroflumethiazide, Benzthiazide, Bretylium, Bumetanide, Canrenoate, Chloral Hydrate, Chloroquine, Chlorpromazine, Chlorthalidone, Ciprofloxacin, Clarithromycin, Clonidine, Clopamide, Cyclothiazide, Desipramine, Diatrizoate, Dibenzepin, Disopyramide, Dofetilide, Dolasetron, Doxepin, Droperidol, Enflurane, Epinephrine, Erythromycin, Ethacrynic Acid, Etozolin, Fenoldopam, Fenquizone, Fentanyl, Flecainide, Fluconazole, Fluoxetine, Foscarnet, Furosemide, Gatifloxacin, Gemifloxacin, Halofantrine, Haloperidol, Halothane, Hydrochlorothiazide, Hydroflumethiazide, Hydroquinidine, Ibutilide, Imipramine, Indapamide, Isoflurane, Isradipine, Levofloxacin, Lidocaine, Lidoflazine, Lorcainide, Mannitol, Mefloquine, Metolazone, Moxifloxacin, Nortriptyline, Octreotide, Ondansetron, Pentamidine, Piretanide, Pirmenol, Polythiazide, Prajmaline, Prilocaine, Probucol, Procainamide, Propafenone, Quetiapine, Quinethazone, Quinidine, Risperidone, Sematilide, Sertindole, Sotalol, Spiramycin, Spironolactone, Sulfamethoxazole, Sultopride, Tedisamil, Telithromycin, Ticrynafen, Torsemide, Triamterene, Trichlormethiazide, Trimethoprim, Trimipramine, Vasopressin, Venlafaxine, Verapamil, Xipamide, Zolmitriptan, Zotepine

Using this medicine with any of the following may cause an increased risk of certain side effects, but using both drugs may be the best treatment for you. If both medicines are prescribed together, your doctor may change the dose or how often you use one or both of the medicines.

Abarelix, Acarbose, Acetohexamide, Alfuzosin, Aluminum Carbonate, Basic, Aluminum Hydroxide, Aluminum Phosphate, Amlodipine, Arbutamine, Benfluorex, Bunazosin, Bupropion, Calcium Carbonate, Chlorpromazine, Chlorpropamide, Cimetidine, Citalopram, Digoxin, Dihydroergotamine, Dihydroxyaluminum Aminoacetate, Dihydroxyaluminum Sodium Carbonate, Diltiazem, Diphenhydramine, Disopyramide, Doxazosin, Enflurane, Epinephrine, Ergotamine, Escitalopram, Felodipine, Flecainide, Fluoxetine, Fluvoxamine, Gliclazide, Glimepiride, Glipizide, Gliquidone, Glyburide, Guar Gum, Guggul, Hydralazine, Insulin, Insulin Aspart, Recombinant, Insulin Glulisine, Insulin Lispro, Recombinant, Iobenguane I 131, Isoflurane, Lacidipine, Lercanidipine, Lidocaine, Magaldrate, Magnesium Sulfate, Manidipine, Metformin, Methyldopa, Mibefradil, Miglitol, Morphine, Morphine Sulfate Liposome, Moxisylyte, Nicardipine, Nifedipine, Nilvadipine, Nimodipine, Nisoldipine, Nitrendipine, Paroxetine, Pentobarbital, Phenelzine, Phenobarbital, Phenoxybenzamine, Phentolamine, Phenylephrine, Piperine, Pranidipine, Prazosin, Propafenone, Propoxyphene, Quinidine, Rifampin, Rifapentine, Ritonavir, Rizatriptan, Sertraline, St John's Wort, Tamsulosin, Telithromycin, Terazosin, Tolazamide, Tolbutamide, Trimazosin, Troglitazone, Tubocurarine, Urapidil, Zileuton

Interactions with Food/Tobacco/Alcohol—Certain medicines should not be used at or around the time of eating food or eating certain types of food since interactions may occur. Using alcohol or tobacco with certain medicines may also cause interactions to occur. The following interactions have been selected on the basis of their potential significance and are not necessarily all-inclusive.

Using medicines in this class with any of the following is usually not recommended, but may be unavoidable in some cases. If used together, your doctor may change the dose or how often you use your medicine, or give you special instructions about the use of food, alcohol, or tobacco.

Orange Juice

Using this medicine with any of the following may cause an increased risk of certain side effects but may be unavoidable in some cases. If used together, your doctor may change the dose or how often you use this medicine, or give you special instructions about the use of food, alcohol, or tobacco.

Grapefruit Juice

Other medical problems—The presence of other medical problems may affect the use of medicines in this class. Make sure you tell your doctor if you have any other medical problems, especially:

- Allergy, history of (asthma, eczema, hay fever, hives), or
- Bronchitis or
- Emphysema—Severity and duration of allergic reactions to other substances may be increased; in addition, beta-blockers can increase trouble in breathing. Carvedilol should not be used in patients with these conditions.
- Bradycardia (unusually slow heartbeat) or
- Heart or blood vessel disease—There is a risk of further decreased heart function; also, if treatment is stopped suddenly, unwanted effects may occur. Carvedilol should not be used in patients with these conditions.
- Diabetes mellitus (sugar diabetes)—Beta-blockers may cause hyperglycemia (high blood sugar) and circulation problems; in addition, if your diabetes medicine causes your blood sugar to be too low, beta-blockers may cover

up some of the symptoms (fast heartbeat), although they will not cover up other symptoms such as dizziness or sweating

- Kidney disease or
- Liver disease—Effects of beta-blockers may be increased because of slower removal from the body
- Major surgery—May increase risks of problems during surgery. Your doctor may want to stop your treatment with a beta-blocker prior to surgery.
- Mental depression (or history of)—May be increased by beta-blockers
- Myasthenia gravis or
- Psoriasis—Beta-blockers may make these conditions worse
- Overactive thyroid—Stopping beta-blockers suddenly may increase symptoms; beta-blockers may cover up fast heartbeat, which is a sign of overactive thyroid

Proper Use of This Medicine

For patients taking the extended-release capsule or tablet form of this medicine:

- Swallow the capsule or tablet whole.
- Do not crush, break (except metoprolol succinate extended-release tablets, which may be broken in half), or chew before swallowing.

For patients taking the concentrated oral solution form of propranolol:

- This medicine is to be taken by mouth even though it comes in a dropper bottle. The amount you should take is to be measured only with the specially marked dropper.
- Mix the medicine with some water, juice, or a carbonated drink. After drinking all the liquid containing the medicine, rinse the glass with a little more liquid and drink that also, to make sure you get all the medicine. If you prefer, you may mix this medicine with applesauce or pudding instead.
- Mix the medicine immediately before you are going to take it. Throw away any mixed medicine that you do not take immediately. Do not save medicine that has been mixed.

Ask your doctor about checking your pulse rate before and after taking beta-blocking agents. If your doctor tells you to check your pulse regularly while you are taking this medicine, and it is much slower than the rate your doctor has designated, check with your doctor. A pulse rate that is too slow may cause circulation problems.

To help you remember to take your medicine, try to get into the habit of taking it at the same time each day.

For patients taking this medicine for high blood pressure:

- In addition to the use of the medicine your doctor has prescribed, treatment for your high blood pressure may include weight control and care in the types of foods you eat, especially foods high in sodium. Your doctor will tell you which of these are most important for you. You should check with your doctor before changing your diet.
- Many patients who have high blood pressure will not notice any signs of the problem. In fact, many may feel normal. However, if high blood pressure is not treated, it can cause serious problems such as heart failure, blood vessel disease, stroke, or kidney disease.

- Remember that this medicine will not cure your high blood pressure but it does help control it. It is very important that you take your medicine exactly as directed, even if you feel well. You must continue to take it as directed if you expect to lower your blood pressure and keep it down. You may have to take high blood pressure medicine for the rest of your life. Also, it is very important to keep your appointments with your doctor, even if you feel well.

Dosing—The dose medicines in this class will be different for different patients. Follow your doctor's orders or the directions on the label. The following information includes only the average doses of these medicines. If your dose is different, do not change it unless your doctor tells you to do so.

The amount of medicine that you take depends on the strength of the medicine. Also, the number of doses you take each day, the time allowed between doses, and the length of time you take the medicine depend on the medical problem for which you are using the medicine.

- For acebutolol:
  - For oral dosage forms (capsules and tablets):
    - For angina (chest pain) or irregular heartbeat:
      — Adults—200 milligrams (mg) two times a day. The dose may be increased up to a total of 1200 mg a day.
      — Children—Dose must be determined by your doctor.
    - For high blood pressure:
      • Adults—200 to 800 mg a day as a single dose or divided into two daily doses.
      • Children—Dose must be determined by your doctor.

- For atenolol:
  - For oral dosage form (tablets):
    - For angina (chest pain):
      — Adults—50 to 100 mg once a day.
    - For high blood pressure:
      — Adults—25 to 100 mg once a day.
      — Children—Dose must be determined by your doctor.
    - For treatment after a heart attack:
      • Adults—50 mg ten minutes after the last intravenous dose, followed by another 50 mg twelve hours later. Then 100 mg once a day or 50 mg two times a day for six to nine days or until discharge from hospital.
  - For injection dosage form:
    - For treatment of heart attacks:
      — Adults—5 mg given over 5 minutes. The dose is repeated ten minutes later.

- For betaxolol:
  - For oral dosage form (tablets):
    - For high blood pressure:
      — Adults—10 mg once a day. Your doctor may double your dose after seven to fourteen days.
      — Children—Dose must be determined by your doctor.

- For bisoprolol:
  - For oral dosage form (tablets):
    - For high blood pressure:
      — Adults—5 to 10 mg once a day.
      — Children—Dose must be determined by your doctor.

- For carvedilol:
  - For oral dosage form (tablets):
    - For heart failure:
      — Adults—3.125 mg two times a day, taken with food. Your doctor may increase your dose if needed.
      — Children—Use and dose must be determined by your doctor.
    - For high blood pressure:
      - Adults—6.25 mg two times a day, taken with food. Your doctor may increase your dose if needed.
      - Children—Use and dose must be determined by your doctor.
    - For treatment after a heart attack:
      - Adults—6.25 mg two times a day, taken with food. Your doctor may increase your dose if needed.
      - Children—Use and dose must be determined by your doctor.
- For carteolol:
  - For oral dosage form (tablets):
    - For high blood pressure:
      — Adults—2.5 to 10 mg once a day.
      — Children—Dose must be determined by your doctor.
- For labetalol:
  - For high blood pressure:
    - For oral dosage form (tablets):
      — Adults—100 to 400 mg two times a day.
      — Children—Dose must be determined by your doctor.
    - For injection dosage form:
      — Adults—20 mg injected slowly over two minutes with additional injections of 40 and 80 mg given every ten minutes if needed, up to a total of 300 mg; may be given instead as an infusion at a rate of 2 mg per minute to a total dose of 50 to 300 mg.
      — Children—Dose must be determined by your doctor.
- For metoprolol:
  - For regular (short-acting) oral dosage form (tablets):
    - For high blood pressure or angina (chest pain):
      — Adults—100 to 450 mg a day, taken as a single dose or in divided doses.
      — Children—Dose must be determined by your doctor.
    - For treatment after a heart attack:
      — Adults—50 mg every six hours starting fifteen minutes after last intravenous dose. Then 100 mg two times a day for three months to 1 to 3 years.
  - For long-acting oral dosage form (extended-release tablets):
    - For heart failure:
      - Adults—Up to 200 mg once a day.
      - Children—Dose must be determined by your doctor.

- For high blood pressure or angina (chest pain):
  - Adults—Up to 400 mg once a day.
  - Children—Dose must be determined by your doctor.
- For injection dosage form:
  - For treatment of a heart attack:
    - Adults—5 mg every two minutes for three doses.
- For nadolol:
  - For oral dosage form (tablets):
    - For angina (chest pain):
      — Adults—40 to 240 mg once a day.
    - For high blood pressure:
      — Adults—40 to 320 mg once a day.
      — Children—Dose must be determined by your doctor.
- For oxprenolol:
  - For high blood pressure:
    - For regular (short-acting) oral dosage form (tablets):
      — Adults—20 mg three times a day. Your doctor may increase your dose up to 480 mg a day.
      — Children—Dose must be determined by your doctor.
    - For long-acting oral dosage form (extended-release tablets):
      — Adults—120 to 320 mg once a day.
      — Children—Dose must be determined by your doctor.
- For penbutolol:
  - For high blood pressure:
    - For oral dosage form (tablets):
      — Adults—20 mg once a day.
      — Children—Dose must be determined by your doctor.
- For pindolol:
  - For high blood pressure:
    - For oral dosage form (tablets):
      — Adults—5 mg two times a day. Your doctor may increase your dose up to 60 mg a day.
      — Children—Dose must be determined by your doctor.
- For propranolol:
  - For angina (chest pain):
    - For regular (short-acting) oral dosage forms (tablets and oral solution):
      — Adults—80 to 320 mg a day taken in two, three, or four divided doses.
    - For long-acting oral dosage form (extended-release capsules):
      — Adults—80 to 320 mg once a day.
  - For irregular heartbeat:
    - For regular (short-acting) oral dosage forms (tablets and oral solution):
      — Adults—10 to 30 mg three or four times a day.
      — Children—500 micrograms (0.5 mg) to 4 mg per kilogram of body weight a day taken in divided doses.

- For injection dosage form:
  - Adults—1 to 3 mg given at a rate not greater than 1 mg per minute. Dose may be repeated after two minutes and again after four hours if needed.
  - Children—10 to 100 micrograms (0.01 to 0.1 mg) per kilogram of body weight given intravenously every six to eight hours.
- For high blood pressure:
  - For regular (short-acting) oral dosage forms (tablets and oral solution):
    - Adults—40 mg two times a day. Your doctor may increase your dose up to 640 mg a day.
    - Children—500 micrograms (0.5 mg) to 4 mg per kilogram of body weight a day taken in divided doses.
  - For long-acting oral dosage form (extended-release capsules):
    - Adults—80 to 160 mg once a day. Doses up to 640 mg once a day may be needed in some patients.
- For diseased heart muscle (cardiomyopathy):
  - For regular (short-acting) oral dosage forms (tablets and oral solution):
    - Adults—20 to 40 mg three or four times a day.
- For treatment after a heart attack:
  - For regular (short-acting) oral dosage forms (tablets and oral solution):
    - Adults—180 to 240 mg a day taken in divided doses.
- For treating pheochromocytoma:
  - For regular (short-acting) oral dosage forms (tablets and oral solution):
    - Adults—30 to 160 mg a day taken in divided doses.
- For preventing migraine headaches:
  - For regular (short-acting) oral dosage forms (tablets and oral solution):
    - Adults—20 mg four times a day. Your doctor may increase your dose up to 240 mg a day.
  - For long-acting oral dosage form (extended-release capsules):
    - Adults—80 to 240 mg once a day.
- For trembling:
  - For regular (short-acting) oral dosage forms (tablets and oral solution):
    - Adults—40 mg two times a day. Your doctor may increase your dose up to 320 mg a day.
- For sotalol:
  - For irregular heartbeat:
    - For oral dosage form (tablets):
      - Adults—80 mg two times a day. Your doctor may increase your dose up to 320 mg per day taken in two or three divided doses.
      - Children—Dose must be determined by your doctor.

- For timolol:
  - For high blood pressure:
    - For oral dosage form (tablets):
      - Adults—10 mg two times a day. Your doctor may increase your dose up 60 mg per day taken as a single dose or in divided doses.
      - Children—Dose must be determined by your doctor.
  - For treatment after a heart attack:
    - For oral dosage form (tablets):
      - Adults—10 mg two times a day.
  - For preventing migraine headaches:
    - For oral dosage form (tablets):
      - Adults—10 mg two times a day. Your doctor may increase your dose up to 30 mg once a day or in divided doses.

Missed dose—If you miss a dose of this medicine, take it as soon as possible. However, if it is almost time for your next dose, skip the missed dose and go back to your regular dosing schedule. Do not double doses.

Storage—Store the medicine in a closed container at room temperature, away from heat, moisture, and direct light. Keep from freezing.

Keep out of the reach of children.

Do not keep outdated medicine or medicine no longer needed.

Precautions While Using This Medicine

It is important that your doctor check your progress at regular visits. This is to make sure the medicine is working for you and to allow the dosage to be changed if needed.

Do not stop taking this medicine without first checking with your doctor. Your doctor may want you to reduce gradually the amount you are taking before stopping completely. Some conditions may become worse when the medicine is stopped suddenly, and the danger of heart attack is increased in some patients.

Make sure that you have enough medicine on hand to last through weekends, holidays, or vacations. You may want to carry an extra written prescription in your billfold or purse in case of an emergency. You can then have it filled if you run out of medicine while you are away from home.

Tell your doctor right away if you have weight gain or increasing shortness of breath. These could be symptoms of worsening heart failure.

Your doctor may want you to carry medical identification stating that you are taking this medicine.

Before having any kind of surgery (including dental surgery) or emergency treatment, tell the medical doctor or dentist in charge that you are taking this medicine.

For diabetic patients:
- This medicine may cause your blood sugar levels to rise. Also, this medicine may cover up signs of hypoglycemia (low blood sugar), such as change in pulse rate.

This medicine may cause some people to become dizzy, drowsy, or lightheaded. Make sure you know how you react to this medicine before you drive, use machines, or do anything else that could be dangerous if you are dizzy or are not alert. If the problem continues or gets worse, check with your doctor.

Beta-blockers may make you more sensitive to cold temperatures, especially if you have blood circulation problems. Beta-blockers tend to decrease blood circulation in the skin, fingers, and toes. Dress warmly during cold weather and be careful during prolonged exposure to cold, such as in winter sports.

Beta-blockers may cause your skin to be more sensitive to sunlight than it is normally. Exposure to sunlight, even for brief periods of time, may cause a skin rash, itching, redness or other discoloration of the skin, or a severe sunburn. When you begin taking this medicine:

- Stay out of direct sunlight, especially between the hours of 10:00 a.m. and 3:00 p.m., if possible.

- Wear protective clothing, including a hat. Also, wear sunglasses.

- Apply a sun block product that has a skin protection factor (SPF) of at least 15. Some patients may require a product with a higher SPF number, especially if they have a fair complexion. If you have any questions about this, check your health care professional.

- Apply a sun block lipstick that has an SPF of at least 15 to protect your lips.

- Do not use a sunlamp or tanning bed or booth.

- If you have a severe reaction from the sun, check with your doctor.

Chest pain resulting from exercise or physical exertion is usually reduced or prevented by this medicine. This may tempt a patient to be overly active. Make sure you discuss with your doctor a safe amount of exercise for your medical problem.

Before you have any medical tests, tell the doctor in charge that you are taking this medicine. The results of some tests may be affected by this medicine.

Before you have any allergy shots, tell the doctor in charge that you are taking a beta-blocker. Beta-blockers may cause you to have a serious reaction to the allergy shot.

For patients with allergies to foods, medicines, or insect stings:

- There is a chance that this medicine will cause allergic reactions to be worse and harder to treat. If you have a severe allergic reaction while you are being treated with this medicine, check with a doctor right away so that it can be treated. Be sure to tell the doctor that you are taking a beta-blocker.

For patients taking this medicine for high blood pressure:

- Do not take other medicines unless they have been discussed with your doctor. This especially includes over-the-counter (nonprescription) medicines for appetite control, asthma, colds, cough, hay fever, or sinus problems since they may tend to increase your blood pressure.

For patients taking labetalol by mouth:

- Dizziness, lightheadedness, or fainting may occur, especially when you get up from a lying or sitting position. This is more likely to occur when you first start taking labetalol or when the dose is increased. Getting up slowly may help. When you get up from lying down, sit on the edge of the bed with your feet dangling for 1 to 2 minutes. Then stand up slowly. If the problem continues or gets worse, check with your doctor.

- The dizziness, lightheadedness, or fainting is also more likely to occur if you drink alcohol, stand for long periods of time, or exercise, or if the weather is hot. While you are taking this medicine, be careful to limit the amount of alcohol you drink. Also, use extra care during exercise or hot weather or if you must stand for long periods of time.

For patients receiving labetalol by injection:

- It is very important that you lie down flat while receiving labetalol and for up to 3 hours afterward. If you try to get up too soon, you may become dizzy or faint. Do not try to sit or stand until your doctor or nurse tells you to do so.

Side Effects of This Medicine

Along with its needed effects, a medicine may cause some unwanted effects. Although not all of these side effects may occur, if they do occur they may need medical attention.

Check with your doctor as soon as possible if any of the following side effects occur:

Less common

Breathing difficulty and/or wheezing; cold hands and feet; mental depression; shortness of breath; slow heartbeat (especially less than 50 beats per minute); swelling of ankles, feet, and/or lower legs

Rare

Back pain or joint pain; chest pain; confusion (especially in elderly patients); dark urine— for acebutolol, bisoprolol, or labetalol; dizziness or lightheadedness when getting up from a lying or sitting position; fever and sore throat; hallucinations (seeing, hearing, or feeling things that are not there); irregular heartbeat; red, scaling, or crusted skin; skin rash; unusual bleeding and bruising; yellow eyes or skin— for acebutolol, bisoprolol, or labetalol

Get emergency help immediately if any of the following symptoms of overdose occur:

Slow heartbeat; dizziness (severe) or fainting; fast or irregular heartbeat; difficulty in breathing; bluish-colored fingernails or palms of hands; convulsions (seizures)

Some side effects may occur that usually do not need medical attention. These side effects may go away during treatment as your body adjusts to the medicine. Also, your health care professional may be able to tell you about ways to prevent or reduce some of these side effects. Check with your health care professional if any of the following side effects continue or are bothersome or if you have any questions about them:

More common

Decreased sexual ability; dizziness or lightheadedness; drowsiness (slight); trouble in sleeping; unusual tiredness or weakness

Less common or rare

Anxiety and/or nervousness; changes in taste— for labetalol only; constipation; diarrhea; dry, sore eyes; frequent urination— for acebutolol and carteolol only; itching of skin; nausea or vomiting; nightmares and vivid dreams; numbness and/or tingling of fingers and/or toes; numbness and/or tingling of skin, especially on scalp— for labetalol only; stomach discomfort; stuffy nose

Although not all of the side effects listed above have been reported for all of these medicines, they have been reported for at least one of them. Since all of the beta-adrenergic blocking agents are very similar, any of the above side effects may occur with any of these medicines. However, they may be more or less common with some agents than with others.

After you have been taking a beta-blocker for a while, it may cause unpleasant or even harmful effects if you stop taking it too suddenly. After you stop taking this medicine or while you are gradually reducing the amount you are taking, check with your doctor right away if any of the following occur:

> Chest pain; fast or irregular heartbeat; general feeling of discomfort or illness or weakness; headache; shortness of breath (sudden); sweating; tremblingFor patients taking labetalol: You may notice a tingling feeling on your scalp when you first begin to take labetalol. This is to be expected and usually goes away after you have been taking labetalol for a while.

Other side effects not listed may also occur in some patients. If you notice any other effects, check with your healthcare professional.

BETAMETHASONE AND CLOTRIMAZOLE (Topical route) - bay-ta-METH-a-sone, kloe-TRIM-a-zole

Commonly used brand name(s)

In the U.S.—
   Lotrisone

Available Dosage Forms:

• Cream

• Lotion

Therapeutic Class: Anti-Infective/Anti-Inflammatory Combination
Pharmacologic Class: Betamethasone

Uses For This Medicine

Betamethasone and clotrimazole combination is used to treat fungus infections. Betamethasone, a corticosteroid (cortisone-like medicine or steroid), is used to help relieve redness, swelling, itching, and other discomfort of fungus infections. Clotrimazole works by killing the fungus or preventing its growth.

Betamethasone and clotrimazole cream is applied to the skin to treat:

• Athlete's foot (ringworm of the foot; tinea pedis);

• Jock itch (ringworm of the groin; tinea cruris); and

• Ringworm of the body (tinea corporis).

This medicine may also be used for other fungus infections of the skin as determined by your doctor.

This medicine is available only with your doctor's prescription.

Before Using This Medicine

In deciding to use a medicine, the risks of taking the medicine must be weighed against the good it will do. This is a decision you and your doctor will make. For this medicine, the following should be considered:

Allergies—Tell your doctor if you have ever had any unusual or allergic reaction to this medicine or any other medicines. Also tell your health care professional if you have any other types of allergies, such as to foods, dyes, preservatives, or animals. For non-prescription products, read the label or package ingredients carefully.

Pediatric—Clotrimazole and betamethasone combination may rarely cause serious side effects. Some of these side effects may be more likely to occur in children, who may absorb greater amounts of this medicine than adults do. Long-term use in children may affect growth and development as well. Therefore, it is especially important that you discuss with the child's doctor the good that this medicine may do, as well as the risks of using it.

Geriatric—Many medicines have not been studied specifically in older people. Therefore, it may not be known whether they work exactly the same way they do in younger adults or if they cause different side effects or problems in older people. There is no specific information comparing use of clotrimazole and betamethasone combination in the elderly with use in other age groups.

Other medicines—

Using this medicine with any of the following medicines is not recommended. Your doctor may decide not to treat you with this medication or change some of the other medicines you take.

Bupropion, Dihydroergotamine, Ergoloid Mesylates, Ergonovine, Ergotamine, Methylergonovine, Rotavirus Vaccine, Live

Interactions with Food/Tobacco/Alcohol—Certain medicines should not be used at or around the time of eating food or eating certain types of food since interactions may occur. Using alcohol or tobacco with certain medicines may also cause interactions to occur. Discuss with your healthcare professional the use of your medicine with food, alcohol, or tobacco.

Other medical problems—The presence of other medical problems may affect the use of this medicine. Make sure you tell your doctor if you have any other medical problems, especially:

• Bacteria infections of the skin or

• Diaper dermatitis (diaper rash) on your child or

• Skin diseases causing impaired circulation, such as stasis dermatitis—Betamethasone may make the condition worse

• Herpes or

• Vaccinia (cowpox) or

• Varicella (chickenpox) or

• Other virus infections of the skin—Betamethasone may speed up the spread of virus infections

• Tuberculosis (TB) of the skin—Betamethasone may make a TB infection worse

Proper Use of This Medicine

Before applying this medicine, wash the affected area with soap and water, and dry thoroughly.

Do not use this medicine in the eyes.

To use:

- Check with your doctor before using this medicine on any other skin problems. It should not be used on bacterial or virus infections or on diaper rash. Also, it should only be used on certain kinds of fungus infections of the skin.
- Apply a thin layer of this medicine to the affected area(s) and surrounding skin. Rub in gently and thoroughly.

The use of any kind of occlusive dressing (airtight covering, such as kitchen plastic wrap) over this medicine may increase absorption of the medicine and the chance of irritation and other side effects. Therefore, do not bandage, wrap, or apply any occlusive dressing over this medicine unless directed by your doctor. Also, wear loose-fitting clothing when using this medicine on the groin area. When using this medicine on the diaper area of children, avoid tight-fitting diapers and plastic pants.

To help clear up your skin infection completely, keep using this medicine for the full time of treatment, even if your symptoms have disappeared. Do not miss any doses. However, do not use this medicine more often or for a longer time than your doctor ordered. To do so may increase absorption through your skin and the chance of side effects. In addition, too much use, especially on thin skin areas (for example, face, armpits, genitals [sex organs], between the toes, groin), may result in thinning of the skin and in stretch marks.

Dosing—The dose of this medicine will be different for different patients. Follow your doctor's orders or the directions on the label. The following information includes only the average doses of this medicine. If your dose is different, do not change it unless your doctor tells you to do so.

The amount of medicine that you take depends on the strength of the medicine. Also, the number of doses you take each day, the time allowed between doses, and the length of time you take the medicine depend on the medical problem for which you are using the medicine.

- For topical cream dosage form:
  - For jock itch (ringworm of the groin; tinea cruris) or ringworm of the body (tinea corporis):
    - Adults and children 12 years of age and over— Apply to the affected skin and surrounding area(s) two times a day, morning and evening, for 2 weeks.
    - Children up to 12 years of age—Use and dose must be determined by your doctor.
  - For athlete's foot (ringworm of the foot; tinea pedis):
    - Adults and children 12 years of age and over— Apply to the affected skin and surrounding area(s) two times a day, morning and evening, for 4 weeks.
    - Children up to 12 years of age—Use and dose must be determined by your doctor.

Missed dose—If you miss a dose of this medicine, apply it as soon as possible. However, if it is almost time for your next dose, skip the missed dose and go back to your regular dosing schedule.

Storage—Store the medicine in a closed container at room temperature, away from heat, moisture, and direct light. Keep from freezing.

Keep out of the reach of children.

Do not keep outdated medicine or medicine no longer needed.

Precautions While Using This Medicine

If your skin infection does not improve within 1 week for jock itch or ringworm of the body and 2 weeks for athlete's foot, or if it becomes worse, check with your doctor. Redness and itching should get better within 3 to 5 days of therapy.

To help clear up your skin infection completely and to help make sure it does not return, the following good health habits are important:

- For patients using this medicine for athlete's foot:
  - Carefully dry the feet, especially between the toes, after bathing.
  - Avoid wearing socks made from wool or synthetic materials (for example, rayon or nylon). Instead, wear clean, cotton socks and change them daily or more often if your feet sweat freely.
  - Wear well-ventilated shoes (for example, shoes with holes) or sandals.
  - Use a bland, absorbent powder (for example, talcum powder) or an antifungal powder freely between the toes, on the feet, and in socks and shoes once or twice a day. Be sure to use the powder after clotrimazole and betamethasone cream has been applied and has disappeared into the skin. Do not use the powder as the only treatment for your fungus infection.

These measures will help keep the feet cool and dry.

- For patients using this medicine for jock itch:
  - Carefully dry the groin area after bathing.
  - Avoid wearing underwear that is tight-fitting or made from synthetic materials (for example, rayon or nylon). Instead, wear loose-fitting, cotton underwear.
  - Use a bland, absorbent powder (for example, talcum powder) or an antifungal powder freely once or twice a day. Be sure to use the powder after clotrimazole and betamethasone cream has been applied and has disappeared into the skin. Do not use the powder as the only treatment for your fungus infection.

These measures will help reduce chafing and irritation and will also help keep the groin area cool and dry.

- For patients using this medicine for ringworm of the body:
  - Carefully dry yourself after bathing.
  - Avoid too much heat and humidity if possible. Try to keep moisture from building up on affected areas of the body.
  - Wear well-ventilated clothing.
  - Use a bland, absorbent powder (for example, talcum powder) or an antifungal powder freely once or twice a day. Be sure to use the powder after clotrimazole and betamethasone cream has been applied and has disappeared into the skin. Do not use the powder as the only treatment for your fungus infection.

These measures will help keep the affected areas cool and dry.

If you have any questions about this, check with your health care professional.

For diabetic patients:
- Rarely, the corticosteroid in this medicine may cause higher blood and urine sugar levels. This is more likely to occur if you have severe diabetes and are using large amounts of this medicine. Check with your doctor before changing your diet or the dosage of your diabetes medicine.

Side Effects of This Medicine

Along with its needed effects, a medicine may cause some unwanted effects. Although not all of these side effects may occur, if they do occur they may need medical attention.

Check with your doctor immediately if any of the following side effects occur:

Rare

Numbness of the hands and feet; rash; secondary infection; swelling

Less common

Blistering, burning, itching, peeling, dryness, redness, or other signs of skin irritation not present before use of this medicine; hives; stinging

Check with your doctor as soon as possible if any of the following side effects occur:

Acne or oily skin; increased hair growth, especially on the face and body; increased loss of hair, especially on the scalp; pus in the hair follicles; reddish purple lines on arms, face, legs, trunk, or groin; redness and scaling around the mouth; softening of the skin; thinning of skin with easy bruising; white spots

Other side effects not listed may also occur in some patients. If you notice any other effects, check with your healthcare professional.

BETHANECHOL (Oral route, Subcutaneous route) - be-THAN-e-kole

Commonly used brand name(s)
In the U.S.—
Urecholine

Available Dosage Forms:
- Tablet
- Elixir
- Solution

Therapeutic Class: Urinary Antispasmodic
Pharmacologic Class: Cholinergic

Uses For This Medicine

Bethanechol is taken to treat certain disorders of the urinary tract or bladder. It helps to cause urination and emptying of the bladder. Bethanechol may also be used for other conditions as determined by your doctor.

Bethanechol is available only with your doctor's prescription.

Once a medicine has been approved for marketing for a certain use, experience may show that it is also useful for other medical problems. Although these uses are not included in product labeling, bethanechol is used in certain patients with the following medical conditions:
- Certain stomach problems
- Gastroesophageal reflux (caused by acid in the stomach washing back up into the esophagus)
- Megacolon (an abnormally large or dilated colon)

Before Using This Medicine

In deciding to use a medicine, the risks of taking the medicine must be weighed against the good it will do. This is a decision you and your doctor will make. For this medicine, the following should be considered:

Allergies—Tell your doctor if you have ever had any unusual or allergic reaction to this medicine or any other medicines. Also tell your health care professional if you have any other types of allergies, such as to foods, dyes, preservatives, or animals. For non-prescription products, read the label or package ingredients carefully.

Pediatric—Although there is no specific information comparing use of bethanechol in children with use in other age groups, this medicine is not expected to cause different side effects or problems in children than it does in adults.

Geriatric—Many medicines have not been studied specifically in older people. Therefore, it may not be known whether they work exactly the same way they do in younger adults. Although there is no specific information comparing use of bethanechol in the elderly with use in other age groups, it is not expected to cause different side effects or problems in older people than it does in younger adults.

Pregnancy—

	Pregnancy Category	Explanation
All Trimesters	C	Animal studies have shown an adverse effect and there are no adequate studies in pregnant women OR no animal studies have been conducted and there are no adequate studies in pregnant women.

Breast Feeding—There are no adequate studies in women for determining infant risk when using this medication during breastfeeding. Weigh the potential benefits against the potential risks before taking this medication while breastfeeding.

Other medicines—

Using this medicine with any of the following medicines may cause an increased risk of certain side effects, but using both drugs may be the best treatment for you. If both medicines are prescribed together, your doctor may change the dose or how often you use one or both of the medicines.

Betel Nut

Interactions with Food/Tobacco/Alcohol—Certain medicines should not be used at or around the time of eating food or eating certain types of food since interactions may occur. Using alcohol or tobacco with certain medicines may also cause interactions to occur. Discuss with your healthcare professional the use of your medicine with food, alcohol, or tobacco.

Other medical problems—The presence of other medical problems may affect the use of this medicine. Make sure you

tell your doctor if you have any other medical problems, especially:

- Asthma or
- Epilepsy or
- Heart or blood vessel disease or
- Intestinal blockage or
- Low blood pressure or
- Parkinson's disease or
- Recent bladder or intestinal surgery or
- Stomach ulcer or other stomach problems or
- Urinary tract blockage or difficult urination—Bethanechol may make these conditions worse
- High blood pressure—Bethanechol may cause a rapid fall in blood pressure
- Overactive thyroid—Bethanechol may further increase the chance of heart problems

Proper Use of This Medicine

Take this medicine on an empty stomach (either 1 hour before or 2 hours after meals) to lessen the possibility of nausea and vomiting, unless otherwise directed by your doctor.

Take this medicine only as directed. Do not take more of it, do not take it more often, and do not take it for a longer time than your doctor ordered. To do so may increase the chance of side effects.

Dosing—The dose of this medicine will be different for different patients. Follow your doctor's orders or the directions on the label. The following information includes only the average doses of this medicine. If your dose is different, do not change it unless your doctor tells you to do so.

The amount of medicine that you take depends on the strength of the medicine. Also, the number of doses you take each day, the time allowed between doses, and the length of time you take the medicine depend on the medical problem for which you are using the medicine.

- To empty the bladder:
  - For oral dosage form (tablets):
    - Adults—25 to 50 milligrams (mg) three or four times a day.
    - Children—Dose is based on body weight and must be determined by your doctor. The usual dose is 0.6 mg per kilogram (kg) (0.27 mg per pound) of body weight a day. This dose is divided into smaller doses and taken three or four times a day.
  - For injection dosage form:
    - Adults—5 mg injected under the skin three or four times a day.
    - Children—Dose is based on body weight and must be determined by your doctor. The usual dose is 0.2 mg per kg (0.09 mg per pound) of body weight a day. This dose is divided into smaller doses, which are injected under the skin three or four times a day.

Missed dose—If you miss a dose of this medicine, take it as soon as possible. However, if it is almost time for your next dose, skip the missed dose and go back to your regular dosing schedule. Do not double doses.

Storage—Store the medicine in a closed container at room temperature, away from heat, moisture, and direct light. Keep from freezing.

Keep out of the reach of children.

Do not keep outdated medicine or medicine no longer needed.

Precautions While Using This Medicine

Dizziness, lightheadedness, or fainting may occur, especially when you get up from a lying or sitting position. Getting up slowly may help lessen this problem.

Side Effects of This Medicine

Along with its needed effects, a medicine may cause some unwanted effects. Although not all of these side effects may occur, if they do occur they may need medical attention.

Check with your doctor as soon as possible if any of the following side effects occur:
> *Rare*—more common with the injection
> Shortness of breath, wheezing, or tightness in chest

Some side effects may occur that usually do not need medical attention. These side effects may go away during treatment as your body adjusts to the medicine. Also, your health care professional may be able to tell you about ways to prevent or reduce some of these side effects. Check with your health care professional if any of the following side effects continue or are bothersome or if you have any questions about them:
> *Less common or rare*—more common with the injection
> Belching; blurred vision or change in near or distance vision; diarrhea; dizziness or lightheadedness; feeling faint; frequent urge to urinate; headache; increased watering of mouth or sweating; nausea or vomiting; redness or flushing of skin or feeling of warmth; seizures; sleeplessness, nervousness, or jitters; stomach discomfort or pain

Other side effects not listed may also occur in some patients. If you notice any other effects, check with your healthcare professional.

BEVACIZUMAB   (Intravenous route) -
be-va-SIZ-yoo-mab

Black Box Warning

- GASTROINTESTINAL PERFORATIONS/WOUND HEALING COMPLICATIONS
  - Bevacizumab administration can result in the development of gastrointestinal perforation and wound dehiscence, in some instances resulting in fatality. Gastrointestinal perforation, sometimes associated with intra-abdominal abscess, occurred throughout treatment with bevacizumab (i.e., was not correlated to duration of exposure). The incidence of gastrointestinal perforation in patients receiving bolus-IFL with bevacizumab was 2%. The typical presentation was reported as abdominal pain associated with symptoms such as constipation and vomiting. Gastrointestinal perforation should be included in the differential diagnosis of patients presenting with abdominal pain on bevacizumab. Bevacizumab therapy should be permanently discontinued in patients with gastroin-

testinal perforation or wound dehiscence requiring medical intervention. The appropriate interval between termination of bevacizumab and subsequent elective surgery required to avoid the risks of impaired wound healing/wound dehiscence has not been determined.

- HEMORRHAGE
  - Serious, and in some cases fatal, hemoptysis has occurred in patients with non-small cell lung cancer treated with chemotherapy and bevacizumab. In a small study, the incidence of serious or fatal hemoptysis was 31% in patients with squamous histology and 4% in patients with adenocarcinoma receiving bevacizumab as compared to no cases in patients treated with chemotherapy alone. Patients with recent hemoptysis should not receive bevacizumab.

Commonly used brand name(s)

In the U.S.—
    Avastin

Available Dosage Forms:
- Solution

Therapeutic Class: Immunological Agent
Pharmacologic Class: Monoclonal Antibody

Uses For This Medicine

Bevacizumab is a substance that helps the body fight cancer. It prevents the growth of certain types of blood vessels to cancer cells. This helps to decrease the growth of cancer cells by starving the cells of nutrients needed to grow.

Bevacizumab is to be administered only by or under the immediate supervision of your doctor.

Once a medicine has been approved for marketing for a certain use, experience may show that it is also useful for other medical problems. Although this use is not included in product labeling, bevacizumab is used in certain patients with the following medical conditions:

- Metastatic breast carcinoma, HER2–negative disease, first line therapy in combination with paclitaxel
- Non-squamous non small cell lung cancer, advanced/metastatic, first-line treatment, in combination with paclitaxel and carboplatin

---

Before Using This Medicine

In deciding to use a medicine, the risks of taking the medicine must be weighed against the good it will do. This is a decision you and your doctor will make. For this medicine, the following should be considered:

Allergies—Tell your doctor if you have ever had any unusual or allergic reaction to this medicine or any other medicines. Also tell your health care professional if you have any other types of allergies, such as to foods, dyes, preservatives, or animals. For non-prescription products, read the label or package ingredients carefully.

Pediatric—Studies on this medicine have been done only in adult patients, and there is no information comparing use of bevacizumab in children with use in other age groups. However, studies of this medicine in animals have shown an increase in side effects.

Geriatric—Specific side effects may be especially likely to occur in elderly patients, who are usually more sensitive than younger adults to the effects of bevacizumab.

Pregnancy—

	Pregnancy Category	Explanation
All Trimesters	C	Animal studies have shown an adverse effect and there are no adequate studies in pregnant women OR no animal studies have been conducted and there are no adequate studies in pregnant women.

Breast Feeding—There are no adequate studies in women for determining infant risk when using this medication during breastfeeding. Weigh the potential benefits against the potential risks before taking this medication while breastfeeding.

Other medicines—Although certain medicines should not be used together at all, in other cases two different medicines may be used together even if an interaction might occur. In these cases, your doctor may want to change the dose, or other precautions may be necessary. Tell your healthcare professional if you are taking any other prescription or nonprescription (over-the-counter [OTC]) medicine.

Interactions with Food/Tobacco/Alcohol—Certain medicines should not be used at or around the time of eating food or eating certain types of food since interactions may occur. Using alcohol or tobacco with certain medicines may also cause interactions to occur. Discuss with your healthcare professional the use of your medicine with food, alcohol, or tobacco.

Other medical problems—The presence of other medical problems may affect the use of this medicine. Make sure you tell your doctor if you have any other medical problems, especially:

- Angina
- Bleeding problems or
- High blood pressure or
- Heart attack or
- Heart failure or
- Hypersensitivity to bevacizumab or
- Kidney problems or
- Liver problems or
- Protein in the urine or
- Stroke or
- Stomach/Intestinal problems or
- Wound healing problems—May be worsened by bevacizumab.

Proper Use of This Medicine

Dosing—The dose of this medicine will be different for different patients. Follow your doctor's orders or the directions on the label. The following information includes only the average doses of this medicine. If your dose is different, do not change it unless your doctor tells you to do so.

The amount of medicine that you take depends on the strength of the medicine. Also, the number of doses you take each day, the time allowed between doses, and the length of time you take the medicine depend on the medical problem for which you are using the medicine.

Be careful when using a regular toothbrush, dental floss, or toothpick. Your medical doctor, dentist, or nurse may recommend other ways to clean your teeth and gums. Check with your medical doctor before having any medical work done.

Bevacizumab is often given together with certain other medicines. If you are using a combination of medicines, make sure that you take each one at the proper time and do not mix them. Ask your health care professional to help you plan a way to remember to take your medicines at the right times.

Storage—Store in the refrigerator. Do not freeze.

Keep out of the reach of children.

Do not keep outdated medicine or medicine no longer needed.

Precautions While Using This Medicine

It is very important that your doctor check your progress at regular visits to make sure that this medicine is working properly and to check for unwanted effects.

Other medicines: Do not take other medicines unless they have been discussed with your doctor.

Surgery: This medicine should not be taken within several weeks before or after surgery.

Side Effects of This Medicine

Along with its needed effects, a medicine may cause some unwanted effects. Although not all of these side effects may occur, if they do occur they may need medical attention.

Check with your doctor immediately if any of the following side effects occur:

More common
Black, tarry stools; bleeding gums; body aches or pain; chest pain; chills; cloudy urine; convulsions; cough; cracks in the skin; decreased urine output; dilated neck veins; ear congestion; extreme fatigue; fever; high blood pressure; irregular breathing; irregular heartbeat; lack or loss of strength; loss of appetite; loss of heat from the body; loss of voice; mood changes; nasal congestion; pain; painful or difficult urination; pinpoint red spots on skin; redness; runny nose; shortness of breath; sore throat; sores, ulcers, or white spots on lips or in mouth; swelling of face, fingers, feet, or lower legs; swollen glands; tightness in chest; troubled breathing; unusual bleeding or bruising; unusual tiredness or weakness; vomiting of blood or material that looks like coffee grounds; watery or bloody diarrhea; weight gain; wheezing; yellow skin

Less common
Difficulty having a bowel movement (stool); fainting; stomach tenderness

Rare
Blisters; coma; confusion; convulsions; decreased urine output; increased thirst; muscle pain or cramps; open sores; pale skin; white spots on lips or in mouth

Some side effects may occur that usually do not need medical attention. These side effects may go away during treatment as your body adjusts to the medicine. Also, your health care professional may be able to tell you about ways to prevent or reduce some of these side effects. Check with your health

care professional if any of the following side effects continue or are bothersome or if you have any questions about them:

More common
Belching; bloody nose; change in walking and balance; clumsiness or unsteadiness; excess flow of tears; hair loss; heartburn; indigestion; low blood pressure; thinning of hair; weight loss

BEXAROTENE   (Oral route) - beks-AIR-oh-teen

Black Box Warning

Bexarotene capsules are a member of the retinoid class of drugs that is associated with birth defects in humans. Bexarotene capsules also caused birth defects when administered orally to pregnant rats. Bexarotene capsules must not be administered to a pregnant woman.

Commonly used brand name(s)

In the U.S.—
Targretin

Available Dosage Forms:
• Capsule

Therapeutic Class: Antineoplastic Agent

Uses For This Medicine

Bexarotene belongs to the group of medicines known as retinoids. It is used to treat a certain type of cancer called cutaneous T-cell lymphoma. It works by interfering with the growth of the cancerous cells.

This medicine is available only with your doctor's prescription.

Before Using This Medicine

In deciding to use a medicine, the risks of taking the medicine must be weighed against the good it will do. This is a decision you and your doctor will make. For this medicine, the following should be considered:

Allergies—Tell your doctor if you have ever had any unusual or allergic reaction to this medicine or any other medicines. Also tell your health care professional if you have any other types of allergies, such as to foods, dyes, preservatives, or animals. For non-prescription products, read the label or package ingredients carefully.

Pediatric—Studies of this medicine have been done only in adult patients, and there is no specific information comparing the use of bexarotene in children with use in other age groups.

Geriatric—This medicine has been tested in patients 60 years of age or older and has not been shown to cause different side effects or problems in older people than it does in younger adults. However, elderly patients may be more sensitive to the effects of bexarotene.

Pregnancy—

	Pregnancy Category	Explanation
All Trimesters	X	Studies in animals or pregnant women have demonstrated positive evidence of fetal abnormalities. This drug should not be used in women who are or may become pregnant because the risk clearly outweighs any possible benefit.

Breast Feeding—There are no adequate studies in women for determining infant risk when using this medication during breastfeeding. Weigh the potential benefits against the potential risks before taking this medication while breastfeeding.

Other medicines—

Using this medicine with any of the following medicines may cause an increased risk of certain side effects, but using both drugs may be the best treatment for you. If both medicines are prescribed together, your doctor may change the dose or how often you use one or both of the medicines.

Desogestrel, Drospirenone, Erythromycin, Estradiol Cypionate, Ethinyl Estradiol, Etonogestrel, Fosphenytoin, Gemfibrozil, Gestodene, Itraconazole, Ketoconazole, Levonorgestrel, Medroxyprogesterone, Mestranol, Norelgestromin, Norethindrone, Norgestimate, Norgestrel, Phenobarbital, Phenytoin, Rifampin, Tamoxifen, Vitamin A

Interactions with Food/Tobacco/Alcohol—Certain medicines should not be used at or around the time of eating food or eating certain types of food since interactions may occur. Using alcohol or tobacco with certain medicines may also cause interactions to occur. The following interactions have been selected on the basis of their potential significance and are not necessarily all-inclusive.

Using this medicine with any of the following may cause an increased risk of certain side effects but may be unavoidable in some cases. If used together, your doctor may change the dose or how often you use this medicine, or give you special instructions about the use of food, alcohol, or tobacco.

Grapefruit Juice

Other medical problems—The presence of other medical problems may affect the use of this medicine. Make sure you tell your doctor if you have any other medical problems, especially:

- Bone marrow depression, existing or
- Infection—There may be an increased risk of infections or worsening of infections because of the body's reduced ability to fight them
- Cataracts—May cause new cataracts or worsen previous cataracts
- Chickenpox (including recent exposure) or
- Herpes zoster (shingles)—Risk of severe disease affecting other parts of the body
- Diabetes mellitus—May be more likely to experience low blood sugar (hypoglycemia).
- High cholesterol—Bexarotene can cause an increase in cholesterol levels.
- Kidney disease—May increase the chance of side effects

- Liver disease—Effects of bexarotene may be increased because of slower removal from the body.
- Pancreatitis or
- Risk factors for pancreatitis, such as:
  - Drinking large quantities of alcohol or
  - Problems with your gallbladder or biliary tract or
  - Type 2 diabetes mellitus that is not well-controlled or
  - High cholesterol that is not well-controlled or
  - Taking medicines that cause high levels of triglycerides (fat-like substances) or
  - Taking medicines that are toxic to the pancreas or
  - Prior pancreatitis—Bexarotene can cause an increase in triglyceride levels which can cause inflammation of the pancreas.
- Photosensitivity—Bexarotene may cause increased sensitivity of the skin to sunlight

Proper Use of This Medicine

Use this medicine exactly as directed by your doctor. Do not use more or less of it, and do not use it more often than your doctor ordered. The exact amount of medicine you need has been carefully worked out. Using too much will increase the risk of side effects, while using too little may not improve your condition.

Dosing—The dose of this medicine will be different for different patients. Follow your doctor's orders or the directions on the label. The following information includes only the average doses of this medicine. If your dose is different, do not change it unless your doctor tells you to do so.

The amount of medicine that you take depends on the strength of the medicine. Also, the number of doses you take each day, the time allowed between doses, and the length of time you take the medicine depend on the medical problem for which you are using the medicine.

- For oral dosage form (capsule):
  - For cutaneous T-cell lymphoma:
    - Adults—Dose is based on body size and must be determined by your doctor. The usual dose is 300 milligrams (mg) for each square meter of body surface area taken once a day with a meal. Your dose may then be adjusted by your doctor.
    - Children—Use and dose must be determined by your doctor.

Missed dose—If you miss a dose of this medicine, take it as soon as possible. However, if it is almost time for your next dose, skip the missed dose and go back to your regular dosing schedule. Do not double doses.

Storage—Store the medicine in a closed container at room temperature, away from heat, moisture, and direct light. Keep from freezing.

Keep out of the reach of children.

Do not keep outdated medicine or medicine no longer needed.

Ask your healthcare professional how you should dispose of any medicine you do not use.

Precautions While Using This Medicine

It is very important that your doctor check your progress at regular visits to make sure that this medicine is working properly and to check for unwanted effects.

While you are being treated with bexarotene, and after you stop treatment with it, do not have any immunizations (vaccinations) without your doctor's approval. Bexarotene may lower your body's resistance, and there is a chance you might get the infection that the immunization is meant to prevent. In addition, other persons living in your household should not take oral polio vaccine, since there is a chance they could pass the polio virus on to you. Also, avoid persons who have taken oral polio vaccine within the last several months. Do not get close to them, and do not stay in the room with them for very long. If you cannot take these precautions, you should consider wearing a protective face mask that covers the nose and mouth.

Bexarotene can temporarily lower the number of white blood cells in your blood, increasing the chance of getting an infection. It can also lower the number of platelets, which are necessary for proper blood clotting. If this occurs, there are certain precautions you can take, especially when your blood count is low, to reduce the risk of infection or bleeding:

- If you can, avoid people with infections. Check with your doctor immediately if you think you are getting an infection or if you get a fever or chills, cough or hoarseness, lower back or side pain, or painful or difficult urination.
- Check with your doctor immediately if you notice any unusual bleeding or bruising; black, tarry stools; blood in urine or stools; or pinpoint red spots on your skin.
- Be careful when using a regular toothbrush, dental floss, or toothpick. Your medical doctor, dentist, or nurse may recommend other ways to clean your teeth and gums. Check with your medical doctor before having any dental work done.
- Do not touch your eyes or the inside of your nose unless you have just washed your hands and have not touched anything else in the meantime.
- Be careful not to cut yourself when you are using sharp objects such as a safety razor or fingernail or toenail cutters.
- Avoid contact sports or other situations where bruising or injury could occur.

Bexarotene may cause your skin to be more sensitive to sunlight than it is normally. Exposure to sunlight, even for brief periods of time, may cause a skin rash, itching, redness or other discoloration of the skin, or a severe sunburn. When you begin taking this medicine:

- Stay out of direct sunlight, especially between the hours of 10:00 a.m. and 3:00 p.m., if possible.
- Wear protective clothing, including a hat. Also, wear sunglasses.
- Apply a sun block product that has a skin protection factor (SPF) of at least 15. Some patients may require a product with a higher SPF number, especially if they have a fair complexion. If you have any questions about this, check with your health care professional.
- Apply a sun block lipstick that has an SPF of at least 15 to protect your lips.
- Do not use a sunlamp or tanning bed or booth.

Side Effects of This Medicine

Along with its needed effects, a medicine may cause some unwanted effects. Although not all of these side effects may occur, if they do occur they may need medical attention.

Since this medication is given in varying doses, the actual frequency of side effects may vary. In general, side effects are less common with lower doses than with higher doses.

Check with your doctor as soon as possible if any of the following side effects occur:

More common
 Unusual tiredness or weakness; skin rash or other skin and mucous membrane lesions; fever; increase in lipid or cholesterol levels; coldness, dry, puffy skin or weight gain; chills, cough, hoarseness, lower back or side pain or painful or difficult urination; swelling of the arms, feet, hands, or legs

Less common
 Severe stomach pain with nausea or vomiting; shortness of breath; yellow eyes or skin

Some side effects may occur that usually do not need medical attention. These side effects may go away during treatment as your body adjusts to the medicine. Also, your health care professional may be able to tell you about ways to prevent or reduce some of these side effects. Check with your health care professional if any of the following side effects continue or are bothersome or if you have any questions about them:

More common
 Abdominal pain; hair loss; loss of appetite; loss of strength or energy, tiredness or weakness; back pain; diarrhea; dry skin; general feeling of discomfort or illness; trouble in sleeping; headache; nausea or vomiting

Other side effects not listed may also occur in some patients. If you notice any other effects, check with your healthcare professional.

BEXAROTENE   (Topical route) - beks-AIR-oh-teen

Commonly used brand name(s)

In the U.S.—
 Targretin

Available Dosage Forms:
- Gel/Jelly

Therapeutic Class: Antineoplastic, Dermatological

Uses For This Medicine

Bexarotene belongs to the group of medicines known as retinoids (RET-i-noyds). When applied to the skin, it is used to treat a form a cancer called cutaneous T-cell lymphoma (CTCL). It acts by interfering with the growth of cells of the tumor. It may be used after other drugs have been tried, and the tumor is still a problem.

This medicine is available only with your doctor's prescription.

Before Using This Medicine

In deciding to use a medicine, the risks of taking the medicine must be weighed against the good it will do. This is a decision you and your doctor will make. For this medicine, the following should be considered:

Allergies—Tell your doctor if you have ever had any unusual or allergic reaction to this medicine or any other medicines. Also tell your health care professional if you have any other types of allergies, such as to foods, dyes, preservatives, or animals. For non-prescription products, read the label or package ingredients carefully.

Pediatric—Studies of this medicine have been done only in adult patients, and there is no specific information comparing the use of bexarotene in children with use in other age groups.

Geriatric—This medicine has been tested in patients 65 years of age or older and has not been shown to cause different side effects or problems in older people than it does in younger adults. However, elderly patients may be more sensitive to the effects of bexarotene.

Pregnancy—

	Pregnancy Category	Explanation
All Trimesters	X	Studies in animals or pregnant women have demonstrated positive evidence of fetal abnormalities. This drug should not be used in women who are or may become pregnant because the risk clearly outweighs any possible benefit.

Breast Feeding—There are no adequate studies in women for determining infant risk when using this medication during breastfeeding. Weigh the potential benefits against the potential risks before taking this medication while breastfeeding.

Other medicines—

Using this medicine with any of the following medicines may cause an increased risk of certain side effects, but using both drugs may be the best treatment for you. If both medicines are prescribed together, your doctor may change the dose or how often you use one or both of the medicines.

Desogestrel, Drospirenone, Erythromycin, Estradiol Cypionate, Ethinyl Estradiol, Etonogestrel, Fosphenytoin, Gemfibrozil, Gestodene, Itraconazole, Ketoconazole, Levonorgestrel, Medroxyprogesterone, Mestranol, Norelgestromin, Norethindrone, Norgestimate, Norgestrel, Phenobarbital, Phenytoin, Rifampin, Tamoxifen, Vitamin A

Interactions with Food/Tobacco/Alcohol—Certain medicines should not be used at or around the time of eating food or eating certain types of food since interactions may occur. Using alcohol or tobacco with certain medicines may also cause interactions to occur. Discuss with your healthcare professional the use of your medicine with food, alcohol, or tobacco.

Other medical problems—The presence of other medical problems may affect the use of this medicine. Make sure you tell your doctor if you have any other medical problems, especially:
- Kidney disease—May increase the risk of side effects

- Liver disease—Effects of bexarotene may be increased because of slower removal from the body
- Photosensitivity—Bexarotene may cause increased sensitivity of the skin to sunlight

Proper Use of This Medicine

Apply enough bexarotene to cover the lesion with a generous coating. Use a cotton tipped applicator or your fingertips to apply the medicine to your skin. If you apply this medicine with your fingertips, make sure you wash your hands immediately afterwards, to prevent any of the medicine from accidentally getting into your eyes or mouth.

Avoid getting the medicine on the surrounding unaffected skin. Do not apply the medicine near mucosal areas (the inside of your mouth, eyes, nose, rectum or vagina).

Do not cover with bandages or dressings, unless directed to do so by your doctor. Allow the bexarotene to dry before covering with clothing.

Dosing—The dose of this medicine will be different for different patients. Follow your doctor's orders or the directions on the label. The following information includes only the average doses of this medicine. If your dose is different, do not change it unless your doctor tells you to do so.

The amount of medicine that you take depends on the strength of the medicine. Also, the number of doses you take each day, the time allowed between doses, and the length of time you take the medicine depend on the medical problem for which you are using the medicine.

Use this medicine exactly as directed by your doctor. Do not use more or less of it, and do not use it more often than your doctor ordered. The exact amount of medicine you need has been carefully worked out. Using too much will increase the risk of side effects, while using too little may not improve your condition.

- For topical dosage form (gel):
  - For cutaneous T-cell lymphoma
    - Adults—The usual dose is started at applying once every other day for the first week. On week two, the dose may be increased to apply once a day. It may be increased to apply twice a day, on week three. On week four, it may be increased to apply three times a day. Finally, increased to apply four times a day on week five.
    - Children—Use and dose must be determined by your doctor.

Missed dose—If you miss a dose of this medicine, take it as soon as possible. However, if it is almost time for your next dose, skip the missed dose and go back to your regular dosing schedule. Do not double doses.

Every Other Day Application: Apply as soon as possible if you remember it on the day it should be used. However, if you do not remember the missed dose until the next day, apply it at that time. Then skip a day and start applying every other day. Do not double doses.

Storage—Store the medicine in a closed container at room temperature, away from heat, moisture, and direct light. Keep from freezing.

Keep out of the reach of children.

Do not keep outdated medicine or medicine no longer needed.

Precautions While Using This Medicine

It is very important that your doctor check you at regular visits to make sure that this medicine is working properly and to check for unwanted effects.

Bexarotene may cause your skin to be more sensitive to sunlight than it is normally. Exposure to sunlight, even for brief periods of time, may cause a skin rash, itching, redness or other discoloration of the skin, or a severe sunburn. When you begin taking this medicine:

- Stay out of direct sunlight, especially between the hours of 10:00 a.m. and 3:00 p.m., if possible.
- Wear protective clothing, including a hat. Also, wear sunglasses.
- Apply a sun block product that has a skin protection factor (SPF) of at least 15. Some patients may require a product with a higher SPF number, especially if they have a fair complexion. If you have any questions about this, check with your health care professional.
- Apply a sun block lipstick that has an SPF of at least 15 to protect your lips.
- Do not use a sunlamp or tanning bed or booth.

Side Effects of This Medicine

Along with its needed effects, a medicine may cause some unwanted effects. Some side effects will have signs or symptoms that you can see or feel. Your doctor may watch for others by doing certain tests. Since the medication is applied externally to the skin, in general, these side effect are less common. Although not all of these side effects may occur, if they do occur they may need medical attention.

Check with your doctor immediately if any of the following side effects occur:

More common

Bloating or swelling of face, hands, lower legs and/or feet; chills, fever, or general feeling of discomfort or illness; decreased urination; lack or loss of strength; rapid or unusual weight gain; skin rash, blisters, redness, or irritation; sticky or tacky sensation; thickened, scaly skin; tingling or "pins and needles" sensation; sore throat; swollen, painful or tender lymph glands in neck, armpit, or groin; unusual bruising; unusual tiredness or weakness.

Some side effects may occur that usually do not need medical attention. These side effects may go away during treatment as your body adjusts to the medicine. Also, your health care professional may be able to tell you about ways to prevent or reduce some of these side effects. Check with your health care professional if any of the following side effects continue or are bothersome or if you have any questions about them:

More common

Abnormal or excessive sweating; blistering, burning, crusting, dryness, flaking, itching, scaling, severe redness, soreness, or swelling of skin or lesion; headache; increased cough; lower back or side pain; painful or difficult urination

Other side effects not listed may also occur in some patients. If you notice any other effects, check with your healthcare professional.

BISMUTH SUBSALICYLATE, METRONIDAZOLE, AND TETRACYCLINE   (Oral route) - BIZmuth sub-sal-IS-i-late, me-troe-NI-da-zole, tet-ra-SYE-kleen

Black Box Warning

Metronidazole has been shown to be carcinogenic in mice and rats. Unnecessary use of the drug should be avoided

Commonly used brand name(s)

In the U.S.—

Helidac

Available Dosage Forms:

- Tablet, Chewable
- Tablet
- Capsule

Uses For This Medicine

Bismuth subsalicylate, metronidazole, and tetracycline are taken together with a histamine H_2–receptor antagonist to treat ulcers related to infection with the H. pylori bacteria (germ).

This package contains a combination of three different medicines. The individual medicines contained in this package should not be used alone or for other purposes than to treat ulcers related to infection with H. pylori.

This combination of medicines is available only with your doctor's prescription.

Before Using This Medicine

In deciding to use a medicine, the risks of taking the medicine must be weighed against the good it will do. This is a decision you and your doctor will make. For this medicine, the following should be considered:

Allergies—Tell your doctor if you have ever had any unusual or allergic reaction to this medicine or any other medicines. Also tell your health care professional if you have any other types of allergies, such as to foods, dyes, preservatives, or animals. For non-prescription products, read the label or package ingredients carefully.

Pediatric—Infants and children up to 8 years of age should not take this combination of medicines unless directed by the child's doctor. Tetracycline may cause permanent discoloration of the teeth.

Children or teenagers who have or who are recovering from chickenpox or influenza should not use this combination of medicines unless directed by the child's doctor. If nausea or vomiting occurs after taking this combination of medicines, check with the child's doctor. Nausea or vomiting could be early signs of Reye's syndrome, a rare but serious illness.

Geriatric—Many medicines have not been studied specifically in older people. Therefore, it may not be known whether they work exactly the same way they do in younger adults or if they cause different side effects or problems in older people. There is no specific information comparing the use of this combination of medicines (bismuth subsalicylate, metronidazole, and tetracycline) in the elderly with its use in other age groups.

Other medicines—

Using this medicine with any of the following medicines is not recommended. Your doctor may decide not to treat you with this medication or change some of the other medicines you take.

Acitretin, Amprenavir, Dihydroergotamine, Disulfiram, Ergoloid Mesylates, Ergonovine, Ergotamine, Methylergonovine

Interactions with Food/Tobacco/Alcohol—Certain medicines should not be used at or around the time of eating food or eating certain types of food since interactions may occur. Using alcohol or tobacco with certain medicines may also cause interactions to occur. The following interactions have been selected on the basis of their potential significance and are not necessarily all-inclusive.

Using this medicine with any of the following is usually not recommended, but may be unavoidable in some cases. If used together, your doctor may change the dose or how often you use this medicine, or give you special instructions about the use of food, alcohol, or tobacco.

Ethanol

Using this medicine with any of the following may cause an increased risk of certain side effects but may be unavoidable in some cases. If used together, your doctor may change the dose or how often you use this medicine, or give you special instructions about the use of food, alcohol, or tobacco.

Dairy Food

Other medical problems—The presence of other medical problems may affect the use of this medicine. Make sure you tell your doctor if you have any other medical problems, especially:

- Kidney disease or
- Liver disease—Higher blood levels of metronidazole and tetracycline in this combination of medicines may occur, resulting in an increased risk of side effects.

Proper Use of This Medicine

This combination of medicines (bismuth subsalicylate, metronidazole, and tetracycline) comes with instructions for the patient included in the package. Make sure you read and understand the instructions, or ask your health care professional if you need additional information or explanation. It is important that you understand and follow the instructions exactly.

Also, it is important that you complete the full course of therapy with this combination of medicines to help clear up the infection from H. pylori related to your ulcer.

Dosing—The dose of this medicine will be different for different patients. Follow your doctor's orders or the directions on the label. The following information includes only the average doses of this medicine. If your dose is different, do not change it unless your doctor tells you to do so.

The amount of medicine that you take depends on the strength of the medicine. Also, the number of doses you take each day, the time allowed between doses, and the length of time you take the medicine depend on the medical problem for which you are using the medicine.

Be sure to swallow the tablet of metronidazole and the capsule of tetracycline with a full glass (eight ounces) of water. This will help prevent irritation of the esophagus (tube between the throat and stomach) or stomach. Each dose of this combination of medicines (bismuth subsalicylate, metronidazole, and tetracycline) is taken four times a day, with meals and at bedtime, for fourteen days. Your doctor will also prescribe for you another medicine, a histamine H$_2$–receptor antagonist, which will come with its own directions and must be taken along with this combination of medicines.

Each day's therapy is packaged on a blister card that contains eight chewable tablets (each containing 262.4 milligrams [mg] of bismuth subsalicylate), four tablets (each containing 250 mg of metronidazole), and four capsules (each containing 500 mg of tetracycline).

- For oral dosage forms (blister card containing chewable tablets, tablets, and capsules):
  - For the treatment of ulcers related to infection with H. pylori:
    - Adults—For each dose of this combination of medicines:
      — Chew and swallow two tablets of bismuth subsalicylate (525 mg)
      — Swallow one tablet of metronidazole (250 mg)
      — Swallow one capsule of tetracycline (500 mg)
    - Children—Use and dose must be determined by your doctor.

Missed dose—If you miss a dose of this medicine, take it as soon as possible. However, if it is almost time for your next dose, skip the missed dose and go back to your regular dosing schedule. Do not double doses.

If you miss more than four doses of this combination of medicines, check with your doctor.

Storage—Store the medicine in a closed container at room temperature, away from heat, moisture, and direct light. Do not refrigerate. Keep from freezing.

Keep out of the reach of children.

Do not keep outdated medicine or medicine no longer needed.

Precautions While Using This Medicine

Check the labels of all over-the-counter (OTC), nonprescription, and prescription medicines you now take. If any contain aspirin or other salicylates, be especially careful. Using other salicylate-containing products while taking bismuth subsalicylate in this combination of medicines may lead to overdose. If you have any questions about this, check with your health care professional.

Do not take milk, milk formulas, or other dairy products within 1 to 2 hours of the time you take tetracycline in this combination of medicines. Milk and other dairy products may keep tetracycline from working properly.

Do not take antacids or sodium bicarbonate within 1 to 2 hours of the time you take tetracycline in this combination of medicines. Also, do not take iron preparations (including vitamin preparations that contain iron) within 2 to 3 hours of the time you take tetracycline in this combination of medicines. To do so may keep tetracycline from working properly.

Drinking alcoholic beverages while taking metronidazole in this combination of medicines may cause stomach pain, nausea, vomiting, headache, or flushing or redness of the face. Other alcohol-containing preparations (for example, elixirs, cough syrups, tonics) may also cause problems. These problems may last for at least a day after you stop taking metronidazole. Also, metronidazole may cause alcoholic beverages to taste different. Therefore, you should not drink alcoholic beverages or take other alcohol-containing preparations while you are taking metronidazole in this combination of medicines and for at least a day after stopping it.

The metronidazole in this combination of medicines may cause some people to become dizzy or lightheaded. Make sure you know how you react to this combination of medicines before you drive, use machines, or do anything else that could be dangerous if you are dizzy or are not alert.

Oral contraceptives (birth control pills) may not work properly if you take them while you are taking tetracycline in this combination of medicines. Unplanned pregnancies may occur. You should use a different or additional means of birth control while you are taking tetracycline in this combination of medicines. If you have any questions about this, check with your health care professional.

The tetracycline in this combination of medicines may cause your skin to be more sensitive to sunlight than it is normally. Exposure to sunlight, even for brief periods of time, may cause a skin rash, itching, redness or other discoloration of the skin, or a severe sunburn. When you begin taking the tetracycline in this combination of medicines:

- Stay out of direct sunlight, especially between the hours of 10:00 a.m. and 3:00 p.m., if possible.
- Wear protective clothing, including a hat. Also, wear sunglasses.
- Apply a sun block product that has a skin protection factor (SPF) of at least 15. Some patients may require a product with a higher SPF number, especially if they have a fair complexion. If you have any questions about this, check with your health care professional.
- Apply a sun block lipstick that has an SPF of at least 15 to protect your lips.
- Do not use a sunlamp or tanning bed or booth.

You may still be more sensitive to sunlight or sunlamps for 2 weeks to several months or more after stopping tetracycline in this combination of medicines. If you have a severe reaction, check with your doctor.

Before having surgery (including dental surgery) with a general anesthetic, tell the medical doctor or dentist in charge that you are taking tetracycline in this combination of medicines.

Side Effects of This Medicine

Along with its needed effects, a medicine may cause some unwanted effects. Although not all of these side effects may occur, if they do occur they may need medical attention.

Check with your doctor as soon as possible if any of the following side effects occur:

More common
Abdominal pain; bloody or black, tarry stools; diarrhea; nausea

Less common
Burning, prickling, or tingling sensations; dizziness; vomiting

Rare
Bloody vomit; convulsions (seizures); fainting; heart attack; high blood pressure; irritation of the mouth; irri-

tation of the tongue; joint pain and swelling; pain; sensitivity of skin to sunlight; skin rash; trouble in swallowing

Symptoms of overdose
Clumsiness or unsteadiness; confusion; continuing ringing or buzzing in ears; convulsions; diarrhea; fast heartbeat; fast or deep breathing; fever; nausea; pain, numbness, or tingling in arms, legs, hands, or feet; unusual tiredness; vomiting

Some side effects may occur that usually do not need medical attention. These side effects may go away during treatment as your body adjusts to the medicine. Also, your health care professional may be able to tell you about ways to prevent or reduce some of these side effects. Check with your health care professional if any of the following side effects continue or are bothersome or if you have any questions about them:

Less common or rare
Burning or itching around anus; constipation; general feeling of discomfort or illness; loss of appetite; nervousness; trouble in sleeping; unusual tiredness or weakness

In some patients, bismuth subsalicylate in this combination of medicines may cause dark tongue and/or grayish black stools. This is only temporary and will go away when you stop taking bismuth subsalicylate.

Other side effects not listed may also occur in some patients. If you notice any other effects, check with your healthcare professional.

BLEOMYCIN (Injection route) - blee-oh-MYE-sin

Black Box Warning

It is recommended that Bleomycin for Injection be administered under the supervision of a qualified physician experienced in the use of cancer chemotherapeutic agents. Appropriate management of therapy and complications is possible only when adequate diagnostic and treatment facilities are readily available.

Pulmonary fibrosis is the most severe toxicity associated with Bleomycin for Injection. The most frequent presentation is pneumonitis occasionally progressing to pulmonary fibrosis. Its occurrence is higher in elderly patients and in those receiving greater than 400 units total dose, but pulmonary toxicity has been observed in young patients and those treated with low doses.

A severe idiosyncratic reaction consisting of hypotension, mental confusion, fever, chills, and wheezing has been reported in approximately 1% of lymphoma patients treated with Bleomycin for Injection.

Commonly used brand name(s)

In the U.S.—
Blenoxane

Available Dosage Forms:
- Powder for Solution

Therapeutic Class: Antibiotic

Uses For This Medicine

Bleomycin belongs to the general group of medicines called antineoplastics. It is used to treat several types of cancer, including cervix and uterus cancer, head and neck cancer, testicle and penile cancer, and certain types of lymphoma. Bleomycin also may used for other conditions, as determined by your doctor.

Bleomycin seems to act by interfering with the growth of cancer cells, which are eventually destroyed. Since the growth of normal body cells may also be affected by bleomycin, other effects will also occur. Some of these may be serious and must be reported to your doctor. Other effects, like darkening of skin or hair loss, may not be serious but may cause concern. Some effects may not occur for months or years after the medicine is used.

Before you begin treatment with bleomycin, you and your doctor should talk about the good this medicine will do as well as the risks of using it.

Bleomycin is to be administered only by or under the immediate supervision of your doctor.

Once a medicine has been approved for marketing for a certain use, experience may show that it is also useful for other medical problems. Although this use is not included in product labeling, bleomycin is used in certain patients with the following medical conditions:

- Bone cancer
- Kaposi's sarcoma
- Malignant melanoma
- Mycosis fungoides (a type of lymphoma)
- Skin cancer
- Thyroid cancer
- Verruca vulgaris (warts)

For patients being treated with bleomycin for warts:

- Bleomycin is used to treat severe cases of warts when other treatments have not worked.
- Before using bleomycin, tell your doctor if you have problems with circulation. Bleomycin can cause paleness or coldness in fingers treated for warts.
- Bleomycin is injected directly into the wart. Because it is not absorbed into the body, it does not cause loss of hair, lung problems, or other unwanted effects described above. However, it may cause burning or pain at the place of injection. Skin rash or itching, nail loss, and pain or coldness in the finger where bleomycin was injected have also been reported.

Before Using This Medicine

In deciding to use a medicine, the risks of taking the medicine must be weighed against the good it will do. This is a decision you and your doctor will make. For this medicine, the following should be considered:

Allergies—Tell your doctor if you have ever had any unusual or allergic reaction to this medicine or any other medicines. Also tell your health care professional if you have any other types of allergies, such as to foods, dyes, preservatives, or animals. For non-prescription products, read the label or package ingredients carefully.

Pediatric—Although there is no specific information comparing use of bleomycin in children with use in other age groups, this medicine is not expected to cause different side effects or problems in children than it does in adults.

Geriatric—Lung problems are more likely to occur in elderly patients (over 70 years of age), who are usually more sensitive to the effects of bleomycin.

Pregnancy—

	Pregnancy Category	Explanation
All Trimesters	D	Studies in pregnant women have demonstrated a risk to the fetus. However, the benefits of therapy in a life threatening situation or a serious disease, may outweigh the potential risk.

Breast Feeding—There are no adequate studies in women for determining infant risk when using this medication during breastfeeding. Weigh the potential benefits against the potential risks before taking this medication while breastfeeding.

Other medicines—Using this medicine with any of the following medicines is not recommended. Your doctor may decide not to treat you with this medication or change some of the other medicines you take.

Rotavirus Vaccine, Live

Interactions with Food/Tobacco/Alcohol—Certain medicines should not be used at or around the time of eating food or eating certain types of food since interactions may occur. Using alcohol or tobacco with certain medicines may also cause interactions to occur. Discuss with your healthcare professional the use of your medicine with food, alcohol, or tobacco.

Other medical problems—The presence of other medical problems may affect the use of this medicine. Make sure you tell your doctor if you have any other medical problems, especially:

- Kidney disease—Effects of bleomycin may be increased because of slower removal from the body
- Liver disease—Bleomycin can cause liver problems
- Lung disease—Bleomycin may worsen the condition

Proper Use of This Medicine

Bleomycin is sometimes given together with certain other medicines. If you are using a combination of medicines, it is important that you receive each medicine at the proper time. If you are taking some of these medicines by mouth, ask your health care professional to help you plan a way to take them at the right times.

Bleomycin often causes nausea, vomiting, and loss of appetite. However, it is very important that you continue to receive the medicine, even if you begin to feel ill. Ask your health care professional for ways to lessen these effects.

Dosing—The dose of this medicine will be different for different patients. Follow your doctor's orders or the directions on the label. The following information includes only the average doses of this medicine. If your dose is different, do not change it unless your doctor tells you to do so.

The amount of medicine that you take depends on the strength of the medicine. Also, the number of doses you take

each day, the time allowed between doses, and the length of time you take the medicine depend on the medical problem for which you are using the medicine.

Precautions While Using This Medicine

It is very important that your doctor check your progress at regular visits to make sure that this medicine is working properly and to check for unwanted effects.

Before having any kind of surgery (including dental surgery) or emergency treatment, tell the medical doctor or dentist in charge that you are receiving or have received this medicine.

Tell your doctor if you smoke. The risk of lung problems is increased in people who smoke.

Side Effects of This Medicine

Along with its needed effects, a medicine may cause some unwanted effects. Although not all of these side effects may occur, if they do occur they may need medical attention.

Also, because of the way these medicines act on the body, there is a chance that they might cause other unwanted effects that may not occur until months or years after the medicine is used. These delayed effects may include certain types of cancer, such as leukemia. Discuss these possible effects with your doctor.

Check with your doctor immediately if any of the following side effects occur:

More common
Fever and chills (occurring within 3 to 6 hours after a dose)

Less common
Confusion; faintness; wheezing

Rare
Chest pain (sudden severe); weakness in arms or legs (sudden)

Check with your doctor as soon as possible if any of the following side effects occur:

More common
Cough; shortness of breath; sores in mouth and on lips

Some side effects may occur that usually do not need medical attention. These side effects may go away during treatment as your body adjusts to the medicine. Also, your health care professional may be able to tell you about ways to prevent or reduce some of these side effects. Check with your health care professional if any of the following side effects continue or are bothersome or if you have any questions about them:

More common
Darkening or thickening of skin; dark stripes on skin; itching of skin; skin rash or colored bumps on fingertips, elbows, or palms; skin redness or tenderness; swelling of fingers; vomiting and loss of appetite

Less common
Changes in fingernails or toenails; weight loss

Bleomycin may cause a temporary loss of hair in some people. After treatment has ended, normal hair growth should return, although it may take several months.

Side effects that affect your lungs (for example, cough and shortness of breath) may be more likely to occur if you smoke.

After you stop using this medicine, it may still produce some side effects that need attention. During this period of time, *check with your doctor immediately* if you notice the following side effects:

Cough; shortness of breath

Other side effects not listed may also occur in some patients. If you notice any other effects, check with your healthcare professional.

BORTEZOMIB (Intravenous route) -
bore-TEZ-oh-mib

Commonly used brand name(s)
In the U.S.—
Velcade

Available Dosage Forms:
• Powder for Solution

Therapeutic Class: Antineoplastic Agent
Pharmacologic Class: Proteasome Inhibitor

Uses For This Medicine

Bortezomib belongs to the general group of medicines known as antineoplastics. It is used to treat multiple myeloma in patients who have received at least one treatment that has not helped.

Bortezomib interferes with the growth of cancer cells, which are then eventually destroyed by the body. Since the growth of normal body cells may also be affected by bortezomib, other effects will also occur. Some of these may be serious and must be reported to your doctor. Other effects may not be serious but may cause concern. Some effects may not occur until months or years after the medicine is used.

Bortezomib is to be administered only by or under the supervision of your doctor.

Once a medicine has been approved for marketing for a certain use, experience may show that it is also useful for other medical problems. Although these uses are not included in the product labeling, bortezomib is used in certain patients with the following medical conditions:
• Mantle cell lymphoma

Before Using This Medicine

In deciding to use a medicine, the risks of taking the medicine must be weighed against the good it will do. This is a decision you and your doctor will make. For this medicine, the following should be considered:

Allergies—Tell your doctor if you have ever had any unusual or allergic reaction to this medicine or any other medicines. Also tell your health care professional if you have any other types of allergies, such as to foods, dyes, preservatives, or animals. For non-prescription products, read the label or package ingredients carefully.

Pediatric—Studies on this medicine have been done only in adult patients, and there is no specific information comparing use of bortezomib in children with use in other age groups.

Pregnancy—

	Pregnancy Category	Explanation
All Trimesters	D	Studies in pregnant women have demonstrated a risk to the fetus. However, the benefits of therapy in a life threatening situation or a serious disease, may outweigh the potential risk.

Breast Feeding—There are no adequate studies in women for determining infant risk when using this medication during breastfeeding. Weigh the potential benefits against the potential risks before taking this medication while breastfeeding.

Other medicines—Although certain medicines should not be used together at all, in other cases two different medicines may be used together even if an interaction might occur. In these cases, your doctor may want to change the dose, or other precautions may be necessary. Tell your healthcare professional if you are taking any other prescription or non-prescription (over-the-counter [OTC]) medicine.

Interactions with Food/Tobacco/Alcohol—Certain medicines should not be used at or around the time of eating food or eating certain types of food since interactions may occur. Using alcohol or tobacco with certain medicines may also cause interactions to occur. Discuss with your healthcare professional the use of your medicine with food, alcohol, or tobacco.

Other medical problems—The presence of other medical problems may affect the use of this medicine. Make sure you tell your doctor if you have any other medical problems, especially:

- Dehydration or
- Syncope, history of—May cause orthostatic/postural hypotension
- Heart disease—Bortezomib may make your heart problems worse or cause new heart problems. Your doctor will watch for this side effect.
- Kidney disease or
- Liver disease—Higher blood levels of bortezomib may result and a smaller dose may be needed
- Peripheral neuropathy—Bortezomib may make the symptoms worse or cause new symptoms
- Tumor lysis syndrome, risk of—Bortezomib may increase your chance of getting this side effect. Your doctor will watch for this side effect.

Proper Use of This Medicine

Dosing—The dose of this medicine will be different for different patients. Follow your doctor's orders or the directions on the label. The following information includes only the average doses of this medicine. If your dose is different, do not change it unless your doctor tells you to do so.

The amount of medicine that you take depends on the strength of the medicine. Also, the number of doses you take each day, the time allowed between doses, and the length of time you take the medicine depend on the medical problem for which you are using the medicine.

- For injection dosage form
  - For treatment of multiple myeloma
    - Adults—
      — Patients without symptoms or with Grade 1 symptoms of peripheral neuropathy (paresthesias and/or loss of reflexes without pain or loss of function)—1.3 milligrams (mg) per m² twice weekly for two weeks (days 1, 4, 8, and 11) followed by a 10– day rest period (days 12–21). For longer treatment of more than 8 cycles, bortezomib may be taken on the regular schedule or on a maintenance schedule of once a week for 4 weeks (days 1, 8, 15, and 22) followed by a 13–day rest period (days 23–35). At least 72 hours should elapse between consecutive dose.
      — Patients with Grade 1 with pain or Grade 2 symptoms of peripheral neuropathy (interfering with function but not with activities of daily living)—1 milligram (mg) per m² twice weekly for two weeks (days 1, 4, 8, and 11) followed by a 10– day rest period (days 12–21). At least 72 hours should elapse between consecutive dose.
      — Patients with Grade 2 with pain or Grade 3 symptoms of peripheral neuropathy (interfering with activities of daily living)—Your doctor will withhold therapy until toxicity resolves. When toxicity resolves your doctor will reduce your dose to 0.7 mg/m² once per week.
      — Patients with Grade 4 symptoms of peripheral neuropathy (permanent sensory loss that interferes with function)—Your doctor will discontinue therapy
      — Your doctor may decrease your dose for severe side effects excluding peripheral neuropathy.
    - Children—Bortezomib is not usually recommended in children.

Missed dose—Call your doctor or pharmacist for instructions.

Precautions While Using This Medicine

It is very important that your doctor check you at regular visits to make sure that this medicine is working properly and to check for unwanted effects.

This medicine may cause some people to become drowsy, dizzy, or less alert than they are normally. Make sure you know how you react to this medicine before you drive, use machines, or do anything else that could be dangerous if you are dizzy or are not alert.

This medicine may cause vomiting and diarrhea, so it is important to drink plenty of fluids. If you experience dizziness or lightheadedness, contact your doctor. These could be symptoms of dehydration (not enough water in your body).

If you are diabetic and you take an oral antidiabetic medicine, you should check your blood sugar level often and report any unusual changes to your doctor.

Side Effects of This Medicine

Along with its needed effects, a medicine may cause some unwanted effects. Although not all of these side effects may occur, if they do occur they may need medical attention.

Also, because of the way these medicines act on the body, there is a chance that they might cause other unwanted effects that may not occur until months or years after the medicine is used. Discuss these possible effects with your doctor.

Check with your doctor immediately if any of the following side effects occur:

More common

Black, tarry stools; bleeding gums; blood in urine or stools; blurred vision; body aches or pain; burning, crawling, itching, numbness, prickling, "pins and needles", or tingling feelings; chest pain; chills; confusion; faintness, or lightheadedness when getting up from a lying or sitting position suddenly; cough; decreased urination; difficult or labored breathing; dry mouth; ear congestion; fainting; fever; headache; increase in heart rate; loss of voice; lower back or side pain; nasal congestion; pale skin; painful or difficult urination; painful blisters on trunk of body; pinpoint red spots on skin; rapid breathing; runny nose; shortness of breath; sneezing; sore throat; sunken eyes; sweating; tightness in chest; thirst; troubled breathing with exertion; wrinkled skin; ulcers, sores, or white spots in mouth; unsteadiness or awkwardness; unusual bleeding or bruising; unusual tiredness or weakness; weakness in arms, hands, legs, or feet; wheezing

Incidence not known

Abdominal pain and tenderness; agitation; back pain; bloating; bruising; coma; constipation; coughing or vomiting blood; dark urine; deafness; dizziness; dizziness or lightheadedness, especially when getting up from a lying or sitting position; drowsiness; fast heartbeat; general tiredness and weakness; hallucinations; irritability; light-colored stools; mood or mental changes; pains in stomach, side, or abdomen, possibly radiating to the back; persistent bleeding or oozing from puncture sites, mouth, or nose; pounding, slow heartbeat; rectal bleeding; seizures; stiff neck; troubled breathing; upper right abdominal pain; yellow eyes or skin

Symptoms of overdose

If you think you or someone else may have taken an overdose get emergency help at once.

Some side effects may occur that usually do not need medical attention. These side effects may go away during treatment as your body adjusts to the medicine. Also, your health care professional may be able to tell you about ways to prevent or reduce some of these side effects. Check with your health care professional if any of the following side effects continue or are bothersome or if you have any questions about them:

More common

Acid or sour stomach; back pain; belching; bone pain; diarrhea; difficulty in moving; difficulty having a bowel movement; fatigue; fear or nervousness; feeling unusually cold; shivering; heartburn; indigestion; itching skin; loss of appetite; loss of taste or change in taste; malaise; muscle cramps; nausea; pain in joints; muscle pain or stiffness; pain in limb; rash; sleeplessness; trouble sleeping; unable to sleep; stomach discomfort, upset or pain; swelling; stomach pain; swollen joints; vomiting

Other side effects not listed may also occur in some patients. If you notice any other effects, check with your healthcare professional.

BOSENTAN   (Oral route) - boe-SEN-tan

Black Box Warning

- Use of bosentan requires attention to two significant concerns: potential for serious liver injury and potential damage to fetus.
- Potential liver injury
  - Bosentan causes at least 3–fold upper limit of normal (ULN); elevation of liver aminotransferases (ALT and AST) in about 11% of patients, accompanied by elevated bilirubin in a small number of cases. Because these changes are a marker for potential serious liver injury, serum aminotransferase levels must be measured prior to initiation of treatment and then monthly. In the post-marketing period, in the setting of close monitoring, rare cases of unexplained hepatic cirrhosis were reported after prolonged (greater than 12 months) therapy with bosentan in patients with multiple co-morbidities and drug therapies. The contribution of bosentan in these cases could not be excluded.
  - In at least one case the initial presentation (after greater than 20 months of treatment) included pronounced elevations in aminotransferases and bilirubin levels accompanied by non-specific symptoms, all of which resolved slowly over time after discontinuation of bosentan. This case reinforces the importance of strict adherence to the monthly monitoring schedule for the duration of treatment and the treatment algorithm, which includes stopping bosentan with a rise of aminotransferases accompanied by signs and symptoms of liver dysfunction.
  - Elevations in aminotransferases require close attention. Bosentan should generally be avoided in patients with elevated aminotransferases (greater than 3 times ULN) at baseline because monitoring liver injury may be more difficult. If liver aminotransferase elevations are accompanied by clinical symptoms of liver injury (such as nausea, vomiting, fever, abdominal pain, jaundice, or unusual lethargy or fatigue) or increases in bilirubin greater than or equal to 2 times ULN, treatment should be stopped. There is no experience with the re-introduction of bosentan in these circumstances.
- Pregnancy
  - Bosentan is very likely to produce major birth defects if used by pregnant women, as this effect has been seen consistently when it is administered to animals. Therefore, pregnancy must be excluded before the start of treatment with bosentan and prevented thereafter by the use of a reliable method of contraception. Hormonal contraceptives, including oral, injectable, transdermal, and implantable contraceptives should not be used as the sole means of contraception because these may not be effective in patients receiving bosentan. Therefore, effective contraception through additional forms of contraception must be practiced. Monthly pregnancy tests should be obtained.
  - Because of potential liver injury and in an effort to make the chance of fetal exposure to bosentan as small as possible, bosentan may be prescribed only through the TRACLEER® Access Program by calling 1 866 228 3546. Adverse events can also be reported directly via this number.

Commonly used brand name(s)

In the U.S.—
Tracleer

Available Dosage Forms:
- Tablet

Therapeutic Class: Antihypertensive
Pharmacologic Class: Endothelin Receptor Antagonist

Uses For This Medicine

Bosentan is used to treat the symptoms of pulmonary arterial hypertension. This is the high blood pressure that occurs in the main artery that carries blood from the right side of the heart (the ventricle) to the lungs. When the smaller blood vessels in the lungs become more resistant to blood flow, the right ventricle must work harder to pump enough blood through the lungs. Bosentan works by blocking a hormone (a naturally occurring substance), that is found in the blood and lungs in large quantities of the people with pulmonary arterial hypertension. Bosentan helps by increasing the supply of blood to the lungs and reducing the workload of the heart.

This medicine is available only with your doctor's prescription.

Before Using This Medicine

In deciding to use a medicine, the risks of taking the medicine must be weighed against the good it will do. This is a decision you and your doctor will make. For this medicine, the following should be considered:

Allergies—Tell your doctor if you have ever had any unusual or allergic reaction to this medicine or any other medicines. Also tell your health care professional if you have any other types of allergies, such as to foods, dyes, preservatives, or animals. For non-prescription products, read the label or package ingredients carefully.

Pediatric—Studies on this medicine have been done only in adult patients, and there is no specific information comparing use of bosentan in children with use in other age groups.

Geriatric—Many medicines have not been studied specifically in older people. Therefore, it may not be known whether they work exactly the same way they do in younger adults or if they cause different side effects or problems in older people. There is no specific information comparing use of bosentan in the elderly with use in other age groups.

Pregnancy—

	Pregnancy Category	Explanation
All Trimesters	X	Studies in animals or pregnant women have demonstrated positive evidence of fetal abnormalities. This drug should not be used in women who are or may become pregnant because the risk clearly outweighs any possible benefit.

Breast Feeding—There are no adequate studies in women for determining infant risk when using this medication during breastfeeding. Weigh the potential benefits against the potential risks before taking this medication while breastfeeding.

Other medicines—
Using this medicine with any of the following medicines is not recommended. Your doctor may decide not to treat you with this medication or change some of the other medicines you take.

Cyclosporine, Glyburide

Interactions with Food/Tobacco/Alcohol—Certain medicines should not be used at or around the time of eating food or eating certain types of food since interactions may occur. Using alcohol or tobacco with certain medicines may also cause interactions to occur. Discuss with your healthcare professional the use of your medicine with food, alcohol, or tobacco.

Other medical problems—The presence of other medical problems may affect the use of this medicine. Make sure you tell your doctor if you have any other medical problems, especially:
- Liver disease—Bosentan may make these conditions worse in patients who have moderate or severe liver disease. Use of bosentan should generally be avoided in patients with liver disease, if possible.

Proper Use of This Medicine

Dosing—The dose of this medicine will be different for different patients. Follow your doctor's orders or the directions on the label. The following information includes only the average doses of this medicine. If your dose is different, do not change it unless your doctor tells you to do so.

The amount of medicine that you take depends on the strength of the medicine. Also, the number of doses you take each day, the time allowed between doses, and the length of time you take the medicine depend on the medical problem for which you are using the medicine.

- For oral dosage form (tablets):
  - For high blood pressure
    - Adults—62.5 milligrams twice daily for 4 weeks, then increased to 125 milligrams twice a day. For patients who weigh less than 40 kilograms (88 pounds) and who are over 12 years of age, the dose is 62.5 milligrams twice a day.

Missed dose—If you miss a dose of this medicine, take it as soon as possible. However, if it is almost time for your next dose, skip the missed dose and go back to your regular dosing schedule. Do not double doses.

Storage—Store the medicine in a closed container at room temperature, away from heat, moisture, and direct light. Keep from freezing.

Keep out of the reach of children.

Do not keep outdated medicine or medicine no longer needed.

Ask your healthcare professional how you should dispose of any medicine you do not use.

Precautions While Using This Medicine

It is very important that your doctor check your progress at regular visits to make sure this medicine is working properly and to check for unwanted effects.

It is also important that your doctor does a blood test to check your liver function before you start bosentan and each month after that.

Do not use hormone-based birth control (pills, injections, patches, and implants) as your only method of birth control while you are taking this medicine.

In addition, check with your doctor immediately if you experience dark urine, light colored stools, loss of appetite, nausea and vomiting, unusual tiredness, yellow eyes or skin, fever with or without chills, or stomach pain.

Side Effects of This Medicine

Along with its needed effects, a medicine may cause some unwanted effects. Although not all of these side effects may occur, if they do occur they may need medical attention.

Check with your doctor immediately if any of the following side effects occur:

More common
   Blurred vision; confusion; dizziness; dark urine; faintness or lightheadedness when getting up from a lying or sitting position; fever with or without chills; light-colored stools; loss of appetite; nausea and vomiting; stomach pain; sudden sweating; unusual tiredness or weakness; yellow eyes or skin

Less common
   Swelling

Frequency not known
   Blue lips and fingernails; chest pain; coughing that sometimes produces a pink frothy sputum; coughing up blood; decrease in amount of urine; difficult, fast, noisy breathing, sometimes with wheezing; fainting; fast heartbeat; fatigue on exertion; fever; hives; hoarseness; increased sweating; irritation; itching; joint pain, stiffness, or swelling; noisy, rattling breathing; pale skin; rash; redness of skin; shortness of breath; swelling of eyelids, face, lips, hands, fingers, legs, ankles, or feet; tightness in chest; troubled breathing at rest; troubled breathing or swallowing; weight gain; wheezing

Symptoms of overdose

   Get emergency help immediately if any of the following symptoms of overdose occur:

   Blurred vision; confusion; dizziness; faintness or lightheadedness when getting up from a lying or sitting position; headache; increased heart rate; nausea; sudden sweating; unusual tiredness or weakness; vomiting

Some side effects may occur that usually do not need medical attention. These side effects may go away during treatment as your body adjusts to the medicine. Also, your health care professional may be able to tell you about ways to prevent or reduce some of these side effects. Check with your health care professional if any of the following side effects continue or are bothersome or if you have any questions about them:

More common
   Fast, irregular, pounding, or racing heartbeat or pulse; feeling of warmth; muscle aches; redness of the face, neck, arms, and occasionally upper chest; stuffy or runny nose; swelling of the legs; sore throat; unusual tiredness or weakness

Less common
   Acid or sour stomach; belching; heartburn; indigestion; itching skin; stomach discomfort, upset or pain

Other side effects not listed may also occur in some patients. If you notice any other effects, check with your healthcare professional.

BOTULINUM TOXIN TYPE A
(Intramuscular route) - BOT-yoo-li-num TOX-in type A

Commonly used brand name(s)

In the U.S.—
   Botox
   Botox Cosmetic

Available Dosage Forms:
   • Powder for Solution

Therapeutic Class: Musculoskeletal Agent
Pharmacologic Class: Neuromuscular Blocker, Non-Depolarizing

Uses For This Medicine

Botulinum toxin type A is used to treat certain eye conditions, such as:

   • Blepharospasm—A condition in which the eyelid will not stay open, because of a spasm of a muscle of the eye.
   • Strabismus—A condition in which the eyes do not line up properly.

Botulinum toxin type A is injected into the surrounding muscle or tissue of the eye, but not into the eye itself. Depending on your condition, more than one treatment may be required.

Botulinum toxin type A is also used to treat muscle spasms of the neck (cervical dystonia) and some types of severe sweating of the armpits (hyperhidrosis).

This medicine is to be administered only by, or under the immediate supervision of, your doctor.

Once a medicine has been approved for marketing for a certain use, experience may show that it is also useful for other medical problems. Although these uses are not included in product labeling, botulinum toxin type A is used in certain patients with the following medical conditions:

   • Deep facial lines or wrinkles
   • Frey's syndrome (gustatory sweating) (red area and sweating on the cheek while eating)
   • Hyperhidrosis (severe sweating of the palms)
   • Spasms of the arms, feet, hands, or legs caused by brain injury, multiple sclerosis, spinal cord injury, or stroke
   • Spasms of the arms and legs in stroke patients
   • Spasms of the face
   • Spasms of the hand, including writer's cramp and musician's cramp
   • Spasms of the arms and legs in patients with multiple sclerosis
   • Spasms of the vocal cords

Before Receiving This Medicine

In deciding to use a medicine, the risks of taking the medicine must be weighed against the good it will do. This is a decision you and your doctor will make. For this medicine, the following should be considered:

In deciding to receive a medicine, the risks of receiving the medicine must be weighed against the good it will do. This is a decision you and your doctor will make. For botulinum toxin type A, the following should be considered:

Allergies—Tell your doctor if you have ever had any unusual or allergic reaction to this medicine or any other medicines. Also tell your health care professional if you have any

other types of allergies, such as to foods, dyes, preservatives, or animals. For non-prescription products, read the label or package ingredients carefully.

Pediatric—Studies on this medicine have been done only in adult patients, and there is no specific information comparing use of botulinum toxin type A in children with use in other age groups.

Geriatric—Many medicines have not been studied specifically in older people. Therefore, it may not be known whether they work exactly the same way they do in younger adults. Elderly people are especially sensitive to the effects of some medicines. This may increase the chance of side effects during treatment.

Pregnancy—

	Pregnancy Category	Explanation
All Trimesters	C	Animal studies have shown an adverse effect and there are no adequate studies in pregnant women OR no animal studies have been conducted and there are no adequate studies in pregnant women.

Breast Feeding—There are no adequate studies in women for determining infant risk when using this medication during breastfeeding. Weigh the potential benefits against the potential risks before taking this medication while breastfeeding.

Other medicines—Although certain medicines should not be used together at all, in other cases two different medicines may be used together even if an interaction might occur. In these cases, your doctor may want to change the dose, or other precautions may be necessary. Tell your healthcare professional if you are taking any other prescription or non-prescription (over-the-counter [OTC]) medicine.

Interactions with Food/Tobacco/Alcohol—Certain medicines should not be used at or around the time of eating food or eating certain types of food since interactions may occur. Using alcohol or tobacco with certain medicines may also cause interactions to occur. Discuss with your healthcare professional the use of your medicine with food, alcohol, or tobacco.

Other medical problems—The presence of other medical problems may affect the use of this medicine. Make sure you tell your doctor if you have any other medical problems, especially:

- Amyotrophic lateral sclerosis (Lou Gehrig's disease) or
- Lambert-Eaton syndrome or
- Motor neuropathy or
- Myasthenia gravis—These medical problems may increase your risk for severe swallowing or breathing problems.
- Heart problems or other medical conditions that may worsen with rapidly increasing activity—Treatment with botulinum toxin type A may give you better vision and the desire to become more active in your daily life; this may put a strain on your heart and body
- Infection where botulinum toxin type A is to be injected— Botulinum toxin type A should not injected into an area that is infected.
- Infection with Clostridium botulinum toxin (botulism poisoning), history of—Persons with a history of infection

with Clostridium botulinum toxin (botulism poisoning) may have produced antibodies that may interfere with botulinum toxin type A therapy and make it less effective

- Nerve problems—May increase your chance of getting side effects.
- Swallowing problems—Treatment with botulinum toxin type A may make this problem worse and increase your risk for serious side effects. Tell your doctor right away if you have severe swallowing problems.
- Swelling where botulinum toxin type A is to be injected or
- Weakness in the muscles where botulinum toxin type A is to be injected—Your doctor may decrease your dose or not inject the botulinum toxin type A until these problems are better.

Proper Use of This Medicine

Dosing—The dose of this medicine will be different for different patients. Follow your doctor's orders or the directions on the label. The following information includes only the average doses of this medicine. If your dose is different, do not change it unless your doctor tells you to do so.

The amount of medicine that you take depends on the strength of the medicine. Also, the number of doses you take each day, the time allowed between doses, and the length of time you take the medicine depend on the medical problem for which you are using the medicine.

- For injection dosage form:
  - For certain eye conditions:
    - Adults and children 12 years of age and older— One or more injections into the muscles around the eyes one or more times, depending on the condition being treated.
    - Children up to 12 years of age—Use and dose must be determined by your doctor.
  - For muscle spasms of the neck (cervical dystonia):
    - Adults and children 16 years of age and older— One or more injections into the muscles of the neck one or more times, depending on the condition being treated.
    - Children up to 16 years of age—Use and dose must be determined by your doctor.
  - For severe sweating of the armpits (hyperhidrosis):
    - Adults and children 16 years of age and older— One or more injections just below the skin in the armpit one or more times.
    - Children up to 16 years of age—Use and dose must be determined by your doctor.

Precautions After Receiving This Medicine

After you have received this medicine and your vision is better, you may find that you are a lot more active than you were before. You should increase your activities slowly and carefully to allow your heart and body time to get stronger. Also, before you start any exercise program, check with your doctor.

Side Effects of This Medicine

Along with its needed effects, a medicine may cause some unwanted effects. Although not all of these side effects may occur, if they do occur they may need medical attention.

Check with your doctor as soon as possible if any of the following side effects occur:

More common—For blepharospasm
   Dryness of the eye; inability to close the eyelid completely

Less common or rare—For blepharospasm
   Decreased blinking; irritation of the cornea (colored portion) of the eye; turning outward or inward of the edge of the eyelid

Some side effects may occur that usually do not need medical attention. These side effects may go away during treatment as your body adjusts to the medicine. Also, your health care professional may be able to tell you about ways to prevent or reduce some of these side effects. Check with your health care professional if any of the following side effects continue or are bothersome or if you have any questions about them:

More common—For blepharospasm
   Blue or purplish bruise on eyelid; drooping of the upper eyelid; irritation or watering of the eye; sensitivity of the eye to light

More common—For cervical dystonia
   Body aches or pain; chills; cough, fever, sneezing, or sore throat; difficulty in breathing; difficulty swallowing; ear congestion; headache; loss of voice; nasal congestion; neck pain; runny nose; unusual tiredness or weakness

More common—For horizontal strabismus
   Drooping of the upper eyelid; eye pointing upward or downward instead of straight ahead

More common—For hyperhidrosis
   Back, neck, or side pain; body aches or pain; chills; congestion; cough; diarrhea; dryness or soreness of throat; fear; fever; general feeling of discomfort or illness; headache; heavy bleeding from place where shot was given; hoarseness; itching skin; joint pain; loss of appetite; muscle aches and pains; nausea; nervousness; painful or difficult urination; runny nose; shivering; sore throat; sweating; tender, swollen glands in neck; trouble sleeping; trouble in swallowing; unusual tiredness or weakness; voice changes; vomiting

Less common or rare—For blepharospasm or strabismus
   Skin rash; swelling of the eyelid skin

Less common or rare—For horizontal strabismus
   Difficulty finding the location of objects; double vision

Other side effects not listed may also occur in some patients. If you notice any other effects, check with your healthcare professional.

BROMOCRIPTINE (Oral route) - broe-moe-KRIP-teen

Commonly used brand name(s)

In the U.S.—
   Parlodel

Available Dosage Forms:
   • Tablet
   • Capsule

Therapeutic Class: Antiparkinsonian
Pharmacologic Class: Dopamine Agonist

Uses For This Medicine

Bromocriptine belongs to the group of medicines known as ergot alkaloids. Bromocriptine blocks release of a hormone called prolactin from the pituitary gland. Prolactin affects the menstrual cycle and milk production. Bromocriptine is used to treat certain menstrual problems or to stop milk production in some women or men who have abnormal milk leakage. It is also used to treat infertility in both men and women that occurs because the body made too much prolactin.

Bromocriptine is also used to treat some people who have Parkinson's disease. It works by stimulating certain parts of the brain and nervous system that are involved in this disease.

Bromocriptine is also used to treat acromegaly (overproduction of growth hormone) and pituitary prolactinomas (tumors of the pituitary gland).

Bromocriptine may also be used for other conditions as determined by your doctor.

Bromocriptine is available only with your doctor's prescription.

Once a medicine has been approved for marketing for a certain use, experience may show that it is also useful for other medical problems. Although these uses are not included in product labeling, bromocriptine is used in certain patients with the following medical conditions:
   • To stop milk production after an abortion or miscarriage or in women after a delivery who should not breast-feed for medical reasons
   • Neuroleptic malignant syndrome

Before Using This Medicine

In deciding to use a medicine, the risks of taking the medicine must be weighed against the good it will do. This is a decision you and your doctor will make. For this medicine, the following should be considered:

Allergies—Tell your doctor if you have ever had any unusual or allergic reaction to this medicine or any other medicines. Also tell your health care professional if you have any other types of allergies, such as to foods, dyes, preservatives, or animals. For non-prescription products, read the label or package ingredients carefully.

Pediatric—This medicine has been tested in a limited number of teenagers 15 years of age and older. In effective doses, the medicine has not been shown to cause different side effects or problems than it does in adults. Appropriate studies have not been done in teenagers younger than 15 years of age, and there is no specific information comparing use of bromocriptine in these teenagers with use in other age groups.

Geriatric—Confusion, hallucinations, or uncontrolled body movements may be more likely to occur in elderly patients, who are usually more sensitive than younger adults to the effects of bromocriptine.

Pregnancy—

	Pregnancy Category	Explanation
All Trimesters	B	Animal studies have revealed no evidence of harm to the fetus, however, there are no adequate studies in pregnant women OR animal studies have shown an adverse effect, but adequate studies in pregnant women have failed to demonstrate a risk to the fetus.

Breast Feeding—Studies suggest that this medication may alter milk production or composition. If an alternative to this medication is not prescribed, you should monitor the infant for side effects and adequate milk intake.

Other medicines—

Using this medicine with any of the following medicines is usually not recommended, but may be required in some cases. If both medicines are prescribed together, your doctor may change the dose or how often you use one or both of the medicines.

Isometheptene, Phenylpropanolamine

Interactions with Food/Tobacco/Alcohol—Certain medicines should not be used at or around the time of eating food or eating certain types of food since interactions may occur. Using alcohol or tobacco with certain medicines may also cause interactions to occur. Discuss with your healthcare professional the use of your medicine with food, alcohol, or tobacco.

Other medical problems—The presence of other medical problems may affect the use of this medicine. Make sure you tell your doctor if you have any other medical problems, especially:

- High blood pressure (or history of) or
- Pregnancy-induced high blood pressure (history of)—Rarely, bromocriptine can make the high blood pressure worse
- Liver disease—Toxic effects of bromocriptine may occur in patients with liver disease because the body is not able to remove bromocriptine from the bloodstream as it normally would
- Mental problems (history of)—Bromocriptine may make certain mental problems worse

Proper Use of This Medicine

If bromocriptine upsets your stomach, it may be taken with meals or milk. Also, taking the dose at bedtime may help to lessen nausea if it occurs. If stomach upset continues, check with your doctor. Your doctor may recommend that you take the first doses vaginally.

Dosing—The dose of this medicine will be different for different patients. Follow your doctor's orders or the directions on the label. The following information includes only the average doses of this medicine. If your dose is different, do not change it unless your doctor tells you to do so.

The amount of medicine that you take depends on the strength of the medicine. Also, the number of doses you take each day, the time allowed between doses, and the length of time you take the medicine depend on the medical problem for which you are using the medicine.

- For oral dosage forms (capsules and tablets):
  - For infertility, male hormone problem (male hypogonadism), starting the menstrual cycle (amenorrhea), or stopping abnormal milk secretion from nipples (galactorrhea):
    - Adults and teenagers 15 years of age or older—At first, 1.25 to 2.5 milligrams (mg) once a day taken at bedtime with a snack. Then your doctor may change your dose by 2.5 mg every three to seven days as needed. Doses greater than 5 mg a day are taken in divided doses with meals or at bedtime with a snack.
    - Teenagers less than 15 years of age and children—Use and dose must be determined by your doctor.
  - For lowering growth hormone (acromegaly):
    - Adults and teenagers 15 years of age or older—At first, 1.25 to 2.5 milligrams (mg) once a day taken at bedtime with a snack for three days. Then your doctor may change your dose by 1.25 or 2.5 mg every three to seven days as needed. Doses greater than 5 mg are divided into smaller doses and taken with meals or at bedtime with a snack.
    - Teenagers less than 15 years of age and children—Use and dose must be determined by your doctor.
  - For Parkinson's disease:
    - Adults and teenagers 15 years of age or older—At first, 1.25 milligrams (mg) one or two times a day taken with meals or at bedtime with a snack. Then your doctor may change your dose over several weeks as needed.
    - Teenagers less than 15 years of age and children—Use and dose must be determined by your doctor.
  - For pituitary tumors:
    - Adults and teenagers 15 years of age or older—At first, 1.25 milligrams (mg) two or three times a day taken with meals. Then your doctor may change your dose over several weeks as needed.
    - Teenagers less than 15 years of age and children—Use and dose must be determined by your doctor.

Missed dose—If you miss a dose of this medicine, take it as soon as possible. However, if it is almost time for your next dose, skip the missed dose and go back to your regular dosing schedule. Do not double doses.

Storage—Store the medicine in a closed container at room temperature, away from heat, moisture, and direct light. Keep from freezing.

Keep out of the reach of children.

Do not keep outdated medicine or medicine no longer needed.

Precautions While Using This Medicine

It is important that your doctor check your progress at regular visits, to make sure that this medicine is working properly and to check for unwanted effects.

This medicine may cause some people to become drowsy, dizzy, or less alert than they are normally. Make sure you know how you react to this medicine before you drive, use machines, or do anything else that could be dangerous if you are dizzy or are not alert.

Dizziness is more likely to occur after the first dose of bromocriptine. Taking the first dose at bedtime or when you are able to lie down may lessen problems. It may also be helpful if you get up slowly from a lying or sitting position. Your doctor may also recommend that you take the first dose vaginally.

Bromocriptine may cause dryness of the mouth. For temporary relief, use sugarless candy or gum, melt bits of ice in your mouth, or use a saliva substitute. However, if dry mouth continues for more than 2 weeks, check with your medical doctor or dentist. Continuing dryness of the mouth may increase the chance of dental disease, including tooth decay, gum disease, and fungus infections.

It may take several weeks for bromocriptine to work. Do not stop taking this medicine or reduce the amount you are taking without first checking with your doctor.

Drinking alcohol while you are taking bromocriptine may cause you to have a certain reaction. Avoid alcoholic beverages until you have discussed this with your doctor. Some of the symptoms you may have if you drink any alcohol while you are taking this medicine are blurred vision, chest pain, confusion, fast or pounding heartbeat, flushing or redness of face, nausea, severe weakness, sweating, throbbing headache, or vomiting.

For females who are able to bear children and who are taking this medicine for menstrual or infertility problems, to stop milk production, or to treat acromegaly or pituitary tumors:

• It is best to use some type of birth control while you are taking bromocriptine. However, do not use oral contraceptives ("the Pill") since they may prevent this medicine from working. For women using bromocriptine for infertility, tell your doctor when your normal menstrual cycle returns. If you wish to become pregnant, you and your doctor should decide on the best time for you to stop using birth control. Tell your doctor right away if you think you have become pregnant while taking this medicine. You and your doctor should discuss whether or not you should continue to take bromocriptine during pregnancy.

• Check with your doctor right away if you develop blurred vision, a sudden headache, or severe nausea and vomiting.

Side Effects of This Medicine

Along with its needed effects, a medicine may cause some unwanted effects. Although not all of these side effects may occur, if they do occur they may need medical attention.

Some serious side effects have occurred during the use of bromocriptine to stop milk flow after pregnancy or abortion. These side effects have included strokes, seizures (convulsions), and heart attacks. Some deaths have also occurred. You should discuss with your doctor the good that this medicine will do as well as the risks of using it.

Check with your doctor immediately if any of the following side effects occur:
> *Rare*
>> Black, tarry stools; bloody vomit; chest pain (severe); convulsions (seizures); fainting; fast heartbeat; headache (unusual); increased sweating; nausea and vomiting (continuing or severe); nervousness; shortness of breath (unexplained); vision changes (such as blurred vision or temporary blindness); weakness (sudden)

Check with your doctor as soon as possible if any of the following side effects occur:
> *Less common—reported more often in patients with Parkinson's disease*
>> Confusion; hallucinations (seeing, hearing, or feeling things that are not there); uncontrolled movements of the body, such as the face, tongue, arms, hands, head, and upper body
>
> *Rare—reported more often in patients taking large doses*
>> Abdominal or stomach pain (continuing or severe); increased frequency of urination; loss of appetite (continuing); lower back pain; runny nose (continuing); weakness

Some side effects may occur that usually do not need medical attention. These side effects may go away during treatment as your body adjusts to the medicine. Also, your health care professional may be able to tell you about ways to prevent or reduce some of these side effects. Check with your health care professional if any of the following side effects continue or are bothersome or if you have any questions about them:
> *More common*
>> Dizziness or lightheadedness, especially when getting up from a lying or sitting position; nausea
>
> *Less common*
>> Constipation; diarrhea; drowsiness or tiredness; dry mouth; leg cramps at night; loss of appetite; mental depression; stomach pain; stuffy nose; tingling or pain in fingers and toes when exposed to cold; vomiting

Some side effects may be more likely to occur in patients who are taking bromocriptine for Parkinson's disease, acromegaly, or pituitary tumors since they may be taking larger doses.

Other side effects not listed may also occur in some patients. If you notice any other effects, check with your healthcare professional.

BRONCHODILATORS, ADRENERGIC (Inhalation)

Some commonly used brand names are:

In the U.S.—

Adrenalin Chloride (3)	Isuprel (7)
Airet (1)	Isuprel Mistometer (7)
Alupent (8)	Maxair (9)
Arm-a-Med Isoetharine (6)	Maxair Autohaler (9)
Arm-a-Med Metaproterenol (8)	Medihaler-Iso (7)
	microNefrin (3)
Asthmahaler Mist (3)	Nephron (3)
AsthmaNefrin (3)	Primatene Mist (3)
Beta-2 (6)	Proventil (1)
Brethaire (12)	Proventil HFA (1)
Bronkaid Mist (3)	S-2 (3)
Bronkaid Suspension Mist (3)	Serevent Diskus (11)
Bronkometer (6)	Vaponefrin (3)
Bronkosol (6)	Ventolin (1)
Dey-Lute Isoetharine (6)	Ventolin HFA (1)
Dey-Lute Metaproterenol (8)	Ventolin Nebules (1)
Foradil (5)	Ventolin Rotacaps (1)

In Canada—

Alupent (8)	Novo-Salmol (1)
Apo-Salvent (1)	Oxeze Turbuhaler (5)
Berotec (4)	Pro-Air (10)
Bricanyl Turbuhaler (12)	Serevent (11)
Bronkaid Mistometer (3)	Serevent Diskhaler (11)
Foradil (5)	Serevent Diskus (11)
Gen-Salbutamol Sterinebs	Vaponefrin (3)
P.F. (1)	Ventodisk (1)
Isuprel (7)	Ventolin (1)
Isuprel Mistometer (7)	Ventolin Nebules P.F. (1)
Maxair (9)	Ventolin Rotacaps (1)

This information applies to the following medicines:

1. Albuterol (al-BYOO-ter-ole)
2. Bitolterol (bye-TOLE-ter-ole)
3. Epinephrine (ep-i-NEF-rin)
4. Fenoterol (fen-OH-ter-ole)
5. Formoterol (for-MOH-ter-ol))
6. Isoetharine (eye-soe-ETH-a-reen)
7. Isoproterenol (eye-soe-proe-TER-e-nole)
8. Metaproterenol (met-a-proe-TER-e-nole)
9. Pirbuterol (peer-BYOO-ter-ole)
10. Procaterol (proe-KAY-ter-ole)
11. Salmeterol (sal-ME-te-role)
12. Terbutaline (ter-BYOO-ta-leen)

Category

- **Bronchodilator**—Albuterol; Bitolterol; Epinephrine; Fenoterol; Formoterol; Isoetharine; Isoproterenol; Metaproterenol; Pirbuterol; Procaterol; Racepinephrine; Salmeterol; Terbutaline
- **Croup therapy agent**—Epinephrine

Description

Adrenergic bronchodilators are medicines that are breathed in through the mouth to open up the bronchial tubes (air passages) of the lungs. Some of these medicines are used to treat the symptoms of asthma, chronic bronchitis, emphysema, and other lung diseases, while others are used to prevent the symptoms.

Salmeterol is a long-acting bronchodilator that is used with anti-inflammatory medication to prevent asthma attacks. *Salmeterol is different from the other adrenergic bronchodilators because it does not act quickly enough to relieve an asthma attack that has already started.*

Some of these medicines are also breathed in through the mouth to prevent bronchospasm (wheezing or difficulty in breathing) caused by exercise. Also, epinephrine may be used in the treatment of croup.

All of these medicines, except some epinephrine preparations, are available only with your doctor's prescription. Although some of the epinephrine preparations are available without a prescription, your doctor may have special instructions on the proper dose of epinephrine for your medical condition.

These medicines are available in the following dosage forms:

Inhalation
- Albuterol
  - ○ Inhalation aerosol
  - ○ Inhalation solution
  - ○ Powder for inhalation
- Bitolterol
  - ○ Inhalation aerosol (Not commercially available)
  - ○ Inhalation solution (Not commercially available)
- Epinephrine
  - ○ Inhalation aerosol
  - ○ Inhalation solution
- Fenoterol
  - ○ Inhalation aerosol
  - ○ Inhalation solution
- Formoterol
  - ○ for inhalation
- Isoetharine
  - ○ Inhalation aerosol
  - ○ Inhalation solution
- Isoproterenol
  - ○ Inhalation aerosol
  - ○ Inhalation solution
- Metaproterenol
  - ○ Inhalation aerosol
  - ○ Inhalation solution
- Pirbuterol
  - ○ Inhalation aerosol
- Procaterol
  - ○ Inhalation aerosol
- Salmeterol
  - ○ Inhalation aerosol
  - ○ Powder for inhalation
- Terbutaline
  - ○ Inhalation aerosol

Before Using This Medicine

In deciding to use a medicine, the risks of taking the medicine must be weighed against the good it will do. This is a decision you and your doctor will make. For inhalation adrenergic bronchodilators, the following should be considered:

Allergies—Tell your doctor if you have ever had any unusual or allergic reaction to albuterol, bitolterol, epinephrine, fenoterol, formoterol, isoetharine, isoproterenol, metaproterenol, pirbuterol, procaterol, salmeterol, terbutaline, or other inhalation medicines. Also tell your health care professional if you are allergic to sulfites, which may be used as a preservative in some of these medicines or to lactose, contained in powders for inhalation.

Pregnancy—
- *For albuterol, bitolterol, formoterol, metaproterenol, and salmeterol:* These medicines are used to treat asthma in pregnant women. Although there are no studies on birth defects in humans, problems have not been reported. Some studies in animals have shown that they cause birth defects when given in doses many times higher than the human dose. Before taking these medicines, make sure your doctor knows if you are pregnant or if you may become pregnant.

- *For epinephrine:* Women given epinephrine subcutaneously (under the skin) during pregnancy have been studied. The babies of these women had more birth defects than expected, although the severity of the mother's asthma may have contributed to this result.

- *For fenoterol, isoproterenol, pirbuterol, procaterol, and terbutaline:* These medicines are used to treat asthma in pregnant women. Although there are no studies on birth defects in humans, problems have not been reported. These medicines have not been shown to cause birth defects in animal studies when given in doses many times higher than the human dose.

- *For isoetharine:* Studies on birth defects have not been done in either humans or animals.

Breast-feeding—
- It is not known whether these medicines pass into the breast milk. Although most medicines pass into breast milk in small amounts, many of them may be used safely while breast-feeding. Mothers who are using these medicines and who wish to breast-feed should discuss this with their doctor.

Children—
Appropriate studies performed to date have not demonstrated pediatrics-specific problems that would limit the usefulness of these medicines in children. However, isoetharine is not recommended for use in children.

Older adults—
- *For albuterol, bitolterol, epinephrine, fenoterol, isoetharine, isoproterenol, metaproterenol, pirbuterol, procaterol, and terbutaline:* These medicines have not been studied specifically in older people. Therefore, it may not be known whether they work exactly the same way they do in younger adults or if they cause different side effects or problems in older people. There is no specific information comparing use of inhalation adrenergic bronchodilators in the elderly with use in other age groups.
- *For salmeterol:* This medicine has been tested in a limited number of patients 65 years of age or older. It has not been shown to cause different side effects or problems in older people than it does in younger adults.

Other medicines—
Although certain medicines should not be used together at all, in other cases two different medicines may be used together even if an interaction might occur. In these cases, your doctor may want to change the dose, or other precautions may be necessary. When you are using inhalation adrenergic bronchodilators, it is especially important that your health care professional know if you are taking any of the following:
- Beta-adrenergic blocking agents (acebutolol [e.g., Sectral], atenolol [e.g., Tenormin], betaxolol [e.g., Kerlone], carteolol [e.g., Cartrol], labetalol [e.g., Normodyne], metoprolol [e.g., Lopressor], nadolol [e.g., Corgard], oxprenolol [e.g., Trasicor], penbutolol [e.g., Levatol], pindolol [e.g., Visken], propranolol [e.g., Inderal], sotalol [e.g., Sotacor], timolol [e.g., Blocadren])—These medicines may make your condition worse and prevent the adrenergic bronchodilators from working properly
- Disopyramide,
- Quinidine,
- Phenothiazines, or
- Procainamide—These medicines may increase the risk of heart problems.

Other medical problems—
The presence of other medical problems may affect the use of inhalation adrenergic bronchodilators. Make sure you tell your doctor if you have any other medical problems, especially:
- Heart or blood vessel disease—These medicines may make these conditions worse.
- High blood pressure, not well controlled—Epinephrine may make this condition worse.

- Overactive thyroid or
- Pheochromocytoma, diagnosed or suspected—The chance of side effects may be increased.

Proper Use of This Medicine

These medicines come with patient directions. Read them carefully before using the medicine. If you do not understand the directions or if you are not sure how to use the medicine, ask your health care professional to show you what to do. Also, ask your health care professional to check regularly how you use the medicine to make sure you are using it properly.

Use this medicine only as directed. Do not use more of it and do not use it more often than recommended on the label, unless otherwise directed by your doctor. Using the medicine more often may increase the chance of serious unwanted effects. Deaths have occurred when too much inhalation bronchodilator medicine was used.

Keep the spray away from your eyes because it may cause irritation.

Salmeterol and formoterol are used to prevent asthma attacks. They are not used to relieve an attack that has already started. For relief of an asthma attack that has already started, you should use another medicine (not formoterol) that starts working faster than salmeterol does. *If you do not have another medicine to use for an attack or if you have any questions about this, check with your doctor.* Because the effects of salmeterol and formoterol usually last about 12 hours, doses should never be taken more than two times a day or less than 12 hours apart.

Salmeterol and formoterol are not substitutes for your oral or inhaled corticosteroid medicine. If you begin taking salmeterol or formoterol, the dosage of your corticosteroid medicine should not be changed or stopped even if you begin to feel better. *If you have any questions about this, check with your doctor.*

Some *epinephrine* preparations are available without a doctor's prescription. However, *do not use this medicine unless you are seeing a doctor about asthma. Do not use this medicine* if you have been hospitalized for asthma treatment or if you are taking a prescription medicine for asthma, unless you have been told to do so by a doctor.

When you use the inhaler for the first time, or if you have not used it in a while, the inhaler may not deliver the right amount of medicine with the first puff. Therefore, before using the inhaler, you may have to test or prime it.

- *To test or prime most inhalers:*
  - Insert the medicine container (canister) firmly into the clean mouthpiece according to the manufacturer's directions. Check to make sure it is placed properly into the mouthpiece.
  - Take the cap off the mouthpiece and shake the inhaler three or four times.
  - Hold the inhaler well away from you at arm's length and press the top of the canister, spraying the medicine into the air *two* times. The inhaler will now be ready to provide the right amount of medicine when you use it.
- *To use most inhalers:*
  - Using your thumb and one or two fingers, hold the inhaler upright, with the mouthpiece end down and pointing toward you.

- Take the cap off the mouthpiece. Check the mouthpiece to make sure it is clear. Then, gently shake the inhaler three or four times.
- Breathe out slowly to the end of a normal breath.
- Use the inhalation method recommended by your doctor:
  - Open-mouth method—Place the mouthpiece about 1 to 2 inches (2 finger widths) in front of your widely opened mouth. Make sure the inhaler is aimed into your mouth so the spray does not hit the roof of your mouth or your tongue.
  - Closed-mouth method—Place the mouthpiece in your mouth between your teeth and over your tongue with your lips closed tightly around it. Make sure your tongue or teeth are not blocking the opening.
- Start to breathe in slowly through your mouth. At the same time, press the top of the canister one time to get 1 puff of medicine. Continue to breathe in slowly for 3 to 5 seconds. Count the seconds while breathing in. It is important to press the canister and breathe in slowly at the same time so the medicine gets into your lungs. This step may be difficult at first. If you are using the closed-mouth method and you see a fine mist coming from your mouth or nose, the inhaler is not being used correctly.
- Hold your breath as long as you can up to 10 seconds. This gives the medicine time to settle into your airways and lungs.
- Take the mouthpiece away from your mouth and breathe out slowly.
- If your doctor has told you to inhale more than 1 puff of medicine at each dose, gently shake the inhaler again and take the next puff following exactly the same steps you used for the first puff. Press the canister one time for each puff of medicine.
- When you are done, wipe off the mouthpiece and replace the cap.

Your doctor, nurse, or pharmacist may want you to use a spacer or holding chamber with the inhaler. A spacer helps get the medicine into the lungs and reduces the amount of medicine that stays in your mouth and throat.

To use a spacer with the inhaler:

- Attach the spacer to the inhaler according to the manufacturer's directions. There are different types of spacers available, but the method of breathing is the same with most spacers.
- Gently shake the inhaler and spacer three or four times.
- Hold the mouthpiece of the spacer away from your mouth and breathe out slowly to the end of a normal breath.
- Place the mouthpiece into your mouth between your teeth and over your tongue with your lips closed around it.
- Press down on the canister top one time to release 1 puff of medicine into the spacer. Within one or two seconds, begin to breathe in slowly through your mouth for three to five seconds. Do not breathe in through your nose. Count the seconds while inhaling.
- Hold your breath as long as you can up to ten seconds (count slowly to ten).
- Breathe out slowly. Do not remove the mouthpiece from your mouth. Breathe in and out slowly two or three times to make sure the spacer is emptied.

- If your doctor has told you to take more than 1 puff of medicine at each dose, gently shake the inhaler and spacer again, and take the next puff, following exactly the same steps you used for the first puff. Do not put more than 1 puff of medicine into the spacer at a time.
- If you rinse your mouth with water after you have finished, be sure to spit out the rinse water. Do not swallow it.
- When you are finished, remove the spacer from the inhaler. Wipe off the mouthpiece and replace the cap.
- Clean the inhaler and mouthpiece at least once a week.
  - To clean the inhaler:
    - Remove the canister from the inhaler and set the canister aside.
    - Wash the mouthpiece and cap with warm, soapy water. Then, rinse well with warm, running water.
    - Shake off the excess water and let the inhaler parts air dry completely before putting the inhaler back together.
- Save your inhaler. Refill units may be available.

For patients using the powder for inhalation dosage form:

- These medicines are used with a special device. If you do not understand the directions that come with the inhaler or if you are not sure how to use the inhaler, ask your health care professional to show you how to use it. Also, ask your health care professional to check regularly how you use the inhaler to make sure you are using it properly.

For patients using the inhalation solution dosage form:

- If you are using this medicine in a nebulizer, make sure you understand exactly how to use it. If you have any questions about this, check with your health care professional.
- Do not use if solution turns pinkish to brownish in color or if it becomes cloudy.
- Do not mix another inhalation medicine with an adrenergic bronchodilator medicine in the nebulizer unless told to do so by your health care professional.

Dosing—The dose of these medicines will be different for different patients. *Follow your doctor's orders or the directions on the label.* The following information includes only the average doses of these medicines. *If your dose is different, do not change it* unless your doctor tells you to do so.

The number of inhalations or the amount of medicine that you use depends on the strength of the medicine. Also, *the number of doses you take each day, the time allowed between doses, and the length of time you take the medicine depend on the medical problem for which you are taking the adrenergic bronchodilator.*

For albuterol
- For *inhalation aerosol* dosage form:
  - For preventing or treating bronchospasm:
    - Adults and children 4 years of age and older— 1 to 2 inhalations (puffs) every four to six hours.
    - Children up to 4 years of age—Dose must be determined by your doctor.
  - For preventing bronchospasm caused by exercise:
    - Adults and children 4 years of age and older— 2 inhalations (puffs) taken fifteen minutes before you start to exercise.

- Children up to 4 years of age—Dose must be determined by your doctor.

For albuterol sulfate

- For *inhalation aerosol* dosage form:
  - For treating bronchospasm:
    - Adults and children 4 years of age and older—1 to 2 inhalations (puffs) every four to six hours.
    - Children up to 4 years of age—Dose must be determined by your doctor.
  - For preventing bronchospasm caused by exercise:
    - Adults and children 4 years of age and older—2 inhalations (puffs) taken fifteen to thirty minutes before you start to exercise.
    - Children up to 4 years of age—Dose must be determined by your doctor.
- For *inhalation solution* dosage form:
  - For preventing or treating bronchospasm:
    - Adults and children 12 years of age and older—This medicine is used in a nebulizer and is taken by inhalation over five to fifteen minutes. The usual dose is 2.5 milligrams (mg) of albuterol taken every four to six hours if needed.
    - Children up to 12 years of age—This medicine is used in a nebulizer and is taken by inhalation over five to fifteen minutes. The usual dose is 1.25 to 2.5 milligrams (mg) of albuterol taken every four to six hours if needed.
- For *capsules (powder) for inhalation* dosage form:
  - For preventing or treating bronchospasm:
    - Adults and children 4 years of age and older—200 or 400 mcg taken by inhalation every four to six hours.
    - Children up to 4 years of age—Dose must be determined by your doctor.
  - For preventing bronchospasm caused by exercise:
    - Adults and children 4 years of age and older—200 mcg taken by inhalation fifteen minutes before you start to exercise.
    - Children up to 4 years of age—Dose must be determined by your doctor.

For bitolterol

- Bitolterol was withdrawn from the U.S. market by Elan Pharmaceuticals in November 2001.
- For *inhalation aerosol* dosage form:
  - For preventing or treating bronchospasm:
    - Adults and children 12 years of age and older—2 inhalations (puffs) every eight hours or 2 inhalations (puffs) at first, allowing one to three minutes between each puff. This dose may be followed by another puff, if needed. However, the dose taken each day should not be more than 2 puffs every four hours or 3 puffs every six hours.
    - Children up to 12 years of age—Dose must be determined by your doctor.
  - For preventing bronchospasm caused by exercise:
    - Adults and teenagers—2 inhalations (puffs) taken five minutes before you start to exercise.
    - Children—1 or 2 inhalations (puffs) taken five minutes before you start to exercise.
- For *inhalation solution* dosage form:
  - For preventing or treating bronchospasm:
    - Adults and children 12 years of age and older—This medicine is used in a nebulizer and is taken

by inhalation over ten to fifteen minutes. The usual dose is 1 to 2.5 milligrams (mg) of bitolterol taken three or four times a day. Doses should be taken at least four hours apart.
    - Children up to 12 years of age—Dose must be determined by your doctor.

For epinephrine

- For treating bronchospasm:
  - For *inhalation aerosol* dosage form:
    - Adults and children 4 years of age and older—1 inhalation (puff). The dose may be repeated after at least one minute, if needed. Doses should be taken at least three hours apart.
    - Children up to 4 years of age—Dose must be determined by your doctor.
  - For *inhalation solution* dosage form:
    - Adults and children 4 years of age and older—This medicine should be used in a hand-bulb nebulizer. The usual dose is 1 to 3 inhalations (puffs) of a 1% solution. Doses should be taken at least three hours apart.
    - Children up to 4 years of age—Dose must be determined by your doctor.

For fenoterol

- For *inhalation aerosol* dosage form:
  - For preventing or treating bronchospasm:
    - Adults and children 12 years of age and older—100 or 200 micrograms (mcg), repeated three or four times a day if needed. This medicine should not be taken more often than every four hours. The total dose should not be more than 8 puffs a day of the 100 mcg per spray product or 6 puffs of the 200 mcg per spray product.
    - Children up to 12 years of age—Dose must be determined by your doctor.
- For *inhalation solution* dosage form:
  - For preventing or treating bronchospasm:
    - Adults and children 12 years of age and older—This medicine is used in a nebulizer and is taken by inhalation over ten to fifteen minutes. The usual dose is 0.5 to 1 milligram (mg) of fenoterol taken every six hours if needed.
    - Children up to 12 years of age—Dose must be determined by your doctor.

For formoterol

- For *powder for inhalation* dosage form:
  - For preventing bronchospasm:
    - Adults and children 5 years of age and older—12 mcg taken by oral inhalation twice daily
    - Children under 5 years of age—Use and dose must be determined by your doctor.
- Canadian product information states that formoterol is used in children 6 years of age and older.

For isoetharine

- For *inhalation solution* dosage form:
  - For treating bronchospasm:
    - Adults—This medicine is used in a nebulizer and is taken by inhalation over fifteen to twenty minutes. The amount of medicine you use and whether it requires dilution depends on the product ordered by your doctor. The usual dose is 2.5 to

10 milligrams (mg). This medicine usually should not be used more often than every four hours.
- Children—Use is not recommended.

- For *inhalation aerosol* dosage form:
  ○ For treating bronchospasm:
    ▪ Adults and teenagers—1 or 2 inhalations (puffs). This dose may be repeated every four hours as necessary.
    ▪ Children—Use is not recommended.

For isoproterenol
- For *inhalation solution* dosage form:
  ○ For treating bronchospasm:
    ▪ Adults and teenagers—This medicine is used in a nebulizer and is taken by inhalation over ten to twenty minutes. The usual dose is 2.5 milligrams (mg). This medicine usually should not be used more often than every four hours.
    ▪ Children—This medicine is used in a nebulizer and is taken by inhalation over ten to twenty minutes. The usual dose is 0.05 to 0.1 milligram (mg) per kilogram (kg) of body weight, up to 1.25 mg, diluted. The dose may be repeated every four hours, if needed.

For isoproterenol hydrochloride
- For *inhalation aerosol* dosage form:
  ○ For treating bronchospasm:
    ▪ Adults and children 12 years of age and older—1 inhalation (puff), repeated after two to five minutes if needed. This dose is taken every three to four hours.
    ▪ Children up to 12 years of age—Use is not recommended.

For isoproterenol sulfate
- For *inhalation aerosol* dosage form:
  ○ For treating bronchospasm:
    ▪ Adults and children 12 years of age and older—1 inhalation (puff), repeated after two to five minutes if needed. This dose is taken every four to six hours.
    ▪ Children up to 12 years of age—Dose must be determined by your doctor.

For metaproterenol
- For *inhalation aerosol* dosage form:
  ○ For preventing and treating bronchospasm:
    ▪ Adults and children 12 years of age and older—2 or 3 inhalations (puffs) every three to four hours. The total dose should not be more than 12 puffs a day.
    ▪ Children up to 12 years of age—1 to 3 inhalations (puffs) every three to four hours. The total dose should not be more than 12 puffs a day.
- For *inhalation solution* dosage form:
  ○ For preventing or treating bronchospasm:
    ▪ Adults and children 6 years of age and older—This medicine is used in a nebulizer and is taken by inhalation. The amount of medicine you use and whether it requires dilution depends on the product ordered by your doctor. The usual dose is 10 to 15 milligrams (mg) taken three or four times a day. Doses should be taken at least four hours apart.
    ▪ Children up to 6 years of age—This medicine is used in a nebulizer and is taken by inhalation. The

amount of medicine you use and whether it requires dilution depends on the product ordered by your doctor. The usual dose is 5 to 15 milligrams (mg) taken three or four times a day, at least four hours apart.

For pirbuterol
- For *inhalation aerosol* dosage form:
  ○ For preventing and treating bronchospasm:
    ▪ Adults and children—1 or 2 inhalations (puffs) every four to six hours. The total dose should not be more than 12 puffs a day.
  ○ For preventing bronchospasm caused by exercise:
    ▪ Adults and children—2 inhalations (puffs) taken five minutes before you start to exercise.

For procaterol
- For *inhalation aerosol* dosage form:
  ○ For preventing and treating bronchospasm:
    ▪ Adults and children 12 years of age and older—1 or 2 inhalations (puffs) three times a day.
    ▪ Children up to 12 years of age—Dose must be determined by your doctor.
  ○ For preventing bronchospasm caused by exercise:
    ▪ Adults and children 12 years of age and older—1 or 2 inhalations (puffs) taken at least fifteen minutes before you start to exercise.

For salmeterol
- For the *inhalation aerosol* dosage form:
  ○ For preventing bronchospasm:
    ▪ Adults and children 12 years of age and older—2 inhalations (puffs) two times a day, in the morning and evening. Doses should be taken about twelve hours apart.
    ▪ Children up to 12 years of age—Dose must be determined by your doctor.
  ○ Canadian manufacturer states that use in children ages 4 years and older is 2 inhalations twice daily.
  ○ For preventing bronchospasm caused by exercise:
    ▪ Adults and children 12 years of age and older—2 inhalations (puffs) taken at least thirty to sixty minutes before you start to exercise. If you are already using salmeterol two times a day to treat your asthma, you do not need to use additional salmeterol before you exercise. If you exercise more than once a day, you should not take more than 2 doses per day, a minimum of 12 hours apart.
    ▪ Children up to 12 years of age—Dose must be determined by your doctor.
- For the *powder for inhalation* dosage form:
  ○ For preventing bronchospasm:
    ▪ Adults and children 4 years of age and older—1 inhalation (the contents of one blister) two times a day, in the morning and evening. Doses should be taken about twelve hours apart.
    ▪ Children up to 4 years of age—Use and dose must be determined by your doctor.
  ○ For preventing bronchospasm caused by exercise:
    ▪ Adults and children 4 years of age and older—1 inhalation (the contents of one blister) at least 30 minutes before exercise
    ▪ Children up to 4 years of age—Use and dose must be determined by your doctor.

For terbutaline
- For *inhalation aerosol* dosage form:
  - For preventing or treating bronchospasm:
    - Adults and children—
      — For the 200 microgram (mcg) per metered spray product: 2 inhalations (puffs) every four to six hours.
      — For the 500 mcg per metered spray product: 1 inhalation (puff), repeated after five minutes if needed. The total dose should not be more than 6 puffs a day.
  - For preventing bronchospasm caused by exercise:
    - Adults and children—
      — For the 200 microgram (mcg) per metered spray product: 2 inhalations (puffs) taken five to fifteen minutes before you start to exercise.

Missed dose—

- *For formoterol:* If you miss a regularly scheduled dose of formoterol and it has been less than 6 hours since the scheduled time, take the dose as soon as possible and then go back to your regular dosing schedule. If it has been longer than 6 hours, skip the dose and take the next dose at the regularly scheduled time. Do not double doses.

- *For all other adrenergic bronchodilators:* If you are using one of these medicines regularly and you miss a dose, use it as soon as possible. Then use any remaining doses for that day at regularly spaced intervals. Do not double doses.

Storage—To store this medicine:
- Keep out of the reach of children.
- Store away from heat.
- Store the solution form of this medicine away from direct light. Store the inhalation aerosol form of this medicine away from direct sunlight.
- Keep the medicine from freezing.
- Store canister with the nozzle end down.
- Do not store the powder for inhalation forms of these medicines in the bathroom, near the kitchen sink, or in other damp places. Moisture may cause the medicine to break down.
- Do not puncture, break, or burn the inhalation aerosol container, even if it is empty.
- Do not keep outdated medicine or medicine no longer needed. Be sure that any discarded medicine is out of the reach of children.

Precautions While Using This Medicine

It is important that your doctor check your progress at regular intervals to make sure that your medicine is working properly.

If you still have trouble breathing after using one of these medicines, or if your condition becomes worse, check with your doctor at once.

You may also be taking an anti-inflammatory medicine for asthma along with this medicine. *Do not stop taking the anti-inflammatory medicine even if your asthma seems better, unless you are told to do so by your doctor.*

For patients using *salmeterol* or *formoterol,* check with your doctor:
- If you need to use 4 or more inhalations (puffs) a day of a fast-acting inhaled bronchodilator for 2 or more days in a row to relieve asthma attacks.
- If you need to use more than 1 canister (a total of 200 inhalations per canister) of a fast-acting inhaled bronchodilator in a 2–month period to relieve asthma attacks.

For patients using *any of these medicines except salmeterol and formoterol, check with your doctor:*
- If you need more inhalations (puffs) than usual of a fast-acting beta-adrenergic bronchodilator to relieve an acute attack
- If not using an anti-inflammatory medicine and using a fast-acting beta-adrenergic bronchodilator to relieve symptoms more than two times per week
- If you are using an anti-inflammatory medicine and you also are using more than 1 canister per month of a fast-acting beta-adrenergic bronchodilator to relieve symptoms

---

Side Effects of This Medicine

Along with its needed effects, a medicine may cause some unwanted effects. Although not all of these side effects may occur, if they do occur they may need medical attention.

Check with your doctor immediately if any of the following side effects occur:
> *Rare*
>> Dizziness, severe; feeling of choking, irritation, or swelling in throat; flushing or redness of skin; hives; increased shortness of breath; skin rash; swelling of face, lips, or eyelids; tightness in chest or wheezing, troubled breathing
> *Incidence not known (for salmeterol)*
>> Difficulty breathing; noisy breathing

Other side effects may occur that usually do not need medical attention. These side effects may go away during treatment as your body adjusts to the medicine. However, check with your doctor if any of the following side effects continue or are bothersome:
> *More common*
>> Fast heartbeat; headache; nervousness; trembling
> *Less common*
>> Coughing or other bronchial irritation; dizziness or light-headedness; dryness or irritation of mouth or throat
> *Rare*
>> Chest discomfort or pain; drowsiness or weakness; irregular heartbeat; irritation of throat or mouth; muscle cramps or twitching; nausea and/or vomiting; restlessness; trouble in sleeping

Not all of the side effects listed above have been reported for each of these medicines, but they have been reported for at least one of them. All of the adrenergic bronchodilators are similar, so any of the above side effects may occur with any of these medicines.

While you are using an adrenergic bronchodilator, you may notice an unusual or unpleasant taste. This may be expected and will go away when you stop using the medicine.

Isoproterenol may cause the saliva to turn pinkish to red. This is to be expected while you are taking this medicine.

Other side effects not listed above may also occur in some patients. If you notice any other effects, check with your doctor.

Additional Information

Once a medicine has been approved for marketing for a certain use, experience may show that it is also useful for other medical problems. Although these uses are not included in product labeling, some of the adrenergic bronchodilators are used in certain patients with the following medical conditions:

- Hyperkalemia (too much potassium in the blood) in children (albuterol)

BRONCHODILATORS, ADRENERGIC (Oral/Injection)

Some commonly used brand names are:

In the U.S.—

Adrenalin (3)	EpiPen Jr. Auto-Injector (3)
Alupent (5)	Isuprel (4)
Ana-Guard (3)	Proventil (1)
Brethine (6)	Proventil Repetabs (1)
Bricanyl (6)	Ventolin (1)
EpiPen Auto-Injector (3)	Volmax (1)

In Canada—

Adrenalin (3)	EpiPen Jr. Auto-Injector (3)
Alupent (5)	Isuprel (4)
Bricanyl (6)	Ventolin (1)
EpiPen Auto-Injector (3)	

This information applies to the following medicines:

1. Albuterol (al-BYOO-ter-ole)
2. Ephedrine (e-FED-rin)
3. Epinephrine (ep-i-NEF-rin)
4. Isoproterenol (eye-soe-proe-TER-e-nole)
5. Metaproterenol (met-a-proe-TER-e-nol)
6. Terbutaline (ter-BYOO-ta-leen)

Category

- **Anesthetic adjunct (local and regional)—**
- **antiallergic, systemic—**
- **antihemorrhagic, dental—**
- **bronchodilator—**
- **priapism reversal agent—**
- **tocolytic agent—**

Description

Adrenergic bronchodilators are medicines that stimulate the nerves in many parts of the body, causing different effects.

Because these medicines open up the bronchial tubes (air passages) of the lungs, they are used to treat the symptoms of asthma, bronchitis, emphysema, and other lung diseases. They relieve cough, wheezing, shortness of breath, and troubled breathing by increasing the flow of air through the bronchial tubes.

Epinephrine injection (including the auto-injector but not the sterile suspension) is used in the emergency treatment of allergic reactions to insect stings, medicines, foods, or other substances. It relieves skin rash, hives, and itching; wheezing; and swelling of the lips, eyelids, tongue, and inside of the nose.

These medicines may be also used for other conditions as determined by your doctor.

Ephedrine capsules are available without a prescription. However, check with your doctor before taking ephedrine.

All of the other adrenergic bronchodilators are available only with your doctor's prescription.

These medicines are available in the following dosage forms:

Oral
- Albuterol
  - Oral solution
  - Syrup
  - Tablets
  - Extended-release tablets
- Ephedrine
  - Capsules
- Metaproterenol
  - Syrup
  - Tablets
- Terbutaline
  - Tablets

Parenteral
- Albuterol
  - Injection
- Ephedrine
  - Injection
- Epinephrine
  - Injection
- Isoproterenol
  - Injection
- Terbutaline
  - Injection

Before Using This Medicine

In deciding to use a medicine, the risks of taking the medicine must be weighed against the good it will do. This is a decision you and your doctor will make. For adrenergic bronchodilators taken by mouth or given by injection, the following should be considered:

Allergies—Tell your doctor if you have ever had any unusual or allergic reaction to albuterol, ephedrine, epinephrine, isoproterenol, metaproterenol, or terbutaline. Also, tell your doctor if you are allergic to any other substances, such as foods, preservatives, or dyes.

Pregnancy—Some of these medicines can increase blood sugar, blood pressure, and heart rate in the mother, and may increase the heart rate and decrease blood sugar in the infant. Before taking any of these medicines, make sure your doctor knows if you are pregnant or may become pregnant.
- *For albuterol:* Albuterol has not been studied in pregnant women. Studies in animals have shown that albuterol causes birth defects when given in doses many times the usual human dose.
- *For ephedrine:* Ephedrine has not been studied in pregnant women or in animals.

- *For epinephrine:* Epinephrine has been shown to cause birth defects in humans. However, this medicine may be needed during allergic reactions that threaten the mother's life.

- *For isoproterenol:* Studies on birth defects with isoproterenol have not been done in humans. However, there is some evidence that it causes birth defects in animals.

- *For metaproterenol:* Metaproterenol has not been studied in pregnant women. However, studies in animals have shown that metaproterenol causes birth defects and death of the animal fetus when given in doses many times the usual human dose.

- *For terbutaline:* Terbutaline has not been shown to cause birth defects in humans using recommended doses or in animal studies when given in doses many times the usual human dose.

Some of these medicines also relax the muscles of the uterus and may delay labor.

- *For albuterol:* Albuterol has not been studied in pregnant women. Studies in animals have shown that albuterol causes birth defects when given in doses many times the usual human dose.

- *For ephedrine:* Ephedrine has not been studied in pregnant women or in animals.

- *For epinephrine:* Epinephrine has been shown to cause birth defects in humans. However, this medicine may be needed during allergic reactions that threaten the mother's life.

- *For isoproterenol:* Studies on birth defects with isoproterenol have not been done in humans. However, there is some evidence that it causes birth defects in animals.

- *For metaproterenol:* Metaproterenol has not been studied in pregnant women. However, studies in animals have shown that metaproterenol causes birth defects and death of the animal fetus when given in doses many times the usual human dose.

- *For terbutaline:* Terbutaline has not been shown to cause birth defects in humans using recommended doses or in animal studies when given in doses many times the usual human dose.

Breast-feeding—

- *For albuterol, isoproterenol, and metaproterenol:* It is not known whether albuterol, isoproterenol, or metaproterenol passes into breast milk. Although most medicines pass into breast milk in small amounts, many of them may be used safely while breast-feeding. Mothers who are taking this medicine and who wish to breast-feed should discuss this with their doctor.

- *For ephedrine:* Ephedrine passes into breast milk and may cause unwanted side effects in babies of mothers using ephedrine.

- *For epinephrine:* Epinephrine passes into breast milk and may cause unwanted side effects in babies of mothers using epinephrine.

- *For terbutaline:* Terbutaline passes into breast milk but has not been shown to cause harmful effects in the infant. Mothers who are taking this medicine and who wish to breast-feed should discuss this with their doctor.

Children—There is no specific information comparing use of isoproterenol, metaproterenol, or terbutaline in children with use in other age groups.

Excitement and nervousness may be more common in children 2 to 6 years of age who take albuterol than in adults and older children.

Infants and children may be especially sensitive to the effects of epinephrine.

Older adults—Older adults may be more sensitive to the side effects of these medicines, such as trembling, high blood pressure, or fast or irregular heartbeats.

Other medicines—Although certain medicines should not be used together at all, in other cases two different medicines may be used together even if an interaction might occur. In these cases, your doctor may want to change the dose, or other precautions may be necessary. When you are taking adrenergic bronchodilators, it is especially important that your health care professional know if you are taking any of the following:

For all adrenergic bronchodilators
- Amphetamines or
- Appetite suppressants (diet pills) or
- Medicine for colds, sinus problems, or hay fever or other allergies (including nose drops or sprays) or
- Other medicines for asthma or other breathing problems—The chance for side effects may be increased

- Beta-adrenergic blocking agents taken orally or by injection (acebutolol [e.g., Sectral], atenolol [e.g., Tenormin], betaxolol [e.g., Kerlone], bisoprolol [e.g., Zebeta], carteolol [e.g., Cartrol], labetalol [e.g., Normodyne], metoprolol [e.g., Lopressor, Toprol XL], nadolol [e.g., Corgard], oxprenolol [e.g., Trasicor], penbutolol [e.g., Levatol], pindolol [e.g., Visken], propranolol [e.g., Inderal], sotalol [e.g., Sotacor], timolol [e.g., Blocadren])—These medicines may prevent the adrenergic bronchodilators from working properly

- Beta-adrenergic blocking agents used in the eye (betaxolol [e.g., Betoptic], levobunolol [e.g., Betagan], metipranolol [e.g., OptiPranolol], timolol [e.g., Timoptic]—Enough of these medicines may be absorbed from the eye into the blood stream to prevent the adrenergic bronchodilators from working properly

- Cocaine—Unwanted effects of both medicines on the heart may be increased

- Digitalis medicines (e.g., Lanoxin) or
- Quinidine (e.g., Quinaglute Dura-Tabs, Quinidex)—The risk of heart rhythm problems may be increased

- Monoamine oxidase (MAO) inhibitor activity (isocarboxazid [e.g., Marplan], phenelzine [e.g., Nardil], procarbazine [e.g., Matulane], selegiline [e.g., Eldepryl], tranylcypromine [e.g., Parnate])—Taking adrenergic bronchodilators while you are taking or within 2 weeks of taking monoamine oxidase (MAO) inhibitors may dramatically increase the effects of MAO inhibitors

- Thyroid hormones—The effect of this medicine may be increased

- Tricyclic antidepressants (amitriptyline [e.g., Elavil], amoxapine [e.g., Asendin], clomipramine [e.g., Anafranil], desipramine [e.g., Norpramin], doxepin [e.g., Sinequan], imipramine [e.g., Tofranil], nortriptyline [e.g.,

Aventyl, Pamelor], protriptyline [e.g., Vivactil], trimipramine [e.g., Surmontil])—The effects of these medicines on the heart and blood vessels may be increased

Other medical problems—The presence of other medical problems may affect the use of these medicines. Make sure you tell your doctor if you have any other medical problems, especially:

- Convulsions (seizures)—These medicines may make this condition worse
- Diabetes mellitus (sugar diabetes)—These medicines may increase blood sugar, which could change the amount of insulin or other diabetes medicine you need
- Enlarged prostate—Ephedrine may make the condition worse
- Gastrointestinal narrowing—Use of the extended-release dosage form of albuterol may result in a blockage in the intestines.
- Glaucoma—Ephedrine or epinephrine may make the condition worse
- High blood pressure or
- Overactive thyroid—Use of ephedrine or epinephrine may cause severe high blood pressure and other side effects may also be increased
- Parkinson's disease—Epinephrine may make stiffness and trembling worse
- Psychiatric problems—Epinephrine may make problems worse
- Reduced blood flow to the brain—Epinephrine further decreases blood flow, which could make the problem worse
- Reduced blood flow to the heart or
- Heart rhythm problems—These medicines may make these conditions worse

Proper Use of This Medicine

Use this medicine only as directed. Do not use more of it and do not use it more often than your doctor ordered, do not use more than recommended on the label unless otherwise directed by your doctor. To do so may increase the chance of side effects.

If you are using this medicine for asthma, you should use another medicine that works faster than this one for an asthma attack that has already started. *If you do not have another medicine to use for an attack or if you have any questions about this, check with your doctor.*

For patients taking *albuterol extended-release tablets:*

- Swallow the tablet whole.
- Do not crush, break, or chew before swallowing.

For patients using *epinephrine injection:*

- This medicine is for injection only. If you will be giving yourself the injections, make sure you understand exactly how to give them. If you have any questions about this, check with your health care professional.
- When injected into the muscle (intramuscular) this medicine should be injected into the thigh. It should not be injected into the buttocks.

- Do not use the epinephrine solution or suspension if it turns pinkish to brownish in color or if the solution becomes cloudy.
- Keep this medicine ready for use at all times. Also, keep the telephone numbers for your doctor and the nearest hospital emergency room readily available.
- Check the expiration date on the injection regularly. Replace the medicine before that date.

For patients using *epinephrine injection* for an *allergic reaction emergency:*

- If a severe allergic reaction occurs, *use the epinephrine injection immediately.*
- *After using the epinephrine injection, notify your doctor immediately or go to the nearest hospital emergency room. Be sure to tell your doctor that you have used the epinephrine injection.*
- If you have been stung by an insect, remove the insect's stinger with your fingernails, if possible. Be careful not to squeeze, pinch, or push it deeper into the skin. Ice packs or sodium bicarbonate (baking soda) soaks, if available, may then be applied to the area stung.
- If you are using the *epinephrine auto-injector* (automatic injection device):
  - The *epinephrine auto-injector* comes with patient directions. Read them carefully before you actually need to use this medicine. Then, when an emergency arises, you will know how to inject the epinephrine.
  - It is important that you do not remove the safety cap on the auto-injector until you are ready to use it. This prevents accidental activation of the device during storage and handling.
  - To use the epinephrine auto-injector:
    - Remove the gray safety cap.
    - Place the black tip on the thigh, at a right angle (90–degree angle) to the leg.
    - Press hard into the thigh until the auto-injector functions. Hold in place for several seconds. Then remove the auto-injector and discard.
    - Massage the injection area for 10 seconds.

Dosing—The dose of these medicines will be different for different patients. *Follow your doctor's orders or the directions on the label.* The following information includes only the average doses of these medicines. *If your dose is different, do not change it* unless your doctor tells you to do so.

The number of capsules or tablets or teaspoonfuls of solution or syrup that you take, or the amount of injection that you use, depends on the strength of the medicine. Also, *the number of doses you take each day, the time allowed between doses, and the length of time you take the medicine depend on the medical problem for which you are taking it.*

For albuterol

- For symptoms of asthma, chronic bronchitis, emphysema, or other lung disease:
  - For *oral* dosage form (solution):
    - Adults and children 12 years of age and older—2 to 4 milligrams (mg) (1 to 2 teaspoonfuls) three or four times a day.
    - Children 6 to 12 years of age—2 mg (1 teaspoonful) three or four times a day.
    - Children 2 to 6 years of age—Dose is based on body weight and must be determined by your

doctor. The usual dose is 0.1 mg per kg (0.045 mg per pound) of body weight up to a maximum dose of 2 mg (1 teaspoonful) three or four times a day..
- Children up to 2 years of age—Use and dose must be determined by your doctor.
  ○ For *oral* dosage form (syrup):
    - Adults and children 14 years of age and older—2 to 4 mg (1 to 2 teaspoonfuls) three or four times a day. Then your doctor may increase your dose, if needed.
    - Children 6 to 14 years of age—At first, 2 mg (1 teaspoonful) of albuterol three or four times a day. Then your doctor may increase your dose, if needed.
    - Children 2 to 6 years of age—Dose is based on body weight and must be determined by your doctor. The usual dose is 0.1 mg per kg (0.045 mg per pound) of body weight up to a maximum dose of 2 mg (1 teaspoonful) three or four times a day.
    - Children up to 2 years of age—Use and dose must be determined by your doctor.
  ○ For *oral* dosage form (tablets):
    - Adults and children 12 years of age and older—At first, 2 to 4 mg three or four times a day. Then your doctor may increase your dose, if needed.
    - Children 6 to 12 years of age—2 mg three or four times a day.
    - Children up to 6 years of age—Use and dose must be determined by your doctor.
  ○ For *oral* dosage form (extended-release tablets):
    - Adults and children 12 years of age and older—4 to 8 mg every twelve hours.
    - Children 6 to 12 years of age—4 mg every twelve hours.
    - Children up to 6 years of age—Use and dose must be determined by your doctor.
  ○ For *injection* dosage form:
    - Dose is usually based on body weight and must be determined by your doctor. Depending on your condition, this medicine is injected into either a muscle or vein or injected slowly into a vein over a period of time.

For epinephrine
- For *injection* dosage form:
  ○ For allergic reactions:
    - Adults—At first, 300 to 500 micrograms (mcg) (0.3 to 0.5 mg) injected into a muscle or under the skin. Then the dose may be repeated, if needed, every ten to twenty minutes for up to three doses. In some cases, it may be necessary for 100 to 250 mcg to be injected slowly into a vein by your doctor instead of injecting the dose into a muscle or under the skin.
    - Children—Dose is based on body weight and must be determined by your doctor. The usual dose is 10 mcg per kg (4.5 mcg per pound) of body weight, up to 300 mcg (0.3 mg) a dose, injected into a muscle or under the skin. The dose may be repeated, if needed, every fifteen minutes for up to three doses.
  ○ For symptoms of bronchial asthma, chronic bronchitis or other lung disease:
    - Adults—Dose is based on body weight and must be determined by your doctor. The usual dose is

10 mcg per kg (4.5 mcg per pound) of body weight, up to 300 to 500 mcg (0.3 to 0.5 mg) a dose, injected under the skin. The dose may be repeated, if needed, every twenty minutes for up to three doses.
- Children—Dose is based on body weight and must be determined by your doctor. The usual dose is 10 mcg per kg (4.5 mcg per pound) of body weight, up to 300 mcg (0.3 mg) a dose, injected under the skin. The dose may be repeated, if needed, every fifteen minutes for three or four doses or every four hours.

For isoproterenol
- For *injection* dosage form:
  ○ For symptoms of asthma, chronic bronchitis, emphysema, or other lung disease:
    - Isoproterenol is given by intravenous injection in a doctor's office or hospital.

For metaproterenol
- For *oral* dosage forms (syrup or tablets):
  ○ For symptoms of asthma, chronic bronchitis, emphysema, or other lung disease:
    - Adults and children 9 years of age and older or weighing 27 kilograms (kg) (59 pounds) or more—20 milligrams (mg) three or four times a day.
    - Children 6 to 9 years of age or weighing up to 27 kg (59 pounds)—10 mg three or four times a day.
    - Children up to 6 years of age—Dose must be determined by your doctor.

For terbutaline
- For symptoms of asthma, chronic bronchitis, emphysema, or other lung disease:
  ○ For *oral* dosage form (tablets):
    - Adults and adolescents 15 years of age and older—5 milligrams (mg) three times a day. The medicine may be taken about every six hours while you are awake, until three doses have been taken.
    - Children 12 to 15 years of age—2.5 mg three times a day, taken about every six hours.
    - Children 6 to 11 years of age—Dose is based on body weight and must be determined by your doctor.
    - Children up to 6 years of age—Use and dose must be determined by your doctor.
  ○ For *injection* dosage form:
    - Adults and children 12 years of age or older—250 micrograms (mcg) injected under the skin. The dose may be repeated after fifteen to thirty minutes, if needed. However, not more than 500 mcg should be taken within a four-hour period.
    - Children 6 to 12 years of age—Dose is based on body weight and must be determined by your doctor. The usual dose is 5 to 10 mcg per kg (2.3 to 4.5 mcg per pound) of body weight injected under the skin. The dose may be repeated after fifteen to twenty minutes for up to a total of three doses.
    - Children up to 6 years of age—Use and dose must be determined by your doctor.

Missed dose—If you are using this medicine regularly and you miss a dose, use it as soon as possible. Then use any remaining doses for that day at regularly spaced intervals. Do not double doses.

Storage—To store this medicine:
- Keep out of the reach of children.
- Store away from heat and direct light.
- Do not store the capsule or tablet form of this medicine in the bathroom, near the kitchen sink, or in other damp places. Heat or moisture may cause the medicine to break down.
- Keep the injection or syrup form of this medicine from freezing.
- Do not keep outdated medicine or medicine no longer needed. Be sure that any discarded medicine is out of the reach of children.

Precautions While Using This Medicine

It is important that your doctor check your progress at regular visits to make sure that this medicine is working properly and to check for unwanted effects.

Do not take other medicines unless they have been discussed with your doctor. This especially includes over-the-counter (nonprescription) medicines for appetite control, asthma, colds, cough, hay fever, or sinus problems, since they could increase the unwanted effects of this medicine.

For patients with diabetes:
- This medicine may cause your blood sugar levels to rise, which could change the amount of insulin or diabetes medicine that you need to take.

For patients taking this medicine for asthma:
- *If you still have trouble breathing or if your condition becomes worse (for example, if you have to use an inhaler more frequently to relieve asthma attacks), check with your doctor right away.*

For patients who are using *epinephrine injection:*
- Because epinephrine reduces blood flow to the area where it is injected, it is possible that it could cause damage to the tissues if it is injected in one spot too often. *Check with your doctor right away if you notice severe pain at the place of injection.*

For patients who are using the *epinephrine auto-injector:*
- Do not inject this medicine into your hands or feet. There is already less blood flow to the hands and feet, and epinephrine could make that worse and cause damage to these tissues. *If you accidentally inject epinephrine into your hands or feet, check with your doctor or go to the hospital emergency room right away.*

Side Effects

Along with its needed effects, a medicine may cause some unwanted effects. Although not all of these side effects may occur, if they do occur they may need medical attention.

Check with your doctor immediately if any of the following side effects occur:
Rare
Possible signs of an allergic reaction
Hoarseness; large hive-like swellings on eyelids, face, genitals, hands or feet, lips, throat, tongue; sudden trouble in swallowing or breathing; tightness in throat

Possible signs of a severe reaction that has occurred in children taking albuterol by mouth
Bleeding or crusting sores on lips; chest pain; chills; fever; general feeling of illness; muscle cramps or pain; nausea; painful eyes; painful sores, ulcers, or white spots in mouth or on lips; red or irritated eyes; skin rash or sores, hives, and/or itching; sore throat; vomiting

Check with your doctor as soon as possible if any of the following side effects occur:
More common
Fast heartbeat; irregular heartbeat

Rare
Chest pain; convulsions (seizures); fainting (with isoproterenol); hives; increase in blood pressure (more common with ephedrine or epinephrine); mental problems; muscle cramps or pain; nausea or vomiting; trouble in urinating; unusual tiredness or weakness

Other side effects may occur that usually do not need medical attention. These side effects may go away during treatment as your body adjusts to the medicine. However, check with your doctor if any of the following side effects continue or are bothersome:
More common
Anxiety (with epinephrine); headache; nervousness; tremor

Less common
Dizziness; feeling of constant movement of self or surroundings; sweating; trouble in sleeping

Although not all of the side effects listed above have been reported for each of these medicines, they have been reported for at least one of them. All of these medicines are similar, so many of the above side effects may occur with any of the medicines.

Other side effects not listed above may also occur in some patients. If you notice any other effects, check with your doctor.

Additional Information

Once a medicine has been approved for marketing for a certain use, experience may show that it is also useful for other medical problems. Although these uses are not included in product labeling, some of the adrenergic bronchodilators are used in certain patients with the following medical conditions:
- Premature labor (terbutaline)
- Bleeding of gums and teeth during dental procedures (epinephrine)
- Priapism (prolonged abnormal erection of penis) (epinephrine)
- Hyperkalemia (too much potassium in the blood) in children (albuterol)

Other than the above information, there is no additional information relating to proper use, precautions, or side effects for these uses.

BRONCHODILATORS, THEOPHYLLINE (Systemic)

Some commonly used brand names are:

In the U.S.—

Aerolate Sr (3)	Theobid Duracaps (3)
Asmalix (3)	Theochron (3)
Choledyl (2)	Theo-Dur (3)
Choledyl SA (2)	Theolair (3)
Elixophyllin (3)	Theolair-SR (3)
Lanophyllin (3)	Theo-Time (3)
Phyllocontin (1)	Theovent Long-Acting (3)
Quibron-T Dividose (3)	Theo-X (3)
Quibron-T/SR Dividose (3)	T-Phyl (3)
Respbid (3)	Truphylline (1)
Slo-Bid Gyrocaps (3)	Truxophyllin (3)
Slo-Phyllin (3)	Uni-Dur (3)
Theo-24 (3)	Uniphyl (3)

In Canada—

Apo-Oxtriphylline (2)	Quibron-T/SR Dividose (3)
Apo-Theo LA (3)	Slo-Bid Gyrocaps (3)
Choledyl (2)	Theochron (3)
Choledyl SA (2)	Theo-Dur (3)
Phyllocontin (1)	Theolair (3)
Phyllocontin-350 (1)	Theolair-SR (3)
PMS Oxtriphylline (2)	Theo-SR (3)
PMS Theophylline (3)	Uniphyl (3)
Pulmophylline (3)	

This information applies to the following medicines:

1. Aminophylline (am-in-OFF-i-lin)
2. Oxtriphylline (ox-TRYE-fi-lin)
3. Theophylline (thee-OFF-i-lin)

Category

- **Bronchodilator**—Aminophylline; Oxtriphylline; Theophylline
- **Asthma prophylactic**—Aminophylline; Oxtriphylline; Theophylline
- **Stimulant, respiratory**—Aminophylline Injection USP; Aminophylline Oral Solution USP; Theophylline Elixir; Theophylline Oral Solution; Theophylline Syrup
- **Antidote (to dipyridamole toxicity)**—Aminophylline Injection USP

Description

Aminophylline, oxtriphylline, and theophylline are used to treat and/or prevent the symptoms of bronchial asthma, chronic bronchitis, and emphysema. These medicines relieve cough, wheezing, shortness of breath, and troubled breathing. They work by opening up the bronchial tubes (air passages of the lungs) and increasing the flow of air through them.

Aminophylline and theophylline may also be used for other conditions as determined by your doctor.

The oral liquid, tablet, and capsule dosage forms of these medicines may be used for treatment of the acute attack or for chronic long-term treatment. The enteric-coated and extended-release dosage forms are usually used only for chronic treatment. Sometimes, aminophylline suppositories may be used but they are generally not recommended because of possible poor absorption.

These medicines are available only with your doctor's prescription, in the following dosage forms:

Oral
- Aminophylline
  - Oral solution
  - Tablets
  - Extended-release tablets
- Oxtriphylline
  - Oral solution
  - Syrup
  - Tablets
  - Delayed-release tablets
  - Extended-release tablets
- Theophylline
  - Capsules
  - Extended-release capsules
  - Elixir
  - Oral solution
  - Syrup
  - Tablets
  - Extended-release tablets

Parenteral
- Aminophylline
  - Injection
- Theophylline
  - Injection

Rectal
- Aminophylline
  - Suppositories

Before Using This Medicine

In deciding to use a medicine, the risks of taking the medicine must be weighed against the good it will do. This is a decision you and your doctor will make. For aminophylline, oxtriphylline, or theophylline, the following should be considered:

Allergies—Tell your doctor if you have ever had any unusual or allergic reaction to aminophylline, ethylenediamine (contained in aminophylline), oxtriphylline, or theophylline.

Diet—Make certain your health care professional knows if you are on any special diet, such as a high-protein, low-carbohydrate or a low-protein, high-carbohydrate diet.

Pregnancy—Aminophylline, oxtriphylline, and theophylline are frequently used to treat asthma in pregnant women. Although there are no studies on birth defects in humans, problems have not been reported. Some studies in animals have shown that aminophylline, oxtriphylline, and theophylline can cause birth defects when given in doses many times the human dose.

Because your ability to clear theophylline from your body may decrease later in pregnancy, your doctor may want to take blood samples during your pregnancy to measure the amount of medicine in the blood. This will help your doctor decide whether the dose of this medicine should be changed.

Theophylline crosses the placenta. Use of aminophylline, oxtriphylline, or theophylline during pregnancy may cause unwanted effects such as fast heartbeat, irritability, jitteriness, or vomiting in the newborn infant if the amount of medicine in your blood is too high.

Breast-feeding—Theophylline passes into the breast milk and may cause irritability in nursing babies of mothers taking aminophylline, oxtriphylline, or theophylline.

Children—Very young children and newborn infants require a lower dose than older children. If the amount of theophylline in the blood is too high, side effects are more likely to occur. Your doctor may want to take blood samples to determine whether a dose change is needed.

Older adults—Patients older than 60 years of age are likely to require a lower dose than younger adults. If the amount of theophylline is too high, side effects are more likely to occur. Your doctor may want to take blood samples to determine whether a dose change is needed.

Other medicines—Although certain medicines should not be used together at all, in other cases two different medicines may be used together even if an interaction might occur. In these cases, your doctor may want to change the dose, or other precautions may be necessary. When you are taking aminophylline, oxtriphylline, or theophylline, it is especially important that your health care professional know if you are taking any of the following:

- Beta-adrenergic blocking agents including those used in the eyes (acebutolol [e.g., Sectral], atenolol [e.g., Tenormin], betaxolol [e.g., Betoptic, Kerlone], bisoprolol [e.g., Zebeta], carteolol [e.g., Cartrol], labetalol [e.g., Normodyne], levobunolol [e.g., Betagan], metipranolol [e.g., OptiPranolol], metoprolol [e.g., Lopressor], nadolol [e.g., Corgard], oxprenolol [e.g., Trasicor], penbutolol [e.g., Levatol], pindolol [e.g., Visken], propranolol [e.g., Inderal], sotalol [e.g., Sotacor], timolol [e.g., Blocadren, Timoptic])—These medicines may prevent aminophylline, oxtriphylline, or theophylline from working properly
- Cimetidine (e.g., Tagamet) or
- Ciprofloxacin (e.g., Cipro) or
- Clarithromycin (e.g., Biaxin) or
- Enoxacin (e.g., Penetrex) or
- Erythromycin (e.g., E-Mycin) or
- Fluvoxamine (e.g., Luvox) or
- Mexiletine (e.g., Mexitil) or
- Pentoxifylline (e.g., Trental) or
- Propranolol (e.g., Inderal) or
- Tacrine (e.g., Cognex) or
- Thiabendazole or
- Ticlopidine (e.g., Ticlid) or
- Troleandomycin (e.g., TAO)—These medicines may increase the effects of aminophylline, oxtriphylline, or theophylline
- Moricizine (e.g., Ethmozine) or
- Phenytoin (e.g., Dilantin) or
- Rifampin (e.g., Rifadin)—These medicines may decrease the effects of aminophylline, oxtriphylline, or theophylline
- Smoking tobacco or marijuana—Starting or stopping smoking may change the effectiveness of these medicines

Other medical problems—The presence of other medical problems may affect the use of aminophylline, oxtriphylline, or theophylline. Make sure you tell your doctor if you have any other medical problems, especially:

- Convulsions (seizures)—Aminophylline, oxtriphylline, or theophylline may make this condition worse

- Heart failure or
- Liver disease or
- Underactive thyroid—The effects of aminophylline, oxtriphylline, or theophylline may be increased

Proper Use of This Medicine

For patients *taking this medicine by mouth:*

- If you are taking the *capsule, tablet, liquid, or extended-release (not including the once-a-day capsule or tablet) form* of this medicine, *it works best when taken with a glass of water on an empty stomach* (either 30 minutes to 1 hour before meals or 2 hours after meals). In some cases your doctor may want you to take this medicine with meals or right after meals to lessen stomach upset. If you have any questions about how you should be taking this medicine, check with your doctor.

- If you are taking the *once-a-day capsule or tablet form* of this medicine, *some products are to be taken each morning after fasting overnight and at least 1 hour before eating. However, other products are to be taken in the morning or evening with or without food. Be sure you understand exactly how to take the medicine prescribed for you.* Try to take the medicine about the same time each day.

- There are several different forms of aminophylline, oxtriphylline, and theophylline capsules and tablets. If you are taking:
    ○ *Enteric-coated or delayed-release tablets,* swallow the tablets whole. Do not crush, break, or chew before swallowing.
    ○ *Extended-release capsules,* swallow the capsule whole. Do not crush, break, or chew before swallowing. Do not open the capsule and sprinkle the beads onto food unless told to do so by your health care professional.
    ○ *Extended-release tablets,* swallow the tablets whole. Do not break (unless tablet is scored for breaking), crush, or chew before swallowing.

Use this medicine only as directed by your doctor. Do not use more of it, do not use it more often, and do not use it for a longer time than your doctor ordered. To do so may increase the chance of serious side effects.

In order for this medicine to help your medical problem, it must be taken every day in regularly spaced doses as ordered by your doctor. This is necessary to keep a constant amount of this medicine in the blood. To help keep the amount constant, do not miss any doses.

Dosing—When you are taking aminophylline, oxtriphylline, or theophylline, it is very important that you get the exact amount of medicine that you need. The dose of these medicines will be different for different patients. Your doctor will determine the proper dose of these medicines for you. *Follow your doctor's orders or the directions on the label.*

After you begin taking aminophylline, oxtriphylline, or theophylline, it is very important that your doctor check the level of medicine in your blood at regular intervals to find out if your dose needs to be changed. *Do not change your dose of aminophylline, oxtriphylline, or theophylline unless your doctor tells you to do so.*

The number of capsules or tablets or teaspoonfuls of solution or syrup that you take depends on the strength of the medicine. Also, *the number of doses you take each day and the time between doses depend on whether you are taking a short-acting or long-acting form of aminophylline, oxtriphylline, or theophylline.*

Missed dose—If you miss a dose of this medicine, take it as soon as possible. However, if it is almost time for your next dose, skip the missed dose and go back to your regular dosing schedule. Do not double doses.

Storage—To store this medicine:

- Keep out of the reach of children.
- Store away from heat and direct light.
- Do not store the capsule or tablet form of this medicine in the bathroom, near the kitchen sink, or in other damp places. Heat or moisture may cause the medicine to break down.
- Keep the liquid form of this medicine from freezing.
- Do not keep outdated medicine or medicine no longer needed. Be sure that any discarded medicine is out of the reach of children.

Precautions While Using This Medicine

Your doctor should check your progress at regular visits, especially for the first few weeks after you begin using this medicine. A blood test may be taken to help your doctor decide whether the dose of this medicine should be changed.

Do not change brands or dosage forms of this medicine without first checking with your doctor. Different products may not work the same way. If you refill your medicine and it looks different, check with your pharmacist.

A change in your usual behavior or physical well-being may affect the way this medicine works in your body. *Check with your doctor if you:*

- have a fever of 102 °F or higher for at least 24 hours or higher than 100 °F for longer than 24 hours.
- start or stop smoking.
- start or stop taking another medicine.
- change your diet for a long time.

This medicine may add to the central nervous system (CNS) stimulant effects of caffeine-containing foods or beverages such as chocolate, cocoa, tea, coffee, and cola drinks. Avoid eating or drinking large amounts of these foods or beverages while using this medicine. If you have questions about this, check with your doctor.

Before you have myocardial perfusion studies (a medical test that shows how well blood is flowing to your heart), tell the medical doctor in charge that you are taking this medicine. The results of the test may be affected by this medicine.

Side Effects of This Medicine

Along with its needed effects, a medicine may cause some unwanted effects. Although not all of these side effects may occur, if they do occur they may need medical attention.

Check with your doctor as soon as possible if any of the following side effects occur:

Less common
    Heartburn and/or vomiting

Rare
    Hives, skin rash, or sloughing of skin (with aminophylline only)

Symptoms of toxicity
    Abdominal pain, continuing or severe; confusion or change in behavior; convulsions (seizures); dark or bloody vomit; diarrhea; dizziness or lightheadedness; fast and/or irregular heartbeat; nervousness or restlessness, continuing; trembling, continuing

Other side effects may occur that usually do not need medical attention. These side effects may go away during treatment as your body adjusts to the medicine. However, check with your doctor if any of the following side effects continue or are bothersome:

Less common
    Headache; fast heartbeat; increased urination; nausea; nervousness; trembling; trouble in sleeping

Other side effects not listed above may also occur in some patients. If you notice any other effects, check with your doctor.

Additional Information

Once a medicine has been approved for marketing for a certain use, experience may show that it is also useful for other medical problems. Although this use is not included in product labeling, aminophylline and theophylline are used in certain patients with the following medical condition:

- Apnea (breathing problem) in newborns

Other than the above information, there is no additional information relating to proper use, precautions, or side effects for this use.

BUPROPION (Oral route) - byoo-PROE-pee-on

Black Box Warning

Antidepressants increased the risk of suicidal thinking and behavior (suicidality) in short-term studies in children and adolescents with Major Depressive Disorder (MDD) and other psychiatric disorders. Anyone considering the use of bupropion hydrochloride or any other antidepressant in a child or adolescent must balance this risk with the clinical need. Patients who are started on therapy should be observed closely for clinical worsening, suicidality, or unusual changes in behavior. Families and caregivers should be advised of the need for close observation and communication with the prescriber. Bupropion hydrochloride is not approved for use in pediatric patients.

Pooled analyses of short-term (4 to 16 weeks) placebo-controlled trials of 9 antidepressant drugs (SSRIs and others) in children and adolescents with major depressive disorder (MDD), obsessive compulsive disorder (OCD), or other psychiatric disorders (a total of 24 trials involving over 4,400 patients) have revealed a greater risk of adverse events representing suicidal thinking or behavior (suicidality) during the first few months of treatment in those receiving antidepressants. The average risk of such events in patients receiving antidepressants was 4%, twice the placebo risk of 2%. No suicides occurred in these trials.

Commonly used brand name(s)

In the U.S.—

Budeprion SR	Wellbutrin SR
Buproban	Wellbutrin XL
Wellbutrin	Zyban

Available Dosage Forms:

- Tablet, Extended Release, 12 HR
- Tablet, Extended Release, 24 HR
- Tablet
- Tablet, Extended Release

Therapeutic Class: Antidepressant

Uses For This Medicine

Bupropion is used to relieve mental depression and is used as part of a support program to help you stop smoking.

Bupropion is sold under different brand names for different uses. If you are already taking medicine for mental depression or to help you stop smoking, discuss this with your health care professional before taking bupropion. It is very important that you receive only one prescription for bupropion at a time.

This medicine is available only with your doctor's prescription.

Before Using This Medicine

In deciding to use a medicine, the risks of taking the medicine must be weighed against the good it will do. This is a decision you and your doctor will make. For this medicine, the following should be considered:

Allergies—Tell your doctor if you have ever had any unusual or allergic reaction to this medicine or any other medicines. Also tell your health care professional if you have any other types of allergies, such as to foods, dyes, preservatives, or animals. For non-prescription products, read the label or package ingredients carefully.

Pediatric—Bupropion must be used with caution in children with depression. Studies have shown occurrences of children thinking about suicide or attempting suicide in clinical trials for this medicine. More study is needed to be sure venlafaxine is safe and effective in children

Geriatric—This medicine has been tested in a limited number of patients 60 years of age and older and has not been shown to cause different side effects or problems in older people than it does in younger adults.

Pregnancy—

	Pregnancy Category	Explanation
All Trimesters	C	Animal studies have shown an adverse effect and there are no adequate studies in pregnant women OR no animal studies have been conducted and there are no adequate studies in pregnant women.

Breast Feeding—There are no adequate studies in women for determining infant risk when using this medication during breastfeeding. Weigh the potential benefits against the potential risks before taking this medication while breastfeeding.

Other medicines—

Using this medicine with any of the following medicines is not recommended. Your doctor may decide not to treat you with this medication or change some of the other medicines you take.

Betamethasone, Budesonide, Clobetasone, Clorgyline, Corticotropin, Cortisone, Cosyntropin, Danazol, Deflazacort, Desonide, Dexamethasone, Fludrocortisone, Flunisolide, Fluticasone, Hydrocortisone, Iproniazid, Isocarboxazid, Methenolone, Methylprednisolone, Methyltestosterone, Moclobemide, Nandrolone, Nialamide, Oxandrolone, Oxymetholone, Paramethasone, Pargyline, Phenelzine, Prednisolone, Prednisone, Procarbazine, Rimexolone, Selegiline, Stanozolol, Testosterone, Toloxatone, Tranylcypromine

Interactions with Food/Tobacco/Alcohol—Certain medicines should not be used at or around the time of eating food or eating certain types of food since interactions may occur. Using alcohol or tobacco with certain medicines may also cause interactions to occur. The following interactions have been selected on the basis of their potential significance and are not necessarily all-inclusive.

Using this medicine with any of the following is usually not recommended, but may be unavoidable in some cases. If used together, your doctor may change the dose or how often you use this medicine, or give you special instructions about the use of food, alcohol, or tobacco.

Ethanol

Other medical problems—The presence of other medical problems may affect the use of this medicine. Make sure you tell your doctor if you have any other medical problems, especially:

- Anorexia nervosa, or history of or
- Brain tumor or
- Bulimia, or history of or
- Drug abuse or
- Head injury, history of or
- Mental retardation or
- Seizure disorders
- Sudden stop in drinking alcohol or using sedatives (medicine that makes you sleepy) or benzodiazepines (alprazolam [e.g., Xanax], diazepam [e.g., Valium], triazolam [e.g., Restoril])—The risk of seizures may be increased when bupropion is taken by patients with these conditions
- Bipolar disorder (manic-depressive illness) or risk of or
- Other nervous, mental, or emotional conditions or
- High blood pressure—Bupropion may make the condition worse
- Heart disease—Higher blood levels of bupropion may result, increasing the chance of side effects, or blood pressure may be increased
- Kidney disease or
- Liver disease—Higher blood levels of bupropion may result, increasing the chance of side effects

Proper Use of This Medicine

Use bupropion only as directed by your doctor. Do not use more of it, do not use it more often, and do not use it for a longer time than your doctor ordered. To do so may increase the chance of side effects.

For patients taking the prompt-release tablet form of this medicine

- Take doses at least 4 hours apart to decrease the chance of seizures.

For patients taking the sustained-release tablet form of this medicine

- Take doses at least 8 hours apart to decrease the chance of seizures.
- Swallow tablets whole. Do not crush, break, or chew them.

For patients taking the extended-release tablet form of this medicine

- Take doses at least 24 hours apart to decrease the chance of seizures.
- Swallow tablets whole. Do not crush, break, or chew them.

To lessen stomach upset, this medicine may be taken with food, unless your doctor has told you to take it on an empty stomach.

For patients taking this medicine for mental depression

- Usually this medicine must be taken for several weeks before you feel better. Your doctor should check your progress at regular visits.
- You will probably need to keep taking bupropion for at least 6 months to help prevent the return of the depression.

Dosing—The dose of this medicine will be different for different patients. Follow your doctor's orders or the directions on the label. The following information includes only the average doses of this medicine. If your dose is different, do not change it unless your doctor tells you to do so.

The amount of medicine that you take depends on the strength of the medicine. Also, the number of doses you take each day, the time allowed between doses, and the length of time you take the medicine depend on the medical problem for which you are using the medicine.

- For oral extended-release dosage form (tablets):
  - For mental depression:
    - Adults—At first, 150 milligrams (mg) once a day in the morning. Your doctor may increase your dose as needed. However, the dose usually is not more than 450 mg one time a day.
    - Children—Use and dose must be determined by your doctor.
- For oral sustained-release dosage form (tablets):
  - For mental depression:
    - Adults—At first, 150 milligrams (mg) once a day in the morning. Your doctor may increase your dose as needed. However, the dose usually is not more than 200 mg two times a day.
    - Children—Use and dose must be determined by your doctor.
  - To help you stop smoking:
    - Adults—At first, 150 mg once a day. Your doctor may increase your dose as needed. However, the dose usually is not more than 150 mg two times a day.
    - Children—Use and dose must be determined by your doctor.

- For oral prompt-release dosage form (tablets):
  - For mental depression:
    - Adults—At first, 100 mg two times a day. Your doctor may increase your dose as needed. However, the dose usually is not more than 150 mg three times a day.
    - Children—Use and dose must be determined by your doctor.

Missed dose—If you miss a dose of this medicine, skip the missed dose and go back to your regular dosing schedule. Do not double doses.

If you are taking the extended-release or the prompt-release form of this medicine and you miss a dose, skip the missed dose and go back to your regular dosing schedule.

Storage—Store the medicine in a closed container at room temperature, away from heat, moisture, and direct light. Keep from freezing.

Keep out of the reach of children.

Do not keep outdated medicine or medicine no longer needed.

Precautions While Using This Medicine

Your doctor should check your progress at regular visits, especially during the first few months of treatment with this medicine. The amount of bupropion you take may have to be changed often to meet the needs of your condition and to help avoid unwanted effects.

Do not take bupropion within 14 days of taking an MAO inhibitor.

Bupropion may cause some people to be agitated, irritable or display other abnormal behaviors. It may also cause some people to have suicidal thoughts and tendencies or to become more depressed. If you or your caregiver notice any of these adverse effects, tell your doctor right away.

Bupropion is sold under different brand names for different uses. If you are already taking medicine for mental depression or to help you stop smoking, discuss this with your health care professional before taking bupropion. It is very important that you receive only one prescription for bupropion at a time.

Drinking of alcoholic beverages should be limited or avoided, if possible, while taking bupropion. This will help prevent seizures.

This medicine may cause some people to feel a false sense of well-being, or to become drowsy, dizzy, or less alert than they are normally. Make sure you know how you react to this medicine before you drive, use machines, or do anything else that could be dangerous if you are dizzy or are not alert and clearheaded.

Side Effects of This Medicine

Along with its needed effects, a medicine may cause some unwanted effects. Although not all of these side effects may occur, if they do occur they may need medical attention.

Check with your doctor as soon as possible if any of the following side effects occur:

More common
 Agitation; anxiety

Less common
 Buzzing or ringing in ears; headache (severe); skin rash, hives, or itching

Rare

Confusion; extreme distrust; fainting; false beliefs that cannot be changed by facts; hallucinations (seeing, hearing, or feeling things that are not there); seizures (convulsions), especially with higher doses; trouble in concentrating

Incidence not determined

Actions that are out of control; anger; assault; attack; being impulsive; chest pain or discomfort; fast or pounding heartbeat; force; inability to sit still; irritability; need to keep moving; nervousness; restlessness; sweating; talking, feeling, and acting with excitement

Symptoms of overdose—may be more severe than side effects seen at regular doses, or two or more may occur together

Fast heartbeat; hallucinations (seeing, hearing, or feeling things that are not there); loss of consciousness; nausea; seizures (convulsions); vomiting

Some side effects may occur that usually do not need medical attention. These side effects may go away during treatment as your body adjusts to the medicine. Also, your health care professional may be able to tell you about ways to prevent or reduce some of these side effects. Check with your health care professional if any of the following side effects continue or are bothersome or if you have any questions about them:

More common

Abdominal pain; constipation; decrease in appetite; dizziness; dryness of mouth; increased sweating; nausea or vomiting; trembling or shaking; trouble in sleeping; weight loss (unusual)

Less common

Blurred vision; change in sense of taste; drowsiness; feeling of fast or irregular heartbeat; frequent need to urinate; muscle pain; sore throat; unusual feeling of well-being

Other side effects not listed may also occur in some patients. If you notice any other effects, check with your healthcare professional.

BUSERELIN (Nasal route, Injection route, Subcutaneous route) - BYOO-se-rel-in

Uses For This Medicine

Buserelin is used to treat cancer of the prostate gland.

It is similar to a hormone normally released from the hypothalamus gland. When given regularly, buserelin decreases testosterone levels. Reducing the amount of testosterone in the body is one way of treating cancer of the prostate.

Buserelin is available only with your doctor's prescription.

Before Using This Medicine

In deciding to use a medicine, the risks of taking the medicine must be weighed against the good it will do. This is a decision you and your doctor will make. For this medicine, the following should be considered:

Allergies—Tell your doctor if you have ever had any unusual or allergic reaction to this medicine or any other medicines. Also tell your health care professional if you have any other types of allergies, such as to foods, dyes, preservatives, or animals. For non-prescription products, read the label or package ingredients carefully.

Geriatric—Many medicines have not been studied specifically in older people. Therefore, it may not be known whether they work exactly the same way they do in younger adults. Although there is no specific information comparing use of buserelin in the elderly to use in other age groups, it has been used mostly in elderly patients and is not expected to cause different side effects or problems in older people than it does in younger adults.

Other medicines—Although certain medicines should not be used together at all, in other cases two different medicines may be used together even if an interaction might occur. In these cases, your doctor may want to change the dose, or other precautions may be necessary. Tell your healthcare professional if you are taking any other prescription or non-prescription (over-the-counter [OTC]) medicine.

Interactions with Food/Tobacco/Alcohol—Certain medicines should not be used at or around the time of eating food or eating certain types of food since interactions may occur. Using alcohol or tobacco with certain medicines may also cause interactions to occur. Discuss with your healthcare professional the use of your medicine with food, alcohol, or tobacco.

Proper Use of This Medicine

Buserelin comes with patient directions. Read these instructions carefully.

For patients using the injection form of this medicine:

- Use the syringes provided in the kit. Other syringes may not provide the correct dose. These disposable syringes and needles are already sterilized and designed to be used one time only and then discarded. If you have any questions about the use of disposable syringes, check with your health care professional.

- After use, dispose of the syringes and needles in a safe manner. If a special container is not provided, ask your health care professional about the best way to dispose of syringes and needles.

For patients using the nasal solution form of this medicine:

- Use the nebulizer (spray pump) provided. Directions about how to use it are included. If you have any questions about the use of the nebulizer, check with your health care professional.

Use this medicine only as directed by your doctor. Do not use more or less of it, and do not use it more often than your doctor ordered. The exact amount of medicine you need has been carefully worked out. Using too much may increase the chance of side effects, while using too little may not improve your condition.

Buserelin sometimes causes unwanted effects such as hot flashes or decreased sexual ability. It may also cause a temporary increase in pain, trouble in urinating, or weakness in your legs when you begin to use it. However, it is very important that you continue to use the medicine, even after you begin to feel better. Do not stop using this medicine without first checking with your doctor.

Dosing—The dose of this medicine will be different for different patients. Follow your doctor's orders or the directions on the label. The following information includes only the average doses of this medicine. If your dose is different, do not change it unless your doctor tells you to do so.

The amount of medicine that you take depends on the strength of the medicine. Also, the number of doses you take each day, the time allowed between doses, and the length of time you take the medicine depend on the medical problem for which you are using the medicine.

- For prostate cancer:
  - For nasal dosage forms:
    - Adults: 200 micrograms (mcg) (2 sprays) into each nostril every eight hours.
  - For injection dosage forms:
    - Adults: In the beginning, 500 mcg (0.5 milligrams [mg]) injected under the skin every eight hours. After a time, your doctor may lower your dose to 200 mcg (0.2 mg) once a day.

Missed dose—If you miss a dose of this medicine, take it as soon as possible. However, if it is almost time for your next dose, skip the missed dose and go back to your regular dosing schedule. Do not double doses.

Storage—Store the medicine in a closed container at room temperature, away from heat, moisture, and direct light. Keep from freezing.

Keep out of the reach of children.

Do not keep outdated medicine or medicine no longer needed.

Dispose of used syringes properly in the container provided.

Precautions While Using This Medicine

It is very important that your doctor check your progress at regular visits to make sure that this medicine is working properly and to check for unwanted effects.

Buserelin causes sterility which may be permanent. If you intend to have children, discuss this with your doctor before receiving this medicine.

Side Effects of This Medicine

Along with its needed effects, a medicine may cause some unwanted effects. Although not all of these side effects may occur, if they do occur they may need medical attention.

Check with your doctor as soon as possible if any of the following side effects occur:

Bone pain; numbness or tingling of hands or feet; trouble in urinating; weakness in legs

Some side effects may occur that usually do not need medical attention. These side effects may go away during treatment as your body adjusts to the medicine. Also, your health care professional may be able to tell you about ways to prevent or reduce some of these side effects. Check with your health care professional if any of the following side effects continue or are bothersome or if you have any questions about them:
  More common
    Decrease in sexual desire; impotence; sudden sweating and feelings of warmth ('hot flashes')

Less common
    Burning, itching, redness, or swelling at place of injection; diarrhea; dry or sore nose (with nasal solution); headache (with nasal solution); increased sweating (with nasal solution); loss of appetite; nausea or vomiting; swelling and increased tenderness of breasts; swelling of feet or lower legs

Other side effects not listed may also occur in some patients. If you notice any other effects, check with your healthcare professional.

BUSPIRONE (Oral route) - byoo-SPYE-rone

Commonly used brand name(s)

In the U.S.—
  Buspar
  Buspar Dividose
  Vanspar

Available Dosage Forms:
  - Tablet

Therapeutic Class: Antianxiety

Uses For This Medicine

Buspirone is used to treat certain anxiety disorders or to relieve the symptoms of anxiety. However, buspirone usually is not used for anxiety or tension caused by the stress of everyday life.

It is not known exactly how buspirone works to relieve the symptoms of anxiety. Buspirone is thought to work by decreasing the amount and actions of a chemical known as serotonin in certain parts of the brain.

Buspirone is available only with your doctor's prescription.

Before Using This Medicine

In deciding to use a medicine, the risks of taking the medicine must be weighed against the good it will do. This is a decision you and your doctor will make. For this medicine, the following should be considered:

Allergies—Tell your doctor if you have ever had any unusual or allergic reaction to this medicine or any other medicines. Also tell your health care professional if you have any other types of allergies, such as to foods, dyes, preservatives, or animals. For non-prescription products, read the label or package ingredients carefully.

Pediatric—Studies on this medicine have been done only in adult patients, and there is no specific information comparing use of buspirone in children up to 18 years of age with use in other age groups.

Geriatric—This medicine has been tested in a limited number of older adults and has not been shown to cause different side effects or problems in older people than it does in younger adults.

Pregnancy—

	Pregnancy Category	Explanation
All Trimesters	B	Animal studies have revealed no evidence of harm to the fetus, however, there are no adequate studies in pregnant women OR animal studies have shown an adverse effect, but adequate studies in pregnant women have failed to demonstrate a risk to the fetus.

Breast Feeding—There are no adequate studies in women for determining infant risk when using this medication during breastfeeding. Weigh the potential benefits against the potential risks before taking this medication while breastfeeding.

Other medicines—

Using this medicine with any of the following medicines is not recommended. Your doctor may decide not to treat you with this medication or change some of the other medicines you take.

Isocarboxazid, Phenelzine, Tranylcypromine

Interactions with Food/Tobacco/Alcohol—Certain medicines should not be used at or around the time of eating food or eating certain types of food since interactions may occur. Using alcohol or tobacco with certain medicines may also cause interactions to occur. The following interactions have been selected on the basis of their potential significance and are not necessarily all-inclusive.

Using this medicine with any of the following may cause an increased risk of certain side effects but may be unavoidable in some cases. If used together, your doctor may change the dose or how often you use this medicine, or give you special instructions about the use of food, alcohol, or tobacco.

Grapefruit Juice

Other medical problems—The presence of other medical problems may affect the use of this medicine. Make sure you tell your doctor if you have any other medical problems, especially:

- Kidney disease or
- Liver disease—Buspirone may be removed from your body more slowly, which may increase the chance of side effects. Your doctor may need to adjust your dose

Proper Use of This Medicine

Take buspirone only as directed by your doctor. Do not take more of it, do not take it more often, and do not take it for a longer time than your doctor ordered. To do so may increase the chance of unwanted effects.

After you begin taking buspirone, 1 to 2 weeks may pass before you begin to feel the effects of this medicine.

Dosing—The dose of this medicine will be different for different patients. Follow your doctor's orders or the directions on the label. The following information includes only the average doses of this medicine. If your dose is different, do not change it unless your doctor tells you to do so.

The amount of medicine that you take depends on the strength of the medicine. Also, the number of doses you take each day, the time allowed between doses, and the length of time you take the medicine depend on the medical problem for which you are using the medicine.

- For oral dosage forms (tablets):
  - Adults: To start, 5 milligrams (mg) two or three times a day, or 7.5 mg two times a day. Your doctor may increase your dose by 5 mg a day every few days if needed. However, the dose usually is not more than 60 mg a day.
  - Children up to 18 years of age: Use and dose must be determined by the doctor.
  - Older adults: To start, 5 milligrams (mg) two or three times a day, or 7.5 mg two times a day. Your doctor may increase your dose by 5 mg a day every few days if needed.

Missed dose—If you miss a dose of this medicine, take it as soon as possible. However, if it is almost time for your next dose, skip the missed dose and go back to your regular dosing schedule. Do not double doses.

Storage—Store the medicine in a closed container at room temperature, away from heat, moisture, and direct light. Keep from freezing.

Keep out of the reach of children.

Do not keep outdated medicine or medicine no longer needed.

Precautions While Using This Medicine

If you will be using buspirone regularly for a long time, your doctor should check your progress at regular visits to make sure the medicine does not cause unwanted effects.

Buspirone may cause some people to become dizzy, lightheaded, drowsy, or less alert than they are normally. Make sure you know how you react to this medicine before you drive, use machines, or do anything else that could be dangerous if you are dizzy or are not alert.

If you think you or someone else may have taken an overdose of buspirone, get emergency help at once. Some symptoms of an overdose are dizziness or lightheadedness; severe drowsiness or loss of consciousness; stomach upset, including nausea or vomiting; or very small pupils of the eyes.

Side Effects of This Medicine

Along with its needed effects, a medicine may cause some unwanted effects. Although not all of these side effects may occur, if they do occur they may need medical attention.

Check with your doctor as soon as possible if any of the following side effects occur:

Rare

Chest pain; confusion; fast or pounding heartbeat; fever; incoordination; mental depression; muscle weakness; numbness, tingling, pain, or weakness in hands or feet; skin rash or hives; stiffness of arms or legs; sore throat; uncontrolled movements of the body

Symptoms of overdose—may be more severe than side effects seen at regular doses or several may occur together

Dizziness or lightheadedness; drowsiness (severe) or loss of consciousness; stomach upset, including nausea or vomiting; very small pupils of the eyes

Some side effects may occur that usually do not need medical attention. These side effects may go away during treatment as your body adjusts to the medicine. Also, your health care professional may be able to tell you about ways to prevent or reduce some of these side effects. Check with your health care professional if any of the following side effects continue or are bothersome or if you have any questions about them:

More common

Dizziness or lightheadedness, especially when getting up from a sitting or lying position; headache; nausea; restlessness, nervousness, or unusual excitement

Less common or rare

Blurred vision; clamminess or sweating; decreased concentration; diarrhea; drowsiness (more common with doses of more than 20 mg per day); dryness of mouth; muscle pain, spasms, cramps, or stiffness; ringing in the ears; trouble in sleeping, nightmares, or vivid dreams; unusual tiredness or weakness

Other side effects not listed may also occur in some patients. If you notice any other effects, check with your healthcare professional.

BUSULFAN (Intravenous route) - byoo-SUL-fan

Black Box Warning

- TABLET
  - ◦ Busulfan is a potent drug. It should not be used unless a diagnosis of chronic myelogenous leukemia has been adequately established and the responsible physician is knowledgeable in assessing response to chemotherapy.
  - ◦ Busulfan can induce severe bone marrow hypoplasia. Reduce or discontinue the dosage immediately at the first sign of any unusual depression of bone marrow function as reflected by an abnormal decrease in any of the formed elements of the blood. A bone marrow examination should be performed if the bone marrow status is uncertain.

- INJECTION
  - ◦ Busulfan injection is a potent cytotoxic drug that causes profound myelosuppression at the recommended dosage. It should be administered under the supervision of a qualified physician who is experienced in allogeneic hematopoietic stem cell transplantation, the use of cancer chemotherapeutic drugs and the management patients with severe pancytopenia. Appropriate management of therapy and complications is only possible when adequate diagnostic and treatment facilities are readily available.

Commonly used brand name(s)

In the U.S.—
Busulfex

Available Dosage Forms:
- Solution

Therapeutic Class: Antineoplastic Agent
Pharmacologic Class: Alkylating Agent

Uses For This Medicine

Busulfan belongs to the group of medicines known as alkylating agents. It is used to treat some kinds of cancer of the blood. It may also be used as a conditioning regimen prior to progenitor cell transplantation for treatment of chronic myelogenous leukemia.

Busulfan seems to act by interfering with the function of the bone marrow. Since the growth of normal body cells may also be affected by busulfan, other effects will also occur. Some of these may be serious and must be reported to your doctor. Other effects may not be serious but may cause concern. Some effects may not occur for months or years after the medicine is used.

Before you begin treatment with busulfan, you and your doctor should talk about the good this medicine will do as well as the risks of using it.

Busulfan is available only with your doctor's prescription.

Before Using This Medicine

In deciding to use a medicine, the risks of taking the medicine must be weighed against the good it will do. This is a decision you and your doctor will make. For this medicine, the following should be considered:

Allergies—Tell your doctor if you have ever had any unusual or allergic reaction to this medicine or any other medicines. Also tell your health care professional if you have any other types of allergies, such as to foods, dyes, preservatives, or animals. For non-prescription products, read the label or package ingredients carefully.

Pediatric—Although there is no specific information comparing use of busulfan in children with use in other age groups, this medicine is not expected to cause different side effects or problems in children than it does in adults.

Geriatric—Many medicines have not been studied specifically in older people. Therefore, it may not be known whether they work exactly the same way they do in younger adults. Although there is no specific information comparing use of busulfan in the elderly with use in other age groups, this medicine is not expected to cause different side effects or problems in older people than it does in younger adults.

Pregnancy—

	Pregnancy Category	Explanation
All Trimesters	D	Studies in pregnant women have demonstrated a risk to the fetus. However, the benefits of therapy in a life threatening situation or a serious disease, may outweigh the potential risk.

Breast Feeding—There are no adequate studies in women for determining infant risk when using this medication during breastfeeding. Weigh the potential benefits against the potential risks before taking this medication while breastfeeding.

Other medicines—

Using this medicine with any of the following medicines is not recommended. Your doctor may decide not to treat you with

this medication or change some of the other medicines you take.

Rotavirus Vaccine, Live

Interactions with Food/Tobacco/Alcohol—Certain medicines should not be used at or around the time of eating food or eating certain types of food since interactions may occur. Using alcohol or tobacco with certain medicines may also cause interactions to occur. Discuss with your healthcare professional the use of your medicine with food, alcohol, or tobacco.

Other medical problems—The presence of other medical problems may affect the use of this medicine. Make sure you tell your doctor if you have any other medical problems, especially:

- Chickenpox (including recent exposure) or
- Herpes zoster (shingles)—Risk of severe disease affecting other parts of the body
- Gout (history of) or
- Kidney stones (or history of)—Busulfan may increase levels of uric acid in the body, which can cause gout or kidney stones
- Head injury or
- Convulsions (seizures, history of)—Busulfan injection and very high doses of oral busulfan can cause convulsions (seizures)
- Infection—Busulfan may decrease your body's ability to fight infection
- Thalassemia—Busulfan may cause increased pressure within the heart in children

Proper Use of This Medicine

Take this medicine only as directed by your doctor. Do not take more or less of it, and do not take it more often than your doctor ordered. The exact amount of medicine you need has been carefully worked out. Taking too much may increase the chance of side effects, while taking too little may not improve your condition.

Take each dose at the same time each day to make sure it has the best effect.

While you are taking this medicine, your doctor may want you to drink extra fluids so that you will pass more urine. This will help prevent kidney problems and keep your kidneys working well.

This medicine sometimes causes nausea and vomiting. However, it is very important that you continue to use the medicine, even if you begin to feel ill. Do not stop taking this medicine without first checking with your doctor. Ask your health care professional for ways to lessen these effects.

If you vomit shortly after taking a dose of busulfan, check with your doctor. You will be told whether to take the dose again or to wait until the next scheduled dose.

Handle and dispose of this medicine with care as directed by your doctor.

Dosing—The dose of this medicine will be different for different patients. Follow your doctor's orders or the directions on the label. The following information includes only the average doses of this medicine. If your dose is different, do not change it unless your doctor tells you to do so.

The amount of medicine that you take depends on the strength of the medicine. Also, the number of doses you take each day, the time allowed between doses, and the length of time you take the medicine depend on the medical problem for which you are using the medicine.

Missed dose—If you miss a dose of this medicine, skip the missed dose and go back to your regular dosing schedule. Do not double doses.

Storage—Store the medicine in a closed container at room temperature, away from heat, moisture, and direct light. Keep from freezing.

Keep out of the reach of children.

Do not keep outdated medicine or medicine no longer needed.

Precautions While Using This Medicine

It is very important that your doctor check your progress at regular visits to make sure that this medicine is working properly and to check for unwanted effects.

While you are being treated with busulfan, and after you stop treatment with it, do not have any immunizations (vaccinations) without your doctor's approval. Busulfan may lower your body's resistance and there is a chance you might get the infection the immunization is meant to prevent. In addition, other persons living in your household should not take oral polio vaccine since there is a chance they could pass the polio virus on to you. Also, avoid persons who have taken oral polio vaccine within the last several months. Do not get close to them, and do not stay in the same room with them for very long. If you cannot take these precautions, you should consider wearing a protective face mask that covers the nose and mouth.

Busulfan can temporarily lower the number of white blood cells in your blood, increasing the chance of getting an infection. It can also lower the number of platelets, which are necessary for proper blood clotting. If this occurs, there are certain precautions you can take, especially when your blood count is low, to reduce the risk of infection or bleeding:

- If you can, avoid people with infections. Check with your doctor immediately if you think you are getting an infection or if you get a fever or chills, cough or hoarseness, lower back or side pain, or painful or difficult urination.
- Check with your doctor immediately if you notice any unusual bleeding or bruising; black, tarry stools; blood in urine or stools; or pinpoint red spots on your skin.
- Be careful when using a regular toothbrush, dental floss, or toothpick. Your medical doctor, dentist, or nurse may recommend other ways to clean your teeth and gums. Check with your medical doctor before having any dental work done.
- Do not touch your eyes or the inside of your nose unless you have just washed your hands and have not touched anything else in the meantime.
- Be careful not to cut yourself when you are using sharp objects such as a safety razor or fingernail or toenail cutters.
- Avoid contact sports or other situations where bruising or injury could occur.

Before you have any medical tests, tell the medical doctor in charge that you are taking this medicine. The results of some body tissue studies may be affected by this medicine.

Side Effects of This Medicine

Along with its needed effects, a medicine may cause some unwanted effects. Although not all of these side effects may occur, if they do occur they may need medical attention.

Also, because of the way these medicines act on the body, there is a chance that they might cause other unwanted effects that may not occur until months or years after the medicine is used. These delayed effects may include certain types of cancer, such as leukemia. Discuss these possible effects with your doctor.

Check with your doctor immediately if any of the following side effects occur:

More common

Black, tarry stools; blood in urine or stools; cough or hoarseness; fever or chills; inflammation of the mouth; lower back or side pain; painful or difficult urination; pinpoint red spots on skin; unusual bleeding or bruising

Less common

Chest pain; dizziness; fast or irregular breathing; joint pain; light-headedness; puffiness or swelling around face; rapid heartbeat; shortness of breath; sudden, severe decrease in blood pressure; sweating; swelling of fingers, hands, arms, lower legs, or feet; sweating; tingling in lower legs, hands, or feet

Rare

Blurred vision; difficulty swallowing; heartburn; severe upper abdominal and back pain; vomiting blood

Some side effects may occur that usually do not need medical attention. These side effects may go away during treatment as your body adjusts to the medicine. Also, your health care professional may be able to tell you about ways to prevent or reduce some of these side effects. Check with your health care professional if any of the following side effects continue or are bothersome or if you have any questions about them:

More common

Abdominal pain; anxiety; diarrhea; general fatigue or muscle pain; headache; missed or irregular menstrual periods; loss of appetite; nausea and vomiting; rash; trouble in sleeping; weight loss (sudden)

Less common

Bloody nose; confusion; constipation; darkening of skin; depression; dry mouth; inflammation at place of injection; itching; sore throat or cough; stuffy nose, runny nose, or sneezing

After you stop using this medicine, it may still produce some side effects that need attention. During this period of time, *check with your doctor immediately* if you notice the following side effects:

Black, tarry stools; blood in urine or stools; cough or hoarseness, accompanied by fever or chills; fever or chills; lower back or side pain, accompanied by fever or chills; painful or difficult urination, accompanied by fever or chills; pinpoint red spots on skin; shortness of breath; unusual bleeding or bruising

Other side effects not listed may also occur in some patients. If you notice any other effects, check with your healthcare professional.

BUTALBITAL AND ACETAMINOPHEN (Systemic)

Some commonly used brand names are:

In the U.S.—

Amaphen (2)	Fioricet (2)
Anolor-300 (2)	Isocet (2)
Anoquan (2)	Medigesic (2)
Arcet (2)	Pacaps (2)
Bancap (1)	Pharmagesic (2)
Bucet (1)	Phrenilin (1)
Butace (2)	Phrenilin Forte (1)
Conten (1)	Repan (2)
Dolmar (2)	Sedapap (1)
Endolor (2)	Tencet (2)
Esgic (2)	Tencon (1)
Esgic-Plus (2)	Triad (2)
Ezol (2)	Triaprin (1)
Femcet (2)	Two-Dyne (2)

This information applies to the following medicines:

1. Butalbital and Acetaminophen (byoo-TAL-bi-tal and a-seat-a-MIN-oh-fen)
2. Butalbital, Acetaminophen, and Caffeine (byoo-TAL-bi-tal, a-seat-a-MIN-oh-fen, and KAF-een)

Category

• Analgesic—

Description

Butalbital and acetaminophen (byoo-TAL-bi-tal and a-seat-a-MIN-oh-fen) combination is a pain reliever and relaxant. It is used to treat tension headaches. Butalbital belongs to the group of medicines called barbiturates (bar-BI-tyoo-rates). Barbiturates act in the central nervous system (CNS) to produce their effects.

When you take butalbital for a long time, your body may get used to it so that larger amounts are needed to produce the same effects. This is called tolerance to the medicine. Also, butalbital may become habit-forming (causing mental or physical dependence) when it is used for a long time or in large doses. Physical dependence may lead to withdrawal side effects when you stop taking the medicine. In patients who get headaches, the first symptom of withdrawal may be new (rebound) headaches.

Some butalbital and acetaminophen combinations also contain caffeine (KAF-een). Caffeine may help to relieve headaches. However, caffeine can also cause physical dependence when it is used for a long time. This may lead to withdrawal (rebound) headaches when you stop taking it.

Butalbital and acetaminophen combination may also be used for other kinds of headaches or other kinds of pain as determined by your doctor.

Butalbital and acetaminophen combinations are available only with your doctor's prescription in the following dosage forms:

Oral

• Butalbital and Acetaminophen
  ○ Capsules
  ○ Tablets
• Butalbital, Acetaminophen, and Caffeine
  ○ Capsules
  ○ Tablets

Before Using This Medicine

In deciding to use a medicine, the risks of taking the medicine must be weighed against the good it will do. This is a decision you and your doctor will make. For butalbital and acetaminophen combinations, the following should be considered:

Allergies—Tell your doctor if you have ever had any unusual or allergic reaction to butalbital or other barbiturates, or to acetaminophen, aspirin, or caffeine. Also tell your health care professional if you are allergic to any other substances, such as foods, preservatives, or dyes.

Pregnancy—
- *For butalbital:* Barbiturates such as butalbital have been shown to increase the chance of birth defects in humans. Also, one study in humans has suggested that barbiturates taken during pregnancy may increase the chance of brain tumors in the baby. Butalbital may cause breathing problems in the newborn baby if taken just before or during delivery.

- *For acetaminophen:* Although studies on birth defects with acetaminophen have not been done in pregnant women, it has not been reported to cause birth defects or other problems.

- *For caffeine:* Studies in humans have not shown that caffeine (contained in some of these combination medicines) causes birth defects. However, use of large amounts of caffeine during pregnancy may cause problems with the heart rhythm and the growth of the fetus. Also, studies in animals have shown that caffeine causes birth defects when given in very large doses (amounts equal to those present in 12 to 24 cups of coffee a day).

Breast-feeding—
- *For butalbital:* Barbiturates such as butalbital pass into the breast milk and may cause drowsiness, unusually slow heartbeat, shortness of breath, or troubled breathing in nursing babies.

- *For acetaminophen:* Although acetaminophen has not been shown to cause problems in nursing babies, it passes into the breast milk in small amounts.

- *For caffeine:* Caffeine (present in some butalbital and acetaminophen combinations) passes into the breast milk in small amounts. Taking caffeine in the amounts present in these medicines has not been shown to cause problems in nursing babies. However, studies have shown that nursing babies may appear jittery and have trouble in sleeping when their mothers drink large amounts of caffeine-containing beverages. Therefore, breast-feeding mothers who use caffeine-containing medicines should probably limit the amount of caffeine they take in from other medicines or from beverages.

Children—
- *For butalbital:* Although barbiturates such as butalbital often cause drowsiness, some children become excited after taking them.

- *For acetaminophen:* Acetaminophen has been tested in children and, in effective doses, has not been shown to cause different side effects or problems than it does in adults.

- *For caffeine:* There is no specific information comparing use of caffeine in children up to 12 years of age with use in other age groups. However, caffeine is not expected to cause different side effects or problems in children than it does in adults.

Older adults—
- *For butalbital:* Certain side effects, such as confusion, excitement, or mental depression, may be especially likely to occur in elderly patients, who are usually more sensitive than younger adults to the effects of the butalbital in this combination medicine.

- *For acetaminophen:* Acetaminophen has been tested and has not been shown to cause different side effects or problems in older people than it does in younger adults.

- *For caffeine:* Many medicines have not been studied specifically in older people. Therefore, it may not be known whether they work exactly the same way they do in younger adults or if they cause different side effects or problems in older people. There is no specific information comparing use of caffeine in the elderly with use in other age groups.

Other medicines—Although certain medicines should not be used together at all, in other cases two different medicines may be used together even if an interaction might occur. In these cases, your doctor may want to change the dose, or other precautions may be necessary. When you are taking a butalbital and acetaminophen combination, it is especially important that your health care professional know if you are taking any of the following:
- Anticoagulants (blood thinners), or
- Carbamazepine (e.g., Tegretol) or
- Contraceptives, oral (birth control pills) containing estrogen, or
- Corticosteroids (cortisone-like medicines) or
- Corticotropin (e.g., ACTH)—Butalbital may make these medicines less effective
- Antidepressants, tricyclic (amitriptyline [e.g., Elavil], amoxapine [e.g., Asendin], clomipramine [e.g., Anafranil], desipramine [e.g., Pertofrane], doxepin [e.g., Sinequan], imipramine [e.g., Tofranil], nortriptyline [e.g., Aventyl], protriptyline [e.g., Vivactil], trimipramine [e.g., Surmontil]) or
- Central nervous system (CNS) depressants (medicines that often cause drowsiness)—These medicines may add to the effects of butalbital and increase the chance of drowsiness or other side effects
- Divalproex (e.g., Depakote) or
- Valproic acid (e.g., Depakene)—The chance of side effects may be increased

Other medical problems—The presence of other medical problems may affect the use of butalbital and acetaminophen combinations. Make sure you tell your doctor if you have any other medical problems, especially:
- Alcohol abuse (or history of) or
- Drug abuse or dependence (or history of)—Dependence on butalbital may develop; also, acetaminophen may cause liver damage in people who abuse alcohol
- Asthma (or history of), emphysema, or other chronic lung disease or
- Hepatitis or other liver disease or
- Hyperactivity (in children) or

- Kidney disease—The chance of serious side effects may be increased
- Diabetes mellitus (sugar diabetes) or
- Mental depression or
- Overactive thyroid or
- Porphyria (or history of)—Butalbital can make these conditions worse
- Heart disease (severe)—The caffeine in some butalbital and acetaminophen combinations can make some kinds of heart disease worse

Proper Use of This Medicine

Take this medicine only as directed by your doctor. Do not take more of it, do not take it more often, and do not take it for a longer time than your doctor ordered. If butalbital and acetaminophen combination is taken regularly (for example, every day), it may become habit-forming (causing mental or physical dependence). The caffeine in some butalbital and acetaminophen combinations can also increase the chance of dependence. Dependence is especially likely to occur in patients who take these medicines to relieve frequent headaches. Taking too much of this medicine may also lead to liver damage or other medical problems.

This medicine will relieve a headache best if you *take it as soon as the headache begins*. If you get warning signs of a migraine, take this medicine as soon as you are sure that the migraine is coming. This may even stop the headache pain from occurring. *Lying down in a quiet, dark room for a while after taking the medicine also helps to relieve headaches*.

People who get a lot of headaches may need to take a different medicine to help prevent headaches. *It is important that you follow your doctor's directions about taking the other medicine, even if your headaches continue to occur*. Headache-preventing medicines may take several weeks to start working. Even after they do start working, your headaches may not go away completely. However, your headaches should occur less often, and they should be less severe and easier to relieve than before. This will reduce the amount of headache relievers that you need. If you do not notice any improvement after several weeks of headache-preventing treatment, check with your doctor.

Dosing—The dose of butalbital and acetaminophen combination medicines will be different for different patients. *Follow your doctor's orders or the directions on the label*. The following information includes only the average doses of these medicines. *If your dose is different, do not change it* unless your doctor tells you to do so.

The number of capsules or tablets that you take depends on the strength of the medicine.

- For *oral* dosage forms (capsules or tablets):
  - For tension headaches:
    - Adults—One or 2 capsules or tablets every four hours as needed. If your medicine contains 325 or 500 milligrams (mg) of acetaminophen in each capsule or tablet, you should not take more than six capsules or tablets a day. If your medicine contains 650 mg of acetaminophen in each capsule or tablet, you should not take more than four capsules or tablets a day.
    - Children—Dose must be determined by your doctor.

Missed dose—If your doctor has ordered you to take this medicine according to a regular schedule and you miss a dose, take it as soon as you remember. However, if it is almost time for your next dose, skip the missed dose and go back to your regular dosing schedule. *Do not double doses*.

Storage—To store this medicine:

- Keep out of the reach of children. Overdose is especially dangerous in young children.
- Store away from heat and direct light.
- Do not store this medicine in the bathroom, near the kitchen sink, or in other damp places. Heat or moisture may cause the medicine to break down.
- Do not keep outdated medicine or medicine no longer needed. Be sure that any discarded medicine is out of the reach of children.

Precautions While Using This Medicine

Check with your doctor:

- If the medicine stops working as well as it did when you first started using it. This may mean that you are in danger of becoming dependent on the medicine. *Do not try to get better pain relief by increasing the dose*.
- *If you are having headaches more often than you did before you started taking this medicine*. This is especially important if a new headache occurs within 1 day after you took your last dose of this medicine, headaches begin to occur every day, or a headache continues for several days in a row. This may mean that you are dependent on the medicine. *Continuing to take this medicine will cause even more headaches later on*. Your doctor can give you advice on how to relieve the headaches.

Check the labels of all nonprescription (over-the-counter [OTC]) or prescription medicines you now take. If any contain a barbiturate or acetaminophen, check with your health care professional. Taking them together with this medicine may cause an overdose.

The butalbital in this medicine will add to the effects of alcohol and other CNS depressants (medicines that slow down the nervous system, possibly causing drowsiness). Some examples of CNS depressants are antihistamines or medicine for hay fever, other allergies, or colds; sedatives, tranquilizers, or sleeping medicine; other prescription pain medicine; narcotics; other barbiturates; medicine for seizures; muscle relaxants; or anesthetics, including some dental anesthetics. Also, drinking large amounts of alcoholic beverages regularly while taking this medicine may increase the chance of liver damage, especially if you take more of this medicine than your doctor ordered or if you take it regularly for a long time. *Therefore, do not drink alcoholic beverages, and check with your doctor before taking any of the medicines listed above, while you are using this medicine*.

This medicine may cause some people to become drowsy, dizzy, or lightheaded. *Make sure you know how you react to this medicine before you drive, use machines, or do anything else that could be dangerous if you are dizzy or are not alert and clearheaded*.

Before you have any medical tests, tell the person in charge that you are taking this medicine. Caffeine (present in some butalbital and acetaminophen combinations) interferes with the results of certain tests that use dipyridamole (e.g., Persantine) to help show how well blood is flowing to your heart.

Caffeine should not be taken for 8 to 12 hours before the test. The results of other tests may also be affected by butalbital and acetaminophen combinations.

Before having any kind of surgery (including dental surgery) or emergency treatment, tell the medical doctor or dentist in charge that you are taking this medicine. Serious side effects can occur if your medical doctor or dentist gives you certain medicines without knowing that you have taken butalbital.

If you have been taking large amounts of this medicine, or if you have been taking it regularly for several weeks or more, *do not suddenly stop taking it without first checking with your doctor*. Your doctor may want you to reduce gradually the amount you are taking before stopping completely in order to lessen the chance of withdrawal side effects.

If you think you or anyone else may have taken an overdose of this medicine, get emergency help at once. Taking an overdose of this medicine or taking alcohol or CNS depressants with this medicine may lead to unconsciousness or possibly death. Signs of butalbital overdose include severe drowsiness, confusion, severe weakness, shortness of breath or unusually slow or troubled breathing, slurred speech, staggering, and unusually slow heartbeat. Signs of severe acetaminophen poisoning may not occur until 2 to 4 days after the overdose is taken, but treatment to prevent liver damage or death must be started within 24 hours or less after the overdose is taken.

Side Effects

Along with its needed effects, a medicine may cause some unwanted effects. Although not all of these side effects may occur, if they do occur they may need medical attention.

Check with your doctor immediately if any of the following side effects occur, especially if several of them occur together:

Rare
Bleeding or crusting sores on lips; chest pain; fever with or without chills; hive-like swellings (large) on eyelids, face, lips, and/or tongue; muscle cramps or pain; red, thickened, or scaly skin; shortness of breath, troubled breathing, tightness in chest, or wheezing; skin rash, itching, or hives; sores, ulcers, or white spots in mouth (painful); sore throat

Symptoms of overdose
Anxiety, confusion, excitement, irritability, nervousness, restlessness, or trouble in sleeping (severe, especially with products containing caffeine); convulsions (seizures) (for products containing caffeine); diarrhea, especially if occurring together with increased sweating, loss of appetite, and stomach cramps or pain; dizziness, lightheadedness, drowsiness, or weakness, (severe); frequent urination (for products containing caffeine); hallucinations (seeing, hearing, or feeling things that are not there); increased sensitivity to touch or pain (for products containing caffeine); muscle trembling or twitching (for products containing caffeine); nausea or vomiting, sometimes with blood; ringing or other sounds in ears (for products containing caffeine); seeing flashes of "zig-zag" lights (for products containing caffeine); shortness of breath or unusually slow or troubled breathing; slow, fast, or irregular heartbeat; slurred speech; staggering; swelling, pain, or tenderness in the upper abdomen or stomach area; unusual movements of the eyes

Also, check with your doctor as soon as possible if any of the following side effects occur:

Less common
Confusion (mild); mental depression; unusual excitement (mild)

Rare
Bloody or black, tarry stools; bloody urine; pinpoint red spots on skin; swollen or painful glands; unusual bleeding or bruising; unusual tiredness or weakness (mild)

Other side effects may occur that usually do not need medical attention. These side effects may go away during treatment as your body adjusts to the medicine. However, check with your doctor if any of the following side effects continue or are bothersome:

More common
Bloated or "gassy" feeling; dizziness or lightheadedness (mild); drowsiness (mild); nausea, vomiting, or stomach pain (occurring without other symptoms of overdose)

Other side effects not listed above may also occur in some patients. If you notice any other effects, check with your doctor.

BUTALBITAL AND ASPIRIN (Systemic)

Some commonly used brand names are:

In the U.S.—

Axotal (1)	Isobutyl (2)
Butalgen (2)	Isolin (2)
Fiorgen (2)	Isollyl (2)
Fiorinal (2)	Laniroif (2)
Fiormor (2)	Lanorinal (2)
Fortabs (2)	Marnal (2)
Isobutal (2)	Vibutal (2)

In Canada—
Fiorinal (2)
Tecnal (2)

This information applies to the following medicines:

1. Butalbital and Aspirin (byoo-TAL-bi-tal and AS-pir-in)
2. Butalbital, Aspirin, and Caffeine (byoo-TAL-bi-tal, AS-pir-in, and kaf-EEN)

Category

Analgesic—

Description

Butalbital and aspirin combination is a pain reliever and relaxant. It is used to treat tension headaches. Butalbital belongs to the group of medicines called barbiturates. Barbiturates act in the central nervous system (CNS) to produce their effects.

When you use butalbital for a long time, your body may get used to it so that larger amounts are needed to produce the same effects. This is called tolerance to the medicine. Also, butalbital may become habit-forming (causing mental or physical dependence) when it is used for a long time or in large doses. Physical dependence may lead to withdrawal side effects when you stop taking the medicine. In patients who get headaches, the first symptom of withdrawal may be new (rebound) headaches.

Some of these medicines also contain caffeine. Caffeine may help to relieve headaches. However, caffeine can also cause physical dependence when it is used for a long time. This may lead to withdrawal (rebound) headaches when you stop taking it.

Butalbital and aspirin combination is sometimes also used for other kinds of headaches or other kinds of pain, as determined by your doctor.

Butalbital and aspirin combination is available only with your doctor's prescription, in the following dosage forms:

Oral
- Butalbital and Aspirin
  - Tablets
- Butalbital, Aspirin, and Caffeine
  - Capsules
  - Tablets

Before Using This Medicine

In deciding to use a medicine, the risks of taking the medicine must be weighed against the good it will do. This is a decision you and your doctor will make. For butalbital and aspirin combinations, the following should be considered:

Allergies—Tell your doctor if you have ever had any unusual or allergic reaction to butalbital or other barbiturates; aspirin or other salicylates, including methyl salicylate (oil of wintergreen); caffeine; or any of the following medicines:

- Diclofenac (e.g., Voltaren)
- Diflunisal (e.g., Dolobid)
- Etodolac (e.g., Lodine)
- Fenoprofen (e.g., Nalfon)
- Floctafenine (e.g., Idarac)
- Flurbiprofen, oral (e.g., Ansaid)
- Ibuprofen (e.g., Motrin)
- Indomethacin (e.g., Indocin)
- Ketoprofen (e.g., Orudis)
- Ketorolac (e.g., Toradol)
- Meclofenamate (e.g., Meclomen)
- Mefenamic acid (e.g., Ponstel)
- Nabumetone (e.g., Relafen)
- Naproxen (e.g., Naprosyn)
- Oxaprozin (e.g., Daypro)
- Oxyphenbutazone (e.g., Tandearil)
- Phenylbutazone (e.g., Butazolidin)
- Piroxicam (e.g., Feldene)
- Sulindac (e.g., Clinoril)
- Suprofen (e.g., Suprol)
- Tenoxicam (e.g., Mobiflex)
- Tiaprofenic acid (e.g., Surgam)
- Tolmetin (e.g., Tolectin)
- Zomepirac (e.g., Zomax)

Also tell your health care professional if you are allergic to any other substances, such as foods, preservatives, or dyes.

Pregnancy—
- *For butalbital:* Barbiturates such as butalbital have been shown to increase the chance of birth defects in humans. Also, one study in humans has suggested that barbiturates taken during pregnancy may increase the chance of brain tumors in the baby. Butalbital may cause breathing problems in the newborn baby if taken just before or during delivery.

- *For aspirin:* Although studies in humans have not shown that aspirin causes birth defects, it has caused birth defects in animal studies. *Do not take aspirin during the last 3 months of pregnancy unless it has been ordered by your doctor.* Some reports have suggested that use of aspirin late in pregnancy may cause a decrease in the newborn's weight and possible death of the fetus or newborn baby. However, the mothers in these reports had been taking much larger amounts of aspirin than are usually recommended. Studies of mothers taking aspirin in the doses that are usually recommended did not show these unwanted effects. There is a chance that regular use of aspirin late in pregnancy may cause unwanted effects on the heart or blood flow in the fetus or in the newborn baby. Also, use of aspirin during the last 2 weeks of pregnancy may cause bleeding problems in the fetus before or during delivery or in the newborn baby. In addition, too much use of aspirin during the last 3 months of pregnancy may increase the length of pregnancy, prolong labor, cause other problems during delivery, or cause severe bleeding in the mother before, during, or after delivery.

- *For caffeine:* Studies in humans have not shown that caffeine causes birth defects. However, use of large amounts of caffeine during pregnancy may cause problems with the heart rhythm and the growth of the fetus. Also, studies in animals have shown that caffeine causes birth defects when given in very large doses (amounts equal to the amount in 12 to 24 cups of coffee a day).

Breast-feeding—Although this combination medicine has not been reported to cause problems, the chance always exists, especially if the medicine is taken for a long time or in large amounts.
- *For butalbital:* Barbiturates such as butalbital pass into the breast milk and may cause drowsiness, unusually slow heartbeat, shortness of breath, or troubled breathing in nursing babies.

- *For aspirin:* Aspirin passes into the breast milk. However, taking aspirin in the amounts present in these combination medicines has not been reported to cause problems in nursing babies.

- *For caffeine:* The caffeine in some of these combination medicines passes into the breast milk in small amounts. Taking caffeine in the amounts present in these medicines has not been reported to cause problems in nursing babies. However, studies have shown that nursing babies may appear jittery and have trouble in sleeping when their mothers drink large amounts of caffeine-containing beverages. Therefore, breast-feeding mothers who use caffeine-containing medicines should probably limit the amount of caffeine they take in from other medicines or from beverages.

Children—
- *For butalbital:* Although barbiturates such as butalbital often cause drowsiness, some children become excited after taking them.

- *For aspirin: Do not give a medicine containing aspirin to a child with fever or other symptoms of a virus infection, especially flu or chickenpox, without first discussing its use with your child's doctor.* This is very important because aspirin may cause a serious illness called Reye's syndrome in children with fever caused by a virus infection, especially flu or chickenpox. Children who do not have a virus infection may also be more sensitive to the effects of aspirin, especially if they have a fever or have lost large amounts of body fluid because of vomiting, diarrhea, or sweating. This may increase the chance of side effects during treatment.

- *For caffeine:* There is no specific information comparing use of caffeine in children up to 12 years of age with use in other age groups. However, caffeine is not expected to cause different side effects or problems in children than it does in adults.

Older adults—
- *For butalbital:* Confusion, depression, or excitement may be especially likely to occur in elderly patients, who are usually more sensitive than younger adults to the effects of butalbital.
- *For aspirin:* Elderly patients are more sensitive than younger adults to the effects of aspirin. This may increase the chance of side effects during treatment.
- *For caffeine:* Many medicines have not been studied specifically in older people. Therefore, it may not be known whether they work exactly the same way they do in younger adults or if they cause different side effects or problems in older people. There is no specific information comparing use of caffeine in the elderly with use in other age groups.

Other medicines—Although certain medicines should not be used together at all, in other cases two different medicines may be used together even if an interaction might occur. In these cases, your doctor may want to change the dose, or other precautions may be necessary. When you are taking a butalbital and aspirin combination, it is especially important that your health care professional know if you are taking any of the following:

- Antacids, large amounts taken regularly, especially calcium- and/or magnesium-containing antacids or sodium bicarbonate (baking soda), or
- Urinary alkalizers (medicine that makes the urine less acid, such as acetazolamide [e.g., Diamox], dichlorphenamide [e.g., Daranide], methazolamide [e.g., Neptazane], potassium or sodium citrate and/or citric acid)— These medicines may cause aspirin to be removed from the body faster than usual, which may shorten the time that aspirin is effective; acetazolamide, dichlorphenamide, and methazolamide may also increase the chance of side effects when taken together with aspirin
- Anticoagulants (blood thinners) or
- Heparin—Use of these medicines together with aspirin may increase the chance of bleeding; also, butalbital may cause anticoagulants to be less effective
- Antidepressants, tricyclic (amitriptyline [e.g., Elavil], amoxapine [e.g., Asendin], clomipramine [e.g., Anafranil], desipramine [e.g., Pertofrane], doxepin [e.g., Sinequan], imipramine [e.g., Tofranil], nortriptyline [e.g., Aventyl], protriptyline [e.g., Vivactil], trimipramine [e.g., Surmontil]) or
- Central nervous system (CNS) depressants (medicines that often cause drowsiness)—These medicines may add to the effects of butalbital and increase the chance of drowsiness or other side effects
- Carbamazepine (e.g., Tegretol) or

- Contraceptives, oral (birth control pills), containing estrogen or
- Corticosteroids (cortisone-like medicines) or
- Corticotropin (e.g., ACTH)—Butalbital may make these medicines less effective
- Divalproex (e.g., Depakote) or
- Methotrexate (e.g., Folex, Mexate) or
- Valproic acid (e.g., Depakene) or
- Vancomycin (e.g., Vancocin)—The chance of serious side effects may be increased
- Probenecid (e.g., Benemid) or
- Sulfinpyrazone (e.g., Anturane)—Aspirin can keep these medicines from working properly for treating gout

Other medical problems—The presence of other medical problems may affect the use of butalbital and aspirin combinations. Make sure you tell your doctor if you have any other medical problems, especially:
- Alcohol abuse (or history of) or
- Drug abuse or dependence (or history of)—Dependence on butalbital may develop
- Asthma, especially if occurring together with other allergies and nasal polyps (or history of), or
- Emphysema or other chronic lung disease or
- Hyperactivity (in children) or
- Kidney disease or
- Liver disease—The chance of serious side effects may be increased
- Diabetes mellitus (sugar diabetes) or
- Mental depression or
- Overactive thyroid or
- Porphyria (or history of)—Butalbital may make these conditions worse
- Gout—Aspirin can make this condition worse and can also lessen the effects of some medicines used to treat gout
- Heart disease (severe)—The caffeine in some of these combination medicines can make some kinds of heart disease worse
- Hemophilia or other bleeding problems or
- Vitamin K deficiency—Aspirin increases the chance of serious bleeding
- Stomach ulcer, especially with a history of bleeding, or other stomach problems—Aspirin can make your condition worse

Proper Use of This Medicine

Take this medicine with food or a full glass (8 ounces) of water to lessen stomach irritation.

Do not take this medicine if it has a strong vinegar-like odor. This odor means the aspirin in it is breaking down. If you have any questions about this, check with your health care professional.

Take this medicine only as directed by your doctor. Do not take more of it, do not take it more often, and do not take it for a longer time than your doctor ordered. If butalbital and aspirin combination is taken regularly (for example, every day), it may become habit-forming (causing mental or physical dependence). The caffeine in some butalbital and aspirin combinations can also increase the chance of dependence. Dependence is especially likely to occur in patients who take this medicine to relieve frequent headaches. Taking too much of this combination medicine can also lead to stomach problems or to other medical problems.

This medicine will relieve a headache best if you *take it as soon as the headache begins*. If you get warning signs of a migraine, take this medicine as soon as you are sure that the migraine is coming. This may even stop the headache pain from occurring. *Lying down in a quiet, dark room for a while after taking the medicine also helps to relieve headaches.*

People who get a lot of headaches may need to take a different medicine to help prevent headaches. *It is important that you follow your doctor's directions about taking the other medicine, even if your headaches continue to occur.* Headache-preventing medicines may take several weeks to start working. Even after they do start working, your headaches may not go away completely. However, your headaches should occur less often, and they should be less severe and easier to relieve than before. This will reduce the amount of headache relievers that you need. If you do not notice any improvement after several weeks of headache-preventing treatment, check with your doctor.

Dosing—The dose of butalbital and aspirin combination medicines will be different for different patients. *Follow your doctor's orders or the directions on the label.* The following information includes only the average doses of the medicine. *If your dose is different, do not change it* unless your doctor tells you to do so.

For Butalbital and Aspirin combination
- For *oral* dosage form (tablets):
  - For tension headaches:
    - Adults—One tablet every four hours as needed. You should not take more than six tablets a day.
    - Children—Dose must be determined by your doctor.

For Butalbital, Aspirin, and Caffeine combination
- For *oral* dosage forms (capsules or tablets):
  - For tension headaches:
    - Adults—One or 2 capsules or tablets every four hours as needed. You should not take more than six capsules or tablets a day.
    - Children—Dose must be determined by your doctor.

Missed dose—If your doctor has ordered you to take this medicine according to a regular schedule and you miss a dose, take it as soon as you remember. However, if it is almost time for your next dose, skip the missed dose and go back to your regular dosing schedule. Do not double doses.

Storage—To store this medicine:
- Keep out of the reach of children. Overdose is especially dangerous in young children.
- Store away from heat and direct light.
- Do not store this medicine in the bathroom, near the kitchen sink, or in other damp places. Heat or moisture may cause the medicine to break down.

- Do not keep outdated medicine or medicine no longer needed. Be sure that any discarded medicine is out of the reach of children.

Precautions While Using This Medicine

Check with your doctor:
- If the medicine stops working as well as it did when you first started using it. This may mean that you are in danger of becoming dependent on the medicine. *Do not try to get better pain relief by increasing the dose.*

- *If you are having headaches more often than you did before you started using this medicine.* This is especially important if a new headache occurs within 1 day after you took your last dose of headache medicine, headaches begin to occur every day, or a headache continues for several days in a row. This may mean that you are dependent on the headache medicine. *Continuing to take this medicine will cause even more headaches later on.* Your doctor can give you advice on how to relieve the headaches.

Check the labels of all nonprescription (over-the-counter [OTC]) and prescription medicines you now take. If any contain a barbiturate, aspirin, or other salicylates, including diflunisal, check with your health care professional. Taking them together with this medicine may cause an overdose.

The butalbital in this medicine will add to the effects of alcohol and other CNS depressants (medicines that slow down the nervous system, possibly causing drowsiness). Some examples of CNS depressants are antihistamines or medicine for hay fever, other allergies, or colds; sedatives, tranquilizers, or sleeping medicine; other prescription pain medicine or narcotics; other barbiturates; medicine for seizures; muscle relaxants; or anesthetics, including some dental anesthetics. Also, stomach problems may be more likely to occur if you drink alcoholic beverages while you are taking aspirin. Therefore, *do not drink alcoholic beverages, and check with your doctor before taking any of the medicines listed above, while you are using this medicine.*

This medicine may cause some people to become drowsy, dizzy, or lightheaded. *Make sure you know how you react to this medicine before you drive, use machines, or do anything else that could be dangerous if you are dizzy or are not alert and clearheaded.*

Before having any kind of surgery (including dental surgery) or emergency treatment, tell the medical doctor or dentist in charge that you are taking this medicine. Serious side effects may occur if your medical doctor or dentist gives you certain other medicines without knowing that you have taken butalbital.

Do not take this medicine for 5 days before any planned surgery, including dental surgery, unless otherwise directed by your medical doctor or dentist. Taking aspirin during this time may cause bleeding problems.

Before you have any medical tests, tell the person in charge that you are taking this medicine. Caffeine (present in some butalbital and aspirin combinations) interferes with the results of certain tests that use dipyridamole (e.g., Persantine) to help show how well blood is flowing to your heart. Caffeine should not be taken for 8 to 12 hours before the test. The results of some other tests may also be affected by butalbital and aspirin combinations.

If you have been taking large amounts of this medicine, or if you have been taking it regularly for several weeks or more, *do not suddenly stop using it without first checking with your doctor*. Your doctor may want you to reduce gradually the amount you are taking before stopping completely, to lessen the chance of withdrawal side effects.

If you think you or anyone else may have taken an overdose of this medicine, get emergency help at once. Taking an overdose of this medicine or taking alcohol or CNS depressants with this medicine may lead to unconsciousness or death. Symptoms of overdose of this medicine include convulsions (seizures); hearing loss; confusion; ringing or buzzing in the ears; severe excitement, nervousness, or restlessness; severe dizziness; severe drowsiness; shortness of breath or troubled breathing; and severe weakness.

Side Effects

Along with its needed effects, a medicine may cause some unwanted effects. Although not all of these side effects may occur, if they do occur they may need medical attention.

The following side effects may mean that a serious allergic reaction is occurring. Check with your doctor or get emergency help immediately if they occur, especially if several of them occur at the same time.
Less common or rare
    Bluish discoloration or flushing or redness of skin (occurring together with other effects listed in this section); coughing, shortness of breath, troubled breathing, tightness in chest, or wheezing; difficulty in swallowing; dizziness or feeling faint (severe); hive-like swellings (large) on eyelids, face, lips, or tongue; skin rash, itching, or hives; stuffy nose (occurring together with other effects listed in this section)

Also check with your doctor immediately if any of the following side effects occur, especially if several of them occur together:
Rare
    Bleeding or crusting sores on lips; chest pain; fever with or without chills; red, thickened, or scaly skin; sores, ulcers, or white spots in mouth (painful); sore throat (unexplained); tenderness, burning, or peeling of skin
Symptoms of overdose
    Anxiety, confusion, excitement, irritability, nervousness, restlessness, or trouble in sleeping (severe, especially with products containing caffeine); convulsions (seizures, with products containing caffeine); diarrhea (severe or continuing); dizziness, lightheadedness, drowsiness, or weakness (severe); frequent urination (for products containing caffeine); hallucinations (seeing, hearing, or feeling things that are not there); increased sensitivity to touch or pain (for products containing caffeine); increased thirst; muscle trembling or twitching (for products containing caffeine); nausea or vomiting (severe or continuing), sometimes with blood; ringing or buzzing in ears (continuing) or hearing loss; seeing flashes of "zig-zag" lights (for products containing caffeine); slow, fast, or irregular heartbeat; slow, fast, irregular, or troubled breathing; slurred speech;

staggering; stomach pain (severe); uncontrollable flapping movements of the hands, especially in elderly patients; unusual movements of the eyes; vision problems

Also, check with your doctor as soon as possible if any of the following side effects occur:
Less common or rare
    Bloody or black, tarry stools; bloody urine; confusion or mental depression; muscle cramps or pain; pinpoint red spots on skin; swollen or painful glands; unusual bleeding or bruising; unusual excitement (mild)

Other side effects may occur that usually do not need medical attention. These side effects may go away during treatment as your body adjusts to the medicine. However, check with your doctor if any of the following side effects continue or are bothersome:
More common
    Bloated or "gassy" feeling; dizziness or lightheadedness (mild); drowsiness (mild); heartburn or indigestion; nausea, vomiting, or stomach pain (occurring without other symptoms of overdose)

Other side effects not listed above may also occur in some patients. If you notice any other effects, check with your doctor.

BUTALBITAL, ACETAMINOPHEN, CAFFEINE, AND CODEINE (Oral route) - byoo-TAL-bi-tal, a-seet-a-MIN-oh-fen, kaf-EEN, KOE-deen

Commonly used brand name(s)

In the U.S.—
    Phrenilin with Caffeine and Codeine

Available Dosage Forms:
• Capsule

Therapeutic Class: Opioid/Barbiturate Combination
Pharmacologic Class: Barbiturate

Uses For This Medicine

Butalbital, acetaminophen, caffeine, and codeine combination is a pain reliever and relaxant. It is used to treat tension headaches. Butalbital belongs to the group of medicines called barbiturates. Barbiturates act in the central nervous system (CNS) to produce their effects.

Codeine is a narcotic analgesic that acts in the CNS to relieve pain. Many of its side effects are also caused by actions in the CNS.

When you take butalbital or codeine for a long time, your body may get used to it so that larger amounts are needed to produce the same effects. This is called tolerance to the medicine. Also, butalbital and codeine may become habit-forming (causing mental or physical dependence) when it is used for a long time or in large doses. Physical dependence may lead to withdrawal side effects when you stop taking the medicine. In patients who get headaches, the first symptom of withdrawal may be new (rebound) headaches.

Caffeine may help to relieve headaches. However, caffeine can also cause physical dependence when it is used for a long time. This may lead to withdrawal (rebound) headaches when you stop taking it.

Butalbital, acetaminophen, caffeine and codeine combination may also be used for other kinds of headaches or other kinds of pain as determined by your doctor.

Butalbital, acetaminophen, caffeine, and codeine combination is available only with your doctor's prescription.

Before Using This Medicine

In deciding to use a medicine, the risks of taking the medicine must be weighed against the good it will do. This is a decision you and your doctor will make. For this medicine, the following should be considered:

Allergies—Tell your doctor if you have ever had any unusual or allergic reaction to this medicine or any other medicines. Also tell your health care professional if you have any other types of allergies, such as to foods, dyes, preservatives, or animals. For non-prescription products, read the label or package ingredients carefully.

Pediatric—

- For butalbital: Although barbiturates such as butalbital often cause drowsiness, some children become excited after taking them.

- For acetaminophen: Acetaminophen has been tested in children and, in effective doses, has not been shown to cause different side effects or problems than it does in adults.

- For caffeine: There is no specific information comparing use of caffeine in children up to 12 years of age with use in other age groups. However, caffeine is not expected to cause different side effects or problems in children than it does in adults.

Geriatric—

- For butalbital: Certain side effects, such as confusion, excitement, or mental depression, may be especially likely to occur in elderly patients, who are usually more sensitive than younger adults to the effects of the butalbital in this combination medicine.

- For acetaminophen: Acetaminophen has been tested and has not been shown to cause different side effects or problems in older people than it does in younger adults.

- For caffeine: Many medicines have not been studied specifically in older people. Therefore, it may not be known whether they work exactly the same way they do in younger adults or if they cause different side effects or problems in older people. There is no specific information comparing use of caffeine in the elderly with use in other age groups.

- For codeine: Breathing problems may be especially likely to occur in elderly patients, who are usually more sensitive than younger adults to the effects of codeine.

Pregnancy—

	Pregnancy Category	Explanation
All Trimesters	C	Animal studies have shown an adverse effect and there are no adequate studies in pregnant women OR no animal studies have been conducted and there are no adequate studies in pregnant women.

Breast Feeding—There are no adequate studies in women for determining infant risk when using this medication during breastfeeding. Weigh the potential benefits against the potential risks before taking this medication while breastfeeding.

Other medicines—

Using this medicine with any of the following medicines is not recommended. Your doctor may decide not to treat you with this medication or change some of the other medicines you take.

Naltrexone

Interactions with Food/Tobacco/Alcohol—Certain medicines should not be used at or around the time of eating food or eating certain types of food since interactions may occur. Using alcohol or tobacco with certain medicines may also cause interactions to occur. The following interactions have been selected on the basis of their potential significance and are not necessarily all-inclusive.

Using this medicine with any of the following is usually not recommended, but may be unavoidable in some cases. If used together, your doctor may change the dose or how often you use this medicine, or give you special instructions about the use of food, alcohol, or tobacco.

Ethanol

Using this medicine with any of the following may cause an increased risk of certain side effects but may be unavoidable in some cases. If used together, your doctor may change the dose or how often you use this medicine, or give you special instructions about the use of food, alcohol, or tobacco.

Cabbage

Other medical problems—The presence of other medical problems may affect the use of this medicine. Make sure you tell your doctor if you have any other medical problems, especially:

- Alcohol abuse (or history of) or

- Drug abuse or dependence (or history of)—Dependence on butalbital and codeine may develop; also, acetaminophen may cause liver damage in people who abuse alcohol

- Asthma (or history of), emphysema, or other chronic lung disease or

- Brain disease or head injury or

- Colitis or

- Convulsions (seizures) (history of) or

- Emphysema or other chronic lung disease or

- Enlarged prostate or problems with urination or

- Gallbladder disease or gallstones or

- Hepatitis or other liver disease or

- Hyperactivity (in children) or

- Kidney disease—The chance of serious side effects may be increased
- Type 2 diabetes mellitus or
- Mental depression or
- Overactive thyroid or
- Porphyria (or history of)—Butalbital can make these conditions worse
- Heart disease (severe)—The caffeine can make some kinds of heart disease worse

Proper Use of This Medicine

Take this medicine only as directed by your doctor. Do not take more of it, do not take it more often, and do not take it for a longer time than your doctor ordered. If butalbital, acetaminophen, caffeine, and codeine combination is taken regularly (for example, every day), it may become habit-forming (causing mental or physical dependence). The caffeine can also increase the chance of dependence. Dependence is especially likely to occur in patients who take these medicines to relieve frequent headaches. Taking too much of this medicine may also lead to liver damage or other medical problems.

This medicine will relieve a headache best if you take it as soon as the headache begins. If you get warning signs of a migraine, take this medicine as soon as you are sure that the migraine is coming. This may even stop the headache pain from occurring. Lying down in a quiet, dark room for a while after taking the medicine also helps to relieve headaches.

People who get a lot of headaches may need to take a different medicine to help prevent headaches. It is important that you follow your doctor's directions about taking the other medicine, even if your headaches continue to occur. Headache-preventing medicines may take several weeks to start working. Even after they do start working, your headaches may not go away completely. However, your headaches should occur less often, and they should be less severe and easier to relieve than before. This will reduce the amount of headache relievers that you need. If you do not notice any improvement after several weeks of headache-preventing treatment, check with your doctor.

Dosing—The dose of this medicine will be different for different patients. Follow your doctor's orders or the directions on the label. The following information includes only the average doses of this medicine. If your dose is different, do not change it unless your doctor tells you to do so.

The amount of medicine that you take depends on the strength of the medicine. Also, the number of doses you take each day, the time allowed between doses, and the length of time you take the medicine depend on the medical problem for which you are using the medicine.

- For oral dosage forms (capsules):
  - For tension headaches:
    - Adults—One or 2 capsules every four hours as needed. You should not take more than six capsules a day.
    - Children—Dose must be determined by your doctor.

Missed dose—If you miss a dose of this medicine, take it as soon as possible. However, if it is almost time for your next dose, skip the missed dose and go back to your regular dosing schedule. Do not double doses.

Storage—Store the medicine in a closed container at room temperature, away from heat, moisture, and direct light. Keep from freezing.

Keep out of the reach of children.

Do not keep outdated medicine or medicine no longer needed.

Precautions While Using This Medicine

Check with your doctor:
- If the medicine stops working as well as it did when you first started using it. This may mean that you are in danger of becoming dependent on the medicine. Do not try to get better pain relief by increasing the dose.
- If you are having headaches more often than you did before you started taking this medicine. This is especially important if a new headache occurs within 1 day after you took your last dose of this medicine, headaches begin to occur every day, or a headache continues for several days in a row. This may mean that you are dependent on the medicine. Continuing to take this medicine will cause even more headaches later on. Your doctor can give you advice on how to relieve the headaches.

Check the labels of all nonprescription (over-the-counter [OTC]) or prescription medicines you now take. If any contain a barbiturate, acetaminophen, caffeine, or codeine, check with your health care professional. Taking them together with this medicine may cause an overdose.

The butalbital and codeine in this medicine will add to the effects of alcohol and other CNS depressants (medicines that slow down the nervous system, possibly causing drowsiness). Some examples of CNS depressants are antihistamines or medicine for hay fever, other allergies, or colds; sedatives, tranquilizers, or sleeping medicine; other prescription pain medicine; narcotics; other barbiturates; medicine for seizures; muscle relaxants; or anesthetics, including some dental anesthetics. Also, drinking large amounts of alcoholic beverages regularly while taking this medicine may increase the chance of liver damage or stomach problems, especially if you take more of this medicine than your doctor ordered or if you take it regularly for a long time. Therefore, do not drink alcoholic beverages, and check with your doctor before taking any of the medicines listed above, while you are using this medicine.

This medicine may cause some people to become drowsy, dizzy, or lightheaded. Make sure you know how you react to this medicine before you drive, use machines, or do anything else that could be dangerous if you are dizzy or are not alert and clearheaded.

Before you have any medical tests, tell the person in charge that you are taking this medicine. Caffeine interferes with the results of certain tests that use dipyridamole (e.g., Persantine) to help show how well blood is flowing to your heart. Caffeine should not be taken for 8 to 12 hours before the test. The results of other tests may also be affected by butalbital, acetaminophen, caffeine and codeine combination.

Before having any kind of surgery (including dental surgery) or emergency treatment, tell the medical doctor or dentist in charge that you are taking this medicine. Serious side effects can occur if your medical doctor or dentist gives you certain medicines without knowing that you have taken butalbital or codeine.

If you have been taking large amounts of this medicine, or if you have been taking it regularly for several weeks or more, do not suddenly stop taking it without first checking with your doctor. Your doctor may want you to reduce gradually the amount you are taking before stopping completely in order to lessen the chance of withdrawal side effects.

If you think you or anyone else may have taken an overdose of this medicine, get emergency help at once. Taking an overdose of this medicine or taking alcohol or CNS depressants with this medicine may lead to unconsciousness or possibly death. Signs of butalbital or codeine overdose include severe drowsiness, confusion, severe weakness, shortness of breath or unusually slow or troubled breathing, slurred speech, staggering, and unusually slow heartbeat. Signs of severe acetaminophen poisoning may not occur until 2 to 4 days after the overdose is taken, but treatment to prevent liver damage or death must be started within 24 hours or less after the overdose is taken.

Side Effects of This Medicine

Along with its needed effects, a medicine may cause some unwanted effects. Although not all of these side effects may occur, if they do occur they may need medical attention.

Check with your doctor immediately if any of the following side effects occur:

Rare

Bleeding or crusting sores on lips; chest pain; fever with or without chills; convulsions, hallucinations, trembling, and/or uncontrolled muscle movements; hive-like swellings (large) on eyelids, face, lips, and/or tongue; mental depression; muscle cramps or pain; red, thickened, or scaly skin; shortness of breath, troubled breathing, tightness in chest, or wheezing; skin rash, itching, or hives; sores, ulcers, or white spots in mouth (painful); sore throat

Symptoms of overdose

Anxiety, confusion, excitement, irritability, nervousness, restlessness, or trouble in sleeping (severe); cold and clammy skin; convulsions (seizures); diarrhea, especially if occurring together with increased sweating, loss of appetite, and stomach cramps or pain; dizziness, lightheadedness, drowsiness, or weakness, (severe); frequent urination; hallucinations (seeing, hearing, or feeling things that are not there); increased sensitivity to touch or pain; muscle trembling or twitching; nausea or vomiting, sometimes with blood; ringing or other sounds in ears; seeing flashes of "zig-zag" lights; shortness of breath or unusually slow or troubled breathing; slow, fast, or irregular heartbeat; slurred speech; staggering; swelling, pain, or tenderness in the upper abdomen or stomach area; unusual movements of the eyes

Check with your doctor as soon as possible if any of the following side effects occur:

Less common

Confusion (mild); mental depression; unusual excitement (mild)

Rare

Bloody or black, tarry stools; bloody urine; pinpoint red spots on skin; swollen or painful glands; unusual bleeding or bruising; unusual tiredness or weakness (mild)

Some side effects may occur that usually do not need medical attention. These side effects may go away during treatment as your body adjusts to the medicine. Also, your health care professional may be able to tell you about ways to prevent or reduce some of these side effects. Check with your health care professional if any of the following side effects continue or are bothersome or if you have any questions about them:

More common

Bloated or "gassy" feeling; dizziness or lightheadedness (mild); drowsiness (mild); nausea, vomiting, or stomach pain (occurring without other symptoms of overdose)

Other side effects not listed may also occur in some patients. If you notice any other effects, check with your healthcare professional.

BUTENAFINE (Topical route) - byoo-TEN-a-feen

Commonly used brand name(s)
In the U.S.—
Mentax

Available Dosage Forms:
• Cream

Therapeutic Class: Antifungal

Uses For This Medicine

Butenafine is used to treat fungus infections. It works by killing the fungus or preventing its growth. Butenafine is applied to the skin to treat:

• Athlete's foot (ringworm of the foot; tinea pedis);
• Jock itch (ringworm of the groin; tinea cruris);
• Ringworm of the body (tinea corporis);
• Fungal infection on the skin of the chest, back and shoulders (tinea versicolor).

This medicine is available only with your doctor's prescription.

Before Using This Medicine

In deciding to use a medicine, the risks of taking the medicine must be weighed against the good it will do. This is a decision you and your doctor will make. For this medicine, the following should be considered:

Allergies—Tell your doctor if you have ever had any unusual or allergic reaction to this medicine or any other medicines. Also tell your health care professional if you have any other types of allergies, such as to foods, dyes, preservatives, or animals. For non-prescription products, read the label or package ingredients carefully.

Pediatric—There is no specific information comparing use of butenafine in children with use in other age groups.

Geriatric—Many medicines have not been studied specifically in older people. Therefore, it may not be known whether they work exactly the same way they do in younger adults. Although there is no specific information comparing use of butenafine in the elderly with use in other age groups, clinical studies included older patients. No differences in effects of butenafine were seen in the elderly compared with younger adults.

Pregnancy—

	Pregnancy Category	Explanation
All Trimesters	B	Animal studies have revealed no evidence of harm to the fetus, however, there are no adequate studies in pregnant women OR animal studies have shown an adverse effect, but adequate studies in pregnant women have failed to demonstrate a risk to the fetus.

Breast Feeding—There are no adequate studies in women for determining infant risk when using this medication during breastfeeding. Weigh the potential benefits against the potential risks before taking this medication while breastfeeding.

Other medicines—Although certain medicines should not be used together at all, in other cases two different medicines may be used together even if an interaction might occur. In these cases, your doctor may want to change the dose, or other precautions may be necessary. Tell your healthcare professional if you are taking any other prescription or nonprescription (over-the-counter [OTC]) medicine.

Interactions with Food/Tobacco/Alcohol—Certain medicines should not be used at or around the time of eating food or eating certain types of food since interactions may occur. Using alcohol or tobacco with certain medicines may also cause interactions to occur. Discuss with your healthcare professional the use of your medicine with food, alcohol, or tobacco.

Proper Use of This Medicine

Apply enough butenafine to cover the affected skin and surrounding areas, and rub in gently.

After applying butenafine, wash your hands to remove any medicine that may be on them.

Keep this medicine away from the eyes and mucous membranes such as the inside of the nose, mouth, or vagina.

Do not bandage or apply an occlusive dressing (airtight covering such as kitchen plastic wrap) over this medicine unless otherwise directed by your doctor. If you have any questions about this, check with your doctor.

To help clear up your skin infection completely, keep using butenafine for the full time of treatment. It may sometimes take quite a while for a fungus infection to be cured. If you stop using this medicine too soon, your symptoms will return.

Dosing—The dose of this medicine will be different for different patients. Follow your doctor's orders or the directions on the label. The following information includes only the average doses of this medicine. If your dose is different, do not change it unless your doctor tells you to do so.

The amount of medicine that you take depends on the strength of the medicine. Also, the number of doses you take each day, the time allowed between doses, and the length of time you take the medicine depend on the medical problem for which you are using the medicine.

- For topical dosage form (cream):
  - For fungus infections:
    - Adults and teenagers—Apply to the affected area(s) of the skin once or twice a day, as ordered by your doctor.
    - Children younger than 12 years of age—Use and dose must be determined by your doctor.

Missed dose—If you miss a dose of this medicine, apply it as soon as possible. However, if it is almost time for your next dose, skip the missed dose and go back to your regular dosing schedule.

Storage—Store the medicine in a closed container at room temperature, away from heat, moisture, and direct light. Keep from freezing.

Keep out of the reach of children.

Do not keep outdated medicine or medicine no longer needed.

Precautions While Using This Medicine

If your skin infection does not improve within 4 weeks, or if it becomes worse, check with your doctor.

Tinea versicolor may cause skin to appear darker or lighter, or spots of both. These changes in color can last for months even when the fungal infection has been eliminated. Continuing treatment longer than recommended will not cause skin color to return to normal faster. Consult your physician if you believe the fungal infection may have returned.

To help clear up your skin infection completely and to help make sure it does not return, the following good health habits are important:

- For patients using butenafine for athlete's foot, these measures will help keep the feet cool and dry:
  - Carefully dry the feet, especially between the toes, after bathing.
  - Avoid wearing socks made from wool or synthetic materials (for example, rayon or nylon). Instead, wear clean, cotton socks and change them daily or more often if your feet sweat very much.
  - Wear well-ventilated shoes (for example, shoes with holes on top or on the side) or sandals.
  - Use a bland, absorbent powder (for example, talcum powder) or an antifungal powder freely between the toes, on the feet, and in socks and shoes once or twice a day. Be sure to use the powder after butenafine has been applied and has disappeared into the skin. Do not use the powder as the only treatment for your fungus infection.

- For patients using butenafine for jock itch, these measures will help reduce chafing and irritation and will also keep the groin area cool and dry:
  - Carefully dry the groin area after bathing.
  - Avoid wearing underwear that is tight-fitting or made from synthetic materials (for example, rayon or nylon). Instead, wear loose-fitting, cotton underwear.
  - Use a bland, absorbent powder (for example, talcum powder) or an antifungal powder freely once or twice a day. Be sure to use the powder after butenafine has been applied and has disappeared into the skin. Do not use the powder as the only treatment for your fungus infection.

- For patients using butenafine for ringworm of the body, these measures will help keep the affected area cool and dry:
  - Carefully dry yourself after bathing.
  - Avoid too much heat and humidity if possible. Try to keep moisture from building up on affected areas of the body.
  - Wear loose-fitting clothing.
  - Use a bland, absorbent powder (for example, talcum powder) or an antifungal powder freely once or twice a day. Be sure to use the powder after butenafine has been applied and has disappeared into the skin. Do not use the powder as the only treatment for your fungus infection.

Side Effects of This Medicine

Along with its needed effects, a medicine may cause some unwanted effects. Although not all of these side effects may occur, if they do occur they may need medical attention.

Check with your doctor as soon as possible if any of the following side effects occur:

Rare

Blistering, burning, itching, oozing, stinging, swelling, or other signs of skin irritation not present before use of this medicine; rash; redness

Other side effects not listed may also occur in some patients. If you notice any other effects, check with your healthcare professional.

BUTORPHANOL   (Nasal route) - byoo-TOR-fa-nole

Commonly used brand name(s)
In the U.S.—
  Stadol NS

Available Dosage Forms:
- Spray

Therapeutic Class: Analgesic
Pharmacologic Class: Opioid Agonist/Antagonist

Uses For This Medicine

Butorphanol is a narcotic analgesic (pain medicine) that is sprayed into the nose. It is used to relieve moderate or severe pain. It is also used to relieve pain that occurs after an operation.

Narcotic analgesics act in the central nervous system (CNS) to relieve pain. Some of their side effects are also caused by actions in the CNS.

If a narcotic is used for a long time, it may become habit-forming (causing mental or physical dependence). Physical dependence may lead to withdrawal side effects when you stop taking the medicine.

This medicine is available only with your doctor's or dentist's prescription.

Before Using This Medicine

In deciding to use a medicine, the risks of taking the medicine must be weighed against the good it will do. This is a decision you and your doctor will make. For this medicine, the following should be considered:

Allergies—Tell your doctor if you have ever had any unusual or allergic reaction to this medicine or any other medicines. Also tell your health care professional if you have any other types of allergies, such as to foods, dyes, preservatives, or animals. For non-prescription products, read the label or package ingredients carefully.

Pediatric—Studies on this medicine have been done only in adult patients, and there is no specific information comparing use of butorphanol in children with use in other age groups.

Geriatric—Elderly people are especially sensitive to the effects of butorphanol. This may increase the chance of side effects, especially dizziness, during treatment. Studies in older adults show that butorphanol stays in the body for a longer time than it does in younger adults. Your doctor will consider this when deciding on your dose.

Pregnancy—

	Pregnancy Category	Explanation
All Trimesters	C	Animal studies have shown an adverse effect and there are no adequate studies in pregnant women OR no animal studies have been conducted and there are no adequate studies in pregnant women.

Breast Feeding—There are no adequate studies in women for determining infant risk when using this medication during breastfeeding. Weigh the potential benefits against the potential risks before taking this medication while breastfeeding.

Other medicines—

Using this medicine with any of the following medicines is usually not recommended, but may be required in some cases. If both medicines are prescribed together, your doctor may change the dose or how often you use one or both of the medicines.

Alfentanil, Alphaprodine, Codeine, Dihydrocodeine, Fentanyl, Hydrocodone, Hydromorphone, Levorphanol, Meperidine, Methadone, Morphine, Morphine Sulfate Liposome, Oxycodone, Oxymorphone, Propoxyphene, Sufentanil

Interactions with Food/Tobacco/Alcohol—Certain medicines should not be used at or around the time of eating food or eating certain types of food since interactions may occur. Using alcohol or tobacco with certain medicines may also cause interactions to occur. Discuss with your healthcare professional the use of your medicine with food, alcohol, or tobacco.

Other medical problems—The presence of other medical problems may affect the use of this medicine. Make sure you tell your doctor if you have any other medical problems, especially:

- CNS disease affecting breathing or
- Emphysema, asthma, or other chronic lung disease or
- Head injury—Some of the side effects of butorphanol can be dangerous if you have any of these conditions
- Drug dependence, especially narcotic abuse, or history of, or
- Emotional problems—The chance of side effects may be increased; also, withdrawal symptoms may occur if a

narcotic you are dependent on is replaced by butorphanol

- Heart disease or
- Kidney disease or
- Liver disease—The chance of side effects may be increased

Proper Use of This Medicine

You will be given an instruction sheet with your prescription for butorphanol that explains how to use the pump spray unit. If you have any questions about using the unit, ask your health care professional.

To use:

- Use this medicine only as directed by your medical doctor or dentist. Do not use more of it, do not use it more often, and do not use it for a longer time than your medical doctor or dentist told you. This is especially important for elderly patients, who may be more sensitive to the effects of butorphanol. If too much is used, the medicine may become habit-forming (causing mental or physical dependence) or lead to medical problems because of an overdose.
- Remove the protective cover and clip. Before you use each new bottle of butorphanol, the spray pump needs to be started. To do this, point the sprayer away from you and other people or pets. Pump the spray unit firmly about 7 or 8 times. A fine, wide spray should come out by the seventh or eighth time you pump the unit. If the unit is not used for 48 hours or longer, the spray pump should be started again by pumping it 1 or 2 times only.
- Before each use, blow your nose gently.
- For a 1–mg dose, insert the spray tip into one nostril. Close off the other nostril by pressing the side of your nose with your index finger. Tilt your head slightly forward and spray one time. Sniff gently with your mouth closed.
- Remove the spray tip from your nostril. Tilt your head back and sniff gently.
- For a 2–mg dose, repeat these steps using the other nostril.
- Replace the protective cover and clip after each use.

Dosing—The dose of this medicine will be different for different patients. Follow your doctor's orders or the directions on the label. The following information includes only the average doses of this medicine. If your dose is different, do not change it unless your doctor tells you to do so.

The amount of medicine that you take depends on the strength of the medicine. Also, the number of doses you take each day, the time allowed between doses, and the length of time you take the medicine depend on the medical problem for which you are using the medicine.

- For nasal dosage form:
  - For pain:
    - Adults—1 mg (one spray in one nostril). If pain is not relieved within sixty to ninety minutes, another spray (1 mg) in one nostril may be used. This dosing procedure may be repeated in three to four hours as needed. However, if pain is severe, a 2–mg dose (one spray in each nostril) may be used every three to four hours, but it is important to remain lying down if drowsiness or dizziness occurs.
    - Children and teenagers—Use and dose must be determined by your doctor.

Missed dose—If you miss a dose of this medicine, take it as soon as possible. However, if it is almost time for your next dose, skip the missed dose and go back to your regular dosing schedule. Do not double doses.

Storage—Store the medicine in a closed container at room temperature, away from heat, moisture, and direct light. Keep from freezing.

Keep out of the reach of children.

Do not keep outdated medicine or medicine no longer needed.

Precautions While Using This Medicine

Butorphanol will add to the effects of alcohol and other CNS depressants (medicines that make you drowsy or less alert). Some examples of CNS depressants are antihistamines or medicine for hay fever, other allergies, or colds; sedatives, tranquilizers, or sleeping medicine; other prescription pain medicines, including other narcotics; barbiturates; medicine for seizures; muscle relaxants; or anesthetics, including some dental anesthetics. Do not drink alcoholic beverages, and check with your medical doctor or dentist before taking any of the medicines listed above, while you are using this medicine.

This medicine may cause some people to become drowsy, dizzy, or lightheaded, or to feel a false sense of well-being. Make sure you know how you react to this medicine before you drive, use machines, or do anything else that could be dangerous if you are dizzy or are not alert and clearheaded.

Dizziness, lightheadedness, or fainting may occur, especially in the first hour after use or when you get up suddenly from a lying or sitting position. Getting up slowly may help lessen this problem.

Before having any kind of surgery (including dental surgery) or emergency treatment, tell the medical doctor or dentist in charge that you are using this medicine.

Butorphanol may cause dryness of the mouth. For temporary relief, use sugarless candy or gum, melt bits of ice in your mouth, or use a saliva substitute. However, if dry mouth continues for more than 2 weeks, check with your dentist. Continuing dryness of the mouth may increase the chance of dental disease, including tooth decay, gum disease, and fungus infections.

If you have been using this medicine regularly for several weeks or more, do not suddenly stop using it without first checking with your doctor. Your doctor may want you to reduce gradually the amount you are using before stopping completely, in order to lessen the chance of withdrawal side effects.

If you think you or someone else may have used an overdose, get emergency help at once. Using an overdose of this medicine or taking alcohol or CNS depressants with this medicine may lead to unconsciousness or death. Signs of overdose include convulsions (seizures), confusion, severe nervousness or restlessness, severe dizziness, severe drowsiness, slow or troubled breathing, and severe weakness.

Side Effects of This Medicine

Along with its needed effects, a medicine may cause some unwanted effects. Although not all of these side effects may occur, if they do occur they may need medical attention.

Get emergency help immediately if any of the following symptoms of overdose occur:

　　Cold, clammy skin; confusion; convulsions (seizures); dizziness (severe); drowsiness (severe); nervousness, restlessness, or weakness (severe); small pupils; slow heartbeat; slow or troubled breathing

Check with your doctor as soon as possible if any of the following side effects occur:

More common

　　Difficulty in breathing; fever; nosebleeds; ringing or buzzing in ears; runny nose; sinus congestion; sneezing; sore throat

Less common or rare

　　Blurred vision; congestion in chest; cough; difficulty in urinating; difficult or painful breathing; ear pain; fainting; hallucinations; itching; sinus congestion with pain; skin rash or hives

Some side effects may occur that usually do not need medical attention. These side effects may go away during treatment as your body adjusts to the medicine. Also, your health care professional may be able to tell you about ways to prevent or reduce some of these side effects. Check with your health care professional if any of the following side effects continue or are bothersome or if you have any questions about them:

More common

　　Confusion; constipation; dizziness; drowsiness; dry mouth; flushing; headache; irritation inside nose; loss of appetite; nasal congestion; nausea or vomiting; sweating or clammy feeling; trouble in sleeping; unpleasant taste; weakness (severe)

Less common or rare

　　Anxious feeling; behavior changes; burning, crawling, or prickling feeling on skin; false sense of well-being; feeling hot; floating feeling; nervousness, sometimes with restlessness; pounding heartbeat; stomach pain; strange dreams; trembling

After you stop using this medicine, it may still produce some side effects that need attention. During this period of time, *check with your doctor immediately* if you notice the following side effects:

　　Anxious feeling; diarrhea; nervousness and restlessness

Other side effects not listed may also occur in some patients. If you notice any other effects, check with your healthcare professional.

CABERGOLINE (Oral route) - ka-BER-goe-leen

Commonly used brand name(s)

In the U.S.—
Dostinex

Available Dosage Forms:
- Tablet

Therapeutic Class: Prolactin Secretion Inhibitor
Pharmacologic Class: Dopamine Agonist

Uses For This Medicine

Cabergoline is used to treat different types of medical problems that occur when too much of the hormone prolactin is produced. It can be used to treat certain menstrual problems, fertility problems in men and women, and pituitary prolactinomas (tumors of the pituitary gland).

It works by stopping the brain from making and releasing the prolactin hormone from the pituitary. Cabergoline use is usually stopped when prolactin levels are normal for 6 months. It may be given again if symptoms of too much prolactin occur again.

This medicine is available only with your doctor's prescription.

Before Using This Medicine

In deciding to use a medicine, the risks of taking the medicine must be weighed against the good it will do. This is a decision you and your doctor will make. For this medicine, the following should be considered:

Allergies—Tell your doctor if you have ever had any unusual or allergic reaction to this medicine or any other medicines. Also tell your health care professional if you have any other types of allergies, such as to foods, dyes, preservatives, or animals. For non-prescription products, read the label or package ingredients carefully.

Pediatric—Studies of this medicine have been done only in adult patients, and there is no specific information comparing use of cabergoline in children with use in other age groups.

Geriatric—Many medicines have not been studied specifically in older people. Therefore, it may not be known whether they work exactly the same way they do in younger adults or if they cause different side effects or problems in older people. There is no specific information comparing use of cabergoline in the elderly with use in other age groups.

Pregnancy—

	Pregnancy Category	Explanation
All Trimesters	B	Animal studies have revealed no evidence of harm to the fetus, however, there are no adequate studies in pregnant women OR animal studies have shown an adverse effect, but adequate studies in pregnant women have failed to demonstrate a risk to the fetus.

Breast Feeding—Studies suggest that this medication may alter milk production or composition. If an alternative to this medication is not prescribed, you should monitor the infant for side effects and adequate milk intake.

Other medicines—Although certain medicines should not be used together at all, in other cases two different medicines may be used together even if an interaction might occur. In these cases, your doctor may want to change the dose, or other precautions may be necessary. Tell your healthcare professional if you are taking any other prescription or nonprescription (over-the-counter [OTC]) medicine.

Interactions with Food/Tobacco/Alcohol—Certain medicines should not be used at or around the time of eating food or eating certain types of food since interactions may occur. Using alcohol or tobacco with certain medicines may

also cause interactions to occur. Discuss with your healthcare professional the use of your medicine with food, alcohol, or tobacco.

Other medical problems—The presence of other medical problems may affect the use of this medicine. Make sure you tell your doctor if you have any other medical problems, especially:

- High blood pressure, untreated or
- High blood pressure of pregnancy (or history of)—Cabergoline usually decreases blood pressure but at times it may increase blood pressure and worsen these conditions
- Liver disease, mild to severe—Cabergoline may worsen this condition; a lower dose of cabergoline may be required

Proper Use of This Medicine

Do not take more or less of it than your doctor ordered.

Dosing—The dose of this medicine will be different for different patients. Follow your doctor's orders or the directions on the label. The following information includes only the average doses of this medicine. If your dose is different, do not change it unless your doctor tells you to do so.

The amount of medicine that you take depends on the strength of the medicine. Also, the number of doses you take each day, the time allowed between doses, and the length of time you take the medicine depend on the medical problem for which you are using the medicine.

- For oral dosage form (tablets):
  - For disorders of high prolactin levels or pituitary tumors:
    - Adults—0.25 mg two times a week. Dose may be increased every four weeks as needed, according to body prolactin levels, up to 1 mg two times a week.
    - Children—Use and dose must be determined by the doctor.

Missed dose—If you miss a dose of this medicine, take it as soon as possible. However, if it is almost time for your next dose, skip the missed dose and go back to your regular dosing schedule. Do not double doses.

However, if it is almost time for your next dose, check with your doctor to see if you can double your dose.

Storage—Store the medicine in a closed container at room temperature, away from heat, moisture, and direct light. Keep from freezing.

Keep out of the reach of children.

Do not keep outdated medicine or medicine no longer needed.

Precautions While Using This Medicine

It is important that your doctor check your progress at regular visits while you are taking this medicine.

This medicine may cause some people to become drowsy, dizzy, or less alert than they are normally. Make sure you know how you react to this medicine before you drive, use machines, or do other jobs that require you to be alert.

Dizziness, lightheadedness, or fainting may occur, especially when you get up from a lying or sitting position. Getting up slowly may help.

Tell your doctor right away if you think you have become pregnant. You and your doctor should discuss whether you should continue to take this medicine during pregnancy.

Check with your doctor right away if you have symptoms of fainting, hallucinations, lightheadedness, stuffy nose, or racing heart.

Side Effects of This Medicine

Along with its needed effects, a medicine may cause some unwanted effects. Although not all of these side effects may occur, if they do occur they may need medical attention.

Check with your doctor as soon as possible if any of the following side effects occur:
More common
    Abdominal pain; sensation that you are moving in space or that objects are moving around you (vertigo)
Rare
    Changes in vision; difficulty in concentrating; dizziness or fainting when getting up suddenly from a lying or sitting position; loss of appetite; swelling of hands, ankles, feet, or lower legs; unusually fast heartbeat; weight gain or loss
Symptoms of overdose
    Fainting; hallucinations; lightheadedness; racing heart; stuffy nose

Some side effects may occur that usually do not need medical attention. These side effects may go away during treatment as your body adjusts to the medicine. Also, your health care professional may be able to tell you about ways to prevent or reduce some of these side effects. Check with your health care professional if any of the following side effects continue or are bothersome or if you have any questions about them:
More common
    Constipation; dizziness; headache; nausea or stomach discomfort; weakness
Less common
    Burning, itching, or stinging of the skin; diarrhea; dry mouth or toothache; gas; general feeling of discomfort or illness; hot flashes; mental depression; muscle or joint pain; runny nose; sleepiness; sore throat; trouble in sleeping; vomiting

Other side effects not listed may also occur in some patients. If you notice any other effects, check with your healthcare professional.

CAFFEINE (Systemic)

Some commonly used brand names are:

In the U.S.—

Caffedrine Caplets (1)	NoDoz Maximum Strength
Cafcit (2)	Caplets (1)
Dexitac Stay Alert Stimulant (1)	Pep-Back (1)
	Quick Pep (1)
Enerjets (1)	Ultra Pep-Back (1)
Keep Alert (1)	Vivarin (1)
Maximum Strength SnapBack Stimulant Powders (1)	

In Canada—
Wake-Up (1)

This information applies to the following medicines:

1. Caffeine (KAF-feen)
2. Citrated Caffeine (SIH-tray-ted KAF-feen)
3. Caffeine and Sodium Benzoate (KAF-feen and SOE-dee-um BEN-zo-ate)

Category

- **Analgesia adjunct**—Caffeine
- **Respiratory stimulant adjunct**—Caffeine; Caffeine, Citrated
- **Stimulant, central nervous system**—Caffeine; Caffeine and Sodium Benzoate; Caffeine, Citrated

Description

Caffeine (KAF-feen) belongs to the group of medicines called central nervous system (CNS) stimulants. It is used to help restore mental alertness when unusual tiredness or weakness or drowsiness occurs. Caffeine's use as an alertness aid should be only occasional. It is not intended to replace sleep and should not be used regularly for this purpose.

Caffeine is also used in combination with ergotamine (for treatment of migraine and cluster headaches) or with certain pain relievers, such as aspirin or aspirin and acetaminophen. When used in this way, caffeine may increase the effectiveness of the other medicines. Caffeine is sometimes used in combination with an antihistamine to overcome the drowsiness caused by the antihistamine.

Citrated caffeine is used to treat breathing problems in premature babies.

Caffeine may also be used for other conditions as determined by your doctor.

Caffeine is present in coffee, tea, soft drinks, cocoa, chocolate, and kola nuts.

Caffeine powder and tablets are available without a prescription; however, your health care professional may have special instructions on its proper use. Citrated caffeine and caffeine and sodium benzoate are to be administered only by or under the supervision of your doctor. Caffeine is available in the following dosage forms:

Oral
- Caffeine
  - Powder
  - Tablets
- Citrated caffeine
  - Oral solution

Parenteral
- Citrated caffeine
  - Injection
- Caffeine and sodium benzoate
  - Injection

Before Using This Medicine

If you are taking this medicine without a prescription, carefully read and follow any precautions on the label. For caffeine, the following should be considered:

Allergies—Tell your doctor if you have ever had any unusual or allergic reactions to aminophylline, caffeine, dyphylline, oxtriphylline, theobromine (also found in cocoa or chocolate), or theophylline. Also tell your health care professional if you are allergic to any other substances, such as foods, preservatives, or dyes.

Pregnancy—Studies in humans have shown that caffeine may cause miscarriage or may slow the growth of a developing fetus when given in doses greater than 300 mg (an amount equal to three cups of coffee) a day. In addition, use of large amounts of caffeine by the mother during pregnancy may cause problems with the heart rhythm of the fetus. Therefore, it is recommended that pregnant women consume less than 300 mg of caffeine a day. Studies in animals have shown that caffeine causes birth defects when given in very large doses (amounts equal to 12 to 24 cups of coffee a day) and problems with bone growth when given in smaller doses.

Breast-feeding—Caffeine passes into breast milk in small amounts and may build up in the nursing baby. Studies have shown that babies may appear jittery and have trouble in sleeping when their mothers drink large amounts of caffeine-containing beverages.

Children—With the exception of infants, there is no specific information comparing use of caffeine in children with use in other age groups. However, this medicine is not expected to cause different side effects or problems in children than it does in adults.

Older adults—Many medicines have not been studied specifically in older people. Therefore, it may not be known whether they work exactly the same way they do in younger adults or if they cause different side effects or problems in older people. There is no specific information comparing use of caffeine in the elderly with use in other age groups.

Other medicines—Although certain medicines should not be used together at all, in other cases two different medicines may be used together even if an interaction might occur. In these cases, your doctor may want to change the dose, or other precautions may be necessary. When you are taking caffeine, it is especially important that your health care professional know if you are taking any of the following:
- Amantadine (e.g., Symmetrel) or
- Amphetamines (e.g., Desoxyn, Dexedrine) or
- Appetite suppressants (diet pills) or
- Bupropion (e.g., Wellbutrin) or
- Chlophedianol (e.g., Ulone) or
- Cocaine or
- Fluoxetine (e.g., Prozac) or
- Medicine for asthma or other breathing problems or
- Medicine for colds, sinus problems, hay fever or other allergies (including nose drops or sprays) or
- Methylphenidate (e.g., Ritalin) or
- Nabilone (e.g., Cesamet) or
- Other medicines or beverages containing caffeine or
- Paroxetine (e.g., Paxil) or
- Pemoline (e.g., Cylert) or
- Sertraline (e.g., Zoloft)—Using these medicines with caffeine may increase the CNS-stimulant effects, such as nervousness, irritability, or trouble in sleeping, or possibly cause convulsions (seizures) or changes in the rhythm of your heart
- Monoamine oxidase (MAO) inhibitors (furazolidone [e.g., Furoxone], isocarboxazid [e.g., Marplan], phenelzine [e.g., Nardil], procarbazine [e.g., Matulane], selegiline [e.g., Eldepryl], tranylcypromine [e.g., Parnate])—Taking large amounts of caffeine while you are taking or within 2 weeks of taking MAO inhibitors may cause extremely high blood pressure or dangerous changes in the rhythm

of your heart; taking small amounts of caffeine may cause mild high blood pressure and fast heartbeat

Other medical problems—The presence of other medical problems may affect the use of caffeine. Make sure you tell your doctor if you have any other medical problems, especially:

- Agoraphobia (fear of being in open places) or
- Anxiety or
- Convulsions (seizures) (in newborn babies) or
- Heart disease, severe or
- High blood pressure or
- Panic attacks or
- Trouble in sleeping—Caffeine may make the condition worse
- Liver disease—Higher blood levels of caffeine may result, increasing the chance of side effects

---

Proper Use of This Medicine

Take caffeine in powder or tablet form only as directed. Do not take more of it, do not take it more often, and do not take it for a longer time than directed. Taking too much of this medicine may increase the chance of side effects. It may also become habit-forming.

For patients taking the *powder* form of this medicine: Each packet contains one dose of medicine. The contents of the packet may be stirred into water or other liquid and drunk. Or, the powder may be placed on the tongue and washed down with water or other liquid drink.

For patients taking the *oral solution* form of this medicine: Throw away any unused portion of the medicine left in the single-use vial (bottle). Follow the manufacturer's instruction for use.

If you think this medicine is not working properly after you have taken it for a long time, *do not increase the dose*. To do so may increase the chance of side effects.

Dosing—The dose of caffeine will be different for different patients. *Follow the directions on the label.*

- For unusual tiredness or weakness, or drowsiness:
  - For *oral* dosage form (powder):
    - Adults and children 12 years of age and older—The usual dose is 200 milligrams (mg) of caffeine (1 packet) repeated no sooner than every three or four hours. You should not take more than 1600 mg in twenty-four hours.
    - Children up to 12 years of age—Use is not recommended.
  - For *oral* dosage form (tablets):
    - Adults and children 12 years of age and older—The usual dose is 100 to 200 mg of caffeine repeated no sooner than every three or four hours. You should not take more than 1000 mg in twenty-four hours.
    - Children up to 12 years of age—Use is not recommended.
- For breathing problems in premature babies:
  - For *oral* dosage form (oral solution):
    - Newborn babies—At first, the dose is 20 mg (1 milliliter [mL]) per kilogram (kg) (9.1 mg per pound) of body weight given one time. Then, the dose is 5 mg (0.25 mL) per kg (2.3 mg per pound) of body weight given once a day.

Storage—To store this medicine:

- Keep out of the reach of children.
- Store away from heat and direct light.
- Do not store in the bathroom, near the kitchen sink, or in other damp places. Heat or moisture may cause the medicine to break down.
- Do not keep outdated medicine or medicine no longer needed. Be sure that any discarded medicine is out of the reach of children.

Precautions While Using This Medicine

Caffeine powder and tablets are for occasional use only. They are not intended to replace sleep and should not be used regularly for this purpose. If unusual tiredness or weakness or drowsiness continues or returns often, check with your doctor.

Before you have any medical tests, tell the doctor in charge that you are taking this medicine. The results of some tests on the heart may be affected by this medicine.

The recommended dose of this medicine contains about the same amount of caffeine as a cup of coffee. Do not drink large amounts of caffeine-containing coffee, tea, or soft drinks while you are taking this medicine. Also, do not take large amounts of other medicines that contain caffeine. To do so may cause unwanted effects.

The amount of caffeine in some common foods and beverages is as follows:

- Coffee, brewed—40 to 180 milligrams (mg) per cup.
- Coffee, instant—30 to 120 mg per cup.
- Coffee, decaffeinated—3 to 5 mg per cup.
- Tea, brewed American—20 to 90 mg per cup.
- Tea, brewed imported—25 to 110 mg per cup.
- Tea, instant—28 mg per cup.
- Tea, canned iced—22 to 36 mg per 12 ounces.
- Cola and other soft drinks, caffeine-containing—36 to 90 mg per 12 ounces.
- Cola and other soft drinks, decaffeinated—0 mg per 12 ounces.
- Cocoa—4 mg per cup.
- Chocolate, milk—3 to 6 mg per ounce.
- Chocolate, bittersweet—25 mg per ounce.

Caffeine may cause nervousness or irritability, trouble in sleeping, dizziness, or a fast or pounding heartbeat. If these effects occur, discontinue the use of caffeine-containing beverages and medicines, and do not eat large amounts of chocolate-containing products.

To prevent trouble in sleeping, do not take caffeine-containing beverages or medicines too close to bedtime.

Side Effects

Along with its needed effects, a medicine may cause some unwanted effects. Although not all of these side effects may occur, they may be more likely to occur if caffeine is taken in large doses or more often than recommended. If they do occur, they may need medical attention.

Check with your doctor as soon as possible if any of the following side effects occur:

More common

Diarrhea; dizziness; fast heartbeat; hyperglycemia, including blurred vision, drowsiness, dry mouth, flushed dry skin, fruit-like breath odor, increased urination, ketones in urine, loss of appetite, nausea, stomachache, tiredness, troubled breathing, unusual thirst, or vomiting (in newborn babies); hypoglycemia, including anxious feeling, blurred vision, cold sweats, confusion, cool pale skin, drowsiness, excessive hunger, fast heartbeat, nausea, nervousness, restless sleep, shakiness, or unusual tiredness or weakness (in newborn babies); irritability, nervousness, or severe jitters (in newborn babies); nausea (severe); tremors; trouble in sleeping; vomiting

Rare

Abdominal or stomach bloating; dehydration; diarrhea (bloody); unusual tiredness or weakness

Symptoms of overdose

Abdominal or stomach pain; agitation, anxiety, excitement, or restlessness; confusion or delirium; convulsions (seizures)— in acute overdose; dehydration; faster breathing rate; fast or irregular heartbeat; fever; frequent urination; headache; increased sensitivity to touch or pain; irritability; muscle trembling or twitching; nausea and vomiting, sometimes with blood; overextending the body with head and heels bent backward and body bowed forward; painful, swollen abdomen or vomiting (in newborn babies); ringing or other sounds in ears; seeing flashes of "zig-zag" lights; trouble in sleeping; whole-body tremors (in newborn babies)

Other side effects may occur that usually do not need medical attention. These side effects may go away during treatment as your body adjusts to the medicine. However, check with your doctor if any of the following side effects continue or are bothersome:

More common

Nausea (mild); nervousness or jitters (mild)

After you stop using this medicine, your body may need time to adjust. The length of time this takes depends on the amount of medicine you were using and how long you used it. During this time, check with your doctor if you notice any of the following side effects:

More common

Anxiety; dizziness; headache; irritability; muscle tension; nausea; nervousness; stuffy nose; unusual tiredness

Other side effects not listed above may also occur in some patients. If you notice any other effects, check with your doctor.

Additional Information

Once a medicine has been approved for marketing for a certain use, experience may show that it is also useful for other medical problems. Although these uses are not included in product labeling, caffeine is used in certain patients with the following medical conditions:

• Postoperative infant apnea (breathing problems after surgery in young babies)

• Psychiatric disorders requiring electroconvulsive or shock therapy (ECT)

Other than the above information, there is no additional information relating to proper use, precautions, or side effects for these uses.

CALCIUM CHANNEL BLOCKING AGENTS   (Systemic)

Some commonly used brand names are:

In the U.S.—

Adalat (8)	Isoptin (10)
Adalat CC (8)	Isoptin SR (10)
Calan (10)	Nimotop (9)
Calan SR (10)	Norvasc (1)
Cardene (7)	Plendil (4)
Cardizem (3)	Procardia (8)
Cardizem CD (3)	Procardia XL (8)
Cardizem LA (3)	Vascor (2)
Cardizem SR (3)	Verelan (10)
Dilacor-XR (3)	Verelan PM (10)
DynaCirc (6)	

In Canada—

Adalat (8)	Norvasc (1)
Adalat PA (8)	Novo-Diltazem (3)
Adalat XL (8)	Novo-Nifedin (8)
Apo-Diltiaz (3)	Novo-Veramil (10)
Apo-Nifed (8)	Nu-Diltiaz (3)
Apo-Verap (10)	Nu-Nifed (8)
Cardizem (3)	Nu-Verap (10)
Cardizem SR (3)	Plendil (4)
Isoptin (10)	Renedil (4)
Isoptin SR (10)	Sibelium (5)
Nimotop (9)	Verelan (10)

This information applies to the following medicines:

1. Amlodipine (am-LOE-di-peen)
2. Bepridil (BE-pri-dil)
3. Diltiazem (dil-TYE-a-zem)
4. Felodipine (fe-LOE-di-peen)
5. Flunarizine (floo-NAR-i-zeen)
6. Isradipine (is-RA-di-peen)
7. Nicardipine (nye-KAR-de-peen)
8. Nifedipine (nye-FED-i-peen)
9. Nimodipine (nye-MOE-di-peen)
10. Verapamil (ver-AP-a-mil)

Category

• **Antianginal**—Amlodipine; Bepridil; Diltiazem; Felodipine; Isradipine; Nicardipine; Nifedipine; Verapamil

• **Antiarrhythmic**—Diltiazem; Verapamil

• **Antihypertensive**—Amlodipine; Diltiazem; Felodipine; Isradipine; Nicardipine; Nifedipine; Verapamil

• **Hypertrophic cardiomyopathy therapy adjunct**—Verapamil

• **Subarachnoid hemorrhage therapy**—Flunarizine; Nicardipine; Nimodipine

• **Vascular headache prophylactic**—Flunarizine; Verapamil

Description

Amlodipine, bepridil, diltiazem, felodipine, flunarizine, isradipine, nicardipine, nifedipine, nimodipine, and verapamil belong to the group of medicines called calcium channel blocking agents.

Calcium channel blocking agents affect the movement of calcium into the cells of the heart and blood vessels. As a result, they relax blood vessels and increase the supply of blood and oxygen to the heart while reducing its workload.

Some of the calcium channel blocking agents are used to relieve and control angina pectoris (chest pain).

Some are also used to treat high blood pressure (hypertension). High blood pressure adds to the workload of the heart and arteries. If it continues for a long time, the heart and arteries may not function properly. This can damage the blood vessels of the brain, heart, and kidneys, resulting in a stroke, heart failure, or kidney failure. High blood pressure may also increase the risk of heart attacks. These problems may be less likely to occur if blood pressure is controlled.

Flunarizine is used to prevent migraine headaches.

Nimodipine is used to prevent and treat problems caused by a burst blood vessel around the brain (also known as a ruptured aneurysm or subarachnoid hemorrhage).

Other calcium channel blocking agents may also be used for these and other conditions as determined by your doctor.

These medicines are available only with your doctor's prescription, in the following dosage forms:

Oral
- Amlodipine
  - Tablets
- Bepridil
  - Tablets
- Diltiazem
  - Extended-release capsules
  - Extended-release tablets
  - Tablets
- Felodipine
  - Extended-release tablets
- Flunarizine
  - Capsules
- Isradipine
  - Capsules
- Nicardipine
  - Capsules
- Nifedipine
  - Capsules
  - Extended-release tablets
- Nimodipine
  - Capsules
- Verapamil
  - Extended-release capsules
  - Tablets
  - Extended-release tablets

Parenteral
- Diltiazem
  - Injection
- Verapamil
  - Injection

Before Using This Medicine

In deciding to use a medicine, the risks of taking the medicine must be weighed against the good it will do. This is a decision you and your doctor will make. For the calcium channel blocking agents, the following should be considered:

Allergies—Tell your doctor if you have ever had any unusual or allergic reaction to amlodipine, bepridil, diltiazem, felodipine, flunarizine, isradipine, nicardipine, nifedipine, nimodipine, or verapamil. Also tell your health care professional if you are allergic to any other substances, such as foods, preservatives, or dyes.

Pregnancy—Calcium channel blocking agents have not been studied in pregnant women. However, studies in animals have shown that large doses of calcium channel blocking agents cause birth defects, prolonged pregnancy, poor bone development in the offspring, and stillbirth.

Breast-feeding—Although bepridil, diltiazem, nifedipine, verapamil, and possibly other calcium channel blocking agents, pass into breast milk, they have not been reported to cause problems in nursing babies.

Children—Although there is no specific information comparing use of this medicine in children with use in other age groups, it is not expected to cause different side effects or problems in children than it does in adults.

Older adults—Elderly people may be especially sensitive to the effects of calcium channel blocking agents. This may increase the chance of side effects during treatment. A lower starting dose may be required.

Other medicines—Although certain medicines should not be used together at all, in other cases two different medicines may be used together even if an interaction might occur. In these cases, your doctor may want to change the dose, or other precautions may be necessary. When taking calcium channel blocking agents it is especially important that your health care professional know if you are taking any of the following:
- Acetazolamide (e.g., Diamox) or
- Amphotericin B by injection (e.g., Fungizone) or
- Corticosteroids (cortisone-like medicine) or
- Dichlorphenamide (e.g., Daranide) or
- Diuretics (water pills) or
- Methazolamide (e.g., Naptazane)—These medicines can cause hypokalemia (low levels of potassium in the body), which can increase the unwanted effects of bepridil
- Beta-adrenergic blocking agents (acebutolol [e.g., Sectral], atenolol [e.g., Tenormin], betaxolol [e.g., Kerlone], carteolol [e.g., Cartrol], labetalol [e.g., Normodyne], metoprolol [e.g., Lopressor], nadolol [e.g., Corgard], oxprenolol [e.g., Trasicor], penbutolol [e.g., Levatol], pindolol [e.g., Visken], propranolol [e.g., Inderal], sotalol [e.g., Sotacor], timolol [e.g., Blocadren])—Effects of both may be increased. In addition, unwanted effects may occur if a calcium channel blocking agent or a beta-blocking agent is stopped suddenly after both have been used together
- Carbamazepine (e.g., Tegretol) or
- Cyclosporine (e.g., Sandimmune) or
- Procainamide (e.g., Pronestyl) or
- Quinidine (e.g., Quinidex)—Effects of these medicines may be increased if they are used with some calcium channel blocking agents
- Digitalis glycosides (heart medicine)—Effects of these medicines may be increased if they are used with some calcium channel blocking agents
- Disopyramide (e.g., Norpace)—Effects of some calcium channel blocking agents on the heart may be increased
- Erythromycin (e.g., Ery-Tab)—Should not be used together with calcium channel blocking agents, especially diltiazem or verapamil; severe heart problems may result.

- Grapefruit juice—Effects of felodipine may be increased. No effects on amlodipine.

Also, tell your health care professional if you are using any of the following medicines in the eye:

- Betaxolol (e.g., Betoptic) or
- Levobunolol (e.g., Betagan) or
- Metipranolol (e.g., OptiPranolol) or
- Timolol (e.g., Timoptic)—Effects on the heart and blood pressure may be increased

Other medical problems—The presence of other medical problems may affect the use of the calcium channel blocking agents. Make sure you tell your doctor if you have any other medical problems, especially:

- Congestive heart failure—Calcium channel blocking agents may make this condition worse. Do not take diltiazem if you have a history of heart attacks.
- Heart rhythm problems (history of)—Bepridil can cause serious heart rhythm problems
- Kidney disease or
- Liver disease—Effects of the calcium channel blocking agent may be increased
- Mental depression (history of)—Flunarizine may cause mental depression
- Parkinson's disease or similar problems—Flunarizine can cause parkinsonian-like effects
- Other heart or blood vessel disorders—Calcium channel blocking agents may make some heart conditions worse

Proper Use of This Medicine

Take this medicine exactly as directed even if you feel well and do not notice any signs of chest pain. Do not take more of this medicine and do not take it more often than your doctor ordered. Do not miss any doses.

For patients taking *amlodipine:*

- Your doctor may suggest that you change your diet and eat foods that are low in salt and fat. Losing weight will help your blood pressure along with your medicine. Talk to your doctor about the best diet for you.

For patients taking *bepridil:*

- If this medicine causes upset stomach, it can be taken with meals or at bedtime.

For patients taking *diltiazem extended-release capsules or tablets:*

- Swallow the capsule or tablet whole, without crushing or chewing it.
- *Do not change to another brand without checking with your physician.* Different brands have different doses. If you refill your medicine and it looks different, check with your pharmacist.
- You should take *Cardizem LA* at about the same time once each day either in the morning or at bedtime. If you have questions about when to take your medicine, ask your doctor.

For patients taking *felodipine:*

- Do not take this medicine with grapefruit juice.

For patients taking *verapamil extended-release capsules:*

- Swallow the capsule whole, without crushing or chewing it.

- If you have trouble swallowing capsules, you may open the verapamil capsule and mix the medicine with applesauce. Mix only one dose at a time just before taking it. *Do not mix any doses to save for later,* because the medicine may change over time and may not work properly.

For patients taking *felodipine* or *nifedipine extended-release tablets:*

- Swallow the tablet whole, without breaking, crushing, or chewing it.
- If you are taking *Adalat XL* or *Procardia XL,* you may sometimes notice what looks like a tablet in your stool. That is just the empty shell that is left after the medicine has been absorbed into your body.
- If you are taking *Adalat CC,* take the medicine on an empty stomach

For patients taking *verapamil extended-release tablets:*

- Swallow the tablet whole, without crushing or chewing it. However, if your doctor tells you to, you may break the tablet in half.
- Take the medicine with food or milk.

For patients taking this medicine *for high blood pressure:*

- In addition to the use of the medicine your doctor has prescribed, appropriate treatment for your high blood pressure may include weight control and care in the types of food you eat, especially foods high in sodium (salt). Your doctor will tell you which factors are most important for you. You should check with your doctor before changing your diet.
- Many patients who have high blood pressure will not notice any signs of the problem. In fact, many may feel normal. It is very important that you *take your medicine exactly as directed* and that you keep your appointments with your doctor even if you feel well.
- Remember that this medicine will not cure your high blood pressure but it does help control it. Therefore, you must continue to take it as directed if you expect to lower your blood pressure and keep it down. *You may have to take high blood pressure medicine for the rest of your life.* If high blood pressure is not treated, it can cause serious problems such as heart failure, blood vessel disease, stroke, or kidney disease.

Dosing—The dose of these medicines will be different for different patients. *Follow your doctor's orders or the directions on the label.* The following information includes only the average doses of these medicines. *If your dose is different, do not change it* unless your doctor tells you to do so.

The number of capsules or tablets that you take depends on the strength of the medicine. Also, *the number of doses you take each day, the time allowed between doses, and the length of time you take the medicine depend on the medical problem for which you are taking calcium channel blocking agents.*

For amlodipine

- For *oral dosage form (tablets):*
  - For angina (chest pain):
    - Adults—5 to 10 milligrams (mg) once a day.
    - Children 6 years of age and older—2.5 to 5 mg once a day.
    - Children younger than 6 years of age—Use must be determined by your doctor.

- Elderly patients or patients determined by your health care professional may be started on a lower dose.
- For high blood pressure:
  - Adults—5 to 10 mg once a day.
  - Children—Use must be determined by your doctor.
- Elderly patients or patients determined by your health care professional may be started on 2.5 mg once a day.

For bepridil
- For *oral* dosage form (tablets):
  - For angina (chest pain):
    - Adults—200 to 300 milligrams (mg) once a day.
    - Children—Use and dose must be determined by your doctor.

For diltiazem
- For *long-acting oral* dosage form (extended-release capsules and tablets):
  - For angina (chest pain):
    - Adults and teenagers:
      — For *Cardizem LA:* 180 mg once a day in the morning or at bedtime.
    - Children—Dose must be determined by your doctor.
  - For high blood pressure:
    - Adults and teenagers:
      — For *Cardizem CD* or *Cardizem LA* or *Dilacor-XR:* 180 to 240 milligrams (mg) once a day.
      — For *Cardizem SR:* 60 to 120 mg two times a day.
    - Children—Dose must be determined by your doctor.
- For *regular (short-acting) oral* dosage form (tablets):
  - For angina (chest pain):
    - Adults and teenagers—30 mg three or four times a day. Your doctor may gradually increase your dose as needed.
    - Children—Dose must be determined by your doctor.
- For *injection* dosage form:
  - For arrhythmias (irregular heartbeat):
    - Adults and teenagers—Dose is based on body weight and must be determined by your doctor.
    - Children—Use and dose must be determined by your doctor.

For felodipine
- For *long-acting oral* dosage form (extended-release tablets):
  - For high blood pressure:
    - Adults—5 to 10 milligrams (mg) once a day.
    - Children—Use and dose must be determined by your doctor.
  - For angina (chest pain):
    - Adults—10 mg once a day.
    - Children—Use and dose must be determined by your doctor.

For flunarizine
- For *oral* dosage form (capsules):
  - To prevent headaches:
    - Adults—10 milligrams (mg) once a day in the evening.
    - Children—Dose must be determined by your doctor.

For isradipine
- For *oral* dosage form (capsules):
  - For high blood pressure:
    - Adults—2.5 milligrams (mg) two times a day. Your doctor may increase your dose as needed.
    - Children—Use and dose must be determined by your doctor.

For nicardipine
- For *oral* dosage form (capsules):
  - For high blood pressure or angina (chest pain):
    - Adults and teenagers—20 milligrams (mg) three times a day.
    - Children—Dose must be determined by your doctor.

For nifedipine
- For *regular (short-acting) oral* dosage form (capsules):
  - For high blood pressure or angina (chest pain):
    - Adults and teenagers—10 milligrams (mg) three times a day. Your doctor may increase your dose as needed.
    - Children—Dose must be determined by your doctor.
- For *long-acting oral* dosage form (extended-release tablets):
  - For high blood pressure or angina (chest pain):
    - Adults and teenagers:
      — For *Adalat CC, Adalat XL* or *Procardia XL:* 30 or 60 mg once a day. Your doctor may increase your dose as needed.
      — For *Adalat PA:* 10 or 20 mg two times a day. Your doctor may increase your dose as needed.
    - Children—Dose must be determined by your doctor.

For nimodipine
- For *oral* dosage form (capsules):
  - To treat a burst blood vessel around the brain:
    - Adults—60 milligrams (mg) every four hours.
    - Children—Dose must be determined by your doctor.

For verapamil
- For *regular (short-acting) oral* dosage form (tablets):
  - For angina (chest pain), arrhythmias (irregular heartbeat), or high blood pressure:
    - Adults and teenagers—40 to 120 milligrams (mg) three times a day. Your doctor may increase your dose as needed.
    - Children—Dose is based on body weight and must be determined by your doctor. The usual dose is 4 to 8 mg per kilogram (kg) (1.82 to 3.64 mg per pound) of body weight a day. This is divided into smaller doses.
- For *long-acting oral* dosage form (extended-release capsules):
  - For high blood pressure:
    - Adults and teenagers
      — For *Verelan:* 240 to 480 mg once a day
      — For *Verelan PM:* 200 mg once a day at bedtime
    - Children—Dose must be determined by your doctor.
- For *long-acting oral* dosage form (extended-release tablets):

○ For high blood pressure:
  ▪ Adults and teenagers—120 mg once a day to 240 mg every twelve hours.
  ▪ Children—Dose must be determined by your doctor.
• For *injection* dosage form:
  ○ For arrhythmias (irregular heartbeat):
    ▪ Adults—5 to 10 mg slowly injected into a vein. The dose may be repeated after thirty minutes.
    ▪ Children—Dose is based on body weight and must be determined by your doctor.
      — Infants up to 1 year of age: 100 to 200 micrograms (mcg) per kg (45.5 to 90.9 mcg per pound) of body weight injected slowly into a vein. The dose may be repeated after thirty minutes.
      — Children 1 to 15 years of age: 100 to 300 mcg per kg (45.5 to 136.4 mcg per pound) of body weight injected slowly into a vein. The dose may be repeated after thirty minutes.

Missed dose—If you miss a dose of this medicine, take it as soon as possible. However, if it is almost time for your next dose, skip the missed dose and go back to your regular dosing schedule. Do not double doses.

Storage—To store this medicine:
• Keep out of the reach of children.
• Store away from heat and direct light.
• Do not store in the bathroom, near the kitchen sink, or in other damp places. Heat or moisture may cause the medicine to break down.
• Do not keep outdated medicine or medicine no longer needed. Be sure that any discarded medicine is out of the reach of children.

Precautions While Using This Medicine

It is important that your doctor check your progress at regular visits. This will allow your doctor to make sure the medicine is working properly and to change the dosage if needed.

If you have been using this medicine regularly for several weeks, do not suddenly stop using it. Stopping suddenly may bring on your previous problem. Check with your doctor for the best way to reduce gradually the amount you are taking before stopping completely.

Chest pain resulting from exercise or physical exertion is usually reduced or prevented by this medicine. This may tempt you to be overly active. *Make sure you discuss with your doctor a safe amount of exercise for your medical problem.*

After taking a dose of this medicine you may get a headache that lasts for a short time. This effect is more common if you are taking felodipine, isradipine, or nifedipine. This should become less noticeable after you have taken this medicine for a while. If this effect continues or if the headaches are severe, check with your doctor.

In some patients, tenderness, swelling, or bleeding of the gums may appear soon after treatment with this medicine is started. Brushing and flossing your teeth carefully and regularly and massaging your gums may help prevent this. *See your dentist regularly to have your teeth cleaned. Check with your medical doctor or dentist if you have any questions about how to take care of your teeth and gums, or if you notice any tenderness, swelling, or bleeding of your gums.*

For patients taking *bepridil, diltiazem,* or *verapamil:*
• *Ask your doctor how to count your pulse rate. Then, while you are taking this medicine, check your pulse regularly.* If it is much slower than your usual rate, or less than 50 beats per minute, check with your doctor. A pulse rate that is too slow may cause circulation problems.

For patients taking *flunarizine:*
• This medicine may cause some people to become drowsy or less alert than they are normally. This is more likely to happen when you begin to take it or when you increase the amount of medicine you are taking. *Make sure you know how you react to this medicine before you drive, use machines, or do anything else that could be dangerous if you are not alert.*

For patients taking this medicine *for high blood pressure:*
• *Do not take other medicines unless they have been discussed with your doctor.* This especially includes over-the-counter (nonprescription) medicines for appetite control, asthma, colds, cough, hay fever, or sinus problems, since they may tend to increase your blood pressure.

Side Effects of This Medicine

Along with its needed effects, a medicine may cause some unwanted effects. Although not all of these side effects may occur, if they do occur they may need medical attention.

Not all of the side effects listed below have been reported for each of these medicines, but they have been reported for at least one of them. Since many of the effects of calcium channel blocking agents are similar, some of these side effects may occur with any of these medicines. However, they may be more common with some of these medicines than with others.

Check with your doctor as soon as possible if any of the following side effects occur:
Less common
  Breathing difficulty, coughing, or wheezing; irregular or fast, pounding heartbeat; skin rash; slow heartbeat (less than 50 beats per minute— bepridil, diltiazem, and verapamil only); swelling of ankles, feet, or lower legs (more common with amlodipine, felodipine and nifedipine)
For flunarizine only—less common
  Loss of balance control; mask-like face; mental depression; shuffling walk; stiffness of arms or legs; trembling and shaking of hands and fingers; trouble in speaking or swallowing
Rare
  Bleeding, tender, or swollen gums; chest pain (may appear about 30 minutes after medicine is taken); fainting; painful, swollen joints (for nifedipine only); trouble in seeing (for nifedipine only)
For flunarizine and verapamil only—rare
  Unusual secretion of milk

Other side effects may occur that usually do not need medical attention. These side effects may go away during treatment as your body adjusts to the medicine. However, check with your doctor if any of the following side effects continue or are bothersome:
More common
  Drowsiness (for flunarizine only); increased appetite and/or weight gain (for flunarizine only)

Less common

Constipation; diarrhea; dizziness or lightheadedness (more common with bepridil and nifedipine); dryness of mouth (for amlodipine and flunarizine only); flushing and feeling of warmth (more common with nicardipine and nifedipine); headache (more common with amlodipine, felodipine, isradipine, and nifedipine); nausea (more common with bepridil and nifedipine); unusual tiredness or weakness

Other side effects not listed above may also occur in some patients. If you notice any other effects, check with your doctor.

Additional Information

Once a medicine has been approved for marketing for a certain use, experience may show that it is also useful for other medical problems. Although these uses are not included in product labeling, calcium channel blocking agents are used in certain patients with the following medical conditions:

- Hypertrophic cardiomyopathy (a heart condition) (verapamil)
- Raynaud's phenomenon (circulation problems) (nicardipine and nifedipine)

Other than the above information, there is no additional information relating to proper use, precautions, or side effects for these uses.

CALCIUM SUPPLEMENTS (Systemic)

Some commonly used brand names are:

In the U.S.—

Alka-Mints (2)	Liquid-Cal (2)
Amitone (2)	Liquid Cal-600 (2)
Calcarb 600 (2)	Maalox Antacid Caplets (2)
Calci-Chew (2)	Mallamint (2)
Calciday 667 (2)	Neo-Calglucon (5)
Calcilac (2)	Nephro-Calci (2)
Calci-Mix (2)	Os-Cal 500 (2)
Calcionate (5)	Os-Cal 500 Chewable (2)
Calcium 600 (2)	Oysco (2)
Calglycine (2)	Oysco 500 Chewable (2)
Calphosan (9)	Oyst-Cal 500 (2)
Cal-Plus (2)	Oystercal 500 (2)
Caltrate 600 (2)	Posture (13)
Caltrate Jr (2)	Rolaids Calcium Rich (2)
Chooz (2)	Titralac (2)
Citracal (4)	Tums (2)
Citracal Liquitabs (4)	Tums 500 (2)
Dicarbosil (2)	Tums E-X (2)
Gencalc 600 (2)	

In Canada—

Apo-Cal (2)	Caltrate 600 (2)
Calciject (3)	Gramcal (11)
Calcite 500 (2)	Nu-Cal (2)
Calcium-Sandoz (5)	Os-Cal (2)
Calcium-Sandoz Forte (11)	Os-Cal Chewable (2)
Calcium Stanley (7)	Tums Extra Strength (2)
Calsan (2)	Tums Regular Strength (2)

This information applies to the following:

1. Calcium Acetate (KAL-see-um ASa-tate)
2. Calcium Carbonate (KAL-see-um KAR-boh-nate)
3. Calcium Chloride (KAL-see-um KLOR-ide)
4. Calcium Citrate (KAL-see-um SIH-trayt)
5. Calcium Glubionate (KAL-see-um gloo-BY-oh-nate)
6. Calcium Gluceptate (KAL-see-um gloo-SEP-tate)
7. Calcium Gluceptate and Calcium Gluconate (KAL-see-um gloo-SEP-tate and KAL-see-um GLOO-coh-nate)
8. Calcium Gluconate (KAL-see-um GLOO-coh-nate)
9. Calcium Glycerophosphate and Calcium Lactate (KAL-see-um gliss-er-o-FOS-fate and KAL-see-um LAK-tate)
10. Calcium Lactate (KAL-see-um LAK-tate)
11. Calcium Lactate-Gluconate and Calcium Carbonate (KAL-see-um LAK-tate GLOO-coh-nate and KAL-see-um KAR-boh-nate)
12. Dibasic Calcium Phosphate (dy-BAY-sic KAL-see-um FOS-fate)
13. Tribasic Calcium Phosphate (try-BAY-sic KAL-see-um FOS-fate)

Category

- **Antacid**—Calcium Carbonate
- **Antihyperkalemic**—Calcium Chloride; Calcium Gluconate Injection
- **Antihypermagnesemic**—Calcium Chloride; Calcium Gluceptate; Calcium Gluconate Injection
- **Antihyperphosphatemic**—Calcium Carbonate; Calcium Citrate
- **Antihypocalcemic**—Calcium Acetate; Calcium Carbonate; Calcium Chloride; Calcium Citrate; Calcium Glubionate; Calcium Gluceptate; Calcium Gluconate; Calcium Glycerophosphate and Calcium Lactate; Calcium Lactate; Calcium Lactate-Gluconate and Calcium Carbonate; Calcium Phosphate, Dibasic; Calcium Phosphate, Tribasic
- **Cardiotonic**—Calcium Chloride; Calcium Gluconate Injection
- **Electrolyte replenisher**—Calcium Acetate; Calcium Chloride; Calcium Gluceptate; Calcium Gluconate Injection
- **Nutritional supplement, mineral**—Calcium Carbonate; Calcium Citrate; Calcium Glubionate, Oral; Calcium Gluceptate and Calcium Gluconate; Calcium Gluconate, Oral; Calcium Lactate; Calcium Lactate-Gluconate and Calcium Carbonate; Calcium Phosphate, Dibasic; Calcium Phosphate, Tribasic

Description

Calcium supplements are taken by individuals who are unable to get enough calcium in their regular diet or who have a need for more calcium. They are used to prevent or treat several conditions that may cause hypocalcemia (not enough calcium in the blood). The body needs calcium to make strong bones. Calcium is also needed for the heart, muscles, and nervous system to work properly.

The bones serve as a storage site for the body's calcium. They are continuously giving up calcium to the bloodstream and then replacing it as the body's need for calcium changes from day to day. When there is not enough calcium in the blood to be used by the heart and other organs, your body will take the needed calcium from the bones. When you eat foods rich in calcium, the calcium will be restored to the bones and the balance between your blood and bones will be maintained.

Pregnant women, nursing mothers, children, and adolescents may need more calcium than they normally get from eating calcium-rich foods. Adult women may take calcium supplements to help prevent a bone disease called osteoporosis. Osteoporosis, which causes thin, porous, easily broken bones, may occur in women after menopause, but may sometimes occur in elderly men also. Osteoporosis in women past menopause is thought to be caused by a reduced amount of ovarian estrogen (a female hormone). However, a diet low in calcium for many years, especially in the younger adult years, may add to the risk of developing it. Other bone diseases in children and adults are also treated with calcium supplements.

Calcium supplements may also be used for other conditions as determined by your health care professional.

Injectable calcium is administered only by or under the supervision of your health care professional. Other forms of calcium are available without a prescription.

Calcium supplements are available in the following dosage forms:

Oral
- Calcium Carbonate
  - Capsules
  - Oral suspension
  - Tablets
  - Chewable tablets
- Calcium Citrate
  - Tablets
  - Tablets for solution
- Calcium Glubionate
  - Syrup
- Calcium Gluceptate and Calcium Gluconate
  - Oral solution
- Calcium Gluconate
  - Tablets
  - Chewable tablets
- Calcium Lactate
  - Tablets
- Calcium Lactate-Gluconate and Calcium Carbonate
  - Tablets for solution
- Dibasic Calcium Phosphate
  - Tablets
- Tribasic Calcium Phosphate
  - Tablets

Parenteral
- Calcium Acetate
  - Injection
- Calcium Chloride
  - Injection
- Calcium Glubionate
  - Injection
- Calcium Gluceptate
  - Injection
- Calcium Gluconate
  - Injection
- Calcium Glycerophosphate and Calcium Lactate
  - Injection

A calcium "salt" contains calcium along with another substance, such as carbonate or gluconate. Some calcium salts have more calcium (elemental calcium) than others. For example, the amount of calcium in calcium carbonate is greater than that in calcium gluconate. To give you an idea of how different calcium supplements vary in calcium content, the following chart explains how many tablets of each type of supplement will provide 1000 milligrams of elemental calcium. When you look for a calcium supplement, be sure the number of milligrams on the label refers to the amount of elemental calcium, and not to the strength of each tablet.

Calcium supplement	Strength of each tablet (in milligrams)	Amount of elemental calcium per tablet (in milligrams)	Number of tablets to provide 1000 milligrams of calcium
Calcium carbonate	625	250	4
	650	260	4
	750	300	4
	835	334	3
	1250	500	2
	1500	600	2
Calcium citrate	950	200	5
Calcium gluconate	500	45	22
	650	58	17
	1000	90	11
Calcium lactate	325	42	24
	650	84	12
Calcium phosphate, dibasic	500	115	9
Calcium phosphate, tribasic	800	304	4
	1600	608	2

Importance of Diet

For good health, it is important that you eat a balanced and varied diet. Follow carefully any diet program your health care professional may recommend. For your specific dietary vitamin and/or mineral needs, ask your health care professional for a list of appropriate foods. If you think that you are not getting enough vitamins and/or minerals in your diet, you may choose to take a dietary supplement.

The daily amount of calcium needed is defined in several different ways.

For U.S.—
- Recommended Dietary Allowances (RDAs) are the amount of vitamins and minerals needed to provide for adequate nutrition in most healthy persons. RDAs for a given nutrient may vary depending on a person's age, sex, and physical condition (e.g., pregnancy).
- Daily Values (DVs) are used on food and dietary supplement labels to indicate the percent of the recommended daily amount of each nutrient that a serving provides. DV replaces the previous designation of United States Recommended Daily Allowances (USRDAs).

For Canada—
- Recommended Nutrient Intakes (RNIs) are used to determine the amounts of vitamins, minerals, and protein needed to provide adequate nutrition and lessen the risk of chronic disease.

Normal daily recommended intakes in milligrams (mg) for calcium are generally defined as follows:

Persons	U.S. (mg)	Canada (mg)
Infants and children		
Birth to 3 years of age	400–800	250–550
4 to 6 years of age	800	600
7 to 10 years of age	800	700–1100
Adolescent and adult males	800–1200	800–1100
Adolescent and adult females	800–1200	700–1100
Pregnant females	1200	1200–1500
Breast-feeding females	1200	1200–1500

Getting the proper amount of calcium in the diet every day and participating in weight-bearing exercise (walking, dancing, bicycling, aerobics, jogging), especially during the early years of life (up to about 35 years of age) is most important in helping to build and maintain bones as dense as possible to prevent the development of osteoporosis in later life.

The following table includes some calcium-rich foods. The calcium content of these foods can supply the daily RDA or RNI for calcium if the foods are eaten regularly in sufficient amounts.

Food (amount)	Milligrams of calcium
Nonfat dry milk, reconstituted (1 cup)	375
Lowfat, skim, or whole milk (1 cup)	290 to 300
Yogurt (1 cup)	275 to 400
Sardines with bones (3 ounces)	370
Ricotta cheese, part skim (½ cup)	340
Salmon, canned, with bones (3 ounces)	285
Cheese, Swiss (1 ounce)	272
Cheese, cheddar (1 ounce)	204
Cheese, American (1 ounce)	174
Cottage cheese, lowfat (1 cup)	154
Tofu (4 ounces)	154
Shrimp (1 cup)	147
Ice milk (¾ cup)	132

Vitamin D helps prevent calcium loss from your bones. It is sometimes called "the sunshine vitamin" because it is made in your skin when you are exposed to sunlight. If you get outside in the sunlight every day for 15 to 30 minutes, you should get all the vitamin D you need. However, in northern locations in winter, the sunlight may be too weak to make vitamin D in the skin. Vitamin D may also be obtained from your diet or from multivitamin preparations. Most milk is fortified with vitamin D.

Do not use bonemeal or dolomite as a source of calcium. The Food and Drug Administration has issued warnings that bonemeal and dolomite could be dangerous because these products may contain lead.

Before Using This Dietary Supplement

If you are taking this dietary supplement without a prescription, carefully read and follow any precautions on the label. For calcium supplements, the following should be considered:

Pregnancy—It is especially important that you are receiving enough calcium when you become pregnant and that you continue to receive the right amount of calcium throughout your pregnancy. The healthy growth and development of the fetus depend on a steady supply of nutrients from the mother. However, taking large amounts of a dietary supplement during pregnancy may be harmful to the mother and/or fetus and should be avoided.

Breast-feeding—It is especially important that you receive the right amount of calcium so that your baby will also get the calcium needed to grow properly. However, taking large amounts of a dietary supplement while breast-feeding may be harmful to the mother and/or baby and should be avoided.

Children—Problems in children have not been reported with intake of normal daily recommended amounts. Injectable forms of calcium should not be given to children because of the risk of irritating the injection site.

Older adults—Problems in older adults have not been reported with intake of normal daily recommended amounts. It is important that older people continue to receive enough calcium in their daily diets. However, some older people may need to take extra calcium or larger doses because they do not absorb calcium as well as younger people. Check with your health care professional if you have any questions about the amount of calcium you should be taking in each day.

Medicines or other dietary supplements—Although certain medicines or dietary supplements should not be used together at all, in other cases they may be used together even if an interaction might occur. In these cases, your health care professional may want to change the dose, or other precautions may be necessary. When you are taking calcium supplements, it is especially important that your health care professional know if you are taking any of the following:

- Calcium-containing medicines, other—Taking excess calcium may cause too much calcium in the blood or urine and lead to medical problems
- Cellulose sodium phosphate (e.g., Calcibind)—Use with calcium supplements may decrease the effects of cellulose sodium phosphate
- Digitalis glycosides (heart medicine)—Use with calcium supplements by injection may increase the chance of irregular heartbeat
- Etidronate (e.g., Didronel)—Use with calcium supplements may decrease the effects of etidronate; etidronate should not be taken within 2 hours of calcium supplements
- Gallium nitrate (e.g., Ganite)—Use with calcium supplements may cause gallium nitrate to not work properly
- Magnesium sulfate (for injection)—Use with calcium supplements may cause either medicine to be less effective
- Phenytoin (e.g., Dilantin)—Use with calcium supplements may decrease the effects of both medicines; calcium supplements should not be taken within 1 to 3 hours of phenytoin
- Tetracyclines (medicine for infection) taken by mouth—Use with calcium supplements may decrease the effects of tetracycline; calcium supplements should not be taken within 1 to 3 hours of tetracyclines

Other medical problems—The presence of other medical problems may affect the use of calcium supplements. Make sure you tell your health care professional if you have any other medical problems, especially:

- Diarrhea or
- Stomach or intestinal problems—Extra calcium or specific calcium preparations may be necessary in these conditions
- Heart disease—Calcium by injection may increase the chance of irregular heartbeat
- Hypercalcemia (too much calcium in the blood) or
- Hypercalciuria (too much calcium in the urine)—Calcium supplements may make these conditions worse
- Hyperparathyroidism or
- Sarcoidosis—Calcium supplements may increase the chance of hypercalcemia (too much calcium in the blood)
- Hypoparathyroidism—Use of calcium phosphate may cause high blood levels of phosphorus which could increase the chance of side effects
- Kidney disease or stones—Too much calcium may increase the chance of kidney stones

Proper Use of This Dietary Supplement

Dosing—The amount of calcium needed to meet normal daily recommended intakes will be different for different individuals. The following information includes only the average amounts of calcium.

- For *oral* dosage form (capsules, chewable tablets, lozenges, oral solution, oral suspension, syrup, tablets, extended-release tablets, tablets for solution):
  - To prevent deficiency, the amount taken by mouth is based on normal daily recommended intakes (Note that the normal daily recommended intakes are expressed as an actual amount of calcium. The salt form [e.g., calcium carbonate, calcium gluconate, etc.] has a different strength):

    For the U.S.
    - Adults and teenagers—800 to 1200 milligrams (mg) per day.
    - Pregnant and breast-feeding females—1200 mg per day.
    - Children 4 to 10 years of age—800 mg per day.
    - Children birth to 3 years of age—400 to 800 mg per day.

    For Canada
    - Adult and teenage males—800 to 1100 mg per day.
    - Adult and teenage females—700 to 1100 mg per day.
    - Pregnant and breast-feeding females—1200 to 1500 mg per day.
    - Children 7 to 10 years of age—700 to 1100 mg per day.
    - Children 4 to 6 years of age—600 mg per day.
    - Children birth to 3 years of age—250 to 550 mg per day.

  - To treat deficiency:
    - Adults, teenagers, and children—Treatment dose is determined by prescriber for each individual based on severity of deficiency.

Drink a full glass (8 ounces) of water or juice when taking a calcium supplement. However, if you are taking calcium carbonate as a phosphate binder in kidney dialysis, it is not necessary to drink a glass of water.

This dietary supplement is best taken 1 to 1½ hours after meals, unless otherwise directed by your health care professional. However, patients with a condition known as achlorhydria may not absorb calcium supplements on an empty stomach and should take them with meals.

For individuals taking *the chewable tablet form* of this dietary supplement:

- Chew the tablets completely before swallowing.

For individuals taking *the syrup form* of this dietary supplement:

- Take the syrup before meals. This will allow the dietary supplement to work faster.
- Mix in water or fruit juice for infants or children.

Take this dietary supplement only as directed. Do not take more of it and do not take it more often than recommended on the label. To do so may increase the chance of side effects.

Missed dose—If you are taking this dietary supplement on a regular schedule and you miss a dose, take it as soon as possible, then go back to your regular dosing schedule.

Storage—To store this dietary supplement:

- Keep out of the reach of children.
- Store away from heat and direct light.
- Do not store in the bathroom, near the kitchen sink, or in other damp places. Heat or moisture may cause the dietary supplement to break down.
- Keep the liquid form of this dietary supplement from freezing.
- Do not keep outdated dietary supplements or those no longer needed. Be sure that any discarded dietary supplement is out of the reach of children.

Precautions While Using This Dietary Supplement

If this dietary supplement has been ordered for you by your health care professional and you will be taking it in large doses or for a long time, your health care professional should check your progress at regular visits. This is to make sure the calcium is working properly and does not cause unwanted effects.

Do not take calcium supplements within 1 to 2 hours of taking other medicine by mouth. To do so may keep the other medicine from working properly.

Unless you are otherwise directed by your health care professional, to make sure that calcium is used properly by your body:

- *Do not take other medicines or dietary supplements containing large amounts of calcium, phosphates, magnesium, or vitamin D unless your health care professional has told you to do so or approved.*
- *Do not take calcium supplements within 1 to 2 hours of eating large amounts of fiber-containing foods, such as bran and whole-grain cereals or breads, especially if you are being treated for hypocalcemia (not enough calcium in your blood).*
- *Do not drink large amounts of alcohol or caffeine-containing beverages (usually more than 8 cups of coffee a day), or use tobacco.*

Some calcium carbonate tablets have been shown to break up too slowly in the stomach to be properly absorbed into the body. If the calcium carbonate tablets you purchase are not specifically labeled as being "USP," check with your pharmacist. He or she may be able to help you determine which tablets are best.

Side Effects of This Dietary Supplement

Along with its needed effects, a dietary supplement may cause some unwanted effects. Although the following side effects occur very rarely when the calcium supplement is taken as recommended, they may be more likely to occur if:

- It is taken in large doses.
- It is taken for a long time.
- It is taken by patients with kidney disease.

Check with your health care professional as soon as possible if any of the following side effects occur:

More common (for injection form only)
  Dizziness; flushing and/or sensation of warmth or heat; irregular heartbeat; nausea or vomiting; skin redness, rash, pain, or burning at injection site; sweating; tingling sensation

Rare

Difficult or painful urination; drowsiness; nausea or vomiting (continuing); weakness

Early signs of overdose

Constipation (severe); dryness of mouth; headache (continuing); increased thirst; irritability; loss of appetite; mental depression; metallic taste; unusual tiredness or weakness

Late signs of overdose

Confusion; drowsiness (severe); high blood pressure; increased sensitivity of eyes or skin to light; irregular, fast, or slow heartbeat; unusually large amount of urine or increased frequency of urination

Other side effects not listed above may also occur in some patients. If you notice any other effects, check with your health care professional.

Additional Information

Once a medicine or dietary supplement has been approved for marketing for a certain use, experience may show that it is also useful for other medical problems. Although this use is not included in product labeling, calcium supplements are used in certain patients with the following medical condition:

- Hyperphosphatemia (too much phosphate in the blood)

Other than the above information, there is no additional information relating to proper use, precautions, or side effects for this use.

CANDESARTAN CILEXETIL (Oral route) - kan-de-SAR-tan sye-LEK-se-til

Black Box Warning

When used in pregnancy during the second and third trimesters, drugs that act directly on the renin-angiotensin system can cause injury and even death to the developing fetus. When pregnancy is detected, candesartan cilexetil should be discontinued as soon as possible.

Commonly used brand name(s)

In the U.S.—

Atacand

Available Dosage Forms:

- Tablet

Therapeutic Class: Cardiovascular Agent

Pharmacologic Class: Angiotensin II Receptor Antagonist

Uses For This Medicine

Candesartan belongs to the class of medicines called angiotensin II inhibitors. It is used to treat high blood pressure (hypertension).

High blood pressure adds to the workload of the heart and arteries. If it continues for a long time, the heart and arteries may not function properly. This can damage the blood vessels of the brain, heart, and kidneys, resulting in a stroke, heart failure, or kidney failure. High blood pressure may also increase the risk of heart attacks. These problems may be less likely to occur if blood pressure is controlled.

Candesartan works by blocking the action of a substance in the body that causes blood vessels to tighten. As a result, candesartan relaxes blood vessels. This lowers blood pressure.

Candesartan is also used to treat heart failure and cut down on the number of hospital visits for heart problems.

This medicine is available only with your doctor's prescription.

Before Using This Medicine

In deciding to use a medicine, the risks of taking the medicine must be weighed against the good it will do. This is a decision you and your doctor will make. For this medicine, the following should be considered:

Allergies—Tell your doctor if you have ever had any unusual or allergic reaction to this medicine or any other medicines. Also tell your health care professional if you have any other types of allergies, such as to foods, dyes, preservatives, or animals. For non-prescription products, read the label or package ingredients carefully.

Pediatric—Studies on this medicine have been done only in adult patients, and there is no specific information comparing use of candesartan in children with use in other age groups.

Geriatric—This medicine has been tested in patients 65 years of age or older and has not been shown to cause different side effects or problems in older people than it does in younger adults. However, blood levels of candesartan are increased in the elderly. Older people may be more sensitive than younger adults to the effects of candesartan. Older adults with heart failure may need to be monitored more carefully for signs of low blood pressure.

Pregnancy—

	Pregnancy Category	Explanation
1st Trimester	C	Animal studies have shown an adverse effect and there are no adequate studies in pregnant women OR no animal studies have been conducted and there are no adequate studies in pregnant women.
2nd Trimester	D	Studies in pregnant women have demonstrated a risk to the fetus. However, the benefits of therapy in a life threatening situation or a serious disease, may outweigh the potential risk.
3rd Trimester	D	Studies in pregnant women have demonstrated a risk to the fetus. However, the benefits of therapy in a life threatening situation or a serious disease, may outweigh the potential risk.

Breast Feeding—There are no adequate studies in women for determining infant risk when using this medication during breastfeeding. Weigh the potential benefits against the potential risks before taking this medication while breastfeeding.

Other medicines—

Using this medicine with any of the following medicines is usually not recommended, but may be required in some cases. If both medicines are prescribed together, your doctor

may change the dose or how often you use one or both of the medicines.

Lithium

Interactions with Food/Tobacco/Alcohol—Certain medicines should not be used at or around the time of eating food or eating certain types of food since interactions may occur. Using alcohol or tobacco with certain medicines may also cause interactions to occur. Discuss with your healthcare professional the use of your medicine with food, alcohol, or tobacco.

Other medical problems—The presence of other medical problems may affect the use of this medicine. Make sure you tell your doctor if you have any other medical problems, especially:

- Dehydration (fluid and electrolyte loss due to excessive perspiration, vomiting, diarrhea, prolonged diuretic therapy, dialysis, or dietary salt restriction)—Blood pressure-lowering effects of candesartan may be increased.

- Heart failure—Lowering of blood pressure by candesartan may make this condition worse. Your doctor may need to lower your dose or take other precautions.

- Kidney disease—Effects of candesartan may make this condition worse.

- Liver disease, severe or moderate—For severe liver disease, effects of candesartan are unknown. For moderate liver disease, your doctor may need to lower your starting dose of candesartan.

Proper Use of This Medicine

Take this medicine only as directed by your doctor. Do not take more of it and do not take it more often than your doctor ordered. This medicine also works best when there is a constant amount in the blood. To help keep the amount constant, do not miss any doses. Also, it is best to take the doses at the same time each day.

Dosing—The dose of this medicine will be different for different patients. Follow your doctor's orders or the directions on the label. The following information includes only the average doses of this medicine. If your dose is different, do not change it unless your doctor tells you to do so.

The amount of medicine that you take depends on the strength of the medicine. Also, the number of doses you take each day, the time allowed between doses, and the length of time you take the medicine depend on the medical problem for which you are using the medicine.

- For oral dosage form (tablets):
  - For heart failure
    - Adults—4 milligrams (mg) once a day. Your doctor may increase your dose as needed.
    - Children—Use and dose must be determined by your doctor.
  - For high blood pressure:
    - Adults—16 milligrams (mg) once a day. Your doctor may increase your dose as needed.
    - Children—Use and dose must be determined by your doctor.

Missed dose—If you miss a dose of this medicine, take it as soon as possible. However, if it is almost time for your next dose, skip the missed dose and go back to your regular dosing schedule. Do not double doses.

Storage—Store the medicine in a closed container at room temperature, away from heat, moisture, and direct light. Keep from freezing.

Keep out of the reach of children.

Do not keep outdated medicine or medicine no longer needed.

Precautions While Using This Medicine

It is important that your doctor check your progress at regular visits to make sure that this medicine is working properly and to check for unwanted effects.

Check with your doctor immediately if you think that you may be pregnant. Candesartan may cause birth defects or other problems in the baby if taken during pregnancy.

Do not take other medicines unless they have been discussed with your doctor. This especially includes over-the-counter (nonprescription) medicines for appetite control, asthma, colds, cough, hay fever, or sinus problems, since they may tend to increase your blood pressure.

Dizziness or lightheadedness may occur, especially if you have been taking a diuretic (water pill). Make sure you know how you react to this medicine before you drive, use machines, or do anything else that could be dangerous if you experience these effects.

Check with your doctor right away if you become sick while taking this medicine, especially with severe or continuing nausea and vomiting or diarrhea. These conditions may cause you to lose too much water and lead to low blood pressure.

Dizziness, lightheadedness, or fainting also may occur if you exercise or if the weather is hot. Heavy sweating can cause loss of too much water and result in low blood pressure. Use extra care during exercise or hot weather.

Black patients may have a smaller response to the blood pressure-lowering effects of candesartan.

Side Effects of This Medicine

Along with its needed effects, a medicine may cause some unwanted effects. Although not all of these side effects may occur, if they do occur they may need medical attention.

Check with your doctor as soon as possible if any of the following side effects occur:
Rare
    Arm, back or jaw pain; bleeding gums; chest pain or discomfort; chest tightness or heaviness; chills; cough or hoarseness; dizziness; fainting; fast or irregular heartbeat; fever; joint pain; large, hive-like swelling on face, eyelids, lips, tongue, throat, hands, legs, feet, sex organs; lightheadedness; lower back or side pain; nausea; nosebleeds; pain or discomfort in arms, jaw, back or neck; painful or difficult urination; shortness of breath; sweating; swelling of feet or lower legs; vomiting
Frequency not known
    Abdominal pain; black, tarry stools; bloody urine; coma; confusion; convulsions; dark urine; decreased urine output; difficult or troubled breathing; general feeling of tiredness or weakness; headache; hives or welts; increased blood pressure; increased thirst; itching; light-colored stools; loss of appetite; muscle pain or cramps; nervousness; numbness or tingling in hands, feet, or

lips; pale skin; redness of skin; skin rash; sore throat; sores, ulcers, or white spots on lips or in mouth; stomach pain; swelling of face, ankles, or hands; unusual bleeding or bruising; unusual tiredness or weakness; upper right abdominal pain; weakness or heaviness of legs; weight gain; yellow eyes or skin

Some side effects may occur that usually do not need medical attention. These side effects may go away during treatment as your body adjusts to the medicine. Also, your health care professional may be able to tell you about ways to prevent or reduce some of these side effects. Check with your health care professional if any of the following side effects continue or are bothersome or if you have any questions about them:

Less common

Ear congestion or pain; head congestion; nasal congestion; runny and/or stuffy nose; sneezing

Other side effects not listed may also occur in some patients. If you notice any other effects, check with your healthcare professional.

CAPECITABINE   (Oral route) - ka-pe-SITE-a-been

Black Box Warning

Capecitabine Warfarin interaction: Patients receiving concomitant capecitabine and oral coumarin-derivative anticoagulant therapy should have their anticoagulant response (INR or prothrombin time) monitored frequently in order to adjust the anticoagulant dose accordingly. A clinically important capecitabine-Warfarin drug interaction was demonstrated in a clinical pharmacology trial. Altered coagulation parameters and/or bleeding, including death, have been reported in patients taking capecitabine concomitantly with coumarin-derivative anticoagulants such as warfarin and phenprocoumon. Postmarketing reports have shown clinically significant increases in prothrombin time (PT) and INR in patients who were stabilized on anticoagulants at the time capecitabine was introduced. These events have occurred within several days and up to several months after initiating capecitabine therapy and, in a few cases, within 1 month after stopping capecitabine. These events occurred in patients with and without liver metastases. Age greater than 60 and a diagnosis of cancer independently predispose patients to an increased risk of coagulopathy.

Commonly used brand name(s)

In the U.S.—
Xeloda

Available Dosage Forms:
• Tablet

Therapeutic Class: Antineoplastic Agent
Pharmacologic Class: Antimetabolite

Uses For This Medicine

Capecitabine belongs to the group of medicines called antimetabolites. It is used to treat breast cancer and colorectal cancer.

Capecitabine interferes with the growth of cancer cells, which are eventually destroyed. Since the growth of normal cells may also be affected by the medicine, other effects will also occur. Some of these may be serious and must be reported to your doctor. Other effects may not be serious but may cause concern.

This medicine is available only with your doctor's prescription.

Before Using This Medicine

In deciding to use a medicine, the risks of taking the medicine must be weighed against the good it will do. This is a decision you and your doctor will make. For this medicine, the following should be considered:

Allergies—Tell your doctor if you have ever had any unusual or allergic reaction to this medicine or any other medicines. Also tell your health care professional if you have any other types of allergies, such as to foods, dyes, preservatives, or animals. For non-prescription products, read the label or package ingredients carefully.

Pediatric—There is no specific information comparing use of capecitabine in children with use in other age groups.

Geriatric—Patients 80 years of age or older may be more sensitive to the effects of capecitabine. Severe diarrhea, nausea, or vomiting may be more likely to occur in these patients. Patients 60 years of age and older and/or who are also taking an anticoagulant (blood thinner), may be more likely to have blood clotting problems.

Pregnancy—

	Pregnancy Category	Explanation
All Trimesters	D	Studies in pregnant women have demonstrated a risk to the fetus. However, the benefits of therapy in a life threatening situation or a serious disease, may outweigh the potential risk.

Breast Feeding—There are no adequate studies in women for determining infant risk when using this medication during breastfeeding. Weigh the potential benefits against the potential risks before taking this medication while breastfeeding.

Other medicines—

Using this medicine with any of the following medicines is not recommended. Your doctor may decide not to treat you with this medication or change some of the other medicines you take.

Rotavirus Vaccine, Live

Interactions with Food/Tobacco/Alcohol—Certain medicines should not be used at or around the time of eating food or eating certain types of food since interactions may occur. Using alcohol or tobacco with certain medicines may also cause interactions to occur. Discuss with your healthcare professional the use of your medicine with food, alcohol, or tobacco.

Other medical problems—The presence of other medical problems may affect the use of this medicine. Make sure you tell your doctor if you have any other medical problems, especially:

- Allergy to capecitabine or to any ingredients in this medicine or
- Allergy to 5–fluorouracil or
- Shortage of an enzyme called dihydropyrimidine dehydrogenase that your body needs—Capecitabine should not be used
- Bone marrow depression or
- Cancer—May increase risk of blood clotting problems
- Chickenpox (including recent exposure) or
- Herpes zoster (shingles)—Risk of severe disease affecting other parts of the body
- Heart disease—The risk of a side effect that affects the heart may be increased
- Kidney disease, moderate or severe—The risk of side effects that affect the kidneys may be increased. Capecitabine should not be used in patients with severe kidney disease.
- Liver disease—The amount of capecitabine in the body may be increased in patients with liver disease. Also, the risk of a side effect that affects the liver may be increased
- Infection—Capecitabine decreases your body's ability to fight infection

Proper Use of This Medicine

Each dose of this medicine should be taken within 30 minutes after the end of a meal.

Swallow the tablets with water.

Dosing—The dose of this medicine will be different for different patients. Follow your doctor's orders or the directions on the label. The following information includes only the average doses of this medicine. If your dose is different, do not change it unless your doctor tells you to do so.

The amount of medicine that you take depends on the strength of the medicine. Also, the number of doses you take each day, the time allowed between doses, and the length of time you take the medicine depend on the medical problem for which you are using the medicine.

- For oral dosage form (tablets):
  - For breast cancer:
    - Adults—The starting dose is usually 2500 milligrams (mg) per square meter of body surface area a day, divided into two doses and taken about twelve hours apart within 30 minutes after the end of a meal. However, the dose may have to be decreased if certain side effects occur.
    - Children—Use and dose must be determined by your doctor.
  - In combination with docetaxel to treat breast cancer:
    - The starting dose of capecitabine is usually 2500 milligrams (mg) per square meter of body surface area a day, divided into two doses and taken about twelve hours apart within 30 minutes after the end of a meal combined with docetaxel at 75 mg per square meter of body surface area as a 1 hour infusion every 3 weeks.
    - Children—Use and dose must be determined by your doctor.

  - For colorectal cancer:
    - Adults—The starting dose is usually 2500 milligrams (mg) per square meter of body surface area a day, divided into two doses and taken about twelve hours apart within 30 minutes after the end of a meal. However, the dose may have to be decreased if certain side effects occur.
    - Children—Use and dose must be determined by your doctor.

Missed dose—If you miss a dose of this medicine, skip the missed dose and go back to your regular dosing schedule. Do not double doses.

Storage—Store the medicine in a closed container at room temperature, away from heat, moisture, and direct light. Keep from freezing.

Keep out of the reach of children.

Do not keep outdated medicine or medicine no longer needed.

Precautions While Using This Medicine

It is very important that your doctor check your progress at regular visits to make sure that this medicine is working properly and to check for unwanted effects.

Your health care professional may request that you have a test to determine if your blood is clotting properly and may preform this test frequently, if you are also taking an anticoagulant (blood thinner).

Check with your doctor immediately if you develop a fever of 100.5 °F or higher, or if you notice any other signs of a possible infection. These signs include cough or hoarseness, lower back or side pain, painful or difficult urination, sneezing, sore throat, stuffy nose, and white spots inside the mouth or throat.

Stop taking this medicine and check with your doctor immediately if any of the following occur:
- Diarrhea, moderately severe (four to six stools a day more than usual, or during the night).
- Pain, blistering, peeling, redness, or swelling of the palms of your hands and/or the bottoms of your feet that is severe enough to interfere with your normal activities.
- Nausea that is severe enough to cause you to eat less than usual.
- Vomiting that occurs two times, or more, in a 24–hour period.
- Pain and redness, swelling, or sores or ulcers in your mouth or on your lips that are severe enough to interfere with eating.

If vomiting occurs less often than mentioned above, or if nausea does not cause you to eat less than usual, it is not necessary for you to stop taking the medicine or to check with your doctor (unless these effects are particularly bothersome). Also, you do not need to stop taking the medicine if diarrhea occurs less often than mentioned above or if the other side effects listed are not severe enough to interfere with eating or other daily activities. However, check with your doctor as soon as possible if they occur.

While you are being treated with capecitabine, and after you stop treatment with it, do not have any immunizations (vaccinations) without your doctor's approval. Capecitabine may lower your body's resistance and there is a chance you might get the infection the immunization is meant to prevent. In addition, other persons living in your household should not take oral polio vaccine since there is a chance they could pass the polio virus on to you. Also, avoid persons who have taken oral polio vaccine within the last several months. Do not get close to them, and do not stay in the same room with them for very long. If you cannot take these precautions, you should consider wearing a protective face mask that covers the nose and mouth.

Capecitabine can temporarily lower the number of white blood cells in your blood, increasing the chance of getting an infection. It can also lower the number of platelets, which are necessary for proper blood clotting. If this occurs, there are certain precautions you can take, especially when your blood count is low, to reduce the risk of infection or bleeding:

- If you can, avoid people with infections. Check with your doctor immediately if you think you are getting an infection or if you get a fever or chills, cough or hoarseness, lower back or side pain, or painful or difficult urination.
- Check with your doctor immediately if you notice any unusual bleeding or bruising; black, tarry stools; blood in urine or stools; or pinpoint red spots on your skin.
- Be careful when using a regular toothbrush, dental floss, or toothpick. Your medical doctor, dentist, or nurse may recommend other ways to clean your teeth and gums. Check with your medical doctor before having any dental work done.
- Do not touch your eyes or the inside of your nose unless you have just washed your hands and have not touched anything else in the meantime.
- Be careful not to cut yourself when you are using sharp objects such as a safety razor or fingernail or toenail cutters.
- Avoid contact sports or other situations where bruising or injury could occur.

Side Effects of This Medicine

Along with its needed effects, a medicine may cause some unwanted effects. Although not all of these side effects may occur, if they do occur they may need medical attention.

Stop taking this medicine and get emergency help immediately if any of the following effects occur:

More common
Diarrhea (moderately severe [four to six stools a day more than usual, or at night]); pain, blistering, peeling, redness, or swelling of palms of hands and/or bottoms of feet (severe enough to interfere with normal activities); pain and redness, swelling, or sores or ulcers in your mouth or on your lips (severe enough to interfere with eating)

Less common
Nausea (severe, accompanied by loss of appetite); vomiting (severe [occurring two times or more in 24 hours])

Check with your doctor immediately if any of the following side effects occur:

Less common or rare
Abdominal or stomach cramping or pain (severe); agitation; back pain; bleeding and bruising; bleeding gums; blood in urine or stools; bloody nose; bloody or black, tarry stools; bloody nose; blurred vision; burning, dry or itching eyes; chest pain; chills; cold; collapse; coma; confusion; constipation (severe); convulsions;

cough or hoarseness (accompanied by fever or chills); cough producing mucus; coughing or spitting up blood; decreased frequency/amount of urine; difficulty breathing; difficulty in swallowing or pain in back of throat or chest when swallowing; discharge from eye; drowsiness; dry mouth; excessive tearing; extra heartbeats; eye redness, irritation, or pain; fainting; fast or irregular heartbeat; fever or chills; flu-like symptoms; hallucinations; headache, sudden and severe; heavier menstrual periods; high fever; hot, red skin on feet or legs; inability to speak; increased blood pressure; increased menstrual flow or vaginal bleeding; increased thirst; irritability; itching in genital or other skin areas; large amount of triglycerides in the blood; lightheadedness; loss of consciousness; lower back or side pain (accompanied by fever or chills); mood or mental changes; muscle aches or cramps; muscle spasms; nosebleeds; numbness or tingling in hands, feet, or lips; painful or difficult urination (accompanied by fever or chills); painful, swollen feet or legs; pain, tenderness, and/or swelling in upper abdominal (stomach) area; pale skin; paralysis; pinpoint red spots on skin; prolonged bleeding from cuts; rapid, shallow breathing; red or dark brown urine; redness, pain, swelling or eye, eyelid or inner lining of eyelid; scaling; seizures; severe constipation; severe vomiting; shortness of breath, troubled breathing, tightness in chest, and/or wheezing; slow or irregular heartbeat; slurred speech; sneezing, sore throat, and/or stuffy nose; sores, ulcers or white spots on lips or in mouth; stiff neck; stomach bloating, burning, cramping, or pain; swelling of lymph nodes; temporary blindness; tiredness or weakness (severe); trouble in speaking; twitching seizures; unusual bleeding or bruising; unusual lump or swelling in the chest; vomiting blood or material that looks like coffee grounds; weakness in arm and/or leg on one side of the body, sudden and severe; weight gain; weight loss; wheezing; white patches in the mouth or throat or on the tongue; white patches with diaper rash; yellow eyes or skin

Incidence not known
Continuing vomiting; dark-colored urine; general feeling of tiredness or weakness

Check with your doctor as soon as possible if any of the following side effects occur:

More common
Abdominal or stomach pain (mild or moderate); blistering, peeling, redness, and/or swelling of palms of hands or bottoms of feet (not severe enough to interfere with daily activities); diarrhea (mild [fewer than four stools a day more than usual]); numbness, pain, tingling, or other unusual sensations in palms of hands or bottoms of feet; pain and redness, swelling, or sores or ulcers in your mouth or on your lips (not severe enough to interfere with eating); unusual tiredness or weakness (mild or moderate); yellow eyes or skin

Less common or rare
Clumsiness or unsteadiness; dark urine; decrease or increase in blood pressure; light-colored stools; problems with coordination; skin rash or itching; swelling of face, fingers, feet, or lower legs; swollen glands; unexplained nosebleeds

Some side effects may occur that usually do not need medical attention. These side effects may go away during treatment as your body adjusts to the medicine. Also, your health care professional may be able to tell you about ways to prevent or reduce some of these side effects. Check with your health care professional if any of the following side effects continue or are bothersome or if you have any questions about them:

More common

Constipation (mild or moderate); loss of appetite (not due to nausea); nausea (not accompanied by loss of appetite); vomiting (mild [once a day or less])

Less common

Burning, crawling, itching, numbness, prickling, "pins and needles" or tingling feelings; changes or discoloration in fingernails or toenails; difficulty in moving; discouragement; dizziness; fatigue; headache; heartburn; increase in heart rate; increased sensitivity of skin to sunlight; muscle pain; pain; pain in joints; pain in limbs; pain and redness of skin at place of earlier radiation (x-ray) treatment; red, sore eyes; sunken eyes; thirst; trouble in sleeping; weakness; wrinkled skin

Rare

Bone pain; change in color of treated skin; difficulty in walking; discouragement; dryness or soreness or throat; feeling of constant movement of self or surroundings; feeling sad or empty; full feeling in abdomen; full or bloated feeling or pressure in the stomach; general feeling of discomfort or illness; hoarseness; hot flushes; impaired balance; increased weight; joint pain; lack of appetite; loss of interest or pleasure; muscle weakness; noisy breathing; pain in rectum; pain, swelling, or redness in joints; passing less gas; rough, scratchy sound to voice; runny nose; sensation of spinning; shakiness in legs, arms, hands, feet; shivering; sleepiness; sores on the skin; sweating increased; swelling of abdominal or stomach area; tremor or shaking of hands or feet; trouble concentrating; voice changes

Other side effects not listed may also occur in some patients. If you notice any other effects, check with your healthcare professional.

CAPREOMYCIN (Injection route) -
kap-ree-oh-MYE-sin

Black Box Warning

The use of capreomycin in patients with renal insufficiency or preexisting auditory impairment must be undertaken with great caution, and the risk of additional cranial nerve VIII impairment or renal injury should be weighed against the benefits to be derived from therapy.

Since other parenteral antituberculosis agents (streptomycin, vancomycin) also have similar and sometimes irreversible toxic effects, particularly on cranial nerve VIII and renal function, simultaneous administration of these agents with capreomycin is not recommended. Use with nonantituberculosis drugs (polymyxin A sulfate, colistin sulfate, amikacin,

gentamicin, tobramycin, vancomycin, kanamycin, and neomycin) having ototoxic or nephrotoxic potential should be undertaken only with great caution.

Usage in Pregnancy: The safety of the use of capreomycin in pregnancy has not been determined.

Pediatric Usage: Safety and effectiveness in pediatric patients have not been established.

Commonly used brand name(s)

In the U.S.—

Capastat Sulfate

Available Dosage Forms:

• Powder for Solution

Therapeutic Class: Antitubercular

Uses For This Medicine

Capreomycin is used to treat tuberculosis (TB). It is given with other medicines for TB.

To help clear up your tuberculosis (TB) completely, you must keep taking this medicine for the full time of treatment, even if you begin to feel better. This is very important. It is also important that you do not miss any doses.

Capreomycin is available only with your doctor's prescription.

Before Receiving This Medicine

In deciding to use a medicine, the risks of taking the medicine must be weighed against the good it will do. This is a decision you and your doctor will make. For this medicine, the following should be considered:

Allergies—Tell your doctor if you have ever had any unusual or allergic reaction to this medicine or any other medicines. Also tell your health care professional if you have any other types of allergies, such as to foods, dyes, preservatives, or animals. For non-prescription products, read the label or package ingredients carefully.

Pediatric—Studies on this medicine have been done only in adult patients, and there is no specific information comparing use of capreomycin in children with use in other age groups.

Geriatric—Many medicines have not been studied specifically in older people. Therefore, it may not be known whether they work exactly the same way they do in younger adults or if they cause different side effects or problems in older people. There is no specific information comparing use of capreomycin in the elderly with use in other age groups.

Pregnancy—

	Pregnancy Category	Explanation
All Trimesters	C	Animal studies have shown an adverse effect and there are no adequate studies in pregnant women OR no animal studies have been conducted and there are no adequate studies in pregnant women.

Breast Feeding—There are no adequate studies in women for determining infant risk when using this medication during

breastfeeding. Weigh the potential benefits against the potential risks before taking this medication while breastfeeding.

Other medicines—

Using this medicine with any of the following medicines may cause an increased risk of certain side effects, but using both drugs may be the best treatment for you. If both medicines are prescribed together, your doctor may change the dose or how often you use one or both of the medicines.

Alcuronium, Atracurium, Cisatracurium, Doxacurium, Fazadinium, Gallamine, Hexafluorenium, Metocurine, Mivacurium, Pancuronium, Pipecuronium, Rapacuronium, Rocuronium, Tubocurarine, Vecuronium

Interactions with Food/Tobacco/Alcohol—Certain medicines should not be used at or around the time of eating food or eating certain types of food since interactions may occur. Using alcohol or tobacco with certain medicines may also cause interactions to occur. Discuss with your healthcare professional the use of your medicine with food, alcohol, or tobacco.

Other medical problems—The presence of other medical problems may affect the use of this medicine. Make sure you tell your doctor if you have any other medical problems, especially:

- Eighth-cranial-nerve disease (loss of hearing and/or balance)—Capreomycin may cause hearing and balance side effects

- Kidney disease—Capreomycin may cause serious side effects affecting the kidneys

- Myasthenia gravis or

- Parkinson's disease—Capreomycin may cause muscular weakness

Proper Use of This Medicine

To help clear up your infection completely, it is very important that you keep taking this medicine for the full time of treatment, even if you begin to feel better after a few weeks. You may have to use it every day for as long as 1 to 2 years or more. If you stop using this medicine too soon, your symptoms may return.

Dosing—The dose of this medicine will be different for different patients. Follow your doctor's orders or the directions on the label. The following information includes only the average doses of this medicine. If your dose is different, do not change it unless your doctor tells you to do so.

The amount of medicine that you take depends on the strength of the medicine. Also, the number of doses you take each day, the time allowed between doses, and the length of time you take the medicine depend on the medical problem for which you are using the medicine.

- For injection dosage form:
  - For treatment of tuberculosis (TB):
    - Adults and adolescents—1 gram of capreomycin injected into the muscle once a day for 60 to 120 days. After this time, 1 gram of capreomycin is injected into the muscle 2 or 3 times a week. This medicine must be given with other medicines to treat tuberculosis (TB).
    - Children—Dose has not been determined.

Side Effects of This Medicine

Along with its needed effects, a medicine may cause some unwanted effects. Although not all of these side effects may occur, if they do occur they may need medical attention.

Check with your doctor as soon as possible if any of the following side effects occur:

More common
> Greatly increased or decreased frequency of urination or amount of urine; increased thirst; loss of appetite; nausea; vomiting

Less common
> Any loss of hearing; clumsiness or unsteadiness; difficulty in breathing; dizziness; drowsiness; fever; irregular heartbeat; itching; muscle cramps or pain; pain, redness, hardness, unusual bleeding, or a sore at the place of injection; ringing or buzzing or a feeling of fullness in the ears; skin rash; swelling; unusual tiredness or weakness

Other side effects not listed may also occur in some patients. If you notice any other effects, check with your healthcare professional.

CAPSAICIN (Topical route) - kap-SAY-sin

Commonly used brand name(s)

In the U.S.—

Arthricare For Women	Pain Enz
Capsagel	Rid-A-Pain
Capsagesic-HP Arthritis Relief	Sportsmed
	Therapatch Warm
Capsin	Trixaicin
Double Cap	Zostrix
Icy Hot Arthritis Therapy	

In Canada—
Axsain
Capsaicin
Capsaicin Hp

Available Dosage Forms:

- Cream
- Ointment
- Stick
- Pad
- Gel/Jelly
- Liquid
- Lotion
- Film

Therapeutic Class: Analgesic

Uses For This Medicine

Capsaicin is used to help relieve a certain type of pain known as neuralgia. Capsaicin is also used to temporarily help relieve the pain from osteoarthritis or rheumatoid arthritis. This medicine will not cure any of these conditions.

Neuralgia is a pain from the nerves near the surface of your skin. This pain may occur after an infection with herpes zoster (shingles). It may also occur if you have diabetic neuropathy. Diabetic neuropathy is a condition that occurs in some persons with diabetes. The condition causes tingling and pain in the feet and toes. Capsaicin will help relieve the pain of diabetic neuropathy, but it will not cure diabetic neuropathy or diabetes.

Capsaicin may also be used for neuralgias or itching of the skin caused by other conditions as determined by your doctor.

Capsaicin is available without a prescription; however, your doctor may have special instructions on the proper use of this medicine.

Before Using This Medicine

In deciding to use a medicine, the risks of taking the medicine must be weighed against the good it will do. This is a decision you and your doctor will make. For this medicine, the following should be considered:

Allergies—Tell your doctor if you have ever had any unusual or allergic reaction to this medicine or any other medicines. Also tell your health care professional if you have any other types of allergies, such as to foods, dyes, preservatives, or animals. For non-prescription products, read the label or package ingredients carefully.

Pediatric—Use is not recommended for infants and children up to 2 years of age, except as directed by your doctor. In children 2 years of age and older, this medicine is not expected to cause different side effects or problems than it does in adults.

Geriatric—Many medicines have not been studied specifically in older people. Therefore, it may not be known whether they work exactly the same way they do in younger adults. Although there is no specific information comparing use of capsaicin in the elderly with use in other age groups, this medicine is not expected to cause different side effects or problems in older people than it does in younger adults.

Other medicines—Although certain medicines should not be used together at all, in other cases two different medicines may be used together even if an interaction might occur. In these cases, your doctor may want to change the dose, or other precautions may be necessary. Tell your healthcare professional if you are taking any other prescription or non-prescription (over-the-counter [OTC]) medicine.

Interactions with Food/Tobacco/Alcohol—Certain medicines should not be used at or around the time of eating food or eating certain types of food since interactions may occur. Using alcohol or tobacco with certain medicines may also cause interactions to occur. Discuss with your healthcare professional the use of your medicine with food, alcohol, or tobacco.

Other medical problems—The presence of other medical problems may affect the use of this medicine. Make sure you tell your doctor if you have any other medical problems, especially:

- Broken or irritated skin on area to be treated with capsaicin

Proper Use of This Medicine

If you are using capsaicin for the treatment of neuralgia caused by herpes zoster, do not apply the medicine until the zoster sores have healed.

It is not necessary to wash the areas to be treated before you apply capsaicin, but doing so will not cause harm.

Apply a small amount of cream and use your fingers to rub it well into the affected area so that little or no cream is left on the surface of the skin afterwards.

Wash your hands with soap and water after applying capsaicin to avoid getting the medicine in your eyes or on other sensitive areas of the body. However, if you are using capsaicin for arthritis in your hands, do not wash your hands for at least 30 minutes after applying the cream.

If a bandage is being used on the treated area, it should not be applied tightly.

When you first begin to use capsaicin, a warm, stinging, or burning sensation (feeling) may occur. This sensation is related to the action of capsaicin on the skin and is to be expected. Although this sensation usually disappears after the first several days of treatment, it may last 2 to 4 weeks or longer. Heat, humidity, clothing, bathing in warm water, or sweating may increase the sensation. However, the sensation usually occurs less often and is less severe the longer you use the medicine. Reducing the number of doses of capsaicin that you use each day will not lessen the sensation and may lengthen the period of time that you get the sensation. Also, reducing the number of doses you use may reduce the amount of pain relief that you get.

Capsaicin must be used regularly every day as directed if it is to work properly. Even then, it may not relieve your pain right away. The length of time it takes to work depends on the type of pain you have. In persons with arthritis, pain relief usually begins within 1 to 2 weeks. In most persons with neuralgia, relief usually begins within 2 to 4 weeks, although with head and neck neuralgias, relief may take as long as 4 to 6 weeks.

Once capsaicin has begun to relieve pain, you must continue to use it regularly 3 or 4 times a day to keep the pain from returning. If you stop using capsaicin and your pain returns, you can begin using it again.

Dosing—The dose of this medicine will be different for different patients. Follow your doctor's orders or the directions on the label. The following information includes only the average doses of this medicine. If your dose is different, do not change it unless your doctor tells you to do so.

The amount of medicine that you take depends on the strength of the medicine. Also, the number of doses you take each day, the time allowed between doses, and the length of time you take the medicine depend on the medical problem for which you are using the medicine.

- For topical dosage form (cream):
  - For neuralgias or itching of the skin:
    - Adults and children 2 years of age or older—Apply regularly 3 or 4 times a day and rub well.
    - Children up to 2 years of age—Use and dose must be determined by your doctor.

Missed dose—If you miss a dose of this medicine, take it as soon as possible. However, if it is almost time for your next dose, skip the missed dose and go back to your regular dosing schedule. Do not double doses.

Storage—Store the medicine in a closed container at room temperature, away from heat, moisture, and direct light. Keep from freezing.

Keep out of the reach of children.

Do not keep outdated medicine or medicine no longer needed.

Precautions While Using This Medicine

If capsaicin gets into your eyes or on other sensitive areas of the body, it will cause a burning sensation. If capsaicin gets into your eyes, flush your eyes with water. If capsaicin gets on other sensitive areas of your body, wash the areas with warm (not hot) soapy water.

If your condition gets worse, or does not improve after 1 month, stop using this medicine and check with your doctor.

Side Effects of This Medicine

Along with its needed effects, a medicine may cause some unwanted effects. Although not all of these side effects may occur, if they do occur they may need medical attention.

Some side effects may occur that usually do not need medical attention. These side effects may go away during treatment as your body adjusts to the medicine. Also, your health care professional may be able to tell you about ways to prevent or reduce some of these side effects. Check with your health care professional if any of the following side effects continue or are bothersome or if you have any questions about them:

More common

Warm, stinging, or burning feeling at the place of treatment

Other side effects not listed may also occur in some patients. If you notice any other effects, check with your healthcare professional.

CARBACHOL (Ophthalmic route) -
KAR-ba-kole

Commonly used brand name(s)

In the U.S.—
Isopto Carbachol

Available Dosage Forms:
• Solution

Therapeutic Class: Direct Acting Miotic
Pharmacologic Class: Cholinergic

Uses For This Medicine

Carbachol is used in the eye to treat glaucoma. Sometimes it is also used in eye surgery.

This medicine is available only with your doctor's prescription.

Before Using This Medicine

In deciding to use a medicine, the risks of taking the medicine must be weighed against the good it will do. This is a decision you and your doctor will make. For this medicine, the following should be considered:

Allergies—Tell your doctor if you have ever had any unusual or allergic reaction to this medicine or any other medicines. Also tell your health care professional if you have any other types of allergies, such as to foods, dyes, preservatives, or animals. For non-prescription products, read the label or package ingredients carefully.

Pediatric—Although there is no specific information comparing use of carbachol in children with use in other age groups, this medicine is not expected to cause different side effects or problems in children than it does in adults.

Geriatric—Many medicines have not been studied specifically in older people. Therefore, it may not be known whether they work exactly the same way they do in younger adults. Although there is no specific information comparing use of carbachol in the elderly with use in other age groups, this medicine is not expected to cause different side effects or problems in older people than it does in younger adults.

Pregnancy—

	Pregnancy Category	Explanation
All Trimesters	C	Animal studies have shown an adverse effect and there are no adequate studies in pregnant women OR no animal studies have been conducted and there are no adequate studies in pregnant women.

Breast Feeding—There are no adequate studies in women for determining infant risk when using this medication during breastfeeding. Weigh the potential benefits against the potential risks before taking this medication while breastfeeding.

Other medicines—Although certain medicines should not be used together at all, in other cases two different medicines may be used together even if an interaction might occur. In these cases, your doctor may want to change the dose, or other precautions may be necessary. Tell your healthcare professional if you are taking any other prescription or nonprescription (over-the-counter [OTC]) medicine.

Interactions with Food/Tobacco/Alcohol—Certain medicines should not be used at or around the time of eating food or eating certain types of food since interactions may occur. Using alcohol or tobacco with certain medicines may also cause interactions to occur. Discuss with your healthcare professional the use of your medicine with food, alcohol, or tobacco.

Other medical problems—The presence of other medical problems may affect the use of this medicine. Make sure you tell your doctor if you have any other medical problems, especially:

• Asthma or
• Eye problems (other) or
• Heart disease or
• Overactive thyroid or
• Parkinson's disease or
• Stomach ulcer or other stomach problems or
• Urinary tract blockage—Carbachol may make the condition worse

Proper Use of This Medicine

Use this medicine only as directed. Do not use more of it and do not use it more often than your doctor ordered. To do so may increase the chance of too much medicine being absorbed into the body and the chance of side effects.

To use:

- First, wash your hands. Tilt the head back and, pressing your finger gently on the skin just beneath the lower eyelid, pull the lower eyelid away from the eye to make a space. Drop the medicine into this space. Let go of the eyelid and gently close the eyes. Do not blink. Keep the eyes closed and apply pressure to the inner corner of the eye with your finger for 1 or 2 minutes to allow the medicine to be absorbed by the eye.
- Immediately after using the eye drops, wash your hands to remove any medicine that may be on them.
- To keep the medicine as germ-free as possible, do not touch the applicator tip to any surface (including the eye). Also, keep the container tightly closed.

Dosing—The dose of this medicine will be different for different patients. Follow your doctor's orders or the directions on the label. The following information includes only the average doses of this medicine. If your dose is different, do not change it unless your doctor tells you to do so.

The amount of medicine that you take depends on the strength of the medicine. Also, the number of doses you take each day, the time allowed between doses, and the length of time you take the medicine depend on the medical problem for which you are using the medicine.

- For glaucoma:
  - For ophthalmic solution (eye drops) dosage form:
    - Adults and children—Use one drop in the eye one to three times a day.
- For use during surgery:
  - For intraocular solution dosage form:
    - Adults and children—Up to 0.5 milliliter (mL), used in the eye during surgery.

Missed dose—If you miss a dose of this medicine, apply it as soon as possible. However, if it is almost time for your next dose, skip the missed dose and go back to your regular dosing schedule.

Storage—Store the medicine in a closed container at room temperature, away from heat, moisture, and direct light. Keep from freezing.

Keep out of the reach of children.

Do not keep outdated medicine or medicine no longer needed.

Precautions While Using This Medicine

Your doctor should check your eye pressure at regular visits.

After you apply this medicine to your eyes, your pupils may become unusually small. This may cause you to see less well at night or in dim light. Be especially careful if you drive, use machines, or do anything else at night or in dim light that could be dangerous if you are not able to see well.

Also, for a short time after you apply this medicine, your vision may be blurred or there may be a change in your near or distance vision. Make sure your vision is clear before you drive, use machines, or do anything else that could be dangerous if you are not able to see well.

Side Effects of This Medicine

Along with its needed effects, a medicine may cause some unwanted effects. Although not all of these side effects may occur, if they do occur they may need medical attention.

Check with your doctor as soon as possible if any of the following side effects occur:

Rare

Veil or curtain appearing across part of vision

Symptoms of too much medicine being absorbed into the body

Diarrhea, stomach cramps or pain, or vomiting; fainting; flushing or redness of face; frequent urge to urinate; increased sweating; irregular heartbeat; shortness of breath, wheezing, or tightness in chest; unusual tiredness or weakness; watering of mouth

Some side effects may occur that usually do not need medical attention. These side effects may go away during treatment as your body adjusts to the medicine. Also, your health care professional may be able to tell you about ways to prevent or reduce some of these side effects. Check with your health care professional if any of the following side effects continue or are bothersome or if you have any questions about them:

More common

Blurred vision or change in near or distance vision; eye pain; stinging or burning of the eye

Less common

Headache; irritation or redness of eyes; twitching of eyelids

Other side effects not listed may also occur in some patients. If you notice any other effects, check with your healthcare professional.

CARBAMAZEPINE   (Oral route) - kar-ba-MAZ-e-peen

Black Box Warning

Aplastic anemia and agranulocytosis have been reported in association with the use of carbamazepine. Data from a population-based case control study demonstrate that the risk of developing these reactions is 5–8 times greater than in the general population. However, the overall risk of these reactions in the untreated general population is low, approximately six patients per one million population per year for agranulocytosis and two patients per one million population per year for aplastic anemia.

Although reports of transient or persistent decreased platelet or white blood cell counts are not uncommon in association with the use of carbamazepine, data are not available to estimate accurately their incidence or outcome. However, the vast majority of the cases of leukopenia have not progressed to the more serious conditions of aplastic anemia or agranulocytosis.

Because of the very low incidence of agranulocytosis and aplastic anemia, the vast majority of minor hematologic changes observed in monitoring of patients on carbamazepine are unlikely to signal the occurrence of either abnormality. Nonetheless, complete pretreatment hematological testing should be obtained as a baseline. If a patient in the course of treatment exhibits low or decreased white blood cell or platelet counts, the patient should be monitored closely. Discontinuation of the drug should be considered if any evidence of significant bone marrow depression develops.

Commonly used brand name(s)

In the U.S.—

Carbatrol	Tegretol
Epitol	Tegretol-XR
Equetro	

Available Dosage Forms:
- Suspension
- Tablet, Extended Release
- Tablet, Chewable
- Capsule, Extended Release
- Tablet

Therapeutic Class: Anticonvulsant

Uses For This Medicine

Carbamazepine is used to control some types of seizures in the treatment of epilepsy. It is also used to relieve pain due to trigeminal neuralgia (tic douloureux). It should not be used for other more common aches or pains. It can also be used in the treatment of bipolar disorder (manic-depressive illness).

Carbamazepine may also be used for other conditions as determined by your doctor.

This medicine is available only with your doctor's prescription.

Once a medicine has been approved for marketing for a certain use, experience may show that it is also useful for other medical problems. Although these uses are not included in product labeling, carbamazepine is used in certain patients with the following medical conditions:
- Neurogenic pain (a type of continuing pain)
- Bipolar disorder (manic-depressive illness) prevention
- Central partial diabetes insipidus (water diabetes)
- Alcohol withdrawal
- Psychotic disorders (severe mental illness)

Before Using This Medicine

In deciding to use a medicine, the risks of taking the medicine must be weighed against the good it will do. This is a decision you and your doctor will make. For this medicine, the following should be considered:

Allergies—Tell your doctor if you have ever had any unusual or allergic reaction to this medicine or any other medicines. Also tell your health care professional if you have any other types of allergies, such as to foods, dyes, preservatives, or animals. For non-prescription products, read the label or package ingredients carefully.

Pediatric—Behavior changes are more likely to occur in children.

Geriatric—Confusion; restlessness and nervousness; irregular, pounding, or unusually slow heartbeat; and chest pain may be especially likely to occur in elderly patients, who are usually more sensitive than younger adults to the effects of carbamazepine.

Pregnancy—

	Pregnancy Category	Explanation
All Trimesters	D	Studies in pregnant women have demonstrated a risk to the fetus. However, the benefits of therapy in a life threatening situation or a serious disease, may outweigh the potential risk.

Breast Feeding—There are no adequate studies in women for determining infant risk when using this medication during breastfeeding. Weigh the potential benefits against the potential risks before taking this medication while breastfeeding.

Other medicines—

Using this medicine with any of the following medicines is not recommended. Your doctor may decide not to treat you with this medication or change some of the other medicines you take.

Clorgyline, Iproniazid, Isocarboxazid, Moclobemide, Nialamide, Pargyline, Phenelzine, Procarbazine, Selegiline, Toloxatone, Tranylcypromine, Voriconazole

Interactions with Food/Tobacco/Alcohol—Certain medicines should not be used at or around the time of eating food or eating certain types of food since interactions may occur. Using alcohol or tobacco with certain medicines may also cause interactions to occur. The following interactions have been selected on the basis of their potential significance and are not necessarily all-inclusive.

Using this medicine with any of the following may cause an increased risk of certain side effects but may be unavoidable in some cases. If used together, your doctor may change the dose or how often you use this medicine, or give you special instructions about the use of food, alcohol, or tobacco.

Grapefruit Juice

Other medical problems—The presence of other medical problems may affect the use of this medicine. Make sure you tell your doctor if you have any other medical problems, especially:
- Alcohol abuse (or history of)—Drinking alcohol may decrease the effectiveness of carbamazepine
- Anemia or other blood problems or
- Behavioral problems or
- Glaucoma or
- Heart or blood vessel disease or
- Problems with urination—Carbamazepine may make the condition worse
- Diabetes mellitus (sugar diabetes)—Carbamazepine may cause increased urine glucose levels
- Kidney disease or
- Liver disease—Higher blood levels of carbamazepine may result, increasing the chance of side effects

Proper Use of This Medicine

Carbamazepine suspension and tablets should be taken with meals to lessen the chance of stomach upset (nausea and vomiting). Carbamazepine extended-release capsules do not need to be taken with meals unless they upset your stomach. The contents of these extended-release capsules may be sprinkled over a teaspoonful of applesauce or other similar food; the capsule or its contents should not be crushed or chewed.

Grapefruit and grapefruit juice may increase the effects of carbamazepine by increasing the amount of this medicine in the body. You should not eat grapefruit or drink grapefruit juice while you are taking this medicine.

It is very important that you take this medicine exactly as directed by your doctor to obtain the best results and lessen the chance of serious side effects. Do not take more of it, do not take it more often, and do not take it for a longer time than your doctor ordered.

If you are taking this medicine for pain relief:

- Carbamazepine is not an ordinary pain reliever. It should be used only when a doctor prescribes it for certain kinds of pain. Do not take carbamazepine for any other aches or pains.

If you are taking this medicine for epilepsy:

- Do not suddenly stop taking this medicine without first checking with your doctor. To keep your seizures under control, it is usually best to gradually reduce the amount of carbamazepine you are taking before stopping completely.

Dosing—The dose of this medicine will be different for different patients. Follow your doctor's orders or the directions on the label. The following information includes only the average doses of this medicine. If your dose is different, do not change it unless your doctor tells you to do so.

The amount of medicine that you take depends on the strength of the medicine. Also, the number of doses you take each day, the time allowed between doses, and the length of time you take the medicine depend on the medical problem for which you are using the medicine.

- For oral dosage form (suspension):
  - For epilepsy:
    - Adults and teenagers—At first, 100 milligrams (mg) taken up to four times a day. Your doctor may increase your dose if needed. However, the dose is usually not more than 1200 mg a day.
    - Children 6 to 12 years of age—At first, 50 mg taken four times a day. Your doctor may increase your dose if needed. However, the dose is usually not more than 1000 mg a day.
    - Children up to 6 years of age—Dose is based on body weight and will be determined by your doctor.
  - For trigeminal neuralgia:
    - Adults and teenagers—At first, 50 mg four times a day. Your doctor may increase your dose if needed. However, the dose is usually not more than 1200 mg a day.
    - Children—Use and dose must be determined by your doctor.
- For oral dosage form (tablets and chewable tablets):
  - For epilepsy:
    - Adults and teenagers—At first, 200 mg taken two times a day. Your doctor may increase your dose if needed. However, the dose is usually not more than 1200 mg a day.
    - Children 6 to 12 years of age—At first, 100 mg taken two times a day. Your doctor may increase your dose if needed. However, the dose is usually not more than 1000 mg a day.
    - Children up to 6 years of age—Dose is based on body weight and will be determined by your doctor.
  - For trigeminal neuralgia:
    - Adults and teenagers—At first, 100 mg taken two times a day. Your doctor may increase your dose if needed. However, the dose is usually not more than 1200 mg a day.
    - Children—Use and dose must be determined by your doctor.

- For oral extended-release capsule dosage form:
  - For bipolar disorder:
    - Adults—At first, 200 mg taken two times a day. Your doctor may increase your dose if needed. However, the dose is usually not more than 1600 mg a day.
    - Children and teenagers—Use and dose must be determined by your doctor.
  - For epilepsy:
    - Adults and teenagers—At first, 200 mg taken one or two times a day. Your doctor may increase your dose if needed. However, the dose is usually not more than 1200 mg a day.
    - Children up to 12 years of age—Dose is based on body weight and will be determined by your doctor. However, the dose is usually not more than 1000 mg a day.
  - For trigeminal neuralgia:
    - Adults and teenagers—At first, 200 mg a day. Your doctor may increase your dose if needed. However, the dose is usually not more than 1200 mg a day.
    - Children—Use and dose must be determined by your doctor.
- For oral extended-release tablet dosage form:
  - For epilepsy:
    - Adults and teenagers—At first, 100 to 200 mg taken one or two times a day with meals. Your doctor may increase your dose if needed. However, the dose is usually not more than 1200 mg a day.
    - Children 6 to 12 years of age—At first, 100 to 200 mg taken in smaller doses during the day. Your doctor may increase your dose if needed. However, the dose is usually not more than 1000 mg a day.
    - Children up to 6 years of age—Use and dose must be determined by your doctor.
  - For trigeminal neuralgia:
    - Adults and teenagers—At first, 100 mg taken two times a day. Your doctor may increase your dose if needed. However, the dose is usually not more than 1200 mg a day.
    - Children—Use and dose must be determined by your doctor.

Missed dose—If you miss a dose of this medicine, take it as soon as possible. However, if it is almost time for your next dose, skip the missed dose and go back to your regular dosing schedule. Do not double doses.

Storage—Store the medicine in a closed container at room temperature, away from heat, moisture, and direct light. Keep from freezing.

Keep out of the reach of children.

Do not keep outdated medicine or medicine no longer needed.

Precautions While Using This Medicine

It is very important that your doctor check your progress at regular visits. Your doctor may want to have certain tests done to see if you are receiving the right amount of medicine or if certain side effects may be occurring without your knowing it. Also, the amount of medicine you are taking may have to be changed often.

Do not take other medicines (prescription, over-the-counter [OTC] or herbal products) unless they have been discussed with your doctor.

Carbamazepine may cause some people to be agitated, irritable or display other abnormal behaviors. It may also cause some people to have suicidal thoughts and tendencies or to become more depressed. If you or your caregiver notice any of these unwanted effects, tell your doctor right away.

Check with your doctor right away if fever, sore throat, rash, ulcers in the mouth, easy bruising, or small red or purple spots on the skin occur. These could be symptoms of a serious blood problem.

This medicine will add to the effects of alcohol and other CNS depressants (medicines that cause drowsiness). Some examples of CNS depressants are antihistamines or medicine for hay fever, other allergies, or colds; sedatives, tranquilizers, or sleeping medicine; prescription pain medicine or narcotics; barbiturates; medicine for seizures; muscle relaxants; or anesthetics, including some dental anesthetics. Check with your doctor before taking any of the above while you are using this medicine.

This medicine may cause some people to become drowsy, dizzy, lightheaded, or less alert than they are normally, especially when they are starting treatment or increasing the dose. It may also cause blurred or double vision, weakness, or loss of muscle control in some people. Make sure you know how you react to this medicine before you drive, use machines, or do anything else that could be dangerous if you are not alert and well-coordinated or able to see well.

Some people who take carbamazepine may become more sensitive to sunlight than they are normally. Exposure to sunlight, even for brief periods of time, may cause a skin rash, itching, redness or other discoloration of the skin, or a severe sunburn. When you begin taking this medicine:

- Stay out of direct sunlight, especially between the hours of 10:00 a.m. and 3:00 p.m., if possible.
- Wear protective clothing, including a hat. Also, wear sunglasses.
- Apply a sun block product that has a skin protection factor (SPF) of at least 15. Some patients may require a product with a higher SPF number, especially if they have a fair complexion. If you have any questions about this, check with your health care professional.
- Apply a sun block lipstick that has an SPF of at least 15 to protect your lips.
- Do not use a sunlamp or tanning bed or booth.

If you have a severe reaction from the sun, check with your doctor.

Oral contraceptives (birth control pills) containing estrogen may not work properly if you take them while you are taking carbamazepine. Unplanned pregnancies may occur. You should use a different or additional means of birth control while you are taking carbamazepine. If you have any questions about this, check with your health care professional.

For diabetic patients:

- Carbamazepine may affect urine sugar levels. While you are using this medicine, be especially careful when testing for sugar in your urine. If you notice a change in the results of your urine sugar tests or have any questions about this, check with your doctor.

For patients taking the oral suspension form of Tegretol:

- Do not take any other liquid medicines at the same time that you take your dose of Tegretol without first checking with your doctor.

Before having any medical tests, tell the medical doctor in charge that you are taking this medicine. The results of some pregnancy tests and the metyrapone test may be affected by this medicine.

Before having any kind of surgery, dental treatment, or emergency treatment, tell the medical doctor or dentist in charge that you are taking this medicine. Taking carbamazepine together with medicines that are used during surgery or dental or emergency treatments may increase the CNS depressant effects and cause other unwanted effects.

Your doctor may want you to carry a medical identification card or bracelet stating that you are taking this medicine.

Side Effects of This Medicine

Along with its needed effects, a medicine may cause some unwanted effects. Although not all of these side effects may occur, if they do occur they may need medical attention.

Check with your doctor immediately if any of the following side effects occur:

Rare

Black, tarry stools; blood in urine or stools; bone or joint pain; cough or hoarseness; darkening of urine; lower back or side pain; nosebleeds or other unusual bleeding or bruising; painful or difficult urination; pain, tenderness, swelling, or bluish color in leg or foot; pale stools; pinpoint red spots on skin; shortness of breath or cough; sores, ulcers, or white spots on lips or in the mouth; sore throat, chills, and fever; swollen or painful glands; unusual tiredness or weakness; wheezing, tightness in chest, or troubled breathing; yellow eyes or skin

Symptoms of overdose

Body spasm in which head and heels are bent backward and body is bowed forward; clumsiness or unsteadiness; convulsions (seizures)— especially in small children; dizziness (severe) or fainting; drowsiness (severe); fast or irregular heartbeat; high or low blood pressure (hypertension or hypotension); irregular, slow, or shallow breathing; large pupils; nausea or vomiting (severe); overactive reflexes followed by underactive reflexes; poor control in body movements (for example, when reaching or stepping); sudden decrease in amount of urine; trembling, twitching, or abnormal body movements

Check with your doctor as soon as possible if any of the following side effects occur:

More common

Blurred vision or double vision; continuous back-and-forth eye movements

Less common

Actions that are out of control; behavioral changes (especially in children); confusion, agitation, or hostility (especially in the elderly); diarrhea (severe); discouragement; drooling; fear; feeling of unreality; feeling sad or empty; headache (continuing); increase in seizures;

irritability; lack of appetite; loss of balance control; loss of interest or pleasure; muscle trembling, jerking or stiffness; nausea and vomiting (severe); other problems with muscle control or coordination; sense of detachment from self or body; shakiness and unsteady walk; shuffling walk; skin rash, hives, or itching; stiffness of limb; sudden, wide mood swings; talking, feeling, and acting with excitement; thoughts or attempts of killing oneself; tiredness; trouble concentrating; trouble sleeping; twisting movements of the body; uncontrolled movements, especially of face, neck, and back; unusual drowsiness

Rare

Chest pain; difficulty in speaking or slurred speech; fainting; frequent urination; irregular, pounding, or unusually slow heartbeat; mental depression with restlessness and nervousness or other mood or mental changes; muscle or stomach cramps; numbness, tingling, pain, or weakness in hands and feet; rapid weight gain; rigidity; ringing, buzzing, or other unexplained sounds in the ears; sudden decrease in amount of urine; swelling of face, hands, feet, or lower legs; trembling; uncontrolled body movements; visual hallucinations (seeing things that are not there)

Some side effects may occur that usually do not need medical attention. These side effects may go away during treatment as your body adjusts to the medicine. Also, your health care professional may be able to tell you about ways to prevent or reduce some of these side effects. Check with your health care professional if any of the following side effects continue or are bothersome or if you have any questions about them:

More common

Clumsiness or unsteadiness; dizziness (mild); drowsiness (mild); lightheadedness; nausea or vomiting (mild)

Less common or rare

Accidental injury; aching joints or muscles; acid sour or stomach; back pain; belching; constipation; diarrhea; dryness of mouth; headache; heartburn; increased sensitivity of skin to sunlight (skin rash, itching, redness or other discoloration of skin, or severe sunburn); increased sweating; indigestion; irritation or soreness of tongue or mouth; itching skin; lack or loss of strength; loss of appetite; loss of hair; loss of memory; problems with memory; sexual problems in males; sleepiness; stomach pain, upset, or discomfort

Other side effects not listed may also occur in some patients. If you notice any other effects, check with your healthcare professional.

CARBIDOPA, ENTACAPONE, AND LEVODOPA (Oral route) - kar-bi-DOE-pa, en-TA-ka-pone, lee-voe-DOE-pa

Commonly used brand name(s)

In the U.S.—
Stalevo 100
Stalevo 150
Stalevo 50

Available Dosage Forms:
• Tablet

Therapeutic Class: Antiparkinsonian
Pharmacologic Class: Dopamine Precursor

Uses For This Medicine

Carbidopa, entacapone and levodopa is used to treat Parkinson's disease, sometimes referred to as shaking palsy. Parkinson's disease is a disorder of the central nervous system (brain and spinal cord).

Dopamine is a naturally occurring substance in the brain that helps provide control of movement and activities such as walking and talking. In patients with Parkinson's disease there is not enough dopamine in some parts of the brain. Levodopa (a component of this medicine) enters the brain and helps replace the missing dopamine, which allows people to function better. By increasing the amount of dopamine in the brain levodopa helps control symptoms and helps you to perform daily activities such as dressing, walking and handling utensils.

This medicine is a combination of three different medicines. This medicine is known as a levodopa therapy. The difference between this medicine and other levodopa therapies is that this medicine also has entacapone in it. Entacapone helps levodopa last longer by blocking a substance called COMT enzyme. This enzyme breaks down levodopa before it reaches the brain. When less levodopa is broken down, more is available to the brain. Increased availability of levodopa may lead to smoother and steadier levels of dopamine in the brain, which may provide better symptom control for longer periods each day. This may lead to improvement in daily activities.

This medicine is available only with your doctor's prescription.

Before Using This Medicine

In deciding to use a medicine, the risks of taking the medicine must be weighed against the good it will do. This is a decision you and your doctor will make. For this medicine, the following should be considered:

Allergies—Tell your doctor if you have ever had any unusual or allergic reaction to this medicine or any other medicines. Also tell your health care professional if you have any other types of allergies, such as to foods, dyes, preservatives, or animals. For non-prescription products, read the label or package ingredients carefully.

Pediatric—Studies on this medicine have been done only in adult patients, and there is no specific information comparing use of carbidopa, entacapone or levodopa in children with use in other age groups.

Geriatric—Many medicines have not been studied specifically in older people. Therefore, it may not be known whether they work the same way in older people as they do in younger adults or if they cause different side effects or problems in older people. There is no specific information comparing the use of carbidopa, entacapone and levodopa combination in the elderly with use in other age groups.

Other medicines—

Using this medicine with any of the following medicines is not recommended. Your doctor may decide not to treat you with

this medication or change some of the other medicines you take.

Clorgyline, Iproniazid, Isocarboxazid, Nialamide, Pargyline, Phenelzine, Procarbazine, Selegiline, Toloxatone, Tranylcypromine

Interactions with Food/Tobacco/Alcohol—Certain medicines should not be used at or around the time of eating food or eating certain types of food since interactions may occur. Using alcohol or tobacco with certain medicines may also cause interactions to occur. Discuss with your healthcare professional the use of your medicine with food, alcohol, or tobacco.

Other medical problems—The presence of other medical problems may affect the use of this medicine. Make sure you tell your doctor if you have any other medical problems, especially:

- Narrow– angle glaucoma (eye pressure problem)—Carbidopa, entacapone and levodopa combination should not be used in patients with this medical problem.

- Melanoma, history of (skin cancer) or

- Skin lesions, undiagnosed (rashes that involve changes in color or texture of the skin)—This medicine may make these medical problems worse.

- Heart attack, history of, with arrhythmias (abnormal heart rhythms)—This medicine should be used with caution with these medical problems.

- Wide-angle glaucoma (eye pressure problem)—This medicine should be used with caution with this medical problem.

Proper Use of This Medicine

Since protein may interfere with the body's response to levodopa, high protein diets should be avoided. Intake of normal amounts of protein should be spaced equally throughout the day, or taken as directed by your doctor.

It is very important that you take your medicine exactly as directed, and every time that you are supposed to take it. It is important that you do not stop taking your medication unless ordered by your doctor. It is also important to not start taking other medicines for your Parkinson's disease without first talking with your doctor.

You may experience a "wearing-off" effect towards the end of the dosing interval. You should tell your doctor if you have problems with this that affect your every day life. Your doctor may want to adjust your dose.

This medicine begins to release its ingredients 30 minutes after you take it.

It is possible that a dark color (red, brown, or black) may appear in saliva, urine, or sweat after taking this medicine. The color may cause some of your garments to become discolored.

It is important to discuss with your doctor any change to your diet. High protein diets or too much acidity in your stomach may cause problems with the way this medicine is absorbed by your body.

If you are taking multi-vitamin tablets or plan to start taking them discuss this with your doctor. Iron salts (in vitamins) may cause this medicine not to work as well.

Dosing—The dose of this medicine will be different for different patients. Follow your doctor's orders or the directions on the label. The following information includes only the average doses of this medicine. If your dose is different, do not change it unless your doctor tells you to do so.

The amount of medicine that you take depends on the strength of the medicine. Also, the number of doses you take each day, the time allowed between doses, and the length of time you take the medicine depend on the medical problem for which you are using the medicine.

- For oral dosage form (capsules):
  - For Parkinson's disease:
    - Adults—The starting dose is usually the same as the current dose you are taking. If you are starting this medicine for the first time your doctor may want to start you on a carbidopa and levodopa combination with entacapone and gradually switch you over to this combination.
    - Children—Use and dose must be determined by your doctor.

Storage—Store the medicine in a closed container at room temperature, away from heat, moisture, and direct light. Do not refrigerate. Keep from freezing.

Keep out of the reach of children.

Do not keep outdated medicine or medicine no longer needed.

Ask your healthcare professional how you should dispose of any medicine you do not use.

Precautions While Using This Medicine

It is important to understand that hypotension (decrease in blood pressure, especially when getting up from a sitting position) may develop. This may occur more frequently when you are beginning treatment with the medicine or when your dosage is increased.

You should get up carefully after sitting or lying down, especially if you have been doing so for long periods of time. You should use extra caution when getting up after sitting or lying down, especially during the beginning of treatment with carbidopa, entacapone and levodopa combination.

It is very important that you discuss new medications with your doctor before starting any new medications.

It is possible that you may experience hallucinations (seeing or hearing things that are not there) or an increase in dyskinesia (trouble in moving). Talk with your doctor if you have any questions about this.

It is possible that you may become nauseous, especially when you are first starting your medicine.

It is important to tell your doctor if you are pregnant or breastfeeding or are planning to become pregnant or planning to breast feed your baby.

This medicine may cause some people to become drowsy, dizzy, or less alert than they are normally. Make sure you know how you react to this medicine before you drive, use machines, or do anything else that could be dangerous if you are dizzy or are not alert.

Side Effects of This Medicine

Along with its needed effects, a medicine may cause some unwanted effects. Although not all of these side effects may occur, if they do occur they may need medical attention.

Also, because of the way these medicines act on the body, there is a chance that they might cause other unwanted effects that may not occur until months or years after the medicine is used. These may include certain types of cancer, such as leukemia or bladder cancer. Discuss these possible effects with your doctor.

Check with your doctor immediately if any of the following side effects occur:

More common-Entacapone
Twitching, twisting, uncontrolled repetitive movements of tongue, lips, face, arms, or legs

Incidence unknown-Carbidopa and Levodopa and/or Levodopa alone
Bleeding gums; bloody or black, tarry stools; bloody or cloudy urine; bluish color; change in size, shape or color of existing mole; changes in skin color; chest pain, discomfort, or tightness; constipation; constricted pupil; convulsions; cough; dark-colored urine; difficult or labored breathing; difficulty in speaking; drooling; drooping eyelid (ptosis); facial dryness; fast, irregular, or pounding heart beat; fever with or without chills; fixed position of eye; general feeling of illness; hallucinations [seeing, hearing, or feeling things that are not there]; hoarseness; high or low blood pressure; large, flat, blue or purplish patches in the skin; large, hive-like swelling on face, eyelids, lips, tongue, throat, hands, legs, feet, sex organs; loss of appetite; loss of bladder control; lower abdominal pain; lower back or side pain; mole that leaks fluid or bleeds; muscle cramps or spasms; muscle pain or stiffness; muscle trembling, jerking, or stiffness; nausea; new mole; pain; painful knees and ankles; pain or discomfort in arms, jaw, back or neck; painful or difficult urination; pale skin; pinpoint red spots on skin; raised red swellings on the skin, the buttocks, legs or ankles; restlessness; seizures; severe mental changes; severe stomach pain; shakiness and unsteady walk; shortness of breath; shuffling walk; sore throat; sores, ulcers, or white spots on lips or in mouth; stomach pain; sweating; swollen glands; tenderness and swelling of foot or leg; trembling, or other problems with muscle control or coordination; uncontrolled movements, especially of face, neck, and back; unusual bleeding or bruising; unusual tiredness or weakness; vomiting; vomiting of blood or material that looks like coffee grounds

Some side effects may occur that usually do not need medical attention. These side effects may go away during treatment as your body adjusts to the medicine. Also, your health care professional may be able to tell you about ways to prevent or reduce some of these side effects. Check with your health care professional if any of the following side effects continue or are bothersome or if you have any questions about them:

More common-Entacapone
Absence of or decrease in body movement; diarrhea; dizziness; urine discoloration

Less common-Entacapone
Acid or sour stomach; anxiety; bacterial infection; belching; bitter, sour or unusual taste in mouth; bloated; burning feeling in chest or stomach; discomfort; dry mouth; excess air or gas in stomach or intestines; fear; full feeling; heartburn; hyperventilation; increased sweating; indigestion; irritability; lack or loss of strength; nervousness; passing gas; restlessness; sleepiness or unusual drowsiness; stomach discomfort, or upset; swollen mouth and tongue; tenderness in stomach area; trouble sleeping; urge to have bowel movement; wheezing

Incidence unknown-Carbidopa and Levodopa and/or Levodopa alone
Being forgetful; bizarre breathing patterns; bladder pain; blurred vision; body aches or pain; burning, crawling, itching, numbness, prickling, "pins and needles", or tingling feelings; burning and upper abdominal pain; burning sensation of the tongue; clenching, gnashing, or grinding teeth; confusion about identity, place, and time; dark saliva; dark sweat; decreased mental acuity; difficulty opening the mouth; difficulty swallowing; discouragement; double vision; ear congestion; enlarged pupils; excessive watering of mouth; fainting; faintness, or lightheadedness when getting up from a lying or sitting position suddenly; false or unusual sense of well-being; feeling like you will pass out; feeling of warmth; feeling sad or empty; flushing; hives or welts; hair loss; increased blinking; headache; hiccups; increased interest in sexual ability, desire, drive, or performance; increased interest in sexual intercourse; lack of appetite; large, hard skin blisters; leg pain; lockjaw; loss of interest or pleasure; loss of voice; muscle spasm, especially of neck and back; nasal congestion; nightmares; numbness; pain in the chest below the breastbone; painful or prolonged erection of the penis; pharyngeal pain; poor insight and judgment; pounding in the ears; problems with memory or speech; redness of skin; redness of the face, neck, arms and occasionally upper chest; runny nose; sense of stimulation; shoulder pain; skin rash; sleeplessness; slow movement; slow or fast heartbeat; slow reflexes; sneezing; swelling; tremor, increased; trouble concentrating; trouble recognizing objects; trouble thinking and planning; twitching of eyelids; urinary frequency; urinary retention; weight gain; weight loss

Other side effects not listed may also occur in some patients. If you notice any other effects, check with your healthcare professional.

CARBOHYDRATES AND ELECTROLYTES (Systemic)

Some commonly used brand names are:

In the U.S.—

Infalyte (3)	Pedialyte (1)
Kao Lectrolyte (1)	Pedialyte Freezer Pops (1)
Naturalyte (1)	Rehydralyte (1)
Oralyte (1)	Resol (1)

In Canada—

Lytren (1)	Pedialyte (1)
Gastrolyte (2)	Rapolyte (2)

This information applies to the following medicines:

1. Dextrose and Electrolytes (DEX-trose and ee-LEK-tro-lites)
2. Oral Rehydration Salts (OR-al ree-hi-DRA-shen solts)
3. Rice Syrup Solids and Electrolytes (RIS SIR-ep SOL-ids and ee-LEK-tro-lites)

Category

- **Electrolyte replenisher**—Dextrose and Electrolytes; Oral Rehydration Salts; Rice Syrup Solids and Electrolytes

Description

Carbohydrate and electrolytes combination is used to treat or prevent dehydration (the loss of too much water from the body) that may occur with severe diarrhea, especially in babies and young children. Although this medicine does not immediately stop the diarrhea, it replaces the water and some important salts (electrolytes), such as sodium and potassium, that are lost from the body during diarrhea, and helps prevent more serious problems. Some carbohydrate and electrolytes solutions may also be used after surgery when food intake has been stopped.

This medicine is available without a prescription; however, your doctor may have special instructions on the proper use and dose for you or your child.

Carbohydrate and electrolytes combination is available in the following dosage forms:

Oral
- Solution
- Powder for oral solution

Before Using This Medicine

If you are taking this medicine without a prescription, carefully read and follow any precautions on the label. For carbohydrate and electrolytes solutions, the following should be considered:

Allergies—Tell your health care professional if you have ever had any unusual or allergic reaction to medicines containing potassium, sodium, citrates, rice, or sugar. Also tell your health care professional if you are allergic to any other substances, such as foods, preservatives, or dyes.

Pregnancy—Carbohydrate and electrolytes solutions have not been shown to cause birth defects or other problems in humans.

Breast-feeding—This medicine has not been reported to cause problems in nursing babies. Breast-feeding should continue, if possible, during treatment with carbohydrate and electrolytes solution.

Children—This medicine has been tested in children and, in effective doses, appears to be safe and effective in children. This medicine has not been tested in premature infants.

Older adults—This medicine has been tested and has been shown to be well tolerated by older people.

Other medicines—Although certain medicines should not be used together at all, in other cases two different medicines may be used together even if an interaction might occur. In these cases, your doctor may want to change the dose, or other precautions may be necessary. Tell your health care professional if you are taking any other prescription or nonprescription (over-the-counter [OTC]) medicine.

Other medical problems—The presence of other medical problems may affect the use of carbohydrate and electrolytes solutions. Make sure you tell your doctor if you have any other medical problems, especially:

- Difficult urination—This condition may prevent the carbohydrate and electrolytes solution from working properly
- Inability to drink or
- Vomiting (severe and continuing)—Treatment by injection may need to be given to patients with these conditions
- Intestinal blockage—Carbohydrate and electrolytes solution may be harmful if given to patients with this condition

Proper Use of This Medicine

For patients using the *commercial powder form* of this medicine:

- Add 7 ounces of boiled, cooled tap water to the entire contents of one powder packet. Shake or stir the container for 2 or 3 minutes until all the powder is dissolved.
- Do not add more water to the solution after it is mixed.
- Do not boil the solution.
- Make and use a fresh solution each day.

For patients using the *freezer pop form* of this medicine:

- Pops should be removed from the box before being placed in the freezer. The pops should be frozen before separating.
- The freezer pop can be eaten without freezing, but tastes best when frozen. To eat the frozen pop, cut the top of the wrapper open and push the pop from the bottom of the plastic sleeve.
- To drink as a liquid, cut the top of the wrapper open and pour the unfrozen pop into a cup or glass.

For patients using the *powder form* of this medicine *distributed by the World Health Organization (WHO)*:

- Add the entire contents of one powder packet to enough drinking water to make one quart (32 ounces) or liter of solution. Shake the container for 2 or 3 minutes until all the powder is dissolved.
- Do not add more water to the solution after it is mixed.
- Do not boil the solution.
- Make and use a fresh solution each day.

Babies and small children should be given the solution slowly, in small amounts, with a spoon, as often as possible, during the first 24 hours of diarrhea.

Take as directed. Do not take it for a longer time than your doctor has recommended. To do so may increase the chance of side effects.

Dosing—The dose of these combination medicines will be different for different patients. *Follow your doctor's orders or the directions on the label*. The following information includes only the average doses of these medicines. *If your dose is different, do not change it* unless your doctor tells you to do so.

For dextrose and electrolytes and for rice syrup solids and electrolytes

- For rehydration (to replace the water and some important salts [electrolytes]):
  - For *oral* dosage form (solution):

- Adults and children over 10 years of age—Dose is based on body weight and must be determined by your doctor. At first, the usual dose is 50 to 100 milliliters (mL) per kilogram (kg) (23 to 45 mL per pound) of body weight taken over four to six hours. Your doctor may change the dose depending on your thirst and your response to the treatment.
- Children up to 2 years of age—The dose is based on body weight and must be determined by your doctor. At first, the usual dose is 75 mL per kg (34 mL per pound) of body weight during the first eight hours and 75 mL per kg (34 mL per pound) of body weight during the next sixteen hours. Your doctor may change the dose depending on your thirst and your response to the treatment. However, the dose is usually not more than 100 mL in any 20-minute period.
- Children 2 to 10 years of age—Dose is based on body weight and must be determined by your doctor. At first, the usual dose is 50 mL per kg (23 mL per pound) of body weight taken over the first four to six hours. Then, the dose is 100 mL per kg (45 mL per pound) of body weight taken over the next eighteen to twenty-four hours. Your doctor may change the dose depending on your thirst and your response to the treatment. However, the dose is usually not more than 100 mL in any 20-minute period.
  - For *oral* dosage form (solution for freezer pop):
    - Children up to 1 year of age—Use must be determined by your doctor.
    - Children older than 1 year of age—Freezer pop may be given as often as desired.

For oral rehydration salts
- For rehydration (to replace the water and some important salts [electrolytes]):
  - For *oral* dosage form (solution):
    - Adults and teenagers—Dose is based on body weight and must be determined by your doctor. At first, the usual dose is 50 to 100 milliliters (mL) of solution per kilogram (kg) (23 to 45 mL per pound) of body weight taken over four to six hours. Your doctor may change the dose depending on your thirst and your response to the treatment.
    - Children—Dose is based on body weight and must be determined by your doctor. At first, the usual dose is 50 to 100 mL per kg (23 to 45 mL per pound) of body weight taken over the first four hours. Your doctor may change the dose depending on your thirst and your response to the treatment.

Storage—To store this medicine:
- Keep out of the reach of children.
- Store away from heat and direct light.
- Do not store the powder packets in the bathroom, near the kitchen sink, or in other damp places. Heat or moisture may cause the medicine to break down.
- Store the liquid in the refrigerator. However, keep the medicine from freezing.
- Make a fresh solution each day. Discard unused solution at the end of each day. Be sure that any discarded medicine is out of the reach of children.

Precautions While Using This Medicine

Eat soft foods, if possible, such as rice cereal, bananas, cooked peas or beans, and potatoes to keep up nutrition until the diarrhea stops and regular food and milk can be taken again. Breast-fed infants should be given breast milk between doses of the solution.

If your diarrhea does not improve in 1 or 2 days, or if it becomes worse, check with your doctor.

Also, *check with your doctor immediately* if your baby or child appears to have severe thirst, doughy skin, sunken eyes, dizziness or lightheadedness, tiredness or weakness, irritability, difficult urination, loss of weight, or convulsions (seizures). These signs may mean that too much water has been lost from the body.

For patients (except nursing babies) using the *powder form* of this medicine:
- Drink plain water whenever thirsty between doses of solution.

For patients taking the *premixed liquid form* of this medicine:
- Do not drink fruit juices or eat foods containing added salt until the diarrhea has stopped.

Side Effects

Along with its needed effects, a medicine may cause some unwanted effects. Although not all of these side effects may occur, if they do occur they may need medical attention.

Check with your doctor as soon as possible if any of the following side effects occur:
Symptoms of too much sodium (salt) in the body
Convulsions (seizures); dizziness; fast heartbeat; high blood pressure; irritability; muscle twitching; restlessness; swelling of feet or lower legs; weakness
Symptoms of too much fluid in the body
Puffy eyelids

Other side effects may occur that usually do not need medical attention. These side effects may go away during treatment as your body adjusts to the medicine. However, check with your doctor if the following side effect continues or is bothersome:
More common
Vomiting (mild)

Other side effects not listed above may also occur in some patients. If you notice any other effects, check with your doctor.

CARBONIC ANHYDRASE INHIBITORS   (Systemic)

Some commonly used brand names are:

In the U.S.—

Ak-Zol (1)	Diamox Sequels (1)
Daranide (2)	MZM (3)
Dazamide (1)	Neptazane (3)
Diamox (1)	Storzolamide (1)

In Canada—

Acetazolam (1)	Diamox Sequels (1)
Apo-Acetazolamide (1)	Neptazane (3)
Diamox (1)	

This information applies to the following medicines:

1. Acetazolamide (a-set-a-ZOLE-a-mide)
2. Dichlorphenamide (dye-klor-FEN-a-mide)
3. Methazolamide (meth-a-ZOLE-a-mide)

Category

- **Altitude sickness, acute, prophylactic and therapeutic agent**—Acetazolamide
- **Anticonvulsant**—Acetazolamide
- **Antiglaucoma agent, systemic**—Acetazolamide; Dichlorphenamide; Methazolamide
- **Antiparalytic, familial periodic paralysis**—Acetazolamide
- **Antiurolithic, cystine calculi**—Acetazolamide
- **Antiurolithic, uric acid calculi**—Acetazolamide
- **Diuretic, urinary alkalinizing**—Acetazolamide

Description

Carbonic anhydrase inhibitors are used to treat glaucoma. Acetazolamide is also used as an anticonvulsant to control certain seizures in the treatment of epilepsy. It is also sometimes used to prevent or lessen some effects in mountain climbers who climb to high altitudes, and to treat other conditions as determined by your doctor.

These medicines are available only with your doctor's prescription, in the following dosage forms:

Oral
- Acetazolamide
  - Extended-release capsules
  - Tablets
- Dichlorphenamide
  - Tablets
- Methazolamide
  - Tablets

Parenteral
- Acetazolamide
  - Injection

Before Using This Medicine

In deciding to use a medicine, the risks of taking the medicine must be weighed against the good it will do. This is a decision you and your doctor will make. For carbonic anhydrase inhibitors, the following should be considered:

Allergies—Tell your doctor if you have ever had any unusual or allergic reaction to carbonic anhydrase inhibitors, sulfonamides (sulfa drugs), or thiazide diuretics (a type of water pill). Also tell your health care professional if you are allergic to any other substances, such as foods, preservatives, or dyes.

Pregnancy—Carbonic anhydrase inhibitors have not been studied in pregnant women. However, studies in animals have shown that carbonic anhydrase inhibitors cause birth defects. Before taking this medicine, make sure your doctor knows if you are pregnant or if you may become pregnant.

Breast-feeding—Carbonic anhydrase inhibitors may pass into the breast milk. These medicines are not recommended during breast-feeding, because they may cause unwanted effects in nursing babies. It may be necessary for you to use another medicine or to stop breast-feeding during treatment. Be sure you have discussed this with your doctor.

Children—Although there is no specific information comparing use of carbonic anhydrase inhibitors in children with use in other age groups, these medicines are not expected to cause different side effects or problems in children than they do in adults.

Older adults—Many medicines have not been studied specifically in older people. Therefore, it may not be known whether they work exactly the same way they do in younger adults. Although there is no specific information comparing use of carbonic anhydrase inhibitors in the elderly with use in other age groups, these medicines are not expected to cause different side effects or problems in older people than they do in younger adults.

Other medicines—Although certain medicines should not be used together at all, in other cases two different medicines may be used together even if an interaction might occur. In these cases, your doctor may want to change the dose, or other precautions may be necessary. When you are using carbonic anhydrase inhibitors, it is especially important that your health care professional know if you are using any of the following:

- Amphetamines or
- Mecamylamine (e.g., Inversine) or
- Quinidine (e.g., Quinidex)—Use of carbonic anhydrase inhibitors may increase the chance of side effects
- Methenamine (e.g., Mandelamine)—Use of carbonic anhydrase inhibitors may decrease the effectiveness of methenamine

Other medical problems—The presence of other medical problems may affect the use of carbonic anhydrase inhibitors. Make sure you tell your doctor if you have any other medical problems, especially:

- Diabetes mellitus (sugar diabetes)—Use of carbonic anhydrase inhibitors may increase the patient's blood and urine sugar concentrations
- Emphysema or other chronic lung disease—Use of carbonic anhydrase inhibitors may increase the risk of acidosis (shortness of breath, troubled breathing)
- Gout or
- Low blood levels of potassium or sodium—Use of carbonic anhydrase inhibitors may make the condition worse
- Kidney disease or stones—Higher blood levels of carbonic anhydrase inhibitors may result, which may increase the chance of side effects; also, these medicines may make the condition worse
- Liver disease—Use of carbonic anhydrase inhibitors may increase the risk of electrolyte imbalance and may make the condition worse
- Underactive adrenal gland (Addison's disease)—Use of carbonic anhydrase inhibitors may increase the risk of electrolyte imbalance

Proper Use of This Medicine

Take this medicine only as directed. Do not take more of it and do not take it more often than your doctor ordered. To do so may increase the chance of side effects without increasing the effectiveness of this medicine.

This medicine may be taken with meals to lessen the chance of stomach upset. However, if stomach upset (nausea or vomiting) continues, check with your doctor.

This medicine may cause an increase in the amount of urine or in your frequency of urination. If you continue to take the medicine every day, these effects should lessen or stop. To keep the increase in urine from affecting your nighttime sleep:

- If you are to take a single dose a day, take it in the morning after breakfast.
- If you are to take more than one dose a day, take the last dose no later than 6 p.m., unless otherwise directed by your doctor.

However, it is best to plan your dose or doses according to a schedule that will least affect your personal activities and sleep. Ask your health care professional to help you plan the best time to take this medicine.

Dosing—The doses of carbonic anhydrase inhibitors will be different for different patients. *Follow your doctor's orders or the directions on the label.* The following information includes only the average doses of these medicines. *If your dose is different, do not change it* unless your doctor tells you to do so.

The number of capsules or tablets that you take depends on the strength of the medicine. Also, *the number of doses you take each day, the time allowed between doses, and the length of time you take the medicine depend on the medical problem for which you are taking the carbonic anhydrase inhibitor.*

For acetazolamide
- For *oral* dosage form (extended-release capsules):
  ○ For glaucoma:
    ▪ Adults—500 milligrams (mg) two times a day, in the morning and evening.
    ▪ Children—Use and dose must be determined by your doctor.
  ○ For altitude sickness:
    ▪ Adults—500 mg one or two times a day.
    ▪ Children—Use and dose must be determined by your doctor.
- For *oral* dosage form (tablets):
  ○ For glaucoma:
    ▪ Adults—250 mg one to four times a day.
    ▪ Children—Dose is based on body weight and must be determined by your doctor. The usual dose is 10 to 15 mg per kilogram (kg) (4.5 to 6.8 mg per pound) of body weight a day in divided doses.
  ○ For epilepsy:
    ▪ Adults and children—Dose is based on body weight and must be determined by your doctor. The usual dose is 10 mg per kg (4.5 mg per pound) of body weight a day in divided doses.
  ○ For altitude sickness:
    ▪ Adults—250 mg two to four times a day.
    ▪ Children—Use and dose must be determined by your doctor.
- For *injection* dosage form:
  ○ For glaucoma:
    ▪ Adults—500 mg, injected into a muscle or vein, for one dose.

  - Children—Dose is based on body weight and must be determined by your doctor. The usual dose is 5 to 10 mg per kg (2.3 to 4.5 mg per pound) of body weight every six hours, injected into a muscle or vein.

For dichlorphenamide
- For *oral* dosage form (tablets):
  ○ For glaucoma:
    ▪ Adults—25 to 50 milligrams (mg) one to three times a day.
    ▪ Children—Use and dose must be determined by your doctor.

For methazolamide
- For *oral* dosage form (tablets):
  ○ For glaucoma:
    ▪ Adults—50 to 100 milligrams (mg) two or three times a day.
    ▪ Children—Use and dose must be determined by your doctor.

Missed dose—If you miss a dose of this medicine, take it as soon as possible. However, if it is almost time for your next dose, skip the missed dose and go back to your regular dosing schedule. Do not double doses.

Storage—To store this medicine:

- Keep out of the reach of children.
- Store away from heat and direct light.
- Do not store the capsule or tablet form of this medicine in the bathroom, near the kitchen sink, or in other damp places. Heat or moisture may cause the medicine to break down.
- Do not keep outdated medicine or medicine no longer needed. Be sure that any discarded medicine is out of the reach of children.

Precautions While Using This Medicine

This medicine may cause some people to feel drowsy, dizzy, lightheaded, or more tired than they are normally. *Make sure you know how you react to this medicine before you drive, use machines, or do anything else that could be dangerous if you are not alert.*

It is important that your doctor check your progress at regular visits. Your doctor may want to do certain tests to see if the medicine is working properly or to see if certain side effects may be occurring without your knowing it.

This medicine may cause a loss of potassium from your body. To help prevent this, your doctor may want you to eat or drink foods that have a high potassium content (for example, orange or other citrus fruit juices) or take a potassium supplement. It is very important to follow these directions. Also, it is important not to change your diet on your own. This is more important if you are already on a special diet (as for diabetes) or if you are taking a potassium supplement. Extra potassium may not be necessary and, in some cases, too much potassium could be harmful.

For diabetic patients:
- This medicine may raise blood and urine sugar levels. While you are using this medicine, be especially careful in testing for sugar in your blood or urine. If you have any questions about this, check with your doctor.

Your doctor may want you to increase the amount of fluids you drink while you are taking this medicine. This is to prevent kidney stones. However, do not increase the amount of fluids you drink without first checking with your doctor.

For patients taking *acetazolamide as an anticonvulsant:*
- *If you have been taking acetazolamide regularly for several weeks or more, do not suddenly stop taking it.* Your doctor may want you to reduce gradually the amount you are taking before stopping completely.

Side Effects

Along with its needed effects, a medicine may cause some unwanted effects. Although not all of these side effects may occur, if they do occur they may need medical attention.

Check with your doctor immediately if either of the following side effects occurs:
  Rare
    Shortness of breath or trouble in breathing

Also, check with your doctor as soon as possible if any of the following side effects occur:
  More common
    Unusual tiredness or weakness

  Less common
    Blood in urine; difficult urination; mental depression; pain in lower back; pain or burning while urinating; sudden decrease in amount of urine

  Rare
    Bloody or black, tarry stools; clumsiness or unsteadiness; confusion; convulsions (seizures); darkening of urine; fever; hives, itching of skin, skin rash, or sores; muscle weakness (severe); pale stools; ringing or buzzing in the ears; sore throat; trembling; unusual bruising or bleeding; yellow eyes or skin

  Symptoms of too much potassium loss
    Dryness of mouth; increased thirst; irregular heartbeats; mood or mental changes; muscle cramps or pain; nausea or vomiting; unusual tiredness or weakness; weak pulse

Also, check with your doctor if you have any changes in your vision (especially problems with seeing faraway objects) when you first begin taking this medicine.

Other side effects may occur that usually do not need medical attention. These side effects may go away during treatment as your body adjusts to the medicine. However, check with your doctor if any of the following side effects continue or are bothersome:
  More common
    Diarrhea; general feeling of discomfort or illness; increase in frequency of urination or amount of urine (rare with methazolamide); loss of appetite; metallic taste in mouth; nausea or vomiting; numbness, tingling, or burning in hands, fingers, feet, toes, mouth, lips, tongue, or anus; weight loss

  Less common or rare
    Constipation; dizziness or lightheadedness; drowsiness; feeling of choking or lump in the throat; headache; increased sensitivity of eyes to sunlight; loss of taste and smell; nervousness or irritability

Other side effects not listed above may also occur in some patients. If you notice any other effects, check with your doctor.

CARBOPLATIN (Intravenous route) -
KAR-boe-pla-tin

Black Box Warning

Carboplatin should be administered under the supervision of a qualified physician experienced in the use of cancer chemotherapeutic agents. Appropriate management of therapy and complications is possible only when adequate treatment facilities are readily available.

Bone marrow suppression is dose related and may be severe, resulting in infection and/or bleeding. Anemia may be cumulative and may require transfusion support. Vomiting is another frequent drug-related side effect.

Anaphylactic-like reactions to carboplatin have been reported and may occur within minutes of carboplatin administration. Epinephrine, corticosteroids, and antihistamines have been employed to alleviate symptoms.

Commonly used brand name(s)

In the U.S.—
  Paraplatin
  Paraplatin NovaPlus

Available Dosage Forms:
- Powder for Solution
- Solution

Therapeutic Class: Antineoplastic Agent
Pharmacologic Class: Platinum Coordination Complex

Uses For This Medicine

Carboplatin belongs to the group of medicines known as alkylating agents. It is used to treat cancer of the ovaries. It may also be used to treat other kinds of cancer, as determined by your doctor.

Carboplatin interferes with the growth of cancer cells, which eventually are destroyed. Since the growth of normal body cells may also be affected by carboplatin, other effects also will occur. Some of these may be serious and must be reported to your doctor. Other effects may not be serious but may cause concern. Some effects may not occur until months or years after the medicine is used.

Before you begin treatment with carboplatin, you and your doctor should talk about the good this medicine will do as well as the risks of using it.

Carboplatin is to be administered only by or under the immediate supervision of your doctor.

Once a medicine has been approved for marketing for a certain use, experience may show that it is also useful for other medical problems. Although these uses are not included in product labeling, carboplatin is used in certain patients with the following medical conditions:
- Cancer of the bladder
- Cancer of the breast
- Cancer of the esophagus, including the junction between the esophagus and stomach
- Cancer of the fallopian tube or lining of the abdomen (spreading from the ovary)
- Cancers of the head and neck
- Cancer of the testicles (including seminoma)
- Cancers of the lymph system

- Cancer of the lung
- Cancer of the endometrium (the lining of the uterus)
- Cancer of unknown origin (primary site)
- Malignant melanoma (a certain type of skin cancer)
- Retinoblastoma (a certain type of eye cancer)
- Tumors in the brain

Before Using This Medicine

In deciding to use a medicine, the risks of taking the medicine must be weighed against the good it will do. This is a decision you and your doctor will make. For this medicine, the following should be considered:

Allergies—Tell your doctor if you have ever had any unusual or allergic reaction to this medicine or any other medicines. Also tell your health care professional if you have any other types of allergies, such as to foods, dyes, preservatives, or animals. For non-prescription products, read the label or package ingredients carefully.

Pediatric—Studies on this medicine have been done only in adult patients and there is no specific information comparing use of carboplatin in children with use in other age groups.

Geriatric—Some side effects of carboplatin (especially blood problems or numbness or tingling in fingers or toes) may be more likely to occur in the elderly.

Pregnancy—

	Pregnancy Category	Explanation
All Trimesters	D	Studies in pregnant women have demonstrated a risk to the fetus. However, the benefits of therapy in a life threatening situation or a serious disease, may outweigh the potential risk.

Breast Feeding—There are no adequate studies in women for determining infant risk when using this medication during breastfeeding. Weigh the potential benefits against the potential risks before taking this medication while breastfeeding.

Other medicines—

Using this medicine with any of the following medicines is not recommended. Your doctor may decide not to treat you with this medication or change some of the other medicines you take.

Rotavirus Vaccine, Live

Interactions with Food/Tobacco/Alcohol—Certain medicines should not be used at or around the time of eating food or eating certain types of food since interactions may occur. Using alcohol or tobacco with certain medicines may also cause interactions to occur. Discuss with your healthcare professional the use of your medicine with food, alcohol, or tobacco.

Other medical problems—The presence of other medical problems may affect the use of this medicine. Make sure you tell your doctor if you have any other medical problems, especially:
- Chickenpox (including recent exposure) or

- Herpes zoster (shingles)—Risk of severe disease affecting other parts of the body
- Hearing problems—May be worsened by carboplatin
- Infection—Carboplatin decreases your body's ability to fight infection
- Kidney disease—Effects may be increased because of slower removal from the body

Proper Use of This Medicine

This medicine is sometimes given together with certain other medicines. If you are using a combination of medicines, it is important that you receive each one at the proper time. If you are taking some of these medicines by mouth, ask your health care professional to help you plan a way to take them at the right times.

This medicine usually causes nausea and vomiting that sometimes may be severe. However, it is very important that you continue to receive the medicine, even if you begin to feel ill. Ask your health care professional for ways to lessen these effects, especially if they are severe.

Dosing—The dose of this medicine will be different for different patients. Follow your doctor's orders or the directions on the label. The following information includes only the average doses of this medicine. If your dose is different, do not change it unless your doctor tells you to do so.

The amount of medicine that you take depends on the strength of the medicine. Also, the number of doses you take each day, the time allowed between doses, and the length of time you take the medicine depend on the medical problem for which you are using the medicine.

Precautions While Using This Medicine

It is very important that your doctor check your progress at regular visits to make sure that this medicine is working properly and to check for unwanted effects.

While you are being treated with carboplatin, and after you stop treatment with it, do not have any immunizations (vaccinations) without your doctor's approval. Carboplatin may lower your body's resistance and there is a chance you might get the infection the immunization is meant to prevent. In addition, other persons living in your household should not take oral polio vaccine since there is a chance they could pass the polio virus on to you. Also, avoid persons who have taken oral polio vaccine within the last several months. Do not get close to them, and do not stay in the same room with them for very long. If you cannot take these precautions, you should consider wearing a protective face mask that covers the nose and mouth.

Carboplatin can temporarily lower the number of white blood cells in your blood, increasing the chance of getting an infection. It can also lower the number of platelets, which are necessary for proper blood clotting. If this occurs, there are certain precautions you can take, especially when your blood count is low, to reduce the risk of infection or bleeding:
- If you can, avoid people with infections. Check with your doctor immediately if you think you are getting an infection or if you get a fever or chills, cough or hoarseness, lower back or side pain, or painful or difficult urination.

- Check with your doctor immediately if you notice any unusual bleeding or bruising; black, tarry stools; blood in urine or stools; or pinpoint red spots on your skin.
- Be careful when using a regular toothbrush, dental floss, or toothpick. Your medical doctor, dentist, or nurse may recommend other ways to clean your teeth and gums. Check with your health care professional before having any dental work done.
- Do not touch your eyes or the inside of your nose unless you have just washed your hands and have not touched anything else in the meantime.
- Be careful not to cut yourself when you are using sharp objects such as a safety razor or fingernail or toenail cutters.
- Avoid contact sports or other situations where bruising or injury could occur.

Side Effects of This Medicine

Along with its needed effects, a medicine may cause some unwanted effects. Although not all of these side effects may occur, if they do occur they may need medical attention.

Also, because of the way these medicines act on the body, there is a chance that they might cause other unwanted effects that may not occur until months or years after the medicine is used. These delayed effects may include certain types of cancer, such as leukemia. Discuss these possible effects with your doctor.

Check with your doctor as soon as possible if any of the following side effects occur:

More common
   Pain at place of injection

Less common
   Black, tarry stools; blood in urine or stools; cough or hoarseness, accompanied by fever or chills; fever or chills; lower back or side pain, accompanied by fever or chills; numbness or tingling in fingers or toes; painful or difficult urination, accompanied by fever or chills; pinpoint red spots on skin; skin rash or itching; unusual bleeding or bruising; unusual tiredness or weakness

Rare
   Blurred vision; ringing in ears; sores in mouth and on lips; wheezing

Some side effects may occur that usually do not need medical attention. These side effects may go away during treatment as your body adjusts to the medicine. Also, your health care professional may be able to tell you about ways to prevent or reduce some of these side effects. Check with your health care professional if any of the following side effects continue or are bothersome or if you have any questions about them:

More common
   Nausea and vomiting; unusual tiredness or weakness

Less common
   Constipation or diarrhea; loss of appetite

This medicine may cause a temporary loss of hair in some people. After treatment with carboplatin has ended, normal hair growth should return.

Other side effects not listed may also occur in some patients. If you notice any other effects, check with your healthcare professional.

CARMUSTINE   (Intravenous route) -
kar-MUS-teen

Black Box Warning

Carmustine for injection should be administered under the supervision of a qualified physician experienced in the use of cancer chemotherapeutic agents.

Bone marrow suppression, notably thrombocytopenia and leukopenia, which may contribute to bleeding and overwhelming infections in an already compromised patient, is the most common and severe of the toxic effects of carmustine.

Since the major toxicity is delayed bone marrow suppression, blood counts should be monitored weekly for at least 6 weeks after a dose. At the recommended dosage, courses of carmustine should not be given more frequently than every 6 weeks.

The bone marrow toxicity of carmustine is cumulative and therefore dosage adjustment must be considered on the basis of nadir blood counts from prior dose.

Pulmonary toxicity from carmustine appears to be dose related. Patients receiving greater than 1400 mg/m(2) cumulative dose are at significantly higher risk than those receiving less.

Delayed pulmonary toxicity can occur years after treatment, and can result in death, particularly in patients treated in childhood.

Commonly used brand name(s)

In the U.S.—
   Bicnu

Available Dosage Forms:
- Powder for Solution

Therapeutic Class: Antineoplastic Agent
Pharmacologic Class: Alkylating Agent

Uses For This Medicine

Carmustine belongs to the group of medicines known as alkylating agents. It is used to treat cancer of the lymph system, cancerous brain tumors, and a certain type of cancer in the bone marrow. It may also be used to treat other kinds of cancer, as determined by your doctor.

Carmustine interferes with the growth of cancer cells, which are eventually destroyed. Since the growth of normal body cells may also be affected by carmustine, other effects will also occur. Some of these may be serious and must be reported to your doctor. Other effects, like hair loss, may not be serious but may cause concern. Some effects may not occur for months or years after the medicine is used.

Before you begin treatment with carmustine, you and your doctor should talk about the good this medicine will do as well as the risks of using it.

Carmustine is to be administered only by or under the immediate supervision of your doctor.

Once a medicine has been approved for marketing for a certain use, experience may show that it is also useful for other medical problems. Although these uses are not included in product labeling, carmustine is used in certain patients with the following conditions:

- Cancer of the colon and rectum
- Cancer of the stomach
- Malignant melanoma (a type of skin cancer)
- Mycosis fungoides (tumors on the skin)
- Waldenströ m's macroglobulinemia (a certain type of cancer of the blood)

Before Using This Medicine

In deciding to use a medicine, the risks of taking the medicine must be weighed against the good it will do. This is a decision you and your doctor will make. For this medicine, the following should be considered:

Allergies—Tell your doctor if you have ever had any unusual or allergic reaction to this medicine or any other medicines. Also tell your health care professional if you have any other types of allergies, such as to foods, dyes, preservatives, or animals. For non-prescription products, read the label or package ingredients carefully.

Pediatric—Although there is no specific information comparing use of carmustine in children with use in other age groups, this medicine is not expected to cause different side effects or problems in children than it does in adults.

Geriatric—Many medicines have not been studied specifically in older people. Therefore, it may not be known whether they work exactly the same way they do in younger adults or if they cause different side effects or problems in older people. There is no specific information comparing use of carmustine in the elderly with use in other age groups.

Pregnancy—

	Pregnancy Category	Explanation
All Trimesters	D	Studies in pregnant women have demonstrated a risk to the fetus. However, the benefits of therapy in a life threatening situation or a serious disease, may outweigh the potential risk.

Breast Feeding—There are no adequate studies in women for determining infant risk when using this medication during breastfeeding. Weigh the potential benefits against the potential risks before taking this medication while breastfeeding.

Other medicines—

Using this medicine with any of the following medicines is not recommended. Your doctor may decide not to treat you with this medication or change some of the other medicines you take.

Rotavirus Vaccine, Live

Interactions with Food/Tobacco/Alcohol—Certain medicines should not be used at or around the time of eating food or eating certain types of food since interactions may occur. Using alcohol or tobacco with certain medicines may also cause interactions to occur. Discuss with your healthcare professional the use of your medicine with food, alcohol, or tobacco.

Other medical problems—The presence of other medical problems may affect the use of this medicine. Make sure you tell your doctor if you have any other medical problems, especially:

- Chickenpox (including recent exposure) or

- Herpes zoster (shingles)—Risk of severe disease affecting other parts of the body
- Infection—Carmustine decreases your body's ability to fight infection
- Kidney disease—Effects of carmustine may be increased because of slower removal from the body
- Liver disease—Carmustine may cause side effects to the liver
- Lung disease—Risk of lung problems caused by carmustine may be increased

Proper Use of This Medicine

Carmustine is sometimes given together with certain other medicines. If you are using a combination of medicines, it is important that you receive each one at the proper time. If you are taking some of these medicines by mouth, ask your health care professional to help you plan a way to take them at the right times.

This medicine often causes nausea and vomiting, which usually last no longer than 4 to 6 hours. It is very important that you continue to receive the medicine, even if you begin to feel ill. Ask your health care professional for ways to lessen these effects.

Dosing—The dose of this medicine will be different for different patients. Follow your doctor's orders or the directions on the label. The following information includes only the average doses of this medicine. If your dose is different, do not change it unless your doctor tells you to do so.

The amount of medicine that you take depends on the strength of the medicine. Also, the number of doses you take each day, the time allowed between doses, and the length of time you take the medicine depend on the medical problem for which you are using the medicine.

Precautions While Using This Medicine

It is very important that your doctor check your progress at regular visits to make sure that this medicine is working properly and to check for unwanted effects.

While you are being treated with carmustine, and after you stop treatment with it, do not have any immunizations (vaccinations) without your doctor's approval. Carmustine may lower your body's resistance and there is a chance you might get the infection the immunization is meant to prevent. In addition, other persons living in your household should not take oral polio vaccine since there is a chance they could pass the polio virus on to you. Also, avoid persons who have taken oral polio vaccine within the last several months. Do not get close to them, and do not stay in the same room with them for very long. If you cannot take these precautions, you should consider wearing a protective face mask that covers the nose and mouth.

Carmustine can temporarily lower the number of white blood cells in your blood, increasing the chance of getting an infection. It can also lower the number of platelets, which are necessary for proper blood clotting. If this occurs, there are certain precautions you can take, especially when your blood count is low, to reduce the risk of infection or bleeding:

- If you can, avoid people with infections. Check with your doctor immediately if you think you are getting an infection or if you get a fever or chills, cough or hoarseness, lower back or side pain, or painful or difficult urination.

- Check with your doctor immediately if you notice any unusual bleeding or bruising; black, tarry stools; blood in urine or stools; or pinpoint red spots on your skin.
- Be careful when using a regular toothbrush, dental floss, or toothpick. Your medical doctor, dentist, or nurse may recommend other ways to clean your teeth and gums. Check with your medical doctor before having any dental work done.
- Do not touch your eyes or the inside of your nose unless you have just washed your hands and have not touched anything else in the meantime.
- Be careful not to cut yourself when you are using sharp objects such as a safety razor or fingernail or toenail cutters.
- Avoid contact sports or other situations where bruising or injury could occur.

If carmustine accidentally seeps out of the vein into which it is injected, it may damage some tissues and cause scarring. Tell the doctor or nurse right away if you notice redness, pain, or swelling at the place of injection.

Increased risk of lung problems while smoking.

Side Effects of This Medicine

Along with its needed effects, a medicine may cause some unwanted effects. Some side effects will have signs or symptoms that you can see or feel. Your doctor may watch for others by doing certain tests. Some of the unwanted effects that may be caused by carmustine are listed below. Although not all of these effects may occur, if they do occur, they may need medical attention.

Also, because of the way these medicines act on the body, there is a chance that they might cause other unwanted effects that may not occur until months or years after the medicine is used. These delayed effects may include certain types of cancer, such as leukemia. Discuss these possible effects with your doctor.

Check with your doctor immediately if any of the following side effects occur:
More common
Cough; pain or redness at place of injection; shortness of breath
Less common
Black, tarry stools; blood in urine or stools; cough or hoarseness, accompanied by fever or chills; fever or chills; lower back or side pain, accompanied by fever or chills; painful or difficult urination, accompanied by fever or chills; pinpoint red spots on skin; unusual bleeding or bruising
Rare
Decrease in urination; swelling of feet or lower legs

Check with your doctor as soon as possible if any of the following side effects occur:
Less common
Flushing of face; sores in mouth and on lips; unusual tiredness or weakness

This medicine may also cause the following side effects that your doctor will watch for:
More common
Low red blood cell count; low white blood cell count; lung problems
Rare
Liver problems

Some side effects may occur that usually do not need medical attention. These side effects may go away during treatment as your body adjusts to the medicine. Also, your health care professional may be able to tell you about ways to prevent or reduce some of these side effects. Check with your health care professional if any of the following side effects continue or are bothersome or if you have any questions about them:
More common
Nausea and vomiting (usually lasting no longer than 4 to 6 hours)
Less common
Diarrhea; discoloration of skin along vein of injection; dizziness; loss of appetite; skin rash and itching; trouble in swallowing; trouble in walking

This medicine may cause a temporary loss of hair in some people. After treatment with carmustine has ended, normal hair growth should return.

Side effects that affect your lungs (for example, cough and shortness of breath) may be more likely to occur if you smoke.

After you stop using this medicine, it may still produce some side effects that need attention. During this period of time, *check with your doctor immediately* if you notice the following side effects:

Black, tarry stools; blood in urine or stools; cough or hoarseness, accompanied by fever or chills; fever or chills; lower back or side pain, accompanied by fever or chills; painful or difficult urination, accompanied by fever or chills; pinpoint red spots on skin; shortness of breath; unusual bleeding or bruising

Other side effects not listed may also occur in some patients. If you notice any other effects, check with your healthcare professional.

CARVEDILOL (Oral route) - KAR-ve-dil-ole

Commonly used brand name(s)
In the U.S.—
Coreg

Available Dosage Forms:
- Tablet

Therapeutic Class: Cardiovascular Agent
Pharmacologic Class: Alpha/Beta-Adrenergic Blocker

Uses For This Medicine

Carvedilol belongs to a group of medicines called beta-adrenergic blocking agents, beta-blocking agents, or, more commonly, beta-blockers. Beta-blockers work by affecting the response to some nerve impulses in certain parts of the body. As a result, they decrease the heart's need for blood and oxygen by reducing its workload. They also help the heart to beat more regularly.

Carvedilol is used to treat high blood pressure (hypertension). High blood pressure adds to the workload of the heart and arteries. If it continues for a long time, the heart and arteries may not function properly. This can damage the blood vessels of the brain, heart, and kidneys, resulting in a stroke, heart failure, or kidney failure. High blood pressure may also increase the risk of heart attacks. These problems may be less likely to occur if blood pressure is controlled.

Carvedilol also is used to prevent further worsening of congestive heart failure. It is used to treat left ventricular dysfunction after a heart attack. Left ventricular dysfunction occurs when the left ventricle (the main pumping chamber of the heart) stiffens and enlarges and can cause the lungs to fill with blood. Carvedilol may also be used for other conditions as determined by your doctor.

This medicine is available only with your doctor's prescription.

Before Using This Medicine

In deciding to use a medicine, the risks of taking the medicine must be weighed against the good it will do. This is a decision you and your doctor will make. For this medicine, the following should be considered:

Allergies—Tell your doctor if you have ever had any unusual or allergic reaction to this medicine or any other medicines. Also tell your health care professional if you have any other types of allergies, such as to foods, dyes, preservatives, or animals. For non-prescription products, read the label or package ingredients carefully.

Pediatric—Studies on this medicine have been done only in adult patients, and there is no specific information comparing use of carvedilol in children with use in other age groups.

Geriatric—Although this medicine has not been shown to cause different side effects or problems in older people than it does in younger adults, blood levels of carvedilol may be increased in the elderly. Elderly patients also may experience dizziness more frequently than will younger adults.

Pregnancy—

	Pregnancy Category	Explanation
All Trimesters	C	Animal studies have shown an adverse effect and there are no adequate studies in pregnant women OR no animal studies have been conducted and there are no adequate studies in pregnant women.

Breast Feeding—There are no adequate studies in women for determining infant risk when using this medication during breastfeeding. Weigh the potential benefits against the potential risks before taking this medication while breastfeeding.

Other medicines—

Using this medicine with any of the following medicines is usually not recommended, but may be required in some cases. If both medicines are prescribed together, your doctor may change the dose or how often you use one or both of the medicines.

Amiodarone, Clonidine, Epinephrine, Fenoldopam, Fentanyl, Verapamil

Interactions with Food/Tobacco/Alcohol—Certain medicines should not be used at or around the time of eating food or eating certain types of food since interactions may occur. Using alcohol or tobacco with certain medicines may also cause interactions to occur. Discuss with your healthcare professional the use of your medicine with food, alcohol, or tobacco.

Other medical problems—The presence of other medical problems may affect the use of this medicine. Make sure you tell your doctor if you have any other medical problems, especially:

- Allergic reaction, severe (that involved facial swelling and/or difficulty breathing), history of or
- Asthma or
- Related bronchospastic conditions, other—Carvedilol may cause a greater reaction to substances that aggravate these conditions and less of a response to treatment of the reaction
- Angina (severe chest pain)—Carvedilol may provoke chest pain
- Bronchial conditions, nonallergic or
- Bronchitis, chronic or
- Emphysema—Carvedilol may aggravate these conditions
- Bradycardia (unusually slow heartbeat) or other heart rate problems or
- Heart or blood vessel disease—Carvedilol may make problems resulting from these conditions worse
- Diabetes mellitus (sugar diabetes) or
- Low blood sugar (hypoglycemia)—Carvedilol may aggravate low blood sugar (hypoglycemia) levels caused by insulin and may delay recovery of blood sugar levels; in patients with diabetes and heart failure, carvedilol may further increase blood sugar levels; in addition, if your diabetes medicine causes your blood sugar to be too low, beta-blockers may cover up some of the symptoms (fast heartbeat)
- Kidney disease or
- Liver disease—Effects of carvedilol may be increased because of slower removal from the body
- Overactive thyroid—Carvedilol may cover up symptoms of this condition, such as a fast heartbeat; suddenly stopping carvedilol may provoke symptoms of this condition

Proper Use of This Medicine

Take this medicine exactly as directed. This medicine works best if you take it at the same time each day; however, do not take more of this medicine and do not take it more often than your doctor ordered. Do not miss any doses.

Take this medicine with food.

Do not interrupt or stop taking this medicine without first checking with your doctor. Your doctor may want you to reduce gradually the amount you are taking before stopping completely. Some conditions may become worse when the medicine is stopped suddenly, which can be dangerous.

Dosing—The dose of this medicine will be different for different patients. Follow your doctor's orders or the directions on the label. The following information includes only the average doses of this medicine. If your dose is different, do not change it unless your doctor tells you to do so.

The amount of medicine that you take depends on the strength of the medicine. Also, the number of doses you take each day, the time allowed between doses, and the length of time you take the medicine depend on the medical problem for which you are using the medicine.

- For oral dosage form (tablets):
  - Congestive heart failure:
    - Adults—3.125 mg two times a day, taken with food. Your doctor may increase your dose if needed.

- Children—Use and dose must be determined by your doctor.
  - Hypertension or left ventricular dysfunction after a heart attack:
    - Adults—6.25 mg two times a day, taken with food. Your doctor may increase your dose if needed.
    - Children—Use and dose must be determined by your doctor.

Missed dose—If you miss a dose of this medicine, take it as soon as possible. However, if it is almost time for your next dose, skip the missed dose and go back to your regular dosing schedule. Do not double doses.

Storage—Store the medicine in a closed container at room temperature, away from heat, moisture, and direct light. Keep from freezing.

Keep out of the reach of children.

Do not keep outdated medicine or medicine no longer needed.

Precautions While Using This Medicine

It is important that your doctor check your progress at regular visits. This is to make sure the medicine is working for you and to allow the dosage to be changed if needed.

Do not take other medicines unless they have been discussed with your doctor.

This medicine may cause dizziness, lightheadedness, or fainting. Make sure you know how you react to this medicine before you drive, use machines, or do anything else that could be dangerous if you experience these effects.

Dizziness, lightheadedness, or fainting can also occur when standing quickly. Sitting or lying down may help alleviate these effects.

Check with your doctor if you become dizzy or if you faint. Your dosage may need to be adjusted.

Before having any kind of surgery (including dental surgery) or emergency treatment, tell the medical doctor or dentist in charge that you are taking this medicine.

For diabetic patients:
- This medicine may cause changes in your blood sugar levels. Also, this medicine may cover up signs of hypoglycemia (low blood sugar), such as a rapid pulse rate. Check with your physician if you experience these problems.

For congestive heart failure patients:
- Check with your physician if you experience weight gain or increased shortness of breath. These may be signs of a worsening of your condition.

For patients who wear contact lenses:
- Carvedilol may cause your eyes to form tears less than they do normally. Check with your physician if you experience dry eyes.

Side Effects of This Medicine

Along with its needed effects, a medicine may cause some unwanted effects. Although not all of these side effects may occur, if they do occur they may need medical attention.

Check with your doctor as soon as possible if any of the following side effects occur:
  More common
    Allergy; chest pain or discomfort, tightness or heaviness; dizziness, lightheadedness or fainting; pain; shortness of breath; slow heartbeat; generalized swelling or swelling of feet, ankles or lower legs; weight gain

  Less common
    Ankle, knee, or great toe joint pain; anxiety; arm, back or jaw pain; blood in urine; bloody, black or tarry stools; chills; cloudy urine; cold sweats; coma; confusion; convulsions; cool pale skin; cough; decreased frequency/amount of urine; depression; difficult breathing; dizziness, faintness, or lightheadedness when getting up from a lying position suddenly; dry mouth; fainting, pounding, slow heartbeat; fast or irregular heartbeat; fatigue; fever; flushed, dry skin; fruit-like breath odor; headache, sudden and severe; inability to speak; increased blood pressure; increased hunger; increased thirst; increased urination; itching; dark urine, decreased appetite, yellow eyes or skin; flu-like symptoms, and/or tenderness on upper right side of body; joint stiffness or swelling; large amount of cholesterol in the blood; loss of appetite; loss of consciousness; lower back, side, or stomach pain; mental depression; muscle pain or cramps; nervousness; nightmares; noisy, rattling breathing; numbness or tingling in hands, feet, or lips; pinpoint red or purple spots on skin; pounding in the ears; rapid breathing; seizures; shakiness; slurred speech; stomachache; sweating; swelling of fingers or hands; temporary blindness; troubled breathing even at rest; unexplained weight loss; unusual bleeding or bruising; weakness in arm and/or leg on one side of the body, sudden and severe; weakness or heaviness of legs

  Incidence not known
    Sores, ulcers, or white spots on lips or in mouth; swollen or painful glands; wheezing

Some side effects may occur that usually do not need medical attention. These side effects may go away during treatment as your body adjusts to the medicine. Also, your health care professional may be able to tell you about ways to prevent or reduce some of these side effects. Check with your health care professional if any of the following side effects continue or are bothersome or if you have any questions about them:
  More common
    Back pain; diarrhea; prickling or tingling sensation; unusual tiredness or weakness

  Less common
    Abdominal pain; bleeding gums; blurred vision; burning, crawling, itching, numbness, prickling, "pins and needles" or tingling feelings; changes in vision; cold hands and feet; decreased interest in sexual intercourse; decreased tearing; difficulty in moving; feeling of constant movement of self or surroundings; general feeling of discomfort or illness; headache; inability to have or keep an erection; increased sweating; joint or muscle pain; lack or loss of strength; loose teeth; loss of sexual inability, desire, or performance; loss of strength or energy; muscle aches, stiffness, or weakness; nausea; persistent breath odor or bad taste in your mouth; redness and swelling of gums; sensation of spinning; sleepiness or unusual drowsiness; small clicking, bubbling or rattling sounds in the lung when listening with a stethoscope; sore throat; stuffy or runny nose; sugar in the urine; trouble sleeping; unusual weak feeling; vomiting; weight loss

Other side effects not listed may also occur in some patients. If you notice any other effects, check with your healthcare professional.

CASPOFUNGIN (Intravenous route) -
kas-poe-FUN-jin

Commonly used brand name(s)
In the U.S.—
Cancidas

Available Dosage Forms:
• Powder for Solution

Therapeutic Class: Antifungal
Pharmacologic Class: Glucan Synthesis Inhibitor

Uses For This Medicine

Caspofungin is an antifungal. It is used to help the body overcome serious fungus infections.

This medicine is available only with your doctor's prescription.

Before Using This Medicine

In deciding to use a medicine, the risks of taking the medicine must be weighed against the good it will do. This is a decision you and your doctor will make. For this medicine, the following should be considered:

Allergies—Tell your doctor if you have ever had any unusual or allergic reaction to this medicine or any other medicines. Also tell your health care professional if you have any other types of allergies, such as to foods, dyes, preservatives, or animals. For non-prescription products, read the label or package ingredients carefully.

Pediatric—Studies on this medicine have been done only in adult patients, and there is no specific information comparing the use of caspofungin in children with use in other age groups.

Geriatric—Many medicines have not been studied specifically in older people. Therefore, it may not be known whether they work exactly the same way they do in younger adults. Although there is no specific information comparing use of caspofungin in the elderly with use in other age groups, this medicine is not expected to cause different side effects or problems in older people than it does in younger adults.

Pregnancy—

	Pregnancy Category	Explanation
All Trimesters	C	Animal studies have shown an adverse effect and there are no adequate studies in pregnant women OR no animal studies have been conducted and there are no adequate studies in pregnant women.

Breast Feeding—There are no adequate studies in women for determining infant risk when using this medication during breastfeeding. Weigh the potential benefits against the potential risks before taking this medication while breastfeeding.

Other medicines—

Using this medicine with any of the following medicines is usually not recommended, but may be required in some cases. If both medicines are prescribed together, your doctor may change the dose or how often you use one or both of the medicines.

Cyclosporine, Tacrolimus

Interactions with Food/Tobacco/Alcohol—Certain medicines should not be used at or around the time of eating food or eating certain types of food since interactions may occur. Using alcohol or tobacco with certain medicines may also cause interactions to occur. Discuss with your healthcare professional the use of your medicine with food, alcohol, or tobacco.

Other medical problems—The presence of other medical problems may affect the use of this medicine. Make sure you tell your doctor if you have any other medical problems, especially:
• Liver disease, moderate to severe—Higher blood levels of caspofungin may result, increasing the chance of side effects

Proper Use of This Medicine

Dosing—The dose of this medicine will be different for different patients. Follow your doctor's orders or the directions on the label. The following information includes only the average doses of this medicine. If your dose is different, do not change it unless your doctor tells you to do so.

The amount of medicine that you take depends on the strength of the medicine. Also, the number of doses you take each day, the time allowed between doses, and the length of time you take the medicine depend on the medical problem for which you are using the medicine.
• For injection dosage form:
  ○ Adults: At first, the dose is 70 milligrams (mg) injected into a vein. After that, the dose is 50 mg a day injected into a vein. For a fungal infection of the esophagus, the dose is 50 mg a day injected into a vein and you do not start with 70 mg on the first day.
  ○ Children: Use and dose must be determined by your doctor.

Side Effects of This Medicine

Along with its needed effects, a medicine may cause some unwanted effects. Although not all of these side effects may occur, if they do occur they may need medical attention.

Check with your doctor as soon as possible if any of the following side effects occur:
More common
Changes in skin color; pain or redness at site of injection; pain, tenderness, or swelling of foot or leg
Less common
Bloody urine; convulsions; decreased frequency/amount of urine; decreased urine; dry mouth; increased thirst; irregular heartbeat; loss of appetite; lower back/side pain; mood changes; muscle pain or cramps; nausea or vomiting; numbness or tingling in hands, feet, or lips; pale skin; shortness of breath; swelling of face, fingers, lower legs; swelling or puffiness of face; troubled breathing with exertion; unusual tiredness or weakness; yellow eyes or skin; weight gain; increased blood pressure
Incidence not known
Bloating or swelling of face, arms, hands, lower legs, or feet; confusion; constipation; dark urine; depression; fever with or without chills; headache; incoherent speech; increased urination; light-colored stools; metallic taste; muscle weakness; rapid weight gain; stomach pain; tingling of hands or feet; unusual weight gain or loss; weight loss

Some side effects may occur that usually do not need medical attention. These side effects may go away during treatment as your body adjusts to the medicine. Also, your health care professional may be able to tell you about ways to prevent or reduce some of these side effects. Check with your health care professional if any of the following side effects continue or are bothersome or if you have any questions about them:

Less common

Fever; flushing or redness of skin; nausea; vomiting

Other side effects not listed may also occur in some patients. If you notice any other effects, check with your healthcare professional.

CEFDITOREN PIVOXIL   (Oral route) -
sef-di-TOE-ren pi-VOX-il

Commonly used brand name(s)

In the U.S.—
Spectracef

Available Dosage Forms:
- Tablet

Therapeutic Class: Antibiotic
Pharmacologic Class: 3rd Generation Cephalosporin

Uses For This Medicine

Cefditoren is used in the treatment of infections caused by bacteria. It works by killing bacteria or preventing their growth.

Cefditoren pivoxil is used to treat some throat and lung infections, including bronchitis and tonsillitis. It is also used to treat some skin infections.

This medicine is available only with your doctor's prescription.

Before Using This Medicine

In deciding to use a medicine, the risks of taking the medicine must be weighed against the good it will do. This is a decision you and your doctor will make. For this medicine, the following should be considered:

Allergies—Tell your doctor if you have ever had any unusual or allergic reaction to this medicine or any other medicines. Also tell your health care professional if you have any other types of allergies, such as to foods, dyes, preservatives, or animals. For non-prescription products, read the label or package ingredients carefully.

Pediatric—Studies on this medicine have been done only in adult patients, and there is no specific information comparing use of cefditoren in children less than 12 years of age with use in other age groups.

Geriatric—This medicine has been tested and has not been shown to cause different side effects or problems in older people than it does in younger adults.

Pregnancy—

	Pregnancy Category	Explanation
All Trimesters	B	Animal studies have revealed no evidence of harm to the fetus, however, there are no adequate studies in pregnant women OR animal studies have shown an adverse effect, but adequate studies in pregnant women have failed to demonstrate a risk to the fetus.

Breast Feeding—Studies in women suggest that this medication poses minimal risk to the infant when used during breastfeeding.

Other medicines—

Using this medicine with any of the following medicines may cause an increased risk of certain side effects, but using both drugs may be the best treatment for you. If both medicines are prescribed together, your doctor may change the dose or how often you use one or both of the medicines.

Aluminum Carbonate, Basic, Aluminum Hydroxide, Aluminum Phosphate, Calcium Carbonate, Dihydroxyaluminum Aminoacetate, Dihydroxyaluminum Sodium Carbonate, Famotidine, Magaldrate, Magnesium Carbonate, Magnesium Hydroxide, Magnesium Oxide, Magnesium Trisilicate, Probenecid

Interactions with Food/Tobacco/Alcohol—Certain medicines should not be used at or around the time of eating food or eating certain types of food since interactions may occur. Using alcohol or tobacco with certain medicines may also cause interactions to occur. Discuss with your healthcare professional the use of your medicine with food, alcohol, or tobacco.

Other medical problems—The presence of other medical problems may affect the use of this medicine. Make sure you tell your doctor if you have any other medical problems, especially:
- Carnitine deficiency—May be worsened by cefditoren
- Kidney disease—Cefditoren may need to be given at a lower dose

Proper Use of This Medicine

To help clear up your infection completely, keep taking this medicine for the full time of treatment, even if you begin to feel better after a few days. Also, if you stop taking this medicine too soon, your symptoms may return.

This medicine works best when there is a constant amount in the blood or urine. To help keep the amount constant, do not miss any doses. Also, it is best to take the doses at evenly spaced times, day and night. For example, if you are to take four doses a day, the doses should be spaced about 6 hours apart. If this interferes with your sleep or other daily activities, or if you need help in planning the best times to take your medicine, check with your health care professional.

Dosing—The dose of this medicine will be different for different patients. Follow your doctor's orders or the directions on the label. The following information includes only the average doses of this medicine. If your dose is different, do not change it unless your doctor tells you to do so.

The amount of medicine that you take depends on the strength of the medicine. Also, the number of doses you take

each day, the time allowed between doses, and the length of time you take the medicine depend on the medical problem for which you are using the medicine.

Cefditoren should be taken with food to increase absorption of the medicine.

- For oral dosage form (tablets):
  ○ For acute bacterial bronchitis:
    ▪ Adults and children 12 years of age and older—400 milligrams (mg) twice a day for ten days.
    ▪ Children under 12 years of age—Use and dose must be determined by your doctor.

- For oral dosage form (tablets):
  ○ For bacterial throat infections or tonsillitis:
    ▪ Adults and children 12 years of age and older—200 mg twice a day for ten days.
    ▪ Children under 12 years of age—Dose must be determined by your doctor.

Missed dose—If you miss a dose of this medicine, take it as soon as possible. However, if it is almost time for your next dose, skip the missed dose and go back to your regular dosing schedule. Do not double doses.

Storage—Store the medicine in a closed container at room temperature, away from heat, moisture, and direct light. Keep from freezing.

Keep out of the reach of children.

Do not keep outdated medicine or medicine no longer needed.

Ask your healthcare professional how you should dispose of any medicine you do not use.

Precautions While Using This Medicine

If your symptoms do not improve within a few days or if they become worse, check with your doctor.

In some patients, cefditoren may cause diarrhea:

- Severe diarrhea may be a sign of a serious side effect. Do not take any diarrhea medicine without first checking with your doctor. Diarrhea medicines may make your diarrhea worse or make it last longer.

- If you have any questions about this or if mild diarrhea continues or gets worse, check with your health care professional.

Side Effects of This Medicine

Along with its needed effects, a medicine may cause some unwanted effects. Although not all of these side effects may occur, if they do occur they may need medical attention.

Check with your doctor immediately if any of the following side effects occur:

Rare

Allergic reaction, such as, itching, pain, redness, or swelling of eye or eyelid, watering of eyes, troubled breathing or wheezing, severe skin rash or hives, flushing, headache, fever, chills, runny nose, increased sensitivity to sunlight, joint pain, swollen glands; leukopenia, such as, black, tarry stools, chest pain, chills, cough, fever, painful or difficult urination, shortness of breath, sore throat, sores, ulcers, or white spots on lips or in mouth, swollen glands, unusual bleeding or bruising, unusual tiredness, or

weakness; pseudomembranous colitis, such as, abdominal or stomach cramps, pain, bloating, abdominal tenderness, diarrhea, watery and severe, which may also be bloody, fever, increased thirst, nausea or vomiting, unusual tiredness or weakness, or unusual weight loss; or thrombocythemia, such as, pain, warmth or burning in fingers, toes, and legs, dizziness, problems with vision or hearing

Some side effects may occur that usually do not need medical attention. These side effects may go away during treatment as your body adjusts to the medicine. Also, your health care professional may be able to tell you about ways to prevent or reduce some of these side effects. Check with your health care professional if any of the following side effects continue or are bothersome or if you have any questions about them:

More common

Diarrhea; nausea; or vaginal moniliasis, such as, thick whitish discharge from the vagina or cervical canal

Less common

Abdominal pain; Dyspepsia, such as, acid or sour stomach, belching, heartburn, indigestion, or stomach discomfort, upset or pain; or headache

Rare

Abnormal dreams; anorexia, such as, loss of appetite; asthenia, such as, lack or loss of strength; constipation; dizziness; dry mouth; dysgeusia, such as, taste perversion; eructation, such as, belching, bloated full feeling, excess air or gas in stomach; fever; flatulence, such as, passing of gas; fungal infection; gastritis, such as, burning feeling in chest or stomach, tenderness in stomach area, stomach upset, or indigestion; headache; hyperglycemia, such as, blurred vision, dry mouth, fatigue, flushed, dry skin, fruit-like breath odor, increased hunger, increased thirst, increased urination, loss of consciousness, nausea, stomachache, sweating, troubled breathing, unexplained weight loss, vomiting; increased appetite; insomnia, such as, sleeplessness; leukorrhea, such as, increase in amount of clear vaginal discharge, white vaginal discharge; mouth ulceration; myalgia, such as, muscle pain; nervousness; oral moniliasis, such as, sore mouth or tongue, white patches in mouth, tongue, or throat; pain; peripheral edema, such as, bloating or swelling of face, arms, hands, lower legs, or feet, rapid weight gain, tingling of hands or feet, unusual weight gain or loss; pharyngitis, such as, body aches or pain, congestion, cough, dryness or soreness of throat, fever, hoarseness, runny nose, tender, swollen glands in neck, trouble in swallowing, or voice changes; pruritus, such as, itching skin; rash; rhinitis, such as, stuffy nose, runny nose, or sneezing; sinusitis, such as, pain or tenderness around eyes and cheekbones, fever, stuffy or runny nose, headache, cough, shortness of breath or troubled breathing, tightness of chest or wheezing; somnolence, such as, sleepiness or unusual drowsiness; stomatitis, such as, swelling or inflammation of the mouth; sweating; urinary frequency; urticaria, such as, hives or welts, itching, redness of skin, or rash; vaginitis; vomiting; or weight loss

Other side effects not listed may also occur in some patients. If you notice any other effects, check with your healthcare professional.

CEFUROXIME (Injection route, Intravenous route) - se-fyoor-OX-eem

Commonly used brand name(s)

In the U.S.—
Zinacef

Available Dosage Forms:
- Powder for Solution
- Solution

Therapeutic Class: Antibiotic
Pharmacologic Class: 2nd Generation Cephalosporin

Uses For This Medicine

Cefuroxime is used in the treatment of infections caused by bacteria. It works by killing bacteria or preventing their growth.

This medicine is available only with your doctor's prescription.

Before Using This Medicine

In deciding to use a medicine, the risks of taking the medicine must be weighed against the good it will do. This is a decision you and your doctor will make. For this medicine, the following should be considered:

Allergies—Tell your doctor if you have ever had any unusual or allergic reaction to this medicine or any other medicines. Also tell your health care professional if you have any other types of allergies, such as to foods, dyes, preservatives, or animals. For non-prescription products, read the label or package ingredients carefully.

Pediatric—This medicine has been tested in children and, in effective doses, has not shown to cause different side effects or problems than it does in adults.

Geriatric—This medicine has been tested in the elderly and has not been shown to cause different side effects or problems in older people than it does in younger adults.

Pregnancy—

	Pregnancy Category	Explanation
All Trimesters	B	Animal studies have revealed no evidence of harm to the fetus, however, there are no adequate studies in pregnant women OR animal studies have shown an adverse effect, but adequate studies in pregnant women have failed to demonstrate a risk to the fetus.

Breast Feeding—There are no adequate studies in women for determining infant risk when using this medication during breastfeeding. Weigh the potential benefits against the potential risks before taking this medication while breastfeeding.

Other medicines—Although certain medicines should not be used together at all, in other cases two different medicines may be used together even if an interaction might occur. In these cases, your doctor may want to change the dose, or other precautions may be necessary. Tell your healthcare professional if you are taking any other prescription or non-prescription (over-the-counter [OTC]) medicine.

Interactions with Food/Tobacco/Alcohol—Certain medicines should not be used at or around the time of eating food or eating certain types of food since interactions may occur. Using alcohol or tobacco with certain medicines may also cause interactions to occur. Discuss with your healthcare professional the use of your medicine with food, alcohol, or tobacco.

Other medical problems—The presence of other medical problems may affect the use of this medicine. Make sure you tell your doctor if you have any other medical problems, especially:
- Colitis, history of or
- Gastrointestinal disease, history of—Cefuroxime may make these worse
- Kidney disease or
- Liver disease or
- Poor nutritional status—These may be worsened by cefuroxime and you may need to have vitamin K
- Kidney problems, temporary or permanent—These may effect how much cefuroxime is in your body, reducing the dose that might be needed.

Proper Use of This Medicine

Dosing—The dose of this medicine will be different for different patients. Follow your doctor's orders or the directions on the label. The following information includes only the average doses of this medicine. If your dose is different, do not change it unless your doctor tells you to do so.

The amount of medicine that you take depends on the strength of the medicine. Also, the number of doses you take each day, the time allowed between doses, and the length of time you take the medicine depend on the medical problem for which you are using the medicine.

- For injection dosage form
  - Adults and teenagers—750 mg to 3 grams every six to eight hours usually for 5 to 14 days, injected into a muscle or vein. Gonorrhea is treated with a single dose of 1.5 grams, injected into a muscle; the total 1.5-gram dose is divided into two doses and injected into muscles at two separate places on the body, and given along with a single, oral 1-gram dose of probenecid.
  - Infants and children 1 month of age and older—12.5 to 150 mg per kg (5.68 to 68 mg per pound) of body weight every six to eight hours, injected into a muscle or vein.
  - Newborns—30 to 100 mg per kg (13.6 to 45.5 mg per pound) of body weight every eight to twelve hours, injected into a vein.

Missed dose—If you miss a dose of this medicine, take it as soon as possible. However, if it is almost time for your next dose, skip the missed dose and go back to your regular dosing schedule. Do not double doses.

Storage—Keep out of the reach of children.

Do not keep outdated medicine or medicine no longer needed.

Ask your healthcare professional how you should dispose of any medicine you do not use.

Consult your health care professional about how to store this medicine.

Precautions While Using This Medicine

If your symptoms do not improve within a few days or if they become worse, check with your doctor.

Side Effects of This Medicine

Along with its needed effects, a medicine may cause some unwanted effects. Although not all of these side effects may occur, if they do occur they may need medical attention.

Check with your doctor immediately if any of the following side effects occur:

More common

Black, tarry stools; chest pain; chills; cough; fever; painful or difficult urination; shortness of breath; sore throat; sores, ulcers, or white spots on lips or in mouth; swollen glands; unusual bleeding or bruising; unusual tiredness or weakness

Less common

Abdominal or stomach cramps; abdominal or stomach tenderness or pain; bloating; bluish color or changes in skin color; diarrhea, watery and severe, which may also be bloody; difficulty in breathing or swallowing, wheezing, shortness of breath; fast heartbeat; fever; hives or welts; increased thirst; muscle spasm or jerking of all extremities; nausea or vomiting; pain; skin itching, rash, or redness; sudden loss of consciousness; swelling of face, throat, or tongue; swelling of foot or leg; tenderness; unusual weight loss

Rare

Blistering, peeling, loosening of skin; bloody or cloudy urine; dizziness; fast heartbeat; greatly decreased frequency of urination or amount of urine; hearing loss, mild to moderate; joint or muscle pain; puffiness or swelling of the eyelids or around the eyes, face, lips or tongue; red or irritated eyes; redness, tenderness, itching, burning, or peeling of skin; red skin lesions, often with a purple center; sore throat; tightness in chest

Some side effects may occur that usually do not need medical attention. These side effects may go away during treatment as your body adjusts to the medicine. Also, your health care professional may be able to tell you about ways to prevent or reduce some of these side effects. Check with your health care professional if any of the following side effects continue or are bothersome or if you have any questions about them:

More common

Gas; loss of appetite

Other side effects not listed may also occur in some patients. If you notice any other effects, check with your healthcare professional.

CELECOXIB   (Oral route) - se-le-KOX-ib

Black Box Warning

- Cardiovascular risk
  - Celecoxib may cause an increased risk of serious cardiovascular thrombotic events, myocardial infarction, and stroke, which can be fatal. All NSAIDs may have a similar risk. This risk may increase with duration of use. Patients with cardiovascular disease or risk factors for cardiovascular disease may be at greater risk.
  - Celecoxib is contraindicated for the treatment of perioperative pain in the setting of coronary artery bypass graft (CABG) surgery.
- Gastrointestinal risk
  - NSAIDs, including celecoxib, cause an increased risk of serious gastrointestinal adverse events including bleeding, ulceration, and perforation of the stomach or intestines, which can be fatal. These events can occur at any time during use and without warning symptoms. Elderly patients are at greater risk for serious gastrointestinal events.

Commonly used brand name(s)

In the U.S.—
Celebrex

Available Dosage Forms:

- Capsule

Therapeutic Class: Analgesic
Pharmacologic Class: Cyclooxygenase-2 Inhibitor

Uses For This Medicine

Celecoxib is used to relieve some symptoms caused by arthritis, such as inflammation, swelling, stiffness, and joint pain. However, this medicine does not cure arthritis and will help you only as long as you continue to take it.

Celecoxib may also be used for the following problems:

- Ankylosing spondylitis;
- Familial adenomatous polyposis (polyps in the intestines);
- Moderate or severe pain, such as after dental or orthopedic procedures;
- Pain during menstruation

This medicine is available only with your doctor's prescription.

Before Using This Medicine

In deciding to use a medicine, the risks of taking the medicine must be weighed against the good it will do. This is a decision you and your doctor will make. For this medicine, the following should be considered:

Allergies—Tell your doctor if you have ever had any unusual or allergic reaction to this medicine or any other medicines. Also tell your health care professional if you have any other types of allergies, such as to foods, dyes, preservatives, or animals. For non-prescription products, read the label or package ingredients carefully.

Pediatric—Studies on this medicine have been done only in adult patients, and there is no specific information com-

paring the use of celecoxib in children with use in older age groups.

Geriatric—This medicine has been tested in a limited number of elderly patients 65 years of age and older and has not been shown to cause different side effects or problems in older people than it does in younger adults. However, elderly patients may be more sensitive to the side effects of celecoxib.

Pregnancy—

	Pregnancy Category	Explanation
All Trimesters	C	Animal studies have shown an adverse effect and there are no adequate studies in pregnant women OR no animal studies have been conducted and there are no adequate studies in pregnant women.

Breast Feeding—There are no adequate studies in women for determining infant risk when using this medication during breastfeeding. Weigh the potential benefits against the potential risks before taking this medication while breastfeeding.

Other medicines—

Using this medicine with any of the following medicines is usually not recommended, but may be required in some cases. If both medicines are prescribed together, your doctor may change the dose or how often you use one or both of the medicines.

Warfarin

Interactions with Food/Tobacco/Alcohol—Certain medicines should not be used at or around the time of eating food or eating certain types of food since interactions may occur. Using alcohol or tobacco with certain medicines may also cause interactions to occur. Discuss with your healthcare professional the use of your medicine with food, alcohol, or tobacco.

Other medical problems—The presence of other medical problems may affect the use of this medicine. Make sure you tell your doctor if you have any other medical problems, especially:

- Alcohol abuse or
- Bleeding problems or
- Stomach ulcer or other stomach or intestinal problems or
- Tobacco use (or recent history of)—The chance of side effects may be increased
- Anemia or
- Asthma or
- Dehydration or
- Fluid retention (swelling of feet or lower legs) or
- Heart disease or
- High blood pressure or
- Kidney disease or
- Liver disease—Celecoxib may make these conditions worse
- Cardiovascular disease—Celecoxib may make this condition worse.

Proper Use of This Medicine

For safe and effective use of this medicine, do not take more of it, do not take it more often, and do not take it for a longer time than ordered by your health care professional. Taking too much of this medicine may increase the chance of unwanted effects.

Dosing—The dose of this medicine will be different for different patients. Follow your doctor's orders or the directions on the label. The following information includes only the average doses of this medicine. If your dose is different, do not change it unless your doctor tells you to do so.

The amount of medicine that you take depends on the strength of the medicine. Also, the number of doses you take each day, the time allowed between doses, and the length of time you take the medicine depend on the medical problem for which you are using the medicine.

- For oral dosage form (capsules):
  - For ankylosing spondylitis:
    - Adults—200 mg once a day or 100 mg twice a day. Dose may be increased to 400 mg a day after 6 weeks if no effect is observed.
    - Children—Use and dose must be determined by your doctor.
  - For familial adenomatous polyposis (polyps in the intestines):
    - Adults—400 mg twice a day with food.
    - Children—Use and dose must be determined by your doctor.
  - For moderate or severe pain, such as after dental or orthopedic procedures:
    - Adults—On the first day take 400 mg for the first dose then 200 mg as needed as a second dose. After the first day take 200 mg twice a day.
    - Children—Use and dose must be determined by your doctor.
  - Pain during menstruation:
    - Adults—On the first day take 400 mg for the first dose then 200 mg as needed as a second dose. After the first day take 200 mg twice a day.
    - Children—Use and dose must be determined by your doctor.
  - For rheumatoid arthritis:
    - Adults—100 to 200 mg twice a day.
    - Children—Use and dose must be determined by your doctor.
  - For osteoarthritis:
    - Adults—200 mg a day as a single dose or 100 mg twice day.
    - Children—Use and dose must be determined by your doctor.

Missed dose—If you miss a dose of this medicine, take it as soon as possible. However, if it is almost time for your next dose, skip the missed dose and go back to your regular dosing schedule. Do not double doses.

Storage—Store the medicine in a closed container at room temperature, away from heat, moisture, and direct light. Keep from freezing.

Keep out of the reach of children.

Do not keep outdated medicine or medicine no longer needed.

Precautions While Using This Medicine

If you will be taking this medicine for a long time, your doctor should check your progress at regular visits.

Stomach problems may be more likely to occur if you drink alcoholic beverages while being treated with this medicine. Therefore, do not regularly drink alcoholic beverages while taking this medicine, unless otherwise directed by your doctor.

Taking two or more of the nonsteroidal anti-inflammatory drugs together on a regular basis may increase the chance of unwanted effects. Also, taking acetaminophen, aspirin or other salicylates, or ketorolac (e.g., Toradol) regularly while you are taking a nonsteroidal anti-inflammatory drug may increase the chance of unwanted effects. The risk will depend on how much of each medicine you take every day, and on how long you take the medicines together. If your health care professional directs you to take these medicines together on a regular basis, follow his or her directions carefully. However, do not take acetaminophen or aspirin or other salicylates together with this medicine for more than a few days, and do not take any ketorolac (e.g., Toradol) while you are taking this medicine, unless your doctor has directed you to do so and is following your progress.

Serious side effects can occur during treatment with this medicine. Sometimes serious side effects can occur without any warning. However, possible warning signs often occur, including swelling of the face, fingers, feet, and/or lower legs; severe stomach pain, black, tarry stools, and/or vomiting of blood or material that looks like coffee grounds; unusual weight gain; and/or skin rash. Also, signs of serious heart problems could occur such as chest pain, tightness in chest, fast or irregular heartbeat, or unusual flushing or warmth of skin. *Stop taking this medicine and check with your doctor immediately if you notice any of these warning signs.*

Check with your doctor immediately if fever, drowsiness, itching of the skin, tiredness, nausea, or stomach pain occurs; these effects may be the first signs of liver toxicity.

Celecoxib may cause a serious type of allergic reaction called anaphylaxis. Although this is rare, it may occur often in patients who are allergic to aspirin, other nonsteroidal anti-inflammatory drugs, or sulfonamide-type drugs. Anaphylaxis requires immediate medical attention. The most serious signs of this reaction are very fast or irregular breathing, gasping for breath, wheezing, or fainting. Other signs may include changes in color of the skin of the face; very fast but irregular heartbeat or pulse; hive-like swellings on the skin; and puffiness or swellings of the eyelids or around the eyes. If these effects occur, get emergency help at once. Ask someone to drive you to the nearest hospital emergency room. If this is not possible, do not try to drive yourself. Call an ambulance, lie down, cover yourself to keep warm, and prop your feet higher than your head. Stay in that position until help arrives.

Side Effects of This Medicine

Along with its needed effects, a medicine may cause some unwanted effects. Although not all of these side effects may occur, if they do occur they may need medical attention.

Check with your doctor as soon as possible if any of the following side effects occur:

More common
Cough; fever; skin rash; sneezing; sore throat; swelling of face, fingers, feet, and/or lower legs

Less common or rare
Abnormal growth in breast; arm, back or jaw pain; bloody or black tarry stools; blurred vision; burning feeling in chest or stomach; burning or stinging of skin; burning, tingling, numbness or pain in the hands, arms, feet, or legs; chest pain or discomfort; chest tightness or heaviness; chills; confusion; congestion in chest; cough; cramps; diarrhea; dry mouth; earache; fast or irregular heartbeat; fatigue; fever; heartburn; heavy bleeding; heavy nonmenstrual vaginal bleeding; high blood pressure; increased hunger; increased thirst; increased urination; loss of appetite; loss of consciousness; muscle aches and pains; nausea; nerve pain; painful blisters on trunk of body; painful cold sores or blisters on lips, nose, eyes, or genitals; pale skin; redness or swelling in ear; sensation of pins and needles; shortness of breath; sore throat; soreness or redness around fingernails and toenails; stabbing pain; stiff neck; stomachache; stomach pain (severe); sweating; tenderness in stomach area; troubled breathing with exertion; unexplained weight loss; unusual bleeding or bruising; unusual tiredness or weakness; unusual weight gain; vomiting; vomiting of blood or material that looks like coffee grounds; weakness; wheezing

Incidence not determined—Observed during clinical practice
Area rash; changes in skin color; clay-colored stools; dilated neck veins; light-colored stools; pale or a bluish color skin of the fingers or toes; seizures; slurred speech; sores, welting or blisters; sudden and severe inability to speak; swelling of face, fingers, feet, or lower legs; unpleasant breath odor; weakness in arm and/or leg on one side of the body; yellow eyes and skin

Symptoms of overdose
Bloody or black, tarry stools; continuing thirst; dizziness; drowsiness; headache, severe or continuing; nausea and/or vomiting; shortness of breath; stomach pain; sudden decrease in the amount of urine; swelling of face, fingers, and/or lower legs; tightness in chest and/or wheezing; troubled breathing; unusual tiredness or weakness; vomiting of blood or material that looks like coffee grounds; weight gain

Some side effects may occur that usually do not need medical attention. These side effects may go away during treatment as your body adjusts to the medicine. Also, your health care professional may be able to tell you about ways to prevent or reduce some of these side effects. Check with your health care professional if any of the following side effects continue or are bothersome or if you have any questions about them:

More common
Back pain; dizziness; gas; headache; heartburn; inability to sleep; nausea; pain or burning in throat; stomach pain; stuffy or runny nose

Less common
Anxiety; bleeding after defecation; bloody or cloudy urine; blurred vision; breast pain; bone deformity; buzzing or ringing noise in ears; change in sense of taste; confusion; constipation; decrease in height; decreased appetite; degenerative disease of the joint; depression; difficult, burning, or painful urination; difficulty in moving or walking; difficulty swallowing; dry mouth; excessive muscle tone, muscle tension or tightness; excessive tearing; fast heartbeat; feeling of pressure; hair loss; hives; hoarseness; increased sweating; infection; inflammation; itching, lumps, numbness, pain,

rash, redness, scarring, soreness, stinging, swelling, tenderness, tingling, ulceration, or warmth at site; itching of the vagina or genital area; joint or muscle pain or stiffness; large amount of cholesterol in the blood; large, flat, blue or purplish patches in the skin; loss of energy or weakness; loss of hearing; muscle pain increased; muscle stiffness; nervousness; numbness or tingling in fingers and/or toes; pain during sexual intercourse; pain in back, ribs, arms, or legs; pain or burning in throat; pounding heartbeat; puffiness or swelling of the eyelids or around the eyes, face, lips or tongue; redness; redness or swelling in arms or legs; sensitivity of skin to sunlight; severe sunburn; sleepiness; straining while passing stool; sudden sweating and feelings of warmth; swelling; swelling or inflammation of the mouth; tenderness; thick, white vaginal discharge with no odor or with a mild odor; thinning of hair; trouble in swallowing; troubled breathing; uncomfortable swelling around anus; unexplained weight loss; unusual tiredness; voice changes; vomiting; warmth on skin; weakness or heaviness of legs

Incidence not determined—Observed during clinical practice

Bleeding gums; blistering, peeling, loosening of skin; bloating; chills; fever and chills, blistering, peeling, loosening of skin; fever, redness, tenderness, itching, burning, or peeling of skin; joint or muscle pain; large, hive-like swelling on face, eyelids, lips, tongue, throat, hands, legs, feet, sex organs; loss of sense of smell; loss of sense of taste; pain; pinpoint red spots on skin; red or irritated eyes; red skin lesions, often with a purple center; shakiness and unsteady walk; sore throat; sores, ulcers, or white spots in mouth or on lips; stomach cramps; swelling of feet or lower legs; swelling of the neck; tenderness; trembling, or other problems with muscle control or coordination; ulcers, or white spots in mouth or on lips; unsteadiness; unusual bleeding or bruising; watery or bloody diarrhea

Other side effects not listed may also occur in some patients. If you notice any other effects, check with your healthcare professional.

CEPHALOSPORIN (Oral route, Injection route, Intravenous route, Intramuscular route)

Commonly used brand name(s)

In the U.S.—

Ancef	Keftab
Bio-Cef	Lorabid
Ceclor	Mandol
Cedax	Maxipime
Cefizox	Mefoxin
Cefobid	Omnicef
Cefotan	Rocephin
Ceftin	Spectracef
Cefzil	Suprax
Claforan	Vantin
Duricef	Velosef
Fortaz	Zinacef
Keflin	

In Canada—

Apo-Cefaclor	Gen-Cefaclor
Cefaclor	Keflex
Cefotaxime	Novo-Lexin
Cefuroxime	Nu-Cefaclor
Ceptaz	

Available Dosage Forms:

- Powder for Solution
- Powder for Suspension
- Tablet
- Solution
- Capsule
- Injectable
- Tablet for Suspension
- Tablet, Chewable
- Tablet, Extended Release

Uses For This Medicine

Cephalosporins are used in the treatment of infections caused by bacteria. They work by killing bacteria or preventing their growth.

Cephalosporins are used to treat infections in many different parts of the body. They are sometimes given with other antibiotics. Some cephalosporins given by injection are also used to prevent infections before, during, and after surgery. However, cephalosporins will not work for colds, flu, or other virus infections.

Once a medicine has been approved for marketing for a certain use, experience may show that it is also useful for other medical problems. Although these uses are not included in product labeling, cephalosporins are used in certain patients with the following medical conditions:

- Amoxicillin-resistant sinusitis (treatment)—Cefaclor
- Bacterial endocarditis (Prophylaxis)—Cefadroxil, cefazolin, and cephalexin
- Melioidosis (treatment)—Ceftazidime

Before Using This Medicine

Allergies—Tell your doctor if you have ever had any unusual or allergic reaction to medicines in this group or any other medicines. Also tell your health care professional if you have any other types of allergies, such as to foods dyes, preservatives, or animals. For non-prescription products, read the label or package ingredients carefully.

Pediatric—Many cephalosporins have been tested in children and, in effective doses, have not been shown to cause different side effects or problems than they do in adults. However, there are some cephalosporins that have not been tested in children up to 12 years of age.

Geriatric—Cephalosporins have been used in the elderly, and they are not expected to cause different side effects or problems in older people than they do in younger adults.

Pregnancy—Studies have not been done in humans. However, most cephalosporins have not been reported to cause birth defects or other problems in animal studies. Studies in rabbits have shown that cefoxitin may increase the risk of miscarriages and cause other problems. Before taking a cephalosporin, make sure your doctor knows if you are pregnant or if you may become pregnant.

Breast Feeding—It is not known if cefditoren passes into breast milk. Most cephalosporins pass into breast milk, usually in small amounts. However, cephalosporins have not been reported to cause problems in nursing babies. Mothers who are taking a cephalosporin and who wish to breast-feed should discuss this with their doctor.

Other medicines—

Using medicines in this class with any of the following medicines is usually not recommended, but may be required in some cases. If both medicines are prescribed together, your doctor may change the dose or how often you use one or both of the medicines.

Heparin

Using this medicine with any of the following may cause an increased risk of certain side effects but using both drugs may be the best treatment for you. If both medicines are prescribed together, your doctor may change the dose or how often you use one or both of the medicines.

Aluminum Carbonate, Basic, Aluminum Hydroxide, Aluminum Phosphate, Calcium Carbonate, Chloramphenicol, Cholestyramine, Cimetidine, Dihydroxyaluminum Aminoacetate, Dihydroxyaluminum Sodium Carbonate, Famotidine, Furosemide, Magaldrate, Magnesium Carbonate, Magnesium Hydroxide, Magnesium Oxide, Magnesium Trisilicate, Metformin, Nizatidine, Probenecid, Ranitidine, Warfarin

Interactions with Food/Tobacco/Alcohol—Certain medicines should not be used at or around the time of eating food or eating certain types of food since interactions may occur. Using alcohol or tobacco with certain medicines may also cause interactions to occur. The following interactions have been selected on the basis of their potential significance and are not necessarily all-inclusive.

Using medicines in this class with any of the following is usually not recommended, but may be unavoidable in some cases. If used together, your doctor may change the dose or how often you use your medicine, or give you special instructions about the use of food, alcohol, or tobacco.

Ethanol

Other medical problems—The presence of other medical problems may affect the use of medicines in this class. Make sure you tell your doctor if you have any other medical problems, especially:

- Bleeding problems, history of (cefamandole, cefditoren, cefoperazone, and cefotetan only)—These medicines may increase the chance of bleeding.
- Carnitine, low levels—Cefditoren may cause carnitine levels to decrease further.
- Kidney disease—Some cephalosporins need to be given at a lower dose to people with kidney disease. Also, cephalothin, and cefuroxime especially, may increase the chance of kidney damage
- Liver disease (cefoperazone and cefuroxime)—Cefoperazone needs to be given at a lower dose to people with liver disease. Condition may be worsened by cefuroxime use.
- Phenylketonuria—Cefprozil oral suspension contains phenylalanine.
- Poor nutritional status—These may be worsened by cefuroxime and you may need to have vitamin K.
- Stomach or gastrointestinal disease, history of (especially colitis, including colitis caused by antibiotics, or enteritis)—Cephalosporins may cause colitis in some patients.

Proper Use of This Medicine

Cephalosporins may be taken on a full or empty stomach. If this medicine upsets your stomach, it may help to take it with food.

Cefaclor extended-release tablets, cefditoren, cefpodoxime, and cefuroxime axetil should be taken with food to increase absorption of the medicine. Ceftibuten oral suspension should be taken on an empty stomach, at least 2 hours before or 1 hour after a meal.

Loracarbef should be taken at least 1 hour before eating or at least 2 hours after eating.

For patients taking the oral liquid form of this medicine:

- This medicine is to be taken by mouth. Use a specially marked measuring spoon or other device to measure each dose accurately. The average household teaspoon may not hold the right amount of liquid.
- Do not use after the expiration date on the label since the medicine may not work properly after that date. Check with your pharmacist if you have any questions about this.

For patients taking cefaclor chewable tablets:

- Chew tablet completely before swallowing. Do not swallow whole.

To help clear up your infection completely, keep taking this medicine for the full time of treatment, even if you begin to feel better after a few days. If you have a "strep" infection, you should keep taking this medicine for at least 10 days. This is especially important in "strep" infections since serious heart or kidney problems could develop later if your infection is not cleared up completely. Also, if you stop taking this medicine too soon, your symptoms may return.

This medicine works best when there is a constant amount in the blood or urine. To help keep the amount constant, do not miss any doses. Also, it is best to take the doses at evenly spaced times, day and night. For example, if you are to take four doses a day, the doses should be spaced about 6 hours apart. If this interferes with your sleep or other daily activities, or if you need help in planning the best times to take your medicine, check with your health care professional.

Dosing—The dose medicines in this class will be different for different patients. Follow your doctor's orders or the directions on the label. The following information includes only the average doses of these medicines. If your dose is different, do not change it unless your doctor tells you to do so.

The amount of medicine that you take depends on the strength of the medicine. Also, the number of doses you take each day, the time allowed between doses, and the length of time you take the medicine depend on the medical problem for which you are using the medicine.

- For cefaclor:
  ○ For bacterial infections:
    ▪ For oral dosage form (capsules or oral suspension):
      — Adults and teenagers—250 to 500 milligrams (mg) every eight hours.
      — Infants and children 1 month of age and older—6.7 to 13.4 mg per kilogram (kg) (3.04 to 6.09 mg per pound) of body weight every eight hours, or 10 to 20 mg per kg (4.54 to 9.09 mg per pound) of body weight every twelve hours.
    ▪ For oral dosage form (chewable tablets):
      — Adults and teenagers—250 to 500 mg every eight hours.
      — Children—20 mg per kg (9.09 mg per pound) of body weight every eight hours.

- For long-acting oral dosage form (extended-release tablets):
  — Adults and teenagers 16 years of age and older—375 to 500 mg every twelve hours for seven to ten days.
  — Children up to 16 years of age—Use and dose must be determined by your doctor.
  ○ For pharyngitis (strep throat):
  ▪ For oral dosage form (chewable tablets):
  — Children—20 mg per kg (9.09 mg per pound) of body weight every twelve hours.
  ○ For otitis media (ear infection):
  ▪ For oral dosage form (chewable tablets):
  — Children—40 mg per kg (18.18 mg per pound) of body weight every eight or twelve hours as directed by the doctor.

- For cefadroxil:
  ○ For bacterial infections:
  ▪ For oral dosage form (capsules, oral suspension, or tablets):
  — Adults and teenagers—500 milligrams (mg) or 1 gram every twelve hours, or 1 or 2 grams once a day.
  — Children—15 mg per kilogram (kg) (6.81 mg per pound) of body weight every twelve hours, or 30 mg per kg (13.63 mg per pound) of body weight once a day.

- For cefamandole:
  ○ For bacterial infections:
  ▪ For injection dosage form:
  — Adults and teenagers—500 milligrams (mg) to 2 grams every four to eight hours, injected into a muscle or vein.
  — Infants and children 1 month of age and older—8.3 to 50 mg per kilogram (kg) (3.77 to 22.72 mg per pound) of body weight every four to eight hours, injected into a muscle or vein.

- For cefazolin:
  ○ For bacterial infections:
  ▪ For injection dosage form:
  — Adults and teenagers—250 milligrams (mg) to 1.5 grams every six to twelve hours, injected into a muscle or vein.
  — Infants and children 1 month of age and older—6.25 to 25 mg per kilogram (kg) (2.84 to 11.36 mg per pound) of body weight every six hours, or 8.3 to 33.3 mg per kg (3.77 to 15.13 mg per pound) of body weight every eight hours, injected into a muscle or vein.
  — Newborns—20 mg per kg (9.09 mg per pound) of body weight every eight to twelve hours, injected into a vein.

- For cefdinir:
  ○ For bacterial infections:
  ▪ For oral dosage form (capsules or oral suspension):
  — Adults and teenagers—300 milligrams (mg) ever twelve hours or 600 mg once a day for 5 to 10 days.
  — Infants and children 6 months of age and older—7 milligrams (mg) per kilogram (3.18 mg per pound) of body weight every twelve hours or 14 mg per kilogram (6.36 mg per pound) once a day for 5 to 10 days.

- For cefditoren:
  ○ For oral dosage form (tablets):
  ▪ For bacterial bronchitis:
  — For oral dosage form (tablets):
  • Adults and children 12 years of age and older—400 milligrams (mg) twice a day for 10 days
  • Children under 12 years of age—Dose must be determined by your doctor
  ▪ For bacterial throat infections or tonsillitis:
  — For oral dosage form (tablets):
  • Adults and children 12 years of age and older—200 milligrams (mg) twice a day for 10 days
  • Children under 12 years of age—Dose must be determined by your doctor

- For cefepime:
  ○ For bacterial infections:
  ▪ For injection dosage form:
  — Adults and teenagers—500 milligrams to 2 grams every eight to twelve hours, injected into a muscle or vein, for seven to ten days.
  — Infants and children 2 months to 16 years of age—50 milligrams per kilogram body weight injected into muscle or vein, every eight to twelve hours, for seven to ten days.

- For cefixime:
  ○ For bacterial infections:
  ▪ For oral dosage form (oral suspension or tablets):
  — Adults and teenagers—200 milligrams (mg) every twelve hours, or 400 mg once a day. Gonorrhea is treated with a single, oral dose of 400 mg.
  — Children 6 months to 12 years of age—4 mg per kilogram (kg) (1.81 mg per pound) of body weight every twelve hours, or 8 mg per kg (3.63 mg per pound) of body weight once a day.
  — Infants up to 6 months of age—Use and dose must be determined by your doctor.

- For cefonicid:
  ○ For bacterial infections:
  ▪ For injection dosage form:
  — Adults and teenagers—500 milligrams (mg) to 2 grams every twenty-four hours, injected into a muscle or vein.
  — Children—Use and dose must be determined by your doctor.

- For cefoperazone:
  ○ For bacterial infections:
  ▪ For injection dosage form:
  — Adults and teenagers—1 to 6 grams every twelve hours, or 2 to 4 grams every eight hours, injected into a muscle or vein.
  — Children—Use and dose must be determined by your doctor.

- For cefotaxime:
  - For bacterial infections:
    - For injection dosage form:
      — Adults and teenagers—1 to 2 grams every four to twelve hours, injected into a muscle or vein. Gonorrhea is usually treated with a single dose of 500 milligrams (mg) or 1 gram, injected into a muscle.
      — Children over 50 kg of body weight (110 pounds)—1 to 2 grams every four to twelve hours, injected into a muscle or vein.
      — Infants and children 1 month of age and older and up to 50 kg of body weight (110 pounds)—8.3 to 30 mg per kg (3.77 to 13.63 mg per pound) of body weight every four hours, or 12.5 to 45 mg per kg (5.68 to 20.45 mg per pound) of body weight every six hours, injected into a muscle or vein.
      — Newborns 1 to 4 weeks of age—50 mg per kg (22.72 mg per pound) of body weight every eight hours, injected into a vein.
      — Newborns up to 1 week of age—50 mg per kilogram (kg) (22.72 mg per pound) of body weight every twelve hours, injected into a vein.

- For cefotetan:
  - For bacterial infections:
    - For injection dosage form:
      — Adults and teenagers—500 milligrams to 3 grams every twelve hours, or 1 or 2 grams every twenty-four hours, injected into a muscle or vein.
      — Children—Use and dose must be determined by your doctor.

- For cefoxitin:
  - For bacterial infections:
    - For injection dosage form:
      — Adults and teenagers—1 to 3 grams every four to eight hours, injected into a vein.
      — Infants and children 3 months of age and older—13.3 to 26.7 milligrams (mg) per kilogram (kg) (6.04 to 12.13 mg per pound) of body weight every four hours, or 20 to 40 mg per kg (9.09 to 18.18 mg per pound) of body weight every six hours, injected into a vein.
      — Infants 1 to 3 months of age—20 to 40 mg per kg (9.09 to 18.18 mg per pound) of body weight every six to eight hours, injected into a vein.
      — Newborns 1 to 4 weeks of age—20 to 40 mg per kg (9.09 to 18.18 mg per pound) of body weight every eight hours, injected into a vein.
      — Premature infants weighing 1500 grams and over to newborns up to 1 week of age—20 to 40 mg per kg (9.09 to 18.18 mg per pound) of body weight every twelve hours, injected into a vein.

- For cefpodoxime:
  - For bacterial infections:
    - For oral dosage form (oral suspension or tablets):
      — Adults and teenagers—100 to 400 milligrams (mg) every twelve hours for

five to fourteen days. Gonorrhea is treated with a single, oral dose of 200 mg.
      — Infants and children 5 months to 12 years of age—5 mg per kilogram (kg) (2.27 mg per pound) of body weight every twelve hours for five to ten days, or 10 mg per kg (4.54 mg per pound) of body weight every twenty-four hours for ten days.
      — Infants up to 5 months of age—Use and dose must be determined by your doctor.

- For cefprozil:
  - For bacterial infections:
    - For oral dosage form (oral suspension or tablets):
      — Adults and teenagers—250 or 500 milligrams (mg) every twelve to twenty-four hours for ten days.
      — Children 2 to 12 years of age—7.5 to 20 mg per kilogram (kg) (3.4 to 9.09 mg per pound) of body weight every twelve to twenty-four hours for ten days.
      — Infants and children 6 months to 12 years of age—7.5 to 15 mg per kg (3.4 to 6.81 mg per pound) of body weight every twelve hours for ten days.
      — Infants up to 6 months of age—Use and dose must be determined by your doctor.

- For ceftazidime:
  - For bacterial infections:
    - For injection dosage form:
      — Adults and teenagers—250 milligrams (mg) to 2 grams every eight to twelve hours, injected into a muscle or vein. Patients with cystic fibrosis may receive 30 to 50 mg per kilogram (kg) (13.63 to 22.72 mg per pound) of body weight every eight hours, injected into a vein.
      — Infants and children 1 month to 12 years of age—30 to 50 mg per kg (13.63 to 22.72 mg per pound) of body weight every eight hours, injected into a vein.
      — Newborns up to 4 weeks of age—30 mg per kg (13.63 mg per pound) of body weight every twelve hours, injected into a vein.

- For ceftibuten:
  - For bacterial infections:
    - For oral dosage form (capsules or oral suspension):
      — Adults and teenagers—400 milligrams (mg) once a day for ten days.
      — Infants and children 6 months to 12 years of age—9 mg per kilogram (4.09 mg per pound) of body weight once a day for ten days.
      — Infants up to 6 months of age—Use and dose must be determined by your doctor.

- For ceftizoxime:
  - For bacterial infections:
    - For injection dosage form:
      — Adults and teenagers—500 milligrams (mg) to 4 grams every eight to twelve hours, injected into a muscle or vein. Gonorrhea is treated with a single dose of 1 gram, injected into a muscle.

— Infants and children 6 months of age and older—50 mg per kilogram (22.72 mg per pound) of body weight every six to eight hours, injected into a muscle or vein.
— Infants up to 6 months of age—Use and dose must be determined by your doctor.

- For ceftriaxone:
  - For bacterial infections:
    - For injection dosage form:
      — Adults and teenagers—1 to 2 grams every twenty-four hours, or 500 milligrams (mg) to 1 gram every twelve hours, injected into a muscle or vein. Gonorrhea is treated with a single 250-mg dose, injected into a muscle.
      — Infants and children—25 to 37.5 mg per kilogram (kg) (11.36 to 17.04 mg per pound) of body weight every twelve hours, or 50 to 75 mg per kg (22.72 to 34.09 mg per pound) of body weight once a day, injected into a muscle or vein. Meningitis is treated with an initial dose of 100 mg per kg, then 100 mg per kg once a day or 50 mg per kg two times a day.

- For cefuroxime:
  - For bacterial infections:
    - For oral dosage form (oral suspension):
      — Adults and teenagers—The oral suspension is usually used only for children. Refer to the dosing for cefuroxime tablets.
      — Infants and children 3 months to 12 years of age—10 to 15 milligrams (mg) per kilogram (kg) (4.54 to 6.81 mg per pound) of body weight every twelve hours for ten days.
    - For oral dosage form (tablets):
      — Adults and teenagers—250 to 500 mg every twelve hours. Gonorrhea is treated with a single, oral 1-gram dose.
      — Children up to 12 years of age who can swallow tablets whole—250 mg every twelve hours for ten days.
    - For injection dosage form:
      — Adults and teenagers—750 mg to 3 grams every six to eight hours usually for 5 to 14 days, injected into a muscle or vein. Gonorrhea is treated with a single dose of 1.5 grams, injected into a muscle; the total 1.5-gram dose is divided into two doses and injected into muscles at two separate places on the body, and given along with a single, oral 1-gram dose of probenecid.
      — Infants and children 1 month of age and older—12.5 to 150 mg per kg (5.68 to mg per pound) of body weight every six to eight hours, injected into a muscle or vein.
      — Newborns—10 to 100 mg per kg (4.54 to 45.5 mg mg per pound) of body weight every eight to twelve hours, injected into a vein.

- For cephalexin:
  - For bacterial infections:
    - For oral dosage form (capsules, oral suspension, or tablets):
      — Adults and teenagers—250 milligrams (mg) to 1 gram every six to twelve hours.

— Children 40 kg (88 pounds) of body weight and over—250 mg to 1 gram every six to twelve hours.
— Children 1 year of age and older and up to 40 kg (88 pounds) of body weight—6.25 to 25 mg per kilogram (kg) (2.84 to 11.36 mg per pound) of body weight every six hours, or 12.5 to 50 mg per kg (5.68 to 22.72 mg per pound) of body weight every twelve hours.
— Infants and children 1 month to 1 year of age—6.25 to 12.5 mg per kg (2.84 to 5.68 mg per pound) of body weight every six hours.

- For cephalothin:
  - For bacterial infections:
    - For injection dosage form:
      — Adults and teenagers—500 milligrams (mg) to 2 grams every four to six hours, injected into a muscle or vein.
      — Children—13.3 to 26.6 mg per kilogram (kg) (6.04 to 12.09 mg per pound) of body weight every four hours, or 20 to 40 mg per kg (9.09 to 18.18 mg per pound) of body weight every six hours, injected into a muscle or vein.

- For cephapirin:
  - For bacterial infections:
    - For injection dosage form:
      — Adults and teenagers—500 milligrams (mg) to 1 gram every four to six hours, injected into a muscle or vein.
      — Infants and children 3 months of age and older—10 to 20 mg per kilogram (kg) (4.54 to 9.09 mg per pound) of body weight every six hours, injected into a muscle or vein.

- For cephradine:
  - For bacterial infections:
    - For oral dosage form (capsules or oral suspension):
      — Adults and teenagers—250 milligrams (mg) to 1 gram every six to twelve hours.
      — Infants and children 9 months of age and older—6.25 mg to 1 gram per kilogram (kg) (2.84 to 454 mg per pound) of body weight every six hours, or 12.5 to 50 mg per kg (5.68 to 22.72 mg per pound) of body weight every twelve hours.

- For loracarbef:
  - For bacterial infections:
    - For oral dosage form (capsules and oral suspension):
      — Adults and teenagers—200 to 400 mg every 12 hours for 7 to 14 days.
      — Infants and children 6 months of age and older—15 to 30 mg per kg (6.81 to 13.62 mg per pound) of body weight every 12 hours for 7 to 10 days.
      — The oral suspension should be taken for an ear infection rather than the capsule form.

Missed dose—If you miss a dose of this medicine, take it as soon as possible. However, if it is almost time for your next dose, skip the missed dose and go back to your regular dosing schedule. Do not double doses.

Storage—Store the medicine in a closed container at room temperature, away from heat, moisture, and direct light. Keep from freezing.

Keep out of the reach of children.

Do not keep outdated medicine or medicine no longer needed.

Store the oral liquid form of most cephalosporins in the refrigerator because heat will cause this medicine to break down. However, keep the medicine from freezing. Follow the directions on the label. Cefixime oral suspension (Suprax), cefuroxime axetil oral suspension (Ceftin), cefdinir oral suspension (Omnicef), and loracarbef oral suspension (Lorabid) do not need to be refrigerated.

Precautions While Using This Medicine

If your symptoms do not improve within a few days, or if they become worse, check with your doctor.

For patients with diabetes:

- This medicine may cause false test results with some urine sugar tests. Check with your doctor before changing your diet or the dosage of your diabetes medicine.

For patients with phenylketonuria (PKU):

- Cefprozil oral suspension (Cefzil) contains phenylalanine. Check with your doctor before taking this medicine.

In some patients, cephalosporins may cause diarrhea:

- Severe diarrhea may be a sign of a serious side effect. Do not take any diarrhea medicine without first checking with your doctor. Diarrhea medicines may make your diarrhea worse or make it last longer.
- For mild diarrhea, diarrhea medicine containing kaolin or attapulgite (e.g., Kaopectate tablets, Diasorb) may be taken. However, other kinds of diarrhea medicine should not be taken. They may make your diarrhea worse or make it last longer.
- If you have any questions about this or if mild diarrhea continues or gets worse, check with your health care professional

For patients receiving cefamandole, cefoperazone, or cefotetan by injection:

- Drinking alcoholic beverages or taking other alcohol-containing preparations (for example, elixirs, cough syrups, tonics, or injections of alcohol) while receiving these medicines may cause problems. The problems may occur if you consume alcohol even several days after you stop taking the cephalosporin. Drinking alcoholic beverages may result in increased side effects such as abdominal or stomach cramps, nausea, vomiting, headache, fainting, fast or irregular heartbeat, difficult breathing, sweating, or redness of the face or skin. These effects usually start within 15 to 30 minutes after you drink alcohol and may not go away for up to several hours. Therefore, you should not drink alcoholic beverages or take other alcohol-containing preparations while you are receiving these medicines and for several days after stopping them.

Side Effects of This Medicine

Along with its needed effects, a medicine may cause some unwanted effects. Although not all of these side effects may occur, if they do occur they may need medical attention.

Check with your doctor immediately if any of the following side effects occur:
  More common
    Black, tarry stools; chest pain; chills; cough; fever; painful or difficult urination; shortness of breath; sore throat; sores, ulcers, or white spots on lips or in mouth; swollen glands; unusual bleeding or bruising (more common for cefamandole, cefoperazone, cefotetan and cefuroxime); unusual tiredness or weakness
  Less common or rare
    Abdominal or stomach cramps and pain (severe); abdominal tenderness; diarrhea (watery and severe, which may also be bloody); hives or welts, itching redness of skin, or skin rash; pain, redness and swelling at site of injection; peeling of skin; seizures

After you stop using this medicine, it may still produce some side effects that need attention. During this period of time, *check with your doctor immediately* if you notice the following side effects:
  Rare
    Blistering, peeling, or loosening of skin; decrease in urine output; hearing loss (more common with cefuroxime treatment for meningitis); joint pain; loss of appetite, nausea, or vomiting (more common with ceftriaxone); red or irritated eyes; trouble in breathing; yellowing of the eyes or skin

Some side effects may occur that usually do not need medical attention. These side effects may go away during treatment as your body adjusts to the medicine. Also, your health care professional may be able to tell you about ways to prevent or reduce some of these side effects. Check with your health care professional if any of the following side effects continue or are bothersome or if you have any questions about them:
  More common (less common with some cephalosporins)
    Diarrhea (mild); headache; sore mouth or tongue; stomach cramps (mild); vaginal itching or discharge

Other side effects not listed may also occur in some patients. If you notice any other effects, check with your healthcare professional.

CETIRIZINE AND PSEUDOEPHEDRINE   (Oral route) -
se-TI-ra-zeen, soo-doe-e-FED-rin

Commonly used brand name(s)

In the U.S.—
  Zyrtec-D

Available Dosage Forms:

- Tablet, Extended Release

Therapeutic Class: Antihistamine/Decongestant Combination
Pharmacologic Class: Cetirizine

Uses For This Medicine

Cetirizine and pseudoephedrine is a combination of an antihistamine and a decongestant used to treat the symptoms of seasonal or yearly allergies. Antihistamines work by preventing the effects of a substance called histamine, which is produced by the body. Histamine can cause itching, sneezing, runny nose, and watery eyes. Decongestants produce a narrowing of blood vessels. This leads to clearing of nasal congestion, but it may also cause an increase in blood pressure in patients who have high blood pressure. This medicine is available only with your doctor's prescription.

Before Using This Medicine

In deciding to use a medicine, the risks of taking the medicine must be weighed against the good it will do. This is a decision you and your doctor will make. For this medicine, the following should be considered:

Allergies—Tell your doctor if you have ever had any unusual or allergic reaction to this medicine or any other medicines. Also tell your health care professional if you have any other types of allergies, such as to foods, dyes, preservatives, or animals. For non-prescription products, read the label or package ingredients carefully.

Pediatric—Use is not recommended in infants and children up to 12 years of age. In children 12 years of age and older, this medicine is not expected to cause different side effects or problems than it does in adults.

Geriatric—Many medicines have not been studied specifically in older people. Therefore, it may not be known whether they work exactly the same way they do in younger adults or if they cause different side effects or problems in older people. There is no specific information comparing use of cetirizine and pseudoephedrine in the elderly with use in other age groups.

Other medicines—

Using this medicine with any of the following medicines is not recommended. Your doctor may decide not to treat you with this medication or change some of the other medicines you take.

Clorgyline, Dihydroergotamine, Furazolidone, Iproniazid, Isocarboxazid, Moclobemide, Nialamide, Pargyline, Phenelzine, Procarbazine, Rasagiline, Selegiline, Toloxatone, Tranylcypromine

Interactions with Food/Tobacco/Alcohol—Certain medicines should not be used at or around the time of eating food or eating certain types of food since interactions may occur. Using alcohol or tobacco with certain medicines may also cause interactions to occur. Discuss with your healthcare professional the use of your medicine with food, alcohol, or tobacco.

Other medical problems—The presence of other medical problems may affect the use of this medicine. Make sure you tell your doctor if you have any other medical problems, especially:
- Kidney disease—Removal of cetirizine and pseudoephedrine from the body may be reduced
   For cetirizine
- Liver disease—May be worsened by cetirizine
   For pseudoephedrine
- Diabetes or
- Heart disease or
- High blood pressure or
- Inner eye pressure or
- Narrow-angle glaucoma or
- Urination difficulties or
- Prostrate, enlarged or
- Thyroid problems—May be worsened by pseudoephedrine

Proper Use of This Medicine

Dosing—The dose of this medicine will be different for different patients. Follow your doctor's orders or the directions on the label. The following information includes only the average doses of this medicine. If your dose is different, do not change it unless your doctor tells you to do so.

The amount of medicine that you take depends on the strength of the medicine. Also, the number of doses you take each day, the time allowed between doses, and the length of time you take the medicine depend on the medical problem for which you are using the medicine.

Swallow the extended-release tablet whole. Do not crush, break, or chew before swallowing.
- For oral dosage form (extended release tablets):
   - For relief of symptoms from seasonal or yearly allergies:
      - Adults and children 12 years of age and older—Take one tablet two times a day with or without food.
      - Children under 12 years of age—Use and dose must be determined by your doctor.

Missed dose—If you miss a dose of this medicine, take it as soon as possible. However, if it is almost time for your next dose, skip the missed dose and go back to your regular dosing schedule. Do not double doses.

Storage—Store the medicine in a closed container at room temperature, away from heat, moisture, and direct light. Keep from freezing.

Keep out of the reach of children.

Do not keep outdated medicine or medicine no longer needed.

Ask your healthcare professional how you should dispose of any medicine you do not use.

Precautions While Using This Medicine

The antihistamine in this medicine will add to the effects of alcohol and other CNS depressants including tricyclic antidepressants (medicines that slow down the nervous system, possibly causing drowsiness). Some examples of CNS depressants are other antihistamines or medicine for hay fever, other allergies, or colds; sedatives, tranquilizers, or sleeping medicine; prescription pain medicine or narcotics; barbiturates; medicine for seizures; muscle relaxants; or anesthetics, including some dental anesthetics. Examples of Tricyclic antidepressants are amitriptyline [e.g. Elavil], amoxapine [e.g. Asendin], clomipramine [e.g. Anafranil], desipramine [e.g. Pertofrane], doxepine [e.g. Sinequan], imipramine [e.g. Tofranil], nortriptyline [e.g. Aventyl], protriptyline [Vivactil], trimipramine [e.g. Surmontil]. Check with your doctor before taking any of the above while you are taking this medicine.

The antihistamine in this medicine may cause some people to become drowsy, dizzy, or less alert than they are normally.

Make sure you know how you react to this medicine before you drive, use machines, or do anything else that could be dangerous if you are dizzy or are not alert.

Antihistamines may cause dryness of the mouth, nose, and throat. For temporary relief, use sugarless candy or gum, melt bits of ice in your mouth, or use a saliva substitute. However, if your mouth continues to feel dry for more than 2 weeks, check with your dentist. Continuing dryness of the mouth may increase the chance of dental disease, including tooth decay, gum disease, and fungus infections.

The decongestant in this medicine may cause some people to be nervous or restless or to have trouble in sleeping. If you have trouble in sleeping, take the last dose of this medicine for each day a few hours before bedtime. If you have any questions about this, check with your doctor.

Side Effects of This Medicine

Along with its needed effects, a medicine may cause some unwanted effects. Although not all of these side effects may occur, if they do occur they may need medical attention.

Get emergency help immediately if any of the following symptoms of overdose occur:
  Symptoms of overdose
    Changes in mood, irrational behavior, depersonalization hallucinations; convulsions (seizures); extreme sleepiness or unusual drowsiness; fast, slow, pounding, or irregular heartbeat or pulse; feeling anxious; giddiness; headache; irritability; muscle weakness or tenderness; nausea; restlessness; shallow, irregular, fast, or slow breathing; sleeplessness or trouble in sleeping; abdominal and/or chest pain; thirst

Check with your doctor as soon as possible if any of the following side effects occur:
  Rare
    Breathing, troubled; back, leg, or stomach pain; blurred vision; bloody, cloudy, or dark urine, sudden decrease in amount of urine; black, tarry stools, diarrhea, light-colored stools; confusion; dizziness, feeling faint, or lightheaded; fever or chills; increased blood pressure; rapid weight gain; skin rash or hives; swelling of face, mouth, throat, fingers, glands, feet, and/or lower legs; stillbirth; twitching, twisting, or uncontrolled repetitive movements of the face; sudden sweating; vomiting blood, bleeding gums, nosebleeds, unusual bleeding or bruising; pale or yellow eyes or skin; unusual tiredness or weakness

Some side effects may occur that usually do not need medical attention. These side effects may go away during treatment as your body adjusts to the medicine. Also, your health care professional may be able to tell you about ways to prevent or reduce some of these side effects. Check with your health care professional if any of the following side effects continue or are bothersome or if you have any questions about them:
  More common
    Sleepiness or unusual drowsiness, extreme tiredness
  Less common
    Dry mouth; weakness
  Rare
    Dizziness; sore throat

Other side effects not listed may also occur in some patients. If you notice any other effects, check with your healthcare professional.

CETRORELIX (Subcutaneous route) -
set-roe-REL-iks

Commonly used brand name(s)

In the U.S.—
  Cetrotide

Available Dosage Forms:
  • Powder for Solution

Therapeutic Class: Endocrine-Metabolic Agent
Pharmacologic Class: Luteinizing Hormone Releasing Hormone Antagonist

Uses For This Medicine

Cetrorelix is a man-made hormone that blocks the effects of Gonadotropin Releasing Hormone (GnRH). GnRH controls another hormone that is called luteinizing hormone (LH), which is the hormone that starts ovulation during the menstrual cycle. When undergoing hormone treatment sometimes premature ovulation can occur, leading to eggs that are not ready for fertilization to be released. Cetrorelix does not allow the premature release of these eggs to occur.

This medicine is available only with your doctor's prescription.

Before Using This Medicine

In deciding to use a medicine, the risks of taking the medicine must be weighed against the good it will do. This is a decision you and your doctor will make. For this medicine, the following should be considered:

Allergies—Tell your doctor if you have ever had any unusual or allergic reaction to this medicine or any other medicines. Also tell your health care professional if you have any other types of allergies, such as to foods, dyes, preservatives, or animals. For non-prescription products, read the label or package ingredients carefully.

Geriatric—Cetrorelix is not intended for use in patients over the age of 65 years.

Pregnancy—

	Pregnancy Category	Explanation
All Trimesters	X	Studies in animals or pregnant women have demonstrated positive evidence of fetal abnormalities. This drug should not be used in women who are or may become pregnant because the risk clearly outweighs any possible benefit.

Breast Feeding—There are no adequate studies in women for determining infant risk when using this medication during breastfeeding. Weigh the potential benefits against the potential risks before taking this medication while breastfeeding.

Other medicines—Although certain medicines should not be used together at all, in other cases two different medicines may be used together even if an interaction might occur. In these cases, your doctor may want to change the dose, or other precautions may be necessary. Tell your healthcare professional if you are taking any other prescription or non-prescription (over-the-counter [OTC]) medicine.

Interactions with Food/Tobacco/Alcohol—Certain medicines should not be used at or around the time of eating food or eating certain types of food since interactions may occur. Using alcohol or tobacco with certain medicines may also cause interactions to occur. Discuss with your healthcare professional the use of your medicine with food, alcohol, or tobacco.

Other medical problems—The presence of other medical problems may affect the use of this medicine. Make sure you tell your doctor if you have any other medical problems, especially:

- Kidney disease—May increase your chance of side effects from cetrorelix.

Proper Use of This Medicine

Take this medicine only as directed by your doctor. If you are to begin on Day 5, count the first day of your menstrual period as Day 1. Beginning on Day 5, take the correct dose every day for as many days as your doctor ordered. To help you to remember to take your dose of medicine, take it at the same time every day.

- Read the paper with information for the patient carefully.
- Understand and use the proper method of safely preparing the medicine.
- Wash your hands with soap and water and use a clean work area to prepare your injection.
- Make sure you clearly understand and carefully follow your doctor's instructions on how to give yourself an injection, including using the proper needle and syringe. Remember to change the site of injection to different areas to prevent skin problems from developing.
- Throw away needles, syringes, bottles, and unused medicine after the injection in a safe manner.

Tell your doctor when you use the last dose of cetrorelix. Cetrorelix often requires that another hormone called human chorionic gonadotropin (hCG) be given as a single dose the day after the last dose of cetrorelix is given. Your doctor will give you this medicine or arrange for you to get this medicine at the right time.

Dosing—The dose of this medicine will be different for different patients. Follow your doctor's orders or the directions on the label. The following information includes only the average doses of this medicine. If your dose is different, do not change it unless your doctor tells you to do so.

The amount of medicine that you take depends on the strength of the medicine. Also, the number of doses you take each day, the time allowed between doses, and the length of time you take the medicine depend on the medical problem for which you are using the medicine.

- For injection dosage form:
  - For treatment of female infertility:
    - Adults—3 milligrams (mg) injected under the skin one time on Day 7 of your menstrual cycle, or 0.25 mg injected under the skin starting on Day 5 or 6 of your menstrual cycle and continuing until HCG administration occurs.

Missed dose—Call your doctor or pharmacist for instructions.

Storage—Store the medicine in a closed container at room temperature, away from heat, moisture, and direct light. Keep from freezing.

Keep out of the reach of children.

Do not keep outdated medicine or medicine no longer needed.

Store the 0.25 mg vials in the refrigerator. Store the 3 mg vials at room temperature.

Precautions While Using This Medicine

It is very important that your doctor check you using ultrasound examination at regular visits to make sure that you are ready for injection with another drug (HCG) to induce ovulation.

Call your doctor immediately if you have taken more of the medication than your doctor ordered

Side Effects of This Medicine

Along with its needed effects, a medicine may cause some unwanted effects. Although not all of these side effects may occur, if they do occur they may need medical attention.

Check with your doctor immediately if any of the following side effects occur:

Less common
> Abdominal or stomach pain; continuing or severe nausea, vomiting or diarrhea; decreased amount of urine; feeling of indigestion; moderate to severe bloating; pelvic pain, severe; rapid weight gain; shortness of breath; swelling of lower legs

Some side effects may occur that usually do not need medical attention. These side effects may go away during treatment as your body adjusts to the medicine. Also, your health care professional may be able to tell you about ways to prevent or reduce some of these side effects. Check with your health care professional if any of the following side effects continue or are bothersome or if you have any questions about them:

More common
> Headache; injection site bruising, itching, swelling, or redness; nausea

Other side effects not listed may also occur in some patients. If you notice any other effects, check with your healthcare professional.

CETUXIMAB (Intravenous route) - se-TUK-see-mab

Black Box Warning

Severe infusion reactions occurred with the administration of cetuximab in approximately 3% of patients, rarely with fatal outcome (less than 1 in 1000). Approximately 90% of severe infusion reactions were associated with the first infusion of cetuximab. Severe infusion reactions are characterized by rapid onset of airway obstruction (bronchospasm, stridor, hoarseness), urticaria, hypotension and/or cardiac arrest. Severe infusion reactions require immediate interruption of the cetuximab infusion and permanent discontinuation from further treatment.

Cardiopulmonary arrest and/or sudden death occurred in 2% (4/208) of patients with squamous cell carcinoma of the head and neck treated with radiation therapy and cetuximab as compared to none of 212 patients treated with radiation therapy alone. Fatal events occurred within 1 to 43 days after the last cetuximab treatment. Cetuximab in combination with radiation therapy should be used with caution in head and neck cancer patients with known coronary artery disease, congestive heart failure, and arrhythmias. Although the etiology of these events is unknown, close monitoring of serum electrolytes, including serum magnesium, potassium, and calcium, during and after cetuximab therapy is recommended.

Commonly used brand name(s)

In the U.S.—
    Erbitux

Available Dosage Forms:
  • Solution

Therapeutic Class: Antineoplastic Agent
Pharmacologic Class: Monoclonal Antibody

Uses For This Medicine

Cetuximab is a monoclonal antibody. It is used to treat cancer of the colon and rectal area and cancers of the head and neck. It may also be used to treat other kinds of cancer, as determined by your doctor. Cetuximab interferes with the growth of cancer cells, which are then eventually destroyed by the body.

Cetuximab is to be administered only by or under the immediate supervision of your doctor.

Before Using This Medicine

In deciding to use a medicine, the risks of taking the medicine must be weighed against the good it will do. This is a decision you and your doctor will make. For this medicine, the following should be considered:

Allergies—Tell your doctor if you have ever had any unusual or allergic reaction to this medicine or any other medicines. Also tell your health care professional if you have any other types of allergies, such as to foods, dyes, preservatives, or animals. For non-prescription products, read the label or package ingredients carefully.

Pediatric—Studies on this medicine have been done only in adult patients, and there is no specific information comparing use of cetuximab in children with use in other age groups.

Geriatric—This medicine has been tested and has not been shown to cause different side effects or problems in older people than it does in younger adults.

Pregnancy—

	Pregnancy Category	Explanation
All Trimesters	C	Animal studies have shown an adverse effect and there are no adequate studies in pregnant women OR no animal studies have been conducted and there are no adequate studies in pregnant women.

Breast Feeding—There are no adequate studies in women for determining infant risk when using this medication during breastfeeding. Weigh the potential benefits against the potential risks before taking this medication while breastfeeding.

Other medicines—Although certain medicines should not be used together at all, in other cases two different medicines may be used together even if an interaction might occur. In these cases, your doctor may want to change the dose, or other precautions may be necessary. Tell your healthcare professional if you are taking any other prescription or non-prescription (over-the-counter [OTC]) medicine.

Interactions with Food/Tobacco/Alcohol—Certain medicines should not be used at or around the time of eating food or eating certain types of food since interactions may occur. Using alcohol or tobacco with certain medicines may also cause interactions to occur. Discuss with your healthcare professional the use of your medicine with food, alcohol, or tobacco.

Other medical problems—The presence of other medical problems may affect the use of this medicine. Make sure you tell your doctor if you have any other medical problems, especially:
  • Fibrotic lung disease, preexisting—May be worsened by cetuximab.
  • Radiation therapy—May increase your chance of getting severe skin reactions.

Proper Use of This Medicine

Dosing—The dose of this medicine will be different for different patients. Follow your doctor's orders or the directions on the label. The following information includes only the average doses of this medicine. If your dose is different, do not change it unless your doctor tells you to do so.

The amount of medicine that you take depends on the strength of the medicine. Also, the number of doses you take each day, the time allowed between doses, and the length of time you take the medicine depend on the medical problem for which you are using the medicine.

Precautions While Using This Medicine

It is very important that your doctor check you at regular visits.

Avoid over exposing your skin to sunlight. Regularly use sunscreen or sun blocking lotions. Also, wear protective clothing and hats.

Side Effects of This Medicine

Along with its needed effects, a medicine may cause some unwanted effects. Although not all of these side effects may occur, if they do occur they may need medical attention.

Check with your doctor immediately if any of the following side effects occur:
  More common
    Blemishes on the skin, pimples; bloating or swelling of face, arms, hands, lower legs, or feet; chills; cough or hoarseness; deep cracks, grooves or lines in skin; difficult or labored breathing; dizziness; facial swelling; fever; headache; lower back or side pain; nausea; painful or difficult urination; pale skin; rapid weight gain; severe dry skin; shortness of breath; skin rash; tightness in chest; tingling of hands or feet; troubled breathing with exertion; unusual bleeding or bruising; unusual tiredness or weakness; unusual weight gain or loss; vomiting; weakness; wheezing
  Less common or rare
    Anxiety; black, tarry stools; chest pain; confusion; decreased urination; dry mouth; fainting; fast heartbeat; increase in heart rate; kidney failure; lightheadedness; rapid, shallow breathing; sore throat; sores, ulcers, or

white spots on lips or in mouth; sunken eyes; swollen glands; thirst; wrinkled skin

Some side effects may occur that usually do not need medical attention. These side effects may go away during treatment as your body adjusts to the medicine. Also, your health care professional may be able to tell you about ways to prevent or reduce some of these side effects. Check with your health care professional if any of the following side effects continue or are bothersome or if you have any questions about them:

More common

Acid or sour stomach; back pain; belching; burning, dry or itching eyes; diarrhea; difficulty having a bowel movement (stool); discharge from eye; discoloration of fingernails or toenails; discouragement; excessive tearing; feeling sad or empty; hair loss, thinning of hair; heartburn; indigestion; irritability; itching skin; lack or loss of appetite; lack or loss of strength; loss of interest or pleasure; pain; redness, pain, swelling of eye, eyelid, or inner lining of eyelid; sleeplessness; stomach discomfort upset or pain; stomach pain; swelling or inflammation of the mouth; trouble concentrating; trouble sleeping; unable to sleep

Other side effects not listed may also occur in some patients. If you notice any other effects, check with your healthcare professional.

CEVIMELINE (Oral route) - se-vi-ME-leen

Commonly used brand name(s)
In the U.S.—
Evoxac

Available Dosage Forms:
• Capsule

Therapeutic Class: Central Nervous System Agent
Pharmacologic Class: Cholinergic

Uses For This Medicine

Cevimeline is used to treat the symptoms of dry mouth often experienced by patients with Sjogren's syndrome. It works by causing certain mouth glands to produce more saliva.

This medicine is available only with your doctor's prescription.

Before Using This Medicine

In deciding to use a medicine, the risks of taking the medicine must be weighed against the good it will do. This is a decision you and your doctor will make. For this medicine, the following should be considered:

Allergies—Tell your doctor if you have ever had any unusual or allergic reaction to this medicine or any other medicines. Also tell your health care professional if you have any other types of allergies, such as to foods, dyes, preservatives, or animals. For non-prescription products, read the label or package ingredients carefully.

Pediatric—Studies on this medicine have been done only in adult patients, and there is no specific information comparing use of cevimeline in children with use in other age groups.

Geriatric—Older adults—Many medicines have not been studied specifically in older people. Therefore, it may not be known whether they work exactly the same way they do in younger adults. Although there is no specific information comparing use of cevimeline in the elderly with use in other age groups, this medicine is not expected to cause different side effects or problems in older people than it does in younger adults.

Pregnancy—

	Pregnancy Category	Explanation
All Trimesters	C	Animal studies have shown an adverse effect and there are no adequate studies in pregnant women OR no animal studies have been conducted and there are no adequate studies in pregnant women.

Breast Feeding—There are no adequate studies in women for determining infant risk when using this medication during breastfeeding. Weigh the potential benefits against the potential risks before taking this medication while breastfeeding.

Other medicines—Although certain medicines should not be used together at all, in other cases two different medicines may be used together even if an interaction might occur. In these cases, your doctor may want to change the dose, or other precautions may be necessary. Tell your healthcare professional if you are taking any other prescription or non-prescription (over-the-counter [OTC]) medicine.

Interactions with Food/Tobacco/Alcohol—Certain medicines should not be used at or around the time of eating food or eating certain types of food since interactions may occur. Using alcohol or tobacco with certain medicines may also cause interactions to occur. Discuss with your healthcare professional the use of your medicine with food, alcohol, or tobacco.

Other medical problems—The presence of other medical problems may affect the use of this medicine. Make sure you tell your doctor if you have any other medical problems, especially:

• Asthma, uncontrolled, or

• Cholelithiasis (gallstones), or

• Heart disease, or

• Nephrolithiasis (kidney stones), or

• Eye conditions in which contraction of the pupils is undesirable (e.g., acute iritis and narrow-angle glaucoma), or

• Pulmonary disease other than asthma

Proper Use of This Medicine

Dosing—The dose of this medicine will be different for different patients. Follow your doctor's orders or the directions on the label. The following information includes only the average doses of this medicine. If your dose is different, do not change it unless your doctor tells you to do so.

The amount of medicine that you take depends on the strength of the medicine. Also, the number of doses you take each day, the time allowed between doses, and the length of time you take the medicine depend on the medical problem for which you are using the medicine.

- For oral dosage form (capsules):
  - For the treatment of dry mouth in patients with Sjogren's syndrome:
    - Adults—30 milligrams three times a day
    - Children—Use and dose must be determined by your doctor.

Missed dose—If you miss a dose of this medicine, take it as soon as possible. However, if it is almost time for your next dose, skip the missed dose and go back to your regular dosing schedule. Do not double doses.

Storage—Store the medicine in a closed container at room temperature, away from heat, moisture, and direct light. Keep from freezing.

Keep out of the reach of children.

Do not keep outdated medicine or medicine no longer needed.

Ask your healthcare professional how you should dispose of any medicine you do not use.

Precautions While Using This Medicine

If you will be taking this medicine for a long time, it is very important that your doctor check you at regular visits for signs of your receiving too much medicine.

If your symptoms do not improve within a few days or if they become worse, check with your doctor.

Do not take other medicines unless they have been discussed with your doctor. This especially includes nonprescription medicines, such as aspirin, and medicines for appetite control, asthma, colds, cough, hay fever, or sinus problems.

This medicine may cause some people to become drowsy, dizzy, or less alert than they are normally. This medicine may also cause a change in vision that could cause you to see less well at night. Make sure you know how you react to this medicine before you drive, use machines, or do anything else that could be dangerous if you are unable to see well, or if you are dizzy or are not alert.

Side Effects of This Medicine

Along with its needed effects, a medicine may cause some unwanted effects. Although not all of these side effects may occur, if they do occur they may need medical attention.

Check with your doctor immediately if any of the following side effects occur:
  Less common
    Difficulty breathing; fast heartbeat; itching
  Rare
    Chest pain; fainting or light-headedness when getting up from a lying or a sitting position; swelling of gums or tongue
  Symptoms of overdose
  Get emergency help immediately if any of the following symptoms of overdose occur:
    Blurring or loss of vision; chest pain; cold, clammy skin; diarrhea, continuous and severe; disturbed color vision; dizziness, faintness, or light-headedness when getting up from a lying or sitting position; difficult or labored breathing; fast, pounding, slow, or irregular heartbeat; fast, weak pulse; headache; mental confusion; nausea; pounding in ears;

shaking or trembling of hands or feet; shortness of breath; stomach cramps or pain; sweating; tearing of the eyes

Check with your doctor as soon as possible if any of the following side effects occur:
  Less common
    Bloody or cloudy urine; blurred vision; chest pain; cough; cracks in skin; difficult, burning, or painful urination; dizziness; dry or itching eyes; earache; feeling of constant movement of self or surroundings; itching of vagina, genital, or other skin area; lower back pain; redness or pain in eye; ringing or buzzing in the ears; scaling of skin; shortness of breath; skin rash; soreness or redness of skin; sores, ulcers, or white spots on tongue, lips, or inside of mouth; stiffness of muscles; swelling of hands, ankles, feet, or lower legs; swelling on side of face and jaw, with or without pain; tense muscles

Some side effects may occur that usually do not need medical attention. These side effects may go away during treatment as your body adjusts to the medicine. Also, your health care professional may be able to tell you about ways to prevent or reduce some of these side effects. Check with your health care professional if any of the following side effects continue or are bothersome or if you have any questions about them:
  More common
    Excessive sweating; nausea; runny or stuffy nose
  Less common
    Abdominal pain; belching; bloating or swelling of face, hands, feet, or lower legs; bloody nose; bone or joint pain; burning, dry, or itching feeling in eye; change in vision; chills; constipation; cough, mucus-producing; decreased touch sensation; depression; diarrhea; dry mouth; eye pain; feelings of warmth in face, neck, arms, and occasionally, chest; fever; heartburn; hiccups; injury; itching; leg cramps; loss of appetite; migraine headache; mood or mental changes; muscle aches, pain, or stiffness; pain and swelling of eye, eyelid, or inner lining of eye; pain on side of face and jaw; pain, swelling, or redness of joints; postoperative pain; rapid weight gain; shortness of breath; skin disorder; tightness in chest; tooth disorders or pain; trembling or shaking of hands or feet; trouble in sleeping; unusual bleeding or bruising; unusual tiredness or weakness; vomiting; watering of mouth; weight loss
  Rare
    Abnormal crying; deep, dark, purple bruise; swelling or puffiness of face; temperature sensation changes

Other side effects not listed may also occur in some patients. If you notice any other effects, check with your healthcare professional.

CHLORAMBUCIL   (Oral route) - klor-AM-byoo-sil

Black Box Warning

Chlorambucil can severely suppress bone marrow function. Chlorambucil is a carcinogen in humans. Chlorambucil is probably mutagenic and teratogenic in humans. Chlorambucil produces human infertility.

Commonly used brand name(s)

In the U.S.—
  Leukeran

Available Dosage Forms:
  • Tablet

Therapeutic Class: Antineoplastic Agent
Pharmacologic Class: Alkylating Agent

Uses For This Medicine

Chlorambucil belongs to the group of medicines called alkylating agents. It is used to treat cancer of the blood and lymph system. It may also be used to treat other kinds of cancer, as determined by your doctor.

Chlorambucil interferes with the growth of cancer cells, which are eventually destroyed. Since the growth of normal body cells may also be affected by chlorambucil, other effects will also occur. Some of these may be serious and must be reported to your doctor. Other effects may not be serious but may cause concern. Some effects may not occur for months or years after the medicine is used.

Before you begin treatment with chlorambucil, you and your doctor should talk about the good this medicine will do as well as the risks of using it.

Chlorambucil may also be used for other conditions as determined by your doctor.

Chlorambucil is available only with your doctor's prescription.

Once a medicine has been approved for marketing for a certain use, experience may show that it is also useful for other medical problems. Although these uses are not included in product labeling, chlorambucil is used in certain patients with the following medical conditions:

  • Cancer of the ovaries
  • Cancer of the lymph system that affects the skin
  • Hairy cell leukemia (a cancer of the blood and bone marrow)
  • Nephrotic syndrome (a kidney disease)
  • Tumors in the uterus (womb)
  • Waldenström's macroglobulinemia (a certain type of cancer of the blood)
  • Histiocytosis X (a certain type of cancer found primarily in children)

Before Using This Medicine

In deciding to use a medicine, the risks of taking the medicine must be weighed against the good it will do. This is a decision you and your doctor will make. For this medicine, the following should be considered:

Allergies—Tell your doctor if you have ever had any unusual or allergic reaction to this medicine or any other medicines. Also tell your health care professional if you have any other types of allergies, such as to foods, dyes, preservatives, or animals. For non-prescription products, read the label or package ingredients carefully.

Pediatric—In general, this medicine has not been shown to cause different side effects or problems in children than it does in adults. However, some children with nephrotic syndrome (a kidney disease) may be more likely to have convulsions (seizures).

Geriatric—Many medicines have not been studied specifically in older people. Therefore, it may not be known whether they work exactly the same way they do in younger adults or if they cause different side effects or problems in older people. There is no specific information comparing use of chlorambucil in the elderly with use in other age groups.

Pregnancy—

	Pregnancy Category	Explanation
All Trimesters	D	Studies in pregnant women have demonstrated a risk to the fetus. However, the benefits of therapy in a life threatening situation or a serious disease, may outweigh the potential risk.

Breast Feeding—There are no adequate studies in women for determining infant risk when using this medication during breastfeeding. Weigh the potential benefits against the potential risks before taking this medication while breastfeeding.

Other medicines—

Using this medicine with any of the following medicines is not recommended. Your doctor may decide not to treat you with this medication or change some of the other medicines you take.

Rotavirus Vaccine, Live

Interactions with Food/Tobacco/Alcohol—Certain medicines should not be used at or around the time of eating food or eating certain types of food since interactions may occur. Using alcohol or tobacco with certain medicines may also cause interactions to occur. Discuss with your healthcare professional the use of your medicine with food, alcohol, or tobacco.

Other medical problems—The presence of other medical problems may affect the use of this medicine. Make sure you tell your doctor if you have any other medical problems, especially:

  • Chickenpox (including recent exposure) or
  • Herpes zoster (shingles)—Risk of severe disease affecting other parts of the body
  • Convulsions (seizures) (history of) or
  • Head injury—Increased risk of seizures
  • Gout or
  • Kidney stones (history of)—Chlorambucil may increase levels of uric acid in the body, which can cause gout or kidney stones
  • Bone marrow depression or
  • Infection—Chlorambucil decreases your body's ability to fight infection
  • Previous failure of chlorambucil therapy—Repeat treatment with chlorambucil not recommended

Proper Use of This Medicine

Take this medicine only as directed by your doctor. Do not take more or less of it, and do not take it more often than your doctor ordered. The exact amount of medicine you need has been carefully worked out. Taking too much may increase the chance of side effects, while taking too little may not improve your condition.

Chlorambucil is sometimes given together with certain other medicines. If you are using a combination of medicines, make sure that you take each one at the proper time and do not mix them. Ask your health care professional to help you plan a way to remember to take your medicines at the right times.

While you are using chlorambucil, your doctor may want you to drink extra fluids so that you will pass more urine. This will help prevent kidney problems and keep your kidneys working well.

This medicine sometimes causes nausea and vomiting. However, it is very important that you continue to use the medicine, even if you begin to feel ill. Do not stop using this medicine without first checking with your doctor. Ask your health care professional for ways to lessen these effects.

If you vomit shortly after taking a dose of chlorambucil, check with your doctor. You will be told whether to take the dose again or to wait until the next scheduled dose.

Dosing—The dose of this medicine will be different for different patients. Follow your doctor's orders or the directions on the label. The following information includes only the average doses of this medicine. If your dose is different, do not change it unless your doctor tells you to do so.

The amount of medicine that you take depends on the strength of the medicine. Also, the number of doses you take each day, the time allowed between doses, and the length of time you take the medicine depend on the medical problem for which you are using the medicine.

Missed dose—If you miss a dose of this medicine, take it as soon as possible. However, if it is almost time for your next dose, skip the missed dose and go back to your regular dosing schedule. Do not double doses.

Storage—Store in the refrigerator. Do not freeze.

Keep out of the reach of children.

Do not keep outdated medicine or medicine no longer needed.

Precautions While Using This Medicine

It is very important that your doctor check your progress at regular visits to make sure this medicine is working properly and to check for unwanted effects.

While you are being treated with chlorambucil, and after you stop treatment with it, do not have any immunizations (vaccinations) without your doctor's approval. Chlorambucil may lower your body's resistance and there is a chance you might get the infection the immunization is meant to prevent. In addition, other persons living in your household should not take oral polio vaccine since there is a chance they could pass the polio virus on to you. Also, avoid persons who have taken oral polio vaccine within the last several months. Do not get close to them, and do not stay in the same room with them for very long. If you cannot take these precautions, you should consider wearing a protective face mask that covers the nose and mouth.

Chlorambucil can temporarily lower the number of white blood cells in your blood, increasing the chance of getting an infection. It can also lower the number of platelets, which are necessary for proper blood clotting. If this occurs, there are cer-

tain precautions you can take, especially when your blood count is low, to reduce the risk of infection or bleeding:

- If you can, avoid people with infections. Check with your doctor immediately if you think you are getting an infection or if you get a fever or chills, cough or hoarseness, lower back or side pain, or painful or difficult urination.
- Check with your doctor immediately if you notice any unusual bleeding or bruising; black, tarry stools; blood in urine or stools; or pinpoint red spots on your skin.
- Be careful when using a regular toothbrush, dental floss, or toothpick. Your medical doctor, dentist, or nurse may recommend other ways to clean your teeth and gums. Check with your medical doctor before having any dental work done.
- Do not touch your eyes or the inside of your nose unless you have just washed your hands and have not touched anything else in the meantime.
- Be careful not to cut yourself when you are using sharp objects such as a safety razor or fingernail or toenail cutters.
- Avoid contact sports or other situations where bruising or injury could occur.

Side Effects of This Medicine

Along with its needed effects, a medicine may cause some unwanted effects. Although not all of these side effects may occur, if they do occur they may need medical attention.

Also, because of the way these medicines act on the body, there is a chance that they might cause other unwanted effects that may not occur until months or years after the medicine is used. These delayed effects may include certain types of cancer, such as leukemia. Discuss these possible effects with your doctor.

Check with your doctor immediately if any of the following side effects occur:
> *More common*
>> Black, tarry stools; blood in urine or stools; cough or hoarseness, accompanied by fever or chills; fever or chills; lower back or side pain, accompanied by fever or chills; painful or difficult urination, accompanied by fever or chills; pinpoint red spots on skin; unusual bleeding or bruising
>
> *Less common*
>> Large, swollen hives; itching; skin rash; sores in mouth and on lips
>
> *Rare*
>> Cough; blisters on skin; muscle twitching or jerking; shortness of breath

Check with your doctor as soon as possible if any of the following side effects occur:
> *Less common*
>> Joint pain; swelling of feet or lower legs
>
> *Rare*
>> Agitation; confusion; convulsions (seizures); hallucinations (seeing, hearing, or feeling things that are not there); tremors; trouble in walking; weakness (severe) or paralysis; yellow eyes or skin
>
> *Symptoms of overdose (in the order of frequency)*
>> Black, tarry stools; blood in urine or stools; cough or hoarseness, accompanied by fever or chills; fever or chills; lower back or side pain, accompanied by fever

or chills; painful or difficult urination, accompanied by fever or chills; pinpoint red spots on skin; unusual bleeding or bruising; agitation; convulsions (seizures); trouble in walking

Some side effects may occur that usually do not need medical attention. These side effects may go away during treatment as your body adjusts to the medicine. Also, your health care professional may be able to tell you about ways to prevent or reduce some of these side effects. Check with your health care professional if any of the following side effects continue or are bothersome or if you have any questions about them:

Less common

Changes in menstrual period; itching of skin; nausea and vomiting

After you stop using this medicine, it may still produce some side effects that need attention. During this period of time, *check with your doctor immediately* if you notice the following side effects:

Black, tarry stools; blood in urine or stools; cough or hoarseness (may be accompanied by fever or chills); fever or chills; lower back or side pain, accompanied by fever or chills; painful or difficult urination, accompanied by fever or chills; pinpoint red spots on skin; shortness of breath; unusual bleeding or bruising

Other side effects not listed may also occur in some patients. If you notice any other effects, check with your healthcare professional.

CHLORAMPHENICOL (Ophthalmic route) - klor-am-FEN-i-kole

Commonly used brand name(s)
In the U.S.—
    Ocu-Chlor

In Canada—

Ak-Chlor	Ophtho-Chloram
Chloromycetin	Pentamycetin Ophthalmic
Chloroptic	Solution 0.25%
Fenicol	Pentamycetin Ophthalmic
Isopto Fenicol	Solution 0.5%
Minims Chloramphenicol	Pms-Chloramphenicol
0.5%	Sopamycetin

Available Dosage Forms:
• Powder for Solution
• Solution
• Ointment

Therapeutic Class: Antibiotic

Uses For This Medicine

Chloramphenicol belongs to the family of medicines called antibiotics. Chloramphenicol ophthalmic preparations are used to treat infections of the eye. This medicine may be given alone or with other medicines that are taken by mouth for eye infections.

Chloramphenicol is available only with your doctor's prescription.

Before Using This Medicine

In deciding to use a medicine, the risks of taking the medicine must be weighed against the good it will do. This is a decision you and your doctor will make. For this medicine, the following should be considered:

Allergies—Tell your doctor if you have ever had any unusual or allergic reaction to this medicine or any other medicines. Also tell your health care professional if you have any other types of allergies, such as to foods, dyes, preservatives, or animals. For non-prescription products, read the label or package ingredients carefully.

Pediatric—Studies on this medicine have been done only in adult patients, and there is no specific information comparing use of this medicine in children with use in other age groups.

Geriatric—Many medicines have not been studied specifically in older people. Therefore, it may not be known whether they work exactly the same way they do in younger adults or if they cause different side effects or problems in older people. There is no specific information comparing use of this medicine in the elderly with use in other age groups.

Breast Feeding—There are no adequate studies in women for determining infant risk when using this medication during breastfeeding. Weigh the potential benefits against the potential risks before taking this medication while breastfeeding.

Other medicines—

Using this medicine with any of the following medicines may cause an increased risk of certain side effects, but using both drugs may be the best treatment for you. If both medicines are prescribed together, your doctor may change the dose or how often you use one or both of the medicines.

Ceftazidime, Chlorpropamide, Cyclosporine, Dicumarol, Fosphenytoin, Phenytoin, Rifampin, Rifapentine, Tacrolimus, Tetanus Toxoid, Tolbutamide

Interactions with Food/Tobacco/Alcohol—Certain medicines should not be used at or around the time of eating food or eating certain types of food since interactions may occur. Using alcohol or tobacco with certain medicines may also cause interactions to occur. Discuss with your healthcare professional the use of your medicine with food, alcohol, or tobacco.

Proper Use of This Medicine

For patients using the eye drop form of chloramphenicol:
• Although the bottle may not be full, it contains exactly the amount of medicine your doctor ordered.
• To use:
    ○ First, wash your hands. Tilt the head back and, pressing your finger gently on the skin just beneath the lower eyelid, pull the lower eyelid away from the eye to make a space. Drop the medicine into this space. Let go of the eyelid and gently close the eyes. Do not blink. Keep the eyes closed and apply pressure to the inner corner of the eye with your finger for 1 or 2 minutes to allow the medicine to come into contact with the infection.
    ○ If you think you did not get the drop of medicine into your eye properly, use another drop.
    ○ To keep the medicine as germ-free as possible, do not touch the applicator tip or dropper to any surface

(including the eye). Also, keep the container tightly closed.

To use the eye ointment form of chloramphenicol:

- First, wash your hands. Tilt the head back and, pressing your finger gently on the skin just beneath the lower eyelid, pull the lower eyelid away from the eye to make a space. Squeeze a thin strip of ointment into this space. A 1–cm (approximately 1/3–inch) strip of ointment is usually enough, unless you have been told by your doctor to use a different amount. Let go of the eyelid and gently close the eyes. Keep the eyes closed for 1 or 2 minutes to allow the medicine to come into contact with the infection.
- To keep the medicine as germ-free as possible, do not touch the applicator tip to any surface (including the eye). After using chloramphenicol eye ointment, wipe the tip of the ointment tube with a clean tissue and keep the tube tightly closed.

To help clear up your infection completely, keep using this medicine for the full time of treatment, even if your symptoms begin to clear up after a few days. If you stop using this medicine too soon, your symptoms may return. Do not miss any doses.

Dosing—The dose of this medicine will be different for different patients. Follow your doctor's orders or the directions on the label. The following information includes only the average doses of this medicine. If your dose is different, do not change it unless your doctor tells you to do so.

The amount of medicine that you take depends on the strength of the medicine. Also, the number of doses you take each day, the time allowed between doses, and the length of time you take the medicine depend on the medical problem for which you are using the medicine.

- For eye infection:
  - For ophthalmic ointment dosage form:
    - Adults and children—Use every three hours.
  - For ophthalmic solution (eye drops) dosage form:
    - Adults and children—One drop every one to four hours.

Missed dose—If you miss a dose of this medicine, apply it as soon as possible. However, if it is almost time for your next dose, skip the missed dose and go back to your regular dosing schedule.

Storage—Store the medicine in a closed container at room temperature, away from heat, moisture, and direct light. Keep from freezing.

Keep out of the reach of children.

Do not keep outdated medicine or medicine no longer needed.

Precautions While Using This Medicine

If your symptoms do not improve within a few days, or if they become worse, check with your doctor.

Side Effects of This Medicine

Along with its needed effects, a medicine may cause some unwanted effects. Although not all of these side effects may occur, if they do occur they may need medical attention.

Check with your doctor immediately if any of the following side effects occur:

Rare—may also occur weeks or months after you stop using this medicine
    Pale skin; sore throat and fever; unusual bleeding or bruising; unusual tiredness or weakness

Check with your doctor as soon as possible if any of the following side effects occur:

Less common
    Itching, redness, skin rash, swelling, or other sign of irritation not present before use of this medicine

Some side effects may occur that usually do not need medical attention. These side effects may go away during treatment as your body adjusts to the medicine. Also, your health care professional may be able to tell you about ways to prevent or reduce some of these side effects. Check with your health care professional if any of the following side effects continue or are bothersome or if you have any questions about them:

Less common
    Burning or stinging

After application, eye ointments may be expected to cause your vision to blur for a few minutes.

Other side effects not listed may also occur in some patients. If you notice any other effects, check with your healthcare professional.

CHLORAMPHENICOL (Oral route, Intravenous route, Injection route) - klor-am-FEN-i-kole

Black Box Warning

Serious and fatal blood dyscrasias (aplastic anemia, hypoplastic anemia, thrombocytopenia, and granulocytopenia) are known to occur after the administration of chloramphenicol. In addition, there have been reports of aplastic anemia attributed to chloramphenicol which later terminated in leukemia. Blood dyscrasias have occurred after both short-term and prolonged therapy with this drug. Chloramphenicol must not be used when less potentially dangerous agents will be effective. It must not be used in the treatment of trivial infections or where it is not indicated, as in colds, influenza, infections of the throat; or as a prophylactic agent to prevent bacterial infections.

Precautions: It is essential that adequate blood studies be made during treatment with the drug. While blood studies may detect early peripheral blood changes, such as leukopenia, reticulocytopenia, or granulocytopenia, before they become irreversible, such studies cannot be relied on to detect bone marrow depression prior to development of aplastic anemia. To facilitate appropriate studies and observation during therapy, it is desirable that patients be hospitalized.

Commonly used brand name(s)

In the U.S.—
    Chloromycetin Sodium Succinate

In Canada—
    Chloromycetin

Available Dosage Forms:
- Powder for Solution
- Capsule
- Suspension

Therapeutic Class: Antibiotic

Uses For This Medicine

Chloramphenicol is used in the treatment of infections caused by bacteria. It works by killing bacteria or preventing their growth.

Chloramphenicol is used to treat serious infections in different parts of the body. It is sometimes given with other antibiotics. However, chloramphenicol should not be used for colds, flu, other virus infections, sore throats or other minor infections, or to prevent infections.

Chloramphenicol should only be used for serious infections in which other medicines do not work. This medicine may cause some serious side effects, including blood problems and eye problems. Symptoms of the blood problems include pale skin, sore throat and fever, unusual bleeding or bruising, and unusual tiredness or weakness. You and your doctor should talk about the good this medicine will do as well as the risks of taking it.

Chloramphenicol is available only with your doctor's prescription.

Before Using This Medicine

In deciding to use a medicine, the risks of taking the medicine must be weighed against the good it will do. This is a decision you and your doctor will make. For this medicine, the following should be considered:

Allergies—Tell your doctor if you have ever had any unusual or allergic reaction to this medicine or any other medicines. Also tell your health care professional if you have any other types of allergies, such as to foods, dyes, preservatives, or animals. For non-prescription products, read the label or package ingredients carefully.

Pediatric—Newborn infants are especially sensitive to the side effects of chloramphenicol because they cannot remove the medicine from their body as well as older children and adults.

Geriatric—Many medicines have not been studied specifically in older people. Therefore, it may not be known whether they work exactly the same way they do in younger adults or if they cause different side effects or problems in older people. There is no specific information comparing use of chloramphenicol in the elderly with use in other age groups.

Breast Feeding—There are no adequate studies in women for determining infant risk when using this medication during breastfeeding. Weigh the potential benefits against the potential risks before taking this medication while breastfeeding.

Other medicines—

Using this medicine with any of the following medicines may cause an increased risk of certain side effects, but using both drugs may be the best treatment for you. If both medicines are prescribed together, your doctor may change the dose or how often you use one or both of the medicines.

Ceftazidime, Chlorpropamide, Cyclosporine, Dicumarol, Fosphenytoin, Phenytoin, Rifampin, Rifapentine, Tacrolimus, Tetanus Toxoid, Tolbutamide

Interactions with Food/Tobacco/Alcohol—Certain medicines should not be used at or around the time of eating food or eating certain types of food since interactions may occur. Using alcohol or tobacco with certain medicines may also cause interactions to occur. Discuss with your healthcare professional the use of your medicine with food, alcohol, or tobacco.

Other medical problems—The presence of other medical problems may affect the use of this medicine. Make sure you tell your doctor if you have any other medical problems, especially:
- Anemia, bleeding, or other blood problems—Chloramphenicol may cause blood problems
- Liver disease—Patients with liver disease may have an increased risk of side effects

Proper Use of This Medicine

Chloramphenicol is best taken with a full glass (8 ounces) of water on an empty stomach (either 1 hour before or 2 hours after meals), unless otherwise directed by your doctor.

For patients taking the oral liquid form of this medicine:
- Use a specially marked measuring spoon or other device to measure each dose accurately. The average household teaspoon may not hold the right amount of liquid.

To help clear up your infection completely, keep taking this medicine for the full time of treatment, even if you begin to feel better after a few days. Do not miss any doses.

Dosing—The dose of this medicine will be different for different patients. Follow your doctor's orders or the directions on the label. The following information includes only the average doses of this medicine. If your dose is different, do not change it unless your doctor tells you to do so.

The amount of medicine that you take depends on the strength of the medicine. Also, the number of doses you take each day, the time allowed between doses, and the length of time you take the medicine depend on the medical problem for which you are using the medicine.
- For infections caused by bacteria:
  - For oral dosage forms (capsules and suspension):
    - Adults and teenagers—Dose is based on body weight. The usual dose is 12.5 milligrams (mg) per kilogram (kg) (5.7 mg per pound) of body weight every six hours.
    - Children—
      — Infants up to 2 weeks of age: Dose is based on body weight. The usual dose is 6.25 mg per kg (2.8 mg per pound) of body weight every six hours.
      — Infants 2 weeks of age and older: Dose is based on body weight. The usual dose is 12.5 mg per kg (5.7 mg per pound) of body weight every six hours; or 25 mg per kg (11.4 mg per pound) of body weight every twelve hours.
  - For injection dosage form:
    - Adults and teenagers—Dose is based on body weight. The usual dose is 12.5 mg per kg (5.7 mg per pound) of body weight every six hours.
    - Children—
      — Infants up to 2 weeks of age: Dose is based on body weight. The usual dose is 6.25 mg per kg (2.8 mg per pound) of body weight every six hours.

— Infants 2 weeks of age and older: Dose is based on body weight. The usual dose is 12.5 mg per kg (5.7 mg per pound) of body weight every six hours; or 25 mg per kg (11.4 mg per pound) of body weight every twelve hours.

Missed dose—If you miss a dose of this medicine, take it as soon as possible. However, if it is almost time for your next dose, skip the missed dose and go back to your regular dosing schedule. Do not double doses.

Storage—Store the medicine in a closed container at room temperature, away from heat, moisture, and direct light. Keep from freezing.

Keep out of the reach of children.

Do not keep outdated medicine or medicine no longer needed.

Precautions While Using This Medicine

If your symptoms do not improve within a few days, or if they become worse, check with your doctor.

It is very important that your doctor check you at regular visits for any blood problems that may be caused by this medicine.

Chloramphenicol may cause blood problems. These problems may result in a greater chance of infection, slow healing, and bleeding of the gums. Therefore, you should be careful when using regular toothbrushes, dental floss, and toothpicks. Dental work, whenever possible, should be done before you begin taking this medicine or delayed until your blood counts have returned to normal. Check with your medical doctor or dentist if you have any questions about proper oral hygiene (mouth care) during treatment.

For diabetic patients:

• This medicine may cause false test results with urine sugar tests. Check with your doctor before changing your diet or the dosage of your diabetes medicine.

Side Effects of This Medicine

Along with its needed effects, a medicine may cause some unwanted effects. Although not all of these side effects may occur, if they do occur they may need medical attention.

Stop taking this medicine and get emergency help immediately if any of the following effects occur:
Rare—in babies only
Bloated stomach; drowsiness; gray skin color; low body temperature; uneven breathing; unresponsiveness

Check with your doctor immediately if any of the following side effects occur:
Less common
Pale skin; sore throat and fever; unusual bleeding or bruising; unusual tiredness or weakness (the above side effects may also occur up to weeks or months after you stop taking this medicine)
Rare
Confusion, delirium, or headache; eye pain, blurred vision, or loss of vision; numbness, tingling, burning pain, or weakness in the hands or feet; skin rash, fever, or difficulty in breathing

Some side effects may occur that usually do not need medical attention. These side effects may go away during treatment as your body adjusts to the medicine. Also, your health care professional may be able to tell you about ways to prevent or reduce some of these side effects. Check with your health care professional if any of the following side effects continue or are bothersome or if you have any questions about them:
Less common
Diarrhea; nausea or vomiting

Other side effects not listed may also occur in some patients. If you notice any other effects, check with your healthcare professional.

CHLORAMPHENICOL (Otic route) -
klor-am-FEN-i-kole

Commonly used brand name(s)
In Canada—
Chloromycetin
Sopamycetin

Available Dosage Forms:
• Solution

Therapeutic Class: Antibacterial

Uses For This Medicine

Chloramphenicol belongs to the family of medicines called antibiotics. Chloramphenicol otic drops are used to treat infections of the ear canal. This medicine may be used alone or with other medicines that are taken by mouth for ear canal infections.

Chloramphenicol is available only with your doctor's prescription.

Before Using This Medicine

In deciding to use a medicine, the risks of taking the medicine must be weighed against the good it will do. This is a decision you and your doctor will make. For this medicine, the following should be considered:

Allergies—Tell your doctor if you have ever had any unusual or allergic reaction to this medicine or any other medicines. Also tell your health care professional if you have any other types of allergies, such as to foods, dyes, preservatives, or animals. For non-prescription products, read the label or package ingredients carefully.

Pediatric—Gray syndrome may be especially likely to occur in children, who are usually more sensitive than adults to the effects of chloramphenicol. Report any of these effects to your health care professional: blue tone to the skin, changes in blood pressure or heart rate, eating problems, irregular breathing, passage of loose green stools, or stomach bloating with or without vomiting. Your health care professional should monitor blood levels of chloramphenicol if possible.

Geriatric—Many medicines have not been studied specifically in older people. Therefore, it may not be known whether they work exactly the same way they do in younger adults or if they cause different side effects or problems in older people. There is no specific information comparing use of this medicine in the elderly with use in other age groups.

Breast Feeding—There are no adequate studies in women for determining infant risk when using this medication during

breastfeeding. Weigh the potential benefits against the potential risks before taking this medication while breastfeeding.

Other medicines—

Using this medicine with any of the following medicines may cause an increased risk of certain side effects, but using both drugs may be the best treatment for you. If both medicines are prescribed together, your doctor may change the dose or how often you use one or both of the medicines.

Ceftazidime, Chlorpropamide, Cyclosporine, Dicumarol, Fosphenytoin, Phenytoin, Rifampin, Rifapentine, Tacrolimus, Tetanus Toxoid, Tolbutamide

Interactions with Food/Tobacco/Alcohol—Certain medicines should not be used at or around the time of eating food or eating certain types of food since interactions may occur. Using alcohol or tobacco with certain medicines may also cause interactions to occur. Discuss with your healthcare professional the use of your medicine with food, alcohol, or tobacco.

Other medical problems—The presence of other medical problems may affect the use of this medicine. Make sure you tell your doctor if you have any other medical problems, especially:

- Opening in your ear drum—This medicine may cause unwanted effects if it goes past the ear drum into the middle ear
- Sensitivity reaction to chloramphenicol

Proper Use of This Medicine

To use:

- Lie down or tilt the head so that the infected ear faces up. Gently pull the earlobe up and back for adults (down and back for children) to straighten the ear canal. Drop the medicine into the ear canal. Keep the ear facing up for about 1 or 2 minutes to allow the medicine to come into contact with the infection. A sterile cotton plug may be gently inserted into the ear opening to prevent the medicine from leaking out.
- To keep the medicine as germ-free as possible, do not touch the dropper to any surface (including the ear). Also, keep the container tightly closed.

To help clear up your infection completely, keep using this medicine for the full time of treatment, even if your symptoms begin to clear up after a few days. If you stop using this medicine too soon, your symptoms may return. Do not miss any doses.

Dosing—The dose of this medicine will be different for different patients. Follow your doctor's orders or the directions on the label. The following information includes only the average doses of this medicine. If your dose is different, do not change it unless your doctor tells you to do so.

The amount of medicine that you take depends on the strength of the medicine. Also, the number of doses you take each day, the time allowed between doses, and the length of time you take the medicine depend on the medical problem for which you are using the medicine.

- For otic solution (ear drops) dosage form:
  - For infections of the ear canal:
    - Adults and children—Use 2 or 3 drops in the affected ear two to three times a day.

Missed dose—If you miss a dose of this medicine, apply it as soon as possible. However, if it is almost time for your next dose, skip the missed dose and go back to your regular dosing schedule.

Storage—Store the medicine in a closed container at room temperature, away from heat, moisture, and direct light. Keep from freezing.

Keep out of the reach of children.

Do not keep outdated medicine or medicine no longer needed.

Precautions While Using This Medicine

If your symptoms do not improve within a few days, or if they become worse, check with your doctor.

Side Effects of This Medicine

Along with its needed effects, a medicine may cause some unwanted effects. Although not all of these side effects may occur, if they do occur they may need medical attention.

Check with your doctor immediately if any of the following side effects occur:

  Rare—may also occur weeks or months after you stop using this medicine
   Bluish tone to the skin; changes in blood pressure or heart rate; eating problems; irregular breathing; pale skin; passage of loose green stools; sore throat and fever; stomach bloating with or without vomiting; unusual bleeding or bruising; unusual tiredness or weakness

Check with your doctor as soon as possible if any of the following side effects occur:

  Less common
   Blindness or changes in vision; burning, itching, redness, skin rash, swelling, or other sign of irritation not present before use of this medicine; diarrhea; fever; hallucinations; headache; mental confusion; mild depression; nausea; stomach pain; swollen mouth and tongue; unpleasant taste; vomiting

Other side effects not listed may also occur in some patients. If you notice any other effects, check with your healthcare professional.

CHLORDIAZEPOXIDE AND AMITRIPTYLINE (Oral route) - klor-dye-az-e-POX-ide, a-mee-TRIP-ti-leen

Commonly used brand name(s)

In the U.S.—
   Limbitrol
   Limbitrol DS

Available Dosage Forms:
- Tablet

Therapeutic Class: Tricyclic Antidepressant/Benzodiazepine Combination
Pharmacologic Class: Benzodiazepine, Long Acting

Uses For This Medicine

Chlordiazepoxide and amitriptyline combination is used to treat mental depression that occurs with anxiety or nervous tension.

This medicine is available only with your doctor's prescription.

Before Using This Medicine

In deciding to use a medicine, the risks of taking the medicine must be weighed against the good it will do. This is a decision you and your doctor will make. For this medicine, the following should be considered:

Allergies—Tell your doctor if you have ever had any unusual or allergic reaction to this medicine or any other medicines. Also tell your health care professional if you have any other types of allergies, such as to foods, dyes, preservatives, or animals. For non-prescription products, read the label or package ingredients carefully.

Pediatric—Children may be especially sensitive to the effects of chlordiazepoxide and amitriptyline combination. This may increase the chance of side effects during treatment.

The chlordiazepoxide and amitriptyline combination must be used with caution in children with depression. Studies have shown occurrences of children thinking about suicide or attempting suicide in clinical trials for this medicine. More study is needed to be sure the chlordiazepoxide and amitriptyline combination is safe and effective in children.

Geriatric—Elderly people are especially sensitive to the effects of chlordiazepoxide and amitriptyline combination. This may increase the chance of side effects during treatment.

Breast Feeding—There are no adequate studies in women for determining infant risk when using this medication during breastfeeding. Weigh the potential benefits against the potential risks before taking this medication while breastfeeding.

Other medicines—

Using this medicine with any of the following medicines is not recommended. Your doctor may decide not to treat you with this medication or change some of the other medicines you take.

Bepridil, Cisapride, Clorgyline, Furazolidone, Grepafloxacin, Iproniazid, Isocarboxazid, Levomethadyl, Mesoridazine, Moclobemide, Nialamide, Pargyline, Phenelzine, Pimozide, Procarbazine, Selegiline, Sparfloxacin, Terfenadine, Thioridazine, Toloxatone, Tranylcypromine, Ziprasidone

Interactions with Food/Tobacco/Alcohol—Certain medicines should not be used at or around the time of eating food or eating certain types of food since interactions may occur. Using alcohol or tobacco with certain medicines may also cause interactions to occur. The following interactions have been selected on the basis of their potential significance and are not necessarily all-inclusive.

Using this medicine with any of the following may cause an increased risk of certain side effects but may be unavoidable in some cases. If used together, your doctor may change the dose or how often you use this medicine, or give you special instructions about the use of food, alcohol, or tobacco.

Ethanol

Other medical problems—The presence of other medical problems may affect the use of this medicine. Make sure you tell your doctor if you have any other medical problems, especially:

- Alcohol abuse (or history of) or

- Drug abuse or dependence (or history of)—Dependence on this medicine may develop
- Bipolar disorder (manic-depressive illness) or
- Blood problems or
- Difficulty in urinating or
- Emphysema, asthma, bronchitis, or other chronic lung disease or
- Enlarged prostate or
- Glaucoma or increased eye pressure or
- Heart disease or
- Mental illness (severe) or
- Myasthenia gravis or
- Porphyria—Chlordiazepoxide and amitriptyline combination may make the condition worse
- Epilepsy or history of seizures—The risk of seizures may be increased
- Hyperactivity—Chlordiazepoxide and amitriptyline combination may cause unexpected effects
- Kidney disease or
- Liver disease—Higher blood levels of chlordiazepoxide and amitriptyline may occur, increasing the chance of side effects
- Overactive thyroid or
- Stomach or intestinal problems—Use of this combination medicine may result in more serious problems

Proper Use of This Medicine

To reduce stomach upset, take this medicine immediately after meals or with food unless your doctor has told you to take it on an empty stomach.

Sometimes this medicine must be taken for several weeks before you begin to feel better. Your doctor should check your progress at regular visits.

Take this medicine only as directed by your doctor. Do not take more of it, do not take it more often, and do not take it for a longer period of time than your doctor ordered. If too much is taken, it may increase unwanted effects or become habit-forming (causing mental or physical dependence).

If you think this medicine is not working properly after you have taken it for a few weeks, do not increase the dose. Instead, check with your doctor.

Dosing—The dose of this medicine will be different for different patients. Follow your doctor's orders or the directions on the label. The following information includes only the average doses of this medicine. If your dose is different, do not change it unless your doctor tells you to do so.

The amount of medicine that you take depends on the strength of the medicine. Also, the number of doses you take each day, the time allowed between doses, and the length of time you take the medicine depend on the medical problem for which you are using the medicine.

- For oral dosage forms (tablets):
  - Adults and adolescents: To start, 5 milligrams of chlordiazepoxide and 12.5 milligrams of amitriptyline or 10 milligrams of chlordiazepoxide and 25 milligrams of amitriptyline, taken three or four times a day. The doctor may adjust your dose if needed. However, the dose is usually not greater than 10 milligrams of

chlordiazepoxide and 25 milligrams of amitriptyline taken six times a day.
- ○ Children up to 12 years of age: Dose must be determined by the doctor.

Missed dose—If you miss a dose of this medicine, skip the missed dose and go back to your regular dosing schedule. Do not double doses.

Storage—Store the medicine in a closed container at room temperature, away from heat, moisture, and direct light. Keep from freezing.

Keep out of the reach of children.

Do not keep outdated medicine or medicine no longer needed.

Precautions While Using This Medicine

It is very important that your doctor check your progress at regular visits to allow dose adjustments and help reduce side effects.

Do not stop taking this medicine without first checking with your doctor. Your doctor may want you to reduce gradually the amount you are using before stopping completely. This may help prevent a possible worsening of your condition and reduce the possibility of withdrawal symptoms such as headache, nausea, and/or an overall feeling of discomfort.

This medicine will add to the effects of alcohol and other CNS depressants (medicines that slow down the nervous system, possibly causing drowsiness). Some examples of CNS depressants are antihistamines or medicine for hay fever, other allergies, or colds; sedatives, tranquilizers, or sleeping medicine; prescription pain medicine or narcotics; barbiturates; medicine for seizures; muscle relaxants; or anesthetics, including some dental anesthetics. This effect may last for a few days after you stop taking this medicine. Check with your doctor before taking any of the above while you are using this medicine.

For diabetic patients:
- This medicine may affect blood sugar levels. If you notice a change in the results of your blood or urine sugar tests or if you have any questions, check with your doctor.

Before you have any medical tests, tell the medical doctor in charge that you are taking this medicine. The results of the metyrapone test may be affected by this medicine.

Chlordiazepoxide and amitriptyline combination may cause some people to be agitated, irritable or display other abnormal behaviors. It may also cause some people to have suicidal thoughts and tendencies or to become more depressed. If you or your caregiver notice any of these adverse effects, tell your doctor right away.

Before having any surgery, any dental treatment, or emergency treatment, tell the medical doctor or dentist in charge that you are using this medicine. Taking chlordiazepoxide and amitriptyline combination together with medicines that are used during surgery or dental or emergency treatments may increase the CNS depressant effects.

This medicine may cause some people to become dizzy, lightheaded, drowsy, or less alert than they are normally. Even if taken at bedtime, it may cause some people to feel drowsy or less alert on arising. Make sure you know how you react to this medicine before you drive, use machines, or do anything else that could be dangerous if you are dizzy or are not alert.

Dizziness, lightheadedness, or fainting may occur when you get up from a lying or sitting position. Getting up slowly may help. If this problem continues or gets worse, check with your doctor.

Chlordiazepoxide and amitriptyline combination may cause dryness of the mouth. For temporary relief, use sugarless candy or gum, melt bits of ice in your mouth, or use a saliva substitute. However, if your mouth continues to feel dry for more than 2 weeks, check with your medical doctor or dentist. Continuing dryness of the mouth may increase the chance of dental disease, including tooth decay, gum disease, and fungus infections.

Chlordiazepoxide and amitriptyline combination may cause your skin to be more sensitive to sunlight than it is normally. Exposure to sunlight, even for brief periods of time, may cause a skin rash, itching, redness or other discoloration of the skin, or a severe sunburn. When you begin taking this medicine:
- Stay out of direct sunlight, especially between the hours of 10:00 a.m. and 3:00 p.m., if possible.
- Wear protective clothing, including a hat. Also, wear sunglasses.
- Apply a sun block product that has a skin protection factor (SPF) of at least 15. Some patients may require a product with a higher SPF number, especially if they have a fair complexion. If you have any questions about this, check with your health care professional.
- Apply a sun block lipstick that has an SPF of at least 15 to protect your lips.
- Do not use a sunlamp or tanning bed or booth.

If you have a severe reaction from the sun, check with your doctor.

Side Effects of This Medicine

Along with its needed effects, a medicine may cause some unwanted effects. Although not all of these side effects may occur, if they do occur they may need medical attention.

Check with your doctor as soon as possible if any of the following side effects occur:

Less common
Blurred vision or other changes in vision; confusion or hallucinations (seeing, hearing, or feeling things that are not there); constipation; difficulty in urinating; eye pain; fainting; irregular heartbeat; mental depression; shakiness; trouble in sleeping; unusual excitement, nervousness, or irritability

Rare
Convulsions (seizures); increased sensitivity to sunlight; skin rash and itching; sore throat and fever; yellow eyes or skin

Symptoms of overdose
Agitation; confusion; convulsions (seizures); dizziness or lightheadedness (severe); drowsiness (severe); enlarged pupils; fast or irregular heartbeat; fever; hallucinations; muscle stiffness or rigidity; vomiting (severe)

Some side effects may occur that usually do not need medical attention. These side effects may go away during treatment as your body adjusts to the medicine. Also, your health care professional may be able to tell you about ways to prevent or reduce some of these side effects. Check with your health

care professional if any of the following side effects continue or are bothersome or if you have any questions about them:

More common

Bloating; clumsiness or unsteadiness; dizziness or lightheadedness; drowsiness; dryness of mouth or unpleasant taste; headache; weight gain

Less common

Diarrhea; nausea or vomiting; unusual tiredness or weakness

After you stop using this medicine, it may still produce some side effects that need attention. During this period of time, *check with your doctor immediately* if you notice the following side effects:

Convulsions (seizures); headache; increased sweating; irritability or restlessness; muscle cramps; nausea or vomiting; stomach cramps; trembling; trouble in sleeping, with vivid dreams

Other side effects not listed may also occur in some patients. If you notice any other effects, check with your healthcare professional.

CHLOROQUINE (Oral route, Intramuscular route) - KLOR-oh-kwin

Commonly used brand name(s)

In the U.S.—

Aralen Phosphate

Available Dosage Forms:

• Tablet
• Solution

Therapeutic Class: Antimalarial

Uses For This Medicine

Chloroquine is a medicine used to prevent and treat malaria, a red blood cell infection transmitted by the bite of a mosquito, and to treat some conditions such as liver disease caused by protozoa (tiny one-celled animals).

Malaria transmission occurs in large areas of Central and South America, Hispaniola, sub-Saharan Africa, the Indian subcontinent, Southeast Asia, the Middle East, and Oceania. Country-specific information on malaria can be obtained from the Centers for Disease Control and Prevention (CDC), or from the CDC's web site at http://www.cdc.gov/travel/yellowbk.

This medicine may be given alone or with one or more other medicines. It may also be used for other conditions as determined by your doctor.

Chloroquine is available only with your doctor's prescription.

Once a medicine has been approved for marketing for a certain use, experience may show that it is also useful for other medical problems. Although these uses are not included in product labeling, chloroquine is used in certain patients with the following medical conditions:

• Arthritis in children
• High levels of calcium in the blood associated with sarcoidosis
• Rheumatoid arthritis

• Systemic lupus erythematosus (lupus; SLE)
• Various skin disorders

For patients taking chloroquine for arthritis or lupus:

• This medicine must be taken regularly as ordered by your doctor in order for it to help you. It may take up to several weeks before you begin to feel better. It may take up to 6 months before you feel the full benefit of this medicine.
• If your symptoms of arthritis do not improve within a few weeks or months, or if they become worse, check with your doctor.

Before Using This Medicine

In deciding to use a medicine, the risks of taking the medicine must be weighed against the good it will do. This is a decision you and your doctor will make. For this medicine, the following should be considered:

Allergies—Tell your doctor if you have ever had any unusual or allergic reaction to this medicine or any other medicines. Also tell your health care professional if you have any other types of allergies, such as to foods, dyes, preservatives, or animals. For non-prescription products, read the label or package ingredients carefully.

Pediatric—Children are especially sensitive to the effects of chloroquine. This may increase the chance of side effects during treatment. Overdose is especially dangerous in children. Taking as little as 1 tablet (300–mg strength) has resulted in the death of a small child. Children should avoid traveling to areas where there is a chance of getting malaria, unless they can take antimalarial medicines that are more effective than chloroquine.

Geriatric—Many medicines have not been studied specifically in older people. Therefore, it may not be known whether they work exactly the same way they do in younger adults or if they cause different side effects or problems in older people. There is no specific information comparing use of chloroquine in the elderly with use in other age groups.

Pregnancy—

	Pregnancy Category	Explanation
All Trimesters	C	Animal studies have shown an adverse effect and there are no adequate studies in pregnant women OR no animal studies have been conducted and there are no adequate studies in pregnant women.

Breast Feeding—There are no adequate studies in women for determining infant risk when using this medication during breastfeeding. Weigh the potential benefits against the potential risks before taking this medication while breastfeeding.

Other medicines—

Using this medicine with any of the following medicines is not recommended. Your doctor may decide not to treat you with this medication or change some of the other medicines you take.

Aurothioglucose, Bepridil, Cisapride, Levomethadyl, Mesoridazine, Pimozide, Terfenadine, Thioridazine, Ziprasidone

Interactions with Food/Tobacco/Alcohol—Certain medicines should not be used at or around the time of eating food or eating certain types of food since interactions may

occur. Using alcohol or tobacco with certain medicines may also cause interactions to occur. Discuss with your healthcare professional the use of your medicine with food, alcohol, or tobacco.

Other medical problems—The presence of other medical problems may affect the use of this medicine. Make sure you tell your doctor if you have any other medical problems, especially:

- Blood disease (severe)—Chloroquine may cause blood disorders
- Eye or vision problems—Chloroquine, especially in high doses, may cause serious side effects affecting the eyes
- Glucose-6–phosphate dehydrogenase (G6PD) deficiency—Chloroquine may cause serious side effects affecting the blood in patients with this deficiency
- Liver disease—May decrease the removal of chloroquine from the blood, increasing the chance of side effects
- Nerve or brain disease (severe), including convulsions (seizures)—Chloroquine may cause muscle weakness and, at high doses, seizures
- Porphyria—Chloroquine may cause episodes of porphyria to occur more frequently
- Psoriasis—Chloroquine may bring on severe attacks of psoriasis
- Stomach or intestinal disease (severe)—Chloroquine may cause stomach or intestinal irritation

Proper Use of This Medicine

Take this medicine with meals or milk to lessen stomach upset, unless otherwise directed by your doctor.

Keep this medicine out of the reach of children. Children are especially sensitive to the effects of chloroquine and overdose is especially dangerous in children. Taking as little as 1 tablet (300–mg strength) has resulted in the death of a small child.

It is very important that you take this medicine only as directed. Do not take more of it, do not take it more often, and do not take it for a longer time than your doctor ordered. To do so may increase the chance of serious side effects.

If you are taking this medicine to help keep you from getting malaria, keep taking it for the full time of treatment. If you already have malaria, you should still keep taking this medicine for the full time of treatment even if you begin to feel better after a few days. This will help to clear up your infection completely. If you stop taking this medicine too soon, your symptoms may return.

Chloroquine works best when you take it on a regular schedule. For example, if you are to take it once a week to prevent malaria, it is best to take it on the same day each week. Or if you are to take two doses a day, one dose may be taken with breakfast and the other with the evening meal. Make sure that you do not miss any doses. If you have any questions about this, check with your health care professional.

For patients taking chloroquine to prevent malaria:

- Your doctor may want you to start taking this medicine 1 to 2 weeks before you travel to an area where there is a chance of getting malaria. This will help you to see how you react to the medicine. Also, it will allow time for your doctor to change to another medicine if you have a reaction to this medicine.

- Also, you should keep taking this medicine while you are in the area and for 4 weeks after you leave the area. No medicine will protect you completely from malaria. However, to protect you as completely as possible, it is important to keep taking this medicine for the full time your doctor ordered. Also, if fever develops during your travels or within 2 months after you leave the area, check with your doctor immediately.

Dosing—The dose of this medicine will be different for different patients. Follow your doctor's orders or the directions on the label. The following information includes only the average doses of this medicine. If your dose is different, do not change it unless your doctor tells you to do so.

The amount of medicine that you take depends on the strength of the medicine. Also, the number of doses you take each day, the time allowed between doses, and the length of time you take the medicine depend on the medical problem for which you are using the medicine.

- For oral dosage form (tablets):
  - For prevention of malaria:
    - Adults—500 milligrams (mg) once every seven days.
    - Children—Dose is based on body weight and must be determined by your doctor. The usual dose is 8.3 mg per kilogram (kg) (3.7 mg per pound) of body weight once every seven days.
  - For treatment of malaria:
    - Adults—Start with 1 gram. Then, 500 mg six to eight hours after the first dose, and 500 mg once a day on the second and third days of treatment.
    - Children—Dose is based on body weight and must be determined by your doctor. The usual dose is 41.7 mg per kg (18.9 mg per pound) of body weight divided up over three days. This dose is given as follows: Start with 16.7 mg per kg (7.5 mg per pound) of body weight, then 8.3 mg per kg (3.7 mg per pound) of body weight six hours, twenty-four hours, and forty-eight hours after the first dose.
  - For treatment of liver disease caused by protozoa:
    - Adults—At first, start with 250 mg four times a day for two days. Then 250 mg two times a day for at least two to three weeks.
    - Children—Dose is based on body weight and must be determined by your doctor. The usual dose is 10 mg per kg (4.5 mg per pound) of body weight a day for three weeks.
- For injection dosage form:
  - For treatment of malaria:
    - Adults—200 to 250 mg injected into a muscle. This dose may be repeated in six hours if needed.
    - Children—Dose is based on body weight and must be determined by your doctor. The usual dose is 4.4 mg per kg (2 mg per pound) of body weight injected into a muscle or under the skin. This dose may be repeated in six hours if needed. Chloroquine may also be injected slowly into a vein. If the medicine is given in this way, the dose must be determined by your doctor.
  - For treatment of liver disease caused by protozoa:
    - Adults—200 to 250 mg a day injected into a muscle for ten to twelve days.
    - Children—Dose is based on body weight and must be determined by your doctor. The usual dose is 7.5 mg per kg (3.4 mg per pound) of body weight a day for ten to twelve days.

Missed dose—If you miss a dose of this medicine, take it as soon as possible. However, if it is almost time for your next dose, skip the missed dose and go back to your regular dosing schedule. Do not double doses.

Storage—Store the medicine in a closed container at room temperature, away from heat, moisture, and direct light. Keep from freezing.

Keep out of the reach of children.

Do not keep outdated medicine or medicine no longer needed.

Precautions While Using This Medicine

If you will be taking this medicine for a long time, it is very important that your doctor check you at regular visits for any blood problems or muscle weakness that may be caused by this medicine. In addition, check with your doctor immediately if blurred vision, difficulty in reading, or any other change in vision occurs during or after treatment. Your doctor may want you to have your eyes checked by an ophthalmologist (eye doctor).

If your symptoms do not improve within a few days or if they become worse, check with your doctor.

Make sure you know how you react to this medicine before you drive, use machines, or do anything else that could be dangerous if you are not able to see well.

Chloroquine may cause blurred vision, difficulty in reading, or other change in vision. It may also cause some people to become lightheaded.

If these reactions are especially bothersome, check with your doctor.

Malaria is spread by mosquitoes. If you are living in, or will be traveling to, an area where there is a chance of getting malaria, the following mosquito-control measures will help to prevent infection:

* Avoid going out between dusk and dawn because it is at these times when mosquitoes most commonly bite.
* If possible, sleep in a screened or air-conditioned room or under mosquito netting, preferably netting coated or soaked with pyrethrum, to avoid being bitten by malaria-carrying mosquitoes.
* Remain in air-conditioned or well-screened rooms to reduce contact with mosquitoes
* Wear long-sleeved shirts or blouses and long trousers to protect your arms and legs, especially from dusk through dawn when mosquitoes are out.
* Apply mosquito repellent, preferably one containing DEET, to uncovered areas of the skin from dusk through dawn when mosquitoes are out.
* Use mosquito coils or sprays to kill mosquitoes in living and sleeping quarters during evening and night-time hours.

Side Effects of This Medicine

Along with its needed effects, a medicine may cause some unwanted effects. Although not all of these side effects may occur, if they do occur they may need medical attention. When this medicine is used for short periods of time, side effects usually are rare. However, when it is used for a long time and/or in high doses, side effects are more likely to occur and may be serious.

Check with your doctor immediately if any of the following side effects occur:
Less common
  Blurred vision; change in vision; eye pain; loss of vision
Rare
  Black, tarry stools; blood in urine or stools; convulsions (seizures); cough or hoarseness; feeling faint or light-headed; fever or chills; increased muscle weakness; lower back or side pain; mood or other mental changes; painful or difficult urination; pinpoint red spots on skin; ringing or buzzing in ears or any loss of hearing; sore throat; unusual bleeding or bruising; unusual tiredness or weakness
Symptoms of overdose
  Drowsiness; headache; increased excitability

Note: The side effects in the Less Common category above may also occur or get worse after you stop taking this medicine.

Some side effects may occur that usually do not need medical attention. These side effects may go away during treatment as your body adjusts to the medicine. Also, your health care professional may be able to tell you about ways to prevent or reduce some of these side effects. Check with your health care professional if any of the following side effects continue or are bothersome or if you have any questions about them:
More common
  Diarrhea; difficulty in seeing to read; headache; itching (more common in black patients); loss of appetite; nausea or vomiting; stomach cramps or pain
Less common
  Bleaching of hair or increased hair loss; blue-black discoloration of skin, fingernails, or inside of mouth; skin rash

Other side effects not listed may also occur in some patients. If you notice any other effects, check with your healthcare professional.

CHLOROXINE   (Topical route) - klor-OX-een

Commonly used brand name(s)

In the U.S.—
  Capitrol

Available Dosage Forms:
  * Shampoo
  * Cream

Therapeutic Class: Dermatological Agent

Uses For This Medicine

Chloroxine is used in the treatment of dandruff and seborrheic dermatitis of the scalp.

This medicine is available only with your doctor's prescription.

Before Using This Medicine

In deciding to use a medicine, the risks of taking the medicine must be weighed against the good it will do. This is a decision you and your doctor will make. For this medicine, the following should be considered:

Allergies—Tell your doctor if you have ever had any unusual or allergic reaction to this medicine or any other medicines. Also tell your health care professional if you have any other types of allergies, such as to foods, dyes, preservatives, or animals. For non-prescription products, read the label or package ingredients carefully.

Pediatric—Studies on this medicine have been done only in adult patients, and there is no specific information comparing use of this medicine in children with use in other age groups.

Geriatric—Many medicines have not been studied specifically in older people. Therefore, it may not be known whether they work exactly the same way they do in younger adults or if they cause different side effects or problems in older people. There is no specific information comparing use of this medicine in the elderly with use in other age groups.

Pregnancy—

	Pregnancy Category	Explanation
All Trimesters	C	Animal studies have shown an adverse effect and there are no adequate studies in pregnant women OR no animal studies have been conducted and there are no adequate studies in pregnant women.

Breast Feeding—There are no adequate studies in women for determining infant risk when using this medication during breastfeeding. Weigh the potential benefits against the potential risks before taking this medication while breastfeeding.

Other medicines—Although certain medicines should not be used together at all, in other cases two different medicines may be used together even if an interaction might occur. In these cases, your doctor may want to change the dose, or other precautions may be necessary. Tell your healthcare professional if you are taking any other prescription or non-prescription (over-the-counter [OTC]) medicine.

Interactions with Food/Tobacco/Alcohol—Certain medicines should not be used at or around the time of eating food or eating certain types of food since interactions may occur. Using alcohol or tobacco with certain medicines may also cause interactions to occur. Discuss with your healthcare professional the use of your medicine with food, alcohol, or tobacco.

Proper Use of This Medicine

Do not use this medicine if blistered, raw, or oozing areas are present on your scalp, unless otherwise directed by your doctor.

Keep this medicine away from the eyes. If you should accidentally get some in your eyes, flush them thoroughly with cool water. Check with your doctor if eye irritation continues or is bothersome.

To use:

- Shake well before using
- Wet the hair and scalp with lukewarm water. Apply enough chloroxine to the scalp to work up a lather, and rub in well. Allow the lather to remain on the scalp for about 3 minutes, then rinse. Apply the medicine again and rinse thoroughly. Use the medicine two times a week or as directed by your doctor.

Dosing—The dose of this medicine will be different for different patients. Follow your doctor's orders or the directions on the label. The following information includes only the average doses of this medicine. If your dose is different, do not change it unless your doctor tells you to do so.

The amount of medicine that you take depends on the strength of the medicine. Also, the number of doses you take each day, the time allowed between doses, and the length of time you take the medicine depend on the medical problem for which you are using the medicine.

- For topical dosage form (shampoo):
  - For dandruff or seborrheic dermatitis of the scalp:
    - Adults—Use two times a week.
    - Children—Use and dose must be determined by your doctor.

Missed dose—If you miss a dose of this medicine, apply it as soon as possible. However, if it is almost time for your next dose, skip the missed dose and go back to your regular dosing schedule.

Storage—Store the medicine in a closed container at room temperature, away from heat, moisture, and direct light. Keep from freezing.

Keep out of the reach of children.

Do not keep outdated medicine or medicine no longer needed.

Precautions While Using This Medicine

This medicine may slightly discolor light-colored hair (for example, bleached, blond, or gray).

Side Effects of This Medicine

Along with its needed effects, a medicine may cause some unwanted effects. Although not all of these side effects may occur, if they do occur they may need medical attention.

Check with your doctor as soon as possible if any of the following side effects occur:

Irritation or burning of scalp not present before use of this medicine; skin rash

Some side effects may occur that usually do not need medical attention. These side effects may go away during treatment as your body adjusts to the medicine. Also, your health care professional may be able to tell you about ways to prevent or reduce some of these side effects. Check with your health care professional if any of the following side effects continue or are bothersome or if you have any questions about them:

Dryness or increased itching of scalp

Other side effects not listed may also occur in some patients. If you notice any other effects, check with your healthcare professional.

CHOLESTYRAMINE   (Oral route) -
koe-less-TEER-a-meen

Commonly used brand name(s)

In the U.S.—
Prevalite   Questran Light
Questran

In Canada—
Novo-Cholamine
Novo-Cholamine Light

Available Dosage Forms:

- Tablet
- Powder for Suspension

Therapeutic Class: Antihyperlipidemic
Pharmacologic Class: Bile Acid Sequestrant

Uses For This Medicine

Cholestyramine is used to lower high cholesterol levels in the blood. This may help prevent medical problems caused by cholesterol clogging the blood vessels. Cholestyramine is also used to remove substances called bile acids from your body. With some liver problems, there is too much bile acid in your body and this can cause severe itching.

Cholestyramine works by attaching to certain substances in the intestine. Since cholestyramine is not absorbed into the body, these substances also pass out of the body without being absorbed.

Cholestyramine may also be used for other conditions as determined by your doctor.

Cholestyramine is available only with your doctor's prescription.

Once a medicine has been approved for marketing for a certain use, experience may show that it is also useful for other medical problems. Although these uses are not included in product labeling, cholestyramine is used in certain patients with the following medical conditions:

- Digitalis glycoside overdose
- Excess oxalate in the urine

Before Using This Medicine

In deciding to use a medicine, the risks of taking the medicine must be weighed against the good it will do. This is a decision you and your doctor will make. For this medicine, the following should be considered:

Allergies—Tell your doctor if you have ever had any unusual or allergic reaction to this medicine or any other medicines. Also tell your health care professional if you have any other types of allergies, such as to foods, dyes, preservatives, or animals. For non-prescription products, read the label or package ingredients carefully.

Pediatric—This medicine has been tested in a limited number of children. In effective doses, the medicine has not been shown to cause different side effects or problems than it does in adults.

Geriatric—Side effects may be more likely to occur in patients over 60 years of age, who are usually more sensitive to the effects of cholestyramine.

Pregnancy—

	Pregnancy Category	Explanation
All Trimesters	C	Animal studies have shown an adverse effect and there are no adequate studies in pregnant women OR no animal studies have been conducted and there are no adequate studies in pregnant women.

Breast Feeding—Studies suggest that this medication may alter milk production or composition. If an alternative to this medication is not prescribed, you should monitor the infant for side effects and adequate milk intake.

Other medicines—

Using this medicine with any of the following medicines is usually not recommended, but may be required in some cases. If both medicines are prescribed together, your doctor may change the dose or how often you use one or both of the medicines.

Mycophenolate Mofetil, Mycophenolate Sodium, Mycophenolic Acid

Interactions   with   Food/Tobacco/Alcohol—Certain medicines should not be used at or around the time of eating food or eating certain types of food since interactions may occur. Using alcohol or tobacco with certain medicines may also cause interactions to occur. Discuss with your healthcare professional the use of your medicine with food, alcohol, or tobacco.

Other medical problems—The presence of other medical problems may affect the use of this medicine. Make sure you tell your doctor if you have any other medical problems, especially:

- Bleeding problems or
- Constipation or
- Gallstones or
- Heart or blood vessel disease or
- Hemorrhoids or
- Stomach ulcer or other stomach problems or
- Underactive thyroid—Cholestyramine may make these conditions worse
- Kidney disease—There is an increased risk of developing electrolyte problems (problems in the blood)
- Phenylketonuria—Phenylalanine in aspartame is included in the sugar-free brand of cholestyramine and should be avoided. Aspartame can cause problems in people with phenylketonuria. Therefore, it is best if you avoid using the sugar-free product.

Proper Use of This Medicine

Take this medicine exactly as directed by your doctor. Try not to miss any doses and do not take more medicine than your doctor ordered.

This medicine should never be taken in its dry form, since it could cause you to choke. Instead, always mix as follows:

- Place the medicine in 2 ounces of any beverage and mix thoroughly. Then add an additional 2 to 4 ounces of beverage and again mix thoroughly (it will not dissolve) before drinking. After drinking all the liquid containing the medicine, rinse the glass with a little more liquid and drink that also, to make sure you get all the medicine.

- You may also mix this medicine with milk in hot or regular breakfast cereals, or in thin soups such as tomato or chicken noodle soup. Or you may add it to some pulpy fruits such as crushed pineapple, pears, peaches, or fruit cocktail.

For patients taking this medicine for high cholesterol:

- Importance of diet—Before prescribing medicine for your condition, your doctor will probably try to control your condition by prescribing a personal diet for you. Such a diet may be low in fats, sugars, and/or cholesterol. Many people are able to control their condition by carefully following their doctor's orders for proper diet and exercise. Medicine is prescribed only when additional help is needed. Follow carefully the special diet your doctor gave you, since the medicine is effective only when a schedule of diet and exercise is properly followed.

- Also, this medicine is less effective if you are greatly overweight. It may be very important for you to go on a reducing diet. However, check with your doctor before going on any diet.

- Remember that this medicine will not cure your cholesterol problem but it will help control it. Therefore, you must continue to take it as directed if you expect to lower your cholesterol level.

Dosing—The dose of this medicine will be different for different patients. Follow your doctor's orders or the directions on the label. The following information includes only the average doses of this medicine. If your dose is different, do not change it unless your doctor tells you to do so.

The amount of medicine that you take depends on the strength of the medicine. Also, the number of doses you take each day, the time allowed between doses, and the length of time you take the medicine depend on the medical problem for which you are using the medicine.

- For oral dosage form (powder for oral suspension):
  - For high cholesterol or pruritus (itching) related to biliary obstruction:
    - Adults—At first, 4 grams one or two times a day before meals. Then, your doctor may increase your dose to 8 to 24 grams a day. This is divided into two to six doses.
    - Children—At first, 4 grams a day. This is divided into two doses and taken before meals. Then, your doctor may increase your dose to 8 to 24 grams a day. This is divided into two or more doses.

Missed dose—If you miss a dose of this medicine, take it as soon as possible. However, if it is almost time for your next dose, skip the missed dose and go back to your regular dosing schedule. Do not double doses.

Storage—Store the medicine in a closed container at room temperature, away from heat, moisture, and direct light. Keep from freezing.

Keep out of the reach of children.

Do not keep outdated medicine or medicine no longer needed.

Precautions While Using This Medicine

It is very important that your doctor check your progress at regular visits. This will allow your doctor to see if the medicine is working properly and to decide if you should continue to take it.

Do not take any other medicine unless prescribed by your doctor since cholestyramine may change the effect of other medicines.

Do not stop taking this medicine without first checking with your doctor. When you stop taking this medicine, your blood cholesterol levels may increase again. Your doctor may want you to follow a special diet to help prevent this from happening.

Side Effects of This Medicine

In some animal studies, cholestyramine was found to cause tumors. It is not known whether cholestyramine causes tumors in humans.

Along with its needed effects, a medicine may cause some unwanted effects. Although not all of these side effects may occur, if they do occur they may need medical attention.

Check with your doctor immediately if any of the following side effects occur:
> *Rare*
>> Black, tarry stools; stomach pain (severe) with nausea and vomiting

Check with your doctor as soon as possible if any of the following side effects occur:
> *More common*
>> Constipation
> *Rare*
>> Loss of weight (sudden)

Some side effects may occur that usually do not need medical attention. These side effects may go away during treatment as your body adjusts to the medicine. Also, your health care professional may be able to tell you about ways to prevent or reduce some of these side effects. Check with your health care professional if any of the following side effects continue or are bothersome or if you have any questions about them:
> *More common*
>> Heartburn or indigestion; nausea or vomiting; stomach pain
> *Less common*
>> Belching; bloating; diarrhea; dizziness; headache

Other side effects not listed may also occur in some patients. If you notice any other effects, check with your healthcare professional.

CHORIONIC GONADOTROPIN (Subcutaneous route, Intramuscular route, Injection route) - kore-ee-ON-ik goe-NAD-oh-troe-pin

Commonly used brand name(s)
In the U.S.—

Chorex	Pregnyl
Novarel	Profasi
Ovidrel	

In Canada—
    Chorionic Gonadotropin

Available Dosage Forms:
  • Powder for Solution
  • Solution

Therapeutic Class: Endocrine-Metabolic Agent
Pharmacologic Class: Gonadotropin

Uses For This Medicine

Chorionic gonadotropin is a drug whose actions are almost the same as those of luteinizing hormone (LH), which is produced by the pituitary gland. It is a hormone also normally produced by the placenta in pregnancy. Chorionic gonadotropin has different uses for females and males.

In females, chorionic gonadotropin is used to help conception occur. It is usually given in combination with other drugs such as menotropins and urofollitropin. Many women being treated with these drugs usually have already tried clomiphene alone (e.g., Serophene) and have not been able to conceive yet. Chorionic gonadotropin is also used in in vitro fertilization (IVF) programs.

In males, LH and chorionic gonadotropin stimulate the testes to produce male hormones such as testosterone. Testosterone causes the enlargement of the penis and testes and the growth of pubic and underarm hair. It also increases the production of sperm.

Although chorionic gonadotropin has been prescribed to help some patients lose weight, it should never be used this way. When used improperly, chorionic gonadotropin can cause serious problems.

Chorionic gonadotropin is to be administered only by or under the immediate supervision of your doctor.

Before Using This Medicine

In deciding to use a medicine, the risks of taking the medicine must be weighed against the good it will do. This is a decision you and your doctor will make. For this medicine, the following should be considered:

Allergies—Tell your doctor if you have ever had any unusual or allergic reaction to this medicine or any other medicines. Also tell your health care professional if you have any other types of allergies, such as to foods, dyes, preservatives, or animals. For non-prescription products, read the label or package ingredients carefully.

Pediatric—Chorionic gonadotropin, when used for treating cryptorchidism (a birth defect where the testes remain inside the body), has caused the sexual organs of some male children to develop too rapidly.

Pregnancy—

	Pregnancy Category	Explanation
All Trimesters	X	Studies in animals or pregnant women have demonstrated positive evidence of fetal abnormalities. This drug should not be used in women who are or may become pregnant because the risk clearly outweighs any possible benefit.

Breast Feeding—There are no adequate studies in women for determining infant risk when using this medication during breastfeeding. Weigh the potential benefits against the potential risks before taking this medication while breastfeeding.

Other medicines—Although certain medicines should not be used together at all, in other cases two different medicines may be used together even if an interaction might occur. In these cases, your doctor may want to change the dose, or other precautions may be necessary. Tell your healthcare professional if you are taking any other prescription or non-prescription (over-the-counter [OTC]) medicine.

Interactions with Food/Tobacco/Alcohol—Certain medicines should not be used at or around the time of eating food or eating certain types of food since interactions may occur. Using alcohol or tobacco with certain medicines may also cause interactions to occur. Discuss with your healthcare professional the use of your medicine with food, alcohol, or tobacco.

Other medical problems—The presence of other medical problems may affect the use of this medicine. Make sure you tell your doctor if you have any other medical problems, especially:
  • Asthma or
  • Epilepsy (seizures) or
  • Heart problems or
  • Kidney problems or
  • Migraine headaches—This medication may worsen these conditions.
  • Cancer of the prostate or
  • Precocious puberty (a condition that causes early puberty in boys before 9 years of age)—Increases in the amount of testosterone in the bloodstream may make these conditions worse.
  • Cyst on ovary or
  • Fibroid tumors of the uterus—Chorionic gonadotropin can cause further growth of cysts on the ovary or fibroid tumors of the uterus
  • Unusual vaginal bleeding—Irregular vaginal bleeding is a sign that the endometrium is growing too much, of endometrial cancer, or of other hormone imbalances; the increases in estrogen production caused by ovulation can aggravate these problems of the endometrium. If other hormone imbalances are present, they should be treated before beginning ovulation induction

Proper Use of This Medicine

Dosing—The dose of this medicine will be different for different patients. Follow your doctor's orders or the directions on the label. The following information includes only the average doses of this medicine. If your dose is different, do not change it unless your doctor tells you to do so.

The amount of medicine that you take depends on the strength of the medicine. Also, the number of doses you take each day, the time allowed between doses, and the length of time you take the medicine depend on the medical problem for which you are using the medicine.
  • For injection dosage form:
    ○ For treating men with problems related to low levels of male hormones:
      ▪ Adults—1000 to 4000 Units injected into the muscle two to three times a week. You may need

to receive this medicine for several weeks, months, or longer. If you are being treated for a low sperm count and have been on this medicine for six months, your doctor may give you another hormone medicine (menotropin or urofollitropin injection). You may need to receive both of these medicines together for up to twelve more months.

- To help pregnancy occur in women:
  - Adults—5000 to 10,000 Units injected into the muscle on a day chosen by your doctor. The dose and day will depend on your hormone levels and the other medicines that you have been using.
- For the treatment of cryptorchidism (condition where testes do not develop properly):
  - Children—1000 to 5000 Units injected into the muscle two to three times a week for up to ten doses.

Precautions While Using This Medicine

It is very important that your doctor check your progress at regular visits to make sure that the medicine is working and to check for unwanted effects.

For women taking this medicine to become pregnant:
- Record your basal body temperature every day if told to do so by your doctor, so that you will know if you have begun to ovulate. It is important that intercourse take place around the time of ovulation to give you the best chance of becoming pregnant. Your doctor will likely want to monitor the development of the ovarian follicle(s) by measuring the amount of estrogen in your bloodstream and by checking the size of the follicle(s) with ultrasound examinations.

Side Effects of This Medicine

Along with its needed effects, a medicine may cause some unwanted effects. Although not all of these side effects may occur, if they do occur they may need medical attention.

Check with your doctor as soon as possible if any of the following side effects occur:
For females only
More common
Bloating (mild); stomach or pelvic pain
Less common or rare
Abdominal or stomach pain (severe); bloating (moderate to severe); decreased amount of urine; feeling of indigestion; nausea, vomiting, or diarrhea (continuing or severe); pelvic pain (severe); shortness of breath; swelling of feet or lower legs; weight gain (rapid)
For boys only
Less common
Acne; enlargement of penis and testes; growth of pubic hair; increase in height (rapid)
Frequency not determined
Difficult or labored breathing; difficulty breathing; flushing of skin; hives or welts; itching of skin; large, hive-like swelling on face, eyelids, lips, tongue, throat, hands, legs, feet, sex organs; pain in chest, groin, or legs, especially the calves; redness of skin; severe, sudden headache; skin rash; slurred speech; sudden loss of coordination; sudden, severe weakness or numbness in arm or leg; sudden, unexplained shortness of breath; tightness in chest; unusually warm skin; vision changes; wheezing

Some side effects may occur that usually do not need medical attention. These side effects may go away during treatment as your body adjusts to the medicine. Also, your health care professional may be able to tell you about ways to prevent or reduce some of these side effects. Check with your health care professional if any of the following side effects continue or are bothersome or if you have any questions about them:
Less common
Discouragement; enlargement of breasts; feeling sad or empty; headache; irritability; lack of appetite; loss of interest or pleasure; pain at place of injection; trouble concentrating; trouble sleeping; tiredness

After you stop using this medicine, it may still produce some side effects that need attention. During this period of time, *check with your doctor immediately* if you notice the following side effects:
For females only
Less common or rare
Abdominal or stomach pain (severe); bloating (moderate to severe); decreased amount of urine; feeling of indigestion; nausea, vomiting, or diarrhea (continuing or severe); pelvic pain (severe); shortness of breath; weight gain (rapid)

Other side effects not listed may also occur in some patients. If you notice any other effects, check with your healthcare professional.

CICLOPIROX (Topical route) - sye-kloe-PEER-ox

Commonly used brand name(s)

In the U.S.—
Loprox
Loprox TS
Penlac

Available Dosage Forms:
- Gel/Jelly
- Lotion
- Solution
- Cream
- Suspension
- Shampoo
- Powder

Therapeutic Class: Antifungal

Uses For This Medicine

Ciclopirox is used to treat infections caused by fungus. It works by killing the fungus or preventing its growth.

Ciclopirox cream, gel, or lotion are applied to the skin to treat:
- ringworm of the body (tinea corporis);
- ringworm of the foot (tinea pedis; athlete's foot);
- ringworm of the groin (tinea cruris; jock itch);
- "sun fungus" (tinea versicolor; pityriasis versicolor); and
- certain other fungus infections, such as Candida (Monilia) infections.

Ciclopirox gel or shampoo may also be applied to the scalp to treat seborrheic dermatitis.

Ciclopirox topical solution (nail lacquer) is applied to the nails to treat ringworm of the nails (tinea unguium).

Ciclopirox is available only with your doctor's prescription.

Before Using This Medicine

In deciding to use a medicine, the risks of taking the medicine must be weighed against the good it will do. This is a decision you and your doctor will make. For this medicine, the following should be considered:

Allergies—Tell your doctor if you have ever had any unusual or allergic reaction to this medicine or any other medicines. Also tell your health care professional if you have any other types of allergies, such as to foods, dyes, preservatives, or animals. For non-prescription products, read the label or package ingredients carefully.

Pediatric—Studies on this medicine have been done only in adult patients, and there is no specific information comparing use of ciclopirox in children under the age of 10 with use in other age groups.

Geriatric—Many medicines have not been studied specifically in older people. Therefore, it may not be known whether they work exactly the same way they do in younger adults. Although there is no specific information comparing use of ciclopirox in the elderly with use in other age groups, this medicine is not expected to cause different side effects or problems in older people than it does in younger adults.

Other medicines—Although certain medicines should not be used together at all, in other cases two different medicines may be used together even if an interaction might occur. In these cases, your doctor may want to change the dose, or other precautions may be necessary. Tell your healthcare professional if you are taking any other prescription or non-prescription (over-the-counter [OTC]) medicine.

Interactions with Food/Tobacco/Alcohol—Certain medicines should not be used at or around the time of eating food or eating certain types of food since interactions may occur. Using alcohol or tobacco with certain medicines may also cause interactions to occur. Discuss with your healthcare professional the use of your medicine with food, alcohol, or tobacco.

Proper Use of This Medicine

For patients using the cream, gel, or lotion form of this medicine:

- Keep this medicine away from the eyes.
- Apply enough ciclopirox to cover the affected and surrounding skin or scalp areas and rub in gently.

For patients using the shampoo form of this medicine:

- Keep this medicine away from the eyes.
- Apply shampoo to wet hair. Lather and leave on hair and scalp for 3 minutes. A timer may be used. Rinse off.

For patients using the topical solution form of this medicine:

- Keep this medicine away from the eyes and mucous membranes
- This medicine comes with a patient instruction sheet. Read this sheet carefully and follow the directions. If you have any questions on how to use this medicine, be sure to ask your health care professional.

- In addition to daily application of this medicine, you will need to trim your nails as directed, and visit your healthcare professional at regular intervals to have the unattached infected nails removed.
- Do not use nail polish or other nail cosmetic products on the treated nails.
- Do not use near heat or open flame.

When ciclopirox is used to treat certain types of fungus infections of the skin, an occlusive dressing (airtight covering, such as kitchen plastic wrap) should not be applied over the medicine. To do so may irritate the skin. Do not apply an airtight covering over this medicine unless you have been directed to do so by your doctor.

To help clear up your infection completely, it is very important that you keep using ciclopirox for the full time of treatment, even if your symptoms begin to clear up after a few days. Since fungus infections may be very slow to clear up, you may have to continue using this medicine every day for several weeks or more. If you stop using this medicine too soon, your symptoms may return. Do not miss any doses.

Dosing—The dose of this medicine will be different for different patients. Follow your doctor's orders or the directions on the label. The following information includes only the average doses of this medicine. If your dose is different, do not change it unless your doctor tells you to do so.

The amount of medicine that you take depends on the strength of the medicine. Also, the number of doses you take each day, the time allowed between doses, and the length of time you take the medicine depend on the medical problem for which you are using the medicine.

- For topical cream and lotion dosage forms:
  - Fungus infections (treatment):
    - Adults and children 10 years of age and over—Apply two times a day, morning and evening.
    - Children up to 10 years of age—Use and dose must be determined by your doctor.

For topical gel dosage form:
  - Fungus infections (treatment) or seborrheic dermatitis (treatment):
    - Adults and children 16 years of age and over—Apply two times a day, morning and evening.
    - Children up to 16 years of age—Use and dose must be determined by your doctor.

For shampoo dosage form:
  - Seborrheic dermatitis (treatment):
    - Adults and children 16 years of age and over—Apply 1 teaspoon (or up to 2 teaspoons for long hair) two times a week for four weeks with at least three days between each application.
    - Children up to 16 years of age—Use and dose must be determined by your doctor.

For topical solution dosage form:
  - Fungus infections (treatment):
    - Adults—Apply once daily, preferably at bedtime or eight hours before washing.
    - Children up to 18 years of age—Use and dose must be determined by your doctor.

Missed dose—If you miss a dose of this medicine, apply it as soon as possible. However, if it is almost time for your next dose, skip the missed dose and go back to your regular dosing schedule.

Storage—Store the medicine in a closed container at room temperature, away from heat, moisture, and direct light. Keep from freezing.

Keep out of the reach of children.

Do not keep outdated medicine or medicine no longer needed.

Precautions While Using This Medicine

If your skin problem does not improve within 2 to 4 weeks, or if it becomes worse, check with your doctor.

Inform your doctor right away if the area where you applied the medicine shows signs of increased irritation (e.g., redness, itching, burning, blistering, swelling, or oozing) because it could be an allergic reaction.

Nail problems treated with the topical solution form of this medicine may take up to 6 months to start improving.

To help clear up your infection completely and to help make sure it does not return, good health habits are also required. The following measures will help reduce chafing and irritation and will also help keep the area cool and dry.

- For patients using ciclopirox for ringworm of the groin (tinea cruris):
  - Avoid wearing underwear that is tight-fitting or made from synthetic materials (for example, rayon or nylon). Instead, wear loose-fitting, cotton underwear.
  - Use a bland, absorbent powder (for example, talcum powder) or an antifungal powder (for example, tolnaftate) on the skin. It is best to use the powder between applications of ciclopirox.
- For patients using ciclopirox for ringworm of the foot (tinea pedis):
  - Carefully dry the feet, especially between the toes, after bathing.
  - Avoid wearing socks made from wool or synthetic materials (for example, rayon or nylon). Instead, wear clean, cotton socks and change them daily or more often if the feet sweat freely.
  - Wear sandals or well-ventilated shoes (for example, shoes with holes on top or on the side).
  - Use a bland, absorbent powder (for example, talcum powder) or an antifungal powder (for example, tolnaftate) between the toes, on the feet, and in socks and shoes freely once or twice a day. It is best to use the powder between applications of ciclopirox.

If you have any questions about these measures, check with your health care professional.

Side Effects of This Medicine

Along with its needed effects, a medicine may cause some unwanted effects. Although not all of these side effects may occur, if they do occur they may need medical attention.

Check with your doctor as soon as possible if any of the following side effects occur:
Less common—with ciclopirox shampoo
Fainting; fast, pounding, or irregular heartbeat or pulse; palpitations
Rare
Burning, itching, redness, swelling, or other signs of irritation not present before use of this medicine

Some side effects may occur that usually do not need medical attention. These side effects may go away during treatment as your body adjusts to the medicine. Also, your health care professional may be able to tell you about ways to prevent or reduce some of these side effects. Check with your health care professional if any of the following side effects continue or are bothersome or if you have any questions about them:
Less common—with ciclopirox shampoo
Dandruff; headache; itching skin or scalp; oily skin; rash; skin disorder

Other side effects not listed may also occur in some patients. If you notice any other effects, check with your healthcare professional.

CIDOFOVIR (Intravenous route) - si-DOF-oh-veer

Black Box Warning

Renal impairment is the major toxicity of cidofovir. Cases of acute renal failure resulting in dialysis and/or contributing to death have occurred with as few as one or two doses of cidofovir. To reduce possible nephrotoxicity, intravenous prehydration with normal saline and administration of probenecid must be used with each cidofovir infusion. Renal function (serum creatinine and urine protein) must be monitored within 48 hours prior to each dose of cidofovir and the dose of cidofovir modified for changes in renal function as appropriate. Cidofovir is contraindicated in patients who are receiving other nephrotoxic agents.

Neutropenia has been observed in association with cidofovir treatment. Therefore, neutrophil counts should be monitored during cidofovir therapy.

Cidofovir is indicated only for the treatment of CMV retinitis in patients with acquired immunodeficiency syndrome.

In animal studies cidofovir was carcinogenic, teratogenic and caused hypospermia.

Commonly used brand name(s)
In the U.S.—
Vistide

Available Dosage Forms:
- Solution

Therapeutic Class: Antiviral

Uses For This Medicine

Cidofovir is an antiviral. It is used to treat infections caused by viruses.

Cidofovir is used to treat the symptoms of cytomegalovirus (CMV) infection of the eyes (CMV retinitis) in patients with acquired immune deficiency syndrome (AIDS). Cidofovir will not cure this eye infection, but it may help to keep the symptoms from becoming worse.

This medicine is available only with your doctor's prescription.

Before Using This Medicine

In deciding to use a medicine, the risks of taking the medicine must be weighed against the good it will do. This is a decision you and your doctor will make. For this medicine, the following should be considered:

Allergies—Tell your doctor if you have ever had any unusual or allergic reaction to this medicine or any other medicines. Also tell your health care professional if you have any other types of allergies, such as to foods, dyes, preservatives, or animals. For non-prescription products, read the label or package ingredients carefully.

Pediatric—Cidofovir can cause serious side effects, including possible cancer and trouble in having children later. Therefore, it is especially important that you discuss with the child's doctor the good that this medicine may do as well as the risks of using it.

Geriatric—Many medicines have not been studied specifically in older people. Therefore, it may not be known whether they work exactly the same way they do in younger adults or if they cause different side effects or problems in older people. There is no specific information comparing use of cidofovir in the elderly with use in other age groups.

Pregnancy—

	Pregnancy Category	Explanation
All Trimesters	C	Animal studies have shown an adverse effect and there are no adequate studies in pregnant women OR no animal studies have been conducted and there are no adequate studies in pregnant women.

Breast Feeding—There are no adequate studies in women for determining infant risk when using this medication during breastfeeding. Weigh the potential benefits against the potential risks before taking this medication while breastfeeding.

Other medicines—

Using this medicine with any of the following medicines is usually not recommended, but may be required in some cases. If both medicines are prescribed together, your doctor may change the dose or how often you use one or both of the medicines.

Amikacin, Dibekacin, Foscarnet, Framycetin, Gentamicin, Kanamycin, Neomycin, Netilmicin, Pentamidine, Streptomycin, Tobramycin

Interactions with Food/Tobacco/Alcohol—Certain medicines should not be used at or around the time of eating food or eating certain types of food since interactions may occur. Using alcohol or tobacco with certain medicines may also cause interactions to occur. Discuss with your healthcare professional the use of your medicine with food, alcohol, or tobacco.

Other medical problems—The presence of other medical problems may affect the use of this medicine. Make sure you tell your doctor if you have any other medical problems, especially:

- Kidney disease—Cidofovir can cause harmful effects on the kidney

Proper Use of This Medicine

To get the best results, cidofovir must be given for the full time of treatment. Also, this medicine works best when there is a constant amount in the blood. To help keep the amount constant, cidofovir must be given on a regular schedule.

Dosing—The dose of this medicine will be different for different patients. Follow your doctor's orders or the directions on the label. The following information includes only the average doses of this medicine. If your dose is different, do not change it unless your doctor tells you to do so.

The amount of medicine that you take depends on the strength of the medicine. Also, the number of doses you take each day, the time allowed between doses, and the length of time you take the medicine depend on the medical problem for which you are using the medicine.

- For injection dosage form:
  - For treatment of cytomegalovirus (CMV) retinitis:
    - Adults—Dose is based on body weight and must be determined by your doctor. At first, 5 milligrams (mg) per kilogram (kg) (2.3 mg per pound) of body weight is injected slowly into a vein once a week for two weeks in a row. Then the dose is reduced to 5 mg per kg (2.3 mg per pound) of body weight injected slowly into a vein once every two weeks. Probenecid is taken along with each dose of cidofovir; follow your doctor's instructions for how much and when to take probenecid.
    - Children—Use and dose must be determined by your doctor.

Precautions While Using This Medicine

It is very important that your doctor check you at regular visits for any blood problems that may be caused by this medicine.

It is very important that your ophthalmologist (eye doctor) check your eyes at regular visits since it is still possible that you may have some loss of eyesight during cidofovir treatment.

Side Effects of This Medicine

Along with its needed effects, a medicine may cause some unwanted effects. Although not all of these side effects may occur, if they do occur they may need medical attention.

Medicines like cidofovir can sometimes cause serious side effects such as blood problems and kidney problems; these are described below. Cidofovir has also been found to cause cancer in animals, and there is a chance it could cause cancer in humans as well. Discuss these possible side effects with your doctor.

Check with your doctor immediately if any of the following side effects occur:
> *More common*
>> Fever, chills, or sore throat

Check with your doctor as soon as possible if any of the following side effects occur:
> *More common*
>> Decreased urination; increased thirst and urination
> *Rare*
>> Decreased vision or any change in vision

Some side effects may occur that usually do not need medical attention. These side effects may go away during treatment as your body adjusts to the medicine. Also, your health care professional may be able to tell you about ways to prevent or reduce some of these side effects. Check with your health care professional if any of the following side effects continue or are bothersome or if you have any questions about them:
> *More common*
>> Diarrhea; headache; loss of appetite; nausea; vomiting
> *Less common*
>> Generalized weakness; loss of strength

Other side effects not listed may also occur in some patients. If you notice any other effects, check with your healthcare professional.

CILOSTAZOL (Oral route) - sil-OH-sta-zol

Commonly used brand name(s)

In the U.S.—
Pletal

Available Dosage Forms:
- Tablet

Therapeutic Class: Platelet Aggregation Inhibitor
Pharmacologic Class: Phosphodiesterase Inhibitor

Uses For This Medicine

Cilostazol improves the flow of blood through blood vessels. It is used to reduce leg pain caused by poor circulation (intermittent claudication). Cilostazol makes it possible to walk farther before having to rest because of leg pain.

Cilostazol works by keeping blood from clotting and by dilating or relaxing the blood vessels.

Cilostazol is available only with your doctor's prescription.

Before Using This Medicine

In deciding to use a medicine, the risks of taking the medicine must be weighed against the good it will do. This is a decision you and your doctor will make. For this medicine, the following should be considered:

Allergies—Tell your doctor if you have ever had any unusual or allergic reaction to this medicine or any other medicines. Also tell your health care professional if you have any other types of allergies, such as to foods, dyes, preservatives, or animals. For non-prescription products, read the label or package ingredients carefully.

Pediatric—Studies on this medicine have been done only in adult patients, and there is no specific information comparing the use of cilostazol in children with use in other age groups.

Geriatric—This medicine has been tested in a limited number of patients and has not been shown to cause different side effects or problems in older people than it does in younger adults.

Pregnancy—

	Pregnancy Category	Explanation
All Trimesters	C	Animal studies have shown an adverse effect and there are no adequate studies in pregnant women OR no animal studies have been conducted and there are no adequate studies in pregnant women.

Breast Feeding—There are no adequate studies in women for determining infant risk when using this medication during breastfeeding. Weigh the potential benefits against the potential risks before taking this medication while breastfeeding.

Other medicines—

Using this medicine with any of the following medicines is usually not recommended, but may be required in some cases. If both medicines are prescribed together, your doctor may change the dose or how often you use one or both of the medicines.

Abciximab, Acenocoumarol, Alteplase, Recombinant, Anisindione, Anistreplase, Argatroban, Bivalirudin, Cilostazol, Clopidogrel, Danaparoid, Defibrotide, Dermatan Sulfate, Desirudin, Dicumarol, Eptifibatide, Fondaparinux, Ginkgo, Heparin, Lamifiban, Phenindione, Phenprocoumon, Reteplase, Recombinant, Sibrafiban, Streptokinase, Tenecteplase, Tirofiban, Urokinase, Warfarin, Xemilofiban

Interactions with Food/Tobacco/Alcohol—Certain medicines should not be used at or around the time of eating food or eating certain types of food since interactions may occur. Using alcohol or tobacco with certain medicines may also cause interactions to occur. The following interactions have been selected on the basis of their potential significance and are not necessarily all-inclusive.

Using this medicine with any of the following may cause an increased risk of certain side effects but may be unavoidable in some cases. If used together, your doctor may change the dose or how often you use this medicine, or give you special instructions about the use of food, alcohol, or tobacco.

Grapefruit Juice

Other medical problems—The presence of other medical problems may affect the use of this medicine. Make sure you tell your doctor if you have any other medical problems, especially:
- Active bleeding (including peptic ulcers and intracranial bleeding [e.g., bleeding on the brain]) or
- Blood or blood clotting disorders or
- Congestive heart failure—This medicine should not be used.
- Kidney disease or
- Liver disease—Special caution should be used.
- Thrombocytopenia (low platelet count in the blood)—Caution should be used.

Proper Use of This Medicine

To help you remember to take your medicine, try to get into the habit of taking it at the same time each day.

Dosing—The dose of this medicine will be different for different patients. Follow your doctor's orders or the directions on the label. The following information includes only the average doses of this medicine. If your dose is different, do not change it unless your doctor tells you to do so.

The amount of medicine that you take depends on the strength of the medicine. Also, the number of doses you take each day, the time allowed between doses, and the length of time you take the medicine depend on the medical problem for which you are using the medicine.
- For oral dosage form (tablets):
  - For treatment of peripheral vascular disease (circulation problems):
    - Adults—100 milligrams (mg) two times a day, taken at least one half hour before or two hours

after breakfast and dinner. In patients who take certain other medicines at the same time as cilostazol, the dose may be 50 mg two times a day.
- Children—Use and dose must be determined by a doctor.

Missed dose—If you miss a dose of this medicine, take it as soon as possible. However, if it is almost time for your next dose, skip the missed dose and go back to your regular dosing schedule. Do not double doses.

Storage—Store the medicine in a closed container at room temperature, away from heat, moisture, and direct light. Keep from freezing.

Keep out of the reach of children.

Do not keep outdated medicine or medicine no longer needed.

Precautions While Using This Medicine

It may take several weeks for this medicine to work. If you feel that cilostazol is not working, do not stop taking it on your own. Instead, check with your doctor.

Smoking tobacco products, such as cigarettes, may worsen your condition since nicotine may further narrow blood vessels and may also affect how this medicine works. Therefore, it is best to avoid smoking.

You should not take cilostazol with grapefruit juice. You may, however, take it with other citrus juices.

Side Effects of This Medicine

Along with its needed effects, a medicine may cause some unwanted effects. Although not all of these side effects may occur, if they do occur they may need medical attention.

Check with your doctor immediately if any of the following side effects occur:

More common
Fast or irregular heartbeat; fever

Less common
Abnormal bleeding; bloody or black tarry stools; bruises and/or red spots on the skin; fainting; nausea, heartburn, and/or indigestion (severe or continuing); nosebleeds; stiff neck; stomach pain, cramping, or burning (severe); swelling of the tongue; vomiting of blood or material that looks like coffee grounds

Incidence not known
Abdominal or stomach pain; area rash; bleeding gums; bleeding tendency; blistering, peeling, loosening of skin; blood in urine or stools; blurred vision; chest pain; chills; clay-colored stools; confusion; cough or hoarseness; coughing up blood; dark urine; diarrhea; difficult breathing; drowsiness; fever with or without chills; general feeling of tiredness or weakness; headache, sudden and severe; inability to speak; irregular heartbeat; itching of eyes; itching of skin; joint or muscle pain; lab results that show problems with the liver; light-colored stools; loss of appetite; loss of consciousness; lower back or side pain; nausea and vomiting; painful or difficult urination; pinpoint red spots on skin; red, irritated eyes; red skin lesions, often with a purple center; seizures; shortness of breath; skin rash; slurred speech; sores, ulcers, or white spots on lips or in mouth; stomach pain; swollen glands; temporary blindness; unpleasant breath odor;

unusual bleeding or bruising; unusual tiredness or weakness; weakness in arm and/or leg on one side of the body, sudden and severe; weakness of part of body; wheezing; yellow eyes or skin

Symptoms of overdose
Diarrhea; dizziness or lightheadedness when getting up from a lying or sitting position; fast or irregular heartbeat; headache (severe)

Some side effects may occur that usually do not need medical attention. These side effects may go away during treatment as your body adjusts to the medicine. Also, your health care professional may be able to tell you about ways to prevent or reduce some of these side effects. Check with your health care professional if any of the following side effects continue or are bothersome or if you have any questions about them:

More common
Back pain; dizziness; gas; headache; increased cough; pain or stiffness in muscles; pounding heartbeat; runny or stuffy nose; sore throat; swelling of arms or legs

Less common
Bone pain; burning feeling in throat or chest; difficulty in swallowing; hives; pain or stiffness in joints; ringing or buzzing in ears; swelling of face, fingers, and/or lower legs

Incidence not known
Bruising; hot flushes; pain

Other side effects not listed may also occur in some patients. If you notice any other effects, check with your healthcare professional.

CINACALCET   (Oral route) - sin-a-KAL-set

Commonly used brand name(s)

In the U.S.—
Sensipar

Available Dosage Forms:
- Tablet

Therapeutic Class: Calcium Regulator
Pharmacologic Class: Calcimimetic

Uses For This Medicine

Cinacalcet is a medicine used to treat hyperparathyroidism in patients with chronic kidney disease who are on dialysis. Hyperparathyroidism is a condition that is caused when the parathyroid glands located in the neck make too much parathyroid hormone (PTH). This hormone controls the concentrations of calcium and phosphorus in your blood. Cinacalcet helps lower the amount of PTH which lowers the calcium and phosphorus concentrations. Cinacalcet is also used to lower calcium in the blood in patients with parathyroid cancer.

This medicine is available only with your doctor's prescription.

Before Using This Medicine

In deciding to use a medicine, the risks of taking the medicine must be weighed against the good it will do. This is a decision you and your doctor will make. For this medicine, the following should be considered:

Allergies—Tell your doctor if you have ever had any unusual or allergic reaction to this medicine or any other medicines. Also tell your health care professional if you have any other types of allergies, such as to foods, dyes, preservatives, or animals. For non-prescription products, read the label or package ingredients carefully.

Pediatric—Studies on this medicine have been done only in adult patients, and there is no specific information comparing use of cinacalcet in children with use in other age groups.

Geriatric—This medicine has been tested in a limited number of patients 65 years of age or older and has not been shown to cause different side effects or problems in older people than it does in younger adults.

Pregnancy—

	Pregnancy Category	Explanation
All Trimesters	C	Animal studies have shown an adverse effect and there are no adequate studies in pregnant women OR no animal studies have been conducted and there are no adequate studies in pregnant women.

Breast Feeding—Studies in women suggest that this medication poses minimal risk to the infant when used during breastfeeding.

Other medicines—

Using this medicine with any of the following medicines may cause an increased risk of certain side effects, but using both drugs may be the best treatment for you. If both medicines are prescribed together, your doctor may change the dose or how often you use one or both of the medicines.

Amitriptyline, Erythromycin, Itraconazole, Ketoconazole

Interactions with Food/Tobacco/Alcohol—Certain medicines should not be used at or around the time of eating food or eating certain types of food since interactions may occur. Using alcohol or tobacco with certain medicines may also cause interactions to occur. Discuss with your healthcare professional the use of your medicine with food, alcohol, or tobacco.

Other medical problems—The presence of other medical problems may affect the use of this medicine. Make sure you tell your doctor if you have any other medical problems, especially:

- Allergy to cinacalcet or any ingredient in the tablet—This medicine should not be used in these patients

- Liver disease—Higher blood levels of cinacalcet may result and your doctor may need to change your dose

- Seizure problems in the past—May increase risk of seizures while taking this medicine

Proper Use of This Medicine

Dosing—The dose of this medicine will be different for different patients. Follow your doctor's orders or the directions on the label. The following information includes only the average doses of this medicine. If your dose is different, do not change it unless your doctor tells you to do so.

The amount of medicine that you take depends on the strength of the medicine. Also, the number of doses you take each day, the time allowed between doses, and the length of time you take the medicine depend on the medical problem for which you are using the medicine.

- For oral dosage form (tablets):
  - For hypercalcemia associated with parathyroid cancer:
    - Adults—Oral, 30 mg twice a day to start. This medicine should be taken with food or shortly after a meal and the tablet should be taken whole, not crushed, divided, or chewed. Your doctor may adjust your dose every two to four weeks.
    - Children—This medicine has not been tested in children under the age of 18. Use and dose must be determined by your doctor.
  - For secondary hyperparathyroidism in those with chronic kidney disease who are on dialysis:
    - Adults—Oral, 30 milligrams (mg) taken once a day to start. This medicine should be taken with food or shortly after a meal and the tablet should be taken whole, not crushed, divided, or chewed. Your doctor may change your dose every two to four weeks.
    - Children—This medicine has not been tested in children under the age of 18. Use and dose must be determined by your doctor.

Missed dose—If you miss a dose of this medicine, take it as soon as possible. However, if it is almost time for your next dose, skip the missed dose and go back to your regular dosing schedule. Do not double doses.

Storage—Store the medicine in a closed container at room temperature, away from heat, moisture, and direct light. Keep from freezing.

Keep out of the reach of children.

Do not keep outdated medicine or medicine no longer needed.

Ask your healthcare professional how you should dispose of any medicine you do not use.

Precautions While Using This Medicine

It is very important that your doctor check your progress at regular visits. This will allow your doctor to see if the medicine is working properly and to decide if you should continue to take it.

Other medicines: Do not take other medicines unless they have been discussed with your doctor. Taking other medicines together with cinacalcet may require your doctor to change the dose of one of the medicines or cinacalcet.

This medicine may lower the calcium in your blood. The symptoms of low calcium may include abdominal cramps; confusion; convulsions; difficulty in breathing; irregular heartbeats; mood or mental changes; muscle cramps in hands, arms, feet, legs, or face; numbness and tingling around the mouth, fingertips, or feet; shortness of breath; and/or tremor. If you experience any of these symptoms, check with your doctor immediately.

This medicine may increase the risk of seizures in people who have had problems with seizures in the past. Your doctor may need to check your progress more often if you have experienced seizures in the past.

Side Effects of This Medicine

Along with its needed effects, a medicine may cause some unwanted effects. Although not all of these side effects may occur, if they do occur they may need medical attention.

Check with your doctor immediately if any of the following side effects occur:

More common
  Blurred vision; chest pain; dizziness; headache; nervousness; pounding in the ears; slow or fast heartbeat

Less common
  Convulsions; cough or hoarseness; fever or chills; loss of bladder control; lower back or side pain; muscle spasm or jerking of all extremities; painful or difficult urination; sudden loss of consciousness

Frequency not known
  Abdominal cramps; confusion; difficulty in breathing; irregular heartbeats; low bone turnover; mood or mental changes; muscle cramps in hands, arms, feet, legs, or face; numbness and tingling around the mouth, fingertips, or feet; shortness of breath; tremor

Get emergency help immediately if any of the following symptoms of overdose occur:

Symptoms of overdose
  Abdominal cramps; confusion; difficulty in breathing; irregular heartbeats; mood or mental changes; muscle cramps in hands, arms, feet, legs, or face; numbness and tingling around the mouth, fingertips, or feet; shortness of breath; tremor

Some side effects may occur that usually do not need medical attention. These side effects may go away during treatment as your body adjusts to the medicine. Also, your health care professional may be able to tell you about ways to prevent or reduce some of these side effects. Check with your health care professional if any of the following side effects continue or are bothersome or if you have any questions about them:

More common
  Diarrhea; difficulty in moving; joint pain; lack or loss of strength; loss of appetite; muscle aching or cramping; muscle pains or stiffness; nausea; swollen joints; vomiting; weight loss

Other side effects not listed may also occur in some patients. If you notice any other effects, check with your healthcare professional.

CIPROFLOXACIN   (Ophthalmic route)
- sip-roe-FLOX-a-sin

Commonly used brand name(s)

In the U.S.—
  Ciloxan

Available Dosage Forms:
  • Solution
  • Ointment

Therapeutic Class: Antibiotic

Uses For This Medicine

Ophthalmic ciprofloxacin is used in the eye to treat bacterial infections of the eye (ophthalmic ointment and solution) and corneal ulcers of the eye (ophthalmic solution). Ophthalmic ciprofloxacin works by killing bacteria.

Ciprofloxacin ophthalmic preparation is available only with your doctor's prescription.

Before Using This Medicine

In deciding to use a medicine, the risks of taking the medicine must be weighed against the good it will do. This is a decision you and your doctor will make. For this medicine, the following should be considered:

Allergies—Tell your doctor if you have ever had any unusual or allergic reaction to this medicine or any other medicines. Also tell your health care professional if you have any other types of allergies, such as to foods, dyes, preservatives, or animals. For non-prescription products, read the label or package ingredients carefully.

Pediatric—Use is not recommended in infants and children up to 2 years of age (ophthalmic ointment) and 1 year of age (ophthalmic solution). In children older than 1 or 2 years of age, this medicine is not expected to cause different side effects or problems than it does in adults.

Geriatric—Many medicines have not been studied specifically in older people. Therefore, it may not be known whether they work exactly the same way they do in younger adults or if they cause different side effects or problems in older people. There is no specific information comparing use of ophthalmic ciprofloxacin in the elderly with use in other age groups.

Pregnancy—

	Pregnancy Category	Explanation
All Trimesters	C	Animal studies have shown an adverse effect and there are no adequate studies in pregnant women OR no animal studies have been conducted and there are no adequate studies in pregnant women.

Breast Feeding—There are no adequate studies in women for determining infant risk when using this medication during breastfeeding. Weigh the potential benefits against the potential risks before taking this medication while breastfeeding.

Other medicines—

Using this medicine with any of the following medicines is not recommended. Your doctor may decide not to treat you with this medication or change some of the other medicines you take.

Tizanidine

Interactions with Food/Tobacco/Alcohol—Certain medicines should not be used at or around the time of eating food or eating certain types of food since interactions may occur. Using alcohol or tobacco with certain medicines may also cause interactions to occur. The following interactions have been selected on the basis of their potential significance and are not necessarily all-inclusive.

Using this medicine with any of the following may cause an increased risk of certain side effects but may be unavoidable in some cases. If used together, your doctor may change the dose or how often you use this medicine, or give you special instructions about the use of food, alcohol, or tobacco.

Caffeine

Proper Use of This Medicine

To use the ophthalmic ointment:

- First, wash your hands. Tilt the head back and, pressing your finger gently on the skin just beneath the lower eyelid, pull the lower eyelid away from the eye to make a space. Squeeze a thin strip of ointment into this space. A ½-inch strip of ointment is usually enough, unless you have been told by your doctor to use a different amount. Let go of the eyelid and gently close the eyes. Keep the eyes closed for 1 or 2 minutes to allow the medicine to come into contact with the infection.
- To keep the medicine as germ-free as possible, do not touch the applicator tip to any surface (including the eye). After using the eye ointment, wipe the tip of the ointment tube with a clean tissue and keep the tube tightly closed.

To use the ophthalmic solution (eye drops):

- First, wash your hands. Then tilt the head back and pull the lower eyelid away from the eye to form a pouch. Drop the medicine into the pouch and gently close the eyes. Do not blink. Keep the eyes closed for 1 or 2 minutes to allow the medicine to come into contact with the infection.
- If you think you did not get the drop of medicine into your eyes properly, use another drop.
- To keep the medicine as germ-free as possible, do not touch the applicator tip to any surface (including the eye). Also, keep the container tightly closed.

To help clear up your eye infection completely, keep using ophthalmic ciprofloxacin for the full time of treatment, even if your symptoms have disappeared. Do not miss any doses.

Dosing—The dose of this medicine will be different for different patients. Follow your doctor's orders or the directions on the label. The following information includes only the average doses of this medicine. If your dose is different, do not change it unless your doctor tells you to do so.

The amount of medicine that you take depends on the strength of the medicine. Also, the number of doses you take each day, the time allowed between doses, and the length of time you take the medicine depend on the medical problem for which you are using the medicine.

- For ophthalmic ointment dosage form:
  - For bacterial conjunctivitis:
    - Adults and children 2 years of age and older— Use a ½-inch strip of eye ointment in each eye three times a day for the first two days, then use a ½-inch strip of eye ointment in each eye two times a day for the next five days.
    - Infants and children up to 2 years of age—Use and dose must be determined by your doctor.
- For ophthalmic solution dosage form:
  - For bacterial conjunctivitis:
    - Adults and children 1 year of age and older—Use 1 drop in each eye every two hours, while you are awake, for two days. Then use 1 drop in each eye every four hours, while you are awake, for the next five days. If you think you did not get the drop of medicine into your eyes properly, use another drop.
    - Infants and children up to 1 year of age—Use and dose must be determined by your doctor.
  - For corneal ulcers:
    - Adults and children 1 year of age and older—On day one, use 2 drops in the affected eye every fifteen minutes for six hours, then 2 drops every thirty minutes for the rest of the day, while you are awake. On day two, use 2 drops every hour, while you are awake. On days three through fourteen, use 2 drops every four hours, while you are awake.
    - Infants and children up to 1 year of age—Use and dose must be determined by your doctor.

Missed dose—If you miss a dose of this medicine, take it as soon as possible. However, if it is almost time for your next dose, skip the missed dose and go back to your regular dosing schedule. Do not double doses.

Storage—Store the medicine in a closed container at room temperature, away from heat, moisture, and direct light. Keep from freezing.

Keep out of the reach of children.

Do not keep outdated medicine or medicine no longer needed.

Precautions While Using This Medicine

If your eye infection does not improve within a few days, or if it becomes worse, check with your doctor.

This medicine may cause your eyes to become more sensitive to light than they are normally. Wearing sunglasses and avoiding too much exposure to bright light may help lessen the discomfort.

Side Effects of This Medicine

Along with its needed effects, a medicine may cause some unwanted effects. Although not all of these side effects may occur, if they do occur they may need medical attention.

Check with your doctor as soon as possible if any of the following side effects occur:

Rare

Allergic reaction, such as skin rash, hives, or itching; blurred vision or other change in vision; eye pain; irritation (severe) or redness of eye; nausea

Some side effects may occur that usually do not need medical attention. These side effects may go away during treatment as your body adjusts to the medicine. Also, your health care professional may be able to tell you about ways to prevent or reduce some of these side effects. Check with your health care professional if any of the following side effects continue or are bothersome or if you have any questions about them:

More common
Burning or other discomfort of eye; crusting or crystals in corner of eye

Less common
Bad taste following use in the eye; feeling of something in eye; itching of eye; redness of the lining of the eyelids

Rare
Dryness of eye; increased sensitivity of eyes to light; swelling of eyelid; tearing of eye

Other side effects not listed may also occur in some patients. If you notice any other effects, check with your healthcare professional.

CIPROFLOXACIN AND DEXAMETHASONE (Otic route) - sip-roe-FLOX-a-sin, dex-a-METH-a-sone

Commonly used brand name(s)

In the U.S.—
Ciprodex

Available Dosage Forms:
• Suspension

Therapeutic Class: Anti-Infective/Anti-Inflammatory Combination
Pharmacologic Class: Adrenal Glucocorticoid

Uses For This Medicine

Ciprofloxacin and dexamethasone is a combination of two medicines used to treat ear infections. One of the medicines is an antibiotic (medicine used to fight infection) and the other is a corticosteroid (cortisone-like medicine). The antibiotic (ciprofloxacin) is used to fight ear infections. The corticosteroid (dexamethasone) is used to relieve the redness, itching, and swelling caused by ear infections.

This medicine is used to treat middle ear infection with drainage through a tube in children 6 months of age and older. A middle ear infection is an infection caused by bacteria behind the eardrum. People who have a tube in the eardrum may notice drainage from the ear canal.

This medicine is also used to treat outer ear canal infections in patients 6 months of age or older. An outer ear canal infection, also known as "Swimmer's Ear," is a bacterial infection of the outer ear canal. The ear canal and outer part of the ear may swell, turn red, and be painful. Also, a fluid discharge may appear in the ear canal.

This medicine is available only with your doctor's prescription.

Before Using This Medicine

In deciding to use a medicine, the risks of taking the medicine must be weighed against the good it will do. This is a decision you and your doctor will make. For this medicine, the following should be considered:

Allergies—Tell your doctor if you have ever had any unusual or allergic reaction to this medicine or any other medicines. Also tell your health care professional if you have any other types of allergies, such as to foods, dyes, preservatives, or animals. For non-prescription products, read the label or package ingredients carefully.

Pediatric—There is no specific information comparing use of ciprofloxacin and dexamethasone combination in children younger than 6 months of age with use in other age groups. This medicine should not be used in children under 6 months of age.

Geriatric—Many medicines have not been studied specifically in older people. Therefore, it may not be known whether they work the same way they do in younger people of if they cause different side effects or problems in older people. It is not expected to cause different side effects or problems in older people than it does in younger adults.

Other medicines—

Using this medicine with any of the following medicines is not recommended. Your doctor may decide not to treat you with this medication or change some of the other medicines you take.

Bupropion, Rotavirus Vaccine, Live, Tizanidine

Interactions with Food/Tobacco/Alcohol—Certain medicines should not be used at or around the time of eating food or eating certain types of food since interactions may occur. Using alcohol or tobacco with certain medicines may also cause interactions to occur. The following interactions have been selected on the basis of their potential significance and are not necessarily all-inclusive.

Using this medicine with any of the following may cause an increased risk of certain side effects but may be unavoidable in some cases. If used together, your doctor may change the dose or how often you use this medicine, or give you special instructions about the use of food, alcohol, or tobacco.

Caffeine

Other medical problems—The presence of other medical problems may affect the use of this medicine. Make sure you tell your doctor if you have any other medical problems, especially:

• Viral ear infections (infections caused by a virus)—This medicine should not be used in patients with viral ear infections of the outer ear canal.

Proper Use of This Medicine

This medicine is to be used in the ear only. It is not approved for use in the eye. Do not take by mouth. If this medicine is accidently swallowed call your doctor right away.

It is important that the infected ear(s) remain clean and dry. When bathing, avoid getting the infected ear(s) wet. Avoid swimming unless your doctor has instructed you otherwise.

To use:

• Wash hands thoroughly with soap and water
• Hold the bottle of ear drops in the hand for one or two minutes to warm the medicine, then shake well.

- Lie down on your side with your infected ear facing up.
- Put drops in infected ear.
- To keep the medicine as germ-free as possible, do not touch the applicator tip to any surface (including the ear). Also, keep the container tightly closed.
- For Patients with Middle Ear Infection with Tubes: While the person getting the ear drops lies on their side the person giving the drops should gently press the small projection in front of the outside opening of the ear 5 times in a pumping motion. This will allow the drops to pass through the tube and into the middle ear.
- For patients with Outer Ear Infection ("Swimmer's Ear"): While the person getting the ear drops lies on their side, the person giving the drops should gently pull the outer ear lobe upward and backward. This will allow the ear drops to flow down into the ear canal.
- The person who just had the ear drops should stay on their side for at least one minute. Repeat the above steps if both ears are infected.
- When you have completed your course of therapy (usually 7 days), throw away the medicine that you did not use.

To help clear up your infection completely, keep using this medicine for the full time of treatment, even if your symptoms have disappeared. Do not miss any doses. If the ear drops are not used for as long as the doctor recommended your infection can return.

Dosing—The dose of this medicine will be different for different patients. Follow your doctor's orders or the directions on the label. The following information includes only the average doses of this medicine. If your dose is different, do not change it unless your doctor tells you to do so.

The amount of medicine that you take depends on the strength of the medicine. Also, the number of doses you take each day, the time allowed between doses, and the length of time you take the medicine depend on the medical problem for which you are using the medicine.

- For ear drops dosage form:
  ○ For ear infections:
    ▪ Adults and children 6 months of age and older—Place four drops in the ear canal of infected ear two times a day for seven days.
    ▪ Children younger than 6 months of age—Use and dose must be determined by your doctor.

Missed dose—If you miss a dose of this medicine, take it as soon as possible. However, if it is almost time for your next dose, skip the missed dose and go back to your regular dosing schedule. Do not double doses.

Storage—Store the medicine in a closed container at room temperature, away from heat, moisture, and direct light. Keep from freezing.

Keep out of the reach of children.

Do not keep outdated medicine or medicine no longer needed.

Precautions While Using This Medicine

If your symptoms do not improve within a week, or if they become worse, check with your doctor.

If you experience a rash or an allergic reaction to this medicine, stop using it and call your doctor immediately.

Side Effects of This Medicine

Along with its needed effects, a medicine may cause some unwanted effects. Although not all of these side effects may occur, if they do occur they may need medical attention.

Some side effects may occur that usually do not need medical attention. These side effects may go away during treatment as your body adjusts to the medicine. Also, your health care professional may be able to tell you about ways to prevent or reduce some of these side effects. Check with your health care professional if any of the following side effects continue or are bothersome or if you have any questions about them:

Less common
  Ear discomfort; ear pain; itching skin on the ear
Rare
  Bitter, sour or unusual taste in mouth; ear congestion; ear debris; ear residue; redness of skin; superimposed ear infection (second ear infection)

Other side effects not listed may also occur in some patients. If you notice any other effects, check with your healthcare professional.

CISPLATIN (Intravenous route) - SIS-pla-tin

Black Box Warning

Cisplatin should be administered under the supervision of a qualified physician experienced in the use of cancer chemotherapeutic agents. Appropriate management of therapy and complications is possible only when adequate diagnostic and treatment facilities are readily available.

Cumulative renal toxicity associated with cisplatin is severe. Other major dose-related toxicities are myelosuppression, nausea and vomiting.

Ototoxicity, which may be more pronounced in children, and is manifested by tinnitus, and/or loss of high frequency hearing and occasionally deafness, is significant.

Anaphylactic-like reactions to cisplatin have been reported. Facial edema, bronchoconstriction, tachycardia, and hypotension may occur within minutes of cisplatin administration. Epinephrine, corticosteroids, and antihistamines have been effectively employed to alleviate symptoms.

Exercise caution to prevent cisplatin overdose. Doses greater than 100 mg/m(2)/cycle once every 3 to 4 weeks are rarely used. Care must be taken to avoid inadvertent cisplatin overdose due to confusion with carboplatin or prescribing practices that fail to differentiate daily doses from total dose per cycle.

Commonly used brand name(s)
In the U.S.—
  Platinol-AQ
Available Dosage Forms:
- Powder for Solution
- Solution

Therapeutic Class: Antineoplastic Agent
Pharmacologic Class: Platinum Coordination Complex

Uses For This Medicine

Cisplatin belongs to the group of medicines known as alkylating agents. It is used to treat cancer of the bladder, ovaries, and testicles. It may also be used to treat other kinds of cancer, as determined by your doctor.

Cisplatin interferes with the growth of cancer cells, which are eventually destroyed. Since the growth of normal body cells may also be affected by cisplatin, other effects will also occur. Some of these may be serious and must be reported to your doctor. Other effects may not be serious but may cause concern. Some effects may not occur for months or years after the medicine is used.

Before you begin treatment with cisplatin, you and your doctor should talk about the good this medicine will do as well as the risks of using it.

Cisplatin is to be administered only by or under the immediate supervision of your doctor.

Once a medicine has been approved for marketing for a certain use, experience may show that it is also useful for other medical problems. Although these uses are not included in product labeling, cisplatin is used in certain patients with the following medical conditions:

- Cancer of the outside layer of the adrenal gland
- Cancer of the breast
- Cancer of the cervix
- Cancer of the endometrium
- Cancer of the fallopian tube or lining of the abdomen (spreading from the ovary)
- Cancer of the esophagus
- Cancer of the stomach
- Cancer of the lung
- Neuroblastoma (a certain type of cancer in nerve tissues that occurs in children)
- Cancer of the prostate
- Cancers of the head and neck
- Cancer of the liver
- Cancer of the thyroid
- Cancer of the anus
- Cancer of the vulva
- Cancer of the bile duct
- Cancer of the skin, including types that spread to other parts of the body
- Cancer of unknown primary site
- Cancer of the lymph system
- Hepatoblastoma (a certain type of liver cancer that occurs in children)
- Thymoma (a cancer of the thymus, which is a small organ that lies under the breastbone)
- Tumors in the ovaries
- Gestational trophoblastic tumors (tumors in the uterus or womb)
- Wilms' tumor (a cancer of the kidneys occurring mainly in children)
- Retinoblastoma (a cancer of the eye occurring mainly in children)
- Cancer of the bones (in children)
- Cancer of the muscles, connective tissues (tendons), vessels that carry blood or lymph, joints, and fat.
- Autoimmune deficiency syndrome (AIDS)– associated Kaposi's sarcoma (a type of cancer of the skin and mucous membranes that is more common in patients with AIDS)

Before Receiving This Medicine

In deciding to use a medicine, the risks of taking the medicine must be weighed against the good it will do. This is a decision you and your doctor will make. For this medicine, the following should be considered:

Allergies—Tell your doctor if you have ever had any unusual or allergic reaction to this medicine or any other medicines. Also tell your health care professional if you have any other types of allergies, such as to foods, dyes, preservatives, or animals. For non-prescription products, read the label or package ingredients carefully.

Pediatric—Hearing problems and loss of balance are more likely to occur in children, who are usually more sensitive to the effects of cisplatin.

Geriatric—Many medicines have not been studied specifically in older people. Therefore, it may not be known whether they work exactly the same way they do in younger adults or if they cause different side effects or problems in older people. There is no specific information comparing use of cisplatin in the elderly with use in other age groups.

Pregnancy—

	Pregnancy Category	Explanation
All Trimesters	D	Studies in pregnant women have demonstrated a risk to the fetus. However, the benefits of therapy in a life threatening situation or a serious disease, may outweigh the potential risk.

Breast Feeding—There are no adequate studies in women for determining infant risk when using this medication during breastfeeding. Weigh the potential benefits against the potential risks before taking this medication while breastfeeding.

Other medicines—

Using this medicine with any of the following medicines is not recommended. Your doctor may decide not to treat you with this medication or change some of the other medicines you take.

Rotavirus Vaccine, Live

Interactions with Food/Tobacco/Alcohol—Certain medicines should not be used at or around the time of eating food or eating certain types of food since interactions may occur. Using alcohol or tobacco with certain medicines may also cause interactions to occur. Discuss with your healthcare professional the use of your medicine with food, alcohol, or tobacco.

Other medical problems—The presence of other medical problems may affect the use of this medicine. Make sure you tell your doctor if you have any other medical problems, especially:

- Chickenpox (including recent exposure) or

- Herpes zoster (shingles)—Risk of severe disease affecting other parts of the body
- Gout (history of) or
- Kidney stones (history of)—Cisplatin may increase levels of uric acid in the body, which can cause gout or kidney stones
- Hearing problems—May be worsened by cisplatin
- Infection—Cisplatin decreases your body's ability to fight infection
- Kidney disease—Effects of cisplatin may be increased because of slower removal from the body

Proper Use of This Medicine

This medicine is sometimes given together with certain other medicines. If you are using a combination of medicines, it is important that you receive each one at the proper time. If you are taking some of these medicines by mouth, ask your health care professional to help you plan a way to take them at the right times.

While you are receiving this medicine, your doctor may want you to drink extra fluids so that you will pass more urine. This will help prevent kidney problems and keep your kidneys working well.

This medicine usually causes nausea and vomiting that may be severe. However, it is very important that you continue to receive the medicine, even if you begin to feel ill. Ask your health care professional for ways to lessen these effects, especially if they are severe.

Dosing—The dose of this medicine will be different for different patients. Follow your doctor's orders or the directions on the label. The following information includes only the average doses of this medicine. If your dose is different, do not change it unless your doctor tells you to do so.

The amount of medicine that you take depends on the strength of the medicine. Also, the number of doses you take each day, the time allowed between doses, and the length of time you take the medicine depend on the medical problem for which you are using the medicine.

Precautions After Receiving This Medicine

It is very important that your doctor check your progress at regular visits to make sure that this medicine is working properly and to check for unwanted effects.

While you are being treated with cisplatin, and after you stop treatment with it, do not have any immunizations (vaccinations) without your doctor's approval. Cisplatin may lower your body's resistance and there is a chance you might get the infection the immunization is meant to prevent. In addition, other persons living in your household should not take oral polio vaccine since there is a chance they could pass the polio virus on to you. Also, avoid persons who have taken oral polio vaccine within the last several months. Do not get close to them, and do not stay in the same room with them for very long. If you cannot take these precautions, you should consider wearing a protective face mask that covers the nose and mouth.

Cisplatin can temporarily lower the number of white blood cells in your blood, increasing the chance of getting an infec-

tion. It can also lower the number of platelets, which are necessary for proper blood clotting. If this occurs, there are certain precautions you can take, especially when your blood count is low, to reduce the risk of infection or bleeding:

- If you can, avoid people with infections. Check with your doctor immediately if you think you are getting an infection or if you get a fever or chills, cough or hoarseness, lower back or side pain, or painful or difficult urination.
- Check with your doctor immediately if you notice any unusual bleeding or bruising; black, tarry stools; blood in urine or stools; or pinpoint red spots on your skin.
- Be careful when using a regular toothbrush, dental floss, or toothpick. Your medical doctor, dentist, or nurse may recommend other ways to clean your teeth and gums. Check with your medical doctor before having any dental work done.
- Do not touch your eyes or the inside of your nose unless you have just washed your hands and have not touched anything else in the meantime.
- Be careful not to cut yourself when you are using sharp objects such as a safety razor or fingernail or toenail cutters.
- Avoid contact sports or other situations where bruising or injury could occur.

If cisplatin accidentally seeps out of the vein into which it is injected, it may damage some tissues and cause scarring. Tell the doctor or nurse right away if you notice redness, pain, or swelling at the place of injection.

Side Effects of This Medicine

Along with its needed effects, a medicine may cause some unwanted effects. Although not all of these side effects may occur, if they do occur they may need medical attention.

Also, because of the way cancer medicines act on the body, there is a chance that they might cause other unwanted effects that may not occur until months or years after the medicine is used. These delayed effects may include certain types of cancer, such as leukemia. Discuss these possible effects with your doctor.

Check with your doctor immediately if any of the following side effects occur:

Less common
   Black, tarry stools; blood in urine or stools; cough or hoarseness accompanied by fever or chills; dizziness or faintness (during or shortly after a dose); fast heartbeat (during or shortly after a dose); fever or chills; lower back or side pain accompanied by fever or chills; painful or difficult urination accompanied by fever or chills; pain or redness at place of injection; pinpoint red spots on skin; swelling of face (during or shortly after a dose); unusual bleeding or bruising; wheezing (during or shortly after a dose)

Check with your doctor as soon as possible if any of the following side effects occur:

More common
   Joint pain; loss of balance; ringing in ears; swelling of feet or lower legs; trouble in hearing; unusual tiredness or weakness

Less common

Convulsions (seizures); loss of reflexes; loss of taste; numbness or tingling in fingers or toes; trouble in walking

Rare

Agitation or confusion; blurred vision; change in ability to see colors (especially blue or yellow); muscle cramps; sores in mouth and on lips

Some side effects may occur that usually do not need medical attention. These side effects may go away during treatment as your body adjusts to the medicine. Also, your health care professional may be able to tell you about ways to prevent or reduce some of these side effects. Check with your health care professional if any of the following side effects continue or are bothersome or if you have any questions about them:

More common

Nausea and vomiting (severe)

Less common

Loss of appetite

After you stop using this medicine, it may still produce some side effects that need attention. During this period of time, *check with your doctor immediately* if you notice the following side effects:

Black, tarry stools; blood in urine or stools; convulsions (seizures); cough or hoarseness; decrease in urination; fever or chills; loss of balance; loss of reflexes; loss of taste; lower back or side pain; numbness or tingling in fingers or toes; painful or difficult urination; pinpoint red spots on skin; ringing in ears; swelling of feet or lower legs; trouble in hearing; trouble in walking; unusual bleeding or bruising

Other side effects not listed may also occur in some patients. If you notice any other effects, check with your healthcare professional.

CITALOPRAM (Oral route) - sye-TAL-oh-pram

Black Box Warning

Antidepressants increased the risk of suicidal thinking and behavior (suicidality) in short-term studies in children and adolescents with Major Depressive Disorder (MDD) and other psychiatric disorders. Anyone considering the use of citalopram hydrobromide or any other antidepressant in a child or adolescent must balance this risk with the clinical need. Patients who are started on therapy should be observed closely for clinical worsening, suicidality, or unusual changes in behavior. Families and caregivers should be advised of the need for close observation and communication with the prescriber. Citalopram hydrobromide is not approved for use in pediatric patients.

Pooled analysis of short-term (4 to 16 weeks) placebo-controlled trials of 9 antidepressant drugs (SSRIs and others) in children and adolescents with major depressive disorder (MDD), obsessive compulsive disorder (OCD), or other psychiatric disorders (a total of 24 trials involving over 4400 patients) have revealed a greater risk of adverse events representing suicidal thinking or behavior (suicidality) during the first few months of treatment in those receiving antidepressants. The average risk of such events in patients receiving antidepressants was 4%, twice the placebo risk of 2%. No suicides occurred in these trials.

Commonly used brand name(s)

In the U.S.—

Celexa

Available Dosage Forms:

- Tablet
- Solution

Therapeutic Class: Antidepressant
Pharmacologic Class: Serotonin Reuptake Inhibitor

Uses For This Medicine

Citalopram is used to treat mental depression.

Citalopram belongs to a group of medicines known as selective serotonin reuptake inhibitors (SSRIs). These medicines are thought to work by increasing the activity of the chemical serotonin in the brain.

This medicine is available only with your doctor's prescription.

Before Using This Medicine

In deciding to use a medicine, the risks of taking the medicine must be weighed against the good it will do. This is a decision you and your doctor will make. For this medicine, the following should be considered:

Allergies—Tell your doctor if you have ever had any unusual or allergic reaction to this medicine or any other medicines. Also tell your health care professional if you have any other types of allergies, such as to foods, dyes, preservatives, or animals. For non-prescription products, read the label or package ingredients carefully.

Pediatric—Citalopram must be used with caution in children with depression. Studies have shown occurrences of children thinking about suicide or attempting suicide in clinical trials for this medicine. More study is needed to be sure citalopram is safe and effective in children.

Geriatric—This medicine has been tested and has not been shown to cause different side effects or problems in older people than it does in younger adults. However, citalopram is removed from the body more slowly in older people and an older person may need a lower dose than a younger adult.

Pregnancy—

	Pregnancy Category	Explanation
All Trimesters	C	Animal studies have shown an adverse effect and there are no adequate studies in pregnant women OR no animal studies have been conducted and there are no adequate studies in pregnant women.

Breast Feeding—Studies in women breastfeeding have demonstrated harmful infant effects. An alternative to this medication should be prescribed or you should stop breast-feeding while using this medicine.

Other medicines—

Using this medicine with any of the following medicines is not recommended. Your doctor may decide not to treat you with this medication or change some of the other medicines you take.

Clorgyline, Furazolidone, Iproniazid, Isocarboxazid, Levomethadyl, Moclobemide, Nialamide, Pargyline, Phenelzine, Procarbazine, Selegiline, Toloxatone, Tranylcypromine

Interactions with Food/Tobacco/Alcohol—Certain medicines should not be used at or around the time of eating food or eating certain types of food since interactions may occur. Using alcohol or tobacco with certain medicines may also cause interactions to occur. The following interactions have been selected on the basis of their potential significance and are not necessarily all-inclusive.

Using this medicine with any of the following may cause an increased risk of certain side effects but may be unavoidable in some cases. If used together, your doctor may change the dose or how often you use this medicine, or give you special instructions about the use of food, alcohol, or tobacco.

Ethanol

Other medical problems—The presence of other medical problems may affect the use of this medicine. Make sure you tell your doctor if you have any other medical problems, especially:

- Bipolar disorder (history of)—May be activated
- Diabetes mellitus (sugar diabetes)—Hypoglycemia has occurred rarely in diabetic patients receiving citalopram
- Heart attack (recent history of) or
- Heart disease (unstable)—Use in patients with these conditions have not been adequately studied
- Kidney disease, severe—Until enough patients have been evaluated, caution is recommended for patients with severe kidney disease
- Liver disease—Higher blood levels of citalopram may occur, increasing the chance of having unwanted effects. You may need to take a lower dose than a person without kidney or liver disease
- Mania (history of)—May be activated
- Seizure disorders (history of)—The risk of having seizures may be increased

Proper Use of This Medicine

Take this medicine only as directed by your doctor to benefit your condition as much as possible. Do not take more of it, do not take it more often, and do not take it for a longer time than your doctor ordered.

Citalopram may be taken with or without food on a full or empty stomach. If your doctor tells you to take it a certain way, follow your doctor's instructions.

You may have to take citalopram for 4 weeks before you begin to feel better. Your doctor should check your progress at regular visits during this time. Also, you may need to keep taking citalopram for 6 months or longer to help prevent the return of the depression.

Do not stop taking this medication without checking first with your doctor

Dosing—The dose of this medicine will be different for different patients. Follow your doctor's orders or the directions on the label. The following information includes only the average doses of this medicine. If your dose is different, do not change it unless your doctor tells you to do so.

The amount of medicine that you take depends on the strength of the medicine. Also, the number of doses you take each day, the time allowed between doses, and the length of time you take the medicine depend on the medical problem for which you are using the medicine.

- For oral dosage form (solution and tablets):
  - For depression:
    - Adults—To start, usually 20 milligrams (mg) once a day, taken either in the morning or evening. Your doctor may increase your dose gradually if needed. However, the dose usually is not more than 60 mg a day.
    - Children—Use and dose must be determined by the doctor.
    - Older adults—Usually 20 milligrams (mg) once a day, taken either in the morning or evening. Your doctor may increase your dose gradually if needed. However, the dose usually is not more than 40 mg a day.

Missed dose—Call your doctor or pharmacist for instructions.

Storage—Store the medicine in a closed container at room temperature, away from heat, moisture, and direct light. Keep from freezing.

Keep out of the reach of children.

Do not keep outdated medicine or medicine no longer needed.

Precautions While Using This Medicine

It is important that your doctor check your progress at regular visits, to allow for changes in your dose and to help reduce any side effects.

Do not take citalopram with or within 14 days of taking an MAO inhibitor (furazolidone, isocarboxazid, phenelzine, procarbazine, selegiline, tranylcypromine). Do not take an MAO inhibitor within 14 days of taking citalopram. If you do, you may develop extremely high blood pressure or convulsions (seizures).

Citalopram may cause some people to be agitated, irritable or display other abnormal behaviors. It may also cause some people to have suicidal thoughts and tendencies or to become more depressed. If you or your caregiver notice any of these adverse effects, tell your doctor right away.

Avoid drinking alcoholic beverages while you are taking citalopram.

This medicine may cause some people to become drowsy, to have trouble thinking, or to have problems with movement. Make sure you know how you react to citalopram before you drive, use machines, or do anything else that could be dangerous if you are not alert or well-coordinated.

Side Effects of This Medicine

Along with its needed effects, a medicine may cause some unwanted effects. Although not all of these side effects may occur, if they do occur they may need medical attention. One rare, but very serious, effect that may occur is the serotonin syndrome. This syndrome (group of symptoms) is more likely to occur shortly after an increase in citalopram dose.

Check with your doctor as soon as possible if any of the following side effects occur:

More common

Decrease in sexual desire or ability

Less common

Agitation; blurred vision; confusion; fever; increase in frequency of urination or amount of urine produced; lack of emotion; loss of memory; menstrual changes; skin rash or itching; trouble in breathing

Rare

Anxiety; behavior change similar to drunkenness; bleeding gums; breast tenderness or enlargement or unusual secretion of milk (in females); difficulty in concentrating; dizziness or fainting; increased hunger; irregular heartbeat; irritability; lethargy; low blood sodium (confusion, convulsions [seizures], drowsiness, dryness of mouth, increased thirst, lack of energy); mood or mental changes; nervousness; nose bleed; painful urination; purple or red spots on skin; sore throat, fever, and chills; rapid weight gain; red or irritated eyes; redness, tenderness, itching, burning, or peeling of skin; seizures; serotonin syndrome (agitation, confusion, diarrhea, fever, overactive reflexes, poor coordination, restlessness, shivering, sweating, talking or acting with excitement you cannot control, trembling or shaking, twitching); shakiness; slow or irregular heartbeat (less than 50 beats per minute); stupor; swelling of face, ankles, or hands; trouble in holding or releasing urine; unusual or sudden body or facial movements or postures; unusual tiredness or weakness

Incidence not determined (observed during clinical practice)

Abdominal or stomach pain; back, leg, or stomach pains; black, tarry stools; bleeding gums; bloating; bloody stools; chest pain; confusion as to time, place, or person; constipation; cough; darkened urine; difficult or fast breathing; difficulty swallowing; drooling; fast, slow or irregular heartbeat; fatigue; general body swelling; hallucinations; hive-like swelling on the face, eyelids, lips, tongue, throat; hives; holding false beliefs that cannot be changed by fact; impaired consciousness, ranging from confusion to coma; indigestion; itching, puffiness or swelling of the eyelids or around the eyes, face, lips or tongue; loss of appetite; loss of bladder control; loss of consciousness; muscle cramps or spasms; muscle tightness; muscle twitching or jerking; nervousness; nosebleeds; pale skin; penile erections, frequent or continuing; restlessness or agitation; redness, tenderness, itching, burning or peeling of skin; recurrent fainting; restlessness; rhythmic movement of muscles; shortness of breath; skin rash; swelling of breasts or unusual milk production; tenderness, pain, swelling, warmth, skin discoloration, and prominent superficial veins over affected area; tightness in chest; total body jerking; twitching, twisting, uncontrolled repetitive movements of tongue, lips, face, arms, or legs; uncontrolled jerking or twisting movements; unusual excitement; vomiting of blood or material that looks like coffee grounds; wheezing; yellowing of the eyes or skin

Symptoms of overdose—more common

Dizziness; drowsiness; fast heartbeat; nausea; sleepiness; sweating; trembling or shaking; vomiting

Symptoms of overdose—rare

Bluish colored skin or lips; confusion; convulsions (seizures); coma; deep or fast breathing with dizziness; fainting; general feeling of discomfort or illness; loss of memory; muscle pain; slow or irregular heartbeat; weakness

Some side effects may occur that usually do not need medical attention. These side effects may go away during treatment as your body adjusts to the medicine. Also, your health care professional may be able to tell you about ways to prevent or reduce some of these side effects. Check with your health care professional if any of the following side effects continue or are bothersome or if you have any questions about them:

More common

Drowsiness; dryness of mouth; nausea; sleepiness or unusual drowsiness; trouble in sleeping

Less common

Abdominal pain; anxiety; body aches or pain; change in sense of taste; chills; diarrhea; difficulty in breathing; gas; headache; headache (severe and throbbing); heartburn; increased sweating; increased yawning; loss of appetite; loss of voice; nasal congestion; pain in muscles or joints; sneezing; sore throat; stuffy or runny nose; tingling, burning, or prickly feelings on skin; tooth grinding; trembling or shaking; unusual increase or decrease in weight; unusual tiredness or weakness; vomiting; watering of mouth

Incidence not determined (observed during clinical practice)

Bruising; inability to sit still; large, flat, blue or purplish patches in the skin; need to keep moving; restlessness; uncontrolled eye movements

After you stop using this medicine, it may still produce some side effects that need attention. During this period of time, *check with your doctor immediately* if you notice the following side effects:

Anxiety; dizziness; nervousness; trembling or shaking

Other side effects not listed may also occur in some patients. If you notice any other effects, check with your healthcare professional.

CITRATES (Systemic)

Some commonly used brand names are:

In the U.S.—

Bicitra (4)	Polycitra-K Crystals (2)
Citrolith (3)	Polycitra-LC (5)
Oracit (4)	Polycitra Syrup (5)
Polycitra-K (2)	Urocit-K (1)

In Canada—

Oracit (4)

This information applies to the following medicines:

1. Potassium Citrate (poe-TASS-ee-um SIH-trayt)
2. Potassium Citrate and Citric Acid (poe-TASS-ee-um SIH-trayt and SIH-trik A-sid)
3. Potassium Citrate and Sodium Citrate (poe-TASS-ee-um SIH-trayt and SOE-dee-um SIH-trayt)
4. Sodium Citrate and Citric Acid (SOE-dee-um SIH-trayt and SIH-trik A-sid)
5. Tricitrates (Try-SIH-trayts)

Category

- **Alkalizer, systemic**—Potassium Citrate and Citric Acid; Sodium Citrate and Citric Acid; Tricitrates

- **Alkalizer, urinary**—Potassium Citrate; Potassium Citrate and Citric Acid; Potassium Citrate and Sodium Citrate; Sodium Citrate and Citric Acid; Tricitrates
- **Antiurolithic, calcium oxalate calculi**—Potassium Citrate; Potassium Citrate and Citric Acid
- **Antiurolithic, calcium phosphate calculi**—Potassium Citrate; Potassium Citrate and Citric Acid
- **Antiurolithic, cystine calculi**—Potassium Citrate; Potassium Citrate and Citric Acid; Potassium Citrate and Sodium Citrate; Sodium Citrate and Citric Acid; Tricitrates
- **Antiurolithic, uric acid calculi**—Potassium Citrate; Potassium Citrate and Citric Acid; Potassium Citrate and Sodium Citrate; Sodium Citrate and Citric Acid; Tricitrates
- **Buffer, neutralizing**—Sodium Citrate and Citric Acid; Tricitrates

Description

Citrates SIH-trayts are used to make the urine more alkaline (less acid). This helps prevent certain kinds of kidney stones. Citrates are sometimes used with other medicines to help treat kidney stones that may occur with gout. They are also used to make the blood more alkaline in certain conditions.

Citrates are available only with your doctor's prescription, in the following dosage forms:

Oral
- Potassium Citrate
  - Tablets
- Potassium Citrate and Citric Acid
  - Oral solution
  - Crystals for oral solution
- Potassium Citrate and Sodium Citrate
  - Tablets
- Sodium Citrate and Citric Acid
  - Oral solution
- Tricitrates
  - Oral solution

Before Using This Medicine

In deciding to use a medicine, the risks of taking the medicine must be weighed against the good it will do. This is a decision you and your doctor will make. For citrates, the following should be considered:

Allergies—Tell your doctor if you have ever had any unusual or allergic reaction to potassium citrate or potassium. Also tell your health care professional if you are allergic to any other substances, such as foods, preservatives, or dyes.

Pregnancy—Studies on effects in pregnancy have not been done in either humans or animals.

Breast-feeding—Although it is not known whether citrates pass into the breast milk, this medicine has not been reported to cause problems in nursing babies.

Children—Although there is no specific information comparing use of citrates in children with use in other age groups, these medicines are not expected to cause different side effects or problems in children than they do in adults.

Older adults—Many medicines have not been studied specifically in older people. Therefore, it may not be known whether they work exactly the same way they do in younger adults or if they cause different side effects or problems in older people. There is no specific information comparing use of citrates in the elderly with use in other age groups.

Other medicines—Although certain medicines should not be used together at all, in other cases two different medicines may be used together even if an interaction might occur. In these cases, your doctor may want to change the dose, or other precautions may be necessary. When you are taking citrates, it is especially important that your health care professional know if you are taking any of the following:

- Amiloride (e.g., Midamor) or
- Benazepril (e.g., Lotensin) or
- Captopril (e.g., Capoten) or
- Digitalis glycosides (heart medicine) or
- Enalapril (e.g., Vasotec) or
- Fosinopril (e.g., Monotril) or
- Heparin (e.g., Panheprin) or
- Lisinopril (e.g., Prinivil; Zestril) or
- Medicines for inflammation or pain (except narcotics) or
- Potassium-containing medicines (other) or
- Quinapril (e.g., Accuprol) or
- Ramipril (e.g., Altase) or
- Salt substitutes, low-salt foods or milk or
- Spironolactone (e.g., Aldactone) or
- Triamterene (e.g., Dyrenium)—Use with potassium-containing citrates may further increase potassium blood levels, possibly leading to serious side effects
- Antacids, especially those containing aluminum or sodium bicarbonate—Use with citrates may increase the risk of kidney stones; also, citrates may increase the amount of aluminum in the blood and cause serious side effects, especially in patients with kidney problems
- Methenamine (e.g., Mandelamine)—Use with citrates may make the methenamine less effective
- Quinidine (e.g., Quinidex)—Use with citrates may cause quinidine to build up in the bloodstream, possibly leading to serious side effects

Other medical problems—The presence of other medical problems may affect the use of citrates. Make sure you tell your doctor if you have any other medical problems, especially:

- Addison's disease (underactive adrenal glands) or
- Diabetes mellitus (sugar diabetes) or
- Kidney disease—The potassium in potassium-containing citrates may worsen or cause heart problems in patients with these conditions
- Diarrhea (chronic)—Treatment with citrates may not be effective; a change in dose of citrate may be needed
- Edema (swelling of the feet or lower legs) or
- High blood pressure or
- Toxemia of pregnancy—The sodium in sodium-containing citrates may cause the body to retain (keep) water
- Heart disease—The sodium in sodium-containing citrates may cause the body to retain (keep) water; the potassium in potassium-containing citrates may make heart disease worse

- Intestinal or esophageal blockage—Potassium citrate tablets may cause irritation of the stomach or intestines

- Stomach ulcer or other stomach problems—Potassium citrate-containing products may make these conditions worse

- Urinary tract infection—Citrates may make conditions worse

Proper Use of This Medicine

For patients taking the *tablet form of this medicine:*

- Swallow the tablets whole. Do not crush, chew, or suck the tablet.

- Take with a full glass (8 ounces) of water.

- *If you have trouble swallowing the tablets or they seem to stick in your throat, check with your doctor at once.* If this medicine is not completely swallowed and not properly dissolved, it can cause severe irritation.

For patients taking the *liquid form of this medicine:*

- Dilute with a full glass (6 ounces) of water or juice and drink; follow with additional water, if desired.

- Chill, but do *not* freeze, this medicine before taking it, for a better taste.

For patients taking the *crystals form of this medicine:*

- Add the contents of one packet to at least 6 ounces of cool water or juice.

- Stir well to make sure the crystals are completely dissolved.

- Drink all the mixture to be sure you are taking the correct dose. Follow with additional water or juice, if desired.

Take each dose immediately after a meal or within 30 minutes after a meal or bedtime snack. This helps prevent the medicine from causing stomach pain or a laxative effect.

Drink at least a full glass (8 ounces) of water or other liquid (except milk) every hour during the day (about 3 quarts a day), unless otherwise directed by your doctor. This will increase the flow of urine and help prevent kidney stones.

Take this medicine only as directed by your doctor. Do not take more of it, do not take it more often, and do not take it for a longer time than your doctor ordered. *This is especially important if you are also taking a diuretic (water pill) or digitalis medicine for your heart.*

Dosing—The dose of these single or combination medicines will be different for different patients. *Follow your doctor's orders or the directions on the label.* The following information includes only the average doses of these medicines. *If your dose is different, do not change it* unless your doctor tells you to do so.

The number of tablets that you take or teaspoonfuls or ounces of solution that you drink depends on the strength of the single or combination medicine. *Also, the number of doses you take each day, the time allowed between doses, and the length of time you take the medicine depend on*

the medical problem for which you are taking this single or combination medicine.

For potassium citrate

- For *oral* dosage form (tablets):
  - To make the urine more alkaline (less acidic) and to prevent kidney stones:
    - Adults—At first, 1.08 to 2.16 grams three times a day with meals. Some people may take 1.62 grams four times a day with meals or within thirty minutes after a meal or bedtime snack. Your doctor may change your dose if needed. However, most people usually will not take more than 10.8 grams a day.
    - Children—Dose must be determined by your doctor.

For potassium citrate and citric acid

- For *oral* dosage form (solution):
  - To make the urine or blood more alkaline (less acidic) and to prevent kidney stones:
    - Adults—At first, 2 to 3 teaspoonfuls of solution, mixed with water or juice, four times a day, after meals and at bedtime. Your doctor may change the dose if needed.
  - To make the urine more alkaline (less acidic):
    - Children—At first, 1 to 3 teaspoonfuls of solution, mixed with water or juice, four times a day after meals and at bedtime. Your doctor may change the dose if needed.

- For *oral* dosage form (crystals for solution):
  - To make the urine or blood more alkaline (less acidic) and to prevent kidney stones:
    - Adults—At first, 3.3 grams of potassium citrate, mixed with water or juice, four times a day, after meals and at bedtime. Your doctor may change the dose if needed.
    - Children—Use is not recommended.

For potassium citrate and sodium citrate

- For *oral* dosage form (tablets):
  - To make the urine more alkaline (less acidic) and to prevent kidney stones:
    - Adults—At first, 1 to 4 tablets after meals and at bedtime.
    - Children—Dose must be determined by your doctor.

For sodium citrate and citric acid

- For *oral* dosage form (solution):
  - To make the urine and blood more alkaline (less acidic) and to prevent kidney stones:
    - Adults—At first, 2 to 6 teaspoonfuls of solution four times a day, after meals and at bedtime. The solution should be mixed in one to three ounces of water. Your doctor may change the dose if needed. However, most people will usually not take more than five ounces a day.
  - To make the contents of the stomach less acidic before surgery:
    - Adults—1 to 2 tablespoonfuls as a single dose. You may mix it in one to two tablespoonfuls of water.
  - To make the blood more alkaline (less acidic):
    - Children—At first, 1 to 3 teaspoonfuls of solution four times a day, after meals and at bedtime. The solution should be mixed in one to three ounces

of water. Your doctor may change the dose if needed.

For tricitrates
- For *oral* dosage form (solution):
  - To make the urine and blood more alkaline (less acidic) and to prevent kidney stones:
    - Adults—At first, 1 to 2 tablespoonfuls of solution four times a day, after meals and at bedtime. Your doctor may change the dose if needed.
  - To make the contents of the stomach less acidic before surgery:
    - Adults—1 tablespoonful as a single dose. You should mix the solution in one tablespoonful of water.
  - To make the urine or blood more alkaline (less acidic):
    - Children—At first, 5 to 10 mL four times a day after meals and at bedtime. Your doctor may change the dose if needed.

Missed dose—If you miss a dose of this medicine, take it as soon as possible if remembered within 2 hours. However, if it is almost time for your next dose, skip the missed dose and go back to your regular dosing schedule. Do not double doses.

Storage—To store this medicine:
- Keep out of the reach of children.
- Store away from heat and direct light.
- Do not store in the bathroom, near the kitchen sink, or in other damp places. Heat or moisture may cause the medicine to break down.
- Keep the liquid form of this medicine from freezing.
- Do not keep outdated medicine or medicine no longer needed. Be sure that any discarded medicine is out of the reach of children.

Precautions While Using This Medicine

It is important that your doctor check your progress at regular visits. This is to make sure the medicine is working properly and to check for unwanted effects.

Do not eat salty foods or use extra table salt on your food while you are taking citrates. This will help prevent kidney stones and unwanted effects.

Check with your doctor before starting any strenuous physical exercise, especially if you are out of condition and are taking any other medication. Exercise and certain medications may increase the amount of potassium in the blood.

For patients taking *potassium citrate-containing medicines:*
- Do not use salt substitutes and low-salt milk unless told to do so by your doctor. They may contain potassium.
- *Check with your doctor at once if you are taking the tablet form and notice black, tarry stools or other signs of stomach or intestinal bleeding.*
- Do not be alarmed if you notice what appears to be a whole tablet in the stool after taking potassium citrate tablets. Your body has received the proper amount of medicine from the tablet and has expelled the tablet shell. However, it is a good idea to check with your doctor also.

- If you are on a potassium-rich or potassium-restricted diet, check with your health care professional. Potassium citrate-containing medicines contain a large amount of potassium.

For patients taking *sodium citrate-containing medicines:*
- If you are on a sodium-restricted diet, check with your health care professional. Sodium citrate-containing medicines contain a large amount of sodium.

Side Effects

Along with its needed effects, a medicine may cause some unwanted effects. Although not all of these side effects may occur, if they do occur they may need medical attention.

Stop taking this medicine and check with your doctor immediately if any of the following side effects occur:
  Rare
    Abdominal or stomach pain or cramping (severe); black, tarry stools; vomiting (severe), sometimes with blood

Also, check with your doctor as soon as possible if any of the following side effects occur:
    Confusion; convulsions (seizures); dizziness; high blood pressure; irregular or fast heartbeat; irritability; mood or mental changes; muscle pain or twitching; nervousness or restlessness; numbness or tingling in hands, feet, or lips; shortness of breath, difficult breathing, or slow breathing; swelling of feet or lower legs; unexplained anxiety; unpleasant taste; unusual tiredness or weakness; weakness or heaviness of legs

Other side effects may occur that usually do not need medical attention. These side effects may go away during treatment as your body adjusts to the medicine. However, check with your doctor if any of the following side effects continue or are bothersome:
  Less common
    Abdominal or stomach soreness or pain (mild); diarrhea or loose bowel movements; nausea or vomiting

Other side effects not listed above may also occur in some patients. If you notice any other effects, check with your doctor.

CLADRIBINE   (Intravenous route) -
KLA-dri-been

Black Box Warning

Cladribine injection should be administered under the supervision of a qualified physician experienced in the use of antineoplastic therapy. Suppression of bone marrow function should be anticipated. This is usually reversible and appears to be dose dependent. Serious neurological toxicity (including irreversible paraparesis and quadraparesis) has been reported in patients who received cladribine injection by continuous infusion at high doses (4 to 9 times the recommended dose for Hairy Cell Leukemia). Neurologic toxicity appears to demonstrate a dose relationship; however, severe neurological toxicity has been reported rarely following treatment with standard cladribine dosing regimen.

Acute nephrotoxicity has been observed with high doses of cladribine (4 to 9 times the recommended dose for Hairy Cell Leukemia), especially when given concomitantly with other nephrotoxic agents/therapies.

Commonly used brand name(s)

In the U.S.—
    Leustatin

Available Dosage Forms:
  • Solution

Therapeutic Class: Antineoplastic Agent
Pharmacologic Class: Antimetabolite

Uses For This Medicine

Cladribine belongs to the group of medicines called antimetabolites. It is used to treat hairy cell leukemia, a cancer of the blood and bone marrow. It is also sometimes used to treat other kinds of cancer, as determined by your doctor.

Cladribine interferes with the growth of cancer cells, which are eventually destroyed. Since the growth of normal body cells may also be affected by cladribine, other effects will also occur. Some of these may be serious and must be reported to your doctor. Other effects may not be serious but may cause concern. Some effects may not occur for months or years after the medicine is used.

Before you begin treatment with cladribine, you and your doctor should talk about the good this medicine will do as well as the risks of using it.

Cladribine is to be administered only by or under the immediate supervision of your doctor.

Once a medicine has been approved for marketing for a certain use, experience may show that it is also useful for other medical problems. Although these uses are not included in product labeling, cladribine is used in certain patients with the following conditions:
  • Cancer of the blood and lymph system
  • Waldenström's macroglobulinemia (a certain type of cancer of the blood)

Before Using This Medicine

In deciding to use a medicine, the risks of taking the medicine must be weighed against the good it will do. This is a decision you and your doctor will make. For this medicine, the following should be considered:

Allergies—Tell your doctor if you have ever had any unusual or allergic reaction to this medicine or any other medicines. Also tell your health care professional if you have any other types of allergies, such as to foods, dyes, preservatives, or animals. For non-prescription products, read the label or package ingredients carefully.

Pediatric—There is no specific information comparing use of cladribine in children with use in other age groups. However, cladribine has been reported to be tested in children with certain types of cancers of the blood.

Geriatric—Many medicines have not been studied specifically in older people. Therefore, it may not be known whether they work exactly the same way they do in younger adults. Although there is no specific information comparing use of cladribine in the elderly with use in other age groups, it is not

expected to cause different side effects or problems in older people than it does in younger adults.

Pregnancy—

	Pregnancy Category	Explanation
All Trimesters	D	Studies in pregnant women have demonstrated a risk to the fetus. However, the benefits of therapy in a life threatening situation or a serious disease, may outweigh the potential risk.

Breast Feeding—There are no adequate studies in women for determining infant risk when using this medication during breastfeeding. Weigh the potential benefits against the potential risks before taking this medication while breastfeeding.

Other medicines—

Using this medicine with any of the following medicines is not recommended. Your doctor may decide not to treat you with this medication or change some of the other medicines you take.

Rotavirus Vaccine, Live

Interactions with Food/Tobacco/Alcohol—Certain medicines should not be used at or around the time of eating food or eating certain types of food since interactions may occur. Using alcohol or tobacco with certain medicines may also cause interactions to occur. Discuss with your healthcare professional the use of your medicine with food, alcohol, or tobacco.

Other medical problems—The presence of other medical problems may affect the use of this medicine. Make sure you tell your doctor if you have any other medical problems, especially:
  • Chickenpox (including recent exposure) or
  • Herpes zoster (shingles)—Risk of severe disease affecting other parts of the body
  • Gout (history of) or
  • Kidney stones (history of)—Cladribine may increase levels of uric acid in the body, which can cause gout or kidney stones
  • Infection—Cladribine may decrease your body's ability to fight infection

Proper Use of This Medicine

This medicine may cause mild nausea and may also cause vomiting. However, it is very important that you continue to receive the medicine even if you begin to feel ill. Ask your health care professional for ways to lessen these effects.

Dosing—The dose of this medicine will be different for different patients. Follow your doctor's orders or the directions on the label. The following information includes only the average doses of this medicine. If your dose is different, do not change it unless your doctor tells you to do so.

The amount of medicine that you take depends on the strength of the medicine. Also, the number of doses you take each day, the time allowed between doses, and the length of time you take the medicine depend on the medical problem for which you are using the medicine.

Precautions While Using This Medicine

It is very important that your doctor check your progress at regular visits to make sure that this medicine is working properly and to check for unwanted effects.

While you are being treated with cladribine, and after you stop treatment with it, do not have any immunizations (vaccinations) without your doctor's approval. Cladribine may lower your body's resistance and there is a chance you might get the infection the immunization is meant to prevent. In addition, other persons living in your household should not take oral polio vaccine since there is a chance they could pass the polio virus on to you. Also, avoid persons who have taken oral polio vaccine within the last several months. Do not get close to them and do not stay in the same room with them for very long. If you cannot take these precautions, you should consider wearing a protective face mask that covers the nose and mouth.

Cladribine can temporarily lower the number of white blood cells in your blood, increasing the chance of getting an infection. It can also lower the number of platelets, which are necessary for proper blood clotting. If this occurs, there are certain precautions you can take, especially when your blood count is low, to reduce the risk of infection or bleeding:

- If you can, avoid people with infections, colds, or flu. Check with your doctor immediately if you think you are getting an infection or if you get a fever or chills, cough or hoarseness, lower back or side pain, or painful or difficult urination.
- Check with your doctor immediately if you notice any unusual bleeding or bruising; black, tarry stools; blood in urine or stools; or pinpoint red spots on your skin.
- Be careful when using a regular toothbrush, dental floss, or toothpick. Your medical doctor, dentist, or nurse may recommend other ways to clean your teeth and gums. Check with your medical doctor before having any dental work done.
- Do not touch your eyes or the inside of your nose unless you have just washed your hands and have not touched anything else in the meantime.
- Be careful not to cut yourself when you are using sharp objects such as a safety razor or fingernail or toenail cutters.
- Avoid contact sports or other situations where bruising or injury could occur.

Side Effects of This Medicine

Along with its needed effects, a medicine may cause some unwanted effects. Some side effects will have signs or symptoms that you can see or feel. Your doctor may watch for others by doing certain tests.

Also, because of the way cancer medicines act on the body, there is a chance that they might cause other unwanted effects that may not occur until months or years after the medicine is used. These delayed effects may include certain types of cancer. Discuss these possible effects with your doctor.

Check with your doctor immediately if any of the following side effects occur:
  More common
    Black, tarry stools; blood in urine; cough or hoarseness, accompanied by fever or chills; fever; lower back or

side pain, accompanied by fever or chills; painful or difficult urination, accompanied by fever or chills; pinpoint red spots on skin; unusual bleeding or bruising

Check with your doctor as soon as possible if any of the following side effects occur:
  More common
    Skin rash
  Less common
    Pain or redness at place of injection; shortness of breath; stomach pain; swelling of feet or lower legs; unusually fast heartbeat

This medicine may also cause the following side effects that your doctor will watch out for:
  More common
    Anemia; low white cell counts in blood

Some side effects may occur that usually do not need medical attention. These side effects may go away during treatment as your body adjusts to the medicine. Also, your health care professional may be able to tell you about ways to prevent or reduce some of these side effects. Check with your health care professional if any of the following side effects continue or are bothersome or if you have any questions about them:
  More common
    Headache; loss of appetite; nausea; unusual tiredness; vomiting
  Less common
    Constipation; diarrhea; dizziness; general feeling of discomfort or illness; itching; muscle or joint pain; sweating; trouble in sleeping; weakness

Other side effects not listed may also occur in some patients. If you notice any other effects, check with your healthcare professional.

CLARITHROMYCIN (Oral route) - kla-RITH-roe-mye-sin

Commonly used brand name(s)

In the U.S.—
  Biaxin
  Biaxin Filmtab
  Biaxin XL

Available Dosage Forms:
- Powder for Suspension
- Tablet
- Tablet, Extended Release

Therapeutic Class: Antibiotic

Uses For This Medicine

Clarithromycin is used to treat bacterial infections in many different parts of the body. It works by killing bacteria or preventing their growth. It is also used to treat and prevent Mycobacterium avium complex (MAC) infection, and to treat duodenal ulcers caused by Helicobacter pylori. However, this medicine will not work for colds, flu, or other virus infections. Clarithromycin also may be used for other problems as determined by your doctor.

Clarithromycin is available only with your doctor's prescription.

Once a medicine has been approved for marketing for a certain use, experience may show that it is also useful for other medical problems. Although this use is not included in product labeling, clarithromycin is used in certain patients with the following medical condition:

• Legionnaires' disease

Before Using This Medicine

In deciding to use a medicine, the risks of taking the medicine must be weighed against the good it will do. This is a decision you and your doctor will make. For this medicine, the following should be considered:

Allergies—Tell your doctor if you have ever had any unusual or allergic reaction to this medicine or any other medicines. Also tell your health care professional if you have any other types of allergies, such as to foods, dyes, preservatives, or animals. For non-prescription products, read the label or package ingredients carefully.

Pediatric—Studies on this medicine have not been done in children up to 6 months of age. In effective doses, the medicine has not been shown to cause different side effects or problems in children over the age of 6 months than it does in adults.

Geriatric—This medicine has been tested in a limited number of elderly patients and has not been shown to cause different side effects or problems in older people than it does in younger adults.

Pregnancy—

	Pregnancy Category	Explanation
All Trimesters	C	Animal studies have shown an adverse effect and there are no adequate studies in pregnant women OR no animal studies have been conducted and there are no adequate studies in pregnant women.

Breast Feeding—There are no adequate studies in women for determining infant risk when using this medication during breastfeeding. Weigh the potential benefits against the potential risks before taking this medication while breastfeeding.

Other medicines—

Using this medicine with any of the following medicines is not recommended. Your doctor may decide not to treat you with this medication or change some of the other medicines you take.

Astemizole, Bepridil, Cisapride, Conivaptan, Dihydroergotamine, Eplerenone, Ergoloid Mesylates, Ergonovine, Ergotamine, Levomethadyl, Mesoridazine, Methylergonovine, Methysergide, Pimozide, Ranolazine, Terfenadine, Thioridazine, Ziprasidone

Interactions with Food/Tobacco/Alcohol—Certain medicines should not be used at or around the time of eating food or eating certain types of food since interactions may occur. Using alcohol or tobacco with certain medicines may also cause interactions to occur. Discuss with your healthcare professional the use of your medicine with food, alcohol, or tobacco.

Other medical problems—The presence of other medical problems may affect the use of this medicine. Make sure you tell your doctor if you have any other medical problems, especially:

• Kidney disease—Patients with severe kidney disease may have an increased chance of side effects.

Proper Use of This Medicine

Clarithromycin may be taken with meals or milk or on an empty stomach, extended release tablets should be taken with food.

If you are taking clarithromycin and zidovudine, these medicines should be taken at least 4 hours apart.

To help clear up your infection completely, keep taking clarithromycin for the full time of treatment, even if you begin to feel better after a few days. If you stop taking this medicine too soon, your symptoms may return.

If you are using clarithromycin oral suspension, use a specially marked measuring spoon or other device to measure each dose accurately. The average household teaspoon may not hold the right amount of liquid.

Dosing—The dose of this medicine will be different for different patients. Follow your doctor's orders or the directions on the label. The following information includes only the average doses of this medicine. If your dose is different, do not change it unless your doctor tells you to do so.

The amount of medicine that you take depends on the strength of the medicine. Also, the number of doses you take each day, the time allowed between doses, and the length of time you take the medicine depend on the medical problem for which you are using the medicine.

• For oral dosage forms (suspension and tablets):
  ○ For bacterial infections:
    ▪ Adults and teenagers—250 to 500 milligrams (mg) every twelve hours for seven to fourteen days.
    ▪ Children 6 months of age and older—7.5 mg per kilogram (kg) (3.4 mg per pound) of body weight every twelve hours for ten days.
    ▪ Infants up to 6 months of age—Use and dose must be determined by your doctor.

    ▪ For community-acquired pneumonia:
      — Adults and teenagers—250 to 500 milligrams (mg) every twelve hours for seven to fourteen days.
      — Children 6 months of age and older—7.5 mg per kilogram (kg) (3.4 mg per pound) of body weight every twelve hours for ten days.
    ▪ For prevention or treatment of Mycobacterium avium complex (MAC) infection:
      — Adults and teenagers—500 mg two times a day.
      — Children 6 months of age and older—7.5 mg per kg (3.4 mg per pound) of body weight, up to 500 mg, two times a day.
      — Infants up to 6 months of age—Use and dose must be determined by your doctor.
    ▪ For treatment of ulcers associated with Helicobacter pylori:
      — Adults and teenagers—500 mg three times a day for fourteen days, in combination with omeprazole or ranitidine bismuth sulfate; or 500 mg every twelve hours in combination

with amoxicillin and lansoprazole for fourteen days.
— Infants and children—Use and dose must be determined by your doctor.
  ○ For long-acting oral dosage form (extended release tablets)
    ▪ For bacterial infections:
      — Adults and teenagers—1000 milligrams (mg) once a day for seven to fourteen days.
    ▪ For community-acquired pneumonia:
      — Adults and teenagers—1000 milligrams (mg) once a day for seven days

Missed dose—If you miss a dose of this medicine, take it as soon as possible. However, if it is almost time for your next dose, skip the missed dose and go back to your regular dosing schedule. Do not double doses.

Storage—Store the medicine in a closed container at room temperature, away from heat, moisture, and direct light. Keep from freezing.

Keep out of the reach of children.

Do not keep outdated medicine or medicine no longer needed.

Do not store suspension in the refrigerator.

Precautions While Using This Medicine

Clarithromycin should not be taken with astemizole, cisapride, dihydroergotamine, ergotamine, pimozide, or terfenadine. Doing so may increase the risk of serious side effects affecting the heart.

If your symptoms do not improve within a few days, or if they become worse, check with your doctor.

Side Effects of This Medicine

Along with its needed effects, a medicine may cause some unwanted effects. Although not all of these side effects may occur, if they do occur they may need medical attention.

Check with your doctor as soon as possible if any of the following side effects occur:
Incidence less frequent
  Cough; fever or chills; hoarseness; lower back or side pain; painful or difficult urination
Rare
  Abdominal tenderness; fever with or without chills; nausea and vomiting; severe abdominal or stomach cramps and pain; shortness of breath; skin rash and itching; unusual bleeding or bruising; watery and severe diarrhea, which may also be bloody; yellow eyes or skin
Incidence not known
  Abdominal pain; anxiety; black, tarry stools; blistering, peeling, loosening of skin; blurred vision; chest pain or discomfort; chills; clay-colored stools; confusion about identity, place, and time; cool pale skin; dark urine; depression; difficulty swallowing; dizziness; fainting; fast, pounding, or irregular heartbeat or pulse; feeling of unreality; feeling that others are watching you or controlling your behavior; feeling that others can hear your thoughts; feeling, seeing, or hearing things that are not there; hives; increased hunger; irregular heartbeat; joint or muscle pain; light-colored stools; loss of appetite; nervousness; nightmares; palpitations; puffiness or

swelling of the eyelids or around the eyes, face, lips or tongue; recurrent fainting; red irritated eyes; red skin lesions, often with a purple center; redness, swelling, or soreness of tongue; seeing, hearing, or feeling things that are not there; seizures; sense of detachment from self or body; severe mood or mental changes; shakiness; slow heartbeat; slurred speech; sore throat; sores, ulcers, or white spots in mouth or on lips; sudden death; swollen glands; tightness in chest; unpleasant breath odor; unusual behavior; unusual tiredness or weakness; vomiting of blood; wheezing

Some side effects may occur that usually do not need medical attention. These side effects may go away during treatment as your body adjusts to the medicine. Also, your health care professional may be able to tell you about ways to prevent or reduce some of these side effects. Check with your health care professional if any of the following side effects continue or are bothersome or if you have any questions about them:
Less common
  Acid or sour stomach; belching; bloated, full feeling; change in sensation of taste; diarrhea (mild); excess air or gas in stomach or intestines; headache; heartburn; indigestion; passing gas; stomach discomfort, upset, or pain
Incidence not known
  Alterations of sense of smell; continuing ringing or buzzing or other unexplained noise in the ears; fear; feeling of constant movement of self or surroundings; hearing loss; lightheadedness; mental depression; mood or mental changes; sensation of spinning; shakiness in legs, arms, hands, feet; skin eruptions; sleeplessness; sore mouth or tongue; swelling or inflammation of the mouth; taste loss; tongue discoloration; tooth discoloration; trembling or shaking of hands or feet; trouble sleeping; unable to sleep; weight loss; white patches in mouth and/or on tongue

Other side effects not listed may also occur in some patients. If you notice any other effects, check with your healthcare professional.

CLINDAMYCIN (Oral route, Injection route, Intravenous route) - klin-da-MYE-sin

Black Box Warning

Pseudomembranous colitis has been reported with nearly all antibacterial agents, including clindamycin, and may range in severity from mild to life-threatening. Therefore, it is important to consider this diagnosis in patients who present with diarrhea subsequent to the administration of antibacterial agents.

Because clindamycin therapy has been associated with severe colitis which may end fatally, it should be reserved for serious infections where less toxic antimicrobial agents are inappropriate. It should not be used in patients with nonbacterial infections such as most upper respiratory tract infections. Treatment with antibacterial agents alters the normal flora of the colon and may permit overgrowth of clostridia. Studies indicate that a toxin produced by *Clostridium difficile* is one primary cause of "antibiotic-associated colitis".

After the diagnosis of pseudomembranous colitis has been established, therapeutic measures should be initiated. Mild cases of pseudomembranous colitis usually respond to drug discontinuation alone. In moderate to severe cases, consideration should be given to management with fluids and electrolytes, protein supplementation and treatment with an antibacterial drug effective against *C. difficile* colitis.

Diarrhea, colitis, and pseudomembranous colitis have been observed to begin up to several weeks following cessation of therapy with clindamycin.

Commonly used brand name(s)

In the U.S.—
Cleocin HCl
Cleocin Pediatric
Cleocin Phosphate

In Canada—
Dalacin C Palmitate

Available Dosage Forms:
- Capsule
- Powder for Solution
- Solution

Therapeutic Class: Antibiotic

Uses For This Medicine

Clindamycin is used to treat bacterial infections. It will not work for colds, flu, or other virus infections.

Clindamycin is available only with your doctor's prescription.

Before Using This Medicine

In deciding to use a medicine, the risks of taking the medicine must be weighed against the good it will do. This is a decision you and your doctor will make. For this medicine, the following should be considered:

Allergies—Tell your doctor if you have ever had any unusual or allergic reaction to this medicine or any other medicines. Also tell your health care professional if you have any other types of allergies, such as to foods, dyes, preservatives, or animals. For non-prescription products, read the label or package ingredients carefully.

Pediatric—This medicine has been tested in children and, in effective doses, has not been reported to cause different side effects or problems than it does in adults.

Geriatric—Many medicines have not been studied specifically in older people. Therefore, it may not be known whether they work exactly the same way they do in younger adults or if they cause different side effects or problems in older people. There is no specific information comparing use of clindamycin in the elderly with use in other age groups.

Pregnancy—

	Pregnancy Category	Explanation
All Trimesters	B	Animal studies have revealed no evidence of harm to the fetus, however, there are no adequate studies in pregnant women OR animal studies have shown an adverse effect, but adequate studies in pregnant women have failed to demonstrate a risk to the fetus.

Breast Feeding—There are no adequate studies in women for determining infant risk when using this medication during breastfeeding. Weigh the potential benefits against the potential risks before taking this medication while breastfeeding.

Other medicines—

Using this medicine with any of the following medicines is usually not recommended, but may be required in some cases. If both medicines are prescribed together, your doctor may change the dose or how often you use one or both of the medicines.

Erythromycin

Interactions with Food/Tobacco/Alcohol—Certain medicines should not be used at or around the time of eating food or eating certain types of food since interactions may occur. Using alcohol or tobacco with certain medicines may also cause interactions to occur. Discuss with your healthcare professional the use of your medicine with food, alcohol, or tobacco.

Other medical problems—The presence of other medical problems may affect the use of this medicine. Make sure you tell your doctor if you have any other medical problems, especially:
- Kidney disease (severe) or
- Liver disease (severe)—Severe kidney or liver disease may increase blood levels of this medicine, increasing the chance of side effects
- Stomach or intestinal disease, history of (especially colitis, including colitis caused by antibiotics, or enteritis)—Patients with a history of stomach or intestinal disease may have an increased chance of side effects

---

Proper Use of This Medicine

For patients taking the capsule form of clindamycin:
- The capsule form of clindamycin should be taken with a full glass (8 ounces) of water or with meals to prevent irritation of the esophagus (tube between the throat and stomach).

For patients taking the oral liquid form of clindamycin:
- Use a specially marked measuring spoon or other device to measure each dose accurately. The average household teaspoon may not hold the right amount of liquid.
- Do not use after the expiration date on the label. The medicine may not work properly after this date. Check with your pharmacist if you have any questions about this.

To help clear up your infection completely, keep taking this medicine for the full time of treatment, even if you begin to feel better after a few days. If you have a "strep" infection, you should keep taking this medicine for at least 10 days. This is especially important in "strep" infections. Serious heart problems could develop later if your infection is not cleared up completely. Also, if you stop taking this medicine too soon, your symptoms may return.

This medicine works best when there is a constant amount in the blood. To help keep the amount constant, do not miss any doses. Also, it is best to take each dose at evenly spaced times day and night. For example, if you are to take 4 doses a day, doses should be spaced about 6 hours apart. If this interferes with your sleep or other daily activities, or if you need help in planning the best times to take your medicine, check with your health care professional.

Dosing—The dose of this medicine will be different for different patients. Follow your doctor's orders or the directions on the label. The following information includes only the average doses of this medicine. If your dose is different, do not change it unless your doctor tells you to do so.

The amount of medicine that you take depends on the strength of the medicine. Also, the number of doses you take each day, the time allowed between doses, and the length of time you take the medicine depend on the medical problem for which you are using the medicine.

- For bacterial infection:
  - For oral dosage forms (capsules and solution):
    - Adults and teenagers—150 to 300 milligrams (mg) every six hours.
    - Children—
      — Infants up to 1 month of age: Use and dose must be determined by your doctor.
      — Infants and children 1 month of age and older: Dose is based on body weight. The usual dose is 2 to 5 mg per kilogram (kg) (0.9 to 2.3 mg per pound) of body weight every six hours; or 2.7 to 6.7 mg per kg (1.2 to 3.0 mg per pound) of body weight every eight hours.
  - For injection dosage form:
    - Adults and teenagers—300 to 600 mg every six to eight hours injected into a muscle or vein; or 900 mg every eight hours injected into a muscle or vein.
    - Children—
      — Infants up to 1 month of age: Dose is based on body weight. The usual dose is 3.75 to 5 mg per kg (1.7 to 2.3 mg per pound) of body weight every six hours injected into a muscle or vein; or 5 to 6.7 mg per kg (2.3 to 3.0 mg per pound) of body weight every eight hours injected into a muscle or vein.
      — Infants and children 1 month of age and older: Dose is based on body weight. The usual dose is 3.75 to 10 mg per kg (1.7 to 4.5 mg per pound) of body weight every six hours injected into a muscle or vein; or 5 to 13.3 mg per kg (2.3 to 6.0 mg per pound) of body weight every eight hours injected into a muscle or vein.

Missed dose—If you miss a dose of this medicine, take it as soon as possible. However, if it is almost time for your next dose, skip the missed dose and go back to your regular dosing schedule. Do not double doses.

Storage—Store the medicine in a closed container at room temperature, away from heat, moisture, and direct light. Keep from freezing.

Keep out of the reach of children.

Do not keep outdated medicine or medicine no longer needed.

Do not refrigerate the oral liquid form of clindamycin. If chilled, the liquid may thicken and be difficult to pour. Follow the directions on the label.

Precautions While Using This Medicine

It is important that your doctor check your progress at regular visits.

If your symptoms do not improve within a few days, or if they become worse, check with your doctor.

In some patients, clindamycin may cause diarrhea.

- Severe diarrhea may be a sign of a serious side effect. Do not take any diarrhea medicine without first checking with your doctor. Diarrhea medicines, such as loperamide (Imodium A-D) or diphenoxylate and atropine (Lomotil), may make your diarrhea worse or make it last longer.
- For mild diarrhea, diarrhea medicine containing attapulgite (e.g., Kaopectate tablets, Diasorb) may be taken. However, attapulgite may keep clindamycin from being absorbed into the body. Therefore, these diarrhea medicines should be taken at least 2 hours before or 3 to 4 hours after you take clindamycin by mouth.
- If you have any questions about this or if mild diarrhea continues or gets worse, check with your health care professional.

Before having surgery (including dental surgery) with a general anesthetic, tell the medical doctor or dentist in charge that you are taking clindamycin.

Side Effects of This Medicine

Along with its needed effects, a medicine may cause some unwanted effects. Although not all of these side effects may occur, if they do occur they may need medical attention.

Check with your doctor immediately if any of the following side effects occur:
More common
    Abdominal or stomach cramps and pain (severe); abdominal tenderness; diarrhea (watery and severe), which may also be bloody; fever(the above side effects may also occur up to several weeks after you stop taking this medicine)
Less common
    Sore throat and fever; skin rash, redness, and itching; unusual bleeding or bruising

Some side effects may occur that usually do not need medical attention. These side effects may go away during treatment as your body adjusts to the medicine. Also, your health care professional may be able to tell you about ways to prevent or reduce some of these side effects. Check with your health care professional if any of the following side effects continue or are bothersome or if you have any questions about them:
More common
    Diarrhea (mild); nausea and vomiting; stomach pain
Less common
    Itching of rectal, or genital (sex organ) areas

Other side effects not listed may also occur in some patients. If you notice any other effects, check with your healthcare professional.

CLINDAMYCIN (Topical route) - klin-da-MYE-sin

Commonly used brand name(s)
In the U.S.—
Cleocin T	Clindets
Clinda-Derm	Evoclin
Clindagel	Z-Clinz 10
ClindaMax	Z-Clinz 5

Available Dosage Forms:
- Lotion
- Gel/Jelly
- Pad
- Foam
- Solution

Therapeutic Class: Antiacne

Uses For This Medicine

Clindamycin belongs to the family of medicines called antibiotics. Topical clindamycin is used to help control acne. It may be used alone or with one or more other medicines that are used on the skin or taken by mouth for acne. Topical clindamycin may also be used for other problems as determined by your doctor.

Clindamycin is available only with your doctor's prescription.

Before Using This Medicine

In deciding to use a medicine, the risks of taking the medicine must be weighed against the good it will do. This is a decision you and your doctor will make. For this medicine, the following should be considered:

Allergies—Tell your doctor if you have ever had any unusual or allergic reaction to this medicine or any other medicines. Also tell your health care professional if you have any other types of allergies, such as to foods, dyes, preservatives, or animals. For non-prescription products, read the label or package ingredients carefully.

Pediatric—Studies on this medicine have been done only in adult patients, and there is no specific information comparing use of this medicine in children up to 12 years of age with use in other age groups.

Geriatric—Many medicines have not been studied specifically in older people. Therefore, it may not be known whether they work exactly the same way they do in younger adults. Although there is no specific information comparing use of this medicine in the elderly with use in other age groups, this medicine is not expected to cause different side effects or problems in older people than it does in younger adults.

Pregnancy—

	Pregnancy Category	Explanation
All Trimesters	B	Animal studies have revealed no evidence of harm to the fetus, however, there are no adequate studies in pregnant women OR animal studies have shown an adverse effect, but adequate studies in pregnant women have failed to demonstrate a risk to the fetus.

Breast Feeding—There are no adequate studies in women for determining infant risk when using this medication during breastfeeding. Weigh the potential benefits against the potential risks before taking this medication while breastfeeding.

Other medicines—

Using this medicine with any of the following medicines is usually not recommended, but may be required in some cases. If both medicines are prescribed together, your doctor may change the dose or how often you use one or both of the medicines.

Erythromycin

Interactions with Food/Tobacco/Alcohol—Certain medicines should not be used at or around the time of eating food or eating certain types of food since interactions may occur. Using alcohol or tobacco with certain medicines may also cause interactions to occur. Discuss with your healthcare professional the use of your medicine with food, alcohol, or tobacco.

Other medical problems—The presence of other medical problems may affect the use of this medicine. Make sure you tell your doctor if you have any other medical problems, especially:
- History of stomach or intestinal disease (especially colitis, including colitis caused by antibiotics, or enteritis)—These conditions may increase the chance of side effects that affect the stomach and intestines

Proper Use of This Medicine

Before applying this medicine, thoroughly wash the affected areas with warm water and soap, rinse well, and pat dry.

When applying the medicine, use enough to cover the affected area lightly. You should apply the medicine to the whole area usually affected by acne, not just to the pimples themselves. This will help keep new pimples from breaking out.

You should avoid washing the acne-affected areas too often. This may dry your skin and make your acne worse. Washing with a mild, bland soap 2 or 3 times a day should be enough, unless you have oily skin. If you have any questions about this, check with your doctor.

Topical clindamycin will not cure your acne. However, to help keep your acne under control, keep using this medicine for the full time of treatment, even if your symptoms begin to clear up after a few days. You may have to continue using this medicine every day for months or even longer in some cases. If you stop using this medicine too soon, your symptoms may return. It is important that you do not miss any doses.

For patients using the topical foam form of clindamycin:
- After washing or shaving, it is best to wait 30 minutes before applying this medicine. The alcohol in it may irritate freshly washed or shaved skin.
- This medicine contains alcohol and is flammable. Do not use near heat, near open flame, or while smoking.
- To apply this medicine:
  - Do not dispense clindamycin topical foam directly onto your hands because the foam will begin to melt on contact with warm skin.
  - Remove the clear cap. Align the black mark with the nozzle of the actuator.
  - Hold the can upright and press firmly to dispense. Dispense amount that will cover the affected area(s) directly into the cap or onto a cool surface.
  - The can may be placed under cold running water if the can seems warm or the foam seems runny.
  - A small amount of topical foam should be picked up with your fingertips and massaged gently into the affected areas until the foam disappears.
  - Unused medicine that was removed from the can should be throw away.
  - Since this medicine contains alcohol, it will sting or burn. In addition, it has an unpleasant taste if it gets on the mouth or lips. Therefore, do not get this medicine in the eyes, nose, or mouth, or on other mucous membranes. Spread the medicine away from these areas when applying. If this medicine does get in the

eyes, wash them out immediately, but carefully, with large amounts of cool tap water. If your eyes still burn or are painful, check with your doctor.

- It is important that you do not use this medicine more often than your doctor ordered. It may cause your skin to become too dry or irritated.

For patients using the topical solution form of clindamycin:

- After washing or shaving, it is best to wait 30 minutes before applying this medicine. The alcohol in it may irritate freshly washed or shaved skin.
- This medicine contains alcohol and is flammable. Do not use near heat, near open flame, or while smoking.
- To apply this medicine:
  - This medicine comes in a bottle with an applicator tip, which may be used to apply the medicine directly to the skin. Use the applicator with a dabbing motion instead of a rolling motion (not like a roll-on deodorant, for example). Tilt the bottle and press the tip firmly against your skin. If needed, you can make the medicine flow faster from the applicator tip by slightly increasing the pressure against the skin. If the medicine flows too fast, use less pressure. If the applicator tip becomes dry, turn the bottle upside down and press the tip several times to moisten it.
  - Since this medicine contains alcohol, it will sting or burn. In addition, it has an unpleasant taste if it gets on the mouth or lips. Therefore, do not get this medicine in the eyes, nose, or mouth, or on other mucous membranes. Spread the medicine away from these areas when applying. If this medicine does get in the eyes, wash them out immediately, but carefully, with large amounts of cool tap water. If your eyes still burn or are painful, check with your doctor.
- It is important that you do not use this medicine more often than your doctor ordered. It may cause your skin to become too dry or irritated.

For patients using the topical suspension form of clindamycin:

- Shake well before applying.

Dosing—The dose of this medicine will be different for different patients. Follow your doctor's orders or the directions on the label. The following information includes only the average doses of this medicine. If your dose is different, do not change it unless your doctor tells you to do so.

The amount of medicine that you take depends on the strength of the medicine. Also, the number of doses you take each day, the time allowed between doses, and the length of time you take the medicine depend on the medical problem for which you are using the medicine.

- For topical dosage form (foam):
  - For acne:
    - Adults and children 12 years of age and over— Apply once a day to areas affected by acne.
    - Infants and children up to 12 years of age—Use and dose must be determined by your doctor.
- For topical dosage forms (gel, solution, and suspension):
  - For acne:
    - Adults and children 12 years of age and over— Apply two times a day to areas affected by acne.
    - Infants and children up to 12 years of age—Use and dose must be determined by your doctor.

Missed dose—If you miss a dose of this medicine, apply it as soon as possible. However, if it is almost time for your next dose, skip the missed dose and go back to your regular dosing schedule.

Storage—Store the medicine in a closed container at room temperature, away from heat, moisture, and direct light. Keep from freezing.

Keep out of the reach of children.

Do not keep outdated medicine or medicine no longer needed.

Precautions While Using This Medicine

If your acne does not improve within about 6 weeks, or if it becomes worse, check with your health care professional. However, treatment of acne may take up to 8 to 12 weeks before full improvement is seen.

If your doctor has ordered another medicine to be applied to the skin along with this medicine, it is best to apply them at different times. This may help keep your skin from becoming too irritated. Also, if the medicines are used at or near the same time, they may not work properly.

For patients using the topical solution form of clindamycin:

- This medicine may cause the skin to become unusually dry, even with normal use. If this occurs, check with your doctor.

In some patients, clindamycin may cause diarrhea.

- Severe diarrhea may be a sign of a serious side effect. Do not take any diarrhea medicine without first checking with your doctor. Diarrhea medicines may make your diarrhea worse or make it last longer.
- For mild diarrhea, only diarrhea medicine containing attapulgite (e.g., Kaopectate, Diasorb) may be taken. Other kinds of diarrhea medicine (e.g., Imodium A.D. or Lomotil) should not be taken. They may make your condition worse or make it last longer.
- If you have any questions about this or if mild diarrhea continues or gets worse, check with your health care professional.

You may continue to use cosmetics (make-up) while you are using this medicine for acne. However, it is best to use only "water-base" cosmetics. Also, it is best not to use cosmetics too heavily or too often. They may make your acne worse. If you have any questions about this, check with your doctor.

Side Effects of This Medicine

Along with its needed effects, a medicine may cause some unwanted effects. Although not all of these side effects may occur, if they do occur they may need medical attention.

Check with your doctor immediately if any of the following side effects occur:
  Rare
    Abdominal or stomach cramps, pain, and bloating (severe); diarrhea (watery and severe), which may also be bloody; fever; increased thirst; nausea or vomiting; unusual tiredness or weakness; weight loss (unusual)— these side effects may also occur up to several weeks after you stop using this medicine

Check with your doctor as soon as possible if any of the following side effects occur:
  Less common
    Skin rash, itching, redness, swelling, or other sign of irritation not present before use of this medicine

Some side effects may occur that usually do not need medical attention. These side effects may go away during treatment as your body adjusts to the medicine. Also, your health care professional may be able to tell you about ways to prevent or reduce some of these side effects. Check with your health care professional if any of the following side effects continue or are bothersome or if you have any questions about them:

More common
 Dryness, scaliness, or peeling of skin (for the topical solution)

Less common
 Abdominal pain; diarrhea (mild); headache; irritation or oiliness of skin; stinging or burning feeling of skin

Other side effects not listed may also occur in some patients. If you notice any other effects, check with your healthcare professional.

CLINDAMYCIN (Vaginal route) - klin-da-MYE-sin

Commonly used brand name(s)

In the U.S.—
 Cleocin Vaginal
 ClindaMax
 Clindesse

Available Dosage Forms:
• Suppository
• Cream

Therapeutic Class: Antibiotic

Uses For This Medicine

Clindamycin is used to treat certain vaginal infections. It works by killing the bacteria. This medicine will not work for vaginal fungus or yeast infections.

Clindamycin is available only with your doctor's prescription.

Before Using This Medicine

In deciding to use a medicine, the risks of taking the medicine must be weighed against the good it will do. This is a decision you and your doctor will make. For this medicine, the following should be considered:

Allergies—Tell your doctor if you have ever had any unusual or allergic reaction to this medicine or any other medicines. Also tell your health care professional if you have any other types of allergies, such as to foods, dyes, preservatives, or animals. For non-prescription products, read the label or package ingredients carefully.

Pediatric—Studies on this medicine have been done only in adult patients, and there is no specific information comparing use of vaginal clindamycin in children with use in other age groups.

Geriatric—Many medicines have not been studied specifically in older people. Therefore, it may not be known whether they work exactly the same way they do in younger adults or if they cause different side effects or problems in older people. There is no specific information comparing use of vaginal clindamycin in the elderly with use in other age groups.

Pregnancy—

	Pregnancy Category	Explanation
All Trimesters	B	Animal studies have revealed no evidence of harm to the fetus, however, there are no adequate studies in pregnant women OR animal studies have shown an adverse effect, but adequate studies in pregnant women have failed to demonstrate a risk to the fetus.

Breast Feeding—There are no adequate studies in women for determining infant risk when using this medication during breastfeeding. Weigh the potential benefits against the potential risks before taking this medication while breastfeeding.

Other medicines—

Using this medicine with any of the following medicines is usually not recommended, but may be required in some cases. If both medicines are prescribed together, your doctor may change the dose or how often you use one or both of the medicines.

Erythromycin

Interactions with Food/Tobacco/Alcohol—Certain medicines should not be used at or around the time of eating food or eating certain types of food since interactions may occur. Using alcohol or tobacco with certain medicines may also cause interactions to occur. Discuss with your healthcare professional the use of your medicine with food, alcohol, or tobacco.

Other medical problems—The presence of other medical problems may affect the use of this medicine. Make sure you tell your doctor if you have any other medical problems, especially:
• Stomach or intestinal disease, history of (especially colitis, including colitis caused by antibiotics, or enteritis)— Patients with a history of stomach or intestinal disease may have an increased chance of side effects including diarrhea

Proper Use of This Medicine

Wash your hands before and after using this medicine.

Avoid getting this medicine in your eyes. If this medicine does get into your eyes, rinse them immediately with large amounts of cool tap water. If your eyes still burn or are painful, check with your doctor.

Vaginal clindamycin usually comes with patient directions. Read them carefully before using this medicine.

Use clindamycin vaginal cream exactly as directed by your doctor.
• To fill the applicator if you are not using a pre-filled applicator
 ○ Remove cap from the tube.
 ○ Screw one of the applicators onto the tube. Always use a new applicator. Never use one that has been used before.
 ○ Squeeze the medicine into the applicator slowly until it is full.
 ○ Remove the applicator from the tube. Replace the cap on the tube.

- To insert the vaginal cream using the applicator
  - Relax while lying on your back with your knees bent.
  - Hold the full applicator in one hand. Insert it slowly into the vagina. Stop before it becomes uncomfortable.
  - Slowly press the plunger until it stops.
  - Withdraw the applicator. The medicine will be left behind in the vagina.
- To care for the applicator
  - Throw the applicator away after you use it.

To help clear up your infection completely, it is very important that you keep using this medicine for the full time of treatment, even if your symptoms begin to clear up after a few days. If you stop using this medicine too soon, your symptoms may return. Do not miss any doses. Also, continue using this medicine even if your menstrual period starts during the time of treatment.

Dosing—The dose of this medicine will be different for different patients. Follow your doctor's orders or the directions on the label. The following information includes only the average doses of this medicine. If your dose is different, do not change it unless your doctor tells you to do so.

The amount of medicine that you take depends on the strength of the medicine. Also, the number of doses you take each day, the time allowed between doses, and the length of time you take the medicine depend on the medical problem for which you are using the medicine.

- For vaginal cream dosage form:
  - For bacterial vaginosis:
    - Adults and teenagers who are not pregnant—One applicatorful (100 milligrams [mg]) inserted into the vagina once a day, usually at bedtime, for three or seven days.
    - Adults and teenagers who are pregnant—One applicatorful (100 milligrams [mg]) inserted into the vagina once a day, usually at bedtime, for seven days.
    - Children—Use and dose must be determined by your doctor.
- For vaginal cream prefilled applicator dosage form:
  - For bacterial vaginosis:
    - Adults and teenagers—One applicatorful (100 milligrams [mg]) inserted into the vagina one time at any time of the day. This is a one-day treatment.
    - Children—Use and dose must be determined by your doctor.

Missed dose—If you miss a dose of this medicine, take it as soon as possible. However, if it is almost time for your next dose, skip the missed dose and go back to your regular dosing schedule. Do not double doses.

Storage—Store the medicine in a closed container at room temperature, away from heat, moisture, and direct light. Keep from freezing.

Keep out of the reach of children.

Do not keep outdated medicine or medicine no longer needed.

Precautions While Using This Medicine

If your symptoms do not improve within a few days, or if they become worse, check with your doctor.

It is important that you visit your doctor after you have used all your medicine to make sure that the infection is gone.

This medicine may cause some people to become dizzy. Make sure you know how you react to this medicine before you drive, use machines, or do anything else that could be dangerous if you are dizzy.

It is important that you tell your doctor right away if diarrhea occurs while you are using this medicine or after you have finished your treatment. It could be a symptom of a serious condition that your doctor will need to diagnose and treat.

Vaginal medicines usually leak out of the vagina during treatment. To keep the medicine from getting on your clothing, wear a minipad or sanitary napkin. Do not use tampons since they may soak up the medicine.

To help clear up your infection completely and make sure it does not return, good health habits are also required.

- Wear cotton panties (or panties or pantyhose with cotton crotches) instead of synthetic (for example, nylon or rayon) panties.
- Wear only freshly washed panties daily.

Do not have sexual intercourse while you are using this medicine. Having sexual intercourse may reduce the strength of the medicine. This may cause the medicine to not work as well.

Do not use latex (rubber) contraceptive products such as condoms, diaphragms, or cervical caps for 72 hours after stopping treatment with vaginal clindamycin cream. The cream contains oils that weaken or harm the latex products, causing them to not work properly to prevent pregnancy. If you have any questions about this, check with your health care professional.

Side Effects of This Medicine

Along with its needed effects, a medicine may cause some unwanted effects. Although not all of these side effects may occur, if they do occur they may need medical attention.

Check with your doctor as soon as possible if any of the following side effects occur:

More common
Itching of the vagina or genital area; pain during sexual intercourse; thick, white vaginal discharge with no odor or with mild odor

Less common
Diarrhea; dizziness; headache; nausea or vomiting; stomach pain or cramps

Rare
Burning, itching, rash, redness, swelling or other signs of skin problems not present before use of this medicine

After you stop using this medicine, it may still produce some side effects that need attention. During this period of time, *check with your doctor immediately* if you notice the following side effects:

Itching of the vagina or genital area; pain during sexual intercourse; thick, white vaginal discharge with no odor or with mild odor

Other side effects not listed may also occur in some patients. If you notice any other effects, check with your healthcare professional.

CLOFARABINE   (Intravenous route) -
kloe-FAR-a-been

Commonly used brand name(s)
In the U.S.—
   Clolar

Available Dosage Forms:
   • Solution

Therapeutic Class: Antineoplastic Agent
Pharmacologic Class: Antimetabolite

Uses For This Medicine

Clofarabine belongs to the general group of medicines known as antineoplastics. It is used to treat some kinds of cancer.

Clofarabine seems to interfere with the growth of cancer cells, which are eventually destroyed. Since the growth of normal body cells also may be affected by clofarabine, other effects also occur. Some of these effects may be serious and must be reported to your doctor.

Clofarabine is to be administered only by or under the immediate supervision of your doctor.

Before Using This Medicine

In deciding to use a medicine, the risks of taking the medicine must be weighed against the good it will do. This is a decision you and your doctor will make. For this medicine, the following should be considered:

Allergies—Tell your doctor if you have ever had any unusual or allergic reaction to this medicine or any other medicines. Also tell your health care professional if you have any other types of allergies, such as to foods, dyes, preservatives, or animals. For non-prescription products, read the label or package ingredients carefully.

Geriatric—Safety and efficacy of clofarabine in adult patients over 21 years of age and geriatric patients have not been established.

Pregnancy—

	Pregnancy Category	Explanation
All Trimesters	D	Studies in pregnant women have demonstrated a risk to the fetus. However, the benefits of therapy in a life threatening situation or a serious disease, may outweigh the potential risk.

Breast Feeding—There are no adequate studies in women for determining infant risk when using this medication during breastfeeding. Weigh the potential benefits against the potential risks before taking this medication while breastfeeding.

Other medicines—Although certain medicines should not be used together at all, in other cases two different medicines may be used together even if an interaction might occur. In these cases, your doctor may want to change the dose, or other precautions may be necessary. Tell your healthcare professional if you are taking any other prescription or non-prescription (over-the-counter [OTC]) medicine.

Interactions with Food/Tobacco/Alcohol—Certain medicines should not be used at or around the time of eating food or eating certain types of food since interactions may occur. Using alcohol or tobacco with certain medicines may also cause interactions to occur. Discuss with your healthcare professional the use of your medicine with food, alcohol, or tobacco.

Other medical problems—The presence of other medical problems may affect the use of this medicine. Make sure you tell your doctor if you have any other medical problems, especially:
   • Kidney disease or
   • Liver disease—Effects of clofarabine may be increased because of slower removal of this medicine from the body

Proper Use of This Medicine

This medicine may cause nausea and vomiting. However, it is very important that you continue to receive the medicine even if you begin to feel ill. Ask your health care professional for ways to lessen these effects.

Dosing—The dose of this medicine will be different for different patients. Follow your doctor's orders or the directions on the label. The following information includes only the average doses of this medicine. If your dose is different, do not change it unless your doctor tells you to do so.

The amount of medicine that you take depends on the strength of the medicine. Also, the number of doses you take each day, the time allowed between doses, and the length of time you take the medicine depend on the medical problem for which you are using the medicine.

Precautions While Using This Medicine

It is very important that your doctor check your progress at regular visits to make sure that this medicine is working properly and to check for unwanted effects.

While you are being treated with clofarabine, and after you stop treatment with it, do not have any immunizations (vaccinations) without your doctor's approval. Clofarabine may lower your body's resistance and there is a chance you might get the infection the immunization is meant to prevent. In addition, other persons living in your household should not take oral polio vaccine since there is a chance they could pass the polio virus on to you. Also, avoid persons who have recently taken oral polio vaccine. Do not get close to them and do not stay in the same room with them for very long. If you cannot take these precautions, you should consider wearing a protective face mask that covers the nose and mouth.

Clofarabine can temporarily lower the number of white blood cells in your blood, increasing the chance of getting an infection. It can also lower the number of platelets, which are necessary for proper blood clotting. If this occurs, there are certain precautions you can take, especially when your blood count is low, to reduce the risk of infection or bleeding:
   • If you can, avoid people with infections. Check with your doctor immediately if you think you are getting an infection or if you get a fever or chills, cough or hoarseness, lower back or side pain, or painful or difficult urination.

- Check with your doctor immediately if you notice any unusual bleeding or bruising; black, tarry stools; blood in urine or stools; or pinpoint red spots on your skin.

- Be careful when using a regular toothbrush, dental floss, or toothpick. Your medical doctor, dentist, or nurse may recommend other ways to clean your teeth and gums. Check with your medical doctor before having any dental work done.

- Do not touch your eyes or the inside of your nose unless you have just washed your hands and have not touched anything else in the meantime.

- Be careful not to cut yourself when you are using sharp objects such as a safety razor or fingernail or toenail cutters.

- Avoid contact sports or other situations where bruising or injury could occur.

- While you are receiving clofarabine, it is important that you drink extra fluids so that you will pass more urine.

- Tell your doctor if you are dizzy, lightheaded, or faint while receiving clofarabine.

- Tell your doctor it the amount of urine you produce is decreased.

- It is important that men and women of child bearing potential should use effective measures of contraception to prevent pregnancy while receiving clofarabine.

Side Effects of This Medicine

Along with its needed effects, a medicine may cause some unwanted effects. Although not all of these side effects may occur, if they do occur they may need medical attention.

Check with your doctor immediately if any of the following side effects occur:
  More common
      Area rash; black, tarry stools; bleeding gums; blood in urine or stools; blurred vision; burning or stinging of skin; chest pain; chills; clay-colored stools; confusion; cough or hoarseness; dark urine; decreased urine output; diarrhea; difficult or labored breathing; dilated neck veins; dizziness; dizziness, faintness, or lightheadedness when getting up from a lying or sitting position suddenly; facial swelling; fainting; fast, pounding, or irregular heartbeat or pulse; fever; headache; irregular breathing; irregular heartbeat; itching; lightheadedness; loss of appetite; lower back or side pain; nausea; nervousness; pain; painful cold sores or blisters on lips, nose, eyes, or genital; painful or difficult urination; pale skin; pinpoint red spots on skin; pounding in the ears; rapid, shallow breathing; redness; shortness of breath; skin rash; slow or fast heartbeat; sneezing; sore throat; sores, ulcers, or white spots on lips or in mouth; Staphylococcal infection; stomach pain; sweating; swelling; swollen glands; tenderness; tightness in chest; troubled breathing with exertion; unpleasant breath odor; unusual bleeding or bruising; unusual tiredness or weakness; vomiting; vomiting of blood; warmth on skin; weight gain; wheezing; yellow eyes or skins
  Frequency unknown
      Cloudy urine; decrease or increase in amount of urine; swelling of hands, ankles, feet, or lower legs

Symptoms of overdose
  Get emergency help immediately if any of the following symptoms of overdose occur:
      Rash with flat lesions or small raised lesions on the skin; vomiting; yellow eyes or skin

Some side effects may occur that usually do not need medical attention. These side effects may go away during treatment as your body adjusts to the medicine. Also, your health care professional may be able to tell you about ways to prevent or reduce some of these side effects. Check with your health care professional if any of the following side effects continue or are bothersome or if you have any questions about them:
  More common
      Back pain; bleeding gums; blistering, crusting, irritation, itching, or reddening of skin; cracked, dry, scaly skin; swelling; bloody nose; contusion; cracked lips; creatinine, elevated; difficulty having a bowel movement (stool); difficulty in moving; difficulty in swallowing; discouragement; dry skin; dullness, tiredness, weakness or feeling of sluggishness; fear; feeling sad or empty; feeling of warmth; feeling unusually cold; flushing, redness of skin; injection site pain; irritability; lack of appetite; loss of appetite; loss of interest or pleasure; muscle aching or cramping; muscle pain or stiffness; pain in joints; pain in limb; redness of the face, neck, arms and occasionally, upper chest; redness, swelling pain of skin; right upper abdominal pain and fullness; scaling of skin on hands and feet; shakiness in legs, arms, hands, feet; shivering; small red or purple spots on skin; swollen joints; tingling of hands and feet; tiredness; trembling or shaking of hands or feet; trouble concentrating; trouble sleeping; unusually warm skin; ulceration of skin; weight loss

Other side effects not listed may also occur in some patients. If you notice any other effects, check with your healthcare professional.

CLOFAZIMINE (Oral route) - kloe-FA-zi-meen

Commonly used brand name(s)
In the U.S.—
  Lamprene

Available Dosage Forms:
  - Capsule

Therapeutic Class: Leprostatic

Uses For This Medicine

Clofazimine is taken to treat leprosy (Hansen's disease). It is sometimes given with other medicines for leprosy. When this medicine is used to treat "flare-ups" of leprosy, it may be given with a cortisone-like medicine. Clofazimine may also be used for other problems as determined by your doctor.

This medicine is available only with your doctor's prescription.

Before Using This Medicine

In deciding to use a medicine, the risks of taking the medicine must be weighed against the good it will do. This is a decision you and your doctor will make. For this medicine, the following should be considered:

Allergies—Tell your doctor if you have ever had any unusual or allergic reaction to this medicine or any other medicines. Also tell your health care professional if you have any other types of allergies, such as to foods, dyes, preservatives, or animals. For non-prescription products, read the label or package ingredients carefully.

Pediatric—Studies on this medicine have been done only in adult patients, and there is no specific information comparing use of clofazimine in children with use in other age groups.

Geriatric—Many medicines have not been studied specifically in older people. Therefore, it may not be known whether they work exactly the same way they do in younger adults or if they cause different side effects or problems in older people. There is no specific information comparing use of clofazimine in the elderly with use in other age groups.

Pregnancy—

	Pregnancy Category	Explanation
All Trimesters	C	Animal studies have shown an adverse effect and there are no adequate studies in pregnant women OR no animal studies have been conducted and there are no adequate studies in pregnant women.

Breast Feeding—There are no adequate studies in women for determining infant risk when using this medication during breastfeeding. Weigh the potential benefits against the potential risks before taking this medication while breastfeeding.

Other medicines—

Using this medicine with any of the following medicines may cause an increased risk of certain side effects, but using both drugs may be the best treatment for you. If both medicines are prescribed together, your doctor may change the dose or how often you use one or both of the medicines.

Aluminum Hydroxide, Magnesium Hydroxide, Phenytoin

Interactions with Food/Tobacco/Alcohol—Certain medicines should not be used at or around the time of eating food or eating certain types of food since interactions may occur. Using alcohol or tobacco with certain medicines may also cause interactions to occur. The following interactions have been selected on the basis of their potential significance and are not necessarily all-inclusive.

Using this medicine with any of the following may cause an increased risk of certain side effects but may be unavoidable in some cases. If used together, your doctor may change the dose or how often you use this medicine, or give you special instructions about the use of food, alcohol, or tobacco.

Orange Juice

Other medical problems—The presence of other medical problems may affect the use of this medicine. Make sure you tell your doctor if you have any other medical problems, especially:

- Liver disease—Clofazimine may on rare occasion cause hepatitis and liver disease
- Stomach or intestinal problems, history of—Clofazimine often causes some stomach upset, but on rare occasion may cause severe, sharp abdominal pain and burning, which may be a sign of a serious side effect

Proper Use of This Medicine

Clofazimine should be taken with meals or milk.

To help clear up your leprosy completely, it is very important that you keep taking clofazimine for the full time of treatment, even if you begin to feel better after a few months. You may have to take it every day for as long as 2 years to life. If you stop taking this medicine too soon, your symptoms may return.

This medicine works best when there is a constant amount in the blood. To help keep the amount constant, do not miss any doses. Also, it is best to take each dose at the same time every day. If you need help in planning the best time to take your medicine, check with your health care professional.

Dosing—The dose of this medicine will be different for different patients. Follow your doctor's orders or the directions on the label. The following information includes only the average doses of this medicine. If your dose is different, do not change it unless your doctor tells you to do so.

The amount of medicine that you take depends on the strength of the medicine. Also, the number of doses you take each day, the time allowed between doses, and the length of time you take the medicine depend on the medical problem for which you are using the medicine.

- For the treatment of leprosy (Hansen's disease):
  - Adults and teenagers: 50 to 100 milligrams once a day. This medicine must be taken with other medicines for the treatment of Hansen's disease.
  - Children: Dose must be determined by the doctor.

Missed dose—If you miss a dose of this medicine, take it as soon as possible. However, if it is almost time for your next dose, skip the missed dose and go back to your regular dosing schedule. Do not double doses.

Storage—Store the medicine in a closed container at room temperature, away from heat, moisture, and direct light. Keep from freezing.

Keep out of the reach of children.

Do not keep outdated medicine or medicine no longer needed.

Precautions While Using This Medicine

If your symptoms do not improve within 1 to 3 months, or if they become worse, check with your doctor. It may take up to 6 months before the full benefit of this medicine is seen.

Clofazimine may cause pink or red to brownish-black discoloration of the skin within a few weeks after you start taking it. Because of the skin discoloration, some patients may become depressed. The discoloration will go away when you stop taking this medicine. However, it may take several months or years for the skin to clear up completely. If skin discoloration causes you to feel very depressed or to have thoughts of suicide, check with your doctor immediately.

This medicine may cause some people to become dizzy, drowsy, or less alert than they are normally. Make sure you know how you react to this medicine before you drive, use machines, or do anything else that could be dangerous if you are dizzy or are not alert or able to see well. If these reactions are especially bothersome, check with your doctor.

Clofazimine may cause your skin to become more sensitive to sunlight than it is normally. Exposure to sunlight, even for brief periods of time, may cause a skin rash, itching, redness or other discoloration of the skin, or a severe sunburn. When you begin taking this medicine:

- Stay out of direct sunlight, especially between the hours of 10:00 a.m. and 3:00 p.m., if possible.
- Wear protective clothing, including a hat. Also, wear sunglasses.
- Apply a sun block product that has a skin protection factor (SPF) of at least 15. Some patients may require a product with a higher SPF number, especially if they have a fair complexion. If you have any questions about this, check with your health care professional.
- Apply a sun block lipstick that has an SPF of at least 15 to protect your lips.
- Do not use a sunlamp or tanning bed or booth.

If you have a severe reaction, check with your doctor.

Clofazimine may also cause dry, rough, or scaly skin. A skin cream, lotion, or oil may help to treat this problem.

Side Effects of This Medicine

Along with its needed effects, a medicine may cause some unwanted effects. Although not all of these side effects may occur, if they do occur they may need medical attention.

Check with your doctor immediately if any of the following side effects occur:

Rare
    Bloody or black, tarry stools; colicky or burning abdominal or stomach pain; mental depression; yellow eyes or skin— may be an orange color if already have a pink to brownish-black skin or eye discoloration

Some side effects may occur that usually do not need medical attention. These side effects may go away during treatment as your body adjusts to the medicine. Also, your health care professional may be able to tell you about ways to prevent or reduce some of these side effects. Check with your health care professional if any of the following side effects continue or are bothersome or if you have any questions about them:

More common
    Diarrhea; dry, rough, or scaly skin; loss of appetite; nausea or vomiting; pink or red to brownish-black discoloration of skin and eyes; skin rash and itching

Less common or rare
    Changes in taste; dryness, burning, itching, or irritation of the eyes; increased sensitivity of skin to sunlight

Clofazimine commonly causes discoloration of the feces, lining of the eyelids, sputum, sweat, tears, and urine. Usually this side effect does not require medical attention, but the discoloration may not go away. However, clofazimine may also cause bloody or black, tarry stools. This side effect may be a symptom of serious bleeding problems that do require medical attention.

Other side effects not listed may also occur in some patients. If you notice any other effects, check with your healthcare professional.

CLOFIBRATE   (Oral route) - kloe-FYE-brate

Uses For This Medicine

Clofibrate is used to lower cholesterol and triglyceride (fat-like substances) levels in the blood. This may help prevent medical problems caused by such substances clogging the blood vessels.

Clofibrate may also be used for other conditions as determined by your doctor.

Clofibrate is available only with your doctor's prescription.

Once a medicine has been approved for marketing for a certain use, experience may show that it is also useful for other medical problems. Although this use is not included in product labeling, clofibrate is used in certain patients with the following medical condition:

- Certain types of diabetes insipidus (water diabetes)

Before Using This Medicine

In deciding to use a medicine, the risks of taking the medicine must be weighed against the good it will do. This is a decision you and your doctor will make. For this medicine, the following should be considered:

In addition to its helpful effects in treating your medical problem, this medicine may have some harmful effects. You may have read or heard about a study called the World Health Organization (WHO) Study. This study compared the effects in patients who used clofibrate with effects in those who used a placebo (sugar pill). The results of this study suggested that clofibrate might increase the patient's risk of cancer, liver disease, and pancreatitis (inflammation of the pancreas), although it might also decrease the risk of heart attack. It may also increase the risk of gallstones and problems from gallbladder surgery. Other studies have not found all of these effects. Be sure you have discussed this with your doctor before taking this medicine.

Allergies—Tell your doctor if you have ever had any unusual or allergic reaction to this medicine or any other medicines. Also tell your health care professional if you have any other types of allergies, such as to foods, dyes, preservatives, or animals. For non-prescription products, read the label or package ingredients carefully.

Pediatric—Studies on this medicine have been done only in adult patients, and there is no specific information comparing use of clofibrate in children with use in other age groups. However, use is not recommended in children under 2 years of age since cholesterol is needed for normal development.

Geriatric—Many medicines have not been studied specifically in older people. Therefore, it may not be known whether they work exactly the same way they do in younger adults. Although there is no specific information comparing use of clofibrate in the elderly with use in other age groups, this medicine is not expected to cause different side effects or problems in older people than it does in younger adults.

Pregnancy—

	Pregnancy Category	Explanation
All Trimesters	C	Animal studies have shown an adverse effect and there are no adequate studies in pregnant women OR no animal studies have been conducted and there are no adequate studies in pregnant women.

Breast Feeding—There are no adequate studies in women for determining infant risk when using this medication during breastfeeding. Weigh the potential benefits against the potential risks before taking this medication while breastfeeding.

Other medicines—

Using this medicine with any of the following medicines is usually not recommended, but may be required in some cases. If both medicines are prescribed together, your doctor may change the dose or how often you use one or both of the medicines.

Atorvastatin, Cerivastatin, Ezetimibe, Fluvastatin, Lovastatin, Pravastatin, Simvastatin

Interactions with Food/Tobacco/Alcohol—Certain medicines should not be used at or around the time of eating food or eating certain types of food since interactions may occur. Using alcohol or tobacco with certain medicines may also cause interactions to occur. Discuss with your healthcare professional the use of your medicine with food, alcohol, or tobacco.

Other medical problems—The presence of other medical problems may affect the use of this medicine. Make sure you tell your doctor if you have any other medical problems, especially:

- Gallstones or
- Stomach or intestinal ulcer—May make these conditions worse
- Heart disease or
- Kidney disease or
- Liver disease—Higher blood levels may result and increase the risk of side effects
- Underactive thyroid—Clofibrate may cause or make muscle disease worse

Proper Use of This Medicine

Before prescribing medicine for your condition, your doctor will probably try to control your condition by prescribing a personal diet for you. Such a diet may be low in fats, sugars, and/or cholesterol. Many people are able to control their condition by carefully following their doctors' orders for proper diet and exercise. Medicine is prescribed only when additional help is needed and is effective only when a schedule of diet and exercise is properly followed.

Also, this medicine is less effective if you are greatly overweight. It may be very important for you to go on a reducing diet. However, check with your doctor before going on any diet.

Make certain your health care professional knows if you are on a low-sodium, low-sugar, or any other special diet. Most medicines contain more than their active ingredient.

Use this medicine only as directed by your doctor. Do not use more or less of it, and do not use it more often or for a longer time than your doctor ordered.

Follow carefully the special diet your doctor gave you. This is the most important part of controlling your condition and is necessary if the medicine is to work properly.

Stomach upset may occur but usually lessens after a few doses. Take this medicine with food or immediately after meals to lessen possible stomach upset.

Dosing—The dose of this medicine will be different for different patients. Follow your doctor's orders or the directions on the label. The following information includes only the average doses of this medicine. If your dose is different, do not change it unless your doctor tells you to do so.

The amount of medicine that you take depends on the strength of the medicine. Also, the number of doses you take each day, the time allowed between doses, and the length of time you take the medicine depend on the medical problem for which you are using the medicine.

- For oral dosage form (capsules):
  - For high cholesterol:
    - Adults—1.5 to 2 grams a day. This is divided into two to four doses.
    - Children—Dose must be determined by your doctor.

Missed dose—If you miss a dose of this medicine, take it as soon as possible. However, if it is almost time for your next dose, skip the missed dose and go back to your regular dosing schedule. Do not double doses.

Storage—Store the medicine in a closed container at room temperature, away from heat, moisture, and direct light. Keep from freezing.

Keep out of the reach of children.

Do not keep outdated medicine or medicine no longer needed.

Precautions While Using This Medicine

It is very important that your doctor check your progress at regular visits. This will allow your doctor to see if the medicine is working properly to lower your cholesterol and triglyceride levels and to decide if you should continue to take it.

Do not stop taking this medicine without first checking with your doctor. When you stop taking this medicine, your blood fat levels may increase again. Your doctor may want you to follow a special diet to help prevent that.

Side Effects of This Medicine

Along with its needed effects, a medicine may cause some unwanted effects. Although not all of these side effects may occur, if they do occur they may need medical attention.

Check with your doctor immediately if any of the following side effects occur:
Rare
   Chest pain; irregular heartbeat; shortness of breath; stomach pain (severe) with nausea and vomiting

Check with your doctor as soon as possible if any of the following side effects occur:

Rare

Blood in urine; cough or hoarseness; decrease in urination; fever or chills; lower back or side pain; painful or difficult urination; swelling of feet or lower legs

Some side effects may occur that usually do not need medical attention. These side effects may go away during treatment as your body adjusts to the medicine. Also, your health care professional may be able to tell you about ways to prevent or reduce some of these side effects. Check with your health care professional if any of the following side effects continue or are bothersome or if you have any questions about them:

More common

Diarrhea; nausea

Less common or rare

Decreased sexual ability; headache; increased appetite or weight gain (slight); muscle aches or cramps; sores in mouth and on lips; stomach pain, gas, or heartburn; unusual tiredness or weakness; vomiting

Other side effects not listed may also occur in some patients. If you notice any other effects, check with your healthcare professional.

CLOMIPHENE (Oral route) - KLOE-mi-feen

Commonly used brand name(s)

In the U.S.—
Clomid
Serophene

Available Dosage Forms:
• Tablet

Therapeutic Class: Female Reproductive Agent
Pharmacologic Class: Gonadotropin

Uses For This Medicine

Clomiphene is used as a fertility medicine in some women who are unable to become pregnant.

Clomiphene probably works by changing the hormone balance of the body. In women, this causes ovulation to occur and prepares the body for pregnancy.

Clomiphene may also be used for other conditions in both females and males as determined by your doctor.

The following information applies only to female patients taking clomiphene. Check with your doctor if you are a male and have any questions about the use of clomiphene.

Clomiphene is available only with your doctor's prescription.

Once a medicine has been approved for marketing for a certain use, experience may show that it is also useful for other medical problems. Although these uses are not included in product labeling, clomiphene is used in certain patients with the following medical conditions:

• Certain problems of the male sexual organs caused by pituitary or hypothalamus gland problems (diagnosis)
• Male infertility caused by low production of sperm
• Problems with the corpus luteum (mature egg)

For males taking this medicine for treatment of infertility caused by low sperm production:
• To help decide on the best treatment for your medical problem, tell your doctor:
  ○ if you have ever had any unusual or allergic reaction to clomiphene.
  ○ if you have any of the following medical problems:
    ▪ Liver disease
    ▪ Mental depression
    ▪ Thrombophlebitis
• If you miss a dose of this medicine, take it as soon as possible. If you do not remember until it is time for the next dose, take both doses together; then go back to your regular dosing schedule. If you miss more than one dose, check with your doctor.
• It is important that your doctor check your progress at regular visits to find out if clomiphene is working and to check for unwanted effects.
• This medicine may cause vision problems, dizziness, or lightheadedness. Make sure you know how you react to this medicine before you drive, use machines, or do anything else that could be dangerous if you are not clear-headed or able to see well.
• Along with its needed effects, a medicine may cause some unwanted effects. Although not all of these side effects may occur, if they do occur they may need medical attention. When this medicine is used for short periods of time at low doses, serious side effects usually are rare. However, check with your doctor if any of the following side effects occur:

Less common or rare
  ○ Blurred vision; decreased or double vision or other vision problems; seeing flashes of light; sensitivity of eyes to light; yellow eyes or skin
  ○ Other side effects may occur that usually do not need medical attention. These side effects may go away during treatment as your body adjusts to the medicine. However, check with your doctor if any of the following side effects continue or are bothersome:

Less common or rare
  ○ Breast enlargement; dizziness or lightheadedness; headache; mental depression; nausea or vomiting; nervousness; restlessness; tiredness; trouble in sleeping

Before Using This Medicine

In deciding to use a medicine, the risks of taking the medicine must be weighed against the good it will do. This is a decision you and your doctor will make. For this medicine, the following should be considered:

Allergies—Tell your doctor if you have ever had any unusual or allergic reaction to this medicine or any other medicines. Also tell your health care professional if you have any other types of allergies, such as to foods, dyes, preservatives, or animals. For non-prescription products, read the label or package ingredients carefully.

Pregnancy—

	Pregnancy Category	Explanation
All Trimesters	X	Studies in animals or pregnant women have demonstrated positive evidence of fetal abnormalities. This drug should not be used in women who are or may become pregnant because the risk clearly outweighs any possible benefit.

Breast Feeding—There are no adequate studies in women for determining infant risk when using this medication during breastfeeding. Weigh the potential benefits against the potential risks before taking this medication while breastfeeding.

Other medicines—Although certain medicines should not be used together at all, in other cases two different medicines may be used together even if an interaction might occur. In these cases, your doctor may want to change the dose, or other precautions may be necessary. Tell your healthcare professional if you are taking any other prescription or non-prescription (over-the-counter [OTC]) medicine.

Interactions with Food/Tobacco/Alcohol—Certain medicines should not be used at or around the time of eating food or eating certain types of food since interactions may occur. Using alcohol or tobacco with certain medicines may also cause interactions to occur. Discuss with your healthcare professional the use of your medicine with food, alcohol, or tobacco.

Other medical problems—The presence of other medical problems may affect the use of this medicine. Make sure you tell your doctor if you have any other medical problems, especially:

- Unusually large ovary or
- Cyst on ovary—Clomiphene may cause the cyst to increase in size
- Endometriosis—Inducing ovulation (including using clomiphene) may worsen endometriosis because the body estrogen level is increased; estrogen can cause growth of endometriosis implants
- Fibroid tumors of the uterus—Clomiphene may cause fibroid tumors to increase in size
- Inflamed veins due to blood clots—Clomiphene may make condition worse
- Liver disease (or history of)—Clomiphene may make any liver disease worse
- Mental depression—Existing depression may become worse because of hormone changes caused by clomiphene
- Unusual vaginal bleeding—Some irregular vaginal bleeding is a sign that the lining of the uterus is growing too much or is a sign of cancer of the uterus lining; these problems must be ruled out before clomiphene is used because clomiphene can make these conditions worse

Proper Use of This Medicine

Take this medicine only as directed by your doctor. If you are to begin on Day 5, count the first day of your menstrual period as Day 1. Beginning on Day 5, take the correct dose every day for as many days as your doctor ordered. To help you to

remember to take your dose of medicine, take it at the same time every day.

Dosing—The dose of this medicine will be different for different patients. Follow your doctor's orders or the directions on the label. The following information includes only the average doses of this medicine. If your dose is different, do not change it unless your doctor tells you to do so.

The amount of medicine that you take depends on the strength of the medicine. Also, the number of doses you take each day, the time allowed between doses, and the length of time you take the medicine depend on the medical problem for which you are using the medicine.

- For oral dosage form (tablets):
  - For treating infertility:
    - Adults—50 milligrams (mg) a day for five days of a menstrual cycle. The treatment is usually started on the fifth day of your menstrual period. If you do not have menstrual cycles, you can begin taking your medicine at any time. If you do not become pregnant after the first course, your doctor may increase your dose a little at a time up to 250 mg a day. Your treatment may be repeated until you do become pregnant or for up to four treatment cycles.

Missed dose—If you miss a dose of this medicine, take it as soon as possible. However, if it is almost time for your next dose, skip the missed dose and go back to your regular dosing schedule. Do not double doses.

If you do not remember until it is time for the next dose, take both doses together; then go back to your regular dosing schedule. If you miss more than one dose, check with your doctor.

Storage—Store the medicine in a closed container at room temperature, away from heat, moisture, and direct light. Keep from freezing.

Keep out of the reach of children.

Do not keep outdated medicine or medicine no longer needed.

Precautions While Using This Medicine

It is very important that your doctor check your progress at regular visits to make sure this medicine is working and to check for unwanted effects.

At certain times in your menstrual cycle, your doctor may want you to use an ovulation prediction test kit. Follow your doctor's instructions carefully. Ovulation is controlled by luteinizing hormone (LH). LH is present in the blood and urine in very small amounts during most of the menstrual cycle but rises suddenly for a short time in the middle of the menstrual cycle. This sharp rise, the LH surge, usually causes ovulation within about 30 hours. A woman is most likely to become pregnant if she has intercourse within the 24 hours after detecting the LH surge. Ovulation prediction test kits are used to test for this large amount of LH in the urine. This method is better for predicting ovulation than measuring daily basal body temperature. It is important that intercourse take place at the correct time to give you the best chance of becoming pregnant.

There is a chance that clomiphene may cause birth defects if it is taken after you become pregnant. Stop taking this medicine and tell your doctor immediately if you think you have become pregnant while still taking clomiphene.

This medicine may cause blurred vision, difficulty in reading, or other changes in vision. It may also cause some people to become dizzy or lightheaded. Make sure you know how you react to this medicine before you drive, use machines, or do anything else that could be dangerous if you are not clear-headed or able to see well. If these reactions are especially bothersome, check with your doctor.

Side Effects of This Medicine

Along with its needed effects, a medicine may cause some unwanted effects. Although not all of these side effects may occur, if they do occur they may need medical attention.

Check with your doctor immediately if any of the following side effects occur:
>   *More common*
>   Bloating; stomach or pelvic pain

Check with your doctor as soon as possible if any of the following side effects occur:
>   *Less common or rare*
>   Blurred vision; decreased or double vision or other vision problems; seeing flashes of light; sensitivity of eyes to light; yellow eyes or skin

Some side effects may occur that usually do not need medical attention. These side effects may go away during treatment as your body adjusts to the medicine. Also, your health care professional may be able to tell you about ways to prevent or reduce some of these side effects. Check with your health care professional if any of the following side effects continue or are bothersome or if you have any questions about them:
>   *More common*
>   Hot flashes
>   *Less common or rare*
>   Breast discomfort; dizziness or lightheadedness; headache; heavy menstrual periods or bleeding between periods; mental depression; nausea or vomiting; nervousness; restlessness; tiredness; trouble in sleeping

Other side effects not listed may also occur in some patients. If you notice any other effects, check with your healthcare professional.

CLONIDINE (Epidural route) - KLOE-ni-deen

Black Box Warning

The 500 microgram/milliliter strength product should be diluted prior to use in an appropriate solution.

Epidural clonidine hydrochloride is not recommended for obstetrical, post-partum, or peri-operative pain management. The risk of hemodynamic instability, especially hypotension and bradycardia, from epidural clonidine hydrochloride may be unacceptable in these patients. However, in a rare obstetrical, post-partum or peri-operative patient, potential benefits may outweigh the possible risks.

Commonly used brand name(s)
In the U.S.—
>   Duraclon

Available Dosage Forms:
- Solution
- Injectable

Therapeutic Class: Analgesic
Pharmacologic Class: Alpha-2 Adrenergic Agonist

Uses For This Medicine

Clonidine injection is used with injected pain medicine to treat pain in cancer patients.

Clonidine is to be started under the immediate supervision of your doctor. After your doctor has seen how you respond to clonidine, you may be able to receive this medicine at home.

This medicine is available only with your doctor's prescription.

Once a medicine has been approved for marketing for a certain use, experience may show that it is also useful for other medical problems. Although these uses are not included in product labeling, clonidine is used in certain patients with the following medical conditions:
- Post-operative shivering (to prevent or treat shivering that occurs after an operation or anesthesia)

Before Using This Medicine

In deciding to use a medicine, the risks of taking the medicine must be weighed against the good it will do. This is a decision you and your doctor will make. For this medicine, the following should be considered:

Allergies—Tell your doctor if you have ever had any unusual or allergic reaction to this medicine or any other medicines. Also tell your health care professional if you have any other types of allergies, such as to foods, dyes, preservatives, or animals. For non-prescription products, read the label or package ingredients carefully.

Pediatric—Although there is no specific information comparing use of clonidine in children with use in other age groups, this medicine is not expected to cause different side effects or problems in children than it does in adults. This medicine is usually used in children only when the pain is severe and other pain medicines did not help.

Geriatric—Many medicines have not been studied specifically in older people. Therefore, it may not be known whether they work exactly the same way they do in younger adults or if they cause different side effects or problems in older people. There is no specific information comparing use of clonidine in the elderly with use in other age groups.

Pregnancy—

	Pregnancy Category	Explanation
All Trimesters	C	Animal studies have shown an adverse effect and there are no adequate studies in pregnant women OR no animal studies have been conducted and there are no adequate studies in pregnant women.

Breast Feeding—Studies suggest that this medication may alter milk production or composition. If an alternative to this medication is not prescribed, you should monitor the infant for side effects and adequate milk intake.

Other medicines—
Using this medicine with any of the following medicines is usually not recommended, but may be required in some cases. If both medicines are prescribed together, your doctor may change the dose or how often you use one or both of the medicines.

Acebutolol, Amitriptyline, Amoxapine, Atenolol, Betaxolol, Bevantolol, Bisoprolol, Carteolol, Carvedilol, Celiprolol, Clomipramine, Desipramine, Dilevalol, Dothiepin, Doxepin, Imipramine, Labetalol, Levobunolol, Lofepramine, Metipranolol, Metoprolol, Mirtazapine, Nadolol, Nebivolol, Nortriptyline, Oxprenolol, Penbutolol, Pindolol, Propranolol, Protriptyline, Sotalol, Tertatolol, Timolol, Trimipramine

Interactions with Food/Tobacco/Alcohol—Certain medicines should not be used at or around the time of eating food or eating certain types of food since interactions may occur. Using alcohol or tobacco with certain medicines may also cause interactions to occur. Discuss with your healthcare professional the use of your medicine with food, alcohol, or tobacco.

Other medical problems—The presence of other medical problems may affect the use of this medicine. Make sure you tell your doctor if you have any other medical problems, especially:

- Anticoagulant therapy or
- Bleeding problems—Bleeding into the area around the spinal cord is possible
- Heart or blood vessel disease—Clonidine may make these conditions worse
- Infection at the place of injection or catheter (tube)—The risk of developing meningitis or an abscess is increased
- Kidney disease—Effects of clonidine may be increased because of slower removal of clonidine from the body
- Pain associated with surgery or
- Pain during or following childbirth—The ability to tolerate some of the potential side effects of clonidine may be decreased

Proper Use of This Medicine

Clonidine is given continuously as an epidural infusion (run around the spinal cord) using an infusion pump. The pump and its tube should be checked regularly to make sure the clonidine flow has not stopped accidentally. The injection or catheter site should also be checked regularly for signs of infection.

If you are using this medicine at home, make sure you understand exactly how to use it.

Dosing—The dose of this medicine will be different for different patients. Follow your doctor's orders or the directions on the label. The following information includes only the average doses of this medicine. If your dose is different, do not change it unless your doctor tells you to do so.

The amount of medicine that you take depends on the strength of the medicine. Also, the number of doses you take each day, the time allowed between doses, and the length of time you take the medicine depend on the medical problem for which you are using the medicine.

- For injection dosage form:
  - For pain:
    - Adults—30 mcg per hour given as a continuous infusion.

- Children—Dosage is based on body weight and must be determined by your doctor.

Missed dose—Call your doctor or pharmacist for instructions.

Tell your doctor immediately if you think the clonidine has stopped for any reason.

Storage—Store the medicine in a closed container at room temperature, away from heat, moisture, and direct light. Keep from freezing.

Keep out of the reach of children.

Do not keep outdated medicine or medicine no longer needed.

Precautions While Using This Medicine

This medicine should not be stopped without the doctor's supervision. Serious side effects may occur if clonidine is stopped suddenly.

This medicine may add to the effects of alcohol and other CNS depressants (medicine that may make you drowsy or less alert). Check with your doctor before taking any such depressants while you are using this medicine.

Dizziness, light-headedness, or fainting may occur, especially when you get up from a lying or sitting position. Getting up slowly may help.

This medicine may cause some people to become drowsy or less alert than they are normally. Make sure you know how you react to this medicine before you drive, use machines, or do other jobs that require you to be alert.

Side Effects of This Medicine

Along with its needed effects, a medicine may cause some unwanted effects. Although not all of these side effects may occur, if they do occur they may need medical attention.

Check with your doctor as soon as possible if any of the following side effects occur:
> *More common*
>> Dizziness, light-headedness, or fainting; slow heartbeat
> *Less common*
>> Chest pain; extremely shallow or slow breathing; fast heartbeat; fever; hallucinations (seeing, feeling, or hearing things that are not there); mental depression; sleepiness (excessive); vomiting

Some side effects may occur that usually do not need medical attention. These side effects may go away during treatment as your body adjusts to the medicine. Also, your health care professional may be able to tell you about ways to prevent or reduce some of these side effects. Check with your health care professional if any of the following side effects continue or are bothersome or if you have any questions about them:
> *More common*
>> Anxiety; confusion; dry mouth; nausea; sleepiness
> *Less common*
>> Constipation; ringing, buzzing, or other unexplained noises in the ears; sweating, unusual; weakness

After you stop using this medicine, it may still produce some side effects that need attention. During this period of time, *check with your doctor immediately* if you notice the following side effects:
> Agitation; headache; nervousness; pounding heartbeat; shaking or trembling

Other side effects not listed may also occur in some patients. If you notice any other effects, check with your healthcare professional.

CLONIDINE (Oral route, Transdermal route) - KLOE-ni-deen

Commonly used brand name(s)

In the U.S.—
Catapres
Catapres-TTS-1

Catapres-TTS-2
Catapres-TTS-3

Available Dosage Forms:
- Patch, Extended Release
- Tablet

Therapeutic Class: Antihypertensive
Pharmacologic Class: Alpha-2 Adrenergic Agonist

Uses For This Medicine

Clonidine belongs to the general class of medicines called antihypertensives. It is used to treat high blood pressure (hypertension).

High blood pressure adds to the work load of the heart and arteries. If it continues for a long time, the heart and arteries may not function properly. This can damage the blood vessels of the brain, heart, and kidneys, resulting in a stroke, heart failure, or kidney failure. Hypertension may also increase the risk of heart attacks. These problems may be less likely to occur if blood pressure is controlled.

Clonidine works by controlling nerve impulses along certain nerve pathways. As a result, it relaxes blood vessels so that blood passes through them more easily. This helps to lower blood pressure.

Clonidine may also be used for other conditions as determined by your doctor.

Clonidine is available only with your doctor's prescription.

Once a medicine has been approved for marketing for a certain use, experience may show that it is also useful for other medical problems. Although these uses are not included in product labeling, clonidine is used in certain patients with the following medical conditions:
- Migraine headache
- Symptoms associated with menopause or menstrual discomfort
- Symptoms of withdrawal associated with alcohol, nicotine, or narcotics
- Gilles de la Tourette's syndrome

Before Using This Medicine

In deciding to use a medicine, the risks of taking the medicine must be weighed against the good it will do. This is a decision you and your doctor will make. For this medicine, the following should be considered:

Allergies—Tell your doctor if you have ever had any unusual or allergic reaction to this medicine or any other medicines. Also tell your health care professional if you have any other types of allergies, such as to foods, dyes, preservatives,

or animals. For non-prescription products, read the label or package ingredients carefully.

Pediatric—Children may be more sensitive than adults to clonidine. Clonidine overdose has been reported when children accidentally took this medicine.

Geriatric—Dizziness or faintness may be more likely to occur in the elderly, who are more sensitive than younger adults to the effects of clonidine.

Pregnancy—

	Pregnancy Category	Explanation
All Trimesters	C	Animal studies have shown an adverse effect and there are no adequate studies in pregnant women OR no animal studies have been conducted and there are no adequate studies in pregnant women.

Breast Feeding—Studies suggest that this medication may alter milk production or composition. If an alternative to this medication is not prescribed, you should monitor the infant for side effects and adequate milk intake.

Other medicines—

Using this medicine with any of the following medicines is usually not recommended, but may be required in some cases. If both medicines are prescribed together, your doctor may change the dose or how often you use one or both of the medicines.

Acebutolol, Amitriptyline, Amoxapine, Atenolol, Betaxolol, Bevantolol, Bisoprolol, Carteolol, Carvedilol, Celiprolol, Clomipramine, Desipramine, Dilevalol, Dothiepin, Doxepin, Imipramine, Labetalol, Levobunolol, Lofepramine, Metipranolol, Metoprolol, Mirtazapine, Nadolol, Nebivolol, Nortriptyline, Oxprenolol, Penbutolol, Pindolol, Propranolol, Protriptyline, Sotalol, Tertatolol, Timolol, Trimipramine

Interactions with Food/Tobacco/Alcohol—Certain medicines should not be used at or around the time of eating food or eating certain types of food since interactions may occur. Using alcohol or tobacco with certain medicines may also cause interactions to occur. Discuss with your healthcare professional the use of your medicine with food, alcohol, or tobacco.

Other medical problems—The presence of other medical problems may affect the use of this medicine. Make sure you tell your doctor if you have any other medical problems, especially:
- Heart or blood vessel disease—Clonidine may make these conditions worse
- Irritated or scraped skin (with transdermal system [skin patch] only)—The effects of clonidine may be increased if the skin patch is placed on an area of scraped or irritated skin because more medicine is absorbed into the body
- Kidney disease—Effects of clonidine may be increased because of slower removal of clonidine from the body
- Mental depression (history of) or
- Raynaud's syndrome—Clonidine may make these conditions worse
- Polyarteritis nodosa or
- Scleroderma or

- Systemic lupus erythematosus (SLE) (with transdermal system [skin patch] only)—Effects of clonidine may be decreased because absorption of this medicine into the body is blocked

Proper Use of This Medicine

For patients taking this medicine for high blood pressure:

- In addition to the use of the medicine your doctor has prescribed, treatment for your high blood pressure may include weight control and care in the types of foods you eat, especially foods high in sodium. Your doctor will tell you which of these are most important for you. You should check with your doctor before changing your diet.
- Many patients who have high blood pressure will not notice any signs of the problem. In fact, many may feel normal. It is very important that you take your medicine exactly as directed and that you keep your appointments with your doctor even if you feel well.
- Remember that this medicine will not cure your high blood pressure but it does help control it. Therefore, you must continue to use it as directed if you expect to lower your blood pressure and keep it down. You may have to take high blood pressure medicine for the rest of your life. If high blood pressure is not treated, it can cause serious problems such as heart failure, blood vessel disease, stroke, or kidney disease.

For patients using the transdermal system (skin patch):

- Use this medicine exactly as directed by your doctor. It will work only if applied correctly. This medicine usually comes with patient instructions. Read them carefully before using.
- Do not try to trim or cut the adhesive patch to adjust the dosage. Check with your doctor if you think the medicine is not working as it should.
- Apply the patch to a clean, dry area of skin on your upper arm or chest. Choose an area with little or no hair and free of scars, cuts, or irritation.
- The system should stay in place even during showering, bathing, or swimming. If the patch becomes loose, cover it with the extra adhesive overlay provided. Apply a new patch if the first one becomes too loose or falls off.
- Each dose is best applied to a different area of skin to prevent skin problems or other irritation.
- After removing a used patch, fold the patch in half with the sticky sides together. Make sure to dispose of it out of the reach of children.

To help you remember to use your medicine, try to get into the habit of using it at regular times. If you are taking the tablets, take them at the same time each day. If you are using the transdermal system (skin patch), try to change it at the same time and day of the week.

Dosing—The dose of this medicine will be different for different patients. Follow your doctor's orders or the directions on the label. The following information includes only the average doses of this medicine. If your dose is different, do not change it unless your doctor tells you to do so.

The amount of medicine that you take depends on the strength of the medicine. Also, the number of doses you take each day, the time allowed between doses, and the length of time you take the medicine depend on the medical problem for which you are using the medicine.

- For oral dosage form (tablets):
  ○ For high blood pressure:
    ▪ Adults and teenagers—100 mcg (0.1 mg) two times a day. Your doctor may increase your dose up to 200 mcg (0.2 mg) to 600 mcg (0.6 mg) a day taken in divided doses.
    ▪ Children—Use and dose must be determined by your doctor.
- For transdermal dosage form (skin patch):
  ○ For high blood pressure:
    ▪ Adults—One transdermal dosage system (skin patch) applied once a week.
    ▪ Children—Use and dose must be determined by your doctor.

Missed dose—If you miss a dose of this medicine, take it as soon as possible. However, if it is almost time for your next dose, skip the missed dose and go back to your regular dosing schedule. Do not double doses.

If you miss two or more doses of the tablets in a row or if you miss changing the transdermal patch for 3 or more days, check with your doctor right away. If your body goes without this medicine for too long, your blood pressure may go up to a dangerously high level and some unpleasant effects may occur.

Storage—Store the medicine in a closed container at room temperature, away from heat, moisture, and direct light. Keep from freezing.

Keep out of the reach of children.

Do not keep outdated medicine or medicine no longer needed.

Precautions While Using This Medicine

It is important that your doctor check your progress at regular visits to make sure that this medicine is working properly.

Check with your doctor before you stop using this medicine. Your doctor may want you to reduce gradually the amount you are using before stopping completely.

Make sure that you have enough clonidine on hand to last through weekends, holidays, or vacations. You should not miss any doses. You may want to ask your doctor for another written prescription for clonidine to carry in your wallet or purse. You can then have it filled if you run out of medicine when you are away from home.

For patients taking this medicine for high blood pressure:

- Do not take other medicines unless they have been discussed with your doctor. This especially includes over-the-counter (nonprescription) medicines for appetite control, asthma, colds, cough, hay fever, or sinus problems, since they may tend to increase your blood pressure.

Clonidine will add to the effects of alcohol and other central nervous system (CNS) depressants (medicines that slow down the nervous system, possibly causing drowsiness). Some examples of CNS depressants are antihistamines or medicine for hay fever, other allergies, or colds; sedatives, tranquilizers, or sleeping medicine; prescription pain medicine or narcotics; barbiturates; medicine for seizures; muscle relaxants; or anesthetics, including some dental anesthetics. Check with your doctor before taking any of the above while you are using this medicine.

Clonidine may cause some people to become drowsy or less alert than they are normally. This is more likely to happen when you begin to take it or when you increase the amount of medicine you are taking. Make sure you know how you react to this medicine before you drive, use machines, or do anything else that could be dangerous if you are not alert.

Before having any kind of surgery (including dental surgery) or emergency treatment, tell the medical doctor or dentist in charge that you are using this medicine.

Dizziness, lightheadedness, or fainting may occur after you take this medicine, especially when you get up from a lying or sitting position. Getting up slowly may help, but if the problem continues or gets worse, check with your doctor.

The dizziness, lightheadedness, or fainting is also more likely to occur if you drink alcohol, stand for long periods of time, exercise, or if the weather is hot. While you are taking clonidine, be careful to limit the amount of alcohol you drink. Also, use extra care during exercise or hot weather or if you must stand for a long time.

Clonidine may cause dryness of the mouth. For temporary relief, use sugarless candy or gum, melt bits of ice in your mouth, or use a saliva substitute. However, if your mouth continues to feel dry for more than 2 weeks, check with your medical doctor or dentist. Continuing dryness of the mouth may increase the chance of dental disease, including tooth decay, gum disease, and fungus infections.

Side Effects of This Medicine

Along with its needed effects, a medicine may cause some unwanted effects. Although not all of these side effects may occur, if they do occur they may need medical attention.

Check with your doctor immediately if any of the following side effects occur:
Signs and symptoms of overdose
  Difficulty in breathing; dizziness (extreme) or faintness; feeling cold; pinpoint pupils of eyes; slow heartbeat; unusual tiredness or weakness (extreme)

Check with your doctor as soon as possible if any of the following side effects occur:
More common—with transdermal system (skin patch) only
  Itching or redness of skin
Less common
  Mental depression; swelling of feet and lower legs
Rare
  Paleness or cold feeling in fingertips and toes; vivid dreams or nightmares

Some side effects may occur that usually do not need medical attention. These side effects may go away during treatment as your body adjusts to the medicine. Also, your health care professional may be able to tell you about ways to prevent or reduce some of these side effects. Check with your health care professional if any of the following side effects continue or are bothersome or if you have any questions about them:
More common
  Constipation; dizziness; drowsiness; dryness of mouth; unusual tiredness or weakness
Less common
  Darkening of skin— with transdermal system (skin patch) only; decreased sexual ability; dizziness, light-

headedness, or fainting, especially when getting up from a lying or sitting position; dry, itching, or burning eyes; loss of appetite; nausea or vomiting; nervousness

After you stop using this medicine, it may still produce some side effects that need attention. During this period of time, *check with your doctor immediately* if you notice the following side effects:

  Anxiety or tenseness; chest pain; fast or pounding heartbeat; headache; increased salivation; nausea; nervousness; restlessness; shaking or trembling of hands and fingers; stomach cramps; sweating; trouble in sleeping; vomiting

Other side effects not listed may also occur in some patients. If you notice any other effects, check with your healthcare professional.

CLONIDINE AND CHLORTHALIDONE (Oral route) -
KLOE-ni-deen, klor-THAL-i-doan

Commonly used brand name(s)

In the U.S.—
  Clorpres

Available Dosage Forms:
  • Tablet

Therapeutic Class: Alpha-Adrenergic Agonist/Thiazide Combination
Pharmacologic Class: Clonidine

Uses For This Medicine

Clonidine and chlorthalidone combinations are used in the treatment of high blood pressure (hypertension).

High blood pressure adds to the work load of the heart and arteries. If it continues for a long time, the heart and arteries may not function properly. This can damage the blood vessels of the brain, heart, and kidneys resulting in a stroke, heart failure, or kidney failure. Hypertension may also increase the risk of heart attacks. These problems may be less likely to occur if blood pressure is controlled.

Clonidine works by controlling nerve impulses along certain body nerve pathways. As a result, it relaxes blood vessels so that blood passes through them more easily. The chlorthalidone in this combination is a diuretic (water pill) that helps reduce the amount of water in the body by increasing the flow of urine.

Clonidine and chlorthalidone combination is available only with your doctor's prescription.

Before Using This Medicine

In deciding to use a medicine, the risks of taking the medicine must be weighed against the good it will do. This is a decision

you and your doctor will make. For this medicine, the following should be considered:

Allergies—Tell your doctor if you have ever had any unusual or allergic reaction to this medicine or any other medicines. Also tell your health care professional if you have any other types of allergies, such as to foods, dyes, preservatives, or animals. For non-prescription products, read the label or package ingredients carefully.

Pediatric—Studies on this medicine have been done only in adult patients, and there is no specific information comparing use of clonidine and chlorthalidone combination in children with use in other age groups. However, children may be more sensitive than adults to clonidine. Clonidine overdose has been reported when children accidentally took this medicine.

Geriatric—Dizziness or lightheadedness and signs of too much potassium loss may be more likely to occur in the elderly, who are more sensitive to the effects of clonidine and chlorthalidone.

Other medicines—

Using this medicine with any of the following medicines is usually not recommended, but may be required in some cases. If both medicines are prescribed together, your doctor may change the dose or how often you use one or both of the medicines.

Acebutolol, Acetyldigoxin, Amitriptyline, Amoxapine, Arsenic Trioxide, Atenolol, Bepridil, Betaxolol, Bevantolol, Bisoprolol, Carteolol, Carvedilol, Celiprolol, Clomipramine, Desipramine, Deslanoside, Digitalis, Digitoxin, Digoxin, Dilevalol, Dofetilide, Dothiepin, Doxepin, Droperidol, Imipramine, Ketanserin, Labetalol, Levobunolol, Levomethadyl, Lithium, Lofepramine, Metildigoxin, Metipranolol, Metoprolol, Mirtazapine, Nadolol, Nebivolol, Nortriptyline, Oxprenolol, Penbutolol, Pindolol, Propranolol, Protriptyline, Sotalol, Tertatolol, Timolol, Trimipramine

Interactions with Food/Tobacco/Alcohol—Certain medicines should not be used at or around the time of eating food or eating certain types of food since interactions may occur. Using alcohol or tobacco with certain medicines may also cause interactions to occur. Discuss with your healthcare professional the use of your medicine with food, alcohol, or tobacco.

Other medical problems—The presence of other medical problems may affect the use of this medicine. Make sure you tell your doctor if you have any other medical problems, especially:

- Type 2 diabetes mellitus—This medicine may change the amount of diabetes medicine needed
- Gout—This medicine may increase the amount of uric acid in the blood, which can lead to gout
- Heart or blood vessel disease or
- Lupus erythematosus (history of) or
- Mental depression (history of) or
- Pancreatitis (inflammation of the pancreas) or
- Raynaud's syndrome—This medicine may make these conditions worse
- Kidney disease—Effects of this medicine may be increased because of slower removal from the body. If kidney disease is severe, the chlorthalidone portion of this medicine may not work

- Liver disease—If this medicine causes loss of too much water from the body, liver disease can become much worse

Proper Use of This Medicine

This medicine may cause you to have an unusual feeling of tiredness when you begin to take it. You may also notice an increase in the amount of urine or in your frequency of urination. After taking the medicine for a while, these effects should lessen. It is best to plan your doses according to a schedule that will least affect your personal activities and sleep. Ask your health care professional to help you plan the best time to take this medicine.

In addition to the use of the medicine your doctor has prescribed, appropriate treatment for your high blood pressure may include weight control and care in the types of foods you eat, especially foods high in sodium. Your doctor will tell you which factors are most important for you. You should check with your doctor before changing your diet.

Many patients who have high blood pressure will not notice any signs of the problem. In fact, many may feel normal. It is very important that you take your medicine exactly as directed and that you keep your appointments with your doctor even if you feel well.

Remember that this medicine will not cure your high blood pressure but it does help control it. Therefore, you must continue to take it as directed if you expect to lower your blood pressure and keep it down. You may have to take high blood pressure medicine for the rest of your life. If high blood pressure is not treated, it can cause serious problems such as heart failure, blood vessel disease, stroke, or kidney disease.

To help you remember to take your medicine, try to get into the habit of taking it at the same time each day.

Dosing—The dose of this medicine will be different for different patients. Follow your doctor's orders or the directions on the label. The following information includes only the average doses of this medicine. If your dose is different, do not change it unless your doctor tells you to do so.

The amount of medicine that you take depends on the strength of the medicine. Also, the number of doses you take each day, the time allowed between doses, and the length of time you take the medicine depend on the medical problem for which you are using the medicine.

- For oral dosage form (tablets):
  - For high blood pressure:
    - Adults—1 tablet one or two times a day.
    - Children—Use and dose must be determined by your doctor.

Missed dose—If you miss a dose of this medicine, take it as soon as possible. However, if it is almost time for your next dose, skip the missed dose and go back to your regular dosing schedule. Do not double doses.

If you miss two or more doses in a row, check with your doctor right away. If your body goes without this medicine for too long, your blood pressure may go up to a dangerously high level and some unpleasant effects may occur.

Storage—Store the medicine in a closed container at room temperature, away from heat, moisture, and direct light. Keep from freezing.

Keep out of the reach of children.

Do not keep outdated medicine or medicine no longer needed.

Precautions While Using This Medicine

It is important that your doctor check your progress at regular visits to make sure that this medicine is working properly.

Check with your doctor before you stop taking this medicine. Your doctor may want you to reduce gradually the amount you are taking before stopping the medicine completely.

Make sure that you have enough medicine on hand to last through weekends, holidays, or vacations. You should not miss taking any doses. You may want to ask your doctor for another written prescription to carry in your wallet or purse. You can then have it filled if you run out of medicine when you are away from home.

Before having any kind of surgery (including dental surgery) or emergency treatment, make sure the medical doctor or dentist in charge knows that you are taking this medicine.

Do not take other medicines unless they have been discussed with your doctor. This especially includes over-the-counter (nonprescription) medicines for appetite control, asthma, colds, cough, hay fever, or sinus problems, since they may tend to increase your blood pressure.

This medicine will add to the effects of alcohol and other central nervous system (CNS) depressants (medicines that slow down the nervous system, possibly causing drowsiness). Some examples of CNS depressants are antihistamines or medicine for hay fever, other allergies, or colds; sedatives, tranquilizers, or sleeping medicine; prescription pain medicine or narcotics; barbiturates; medicine for seizures; muscle relaxants; or anesthetics, including some dental anesthetics. Check with your doctor before taking any of the above while you are using this medicine.

This medicine may cause some people to become drowsy or less alert than they are normally. This is more likely to happen when you begin to take it or when you increase the amount of medicine you are taking. Make sure you know how you react to this medicine before you drive, use machines, or do anything else that could be dangerous if you are not alert.

Dizziness, lightheadedness, or fainting may occur, especially when you get up from a lying or sitting position. Getting up slowly may help, but if the problem continues or gets worse, check with your doctor.

The dizziness, lightheadedness, or fainting is also more likely to occur if you drink alcohol, stand for long periods of time, exercise, or if the weather is hot. Drinking alcoholic beverages may also make the drowsiness worse. While you are taking this medicine, be careful to limit the amount of alcohol you drink. Also, use extra care during exercise or hot weather or if you must stand for long periods of time.

This medicine may cause a loss of potassium from your body.
- To help prevent this, your doctor may want you to:
  - eat or drink foods that have a high potassium content (for example, orange or other citrus fruit juices), or
  - take a potassium supplement, or
  - take another medicine to help prevent the loss of the potassium in the first place.
- It is very important to follow these directions. Also, it is important not to change your diet on your own. This is more important if you are already on a special diet (as for diabetes), or if you are taking a potassium supple-

ment or a medicine to reduce potassium loss. Extra potassium may not be necessary and, in some cases, too much potassium could be harmful.

Check with your doctor if you become sick and have severe or continuing vomiting or diarrhea. These problems may cause you to lose additional water and potassium.

For patients with diabetes:
- The chlorthalidone contained in this medicine may raise blood sugar levels. While you are using this medicine, be sure to test your blood sugar (glucose) level, or test for sugar in your urine.

This medicine may cause your skin to be more sensitive to sunlight than it is normally. Exposure to sunlight, even for brief periods of time, may cause a skin rash, itching, redness or other discoloration of the skin, or a severe sunburn. When you begin taking this medicine:
- Stay out of direct sunlight, especially between the hours of 10:00 a.m. and 3:00 p.m., if possible.
- Wear protective clothing, including a hat. Also, wear sunglasses.
- Apply a sun block product that has a skin protection factor (SPF) of at least 15. Some patients may require a product with a higher SPF number, especially if they have a fair complexion. If you have any questions about this, check with your health care professional.
- Apply a sun block for lips that has an SPF of at least 15 to protect your lips.
- Do not use a sunlamp or tanning bed or booth.

If you have a severe reaction from the sun, check with your doctor.

This medicine may cause dryness of the mouth. For temporary relief, use sugarless candy or gum, melt bits of ice in your mouth, or use a saliva substitute. However, if your mouth continues to feel dry for more than 2 weeks, check with your medical doctor or dentist. Continuing dryness of the mouth may increase the chance of dental disease, including tooth decay, gum disease, and fungus infections.

Side Effects of This Medicine

Along with its needed effects, a medicine may cause some unwanted effects. Although not all of these side effects may occur, if they do occur they may need medical attention.

Check with your doctor immediately if any of the following side effects occur:
Signs and symptoms of overdose
Difficulty in breathing; dizziness (extreme) or faintness; feeling cold; pinpoint pupils of eyes; slow heartbeat; unusual tiredness or weakness (extreme)

Check with your doctor as soon as possible if any of the following side effects occur:
Signs and symptoms of too much potassium loss
Dryness of mouth; increased thirst; irregular heartbeat; mood or mental changes; muscle cramps or pain; nausea or vomiting; weak pulse
Signs and symptoms of too much sodium loss
Confusion; convulsions (seizures); decreased mental activity; irritability; muscle cramps; unusual tiredness or weakness
Less common
Mental depression; swelling of feet and lower legs

Rare

Black, tarry stools; blood in urine or stools; cough or hoarseness; fever or chills; joint pain; lower back or side pain; paleness or cold feeling in fingertips and toes; pinpoint red spots on skin; skin rash or hives; stomach pain (severe) with nausea and vomiting; unusual bleeding or bruising; vivid dreams or nightmares; yellow eyes or skin

Some side effects may occur that usually do not need medical attention. These side effects may go away during treatment as your body adjusts to the medicine. Also, your health care professional may be able to tell you about ways to prevent or reduce some of these side effects. Check with your health care professional if any of the following side effects continue or are bothersome or if you have any questions about them:

More common

Constipation; dizziness; drowsiness; dryness of mouth; unusual tiredness or weakness

Less common

Decreased sexual ability; diarrhea; dizziness or light-headedness when getting up from a lying or sitting position; dry, itching, or burning eyes; increased sensitivity of skin to sunlight; loss of appetite; nausea or vomiting; nervousness; upset stomach

After you stop using this medicine, it may still produce some side effects that need attention. During this period of time, *check with your doctor immediately* if you notice the following side effects:

Anxiety or tenseness; chest pain; fast or pounding heartbeat; headache; increased salivation; nausea; nervousness; restlessness; shaking or trembling of hands and fingers; stomach cramps; sweating; trouble in sleeping; vomiting

Other side effects not listed may also occur in some patients. If you notice any other effects, check with your healthcare professional.

CLOPIDOGREL (Oral route) - kloh-PID-oh-grel

Commonly used brand name(s)

In the U.S.—
Plavix

Available Dosage Forms:
• Tablet

Therapeutic Class: Platelet Aggregation Inhibitor
Pharmacologic Class: ADP-Induced Aggregation Inhibitor

Uses For This Medicine

Clopidogrel is used to lessen the chance of heart attack or stroke. It is given to people who have already had a heart attack or stroke or to people with other blood circulation problems that could lead to a stroke or heart attack.

A heart attack or stroke may occur when a blood vessel in the heart or brain is blocked by a blood clot. Clopidogrel reduces the chance that a harmful blood clot will form by preventing certain cells in the blood from clumping together. This effect of clopidogrel may also increase the chance of serious bleeding in some people.

This medicine is available only with your doctor's prescription.

Before Using This Medicine

In deciding to use a medicine, the risks of taking the medicine must be weighed against the good it will do. This is a decision you and your doctor will make. For this medicine, the following should be considered:

Allergies—Tell your doctor if you have ever had any unusual or allergic reaction to this medicine or any other medicines. Also tell your health care professional if you have any other types of allergies, such as to foods, dyes, preservatives, or animals. For non-prescription products, read the label or package ingredients carefully.

Pediatric—There is no specific information comparing use of clopidogrel in children with use in other age groups.

Geriatric—Although blood levels of clopidogrel may be higher in elderly patients than in younger adults, it is not expected to cause different side effects or problems in older people than it does in other adults.

Pregnancy—

	Pregnancy Category	Explanation
All Trimesters	B	Animal studies have revealed no evidence of harm to the fetus, however, there are no adequate studies in pregnant women OR animal studies have shown an adverse effect, but adequate studies in pregnant women have failed to demonstrate a risk to the fetus.

Breast Feeding—There are no adequate studies in women for determining infant risk when using this medication during breastfeeding. Weigh the potential benefits against the potential risks before taking this medication while breastfeeding.

Other medicines—

Using this medicine with any of the following medicines is usually not recommended, but may be required in some cases. If both medicines are prescribed together, your doctor may change the dose or how often you use one or both of the medicines.

Abciximab, Acenocoumarol, Alteplase, Recombinant, Anisindione, Anistreplase, Ardeparin, Argatroban, Bivalirudin, Certoparin, Cilostazol, Clopidogrel, Dalteparin, Danaparoid, Defibrotide, Dermatan Sulfate, Desirudin, Dicumarol, Enoxaparin, Eptifibatide, Fondaparinux, Ginkgo, Heparin, Lamifiban, Nadroparin, Parnaparin, Phenindione, Phenprocoumon, Reteplase, Recombinant, Reviparin, Sibrafiban, Streptokinase, Tenecteplase, Tinzaparin, Tirofiban, Urokinase, Warfarin, Xemilofiban

Interactions with Food/Tobacco/Alcohol—Certain medicines should not be used at or around the time of eating food or eating certain types of food since interactions may occur. Using alcohol or tobacco with certain medicines may also cause interactions to occur. Discuss with your healthcare professional the use of your medicine with food, alcohol, or tobacco.

Other medical problems—The presence of other medical problems may affect the use of this medicine. Make sure you tell your doctor if you have any other medical problems, especially:

- Bleeding problems or
- Liver disease (severe) or
- Stomach ulcers—The chance of serious bleeding may be increased

Proper Use of This Medicine

Take this medicine only as directed by your doctor. Clopidogrel will not work properly if you take less of it than directed. Taking more clopidogrel than directed may increase the chance of serious side effects without increasing the helpful effects.

Dosing—The dose of this medicine will be different for different patients. Follow your doctor's orders or the directions on the label. The following information includes only the average doses of this medicine. If your dose is different, do not change it unless your doctor tells you to do so.

The amount of medicine that you take depends on the strength of the medicine. Also, the number of doses you take each day, the time allowed between doses, and the length of time you take the medicine depend on the medical problem for which you are using the medicine.

- For oral dosage form (tablets):
  - For prevention of heart attacks or strokes:
    - Adults—1 tablet (75 milligrams [mg]) once a day.
    - Children—It is not likely that clopidogrel would be used to help prevent heart attacks or strokes in children. If a child needs this medicine, however, the dose would have to be determined by the doctor.

Missed dose—If you miss a dose of this medicine, take it as soon as possible. However, if it is almost time for your next dose, skip the missed dose and go back to your regular dosing schedule. Do not double doses.

Storage—Store the medicine in a closed container at room temperature, away from heat, moisture, and direct light. Keep from freezing.

Keep out of the reach of children.

Do not keep outdated medicine or medicine no longer needed.

Precautions While Using This Medicine

Tell all medical doctors, dentists, nurses, and pharmacists you go to that you are taking this medicine. Clopidogrel may increase the risk of serious bleeding during an operation or some kinds of dental work. Therefore, treatment may have to be stopped about 7 days before the operation or dental work is done.

Check with your doctor immediately if you notice bruising or bleeding, especially bleeding that is hard to stop. Bleeding inside the body sometimes appears as bloody or black, tarry stools, or faintness.

Side Effects of This Medicine

Along with its needed effects, a medicine may cause some unwanted effects. Although not all of these side effects may occur, if they do occur they may need medical attention.

Check with your doctor immediately if any of the following side effects occur:
  More common
    Red or purple spots on skin, varying in size from pinpoint to large bruises
  Less common
    Nosebleed; vomiting of blood or material that looks like coffee grounds
  Rare
    Black, tarry stools; blistering, flaking, or peeling of skin; blood in urine or stools; fever, chills, or sore throat; headache (sudden, severe); stomach pain (severe); ulcers, sores, or white spots in mouth; unusual bleeding or bruising; weakness (sudden)

Check with your doctor as soon as possible if any of the following side effects occur:
  More common
    Chest pain; cough; generalized pain; runny nose; sneezing
  Less common
    Fainting; frequent urination; irregular heartbeat; joint pain; painful or difficult urination; shortness of breath; swelling of feet or lower legs

Some side effects may occur that usually do not need medical attention. These side effects may go away during treatment as your body adjusts to the medicine. Also, your health care professional may be able to tell you about ways to prevent or reduce some of these side effects. Check with your health care professional if any of the following side effects continue or are bothersome or if you have any questions about them:
  More common
    Abdominal or stomach pain (mild); aching muscles; back pain; dizziness; general feeling of discomfort or illness; headache; heartburn
  Less common
    Anxiety; constipation; diarrhea; itching; leg cramps; mental depression; numbness or tingling; nausea; skin rash; trouble in sleeping; unusual tiredness; vomiting; weakness

Other side effects not listed may also occur in some patients. If you notice any other effects, check with your healthcare professional.

CLOTRIMAZOLE (Mucous membrane, oral route) - kloe-TRIM-a-zole

Commonly used brand name(s)
In the U.S.—
  Mycelex Troche

Available Dosage Forms:
- Lozenge/Troche

Therapeutic Class: Antifungal

Uses For This Medicine

Clotrimazole lozenges are dissolved slowly in the mouth to prevent and treat thrush. Thrush, also called candidiasis or white mouth, is a fungus infection of the mouth and throat.

This medicine may also be used for other problems as determined by your doctor.

Clotrimazole is available only with your doctor's prescription.

Before Using This Medicine

In deciding to use a medicine, the risks of taking the medicine must be weighed against the good it will do. This is a decision you and your doctor will make. For this medicine, the following should be considered:

Allergies—Tell your doctor if you have ever had any unusual or allergic reaction to this medicine or any other medicines. Also tell your health care professional if you have any other types of allergies, such as to foods, dyes, preservatives, or animals. For non-prescription products, read the label or package ingredients carefully.

Pediatric—Although this medicine has not been shown to cause different side effects or problems in children than it does in adults, it should not be given to children under 3 years of age since they may be too young to use the lozenges safely.

Geriatric—Many medicines have not been studied specifically in older people. Therefore, it may not be known whether they work exactly the same way they do in younger adults. Although there is no specific information comparing use of clotrimazole lozenges in the elderly with use in other age groups, this medicine is not expected to cause different side effects or problems in older people than it does in younger adults.

Pregnancy—

	Pregnancy Category	Explanation
All Trimesters	C	Animal studies have shown an adverse effect and there are no adequate studies in pregnant women OR no animal studies have been conducted and there are no adequate studies in pregnant women.

Breast Feeding—There are no adequate studies in women for determining infant risk when using this medication during breastfeeding. Weigh the potential benefits against the potential risks before taking this medication while breastfeeding.

Other medicines—

Using this medicine with any of the following medicines is not recommended. Your doctor may decide not to treat you with this medication or change some of the other medicines you take.

Dihydroergotamine, Ergoloid Mesylates, Ergonovine, Ergotamine, Methylergonovine

Interactions with Food/Tobacco/Alcohol—Certain medicines should not be used at or around the time of eating food or eating certain types of food since interactions may occur. Using alcohol or tobacco with certain medicines may also cause interactions to occur. Discuss with your healthcare professional the use of your medicine with food, alcohol, or tobacco.

Other medical problems—The presence of other medical problems may affect the use of this medicine. Make sure you tell your doctor if you have any other medical problems, especially:

The presence of other medical problems may affect the use of clotrimazole. Make sure you tell your doctor if you have the following medical condition:

- Liver disease—Your doctor may want to monitor your liver function while you are taking this medicine.

Proper Use of This Medicine

Clotrimazole lozenges should be held in the mouth and allowed to dissolve slowly and completely. This may take 15 to 30 minutes. Swallow saliva during this time. Do not chew the lozenges or swallow them whole.

Do not give clotrimazole lozenges to infants or children under 3 years of age. They may be too young to use the lozenges safely.

To help clear up your infection completely, it is very important that you keep using clotrimazole for the full time of treatment, even if your symptoms begin to clear up after a few days. Since fungus infections may be very slow to clear up, you may have to continue using this medicine every day for two weeks or more. If you stop using this medicine too soon, your symptoms may return. Do not miss any doses.

Dosing—The dose of this medicine will be different for different patients. Follow your doctor's orders or the directions on the label. The following information includes only the average doses of this medicine. If your dose is different, do not change it unless your doctor tells you to do so.

The amount of medicine that you take depends on the strength of the medicine. Also, the number of doses you take each day, the time allowed between doses, and the length of time you take the medicine depend on the medical problem for which you are using the medicine.

- For the treatment of thrush:
  - Adults and children 3 years of age and older: Dissolve one 10–milligram lozenge slowly and completely in your mouth; this dose should be taken five times a day for at least fourteen days.
  - Children up to 3 years of age: This medicine is not recommended in children under 3 years of age since they may be too young to use the lozenges safely.

- For the prevention of thrush:
  - Adults and children 3 years of age and older: Dissolve one 10–milligram lozenge slowly and completely in your mouth; this dose should be taken three times a day.
  - Children up to 3 years of age: This medicine is not recommended in children under 3 years of age since they may be too young to use the lozenges safely.

Missed dose—If you miss a dose of this medicine, take it as soon as possible. However, if it is almost time for your next dose, skip the missed dose and go back to your regular dosing schedule. Do not double doses.

Storage—Store the medicine in a closed container at room temperature, away from heat, moisture, and direct light. Keep from freezing.

Keep out of the reach of children.

Do not keep outdated medicine or medicine no longer needed.

Precautions While Using This Medicine

If your symptoms do not improve within 1 week, or if they become worse, check with your doctor.

Side Effects of This Medicine

Along with its needed effects, a medicine may cause some unwanted effects. Although not all of these side effects may occur, if they do occur they may need medical attention.

Some side effects may occur that usually do not need medical attention. These side effects may go away during treatment as your body adjusts to the medicine. Also, your health care professional may be able to tell you about ways to prevent or reduce some of these side effects. Check with your health care professional if any of the following side effects continue or are bothersome or if you have any questions about them:

More common

Abdominal or stomach cramping or pain; diarrhea; itching; nausea or vomiting; unpleasant mouth sensations

Note: Some of the side effects, such as abdominal or stomach cramping or pain or diarrhea, usually occur only when the medicine is swallowed

Other side effects not listed may also occur in some patients. If you notice any other effects, check with your healthcare professional.

CLOTRIMAZOLE (Topical route) -
kloe-TRIM-a-zole

Commonly used brand name(s)

In the U.S.—

Clotrim Antifungal   Lotrimin AF
Cruex Prescription Strength   Mycelex
Lotrimin

In Canada—

Canesten   Myclo-Derm
Clotrimaderm   Neo-Zol
Desenex

Available Dosage Forms:

• Cream
• Solution
• Lotion

Therapeutic Class: Antifungal

Uses For This Medicine

Clotrimazole topical preparations are used to treat fungus infections.

Some of these preparations are available only with your doctor's prescription.

Before Using This Medicine

In deciding to use a medicine, the risks of taking the medicine must be weighed against the good it will do. This is a decision you and your doctor will make. For this medicine, the following should be considered:

Allergies—Tell your doctor if you have ever had any unusual or allergic reaction to this medicine or any other medicines. Also tell your health care professional if you have any other types of allergies, such as to foods, dyes, preservatives, or animals. For non-prescription products, read the label or package ingredients carefully.

Pediatric—This medicine has been tested in children and, in effective doses, has not been shown to cause different side effects or problems than it does in adults.

Geriatric—Many medicines have not been studied specifically in older people. Therefore, it may not be known whether they work exactly the same way they do in younger adults. Although there is no specific information comparing use of topical clotrimazole in the elderly with use in other age groups, this medicine is not expected to cause different side effects or problems in older people than it does in younger adults.

Pregnancy—

	Pregnancy Category	Explanation
All Trimesters	C	Animal studies have shown an adverse effect and there are no adequate studies in pregnant women OR no animal studies have been conducted and there are no adequate studies in pregnant women.

Breast Feeding—There are no adequate studies in women for determining infant risk when using this medication during breastfeeding. Weigh the potential benefits against the potential risks before taking this medication while breastfeeding.

Other medicines—

Using this medicine with any of the following medicines is not recommended. Your doctor may decide not to treat you with this medication or change some of the other medicines you take.

Dihydroergotamine, Ergoloid Mesylates, Ergonovine, Ergotamine, Methylergonovine

Interactions with Food/Tobacco/Alcohol—Certain medicines should not be used at or around the time of eating food or eating certain types of food since interactions may occur. Using alcohol or tobacco with certain medicines may also cause interactions to occur. Discuss with your healthcare professional the use of your medicine with food, alcohol, or tobacco.

Proper Use of This Medicine

Apply enough clotrimazole to cover the affected and surrounding skin areas, and rub in gently.

Keep this medicine away from the eyes.

When clotrimazole is used to treat certain types of fungus infections of the skin, an occlusive dressing (airtight covering, such as kitchen plastic wrap) should not be applied over the medicine. To do so may cause irritation of the skin. Do not apply an occlusive dressing over this medicine unless you have been directed to do so by your doctor.

To help clear up your infection completely, it is very important that you keep using this medicine for the full time of treatment, even if your symptoms begin to clear up after a few days. Since fungus infections may be very slow to clear up, you may have to continue using this medicine every day for several weeks or more. If you stop using this medicine too soon, your symptoms may return. Do not miss any doses.

Dosing—The dose of this medicine will be different for different patients. Follow your doctor's orders or the directions on the label. The following information includes only the average doses of this medicine. If your dose is different, do not change it unless your doctor tells you to do so.

The amount of medicine that you take depends on the strength of the medicine. Also, the number of doses you take each day, the time allowed between doses, and the length of time you take the medicine depend on the medical problem for which you are using the medicine.

- For topical dosage forms (cream, lotion, and solution):
  - Fungal infections (treatment):
    - Adults and children—Use two times a day, morning and evening.

Missed dose—If you miss a dose of this medicine, apply it as soon as possible. However, if it is almost time for your next dose, skip the missed dose and go back to your regular dosing schedule.

Storage—Store the medicine in a closed container at room temperature, away from heat, moisture, and direct light. Keep from freezing.

Keep out of the reach of children.

Do not keep outdated medicine or medicine no longer needed.

Precautions While Using This Medicine

If your skin problem does not improve within 4 weeks, or if it becomes worse, check with your doctor.

Side Effects of This Medicine

Along with its needed effects, a medicine may cause some unwanted effects. Although not all of these side effects may occur, if they do occur they may need medical attention.

Check with your doctor as soon as possible if any of the following side effects occur:

Skin rash, hives, blistering, burning, itching, peeling, redness, stinging, swelling, or other sign of skin irritation not present before use of this medicine

Other side effects not listed may also occur in some patients. If you notice any other effects, check with your healthcare professional.

CLOZAPINE (Oral route) - KLOE-za-peen

Black Box Warning

- Agranulocytosis
  - Clozaril(R):
    - Because of a significant risk of agranulocytosis, a potentially life-threatening adverse event, Clozaril(R) should be reserved for use in (1) the treat-ment of severely ill patients with schizophrenia who fail to show an acceptable response to adequate courses of standard antipsychotic drug treatment, or (2) for reducing the risk of recurrent suicidal behavior in patients with schizophrenia or schizoaffective disorder who are judged to be at risk of reexperiencing suicidal behavior.
  - FazaClo(R):
    - Because of a significant risk of agranulocytosis, a potentially life-threatening adverse event, FazaClo(R) should be reserved for use in the treatment of severely ill patients with schizophrenia who fail to show an acceptable response to adequate courses of standard antipsychotic drug treatment.
  - Patients being treated with clozapine must have a baseline white blood cell (WBC) count and absolute neutrophil count (ANC) before initiation of treatment as well as regular WBC counts and ANCs during treatment and for at least 4 weeks after discontinuation of treatment.
  - Clozapine is available only through a distribution system that ensures monitoring of WBC count and ANC according to the schedule described below prior to delivery of the next supply of medication.
- Seizures
  - Seizures have been associated with the use of clozapine. Dose appears to be an important predictor of seizure, with a greater likelihood at higher clozapine doses. Caution should be used when administering clozapine to patients having a history of seizures or other predisposing factors. Patients should be advised not to engage in any activity where sudden loss of consciousness could cause serious risk to themselves or others.
- Myocarditis
  - Analyses of post-marketing safety databases suggest that clozapine is associated with an increased risk of fatal myocarditis, especially during, but not limited to, the first month of therapy. In patients in whom myocarditis is suspected, clozapine treatment should be promptly discontinued.
- Other Adverse Cardiovascular and Respiratory Effects
  - Orthostatic hypotension, with or without syncope, can occur with clozapine treatment. Rarely, collapse can be profound and be accompanied by respiratory and/or cardiac arrest. Orthostatic hypotension is more likely to occur during initial titration in association with rapid dose escalation. In patients who have had even a brief interval off clozapine, i.e., 2 or more days since the last dose, treatment should be started with 12.5 mg once or twice daily.
  - Since collapse, respiratory arrest and cardiac arrest during initial treatment has occurred in patients who were being administered benzodiazepines or other psychotropic drugs, caution is advised when clozapine is initiated in patients taking a benzodiazepine or any other psychotropic drug.
- Increased Mortality in Elderly Patients with Dementia-related Psychosis
  - Elderly patients with dementia-related psychosis treated with atypical antipsychotic drugs are at an increased risk of death compared to placebo. Analysis of seventeen placebo-controlled trials (modal duration of 10 weeks) in these patients revealed a risk of

death in the drug-treated patients of between 1.6 to 1.7 times that seen in placebo-treated patients. Over the course of a typical 10–week controlled trial, the rate of death in drug-treated patients was about 4.5%, compared to a rate of about 2.6% in the placebo group. Although the causes of death were varied, most of the deaths appeared to be either cardiovascular (e.g., heart failure, sudden death) or infectious (e.g., pneumonia) in nature. Clozapine is not approved for the treatment of patients with dementia-related psychosis.

Commonly used brand name(s)

In the U.S.—
　Clozaril
　FazaClo

Available Dosage Forms:

- Tablet, Disintegrating
- Tablet

Therapeutic Class: Antipsychotic

Uses For This Medicine

Clozapine is used to treat schizophrenia in patients who have not been helped by or are unable to take other medicines. This medicine should NOT be used to treat behavioral problems in older adult patients who have dementia.

Clozapine is available only from pharmacies that agree to participate with your doctor in a plan to monitor your blood tests. You will need to have blood tests done every week for at least 6 months. After that, your doctor will decide if it is safe for you to have blood tests every other week. You will receive enough clozapine to last until your next blood test, but only if the results of your blood tests show that it is safe for you to take this medicine. If any of your blood tests are not normal, you may need to have blood tests more often than every week until they return to normal.

Before Using This Medicine

In deciding to use a medicine, the risks of taking the medicine must be weighed against the good it will do. This is a decision you and your doctor will make. For this medicine, the following should be considered:

Allergies—Tell your doctor if you have ever had any unusual or allergic reaction to this medicine or any other medicines. Also tell your health care professional if you have any other types of allergies, such as to foods, dyes, preservatives, or animals. For non-prescription products, read the label or package ingredients carefully.

Pediatric—Studies on this medicine have been done only in adult patients, and there is no specific information comparing use of clozapine in children with use in other age groups.

Geriatric—Many medicines have not been tested in older people. Therefore, it may not be known whether they work exactly the same way they do in younger adults. Clozapine may be more likely to cause side effects in the elderly, including dizziness and fainting, low blood pressure, and confusion or excitement. This medicine should not be used for behavioral problems in older adults with dementia.

Pregnancy—

	Pregnancy Category	Explanation
All Trimesters	B	Animal studies have revealed no evidence of harm to the fetus, however, there are no adequate studies in pregnant women OR animal studies have shown an adverse effect, but adequate studies in pregnant women have failed to demonstrate a risk to the fetus.

Breast Feeding—There are no adequate studies in women for determining infant risk when using this medication during breastfeeding. Weigh the potential benefits against the potential risks before taking this medication while breastfeeding.

Other medicines—

Using this medicine with any of the following medicines is not recommended. Your doctor may decide not to treat you with this medication or change some of the other medicines you take.

Droperidol

Interactions with Food/Tobacco/Alcohol—Certain medicines should not be used at or around the time of eating food or eating certain types of food since interactions may occur. Using alcohol or tobacco with certain medicines may also cause interactions to occur. The following interactions have been selected on the basis of their potential significance and are not necessarily all-inclusive.

Using this medicine with any of the following may cause an increased risk of certain side effects but may be unavoidable in some cases. If used together, your doctor may change the dose or how often you use this medicine, or give you special instructions about the use of food, alcohol, or tobacco.

Caffeine

Other medical problems—The presence of other medical problems may affect the use of this medicine. Make sure you tell your doctor if you have any other medical problems, especially:

- Blood diseases or
- Enlarged prostate or difficult urination or
- Gastrointestinal problems or
- Glaucoma, narrow angle or
- Heart or blood vessel problems—Clozapine may make these conditions worse
- Epilepsy or other seizure disorder—Clozapine may increase the chance that seizures will occur
- Kidney or liver disease—Higher blood levels of clozapine may occur, increasing the chance that unwanted effects will occur

Proper Use of This Medicine

Take this medicine exactly as directed. Do not take more of this medicine and do not take it more often than your doctor ordered. Do not miss any doses.

This medicine has been prescribed for your current medical problem only. It must not be given to other people or used for other problems unless you are directed to do so by your doctor.

Dosing—The dose of this medicine will be different for different patients. Follow your doctor's orders or the directions on the label. The following information includes only the average doses of this medicine. If your dose is different, do not change it unless your doctor tells you to do so.

The amount of medicine that you take depends on the strength of the medicine. Also, the number of doses you take each day, the time allowed between doses, and the length of time you take the medicine depend on the medical problem for which you are using the medicine.

- For oral dosage form (tablets):
  - For schizophrenia:
    - Adults—At first, 12.5 milligrams (mg) (one half of a 25–mg tablet) once or twice a day. Your doctor may increase your dose as needed. However, the dose usually is not more than 900 mg a day.
    - Children younger than 16 years of age—Use and dose must be determined by your doctor.

Missed dose—If you miss a dose of this medicine, take it as soon as possible. However, if it is almost time for your next dose, skip the missed dose and go back to your regular dosing schedule. Do not double doses.

If you miss 2 or more days of clozapine doses, talk to your doctor before you start taking it again. You may need to restart this medicine at a lower dose than you were taking before.

Storage—Store the medicine in a closed container at room temperature, away from heat, moisture, and direct light. Keep from freezing.

Keep out of the reach of children.

Do not keep outdated medicine or medicine no longer needed.

Precautions While Using This Medicine

It is important that you have your blood tests done when they are scheduled, and that your doctor check your progress at regular visits. Clozapine can cause some very serious blood problems that you may not be able to feel or see. The pharmacy will give you this medicine only if your blood tests show that it is safe for you to take clozapine. Also, your doctor will make sure the medicine is working properly and change the dosage if needed.

If you do not take clozapine for 2 or more days, talk to your doctor about what to do. You may need to take a lower dose when you first start taking this medicine again.

If you have been using this medicine regularly, do not stop taking it without first checking with your doctor. Your doctor may want you to reduce gradually the amount you are taking before stopping completely. This is to help prevent the illness from suddenly returning.

This medicine will add to the effects of alcohol and other CNS depressants (medicines that slow down the nervous system, possibly causing drowsiness). Some examples of CNS depressants are antihistamines or medicine for hay fever, other allergies, or colds; sedatives, tranquilizers, or sleeping medicine; prescription pain medicine or narcotics; barbiturates; medicine for seizures; muscle relaxants; or anesthetics, including some dental anesthetics. Check with your doctor before taking any of the above while you are using this medicine.

Contact your doctor as soon as possible if you develop unusual tiredness or weakness, fever, sore throat, or other symptoms of infection. These can be symptoms of a very serious blood problem.

Contact your doctor as soon as possible if you have chest pain or discomfort, a fast heartbeat, trouble breathing, or fever and chills. These can be symptoms of a very serious problem with your heart.

Clozapine may cause drowsiness, blurred vision or convulsions (seizures). Do not drive, climb, swim, operate machines or do anything else that could be dangerous while you are taking this medicine.

Dizziness, lightheadedness, or fainting may occur, especially when you get up from a lying or sitting position. Getting up slowly may help. If this problem continues or gets worse, check with your doctor.

In some patients, clozapine may cause increased watering of the mouth. Other patients, however, may get dryness of the mouth. For temporary relief of mouth dryness, use sugarless gum or candy, melt bits of ice in your mouth, or use a saliva substitute. However, if your mouth continues to feel dry for more than 2 weeks, check with your medical doctor or dentist. Continuing dryness of the mouth may increase the chance of dental disease, including tooth decay, gum disease, and fungus infections.

Side Effects of This Medicine

Along with its needed effects, a medicine may cause some unwanted effects. Some side effects may not have signs or symptoms that you can see or feel. Clozapine can cause some very serious blood problems. Your doctor will watch for these by doing blood tests every week or two for as long as you are taking clozapine and for 4 weeks after you stop taking it. Although not all of these side effects may occur, if they do occur they may need medical attention.

Check with your doctor immediately if any of the following side effects occur:
  More common
    Fast or irregular heartbeat; fever; low blood pressure
  Less common
    High blood pressure (severe or continuing headache)
  Rare
    Chest pain or discomfort; chills; convulsions (seizures); cough; difficult or fast breathing or sudden shortness of breath; fainting; increased sweating; loss of bladder control; muscle stiffness (severe); sore throat; sores, ulcers, or white spots on lips or in mouth; swelling or pain in leg; trouble breathing; unusual bleeding or bruising; unusual tiredness or weakness; unusually pale skin

Check with your doctor as soon as possible if any of the following side effects occur:
  More common
    Dizziness, especially when getting up from a lying or sitting position
  Less common
    Blurred vision; confusion; restlessness or need to keep moving; unusual anxiety, nervousness, or irritability
  Rare
    Absence of or decrease in movement; decreased sexual ability; high blood sugar (increased appetite, increased thirst, increased urination, weakness); lip smacking or puckering; liver problems (dark urine, decreased appetite, nausea, vomiting, yellow eyes or skin); mental depression; puffing of cheeks; rapid or worm-like movements of tongue; trembling or shaking;

trouble in sleeping; trouble in urinating; uncontrolled chewing movements; uncontrolled movements of arms and legs

Symptoms of overdose

Convulsions (seizures); dizziness or fainting; drowsiness (severe) or coma; fast, slow, or irregular heartbeat; hallucinations (seeing, hearing, or feeling things that are not there); increased watering of mouth (severe); slow, irregular, or troubled breathing; unusual excitement, nervousness, or restlessness

Some side effects may occur that usually do not need medical attention. These side effects may go away during treatment as your body adjusts to the medicine. Also, your health care professional may be able to tell you about ways to prevent or reduce some of these side effects. Check with your health care professional if any of the following side effects continue or are bothersome or if you have any questions about them:

More common

Constipation; dizziness or lightheadedness (mild); drowsiness; headache (mild); increased watering of mouth; nausea or vomiting; unusual weight gain

Less common

Abdominal discomfort or heartburn; dryness of mouth

Other side effects not listed may also occur in some patients. If you notice any other effects, check with your healthcare professional.

COAL TAR (Topical route) - kole tar

Commonly used brand name(s)

In the U.S.—

Betatar Gel	Fototar
Cutar Emulsion	Ionil-T Plus
Denorex	Medotar
DHS Tar	MG 217
Doak Tar	Neutrogena T/Derm
Duplex T	Neutrogena T/Gel

In Canada—

Estar	Spectro Tar Skin Wash
Liquor Carbonis Detergens	Tar Distillate
Psorigel	

Available Dosage Forms:

- Liquid
- Shampoo
- Solution
- Soap
- Gel/Jelly
- Ointment
- Lotion
- Cream
- Kit
- Emulsion
- Bar

Therapeutic Class: Keratolytic

Uses For This Medicine

Coal tar is used to treat eczema, psoriasis, seborrheic dermatitis, and other skin disorders.

Some of these preparations are available only with your doctor's prescription.

Before Using This Medicine

In deciding to use a medicine, the risks of taking the medicine must be weighed against the good it will do. This is a decision you and your doctor will make. For this medicine, the following should be considered:

Allergies—Tell your doctor if you have ever had any unusual or allergic reaction to this medicine or any other medicines. Also tell your health care professional if you have any other types of allergies, such as to foods, dyes, preservatives, or animals. For non-prescription products, read the label or package ingredients carefully.

Pediatric—Coal tar products should not be used on infants, unless otherwise directed by your doctor. Studies on this medicine have been done only in adult patients, and there is no specific information comparing use of this medicine in children with use in other age groups.

Geriatric—Many medicines have not been studied specifically in older people. Therefore, it may not be known whether they work exactly the same way they do in younger adults or if they cause different side effects or problems in older people. There is no specific information comparing use of this medicine in the elderly with use in other age groups.

Breast Feeding—There are no adequate studies in women for determining infant risk when using this medication during breastfeeding. Weigh the potential benefits against the potential risks before taking this medication while breastfeeding.

Other medicines—Although certain medicines should not be used together at all, in other cases two different medicines may be used together even if an interaction might occur. In these cases, your doctor may want to change the dose, or other precautions may be necessary. Tell your healthcare professional if you are taking any other prescription or non-prescription (over-the-counter [OTC]) medicine.

Interactions with Food/Tobacco/Alcohol—Certain medicines should not be used at or around the time of eating food or eating certain types of food since interactions may occur. Using alcohol or tobacco with certain medicines may also cause interactions to occur. Discuss with your healthcare professional the use of your medicine with food, alcohol, or tobacco.

Proper Use of This Medicine

Use this medicine only as directed. Do not use more of it and do not use it more often than recommended on the label, unless otherwise directed by your doctor. To do so may increase the chance of side effects.

After applying coal tar, protect the treated area from direct sunlight and do not use a sunlamp for 72 hours, unless otherwise directed by your doctor, since a severe reaction may occur. Also, make sure you have removed all the coal tar medicine from your skin before you go back into direct sunlight or use a sunlamp.

Do not apply this medicine to infected, blistered, raw, or oozing areas of the skin.

Keep this medicine away from the eyes. If you should accidentally get some in your eyes, flush them thoroughly with water at once.

To use the cream or ointment form of this medicine:

- Apply enough medicine to cover the affected area, and rub in gently.

To use the gel form of this medicine:

- Apply enough gel to cover the affected area, and rub in gently. Allow the gel to remain on the affected area for 5 minutes, then remove excess gel by patting with a clean tissue.

To use the shampoo form of this medicine:

- Wet the scalp and hair with lukewarm water. Apply a generous amount of shampoo and rub into the scalp, then rinse. Apply the shampoo again, working up a rich lather, and allow to remain on the scalp for 5 minutes. Then rinse thoroughly.

To use the nonshampoo liquid form of this medicine:

- Some of these preparations are to be applied directly to dry or wet skin, some are to be added to lukewarm bath water, and some may be applied directly to dry or wet skin or added to lukewarm bath water. Make sure you know exactly how you should use this medicine. If you have any questions about this, check with your health care professional.
- If this medicine is to be applied directly to the skin, apply enough to cover the affected area, and rub in gently.
- Some of these preparations contain alcohol and are flammable. Do not use near heat, near open flame, or while smoking.

Dosing—The dose of this medicine will be different for different patients. Follow your doctor's orders or the directions on the label. The following information includes only the average doses of this medicine. If your dose is different, do not change it unless your doctor tells you to do so.

The amount of medicine that you take depends on the strength of the medicine. Also, the number of doses you take each day, the time allowed between doses, and the length of time you take the medicine depend on the medical problem for which you are using the medicine.

- For eczema, psoriasis, seborrheic dermatitis, and other skin disorders:
  - For cleansing bar dosage form:
    - Adults—Use one or two times a day, or as directed by your doctor.
    - Children—Use and dose must be determined by your doctor.
  - For cream dosage form:
    - Adults—Apply to the affected area(s) of the skin up to four times a day.
    - Children—Use and dose must be determined by your doctor.
  - For gel dosage form:
    - Adults—Apply to the affected area(s) of the skin one or two times a day.
    - Children—Use and dose must be determined by your doctor.
  - For lotion dosage form:
    - Adults—Apply directly to the affected area(s) of the skin or use as a bath, hand or foot soak, or as a hair rinse, depending on the product.
    - Children—Use and dose must be determined by your doctor.
  - For ointment dosage form:
    - Adults—Apply to the affected area(s) of the skin two or three times a day.
    - Children—Use and dose must be determined by your doctor.
  - For shampoo dosage form:
    - Adults—Use once a day to once a week or as directed by your doctor.
    - Children—Use and dose must be determined by your doctor.
  - For topical solution dosage form:
    - Adults—Apply to wet the skin or scalp, or use as a bath, depending on the product.
    - Children—Use and dose must be determined by your doctor.
  - For topical suspension dosage form:
    - Adults—Use as a bath.
    - Children—Use and dose must be determined by your doctor.

Missed dose—If you miss a dose of this medicine, apply it as soon as possible. However, if it is almost time for your next dose, skip the missed dose and go back to your regular dosing schedule.

Storage—Store the medicine in a closed container at room temperature, away from heat, moisture, and direct light. Keep from freezing.

Keep out of the reach of children.

Do not keep outdated medicine or medicine no longer needed.

Precautions While Using This Medicine

If this medicine is used on the scalp, it may temporarily discolor blond, bleached, or tinted hair.

Coal tar may stain the skin or clothing. Avoid getting it on your clothing. The stain on the skin will wear off after you stop using the medicine.

Side Effects of This Medicine

In animal studies, coal tar has been shown to increase the chance of skin cancer.

Along with its needed effects, a medicine may cause some unwanted effects. Although not all of these side effects may occur, if they do occur they may need medical attention.

Check with your doctor as soon as possible if any of the following side effects occur:

Rare

Skin irritation not present before use of this medicine; skin rash

Some side effects may occur that usually do not need medical attention. These side effects may go away during treatment as your body adjusts to the medicine. Also, your health care professional may be able to tell you about ways to prevent or reduce some of these side effects. Check with your health care professional if any of the following side effects continue or are bothersome or if you have any questions about them:

More common

Stinging (mild)— especially for gel and solution dosage forms

Other side effects not listed may also occur in some patients. If you notice any other effects, check with your healthcare professional.

COLCHICINE   (Oral route, Intravenous route) - KOL-chi-seen

Commonly used brand name(s)

In the U.S.—
    Colsalide

Available Dosage Forms:
* Solution
* Tablet

Therapeutic Class: Antigout

Uses For This Medicine

Colchicine is used to prevent or treat attacks of gout (also called gouty arthritis). People with gout have too much uric acid in their blood and joints. An attack of gout occurs when uric acid causes inflammation (pain, redness, swelling, and heat) in a joint. Colchicine does not cure gout or take the place of other medicines that lower the amount of uric acid in the body. It prevents or relieves gout attacks by reducing inflammation. Colchicine is not an ordinary pain reliever and will not relieve most kinds of pain.

Colchicine may also be used for other conditions as determined by your doctor.

Colchicine may be used in 2 ways. Most people take small amounts of it regularly for a long time (months or even years) to prevent severe attacks or other problems caused by inflammation. Other people take large amounts of colchicine during a short period of time (several hours) only when the medicine is needed to relieve an attack that is occurring. The chance of serious side effects is much lower with the first (preventive) kind of treatment.

Because some of colchicine's side effects can be very serious, you should discuss with your doctor the good that this medicine can do as well as the risks of using it. Make sure you understand exactly how you are to use it, and follow the instructions carefully, to lessen the chance of unwanted effects.

This medicine is available only with your doctor's prescription.

Once a medicine has been approved for marketing for a certain use, experience may show that it is also useful for other medical problems. Although these uses are not included in product labeling, colchicine is used in certain patients with the following medical conditions:
* Amyloidosis
* Behçet's syndrome
* Calcium pyrophosphate deposition disease (pseudogout)
* Cirrhosis of the liver
* Familial Mediterranean fever
* Pericarditis
* Sarcoid arthritis

If you are taking colchicine for any of these conditions, the following information may apply:
* For all of these conditions, colchicine is usually given regularly in small amounts to reduce inflammation (preventive treatment). This usually decreases the occurrence of severe attacks or other problems caused by inflammation.
* Colchicine is not a cure for these conditions. It will help prevent problems caused by inflammation only as long as you continue to take it.
* Some patients with calcium pyrophosphate deposition disease (pseudogout) or familial Mediterranean fever may take larger amounts of colchicine only when an attack occurs, to relieve the attack.

For patients taking colchicine for familial Mediterranean fever:
* Preventive treatment with colchicine may be helping you even if it does not reduce the number of severe attacks. Colchicine helps prevent other serious problems, such as kidney disease, that can occur in people with this condition. Therefore, even if you think that the colchicine isn't working, do not stop taking it. Check with your doctor instead.

Before Receiving This Medicine

In deciding to use a medicine, the risks of taking the medicine must be weighed against the good it will do. This is a decision you and your doctor will make. For this medicine, the following should be considered:

Allergies—Tell your doctor if you have ever had any unusual or allergic reaction to this medicine or any other medicines. Also tell your health care professional if you have any other types of allergies, such as to foods, dyes, preservatives, or animals. For non-prescription products, read the label or package ingredients carefully.

Pediatric—Studies on the effects of colchicine in patients with gout have been done only in adults. Gout is very rare in children. However, colchicine is used in children 3 years of age and older who need preventive treatment for other medical conditions. It has not been reported to cause different side effects or problems in these children than it does in adults.

Geriatric—Elderly people are especially sensitive to the effects of colchicine. Also, colchicine may stay in the body longer in older patients than it does in younger adults. This may increase the chance of side effects during treatment.

Pregnancy—

	Pregnancy Category	Explanation
All Trimesters	D	Studies in pregnant women have demonstrated a risk to the fetus. However, the benefits of therapy in a life threatening situation or a serious disease, may outweigh the potential risk.

Breast Feeding—Studies in women suggest that this medication poses minimal risk to the infant when used during breastfeeding.

Other medicines—

Using this medicine with any of the following medicines is usually not recommended, but may be required in some cases. If both medicines are prescribed together, your doctor may change the dose or how often you use one or both of the medicines.

Clarithromycin, Cyclosporine, Erythromycin, Interferon Alfa-2a

Interactions with Food/Tobacco/Alcohol—Certain medicines should not be used at or around the time of eating food or eating certain types of food since interactions may occur. Using alcohol or tobacco with certain medicines may also cause interactions to occur. The following interactions have been selected on the basis of their potential significance and are not necessarily all-inclusive.

Using this medicine with any of the following is usually not recommended, but may be unavoidable in some cases. If used together, your doctor may change the dose or how often you use this medicine, or give you special instructions about the use of food, alcohol, or tobacco.

Grapefruit Juice

Other medical problems—The presence of other medical problems may affect the use of this medicine. Make sure you tell your doctor if you have any other medical problems, especially:

- Alcohol abuse or
- Intestinal disease or
- Stomach ulcer or other stomach problems—The chance of stomach upset may be increased. Also, colchicine can make some kinds of stomach or intestinal problems worse
- Heart disease or
- Kidney disease or
- Liver disease—The chance of serious side effects may be increased because these conditions can cause colchicine to build up in the body
- Low white blood cell count or
- Low platelet count—The chance of serious side effects may be increased because colchicine can make these conditions worse

Proper Use of This Medicine

Colchicine can build up in the body and cause serious side effects if too much of it is taken or if it is taken too often. Therefore, do not take more of this medicine, and do not take it more often, than directed by your doctor. This is especially important for elderly patients, who are more likely than younger adults to have colchicine build up in the body and who are also more sensitive to its effects.

For patients taking small amounts of colchicine regularly (preventive treatment):

- Take this medicine regularly as directed by your doctor, even if you feel well. If you are taking colchicine to prevent gout attacks, and you are also taking another medicine to reduce the amount of uric acid in your body, you probably will be able to stop taking colchicine after a while. However, if you stop taking it too soon, your attacks may return or get worse. If you are taking colchicine for certain other medical conditions, you may need to keep taking it for the rest of your life.
- If you are taking colchicine to prevent gout attacks, ask your doctor to recommend other medicine to be taken if an attack occurs. Most people receiving preventive amounts of colchicine should not take extra colchicine to relieve an attack. However, some people cannot take the other medicines that are used for gout attacks and will have to take extra colchicine. If you are one of these people, ask your doctor to tell you the largest amount of

colchicine you should take for an attack and how long you should wait before starting to take the smaller preventive amounts again. Be sure to follow these directions carefully.

For patients taking large amounts of colchicine only when needed to relieve an attack:

- Start taking this medicine at the first sign of the attack for best results.
- Stop taking this medicine as soon as the pain is relieved or at the first sign of nausea, vomiting, stomach pain, or diarrhea. Also, stop taking colchicine when you have taken the largest amount that your doctor ordered for each attack, even if the pain is not relieved or none of these side effects occurs.
- The first few times you take colchicine, keep a record of each dose as you take it. Then, whenever stomach upset (nausea, vomiting, stomach pain, or diarrhea) occurs, count the number of doses you have taken. The next time you need colchicine, stop taking it before that number of doses is reached. For example, if diarrhea occurs after your fifth dose of medicine, take no more than four doses the next time. If taking fewer doses does not prevent stomach upset from occurring after a few treatments, check with your doctor.
- After taking colchicine tablets to treat an attack, do not take any more colchicine for at least 3 days. Also, after receiving the medicine by injection for an attack, do not take any more colchicine (tablets or injection) for at least 7 days. Elderly patients may have to wait even longer between treatments and should check with their doctor for directions.
- If you are taking colchicine for an attack of gout, and you are also taking other medicine to reduce the amount of uric acid in your body, do not stop taking the other medicine. Continue taking the other medicine as directed by your doctor.

Dosing—The dose of this medicine will be different for different patients. Follow your doctor's orders or the directions on the label. The following information includes only the average doses of this medicine. If your dose is different, do not change it unless your doctor tells you to do so.

The amount of medicine that you take depends on the strength of the medicine. Also, the number of doses you take each day, the time allowed between doses, and the length of time you take the medicine depend on the medical problem for which you are using the medicine.

The number of doses you take each day, the time allowed between doses, and the length of time you take the medicine depend on how often your attacks occur and on whether you are taking the medicine to prevent or to relieve attacks. The amount of medicine you take will also depend on how you react to the medicine.

- For oral dosage form (tablets):
  ○ Adults:
    ▪ For preventing gout attacks—Most people start with one 0.5–milligram (mg) or 0.6–mg tablet a day. If gout attacks continue to occur, the doctor may direct you to increase the dose to one tablet two or even three times a day for a while. Some people with mild gout may need only one tablet every other day, or even less.

- For treating a gout attack that has already started—Your doctor will probably recommend one of the following treatment plans:
  - One or two 0.5–mg or 0.6–mg tablets for the first dose, then one 0.5–mg or 0.6–mg tablet every one or two hours, OR
  - Two 0.5–mg or 0.6–mg tablets or one 1–mg tablet every two hours.
  - For both plans, stop taking this medicine after you have taken the largest amount ordered by your doctor. If your doctor has not told you the largest amount that you should take for one attack, do not take more than 6 mg of this medicine (a total of twelve 0.5–mg tablets, ten 0.6–mg tablets, or six 1–mg tablets, spread over a period of several hours).
  - Children: Use and dose must be determined by the doctor.
- For parenteral dosage form (injection):
  - Adults:
    - For preventing gout attacks—0.5 or 1 mg one or two times a day, injected into a vein.
    - For treating an attack of gout that has already started—1 or 2 mg for the first dose, then 0.5 mg or 1 mg every six to twelve hours, injected into a vein. After a total of 4 mg has been given, no more colchicine (tablets or injections) should be given for at least seven days.
  - Children: Use and dose must be determined by the doctor.

Missed dose—If you miss a dose of this medicine, take it as soon as possible. However, if it is almost time for your next dose, skip the missed dose and go back to your regular dosing schedule. Do not double doses.

Storage—Store the medicine in a closed container at room temperature, away from heat, moisture, and direct light. Keep from freezing.

Keep out of the reach of children.

Do not keep outdated medicine or medicine no longer needed.

Precautions After Receiving This Medicine

If you must take colchicine for a long time (preventive treatment), your doctor may want to check your progress at regular visits. He or she may also want to check for certain side effects. Finding these side effects early can help to keep them from becoming serious.

Stomach problems may be more likely to occur if you drink large amounts of alcoholic beverages while taking colchicine. Also, drinking too much alcohol may increase the amount of uric acid in your blood. This may lessen the effects of colchicine when it is used to prevent gout attacks. Therefore, people who take colchicine should be careful to limit the amount of alcohol they drink.

For patients taking small amounts of colchicine regularly (preventive treatment):

- Attacks of gout or other problems caused by inflammation may continue to occur during treatment. However, the attacks or other problems should occur less often, and they should not be as severe as they were before

you started taking colchicine. Even if you think the colchicine is not working, do not stop taking it and do not increase the dose. Check with your doctor instead.

Side Effects of This Medicine

Along with its needed effects, a medicine may cause some unwanted effects. Although not all of these side effects may occur, if they do occur they may need medical attention.

Stop taking this medicine and get emergency help immediately if any of the following effects occur:

More common

Diarrhea; nausea or vomiting; stomach pain

If any of these side effects continue for 3 hours or longer after you have stopped taking colchicine, check with your doctor.

Check with your doctor immediately if any of the following side effects occur:

Rare

Black, tarry stools; blood in urine or stools; difficulty in breathing when exercising; fever with or without chills; headache; large, hive-like swellings on the face, eyelids, mouth, lips, and/or tongue; pinpoint red spots on skin; sores, ulcers, or white spots on lips or in mouth; sore throat; unusual bleeding or bruising; unusual tiredness or weakness

Signs and symptoms of overdose

Burning feeling in the stomach, throat, or skin; diarrhea (severe or bloody); nausea, stomach pain, or vomiting (severe)Note: These side effects are usually the first signs of an overdose of colchicine tablets. They are not likely to occur when too much colchicine has been given by injection. Other signs and symptoms that may occur after an overdose of either the tablets or the injection include bleeding; fast, shallow breathing; convulsions (seizures); fever; and very severe muscle weakness. An overdose of colchicine can cause damage to the blood, heart, intestines, kidneys, liver, lungs, and muscles.

Check with your doctor as soon as possible if any of the following side effects occur:

Rare

Burning, "crawling", or tingling feeling in the skin; pain; peeling of skin; redness; swelling; tenderness

Check with your doctor as soon as possible if any of the following side effects occur:

Rare

Muscle weakness; numbness in fingers or toes (usually mild); skin rash or hives

Some side effects may occur that usually do not need medical attention. These side effects may go away during treatment as your body adjusts to the medicine. Also, your health care professional may be able to tell you about ways to prevent or reduce some of these side effects. Check with your health care professional if any of the following side effects continue or are bothersome or if you have any questions about them:

Less common

Loss of appetite

With long-term use

Loss of hair

Other side effects not listed may also occur in some patients. If you notice any other effects, check with your healthcare professional.

COLESEVELAM (Oral route) - koh-le-SEV-e-lam

Commonly used brand name(s)

In the U.S.—
Welchol

Available Dosage Forms:
- Tablet

Therapeutic Class: Antihyperlipidemic
Pharmacologic Class: Bile Acid Sequestrant

Uses For This Medicine

Colesevelam is used to lower high cholesterol levels in the blood. This may help prevent medical problems caused by cholesterol clogging the blood vessels.

Colesevelam works by attaching to certain substances in the intestine. Since colesevelam is not absorbed into the body, these substances also pass out of the body without being absorbed.

This medicine is available only with your doctor's prescription.

Before Using This Medicine

In deciding to use a medicine, the risks of taking the medicine must be weighed against the good it will do. This is a decision you and your doctor will make. For this medicine, the following should be considered:

Allergies—Tell your doctor if you have ever had any unusual or allergic reaction to this medicine or any other medicines. Also tell your health care professional if you have any other types of allergies, such as to foods, dyes, preservatives, or animals. For non-prescription products, read the label or package ingredients carefully.

Pediatric—Studies on this medicine have been done only in adult patients, and there is no specific information comparing use of colesevelam in children with use in other age groups.

Geriatric—This medicine has not been shown to cause different side effects or problems in older people than it does in younger adults.

Pregnancy—

	Pregnancy Category	Explanation
All Trimesters	B	Animal studies have revealed no evidence of harm to the fetus, however, there are no adequate studies in pregnant women OR animal studies have shown an adverse effect, but adequate studies in pregnant women have failed to demonstrate a risk to the fetus.

Breast Feeding—There are no adequate studies in women for determining infant risk when using this medication during breastfeeding. Weigh the potential benefits against the potential risks before taking this medication while breastfeeding.

Other medicines—

Using this medicine with any of the following medicines is usually not recommended, but may be required in some cases. If both medicines are prescribed together, your doctor may change the dose or how often you use one or both of the medicines.

Mycophenolate Mofetil, Mycophenolate Sodium, Mycophenolic Acid

Interactions with Food/Tobacco/Alcohol—Certain medicines should not be used at or around the time of eating food or eating certain types of food since interactions may occur. Using alcohol or tobacco with certain medicines may also cause interactions to occur. Discuss with your healthcare professional the use of your medicine with food, alcohol, or tobacco.

Other medical problems—The presence of other medical problems may affect the use of this medicine. Make sure you tell your doctor if you have any other medical problems, especially:
- Bowel obstruction or
- Difficulty swallowing or
- Major gastrointestinal surgery (recent) or
- Severe gastrointestinal motility disorders—Colesevelam may make these conditions worse
- Hypersensitivity

Proper Use of This Medicine

Dosing—The dose of this medicine will be different for different patients. Follow your doctor's orders or the directions on the label. The following information includes only the average doses of this medicine. If your dose is different, do not change it unless your doctor tells you to do so.

The amount of medicine that you take depends on the strength of the medicine. Also, the number of doses you take each day, the time allowed between doses, and the length of time you take the medicine depend on the medical problem for which you are using the medicine.

Before prescribing medicine for your condition, your doctor will probably try to control your condition by prescribing a personal diet for you. Such a diet may be low in fats, sugars, and/or cholesterol. Many people are able to control their condition by carefully following their doctor's orders for proper diet and exercise. Medicine is prescribed only when additional help is needed and is effective only when a schedule of diet and exercise is properly followed.

Also, this medicine is less effective if you are greatly overweight. It may be very important for you to go on a reducing diet. However, check with your doctor before going on any diet.

Make certain your health care professional knows if you are on any special diet, such as a low-sodium or low-sugar diet. Most medicines contain more than their active ingredient.
- For high cholesterol:
  - Adults—6 tablets a day. This may be taken as one dose or divided into two doses. The dose should be taken with a meal and liquid.

○ Children—Use and dose must be determined by your doctor.

Missed dose—If you miss a dose of this medicine, skip the missed dose and go back to your regular dosing schedule. Do not double doses.

Storage—Store the medicine in a closed container at room temperature, away from heat, moisture, and direct light. Keep from freezing.

Keep out of the reach of children.

Do not keep outdated medicine or medicine no longer needed.

Ask your healthcare professional how you should dispose of any medicine you do not use.

Precautions While Using This Medicine

Your doctor will want to check your progress at regular visits. This will allow your doctor to see if the medicine is working properly to lower your cholesterol levels and to decide if you should continue to take it.

Do not stop taking this medicine without first checking with your doctor. When you stop taking this medicine, your blood cholesterol levels may increase again. Your doctor may want you to follow a special diet to help prevent this from happening.

Side Effects of This Medicine

Along with its needed effects, a medicine may cause some unwanted effects. Although not all of these side effects may occur, if they do occur they may need medical attention.

Check with your doctor as soon as possible if any of the following side effects occur:

Less common

Congestion; cough; dryness or soreness of throat; hoarseness; muscle aches or pain; trouble in swallowing

Some side effects may occur that usually do not need medical attention. These side effects may go away during treatment as your body adjusts to the medicine. Also, your health care professional may be able to tell you about ways to prevent or reduce some of these side effects. Check with your health care professional if any of the following side effects continue or are bothersome or if you have any questions about them:

More common

Acid or sour stomach; belching; constipation; indigestion; stomach discomfort, upset, or pain

Other side effects not listed may also occur in some patients. If you notice any other effects, check with your healthcare professional.

COLESTIPOL (Oral route) - koe-LES-ti-pole

Commonly used brand name(s)

In the U.S.—
Colestid

Available Dosage Forms:
• Powder for Suspension
• Tablet

Therapeutic Class: Antihyperlipidemic
Pharmacologic Class: Bile Acid Sequestrant

Uses For This Medicine

Colestipol is used to lower high cholesterol levels in the blood. This may help prevent medical problems caused by cholesterol clogging the blood vessels.

Colestipol works by attaching to certain substances in the intestine. Since colestipol is not absorbed into the body, these substances also pass out of the body without being absorbed.

Colestipol may also be used for other conditions as determined by your doctor.

Colestipol is available only with your doctor's prescription.

Once a medicine has been approved for marketing for a certain use, experience may show that it is also useful for other medical problems. Although these uses are not included in product labeling, colestipol is used in certain patients with the following medical conditions:
• Diarrhea caused by bile acids
• Digitalis glycoside overdose
• Excess oxalate in the urine
• Itching (pruritus) associated with partial biliary obstruction

Before Using This Medicine

In deciding to use a medicine, the risks of taking the medicine must be weighed against the good it will do. This is a decision you and your doctor will make. For this medicine, the following should be considered:

Allergies—Tell your doctor if you have ever had any unusual or allergic reaction to this medicine or any other medicines. Also tell your health care professional if you have any other types of allergies, such as to foods, dyes, preservatives, or animals. For non-prescription products, read the label or package ingredients carefully.

Pediatric—There is no specific information comparing use of colestipol in children with use in other age groups. However, use is not recommended in children under 2 years of age since cholesterol is needed for normal development.

Geriatric—Side effects may be more likely to occur in patients over 60 years of age, who are usually more sensitive to the effects of colestipol.

Breast Feeding—Studies suggest that this medication may alter milk production or composition. If an alternative to this medication is not prescribed, you should monitor the infant for side effects and adequate milk intake.

Other medicines—

Using this medicine with any of the following medicines is usually not recommended, but may be required in some cases. If both medicines are prescribed together, your doctor may change the dose or how often you use one or both of the medicines.

Mycophenolate Mofetil, Mycophenolate Sodium, Mycophenolic Acid

Interactions with Food/Tobacco/Alcohol—Certain medicines should not be used at or around the time of eating

food or eating certain types of food since interactions may occur. Using alcohol or tobacco with certain medicines may also cause interactions to occur. Discuss with your healthcare professional the use of your medicine with food, alcohol, or tobacco.

Other medical problems—The presence of other medical problems may affect the use of this medicine. Make sure you tell your doctor if you have any other medical problems, especially:

- Bleeding problems or
- Constipation or
- Gallstones or
- Heart or blood vessel disease or
- Hemorrhoids or
- Stomach ulcer or other stomach problems or
- Underactive thyroid—Colestipol may make these conditions worse
- Kidney disease—There is an increased risk of developing electrolyte problems
- Liver disease—Cholesterol levels may be raised

Proper Use of This Medicine

Before prescribing medicine for your condition, your doctor will probably try to control your condition by prescribing a personal diet for you. Such a diet may be low in fats, sugars, and/or cholesterol. Many people are able to control their condition by carefully following their doctor's orders for proper diet and exercise. Medicine is prescribed only when additional help is needed and is effective only when a schedule of diet and exercise is properly followed.

Also, this medicine is less effective if you are greatly overweight. It may be very important for you to go on a reducing diet. However, check with your doctor before going on any diet.

Make certain your health care professional knows if you are on a low-sodium, low-sugar, or any other special diet.

Take this medicine exactly as directed by your doctor. Try not to miss any doses and do not take more medicine than your doctor ordered.

Follow carefully the special diet your doctor gave you. This is the most important part of controlling your condition and is necessary if the medicine is to work properly.

This medicine should never be taken in its dry form, since it could cause you to choke. Instead, always mix as follows:

- Add this medicine to 3 ounces or more of water, milk, flavored drink, or your favorite juice or carbonated drink. If you use a carbonated drink, slowly mix in the powder in a large glass to prevent too much foaming. Stir until it is completely mixed (it will not dissolve) before drinking. After drinking all the liquid containing the medicine, rinse the glass with a little more liquid and drink that also, to make sure you get all the medicine.
- You may also mix this medicine with milk in hot or regular breakfast cereals, or in thin soups such as tomato or chicken noodle soup. Or you may add it to some pulpy fruits such as crushed pineapple, pears, peaches, or fruit cocktail.

Dosing—The dose of this medicine will be different for different patients. Follow your doctor's orders or the directions on the label. The following information includes only the average doses of this medicine. If your dose is different, do not change it unless your doctor tells you to do so.

The amount of medicine that you take depends on the strength of the medicine. Also, the number of doses you take each day, the time allowed between doses, and the length of time you take the medicine depend on the medical problem for which you are using the medicine.

- For oral dosage form (powder for oral suspension):
  - For high cholesterol:
    - Adults—15 to 30 grams a day. This is divided into two to four doses and taken before meals.
    - Children—Use and dose must be determined by your doctor.

Missed dose—If you miss a dose of this medicine, take it as soon as possible. However, if it is almost time for your next dose, skip the missed dose and go back to your regular dosing schedule. Do not double doses.

Storage—Store the medicine in a closed container at room temperature, away from heat, moisture, and direct light. Keep from freezing.

Keep out of the reach of children.

Do not keep outdated medicine or medicine no longer needed.

Precautions While Using This Medicine

It is very important that your doctor check your progress at regular visits. This will allow your doctor to see if the medicine is working properly to lower your cholesterol levels and to decide if you should continue to take it.

Do not stop taking this medicine without first checking with your doctor. When you stop taking this medicine, your blood cholesterol levels may increase again. Your doctor may want you to follow a special diet to help prevent this from happening.

Do not take any other medicine unless prescribed by your doctor since colestipol may interfere with other medicines.

Side Effects of This Medicine

Along with its needed effects, a medicine may cause some unwanted effects. Although not all of these side effects may occur, if they do occur they may need medical attention.

Check with your doctor immediately if any of the following side effects occur:
  Rare
     Black, tarry stools; stomach pain (severe) with nausea and vomiting

Check with your doctor as soon as possible if any of the following side effects occur:
  More common
     Constipation
  Rare
     Loss of weight (sudden)

Some side effects may occur that usually do not need medical attention. These side effects may go away during treatment as your body adjusts to the medicine. Also, your health care professional may be able to tell you about ways to prevent or reduce some of these side effects. Check with your health

care professional if any of the following side effects continue or are bothersome or if you have any questions about them:

Less common

Belching; bloating; diarrhea; dizziness; headache; nausea or vomiting; stomach pain

Other side effects not listed may also occur in some patients. If you notice any other effects, check with your healthcare professional.

COLONY STIMULATING FACTOR
(Injection route, Intravenous route, Subcutaneous route)

Commonly used brand name(s)

In the U.S.—
Leukine
Neulasta
Neupogen

Available Dosage Forms:
- Solution
- Powder for Solution
- Injectable

Uses For This Medicine

Filgrastim, pegfilgrastim, and sargramostim are synthetic (man-made) versions of substances naturally produced in your body. These substances, called colony stimulating factors, help the bone marrow to make new white blood cells.

When certain cancer medicines fight your cancer cells, they also affect those white blood cells that fight infection. To help prevent infections when these cancer medicines are used, colony stimulating factors may be given. Colony stimulating factors also may be used to help the bone marrow recover after bone marrow transplantation and stem cell transplantation.

Once a medicine has been approved for marketing for a certain use, experience may show that it also is useful for other medical problems. Although not specifically included in the product labeling, colony stimulating factors are used in certain patients with the following medical conditions:
- Failure or delay of myeloid engraftment after hematopoietic stem cell transplantation
- Myelodysplastic syndromes
- Neutropenia, AIDS-associated
- Neutropenia, drug-induced

Before Using This Medicine

Allergies—Tell your doctor if you have ever had any unusual or allergic reaction to medicines in this group or any other medicines. Also tell your health care professional if you have any other types of allergies, such as to foods dyes, preservatives, or animals. For non-prescription products, read the label or package ingredients carefully.

Pediatric—Although there is no specific information comparing use of colony stimulating factors in children with use in other age groups, this medicine is not expected to cause

different side effects or problems in children than it does in adults. In Canada, data from clinical trials in children indicate that the safety of filgrastim is similar in both adults and children receiving certain cancer medicines. Sargramostim may contain benzyl alcohol and should not be given to infants because it could cause serious adverse effects. The pegfilgrastim 6–mg syringe should not be used in infants, children, and small teenagers who weigh less than 45 kg (99.2 lbs).

Geriatric—Many medicines have not been studied specifically in older people. Therefore, it may not be known whether they work exactly the same way they do in younger adults. Although there is no specific information comparing use of colony stimulating factors in the elderly with use in other age groups, this medicine has been used in many elderly patients and is not expected to cause different side effects or problems in older people than it does in younger adults.

Pregnancy—Colony stimulating factors have not been studied in pregnant women. Before you take a colony stimulating factor, make sure your doctor knows if you are pregnant of if you may become pregnant.

Breast Feeding—It is not known whether colony stimulating factors pass into human breast milk. However, these medicines have not been reported to cause problems in nursing babies. Mothers who are taking a colony stimulating factor and who wish to breast-feed should discuss this with their doctor.

Other medicines—

Using medicines in this class with any of the following medicines is usually not recommended, but may be required in some cases. If both medicines are prescribed together, your doctor may change the dose or how often you use one or both of the medicines.

Topotecan, Vincristine, Vincristine Liposome

Interactions with Food/Tobacco/Alcohol—Certain medicines should not be used at or around the time of eating food or eating certain types of food since interactions may occur. Using alcohol or tobacco with certain medicines may also cause interactions to occur. Discuss with your healthcare professional the use of your medicine with food, alcohol, or tobacco.

Other medical problems—The presence of other medical problems may affect the use of medicines in this class. Make sure you tell your doctor if you have any other medical problems, especially:
- Radiation therapy—You should not use filgrastim close to the time you are undergoing chemotherapy or radiation therapy for cancer treatment.
- Conditions caused by inflammation or immune system problems—There is a chance these may be worsened by colony stimulating factor
- Heart disease—Risk of some unwanted effects (heart rhythm problems, retaining water) may be increased
- Kidney disease or
- Liver disease—May sometimes be worsened by colony stimulating factor
- Leukemia (cancer of the blood-forming organs)—May make condition worse
- Lung disease—Colony stimulating factor may cause shortness of breath

- Sickle cell disease (condition that affects the cells in your blood)—May make condition worse

Proper Use of This Medicine

If you are injecting this medicine yourself, use it exactly as directed by your doctor. Do not use more or less of it, and do not use it more often than your doctor ordered. The exact amount of medicine you need has been carefully worked out. Using too much will increase the risk of side effects, while using too little may not improve your condition.

If you are injecting this medicine yourself, each package of colony stimulating factor will contain a patient instruction sheet. Read this sheet carefully and make sure you understand:

- How to prepare the injection
- Proper use of disposable syringes.
- How to give the injection.
- How long the injection is stable.

If you have any questions about any of this, check with your health care professional.

Dosing—The dose medicines in this class will be different for different patients. Follow your doctor's orders or the directions on the label. The following information includes only the average doses of these medicines. If your dose is different, do not change it unless your doctor tells you to do so.

The amount of medicine that you take depends on the strength of the medicine. Also, the number of doses you take each day, the time allowed between doses, and the length of time you take the medicine depend on the medical problem for which you are using the medicine.

Missed dose—Call your doctor or pharmacist for instructions.

Storage—Store in the refrigerator. Do not freeze.

Keep out of the reach of children.

Do not keep outdated medicine or medicine no longer needed.

Precautions While Using This Medicine

It is very important that your doctor check your progress at regular visits to make sure that this medicine is working properly and to check for unwanted effects.

Colony stimulating factors are used to prevent or reduce the risk of infection while you are being treated with cancer medicines. Because your body's ability to fight infection is reduced, it is very important that you call your doctor at the first sign of any infection (for example, if you get a fever or chills) so you can start antibiotic treatment right away.

Contact your doctor if you develop shortness of breath, tightness in chest. troubled breathing, or wheezing. These could be symptoms of a serious lung condition called adult respiratory distress syndrome (ARDS).

If you experience left upper abdominal or shoulder tip pain, contact your doctor right away. These could be symptoms of an enlarged or ruptured spleen.

Colony stimulating factors commonly cause mild bone pain, usually in the lower back or pelvis, about the time the white blood cells start to come back in your bone marrow. The pain is usually mild and lasts only a few days. Your doctor will probably prescribe a mild analgesic (painkiller) for you to take during that time. If you find that the analgesic is not strong enough, talk with your doctor about using something that will make you more comfortable.

Side Effects of This Medicine

Along with its needed effects, a medicine may cause some unwanted effects. Although not all of these side effects may occur, if they do occur they may need medical attention.

The side effects listed below include only those that might be caused by colony stimulating factors. To find out about other side effects that may be caused by the cancer medicines you are also receiving, look under the information about those specific medicines.

Check with your doctor as soon as possible if any of the following side effects occur:
  For filgrastim: Less common
    Redness or pain at the site of subcutaneous (under the skin) injection
  For filgrastim: Rare
    Fever; rapid or irregular heartbeat; sores on skin; wheezing
  For sargramostim: Less common
    Fever; redness or pain at the site of subcutaneous (under the skin) injection; shortness of breath; swelling of feet or lower legs; weight gain (sudden)
  For sargramostim: Rare
    Chest pain; rapid or irregular heartbeat; sores on skin; wheezing

Some side effects may occur that usually do not need medical attention. These side effects may go away during treatment as your body adjusts to the medicine. Also, your health care professional may be able to tell you about ways to prevent or reduce some of these side effects. Check with your health care professional if any of the following side effects continue or are bothersome or if you have any questions about them:
  For filgrastim, pegfilgrastim, and sargramostim: More common
    Headache; pain in arms or legs; pain in joints or muscles; pain in lower back or pelvis; skin rash or itching
  For sargramostim only (in addition to the above): Less common or rare
    Dizziness or faintness after first dose of medicine; flushing of face after first dose of medicine; weakness

Other side effects not listed may also occur in some patients. If you notice any other effects, check with your healthcare professional.

CONJUGATED ESTROGENS AND MEDROXYPROGESTERONE FOR OVARIAN HORMONE THERAPY (OHT) (Systemic)

Some commonly used brand names are:
In the U.S.—
  Premphase (1)
  Prempro (2)

In Canada—
  Premplus (2)

This information applies to the following medicines

1. Conjugated Estrogens, and Conjugated Estrogens and Medroxyprogesterone (CON-ju-gate-ed ES-troe-jenz, and CON-ju-gate-ed ES-troe-jenz and me-DROX-ee-proe-JES-te-rone)
2. Conjugated Estrogens and Medroxyprogesterone (CON-ju-gate-ed ES-troe-jenz and me-DROX-ee-proe-JES-te-rone)

Category

- **Estrogen-progestin—**
- **Osteoporosis prophylactic—**
- **Ovarian hormone therapy agent—**

Description

Conjugated estrogens and medroxyprogesterone (CON-ju-gate-ed ES-troe-jenz and me-DROX-ee-proe-JES-te-rone) are estrogen and progestin hormones. Along with other effects, estrogens help females develop sexually at puberty and regulate the menstrual cycle. Progestin lowers the effect of estrogen on the uterus and keeps estrogen-related problems from developing.

Around the time of menopause, the ovaries produce less estrogen. Estrogens are given to:

- Relieve the signs of menopause (vasomotor symptoms of menopause), such as hot flashes and unusual sweating, chills, faintness, or dizziness.
- Treat inflammation of the vagina (atrophic vaginitis) and of the genital area (atrophy of the vulva) by keeping these areas from becoming too dry, itchy, or painful.
- Prevent the loss of bone that begins at the time of menopause. Keeping bones strong decreases the chance of developing weak bones that easily break (osteoporosis). Estrogen use is most effective when it is taken for more than 7 years while you are getting regular exercise and extra calcium. Protection from bone loss can then last for many years after you stop taking the medicine.

There is *no* medical evidence to support the belief that the use of estrogens will keep the patient feeling young, keep the skin soft, or delay the appearance of wrinkles. Nor has it been proven that the use of estrogens during menopause will relieve emotional and nervous symptoms, unless these symptoms are related to the menopausal symptoms, such as hot flashes.

Progestins are not needed if the uterus has been removed (by a surgical method called hysterectomy). In that case, it may be better to receive estrogens alone without the progestin.

Conjugated estrogens and medroxyprogesterone are available only with your doctor's prescription, in the following dosage forms:

Oral
- Conjugated Estrogens; Conjugated Estrogens and Medroxyprogesterone
  - Tablets (U.S.)
- Conjugated Estrogens and Medroxyprogesterone
  - Tablets and Canada

Before Using This Medicine

In deciding to use a medicine, the risks of taking the medicine must be weighed against the good it will do. This is a decision you and your doctor will make. For conjugated estrogens and medroxyprogesterone, the following should be considered:

Allergies—Tell your doctor if you have ever had any unusual or allergic reaction to estrogens or progestins. Also tell your health care professional if you are allergic to any other substances, such as foods, preservatives, or dyes.

Pregnancy—Conjugated estrogens and medroxyprogesterone are not recommended for use during pregnancy. Becoming pregnant or maintaining a pregnancy is not likely to occur around the time of menopause. Tell your doctor right away if you suspect you are pregnant.

Breast-feeding—Conjugated estrogens and medroxyprogesterone pass into the breast milk. This medicine is not recommended for use during breast-feeding.

Older adults—Conjugated estrogens and medroxyprogesterone may increase your chance of having a stroke, memory problems, or breast cancer that spreads to other parts of your body.

Other medicines—Although certain medicines should not be used together at all, in other cases two different medicines may be used together even if an interaction might occur. In these cases, your doctor may want to change the dose, or other precautions may be necessary. When you are taking conjugated estrogens and medroxyprogesterone, it is especially important that your health care professional know if you are taking any of the following:

- Acetaminophen (e.g., Tylenol) (with long-term, high-dose use) or
- Amiodarone (e.g., Cordarone) or
- Anabolic steroids (nandrolone [e.g., Anabolin], oxandrolone [e.g., Anavar], oxymetholone [e.g., Anadrol], stanozolol [e.g., Winstrol]) or
- Androgens (male hormones) or
- Anti-infectives by mouth or by injection (medicine for infection) or
- Antithyroid agents (medicine for overactive thyroid) or
- Carmustine (e.g., BiCNU) or
- Chloroquine (e.g., Aralen) or
- Dantrolene (e.g., Dantrium) or
- Daunorubicin (e.g., Cerubidine) or
- Disulfiram (e.g., Antabuse) or
- Divalproex (e.g., Depakote) or
- Etretinate (e.g., Tegison) or
- Gold salts (medicine for arthritis) or
- Hydroxychloroquine (e.g., Plaquenil) or
- Isoniazid or
- Mercaptopurine (e.g., Purinethol) or
- Methotrexate (e.g., Mexate) or
- Methyldopa (e.g., Aldomet) or
- Naltrexone (e.g., Trexan) (with long-term, high-dose use) or
- Phenothiazines (acetophenazine [e.g., Tindal], chlorpromazine [e.g., Thorazine], fluphenazine [e.g., Prolixin], mesoridazine [e.g., Serentil], perphenazine [e.g., Trilafon], prochlorperazine [e.g., Compazine], promazine [e.g., Sparine], promethazine [e.g., Phenergan], thioridazine [e.g., Mellaril], trifluoperazine [e.g., Stela-

zine], triflupromazine [e.g., Vesprin], trimeprazine [e.g., Temaril]) or

- Plicamycin (e.g., Mithracin)—Use of these medicines with conjugated estrogens and medroxyprogesterone may increase the chance of problems occurring that affect the liver
- Aminoglutethimide (e.g., Cytadren) or
- Barbiturates, especially phenobarbital or
- Carbamazepine (e.g., Tegretol) or
- Phenytoin (e.g., Dilantin) or
- Rifampin (e.g., Rifadin) or
- St. John's wort (*Hypericum perforatum*—These medicines may decrease the effect of conjugated estrogens or medroxyprogesterone
- Cyclosporine (e.g., Sandimmune)—Conjugated estrogens can prevent cyclosporine's removal from the body; this can lead to cyclosporine causing kidney or liver problems

Other medical problems—The presence of other medical problems may affect the use of conjugated estrogens and medroxyprogesterone. Make sure you tell your doctor if you have any other medical problems, especially:

- Asthma or
- Heart problems or
- Epilepsy or
- High blood pressure or
- Kidney problems, severe or
- Migraine headaches—Rarely, water retention caused by conjugated estrogens or medroxyprogesterone may worsen these conditions; on the other hand, blood pressure and some heart or blood vessel problems can improve for most patients
- Blood clotting problems (or history of during previous estrogen therapy)—Estrogens usually are not used until blood clotting problems stop; using estrogens is usually not a problem for most patients without a history of blood clotting problems due to estrogen use
- Bone cancer or
- Breast cancer or
- Cancer of the uterus (active or suspected) or
- Fibroid tumors of the uterus—Estrogens may interfere with the treatment of breast or bone cancer, worsen cancer of the uterus, or increase the size of fibroid tumors
- Changes in genital or vaginal bleeding of unknown causes—Estrogens may make these conditions worse; some irregular vaginal bleeding may be a sign that the lining of the uterus may be growing too much or is a sign of cancer of the uterus lining
- Changes in vision—This medicine may make cause changes in vision; your medicine may need to be stopped if these conditions become worse
- Diabetes mellitus (sugar diabetes)—Conjugated estrogens or medroxyprogesterone may slightly change the amount of blood sugar for some patients, but for most patients with sugar diabetes, there is no change in blood sugar
- Endometriosis or
- Gallbladder disease or gallstones (or history of) or

- High cholesterol or triglycerides (or family history of) or
- Jaundice (yellow skin) or
- Liver disease, including jaundice (or history of) or
- Pancreatitis (inflammation of pancreas) or
- Porphyria (liver problem)—Conjugated estrogens or medroxyprogesterone may worsen these conditions; using estrogens can lower blood cholesterol in many patients with high cholesterol
- Low blood calcium, severe—Estrogens should be used with caution in patients with this condition
- Low blood calcium, severe—Estrogens should be used with caution in patients with this condition
- Underactive thyroid—A change in dose of thyroid medication may be needed. Your doctor will watch for this.

Proper Use of This Medicine

Conjugated estrogens and medroxyprogesterone usually come with patient directions. Read them carefully before taking this medicine.

Take this medicine only as directed by your doctor. Do not take more of it and do not take it for a longer period of time than your doctor ordered. The length of time you take the medicine will depend on the medical problem for which you are taking conjugated estrogens and medroxyprogesterone. Discuss with your doctor how long you will need to take these medicines.

If you are taking the estrogen or progestin hormones in a certain order (i.e., conjugated estrogens tablets followed by conjugated estrogens and medroxyprogesterone tablets), *be sure you know in which order you need to take the medicines*. If you have questions about this, ask your health care professional.

Nausea may occur during the first few weeks after you start taking estrogens. This effect usually disappears with continued use. If the nausea is bothersome, it can usually be prevented or reduced by taking each dose with food or immediately after food.

Dosing—The dose of these medicines will be different for different patients. *Follow your doctor's orders or the directions on the label.* The following information includes only the average doses of these medicines. *If your dose is different, do not change it* unless your doctor tells you to do so.

For conjugated estrogens, and conjugated estrogens and medroxyprogesterone
- For *oral* dosage form (tablets):
  - To prevent loss of bone (osteoporosis) or for treating itching or dryness of the genital area (atrophy of the vulva), inflammation of the vagina (atrophic vaginitis), or symptoms of menopause:
    - Adults—One tablet (containing 0.625 mg conjugated estrogens) once a day on Days 1 through 14; then, one tablet (containing 0.625 mg conjugated estrogens and 5 mg medroxyprogesterone) once a day on Days 15 through 28. Repeat cycle.

For conjugated estrogens and medroxyprogesterone
- For *oral* dosage form (tablets):
  - To prevent loss of bone (osteoporosis) or for treating itching or dryness of the genital area (atrophy of the

vulva), inflammation of the vagina (atrophic vaginitis), or symptoms of menopause:

- Adults—One tablet (containing 0.3 mg conjugated estrogens and 1.5 mg medroxyprogesterone) once a day for twenty-eight days. Repeat cycle. If vaginal bleeding or spotting continues and it is undesired, your doctor may increase your dose to the next highest strength tablet (0.45 mg conjugated estrogens and 1.5 mg medroxyprogesterone). It should be taken once a day for twenty-eight days. Repeat cycle.

Missed dose—If you miss a dose of this medicine, take it as soon as possible. However, if it is almost time for your next dose, skip the missed dose and go back to your regular dosing schedule. Do not double doses.

Storage—To store this medicine:

- Keep out of the reach of children.
- Store away from heat and direct light.
- Do not store in the bathroom, near the kitchen sink, or in other damp places. Heat or moisture may cause the medicine to break down.
- Do not keep outdated medicine or medicine no longer needed. Be sure that any discarded medicine is out of the reach of children.

Precautions While Using This Medicine

It is very important that your doctor check your progress at regular visits to make sure this medicine does not cause unwanted effects. Plan on going to see your doctor every year, but some doctors require visits more often.

Although the risk for developing breast problems or breast cancer is low, it is still important that you regularly check your breasts for any unusual lumps or discharge, and report any problems to your doctor. You should also have a mammogram (x-ray pictures of the breasts) and breast examination done by your doctor whenever your doctor recommends it.

If your menstrual periods have stopped, they may start again once you begin taking this medicine. This effect will continue for as long as the medicine is taken. However, if taking the continuous treatment (0.625 mg conjugated estrogens and 2.5 mg medroxyprogesterone once a day), monthly bleeding usually stops within 10 months.

Also, vaginal bleeding between your regular menstrual periods may occur during the first 3 months of use. *Do not stop taking your medicine. Check with your doctor* if bleeding continues for an unusually long time, if your period has not started within 45 days of your last period, or if you think you are pregnant.

Tell the doctor in charge that you are taking this medicine before having any laboratory test, because some test results may be affected.

You may need to stop taking this medicine before having some kinds of surgery or while your doctor has ordered a long period of bedrest. Talk with your doctor about this.

Side Effects of This Medicine

Healthy women rarely have severe side effects from taking conjugated estrogens or medroxyprogesterone to replace estrogen.

Check with your doctor as soon as possible if any of the following side effects occur:

More common
Itching of the vagina or genital area; menstrual periods beginning again, including changing menstrual bleeding pattern for up to 6 months (spotting, breakthrough bleeding, prolonged or heavier vaginal bleeding, or vaginal bleeding completely stopping by 10 months); pain during sexual intercourse; thick, white vaginal discharge

Less common
Blurred vision; breast lumps; chest pain; discharge from breast; dizziness; feeling faint, dizzy, or light-headed; feeling of warmth or heat; flushing or redness of skin, especially on face and neck; headache; heavy nonmenstrual vaginal bleeding; nervousness; pounding in the ears; severe cramping of the uterus; skin rash; slow or fast heartbeat; sweating

Rare
Change in vaginal discharge; pain or feeling of pressure in pelvis; pain or tenderness in stomach, side, or abdomen; yellow eyes or skin

Unknown
acid or sour stomach; belching; backache; full or bloated feeling or pressure in the stomach; heartburn; indigestion; loss of appetite; stomach discomfort, upset or pain; swelling of abdominal or stomach area; abdominal bloating; pelvic pain; stomach pain

Other side effects may occur that usually do not need medical attention. These side effects may go away during treatment as your body adjusts to the medicine. However, check with your doctor if any of the following side effects continue or are bothersome:

More common
Abdominal cramps; back pain; body aches or pain; breast pain or tenderness; congestion; chills; cough; crying; diarrhea; depersonalization; dryness or soreness of throat; dysphoria; enlarged breasts; euphoria; feeling faint, dizzy, or light-headedness; feeling of warmth or heat; fever; flushing or redness of skin, especially on face and neck; general feeling of discomfort or illness; headache, severe and throbbing; hoarseness; increase in amount of clear vaginal discharge; itching; joint pain; lack or loss of strength; mental depression; muscle aches and pains; nausea; pain; pain or tenderness around eyes and cheekbones; painful menstrual periods; painful or difficult urination; paranoia; passing of gas; quick to react or overreact emotionally; rapidly changing moods; runny nose; shivering; shortness of breath or troubled breathing; sneezing; sore throat; stuffy nose; stomach discomfort following meals; tender, swollen glands in neck; tightness of chest or wheezing; trouble sleeping; trouble in swallowing; unusual tiredness; voice changes; vomiting

Less common
Acne; bloating or swelling of face, ankles, or feet; cervix disorder; crying; depersonalization; dysphoria; euphoria; increase in sexual desire; leg cramps; mental depression; paranoia; quick to react or overreact emotionally; rapidly changing moods; sleeplessness; tense muscles; trouble sleeping; unable to sleep; unusual weight gain or loss

Unknown
light vaginal bleeding between periods and after intercourse; bloody vaginal discharge; bloody or cloudy

urine; difficult, burning, or painful urination; frequent urge to urinate; abdominal cramping

Other side effects not listed above may also occur in some patients. If you notice any other effects, check with your doctor.

CORTICOSTEROIDS (Inhalation)

Some commonly used brand names are:

In the U.S.—

AeroBid (3)	Pulmicort Turbuhaler (2)
AeroBid-M (3)	Qvar (1)
Azmacort (4)	Vanceril (1)
Beclovent (1)	Vanceril 84 mcg Double
Pulmicort Respules (2)	Strength (1)

In Canada—

Azmacort (4)	
Beclodisk (1)	Bronalide (3)
Becloforte (1)	Qvar (1)
Beclovent (1)	Pulmicort Nebuamp (2)
Beclovent Rotacaps (1)	Pulmicort Turbuhaler (2)
	Vanceril (1)

This information applies to the following medicines:

1. Beclomethasone (be-kloe-METH-a-sone)
2. Budesonide (byoo-DES-oh-nide)
3. Flunisolide (floo-NISS-oh-lide)
4. Triamcinolone (try-am-SIN-oh-lone)

Category

- **Anti-inflammatory, inhalation**—Beclomethasone; Budesonide; Flunisolide; Triamcinolone
- **Antiasthmatic**—Beclomethasone; Budesonide; Flunisolide; Triamcinolone

Description

Inhalation corticosteroids (kor-ti-koe-STER-oids) are cortisone-like medicines. They are used to help prevent the symptoms of asthma. When used regularly every day, inhalation corticosteroids decrease the number and severity of asthma attacks. However, they will not relieve an asthma attack that has already started.

Inhaled corticosteroids work by preventing certain cells in the lungs and breathing passages from releasing substances that cause asthma symptoms.

This medicine may be used with other asthma medicines, such as bronchodilators (medicines that open up narrowed breathing passages) or other corticosteroids taken by mouth.

Inhalation corticosteroids are available only with your doctor's prescription, in the following dosage forms:

Inhalation

- Beclomethasone
  - Aerosol
  - Capsules for inhalation
  - Powder for inhalation
- Beclomethasone dipropionate HFA
  - Aerosol
- Budesonide
  - Powder for inhalation
  - Suspension for inhalation

- Flunisolide
  - Aerosol
- Triamcinolone
  - Aerosol

Before Using This Medicine

In deciding to use a medicine, the risks of taking the medicine must be weighed against the good it will do. This is a decision you and your doctor will make. For inhalation corticosteroids, the following should be considered:

Allergies—Tell your doctor if you have ever had any unusual or allergic reaction to corticosteroids. Also tell your health care professional if you are allergic to any other substances, such as foods, preservatives, or dyes.

Pregnancy—Although studies in animals have shown that inhaled corticosteroids cause birth defects and other problems, in humans these medicines, when used in regular daily doses during pregnancy to keep the mother's asthma under control, have not been reported to cause breathing problems or birth defects in the newborn. Also, corticosteroids may prevent the effects of poorly controlled asthma, which are known to be harmful to the baby. Before taking an inhaled corticosteroid, make sure your doctor knows if you are pregnant or if you may become pregnant.

Breast-feeding—It is not known whether inhaled corticosteroids pass into breast milk. Although most medicines pass into breast milk in small amounts, many of them may be used safely while breast-feeding. Mothers who are using this medicine and who wish to breast-feed should discuss this with their doctor.

Children—Inhalation corticosteroids have been tested in children and, except for the possibility of slowed growth, in low effective doses, have not been shown to cause different side effects or problems than they do in adults.

Studies have shown that slowed growth or reduced adrenal gland function may occur in some children using inhaled corticosteroids in recommended doses. However, poorly controlled asthma may cause slowed growth, especially when corticosteroids taken by mouth are needed often. Your doctor will want you to use the lowest possible dose of an inhaled corticosteroid that controls asthma. This will lessen the chance of an effect on growth or adrenal gland function. *It is also important that children taking inhaled corticosteroids visit their doctors regularly so that their growth rates may be monitored.*

Regular use of inhaled corticosteroids may allow some children to stop using or decrease the amount of corticosteroids taken by mouth. This also will reduce the risk of slowed growth or reduced adrenal function.

Children who are using inhaled corticosteroids in large doses should avoid exposure to chickenpox or measles. When a child is exposed or the disease develops, the doctor should be contacted and his or her directions should be followed carefully.

Before this medicine is given to a child, you and your child's doctor should talk about the good this medicine will do as well as the risks of using it. Follow the doctor's directions very carefully to lessen the chance that unwanted effects will occur.

Older adults—Many medicines have not been studied specifically in older people. Therefore, it may not be known whether they work exactly the same way they do in younger adults. Although there is no specific information comparing use of inhaled corticosteroids in the elderly with use in other age groups, this medicine is not expected to cause different side effects or problems in older people than it does in younger adults.

Other medicines—Although certain medicines should not be used together at all, in other cases two different medicines may be used together even if an interaction might occur. In these cases, your doctor may want to change the dose, or other precautions may be necessary. Tell your health care professional if you are taking any other prescription or non-prescription (over-the-counter [OTC]) medicine.

Other medical problems—The presence of other medical problems may affect the use of inhaled corticosteroids. Make sure you tell your doctor if you have any other medical problems, especially:

- Cirrhosis (liver disease)—The effect of inhaled corticosteroids may be stronger in patients with this disease
- Glaucoma—Use of this medicine may cause the pressure in the eye to be increased
- Hypothyroidism (decreased production of thyroid hormone)—The effect of inhaled corticosteroids may be stronger in patients with this condition
- Infections, untreated—Using this medicine while an infection is present and is not being treated may cause the infection to get worse.
- Osteoporosis (bone disease)—Inhaled corticosteroids in high doses may make this condition worse in women who are past menopause and who are not receiving an estrogen replacement
- Tuberculosis (history of)—Use of this medicine may cause a tuberculosis infection to occur again

Proper Use of This Medicine

Inhaled corticosteroids will not relieve an asthma attack that has already started. However, your doctor may want you to continue taking this medicine at the usual time, even if you use another medicine to relieve the asthma attack.

Use this medicine only as directed. Do not use more of it and do not use it more often than your doctor ordered. To do so may increase the chance of side effects. Do not stop taking this medicine abruptly. This medicine should be discontinued only under the supervision of your doctor.

In order for this medicine to help prevent asthma attacks, it must be used every day in regularly spaced doses, as ordered by your doctor. Up to 4 to 6 weeks may pass before you begin to notice improvement in your condition. It may take several months before you feel the full effects of this medicine. This may not take as long if you have already been taking certain other medicines for your asthma.

Gargling and rinsing your mouth with water after each dose may help prevent hoarseness, throat irritation, and infection in the mouth. However, do not swallow the water after rinsing. Your doctor may also want you to use a spacer device to lessen these problems.

Inhaled corticosteroids are used with a special inhaler and usually come with patient directions. *Read the directions carefully before using this medicine.* If you do not understand the directions or you are not sure how to use the inhaler, ask your health care professional to show you what to do. Also, *ask your health care professional to check regularly how you use the inhaler to make sure you are using it properly.*

For patients using *beclomethasone, flunisolide, or triamcinolone inhalation aerosol:*

- When you use the inhaler for the first time, or if you have not used it in a while, it may not deliver the right amount of medicine with the first puff. Therefore, before using the inhaler, test or prime it.
- *To test or prime most inhalers:*
  ○ Insert the metal canister firmly into the clean mouthpiece according to the manufacturer's instructions. Check to make sure the canister is placed properly into the mouthpiece.
  ○ Take the cover off the mouthpiece and shake the inhaler three or four times.
  ○ Hold the inhaler well away from you at arm's length and press the top of the canister, spraying the medicine into the air *two* times. The inhaler will now be ready to provide the right amount of medicine when you use it.
- *To use most inhalers:*
  ○ Using your thumb and one or two fingers, hold the inhaler upright with the mouthpiece end down and pointing toward you.
  ○ Take the cover off the mouthpiece. Check the mouthpiece and remove any foreign objects. Then gently shake the inhaler three or four times.
  ○ Hold the mouthpiece away from your mouth and breathe out slowly to the end of a normal breath.
  ○ Use the inhalation method recommended by your doctor:
    ▪ Open-mouth method—Place the mouthpiece about 1 or 2 inches (2 finger widths) in front of your widely opened mouth. Make sure the inhaler is aimed into your mouth so that the spray does not hit the roof of your mouth or your tongue.
    ▪ Closed-mouth method—Place the mouthpiece in your mouth between your teeth and over your tongue with your lips closed tightly around it. Do not block the mouthpiece with your teeth or tongue.
  ○ Start to breathe in slowly through your mouth and, at the same time, press the top of the canister one time to get 1 puff of medicine. Continue to breathe in slowly for 3 to 5 seconds. Count the seconds while inhaling. It is important to press the top of the canister and breathe in slowly at the same time so the medicine gets into your lungs. This step may be difficult at first. If you are using the closed-mouth method and you see a fine mist coming from your mouth or nose, the inhaler is not being used correctly.
  ○ Hold your breath as long as you can up to 10 seconds. This gives the medicine time to settle in your airways and lungs.
  ○ Take the mouthpiece away from your mouth and breathe out slowly.
  ○ If your doctor has told you to inhale more than 1 puff of medicine at each dose, gently shake the inhaler again, and take the next puff, following exactly the same steps you used for the first puff. Press the canister one time for each puff of medicine.
  ○ When you are finished, wipe off the mouthpiece and replace the cap.

- Your doctor, nurse, or pharmacist may want you to use a spacer device with the inhaler. A spacer helps get the medicine into the lungs and reduces the amount of medicine that stays in your mouth and throat.
  - *To use a spacer device with the inhaler:*
    - Attach the spacer to the inhaler according to the manufacturer's directions. There are different types of spacers available, but the method of breathing remains the same with most spacers.
    - Gently shake the inhaler and spacer three or four times.
    - Hold the mouthpiece of the spacer away from your mouth and breathe out slowly to the end of a normal breath.
    - Place the mouthpiece into your mouth between your teeth and over your tongue with your lips closed around it.
    - Press down on the canister top once to release 1 puff of medicine into the spacer. Within one or two seconds, start to breathe in slowly through your mouth for 3 to 5 seconds. Count the seconds while inhaling. Do not breathe in through your nose.
    - Hold your breath as long as you can up to 10 seconds.
    - Breathe out slowly. Do not remove the mouthpiece from your mouth. Breathe in and out slowly two or three times to make sure the spacer device is emptied.
    - If your doctor has told you to take more than 1 puff of medicine at each dose, gently shake the inhaler and spacer again and take the next puff, following exactly the same steps you used for the first puff. Do not spray more than 1 puff at a time into the spacer.
    - When you are finished, remove the spacer device from the inhaler and replace the cover of the mouthpiece.
- Clean the inhaler mouthpiece, and spacer at least once a week.
  - *To clean the inhaler:*
    - Remove the canister from the inhaler and set the canister aside.
    - Wash the mouthpiece, cap, and spacer with warm, soapy water. Then, rinse well with warm, running water.
    - Shake off the excess water and let the inhaler parts air-dry completely before putting the inhaler back together.
- Check with your pharmacist to see if you should save the inhaler piece that comes with this medicine after the medicine is used up. Refill units may be available at a lower cost. However, remember that the inhaler is meant to be used only for the medicine that comes with it. Do not use the inhaler for any other inhalation aerosol medicine, even if the cartridge fits.

For patients using *beclomethasone capsules for inhalation:*

- *Do not swallow the capsules. The medicine will not work if you swallow it.*
- *To load the inhaler:*
  - Make sure your hands are clean and dry.
  - Do not insert the capsule into the inhaler until just before you are ready to use this medicine.
  - Take the inhaler from its container. Hold the inhaler by the mouthpiece and twist the barrel in either direction until it stops.
  - Take a capsule from its container. Hold the inhaler upright with the mouthpiece pointing downward. Press the capsule, with the clear end first, firmly into the raised small hole.
  - Make sure the top of the capsule is even with the top of the hole. This will push the old used capsule shell, if there is one, into the inhaler.
  - Hold the inhaler on its side with the white dot facing up. Twist the barrel quickly until it stops. This will break the capsule into two halves so the powder can be inhaled.
- *To use the inhaler:*
  - Hold the inhaler away from your mouth and breathe out slowly to the end of a normal breath.
  - Keep the inhaler on its side and place the mouthpiece in your mouth. Close your lips around it, and tilt your head slightly back. Do not block the mouthpiece with your teeth or tongue.
  - Breathe in slowly through your mouth until you have taken a full deep breath.
  - Take the inhaler from your mouth and hold your breath as long as you can up to 10 seconds. This gives the medicine time to settle in your airways and lungs.
  - Hold the inhaler well away from your mouth and breathe out to the end of a normal breath.
  - If your doctor has told you to use a second capsule, follow the same steps you used for the first capsule.
  - When you have finished using the inhaler, pull the two halves of the inhaler apart and throw away the empty capsule shells. There is no need to remove the shell left in the small hole, except before cleaning.
  - Put the two halves of the inhaler back together again and place it into its container to keep it clean.
- *To clean the inhaler:*
  - Every two weeks, take the inhaler apart and wash the two halves of the inhaler in clean, warm water. Make sure the empty capsule shell is removed from the small raised hole.
  - Shake out the excess water.
  - Allow all parts of the inhaler to dry before you put it back together.
- The inhaler should be replaced every 6 months.

For patients using *beclomethasone powder for inhalation:*

- *To load the inhaler:*
  - Make sure your hands are clean and dry.
  - Do not insert the cartridge until just before you are ready to use this medicine.
  - Take off the dark brown mouthpiece cover and make sure the mouthpiece is clean.
  - Hold the white cartridge by the exposed corners and gently pull it out until you see the ribbed sides of the cartridge.
  - Squeeze the ribbed sides and take out the cartridge unit from the body of the inhaler.
  - Place the disk containing the medicine onto the white wheel with the numbers facing up. Allow the underside of the disk to fit into the holes of the wheel.
  - Slide the cartridge unit with wheel and disk back into the body of the inhaler. Gently push the cartridge in and pull it out again. The disk will turn.

- Continue to turn the disk in this way until the number 8 appears in the side indicator window. Each disk has eight blisters containing the medicine. The window will display how many doses you have left after you use it each time, by counting down from 8. For example, when you see the number 1, you have one dose left.
- To replace the empty disk with a full disk, follow the same steps you used to load the inhaler. Do not throw away the wheel when you discard the empty disk.

- *To use the inhaler:*
  - Hold the inhaler flat in your hand. Lift the rear edge of the lid until it is fully upright.
  - The plastic needle on the front of the lid will break the blister containing one inhalation of medicine. When the lid is raised as far as it will go, both the upper and the lower surfaces of the blister will be pierced. Do not lift the lid if the cartridge is not in the inhaler. Doing this will break the needle and you will need a new inhaler.
  - After the blister is broken open, close the lid. Keeping the inhaler flat and well away from your mouth, breathe out to the end of a normal breath.
  - Raise the inhaler to your mouth, and place the mouthpiece in your mouth.
  - Close your lips around the mouthpiece and tilt your head slightly back. Do not block the mouthpiece with your teeth or tongue. Do not cover the air holes on the side of the mouthpiece.
  - Breathe in through your mouth as fast as you can until you have taken a full deep breath.
  - Hold your breath and remove the mouthpiece from your mouth. Continue holding your breath as long as you can up to 10 seconds before breathing out. This gives the medicine time to settle in your airways and lungs.
  - Hold the inhaler well away from your mouth and breathe out to the end of a normal breath.
  - Prepare the cartridge for your next inhalation. Pull the cartridge out once and push it in once. The disk will turn to the next numbered dose as seen in the indicator window. Do not pierce the blister until just before the inhalation.
- *To clean the inhaler:* Brush away the loose powder each day with the brush provided.
- The inhaler should be replaced every 6 months.

For patients using *budesonide powder for inhalation:*
- *To prime the inhaler:*
  - Unscrew the cover of the inhaler and lift it off.
  - Hold the inhaler *upright* with the brown piece pointing downward. Turn the brown piece of the inhaler in one direction as far as it will go. Then twist it back until it clicks. Repeat this step one more time and the inhaler will be primed.
  - Prime each new inhaler before using it the first time. After it has been primed, it is not necessary to prime it again, even if you put it aside for a long period of time.
- *To load the inhaler:*
  - Unscrew the cover of the inhaler and lift it off.
  - Hold the inhaler *upright* with the brown piece pointing downward. Turn the brown piece of the inhaler in one direction as far as it will go. Then twist it back until it clicks.

- *To use the inhaler:*
  - Hold the inhaler away from your mouth and breathe out slowly to the end of a normal breath.
  - Place the mouthpiece in your mouth and close your lips around it. Tilt your head slightly back. Do not block the mouthpiece with your teeth or tongue.
  - Breathe in quickly and evenly through your mouth until you have taken a full deep breath.
  - Hold your breath and remove the inhaler from your mouth. Continue holding your breath as long as you can up to 10 seconds before breathing out. This gives the medicine time to settle in your airways and lungs.
  - Hold the inhaler well away from your mouth and breathe out to the end of a normal breath.
  - Replace the cover on the mouthpiece to keep it clean.
- This inhaler delivers the medicine as a very fine powder. You may not taste, smell, or feel this medicine.
- This inhaler should not be used with a spacer.
- When the indicator window begins to show a red mark, there are about 20 doses left. When the red mark covers the window, the inhaler is empty.

For patients using *budesonide suspension for inhalation:*
- This medicine is to be used in a power-operated nebulizer equipped with a face mask or mouthpiece. Your doctor will advise you on which nebulizer to use. Make sure you understand how to use the nebulizer. If you have any questions about this, check with your doctor.
- Any opened ampul should be protected from light. The medicine in an open ampul must be used promptly after the ampul is opened. Ampuls should be used within 2 weeks after the envelope containing them is opened.
- *To prepare the medicine for use in the nebulizer:*
  - Remove one ampul from the sheet of five units and shake it gently.
  - Hold the ampul upright. Open it by twisting off the wing.
  - Squeeze the contents of the ampul into the cup of the nebulizer. If you use only half of the contents of an ampul, add enough of the sodium chloride solution provided to dilute the solution.
  - Gently shake the nebulizer. Then attach the face mask to the nebulizer and connect the nebulizer to the air pump.
- *To use the medicine in the nebulizer:*
  - This medicine should be inhaled over a period of 10 to 15 minutes.
  - Breathe slowly and evenly, in and out, until no more mist is left in the nebulizer cup.
  - Rinse your mouth when you are finished with the treatment. Wash your face if you used a face mask.
- *To clean the nebulizer:*
  - After each treatment, wash the cup of the nebulizer and the mask or mouthpiece in warm water with a mild detergent.
  - Allow the nebulizer parts to dry before putting them back together again.

Dosing—The dose of these medicines will be different for different patients. *Follow your doctor's orders or the directions on the label.* The following information includes only the average doses of these medicines. *If your dose is different, do not change it* unless your doctor tells you to do so.

For beclomethasone
- For inhalation *aerosol:*
  - For bronchial asthma:
    - Adults and children 12 years of age and older—For the 42– or 50–mcg-per-metered-spray products: 2 puffs (84 to 100 micrograms [mcg]) three or four times a day, or 4 puffs (168 to 200 mcg) two times a day. In severe asthma, your doctor may want you to take a higher dose. For the 84–mcg-per-metered-spray product: 2 puffs (168 mcg) two times a day. In severe asthma, your doctor may want you to take a higher dose.
    - Children 6 to 12 years of age—For the 42– or 50–mcg-per-metered-spray products: 1 or 2 puffs (42 to 100 mcg) three or four times a day, or 4 puffs (168 to 200 mcg) two times a day. For the 84–mcg-per-metered-spray product: 2 puffs (168 mcg) two times a day.
    - Children up to 6 years of age—Use and dose must be determined by your doctor.
- For *capsules* for inhalation or *powder* for inhalation:
  - For bronchial asthma:
    - Adults and teenagers 14 years of age and older—At first, 200 mcg three or four times a day. Then your doctor may reduce the dose, based on your condition.
    - Children 6 to 14 years of age—At first, 100 mcg two to four times a day. Then your doctor may reduce the dose, based on your condition.
    - Children up to 6 years of age—Use and dose must be determined by the doctor.

For beclomethasone dipropionate HFA
- For inhalation *aerosol:*
  - For bronchial asthma:
    - Adults and children 12 years of age and older—For the 40–mcg-per-metered-spray products: 1 to 4 puffs (40 to 160 micrograms [mcg]) two times a day. The higher doses generally are used for patients previously treated with other corticosteroids.For the 50–mcg-per-metered-spray products: 1 to 2 puffs (50 to 100 mcg) two times a day if your asthma is mild or 2 to 5 puffs (100 to 250 mcg) two times a day if your asthma is more severe. For the 80–mcg-per-metered-spray products: 1 or 2 puffs (80 to 160 mcg) two times a day. The higher dose generally is used for patients previously treated with other corticosteroids. For the 100–mcg-per-metered-spray product: 3 to 4 puffs (300 to 400 mcg) two times a day.
    - Children up to 5 years of age—Use and dose must be determined by your doctor.
    - Children 5 to 11 years of age—1 puff (40 mcg) two times a day.

For budesonide
- For *powder* for inhalation:
  - For bronchial asthma:
    - Adults—200 to 800 micrograms (mcg) two times a day. A lower dose of 200 mcg or 400 mcg once daily, either in the morning or in the evening, may sometimes be used for mild to moderate asthma when the symptoms are well controlled. The higher doses generally are used for patients previously treated with other corticosteroids. Then your doctor may increase or decrease the dose, depending on your condition.

- Children 6 years of age and older—At first, 200 mcg two times a day. Then your doctor may increase the dose to 400 mcg two times a day, depending on your condition. A lower dose of 200 mcg or 400 mcg once daily, either in the morning or in the evening, may sometimes be used for mild to moderate asthma when the symptoms are well controlled.
- Children up to 6 years of age—Use and dose must be determined by the doctor.
- For *suspension* for inhalation:
  - For bronchial asthma:
    - Adults and children 8 years of age and older—1000 to 2000 micrograms (mcg) mixed with enough sterile sodium chloride solution for inhalation, if necessary, to make 2 to 4 milliliters (mL). This solution is used in a nebulizer for a period of ten to fifteen minutes. The medicine should be used two times a day.
    - Children 12 months to 8 years of age—250 to 500 mcg mixed with enough sterile sodium chloride solution for inhalation, if necessary, to make 2 to 4 mL. This solution is used in a nebulizer for a period of ten to fifteen minutes. The medicine should be used two times a day.
    - Children up to 12 months of age—Use and dose must be determined by the doctor.

For flunisolide
- For inhalation *aerosol:*
  - For bronchial asthma:
    - Adults and children 4 years of age and older—500 micrograms (mcg) (2 puffs) two times a day, morning and evening.
    - Children up to 4 years of age—Use and dose must be determined by the doctor.

For triamcinolone
- For inhalation *aerosol:*
  - For bronchial asthma:
    - Adults and children 12 years of age and older—At first, 200 micrograms (mcg) (2 puffs) two to four times a day. Then your doctor may reduce the dose, based on your condition. In severe asthma, your doctor may want you to take a higher dose.
    - Children 6 to 12 years of age—At first, 100 to 200 mcg (1 or 2 puffs) three or four times a day. Then your doctor may adjust your dose, based on your condition.
    - Children up to 6 years of age—Use and dose must be determined by the doctor.

Missed dose—If you miss a dose of this medicine, use it as soon as possible. Then use any remaining doses for that day at regularly spaced times.

Storage—To store this medicine:
- Keep out of the reach of children.
- Store away from heat and direct light.
- Do not store the capsule form of this medicine in the bathroom, near the kitchen sink, or in other damp places. Heat or moisture may cause the medicine to break down.
- Keep the aerosol or suspension form of this medicine from getting too cold or freezing. This medicine may be less effective if the container is cold when you use it.

- The 84–mcg-per-metered-spray product of beclomethasone should not be stored for longer than 6 months after it has been removed from its moisture-protective pouch. After 6 months, any remaining medicine should be discarded.
- Do not puncture, break, or burn the aerosol container, even after it is empty.
- Do not keep outdated medicine or medicine no longer needed. Be sure that any discarded medicine is out of the reach of children.

Precautions While Using This Medicine

Check with your doctor if:
- *You go through a period of unusual stress to your body, such as surgery, injury, or infection.*
- *You have an asthma attack that does not improve after you take a bronchodilator medicine.*
- *You are exposed to viral infections, such as chickenpox or measles.*
- *Signs of infection occur, especially in your mouth, throat, or lung.*
- *Your symptoms do not improve or if your condition gets worse.*

Your doctor may want you to carry a medical identification card stating that you are using this medicine and that you may need additional medicine during times of emergency, a severe asthma attack or other illness, or unusual stress.

Before you have any kind of surgery (including dental surgery) or emergency treatment, tell the medical doctor or dentist in charge that you are using this medicine.

For patients who are also regularly taking a corticosteroid by mouth in tablet or liquid form:
- *Do not stop taking the corticosteroid taken by mouth without your doctor's advice, even if your asthma seems better.* Your doctor may want you to reduce gradually the amount you are taking before stopping completely to lessen the chance of unwanted effects.
- When your doctor tells you to reduce the dose, or to stop taking the corticosteroid taken by mouth, follow the directions carefully. Your body may need time to adjust to the change. The length of time this takes may depend on the amount of medicine you were taking and how long you took it. *It is especially important that your doctor check your progress at regular visits during this time.* Ask your doctor if there are special directions you should follow if you have a severe asthma attack, if you need any other medical or surgical treatment, or if certain side effects occur. Be certain that you understand these directions, and follow them carefully.

Side Effects

Along with its needed effects, a medicine may cause some unwanted effects. Although not all of these side effects may occur, if they do occur they may need medical attention.

Check with your doctor immediately if any of the following side effects occur just after you use this medicine:
Rare
   Shortness of breath, troubled breathing, tightness in chest, or wheezing; signs of hypersensitivity reactions, such as swelling of face, lips, or eyelids

Also, check with your doctor as soon as possible if any of the following side effects occur:
Less common
   Bruising; burning or pain while urinating, blood in urine, or frequent urge to urinate; chest pain; creamy white, curd-like patches in the mouth or throat and/or pain when eating or swallowing; dizziness or sense of constant movement or surroundings; general feeling of discomfort or illness; irregular or fast heartbeat; itching, rash, or hives; sinus problems; stomach or abdominal pain; swelling of fingers, ankles, feet, or lower legs; unusual tiredness or weakness; weight gain

Rare
   Bleeding from rectum or bloody stools; blurred vision or other changes in vision; diarrhea or nausea; fainting or feeling faint; fever; frequent urination or unusual thirst; growth inhibition in children; high blood pressure; increased fat deposits in face, neck, and trunk; increased skin pigmentation; loss of appetite; menstrual changes; mood or mental changes; numbness; pain or burning in chest; vomiting

Additional side effects may occur if you take this medicine for a long time. Check with your doctor if any of the following side effects occur:
   Pain in back, ribs, arms, or legs (osteoporosis)

Other side effects may occur that usually do not need medical attention. These side effects may go away during treatment as your body adjusts to the medicine. However, check with your doctor if any of the following side effects continue or are bothersome:
More common
   Cold-like symptoms; cough; dry mouth or throat; headache; sore throat, hoarseness or voice changes

Less common or rare
   Constipation; nosebleeds; trouble in sleeping

Other side effects not listed above may also occur in some patients. If you notice any other effects, check with your doctor.

Additional Information

Once a medicine has been approved for marketing for a certain use, experience may show that it is also useful for other medical problems. Although this use is not included in product labeling, some of the inhaled corticosteroids are used in certain patients with the following medical condition:

- Croup in children (budesonide)

CORTICOSTEROIDS (Nasal)

Some commonly used brand names are:

In the U.S.—

Beconase (1)	Nasarel (4)
Beconase AQ (1)	Nasonex (6)
Dexacort Turbinaire (3)	Rhinocort (2)
Flonase (5)	Vancenase (1)
Nasacort (7)	Vancenase AQ 84 mcg (1)
Nasacort AQ (7)	Vancenase pockethaler (1)
Nasalide (4)	

Beconase (1)	Rhinalar (4)
Flonase (5)	Rhinocort Aqua (2)
Nasacort (7)	Rhinocort Turbuhaler (2)
Nasacort AQ (7)	Vancenase (1)
Nasonex (6)	

This information applies to the following medicines:

1. Beclomethasone (be-kloe-METH-a-sone)
2. Budesonide (byoo-DES-oh-nide)
3. Dexamethasone (dex-a-METH-a-sone)
4. Flunisolide (floo-NISS-oh-lide)
5. Fluticasone (floo-TIC-a-sone)
6. Mometasone (mo-MET-a-sone)
7. Triamcinolone (trye-am-SIN-oh-lone)

Category

- **Anti-inflammatory, steroidal, nasal**—Beclomethasone; Budesonide; Dexamethasone; Flunisolide; Fluticasone; Mometasone; Triamcinolone

- **Corticosteroid, nasal**—Beclomethasone; Budesonide; Dexamethasone; Flunisolide; Fluticasone; Mometasone; Triamcinolone

Description

Nasal corticosteroids (kor-ti-ko-STER-oids) are cortisone-like medicines. They belong to the family of medicines called steroids. These medicines are sprayed or inhaled into the nose to help relieve the stuffy nose, irritation, and discomfort of hay fever, other allergies, and other nasal problems. These medicines are also used to prevent nasal polyps from growing back after they have been removed by surgery.

These medicines are available only with your doctor's prescription, in the following dosage forms:

Nasal
- Beclomethasone
  - Aerosol
  - Suspension
- Budesonide
  - Aerosol
  - Powder
  - Suspension
- Dexamethasone
  - Aerosol
- Flunisolide
  - Solution
- Fluticasone
  - Suspension
- Mometasone
  - Suspension
- Triamcinolone
  - Aerosol
  - Suspension

Before Using This Medicine

In deciding to use a medicine, the risks of taking the medicine must be weighed against the good it will do. This is a decision you and your doctor will make. For corticosteroids, the following should be considered:

Allergies—Tell your doctor if you have ever had any unusual or allergic reaction to corticosteroids. Also tell your health care professional if you are allergic to any other substances, such as foods, preservatives, or dyes.

Pregnancy—In one human study, use of beclomethasone oral inhalation by pregnant women did not cause birth defects or other problems. Other studies on birth defects with beclomethasone, budesonide, dexamethasone, flunisolide, fluticasone, mometasone or triamcinolone have not been done in humans.

In animal studies, corticosteroids taken by mouth or injection during pregnancy were shown to cause birth defects. Also, too much use of corticosteroids during pregnancy, especially during the first trimester, may cause other unwanted effects in the infant, such as slower growth and reduced adrenal gland function.

If corticosteroids are medically necessary during pregnancy to control nasal problems, nasal corticosteroids are generally considered safer than corticosteroids taken by mouth or injection. Also, use of nasal corticosteroids may allow some patients to stop using or decrease the amount of corticosteroids taken by mouth or injection.

Breast-feeding—Use of dexamethasone is not recommended in nursing mothers, since dexamethasone passes into breast milk and may affect the infant's growth.

It is not known whether beclomethasone, budesonide, flunisolide, fluticasone or triamcinolone passes into breast milk. Although most medicines pass into breast milk in small amounts, many of them may be used safely while breast-feeding. Levels of mometasone are not measurable in breast milk, thus exposure is expected to be low. Mothers who are taking these medicines and wish to breast-feed should discuss them with their doctor.

Children—Corticosteroids taken by mouth or injection have been shown to slow or stop growth in children and cause reduced adrenal gland function. If corticosteroids are medically necessary to control nasal problems in a child, nasal corticosteroids are generally considered to be safer than corticosteroids taken by mouth or injection. Prolonged or high-dose use of nasal corticosteroids may potentially affect growth; although, most nasal corticosteroids have not been shown to affect growth. Also, use of most nasal corticosteroids may allow some children to stop using or decrease the amount of corticosteroids taken by mouth or injection.

Before this medicine is given to a child, you and your child's doctor should talk about the good this medicine will do as well as the risks of using it. Follow the doctor's directions very carefully to lessen the chance of unwanted effects.

Older adults—Although there is no specific information comparing use of nasal corticosteroids in the elderly with use in other age groups, they are not expected to cause different side effects or problems in older people than they do in younger adults.

Other medicines—Although certain medicines should not be used together at all, in other cases two different medicines may be used together even if an interaction might occur. In these cases, your doctor may want to change the dose, or other precautions may be necessary. Tell your health care professional if you are taking any prescription or nonprescription (over-the-counter [OTC]) medicines, such as:

- Ephedrine or
- Phenobarbital or
- Rifampin (e.g., Rifadin)—Ephedrine, phenobarbital, and rifampin may decrease the blood levels of nasal corticosteroids, such as dexamethasone, warranting an increase in corticosteroid dose
- Ephedrine or
- Phenobarbital or
- Rifampin (e.g., Rifadin)—Ephedrine, phenobarbital, and rifampin may decrease the blood levels of nasal corticosteroids, such as dexamethasone, warranting an increase in corticosteroid dose

Other medical problems—The presence of other medical problems may affect the use of corticosteroids. Make sure you tell your doctor if you have any other medical problems, especially:

- Amebiasis—Nasal corticosteroids may make this condition worse
- Asthma—Nasal corticosteroids may make this condition worse
- Diabetes mellitus (sugar diabetes)—Use of dexamethasone may decrease carbohydrate tolerance, worsening blood glucose control and warranting an increase in insulin dosage
- Glaucoma—Long-term use of nasal corticosteroids may worsen glaucoma by increasing the pressure within the eye
- Herpes simplex (virus) infection of the eye or
- Infections (virus, bacteria, or fungus)—Nasal corticosteroids may cover up the signs of these conditions
- Injury to the nose (recent) or
- Nose surgery (recent) or
- Sores in the nose—Nasal corticosteroids may prevent proper healing of these conditions
- Liver disease
- Tuberculosis (active or history of)
- Underactive thyroid
- Weak heart or
- Recent heart attack—Use of dexamethasone may worsen these conditions

Proper Use of This Medicine

This medicine usually comes with patient directions. *Read them carefully before using the medicine.* Beclomethasone, budesonide, dexamethasone, and triamcinolone are used with a special inhaler. If you do not understand the directions, or if you are not sure how to use the inhaler, check with your health care professional.

Before using this medicine, clear the nasal passages by blowing your nose. Then, with the nosepiece inserted into the nostril, aim the spray towards the inner corner of the eye.

In order for this medicine to help you, it must be used regularly as ordered by your doctor. This medicine usually begins to work in about 1 week (for dexamethasone), but up to 3 weeks may pass before you feel its full effects.

Use this medicine only as directed. Do not use more of it and do not use it more often than your doctor ordered. To do so may increase the chance of absorption through the lining of the nose and the chance of unwanted effects.

Check with your doctor before using this medicine for nasal problems other than the one for which it was prescribed, since it should not be used on many bacterial, virus, or fungus nasal infections.

Save the inhaler that comes with beclomethasone or dexamethasone, since refill units may be available at lower cost.

Dosing—The dose of nasal corticosteroids will be different for different patients. *Follow your doctor's orders or the directions on the label.* The following information includes only the average doses of nasal corticosteroids. *If your dose is different, do not change it* unless your doctor tells you to do so.

For beclomethasone
- For allergies or other nasal conditions:
  - For *nasal aerosol* dosage form:
    - Adults and children 6 years of age and older— One spray in each nostril two to four times a day.
    - Children up to 6 years of age—Use and dose must be determined by your doctor.
  - For *nasal suspension* dosage form:
    - Adults and children 6 years of age and older— One or two sprays in each nostril two times a day.
    - Children up to 6 years of age—Use and dose must be determined by your doctor.

For budesonide
- For allergies or other nasal conditions:
  - For *nasal powder* dosage form:
    - Adults and children 6 years of age and older— Two inhalations in each nostril once a day in the morning.
    - Children up to 6 years of age—Use and dose must be determined by your doctor.
  - For *nasal suspension* dosage form:
    - Adults and children 6 years of age and older— One or two sprays in each nostril one or two times a day.
    - Children up to 6 years of age—Use and dose must be determined by your doctor.

For dexamethasone
- For allergies or other nasal conditions:
  - For *nasal aerosol* dosage form:
    - Adults and children 12 years of age and older— Two sprays in each nostril two or three times a day for up to two weeks.
    - Children 6 to 12 years of age—One to two sprays in each nostril two times a day for up to two weeks.
    - Children up to 6 years of age—Use and dose must be determined by your doctor.

For flunisolide
- For allergies or other nasal conditions:
  - For *nasal solution* dosage form:
    - Adults and children 6 years of age and older— One or two sprays in each nostril one to three times a day.
    - Children up to 6 years of age—Use and dose must be determined by your doctor.

For fluticasone
- For allergies or other nasal conditions:
  - For *nasal suspension* dosage form:
    - Adults and children 4 years of age and older—One or two sprays in each nostril one or two times a day.
    - Children up to 4 years of age—Use and dose must be determined by your doctor.

For mometasone
- For allergies or other nasal conditions:
  - For *nasal suspension* dosage form:
    - Adults and children 12 years of age and older—One or two sprays in each nostril one time a day.
    - Children up to 12 years of age—Use and dose must be determined by your doctor.

For triamcinolone
- For allergies or other nasal conditions:
  - For *nasal aerosol* dosage form:
    - Adults and children 6 years of age and older (In Canada, children 12 years of age and older)—One or two sprays in each nostril once a day.
    - Children up to 6 years of age (In Canada, children up to 12 years of age)—Use and dose must be determined by your doctor.
  - For *nasal suspension* dosage form:
    - Adults and children 6 years of age and older—One or two sprays in each nostril one time a day.
    - Children up to 6 years of age—Use and dose must be determined by your doctor.

Missed dose—If you miss a dose of this medicine and remember within an hour or so, use it right away. However, if you do not remember until later, skip the missed dose and go back to your regular dosing schedule. Do not double doses.

Storage—To store this medicine:
- Keep out of the reach of children.
- Store away from heat and direct light.
- Do not store budesonide powder in the bathroom, near the kitchen sink, or in other damp places, especially if the cap has not been tightly screwed back on. Moisture may cause the medicine to break down.
- Keep the medicine from getting too cold or freezing. This medicine may be less effective if it is too cold when you use it.
- Do not puncture, break, or burn the beclomethasone, dexamethasone, or triamcinolone aerosol container, even after it is empty.
- Do not keep outdated medicine or medicine no longer needed. Also, discard any unused beclomethasone or flunisolide solution 3 months after you open the package. Be sure that any discarded medicine is out of the reach of children.

Precautions While Using This Medicine

If you will be using this medicine for more than a few weeks, your doctor should check your progress at regular visits.

Check with your doctor:
- if signs of a nose, sinus, or throat infection occur.
- if your symptoms do not improve within 7 days (for dexamethasone) or within 3 weeks (for beclomethasone, budesonide, flunisolide, fluticasone, mometasone, or triamcinolone).
- if your condition gets worse.

When you are being treated with dexamethasone, and after you stop treatment with it, do not have any immunizations (vaccinations) without your doctor's approval. Dexamethasone may lower your body's resistance and there is a chance you may get the infection the immunization is meant to prevent. In addition, other persons living in your household should not take or have recently taken oral polio vaccine since there is a chance they could pass the polio virus on to you. Also, avoid other persons who have taken oral polio vaccine. Don't get close to them, and do not stay in the same room with them for very long. If you cannot take these precautions, you should consider wearing a protective face mask that covers the nose and mouth.

Side Effects

Along with its needed effects, a medicine may cause some unwanted effects. Although not all of these side effects may occur, if they do occur they may need medical attention.

Check with your doctor as soon as possible if any of the following side effects occur:

Less common or rare
Bad smell; blindness; bloody mucus or unexplained nosebleeds; blurred or gradual loss of vision; burning or stinging after use of spray or irritation inside nose (continuing); crusting, white patches, or sores inside nose; discharge or redness in eye, eyelid, or inner lining of the eyelid; eye pain; headache; hives; light-headedness or dizziness; loss of sense of taste or smell; muscle pain; nausea or vomiting; ringing in the ears; shortness of breath; skin rash; sore throat, cough, or hoarseness; stomach pains; stuffy, dry, or runny nose or watery eyes (continuing); swelling of eyelids, face, or lips; tightness in chest; troubled breathing; unusual tiredness or weakness; wheezing; white patches in throat

Symptoms of overdose
Acne; blurred vision; bone fractures; excess hair growth in females; fullness or rounding of the face, neck, and trunk; high blood pressure; impotence in males; increased urination or thirst; lack of menstrual periods; menstrual changes; muscle wasting and weakness

Other side effects may occur that usually do not need medical attention. These side effects may go away during treatment as your body adjusts to the medicine. However, check with your doctor if any of the following side effects continue or are bothersome:

More common
Burning, dryness, or other irritation inside the nose (mild, lasting only a short time); increase in sneezing; irritation of throat

Less common
Sneezing; itching of throat

Not all of the side effects listed above have been reported for each of these medicines, but they have been reported for at least one of them. All of the nasal corticosteroids are very similar, so any of the above side effects may occur with any of these medicines.

Other side effects not listed above may also occur in some patients. If you notice any other effects, check with your doctor.

CORTICOSTEROIDS   (Systemic)

Some commonly used brand names are:

In the U.S.—

Acetocot (9)	Meprolone (6)
A-hydroCort (5)	Meticorten (8)
Amcort (9)	Nor-Pred T.B.A. (7)
A-MethaPred (6)	Orasone 1 (8)
Aristocort (9)	Orasone 5 (8)
Aristocort Forte (9)	Orasone 10 (8)
Aristopak (9)	Orasone 20 (8)
Aristospan (9)	Orasone 50 (8)
Articulose-50 (7)	Pediapred (7)
Articulose-L.A. (9)	Predacort 50 (7)
Celestone (1)	Predalone 50 (7)
Celestone Phosphate (1)	Predalone T.B.A. (7)
Celestone Soluspan (1)	Predate-50 (7)
Cinalone 40 (9)	Predate S (7)
Cinonide 40 (9)	Predate TBA (7)
Clinacort (9)	Predcor-25 (7)
Clinalog (9)	Predcor-50 (7)
Cordrol (8)	Predcor-TBA (7)
Cortastat (4)	Predicort-RP (7)
Cortastat 10 (4)	Pred-Ject-50 (7)
Cortastat LA (4)	Prednicot (8)
Cortef (5)	Prednisone Intensol (8)
Cortone Acetate (3)	Pred-Pak 45 (8)
Cotolone (7)	Pred-Pak 79 (8)
Decadron (4)	Prelone (7)
Delta-Cortef (7)	Robalog (9)
Deltasone (8)	Selestoject (1)
Depo-Medrol (6)	Solu-Cortef (5)
Dexamethasone Intensol (4)	Solu-Medrol (6)
Dexasone (4)	Solurex (4)
Dexasone L.A. (4)	Solurex LA (4)
Hydrocortone (5)	Sterapred (8)
Hydrocortone Acetate (5)	Sterapred DS (8)
Hydrocortone Phosphate (5)	Tac-3 (9)
Kenacort (9)	Tramacort-D (9)
Kenacort Diacetate (9)	Triam-A (9)
Kenaject-40 (9)	Triam-Forte (9)
Kenalog-10 (9)	Triamolone 40 (9)
Kenalog-40 (9)	Triamonide 40 (9)
Ken-Jec 40 (9)	Tri-Kort (9)
Key-Pred (7)	Trilog (9)
Key-Pred SP (7)	Trilone (9)
Liquid Pred (8)	Tristoject (9)
Medrol (6)	

In Canada—

A-Hydrocort (5)	Deronil (4)
Apo-Prednisone (8)	Dexasone (4)
Aristocort (9)	Entocort (2)
Aristocort Forte (9)	Hexadrol Phosphate (4)
Aristocort Intralesional (9)	Kenacort (9)
Aristospan (9)	Kenalog-10 (9)
Betnesol (1)	Kenalog-40 (9)
Celestone Soluspan (1)	Medrol (6)
Cortef (5)	Oradexon (4)
Cortisone Acetate-ICN (3)	Pediapred (7)
Cortone (3)	Scheinpharm Triamcine-A (9)
Decadron (4)	Solu-Cortef (5)
Decadron Phosphate (4)	Solu-Medrol (6)
Deltasone (8)	Winpred (8)
Depo-Medrol (6)	

This information applies to the following medicines:

1. Betamethasone (bay-ta-METH-a-sone)
2. Budesonide (byoo-DES-oh-nide)
3. Cortisone (KOR-ti-sone)
4. Dexamethasone (dex-a-METH-a-sone)
5. Hydrocortisone (hye-droe-KOR-ti-sone)
6. Methylprednisolone (meth-il-pred-NIS-oh-lone)
7. Prednisolone (pred-NISS-oh-lone)
8. Prednisone (PRED-ni-sone)
9. Triamcinolone (trye-am-SIN-oh-lone)

Category

- **Anti-inflammatory, steroidal**—Betamethasone; Budesonide; Cortisone; Dexamethasone; Hydrocortisone; Methylprednisolone; Prednisolone; Prednisone; Triamcinolone

- **Antiemetic, in cancer chemotherapy**—Dexamethasone; Hydrocortisone; Prednisone

- **Corticosteroid**—Betamethasone; Budesonide; Cortisone; Dexamethasone; Hydrocortisone; Methylprednisolone; Prednisolone; Prednisone; Triamcinolone

- **Diagnostic aid, Cushing's syndrome**—Dexamethasone

- **Diagnostic aid, endogenous depression**—Dexamethasone

- **Immunosuppressant**—Betamethasone;   Cortisone; Dexamethasone; Hydrocortisone; Methylprednisolone; Prednisolone; Prednisone; Triamcinolone

Description

Corticosteroids (kor-ti-koe-STER-oyds) (cortisone-like medicines) are used to provide relief for inflamed areas of the body. They lessen swelling, redness, itching, and allergic reactions. They are often used as part of the treatment for a number of different diseases, such as severe allergies or skin problems, asthma, or arthritis. Corticosteroids may also be used for other conditions as determined by your doctor.

Your body naturally produces certain cortisone-like hormones that are necessary to maintain good health. If your body does not produce enough, your doctor may have prescribed this medicine to help make up the difference.

Corticosteroids are very strong medicines. In addition to their helpful effects in treating your medical problem, they have side effects that can be very serious. If your adrenal glands are not producing enough cortisone-like hormones, taking this medicine is not likely to cause problems unless you take too much of it. If you are taking this medicine to treat another medical problem, be sure that you discuss the risks and benefits of this medicine with your doctor.

These medicines are available only with your doctor's prescription, in the following dosage forms:

Oral
- Betamethasone
  - Syrup
  - Tablets
  - Effervescent tablets
  - Extended-release tablets
- Budesonide
  - Extended-release capsules
- Cortisone
  - Tablets
- Dexamethasone
  - Elixir
  - Oral solution
  - Tablets
- Hydrocortisone
  - Oral suspension
  - Tablets

- Methylprednisolone
  - Tablets
- Prednisolone
  - Oral solution
  - Syrup
  - Tablets
- Prednisone
  - Oral solution
  - Syrup
  - Tablets
- Triamcinolone
  - Syrup
  - Tablets

Parenteral
- Betamethasone
  - Injection
- Cortisone
  - Injection
- Dexamethasone
  - Injection
- Hydrocortisone
  - Injection
- Methylprednisolone
  - Injection
- Prednisolone
  - Injection
- Triamcinolone
  - Injection

Before Using This Medicine

In deciding to use a medicine, the risks of taking the medicine must be weighed against the good it will do. This is a decision you and your doctor will make. For corticosteroids, the following should be considered:

Allergies—Tell your doctor if you have ever had any unusual or allergic reaction to corticosteroids. Also tell your health care professional if you are allergic to any other substances, such as foods, preservatives, or dyes.

Diet—If you will be using this medicine for a long time, your doctor may want you to:
- Follow a low-salt diet and/or a potassium-rich diet.
- Watch your calories to prevent weight gain.
- Add extra protein to your diet.

Make certain your health care professional knows if you are already on any special diet, such as a low-sodium or low-sugar diet.

Pregnancy—Studies on birth defects with corticosteroids have not been done in humans. However, studies in animals have shown that corticosteroids cause birth defects.

Breast-feeding—Corticosteroids pass into breast milk and may cause problems with growth or other unwanted effects in nursing babies. Depending on the amount of medicine you are taking every day, it may be necessary for you to take another medicine or to stop breast-feeding during treatment.

Children—Corticosteroids may cause infections such as chickenpox or measles to be more serious in children who catch them. These medicines can also slow or stop growth in children and in growing teenagers, especially when they are used for a long time. Before this medicine is given to children or teenagers, you should discuss its use with your child's doctor and then carefully follow the doctor's instructions.

Older adults—Older patients may be more likely to develop high blood pressure or osteoporosis (bone disease) from corticosteroids. Women are especially at risk of developing bone disease.

Other medicines—Although certain medicines should not be used together at all, in other cases two different medicines may be used together even if an interaction might occur. In these cases, your doctor may want to change the dose, or other precautions may be necessary. When you are taking corticosteroids, it is especially important that your health care professional know if you are taking any of the following:
- Ambenonium (e.g., Mytelase) or
- Neostigmine (e.g., Prostigmin) or
- Pyridostigmine (e.g., Mestinon)—May produce severe weakness in patients with myasthenia gravis.
- Aminoglutethimide (e.g., Cytadren) or
- Antacids (in large amounts) or
- Barbiturates, except butalbital, or
- Carbamazepine (e.g., Tegretol) or
- Griseofulvin (e.g., Fulvicin) or
- Mitotane (e.g., Lysodren) or
- Phenylbutazone (e.g., Butazolidin) or
- Phenytoin (e.g., Dilantin) or
- Primidone (e.g., Mysoline) or
- Rifampin (e.g., Rifadin)—Use of these medicines may make certain corticosteroids less effective
- Amphotericin B by injection (e.g., Fungizone)—Using corticosteroids with this medicine may decrease the amount of potassium in the blood. Serious side effects could occur if the level of potassium gets too low
- Antidiabetic agents, oral (diabetes medicine taken by mouth) or
- Insulin—Corticosteroids may increase blood glucose (sugar) levels
- Clarithromycin (e.g., Biaxin) or
- Erythromycin (e.g., E-Mycin, Erythrocin)—These medications may increase the amount of corticosteroid removed from your body.
- Cyclosporine (e.g., Sandimmune)—Use of this medicine with high doses of methylprednisolone may cause convulsions (seizures)
- Digitalis glycosides (heart medicine)—Corticosteroids decrease the amount of potassium in the blood. Digitalis can increase the risk of having an irregular heartbeat or other problems if the amount of potassium in the blood gets too low
- Diuretics (water pills) or
- Medicine containing potassium—Using corticosteroids with diuretics may cause the diuretic to be less effective. Also, corticosteroids may increase the risk of low blood potassium, which is also a problem with certain diuretics. Potassium supplements or a different type of diuretic is used in treating high blood pressure in those people who have problems keeping their blood potassium at a normal level. Corticosteroids may make these medicines less able to do this
- Immunizations (vaccinations)—While you are being treated with this medicine, and even after you stop taking it, do not have any immunizations without your doctor's

approval. Also, other people living in your home should not receive the oral polio vaccine, since there is a chance they could pass the polio virus on to you. In addition, you should avoid close contact with other people at school or work who have recently taken the oral polio vaccine

- Ketoconazole (e.g., Nizoral)—May increase your risk of steroid side effects.

- Ritodrine (e.g., Yutopar)—Serious side effects could occur

- Skin test injections—Corticosteroids may cause false results in skin tests

- Sodium-containing medicine—Corticosteroids cause the body to retain (keep) more sodium (salt) and water. Too much sodium may cause high blood sodium, high blood pressure, and excess body water

- Somatrem (e.g., Protropin) or

- Somatropin (e.g., Humatrope)—Corticosteroids can interfere with the effects of these medicines

There are many other medicines that may interact with corticosteroids. Tell your health care professional if you are taking any other prescription or nonprescription (over-the-counter [OTC]) medicine.

Other medical problems—The presence of other medical problems may affect the use of corticosteroids. Make sure you tell your doctor if you have any other medical problems, especially:

- Acquired immunodeficiency syndrome (AIDS) or

- Fungus infection or

- Herpes simplex infection of the eye or

- Human immunodeficiency virus (HIV) infection or

- Infection at the place of treatment or

- Other infection or

- Recent surgery or serious injury or

- Strongyloides (worm) infestation or

- Tuberculosis (active TB, nonactive TB, or past history of)—Corticosteroids can cause slower healing, worsen existing infections, or cause new infections

- Chickenpox (including recent exposure) or

- Measles (including recent exposure)—Risk of severe disease affecting other parts of the body

- Diabetes mellitus (sugar diabetes)—Corticosteroids may cause a loss of control of diabetes by increasing blood glucose (sugar)

- Diverticulitis or

- Stomach ulcer or other stomach or intestine problems or

- Ulcerative colitis, severe—Corticosteroids may cover up symptoms of a worsening stomach or intestinal condition. A patient would not know if his or her condition was getting worse and would not get medical help when needed

- Glaucoma—Corticosteroids may cause the pressure within the eye to increase

- Heart disease or

- High blood pressure or

- Kidney disease (especially if you are receiving dialysis) or

- Kidney stones—Corticosteroids cause the body to retain (keep) more salt and water. These conditions may be made worse by this extra body water

- High cholesterol levels—Corticosteroids may increase blood cholesterol levels

- Liver disease or

- Overactive thyroid or

- Underactive thyroid—With these conditions, the body may not eliminate the corticosteroid at the usual rate, which may change the medicine's effect

- Myasthenia gravis—When you first start taking corticosteroids, muscle weakness may occur. Your doctor may want to take special precautions because this could cause problems with breathing

- Osteoporosis (bone disease)—Corticosteroids may worsen bone disease because they cause the body to lose more calcium

- Psychosis—This condition may be made worse

- Systemic lupus erythematosus (SLE)—This condition may cause certain side effects of corticosteroids to occur more easily

Proper Use of This Medicine

For patients taking this medicine by mouth:

- *Take this medicine with food* to help prevent stomach upset. If stomach upset, burning, or pain continues, check with your doctor.

- Stomach problems may be more likely to occur if you drink alcoholic beverages while being treated with this medicine. You should not drink alcoholic beverages while taking this medicine, unless you have first checked with your doctor.

For patients taking *budesonide extended-release capsules:*

- Swallow the capsule whole, without breaking, crushing, or chewing it.

Use this medicine only as directed by your doctor. Do not use more or less of it, do not use it more often, and do not use it for a longer time than your doctor ordered. To do so may increase the chance of side effects.

Dosing—The dose of these medicines will be different for different patients. *Follow your doctor's orders or the directions on the label.* The following information gives the range of doses of these medicines for all uses, which can vary widely. The dose that you are receiving may be very different. *If your dose is different, do not change it* unless your doctor tells you to do so.

The number of capsules, tablets, teaspoonfuls of liquid or amount of injection that you use depends on the strength of the medicine. Also, *the number of doses you take each day, the time allowed between doses, and the length of time you take the medicine depend on the medical problem for which you are taking the corticosteroid. In addition, your doctor may need to change the dose from time to time.*

For betamethasone
- For *oral* dosage forms:
  - Syrup, tablets, effervescent tablets:
    - Adults and teenagers—Dose may range from 0.25 to 7.2 milligrams (mg) a day, as a single dose or divided into several doses.

- Children—Dose is based on body weight or size and must be determined by your doctor.
  - Extended-release tablets:
    - Adults and teenagers—2 to 6 mg a day.
    - Children—Dose is based on body weight or size and must be determined by your doctor.
- For *injection* dosage form:
  - Adults and teenagers: Dose may range from 1.2 to 12 mg injected into a joint, lesion, muscle, or vein as often as necessary, as determined by your doctor.
  - Children: Dose is based on body weight or size and must be determined by your doctor.

For budesonide
- For *oral* dosage form (extended-release capsules):
  - Adults: At first, the dose is 9 milligrams (mg) a day for up to eight weeks. Then your doctor may decrease the dose to 6 mg a day. Each dose should be taken in the morning before breakfast.
  - Children: Use and dose must be determined by your doctor.

For cortisone
- For *oral* dosage form (tablets):
  - Adults and teenagers: 25 to 300 milligrams (mg) a day, as a single dose or divided into several doses.
  - Children: Dose is based on body weight or size and must be determined by your doctor.
- For *injection* dosage form:
  - Adults and teenagers: 20 to 300 mg a day, injected into a muscle.
  - Children: Dose is based on body weight or size and must be determined by your doctor.

For dexamethasone
- For *oral* dosage forms (elixir, oral solution, tablets):
  - Adults and teenagers: 0.5 to 10 milligrams (mg) taken as often as necessary, as determined by your doctor.
  - Children: Dose is based on body weight or size and must be determined by your doctor.
- For *injection* dosage form:
  - Adults and teenagers: 0.2 to 40 mg injected into a joint, lesion, muscle, or vein as often as necessary, as determined by your doctor.
  - Children: Dose is based on body weight or size and must be determined by your doctor.

For hydrocortisone
- For *oral* dosage forms (oral suspension, tablets):
  - Adults and teenagers: 20 to 800 milligrams (mg) every one or two days, as a single dose or divided into several doses.
  - Children: Dose is based on body weight or size and must be determined by your doctor.
- For *injection* dosage form:
  - Adults and teenagers: 5 to 500 mg injected into a joint, lesion, muscle, or vein, or under the skin as often as necessary, as determined by your doctor.
  - Children: Dose is based on body weight or size and must be determined by your doctor.

For methylprednisolone
- For *oral* dosage form (tablets):
  - Adults and teenagers: 4 to 160 milligrams (mg) every one or two days, as a single dose or divided into several doses.
  - Children: Dose is based on body weight or size and must be determined by your doctor.

- For *injection* dosage form:
  - Adults and teenagers: 4 to 160 mg injected into a joint, lesion, muscle, or vein as often as necessary, as determined by your doctor.
  - Children: Dose is based on body weight or size and must be determined by your doctor.

For prednisolone
- For *oral* dosage forms (oral solution, syrup, tablets):
  - Adults and teenagers: 5 to 200 milligrams (mg) taken as often as necessary, as determined by your doctor.
  - Children: Dose is based on body weight or size and must be determined by your doctor.
- For *injection* dosage form:
  - Adults and teenagers: 2 to 100 mg injected into a joint, lesion, muscle, or vein as often as necessary, as determined by your doctor.
  - Children: Dose is based on body weight or size and must be determined by your doctor.

For prednisone
- For *oral* dosage forms (oral solution, syrup, tablets):
  - Adults and teenagers: 5 to 200 milligrams (mg) every one or two days, as a single dose or divided into several doses.
  - Children: Dose is based on body weight or size and must be determined by your doctor.

For triamcinolone
- For *oral* dosage forms (syrup, tablets):
  - Adults and teenagers: 2 to 60 milligrams (mg) a day, as a single dose or divided into several doses.
  - Children: Dose is based on body weight or size and must be determined by your doctor.
- For *injection* dosage form:
  - Adults and teenagers: 0.5 to 100 mg injected into a joint, lesion, or muscle, or under the skin as often as necessary, as determined by your doctor.
  - Children: Dose is based on body weight or size and must be determined by your doctor.

Missed dose—If you miss a dose of this medicine and your dosing schedule is:

- One dose every other day—Take the missed dose as soon as possible if you remember it the same morning, then go back to your regular dosing schedule. If you do not remember the missed dose until later, wait and take it the following morning. Then skip a day and start your regular dosing schedule again.
- One dose a day—Take the missed dose as soon as possible, then go back to your regular dosing schedule. If you do not remember until the next day, skip the missed dose and do not double the next one.
- Several doses a day—Take the missed dose as soon as possible, then go back to your regular dosing schedule. If you do not remember until your next dose is due, double the next dose.

If you have any questions about this, check with your health care professional.

Storage—To store this medicine:

- Keep out of the reach of children.
- Store away from heat and direct light.
- Do not store capsules or tablets in the bathroom, near the kitchen sink, or in other damp places. Heat or moisture may cause the medicine to break down.

- Keep the liquid dosage forms of this medicine from freezing.
- Do not keep outdated medicine or medicine no longer needed. Be sure that any discarded medicine is out of the reach of children.

Precautions While Using This Medicine

Your doctor should check your progress at regular visits. Also, your progress may have to be checked after you have stopped using this medicine, since some of the effects may continue.

Do not stop using this medicine without first checking with your doctor. Your doctor may want you to reduce gradually the amount you are using before stopping the medicine completely.

Check with your doctor if your condition reappears or worsens after the dose has been reduced or treatment with this medicine is stopped.

If you will be using corticosteroids for a long time:
- *Your doctor may want you to follow a low-salt diet and/or a potassium-rich diet.*
- Your doctor may have you take a bisphosphonate (alendronate [e.g., Fosamax], risedronate [e.g., Actonel]) to help prevent and treat bone problems while you are taking a corticosteroid.
- Your doctor may want you to watch your calories to prevent weight gain.
- Your doctor may want you to add extra protein to your diet.
- Your doctor may want you to have your eyes examined by an ophthalmologist (eye doctor) before, and also sometime later during treatment.
- Your doctor may want you to carry a medical identification card stating that you are using this medicine.

Tell the doctor in charge that you are using this medicine:
- *Before having skin tests.*
- *Before having any kind of surgery (including dental surgery) or emergency treatment.*
- *If you get a serious infection or injury.*

Avoid close contact with anyone who has chickenpox or measles. This is especially important for children. *Tell your doctor right away if you think you have been exposed to chickenpox or measles.*

While you are being treated with this medicine, and after you stop taking it, *do not have any immunizations without your doctor's approval.* Also, other people living in your home should not receive the oral polio vaccine, since there is a chance they could pass the polio virus on to you. In addition, you should avoid close contact with other people at school or work who have recently taken the oral polio vaccine.

For *patients with diabetes:*
- This medicine may affect blood glucose (sugar) levels. If you notice a change in the results of your blood or urine sugar tests or if you have any questions, check with your doctor.

For patients having this medicine *injected into their joints:*
- If this medicine is injected into one of your joints, you should be careful not to put too much stress or strain on that joint for a while, even if it begins to feel better. Make sure your doctor has told you how much you are allowed to move this joint while it is healing.

- If redness or swelling occurs at the place of injection, and continues or gets worse, check with your doctor.

Side Effects of This Medicine

Corticosteroids may lower your resistance to infections. Also, any infection you get may be harder to treat. Always check with your doctor as soon as possible if you notice any signs of a possible infection, such as sore throat, fever, sneezing, or coughing.

Along with its needed effects, a medicine may cause some unwanted effects. Although not all of these side effects may occur, if they do occur they may need medical attention. When this medicine is used for short periods of time, side effects usually are rare. However, check with your doctor as soon as possible if any of the following side effects occur:

Less common
> Decreased or blurred vision; frequent urination; increased thirst

Rare
> Blindness (sudden, when injected in the head or neck area); burning, numbness, pain, or tingling at or near place of injection; confusion; excitement; false sense of well-being; hallucinations (seeing, hearing, or feeling things that are not there); mental depression; mistaken feelings of self-importance or being mistreated; mood swings (sudden and wide); redness, swelling, or other sign of allergy or infection at place of injection; restlessness; skin rash or hives

Additional side effects may occur if you take this medicine for a long time. Check with your doctor if any of the following side effects occur:
> Abdominal or stomach pain or burning (continuing); acne; bloody or black, tarry stools; changes in vision; eye pain; filling or rounding out of the face; headache; irregular heartbeat; menstrual problems; muscle cramps or pain; muscle weakness; nausea; pain in arms, back, hips, legs, ribs, or shoulders; pitting, scarring, or depression of skin at place of injection; reddish purple lines on arms, face, groin, legs, or trunk; redness of eyes; sensitivity of eyes to light; stunting of growth (in children); swelling of feet or lower legs; tearing of eyes; thin, shiny skin; trouble in sleeping; unusual bruising; unusual increase in hair growth; unusual tiredness or weakness; vomiting; weight gain (rapid); wounds that will not heal

Other side effects may occur that usually do not need medical attention. These side effects may go away during treatment as your body adjusts to the medicine. However, check with your doctor if any of the following side effects continue or are bothersome:

More common
> Increased appetite; indigestion; loss of appetite (for triamcinolone only); nervousness or restlessness

Less common or rare
> Darkening or lightening of skin color; dizziness or lightheadedness; flushing of face or cheeks; hiccups; increased joint pain (after injection into a joint); increased sweating; nosebleeds (after injection into the nose); sensation of spinning

After you stop using this medicine, your body may need time to adjust. The length of time this takes depends on the amount of medicine you were using and how long you used it. If you have taken large doses of this medicine for a long time, your body may need one year to adjust. During this time, *check with your doctor immediately if any of the following side effects occur:*

Abdominal, stomach, or back pain; dizziness; fainting; fever; loss of appetite (continuing); muscle or joint pain; nausea; reappearance of disease symptoms; shortness of breath; unexplained headaches (frequent or continuing); unusual tiredness or weakness; vomiting; weight loss (rapid)

Other side effects not listed above may also occur in some patients. If you notice any other effects, check with your doctor.

Additional Information

Once a medicine has been approved for marketing for a certain use, experience may show that it is also useful for other medical problems. Although this use is not included in product labeling, some corticosteroids are used in certain patients with the following medical condition:

- Croup in children (dexamethasone)

CORTICOSTEROIDS—LOW POTENCY (Topical)

Some commonly used brand names are:

In the U.S.—

Aclovate (1)	Dermtex HC (7)
Acticort 100 (7)	DesOwen (3)
Aeroseb-Dex (4)	Epifoam (9)
Aeroseb-HC (7)	FoilleCort (9)
Ala-Cort (7)	Gly-Cort (7)
Ala-Scalp HP (7)	Gynecort (9)
Allercort (7)	Gynecort 10 (9)
Alphaderm (7)	Hi-Cor 1.0 (7)
Bactine (7)	Hi-Cor 2.5 (7)
Beta-HC (7)	Hydro-Tex (7)
CaldeCORT Anti-Itch (8)	Hytone (7)
CaldeCORT Light (9)	LactiCare-HC (7)
Carmol-HC (9)	Lanacort (9)
Cetacort (7)	Lanacort 10 (9)
Cloderm (2)	Lemoderm (7)
Cortaid (8)	Maximum Strength Cortaid (7)
Cort-Dome (7)	MyCort (7)
Cortef Feminine Itch (9)	9-1-1 (9)
Corticaine (9)	Nutracort (7)
Cortifair (7)	Penecort (7)
Cortril (7)	Pentacort (7)
Decaderm (4)	Pharma-Cort (9)
Decadron (4)	Rederm (7)
Decaspray (4)	Rhulicort (9)
Delacort (7)	S-T Cort (7)
Dermacort (7)	Synacort (7)
Dermarest DriCort (7)	Texacort (7)
DermiCort (7)	Tridesilon (3)

In Canada—

Barriere-HC (7)	Hyderm (9)
Cortacet (9)	Locacorten (5)
Cortate (7)	Novohydrocort (9)
Cortef (8)	Prevex HC (7)
Corticreme (9)	Sarna HC 1.0% (7)
Cortoderm (9)	Sential (7)
Drenison-¼ (6)	Tridesilon (3)
Emo-Cort (7)	Unicort (7)
Emo-Cort Scalp Solution (7)	

This information applies to the following medicines:

1. Alclometasone (al-kloe-MET-a-sone)
2. Clocortolone (kloe-KOR-toe-lone)
3. Desonide (DESS-oh-nide)
4. Dexamethasone (dex-a-METH-a-sone)
5. Flumethasone (floo-METH-a-sone)
6. Flurandrenolide (flure-an-DREN-oh-lide)
7. Hydrocortisone (hye-droe-KOR-ti-sone)
8. Hydrocortisone or hydrocortisone acetate (hye-droe-KOR-ti-son or hye-droe-KOR-ti-sonee AS-a-tate)
9. Hydrocortisone acetate (hye-droe-KOR-ti-sone AS-a-tate)

Category

- **Anti-inflammatory, steroidal, topical—**
- **Corticosteroid, topical—**

Description

Topical corticosteroids (kor-ti-ko-STER-oyds) are used to help relieve redness, swelling, itching, and discomfort of many skin problems. These medicines are like cortisone. They belong to the general family of medicines called steroids.

Most corticosteroids are available only with your doctor's prescription. Some strengths of hydrocortisone are available without a prescription. However, your doctor may have special instructions on the proper use for your medical condition.

Topical corticosteroids are available in the following dosage forms:

Topical
- Alclometasone
  - Cream
  - Ointment
- Clocortolone
  - Cream
- Desonide
  - Cream
  - Lotion
  - Ointment
- Dexamethasone
  - Cream
  - Gel
  - Topical aerosol
- Flumethasone
  - Cream
  - Ointment
- Flurandrenolide
  - Cream 0.0125%
  - Ointment 0.0125%
- Hydrocortisone
  - Cream
  - Lotion
  - Ointment
  - Topical solution
- Hydrocortisone acetate
  - Cream
  - Topical aerosol foam
  - Lotion
  - Ointment

Before Using This Medicine

In deciding to use a medicine, the risks of taking the medicine must be weighed against the good it will do. This is a decision you and your doctor will make. For topical corticosteroids, the following should be considered:

Allergies—Tell your doctor if you have ever had any unusual or allergic reaction to corticosteroids. Also tell your health care professional if you are allergic to any other substances, such as foods, preservatives, or dyes.

Pregnancy—When used properly, these medicines have not been shown to cause problems in humans. Studies on birth defects have not been done in humans. However, studies in animals have shown that topical corticosteroids, when applied to the skin in large amounts or used for a long time, could cause birth defects.

Breast-feeding—Topical corticosteroids have not been reported to cause problems in nursing babies when used properly. However, corticosteroids should not be applied to the breasts just before nursing.

Children—Children and teenagers who must use this medicine for a long time should be checked often by their doctor. Other, more potent corticosteroids are absorbed through the skin and can affect growth or cause other unwanted effects. Topical corticosteroids also can be absorbed if they are applied to large areas of skin. These effects are less likely to occur with the use of the lower potency corticosteroids. However, before using this medicine in children, you should discuss its use with your child's doctor.

Older adults—This medicine is not expected to cause different side effects or problems in older people than it does in younger adults.

Other medicines—Although certain medicines should not be used together at all, in other cases two different medicines may be used together even if an interaction might occur. In these cases, your doctor may want to change the dose, or other precautions may be necessary. Tell your health care professional if you are using any other topical prescription or nonprescription (over-the-counter [OTC]) medicine that is to be applied to the same area of the skin.

Other medical problems—The presence of other medical problems may affect the use of topical corticosteroids. Make sure you tell your doctor if you have any other medical problems, especially:

- Diabetes mellitus (sugar diabetes)—Too much use of corticosteroids may cause a loss of control of diabetes by increasing blood and urine glucose. However, this is not likely to happen when topical corticosteroids are used for a short time
- Infection or sores at the place of treatment or
- Tuberculosis—Corticosteroids may make existing infections worse or cause new infections
- Skin conditions that cause thinning of skin with easy bruising—Corticosteroids may make thinning of the skin worse

Proper Use of This Medicine

Be very careful not to get this medicine in your eyes. Wash your hands after using your finger to apply the medicine. If you accidentally get this medicine in your eyes, flush them with water.

Do not bandage or otherwise wrap the skin being treated unless directed to do so by your doctor.

If your doctor has ordered an occlusive dressing (airtight covering, such as kitchen plastic wrap or a special patch) to be applied over this medicine, make sure you know how to apply it. Since occlusive dressings increase the amount of medicine absorbed through your skin and the possibility of side effects, use them only as directed. If you have any questions about this, check with your doctor.

For patients using the *topical aerosol form* of this medicine:

- This medicine usually comes with patient directions. Read them carefully before using this medicine.
- It is important to avoid breathing in the vapors from the spray or getting them in your eyes. If you accidentally get this medicine in your eyes, flush them with water.
- Do not use near heat, near an open flame, or while smoking.

Do not use this medicine more often or for a longer time than your doctor ordered or than recommended on the package label. To do so may increase the chance of absorption through the skin and the chance of side effects.

If this medicine has been prescribed for you, it is meant to treat a specific skin problem. *Do not use it for other skin problems, and do not use nonprescription hydrocortisone for skin problems that are not listed on the package label, without first checking with your doctor.* Topical corticosteroids should not be used on many kinds of bacterial, viral, or fungal skin infections.

Dosing—The dose of topical corticosteroid will be different for different patients and products. *Follow your doctor's orders or the directions on the label.*

Missed dose—If your doctor has ordered you to use this medicine on a regular schedule and you miss a dose, apply it as soon as possible. But if it is almost time for your next dose, skip the missed dose and apply it at the next regularly scheduled time.

Storage—To store this medicine:

- Keep out of the reach of children.
- Store away from heat and direct light.
- Keep the medicine from freezing.
- Do not puncture, break, or burn aerosol containers, even after they are empty.
- Do not keep outdated medicine or medicine no longer needed. Be sure that any discarded medicine is out of the reach of children.

Precautions While Using This Medicine

Check with your doctor if your symptoms do not improve within 1 week or if your condition gets worse.

Avoid using tight-fitting diapers or plastic pants on a child if this medicine is being used on the child's diaper area. Plastic pants and tight-fitting diapers may increase the chance of absorption of the medicine through the skin and the chance of side effects.

Side Effects

Along with its needed effects, a medicine may cause some unwanted effects. Although not all of these side effects may occur, if they do occur they may need medical attention.

Check with your doctor as soon as possible if any of the following side effects occur:

Less common or rare
   Blood-containing blisters on skin; burning and itching of skin; increased skin sensitivity; lack of healing of skin condition; numbness in fingers; painful, red or itchy, pus-containing blisters in hair follicles; raised, dark red, wart-like spots on skin, especially when used on the face; skin infection; thinning of skin with easy bruising

Some side effects may occur that usually do not need medical attention. These side effects may go away during treatment as your body adjusts to the medicine. However, check with your doctor if any of the following side effects continue or are bothersome:

Less common or rare—usually mild and transient
Burning, dryness, irritation, itching, or redness of skin; increased redness or scaling of skin sores; skin rash

When the gel, lotion, solution, or aerosol form of this medicine is applied, a mild, temporary stinging may be expected.

Other side effects not listed above may also occur in some patients. If you notice any other effects, check with your doctor.

CORTICOSTEROIDS—MEDIUM TO VERY HIGH POTENCY (Topical)

Some commonly used brand names are:

In the U.S.—

Alphatrex (3)	Licon (10)
Aristocort (20)	Lidex (10)
Aristocort A (20)	Lidex-E (10)
Betatrex (3)	Locoid (15)
Beta-Val (3)	Luxiq (3)
Bio-Syn (9)	Maxiflor (7)
Cordran (11)	Maxivate (3)
Cordran SP (11)	Olux (4)
Cormax (4)	Pandel (16)
Cutivate (12)	Psorcon (7)
Cyclocort (1)	Synalar (9)
Delta-Tritex (20)	Synalar-HP (9)
Dermabet (3)	Synemol (9)
Dermatop (19)	Teladar (3)
Diprolene (3)	Temovate (4)
Diprolene AF (3)	Temovate E (4)
Diprosone (3)	Temovate Scalp Application
Elocon (18)	(4)
Florone (7)	Topicort (6)
Florone E (7)	Topicort LP (6)
Fluocet (9)	Triacet (20)
Fluocin (10)	Triderm (20)
Fluonid (9)	Ultravate (14)
Flurosyn (9)	Uticort (3)
Flutex (20)	Valisone (3)
Halog (13)	Valisone Reduced Strength
Halog-E (13)	(3)
Kenac (20)	Valnac (3)
Kenalog (20)	Vanos (10)
Kenalog-H (20)	Westcort (17)
Kenonel (20)	

In Canada—

Aristocort C (20)	Dermovate Scalp Lotion (4)
Aristocort D (20)	Diprolene (3)
Aristocort R (20)	Diprosone (3)
Beben (3)	Drenison (11)
Betacort Scalp Lotion (3)	Ectosone Mild (3)
Betaderm (3)	Ectosone Regular (3)
Betaderm Scalp Lotion (3)	Ectosone Scalp Lotion (3)
Betnovate (3)	Elocom (18)
Betnovate-½ (3)	Eumovate (5)
Celestoderm-V (3)	Florone (7)
Celestoderm-V/2 (3)	Fluoderm (9)
Cyclocort (1)	Fluolar (9)
Dermovate (4)	Fluonide (9)

Halog (13)	Synalar (9)
Kenalog (20)	Synamol (9)
Lidemol (10)	Topicort (6)
Lidex (10)	Topicort Mild (6)
Lyderm (10)	Topilene (3)
Metaderm Mild (3)	Topisone (3)
Metaderm Regular (3)	Topsyn (10)
Nerisone (8)	Triaderm (20)
Nerisone Oily (8)	Trianide Mild (20)
Novobetamet (3)	Trianide Regular (20)
Occulocort (3)	Valisone Scalp Lotion (3)
Prevex B (3)	Westcort (17)
Propaderm (2)	

This information applies to the following medicines:

1. Amcinonide (am-SIN-oh-nide)
2. Beclomethasone (be-kloe-METH-a-sone)
3. Betamethasone (bay-ta-METH-a-sone)
4. Clobetasol (kloe-BAY-ta-sol)
5. Clobetasone (kloe-BAY-ta-sone)
6. Desoximetasone (des-ox-i-MET-a-sone)
7. Diflorasone (dye-FLOR-a-sone)
8. Diflucortolone (dye-floo-KOR-toe-lone)
9. Fluocinolone (floo-oh-SIN-oh-lone)
10. Fluocinonide (floo-oh-SIN-oh-nide)
11. Flurandrenolide (flure-an-DREN-oh-lide)
12. Fluticasone (floo-TIK-a-sone)
13. Halcinonide (hal-SIN-oh-nide)
14. Halobetasol (hal-oh-BAY-ta-sol)
15. Hydrocortisone butyrate (hye-droe-KOR-ti-sone bue-TEAR-ate)
16. Hydrocortisone probutate (hye-droe-KOR-ti-sone proe-BYOE-tate)
17. Hydrocortisone valerate (hye-droe-KOR-ti-sone val-AIR-ate)
18. Mometasone (moe-MET-a-sone)
19. Prednicarbate (PRED-ni-kar-bate)
20. Triamcinolone (trye-am-SIN-oh-lone)

Category

- **Anti-inflammatory, steroidal, topical—**
- **Corticosteroid, topical—**

Description

Topical corticosteroids (kor-ti-ko-STER-oyds) are used to help relieve redness, swelling, itching, and discomfort of many skin problems. These medicines are like cortisone. They belong to the general family of medicines called steroids.

These corticosteroids are available only with your doctor's prescription. Topical corticosteroids are available in the following dosage forms:

Topical
- Amcinonide
  - Cream
  - Lotion
  - Ointment
- Beclomethasone
  - Cream
  - Lotion
- Betamethasone
  - Cream
  - Foam
  - Gel
  - Lotion
  - Ointment
  - Topical aerosol
- Clobetasol
  - Cream
  - Foam

- ○ Ointment
- ○ Topical solution
- Clobetasone
  - ○ Cream
  - ○ Ointment
- Desoximetasone
  - ○ Cream
  - ○ Gel
  - ○ Ointment
- Diflorasone
  - ○ Cream
  - ○ Ointment
- Diflucortolone
  - ○ Cream
  - ○ Ointment
- Fluocinolone
  - ○ Cream
  - ○ Ointment
  - ○ Topical solution
- Fluocinonide
  - ○ Cream
  - ○ Gel
  - ○ Ointment
  - ○ Topical solution
- Flurandrenolide
  - ○ Cream
  - ○ Lotion
  - ○ Ointment
  - ○ Tape
- Fluticasone
  - ○ Cream
  - ○ Ointment
- Halcinonide
  - ○ Cream
  - ○ Ointment
  - ○ Topical solution
- Halobetasol
  - ○ Cream
  - ○ Ointment
- Hydrocortisone butyrate
  - ○ Cream
  - ○ Ointment
- Hydrocortisone probutate
  - ○ Cream
- Hydrocortisone valerate
  - ○ Cream
  - ○ Ointment
- Mometasone
  - ○ Cream
  - ○ Lotion
  - ○ Ointment
- Prednicarbate
  - ○ Cream
- Triamcinolone
  - ○ Cream
  - ○ Lotion
  - ○ Ointment
  - ○ Topical aerosol

Before Using This Medicine

In deciding to use a medicine, the risks of taking the medicine must be weighed against the good it will do. This is a decision you and your doctor will make. For corticosteroids, the following should be considered:

Allergies—Tell your doctor if you have ever had any unusual or allergic reaction to corticosteroids. Also tell your health care professional if you are allergic to any other substances, such as foods, preservatives, or dyes.

Pregnancy—When used properly, these medicines have not been shown to cause problems in humans. Studies on birth defects have not been done in humans. However, studies in animals have shown that topical corticosteroids, when applied to the skin in large amounts or used for a long time, could cause birth defects.

Breast-feeding—Topical corticosteroids have not been reported to cause problems in nursing babies when used properly. However, corticosteroids should not be applied to the breasts before nursing.

Children—Children and teenagers who must use this medicine should be checked often by their doctor since this medicine may be absorbed through the skin and can affect growth or cause other unwanted effects.

Older adults—Certain side effects may be more likely to occur in elderly patients since the skin of older adults may be naturally thin. These unwanted effects may include tearing of the skin or blood-containing blisters on the skin.

Other medicines—Although certain medicines should not be used together at all, in other cases two different medicines may be used together even if an interaction might occur. In these cases, your doctor may want to change the dose, or other precautions may be necessary. Tell your health care professional if you are using any other topical prescription or nonprescription (over-the-counter [OTC]) medicine that is to be applied to the same area of the skin.

Other medical problems—The presence of other medical problems may affect the use of topical corticosteroids. Make sure you tell your doctor if you have any other medical problems, especially:
- Cataracts or
- Glaucoma—Corticosteroids may make these medical problems worse, especially when stronger corticosteroids are used in the eye area
- Diabetes mellitus (sugar diabetes)—Too much use of corticosteroids may cause a loss of control of diabetes by increasing blood and urine glucose. However, this is not likely to happen when topical corticosteroids are used for a short time
- Infection or sores at the place of treatment (unless your doctor also prescribed medicine for the infection) or
- Tuberculosis—Corticosteroids may make existing infections worse or cause new infections
- Skin conditions that cause thinning of skin with easy bruising—Corticosteroids may make thinning of the skin worse

Proper Use of This Medicine

Be very careful not to get this medicine in your eyes. Wash your hands after using your finger to apply the medicine. If you accidentally get this medicine in your eyes, flush them with water.

Do not bandage or otherwise wrap the skin being treated unless directed to do so by your doctor.

If your doctor has ordered an occlusive dressing (airtight covering, such as kitchen plastic wrap or a special patch) to be applied over this medicine, make sure you know how to apply it. Since occlusive dressings increase the amount of medicine absorbed through your skin and the possibility of side effects, use them only as directed. If you have any questions about this, check with your doctor.

Do not use on face, groin, or armpits unless directed to do so by your doctor.

For patients using the *foam form* of this medicine:

- This medicine usually comes with patient directions. Read them carefully before using this medicine.
- Do not use near heat, near an open flame, or while smoking.

For patients using the *topical aerosol form* of this medicine:

- This medicine usually comes with patient directions. Read them carefully before using this medicine.
- It is important to avoid breathing in the vapors from the spray or getting them in your eyes. If you accidentally get this medicine in your eyes, flush them with water.
- Do not use near heat, near an open flame, or while smoking.

For patients using *flurandrenolide tape:*

- This medicine usually comes with patient directions. Read them carefully before using this medicine.

Do not use this medicine more often or for a longer time than your doctor ordered. To do so may increase the chance of absorption through the skin and the chance of side effects. In addition, too much use, especially on areas with thinner skin (for example, face, armpits, groin), may result in thinning of the skin and stretch marks or other unwanted effects.

Do not use this medicine for other skin problems without first checking with your doctor. Topical corticosteroids should not be used on many kinds of bacterial, viral, or fungal skin infections.

Dosing—The dose of topical corticosteroid will be different for different patients and products. *Follow your doctor's orders or the directions on the label.*

Missed dose—If your doctor has ordered you to use this medicine on a regular schedule and you miss a dose, apply it as soon as possible. However, if it is almost time for your next dose, skip the missed dose and apply it at the next regularly scheduled time.

Storage—To store this medicine:

- Keep out of the reach of children.
- Store away from heat and direct light.
- Keep the medicine from freezing.
- Do not puncture, break, or burn aerosol containers, even after they are empty.
- Do not keep outdated medicine or medicine no longer needed. Be sure that any discarded medicine is out of the reach of children.

Precautions While Using This Medicine

Check with your doctor if your symptoms do not improve within 1 week or if your condition gets worse.

Avoid using tight-fitting diapers or plastic pants on a child if this medicine is being used on the child's diaper area. Plastic pants or tight-fitting diapers may increase the chance of absorption of the medicine through the skin and the chance of side effects.

Side Effects

Along with its needed effects, a medicine may cause some unwanted effects. Although not all of these side effects may occur, if they do occur they may need medical attention.

Check with your doctor as soon as possible if any of the following side effects occur:
    Less frequent or rare
        Blood-containing blisters on skin; burning and itching of skin; increased skin sensitivity (for some brands of betamethasone lotion); lack of healing of skin condition; loss of top skin layer (for tape dosage forms); numbness in fingers; painful, red or itchy, pus-containing blisters in hair follicles; raised, dark red, wart-like spots on skin, especially when used on the face; skin infection; thinning of skin with easy bruising

Additional side effects may occur if you use this medicine improperly or for a long time. Check with your doctor if any of the following side effects occur:
    Rare
        Acne or oily skin; backache; blurring or loss of vision (occurs gradually if certain products have been used near the eye); burning and itching of skin with pinhead-sized red blisters; eye pain (if certain products have been used near the eye); filling or rounding out of the face; increased blood pressure; irregular heartbeat; irregular menstrual periods; irritability; irritation of skin around mouth; loss of appetite; mental depression; muscle cramps, pain, or weakness; nausea; rapid weight gain or loss; reddish purple lines (stretch marks) on arms, face, legs, trunk, or groin; skin color changes; softening of skin; stomach bloating, burning, cramping, or pain; swelling of feet or lower legs; tearing of the skin; unusual bruising; unusual decrease in sexual desire or ability (in men); unusual increase in hair growth, especially on the face; unusual loss of hair, especially on the scalp; unusual tiredness or weakness; vomiting; weakness of the arms, legs, or trunk (severe); worsening of infections

Some side effects may occur that usually do not need medical attention. These side effects may go away during treatment as your body adjusts to the medicine. However, check with your doctor if any of the following side effects continue or are bothersome:
    Less frequent or rare—usually mild and transient
        Burning, dryness, irritation, itching, or redness of skin; increased redness or scaling of skin sores; skin rash

When the foam, gel, lotion, solution, or aerosol form of this medicine is applied, a mild, temporary stinging may be expected.

Other side effects not listed above may also occur in some patients. If you notice any other effects, check with your doctor.

Additional Information

Once a medicine has been approved for marketing for a certain use, experience may show that it is also useful for other medical problems. Although this use is not included in product labeling, topical corticosteroids may be used in certain patients with the following medical conditions:

- Phimosis

COUGH/COLD COMBINATIONS (Systemic)

Some commonly used brand names are:

In the U.S.—

Alka-Seltzer Plus Cold and Cough (21)
Alka-Seltzer Plus Cold and Cough Medicine Liqui-Gels (34)
Alka-Seltzer Plus Night-Time Cold Liqui-Gels (35)
Ami-Tex LA (69)
Anatuss LA (70)
Benylin Expectorant (54)
Bromfed-DM (17)
Broncholate (68)
Carbinoxamine Compound-Drops (18)
Cardec DM (18)
Children's Tylenol Cold Plus Cough Multi Symptom (34)
Co-Apap (34)
Codeprex (1)
Comtrex Daytime Maximum Strength Cold, Cough, and Flu Relief (60)
Comtrex Daytime Maximum Strength Cold and Flu Relief (60)
Comtrex Multi-Symptom Maximum Strength Non-Drowsy Caplets (60)
Comtrex Nighttime Maximum Strength Cold and Flu Relief (34)
Congestac Caplets (70)
Contac Cold/Flu Day Caplets (60)
Contac Severe Cold and Flu Caplets (34)
Co-Tuss V (56)
Deconsal II (70)
Despec (69)
Despec-SR Caplets (70)
Donatussin (42)
Donatussin DC (62)
Duratuss (70)
Duratuss HD (65)
ED-TLC (22)
ED Tuss HC (22)
Endagen-HD (22)
Endal Expectorant (61)
Entex LA (69)
Father John's Medicine Plus (43)
Genatuss DM (54)
GP-500 (70)
Guaifed (70)
Guaifenex PSE 60 (70)
Guaifenex PSE 120 (70)
GuaiMAX-D (70)
Guai-Vent/PSE (70)
Guiatuss A.C. (53)
Guiatuss CF (64)
Guiatuss DAC (63)
Guiatuss PE (70)
Histinex HC (22)
Histinex PV (25)
Hycodan (51)

Hycomine Compound (32)
Hydropane (51)
Iobid DM (54)
Iodal HD (22)
Iosal II (70)
Iotussin HC (22)
Kolephrin/DM Cough and Cold Medication (34)
Kolephrin GG/DM (54)
Kwelcof Liquid (56)
Mapap Cold Formula (34)
Marcof Expectorant (57)
Nalex DH (58)
Novahistine DH Liquid (23)
Nucofed Expectorant (63)
Nucofed Pediatric Expectorant (63)
Nucotuss Expectorant (63)
Nucotuss Pediatric Expectorant (63)
Nytcold Medicine (35)
Nytime Cold Medicine Liquid (35)
Ornex Severe Cold No Drowsiness Caplets (60)
PanMist-JR (70)
PediaCare Cough-Cold (24)
PediaCare Night Rest Cough-Cold Liquid (24)
Pediacof Cough (41)
Phanatuss (54)
Phenameth VC (14)
Phenergan with Codeine (5)
Phenergan with Dextromethorphan (6)
Phenergan VC with Codeine (29)
Pneumotussin HC (56)
Poly-Histine (15)
Primatuss Cough Mixture 4 (2)
Primatuss Cough Mixture 4D (64)
Profen II (70)
Promethazine DM (6)
Promethazine VC w/Codeine (29)
Prometh VC with Codeine (29)
Protuss-D (66)
Pseudo-Car DM (18)
P-V-Tussin (26)
Quelidrine Cough (39)
Rentamine Pediatric (20)
Rescon-DM (24)
Rescon-GG (69)
Respa-1st (70)
Respa-DM (54)
Respaire-60 SR (70)
Respaire-120 SR (70)
Rhinosyn-DM (24)
Rhinosyn-DMX Expectorant (54)
Rhinosyn-X (64)
Robafen AC Cough (53)
Robafen DAC (63)
Robafen DM (54)

Robitussin A-C (53)
Robitussin Cold and Cough Liqui-Gels (64)
Robitussin Cold, Cough and Flu Liqui-Gels (67)
Robitussin-DAC (63)
Robitussin-DM (54)
Robitussin Night Relief (36)
Robitussin Night-Time Cold Formula (35)
Robitussin-PE (70)
Robitussin Pediatric Cough and Cold (59)
Robitussin Severe Congestion Liqui-Gels (70)
Rondamine-DM Drops (18)
Rondec-DM (18)
Rondec-DM Drops (18)
Ru-Tuss DE (70)
Ru-Tuss Expectorant (64)
Ryna-C Liquid (23)
Ryna-CX Liquid (63)
Rynatuss (20)
Rynatuss Pediatric (20)
Safe Tussin 30 (54)
Scot-Tussin DM (2)
Scot-Tussin Senior Clear (54)
Sildec-DM (17)
Silexin Cough (54)
Siltussin DM (54)
Sinufed Timecelles (70)
Sinutab Non-Drying No Drowsiness Liquid Caps (70)
Stamoist E (70)
Statuss Green (19)
S-T Forte 2 (3)
Sudafed Children's Non-Drowsy Cold and Cough (64)
Sudafed Cold and Cough Liquid Caps (67)
Sudafed Children's Cold and Cough (64)
Sudal 60/500 (70)
Syracol CF (54)
TheraFlu Flu, Cold and Cough Medicine (34)
TheraFlu Maximum Strength Non-Drowsy Formula Flu, Cold and Cough Medicine (60)
TheraFlu Maximum Strength Non-Drowsy Formula Flu, Cold and Cough Medicine Caplets (60)
TheraFlu Nighttime Maximum Strength Flu, Cold and Cough (34)
Tolu-Sed DM (54)
Touro DM (54)
Touro LA Caplets (70)
Triacin C Cough (30)
Triafed w/Codeine (30)
Triaminic AM Non-Drowsy Cough and Decongestant (59)
Triaminic Night Time (24)

Triaminic Sore Throat Formula (60)
Tri-Tannate Plus Pediatric (20)
Tussafed (18)
Tussafed Drops (18)
Tussar DM (21)
Tussigon (51)
Tussionex Pennkinetic (3)
Tussi-Organidin DM NR Liquid (54)
Tussi-Organidin DM-S NR Liquid (54)
Tussi-Organidin NR Liquid (53)
Tussi-Organidin-S NR Liquid (53)
Tussirex (47)
Tuss-LA (70)
Tusso-DM (55)
Tylenol Cold and Flu No Drowsiness Powder (60)
Tylenol Cold Medication (34)
Tylenol Cold Medication Caplets (34)
Tylenol Cold Medication, Non-Drowsy Caplets (60)
Tylenol Cold Medication, Non-Drowsy Gelcaps (60)
Tylenol Cold Multi-Symptom (34)
Tylenol Maximum Strength Flu Gelcaps (60)
Tylenol Multi-Symptom Cough (60)
Uni-tussin DM (54)
Vanex-HD (22)
V-Dec-M (70)
Versacaps (70)
Vicks Children's NyQuil Cold/Cough Relief (24)
Vicks 44 Cough and Cold Relief Non-Drowsy LiquiCaps (59)
Vicks 44D Cough and Head Congestion (59)
Vicks DayQuil Multi-Symptom Cold/Flu LiquiCaps (60)
Vicks DayQuil Multi-Symptom Cold/Flu Relief (60)
Vicks 44E Cough and Chest Congestion (54)
Vicks 44M Cough, Cold and Flu Relief (34)
Vicks NyQuil Hot Therapy (35)
Vicks NyQuil Multi-Symptom Cold/Flu LiquiCaps (35)
Vicks NyQuil Multi-Symptom Cold/Flu Relief (35)
Vicks Pediatric 44D Cough and Head Decongestion (59)
Vicks Children's Cough Syrup (54)
Vicks Pediatric 44M Multi-Symptom Cough and Cold (24)
Vicodin Tuss (56)
Zephrex (70)
Zephrex-LA (70 In Canada)

In Canada—

Benylin DM-D (59)
Benylin DM-D for Children (59)
Benylin DM-D-E (64)
Benylin DM-D-E Extra Strength (64)
Benylin DM-E (54)
Benylin DM-E Extra Strength (54)

Benylin 4 Flu (67)
Calmydone (27)
Calmylin #2 (59)
Calmylin #3 (64)
Calmylin #4 (10)
Calmylin Cough and Flu (67)
Calmylin DM-D-E Extra Strength (64)

Calmylin Original with Codeine (9)
Calmylin Pediatric (59)
Cheracol (52)
CoActifed (30)
CoActifed Expectorant (46)
Coristex-DH (58)
Coristine-DH (58)
Cotridin (30)
Cotridin Expectorant (46)
Dimetane Expectorant-C (37)
Dimetane Expectorant-DC (38)
Dimetapp-C (16)
Entex LA (69)
Histenol (60)
Hycodan (51)
Hycomine (45)
Mersyndol with Codeine (8)
NeoCitran DM Coughs and Colds (28)
Novahistex DH (58)
Novahistex DH Expectorant (62)
Novahistine DH (58)
Novahistine DM w/ Decongestant (59)
Novahistine DM Expectorant w/ Decongestant (64)
Penntuss (1)
Pharmasave Children's Cough Syrup (59)
Phenergan Expectorant w/ Codeine (13)
Robitussin A-C (11)
Robitussin with Codeine (11)
Robitussin Cough and Cold (64)
Robitussin Cough and Cold Liqui-Fills (64)
Robitussin-DM (54)
Robitussin-PE (70)
Robitussin Pediatric Cough and Cold (59)
Sinutab with Codeine (33)

Sudafed Cold and Flu Gelcaps (67)
Sudafed Cough and Cold Extra Strength Caplets (60)
Sudafed DM (59)
Tanta Cough Syrup (54)
Triaminic-DM Expectorant (44)
Triaminic DM NightTime for Children (24)
Tussilyn DM (24)
Tussionex (4)
Tylenol Children's Cold DM Medication (34)
Tylenol Cold and Flu (34)
Tylenol Cold Medication Extra Strength Daytime Caplets (60)
Tylenol Cold Medication Extra Strength Nighttime Caplets (34)
Tylenol Cold Medication Regular Strength Daytime Caplets (60)
Tylenol Cold Medication Regular Strength Nighttime Caplets (34)
Tylenol Cough Extra Strength Caplets (50)
Tylenol Cough Medication with Decongestant, Regular Strength (60)
Tylenol Cough Medication Regular Strength (50)
Tylenol Extra Strength Cold and Flu Medication Powder (34)
Tylenol Junior Strength Cold DM Medication (34)
Vicks Children's NyQuil (24)
Vicks DayQuil Liquicaps (60)
Vicks Formula 44-D (59)
Vicks Formula 44-D Pediatric (59)
Vicks Formula 44E (54)
Vicks Formula 44E Pediatric (54)
Vicks Formula 44M (34)
Vicks NyQuil (35)
Vicks NyQuil LiquiCaps (35)

Note: For quick reference the following cough/cold combinations are numbered to match the preceding corresponding brand names.

Note: Products containing phenylpropanolamine were removed from the U.S. and Canadian Markets in November 2000.

Antihistamine and antitussive combinations—
1. Chlorpheniramine and Codeine (klor-fen-EER-a-meen and KOE-deen)
2. Chlorpheniramine and Dextromethorphan (klor-fen-EER-a-meen and dex-troe-meth-OR-fan)
3. Chlorpheniramine and Hydrocodone (klor-fen-EER-a-meen and hye-droe-KOE-done)
4. Phenyltoloxamine and Hydrocodone (fen-ill-tole-OX-a-meen and hye-droe-KOE-done)
5. Promethazine and Codeine (proe-METH-a-zeen and KOE-deen)
6. Promethazineand Dextromethorphan (proe-METH-a-zeen and dex-troe-meth-OR-fan)
7. Pyrilamine and Codeine (peer-ILL-a-meen and KOE-deen)

Antihistamine, antitussive, and analgesic combinations—
8. Doxylamine, Codeine, and Acetaminophen (dox-ILL-a-meen, KOE-deen, and a-seat-a-MIN-oh-fen)

Antihistamine, antitussive, and expectorant combinations—
9. Diphenhydramine, Codeine, and Ammonium Chloride (dye-fen-HYE-dra-meen, KOE-deen, and a-MOE-nee-um KLOR-ide)
10. Diphenhydramine, Dextromethorphan, and Ammonium Chloride (dye-fen-HYE-dra-meen, dex-troe-meth-OR-fan, and a-MOE-nee-um KLOR-ide)
11. Pheniramine, Codeine, and Guaifenesin (fen-EER-a-meen, KOE-deen, and gwye-FEN-e-sin)

12. Pheniramine, Pyrilamine, Hydrocodone, Potassium Citrate, and Ascorbic Acid (fen-EER-a-meen, peer-ILL-a-meen,hye-droe-KOE-done, poe-TAS-ee-um SI-trate, and a-SKOR-bik AS-id)
13. Promethazine, Codeine, and Potassium Guaiacolsulfonate (proe-METH-a-zeen, KOE-deen, and poe-TAS-ee-um gwye-a-kol-SUL-fon-ate)

Antihistamine, and decongestant combinations—
14. Promethazine, and Phenylephrine (proe-METH-a-zeen,and fen-ill-EF-rin)
15. Pheniramine, Pyrilamine and Phenyltoloxamine (fen-EER-a-meen, peer-ILL-a-meen, and fen-ill-tole-OX-a-meen)

Antihistamine, decongestant, and antitussive combinations—
16. Brompheniramine, Phenylephrine, and Codeine (brome-fen-EER-a-meen, fen-ill-EF-rin, and KOE-deen)
17. Brompheniramine, Pseudoephedrine, and Dextromethorphan (brome-fen-EER-a-meen, soo-doe-e-FED-rin, and dex-troe-meth-OR-fan)
18. Carbinoxamine, Pseudoephedrine, and Dextromethorphan (kar-bi-NOX-a-meen, soo-doe-e-FED-rin, and dex-troe-meth-OR-fan)
19. Chlorpheniramine, Pyrilamine, Phenylephrine, Pseudoephedrine and Hydrocodone (klor-fen-EER-a-meen, peer-ILL-a-meen,fen-ill-EF-rin, soo-doe-e-FED-rin and hye-droe-KOE-done)
20. Chlorpheniramine, Ephedrine, Phenylephrine, and Carbetapentane (klor-fen-EER-a-meen, e-FED-rin, fen-ill-EF-rin, and kar-bay-ta-PEN-tane)
21. Chlorpheniramine, Phenylephrine, and Dextromethorphan (klor-fen-EER-a-meen, fen-ill-EF-rin, and dex-troe-meth-OR-fan)
22. Chlorpheniramine, Phenylephrine, and Hydrocodone (klor-fen-EER-a-meen, fen-ill-EF-rin, and hye-droe-KOE-done)
23. Chlorpheniramine, Pseudoephedrine, and Codeine (klor-fen-EER-a-meen, soo-doe-e-FED-rin, and KOE-deen)
24. Chlorpheniramine, Pseudoephedrine, and Dextromethorphan (klor-fen-EER-a-meen, soo-doe-e-FED-rin, and dex-troe-meth-OR-fan)
25. Chlorpheniramine, Pseudoephedrine, and Hydrocodone (klor-fen-EER-a-meen, soo-doe-e-FED-rin, and hye-droe-KOE-done)
26. Chlorpheniramine, Pseudoephedrine, and Hydrocodone or Pseudoephedrine andHydrocodone (klor-fen-EER-a-meen,soo-doe-e-FED-rin, and hye-droe-KOE-done or soo-doe-e-FED-rin and hye-droe-KOE-done)
27. Doxylamine, Etafedrine, and Hydrocodone (dox-ILL-a-meen, et-a-FED-rin, and hye-droe-KOE-done)
28. Pheniramine, Phenylephrine, and Dextromethorphan (fen-EER-a-meen, fen-ill-EF-rin, and dex-troe-meth-OR-fan)
29. Promethazine, Phenylephrine, and Codeine (proe-METH-a-zeen, fen-ill-EF-rin, and KOE-deen)
30. Triprolidine, Pseudoephedrine, and Codeine (trye-PROE-li-deen, soo-doe-e-FED-rin, and KOE-deen)

Antihistamine, decongestant, antitussive, and analgesic combinations—
31. Chlorpheniramine, Pheniramine, Pyrilamine, Phenylephrine, Hydrocodone, Salicylamide,Caffeine, and Ascorbic Acid (klor-fen-EER-a-meen,fen-EER-a-meen, peer-ILL-a-meen, fen-ill-EF-rin, hye-droe-KOE-done, sal-i-SILL-a-mide,kaf-EEN, and a-SKOR-bik AS-id)
32. Chlorpheniramine,Phenylephrine, Hydrocodone, Acetaminophen, and Caffeine (klor-fen-EER-a-meen, fen-ill-EF-rin, hye-droe-KOE-done, a-seat-a-MIN-oh-fen,and kaf-EEN)
33. Chlorpheniramine, Pseudoephedrine, Codeine, and Acetaminophen (klor-fen-EER-a-meen, soo-doe-e-FED-rin,KOE-deen, and a-seat-a-MIN-oh-fen)
34. Chlorpheniramine,Pseudoephedrine, Dextromethorphan, and Acetaminophen (klor-fen-EER-a-meen, soo-doe-e-FED-rin, dex-troe-meth-OR-fan, and a-seat-a-MIN-oh-fen)
35. Doxylamine, Pseudoephedrine, Dextromethorphan, andAcetaminophen (dox-ILL-a-meen, soo-doe-e-FED-rin,dex-troe-meth-OR-fan, and a-seat-a-MIN-oh-fen)
36. Pyrilamine, Pseudoephedrine, Dextromethorphan, and Acetaminophen (peer-ILL-a-meen, soo-doe-e-FED-rin, dex-troe-meth-OR-fan, and a-seat-a-MIN-oh-fen)

Antihistamine, decongestant, antitussive, and expectorant combinations—

37. Brompheniramine, Phenylephrine, Codeine, and Guaifenesin (brome-fen-EER-a-meen, fen-ill-EF-rin, KOE-deen, and gwye-FEN-e-sin)
38. Brompheniramine, Phenylephrine, Hydrocodone, and Guaifenesin (brome-fen-EER-a-meen, fen-ill-EF-rin, hye-droe-KOE-done, and gwye-FEN-e-sin)
39. Chlorpheniramine, Ephedrine, Phenylephrine, Dextromethorphan,Ammonium Chloride, and Ipecac (klor-fen-EER-a-meen,e-FED-rin, fen-ill-EF-rin, dex-troe-meth-OR-fan, a-MOE-nee-um KLOR-ide, andIP-e-kak)
40. Chlorpheniramine, Phenylephrine, Codeine and Ammonium Chloride (klor-fen-EER-a-meen, fen-ill-EF-rin,KOE-deen, and a-MOE-nee-um KLOR-ide)
41. Chlorpheniramine,Phenylephrine, Codeine, and Potassium Iodide (klor-fen-EER-a-meen, fen-ill-EF-rin, KOE-deen, and por-TAS-ee-um EYE-oh-dyed)
42. Chlorpheniramine, Phenylephrine, Dextromethorphan,and Guaifenesin (klor-fen-EER-a-meen,fen-ill-EF-rin, dex-troe-meth-OR-fan, and gwye-FEN-e-sin)
43. Chlorpheniramine, Phenylephrine, Dextromethorphan, Guaifenesin, and Ammonium Chloride (klor-fen-EER-a-meen, fen-ill-EF-rin,dex-troe-meth-OR-fan, gwye-FEN-e-sin, and a-MOE-nee-um KLOR-ide)
44. Chlorpheniramine, Pseudoephedrine, Dextromethorphan, and Guaifenesin (klor-fen-EER-a-meen, soo-doe-e-FED-rin, dex-troe-meth-OR-fan, and gwye-FEN-e-sin)
45. Pyrilamine, Phenylephrine, Hydrocodone, and Ammonium Chloride (peer-ILL-a-meen, fen-ill-EF-rin,hye-droe-KOE-done, and a-MOE-nee-um KLOR-ide)
46. Triprolidine, Pseudoephedrine, Codeine, and Guaifenesin (trye-PROE-li-deen, soo-doe-e-FED-rin, KOE-deen, and gwye-FEN-e-sin)

Antihistamine, decongestant, antitussive, expectorant,and analgesic combinations—

47. Pheniramine, Phenylephrine, Codeine, Sodium Citrate, Sodium Salicylate, and Caffeine (fen-EER-a-meen, fen-ill-EF-rin,KOE-deen, SOE-dee-um SI-trate, SOE-dee-um sa-LI-sill-ate, and kaf-EEN)

Antihistamine, decongestant, and expectorant combinations—

48. Chlorpheniramine, Ephedrine, and Guaifenesin (klor-fen-EER-a-meen, e-FED-rin, and gwye-FEN-e-sin)
49. Promethazine, Phenylephrine, and Potassium Guaiacolsulfonate (pro-METH-a-zeen, fen-ill-EF-rin, and poe-TAS-see-um gwye-a-kol-SUL-fon-ate)

Antitussive and analgesic combination—

50. Dextromethorphan and Acetaminophen (dex-troe-meth-OR-fan and a-seat-a-MIN-oh-fen)

Antitussive and anticholinergic combination—

51. Hydrocodone and Homatropine (hye-droe-KOE-done and hoe-MA-troe-peen)

Antitussive and expectorant combinations—

52. Codeine, Ammonium Chloride, and Guaifenesin (KOE-deen, a-MOE-nee-um KLOR-ide, and gwye-FEN-e-sin)
53. Codeine and Guaifenesin (KOE-deen and gwye-FEN-e-sin)
54. Dextromethorphanand Guaifenesin (dex-troe-meth-OR-fan and gwye-FEN-e-sin)
55. Dextromethorphan and Iodinated Glycerol (dex-troe-meth-OR-fan and EYE-oh-di-nay-ted GLI-ser-ole)
56. Hydrocodone and Guaifenesin (hye-droe-KOE-done and gwye-FEN-e-sin)
57. Hydrocodoneand Potassium Guaiacolsulfonate (hye-droe-KOE-done and poe-TAS-see-um gwye-a-kol-SUL-fon-ate)

Decongestant and antitussive combinations—

58. Phenylephrine and Hydrocodone (fen-ill-EF-rinand hye-droe-KOE-done)
59. Pseudoephedrine and Dextromethorphan (soo-doe-e-FED-rin and dex-troe-meth-OR-fan)

Decongestant, antitussive, and analgesic combinations—

60. Pseudoephedrine, Dextromethorphan, and Acetaminophen (soo-doe-e-FED-rin, dex-troe-meth-OR-fan, and a-seat-a-MIN-oh-fen)

Decongestant, antitussive, and expectorant combinations—

61. Phenylephrine, Codeine, and Guaifenesin (fen-ill-EF-rin, KOE-deen, and gwye-FEN-e-sin)
62. Phenylephrine, Hydrocodone, and Guaifenesin (fen-ill-EF-rin, hye-droe-KOE-done, and gwye-FEN-e-sin)
63. Pseudoephedrine, Codeine, and Guaifenesin (soo-doe-e-FED-rin, KOE-deen, and gwye-FEN-e-sin)
64. Pseudoephedrine, Dextromethorphan, and Guaifenesin (soo-doe-e-FED-rin, dex-troe-meth-OR-fan, and gwye-FEN-e-sin)
65. Pseudoephedrine, Hydrocodone, and Guaifenesin (soo-doe-e-FED-rin, hye-droe-KOE-done, and gwye-FEN-e-sin)
66. Pseudoephedrine, Hydrocodone, and Potassium Guaiacolsulfonate (soo-doe-e-FED-rin, hye-droe-KOE-done, and poe-TAS-ee-um gwye-a-kol-SUL-fon-ate)

Decongestant, antitussive, expectorant, and analgesic combinations—

67. Pseudoephedrine, Dextromethorphan, Guaifenesin, and Acetaminophen (soo-doe-e-FED-rin, dex-troe-meth-OR-fan, gwye-FEN-e-sin, and a-seat-a-MIN-oh-fen)

Decongestant and expectorant combinations—

68. Ephedrine and Guaifenesin (e-FED-rinand gwye-FEN-e-sin)
69. Phenylephrine and Guaifenesin (fen-ill-EF-rin and gwye-FEN-e-sin)
70. Pseudoephedrine and Guaifenesin (soo-doe-e-FED-rin and gwye-FEN-e-sin)

Category

- **Antihistaminic (H$_1$-receptor)-antitussive**—Chlorpheniramine and Dextromethorphan; Chlorpheniramine and Hydrocodone; Phenyltoloxamine and Hydrocodone; Promethazine and Codeine; Promethazine and Dextromethorphan; Pyrilamine and Codeine

- **Antihistaminic (H$_1$-receptor)-antitussive-analgesic**—Doxylamine, Codeine and Acetaminophen

- **Antihistaminic (H$_1$-receptor)-antitussive-expectorant**—Diphenhydramine, Codeine, and Ammonium Chloride; Diphenhydramine, Dextromethorphan, and Ammonium Chloride; Pheniramine, Codeine, and Guaifenesin; Pheniramine, Pyrilamine, Hydrocodone, Potassium Citrate, and Ascorbic Acid; Promethazine, Codeine, and Potassium Guaiacolsulfonate

- **Antihistaminic (H$_1$-receptor) and decongestant**—Promethazine and Phenylephrine; Pheniramine, Pyrilamine, and Phenyltoloxamine

- **Antihistaminic (H$_1$-receptor)-decongestant-antitussive**—Brompheniramine, Phenylephrine and Codeine; Brompheniramine, Pseudoephedrine, and Dextromethorphan; Carbinoxamine, Pseudoephedrine, and Dextromethorphan; Chlorpheniramine, Pyrilamine, Phenylephrine, Pseudoephedrine and Hydrocodone; Chlorpheniramine, Ephedrine, Phenylephrine, and Carbetapentane; Chlorpheniramine, Phenylephrine, and Dextromethorphan; Chlorpheniramine, Phenylephrine, and Hydrocodone; Chlorpheniramine, Pseudoephedrine, and Codeine; Chlorpheniramine, Pseudoephedrine, and Dextromethorphan; Chlorpheniramine, Pseudoephedrine, and Hydrocodone; Chlorpheniramine, Pseudoephedrine and Hydrocodone; Doxylamine, Etafedrine and Hydrocodone; Pheniramine, Phenylephrine, and Dextromethorphan; Promethazine, Phenylephrine, and Codeine; Triprolidine, Pseudoephedrine, and Codeine

- **Antihistaminic (H$_1$-receptor)-decongestant-antitussive-analgesic**—Chlorpheniramine, Pheniramine, Pyrilamine, Phenylephrine, Hydrocodone, Salicylamide, Caffeine, and Ascorbic Acid; Chlorpheniramine, Phenylephrine, Hydrocodone, Acetaminophen, and Caffeine; Chlorpheniramine, Pseudoephedrine, Codeine and Acetaminophen; Chlorpheniramine, Pseudoephedrine,

Dextromethorphan, and Acetaminophen,; Doxylamine, Pseudoephedrine, Dextromethorphan, and Acetaminophen; Pyrilamine, Pseudoephedrine, Dextromethorphan, and Acetaminophen

- **Antihistaminic (H₁-receptor)-decongestant-antitussive-expectorant**—Brompheniramine, Phenylephrine, Codeine and Guaifenesin; Brompheniramine, Phenylephrine, Hydrocodone and Guaifenesin; Chlorpheniramine, Ephedrine, Phenylephrine, Dextromethorphan, Ammonium Chloride, and Ipecac; Chlorpheniramine, Phenylephrine, Codeine, and Ammonium Chloride; Chlorpheniramine, Phenylephrine, Codeine, and Potassium Iodide; Chlorpheniramine, Phenylephrine, Dextromethorphan, and Guaifenesin; Chlorpheniramine, Phenylephrine, Dextromethorphan, Guaifenesin, and Ammonium Chloride; Chlorpheniramine, Pseudoephedrine, Dextromethorphan and Guaifenesin; Pyrilamine, Phenylephrine, Hydrocodone, and Ammonium Chloride; Triprolidine, Pseudoephedrine, Codeine, and Guaifenesin
- **Antihistaminic (H₁-receptor)-decongestant-antitussive-expectorant-analgesic**—Pheniramine, Phenylephrine, Codeine, Sodium Citrate, Sodium Salicylate, and Caffeine
- **Antihistaminic (H₁-receptor)-decongestant-expectorant**—Chlorpheniramine, Ephedrine, and Guaifenesin; Promethazine, Phenylephrine, and Potassium Guaiacolsulfonate
- **Antitussive-analgesic**—Dextromethorphan and Acetaminophen
- **Antitussive-anticholinergic**—Hydrocodone and Homatropine
- **Antitussive-expectorant**—Codeine, Ammonium Chloride, and Guaifenesin; Codeine and Guaifenesin; Dextromethorphan and Guaifenesin; Dextromethorphan and Iodinated Glycerol; Hydrocodone and Guaifenesin; Hydrocodone and Potassium Guaiacolsulfonate
- **Decongestant-antitussive**—Phenylephrine and Hydrocodone; Pseudoephedrine and Dextromethorphan
- **Decongestant-antitussive-analgesic**—Pseudoephedrine, Dextromethorphan, and Acetaminophen
- **Decongestant-antitussive-expectorant**—Phenylephrine, Codeine and Guaifenesin; Phenylephrine, Hydrocodone, and Guaifenesin; Pseudoephedrine, Codeine, and Guaifenesin; Pseudoephedrine, Dextromethorphan, and Guaifenesin; Pseudoephedrine, Hydrocodone, and Guaiacolsulfonate; Pseudoephedrine, Hydrocodone, and Guaifenesin
- **Decongestant-antitussive-expectorant-analgesic**—Pseudoephedrine, Dextromethorphan, Guaifenesin, and Acetaminophen
- **Decongestant-expectorant**—Ephedrine and Guaifenesin; Ephedrine and Potassium Iodide; Phenylephrine and Guaifenesin; Pseudoephedrine and Guaifenesin

Description

Cough/cold combinations are used mainly to relieve the cough due to colds, influenza, or hay fever. They are not to be used for the chronic cough that occurs with smoking, asthma, or emphysema or when there is an unusually large amount of mucus or phlegm (pronounced flem) with the cough.

Cough/cold combination products contain more than one ingredient. For example, some products may contain an antihistamine, a decongestant, and an analgesic, in addition to a medicine for coughing. If you are treating yourself, it is important to select a product that is best for your symptoms. Also, in general, it is best to buy a product that includes only those medicines you really need. If you have questions about which product to buy, check with your pharmacist.

Since different products contain ingredients that will have different precautions and side effects, it is important that you know the ingredients of the medicine you are taking. The different kinds of ingredients that may be found in cough/cold combinations include:

Antihistamines—Antihistamines are used to relieve or prevent the symptoms of hay fever and other types of allergy. They also help relieve some symptoms of the common cold, such as sneezing and runny nose. They work by preventing the effects of a substance called histamine, which is produced by the body. Some examples of antihistamines contained in these combinations are: bromodiphenhydramine broe-moe-dye-fen-HYE-dra-meen, brompheniramine brome-fen-EER-a-meen, carbinoxamine kar-bi-NOX-a-meen, chlorpheniramine klor-fen-EER-a-meen, dexchlorpheniramine dex-klor-fen-EER-a-meen, diphenhydramine dye-fen-HYE-dra-meen, doxylamine dox-ILL-a-meen, phenindamine fen-IN-da-meen, pheniramine fen-EER-a-meen, phenyltoloxamine fen-ill-tole-OX-a-meen, pyrilamine peer-ILL-a-meen, promethazine proe-METH-a-zeen, and triprolidine trye-PROE-li-deen.

Decongestants—Decongestants, such as ephedrine e-FED-rin, phenylephrine fen-ill-EF-rin, and pseudoephedrine soo-doe-e-FED-rin, produce a narrowing of blood vessels. This leads to clearing of nasal congestion. However, this effect may also increase blood pressure in patients who have high blood pressure.

Antitussives—To help relieve coughing these combinations contain either a narcotic [codeine KOE-deen, dihydrocodeine dye-hye-droe-KOE-deen, hydrocodone hye-droe-KOE-done or hydromorphone hye-droe-MOR-fone] or a nonnarcotic [carbetapentane kar-bay-ta-PEN-tane, caramiphen kar-AM-i-fen, or dextromethorphan dex-troe-meth-OR-fan] antitussive. These antitussives act directly on the cough center in the brain. Narcotics may become habit-forming, causing mental or physical dependence, if used for a long time. Physical dependence may lead to withdrawal side effects when you stop taking the medicine.

Expectorants—Guaifenesin gwye-FEN-e-sin works by loosening the mucus or phlegm in the lungs. Other ingredients added as expectorants (for example, ammonium chloride, calcium iodide, iodinated glycerol, ipecac, potassium guaiacolsulfonate, potassium iodide, and sodium citrate) have not been proven to be effective. In general, the best thing you can do to loosen mucus or phlegm is to drink plenty of water.

Analgesics—Analgesics, such as acetaminophen a-seat-a-MIN-oh-fen, aspirin, and other salicylates [such as salicylamide sal-i-SILL-a-mide and sodium salicylate SOE-dee-um sa-LI-sill-ate] are used in these combination medicines to help relieve the aches and pain that may occur with the common cold.

The use of too much acetaminophen and salicylates at the same time may cause kidney damage or cancer of the kidney or urinary bladder. This may occur if large amounts of both medicines are taken together for a long time. However, taking the recommended amounts of combination medicines that contain both acetaminophen and a salicylate for short periods of time has not been shown to cause these unwanted effects.

Anticholinergics—Anticholinergics such as homatropine hoe-MA-troe-peen may help produce a drying effect in the nose and chest.

Some of these combinations are available only with your doctor's prescription. Others are available without a prescription; however, your health care professional may have special instructions on the proper dose of the medicine for your medical condition.

Cough/cold combinations are available in the following dosage forms:

- **Antihistamine and antitussive combinations—**
  Oral
  - Chlorpheniramine and Codeine
    - Oral suspension
  - Chlorpheniramine and Dextromethorphan
    - Oral solution
  - Chlorpheniramine and Hydrocodone
    - Oral solution
    - Oral suspension
  - Phenyltoloxamine and Hydrocodone
    - Oral suspension
    - Tablets
  - Promethazine and Codeine
    - Oral solution
    - Syrup
  - Promethazine and Dextromethorphan
    - Oral solution
    - Syrup
  - Pyrilamine and Codeine
    - Oral solution
- **Antihistamine, antitussive, and analgesic combinations—**
  Oral
  - Doxylamine, Codeine, and Acetaminophen
    - Tablets
- **Antihistamine, antitussive, and expectorant combinations—**
  Oral
  - Diphenhydramine, Codeine, and Ammonium Chloride
    - Syrup
  - Diphenhydramine, Dextromethorphan, and Ammonium Chloride
    - Syrup
  - Pheniramine, Codeine, and Guaifenesin
    - Syrup
  - Pheniramine, Pyrilamine, Hydrocodone, Potassium Citrate, and Ascorbic Acid
    - Syrup
  - Promethazine, Codeine, and Potassium Guaiacolsulfonate
    - Syrup
- **Antihistamine, and decongestant combinations—**
  Oral
  - Promethazine, and phenylephrine
    - Syrup
  - Pheniramine, Pyrilamine and Phenyltoloxamine
    - Syrup
- **Antihistamine, decongestant, and antitussive combinations—**
  Oral
  - Brompheniramine, Phenylephrine, and Codeine
    - Syrup
  - Brompheniramine, Pseudoephedrine, and Dextromethorphan
    - Syrup

- Carbinoxamine, Pseudoephedrine, and Dextromethorphan
  - Oral solution
  - Syrup
- Chlorpheniramine, Pyrilamine, Phenylephrine, Pseudoephedrine, and Hydrocodone
  - Oral solution
- Chlorpheniramine, Ephedrine, Phenylephrine, and Carbetapentane
  - Oral suspension
  - Tablets
- Chlorpheniramine, Phenylephrine, and Dextromethorphan
  - Oral solution
  - Syrup
  - Tablets
- Chlorpheniramine, Phenylephrine, and Hydrocodone
  - Oral solution
  - Syrup
- Chlorpheniramine, Pseudoephedrine, and Codeine
  - Elixir
  - Oral solution
- Chlorpheniramine, Pseudoephedrine, and Dextromethorphan
  - Chewable tablets
  - Oral solution
  - Syrup
- Chlorpheniramine, Pseudoephedrine, and Hydrocodone
  - Oral solution
  - Syrup
- Chlorpheniramine, Pseudoephedrine, and Hydrocodone
  - Syrup
- Doxylamine, Etadrine, and Hydrocodone
  - Syrup
- Pheniramine, Phenylephrine, and Dextromethorphan
  - Oral solution
- Promethazine, Phenylephrine, and Codeine
  - Oral solution
  - Syrup
- Triprolidine, Pseudoephedrine, and Codeine
  - Oral solution
  - Syrup
  - Tablets
- **Antihistamine, decongestant, antitussive, and analgesic combinations—**
  Oral
  - Chlorpheniramine, Pheniramine, Pyrilamine, Phenylephrine, Hydrocodone, Salicylamide, Caffeine, and Ascorbic Acid
    - Capsules
  - Chlorpheniramine, Phenylephrine, Hydrocodone, Acetaminophen, and Caffeine
    - Tablets
  - Chlorpheniramine, Pseudoephedrine, Codeine, and Acetaminophen
    - Tablets
  - Chlorpheniramine, Pseudoephedrine, Dextromethorphan, and Acetaminophen
    - Capsules
    - Chewable tablets

- Oral solution
- Syrup
- Tablets
  - Doxylamine, Pseudoephedrine, Dextromethorphan, and Acetaminophen
    - Capsules
    - Oral solution
  - Pyrilamine, Pseudoephedrine, Dextromethorphan, and Acetaminophen
    - Oral solution
- **Antihistamine, decongestant, antitussive, and expectorant combinations—**
  - *Oral*
    - Brompheniramine, Phenylephrine, Codeine, and Guaifenesin
      - Oral solution
    - Brompheniramine, Phenylephrine, Hydrocodone, and Guaifenesin
      - Oral solution
    - Chlorpheniramine, Ephedrine, Phenylephrine, Dextromethorphan, Ammonium Chloride, and Ipecac
      - Syrup
    - Chlorpheniramine, Phenylephrine, Codeine, and Ammonium Chloride
      - Oral solution
    - Chlorpheniramine, Phenylephrine, Codeine, and Potassium Iodide
      - Syrup
    - Chlorpheniramine, Phenylephrine, Dextromethorphan, and Guaifenesin
      - Syrup
    - Chlorpheniramine, Phenylephrine, Dextromethorphan, Guaifenesin, and Ammonium Chloride
      - Oral solution
    - Chlorpheniramine, Pseudoephedrine, Dextromethorphan and Guaifenesin
      - Oral solution
    - Pyrilamine, Phenylephrine, Hydrocodone, and Ammonium Chloride
      - Syrup
    - Triprolidine, Pseudoephedrine, Codeine, and Guaifenesin
      - Oral solution
- **Antihistamine, decongestant, antitussive, expectorant, and analgesic combinations—**
  - *Oral*
    - Pheniramine, Phenylephrine, Codeine, Sodium Citrate, Sodium Salicylate, and Caffeine
      - Oral solution
- **Antihistamine, decongestant, and expectorant combinations—**
  - *Oral*
    - Chlorpheniramine, Ephedrine, and Guaifenesin
      - Oral solution
    - Promethazine, Phenylephrine, and Potassium Guaiacolsulfonate
      - Syrup
- **Antitussive and analgesic combination—**
  - *Oral*
    - Dextromethorphan and Acetaminophen
      - Capsules
      - Oral solution

- Oral suspension
- Tablets
- **Antitussive and anticholinergic combination—**
  - *Oral*
    - Hydrocodone and Homatropine (Canadian product does not contain homatropine)
      - Syrup
      - Tablets
- **Antitussive and expectorant combinations—**
  - *Oral*
    - Codeine, Ammonium Chloride, and Guaifenesin
      - Syrup
    - Codeine and Guaifenesin
      - Oral solution
      - Syrup
      - Tablets
    - Dextromethorphan and Guaifenesin
      - Capsules
      - Extended-release capsules
      - Oral solution
      - Syrup
      - Tablets
      - Extended-release tablets
    - Dextromethorphan and Iodinated Glycerol
      - Oral solution
    - Hydrocodone and Guaifenesin
      - Oral solution
      - Syrup
      - Tablets
    - Hydrocodone and Potassium Guaiacolsulfonate
      - Oral solution
      - Syrup
- **Decongestant and antitussive combinations—**
  - *Oral*
    - Phenylephrine and Hydrocodone
      - Oral solution
      - Syrup
    - Pseudoephedrine and Dextromethorphan
      - Capsules
      - Oral solution
      - Syrup
- **Decongestant, antitussive, and analgesic combinations—**
  - *Oral*
    - Pseudoephedrine, Dextromethorphan, and Acetaminophen
      - Capsules
      - Oral solution
      - Oral suspension
      - Tablets
- **Decongestant, antitussive, and expectorant combinations—**
  - *Oral*
    - Phenylephrine, Hydrocodone, and Guaifenesin
      - Syrup
    - Phenylephrine, Hydrocodone, and Guaifenesin
      - Oral solution
      - Syrup
    - Pseudoephedrine, Codeine, and Guaifenesin
      - Oral solution
      - Syrup

      ○ Pseudoephedrine, Dextromethorphan, and Guaifenesin
- Capsules
- Oral solution
- Syrup
- Tablets

      ○ Pseudoephedrine, Hydrocodone, and Guaifenesin
- Elixir
- Oral solution
- Syrup
- Tablets

      ○ Pseudoephedrine, Hydrocodone, and Potassium Guaiacolsulfonate
- Oral solution

- **Decongestant, antitussive, expectorant, and analgesic combinations—**

Oral

      ○ Pseudoephedrine, Dextromethorphan, Guaifenesin, and Acetaminophen
- Capsules
- Oral solution
- Syrup
- Tablets

- **Decongestant and expectorant combinations—**

Oral

      ○ Ephedrine and Guaifenesin
- Syrup

      ○ Phenylephrine and Guaifenesin
- Oral solution
- Extended-release capsules
- Extended-release tablets

      ○ Pseudoephedrine and Guaifenesin
- Capsules
- Extended-release capsules
- Oral solution
- Syrup
- Tablets
- Extended-release tablets

Before Using This Medicine

If you are taking this medicine without a prescription, carefully read and follow any precautions on the label. For cough/cold combinations, the following should be considered:

Allergies—Tell your doctor if you have ever had any unusual or allergic reaction to any of the ingredients contained in this medicine. Also tell your health care professional if you are allergic to any other substances, such as foods, preservatives, or dyes. In addition, if this medicine contains *aspirin or other salicylates*, before taking it, check with your doctor if you have ever had any unusual or allergic reaction to any of the following medicines:
- Aspirin or other salicylates
- Diclofenac (e.g., Voltaren)
- Diflunisal (e.g., Dolobid)
- Fenoprofen (e.g., Nalfon)
- Floctafenine
- Flurbiprofen, by mouth (e.g., Ansaid)
- Ibuprofen (e.g., Motrin)
- Indomethacin (e.g., Indocin)
- Ketoprofen (e.g., Orudis)
- Ketorolac (e.g., Toradol)
- Meclofenamate (e.g., Meclomen)
- Mefenamic acid (e.g., Ponstel)
- Methyl salicylate (oil of wintergreen)
- Naproxen (e.g., Naprosyn)
- Oxyphenbutazone (e.g., Tandearil)
- Phenylbutazone (e.g., Butazolidin)
- Piroxicam (e.g., Feldene)
- Sulindac (e.g., Clinoril)
- Suprofen (e.g., Suprol)
- Tiaprofenic acid (e.g., Surgam)
- Tolmetin (e.g., Tolectin)
- Zomepirac (e.g., Zomax)

Diet—Make certain your health care professional knows if you are on any special diet, such as a low-sodium or low-sugar diet.

Pregnancy—The occasional use of a cough/cold combination is not likely to cause problems in the fetus or in the newborn baby. However, when these medicines are used at higher doses and/or for a long time, the chance that problems might occur may increase. For the individual ingredients of these combinations, the following information should be considered before you decide to use a particular cough/cold combination:

- *Acetaminophen*—Studies on birth defects have not been done in humans. However, acetaminophen has not been shown to cause birth defects or other problems in humans.

- *Alcohol*—Some of these combination medicines contain a large amount of alcohol. Too much use of alcohol during pregnancy may cause birth defects.

- *Antihistamines*—Antihistamines have not been shown to cause problems in humans.

- *Caffeine*—Studies in humans have not shown that caffeine causes birth defects. However, studies in animals have shown that caffeine causes birth defects when given in very large doses (amounts equal to the amount of caffeine contained in 12 to 24 cups of coffee a day).

- *Codeine*—Although studies on birth defects with codeine have not been done in humans, it has not been reported to cause birth defects in humans. Codeine has not been shown to cause birth defects in animal studies, but it caused other unwanted effects. Also, regular use of narcotics during pregnancy may cause the baby to become dependent on the medicine. This may lead to withdrawal side effects after birth. In addition, narcotics may cause breathing problems in the newborn baby if taken by the mother just before delivery.

- *Hydrocodone*—Although studies on birth defects with hydrocodone have not been done in humans, it has not been reported to cause birth defects in humans. However, hydrocodone has been shown to cause birth defects in animals when given in very large doses. Also, regular use of narcotics during pregnancy may cause the baby to become dependent on the medicine. This may lead to withdrawal side effects after birth. In addition, narcotics may cause breathing problems in the newborn baby if taken by the mother just before delivery.

- *Iodides (e.g., calcium iodide and iodinated glycerol)*—Not recommended during pregnancy. Iodides have caused enlargement of the thyroid gland in the fetus and resulted in breathing problems in newborn babies whose mothers took iodides in large doses for a long period of time.

- *Phenylephrine*—Studies on birth defects with phenylephrine have not been done in either humans or animals.
- *Pseudoephedrine*—Studies on birth defects with pseudoephedrine have not been done in humans. In animal studies pseudoephedrine did not cause birth defects but did cause a decrease in average weight, length, and rate of bone formation in the animal fetus when given in high doses.
- *Salicylates (e.g., aspirin)*—Studies on birth defects in humans have been done with aspirin, but not with salicylamide or sodium salicylate. Salicylates have not been shown to cause birth defects in humans. However, salicylates have been shown to cause birth defects in animals.Some reports have suggested that too much use of aspirin late in pregnancy may cause a decrease in the newborn's weight and possible death of the fetus or newborn infant. However, the mothers in these reports had been taking much larger amounts of aspirin than are usually recommended. Studies of mothers taking aspirin in the doses that are usually recommended did not show these unwanted effects. However, there is a chance that regular use of salicylates late in pregnancy may cause unwanted effects on the heart or blood flow in the fetus or newborn baby.Use of salicylates, especially aspirin, during the last 2 weeks of pregnancy may cause bleeding problems in the fetus before or during delivery, or in the newborn baby. Also, too much use of salicylates during the last 3 months of pregnancy may increase the length of pregnancy, prolong labor, cause other problems during delivery, or cause severe bleeding in the mother before, during, or after delivery. *Do not take aspirin during the last 3 months of pregnancy unless it has been ordered by your doctor.*

Breast-feeding—If you are breast-feeding, the chance that problems might occur depends on the ingredients of the combination. For the individual ingredients of these combinations, the following apply:
- *Acetaminophen*—Acetaminophen passes into the breast milk. However, it has not been reported to cause problems in nursing babies.
- *Alcohol*—Alcohol passes into the breast milk. However, the amount of alcohol in recommended doses of this medicine does not usually cause problems in nursing babies.
- *Antihistamines*—Small amounts of antihistamines pass into the breast milk. Antihistamine-containing medicine is not recommended for use while breast-feeding since most antihistamines are especially likely to cause side effects, such as unusual excitement or irritability, in the baby. Also, since antihistamines tend to decrease the secretions of the body, the flow of breast milk may be reduced in some patients.
- *Caffeine*—Small amounts of caffeine pass into the breast milk and may build up in the nursing baby. However, the amount of caffeine in recommended doses of this medicine does not usually cause problems in nursing babies.
- *Decongestants (e.g., ephedrine, phenylephrine, pseudoephedrine)*—Phenylephrine has not been re-

ported to cause problems in nursing babies. Ephedrine and pseudoephedrine pass into the breast milk and may cause unwanted effects in nursing babies (especially newborn and premature babies).
- *Iodides (e.g., calcium iodide and iodinated glycerol)*—These medicines pass into the breast milk and may cause unwanted effects, such as underactive thyroid, in the baby.
- *Narcotic antitussives (e.g., codeine, dihydrocodeine, hydrocodone, and hydromorphone)*—Small amounts of codeine have been shown to pass into the breast milk. However, the amount of codeine or other narcotic antitussives in recommended doses of this medicine has not been reported to cause problems in nursing babies.
- *Salicylates (e.g., aspirin)*—Salicylates pass into the breast milk. Although salicylates have not been reported to cause problems in nursing babies, it is possible that problems may occur if large amounts are taken regularly.

Children—Very young children are usually more sensitive to the effects of this medicine. *Before giving any of these combination medicines to a child, check the package label very carefully. Some of these medicines are too strong for use in children.* If you are not certain whether a specific product can be given to a child, or if you have any questions about the amount to give, check with your health care professional, especially if it contains:
- *Antihistamines*—Nightmares, unusual excitement, nervousness, restlessness, or irritability may be more likely to occur in children taking antihistamines.
- *Decongestants (e.g., ephedrine, phenylephrine, pseudoephedrine)*—Increases in blood pressure may be more likely to occur in children taking decongestants.
- *Narcotic antitussives (e.g., codeine, hydrocodeine, hydrocodone, and hydromorphone)*—Breathing problems may be especially likely to occur in children younger than 2 years of age taking narcotic antitussives. Also, unusual excitement or restlessness may be more likely to occur in children receiving these medicines.
- *Salicylates (e.g., aspirin)*—Do not give medicines containing aspirin or other salicylates to a child with a fever or other symptoms of a virus infection, especially flu or chickenpox, without first discussing its use with your child's doctor.* This is very important because salicylates may cause a serious illness called Reye's syndrome in children with fever caused by a virus infection, especially flu or chickenpox. Also, children may be more sensitive to the aspirin or other salicylates contained in some of these medicines, especially if they have a fever or have lost large amounts of body fluid because of vomiting, diarrhea, or sweating.

Teenagers—*Do not give medicines containing aspirin or other salicylates to a teenager with a fever or other symptoms of a virus infection, especially flu or chickenpox, without first discussing its use with your child's doctor.* This is very important because salicylates may cause a serious illness called Reye's syndrome in teenagers with fever caused by a virus infection, especially flu or chickenpox.

Older adults—The elderly are usually more sensitive to the effects of this medicine, especially if it contains:
- *Antihistamines*—Confusion, difficult or painful urination, dizziness, drowsiness, feeling faint, or dryness of mouth, nose, or throat may be more likely to occur in elderly patients. Also, nightmares or unusual excitement,

nervousness, restlessness, or irritability may be more likely to occur in the elderly taking antihistamines.

- *Decongestants (e.g., ephedrine, phenylephrine, pseudoephedrine)*—Confusion, hallucinations, drowsiness, or convulsions (seizures) may be more likely to occur in the elderly, who are usually more sensitive to the effects of this medicine. Also, increases in blood pressure may be more likely to occur in elderly persons taking decongestants.

Other medicines—Although certain medicines should not be used together at all, in other cases two different medicines may be used together even if an interaction might occur. In these cases, your doctor may want to change the dose, or other precautions may be necessary. Tell your health care professional if you are taking *any* other prescription or non-prescription (over-the-counter [OTC]) medicine, for example, aspirin or other medicine for allergies. Some medicines may change the way this medicine affects your body. Also, the effect of other medicines may be increased or reduced by some of the ingredients in this medicine. Check with your health care professional about which medicines you should not take with this medicine.

Other medical problems—The presence of other medical problems may affect the use of the cough/cold combination medicine. Make sure you tell your doctor if you have any other medical problems, especially:

- Alcohol abuse (or history of)—Acetaminophen-containing medicines increase the chance of liver damage; also, some of the liquid medicines contain a large amount of alcohol
- Anemia or
- Gout or
- Hemophilia or other bleeding problems or
- Stomach ulcer or other stomach problems—These conditions may become worse if you are taking a combination medicine containing aspirin or another salicylate
- Brain disease or injury or
- Colitis or
- Convulsions (seizures) (history of) or
- Diarrhea or
- Gallbladder disease or gallstones—These conditions may become worse if you are taking a combination medicine containing codeine, dihydrocodeine, hydrocodone, or hydromorphone
- Cystic fibrosis (in children)—Side effects of iodinated glycerol may be more likely in children with cystic fibrosis
- Diabetes mellitus (sugar diabetes)—Decongestants may put diabetic patients at greater risk of having heart or blood vessel disease
- Emphysema, asthma, or chronic lung disease (especially in children)—Salicylate-containing medicine may cause an allergic reaction in which breathing becomes difficult
- Enlarged prostate or
- Urinary tract blockage or difficult urination—Some of the effects of anticholinergics (e.g., homatropine) or antihistamines may make urinary problems worse
- Glaucoma—A slight increase in inner eye pressure may occur with the use of anticholinergics (e.g., homatropine) or antihistamines, which may make the condition worse

- Heart or blood vessel disease or
- High blood pressure—Decongestant-containing medicine may increase the blood pressure and speed up the heart rate; also, caffeine-containing medicine, if taken in large amounts, may speed up the heart rate
- Kidney disease—This condition may increase the chance of side effects of this medicine because the medicine may build up in the body
- Liver disease—Liver disease increases the chance of side effects because the medicine may build up in the body; also, if liver disease is severe, there is a greater chance that aspirin-containing medicine may cause bleeding
- Thyroid disease—If an overactive thyroid has caused a fast heart rate, the decongestant in this medicine may cause the heart rate to speed up further; also, if the medicine contains narcotic antitussives (e.g., codeine), iodides (e.g., iodinated glycerol), or salicylates, the thyroid problem may become worse

---

Proper Use of This Medicine

To help loosen mucus or phlegm in the lungs, *drink a glass of water after each dose of this medicine,* unless otherwise directed by your doctor.

Take this medicine only as directed. Do not take more of it and do not take it more often than recommended on the label, unless otherwise directed by your doctor. To do so may increase the chance of side effects.

For patients *taking the extended-release capsule or tablet form of this medicine:*

- Swallow the capsule or tablet whole.
- Do not crush, break, or chew before swallowing.
- If the capsule is too large to swallow, you may mix the contents of the capsule with applesauce, jelly, honey, or syrup and swallow without chewing.

For patients *taking the extended-release oral solution or oral suspension form of this medicine:*

- Do not dilute with fluids or mix with other drugs.

For patients *taking a combination medicine containing an antihistamine and/or aspirin or other salicylate:*

- Take with food or a glass of water or milk to lessen stomach irritation, if necessary.

If a combination medicine containing aspirin has a strong vinegar-like odor, do not use it. This odor means the medicine is breaking down. If you have any questions about this, check with your pharmacist.

Missed dose—If you must take this medicine regularly and you miss a dose, take it as soon as possible. However, if it is almost time for your next dose, skip the missed dose and go back to your regular dosing schedule. Do not double doses.

Storage—To store this medicine:

- Keep this medicine out of the reach of children. Overdose is very dangerous in young children.
- Store away from heat and direct light.
- Do not store the capsule or tablet form of this medicine in the bathroom, near the kitchen sink, or in other damp places. Heat or moisture may cause the medicine to break down.

- Keep the liquid form of this medicine from freezing. Do not refrigerate the syrup.
- Do not keep outdated medicine or medicine no longer needed. Be sure that any discarded medicine is out of the reach of children.

Precautions While Using This Medicine

If your cough has not improved after 7 days or if you have a high fever, skin rash, continuing headache, or sore throat with the cough, check with your doctor. These signs may mean that you have other medical problems.

For patients *taking antihistamine-containing medicine:*
- Before you have any skin tests for allergies, tell the doctor in charge that you are taking this medicine. The results of the test may be affected by the antihistamine in this medicine.
- This medicine will add to the effects of alcohol and other CNS depressants (medicines that slow down the nervous system, possibly causing drowsiness). Some examples of CNS depressants are antihistamines or medicine for hay fever, other allergies, or colds; sedatives, tranquilizers, or sleeping medicine; prescription pain medicine or narcotics; barbiturates; medicine for seizures; muscle relaxants; or anesthetics, including some dental anesthetics. *Check with your doctor before taking any of the above while you are taking this medicine.*
- This medicine may cause some people to become drowsy, dizzy, or less alert than they are normally. *Make sure you know how you react to this medicine before you drive, use machines, or do anything else that could be dangerous if you are dizzy or are not alert.*
- When taking antihistamines on a regular basis, make sure your doctor knows if you are taking large amounts of aspirin at the same time (as in arthritis or rheumatism). Effects of too much aspirin, such as ringing in the ears, may be covered up by the antihistamine.
- Antihistamines may cause dryness of the mouth. For temporary relief, use sugarless candy or gum, melt bits of ice in your mouth, or use a saliva substitute. However, if your mouth continues to feel dry for more than 2 weeks, check with your medical doctor or dentist. Continuing dryness of the mouth may increase the chance of dental disease, including tooth decay, gum disease, and fungus infections.

For patients *taking decongestant-containing medicine:*
- This medicine may add to the central nervous system (CNS) stimulant effects of diet aids. *Do not use medicines for diet or appetite control while taking this medicine unless you have checked with your doctor.*
- This medicine may cause some people to be nervous or restless or to have trouble in sleeping. If you have trouble in sleeping, *take the last dose of this medicine for each day a few hours before bedtime.* If you have any questions about this, check with your doctor.
- Before having any kind of surgery (including dental surgery) or emergency treatment, tell the medical doctor or dentist in charge that you are taking this medicine.

For patients *taking narcotic antitussive (codeine, dihydrocodeine, hydrocodone, or hydromorphone)–containing medicine:*
- This medicine will add to the effects of alcohol and other CNS depressants (medicines that slow down the nervous system, possibly causing drowsiness). Some examples of CNS depressants are antihistamines or medicine for hay fever, other allergies, or colds; sedatives, tranquilizers, or sleeping medicine; prescription pain medicine or narcotics; barbiturates; medicine for seizures; muscle relaxants; or anesthetics, including some dental anesthetics. *Check with your doctor before taking any of the above while you are taking this medicine.*
- This medicine may cause some people to become drowsy, dizzy, less alert than they are normally, or to feel a false sense of well-being. *Make sure you know how you react to this medicine before you drive, use machines, or do anything else that could be dangerous if you are dizzy or are not alert and clearheaded.*
- Nausea or vomiting may occur after taking a narcotic antitussive. This effect may go away if you lie down for a while. However, if nausea or vomiting continues, check with your doctor.
- Dizziness, lightheadedness, or fainting may be especially likely to occur when you get up suddenly from a lying or sitting position. Getting up slowly may help lessen this problem.
- Before having any kind of surgery (including dental surgery) or emergency treatment, tell the medical doctor or dentist in charge that you are taking this medicine.

For patients *taking iodide (calcium iodide, iodinated glycerol, or potassium iodide)-containing medicine:*
- Make sure your doctor knows if you are planning to have any future thyroid tests. The results of the thyroid test may be affected by the iodine in this medicine.

For patients *taking analgesic-containing medicine:*
- *Check the label of all nonprescription (over-the-counter [OTC]), and prescription medicines you now take.* If any contain acetaminophen or aspirin or other salicylates, including diflunisal or bismuth subsalicylate, be especially careful. Taking them while taking a cough/cold combination medicine that already contains them may lead to overdose. If you have any questions about this, check with your health care professional.
- Do not take aspirin-containing medicine for 5 days before any surgery, including dental surgery, unless otherwise directed by your medical doctor or dentist. Taking aspirin during this time may cause bleeding problems.

For *diabetic patients taking aspirin- or sodium salicylate–containing medicine:*
- False urine sugar test results may occur:
  - If you take 8 or more 325–mg (5–grain) doses of aspirin every day for several days in a row.
  - If you take 8 or more 325–mg (5–grain), or 4 or more 500–mg (10–grain) doses of sodium salicylate.
- Smaller doses or occasional use of aspirin or sodium salicylate usually will not affect urine sugar tests. If you have any questions about this, check with your health care professional, especially if your diabetes is not well controlled.

For patients *taking homatropine-containing medicine:*
- This medicine may make you sweat less, causing your body temperature to increase. *Use extra care not to become overheated during exercise or hot weather while you are taking this medicine,* since overheating may result in heat stroke. Also, hot baths or saunas may

make you feel dizzy or faint while you are taking this medicine.

Side Effects of This Medicine

Along with its needed effects, a medicine may cause some unwanted effects. Although serious side effects occur rarely when this medicine is taken as recommended, they may be more likely to occur if:

- too much medicine is taken.
- it is taken in large doses.
- it is taken for a long period of time.

Get emergency help immediately if any of the following symptoms of overdose occur:

For narcotic antitussive (codeine, dihydrocodeine, hydrocodone, or hydromorphone)–containing
Cold, clammy skin; confusion (severe); convulsions (seizures); drowsiness or dizziness (severe); nervousness or restlessness (severe); pinpoint pupils of eyes; slow heartbeat; slow or troubled breathing; weakness (severe)

For acetaminophen-containing
Diarrhea; increased sweating; loss of appetite; nausea or vomiting; stomach cramps or pain; swelling or tenderness in the upper abdomen or stomach area

For salicylate-containing
Any loss of hearing; bloody urine; confusion; convulsions (seizures); diarrhea (severe or continuing); dizziness or lightheadedness; drowsiness (severe); excitement or nervousness (severe); fast or deep breathing; fever; hallucinations (seeing, hearing, or feeling things that are not there); increased sweating; nausea or vomiting (severe or continuing); shortness of breath or troubled breathing (for salicylamide only); stomach pain (severe or continuing); uncontrollable flapping movements of the hands, especially in elderly patients; unusual thirst; vision problems

For decongestant-containing
Fast, pounding, or irregular heartbeat; headache (continuing and severe); nausea or vomiting (severe); nervousness or restlessness (severe); shortness of breath or troubled breathing (severe or continuing)

Also, check with your doctor as soon as possible if any of the following side effects occur:

For all combinations
Skin rash, hives, and/or itching

For antihistamine- or anticholinergic-containing
Clumsiness or unsteadiness; convulsions (seizures); drowsiness (severe); dryness of mouth, nose, or throat (severe); flushing or redness of face; hallucinations (seeing, hearing, or feeling things that are not there); restlessness (severe); shortness of breath or troubled breathing; slow or fast heartbeat

For iodine-containing
Headache (continuing); increased watering of mouth; loss of appetite; metallic taste; skin rash, hives, or redness; sore throat; swelling of face, lips, or eyelids

For acetaminophen-containing
Unexplained sore throat and fever; unusual tiredness or weakness; yellow eyes or skin

Other side effects may occur that usually do not need medical attention. These side effects may go away during treatment as your body adjusts to the medicine. However, check with your doctor if any of the following side effects continue or are bothersome:

Not all of the side effects listed above have been reported for each of these medicines, but they have been reported for at least one of them. There are some similarities among these combination medicines, so many of the above side effects may occur with any of these medicines.

Constipation; decreased sweating; difficult or painful urination; dizziness or lightheadedness; drowsiness; dryness of mouth, nose, or throat; false sense of well-being; increased sensitivity of skin to sun; nausea or vomiting; nightmares; stomach pain; thickening of mucus; trouble in sleeping; unusual excitement, nervousness, restlessness, or irritability; unusual tiredness or weakness

Other side effects not listed above may also occur in some patients. If you notice any other effects, check with your doctor.

CROMOLYN (Inhalation, oral/nebulization route) - KROE-moe-lin

Commonly used brand name(s)

In the U.S.—
Intal
Intal Inhaler

Available Dosage Forms:

- Aerosol Powder
- Aerosol Liquid
- Capsule
- Solution

Therapeutic Class: Antiasthma
Pharmacologic Class: Mast Cell Stabilizer

Uses For This Medicine

Cromolyn is used to prevent the symptoms of asthma. When it is used regularly, cromolyn lessens the number and severity of asthma attacks by reducing inflammation in the lungs. Cromolyn is also used just before exposure to conditions or substances (for example, exercise, allergens, such as pollen, aspirin, chemicals, cold air, or air pollutants) that cause bronchospasm (wheezing or difficulty in breathing). Cromolyn will not help an asthma or bronchospasm attack that has already started.

Cromolyn may be used alone or with other asthma medicines, such as bronchodilators (medicines that open up narrowed breathing passages) or corticosteroids (cortisone-like medicines).

Cromolyn inhalation works by acting on certain inflammatory cells in the lungs to prevent them from releasing substances that cause asthma symptoms or bronchospasm.

This medicine is available only with your doctor's prescription.

It is very important that you read and understand the following information. If any of it causes you special concern, check with your doctor. Also, if you have any questions or if you want more information about this medicine or your medical problem, ask your doctor, nurse, or pharmacist.

Before Using This Medicine

In deciding to use a medicine, the risks of taking the medicine must be weighed against the good it will do. This is a decision you and your doctor will make. For this medicine, the following should be considered:

Allergies—Tell your doctor if you have ever had any unusual or allergic reaction to this medicine or any other medicines. Also tell your health care professional if you have any other types of allergies, such as to foods, dyes, preservatives, or animals. For non-prescription products, read the label or package ingredients carefully.

Pediatric—Although there is no specific information comparing the use of cromolyn in children with use in other age groups, this medicine is not expected to cause different side effects or problems in children than it does in adults. The inhalation solution form of this medicine should not be used in children younger than 2 years of age, and the inhalation aerosol should not be used in children younger than 5 years of age.

Geriatric—Many medicines have not been studied specifically in older people. Therefore, it may not be known whether they work exactly the same way they do in younger adults. Although there is no specific information comparing the use of cromolyn inhalation in the elderly with use in other age groups, this medicine is not expected to cause different side effects or problems in older people than it does in younger adults.

Pregnancy—

	Pregnancy Category	Explanation
All Trimesters	B	Animal studies have revealed no evidence of harm to the fetus, however, there are no adequate studies in pregnant women OR animal studies have shown an adverse effect, but adequate studies in pregnant women have failed to demonstrate a risk to the fetus.

Breast Feeding—There are no adequate studies in women for determining infant risk when using this medication during breastfeeding. Weigh the potential benefits against the potential risks before taking this medication while breastfeeding.

Other medicines—Although certain medicines should not be used together at all, in other cases two different medicines may be used together even if an interaction might occur. In these cases, your doctor may want to change the dose, or other precautions may be necessary. Tell your healthcare professional if you are taking any other prescription or non-prescription (over-the-counter [OTC]) medicine.

Interactions with Food/Tobacco/Alcohol—Certain medicines should not be used at or around the time of eating food or eating certain types of food since interactions may occur. Using alcohol or tobacco with certain medicines may also cause interactions to occur. Discuss with your healthcare professional the use of your medicine with food, alcohol, or tobacco.

Other medical problems—The presence of other medical problems may affect the use of this medicine. Make sure you tell your doctor if you have any other medical problems, especially:

- Heart disease or
- Irregular heartbeat—The propellants used to deliver the medicine in the aerosol inhaler may worsen these conditions

Proper Use of This Medicine

Cromolyn oral inhalation is used to help prevent symptoms of asthma or bronchospasm (wheezing or difficulty in breathing). Cromolyn will not relieve an asthma or a bronchospasm attack that has already started. It is important to use cromolyn at regular times as directed by your doctor.

Use cromolyn inhalation only as directed. Do not use more of it and do not use it more often than your doctor ordered. To do so may increase the chance of side effects.

Cromolyn inhalation usually comes with patient directions. Read them carefully before using this medicine. If you do not understand the directions that come with the inhaler or if you are not sure how to use the inhaler, ask your health care professional to show you how to use it. Also, ask your health care professional to check regularly how you use the inhaler to make sure you are using it properly.

For patients using cromolyn inhalation aerosol:

- The cromolyn aerosol canister provides about 112 or 200 inhalations, depending on the size of the canister your doctor ordered. You should try to keep a record of the number of inhalations you use so you will know when the canister is almost empty. This canister, unlike some other aerosol canisters, cannot be floated in water to test its fullness.

- When you use the inhaler for the first time, or if you have not used it in a while, the inhaler may not deliver the right amount of medicine with the first puff. Therefore, before using the inhaler, test or prime it.

- To test or prime the inhaler:
  - Insert the medicine container (canister) firmly into the clean mouthpiece according to the manufacturer's directions. Check to make sure the canister is placed properly into the mouthpiece.
  - Take the cap off the mouthpiece and shake the inhaler three or four times.
  - Hold the inhaler well away from you at arm's length and press the top of the canister, spraying the medicine one time into the air. The inhaler will now be ready to provide the right amount of medicine when you use it.

- To use the inhaler:
  - Using your thumb and one or two fingers, hold the inhaler upright, with the mouthpiece end down and pointing toward you.
  - Take the cap off the mouthpiece. Check the mouthpiece to make sure it is clear. Do not use the inhaler with any other mouthpieces.
  - Gently shake the inhaler three or four times.
  - Hold the mouthpiece away from your mouth and breathe out slowly and completely to the end of a normal breath.
  - Use the inhalation method recommended by your doctor.
    - Open-mouth method: Place the mouthpiece about 1 to 2 inches (2 fingerwidths) in front of your widely opened mouth. Make sure the inhaler is aimed into

your mouth so the spray does not hit the roof of your mouth or your tongue. Avoid spraying in eyes.

- Closed-mouth method: Place the mouthpiece in your mouth between your teeth and over your tongue with your lips closed tightly around it. Make sure your tongue or teeth are not blocking the opening.
  - Tilt your head back a little. Start to breathe in slowly through your mouth. At the same time, press the top of the canister once to get one puff of medicine. Continue to breathe in slowly for 3 to 4 seconds until you have taken a full deep breath. It is important to press down on the canister and breathe in slowly at the same time so the medicine gets into your lungs. This step may be difficult at first. If you are using the closed-mouth method and you see a fine mist coming from your mouth or nose, the inhaler is not being used correctly.
  - Hold your breath as long as you can up to 10 seconds (count slowly to ten). This gives the medicine time to settle into your airways and lungs.
  - Take the mouthpiece away from your mouth and breathe out slowly.
  - If your doctor has told you to inhale more than 1 puff of medicine at each dose, wait about 1 minute between puffs. Then, gently shake the inhaler again, and take the second puff following exactly the same steps you used for the first puff. Breathe in only one puff at a time.
  - When you are finished using the inhaler, wipe off the mouthpiece and replace the cap.
  - Keep track of the number of sprays you have used from the inhaler, and discard the inhaler after the labeled maximum number of sprays has been used.

Your doctor may want you to use a spacer device with the inhaler. A spacer makes the inhaler easier to use. It allows more of the medicine to reach your lungs, rather than staying in your mouth and throat.

- To use a spacer device with the inhaler:
  - Attach the spacer to the inhaler according to the manufacturer's directions. There are different types of spacers available, but the method of breathing remains the same with most spacers.
  - Gently shake the inhaler and spacer well.
  - Hold the mouthpiece of the spacer away from your mouth and breathe out slowly and completely.
  - Place the mouthpiece of the spacer into your mouth between your teeth and over your tongue with your lips closed around it.
  - Press down on the canister top once to release one puff of medicine into the spacer. Then, within 1 or 2 seconds, begin to breathe in slowly and deeply through your mouth for 5 to 10 seconds. Count the seconds while inhaling.
  - Hold your breath as long as you can up to 10 seconds (count slowly to 10).
  - Breathe out slowly.
  - Wait a minute between puffs. Then, gently shake the inhaler and spacer again and take the second puff, following exactly the same steps you used for the first puff. Do not spray more than one puff at a time into the spacer.
  - When you are finished using the inhaler, remove the spacer device from the inhaler and replace the cap.

Clean the inhaler, mouthpiece, and spacer at least once a week.

- To clean the inhaler:
  - Remove the canister from the inhaler and set the canister aside. Do not get the canister wet.
  - Wash the mouthpiece, cap, and the spacer in warm soapy water. Rinse well with warm, running water.
  - Shake off the excess water and let the inhaler parts air dry completely before putting the inhaler back together.

For patients using cromolyn capsules for inhalation:

- Do not swallow the capsules. The medicine will not work if you swallow it.
- This medicine is used with a special inhaler, either the Spinhaler or the Halermatic. If you do not understand the directions that come with the inhaler or if you are not sure how to use the inhaler, ask your health care professional to show you how to use it. Also, ask your health care professional to check regularly how you use the inhaler to make sure you are using it properly.
- If you are using cromolyn capsules for inhalation with the Spinhaler:
  - To load the Spinhaler:
    - Make sure your hands are clean and dry.
    - Insert the capsule into the inhaler just before using this medicine.
    - Hold the inhaler upright with the mouthpiece pointing down. Unscrew the body of the inhaler from the mouthpiece.
    - Keep the mouthpiece pointing down and the propeller on the spindle. Remove the foil from the capsule and insert the colored end of the cromolyn capsule firmly into the cup of the propeller. Avoid too much handling of the capsule, because moisture from your hands may make the capsule soft.
    - Make sure the propeller moves freely.
    - Screw the body of the inhaler back into the mouthpiece and make certain that it is fastened well.
    - While keeping the inhaler upright with the mouthpiece pointing down, slide the grey outer sleeve down firmly until it stops. This will puncture the capsule. Then slide the sleeve up as far as it will go. This step may be repeated a second time to make sure the capsule is punctured.
  - To use the Spinhaler:
    - Check to make sure the mouthpiece is properly attached to the body of the inhaler.
    - Hold the inhaler away from your mouth and breathe out slowly to the end of a normal breath.
    - Place the mouthpiece in your mouth, close your lips around it, and tilt your head back. Do not block the mouthpiece with your teeth or tongue.
    - Take a deep and rapid breath. You should hear and feel the vibrations of the rotating propeller as you breathe in.
    - Take the inhaler from your mouth and hold your breath for a few seconds or as long as possible.
    - Hold the inhaler away from your mouth and breathe out slowly and completely to the end of a normal breath. Do not breathe out through the inhaler because this may prevent the inhaler from working properly.
    - Keep taking inhalations of this medicine until all the powder from the capsule is inhaled. A light

dusting of powder remaining in the capsule is normal and is not a sign that the inhaler is not working properly.

- Throw away the empty capsule. Then return the inhaler to the container and replace the lid on the container.

  ○ To clean the Spinhaler:
  - At least once a week, brush off any powder left sticking to the propeller.
  - Take the inhaler apart and wash the parts of the inhaler with clean, warm water.
  - Wash the inside of the propeller shaft by moving the propeller on and off the steel spindle under water.
  - Shake out the excess water.
  - Allow all parts of the inhaler to dry completely before putting it back together.
  - The Spinhaler should be replaced after 6 months.

- If you are using cromolyn capsules for inhalation with the Halermatic:
  ○ To load the Halermatic:
  - Make sure your hands are clean and dry.
  - Insert the capsule cartridge into the inhaler just before using this medicine.
  - Remove the mouthpiece cover. Then pull off the mouthpiece.
  - Push a cromolyn capsule cartridge firmly down to the bottom of the slot.
  - Slide the mouthpiece back on the body of the inhaler. Push down slowly as far as the mouthpiece will go. This punctures the capsule cartridge and lifts it into the rotation chamber. Do not repeat this step because the capsule cartridge needs to be punctured only once.

  ○ To use the Halermatic:
  - Hold the inhaler away from your mouth and breathe out slowly to the end of a normal breath.
  - Place the mouthpiece in your mouth, close your lips around it, and tilt your head back. Do not block the flow of medicine into the lungs with your teeth or tongue.
  - Breathe in quickly and steadily through the mouthpiece.
  - Hold your breath for a few seconds to keep the medicine in the lungs as long as possible. Then take the inhaler away from your mouth.
  - Hold the inhaler well away from your mouth and breathe out to the end of a normal breath. Do not breathe out through the inhaler because this may prevent the inhaler from working properly.
  - Keep taking inhalations of this medicine until all the powder from the capsule is inhaled. A light dusting of powder remaining in the capsule is normal and is not a sign that the inhaler is not working properly.
  - Throw away the empty capsule cartridge.

  ○ To clean the Halermatic:
  - Brush away powder deposits each day with a brush.
  - When powder deposits build up, wipe them away with a slightly damp cloth.
  - The mouthpiece may be washed separately if necessary. However, do not wet the blue-based body of the inhaler. Be sure the mouthpiece grid is dry before putting the inhaler back together.

- The Halermatic should be replaced every 6 months.

For patients using cromolyn inhalation solution:

- Cromolyn inhalation solution comes in a small glass container called an ampul. The ampul must be broken gently to empty the contents. If you do not understand the manufacturer's directions, ask your health care professional to show you what to do.
- Do not use the solution in the ampul if it is cloudy or contains particles.
- To break and empty the ampul:
  ○ The glass ampul is weak at each end so the ends can be broken easily by hand.
  ○ Hold the ampul away from the nebulizer and your face when you break it. Hold the ampul at an angle and carefully break off the lower end. No solution will come out.
  ○ Turn the ampul over so the open end faces up. Place a forefinger carefully over the open end.
  ○ Keep your finger firmly in place and break off the lower end of the ampul.
  ○ To empty the ampul, hold it over the bowl of the nebulizer unit and remove your finger to let the solution flow out.
  ○ Throw away any solution left in the nebulizer after you have taken your treatment.
- Use this medicine only in a power-operated nebulizer that has an adequate flow rate and is equipped with a face mask or mouthpiece. Your doctor will advise you on which nebulizer to use. Make sure you understand exactly how to use it. Hand-squeezed bulb nebulizers cannot be used with this medicine. If you have any questions about this, check with your doctor.

For patients using cromolyn oral inhalation regularly (for example, every day):

- In order for cromolyn to work properly, it must be inhaled every day in regularly spaced doses as ordered by your doctor. Up to 4 weeks may pass before you feel the full effects of the medicine.

Dosing—The dose of this medicine will be different for different patients. Follow your doctor's orders or the directions on the label. The following information includes only the average doses of this medicine. If your dose is different, do not change it unless your doctor tells you to do so.

The amount of medicine that you take depends on the strength of the medicine. Also, the number of doses you take each day, the time allowed between doses, and the length of time you take the medicine depend on the medical problem for which you are using the medicine.

- For inhalation aerosol dosage form:
  ○ For prevention of asthma symptoms:
  - Adults and children 5 years of age or older—2 inhalations (puffs) taken four times a day with doses spaced four to six hours apart.
  - Children up to 5 years of age—Cromolyn inhalation aerosol should not be used in children younger than 5 years of age.
  ○ For prevention of bronchospasm caused by exercise or a condition or substance:
  - Adults and children 5 years of age or older—2 inhalations (puffs) taken at least ten to fifteen (but not more than sixty) minutes before exercise

or exposure to any condition or substance that may cause an attack.

- Children up to 5 years of age—Cromolyn inhalation aerosol should not be used in children younger than 5 years of age.

- For capsule for inhalation dosage form:
  - For prevention of asthma symptoms:
    - Adults and children 2 years of age or older—20 mg (contents of 1 capsule) used in an inhaler, taken four times a day with doses spaced four to six hours apart.
    - Children up to 2 years of age—The capsule for inhalation should not be used in children younger than 2 years of age.
  - For prevention of bronchospasm caused by exercise or a condition or substance:
    - Adults and children 2 years of age or older—20 mg (contents of 1 capsule) used in an inhaler, taken at least ten to fifteen (but not more than sixty) minutes before exercise or exposure to any condition or substance that may cause an attack.
    - Children up to 2 years of age—The capsule for inhalation should not be used in children younger than 2 years of age.

- For inhalation solution dosage form:
  - For prevention of asthma symptoms:
    - Adults and children 2 years of age or older—20 mg (contents of 1 ampul) used in a nebulizer. This medicine should be used four times a day with doses spaced four to six hours apart. Use a new ampul of solution for each dose.
    - Children up to 2 years of age—Cromolyn inhalation solution should not be used in children younger than 2 years of age.
  - For prevention of bronchospasm caused by exercise or a condition or substance:
    - Adults and children 2 years of age or older—20 mg (contents of 1 ampul) used in a nebulizer. This medicine should be used at least ten to fifteen (but not more than sixty) minutes before exercise or exposure to any condition or substance that may cause an attack. Use a new ampul of solution for each dose.
    - Children up to 2 years of age—Cromolyn inhalation solution should not be used in children younger than 2 years of age.

Missed dose—If you miss a dose of this medicine, take it as soon as possible. However, if it is almost time for your next dose, skip the missed dose and go back to your regular dosing schedule. Do not double doses.

Storage—Store the medicine in a closed container at room temperature, away from heat, moisture, and direct light. Keep from freezing.

Store the canister at room temperature, away from heat and direct light. Do not freeze. Do not keep this medicine inside a car where it could be exposed to extreme heat or cold. Do not poke holes in the canister or throw it into a fire, even if the canister is empty.

Keep out of the reach of children.

Do not keep outdated medicine or medicine no longer needed.

Precautions While Using This Medicine

If your symptoms do not improve within 4 weeks or if your condition becomes worse after you begin using cromolyn, check with your doctor.

If you are also taking a corticosteroid or a bronchodilator for your asthma along with this medicine, do not stop taking the corticosteroid or bronchodilator even if your asthma seems better, unless you are told to do so by your doctor.

Dryness of the mouth or throat or throat irritation may occur after you use this medicine. Gargling and rinsing your mouth or taking a drink of water after each dose may help prevent these effects.

Side Effects of This Medicine

Along with its needed effects, a medicine may cause some unwanted effects. Although not all of these side effects may occur, if they do occur they may need medical attention.

Check with your doctor as soon as possible if any of the following side effects occur:

Rare
> Difficulty in swallowing; hives; increased wheezing or difficulty in breathing; itching of skin; low blood pressure; shortness of breath; swelling of face, lips, or eyelids; tightness in chest

Some side effects may occur that usually do not need medical attention. These side effects may go away during treatment as your body adjusts to the medicine. Also, your health care professional may be able to tell you about ways to prevent or reduce some of these side effects. Check with your health care professional if any of the following side effects continue or are bothersome or if you have any questions about them:

More common
> Coughing; nausea; throat irritation or dryness

If you are using the cromolyn inhalation aerosol, you may notice an unpleasant taste. This may be expected and will go away when you stop using the medicine.

Other side effects not listed may also occur in some patients. If you notice any other effects, check with your healthcare professional.

CROMOLYN   (Nasal route) - KROE-moe-lin

Commonly used brand name(s)
In the U.S.—
  Nasalcrom

Available Dosage Forms:
- Spray

Therapeutic Class: Nasal Agent
Pharmacologic Class: Mast Cell Stabilizer

Uses For This Medicine

Cromolyn nasal solution is used to help prevent or treat the symptoms (sneezing, wheezing, runny nose, itching) of seasonal (short-term) or chronic (long-term) allergic rhinitis.

Cromolyn powder for nasal inhalation is used to help prevent seasonal (short-term) allergic rhinitis.

This medicine works by acting on certain cells in the body, called mast cells, to prevent them from releasing substances that cause the allergic reaction.

When cromolyn is used to treat chronic (long-term) allergic rhinitis, an antihistamine and/or a nasal decongestant may be used with this medicine, especially during the first few weeks of treatment.

Nasal cromolyn is available without a prescription.

Before Using This Medicine

In deciding to use a medicine, the risks of taking the medicine must be weighed against the good it will do. This is a decision you and your doctor will make. For this medicine, the following should be considered:

Allergies—Tell your doctor if you have ever had any unusual or allergic reaction to this medicine or any other medicines. Also tell your health care professional if you have any other types of allergies, such as to foods, dyes, preservatives, or animals. For non-prescription products, read the label or package ingredients carefully.

Pediatric—Studies on this medicine have been done only in adult patients, and there is no specific information comparing use of nasal cromolyn in children up to 6 years of age (in Canada, up to 5 years of age) with use in other age groups. In older children, this medicine is not expected to cause different side effects or problems than it does in adults.

Geriatric—Many medicines have not been studied specifically in older people. Therefore, it may not be known whether they work exactly the same way they do in younger adults. Although there is no specific information comparing use of nasal cromolyn in the elderly with use in other age groups, this medicine is not expected to cause different side effects or problems in older people than it does in younger adults.

Pregnancy—

	Pregnancy Category	Explanation
All Trimesters	B	Animal studies have revealed no evidence of harm to the fetus, however, there are no adequate studies in pregnant women OR animal studies have shown an adverse effect, but adequate studies in pregnant women have failed to demonstrate a risk to the fetus.

Breast Feeding—There are no adequate studies in women for determining infant risk when using this medication during breastfeeding. Weigh the potential benefits against the potential risks before taking this medication while breastfeeding.

Other medicines—Although certain medicines should not be used together at all, in other cases two different medicines may be used together even if an interaction might occur. In these cases, your doctor may want to change the dose, or other precautions may be necessary. Tell your healthcare professional if you are taking any other prescription or nonprescription (over-the-counter [OTC]) medicine.

Interactions with Food/Tobacco/Alcohol—Certain medicines should not be used at or around the time of eating food or eating certain types of food since interactions may occur. Using alcohol or tobacco with certain medicines may also cause interactions to occur. Discuss with your healthcare professional the use of your medicine with food, alcohol, or tobacco.

Other medical problems—The presence of other medical problems may affect the use of this medicine. Make sure you tell your doctor if you have any other medical problems, especially:
- Kidney disease or
- Liver disease—Diseases of these body systems may alter the concentration of nasal cromolyn in the body
- Polyps or growths inside the nose—Cromolyn may not work if nasal passages are blocked

Proper Use of This Medicine

This medicine usually comes with patient directions. Read them carefully before using the medicine.

Before using this medicine, clear the nasal passages by blowing your nose.

To use:
- Cromolyn solution is used with a special spray device.
- To keep clean, wipe the nosepiece with a clean tissue and replace the dust cap after use.
- To avoid spreading an infection, do not use the container for more than one person.

Use this medicine only as directed. Do not use more of it and do not use it more often than your doctor ordered. To do so may increase the chance of side effects.

In order for this medicine to work properly, it must be used every day in regularly spaced doses as ordered by your doctor:
- For patients using cromolyn for seasonal (short-term) allergic rhinitis, up to 1 week may pass before you begin to feel better.
- For patients using cromolyn for chronic (long-term) allergic rhinitis, up to 2 to 4 weeks may pass before you feel the full effects of this medicine, although you may begin to feel better after 1 week.

Dosing—The dose of this medicine will be different for different patients. Follow your doctor's orders or the directions on the label. The following information includes only the average doses of this medicine. If your dose is different, do not change it unless your doctor tells you to do so.

The amount of medicine that you take depends on the strength of the medicine. Also, the number of doses you take each day, the time allowed between doses, and the length of time you take the medicine depend on the medical problem for which you are using the medicine.
- For nasal solution dosage form:
  - For allergic rhinitis:
    - Adults and children 6 years of age (in Canada, 5 years of age) and older—One spray into each nostril three to six times a day until condition is better; then, one spray in each nostril every eight to twelve hours.
    - Children up to 6 years of age (in Canada, up to 5 years of age)—Use and dose must be determined by your doctor.

Missed dose—If you miss a dose of this medicine, take it as soon as possible. However, if it is almost time for your next

dose, skip the missed dose and go back to your regular dosing schedule. Do not double doses.

Storage—Store the medicine in a closed container at room temperature, away from heat, moisture, and direct light. Keep from freezing.

Keep out of the reach of children.

Do not keep outdated medicine or medicine no longer needed.

Precautions While Using This Medicine

If your symptoms do not improve or if your condition becomes worse, check with your doctor.

Side Effects of This Medicine

Along with its needed effects, a medicine may cause some unwanted effects. Although not all of these side effects may occur, if they do occur they may need medical attention.

Check with your doctor as soon as possible if any of the following side effects occur:

Rare

Allergic reaction (coughing; difficulty in swallowing; hives or itching; swelling of face, lips, or eyelids; wheezing or difficulty in breathing); nosebleeds; skin rash

Some side effects may occur that usually do not need medical attention. These side effects may go away during treatment as your body adjusts to the medicine. Also, your health care professional may be able to tell you about ways to prevent or reduce some of these side effects. Check with your health care professional if any of the following side effects continue or are bothersome or if you have any questions about them:

More common

Burning, stinging, or irritation inside of nose; flushing; increase in sneezing

Less common

Cough; headache; postnasal drip; unpleasant taste

Other side effects not listed may also occur in some patients. If you notice any other effects, check with your healthcare professional.

CROMOLYN (Ophthalmic route) -
KROE-moe-lin

Commonly used brand name(s)
In the U.S.—
Crolom

Available Dosage Forms:
• Solution

Therapeutic Class: Ophthalmologic Agent
Pharmacologic Class: Mast Cell Stabilizer

Uses For This Medicine

Cromolyn ophthalmic solution is used in the eye to treat certain disorders of the eye caused by allergies. It works by acting on certain cells, called mast cells, to prevent them from releasing substances that cause the allergic reaction.

Cromolyn is available only with your doctor's prescription.

Before Using This Medicine

In deciding to use a medicine, the risks of taking the medicine must be weighed against the good it will do. This is a decision you and your doctor will make. For this medicine, the following should be considered:

Allergies—Tell your doctor if you have ever had any unusual or allergic reaction to this medicine or any other medicines. Also tell your health care professional if you have any other types of allergies, such as to foods, dyes, preservatives, or animals. For non-prescription products, read the label or package ingredients carefully.

Pediatric—Studies on this medicine have been done only in adult patients, and there is no specific information comparing use of cromolyn in children up to 4 years of age with use in other age groups. For older children, this medicine is not expected to cause different side effects or problems than it does in adults.

Geriatric—Many medicines have not been studied specifically in older people. Therefore, it may not be known whether they work exactly the same way they do in younger adults. Although there is no specific information comparing use of ophthalmic cromolyn in the elderly with use in other age groups, this medicine is not expected to cause different side effects or problems in older people than it does in younger adults.

Other medicines—Although certain medicines should not be used together at all, in other cases two different medicines may be used together even if an interaction might occur. In these cases, your doctor may want to change the dose, or other precautions may be necessary. Tell your healthcare professional if you are taking any other prescription or non-prescription (over-the-counter [OTC]) medicine.

Interactions with Food/Tobacco/Alcohol—Certain medicines should not be used at or around the time of eating food or eating certain types of food since interactions may occur. Using alcohol or tobacco with certain medicines may also cause interactions to occur. Discuss with your healthcare professional the use of your medicine with food, alcohol, or tobacco.

Proper Use of This Medicine

To use the eye drops:
• First, wash your hands. Tilt the head back and, pressing your finger gently on the skin just beneath the lower eyelid, pull the lower eyelid away from the eye to make a space. Drop the medicine into this space. Let go of the eyelid and gently close the eyes. Do not blink. Keep the eyes closed for 1 or 2 minutes to allow the medicine to be absorbed by the eye.
• If you think you did not get the drop of medicine into your eye properly, use another drop.
• To keep the medicine as germ-free as possible, do not touch the applicator tip to any surface (including the eye). Also, keep the container tightly closed.

Use cromolyn eye drops only as directed. Do not use more of this medicine and do not use it more often than your doctor ordered. To do so may increase the chance of side effects.

In order for this medicine to work properly, it must be used every day in regularly spaced doses as ordered by your doctor. A few days may pass before you begin to feel better. However, in some conditions, it may take several weeks before you begin to feel better.

Dosing—The dose of this medicine will be different for different patients. Follow your doctor's orders or the directions on the label. The following information includes only the average doses of this medicine. If your dose is different, do not change it unless your doctor tells you to do so.

The amount of medicine that you take depends on the strength of the medicine. Also, the number of doses you take each day, the time allowed between doses, and the length of time you take the medicine depend on the medical problem for which you are using the medicine.

- For ophthalmic solution (eye drops) dosage form:
  - For eye allergies:
    - Adults and children 4 years of age and older— Use one drop four to six times a day in regularly spaced doses.
    - Children up to 4 years of age—Use and dose must be determined by your doctor.

Missed dose—If you miss a dose of this medicine, take it as soon as possible. However, if it is almost time for your next dose, skip the missed dose and go back to your regular dosing schedule. Do not double doses.

Storage—Store the medicine in a closed container at room temperature, away from heat, moisture, and direct light. Keep from freezing.

Keep out of the reach of children.

Do not keep outdated medicine or medicine no longer needed.

Precautions While Using This Medicine

If your symptoms do not improve or if your condition becomes worse, check with your doctor.

Side Effects of This Medicine

Along with its needed effects, a medicine may cause some unwanted effects. Although not all of these side effects may occur, if they do occur they may need medical attention.

Check with your doctor as soon as possible if any of the following side effects occur:

Rare

Rash or redness around the eyes; swelling of the membrane covering the white part of the eye, redness of the white part of the eye, styes, or other eye irritation not present before therapy

Some side effects may occur that usually do not need medical attention. These side effects may go away during treatment as your body adjusts to the medicine. Also, your health care professional may be able to tell you about ways to prevent or reduce some of these side effects. Check with your health care professional if any of the following side effects continue or are bothersome or if you have any questions about them:

More common

Burning or stinging of eye (mild and temporary)

Less common or rare

Dryness or puffiness around the eye; watering or itching of eye (increased)

Other side effects not listed may also occur in some patients. If you notice any other effects, check with your healthcare professional.

CROMOLYN (Oral route) - KROE-moe-lin

Commonly used brand name(s)
In the U.S.—
Gastrocrom

Available Dosage Forms:
- Capsule
- Solution

Therapeutic Class: Gastrointestinal Agent
Pharmacologic Class: Mast Cell Stabilizer

Uses For This Medicine

Cromolyn is used to treat the symptoms of mastocytosis. Mastocytosis is a rare condition caused by too many mast cells in the body. These mast cells release substances that cause the symptoms of the disease, such as abdominal pain, nausea, vomiting, diarrhea, headache, flushing or itching of skin, or hives.

Cromolyn works by acting on the mast cells in the body to prevent them from releasing substances that cause the symptoms of mastocytosis.

Cromolyn is available only with your doctor's prescription.

Before Using This Medicine

In deciding to use a medicine, the risks of taking the medicine must be weighed against the good it will do. This is a decision you and your doctor will make. For this medicine, the following should be considered:

Allergies—Tell your doctor if you have ever had any unusual or allergic reaction to this medicine or any other medicines. Also tell your health care professional if you have any other types of allergies, such as to foods, dyes, preservatives, or animals. For non-prescription products, read the label or package ingredients carefully.

Pediatric—Although there is no specific information comparing use of oral cromolyn in children with use in other age groups, this medicine is not expected to cause different side effects or problems in children than it does in adults. This medicine is usually used in children two years of age and older. However, it may be used in children younger than two years of age if their disease is severe.

Geriatric—Many medicines have not been studied specifically in older people. Therefore, it may not be known whether they work exactly the same way they do in younger adults. Although there is no specific information comparing use of oral cromolyn in the elderly with use in other age groups, this medicine is not expected to cause different side effects or problems in older people than it does in younger adults.

Pregnancy—

	Pregnancy Category	Explanation
All Trimesters	B	Animal studies have revealed no evidence of harm to the fetus, however, there are no adequate studies in pregnant women OR animal studies have shown an adverse effect, but adequate studies in pregnant women have failed to demonstrate a risk to the fetus.

Breast Feeding—There are no adequate studies in women for determining infant risk when using this medication during breastfeeding. Weigh the potential benefits against the potential risks before taking this medication while breastfeeding.

Other medicines—Although certain medicines should not be used together at all, in other cases two different medicines may be used together even if an interaction might occur. In these cases, your doctor may want to change the dose, or other precautions may be necessary. Tell your healthcare professional if you are taking any other prescription or non-prescription (over-the-counter [OTC]) medicine.

Interactions with Food/Tobacco/Alcohol—Certain medicines should not be used at or around the time of eating food or eating certain types of food since interactions may occur. Using alcohol or tobacco with certain medicines may also cause interactions to occur. Discuss with your healthcare professional the use of your medicine with food, alcohol, or tobacco.

Other medical problems—The presence of other medical problems may affect the use of this medicine. Make sure you tell your doctor if you have any other medical problems, especially:
- Kidney disease or
- Liver disease—The effects of cromolyn may be increased, which may increase the chance of side effects

---

Proper Use of This Medicine

Make certain your health care professional knows if you are on any special diet, such as a low-sodium diet. This medicine contains sodium.

Unless otherwise directed by your doctor, it is best to take oral cromolyn as follows:

Capsules
- Open the cromolyn capsule(s) and pour all of the powder into one-half glass (4 ounces) of hot water. Stir the solution until the powder is completely dissolved and the solution is clear. Then add an equal amount (one-half glass) of cold water to the solution while stirring.
- Be sure to drink all of the liquid to get the full dose of medicine.
- Do not mix this medicine with fruit juice, milk, or food because they may keep the medicine from working properly.
- It is important to take this medicine at regular intervals for best results.

Ampuls
- Break open the ampul(s) and squeeze contents into a glass of water and stir well.
- Be sure to drink all of the liquid to get the full dose of medicine.
- It is important to take this medicine at regular intervals for best results.
- Do not use the ampul if it appears cloudy or discolored.

Take cromolyn only as directed. Do not take more of it and do not take it more often than your doctor ordered. To do so may increase the chance of side effects.

Dosing—The dose of this medicine will be different for different patients. Follow your doctor's orders or the directions on the label. The following information includes only the average doses of this medicine. If your dose is different, do not change it unless your doctor tells you to do so.

The amount of medicine that you take depends on the strength of the medicine. Also, the number of doses you take each day, the time allowed between doses, and the length of time you take the medicine depend on the medical problem for which you are using the medicine.

- For oral dosage form (capsules and ampuls):
  - For symptoms of mastocytosis:
    - Adults and children 12 years of age and older—200 milligrams (mg) dissolved or mixed in water and taken four times a day, thirty minutes before meals and at bedtime.
    - Children 2 to 12 years of age—100 mg dissolved or mixed in water and taken four times a day, thirty minutes before meals and at bedtime. Your doctor may increase the dose if your symptoms are not under control within two to three weeks after you begin taking this medicine.
    - Infants and children up to 2 years of age—Dose is based on body weight and must be determined by your doctor. The dose is usually 20 mg per kilogram (kg) (9.1 mg per pound) of body weight a day. This dose is divided into four doses. Your doctor may increase the dose if your symptoms are not under control within two to three weeks after you begin taking this medicine.
    - Premature infants—Use is not recommended.

Missed dose—If you miss a dose of this medicine, take it as soon as possible. However, if it is almost time for your next dose, skip the missed dose and go back to your regular dosing schedule. Do not double doses.

Storage—Store the medicine in a closed container at room temperature, away from heat, moisture, and direct light. Keep from freezing.

Keep the medicine in the foil pouch until you are ready to use it. Store at room temperature, away from heat and direct light. Do not freeze.

Keep out of the reach of children.

Do not keep outdated medicine or medicine no longer needed.

Precautions While Using This Medicine

If your symptoms do not improve or if your condition becomes worse, check with your doctor.

Side Effects of This Medicine

Along with its needed effects, a medicine may cause some unwanted effects. Although not all of these side effects may occur, if they do occur they may need medical attention.

Check with your doctor immediately if any of the following side effects occur:

Rare
Coughing; difficulty in swallowing; hives or itching of skin; swelling of face, lips, or eyelids; wheezing or difficulty in breathing

Check with your doctor as soon as possible if any of the following side effects occur:

Less common
Skin rash

Some side effects may occur that usually do not need medical attention. These side effects may go away during treatment as your body adjusts to the medicine. Also, your health care professional may be able to tell you about ways to prevent or reduce some of these side effects. Check with your health care professional if any of the following side effects continue or are bothersome or if you have any questions about them:

More common
Diarrhea; headache

Less common
Abdominal pain; irritability; muscle pain; nausea; trouble in sleepingNote: If the above side effects occur in patients with mastocytosis, they are usually only temporary and could be symptoms of the disease.

Other side effects not listed may also occur in some patients. If you notice any other effects, check with your healthcare professional.

CROTAMITON (Topical route) - kroe-TAM-i-ton

Commonly used brand name(s)
In the U.S.—
Eurax

Available Dosage Forms:
• Cream
• Lotion

Therapeutic Class: Scabicide

Uses For This Medicine

Crotamiton is used to treat scabies infection. It is also used to relieve the itching of certain skin conditions.

This medicine is available only with your doctor's prescription.

Before Using This Medicine

In deciding to use a medicine, the risks of taking the medicine must be weighed against the good it will do. This is a decision you and your doctor will make. For this medicine, the following should be considered:

Allergies—Tell your doctor if you have ever had any unusual or allergic reaction to this medicine or any other medicines. Also tell your health care professional if you have any other types of allergies, such as to foods, dyes, preservatives, or animals. For non-prescription products, read the label or package ingredients carefully.

Pediatric—Studies on this medicine have been done only in adult patients, and there is no specific information comparing use of this medicine in children with use in other age groups.

Geriatric—Many medicines have not been studied specifically in older people. Therefore, it may not be known whether they work exactly the same way they do in younger adults or if they cause different side effects or problems in older people. There is no specific information comparing use of crotamiton in the elderly with use in other age groups.

Pregnancy—

	Pregnancy Category	Explanation
All Trimesters	C	Animal studies have shown an adverse effect and there are no adequate studies in pregnant women OR no animal studies have been conducted and there are no adequate studies in pregnant women.

Breast Feeding—There are no adequate studies in women for determining infant risk when using this medication during breastfeeding. Weigh the potential benefits against the potential risks before taking this medication while breastfeeding.

Other medicines—Although certain medicines should not be used together at all, in other cases two different medicines may be used together even if an interaction might occur. In these cases, your doctor may want to change the dose, or other precautions may be necessary. Tell your healthcare professional if you are taking any other prescription or non-prescription (over-the-counter [OTC]) medicine.

Interactions with Food/Tobacco/Alcohol—Certain medicines should not be used at or around the time of eating food or eating certain types of food since interactions may occur. Using alcohol or tobacco with certain medicines may also cause interactions to occur. Discuss with your healthcare professional the use of your medicine with food, alcohol, or tobacco.

Other medical problems—The presence of other medical problems may affect the use of this medicine. Make sure you tell your doctor if you have any other medical problems, especially:
• Severely inflamed skin or raw oozing areas of the skin—Use of crotamiton on these areas may make the condition worse

Proper Use of This Medicine

Keep crotamiton away from the mouth. It may be harmful if swallowed.

Use this medicine only as directed. Do not use it more often than your doctor ordered. To do so may increase the chance of side effects.

Keep crotamiton away from the eyes and other mucous membranes, such as the inside of the nose. It may cause irritation. If you should accidentally get some in your eyes, flush them thoroughly with water at once.

This medicine usually comes with patient directions. Read them carefully before using.

If you take a bath or shower before using this medicine, dry the skin well before applying crotamiton.

For patients using this medicine for scabies:

- Apply enough medicine to cover the entire skin surface from the chin down, and rub in well. This applies especially to folds and creases in the skin and to the hands, feet (including the soles), between fingers and toes, and moist areas (such as underarms and groin).
- Do not wash off the first coat of this medicine.
- Apply a second coat of this medicine 24 hours after the first one.
- The next day, put on freshly washed or dry-cleaned clothing and change bedding in order to prevent reinfection.
- Then, 48 hours after the second application of this medicine, take a cleansing bath to remove the medicine.
- Your sexual partners, especially, and all members of your household may need to be treated also, since the infection may spread to persons in close contact. If these persons are not being treated or if you have any questions about this, check with your doctor.

Dosing—The dose of this medicine will be different for different patients. Follow your doctor's orders or the directions on the label. The following information includes only the average doses of this medicine. If your dose is different, do not change it unless your doctor tells you to do so.

The amount of medicine that you take depends on the strength of the medicine. Also, the number of doses you take each day, the time allowed between doses, and the length of time you take the medicine depend on the medical problem for which you are using the medicine.

- For topical dosage forms (cream and lotion):
  - For scabies:
    - Adults—Use two times. Apply one time the first day, and one time the second day. For severe cases, treatment may be repeated one time after one week.
    - Children—Use and dose must be determined by your doctor.
  - For pruritus:
    - Adults—Use when necessary according to the directions on the label or your doctor's instructions.
    - Children—Use and dose must be determined by your doctor.

Storage—Store the medicine in a closed container at room temperature, away from heat, moisture, and direct light. Keep from freezing.

Keep out of the reach of children.

Do not keep outdated medicine or medicine no longer needed.

Precautions While Using This Medicine

If your condition does not improve or if it becomes worse, check with your doctor.

For patients using this medicine for scabies:

- To prevent reinfection or spreading of the infection to other people, good health habits are also required. These include machine washing all underwear, pajamas, sheets, pillowcases, towels, and washcloths in

very hot water and drying them using the hot cycle of a dryer. Clothing or bedding that cannot be washed in this way should be dry cleaned.

Side Effects of This Medicine

Along with its needed effects, a medicine may cause some unwanted effects. Although not all of these side effects may occur, if they do occur they may need medical attention.

Check with your doctor as soon as possible if any of the following side effects occur:

Rare

Skin irritation or rash not present before use of this medicine

Other side effects not listed may also occur in some patients. If you notice any other effects, check with your healthcare professional.

CYCLOBENZAPRINE   (Oral route) -
sye-kloe-BEN-za-preen

Commonly used brand name(s)

In the U.S.—
Flexeril

Available Dosage Forms:

- Tablet

Therapeutic Class: Skeletal Muscle Relaxant, Centrally Acting

Uses For This Medicine

Cyclobenzaprine is used to help relax certain muscles in your body. It helps relieve the pain, stiffness, and discomfort caused by strains, sprains, or injuries to your muscles. However, this medicine does not take the place of rest, exercise or physical therapy, or other treatment that your doctor may recommend for your medical problem. Cyclobenzaprine acts on the central nervous system (CNS) to produce its muscle relaxant effects. Its actions on the CNS may also cause some of this medicine's side effects.

Cyclobenzaprine may also be used for other conditions as determined by your doctor.

Cyclobenzaprine is available only with your doctor's prescription.

Once a medicine has been approved for marketing for a certain use, experience may show that it is also useful for other medical problems. Although this use is not included in product labeling, cyclobenzaprine is used in certain patients with fibromyalgia syndrome (also called fibrositis or fibrositis syndrome).

Before Using This Medicine

In deciding to use a medicine, the risks of taking the medicine must be weighed against the good it will do. This is a decision you and your doctor will make. For this medicine, the following should be considered:

Allergies—Tell your doctor if you have ever had any unusual or allergic reaction to this medicine or any other medicines. Also tell your health care professional if you have any

other types of allergies, such as to foods, dyes, preservatives, or animals. For non-prescription products, read the label or package ingredients carefully.

Pediatric—Studies on this medicine have been done only in adult patients, and there is no specific information comparing use of cyclobenzaprine in children with use in other age groups.

Geriatric—Many medicines have not been studied specifically in older people. Therefore, it may not be known whether they work exactly the same way they do in younger adults or if they cause different side effects or problems in older people. There is no specific information comparing use of cyclobenzaprine in the elderly with use in other age groups.

Pregnancy—

	Pregnancy Category	Explanation
All Trimesters	B	Animal studies have revealed no evidence of harm to the fetus, however, there are no adequate studies in pregnant women OR animal studies have shown an adverse effect, but adequate studies in pregnant women have failed to demonstrate a risk to the fetus.

Breast Feeding—There are no adequate studies in women for determining infant risk when using this medication during breastfeeding. Weigh the potential benefits against the potential risks before taking this medication while breastfeeding.

Other medicines—

Using this medicine with any of the following medicines is not recommended. Your doctor may decide not to treat you with this medication or change some of the other medicines you take.

Clorgyline, Iproniazid, Isocarboxazid, Moclobemide, Nialamide, Pargyline, Phenelzine, Procarbazine, Rasagiline, Selegiline, Toloxatone, Tranylcypromine

Interactions with Food/Tobacco/Alcohol—Certain medicines should not be used at or around the time of eating food or eating certain types of food since interactions may occur. Using alcohol or tobacco with certain medicines may also cause interactions to occur. Discuss with your healthcare professional the use of your medicine with food, alcohol, or tobacco.

Other medical problems—The presence of other medical problems may affect the use of this medicine. Make sure you tell your doctor if you have any other medical problems, especially:
- Glaucoma or
- Problems with urination—Cyclobenzaprine can make your condition worse
- Heart or blood vessel disease or
- Overactive thyroid—The chance of side effects may be increased

Proper Use of This Medicine

Take this medicine only as directed by your doctor. Do not take more of it and do not take it more often than your doctor ordered. To do so may increase the chance of serious side effects.

Dosing—The dose of this medicine will be different for different patients. Follow your doctor's orders or the directions on the label. The following information includes only the average doses of this medicine. If your dose is different, do not change it unless your doctor tells you to do so.

The amount of medicine that you take depends on the strength of the medicine. Also, the number of doses you take each day, the time allowed between doses, and the length of time you take the medicine depend on the medical problem for which you are using the medicine.

- For the oral dosage form (tablets):
    - For relaxing stiff muscles:
        - Adults and teenagers 15 years of age and older— The usual dose is 10 milligrams (mg) three times a day. The largest amount should be no more than 60 mg (six 10–mg tablets) a day.
        - Children and teenagers up to 15 years of age— Dose must be determined by your doctor.

Missed dose—If you miss a dose of this medicine, take it as soon as possible. However, if it is almost time for your next dose, skip the missed dose and go back to your regular dosing schedule. Do not double doses.

Storage—Store the medicine in a closed container at room temperature, away from heat, moisture, and direct light. Keep from freezing.

Keep out of the reach of children.

Do not keep outdated medicine or medicine no longer needed.

Precautions While Using This Medicine

This medicine will add to the effects of alcohol and other CNS depressants (medicines that slow down the nervous system, possibly causing drowsiness). Some examples of CNS depressants are antihistamines or medicine for hay fever, other allergies, or colds; sedatives, tranquilizers, or sleeping medicine; prescription pain medicine or narcotics; barbiturates; medicine for seizures; other muscle relaxants; or anesthetics, including some dental anesthetics. Check with your doctor before taking any of the above while you are using this medicine.

This medicine may cause some people to have blurred vision or to become drowsy, dizzy, or less alert than they are normally. Make sure you know how you react to this medicine before you drive, use machines, or do anything else that could be dangerous if you are dizzy or are not alert and able to see well.

Cyclobenzaprine may cause dryness of the mouth. For temporary relief, use sugarless candy or gum, melt bits of ice in your mouth, or use a saliva substitute. However, if your mouth continues to feel dry for more than 2 weeks, check with your medical doctor or dentist. Continuing dryness of the mouth may increase the chance of dental disease, including tooth decay, gum disease, and fungus infections.

Side Effects of This Medicine

Along with its needed effects, a medicine may cause some unwanted effects. Although not all of these side effects may occur, if they do occur they may need medical attention.

Stop taking this medicine and get emergency help immediately if any of the following effects occur:
Rare

   Changes in the skin color of the face; fast or irregular breathing; large swellings that look like hives on the face, eyelids, mouth, lips, and/or tongue; puffiness or swelling of the eyelids or the area around the eyes; shortness of breath, troubled breathing, tightness in chest, and/or wheezing; skin rash, hives, or itching

Check with your doctor immediately if any of the following side effects occur:

Rare

Fainting

Symptoms of overdose

Convulsions (seizures); drowsiness (severe); dry, hot, flushed skin; fast or irregular heartbeat; hallucinations (seeing, hearing, or feeling things that are not there); increase or decrease in body temperature; troubled breathing; unexplained muscle stiffness; unusual nervousness or restlessness (severe); vomiting (occurring together with other symptoms of overdose)

Check with your doctor as soon as possible if any of the following side effects occur:

Rare

Clumsiness or unsteadiness; confusion; mental depression or other mood or mental changes; problems in urinating; ringing or buzzing in the ears; skin rash, hives, or itching occurring without other symptoms of an allergic reaction listed above; unusual thoughts or dreams; yellow eyes or skin

Some side effects may occur that usually do not need medical attention. These side effects may go away during treatment as your body adjusts to the medicine. Also, your health care professional may be able to tell you about ways to prevent or reduce some of these side effects. Check with your health care professional if any of the following side effects continue or are bothersome or if you have any questions about them:

More common

Blurred vision; dizziness or lightheadedness; drowsiness; dryness of mouth

Less common or rare

Bloated feeling or gas, indigestion, nausea or vomiting, or stomach cramps or pain; constipation; diarrhea; excitement or nervousness; frequent urination; general feeling of discomfort or illness; headache; muscle twitching; numbness, tingling, pain, or weakness in hands or feet; pounding heartbeat; problems in speaking; trembling; trouble in sleeping; unpleasant taste or other taste changes; unusual muscle weakness; unusual tiredness

Other side effects not listed may also occur in some patients. If you notice any other effects, check with your healthcare professional.

CYCLOPENTOLATE (Ophthalmic route) - sye-kloe-PEN-toe-late

Commonly used brand name(s)

In the U.S.—

| AK-Pentolate | Cylate |
| Cyclogyl | Ocu-Pentolate |

In Canada—

Minims Cyclopentolate 0.5%
Minims Cyclopentolate 1%

Available Dosage Forms:
• Solution

Therapeutic Class: Mydriatic-Cycloplegic
Pharmacologic Class: Antimuscarinic

Uses For This Medicine

Cyclopentolate is used to dilate (enlarge) the pupil. It is used before eye examinations (such as cycloplegic refraction or ophthalmoscopy).

This medicine is available only with your doctor's prescription.

Once a medicine has been approved for marketing for a certain use, experience may show that it is also useful for other medical problems. Although this use is not included in product labeling, cyclopentolate is used in certain patients with the following medical conditions:
• Posterior synechiae
• Uveitis

Before Using This Medicine

In deciding to use a medicine, the risks of taking the medicine must be weighed against the good it will do. This is a decision you and your doctor will make. For this medicine, the following should be considered:

Allergies—Tell your doctor if you have ever had any unusual or allergic reaction to this medicine or any other medicines. Also tell your health care professional if you have any other types of allergies, such as to foods, dyes, preservatives, or animals. For non-prescription products, read the label or package ingredients carefully.

Pediatric—Infants and young children and children with blond hair or blue eyes may be especially sensitive to the effects of cyclopentolate. This may increase the chance of side effects during treatment.

Geriatric—Elderly people are especially sensitive to the effects of cyclopentolate. This may increase the chance of side effects during treatment.

Pregnancy—

	Pregnancy Category	Explanation
All Trimesters	C	Animal studies have shown an adverse effect and there are no adequate studies in pregnant women OR no animal studies have been conducted and there are no adequate studies in pregnant women.

Breast Feeding—There are no adequate studies in women for determining infant risk when using this medication during breastfeeding. Weigh the potential benefits against the potential risks before taking this medication while breastfeeding.

Other medicines—Although certain medicines should not be used together at all, in other cases two different medicines may be used together even if an interaction might occur. In these cases, your doctor may want to change the dose, or other precautions may be necessary. Tell your healthcare professional if you are taking any other prescription or nonprescription (over-the-counter [OTC]) medicine.

Interactions with Food/Tobacco/Alcohol—Certain medicines should not be used at or around the time of eating food or eating certain types of food since interactions may

occur. Using alcohol or tobacco with certain medicines may also cause interactions to occur. Discuss with your healthcare professional the use of your medicine with food, alcohol, or tobacco.

Other medical problems—The presence of other medical problems may affect the use of this medicine. Make sure you tell your doctor if you have any other medical problems, especially:

- Brain damage (in children) or
- Down's syndrome (mongolism) (in children and adults) or
- Glaucoma or
- Spastic paralysis (in children)—Cyclopentolate may make the condition worse

Proper Use of This Medicine

To use:

- First, wash your hands. Tilt the head back and with the index finger of one hand, press gently on the skin just beneath the lower eyelid and pull the lower eyelid away from the eye to make a space. Drop the medicine into this space. Let go of the eyelid and gently close the eyes. Do not blink. Keep the eyes closed and apply pressure to the inner corner of the eye with your finger for 2 or 3 minutes, to allow the medicine to be absorbed. This is especially important in infants.
- Immediately after using the eye drops, wash your hands to remove any medicine that may be on them. If you are using the eye drops for an infant or child, be sure to wash the infant's or child's hands also, and do not let any of the medicine get in the infant's or child's mouth.
- To keep the medicine as germ-free as possible, do not touch the applicator tip to any surface (including the eye). Also, keep the container tightly closed.

Use this medicine only as directed. Do not use more of it and do not use it more often than your doctor ordered. To do so may increase the chance of too much medicine being absorbed into the body and the chance of side effects.

Dosing—The dose of this medicine will be different for different patients. Follow your doctor's orders or the directions on the label. The following information includes only the average doses of this medicine. If your dose is different, do not change it unless your doctor tells you to do so.

The amount of medicine that you take depends on the strength of the medicine. Also, the number of doses you take each day, the time allowed between doses, and the length of time you take the medicine depend on the medical problem for which you are using the medicine.

- For ophthalmic solution (eye drops) dosage form:
  - For eye examinations:
    - Adults—One drop 40 to 50 minutes before the exam. Dose may be repeated in five to ten minutes.
    - Children—One drop 40 to 50 minutes before the exam. After five to ten minutes, another drop may be used.
    - Babies—One drop of 0.5% solution.

Missed dose—If you miss a dose of this medicine, apply it as soon as possible. However, if it is almost time for your next dose, skip the missed dose and go back to your regular dosing schedule.

Storage—Store the medicine in a closed container at room temperature, away from heat, moisture, and direct light. Keep from freezing.

Keep out of the reach of children.

Do not keep outdated medicine or medicine no longer needed.

Precautions While Using This Medicine

After you apply this medicine to your eyes:

- Your pupils will become unusually large and you will have blurring of vision, especially for close objects. Make sure your vision is clear before you drive, use machines, or do anything else that could be dangerous if you are not able to see well.
- Your eyes will become more sensitive to light than they are normally. When you go out during the daylight hours, even on cloudy days, wear sunglasses that block ultraviolet (UV) light to protect your eyes from sunlight and other bright lights. Ordinary sunglasses may not protect your eyes. If you have any questions about the kind of sunglasses to wear, check with your doctor.

If these side effects continue for longer than 36 hours after you have stopped using this medicine, check with your doctor.

Side Effects of This Medicine

Along with its needed effects, a medicine may cause some unwanted effects. Although not all of these side effects may occur, if they do occur they may need medical attention.

Check with your doctor as soon as possible if any of the following side effects occur:

Symptoms of too much medicine being absorbed into the body

Clumsiness or unsteadiness; confusion; constipation, full feeling, passing gas, or stomach cramps or pain; fast or irregular heartbeat; convulsions (seizures); fever; flushing or redness of face; hallucinations (seeing, hearing, or feeling things that are not there); passing urine less often; skin rash; slurred speech; swollen stomach (in infants); thirst or dryness of mouth; unusual behavior, such as disorientation to time or place, failure to recognize people, hyperactivity, or restlessness, especially in children; unusual drowsiness, tiredness, or weakness

Some side effects may occur that usually do not need medical attention. These side effects may go away during treatment as your body adjusts to the medicine. Also, your health care professional may be able to tell you about ways to prevent or reduce some of these side effects. Check with your health care professional if any of the following side effects continue or are bothersome or if you have any questions about them:

Blurred vision; burning of eye; eye irritation not present before therapy; increased sensitivity of eyes to light

Other side effects not listed may also occur in some patients. If you notice any other effects, check with your healthcare professional.

CYCLOPHOSPHAMIDE (Oral route, Intravenous route) - sye-kloe-FOS-fa-mide

Commonly used brand name(s)

In the U.S.—
Cytoxan
Cytoxan Lyophilized

Available Dosage Forms:

• Tablet

• Powder for Solution

Therapeutic Class: Antineoplastic Agent
Pharmacologic Class: Alkylating Agent

Uses For This Medicine

Cyclophosphamide belongs to the group of medicines called alkylating agents. It is used to treat cancer of the ovaries, breast, blood and lymph system, nerves (found primarily in children), retinoblastoma (a cancer of the eye found primarily in children), multiple myeloma (cancer in the bone marrow), and mycosis fungoides (tumors on the skin).

Cyclophosphamide is also used for treatment of some kinds of kidney disease.

Cyclophosphamide may also be used for other conditions as determined by your doctor.

Cyclophosphamide interferes with the growth of cancer cells, which are eventually destroyed. Since the growth of normal body cells may also be affected by cyclophosphamide, other effects will also occur. Some of these may be serious and must be reported to your doctor. Other effects, like hair loss, may not be serious but may cause concern. Some effects may not occur for months or years after the medicine is used.

Before you begin treatment with cyclophosphamide, you and your doctor should talk about the good this medicine will do as well as the risks of using it.

Cyclophosphamide is available only with your doctor's prescription.

Once a medicine has been approved for marketing for a certain use, experience may show that it is also useful for other medical problems. Although these uses are not included in product labeling, cyclophosphamide is used in certain patients with the following medical conditions:

• Cancer of the bladder

• Cancer in the bones

• Cancer of the cervix

• Cancer of the endometrium

• Cancers of the lungs

• Cancer of the prostate

• Cancer of the testicles

• Cancer of the adrenal cortex (the outside layer of the adrenal gland)

• Ewing's sarcoma (a certain type of bone cancer)

• Germ cell tumors in the ovaries (a cancer in the egg-making cells in the ovary)

• Gestational trophoblastic tumors (a certain type of tumor in the uterus/womb)

• Soft tissue sarcomas (a cancer of the muscles, tendons, vessels that carry blood or lymph, joints, and fat)

• Thymoma (a cancer in the thymus, a small organ beneath the breastbone)

• Tumors in the brain

• Waldenströ m's macroglobulinemia (a certain type of cancer of the blood)

• Wilms' tumor (a cancer of the kidney found primarily in children)

• Histiocytosis X (a certain type of cancer found primarily in children)

• Organ transplant rejection (prevention)

• Rheumatoid arthritis

• Wegener's granulomatosis

• Systemic lupus erythematosus

• Systemic dermatomyositis or

• Multiple sclerosis (a disease of the nervous system)

Before Using This Medicine

In deciding to use a medicine, the risks of taking the medicine must be weighed against the good it will do. This is a decision you and your doctor will make. For this medicine, the following should be considered:

Allergies—Tell your doctor if you have ever had any unusual or allergic reaction to this medicine or any other medicines. Also tell your health care professional if you have any other types of allergies, such as to foods, dyes, preservatives, or animals. For non-prescription products, read the label or package ingredients carefully.

Pediatric—This medicine has been tested in children and has not been shown to cause different side effects or problems than it does in adults.

Geriatric—Many medicines have not been studied specifically in older people. Therefore, it may not be known whether they work exactly the same way they do in younger adults. Although there is no specific information comparing use of cyclophosphamide in the elderly with use in other age groups, it is not expected to cause different side effects or problems in older people than it does in younger adults.

Pregnancy—

	Pregnancy Category	Explanation
All Trimesters	D	Studies in pregnant women have demonstrated a risk to the fetus. However, the benefits of therapy in a life threatening situation or a serious disease, may outweigh the potential risk.

Breast Feeding—Studies in women breastfeeding have demonstrated harmful infant effects. An alternative to this medication should be prescribed or you should stop breast-feeding while using this medicine.

Other medicines—

Using this medicine with any of the following medicines is not recommended. Your doctor may decide not to treat you with this medication or change some of the other medicines you take.

Rotavirus Vaccine, Live

Interactions with Food/Tobacco/Alcohol—Certain medicines should not be used at or around the time of eating

food or eating certain types of food since interactions may occur. Using alcohol or tobacco with certain medicines may also cause interactions to occur. Discuss with your healthcare professional the use of your medicine with food, alcohol, or tobacco.

Other medical problems—The presence of other medical problems may affect the use of this medicine. Make sure you tell your doctor if you have any other medical problems, especially:

- Chickenpox (including recent exposure) or
- Herpes zoster (shingles)—Risk of severe disease affecting other parts of the body
- Gout (history of) or
- Kidney stones (history of)—Cyclophosphamide may increase levels of uric acid in the body, which can cause gout or kidney stones
- Infection—Cyclophosphamide can decrease your body's ability to fight infection
- Kidney disease—Effects of cyclophosphamide may be increased because of slower removal from the body
- Liver disease—The effect of cyclophosphamide may be decreased
- Prior removal of adrenal gland(s)—Toxic effects of cyclophosphamide may be increased, dosage adjustment may be necessary
- Tumor cell accumulation—Increased risk of tumor cells entering the bone marrow, due to bone marrow depression from high doses of cyclophosphamide

Proper Use of This Medicine

Take this medicine only as directed by your doctor. Do not take more or less of it, and do not take it more often than your doctor ordered. The exact amount of medicine you need has been carefully worked out. Taking too much may increase the chance of side effects, while taking too little may not improve your condition.

Cyclophosphamide is sometimes given together with certain other medicines. If you are using a combination of medicines, make sure that you take each one at the proper time and do not mix them. Ask your health care professional to help you plan a way to remember to take your medicines at the right times.

While you are using cyclophosphamide, it is important that you drink extra fluids so that you will pass more urine. Also, empty your bladder frequently, including at least once during the night. This will help prevent kidney and bladder problems and keep your kidneys working well. Cyclophosphamide passes from the body in the urine. If too much of it appears in the urine or if the urine stays in the bladder too long, it can cause dangerous irritation. Follow your doctor's instructions carefully about how much fluid to drink every day. Some patients may have to drink up to 7 to 12 cups (3 quarts) of fluid a day.

Usually it is best to take cyclophosphamide first thing in the morning, to reduce the risk of bladder problems. However, your doctor may want you to take it with food in smaller doses over the day, to lessen stomach upset or help the medicine work better. Follow your doctor's instructions carefully about when to take cyclophosphamide.

Cyclophosphamide often causes nausea, vomiting, and loss of appetite. However, it is very important that you continue to use the medicine even if you begin to feel ill. Do not stop

taking this medicine without first checking with your doctor. Ask your health care professional for ways to lessen these effects.

If you vomit shortly after taking a dose of cyclophosphamide, check with your doctor. You will be told whether to take the dose again or to wait until the next scheduled dose.

Dosing—The dose of this medicine will be different for different patients. Follow your doctor's orders or the directions on the label. The following information includes only the average doses of this medicine. If your dose is different, do not change it unless your doctor tells you to do so.

The amount of medicine that you take depends on the strength of the medicine. Also, the number of doses you take each day, the time allowed between doses, and the length of time you take the medicine depend on the medical problem for which you are using the medicine.

Missed dose—If you miss a dose of this medicine, take it as soon as possible. However, if it is almost time for your next dose, skip the missed dose and go back to your regular dosing schedule. Do not double doses.

Call your doctor or pharmacist for instructions.

Storage—Store the medicine in a closed container at room temperature, away from heat, moisture, and direct light. Keep from freezing.

Keep out of the reach of children.

Do not keep outdated medicine or medicine no longer needed.

Store the oral solution form of this medicine in the refrigerator. Keep it from freezing.

Precautions While Using This Medicine

It is very important that your doctor check your progress at regular visits to make sure that this medicine is working properly and to check for unwanted effects.

While you are being treated with cyclophosphamide, and after you stop treatment with it, do not have any immunizations (vaccinations) without your doctor's approval. Cyclophosphamide may lower your body's resistance and there is a chance you might get the infection the immunization is meant to prevent. In addition, other persons living in your house should not take oral polio vaccine since there is a chance they could pass the polio virus on to you. Also, avoid persons who have recently taken oral polio vaccine within the last several months. Do not get close to them, and do not stay in the same room with them for very long. If you cannot take these precautions, you should consider wearing a protective face mask that covers the nose and mouth.

Before having any kind of surgery, including dental surgery, or emergency treatment, make sure the medical doctor or dentist in charge knows that you are taking this medicine, especially if you have taken it within the last 10 days.

Cyclophosphamide can temporarily lower the number of white blood cells in your blood, increasing the chance of getting an infection. It can also lower the number of platelets, which are necessary for proper blood clotting. If this occurs, there are certain precautions you can take, especially when your blood count is low, to reduce the risk of infection or bleeding:

- If you can, avoid people with infections. Check with your doctor immediately if you think you are getting an infection or if you get a fever or chills, cough or hoarseness, lower back or side pain, or painful or difficult urination.

- Check with your doctor immediately if you notice any unusual bleeding or bruising; black, tarry stools; blood in urine or stools; or pinpoint red spots on your skin.
- Be careful when using a regular toothbrush, dental floss, or toothpick. Your medical doctor, dentist, or nurse may recommend other ways to clean your teeth and gums. Check with your medical doctor before having any dental work done.
- Do not touch your eyes or the inside of your nose unless you have just washed your hands and have not touched anything else in the meantime.
- Be careful not to cut yourself when you are using sharp objects such as a safety razor or fingernail or toenail cutters.
- Avoid contact sports or other situations where bruising or injury could occur.

Before you have any medical tests, tell the medical doctor in charge that you are taking this medicine. The results of some tests may be affected by this medicine.

Side Effects of This Medicine

Along with its needed effects, a medicine may cause some unwanted effects. Although not all of these side effects may occur, if they do occur they may need medical attention.

Also, because of the way these medicines act on the body, there is a chance that they might cause other unwanted effects that may not occur until months or years after the medicine is used. These may include certain types of cancer, such as leukemia or bladder cancer. Discuss these possible effects with your doctor.

Check with your doctor immediately if any of the following side effects occur:

More common
Cough or hoarseness; fever or chills; lower back or side pain; missing menstrual periods; painful or difficult urination

With high doses and/or long-term treatment
Blood in urine; dizziness, confusion, or agitation; fast heartbeat; joint pain; shortness of breath; swelling of feet or lower legs; unusual tiredness or weakness

Less common
Black, tarry stools or blood in stools; pinpoint red spots on skin; unusual bleeding or bruising

Rare
Frequent urination; redness, swelling, or pain at site of injection; sores in mouth and on lips; sudden shortness of breath; unusual thirst; yellow eyes or skin

Some side effects may occur that usually do not need medical attention. These side effects may go away during treatment as your body adjusts to the medicine. Also, your health care professional may be able to tell you about ways to prevent or reduce some of these side effects. Check with your health care professional if any of the following side effects continue or are bothersome or if you have any questions about them:

More common
Darkening of skin and fingernails; loss of appetite; nausea or vomiting

Less common
Diarrhea or stomach pain; flushing or redness of face; headache; increased sweating; skin rash, hives, or itching; swollen lips

Cyclophosphamide may cause a temporary loss of hair in some people. After treatment has ended, normal hair growth should return, although the new hair may be a slightly different color or texture.

After you stop using this medicine, it may still produce some side effects that need attention. During this period of time, *check with your doctor immediately* if you notice the following side effects:

Blood in urine

Other side effects not listed may also occur in some patients. If you notice any other effects, check with your healthcare professional.

CYCLOSERINE (Oral route) - sye-kloe-SER-een

Commonly used brand name(s)
In the U.S.—
Seromycin

Available Dosage Forms:
- Capsule

Therapeutic Class: Antitubercular

Uses For This Medicine

Cycloserine belongs to the family of medicines called antibiotics. It is used to treat tuberculosis (TB). When cycloserine is used for TB, it is given with other medicines for TB. Cycloserine may also be used for other conditions as determined by your doctor.

To help clear up your tuberculosis (TB) completely, you must keep taking this medicine for the full time of treatment, even if you begin to feel better. This is very important. It is also important that you do not miss any doses.

Cycloserine is available only with your doctor's prescription.

Once a medicine has been approved for marketing for a certain use, experience may show that it is also useful for other medical problems. Although this use is not included in product labeling, cycloserine is used in certain patients with the following medical condition:
- Atypical mycobacterial infections, such as Mycobacterium avium complex (MAC)

Before Using This Medicine

In deciding to use a medicine, the risks of taking the medicine must be weighed against the good it will do. This is a decision you and your doctor will make. For this medicine, the following should be considered:

Allergies—Tell your doctor if you have ever had any unusual or allergic reaction to this medicine or any other medicines. Also tell your health care professional if you have any other types of allergies, such as to foods, dyes, preservatives, or animals. For non-prescription products, read the label or package ingredients carefully.

Pediatric—Although there is no specific information comparing use of cycloserine in children with use in other age groups, this medicine is not expected to cause different side effects or problems in children than it does in adults.

Geriatric—Many medicines have not been studied specifically in older people. Therefore, it may not be known whether

they work exactly the same way they do in younger adults. Although there is no specific information comparing use of cycloserine in the elderly with use in other age groups, this medicine is not expected to cause different side effects or problems in older people than it does in younger adults.

Pregnancy—

	Pregnancy Category	Explanation
All Trimesters	C	Animal studies have shown an adverse effect and there are no adequate studies in pregnant women OR no animal studies have been conducted and there are no adequate studies in pregnant women.

Breast Feeding—There are no adequate studies in women for determining infant risk when using this medication during breastfeeding. Weigh the potential benefits against the potential risks before taking this medication while breastfeeding.

Other medicines—Although certain medicines should not be used together at all, in other cases two different medicines may be used together even if an interaction might occur. In these cases, your doctor may want to change the dose, or other precautions may be necessary. Tell your healthcare professional if you are taking any other prescription or non-prescription (over-the-counter [OTC]) medicine.

Interactions with Food/Tobacco/Alcohol—Certain medicines should not be used at or around the time of eating food or eating certain types of food since interactions may occur. Using alcohol or tobacco with certain medicines may also cause interactions to occur. The following interactions have been selected on the basis of their potential significance and are not necessarily all-inclusive.

Using this medicine with any of the following is not recommended. Your doctor may decide not to treat you with this medication, change some of the other medicines you take, or give you special instructions about the use of food, alcohol, or tobacco.

Ethanol

Other medical problems—The presence of other medical problems may affect the use of this medicine. Make sure you tell your doctor if you have any other medical problems, especially:

- Alcohol abuse (or history of) or
- Convulsive disorders such as seizures or epilepsy—Cycloserine may increase the risk of seizures in patients who drink alcohol or have a history of seizures
- Kidney disease—Cycloserine is removed from the body through the kidneys, and patients with kidney disease may need an adjustment in dose or the medicine may need to be discontinued
- Mental disorders such as mental depression, psychosis, or severe anxiety—Cycloserine may cause anxiety, mental depression, or psychosis

Proper Use of This Medicine

Cycloserine may be taken after meals if it upsets your stomach.

To help clear up your infection completely, it is very important that you keep taking this medicine for the full time of treat-

ment, even if you begin to feel better after a few weeks. If you are taking this medicine for TB, you may have to take it every day for as long as 1 to 2 years or more. If you stop taking this medicine too soon, your symptoms may return.

This medicine works best when there is a constant amount in the blood or urine. To help keep the amount constant, do not miss any doses. Also, it is best to take the doses at evenly spaced times day and night. For example, if you are to take 2 doses a day, the doses should be spaced about 12 hours apart. If this interferes with your sleep or other daily activities, or if you need help in planning the best times to take your medicine, check with your health care professional.

Dosing—The dose of this medicine will be different for different patients. Follow your doctor's orders or the directions on the label. The following information includes only the average doses of this medicine. If your dose is different, do not change it unless your doctor tells you to do so.

The amount of medicine that you take depends on the strength of the medicine. Also, the number of doses you take each day, the time allowed between doses, and the length of time you take the medicine depend on the medical problem for which you are using the medicine.

- For the oral dosage form (capsules):
  - For treatment of tuberculosis:
    - Adults and teenagers—250 milligrams (mg) two times a day to start. Your doctor may slowly increase your dose up to 250 mg three or four times a day. This medicine must be taken along with other medicines to treat tuberculosis.
    - Children—Use and dose must be determined by your doctor. Doses of 10 to 20 mg per kilogram (4.5 to 9.1 mg per pound) of body weight per day have been used. This medicine must be taken along with other medicines to treat tuberculosis.

Missed dose—If you miss a dose of this medicine, take it as soon as possible. However, if it is almost time for your next dose, skip the missed dose and go back to your regular dosing schedule. Do not double doses.

Storage—Store the medicine in a closed container at room temperature, away from heat, moisture, and direct light. Keep from freezing.

Keep out of the reach of children.

Do not keep outdated medicine or medicine no longer needed.

Precautions While Using This Medicine

It is very important that your doctor check your progress at regular visits.

If your symptoms do not improve within 2 to 3 weeks, or if they become worse, check with your doctor.

If cycloserine causes you to feel very depressed or to have thoughts of suicide, check with your doctor immediately. Your doctor will probably want to change your medicine.

This medicine may cause some people to become dizzy, drowsy, or less alert than they are normally. Make sure you know how you react to this medicine before you drive, use machines, or do anything else that could be dangerous if you are dizzy or are not alert. If these reactions are especially bothersome, check with your doctor.

Some of cycloserine's side effects (for example, convulsions [seizures]) may be more likely to occur if you drink alcoholic beverages regularly while you are taking this medicine. Therefore, you should not drink alcoholic beverages while you are taking this medicine.

Side Effects of This Medicine

Along with its needed effects, a medicine may cause some unwanted effects. Although not all of these side effects may occur, if they do occur they may need medical attention.

Check with your doctor immediately if any of the following side effects occur:

More common

Anxiety; confusion; dizziness; drowsiness; increased irritability; increased restlessness; mental depression; muscle twitching or trembling; nervousness; nightmares; other mood or mental changes; speech problems; thoughts of suicide

Less common

Convulsions (seizures); numbness, tingling, burning pain, or weakness in the hands or feet; skin rash

Some side effects may occur that usually do not need medical attention. These side effects may go away during treatment as your body adjusts to the medicine. Also, your health care professional may be able to tell you about ways to prevent or reduce some of these side effects. Check with your health care professional if any of the following side effects continue or are bothersome or if you have any questions about them:

More common

Headache

Other side effects not listed may also occur in some patients. If you notice any other effects, check with your healthcare professional.

CYCLOSPORINE (Ophthalmic route) - SYE-kloe-spor-een

Commonly used brand name(s)

In the U.S.—

Restasis

Available Dosage Forms:

• Emulsion

Therapeutic Class: Anti-Inflammatory

Uses For This Medicine

Cyclosporine belongs to a class of medicines known as immunosuppressants. It is used to increase tear production in people who have a certain eye condition.

This medicine is available only with your doctor's prescription.

Before Using This Medicine

In deciding to use a medicine, the risks of taking the medicine must be weighed against the good it will do. This is a decision you and your doctor will make. For this medicine, the following should be considered:

Allergies—Tell your doctor if you have ever had any unusual or allergic reaction to this medicine or any other medicines. Also tell your health care professional if you have any

other types of allergies, such as to foods, dyes, preservatives, or animals. For non-prescription products, read the label or package ingredients carefully.

Pediatric—Cyclosporine eye drops have only been studied in children age 16 and older. Discuss with your child's doctor the good that this medicine may do as well as the risks of using it.

Geriatric—This medicine has been tested and has not been shown to cause different side effects or problems in older people than it does in younger adults.

Other medicines—Although certain medicines should not be used together at all, in other cases two different medicines may be used together even if an interaction might occur. In these cases, your doctor may want to change the dose, or other precautions may be necessary. Tell your healthcare professional if you are taking any other prescription or non-prescription (over-the-counter [OTC]) medicine.

Interactions with Food/Tobacco/Alcohol—Certain medicines should not be used at or around the time of eating food or eating certain types of food since interactions may occur. Using alcohol or tobacco with certain medicines may also cause interactions to occur. Discuss with your healthcare professional the use of your medicine with food, alcohol, or tobacco.

Other medical problems—The presence of other medical problems may affect the use of this medicine. Make sure you tell your doctor if you have any other medical problems, especially:

• Current eye infections or

• Hypersensitivity to cyclosporine or any ingredients in cyclosporine—This medicine should not be used if you have these conditions.

• History of herpes infection of your cornea—Caution should be used with this medicine if you have this condition.

• If you are a contact lens user—Patients with decreased tear production should not wear contacts.

Proper Use of This Medicine

Dosing—The dose of this medicine will be different for different patients. Follow your doctor's orders or the directions on the label. The following information includes only the average doses of this medicine. If your dose is different, do not change it unless your doctor tells you to do so.

The amount of medicine that you take depends on the strength of the medicine. Also, the number of doses you take each day, the time allowed between doses, and the length of time you take the medicine depend on the medical problem for which you are using the medicine.

You should not use cyclosporine eye drops if you have contact lenses in your eyes. Remove your contact lenses before putting the medicine in your eyes. You can reinsert your contacts 15 minutes after you put the medicine in your eyes.

You may use cyclosporine eye drops if you use artificial tears. However, after putting in your artificial tears, you must wait 15 minutes before putting the cyclosporine eye drops into your eyes.

Do not shake the vial. Instead, rotate the vial gently back and forth before use.

Use this medicine only once, then throw away any unused drug.

To use:

- First, wash your hands. Tilt the head back and pressing your finger gently on the skin just beneath the lower eyelid, pull the lower eyelid away from the eye to make a space. Drop the medicine into this space. Let go of the eyelid and gently close the eyes. Do not blink.
- If you think you did not get the drop of medicine into your eye properly, use another drop.
- Immediately after using the eye drops, wash your hands to remove any medicine that may be on them.
- To keep the medicine as germ free as possible, do not touch the applicator tip to any surface (including the eye).
- For ophthalmic emulsion (eye drops) dosage form:
  - For dry eyes:
    - Adults—Instill one drop into the eye every 12 hours.
    - Children—Use and dose must be determined by your doctor.

Missed dose—If you miss a dose of this medicine, take it as soon as possible. However, if it is almost time for your next dose, skip the missed dose and go back to your regular dosing schedule. Do not double doses.

Storage—Keep out of the reach of children.

Do not keep outdated medicine or medicine no longer needed.

Ask your healthcare professional how you should dispose of any medicine you do not use.

Precautions While Using This Medicine

It is very important that your doctor check you at regular visits. This will allow your doctor to see if the medicine is working properly and to decide if you should continue to take it.

If your symptoms do not improve or if they become worse, check with your doctor.

This medicine may cause blurred vision or other vision problems. If any of these occur, do not drive, use machines, or do anything else that could be dangerous if you are not able to see well.

Side Effects of This Medicine

Along with its needed effects, a medicine may cause some unwanted effects. Although not all of these side effects may occur, if they do occur they may need medical attention.

Some side effects may occur that usually do not need medical attention. These side effects may go away during treatment as your body adjusts to the medicine. Also, your health care professional may be able to tell you about ways to prevent or reduce some of these side effects. Check with your health care professional if any of the following side effects continue or are bothersome or if you have any questions about them:

More common
Burning or other discomfort of the eye

Less common
Blurred vision; clear or yellow fluid from eye; difficulty reading; eye pain; feeling of having something in the eye; halos around lights; itching skin; redness of the white part of your eyes or inside of your eyelids; sticky or matted eyelashes; stinging; watery eye

Other side effects not listed may also occur in some patients. If you notice any other effects, check with your healthcare professional.

CYCLOSPORINE   (Oral route, Intravenous route) - SYE-kloe-spor-een

Black Box Warning

Only physicians experienced in immunosuppressive therapy and management of organ transplant patients should prescribe Sandimmune(R) (cyclosporine). Patients receiving the drug should be managed in facilities equipped and staffed with adequate laboratory and supportive medical resources. The physician responsible for maintenance therapy should have complete information requisite for the follow-up of the patient.

Sandimmune(R) (cyclosporine) should be administered with adrenal corticosteroids but not with other immunosuppressive agents. Increased susceptibility to infection and the possible development of lymphoma may result from immunosuppression.

Sandimmune(R) soft gelatin capsules (cyclosporine capsules, USP) and Sandimmune(R) oral solution (cyclosporine oral solution, USP) have decreased bioavailability in comparison to Neoral(R) soft gelatin capsules (cyclosporine capsules, USP) MODIFIED and Neoral(R) oral solution (cyclosporine oral solution, USP) MODIFIED.

Sandimmune(R) and Neoral(R) are not bioequivalent and cannot be used interchangeably without physician supervision.

The absorption of cyclosporine during chronic administration of Sandimmune(R) Soft Gelatin Capsules and Oral Solution was found to be erratic. It is recommended that patients taking the soft gelatin capsules or oral solution over a period of time be monitored at repeated intervals for cyclosporine blood levels and subsequent dose adjustments be made in order to avoid toxicity due to high levels and possible organ rejection due to low absorption of cyclosporine. This is of special importance in liver transplants. Numerous assays are being developed to measure blood levels of cyclosporine. Comparison of levels in published literature to patient levels using current assays must be done with detailed knowledge of the assay methods employed.

Commonly used brand name(s)

In the U.S.—
Gengraf
Neoral
Sandimmune

In Canada—
Apo-Cyclosporine

Available Dosage Forms:
- Capsule, Liquid Filled
- Capsule
- Solution

Therapeutic Class: Immune Suppressant

Uses For This Medicine

Cyclosporine belongs to the group of medicines known as immunosuppressive agents. It is used to reduce the body's natural immunity in patients who receive organ (for example, kidney, liver, and heart) transplants.

When a patient receives an organ transplant, the body's white blood cells will try to get rid of (reject) the transplanted organ. Cyclosporine works by preventing the white blood cells from doing this.

Cyclosporine also is used to treat severe cases of psoriasis and rheumatoid arthritis.

Cyclosporine may also be used for other conditions, as determined by your doctor.

Cyclosporine is a very strong medicine. It may cause side effects that could be very serious, such as high blood pressure and kidney and liver problems. It may also reduce the body's ability to fight infections. You and your doctor should talk about the good this medicine will do as well as the risks of using it.

Cyclosporine is available only with your doctor's prescription.

Once a medicine has been approved for marketing for a certain use, experience may show that it is also useful for other medical problems. Although not specifically included in the product labeling, cyclosporine is used in certain patients with the following medical conditions:
- Bone marrow transplantation
- Nephrotic syndrome

For patients receiving bone marrow transplantation, cyclosporine may work by preventing the cells from the transplanted bone marrow from attacking the cells of the patient's own body.

The doses of cyclosporine for patients receiving bone marrow transplantation and for patients with nephrotic syndrome are based on the patients' body weight. The usual starting dose for patients receiving bone marrow transplantation is 12.5 milligrams (mg) per kilogram (kg) (5.7 mg per pound) of body weight a day. The dose of cyclosporine for patients with nephrotic syndrome is 3.5 to 5 mg per kg (1.6 to 2.3 mg per pound) of body weight a day.

The side effects that patients experience when they receive cyclosporine for bone marrow transplantation or nephrotic syndrome are similar to those side effects experienced by patients receiving cyclosporine for organ transplantation.

Before Using This Medicine

In deciding to use a medicine, the risks of taking the medicine must be weighed against the good it will do. This is a decision you and your doctor will make. For this medicine, the following should be considered:

Allergies—Tell your doctor if you have ever had any unusual or allergic reaction to this medicine or any other medicines. Also tell your health care professional if you have any other types of allergies, such as to foods, dyes, preservatives, or animals. For non-prescription products, read the label or package ingredients carefully.

Pediatric—This medicine has been tested in children receiving organ transplants and, in effective doses, has not been shown to cause different side effects or problems than it does in adults.

Studies of this medicine have been done only in adult patients with rheumatoid arthritis and psoriasis, and there is no specific information comparing use of cyclosporine for rheumatoid arthritis or psoriasis in children with use in other age groups.

Geriatric—Older people are more likely to experience some side effects (e.g., high blood pressure and kidney problems) than are younger adults.

Pregnancy—

	Pregnancy Category	Explanation
All Trimesters	C	Animal studies have shown an adverse effect and there are no adequate studies in pregnant women OR no animal studies have been conducted and there are no adequate studies in pregnant women.

Breast Feeding—There are no adequate studies in women for determining infant risk when using this medication during breastfeeding. Weigh the potential benefits against the potential risks before taking this medication while breastfeeding.

Other medicines—

Using this medicine with any of the following medicines is not recommended. Your doctor may decide not to treat you with this medication or change some of the other medicines you take.

Bosentan, St John's Wort

Interactions with Food/Tobacco/Alcohol—Certain medicines should not be used at or around the time of eating food or eating certain types of food since interactions may occur. Using alcohol or tobacco with certain medicines may also cause interactions to occur. The following interactions have been selected on the basis of their potential significance and are not necessarily all-inclusive.

Using this medicine with any of the following may cause an increased risk of certain side effects but may be unavoidable in some cases. If used together, your doctor may change the dose or how often you use this medicine, or give you special instructions about the use of food, alcohol, or tobacco.

Grapefruit Juice

Other medical problems—The presence of other medical problems may affect the use of this medicine. Make sure you tell your doctor if you have any other medical problems, especially:
- Cancer or
- Precancerous skin changes—Cyclosporine can make these conditions worse
- Chickenpox (including recent exposure) or
- Herpes zoster (shingles)—Risk of severe disease affecting other parts of the body
- High blood pressure—Cyclosporine can cause high blood pressure. Patients with high blood pressure who have psoriasis or rheumatoid arthritis should not receive cyclosporine.
- Hyperkalemia (too much potassium in the blood)—Cyclosporine can make this condition worse
- Infection—Cyclosporine decreases the body's ability to fight infection
- Intestine problems—Effects may be decreased because cyclosporine cannot be absorbed into the body

- Kidney disease—Cyclosporine can have harmful effects on the kidney when it is taken for long periods of time. Patients with psoriasis or rheumatoid arthritis who have kidney disease should not receive cyclosporine
- Liver disease—Effects of cyclosporine may be increased because of slower removal of the medicine from the body

Proper Use of This Medicine

Take this medicine only as directed by your doctor. Do not take more or less of it and do not take it more often than your doctor ordered. The exact amount of medicine you need has been carefully worked out. Taking too much may increase the chance of side effects, while taking too little may not improve your condition.

To help you remember to take your medicine, try to get into the habit of taking it at the same time each day. This will also help cyclosporine work better by keeping a constant amount in the blood.

Absorption of this medicine may be changed if you change your diet. This medicine should be taken consistently with respect to meals. You should not change the type or amount of food you eat unless you discuss it with your health care professional. If this medicine upsets your stomach, your doctor may recommend that you take it with meals. However, check with your doctor before you decide to do this on your own.

Grapefruit and grapefruit juice may increase the effects of cyclosporine by increasing the amount of this medicine in the body. You should not eat grapefruit or drink grapefruit juice while you are taking this medicine.

This medicine is to be taken by mouth even if it comes in a dropper bottle. The amount you should take is to be measured only with the specially marked dropper provided with your prescription. The dropper should be wiped with a clean towel after it is used, and stored in its container.

To make Sandimmune® taste better, mix it in a glass container with milk, chocolate milk, or orange juice (preferably at room temperature). To make Neoral® taste better, mix it in a glass container with apple juice or orange juice (preferably at room temperature). Do not use a wax-lined or plastic disposable container. Stir it well, then drink it immediately. After drinking all the liquid containing the medicine, rinse the glass with a little more liquid and drink that also, to make sure you get all the medicine. Dry the dropper used to measure the cyclosporine, but do not rinse it with water.

Do not stop taking this medicine without first checking with your doctor. You may have to take medicine for the rest of your life to prevent your body from rejecting the transplant.

Dosing—The dose of this medicine will be different for different patients. Follow your doctor's orders or the directions on the label. The following information includes only the average doses of this medicine. If your dose is different, do not change it unless your doctor tells you to do so.

The amount of medicine that you take depends on the strength of the medicine. Also, the number of doses you take each day, the time allowed between doses, and the length of time you take the medicine depend on the medical problem for which you are using the medicine.

- For oral dosage forms (capsules, oral solution):
  - For transplant rejection:
    - Adults, teenagers, or children: Dose is based on body weight. The usual dose in the beginning is 12 to 15 milligrams (mg) per kilogram (kg) (5.5 to 6.8 mg per pound) of body weight a day. After a period of time, the dose may be decreased to 5 to 10 mg per kg (2.3 to 4.5 mg per pound) of body weight a day.
  - For rheumatoid arthritis:
    - Adults or teenagers: Dose is based on body weight. The usual dose is 2.5 to 4 mg per kg (1.1 to 1.8 mg per pound) of body weight a day.
    - Children—Use and dose must be determined by your doctor.
  - For psoriasis:
    - Adults or teenagers: Dose is based on body weight. The usual dose is 2.5 to 4 mg per kg (1.1 to 1.8 mg per pound) of body weight a day.
    - Children—Use and dose must be determined by your doctor.
- For injection dosage form:
  - For transplant rejection:
    - Adults, teenagers, or children: Dose is based on body weight. The usual dose is 2 to 6 mg per kg (0.9 to 2.7 mg per pound) of body weight a day.

Missed dose—If you miss a dose of this medicine, take it as soon as possible. However, if it is almost time for your next dose, skip the missed dose and go back to your regular dosing schedule. Do not double doses.

Call your doctor or pharmacist for instructions.

If you miss a dose of cyclosporine and remember it within 12 hours, take the missed dose as soon as you remember.

Storage—Store the medicine in a closed container at room temperature, away from heat, moisture, and direct light. Keep from freezing.

Keep out of the reach of children.

Do not keep outdated medicine or medicine no longer needed.

Do not store the oral solution in the refrigerator.

Precautions While Using This Medicine

It is very important that your doctor check your progress at regular visits. Your doctor will want to do laboratory tests to make sure that cyclosporine is working properly and to check for unwanted effects.

While you are being treated with cyclosporine, and after you stop treatment with it, it is important to see your doctor about the immunizations (vaccinations) you should receive. Do not have any immunizations without your doctor's approval. Cyclosporine lowers your body's resistance and there is a chance you might get the infection the immunization is meant to prevent. However, it may be especially important to receive certain immunizations to prevent a disease. In addition, other persons living in your house should not take oral polio vaccine since there is a chance they could pass the polio virus on to you. Also, avoid persons who have recently taken oral polio vaccine. Do not get close to them, and do not stay in the same room with them for very long. If you cannot take these precautions, you should consider wearing a protective face mask that covers the nose and mouth.

In some patients (usually younger patients), tenderness, swelling, or bleeding of the gums may appear soon after treatment with cyclosporine is started. Brushing and flossing your teeth, carefully and regularly, and massaging your gums may help prevent this. See your dentist regularly to have your teeth cleaned. Check with your medical doctor or dentist if you have any questions about how to take care of your teeth and gums, or if you notice any tenderness, swelling, or bleeding of your gums.

Side Effects of This Medicine

Along with its needed effects, a medicine may cause some unwanted effects. Some side effects will have signs or symptoms that you can see or feel. Your doctor will watch for others by doing certain tests.

Also, because of the way that cyclosporine acts on the body, there is a chance that it may cause effects that may not occur until years after the medicine is used. These delayed effects may include certain types of cancer, such as lymphomas or skin cancers. You and your doctor should discuss the good this medicine will do as well as the risks of using it.

Check with your doctor immediately if any of the following side effects occur:

Rare

Blood in urine; flushing of face and neck (for injection only); wheezing or shortness of breath (for injection only)

Check with your doctor as soon as possible if any of the following side effects occur:

More common

Bleeding, tender, or enlarged gums

Less common

Convulsions (seizures); fever or chills; frequent urge to urinate; vomiting

Rare

Confusion; general feeling of discomfort and illness; irregular heartbeat; numbness or tingling in hands, feet, or lips; shortness of breath or difficult breathing; stomach pain (severe) with nausea and vomiting; unexplained nervousness; unusual tiredness or weakness; weakness or heaviness of legs; weight loss

Incidence not known

Agitation; back pain; blurred vision; coma; dizziness; drowsiness; hallucinations; irritability; mood or mental changes; seizures; stiff neck

This medicine may also cause the following side effects that your doctor will watch for:

More common

High blood pressure; kidney problems

Less common

Liver problems; changes in blood chemistry

Some side effects may occur that usually do not need medical attention. These side effects may go away during treatment as your body adjusts to the medicine. Also, your health care professional may be able to tell you about ways to prevent or reduce some of these side effects. Check with your health care professional if any of the following side effects continue or are bothersome or if you have any questions about them:

More common

Increase in hair growth; trembling and shaking of hands

Less common

Acne or oily skin; headache; leg cramps; nausea

Other side effects not listed may also occur in some patients. If you notice any other effects, check with your healthcare professional.

CYTARABINE   (Oral route) - sye-TARE-a-been

Uses For This Medicine

Cytarabine belongs to the group of medicines called antimetabolites. It is used to treat some kinds of cancers of the blood. It may also be used to treat other kinds of cancer, as determined by your doctor.

Cytarabine interferes with the growth of cancer cells, which are eventually destroyed. Since the growth of normal body cells may also be affected by cytarabine, other effects will also occur. Some of these may be serious and must be reported to your doctor. Other effects, like hair loss, may not be serious but may cause concern. Some effects may not occur for months or years after the medicine is used.

Before you begin treatment with cytarabine, you and your doctor should talk about the good this medicine will do as well as the risks of using it.

Cytarabine is to be administered only by or under the immediate supervision of your doctor.

Once a medicine has been approved for marketing for a certain use, experience may show that it is also useful for other medical problems. Although these uses are not included in product labeling, cytarabine is used in certain patients with the following medical conditions:

• Cancer of the lymph system
• Cancer of the brain and spinal cord
• Myelodysplastic syndromes (MDS)

Before Using This Medicine

In deciding to use a medicine, the risks of taking the medicine must be weighed against the good it will do. This is a decision you and your doctor will make. For this medicine, the following should be considered:

Allergies—Tell your doctor if you have ever had any unusual or allergic reaction to this medicine or any other medicines. Also tell your health care professional if you have any other types of allergies, such as to foods, dyes, preservatives, or animals. For non-prescription products, read the label or package ingredients carefully.

Pediatric—Although there is no specific information comparing use of cytarabine in children with use in other age groups, this medicine is not expected to cause different side effects or problems in children than it does in adults.

Geriatric—Many medicines have not been studied specifically in older people. Therefore, it may not be known whether they work exactly the same way they do in younger adults. Although there is no specific information comparing use of cytarabine in the elderly with use in other age groups, this medicine is not expected to cause different side effects or problems in older people than it does in younger adults.

Pregnancy—

	Pregnancy Category	Explanation
All Trimesters	D	Studies in pregnant women have demonstrated a risk to the fetus. However, the benefits of therapy in a life threatening situation or a serious disease, may outweigh the potential risk.

Breast Feeding—There are no adequate studies in women for determining infant risk when using this medication during breastfeeding. Weigh the potential benefits against the potential risks before taking this medication while breastfeeding.

Other medicines—

Using this medicine with any of the following medicines is not recommended. Your doctor may decide not to treat you with this medication or change some of the other medicines you take.

Rotavirus Vaccine, Live

Interactions with Food/Tobacco/Alcohol—Certain medicines should not be used at or around the time of eating food or eating certain types of food since interactions may occur. Using alcohol or tobacco with certain medicines may also cause interactions to occur. Discuss with your healthcare professional the use of your medicine with food, alcohol, or tobacco.

Other medical problems—The presence of other medical problems may affect the use of this medicine. Make sure you tell your doctor if you have any other medical problems, especially:

- Chickenpox (including recent exposure) or
- Herpes zoster (shingles)—Risk of severe disease affecting other parts of the body
- Gout (history of) or
- Kidney stones (history of)—Cytarabine may increase levels of uric acid in the body, which can cause gout or kidney stones
- Infection—Cytarabine can decrease your body's ability to fight infection
- Kidney disease or
- Liver disease—Effects of cytarabine may be increased because of slower removal from the body

Proper Use of This Medicine

This medicine is sometimes given together with certain other medicines. If you are using a combination of medicines, it is important that you receive each one at the proper time. If you are taking some of these medicines by mouth, ask your health care professional to help you plan a way to take them at the right times.

While you are receiving this medicine, your doctor may want you to drink extra fluids so that you will pass more urine. This will help prevent kidney problems and keep your kidneys working well.

This medicine often causes nausea and vomiting. However, it is very important that you continue to receive the medicine even if you begin to feel ill. Ask your health care professional for ways to lessen these effects.

Dosing—The dose of this medicine will be different for different patients. Follow your doctor's orders or the directions on the label. The following information includes only the average doses of this medicine. If your dose is different, do not change it unless your doctor tells you to do so.

The amount of medicine that you take depends on the strength of the medicine. Also, the number of doses you take each day, the time allowed between doses, and the length of time you take the medicine depend on the medical problem for which you are using the medicine.

Precautions While Using This Medicine

It is very important that your doctor check your progress at regular visits to make sure that this medicine is working properly and to check for unwanted effects.

While you are being treated with cytarabine, and after you stop treatment with it, do not have any immunizations (vaccinations) without your doctor's approval. Cytarabine may lower your body's resistance and there is a chance you might get the infection the immunization is meant to prevent. In addition, other persons living in your household should not take oral polio vaccine since there is a chance they could pass the polio virus on to you. Also, avoid persons who have taken oral polio vaccine. Do not get close to them and do not stay in the same room with them for very long. If you cannot take these precautions, you should consider wearing a protective face mask that covers the nose and mouth.

Cytarabine can temporarily lower the number of white blood cells in your blood, increasing the chance of getting an infection. It can also lower the number of platelets, which are necessary for proper blood clotting. If this occurs, there are certain precautions you can take, especially when your blood count is low, to reduce the risk of infection or bleeding:

- If you can, avoid people with infections. Check with your doctor immediately if you think you are getting an infection or if you get a fever or chills, cough or hoarseness, lower back or side pain, or painful or difficult urination.
- Check with your doctor immediately if you notice any unusual bleeding or bruising; black, tarry stools; blood in urine or stools; or pinpoint red spots on your skin.
- Be careful when using a regular toothbrush, dental floss, or toothpick. Your medical doctor, dentist, or nurse may recommend other ways to clean your teeth and gums. Check with your medical doctor before having any dental work done.
- Do not touch your eyes or the inside of your nose unless you have just washed your hands and have not touched anything else in the meantime.
- Be careful not to cut yourself when you are using sharp objects such as a safety razor or fingernail or toenail cutters.
- Avoid contact sports or other situations where bruising or injury could occur.

Side Effects of This Medicine

Along with its needed effects, a medicine may cause some unwanted effects. Although not all of these side effects may occur, if they do occur they may need medical attention.

Also, because of the way these medicines act on the body, there is a chance that they might cause other unwanted effects that may not occur until months or years after the medicine is used. These delayed effects may include certain types of cancer, such as leukemia. Discuss these possible effects with your doctor.

Check with your doctor immediately if any of the following side effects occur:

Less common

Black, tarry stools; blood in urine; cough or hoarseness; fever or chills; lower back or side pain; painful or difficult urination; pinpoint red spots on skin; unusual bleeding or bruising

Check with your doctor as soon as possible if any of the following side effects occur:

More common

Sores in mouth and on lips

Less common

Joint pain; numbness or tingling in fingers, toes, or face; swelling of feet or lower legs; unusual tiredness

Rare

Bone or muscle pain; chest pain; decrease in urination; difficulty in swallowing; fainting spells; general feeling of discomfort or illness or weakness; heartburn; irregular heartbeat; pain at place of injection; reddened eyes; shortness of breath; skin rash; weakness; yellow eyes or skin

Some side effects may occur that usually do not need medical attention. These side effects may go away during treatment as your body adjusts to the medicine. Also, your health care professional may be able to tell you about ways to prevent or reduce some of these side effects. Check with your health care professional if any of the following side effects continue or are bothersome or if you have any questions about them:

More common

Loss of appetite; nausea and vomiting

Less common or rare

Diarrhea; dizziness; headache; itching of skin; skin freckling

This medicine may cause a temporary loss of hair in some people. After treatment with cytarabine has ended, normal hair growth should return.

After you stop using this medicine, it may still produce some side effects that need attention. During this period of time, *check with your doctor immediately* if you notice the following side effects:

Black, tarry stools; blood in urine or stools; cough or hoarseness; fever or chills; lower back or side pain; painful or difficult urination; pinpoint red spots on skin; unusual bleeding or bruising

Other side effects not listed may also occur in some patients. If you notice any other effects, check with your healthcare professional.

CYTARABINE LIPOSOME
(Intrathecal route) - sye-TARE-a-been LYE-poh-some

Black Box Warning

Cytarabine liposome injection should be administered only under the supervision of a qualified physician experienced in the use of intrathecal cancer chemotherapeutic agents. Appropriate management of complications is possible only when adequate diagnostic and treatment facilities are readily available. In all clinical studies, chemical arachnoiditis, a syndrome manifested primarily by nausea, vomiting, headache, and fever was a common adverse event. If left untreated, chemical arachnoiditis may be fatal. The incidence and severity of chemical arachnoiditis can be reduced by coadministration of dexamethasone. Patients receiving cytarabine li-

posome should be treated concurrently with dexamethasone to mitigate the symptoms of chemical arachnoiditis.

Commonly used brand name(s)

In the U.S.—
Depocyt

Available Dosage Forms:

• Suspension

Therapeutic Class: Antineoplastic Agent
Pharmacologic Class: Antimetabolite

Uses For This Medicine

Liposomal cytarabine belongs to the group of medicines known as antineoplastics. It is used to treat cancer of the lymph system that has spread to the brain.

Liposomal cytarabine interferes with the growth of cancer cells, which are eventually destroyed. Since the growth of normal cells may also be affected by the medicine, other effects may also occur. Some of these may be serious and must be reported to your doctor. Some effects may occur after treatment with liposomal cytarabine has been stopped.

Before you begin treatment with liposomal cytarabine, you and your doctor should talk about the good this medicine will do as well as the risks of using it.

Liposomal cytarabine is to be administered only by or under the immediate supervision of your doctor.

Before Using This Medicine

In deciding to use a medicine, the risks of taking the medicine must be weighed against the good it will do. This is a decision you and your doctor will make. For this medicine, the following should be considered:

Allergies—Tell your doctor if you have ever had any unusual or allergic reaction to this medicine or any other medicines. Also tell your health care professional if you have any other types of allergies, such as to foods, dyes, preservatives, or animals. For non-prescription products, read the label or package ingredients carefully.

Pediatric—Studies on this medicine have been done only in adult patients, and there is no specific information comparing use of liposomal cytarabine in children with use in other age groups.

Geriatric—Many medicines have not been studied specifically in older people. Therefore, it may not be known whether they work exactly the same way they do in younger adults or if they cause different side effects or problems in older people. There is no specific information comparing use of liposomal cytarabine in the elderly with use in other age groups.

Pregnancy—

	Pregnancy Category	Explanation
All Trimesters	D	Studies in pregnant women have demonstrated a risk to the fetus. However, the benefits of therapy in a life threatening situation or a serious disease, may outweigh the potential risk.

Breast Feeding—There are no adequate studies in women for determining infant risk when using this medication during breastfeeding. Weigh the potential benefits against the potential risks before taking this medication while breastfeeding.

Other medicines—

Using this medicine with any of the following medicines is not recommended. Your doctor may decide not to treat you with this medication or change some of the other medicines you take.

Rotavirus Vaccine, Live

Interactions with Food/Tobacco/Alcohol—Certain medicines should not be used at or around the time of eating food or eating certain types of food since interactions may occur. Using alcohol or tobacco with certain medicines may also cause interactions to occur. Discuss with your healthcare professional the use of your medicine with food, alcohol, or tobacco.

Other medical problems—The presence of other medical problems may affect the use of this medicine. Make sure you tell your doctor if you have any other medical problems, especially:

- Active meningitis—Use is not recommended
- Blockage to cerebrospinal fluid flow—Increased risk of neurotoxicity

Proper Use of This Medicine

This medicine often causes nausea and vomiting. However, it is very important that you continue to receive the medicine, even if you begin to feel ill. Ask your health care professional for ways to lessen these effects.

Dosing—The dose of this medicine will be different for different patients. Follow your doctor's orders or the directions on the label. The following information includes only the average doses of this medicine. If your dose is different, do not change it unless your doctor tells you to do so.

The amount of medicine that you take depends on the strength of the medicine. Also, the number of doses you take each day, the time allowed between doses, and the length of time you take the medicine depend on the medical problem for which you are using the medicine.

Precautions While Using This Medicine

It is very important that your doctor check your progress at regular visits to make sure that this medicine is working properly and to check for unwanted effects.

Side Effects of This Medicine

Along with its needed effects, a medicine may cause some unwanted effects. Although not all of these side effects may occur, if they do occur they may need medical attention.

Check with your doctor as soon as possible if any of the following side effects occur:

More common
Back pain; fever; headache; nausea; neck pain or rigidity; sleepiness; vomiting; weakness

Less common
Black, tarry stools; blood in urine or stools; chills; cough or hoarseness; lower back or side pain; painful or difficult urination; pinpoint red spots on skin; sore throat; swelling of fingers, hands, arms, lower legs, or feet; unusual bleeding or bruising

Rare
Fast or irregular breathing; puffiness or swelling around the face; shortness of breath; sudden, severe decrease in blood pressure; unusual tiredness

Some side effects may occur that usually do not need medical attention. These side effects may go away during treatment as your body adjusts to the medicine. Also, your health care professional may be able to tell you about ways to prevent or reduce some of these side effects. Check with your health care professional if any of the following side effects continue or are bothersome or if you have any questions about them:

Less common
Constipation; urinary incontinence

Other side effects not listed may also occur in some patients. If you notice any other effects, check with your healthcare professional.

DACARBAZINE (Intravenous route, Injection route) - da-KAR-be-zeen

Black Box Warning

It is recommended that dacarbazine for injection be administered under the supervision of a qualified physician experienced in the use of cancer chemotherapeutic agents.

Hemopoietic depression is the most common toxicity with dacarbazine for injection.

Hepatic necrosis has been reported.

Studies have demonstrated this agent to have a carcinogenic and teratogenic effect when used in animals.

In treatment of each patient, the physician must weigh carefully the possibility of achieving therapeutic benefit against the risk of toxicity.

Commonly used brand name(s)

In the U.S.—
Dtic-Dome

In Canada—
Dacarbazine

Available Dosage Forms:
- Powder for Solution
- Powder for Suspension

Therapeutic Class: Antineoplastic Agent
Pharmacologic Class: Alkylating Agent

Uses For This Medicine

Dacarbazine belongs to the group of medicines called alkylating agents. It is used to treat cancer of the lymph system and malignant melanoma (a type of skin cancer). It may also be used to treat other kinds of cancer, as determined by your doctor.

Dacarbazine interferes with the growth of cancer cells, which are eventually destroyed. Since the growth of normal body cells may also be affected by dacarbazine, other effects will also occur. Some of these may be serious and must be reported to your doctor. Other effects, like hair loss, may not be serious but may cause concern. Some effects may not occur for months or years after the medicine is used.

Before you begin treatment with dacarbazine, you and your doctor should talk about the good this medicine will do as well as the risks of using it.

Dacarbazine is to be administered only by or under the immediate supervision of your doctor.

Once a medicine has been approved for marketing for a certain use, experience may show that it is also useful for other medical problems. Although these uses are not included in product labeling, dacarbazine is used in certain patients with the following medical conditions:

- Cancer of the islet cells (a part of the pancreas)
- Soft tissue sarcomas (a cancer of the muscles, tendons, vessels that carry blood or lymph, joints, and fat)

Before Using This Medicine

In deciding to use a medicine, the risks of taking the medicine must be weighed against the good it will do. This is a decision you and your doctor will make. For this medicine, the following should be considered:

Allergies—Tell your doctor if you have ever had any unusual or allergic reaction to this medicine or any other medicines. Also tell your health care professional if you have any other types of allergies, such as to foods, dyes, preservatives, or animals. For non-prescription products, read the label or package ingredients carefully.

Pediatric—Studies on this medicine have been done only in adult patients and there is no specific information comparing use of dacarbazine in children with use in other age groups.

Geriatric—Many medicines have not been studied specifically in older people. Therefore, it may not be known whether they work exactly the same way they do in younger adults or if they cause different side effects or problems in older people. There is no specific information about the use of dacarbazine in the elderly.

Pregnancy—

	Pregnancy Category	Explanation
All Trimesters	C	Animal studies have shown an adverse effect and there are no adequate studies in pregnant women OR no animal studies have been conducted and there are no adequate studies in pregnant women.

Breast Feeding—There are no adequate studies in women for determining infant risk when using this medication during breastfeeding. Weigh the potential benefits against the potential risks before taking this medication while breastfeeding.

Other medicines—

Using this medicine with any of the following medicines is not recommended. Your doctor may decide not to treat you with this medication or change some of the other medicines you take.

Rotavirus Vaccine, Live

Interactions with Food/Tobacco/Alcohol—Certain medicines should not be used at or around the time of eating food or eating certain types of food since interactions may occur. Using alcohol or tobacco with certain medicines may also cause interactions to occur. Discuss with your healthcare professional the use of your medicine with food, alcohol, or tobacco.

Other medical problems—The presence of other medical problems may affect the use of this medicine. Make sure you tell your doctor if you have any other medical problems, especially:

- Chickenpox (including recent exposure) or
- Herpes zoster (shingles)—Risk of severe disease affecting other parts of the body
- Infection—Dacarbazine can decrease your body's ability to fight infection
- Kidney disease or
- Liver disease—Effects of dacarbazine may be increased because of slower removal from the body

Proper Use of This Medicine

Dacarbazine is sometimes given together with certain other medicines. If you are using a combination of medicines, it is important that you receive each one at the proper time. If you are taking some of these medicines by mouth, ask your health care professional to help you plan a way to remember to take them at the right times.

This medicine often causes nausea, vomiting, and loss of appetite. The injection may also cause a feeling of burning or pain. However, it is very important that you continue to receive the medicine, even if you have discomfort or begin to feel ill. After 1 or 2 days, your stomach upset should lessen. Ask your health care professional for ways to lessen these effects.

Dosing—The dose of this medicine will be different for different patients. Follow your doctor's orders or the directions on the label. The following information includes only the average doses of this medicine. If your dose is different, do not change it unless your doctor tells you to do so.

The amount of medicine that you take depends on the strength of the medicine. Also, the number of doses you take each day, the time allowed between doses, and the length of time you take the medicine depend on the medical problem for which you are using the medicine.

Precautions While Using This Medicine

It is very important that your doctor check your progress at regular visits to make sure that this medicine is working properly and to check for unwanted effects.

While you are being treated with dacarbazine, and after you stop treatment with it, do not have any immunizations (vaccinations) without your doctor's approval. Dacarbazine may lower your body's resistance and there is a chance you might get the infection the immunization is meant to prevent. In addition, other persons living in your household should not take oral polio vaccine since there is a chance they could pass the polio virus on to you. Also, avoid persons who have taken oral polio vaccine within the last several months. Do not get close to them, and do not stay in the same room with them for very long. If you cannot take these precautions, you should consider wearing a protective face mask that covers the nose and mouth.

Dacarbazine can temporarily lower the number of white blood cells in your blood, increasing the chance of getting an infection. It can also lower the number of platelets, which are necessary for proper blood clotting. If this occurs, there are certain precautions you can take, especially when your blood count is low, to reduce the risk of infection or bleeding:

- If you can, avoid people with infections. Check with your doctor immediately if you think you are getting an infection or if you get a fever or chills, cough or hoarseness, lower back or side pain, or painful or difficult urination.
- Check with your doctor immediately if you notice any unusual bleeding or bruising; black, tarry stools; blood in urine or stools; or pinpoint red spots on your skin.
- Be careful when using a regular toothbrush, dental floss, or toothpick. Your medical doctor, dentist, or nurse may recommend other ways to clean your teeth and gums. Check with your medical doctor before having any dental work done.
- Do not touch your eyes or the inside of your nose unless you have just washed your hands and have not touched anything else in the meantime.
- Be careful not to cut yourself when you are using sharp objects such as a safety razor or fingernail or toenail cutters.
- Avoid contact sports or other situations where bruising or injury could occur.

If dacarbazine accidentally seeps out of the vein into which it is injected, it may damage some tissues and cause scarring. Tell the doctor or nurse right away if you notice redness, pain, or swelling at the place of injection.

Side Effects of This Medicine

Along with its needed effects, a medicine may cause some unwanted effects. Although not all of these side effects may occur, if they do occur they may need medical attention.

Also, because of the way these medicines act on the body, there is a chance that they might cause other unwanted effects that may not occur until months or years after the medicine is used. These delayed effects may include certain types of cancer, such as leukemia. Discuss these possible effects with your doctor.

Check with your doctor immediately if any of the following side effects occur:

More common
   Redness, pain, or swelling at place of injection
Less common
   Black, tarry stools; blood in urine or stools; cough or hoarseness, accompanied by fever or chills; fever or chills; lower back or side pain, accompanied by fever or chills; painful or difficult urination, accompanied by fever or chills; pinpoint red spots on skin; unusual bleeding or bruising
Rare
   Shortness of breath; stomach pain; swelling of face; yellow eyes or skin

Check with your doctor as soon as possible if any of the following side effects occur:

Rare
   Sores in mouth and on lips

Some side effects may occur that usually do not need medical attention. These side effects may go away during treatment as your body adjusts to the medicine. Also, your health care

professional may be able to tell you about ways to prevent or reduce some of these side effects. Check with your health care professional if any of the following side effects continue or are bothersome or if you have any questions about them:

More common
   Loss of appetite; nausea or vomiting (should lessen after 1 or 2 days)
Less common
   Feelings of uneasiness; flushing of face; muscle pain; numbness of face

This medicine may cause a temporary loss of hair in some people. After treatment with dacarbazine has ended, normal hair growth should return.

After you stop using this medicine, it may still produce some side effects that need attention. During this period of time, *check with your doctor immediately* if you notice the following side effects:

   Black, tarry stools; blood in urine or stools; cough or hoarseness, accompanied by fever or chills; fever or chills; lower back or side pain, accompanied by fever or chills; painful or difficult urination, accompanied by fever or chills; pinpoint red spots on skin; unusual bleeding or bruising

Other side effects not listed may also occur in some patients. If you notice any other effects, check with your healthcare professional.

DACLIZUMAB   (Intravenous route) -
dac-KLYE-zue-mab

Black Box Warning

Only physicians experienced in immunosuppressive therapy and management of organ transplant patients should prescribe daclizumab. The physician responsible for daclizumab administration should have complete information requisite for the follow-up of the patient. Daclizumab should only be administered by healthcare personnel trained in the administration of the drug who have available adequate laboratory and supportive medical resources.

Commonly used brand name(s)

In the U.S.—
   Zenapax

Available Dosage Forms:
- Solution

Therapeutic Class: Immune Suppressant
Pharmacologic Class: Monoclonal Antibody

Uses For This Medicine

Daclizumab belongs to a group of medicines known as immunosuppressive agents. It is used to lower the body's natural immunity in patients who receive kidney transplants.

When a patient receives a kidney transplant, the body's white blood cells will try to get rid of (reject) the transplanted kidney. Daclizumab works by preventing the white blood cells from getting rid of the transplanted kidney. The effect of daclizumab on the white blood cells may also reduce the body's ability to fight infections.

Daclizumab is to be administered only by or under the immediate supervision of your doctor.

Before Using This Medicine

In deciding to use a medicine, the risks of taking the medicine must be weighed against the good it will do. This is a decision you and your doctor will make. For this medicine, the following should be considered:

Allergies—Tell your doctor if you have ever had any unusual or allergic reaction to this medicine or any other medicines. Also tell your health care professional if you have any other types of allergies, such as to foods, dyes, preservatives, or animals. For non-prescription products, read the label or package ingredients carefully.

Pediatric—Studies on the use of daclizumab in children have not been completed. However, daclizumab may cause high blood pressure and dehydration more often in children than it does in adults.

Geriatric—Many medicines have not been studied specifically in older people. Therefore, it may not be known whether they work exactly the same way they do in younger adults or if they cause different side effects or problems in older people. There is no specific information comparing use of daclizumab in the elderly with use in other age groups.

Pregnancy—

	Pregnancy Category	Explanation
All Trimesters	C	Animal studies have shown an adverse effect and there are no adequate studies in pregnant women OR no animal studies have been conducted and there are no adequate studies in pregnant women.

Breast Feeding—There are no adequate studies in women for determining infant risk when using this medication during breastfeeding. Weigh the potential benefits against the potential risks before taking this medication while breastfeeding.

Other medicines—Although certain medicines should not be used together at all, in other cases two different medicines may be used together even if an interaction might occur. In these cases, your doctor may want to change the dose, or other precautions may be necessary. Tell your healthcare professional if you are taking any other prescription or non-prescription (over-the-counter [OTC]) medicine.

Interactions with Food/Tobacco/Alcohol—Certain medicines should not be used at or around the time of eating food or eating certain types of food since interactions may occur. Using alcohol or tobacco with certain medicines may also cause interactions to occur. Discuss with your healthcare professional the use of your medicine with food, alcohol, or tobacco.

Other medical problems—The presence of other medical problems may affect the use of this medicine. Make sure you tell your doctor if you have any other medical problems, especially:

- Cancer—Daclizumab may make this condition worse

- Diabetes mellitus (sugar diabetes)—Daclizumab can increase the amount of sugar in the blood
- Infection—Daclizumab may decrease the body's ability to fight infection

Proper Use of This Medicine

Dosing—The dose of this medicine will be different for different patients. Follow your doctor's orders or the directions on the label. The following information includes only the average doses of this medicine. If your dose is different, do not change it unless your doctor tells you to do so.

The amount of medicine that you take depends on the strength of the medicine. Also, the number of doses you take each day, the time allowed between doses, and the length of time you take the medicine depend on the medical problem for which you are using the medicine.

- For injection dosage form:
  - To prevent kidney transplant rejection:
    - Adults or children—1 milligram (mg) per kilogram (kg) (0.45 mg per pound) of body weight.

Precautions While Using This Medicine

If you are continuing your course of therapy with daclizumab after you are discharged from the hospital, it is very important that your doctor check your progress at regular visits. Your doctor will want to do laboratory tests to make sure daclizumab is working properly.

Dental—It is important to maintain good dental hygiene and see a dentist regularly for teeth cleaning.

If you are a woman of childbearing age, you should use effective contraception while receiving this medicine.

Side Effects of This Medicine

Along with its needed effects, a medicine may cause some unwanted effects. Although not all of these side effects may occur, if they do occur they may need medical attention.

Check with your doctor immediately if any of the following side effects occur:
  Less common
    Chest pain; coughing; dizziness; fever; nausea; rapid heart rate; red, tender, oozing skin at incision; shortness of breath; swelling of the feet or lower legs; trembling or shaking of the hands or feet; vomiting; weakness
  Rare
  Frequent urination

Some side effects may occur that usually do not need medical attention. These side effects may go away during treatment as your body adjusts to the medicine. Also, your health care professional may be able to tell you about ways to prevent or reduce some of these side effects. Check with your health care professional if any of the following side effects continue or are bothersome or if you have any questions about them:
  Less common
    Constipation; diarrhea; headache; heartburn; joint pain; muscle pain; slow wound healing; trouble in sleeping

Other side effects not listed may also occur in some patients. If you notice any other effects, check with your healthcare professional.

DACTINOMYCIN (Intravenous route) -
dak-ti-noe-MYE-sin

Commonly used brand name(s)

In the U.S.—
Cosmegen

Available Dosage Forms:
- Powder for Solution

Therapeutic Class: Antibiotic

Uses For This Medicine

Dactinomycin belongs to the group of medicines known as antineoplastics. It is used to treat some kinds of cancer of the bones and soft tissue, including muscles and tendons; Wilms' tumor (a cancer of the kidney found primarily in children); tumors in the uterus or womb; and cancer of the testicles.

Dactinomycin interferes with the growth of cancer cells, which are eventually destroyed. Since the growth of normal body cells may also be affected by dactinomycin, other effects will also occur. Some of these may be serious and must be reported to your doctor. Other effects, like hair loss, may not be serious but may cause concern. Some effects may not occur for months or years after the medicine is used.

Before you begin treatment with dactinomycin, you and your doctor should talk about the good this medicine will do as well as the risks of using it.

Dactinomycin is to be administered only by or under the immediate supervision of your doctor.

Once a medicine has been approved for marketing for a certain use, experience may show that it is also useful for other medical problems. Although these uses are not included in product labeling, dactinomycin is used in certain patients with the following medical conditions:

- Kaposi's sarcoma (a type of cancer of the skin and mucous membranes)
- Osteosarcoma (a type of bone cancer found primarily in children)

Before Using This Medicine

In deciding to use a medicine, the risks of taking the medicine must be weighed against the good it will do. This is a decision you and your doctor will make. For this medicine, the following should be considered:

Allergies—Tell your doctor if you have ever had any unusual or allergic reaction to this medicine or any other medicines. Also tell your health care professional if you have any other types of allergies, such as to foods, dyes, preservatives, or animals. For non-prescription products, read the label or package ingredients carefully.

Pediatric—Because of increased toxicity, use of dactinomycin in infants less than 6 to 12 months of age is not recommended.

Geriatric—Many medicines have not been studied specifically in older people. Therefore, it may not be known whether they work exactly the same way they do in younger adults or if they cause different side effects or problems in older people. There is no specific information about the use of dactinomycin in the elderly.

Pregnancy—

	Pregnancy Category	Explanation
All Trimesters	D	Studies in pregnant women have demonstrated a risk to the fetus. However, the benefits of therapy in a life threatening situation or a serious disease, may outweigh the potential risk.

Breast Feeding—There are no adequate studies in women for determining infant risk when using this medication during breastfeeding. Weigh the potential benefits against the potential risks before taking this medication while breastfeeding.

Other medicines—

Using this medicine with any of the following medicines is not recommended. Your doctor may decide not to treat you with this medication or change some of the other medicines you take.

Rotavirus Vaccine, Live

Interactions with Food/Tobacco/Alcohol—Certain medicines should not be used at or around the time of eating food or eating certain types of food since interactions may occur. Using alcohol or tobacco with certain medicines may also cause interactions to occur. Discuss with your healthcare professional the use of your medicine with food, alcohol, or tobacco.

Other medical problems—The presence of other medical problems may affect the use of this medicine. Make sure you tell your doctor if you have any other medical problems, especially:

- Cancer treatment, past or
- Radiation treatment, past—Caution should be used
- Chickenpox (including recent exposure) or
- Herpes zoster (shingles)—Risk of severe disease affecting other parts of the body
- Gout (or history of) or
- Kidney stones—Dactinomycin may increase levels of uric acid in the body, which can cause gout or kidney stones
- Infection—Dactinomycin can decrease your body's ability to fight infection
- Liver disease—Effects of dactinomycin may be increased
- Radiation treatment—If you are taking this medicine for Wilms' tumor and you are having radiation treatment or you have in the past two months, tell your doctor right away.

Proper Use of This Medicine

Dactinomycin is sometimes given together with certain other medicines. If you are receiving a combination of medicines, it is important that you receive each one at the proper time. If you are taking some of these medicines by mouth, ask your health care professional to help you plan a way to remember to take them at the right times.

This medicine often causes nausea and vomiting. However, it is very important that you continue to receive the medicine, even if you begin to feel ill. Ask your health care professional for ways to lessen these effects.

This medicine is very toxic and can cause severe damage to your skin, eyes, nose, throat, or lungs. The medicine must NOT come into contact with your skin, eyes, or any other part of your body. Ask your doctor about instructions for handling this medicine, especially if you will be receiving dactinomycin at home. The doctor will have specific instructions for protective clothing to be worn and what to do if you inhale this medicine, or if it comes into contact with your eyes or skin.

Dosing—The dose of this medicine will be different for different patients. Follow your doctor's orders or the directions on the label. The following information includes only the average doses of this medicine. If your dose is different, do not change it unless your doctor tells you to do so.

The amount of medicine that you take depends on the strength of the medicine. Also, the number of doses you take each day, the time allowed between doses, and the length of time you take the medicine depend on the medical problem for which you are using the medicine.

Precautions While Using This Medicine

It is very important that your doctor check your progress at regular visits to make sure that this medicine is working properly and to check for unwanted effects.

While you are being treated with dactinomycin, and after you stop treatment with it, do not have any immunizations (vaccinations) without your doctor's approval. Dactinomycin may lower your body's resistance, and there is a chance you might get the infection the immunization is meant to prevent. In addition, other persons living in your household should not take oral polio vaccine since there is a chance they could pass the polio virus on to you. Also, avoid persons who have taken oral polio vaccine within the last several months. Do not get close to them, and do not stay in the same room with them for very long. If you cannot take these precautions, you should consider wearing a protective face mask that covers the nose and mouth.

Dactinomycin can temporarily lower the number of white blood cells in your blood increasing the chance of getting an infection. It can also lower the number of platelets, which are necessary for proper blood clotting. If this occurs, there are certain precautions you can take, especially when your blood count is low, to reduce the risk of infection or bleeding:

- If you can, avoid people with infections. Check with your doctor immediately if you think you are getting an infection or if you get a fever or chills, cough or hoarseness, lower back or side pain, or painful or difficult urination.
- Check with your doctor immediately if you notice any unusual bleeding or bruising; black, tarry stools; blood in urine or stools; or pinpoint red spots on your skin.
- Be careful when using a regular toothbrush, dental floss, or toothpick. Your medical doctor, dentist, or nurse may recommend other ways to clean your teeth and gums. Check with your medical doctor before having any dental work done.
- Do not touch your eyes or the inside of your nose unless you have just washed your hands and have not touched anything else in the meantime.
- Be careful not to cut yourself when you are using sharp objects such as a safety razor or fingernail or toenail cutters.
- Avoid contact sports or other situations where bruising or injury could occur.

If dactinomycin accidentally seeps out of the vein into which it is injected, it may severely damage some tissues and cause scarring. Tell the health care professional right away if you notice redness, pain, or swelling at the place of injection.

Side Effects of This Medicine

Along with its needed effects, a medicine may cause some unwanted effects. Although not all of these side effects may occur, if they do occur they may need medical attention.

Also, because of the way these medicines act on the body, there is a chance that they might cause other unwanted effects that may not occur until months or years after the medicine is used. These delayed effects may include certain types of cancer, such as leukemia. Discuss these possible effects with your doctor.

Check with your doctor immediately if any of the following side effects occur:

More common
Black, tarry stools; blood in urine or stools; cough or hoarseness accompanied by fever or chills; fever or chills; lower back or side pain accompanied by fever or chills; painful or difficult urination accompanied by fever or chills; pinpoint red spots on skin; unusual bleeding or bruising

Rare
Pain at place of injection; wheezing

Incidence not known
Abdominal cramps; confusion; convulsions; difficulty in breathing; growth retardation; irregular heartbeats; mood or mental changes; muscle cramps in hands, arms, feet, legs, or face; numbness and tingling around the mouth, fingertips, or feet; shortness of breath; tremor

Check with your doctor as soon as possible if any of the following side effects occur:

More common
Diarrhea (continuing); difficulty in swallowing; heartburn; sores in mouth and on lips; stomach pain (continuing); unusual tiredness or weakness

Rare
Joint pain; swelling of feet or lower legs; yellow eyes or skin

Incidence not known
Blisters; body aches or pain; chapped, red, or swollen lips; congestion; cough; diarrhea; difficulty in moving; difficulty swallowing; dryness or soreness of throat; fever; flushing, redness of skin; hoarseness; joint pain; muscle aching or cramping; muscle pains or stiffness; runny nose; scaling, redness, burning, pain, or other signs of inflammation of lips; swollen joints; tender, swollen glands in neck; trouble in swallowing; unusually warm skin; voice changes

Some side effects may occur that usually do not need medical attention. These side effects may go away during treatment as your body adjusts to the medicine. Also, your health care professional may be able to tell you about ways to prevent or reduce some of these side effects. Check with your health

care professional if any of the following side effects continue or are bothersome or if you have any questions about them:

More common

> Darkening of skin; infection; unusual feeling of dullness or sluggishness; general feeling of discomfort or weakness; nausea and vomiting; redness of skin; skin rash or acne

This medicine often causes a temporary loss of hair, sometimes including the eyebrows. After treatment with dactinomycin has ended, normal hair growth should return.

After you stop using this medicine, it may still produce some side effects that need attention. During this period of time, *check with your doctor immediately* if you notice the following side effects:

> Black, tarry stools; blood in urine or stools; cough or hoarseness accompanied by fever or chills; diarrhea; fever or chills; lower back or side pain accompanied by fever or chills; painful or difficult urination accompanied by fever or chills; pinpoint red spots on skin; sores in mouth and on lips; stomach pain; unusual bleeding or bruising; yellow eyes or skin

Other side effects not listed may also occur in some patients. If you notice any other effects, check with your healthcare professional.

DALTEPARIN (Subcutaneous route, Injection route) - dal-TE-pa-rin

Black Box Warning

When neuraxial anesthesia (epidural/spinal anesthesia) or spinal puncture is employed, patients anticoagulated or scheduled to be anticoagulated with low molecular weight heparins or heparinoids for prevention of thromboembolic complications are at risk of developing an epidural or spinal hematoma which can result in long-term or permanent paralysis.

The risk of these events is increased by the use of indwelling epidural catheters for administration of analgesia or by the concomitant use of drugs affecting hemostasis such as non steroidal anti-inflammatory drugs (NSAIDS), platelet inhibitors, or other anticoagulants. The risk also appears to be increased by traumatic or repeated epidural or spinal puncture.

Patients should be frequently monitored for signs and symptoms of neurological impairment. If neurological compromise is noted, urgent treatment is necessary.

The physician should consider the potential benefit versus risk before neuraxial intervention in patients anticoagulated or to be anticoagulated for thromboprophylaxis.

Commonly used brand name(s)

In the U.S.—
> Fragmin

Available Dosage Forms:
- Injectable
- Solution

Therapeutic Class: Anticoagulant
Pharmacologic Class: Low Molecular Weight Heparin

Uses For This Medicine

Dalteparin is used to prevent deep venous thrombosis, a condition in which harmful blood clots form in the blood vessels of the legs. These blood clots can travel to the lungs and can become lodged in the blood vessels of the lungs, causing a condition called pulmonary embolism. Dalteparin is used for several days after abdominal surgery, while you are unable to walk. It is during this time that blood clots are most likely to form. Dalteparin also may be used for other conditions as determined by your doctor.

Dalteparin is available only with your doctor's prescription.

Before Using This Medicine

In deciding to use a medicine, the risks of taking the medicine must be weighed against the good it will do. This is a decision you and your doctor will make. For this medicine, the following should be considered:

Allergies—Tell your doctor if you have ever had any unusual or allergic reaction to this medicine or any other medicines. Also tell your health care professional if you have any other types of allergies, such as to foods, dyes, preservatives, or animals. For non-prescription products, read the label or package ingredients carefully.

Pediatric—Studies on this medicine have been done only in adult patients, and there is no specific information comparing use of dalteparin in children with use in other age groups.

Geriatric—This medicine has been tested and has not been shown to cause different side effects or problems in older people than it does in younger adults.

Pregnancy—

	Pregnancy Category	Explanation
All Trimesters	B	Animal studies have revealed no evidence of harm to the fetus, however, there are no adequate studies in pregnant women OR animal studies have shown an adverse effect, but adequate studies in pregnant women have failed to demonstrate a risk to the fetus.

Breast Feeding—There are no adequate studies in women for determining infant risk when using this medication during breastfeeding. Weigh the potential benefits against the potential risks before taking this medication while breastfeeding.

Other medicines—

Using this medicine with any of the following medicines is usually not recommended, but may be required in some cases. If both medicines are prescribed together, your doctor may change the dose or how often you use one or both of the medicines.

Abciximab, Aceclofenac, Acemetacin, Acenocoumarol, Alclofenac, Alteplase, Recombinant, Ancrod, Anisindione, Anistreplase, Antithrombin III Human, Apazone, Ardeparin, Argatroban, Benoxaprofen, Bivalirudin, Bromfenac, Bufexamac, Carprofen, Certoparin, Clometacin, Clonixin, Clopidogrel, Dalteparin, Danaparoid, Defibrotide, Dermatan Sulfate, Desirudin, Dexketoprofen, Diclofenac, Dicumarol, Diflunisal, Dipyrone, Droxicam, Enoxaparin, Eptifibatide, Etodolac, Etofenamate, Felbinac, Fenbufen, Fenoprofen, Fentiazac, Floctafenine, Flufenamic Acid, Flurbiprofen, Fondaparinux, Heparin, Ibuprofen, Indomethacin, Indoprofen, Isoxicam, Ketoprofen, Ketorolac, Lamifiban, Lornoxicam, Meclofenamate, Mefenamic Acid, Meloxicam, Nabumetone, Nadroparin, Naproxen, Niflumic Acid, Nimesulide, Oxaprozin, Oxyphenbutazone, Parnaparin, Pentosan Polysulfate Sodium, Phenindione, Phenprocoumon, Phenylbutazone, Pirazolac, Piroxicam, Pirprofen, Propyphenazone, Proquazone, Reteplase, Recombinant, Reviparin, Sibrafiban, Streptokinase, Sulindac, Suprofen, Tenecteplase, Tenidap, Tenoxicam, Tiaprofenic Acid, Tinzaparin, Tirofiban, Tolmetin, Urokinase, Warfarin, Xemilofiban, Zomepirac

Interactions with Food/Tobacco/Alcohol—Certain medicines should not be used at or around the time of eating food or eating certain types of food since interactions may occur. Using alcohol or tobacco with certain medicines may also cause interactions to occur. Discuss with your healthcare professional the use of your medicine with food, alcohol, or tobacco.

Other medical problems—The presence of other medical problems may affect the use of this medicine. Make sure you tell your doctor if you have any other medical problems, especially:

- Bleeding problems or
- Eye problems caused by diabetes or high blood pressure or
- Heart infection or
- High blood pressure (hypertension) or
- Kidney disease or
- Liver disease or
- Stomach or intestinal ulcer (active) or
- Stroke—The risk of bleeding may be increased
- Also, tell your doctor if you have received dalteparin or heparin before and had a reaction to either of them called thrombocytopenia (a low platelet count in the blood), or if new blood clots formed while you were receiving the medicine.
- In addition, tell your doctor if you have recently had medical surgery. This may increase the risk of serious bleeding when you are taking dalteparin.

Proper Use of This Medicine

If you are using dalteparin at home, your health care professional will teach you how to inject yourself with the medicine. Be sure to follow the directions carefully. Check with your health care professional if you have any problems using the medicine.

Put used syringes in a puncture-resistant, disposable container, or dispose of them as directed by your health care professional.

Dosing—The dose of this medicine will be different for different patients. Follow your doctor's orders or the directions on the label. The following information includes only the average doses of this medicine. If your dose is different, do not change it unless your doctor tells you to do so.

The amount of medicine that you take depends on the strength of the medicine. Also, the number of doses you take each day, the time allowed between doses, and the length of time you take the medicine depend on the medical problem for which you are using the medicine.

- For injection dosage form:
  - For prevention of deep venous thrombosis (leg clots) and pulmonary embolism (lung clots):
    - Adults—The dose will be determined by your doctor, based on your condition.
    - Children—Use and dose must be determined by your doctor.
- For prevention of blood clots after unstable angina (chest pain) or non–Q-wave myocardial infarction (a type of heart attack)
  - Adults—120 International Units (IU) per kilogram of body weight injected under the skin (but no more than 10,000 IU) given every 12 hours for 5 to 8 days. Unless your doctor recommends otherwise, aspirin should be given 75 to 165 milligrams daily.
  - Children—Use and dose must be determined by your doctor.

Missed dose—If you miss a dose of this medicine, take it as soon as possible. However, if it is almost time for your next dose, skip the missed dose and go back to your regular dosing schedule. Do not double doses.

Storage—Store the medicine in a closed container at room temperature, away from heat, moisture, and direct light. Keep from freezing.

Keep out of the reach of children.

Do not keep outdated medicine or medicine no longer needed.

Precautions While Using This Medicine

Tell all your medical doctors and dentists that you are using this medicine.

Check with your doctor immediately if you notice any of the following side effects:

- Bruising or bleeding, especially bleeding that is hard to stop. (Bleeding inside the body sometimes appears as bloody or black, tarry stools or causes faintness.)
- Back pain; burning, pricking, tickling, or tingling sensation; leg weakness; numbness; paralysis; or problems with bowel or bladder function.

Side Effects of This Medicine

Along with its needed effects, a medicine may cause some unwanted effects. Although not all of these side effects may occur, if they do occur they may need medical attention.

Stop taking this medicine and get emergency help immediately if any of the following effects occur:

More common
    Deep, dark purple bruise, pain, or swelling at place of injection

Less common
    Bleeding of gums; coughing up blood; difficulty in breathing or swallowing; dizziness; headache; increased menstrual flow or vaginal bleeding; nosebleeds; paralysis; prolonged bleeding from cuts; red or dark brown urine; red or black, tarry stools; shortness of breath; unexplained pain, swelling, or discomfort, especially in the chest, abdomen, joints, or muscles; un-

usual bruising; vomiting of blood or coffee ground-like material; weakness

Rare

Back pain; bleeding from mucous membranes; bluish or black discoloration, flushing, or redness of skin; burning, pricking, tickling, or tingling sensation; coughing; feeling faint; fever; leg weakness; numbness; problems with bowel or bladder function; skin rash (which may consist of pinpoint, purple-red spots), hives, or itching; sloughing of skin at place of injection; swelling of eyelids, face, or lips; tightness in chest or wheezing

Other side effects not listed may also occur in some patients. If you notice any other effects, check with your healthcare professional.

DANAPAROID (Subcutaneous route)

Commonly used brand name(s)
In the U.S.—
Orgaran

Available Dosage Forms:
• Solution

Therapeutic Class: Anticoagulant
Pharmacologic Class: Low Molecular Weight Heparin

Uses For This Medicine

Danaparoid is used to prevent deep venous thrombosis, a condition in which harmful blood clots form in the blood vessels of the legs. These blood clots can travel to the lungs and can become lodged in the blood vessels of the lungs, causing a condition called pulmonary embolism. Danaparoid is used for several days after hip replacement surgery, while you are unable to walk. It is during this time that blood clots are most likely to form. Danaparoid also may be used for other conditions as determined by your doctor.

Danaparoid is available only with your doctor's prescription.

Before Using This Medicine

In deciding to use a medicine, the risks of taking the medicine must be weighed against the good it will do. This is a decision you and your doctor will make. For this medicine, the following should be considered:

Allergies—Tell your doctor if you have ever had any unusual or allergic reaction to this medicine or any other medicines. Also tell your health care professional if you have any other types of allergies, such as to foods, dyes, preservatives, or animals. For non-prescription products, read the label or package ingredients carefully.

Pediatric—Studies on this medicine have been done only in adult patients, and there is no specific information comparing use of danaparoid in children with use in other age groups.

Geriatric—Many medicines have not been studied specifically in older people. Therefore, it may not be known whether they work exactly the same way they do in younger adults or if they cause different side effects or problems in older people.

There is no specific information comparing use of danaparoid in the elderly with use in other age groups.

Pregnancy—

	Pregnancy Category	Explanation
All Trimesters	B	Animal studies have revealed no evidence of harm to the fetus, however, there are no adequate studies in pregnant women OR animal studies have shown an adverse effect, but adequate studies in pregnant women have failed to demonstrate a risk to the fetus.

Breast Feeding—There are no adequate studies in women for determining infant risk when using this medication during breastfeeding. Weigh the potential benefits against the potential risks before taking this medication while breastfeeding.

Other medicines—

Using this medicine with any of the following medicines is usually not recommended, but may be required in some cases. If both medicines are prescribed together, your doctor may change the dose or how often you use one or both of the medicines.

Abciximab, Aceclofenac, Acemetacin, Acenocoumarol, Alclofenac, Alteplase, Recombinant, Anisindione, Anistreplase, Apazone, Ardeparin, Argatroban, Benoxaprofen, Bivalirudin, Bromfenac, Bufexamac, Carprofen, Certoparin, Cilostazol, Clometacin, Clonixin, Clopidogrel, Dalteparin, Danaparoid, Defibrotide, Dermatan Sulfate, Desirudin, Dexketoprofen, Diclofenac, Dicumarol, Diflunisal, Dipyrone, Droxicam, Enoxaparin, Eptifibatide, Etodolac, Etofenamate, Felbinac, Fenbufen, Fenoprofen, Fentiazac, Floctafenine, Flufenamic Acid, Flurbiprofen, Fondaparinux, Garlic, Ginkgo, Heparin, Ibuprofen, Indomethacin, Indoprofen, Isoxicam, Ketoprofen, Ketorolac, Lamifiban, Lornoxicam, Meclofenamate, Mefenamic Acid, Meloxicam, Nabumetone, Nadroparin, Naproxen, Niflumic Acid, Nimesulide, Oxaprozin, Oxyphenbutazone, Papaya, Parnaparin, Phenindione, Phenprocoumon, Phenylbutazone, Pirazolac, Piroxicam, Pirprofen, Propyphenazone, Proquazone, Reteplase, Recombinant, Reviparin, Sibrafiban, St John's Wort, Streptokinase, Sulindac, Suprofen, Tan-Shen, Tenecteplase, Tenidap, Tenoxicam, Tiaprofenic Acid, Tinzaparin, Tirofiban, Tolmetin, Urokinase, Warfarin, Xemilofiban, Zomepirac

Interactions with Food/Tobacco/Alcohol—Certain medicines should not be used at or around the time of eating food or eating certain types of food since interactions may occur. Using alcohol or tobacco with certain medicines may also cause interactions to occur. Discuss with your healthcare professional the use of your medicine with food, alcohol, or tobacco.

Other medical problems—The presence of other medical problems may affect the use of this medicine. Make sure you tell your doctor if you have any other medical problems, especially:
• Bleeding problems or
• Heart infection or
• High blood pressure (hypertension) or
• Kidney disease or

- Stomach or intestinal ulcer (active) or
- Stroke—The risk of bleeding may be increased

Also, tell your doctor if you have received danaparoid before and had a reaction to it called thrombocytopenia (a low platelet count in the blood), or if new blood clots formed while you were receiving the medicine.

In addition, tell your doctor if you have recently had medical surgery. This may increase the risk of serious bleeding when you are taking danaparoid.

Proper Use of This Medicine

If you are using danaparoid at home, your health care professional will teach you how to inject yourself with the medicine. Be sure to follow the directions carefully. Check with your health care professional if you have any problems using the medicine.

Put used syringes in a puncture-resistant, disposable container, or dispose of them as directed by your health care professional.

Dosing—The dose of this medicine will be different for different patients. Follow your doctor's orders or the directions on the label. The following information includes only the average doses of this medicine. If your dose is different, do not change it unless your doctor tells you to do so.

The amount of medicine that you take depends on the strength of the medicine. Also, the number of doses you take each day, the time allowed between doses, and the length of time you take the medicine depend on the medical problem for which you are using the medicine.

- For injection dosage form:
  - For prevention of deep venous thrombosis (leg clots) and pulmonary embolism (lung clots):
    - Adults—750 anti-factor Xa units, injected under the skin, two times a day for up to fourteen days after surgery.
    - Children—Use and dose must be determined by your doctor.

Missed dose—If you miss a dose of this medicine, take it as soon as possible. However, if it is almost time for your next dose, skip the missed dose and go back to your regular dosing schedule. Do not double doses.

Storage—Store the medicine in a closed container at room temperature, away from heat, moisture, and direct light. Keep from freezing.

Keep out of the reach of children.

Do not keep outdated medicine or medicine no longer needed.

Precautions While Using This Medicine

Tell all your medical doctors and dentists that you are using this medicine.

Check with your doctor immediately if you notice any of the following side effects:

- Bruising or bleeding, especially bleeding that is hard to stop. Bleeding inside the body sometimes appears as bloody or black, tarry stools, or faintness.
- Back pain; burning, pricking, tickling, or tingling sensation; leg weakness; numbness; paralysis; or problems with bowel or bladder function.

Side Effects of This Medicine

Along with its needed effects, a medicine may cause some unwanted effects. Although not all of these side effects may occur, if they do occur they may need medical attention.

Stop taking this medicine and get emergency help immediately if any of the following effects occur:
Less common
> Bleeding gums; coughing up blood; difficulty in breathing or swallowing; dizziness; headache; increased menstrual flow or vaginal bleeding; nosebleeds; paralysis; prolonged bleeding from cuts; red or dark brown urine; red or black, tarry stools; shortness of breath; unexplained pain, swelling, or discomfort, especially in the chest, abdomen, joints, or muscles; unusual bruising; vomiting of blood or coffee ground-like material; weakness

Rare
> Back pain; burning, pricking, tickling, or tingling sensation; leg weakness; numbness; problems with bowel or bladder function

Check with your doctor as soon as possible if any of the following side effects occur:
Less common
> Fever

Rare
> Skin rash

Some side effects may occur that usually do not need medical attention. These side effects may go away during treatment as your body adjusts to the medicine. Also, your health care professional may be able to tell you about ways to prevent or reduce some of these side effects. Check with your health care professional if any of the following side effects continue or are bothersome or if you have any questions about them:
More common
> Pain at injection site

Less common
> Constipation; nausea

Other side effects not listed may also occur in some patients. If you notice any other effects, check with your healthcare professional.

DANAZOL   (Oral route) - DA-na-zole

Commonly used brand name(s)
In the U.S.—
> Danocrine

Available Dosage Forms:
- Capsule

Therapeutic Class: Endocrine-Metabolic Agent
Pharmacologic Class: Androgen

Uses For This Medicine

Danazol may be used for a number of different medical problems. These include treatment of:
- Pain and/or infertility due to endometriosis;

- A tendency for females to develop cysts in the breasts (fibrocystic breast disease); or
- Hereditary angioedema, which causes swelling of the face, arms, legs, throat, windpipe, bowels, or sexual organs.

Danazol may also be used for other conditions as determined by your doctor.

This medicine is available only with your doctor's prescription.

Once a medicine has been approved for marketing for a certain use, experience may show that it is also useful for other medical problems. Although these uses may not be included in product labeling, danazol is used in certain patients with the following medical conditions:

- Gynecomastia (excess breast development in males)
- Menorrhagia (excessively long menstrual periods)
- Precocious puberty in females (premature sexual development)

Before Using This Medicine

In deciding to use a medicine, the risks of taking the medicine must be weighed against the good it will do. This is a decision you and your doctor will make. For this medicine, the following should be considered:

Allergies—Tell your doctor if you have ever had any unusual or allergic reaction to this medicine or any other medicines. Also tell your health care professional if you have any other types of allergies, such as to foods, dyes, preservatives, or animals. For non-prescription products, read the label or package ingredients carefully.

Pediatric—Danazol may cause male-like changes in female children and cause premature sexual development in male children. It may also slow or stop growth in any child.

Geriatric—Many medicines have not been studied specifically in older people. Therefore, it may not be known whether they work exactly the same way they do in younger adults. Although there is no specific information comparing use of danazol in the elderly with use in other age groups, danazol has effects similar to androgens (male hormones). Androgens used in older males may increase the risk of developing prostate enlargement or cancer.

Pregnancy—

	Pregnancy Category	Explanation
All Trimesters	X	Studies in animals or pregnant women have demonstrated positive evidence of fetal abnormalities. This drug should not be used in women who are or may become pregnant because the risk clearly outweighs any possible benefit.

Breast Feeding—There are no adequate studies in women for determining infant risk when using this medication during breastfeeding. Weigh the potential benefits against the potential risks before taking this medication while breastfeeding.

Other medicines—

Using this medicine with any of the following medicines is not recommended. Your doctor may decide not to treat you with this medication or change some of the other medicines you take.

Bupropion

Interactions with Food/Tobacco/Alcohol—Certain medicines should not be used at or around the time of eating food or eating certain types of food since interactions may occur. Using alcohol or tobacco with certain medicines may also cause interactions to occur. Discuss with your healthcare professional the use of your medicine with food, alcohol, or tobacco.

Other medical problems—The presence of other medical problems may affect the use of this medicine. Make sure you tell your doctor if you have any other medical problems, especially:

- Blood clotting disorders or
- Severe liver disease or
- Tumor caused by too much male hormones or
- Tumor on the genitals or
- Unusual bleeding from the vagina—Danazol should not be used when these conditions exist
- Porphyria—This condition may be made worse
- Type 2 diabetes mellitus—Danazol may increase blood glucose (sugar) levels
- Epilepsy or
- Heart disease or
- Kidney disease or
- Migraine headaches—These conditions can be made worse by the fluid retention (keeping too much body water) that can be caused by danazol

Proper Use of This Medicine

In order for danazol to help you, it must be taken regularly for the full time of treatment as ordered by your doctor.

Dosing—The dose of this medicine will be different for different patients. Follow your doctor's orders or the directions on the label. The following information includes only the average doses of this medicine. If your dose is different, do not change it unless your doctor tells you to do so.

The amount of medicine that you take depends on the strength of the medicine. Also, the number of doses you take each day, the time allowed between doses, and the length of time you take the medicine depend on the medical problem for which you are using the medicine.

- For capsules dosage form:
  - Adults and teenagers:
    - For treatment of endometriosis: 100 to 400 milligrams (mg) two times a day for at least three to six months, and possibly for nine months.
    - For treatment of fibrocystic breast disease: 50 to 200 mg two times a day for six months or until signs of the disease go away, whichever comes first.
    - For prevention of attacks of hereditary angioedema: 200 mg two or three times a day. The dose may be lowered, depending upon your condition.
  - Children: Dose must be determined by your doctor.

Missed dose—If you miss a dose of this medicine, take it as soon as possible. However, if it is almost time for your next

dose, skip the missed dose and go back to your regular dosing schedule. Do not double doses.

Storage—Store the medicine in a closed container at room temperature, away from heat, moisture, and direct light. Keep from freezing.

Keep out of the reach of children.

Do not keep outdated medicine or medicine no longer needed.

Precautions While Using This Medicine

Your doctor should check your progress at regular visits to make sure that this medicine does not cause unwanted effects.

Contact your doctor if you are a female and have a larger clitoris (sexual organ), deepening of your voice, or unnatural hair growth after taking danazol. Your doctor may advise you to stop taking the medicine so these effects do not get worse.

For patients with diabetes:

- This medicine may affect blood glucose (sugar) levels. If you notice a change in the results of your blood or urine glucose test or if you have any questions about this, check with your doctor.

Danazol may cause your skin to be more sensitive to sunlight than it is normally. Exposure to sunlight, even for brief periods of time, may cause a skin rash, itching, redness, or other discoloration of the skin, or a severe sunburn. When you begin taking this medicine:

- Stay out of direct sunlight, especially between the hours of 10:00 a.m. and 3:00 p.m., if possible.
- Wear protective clothing, including a hat. Also, wear sunglasses.
- Apply a sun block product that has a skin protection factor (SPF) of a least 15. Some patients may require a product with a higher SPF number, especially if they have a fair complexion. If you have questions about this, check with your health care professional.
- Apply a sun block lipstick that has an SPF of at least 15 to protect your lips.
- Do not use a sunlamp or tanning bed or booth.

If you have a severe reaction from the sun, check with your doctor.

If you are taking danazol for endometriosis or fibrocystic breast disease:

- During the time you are taking danazol, your menstrual period may not be regular or you may not have a menstrual period at all. This is to be expected when you are taking this medicine. If regular menstruation does not begin within 60 to 90 days after you stop taking this medicine, check with your doctor.
- During the time you are taking danazol, you should use birth control methods that do not contain hormones. If you have any questions about this, check with your health care professional.
- If you suspect that you may have become pregnant, stop taking this medicine and check with your doctor. Continued use of danazol during pregnancy may cause male-like changes in female babies.

Side Effects of This Medicine

Along with its needed effects, a medicine may cause some unwanted effects. Although not all of these side effects may occur, if they do occur they may need medical attention.

Check with your doctor as soon as possible if any of the following side effects occur:
For both females and males
Less common
 Acne; dark-colored urine; increased oiliness of hair or skin; muscle cramps or spasms; swelling of feet or lower legs; unusual tiredness or weakness; weight gain (rapid)
Rare
 Bleeding gums; bloating, pain or tenderness of abdomen or stomach; blood in urine; burning, numbness, pain, or tingling in all fingers except the smallest finger; changes in vision; chest pain; chills; complete or partial numbness or weakness on one side of body; cough; coughing up blood; diarrhea; difficulty in speaking; difficulty in swallowing; discharge from nipple; eye pain; fast heartbeat; fever; headache; hives or other skin rash; joint pain; light-colored stools; loss of appetite (continuing); loss of muscle coordination; more frequent nosebleeds; muscle aches; nausea; purple- or red-colored, or other spots on body or inside the mouth or nose; restlessness; shortness of breath; sore throat; sweating; tingling, numbness, or weakness in legs, which may move upward to arms, trunk, or face; unusual bruising or bleeding; unusual tiredness, weakness, or general feeling of illness; vomiting; yellow eyes or skin

For females only
More common
 Decrease in breast size; irregular menstrual periods; weight gain
Rare
 Enlarged clitoris; hoarseness or deepening of voice; unnatural hair growth

For males only
Rare
 Changes in semen; decrease in size of testicles

Some side effects may occur that usually do not need medical attention. These side effects may go away during treatment as your body adjusts to the medicine. Also, your health care professional may be able to tell you about ways to prevent or reduce some of these side effects. Check with your health care professional if any of the following side effects continue or are bothersome or if you have any questions about them:
For both females and males
Less common
 Flushing or redness of skin; mood or mental changes; nervousness
Rare
 Increased sensitivity of skin to sunlight
For females only
Less common
 Burning, dryness, or itching of vagina; vaginal bleeding

Other side effects not listed may also occur in some patients. If you notice any other effects, check with your healthcare professional.

DANTROLENE (Oral route, Intravenous route) - DAN-troe-leen

Black Box Warning

Dantrolene sodium has a potential for hepatotoxicity, and should not be used in conditions other than those recommended. Symptomatic hepatitis (fatal and non-fatal) has been reported at various dose levels of the drug. The incidence reported in patients taking up to 400 mg per day is much lower than in those taking doses of 800 mg or more per day. Even sporadic short courses of these higher dose levels within a treatment regimen markedly increased the risk of serious hepatic injury. Liver dysfunction as evidenced by blood chemical abnormalities alone (liver enzyme elevations) has been observed in patients exposed to dantrolene sodium for varying periods of time. Overt hepatitis has occurred at varying intervals after initiation of therapy, but has been most frequently observed between the third and twelfth month of therapy. The risk of hepatic injury appears to be greater in females, in patients over 35 years of age, and in patients taking other medication(s) in addition to dantrolene sodium. Dantrolene sodium should be used only in conjunction with appropriate monitoring of hepatic function including frequent determination of SGOT or SGPT. If no observable benefit is derived from the administration of dantrolene sodium after a total of 45 days, therapy should be discontinued. The lowest possible effective dose for the individual patient should be prescribed.

Commonly used brand name(s)

In the U.S.—
Dantrium
Dantrium Intravenous

Available Dosage Forms:
* Capsule
* Powder for Solution

Therapeutic Class: Skeletal Muscle Relaxant, Direct Acting

Uses For This Medicine

Dantrolene is used to help relax certain muscles in your body. It relieves the spasms, cramping, and tightness of muscles caused by certain medical problems such as multiple sclerosis (MS), cerebral palsy, stroke, or injury to the spine. Dantrolene does not cure these problems, but it may allow other treatment, such as physical therapy, to be more helpful in improving your condition. Dantrolene acts directly on the muscles to produce its relaxant effects.

Dantrolene is also used to prevent or treat a medical problem called malignant hyperthermia that may occur in some people during or following surgery or anesthesia. Malignant hyperthermia consists of a group of symptoms including very high fever, fast and irregular heartbeat, and breathing problems. It is believed that the tendency to develop malignant hyperthermia is inherited.

Dantrolene has been shown to cause cancer and noncancerous tumors in some animals (but not in others) when given in large doses for a long time. It is not known whether long-term use of dantrolene causes cancer or tumors in humans. Before taking this medicine, be sure that you have discussed this with your doctor.

This medicine is available only with your doctor's prescription.

Before Using This Medicine

In deciding to use a medicine, the risks of taking the medicine must be weighed against the good it will do. This is a decision you and your doctor will make. For this medicine, the following should be considered:

Allergies—Tell your doctor if you have ever had any unusual or allergic reaction to this medicine or any other medicines. Also tell your health care professional if you have any other types of allergies, such as to foods, dyes, preservatives, or animals. For non-prescription products, read the label or package ingredients carefully.

Pediatric—This medicine has been tested in children 5 years of age and older and has not been shown to cause different side effects or problems than it does in adults.

Geriatric—Many medicines have not been studied specifically in older people. Therefore, it may not be known whether they work exactly the same way they do in younger adults or if they cause different side effects or problems in older people. There is no specific information comparing use of dantrolene in the elderly with use in other age groups.

Pregnancy—

	Pregnancy Category	Explanation
All Trimesters	C	Animal studies have shown an adverse effect and there are no adequate studies in pregnant women OR no animal studies have been conducted and there are no adequate studies in pregnant women.

Breast Feeding—There are no adequate studies in women for determining infant risk when using this medication during breastfeeding. Weigh the potential benefits against the potential risks before taking this medication while breastfeeding.

Other medicines—

Using this medicine with any of the following medicines is usually not recommended, but may be required in some cases. If both medicines are prescribed together, your doctor may change the dose or how often you use one or both of the medicines.

Adinazolam, Alfentanil, Alprazolam, Amobarbital, Anileridine, Aprobarbital, Bromazepam, Brotizolam, Butabarbital, Butalbital, Carisoprodol, Chloral Hydrate, Chlordiazepoxide, Chlorzoxazone, Clobazam, Clonazepam, Clorazepate, Codeine, Dantrolene, Diazepam, Estazolam, Ethchlorvynol, Fentanyl, Flunitrazepam, Flurazepam, Halazepam, Hydrocodone, Hydromorphone, Ketazolam, Levorphanol, Lorazepam, Lormetazepam, Medazepam, Meperidine, Mephenesin, Mephobarbital, Meprobamate, Metaxalone, Methocarbamol, Methohexital, Midazolam, Morphine, Morphine Sulfate Liposome, Nitrazepam, Nordazepam, Oxazepam, Oxycodone, Oxymorphone, Pentobarbital, Phenobarbital, Prazepam, Primidone, Propoxyphene, Quazepam, Remifentanil, Secobarbital, Sodium Oxybate, Sufentanil, Temazepam, Thiopental, Triazolam, Verapamil

Interactions with Food/Tobacco/Alcohol—Certain medicines should not be used at or around the time of eating food or eating certain types of food since interactions may occur. Using alcohol or tobacco with certain medicines may also cause interactions to occur. Discuss with your healthcare

professional the use of your medicine with food, alcohol, or tobacco.

Other medical problems—The presence of other medical problems may affect the use of this medicine. Make sure you tell your doctor if you have any other medical problems, especially:

- Emphysema, asthma, bronchitis, or other chronic lung disease or
- Heart disease or
- Liver disease, such as hepatitis or cirrhosis (or history of)—The chance of serious side effects may be increased

Proper Use of This Medicine

If you are unable to swallow the capsules, you may empty the number of capsules needed for one dose into a small amount of fruit juice or other liquid. Stir gently to mix the powder with the liquid before drinking. Drink the medicine right away. Rinse the glass with a little more liquid and drink that also to make sure that you have taken all of the medicine.

Dantrolene may be taken with or without food or on a full or empty stomach. However, if your doctor tells you to take the medicine a certain way, take it exactly as directed.

Take this medicine only as directed by your doctor. Do not take more of it and do not take it more often than your doctor ordered. Dantrolene may cause liver damage or other unwanted effects if too much is taken.

Dosing—The dose of this medicine will be different for different patients. Follow your doctor's orders or the directions on the label. The following information includes only the average doses of this medicine. If your dose is different, do not change it unless your doctor tells you to do so.

The amount of medicine that you take depends on the strength of the medicine. Also, the number of doses you take each day, the time allowed between doses, and the length of time you take the medicine depend on the medical problem for which you are using the medicine.

- For oral dosage form (capsules):
  - For prevention or treatment of a malignant hyperthermic crisis:
    - Adults—Dose is based on body weight and must be determined by your doctor. The usual dose is 4 to 8 milligrams (mg) per kilogram (kg) (1.8 to 3.6 mg per pound) of body weight. The doctor will instruct you exactly when and how often to take your medicine.
  - To relieve spasms:
    - Adults—To start, 25 mg once a day. The doctor may increase your dose as needed and tolerated. However, the dose is usually not more than 100 mg four times a day.
    - Children—Dose is based on body weight and must be determined by your doctor. To start, the dose is usually 0.5 mg per kg (0.23 mg per pound) of body weight twice a day. The doctor may increase the dose as needed and tolerated. However, the dose is usually not more than 3 mg per kg or 100 mg four times a day.
- For injection dosage form:
  - For prevention or treatment of a malignant hyperthermia crisis:
    - Adults, teenagers, and children—Dose is based on body weight and must be determined by your doctor.

Missed dose—If you miss a dose of this medicine, take it as soon as possible. However, if it is almost time for your next dose, skip the missed dose and go back to your regular dosing schedule. Do not double doses.

Storage—Store the medicine in a closed container at room temperature, away from heat, moisture, and direct light. Keep from freezing.

Keep out of the reach of children.

Do not keep outdated medicine or medicine no longer needed.

Precautions While Using This Medicine

If you will be taking dantrolene for a long time (for example, for several months at a time), your doctor should check your progress at regular visits. It may be necessary to have certain blood tests to check for unwanted effects while you are taking dantrolene.

This medicine will add to the effects of alcohol and other CNS depressants (medicines that slow down the nervous system, possibly causing drowsiness). Some examples of CNS depressants are antihistamines or medicine for hay fever, other allergies, or colds; sedatives, tranquilizers, or sleeping medicine; prescription pain medicine or narcotics; barbiturates; medicine for seizures; other muscle relaxants; or anesthetics, including some dental anesthetics. Therefore, do not drink alcoholic beverages, and check with your doctor before taking any of the medicines listed above, while you are using this medicine.

This medicine may cause drowsiness, dizziness or lightheadedness, vision problems, or muscle weakness in some people. Make sure you know how you react to this medicine before you drive, use machines, or do anything else that could be dangerous if you are dizzy or are not alert, well-coordinated, and able to see well.

Side Effects of This Medicine

Along with its needed effects, a medicine may cause some unwanted effects. Although not all of these side effects may occur, if they do occur they may need medical attention. Serious side effects are very rare when dantrolene is taken for a short time (for example, when it is used for a few days before, during, or after surgery or anesthesia to prevent or treat malignant hyperthermia). However, serious side effects may occur, especially when the medicine is taken for a long time.

Check with your doctor immediately if any of the following side effects occur:
> *Less common*
>> Convulsions (seizures); pain, tenderness, changes in skin color, or swelling of foot or leg; shortness of breath or slow or troubled breathing

Check with your doctor as soon as possible if any of the following side effects occur:
> *Less common*
>> Bloody or dark urine; chest pain; confusion; constipation (severe); diarrhea (severe); difficult urination; mental depression; skin rash, hives, or itching; yellow eyes or skin

Some side effects may occur that usually do not need medical attention. These side effects may go away during treatment as your body adjusts to the medicine. Also, your health care

professional may be able to tell you about ways to prevent or reduce some of these side effects. Check with your health care professional if any of the following side effects continue or are bothersome or if you have any questions about them:

More common

Diarrhea (mild); dizziness or lightheadedness; drowsiness; general feeling of discomfort or illness; muscle weakness; nausea or vomiting; unusual tiredness

Less common

Abdominal or stomach cramps or discomfort; blurred or double vision or any change in vision; chills and fever; constipation (mild); difficulty in swallowing; frequent urge to urinate or uncontrolled urination; headache; loss of appetite; slurring of speech or other speech problems; sudden decrease in amount of urine; trouble in sleeping; unusual nervousness

Other side effects not listed may also occur in some patients. If you notice any other effects, check with your healthcare professional.

DAPIPRAZOLE (Ophthalmic route) - DA-pi-pray-zole

Commonly used brand name(s)

In the U.S.—
Rev-Eyes

Available Dosage Forms:
• Powder for Solution

Therapeutic Class: Ophthalmologic Agent
Pharmacologic Class: Alpha-Adrenergic Blocker

Uses For This Medicine

Dapiprazole is used in the eye to reduce the size of the pupil after certain kinds of eye examinations.

Some eye examinations are best done when your pupil (the black center of the colored part of your eye) is very large, so the doctor can see into your eye better. This medicine helps to reduce the size of your pupil back to its normal size after the eye examination.

Before Using This Medicine

In deciding to use a medicine, the risks of taking the medicine must be weighed against the good it will do. This is a decision you and your doctor will make. For this medicine, the following should be considered:

Allergies—Tell your doctor if you have ever had any unusual or allergic reaction to this medicine or any other medicines. Also tell your health care professional if you have any other types of allergies, such as to foods, dyes, preservatives, or animals. For non-prescription products, read the label or package ingredients carefully.

Pediatric—Studies on this medicine have been done only in adult patients, and there is no specific information comparing use of dapiprazole in children with use in other age groups.

Geriatric—Many medicines have not been studied specifically in older people. Therefore, it may not be known whether they work exactly the same way they do in younger adults.

Although there is no specific information comparing use of dapiprazole in the elderly with use in other age groups, this medicine is not expected to cause different side effects or problems in older people than it does in younger adults.

Pregnancy—

	Pregnancy Category	Explanation
All Trimesters	B	Animal studies have revealed no evidence of harm to the fetus, however, there are no adequate studies in pregnant women OR animal studies have shown an adverse effect, but adequate studies in pregnant women have failed to demonstrate a risk to the fetus.

Breast Feeding—There are no adequate studies in women for determining infant risk when using this medication during breastfeeding. Weigh the potential benefits against the potential risks before taking this medication while breastfeeding.

Other medicines—Although certain medicines should not be used together at all, in other cases two different medicines may be used together even if an interaction might occur. In these cases, your doctor may want to change the dose, or other precautions may be necessary. Tell your healthcare professional if you are taking any other prescription or non-prescription (over-the-counter [OTC]) medicine.

Interactions with Food/Tobacco/Alcohol—Certain medicines should not be used at or around the time of eating food or eating certain types of food since interactions may occur. Using alcohol or tobacco with certain medicines may also cause interactions to occur. Discuss with your healthcare professional the use of your medicine with food, alcohol, or tobacco.

Other medical problems—The presence of other medical problems may affect the use of this medicine. Make sure you tell your doctor if you have any other medical problems, especially:
• Eye problems, other—Use of dapiprazole may make the condition worse

Proper Use of This Medicine

Dosing—The dose of this medicine will be different for different patients. Follow your doctor's orders or the directions on the label. The following information includes only the average doses of this medicine. If your dose is different, do not change it unless your doctor tells you to do so.

The amount of medicine that you take depends on the strength of the medicine. Also, the number of doses you take each day, the time allowed between doses, and the length of time you take the medicine depend on the medical problem for which you are using the medicine.
• For ophthalmic solution (eye drops) dosage form:
  ○ For reduction of size of pupil of eye:
    ▪ Adults—One drop, then one drop in five minutes, following eye examination.
    ▪ Children—Use and dose must be determined by your doctor.

Precautions While Using This Medicine

Even after using this medicine, you may have blurred vision or other vision problems. If any of these occur, do not drive, use machines, or do anything else that could be dangerous if you are not able to see well.

This medicine may cause your eyes to become more sensitive to light than they are normally. Wearing sunglasses and avoiding too much exposure to bright light may help lessen the discomfort.

Side Effects of This Medicine

Along with its needed effects, a medicine may cause some unwanted effects. Although not all of these side effects may occur, if they do occur they may need medical attention.

Check with your doctor as soon as possible if any of the following side effects occur:

Less common
Irritation (severe) or swelling of the clear part of the eye

Some side effects may occur that usually do not need medical attention. These side effects may go away during treatment as your body adjusts to the medicine. Also, your health care professional may be able to tell you about ways to prevent or reduce some of these side effects. Check with your health care professional if any of the following side effects continue or are bothersome or if you have any questions about them:

More common
Burning of eye when medicine is applied; redness of the white part of the eye

Less common
Blurring of vision; browache; drooping of upper eyelid; dryness of eye; headache; increased sensitivity of eye to light; itching of eye; redness of eyelid; swelling of eyelid; swelling of the membrane covering the white part of the eye; tearing of eye

Other side effects not listed may also occur in some patients. If you notice any other effects, check with your healthcare professional.

DAPSONE (Topical route) - DAP-sone

Uses For This Medicine

Dapsone belongs to the family of medicines called antibiotics. Topical dapsone preparations are used on the skin to help control acne. They may be used alone or with one or more other medicines that are applied to the skin or taken by mouth for acne. They may also be used for other problems, such as skin infections, as determined by your doctor.

This medicine is available only with your doctor's prescription.

Before Using This Medicine

In deciding to use a medicine, the risks of taking the medicine must be weighed against the good it will do. This is a decision you and your doctor will make. For this medicine, the following should be considered:

Allergies—Tell your doctor if you have ever had any unusual or allergic reaction to this medicine or any other medicines. Also tell your health care professional if you have any other types of allergies, such as to foods, dyes, preservatives, or animals. For non-prescription products, read the label or package ingredients carefully.

Pediatric—Studies on this medicine have been done only in adult and teenager patients, and there is no specific information comparing use of topical dapsone in children less than 12 years of age with use in other age groups.

Geriatric—Many medicines have not been studied specifically in older people. Therefore, it may not be known whether they work exactly the same way they do in younger adults or if they cause different side effects or problems in older people. There is no specific information comparing use of topical dapsone in the elderly with use in other age groups.

Pregnancy—

	Pregnancy Category	Explanation
All Trimesters	C	Animal studies have shown an adverse effect and there are no adequate studies in pregnant women OR no animal studies have been conducted and there are no adequate studies in pregnant women.

Breast Feeding—There are no adequate studies in women for determining infant risk when using this medication during breastfeeding. Weigh the potential benefits against the potential risks before taking this medication while breastfeeding.

Other medicines—

Using this medicine with any of the following medicines is usually not recommended, but may be required in some cases. If both medicines are prescribed together, your doctor may change the dose or how often you use one or both of the medicines.

Zidovudine

Interactions with Food/Tobacco/Alcohol—Certain medicines should not be used at or around the time of eating food or eating certain types of food since interactions may occur. Using alcohol or tobacco with certain medicines may also cause interactions to occur. Discuss with your healthcare professional the use of your medicine with food, alcohol, or tobacco.

Other medical problems—The presence of other medical problems may affect the use of this medicine. Make sure you tell your doctor if you have any other medical problems, especially:

- Anemia (history of) or
- Glucose-6–phosphate dehydrogenase (G6PD) deficiency or
- Hemoglobin M or
- Methemoglobin reductase deficiency—May increase chance of severe blood disorder.

Proper Use of This Medicine

Proper laboratory evaluation prior to starting dapsone treatment.

Not using for any other disorder other than that for which it was prescribed.

Gently washing the affected area with warm water and patting dry before applying this medicine.

Dosing—The dose of this medicine will be different for different patients. Follow your doctor's orders or the directions on the label. The following information includes only the av-

erage doses of this medicine. If your dose is different, do not change it unless your doctor tells you to do so.

The amount of medicine that you take depends on the strength of the medicine. Also, the number of doses you take each day, the time allowed between doses, and the length of time you take the medicine depend on the medical problem for which you are using the medicine.

- For gel dosage form:
  - For acne
    - Adults and teenagers—Apply a thin layer to the affected area(s) of the skin twice daily, morning and evening.
    - Children—Use and dose must be determined by your doctor.

Missed dose—If you miss a dose of this medicine, take it as soon as possible. However, if it is almost time for your next dose, skip the missed dose and go back to your regular dosing schedule. Do not double doses.

Storage—Keep out of the reach of children.

Store the medicine in a closed container at room temperature, away from heat, moisture, and direct light. Keep from freezing.

Do not keep outdated medicine or medicine no longer needed.

Precautions While Using This Medicine

Report any side effects to your physician for any blood problems that may be caused by this medicine.

Tell your doctor if you have history of anemia or an enzyme deficiency (such as G6PD).

Side Effects of This Medicine

Along with its needed effects, a medicine may cause some unwanted effects. Although not all of these side effects may occur, if they do occur they may need medical attention.

Check with your doctor as soon as possible if any of the following side effects occur:

Incidence not known
Attempts at killing oneself; bloating; body aches or pain; chills; congestion; constipation; cough; darkened urine; dryness or soreness of throat; fast heartbeat; fever; hoarseness; indigestion; loss of appetite; nausea; pains in stomach, side, or abdomen, possibly radiating to the back; runny nose; stomach pain; tender, swollen glands in neck; tonic and clonic muscle movements; trouble swallowing; voice changes; vomiting, severe

Reported in clinical trials
Discouragement; feeling sad or empty; feeling that others are watching you or controlling your behavior; feeling that others can hear your thoughts; feeling, seeing, or hearing things that are not there; irritability; loss of interest or pleasure; severe mood or mental changes; tiredness; trouble concentrating; unusual behavior

Some side effects may occur that usually do not need medical attention. These side effects may go away during treatment as your body adjusts to the medicine. Also, your health care professional may be able to tell you about ways to prevent or reduce some of these side effects. Check with your health care professional if any of the following side effects continue or are bothersome or if you have any questions about them:

More common
Dryness; flushing, redness of skin; oiliness/peeling; unusually warm skin

Less common
Burning; diarrhea; difficulty breathing; ear congestion; headache; itching skin; general feeling of discomfort or illness; headache; joint pain; joint sprain; muscle aches and pains; pain or tenderness around eyes and cheekbones; shivering; shortness of breath or trouble breathing; sneezing; sore throat; stuffy nose; sweating; tightness of chest or wheezing; trouble sleeping; unusual tiredness or weakness

Incidence not known
Facial swelling

Other side effects not listed may also occur in some patients. If you notice any other effects, check with your healthcare professional.

DAPTOMYCIN   (Intravenous route) -
DAP-toe-mye-sin

Commonly used brand name(s)

In the U.S.—
Cubicin

Available Dosage Forms:
- Powder for Solution

Therapeutic Class: Antibiotic

Uses For This Medicine

Daptomycin belongs to the family of medicines called antibiotics. Antibiotics are medicines used in the treatment of infections caused by bacteria. They work by killing bacteria or preventing their growth. Daptomycin will not work for colds, flu, or other virus infections.

Daptomycin is used to treat complicated skin infections. It is also used to treat infections in the bloodstream caused by a bacteria called *Staphylococcus aureus*.

This medicine is available only with your doctor's prescription.

Before Receiving This Medicine

In deciding to use a medicine, the risks of taking the medicine must be weighed against the good it will do. This is a decision you and your doctor will make. For this medicine, the following should be considered:

Allergies—Tell your doctor if you have ever had any unusual or allergic reaction to this medicine or any other medicines. Also tell your health care professional if you have any other types of allergies, such as to foods, dyes, preservatives, or animals. For non-prescription products, read the label or package ingredients carefully.

Pediatric—Studies on this medicine have been done only in adult patients, and there is no specific information comparing use of daptomycin in children with use in other age groups.

Geriatric—Elderly people are especially sensitive to the effects of daptomycin. This may increase the chance of side effects during treatment.

Pregnancy—

	Pregnancy Category	Explanation
All Trimesters	B	Animal studies have revealed no evidence of harm to the fetus, however, there are no adequate studies in pregnant women OR animal studies have shown an adverse effect, but adequate studies in pregnant women have failed to demonstrate a risk to the fetus.

Breast Feeding—There are no adequate studies in women for determining infant risk when using this medication during breastfeeding. Weigh the potential benefits against the potential risks before taking this medication while breastfeeding.

Other medicines—Although certain medicines should not be used together at all, in other cases two different medicines may be used together even if an interaction might occur. In these cases, your doctor may want to change the dose, or other precautions may be necessary. Tell your healthcare professional if you are taking any other prescription or non-prescription (over-the-counter [OTC]) medicine.

Interactions with Food/Tobacco/Alcohol—Certain medicines should not be used at or around the time of eating food or eating certain types of food since interactions may occur. Using alcohol or tobacco with certain medicines may also cause interactions to occur. Discuss with your healthcare professional the use of your medicine with food, alcohol, or tobacco.

Other medical problems—The presence of other medical problems may affect the use of this medicine. Make sure you tell your doctor if you have any other medical problems, especially:

- Kidney disease—Your doctor may need to lower your dose
- Liver disease—Studies on this medicine have not been done in patients with severe liver disease.
- Muscle problems—May be worsened by daptomycin.

Proper Use of This Medicine

Dosing—The dose of this medicine will be different for different patients. Follow your doctor's orders or the directions on the label. The following information includes only the average doses of this medicine. If your dose is different, do not change it unless your doctor tells you to do so.

The amount of medicine that you take depends on the strength of the medicine. Also, the number of doses you take each day, the time allowed between doses, and the length of time you take the medicine depend on the medical problem for which you are using the medicine.

To help clear up your infection completely, daptomycin must be given for the full time of treatment, even if you begin to feel better after a few days. Also, this medicine works best when there is a constant amount in the blood. To help keep the amount constant, daptomycin must be given on a regular schedule.

- For injection dosage form:
  - For complicated skin infections caused by bacteria:
    - Adults—4 milligrams (mg) per kilogram (kg) (1.82 mg per pound) of body weight injected into a vein every 24 hours.
    - Children—Use and dose must be determined by your doctor.
  - For bloodstream infections caused by bacteria:
    - Adults—6 mg per kg (2.73 mg per pound) of body weight injected into a vein every 24 hours.
    - Children—Use and dose must be determined by your doctor.

Missed dose—If you miss a dose of this medicine, take it as soon as possible. However, if it is almost time for your next dose, skip the missed dose and go back to your regular dosing schedule. Do not double doses.

Do not take more than one dose each day.

Storage—Store in the refrigerator. Do not freeze.

Keep out of the reach of children.

Do not keep outdated medicine or medicine no longer needed.

Ask your healthcare professional how you should dispose of any medicine you do not use.

Precautions After Receiving This Medicine

If you have muscle pain or weakness while receiving this medicine, check with your doctor right away.

If your symptoms do not improve within a few days or if they become worse, check with your doctor.

Do not take other medicines unless they have been discussed with your doctor. This especially includes nonprescription medicines, such as aspirin, and medicines for appetite control, asthma, colds, cough, hay fever, or sinus problems.

Side Effects of This Medicine

Along with its needed effects, a medicine may cause some unwanted effects. Although not all of these side effects may occur, if they do occur they may need medical attention.

Check with your doctor immediately if any of the following side effects occur:

Less common
   Agitation; bladder pain; bloody or cloudy urine; blurred vision; coma; confusion; decreased urine output; depression; difficult, burning, or painful urination; dizziness; faintness, or lightheadedness when getting up from a lying or sitting position suddenly; frequent urge to urinate; headache; hostility; irritability; itching in genital or other skin areas; lethargy; lower back or side pain; muscle twitching; nausea; nervousness; pale skin; pounding in the ears; rapid weight gain; scaling; seizures; slow or fast heartbeat; stupor; sweating; swelling of face, ankles, or hands; troubled breathing with exertion; unusual bleeding or bruising; usual tiredness or weakness

Frequency not determined
   Abdominal or stomach cramps; abdominal tenderness; bloating; diarrhea, watery and severe, which may also

be bloody; fever; increased thirst; pain; unusual weight loss; vomiting

Some side effects may occur that usually do not need medical attention. These side effects may go away during treatment as your body adjusts to the medicine. Also, your health care professional may be able to tell you about ways to prevent or reduce some of these side effects. Check with your health care professional if any of the following side effects continue or are bothersome or if you have any questions about them:

More common
Bleeding, blistering, burning, coldness, discoloration of skin, feeling of pressure, hives, infection, inflammation, itching, lumps, numbness, pain, rash, redness, scarring, soreness, stinging, swelling, tenderness, tingling, ulceration, or warmth at site of injection; diarrhea, mild; difficulty having a bowel movement (stool)

Less common
Difficult or labored breathing; itching skin; limb pain; shortness of breath; skin rash; sleeplessness; tightness in chest; trouble sleeping; unable to sleep; wheezing

Rare
Acid or sour stomach; belching; difficulty in moving; heartburn; indigestion; muscle pain or stiffness; pain in joints

Other side effects not listed may also occur in some patients. If you notice any other effects, check with your healthcare professional.

Other side effects not listed may also occur in some patients. If you notice any other effects, check with your healthcare professional.

DARBEPOETIN ALFA (Injection route) - dar-be-POE-e-tin AL-fa

Commonly used brand name(s)

In the U.S.—
Aranesp

Available Dosage Forms:
• Solution

Therapeutic Class: Hematopoietic
Pharmacologic Class: Erythropoietic

Uses For This Medicine

Darbepoetin alfa stimulates the bone marrow to produce red blood cells. If the body does not produce enough red blood cells, severe anemia can occur. This often occurs in people with chronic kidney failure whose kidneys are not working properly. Anemia can also occur in people who have cancer and are receiving chemotherapy to treat their cancer. Darbepoetin alfa is used to treat severe anemia in these people. Darbepoetin may be used for patients on dialysis and for patients not on dialysis.

Darbepoetin alfa is given by injection. It is available only with your doctor's prescription.

Once a medicine has been approved for marketing for a certain use, experience may show that it is also useful for other medical problems. Although this use is not included in product

labeling, darbepoetin alfa is used in certain patients with the following medical condition:
• Anemia associated with cancer (in patients not receiving chemotherapy)

Before Receiving This Medicine

In deciding to use a medicine, the risks of taking the medicine must be weighed against the good it will do. This is a decision you and your doctor will make. For this medicine, the following should be considered:

Allergies—Tell your doctor if you have ever had any unusual or allergic reaction to this medicine or any other medicines. Also tell your health care professional if you have any other types of allergies, such as to foods, dyes, preservatives, or animals. For non-prescription products, read the label or package ingredients carefully.

Pediatric—Appropriate studies performed to date have not demonstrated pediatrics-specific problems that would limit the usefulness of darbepoetin alfa in children with chronic kidney failure who are over 1 year of age. Safety and efficacy have not been established in children with chronic kidney failure who are less than 1 year of age.

No information is available on the relationship of age to the effects of darbepoetin alfa in children with cancer. Safety and efficacy have not been established.

Geriatric—This medicine has been tested and has not been shown to cause different side effects or problems in older people than it does in younger adults.

Pregnancy—

	Pregnancy Category	Explanation
All Trimesters	C	Animal studies have shown an adverse effect and there are no adequate studies in pregnant women OR no animal studies have been conducted and there are no adequate studies in pregnant women.

Breast Feeding—There are no adequate studies in women for determining infant risk when using this medication during breastfeeding. Weigh the potential benefits against the potential risks before taking this medication while breastfeeding.

Other medicines—
Using this medicine with any of the following medicines is usually not recommended, but may be required in some cases. If both medicines are prescribed together, your doctor may change the dose or how often you use one or both of the medicines.

Thalidomide

Interactions with Food/Tobacco/Alcohol—Certain medicines should not be used at or around the time of eating food or eating certain types of food since interactions may occur. Using alcohol or tobacco with certain medicines may also cause interactions to occur. Discuss with your healthcare professional the use of your medicine with food, alcohol, or tobacco.

Other medical problems—The presence of other medical problems may affect the use of this medicine. Make sure you tell your doctor if you have any other medical problems, especially:
• Aluminum poisoning or

- Bone marrow problems or
- Bone problems or
- Cancer or
- Folic acid deficiency or
- Infection or
- Inflammation or
- Vitamin B 12 deficiency—May cause a decrease or delay in response to treatment with darbepoetin alfa.
- Blood or bleeding problems (history of)—The safe use of darbepoetin has not been determined for patients with a history of bleeding problems.
- Heart or blood vessel disease—May be worsened by taking darbepoetin alfa.
- High blood pressure—May become worse when taking darbepoetin.
- Pure red cell aplasia (rare bone marrow disorder resulting in less red blood cells than normal)—Darbepoetin should not be used if you have this condition because it could cause this medicine to not work.

Proper Use of This Medicine

Darbepoetin alfa is usually given by a health care professional. However, medicines given by injection are sometimes used at home. If you will be using darbepoetin alfa at home, your health care professional will teach you how the injections are to be given. You will also have a chance to practice giving them. Be certain that you understand exactly how the medicine is to be injected. Do not reuse needles and syringes.

Put used needles and syringes in a puncture-resistant disposable container, or dispose of them as directed by your health care professional.

Dosing—The dose of this medicine will be different for different patients. Follow your doctor's orders or the directions on the label. The following information includes only the average doses of this medicine. If your dose is different, do not change it unless your doctor tells you to do so.

The amount of medicine that you take depends on the strength of the medicine. Also, the number of doses you take each day, the time allowed between doses, and the length of time you take the medicine depend on the medical problem for which you are using the medicine.

- For injection dosage form
  - For anemia from chronic kidney failure:
    - Adults—Dose is based on body weight and must be determined by your doctor. Darbepoetin alfa is injected into a vein or under the skin. How often you take this medicine must be determined by your doctor. Your doctor may need to adjust the dose to determine the best dose for you.
    - Children—Use and dose must be determined by your doctor.
  - For anemia from cancer chemotherapy:
    - Adults—Dose is based on body weight and must be determined by your doctor. Darbepoetin alfa is injected into a vein or under the skin. How often you take this medicine must be determined by your doctor. Your doctor may need to adjust the dose to determine the best dose for you.
    - Children—Use and dose must be determined by your doctor.

Missed dose—Call your doctor or pharmacist for instructions.

Storage—Store in the refrigerator. Do not freeze.

Keep out of the reach of children.

Do not keep outdated medicine or medicine no longer needed.

Precautions After Receiving This Medicine

People with severe anemia usually feel very tired and sick. When darbepoetin alfa begins to work, usually in about 6 weeks, most people start to feel better. Some people are able to be more active. However, darbepoetin alfa only corrects anemia. It has no effect on kidney disease, cancer or any other medical problem that needs regular medical attention. Therefore, even if you are feeling much better, it is very important that you do not miss any appointments with your doctor or any dialysis treatments.

It is very important that your doctor check your blood regularly while you are taking this medicine. Be sure and keep all of your appointments.

Many people with kidney problems need to be on a special diet. Also, people with high blood pressure (which may be caused by kidney disease or by darbepoetin alfa treatment) may need to be on a special diet and/or to take medicine to keep their blood pressure under control. After their anemia has been corrected, some people feel so much better that they want to eat more than before. To keep your kidney disease or your high blood pressure from getting worse, it is very important that you follow your special diet and take your medicines regularly, even if you are feeling better.

If you are giving this medicine at home:
- Use a new needle and syringe each time you inject your medicine.
- Do not use more medicine or use it more often than your doctor tells you to.
- You will be shown the body areas where this shot can be given.
- Throw away used needles in a hard closed container that the needles cannot poke through. Keep this container away from children and pets.

In addition to darbepoetin alfa, your body needs iron to make red blood cells. Your doctor may direct you to take iron supplements. He or she may also direct you to take certain vitamins that help the iron work better. Be sure to follow your doctor's orders carefully, because darbepoetin alfa will not work properly if there is not enough iron in your body.

Side Effects of This Medicine

Along with its needed effects, a medicine may cause some unwanted effects. Although not all of these side effects may occur, if they do occur they may need medical attention.

Check with your doctor immediately if any of the following side effects occur:
  More common
    Abdominal or stomach pain; accumulation of pus; arm, back or jaw pain; blurred vision; breathing difficulties (irregular, noisy, trouble at rest); chest pain, discomfort, tightness, or heaviness; chills; confusion; cough producing mucus; decrease in amount of urine; diarrhea; dilated neck veins; dizziness or lightheadedness; fainting or lightheadedness; fast, slow, or irregular heartbeat; fatigue or tiredness (extreme or unusual); fever; headache; nausea; pain, tenderness, swelling or

warmth over injection site; shortness of breath or troubled breathing; pounding in the ears; rapid breathing; rapid or pounding pulse; skin discoloration at injection site; sweating; swelling of ankles, face, fingers, feet, hands, or lower legs; unconsciousness; vomiting; weight gain; wheezing

Less common

Anxiety; convulsions; difficulty in speaking (slow speech or inability to speak); double vision; inability to move arms, legs, or facial muscles (including numbness and tingling); trouble thinking or walking

Rare

Fever and sore throat; hives; itching; pale skin; skin rash; unusual bleeding or bruising; unusual tiredness or weaknessSome side effects may occur that usually do not need medical attention. These side effects may go away during treatment as your body adjusts to the medicine. Also, your health care professional may be able to tell you about ways to prevent or reduce some of these side effects. Check with your health care professional if any of the following side effects continue or are bothersome or if you have any questions about them:

More common

Constipation; general feeling of discomfort or illness; lack or loss of strength; loss of appetite; muscle aches, pains, or stiffness; runny nose; pain in joints; shivering; sneezing; sore throat; trouble sleeping

Less common

Confusion; decreased urination; dry mouth; lightheadedness; sunken eyes; thirst; wrinkled skin

Other side effects not listed may also occur in some patients. If you notice any other effects, check with your healthcare professional.

DARIFENACIN (Oral route) - dar-i-FEN-a-sin

Commonly used brand name(s)

In the U.S.—
Enablex

Available Dosage Forms:
• Tablet, Extended Release

Therapeutic Class: Urinary Antispasmodic
Pharmacologic Class: Antimuscarinic

Uses For This Medicine

Darifenacin is used to treat bladder problems such as frequent need to urinate or loss of control of urinary function.

This medicine is available only with your doctor's prescription.

Before Using This Medicine

In deciding to use a medicine, the risks of taking the medicine must be weighed against the good it will do. This is a decision you and your doctor will make. For this medicine, the following should be considered:

Allergies—Tell your doctor if you have ever had any unusual or allergic reaction to this medicine or any other medicines. Also tell your health care professional if you have any other types of allergies, such as to foods, dyes, preservatives, or animals. For non-prescription products, read the label or package ingredients carefully.

Pediatric—Studies on this medicine have been done only in adult patients, and there is no specific information comparing use of darifenacin in children with use in other age groups.

Geriatric—This medicine has been tested and has not been shown to cause different side effects or problems in older people than it does in younger adults.

Pregnancy—

	Pregnancy Category	Explanation
All Trimesters	C	Animal studies have shown an adverse effect and there are no adequate studies in pregnant women OR no animal studies have been conducted and there are no adequate studies in pregnant women.

Breast Feeding—There are no adequate studies in women for determining infant risk when using this medication during breastfeeding. Weigh the potential benefits against the potential risks before taking this medication while breastfeeding.

Other medicines—

Using this medicine with any of the following medicines is usually not recommended, but may be required in some cases. If both medicines are prescribed together, your doctor may change the dose or how often you use one or both of the medicines.

Desipramine, Flecainide, Imipramine, Thioridazine

Interactions with Food/Tobacco/Alcohol—Certain medicines should not be used at or around the time of eating food or eating certain types of food since interactions may occur. Using alcohol or tobacco with certain medicines may also cause interactions to occur. Discuss with your healthcare professional the use of your medicine with food, alcohol, or tobacco.

Other medical problems—The presence of other medical problems may affect the use of this medicine. Make sure you tell your doctor if you have any other medical problems, especially:
• Glaucoma or
• Stomach problems or
• Urinary retention—You should not use darifenacin; it will make these conditions worse.
• Liver problems—You should not use darifenacin if you have severe liver problems.

Proper Use of This Medicine

Dosing—The dose of this medicine will be different for different patients. Follow your doctor's orders or the directions on the label. The following information includes only the average doses of this medicine. If your dose is different, do not change it unless your doctor tells you to do so.

The amount of medicine that you take depends on the strength of the medicine. Also, the number of doses you take each day, the time allowed between doses, and the length of

time you take the medicine depend on the medical problem for which you are using the medicine.

- For oral dosage form (tablets):
  - To treat bladder problems:
    - Adults—7.5 milligrams (mg) once a day.
    - Children—Use and dose must be determined by your doctor.

Missed dose—If you miss a dose of this medicine, skip the missed dose and go back to your regular dosing schedule. Do not double doses.

Storage—Store the medicine in a closed container at room temperature, away from heat, moisture, and direct light. Keep from freezing.

Keep out of the reach of children.

Do not keep outdated medicine or medicine no longer needed.

Ask your healthcare professional how you should dispose of any medicine you do not use.

Precautions While Using This Medicine

This medicine may cause some people to have vision problems. Make sure your vision is clear before you drive or do anything else that could be dangerous if you are not able to see well.

Use caution during exercise or hot weather. Overheating may result in heat exhaustion.

This medicine may cause constipation, call your doctor if you get severe stomach pain or become constipated.

This medicine may cause dryness of the mouth. For temporary relief of mouth dryness, use sugarless candy or gum, melt bits of ice in your mouth, or use a saliva substitute. However, if your mouth continues to feel dry for more than 2 weeks, check with your medical doctor or dentist.

Side Effects of This Medicine

Along with its needed effects, a medicine may cause some unwanted effects. Although not all of these side effects may occur, if they do occur they may need medical attention.

Check with your doctor immediately if any of the following side effects occur:

Frequency unknown
Decrease in frequency of urination; decrease in urine volume; difficulty in passing urine; dribbling, painful urination

Symptoms of overdose

Get emergency help immediately if any of the following symptoms of overdose occur:

Changes in vision

Some side effects may occur that usually do not need medical attention. These side effects may go away during treatment as your body adjusts to the medicine. Also, your health care professional may be able to tell you about ways to prevent or reduce some of these side effects. Check with your health care professional if any of the following side effects continue or are bothersome or if you have any questions about them:

More common
Acid or sour stomach; belching; difficulty having a bowel movement (stool); dry mouth; heartburn; indigestion; stomach discomfort upset or pain

Less common
Bladder pain; bloody or cloudy urine; diarrhea; difficult, burning, or painful urination; dizziness; dry eyes; frequent urge to urinate; lack or loss of strength; lower back or side pain; nausea

Frequency unknown
Accidental injury; bloating or swelling of face, arms, hands, lower legs, or feet; blurred vision; changes in vision; chills; congestion; cough producing mucus; difficulty breathing; difficulty in moving; dry skin; dryness or soreness of throat; fever; general feeling of discomfort or illness; headache; hoarseness; itching of the vagina or genital area; itching skin; joint pain; loss of appetite; muscle aches and pains; muscle pain or stiffness; nervousness; pain during sexual intercourse; pain in joints; pain or tenderness around eyes and cheekbones; pounding in the ears; rash; runny nose; shortness of breath or troubled breathing; slow or fast heartbeat; sneezing; stuffy nose; tender, swollen glands in neck; thick, white vaginal discharge with no odor or with a mild odor; tightness in chest; tingling of hands or feet; trouble in swallowing; unusual weight gain or loss; voice changes; vomiting; wheezing

Other side effects not listed may also occur in some patients. If you notice any other effects, check with your healthcare professional.

DAUNORUBICIN (Intravenous route) - daw-noe-ROO-bi-sin

Black Box Warning

Daunorubicin hydrochloride injection must be given into a rapidly flowing intravenous infusion. It must never be given by the intramuscular or subcutaneous route. Severe local tissue necrosis will occur if there is extravasation during administration.

Myocardial toxicity manifested in its most severe form by potentially fatal congestive heart failure may occur either during therapy or months to years after termination of therapy. The incidence of myocardial toxicity increases after a total cumulative dose exceeding 400 to 550 mg/m(2) in adults, 300 mg/m(2) in children more than 2 years of age, or 10 mg/kg in children less than 2 years of age.

Severe myelosuppression occurs when used in therapeutic doses; this may lead to infection or hemorrhage.

It is recommended that daunorubicin hydrochloride be administered only by physicians who are experienced in leukemia chemotherapy and in facilities with laboratory and supportive resources adequate to monitor drug tolerance and protect and maintain a patient compromised by drug toxicity. The physician and institution must be capable of responding rapidly and completely to severe hemorrhagic conditions and/or overwhelming infection.

Dosage should be reduced in patients with impaired hepatic or renal function.

Commonly used brand name(s)

In the U.S.—
Cerubidine

Available Dosage Forms:
- Solution
- Powder for Solution

Therapeutic Class: Antineoplastic Agent

Uses For This Medicine

Daunorubicin belongs to the general group of medicines known as antineoplastics. It is used to treat some kinds of cancer.

Daunorubicin seems to interfere with the growth of cancer cells, which are eventually destroyed. Since the growth of normal body cells may also be affected by daunorubicin, other effects will also occur. Some of these may be serious and must be reported to your doctor. Other effects, like hair loss, may not be serious but may cause concern. Some effects may not occur for months or years after the medicine is used.

Before you begin treatment with daunorubicin, you and your doctor should talk about the good this medicine will do as well as the risks of using it.

Daunorubicin is to be administered only by or under the immediate supervision of your doctor.

Before Using This Medicine

In deciding to use a medicine, the risks of taking the medicine must be weighed against the good it will do. This is a decision you and your doctor will make. For this medicine, the following should be considered:

Allergies—Tell your doctor if you have ever had any unusual or allergic reaction to this medicine or any other medicines. Also tell your health care professional if you have any other types of allergies, such as to foods, dyes, preservatives, or animals. For non-prescription products, read the label or package ingredients carefully.

Pediatric—Although daunorubicin is used in children, there is no specific information comparing use in children with use in other age groups.

Geriatric—Heart problems are more likely to occur in the elderly, who are usually more sensitive to the effects of daunorubicin. The elderly may also be more likely to have blood problems.

Pregnancy—

	Pregnancy Category	Explanation
All Trimesters	D	Studies in pregnant women have demonstrated a risk to the fetus. However, the benefits of therapy in a life threatening situation or a serious disease, may outweigh the potential risk.

Breast Feeding—There are no adequate studies in women for determining infant risk when using this medication during breastfeeding. Weigh the potential benefits against the potential risks before taking this medication while breastfeeding.

Other medicines—

Using this medicine with any of the following medicines is not recommended. Your doctor may decide not to treat you with this medication or change some of the other medicines you take.

Rotavirus Vaccine, Live

Interactions with Food/Tobacco/Alcohol—Certain medicines should not be used at or around the time of eating food or eating certain types of food since interactions may occur. Using alcohol or tobacco with certain medicines may also cause interactions to occur. Discuss with your healthcare professional the use of your medicine with food, alcohol, or tobacco.

Other medical problems—The presence of other medical problems may affect the use of this medicine. Make sure you tell your doctor if you have any other medical problems, especially:
- Chickenpox (including recent exposure) or
- Herpes zoster (shingles)—Risk of severe disease affecting other parts of the body
- Gout (history of) or
- Kidney stones—Daunorubicin may increase uric acid in the body, which can cause gout or kidney stones
- Heart disease—Risk of heart problems caused by daunorubicin may be increased
- Infection—Daunorubicin can decrease your body's ability to fight infection
- Kidney disease or
- Liver disease—Effects of daunorubicin may be increased because of slower removal from the body

Proper Use of This Medicine

Daunorubicin is sometimes given together with certain other medicines. If you are using a combination of medicines, it is important that you receive each one at the proper time. If you are taking some of these medicines by mouth, ask your health care professional to help you plan a way to take them at the right times.

While you are receiving daunorubicin, your doctor may want you to drink extra fluids so that you will pass more urine. This will help prevent kidney problems and keep your kidneys working well.

This medicine often causes nausea and vomiting. However, it is very important that you continue to receive it, even if you begin to feel ill. Ask your health care professional for ways to lessen these effects.

Dosing—The dose of this medicine will be different for different patients. Follow your doctor's orders or the directions on the label. The following information includes only the average doses of this medicine. If your dose is different, do not change it unless your doctor tells you to do so.

The amount of medicine that you take depends on the strength of the medicine. Also, the number of doses you take each day, the time allowed between doses, and the length of time you take the medicine depend on the medical problem for which you are using the medicine.

Precautions While Using This Medicine

It is very important that your doctor check your progress at regular visits to make sure that this medicine is working properly and to check for unwanted effects.

While you are being treated with daunorubicin, and after you stop treatment with it, do not have any immunizations (vaccinations) without your doctor's approval. Daunorubicin may lower your body's resistance and there is a chance you might get the infection the immunization is meant to prevent. In addition, other persons living in your household should not take oral polio vaccine since there is a chance they could pass the polio virus on to you. Also, avoid persons who have taken oral polio vaccine. Do not get close to them, and do not stay in the same room with them for very long. If you cannot take these precautions, you should consider wearing a protective face mask that covers the nose and mouth.

Daunorubicin can temporarily lower the number of white blood cells in your blood, increasing the chance of getting an infection. It can also lower the number of platelets, which are necessary for proper blood clotting. If this occurs, there are certain precautions you can take, especially when your blood count is low, to reduce the risk of infection or bleeding:

- If you can, avoid people with infections. Check with your doctor immediately if you think you are getting an infection or if you get a fever or chills, cough or hoarseness, lower back or side pain, or painful or difficult urination.
- Check with your doctor immediately if you notice any unusual bleeding or bruising; black, tarry stools; blood in urine or stools; or pinpoint red spots on your skin.
- Be careful when using a regular toothbrush, dental floss, or toothpick. Your medical doctor, dentist, or nurse may recommend other ways to clean your teeth and gums. Check with your medical doctor before having any dental work done.
- Do not touch your eyes or the inside of your nose unless you have just washed your hands and have not touched anything else in the meantime.
- Be careful not to cut yourself when you are using sharp objects such as a safety razor or fingernail or toenail cutters.
- Avoid contact sports or other situations where bruising or injury could occur.

If daunorubicin accidentally seeps out of the vein into which it is injected, it may damage some tissues and cause scarring. Tell the doctor or nurse right away if you notice redness, pain, or swelling at the place of injection.

Side Effects of This Medicine

Along with its needed effects, a medicine may cause some unwanted effects. Although not all of these side effects may occur, if they do occur they may need medical attention.

Also, because of the way these medicines act on the body, there is a chance that they might cause other unwanted effects that may not occur until months or years after the medicine is used. These delayed effects may include certain types of cancer, such as leukemia. Discuss these possible effects with your doctor.

Check with your doctor immediately if any of the following side effects occur:

Less common
Cough or hoarseness; fever or chills; irregular heartbeat; lower back or side pain; pain at place of injection; painful or difficult urination; shortness of breath; swelling of feet and lower legs

Rare
Black, tarry stools; blood in urine or stools; pinpoint red spots on skin; unusual bleeding or bruising

Check with your doctor as soon as possible if any of the following side effects occur:

More common
Sores in mouth and on lips

Less common
Joint pain

Rare
Skin rash or itching

Some side effects may occur that usually do not need medical attention. These side effects may go away during treatment as your body adjusts to the medicine. Also, your health care professional may be able to tell you about ways to prevent or reduce some of these side effects. Check with your health care professional if any of the following side effects continue or are bothersome or if you have any questions about them:

More common
Nausea and vomiting

Less common or rare
Darkening or redness of skin; diarrhea

Daunorubicin causes the urine to turn reddish in color, which may stain clothes. This is not blood. It is perfectly normal and lasts for only 1 or 2 days after each dose is given.

This medicine often causes a temporary and total loss of hair. After treatment with daunorubicin has ended, normal hair growth should return.

After you stop using this medicine, it may still produce some side effects that need attention. During this period of time, *check with your doctor immediately* if you notice the following side effects:

Irregular heartbeat; shortness of breath; swelling of feet and lower legs

Other side effects not listed may also occur in some patients. If you notice any other effects, check with your healthcare professional.

DECONGESTANTS AND ANALGESICS (Systemic)

Some commonly used brand names are:

In the U.S.—

Actifed Sinus Daytime (2)
Actifed Sinus Daytime Caplets (2)
Advil Cold and Sinus (3)
Advil Cold and Sinus Caplets (3)
Allerest No-Drowsiness Caplets (2)
Coldrine (2)
Contac Allergy/Sinus Day Caplets (2)
Dristan Cold Caplets (2)
Dristan Sinus Caplets (2)
Motrin IB Sinus (3)
Motrin IB Sinus Caplets (3)
Ornex Maximum Strength Caplets (2)
PhenAPAP Without Drowsiness (2)
Sinarest No-Drowsiness Caplets (2)
Sine-Aid Maximum Strength (2)
Sine-Aid Maximum Strength Caplets (2)
Sine-Off Maximum Strength No Drowsiness Formula Caplets (2)
Sinus-Relief (2)
Sinutab Sinus Maximum Strength Without Drowsiness (2)
Sudafed Sinus Maximum Strength Without Drowsiness (2)
Sudafed Sinus Maximum Strength Without Drowsiness Caplets (2)
Tylenol Sinus Maximum Strength (2)
Tylenol Sinus Maximum Strength Caplets (2)
Tylenol Sinus Maximum Strength Gelcaps (2)
Tylenol Sinus Maximum Strength Geltabs (2)

In Canada—

Dristan N.D. Caplets (2)
Dristan N.D. Extra Strength
    Caplets (2)
Neo Citran Extra Strength
    Sinus (1)
Sinutab No Drowsiness
    Caplets (2)
Sinutab No Drowsiness Extra
    Strength Caplets (2)

Sudafed Head Cold and
    Sinus Extra Strength Caplets
    (2)
Tylenol Sinus Medication
    Regular Strength Caplets (2)
Tylenol Sinus Medication
    Extra Strength Caplets (2)

This information applies to the following medicines:

1. Phenylephrine and Acetaminophen (fen-ill-EF-rin and a-seat-a-MIN-oh-fen)
2. Pseudoephedrine and Acetaminophen (soo-doe-e-FED-rin and a-seat-a-MIN-oh-fen)
3. Pseudoephedrine and Ibuprofen (soo-doe-e-FED-rin and eye-byoo-PRO-fen)

Category

• Decongestant-analgesic—

Description

Decongestant and analgesic combinations are taken by mouth to relieve sinus and nasal congestion (stuffy nose) and headache of colds, allergy, and hay fever.

Decongestants, such as phenylephrine, and pseudoephedrine produce a narrowing of blood vessels. This leads to clearing of nasal congestion, but it may also cause an increase in blood pressure in patients who have high blood pressure.

Analgesics, such as acetaminophen, ibuprofen, and salicylates (e.g., aspirin, salicylamide), are used in these combination medicines to help relieve headache and sinus pain.

Acetaminophen and salicylates may cause kidney damage or cancer of the kidney or urinary bladder if large amounts of both medicines are taken together for a long time. However, taking the recommended amounts of combination medicines that contain both acetaminophen and a salicylate for short periods of time has not been shown to cause these unwanted effects.

These medicines are available without a prescription. However, your doctor may have special instructions on the proper dose of these medicines for your medical condition. They are available in the following dosage forms:

Oral
  • Phenylephrine and Acetaminophen
    ○ For oral solution
  • Pseudoephedrine and Acetaminophen
    ○ Capsules
    ○ Tablets
  • Pseudoephedrine and Ibuprofen
    ○ Tablets

Before Using This Medicine

If you are taking this medicine without a prescription, carefully read and follow any precautions on the label. For decongestant and analgesic combinations, the following should be considered:

Allergies—Tell your doctor if you have ever had any unusual or allergic reaction to any of the ingredients contained in this medicine.

If this medicine contains *aspirin, salicylamide*, or *ibuprofen*, before taking it check with your doctor if you have ever had any unusual or allergic reaction to any of the following medicines:

  • Aspirin or other salicylates
  • Diclofenac (e.g., Voltaren)
  • Diflunisal (e.g., Dolobid)
  • Etodolac (e.g., Lodine)
  • Fenoprofen (e.g., Nalfon)
  • Floctafenine (e.g., Idarac)
  • Flurbiprofen, by mouth (e.g., Ansaid)
  • Ibuprofen (e.g., Motrin)
  • Indomethacin (e.g., Indocin)
  • Ketoprofen (e.g., Orudis)
  • Ketorolac (e.g., Toradol)
  • Meclofenamate (e.g., Meclomen)
  • Mefenamic acid (e.g., Ponstel)
  • Methyl salicylate (oil of wintergreen)
  • Nabumetone (e.g., Relafen)
  • Naproxen (e.g., Naprosyn)
  • Oxaprozin (e.g., Daypro)
  • Oxyphenbutazone (e.g., Tandearil)
  • Phenylbutazone (e.g., Butazolidin)
  • Piroxicam (e.g., Feldene)
  • Sulindac (e.g., Clinoril)
  • Suprofen (e.g., Suprol)
  • Tenoxicam (e.g., Mobiflex)
  • Tiaprofenic acid (e.g., Surgam)
  • Tolmetin (e.g., Tolectin)
  • Zomepirac (e.g., Zomax)

Also tell your health care professional if you are allergic to any other substances, such as foods, preservatives, or dyes.

Pregnancy—The occasional use of decongestant and analgesic combinations at the doses recommended on the label is not likely to cause problems in the fetus or in the newborn baby. However, for the individual ingredients of these combinations, the following information applies:

  • *Alcohol*—Some of these combination medicines contain large amounts of alcohol. Too much use of alcohol during pregnancy may cause birth defects.
  • *Caffeine*—Studies in humans have not shown that caffeine causes birth defects. However, studies in animals have shown that caffeine causes birth defects when given in very large doses (amounts equal to the amount of caffeine contained in 12 to 24 cups of coffee a day).
  • *Ibuprofen*—Studies on birth defects have not been done in humans. However, there is a chance that ibuprofen may cause unwanted effects on the heart or blood flow of the fetus or newborn baby if it is taken regularly during the last few months of pregnancy.
  • *Phenylephrine*—Studies on birth defects have not been done in either humans or animals with phenylephrine.
  • *Pseudoephedrine*—Studies on birth defects with pseudoephedrine have not been done in humans. In animal studies pseudoephedrine did not cause birth defects.

However, when given to animals in high doses, pseudoephedrine did cause a decrease in average weight, length, and rate of bone formation in the animal fetus.

- *Salicylates (e.g., aspirin)*—Studies on birth defects in humans have been done with aspirin, but not with salicylamide. Although salicylates have been shown to cause birth defects in animals, they have not been shown to cause birth defects in humans. Regular use of salicylates late in pregnancy may cause unwanted effects on the heart or blood flow in the fetus or newborn baby. Use of salicylates during the last 2 weeks of pregnancy may cause bleeding problems in the fetus before or during delivery, or in the newborn baby. Also, too much use of salicylates during the last 3 months of pregnancy may increase the length of pregnancy, prolong labor and cause other problems during delivery, or cause severe bleeding in the mother before, during, or after delivery. *Do not take aspirin during the last 3 months of pregnancy unless it has been ordered by your doctor.*

Breast-feeding—If you are breast-feeding the chance that problems might occur depends on the ingredients of the combination. For the individual ingredients of these combinations, the following apply:

- *Acetaminophen*—Acetaminophen passes into the breast milk. However, it has not been reported to cause problems in nursing babies.
- *Alcohol*—Alcohol passes into the breast milk. However, the amount of alcohol in recommended doses of this medicine does not usually cause problems in nursing babies.
- *Caffeine*—Small amounts of caffeine pass into the breast milk and may build up in the nursing baby. However, the amount of caffeine in recommended doses of this medicine does not usually cause problems in nursing babies.
- *Decongestants (e.g., phenylephrine, pseudoephedrine)*—Decongestants may pass into the breast milk and may cause unwanted effects in nursing babies of mothers taking this medicine.
- *Salicylates (e.g., aspirin, salicylamide)*—Salicylates pass into the breast milk. Although salicylates have not been reported to cause problems in nursing babies, it is possible that problems may occur if large amounts are taken regularly.

Children—Very young children are usually more sensitive to the effects of this medicine. *Before giving any of these combination medicines to a child, check the package label very carefully. Some of these medicines are too strong for use in children.* If you are not certain whether a specific product can be given to a child, or if you have any questions about the amount to give, check with your health care professional, especially if it contains:

- *Decongestants (e.g., phenylephrine, pseudoephedrine)*—Increases in blood pressure may be more likely to occur in children taking decongestants.
- *Salicylates (e.g., aspirin)*—Do not give aspirin or other salicylates to a child with a fever or other symptoms of a virus infection, especially flu or chickenpox, without first discussing its use with your child's doctor. This is very important because salicylates may cause a serious illness called Reye's syn-

drome in these children. Also, children may be more sensitive to the aspirin or other salicylates contained in some of these medicines, especially if they have a fever or have lost large amounts of body fluid because of vomiting, diarrhea, or sweating.

Teenagers—*Do not give aspirin or other salicylates to a teenager with a fever or other symptoms of a virus infection, especially flu or chickenpox, without first discussing its use with your child's doctor.* This is very important because salicylates may cause a serious illness called Reye's syndrome in these individuals.

Older adults—The elderly are usually more sensitive to the effects of this medicine.

Other medicines—Although certain medicines should not be used together at all, in other cases two different medicines may be used together even if an interaction might occur. In these cases, your doctor may want to change the dose, or other precautions may be necessary. Tell your health care professional if you are taking *any* other prescription or non-prescription (over-the-counter [OTC]) medicine, for example, aspirin or other medicine for allergies. Some medicines may change the way this medicine affects your body. Also, the effect of other medicines may be increased or reduced by some of the ingredients in this medicine. Check with your health care professional about which medicines you should not take together with this medicine.

Other medical problems—The presence of other medical problems may affect the use of decongestant and analgesic combinations. Make sure you tell your doctor if you have any other medical problems, especially:

- Alcohol abuse—Acetaminophen-containing medicine increases the chance of liver damage
- Anemia—Taking aspirin-, salicylamide-, or ibuprofen-containing medicine may make the anemia worse
- Asthma, allergies, and nasal polyps, history of—Taking salicylate- or ibuprofen-containing medicine may cause an allergic reaction in which breathing becomes difficult
- Diabetes mellitus (sugar diabetes)—The decongestant in this medicine may put the patient with diabetes at a greater risk of having heart or blood vessel disease
- Gout—Aspirin-containing medicine may make the gout worse and reduce the benefit of the medicines used for gout
- Hepatitis or other liver disease—Liver disease increases the chance of side effects because the medicine is not broken down and may build up in the body; also, if liver disease is severe there is a greater chance that aspirin-containing medicine may cause bleeding, and that ibuprofen-containing medicine may cause serious kidney damage
- Heart or blood vessel disease or
- High blood pressure—The decongestant in this medicine may cause the blood pressure to increase and may also speed up the heart rate; also, caffeine-containing medicine if taken in large amounts may increase the heart rate; ibuprofen-containing medicine may cause the blood pressure to increase
- Hemophilia or other bleeding problems—Aspirin- or ibuprofen-containing medicine increases the chance of bleeding

- Kidney disease—The kidneys may be affected, especially if too much of this medicine is taken for a long time
- Mental illness (history of)—The decongestant in this medicine may increase the chance of mental side effects
- Overactive thyroid—If an overactive thyroid has caused a fast heart rate, the decongestant in this medicine may cause the heart rate to speed up further
- Stomach ulcer or other stomach problems—Salicylate- or ibuprofen-containing medicine may make the ulcer worse or cause bleeding of the stomach
- Systemic lupus erythematosus (SLE)—Ibuprofen-containing medicine may put the patient with SLE at a greater risk of having unwanted effects on the central nervous system and/or kidneys
- Ulcers, sores, or white spots in the mouth—This may be a sign of a serious side effect of ibuprofen-containing medicine; if you already have ulcers or sores in the mouth you and your doctor may not be able to tell when this side effect occurs

Proper Use of This Medicine

Take this medicine only as directed. Do not take more of it and do not take it more often than recommended on the label, unless otherwise directed by your doctor. To do so may increase the chance of side effects.

For *aspirin- or salicylamide-containing medicines:*

- If this medicine irritates your stomach, you may take it with food or a glass of water or milk to lessen the irritation.
- *If a combination medicine containing aspirin has a strong vinegar-like odor, do not use it.* This odor means the medicine is breaking down. If you have any questions about this, check with your pharmacist.

For *ibuprofen-containing medicines:*

- To lessen stomach upset, these medicines may be taken with food or an antacid.
- Take with a full glass (8 ounces) of water. Also, do not lie down for about 15 to 30 minutes after taking the medicine. Doing so may cause irritation that may lead to trouble in swallowing.

Dosing—The dose of these combination medicines will be different for different products. *Follow the directions on the box if you are buying this medicine without a prescription. Or, follow your doctor's orders if this medicine was prescribed.* The following information includes only the average doses for these combinations.

The number of capsules or tablets or teaspoonfuls of liquid that you take depends on the strengths of the medicines.

There is a large variety of decongestant and analgesic combination products on the market. Some products are for use in adults only, while others may be used in children. If you have any questions about this, check with your health care professional.

- For *oral* dosage forms (capsules, liquid, or tablets):
  - For sinus pain and congestion:
    - Adults and children 12 years of age and older: 1 to 2 capsules or tablets every four to six hours.
    - Children up to 6 years of age: Use and dose must be determined by your doctor.
    - Children 6 to 12 years of age: 1 tablet, 4 to 6 chewable tablets, or 1 to 2 teaspoonfuls of liquid every four hours.

Missed dose—If you must take this medicine regularly and you miss a dose, take it as soon as possible. However, if it is almost time for your next dose, skip the missed dose and go back to your regular dosing schedule. Do not double doses.

Storage—To store this medicine:

- Keep this medicine out of the reach of children. Overdose is very dangerous in young children.
- Store away from heat and direct light.
- Do not store the capsule or tablet form of this medicine in the bathroom, near the kitchen sink, or in other damp places. Heat or moisture may cause the medicine to break down.
- Keep the liquid form of this medicine from freezing.
- Do not keep outdated medicine or medicine no longer needed. Be sure that any discarded medicine is out of the reach of children.

Precautions While Using This Medicine

Check with your doctor if your symptoms do not improve or become worse, or if you have a high fever.

This medicine may cause some people to become nervous or restless or to have trouble in sleeping. If you have trouble in sleeping, *take the last dose of this medicine for each day a few hours before bedtime.* If you have any questions about this, check with your doctor.

Before having any kind of surgery (including dental surgery) or emergency treatment, tell the medical doctor or dentist in charge that you are taking this medicine.

Check the label of all over-the-counter (OTC), nonprescription, and prescription medicines you now take. If any of them contain acetaminophen, aspirin, other salicylates such as bismuth subsalicylate (e.g., Pepto Bismol) or magnesium salicylate (e.g., Nuprin Backache Caplets), or salicylic acid (present in some shampoos and skin products), *check with your health care professional. Using any of them together with this medicine may cause an overdose.*

Do not drink alcoholic beverages while taking this medicine. Stomach problems may be more likely to occur if you drink alcoholic beverages while you are taking aspirin or ibuprofen. Also, liver damage may be more likely to occur if you drink large amounts of alcoholic beverages while you are taking acetaminophen.

If you think that you or anyone else may have taken an overdose of this medicine, get emergency help at once. Taking an overdose of a salicylate may cause unconsciousness or death. The first sign of an aspirin overdose may be ringing or buzzing in the ears. Other signs include convulsions (seizures), hearing loss, confusion, severe drowsiness or tiredness, severe excitement or nervousness, and unusually fast or deep breathing. Signs of severe acetaminophen overdose may not appear until 2 to 4 days after the overdose is taken, but treatment to prevent liver damage or death must be started within 24 hours or less after the overdose is taken.

For patients *taking aspirin-containing medicine:*

- Do not take aspirin-containing medicine for 5 days before any surgery, including dental surgery, unless otherwise directed by your medical doctor or dentist. Taking aspirin during this time may cause bleeding problems.

For diabetic patients *taking salicylate-containing medicine:*

- False urine sugar test results may occur if you take 8 or more 325–mg (5–grain) doses of aspirin every day for several days in a row. Smaller doses or occasional use of aspirin usually will not affect urine sugar tests. If you have any questions about this, check with your health care professional, especially if your diabetes is not well controlled.

For patients *taking ibuprofen-containing medicine:*

- This medicine may cause some people to become confused, drowsy, dizzy, lightheaded, or less alert than they are normally. It may also cause blurred vision or other vision problems in some people. *Make sure you know how you react to this medicine before you drive, use machines, or do anything else that could be dangerous if you are dizzy or are not alert and able to see well.*

- Serious side effects can occur during treatment with this medicine. Sometimes serious side effects can occur without any warning. However, possible warning signs often occur, including swelling of the face, fingers, feet, and/or lower legs; severe stomach pain, black, tarry stools, and/or vomiting of blood or material that looks like coffee grounds; unusual weight gain; and/or skin rash. Also, signs of serious heart problems could occur such as chest pain, tightness in chest, fast or irregular heartbeat, or unusual flushing or warmth of skin. *Stop taking this medicine and check with your doctor immediately if you notice any of these warning signs.*

Side Effects of This Medicine

Along with its needed effects, a medicine may cause some unwanted effects. Although serious side effects occur rarely when this medicine is taken as recommended, they may be more likely to occur if:

- Too much medicine is taken
- It is taken in large doses
- It is taken for a long period of time

Get emergency help immediately if any of the following symptoms of overdose occur:

For all combinations
Convulsions (seizures); dizziness or lightheadedness (severe); fast, slow, or irregular heartbeat; hallucinations (seeing, hearing, or feeling things that are not there); headache (continuing and severe); increased sweating; mood or mental changes; nausea or vomiting (severe or continuing); nervousness or restlessness (severe); shortness of breath or troubled breathing; stomach cramps or pain (severe or continuing); swelling or tenderness in the upper abdomen or stomach area; trouble in sleeping

For acetaminophen-containing only
Diarrhea; loss of appetite

For aspirin- or salicylamide-containing only
Any loss of hearing; changes in behavior (in children); confusion; diarrhea (severe or continuing); drowsiness or tiredness (severe, especially in children); fast or deep breathing (especially in children); ringing or buzzing in ears (continuing); uncontrollable flapping

movements of the hands, (especially in elderly patients); unexplained fever; unusual thirst; vision problems

Also, check with your doctor as soon as possible if any of the following side effects occur:

More common
Nausea, vomiting, or stomach pain (mild— for combinations containing aspirin or ibuprofen)

Less common or rare
Bloody or black, tarry stools; bloody or cloudy urine; blurred vision or any changes in vision or eyes; changes in facial skin color; changes in hearing; changes or problems with urination; difficult or painful urination; fever; headache, severe, with fever and stiff neck; increased blood pressure; muscle cramps or pain; skin rash, hives, or itching; sores, ulcers, or white spots on lips or in mouth; swelling of face, fingers, feet, or lower legs; swollen and/or painful glands; unexplained sore throat and fever; unusual bleeding or bruising; unusual tiredness or weakness; vomiting of blood or material that looks like coffee grounds; weight gain (unusual); yellow eyes or skin

Other side effects may occur that usually do not need medical attention. These side effects may go away during treatment as your body adjusts to the medicine. However, check with your doctor if any of the following side effects continue or are bothersome:

More common
Heartburn or indigestion (for medicines containing salicylate or ibuprofen); nervousness or restlessness

Less common
Drowsiness (for medicines containing salicylamide)

Not all of the side effects listed above have been reported for each of these medicines, but they have been reported for at least one of them. There are some similarities among these combination medicines, so many of the above side effects may occur with any of these medicines.

Other side effects not listed above may also occur in some patients. If you notice any other effects, check with your doctor.

DEFEROXAMINE (Injection route) -
de-fer-OX-a-meen

Commonly used brand name(s)
In the U.S.—
Desferal

Available Dosage Forms:
- Powder for Solution

Therapeutic Class: Heavy Metal Chelator-Antagonist

Uses For This Medicine

Deferoxamine is used to remove excess iron from the body. This may be necessary in certain patients with anemia who must receive many blood transfusions. It is also used to treat acute iron poisoning, especially in small children.

Deferoxamine combines with iron in the bloodstream. The combination of iron and deferoxamine is then removed from the body by the kidneys. By removing the excess iron, the medicine lessens damage to various organs and tissues of the body. This medicine may be used for other conditions as determined by your doctor.

Deferoxamine is to be administered only by or under the immediate supervision of your doctor.

Once a medicine has been approved for marketing for a certain use, experience may show that it is also useful for other medical problems. Although this use is not included in product labeling, deferoxamine is used in certain patients with the following medical condition:

- Aluminum toxicity (too much aluminum in the body)

Before Receiving This Medicine

In deciding to use a medicine, the risks of taking the medicine must be weighed against the good it will do. This is a decision you and your doctor will make. For this medicine, the following should be considered:

Allergies—Tell your doctor if you have ever had any unusual or allergic reaction to this medicine or any other medicines. Also tell your health care professional if you have any other types of allergies, such as to foods, dyes, preservatives, or animals. For non-prescription products, read the label or package ingredients carefully.

Pediatric—Deferoxamine is not used for long-term treatment of children up to 3 years of age. Also, younger patients are more likely to develop hearing and vision problems with the use of deferoxamine in high doses for a long time.

Geriatric—The combination of deferoxamine and vitamin C should be used with caution in older patients, since this combination may be more likely to cause heart problems in these patients than in younger adults.

Pregnancy—

	Pregnancy Category	Explanation
All Trimesters	C	Animal studies have shown an adverse effect and there are no adequate studies in pregnant women OR no animal studies have been conducted and there are no adequate studies in pregnant women.

Breast Feeding—There are no adequate studies in women for determining infant risk when using this medication during breastfeeding. Weigh the potential benefits against the potential risks before taking this medication while breastfeeding.

Other medicines—Although certain medicines should not be used together at all, in other cases two different medicines may be used together even if an interaction might occur. In these cases, your doctor may want to change the dose, or other precautions may be necessary. Tell your healthcare professional if you are taking any other prescription or nonprescription (over-the-counter [OTC]) medicine.

Interactions with Food/Tobacco/Alcohol—Certain medicines should not be used at or around the time of eating food or eating certain types of food since interactions may occur. Using alcohol or tobacco with certain medicines may also cause interactions to occur. Discuss with your healthcare professional the use of your medicine with food, alcohol, or tobacco.

Other medical problems—The presence of other medical problems may affect the use of this medicine. Make sure you tell your doctor if you have any other medical problems, especially:

- Kidney disease—Patients with kidney disease may be more likely to have side effects

Proper Use of This Medicine

Deferoxamine may sometimes be given at home to patients who do not need to be in the hospital. If you are receiving this medicine at home, make sure you clearly understand and carefully follow your doctor's instructions.

Dosing—The dose of this medicine will be different for different patients. Follow your doctor's orders or the directions on the label. The following information includes only the average doses of this medicine. If your dose is different, do not change it unless your doctor tells you to do so.

The amount of medicine that you take depends on the strength of the medicine. Also, the number of doses you take each day, the time allowed between doses, and the length of time you take the medicine depend on the medical problem for which you are using the medicine.

- For injection dosage form:
  - For acute iron toxicity:
    - Adults and children over 3 years of age—Dose is based on body weight and must be determined by your doctor. The usual dose is 90 milligrams (mg) per kilogram (kg) (41 mg per pound) of body weight, followed by 45 mg per kg (20 mg per pound) of body weight, injected into a muscle every four to twelve hours. If it is injected into a vein, the usual dose is 15 mg per kg (7 mg per pound) of body weight per hour every eight hours.
    - Children up to 3 years of age—The usual dose is 15 mg per kg (7 mg per pound) of body weight per hour, injected into a vein.
  - For chronic iron toxicity:
    - Adults and children over 3 years of age—The usual dose is 500 mg to 1 gram a day, injected into a muscle. Or, the medicine may be injected under the skin by an infusion pump. The usual dose is 1 to 2 grams (20 to 40 mg per kg [9 to 18 mg per pound] of body weight) a day, injected under the skin, over a period of eight to twenty-four hours. If you are receiving blood transfusions, the usual dose is 500 mg to 1 gram a day, injected into a muscle. An extra 2 grams of the medicine is injected into a vein with each unit of blood at a rate of 15 mg per kg of body weight per hour.
    - Children up to 3 years of age—Use and dose must be determined by your doctor. The usual dose is 10 mg per kg (5 mg per pound) of body weight a day, injected under the skin.

Storage—Store the medicine in a closed container at room temperature, away from heat, moisture, and direct light. Do not refrigerate. Keep from freezing.

Keep out of the reach of children.

Do not keep outdated medicine or medicine no longer needed.

Store the mixed medicine at room temperature for no longer than recommended by your doctor or the manufacturer.

Precautions After Receiving This Medicine

It is important that your doctor check your progress at regular visits to make sure that this medicine is working properly and to prevent unwanted effects. Certain blood and urine tests must be done regularly to check for the need for dosage changes.

Deferoxamine may cause some people, especially younger patients, to have hearing and vision problems within a few weeks after they start taking it. If you notice any problems with your vision, such as blurred vision, difficulty in seeing at night, or difficulty in seeing colors, or difficulty with your hearing, check with your doctor as soon as possible. The dose of deferoxamine may need to be adjusted.

Do not take vitamin C unless your doctor has told you to do so.

Side Effects of This Medicine

Along with its needed effects, a medicine may cause some unwanted effects. Although not all of these side effects may occur, if they do occur they may need medical attention.

Check with your doctor as soon as possible if any of the following side effects occur:

More common
Bluish fingernails, lips, or skin; blurred vision or other problems with vision; convulsions (seizures); difficulty in breathing (wheezing), or fast breathing; fast heartbeat; hearing problems; pain or swelling at place of injection; redness or flushing of skin; skin rash, hives, or itching

Less common
Diarrhea; difficult urination; fever; leg cramps; stomach and muscle cramps; stomach discomfort; unusual bleeding or bruising

Hearing and vision problems are more likely to occur in younger patients taking high doses and on long-term treatment.

Deferoxamine may cause the urine to turn orange-rose in color. This is to be expected while you are using this medicine.

Other side effects not listed may also occur in some patients. If you notice any other effects, check with your healthcare professional.

DELAVIRDINE (Oral route) - de-la-VIR-deen

Commonly used brand name(s)
In the U.S.—
Rescriptor

Available Dosage Forms:
- Tablet

Therapeutic Class: Antiretroviral Agent
Pharmacologic Class: Non-Nucleoside Reverse Transcriptase Inhibitor

Uses For This Medicine

Delavirdine is used, in combination with other medicines, in the treatment of the infection caused by the human immunodeficiency virus (HIV). HIV is the virus that causes acquired immune deficiency syndrome (AIDS).

Delavirdine will not cure or prevent HIV infection or AIDS; however, it helps keep HIV from reproducing and appears to slow down the destruction of the immune system. This may help delay the development of problems usually related to AIDS or HIV disease. Delavirdine will not keep you from spreading HIV to other people. People who receive this medicine may continue to have other problems usually related to AIDS or HIV disease.

This medicine is available only with your doctor's prescription.

Before Using This Medicine

In deciding to use a medicine, the risks of taking the medicine must be weighed against the good it will do. This is a decision you and your doctor will make. For this medicine, the following should be considered:

Allergies—Tell your doctor if you have ever had any unusual or allergic reaction to this medicine or any other medicines. Also tell your health care professional if you have any other types of allergies, such as to foods, dyes, preservatives, or animals. For non-prescription products, read the label or package ingredients carefully.

Geriatric—Delavirdine has not been studied specifically in older people. Therefore, it is not known whether it causes different side effects or problems in the elderly than it does in younger adults.

Pregnancy—

	Pregnancy Category	Explanation
All Trimesters	C	Animal studies have shown an adverse effect and there are no adequate studies in pregnant women OR no animal studies have been conducted and there are no adequate studies in pregnant women.

Breast Feeding—There are no adequate studies in women for determining infant risk when using this medication during breastfeeding. Weigh the potential benefits against the potential risks before taking this medication while breastfeeding.

Other medicines—

Using this medicine with any of the following medicines is not recommended. Your doctor may decide not to treat you with this medication or change some of the other medicines you take.

Alprazolam, Astemizole, Cisapride, Dihydroergotamine, Ergonovine, Ergotamine, Methylergonovine, Midazolam, Pimozide, St John's Wort, Terfenadine, Triazolam

Interactions with Food/Tobacco/Alcohol—Certain medicines should not be used at or around the time of eating food or eating certain types of food since interactions may occur. Using alcohol or tobacco with certain medicines may also cause interactions to occur. Discuss with your healthcare professional the use of your medicine with food, alcohol, or tobacco.

Other medical problems—The presence of other medical problems may affect the use of this medicine. Make sure you tell your doctor if you have any other medical problems, especially:

- Achlorhydria (absence of stomach acid)—Delavirdine should be taken with an acidic beverage such as orange or cranberry juice
- Liver disease—Effects of delavirdine may be increased because of slower removal from the body

Proper Use of This Medicine

This medicine can be taken with our without food.

It is very important that you find out about medicines that can not be taken with delavirdine.

It is best to swallow both the 100 milligram (mg) and 200 milligram (mg) tablets whole. However, if swallowing is difficult, the 100 milligram (mg) tablet can be put in a glass of water (at least 3 ounces), allowed to sit for a few minutes, and then stirred to mix. Drink the mixture right away. Then rinse the glass with water and drink that rinse to make sure the full dose is taken.

Note: Only the 100 milligram (mg) tablets can be put into a glass of water to dissolve. The 200 milligram (mg) tablets must be swallowed whole.

Do not take any antacid medications within 1 hour of the time you take delavirdine. They may prevent delavirdine from being absorbed into the body.

For patients with achlorhydria (absence of stomach acid) they should take delavirdine with a glass of orange juice or cranberry juice.

Take this medicine exactly as directed by your doctor. Do not take it more often, and do not take it for a longer time than your doctor ordered. Also, do not stop taking this medicine without checking with your doctor first.

Keep taking delavirdine for the full time of treatment, even if you begin to feel better.

Dosing—The dose of this medicine will be different for different patients. Follow your doctor's orders or the directions on the label. The following information includes only the average doses of this medicine. If your dose is different, do not change it unless your doctor tells you to do so.

The amount of medicine that you take depends on the strength of the medicine. Also, the number of doses you take each day, the time allowed between doses, and the length of time you take the medicine depend on the medical problem for which you are using the medicine.

- For oral dosage form (tablets):
  - For treatment of HIV infection:
    - Adults—400 mg three times a day in combination with other antiretroviral medicines. Your healthcare professional will decide on the other medicines needed and how much you will use.
    - Children younger than 16 years of age—Use and dose must be determined by your doctor.

Missed dose—If you miss a dose of this medicine, take it as soon as possible. However, if it is almost time for your next dose, skip the missed dose and go back to your regular dosing schedule. Do not double doses.

Storage—Store the medicine in a closed container at room temperature, away from heat, moisture, and direct light. Keep from freezing.

Keep out of the reach of children.

Do not keep outdated medicine or medicine no longer needed.

Precautions While Using This Medicine

It is very important that your doctor check your progress at regular visits.

Side Effects of This Medicine

Along with its needed effects, a medicine may cause some unwanted effects. Although not all of these side effects may occur, if they do occur they may need medical attention.

Check with your doctor as soon as possible if any of the following side effects occur:

More common
    Skin rash (severe) with itching

Less common
    Skin rash with symptoms such as fever, blistering, oral lesions, conjunctivitis, swelling, muscle aches, or joint aches

Rare
    Difficulty in breathing

Incidence unknown
    Agitation; back, leg, or stomach pains; bleeding gums; chills; coma; confusion; dark urine; decreased urine output; depression; difficulty breathing; dizziness; fatigue; fever; general body swelling; headache; hostility; irritability; lethargy; loss of appetite; muscle twitching; nausea; nosebleeds; pale skin; rapid weight gain; seizures (convulsions); sore throat; stupor; swelling of face, ankles, or hands; unusual tiredness or weakness; vomiting; yellowing of the eyes or skin

Some side effects may occur that usually do not need medical attention. These side effects may go away during treatment as your body adjusts to the medicine. Also, your health care professional may be able to tell you about ways to prevent or reduce some of these side effects. Check with your health care professional if any of the following side effects continue or are bothersome or if you have any questions about them:

More common
    Body aches or pain; cough; diarrhea; discouragement; ear congestion; fear; feeling sad or empty; general feeling of discomfort or illness; joint pain; lack or loss of strength; loss of interest or pleasure; loss of voice; muscle aches and pains; nasal congestion; nervousness; pain, localized; pain or tenderness around eyes and cheekbones; runny nose; shivering; shortness of breath; sneezing; sweating; tightness in chest; tiredness; trouble concentrating; trouble sleeping; wheezing

Less common
    Abdominal pain, generalized; dryness or soreness of throat; hoarseness; sleeplessness; tender, swollen glands in neck; trouble in swallowing; unable to sleep; voice changes

Other side effects not listed may also occur in some patients. If you notice any other effects, check with your healthcare professional.

DENILEUKIN DIFTITOX (Intravenous route) - de-ni-LOO-kin DIF-ti-toks

Black Box Warning

Only physicians experienced in the use of antineoplastic therapy and management of patients with cancer should use denileukin diftitox. Patients treated with denileukin diftitox must be managed in a facility equipped and staffed for cardiopulmonary resuscitation and where the patient can be closely monitored for an appropriate period based on his or her health status.

Commonly used brand name(s)

In the U.S.—
 Ontak

Available Dosage Forms:
 • Injectable
 • Solution

Therapeutic Class: Antineoplastic Agent
Pharmacologic Class: Interleukin

Uses For This Medicine

Denileukin diftitox is used to treat cutaneous T-cell lymphoma, a rare type of cancer that affects certain white blood cells and causes lesions to develop on the skin.

Denileukin diftitox interferes with the growth of cancer cells, which are eventually destroyed. Since the growth of normal cells may also be affected by the medicine, other effects may also occur. Some of these may be serious and must be reported to your doctor. Some effects may occur after treatment with denileukin diftitox.

Denileukin diftitox is to be administered only by or under the supervision of your doctor or other health care professional.

Before Using This Medicine

In deciding to use a medicine, the risks of taking the medicine must be weighed against the good it will do. This is a decision you and your doctor will make. For this medicine, the following should be considered:

Allergies—Tell your doctor if you have ever had any unusual or allergic reaction to this medicine or any other medicines. Also tell your health care professional if you have any other types of allergies, such as to foods, dyes, preservatives, or animals. For non-prescription products, read the label or package ingredients carefully.

Pediatric—Studies on this medicine have been done only in adult patients, and there is no specific information comparing use of denileukin diftitox in children with use in other age groups.

Geriatric—Adverse effects such as anorexia, hypotension, anemia, confusion, rash, nausea, and/or vomiting may be especially likely to occur in elderly patients who may be more sensitive than younger adults to the effects of denileukin diftitox.

Pregnancy—

	Pregnancy Category	Explanation
All Trimesters	C	Animal studies have shown an adverse effect and there are no adequate studies in pregnant women OR no animal studies have been conducted and there are no adequate studies in pregnant women.

Breast Feeding—There are no adequate studies in women for determining infant risk when using this medication during breastfeeding. Weigh the potential benefits against the potential risks before taking this medication while breastfeeding.

Other medicines—Although certain medicines should not be used together at all, in other cases two different medicines may be used together even if an interaction might occur. In these cases, your doctor may want to change the dose, or other precautions may be necessary. Tell your healthcare professional if you are taking any other prescription or nonprescription (over-the-counter [OTC]) medicine.

Interactions with Food/Tobacco/Alcohol—Certain medicines should not be used at or around the time of eating food or eating certain types of food since interactions may occur. Using alcohol or tobacco with certain medicines may also cause interactions to occur. Discuss with your healthcare professional the use of your medicine with food, alcohol, or tobacco.

Other medical problems—The presence of other medical problems may affect the use of denileukin diftitox. Make sure to tell your doctor if you have any other medical problems, especially heart disease.

Proper Use of This Medicine

Dosing—The dose of this medicine will be different for different patients. Follow your doctor's orders or the directions on the label. The following information includes only the average doses of this medicine. If your dose is different, do not change it unless your doctor tells you to do so.

The amount of medicine that you take depends on the strength of the medicine. Also, the number of doses you take each day, the time allowed between doses, and the length of time you take the medicine depend on the medical problem for which you are using the medicine.

Precautions While Using This Medicine

It is very important that your doctor check your progress at regular visits to make sure that this medicine is working properly and to check for unwanted effects.

Side Effects of This Medicine

Along with its needed effects, a medicine may cause some unwanted effects. Although not all of these side effects may occur, if they do occur they may need medical attention.

Check with your doctor immediately if any of the following side effects occur:
 More common
  Back pain; chest pain; dizziness or faintness; difficulty swallowing; fast or irregular heartbeat; fever or chills; infection; rash; shortness of breath; swelling of face, feet, or lower legs; warmth and flushing of skin

Less common

Abdominal pain, severe; black, tarry stools; cloudy urine; blood in urine or stools; cloudy urine; cough or hoarseness accompanied by fever or chills; headache, severe; loss of coordination; lower back pain or side pain accompanied by fever or chills; painful or difficult urination accompanied by fever or chills; pain in groin or leg; pinpoint red spots on skin; slurring of speech; sudden vision changes; swelling or pain at injection site; unusual bleeding or bruising; weakness of arm and leg

Rare

Decreased urination, accompanied by nausea and loss of appetite

Check with your doctor as soon as possible if any of the following side effects occur:

More common

Difficulty swallowing; loss of strength or energy; nausea; pain in joints and muscles; unusual tiredness or weakness; vomiting

Rare

Dry, puffy skin; increased heart rate; loss of appetite; weight gain

Some side effects may occur that usually do not need medical attention. These side effects may go away during treatment as your body adjusts to the medicine. Also, your health care professional may be able to tell you about ways to prevent or reduce some of these side effects. Check with your health care professional if any of the following side effects continue or are bothersome or if you have any questions about them:

More common

Cough; diarrhea; skin rash; sore throat

Less common or rare

Confusion; constipation; indigestion; numbness or tingling of fingers, toes, or face; runny nose; trouble in sleeping

Some side effects of denileukin diftitox may not develop until long after you have received the medicine, sometimes up to two weeks later.

Other side effects not listed may also occur in some patients. If you notice any other effects, check with your healthcare professional.

DESLORATADINE (Oral route) - des-lor-AT-a-deen

Commonly used brand name(s)

In the U.S.—
Clarinex
Clarinex Reditabs

Available Dosage Forms:
- Tablet, Disintegrating
- Tablet
- Syrup

Therapeutic Class: Respiratory Agent
Pharmacologic Class: Antihistamine, Less-Sedating

Uses For This Medicine

Desloratadine is an antihistamine. It is used to relieve the symptoms of hay fever and hives of the skin.

Antihistamines work by preventing the effects of a substance called histamine, which is produced by the body. Histamine can cause itching, sneezing, runny nose, and watery eyes. Also, in some persons histamine can close up the bronchial tubes (air passages of the lungs) and make breathing difficult. Histamine can also cause some persons to have hives, with severe itching of the skin.

This medicine is available only with your doctor's prescription.

Before Using This Medicine

In deciding to use a medicine, the risks of taking the medicine must be weighed against the good it will do. This is a decision you and your doctor will make. For this medicine, the following should be considered:

Allergies—Tell your doctor if you have ever had any unusual or allergic reaction to this medicine or any other medicines. Also tell your health care professional if you have any other types of allergies, such as to foods, dyes, preservatives, or animals. For non-prescription products, read the label or package ingredients carefully.

Pediatric—This medicine has been tested in children 6 months of age and older. In effective doses, the medicine has not been shown to cause different side effects or problems than it does in adults.

Geriatric—Desloratadine has been tested in patients 65 years of age and older and has not been shown to cause different side effects or problems in older people than it does in younger adults. However, older patients are more likely to have kidney or liver problems which may make them more sensitive to the effects of desloratadine. Your doctor may give you a different desloratadine dose if you have kidney or liver problems.

Pregnancy—

	Pregnancy Category	Explanation
All Trimesters	C	Animal studies have shown an adverse effect and there are no adequate studies in pregnant women OR no animal studies have been conducted and there are no adequate studies in pregnant women.

Breast Feeding—There are no adequate studies in women for determining infant risk when using this medication during breastfeeding. Weigh the potential benefits against the potential risks before taking this medication while breastfeeding.

Other medicines—Although certain medicines should not be used together at all, in other cases two different medicines may be used together even if an interaction might occur. In these cases, your doctor may want to change the dose, or other precautions may be necessary. Tell your healthcare professional if you are taking any other prescription or non-prescription (over-the-counter [OTC]) medicine.

Interactions with Food/Tobacco/Alcohol—Certain medicines should not be used at or around the time of eating food or eating certain types of food since interactions may

occur. Using alcohol or tobacco with certain medicines may also cause interactions to occur. Discuss with your healthcare professional the use of your medicine with food, alcohol, or tobacco.

Other medical problems—The presence of other medical problems may affect the use of this medicine. Make sure you tell your doctor if you have any other medical problems, especially:

- Liver disease or
- Kidney disease—Effects of desloratadine may be increased because of slower removal from the body.
- Phenylketonuria (PKU)—The oral disintegrating tablets may contain aspartame, which can make your condition worse.
- Slow metabolizers of desloratadine—May increase chances of unwanted effects

Proper Use of This Medicine

Dosing—The dose of this medicine will be different for different patients. Follow your doctor's orders or the directions on the label. The following information includes only the average doses of this medicine. If your dose is different, do not change it unless your doctor tells you to do so.

The amount of medicine that you take depends on the strength of the medicine. Also, the number of doses you take each day, the time allowed between doses, and the length of time you take the medicine depend on the medical problem for which you are using the medicine.

For patients using the oral disintegrating tablet form of this medicine:

- Make sure your hands are dry.
- Do not push the tablet through the foil backing of the package. Instead, gently peel back the foil backing and remove the tablet.
- Immediately place the tablet on top of the tongue.
- The tablet will dissolve in seconds, and you may swallow it with your saliva. You do not need to drink water or other liquid to swallow the tablet.

For patients using the syrup form of this medicine: Use a calibrated measuring dropper or syringe to measure the direct dose for your child based on your doctor's instructions. Do not use a regular teaspoon. If you are unsure about how much of the syrup to give to your child, ask your doctor or pharmacist.

- For oral dosage form (oral disintegrating tablets):
  - For symptoms of chronic hives:
    - Adults and children 12 years of age and older— 5 milligrams (mg) once a day.
    - Children 6 to 11 years of age—2.5 mg once a day.
    - Children younger than 6 years of age—Use and dose must be determined by your doctor.
  - For symptoms of hay fever:
    - Adults and children 12 years of age and older— 5 mg once a day.
    - Children 6 to 11 years of age—2.5 mg once a day.
    - Children younger than 6 years of age—Use and dose must be determined by your doctor.
- For oral dosage form (tablets):
  - For symptoms of chronic hives:
    - Adults and children 12 years of age and older— 5 mg once a day.

- Children younger than 12 years of age—Use and dose must be determined by your doctor.
  - For symptoms of hay fever:
    - Adults and children 12 years of age and older— 5 mg once a day.
    - Children younger than 12 years of age—Use and dose must be determined by your doctor.
- For oral dosage form (syrup):
  - For symptoms of chronic hives:
    - Adults and children 12 years of age and older— 2 teaspoonfuls (5 milligrams [mg] in 10 milliliters [mL]) once a day.
    - Children 6 to 11 years of age—1 teaspoonful (2.5 mg in 5 mL) once a day
    - Children 12 months to 5 years of age—½ teaspoonful (1.25 mg in 2.5 mL) once a day
    - Children 6 to 11 months of age—2 mL (1 mg) once a day
  - For symptoms of hay fever:
    - Adults and children 12 years of age and older— 2 teaspoonfuls (5 milligrams [mg] in 10 milliliters [mL]) once a day.
    - Children 6 to 11 years of age—1 teaspoonful (2.5 mg in 5 mL) once a day
    - Children 12 months to 5 years of age—½ teaspoonful (1.25 mg in 2.5 mL) once a day
    - Children 6 to 11 months of age—2 mL (1 mg) once a day

Missed dose—If you miss a dose of this medicine, take it as soon as possible. However, if it is almost time for your next dose, skip the missed dose and go back to your regular dosing schedule. Do not double doses.

Storage—Store the medicine in a closed container at room temperature, away from heat, moisture, and direct light. Keep from freezing.

Keep out of the reach of children.

Do not keep outdated medicine or medicine no longer needed.

Ask your healthcare professional how you should dispose of any medicine you do not use.

Precautions While Using This Medicine

If your symptoms do not improve within a few days or if they become worse, check with your doctor.

This medicine may cause some people to become drowsy, dizzy, or less alert than they are normally. Make sure you know how you react to this medicine before you drive, use machines, or do anything else that could be dangerous if you are dizzy or are not alert.

Side Effects of This Medicine

Along with its needed effects, a medicine may cause some unwanted effects. Although not all of these side effects may occur, if they do occur they may need medical attention.

Check with your doctor immediately if any of the following side effects occur:
> *Rare*
>> Anaphylaxis, such as, cough, difficulty swallowing, dizziness, fast heartbeat, hives, itching, puffiness or swelling of eyelids or around the eyes or face or lips or tongue, shortness of breath, skin rash, tightness in

chest, unusual tiredness or weakness, wheezing; dyspnea, such as, shortness of breath, difficult or labored breathing, tightness in chest, wheezing; edema, such as, swelling; pruritus, such as, itching skin; rash; tachycardia, such as, fast, pounding, or irregular heartbeat or pulse; urticaria, such as, hives or welts, itching, redness of skin, skin rash.

Some side effects may occur that usually do not need medical attention. These side effects may go away during treatment as your body adjusts to the medicine. Also, your health care professional may be able to tell you about ways to prevent or reduce some of these side effects. Check with your health care professional if any of the following side effects continue or are bothersome or if you have any questions about them:

More common
  Headache

Less common
  Dizziness; dry mouth; dysmenorrhea, such as, difficult or painful menstruation; dyspepsia, such as, acid or sour stomach, belching, heartburn, indigestion, stomach discomfort, upset or pain,; fatigue, such as, unusual tiredness or weakness; myalgia, such as, joint pain, swollen joints, muscle aching or cramping, muscle pains or stiffness, difficulty in moving; pharyngitis, such as, body aches or pain, congestion, cough, dryness or soreness of throat, fever, hoarseness, runny nose, tender swollen glands in neck, trouble in swallowing, voice changes.; somnolence, such as, sleepiness or unusual drowsiness; nausea

Other side effects not listed may also occur in some patients. If you notice any other effects, check with your healthcare professional.

DESLORATADINE AND PSEUDOEPHEDRINE (Oral route) -
des-lor-AT-a-deen, soo-doe-e-FED-rin

Commonly used brand name(s)

In the U.S.—
  Clarinex-D

Available Dosage Forms:
- Tablet, Extended Release, 24 HR
- Tablet, Extended Release, 12 HR

Therapeutic Class: Antihistamine, Less-Sedating/Decongestant Combination
Pharmacologic Class: Antihistamine, Less-Sedating

Uses For This Medicine

Desloratadine and pseudoephedrine is a combination of two medicines used to treat nasal congestion (stuffy nose), sneezing, and runny nose caused by hay fever.

Desloratadine works by preventing the effects of a substance called histamine, which is produced by the body. Histamine can cause itching, sneezing, runny nose, and watery eyes.

The pseudoephedrine causes narrowing of blood vessels. This leads to clearing of nasal congestion, but it may also cause an increase in blood pressure in patients who have high blood pressure.

This medicine is available only with your doctor's prescription.

Before Using This Medicine

In deciding to use a medicine, the risks of taking the medicine must be weighed against the good it will do. This is a decision you and your doctor will make. For this medicine, the following should be considered:

Allergies—Tell your doctor if you have ever had any unusual or allergic reaction to this medicine or any other medicines. Also tell your health care professional if you have any other types of allergies, such as to foods, dyes, preservatives, or animals. For non-prescription products, read the label or package ingredients carefully.

Pediatric—Desloratadine and pseudoephedrine combination is not recommended for use in pediatric patients under 12 years of age.

Geriatric—Many medicines have not been studied specifically in older people. Therefore, it may not be known whether they work exactly the same way they do in younger adults. Although there is no specific information comparing use of desloratadine and pseudoephedrine combination in the elderly with use in other age groups, elderly patients are more likely to be sensitive to the effects of this drug.

Pregnancy—

	Pregnancy Category	Explanation
All Trimesters	C	Animal studies have shown an adverse effect and there are no adequate studies in pregnant women OR no animal studies have been conducted and there are no adequate studies in pregnant women.

Breast Feeding—There are no adequate studies in women for determining infant risk when using this medication during breastfeeding. Weigh the potential benefits against the potential risks before taking this medication while breastfeeding.

Other medicines—

Using this medicine with any of the following medicines is not recommended. Your doctor may decide not to treat you with this medication or change some of the other medicines you take.

Clorgyline, Dihydroergotamine, Furazolidone, Iproniazid, Isocarboxazid, Moclobemide, Nialamide, Pargyline, Phenelzine, Procarbazine, Rasagiline, Selegiline, Toloxatone, Tranylcypromine

Interactions with Food/Tobacco/Alcohol—Certain medicines should not be used at or around the time of eating food or eating certain types of food since interactions may occur. Using alcohol or tobacco with certain medicines may also cause interactions to occur. Discuss with your healthcare professional the use of your medicine with food, alcohol, or tobacco.

Other medical problems—The presence of other medical problems may affect the use of this medicine. Make sure you

tell your doctor if you have any other medical problems, especially:

- Diabetes mellitus (sugar diabetes)—The decongestant in this medicine may put diabetic patients at a greater risk of having heart or blood vessel disease.

- Enlarged prostate or

- Urinary tract blockage or difficult urination—Some of the effects of antihistamines may make urinary problems worse.

- Glaucoma—A slight increase in inner eye pressure may occur.

- Heart or blood vessel disease or

- High blood pressure—The decongestant in this medicine may cause blood pressure to increase and may also speed up the heart rate.

- Kidney disease—Higher blood levels of desloratadine may result, which may increase the chance of side effects. If you are taking the 24 hour extended-release tablets, the dosage may need to be reduced. The 12 hour extended-release tablets should generally be avoided if you have kidney disease.

- Liver disease—Higher blood levels of desloratadine may result, which may increase the chance of side effects. This medicine should generally be avoided if you have liver disease.

- Overactive thyroid—If an overactive thyroid has caused a fast heart rate, desloratadine in this medicine may cause the heart rate to speed up further.

- Urinary retention—Condition may be worsened with use of pseudoephedrine

Proper Use of This Medicine

Take this medicine only as directed. Do not take more of it and do not take it more often than recommended on the label, unless otherwise directed by your doctor. To do so may increase the chance of side effects.

Not taking over-the-counter antihistamines and decongestants while taking desloratadine and pseudoephedrine combination.

When taking desloratadine and pseudoephedrine extended-release tablet:

- Swallow it whole.
- Do not crush, break, or chew before swallowing.

Dosing—The dose of this medicine will be different for different patients. Follow your doctor's orders or the directions on the label. The following information includes only the average doses of this medicine. If your dose is different, do not change it unless your doctor tells you to do so.

The amount of medicine that you take depends on the strength of the medicine. Also, the number of doses you take each day, the time allowed between doses, and the length of time you take the medicine depend on the medical problem for which you are using the medicine.

- For oral dosage form (extended-release tablets [12 hour]):
  - For nasal congestion or rhinorrhea
    - Adults and teenagers—Oral, one tablet (2.5 milligrams desloratadine, 120 milligrams pseudo-

ephedrine) two times a day 12 hours apart, taken with or without a meal
    - Children—Use and dose must be determined by your doctor.

- For oral dosage form (extended-release tablets [24 hour]):
  - For nasal congestion or rhinorrhea
    - Adults and teenagers—Oral, one tablet (5 milligrams desloratadine, 240 milligrams pseudoephedrine) daily, taken with or without a meal
    - Children—Use and dose must be determined by your doctor.

Missed dose—If you miss a dose of this medicine, take it as soon as possible. However, if it is almost time for your next dose, skip the missed dose and go back to your regular dosing schedule. Do not double doses.

Storage—Store the medicine in a closed container at room temperature, away from heat, moisture, and direct light. Keep from freezing.

Keep out of the reach of children.

Do not keep outdated medicine or medicine no longer needed.

Ask your healthcare professional how you should dispose of any medicine you do not use.

Precautions While Using This Medicine

Desloratadine may cause dryness of the mouth, nose, and throat. For temporary relief, use sugarless candy or gum, melt bits of ice in your mouth, or use a saliva substitute. However, if your mouth continues to feel dry for more than 2 weeks, check with your dentist. Continuing dryness of the mouth may increase the chance of dental disease, including tooth decay, gum disease, and fungus infections.

Side Effects of This Medicine

Along with its needed effects, a medicine may cause some unwanted effects. Although not all of these side effects may occur, if they do occur they may need medical attention.

Check with your doctor immediately if any of the following side effects occur:

Observed during clinical practice

Abdominal or stomach pain area; chills; clay-colored stools; cough; dark urine; difficult or labored breathing; difficulty swallowing; dizziness; elevated liver enzymes; fast heartbeat; fast, pounding, or irregular heartbeat or pulse; fever; general tiredness and weakness; headache; hives; irregular heartbeat; itching; light-colored stools; loss of appetite; nausea; puffiness or swelling of the eyelids or around the eyes, face, lips or tongue; rash; redness of skin; shortness of breath; skin rash; swelling; tightness in chest; unpleasant breath odor; unusual tiredness or weakness; upper right abdominal pain; vomiting of blood; vomiting; welts; wheezing; yellow eyes or skin

Symptoms of overdose

Get emergency help immediately if any of the following symptoms of overdose occur:

Increased heart rate; sleepiness or unusual drowsiness

Some side effects may occur that usually do not need medical attention. These side effects may go away during treatment as your body adjusts to the medicine. Also, your health care professional may be able to tell you about ways to prevent or reduce some of these side effects. Check with your health care professional if any of the following side effects continue or are bothersome or if you have any questions about them:

More common

Dry mouth; sleeplessness; trouble sleeping; unable to sleep

Less common

Body aches or pain; congestion; dryness or soreness of throat; hoarseness; nervousness; restlessness; runny nose; sleepiness or unusual drowsiness; tender, swollen glands in neck; trouble sitting still; voice changes; weight loss

Other side effects not listed may also occur in some patients. If you notice any other effects, check with your healthcare professional.

DESMOPRESSIN (Nasal route, Oral route, Injection route) - des-moe-PRES-in

Commonly used brand name(s)

In the U.S.—

DDAVP
DDAVP Rhinal Tube

Minirin
Stimate

Available Dosage Forms:

- Tablet
- Solution
- Spray

Therapeutic Class: Endocrine-Metabolic Agent
Pharmacologic Class: Vasopressin (class)

Uses For This Medicine

Desmopressin is a hormone taken through the nose, by mouth, or given by injection to prevent or control the frequent urination, increased thirst, and loss of water associated with diabetes insipidus (water diabetes). It is used also to control bed-wetting and frequent urination and increased thirst associated with certain types of brain injuries or brain surgery. Desmopressin works by acting on the kidneys to reduce the flow of urine.

Desmopressin is also given by injection to treat some patients with certain bleeding problems such as hemophilia or von Willebrand's disease.

Desmopressin is available only with your doctor's prescription.

Once a medicine has been approved for marketing for a certain use, experience may show that it is also useful for other medical problems. Although this use is not included in product labeling, desmopressin is used in certain patients to determine the cause of Cushing's syndrome.

Before Using This Medicine

In deciding to use a medicine, the risks of taking the medicine must be weighed against the good it will do. This is a decision you and your doctor will make. For this medicine, the following should be considered:

Allergies—Tell your doctor if you have ever had any unusual or allergic reaction to this medicine or any other medicines. Also tell your health care professional if you have any other types of allergies, such as to foods, dyes, preservatives, or animals. For non-prescription products, read the label or package ingredients carefully.

Pediatric—Infants may be more sensitive to the effects of desmopressin.

Geriatric—Some side effects (confusion, continuing headache, drowsiness, problem with urination, weight gain) may be especially likely to occur in elderly patients, who are usually more sensitive than younger adults to the effects of desmopressin.

Pregnancy—

	Pregnancy Category	Explanation
All Trimesters	B	Animal studies have revealed no evidence of harm to the fetus, however, there are no adequate studies in pregnant women OR animal studies have shown an adverse effect, but adequate studies in pregnant women have failed to demonstrate a risk to the fetus.

Breast Feeding—There are no adequate studies in women for determining infant risk when using this medication during breastfeeding. Weigh the potential benefits against the potential risks before taking this medication while breastfeeding.

Other medicines—Although certain medicines should not be used together at all, in other cases two different medicines may be used together even if an interaction might occur. In these cases, your doctor may want to change the dose, or other precautions may be necessary. Tell your healthcare professional if you are taking any other prescription or non-prescription (over-the-counter [OTC]) medicine.

Interactions with Food/Tobacco/Alcohol—Certain medicines should not be used at or around the time of eating food or eating certain types of food since interactions may occur. Using alcohol or tobacco with certain medicines may also cause interactions to occur. Discuss with your healthcare professional the use of your medicine with food, alcohol, or tobacco.

Other medical problems—The presence of other medical problems may affect the use of this medicine. Make sure you tell your doctor if you have any other medical problems, especially:

- Cystic fibrosis or
- Dehydration—Loss of sodium from the blood and serious side effects may be more likely to occur in patients with these conditions
- Headache, severe, or migraine or
- Heart or blood vessel disease or

- High blood pressure—Large doses of desmopressin can cause an increase or decrease in blood pressure
- Kidney problems—Desmopressin should NOT be used.
- Stuffy nose caused by cold or allergy—May prevent nasal desmopressin from being absorbed through the lining of the nose into the blood stream

Proper Use of This Medicine

Use this medicine only as directed. Do not use more of it and do not use it more often than your doctor ordered. To do so may increase the chance of side effects.

For patients using the nasal solution form of this medicine:

- This medicine usually comes with patient directions. Read them carefully before using this medicine.
- Do not use the nasal spray more times than the number indicated on the label. If you do, you may not receive the correct amount of medicine.

Dosing—The dose of this medicine will be different for different patients. Follow your doctor's orders or the directions on the label. The following information includes only the average doses of this medicine. If your dose is different, do not change it unless your doctor tells you to do so.

The amount of medicine that you take depends on the strength of the medicine. Also, the number of doses you take each day, the time allowed between doses, and the length of time you take the medicine depend on the medical problem for which you are using the medicine.

- For nasal dosage form (nasal solution):
  - For preventing or controlling diabetes insipidus (water diabetes):
    - Adults and teenagers—10 to 40 mcg - used as a single dose or it may be divided into two or three doses a day.
    - Children 3 months to 12 years of age—The dose is usually 0.05 to 0.3 milliliters (mL) inhaled in each nostril one or two times a day.
    - Children up to 3 months of age—Dose must be determined by your doctor.
  - For controlling bed-wetting:
    - Adults, teenagers, and children 6 years of age or older—At first, 20 mcg inhaled into each nostril at bedtime. Then, your doctor may change the dose to 10 to 40 mcg a day.
    - Children up to 6 years of age—Dose must be determined by your doctor.
- For oral dosage form (tablets):
  - For preventing or controlling diabetes insipidus (water diabetes):
    - Adults, teenagers, and children—At first, 0.05 milligram (mg) two times a day. Then, your doctor may change the dose to 0.1 to 0.8 mg. The dose may be divided into several doses a day.
  - For controlling bed-wetting:
    - Adults, teenagers, and children 6 years of age or older—At first, 0.2 mg once a day at bedtime. Then, your doctor may increase the dose to as much as 0.6 mg a day.
    - Children up to 6 years of age—Dose must be determined by your doctor.

- For parenteral dosage form (injection):
  - For preventing or controlling frequent urination:
    - Adults and teenagers—2 to 4 mcg injected into a muscle, vein, or under the skin. This dose is usually divided into two doses a day, one given in the morning, and the other given in the evening.
    - Children—0.4 mcg or 0.025 mcg per kg (0.011 mcg per pound) of body weight injected into a muscle, vein, or under the skin once a day.
  - For treating some bleeding problems such as hemophilia or von Willebrand's disease:
    - Adults, teenagers, and children 11 months of age or older weighing more than 10 kg (22 pounds)—The dose is based on body weight and must be determined by your doctor. It is usually 0.3 mcg per kg (0.14 mcg per pound) of body weight mixed in 50 milliliters (mL) of 0.9% sodium chloride. This solution is injected into a vein slowly over fifteen to thirty minutes. Your doctor may repeat this treatment if needed.
    - Children 3 months of age or older weighing 10 kg (22 pounds) or less—The dose is based on body weight and must be determined by your doctor. It is usually 0.3 mcg per kg (0.14 mcg per pound) of body weight mixed in 10 mL of 0.9% sodium chloride. This solution is injected into a vein slowly over fifteen to thirty minutes. Your doctor may repeat this treatment if needed.
    - Children up to 11 months of age—Use is not recommended.

Missed dose—If you miss a dose of this medicine, take it as soon as possible. However, if it is almost time for your next dose, skip the missed dose and go back to your regular dosing schedule. Do not double doses.

Has a bulleted list describing how to handle missed doses for various possible dosing schedules.

Storage—Keep out of the reach of children.

Do not keep outdated medicine or medicine no longer needed.

Store as directed on the label or by your health care professional.

Side Effects of This Medicine

Along with its needed effects, a medicine may cause some unwanted effects. Although not all of these side effects may occur, if they do occur they may need medical attention.

Check with your doctor immediately if any of the following side effects occur:
  Rare
    Chills; confusion; convulsions (seizures); decreased urination; drowsiness; fever; headache (continuing); shortness of breath, tightness in chest, trouble in breathing, or wheezing; skin rash, hives, or itching; weight gain (rapid)

Check with your doctor as soon as possible if any of the following side effects occur:
  Rare
    Fast heartbeat

Some side effects may occur that usually do not need medical attention. These side effects may go away during treatment as your body adjusts to the medicine. Also, your health care

professional may be able to tell you about ways to prevent or reduce some of these side effects. Check with your health care professional if any of the following side effects continue or are bothersome or if you have any questions about them:

Less common or rare

Abdominal or stomach cramps; flushing or redness of skin; nausea; pain in the vulva (genital area outside of the vagina)

With intranasal (through the nose) use

Cough; nosebleed; runny or stuffy nose; sneezing; sore throat

With intravenous use

Pain, redness, or swelling at place of injection

Other side effects not listed may also occur in some patients. If you notice any other effects, check with your healthcare professional.

DEXMETHYLPHENIDATE (Oral route) - dex-meth-il-FEN-a-date

Black Box Warning

Dexmethylphenidate hydrochloride should be given cautiously to patients with a history of drug dependence or alcoholism. Chronic, abusive use can lead to marked tolerance and psychological dependence with varying degrees of abnormal behavior. Frank psychotic episodes can occur, especially with parenteral abuse. Careful supervision is required during drug withdrawal from abusive use since severe depression may occur. Withdrawal following chronic therapeutic use may unmask symptoms of the underlying disorder that may require follow-up.

Commonly used brand name(s)

In the U.S.—

Focalin

Focalin XR

Available Dosage Forms:

- Capsule, Extended Release
- Tablet

Therapeutic Class: CNS Stimulant

Uses For This Medicine

Dexmethylphenidate belongs to the group of medicines called central nervous system (CNS) stimulants. It is used to treat Attention Deficit Hyperactivity Disorder (ADHD) in patients 6 years of age and older.

Dexmethylphenidate works in the treatment of ADHD by increasing attention and decreasing restlessness in children and adults who are overactive, cannot concentrate for very long or are easily distracted, and are impulsive. This medicine is used as part of a total treatment program that also includes social, educational, and psychological treatment.

This medicine is available only with your doctor's prescription.

Before Using This Medicine

In deciding to use a medicine, the risks of taking the medicine must be weighed against the good it will do. This is a decision you and your doctor will make. For this medicine, the following should be considered:

Allergies—Tell your doctor if you have ever had any unusual or allergic reaction to this medicine or any other medicines. Also tell your health care professional if you have any other types of allergies, such as to foods, dyes, preservatives, or animals. For non-prescription products, read the label or package ingredients carefully.

Pediatric—Side effects such as loss of appetite, stomach pain, weight loss (during prolonged treatment), trouble sleeping, and a fast heartbeat may be especially likely to occur in children, who are usually more sensitive than adults to the effects of dexmethylphenidate. Some children who used medicines like dexmethylphenidate for a long time grew more slowly than expected. It is not known whether long-term use of dexmethylphenidate causes slowed growth. The doctor should regularly measure the height and weight of children who are taking methylphenidate.

Studies on this medicine have been done only in children 6 years of age and older and there is no specific information comparing use of dexmethylphenidate in children less than 6 years of age with use in other age groups.

Geriatric—Many medicines have not been studied specifically in older people. Therefore, it may not be known whether they work exactly the same way they do in younger adults or if they cause different side effects or problems in older people. There is no specific information comparing use of dexmethylphenidate with use in other age groups.

Pregnancy—

	Pregnancy Category	Explanation
All Trimesters	C	Animal studies have shown an adverse effect and there are no adequate studies in pregnant women OR no animal studies have been conducted and there are no adequate studies in pregnant women.

Breast Feeding—There are no adequate studies in women for determining infant risk when using this medication during breastfeeding. Weigh the potential benefits against the potential risks before taking this medication while breastfeeding.

Other medicines—

Using this medicine with any of the following medicines is not recommended. Your doctor may decide not to treat you with this medication or change some of the other medicines you take.

Clorgyline, Iproniazid, Isocarboxazid, Lazabemide, Moclobemide, Nialamide, Pargyline, Phenelzine, Procarbazine, Selegiline, Toloxatone, Tranylcypromine

Interactions with Food/Tobacco/Alcohol—Certain medicines should not be used at or around the time of eating food or eating certain types of food since interactions may occur. Using alcohol or tobacco with certain medicines may also cause interactions to occur. Discuss with your healthcare professional the use of your medicine with food, alcohol, or tobacco.

Other medical problems—The presence of other medical problems may affect the use of this medicine. Make sure you

tell your doctor if you have any other medical problems, especially:

- Alcohol abuse (or history of) or
- Drug abuse or dependence (or history of)—Dependence on dexmethylphenidate may be more likely to develop
- Agitation or
- Anxiety or
- Tension—Dexmethylphenidate may make the condition worse and should not be used.
- Depression, severe or
- Glaucoma or
- Motor tics or
- Tourette's syndrome, family history or diagnosis—Dexmethylphenidate should not be used when these conditions exist.
- Growth rate slowed, long-term—Reported with long-term use of stimulant medicines similar to dexmethylphenidate.
- Heart failure or
- Hypertension or
- Hyperthyroidism or
- Recent heart attack—May increase blood pressure or heart rate.
- Psychosis—Dexmethylphenidate may make behavior problems and thought disorder symptoms in children worse.
- Seizures (history of) or
- EEG abnormalities or—The risk of having seizures may be increased.

Proper Use of This Medicine

Take this medicine only as directed by your doctor. Do not take more of it, do not take it more often, and do not take it for a longer time than your doctor ordered. If too much is taken, it may become habit-forming.

Dexmethylphenidate may be taken with or without food or on a full or empty stomach. However, if your doctor tells you to take the medicine a certain way, take it exactly as directed.

You should take the extended-release capsule one time per day in the morning.

The extended-release capsule should be swallowed whole and not crushed, divided, or chewed.

If you are unable to swallow the capsule whole, you may sprinkle the contents of the capsule. Open the capsule carefully and sprinkle the beads over a spoonful of applesauce. The mixture of drug and applesauce should be taken immediately in its entirety. The drug and applesauce should not be stored for future use.

While your are taking dexmethylphenidate, your doctor may require different tests for monitoring of your condition, such as blood pressure, heart rate, complete blood cell counts, and growth rates.

Dosing—The dose of this medicine will be different for different patients. Follow your doctor's orders or the directions on the label. The following information includes only the average doses of this medicine. If your dose is different, do not change it unless your doctor tells you to do so.

The amount of medicine that you take depends on the strength of the medicine. Also, the number of doses you take each day, the time allowed between doses, and the length of time you take the medicine depend on the medical problem for which you are using the medicine.

- For oral dosage form (long-acting capsules):
  - For attention deficit hyperactivity disorder (ADHD):
    - Children 6 years of age and older—
      - Patients not taking dexmethylphenidate, methylphenidate, or taking other stimulant medicines other than methylphenidate— 5 milligrams (mg) one time a day in the morning. If needed, your doctor may increase the dose once a week by 5 mg a day until symptoms improve or a maximum dose is reached.
      - Patients taking methylphenidate—Your doctor will start the dose at half the dose of methylphenidate you are taking, one time a day. If needed, your doctor will adjust your dose once a week to a maximum dose of 20 mg one time a day.
    - Children up to 6 years of age—Use and dose must be determined by your doctor.

- For oral dosage form (tablets):
  - For attention deficit hyperactivity disorder (ADHD):
    - Adults, teenagers, and children 6 years of age and older—
      - Patients not taking methylphenidate or taking other stimulant medicines other than methylphenidate—2.5 milligrams (mg) two times a day, at least 4 hours apart. If needed, your doctor may increase the dose once a week by 2.5 to 5 mg a day until symptoms improve or a maximum dose is reached.
      - Patients taking methylphenidate—Your doctor will start the dose at half the dose of methylphenidate you are taking, at least 4 hours apart. If needed, your doctor will adjust your dose once a week to a maximum dose of 10 mg two times a day.
    - Children up to 6 years of age—Use and dose must be determined by your doctor.

Missed dose—If you miss a dose of this medicine, take it as soon as possible. However, if it is almost time for your next dose, skip the missed dose and go back to your regular dosing schedule. Do not double doses.

Then take any remaining doses for that day at regularly spaced intervals that are at least 4 hours apart for the tablets and 24 apart for the extended-release capsules.

Storage—Store the medicine in a closed container at room temperature, away from heat, moisture, and direct light. Keep from freezing.

Do not keep outdated medicine or medicine no longer needed.

Precautions While Using This Medicine

Your doctor should check your progress at regular visits and make sure that your dose is right and that the medicine is helping you.

Do not take other medicines unless they have been discussed with your doctor. This especially includes nonprescription medicines, such as aspirin, and medicines for appetite control, asthma, colds, cough, hay fever, or sinus problems.

This medicine may cause some people to become drowsy, dizzy, or less alert than they are normally. Make sure you know how you react to this medicine before you drive, use machines, or do anything else that could be dangerous if you are dizzy or are not alert.

Side Effects of This Medicine

Along with its needed effects, a medicine may cause some unwanted effects. Although not all of these side effects may occur, if they do occur they may need medical attention.

Check with your doctor as soon as possible if any of the following side effects occur:

Less common
Fast, pounding, or irregular heartbeat or pulse

Rare
Blurred vision; change in near or distance vision; difficulty in focusing eyes

Incidence not known
Convulsions; muscle spasm or jerking of arms and legs; sudden loss of consciousness

Some side effects may occur that usually do not need medical attention. These side effects may go away during treatment as your body adjusts to the medicine. Also, your health care professional may be able to tell you about ways to prevent or reduce some of these side effects. Check with your health care professional if any of the following side effects continue or are bothersome or if you have any questions about them:

More common
Acid or sour stomach; belching; dry mouth; headache; heartburn; indigestion; stomach discomfort, upset or pain; loss of appetite; nausea; throat pain; weight loss

Less common
Fever; sleeplessness; trouble sleeping; twitching; unable to sleep

Symptoms of overdose
Get emergency help immediately if any of the following symptoms of overdose occur:
Anxiety; bigger, dilated, or enlarged pupils (black part of eye); blurred vision; change in consciousness; chest pain or discomfort; confusion as to time, place, or person; dizziness; dry mouth; dryness of mucous membranes; fainting; false or unusual sense of well-being; fast, slow, or irregular heartbeat; feeling of warmth; fever; hallucinations; headache; holding false beliefs that cannot be changed by fact; hyperventilation; increased sensitivity of eyes to light; irregular heartbeats; irritability; lightheadedness; loss of consciousness; mood or mental changes; muscle twitching; nervousness; overactive reflexes; pounding in the ears; pounding or rapid pulse; redness of the face, neck, arms and occasionally upper chest; restlessness; shaking; seeing, hearing, or feeling things that are not there; seizures; shortness of breath; slow or fast heartbeat; sweating; tremors such as shakiness; trouble sleeping; unusual excitement; vomiting

Some side effects may occur that usually do not need medical attention. These side effects may go away during treatment as your body adjusts to the medicine. Also, your health care professional may be able to tell you about ways to prevent or reduce some of these side effects. Check with your health care professional if any of the following side effects continue or are bothersome or if you have any questions about them:

Other side effects not listed may also occur in some patients. If you notice any other effects, check with your healthcare professional.

DEXRAZOXANE (Intravenous route) - dex-ray-ZOKS-ane

Commonly used brand name(s)

In the U.S.—
Zinecard

Available Dosage Forms:
• Powder for Solution

Therapeutic Class: Cardioprotective Agent

Uses For This Medicine

Dexrazoxane is used to help prevent or lessen a toxic effect to your heart that is caused by certain medicines that are used to treat cancer.

This medicine is available only with your doctor's prescription.

Before Using This Medicine

In deciding to use a medicine, the risks of taking the medicine must be weighed against the good it will do. This is a decision you and your doctor will make. For this medicine, the following should be considered:

Allergies—Tell your doctor if you have ever had any unusual or allergic reaction to this medicine or any other medicines. Also tell your health care professional if you have any other types of allergies, such as to foods, dyes, preservatives, or animals. For non-prescription products, read the label or package ingredients carefully.

Pediatric—Studies on this medicine have been done only in adult patients, and there is no specific information comparing use of dexrazoxane in children with use in other age groups.

Geriatric—Many medicine have not been studies specifically on older people. Therefore, it may not be known whether they work exactly the same way they do in younger adults or if they cause different side effects or problems in older people. There is no specific information comparing the use of dexrazoxane in the elderly with use in other age groups.

Pregnancy—

	Pregnancy Category	Explanation
All Trimesters	C	Animal studies have shown an adverse effect and there are no adequate studies in pregnant women OR no animal studies have been conducted and there are no adequate studies in pregnant women.

Breast Feeding—There are no adequate studies in women for determining infant risk when using this medication during breastfeeding. Weigh the potential benefits against the potential risks before taking this medication while breastfeeding.

Other medicines—Although certain medicines should not be used together at all, in other cases two different medicines may be used together even if an interaction might occur. In these cases, your doctor may want to change the dose, or other precautions may be necessary. Tell your healthcare professional if you are taking any other prescription or non-prescription (over-the-counter [OTC]) medicine.

Interactions with Food/Tobacco/Alcohol—Certain medicines should not be used at or around the time of eating food or eating certain types of food since interactions may occur. Using alcohol or tobacco with certain medicines may also cause interactions to occur. Discuss with your healthcare professional the use of your medicine with food, alcohol, or tobacco.

Proper Use of This Medicine

Dosing—The dose of this medicine will be different for different patients. Follow your doctor's orders or the directions on the label. The following information includes only the average doses of this medicine. If your dose is different, do not change it unless your doctor tells you to do so.

The amount of medicine that you take depends on the strength of the medicine. Also, the number of doses you take each day, the time allowed between doses, and the length of time you take the medicine depend on the medical problem for which you are using the medicine.

Side Effects of This Medicine

Along with its needed effects, a medicine may cause some unwanted effects. Although not all of these side effects may occur, if they do occur they may need medical attention.

Check with your doctor immediately if any of the following side effects occur:
> *Less common*
>> Pain at place of injection

Other side effects not listed may also occur in some patients. If you notice any other effects, check with your healthcare professional.

DEXTROMETHORPHAN (Oral route)
- dex-troe-meth-OR-fan

Commonly used brand name(s)

In the U.S.—

Babee Cof Syrup	Miltuss
Benylin Pediatric Formula	Nycoff
Creomulsion	Pediacare
Creo-Terpin	Robitussin
Delsym	Silphen DM
Dexalone	Simply Cough
ElixSure Cough Children's	St. Joseph
Father John's Medicine	Vicks 44 Cough Relief

Available Dosage Forms:
- Suspension, Extended Release
- Solution
- Syrup
- Liquid
- Tablet
- Lozenge/Troche
- Capsule

Therapeutic Class: Antitussive

Uses For This Medicine

Dextromethorphan is used to relieve coughs due to colds or influenza (flu). It should not be used for chronic cough that occurs with smoking, asthma, or emphysema or when there is an unusually large amount of mucus or phlegm (flem) with the cough.

Dextromethorphan relieves cough by acting directly on the cough center in the brain.

This medicine is available without a prescription.

Before Using This Medicine

In deciding to use a medicine, the risks of taking the medicine must be weighed against the good it will do. This is a decision you and your doctor will make. For this medicine, the following should be considered:

Allergies—Tell your doctor if you have ever had any unusual or allergic reaction to this medicine or any other medicines. Also tell your health care professional if you have any other types of allergies, such as to foods, dyes, preservatives, or animals. For non-prescription products, read the label or package ingredients carefully.

Pediatric—Although there is no specific information comparing use of dextromethorphan in children with use in other age groups, this medicine is not expected to cause different side effects or problems in children than it does in adults.

Geriatric—Many medicines have not been studied specifically in older people. Therefore, it may not be known whether they work exactly the same way they do in younger adults or if they cause different side effects or problems in older people. There is no specific information comparing use of dextromethorphan in the elderly with use in other age groups.

Breast Feeding—Studies in women suggest that this medication poses minimal risk to the infant when used during breastfeeding.

Other medicines—

Using this medicine with any of the following medicines is not recommended. Your doctor may decide not to treat you with this medication or change some of the other medicines you take.

Clorgyline, Iproniazid, Isocarboxazid, Moclobemide, Nialamide, Pargyline, Phenelzine, Procarbazine, Rasagiline, Selegiline, Toloxatone, Tranylcypromine

Interactions with Food/Tobacco/Alcohol—Certain medicines should not be used at or around the time of eating food or eating certain types of food since interactions may occur. Using alcohol or tobacco with certain medicines may also cause interactions to occur. Discuss with your healthcare professional the use of your medicine with food, alcohol, or tobacco.

Other medical problems—The presence of other medical problems may affect the use of this medicine. Make sure you tell your doctor if you have any other medical problems, especially:

- Asthma—Since dextromethorphan decreases coughing, it makes it difficult to get rid of the mucus that collects in the lungs and airways during asthma
- Diabetes (sugar diabetes)—Some products contain sugar and may affect control of blood glucose monitoring
- Liver disease—Dextromethorphan may build up in the body and cause unwanted effects
- Chronic bronchitis or
- Emphysema or
- Mucus or phlegm with cough—Since dextromethorphan decreases coughing, it makes it difficult to get rid of the mucus that may collect in the lungs and airways with some diseases
- Slowed breathing—Dextromethorphan may slow the rate of breathing even further

Proper Use of This Medicine

Make certain your health care professional knows if you are on a low-sodium, low-sugar, or any other special diet. Most medicines contain more than their active ingredient, and many liquid medicines contain alcohol.

Use this medicine only as directed by your doctor or the directions on the label. Do not use more of it, do not use it more often, and do not use it for a longer time than your doctor or the label says. Although this effect has happened only rarely, dextromethorphan has become habit-forming (causing mental or physical dependence) in some persons who used too much for a long time.

Dosing—The dose of this medicine will be different for different patients. Follow your doctor's orders or the directions on the label. The following information includes only the average doses of this medicine. If your dose is different, do not change it unless your doctor tells you to do so.

The amount of medicine that you take depends on the strength of the medicine. Also, the number of doses you take each day, the time allowed between doses, and the length of time you take the medicine depend on the medical problem for which you are using the medicine.

- For lozenge dosage form:
  - For cough:
    - Adults and children 12 years of age and older—5 to 15 mg every two to four hours, as needed.
    - Children younger than 2 years of age—Use and dose must be determined by your doctor.
    - Children 2 to 6 years of age—5 mg every four hours, as needed.
    - Children 6 to 12 years of age—5 to 15 mg every two to six hours, as needed.
- For syrup dosage form:
  - For cough:
    - Adults and children 12 years of age and older—30 mg every six to eight hours, as needed.
    - Children younger than 2 years of age—Use and dose must be determined by your doctor.
    - Children 2 to 6 years of age—3.5 mg every four hours or 7.5 mg every six to eight hours, as needed.
    - Children 6 to 12 years of age—7 mg every four hours or 15 mg every six to eight hours, as needed.
- For extended-release oral suspension dosage form:
  - For cough:
    - Adults and children 12 years of age and older—60 mg every twelve hours, as needed.
    - Children younger than 2 years of age—Use and dose must be determined by your doctor.
    - Children 2 to 6 years of age—15 mg every twelve hours, as needed.
    - Children 6 to 12 years of age—30 mg every twelve hours, as needed.

Missed dose—If you miss a dose of this medicine, take it as soon as possible. However, if it is almost time for your next dose, skip the missed dose and go back to your regular dosing schedule. Do not double doses.

Storage—Store the medicine in a closed container at room temperature, away from heat, moisture, and direct light. Keep from freezing.

Keep out of the reach of children.

Do not keep outdated medicine or medicine no longer needed.

Precautions While Using This Medicine

If your cough has not improved after 7 days, if sore throat has not improved after 2 days, if you have a high fever, skin rash, or continuing headache with the cough, or if asthma or high blood pressure is present, check with your doctor. These signs may mean that you have other medical problems.

Dissolve lozenges in the mouth with caution, to lessen the risk of choking.

Side Effects of This Medicine

Along with its needed effects, a medicine may cause some unwanted effects. Although not all of these side effects may occur, if they do occur they may need medical attention.

Check with your doctor as soon as possible if any of the following side effects occur:

Symptoms of overdose

Blurred vision; confusion; difficulty in urination; drowsiness or dizziness; nausea or vomiting (severe); shakiness and unsteady walk; slowed breathing; unusual excitement, nervousness, restlessness, or irritability (severe)

Some side effects may occur that usually do not need medical attention. These side effects may go away during treatment as your body adjusts to the medicine. Also, your health care professional may be able to tell you about ways to prevent or reduce some of these side effects. Check with your health care professional if any of the following side effects continue or are bothersome or if you have any questions about them:

Less common or rare

Confusion; constipation; dizziness (mild); drowsiness (mild); headache; nausea or vomiting; stomach pain

Other side effects not listed may also occur in some patients. If you notice any other effects, check with your healthcare professional.

DIAZOXIDE (Oral route) - dye-az-OX-ide

Commonly used brand name(s)

In the U.S.—
Proglycem

Available Dosage Forms:
- Capsule
- Suspension

Therapeutic Class: Glucose Regulation, Antihypoglycemic

Uses For This Medicine

Diazoxide when taken by mouth is used in the treatment of hypoglycemia (low blood sugar). It works by preventing release of insulin from the pancreas.

Diazoxide is available only with your doctor's prescription.

Before Using This Medicine

In deciding to use a medicine, the risks of taking the medicine must be weighed against the good it will do. This is a decision you and your doctor will make. For this medicine, the following should be considered:

Allergies—Tell your doctor if you have ever had any unusual or allergic reaction to this medicine or any other medicines. Also tell your health care professional if you have any other types of allergies, such as to foods, dyes, preservatives, or animals. For non-prescription products, read the label or package ingredients carefully.

Pediatric—Infants are more likely to retain (keep) body water because of diazoxide. In some infants, this may lead to certain types of heart problems. Also, a few children who received diazoxide for prolonged periods (longer than 4 years) developed changes in their facial structure.

Geriatric—Many medicines have not been tested in older people. Therefore, it may not be known whether they work exactly the same way they do in younger adults or if they cause different side effects or problems in older people. There is no specific information comparing use of oral diazoxide in the elderly with use in other age groups.

Pregnancy—

	Pregnancy Category	Explanation
All Trimesters	C	Animal studies have shown an adverse effect and there are no adequate studies in pregnant women OR no animal studies have been conducted and there are no adequate studies in pregnant women.

Breast Feeding—There are no adequate studies in women for determining infant risk when using this medication during breastfeeding. Weigh the potential benefits against the potential risks before taking this medication while breastfeeding.

Other medicines—

Using this medicine with any of the following medicines is usually not recommended, but may be required in some cases. If both medicines are prescribed together, your doctor may change the dose or how often you use one or both of the medicines.

Dofetilide

Interactions with Food/Tobacco/Alcohol—Certain medicines should not be used at or around the time of eating food or eating certain types of food since interactions may occur. Using alcohol or tobacco with certain medicines may also cause interactions to occur. Discuss with your healthcare professional the use of your medicine with food, alcohol, or tobacco.

Other medical problems—The presence of other medical problems may affect the use of this medicine. Make sure you tell your doctor if you have any other medical problems, especially:
- Angina (chest pain)
- Gout—Diazoxide may make this condition worse
- Heart attack (recent)
- Heart or blood vessel disease
- Kidney disease—The effects of diazoxide may last longer because the kidney may not be able to get the medicine out of the bloodstream as it normally would
- Liver disease
- Stroke (recent)

Proper Use of This Medicine

Take this medicine only as directed by your doctor. Do not take more or less of it than your doctor ordered, and take it at the same time each day.

Follow carefully the special diet your doctor gave you. This is an important part of controlling your condition, and is necessary if the medicine is to work properly.

Test for sugar in your urine or blood with a diabetic urine or blood test kit as directed by your doctor. This is a convenient way to make sure your condition is being controlled, and it provides an early warning when it is not. Your doctor may also want you to test your urine for acetone.

Dosing—The dose of this medicine will be different for different patients. Follow your doctor's orders or the directions on the label. The following information includes only the average doses of this medicine. If your dose is different, do not change it unless your doctor tells you to do so.

The amount of medicine that you take depends on the strength of the medicine. Also, the number of doses you take each day, the time allowed between doses, and the length of time you take the medicine depend on the medical problem for which you are using the medicine.

- For oral dosage forms (capsules or suspension):
  - For treating hypoglycemia (low blood sugar):
    - Adults, teenagers, and children—Dose is based on body weight and must be determined by your doctor. At first, the usual dose is 1 milligram (mg) per kilogram (kg) (0.45 mg per pound) of body weight every eight hours. Then, your doctor may increase your dose to 3 to 8 mg per kg (1.4 to 3.6 mg per pound) of body weight a day. This dose may be divided into two or three doses.
    - Newborn babies and infants—Dose is based on body weight and must be determined by your doctor. At first, the usual dose is 3.3 mg per kg (1.5 mg per pound) of body weight every eight hours. Then, your doctor may increase the dose

to 8 to 15 mg per kg (3.6 to 6.8 mg per pound) of body weight a day. This dose may be divided into two or three doses.

Missed dose—If you miss a dose of this medicine, take it as soon as possible. However, if it is almost time for your next dose, skip the missed dose and go back to your regular dosing schedule. Do not double doses.

Storage—Store the medicine in a closed container at room temperature, away from heat, moisture, and direct light. Keep from freezing.

Keep out of the reach of children.

Do not keep outdated medicine or medicine no longer needed.

Precautions While Using This Medicine

It is very important that your doctor check your progress at regular visits, especially during the first few weeks of treatment, to make sure that this medicine is working properly.

Before you have any kind of surgery, dental treatment, or emergency treatment, tell the medical doctor or dentist in charge that you are using this medicine.

Do not take any other medicine, unless prescribed or approved by your doctor, since some may interfere with this medicine's effects. This especially includes over-the-counter (OTC) or nonprescription medicine such as that for colds, cough, asthma, hay fever, or appetite control.

Check with your doctor right away if symptoms of high blood sugar (hyperglycemia) occur. These symptoms usually include:

- Drowsiness
- Flushed, dry skin
- Fruit-like breath odor
- Increased urination
- Loss of appetite (continuing)
- Unusual thirst

These symptoms may occur if the dose of the medicine is too high, or if you have a fever or infection or are experiencing unusual stress.

Check with your doctor as soon as possible also if these symptoms of low blood sugar (hypoglycemia) occur:

- Anxiety
- Chills
- Cold sweats
- Cool pale skin
- Drowsiness
- Excessive hunger
- Fast pulse
- Headache
- Nausea
- Nervousness
- Shakiness
- Unusual tiredness or weakness

Symptoms of both low blood sugar and high blood sugar must be corrected before they progress to a more serious condition. In either situation, you should check with your doctor immediately.

Side Effects of This Medicine

Along with its needed effects, a medicine may cause some unwanted effects. Although not all of these side effects may occur, if they do occur they may need medical attention.

Stop taking this medicine and get emergency help immediately if any of the following effects occur:

Rare

Chest pain caused by exercise or activity; confusion; numbness of the hands; shortness of breath (unexplained)

Check with your doctor as soon as possible if any of the following side effects occur:

More common

Decreased urination; swelling of feet or lower legs; weight gain (rapid)

Less common

Fast heartbeat

Rare

Fever; skin rash; stiffness of arms or legs; trembling and shaking of hands and fingers; unusual bleeding or bruising

Some side effects may occur that usually do not need medical attention. These side effects may go away during treatment as your body adjusts to the medicine. Also, your health care professional may be able to tell you about ways to prevent or reduce some of these side effects. Check with your health care professional if any of the following side effects continue or are bothersome or if you have any questions about them:

Less common

Changes in ability to taste; constipation; increased hair growth on forehead, back, arms, and legs; loss of appetite; nausea and vomiting; stomach pain

This medicine may cause a temporary increase in hair growth in some people when it is used for a long time. After treatment with diazoxide has ended, normal hair growth should return.

Other side effects not listed may also occur in some patients. If you notice any other effects, check with your healthcare professional.

DICLOFENAC   (Topical route) - di-KLO-fen-ack

Black Box Warning

- CARDIOVASCULAR RISK
  - NSAIDs may cause an increased risk of serious cardiovascular thrombotic events, myocardial infarction, and stroke, which can be fatal. This risk may increase with duration of use. Patients with cardiovascular disease or risk factors for cardiovascular disease may be at greater risk
- Diclofenac is contraindicated for the treatment of perioperative pain in the setting of coronary artery bypass graft (CABG) surgery.
- GASTROINTESTINAL RISK
  - NSAIDs cause an increased risk of serious gastrointestinal adverse events including bleeding, ulcer-

ation, and perforation of the stomach or intestines, which can be fatal. These events can occur at any time during use and without warning symptoms. Elderly patients are at greater risk for serious gastrointestinal events.

Commonly used brand name(s)

In the U.S.—
Solaraze

Available Dosage Forms:
• Gel/Jelly

Therapeutic Class: Analgesic
Pharmacologic Class: NSAID

Uses For This Medicine

Diclofenac belongs to the family of medicines called antineoplastics. Antineoplastics are used to treat cancer by killing cancer cells.

When applied to the skin, diclofenac is used to treat actinic keratosis, a skin problem that may be cancer or may become cancerous if not treated. The exact way that topical diclofenac helps this condition is unknown.

This medicine is available only with your doctor's prescription.

Before Using This Medicine

In deciding to use a medicine, the risks of taking the medicine must be weighed against the good it will do. This is a decision you and your doctor will make. For this medicine, the following should be considered:

Allergies—Tell your doctor if you have ever had any unusual or allergic reaction to this medicine or any other medicines. Also tell your health care professional if you have any other types of allergies, such as to foods, dyes, preservatives, or animals. For non-prescription products, read the label or package ingredients carefully.

Pediatric—Studies on this medicine have been done only in adult patients, and there is no specific information comparing use of diclofenac on the skin in children with use in other age groups.

Geriatric—Many medicines have not been studied specifically in older people. Therefore, it may not be known whether they work exactly the same way they do in younger adults. Although there is no specific information comparing use of diclofenac on the skin in the elderly with use in other age groups, this medicine is not expected to cause different side effects or problems in older people than it does in younger adults.

Pregnancy—

	Pregnancy Category	Explanation
All Trimesters	C	Animal studies have shown an adverse effect and there are no adequate studies in pregnant women OR no animal studies have been conducted and there are no adequate studies in pregnant women.

Breast Feeding—There are no adequate studies in women for determining infant risk when using this medication during breastfeeding. Weigh the potential benefits against the potential risks before taking this medication while breastfeeding.

Other medicines—

Using this medicine with any of the following medicines is not recommended. Your doctor may decide not to treat you with this medication or change some of the other medicines you take.

Ketorolac

Interactions with Food/Tobacco/Alcohol—Certain medicines should not be used at or around the time of eating food or eating certain types of food since interactions may occur. Using alcohol or tobacco with certain medicines may also cause interactions to occur. Discuss with your healthcare professional the use of your medicine with food, alcohol, or tobacco.

Other medical problems—The presence of other medical problems may affect the use of this medicine. Make sure you tell your doctor if you have any other medical problems, especially:

• Stomach or intestinal ulcers or bleeding—Diclofenac may make these conditions worse

• Kidney disease or

• Liver disease—Effects of this medicine may be increased because of slower removal of the medicine from the body

Proper Use of This Medicine

Keep using this medicine for the full time of treatment. However, do not use this medicine more often or for a longer time than your doctor ordered. Apply enough medicine each time to cover the entire affected area.

Diclofenac may cause redness, soreness, scaling, and peeling of the affected skin. Do not stop using this medicine without first checking with your doctor. If the reaction is very uncomfortable, check with your doctor.

Apply this medicine very carefully, and avoid getting any in your eyes. Do not apply this medicine to areas with broken skin or open wounds, infection, or severely peeling skin.

Dosing—The dose of this medicine will be different for different patients. Follow your doctor's orders or the directions on the label. The following information includes only the average doses of this medicine. If your dose is different, do not change it unless your doctor tells you to do so.

The amount of medicine that you take depends on the strength of the medicine. Also, the number of doses you take each day, the time allowed between doses, and the length of time you take the medicine depend on the medical problem for which you are using the medicine.

• For topical dosage form (gel):
  ○ For actinic keratosis:
    ▪ Adults—Apply to affected skin 2 times a day

Missed dose—If you miss a dose of this medicine, take it as soon as possible. However, if it is almost time for your next dose, skip the missed dose and go back to your regular dosing schedule. Do not double doses.

Storage—Store the medicine in a closed container at room temperature, away from heat, moisture, and direct light. Keep from freezing.

Keep out of the reach of children.

Do not keep outdated medicine or medicine no longer needed.

Ask your healthcare professional how you should dispose of any medicine you do not use.

Precautions While Using This Medicine

It is very important that your doctor check your progress at regular visits to make sure that this medicine is working properly and to check for unwanted effects.

If your symptoms become worse, check with your doctor.

While using this medicine, your skin may become more sensitive to sunlight than usual, and too much sunlight may increase the effects of the medicine. During this period of time:

- Stay out of direct sunlight, especially between the hours of 10:00 a.m. and 3:00 p.m., if possible.
- Wear protective clothing, including a hat and sunglasses.
- Do not use a sunlamp or tanning bed or booth.
- Make sure you have discussed the use of a sun block product with your doctor.

If you have a severe reaction from the sun, check with your doctor.

Side Effects of This Medicine

Along with its needed effects, a medicine may cause some unwanted effects. Although not all of these side effects may occur, if they do occur they may need medical attention.

Check with your doctor as soon as possible if any of the following side effects occur:

More common
Application site reactions, including skin rash, pain, tingling or burning sensation; itching skin; flu-like syndrome (bodyache; headache; fever, with or without chills)

Less common or rare
Application site reactions, including swelling; increased skin sensitivity; or skin rash, itching, redness, or pain caused by reaction from exposure to sun; blood in the urine; cough; decrease in body movement; dry, itching, or burning eyes; eye pain; fever; headaches, including migraines; high blood pressure; increased sensitivity of eyes to light; infection; nasal congestion; pain or tenderness around eyes and cheekbones; redness or swelling of eyes; shortness of breath; skin rash other than at the application site; sore throat; tightness in chest; troubled breathing; ulcers or sores on skin, other than at the application site; wheezing

Some side effects may occur that usually do not need medical attention. These side effects may go away during treatment as your body adjusts to the medicine. Also, your health care professional may be able to tell you about ways to prevent or reduce some of these side effects. Check with your health care professional if any of the following side effects continue or are bothersome or if you have any questions about them:

More common
burning skin; dry skin; red skin; scaly skin; thickened skin; tingling skin

Less common
Acne; back pain; belching; bleeding skin; chest pain; diarrhea; heartburn; indigestion; joint pain; lack or loss

of strength; loss or thinning of hair; muscle pain; neck pain; runny nose; stomach upset or pain

Other side effects not listed may also occur in some patients. If you notice any other effects, check with your healthcare professional.

DICLOFENAC AND MISOPROSTOL
(Oral route) - di-KLO-fen-ack, mye-soe-PROST-ole

Black Box Warning

Administration of misoprostol to women who are pregnant can cause abortion, premature birth, or birth defects. Uterine rupture has been reported when misoprostol was administered in pregnant women to induce labor or to induce abortion beyond the eighth week of pregnancy. Diclofenac sodium/misoprostol should not be taken by pregnant women.

Patients must be advised of the abortifacient property and warned not to give the drug to others.

Diclofenac sodium/misoprostol should not be used in women of childbearing potential unless the patient requires nonsteroidal anti-inflammatory drug (NSAID) therapy and is at high risk of developing gastric or duodenal ulceration or for developing complications from gastric or duodenal ulcers associated with the use of the NSAID. In such patients, diclofenac sodium/misoprostol may be prescribed if the patient:

- has had a negative serum pregnancy test within 2 weeks prior to beginning therapy.
- is capable of complying with effective contraceptive measures.
- has received both oral and written warnings of the hazards of misoprostol, the risk of possible contraception failure, and the danger to other women of childbearing potential should the drug be taken by mistake.
- will begin diclofenac sodium/misoprostol only on the third day of the next normal menstrual period.

Commonly used brand name(s)
In the U.S.—
Arthrotec

Available Dosage Forms:
- Tablet
- Tablet, Enteric Coated

Therapeutic Class: Analgesic
Pharmacologic Class: Diclofenac

Uses For This Medicine

Diclofenac and misoprostol combination is used for patients with arthritis who may develop stomach ulcers from taking nonsteroidal anti-inflammatory drugs (NSAIDs) alone.

Diclofenac is a NSAID used in this combination medicine to help relieve some symptoms of arthritis, such as inflammation, swelling, stiffness, and joint pain.

Misoprostol is used in this combination medicine to prevent stomach ulcers.

This medicine is available only with your doctor's prescription.

Before Using This Medicine

In deciding to use a medicine, the risks of taking the medicine must be weighed against the good it will do. This is a decision you and your doctor will make. For this medicine, the following should be considered:

Allergies—Tell your doctor if you have ever had any unusual or allergic reaction to this medicine or any other medicines. Also tell your health care professional if you have any other types of allergies, such as to foods, dyes, preservatives, or animals. For non-prescription products, read the label or package ingredients carefully.

Pediatric—Studies on this medicine have been done only in adult patients, and there is no specific information comparing use of diclofenac and misoprostol combination in children with use in other age groups.

Geriatric—Certain side effects, such as confusion, swelling of the face, feet, or lower legs, or sudden decrease in the amount of urine, may be especially likely to occur in elderly patients, who are usually more sensitive than younger adults to the effects of nonsteroidal anti-inflammatory drugs. Also, elderly people are more likely than younger adults to get sick if this medicine causes stomach problems.

Pregnancy—

	Pregnancy Category	Explanation
All Trimesters	X	Studies in animals or pregnant women have demonstrated positive evidence of fetal abnormalities. This drug should not be used in women who are or may become pregnant because the risk clearly outweighs any possible benefit.

Breast Feeding—There are no adequate studies in women for determining infant risk when using this medication during breastfeeding. Weigh the potential benefits against the potential risks before taking this medication while breastfeeding.

Other medicines—

Using this medicine with any of the following medicines is not recommended. Your doctor may decide not to treat you with this medication or change some of the other medicines you take.

Ketorolac

Interactions with Food/Tobacco/Alcohol—Certain medicines should not be used at or around the time of eating food or eating certain types of food since interactions may occur. Using alcohol or tobacco with certain medicines may also cause interactions to occur. Discuss with your healthcare professional the use of your medicine with food, alcohol, or tobacco.

Other medical problems—The presence of other medical problems may affect the use of this medicine. Make sure you tell your doctor if you have any other medical problems, especially:

- Alcohol abuse or
- Bleeding problems or
- Hepatitis or other liver disease or
- Kidney disease (or history of) or
- Tobacco use (or recent history of) or
- Stomach ulcer, or other stomach or intestinal problems or
- Systemic lupus erythematosus—The chance of side effects may be increased
- Anemia or
- Asthma or
- Dehydration or
- Fluid retention (swelling of feet or lower legs) or
- Heart disease or
- High blood pressure or
- Low platelet count or
- Low white blood cell count or
- Porphyria (liver) or
- Volume depletion—Diclofenac and misoprostol combination may make these conditions worse

Proper Use of This Medicine

For safe and effective use of this medicine, do not take more of it, do not take it more often, and do not take it for a longer time than ordered by your health care professional. Taking too much of this medicine may increase the chance of unwanted effects.

Do not take diclofenac and misoprostol combination with magnesium-containing antacids. Antacids may be taken with diclofenac and misoprostol combination, if needed, to help relieve stomach pain, unless you are otherwise directed by your doctor. However, do not take magnesium-containing antacids, since they may cause diarrhea or worsen the diarrhea that is sometimes caused by the diclofenac and misoprostol combination.

Do not chew, crush, or dissolve tablets.

Do not give this medication to another person.

Diclofenac and misoprostol combination should be taken with meals.

Dosing—The dose of this medicine will be different for different patients. Follow your doctor's orders or the directions on the label. The following information includes only the average doses of this medicine. If your dose is different, do not change it unless your doctor tells you to do so.

The amount of medicine that you take depends on the strength of the medicine. Also, the number of doses you take each day, the time allowed between doses, and the length of time you take the medicine depend on the medical problem for which you are using the medicine.

- For oral dosage form (tablets):
  - For osteoarthritis:
    - Adults—1 tablet of Arthrotec 50 three times a day.
    - Children—Use and dose must be determined by your doctor.
  - For rheumatoid arthritis:
    - Adults—1 tablet of Arthrotec 50 three or four times a day.
    - Children—Use and dose must be determined by your doctor.
  - For osteoarthritis or rheumatoid arthritis (for patients who are unable to tolerate other doses):
    - Adults—1 tablet of Arthrotec 50 two times a day or 1 tablet of Arthrotec 75 two times a day.
    - Children—Use and dose must be determined by your doctor.

Missed dose—If you miss a dose of this medicine, take it as soon as possible. However, if it is almost time for your next dose, skip the missed dose and go back to your regular dosing schedule. Do not double doses.

Storage—Store the medicine in a closed container at room temperature, away from heat, moisture, and direct light. Keep from freezing.

Keep out of the reach of children.

Do not keep outdated medicine or medicine no longer needed.

Precautions While Using This Medicine

Misoprostol may cause miscarriage if taken during pregnancy. Therefore, if you suspect that you may have become pregnant, stop taking this medicine immediately and check with your doctor.

This medicine may cause diarrhea in some people. The diarrhea will usually disappear within a few days as your body adjusts to the medicine. However, check with your doctor if the diarrhea is severe and/or does not stop after a week.

If you will be taking this medicine for a long time, your doctor should check your progress at regular visits. Your doctor may want to do certain tests to find out if unwanted effects are occurring. The tests are very important because serious side effects, including ulcers, bleeding, blood, or liver problems, can occur without any warning.

Stomach problems may be more likely to occur if you drink alcoholic beverages while being treated with this medicine. Therefore, do not regularly drink alcoholic beverages while taking this medicine, unless otherwise directed by your doctor.

Taking nonsteroidal anti-inflammatory drugs together with this medicine on a regular basis may increase the chance of unwanted effects. Also, taking acetaminophen, aspirin or other salicylates, or ketorolac (e.g.,Toradol) regularly while you are taking a diclofenac and misoprostol combination may increase the chance of unwanted effects. The risk will depend on how much of each medicine you take every day, and on how long you take the medicine together. If your health care professional directs you to take these medicines together on a regular basis, follow his or her directions carefully. However, do not take acetaminophen or aspirin or other salicylates together with this medicine for more than a few days, and do not take any ketorolac (e.g., Toradol) while you are taking this medicine, unless your doctor has directed you to do so and is following your progress.

Side Effects of This Medicine

Along with its needed effects, a medicine may cause some unwanted effects. Although not all of these side effects may occur, if they do occur they may need medical attention.

Check with your doctor as soon as possible if any of the following side effects occur:

Less common

Black, tarry stools; bleeding or crusting sores on lips; blood in urine or stools; bruises and/or red spots on the skin; chest pain; chills; confusion; continuing thirst; convulsions (seizures); cough or hoarseness; disorientation; drowsiness; fainting; fever with or without chills; fluid retention; general feeling of illness; heartburn and/or indigestion; increased blood pressure; increased heart rate; increased weight gain; itching of the skin; irregular heartbeat; large, flat, blue or purplish patches on the skin; light-headedness or dizziness; lower back or side pain; mental depression; muscle cramps; nausea; painful or difficult urination; pounding heartbeat; psychotic reaction; rectal bleeding; seeing, hearing, or feeling things that are not there; severe headache; severe hepatic reactions; severe stomach pain, cramping or burning; shortness of breath, troubled breathing, tightness in chest, and/or wheezing; skin rash; sores, ulcers, or white spots on lips or in mouth; sore throat; stiff neck and/or back; sudden decrease in the amount of urine; swelling and/or tenderness in upper stomach; swelling of face, fingers, feet, and/or lower legs; unusual bleeding or bruising; unusual tiredness or weakness; vomiting of material that looks like coffee grounds; yellow eyes or skin

Rare

Changes in facial skin color; fast or irregular breathing; puffiness or swelling of the eyelids or around the eyes

Symptoms of overdose

Confusion; diarrhea; drowsiness; fever; nausea and/or vomiting; pounding heartbeat; convulsions (seizures); shortness of breath; slow heartbeat; stomach pain; trembling or shaking

Some side effects may occur that usually do not need medical attention. These side effects may go away during treatment as your body adjusts to the medicine. Also, your health care professional may be able to tell you about ways to prevent or reduce some of these side effects. Check with your health care professional if any of the following side effects continue or are bothersome or if you have any questions about them:

More common

Diarrhea; gas; heartburn

Less common

Abnormal vision; acne; change in sense of taste; decreased appetite; dry mouth; irritability or nervousness; loss of hair; muscle pain; decrease in sexual ability; tingling, burning, or prickling sensations; trembling or shaking; trouble swallowing; vaginal bleeding

Other side effects not listed may also occur in some patients. If you notice any other effects, check with your healthcare professional.

DIDANOSINE   (Oral route) - dye-DAN-oh-seen

Black Box Warning

Fatal and nonfatal pancreatitis have occurred during therapy with didanosine used alone or in combination regimens in both treatment-naive and treatment-experienced patients, regardless of degree of immunosuppression. Didanosine should be suspended in patients with suspected pancreatitis and discontinued in patients with confirmed pancreatitis.

Lactic acidosis and severe hepatomegaly with steatosis, including fatal cases, have been reported with the use of nucleoside analogues alone or in combination, including didanosine and other antiretrovirals. Fatal lactic acidosis has been reported in pregnant women who received the combination of didanosine and stavudine with other antiretroviral agents. The combination of didanosine and stavudine should be used with caution during pregnancy and is recommended only if the potential benefit clearly outweighs the potential risk.

Commonly used brand name(s)

In the U.S.—
    Videx
    Videx EC
    Videx Pediatric

Available Dosage Forms:
- Powder for Solution
- Powder for Suspension
- Tablet, Chewable
- Capsule, Delayed Release

Therapeutic Class: Antiretroviral Agent
Pharmacologic Class: Nucleoside Reverse Transcriptase Inhibitor

Uses For This Medicine

Didanosine (also known as ddI) is used in the treatment of the infection caused by the human immunodeficiency virus (HIV). HIV is the virus responsible for acquired immune deficiency syndrome (AIDS).

Didanosine (ddI) will not cure or prevent HIV infection or AIDS; however, it helps keep HIV from reproducing and appears to slow down the destruction of the immune system. This may help delay the development of problems usually related to AIDS or HIV disease. Didanosine will not keep you from spreading HIV to other people. People who receive this medicine may continue to have the problems usually related to AIDS or HIV disease.

Didanosine may cause some serious side effects, including pancreatitis (inflammation of the pancreas). Symptoms of pancreatitis include stomach pain, and nausea and vomiting. Didanosine may also cause peripheral neuropathy. Symptoms of peripheral neuropathy include tingling, burning, numbness, and pain in the hands or feet. Check with your doctor if any new health problems or symptoms occur while you are taking didanosine.

Didanosine is available only with your doctor's prescription.

Before Using This Medicine

In deciding to use a medicine, the risks of taking the medicine must be weighed against the good it will do. This is a decision you and your doctor will make. For this medicine, the following should be considered:

Allergies—Tell your doctor if you have ever had any unusual or allergic reaction to this medicine or any other medicines. Also tell your health care professional if you have any other types of allergies, such as to foods, dyes, preservatives, or animals. For non-prescription products, read the label or package ingredients carefully.

Pediatric—Didanosine can cause serious side effects in any patient. Therefore, it is especially important that you discuss with your child's doctor the good that this medicine may do as well as the risks of using it. Your child must be carefully followed, and frequently seen, by the doctor while taking didanosine.

Geriatric—Many medicines have not been studied specifically in older people. Therefore, it may not be known whether they work exactly the same way they do in younger adults or

if they cause different side effects or problems in older people. There is no specific information comparing use of didanosine in the elderly with use in other age groups.

Pregnancy—

	Pregnancy Category	Explanation
All Trimesters	B	Animal studies have revealed no evidence of harm to the fetus, however, there are no adequate studies in pregnant women OR animal studies have shown an adverse effect, but adequate studies in pregnant women have failed to demonstrate a risk to the fetus.

Breast Feeding—There are no adequate studies in women for determining infant risk when using this medication during breastfeeding. Weigh the potential benefits against the potential risks before taking this medication while breastfeeding.

Other medicines—

Using this medicine with any of the following medicines is usually not recommended, but may be required in some cases. If both medicines are prescribed together, your doctor may change the dose or how often you use one or both of the medicines.

Hydroxyurea, Ribavirin, Stavudine, Tenofovir Disoproxil Fumarate, Zalcitabine

Interactions with Food/Tobacco/Alcohol—Certain medicines should not be used at or around the time of eating food or eating certain types of food since interactions may occur. Using alcohol or tobacco with certain medicines may also cause interactions to occur. Discuss with your healthcare professional the use of your medicine with food, alcohol, or tobacco.

Other medical problems—The presence of other medical problems may affect the use of this medicine. Make sure you tell your doctor if you have any other medical problems, especially:
- Alcoholism, active, or
- Increased blood triglycerides (substance formed in the body from fats in foods) or
- Pancreatitis (or a history of)—Patients with these medical problems may be at increased risk of pancreatitis (inflammation of the pancreas)
- Edema or
- Heart disease or
- High blood pressure or
- Kidney disease or
- Liver disease or
- Toxemia of pregnancy—The salt contained in the didanosine tablets and the oral solution packets may make these conditions worse
- Gouty arthritis—Didanosine may cause an attack or worsen gout
- Peripheral neuropathy—Didanosine may make this condition worse

- Phenylketonuria (PKU)—Didanosine tablets contain phenylalanine, which must be restricted in patients with PKU

Proper Use of This Medicine

Make certain your health care professional knows if you are on any special diet, such as a low-sodium (low-salt) diet. Didanosine chewable tablets and the oral solution packets contain a large amount of sodium. Also, didanosine tablets contain phenylalanine, which must be restricted in patients with phenylketonuria.

Take this medicine exactly as directed by your doctor. Do not take more of it, do not take it more often, and do not take it for a longer time than your doctor ordered. Also, do not stop taking this medicine without checking with your doctor first. However, stop taking didanosine and call your doctor right away if you get severe nausea, vomiting, and stomach pain.

Otherwise, keep taking didanosine for the full time of treatment, even if you begin to feel better.

For patients taking didanosine delayed-release capsules:

- Capsules should be swallowed intact.

For patients taking didanosine for oral solution, buffered powder:

- Open the foil packet and pour its contents into approximately 1/2 glass (4 ounces) of water. Do not mix with fruit juice or other acid-containing drinks.
- Stir for approximately 2 to 3 minutes until the powder is dissolved.
- Drink at once.

For patients taking didanosine for oral suspension, pediatric powder:

- Use a specially marked measuring spoon or other device to measure each dose accurately. The average household teaspoon may not hold the right amount of liquid.

For patients taking didanosine tablets, buffered— chewable and for oral suspension:

- Tablets should be thoroughly chewed or crushed or mixed in at least 1 ounce of water before swallowing. The tablets are hard and some people may find them difficult to chew. If the tablets are mixed in water, stir well until a uniform suspension is formed and take at once. For additional flavoring, mix the prepared suspension with 1 ounce of clear apple juice.
- Two tablets must be taken together by patients over 1 year of age. These tablets contain a special buffer to keep didanosine from being destroyed in the stomach. In order to get the correct amount of buffer, 2 tablets always need to be taken together. Infants from 6 to 12 months of age will get enough buffer from just 1 tablet. For 1–tablet dose, a ½ ounce of clear apple juice may be added as a flavor enhancer.

Didanosine should be taken on an empty stomach since food may decrease the absorption in the stomach and keep it from working properly. Didanosine should be taken at least 2 hours before or 2 hours after you eat.

This medicine works best when there is a constant amount in the blood. To help keep the amount constant, do not miss any doses. If you need help in planning the best times to take your medicine, check with your health care professional.

Dosing—The dose of this medicine will be different for different patients. Follow your doctor's orders or the directions on the label. The following information includes only the average doses of this medicine. If your dose is different, do not change it unless your doctor tells you to do so.

The amount of medicine that you take depends on the strength of the medicine. Also, the number of doses you take each day, the time allowed between doses, and the length of time you take the medicine depend on the medical problem for which you are using the medicine.

- For the treatment of advanced HIV infection or AIDS:
  - For oral dosage form (capsules, delayed-release):
    - Adults and teenagers—Dose is based on body weight.
      — For patients weighing less than 60 kilograms (kg) (132 pounds): 250 milligrams (mg) once daily.
      — For patients weighing 60 kg (132 pounds) or more: 400 mg once daily.
    - Children—The oral capsules are usually not used for small children.
  - For oral dosage form (solution, buffered powder):
    - Adults and teenagers—Dose is based on body weight.
      — For patients weighing less than 60 kilograms (kg) (132 pounds): 167 mg every twelve hours.
      — For patients weighing 60 kg (132 pounds) or more: 250 mg every twelve hours.
    - Children—The oral solution is usually not used for small children.
  - For oral dosage form (suspension, pediatric powder):
    - Adults and teenagers—The pediatric oral suspension is usually not used in adults and teenagers.
    - Children—Dose is based on body size and must be determined by your doctor.
  - For oral dosage form (tablets):
    - Adults and teenagers—Dose is based on body weight.
      — For patients weighing less than 60 kg (132 pounds): 125 mg every twelve hours, or 250 mg once daily.
      — For patients weighing 60 kg (132 pounds) or more: 200 mg every twelve hours, or 400 mg once daily.
    - Children—Dose is based on body size and must be determined by your doctor.

Missed dose—If you miss a dose of this medicine, take it as soon as possible. However, if it is almost time for your next dose, skip the missed dose and go back to your regular dosing schedule. Do not double doses.

Storage—Store the medicine in a closed container at room temperature, away from heat, moisture, and direct light. Keep from freezing.

Keep out of the reach of children.

Do not keep outdated medicine or medicine no longer needed.

Precautions While Using This Medicine

It is very important that your doctor check your progress at regular visits.

Do not take any other medicines without checking with your doctor first. To do so may increase the chance of side effects from didanosine.

HIV may be acquired from or spread to other people through infected body fluids, including blood, vaginal fluid, or semen.

If you are infected, it is best to avoid any sexual activity involving an exchange of body fluids with other people. If you do have sex, always wear (or have your partner wear) a condom ("rubber"). Only use condoms made of latex, and use them every time you have vaginal, anal, or oral sex. The use of a spermicide (such as nonoxynol-9) may also help prevent transmission of HIV if it is not irritating to the vagina, rectum, or mouth. Spermicides have been shown to kill HIV in lab tests. Do not use oil-based jelly, cold cream, baby oil, or shortening as a lubricant— these products can cause the condom to break. Lubricants without oil, such as K-Y jelly, are recommended. Women may wish to carry their own condoms. Birth control pills and diaphragms will help protect against pregnancy, but they will not prevent someone from giving or getting the AIDS virus. If you inject drugs, get help to stop. Do not share needles or equipment with anyone. In some cities, more than half of the drug users are infected and sharing even 1 needle or syringe can spread the virus. If you have any questions about this, check with your health care professional.

Side Effects of This Medicine

Along with its needed effects, a medicine may cause some unwanted effects. Although not all of these side effects may occur, if they do occur they may need medical attention.

Check with your doctor immediately if any of the following side effects occur:

Less common
>   Nausea and vomiting; stomach pain; tingling, burning, numbness, and pain in the hands or feet

Rare
>   Convulsions (seizures); fever and chills; shortness of breath; skin rash and itching; sore throat; swelling of feet or lower legs; unusual bleeding and bruising; unusual tiredness and weakness; yellow skin and eyes

Some side effects may occur that usually do not need medical attention. These side effects may go away during treatment as your body adjusts to the medicine. Also, your health care professional may be able to tell you about ways to prevent or reduce some of these side effects. Check with your health care professional if any of the following side effects continue or are bothersome or if you have any questions about them:

More common
>   Anxiety; diarrhea; difficulty in sleeping; dryness of mouth; headache; irritability; restlessness

Other side effects not listed may also occur in some patients. If you notice any other effects, check with your healthcare professional.

DIGITALIS MEDICINES (Systemic)

Some commonly used brand names are:

In the U.S.—
Lanoxicaps (2)	Lanoxin Injection (2)
Lanoxin (2)	Lanoxin Injection Pediatric (2)
Lanoxin Elixir Pediatric (2)	

In Canada—
Digitaline (1)	Lanoxin Injection (2)
Lanoxin (2)	Lanoxin Pediatric Injection (2)
Lanoxin Pediatric Elixir (2)	Novo-Digoxin (2)

This information applies to the following medicines:
1. Digitoxin (di-ji-TOX-in)
2. Digoxin (di-JOX-in)

Category

- **Antiarrhythmic—**
- **cardiotonic—**

Description

Digitalis medicines are used to improve the strength and efficiency of the heart, or to control the rate and rhythm of the heartbeat. This leads to better blood circulation and reduced swelling of hands and ankles in patients with heart problems.

Although digitalis has been prescribed to help some patients lose weight, it should *never* be used in this way. When used improperly, digitalis can cause serious problems.

Digitalis medicines are available only with your doctor's prescription, in the following dosage forms:

Oral
- Digitoxin
    - Tablets
- Digoxin
    - Capsules
    - Elixir
    - Tablets

Parenteral
- Digoxin
    - Injection

Before Using This Medicine

In deciding to use a medicine, the risks of taking the medicine must be weighed against the good it will do. This is a decision you and your doctor will make. For digitalis medicines, the following should be considered:

Allergies—Tell your doctor if you have ever had any unusual or allergic reaction to digitalis medicines. Also tell your health care professional if you are allergic to any other substances, such as foods, preservatives, or dyes.

Pregnancy—Digitalis medicines pass from the mother to the fetus. However, studies on effects in pregnancy have not been done in either humans or animals. Make sure your doctor knows if you are pregnant or if you may become pregnant before taking digitalis medicines.

Breast-feeding—Digoxin passes into breast milk; it is not known if digitoxin passes into breast milk. Although most medicines pass into breast milk in small amounts, many of them may be used safely while breast-feeding. Mothers who are taking this medicine and who wish to breast-feed should discuss this with their doctor.

Children—This medicine has been tested in children and, in effective doses, has not been shown to cause different side effects or problems than it does in adults. However, the dose is very different for babies and children, and it is important to follow your doctor's instructions exactly.

Older adults—Signs and symptoms of overdose may be especially likely to occur in elderly patients, who are usually more sensitive than younger adults to the effects of digitalis medicines.

Other medicines—Although certain medicines should not be used together at all, in other cases two different medicines may be used together even if an interaction might occur. In these cases, your doctor may want to change the dose, or other precautions may be necessary. When you are taking or receiving digitalis medicines it is especially important that your health care professional know if you are taking any other medicines because they may affect the levels of digitalis in the body and cause side effects. The following medicines are especially important:

- Amphetamines or
- Appetite suppressants (diet pills) or
- Medicine for asthma or other breathing problems or
- Medicine for colds, sinus problems, or hay fever or other allergies (including nose drops or sprays)—May increase the risk of heart rhythm problems
- Antiarrhythmic or other heart medicine, such as amiodarone (e.g., Cordarone) taken within the last 3 months or
- Calcium channel blocking agents (bepridil [e.g., Bepadin, Vascor], diltiazem [e.g., Cardizem, Cardizem CD, Cardizem SR], felodipine [e.g., Plendil], flunarizine [e.g., Sibelium], isradipine [e.g., DynaCirc], nicardipine [e.g., Cardene], nifedipine [e.g., Adalat, Procardia, Procardia XL], nimodipine [e.g., Nimotop], nisoldipine [e.g., Sular], verapamil [e.g., Calan, Calan SR, Isoptin, Isoptin SR, Verelan]) or
- Propafenone (e.g., Rythmol) or
- Quinidine (e.g., Quinidex)—May cause levels of digitalis medicines in the body to be higher than usual, which could lead to overdose
- Beta-adrenergic blocking agents (acebutolol [e.g., Sectral], atenolol [e.g., Tenormin], betaxolol [e.g., Kerlone], bisoprolol [e.g., Zebeta], carteolol [e.g., Cartrol], carvedilol [e.g., Coreg], labetalol [e.g., Normodyne], metoprolol [e.g., Lopressor], nadolol [e.g., Corgard], oxprenolol [e.g., Trasicor], penbutolol [e.g., Levatol], pindolol [e.g., Visken], propranolol [e.g., Inderal], sotalol [e.g., Sotacor], timolol [e.g., Blocadren])—Effects on slowing the heartbeat may be increased
- Diuretics (water pills)—These medicines can cause hypokalemia (low levels of potassium in the body), which can increase the unwanted effects of digitalis medicines

Other medical problems—The presence of other medical problems may affect the use of digitalis medicines. Make sure you tell your doctor if you have any other medical problems, especially:

- Electrolyte disorders or
- Heart disease or
- Lung disease (severe)—The heart may be more sensitive to the effects of digitalis medicines
- Heart rhythm problems—Digitalis medicines may make certain heart rhythm problems worse
- Kidney disease or
- Liver disease—Effects may be increased because of slower removal of digitalis medicines from the body
- Thyroid disease—Patients with low or high thyroid gland activity may be more or less sensitive to the effects of digitalis medicines

Proper Use of This Medicine

To keep your heart working properly, *take this medicine exactly as directed even though you may feel well.* Do not take more of it than your doctor ordered and do not miss any doses. Take the medicine at the same time each day. This medicine works best when there is a constant amount in the blood.

For patients taking the *liquid form of digoxin:*

- This medicine is to be taken by mouth even if it comes in a dropper bottle. The amount you should take is to be measured only with the specially marked dropper.

Dosing—When you are taking digitalis medicines, it is very important that you get the exact amount of medicine that you need. The dose of digitalis medicine will be different for different patients. Your doctor will determine the proper dose of digitalis medicine for you. *Follow your doctor's orders or the directions on the label.*

After you begin taking digitalis medicines, your doctor may sometimes check your blood level of digitalis medicine to find out if your dose needs to be changed. *Do not change your dose of digitalis medicine* unless your doctor tells you to do so.

The number of capsules, tablets, drops, or dropperfuls of solution that you take depends on the strength of the medicine.

Missed dose—If you miss a dose of this medicine, and you remember it within 12 hours, take it as soon as you remember. However, if you do not remember until later, do not take the missed dose at all and do not double the next one. Instead, go back to your regular dosing schedule. If you have any questions about this or if you miss doses for 2 or more days in a row, check with your doctor.

Storage—To store this medicine:

- Keep out of the reach of children.
- Store away from heat and direct light.
- Do not store in the bathroom, near the kitchen sink, or in other damp places. Heat or moisture may cause the medicine to break down.
- Do not keep outdated medicine or medicine no longer needed. Be sure that any discarded medicine is out of the reach of children.

Precautions While Using This Medicine

It is important that your doctor check your progress at regular visits to make sure the medicine is working properly. This will allow your doctor to make any changes in directions for taking it, if necessary.

Do not stop taking this medicine without first checking with your doctor. Stopping suddenly may cause a serious change in heart function.

Keep this medicine out of the reach of children. Digitalis medicines are a major cause of poisoning in children.

Watch for signs and symptoms of overdose while you are taking digitalis medicine. Follow your doctor's directions carefully. The amount of this medicine needed to help most people is very close to the amount that could cause serious problems from overdose. Some early warning signs of overdose are loss of appetite, nausea, vomiting, diarrhea, or problems in seeing. Other signs of overdose are changes in the rate or rhythm of the heartbeat (becoming irregular or slow), palpitations (feeling of pounding in the chest), and/or fainting. In infants and small children, the earliest signs of overdose are changes in the rate and rhythm of the heartbeat. Children may not show the other symptoms as soon as adults.

Your doctor may want you to carry a medical identification card or bracelet stating that you are taking this medicine.

Do not take any other medicine without consulting your doctor. Many over-the-counter (OTC) or nonprescription medicines contain ingredients that interfere with digitalis medicines or that may make your condition worse. These medicines include antacids; laxatives; asthma remedies; cold, cough, or sinus preparations; medicine for diarrhea; and weight reducing or diet medicines.

For patients taking the *tablet or capsule* form of this medicine:

- This medicine may look like other tablets or capsules you now take. It is very important that you do not get the medicines mixed up since this may have serious results. Ask your pharmacist for ways to avoid mix-ups with medicines that look alike.

Side Effects

Along with its needed effects, a medicine may cause some unwanted effects. Although not all of these side effects may occur, if they do occur they may need medical attention.

Check with your doctor as soon as possible if any of the following side effects or symptoms occur:

In adults
Anxiety, blurred or yellow vision, confusion, dizziness, mental depression, feeling of not caring, headache, loss of appetite, seeing or hearing things that are not there, and/or weakness; diarrhea, loss of appetite, lower stomach pain, nausea, and/or vomiting; irregular or slow heartbeat, palpitations (feeling of pounding in the chest), and/or fainting

Rare
Skin rash; nosebleeds or bleeding gums

With long-term use
Breast enlargement in males

In infants and children

The above signs and symptoms also can occur in infants and children, but heartbeat rate or rhythm side effects are more common initially than stomach upset, loss of appetite, changes in vision, or other side effects.

Other side effects not listed above may also occur in some patients. If you notice any other effects, check with your doctor.

DIHYDROERGOTAMINE (Nasal route) - dye-hye-droe-er-GOT-a-meen

Black Box Warning

Serious and/or life-threatening peripheral ischemia has been associated with the coadministration of dihydroergotamine with potent CYP3A4 inhibitors including protease inhibitors and macrolide antibiotics. Because CYP3A4 inhibition elevates the serum levels of dihydroergotamine, the risk for vasospasm leading to cerebral ischemia and/or ischemia of the extremities is increased. Hence, concomitant use of these medications is contraindicated.

Commonly used brand name(s)

In the U.S.—
Migranal

Available Dosage Forms:
- Spray

Therapeutic Class: Antimigraine

Uses For This Medicine

Dihydroergotamine belongs to the group of medicines called ergot alkaloids. It is a nasal solution used to help relieve migraine headaches. Nasal dihydroergotamine is not an ordinary pain reliever. It will not relieve any kind of pain other than throbbing headaches.

Nasal dihydroergotamine may cause blood vessels in the body to constrict (become narrower). This action can lead to serious effects that are caused by a decrease in the flow of blood (blood circulation) to many parts of the body. Be sure that you discuss with your doctor the risks of using this medicine as well as the good it can do.

This medicine is available only with your doctor's prescription.

Before Using This Medicine

In deciding to use a medicine, the risks of taking the medicine must be weighed against the good it will do. This is a decision you and your doctor will make. For this medicine, the following should be considered:

Allergies—Tell your doctor if you have ever had any unusual or allergic reaction to this medicine or any other medicines. Also tell your health care professional if you have any other types of allergies, such as to foods, dyes, preservatives, or animals. For non-prescription products, read the label or package ingredients carefully.

Pediatric—There is no specific information comparing use of nasal dihydroergotamine in children with use in other age groups.

Geriatric—There is no specific information comparing use of nasal dihydroergotamine in older adults with use in other age groups.

Breast Feeding—Studies in women breastfeeding have demonstrated harmful infant effects. An alternative to this medication should be prescribed or you should stop breast-feeding while using this medicine.

Other medicines—

Using this medicine with any of the following medicines is not recommended. Your doctor may decide not to treat you with this medication or change some of the other medicines you take.

Almotriptan, Amprenavir, Atazanavir, Azithromycin, Clarithromycin, Clotrimazole, Cocaine, Darunavir, Delavirdine, Dirithromycin, Efavirenz, Epinephrine, Erythromycin, Fluconazole, Fluoxetine, Fluvoxamine, Fosamprenavir, Frovatriptan, Indinavir, Itraconazole, Josamycin, Ketoconazole, Lidocaine, Lopinavir, Mepartricin, Metronidazole, Midodrine, Miokamycin, Naratriptan, Nefazodone, Nelfinavir, Norepinephrine, Phenylpropanolamine, Propylhexedrine, Pseudoephedrine, Ritonavir, Rizatriptan, Rokitamycin, Roxithromycin, Saquinavir, Saralasin, Spiramycin, Sumatriptan, Tipranavir, Troleandomycin, Voriconazole, Zileuton, Zolmitriptan

Interactions with Food/Tobacco/Alcohol—Certain medicines should not be used at or around the time of eating food or eating certain types of food since interactions may

occur. Using alcohol or tobacco with certain medicines may also cause interactions to occur. The following interactions have been selected on the basis of their potential significance and are not necessarily all-inclusive.

Using this medicine with any of the following is not recommended. Your doctor may decide not to treat you with this medication, change some of the other medicines you take, or give you special instructions about the use of food, alcohol, or tobacco.

Grapefruit Juice

Other medical problems—The presence of other medical problems may affect the use of this medicine. Make sure you tell your doctor if you have any other medical problems, especially:

- Heart or blood vessel disease or

- Hypertension (high blood pressure) or

- Kidney disease or

- Liver disease or

- Infection—The chance of serious side effects caused by nasal dihydroergotmine may be increased. Heart or blood vessel disease and high blood pressure sometimes do not cause any symptoms, so some people do not know that they have these problems. Before deciding whether you should use nasal dihydroergotamine, your doctor may need to do some tests to make sure that you do not have any of these conditions.

Proper Use of This Medicine

It is important to use this medicine properly. Make sure that you read the patient directions carefully before using this medicine.

Do not use nasal dihydroergotamine for a headache that is different from your usual migraine. Instead, check with your doctor.

To relieve your migraine as soon as possible, use nasal dihydroergotamine as soon as the headache begins. Even if you get warning signals of a coming migraine (an aura), you should wait until the headache pain starts before using nasal dihydroergotamine.

Lying down in a quiet, dark room for a while after you use this medicine may help relieve your migraine.

If you feel much better after a dose of nasal dihydroergotamine, but your headache comes back or gets worse after a while, you may use more nasal dihydroergotamine. However, use this medicine only as directed by your doctor. Do not use more of it, and do not use it more often, than directed.

Your doctor may direct you to take another medicine to help prevent headaches. It is important that you follow your doctor's directions, even if your headaches continue to occur. Headache-preventing medicines may take several weeks to start working. Even after they do start working, your headaches should occur less often, and they should be less severe, and easier to relieve. This can reduce the amount of nasal dihydroergotamine or other pain medicines that you need. If you do not notice any improvement after several weeks of headache-preventing treatment, check with your doctor.

Dosing—The dose of this medicine will be different for different patients. Follow your doctor's orders or the directions on the label. The following information includes only the av-

erage doses of this medicine. If your dose is different, do not change it unless your doctor tells you to do so.

The amount of medicine that you take depends on the strength of the medicine. Also, the number of doses you take each day, the time allowed between doses, and the length of time you take the medicine depend on the medical problem for which you are using the medicine.

- For nasal dosage form (nasal solution):
  - For migraine headaches:
    - Adults—One spray (0.5 mg) in each nostril. After 15 minutes, another spray (0.5 mg) in each nostril should be used.
    - Children—Use and dose must be determined by your doctor.

Storage—Store the medicine in a closed container at room temperature, away from heat, moisture, and direct light. Keep from freezing.

Keep out of the reach of children.

Do not keep outdated medicine or medicine no longer needed.

Precautions While Using This Medicine

Drinking alcoholic beverages can make headaches worse or cause new headaches to occur. People who suffer from severe headaches should probably avoid alcoholic beverages, especially during a headache.

Some people feel drowsy or dizzy during or after a migraine attack, or after taking nasal dihydroergotamine to relieve a migraine headache. As long as you are feeling drowsy or dizzy, do not drive, use machines or do anything else that could be dangerous if you are dizzy or are not alert.

Side Effects of This Medicine

Along with its needed effects, a medicine may cause some unwanted effects. Although not all of these side effects may occur, if they do occur they may need medical attention.

Check with your doctor as soon as possible if any of the following side effects occur:

Less common or rare
Chest pain; cough, fever, sneezing, or sore throat; feeling of heaviness in chest; irregular heartbeat; itching of the skin; numbness and tingling of face, fingers, or toes; pain in arms, legs, or lower back; pain in back, chest or left arm; pale bluish-colored or cold hands or feet; shortness of breath or troubled breathing; weak or absent pulses in legs

Symptoms of overdose
Confusion; convulsions (seizures); delirium; dizziness; headaches; nausea and/or vomiting; numbness, tingling, and/or pain in the legs or arms; shortness of breath; stomach pain

Some side effects may occur that usually do not need medical attention. These side effects may go away during treatment as your body adjusts to the medicine. Also, your health care professional may be able to tell you about ways to prevent or reduce some of these side effects. Check with your health care professional if any of the following side effects continue or are bothersome or if you have any questions about them:

More common
Burning or tingling sensation, dryness, soreness, or pain in the nose; change in sense of taste; diarrhea;

dizziness; dry mouth; fatigue; headache; increased sweating; nausea and or vomiting; muscle stiffness; runny and or stuffy nose; sudden sweatings and feelings of warmth; sensation of burning, warmth, or heat; sore throat; sleepiness; unexplained nose bleeds; unusual tiredness or weakness

Less common

Anxiety; blurred vision; cold clammy skin; confusion; congestion in chest; cough; decreased appetite; depression; difficulty swallowing; dizziness or lightheadedness when getting up from a lying or sitting position; ear pain; eye pain; fever; heartburn; increased watering of eyes; increased watering of the mouth; increased yawning; muscle weakness; nervousness; pinpoint red spots on skin; pounding heartbeat; red or irritated eyes; ringing or buzzing in ears; skin rash; stomach pain; sudden fainting; swelling of face, fingers, feet, or lower legs; trembling or shaking of hands or feet; trouble in sleeping; unusual feeling of well being

Other side effects not listed may also occur in some patients. If you notice any other effects, check with your healthcare professional.

DIMETHYL SULFOXIDE (Intravesical route) - dye-METH-il sul-FOX-ide

Commonly used brand name(s)

In the U.S.—
Rimso-50

Available Dosage Forms:
- Solution

Therapeutic Class: Renal-Urologic Agent

Uses For This Medicine

Dimethyl sulfoxide is a purified preparation used in the bladder to relieve the symptoms of the bladder condition called interstitial cystitis. A catheter (tube) or syringe is used to put the solution into the bladder where it is allowed to remain for about 15 minutes. Then, the solution is expelled by urinating.

Interstitial cystitis is the only human use for dimethyl sulfoxide that is approved by the U.S. Food and Drug Administration (FDA).

Claims that dimethyl sulfoxide is effective for treating various types of arthritis, ulcers in scleroderma, muscle sprains and strains, bruises, infections of the skin, burns, wounds, and mental conditions have not been proven.

Although other preparations of dimethyl sulfoxide are available for industrial and veterinary (animal) use, they must not be used by humans, because of their unknown purity. Impurities in these preparations may cause serious unwanted effects in humans. Even if dimethyl sulfoxide is applied to the skin, it is absorbed into the body through the skin and mucous membranes.

This medicine is available only with your doctor's prescription.

Before Using This Medicine

In deciding to use a medicine, the risks of taking the medicine must be weighed against the good it will do. This is a decision you and your doctor will make. For this medicine, the following should be considered:

Allergies—Tell your doctor if you have ever had any unusual or allergic reaction to this medicine or any other medicines. Also tell your health care professional if you have any other types of allergies, such as to foods, dyes, preservatives, or animals. For non-prescription products, read the label or package ingredients carefully.

Pediatric—Studies on this medicine have been done only in adult patients, and there is no specific information comparing use of this medicine in children with use in other age groups.

Geriatric—Many medicines have not been studied specifically in older people. Therefore, it may not be known whether they work exactly the same way they do in younger adults or if they cause different side effects or problems in older people. There is no specific information comparing use of this medicine in the elderly with use in other age groups.

Pregnancy—

	Pregnancy Category	Explanation
All Trimesters	C	Animal studies have shown an adverse effect and there are no adequate studies in pregnant women OR no animal studies have been conducted and there are no adequate studies in pregnant women.

Breast Feeding—There are no adequate studies in women for determining infant risk when using this medication during breastfeeding. Weigh the potential benefits against the potential risks before taking this medication while breastfeeding.

Other medicines—Although certain medicines should not be used together at all, in other cases two different medicines may be used together even if an interaction might occur. In these cases, your doctor may want to change the dose, or other precautions may be necessary. Tell your healthcare professional if you are taking any other prescription or non-prescription (over-the-counter [OTC]) medicine.

Interactions with Food/Tobacco/Alcohol—Certain medicines should not be used at or around the time of eating food or eating certain types of food since interactions may occur. Using alcohol or tobacco with certain medicines may also cause interactions to occur. Discuss with your healthcare professional the use of your medicine with food, alcohol, or tobacco.

Proper Use of This Medicine

Dosing—The dose of this medicine will be different for different patients. Follow your doctor's orders or the directions on the label. The following information includes only the average doses of this medicine. If your dose is different, do not change it unless your doctor tells you to do so.

The amount of medicine that you take depends on the strength of the medicine. Also, the number of doses you take each day, the time allowed between doses, and the length of

time you take the medicine depend on the medical problem for which you are using the medicine.

- For bladder irrigation dosage form:
  - For interstitial cystitis of bladder:
    - Adults—50 mL (milliliters) of a 50% solution is instilled into the bladder and left there for fifteen minutes. The treatment is repeated every two weeks until relief is obtained; then the treatment is repeated less often.
    - Children—Use and dose must be determined by your doctor.

Side Effects of This Medicine

Along with its needed effects, a medicine may cause some unwanted effects. Although not all of these side effects may occur, if they do occur they may need medical attention.

Check with your doctor immediately if any of the following side effects occur:

Nasal congestion; shortness of breath or troubled breathing; skin rash, hives, or itching; swelling of face

Some patients may have some discomfort during the time this medicine is being put into the bladder. However, the discomfort usually becomes less each time the medicine is used.

Dimethyl sulfoxide may cause you to have a garlic-like taste within a few minutes after the medicine is put into the bladder. This effect may last for several hours. It may also cause your breath and skin to have a garlic-like odor, which may last up to 72 hours.

Other side effects not listed may also occur in some patients. If you notice any other effects, check with your healthcare professional.

DINOPROSTONE (Vaginal route) -
dye-noe-PROST-one

Black Box Warning

Dinoprostone, as with other potent oxytocic agents, should be used only with strict adherence to recommended dosages. Dinoprostone should be used by medically trained personnel in a hospital which can provide immediate intensive care and acute surgical facilities.

Commonly used brand name(s)

In the U.S.—
Cervidil
Prepidil
Prostin E2

Available Dosage Forms:

- Gel/Jelly
- Tampon
- Insert, Extended Release
- Suppository

Therapeutic Class: Uterine Stimulant
Pharmacologic Class: Prostaglandin

Uses For This Medicine

Dinoprostone works by causing the cervix to thin and dilate (open) and the uterus to contract (cramp) the way it does during labor.

Dinoprostone may also be used for other purposes as determined by your doctor.

Dinoprostone is to be administered only by or under the immediate care of your doctor.

Once a medicine has been approved for marketing for a certain use, experience may show that it is also useful for other medical problems. Although these uses are not included in product labeling, dinoprostone is used in certain patients with the following medical condition:

- Unusual increase in bleeding of the uterus after delivery (postpartum hemorrhage)

Before Receiving This Medicine

In deciding to use a medicine, the risks of taking the medicine must be weighed against the good it will do. This is a decision you and your doctor will make. For this medicine, the following should be considered:

Allergies—Tell your doctor if you have ever had any unusual or allergic reaction to this medicine or any other medicines. Also tell your health care professional if you have any other types of allergies, such as to foods, dyes, preservatives, or animals. For non-prescription products, read the label or package ingredients carefully.

Pregnancy—

	Pregnancy Category	Explanation
All Trimesters	C	Animal studies have shown an adverse effect and there are no adequate studies in pregnant women OR no animal studies have been conducted and there are no adequate studies in pregnant women.

Breast Feeding—There are no adequate studies in women for determining infant risk when using this medication during breastfeeding. Weigh the potential benefits against the potential risks before taking this medication while breastfeeding.

Other medicines—Although certain medicines should not be used together at all, in other cases two different medicines may be used together even if an interaction might occur. In these cases, your doctor may want to change the dose, or other precautions may be necessary. Tell your healthcare professional if you are taking any other prescription or non-prescription (over-the-counter [OTC]) medicine.

Interactions with Food/Tobacco/Alcohol—Certain medicines should not be used at or around the time of eating food or eating certain types of food since interactions may occur. Using alcohol or tobacco with certain medicines may also cause interactions to occur. Discuss with your healthcare professional the use of your medicine with food, alcohol, or tobacco.

Other medical problems—The presence of other medical problems may affect the use of this medicine. Make sure you tell your doctor if you have any other medical problems, especially:

- Anemia (or history of)—Dinoprostone, when used in doses that stimulate the uterus to contract, may result in loss of blood in some patients that may require a blood transfusion

- Asthma (or history of, including childhood asthma) or
- Lung disease—Dinoprostone may cause narrowing of the blood vessels in the lungs or narrowing of the lung passages, especially when it is used in doses that stimulate the uterus to contract
- Epilepsy (or history of)—Rarely, seizures have occurred with dinoprostone when it is used in doses that stimulate the uterus to contract
- Glaucoma—Rarely, the pressure within the eye has increased and constriction of the pupils has occurred during the use of medicines like dinoprostone; this may also be a problem with dinoprostone when it is used in doses that stimulate the uterus to contract
- Heart or blood vessel disease (or history of) or
- High blood pressure (or history of) or
- Low blood pressure (history of)—Dinoprostone may cause changes in heart function or blood pressure changes; two patients with a history of heart disease had heart attacks when dinoprostone was used in doses that stimulated the uterus to contract
- Kidney disease (or history of) or
- Liver disease (or history of)—The body may not remove dinoprostone from the blood stream at the usual rate, which may make the dinoprostone work longer or cause an increased chance of side effects, especially when dinoprostone is used in doses that stimulate the uterus to contract
- Problems during delivery, history of or
- Surgery of uterus (history of) or
- Unusual vaginal bleeding—There is an increased risk of problems occurring with dinoprostone when it is used in doses that stimulate the uterus to contract

Proper Use of This Medicine

After dinoprostone is given, you will need to lie down for 10 minutes to 2 hours so that the medicine can be absorbed. The length of time you must remain lying down will depend on what form of the medicine you are using.

Dosing—The dose of this medicine will be different for different patients. Follow your doctor's orders or the directions on the label. The following information includes only the average doses of this medicine. If your dose is different, do not change it unless your doctor tells you to do so.

The amount of medicine that you take depends on the strength of the medicine. Also, the number of doses you take each day, the time allowed between doses, and the length of time you take the medicine depend on the medical problem for which you are using the medicine.

- For cervical dosage form (gel):
  - To thin and widen the opening of the cervix just before labor:
    - Adults and teenagers—Your doctor will insert 0.5 milligram (mg) (one application) of dinoprostone into the canal of your cervix. You should remain lying on your back for at least ten to thirty minutes after it has been applied.
- For vaginal dosage form (gel):
  - To cause the uterus to contract for labor:
    - Adults and teenagers—Your doctor will insert 1 milligram (mg) (one applicatorful) of dinoprostone into your vagina. You should remain lying on your back for at least thirty minutes after it has been applied. You may need another dose of 1 to 2 mg six hours after the first dose.
- For vaginal dosage form (suppositories):
  - To cause the uterus to contract to abort a pregnancy:
    - Adults and teenagers—Your doctor will insert 20 milligrams (mg) (one suppository) into your vagina every three to five hours as needed. You should remain lying on your back for at least ten minutes after it has been inserted.
- For vaginal dosage form (system):
  - To thin and widen the opening of the cervix just before labor:
    - Adults and teenagers—Your doctor will insert 10 milligrams (mg) (one system) into your vagina. You should remain lying on your back for at least two hours after it has been inserted.

Side Effects of This Medicine

Along with its needed effects, a medicine may cause some unwanted effects. Although not all of these side effects may occur, if they do occur they may need medical attention.

Check with your doctor immediately if any of the following side effects occur:

Less common or rare
Fast or slow heartbeat; hives; increased pain of the uterus; pale, cool, blotchy skin on arms or legs; pressing or painful feeling in chest; shortness of breath; swelling of face, inside the nose, and eyelids; tightness in chest; trouble in breathing; weak or absent pulse in arms or legs; wheezing

Some side effects may occur that usually do not need medical attention. These side effects may go away during treatment as your body adjusts to the medicine. Also, your health care professional may be able to tell you about ways to prevent or reduce some of these side effects. Check with your health care professional if any of the following side effects continue or are bothersome or if you have any questions about them:

More common
Abdominal or stomach cramps; diarrhea; fever; nausea; vomiting

Less common or rare
Chills or shivering; constipation; flushing; headache; swelling of the genital area (vulva); tender or mildly bloated abdomen or stomach

This procedure may still result in some effects, which occur after the procedure is completed, that need medical attention. Check with your doctor if any of the following side effects occur:

Chills or shivering (continuing); fever (continuing); foul-smelling vaginal discharge; pain in lower abdomen; unusual increase in bleeding of the uterus

Other side effects not listed may also occur in some patients. If you notice any other effects, check with your healthcare professional.

DIPHENOXYLATE AND ATROPINE
(Oral route) - dye-fen-OX-i-ilate hye-droe-KLOR-ide, A-troe-peen SUL-fate

Commonly used brand name(s)
In the U.S.—

Lomocot	Lonox
Lomotil	Vi-Atro

Available Dosage Forms:
- Solution
- Tablet

Therapeutic Class: Antidiarrheal
Pharmacologic Class: Atropine

Uses For This Medicine

Diphenoxylate and atropine is a combination medicine used along with other measures to treat severe diarrhea in adults. Diphenoxylate helps stop diarrhea by slowing down the movements of the intestines.

Since diphenoxylate is chemically related to some narcotics, it may be habit-forming if taken in doses that are larger than prescribed. To help prevent possible abuse, atropine (an anticholinergic) has been added. If higher than normal doses of the combination are taken, the atropine will cause unpleasant effects, making it unlikely that such doses will be taken again.

Diphenoxylate and atropine combination medicine should not be used in children. Children with diarrhea should be given solutions of carbohydrates (sugars) and important salts (electrolytes) to replace the water, sugars, and important salts that are lost from the body during diarrhea. For more information on these solutions, see the Carbohydrates and Electrolytes (Systemic) monograph.

This medicine is available only with your doctor's prescription.

Before Using This Medicine

In deciding to use a medicine, the risks of taking the medicine must be weighed against the good it will do. This is a decision you and your doctor will make. For this medicine, the following should be considered:

Allergies—Tell your doctor if you have ever had any unusual or allergic reaction to this medicine or any other medicines. Also tell your health care professional if you have any other types of allergies, such as to foods, dyes, preservatives, or animals. For non-prescription products, read the label or package ingredients carefully.

Pediatric—This medicine should not be used in children. Children, especially very young children, are very sensitive to the effects of diphenoxylate and atropine. This may increase the chance of side effects during treatment. Also, the fluid loss caused by diarrhea may result in a severe condition. For this reason, it is very important that a sufficient amount of liquids be given to replace the fluid lost by the body. If you have any questions about this, check with your health care professional.

Geriatric—Shortness of breath or difficulty in breathing may be especially likely to occur in elderly patients, who are usually more sensitive than younger adults to the effects of diphenoxylate. Also, the fluid loss caused by diarrhea may result in a severe condition. For this reason, elderly persons should not take this medicine without first checking with their doctor. It is also very important that a sufficient amount of liquids be taken to replace the fluid lost by the body. If you have any questions about this, check with your health care professional.

Pregnancy—

	Pregnancy Category	Explanation
All Trimesters	C	Animal studies have shown an adverse effect and there are no adequate studies in pregnant women OR no animal studies have been conducted and there are no adequate studies in pregnant women.

Breast Feeding—There are no adequate studies in women for determining infant risk when using this medication during breastfeeding. Weigh the potential benefits against the potential risks before taking this medication while breastfeeding.

Other medicines—

Using this medicine with any of the following medicines is not recommended. Your doctor may decide not to treat you with this medication or change some of the other medicines you take.

Ambenonium

Interactions with Food/Tobacco/Alcohol—Certain medicines should not be used at or around the time of eating food or eating certain types of food since interactions may occur. Using alcohol or tobacco with certain medicines may also cause interactions to occur. Discuss with your healthcare professional the use of your medicine with food, alcohol, or tobacco.

Other medical problems—The presence of other medical problems may affect the use of this medicine. Make sure you tell your doctor if you have any other medical problems, especially:
- Alcohol abuse (or history of) or
- Drug abuse (history of)—There is a greater chance that this medicine will become habit-forming
- Colitis (severe)—A more serious problem of the colon may develop if you use this medicine
- Down's syndrome—Side effects may be more likely and severe in these patients
- Dysentery—This condition may get worse; a different kind of treatment may be needed
- Emphysema, asthma, bronchitis, or other chronic lung disease—There is a greater chance that this medicine may cause serious breathing problems in patients who have any of these conditions
- Enlarged prostate or
- Urinary tract blockage or difficult urination—Severe problems with urination may develop with the use of this medicine
- Gallbladder disease or gallstones—Use of this medicine may cause spasms of the biliary tract and make the condition worse
- Glaucoma—Severe pain in the eye may occur with the use of this medicine; however, the chance of this happening is small
- Heart disease—This medicine may have some effects on the heart, which may make the condition worse

- Hiatal hernia—The atropine in this medicine may make this condition worse; however, the chance of this happening is small
- High blood pressure (hypertension)—The atropine in this medicine may cause an increase in blood pressure; however, the chance of this happening is small
- Intestinal blockage—This medicine may make the condition worse
- Kidney disease—The atropine in this medicine may build up in the body and cause side effects
- Liver disease—The chance of central nervous system (CNS) side effects, including coma, may be greater in patients who have this condition
- Myasthenia gravis—This medicine may make the condition worse
- Overactive or underactive thyroid—Unwanted effects on breathing and heart rate may occur
- Overflow incontinence—This medicine may make the condition worse

Proper Use of This Medicine

If this medicine upsets your stomach, your doctor may want you to take it with food.

Take this medicine only as directed by your doctor. Do not take more of it, do not take it more often, and do not take it for a longer time than your doctor ordered. If too much is taken, it may become habit-forming.

For patients taking the liquid form of this medicine:

- This medicine is to be taken by mouth even if it comes in a dropper bottle. The amount to be taken is to be measured with the specially marked dropper.

Importance of diet and fluids while treating diarrhea:

- In addition to using medicine for diarrhea, it is very important that you replace the fluid lost by the body and follow a proper diet. For the first 24 hours you should eat gelatin and drink plenty of caffeine-free clear liquids, such as ginger ale, decaffeinated cola, decaffeinated tea, and broth. During the next 24 hours you may eat bland foods, such as cooked cereals, bread, crackers, and applesauce. Fruits, vegetables, fried or spicy foods, bran, candy, caffeine, and alcoholic beverages may make the condition worse.
- If too much fluid has been lost by the body due to the diarrhea a serious condition may develop. Check with your doctor as soon as possible if any of the following signs or symptoms of too much fluid loss occur:
  - Decreased urination
  - Dizziness and light-headedness
  - Dryness of mouth
  - Increased thirst
  - Wrinkled skin

Dosing—The dose of this medicine will be different for different patients. Follow your doctor's orders or the directions on the label. The following information includes only the average doses of this medicine. If your dose is different, do not change it unless your doctor tells you to do so.

The amount of medicine that you take depends on the strength of the medicine. Also, the number of doses you take each day, the time allowed between doses, and the length of time you take the medicine depend on the medical problem for which you are using the medicine.

- For severe diarrhea:
  - For oral dosage form (oral solution):
    - Adults and teenagers—At first, the dose is 5 milligrams (mg) (2 teaspoonfuls) three or four times a day. Then, the dose is usually 5 mg (2 teaspoonfuls) once a day, as needed.
    - Children up to 12 years of age—Use is not recommended.
  - For oral dosage form (tablets):
    - Adults and teenagers—At first, the dose is 5 mg (2 tablets) three or four times a day. Then, the dose is usually 5 mg (2 tablets) once a day, as needed.
    - Children up to 12 years of age—Use is not recommended.

Missed dose—If you miss a dose of this medicine, take it as soon as possible. However, if it is almost time for your next dose, skip the missed dose and go back to your regular dosing schedule. Do not double doses.

Storage—Store the medicine in a closed container at room temperature, away from heat, moisture, and direct light. Keep from freezing.

Keep out of the reach of children.

Do not keep outdated medicine or medicine no longer needed.

Precautions While Using This Medicine

Your doctor should check your progress at regular visits if you will be taking this medicine regularly for a long time.

Check with your doctor if your diarrhea does not stop after two days or if you develop a fever.

This medicine will add to the effects of alcohol and other CNS depressants (medicines that slow down the nervous system, possibly causing drowsiness). Some examples of CNS depressants are antihistamines or medicine for hay fever, other allergies, or colds; sedatives, tranquilizers, or sleeping medicine; prescription pain medicine or narcotics; barbiturates; medicine for seizures; muscle relaxants; or anesthetics, including some dental anesthetics. Check with your doctor before taking any of the above while you are taking this medicine.

If you think you or anyone else may have taken an overdose, get emergency help at once. Taking an overdose of this medicine may lead to unconsciousness and possibly death. Signs or symptoms of overdose include severe drowsiness; shortness of breath or troubled breathing; fast heartbeat; and unusual warmth, dryness, and flushing of the skin.

Before having any kind of surgery (including dental surgery) or emergency treatment, tell the medical doctor or dentist in charge that you are taking this medicine.

This medicine may cause some people to become dizzy, drowsy, or less alert than they are normally. Even if taken at bedtime, it may cause some people to feel drowsy or less alert on arising. Make sure you know how you react to this medicine before you drive, use machines, or do anything else that could be dangerous if you are dizzy or are not alert.

Side Effects of This Medicine

Along with its needed effects, a medicine may cause some unwanted effects. Although not all of these side effects may occur, if they do occur they may need medical attention.

Check with your doctor immediately if any of the following side effects occur:

> Bloating; constipation; loss of appetite; stomach pain (severe) with nausea and vomiting

Check with your doctor immediately if any of the following side effects occur:

> Blurred vision (continuing) or changes in near vision; drowsiness (severe); dryness of mouth, nose, and throat (severe); fast heartbeat; shortness of breath or troubled breathing (severe); unusual excitement, nervousness, restlessness, or irritability; unusual warmth, dryness, and flushing of the skin

Some side effects may occur that usually do not need medical attention. These side effects may go away during treatment as your body adjusts to the medicine. Also, your health care professional may be able to tell you about ways to prevent or reduce some of these side effects. Check with your health care professional if any of the following side effects continue or are bothersome or if you have any questions about them:

> *Less common or rare*
> Blurred vision; confusion; difficult urination; dizziness or light-headedness; drowsiness; dryness of skin and mouth; fever; headache; increased body temperature; mental depression; numbness of hands or feet; skin rash or itching; swelling of the gums

After you stop using this medicine, it may still produce some side effects that need attention. During this period of time, *check with your doctor immediately* if you notice the following side effects:

> *Rare*
> Increased sweating; muscle cramps; nausea or vomiting; shivering or trembling; stomach cramps

Other side effects not listed may also occur in some patients. If you notice any other effects, check with your healthcare professional.

DIPHTHERIA AND TETANUS TOXOIDS   (Systemic)

This information applies to the following medicines:

1. Diphtheria and Tetanus Toxoids for Pediatric Use (dif-THEE-ree-a and TET-n-us)
2. Tetanus and Diphtheria Toxoids for Adult Use (TET-n-us and dif-THEE-ree-a)

Category

• **Immunizing agent, active—**

Description

Diphtheria and Tetanus Toxoids (also known as DT and Td) is a combination immunizing agent given by injection to prevent diphtheria and tetanus.

Diphtheria is a serious illness that can cause breathing difficulties, heart problems, nerve damage, pneumonia, and possibly death. The risk of serious complications and death is greatest in very young children and in the elderly.

Tetanus (also known as lockjaw) is a serious illness that causes convulsions (seizures) and severe muscle spasms that can be strong enough to cause bone fractures of the spine. Tetanus causes death in 30 to 40 percent of cases.

Immunization with diphtheria and tetanus toxoids for pediatric use (DT) is recommended for infants and children from 6 weeks of age (8 weeks in Canada) up until their 7th birthday.

Children 7 years of age and older and adults should be immunized with tetanus and diphtheria toxoids for adult use (Td). In addition, these children and adults should receive booster doses of Td every 10 years for the rest of their lives.

Diphtheria and tetanus are serious diseases that can cause life-threatening illnesses. Although some serious side effects can occur after a dose of DT or Td, these are rare. The chance of your child catching one of these diseases and being permanently injured or dying as a result is much greater than the chance of your child getting a serious side effect from the DT or Td vaccine.

DT and Td are available in the following dosage form:

> *Parenteral*
> • Injection

Before Receiving This Vaccine

In deciding to use a vaccine, the risks of using the vaccine must be weighed against the good it will do. This is a decision you and your doctor will make. For DT and Td, the following should be considered:

Allergies—Tell your doctor if you have ever had any unusual or allergic reaction to diphtheria toxoid, tetanus toxoid, DT, or Td. Also tell your health care professional if you are allergic to any other substances, such as preservatives.

Pregnancy—This vaccine has not been shown to cause birth defects or other problems in humans. Immunization of a pregnant woman can prevent her newborn baby from getting tetanus at birth.

Breast-feeding—This vaccine has not been shown to cause problems in nursing babies.

Children—For infants up to 6 weeks of age, use of DT or Td is not recommended.

For infants and children 6 weeks up to 7 years of age, Td is not recommended. DT is used instead.

For children 7 years of age and older, DT is not recommended. Td is used instead.

Older adults—DT is not recommended. Td is used instead. Td is not expected to cause different side effects or problems in older people than it does in younger adults. However, Td may be slightly less effective in older people than in younger adults.

Other medical problems—The presence of other medical problems may affect the use of DT or Td. Make sure you tell your doctor if you have any other medical problems, especially:

> • Fever or
>
> • Infection or illness (severe)—Use of DT or Td may make the condition worse or may increase the chance of side effects

Proper Use of This Vaccine

Dosing—The doses of DT and Td will be different for different patients. The following information includes only the average doses of DT and Td.

For DT
- For *injection* dosage form:
  - For prevention of diphtheria and tetanus:
    - Children up to 6 weeks of age—Use is not recommended.
    - Children 6 weeks to 1 year of age—One dose is given every four to eight weeks for a total of three doses. A fourth dose is given six to twelve months after the third dose. A booster (fifth) dose is given when the child is four to six years of age. The booster (fifth) dose is given only if the fourth dose was given before the child's fourth birthday. The doses are injected into a muscle.
    - Children 1 to 7 years of age—One dose is given at the first visit to the doctor, followed by a second dose four to eight weeks later. A third dose is given six to twelve months after the second dose. A booster (fourth) dose is given when the child is four to six years of age. The booster (fourth dose) is given only if the third dose was given before the child's fourth birthday. The doses are injected into a muscle.
    - Adults and children 7 years of age and over—Use is not recommended. Td should be used instead.

For Td
- For *injection* dosage form:
  - For prevention of diphtheria and tetanus:
    - Children up to 7 years of age—Use is not recommended. DT should be used instead.
    - Adults and children 7 years of age and over—One dose is given at the first visit to the doctor, followed by a second dose four to eight weeks later. A third dose is given six to twelve months after the second dose. You should receive a booster dose every ten years. In addition, if you get a wound that is unclean or hard to clean, you may need an emergency booster injection if it has been more than five years since your last booster dose. The doses are injected into a muscle.

Side Effects

Along with its needed effects, a medicine may cause some unwanted effects. Although not all of these side effects may occur, if they do occur they may need medical attention. *It is very important that you tell your doctor about any side effect that occurs after a dose of DT or Td*, even if the side effect has gone away without treatment. Some types of side effects may mean that you should not receive any more doses of DT or Td.

Get emergency help immediately if any of the following side effects occur:
  Rare—Symptoms of allergic reaction
    Difficulty in breathing or swallowing; hives; itching, especially of feet or hands; reddening of skin, especially around ears; swelling of eyes, face, or inside of nose; unusual tiredness or weakness (sudden and severe)

Check with your doctor as soon as possible if any of the following side effects occur:
  Rare
    Confusion; convulsions (seizures); excessive sleepiness; fever over 39.4 °C (103 °F); headache or vomiting (severe or continuing); hives; itching; joint aches or pain; skin rash; swelling, blistering, pain, or other severe reaction at the place of injection (generally starts within 2 to 8 hours after the injection); unusual irritability

Other side effects may occur that usually do not need medical attention. However, check with your doctor if any of the following side effects continue or are bothersome:
  More common—For DT and Td
    Redness or hard lump at the place of injection (this may last for a few days; however, less often, the hard lump may last for a few weeks)
  More common—For DT only
    Fever under 39.4 °C (103 °F); swelling, pain, or tenderness at the place of injection (this may last for a few days)
  Less common—For DT and Td
    Dent or indentation at the place of injection
  Less common—For DT only
    Crying (continuing); drowsiness; fretfulness; loss of appetite; vomiting
  Less common—For Td only
    Chills; fast heartbeat; fever under 39.4 °C (103 °F); general feeling of discomfort or illness; headache; muscle aches; swelling of glands in armpit; unusual tiredness or weakness

Other side effects not listed above may also occur in some patients. If you notice any other effects, check with your doctor.

DIPHTHERIA AND TETANUS TOXOIDS AND PERTUSSIS VACCINE ADSORBED AND HAEMOPHILUS B CONJUGATE VACCINE   (Systemic)

Some commonly used brand names are:

In the U.S.—
  Tetramune

In Canada—
  DPT-Hib
  Tetramune

Category

- **Immunizing agent, active—**

Description

Diphtheria and tetanus toxoids and pertussis (dif-THEER-ee-a and TET-n-us and per-TUSS-iss) vaccine (also known as DTP vaccine) combined with Haemophilus b conjugate (hem-OFF-fil-us BEE KON-ja-gat) vaccine (also known as Hib vaccine) is a combination immunizing agent used to prevent illness caused by diphtheria, tetanus, pertussis, and Haemophilus influenzae type b (Hib) bacteria. The vaccine works by causing the body to produce its own protection (antibodies) against these diseases. This combination vaccine is also known as DTP-Hib vaccine.

Diphtheria is a serious illness that can cause breathing difficulties, heart problems, nerve damage, pneumonia, and possibly death. The risk of serious complications and death is greater in very young children and in the elderly.

Tetanus (also known as lockjaw) is a serious illness that causes convulsions (seizures) and severe muscle spasms that can be strong enough to cause bone fractures of the spine. Tetanus causes death in 30 to 40 percent of cases.

Pertussis (also known as whooping cough) is a serious disease that causes severe spells of coughing that can interfere with breathing. Pertussis can also cause pneumonia, long-lasting bronchitis, seizures, brain damage, and death.

Infection by Haemophilus influenzae type b (Hib) bacteria can cause life-threatening illnesses, such as meningitis, which affects the brain; epiglottitis, which can cause death by suffocation; pericarditis, which affects the heart; pneumonia, which affects the lungs; and septic arthritis, which affects the bones and joints. Hib meningitis causes death in 5 to 10% of children who are infected. Also, approximately 30% of children who survive Hib meningitis are left with some type of serious permanent damage, such as mental retardation, deafness, epilepsy, or partial blindness.

DTP-Hib vaccine is available in the following dosage form:

Parenteral
• Injection

Before Receiving This Vaccine

In deciding to use a vaccine, the risks of receiving the vaccine must be weighed against the good it will do. This is a decision you and your doctor will make. For DTP-Hib vaccine, the following should be considered:

Allergies—Tell your doctor if your child has ever had any unusual or allergic reaction to diphtheria toxoid, tetanus toxoid, pertussis vaccine, DTP vaccine, Haemophilus b conjugate vaccine, Hib vaccine, or Haemophilus b polysaccharide vaccine. Also tell your health care professional if your child is allergic to any other substances, such as thimerosal or other preservatives.

Children—This vaccine is not recommended for children younger than 2 months of age or older than 7 years of age.

Other medical problems—The presence of other medical problems may affect the use of DTP-Hib vaccine. Make sure you tell your doctor if your child has any other medical problems, especially:

• Brain disease or

• Central nervous system (CNS) disease or family history of or

• Convulsions (seizures) or family history of—Use of the vaccine may make the condition worse or may increase the chance of side effects

• Fever or

• Serious illness—The symptoms of the condition may be confused with some of the possible side effects of the vaccine

Proper Use of This Vaccine

Dosing—The number of doses of DTP-Hib vaccine will be different for different patients. The following information includes only the average doses of DTP-Hib vaccine.

• For *injection* dosage form:
  ○ For prevention of diphtheria, tetanus, pertussis, and Haemophilus influenzae type b illnesses:
    ▪ Children up to 2 months of age—Use is not recommended.
    ▪ Children 2 to 6 months of age at the first dose—Three doses, at least two months apart. Then a fourth dose at 12 to 18 months of age after at least 6 months have passed since the third dose. The doses are injected into a muscle.
    ▪ Children 7 to 11 months of age at the first dose—Two doses, at least two months apart, followed by additional doses of either this vaccine, DTP vaccine, or Hib vaccine, depending on the immunization schedule. The doses are injected into a muscle.
    ▪ Children 12 to 14 months of age at the first dose—One dose, followed by additional doses of either this vaccine, DTP vaccine, or Hib vaccine, depending on the immunization schedule. The doses are injected into a muscle.
    ▪ Children 15 to 59 months of age at the first dose—One dose, followed by additional doses of DTP vaccine to complete the immunization schedule for DTP. The doses are injected into a muscle.
    ▪ Adults and children 7 years of age and older—Use is not recommended.

After Receiving This Vaccine

At the time of the DTP-Hib vaccine injection, your doctor may give your child a dose of acetaminophen (or another medicine that helps prevent fever). This is to help prevent some of the side effects of this vaccine. Your doctor may also want your child to take the acetaminophen every 4 hours for 24 hours after your child receives this vaccine. Check with your doctor if you have any questions.

This vaccine may interfere with laboratory tests that check for Hib disease. Make sure your doctor knows that your child has received DTP-Hib vaccine if your child is treated for a severe infection during the 2 weeks after your child receives this vaccine.

Side Effects of This Vaccine

Along with its needed effects, a vaccine may cause some unwanted effects. Although not all of these side effects may occur, if they do occur they may need medical attention. *It is very important that you tell your doctor about any side effect that occurs after a dose of DTP-Hib vaccine*, even if the side effect goes away without treatment. Some types of side effects may mean that your child should not receive any more doses of DTP-Hib vaccine.

Get emergency help immediately if any of the following side effects occur:
  Rare
    Collapse; confusion; convulsions (seizures); crying for three or more hours; fever of 40.5 °C (105 °F) or more; headache (severe or continuing); irritability (unusual and continuing); periods of unconsciousness or lack of

awareness; sleepiness (unusual and continuing); vomiting (severe or continuing)

Check with your doctor immediately if any of the following side effects occur:

Rare

Symptoms of allergic reactions—Difficulty in breathing or swallowing; hives; itching (especially of feet or hands); reddening of skin (especially around ears); swelling of eyes, face, or inside of nose; unusual tiredness or weakness (sudden and severe)

Other side effects may occur that usually do not need medical attention. These side effects may go away as your child's body adjusts to the vaccine. However, check with your doctor if any of the following side effects continue or are bothersome:

More common

Drowsiness; fever of up to 102.2 °F (39 °C) (usually lasts less than 48 hours and may occur with fretfulness, drowsiness, vomiting, and loss of appetite); fretfulness; irritability; lump at place of injection (may be present for a few weeks after injection); redness, warm feeling, swelling, tenderness, or pain at place of injection

Less common

Diarrhea; fever between 102.2 and 104 °F (39 and 40 °C) (usually lasts less than 48 hours and may occur with fretfulness, drowsiness, vomiting, and loss of appetite); hard lump at place of injection (may be present for a few days after injection); loss of appetite; vomiting

Rare

Fever between 104 and 104.8 °F (40 and 40.4 °C) (usually lasts less than 48 hours and may occur with fretfulness, drowsiness, vomiting, and loss of appetite); lack of interest; reduced physical activity; skin rash

Other side effects not listed above may also occur in some patients. If you notice any other effects, check with your doctor.

DIPHTHERIA TOXOID, TETANUS TOXOID, ACELLULAR PERTUSSIS VACCINE, HEPATITIS B VACCINE RECOMBINANT, AND INACTIVATED POLIOVIRUS VACCINE (Intramuscular Route) - dif-THEER-ee-a TOX-oyd, TET-n-us TOX-oyd, a-SELL-yoo-lar per-TUS-iss vak-seen, hep-ah-TY-tiss B vak-seen re-KOM-bin-ant, in-AK-ti-vated POE-lee-oh VYE-rus vak-SEEN

Commonly used brand name(s)

In the U.S.—
Pediarix

Available Dosage Forms:
• Suspension

Therapeutic Class: Vaccine

Uses For This Vaccine

Diphtheria and tetanus toxoids and pertussis vaccine (also known as DTP vaccine) combined with hepatitis B and poliovirus vaccine (also known as HepB and IPV) is a combination immunizing agent used to prevent illness caused by diphtheria, tetanus, pertussis, hepatitis B, and poliovirus. The vaccine works by causing the body to produce its own protection (antibodies) against these diseases.

This vaccine combines five agents into one vaccine. In order to complete the series, you must get three injections of this vaccine at separate intervals. Because there are many different diseases you will need to be vaccinated against, be sure to follow your doctor's directions about your vaccination schedule.

Diphtheria is a serious illness that can cause breathing difficulties, heart problems, nerve damage, pneumonia, and possibly death. The risk of serious complications is greater in very young children and the elderly.

Tetanus (also known as lockjaw) is a very serious illness that causes seizures and severe muscle spasms that can be strong enough to cause bone fractures of the spine. The disease continues to occur almost exclusively among people who do not get vaccinated or do not have enough protection from previous vaccines.

Pertussis (also known as whooping cough) is a serious disease that causes severe spells of coughing that can interfere with breathing. Pertussis can also cause pneumonia, long lasting bronchitis, seizures, brain damage, and death.

Hepatitis B infection is a major cause of serious liver diseases including liver cancer. You get hepatitis B by being exposed to someone else's body fluids. Pregnant women can also give hepatitis B to their unborn child. People who have the virus can give it to others without them knowing it.

Polio is a very serious infection that causes paralysis of the muscles, including the muscles that enable you to walk and breathe. A polio infection may leave a person unable to breathe without the help of a breathing machine. It may also leave a person unable to walk without leg braces or being confined to a wheelchair. There is no cure for polio.

Before Receiving This Vaccine

In deciding to use a vaccine, the risks of taking the vaccine must be weighed against the good it will do. This is a decision you and your doctor will make. For this vaccine, the following should be considered:

In deciding to use a vaccine, the risks of taking the vaccine must be weighed against the good it will do. This is a decision you and your doctor will make. For DTaP-HepB-IPV vaccine, the following should be considered:

Allergies—Tell your doctor if you have ever had any unusual or allergic reaction to this medicine or any other medicines. Also tell your health care professional if you have any other types of allergies, such as to foods, dyes, preservatives, or animals. For non-prescription products, read the label or package ingredients carefully.

Pediatric—Safety and effectiveness have not been established in children younger than six weeks of age. This vaccine is also not recommended for children over seven years of age.

Geriatric—DTaP-HepB-IPV is not approved for use in older adults.

Other medicines—Although certain medicines should not be used together at all, in other cases two different medicines may be used together even if an interaction might occur. In these cases, your doctor may want to change the dose, or other precautions may be necessary. Tell your healthcare professional if you are taking any other prescription or non-prescription (over-the-counter [OTC]) medicine.

Interactions with Food/Tobacco/Alcohol—Certain medicines should not be used at or around the time of eating food or eating certain types of food since interactions may occur. Using alcohol or tobacco with certain medicines may also cause interactions to occur. Discuss with your healthcare professional the use of your medicine with food, alcohol, or tobacco.

Other medical problems—The presence of other medical problems may affect the use of this vaccine. Make sure you tell your doctor if you have any other medical problems, especially:

- Bleeding disorders (hemophilia or thrombocytopenia)—You may develop a formation of blood at the injection site. Your doctor should take steps to avoid this.

- Central nervous system disorders—If your child has certain disorders, you will need to look at the potential risks and benefits of getting DTaP-HepB-IPV. You should talk to your child's doctor to find out if your child should receive this vaccine.

- Disease of the brain—This includes coma, decreased level of consciousness, or seizures. People who have these symptoms within seven days of receiving a vaccine with pertussis in it should not get DTaP-HepB-IPV vaccine.

- Guillain-Barre syndrome—If you have ever had this condition after getting a vaccine with tetanus in it, you should weigh the potential benefits and possible risks of getting DTaP-HepB-IPV.

- Immunodeficiency disorder—If you have an immune system disorder, this vaccine may not work well for you

- Life threatening allergic reaction—You should not take this vaccine if you have had a severe allergic reaction to a previous dose of this vaccine or any ingredients in the vaccine. This includes polymyxin B, neomycin, and yeast.

- Moderate or severe illness, with or without fever—You should not get DTaP-HepB-IPV until the illness is gone and you feel better.

- Previous adverse reaction to this vaccine or any of its ingredients—If you have ever had an adverse reaction after getting a DTaP-HepB-IPV vaccine or another vaccine with pertussis in it, you should weigh the potential benefits and possible risks of getting DTaP-HepB-IPV. Adverse reactions include being unresponsive, crying continually without being able to stop for 3 hours or more, seizures with or without a fever, or a fever that is 105°F or higher.

- Progressive neurologic disorder—This includes infantile spasms, progressive brain disease, or uncontrolled epilepsy (seizures). DTaP-HepB-IPV should not be given until these conditions are treated and stabilized.

- Seizures, higher risk—Children at higher risk for seizures may be given a fever reducing medicine at the time the vaccine is given and for 24 hours after. By giving a fever reducing medicine, this may decrease the chance a fever may occur and cause a seizure.

Proper Use of This Vaccine

Dosing—The dose of this medicine will be different for different patients. Follow your doctor's orders or the directions on the label. The following information includes only the average doses of this medicine. If your dose is different, do not change it unless your doctor tells you to do so.

The amount of medicine that you take depends on the strength of the medicine. Also, the number of doses you take each day, the time allowed between doses, and the length of time you take the medicine depend on the medical problem for which you are using the medicine.

- For injection dosage form:
  - For prevention of diphtheria, tetanus, pertussis, hepatitis B, and poliovirus:
    - Adults and children greater than 7 years of age—Use is not approved.
    - Children up to 6 weeks—Use is not approved.
    - Children 6 weeks to 7 years of age—Three doses, 6 to 8 weeks apart. These doses are given into a muscle.
    - Children already vaccinated with one or more doses of hepatitis B vaccine—Infants vaccinated with hepatitis B at or shortly after birth should be given 3 doses according to the recommended schedule. The doses are given into a muscle.
    - Children previously vaccinated with Infanrix®—DTaP-HepB-IPV may be used to complete the first three doses of the DTaP and IPV series in infants who have received 1 or 2 doses of Infanrix® and are also due to get other components of DTaP-HepB-IPV.
    - Geriatric—Use is not approved for this group.

Precautions While Using This Vaccine

It is very important that your doctor check you at regular visits. Be sure to notify your doctor or clinic of any side effects that occur after you have received the vaccination. It is very important that you return to your doctor for the next dose in the series.

Side Effects of This Vaccine

Along with its needed effects, a vaccine may cause some unwanted effects. Although not all of these side effects may occur, if they do occur they may need medical attention. It is very important that you tell your doctor about any side effect that occurs after a dose of DTaP-HepB-IPV vaccine, even if the side effect goes away without treatment. Some types of side effects may mean that your child should not receive any more doses of DTaP-HepB-IPV vaccine.

Check with your doctor immediately if any of the following side effects occur:

Incidence not determined

Abdominal or stomach pain; agitation; back pain; black, tarry stools; bleeding gums; blood in urine or stools; bluish color of fingernails, lips, skin, palms, or nail beds; blurred vision; chills; clay colored stools; collapse or shock-like state; coma; confusion; cough; dark urine; diarrhea; difficulty swallowing; dizziness; drowsiness; fast heartbeat; fever; hallucinations; headache; heavier menstrual periods; hives or hive like swelling on face, eyelids, lips, tongue, throat, hands, legs, feet, or sex organs; hoarseness; irritability; irritation; itchiness, puffiness or swelling of the eyelids or around the eyes, face, lips or tongue, hands, or feet; itching; joint pain; loosening of skin; mood or mental changes; nausea; pain or cramping in abdomen; pinpoint red spots on skin; red irritated eyes; redness of skin; seizures; skin rash; shortness of breath; sore throat; sores, ulcers, or white spots in mouth or on lips; stiff neck; stiffness or swelling; Sudden Infant Death Syndrome (SIDS); swelling; tightness in chest; troubled breathing; unpleasant breath odor; unusual bleeding or bruising; unusual tiredness or weakness; vomiting or vomiting of blood; weight loss; wheezing; yellow eyes or skin

Some side effects may occur that usually do not need medical attention. These side effects may go away during treatment as your body adjusts to the medicine. Also, your health care professional may be able to tell you about ways to prevent or reduce some of these side effects. Check with your health care professional if any of the following side effects continue or are bothersome or if you have any questions about them:

More common

Bleeding; blistering; burning; coldness; discoloration of skin; fussiness; feeling of pressure; infection; inflammation; lumps; numbness; pain; restlessness; scarring; sleeping more than usual; soreness; stinging; tenderness; tingling; ulceration; unusual cry; warmth on skin

Incidence not determined

Arm or leg swelling; difficulty in moving; dullness, tiredness, weakness or feeling of sluggishness; flushing; itching skin; lack or loss of strength; loss of appetite; loss of strength or energy; malaise; muscle pain, weakness, or stiffness; pain in joints; sneezing; sores, ulcers, or white spots in mouth or on lips; swollen, painful, or tender lymph glands in neck, armpit, or groin

Some side effects may occur that usually do not need medical attention. These side effects may go away during treatment as your body adjusts to the medicine. Also, your health care professional may be able to tell you about ways to prevent or reduce some of these side effects. Check with your health care professional if any of the following side effects continue or are bothersome or if you have any questions about them:

Incidence not determined

Hair loss; paleness of skin; thinning of hair

Other side effects not listed may also occur in some patients. If you notice any other effects, check with your healthcare professional.

DIPHTHERIA TOXOID, TETANUS TOXOID, AND ACELLULAR PERTUSSIS VACCINE

(Intramuscular route) - dif-THEER-ee-a TOX-oyd, TET-n-us TOX-oyd, a-SELL-yoo-lar per-TUS-iss vak-seen

Commonly used brand name(s)

In the U.S.—

Adacel	Infanrix
Boostrix	Tripedia
Daptacel	

Available Dosage Forms:
- Suspension

Therapeutic Class: Vaccine

Uses For This Vaccine

Diphtheria and tetanus toxoids and pertussis vaccine (also known as DTP) is a combination immunizing agent given by injection to prevent diphtheria, tetanus, and pertussis.

Diphtheria is a serious illness that can cause breathing difficulties, heart problems, nerve damage, pneumonia, and possibly death. The risk of serious complications and death is greater in very young children and in the elderly.

Tetanus (also known as lockjaw) is a serious illness that causes convulsions (seizures) and severe muscle spasms that can be strong enough to cause bone fractures of the spine. Tetanus causes death in 30 to 40 percent of cases.

Pertussis (also known as whooping cough) is a serious disease that causes severe spells of coughing that can interfere with breathing. Pertussis also can cause pneumonia, longlasting bronchitis, seizures, brain damage, and death.

Immunization against diphtheria, tetanus, and pertussis is recommended for all infants and children from 2 months of age up to their 7th birthday. Children 10 years of age and older and adults may need an additional immunization against diphtheria, tetanus, and pertussis. Adults and teenagers should receive DTP instead of the diphtheria and tetanus injection if it has been 10 years or more since their last diphtheria and tetanus vaccination. DTP vaccination is recommended for adults who are in close contact with a baby who is less than a year old and for adults who work in the healthcare field.

Diphtheria, tetanus, and pertussis are serious diseases that can cause life-threatening illnesses. Although some serious side effects can occur after a dose of DTP (usually from the pertussis vaccine in DTP), this rarely happens. The chance of your child catching one of these diseases and being permanently injured or dying as a result is much greater than the chance of your child getting a serious side effect from the DTP vaccine.

Before Receiving This Vaccine

In deciding to use a vaccine, the risks of taking the vaccine must be weighed against the good it will do. This is a decision you and your doctor will make. For this vaccine, the following should be considered:

Allergies—Tell your doctor if you have ever had any unusual or allergic reaction to this medicine or any other medicines. Also tell your health care professional if you have any other types of allergies, such as to foods, dyes, preservatives, or animals. For non-prescription products, read the label or package ingredients carefully.

Pediatric—Use is not recommended for infants up to 2 months of age.

The Advisory Committee on Immunization Practices (ACIP) has recommended that teenagers be given a DTP vaccination instead of the tetanus-diphtheria (Td) vaccination. The committee is also encouraging all teenagers, even those who have already received Td, to get a DTP booster to help protect against pertussis (e.g., whooping cough). If you have questions about whether your teenager should receive DTP, contact your doctor.

Geriatric—Use is not recommended for persons older than 64 years of age.

Pregnancy—

	Pregnancy Category	Explanation
All Trimesters	C	Animal studies have shown an adverse effect and there are no adequate studies in pregnant women OR no animal studies have been conducted and there are no adequate studies in pregnant women.

Breast Feeding—There are no adequate studies in women for determining infant risk when using this medication during breastfeeding. Weigh the potential benefits against the potential risks before taking this medication while breastfeeding.

Other medicines—Although certain medicines should not be used together at all, in other cases two different medicines may be used together even if an interaction might occur. In these cases, your doctor may want to change the dose, or other precautions may be necessary. Tell your healthcare professional if you are taking any other prescription or non-prescription (over-the-counter [OTC]) medicine.

Interactions with Food/Tobacco/Alcohol—Certain medicines should not be used at or around the time of eating food or eating certain types of food since interactions may occur. Using alcohol or tobacco with certain medicines may also cause interactions to occur. Discuss with your healthcare professional the use of your medicine with food, alcohol, or tobacco.

Other medical problems—The presence of other medical problems may affect the use of this vaccine. Make sure you tell your doctor if you have any other medical problems, especially:

- Allergic reaction to a previous dose of DTP or
- Brain disease or
- Fever—Use of DTP may make the condition worse or may increase the chance of side effects.
- Bleeding disorders—This vaccine should not be given to anyone who has a bleeding disorder.
- Epilepsy or
- Guillain-Barr C syndrome (inflammatory disorder which causes paralysis) or
- Nervous system disorder—Your doctor will decide if you should receive this vaccine.

Proper Use of This Vaccine

Only the *Adacel* brand of DTaP vaccine should be given to adults and teenagers 11 to 64 years of age.

Only the *Boostrix* brand of DTaP vaccine should be given to children and teenagers 10 to 18 years of age.

Dosing—The dose of this medicine will be different for different patients. Follow your doctor's orders or the directions on the label. The following information includes only the average doses of this medicine. If your dose is different, do not change it unless your doctor tells you to do so.

The amount of medicine that you take depends on the strength of the medicine. Also, the number of doses you take each day, the time allowed between doses, and the length of time you take the medicine depend on the medical problem for which you are using the medicine.

- For injection dosage form:
  - For prevention of diphtheria, tetanus, and pertussis:
    - Adults and children 11 years of age and older— One single dose of Adacel brand vaccine.
    - Teenagers and children 10 to 18 years of age— One single dose of Boostrix brand vaccine.
    - Children 2 months to 7 years of age—One dose every four to eight weeks for a total of three doses, then a fourth dose six to twelve months after the third dose. A booster dose should be given at 4, 5, or 6 years of age. (The booster dose is given only if the fourth dose was given before the child's 4th birthday.)

Precautions While Using This Vaccine

At the time of the DTP injection, your doctor may give your child a dose of acetaminophen (or another medicine that helps prevent fever). This is to help prevent some of the side effects of DTP. Your doctor may also want your child to take this medicine every 4 hours for 24 hours after your child receives the DTP injection. Check with your doctor if you have any questions.

Side Effects of This Vaccine

Along with its needed effects, a vaccine may cause some unwanted effects. Although not all of these side effects may occur, if they do occur they may need medical attention. It is very important that you tell your doctor about any side effect that occurs after a dose of DTP, even though the side effect may have gone away without treatment. Some types of side effects may mean that your child should not receive any more doses of DTP.

Check with your doctor immediately if any of the following side effects occur:

Less frequent
Collapse; crying for 3 or more hours

Rare
Confusion; convulsions (seizures); difficulty in breathing or swallowing; fever of 105 °F (40.5 °C) or more; headache (severe or continuing); hives; irritability (unusual); itching, especially of feet or hands; periods of unconsciousness or lack of awareness; reddening of skin, especially around ears; sleepiness (unusual and continuing); swelling of eyes, face, or inside of nose; unusual tiredness, weakness (sudden and severe); vomiting (severe or continuing)

Some side effects may occur that usually do not need medical attention. These side effects may go away during treatment as your body adjusts to the medicine. Also, your health care professional may be able to tell you about ways to prevent or reduce some of these side effects. Check with your health care professional if any of the following side effects continue or are bothersome or if you have any questions about them:

More common
Fever between 100.4 and 102.2 °F (38 and 39 °C) (may occur with fretfulness, drowsiness, vomiting, and loss of appetite); lump at place of injection (may be present for a few weeks after injection); redness, swelling, tenderness, or pain at place of injection

Less common

Fever between 102.2 and 104 °F (39 and 40 °C) (may occur with fretfulness, drowsiness, vomiting, and loss of appetite)

Rare

Fever between 104 and 105 °F (40 and 40.5 °C) (may occur with fretfulness, drowsiness, vomiting, and loss of appetite); skin rash; swollen glands on side of neck (following DTP injection into arm)

Incidence not known

Injection site bruising; itching skin; redness of skin; welts

Other side effects not listed may also occur in some patients. If you notice any other effects, check with your healthcare professional.

DIPIVEFRIN (Ophthalmic route) - dye-PI-ve-frin

Commonly used brand name(s)

In the U.S.—
Propine

Available Dosage Forms:
- Solution

Therapeutic Class: Antiglaucoma
Pharmacologic Class: Adrenergic

Uses For This Medicine

Dipivefrin is used to treat certain types of glaucoma.

This medicine is available only with your doctor's prescription.

Before Using This Medicine

In deciding to use a medicine, the risks of taking the medicine must be weighed against the good it will do. This is a decision you and your doctor will make. For this medicine, the following should be considered:

Allergies—Tell your doctor if you have ever had any unusual or allergic reaction to this medicine or any other medicines. Also tell your health care professional if you have any other types of allergies, such as to foods, dyes, preservatives, or animals. For non-prescription products, read the label or package ingredients carefully.

Pediatric—Studies on this medicine have been done only in adult patients, and there is no specific information comparing use of this medicine in children with use in other age groups.

Geriatric—Many medicines have not been studied specifically in older people. Therefore, it may not be known whether they work exactly the same way they do in younger adults. Although there is no specific information comparing use of this medicine in the elderly with use in other age groups, this medicine is not expected to cause different side effects or problems in older people than it does in younger adults.

Pregnancy—

	Pregnancy Category	Explanation
All Trimesters	B	Animal studies have revealed no evidence of harm to the fetus, however, there are no adequate studies in pregnant women OR animal studies have shown an adverse effect, but adequate studies in pregnant women have failed to demonstrate a risk to the fetus.

Breast Feeding—There are no adequate studies in women for determining infant risk when using this medication during breastfeeding. Weigh the potential benefits against the potential risks before taking this medication while breastfeeding.

Other medicines—Although certain medicines should not be used together at all, in other cases two different medicines may be used together even if an interaction might occur. In these cases, your doctor may want to change the dose, or other precautions may be necessary. Tell your healthcare professional if you are taking any other prescription or non-prescription (over-the-counter [OTC]) medicine.

Interactions with Food/Tobacco/Alcohol—Certain medicines should not be used at or around the time of eating food or eating certain types of food since interactions may occur. Using alcohol or tobacco with certain medicines may also cause interactions to occur. Discuss with your healthcare professional the use of your medicine with food, alcohol, or tobacco.

Other medical problems—The presence of other medical problems may affect the use of this medicine. Make sure you tell your doctor if you have any other medical problems, especially:
- Eye disease or problems (other)—Dipivefrin may make the condition worse

Proper Use of This Medicine

Use this medicine only as directed. Do not use more of it and do not use it more often than your doctor ordered. To do so may increase the chance of too much medicine being absorbed into the body and the chance of side effects.

To use:
- First, wash your hands. Tilt the head back and, pressing your finger gently on the skin just beneath the lower eyelid, pull the lower eyelid away from the eye to make a space. Drop the medicine into this space. Let go of the eyelid and gently close the eyes. Do not blink. Keep the eyes closed and apply pressure to the inner corner of the eye with your finger for 1 or 2 minutes to allow the medicine to be absorbed by the eye.
- Immediately after using the eye drops, wash your hands to remove any medicine that may be on them.
- To keep the medicine as germ-free as possible, do not touch the applicator tip to any surface (including the eye). Also, keep the container tightly closed.
- If you are using the medicine with the compliance cap (C Cap):
  - Before using the eye drops for the first time, make sure the number 1 or the correct day of the week appears in the window on the cap.

○ Remove the cap and use the eye drops as directed.
○ Replace the cap. Holding the cap between your thumb and forefinger, rotate the bottle until the cap clicks to the next station. This will tell you your next dose.
○ After every dose, rotate the bottle until the cap clicks to the position that tells you your next dose.

Dosing—The dose of this medicine will be different for different patients. Follow your doctor's orders or the directions on the label. The following information includes only the average doses of this medicine. If your dose is different, do not change it unless your doctor tells you to do so.

The amount of medicine that you take depends on the strength of the medicine. Also, the number of doses you take each day, the time allowed between doses, and the length of time you take the medicine depend on the medical problem for which you are using the medicine.

- For ophthalmic solution (eye drops) dosage form:
  ○ For glaucoma:
    ▪ Adults—One drop every twelve hours.
    ▪ Children—Use and dose must by determined by your doctor.

Missed dose—If you miss a dose of this medicine, apply it as soon as possible. However, if it is almost time for your next dose, skip the missed dose and go back to your regular dosing schedule.

Storage—Store the medicine in a closed container at room temperature, away from heat, moisture, and direct light. Keep from freezing.

Keep out of the reach of children.

Do not keep outdated medicine or medicine no longer needed.

Precautions While Using This Medicine

Your doctor should check your eye pressure at regular visits.

Side Effects of This Medicine

Along with its needed effects, a medicine may cause some unwanted effects. Although not all of these side effects may occur, if they do occur they may need medical attention.

Check with your doctor as soon as possible if any of the following side effects occur:
  Rare
    Fast or irregular heartbeat; increase in blood pressure; itching, pain, redness, or swelling of eye or eyelid (severe), or other irritation of the eye; skin rash or hives; watering of eyes (severe and continuing)

Some side effects may occur that usually do not need medical attention. These side effects may go away during treatment as your body adjusts to the medicine. Also, your health care professional may be able to tell you about ways to prevent or reduce some of these side effects. Check with your health care professional if any of the following side effects continue or are bothersome or if you have any questions about them:
  Less common
    Blurred vision; burning or stinging of the eye; headache; increased sensitivity of eyes to light; large pupils

Other side effects not listed may also occur in some patients. If you notice any other effects, check with your healthcare professional.

DIPYRIDAMOLE (Oral route, Intravenous route) - dye-peer-ID-a-mole

Commonly used brand name(s)

In the U.S.—
  Persantine

Available Dosage Forms:
  - Tablet
  - Tablet, Extended Release
  - Solution
  - Capsule, Extended Release

Therapeutic Class: Platelet Aggregation Inhibitor
Pharmacologic Class: Phosphodiesterase Inhibitor

Uses For This Medicine

Dipyridamole is used to lessen the chance of stroke or other serious medical problems that may occur when a blood vessel is blocked by blood clots. It is given only when there is a larger-than-usual chance that these problems may occur. For example, it is given to people who have had diseased heart valves replaced by mechanical valves, because dangerous blood clots are especially likely to occur in these patients. Dipyridamole works by helping to prevent dangerous blood clots from forming.

Dipyridamole may also be used for other heart and blood conditions as determined by your doctor.

Dipyridamole is also sometimes used as part of a medical test that shows how well blood is flowing to your heart. For information on this use of dipyridamole, see Dipyridamole—Diagnostic (Systemic).

Dipyridamole is available only with your doctor's prescription.

Before Using This Medicine

In deciding to use a medicine, the risks of taking the medicine must be weighed against the good it will do. This is a decision you and your doctor will make. For this medicine, the following should be considered:

Allergies—Tell your doctor if you have ever had any unusual or allergic reaction to this medicine or any other medicines. Also tell your health care professional if you have any other types of allergies, such as to foods, dyes, preservatives, or animals. For non-prescription products, read the label or package ingredients carefully.

Pediatric—This medicine has been tested only in adults and in children older than 12 years of age. There is no specific information comparing use of dipyridamole in children younger than 12 years of age with use in other age groups.

Geriatric—Dipyridamole has not been studied specifically in older people taking the medicine regularly to prevent blood clots from forming. Although there is no specific information comparing this use of dipyridamole in the elderly with use in other age groups, it is not expected to cause different side effects or problems in older people than it does in younger adults.

Pregnancy—

	Pregnancy Category	Explanation
All Trimesters	B	Animal studies have revealed no evidence of harm to the fetus, however, there are no adequate studies in pregnant women OR animal studies have shown an adverse effect, but adequate studies in pregnant women have failed to demonstrate a risk to the fetus.

Breast Feeding—There are no adequate studies in women for determining infant risk when using this medication during breastfeeding. Weigh the potential benefits against the potential risks before taking this medication while breastfeeding.

Other medicines—

Using this medicine with any of the following medicines is usually not recommended, but may be required in some cases. If both medicines are prescribed together, your doctor may change the dose or how often you use one or both of the medicines.

Ginkgo, Streptokinase

Interactions with Food/Tobacco/Alcohol—Certain medicines should not be used at or around the time of eating food or eating certain types of food since interactions may occur. Using alcohol or tobacco with certain medicines may also cause interactions to occur. Discuss with your healthcare professional the use of your medicine with food, alcohol, or tobacco.

Other medical problems—The presence of other medical problems may affect the use of this medicine. Make sure you tell your doctor if you have any other medical problems, especially:

- Chest pain—The chance of side effects may be increased
- Low blood pressure—Large amounts of dipyridamole can make your condition worse

Proper Use of This Medicine

This medicine works best when there is a constant amount in the blood. To help keep the amount constant, dipyridamole must be taken in regularly spaced doses, as ordered by your doctor.

This medicine works best when taken with a full glass (8 ounces) of water at least 1 hour before or 2 hours after meals. However, to lessen stomach upset, your doctor may want you to take the medicine with food or milk.

Dosing—The dose of this medicine will be different for different patients. Follow your doctor's orders or the directions on the label. The following information includes only the average doses of this medicine. If your dose is different, do not change it unless your doctor tells you to do so.

The amount of medicine that you take depends on the strength of the medicine. Also, the number of doses you take each day, the time allowed between doses, and the length of time you take the medicine depend on the medical problem for which you are using the medicine.

- For preventing blood clots:
  - For oral dosage form (tablets):
    - Adults—The usual dose is 75 to 100 milligrams (mg) four times a day taken together with an anticoagulant (blood-thinning) medicine.
    - Children—Use and dose must be determined by your doctor.

Missed dose—If you miss a dose of this medicine, take it as soon as possible. However, if it is almost time for your next dose, skip the missed dose and go back to your regular dosing schedule. Do not double doses.

Storage—Store the medicine in a closed container at room temperature, away from heat, moisture, and direct light. Keep from freezing.

Keep out of the reach of children.

Do not keep outdated medicine or medicine no longer needed.

Precautions While Using This Medicine

Dipyridamole is sometimes used together with an anticoagulant (blood thinner) or aspirin. The combination of medicines may provide better protection against the formation of blood clots than any of the medicines used alone. However, the risk of bleeding may also be increased when dipyridamole is taken with aspirin. To reduce the risk of bleeding:

- Do not take aspirin, or any combination medicine containing aspirin, unless the same doctor who directed you to take dipyridamole also directs you to take aspirin. This is especially important if you are taking an anticoagulant together with dipyridamole.
- If you have been directed to take aspirin together with dipyridamole, take only the amount of aspirin ordered by your doctor. If you need a medicine to relieve pain or a fever, your doctor may not want you to take extra aspirin. It is a good idea to discuss this with your doctor, so that you will know ahead of time what medicine to take.
- Your doctor should check your progress at regular visits.

Tell all medical doctors and dentists you go to that you are taking dipyridamole, and whether or not you are taking an anticoagulant (blood thinner) or aspirin together with it.

Dizziness, lightheadedness, or fainting may occur, especially when you get up from a lying or sitting position. Getting up slowly may help. If this problem continues or gets worse, check with your doctor.

Side Effects of This Medicine

Along with its needed effects, a medicine may cause some unwanted effects. Although not all of these side effects may occur, if they do occur they may need medical attention.

Check with your doctor as soon as possible if any of the following side effects occur:

Rare

   Chest pain; gallstones; tightness or swelling of neck; yellow eyes or skin

Some side effects may occur that usually do not need medical attention. These side effects may go away during treatment as your body adjusts to the medicine. Also, your health care professional may be able to tell you about ways to prevent or reduce some of these side effects. Check with your health

care professional if any of the following side effects continue or are bothersome or if you have any questions about them:

More common
   Abdominal or stomach cramps; diarrhea; dizziness or lightheadedness

Less common
   Flushing; headache; nausea or vomiting; weakness

Rare
   General discomfort and/or unusual tiredness or weakness; hair loss; joint pain or swelling; muscle pain; runny nose; sneezing

Other side effects not listed may also occur in some patients. If you notice any other effects, check with your healthcare professional.

DISOPYRAMIDE (Oral route) - dye-soe-PEER-a-mide

Black Box Warning

In the National Heart, Lung and Blood Institute's Cardiac Arrhythmia Suppression Trial (CAST), a long-term, multi-center, randomized, double-blind study in patients with asymptomatic non-life-threatening ventricular arrhythmias who had had a myocardial infarction more than 6 days but less than 2 years previously, an excessive mortality or non-fatal cardiac arrest rate (7.7%) was seen in patients treated with encainide or flecainide compared with that seen in patients assigned to carefully matched placebo-treated groups (3%). The average duration of treatment with encainide or flecainide in this study was 10 months.

The applicability of the CAST results to other populations (eg, those without recent myocardial infarction) is uncertain. Considering the known proarrhythmic properties of disopyramide phosphate and the lack of evidence of improved survival for any antiarrhythmic drug in patients without life-threatening arrhythmias, the use of disopyramide phosphate as well as other antiarrhythmic agents should be reserved for patients with life-threatening ventricular arrhythmias.

Commonly used brand name(s)

In the U.S.—
   Norpace
   Norpace CR

Available Dosage Forms:
   • Capsule
   • Tablet, Extended Release
   • Capsule, Extended Release

Therapeutic Class: Antiarrhythmic, Group IA

Uses For This Medicine

Disopyramide is used to treat abnormal heart rhythms.

It is available only with your doctor's prescription.

Before Using This Medicine

In deciding to use a medicine, the risks of taking the medicine must be weighed against the good it will do. This is a decision you and your doctor will make. For this medicine, the following should be considered:

Allergies—Tell your doctor if you have ever had any unusual or allergic reaction to this medicine or any other medicines. Also tell your health care professional if you have any other types of allergies, such as to foods, dyes, preservatives, or animals. For non-prescription products, read the label or package ingredients carefully.

Pediatric—This medicine has been tested in children and has not been shown to cause different side effects or problems than it does in adults.

Geriatric—Some side effects, such as difficult urination and dry mouth, may be especially likely to occur in elderly patients, who are usually more sensitive than younger adults to the effects of disopyramide.

Pregnancy—

	Pregnancy Category	Explanation
All Trimesters	C	Animal studies have shown an adverse effect and there are no adequate studies in pregnant women OR no animal studies have been conducted and there are no adequate studies in pregnant women.

Breast Feeding—There are no adequate studies in women for determining infant risk when using this medication during breastfeeding. Weigh the potential benefits against the potential risks before taking this medication while breastfeeding.

Other medicines—

Using this medicine with any of the following medicines is not recommended. Your doctor may decide not to treat you with this medication or change some of the other medicines you take.

Bepridil, Cisapride, Levomethadyl, Mesoridazine, Pimozide, Ranolazine, Sparfloxacin, Terfenadine, Thioridazine, Ziprasidone

Interactions with Food/Tobacco/Alcohol—Certain medicines should not be used at or around the time of eating food or eating certain types of food since interactions may occur. Using alcohol or tobacco with certain medicines may also cause interactions to occur. Discuss with your healthcare professional the use of your medicine with food, alcohol, or tobacco.

Other medical problems—The presence of other medical problems may affect the use of this medicine. Make sure you tell your doctor if you have any other medical problems, especially:
   • Diabetes mellitus (sugar diabetes)—Disopyramide may cause low blood sugar
   • Difficult urination or
   • Enlarged prostate—Disopyramide may cause difficult urination
   • Electrolyte disorders—Disopyramide may worsen heart rhythm problems
   • Glaucoma (history of) or
   • Myasthenia gravis—Disopyramide may aggravate these conditions

- Kidney disease or
- Liver disease—Effects may be increased because of slower removal of disopyramide from the body
- Low blood pressure or
- Other heart disorders—Effects of disopyramide on the heart may make these conditions worse
- Malnutrition, long term—Disopyramide may cause low blood sugar

Proper Use of This Medicine

Take disopyramide exactly as directed by your doctor even though you may feel well. Do not take more medicine than ordered.

For patients taking the extended-release capsules:

- Swallow the capsule whole without breaking, crushing, or chewing.

For patients taking the extended-release tablets:

- Do not crush or chew the tablet.

This medicine works best when there is a constant amount in the blood. To help keep the amount constant, do not miss any doses. Also, it is best to take the doses at evenly spaced times day and night. For example, if you are to take four doses a day, the doses should be spaced about 6 hours apart. If this interferes with your sleep or other daily activities, or if you need help in planning the best times to take your medicine, check with your health care professional.

Dosing—The dose of this medicine will be different for different patients. Follow your doctor's orders or the directions on the label. The following information includes only the average doses of this medicine. If your dose is different, do not change it unless your doctor tells you to do so.

The amount of medicine that you take depends on the strength of the medicine. Also, the number of doses you take each day, the time allowed between doses, and the length of time you take the medicine depend on the medical problem for which you are using the medicine.

- For treatment of arrhythmias:
  - For short-acting oral dosage form (capsules):
    - Adults—100 to 150 mg taken every six to eight hours.
    - Children—Dose is based on body weight and age and must be determined by your doctor. The dose is usually 6 to 30 mg per kilogram (kg) (2.73 to 13.64 mg per pound) of body weight per day. This dose is evenly divided and taken every six hours.
  - For long-acting oral dosage forms (extended-release capsules or tablets):
    - Adults—200 or 400 mg every twelve hours.
    - Children—Use is not recommended.

Missed dose—If you miss a dose of this medicine, take it as soon as possible. However, if it is almost time for your next dose, skip the missed dose and go back to your regular dosing schedule. Do not double doses.

Storage—Store the medicine in a closed container at room temperature, away from heat, moisture, and direct light. Keep from freezing.

Keep out of the reach of children.

Do not keep outdated medicine or medicine no longer needed.

Precautions While Using This Medicine

Your doctor should check your progress at regular visits to make sure the medicine is working properly.

Do not stop taking this medicine without first checking with your doctor. Stopping suddenly may cause a serious change in heart function.

Dizziness, lightheadedness, or fainting may occur, especially when you get up from a lying or sitting position. This is due to lowered blood pressure. Getting up slowly may help. This effect does not occur often at doses of disopyramide usually used; however, make sure you know how you react to this medicine before you drive, use machines, or do anything else that could be dangerous if you are not alert. If the problem continues or gets worse, check with your doctor.

Disopyramide may rarely cause hypoglycemia (low blood sugar) in some people. (See the Side Effects of This Medicine section below.) If these signs appear, eat or drink a food containing sugar and call your doctor right away.

This medicine may cause blurred vision or other vision problems. If any of these occur, do not drive, use machines, or do anything else that could be dangerous if you are not able to see well.

Disopyramide may cause dryness of the eyes, mouth, and nose. For temporary relief of mouth dryness, use sugarless candy or gum, melt bits of ice in your mouth, or use a saliva substitute. However, if dry mouth continues for more than 2 weeks, check with your medical doctor or dentist. Continuing dryness of the mouth may increase the chance of dental disease, including tooth decay, gum disease, and oral yeast infections.

This medicine often will make you sweat less, allowing your body temperature to increase. Use extra care not to become overheated during exercise or hot weather while you are taking this medicine, since becoming overheated could possibly result in heatstroke.

Side Effects of This Medicine

Along with its needed effects, a medicine may cause some unwanted effects. Although not all of these side effects may occur, if they do occur they may need medical attention.

Check with your doctor as soon as possible if any of the following side effects occur:

More common
    Dizziness, feeling of faintness; fainting; heartbeat sensations; shortness of breath; unusual tiredness

Less common
    Chest pain; fast or slow heartbeat, rapid weight gain, swelling of feet or lower legs; lightheadedness; rash and/or itching

Rare
    Enlargement of breasts in men; fever; mental depression; nosebleeds or bleeding gums; sore throat and fever; yellow eyes or skin

Signs and symptoms of hypoglycemia (low blood sugar)
    Anxious feeling; chills; cold sweats; confusion; cool, pale skin; drowsiness; fast heartbeat; headache; hunger (excessive); nausea; nervousness; shakiness; unsteady walk; unusual tiredness or weakness

Some side effects may occur that usually do not need medical attention. These side effects may go away during treatment as your body adjusts to the medicine. Also, your health care professional may be able to tell you about ways to prevent or reduce some of these side effects. Check with your health care professional if any of the following side effects continue or are bothersome or if you have any questions about them:

More common

Blurred vision; constipation; dry eyes, mouth, nose, or throat; problems with urination

Less common

Bloating or stomach pain; diarrhea; headache; impotence; loss of appetite; muscle weakness; nausea; nervousness; trouble in sleeping

Other side effects not listed may also occur in some patients. If you notice any other effects, check with your healthcare professional.

DISULFIRAM (Oral route) - dye-SUL-fi-ram

Black Box Warning

Disulfiram should never be administered to a patient when he is in a state of alcohol intoxication, or without his full knowledge. The physician should instruct relatives accordingly.

Commonly used brand name(s)

In the U.S.—

Antabuse

Available Dosage Forms:

• Tablet

Therapeutic Class: Ethanol Dependency

Uses For This Medicine

Disulfiram is used to help overcome your drinking problem. It is not a cure for alcoholism, but rather will discourage you from drinking.

Disulfiram is available only with your doctor's prescription.

Before Using This Medicine

In deciding to use a medicine, the risks of taking the medicine must be weighed against the good it will do. This is a decision you and your doctor will make. For this medicine, the following should be considered:

Allergies—Tell your doctor if you have ever had any unusual or allergic reaction to this medicine or any other medicines. Also tell your health care professional if you have any other types of allergies, such as to foods, dyes, preservatives, or animals. For non-prescription products, read the label or package ingredients carefully.

Pediatric—Studies on this medicine have been done only in adult patients, and there is no specific information comparing use of disulfiram in children with use in other age groups.

Geriatric—Many medicines have not been studied specifically in older people. Therefore, it may not be known whether they work exactly the same way they do in younger adults or

if they cause different side effects or problems in older people. There is no specific information comparing use of disulfiram in the elderly with use in other age groups.

Breast Feeding—There are no adequate studies in women for determining infant risk when using this medication during breastfeeding. Weigh the potential benefits against the potential risks before taking this medication while breastfeeding.

Other medicines—

Using this medicine with any of the following medicines is not recommended. Your doctor may decide not to treat you with this medication or change some of the other medicines you take.

Amprenavir, Metronidazole, Paraldehyde

Interactions with Food/Tobacco/Alcohol—Certain medicines should not be used at or around the time of eating food or eating certain types of food since interactions may occur. Using alcohol or tobacco with certain medicines may also cause interactions to occur. The following interactions have been selected on the basis of their potential significance and are not necessarily all-inclusive.

Using this medicine with any of the following is not recommended. Your doctor may decide not to treat you with this medication, change some of the other medicines you take, or give you special instructions about the use of food, alcohol, or tobacco.

Ethanol

Other medical problems—The presence of other medical problems may affect the use of this medicine. Make sure you tell your doctor if you have any other medical problems, especially:

• Asthma or other lung disease, severe, or
• Diabetes mellitus (sugar diabetes) or
• Epilepsy or other seizure disorder or
• Heart or blood vessel disease or
• Kidney disease or
• Liver disease or cirrhosis of the liver or
• Underactive thyroid—A disulfiram-alcohol reaction may make the condition worse
• Depression or
• Severe mental illness—Disulfiram may make the condition worse
• Skin allergy—Disulfiram may cause an allergic reaction

Proper Use of This Medicine

In addition to beverages, alcohol is found in many other products. Reading the list of ingredients on foods and other products before using them will help you to avoid alcohol. Do not use alcohol-containing foods such as sauces and vinegars.

Before you take the first dose of this medicine, make sure you have not taken any alcoholic beverage or alcohol-containing product or medicine (for example, tonics, elixirs, and cough syrups) during the past 12 hours. If you are not sure about the alcohol content of medicines you may have taken, check with your health care professional.

Take this medicine every day as directed by your doctor. The medicine is usually taken each morning. However, if it makes you drowsy, ask your doctor if you may take it at bedtime instead.

Dosing—The dose of this medicine will be different for different patients. Follow your doctor's orders or the directions on the label. The following information includes only the average doses of this medicine. If your dose is different, do not change it unless your doctor tells you to do so.

The amount of medicine that you take depends on the strength of the medicine. Also, the number of doses you take each day, the time allowed between doses, and the length of time you take the medicine depend on the medical problem for which you are using the medicine.

- For oral dosage form (tablets):
  - To help overcome drinking problems:
    - Adults and teenagers—At first, the dose is 500 milligrams (mg) or less, once a day for one or two weeks. Then, your doctor may lower your dose to 125 to 500 mg (usually to 250 mg) once a day.
    - Children—Use and dose must be determined by your doctor.

Storage—Store the medicine in a closed container at room temperature, away from heat, moisture, and direct light. Keep from freezing.

Keep out of the reach of children.

Do not keep outdated medicine or medicine no longer needed.

Precautions While Using This Medicine

Do not drink any alcohol, even small amounts, while you are taking this medicine and for 14 days after you stop taking it, because the alcohol may make you very sick. In addition to beverages, alcohol is found in many other products. Reading the list of ingredients on foods and other products before using them will help you to avoid alcohol. You can also avoid alcohol if you:

- Do not use alcohol-containing foods, products, or medicines, such as elixirs, tonics, sauces, vinegars, cough syrups, mouth washes, or gargles.
- Do not come in contact with or breathe in the fumes of chemicals that may contain alcohol, acetaldehyde, paraldehyde, or other related chemicals, such as paint thinner, paint, varnish, or shellac.
- Use caution when using alcohol-containing products that are applied to the skin, such as some transdermal (stick-on patch) medicines or rubbing alcohol, back rubs, after-shave lotions, colognes, perfumes, toilet waters, or after-bath preparations. Using such products while you are taking disulfiram may cause headache, nausea, or local redness or itching because the alcohol in these products may be absorbed into your body. Before using alcohol-containing products on your skin, first test the product by applying some to a small area of your skin. Allow the product to remain on your skin for 1 or 2 hours. If no redness, itching, or other unwanted effects occur, you should be able to use the product.
- Do not use any alcohol-containing products on raw skin or open wounds.

Check with your doctor if you have any questions.

Some of the symptoms you may experience if you use any alcohol while taking this medicine are:

- Blurred vision
- Chest pain
- Confusion
- Dizziness or fainting
- Fast or pounding heartbeat
- Flushing or redness of face
- Increased sweating
- Nausea and vomiting
- Throbbing headache
- Troubled breathing
- Weakness

These symptoms will last as long as there is any alcohol left in your system, from 30 minutes to several hours. On rare occasions, if you have a severe reaction or have taken a large enough amount of alcohol, a heart attack, unconsciousness, convulsions (seizures), and death may occur.

Your doctor may want you to carry an identification card stating that you are using this medicine. This card should list the symptoms most likely to occur if alcohol is taken, and the doctor, clinic, or hospital to be contacted in case of an emergency. These cards may be available from the manufacturer. Ask your health care professional if you have any questions about this.

If you will be taking this medicine for a long period of time (for example, for several months at a time), your doctor should check your progress at regular visits.

Before buying or using any liquid prescription or nonprescription medicine, check with your pharmacist to see if it contains any alcohol.

This medicine may cause some people to become drowsy or less alert than they are normally. If this occurs, do not drive, use machines, or do anything else that could be dangerous if you are not alert.

Disulfiram will add to the effects of other CNS depressants (medicines that slow down the nervous system, possibly causing drowsiness). Some examples of CNS depressants are antihistamines or medicine for hay fever, other allergies, or colds; sedatives, tranquilizers, or sleeping medicine; prescription pain medicine or narcotics; barbiturates; medicine for seizures; muscle relaxants; or anesthetics, including some dental anesthetics. Check with your doctor before taking any of the above while you are using this medicine.

Side Effects of This Medicine

Along with its needed effects, a medicine may cause some unwanted effects. Although not all of these side effects may occur, if they do occur they may need medical attention.

Check with your doctor as soon as possible if any of the following side effects occur:
Less common
Eye pain or tenderness or any change in vision; mood or mental changes; numbness, tingling, pain, or weakness in hands or feet
Rare
Darkening of urine; light gray-colored stools; severe stomach pain; yellow eyes or skin

Some side effects may occur that usually do not need medical attention. These side effects may go away during treatment as your body adjusts to the medicine. Also, your health care professional may be able to tell you about ways to prevent or reduce some of these side effects. Check with your health care professional if any of the following side effects continue or are bothersome or if you have any questions about them:
More common
Drowsiness

Less common or rare

Decreased sexual ability in males; headache; metallic or garlic-like taste in mouth; skin rash; unusual tiredness

Other side effects not listed may also occur in some patients. If you notice any other effects, check with your healthcare professional.

DIURETIC, LOOP (Oral route, Injection route, Intravenous route)

Commonly used brand name(s)

In the U.S.—

Bumex	Furocot
Demadex	Furomide M.D.
Edecrin	Lasix
Edecrin Sodium	

Available Dosage Forms:

- Tablet
- Powder for Solution
- Solution
- Injectable

Uses For This Medicine

Loop diuretics are given to help reduce the amount of water in the body. They work by acting on the kidneys to increase the flow of urine.

Furosemide and torsemide are also used to treat high blood pressure (hypertension) in those patients who are not helped by other medicines or in those patients who have kidney problems.

Loop diuretics may also be used for other conditions as determined by your doctor.

Once a medicine has been approved for marketing for a certain use, experience may show that it is also useful for other medical problems. Although these uses are not included in product labeling, loop diuretics are used in certain patients with the following medical conditions:

- Hypercalcemia (too much calcium in the blood)
- Diagnostic aid for kidney disease

Before Using This Medicine

Allergies—Tell your doctor if you have ever had any unusual or allergic reaction to medicines in this group or any other medicines. Also tell your health care professional if you have any other types of allergies, such as to foods dyes, preservatives, or animals. For non-prescription products, read the label or package ingredients carefully.

Pediatric—Although there is no specific information comparing the use of loop diuretics in children with use in any other age group, these medicines are not expected to cause different side effects in children than they do in adults.

Geriatric—Dizziness, lightheadedness, or signs of too much potassium loss may be more likely to occur in the elderly, who are more sensitive to the effects of this medicine. Elderly patients may also be more likely to develop blood clots.

Pregnancy—Studies have not been done in pregnant women. However, studies in animals have shown this medicine to cause harmful effects. Before taking this medicine, make sure your doctor knows if you are pregnant or if you may become pregnant.

In general, diuretics are not useful for normal swelling of feet and hands that occurs during pregnancy. Diuretics should not be taken during pregnancy unless recommended by your doctor.

Breast Feeding—These medicines have not been reported to cause problems in nursing babies. Furosemide passes into breast milk; it is not known whether bumetanide, ethacrynic acid, or torsemide passes into breast milk. Although most medicines pass into breast milk in small amounts, many of them may be used safely while breast-feeding. Mothers who are taking a diuretic and who wish to breast-feed should discuss this with their doctor.

Other medicines—

Using medicines in this class with any of the following medicines is usually not recommended, but may be required in some cases. If both medicines are prescribed together, your doctor may change the dose or how often you use one or both of the medicines.

Arsenic Trioxide, Bepridil, Digitoxin, Dofetilide, Droperidol, Ethacrynic Acid, Furosemide, Ketanserin, Levomethadyl, Lithium, Sotalol

Using this medicine with any of the following may cause an increased risk of certain side effects but using both medicines may be the best treatment for you. If both medicines are prescribed together, your doctor may change the dose or how often you use one or both of the medicines.

Aceclofenac, Acemetacin, Alacepril, Alclofenac, Apazone, Aspirin, Benazepril, Benoxaprofen, Bromfenac, Bufexamac, Captopril, Carprofen, Celecoxib, Cephaloridine, Cholestyramine, Cilazapril, Clofibrate, Clometacin, Clonixin, Colestipol, Cortisone, Delapril, Dexketoprofen, Dibekacin, Diclofenac, Diflunisal, Digoxin, Dipyrone, Droxicam, Enalaprilat, Enalapril Maleate, Etodolac, Etofenamate, Felbinac, Fenbufen, Fenoprofen, Fentiazac, Floctafenine, Fludrocortisone, Flufenamic Acid, Flurbiprofen, Fosinopril, Gentamicin, Germanium, Ginseng, Gossypol, Ibuprofen, Imidapril, Indomethacin, Indoprofen, Isoxicam, Kanamycin, Ketoprofen, Ketorolac, Licorice, Lisinopril, Lornoxicam, Meclofenamate, Mefenamic Acid, Meloxicam, Moexipril, Nabumetone, Naproxen, Neomycin, Niflumic Acid, Nimesulide, Oxaprozin, Oxyphenbutazone, Pancuronium, Pentopril, Perindopril, Phenylbutazone, Pirazolac, Piroxicam, Pirprofen, Probenecid, Propyphenazone, Proquazone, Quinapril, Ramipril, Rofecoxib, Spirapril, Streptomycin, Sulindac, Suprofen, Temocapril, Tenidap, Tenoxicam, Tiaprofenic Acid, Tobramycin, Tolmetin, Trandolapril, Tubocurarine, Valdecoxib, Vecuronium, Zofenopril, Zomepirac

Interactions with Food/Tobacco/Alcohol—Certain medicines should not be used at or around the time of eating food or eating certain types of food since interactions may occur. Using alcohol or tobacco with certain medicines may also cause interactions to occur. Discuss with your healthcare professional the use of your medicine with food, alcohol, or tobacco.

Other medical problems—The presence of other medical problems may affect the use of medicines in this class. Make sure you tell your doctor if you have any other medical problems, especially:

- Anuric (inability to urinate)—Torsemide should NOT be used if you have this condition.
- Diabetes mellitus (sugar diabetes)—Loop diuretics may increase the amount of sugar in the blood
- Gout or
- Hearing problems or

- Pancreatitis (inflammation of the pancreas)—Loop diuretics may make these conditions worse
- Heart attack, recent—Use of loop diuretics after a recent heart attack may increase the chance of side effects
- Liver disease—Higher blood levels of the loop diuretic may occur, which may increase the chance of side effects
- Lupus erythematosus (history of)—Ethacrynic acid and furosemide may make this condition worse

Proper Use of This Medicine

This medicine may cause you to have an unusual feeling of tiredness when you begin to take it. You may also notice an increase in the amount of urine or in your frequency of urination. After you have taken the medicine for a while, these effects should lessen. In general, to keep the increase in urine from affecting your sleep:

- If you are to take a single dose a day, take it in the morning after breakfast.
- If you are to take more than one dose a day, take the last dose no later than 6 p.m., unless otherwise directed by your doctor.

However, it is best to plan your dose or doses according to a schedule that will least affect your personal activities and sleep. Ask your health care professional to help you plan the best time to take this medicine.

To help you remember to take your medicine, try to get into the habit of taking it at the same time each day.

For patients taking the oral liquid form of furosemide:

- This medicine is to be taken by mouth even if it comes in a dropper bottle. If this medicine does not come in a dropper bottle, use a specially marked measuring spoon or other device to measure each dose accurately, since the average household teaspoon may not hold the right amount of liquid.

For patients taking this medicine for high blood pressure:

- In addition to the use of the medicine your doctor has prescribed, appropriate treatment for your high blood pressure may include weight control and care in the types of foods you eat, especially foods high in sodium. Your doctor will tell you which factors are most important for you. You should check with your doctor before changing your diet.

Many patients who have high blood pressure will not notice any signs of the problem. In fact, many may feel normal. It is very important that you take your medicine exactly as directed and that you keep your appointments with your doctor even if you feel well.

Remember that this medicine will not cure your high blood pressure but it does help control it. Therefore, you must continue to take it as directed if you expect to lower your blood pressure and keep it down. You may have to take high blood pressure medicine for the rest of your life. If high blood pressure is not treated, it can cause serious problems such as heart failure, blood vessel disease, stroke, or kidney disease.

If this medicine upsets your stomach, it may be taken with meals or milk. If stomach upset (nausea, vomiting, or stomach pain) continues or gets worse, or if you suddenly get severe diarrhea, check with your doctor.

Dosing—The dose medicines in this class will be different for different patients. Follow your doctor's orders or the directions on the label. The following information includes only the average doses of these medicines. If your dose is different, do not change it unless your doctor tells you to do so.

The amount of medicine that you take depends on the strength of the medicine. Also, the number of doses you take each day, the time allowed between doses, and the length of time you take the medicine depend on the medical problem for which you are using the medicine.

- For bumetanide:
  - To lower the amount of water in the body:
    - For oral dosage form (tablets):
      - Adults-0.5 to 2 milligrams (mg) once a day. Your doctor may increase your dose if needed.
      - Children-Dose must be determined by your doctor.
    - For injection dosage form:
      - Adults—0.5 to 1 mg injected into a muscle or a vein every two to three hours as needed.
      - Children—Dose must be determined by your doctor.

- For ethacrynic acid:
  - To lower the amount of water in the body:
    - For oral dosage form (oral solution or tablets):
      - Adults-50 to 200 milligrams (mg) a day. This may be taken as a single dose or divided into smaller doses.
      - Children—At first, 25 mg a day. Your doctor may increase your dose as needed.
    - For injection dosage form:
      - Adults—50 mg injected into a vein every two to six hours as needed.
      - Children—Dose is based on body weight and must be determined by your doctor. The usual dose is 1 mg per kilogram (kg) (0.45 mg per pound) of body weight injected into a vein.

- For furosemide:
  - To lower the amount of water in the body:
    - For oral dosage form (oral solution or tablets):
      - Adults—At first, 20 to 80 milligrams (mg) once a day. Then, your doctor may increase your dose as needed. Your doctor may tell you to take a dose once a day, two or three times a day, or every other day.
      - Children—Dose is based on body weight and must be determined by your doctor. The usual dose is 2 mg per kilogram (kg) (0.91 mg per pound) of body weight for one dose. Then, your doctor may increase your dose every six to eight hours as needed.
    - For injection dosage form:
      - Adults—At first, 20 to 40 mg injected into a muscle or a vein for one dose. Then, your doctor may increase your dose every two hours as needed. Once the medicine is working, the dose is injected into a muscle or a vein one or two times a day.
      - Children—Dose is based on body weight and must be determined by your doctor. The usual dose is 1 mg per kg (0.45 mg per pound) of body weight injected into a muscle or a vein for one dose. Your doctor may increase your dose every two hours as needed.

○ For high blood pressure:
  ▪ For oral dosage form (oral solution or tablets):
    — Adults—40 mg two times a day. Your doctor may increase your dose.
○ For very high blood pressure:
  ▪ For injection dosage form:
    — Adults—40 to 200 mg injected into a vein.

• For torsemide:
  ○ For lowering the amount of water in the body:
    ▪ For oral dosage form (tablets):
      — Adults—Dose is usually 5 to 20 milligrams (mg) once a day. However, your doctor may increase your dose as needed.
      — Children—Use and dose must be determined by your doctor.
    ▪ For injection dosage form:
      — Adults—Dose is usually 5 to 20 mg injected into a vein once a day. However, your doctor may increase your dose as needed.
      — Children—Use and dose must be determined by your doctor.
  ○ For high blood pressure:
    ▪ For oral dosage form (tablets):
      — Adults—5 to 10 mg once a day.
      — Children—Use and dose must be determined by your doctor.

Missed dose—If you miss a dose of this medicine, take it as soon as possible. However, if it is almost time for your next dose, skip the missed dose and go back to your regular dosing schedule. Do not double doses.

Storage—Store the medicine in a closed container at room temperature, away from heat, moisture, and direct light. Keep from freezing.

Keep out of the reach of children.

Do not keep outdated medicine or medicine no longer needed.

Precautions While Using This Medicine

It is important that your doctor check your progress at regular visits to make sure that this medicine is working properly.

This medicine may cause a loss of potassium from your body.
• To help prevent this, your doctor may want you to:
  ○ eat or drink foods that have a high potassium content (for example, orange or other citrus fruit juices), or
  ○ take a potassium supplement, or
  ○ take another medicine to help prevent the loss of the potassium in the first place.
    ▪ It is very important to follow these directions. Also, it is important not to change your diet on your own. This is more important if you are already on a special diet (as for diabetes), or if you are taking a potassium supplement or a medicine to reduce potassium loss. Extra potassium may not be necessary and, in some cases, too much potassium could be harmful.

To prevent the loss of too much water and potassium, tell your doctor if you become sick, especially with severe or continuing nausea and vomiting or diarrhea.

Before having any kind of surgery (including dental surgery) or emergency treatment, make sure the medical doctor or dentist in charge knows that you are taking this medicine.

Dizziness, lightheadedness, or fainting may occur, especially when you get up from a lying or sitting position. This is more likely to occur in the morning. Getting up slowly may help. When you get up from lying down, sit on the edge of the bed with your feet dangling for 1 or 2 minutes. Then stand up slowly. If the problem continues or gets worse, check with your doctor.

The dizziness, lightheadedness, or fainting is also more likely to occur if you drink alcohol, stand for long periods of time, exercise, or if the weather is hot. While you are taking this medicine, be careful to limit the amount of alcohol you drink. Also, use extra care during exercise or hot weather or if you must stand for long periods of time.

For diabetic patients:
• This medicine may affect blood sugar levels. While you are using this medicine, be especially careful in testing for sugar in your blood or urine.

Do not take other medicines unless they have been discussed with your doctor. This especially includes over-the-counter (nonprescription) medicines for appetite control, asthma, colds, cough, hay fever, or sinus problems, since they may tend to increase your blood pressure.

For patients taking furosemide:
• Furosemide may cause your skin to be more sensitive to sunlight than it is normally. Exposure to sunlight, even for brief periods of time, may cause a skin rash, itching, redness or other discoloration of the skin, or a severe sunburn. When you begin taking this medicine:
  ○ Stay out of direct sunlight, especially between the hours of 10:00 a.m. and 3:00 p.m., if possible
  ○ Wear protective clothing, including a hat. Also, wear sunglasses.
  ○ Apply a sun block product that has a skin protection factor (SPF) of at least 15. Some patients may require a product with a higher SPF number, especially if they have a fair complexion. If you have any questions about this, check with your health care professional.
  ○ Apply a sun block lipstick that has an SPF of at least 15 to protect your lips.
  ○ Do not use a sunlamp or tanning bed or booth.

If you have a severe reaction from the sun, check with your doctor.

Side Effects of This Medicine

Along with its needed effects, a medicine may cause some unwanted effects. Although not all of these side effects may occur, if they do occur they may need medical attention.

Check with your doctor as soon as possible if any of the following side effects occur:

More common
  ECG abnormality— with torsemide only

Rare
  Black, tarry stools; blood in urine or stools; cough or hoarseness; fever or chills; joint pain; lower back or side pain; painful or difficult urination; pinpoint red spots on skin; ringing or buzzing in ears or any loss of hearing— more common with ethacrynic acid; skin rash or hives; stomach pain (severe) with nausea and vomiting; unusual bleeding or bruising; yellow eyes or skin; yellow vision—for furosemide only

Signs and symptoms of too much potassium loss
Dryness of mouth; increased thirst; irregular heartbeat; mood or mental changes; muscle cramps or pain; nausea or vomiting; unusual tiredness or weakness; weak pulse

Some side effects may occur that usually do not need medical attention. These side effects may go away during treatment as your body adjusts to the medicine. Also, your health care professional may be able to tell you about ways to prevent or reduce some of these side effects. Check with your health care professional if any of the following side effects continue or are bothersome or if you have any questions about them:

More common
Dizziness or lightheadedness when getting up from a lying or sitting position; excessive urination— with torsemide only

Less common
Acid or sour stomach—with torsemide only; belching—with torsemide only; blurred vision; chest pain—with bumetanide and torsemide only; confusion—with ethacrynic acid only; cough increase—with torsemide only; diarrhea—more common with ethacrynic acid; difficulty having a bowel movement (stool)—with torsemide only; difficulty in moving—with torsemide only; headache; heartburn—with torsemide only; increased sensitivity of skin to sunlight—with furosemide only; indigestion—with torsemide only; lack or loss of strength—with torsemide only; loss of appetite—more common with ethacrynic acid; muscle aching or stiffness—with torsemide only; nervousness—with ethacrynic acid and torsemide only; premature ejaculation or difficulty in keeping an erection—with bumetanide only; redness or pain at place of injection; runny nose—with torsemide only; sneezing—with torsemide only; sore throat—with torsemide only; stomach cramps or pain; stomach discomfort or upset—with torsemide only; stuffy nose—with torsemide only; swollen joints—with torsemide only

Other side effects not listed may also occur in some patients. If you notice any other effects, check with your healthcare professional.

DIURETICS, POTASSIUM-SPARING (Systemic)

Some commonly used brand names are:

In the U.S.—
Aldactone (2)
Dyrenium (3)
Midamor (1)

In Canada—
Aldactone (2)   Midamor (1)
Dyrenium (3)   Novospiroton (2)

This information applies to the following medicines:
1. Amiloride (a-MILL-oh-ride)
2. Spironolactone (speer-on-oh-LAK-tone)
3. Triamterene (trye-AM-ter-een)

Category

- **Aldosterone antagonist—**Spironolactone
- **Antihypertensive—**Amiloride; Spironolactone; Triamterene
- **Antihypokalemic—**Amiloride; Spironolactone; Triamterene
- **Diagnostic aid, primary hyperaldosteronism—**Spironolactone
- **Diuretic—**Amiloride; Spironolactone; Triamterene

Description

Potassium-sparing diuretics are commonly used to help reduce the amount of water in the body. Unlike some other diuretics, these medicines do not cause your body to lose potassium.

Amiloride and spironolactone are also used to treat high blood pressure (hypertension). High blood pressure adds to the workload of the heart and arteries. If the condition continues for a long time, the heart and arteries may not function properly. This can damage the blood vessels of the brain, heart, and kidneys, resulting in a stroke, heart failure, or kidney failure. High blood pressure may also increase the risk of heart attacks. These problems may be less likely to occur if blood pressure is controlled.

Spironolactone is also used to help increase the amount of potassium in the body when it is getting too low.

Potassium-sparing diuretics help to reduce the amount of water in the body by acting on the kidneys to increase the flow of urine. This also helps to lower blood pressure.

These medicines can also be used for other conditions as determined by your doctor.

Potassium-sparing diuretics are available only with your doctor's prescription, in the following dosage forms:

Oral
- Amiloride
  - Tablets
- Spironolactone
  - Tablets
- Triamterene
  - Capsules
  - Tablets

Before Using This Medicine

In deciding to use a medicine, the risks of taking the medicine must be weighed against the good it will do. This is a decision you and your doctor will make. For potassium-sparing diuretics, the following should be considered:

Allergies—Tell your doctor if you have ever had any unusual or allergic reaction to amiloride, spironolactone, or triamterene. Also tell your health care professional if you are allergic to any other substances, such as foods, preservatives, or dyes.

Pregnancy—Studies have not been done in pregnant women. However, this medicine has not been shown to cause birth defects or other problems in animals.

In general, diuretics are not useful for normal swelling of feet and hands that occurs during pregnancy. Diuretics should not be taken during pregnancy unless recommended by your doctor.

Breast-feeding—Although amiloride, spironolactone, and triamterene may pass into breast milk, these medicines have not been reported to cause problems in nursing babies.

Children—This medicine has been tested in children and, in effective doses, has not been shown to cause different side effects or problems in children than it does in adults.

Older adults—Signs and symptoms of too much potassium are more likely to occur in the elderly, who are more sensitive than younger adults to the effects of this medicine.

Other medicines—Although certain medicines should not be used together at all, in other cases two different medicines may be used together even if an interaction might occur. In these cases, your doctor may want to change the dose, or other precautions may be necessary. When you are taking potassium-sparing diuretics, it is especially important that your health care professional know if you are taking any of the following:

- Angiotensin-converting enzyme (ACE) inhibitors (benazepril [e.g., Lotensin], captopril [e.g., Capoten], enalapril [e.g., Vasotec], fosinopril [e.g., Monopril], lisinopril [e.g., Prinivil, Zestril], quinapril [e.g., Accupril], ramipril [e.g., Altace]) or
- Cyclosporine (e.g., Sandimmune) or
- Potassium-containing medicines or supplements—Use with potassium-sparing diuretics may cause high blood levels of potassium, which may increase the chance of side effects
- Digoxin—Use with spironolactone may cause high blood levels of digoxin, which may increase the chance of side effects
- Lithium (e.g., Lithane)—Use with potassium-sparing diuretics may cause high blood levels of lithium, which may increase the chance of side effects

Other medical problems—The presence of other medical problems may affect the use of potassium-sparing diuretics. Make sure you tell your doctor if you have any other medical problems, especially:

- Diabetes mellitus (sugar diabetes) or
- Kidney disease or
- Liver disease—Higher blood levels of potassium may occur, which may increase the chance of side effects
- Gout or
- Kidney stones (history of)—Triamterene may make these conditions worse
- Menstrual problems or breast enlargement—Spironolactone may make these conditions worse

Proper Use of This Medicine

This medicine may cause you to have an unusual feeling of tiredness when you begin to take it. You may also notice an increase in the amount of urine or in your frequency of urination. After you have taken the medicine for a while, these effects should lessen. In general, to keep the increase in urine from affecting your sleep:

- If you are to take a single dose a day, take it in the morning after breakfast.
- If you are to take more than one dose a day, take the last dose no later than 6 p.m., unless otherwise directed by your doctor.

However, it is best to plan your dose or doses according to a schedule that will least affect your personal activities and sleep. Ask your health care professional to help you plan the best time to take this medicine.

To help you remember to take your medicine, try to get into the habit of taking it at the same time each day.

If this medicine upsets your stomach, it may be taken with meals or milk. If stomach upset (nausea, vomiting, stomach pain or cramps) continues, check with your doctor.

For patients taking this medicine for *high blood pressure:*

- In addition to the use of the medicine your doctor has prescribed, treatment for your high blood pressure may include weight control and care in the types of foods you eat, especially foods high in sodium. Your doctor will tell you which of these are most important for you. You should check with your doctor before changing your diet.
- Many patients who have high blood pressure will not notice any signs of the problem. In fact, many may feel normal. It is very important that you *take your medicine exactly as directed* and that you keep your appointments with your doctor even if you feel well.
- Remember that this medicine will not cure your high blood pressure but it does help control it. Therefore, you must continue to take it as directed if you expect to lower your blood pressure and keep it down. *You may have to take high blood pressure medicine for the rest of your life.* If high blood pressure is not treated, it can cause serious problems such as heart failure, blood vessel disease, stroke, or kidney disease.

Dosing—The dose of potassium-sparing diuretics will be different for different patients. *Follow your doctor's orders or the directions on the label.* The following information includes only the average doses of potassium-sparing diuretics. *If your dose is different, do not change it* unless your doctor tells you to do so.

The number of capsules or tablets that you take depends on the strength of the medicine. Also, *the number of doses you take each day, the time allowed between doses, and the length of time you take the medicine depend on the medical problem for which you are taking potassium-sparing diuretics.*

For amiloride
- For *oral* dosage form (tablets):
  - For high blood pressure or to lower the amount of water in the body:
    - Adults—5 to 10 milligrams (mg) once a day.
    - Children—Dose must be determined by your doctor.

For spironolactone
- For *oral* dosage form (tablets):
  - To lower the amount of water in the body:
    - Adults—At first, 25 to 200 milligrams (mg) a day. This is divided into two to four doses. Your doctor may increase your dose as needed.
    - Children—Dose is based on body weight and must be determined by your doctor. The usual dose is 1 to 3 mg per kilogram (kg) (0.45 to 1.36 mg per pound) of body weight a day. The dose may be taken as a single dose or divided into two to four doses. Your doctor may increase your dose as needed.
  - For high blood pressure:
    - Adults—At first, 50 to 100 milligrams (mg) a day. This may be taken as a single dose or divided into two to four doses. Your doctor may gradually increase your dose up to 200 mg a day.

- Children—Dose is based on body weight and must be determined by your doctor. The usual dose is 1 to 3 mg per kg (0.45 to 1.36 mg per pound) of body weight a day. The dose may be taken as a single dose or divided into two to four doses. Your doctor may increase your dose as needed.
  - To treat high aldosterone levels in the body:
    - Adults—100 to 400 mg a day. This is divided into two to four doses and taken until you have surgery. If you are not having surgery, your doses may be smaller.
  - For detecting high aldosterone levels in the body:
    - Adults—400 mg a day, taken in two to four divided doses. Your doctor may want you to take this dose for as little as four days or as long as three to four weeks. Follow your doctor's instructions.
  - To treat low potassium levels in the blood:
    - Adults—25 to 100 mg a day. This may be taken as a single dose or divided into two to four doses.

For triamterene
- For *oral* dosage form (capsules or tablets):
  - To lower the amount of water in the body:
    - Adults—100 mg twice a day. Your doctor may gradually increase your dose.
    - Children—Dose is based on body weight and must be determined by your doctor. To start, the usual dose is 2 to 4 mg per kilogram (kg) (0.9 to 1.82 mg per pound) of body weight a day or every other day. This is divided into smaller doses. Your doctor may increase your dose as needed.

Missed dose—If you miss a dose of this medicine, take it as soon as possible. However, if it is almost time for your next dose, skip the missed dose and go back to your regular dosing schedule. Do not double doses.

Storage—To store this medicine:
- Keep out of the reach of children.
- Store away from heat and direct light.
- Do not store in the bathroom, near the kitchen sink, or in other damp places. Heat or moisture may cause the medicine to break down.
- Do not keep outdated medicine or medicine no longer needed. Be sure that any discarded medicine is out of the reach of children.

Precautions While Using This Medicine

It is important that your doctor check your progress at regular visits to make sure that this medicine is working properly.

This medicine does not cause a loss of potassium from your body as some other diuretics (water pills) do. Therefore, it is not necessary for you to get extra potassium in your diet, and too much potassium could even be harmful. Since salt substitutes and low-sodium milk may contain potassium, do not use them unless told to do so by your doctor.

Check with your doctor if you become sick and have severe or continuing nausea, vomiting, or diarrhea. These problems may cause you to lose additional water, which could be harmful, or to lose potassium, which could lessen the medicine's helpful effects.

Before having any kind of surgery (including dental surgery) or emergency treatment, tell the medical doctor or dentist in charge that you are taking this medicine.

Before you have any medical tests, tell the doctor in charge that you are taking this medicine. The results of some tests may be affected by this medicine.

For patients taking this medicine for *high blood pressure:*
- *Do not take other medicines unless they have been discussed with your doctor.* This especially includes over-the-counter (nonprescription) medicines for appetite control, asthma, colds, cough, hay fever, or sinus problems, since these medicines may tend to increase your blood pressure.

For patients taking *triamterene:*
- This medicine may cause your skin to be more sensitive to sunlight than it is normally. Exposure to sunlight, even for brief periods of time, may cause a skin rash, itching, redness or other discoloration of the skin, or a severe sunburn. When you begin taking this medicine:
  - Stay out of direct sunlight, especially between the hours of 10:00 a.m. and 3:00 p.m., if possible.
  - Wear protective clothing, including a hat. Also, wear sunglasses.
  - Apply a sun block product that has a skin protection factor (SPF) of at least 15. Some patients may require a product with a higher SPF number, especially if they have a fair complexion. If you have any questions about this, check with your health care professional.
  - Apply a sun block lipstick that has an SPF of at least 15 to protect your lips.
  - Do not use a sunlamp or tanning bed or booth.
  - If you have a severe reaction from the sun, check with your doctor.

Side Effects

In rats, spironolactone has been found to increase the risk of tumors. It is not known if spironolactone increases the chance of tumors in humans.

Check with your doctor as soon as possible if any of the following side effects occur:
Rare
For amiloride, spironolactone, and triamterene
  Skin rash or itching; shortness of breath
For spironolactone and triamterene only (in addition to effects listed above)
  Cough or hoarseness; fever or chills; lower back or side pain; painful or difficult urination
For triamterene only (in addition to effects listed above)
  Black, tarry stools; blood in urine or stools; bright red tongue; burning, inflamed feeling in tongue; cracked corners of mouth; lower back pain (severe); pinpoint red spots on skin; unusual bleeding or bruising; weakness
Signs and symptoms of too much potassium
  Confusion; irregular heartbeat; nervousness; numbness or tingling in hands, feet, or lips; shortness of breath or difficult breathing; unusual tiredness or weakness; weakness or heaviness of legs

Other side effects may occur that usually do not need medical attention. These side effects may go away during treatment as your body adjusts to the medicine. However, check with your doctor if any of the following side effects continue or are bothersome:
More common (less common with amiloride and triamterene)
  Nausea and vomiting; stomach cramps and diarrhea

Less common
For amiloride, spironolactone, and triamterene
   Dizziness; headache
For amiloride and spironolactone only (in addition to effects listed above)
   Decreased sexual ability
For amiloride only (in addition to effects listed above)
   Constipation; muscle cramps
For spironolactone only (in addition to effects listed above for spironolactone)
   Breast tenderness in females; clumsiness; deepening of voice in females; enlargement of breasts in males; inability to have or keep an erection; increased hair growth in females; irregular menstrual periods; sweating
For triamterene only (in addition to effects listed above for triamterene)
   Increased sensitivity of skin to sunlight
Signs and symptoms of too little sodium
   Drowsiness; dryness of mouth; increased thirst; lack of energy

For *male patients:*

• Spironolactone sometimes causes enlarged breasts in males, especially when they take large doses of it for a long time. Breasts usually decrease in size gradually over several months after this medicine is stopped. If you have any questions about this, check with your doctor.

Other side effects not listed above may also occur in some patients. If you notice any other effects, check with your doctor.

Additional Information

Once a medicine has been approved for marketing for a certain use, experience may show that it is also useful for other medical problems. Although these uses are not included in product labeling, spironolactone is used in certain patients with the following medical conditions:

• Polycystic ovary syndrome
• Hirsutism, female (increased hair growth)
• Congestive heart failure, severe

Other than the above information, there is no additional information relating to proper use, precautions, or side effects for these uses.

DIURETICS, POTASSIUM-SPARING, AND HYDROCHLOROTHIAZIDE (Systemic)

Some commonly used brand names are:

In the U.S.—

Aldactazide (2)	Moduretic (1)
Dyazide (3)	Spirozide (2)
Maxzide (3)	

In Canada—

Aldactazide (2)	Moduret (1)
Apo-Triazide (3)	Novo-Spirozine (2)
Dyazide (3)	Novo-Triamzide (3)

This information applies to the following medicines:

1. Amiloride and Hydrochlorothiazide (a-MILL-oh-ride and hye-droe-klor-oh-THYE-a-zide)
2. Spironolactone and Hydrochlorothiazide (speer-on-oh-LAK-tone and hye-droe-klor-oh-THYE-a-zide)
3. Triamterene and Hydrochlorothiazide (trye-AM-ter-een and hye-droe-klor-oh-THYE-a-zide)

Category

• **Antihypertensive**—Amiloride and Hydrochlorothiazide; Spironolactone and Hydrochlorothiazide; Triamterene and Hydrochlorothiazide

• **Antihypokalemic**—Amiloride and Hydrochlorothiazide; Spironolactone and Hydrochlorothiazide; Triamterene and Hydrochlorothiazide

• **Diuretic**—Amiloride and Hydrochlorothiazide; Spironolactone and Hydrochlorothiazide; Triamterene and Hydrochlorothiazide

Description

This medicine is a combination of two diuretics (water pills). It is commonly used to help reduce the amount of water in the body.

This combination is also used to treat high blood pressure (hypertension). High blood pressure adds to the work load of the heart and arteries. If it continues for a long time, the heart and arteries may not function properly. This can damage the blood vessels of the brain, heart, and kidneys, resulting in a stroke, heart failure, or kidney failure. High blood pressure may also increase the risk of heart attacks. These problems may be less likely to occur if blood pressure is controlled.

Diuretics help to reduce the amount of water in the body by acting on the kidneys to increase the flow of urine. This also helps to lower blood pressure.

This combination is also used to treat problems caused by too little potassium in the body.

This medicine is available only with your doctor's prescription, in the following dosage forms:

Oral

• Amiloride and Hydrochlorothiazide
   ◦ Tablets
• Spironolactone and Hydrochlorothiazide
   ◦ Tablets
• Triamterene and Hydrochlorothiazide
   ◦ Capsules
   ◦ Tablets

Before Using This Medicine

In deciding to use a medicine, the risks of taking the medicine must be weighed against the good it will do. This is a decision you and your doctor will make. For potassium-sparing diuretics and hydrochlorothiazide, the following should be considered:

Allergies—Tell your doctor if you have ever had any unusual or allergic reaction to amiloride, spironolactone, triamterene, sulfonamides (sulfa drugs), bumetanide, furosemide, acetazolamide, dichlorphenamide, methazolamide, or to hydrochlorothiazide or any of the other thiazide diuretics. Also tell your health care professional if you are allergic to any other substances, such as foods, preservatives, or dyes.

Pregnancy—In general, diuretics are not useful for normal swelling of feet and hands that occurs during pregnancy. They should not be taken during pregnancy unless recommended by your doctor.

Breast-feeding—Hydrochlorothiazide and spironolactone pass into breast milk. It is not known whether amiloride or triamterene passes into breast milk. Hydrochlorothiazide may also decrease the flow of breast milk. Therefore, you should avoid use of potassium-sparing diuretic and hydrochlorothiazide combinations during the first month of breast-feeding.

Children—Studies on this combination medicine have been done only in adult patients, and there is no specific information comparing use of potassium-sparing diuretic and hydrochlorothiazide combinations in children with use in other age groups.

Older adults—Dizziness or lightheadedness and signs and symptoms of too much potassium in the body or too little potassium in the body may be more likely to occur in the elderly, who are more sensitive than younger adults to the effects of this medicine.

Other medicines—Although certain medicines should not be used together at all, in other cases two different medicines may be used together even if an interaction might occur. In these cases, your doctor may want to change the dose, or other precautions may be necessary. When you are taking potassium-sparing diuretics and hydrochlorothiazide, it is especially important that your health care professional know if you are taking any of the following:

- Angiotensin-converting enzyme (ACE) inhibitors (benazepril [e.g., Lotensin], captopril [e.g., Capoten], enalapril [e.g., Vasotec], fosinopril [e.g., Monopril], lisinopril [e.g., Prinivil, Zestril], quinapril [e.g., Accupril], ramipril [e.g., Altace]) or
- Cyclosporine (e.g., Sandimmune) or
- Potassium-containing medicines or supplements—Use with potassium-sparing diuretic and hydrochlorothiazide combinations may cause high blood levels of potassium, which may increase the chance of side effects
- Cholestyramine or
- Colestipol—Use with potassium-sparing diuretic and hydrochlorothiazide combinations may prevent the diuretic from working properly; take the diuretic at least 1 hour before or 4 hours after cholestyramine or colestipol
- Digitalis glycosides (heart medicine)—Use with diuretics may cause high blood levels of digoxin, which may increase the chance of side effects
- Lithium (e.g., Lithane)—Use with diuretics may cause high blood levels of lithium, which may increase the chance of side effects

Other medical problems—The presence of other medical problems may affect the use of potassium-sparing diuretics and hydrochlorothiazide. Make sure you tell your doctor if you have any other medical problems, especially:

- Diabetes mellitus (sugar diabetes) or
- Kidney disease or
- Liver disease—Higher blood levels of potassium may occur, which may increase the chance of side effects
- Gout (history of) or
- Kidney stones (history of)—Triamterene and hydrochlorothiazide combination may make these conditions worse

- Heart or blood vessel disease—These medicines may cause high cholesterol levels or high triglyceride levels
- Lupus erythematosus (history of) or
- Pancreatitis (inflammation of pancreas)—Potassium-sparing diuretic and hydrochlorothiazide combinations may make these conditions worse
- Menstrual problems in women or breast enlargement in men—Spironolactone and hydrochlorothiazide combination may make these conditions worse

Proper Use of This Medicine

This medicine may cause you to have an unusual feeling of tiredness when you begin to take it. You may also notice an increase in the amount of urine or in your frequency of urination. After you have taken the medicine for a while, these effects should lessen. In general, to keep the increase in urine from affecting your sleep:

- If you are to take a single dose a day, take it in the morning after breakfast.
- If you are to take more than one dose a day, take the last dose no later than 6 p.m., unless otherwise directed by your doctor.

However, it is best to plan your dose or doses according to a schedule that will least affect your personal activities and sleep. Ask your health care professional to help you plan the best time to take this medicine.

To help you remember to take your medicine, try to get into the habit of taking it at the same time each day.

If this medicine upsets your stomach, it may be taken with meals or milk. If stomach upset (nausea, vomiting, stomach pain, or cramps) continues, check with your doctor.

For patients taking this medicine for *high blood pressure:*

- In addition to the use of the medicine your doctor has prescribed, treatment for your high blood pressure may include weight control and care in the types of foods you eat, especially foods high in sodium. Your doctor will tell you which of these are most important for you. You should check with your doctor before changing your diet.
- Many patients who have high blood pressure will not notice any signs of the problem. In fact, many may feel normal. It is very important that you *take your medicine exactly as directed* and that you keep your appointments with your doctor even if you feel well.
- Remember that this medicine will not cure your high blood pressure but it does help control it. Therefore, you must continue to take it as directed if you expect to lower your blood pressure and keep it down. *You may have to take high blood pressure medicine for the rest of your life.* If high blood pressure is not treated, it can cause serious problems such as heart failure, blood vessel disease, stroke, or kidney disease.

Dosing—The dose of potassium-sparing diuretic and hydrochlorothiazide combinations will be different for different patients. *Follow your doctor's orders or the directions on the label.* The following information includes only the average doses of potassium-sparing diuretic and hydrochlorothiazide combinations. *If your dose is different, do not change it* unless your doctor tells you to do so.

The number of capsules or tablets that you take depends on the strength of the medicine. Also, *the number of doses you take each day depends on the strength of the medicine and the medical problem for which you are taking potassium-sparing diuretic and hydrochlorothiazide combinations.*

For amiloride and hydrochlorothiazide combination
- For *oral* dosage form (tablets):
  - For high blood pressure or lowering the amount of water in the body:
    - Adults—1 or 2 tablets a day.
    - Children—Dose must be determined by your doctor.

For spironolactone and hydrochlorothiazide combination
- For *oral* dosage form (tablets):
  - For high blood pressure or lowering the amount of water in the body:
    - Adults—1 to 4 tablets a day.
    - Children—Dose is based on body weight and must be determined by your doctor.

For triamterene and hydrochlorothiazide combination
- For *oral* dosage form (capsules):
  - For high blood pressure or lowering the amount of water in the body:
    - Adults—1 or 2 capsules once a day.
    - Children—Dose must be determined by your doctor.
- For *oral* dosage form (tablets):
  - For high blood pressure or lowering the amount of water in the body:
    - Adults—1 to 4 tablets a day, depending on the strength of your tablet.
    - Children—Dose must be determined by your doctor.

Missed dose—If you miss a dose of this medicine, take it as soon as possible. However, if it is almost time for your next dose, skip the missed dose and go back to your regular dosing schedule. Do not double doses.

Storage—To store this medicine:
- Keep out of the reach of children.
- Store away from heat and direct light.
- Do not store in the bathroom, near the kitchen sink, or in other damp places. Heat or moisture may cause the medicine to break down.
- Do not keep outdated medicine or medicine no longer needed. Be sure that any discarded medicine is out of the reach of children.

Precautions While Using This Medicine

It is important that your doctor check your progress at regular visits to make sure that this medicine is working properly.

This medicine may cause a loss or increase of potassium in your body. Your doctor may have special instructions about whether or not you need to eat or drink foods or beverages that have a high potassium content (for example, orange or other citrus fruit juices), taking a potassium supplement, or using salt substitutes. Since too much potassium can be harmful, it is important not to change your diet on your own. Tell your doctor if you are already on a special diet (as for diabetes). Since salt substitutes and low-sodium milk may contain potassium, do not use them unless told to do so by your doctor. Check with your health care professional if you need a list of foods that are high in potassium or if you have any questions.

Check with your doctor if you become sick and have severe or continuing vomiting or diarrhea. These problems may cause you to lose additional water and potassium and lead to low blood pressure.

For *diabetic patients:*
- Hydrochlorothiazide (contained in this combination medicine) may raise blood sugar levels. While you are taking this medicine, be especially careful in testing for sugar in your blood or urine.

Potassium-sparing diuretics and hydrochlorothiazide may cause your skin to be more sensitive to sunlight than it is normally. Exposure to sunlight, even for brief periods of time, may cause a skin rash, itching, redness or other discoloration of the skin, or a severe sunburn. When you begin taking this medicine:
- Stay out of direct sunlight, especially between the hours of 10:00 a.m. and 3:00 p.m., if possible.
- Wear protective clothing, including a hat. Also, wear sunglasses.
- Apply a sun block product that has a skin protection factor (SPF) of at least 15. Some patients may require a product with a higher SPF number, especially if they have a fair complexion. If you have any questions about this, check with your health care professional.
- Apply a sun block lipstick that has an SPF of at least 15 to protect your lips.
- Do not use a sunlamp or tanning bed or booth.

If you have a severe reaction from the sun, check with your doctor.

Before having any kind of surgery (including dental surgery) or emergency treatment, tell the medical doctor or dentist in charge that you are taking this medicine.

For patients taking *triamterene and hydrochlorothiazide combination:*
- Do not change brands of triamterene and hydrochlorothiazide without first checking with your doctor. Different products may not work the same way. If you refill your medicine and it looks different, check with your pharmacist.

For patients taking this medicine for *high blood pressure:*
- *Do not take other medicines unless they have been discussed with your doctor.* This especially includes over-the-counter (nonprescription) medicines for appetite control, asthma, colds, cough, hay fever, or sinus problems, since they may tend to increase your blood pressure.

Tell the doctor in charge that you are taking this medicine before you have any medical tests. The results of some tests may be affected by this medicine.

Side Effects

In rats, spironolactone has been found to increase the risk of development of tumors. However, the doses given were many times the dose of spironolactone given to humans. It is not known whether spironolactone causes tumors in humans.

Along with its needed effects, a medicine may cause some unwanted effects. Although not all of these side effects may occur, if they do occur they may need medical attention.

Check with your doctor as soon as possible if any of the following side effects occur:

Rare

Black, tarry stools; blood in urine or stools; cough or hoarseness; fever or chills; joint pain; lower back or side pain; painful or difficult urination; pinpoint red spots on skin; skin rash or hives; stomach pain (severe) with nausea and vomiting; unusual bleeding or bruising; yellow eyes or skin

Signs and symptoms of changes in potassium

Confusion; dryness of mouth; increased thirst; irregular heartbeat; mood or mental changes; muscle cramps or pain; numbness or tingling in hands, feet, or lips; shortness of breath or difficulty breathing; unusual tiredness or weakness; weak pulse; weakness or heaviness of legs

Reported for triamterene only (rare)

Bright red tongue; burning, inflamed feeling in tongue; cracked corners of mouth

Other side effects may occur that usually do not need medical attention. These side effects may go away during treatment as your body adjusts to the medicine. However, check with your doctor if any of the following side effects continue or are bothersome:

More common (less common with triamterene)

Loss of appetite; nausea and vomiting; stomach cramps and diarrhea; upset stomach

Less common

Decreased sexual ability; dizziness or lightheadedness when getting up from a lying or sitting position; headache; increased sensitivity of skin to sunlight

Reported for amiloride only (less common)

Constipation

Reported for spironolactone only (less common)

Breast tenderness in females; deepening of voice in females; enlargement of breasts in males; increased hair growth in females; irregular menstrual periods; sweating

Spironolactone sometimes causes enlarged breasts in males, especially when they take large doses of it for a long time. Breasts usually decrease in size gradually over several months after this medicine is stopped. If you have any questions about this, check with your doctor.

Other side effects not listed above may also occur in some patients. If you notice any other effects, check with your doctor.

DIURETICS, THIAZIDE (Systemic)

Some commonly used brand names are:

In the U.S.—

Aquatensen (6)	Hydro-chlor (4)
Diucardin (5)	Hydro-D (4)
Diulo (7)	HydroDIURIL (4)
Diuril (2)	Hydromox (9)
Enduron (6)	Hygroton (3)
Esidrix (4)	Metahydrin (10)
Microzide (4)	Renese (8)
Mykrox (7)	Saluron (5)
Naqua (10)	Thalitone (3)
Naturetin (1)	Trichlorex (10)
Oretic (4)	Zaroxolyn (7)

In Canada—

Apo-Chlorthalidone (3)	Neo-Codema (4)
Apo-Hydro (4)	Novo-Hydrazide (4)
Diuchlor H (4)	Novo-Thalidone (3)
Duretic (6)	Uridon (3)
HydroDIURIL (4)	Urozide (4)
Hygroton (3)	Zaroxolyn (7)
Naturetin (1)	

This information applies to the following medicines:

1. Bendroflumethiazide (ben-droe-floo-meth-EYE-a-zide)
2. Chlorothiazide (klor-oh-THYE-a-zide)
3. Chlorthalidone (klor-THAL-i-doan)
4. Hydrochlorothiazide (hye-droe-klor-oh-THYE-a-zide)
5. Hydroflumethiazide (hye-droe-floo-meth-EYE-a-zide)
6. Methyclothiazide (meth-ee-kloe-THYE-a-zide)
7. Metolazone (me-TOLE-a-zone)
8. Polythiazide (pol-i-THYE-a-zide)
9. Quinethazone (kwin-ETH-a-zone)
10. Trichlormethiazide (trye-klor-meth-EYE-a-zide)

Category

- **Antidiuretic, central and nephrogenic diabetes insipidus—**Bendroflumethiazide; Chlorothiazide; Chlorthalidone; Hydrochlorothiazide; Hydroflumethiazide; Methyclothiazide; Metolazone; Polythiazide; Quinethazone; Trichlormethiazide

- **Antihypertensive—**Bendroflumethiazide; Chlorothiazide; Chlorthalidone; Hydrochlorothiazide; Hydroflumethiazide; Methyclothiazide; Metolazone; Polythiazide; Quinethazone; Trichlormethiazide

- **Antiurolithic, calcium calculi—**Bendroflumethiazide; Chlorothiazide; Chlorthalidone; Hydrochlorothiazide; Hydroflumethiazide; Methyclothiazide; Metolazone; Polythiazide; Quinethazone; Trichlormethiazide

- **Diuretic—**Bendroflumethiazide; Chlorothiazide; Chlorthalidone; Hydrochlorothiazide; Hydroflumethiazide; Methyclothiazide; Metolazone; Polythiazide; Quinethazone; Trichlormethiazide

Description

Thiazide or thiazide-like diuretics are commonly used to treat high blood pressure (hypertension). High blood pressure adds to the workload of the heart and arteries. If it continues for a long time, the heart and arteries may not function properly. This can damage the blood vessels of the brain, heart, and kidneys, resulting in a stroke, heart failure, or kidney failure. High blood pressure may also increase the risk of heart attacks. These problems may be less likely to occur if blood pressure is controlled.

Thiazide diuretics are also used to help reduce the amount of water in the body by increasing the flow of urine. They may also be used for other conditions as determined by your doctor.

Thiazide diuretics are available only with your doctor's prescription, in the following dosage forms:

Oral
- Bendroflumethiazide
  - Tablets

89

- Chlorothiazide
  - Oral suspension
  - Tablets
- Chlorthalidone
  - Tablets
- Hydrochlorothiazide
  - Capsules
  - Oral solution
  - Tablets
- Hydroflumethiazide
  - Tablets
- Methyclothiazide
  - Tablets
- Metolazone
  - Tablets
- Polythiazide
  - Tablets
- Quinethazone
  - Tablets
- Trichlormethiazide
  - Tablets

Parenteral
- Chlorothiazide
  - Injection

Before Using This Medicine

In deciding to use a medicine, the risks of taking the medicine must be weighed against the good it will do. This is a decision you and your doctor will make. For thiazide diuretics, the following should be considered:

Allergies—Tell your doctor if you have ever had any unusual or allergic reaction to sulfonamides (sulfa drugs), bumetanide, furosemide, acetazolamide, dichlorphenamide, methazolamide, or to any of the thiazide diuretics. Also tell your health care professional if you are allergic to any other substances, such as foods, preservatives, or dyes.

Pregnancy—When this medicine is used during pregnancy, it may cause side effects including jaundice, blood problems, and low potassium in the newborn infant. In addition, although this medicine has not been shown to cause birth defects or other problems in animals, studies have not been done in humans.

In general, diuretics are not useful for normal swelling of feet and hands that occurs during pregnancy. They should not be taken during pregnancy unless recommended by your doctor.

Breast-feeding—Thiazide diuretics pass into breast milk. These medicines also may decrease the flow of breast milk. Therefore, you should avoid use of thiazide diuretics during the first month of breast-feeding.

Children—Although there is no specific information comparing the use of thiazide diuretics in children with use in other age groups, these medicines are not expected to cause different side effects or problems in children than they do in adults. However, extra caution may be necessary in infants with jaundice, because these medicines can make the condition worse.

Older adults—Dizziness or lightheadedness and signs of too much potassium loss may be more likely to occur in the elderly, who are more sensitive than younger adults to the effects of thiazide diuretics.

Other medicines—Although certain medicines should not be used together at all, in other cases two different medicines may be used together even if an interaction might occur. In these cases, your doctor may want to change the dose, or other precautions may be necessary. When you are taking thiazide diuretics, it is especially important that your health care professional know if you are taking any of the following:
- Cholestyramine or
- Colestipol—Use with thiazide diuretics may prevent the diuretic from working properly; take the diuretic at least 1 hour before or 4 hours after cholestyramine or colestipol
- Digitalis glycosides (heart medicine)—Use with thiazide diuretics may cause high blood levels of digoxin, which may increase the chance of side effects
- Lithium (e.g., Lithane)—Use with thiazide diuretics may cause high blood levels of lithium, which may increase the chance of side effects

Other medical problems—The presence of other medical problems may affect the use of thiazide diuretics. Make sure you tell your doctor if you have any other medical problems, especially:
- Diabetes mellitus (sugar diabetes)—Thiazide diuretics may increase the amount of sugar in the blood
- Gout (history of) or
- Lupus erythematosus (history of) or
- Pancreatitis (inflammation of the pancreas)—Thiazide diuretics may make these conditions worse
- Heart or blood vessel disease—Thiazide diuretics may cause high cholesterol levels or high triglyceride levels
- Liver disease or
- Kidney disease (severe)—Higher blood levels of the thiazide diuretic may occur, which may prevent the thiazide diuretic from working properly

Proper Use of This Medicine

This medicine may cause you to have an unusual feeling of tiredness when you begin to take it. You may also notice an increase in the amount of urine or in your frequency of urination. After you have taken the medicine for a while, these effects should lessen. In general, to keep the increase in urine from affecting your sleep:
- If you are to take a single dose a day, take it in the morning after breakfast.
- If you are to take more than one dose a day, take the last dose no later than 6 p.m., unless otherwise directed by your doctor.

However, it is best to plan your dose or doses according to a schedule that will least affect your personal activities and sleep. Ask your health care professional to help you plan the best time to take this medicine.

Take each dose at the same time each day. This medicine works best if there is a constant amount in the blood.

For patients taking this medicine for *high blood pressure:*
- In addition to the use of the medicine your doctor has prescribed, appropriate treatment for your high blood pressure may include weight control and care in the types of foods you eat, especially foods high in sodium.

Your doctor will tell you which factors are most important for you. You should check with your doctor before changing your diet.

- Many patients who have high blood pressure will not notice any signs of the problem. In fact, many may feel normal. It is very important that you *take your medicine exactly as directed* and that you keep your appointments with your doctor even if you feel well.

- Remember that this medicine will not cure your high blood pressure but it does help control it. Therefore, you must continue to take it as directed if you expect to lower your blood pressure and keep it down. *You may have to take high blood pressure medicine for the rest of your life.* If high blood pressure is not treated, it can cause serious problems such as heart failure, blood vessel disease, stroke, or kidney disease.

For patients taking the *oral liquid form of hydrochlorothiazide*, which comes in a dropper bottle:

- This medicine is to be taken by mouth. The amount you should take is to be measured only with the specially marked dropper.

Dosing—The dose of these medicines will be different for different patients. *Follow your doctor's orders or the directions on the label.* The following information includes only the average doses of these medicines. *If your dose is different, do not change it* unless your doctor tells you to do so.

The number of tablets or teaspoonfuls of solution or suspension that you take depends on the strength of the medicine. Also, *the number of doses you take each day, the time allowed between doses, and the length of time you take the medicine depend on the medical problem for which you are taking thiazide diuretics.*

For bendroflumethiazide
- For *oral* dosage form (tablets):
  - To lower the amount of water in the body:
    - Adults—At first, 2.5 to 10 milligrams (mg) one or two times a day. Then, your doctor may lower your dose to 2.5 to 5 mg once a day. Or your doctor may want you to take this dose once every other day or once a day for only three to five days out of the week.
    - Children—Dose is based on body weight and must be determined by your doctor. The usual dose is 50 to 100 micrograms (mcg) per kilogram (kg) (22.7 to 45.4 mcg per pound) of body weight once a day.
  - For high blood pressure:
    - Adults—2.5 to 20 mg a day. This may be taken as a single dose or divided into two doses.
    - Children—Dose is based on body weight and must be determined by your doctor. The usual dose is 50 to 400 mcg per kg (22.7 to 181.8 mcg per pound) of body weight a day. This may be taken as a single dose or divided into two doses.

For chlorothiazide
- For *oral* dosage forms (oral suspension or tablets):
  - To lower the amount of water in the body:
    - Adults—250 milligrams (mg) every six to twelve hours.
    - Children—Dose is based on body weight and must be determined by your doctor.

- For high blood pressure:
  - Adults—250 to 1000 mg a day. This may be taken as a single dose or divided into smaller doses.
  - Children—Dose is based on body weight and must be determined by your doctor.
- For *injection* dosage form:
  - To lower the amount of water in the body:
    - Adults—250 mg injected into a vein every six to twelve hours.
    - Children—Use and dose must be determined by your doctor.
  - For high blood pressure:
    - Adults—500 to 1000 mg a day, injected into a vein. This dose may be given as a single dose or divided into two doses.
    - Children—Use and dose must be determined by your doctor.

For chlorthalidone
- For *oral* dosage form (tablets):
  - To lower the amount of water in the body:
    - Adults—25 to 100 milligrams (mg) once a day. Or 100 to 200 mg taken once every other day or once a day for three days out of the week.
    - Children—Dose is based on body weight and must be determined by your doctor.
  - For high blood pressure:
    - Adults—25 to 100 mg once a day.
    - Children—Dose is based on body weight and must be determined by your doctor.

For hydrochlorothiazide
- For *oral* dosage forms (oral solution or tablets):
  - To lower the amount of water in the body:
    - Adults—25 to 100 milligrams (mg) one or two times a day. Or your doctor may want you to take this dose once every other day or once a day for three to five days out of the week.
    - Children—Dose is based on body weight and must be determined by your doctor.
  - For high blood pressure:
    - Adults—25 to 100 mg a day. This may be taken as a single dose or divided into two doses.
    - Children—Dose is based on body weight and must be determined by your doctor.

For hydroflumethiazide
- For *oral* dosage form (tablets):
  - To lower the amount of water in the body:
    - Adults—25 to 100 milligrams (mg) one or two times a day. Or your doctor may want you to take this dose once every other day or once a day for three to five days out of the week.
    - Children—Dose is based on body weight and must be determined by your doctor.
  - For high blood pressure:
    - Adults—50 to 100 mg a day. This may be taken as a single dose or divided into two doses.
    - Children—Dose is based on body weight and must be determined by your doctor.

For methyclothiazide
- For *oral* dosage form (tablets):
  - To lower the amount of water in the body:
    - Adults—2.5 to 10 milligrams (mg) once a day. Or your doctor may want you to take this dose once every other day or once a day for three to five days out of the week.

Children—Dose is based on body weight and must be determined by your doctor.
- For high blood pressure:
  - Adults—2.5 to 5 mg once a day.
  - Children—Dose is based on body weight and must be determined by your doctor.

For metolazone
- For *oral* dosage form (*extended* metolazone tablets):
  - To lower the amount of water in the body:
    - Adults—5 to 20 milligrams (mg) once a day.
    - Children—Dose must be determined by your doctor.
  - For high blood pressure:
    - Adults—2.5 to 5 mg once a day.
    - Children—Dose must be determined by your doctor.
- For *oral* dosage form (*prompt* metolazone tablets):
  - For high blood pressure:
    - Adults—At first, 500 micrograms (mcg) once a day. Then, 500 to 1000 mcg once a day.
    - Children—Dose must be determined by your doctor.

For polythiazide
- For *oral* dosage form (tablets):
  - To lower the amount of water in the body:
    - Adults—1 to 4 milligrams (mg) once a day. Or your doctor may want you to take this dose once every other day or once a day for three to five days out of the week.
    - Children—Dose is based on body weight and must be determined by your doctor.
  - For high blood pressure:
    - Adults—2 to 4 mg once a day.
    - Children—Dose is based on body weight and must be determined by your doctor.

For quinethazone
- For *oral* dosage form (tablets):
  - To lower the amount of water in the body or for high blood pressure:
    - Adults—50 to 200 milligrams (mg) a day. This may be taken as a single dose or divided into two doses.
    - Children—Dose must be determined by your doctor.

For trichlormethiazide
- For *oral* dosage form (tablets):
  - To lower the amount of water in the body:
    - Adults—1 to 4 milligrams (mg) once a day. Or your doctor may want you to take this dose once every other day or once a day for three to five days out of the week.
    - Children—Dose is based on body weight and must be determined by your doctor.
  - For high blood pressure:
    - Adults—2 to 4 mg once a day.
    - Children—Dose is based on body weight and must be determined by your doctor.

Missed dose—If you miss a dose of this medicine, take it as soon as possible. However, if it is almost time for your next dose, skip the missed dose and go back to your regular dosing schedule. Do not double doses.

Storage—To store this medicine:
- Keep out of the reach of children.
- Store away from heat and direct light.
- Do not store in the bathroom, near the kitchen sink, or in other damp places. Heat or moisture may cause the medicine to break down.
- Keep the oral liquid form of this medicine from freezing.
- Do not keep outdated medicine or medicine no longer needed. Be sure that any discarded medicine is out of the reach of children.

Precautions While Using This Medicine

It is important that your doctor check your progress at regular visits to make sure that this medicine is working properly.

This medicine may cause a loss of potassium from your body:
- To help prevent this, your doctor may want you to:
  - eat or drink foods that have a high potassium content (for example, orange or other citrus fruit juices), or
  - take a potassium supplement, or
  - take another medicine to help prevent the loss of the potassium in the first place.

- It is very important to follow these directions. Also, it is important not to change your diet on your own. This is more important if you are already on a special diet (as for diabetes), or if you are taking a potassium supplement or a medicine to reduce potassium loss. Extra potassium may not be necessary and, in some cases, too much potassium could be harmful.

Check with your doctor if you become sick and have severe or continuing vomiting or diarrhea. These problems may cause you to lose additional water and potassium.

For *diabetic patients:*
- Thiazide diuretics may raise blood sugar levels. While you are using this medicine, be especially careful in testing for sugar in your blood or urine.

Thiazide diuretics may cause your skin to be more sensitive to sunlight than it is normally. Exposure to sunlight, even for brief periods of time, may cause a skin rash, itching, redness or other discoloration of the skin, or a severe sunburn. When you begin taking this medicine:
- Stay out of direct sunlight, especially between the hours of 10:00 a.m. and 3:00 p.m., if possible.
- Wear protective clothing, including a hat. Also, wear sunglasses.
- Apply a sun block product that has a skin protection factor (SPF) of at least 15. Some patients may require a product with a higher SPF number, especially if they have a fair complexion. If you have any questions about this, check with your health care professional.
- Apply a sun block lipstick that has an SPF of at least 15 to protect your lips.
- Do not use a sunlamp or tanning bed or booth.

If you have a severe reaction from the sun, check with your doctor.

For patients taking this medicine for *high blood pressure:*
- *Do not take other medicines unless they have been discussed with your doctor.* This especially includes

over-the-counter (nonprescription) medicines for appetite control, asthma, colds, cough, hay fever, or sinus problems, since they may tend to increase your blood pressure.

Side Effects

Along with its needed effects, a medicine may cause some unwanted effects. Although not all of these side effects may occur, if they do occur they may need medical attention.

Check with your doctor as soon as possible if any of the following side effects occur:

Rare

Black, tarry stools; blood in urine or stools; cough or hoarseness; fever or chills; joint pain; lower back or side pain; painful or difficult urination; pinpoint red spots on skin; skin rash or hives; stomach pain (severe) with nausea and vomiting; unusual bleeding or bruising; yellow eyes or skin

Signs and symptoms of too much potassium loss

Dryness of mouth; increased thirst; irregular heartbeat; mood or mental changes; muscle cramps or pain; nausea or vomiting; unusual tiredness or weakness; weak pulse

Signs and symptoms of too much sodium loss

Confusion; convulsions; decreased mental activity; irritability; muscle cramps; unusual tiredness or weakness

Other side effects may occur that usually do not need medical attention. These side effects may go away during treatment as your body adjusts to the medicine. However, check with your doctor if any of the following side effects continue or are bothersome:

Less common

Decreased sexual ability; diarrhea; dizziness or lightheadedness when getting up from a lying or sitting position; increased sensitivity of skin to sunlight; loss of appetite; upset stomach

Other side effects not listed above may also occur in some patients. If you notice any other effects, check with your doctor.

Additional Information

Once a medicine has been approved for marketing for a certain use, experience may show that it is also useful for other medical problems. Although these uses are not specifically included in product labeling, thiazide diuretics are used in certain patients with the following medical conditions:

- Diabetes insipidus (water diabetes)
- Kidney stones (calcium-containing)

For patients taking this medicine for *diabetes insipidus (water diabetes):*

- Some thiazide diuretics are used in the treatment of diabetes insipidus (water diabetes). In patients with water diabetes, this medicine causes a decrease in the flow of urine and helps the body hold water. Thus, the information given above about increased urine flow will not apply to you.

Other than the above information, there is no additional information relating to proper use, precautions, or side effects for these uses.

DOCETAXEL (Intravenous route) -
doe-se-TAX-el

Black Box Warning

Docetaxel should be administered under the supervision of a qualified physician experienced in the use of antineoplastic agents. Appropriate management of complications is possible only when adequate diagnostic and treatment facilities are readily available.

The incidence of treatment-related mortality associated with docetaxel therapy is increased in patients with abnormal liver function, in patients receiving higher doses, and in patients with non-small cell lung carcinoma and a history of prior treatment with platinum-based chemotherapy who receive docetaxel as a single agent at a dose of 100 mg/m(2).

Docetaxel should generally not be given to patients with bilirubin greater than the upper limit of normal (ULN), or to patients with SGOT and/or SGPT greater than 1.5 times ULN concomitant with alkaline phosphatase greater than 2.5 times ULN. Patients with elevations of bilirubin or abnormalities of transaminase concurrent with alkaline phosphatase are at increased risk for the development of grade 4 neutropenia, febrile neutropenia, infections, severe thrombocytopenia, severe stomatitis, severe skin toxicity, and toxic death. Patients with isolated elevations of transaminase greater than 1.5 times ULN also had a higher rate of febrile neutropenia grade 4 but did not have an increased incidence of toxic death. Bilirubin, SGOT or SGPT, and alkaline phosphatase values should be obtained prior to each cycle of docetaxel therapy and reviewed by the treating physician.

Docetaxel therapy should not be given to patients with neutrophil counts of less than 1500 cells/mm(3). In order to monitor the occurrence of neutropenia, which may be severe and result in infection, frequent blood cell counts should be performed on all patients receiving docetaxel.

Severe hypersensitivity reactions characterized by generalized rash/erythema, hypotension and/or bronchospasm, or very rarely fatal anaphylaxis, have been reported in patients who received the recommended 3–day dexamethasone premedication. Hypersensitivity reactions require immediate discontinuation of the docetaxel infusion and administration of appropriate therapy. Docetaxel must not be given to patients who have a history of severe hypersensitivity reactions to docetaxel or to other drugs formulated with polysorbate 80.

Severe fluid retention occurred in 6.5% (6/92) of patients despite use of a 3–day dexamethasone premedication regimen. It was characterized by one or more of the following events: poorly tolerated peripheral edema, generalized edema, pleural effusion requiring urgent drainage, dyspnea at rest, cardiac tamponade, or pronounced abdominal distention (due to ascites).

Commonly used brand name(s)

In the U.S.—
Taxotere

Available Dosage Forms:
- Powder for Solution
- Solution

Therapeutic Class: Antineoplastic Agent
Pharmacologic Class: Mitotic Inhibitor

Uses For This Medicine

Docetaxel belongs to the group of medicines called antineoplastics. It is used to treat breast cancer, non-small cell lung cancer, gastrointestinal (stomach) and prostate cancer. Docetaxel is sometimes used in combination with other medicines for certain types of cancer.

Docetaxel interferes with the growth of cancer cells, which are eventually destroyed. Since the growth of normal body cells may also be affected by docetaxel, other effects will also occur. Some of these may be serious and must be reported to your doctor. Other effects may not be serious but may cause concern. Some effects may not occur for months or years after the medicine is used.

Docetaxel may also be used to treat other conditions as determined by your doctor.

Before you begin treatment with docetaxel, you and your doctor should talk about the good this medicine will do as well as the risks of using it.

Docetaxel is to be administered only by or under the immediate supervision of your doctor.

Once a medicine has been approved for marketing for a certain use, experience may show that it is also useful for other medical problems. Although these uses are not included in the product labeling, docetaxel is used in certain patients with the following medical conditions:

- Bladder cancer
- Esophageal cancer
- Head and neck cancer
- Lung cancer, small cell
- Ovarian cancer

Before Using This Medicine

In deciding to use a medicine, the risks of taking the medicine must be weighed against the good it will do. This is a decision you and your doctor will make. For this medicine, the following should be considered:

Allergies—Tell your doctor if you have ever had any unusual or allergic reaction to this medicine or any other medicines. Also tell your health care professional if you have any other types of allergies, such as to foods, dyes, preservatives, or animals. For non-prescription products, read the label or package ingredients carefully.

Pediatric—Docetaxel has been studied in a limited number of children. The study showed that children are especially sensitive to the effects of docetaxel and cannot be given usual doses of the medicine.

Geriatric—Elderly people are especially sensitive to the effects of docetaxel. This may increase the chance of side effects during treatment.

Pregnancy—

	Pregnancy Category	Explanation
All Trimesters	D	Studies in pregnant women have demonstrated a risk to the fetus. However, the benefits of therapy in a life threatening situation or a serious disease, may outweigh the potential risk.

Breast Feeding—There are no adequate studies in women for determining infant risk when using this medication during breastfeeding. Weigh the potential benefits against the potential risks before taking this medication while breastfeeding.

Other medicines—

Using this medicine with any of the following medicines is not recommended. Your doctor may decide not to treat you with this medication or change some of the other medicines you take.

Rotavirus Vaccine, Live

Interactions with Food/Tobacco/Alcohol—Certain medicines should not be used at or around the time of eating food or eating certain types of food since interactions may occur. Using alcohol or tobacco with certain medicines may also cause interactions to occur. Discuss with your healthcare professional the use of your medicine with food, alcohol, or tobacco.

Other medical problems—The presence of other medical problems may affect the use of this medicine. Make sure you tell your doctor if you have any other medical problems, especially:

- Alcohol abuse or history of—The risk of some side effects affecting the muscles and nerves may be increased.
- Chickenpox (including recent exposure) or
- Herpes zoster (shingles)—The risk of severe disease affecting other parts of the body may be increased.
- Fluid in lungs—Docetaxel may make your condition worse.
- Infection—Docetaxel may decrease your body's ability to fight infection.
- Liver disease—The chance of serious side effects is greatly increased.

Proper Use of This Medicine

This medicine often causes nausea and vomiting, which is usually mild. However, it is very important that you continue to receive the medicine even if you begin to feel ill. Ask your health care professional for ways to lessen these effects.

Your doctor may direct you to take a corticosteroid medicine such as dexamethasone (e.g., Decadron), starting the day before you receive an injection of docetaxel and may continue for a few days after a docetaxel treatment. This other medicine decreases the chance of an allergic reaction to docetaxel and certain other side effects. It is very important that you take each dose of the corticosteroid medicine as directed.

Dosing—The dose of this medicine will be different for different patients. Follow your doctor's orders or the directions on the label. The following information includes only the average doses of this medicine. If your dose is different, do not change it unless your doctor tells you to do so.

The amount of medicine that you take depends on the strength of the medicine. Also, the number of doses you take each day, the time allowed between doses, and the length of time you take the medicine depend on the medical problem for which you are using the medicine.

Precautions While Using This Medicine

It is very important that your doctor check your progress at regular visits to make sure that this medicine is working properly and to check for unwanted effects.

While you are being treated with docetaxel, and after you stop treatment with it, do not have any immunizations (vaccinations) without your doctor's approval. Docetaxel may lower your body's resistance and there is a chance you might get the infection the immunization is meant to prevent. In addition, other persons living in your household should not take oral polio vaccine since there is a chance they could pass the polio virus on to you. Also, avoid persons who have taken oral polio vaccine within the past several months. Do not get close to them and do not stay in the same room with them for very long. If you cannot take these precautions, you should consider wearing a protective face mask that covers the nose and mouth.

Docetaxel can temporarily lower the number of white blood cells in your blood, increasing the chance of getting an infection. It can also lower the number of platelets, which are necessary for proper blood clotting. If this occurs, there are certain precautions you can take, especially when your blood count is low, to reduce the risk of infection or bleeding:

- If you can, avoid people with infections. Check with your doctor immediately if you think you are getting an infection or if you get a fever or chills, cough or hoarseness, lower back or side pain, or painful or difficult urination.
- Check with your doctor immediately if you notice any unusual bleeding or bruising; black, tarry stools; blood in urine or stools; or pinpoint red spots on your skin.
- Be careful when using a regular toothbrush, dental floss, or toothpick. Your medical doctor, dentist, or nurse may recommend other ways to clean your teeth and gums. Check with your medical doctor before having any dental work done.
- Do not touch your eyes or the inside of your nose unless you have just washed your hands and have not touched anything else in the meantime.
- Be careful not to cut yourself when you are using sharp objects such as a safety razor or fingernail or toenail cutters.
- Avoid contact sports or other situations where bruising or injury could occur.

Side Effects of This Medicine

Along with its needed effects, a medicine may cause some unwanted effects. Some side effects will have signs or symptoms that you can see or feel. Your doctor may watch for others by doing certain tests.

Also, because of the way these medicines act on the body, there is a chance that they might cause other unwanted effects that may not occur until months or years after the medicine is used. These delayed effects may include certain types of cancer. Discuss these possible effects with your doctor.

Check with your doctor immediately if any of the following side effects occur:

Less common
Black, tarry stools; blood in urine or stools; cough or hoarseness (accompanied by fever or chills); difficult or labored breathing; difficult or painful urination (accompanied by fever or chills); difficulty swallowing; dizziness; fast heartbeat; fever or chills; heart problems; hives; itching, puffiness or swelling of the eyelids or around the eyes, face, lips, or tongue; lower back or side pain (accompanied by fever or chills); noisy, rattling breathing; pinpoint red spots on skin; shortness of breath; skin rash; tightness in chest; troubled breathing

while at rest; unusual bleeding or bruising; unusual tiredness or weakness; wheezing

Rare
Chest pain or discomfort; fast or irregular heartbeat; shortness of breath

Docetaxel sometimes causes allergic reactions, especially during the first few treatments. Tell your doctor or nurse right away if you notice back pain or itching during an injection. Your doctor or nurse will be watching out for other signs of an allergic reaction while you are receiving this medicine, and will be ready to treat any serious effects right away.

A kind of leukemia called acute myeloid leukemia [AML] can occur if you are taking a combination of docetaxel and cyclophosphamide to treat your breast cancer. Tell your doctor right away if you develop a lot of infections, experience bone or joint pain, or have a fever.

Check with your doctor as soon as possible if any of the following side effects occur:

More common
Swelling of abdomen, face, fingers, hands, feet, or lower legs; unusual tiredness or weakness; weight gain

Less common
Red, scaly, swollen, or peeling areas of skin (severe)

Rare
Decrease in blood pressure, sometimes with dizziness or fainting; increase in blood pressure, sometimes with dizziness or headaches

This medicine may also cause the following side effects that your doctor will watch out for:

More common
Anemia; low white blood cell count

Less common
High or low blood pressure; low platelet count in blood

Some side effects may occur that usually do not need medical attention. These side effects may go away during treatment as your body adjusts to the medicine. Also, your health care professional may be able to tell you about ways to prevent or reduce some of these side effects. Check with your health care professional if any of the following side effects continue or are bothersome or if you have any questions about them:

More common
Burning, numbness, tingling, or pain in arms, hands, legs, or feet; congestion; diarrhea; dryness or soreness of throat; nausea; skin rash or redness (mild); sores or ulcers on the lips or tongue or inside the mouth; weakness in arms, hands, legs, or feet

Less common
Bloody nose; body aches or pain; change in color of fingernails or toenails; congestion; dry, red, hot, or irritated skin at place of injection; headache; hoarseness; loosening or loss of fingernails or toenails, sometimes painful; pain in joints or muscles; pain, swelling, or lump under the skin at place of injection; runny nose; tender, swollen glands in neck; trouble in swallowing; voice changes; vomiting

Incidence not known
Burning, dry or itching eyes; burning upper abdominal pain; confusion; difficulty having a bowel movement [stool] discharge from eyes; excessive tearing; mood or mental changes; pain all over body; pain and redness of skin at place of earlier radiation treatment; rapid breathing; redness, pain, swelling of eye, eyelid,

or inner lining of eyelid; stomach pain; sunken eyes; tearing of the eyes; wrinkled skin

This medicine usually causes a temporary loss of hair. After treatment with docetaxel has ended, normal hair growth should return.

Other side effects not listed may also occur in some patients. If you notice any other effects, check with your healthcare professional.

DOCOSANOL (Topical route) - doe-KOE-san-ole

Commonly used brand name(s)

In the U.S.—
    Abreva

Available Dosage Forms:
- Cream

Therapeutic Class: Antiviral

Uses For This Medicine

Docosanol belongs to the family of medicines called antivirals. Antivirals are used to treat infections caused by viruses. Usually they work for only one kind or group of virus infections.

Topical docosanol is used to treat the symptoms of herpes simplex virus infections around the mouth. Although topical docosanol will not cure herpes simplex, it may help relieve the pain and discomfort and may help the sores (if any) heal faster.

Docosanol is available over the counter.

Before Using This Medicine

In deciding to use a medicine, the risks of taking the medicine must be weighed against the good it will do. This is a decision you and your doctor will make. For this medicine, the following should be considered:

Allergies—Tell your doctor if you have ever had any unusual or allergic reaction to this medicine or any other medicines. Also tell your health care professional if you have any other types of allergies, such as to foods, dyes, preservatives, or animals. For non-prescription products, read the label or package ingredients carefully.

Pediatric—Although there is no specific information comparing use of docosanol in children with use in other age groups, this medicine is not expected to cause different side effects or problems in children than it does in adults.

Geriatric—Many medicines have not been studied specifically in older people. Therefore, it may not be known whether they work exactly the same way they do in younger adults or if they cause different side effects or problems in older people. There is no specific information comparing use of docosanol in the elderly with use in other age groups.

Other medicines—Although certain medicines should not be used together at all, in other cases two different medicines may be used together even if an interaction might occur. In these cases, your doctor may want to change the dose, or

other precautions may be necessary. Tell your healthcare professional if you are taking any other prescription or non-prescription (over-the-counter [OTC]) medicine.

Interactions with Food/Tobacco/Alcohol—Certain medicines should not be used at or around the time of eating food or eating certain types of food since interactions may occur. Using alcohol or tobacco with certain medicines may also cause interactions to occur. Discuss with your healthcare professional the use of your medicine with food, alcohol, or tobacco.

Proper Use of This Medicine

Do not use this medicine in or around the eyes or on the genitalia.

Docosanol is best used as soon as possible after the signs and symptoms of herpes infection (for example, pain, burning, or blisters) begin to appear.

Apply the medication to the sores (blisters); rub in gently and completely.

To help clear up your herpes infection, continue using docosanol for the full time of treatment. Do not miss any doses. However, do not use this medicine more often or for a longer time than your health care professional or the OTC label indicates.

Dosing—The dose of this medicine will be different for different patients. Follow your doctor's orders or the directions on the label. The following information includes only the average doses of this medicine. If your dose is different, do not change it unless your doctor tells you to do so.

The amount of medicine that you take depends on the strength of the medicine. Also, the number of doses you take each day, the time allowed between doses, and the length of time you take the medicine depend on the medical problem for which you are using the medicine.

- For topical dosage form (cream):
  - Adults and adolescents:
    - Apply to the affected area(s), five times a day until sore is healed.
    - Rub in gently and completely
  - Children under 12 years of age
    - Use and dosage must be determined by your doctor.

Storage—Keep out of the reach of children.

Do not keep outdated medicine or medicine no longer needed.

Ask your healthcare professional how you should dispose of any medicine you do not use.

Side Effects of This Medicine

Along with its needed effects, a medicine may cause some unwanted effects. Although not all of these side effects may occur, if they do occur they may need medical attention.

Some side effects may occur that usually do not need medical attention. These side effects may go away during treatment as your body adjusts to the medicine. Also, your health care professional may be able to tell you about ways to prevent or reduce some of these side effects. Check with your health care professional if any of the following side effects continue or are bothersome or if you have any questions about them:

More common
    Headache

Less common

 Surface problems including:; acne; burning; dryness; itching; rash; redness; soreness; swelling

Other side effects not listed may also occur in some patients. If you notice any other effects, check with your healthcare professional.

DOFETILIDE (Oral route) - doe-FET-il-ide

Black Box Warning

To minimize the risk of induced arrhythmia, patients initiated or re-initiated on dofetilide should be placed for a minimum of 3 days in a facility that can provide calculations of creatinine clearance, continuous electrocardiographic monitoring, and cardiac resuscitation. Dofetilide is available only to hospitals and prescribers who have received appropriate dofetilide dosing and treatment initiation education.

Commonly used brand name(s)

In the U.S.—
 Tikosyn

Available Dosage Forms:
• Capsule

Therapeutic Class: Antiarrhythmic, Group III

Uses For This Medicine

Dofetilide belongs to the group of medicines known as antiarrhythmics. It is used to correct irregular heartbeats to a normal rhythm

Dofetilide produces its helpful effects by slowing nerve impulses in the heart.

This medicine is available only with your doctor's prescription.

Before Using This Medicine

In deciding to use a medicine, the risks of taking the medicine must be weighed against the good it will do. This is a decision you and your doctor will make. For this medicine, the following should be considered:

Allergies—Tell your doctor if you have ever had any unusual or allergic reaction to this medicine or any other medicines. Also tell your health care professional if you have any other types of allergies, such as to foods, dyes, preservatives, or animals. For non-prescription products, read the label or package ingredients carefully.

Pediatric—Studies on this medicine have been done only in adult patients, and there is no specific information comparing use of dofetilide in children less than 18 years of age with use in other age groups.

Geriatric—This medicine has been tested in patients 65 to 89 years old and has not been shown to cause different side effects or problems in older people than it does in younger adults.

Pregnancy—

	Pregnancy Category	Explanation
All Trimesters	C	Animal studies have shown an adverse effect and there are no adequate studies in pregnant women OR no animal studies have been conducted and there are no adequate studies in pregnant women.

Breast Feeding—There are no adequate studies in women for determining infant risk when using this medication during breastfeeding. Weigh the potential benefits against the potential risks before taking this medication while breastfeeding.

Other medicines—

Using this medicine with any of the following medicines is not recommended. Your doctor may decide not to treat you with this medication or change some of the other medicines you take.

Bepridil, Cimetidine, Cisapride, Hydrochlorothiazide, Itraconazole, Ketoconazole, Levomethadyl, Megestrol, Mesoridazine, Pimozide, Prochlorperazine, Ranolazine, Sparfloxacin, Sulfamethoxazole, Terfenadine, Thioridazine, Trimethoprim, Verapamil, Ziprasidone

Interactions with Food/Tobacco/Alcohol—Certain medicines should not be used at or around the time of eating food or eating certain types of food since interactions may occur. Using alcohol or tobacco with certain medicines may also cause interactions to occur. Discuss with your healthcare professional the use of your medicine with food, alcohol, or tobacco.

Other medical problems—The presence of other medical problems may affect the use of this medicine. Make sure you tell your doctor if you have any other medical problems, especially:
• Electrolyte disorders, such as low potassium or magnesium levels or
• Heart rhythm problems—May cause irregular heartbeats
• Liver disease (severe)—Safety with this condition is unknown
• Kidney disease—Higher blood levels may occur, which may increase the chance of side effects. Your doctor may need to change your dose.

Proper Use of This Medicine

Patient information about dofetilide is available. Read this information carefully.

Use this medicine exactly as directed by your doctor. Do not use more or less of it, and do not use it more often than your doctor ordered. This medicine works best when there is a constant amount in the body. To help keep the amount constant, it is best to take the doses at the same time every day.

Dosing—The dose of this medicine will be different for different patients. Follow your doctor's orders or the directions on the label. The following information includes only the average doses of this medicine. If your dose is different, do not change it unless your doctor tells you to do so.

The amount of medicine that you take depends on the strength of the medicine. Also, the number of doses you take

each day, the time allowed between doses, and the length of time you take the medicine depend on the medical problem for which you are using the medicine.

- For oral dosage form (capsules):
  - For abnormal heart rhythm:
    - Adults—125 to 500 micrograms (mcg) two times a day.
    - Children—Use and dose must be determined by your doctor.

Missed dose—If you miss a dose of this medicine, skip the missed dose and go back to your regular dosing schedule. Do not double doses.

Storage—Store the medicine in a closed container at room temperature, away from heat, moisture, and direct light. Keep from freezing.

Keep out of the reach of children.

Do not keep outdated medicine or medicine no longer needed.

Precautions While Using This Medicine

It is very important that your doctor check your progress at regular visits to make sure that this medicine is working properly and to check for unwanted effects. This will allow for changes to be made in the amount of medicine you are taking, if necessary.

Other medicines: Do not take other medicines unless they have been discussed with your doctor. This especially includes nonprescription medicines, such as Tagamet and Tagamet HB.

Side Effects of This Medicine

Along with its needed effects, a medicine may cause some unwanted effects. Although not all of these side effects may occur, if they do occur they may need medical attention.

Check with your doctor as soon as possible if any of the following side effects occur:

More common
  dizziness; fainting; fast or irregular heartbeat

Less common
  Chest pain; confusion; facial or flaccid paralysis; numbness or tingling of the hands, feet or face; paralysis; pounding, slow heartbeat; slurred speech; swelling of the ankles, arms, face, feet, fingers, legs, lips, tongue, and/or throat; troubled breathing; unexplained shortness of breath; unusual tiredness or weakness; weight gain; yellow eyes or skin

Some side effects may occur that usually do not need medical attention. These side effects may go away during treatment as your body adjusts to the medicine. Also, your health care professional may be able to tell you about ways to prevent or reduce some of these side effects. Check with your health care professional if any of the following side effects continue or are bothersome or if you have any questions about them:

Less common
  Abdominal or stomach pain; accidental injury; back pain; chills; cough; diarrhea; fever; flu-like symptoms; general feeling of discomfort or illness; headache; joint pain; loss of appetite; migraine; muscle aches and pains; nausea; rash; runny nose; shivering; sneezing; sore throat; sweating; trouble sleeping; vomiting

Other side effects not listed may also occur in some patients. If you notice any other effects, check with your healthcare professional.

DOLASETRON   (Oral route, Intravenous route) - dol-A-se-tron

Commonly used brand name(s)

In the U.S.—
  Anzemet

Available Dosage Forms:
- Tablet
- Solution

Therapeutic Class: Antiemetic
Pharmacologic Class: Serotonin Receptor Antagonist, 5–HT3

Uses For This Medicine

Dolasetron is used to prevent and treat the nausea and vomiting that may occur after treatment with anticancer medicines (chemotherapy) or after surgery.

This medicine is available only with your doctor's prescription.

Before Using This Medicine

In deciding to use a medicine, the risks of taking the medicine must be weighed against the good it will do. This is a decision you and your doctor will make. For this medicine, the following should be considered:

Allergies—Tell your doctor if you have ever had any unusual or allergic reaction to this medicine or any other medicines. Also tell your health care professional if you have any other types of allergies, such as to foods, dyes, preservatives, or animals. For non-prescription products, read the label or package ingredients carefully.

Pediatric—This medicine has been tested in a limited number of children between 2 and 17 years of age with cancer. In effective doses, this medicine has not been shown to cause different side effects or problems than it does in adults.

Geriatric—This medicine has not been shown to cause different side effects or problems in older people than it does in younger adults.

Pregnancy—

	Pregnancy Category	Explanation
All Trimesters	B	Animal studies have revealed no evidence of harm to the fetus, however, there are no adequate studies in pregnant women OR animal studies have shown an adverse effect, but adequate studies in pregnant women have failed to demonstrate a risk to the fetus.

Breast Feeding—There are no adequate studies in women for determining infant risk when using this medication during

breastfeeding. Weigh the potential benefits against the potential risks before taking this medication while breastfeeding.

Other medicines—

Using this medicine with any of the following medicines is not recommended. Your doctor may decide not to treat you with this medication or change some of the other medicines you take.

Apomorphine, Bepridil, Cisapride, Levomethadyl, Mesoridazine, Pimozide, Thioridazine, Ziprasidone

Interactions with Food/Tobacco/Alcohol—Certain medicines should not be used at or around the time of eating food or eating certain types of food since interactions may occur. Using alcohol or tobacco with certain medicines may also cause interactions to occur. Discuss with your healthcare professional the use of your medicine with food, alcohol, or tobacco.

Other medical problems—The presence of other medical problems may affect the use of dolasetron. Make sure you tell your doctor if you have any other medical problems.

Proper Use of This Medicine

Dosing—The dose of this medicine will be different for different patients. Follow your doctor's orders or the directions on the label. The following information includes only the average doses of this medicine. If your dose is different, do not change it unless your doctor tells you to do so.

The amount of medicine that you take depends on the strength of the medicine. Also, the number of doses you take each day, the time allowed between doses, and the length of time you take the medicine depend on the medical problem for which you are using the medicine.

- For oral dosage form (tablets):
  - For prevention of nausea and vomiting after anticancer medicine:
    - Adults—100 milligrams (mg) given within one hour before the anticancer medicine is given.
    - Children 2 to 16 years of age—1.8 mg per kilogram (kg) (0.82 mg per pound) of body weight given within one hour before the anticancer medicine is given. The dose generally is not greater than 100 mg.
    - Children up to 2 years of age—Use and dose must be determined by your doctor.
  - For prevention of nausea and vomiting after surgery:
    - Adults—100 mg given within two hours before surgery.
    - Children 2 to 16 years of age—1.2 mg per kg (0.55 mg per pound) of body weight given within two hours before surgery. The dose generally is not greater than 100 mg.
    - Children up to 2 years of age—Use and dose must be determined by your doctor.
- For injection dosage form:
  - For prevention of nausea and vomiting after anticancer medicine:
    - Adults—100 milligrams (mg) given into a vein approximately 30 minutes before the anticancer medicine is given.
    - Children 2 to 16 years of age—1.8 mg per kilogram (kg) (0.82 mg per pound) of body weight given into a vein approximately 30 minutes before

the anticancer medicine is given. The dose generally is not greater than 100 mg.
    - Children up to 2 years of age—Use and dose must be determined by your doctor.
  - For prevention of nausea and vomiting after surgery:
    - Adults—12.5 mg given into a vein approximately 15 minutes before anesthesia (medicine to put you to sleep during surgery) is ended.
    - Children 2 to 16 years of age—0.35 mg per kg (0.16 mg per pound) of body weight given into a vein approximately 15 minutes before anesthesia (medicine to put you to sleep during surgery) is ended. The dose generally is not greater than 12.5 mg.
    - Children up to 2 years of age—Use and dose must be determined by your doctor.
  - For treatment of nausea and vomiting after surgery:
    - Adults—12.5 mg given into a vein as soon as nausea and vomiting start.
    - Children 2 to 16 years of age—0.35 mg per kg (0.16 mg per pound) of body weight given into a vein as soon as nausea and vomiting start. The dose generally is not greater than 12.5 mg.
    - Children up to 2 years of age—Use and dose must be determined by your doctor.

Storage—Store the medicine in a closed container at room temperature, away from heat, moisture, and direct light. Keep from freezing.

Keep out of the reach of children.

Do not keep outdated medicine or medicine no longer needed.

Side Effects of This Medicine

Along with its needed effects, a medicine may cause some unwanted effects. Although not all of these side effects may occur, if they do occur they may need medical attention.

Check with your doctor as soon as possible if any of the following side effects occur:
Less common
　High or low blood pressure
Rare
　Blood in the urine; chest pain; decrease in amount of urine; fast heartbeat; pain; painful urination or trouble in urinating; severe stomach pain with nausea or vomiting; skin rash, hives, and/or itching; slow or irregular heartbeat; swelling of face; swelling of feet or lower legs; troubled breathing

Some side effects may occur that usually do not need medical attention. These side effects may go away during treatment as your body adjusts to the medicine. Also, your health care professional may be able to tell you about ways to prevent or reduce some of these side effects. Check with your health care professional if any of the following side effects continue or are bothersome or if you have any questions about them:
More common
　Diarrhea; headache

Less common
　Abdominal or stomach pain; dizziness or lightheadedness; fever or chills; unusual tiredness

Other side effects not listed may also occur in some patients. If you notice any other effects, check with your healthcare professional.

DONEPEZIL (Oral route) - doh-NEP-e-zil

Commonly used brand name(s)

In the U.S.—
   Aricept

Available Dosage Forms:
   • Tablet
   • Tablet, Disintegrating

Therapeutic Class: Central Nervous System Agent
Pharmacologic Class: Cholinesterase Inhibitor, Centrally Acting

Uses For This Medicine

Donepezil is used to treat the symptoms of mild to moderate Alzheimer's disease. Donepezil will not cure Alzheimer's disease, and it will not stop the disease from getting worse. However, it can improve thinking ability in some patients.

This medicine is available only with your doctor's prescription.

Before Using This Medicine

In deciding to use a medicine, the risks of taking the medicine must be weighed against the good it will do. This is a decision you and your doctor will make. For this medicine, the following should be considered:

Allergies—Tell your doctor if you have ever had any unusual or allergic reaction to this medicine or any other medicines. Also tell your health care professional if you have any other types of allergies, such as to foods, dyes, preservatives, or animals. For non-prescription products, read the label or package ingredients carefully.

Pediatric—Studies on this medicine have been done only in adult patients, and there is no specific information comparing use of donepezil in children with use in other age groups.

Geriatric—In studies done to date that have included older adults, some side effects of donepezil have been shown to occur more frequently in older people than in younger adults.

Pregnancy—

	Pregnancy Category	Explanation
All Trimesters	C	Animal studies have shown an adverse effect and there are no adequate studies in pregnant women OR no animal studies have been conducted and there are no adequate studies in pregnant women.

Breast Feeding—There are no adequate studies in women for determining infant risk when using this medication during breastfeeding. Weigh the potential benefits against the potential risks before taking this medication while breastfeeding.

Other medicines—

Using this medicine with any of the following medicines is usually not recommended, but may be required in some cases. If both medicines are prescribed together, your doctor may change the dose or how often you use one or both of the medicines.

Succinylcholine

Interactions with Food/Tobacco/Alcohol—Certain medicines should not be used at or around the time of eating food or eating certain types of food since interactions may occur. Using alcohol or tobacco with certain medicines may also cause interactions to occur. Discuss with your healthcare professional the use of your medicine with food, alcohol, or tobacco.

Other medical problems—The presence of other medical problems may affect the use of this medicine. Make sure you tell your doctor if you have any other medical problems, especially:
   • Asthma or
   • Lung disease or
   • Peptic ulcers, or history of or
   • Seizures, or history of or
   • Urinary tract blockage—Donepezil may make these conditions worse
   • Heart problems—Donepezil may have unwanted effects on heart rate
   • Liver problems—Higher blood levels of donepezil may result and increase the chance of side effects

Proper Use of This Medicine

Take this medicine exactly as directed by your doctor in order to improve your condition as much as possible. Do not take more of it or less of it, and do not take it more or less often than your doctor ordered.

Donepezil should be taken at bedtime unless otherwise directed by your doctor. It may be taken with or without food, on a full or empty stomach.

For patients using the oral disintegrating tablet form of this medicine:
   • Make sure your hands are dry.
   • Do not push the tablet through the foil backing of the package. Instead, gently peel back the foil backing and remove the tablet.
   • Immediately place the tablet on top of the tongue.
   • The tablet will dissolve in seconds, and you may swallow it with your saliva. You should drink a glass of water after the tablet has dissolved.

For patients taking the oral solution form of this medicine:
   • Shake the bottle well before measuring the dose.
   • Use a specially marked measuring spoon, a plastic syringe, or a small marked measuring cup to measure each dose accurately. The average household teaspoon may not hold the right amount of liquid.
   • If your dose is 5 mg, you should take 5 mL of this medicine.
   • If your dose is 10 mg, you should take 10 mL of this medicine.

Dosing—The dose of this medicine will be different for different patients. Follow your doctor's orders or the directions on the label. The following information includes only the av-

erage doses of this medicine. If your dose is different, do not change it unless your doctor tells you to do so.

The amount of medicine that you take depends on the strength of the medicine. Also, the number of doses you take each day, the time allowed between doses, and the length of time you take the medicine depend on the medical problem for which you are using the medicine.

- For oral dosage forms (oral disintegrating tablets, oral solution, and tablets):
  - For Alzheimer's disease:
    - Adults—5 milligrams (mg) taken at bedtime. Your doctor may increase your dose as needed. However, the dose usually is not more than 10 mg a day.
    - Children—Use and dose must be determined by your doctor.

Missed dose—If you miss a dose of this medicine, skip the missed dose and go back to your regular dosing schedule. Do not double doses.

Storage—Store the medicine in a closed container at room temperature, away from heat, moisture, and direct light. Keep from freezing.

Keep out of the reach of children.

Do not keep outdated medicine or medicine no longer needed.

Precautions While Using This Medicine

It is important that your doctor check your progress at regular visits. This is necessary to allow dose adjustments and to reduce any unwanted effects.

Before you have any kind of surgery, dental treatment, or emergency treatment, tell the medical doctor or dentist in charge that you are using this medicine. Taking donepezil together with certain medicines that are used during surgery or dental or emergency treatments may increase the effects of those medicines and cause unwanted effects.

This medicine may cause some people to become dizzy or drowsy, to have blurred vision, or to have problems with clumsiness or unsteadiness. Make sure you know how you react to this medicine before you drive, use machines, or do anything else that could be dangerous if you are not alert, well-coordinated, and able to see clearly.

If you think that you or someone else may have taken an overdose of this medicine, get emergency help at once. Taking an overdose of this medicine may cause convulsions (seizures) or serious effects on your heart and your breathing. Signs of overdose include increased watering of mouth, increased sweating, low blood pressure, muscle weakness, severe nausea, severe vomiting, slow heartbeat, and troubled breathing.

Side Effects of This Medicine

Along with its needed effects, a medicine may cause some unwanted effects. Although not all of these side effects may occur, if they do occur they may need medical attention.

Check with your doctor as soon as possible if any of the following side effects occur:

More common
Diarrhea; loss of appetite; muscle cramps; nausea; trouble in sleeping; unusual tiredness or weakness; vomiting

Less common
Abnormal dreams; constipation; dizziness; drowsiness; fainting; frequent urination; headache; joint pain, stiffness, or swelling; mental depression; pain; unusual bleeding or bruising; weight loss

Rare
Black, tarry stools; bloating; bloody or cloudy urine; blurred vision; burning, prickling, or tingling sensations; cataract; chills; clumsiness or unsteadiness; confusion; cough; decreased urination; difficult or painful urination; dryness of mouth; eye irritation; fever; flushing of skin; frequent urge to urinate; high or low blood pressure; hives; hot flashes; increased heart rate and breathing; increase in sexual desire or performance; increased sweating; increased urge to urinate during the night; irregular heartbeat; itching; loss of bladder control; loss of bowel control; mood or mental changes, including abnormal crying, aggression, agitation, delusions, irritability, nervousness, or restlessness; nasal congestion; pain in chest, upper stomach, or throat; problems with speech; runny nose; severe thirst; shortness of breath; sneezing; sore throat; sunken eyes; tightness in chest; tremor; troubled breathing; wheezing; wrinkled skin

Incidence not known
Back, leg, or stomach pains; bleeding gums; chest pain or discomfort; coma; convulsions; dark urine; difficulty breathing; fast or irregular heartbeat; fatigue; general body swelling; general tiredness and weakness; high fever; increased thirst; indigestion; light-colored stools; muscle pain or cramps; nausea and vomiting; nosebleeds; pains in stomach, side, or abdomen, possibly radiating to the back; pale skin; rash; seeing, hearing, or feeling things that are not there; seizures; severe muscle stiffness; severe nausea; slow or irregular heartbeat; stomach pain; sweating; swelling of face, ankles, or hands; tiredness; unusually pale skin; upper right abdominal pain; yellow eyes and skin

Symptoms of overdose
Convulsions (seizures); increased sweating; increased watering of mouth; increasing muscle weakness; low blood pressure; severe nausea; severe vomiting; slow heartbeat; troubled breathing

Other side effects not listed may also occur in some patients. If you notice any other effects, check with your healthcare professional.

DORNASE ALFA (Inhalation, oral/nebulization route) - DOR-nase AL-fa

Commonly used brand name(s)

In the U.S.—
Pulmozyme

Available Dosage Forms:
- Solution

Therapeutic Class: Mucolytic
Pharmacologic Class: Mucolytic Enzyme

Uses For This Medicine

Dornase alfa is used in the management of cystic fibrosis. It is used every day with other cystic fibrosis medicines, especially antibiotics, bronchodilators (medicines that open up narrowed breathing passages), and corticosteroids (cortisone-like medicines).

Cystic fibrosis is a condition in which thick mucus is formed in the lungs and breathing passages. The mucus blocks the airways and increases the chance of lung infections. The infections then cause the mucus to become even thicker, making it more difficult to breathe.

Dornase alfa will not cure cystic fibrosis. However, when it is used every day, it helps make breathing easier and reduces the number of serious lung infections that require treatment with antibiotics.

Dornase alfa is available only with your doctor's prescription.

Before Using This Medicine

In deciding to use a medicine, the risks of taking the medicine must be weighed against the good it will do. This is a decision you and your doctor will make. For this medicine, the following should be considered:

Allergies—Tell your doctor if you have ever had any unusual or allergic reaction to this medicine or any other medicines. Also tell your health care professional if you have any other types of allergies, such as to foods, dyes, preservatives, or animals. For non-prescription products, read the label or package ingredients carefully.

Pediatric—Dornase alfa has been studied in children 3 months of age and older and has not been shown to cause different side effects or problems in children than it does in adults, although coughing, runny or stuffy nose, and skin rashes were more common in children 3 months to 5 years of age than in other age groups.

Geriatric—Dornase alfa has not been tested on enough patients 65 years and older. Cystic fibrosis is a disease that usually affects children and young adults. Although there is no specific information comparing use of dornase alfa in the elderly with use in other age groups, this medicine is not expected to cause different side effects or problems in older people than it does in younger adults.

Other medicines—Although certain medicines should not be used together at all, in other cases two different medicines may be used together even if an interaction might occur. In these cases, your doctor may want to change the dose, or other precautions may be necessary. Tell your healthcare professional if you are taking any other prescription or non-prescription (over-the-counter [OTC]) medicine.

Interactions with Food/Tobacco/Alcohol—Certain medicines should not be used at or around the time of eating food or eating certain types of food since interactions may occur. Using alcohol or tobacco with certain medicines may also cause interactions to occur. Discuss with your healthcare professional the use of your medicine with food, alcohol, or tobacco.

Proper Use of This Medicine

Dornase alfa usually comes with patient instructions. Read them carefully before using this medicine.

Dornase alfa is packaged in small plastic containers called ampules. Each ampule contains one full dose of dornase alfa. Do not use an ampule that has already been opened. Also, do not use an ampule of this medicine after the expiration date printed on the package.

Do not use dornase alfa solution if it is cloudy or discolored.

Dornase alfa must be used in a nebulizer with a compressor. Only the following nebulizers and compressors should be used with this medicine:

- Hudson T Up-draft II disposable jet nebulizer used with the Pulmo-Aide compressor
- Marquest Acorn II disposable jet nebulizer used with the Pulmo-Aide compressor
- Reusable PARI LC Jet+ nebulizer used with the PARI PRONEB compressor
- Reusable PARI BABY nebulizer used with the PARI PRONEB compressor
- Reusable Durable Sidestream jet nebulizer with the MOBILAIRE or the Porta-Neb compressor

Your health care professional will help you decide which nebulizer and compressor to use.

It is very important that you use dornase alfa only as directed. Use the mouthpiece provided with the nebulizer. Do not use a face mask with the nebulizer because less medicine will get into your lungs. Patients who are unable to inhale and exhale through the mouth for the entire nebulizer treatment may use the PARI BABY nebulizer with the supplied face mask. Make sure you understand exactly how to use this medicine in the nebulizer.

In order to receive the full effects of this medicine, you must use it every day as ordered by your doctor. If possible, dornase alfa should be used at about the same time each day. You may notice some improvement in your condition within the first week of treatment. However, some patients may not feel the full effects of this medicine for weeks or months.

If you are taking any other medicines for cystic fibrosis, keep taking them as you did before you started using dornase alfa, unless otherwise directed by your doctor. However, do not put any other inhaled medicine in the nebulizer at the same time that you use dornase alfa. Other inhaled medicines may be used in a clean nebulizer before or after your treatment with dornase alfa.

To prepare the nebulizer for use:

- Wash your hands well with soap and water before putting the nebulizer together and preparing the medicine. This will help prevent infection.
- Put the nebulizer together only on a clean surface. If dirt or germs get on the nebulizer or in the medicine, they may cause infection.
- After you put the nebulizer together, test the compressor (following the manufacturer's directions) to make sure it works properly. If you have any questions about this, ask your health care professional.
- If you are using the Durable Sidestream jet nebulizer with the MOBILAIRE compressor, turn the compressor control knob all the way to the right and then turn on the compressor. The needle on the gauge vibrates between 35 and 45, which is the highest amount of pressure.

To prepare the medicine for use in the nebulizer:

- Remove one ampule of dornase alfa from the refrigerator. Squeeze the ampule before opening to make sure there are no leaks. Hold the tab at the base of the ampule firmly. Twist off the top of the ampule, but do not squeeze the body of the ampule while doing so.
- Take the cap off the nebulizer cup. Turn the opened ampule upside down over the cup. Squeeze the ampule gently until all the contents are emptied into the cup. It is very important that you use the full dose of this medicine.
- Replace the cap on the nebulizer cup. Connect the nebulizer and compressor, following the manufacturer's directions.
- Turn on the compressor. Make sure there is mist coming from the nebulizer.

To use the medicine in the nebulizer:

- Place the mouthpiece between your teeth and on top of your tongue. Close your lips around the mouthpiece. Be sure that you do not block the airflow with your tongue or teeth.
- Breathe normally, in and out, through your mouth. Do not breathe through your nose. If you have trouble breathing only through your mouth, use a nose clip.
- During treatment, moisture may collect in the long connecting tube of the nebulizer. This should be expected. However, if you notice a leak or feel moisture coming from the nebulizer during the treatment, turn off the compressor. Then check to make sure the nebulizer cap is sealed correctly before you continue the treatment.
- When the nebulizer begins 'spitting' gently tap the nebulizer cup. Continue breathing until the cup is empty or no more mist comes from the nebulizer.
- If you have to stop the treatment for some reason or if you start coughing during the treatment, turn off the compressor. To begin the treatment again, turn on the compressor and continue as before.
- The complete treatment usually takes 10 to 15 minutes. Be sure to inhale the full dose of dornase alfa.

After using dornase alfa:

- Turn off the compressor. Then take apart the nebulizer system.
- Follow the manufacturer's directions for care and cleaning of your nebulizer and compressor.

Dosing—The dose of this medicine will be different for different patients. Follow your doctor's orders or the directions on the label. The following information includes only the average doses of this medicine. If your dose is different, do not change it unless your doctor tells you to do so.

The amount of medicine that you take depends on the strength of the medicine. Also, the number of doses you take each day, the time allowed between doses, and the length of time you take the medicine depend on the medical problem for which you are using the medicine.

- For inhalation dosage form (inhalation solution):
  - For cystic fibrosis:
    - Adults and children 5 years of age and older—The usual dose is 2.5 milligrams (mg) (one ampule), used in a nebulizer once a day for about 10 to 15 minutes. However, your doctor may want you to use this medicine two times a day at regularly spaced times.
    - Children 3 months to 5 years of age—The usual dose is 2.5 milligrams (mg) (one ampule), used in a nebulizer once a day for about 10 to 15 minutes.
    - Children up to 3 months of age—Use and dose must be determined by your doctor.

Missed dose—If you miss a dose of this medicine, take it as soon as possible. However, if it is almost time for your next dose, skip the missed dose and go back to your regular dosing schedule. Do not double doses.

Storage—Keep out of the reach of children.

Do not keep outdated medicine or medicine no longer needed.

Store the medicine in the refrigerator in the foil pouches. However, keep the medicine from freezing. Do not leave this medicine out of the refrigerator for longer than 24 hours. If an ampule of medicine is left out for longer than this, it should be thrown away and a new ampule should be used.

Precautions While Using This Medicine

If your condition becomes worse while you are using this medicine, check with your doctor.

Side Effects of This Medicine

Along with its needed effects, a medicine may cause some unwanted effects. Although not all of these side effects may occur, if they do occur they may need medical attention.

Check with your doctor as soon as possible if any of the following side effects occur:

Rare
  Hives or welts; itching; redness of skin; skin rash

Some side effects may occur that usually do not need medical attention. These side effects may go away during treatment as your body adjusts to the medicine. Also, your health care professional may be able to tell you about ways to prevent or reduce some of these side effects. Check with your health care professional if any of the following side effects continue or are bothersome or if you have any questions about them:

More common
  Chest pain or discomfort; hoarseness; sore throat

Less common
  Difficulty breathing; fever; redness, itching, pain, swelling, or other irritation of eyes; runny or stuffy nose; upset stomach

Other side effects not listed may also occur in some patients. If you notice any other effects, check with your healthcare professional.

DORZOLAMIDE (Ophthalmic route) -
dor-ZOLE-a-mide

Commonly used brand name(s)

In the U.S.—
Trusopt Ocumeter
Trusopt Ocumeter Plus

Available Dosage Forms:
- Solution

Therapeutic Class: Antiglaucoma

Pharmacologic Class: Carbonic Anhydrase Inhibitor

Uses For This Medicine

Dorzolamide is a carbonic anhydrase inhibitor that is used in the eye. It is used to treat increased pressure in the eye caused by open-angle glaucoma. It is also used to treat a condition called hypertension of the eye.

Dorzolamide is available only with your doctor's prescription.

Before Using This Medicine

In deciding to use a medicine, the risks of taking the medicine must be weighed against the good it will do. This is a decision you and your doctor will make. For this medicine, the following should be considered:

Allergies—Tell your doctor if you have ever had any unusual or allergic reaction to this medicine or any other medicines. Also tell your health care professional if you have any other types of allergies, such as to foods, dyes, preservatives, or animals. For non-prescription products, read the label or package ingredients carefully.

Pediatric—This medicine has been tested in children and, in effective doses, has not been shown to cause different side effects or problems than it does in adults.

Geriatric—This medicine has been tested in a limited number of patients 65 years of age or older and has not been shown to cause different side effects or problems in older people than it does in younger adults.

Pregnancy—

	Pregnancy Category	Explanation
All Trimesters	C	Animal studies have shown an adverse effect and there are no adequate studies in pregnant women OR no animal studies have been conducted and there are no adequate studies in pregnant women.

Breast Feeding—There are no adequate studies in women for determining infant risk when using this medication during breastfeeding. Weigh the potential benefits against the potential risks before taking this medication while breastfeeding.

Other medicines—Although certain medicines should not be used together at all, in other cases two different medicines may be used together even if an interaction might occur. In these cases, your doctor may want to change the dose, or other precautions may be necessary. Tell your healthcare professional if you are taking any other prescription or non-prescription (over-the-counter [OTC]) medicine.

Interactions with Food/Tobacco/Alcohol—Certain medicines should not be used at or around the time of eating food or eating certain types of food since interactions may occur. Using alcohol or tobacco with certain medicines may also cause interactions to occur. Discuss with your healthcare professional the use of your medicine with food, alcohol, or tobacco.

Other medical problems—The presence of other medical problems may affect the use of this medicine. Make sure you tell your doctor if you have any other medical problems, especially:

- Acute angle-closure glaucoma—Use of ophthalmic dorzolamide in these patients has not been studied. This condition may need other medicine or treatment besides dorzolamide.

- Kidney disease, severe, or

- Liver disease—Use of ophthalmic dorzolamide may lead to increased side effects from the medication

- Kidney stones—Use of ophthalmic dorzolamide may make this condition worse

---

Proper Use of This Medicine

To use: First, wash your hands. Tilt the head back and, pressing your finger gently on the skin just beneath the lower eyelid, pull the lower eyelid away from the eye to make a space. Drop the medicine into this space. Let go of the eyelid and gently close the eyes. Do not blink. Keep the eyes closed and apply pressure to the inner corner of the eye with your finger for 1 or 2 minutes to allow the medicine to be absorbed by the eye.

Do not touch or contaminate the tip of the container.

Use this medicine only as directed. Do not use more of it and do not use it more often than your doctor ordered. To do so may increase the chance of too much medicine being absorbed into the body and the chance of side effects.

If your doctor ordered two different eye drops to be used together, wait at least 10 minutes between the times you apply the medicines. This will help to keep the second medicine from "washing out" the first one.

Dosing—The dose of this medicine will be different for different patients. Follow your doctor's orders or the directions on the label. The following information includes only the average doses of this medicine. If your dose is different, do not change it unless your doctor tells you to do so.

The amount of medicine that you take depends on the strength of the medicine. Also, the number of doses you take each day, the time allowed between doses, and the length of time you take the medicine depend on the medical problem for which you are using the medicine.

- For ophthalmic dosage form (eye drops):
  - For glaucoma or hypertension of the eye:
    - Adults and teenagers—Use one drop in the eye three times a day.
    - Children—Use and dose must be determined by your doctor.

Missed dose—If you miss a dose of this medicine, take it as soon as possible. However, if it is almost time for your next dose, skip the missed dose and go back to your regular dosing schedule. Do not double doses.

Storage—Store the medicine in a closed container at room temperature, away from heat, moisture, and direct light. Keep from freezing.

Keep out of the reach of children.

Do not keep outdated medicine or medicine no longer needed.

Precautions While Using This Medicine

It is important that your doctor check your progress at regular visits. Your doctor may want to do certain tests to see if the medicine is working properly or to see if certain side effects may be occurring without your knowing it.

If itching, redness, swelling, or other signs of eye or eyelid irritation occur, check with your doctor. These signs may mean that you are allergic to ophthalmic dorzolamide.

This medicine may cause some people to have blurred vision for a short time. Make sure you know how you react to this medicine before you drive, use machines, or do anything else that could be dangerous if you cannot see properly. Also, since blurred vision may be a sign of a side effect that needs medical attention, check with your doctor if it continues.

Ophthalmic dorzolamide may cause your eyes to become more sensitive to light than they are normally. Wearing sunglasses and avoiding too much exposure to bright light may help lessen the discomfort. If the discomfort continues, check with your doctor.

Side Effects of This Medicine

Along with its needed effects, a medicine may cause some unwanted effects. Although not all of these side effects may occur, if they do occur they may need medical attention.

Check with your doctor as soon as possible if any of the following side effects occur:
  More common
    Itching, redness, swelling, or other sign of eye or eyelid irritation
  Less common
    Burning, dry or itching eyes; discharge from the eye; excessive tearing; redness, pain, or swelling of eye, eyelid, or inner lining of eyelid
  Rare
    Blurred vision; eye pain; skin rash; symptoms of kidney stone (blood in urine, nausea or vomiting, or pain in side, back, or abdomen); tearing
  Incidence not known—occurred during clinical practice
    Change in vision; cough; difficult or labored breathing; flashes of light; floaters in vision; hives or welts; itching skin; large, hive-like swelling on face, eyelids, lips, tongue, throat, hands, legs, feet, sex organs; noisy breathing; redness of skin; shortness of breath; tightness in chest; wheezing

Some side effects may occur that usually do not need medical attention. These side effects may go away during treatment as your body adjusts to the medicine. Also, your health care professional may be able to tell you about ways to prevent or reduce some of these side effects. Check with your health care professional if any of the following side effects continue or are bothersome or if you have any questions about them:
  More common
    Bitter taste; burning, stinging, or discomfort when medicine is applied; feeling of something in eye; sensitivity of eyes to light
  Less common
    Dryness of eyes; eyelid reactions; headache; nausea; unusual tiredness or weakness

Incidence not known—occurred during clinical practice
    Blistering, burning, crusting, dryness, flaking of skin; bloody nose; burning, crawling, itching, numbness, prickling, "pins and needles", or tingling feelings; change in distance vision; difficulty in focusing eyes; dizziness; dry mouth; eyelid crusting; scaling of skin; severe redness, soreness, swelling of skin

Other side effects not listed may also occur in some patients. If you notice any other effects, check with your healthcare professional.

DORZOLAMIDE AND TIMOLOL
(Ophthalmic route) - dor-ZOLE-a-mide, TYE-moe-lole

Commonly used brand name(s)

In the U.S.—
    Cosopt Ocumeter
    Cosopt Ocumeter Plus

Available Dosage Forms:
  • Solution

Therapeutic Class: Antiglaucoma, Beta-Adrenergic Blocker/ Carbonic Anhydrase Inhibitor Combination
Pharmacologic Class: Dorzolamide

Uses For This Medicine

Dorzolamide and timolol combination medicine contains a carbonic anhydrase inhibitor (dorzolamide) and a beta-adrenergic blocking agent (timolol). It is used in the eye to treat increased pressure in the eye caused by open-angle glaucoma and a condition called hypertension of the eye.

This medicine is available only with your doctor's prescription.

Before Using This Medicine

In deciding to use a medicine, the risks of taking the medicine must be weighed against the good it will do. This is a decision you and your doctor will make. For this medicine, the following should be considered:

Allergies—Tell your doctor if you have ever had any unusual or allergic reaction to this medicine or any other medicines. Also tell your health care professional if you have any other types of allergies, such as to foods, dyes, preservatives, or animals. For non-prescription products, read the label or package ingredients carefully.

Pediatric—This medicine has been tested in children 2 years of age and older and, in effective doses, has not been shown to cause different side effects or problems than it does in adults.

Geriatric—Many medicines have not been studied specifically in older people. Therefore, it may not be known whether they work exactly the same way they do in younger adults or if they cause different side effects or problems in older people. There is no specific information comparing use of this medicine in the elderly with use in other age groups.

Other medicines—

Using this medicine with any of the following medicines is usually not recommended, but may be required in some cases. If both medicines are prescribed together, your doctor may change the dose or how often you use one or both of the medicines.

Amiodarone, Clonidine, Epinephrine, Fenoldopam, Fentanyl, Verapamil

Interactions with Food/Tobacco/Alcohol—Certain medicines should not be used at or around the time of eating food or eating certain types of food since interactions may occur. Using alcohol or tobacco with certain medicines may also cause interactions to occur. Discuss with your healthcare professional the use of your medicine with food, alcohol, or tobacco.

Other medical problems—The presence of other medical problems may affect the use of this medicine. Make sure you tell your doctor if you have any other medical problems, especially:

- Allergy, history of—Severity and duration of allergic reactions to other substances may be increased
- Asthma or
- Bronchitis or
- Emphysema or
- Lung problems, other—This medicine can increase trouble in breathing
- Bradycardia (unusually slow heartbeat) or
- Heart problems, other—There is a risk of further decreased heart function
- Diabetes mellitus (sugar diabetes) or
- Hypoglycemia—If your blood sugar becomes too low, this medicine may cover up some of the symptoms
- Kidney disease, severe—Effects of this medicine may be increased because of its slower removal from the body
- Myasthenia gravis—This medicine may make this condition worse
- Overactive thyroid—This medicine may cover up fast heartbeat, which is a sign of overactive thyroid

Proper Use of This Medicine

To use:

- The bottle is only partially full to provide proper drop control.
- First, wash your hands. Tilt the head back and, pressing your finger gently on the skin just beneath the lower eyelid, pull the lower eyelid away from the eye to make a space. Drop the medicine into this space. Let go of the eyelid and gently close the eyes. Do not blink. Keep the eyes closed and apply pressure to the inner corner of the eye with your finger for 1 or 2 minutes to allow the medicine to be absorbed by the eye.
- Immediately after using the eye drops, wash your hands to remove any medicine that may be on them.
- To keep the medicine as germ-free as possible, do not touch the applicator tip to any surface (including the eye). Also, keep the container tightly closed. Serious damage to the eye and possible loss of vision may result from using contaminated eye drops.

Use this medicine only as directed by your doctor. Do not use more of it and do not use it more often than your doctor ordered. To do so may increase the chance of too much medicine being absorbed into the body and the chance of side effects.

If your doctor ordered two different eye drops to be used together, wait at least 10 minutes between the times you apply the medicines. This will help to keep the second medicine from "washing out" the first one.

Dosing—The dose of this medicine will be different for different patients. Follow your doctor's orders or the directions on the label. The following information includes only the average doses of this medicine. If your dose is different, do not change it unless your doctor tells you to do so.

The amount of medicine that you take depends on the strength of the medicine. Also, the number of doses you take each day, the time allowed between doses, and the length of time you take the medicine depend on the medical problem for which you are using the medicine.

- For ophthalmic dosage form (eye drops):
  - For glaucoma or hypertension of the eye:
    - Adults—Use 1 drop of the medicine in the affected eye(s) two times a day.
    - Children—Use and dose must be determined by your doctor.

Missed dose—If you miss a dose of this medicine, take it as soon as possible. However, if it is almost time for your next dose, skip the missed dose and go back to your regular dosing schedule. Do not double doses.

Storage—Store the medicine in a closed container at room temperature, away from heat, moisture, and direct light. Keep from freezing.

Keep out of the reach of children.

Do not keep outdated medicine or medicine no longer needed.

Precautions While Using This Medicine

It is important that your doctor check your progress at regular visits to make sure that this medicine is working properly and is not causing unwanted effects.

If itching, redness, swelling, or other signs of eye or eyelid irritation occur, stop using this medicine and check with your doctor. These signs may mean that you are allergic to this medicine.

Before you have any kind of surgery, dental treatment, or emergency treatment, tell the medical doctor or dentist in charge that you are using this medicine. This medicine contains an ophthalmic beta-adrenergic blocking agent. Using an ophthalmic beta-adrenergic blocking agent during this time may cause an increased risk of side effects.

It is very important that you check with your doctor if you get an injury or infection in your eye or if you are scheduled to have eye surgery. Your doctor will tell you whether to keep using the same container of eye drops or whether you should start using a fresh bottle of eye drops.

For diabetic patients:

- This medicine may cover up some signs of hypoglycemia (low blood sugar). If you notice a change in the results of your blood or urine sugar tests or if you have any questions, check with your doctor.

This medicine contains benzalkonium chloride, which may be absorbed by contact lenses. Take soft contact lenses out before using this medicine. Lenses may be put back in 15 minutes after using the medicine.

Side Effects of This Medicine

Along with its needed effects, a medicine may cause some unwanted effects. Although not all of these side effects may occur, if they do occur they may need medical attention.

Check with your doctor as soon as possible if any of the following side effects occur:

More common
Blurred vision; feeling of something in eye; itching of the eye; redness of eye and lining of eyelid; sensitivity of eyes to light

Less common
Back, abdominal, or stomach pain; change in vision; coughing, shortness of breath, troubled breathing, tightness in chest, or wheezing; discharge from eye; dizziness; eye or eyelid pain, swelling, discomfort, or irritation; increased blood pressure; increased frequency of urination or painful urination; itching of eyelid; seeing flashes or sparks of light; seeing floating spots before the eyes; swelling of lining of eyelid; tiny bumps on lining of eyelid

Rare
Blood in urine; blue lips, fingernails, or skin; chest pain or discomfort; diarrhea; difficult or troubled breathing; fainting; lightheadedness or fainting; headache or weakness, severe and sudden; irregular, fast or slow, or shallow breathing; mental depression; nausea or vomiting; pain, numbness, tingling, or burning feeling in hands or feet; shortness of breath; skin rash; slow or irregular heartbeat; sweating; unusual tiredness or weakness

Some side effects may occur that usually do not need medical attention. These side effects may go away during treatment as your body adjusts to the medicine. Also, your health care professional may be able to tell you about ways to prevent or reduce some of these side effects. Check with your health care professional if any of the following side effects continue or are bothersome or if you have any questions about them:

More common
Bitter, sour, or unusual taste; burning or stinging of the eye (when medicine is applied)

Less common
Cold- or flu-like symptoms; crusting or scales on eyelid; dryness of eyes; headache; indigestion or upset stomach; sore throat; stuffy or runny nose; tearing of eye

Other side effects not listed may also occur in some patients. If you notice any other effects, check with your healthcare professional.

DOXAZOSIN (Oral route) - dox-AY-zoe-sin

Commonly used brand name(s)

In the U.S.—
Cardura
Cardura XL

Available Dosage Forms:
- Tablet, Extended Release
- Tablet

Therapeutic Class: Cardiovascular Agent
Pharmacologic Class: Alpha-1 Adrenergic Blocker

Uses For This Medicine

Doxazosin belongs to the general class of medicines called antihypertensives. It is used to treat high blood pressure (hypertension).

High blood pressure adds to the workload of the heart and arteries. If it continues for a long time, the heart and arteries may not function properly. This can damage the blood vessels of the brain, heart, and kidneys, resulting in a stroke, heart failure, or kidney failure. High blood pressure may also increase the risk of heart attacks. These problems may be less likely to occur if blood pressure is controlled.

Doxazosin works by relaxing blood vessels so that blood passes through them more easily. This helps to lower blood pressure.

Doxazosin is also used to treat benign (noncancerous) enlargement of the prostate (benign prostatic hyperplasia [BPH]). Benign enlargement of the prostate is a problem that can occur in men as they get older. The prostate gland is located below the bladder. As the prostate gland enlarges, certain muscles in the gland may become tight and get in the way of the tube that drains urine from the bladder. This can cause problems in urinating, such as a need to urinate often, a weak stream when urinating, or a feeling of not being able to empty the bladder completely.

Doxazosin helps relax the muscles in the prostate and the opening of the bladder. This may help increase the flow of urine and/or decrease the symptoms. However, doxazosin will not shrink the prostate. The prostate may continue to get larger. This may cause the symptoms to become worse over time. Therefore, even though doxazosin may lessen the problems caused by enlarged prostate now, surgery still may be needed in the future.

Doxazosin is available only with your doctor's prescription.

Before Using This Medicine

In deciding to use a medicine, the risks of taking the medicine must be weighed against the good it will do. This is a decision you and your doctor will make. For this medicine, the following should be considered:

Allergies—Tell your doctor if you have ever had any unusual or allergic reaction to this medicine or any other medicines. Also tell your health care professional if you have any other types of allergies, such as to foods, dyes, preservatives, or animals. For non-prescription products, read the label or package ingredients carefully.

Pediatric—Studies on this medicine have been done only in adult patients, and there is no specific information comparing use of doxazosin in children with use in other age groups.

Geriatric—Dizziness, lightheadedness, or fainting may be especially likely to occur in elderly patients with high blood pressure, because these patients are usually more sensitive than younger adults to the effects of doxazosin.

Pregnancy—

	Pregnancy Category	Explanation
All Trimesters	C	Animal studies have shown an adverse effect and there are no adequate studies in pregnant women OR no animal studies have been conducted and there are no adequate studies in pregnant women.

Breast Feeding—

There are no adequate studies in women for determining infant risk when using this medication during breastfeeding. Weigh the potential benefits against the potential risks before taking this medication while breastfeeding.

Other medicines—

Using this medicine with any of the following medicines is usually not recommended, but may be required in some cases. If both medicines are prescribed together, your doctor may change the dose or how often you use one or both of the medicines.

Tadalafil, Vardenafil

Interactions with Food/Tobacco/Alcohol—

Certain medicines should not be used at or around the time of eating food or eating certain types of food since interactions may occur. Using alcohol or tobacco with certain medicines may also cause interactions to occur. Discuss with your healthcare professional the use of your medicine with food, alcohol, or tobacco.

Other medical problems—

The presence of other medical problems may affect the use of this medicine. Make sure you tell your doctor if you have any other medical problems, especially:

- Gastrointestinal (stomach and intestines) blockage—May increase the effect of doxazosin which could increase the chance of side effects.
- Heart problems—May make condition worse.
- Hypotension (decrease in blood pressure)—Possible increased chance of fainting, especially after the first dose or a dose increase of this medicine.
- Kidney disease—Possible increased sensitivity to the effects of doxazosin
- Liver disease—The effects of doxazosin may be increased, which may increase the chance of side effects
- Prostate cancer—Your doctor will want to make sure that you do not have prostate cancer before starting you on this medicine.

Proper Use of This Medicine

For the regular tablet—To help you remember to take your medicine, try to get into the habit of taking it at the same time each day.

For the extended-release tablet—

- Take in the morning with breakfast each day.
- Swallow whole. Do not crush or chew.
- Your doctor will not prescribe the extended-release tablet form of this medicine for high blood pressure. It can only be used in men for benign enlargement of the prostate.

For patients taking this medicine for high blood pressure:

- In addition to the use of the medicine your doctor has prescribed, treatment for your high blood pressure may include weight control and care in the types of foods you eat, especially foods high in sodium. Your doctor will tell you which of these are most important for you. You should check with your doctor before changing your diet.
- Many patients who have high blood pressure will not notice any signs of the problem. In fact, many may feel normal. It is very important that you take your medicine exactly as directed and that you keep your appointments with your doctor even if you feel well.
- Remember that doxazosin will not cure your high blood pressure but it does help control it. Therefore, you must continue to take it as directed if you expect to lower your blood pressure and keep it down. You may have to take high blood pressure medicine for the rest of your life. If high blood pressure is not treated, it can cause serious problems such as heart failure, blood vessel disease, stroke, or kidney disease.

For patients taking this medicine for benign enlargement of the prostate:

- Remember that doxazosin will not shrink the size of your prostate but it does help to relieve the symptoms of this condition. You may still need to have surgery later.
- It may take up to 2 weeks before your symptoms improve.

Dosing—

The dose of this medicine will be different for different patients. Follow your doctor's orders or the directions on the label. The following information includes only the average doses of this medicine. If your dose is different, do not change it unless your doctor tells you to do so.

The amount of medicine that you take depends on the strength of the medicine. Also, the number of doses you take each day, the time allowed between doses, and the length of time you take the medicine depend on the medical problem for which you are using the medicine.

- For oral dosage form (tablets):
  - For benign enlargement of the prostate:
    - Adults—At first, 1 milligram (mg) once a day, in the morning or in the evening. Your doctor may increase your dose slowly up to 8 mg once a day.
  - For high blood pressure:
    - Adults—1 mg once a day to start. Your doctor may increase your dose slowly to as much as 16 mg once a day.
    - Children—Use and dose must be determined by your doctor.

- For oral dosage form (extended-release tablets):
  - For benign enlargement of the prostate:
    - Adults—At first, 4 milligram (mg) once a day, in the morning with breakfast. Your doctor may increase your dose slowly up to 8 mg once a day.

Missed dose—

If you miss a dose of this medicine, take it as soon as possible. However, if it is almost time for your next dose, skip the missed dose and go back to your regular dosing schedule. Do not double doses.

Storage—

Store the medicine in a closed container at room temperature, away from heat, moisture, and direct light. Keep from freezing.

Keep out of the reach of children.

Do not keep outdated medicine or medicine no longer needed.

Precautions While Using This Medicine

It is important that your doctor check your progress at regular visits to make sure that this medicine is working properly. This is especially important for elderly patients, who may be more sensitive to the effects of this medicine.

For patients taking this medicine for high blood pressure:
- Do not take other medicines unless they have been discussed with your doctor. This especially includes over-the-counter (nonprescription) medicines for appetite control, asthma, colds, cough, hay fever, or sinus problems, since they may tend to increase your blood pressure.

Dizziness, lightheadedness, or sudden fainting may occur after you take this medicine, especially when you get up from a lying or sitting position. These effects are more likely to occur when you take the first dose of this medicine. Taking the first dose at bedtime may prevent problems. However, be especially careful if you need to get up during the night. These effects may also occur with any doses you take after the first dose. Getting up slowly may help lessen this problem. If you feel dizzy, lie down so that you do not faint. Then sit for a few moments before standing to prevent the dizziness from returning.

The dizziness, lightheadedness, or sudden fainting is more likely to occur if you drink alcohol, stand for a long time, exercise, or if the weather is hot. While you are taking this medicine, be careful to limit the amount of alcohol you drink. Also, use extra care during exercise or hot weather or if you must stand for a long time.

Doxazosin may cause some people to become drowsy or less alert than they are normally. Make sure you know how you react to this medicine before you drive, use machines, or do anything else that could be dangerous if you are dizzy, drowsy, or are not alert. After you have taken several doses of this medicine, these effects should lessen.

The possibility of priapism, a painful or prolonged erection of the penis, is a rare side effect that can occur when taking doxazosin and must have immediate medical attention.

Side Effects of This Medicine

Along with its needed effects, a medicine may cause some unwanted effects. Although not all of these side effects may occur, if they do occur they may need medical attention.

Check with your doctor as soon as possible if any of the following side effects occur:

More common
Dizziness or lightheadedness

Less common
Blurred vision; confusion; dizziness, faintness, or light-headedness when getting up from a lying or sitting position; fainting (sudden); fast and pounding heartbeat; irregular heartbeat; shortness of breath; sweating; swelling of feet or lower legs

Rare
Painful or prolonged erection of the penis (called priapism), although extremely rare, must have immediate medical attention. If painful or prolonged erection occurs, call your doctor or go to an emergency room as soon as possible

Incidence not known
Abdominal or stomach pain; area rash; black, tarry stools; bleeding gums; blood in urine or stools; chest pain or discomfort; chills; clay-colored stools; cough; dark urine; diarrhea; difficulty breathing; difficult, burning, or painful urination; fever; general tiredness and weakness; headache, sudden and severe; inability to speak; itching; lab results that show problems with liver; light-colored stools; loss of appetite; noisy breathing; pain or discomfort in arms, jaw, back or neck; pinpoint red or purple spots on skin; rash; seizures; slow or irregular heartbeat; slurred speech; sore throat; sores, ulcers, or white spots on lips or in mouth; swollen glands; temporary blindness; tightness in chest; unpleasant breath odor; unusual bleeding or bruising; upper right abdominal pain; vomiting; vomiting of blood; weakness in arm and/or leg on one side of the body, sudden and severe; wheezing; yellow eyes and skin

Some side effects may occur that usually do not need medical attention. These side effects may go away during treatment as your body adjusts to the medicine. Also, your health care professional may be able to tell you about ways to prevent or reduce some of these side effects. Check with your health care professional if any of the following side effects continue or are bothersome or if you have any questions about them:

More common
Headache; lack or loss of strength; unusual tiredness or weakness

Less common
Acid or sour stomach; back pain; belching; bladder pain; cloudy urine; difficulty in moving; frequent urge to urinate; heartburn; indigestion; joint pain; lower back or side pain; muscle aching, cramping, or weakness; muscle pains or stiffness; nausea; nervousness, restlessness, unusual irritability; runny nose; sleepiness or drowsiness; sneezing; sore throat; stomach discomfort, upset or pain; swollen joints

Incidence not known
Anxiety; burning, crawling, itching, numbness, prickling, "pins and needles", or tingling feeling; change in frequency or urination; dry mouth; feeling of warmth; frequent urination; general feeling of discomfort or illness; hair loss; hives or welts; hyperventilation; increased urge to urinate during the night; increased volume of pale dilute urine; loss of appetite; painful urination; redness of skin; redness of the face, neck, arms and occasionally upper chest; shaking; swelling of the breasts or breast soreness in both females and males; thinning of hair; trouble in holding or releasing urine; trouble sleeping; waking to urinate at night; weight loss

Other side effects not listed may also occur in some patients. If you notice any other effects, check with your healthcare professional.

DOXEPIN   (Topical route) - DOX-e-pin

Commonly used brand name(s)

In the U.S.—
Prudoxin
Zonalon

Available Dosage Forms:
- Cream

Therapeutic Class: Dermatological Agent
Pharmacologic Class: Antidepressant, Tricyclic

Uses For This Medicine

Topical doxepin is used to relieve itching in patients with certain types of eczema. It appears to work by preventing the effects of histamine, which is a substance produced by the body that causes itching.

Doxepin is available only with your doctor's prescription.

Before Using This Medicine

In deciding to use a medicine, the risks of taking the medicine must be weighed against the good it will do. This is a decision you and your doctor will make. For this medicine, the following should be considered:

Allergies—Tell your doctor if you have ever had any unusual or allergic reaction to this medicine or any other medicines. Also tell your health care professional if you have any other types of allergies, such as to foods, dyes, preservatives, or animals. For non-prescription products, read the label or package ingredients carefully.

Pediatric—Studies on this medicine have been done only in adult patients, and there is no specific information comparing use of doxepin in children with use in other age groups.

Geriatric—Many medicines have not been studied specifically in older people. Therefore, it may not be known whether they work exactly the same way they do in younger adults. Although there is no specific information comparing use of doxepin in the elderly with use in other age groups, this medicine is not expected to cause different side effects or problems in older people than it does in younger adults.

Pregnancy—

	Pregnancy Category	Explanation
All Trimesters	B	Animal studies have revealed no evidence of harm to the fetus, however, there are no adequate studies in pregnant women OR animal studies have shown an adverse effect, but adequate studies in pregnant women have failed to demonstrate a risk to the fetus.

Breast Feeding—Studies in women breastfeeding have demonstrated harmful infant effects. An alternative to this medication should be prescribed or you should stop breastfeeding while using this medicine.

Other medicines—

Using this medicine with any of the following medicines is not recommended. Your doctor may decide not to treat you with this medication or change some of the other medicines you take.

Bepridil, Cisapride, Grepafloxacin, Isocarboxazid, Levomethadyl, Mesoridazine, Moclobemide, Pimozide, Sparfloxacin, Terfenadine, Thioridazine, Tranylcypromine, Ziprasidone

Interactions with Food/Tobacco/Alcohol—Certain medicines should not be used at or around the time of eating food or eating certain types of food since interactions may occur. Using alcohol or tobacco with certain medicines may also cause interactions to occur. The following interactions have been selected on the basis of their potential significance and are not necessarily all-inclusive.

Using this medicine with any of the following may cause an increased risk of certain side effects but may be unavoidable in some cases. If used together, your doctor may change the dose or how often you use this medicine or give you special instructions about the use of food, alcohol, or tobacco.

Ethanol

Other medical problems—The presence of other medical problems may affect the use of this medicine. Make sure you tell your doctor if you have any other medical problems, especially:
- Glaucoma or
- Urinary tract blockage or difficult urination—Using topical doxepin may make these conditions worse

Proper Use of This Medicine

Topical doxepin is for external use only. Do not use this medicine orally, do not use it on the eyes, or inside of the vagina.

Use this medicine exactly as directed. Do not use more of it, do not use it more often, and do not use it for more than 8 days. Also, do not apply it to an area of skin larger than recommended by your doctor. To do so may increase the chance of side effects.

Apply a thin layer of doxepin cream to only the affected area(s) of the skin and rub in gently.

To help clear up your skin problem it is very important that you keep using topical doxepin for the full time of treatment. Do not miss any doses.

Do not cover with a bandage or otherwise wrap the area of skin being treated. This may increase the amount of medicine that gets into the bloodstream, thereby increasing the chance of side effects.

Dosing—The dose of this medicine will be different for different patients. Follow your doctor's orders or the directions on the label. The following information includes only the average doses of this medicine. If your dose is different, do not change it unless your doctor tells you to do so.

The amount of medicine that you take depends on the strength of the medicine. Also, the number of doses you take each day, the time allowed between doses, and the length of time you take the medicine depend on the medical problem for which you are using the medicine.

- For topical dosage form (cream):
  - For itching due to eczema:
    - Adults—Apply a thin layer to the affected area(s) of the skin four times a day. Space the doses or applications at least three or four hours apart. Treatment may be continued for up to eight days.
    - Children—Use and dose must be determined by your doctor.

Missed dose—If you miss a dose of this medicine, apply it as soon as possible. However, if it is almost time for your next dose, skip the missed dose and go back to your regular dosing schedule.

Storage—Store the medicine in a closed container at room temperature, away from heat, moisture, and direct light. Keep from freezing.

Keep out of the reach of children.

Do not keep outdated medicine or medicine no longer needed.

Precautions While Using This Medicine

If your skin problem does not improve after 8 days or if it becomes worse, check with your doctor.

This medicine will add to the effects of alcohol (alcoholic beverages or other alcohol-containing preparations [e.g., elixirs, cough syrups, tonics]) and other CNS depressants (medicines that slow down the nervous system, possibly causing drowsiness). Some examples of CNS depressants are antihistamines or medicine for hay fever, other allergies, or colds; sedatives, tranquilizers, or sleeping medicine; prescription pain medicine or narcotics; barbiturates; medicine for seizures; muscle relaxants; or anesthetics, including some dental anesthetics. Check with your doctor before taking any of the above while you are using this medicine.

Topical doxepin may cause some people to become drowsy. Make sure you know how to react to this medicine before you drive, use machines, or do other jobs that require you to be alert. If too much drowsiness occurs, it may be necessary to use less medicine, use it less often, or stop using it completely. However, check with your doctor first before lessening your dose or stopping use of this medicine.

This medicine may cause dryness of the mouth. For temporary relief, use sugarless gum or candy, or melt bits of ice in your mouth, or use a saliva substitute. However, if your mouth continues to feel dry for more than 2 weeks, check with your medical doctor or dentist. Continuing dryness of the mouth may increase the chance of dental disease, including tooth decay, gum disease, and fungus infections.

Side Effects of This Medicine

Along with its needed effects, a medicine may cause some unwanted effects. Although not all of these side effects may occur, if they do occur they may need medical attention.

Check with your doctor as soon as possible if any of the following side effects occur:

More common
   Burning, crawling, or tingling sensation of the skin; swelling at the site of application; worsening of eczema and itching

Rare
   Fever

Symptoms of overdose
   Abdominal pain and swelling; blurring of vision; convulsions (seizures); decreased awareness or responsiveness; difficulty in breathing; difficulty in passing urine; dizziness, fainting, or lightheadedness; drowsiness; enlarged pupils; excessive dryness of mouth; extremely high fever or body temperature; extremely low body temperature; fast heartbeat; increased or excessive unconscious or jerking movements; incurable constipation; irregular heartbeat; unconsciousness; vomiting; weak pulse

Some side effects may occur that usually do not need medical attention. These side effects may go away during treatment as your body adjusts to the medicine. Also, your health care professional may be able to tell you about ways to prevent or reduce some of these side effects. Check with your health care professional if any of the following side effects continue or are bothersome or if you have any questions about them:

More common
   Burning and/or stinging at the site of application; changes in taste; dizziness; drowsiness; dryness and tightness of skin; dryness of mouth and/or lips; emotional changes; headache; thirst; unusual tiredness or weakness

Less common
   Anxiety; irritation, tingling, scaling, and cracking of skin; nausea

Other side effects not listed may also occur in some patients. If you notice any other effects, check with your healthcare professional.

DOXORUBICIN   (Intravenous route) -
dox-oh-ROO-bi-sin

Black Box Warning

Severe local tissue necrosis will occur if there is extravasation during administration. Doxorubicin must not be given by the intramuscular or subcutaneous route.

Myocardial toxicity manifested in its most severe form by potentially fatal congestive heart failure may occur either during therapy or months to years after termination of therapy. The probability of developing impaired myocardial function based on a combined index of signs, symptoms and decline in left ventricular ejection fraction (LVEF) is estimated to be 1% to 2% at a total cumulative dose of 300 mg/m(2) of doxorubicin, 3% to 5% at a dose of 400 mg/m(2), 5% to 8% at 450 mg/m(2) and 6% to 20% at 500 mg/m(2). The risk of developing congestive heart failure (CHF) increases rapidly with increasing total cumulative doses of doxorubicin in excess of 450 mg/m(2). Risk factors (active or dormant cardiovascular disease, prior or concomitant radiotherapy to the mediastinal/pericardial area, previous therapy with other anthracyclines or anthracenediones, concomitant use of other cardiotoxic drugs) may increase the risk of cardiac toxicity. Cardiac toxicity with doxorubicin may occur at lower cumulative doses whether or not cardiac risk factors are present. Pediatric patients are at increased risk for developing delayed cardiotoxicity.

Secondary acute myelogenous leukemia (AML) has been reported in patients treated with anthracyclines, including doxorubicin. The occurrence of refractory secondary leukemia is more common when such drugs are given in combination with DNA-damaging anti-neoplastic agents, when patients have been heavily pretreated with cytotoxic drugs, or when doses of anthracyclines have been escalated. The rate of developing treatment-related leukemia was estimated in an analysis of 1474 breast cancer patients who received adjuvant treatment with doxorubicin-containing regimens (i.e., FAC) in clinical trials. The estimated risk of developing treatment-related leukemia at 10 years was 2.5% for the 810 patients receiving radiotherapy plus chemotherapy and 0.5% for the 664 patients receiving chemotherapy alone. The overall risk was estimated at 1.5% at 10 years for the entire patient population. Pediatric patients are also at risk of developing secondary AML.

Dosage should be reduced in patients with impaired hepatic function.

Severe myelosuppression may occur.

Doxorubicin should be administered only under the supervision of a physician who is experienced in the use of cancer chemotherapeutic agents.

Commonly used brand name(s)

In the U.S.—
  Adriamycin

Available Dosage Forms:
  • Solution
  • Powder for Solution

Therapeutic Class: Antineoplastic Agent

Uses For This Medicine

Doxorubicin belongs to the general group of medicines known as antineoplastics. It is used to treat some kinds of cancers of the blood; lymph system; bladder; breast; stomach; lung; ovaries; thyroid; nerves; kidneys; bones; and soft tissues, including muscles and tendons. It may also be used to treat other kinds of cancer, as determined by your doctor.

Doxorubicin seems to interfere with the growth of cancer cells, which are then eventually destroyed by the body. Since the growth of normal body cells may also be affected by doxorubicin, other effects will also occur. Some of these may be serious and must be reported to your doctor. Other effects, like hair loss, may not be serious but may cause concern. Some effects may not occur until months or years after the medicine is used.

Before you begin treatment with doxorubicin, you and your doctor should talk about the good this medicine will do as well as the risks of using it.

Doxorubicin is to be administered only by or under the supervision of your doctor.

Once a medicine has been approved for marketing for a certain use, experience may show that it is also useful for other medical problems. Although these uses are not included in product labeling, doxorubicin is used in certain patients with the following medical conditions:
  • Autoimmune deficiency syndrome (AIDS)–associated Kaposi's sarcoma (a type of cancer of the skin and mucous membranes that is more common in patients with AIDS)
  • Cancer of the adrenal cortex (the outside layer of the adrenal gland)
  • Cancer of the cervix
  • Cancer of the endometrium
  • Cancer of the esophagus
  • Cancers of the head and neck
  • Cancer of the liver
  • Cancer of the pancreas
  • Cancer of the prostate
  • Cancer of the thymus (a small organ found under the breast bone)
  • Carcinoid tumors
  • Chronic lymphocytic leukemia (a type of cancer of the blood and lymph system)
  • Ewing's sarcoma (a type of cancer found in the bone)
  • Gestational trophoblastic tumors (tumors in the uterus or womb)
  • Hepatoblastoma (a certain type of liver cancer that occurs in children)
  • Multiple myeloma (a certain type of cancer of the blood)
  • Non–small cell lung cancer (a certain type of lung cancer usually associated with prior smoking, passive smoking, or radon exposure)
  • Retinoblastoma (a type of eye cancer found primarily in children)
  • Tumors in the ovaries

Before Receiving This Medicine

In deciding to use a medicine, the risks of taking the medicine must be weighed against the good it will do. This is a decision you and your doctor will make. For this medicine, the following should be considered:

Allergies—Tell your doctor if you have ever had any unusual or allergic reaction to this medicine or any other medicines. Also tell your health care professional if you have any other types of allergies, such as to foods, dyes, preservatives, or animals. For non-prescription products, read the label or package ingredients carefully.

Pediatric—Heart problems are more likely to occur in children younger than 2 years of age, who are usually more sensitive to the effects of doxorubicin.

Geriatric—Heart problems are more likely to occur in the elderly, who are usually more sensitive to the effects of doxorubicin. The elderly may also be more likely to have blood problems.

Pregnancy—

	Pregnancy Category	Explanation
All Trimesters	D	Studies in pregnant women have demonstrated a risk to the fetus. However, the benefits of therapy in a life threatening situation or a serious disease, may outweigh the potential risk.

Breast Feeding—Studies in women breastfeeding have demonstrated harmful infant effects. An alternative to this medication should be prescribed or you should stop breast-feeding while using this medicine.

Other medicines—

Using this medicine with any of the following medicines is not recommended. Your doctor may decide not to treat you with this medication or change some of the other medicines you take.

Rotavirus Vaccine, Live

Interactions with Food/Tobacco/Alcohol—Certain medicines should not be used at or around the time of eating food or eating certain types of food since interactions may occur. Using alcohol or tobacco with certain medicines may also cause interactions to occur. Discuss with your healthcare professional the use of your medicine with food, alcohol, or tobacco.

Other medical problems—The presence of other medical problems may affect the use of this medicine. Make sure you tell your doctor if you have any other medical problems, especially:
  • Chickenpox (including recent exposure) or
  • Herpes zoster (shingles)—Risk of severe disease affecting other parts of the body
  • Gout or
  • Kidney stones—Doxorubicin may increase levels of uric acid in the body, which can cause gout or kidney stones

- Heart disease—Risk of heart problems caused by doxorubicin may be increased
- Liver disease—Effects of doxorubicin may be increased because of its slower removal from the body

Proper Use of This Medicine

Doxorubicin is sometimes given together with certain other medicines. If you are receiving a combination of medicines, it is important that you receive each one at the proper time. If you are taking some of these medicines by mouth, ask your health care professional to help you plan a way to take them at the right times.

While you are using this medicine, your doctor may want you to drink extra fluids so that you will pass more urine. This will help prevent kidney problems and keep your kidneys working well.

Doxorubicin often causes nausea and vomiting. However, it is very important that you continue to receive the medication, even if you begin to feel ill. Ask your health care professional for ways to lessen these effects.

Dosing—The dose of this medicine will be different for different patients. Follow your doctor's orders or the directions on the label. The following information includes only the average doses of this medicine. If your dose is different, do not change it unless your doctor tells you to do so.

The amount of medicine that you take depends on the strength of the medicine. Also, the number of doses you take each day, the time allowed between doses, and the length of time you take the medicine depend on the medical problem for which you are using the medicine.

Precautions After Receiving This Medicine

It is very important that your doctor check your progress at regular visits to make sure that this medicine is working properly and to check for unwanted effects.

While you are being treated with doxorubicin, and after you stop treatment with it, do not have any immunizations (vaccinations) without your doctor's approval. Doxorubicin may lower your body's resistance, and there is a chance you might get the infection the immunization is meant to prevent. In addition, other persons living in your household should not take oral polio vaccine, since there is a chance they could pass the polio virus on to you. Also, avoid persons who have taken oral polio vaccine within the last several months. Do not get close to them, and do not stay in the same room with them for very long. If you cannot take these precautions, you should consider wearing a protective face mask that covers the nose and mouth.

Doxorubicin can temporarily lower the number of white blood cells in your blood, increasing the chance of getting an infection. It can also lower the number of platelets, which are necessary for proper blood clotting. If this occurs, there are certain precautions you can take, especially when your blood count is low, to reduce the risk of infection or bleeding:

- If you can, avoid people with infections. Check with your doctor immediately if you think you are getting an infection or if you get a fever or chills, cough or hoarseness, lower back or side pain, or painful or difficult urination.
- Check with your doctor immediately if you notice any unusual bleeding or bruising; black, tarry stools; blood in urine or stools; or pinpoint red spots on your skin.

- Be careful when using a regular toothbrush, dental floss, or toothpick. Your medical doctor, dentist, or nurse may recommend other ways to clean your teeth and gums. Check with your medical doctor before having any dental work done.
- Do not touch your eyes or the inside of your nose unless you have just washed your hands and have not touched anything else in the meantime.
- Be careful not to cut yourself when you are using sharp objects such as a safety razor or fingernail or toenail cutters.
- Avoid contact sports or other situations where bruising or injury could occur.

If doxorubicin accidentally seeps out of the vein into which it is injected, it may damage some tissues and cause scarring. Tell the doctor or nurse right away if you notice redness, pain, or swelling at the place of injection.

Side Effects of This Medicine

Along with its needed effects, a medicine may cause some unwanted effects. Although not all of these side effects may occur, if they do occur they may need medical attention.

Also, because of the way these medicines act on the body, there is a chance that they might cause other unwanted effects that may not occur until months or years after the medicine is used. These delayed effects may include certain types of cancer, such as leukemia. Discuss these possible effects with your doctor.

Check with your doctor immediately if any of the following side effects occur:
> *Less common*
>> Fast or irregular heartbeat; pain at place of injection; shortness of breath; swelling of feet and lower legs
> *Rare*
>> Black, tarry stools; blood in urine; pinpoint red spots on skin; unusual bleeding or bruising; wheezing

Check with your doctor as soon as possible if any of the following side effects occur:
> *More common*
>> Sores in mouth and on lips
> *Less common*
>> Cough or hoarseness accompanied by fever or chills; darkening or redness of skin (if you recently had radiation treatment); fever or chills; joint pain; lower back or side pain accompanied by fever or chills; painful or difficult urination accompanied by fever or chills; red streaks along injected vein; stomach pain
> *Rare*
>> Skin rash or itching

Some side effects may occur that usually do not need medical attention. These side effects may go away during treatment as your body adjusts to the medicine. Also, your health care professional may be able to tell you about ways to prevent or reduce some of these side effects. Check with your health care professional if any of the following side effects continue or are bothersome or if you have any questions about them:
> *More common*
>> Nausea and vomiting
> *Less common*
>> Darkening of soles, palms, or nails; diarrhea

Doxorubicin causes the urine to turn reddish in color, which may stain clothes. This is not blood. It is to be expected and only lasts for 1 or 2 days after each dose is given.

This medicine often causes a temporary and total loss of hair. After treatment with doxorubicin has ended, normal hair growth should return.

After you stop using this medicine, it may still produce some side effects that need attention. During this period of time, *check with your doctor immediately* if you notice the following side effects:

Fast or irregular heartbeat; shortness of breath; swelling of feet and lower legs

Other side effects not listed may also occur in some patients. If you notice any other effects, check with your healthcare professional.

DOXORUBICIN HYDROCHLORIDE LIPOSOME (Intravenous route) - dox-oh-ROO-bi-sin hye-droe-KLOR-ide LYE-poh-some

Black Box Warning

Myocardial damage may lead to congestive heart failure and may be encountered as the total cumulative dose of doxorubicin hydrochloride (HCl) approaches 550 mg/m(2). The use of doxorubicin HCl liposome injection may lead to cardiac toxicity. In a large clinical study in patients with advanced breast cancer, 250 patients received doxorubicin HCl liposome at a starting dose of 50 mg/m(2) every 4 weeks. At all cumulative anthracycline doses between 450 mg/m(2) to 500 mg/m(2) or between 500 mg/m(2) to 550 mg/m(2), the risk of cardiac toxicity for patients treated with doxorubicin HCl liposome was 11%. Prior use of other anthracyclines or anthracenediones should be included in calculations of total cumulative dosage. Cardiac toxicity may also occur at lower cumulative doses in patients with prior mediastinal irradiation or who are receiving concurrent cyclophosphamide therapy.

Acute infusion-related reactions including, but not limited to, flushing, shortness of breath, facial swelling, headache, chills, back pain, tightness in the chest or throat, and/or hypotension have occurred in up to 10% of patients treated with doxorubicin HCl liposome. In most patients, these reactions resolve over the course of several hours to a day once the infusion is terminated. In some patients, the reaction has resolved with slowing of the infusion rate. Serious and sometimes life-threatening or fatal allergic/anaphylactoid-like infusion reactions have been reported. Medications to treat such reactions, as well as emergency equipment, should be available for immediate use. Doxorubicin HCl liposome should be administered at an initial rate of 1 mg/min to minimize the risk of infusion reactions.

Severe myelosuppression may occur.

Dosage should be reduced in patients with impaired hepatic function.

Accidental substitution of doxorubicin HCl liposome for doxorubicin HCl has resulted in severe side effects. Doxorubicin HCl liposome should not be substituted for doxorubicin HCl on a mg per mg basis.

Doxorubicin HCl liposome should be administered only under the supervision of a physician who is experienced in the use of cancer chemotherapeutic agents.

Commonly used brand name(s)

In the U.S.—
Doxil

Available Dosage Forms:
• Solution

Therapeutic Class: Antineoplastic Agent

Uses For This Medicine

Liposomal doxorubicin belongs to the general group of medicines known as antineoplastics. It is used to treat some kinds of cancer.

Liposomal doxorubicin seems to interfere with the growth of cancer cells, which are eventually destroyed. Since the growth of normal body cells may also be affected by liposomal doxorubicin, other effects will also occur. Some of these may be serious and must be reported to your doctor. Other effects, like hair loss, may not be serious but may cause concern. Some effects may not occur for months or years after the medicine is used.

Before you begin treatment with liposomal doxorubicin, you and your doctor should talk about the good this medicine will do as well as the risks of using it.

Liposomal doxorubicin is to be administered only by or under the immediate supervision of your doctor.

Once a medicine has been approved for marketing for a certain use, experience may show that it is also useful for other medical problems. Although these uses are not included in product labeling, liposomal doxorubicin is used in certain patients with the following medical conditions:
• Cancer of the breast
• Multiple myeloma

Before Receiving This Medicine

In deciding to use a medicine, the risks of taking the medicine must be weighed against the good it will do. This is a decision you and your doctor will make. For this medicine, the following should be considered:

Allergies—Tell your doctor if you have ever had any unusual or allergic reaction to this medicine or any other medicines. Also tell your health care professional if you have any other types of allergies, such as to foods, dyes, preservatives, or animals. For non-prescription products, read the label or package ingredients carefully.

Pediatric—There is no specific information comparing the use of liposomal doxorubicin in children with use in any other age group. Safety and efficacy of liposomal doxorubicin in children have not been established. However, problems are more likely to occur in children younger than 2 years of age, who are usually more sensitive to the effects of the active ingredient, doxorubicin.

Geriatric—This medicine has been tested in a limited number of patients 60 years of age or older and has not been shown to cause different side effects in older people than it does in younger adults. However, problems are more likely to occur in the elderly, who are usually more sensitive to the effects of the active ingredient, doxorubicin. The elderly are also more likely to have blood problems.

Other medicines—

Using this medicine with any of the following medicines is not recommended. Your doctor may decide not to treat you with this medication or change some of the other medicines you take.

Rotavirus Vaccine, Live

Interactions with Food/Tobacco/Alcohol—Certain medicines should not be used at or around the time of eating food or eating certain types of food since interactions may occur. Using alcohol or tobacco with certain medicines may also cause interactions to occur. Discuss with your healthcare professional the use of your medicine with food, alcohol, or tobacco.

Other medical problems—The presence of other medical problems may affect the use of this medicine. Make sure you tell your doctor if you have any other medical problems, especially:

- Chickenpox (including recent exposure) or
- Herpes zoster (shingles)—Risk of severe disease affecting other parts of the body
- Heart disease—Risk of heart problems caused by liposomal doxorubicin may be increased
- Infection—Liposomal doxorubicin can decrease your body's ability to fight infection
- Liver disease—Effects of liposomal doxorubicin may be increased because of slower removal from the body

Proper Use of This Medicine

Liposomal doxorubicin is sometimes given together with certain other medicines. If you are using a combination of medicines, it is important that you receive each one at the proper time. If you are taking some of these medicines by mouth, ask your health care professional to help you plan a way to take them at the right times.

While you are receiving liposomal doxorubicin, your doctor may want you to drink extra fluids so that you will pass more urine. This will help prevent kidney problems and keep your kidneys working well.

This medicine often causes nausea and vomiting. However, it is very important that you continue to receive it, even if you begin to feel ill. Ask your health care professional for ways to lessen these effects.

Dosing—The dose of this medicine will be different for different patients. Follow your doctor's orders or the directions on the label. The following information includes only the average doses of this medicine. If your dose is different, do not change it unless your doctor tells you to do so.

The amount of medicine that you take depends on the strength of the medicine. Also, the number of doses you take each day, the time allowed between doses, and the length of time you take the medicine depend on the medical problem for which you are using the medicine.

Precautions After Receiving This Medicine

It is very important that your doctor check your progress at regular visits to make sure that this medicine is working properly and to check for unwanted effects.

While you are being treated with liposomal doxorubicin, and after you stop treatment with it, do not have any immunizations (vaccinations) without your doctor's approval. Liposomal doxorubicin may lower your body's resistance and there is a chance you might get the infection the immunization is meant to prevent. In addition, other persons living in your household should not take oral poliovirus vaccine since there is a chance they could pass the poliovirus on to you. Also, avoid persons who have taken oral poliovirus vaccine. Do not get close to them, and do not stay in the same room with them for very long. If you cannot take these precautions, you should consider wearing a protective face mask that covers the nose and the mouth.

Liposomal doxorubicin can temporarily lower the number of white blood cells in your blood, increasing the chance of getting an infection. It can also lower the number of platelets, which are necessary for proper blood clotting. If this occurs, there are certain precautions you can take, especially when your blood count is low, to reduce the risk of infection or bleeding:

- If you can, avoid people with infections. Check with your doctor immediately if you think you are getting an infection or if you get a fever or chills, cough or hoarseness, lower back or side pain, or painful or difficult urination.
- Check with your doctor immediately if you notice any unusual bleeding or bruising; black, tarry stools; blood in urine or stools; or pinpoint red spots on your skin.
- Do not touch your eyes or the inside of your nose unless you have just washed your hands and have not touched anything else in the meantime.
- Be careful not to cut yourself when you are using sharp objects such as a safety razor or fingernail or toenail cutters.
- Avoid contact sports or other situations where bruising or injury can occur.

If liposomal doxorubicin accidentally seeps out of the vein into which it is injected, it may damage some tissues and cause scarring. Tell the doctor or nurse right away if you notice redness, pain, or swelling at the place of injection.

Be careful when using a regular toothbrush, dental floss, or toothpick. Your medical doctor, dentist, or nurse may recommend other ways to clean your teeth and gums. Check with your medical doctor before having any dental work done.

Side Effects of This Medicine

Along with its needed effects, a medicine may cause some unwanted effects. Although not all of these side effects may occur, if they do occur they may need medical attention.

Check with your doctor as soon as possible if any of the following side effects occur:

More common—in any treatment group
   Black, tarry stools; blistering, peeling, redness, and/or swelling of palms of hands or bottoms of feet; blood in urine or stools; chills; cough or hoarseness; facial swelling; fever; headache; loss of strength and energy; low blood pressure; lower back or side pain; numbness, pain, tingling, or unusual sensations in palms of hands or bottoms of feet; painful or difficult urination; pinpoint red spots on skin; shortness of breath; sore throat; sores in mouth and on lips; unusual bleeding or bruising; unusual tiredness or weakness

Less common—in any treatment group
   Skin rash or itching

Rare—in any treatment group
   chest pain; decreased urine output; dilated neck veins; extreme fatigue; irregular breathing; irregular heart-

beat; shortness of breath; swelling of face, fingers, feet, or lower legs; tightness in chest; troubled breathing; weight gain; wheezing; Yellowing of the eyes and skin

Less common— for patients being treated for Kaposi's sarcoma
Cough; fever; pain at place of injection; troubled breathing; wheezing

Rare— for patients being treated for Kaposi's sarcoma
Blurred or loss of vision; eye pain; flushed, dry skin; frequent urination; fruit-like breath odor; unusual thirst

Less common— for patients being treated for ovarian cancer
Chest pain; decreased urination; rapid weight gain; bloating or swelling of face, hands, lower legs, and/or feet; fever or chills; cough or hoarseness; lower back or side pain; painful or difficult urination

Rare— for patients being treated for ovarian cancer
Cough; difficulty swallowing; hives; pain at place of injection; puffiness or swelling of the eyelids or around the eyes, face, lips or tongue; shortness of breath; tightness in chest; wheezing

Symptoms of overdose
Black, tarry stools; blood in urine or stools; cough or hoarseness accompanied by fever or chills; fever or chills; lower back or side pain accompanied by fever or chills; painful or difficult urination accompanied by fever or chills; pinpoint red spots on skin; sores in mouth and on lips; unusual bleeding or bruising

Some side effects may occur that usually do not need medical attention. These side effects may go away during treatment as your body adjusts to the medicine. Also, your health care professional may be able to tell you about ways to prevent or reduce some of these side effects. Check with your health care professional if any of the following side effects continue or are bothersome or if you have any questions about them:

More common—in any treatment group
Diarrhea; nausea; vomiting

Less common—in any treatment group
Back pain; difficulty swallowing; dizziness

More common—for patients being treated for Kaposi's sarcoma
Creamy white, curd-like patches in mouth or throat; pain when eating or swallowing

Less common—for patients being treated for Kaposi's sarcoma
Constipation; headache

More common—for patients being treated for ovarian cancer
Abdominal or stomach pain; loss of appetite; changes in the lining of the mouth or nose; constipation; headache; pain; rash; sore throat; tingling, burning, or prickly sensations

Less common—for patients being treated for ovarian cancer
Anxiety; bad, unusual, or unpleasant (after)taste; burning, dry, or itching eyes; difficulty swallowing; change in taste; excessive tearing; itching skin; muscle aches; redness, pain, swelling of eye, eyelid, or inner lining of eyelid; trouble sleeping

Rare—for patients being treated for ovarian cancer
Shakiness and unsteady walk; clumsiness, unsteadiness, trembling, or other problems with muscle control

or coordination; change in sense of smell; chills; cough; fever; general feeling of discomfort or illness; increased white vaginal discharge; joint pain; nausea; shivering; sore throat; sweating; thinking abnormal; vomiting

Liposomal doxorubicin causes the urine to turn reddish in color, which may stain clothes. This is not blood. It is to be expected and only lasts for 1 or 2 days after each dose is given.

Some side effects may occur that usually do not need medical attention. These side effects may go away during treatment as your body adjusts to the medicine. Also, your health care professional may be able to tell you about ways to prevent or reduce some of these side effects. Check with your health care professional if any of the following side effects continue or are bothersome or if you have any questions about them:

More common—for patients being treated for ovarian cancer
Dry skin

Less common—for patients being treated for ovarian cancer
Change in skin color

This medicine often causes a temporary and total loss of hair. After treatment with liposomal doxorubicin has ended, normal hair growth should return.

After you stop using this medicine, it may still produce some side effects that need attention. During this period of time, *check with your doctor immediately* if you notice the following side effects:
Fast or irregular heartbeat; shortness of breath; swelling of feet and lower legs

Other side effects not listed may also occur in some patients. If you notice any other effects, check with your healthcare professional.

DRONABINOL (Oral route) - droe-NAB-i-nol

Commonly used brand name(s)
In the U.S.—
Marinol

Available Dosage Forms:
- Capsule, Liquid Filled
- Capsule

Therapeutic Class: Antiemetic

Uses For This Medicine

Dronabinol is used to prevent the nausea and vomiting that may occur after treatment with cancer medicines. It is used only when other kinds of medicine for nausea and vomiting do not work. Dronabinol is also used to increase appetite in patients with acquired immunodeficiency syndrome (AIDS).

Dronabinol is available only with your doctor's prescription.

Before Using This Medicine

In deciding to use a medicine, the risks of taking the medicine must be weighed against the good it will do. This is a decision

you and your doctor will make. For this medicine, the following should be considered:

Allergies—Tell your doctor if you have ever had any unusual or allergic reaction to this medicine or any other medicines. Also tell your health care professional if you have any other types of allergies, such as to foods, dyes, preservatives, or animals. For non-prescription products, read the label or package ingredients carefully.

Pediatric—Although there is no specific information comparing use of dronabinol in children with use in other age groups, the effects that this medicine may have on the mind may be of special concern in children. Children should be watched closely while they are taking this medicine.

Geriatric—This medicine has been tested in a limited number of patients up to 82 years of age and has not been shown to cause different side effects or problems in older people than it does in younger adults. However, the effects this medicine may have on the mind may be of special concern in the elderly. Therefore, older people should be watched closely while they are taking this medicine.

Pregnancy—

	Pregnancy Category	Explanation
All Trimesters	C	Animal studies have shown an adverse effect and there are no adequate studies in pregnant women OR no animal studies have been conducted and there are no adequate studies in pregnant women.

Breast Feeding—There are no adequate studies in women for determining infant risk when using this medication during breastfeeding. Weigh the potential benefits against the potential risks before taking this medication while breastfeeding.

Other medicines—Although certain medicines should not be used together at all, in other cases two different medicines may be used together even if an interaction might occur. In these cases, your doctor may want to change the dose, or other precautions may be necessary. Tell your healthcare professional if you are taking any other prescription or non-prescription (over-the-counter [OTC]) medicine.

Interactions with Food/Tobacco/Alcohol—Certain medicines should not be used at or around the time of eating food or eating certain types of food since interactions may occur. Using alcohol or tobacco with certain medicines may also cause interactions to occur. Discuss with your healthcare professional the use of your medicine with food, alcohol, or tobacco.

Other medical problems—The presence of other medical problems may affect the use of this medicine. Make sure you tell your doctor if you have any other medical problems, especially:

- Alcohol abuse (or history of) or
- Drug abuse or dependence (or history of)—Dependence on dronabinol may develop
- Bipolar disorder (manic or depressive states) or
- Heart disease or
- High blood pressure (hypertension) or
- Severe mental illness—Dronabinol may make the condition worse

Proper Use of This Medicine

Take this medicine only as directed by your physician. Do not take more of it, do not take it more often, and do not take it for a longer time than your doctor ordered. If too much is taken, it may lead to medical problems because of an overdose.

Dosing—The dose of this medicine will be different for different patients. Follow your doctor's orders or the directions on the label. The following information includes only the average doses of this medicine. If your dose is different, do not change it unless your doctor tells you to do so.

The amount of medicine that you take depends on the strength of the medicine. Also, the number of doses you take each day, the time allowed between doses, and the length of time you take the medicine depend on the medical problem for which you are using the medicine.

- For oral dosage form (capsules):
  - For nausea and vomiting caused by cancer medicines:
    - Adults and teenagers—Dose is based on body surface area. Your doctor will tell you how much medicine to take and when to take it.
    - Children—Dose is based on body surface area and must be determined by your doctor.
  - For increasing appetite in patients with AIDS:
    - Adults and teenagers—To start, 2.5 milligrams (mg) two times a day, taken before lunch and supper. Your doctor may change your dose depending on your condition. However, the dose is usually not more than 20 mg a day.
    - Children—Use and dose must be determined by your doctor.

Missed dose—If you miss a dose of this medicine, take it as soon as possible. However, if it is almost time for your next dose, skip the missed dose and go back to your regular dosing schedule. Do not double doses.

Storage—Store in the refrigerator. Do not freeze.

Keep out of the reach of children.

Do not keep outdated medicine or medicine no longer needed.

Precautions While Using This Medicine

Dronabinol will add to the effects of alcohol and other CNS depressants (medicines that make you drowsy or less alert). Some examples of CNS depressants are antihistamines or medicine for hay fever, other allergies, or colds; sedatives, tranquilizers, or sleeping medicine; prescription pain medicines including other narcotics; barbiturates; medicine for seizures; muscle relaxants; or anesthetics, including some dental anesthetics. Check with your doctor before taking any of the above while you are taking this medicine.

This medicine may cause some people to become drowsy, dizzy, or lightheaded, or to feel a false sense of well-being. Make sure you know how you react to this medicine before you drive, use machines, or do anything else that could be dangerous if you are dizzy or are not alert and clearheaded.

Dizziness, lightheadedness, or fainting may occur, especially when you get up suddenly from a lying or sitting position. Getting up slowly may help lessen this problem.

If you think you or someone else may have taken an overdose of dronabinol, get emergency help at once. Taking an overdose of this medicine or taking alcohol or CNS depressants with this medicine may lead to severe mental effects. Signs of overdose include changes in mood, confusion, hallucinations, mental depression, nervousness or anxiety, and fast or pounding heartbeat.

Side Effects of This Medicine

Along with its needed effects, a medicine may cause some unwanted effects. Although not all of these side effects may occur, if they do occur they may need medical attention.

Check with your doctor as soon as possible if any of the following side effects occur:

Less common (may also be signs of overdose)
Amnesia (memory loss); changes in mood; confusion; delusions; feelings of unreality; hallucinations (seeing, hearing, or feeling things that are not there); mental depression; nervousness or anxiety; fast or pounding heartbeat

Symptoms of overdose
Being forgetful; change in your sense of smell, taste, sight, sound, or touch; change in how fast you think time is passing; constipation; decrease in motor coordination; drowsiness (severe); dryness of mouth (severe); false sense of well-being; fast or pounding heartbeat; feeling dizzy or lightheaded, especially when getting up from a lying or sitting position; feeling sluggish; mood changes; panic reaction; problems in urinating; redness of eyes; seizures; slurred speech; unusual drowsiness or dullness

Some side effects may occur that usually do not need medical attention. These side effects may go away during treatment as your body adjusts to the medicine. Also, your health care professional may be able to tell you about ways to prevent or reduce some of these side effects. Check with your health care professional if any of the following side effects continue or are bothersome or if you have any questions about them:

More common
Clumsiness or unsteadiness; dizziness; drowsiness; false sense of well-being; nausea; trouble thinking; vomiting

Less common or rare
Blurred vision or any changes in vision; dryness of mouth; feeling faint or lightheaded, especially when getting up from a lying or sitting position; flushing of face; restlessness; unusual tiredness or weakness

Other side effects not listed may also occur in some patients. If you notice any other effects, check with your healthcare professional.

DROPERIDOL   (Injection route) - droe-PER-i-dole

Commonly used brand name(s)

In the U.S.—
Inapsine

Available Dosage Forms:
- Solution
- Injectable

Therapeutic Class: Antiemetic
Pharmacologic Class: Dopamine Antagonist

Uses For This Medicine

Droperidol is used to reduce the amount of nausea and vomiting you may have after surgery or other procedures.

This medicine is available only with your doctor's prescription.

Once a medicine has been approved for marketing for a certain use, experience may show that it is also useful for other medical problems. Although these uses are not included in product labeling, droperidol is used
- In certain patients with severe agitation and combativeness
- To produce sleepiness or drowsiness before surgery or certain procedures

For patients receiving this medicine for severe agitation and combativeness, the dose administered will depend on the degree of agitation and the size of the patient.

Before Receiving This Medicine

In deciding to use a medicine, the risks of taking the medicine must be weighed against the good it will do. This is a decision you and your doctor will make. For this medicine, the following should be considered:

Allergies—Tell your doctor if you have ever had any unusual or allergic reaction to this medicine or any other medicines. Also tell your health care professional if you have any other types of allergies, such as to foods, dyes, preservatives, or animals. For non-prescription products, read the label or package ingredients carefully.

Pediatric—Droperidol has not been studied in children up to 2 years of age. There is no specific information comparing the use of droperidol in children with use in other age groups. However, based on experience with similar drugs, children may be more likely than older patients to experience side effects after receiving droperidol, such as muscle spasms in the tongue, face, neck, and back, and inability to move the eyes.

Geriatric—Older patients may be more likely than younger adult patients to experience dizziness and excessive sleepiness from droperidol. Older patients may also have problems with unusual heartbeats from droperidol

Pregnancy—

	Pregnancy Category	Explanation
All Trimesters	C	Animal studies have shown an adverse effect and there are no adequate studies in pregnant women OR no animal studies have been conducted and there are no adequate studies in pregnant women.

Breast Feeding—There are no adequate studies in women for determining infant risk when using this medication during breastfeeding. Weigh the potential benefits against the potential risks before taking this medication while breastfeeding.

Other medicines—

Using this medicine with any of the following medicines is not recommended. Your doctor may decide not to treat you with this medication or change some of the other medicines you take.

Acetophenazine, Bepridil, Bromperidol, Cisapride, Clozapine, Levomethadyl, Mesoridazine, Molindone, Perphenazine, Pimozide, Pipamperone, Remoxipride, Thioridazine, Tiapride, Triflupromazine, Ziprasidone

Interactions with Food/Tobacco/Alcohol—Certain medicines should not be used at or around the time of eating food or eating certain types of food since interactions may occur. Using alcohol or tobacco with certain medicines may also cause interactions to occur. Discuss with your healthcare professional the use of your medicine with food, alcohol, or tobacco.

Other medical problems—The presence of other medical problems may affect the use of this medicine. Make sure you tell your doctor if you have any other medical problems, especially:

- Age over 65 or
- Alcoholism or
- Congestive heart failure or
- Enlargement of the heart or
- Hypokalemia (too little potassium in the blood) or
- Hypomagnesemia (too little magnesium in the blood) or
- Irregular heartbeat
- Slow heartbeat—Droperidol may increase the risk of irregular heartbeats
- Epilepsy—The risk of seizures may be increased
- Heart disease or
- Mental depression or
- Parkinsonism—Droperidol may worsen these conditions
- Hypovolemia—The risk of dizziness may be increased
- Liver disease—The risk of side effects may be increased
- Pheochromocytoma—High blood pressure and rapid heart rate may occur

Proper Use of This Medicine

Dosing—The dose of this medicine will be different for different patients. Follow your doctor's orders or the directions on the label. The following information includes only the average doses of this medicine. If your dose is different, do not change it unless your doctor tells you to do so.

The amount of medicine that you take depends on the strength of the medicine. Also, the number of doses you take each day, the time allowed between doses, and the length of time you take the medicine depend on the medical problem for which you are using the medicine.

- Your age;
- Your general physical condition;
- The reason you are receiving droperidol; and
- Other medicines you are taking or will receive before or after droperidol is given.

Precautions After Receiving This Medicine

For patients going home within a few hours after surgery:
- Droperidol and other medicines that may be given during surgery may cause some people to feel drowsy, tired, or

weak for up to a few days afterwards. Therefore, for at least 24 hours (or longer if necessary) after receiving this medicine, do not drive, use machines, or do anything else that could be dangerous if you are dizzy or are not alert.
- Unless otherwise directed by your medical doctor, do not drink alcoholic beverages or take other central nervous system (CNS) depressants (medicines that slow down the nervous system, possibly causing drowsiness) for about 24 hours after you have received this medicine. To do so may add to the effects of droperidol. Some examples of CNS depressants are antihistamines or medicine for hay fever, other allergies, or colds; sedatives, tranquilizers, or sleeping medicine; prescription pain medicine or narcotics; barbiturates; medicine for seizures; and muscle relaxants.

Side Effects of This Medicine

Along with its needed effects, a medicine may cause some unwanted effects. Although not all of these side effects may occur, if they do occur they may need medical attention.

Check with your doctor as soon as possible if any of the following side effects occur:
Less common
> Anxiety; high blood pressure; restlessness

Rare
> Fainting; fever; fixed upward position of the eyeballs; irregular or slow heart rate; spasm of the muscles of the tongue, face, neck, and back; sudden death

Other side effects not listed may also occur in some patients. If you notice any other effects, check with your healthcare professional.

Symptoms of overdose
> Dizziness; fixed upward position of the eyeballs; restlessness; slowed breathing; spasm of the muscles of the tongue, face, neck, and back

Some side effects may occur that usually do not need medical attention. These side effects may go away during treatment as your body adjusts to the medicine. Also, your health care professional may be able to tell you about ways to prevent or reduce some of these side effects. Check with your health care professional if any of the following side effects continue or are bothersome or if you have any questions about them:
More common
> Drowsiness; lightheadedness; rapid heart rate

Other side effects not listed may also occur in some patients. If you notice any other effects, check with your healthcare professional.

DROSPIRENONE AND ESTRADIOL
(Oral route) - droh-SPYE-re-none, es-tra-DYE-ole

Black Box Warning

Estrogens with or without progestins should not be used for the prevention of cardiovascular disease or dementia.

The Women's Health Initiative (WHI) study reported increased risks of myocardial infarction, stroke, invasive breast cancer, pulmonary emboli, and deep vein thrombosis in post-menopausal women (50 to 79 years of age) during 5 years of treatment with oral conjugated equine estrogens (CE 0.625mg) combined with medroxyprogesterone acetate (MPA 2.5mg) relative to placebo.

The Women's Health Initiative Memory Study (WHIMS), a substudy of WHI, reported increased risk of developing probable dementia in postmenopausal women 65 years of age or older during 5.2 years of treatment with conjugated estrogens alone and during 4 years of treatment with oral conjugated estrogens plus medroxyprogesterone acetate, relative to placebo. It is unknown whether this finding applies to younger postmenopausal women.

Other doses of oral conjugated estrogens with medroxyprogesterone acetate, and other combinations and dosage forms of estrogens and progestins were not studied in the WHI clinical trials, and, in the absence of comparable data, these risks should be assumed to be similar. Because of these risks, estrogens with or without progestins should be prescribed at the lowest effective doses and for the shortest duration consistent with treatment goals and risks for the individual woman.

Uses For This Medicine

Drospirenone and estradiol are female hormones called progestins and estrogens that make up this combination medicine. These female hormones are produced by the body and are necessary for the normal sexual development of the female and for the regulation of the menstrual cycle during the childbearing years.

The ovaries begin to produce less estrogen after menopause (the change of life). This medicine is prescribed to make up for the lower amount of estrogen in postmenopausal women who still have a uterus. Estrogen helps relieve signs of menopause, such as hot flashes and unusual sweating, chills, faintness, or dizziness. Estrogen can also help to relieve a genital skin condition called vaginal or vulvar atrophy. Progestin helps to regulate the effects of estradiol.

This medicine is available only with your doctor's prescription.

Before Using This Medicine

In deciding to use a medicine, the risks of taking the medicine must be weighed against the good it will do. This is a decision you and your doctor will make. For this medicine, the following should be considered:

Allergies—Tell your doctor if you have ever had any unusual or allergic reaction to this medicine or any other medicines. Also tell your health care professional if you have any other types of allergies, such as to foods, dyes, preservatives, or animals. For non-prescription products, read the label or package ingredients carefully.

Geriatric—Many medicines have not been studied specifically in older people. Therefore, it may not be known whether they work exactly the same way they do in younger adults or if they cause different side effects or problems in older people. However, use of drospirenone/estradiol by postmenopausal women 65 years of age and older may increase the chances of dementia.

Pregnancy—

	Pregnancy Category	Explanation
All Trimesters	X	Studies in animals or pregnant women have demonstrated positive evidence of fetal abnormalities. This drug should not be used in women who are or may become pregnant because the risk clearly outweighs any possible benefit.

Breast Feeding—

Drospirenone
- Studies in women breastfeeding have demonstrated harmful infant effects. An alternative to this medication should be prescribed or you should stop breastfeeding while using this medicine.

Estradiol
- Studies suggest that this medication may alter milk production or composition. If an alternative to this medication is not prescribed, you should monitor the infant for side effects and adequate milk intake.

Other medicines—

Using this medicine with any of the following medicines may cause an increased risk of certain side effects, but using both drugs may be the best treatment for you. If both medicines are prescribed together, your doctor may change the dose or how often you use one or both of the medicines.

Alprazolam, Aprepitant, Bexarotene, Bosentan, Clarithromycin, Fosamprenavir, Ginseng, Itraconazole, Ketoconazole, Lamotrigine, Levothyroxine, Licorice, Prednisolone, St John's Wort, Tacrine, Tipranavir

Interactions with Food/Tobacco/Alcohol—Certain medicines should not be used at or around the time of eating food or eating certain types of food since interactions may occur. Using alcohol or tobacco with certain medicines may also cause interactions to occur. The following interactions have been selected on the basis of their potential significance and are not necessarily all-inclusive.

Using this medicine with any of the following may cause an increased risk of certain side effects but may be unavoidable in some cases. If used together, your doctor may change the dose or how often you use this medicine, or give you special instructions about the use of food, alcohol, or tobacco.

Grapefruit Juice

Other medical problems—The presence of other medical problems may affect the use of this medicine. Make sure you tell your doctor if you have any other medical problems, especially:
- Abnormal genital or vaginal bleeding of unknown causes or
- Adrenal gland problems or
- Breast cancer, known, suspected or history of, or
- Cancer of the uterus or
- Liver problems or disease—This medicine should NOT be used.
- Asthma or
- Diabetes or
- Endometriosis or

- Epilepsy (seizures) or
- High cholesterol or triglycerides (or history of) or
- Hypocalcemia (too little calcium in the blood) or
- Hyponatremia (too little sodium in the blood) or
- Liver tumor, benign, or
- Lupus or
- Migraine or
- Porphyria (problem with metabolism causing stomach pain and mental confusion)—This medicine should be used with caution. It can cause these conditions to become worse.
- Blood clots in deep veins or the pulmonary artery or
- Heart attack, active or recent (within the past year) or
- Stroke, active or recent—This medicine should NOT be used.
- Blood clot risk factors (e.g., obesity, personal or family history of blood clots, or lupus) or
- Heart disease risk factors (e.g., diabetes, high cholesterol, high blood pressure, obesity, tobacco use)—Your doctor will help you lower your chances of having heart disease.
- Heart problems or
- Liver problems—These conditions could be affected by fluid retention (e.g., water weight gain). The patient should be observed when taking this medicine because estradiol may cause some fluid retention.
- Hypothyroid (too little thyroid hormone)—Dose of thyroid medicine may need to be increased.

Proper Use of This Medicine

Read the enclosed patient leaflet carefully before taking this medicine.

You should not take this medicine if you have had a hysterectomy.

You should not take this medicine to prevent heart disease or dementia.

Tell your doctor if you take any medicine or supplement that increases potassium levels. Your doctor may want to prescribe a different medicine for you or have your blood tested to check potassium levels.

Swallow the tablet whole. Do not crush or chew.

Dosing—The dose of this medicine will be different for different patients. Follow your doctor's orders or the directions on the label. The following information includes only the average doses of this medicine. If your dose is different, do not change it unless your doctor tells you to do so.

The amount of medicine that you take depends on the strength of the medicine. Also, the number of doses you take each day, the time allowed between doses, and the length of time you take the medicine depend on the medical problem for which you are using the medicine.

- For oral dosage forms (tablets):
  - For treating a genital skin condition (vaginal or vulvar atrophy), or vasomotor symptoms of menopause:
    - Adults—Oral, 1 tablet (drospirenone 0.5 milligram (mg)/estradiol 1 mg) once a day.

Missed dose—Call your doctor or pharmacist for instructions.

Storage—Keep out of the reach of children.

Store the medicine in a closed container at room temperature, away from heat, moisture, and direct light. Keep from freezing.

Do not keep outdated medicine or medicine no longer needed.

Precautions While Using This Medicine

It is very important that your doctor check you at regular visits every 3 to 6 months to discuss whether you need to continue taking this medicine.

If you are going to have surgery or will be on bed rest, you need to inform your doctor. You may need to stop taking drospirenone/estradiol during this time.

Check with your doctor immediately if vaginal bleeding occurs.

It is important that you check your breasts by self-examination regularly and have clinical examinations and mammographies as required by your doctor. Report unusual breast lumps or discharge right away.

If you are scheduled for any lab tests, tell your doctor or lab technician that you are taking this medicine. Certain blood tests are affected by estradiol.

Tell your doctor about any risk factors for heart disease that you may have, such as high blood pressure, diabetes, tobacco use, high cholesterol, and obesity. It is important that you work with your doctor to lower these risk factors.

Side Effects of This Medicine

Along with its needed effects, a medicine may cause some unwanted effects. Although not all of these side effects may occur, if they do occur they may need medical attention.

Also, because of the way these medicines act on the body, there is a chance that they might cause other unwanted effects that may not occur until months or years after the medicine is used. These may include certain types of cancer, such as leukemia or bladder cancer. Discuss these possible effects with your doctor.

Check with your doctor immediately if any of the following side effects occur:

More common
  Breast pain; full or bloated feeling; heavy nonmenstrual vaginal bleeding; pressure in the stomach; surgery; swelling of abdominal or stomach area

Less common
  Bloating or swelling of face, arms, hands, legs, or feet; change in vaginal discharge; increased clear or white vaginal discharge; pain or feeling of pressure in pelvis; rapid weight gain; tingling of hands or feet; unusual weight gain or loss; vaginal bleeding

Incidence not known
  Abdominal pain; anxiety; blurred vision; change in vision; chest pain or discomfort; clear or bloody discharge from nipple; confusion; constipation; cough; coughing up blood; depression; difficulty in speaking; dimpling of breast skin; dizziness or lightheadedness; double vision; dry mouth; fainting; fast heartbeat; headache; headache, severe and throbbing; inability to move arms, legs, or facial muscles; inability to speak; incoherent speech; increased urination; inverted nipple; loss of appetite; lump in breast or under the arm;

metallic taste; muscle weakness; nausea and vomiting; numbness or weakness in your arm or leg, or on one side of your body; pain or discomfort in arms, jaw, back, or neck; pain or redness in your lower leg (calf); persistent crusting or scaling of nipple; poor insight and judgment; problems with memory, vision, speech, or walking; redness or swelling of breast; seeing double; shortness of breath; slow speech; sore on the skin of the breast that does not heal; sudden or severe headache; sudden shortness of breath or troubled breathing; sweating; thirst; trouble recognizing objects; trouble thinking and planning; trouble walking; unusual tiredness or weakness; weight loss

Some side effects may occur that usually do not need medical attention. These side effects may go away during treatment as your body adjusts to the medicine. Also, your health care professional may be able to tell you about ways to prevent or reduce some of these side effects. Check with your health care professional if any of the following side effects continue or are bothersome or if you have any questions about them:

More common

Accidental injury; back pain; body aches or pain; chills; diarrhea; difficulty in breathing; ear congestion; fever, sneezing, or sore throat; general feeling of discomfort or illness; joint pain; loss of voice; muscle aches and pains; nasal congestion; pain in arms or legs; pain or tenderness around eyes and cheekbones; runny nose; shivering; stuffy or runny nose; sweating; tightness of chest or wheezing; trouble sleeping

Other side effects not listed may also occur in some patients. If you notice any other effects, check with your healthcare professional.

DROTRECOGIN ALFA (Intravenous route) - droe-tre-KOH-jen AL-fa

Commonly used brand name(s)

In the U.S.—
Xigris

Available Dosage Forms:
• Powder for Solution

Therapeutic Class: Anticoagulant
Pharmacologic Class: Profibrinolytic

Uses For This Medicine

Drotrecogin alfa is used to treat severe cases of sepsis, a life threatening infection in the blood. This medicine has been shown to reduce the risk of death in patients with severe sepsis who are at high risk of death. This medicine works by decreasing inflammation and the formation of blood clots in blood vessels.

This medicine is available only with your doctor's prescription.

Before Using This Medicine

In deciding to use a medicine, the risks of taking the medicine must be weighed against the good it will do. This is a decision you and your doctor will make. For this medicine, the following should be considered:

Allergies—Tell your doctor if you have ever had any unusual or allergic reaction to this medicine or any other medicines. Also tell your health care professional if you have any other types of allergies, such as to foods, dyes, preservatives, or animals. For non-prescription products, read the label or package ingredients carefully.

Pediatric—Studies on this medicine have been done only in adult patients, and there is no specific information on the safety and effectiveness of drotrecogin alfa in children.

Geriatric—This medicine has been tested and has not been shown to cause different side effects or problems in older people than it does in younger adults.

Pregnancy—

	Pregnancy Category	Explanation
All Trimesters	C	Animal studies have shown an adverse effect and there are no adequate studies in pregnant women OR no animal studies have been conducted and there are no adequate studies in pregnant women.

Breast Feeding—There are no adequate studies in women for determining infant risk when using this medication during breastfeeding. Weigh the potential benefits against the potential risks before taking this medication while breastfeeding.

Other medicines—Although certain medicines should not be used together at all, in other cases two different medicines may be used together even if an interaction might occur. In these cases, your doctor may want to change the dose, or other precautions may be necessary. Tell your healthcare professional if you are taking any other prescription or non-prescription (over-the-counter [OTC]) medicine.

Interactions with Food/Tobacco/Alcohol—Certain medicines should not be used at or around the time of eating food or eating certain types of food since interactions may occur. Using alcohol or tobacco with certain medicines may also cause interactions to occur. Discuss with your healthcare professional the use of your medicine with food, alcohol, or tobacco.

Other medical problems—The presence of other medical problems may affect the use of this medicine. Make sure you tell your doctor if you have any other medical problems, especially:

• Aneurysm (swelling in a blood vessel) especially in the head or

• Blood disease or a history of unusual bleeding or

• Brain problems which may include bleeding, disease, injury or tumor or

• Injury to any part of the body or

• Liver disease or

• Recent spinal anesthesia

• Severe head injury

• Stroke or

• Thrombocytopenia (a low platelet count in the blood)— The risk of bleeding may be increased

- Recent surgery or
- Single organ dysfunction—May cause serious problems; caution should be used

Proper Use of This Medicine

Dosing—The dose of this medicine will be different for different patients. Follow your doctor's orders or the directions on the label. The following information includes only the average doses of this medicine. If your dose is different, do not change it unless your doctor tells you to do so.

The amount of medicine that you take depends on the strength of the medicine. Also, the number of doses you take each day, the time allowed between doses, and the length of time you take the medicine depend on the medical problem for which you are using the medicine.

- For injection dosage form:
  - To treat the most severe cases of sepsis (infection in the blood):
    - Adults—The dose is usually 24 micrograms (mcg) per kilogram (10.9 mcg per pound) of body weight per hour injected into a vein over a period of 4 days (96 hours).
    - Children—Use and dose must be determined by your doctor.

Precautions While Using This Medicine

Drotrecogin alfa can cause bleeding that usually is not serious. However, serious bleeding may occur in some people. To help prevent serious bleeding, carefully follow any instructions given by your health care professional. Move around as little as possible, and do not get out of bed on your own, unless your health care professional tells you it is okay.

Side Effects of This Medicine

Along with its needed effects, a medicine may cause some unwanted effects. Although not all of these side effects may occur, if they do occur they may need medical attention.

Check with your doctor immediately if any of the following side effects occur:

More common
　Bleeding Other side effects not listed may also occur in some patients. If you notice any other effects, check with your healthcare professional.

DULOXETINE   (Oral route) - doo-LOX-e-teen

Black Box Warning

Antidepressants increased the risk of suicidal thinking and behavior (suicidality) in short-term studies in children and adolescents with major depressive disorder (MDD) and other psychiatric disorders. Anyone considering the use of duloxetine hydrochloride or any other antidepressant in a child or adolescent must balance this risk with the clinical need. Patients who are started on therapy should be observed closely for clinical worsening, suicidality, or unusual changes in be-

havior. Families and caregivers should be advised of the need for close observation and communication with the prescriber. Duloxetine hydrochloride is not approved for use in pediatric patients.

Pooled analyses of short-term (4 to 16 weeks) placebo-controlled trials of 9 antidepressant drugs (SSRIs and others) in children and adolescents with major depressive disorder (MDD), obsessive compulsive disorder (OCD), or other psychiatric disorders (a total of 24 trials involving over 4400 patients) have revealed a greater risk of adverse events representing suicidal thinking or behavior (suicidality) during the first few months of treatment in those receiving antidepressants. The average risk of such events in patients receiving antidepressants was 4%, twice the placebo risk of 2%. No suicides occurred in these trials.

Commonly used brand name(s)

In the U.S.—
　Cymbalta

Available Dosage Forms:

- Capsule, Delayed Release
- Capsule

Therapeutic Class: Antidepressant
Pharmacologic Class: Serotonin/Norepinephrine Reuptake Inhibitor

Uses For This Medicine

Duloxetine is used to treat mental depression. It is also used for pain caused by nerve damage associated with diabetes.

Duloxetine belongs to a group of medicines known as selective serotonin and norepinephrine reuptake inhibitors (SSNRIs). These medicines are thought to work by increasing the activity of chemicals called serotonin and norepinephrine in the brain.

This medicine is available only with your doctor's prescription.

Before Using This Medicine

In deciding to use a medicine, the risks of taking the medicine must be weighed against the good it will do. This is a decision you and your doctor will make. For this medicine, the following should be considered:

Allergies—Tell your doctor if you have ever had any unusual or allergic reaction to this medicine or any other medicines. Also tell your health care professional if you have any other types of allergies, such as to foods, dyes, preservatives, or animals. For non-prescription products, read the label or package ingredients carefully.

Pediatric—Children should not usually take duloxetine. However, if your doctor prescribes duloxetine for your child to treat depression, caution must be used. Studies have shown occurrences of children thinking about suicide or attempting suicide in clinical trials for this medicine. More study is needed to be sure duloxetine is safe and effective in children

Geriatric—This medicine has been tested and has not been shown to cause different side effects or problems in older people than it does in younger adults. However, elderly patients are more likely to be sensitive than younger adults to the effects of duloxetine.

Pregnancy—

	Pregnancy Category	Explanation
All Trimesters	C	Animal studies have shown an adverse effect and there are no adequate studies in pregnant women OR no animal studies have been conducted and there are no adequate studies in pregnant women.

Breast Feeding—There are no adequate studies in women for determining infant risk when using this medication during breastfeeding. Weigh the potential benefits against the potential risks before taking this medication while breastfeeding.

Other medicines—

Using this medicine with any of the following medicines is not recommended. Your doctor may decide not to treat you with this medication or change some of the other medicines you take.

Clorgyline, Isocarboxazid, Lazabemide, Moclobemide, Phenelzine, Rasagiline, Selegiline, Thioridazine, Tranylcypromine

Interactions with Food/Tobacco/Alcohol—Certain medicines should not be used at or around the time of eating food or eating certain types of food since interactions may occur. Using alcohol or tobacco with certain medicines may also cause interactions to occur. Discuss with your healthcare professional the use of your medicine with food, alcohol, or tobacco.

Other medical problems—The presence of other medical problems may affect the use of this medicine. Make sure you tell your doctor if you have any other medical problems, especially:

- Bipolar disorder (mood disorder with alternating episodes of mania and depression) or risk of—May make condition worse. Your doctor will check you for this condition.
- Diabetes mellitus (sugar diabetes)—May increase your blood sugar.
- Kidney disease, severe, or
- Liver disease, severe—Higher blood levels of duloxetine may occur, increasing the chance of side effects.
- Mania (history of)—The condition may be activated.
- Narrow-angle glaucoma—May increase your chance of getting blurred vision.
- Seizures (history of)—The risk of seizures may be increased.

Proper Use of This Medicine

Take this medicine only as directed by your doctor to benefit your condition as much as possible. Do not take more of it, do not take it more often, and do not take it for a longer time than your doctor ordered.

Swallow the capsule whole. Do not chew, crush or sprinkle the contents on food or mix with liquids before swallowing.

Dosing—The dose of this medicine will be different for different patients. Follow your doctor's orders or the directions on the label. The following information includes only the average doses of this medicine. If your dose is different, do not change it unless your doctor tells you to do so.

The amount of medicine that you take depends on the strength of the medicine. Also, the number of doses you take each day, the time allowed between doses, and the length of time you take the medicine depend on the medical problem for which you are using the medicine.

- For oral dosage form (capsule):
  - For treatment of depression:
    - Adults—40 milligrams (mg) a day (given as 20 mg twice a day) to 60 mg a day (given either once a day or as 30 mg twice a day) with or without meals.
    - Children—Use and dose must be determined by your doctor.
  - For treatment of pain associated with diabetic peripheral neuropathy
    - Adults—60 milligrams (mg) a day with or without meals.
    - Children—Dose must be determined by your doctor.

Missed dose—If you miss a dose of this medicine, take it as soon as possible. However, if it is almost time for your next dose, skip the missed dose and go back to your regular dosing schedule. Do not double doses.

Storage—Store the medicine in a closed container at room temperature, away from heat, moisture, and direct light. Keep from freezing.

Keep out of the reach of children.

Do not keep outdated medicine or medicine no longer needed.

Ask your healthcare professional how you should dispose of any medicine you do not use.

Precautions While Using This Medicine

It is important that your doctor check your progress at regular visits, to allow for changes in your dose and to help reduce any side effects.

Duloxetine has not been shown to add to the effects of alcohol. However, use of alcohol is not recommended in patients who are taking duloxetine.

Duloxetine may cause some people to be agitated, irritable or display other abnormal behaviors. It may also cause some people to have suicidal thoughts and tendencies or to become more depressed. If you or your caregiver notice any of these adverse effects, tell your doctor right away.

This medicine can cause serious liver problems. If you experience symptoms such as dark urine, general tiredness and weakness, light-colored stools, nausea and vomiting, upper right abdominal pain, or yellow eyes and skin, *contact your doctor immediately.*

Four weeks of duloxetine may be required before your symptoms improve. It is important to continue duloxetine after symptoms of depression are relieved.

Do not suddenly stop taking your duloxetine. If you have been instructed to stop taking duloxetine, ask your healthcare professional how to slowly decrease the dose. This is to decrease the chance of having discontinuation symptoms such as dizziness, nausea, headache, vomiting, irritability, nightmares, prickling or tingling feelings.

Do not take duloxetine if you have taken a monoamine oxidase (MAO) inhibitor (furazolidone, phenelzine, procarbazine, selegiline, tranylcypromine) in the past 2 weeks. Do not start taking an MAO inhibitor within 5 days of stopping duloxetine. If you do, you may develop confusion, agitation, restlessness, stomach or intestinal symptoms, sudden high body temperature, extremely high blood pressure, severe convulsions, or the serotonin syndrome.

For diabetic patients:

- This medicine may affect blood sugar levels. If you notice a change in the results of your blood or urine sugar tests or if you have any questions, check with your doctor.

Duloxetine may cause some people to become drowsy or have blurred vision. Make sure you know how you react to this medicine before you drive, use machines, or do anything else that could be dangerous if you are not alert or able to see clearly.

Side Effects of This Medicine

Along with its needed effects, a medicine may cause some unwanted effects. Although not all of these side effects may occur, if they do occur they may need medical attention.

Check with your doctor as soon as possible if any of the following side effects occur:

Incidence not known

Abdominal or stomach pain; area rash; blindness; blistering, peeling, loosening of skin; blurred vision; chills; clay-colored stools; cold sweats; coma; confusion; convulsions; dark urine; decreased urine output; decreased vision; difficulty swallowing; dizziness, faintness, or lightheadedness when getting up from a lying or sitting position; eye pain; fainting; fast or irregular heartbeat; general tiredness or weakness; hives or welts; hives, itching, puffiness, or swelling of the eyelids or around the eyes, face, lips, or tongue; increased thirst; itching; joint or muscle pain; large, hive-like swelling on face, eyelids, lips, tongue, throat, hands, legs, feet, sex organs; light-colored stools; red, irritated eyes; red skin lesions, often with a purple center; redness of skin; shortness of breath; skin rash; sores, ulcers, or white spots in mouth or on lips; swelling of face, ankles or hands; tearing; tightness in chest; unpleasant breath odor; upper right abdominal pain; vomiting of blood; wheezing; yellow eyes and skin

Some side effects may occur that usually do not need medical attention. These side effects may go away during treatment as your body adjusts to the medicine. Also, your health care professional may be able to tell you about ways to prevent or reduce some of these side effects. Check with your health care professional if any of the following side effects continue or are bothersome or if you have any questions about them:

More common

Cough; diarrhea; difficulty having a bowel movement (stool); dizziness; dry mouth; fever; frequent urination; headache; lack or loss of strength; loss of appetite; muscle aches; nausea; sleepiness or unusual drowsiness; sleeplessness; sore throat; stuffy or runny nose; sweating increased; trouble sleeping; unable to sleep; unusual tiredness or weakness; vomiting; weight loss

Less common

Abnormal orgasm; acid or sour stomach; belching; change or problem with discharge of semen; decreased interest in sexual intercourse; difficulty in

moving; erectile dysfunction; fear; feeling of warmth redness of the face, neck, arms and occasionally, upper chest; heartburn; inability to have or keep an erection; indigestion; joint pain; longer than usual time to ejaculation of semen; loose stools; loss in sexual ability, desire, drive, or performance; muscle aching or cramping; muscle pains or stiffness; nervousness; shakiness in legs, arms, hands, feet; stomach discomfort upset or pain; sudden sweating; swollen joints; trembling or shaking of hands or feet; vision blurred

Other side effects not listed may also occur in some patients. If you notice any other effects, check with your healthcare professional.

DUTASTERIDE (Oral route) - doo-TAS-teer-ide

Commonly used brand name(s)

In the U.S.—
Avodart

Available Dosage Forms:

- Capsule, Liquid Filled

Therapeutic Class: Benign Prostatic Hypertrophy Agent
Pharmacologic Class: 5–Alpha Reductase Inhibitor

Uses For This Medicine

Note: Women of childbearing potential should not use or handle dutasteride capsules. Dutasteride can cause birth defects in male fetuses.

Dutasteride is used to treat men who have symptoms of an enlarged prostate gland.

Dutasteride blocks an enzyme called 5–alpha-reductase, which is necessary to change testosterone to another hormone that causes the prostate to grow. As a result, the size of the prostate is decreased. The effect of dutasteride on the prostate lasts only as long as the medicine is taken. If it is stopped, the prostate begins to grow again.

This medicine is available only with your doctor's prescription.

Before Using This Medicine

In deciding to use a medicine, the risks of taking the medicine must be weighed against the good it will do. This is a decision you and your doctor will make. For this medicine, the following should be considered:

Allergies—Tell your doctor if you have ever had any unusual or allergic reaction to this medicine or any other medicines. Also tell your health care professional if you have any other types of allergies, such as to foods, dyes, preservatives, or animals. For non-prescription products, read the label or package ingredients carefully.

Pediatric—Dutasteride should not be used in children.

Geriatric—This medicine has been tested and has not been shown to cause different side effects or problems in older people than it does in younger adults.

Pregnancy—

	Pregnancy Category	Explanation
All Trimesters	X	Studies in animals or pregnant women have demonstrated positive evidence of fetal abnormalities. This drug should not be used in women who are or may become pregnant because the risk clearly outweighs any possible benefit.

Breast Feeding—There are no adequate studies in women for determining infant risk when using this medication during breastfeeding. Weigh the potential benefits against the potential risks before taking this medication while breastfeeding.

Other medicines—

Using this medicine with any of the following medicines may cause an increased risk of certain side effects, but using both drugs may be the best treatment for you. If both medicines are prescribed together, your doctor may change the dose or how often you use one or both of the medicines.

Cimetidine, Ciprofloxacin, Diltiazem, Ketoconazole, Ritonavir, Verapamil

Interactions with Food/Tobacco/Alcohol—Certain medicines should not be used at or around the time of eating food or eating certain types of food since interactions may occur. Using alcohol or tobacco with certain medicines may also cause interactions to occur. Discuss with your healthcare professional the use of your medicine with food, alcohol, or tobacco.

Other medical problems—The presence of other medical problems may affect the use of this medicine. Make sure you tell your doctor if you have any other medical problems, especially:

- Cancer of the prostate—Your doctor will check you for prostate cancer before beginning treatment with this medicine.
- Liver disease—Dutasteride should be used with caution. Effects of this medicine may be increased.
- Problems with urination—Your doctor may want to choose another medicine for you or monitor your kidneys for blockage.

Proper Use of This Medicine

Dosing—The dose of this medicine will be different for different patients. Follow your doctor's orders or the directions on the label. The following information includes only the average doses of this medicine. If your dose is different, do not change it unless your doctor tells you to do so.

The amount of medicine that you take depends on the strength of the medicine. Also, the number of doses you take each day, the time allowed between doses, and the length of time you take the medicine depend on the medical problem for which you are using the medicine.

- For oral dosage form (capsules):
  - For benign prostatic hyperplasia:
    - Adults—0.5 milligram (mg) once a day. May take with or without food. Capsules should be swallowed whole. Dutasteride is not for use in women.
    - Children—Dutasteride is not for use in children.

Missed dose—If you miss a dose of this medicine, take it as soon as possible. However, if it is almost time for your next dose, skip the missed dose and go back to your regular dosing schedule. Do not double doses.

Storage—Store the medicine in a closed container at room temperature, away from heat, moisture, and direct light. Do not refrigerate. Keep from freezing.

Keep out of the reach of children.

Do not keep outdated medicine or medicine no longer needed.

Ask your healthcare professional how you should dispose of any medicine you do not use.

Precautions While Using This Medicine

It is very important that your doctor check you at regular visits for any problems that may be caused by this medicine.

Do not take other medicines unless they have been discussed with your doctor. It is very important that you take all of your medicine. Your doctor will discuss with you any changes in your medicine. Ask your doctor if you have any questions.

Pregnant women or women who may become pregnant should not handle or touch the capsules. Dutasteride can be absorbed through the skin and can cause a risk to the developing male baby. It is very important that pregnant women or women who could become pregnant use caution in handling dutasteride capsules or avoid handling them at all. If a woman does come into contact with this medicine, the affected area should be washed right away with soap and water, especially if the capsule is leaking.

Men who have taken dutasteride should not donate blood until 6 months has passed since their last dose. Dutasteride can remain in your blood for a long time, and can be passed on to a pregnant woman receiving a blood transfusion.

Side Effects of This Medicine

Along with its needed effects, a medicine may cause some unwanted effects. Although not all of these side effects may occur, if they do occur they may need medical attention.

Check with your doctor as soon as possible if any of the following side effects occur:
Incidence not known
  Cough; difficulty swallowing; dizziness; fast heartbeat; hives or welts; itching skin; puffiness or swelling of the eyelids or around the eyes, face, lips, or tongue; redness of skin; shortness of breath; skin rash; swelling of face, fingers, feet, and/or lower legs; tightness in chest; unusual tiredness or weakness; wheezing

Some side effects may occur that usually do not need medical attention. These side effects may go away during treatment as your body adjusts to the medicine. Also, your health care professional may be able to tell you about ways to prevent or reduce some of these side effects. Check with your health care professional if any of the following side effects continue or are bothersome or if you have any questions about them:
Less common
  Abnormal ejaculation; decreased interest in sexual intercourse; decreased sexual performance or desire; impotence; inability to have or keep an erection; loss in

sexual ability, desire, drive, or performance; swelling of the breasts or breast soreness

Amount of semen in ejaculate may be decreased in some patients. This decrease does not interfere with normal sexual function.

Other side effects not listed may also occur in some patients. If you notice any other effects, check with your healthcare professional.

ECONAZOLE (Topical route) -
e-KONE-a-zole

Commonly used brand name(s)

In the U.S.—
   Spectazole

Available Dosage Forms:
- Powder
- Solution
- Cream

Therapeutic Class: Antifungal

Uses For This Medicine

Econazole belongs to the family of medicines called antifungals, which are used to treat infections caused by a fungus. They work by killing the fungus or preventing its growth.

Econazole cream is applied to the skin to treat fungus infections. These include:
- Ringworm of the body (tinea corporis);
- Ringworm of the foot (tinea pedis; athlete's foot);
- Ringworm of the groin (tinea cruris; jock itch);
- Tinea versicolor (sometimes called "sun fungus"); and
- Certain other fungus infections, such as Candida (Monilia) infections.

Econazole is available only with your doctor's prescription.

Before Using This Medicine

In deciding to use a medicine, the risks of taking the medicine must be weighed against the good it will do. This is a decision you and your doctor will make. For this medicine, the following should be considered:

Allergies—Tell your doctor if you have ever had any unusual or allergic reaction to this medicine or any other medicines. Also tell your health care professional if you have any other types of allergies, such as to foods, dyes, preservatives, or animals. For non-prescription products, read the label or package ingredients carefully.

Pediatric—Although there is no specific information comparing use of this medicine in children with use in other age groups, this medicine is not expected to cause different side effects or problems in children than it does in adults.

Geriatric—Many medicines have not been studied specifically in older people. Therefore, it may not be known whether they work exactly the same way they do in younger adults. Although there is no specific information comparing use of econazole in the elderly with use in other age groups, this medicine is not expected to cause different side effects or problems in older people than it does in younger adults.

Other medicines—Although certain medicines should not be used together at all, in other cases two different medicines may be used together even if an interaction might occur. In these cases, your doctor may want to change the dose, or other precautions may be necessary. Tell your healthcare professional if you are taking any other prescription or non-prescription (over-the-counter [OTC]) medicine.

Interactions with Food/Tobacco/Alcohol—Certain medicines should not be used at or around the time of eating food or eating certain types of food since interactions may occur. Using alcohol or tobacco with certain medicines may also cause interactions to occur. Discuss with your healthcare professional the use of your medicine with food, alcohol, or tobacco.

Proper Use of This Medicine

Apply enough econazole to cover the affected and surrounding skin areas, and massage in gently.

Keep this medicine away from the eyes.

When econazole is used to treat certain types of fungus infections of the skin, an occlusive dressing (airtight covering, such as kitchen plastic wrap) should not be applied over the medicine. To do so may cause irritation of the skin. Do not apply an airtight covering over this medicine unless you have been directed to do so by your doctor.

To help clear up your infection completely, it is very important that you keep using econazole for the full time of treatment, even if your symptoms begin to clear up after a few days. Since fungus infections may be very slow to clear up, you may have to continue using this medicine every day for several weeks or more. If you stop using this medicine too soon, your symptoms may return. Do not miss any doses.

Dosing—The dose of this medicine will be different for different patients. Follow your doctor's orders or the directions on the label. The following information includes only the average doses of this medicine. If your dose is different, do not change it unless your doctor tells you to do so.

The amount of medicine that you take depends on the strength of the medicine. Also, the number of doses you take each day, the time allowed between doses, and the length of time you take the medicine depend on the medical problem for which you are using the medicine.

- For topical dosage form (cream):
  - For fungus infections:
    - Adults and children—Apply to the affected skin and surrounding areas, one or two times a day, for two to four weeks. If you have to use the cream two times a day, apply it in the morning and evening.

Missed dose—If you miss a dose of this medicine, apply it as soon as possible. However, if it is almost time for your next dose, skip the missed dose and go back to your regular dosing schedule.

Storage—Store the medicine in a closed container at room temperature, away from heat, moisture, and direct light. Keep from freezing.

Keep out of the reach of children.

Do not keep outdated medicine or medicine no longer needed.

Precautions While Using This Medicine

If your skin problem does not improve within 2 weeks or more, or if it becomes worse, check with your doctor.

To help clear up your infection completely and to help make sure it does not return, good health habits are also required.

- For patients using econazole for ringworm of the groin (tinea cruris; jock itch):
  - Avoid wearing underwear that is tight-fitting or made from synthetic materials (for example, rayon or nylon). Instead, wear loose-fitting, cotton underwear.
  - Use a bland, absorbent powder (for example, talcum powder) or an antifungal powder (for example, tolnaftate) on the skin. It is best not to use econazole cream or any other antifungal cream at the same time that you use the powder.

These measures will help reduce chafing and irritation and will also help keep the groin area cool and dry.

- For patients using econazole for ringworm of the foot (tinea pedis; athlete's foot):
  - Carefully dry the feet, especially between the toes, after bathing.
  - Avoid wearing socks made from wool or synthetic materials (for example, rayon or nylon). Instead, wear clean, cotton socks and change them daily or more often if the feet sweat freely.
  - Wear well-ventilated shoes (for example, shoes with holes) or sandals.
  - Use a bland, absorbent powder (for example, talcum powder) or an antifungal powder (for example, tolnaftate) between the toes, on the feet, and in socks and shoes freely once or twice a day. It is best not to use econazole cream or any other antifungal cream at the same time that you use the powder.

These measures will help keep the feet cool and dry.

If you have any questions about this, check with your health care professional.

Side Effects of This Medicine

Along with its needed effects, a medicine may cause some unwanted effects. Although not all of these side effects may occur, if they do occur they may need medical attention.

Check with your doctor as soon as possible if any of the following side effects occur:

Less common
  Burning, itching, stinging, redness, or other sign of irritation not present before use of this medicine

Rare
  Skin rash with itching

Other side effects not listed may also occur in some patients. If you notice any other effects, check with your healthcare professional.

EFALIZUMAB (Subcutaneous route) -
e-fa-li-ZOO-mab

Commonly used brand name(s)
In the U.S.—
  Raptiva

Available Dosage Forms:
- Powder for Solution

Therapeutic Class: Immune Suppressant
Pharmacologic Class: Monoclonal Antibody

Uses For This Medicine

Efalizumab is used in adult patients to treat moderate to severe psoriasis.

This medicine is available only with your doctor's prescription.

Before Using This Medicine

In deciding to use a medicine, the risks of taking the medicine must be weighed against the good it will do. This is a decision you and your doctor will make. For this medicine, the following should be considered:

Allergies—Tell your doctor if you have ever had any unusual or allergic reaction to this medicine or any other medicines. Also tell your health care professional if you have any other types of allergies, such as to foods, dyes, preservatives, or animals. For non-prescription products, read the label or package ingredients carefully.

Pediatric—Studies on this medicine have been done only in adult patients, and there is no specific information comparing the use of efalizumab in children with use in other age groups.

Geriatric—Many medicines have not been studied specifically in older people and it may not be known if they work the same way they do in younger adults. Elderly people may have more age-related problems than younger people and may need less of this medicine.

Pregnancy—

	Pregnancy Category	Explanation
All Trimesters	C	Animal studies have shown an adverse effect and there are no adequate studies in pregnant women OR no animal studies have been conducted and there are no adequate studies in pregnant women.

Breast Feeding—There are no adequate studies in women for determining infant risk when using this medication during breastfeeding. Weigh the potential benefits against the potential risks before taking this medication while breastfeeding.

Other medicines—Although certain medicines should not be used together at all, in other cases two different medicines may be used together even if an interaction might occur. In these cases, your doctor may want to change the dose, or other precautions may be necessary. Tell your healthcare professional if you are taking any other prescription or nonprescription (over-the-counter [OTC]) medicine.

Interactions with Food/Tobacco/Alcohol—Certain medicines should not be used at or around the time of eating food or eating certain types of food since interactions may occur. Using alcohol or tobacco with certain medicines may also cause interactions to occur. Discuss with your healthcare professional the use of your medicine with food, alcohol, or tobacco.

Other medical problems—The presence of other medical problems may affect the use of this medicine. Make sure you tell your doctor if you have any other medical problems, especially:

- Cancer, history of—This medicine should not be used in patients with a history of cancer and it should be used with caution in patients at risk for cancer
- Infection, moderate to severe—Efalizumab could make your infection worse; your doctor may want to stop this medicine if you get an infection
- Thrombocytopenia (not enough platelets in your blood)—May give you a higher chance for bleeding; your doctor may want to stop this medicine if you have a low platelet count

---

Proper Use of This Medicine

Dosing—The dose of this medicine will be different for different patients. Follow your doctor's orders or the directions on the label. The following information includes only the average doses of this medicine. If your dose is different, do not change it unless your doctor tells you to do so.

The amount of medicine that you take depends on the strength of the medicine. Also, the number of doses you take each day, the time allowed between doses, and the length of time you take the medicine depend on the medical problem for which you are using the medicine.

- For parenteral dosage form
  - Psoriasis
    - Adults—The dose is based on your body weight and must be determined by your doctor. This medicine is injected under your skin of your upper leg (thigh), upper arm, abdomen or buttocks once a week. Change (rotate) your skin injection site with each injection.
    - Children—Use and dose must be determined by your doctor.

Missed dose—Call your doctor or pharmacist for instructions.

Storage—Store in the refrigerator. Do not freeze.

Keep out of the reach of children.

Do not keep outdated medicine or medicine no longer needed.

Ask your healthcare professional how you should dispose of any medicine you do not use.

Precautions While Using This Medicine

It is very important that your doctor check you at regular visits for any blood problems or any other side effects that may be caused by this medicine.

While you are being treated with efalizumab, and after you stop treatment with it, do not have any immunizations (vaccinations) without your doctor's approval. Efalizumab may lower your body's resistance and there is a chance you might get the infection the immunization is meant to prevent. In addition, the other persons living in your household should not take oral polio vaccine since there is a chance they could pass the polio virus on to you. Also avoid persons who have recently taken oral polio vaccine. Do not get close to them or stay in the same room with them for very long. If you cannot take these precautions, you should consider wearing a protective mask that covers the nose and mouth.

It is important to check with your doctor if you have any symptoms of an infection such as fever or chills, cough or hoarseness, lower back or side pain, painful or difficult urination. If your symptoms do not improve within a few days or if they become worse, check with your doctor.

Check with you doctor immediately if you notice an unusual bleeding or busing, black, tarry stools, blood in urine, or stools, or pinpoint red spots on your skin

It is important to tell your doctor if you become pregnant. Your doctor may want you join a pregnancy registry for patients taking this medicine.

Side Effects of This Medicine

Along with its needed effects, a medicine may cause some unwanted effects. Although not all of these side effects may occur, if they do occur they may need medical attention.

Check with your doctor immediately if any of the following side effects occur:

Less common
> Accumulation of pus; chest pain; cough; cough producing mucus; diarrhea; difficulty in breathing or swallowing; fast heartbeat; fever or chills; headache; increase bone pain in vertebrae; itching, pain, redness, swelling, tenderness, warmth on skin; loss of appetite; muscle or joint stiffness, tightness, or rigidity; nausea; pain or tenderness around eyes and cheekbones; rash or redness; shortness of breath; skin itching; sneezing; sore throat; stiff neck or back; stomach pain; stuffy or runny nose; swelling of face, throat, or tongue; swollen, red, tender area of infection; tightness in chest; vomiting; weakness; wheezing

Rare
> Back pain; black, tarry stools; bleeding gums; blood in urine or stools; dark urine; difficulty in moving; general tiredness and weakness; hearing loss; light-colored stools; muscle pain; pain, swelling, or redness in joints; pinpoint red spots on skin; spots on your skin resembling a blister or pimple; small usually colored spots on skin; sudden and severe muscle weakness, sudden and progressing; swollen salivary glands; unusual bleeding or bruising; unusual lumps or skin changes; upper right abdominal pain; yellow eyes and skin

Some side effects may occur that usually do not need medical attention. These side effects may go away during treatment as your body adjusts to the medicine. Also, your health care professional may be able to tell you about ways to prevent or reduce some of these side effects. Check with your health care professional if any of the following side effects continue or are bothersome or if you have any questions about them:

More common
> Difficulty in moving; general feeling of discomfort or illness; joint pain; loss of appetite; muscle cramping; shivering; sweating; swollen joints; trouble sleeping; unusual tiredness or weakness

Less common
> Blemishes on the skin; lack or loss of strength; pimples; swelling of hands, ankles, feet, or lower legs

Other side effects not listed may also occur in some patients. If you notice any other effects, check with your healthcare professional.

EFAVIRENZ (Oral route) - ef-a-VYE-renz

Commonly used brand name(s)
In the U.S.—
    Sustiva

Available Dosage Forms:
- Capsule
- Tablet

Therapeutic Class: Antiretroviral Agent
Pharmacologic Class: Non-Nucleoside Reverse Transcriptase Inhibitor

Uses For This Medicine

Efavirenz is used with other medicines in the treatment of the infection caused by the human immunodeficiency virus (HIV). HIV is the virus that causes acquired immune deficiency syndrome (AIDS).

Efavirenz will not cure or prevent HIV infection or AIDS; however, it helps keep HIV from reproducing and appears to slow down the destruction of the immune system. This may help delay the development of problems that usually result from AIDS or HIV disease. Efavirenz will not keep you from spreading HIV to other people. People who receive this medicine may continue to have some of the problems usually related to AIDS or HIV disease.

This medicine is available only with your doctor's prescription.

Before Using This Medicine

In deciding to use a medicine, the risks of taking the medicine must be weighed against the good it will do. This is a decision you and your doctor will make. For this medicine, the following should be considered:

Allergies—Tell your doctor if you have ever had any unusual or allergic reaction to this medicine or any other medicines. Also tell your health care professional if you have any other types of allergies, such as to foods, dyes, preservatives, or animals. For non-prescription products, read the label or package ingredients carefully.

Pediatric—Children have a higher risk of developing a rash, which is sometimes severe, while taking this medicine. Your doctor may suggest that an additional medicine, an antihistamine, be taken to prevent a rash from occurring. The appearance of a rash should be reported to your doctor as soon as possible.

Geriatric—Many medicines have not been studied specifically in older people. Therefore, it may not be known whether they work exactly the same way they do in younger adults or if they cause different side effects or problems in older people. There is no specific information comparing use of efavirenz in the elderly with use in other age groups.

Pregnancy—

	Pregnancy Category	Explanation
All Trimesters	D	Studies in pregnant women have demonstrated a risk to the fetus. However, the benefits of therapy in a life threatening situation or a serious disease, may outweigh the potential risk.

Breast Feeding—There are no adequate studies in women for determining infant risk when using this medication during breastfeeding. Weigh the potential benefits against the potential risks before taking this medication while breastfeeding.

Other medicines—

Using this medicine with any of the following medicines is not recommended. Your doctor may decide not to treat you with this medication or change some of the other medicines you take.

Astemizole, Cisapride, Dihydroergotamine, Ergoloid Mesylates, Ergonovine, Ergotamine, Methylergonovine, Methysergide, Midazolam, St John's Wort, Triazolam, Voriconazole

Interactions with Food/Tobacco/Alcohol—Certain medicines should not be used at or around the time of eating food or eating certain types of food since interactions may occur. Using alcohol or tobacco with certain medicines may also cause interactions to occur. Discuss with your healthcare professional the use of your medicine with food, alcohol, or tobacco.

Other medical problems—The presence of other medical problems may affect the use of this medicine. Make sure you tell your doctor if you have any other medical problems, especially:
- Alcohol or drug abuse history or
- Mental illness history—May increase the chance of having serious psychiatric side effects.
- Hepatitis B or C (history of) or
- Liver disease—Efavirenz may cause unwanted effects in the liver
- Seizures history—May increase chances of convulsions occurring

Proper Use of This Medicine

Take this medicine exactly as directed by your doctor. Do not take it more often, and do not take it for a longer time than your doctor ordered. Also, do not stop taking this medicine without checking with your doctor first.

Keep taking efavirenz for the full time of treatment even if you begin to feel better. It is also important that you continue taking all other medicines for HIV infection your doctor has instructed you to take. Efavirenz will not work if it is taken alone. It must be taken with other HIV medication.

Efavirenz should be taken on an empty stomach because the amount of efavirenz absorbed into the body may be increased when taken with food, which might increase the chance of side effects.

Take efavirenz at bedtime, especially during the first 2 to 4 weeks, to lessen central nervous system (CNS) side effects that may occur with this medicine. These effects usually lessen after you have been taking this medicine for awhile.

Dosing—The dose of this medicine will be different for different patients. Follow your doctor's orders or the directions on the label. The following information includes only the av-

erage doses of this medicine. If your dose is different, do not change it unless your doctor tells you to do so.

The amount of medicine that you take depends on the strength of the medicine. Also, the number of doses you take each day, the time allowed between doses, and the length of time you take the medicine depend on the medical problem for which you are using the medicine.

- For oral dosage form (capsules or tablets):
  - For treatment of HIV infection:
    - Adults—600 milligrams (mg) once a day, taken with other medicines.
    - Children 3 years of age and older (by weight)—
      - 10 to 15 kilograms (22 to 33 pounds) of body weight: 200 mg once a day, taken with other medicines.
      - 15 to 20 kilograms (33 to 44 pounds) of body weight: 250 mg once a day, taken with other medicines.
      - 20 to 25 kilograms (44 to 55 pounds) of body weight: 300 mg once a day, taken with other medicines.
      - 25 to 32.5 kilograms (55 to 71.5 pounds) of body weight: 350 mg once a day, taken with other medicines.
      - 32.5 to 40 kilograms (71.5 to 88 pounds) of body weight: 400 mg once a day, taken with other medicines.
      - 40 kilograms (88 pounds) of body weight or over: 600 mg once a day, taken with other medicines.
    - Children up to 3 years of age—Use and dose must be determined by your doctor.

Missed dose—If you miss a dose of this medicine, take it as soon as possible. However, if it is almost time for your next dose, skip the missed dose and go back to your regular dosing schedule. Do not double doses.

Storage—Store the medicine in a closed container at room temperature, away from heat, moisture, and direct light. Keep from freezing.

Keep out of the reach of children.

Do not keep outdated medicine or medicine no longer needed.

Precautions While Using This Medicine

Efavirenz may cause dizziness, difficulty in concentrating, or drowsiness. Make sure you know how you react to this medicine before you drive, use machines, or do anything else that could be dangerous if you are dizzy or are not alert.

Check with your physician before taking efavirenz with alcohol or other medicines that affect the central nervous system (CNS). The use of alcohol or other medicines that affect the CNS with efavirenz may worsen the side effects of this medicine, such as dizziness, poor concentration, drowsiness, unusual dreams, and trouble in sleeping. Some examples of medicines that affect the CNS are antihistamines or medicine for hay fever, other allergies, or colds; sedatives, tranquilizers, or sleeping medicine; medicine for depression; medicine for anxiety; prescription pain medicine or narcotics; barbiturates; medicine for attention deficit and hyperactivity disorder; medicine for seizures; muscle relaxants; or anesthetics, including some dental anesthetics.

Check with your doctor right away if you have serious psychiatric problems, such as severe depression, strange thoughts, or angry behavior.

Efavirenz does not decrease the risk of transmitting the HIV infection to others through sexual contact or by contamination through blood.

Women of childbearing potential should use two forms of birth control while taking this medicine, a barrier method of contraception and an oral or other hormonal method of contraception.

Check with your doctor promptly, if you develop a skin rash.

Side Effects of This Medicine

Along with its needed effects, a medicine may cause some unwanted effects. Although not all of these side effects may occur, if they do occur they may need medical attention.

Check with your doctor as soon as possible if any of the following side effects occur:

More common
  Depression; skin rash or itching

Less common
  Blood in urine; difficult or painful urination; pain in lower back and/or side

Rare
  Abdominal pain; changes in vision; blistering; clumsiness or unsteadiness; confusion; convulsions (seizures); cough; dark urine; delusions; double vision; fainting; fast or pounding heartbeat; fever or chills; headache (severe and throbbing); hives; inappropriate behavior; loss of appetite; mood or mental changes (severe); muscle cramps or pain; nausea or vomiting; nerve pain; open sores; pain, tenderness, bluish color, or swelling of leg or foot; rapid weight gain; seeing, hearing, or feeling things that are not there; sense of constant movement of self or surroundings; sores, ulcers, or white spots in mouth or on lips; speech disorder; swelling and/or tenderness in upper abdominal or stomach area; swelling of hands, arms, feet, or legs; thoughts of suicide or attempts at suicide; tightness in chest; tingling, burning, or prickling sensations; tingling, burning, numbness, or pain in the hands, arms, feet, or legs; tremor; troubled breathing; unusual tiredness; weight loss; wheezing; yellow eyes or skin

Incidence not known
  Actions that are out of control; attack, assault, force; continuing vomiting; delusions of persecution, mistrust, suspiciousness, and/or combativeness; difficult or labored breathing; early appearance of redness or swelling of the skin; general feeling of tiredness or weakness; irritability; late appearance of rash with or without weeping blisters that become crusted, especially in sun-exposed areas of skin, may extend to unexposed areas; light-colored stools; nervousness; neurosis; shortness of breath; stomach pain; talking, feeling, and acting with excitement

Some side effects may occur that usually do not need medical attention. These side effects may go away during treatment as your body adjusts to the medicine. Also, your health care professional may be able to tell you about ways to prevent or reduce some of these side effects. Check with your health

care professional if any of the following side effects continue or are bothersome or if you have any questions about them:

More common

Diarrhea; dizziness; drowsiness; fatigue; headache; increased sweating; poor concentration; trouble in sleeping

Less common or rare

Abnormally decreased sensitivity, particularly to touch; agitation or anxiety; belching; change in sense of taste or smell; dry mouth; excessive gas; false sense of well-being; flaking and falling off of skin; flushing; general feeling of discomfort; heartburn; indigestion; joint pain; lack of feeling or emotion; loss of hair; loss of memory; loss of sense of reality; mood changes; nervousness; pain; painful, red, hot or irritated hair follicles; ringing in the ears; stomach discomfort; unusual dreams; weakness

Incidence not known

Difficulty having a bowel movement (stool); discoloration of fingernails or toenails; large amount of triglyceride in the blood; malabsorption; redistribution/accumulation of body fat; swelling of the breasts or breast soreness in both females and males

Other side effects not listed may also occur in some patients. If you notice any other effects, check with your healthcare professional.

EFLORNITHINE (Topical route) - ee-FLOR-ni-theen

Commonly used brand name(s)

In the U.S.—

Vaniqa

Available Dosage Forms:

- Cream

Therapeutic Class: Hair Growth Retardant

Pharmacologic Class: Ornithine Decarboxylase Inhibitor

Uses For This Medicine

Eflornithine is used to slow down bodily substances called enzymes that help hair grow. The effect is slower facial hair growth.

This medicine is available only with your doctor's prescription.

Before Using This Medicine

In deciding to use a medicine, the risks of taking the medicine must be weighed against the good it will do. This is a decision you and your doctor will make. For this medicine, the following should be considered:

Allergies—Tell your doctor if you have ever had any unusual or allergic reaction to this medicine or any other medicines. Also tell your health care professional if you have any other types of allergies, such as to foods, dyes, preservatives, or animals. For non-prescription products, read the label or package ingredients carefully.

Pediatric—There is no specific information comparing use of eflornithine in children under the age of 12 years with use in other age groups. However, this medicine is not expected to cause different side effects or problems in older children than it does in adults.

Geriatric—This medicine has been tested and has not been shown to cause different side effects or problems in older people than it does in younger adults.

Other medicines—Although certain medicines should not be used together at all, in other cases two different medicines may be used together even if an interaction might occur. In these cases, your doctor may want to change the dose, or other precautions may be necessary. Tell your healthcare professional if you are taking any other prescription or non-prescription (over-the-counter [OTC]) medicine.

Interactions with Food/Tobacco/Alcohol—Certain medicines should not be used at or around the time of eating food or eating certain types of food since interactions may occur. Using alcohol or tobacco with certain medicines may also cause interactions to occur. Discuss with your healthcare professional the use of your medicine with food, alcohol, or tobacco.

Proper Use of This Medicine

This medicine comes with a patient instruction sheet. Read this sheet carefully and follow the directions. If you have any questions on how to use this medicine, be sure to ask your health care professional.

This medicine is usually used on the face and nearby involved areas under the chin only. Do not get the medicine in your eyes, nose, or mouth. Rinse thoroughly with water and contact your doctor if the medicine gets in the eyes

You need to continue your normal hair removal procedures while using this medicine, and the medicine should be applied at least five minutes after the unwanted hair has been removed. You should wait until the medicine dries before applying cosmetics or sunscreen.

Do not wash the treated areas for at least 4 hours after applying the medicine.

Dosing—The dose of this medicine will be different for different patients. Follow your doctor's orders or the directions on the label. The following information includes only the average doses of this medicine. If your dose is different, do not change it unless your doctor tells you to do so.

The amount of medicine that you take depends on the strength of the medicine. Also, the number of doses you take each day, the time allowed between doses, and the length of time you take the medicine depend on the medical problem for which you are using the medicine.

- For topical dosage form (cream):
  - For reduced rate of facial hair growth in women.
    - Adults and children 12 years of age or older—Coat the problem areas on the face and nearby areas under the chin with the medicine two times a day with the second treatment coming at least eight hours after the first.
    - Children under 12 years of age—Use and dose must be determined by your doctor.

Missed dose—If you miss a dose of this medicine, apply it as soon as possible. However, if it is almost time for your next dose, skip the missed dose and go back to your regular dosing schedule.

Storage—Store the medicine in a closed container at room temperature, away from heat, moisture, and direct light. Keep from freezing.

Keep out of the reach of children.

Do not keep outdated medicine or medicine no longer needed.

Precautions While Using This Medicine

If skin irritation occurs, reduce the frequency of treatments. If irritation continues, stop using the medicine and contact your doctor.

If no improvement is seen after six months of treatment, stop using the medicine and contact your doctor.

If condition gets worse while you use the medicine, stop the medicine and contact your doctor.

Side Effects of This Medicine

Some side effects may occur that usually do not need medical attention. These side effects may go away during treatment as your body adjusts to the medicine. Also, your health care professional may be able to tell you about ways to prevent or reduce some of these side effects. Check with your health care professional if any of the following side effects continue or are bothersome or if you have any questions about them:

More common
Acne; stinging skin

Less common
Burning or bleeding skin; chapped, red lips; chronic acne; hair bumps; numbness; rash; reddening of skin; swelling of lips; tingling skin

Other side effects not listed may also occur in some patients. If you notice any other effects, check with your healthcare professional.

ELETRIPTAN   (Oral route) - el-e-TRIP-tan

Commonly used brand name(s)

In the U.S.—
Relpax

Available Dosage Forms:
• Tablet

Therapeutic Class: Antimigraine
Pharmacologic Class: Serotonin Receptor Agonist, 5–HT1

Uses For This Medicine

Eletriptan is used to treat severe migraine headaches. Many people find that their headaches go away completely after they take eletriptan. Other people find that their headaches are much less painful, and that they are able to go back to their normal activities even though their headaches are not completely gone. Eletriptan often relieves other symptoms that occur together with a migraine headache, such as nausea, vomiting, sensitivity to light, and sensitivity to sound.

Eletriptan is not an ordinary pain reliever. It will not relieve any kind of pain other than migraine headaches. This medicine is usually used for people whose headaches are not relieved by acetaminophen, aspirin, or other pain relievers.

Eletriptan has caused serious side effects in some people, especially people who have heart or blood vessel disease. Be sure that you discuss with your doctor the risks of using this medicine as well as the good that it can do.

This medicine is available only with your doctor's prescription.

Before Using This Medicine

In deciding to use a medicine, the risks of taking the medicine must be weighed against the good it will do. This is a decision you and your doctor will make. For this medicine, the following should be considered:

Allergies—Tell your doctor if you have ever had any unusual or allergic reaction to this medicine or any other medicines. Also tell your health care professional if you have any other types of allergies, such as to foods, dyes, preservatives, or animals. For non-prescription products, read the label or package ingredients carefully.

Pediatric—Studies on this medicine have been done only on a small number of adolescents (11 to 17 years of age). However, eletriptan is not recommended for use in patients younger than 18 years of age.

Geriatric—Many medicines have not been studied specifically in older people. Therefore, it may not be known whether they work exactly the same way they do in younger adults. However, eletriptan has been shown to remain in the body longer in elderly patients. It has also been shown to increase blood pressure.

Pregnancy—

	Pregnancy Category	Explanation
All Trimesters	C	Animal studies have shown an adverse effect and there are no adequate studies in pregnant women OR no animal studies have been conducted and there are no adequate studies in pregnant women.

Breast Feeding—There are no adequate studies in women for determining infant risk when using this medication during breastfeeding. Weigh the potential benefits against the potential risks before taking this medication while breastfeeding.

Other medicines—

Using this medicine with any of the following medicines is not recommended. Your doctor may decide not to treat you with this medication or change some of the other medicines you take.

Frovatriptan

Interactions with Food/Tobacco/Alcohol—Certain medicines should not be used at or around the time of eating food or eating certain types of food since interactions may occur. Using alcohol or tobacco with certain medicines may also cause interactions to occur. The following interactions have been selected on the basis of their potential significance and are not necessarily all-inclusive.

Using this medicine with any of the following may cause an increased risk of certain side effects but may be unavoidable in some cases. If used together, your doctor may change the dose or how often you use this medicine or give you special instructions about the use of food, alcohol, or tobacco.

Grapefruit Juice

Other medical problems—The presence of other medical problems may affect the use of this medicine. Make sure you tell your doctor if you have any other medical problems, especially:
• Basilar migraine or
• Cerebrovascular syndrome, such as
• Stroke or
• Transient ischemic attack (TIA) or

- Coronary artery disease, such as
- Angina (chest pain) or
- Decreased blood flow to your heart or
- Heart attack, history of, or
- Other heart conditions or
- Hemiplegic migraine or
- High blood pressure, not treated or
- Liver problems, severe or
- Peripheral vascular disease, such as
- Bowel disease or
- Raynaud's syndrome—Eletriptan should not be used if you have any of these conditions.
- Cerebrovascular event—Eletriptan should be used with caution in patients who have an increased risk of bleeding in the brain, stroke, or transient ischemic attack (TIA).
- Coronary artery disease, predisposition to—Eletriptan and similar medicines may cause serious heart problems, especially if you have a predisposition for heart problems.
- High blood pressure, treated—Eletriptan may cause high blood pressure in patients already being treated for high blood pressure.
- Kidney problems—Eletriptan may cause increased blood pressure in patients who have kidney problems.
- Liver problems, mild or moderate—This could cause higher blood levels of eletriptan.

Proper Use of This Medicine

Do not use eletriptan for a headache that is different from your usual migraines. Instead, check with your doctor.

To relieve your migraine as soon as possible, use eletriptan as soon as the headache pain begins.

You may get additional benefit from eletriptan if you lie down in a quiet, dark room after taking eletriptan.

Ask your doctor ahead of time about any other medicine you may take if eletriptan does not work. After you take the other medicine, check with your doctor as soon as possible.

If you feel much better after a dose of eletriptan, but your headache comes back or gets worse after 2 or more hours, you may use one additional dose of eletriptan. Do not take a second tablet if the first did not help your headache at all. However, use this medicine only as directed by your doctor. Do not use more of it, and do not use it more often than directed.

Dosing—The dose of this medicine will be different for different patients. Follow your doctor's orders or the directions on the label. The following information includes only the average doses of this medicine. If your dose is different, do not change it unless your doctor tells you to do so.

The amount of medicine that you take depends on the strength of the medicine. Also, the number of doses you take each day, the time allowed between doses, and the length of time you take the medicine depend on the medical problem for which you are using the medicine.

- For oral dosage form (tablets):
  - For migraine headaches:
    - Adults—20 milligrams (mg) or 40 mg as a single dose. If the migraine comes back after being re-

lieved, another dose be taken two hours or more after the first dose. Do not take more than 2 doses in any twenty-four-hour period
    - Children—Use and dose must be determined by your doctor.

Storage—Store the medicine in a closed container at room temperature, away from heat, moisture, and direct light. Keep from freezing.

Keep out of the reach of children.

Do not keep outdated medicine or medicine no longer needed.

Precautions While Using This Medicine

Drinking alcoholic beverages may make headaches worse or cause new headaches to occur. People who suffer from severe headaches should probably avoid alcoholic beverages.

Call your doctor if your usual dose of eletriptan does not relieve three consecutive headaches, or the frequency or severity of headaches increases.

Call your doctor right away if you have severe chest pains or shortness of breath.

This medicine may cause some people to become drowsy, dizzy, or less alert than they are normally. Make sure you know how you react to this medicine before you drive, use machines, or do anything else that could be dangerous if you are dizzy or are not alert.

Side Effects of This Medicine

Along with its needed effects, a medicine may cause some unwanted effects. Although not all of these side effects may occur, if they do occur they may need medical attention.

Check with your doctor immediately if any of the following side effects occur:
> *Less common*
> > Chest pain or tightness; difficulty swallowing

Some side effects may occur that usually do not need medical attention. These side effects may go away during treatment as your body adjusts to the medicine. Also, your health care professional may be able to tell you about ways to prevent or reduce some of these side effects. Check with your health care professional if any of the following side effects continue or are bothersome or if you have any questions about them:
> *More common*
> > Dizziness; lack or loss of strength; nausea; sleepiness or unusual drowsiness
>
> *Less common*
> > Acid or sour stomach; belching; burning, crawling, itching, numbness, prickling, "pins and needles", or tingling feelings; dry mouth; feeling of warmth; headache; heartburn; indigestion; redness of the face, neck, arms, and occasionally upper chest; stomach soreness or discomfort; stomach upset or pain

Other side effects not listed may also occur in some patients. If you notice any other effects, check with your healthcare professional.

EMEDASTINE (Ophthalmic route) -
em-e-DAS-teen

Commonly used brand name(s)
In the U.S.—
Emadine

Available Dosage Forms:
- Solution

Therapeutic Class: Ophthalmologic Agent
Pharmacologic Class: Antihistamine

Uses For This Medicine

Emedastine ophthalmic solution is used to treat symptoms of the eye caused by allergic conjunctivitis. It works by preventing the effects of a substance called histamine, which is produced in certain cells in your eyes and which causes the allergic reaction.

This medicine is available only with your doctor's prescription.

Before Using This Medicine

In deciding to use a medicine, the risks of taking the medicine must be weighed against the good it will do. This is a decision you and your doctor will make. For this medicine, the following should be considered:

Allergies—Tell your doctor if you have ever had any unusual or allergic reaction to this medicine or any other medicines. Also tell your health care professional if you have any other types of allergies, such as to foods, dyes, preservatives, or animals. For non-prescription products, read the label or package ingredients carefully.

Pediatric—Studies on this medicine have been done only in adult patients, and there is no specific information comparing use of ophthalmic emedastine in children younger than 3 years of age with use in other age groups.

Geriatric—Many medicines have not been studied specifically in older people. Therefore, it may not be known whether they work exactly the same way they do in younger adults or if they cause different side effects or problems in older people. There is no specific information comparing use of ophthalmic emedastine in the elderly with use in other age groups.

Pregnancy—

	Pregnancy Category	Explanation
All Trimesters	B	Animal studies have revealed no evidence of harm to the fetus, however, there are no adequate studies in pregnant women OR animal studies have shown an adverse effect, but adequate studies in pregnant women have failed to demonstrate a risk to the fetus.

Breast Feeding—There are no adequate studies in women for determining infant risk when using this medication during breastfeeding. Weigh the potential benefits against the potential risks before taking this medication while breastfeeding.

Other medicines—Although certain medicines should not be used together at all, in other cases two different medicines may be used together even if an interaction might occur. In these cases, your doctor may want to change the dose, or other precautions may be necessary. Tell your healthcare professional if you are taking any other prescription or non-prescription (over-the-counter [OTC]) medicine.

Interactions with Food/Tobacco/Alcohol—Certain medicines should not be used at or around the time of eating food or eating certain types of food since interactions may occur. Using alcohol or tobacco with certain medicines may also cause interactions to occur. Discuss with your healthcare professional the use of your medicine with food, alcohol, or tobacco.

Proper Use of This Medicine

Do not wear contact lenses if your eyes are red. If your eyes are not red, contact lenses should be removed before you use this medicine. Also, you should wait at least 10 minutes after using this medicine before putting the contact lenses back in.

To use:
- First, wash your hands. Tilt the head back and, pressing your finger gently on the skin just beneath the lower eyelid, pull the lower eyelid away from the eye to make a space. Drop the medicine into this space. Let go of the eyelid and gently close the eyes. Do not blink. Keep the eyes closed for 1 to 2 minutes to allow the medicine to be absorbed by the eye.
- If you think you did not get the drop of medicine into your eye properly, use another drop.
- To keep the medicine as germ-free as possible, do not touch the applicator tip to any surface (including the eye). Also, keep the container tightly closed.

Dosing—The dose of this medicine will be different for different patients. Follow your doctor's orders or the directions on the label. The following information includes only the average doses of this medicine. If your dose is different, do not change it unless your doctor tells you to do so.

The amount of medicine that you take depends on the strength of the medicine. Also, the number of doses you take each day, the time allowed between doses, and the length of time you take the medicine depend on the medical problem for which you are using the medicine.
- For ophthalmic dosage form (eye drops):
  - For eye allergy:
    - Adults and children 3 years of age and older—Use one drop in the affected eye one to four times a day.
    - Children younger than 3 years of age—Use and dose must be determined by your doctor.

Missed dose—If you miss a dose of this medicine, take it as soon as possible. However, if it is almost time for your next dose, skip the missed dose and go back to your regular dosing schedule. Do not double doses.

Storage—Store the medicine in a closed container at room temperature, away from heat, moisture, and direct light. Do not refrigerate. Keep from freezing.

Keep out of the reach of children.

Do not keep outdated medicine or medicine no longer needed.

Precautions While Using This Medicine

If your symptoms do not improve or if your condition becomes worse, check with your doctor.

Side Effects of This Medicine

Along with its needed effects, a medicine may cause some unwanted effects. Although not all of these side effects may occur, if they do occur they may need medical attention.

Check with your doctor as soon as possible if any of the following side effects occur:

Less common

Abnormal dreams; blurred vision or other change in vision; eye redness, irritation, or pain; tearing, discomfort, or other eye irritation not present before therapy or becoming worse during therapy; weakness

Some side effects may occur that usually do not need medical attention. These side effects may go away during treatment as your body adjusts to the medicine. Also, your health care professional may be able to tell you about ways to prevent or reduce some of these side effects. Check with your health care professional if any of the following side effects continue or are bothersome or if you have any questions about them:

More common

Headache

Less common

Bad taste; burning or stinging of the eye; dry eye; feeling of something in the eye; itching; skin rash; stuffy or runny nose

Other side effects not listed may also occur in some patients. If you notice any other effects, check with your healthcare professional.

EMTRICITABINE   (Oral route) - em-trye-SYE-ta-been

Black Box Warning

Lactic acidosis and severe hepatomegaly with steatosis, including fatal cases, have been reported with the use of nucleoside analogues alone or in combination with other antiretrovirals.

Emtricitabine is not indicated for the treatment of chronic hepatitis B virus (HBV) infection and the safety and efficacy of emtricitabine have not been established in patients co-infected with HBV and HIV. Severe acute exacerbations of hepatitis B have been reported in patients after the discontinuation of emtricitabine. Hepatic function should be monitored closely with both clinical and laboratory follow-up at least several months in patients who discontinue emtricitabine and are co-infected with HIV and HBV. If appropriate, initiation of anti-hepatitis B therapy may be warranted.

Commonly used brand name(s)

In the U.S.—
Emtriva

Available Dosage Forms:
• Capsule
• Solution

Therapeutic Class: Antiretroviral Agent
Pharmacologic Class: Nucleoside Reverse Transcriptase Inhibitor

Uses For This Medicine

Emtricitabine is a type of medicine called an HIV (human immunodeficiency virus) nucleoside reverse transcriptase inhibitor (NRTI). Emtricitabine is always used with other anti-HIV medicines to treat people with HIV infection.

HIV infection destroys CD4 (T) cells, which are important to the immune system in your body. The immune system helps fight infection. After a large number of T cells are destroyed, acquired immune deficiency syndrome (AIDS) develops.

Emtricitabine helps to block HIV reverse transcriptase, a chemical in your body (enzyme) that is needed for HIV to multiply. Emtricitabine may lower the amount of HIV in your blood (viral load). Emtricitabine may also help to increase the number of T cells called CD4 cells. Lowering the amount of HIV in your blood lowers the chance of you having problems that happens when your immune system is weak.

Emtricitabine will not cure or prevent HIV infection or AIDS; however, it helps keep HIV from reproducing and appears to slow down the destruction of the immune system.

Emtricitabine will not keep you from spreading HIV to other people. People who receive this medicine may continue to have the problems usually related to AIDS or HIV disease

This medicine is available only with your doctor's prescription.

Before Using This Medicine

In deciding to use a medicine, the risks of taking the medicine must be weighed against the good it will do. This is a decision you and your doctor will make. For this medicine, the following should be considered:

Allergies—Tell your doctor if you have ever had any unusual or allergic reaction to this medicine or any other medicines. Also tell your health care professional if you have any other types of allergies, such as to foods, dyes, preservatives, or animals. For non-prescription products, read the label or package ingredients carefully.

Pediatric—This medicine has been tested in children 3 months of age and older and, in effective doses, has not been shown to cause different side effects or problems than it does in adults.

Geriatric—Many medicines have not been studied specifically in older people. Therefore, it may not be known whether they work exactly the same way they do in younger adults or if they cause different side effects or problems in older people. Elderly patients are more likely to have other medical problems and they may take a lower dose than some younger adults.

Pregnancy—

	Pregnancy Category	Explanation
All Trimesters	B	Animal studies have revealed no evidence of harm to the fetus, however, there are no adequate studies in pregnant women OR animal studies have shown an adverse effect, but adequate studies in pregnant women have failed to demonstrate a risk to the fetus.

Breast Feeding—There are no adequate studies in women for determining infant risk when using this medication during

breastfeeding. Weigh the potential benefits against the potential risks before taking this medication while breastfeeding.

Other medicines—Although certain medicines should not be used together at all, in other cases two different medicines may be used together even if an interaction might occur. In these cases, your doctor may want to change the dose, or other precautions may be necessary. Tell your healthcare professional if you are taking any other prescription or non-prescription (over-the-counter [OTC]) medicine.

Interactions with Food/Tobacco/Alcohol—Certain medicines should not be used at or around the time of eating food or eating certain types of food since interactions may occur. Using alcohol or tobacco with certain medicines may also cause interactions to occur. Discuss with your healthcare professional the use of your medicine with food, alcohol, or tobacco.

Other medical problems—The presence of other medical problems may affect the use of this medicine. Make sure you tell your doctor if you have any other medical problems, especially:

- Hepatitis B virus (HBV) infection—Emtricitabine is not used to treat patients with hepatitis B virus infection. Therefore, it is recommended that everyone with HIV be tested for hepatitis B before taking emtricitabine. You may receive emtricitabine to treat your HIV infection even if you also have hepatitis B virus infection. Your doctor will want to follow you closely for several months and do regular medical exams once you stop taking emtricitabine.

- Kidney problems—Your doctor may want to lower your dose if you have kidney problems.

- Obesity (overweight) or

- Using nucleoside medicine for a long time—These conditions might increase your chances of getting lactic acidosis (buildup of acid in your blood) or liver problems. This is more common in females.

Proper Use of This Medicine

Dosing—The dose of this medicine will be different for different patients. Follow your doctor's orders or the directions on the label. The following information includes only the average doses of this medicine. If your dose is different, do not change it unless your doctor tells you to do so.

The amount of medicine that you take depends on the strength of the medicine. Also, the number of doses you take each day, the time allowed between doses, and the length of time you take the medicine depend on the medical problem for which you are using the medicine.

It is important to take this medicine in combination with another anti-HIV medicine and to take it exactly as your doctor tells you to. You should take your medicine at the same time every day to avoid missing doses. It is very important that you do not miss any doses of this medicine or of your other anti-HIV medicines.

Do not take other medicines unless they have been discussed with your doctor. Tell your healthcare professional about all of the medicines and dietary supplements that you take. Keep a complete list of all the medications that you take. Make a new list when medications are added or stopped. Make sure you show this list to your doctor or pharmacist each time you have a visit or refill a prescription.

When your emtricitabine supply runs low, get more from your pharmacy or from your healthcare provider. This is very im-

portant because the amount of virus in your blood may increase if the medicine is stopped, even for a short time. The virus may develop resistance to emtricitabine and be harder to treat.

- For oral dosage form (capsules):
  - For treatment of HIV infection
    - Adults—Oral, 200 milligrams (mg) taken once a day. This medicine can be taken with or without food. Your doctor may want to change the dose if you have certain medical problems.
    - Children weighing more than 33 kg (73 lbs) who are able to swallow a capsule whole—Oral, 200 mg taken once a day.

- For oral dosage form (solution):
  - For treatment of HIV infection
    - Adults—Oral, 240 mg (24 milliliters [mL]) taken once a day. This medicine can be taken with or without food. Your doctor may want to change the dose if you have certain medical problems.
    - Children (3 months through 17 years of age)—Oral, 6 mg per kg (2.72 mg per lb) of body weight up to 240 mg (24 mL) taken once a day.

Missed dose—If you miss a dose of this medicine, take it as soon as possible. However, if it is almost time for your next dose, skip the missed dose and go back to your regular dosing schedule. Do not double doses.

Call your doctor or pharmacist for instructions.

Do not take more than 1 dose of emtricitabine in a day. Do not take 2 doses at the same time.

Storage—Store the medicine in a closed container at room temperature, away from heat, moisture, and direct light. Keep from freezing.

Keep out of the reach of children.

Do not keep outdated medicine or medicine no longer needed.

Precautions While Using This Medicine

It is very important that you read the patient information when you start taking this medicine and each time you get a refill. There may be new information for you.

It is very important that your doctor check you at regular visits to be sure this medicine is working properly. You should remain under the care of a doctor while taking emtricitabine.

Emtricitabine does not decrease the risk of transmitting the HIV infection to others through sexual contact or by contamination through blood. HIV may be acquired from or spread to others through infected body fluids, including blood, vaginal fluid, or semen. If you are infected, it is best to avoid any sexual activity involving an exchange of body fluids with other people. If you do have sex, always wear (or have your partner wear) a condom ("rubber"). Only use condoms made of latex or polyurethane and use them every time you have contact with semen, vaginal secretions, or blood. Also, do not share needles or equipment with anyone or use dirty needles. If you have any questions about this, check with your health care professional.

Side Effects of This Medicine

Along with its needed effects, a medicine may cause some unwanted effects. Although not all of these side effects may occur, if they do occur they may need medical attention.

Check with your doctor immediately if any of the following side effects occur:

Incidence unknown

Abdominal discomfort; decreased appetite; diarrhea; fast, shallow breathing; general feeling of discomfort; muscle pain or cramping; nausea; shortness of breath; sleepiness; unusual tiredness or weakness

Along with its needed effects, a medicine may cause some unwanted effects. Although not all of these side effects may occur, if they do occur they may need medical attention.

More common

Cough; diarrhea; headache; lack or loss of strength; nausea; runny nose; sneezing; stuffy nose

Less common

Abdominal pain; abnormal dreams; acid or sour stomach; belching; burning, crawling, itching, numbness, prickling, "pins and needles", or tingling feelings; depression problems; difficulty in moving; dizziness; heartburn; indigestion; joint pain; muscle aching or cramping; muscle pain or stiffness; numbness or tingling of hands, feet, or face; pain in joints; rash; stomach discomfort, upset, or pain; sleeplessness; swollen joints; trouble sleeping; unable to sleep; unsteadiness or awkwardness; vomiting; weakness in arms, hands, legs, or feet

Other side effects not listed may also occur in some patients. If you notice any other effects, check with your healthcare professional.

EMTRICITABINE AND TENOFOVIR DISOPROXIL FUMARATE (Oral route) - em-trye-SYE-ta-been, te-NOE-fo-veer dye-soe-PROX-il FOO-ma-rate

Black Box Warning

Lactic acidosis and severe hepatomegaly with steatosis, including fatal cases, have been reported with the use of nucleoside analogs alone or in combination with other antiretrovirals.

Emtricitabine/tenofovir disoproxil fumarate is not indicated for the treatment of chronic hepatitis B virus (HBV) infection and the safety and efficacy of emtricitabine/tenofovir disoproxil fumarate have not been established in patients coinfected with HBV and HIV. Severe acute exacerbations of hepatitis B have been reported in patients who have discontinued emtricitabine or tenofovir. Hepatic function should be monitored closely with both clinical and laboratory follow-up for at least several months in patients who discontinue emtricitabine/tenofovir disoproxil fumarate and are coinfected with HIV and HBV. If appropriate, initiation of anti-hepatitis B therapy may be warranted.

Commonly used brand name(s)

In the U.S.—
   Truvada

Available Dosage Forms:
- Tablet

Therapeutic Class: Antiretroviral Agent
Pharmacologic Class: Nucleoside Reverse Transcriptase Inhibitor

Uses For This Medicine

Emtricitabine and tenofovir combination is used with other anti-HIV medicines in the treatment of human immunodeficiency virus (HIV) infection. HIV is the virus that causes acquired immune deficiency syndrome (AIDS).

Emtricitabine and tenofovir combination will not cure or prevent HIV infection or the symptoms of AIDS; however, it helps keep HIV from reproducing, and appears to slow down the destruction of the immune system. This may help delay the development of serious health problems usually related to AIDS or HIV infection. Emtricitabine and tenofovir combination will not keep you from spreading HIV to other people. People who receive this medicine may continue to have other problems usually related to AIDS or HIV infection.

This medicine is available only with your doctor's prescription.

Before Using This Medicine

In deciding to use a medicine, the risks of taking the medicine must be weighed against the good it will do. This is a decision you and your doctor will make. For this medicine, the following should be considered:

Allergies—Tell your doctor if you have ever had any unusual or allergic reaction to this medicine or any other medicines. Also tell your health care professional if you have any other types of allergies, such as to foods, dyes, preservatives, or animals. For non-prescription products, read the label or package ingredients carefully.

Pediatric—Studies on this medicine have been done only in adult patients, and there is no specific information comparing use of emtricitabine and tenofovir combination in children with use in other age groups.

Geriatric—Many medicines have not been studied specifically in older people. Therefore, it may not be known whether they work exactly the same way they do in younger adults or if they cause different side effects or problems in older people. Elderly patients are more likely to have other medical problems and they may need to take a lower dose than some younger adults.

Other medicines—

Using this medicine with any of the following medicines is usually not recommended, but may be required in some cases. If both medicines are prescribed together, your doctor may change the dose or how often you use one or both of the medicines.

Atazanavir, Didanosine

Interactions with Food/Tobacco/Alcohol—Certain medicines should not be used at or around the time of eating food or eating certain types of food since interactions may occur. Using alcohol or tobacco with certain medicines may also cause interactions to occur. Discuss with your healthcare professional the use of your medicine with food, alcohol, or tobacco.

Other medical problems—The presence of other medical problems may affect the use of this medicine. Make sure you tell your doctor if you have any other medical problems, especially:

- Hepatitis B virus (HBV) infection—Emtricitabine and tenofovir combination is not used to treat patients with hepatitis B virus infection. You may receive emtricitabine and tenofovir combination to treat your HIV infection even if you also have hepatitis B virus infection. Your doctor will want to follow you closely for several months and do regular medical exams once you stop taking emtricitabine and tenofovir combination.

- Kidney problems or
- Risk factors for kidney disease—Your doctor may want to lower your dose if you have kidney problems or are at risk for having kidney problems.
- Liver disease or
- Risk factors for liver disease or
- Obesity (being overweight)—This medicine may make liver disease worse in patients with liver disease, obesity and other HIV medicine use.

Proper Use of This Medicine

Dosing—The dose of this medicine will be different for different patients. Follow your doctor's orders or the directions on the label. The following information includes only the average doses of this medicine. If your dose is different, do not change it unless your doctor tells you to do so.

The amount of medicine that you take depends on the strength of the medicine. Also, the number of doses you take each day, the time allowed between doses, and the length of time you take the medicine depend on the medical problem for which you are using the medicine.

It is important to take this medicine in combination with another anti-HIV medicine and to take it exactly as your doctor tells you to. You should take your medicine at the same time every day to avoid missing doses. It is very important that you do not miss any doses of this medicine or of your other anti-HIV medicines.

Do not take other medicines unless they have been discussed with your doctor. Tell your healthcare professional about all of the medicines and dietary supplements that you take. Keep a complete list of all the medications that you take. Make a new list when medications are added or stopped. Make sure you show this list to your doctor or pharmacist each time you have a visit or refill a prescription.

When your emtricitabine and tenofovir combination supply runs low, get more from your pharmacy or from your healthcare provider. This is very important because the amount of virus in your blood may increase if the medicine is stopped, even for a short time. The virus may develop resistance to emtricitabine or tenofovir and be harder to treat.

- For oral dosage form (capsules):
  - For treatment of HIV infection
    - Adults—Oral, one tablet (200 milligrams [mg] of emtricitabine and 300 mg of tenofovir) taken once a day. This medicine can be taken with or without food. Your doctor may want to change the dose if you have certain medical problems.
    - Children—Use and dose must be determined by your doctor.

Missed dose—If you miss a dose of this medicine, take it as soon as possible. However, if it is almost time for your next dose, skip the missed dose and go back to your regular dosing schedule. Do not double doses.

Call your healthcare provider or pharmacy if you are not sure what to do.

Storage—Store the medicine in a closed container at room temperature, away from heat, moisture, and direct light. Keep from freezing.

Keep out of the reach of children.

Do not keep outdated medicine or medicine no longer needed.

Ask your healthcare professional how you should dispose of any medicine you do not use.

Precautions While Using This Medicine

It is very important that you read the patient information when you start taking this medicine and each time you get a refill. There may be new information for you.

It is very important that your doctor check you at regular visits to be sure this medicine is working properly. You should remain under the care of a doctor while taking emtricitabine.

This medicine may cause serious problems with your liver or cause too much acid in your blood. If untreated, it can lead to severe low blood pressure and even death. Check with your doctor immediately if you notice abdominal discomfort; decreased appetite; diarrhea; fast, shallow breathing; general feeling of discomfort; muscle pain or cramping; nausea; shortness of breath; sleepiness; or unusual tiredness or weakness.

This medicine is not for the treatment of hepatitis B virus infection. Patients infected with both HBV and HIV who take emtricitabine and tenofovir combination need close medical follow-up for several months after stopping treatment to make sure their hepatitis B does not get worse.

Emtricitabine and tenofovir combination does not decrease the risk of transmitting the HIV infection to others through sexual contact or by contamination through blood. HIV may be acquired from or spread to others through infected body fluids, including blood, vaginal fluid, or semen. If you are infected, it is best to avoid any sexual activity involving an exchange of body fluids with other people. If you do have sex, always wear (or have your partner wear) a condom ("rubber"). Only use condoms made of latex or polyurethane and use them every time you have contact with semen, vaginal secretions, or blood. Also, do not share needles or equipment with anyone or use dirty needles. If you have any questions about this, check with your health care professional.

Side Effects of This Medicine

Along with its needed effects, a medicine may cause some unwanted effects. Although not all of these side effects may occur, if they do occur they may need medical attention.

Check with your doctor immediately if any of the following side effects occur:

Less common

Blisters under the skin; hives or welts; itching skin; rash with flat lesions or small raised lesions on the skin; redness of skin; spots on your skin resembling a blister or pimple; skin rash

Rare

Blindness or vision changes; burning of face or mouth; burning, crawling, itching, numbness, painful, prickling, "pins and needles", or tingling feelings in the hands, arms, feet, or legs; chest pain; clumsiness or unsteadiness; sensation of pins and needles; sneezing; sore throat; stabbing pain; weakness in hands or feet

Incidence not known

Abdominal discomfort; agitation; bloating; bloody or cloudy urine; bone pain; chills; coma; confusion; constipation; convulsions or seizures; cough; darkened urine; decreased appetite; decreased frequency or amount of urine; depression; difficult or labored breathing; difficult or painful urination; difficulty swallowing; diarrhea; dizziness; fast heartbeat; fast, shallow breathing; fever; general feeling of discomfort; headache; hostility; increase in amount of urine; increased blood pressure; increased thirst; indigestion; irritability; lethargy; loss of appetite; lower back or side pain; muscle pain or cramping; muscle twitching; nausea; pains in stomach, side, or abdomen, possibly radiating to the back; puffiness or swelling of the eyelids or around the eyes, face, lips or tongue; rapid weight gain; sleepiness; shortness of breath; stupor; sudden decrease in amount of urine; swelling of face, fingers, hands, lower legs, or ankles; tightness in chest; troubled breathing; unusual tiredness or weakness; vomiting; weight gain; wheezing; yellow eyes or skin

Some side effects may occur that usually do not need medical attention. These side effects may go away during treatment as your body adjusts to the medicine. Also, your health care professional may be able to tell you about ways to prevent or reduce some of these side effects. Check with your health care professional if any of the following side effects continue or are bothersome or if you have any questions about them:

Less common

Lack or loss of strength; passing of gas; weight loss

Rare

Acid or sour stomach; back pain; belching; difficulty in moving; discouragement; feeling sad or empty; heartburn; increased cough; joint pain; lack of appetite; loss of interest or pleasure; muscle aching or cramping; muscle pain or stiffness; pain; pain in joints; runny nose; shortness of breath; sleeplessness; stomach discomfort, upset, or pain; stuffy nose; sweating; swollen joints; tiredness; trouble concentrating; trouble sleeping; unable to sleep

Other side effects not listed may also occur in some patients. If you notice any other effects, check with your healthcare professional.

ENALAPRIL AND FELODIPINE
(Oral route) - e-NAL-a-pril MAL-ee-ate, fe-LOE-di-peen

Black Box Warning

When used in pregnancy during the second and third trimesters, ACE inhibitors can cause injury and even death to the developing fetus. When pregnancy is detected, enalapril maleate/felodipine should be discontinued as soon as possible.

Commonly used brand name(s)

In the U.S.—
Lexxel

Available Dosage Forms:
- Tablet, Extended Release

Therapeutic Class: ACE Inhibitor/Calcium Channel Blocker Combination
Pharmacologic Class: Enalapril

Uses For This Medicine

Enalapril and felodipine combination belongs to the class of medicines called high blood pressure medicines (antihypertensives). This medicine is used to treat high blood pressure (hypertension).

High blood pressure adds to the workload of the heart and arteries. If it continues for a long time, the heart and arteries may not function properly. This can damage the blood vessels of the brain, heart, and kidneys, resulting in a stroke, heart failure, or kidney failure. High blood pressure may also increase the risk of heart attacks. These problems may be less likely to occur if blood pressure is controlled.

The exact way in which this medicine works is not known. Enalapril is a type of medicine known as an angiotensin-converting enzyme (ACE) inhibitor. It blocks an enzyme in the body that is necessary in producing a substance that causes blood vessels to tighten. Felodipine is a type of medicine known as a calcium channel blocker. Calcium channel blocking agents affect the movement of calcium into the cells of the heart and blood vessels. The actions of both medicines relax blood vessels, lower blood pressure, and increase the supply of blood and oxygen to the heart.

This medicine is available only with your doctor's prescription.

Before Using This Medicine

In deciding to use a medicine, the risks of taking the medicine must be weighed against the good it will do. This is a decision you and your doctor will make. For this medicine, the following should be considered:

Allergies—Tell your doctor if you have ever had any unusual or allergic reaction to this medicine or any other medicines. Also tell your health care professional if you have any other types of allergies, such as to foods, dyes, preservatives, or animals. For non-prescription products, read the label or package ingredients carefully.

Pediatric—Studies on this medicine have been done only in adult patients, and there is no specific information comparing use of enalapril and felodipine in children with use in other age groups.

Geriatric—Although this medicine has not been shown to cause different side effects or problems in older people than it does in younger adults, blood levels of the felodipine component may be increased in the elderly.

Other medicines—

Using this medicine with any of the following medicines is usually not recommended, but may be required in some cases. If both medicines are prescribed together, your doctor may change the dose or how often you use one or both of the medicines.

Allopurinol, Amiloride, Amiodarone, Atazanavir, Azathioprine, Canrenoate, Cyclosporine, Droperidol, Fentanyl, Interferon Alfa-2a, Mibefradil, Potassium, Spironolactone, Triamterene

Interactions with Food/Tobacco/Alcohol—Certain medicines should not be used at or around the time of eating

food or eating certain types of food since interactions may occur. Using alcohol or tobacco with certain medicines may also cause interactions to occur. The following interactions have been selected on the basis of their potential significance and are not necessarily all-inclusive.

Using this medicine with any of the following may cause an increased risk of certain side effects but may be unavoidable in some cases. If used together, your doctor may change the dose or how often you use this medicine, or give you special instructions about the use of food, alcohol, or tobacco.

Grapefruit Juice

Other medical problems—The presence of other medical problems may affect the use of this medicine. Make sure you tell your doctor if you have any other medical problems, especially:

- Angioedema (an allergic skin disease), family history of or unknown cause—This medicine should not be used in patients with this condition.
- Bee-sting allergy treatments or
- Dialysis—Increased risk of serious allergic reaction occurring
- Dehydration—Lowering effects on blood pressure may be increased
- Diabetes mellitus (sugar diabetes)—Increased risk of potassium levels in the body becoming too high
- Heart attack or stroke or
- Heart or blood vessel disease or
- Hypotension (low blood pressure)—Further lowering of blood pressure may make problems resulting from these conditions worse
- Kidney disease or
- Liver disease—Effects may be increased because of slower removal from the body
- Previous reaction to any ACE inhibitor involving hoarseness; swelling of the face, mouth, hands, or feet; or sudden trouble in swallowing or breathing—Reaction is more likely to occur again
- Scleroderma or
- Systemic lupus erythematosus (SLE) (or history of)—Increased risk of blood problems caused by ACE inhibitors

Proper Use of This Medicine

Take this medicine exactly as directed by your doctor, at the same time each day. Do not take more of it and do not take it more often than directed.

Swallow the tablets whole, without breaking, crushing, or chewing them.

If felodipine is taken with grapefruit juice, its effects may be increased. Check with your doctor before taking this medicine with grapefruit juice.

Dosing—The dose of this medicine will be different for different patients. Follow your doctor's orders or the directions on the label. The following information includes only the average doses of this medicine. If your dose is different, do not change it unless your doctor tells you to do so.

The amount of medicine that you take depends on the strength of the medicine. Also, the number of doses you take each day, the time allowed between doses, and the length of time you take the medicine depend on the medical problem for which you are using the medicine.

- For oral dosage form (tablets):
  - For high blood pressure:
    - Adults—1 tablet once a day to start. Your doctor may increase your dose up to 4 tablets once a day if needed, to equal 20 mg enalapril and 10 mg felodipine extended-release.
    - Children—Use and dose must be determined by your doctor.

Missed dose—If you miss a dose of this medicine, take it as soon as possible. However, if it is almost time for your next dose, skip the missed dose and go back to your regular dosing schedule. Do not double doses.

Storage—Store the medicine in a closed container at room temperature, away from heat, moisture, and direct light. Keep from freezing.

Keep out of the reach of children.

Do not keep outdated medicine or medicine no longer needed.

Precautions While Using This Medicine

It is very important that your doctor check your progress at regular visits. This will allow your doctor to make sure the medicine is working properly, to check for unwanted effects, and to change the dosage if needed.

If you think that you may have become pregnant, check with your doctor immediately. Use of this medicine, especially during the second and third trimesters (after the first 3 months) of pregnancy, may cause serious injury or even death to the unborn child.

Do not take any other medicines, potassium supplements, or salt substitutes that contain potassium unless approved or prescribed by your doctor.

Dizziness, lightheadedness, or fainting may occur after the first dose, especially if you have been taking a diuretic (water pill). Make sure you know how you react to the medicine before you drive, use machines, or do other things that could be dangerous if you experience these effects.

Call your doctor if you faint or feel lightheaded while you are taking this medicine.

Check with your doctor if you notice any signs of fever, sore throat, or chills. These could be symptoms of an infection developing as a result of low white blood cell counts.

Check with your doctor if you notice difficult breathing or swelling of the face, arms, or legs. These could be symptoms of a serious allergic reaction.

Check with your doctor if you become sick while taking this medicine, especially with severe or continuing vomiting or diarrhea. These conditions may cause you to lose too much water, possibly resulting in low blood pressure.

Dizziness, lightheadedness, or fainting may also occur if you exercise or if the weather is hot. Heavy sweating can cause loss of too much water and result in low blood pressure. Use extra care during exercise or hot weather.

Black patients may be less sensitive to the blood pressure-lowering effects of this medicine. In addition, the risk of a serious allergic reaction involving swelling of the face, mouth, hands, or feet may be increased.

Before having any kind of surgery (including dental surgery) or emergency treatment, tell the medical doctor or dentist in charge that you are taking this medicine.

Side Effects of This Medicine

Along with its needed effects, a medicine may cause some unwanted effects. Although not all of these side effects may occur, if they do occur they may need medical attention.

Check with your doctor immediately if any of the following side effects occur:

Rare
   Swelling of face, mouth, hands, or feet; trouble in swallowing or breathing (sudden), accompanied by hoarseness

Check with your doctor as soon as possible if any of the following side effects occur:

Less common
   Dizziness, lightheadedness, or fainting; swelling of ankles, feet, or lower legs
Rare
   Chills, fever, and sore throat; unusual bleeding or bruising; yellow eyes or skin
Signs and symptoms of too much potassium in the body
   Confusion; irregular heartbeat; nervousness; numbness or tingling in hands, feet, or lips; shortness of breath; weakness or heaviness of legs

Some side effects may occur that usually do not need medical attention. These side effects may go away during treatment as your body adjusts to the medicine. Also, your health care professional may be able to tell you about ways to prevent or reduce some of these side effects. Check with your health care professional if any of the following side effects continue or are bothersome or if you have any questions about them:

More common
   Headache
Less common
   Cough (dry, persistent); flushing; swelling of the gums; unusual tiredness

Other side effects not listed may also occur in some patients. If you notice any other effects, check with your healthcare professional.

ENFUVIRTIDE (Subcutaneous route) - en-FYOO-vir-tide

Commonly used brand name(s)

In the U.S.—
   Fuzeon

Available Dosage Forms:
   • Powder for Solution

Therapeutic Class: Antiretroviral Agent
Pharmacologic Class: HIV Fusion Inhibitor

Uses For This Medicine

Enfuvirtide is used, in combination with other medicines, in the treatment of the infection caused by the human immu-nodeficiency virus (HIV). HIV is the virus that causes acquired immunodeficiency syndrome (AIDS).

Enfuvirtide will not cure or prevent HIV infection or AIDS; however, it helps keep HIV from reproducing and appears to slow down the destruction of the immune system. This may help delay the development of problems usually related to AIDS or HIV disease. Enfuvirtide will not keep you from spreading HIV to other people. People who receive this medicine may continue to have other problems usually related to AIDS or HIV disease.

This medicine is available only with your doctor's prescription.

Before Using This Medicine

In deciding to use a medicine, the risks of taking the medicine must be weighed against the good it will do. This is a decision you and your doctor will make. For this medicine, the following should be considered:

Allergies—Tell your doctor if you have ever had any unusual or allergic reaction to this medicine or any other medicines. Also tell your health care professional if you have any other types of allergies, such as to foods, dyes, preservatives, or animals. For non-prescription products, read the label or package ingredients carefully.

Pediatric—This medicine has been studied in children ages 6 to 16 years old and it is not expected to cause different effects than it does in adult patients.

Geriatric—Many medicines have not been studied specifically in older people and it may not be known if they work the same way they do in younger adults.

Pregnancy—

	Pregnancy Category	Explanation
All Trimesters	B	Animal studies have revealed no evidence of harm to the fetus, however, there are no adequate studies in pregnant women OR animal studies have shown an adverse effect, but adequate studies in pregnant women have failed to demonstrate a risk to the fetus.

Breast Feeding—There are no adequate studies in women for determining infant risk when using this medication during breastfeeding. Weigh the potential benefits against the potential risks before taking this medication while breastfeeding.

Other medicines—Although certain medicines should not be used together at all, in other cases two different medicines may be used together even if an interaction might occur. In these cases, your doctor may want to change the dose, or other precautions may be necessary. Tell your healthcare professional if you are taking any other prescription or non-prescription (over-the-counter [OTC]) medicine.

Interactions with Food/Tobacco/Alcohol—Certain medicines should not be used at or around the time of eating food or eating certain types of food since interactions may occur. Using alcohol or tobacco with certain medicines may also cause interactions to occur. Discuss with your healthcare professional the use of your medicine with food, alcohol, or tobacco.

Other medical problems—The presence of other medical problems may affect the use of this medicine. Make sure you tell your doctor if you have any other medical problems, especially:

- Pneumonia risk factors, such as
- Immune system blood tests (abnormal) or
- Cigarette smoking
- Intravenous drug use or
- Lung disease (history of)—Patients with these conditions may have an increased chance of getting bacterial pneumonia

Proper Use of This Medicine

It is very important that you read the information for patients and the injection instructions very carefully. Ask your healthcare professional if you have any questions.

Enfuvirtide can be given by a health care professional. However, medicines given by injection are sometimes used at home. If you will be using enfuvirtide at home, your health care professional will teach you how get the medicine ready for injection and how the injections are to be given. Be certain that you understand exactly how to get the medicine ready for injection and how the medicine is to be injected. Do not reuse needles and syringes.

Put used needles and syringes in a puncture-resistant disposable container, or dispose of them as directed by your health care professional.

It is important to take enfuvirtide as part of a combination treatment. Be sure to take all the medicines your doctor has prescribed for you, including enfuvirtide.

Do not stop taking this medicine without checking with your doctor first.

This medicine may cause a severe allergic reaction in some patients. Stop taking this medicine and check with your doctor immediately if you notice cough; difficulty breathing; fever; skin rash; unusual tiredness or weakness.

This medicine may increase the chance of bacterial pneumonia in some patients. Stop taking this medicine and check with your doctor immediately if you notice cough with fever; difficulty breathing; fast breathing; shortness of breath.

This medicine can cause reactions at the place on your body where it was injected. Almost all people get injection site reactions with enfuvirtide. These reactions hurt and itch, and they are usually mild to moderate but can occasionally be severe. These reactions generally happen within the first week of treatment and usually happen again as you keep using enfuvirtide. If the injection site nodules drain pus or cause redness that spreads or streaks from the sites, or you are worried about the reaction you are having, call your healthcare provider right away.

Dosing—The dose of this medicine will be different for different patients. Follow your doctor's orders or the directions on the label. The following information includes only the average doses of this medicine. If your dose is different, do not change it unless your doctor tells you to do so.

The amount of medicine that you take depends on the strength of the medicine. Also, the number of doses you take each day, the time allowed between doses, and the length of time you take the medicine depend on the medical problem for which you are using the medicine.

- For parenteral dosage form (injection):
  - For treatment of HIV infection:
    - Adults—90 milligrams (mg) twice a day given by injection
    - Children—Dose must be determined by your doctor.

Missed dose—If you miss a dose of this medicine, take it as soon as possible. However, if it is almost time for your next dose, skip the missed dose and go back to your regular dosing schedule. Do not double doses.

Storage—Keep out of the reach of children.

Do not keep outdated medicine or medicine no longer needed.

Store reconstituted solution (mixed with water) in the refrigerator and use within 24 hours.

Precautions While Using This Medicine

It is very important that your doctor check you at regular visits.

Enfuvirtide does not reduce the risk of giving HIV to other people. Caution should be taken to avoid spreading HIV.

This medicine may make you dizzy. Avoid driving, using machines, or doing anything else that could be dangerous if you are not alert.

Side Effects of This Medicine

Along with its needed effects, a medicine may cause some unwanted effects. Although not all of these side effects may occur, if they do occur they may need medical attention.

Check with your doctor immediately if any of the following side effects occur:

More common
Awkwardness; burning, numbness, tingling, or painful sensations or weakness in arms, hands, legs, or feet; cough; headache; pain or tenderness around eyes and cheekbones; shortness of breath or troubled breathing; stuffy or runny nose; tightness of chest; unsteadiness; wheezing

Less common
Bloating; chills; constipation; darkened urine; dry or itching eyes; excessive tearing; eye discharge; fast heartbeat; fever; indigestion; itching, pain, redness, swelling, tenderness, or warmth on skin at injection site; loss of appetite; lump or growth on skin; nausea; pains in stomach, side, or abdomen, possibly radiating to the back; redness, pain, swelling of eye, eyelid, or inner lining of eyelid burning; vomiting; yellow eyes or skin

Rare
Difficulty in breathing or swallowing; fast heartbeat; skin itching, rash, or redness; swelling of face, throat, or tongue

Incidence not known
Black, tarry stools; bleeding gums; blood in urine or stools; bloody urine; chest pain; decreased frequency or amount of urine; inability to move arms and legs; increased blood pressure; increased thirst; lower back or side pain; painful or difficult urination; pale skin; pinpoint red spots on skin; sneezing; sore throat; sudden numbness and weakness in the arms and legs; swelling of face, fingers, lower legs; weight gain; ulcers, sores,

or white spots in mouth; unusual bleeding or bruising; unusual tiredness or weakness

Some side effects may occur that usually do not need medical attention. These side effects may go away during treatment as your body adjusts to the medicine. Also, your health care professional may be able to tell you about ways to prevent or reduce some of these side effects. Check with your health care professional if any of the following side effects continue or are bothersome or if you have any questions about them:

More common

Abnormal growth filled with fluid or semisolid material; bruising; burning or stinging of skin; decreased appetite; diarrhea; discouragement; dry mouth; fear; feeling sad or empty; flushing; hard lump; itching skin; irritability; lack of appetite; lack or loss of strength; large, flat, blue or purplish patches in the skin; muscle pain; nervousness; painful cold sores or blisters on lips, nose, eyes, or genitals; redness of skin; small lumps under the skin; tiredness; trouble concentrating; trouble sleeping; unusually warm skin; weight loss

Less common

Bad, unusual or unpleasant (after) taste; burning, itching, and pain in hairy areas; change in taste; diarrhea; general feeling of discomfort or illness; joint pain; pus at root of hair; stomach pain; swollen, painful, or tender lymph glands in neck, armpit, or groin

Other side effects not listed may also occur in some patients. If you notice any other effects, check with your healthcare professional.

ENOXAPARIN (Subcutaneous route) - ee-nox-a-PA-rin

Black Box Warning

When neuraxial anesthesia (epidural/spinal anesthesia) or spinal puncture is employed, patients anticoagulated or scheduled to be anticoagulated with low molecular weight heparins or heparinoids for prevention of thromboembolic complications are at risk of developing an epidural or spinal hematoma which can result in long-term or permanent paralysis.

The risk of these events is increased by the use of indwelling epidural catheters for administration of analgesia or by the concomitant use of drugs affecting hemostasis such as non steroidal anti-inflammatory drugs (NSAIDs), platelet inhibitors, or other anticoagulants. The risk also appears to be increased by traumatic or repeated epidural or spinal puncture.

Patients should be frequently monitored for signs and symptoms of neurological impairment. If neurologic compromise is noted, urgent treatment is necessary.

The physician should consider the potential benefit versus risk before neuraxial intervention in patients anticoagulated or to be anticoagulated for thromboprophylaxis.

Commonly used brand name(s)

In the U.S.—
Lovenox

Available Dosage Forms:

- Solution
- Injectable

Therapeutic Class: Anticoagulant
Pharmacologic Class: Low Molecular Weight Heparin

Uses For This Medicine

Enoxaparin is used to prevent deep venous thrombosis, a condition in which harmful blood clots form in the blood vessels of the legs. This medicine is used for several days after hip or knee replacement surgery, and in some cases following abdominal surgery, while you are unable to walk. It is during this time that blood clots are most likely to form. Enoxaparin is also used if you are unable to get out of bed because of a serious illness. In addition, enoxaparin is used to prevent blood clots from forming in the arteries of the heart during certain types of chest pain and heart attacks. Enoxaparin also may be used for other conditions as determined by your doctor.

Enoxaparin is available only with your doctor's prescription.

Before Using This Medicine

In deciding to use a medicine, the risks of taking the medicine must be weighed against the good it will do. This is a decision you and your doctor will make. For this medicine, the following should be considered:

Allergies—Tell your doctor if you have ever had any unusual or allergic reaction to this medicine or any other medicines. Also tell your health care professional if you have any other types of allergies, such as to foods, dyes, preservatives, or animals. For non-prescription products, read the label or package ingredients carefully.

Pediatric—Studies on this medicine have been done only in adult patients, and there is no specific information comparing use of enoxaparin in children with use in other age groups.

Geriatric—This medicine has been tested and has been shown to cause an increased risk of side effects or problems in older people than it does in younger adults. You doctor may adjust your dose, especially if you are less than 45 kg (99 lbs.) of body weight or in elderly patients with decreased kidney function.

Pregnancy—

	Pregnancy Category	Explanation
All Trimesters	B	Animal studies have revealed no evidence of harm to the fetus, however, there are no adequate studies in pregnant women OR animal studies have shown an adverse effect, but adequate studies in pregnant women have failed to demonstrate a risk to the fetus.

Breast Feeding—There are no adequate studies in women for determining infant risk when using this medication during breastfeeding. Weigh the potential benefits against the potential risks before taking this medication while breastfeeding.

Other medicines—

Using this medicine with any of the following medicines is usually not recommended, but may be required in some cases. If both medicines are prescribed together, your doctor may change the dose or how often you use one or both of the medicines.

Abciximab, Aceclofenac, Acemetacin, Acenocoumarol, Alclofenac, Alteplase, Recombinant, Ancrod, Anisindione, Anistreplase, Antithrombin III Human, Apazone, Ardeparin, Argatroban, Benoxaprofen, Bivalirudin, Bromfenac, Bufexamac, Carprofen, Certoparin, Clometacin, Clonixin, Clopidogrel, Dalteparin, Danaparoid, Defibrotide, Dermatan Sulfate, Desirudin, Dexketoprofen, Diclofenac, Dicumarol, Diflunisal, Dipyrone, Droxicam, Enoxaparin, Eptifibatide, Etodolac, Etofenamate, Felbinac, Fenbufen, Fenoprofen, Fentiazac, Floctafenine, Flufenamic Acid, Flurbiprofen, Fondaparinux, Heparin, Ibuprofen, Indomethacin, Indoprofen, Isoxicam, Ketoprofen, Ketorolac, Lamifiban, Lornoxicam, Meclofenamate, Mefenamic Acid, Meloxicam, Nabumetone, Nadroparin, Naproxen, Niflumic Acid, Nimesulide, Oxaprozin, Oxyphenbutazone, Parnaparin, Pentosan Polysulfate Sodium, Phenindione, Phenprocoumon, Phenylbutazone, Pirazolac, Piroxicam, Pirprofen, Propyphenazone, Proquazone, Reteplase, Recombinant, Reviparin, Sibrafiban, Streptokinase, Sulindac, Suprofen, Tenecteplase, Tenidap, Tenoxicam, Tiaprofenic Acid, Tinzaparin, Tirofiban, Tolmetin, Urokinase, Warfarin, Xemilofiban, Zomepirac

Interactions with Food/Tobacco/Alcohol—Certain medicines should not be used at or around the time of eating food or eating certain types of food since interactions may occur. Using alcohol or tobacco with certain medicines may also cause interactions to occur. Discuss with your healthcare professional the use of your medicine with food, alcohol, or tobacco.

Other medical problems—The presence of other medical problems may affect the use of this medicine. Make sure you tell your doctor if you have any other medical problems, especially:

- Blood disease or bleeding problems or
- Blood vessel problems or
- Heart infection or
- Heart valves, prosthetic or
- High blood pressure (hypertension) or
- Kidney disease or
- Liver disease or
- Septic shock or
- Stomach ulcer (active) or
- Threatened miscarriage—The risk of bleeding may be increased

Also, tell your doctor if you have received enoxaparin or heparin before and had a reaction to either of them called thrombocytopenia, or if new blood clots formed while you were receiving the medicine.

In addition, tell your doctor if you have recently given birth, fallen or suffered a blow to the body or head, or had medical or dental surgery. These events may increase the risk of serious bleeding when you are taking enoxaparin.

Proper Use of This Medicine

If you are using enoxaparin at home, your health care professional will teach you how to inject yourself with the medicine. Be sure to follow the directions carefully. Check with your health care professional if you have any problems using the medicine.

Put used syringes in a puncture-resistant, disposable container, or dispose of them as directed by your health care professional.

Dosing—The dose of this medicine will be different for different patients. Follow your doctor's orders or the directions on the label. The following information includes only the average doses of this medicine. If your dose is different, do not change it unless your doctor tells you to do so.

The amount of medicine that you take depends on the strength of the medicine. Also, the number of doses you take each day, the time allowed between doses, and the length of time you take the medicine depend on the medical problem for which you are using the medicine.

- For injection dosage form:
  - For prevention of deep venous thrombosis (hip or knee replacement surgery):
    - Adults—30 milligrams (mg) injected under the skin every twelve hours for seven to ten days. Alternatively, for hip replacement surgery, the dose may be 40 mg injected under the skin once a day for three weeks. 30 mg once a day if you have a poorly performing kidney
    - Children—Use and dose must be determined by your doctor.
  - For prevention of deep venous thrombosis (abdominal surgery):
    - Adults—40 mg injected under the skin once a day for seven to ten days. 30 mg once a day if you have a poorly performing kidney
    - Children—Use and dose must be determined by your doctor.
  - For prevention of certain types of chest pain and heart attack:
    - Adults—1 mg per kilogram (kg) (0.45 mg per pound) of body weight injected under the skin every twelve hours for two to eight days. 1 mg per kg once a day if you have a poorly performing kidney
    - Children—Use and dose must be determined by your doctor.
  - For prevention of deep venous thrombosis (in patients with a serious illness who cannot get out of bed):
    - Adults—40 mg injected under the skin once a day for six to eleven days. 30 mg once a day if you have a poorly performing kidney
    - Children—Use and dose must be determined by your doctor.
  - For treatment of certain types of chest pain and heart attack
    - Adults—1 mg per kg (2.2 lbs) of body weight every 12 hours injected under the skin for two to eight days. Aspirin 100 to 325 mg orally once a day may also be given.
    - Children—Use and dose must be determined by your doctor.

Missed dose—If you miss a dose of this medicine, take it as soon as possible. However, if it is almost time for your next dose, skip the missed dose and go back to your regular dosing schedule. Do not double doses.

Storage—Store the medicine in a closed container at room temperature, away from heat, moisture, and direct light. Keep from freezing.

Keep out of the reach of children.

Do not keep outdated medicine or medicine no longer needed.

Precautions While Using This Medicine

Tell all your medical doctors and dentists that you are using this medicine.

Check with your doctor immediately if you notice any of the following side effects:

- Bruising or bleeding, especially bleeding that is hard to stop. Bleeding inside the body sometimes appears as bloody or black, tarry stools, or faintness.
- Back pain; burning, pricking, tickling, or tingling sensation; leg weakness; numbness; paralysis; or problems with bowel or bladder function.

Side Effects of This Medicine

Along with its needed effects, a medicine may cause some unwanted effects. Although not all of these side effects may occur, if they do occur they may need medical attention.

Stop taking this medicine and get emergency help immediately if any of the following effects occur:

More common
Black, tarry stools; bleeding gums; blood in urine or stools; coughing up blood; difficulty in breathing or swallowing; dizziness; headache; increased menstrual flow or vaginal bleeding; moderate to severe pain or numbness in the arms, legs, hands, feet; nosebleeds; pale skin; paralysis; pinpoint red spots on skin; prolonged bleeding from cuts; red or black, tarry stools; red or dark brown urine; shortness of breath; swelling of ankles, feet, fingers; troubled breathing with exertion; unusual bleeding or bruising; unusual tiredness or weakness

Less common
Bruising; chest discomfort; collection of blood under the skin; confusion; continuing bleeding or oozing from the nose and/or mouth, or surgical wound; convulsions; difficult or labored breathing; fever; irritability; lightheadedness; lower back pain; pain or burning while urinating; swelling of hands and/or feet; tightness in chest; uncontrolled bleeding at site of injection; wheezing; vomiting of blood or material that looks like coffee grounds

Rare
Back pain; burning, pricking, tickling, or tingling sensation; chest pain; chills; cough; dizziness or lightheadedness when getting up from a lying or sitting position; fainting; fast or irregular heartbeat; fever; general feeling of discomfort or illness; leg weakness; paralysis; problems with bowel or bladder function; shortness of breath; skin rash or hives; sneezing; sore throat; sudden fainting; swelling of the face, genitals, mouth, or tongue; thickening of bronchial secretions; troubled breathing

Some side effects may occur that usually do not need medical attention. These side effects may go away during treatment as your body adjusts to the medicine. Also, your health care professional may be able to tell you about ways to prevent or reduce some of these side effects. Check with your health care professional if any of the following side effects continue or are bothersome or if you have any questions about them:

Less common
Diarrhea; irritation, pain, or redness at place of injection; nausea; vomiting

Other side effects not listed may also occur in some patients. If you notice any other effects, check with your healthcare professional.

ENTACAPONE (Oral route) - en-TA-ka-pone

Commonly used brand name(s)

In the U.S.—
Comtan

Available Dosage Forms:
- Tablet

Therapeutic Class: Antiparkinsonian
Pharmacologic Class: Catechol-O-Methyltransferase Inhibitor

Uses For This Medicine

Entacapone is used in combination with levodopa/carbidopa to treat Parkinson's disease, sometimes referred to as shaking palsy. Some patients experience signs and symptoms of end-of-dose "wearing-off" effect despite taking levodopa/carbidopa. Entacapone enhances the effect of levodopa/carbidopa. By improving muscle control, this medicine allows more normal movements of the body.

This medicine is available only with your doctor's prescription.

Before Using This Medicine

In deciding to use a medicine, the risks of taking the medicine must be weighed against the good it will do. This is a decision you and your doctor will make. For this medicine, the following should be considered:

Allergies—Tell your doctor if you have ever had any unusual or allergic reaction to this medicine or any other medicines. Also tell your health care professional if you have any other types of allergies, such as to foods, dyes, preservatives, or animals. For non-prescription products, read the label or package ingredients carefully.

Pediatric—Studies on this medicine have been done only in adult patients. There is no identified potential use of entacapone in children.

Geriatric—Many medicines have not been tested in older people. Therefore, it may not be known whether they work exactly the same way they do in younger adults or if they cause different side effects or problems in older people. In studies done to date that included elderly people, entacapone did not cause different side effects or problems in older people than it did in younger adults.

Pregnancy—

	Pregnancy Category	Explanation
All Trimesters	C	Animal studies have shown an adverse effect and there are no adequate studies in pregnant women OR no animal studies have been conducted and there are no adequate studies in pregnant women.

Breast Feeding—There are no adequate studies in women for determining infant risk when using this medication during breastfeeding. Weigh the potential benefits against the potential risks before taking this medication while breastfeeding.

Other medicines—

Using this medicine with any of the following medicines is usually not recommended, but may be required in some cases. If both medicines are prescribed together, your doctor may change the dose or how often you use one or both of the medicines.

Apomorphine, Bitolterol, Desipramine, Dobutamine, Dopamine, Epinephrine, Iproniazid, Isocarboxazid, Isoetharine, Isoproterenol, Methyldopa, Nialamide, Norepinephrine, Pargyline, Phenelzine, Procarbazine, Tranylcypromine, Venlafaxine

Interactions with Food/Tobacco/Alcohol—Certain medicines should not be used at or around the time of eating food or eating certain types of food since interactions may occur. Using alcohol or tobacco with certain medicines may also cause interactions to occur. Discuss with your healthcare professional the use of your medicine with food, alcohol, or tobacco.

Other medical problems—The presence of other medical problems may affect the use of this medicine. Make sure you tell your doctor if you have any other medical problems, especially:

• Liver problems—Side effects of entacapone may be increased because of a slower removal from the body.

Proper Use of This Medicine

Take this medicine only as directed by your doctor, to help your condition as much as possible. Do not take more or less of it, and do not take it more or less often than your doctor ordered.

Dosing—The dose of this medicine will be different for different patients. Follow your doctor's orders or the directions on the label. The following information includes only the average doses of this medicine. If your dose is different, do not change it unless your doctor tells you to do so.

The amount of medicine that you take depends on the strength of the medicine. Also, the number of doses you take each day, the time allowed between doses, and the length of time you take the medicine depend on the medical problem for which you are using the medicine.

Entacapone is always used in combination with levodopa/carbidopa (Sinemet); never alone.

The number of times a day you take the tablets depends on how often you take levodopa/carbidopa (Sinemet).

• For oral dosage form (tablets):
  ○ For Parkinson's disease:
    ▪ Adults—200 mg with each levodopa/carbidopa (Sinemet) dose. Entacapone may be taken up to 8 times a day, but the total daily dose is usually not more than 1600 mg..
    ▪ Children—Use and dose must be determined by your doctor.

Missed dose—If you miss a dose of this medicine, take it as soon as possible. However, if it is almost time for your next dose, skip the missed dose and go back to your regular dosing schedule. Do not double doses.

Storage—Store the medicine in a closed container at room temperature, away from heat, moisture, and direct light. Keep from freezing.

Keep out of the reach of children.

Do not keep outdated medicine or medicine no longer needed.

Ask your healthcare professional how you should dispose of any medicine you do not use.

Precautions While Using This Medicine

It is important that your doctor check your progress at regular visits to make sure that this medicine is working properly and to check for unwanted effects.

Do not stop taking entacapone without first checking with your doctor. Your doctor may want you to gradually reduce the amount you are taking before stopping completely.

Nausea may occur, especially when you first start taking this medicine. Also, an increase in body movements and twitching, twisting, or uncontrolled movements of the tongue, lips, face, arms or legs may occur. Your doctor may need to adjust your dose of levodopa/carbidopa if these movements occur.

This medicine may cause some people to become dizzy or drowsy. Make sure you know how you react to this medicine before you drive, use machines, or do anything else that could be dangerous if you are not alert.

Dizziness, lightheadedness, or fainting may occur, especially when you get up from a lying or sitting position. Getting up slowly may help. If you should have this problem, check with your doctor.

Hallucinations (seeing, hearing, or feeling things that are not there) may occur in some patients.

Entacapone may cause your urine to turn brownish orange. This effect is harmless and will go away after you stop taking the medicine.

Side Effects of This Medicine

Along with its needed effects, a medicine may cause some unwanted effects. Although not all of these side effects may occur, if they do occur they may need medical attention.

Check with your doctor as soon as possible if any of the following side effects occur:

More common

Absence of or decrease in body movements; hyperactivity; increase in body movements; seeing, hearing, or feeling things that are not there; twitching; twisting; uncontrolled repetitive movements of tongue, lips, face, arms, or legs

Less common

Fever or chills; cough or hoarseness; lower back or side pain; painful or difficult urination

Rare

Confusion; muscle cramps; pain; shortness of breath; stiffness; weakness; unusual tiredness

Some side effects may occur that usually do not need medical attention. These side effects may go away during treatment as your body adjusts to the medicine. Also, your health care professional may be able to tell you about ways to prevent or reduce some of these side effects. Check with your health care professional if any of the following side effects continue or are bothersome or if you have any questions about them:

More common

Abdominal pain; constipation; diarrhea; dizziness; fatigue; nausea

Less common

Acid or sour stomach; anxiety; belching; bruising; burning feeling in chest or stomach; heartburn; difficult or labored breathing; dry mouth; indigestion; insomnia; irritability; loss of strength or energy; muscle pain or weakness; nervousness; passing gas; sleepiness or unusual drowsiness; small, red spots on skin; stomach discomfort, upset or pain; sweating increased; restlessness; tenderness in stomach area; tightness in chest; tremor; shortness of breath; unusual or unpleasant (after) taste; unusual weak feeling; wheezing

This medicine may cause your urine to turn brownish orange. This effect is harmless and will go away after you stop taking the medicine.

Other side effects not listed may also occur in some patients. If you notice any other effects, check with your healthcare professional.

ENTECAVIR (Oral route) - en-TE-ka-veer

Black Box Warning

Lactic acidosis and severe hepatomegaly with steatosis, including fatal cases, have been reported with the use of nucleoside analogues alone or in combination with antiretrovirals.

Severe acute exacerbations of hepatitis B have been reported in patients who have discontinued anti-hepatitis B therapy, including entecavir. Hepatic function should be monitored closely with both clinical and laboratory follow-up for at least several months in patients who discontinue anti-hepatitis B therapy. If appropriate, initiation of anti-hepatitis B therapy may be warranted.

Commonly used brand name(s)

In the U.S.—

Baraclude

Available Dosage Forms:

• Solution
• Tablet

Therapeutic Class: Antiviral

Uses For This Medicine

Entecavir is used in the treatment of the infection caused by hepatitis B virus. Entecavir is not a cure for the hepatitis B virus; the long-term effects of the drug on the infection and the liver are unknown at this time.

This medicine is available only with your doctor's prescription.

Before Using This Medicine

In deciding to use a medicine, the risks of taking the medicine must be weighed against the good it will do. This is a decision you and your doctor will make. For this medicine, the following should be considered:

Allergies—Tell your doctor if you have ever had any unusual or allergic reaction to this medicine or any other medicines. Also tell your health care professional if you have any other types of allergies, such as to foods, dyes, preservatives, or animals. For non-prescription products, read the label or package ingredients carefully.

Pediatric—Studies on this medicine have been done only in adult patients, and there is no specific information comparing use of entecavir in children with use in other age groups.

Geriatric—Many medicines have not been studied specifically in older people. Therefore, it may not be known whether they work exactly the same way they do in younger adults. Although there is no specific information comparing use of entecavir in the elderly with use in other age groups, the elderly may be more sensitive to the effects of entecavir.

Pregnancy—

	Pregnancy Category	Explanation
All Trimesters	C	Animal studies have shown an adverse effect and there are no adequate studies in pregnant women OR no animal studies have been conducted and there are no adequate studies in pregnant women.

Breast Feeding—There are no adequate studies in women for determining infant risk when using this medication during breastfeeding. Weigh the potential benefits against the potential risks before taking this medication while breastfeeding.

Other medicines—Although certain medicines should not be used together at all, in other cases two different medicines may be used together even if an interaction might occur. In these cases, your doctor may want to change the dose, or other precautions may be necessary. Tell your healthcare professional if you are taking any other prescription or non-prescription (over-the-counter [OTC]) medicine.

Interactions with Food/Tobacco/Alcohol—Certain medicines should not be used at or around the time of eating food or eating certain types of food since interactions may occur. Using alcohol or tobacco with certain medicines may also cause interactions to occur. Discuss with your healthcare professional the use of your medicine with food, alcohol, or tobacco.

Other medical problems—The presence of other medical problems may affect the use of this medicine. Make sure you tell your doctor if you have any other medical problems, especially:

- Kidney disease—Your doctor may need to adjust your dose
- Liver transplant—Your doctor will need to monitor your kidney function

Proper Use of This Medicine

Take this medicine exactly as directed by your doctor. Do not take it more often, and do not take it for a longer time than your doctor ordered. Also, do not stop taking this medicine without checking with your doctor first.

Importance of taking on an empty stomach.

The importance of reading the patient information leaflet before starting entecavir treatment and each time you refill.

Correctly measuring the oral solution and rinsing the dosing spoon with water after each use.

Dosing—The dose of this medicine will be different for different patients. Follow your doctor's orders or the directions on the label. The following information includes only the average doses of this medicine. If your dose is different, do not change it unless your doctor tells you to do so.

The amount of medicine that you take depends on the strength of the medicine. Also, the number of doses you take each day, the time allowed between doses, and the length of time you take the medicine depend on the medical problem for which you are using the medicine.

- For oral dosage form (tablets):
  - For chronic hepatitis B infection
  - For oral dosage form (oral solution):
    - Adults—0.5 to 1 milligram once daily. You may take less of this medicine or less often if you have kidney problems.
    - Children—Dose must be determined by your doctor.
  - For oral dosage form (tablets):
    - Adults—0.5 to 1 milligram once daily. You may take less of this medicine or less often if you have kidney problems.
    - Children—Use and dose must be determined by your doctor.

Missed dose—If you miss a dose of this medicine, take it as soon as possible. However, if it is almost time for your next dose, skip the missed dose and go back to your regular dosing schedule. Do not double doses.

Storage—Store the medicine in a closed container at room temperature, away from heat, moisture, and direct light. Keep from freezing.

Keep out of the reach of children.

Do not keep outdated medicine or medicine no longer needed.

Ask your healthcare professional how you should dispose of any medicine you do not use.

Precautions While Using This Medicine

It is very important that your doctor check your progress at regular visits. This will allow your doctor to see if the medicine is working properly.

Consulting physician immediately if symptoms of hepatomegaly or lactic acidosis occur

Liver disease may become worse if treatment with entecavir is stopped. Do not stop taking entecavir unless your doctor tells you to stop.

Treatment with entecavir has not been shown to decrease the chance of giving hepatitis B virus infection to other people through sexual contact or blood contamination.

Side Effects of This Medicine

Along with its needed effects, a medicine may cause some unwanted effects. Although not all of these side effects may occur, if they do occur they may need medical attention.

Check with your doctor immediately if any of the following side effects occur:

Frequency unknown
  Abdominal discomfort; decreased appetite; diarrhea; fast, shallow breathing; general feeling of discomfort; muscle pain or cramping; nausea; right upper abdominal pain and fullness; shortness of breath; sleepiness; unusual tiredness or weakness

Some side effects may occur that usually do not need medical attention. These side effects may go away during treatment as your body adjusts to the medicine. Also, your health care professional may be able to tell you about ways to prevent or reduce some of these side effects. Check with your health care professional if any of the following side effects continue or are bothersome or if you have any questions about them:

Less common
  Headache
Rare
  Acid or sour stomach; belching; dizziness; heartburn; indigestion; nausea; sleepiness or unusual drowsiness; sleeplessness; stomach discomfort upset or pain; trouble sleeping; vomiting

Other side effects not listed may also occur in some patients. If you notice any other effects, check with your healthcare professional.

EPINASTINE (Ophthalmic route) - ep-i-NAS-teen

Commonly used brand name(s)

In the U.S.—
  Elestat

Available Dosage Forms:
- Solution

Therapeutic Class: Ophthalmologic Agent
Pharmacologic Class: Antihistamine, Less-Sedating

Uses For This Medicine

Epinastine ophthalmic (eye) solution is used to treat itching of the eye caused by a condition known as allergic conjunctivitis. It works by preventing the effects of certain inflammatory substances, which are produced by cells in your eyes and sometimes cause allergic reactions.

This medicine is available only with your doctor's prescription.

Before Using This Medicine

In deciding to use a medicine, the risks of taking the medicine must be weighed against the good it will do. This is a decision you and your doctor will make. For this medicine, the following should be considered:

Allergies—Tell your doctor if you have ever had any unusual or allergic reaction to this medicine or any other medicines. Also tell your health care professional if you have any other types of allergies, such as to foods, dyes, preservatives, or animals. For non-prescription products, read the label or package ingredients carefully.

Pediatric—Studies on this medicine have been done only in adult patients, and there is no specific information comparing use of epinastine in children under the age of 3 years with use in other age groups.

Geriatric—This medicine has been tested and has not been shown to cause different side effects or problems in older people than it does in younger adults.

Pregnancy—

	Pregnancy Category	Explanation
All Trimesters	C	Animal studies have shown an adverse effect and there are no adequate studies in pregnant women OR no animal studies have been conducted and there are no adequate studies in pregnant women.

Breast Feeding—There are no adequate studies in women for determining infant risk when using this medication during breastfeeding. Weigh the potential benefits against the potential risks before taking this medication while breastfeeding.

Other medicines—Although certain medicines should not be used together at all, in other cases two different medicines may be used together even if an interaction might occur. In these cases, your doctor may want to change the dose, or other precautions may be necessary. Tell your healthcare professional if you are taking any other prescription or non-prescription (over-the-counter [OTC]) medicine.

Interactions with Food/Tobacco/Alcohol—Certain medicines should not be used at or around the time of eating food or eating certain types of food since interactions may occur. Using alcohol or tobacco with certain medicines may also cause interactions to occur. Discuss with your healthcare professional the use of your medicine with food, alcohol, or tobacco.

Proper Use of This Medicine

Do not wear contact lenses if your eyes are red. If your eyes are not red, contact lenses should be removed before you use this medicine. Also, you should wait at least 10 minutes after using this medicine before putting the contact lenses back in.

To keep the medicine as germ-free as possible, do not touch the applicator tip to any surface (including the eye). Also, keep the container tightly closed. Serious damage to the eye and possible loss of vision may result from using contaminated eye drops.

The dose of epinastine will be different for different patients. Follow your doctor's orders or the directions on the label. The

following information includes only the average doses of epinastine. If your dose is different, do not change it unless your doctor tells you to do so.

- For ophthalmic dosage form (eye drops):
  - For eye allergy:
    - Adults and children 3 years of age and older—Use one drop in each eye twice a day.
    - Children younger than 3 years of age—Use and dose must be determined by your doctor.

Dosing—The dose of this medicine will be different for different patients. Follow your doctor's orders or the directions on the label. The following information includes only the average doses of this medicine. If your dose is different, do not change it unless your doctor tells you to do so.

The amount of medicine that you take depends on the strength of the medicine. Also, the number of doses you take each day, the time allowed between doses, and the length of time you take the medicine depend on the medical problem for which you are using the medicine.

Missed dose—If you miss a dose of this medicine, take it as soon as possible. However, if it is almost time for your next dose, skip the missed dose and go back to your regular dosing schedule. Do not double doses.

Storage—Store the medicine in a closed container at room temperature, away from heat, moisture, and direct light. Keep from freezing.

Keep out of the reach of children.

Do not keep outdated medicine or medicine no longer needed.

Precautions While Using This Medicine

If your symptoms do not improve within a few days or if they become worse, check with your doctor.

Side Effects of This Medicine

Some side effects may occur that usually do not need medical attention. These side effects may go away during treatment as your body adjusts to the medicine. Also, your health care professional may be able to tell you about ways to prevent or reduce some of these side effects. Check with your health care professional if any of the following side effects continue or are bothersome or if you have any questions about them:

More common—some side effects were similar to problem being treated
  Cough; fever; runny nose; sneezing; sore throat

Less common—some side effects were similar to problem being treated
  Body aches or pain; burning eyes; congestion; dryness or soreness of throat; headache; hoarseness; increased cough; increase in blood flow to an area of the body; itching skin; pain or tenderness around eyes and cheekbones; redness, itching, pain, swelling, or other irritation of the eye; shortness of breath; stuffy nose; tender, swollen glands in neck; tightness of chest or wheezing; trouble in swallowing; troubled breathing; voice changes

Other side effects not listed may also occur in some patients. If you notice any other effects, check with your healthcare professional.

EPIRUBICIN (Intravenous route, Injection route) - ep-i-ROO-bi-sin

Black Box Warning

Severe local tissue necrosis will occur if there is extravasation during administration. Epirubicin must not be given by the intramuscular or subcutaneous route.

Myocardial toxicity, manifested in its most severe form by potentially fatal congestive heart failure (CHF), may occur either during therapy with epirubicin or months to years after termination of therapy. The probability of developing clinically evident CHF is estimated as approximately 0.9% at a cumulative dose of 550 mg/m(2), 1.6% at 700 mg/m(2), and 3.3% at 900 mg/m(2). In the adjuvant treatment of breast cancer, the maximum cumulative dose used in clinical trials was 720 mg/m(2). The risk of developing CHF increases rapidly with increasing total cumulative doses of epirubicin in excess of 900 mg/m(2); this cumulative dose should only be exceeded with extreme caution. Active or dormant cardiovascular disease, prior or concomitant radiotherapy to the mediastinal/pericardial area, previous therapy with other anthracyclines or anthracenediones, or concomitant use of other cardiotoxic drugs may increase the risk of cardiac toxicity. Cardiac toxicity with epirubicin hydrochloride may occur at lower cumulative doses whether or not cardiac risk factors are present.

Secondary acute myelogenous leukemia (AML) has been reported in patients with breast cancer treated with anthracyclines, including epirubicin. The occurrence of refractory secondary leukemia is more common when such drugs are given in combination with DNA-damaging antineoplastic agents, when patients have been heavily pretreated with cytotoxic drugs, or when doses of anthracyclines have been escalated. The cumulative risk of developing treatment-related AML or myelodysplastic syndrome (MDS), in 7110 patients with breast cancer who received adjuvant treatment with epirubicin-containing regimens, was estimated as 0.27% at 3 years, 0.46% at 5 years and 0.55% at 8 years.

Dosage should be reduced in patients with impaired hepatic function.

Severe myelosuppression may occur.

Epirubicin should be administered only under the supervision of a physician who is experienced in the use of cancer chemotherapeutic agents.

Commonly used brand name(s)

In the U.S.—
    Ellence

Available Dosage Forms:
- Powder for Solution
- Injectable
- Solution

Therapeutic Class: Antineoplastic Agent

Uses For This Medicine

Epirubicin belongs to the general group of medicines known as antineoplastics. It is used to treat some kinds of cancers of the breast; lung; lymph system; stomach; and ovaries. It may also be used to treat other kinds of cancer, as determined by your doctor.

Epirubicin seems to interfere with the growth of cancer cells, which are then eventually destroyed by the body. Since the growth of normal body cells may also be affected by epirubicin, other effects will also occur. Some of these may be serious and must be reported to your doctor. Other effects, like hair loss, may not be serious but may cause concern. Some effects may not occur until months or years after the medicine is used.

Before you begin treatment with epirubicin, you and your doctor should talk about the good this medicine will do as well as the risks of using it.

Epirubicin is to be administered only by or under the supervision of your doctor.

Once a medicine has been approved for marketing for a certain use, experience may show that it is also useful for other medical problems. Although these uses are not included in the product labeling, epirubicin is used in certain patients with the following medical condition:
- Cancer of the muscles, connective tissues (tendons), vessels that carry blood or lymph, joints, and fat
- Cancer of the esophagus

Before Using This Medicine

In deciding to use a medicine, the risks of taking the medicine must be weighed against the good it will do. This is a decision you and your doctor will make. For this medicine, the following should be considered:

Allergies—Tell your doctor if you have ever had any unusual or allergic reaction to this medicine or any other medicines. Also tell your health care professional if you have any other types of allergies, such as to foods, dyes, preservatives, or animals. For non-prescription products, read the label or package ingredients carefully.

Pediatric—Studies on this medicine have been done only in adult patients, and there is no specific information comparing use of epirubicin in children with use in other age groups. Heart problems are more likely to occur in children younger than 2 years of age.

Geriatric—Heart problems are more likely to occur in the elderly, who may have existing heart disease. The elderly may also be more likely to have blood problems. Also, elderly patients may not be able to metabolize the medication as quickly as younger patients, which may put them at risk for added toxicity.

Pregnancy—

	Pregnancy Category	Explanation
All Trimesters	D	Studies in pregnant women have demonstrated a risk to the fetus. However, the benefits of therapy in a life threatening situation or a serious disease, may outweigh the potential risk.

Breast Feeding—There are no adequate studies in women for determining infant risk when using this medication during breastfeeding. Weigh the potential benefits against the potential risks before taking this medication while breastfeeding.

Other medicines—

Using this medicine with any of the following medicines is not recommended. Your doctor may decide not to treat you with

this medication or change some of the other medicines you take.

Rotavirus Vaccine, Live

Interactions with Food/Tobacco/Alcohol—Certain medicines should not be used at or around the time of eating food or eating certain types of food since interactions may occur. Using alcohol or tobacco with certain medicines may also cause interactions to occur. Discuss with your healthcare professional the use of your medicine with food, alcohol, or tobacco.

Other medical problems—The presence of other medical problems may affect the use of this medicine. Make sure you tell your doctor if you have any other medical problems, especially:

- Bone marrow depression or
- Viral, fungal, or bacterial infection—There may be an increased risk of infections or worsening infections because of the body's reduced ability to fight them
- Heart disease—Risk of heart problems caused by epirubicin may be increased
- Kidney disease or
- Liver disease—Effects of epirubicin may be increased because of its slower removal from the body
- Tumor cell infiltration of bone marrow—Increased susceptibility for cancer to spread to bone marrow

Proper Use of This Medicine

Epirubicin is sometimes given together with certain other medicines. If you are receiving a combination of medicines, it is important that you receive each one at the proper time. If you are taking some of these medicines by mouth, ask your health care professional to help you plan a way to take them at the right times.

While you are using this medicine, your doctor may want you to drink extra fluids so that you will pass more urine. This will help prevent kidney problems and keep your kidneys working well.

Epirubicin often causes nausea and vomiting. However, it is very important that you continue to receive the medication, even if you begin to feel ill. Ask your health care professional for ways to lessen these effects.

Dosing—The dose of this medicine will be different for different patients. Follow your doctor's orders or the directions on the label. The following information includes only the average doses of this medicine. If your dose is different, do not change it unless your doctor tells you to do so.

The amount of medicine that you take depends on the strength of the medicine. Also, the number of doses you take each day, the time allowed between doses, and the length of time you take the medicine depend on the medical problem for which you are using the medicine.

Precautions While Using This Medicine

It is very important that your doctor check your progress at regular visits to make sure that this medicine is working properly and to check for unwanted effects.

While you are being treated with epirubicin, and after you stop treatment with it, do not have any immunizations (vaccinations) without your doctor's approval. Epirubicin may lower your body's resistance, and there is a chance you might get the infection the immunization is meant to prevent. In addition, other persons living in your household should not take oral polio vaccine, since there is a chance they could pass the polio virus on to you. Also, avoid persons who have taken oral polio vaccine within the last several months. Do not get close to them, and do not stay in the same room with them for very long. If you cannot take these precautions, you should consider wearing a protective face mask that covers the nose and mouth.

Epirubicin can temporarily lower the number of white blood cells in your blood, increasing the chance of getting an infection. It can also lower the number of platelets, which are necessary for proper blood clotting. If this occurs, there are certain precautions you can take, especially when your blood count is low, to reduce the risk of infection or bleeding:

- If you can, avoid people with infections. Check with your doctor immediately if you think you are getting an infection or if you get a fever or chills, cough or hoarseness, lower back or side pain, or painful or difficult urination.
- Check with your doctor immediately if you notice any unusual bleeding or bruising; black, tarry stools; blood in urine or stools; or pinpoint red spots on your skin.
- Be careful when using a regular toothbrush, dental floss, or toothpick. Your medical doctor, dentist, or nurse may recommend other ways to clean your teeth and gums. Check with your medical doctor before having any dental work done.
- Do not touch your eyes or the inside of your nose unless you have just washed your hands and have not touched anything else in the meantime.
- Be careful not to cut yourself when you are using sharp objects such as a safety razor or fingernail or toenail cutters.
- Avoid contact sports or other situations where bruising or injury could occur.

If epirubicin accidentally leaks out of the vein into which it is injected, it may damage some tissues and cause scarring. Tell the doctor or nurse right away if you notice redness, pain, or swelling at the place of injection.

Side Effects of This Medicine

Along with its needed effects, a medicine may cause some unwanted effects. Although not all of these side effects may occur, if they do occur they may need medical attention.

Also, because of the way these medicines act on the body, there is a chance that they might cause other unwanted effects that may not occur until months or years after the medicine is used. These delayed effects may include certain types of cancer, such as leukemia. Discuss these possible effects with your doctor.

Check with your doctor immediately if any of the following side effects occur:

More common
> Bleeding, redness, or ulcers in mouth or throat; cough or hoarseness; fever or chills; lower back or side pain; painful or difficult urination; pain or burning in mouth or throat; sores in mouth or on lips

Less common
> Black, tarry stools; blood in urine or stools; pinpoint red spots on skin; redness or discharge of the eye, eyelid,

or lining of the eyelid; red streaks along injected vein; unusual bleeding or bruising

Rare

Darkening or redness of skin at place of irradiation; fast or irregular heartbeat; joint pain; pain, redness, or warmth at place of injection; skin rash or itching; swelling of abdomen, lower legs, and feet; swelling or tenderness of lymph nodes, abdomen, side or lower back; wheezing, difficulty breathing or shortness of breath

Symptoms of overdose

Abdominal swelling or tenderness; black, tarry stools or blood in stools; difficulty in urination; fast or irregular heartbeat; high fever; shortness of breath; stomach pain; swelling of the lining of the mouth, nose or throat; vomiting

Some side effects may occur that usually do not need medical attention. These side effects may go away during treatment as your body adjusts to the medicine. Also, your health care professional may be able to tell you about ways to prevent or reduce some of these side effects. Check with your health care professional if any of the following side effects continue or are bothersome or if you have any questions about them:

More common

Lack of menstrual periods; nausea and vomiting

Less common

Diarrhea; hot flashes

Rare

Darkening of soles, palms, or nails; loss of appetite or weight loss

Epirubicin causes the urine to turn reddish in color, which may stain clothes. This is not blood. It is to be expected and only lasts for 1 or 2 days after each dose is given.

This medicine often causes a temporary and total loss of hair. After treatment with epirubicin has ended, normal hair growth should return.

After you stop using this medicine, it may still produce some side effects that need attention. During this period of time, *check with your doctor immediately* if you notice the following side effects:

Fast or irregular heartbeat; shortness of breath; swelling of abdomen, feet, and lower legs

Other side effects not listed may also occur in some patients. If you notice any other effects, check with your healthcare professional.

EPLERENONE (Oral route) - e-PLER-en-one

Commonly used brand name(s)

In the U.S.—
Inspra

Available Dosage Forms:
- Tablet

Therapeutic Class: Cardiovascular Agent
Pharmacologic Class: Aldosterone Receptor Antagonist

Uses For This Medicine

Eplerenone belongs to the general class of medicines called antihypertensives. It is used to treat high blood pressure (hypertension).

High blood pressure adds to the work load of the heart and arteries. If it continues for a long time, the heart and arteries may not function properly. This can damage the blood vessels of the brain, heart, and kidneys, resulting in a stroke, heart failure, or kidney failure. Hypertension may also increase the risk of heart attacks. These problems may be less likely to occur if blood pressure is controlled.

This medicine is available only with your healthcare professional's prescription.

Before Using This Medicine

In deciding to use a medicine, the risks of taking the medicine must be weighed against the good it will do. This is a decision you and your doctor will make. For this medicine, the following should be considered:

Allergies—Tell your doctor if you have ever had any unusual or allergic reaction to this medicine or any other medicines. Also tell your health care professional if you have any other types of allergies, such as to foods, dyes, preservatives, or animals. For non-prescription products, read the label or package ingredients carefully.

Pediatric—Studies on this medicine have been done only in adult patients, and there is no specific information comparing use of eplerenone in children with use in other age groups.

Geriatric—Many medicines have not been studied specifically in older people. Therefore, it may not be known whether they work exactly the same way they do in younger adults or if they cause different side effects or problems in older people. Although eplerenone has been given to a limited number of elderly people and has not been shown to cause different side effects in the elderly than in other age groups. Some elderly people may have a greater sensitivity to certain medicines.

Pregnancy—

	Pregnancy Category	Explanation
All Trimesters	B	Animal studies have revealed no evidence of harm to the fetus, however, there are no adequate studies in pregnant women OR animal studies have shown an adverse effect, but adequate studies in pregnant women have failed to demonstrate a risk to the fetus.

Breast Feeding—There are no adequate studies in women for determining infant risk when using this medication during breastfeeding. Weigh the potential benefits against the potential risks before taking this medication while breastfeeding.

Other medicines—

Using this medicine with any of the following medicines is not recommended. Your doctor may decide not to treat you with this medication or change some of the other medicines you take.

Amiloride, Clarithromycin, Itraconazole, Ketoconazole, Nefazodone, Nelfinavir, Ritonavir, Spironolactone, Triamterene, Troleandomycin

Interactions with Food/Tobacco/Alcohol—Certain medicines should not be used at or around the time of eating food or eating certain types of food since interactions may occur. Using alcohol or tobacco with certain medicines may also cause interactions to occur. Discuss with your healthcare professional the use of your medicine with food, alcohol, or tobacco.

Other medical problems—The presence of other medical problems may affect the use of this medicine. Make sure you tell your doctor if you have any other medical problems, especially:

- Diabetes mellitus (sugar diabetes), Type II with microalbuminuria—Use of eplerenone may cause serious side effects in patients with type 2 diabetes and microalbuminuria.
- Kidney disease or
- Liver disease—These conditions may affect how much eplerenone is in your body. Your healthcare professional will decide if eplerenone can be used if you have kidney or liver disease.
- Potassium, serum high (a blood test)— this medicine may cause serious side effects if used in patients with high levels of potassium in thier blood

Proper Use of This Medicine

Dosing—The dose of this medicine will be different for different patients. Follow your doctor's orders or the directions on the label. The following information includes only the average doses of this medicine. If your dose is different, do not change it unless your doctor tells you to do so.

The amount of medicine that you take depends on the strength of the medicine. Also, the number of doses you take each day, the time allowed between doses, and the length of time you take the medicine depend on the medical problem for which you are using the medicine.

- For oral (tablets):
  - For high blood pressure:
    - Adults—50 milligrams (mg) once a day, may be increased by your healthcare professional as needed to 50 milligrams (mg) two times a day.

Missed dose—If you miss a dose of this medicine, take it as soon as possible. However, if it is almost time for your next dose, skip the missed dose and go back to your regular dosing schedule. Do not double doses.

Storage—Store the medicine in a closed container at room temperature, away from heat, moisture, and direct light. Keep from freezing.

Keep out of the reach of children.

Do not keep outdated medicine or medicine no longer needed.

Ask your healthcare professional how you should dispose of any medicine you do not use.

Precautions While Using This Medicine

It is very important that your healthcare professional check your progress at regular visits. This will allow your healthcare professional to see if the medicine is working properly and to decide if you should continue to take it.

Do not take other medicines unless they have been discussed with your healthcare professional. This especially includes potassium supplements or salt substitutes containing potassium. Check with your healthcare professional before taking amiloride, spironolactone, triamterene, ketoconazole, or itraconazole.

Side Effects of This Medicine

Along with its needed effects, a medicine may cause some unwanted effects. Although not all of these side effects may occur, if they do occur they may need medical attention.

Check with your doctor immediately if any of the following side effects occur:

Less common
Excess of cholesterol in the blood; excess of triglycerides in the blood

Incidence unknown
Abdominal pain; arm, back or jaw pain; chest pain or discomfort; chest tightness or heaviness; confusion; difficult breathing; dizziness; fast or irregular heartbeat; headache; irregular heartbeat; nausea; nervousness; numbness or tingling in hands, feet, or lips; pain or discomfort in arms, jaw, back or neck; shortness of breath; sweating; vomiting; weakness or heaviness of legs

Some side effects may occur that usually do not need medical attention. These side effects may go away during treatment as your body adjusts to the medicine. Also, your health care professional may be able to tell you about ways to prevent or reduce some of these side effects. Check with your health care professional if any of the following side effects continue or are bothersome or if you have any questions about them:

Less common
Abnormal vaginal bleeding; breast pain; chills; cloudy urine; cough; diarrhea; fever; general feeling of discomfort or illness; joint pain; loss of appetite; muscle aches and pains; stomach pain; swelling of the breasts or breast soreness in both females and males; unusual tiredness or weakness

Other side effects not listed may also occur in some patients. If you notice any other effects, check with your healthcare professional.

EPROSARTAN (Oral route) - ep-roe-SAR-tan

Black Box Warning

When used in pregnancy during the second and third trimesters, drugs that act directly on the renin-angiotensin system can cause injury and even death to the developing fetus. When pregnancy is detected, eprosartan mesylate should be discontinued as soon as possible.

Commonly used brand name(s)

In the U.S.—
Teveten

Available Dosage Forms:
- Tablet

Therapeutic Class: Cardiovascular Agent
Pharmacologic Class: Angiotensin II Receptor Antagonist

Uses For This Medicine

Eprosartan belongs to the class of medicines called angiotensin II inhibitors. It is used to treat high blood pressure (hypertension).

High blood pressure adds to the workload of the heart and arteries. If it continues for a long time, the heart and arteries may not function properly. This can damage the blood vessels of the brain, heart, and kidneys, resulting in a stroke, heart failure, or kidney failure. High blood pressure may also increase the risk of heart attacks. These problems may be less likely to occur if blood pressure is controlled.

Eprosartan works by blocking the action of a substance in the body that causes blood vessels to tighten. As a result, eprosartan relaxes blood vessels. This lowers blood pressure.

This medicine is available only with your doctor's prescription.

Before Using This Medicine

In deciding to use a medicine, the risks of taking the medicine must be weighed against the good it will do. This is a decision you and your doctor will make. For this medicine, the following should be considered:

Allergies—Tell your doctor if you have ever had any unusual or allergic reaction to this medicine or any other medicines. Also tell your health care professional if you have any other types of allergies, such as to foods, dyes, preservatives, or animals. For non-prescription products, read the label or package ingredients carefully.

Pediatric—Studies on this medicine have been done only in adult patients, and there is no specific information comparing use of eprosartan in children with use in other age groups.

Geriatric—This medicine has been tested in patients 65 years of age or older and has not been shown to cause different side effects or problems in older people than it does in younger adults.

Pregnancy—

	Pregnancy Category	Explanation
1st Trimester	C	Animal studies have shown an adverse effect and there are no adequate studies in pregnant women OR no animal studies have been conducted and there are no adequate studies in pregnant women.
2nd Trimester	D	Studies in pregnant women have demonstrated a risk to the fetus. However, the benefits of therapy in a life threatening situation or a serious disease, may outweigh the potential risk.
3rd Trimester	D	Studies in pregnant women have demonstrated a risk to the fetus. However, the benefits of therapy in a life threatening situation or a serious disease, may outweigh the potential risk.

Breast Feeding—There are no adequate studies in women for determining infant risk when using this medication during breastfeeding. Weigh the potential benefits against the potential risks before taking this medication while breastfeeding.

Other medicines—Although certain medicines should not be used together at all, in other cases two different medicines may be used together even if an interaction might occur. In these cases, your doctor may want to change the dose, or other precautions may be necessary. Tell your healthcare professional if you are taking any other prescription or non-prescription (over-the-counter [OTC]) medicine.

Interactions with Food/Tobacco/Alcohol—Certain medicines should not be used at or around the time of eating food or eating certain types of food since interactions may occur. Using alcohol or tobacco with certain medicines may also cause interactions to occur. Discuss with your healthcare professional the use of your medicine with food, alcohol, or tobacco.

Other medical problems—The presence of other medical problems may affect the use of this medicine. Make sure you tell your doctor if you have any other medical problems, especially:

- Congestive heart failure (severe)—Lowering of blood pressure by eprosartan may make this condition worse
- Dehydration or salt depletion—Blood pressure-lowering effects of eprosartan may be increased
- Kidney disease—Effects of eprosartan may make this condition worse

Proper Use of This Medicine

Take this medicine only as directed by your doctor. Do not take more of it and do not take it more often than your doctor ordered. This medicine also works best when there is a constant amount in the blood. To help keep the amount constant, do not miss any doses. Also, it is best to take the doses at the same time each day.

Dosing—The dose of this medicine will be different for different patients. Follow your doctor's orders or the directions on the label. The following information includes only the average doses of this medicine. If your dose is different, do not change it unless your doctor tells you to do so.

The amount of medicine that you take depends on the strength of the medicine. Also, the number of doses you take each day, the time allowed between doses, and the length of time you take the medicine depend on the medical problem for which you are using the medicine.

- For oral dosage form (tablets):
  - For high blood pressure:
    - Adults—400 to 800 milligrams (mg) a day. The dose may be taken once a day or divided into two doses.
    - Children—Use and dose must be determined by your doctor.

Missed dose—If you miss a dose of this medicine, take it as soon as possible. However, if it is almost time for your next dose, skip the missed dose and go back to your regular dosing schedule. Do not double doses.

Storage—Store the medicine in a closed container at room temperature, away from heat, moisture, and direct light. Keep from freezing.

Keep out of the reach of children.

Do not keep outdated medicine or medicine no longer needed.

Precautions While Using This Medicine

It is important that your doctor check your progress at regular visits to make sure that this medicine is working properly and to check for unwanted effects.

Check with your doctor immediately if you think that you may be pregnant. Eprosartan may cause birth defects or other problems in the baby if taken during pregnancy.

Do not take other medicines unless they have been discussed with your doctor. This especially includes over-the-counter (nonprescription) medicines for appetite control, asthma, colds, cough, hay fever, or sinus problems, since they may increase your blood pressure.

Dizziness or light-headedness may occur, especially if you have been taking a diuretic (water pill). Make sure you know how you react to this medicine before you drive, use machines, or do anything else that could be dangerous if you experience these effects.

Check with your doctor right away if you become sick while taking this medicine, especially with severe or continuing nausea and vomiting or diarrhea. These conditions may cause you to lose too much water and lead to low blood pressure.

Dizziness, light-headedness, or fainting also may occur if you exercise or if the weather is hot. Heavy sweating can cause loss of too much water and result in low blood pressure. Use extra care during exercise or hot weather.

Side Effects of This Medicine

Side Effects of This Medicine

Along with its needed effects, a medicine may cause some unwanted effects. Although not all of these side effects may occur, if they do occur they may need medical attention.

Check with your doctor as soon as possible if any of the following side effects occur:

Less common
Burning or painful urination or changes in urinary frequency; cough, fever, or sore throat

Rare
Dizziness, light-headedness, or fainting; swollen face, lips, limbs, or tongue

Some side effects may occur that usually do not need medical attention. These side effects may go away during treatment as your body adjusts to the medicine. Also, your health care professional may be able to tell you about ways to prevent or reduce some of these side effects. Check with your health care professional if any of the following side effects continue or are bothersome or if you have any questions about them:

Less common or rare
Abdominal pain; joint pain; unusual tiredness

Other side effects not listed may also occur in some patients. If you notice any other effects, check with your healthcare professional.

ERGOLOID MESYLATES (Oral route, Sublingual route) - ER-goe-loid MES-i-lates

Commonly used brand name(s)

In the U.S.—
  Hydergine

Available Dosage Forms:
- Tablet
- Capsule, Liquid Filled
- Solution

Therapeutic Class: Antimigraine

Uses For This Medicine

Ergoloid mesylates belongs to the group of medicines known as ergot alkaloids. It is used to treat some mood, behavior, or other problems that may be due to changes in the brain from Alzheimer's disease or multiple small strokes.

This medicine is different from other ergot alkaloids such as ergotamine and methysergide. It is not useful for treating migraine headache. The exact way ergoloid mesylates acts on the body is not known.

This medicine is available only with your doctor's prescription.

Before Using This Medicine

In deciding to use a medicine, the risks of taking the medicine must be weighed against the good it will do. This is a decision you and your doctor will make. For this medicine, the following should be considered:

Allergies—Tell your doctor if you have ever had any unusual or allergic reaction to this medicine or any other medicines. Also tell your health care professional if you have any other types of allergies, such as to foods, dyes, preservatives, or animals. For non-prescription products, read the label or package ingredients carefully.

Breast Feeding—There are no adequate studies in women for determining infant risk when using this medication during breastfeeding. Weigh the potential benefits against the potential risks before taking this medication while breastfeeding.

Other medicines—

Using this medicine with any of the following medicines is not recommended. Your doctor may decide not to treat you with this medication or change some of the other medicines you take.

Almotriptan, Atazanavir, Azithromycin, Clarithromycin, Clotrimazole, Dirithromycin, Efavirenz, Erythromycin, Fluconazole, Fluoxetine, Fluvoxamine, Fosamprenavir, Frovatriptan, Indinavir, Itraconazole, Josamycin, Ketoconazole, Mepartricin, Metronidazole, Miokamycin, Naratriptan, Nefazodone, Nelfinavir, Ritonavir, Rizatriptan, Rokitamycin, Roxithromycin, Saquinavir, Spiramycin, Sumatriptan, Troleandomycin, Voriconazole, Zileuton, Zolmitriptan

Interactions with Food/Tobacco/Alcohol—Certain medicines should not be used at or around the time of eating food or eating certain types of food since interactions may occur. Using alcohol or tobacco with certain medicines may also cause interactions to occur. The following interactions have been selected on the basis of their potential significance and are not necessarily all-inclusive.

Using this medicine with any of the following is not recommended. Your doctor may decide not to treat you with this medication, change some of the other medicines you take, or give you special instructions about the use of food, alcohol, or tobacco.

Grapefruit Juice

Other medical problems—The presence of other medical problems may affect the use of this medicine. Make sure you tell your doctor if you have any other medical problems, especially:

- Liver disease—Higher blood levels of ergoloid mesylates may occur, increasing the chance of side effects
- Low blood pressure or
- Other mental problems or
- Slow heartbeat—Ergoloid mesylates may make the condition worse

Proper Use of This Medicine

Take this medicine only as directed by your doctor. Do not take more or less of it, and do not take it more often or for a longer period of time than your doctor ordered. To do so may increase the chance of unwanted effects.

For patients taking the sublingual (under-the-tongue) tablets:

- Dissolve the tablet under your tongue. The sublingual tablet should not be chewed or swallowed, since it works much faster when absorbed through the lining of the mouth. Do not eat, drink, or smoke while a tablet is dissolving.

Dosing—The dose of this medicine will be different for different patients. Follow your doctor's orders or the directions on the label. The following information includes only the average doses of this medicine. If your dose is different, do not change it unless your doctor tells you to do so.

The amount of medicine that you take depends on the strength of the medicine. Also, the number of doses you take each day, the time allowed between doses, and the length of time you take the medicine depend on the medical problem for which you are using the medicine.

- For oral dosage forms (capsules, tablets, sublingual tablets, or oral solution):
  - Adults: 1 to 2 milligrams (mg) three times a day.

Storage—Store the medicine in a closed container at room temperature, away from heat, moisture, and direct light. Keep from freezing.

Keep out of the reach of children.

Do not keep outdated medicine or medicine no longer needed.

Precautions While Using This Medicine

It is important that your doctor check your progress at regular visits to make sure this medicine is working and to check for unwanted effects.

It may take several weeks for this medicine to work. However, do not stop taking this medicine without first checking with your doctor.

Side Effects of This Medicine

Along with its needed effects, a medicine may cause some unwanted effects. Although not all of these side effects may occur, if they do occur they may need medical attention.

Check with your doctor as soon as possible if any of the following side effects occur:

Less common or rare
Dizziness or lightheadedness when getting up from a lying or sitting position; drowsiness; skin rash; slow pulse

Signs and symptoms of overdose
Blurred vision; dizziness; fainting; flushing; headache; loss of appetite; nausea or vomiting; stomach cramps; stuffy nose

Some side effects may occur that usually do not need medical attention. These side effects may go away during treatment as your body adjusts to the medicine. Also, your health care professional may be able to tell you about ways to prevent or reduce some of these side effects. Check with your health care professional if any of the following side effects continue or are bothersome or if you have any questions about them:

Less common or rare
Soreness under tongue (with sublingual use)

Other side effects not listed may also occur in some patients. If you notice any other effects, check with your healthcare professional.

ERGONOVINE/ METHYLERGONOVINE (Systemic)

Some commonly used brand names are:

In the U.S.—
Ergotrate (1)
Methergine (2)

In Canada—
Ergotrate Maleate (1)

This information applies to the following medicines

1. Ergonovine (er-goe-NOE-veen)
2. Methylergonovine (meth-ill-er-goe-NOE-veen)

Category

- **Diagnostic aid, coronary vasospasm**—Ergonovine
- **Uterine stimulant**—Ergonovine; Methylergonovine

Description

Ergonovine and methylergonovine belong to the group of medicines known as ergot alkaloids. These medicines are usually given to stop excessive bleeding that sometimes occurs after abortion or a baby is delivered. They work by causing the muscle of the uterus to contract.

Ergonovine and methylergonovine may also be used for other conditions as determined by your doctor.

These medicines are available only on prescription and are to be administered only by or under the supervision of your doctor. They are available in the following dosage forms:

Oral
- Ergonovine
  - Tablets
- Methylergonovine
  - Tablets

Parenteral
- Ergonovine
  - Injection
- Methylergonovine
  - Injection

Before Using This Medicine

In deciding to use a medicine, the risks of taking the medicine must be weighed against the good it will do. This is a decision you and your doctor will make. For ergonovine and methylergonovine, the following should be considered:

Allergies—Tell your doctor if you have ever had any unusual or allergic reaction to ergonovine, methylergonovine, or other ergot medicines. Also tell your health care professional if you are allergic to any other substances, such as foods, preservatives, or dyes.

Breast-feeding—This medicine passes into the breast milk and may cause unwanted effects, such as vomiting; decreased circulation in the hands, lower legs, and feet; diarrhea; weak pulse; unstable blood pressure; or convulsions (seizures) in infants of mothers taking large doses.

Children—Although there is no specific information comparing use of ergonovine or methylergonovine in children with use in other age groups, these medicines are not expected to cause different problems in children than they do in adults.

Older adults—Many medicines have not been studied specifically in older people. Therefore, it may not be known whether they work exactly the same way they do in younger adults or if they cause different side effects or problems in older people. There is no specific information comparing use of ergonovine or methylergonovine in the elderly with use in other age groups.

Other medicines—Although certain medicines should not be used together at all, in other cases two different medicines may be used together even if an interaction might occur. In these cases, your doctor may want to change the dose, or other precautions may be necessary. When you are taking ergonovine or methylergonovine it is especially important that your health care professional know if you are taking any of the following:
- Bromocriptine (e.g., Parlodel) or
- Other ergot alkaloids (dihydroergotamine [e.g., D.H.E. 45], ergoloid mesylates [e.g., Hydergine], ergotamine [e.g., Gynergen], methysergide [e.g., Sansert])—Use of these medicines with ergonovine or methylergonovine may increase the chance of side effects of these medicines.
- Nitrates or
- Other medicines for angina—Use of these medicines with ergonovine or methylergonovine may keep these medicines from working properly

Other medical problems—The presence of other medical problems may affect the use of ergonovine or methylergonovine. Make sure you tell your doctor if you have any other medical problems, especially:
- Angina (chest pain) or other heart problems or
- Blood vessel disease or
- High blood pressure (or history of) or

- Stroke (history of)—These medicines may cause changes in how the heart works or blood pressure changes
- Infection—Infections may cause an increased sensitivity to the effect of these medicines
- Kidney disease
- Liver disease—The body may not remove these medicines from the bloodstream at the usual rate, which may make the medicine work longer or increase the chance for side effects
- Raynaud's phenomenon—Use of these medicines may cause worsening of the blood vessel narrowing that occurs with this disease

Proper Use of This Medicine

Take this medicine only as directed by your doctor. Do not take more of it, do not take it more often, and do not take it for a longer time than your doctor ordered. If too much is taken or if it is taken for a longer time than your doctor ordered, it may cause serious effects.

Dosing—The dose of ergonovine or methylergonovine will be different for different patients. *Follow your doctor's orders or the directions on the label.* The following information includes only the average doses of ergonovine and methylergonovine. *If your dose is different, do not change it unless your doctor tells you to do so.*

For ergonovine
- For *oral* dosage forms (tablets):
  - For treatment of excessive uterine bleeding:
    - Adults—0.2 to 0.4 milligram, swallowed or placed under the tongue every six to twelve hours. Usually this medicine is taken for forty-eight hours or less.
- For *injection* dosage form:
  - For treatment of excessive uterine bleeding:
    - Adults—0.2 milligram, injected into a muscle or vein. This dose can be repeated up to five times if needed, with a two- to four-hour wait between doses.

For methylergonovine
- For *oral* dosage forms (tablets):
  - For treatment of excessive uterine bleeding:
    - Adults—0.2 to 0.4 milligram, taken every six to twelve hours. Usually this medicine is taken for forty-eight hours or less.
- For *injection* dosage form:
  - For treatment of excessive uterine bleeding:
    - Adults—0.2 milligram, injected into a muscle or vein. This dose can be repeated up to five times if needed, with a two- to four-hour wait between doses.

Missed dose—If you miss a dose of this medicine, do not take the missed dose at all and do not double the next one. Instead, go back to your regular dosing schedule. If you have any questions about this, check with your doctor.

Storage—To store this medicine:
- Keep out of the reach of children.
- Store away from heat and direct light.

- Do not store in the bathroom, near the kitchen sink, or in other damp places. Heat or moisture may cause the medicine to break down.
- Do not keep outdated medicine or medicine no longer needed. Be sure that any discarded medicine is out of the reach of children.

Precautions While Using This Medicine

If you have an infection or illness of any kind, check with your doctor before taking this medicine, since you may be more sensitive to its effects.

Side Effects

Along with its needed effects, a medicine may cause some unwanted effects. Although not all of these side effects may occur, if they do occur they may need medical attention.

Check with the health care professional immediately if any of the following side effects occur:

Less common
    Chest pain

Rare
    Blurred vision; convulsions (seizures); crushing chest pain; headache (sudden and severe); irregular heartbeat; unexplained shortness of breath

Check with your doctor as soon as possible if any of the following side effects occur:

Less common
    Slow heartbeat

Rare
    Itching of skin; pain in arms, legs, or lower back; pale or cold hands or feet; weakness in legs

Symptoms of overdose
    Bluish color of skin or inside of nose or mouth; chest pain; cool, pale, or numb arms or legs; confusion; cramping of the uterus (severe); decreased breathing rate; drowsiness; heartbeat changes; muscle pain; small pupils; tingling, itching, and cool skin; trouble in breathing; unconsciousness; unusual thirst; weak or absent pulse in arms or legs; weak pulse

With long-term use
    Dry, shriveled-looking skin on hands, lower legs, or feet; false feeling of insects crawling on the skin; pain and redness in an arm or leg; paralysis of one side of the body

Other side effects may occur that usually do not need medical attention. These side effects may go away during treatment as your body adjusts to the medicine. However, check with your doctor if any of the following side effects continue or are bothersome:

More common
    Cramping of the uterus; nausea; vomiting

Less common
    Abdominal or stomach pain; diarrhea; dizziness; headache (mild and temporary); ringing in the ears; stuffy nose; sweating; unpleasant taste

Other side effects not listed above may also occur in some patients. If you notice any other effects, check with your doctor.

ERLOTINIB (Oral route) - er-LOE-tye-nib

Commonly used brand name(s)
In the U.S.—
    Tarceva

Available Dosage Forms:
- Tablet

Therapeutic Class: Antineoplastic Agent
Pharmacologic Class: Tyrosine Kinase Inhibitor

Uses For This Medicine

Erlotinib belongs to the group of medicines called antineoplastics. It is used to treat non-small cell lung cancer after the failure of other chemotherapy treatment. It is also used together with another medicine called gemcitabine (e.g., Gemzar) to treat cancer of the pancreas.

This medicine is available only with your doctor's prescription.

Before Using This Medicine

In deciding to use a medicine, the risks of taking the medicine must be weighed against the good it will do. This is a decision you and your doctor will make. For this medicine, the following should be considered:

Allergies—Tell your doctor if you have ever had any unusual or allergic reaction to this medicine or any other medicines. Also tell your health care professional if you have any other types of allergies, such as to foods, dyes, preservatives, or animals. For non-prescription products, read the label or package ingredients carefully.

Pediatric—Studies on this medicine have been done only in adult patients, and there is no specific information comparing use of erlotinib in children with use in other age groups.

Geriatric—This medicine has been tested in elderly patients and has not been shown to cause different side effects or problems in older people than it does in younger adults.

Pregnancy—

	Pregnancy Category	Explanation
All Trimesters	D	Studies in pregnant women have demonstrated a risk to the fetus. However, the benefits of therapy in a life threatening situation or a serious disease, may outweigh the potential risk.

Breast Feeding—There are no adequate studies in women for determining infant risk when using this medication during breastfeeding. Weigh the potential benefits against the potential risks before taking this medication while breastfeeding.

Other medicines—

Using this medicine with any of the following medicines is usually not recommended, but may be required in some cases. If both medicines are prescribed together, your doctor may change the dose or how often you use one or both of the medicines.

Carbamazepine, Fosphenytoin, Phenobarbital, Phenytoin, Rifabutin, Rifampin, Rifapentine, St John's Wort

Interactions with Food/Tobacco/Alcohol—Certain medicines should not be used at or around the time of eating food or eating certain types of food since interactions may occur. Using alcohol or tobacco with certain medicines may also cause interactions to occur. The following interactions have been selected on the basis of their potential significance and are not necessarily all-inclusive.

Using this medicine with any of the following may cause an increased risk of certain side effects but may be unavoidable in some cases. If used together, your doctor may change the dose or how often you use this medicine or give you special instructions about the use of food, alcohol, or tobacco.

Tobacco

Other medical problems—The presence of other medical problems may affect the use of this medicine. Make sure you tell your doctor if you have any other medical problems, especially:

- Liver disease—The chance of serious side effects is greatly increased.

Proper Use of This Medicine

It is important that you take erlotinib one hour before or at least two hours after the ingestion of food

Dosing—The dose of this medicine will be different for different patients. Follow your doctor's orders or the directions on the label. The following information includes only the average doses of this medicine. If your dose is different, do not change it unless your doctor tells you to do so.

The amount of medicine that you take depends on the strength of the medicine. Also, the number of doses you take each day, the time allowed between doses, and the length of time you take the medicine depend on the medical problem for which you are using the medicine.

- For oral dosage form (tablets):
    - For lung cancer, non-small cell:
        - Adults—150 milligrams (mg) daily.
        - Children—Use and dose must be determined by your doctor.
    - For cancer of the pancreas:
        - Adults—100 mg daily.
        - Children—Use and dose must be determined by your doctor.

Missed dose—If you miss a dose of this medicine, take it as soon as possible. However, if it is almost time for your next dose, skip the missed dose and go back to your regular dosing schedule. Do not double doses.

Storage—Store the medicine in a closed container at room temperature, away from heat, moisture, and direct light. Keep from freezing.

Keep out of the reach of children.

Do not keep outdated medicine or medicine no longer needed.

Ask your healthcare professional how you should dispose of any medicine you do not use.

Precautions While Using This Medicine

It is very important that your doctor check you at regular visits.

It is important that you seek prompt medical attention should severe or persistent diarrhea, nausea, anorexia, or vomiting occur.

You should seek prompt medical attention if onset or worsening of unexplained shortness of breath or cough occur.

Contact your doctor if you develop eye irritation.

Side Effects of This Medicine

Along with its needed effects, a medicine may cause some unwanted effects. Although not all of these side effects may occur, if they do occur they may need medical attention.

Check with your doctor immediately if any of the following side effects occur:

More common

Burning, tingling, numbness or pain in the hands, arms, feet, or legs; cough; diarrhea, severe; difficult or labored breathing; fever; rash, severe; sensation of pins and needles; shortness of breath; stabbing pain; tightness in chest; wheezing

Rare

Bloody or black, tarry stool; blurred vision; chest pain or discomfort; constipation; eye irritation or redness; inability to speak; pain or discomfort in arms, jaw, back, or neck; seizures; severe stomach pain; shortness of breath; slurred speech; sudden and severe headache; sudden and severe weakness in arm and/or leg on one side of the body; sudden, severe chest pain; sudden weakness in arms or legs; sweating; temporary blindness; vomiting of blood or material that looks like coffee grounds

Symptoms of overdose

Get emergency help immediately if any of the following symptoms of overdose occur:

Diarrhea; rash

Some side effects may occur that usually do not need medical attention. These side effects may go away during treatment as your body adjusts to the medicine. Also, your health care professional may be able to tell you about ways to prevent or reduce some of these side effects. Check with your health care professional if any of the following side effects continue or are bothersome or if you have any questions about them:

More common

Acid or sour stomach; belching; bloated full feeling; bone pain; burning, dry or itching eyes; diarrhea, mild; difficulty in moving; discharge; discouragement; dizziness; dry skin; dryness of the eye; excess air or gas in stomach or intestines; excessive tearing; fear; feeling sad or empty; feeling unusually cold; fever or chills; hair loss; headache; heartburn; hoarseness; indigestion; irritability; itching skin; joint pain; lack or loss of appetite; loss of interest or pleasure; lower back or side pain; muscle aching or cramping; muscle pains or stiffness; nausea; nervousness; painful or difficult urination; passing gas; rash, mild; redness, pain, swelling of eye, eyelid, or inner lining of eyelid; shivering; sleeplessness; stomach discomfort, upset or pain; swelling; swelling or inflammation of the mouth; swollen joints; thinning of hair; tiredness; trouble concentrating; trouble or inability to sleep; unusual tiredness or weakness; vomiting; weight loss

Other side effects not listed may also occur in some patients. If you notice any other effects, check with your healthcare professional.

ERTAPENEM (Injection route) - er-ta-PEN-em

Commonly used brand name(s)

In the U.S.—
Invanz

Available Dosage Forms:
• Powder for Solution

Therapeutic Class: Antibiotic
Pharmacologic Class: Beta-Lactam

Uses For This Medicine

Ertapenem is used alone or in combination with other antibiotics to treat infections caused by bacteria in many different parts of the body. It works by killing bacteria or preventing their growth. This medicine will not work for colds, flu, or other virus infections. Ertapenem is also used to prevent infections after having surgery of the colon and rectum.

This medicine is available only with your doctor's prescription.

Before Using This Medicine

In deciding to use a medicine, the risks of taking the medicine must be weighed against the good it will do. This is a decision you and your doctor will make. For this medicine, the following should be considered:

Allergies—Tell your doctor if you have ever had any unusual or allergic reaction to this medicine or any other medicines. Also tell your health care professional if you have any other types of allergies, such as to foods, dyes, preservatives, or animals. For non-prescription products, read the label or package ingredients carefully.

Pediatric—This medicine has been tested in infants and children 3 months to 17 years of age and, in effective doses, and has not been shown to cause different side effects or problems than it does in adults. Use in infants less than 3 months of age is not recommended.

Geriatric—Appropriate studies performed to date have not demonstrated geriatrics-specific problems that would limit the usefulness of ertapenem in the elderly. However, elderly patients are more likely to have age-related kidney problems, which may require caution or adjustment of dosage in patients receiving ertapenem.

Pregnancy—

	Pregnancy Category	Explanation
All Trimesters	B	Animal studies have revealed no evidence of harm to the fetus, however, there are no adequate studies in pregnant women OR animal studies have shown an adverse effect, but adequate studies in pregnant women have failed to demonstrate a risk to the fetus.

Breast Feeding—There are no adequate studies in women for determining infant risk when using this medication during breastfeeding. Weigh the potential benefits against the potential risks before taking this medication while breastfeeding.

Other medicines—

Using this medicine with any of the following medicines may cause an increased risk of certain side effects, but using both drugs may be the best treatment for you. If both medicines are prescribed together, your doctor may change the dose or how often you use one or both of the medicines.

Probenecid

Interactions with Food/Tobacco/Alcohol—Certain medicines should not be used at or around the time of eating food or eating certain types of food since interactions may occur. Using alcohol or tobacco with certain medicines may also cause interactions to occur. Discuss with your healthcare professional the use of your medicine with food, alcohol, or tobacco.

Other medical problems—The presence of other medical problems may affect the use of this medicine. Make sure you tell your doctor if you have any other medical problems, especially:

• Gastrointestinal disease (for example, stomach or intestinal problems, especially diarrhea)—Patients with stomach or intestinal problems, especially diarrhea, may be more likely to have side effects

• Central nervous system (CNS) disorders (for example, brain disease or history of seizures)—Patients with nervous system disorders, including seizures, may be more likely to have side effects

• Kidney disease—Patients with kidney disease may be more likely to have side effects

Proper Use of This Medicine

To help clear up your infection completely, ertapenem must be given for the full time of treatment, even if you begin to feel better after a few days. Skipping doses or not completing the full course of therapy may decrease the usefulness of this medicine. It may also increase the likelihood that the bacteria causing your infection will develop resistance. If this happens, ertapenem and other medicines used to treat infections will not work in the future. Also, this medicine works best when there is a constant amount in the blood or urine. To help keep the amount constant, it must be given on a regular schedule.

Dosing—The dose of this medicine will be different for different patients. Follow your doctor's orders or the directions on the label. The following information includes only the average doses of this medicine. If your dose is different, do not change it unless your doctor tells you to do so.

The amount of medicine that you take depends on the strength of the medicine. Also, the number of doses you take each day, the time allowed between doses, and the length of time you take the medicine depend on the medical problem for which you are using the medicine.

• For injection dosage form:
  ◦ For bacterial infections:
    ▪ Adults and teenagers—1 gram injected into a vein or injected into a muscle once a day. Your doctor will determine whether the medication is injected into a vein or injected into a muscle and the length of time that you will take it.
    ▪ Children 3 months to 12 years of age—15 mg per kg (6.8 mg per pound [lb]) of body weight injected

into a vein or injected into a muscle twice a day. Your doctor will determine whether the medication is injected into a vein or injected into a muscle and the length of time you will take it.

Missed dose—If you miss a dose of this medicine, take it as soon as possible. However, if it is almost time for your next dose, skip the missed dose and go back to your regular dosing schedule. Do not double doses.

Storage—Keep out of the reach of children.

Do not keep outdated medicine or medicine no longer needed.

Ask your healthcare professional how you should dispose of any medicine you do not use.

Precautions While Using This Medicine

Some patients may develop tremors or seizures while receiving this medicine. If you already have a history of seizures and you are taking anticonvulsants, you should continue to take them unless otherwise directed by your doctor.

In some patients, ertapenem may cause diarrhea.

- Severe diarrhea may be a sign of a serious side effect. Do not take any diarrhea medicine without first checking with your doctor. Diarrhea medicines may make your diarrhea worse or make it last longer.
- For mild diarrhea, diarrhea medicine containing kaolin (e.g., Kaopectate liquid) or attapulgite (e.g., Kaopectate tablets, Diasorb) may be taken. However, other kinds of diarrhea medicine should not be taken. They may make your diarrhea worse or make it last longer.
- If you have any questions about this or if mild diarrhea continues or gets worse, check with your health care professional.

If your symptoms do not improve within a few days or if they become worse, check with your doctor.

Do not take other medicines unless they have been discussed with your doctor.

Side Effects of This Medicine

Along with its needed effects, a medicine may cause some unwanted effects. Although not all of these side effects may occur, if they do occur they may need medical attention.

Check with your doctor immediately if any of the following side effects occur:

More common
Bleeding; blistering; burning; coldness; discoloration of skin; feeling of pressure; hives; infection; inflammation; itching skin; lumps; numbness; pain; skin rash; redness of skin; scarring; soreness; stinging; swelling; tenderness; tingling; ulceration; unusually warm skin

Less common
Bluish color changes in skin color; fast, pounding, or irregular heartbeat or pulse; pain, tenderness, swelling of foot or leg

Rare
Abdominal or stomach cramps; abdominal tenderness; bloating; convulsions; diarrhea, watery and severe, which may also be bloody; fainting or loss of consciousness; fast or irregular breathing; fever; increased thirst; loss of bladder control; muscle spasm or jerking of all extremities; nausea; sudden loss of consciousness;

swelling of eyes or eyelids; tightness in chest; trouble in breathing; unusual tiredness or weakness; unusual weight loss; vomiting; wheezing

Incidence not known—occurred during clinical practice
Cough; difficulty swallowing; fast heartbeat; hives; itching, puffiness or swelling of the eyelids or around the eyes, face, lips or tongue; seeing, hearing, or feeling things that are not there; shortness of breath; skin rash; tightness in chest; wheezing

Some side effects may occur that usually do not need medical attention. These side effects may go away during treatment as your body adjusts to the medicine. Also, your health care professional may be able to tell you about ways to prevent or reduce some of these side effects. Check with your health care professional if any of the following side effects continue or are bothersome or if you have any questions about them:

More common
Agitation; chest pain; confusion about identity, place, and time; drowsiness; headache; mental depression

Less common
Acid or sour stomach; belching; blurred vision; body aches or pain; congestion; cough; difficult or labored breathing; difficulty having a bowel movement (stool); dizziness; dryness or soreness of throat; fear; faintness or lightheadedness when getting up from a lying or sitting position; flushing; heartburn; hoarseness; indigestion; itching of the vagina or genital area; itching skin; lack or loss of strength; leg pain; nervousness; pain during sexual intercourse; pounding in the ears; runny nose; shortness of breath; sleeplessness; slow heartbeat; sore mouth or tongue; stomach discomfort, upset, or pain; sudden sweating; tender, swollen glands in neck; thick, white vaginal discharge with no odor or with a mild odor; tightness in chest; trouble in swallowing; trouble sleeping; unable to sleep; voice changes; white patches in mouth and/or on tongue

Other side effects not listed may also occur in some patients. If you notice any other effects, check with your healthcare professional.

ERYTHROMYCIN (Ophthalmic route) -
er-ith-roe-MYE-sin

Commonly used brand name(s)

In the U.S.—
Romycin

In Canada—

Diomycin	Ilotycin
Erythromycin	Pms-Erythromycin

Available Dosage Forms:
- Ointment

Therapeutic Class: Antibiotic

Uses For This Medicine

Erythromycin belongs to the family of medicines called antibiotics. Erythromycin ophthalmic preparations are used to treat infections of the eye. They also may be used to prevent certain eye infections of newborn babies, such as neonatal conjunctivitis and ophthalmia neonatorum. They may be used with other medicines for some eye infections.

Erythromycin is available only with your doctor's prescription.

Before Using This Medicine

In deciding to use a medicine, the risks of taking the medicine must be weighed against the good it will do. This is a decision you and your doctor will make. For this medicine, the following should be considered:

Allergies—Tell your doctor if you have ever had any unusual or allergic reaction to this medicine or any other medicines. Also tell your health care professional if you have any other types of allergies, such as to foods, dyes, preservatives, or animals. For non-prescription products, read the label or package ingredients carefully.

Pediatric—Studies on this medicine have been done only in adult patients, and there is no specific information comparing use of this medicine in children with use in other age groups.

Geriatric—Many medicines have not been studied specifically in older people. Therefore, it may not be known whether they work exactly the same way they do in younger adults or if they cause different side effects or problems in older people. There is no specific information comparing use of this medicine in the elderly with use in other age groups.

Other medicines—Although certain medicines should not be used together at all, in other cases two different medicines may be used together even if an interaction might occur. In these cases, your doctor may want to change the dose, or other precautions may be necessary. Tell your healthcare professional if you are taking any other prescription or non-prescription (over-the-counter [OTC]) medicine.

Interactions with Food/Tobacco/Alcohol—Certain medicines should not be used at or around the time of eating food or eating certain types of food since interactions may occur. Using alcohol or tobacco with certain medicines may also cause interactions to occur. Discuss with your healthcare professional the use of your medicine with food, alcohol, or tobacco.

Proper Use of This Medicine

To use:

- First, wash your hands. Tilt the head back and, pressing your finger gently on the skin just beneath the lower eyelid, pull the lower eyelid away from the eye to make a space. Squeeze a thin strip of ointment into this space. A 1–cm (approximately 1/3–inch) strip of ointment is usually enough, unless you have been told by your doctor to use a different amount. Let go of the eyelid and gently close the eyes. Keep the eyes closed for 1 or 2 minutes to allow the medicine to come into contact with the infection.

- To keep the medicine as germ-free as possible, do not touch the applicator tip to any surface (including the eye). After using erythromycin eye ointment, wipe the tip of the ointment tube with a clean tissue and keep the tube tightly closed.

To help clear up your infection completely, keep using this medicine for the full time of treatment, even if your symptoms begin to clear up after a few days. If you stop using this medicine too soon, your symptoms may return. Do not miss any doses.

Dosing—The dose of this medicine will be different for different patients. Follow your doctor's orders or the directions on the label. The following information includes only the average doses of this medicine. If your dose is different, do not change it unless your doctor tells you to do so.

The amount of medicine that you take depends on the strength of the medicine. Also, the number of doses you take each day, the time allowed between doses, and the length of time you take the medicine depend on the medical problem for which you are using the medicine.

- For ophthalmic ointment dosage form:
  - For treatment of eye infections:
    - Adults and children—Use in the eyes up to six times a day as directed by your doctor.
  - For prevention of neonatal conjunctivitis and ophthalmia neonatorum:
    - Newborn babies—Use in the eyes once at birth.

Missed dose—If you miss a dose of this medicine, apply it as soon as possible. However, if it is almost time for your next dose, skip the missed dose and go back to your regular dosing schedule.

Storage—Store the medicine in a closed container at room temperature, away from heat, moisture, and direct light. Keep from freezing.

Keep out of the reach of children.

Do not keep outdated medicine or medicine no longer needed.

Precautions While Using This Medicine

If your symptoms do not improve within a few days, or if they become worse, check with your doctor.

After application, eye ointments usually cause your vision to blur for a few minutes.

Side Effects of This Medicine

Along with its needed effects, a medicine may cause some unwanted effects. Although not all of these side effects may occur, if they do occur they may need medical attention.

Check with your doctor as soon as possible if any of the following side effects occur:
> *Rare*
>> Eye irritation not present before therapy

Other side effects not listed may also occur in some patients. If you notice any other effects, check with your healthcare professional.

ERYTHROMYCIN (Topical route) - er-ith-roe-MYE-sin

Commonly used brand name(s)

In the U.S.—

A/T/S	Erycette
Akne-Mycin	Eryderm
Emcin	Erygel
Emgel	Theramycin Z

In Canada—
Sans-Acne
Staticin

Available Dosage Forms:

- Gel/Jelly
- Pad
- Lotion
- Ointment
- Swab
- Solution

Therapeutic Class: Antiacne

Uses For This Medicine

Erythromycin belongs to the family of medicines called antibiotics. Erythromycin topical preparations are used on the skin to help control acne. They may be used alone or with one or more other medicines that are applied to the skin or taken by mouth for acne. They may also be used for other problems, such as skin infections, as determined by your doctor.

Erythromycin is available only with your doctor's prescription.

Before Using This Medicine

In deciding to use a medicine, the risks of taking the medicine must be weighed against the good it will do. This is a decision you and your doctor will make. For this medicine, the following should be considered:

Allergies—Tell your doctor if you have ever had any unusual or allergic reaction to this medicine or any other medicines. Also tell your health care professional if you have any other types of allergies, such as to foods, dyes, preservatives, or animals. For non-prescription products, read the label or package ingredients carefully.

Pediatric—Erythromycin topical solution has been tested in children 12 years of age and older and, in effective doses, has not been shown to cause different side effects or problems than it does in adults.

Geriatric—Many medicines have not been studied specifically in older people. Therefore, it may not be known whether they work exactly the same way they do in younger adults. Although there is no specific information comparing use of topical erythromycin in the elderly with use in other age groups, this medicine is not expected to cause different side effects or problems in older people than it does in younger adults.

Other medicines—Although certain medicines should not be used together at all, in other cases two different medicines may be used together even if an interaction might occur. In these cases, your doctor may want to change the dose, or other precautions may be necessary. Tell your healthcare professional if you are taking any other prescription or non-prescription (over-the-counter [OTC]) medicine.

Interactions with Food/Tobacco/Alcohol—Certain medicines should not be used at or around the time of eating food or eating certain types of food since interactions may occur. Using alcohol or tobacco with certain medicines may also cause interactions to occur. Discuss with your healthcare professional the use of your medicine with food, alcohol, or tobacco.

Proper Use of This Medicine

Before applying this medicine, thoroughly wash the affected area with warm water and soap, rinse well, and pat dry. After washing or shaving, it is best to wait 30 minutes before applying the pledget (swab), topical gel, or topical liquid form. The alcohol in them may irritate freshly washed or shaved skin.

For patients using the pledget (swab), topical gel, or topical liquid form of erythromycin:

- These forms contain alcohol and are flammable. Do not use near heat, near open flame, or while smoking.

- It is important that you do not use this medicine more often than your doctor ordered. It may cause your skin to become too dry or irritated.

- Also, you should avoid washing the acne-affected areas too often. This may dry your skin and make your acne worse. Washing with a mild, bland soap 2 or 3 times a day should be enough, unless you have oily skin. If you have any questions about this, check with your doctor.

- To use:
  - The topical liquid form of this medicine may come in a bottle with an applicator tip, which may be used to apply the medicine directly to the skin. Use the applicator with a dabbing motion instead of a rolling motion (not like a roll-on deodorant, for example). If the medicine does not come in an applicator bottle, you may moisten a pad with the medicine and then rub the pad over the whole affected area. Or you may also apply this medicine with your fingertips. Be sure to wash the medicine off your hands afterward.
  - Apply a thin film of medicine, using enough to cover the affected area lightly. You should apply the medicine to the whole area usually affected by acne, not just the pimples themselves. This will help keep new pimples from breaking out.
  - The pledget (swab) form should be rubbed over the whole affected area. You may use extra pledgets (swabs), if needed, to cover larger areas.
  - Since these medicines contain alcohol, they may sting or burn. Therefore, do not get these medicines in the eyes, nose, mouth, or on other mucous membranes. Spread the medicine away from these areas when applying. If these medicines do get in the eyes, wash them out immediately, but carefully, with large amounts of cool tap water. If your eyes still burn or are painful, check with your doctor.

This medicine will not cure your acne. However, to help keep your acne under control, keep using this medicine for the full time of treatment, even if your symptoms begin to clear up after a few days. You may have to continue using this medicine every day for months or even longer in some cases. If you stop using this medicine too soon, your symptoms may return. It is important that you do not miss any doses.

Dosing—The dose of this medicine will be different for different patients. Follow your doctor's orders or the directions on the label. The following information includes only the average doses of this medicine. If your dose is different, do not change it unless your doctor tells you to do so.

The amount of medicine that you take depends on the strength of the medicine. Also, the number of doses you take each day, the time allowed between doses, and the length of time you take the medicine depend on the medical problem for which you are using the medicine.

- For acne:
  - For gel dosage form:
    - Adults—Apply to the affected area(s) of the skin two times a day, morning and evening.
    - Children—Dose must be determined by your doctor.
  - For ointment dosage form:
    - Adults, teenagers, and children—Apply to the affected area(s) of the skin two times a day, morning and evening.
  - For pledgets dosage form:
    - Adults, teenagers, and children—Apply to the affected area(s) of the skin two times a day.
  - For topical solution dosage form:
    - Adults, teenagers, and children 12 years of age and over—Apply to the affected area(s) of the skin two times a day, morning and evening.
    - Children up to 12 years of age—Dose must be determined by your doctor.

Missed dose—If you miss a dose of this medicine, take it as soon as possible. However, if it is almost time for your next dose, skip the missed dose and go back to your regular dosing schedule. Do not double doses.

Storage—Store the medicine in a closed container at room temperature, away from heat, moisture, and direct light. Keep from freezing.

Keep out of the reach of children.

Do not keep outdated medicine or medicine no longer needed.

Precautions While Using This Medicine

If your acne does not improve within 3 to 4 weeks, or if it becomes worse, check with your health care professional. However, treatment of acne may take up to 8 to 12 weeks before you see full improvement.

For patients using the pledget (swab), topical gel, or topical liquid form of erythromycin:

- If your doctor has ordered another medicine to be applied to the skin along with this medicine, it is best to wait at least 1 hour before you apply the second medicine. This may help keep your skin from becoming too irritated. Also, if the medicines are used too close together, they may not work properly.
- After application of this medicine to the skin, mild stinging or burning may be expected and may last up to a few minutes or more.
- This medicine may also cause the skin to become unusually dry, even with normal use. If this occurs, check with your doctor.
- You may continue to use cosmetics (make-up) while you are using this medicine for acne. However, it is best to use only "water-base" cosmetics. Also, it is best not to use cosmetics too heavily or too often. They may make your acne worse. If you have any questions about this, check with your doctor.

Side Effects of This Medicine

Along with its needed effects, a medicine may cause some unwanted effects. Although not all of these side effects may occur, if they do occur they may need medical attention.

Some side effects may occur that usually do not need medical attention. These side effects may go away during treatment as your body adjusts to the medicine. Also, your health care professional may be able to tell you about ways to prevent or reduce some of these side effects. Check with your health care professional if any of the following side effects continue or are bothersome or if you have any questions about them:

For erythromycin ointment
Less common
Peeling; redness
For erythromycin pledget (swab), topical gel, or topical liquid form
More common
Dry or scaly skin; irritation; itching; stinging or burning feeling
Less common
Peeling; redness

Other side effects not listed may also occur in some patients. If you notice any other effects, check with your healthcare professional.

ERYTHROMYCIN AND BENZOYL PEROXIDE (Topical route) - er-ith-roe-MYE-sin, BEN-zoe-ill per-OX-ide

Available Dosage Forms:
- Gel/Jelly

Therapeutic Class: Antiacne

Uses For This Medicine

Erythromycin and benzoyl peroxide combination is used to help control acne.

This medicine is applied to the skin. It may be used alone or with other medicines that are applied to the skin or taken by mouth for acne.

Erythromycin and benzoyl peroxide combination is available only with your doctor's prescription.

Before Using This Medicine

In deciding to use a medicine, the risks of taking the medicine must be weighed against the good it will do. This is a decision you and your doctor will make. For this medicine, the following should be considered:

Allergies—Tell your doctor if you have ever had any unusual or allergic reaction to this medicine or any other medicines. Also tell your health care professional if you have any other types of allergies, such as to foods, dyes, preservatives, or animals. For non-prescription products, read the label or package ingredients carefully.

Pediatric—Studies on this medicine have been done only in adult patients, and there is no specific information comparing use of this medicine in children up to 12 years of age with use in other age groups.

Geriatric—Many medicines have not been studied specifically in older people. Therefore, it may not be known whether they work exactly the same way they do in younger adults or if they cause different side effects or problems in older people. There is no specific information comparing use of this medicine in the elderly with use in other age groups.

Other medicines—

Using this medicine with any of the following medicines is not recommended. Your doctor may decide not to treat you with this medication or change some of the other medicines you take.

Astemizole, Bepridil, Cisapride, Dihydroergotamine, Ergoloid Mesylates, Ergonovine, Ergotamine, Grepafloxacin, Levomethadyl, Mesoridazine, Methylergonovine, Methysergide, Pimozide, Ranolazine, Sparfloxacin, Terfenadine, Thioridazine, Ziprasidone

Interactions with Food/Tobacco/Alcohol—Certain medicines should not be used at or around the time of eating food or eating certain types of food since interactions may occur. Using alcohol or tobacco with certain medicines may also cause interactions to occur. Discuss with your healthcare professional the use of your medicine with food, alcohol, or tobacco.

Proper Use of This Medicine

Do not use this medicine on raw or irritated skin.

Before applying this medicine, thoroughly wash the affected area(s) with warm water and soap, rinse well, and gently pat dry. After washing or shaving, it is best to wait 30 minutes before applying the medicine. The alcohol in it may irritate freshly washed or shaved skin.

Avoid washing the acne-affected area(s) too often. This may dry your skin and make your acne worse. Washing with a mild, bland soap 2 or 3 times a day should be enough, unless you have oily skin. If you have any questions about this, check with your doctor.

To use:

- Use this medicine only as directed. Do not use more of it and do not use it more often than your doctor ordered. To do so may cause your skin to become too dry or irritated.

- After washing the affected area(s), you may apply this medicine with your fingertips. However, be sure to wash the medicine off your hands afterward.

- Apply and rub in a thin film of medicine, using enough to cover the affected area(s) lightly. You should apply the medicine to the whole area usually affected by acne, not just to the pimples themselves.

- Since this medicine contains alcohol, it may sting or burn. Therefore, do not get this medicine in or around your eyes, nose, or mouth, or on other mucous membranes. Spread the medicine away from these areas when applying. If this medicine does get in your eyes, wash them out immediately, but carefully, with large amounts of cool tap water. If your eyes still burn or are painful, check with your doctor.

Do not use this medicine after the expiration date on the label. The medicine may not work properly. Get a fresh supply from your pharmacist. Check with your pharmacist if you have any questions about this.

To help keep your acne under control, keep using this medicine for the full time of treatment. You may have to continue using this medicine every day for months or even longer in some cases.

Dosing—The dose of this medicine will be different for different patients. Follow your doctor's orders or the directions on the label. The following information includes only the average doses of this medicine. If your dose is different, do not change it unless your doctor tells you to do so.

The amount of medicine that you take depends on the strength of the medicine. Also, the number of doses you take each day, the time allowed between doses, and the length of time you take the medicine depend on the medical problem for which you are using the medicine.

- For gel dosage form:
  ○ For acne:
    ▪ Adults and children 12 years of age and over— Apply to the affected area(s) of the skin two times a day, morning and evening, or as directed by your doctor.
    ▪ Children up to 12 years of age—Dose must be determined by your doctor.

Missed dose—If you miss a dose of this medicine, apply it as soon as possible. However, if it is almost time for your next dose, skip the missed dose and go back to your regular dosing schedule.

Storage—Store in the refrigerator. Do not freeze.

Keep out of the reach of children.

Do not keep outdated medicine or medicine no longer needed.

Precautions While Using This Medicine

If your acne does not improve within 3 to 4 weeks, or if it becomes worse, check with your health care professional. However, treatment of acne may take up to 8 to 12 weeks before you see full improvement.

If your doctor has ordered another medicine to be applied to the skin along with this medicine, it is best to apply the second medicine at least 1 hour after you apply the first medicine. This may help keep your skin from becoming too irritated. Also, if the medicines are used too close together, they may not work properly.

Mild stinging or burning of the skin may be expected after this medicine is applied. These effects may last up to a few minutes or more. If irritation continues, check with your doctor. You may have to use the medicine less often. Follow your doctor's directions.

This medicine may also cause the skin to become unusually dry, even with normal use. If this occurs, check with your doctor.

This medicine may bleach hair or colored fabrics.

You may continue to use cosmetics (make-up) while you are using this medicine for acne. However, it is best to use only "oil-free" cosmetics. Also, it is best not to use cosmetics too heavily or too often. They may make your acne worse. If you have any questions about this, check with your doctor.

Side Effects of This Medicine

Along with its needed effects, a medicine may cause some unwanted effects. Although not all of these side effects may occur, if they do occur they may need medical attention.

Check with your doctor as soon as possible if any of the following side effects occur:

Less common or rare
Burning, blistering, crusting, itching, severe redness, or swelling of the skin; painful irritation of the skin; skin rash

Symptoms of topical overdose
Burning, itching, scaling, redness, or swelling of the skin (severe)

Some side effects may occur that usually do not need medical attention. These side effects may go away during treatment as your body adjusts to the medicine. Also, your health care professional may be able to tell you about ways to prevent or reduce some of these side effects. Check with your health care professional if any of the following side effects continue or are bothersome or if you have any questions about them:

Less common
Dryness or peeling of the skin; feeling of warmth, mild stinging, or redness of the skin

Other side effects not listed may also occur in some patients. If you notice any other effects, check with your healthcare professional.

ERYTHROMYCIN AND SULFISOXAZOLE (Oral route) - er-ith-roe-MYE-sin, sul-fi-SOX-a-zole

Commonly used brand name(s)
In the U.S.—
Eryzole
Pediazole

Available Dosage Forms:
• Powder for Suspension

Therapeutic Class: Antibiotic Combination

Uses For This Medicine

Erythromycin and sulfisoxazole is a combination antibiotic used to treat ear infections in children. It also may be used for other problems as determined by your doctor. It will not work for colds, flu, or other virus infections.

Erythromycin and sulfisoxazole combination is available only with your doctor's prescription.

Once a medicine has been approved for marketing for a certain use, experience may show that it is also useful for other medical problems. Although this use is not specifically included in product labeling, erythromycin and sulfisoxazole combination is used in certain patients with the following medical condition:
• Sinusitis (sinus infection)

Before Using This Medicine

In deciding to use a medicine, the risks of taking the medicine must be weighed against the good it will do. This is a decision you and your doctor will make. For this medicine, the following should be considered:

Allergies—Tell your doctor if you have ever had any unusual or allergic reaction to this medicine or any other medicines. Also tell your health care professional if you have any other types of allergies, such as to foods, dyes, preservatives, or animals. For non-prescription products, read the label or package ingredients carefully.

Pediatric—This medicine has been tested in children over the age of 2 months and has not been shown to cause different side effects or problems than it does in adults. This medicine should not be given to infants under 2 months of age unless directed by the child's doctor, because it may cause unwanted effects.

Geriatric—This medicine is intended for use in children and is not generally used in adult patients.

Pregnancy—

	Pregnancy Category	Explanation
All Trimesters	C	Animal studies have shown an adverse effect and there are no adequate studies in pregnant women OR no animal studies have been conducted and there are no adequate studies in pregnant women.

Breast Feeding—There are no adequate studies in women for determining infant risk when using this medication during breastfeeding. Weigh the potential benefits against the potential risks before taking this medication while breastfeeding.

Other medicines—

Using this medicine with any of the following medicines is not recommended. Your doctor may decide not to treat you with this medication or change some of the other medicines you take.

Astemizole, Bepridil, Cisapride, Dihydroergotamine, Ergoloid Mesylates, Ergonovine, Ergotamine, Grepafloxacin, Levomethadyl, Mesoridazine, Methylergonovine, Methysergide, Pimozide, Ranolazine, Sparfloxacin, Terfenadine, Thioridazine, Ziprasidone

Interactions with Food/Tobacco/Alcohol—Certain medicines should not be used at or around the time of eating food or eating certain types of food since interactions may occur. Using alcohol or tobacco with certain medicines may also cause interactions to occur. Discuss with your healthcare professional the use of your medicine with food, alcohol, or tobacco.

Other medical problems—The presence of other medical problems may affect the use of this medicine. Make sure you tell your doctor if you have any other medical problems, especially:
• Anemia or other blood problems or

- Glucose-6–phosphate dehydrogenase (G6PD) deficiency—Erythromycin and sulfisoxazole may increase the chance of blood problems
- Heart disease—High doses of erythromycin and sulfisoxazole may increase the chance of side effects in patients with a history of an irregular heartbeat
- Kidney disease or
- Liver disease—Patients with liver or kidney disease may have an increased chance of side effects
- Loss of hearing—High doses of erythromycin and sulfisoxazole may increase the chance for hearing loss in some patients
- Porphyria—Erythromycin and sulfisoxazole may increase the chance of a porphyria attack

Proper Use of This Medicine

Erythromycin and sulfisoxazole combination is best taken with extra amounts of water and may be taken with food. Additional amounts of water should be taken several times every day, unless otherwise directed by your doctor. Drinking extra water will help to prevent some unwanted effects (e.g., kidney stones) of sulfa medicines.

Do not give this medicine to infants under 2 months of age, unless otherwise directed by your doctor. Sulfa medicines may cause liver problems in these infants.

Use a specially marked measuring spoon or other device to measure each dose accurately. The average household teaspoon may not hold the right amount of liquid.

Do not use after the expiration date on the label. The medicine may not work properly after that date. Check with your pharmacist if you have any questions about this.

To help clear up your infection completely, keep taking this medicine for the full time of treatment, even if you begin to feel better after a few days. If you stop taking this medicine too soon, your symptoms may return.

This medicine works best when there is a constant amount in the blood. To help keep the amount constant, do not miss any doses. Also, it is best to take the doses at evenly spaced times, day and night. For example, if you are to take 4 doses a day, the doses should be spaced about 6 hours apart. If this interferes with your sleep or other daily activities, or if you need help in planning the best times to take your medicine, check with your health care professional.

Dosing—The dose of this medicine will be different for different patients. Follow your doctor's orders or the directions on the label. The following information includes only the average doses of this medicine. If your dose is different, do not change it unless your doctor tells you to do so.

The amount of medicine that you take depends on the strength of the medicine. Also, the number of doses you take each day, the time allowed between doses, and the length of time you take the medicine depend on the medical problem for which you are using the medicine.

- For oral dosage form (suspension):
  - For infections caused by bacteria:
    - Adults and teenagers—This medicine is used only in children.
    - Children up to 2 months of age—Use is not recommended.

- Children 2 months of age and older—Dose is based on body weight:

For the four-times-a-day dosing schedule
- — Children weighing less than 8 kilograms (kg) (under 18 pounds): Dose must be determined by your doctor.
- — Children weighing 8 to 16 kg (18 to 35 pounds): 1/2 teaspoonful (2.5 milliliters [mL]) every six hours for ten days.
- — Children weighing 16 to 24 kg (35 to 53 pounds): 1 teaspoonful (5 mL) every six hours for ten days.
- — Children weighing 24 to 32 kg (53 to 70 pounds): 1 1/2 teaspoonfuls (7.5 mL) every six hours for ten days.
- — Children weighing more than 32 kg (over 70 pounds): 2 teaspoonfuls (10 mL) every six hours for ten days.

For the three-times-a-day dosing schedule
- — Children weighing less than 6 kg (under 13 pounds): Dose must be determined by your doctor.
- — Children weighing 6 to 12 kg (13 to 26 pounds): 1/2 teaspoonful (2.5 mL) every eight hours for ten days.
- — Children weighing 12 to 18 kg (26 to 40 pounds): 1 teaspoonful (5 mL) every eight hours for ten days.
- — Children weighing 18 to 24 kg (40 to 53 pounds): 1 1/2 teaspoonfuls (7.5 mL) every eight hours for ten days.
- — Children weighing 24 to 30 kg (53 to 66 pounds): 2 teaspoonfuls (10 mL) every eight hours for ten days.
- — Children weighing more than 30 kg (over 66 pounds): 2 1/2 teaspoonfuls (12.5 mL) every eight hours for ten days.

Missed dose—If you miss a dose of this medicine, take it as soon as possible. However, if it is almost time for your next dose, skip the missed dose and go back to your regular dosing schedule. Do not double doses.

Storage—Store in the refrigerator. Do not freeze.

Keep out of the reach of children.

Do not keep outdated medicine or medicine no longer needed.

Precautions While Using This Medicine

It is very important that your doctor check you at regular visits for any blood problems that may be caused by this medicine, especially if you will be taking this medicine for a long time.

If your symptoms do not improve within a few days, or if they become worse, check with your doctor.

Erythromycin and sulfisoxazole may cause your skin to be more sensitive to sunlight than it is normally. Exposure to sunlight, even for brief periods of time, may cause a skin rash, itching, redness or other discoloration of the skin, or a severe sunburn. When you begin taking this medicine:

- Stay out of direct sunlight, especially between the hours of 10:00 a.m. and 3:00 p.m., if possible.
- Wear protective clothing, including a hat. Also, wear sunglasses.

- Apply a sun block product that has a skin protection factor (SPF) of at least 15. Some patients may require a product with a higher SPF number, especially if they have a fair complexion. If you have any questions about this, check with your health care professional.
- Apply a sun block lipstick that has an SPF of at least 15 to protect your lips.
- Do not use a sunlamp or tanning bed or booth.

If you have a severe reaction from the sun, check with your doctor.

Erythromycin and sulfisoxazole combination may cause blood problems. These problems may result in a greater chance of infection, slow healing, and bleeding of the gums. Therefore, you should be careful when using regular toothbrushes, dental floss, and toothpicks. Dental work should be delayed until your blood counts have returned to normal. Check with your medical doctor or dentist if you have any questions about proper oral hygiene (mouth care) during treatment.

Side Effects of This Medicine

Along with its needed effects, a medicine may cause some unwanted effects. Although not all of these side effects may occur, if they do occur they may need medical attention.

Check with your doctor immediately if any of the following side effects occur:

More common
   Itching; skin rash

Less common
   Aching of joints and muscles; difficulty in swallowing; nausea or vomiting; pale skin; redness, blistering, peeling, or loosening of skin; skin rash; sore throat and fever; stomach pain, severe; unusual bleeding or bruising; unusual tiredness or weakness; yellow eyes or skin

Rare
   Blood in urine; dark or amber urine; irregular or slow heartbeat; temporary loss of hearing (with kidney disease and high doses); lower back pain; pain or burning while urinating; pale stools; recurrent fainting; severe stomach pain; swelling of front part of neck

Check with your doctor as soon as possible if any of the following side effects occur:

More common
   Increased sensitivity to sunlight

Some side effects may occur that usually do not need medical attention. These side effects may go away during treatment as your body adjusts to the medicine. Also, your health care professional may be able to tell you about ways to prevent or reduce some of these side effects. Check with your health care professional if any of the following side effects continue or are bothersome or if you have any questions about them:

More common
   Abdominal or stomach cramping and discomfort; diarrhea; headache; loss of appetite; nausea or vomiting

Less common
   Sore mouth or tongue

Other side effects not listed may also occur in some patients. If you notice any other effects, check with your healthcare professional.

ERYTHROMYCINS   (Systemic)

Some commonly used brand names are:

In the U.S.—

E-Base (1)	Erythrocin (6)
E-Mycin (1)	Erythrocot (6)
ERYC (1)	Ilotycin (1)
Ery-Tab (1)	Ilosone (2)
E.E.S. (3)	My-E (6)
EryPed (3)	PCE (1)
Erythro (3)	Wintrocin (6)

In Canada—

Apo-Erythro (1)	Erythrocin (5)
Apo-Erythro E-C (1)	Erythrocin (6)
Apo-Erythro-ES (3)	Erythromid (1)
Apo-Erythro-S (6)	Ilosone (2)
E-Mycin (1)	Ilotycin (4)
E.E.S. (3)	Novo-rythro (2)
Erybid (1)	Novo-rythro (6)
EryPed (3)	Novo-rythro Encap (1)
ERYC-250 (1)	PCE (1)
ERYC-333 (1)	

This information applies to the following medicines:

1. Erythromycin Base (er-ith-roe-MYE-sin)
2. Erythromycin Estolate (er-ith-roe-MYE-sin ESS-toe-layt)
3. Erythromycin Ethylsuccinate (er-ith-roe-MYE-sin eth-ill-SUK-sin-ayt)
4. Erythromycin Gluceptate (er-ith-roe-MYE-sin gloo-SEP-tayt)
5. Erythromycin Lactobionate (er-ith-roe-MYE-sin lak-toe-BYE-oh-nayt)
6. Erythromycin Stearate (er-ith-roe-MYE-sin STEER-ate)

Category

- **Antiacne agent, systemic**—Erythromycin Base; Erythromycin Estolate; Erythromycin Ethylsuccinate; Erythromycin Stearate
- **Antibacterial, systemic**—Erythromycin Base; Erythromycin Estolate; Erythromycin Ethylsuccinate; Erythromycin Gluceptate; Erythromycin Lactobionate; Erythromycin Stearate
- **Bowel preparation, preoperative, adjunct**—Erythromycin Base

Description

Erythromycins (eh-rith-roe-MYE-sins) are used to treat many kinds of infections. Erythromycins are also used to prevent "strep" infections in patients with a history of rheumatic heart disease who may be allergic to penicillin.

These medicines may also be used to treat Legionnaires' disease and for other problems as determined by your doctor. They will not work for colds, flu, or other virus infections.

Erythromycins are available only with your doctor's prescription, in the following dosage forms:

Oral
- Erythromycin Base
  - Delayed-release capsules
  - Delayed-release tablets
  - Tablets
- Erythromycin Estolate
  - Capsules
  - Oral suspension
  - Tablets

- Erythromycin Ethylsuccinate
  - Chewable tablets
  - Oral suspension
  - Tablets
- Erythromycin Stearate
  - Oral suspension
  - Tablets

Parenteral
- Erythromycin Gluceptate
  - Injection
- Erythromycin Lactobionate
  - Injection

Before Using This Medicine

In deciding to use a medicine, the risks of taking the medicine must be weighed against the good it will do. This is a decision you and your doctor will make. For erythromycins, the following should be considered:

Allergies—Tell your doctor if you have ever had any unusual or allergic reaction to erythromycins, or any related medicines, such as azithromycin or clarithromycin. Also tell your health care professional if you are allergic to any other substances, such as foods, preservatives, or dyes.

Pregnancy—Erythromycin estolate has caused side effects involving the liver in some pregnant women. However, none of the erythromycins has been shown to cause birth defects or other problems in human babies.

Breast-feeding—Erythromycins pass into the breast milk. However, erythromycins have not been shown to cause problems in nursing babies.

Children—This medicine has been tested in children and, in effective doses, has not been shown to cause different side effects or problems in children than it does in adults.

Older adults—This medicine has been tested and has not been shown to cause different side effects or problems in older people than it does in younger adults. However, older adults may be at increased risk of hearing loss, especially if they are taking high doses of erythromycin and/or have kidney or liver disease.

Other medicines—Although certain medicines should not be used together at all, in other cases two different medicines may be used together even if an interaction might occur. In these cases, your doctor may want to change the dose, or other precautions may be necessary. When you are taking or receiving erythromycins, it is especially important that your health care professional know if you are taking any of the following:

- Acetaminophen (e.g., Tylenol) (with long-term, high-dose use) or
- Amiodarone (e.g., Cordarone) or
- Anabolic steroids (nandrolone [e.g., Anabolin], oxandrolone [e.g., Anavar], oxymetholone [e.g., Anadrol], stanozolol [e.g., Winstrol]) or
- Androgens (male hormones) or
- Antithyroid agents (medicine for overactive thyroid) or
- Carmustine (e.g., BiCNU) or
- Chloroquine (e.g., Aralen) or
- Dantrolene (e.g., Dantrium) or
- Daunorubicin (e.g., Cerubidine) or

- Disulfiram (e.g., Antabuse) or
- Divalproex (e.g., Depakote) or
- Estrogens (female hormones) or
- Etretinate (e.g., Tegison) or
- Gold salts (medicine for arthritis) or
- Hydroxychloroquine (e.g., Plaquenil) or
- Mercaptopurine (e.g., Purinethol) or
- Methotrexate (e.g., Mexate) or
- Methyldopa (e.g., Aldomet) or
- Naltrexone (e.g., Trexan) (with long-term, high-dose use) or
- Oral contraceptives (birth control pills) containing estrogen or
- Other anti-infectives by mouth or by injection (medicine for infection) or
- Phenothiazines (acetophenazine [e.g., Tindal], chlorpromazine [e.g., Thorazine], fluphenazine [e.g., Prolixin], mesoridazine [e.g., Serentil], perphenazine [e.g., Trilafon], prochlorperazine [e.g., Compazine], promazine [e.g., Sparine], promethazine [e.g., Phenergan], thioridazine [e.g., Mellaril], trifluoperazine [e.g., Stelazine], triflupromazine [e.g., Vesprin], trimeprazine [e.g., Temaril]) or
- Phenytoin (e.g., Dilantin) or
- Plicamycin (e.g., Mithracin) or
- Valproic acid (e.g., Depakene)—Use of these medicines with erythromycins, especially erythromycin estolate, may increase the chance of liver problems
- Aminophylline (e.g., Somophyllin) or
- Caffeine (e.g., NoDoz) or
- Oxtriphylline (e.g., Choledyl) or
- Theophylline (e.g., Somophyllin-T, Theo-Dur)—Use of these medicines with erythromycins may increase the chance of side effects from aminophylline, caffeine, oxtriphylline, or theophylline
- Astemizole (e.g., Hismanal) or
- Terfenadine (e.g., Seldane)—Use of astemizole or terfenadine with erythromycins may cause heart problems, such as an irregular heartbeat; these medicines should not be used together
- Carbamazepine (e.g., Tegretol)—Use of carbamazepine with erythromycin may increase the side effects of carbamazepine or increase the chance of liver problems
- Chloramphenicol (e.g., Chloromycetin) or
- Clindamycin (e.g., Cleocin) or
- Lincomycin (e.g., Lincocin)—Use of these medicines with erythromycins may decrease the effectiveness of these other antibiotics
- Cyclosporine (e.g., Sandimmune) or
- Warfarin (e.g., Coumadin)—Use of any of these medicines with erythromycins may increase the side effects of these medicines

Other medical problems—The presence of other medical problems may affect the use of erythromycins. Make sure you

tell your doctor if you have any other medical problems, especially:

- Heart disease—High doses of erythromycin may increase the chance of side effects in patients with a history of an irregular heartbeat
- Liver disease—Erythromycins, especially erythromycin estolate, may increase the chance of side effects involving the liver
- Loss of hearing—High doses of erythromycins may, on rare occasion, cause hearing loss, especially if you have kidney or liver disease

Proper Use of This Medicine

Generally, erythromycins are best taken with a full glass (8 ounces) of water on an empty stomach (at least 1 hour before or 2 hours after meals). If stomach upset occurs, these medicines may be taken with food. If you have questions about the erythromycin medicine you are taking, check with your health care professional.

For patients taking the *oral liquid form* of this medicine:

- This medicine is to be taken by mouth even if it comes in a dropper bottle. If this medicine does not come in a dropper bottle, use a specially marked measuring spoon or other device to measure each dose accurately. The average household teaspoon may not hold the right amount of liquid.
- Do not use after the expiration date on the label. The medicine may not work properly after that date. Check with your pharmacist if you have any questions about this.

For patients taking the *chewable tablet form* of this medicine:

- Tablets must be chewed or crushed before they are swallowed.

For patients taking the *delayed-release capsule form (with enteric-coated pellets) or the delayed-release tablet form* of this medicine:

- Swallow capsules or tablets whole. Do not break or crush. If you are not sure about which type of capsule or tablet you are taking, check with your pharmacist.

To help clear up your infection completely, *keep taking this medicine for the full time of treatment,* even if you begin to feel better after a few days. *If you have a" strep" infection, you should keep taking this medicine for at least 10 days. This is especially important in" strep" infections. Serious heart problems could develop later* if your infection is not cleared up completely. Also, if you stop taking this medicine too soon, your symptoms may return.

This medicine works best when there is a constant amount in the blood. *To help keep the amount constant, do not miss any doses. Also, it is best to take the doses at evenly spaced times day and night.* For example, if you are to take 4 doses a day, the doses should be spaced about 6 hours apart. If this interferes with your sleep or other daily activities, or if you need help in planning the best times to take your medicine, check with your health care professional.

Dosing—The dose of erythromycin will be different for different patients. *Follow your doctor's orders or the directions on the label.* The following information includes only the average doses of erythromycin. *If your dose is different, do not change it* unless your doctor tells you to do so.

The number of capsules or tablets or teaspoonfuls of suspension that you take depends on the strength of the medicine. Also, *the number of doses you take each day, the time allowed between doses, and the length of time you take the medicine depend on the medical problem for which you are taking erythromycin.*

For erythromycin base

- For *oral* dosage forms (capsules, tablets):
  - For treatment of infections:
    - Adults and teenagers—250 to 500 milligrams (mg) two to four times a day.
    - Children—Dose is based on body weight. The usual dose is 7.5 to 12.5 mg per kilogram (kg) (3.4 to 5.6 mg per pound) of body weight four times a day, or 15 to 25 mg per kg (6.8 to 11.4 mg per pound) of body weight two times a day.
  - For prevention of heart infections:
    - Adults and teenagers—Take 1 gram two hours before your dental appointment or surgery, then 500 mg six hours after taking the first dose.
    - Children—Dose is based on body weight. The usual dose is 20 mg per kg (9.1 mg per pound) of body weight two hours before the dental appointment or surgery, then 10 mg per kg (4.5 mg per pound) of body weight six hours after taking the first dose.

For erythromycin estolate

- For *oral* dosage forms (capsules, oral suspension, tablets):
  - For treatment of infections:
    - Adults and teenagers—250 to 500 milligrams (mg) two to four times a day.
    - Children—Dose is based on body weight. The usual dose is 7.5 to 12.5 mg per kilogram (kg) (3.4 to 5.6 mg per pound) of body weight four times a day, or 15 to 25 mg per kg (6.8 to 11.4 mg per pound) of body weight two times a day.
  - For prevention of heart infections:
    - Adults and teenagers—Take 1 gram two hours before your dental appointment or surgery, then 500 mg six hours after taking the first dose.
    - Children—Dose is based on body weight. The usual dose is 20 mg per kg (9.1 mg per pound) of body weight two hours before the dental appointment or surgery, then 10 mg per kg (4.5 mg per pound) of body weight six hours after taking the first dose.

For erythromycin ethylsuccinate

- For *oral* dosage forms (oral suspension, tablets):
  - For treatment of infections:
    - Adults and teenagers—400 to 800 milligrams (mg) two to four times a day.
    - Children—Dose is based on body weight. The usual dose is 7.5 to 12.5 mg per kilogram (kg) (3.4 to 5.6 mg per pound) of body weight four times a day, or 15 to 25 mg per kg (6.8 to 11.4 mg per pound) of body weight two times a day.
  - For prevention of heart infections:
    - Adults and teenagers—Take 1.6 grams two hours before your dental appointment or surgery, then 800 mg six hours after taking the first dose.

- Children—Dose is based on body weight. The usual dose is 20 mg per kg (9.1 mg per pound) of body weight two hours before the dental appointment or surgery, then 10 mg per kg (4.5 mg per pound) of body weight six hours after taking the first dose.

For erythromycin gluceptate
- For *injection* dosage forms:
  ○ For treatment of infections:
    ▪ Adults and teenagers—250 to 500 milligrams (mg) injected into a vein every six hours; or 3.75 to 5 mg per kilogram (kg) (1.7 to 2.3 mg per pound) of body weight injected into a vein every six hours.
    ▪ Children—Dose is based on body weight. The usual dose is 3.75 to 5 mg per kg (1.7 to 2.3 mg per pound) of body weight injected into a vein every six hours.

For erythromycin lactobionate
- For *injection* dosage forms:
  ○ For treatment of infections:
    ▪ Adults and teenagers—250 to 500 milligrams (mg) injected into a vein every six hours; or 3.75 to 5 mg per kilogram (kg) (1.7 to 2.3 mg per pound) of body weight injected into a vein every six hours.
    ▪ Children—Dose is based on body weight. The usual dose is 3.75 to 5 mg per kg (1.7 to 2.3 mg per pound) of body weight injected into a vein every six hours.

For erythromycin stearate
- For *oral* dosage forms (oral suspension, tablets):
  ○ For treatment of infections:
    ▪ Adults and teenagers—250 to 500 milligrams (mg) two to four times a day.
    ▪ Children—Dose is based on body weight. The usual dose is 7.5 to 12.5 mg per kilogram (kg) (3.4 to 5.6 mg per pound) of body weight four times a day; or 15 to 25 mg per kg (6.8 to 11.4 mg per pound) of body weight two times a day.
  ○ For prevention of heart infections:
    ▪ Adults and teenagers—Take 1 gram two hours before your dental appointment or surgery, then 500 mg six hours after taking the first dose.
    ▪ Children—Dose is based on body weight. The usual dose is 20 mg per kg (9.1 mg per pound) of body weight two hours before the dental appointment or surgery, then 10 mg per kg (4.5 mg per pound) of body weight six hours after taking the first dose.

Missed dose—If you miss a dose of this medicine, take it as soon as possible. This will help to keep a constant amount of medicine in the blood. However, if it is almost time for your next dose, skip the missed dose and go back to your regular dosing schedule. Do not double doses.

Storage—To store this medicine:
- Keep out of the reach of children.
- Store away from heat and direct light.
- Do not store the capsule or tablet form of erythromycins in the bathroom, near the kitchen sink, or in other damp places. Heat or moisture may cause the medicine to break down.

- Store the oral liquid form of some erythromycins in the refrigerator because heat will cause this medicine to break down. However, keep the medicine from freezing. Follow the directions on the label.
- Do not keep outdated medicine or medicine no longer needed. Be sure that any discarded medicine is out of the reach of children.

Precautions While Using This Medicine

If your symptoms do not improve within a few days, or if they become worse, check with your doctor.

Side Effects of This Medicine

Along with its needed effects, a medicine may cause some unwanted effects. Although not all of these side effects may occur, if they do occur they may need medical attention.

Check with your doctor immediately if any of the following side effects occur:
  Less common
    Fever; nausea; skin rash, redness, or itching; stomach pain (severe); unusual tiredness or weakness; vomiting; yellow eyes or skin– with erythromycin estolate (rare with other erythromycins)

  Less common—with erythromycin injection only
    Pain, swelling, or redness at place of injection

  Rare
    Fainting (repeated); irregular or slow heartbeat; loss of hearing (temporary)

Other side effects may occur that usually do not need medical attention. These side effects may go away during treatment as your body adjusts to the medicine. However, check with your doctor if any of the following side effects continue or are bothersome:
  More common
    Abdominal or stomach cramping and discomfort; diarrhea; nausea or vomiting
  Less common
    Sore mouth or tongue; vaginal itching and discharge

Other side effects not listed above may also occur in some patients. If you notice any other effects, check with your doctor.

Additional Information

Once a medicine has been approved for marketing for a certain use, experience may show that it is also useful for other medical problems. Although these uses are not included in product labeling, erythromycins are used in certain patients with the following medical conditions:

- Acne
- Actinomycosis
- Anthrax
- Chancroid
- Gastroparesis
- Lyme disease
- Lymphogranuloma venereum
- Relapsing fever

Other than the above information, there is no additional information relating to proper use, precautions, or side effects for these uses.

ERYTHROPOIETIN (Injection route) -
er-ith-roe-POE-e-tin

Commonly used brand name(s)

In the U.S.—
    Epogen
    Procrit

Available Dosage Forms:
  • Solution

Therapeutic Class: Hematopoietic
Pharmacologic Class: Erythropoietic

Uses For This Medicine

Epoetin is a man-made version of human erythropoietin (EPO). EPO is produced naturally in the body, mostly by the kidneys. It stimulates the bone marrow to produce red blood cells. If the body does not produce enough EPO, severe anemia can occur. This often occurs in people whose kidneys are not working properly. Epoetin is used to treat severe anemia in these people.

Epoetin may also be used to prevent or treat anemia caused by other conditions, such as AIDS, cancer, or surgery, as determined by your doctor.

Epoetin is given by injection. It is available only with your doctor's prescription.

For patients receiving epoetin who do not have anemia caused by kidney disease:
  • The information about the importance of keeping dialysis appointments and following a special diet for people with kidney problems does not apply to you. However, your doctor may have other special directions for you to follow. Be sure to follow these directions carefully, even if you feel much better after receiving epoetin for a while.

Before Using This Medicine

In deciding to use a medicine, the risks of taking the medicine must be weighed against the good it will do. This is a decision you and your doctor will make. For this medicine, the following should be considered:

Allergies—Tell your doctor if you have ever had any unusual or allergic reaction to this medicine or any other medicines. Also tell your health care professional if you have any other types of allergies, such as to foods, dyes, preservatives, or animals. For non-prescription products, read the label or package ingredients carefully.

Pediatric—This medicine has been tested in children and teenagers and, in effective doses, has not been shown to cause different side effects or problems than it does in adults.

Geriatric—Epoetin has been given to elderly people. However, there is no specific information about whether epoetin works the same way it does in younger adults or whether it causes different side effects or problems in older people.

Pregnancy—

	Pregnancy Category	Explanation
All Trimesters	C	Animal studies have shown an adverse effect and there are no adequate studies in pregnant women OR no animal studies have been conducted and there are no adequate studies in pregnant women.

Breast Feeding—There are no adequate studies in women for determining infant risk when using this medication during breastfeeding. Weigh the potential benefits against the potential risks before taking this medication while breastfeeding.

Other medicines—Although certain medicines should not be used together at all, in other cases two different medicines may be used together even if an interaction might occur. In these cases, your doctor may want to change the dose, or other precautions may be necessary. Tell your healthcare professional if you are taking any other prescription or non-prescription (over-the-counter [OTC]) medicine.

Interactions with Food/Tobacco/Alcohol—Certain medicines should not be used at or around the time of eating food or eating certain types of food since interactions may occur. Using alcohol or tobacco with certain medicines may also cause interactions to occur. Discuss with your healthcare professional the use of your medicine with food, alcohol, or tobacco.

Other medical problems—The presence of other medical problems may affect the use of this medicine. Make sure you tell your doctor if you have any other medical problems, especially:
  • Aluminum poisoning
  • Blood clots (history of) or other problems with the blood or
  • Folic acid, iron, or vitamin B12 deficiencies
  • Heart or blood vessel disease or
  • Heart attacks, history of or
  • Heart bypass surgery or
  • High blood pressure or
  • Thrombosis, at risk for—The chance of side effects may be increased
  • Infection, inflammation, or cancer
  • Bone problems or
  • Porphyrin (red blood cell pigment) metabolism disorder—Symptoms include change in color of urine, increased sun sensitivity, abdominal pain, and nerve swelling
  • Sickle cell anemia—Epoetin may not work properly
  • Seizures (history of)—The chance of seizures may be increased

Proper Use of This Medicine

Epoetin is usually given by a health care professional after a dialysis treatment. However, medicines given by injection are sometimes used at home. If you will be using epoetin at home, your health care professional will teach you how the injections are to be given. You will also have a chance to practice giving them. Be certain that you understand exactly how the medicine is to be injected.

Your doctor will need to check your blood at regular visits while you are using this medicine. Be sure to keep all appointments.

Dosing—The dose of this medicine will be different for different patients. Follow your doctor's orders or the directions on the label. The following information includes only the average doses of this medicine. If your dose is different, do not change it unless your doctor tells you to do so.

The amount of medicine that you take depends on the strength of the medicine. Also, the number of doses you take each day, the time allowed between doses, and the length of time you take the medicine depend on the medical problem for which you are using the medicine.

- For injection dosage form:
  - For severe anemia:
    - Adults and teenagers—Dose is based on body weight and must be determined by your doctor. Epoetin is injected into a vein or under the skin. How often you take this medicine must be determined by your doctor. Your doctor may need to adjust the dose to determine the best dose for you.
    - Children 1 month to 12 years of age—Dose is based on body weight and must be determined by your doctor. Epoetin is injected into a vein or under the skin. How often you take this medicine must be determined by your doctor. Your doctor may need to adjust the dose to determine the best dose for you.
    - Children up to 1 month of age—Use and dose must be determined by your doctor.

Missed dose—If you miss a dose of this medicine, take it as soon as possible. However, if it is almost time for your next dose, skip the missed dose and go back to your regular dosing schedule. Do not double doses.

Storage—Store in the refrigerator. Do not freeze.

Keep out of the reach of children.

Do not keep outdated medicine or medicine no longer needed.

Precautions While Using This Medicine

Epoetin sometimes causes convulsions (seizures), especially during the first 90 days of treatment. During this time, it is best to avoid driving, operating heavy machinery, or other activities that could cause a serious injury if a seizure occurs while you are performing them.

People with severe anemia usually feel very tired and sick. When epoetin begins to work, usually in about 6 weeks, most people start to feel better. Some people are able to be more active. However, epoetin only corrects anemia. It has no effect on kidney disease or any other medical problem that needs regular medical attention. Therefore, even if you are feeling much better, it is very important that you do not miss any appointments with your doctor or any dialysis treatments.

Many people with kidney problems need to be on a special diet. Also, people with high blood pressure (which may be caused by kidney disease or by epoetin treatment) may need to be on a special diet and/or to take medicine to keep their blood pressure under control. After their anemia has been corrected, some people feel so much better that they want to eat more than before. To keep your kidney disease or your high blood pressure from getting worse, it is very important that you follow your special diet and take your medicines regularly, even if you are feeling better.

In addition to epoetin, your body needs iron to make red blood cells. Your doctor may direct you to take iron supplements. He or she may also direct you to take certain vitamins that help the iron work better. Be sure to follow your doctor's orders carefully, because epoetin will not work properly if there is not enough iron in your body.

If you are giving this medicine at home:

- Use a new needle and syringe each time you inject your medicine.
- Do not use more medicine or use it more often than your doctor tells you to.
- You will be shown the body areas where this shot can be given.
- Throw away used needles in a hard closed container that the needles cannot poke through. Keep this container away from children and pets.

Side Effects of This Medicine

Along with its needed effects, a medicine may cause some unwanted effects. Although not all of these side effects may occur, if they do occur they may need medical attention.

Check with your doctor immediately if any of the following side effects occur:

More common—in any treatment group
Chest pain; shortness of breath

Less common—in any treatment group
Anxiety; blurred vision; convulsions (seizures); cough; dizziness or lightheadedness; fainting; fast heartbeat; nausea; pain or discomfort in arms, jaw, back or neck; pains in chest, groin, or legs, especially calves of legs; severe headaches of sudden onset; sudden loss of coordination; sudden and severe inability to speak; slurred speech; sudden vision changes; sweating; temporary blindness; vomiting; weakness in arm and/or leg on one side of the body, sudden and severe

Check with your doctor as soon as possible if any of the following side effects occur:

More common— for patients being treated for anemia due to chronic kidney failure
Fever; headache; increased blood pressure; swelling of face, fingers, ankles, feet, or lower legs; vision problems; weight gain

Rare— for patients being treated for anemia due to chronic kidney failure
Changes in skin color; changes in vision; double vision; migraine headache; pain, tenderness, swelling of foot or leg; pale skin; partial or complete loss of vision in eye; skin rash or hives; sore throat; tenderness, pain, swelling, warmth, skin discoloration, and prominent superficial veins over affected area; unusual bleeding or bruising; unusual tiredness or weakness

More common—for patients being treated for anemia due to chronic kidney failure who require dialysis (in addition to those listed above)
Cough; fast heartbeat; fever; redness or pain at the dialysis access site; sneezing; sore throat

More common—for zidovudine-treated HIV-infected patients
    Fever; headache; skin rash or hives

More common—for cancer patients on chemotherapy
    Cough, sneezing or sore throat; fever; swelling of face, fingers, ankles, feet or lower legs; weight gain

More common—for surgical patients
    Blood in urine, lower back pain, or pain or burning while urinating; fever; headache; increased blood pressure; skin rash or hives; swelling of face, fingers, ankles, feet or lower legs; swelling or pain in legs; weight gain

Some side effects may occur that usually do not need medical attention. These side effects may go away during treatment as your body adjusts to the medicine. Also, your health care professional may be able to tell you about ways to prevent or reduce some of these side effects. Check with your health care professional if any of the following side effects continue or are bothersome or if you have any questions about them:

More common—in all treatment groups
    Diarrhea; dizziness; nausea or vomiting

More common—for patients being treated for anemia due to chronic kidney failure (in addition to those listed above)
    Bone or joint pain, muscle aches, chills, shivering, sweating; general feeling of tiredness or weakness; itching or stinging at site of injection; loss of strength or energy; muscle pain or weakness

More common—for patients being treated for anemia due to chronic kidney failure who require dialysis (in addition to those listed above)
    Abdominal pain and swelling; constipation; cough; fever; sore throat; weight loss

More common—for zidovudine-treated HIV-infected patients
    Congestion in the lungs; cough; general feeling of tiredness or weakness; itching or stinging at site of injection; loss of strength or energy; muscle pain or weakness

More common—for cancer patients on chemotherapy
    General feeling of tiredness or weakness; loss of strength or energy; muscle pain or weakness; tingling, burning or prickly sensation

More common—for surgical patients
    Anxiety; constipation; heartburn or belching, acid or sour stomach; inability to sleep; itching or stinging at site of injection; skin pain; stomach discomfort, upset or pain

Other side effects not listed may also occur in some patients. If you notice any other effects, check with your healthcare professional.

ESCITALOPRAM (Oral route) - es-sye-TAL-oh-pram

Black Box Warning

Suicidality in children and adolescents: Antidepressants increased the risk of suicidal thinking and behavior (suicidality) in short-term studies in children and adolescents with Major Depressive Disorder (MDD) and other psychiatric disorders. Anyone considering the use of escitalopram oxalate or any other antidepressant in a child or adolescent must balance this risk with the clinical need. Patients who are started on therapy should be observed closely for clinical worsening, suicidality, or unusual changes in behavior. Families and caregivers should be advised of the need for close observation and communication with the prescriber. Escitalopram oxalate is not approved for use in pediatric patients.

Pooled analyses of short-term (4 to 16 weeks) placebo-controlled trials of 9 antidepressant drugs (SSRIs and others) in children and adolescents with major depressive disorder (MDD), obsessive compulsive disorder (OCD), or other psychiatric disorders (a total of 24 trials involving over 4,400 patients) have revealed a greater risk of adverse events representing suicidal thinking or behavior (suicidality) during the first few months of treatment in those receiving antidepressants. The average risk of such events in patients receiving antidepressants was 4%, twice the placebo risk of 2%. No suicides occurred in these trials.

Commonly used brand name(s)

In the U.S.—
    Lexapro

Available Dosage Forms:
- Solution
- Tablet

Therapeutic Class: Antidepressant
Pharmacologic Class: Serotonin Reuptake Inhibitor

Uses For This Medicine

Escitalopram is used to treat mental depression.

Escitalopram belongs to a group of medicines known as selective serotonin reuptake inhibitors (SSRIs). These medicines are thought to work by increasing the activity of the chemical serotonin in the brain.

This medicine is available only with your doctor's prescription.

Before Using This Medicine

In deciding to use a medicine, the risks of taking the medicine must be weighed against the good it will do. This is a decision you and your doctor will make. For this medicine, the following should be considered:

Allergies—Tell your doctor if you have ever had any unusual or allergic reaction to this medicine or any other medicines. Also tell your health care professional if you have any other types of allergies, such as to foods, dyes, preservatives, or animals. For non-prescription products, read the label or package ingredients carefully.

Pediatric—Escitalopram must be used with caution in children with depression. Studies have shown occurrences of children thinking about suicide or attempting suicide in clinical trials for this medicine. More study is needed to be sure escitalopram is safe and effective in children

Geriatric—This medicine has been tested in elderly patients and has not been shown to cause different side effects or problems in older people than it does in younger adults. However, escitalopram is removed from the body more slowly in older people and an older person may need a lower dose than a younger adult.

Pregnancy—

	Pregnancy Category	Explanation
All Trimesters	C	Animal studies have shown an adverse effect and there are no adequate studies in pregnant women OR no animal studies have been conducted and there are no adequate studies in pregnant women.

Breast Feeding—Studies in women breastfeeding have demonstrated harmful infant effects. An alternative to this medication should be prescribed or you should stop breastfeeding while using this medicine.

Other medicines—

Using this medicine with any of the following medicines is not recommended. Your doctor may decide not to treat you with this medication or change some of the other medicines you take.

Clorgyline, Furazolidone, Isocarboxazid, Lazabemide, Moclobemide, Phenelzine, Selegiline, Tranylcypromine

Interactions with Food/Tobacco/Alcohol—Certain medicines should not be used at or around the time of eating food or eating certain types of food since interactions may occur. Using alcohol or tobacco with certain medicines may also cause interactions to occur. The following interactions have been selected on the basis of their potential significance and are not necessarily all-inclusive.

Using this medicine with any of the following may cause an increased risk of certain side effects but may be unavoidable in some cases. If used together, your doctor may change the dose or how often you use this medicine or give you special instructions about the use of food, alcohol, or tobacco.

Ethanol

Other medical problems—The presence of other medical problems may affect the use of this medicine. Make sure you tell your doctor if you have any other medical problems, especially:

- Diseases affecting metabolism or diseases involving blood circulation—caution should be used in patients with these medical problems
- Drug abuse, history of—potential for increased dependence on medicine
- Heart disease (unstable) or
- Myocardial infarction (heart attack) recent history of—The effects of escitalopram in patients with these conditions are not known.
- Kidney disease, severe—Until enough patients have been evaluated, caution is recommended for patients with severe kidney disease.
- Liver disease—Higher blood levels of escitalopram may occur, increasing the chance of having unwanted effects. You may need to take a lower dose than a person without liver disease.
- Mania or hypomania (history of)—Use of escitalopram may activate these conditions.
- Seizure disorders (history of)—The risk of having seizures may be increased.

Proper Use of This Medicine

Take this medicine only as directed by your doctor to help your condition as much as possible. Do not take more of it,

do not take it more often, and do not take it for a longer time than your doctor ordered.

Escitalopram may be taken with or without food on a full or empty stomach. If your doctor tells you to take it a certain way, follow your doctor's instructions.

You may have to take escitalopram for 1 to 4 weeks before you begin to feel better.

Do not stop taking this medication without checking first with your doctor

Dosing—The dose of this medicine will be different for different patients. Follow your doctor's orders or the directions on the label. The following information includes only the average doses of this medicine. If your dose is different, do not change it unless your doctor tells you to do so.

The amount of medicine that you take depends on the strength of the medicine. Also, the number of doses you take each day, the time allowed between doses, and the length of time you take the medicine depend on the medical problem for which you are using the medicine.

- For oral dosage form (oral solution):
  - For depression:
    - Adults—To start, usually 10 milligrams (mg) once a day, taken either in the morning or evening. Your doctor may increase your dose gradually if needed. However, the dose usually is not more than 20 mg a day.
    - Older adults and patients with liver problems—Usually 10 milligrams (mg) once a day, taken either in the morning or evening.
    - Children—Use and dose must be determined by your doctor.
  - For anxiety:
    - Adults—To start, usually 10 milligrams (mg) once a day, taken either in the morning or evening. Your doctor may increase your dose gradually if needed. However, the dose usually is not more than 20 mg a day.
    - Older adults and patients with liver problems—Usually 10 milligrams (mg) once a day, taken either in the morning or evening.
    - Children—Use and dose must be determined by your doctor.
- For oral dosage form (tablets):
  - For depression:
    - Adults—To start, usually 10 milligrams (mg) once a day, taken either in the morning or evening. Your doctor may increase your dose gradually if needed. However, the dose usually is not more than 20 mg a day.
    - Older adults and patients with liver problems—Usually 10 milligrams (mg) once a day, taken either in the morning or evening.
    - Children—Use and dose must be determined by your doctor.
  - For anxiety:
    - Adults—To start, usually 10 milligrams (mg) once a day, taken either in the morning or evening. Your doctor may increase your dose gradually if needed. However, the dose usually is not more than 20 mg a day.
    - Older adults and patients with liver problems—Usually 10 milligrams (mg) once a day, taken either in the morning or evening.
    - Children—Use and dose must be determined by your doctor.

Missed dose—Call your doctor or pharmacist for instructions.

Because escitalopram may be taken by different patients at different times of the day, you and your doctor should discuss what to do if you miss any doses.

Storage—Store the medicine in a closed container at room temperature, away from heat, moisture, and direct light. Keep from freezing.

Keep out of the reach of children.

Do not keep outdated medicine or medicine no longer needed.

Precautions While Using This Medicine

It is important that your doctor check your progress at regular visits, to allow for changes in your dose and to help reduce any side effects.

Do not take escitalopram with or within 14 days of taking a drug with Monoamine oxidase (MAO) inhibitor activity (isocarboxazid [e.g., Marplan], phenelzine [e.g., Nardil], procarbazine [e.g., Matulane], selegiline [e.g., Eldepryl], tranylcypromine [e.g., Parnate]). Do not take an MAO inhibitor within 14 days of taking escitalopram. If you do, you may develop extremely high blood pressure or convulsions (seizures).

Escitalopram may cause some people to be agitated, irritable or display other abnormal behaviors. It may also cause some people to have suicidal thoughts and tendencies or to become more depressed. If you or your caregiver notice any of these adverse effects, tell your doctor right away.

Avoid drinking alcoholic beverages while you are taking escitalopram.

This medicine may cause some people to become drowsy, to have trouble thinking, or to have problems with movement. Make sure you know how you react to citalopram before you drive, use machines, or do anything else that could be dangerous if you are not alert or well-coordinated.

Contact your doctor right away if you are unusually agitated, irritable, or have thoughts about hurting or killing yourself.

Side Effects of This Medicine

Along with its needed effects, a medicine may cause some unwanted effects. Although not all of these side effects may occur, if they do occur they may need medical attention.

Check with your doctor immediately if any of the following side effects occur:
> *Rare*
>> Coma; confusion; convulsions; decreased urine output; dizziness; fast or irregular heartbeat; headache; increased thirst; muscle pain or cramps; nausea or vomiting; shortness of breath; swelling of face, ankles, or hands; unusual tiredness or weakness

Some side effects may occur that usually do not need medical attention. These side effects may go away during treatment as your body adjusts to the medicine. Also, your health care professional may be able to tell you about ways to prevent or reduce some of these side effects. Check with your health care professional if any of the following side effects continue or are bothersome or if you have any questions about them:
> *More common*
>> Constipation; decreased interest in sexual intercourse; diarrhea; dizziness; dry mouth; ejaculation delay; gas

in stomach; heartburn; inability to have or keep an erection; impotence; increased sweating; loss in sexual ability desire, drive, or performance; nausea; stomach pain; sleeplessness; trouble sleeping; unable to sleep; sleepiness or unusual drowsiness
> *Less common*
>> Abdominal pain; chills; cough; decreased appetite; diarrhea; fever; general feeling of discomfort or illness; headache; joint pain; loss of appetite; muscle aches and pains; nausea; not able to have an orgasm; pain or tenderness around eyes and cheekbones; runny nose; shivering; shortness of breath or troubled breathing; sneezing; sore throat; stuffy nose; sweating; tightness of chest or wheezing; trouble sleeping; unusual tiredness or weakness; vomiting

After you stop using this medicine, it may still produce some side effects that need attention. During this period of time, *check with your doctor immediately* if you notice the following side effects:
> *Less common*
>> Ejaculation delay; nausea

Other side effects not listed may also occur in some patients. If you notice any other effects, check with your healthcare professional.

ESOMEPRAZOLE (Oral route) - es-oh-ME-pray-zole

Commonly used brand name(s)

In the U.S.—
> Nexium

Available Dosage Forms:
- Capsule, Delayed Release

Therapeutic Class: Antiulcer
Pharmacologic Class: Proton Pump Inhibitor

Uses For This Medicine

Esomeprazole is used to treat conditions in which there is too much acid in the stomach. It is used to treat duodenal ulcers and gastroesophageal reflux disease (GERD). This is a condition in which the acid in the stomach washes back up into the esophagus. It also reduces the chance of gastric ulcers in patients who use a group of medicines called NSAIDs and who may be at greater risk (i.e., patients 60 years of age or older or patients who have a history of gastric ulcers). Sometimes esomeprazole is used along with antibiotics to treat ulcers associated with infection caused by the H. pylori bacteria (germ).

Esomeprazole works by decreasing the amount of acid produced by the stomach.

This medicine is available only with your doctor's prescription.

Before Using This Medicine

In deciding to use a medicine, the risks of taking the medicine must be weighed against the good it will do. This is a decision you and your doctor will make. For this medicine, the following should be considered:

Allergies—Tell your doctor if you have ever had any unusual or allergic reaction to this medicine or any other medicines. Also tell your health care professional if you have any other types of allergies, such as to foods, dyes, preservatives, or animals. For non-prescription products, read the label or package ingredients carefully.

Pediatric—Studies on this medicine for uses other than GERD have been done only in adult patients, and there is no specific information comparing the use of esomeprazole in children with use in other age groups.

For the short-term treatment (up to 8 weeks) of GERD—This medicine has been tested in children and teenagers 12 to 17 years of age and, in effective doses, has not been shown to cause any different side effects or problems than it does in adults.

Geriatric—This medicine has been tested and has not been shown to cause different side effects or problems in older people than it does in younger adults.

Pregnancy—

	Pregnancy Category	Explanation
All Trimesters	B	Animal studies have revealed no evidence of harm to the fetus, however, there are no adequate studies in pregnant women OR animal studies have shown an adverse effect, but adequate studies in pregnant women have failed to demonstrate a risk to the fetus.

Breast Feeding—There are no adequate studies in women for determining infant risk when using this medication during breastfeeding. Weigh the potential benefits against the potential risks before taking this medication while breastfeeding.

Other medicines—

Using this medicine with any of the following medicines is usually not recommended, but may be required in some cases. If both medicines are prescribed together, your doctor may change the dose or how often you use one or both of the medicines.

Atazanavir

Interactions with Food/Tobacco/Alcohol—Certain medicines should not be used at or around the time of eating food or eating certain types of food since interactions may occur. Using alcohol or tobacco with certain medicines may also cause interactions to occur. Discuss with your healthcare professional the use of your medicine with food, alcohol, or tobacco.

Other medical problems—The presence of other medical problems may affect the use of this medicine. Make sure you tell your doctor if you have any other medical problems, especially:

- Liver disease or a history of liver disease—This condition may cause esomeprazole to build up in the body.

Proper Use of This Medicine

If you are taking the capsule form of this medicine: *Take esomeprazole at least one hour before a meal.*

Swallow the capsule whole. Do not crush, break, or chew the capsule. If you cannot swallow the capsule whole, you may open it and sprinkle the granules contained in the capsule on one tablespoonful of applesauce or yogurt and swallow it immediately; or you may mix the granules in some tap water or fruit juice and drink it immediately. The applesauce should not be hot, and the juices you may use include apple or orange juice. Do not chew or crush the granules.

Take this medicine for the full time of treatment, even if you begin to feel better. Also, keep your appointments with your doctor for check-ups so that your doctor will be better able to tell you when to stop taking this medicine.

Follow your doctor's instructions for switching from the injectable form of esomeprazole to the capsule form.

Dosing—The dose of this medicine will be different for different patients. Follow your doctor's orders or the directions on the label. The following information includes only the average doses of this medicine. If your dose is different, do not change it unless your doctor tells you to do so.

The amount of medicine that you take depends on the strength of the medicine. Also, the number of doses you take each day, the time allowed between doses, and the length of time you take the medicine depend on the medical problem for which you are using the medicine.

- For oral dosage form (delayed-release capsule):
  - To treat gastroesophageal reflux disease (GERD):
    - Adults—20 or 40 milligrams (mg) taken once a day for 4 to 8 weeks.
    - Children up to 18 years of age—Use and dose must be determined by your doctor
  - To treat gastroesophageal reflux disease (GERD) short-term (up to 8 weeks):
    - Children 12 to 17 years of age—20 or 40 mg taken once a day for up to 8 weeks.
    - Children up to 12 years of age—Use and dose must be determined by your doctor.
  - To prevent gastroesophageal reflux disease (GERD)
    - Adults—20 mg taken once a day.
    - Children up to 18 years of age—Use and dose must be determined by your doctor
  - To treat ulcer related infection with H. pylori
    - Adults—40 mg once daily, plus amoxicillin 1000 mg (1 gram) plus clarithromycin 500 mg, taken together before meals twice a day for 10 days.
    - Children up to 18 years of age—Use and dose must be determined by your doctor.
- For injection dosage form:
  - To treat gastroesophageal reflux disease (GERD):
    - Adults—20 or 40 milligrams (mg) once a day for no more than 10 days.
    - Children up to 18 years of age—Use and dose must be determined by your doctor.

Missed dose—If you miss a dose of this medicine, take it as soon as possible. However, if it is almost time for your next dose, skip the missed dose and go back to your regular dosing schedule. Do not double doses.

Storage—Store the medicine in a closed container at room temperature, away from heat, moisture, and direct light. Keep from freezing.

Keep out of the reach of children.

Do not keep outdated medicine or medicine no longer needed.

Ask your healthcare professional how you should dispose of any medicine you do not use.

Precautions While Using This Medicine

It is very important that your doctor check you at regular visits. If your condition does not improve, or if it becomes worse, discuss this with your doctor.

Side Effects of This Medicine

Along with its needed effects, a medicine may cause some unwanted effects. Although not all of these side effects may occur, if they do occur they may need medical attention.

Check with your doctor immediately if any of the following side effects occur:
> *Incidence not known*
>> Blistering, peeling, loosening of skin; bloating; chills; cough; darkened urine; difficulty swallowing; dizziness; fast heartbeat; fever; hives; indigestion; itching; joint or muscle pain; loss of appetite; pains in stomach, side, or abdomen, possibly radiating to the back; puffiness or swelling of the eyelids or around the eyes, face, lips or tongue; red, irritated eyes; red skin lesions, often with a purple center; shortness of breath; skin rash; sore throat; sores, ulcers, or white spots in mouth or on lips; tightness in chest; unusual tiredness or weakness; vomiting; wheezing; yellow eyes or skin

Some side effects may occur that usually do not need medical attention. These side effects may go away during treatment as your body adjusts to the medicine. Also, your health care professional may be able to tell you about ways to prevent or reduce some of these side effects. Check with your health care professional if any of the following side effects continue or are bothersome or if you have any questions about them:
> *More common*
>> Acid or sour stomach; belching; heartburn; indigestion; stomach discomfort, upset, or pain
> *Less common*
>> Abdominal pain; burning, itching, redness, skin rash, swelling or soreness at injection site; constipation; diarrhea; dryness of mouth; gas; headache; nausea; pain or tenderness around eyes and cheekbones; sneezing; stuffy or runny nose; tightness of chest or wheezing

Other side effects not listed may also occur in some patients. If you notice any other effects, check with your healthcare professional.

ESTRADIOL AND MEDROXYPROGESTERONE
(Intramuscular route) - es-tra-DYE-ole, me-DROKS-ee-proe-JES-te-rone

Commonly used brand name(s)
In the U.S.—
> Lunelle Monthly Contraceptive

Available Dosage Forms:
• Oil

Therapeutic Class: Estrogen/Progestin Combination
Pharmacologic Class: Medroxyprogesterone

Uses For This Medicine

Contraceptives are designed to prevent pregnancy. The combination of estradiol and medroxyprogesterone are two types of hormones that work by stopping a women's egg from fully developing each month. The egg can no longer accept sperm and fertilization is prevented. Although contraceptives have other effects that help prevent a pregnancy from occurring, this is the main action

This medicine is available only with your doctor's prescription.

Before Using This Medicine

In deciding to use a medicine, the risks of taking the medicine must be weighed against the good it will do. This is a decision you and your doctor will make. For this medicine, the following should be considered:

Allergies—Tell your doctor if you have ever had any unusual or allergic reaction to this medicine or any other medicines. Also tell your health care professional if you have any other types of allergies, such as to foods, dyes, preservatives, or animals. For non-prescription products, read the label or package ingredients carefully.

Pediatric—This medicine can be used for birth control in teenage females and is not expected to cause different side effects or problems than it does in adults. Some teenagers may need extra information on the importance of taking this medication exactly as prescribed.

Other medicines—

Using this medicine with any of the following medicines may cause an increased risk of certain side effects, but using both drugs may be the best treatment for you. If both medicines are prescribed together, your doctor may change the dose or how often you use one or both of the medicines.

Alprazolam, Aprepitant, Bexarotene, Bosentan, Clarithromycin, Ginseng, Itraconazole, Ketoconazole, Levothyroxine, Licorice, St John's Wort, Tacrine, Tipranavir

Interactions with Food/Tobacco/Alcohol—Certain medicines should not be used at or around the time of eating food or eating certain types of food since interactions may occur. Using alcohol or tobacco with certain medicines may also cause interactions to occur. The following interactions have been selected on the basis of their potential significance and are not necessarily all-inclusive.

Using this medicine with any of the following may cause an increased risk of certain side effects but may be unavoidable in some cases. If used together, your doctor may change the dose or how often you use this medicine, or give you special instructions about the use of food, alcohol, or tobacco.

Grapefruit Juice

Other medical problems—The presence of other medical problems may affect the use of this medicine. Make sure you tell your doctor if you have any other medical problems, especially:
• Abnormal changes in menstrual or uterine bleeding
• Blood clots (or history of) or
• Gallbladder disease or gallstones (or history of) or

- Heart or circulation problems or
- High blood cholesterol or
- High blood pressure (hypertension) or
- Liver disease (or history of) or
- Mental problems—Combination contraceptives may make these conditions worse or, rarely, cause them to occur again.
- Cancer, including breast cancer—Contraceptives may worsen some cancers, especially when breast, cervical, or uterine cancers already exist. Use of monthly injectable contraceptives is not recommended if you have any of these conditions. If you have a family history of breast disease, injectable contraceptives may still be a good choice but you may need to be tested more often
- Diabetes mellitus (sugar diabetes)—Use of combination contraceptives may cause an increase, usually only a small increase, in your blood sugar and usually does not affect the amount of diabetes medicine that you take.
- Migraine headaches—Combination contraceptives may cause fluid build-up and may cause these conditions to become worse; however, some people have fewer migraine headaches when they use contraceptives

Proper Use of This Medicine

Dosing—The dose of this medicine will be different for different patients. Follow your doctor's orders or the directions on the label. The following information includes only the average doses of this medicine. If your dose is different, do not change it unless your doctor tells you to do so.

The amount of medicine that you take depends on the strength of the medicine. Also, the number of doses you take each day, the time allowed between doses, and the length of time you take the medicine depend on the medical problem for which you are using the medicine.

- For injection dosage form:
  - For contraception
    - Adults—0.5 milliliters (mL) injected into a muscle in the upper arm, upper thigh or in the buttocks every 28 to 30 days.

Missed dose—Call your doctor or pharmacist for instructions.

If you miss having your next injection by day 33 your doctor will want to rule out pregnancy before the medicine is given to you again. Another method of birth control should be used until your period begins or until your doctor determines that you are not pregnant, and you are able to have the medicine again.

Precautions While Using This Medicine

It is very important that your health care professional check your progress at regular visits to make sure this medicine does not cause unwanted effects. These physical exams will usually be every 12 months, but you need to visit your doctor every 28 to 30 days to get your injection.

This medicine does not protect a woman from sexually transmitted diseases (STDs), including human immunodeficiency virus (HIV), or acquired immunodeficiency syndrome (AIDS).

Side Effects of This Medicine

Along with its needed effects, a medicine may cause some unwanted effects. Although not all of these side effects may occur, if they do occur they may need medical attention.

Check with your doctor immediately if any of the following side effects occur:

More common
> Bloating or swelling of face, hands, lower legs and/or feet; cough; difficulty swallowing; dizziness; fast heartbeat; hives; itching; loss of appetite and nausea; puffiness or swelling of the eyelids or around the eyes, face, lips or tongue; rapid weight gain; shortness of breath; tightness in chest; unusual tiredness or weakness; vomiting blood; wheezing; yellow eyes or skin

Symptoms of overdose—More common
> Nausea; menstrual irregularities; vaginal bleeding; vomiting

Some side effects may occur that usually do not need medical attention. These side effects may go away during treatment as your body adjusts to the medicine. Also, your health care professional may be able to tell you about ways to prevent or reduce some of these side effects. Check with your health care professional if any of the following side effects continue or are bothersome or if you have any questions about them:

More common
> Abdominal pain or enlarged abdomen; absent or missed menstrual periods; acne; allergic rash; brown, blotchy spots on skin; decreased sex drive; depression; hair loss/thinning of hair; headache; increased amount of menstrual bleeding, or normal bleeding that comes earlier; lack or loss of strength
> nervousness; quick to react or overact emotionally; rapidly changing moods; stopping of menstrual bleeding over several months; vaginal yeast infection; weight change

ESTRAMUSTINE   (Oral route) - es-tra-MUS-teen

Commonly used brand name(s)
In the U.S.—
    Emcyt

Available Dosage Forms:
- Capsule

Therapeutic Class: Antineoplastic Agent
Pharmacologic Class: Estrogen

Uses For This Medicine

Estramustine belongs to the general group of medicines called antineoplastics. It is used to treat some cases of prostate cancer.

Estramustine is a combination of two medicines, an estrogen and mechlorethamine. The way that estramustine works against cancer is not completely understood. However, it seems to interfere with the growth of cancer cells, which are eventually destroyed.

Estramustine is available only with your doctor's prescription.

Before Using This Medicine

In deciding to use a medicine, the risks of taking the medicine must be weighed against the good it will do. This is a decision you and your doctor will make. For this medicine, the following should be considered:

Allergies—Tell your doctor if you have ever had any unusual or allergic reaction to this medicine or any other medicines. Also tell your health care professional if you have any other types of allergies, such as to foods, dyes, preservatives, or animals. For non-prescription products, read the label or package ingredients carefully.

Geriatric—Many medicines have not been studied specifically in older people. Therefore, it may not be known whether they work exactly the same way they do in younger adults or if they cause different side effects or problems in older people. There is no specific information comparing use of estramustine in the elderly with use in other age groups.

Breast Feeding—There are no adequate studies in women for determining infant risk when using this medication during breastfeeding. Weigh the potential benefits against the potential risks before taking this medication while breastfeeding.

Other medicines—

Using this medicine with any of the following medicines is not recommended. Your doctor may decide not to treat you with this medication or change some of the other medicines you take.

Rotavirus Vaccine, Live

Interactions with Food/Tobacco/Alcohol—Certain medicines should not be used at or around the time of eating food or eating certain types of food since interactions may occur. Using alcohol or tobacco with certain medicines may also cause interactions to occur. The following interactions have been selected on the basis of their potential significance and are not necessarily all-inclusive.

Using this medicine with any of the following may cause an increased risk of certain side effects but may be unavoidable in some cases. If used together, your doctor may change the dose or how often you use this medicine, or give you special instructions about the use of food, alcohol, or tobacco.

Dairy Food

Other medical problems—The presence of other medical problems may affect the use of this medicine. Make sure you tell your doctor if you have any other medical problems, especially:

- Asthma or
- Epilepsy or
- Mental depression (or history of) or
- Migraine headaches or
- Kidney disease—Fluid retention sometimes caused by estramustine may worsen these conditions
- Blood clots (or history of) or
- Stroke (or history of) or
- Recent heart attack or stroke—May be worsened because of blood vessel problems caused by estramustine
- Chickenpox (including recent exposure) or
- Herpes zoster (shingles)—Risk of severe disease affecting other parts of the body

- Diabetes mellitus (sugar diabetes)—Estramustine may change the amount of antidiabetic medicine needed
- Gallbladder disease (or history of)—May be worsened by estramustine
- Heart or blood vessel disease—Estramustine can cause circulation problems
- Jaundice or hepatitis (or history of) or other liver disease—Effects, including liver problems, may be increased
- Stomach ulcer—May be aggravated by estramustine

Proper Use of This Medicine

Use this medicine only as directed by your doctor. Do not use more or less of it, and do not use it more often than your doctor ordered. The exact amount of medicine you need has been carefully worked out. Taking too much may increase the chance of side effects, while taking too little may not improve your condition.

Do not take estramustine within 1 hour before or 2 hours after meals or after the time you take milk, milk formulas, or other dairy products, since they may keep the medicine from working properly.

This medicine commonly causes nausea and sometimes causes vomiting. However, it may have to be taken for several weeks to months to be effective. Even if you begin to feel ill, do not stop using this medicine without first checking with your doctor. Ask your health care professional for ways to lessen these effects.

If you vomit shortly after taking a dose of estramustine, check with your doctor. You will be told whether to take the dose again or to wait until the next scheduled dose.

Dosing—The dose of this medicine will be different for different patients. Follow your doctor's orders or the directions on the label. The following information includes only the average doses of this medicine. If your dose is different, do not change it unless your doctor tells you to do so.

The amount of medicine that you take depends on the strength of the medicine. Also, the number of doses you take each day, the time allowed between doses, and the length of time you take the medicine depend on the medical problem for which you are using the medicine.

Missed dose—If you miss a dose of this medicine, skip the missed dose and go back to your regular dosing schedule. Do not double doses.

Storage—Store in the refrigerator. Do not freeze.

Keep out of the reach of children.

Do not keep outdated medicine or medicine no longer needed.

Precautions While Using This Medicine

It is very important that your doctor check your progress at regular visits to make sure that the medicine is working properly and does not cause unwanted effects.

While you are being treated with estramustine, and after you stop treatment with it, do not have any immunizations (vaccinations) without your doctor's approval. Estramustine may lower your body's resistance and there is a chance you might get the infection the immunization is meant to prevent. In addition, other persons living in your household should not take oral polio vaccine since there is a chance they could pass the polio virus on to you. Also, avoid persons who have recently taken oral polio vaccine. Do not get close to them and do not stay in the same room with them for very long. If you cannot take these precautions, you should consider wearing a protective face mask that covers the nose and mouth.

Side Effects of This Medicine

Along with its needed effects, a medicine may cause some unwanted effects. Although not all of these side effects may occur, if they do occur they may need medical attention.

Check with your doctor immediately if any of the following side effects occur:

Rare

Black, tarry stools; blood in urine or stools; cough or hoarseness; fever or chills; headaches (severe or sudden); loss of coordination (sudden); lower back or side pain; painful or difficult urination; pains in chest, groin, or leg (especially calf of leg); pinpoint red spots on skin; shortness of breath (sudden, for no apparent reason); slurred speech (sudden); unusual bleeding or bruising; vision changes (sudden); weakness or numbness in arm or leg

Check with your doctor as soon as possible if any of the following side effects occur:

More common

Swelling of feet or lower legs

Rare

Skin rash or fever; unusual tiredness or weakness

Some side effects may occur that usually do not need medical attention. These side effects may go away during treatment as your body adjusts to the medicine. Also, your health care professional may be able to tell you about ways to prevent or reduce some of these side effects. Check with your health care professional if any of the following side effects continue or are bothersome or if you have any questions about them:

More common

Breast tenderness or enlargement; decreased interest in sex; diarrhea; nausea

Less common

Trouble in sleeping; vomiting

Other side effects not listed may also occur in some patients. If you notice any other effects, check with your healthcare professional.

ESTROGENS (Systemic)

Some commonly used brand names are:

In the U.S.—

Alora (4)	Estraderm (4)
Climara (4)	Estragyn 5 (5)
Congest (1)	Estragyn LA 5 (4)
Delestrogen (4)	Estrasorb (4)
Depo-Estradiol (4)	Estro-L.A. (4)
Depogen (4)	Kestrone-5 (5)
Estinyl (7)	Neo-Estrone (4)
Estrace (4)	Menest (3)

Ogen.625 (6)	Premarin Intravenous (1)
Ogen 1.25 (6)	Valergen-10 (4)
Ogen 2.5 (6)	Valergen-20 (4)
Ortho-Est.625 (6)	Valergen-40 (4)
Ortho-Est 1.25 (6)	Vivelle (4)
Premarin (1)	Vivelle-Dot (4)

In Canada—

C.E.S. (1)	Ogen (6)
Delestrogen (4)	Premarin (1)
Estradot (4)	Premarin Intravenous (1)
Estraderm (4)	Vivelle (4)

This information applies to the following medicines

1. Conjugated Estrogens (CON-ju-gate-ed ES-troe-jenz)
2. Diethylstilbestrol (dye-eth-il-stil-BES-trole)
3. Esterified Estrogens (es-TAIR-i-fyed ES-troe-jenz)
4. Estradiol (es-tra-DYE-ole)
5. Estrone (ES-trone)
6. Estropipate (es-troe-PIH-pate)
7. Ethinyl Estradiol (ETH-in-il es-tra-DYE-ole)

Category

- **Antineoplastic**—Conjugated–Estrogens; Diethylstilbestrol; Esterified Estrogens; Estradiol; Estradiol valerate; Estrone; Ethinyl Estradiol

- **Estrogen, systemic**—Conjugated Estrogens; Diethylstilbestrol; Esterified Estrogens; Estradiol; Estrone; Estropipate; Ethinyl Estradiol

- **Osteoporosis prophylactic**—Conjugated Estrogens; Esterified Estrogens; Estradiol; Estropipate

- **Ovarian hormone therapy**—Conjugated Estrogens; Esterified Estrogens; Estradiol; Estropipate

---

Description

Estrogens ES-troe-jenz are female hormones. They are produced by the body and are necessary for the normal sexual development of the female and for the regulation of the menstrual cycle during the childbearing years.

The ovaries begin to produce less estrogen after menopause (the change of life). This medicine is prescribed to make up for the lower amount of estrogen. Estrogens help relieve signs of menopause, such as hot flashes and unusual sweating, chills, faintness, or dizziness.

Estrogens are prescribed for several reasons:

- to provide additional hormone when the body does not produce enough of its own, such as during menopause or when female puberty (development of female sexual organs) does not occur on time. Other conditions include a genital skin condition (vulvar atrophy), inflammation of the vagina (atrophic vaginitis), or ovary problems (female hypogonadism or failure or removal of both ovaries).

- to help prevent weakening of bones (osteoporosis) in women past menopause.

- in the treatment of selected cases of breast cancer in men and women.

- in the treatment of cancer of the prostate in men.

Estrogens may also be used for other conditions as determined by your doctor.

There is *no* medical evidence to support the belief that the use of estrogens will keep the patient feeling young, keep the skin soft, or delay the appearance of wrinkles. Nor has it been proven that the use of estrogens during menopause will relieve emotional and nervous symptoms, unless these symptoms are caused by other menopausal symptoms, such as hot flashes or hot flushes.

Estrogens are available only with your doctor's prescription, in the following dosage forms:

Oral
- Conjugated Estrogens
  - Tablets
- Esterified Estrogens
  - Tablets
- Estradiol
  - Tablets
- Estropipate
  - Tablets
- Ethinyl Estradiol
  - Tablets

Parenteral
- Conjugated Estrogens
  - Injection
- Estradiol
  - Injection
- Estrone
  - Injection

Topical
- Estradiol
  - Emulsion
  - Transdermal system (skin patch)

Before Using This Medicine

In deciding to use a medicine, the risks of taking the medicine must be weighed against the good it will do. This is a decision you and your doctor will make. For estrogens, the following should be considered:

Allergies—Tell your doctor if you have ever had any unusual or allergic reaction to estrogens. Also tell your health care professional if you are allergic to any other substances, such as foods, preservatives, or dyes.

Pregnancy—Estrogens are not recommended for use during pregnancy or right after giving birth. Becoming pregnant or maintaining a pregnancy is not likely to occur around the time of menopause.

Certain estrogens have been shown to cause serious birth defects in humans and animals. Some daughters of women who took diethylstilbestrol (DES) during pregnancy have developed reproductive (genital) tract problems and, rarely, cancer of the vagina or cervix (opening to the uterus) when they reached childbearing age. Some sons of women who took DES during pregnancy have developed urinary-genital tract problems.

Breast-feeding—Use of this medicine is not recommended in nursing mothers. Estrogens pass into the breast milk and their possible effect on the baby is not known.

Children—Use of this medicine before puberty is not recommended. Growth of bones can be stopped early. Girls and boys may develop growth of breasts. Girls may have vaginal changes, including vaginal bleeding.

Teenagers—This medicine may be used to start puberty in teenagers with some types of delayed puberty.

Older adults—Elderly people are especially sensitive to the effects of estrogens. This may increase the chance of side

effects during treatment, especially stroke, invasive breast cancer, and memory problems.

Other medicines—Although certain medicines should not be used together at all, in other cases two different medicines may be used together even if an interaction might occur. In these cases, your doctor may want to change the dose, or other precautions may be necessary. When you are taking estrogens, it is especially important that your health care professional know if you are taking any of the following:

- Acetaminophen (e.g., Tylenol) (with long-term, high-dose use) or
- Amiodarone (e.g., Cordarone) or
- Anabolic steroids (nandrolone [e.g., Anabolin], oxandrolone [e.g., Anavar], oxymetholone [e.g., Anadrol], stanozolol [e.g., Winstrol]) or
- Androgens (male hormones) or
- Anti-infectives by mouth or by injection (medicine for infection) or
- Antithyroid agents (medicine for overactive thyroid) or
- Carbamazepine (e.g., Tegretol) or
- Carmustine (e.g., BiCNU) or
- Chloroquine (e.g., Aralen) or
- Dantrolene (e.g., Dantrium) or
- Daunorubicin (e.g., Cerubidine) or
- Disulfiram (e.g., Antabuse) or
- Divalproex (e.g., Depakote) or
- Etretinate (e.g., Tegison) or
- Gold salts (medicine for arthritis) or
- Hydroxychloroquine (e.g., Plaquenil) or
- Isoniazid or
- Mercaptopurine (e.g., Purinethol) or
- Methotrexate (e.g., Mexate) or
- Methyldopa (e.g., Aldomet) or
- Naltrexone (e.g., Trexan) (with long-term, high-dose use) or
- Oral contraceptives (birth control pills) containing estrogen or
- Phenothiazines (acetophenazine [e.g., Tindal], chlorpromazine [e.g., Thorazine], fluphenazine [e.g., Prolixin], mesoridazine [e.g., Serentil], perphenazine [e.g., Trilafon], prochlorperazine [e.g., Compazine], promazine [e.g., Sparine], promethazine [e.g., Phenergan], thioridazine [e.g., Mellaril], trifluoperazine [e.g., Stelazine], triflupromazine [e.g., Vesprin], trimeprazine [e.g., Temaril]) or
- Phenytoin (e.g., Dilantin) or
- Plicamycin (e.g., Mithracin) or
- Valproic acid (e.g., Depakene)—Use of these medicines with estrogens may increase the chance of problems occurring that affect the liver
- Cyclosporine (e.g., Sandimmune)—Estrogens can prevent cyclosporine's removal from the body; this can lead to cyclosporine causing kidney or liver problems

Other medical problems—The presence of other medical problems may affect the use of estrogens. Make sure you tell your doctor if you have any other medical problems, especially:

For all patients
- Blood clotting problems (or history of during previous estrogen therapy)—Estrogens usually are not used until blood clotting problems stop; using estrogens is not a problem for most patients without a history of blood clotting problems due to estrogen use
- Asthma or
- Calcium, too much or too little in blood or
- Diabetes mellitus (sugar diabetes)
- Epilepsy (seizures) or
- Heart problems or
- Kidney problems or
- Liver tumors, benign or
- Lupus erythematosus, systemic or
- Migraine headaches—Estrogens may worsen these conditions.
- Breast cancer or
- Bone cancer or
- Cancer of the uterus or
- Fibroid tumors of the uterus—Estrogens may interfere with the treatment of breast or bone cancer or worsen cancer of the uterus when these conditions are present
- Changes in genital or vaginal bleeding of unknown causes—Use of estrogens may delay diagnosis or worsen condition. The reason for the bleeding should be determined before estrogens are used
- Endometriosis or
- High cholesterol or triglycerides (or history of) or
- Gallbladder disease or gallstones (or history of) or
- Liver disease (or history of) or
- Pancreatitis (inflammation of pancreas) or
- Porphyria—Estrogens may worsen these conditions. Although estrogens can improve blood cholesterol, they can worsen blood triglycerides for some people
- Hypothyroid (too little thyroid hormone)—Dose of thyroid medicine may need to be increased.
- Vision changes, sudden onset including
- Bulging eyes or
- Double vision or
- Migraine headache or
- Vision loss, partial or complete—Estrogens may cause these problems. Tell your doctor if you have had any of these problems, especially while taking estrogen or oral contraceptives ("birth control pills").

For males treated for breast or prostate cancer
- Blood clots or
- Heart or circulation disease or
- Stroke—Males with these medical problems may be more likely to have clotting problems while taking estrogens; the high doses of estrogens used to treat male breast or prostate cancer have been shown to increase the chances of heart attack, phlebitis (inflamed veins) caused by a blood clot, or blood clots in the lungs

Proper Use of This Medicine

Estrogens usually come with patient information or directions. Read them carefully before taking this medicine.

Take this medicine only as directed by your doctor. Do not take more of it and do not take or use it for a longer time than your doctor ordered. For patients taking any of the estrogens by mouth, try to take the medicine at the same time each day to reduce the possibility of side effects and to allow it to work better.

For patients taking any of the estrogens by mouth or by injection:
- Nausea may occur during the first few weeks after you start taking estrogens. This effect usually disappears with continued use. If the nausea is bothersome, it can usually be prevented or reduced by taking each dose with food or immediately after food.

For patients using the transdermal (skin patch) form of estradiol:
- Wash and dry your hands thoroughly before and after handling the patch.
- Apply the patch to a clean, dry, nonoily skin area of your lower abdomen, hips below the waist, or buttocks that has little or no hair and is free of cuts or irritation. The manufacturer of the 0.025–mg patch recommends that its patch be applied to the buttocks only. Furthermore, each new patch should be applied to a new site of application. For instance, if the old patch is taken off the left buttock, then apply the new patch to the right buttock.
- *Do not apply to the breasts.* Also, do not apply to the waistline or anywhere else where tight clothes may rub the patch loose.
- Press the patch firmly in place with the palm of your hand for about 10 seconds. Make sure there is good contact, especially around the edges.
- If a patch becomes loose or falls off, you may reapply it or discard it and apply a new patch.
- Each dose is best applied to a different area of skin on your lower abdomen, hips below the waist, or buttocks so that at least 1 week goes by before the same area is used again. This will help prevent skin irritation.

For patients using the topical emulsion (skin lotion) form of estradiol:
- Washing and drying hands thoroughly before each application.
- Apply while you are sitting comfortably. Apply one pouch to each leg every morning.
- Apply the entire contents of one pouch to clean, dry skin on the left thigh. Rub the emulsion into the entire thigh and calf for 3 minutes until thoroughly absorbed.
- Apply entire contents of the second pouch to clean, dry skin on the right thigh. Rub the emulsion into the entire thigh and calf for 3 minutes until thoroughly absorbed.
- Rub any remaining emulsion on both hands on the buttocks.
- Washing and drying hands thoroughly after application.
- To avoid transfer to other individuals, allow the application areas to dry completely before covering with clothing.

Dosing—The dose of these medicines will be different for different patients. *Follow your doctor's orders or the di-*

rections on the label. The following information includes only the average doses of these medicines. *If your dose is different, do not change it* unless your doctor tells you to do so.

The number of tablets that you take or the amount of injection you use depends on the strength of the medicine. Also, *the number of doses you take or use each day or patches you apply each week, the time allowed between doses, and the length of time you take or use the medicine depend on the medical problem for which you are taking, using, or applying estrogen.*

For conjugated estrogens
- For *oral* dosage form (tablets):
  - For treating breast cancer in women after menopause and in men:
    - Adults—10 milligrams (mg) three times a day for at least three months.
  - For treating a genital skin condition (vulvar atrophy), inflammation of the vagina (atrophic vaginitis), or symptoms of menopause:
    - Adults—0.3 mg a day. Your doctor may want you to take the medicine each day or only on certain days of the month. Your doctor may change the dose based on how your body responds to the medication.
  - To prevent loss of bone (osteoporosis):
    - Adults—0.3 mg a day. Your doctor may want you to take the medicine each day or only on certain days of the month. Your doctor may change the dose based on how your body responds to the medication.
  - For treating ovary problems (female hypogonadism or for starting puberty):
    - Adults and teenagers—0.3 to 0.625 mg a day. Your doctor may want you to take the medicine only on certain days of the month.
  - For treating ovary problems (failure or removal of both ovaries):
    - Adults—1.25 mg a day. Your doctor may want you to take the medicine each day or only on certain days of the month.
  - For treating prostate cancer:
    - Adults—1.25 to 2.5 mg three times a day.
- For *injection* dosage form:
  - For controlling abnormal bleeding of the uterus:
    - Adults—25 mg injected into a muscle or vein. This may be repeated in six to twelve hours if needed.

For esterified estrogens
- For *oral* dosage form (tablets):
  - For treating breast cancer in women after menopause and in men:
    - Adults—10 milligrams (mg) three times a day for at least three months.
  - For treating a genital skin condition (vulvar atrophy) or inflammation of the vagina (atrophic vaginitis), or to prevent loss of bone (osteoporosis):
    - Adults—0.3 to 1.25 mg a day. Your doctor may want you to take the medicine each day or only on certain days of the month.
  - For treating ovary problems (failure or removal of both ovaries):
    - Adults—1.25 mg a day. Your doctor may want you to take the medicine each day or only on certain days of the month.
  - For treating ovary problems (female hypogonadism):
    - Adults—2.5 to 7.5 mg a day. This dose may be divided up and taken in smaller doses. Your doctor may want you to take the medicine each day or only on certain days of the month.
  - For treating symptoms of menopause:
    - Adults—0.625 to 1.25 mg a day. Your doctor may want you to take the medicine each day or only on certain days of the month.
  - For treating prostate cancer:
    - Adults—1.25 to 2.5 mg three times a day.

For estradiol
- For *oral* dosage form (tablets):
  - For treating breast cancer in women after menopause and in men:
    - Adults—10 milligrams (mg) three times a day for at least three months.
  - For treating a genital skin condition (vulvar atrophy), inflammation of the vagina (atrophic vaginitis), ovary problems (female hypogonadism or failure or removal of both ovaries), or symptoms of menopause:
    - Adults—0.5 to 2 mg a day. Your doctor may want you to take the medicine each day or only on certain days of the month.
  - For treating prostate cancer:
    - Adults—1 to 2 mg three times a day.
  - To prevent loss of bone (osteoporosis):
    - Adults—0.5 mg a day. Your doctor may want you to take the medicine each day or only on certain days of the month.
- For *topical emulsion* dosage form (skin lotion):
  - For treating symptoms of menopause:
    - Adults—1.74 grams (one pouch) applied to the skin of each leg (thigh and calf) once a day in the morning.
- For *transdermal* dosage form (skin patches):
  - For treating a genital skin condition (vulvar atrophy), inflammation of the vagina (atrophic vaginitis), symptoms of menopause, ovary problems (female hypogonadism or failure or removal of both ovaries), or to prevent loss of bone (osteoporosis):

  For the Climara patches
    - Adults—0.025 to 0.1 milligram (mg) (one patch) applied to the skin and worn for one week. Then, remove that patch and apply a new one. A new patch should be applied once a week for three weeks. During the fourth week, you may or may not wear a patch. Your health care professional will tell you what you should do for this fourth week. After the fourth week, you will repeat the cycle.

  For the Alora, Estraderm, Estradot, Vivelle, or Vivelle-Dot patches
    - Adults—0.025 to 0.1 mg (one patch) applied to the skin and worn for one half of a week. Then, remove that patch and apply and wear a new patch for the rest of the week. A new patch should be applied two times a week for three weeks. During the fourth week, you may or may not apply new patches. Your health care professional will tell you what you should do for this fourth week. After the fourth week, you will repeat the cycle.

For estradiol cypionate
- For *injection* dosage form:
  - For treating ovary problems (female hypogonadism):
    - Adults—1.5 to 2 milligrams (mg) injected into a muscle once a month.
  - For treating symptoms of menopause:
    - Adults—1 to 5 mg injected into a muscle every three to four weeks.

For estradiol valerate
- For *injection* dosage form:
  - For treating a genital skin condition (vulvar atrophy), inflammation of the vagina (atrophic vaginitis), symptoms of menopause, or ovary problems (female hypogonadism or failure or removal of both ovaries):
    - Adults—10 to 20 milligrams (mg) injected into a muscle every four weeks as needed.
  - For treating prostate cancer:
    - Adults—30 mg injected into a muscle every one or two weeks.

For estrone
- For *injection* dosage form:
  - For controlling abnormal bleeding of the uterus:
    - Adults—2 to 5 milligrams (mg) a day, injected into a muscle for several days.
  - For treating a genital skin condition (vulvar atrophy), inflammation of the vagina (atrophic vaginitis), or symptoms of menopause:
    - Adults—0.1 to 0.5 mg injected into a muscle two or three times a week. Your doctor may want you to receive the medicine each week or only during certain weeks of the month.
  - For treating ovary problems (female hypogonadism or failure or removal of both ovaries):
    - Adults—0.1 to 1 mg a week. This is injected into a muscle as a single dose or divided into more than one dose. Your doctor may want you to receive the medicine each week or only during certain weeks of the month.
  - For treating prostate cancer:
    - Adults—2 to 4 mg injected into a muscle two or three times a week.

For estropipate
- For *oral* dosage form (tablets):
  - For treating a genital skin condition (vulvar atrophy), inflammation of the vagina (atrophic vaginitis), or symptoms of menopause:
    - Adults—0.75 to 6 milligrams (mg) a day. Your doctor may want you to take the medicine each day or only on certain days of the month.
  - For treating ovary problems (female hypogonadism or failure or removal of both ovaries):
    - Adults—1.5 to 9 mg a day. Your doctor may want you to take the medicine each day or only on certain days of the month.
  - To prevent loss of bone (osteoporosis):
    - Adults—0.75 mg a day. Your doctor may want you to take the medicine each day for twenty-five days of a thirty-one-day cycle.

For ethinyl estradiol
- For *oral* dosage form (tablets):
  - For treating breast cancer in women after menopause and in men:
    - Adults—1 milligram (mg) three times a day.

  - For treating ovary problems (female hypogonadism or failure or removal of both ovaries):
    - Adults—0.05 mg one to three times a day for three to six months. Your doctor may want you to take the medicine each day or only on certain days of the month.
  - For treating prostate cancer:
    - Adults—0.15 to 3 mg a day.
  - For treating symptoms of menopause:
    - Adults—0.02 to 0.05 mg a day. Your doctor may want you to take the medicine each day or only on certain days of the month.

For ethinyl estradiol and norethindrone
- For *oral* dosage form (tablets):
  - For treating symptoms of menopause:
    - Adults—1 tablet (5 mcg ethinyl estradiol and 1 mg of norethindrone) each day
  - To prevent loss of bone (osteoporosis):
    - Adults—1 tablet (5 mcg ethinyl estradiol and 1 mg of norethindrone) each day

Missed dose—

- For patients taking any of the estrogens by mouth: If you miss a dose of this medicine, take it as soon as possible. However, if it is almost time for your next dose, skip the missed dose and go back to your regular dosing schedule. Do not double doses.

- For patients using the topical emulsion (skin lotion) form of estradiol: If you forget to apply the emulsion when you are suppose to, apply it as soon as possible. However, if it is almost time for the next dose, skip the missed one and go back to your regular schedule. Do not apply more than once a day.

- For patients using the transdermal (skin patch) form of estradiol: If you forget to apply a new patch when you are supposed to, apply it as soon as possible. However, if it is almost time for the next patch, skip the missed one and go back to your regular schedule. Always remove the old patch before applying a new one. Do not apply more than one patch at a time.

Storage—To store this medicine:

- Keep out of the reach of children.
- Store away from heat and direct light.
- Do not store in the bathroom medicine cabinet because the heat or moisture may cause the medicine to break down.
- Keep the injection form of this medicine from freezing.
- Do not keep outdated medicine or medicine no longer needed. Be sure that any discarded medicine is out of the reach of children.

Precautions While Using This Medicine

It is very important that your doctor check your progress at regular visits to make sure this medicine does not cause unwanted effects. These visits will usually be every year, but some doctors require them more often.

In some patients using estrogens, tenderness, swelling, or bleeding of the gums may occur. Brushing and flossing your teeth carefully and regularly and massaging your gums may help prevent this. See your dentist regularly to have your teeth cleaned. Check with your medical doctor or dentist if you have any questions about how to take care of your teeth and gums, or if you notice any tenderness, swelling, or bleeding of your gums.

Although the incidence is low, the use of estrogens may increase you chance of getting cancer of the breast, ovaries, or uterus (womb).. Therefore, it is very important that you regularly check your breasts for any unusual lumps or discharge. Report any problems to your doctor. You should also have a mammogram (x-ray pictures of the breasts) done if your doctor recommends it. Because breast cancer has occurred in men taking estrogens, regular breast self-exams and exams by your doctor for any unusual lumps or discharge should be done.

If your menstrual periods have stopped, they may start again. This effect will continue for as long as the medicine is taken. However, if taking the continuous treatment (0.625 mg conjugated estrogens and 2.5 mg medroxyprogesterone once a day), monthly bleeding usually stops within 10 months.

Also, vaginal bleeding between your regular menstrual periods may occur during the first 3 months of use. Do not stop taking your medicine. *Check with your doctor if bleeding continues for an unusually long time, if your period has not started within 45 days of your last period, or if you think you are pregnant.*

Tell the doctor in charge that you are taking this medicine before having any laboratory test because some results may be affected.

Side Effects of This Medicine

Women rarely have severe side effects from taking estrogens to replace estrogen. Discuss these possible effects with your doctor:

- The prolonged use of estrogens has been reported to increase the risk of endometrial cancer (cancer of the lining of the uterus) in women after menopause. This risk seems to increase as the dose and the length of use increase. When estrogens are used in low doses for less than 1 year, there is less risk. The risk is also reduced if a progestin (another female hormone) is added to, or replaces part of, your estrogen dose. If the uterus has been removed by surgery (total hysterectomy), there is no risk of endometrial cancer.

- Although the incidence is low, the use of estrogens may increase you chance of getting cancer of the breast. Breast cancer has been reported in men taking estrogens.

The following side effects may be caused by blood clots, which could lead to stroke, heart attack, or death. These side effects occur rarely, and, when they do occur, they occur in men treated for cancer using high doses of estrogens. *Get emergency help immediately* if any of the following side effects occur:

Rare—for males being treated for breast or prostate cancer only

Headache (sudden or severe); loss of coordination (sudden); loss of vision or change of vision (sudden); pains in chest, groin, or leg, especially in calf of leg; shortness of breath (sudden and unexplained); slurring of speech (sudden); weakness or numbness in arm or leg

Also, check with your doctor as soon as possible if any of the following side effects occur:

More common

Breast pain (in females and males); fast heartbeat; fever; hives; hoarseness; increased breast size (in females and males); irritation of skin; itching of skin; joint pain, stiffness or swelling; rash; redness of skin; shortness of breath; swelling of eyelids, face, lips, hands, or feet; swelling of feet and lower legs; tightness in chest; troubled breathing or swallowing; weight gain (rapid); wheezing

Less common or rare

Changes in vaginal bleeding (spotting, breakthrough bleeding, prolonged or heavier bleeding, or complete stoppage of bleeding); chest pain; chills; cough; heavy nonmenstrual vaginal bleeding; lumps in, or discharge from, breast (in females and males); pains in stomach, side, or abdomen; yellow eyes or skin

Frequency not determined

Abdominal bloating; abdominal cramps; acid or sour stomach; anxiety; backache; belching; blindness; blistering, peeling, loosening of skin; blue-yellow color blindness; blurred vision; change in vaginal discharge; changes in vision; changes in skin color; chest discomfort; clay-colored stools; clear or bloody discharge from nipple; confusion; constipation; convulsions; dark urine; decrease in amount of urine; decreased vision; depression; diarrhea; difficulty breathing; difficulty in speaking; dimpling of breast skin; dizziness; double vision; dry mouth; eye pain; fainting; fluid-filled skin blisters; full feeling in upper abdomen; full or bloated feeling or pressure in the stomach; headache; heartburn; inability to move arms, legs, or facial muscles; inability to speak; incoherent speech; increased urination; indigestion; inverted nipple; irregular heartbeats; light-colored stools; lightheadedness; loss of appetite; loss of bladder control; lump under the arm; metallic taste; migraine headache; mood or mental changes; muscle cramps in hands, arms, feet, legs, or face; muscle pain; muscle spasm or jerking of all extremities; muscle weakness; nausea; noisy breathing; numbness or tingling of hands, feet, or face; pain in ankles or knees; pains in chest, groin, or legs, especially calves of legs; pain or discomfort in arms, jaw, back or neck; pain or feeling of pressure in pelvis; painful or tender cysts in the breasts; painful, red lumps under the skin, mostly on the legs; pain; tenderness; swelling of foot or leg; partial or complete loss of vision in eye; pelvic pain; persistent crusting or scaling of nipple; pinpoint red or purple spots on skin; prominent superficial veins over affected area; red, irritated eyes; redness or swelling of breast; sensitivity to the sun; severe headaches of sudden onset; skin thinness; skin warmth; slow speech; sore on the skin of the breast that does not heal; sore throat; sores, ulcers, or white spots in mouth or on lips; stomach discomfort, upset or pain; sudden loss of consciousness; sudden loss of coordination; sudden onset of shortness of breath for no apparent reason; sudden onset of slurred speech; sudden vision changes; sweating; swelling of abdominal or stomach area; swelling of fingers or hands; thirst; tremor; unpleasant breath odor; unusual tiredness or weakness; vomiting; vomiting of blood; weight loss

Other side effects may occur that usually do not need medical attention. These side effects may go away during treatment

---

as your body adjusts to the medicine. However, check with your doctor if any of the following side effects continue or are bothersome:

More common

Abnormal growth filled with fluid or semisolid material; accidental injury; bladder pain; bloated full feeling; bloody or cloudy urine; body aches or pain; coating or white patches on tongue; congestion; cough producing mucus; decrease in amount of urine; difficult, burning, or painful urination; discouragement; dryness of throat; ear congestion or pain; excess air or gas in stomach or intestines; fear; feeling of warmth; feeling sad or empty; frequent urge to urinate; general feeling of discomfort or illness; headache, severe and throbbing; increased clear or white vaginal discharge; irritability; itching of the vaginal, rectal or genital areas; lack of appetite; lack or loss of strength; loss of interest or pleasure; mild dizziness; neck pain; nervousness; pain; pain during sexual intercourse; painful or difficult urination; pain or tenderness around eyes and cheekbones; passing gas; redness of the face, neck, arms and occasionally, upper chest; runny nose; skin irritation or redness where skin patch was worn; shivering; sleeplessness; sneezing; sore mouth or tongue; stuffy nose; sudden sweating; tender, swollen glands in neck; thick, white vaginal discharge with no odor or with a mild odor; tiredness; trouble concentrating; trouble sleeping; unable to sleep; voice changes

Less common

Blemishes on the skin; burning, crawling, itching, numbness, prickling, "pins and needles", or tingling feelings; burning or stinging of skin; diarrhea (mild); dizziness (mild); increased hair growth, especially on the face; lower abdominal pain or pressure; mood or mental changes; muscle stiffness; difficulty in moving; painful cold sores or blisters on lips, nose, eyes, or genitals; pimples; pounding in the ears; slow heartbeat; problems in wearing contact lenses; tooth or gum pain; unusual decrease in sexual desire (in males); unusual increase in sexual desire (in females); white or brownish vaginal discharge

Frequency not determined

abdominal pain; abnormal turning out of cervix; changes in appetite; dull ache or feeling of pressure or heaviness in legs; fatigue; flushed, dry skin; fruit-like breath odor; increased hunger; irritability; large amount of triglyceride in the blood; leg cramps; patchy brown or dark brown discoloration of skin; poor insight and judgment; problems with memory or speech; trouble recognizing objects; trouble thinking and planning; trouble walking; twitching, uncontrolled movements of tongue, lips, face, arms, or legs; unexpected or excess milk flow from breasts

Also, many women who are taking estrogens with a progestin (another female hormone) will start having monthly vaginal bleeding, similar to menstrual periods, again. This effect will continue for as long as the medicine is taken. However, monthly bleeding will not occur in women who have had the uterus removed by surgery (total hysterectomy).

This medicine may cause loss or thinning of scalp hair in some people.

Other side effects not listed above may also occur in some patients. If you notice any other effects, check with your doctor.

Additional Information

Once a medicine has been approved for marketing for a certain use, experience may show that it is also useful for other medical problems. Although these uses are not included in product labeling, estrogen is used in certain patients with the following medical conditions:

- Osteoporosis caused by lack of estrogen before menopause
- Turner's syndrome (a genetic disorder)

Other than the above information, there is no additional information relating to proper use, precautions, or side effects for these uses.

ESTROGENS (Vaginal)

Some commonly used brand names are:

In the U.S.—
Estrace (3)
Estring (3)
Premarin (1)

In Canada—
Estring (3)
Oestrilin (4)
Premarin (1)

This information applies to the following medicines

1. Conjugated Estrogens (CON-ju-gate-ed ES-troe-jenz)
2. Dienestrol (dye-en-ES-trole)
3. Estradiol (es-tra-DYE-ole)
4. Estrone (ES-trone)
5. Estropipate (es-troe-PIH-pate)

Category

- **Urogenital symptoms suppressant**—Conjugated Estrogens; Dienestrol; Estradiol; Estrone; Estropipate

Description

Estrogens (ES-troe-jenz) are hormones produced by the body. Among other things, estrogens help develop and maintain female organs.

When your body is in short supply of this hormone, replacing it can ease uncomfortable changes that occur in the vagina, vulva (female genitals), and urethra (part of the urinary system). Conditions that are treated with vaginal estrogens include a genital skin condition (vulvar atrophy), inflammation of the vagina (atrophic vaginitis), and inflammation of the urethra (atrophic urethritis).

Estrogens work partly by increasing a normal clear discharge from the vagina and making the vulva and urethra healthy. Using or applying an estrogen relieves or lessens:

- Dryness and soreness in the vagina
- Itching, redness, or soreness of the vulva
- Feeling an urge to urinate more often then is needed or experiencing pain while urinating
- Pain during sexual intercourse

When used vaginally or on the skin, most estrogens are absorbed into the bloodstream and cause some, but not all, of the same effects as when they are taken by mouth. Estrogens used vaginally at very low doses for treating local problems of the genitals and urinary system will not protect against osteoporosis or stop the hot flushes caused by menopause.

Estrogens for vaginal use are available only with your doctor's prescription, in the following dosage forms:

Vaginal
- Conjugated Estrogens
  - Cream
- Estradiol
  - Cream
  - Insert (or ring)
- Estrone
  - Cream
  - Suppositories

Before Using This Medicine

In deciding to use a medicine, the risks of using the medicine must be weighed against the good it will do. This is a decision you and your doctor will make. For vaginal estrogens, the following should be considered:

Allergies—Tell your doctor if you have ever had any unusual or allergic reaction to estrogens or to parabens. Also tell your health care professional if you are allergic to any other substances, such as foods, preservatives, or dyes.

Pregnancy—Estrogens are not recommended for use during pregnancy, since an estrogen called diethylstilbestrol (DES) that is no longer taken for hormone replacement has caused serious birth defects in humans and animals.

Breast-feeding—Use of this medicine is not recommended in nursing mothers. Estrogens pass into the breast milk and may decrease the amount and quality of breast milk.

Children—Estrogen therapy has been used for the induction of puberty in adolescents with some forms of pubertal delay. Safety and effectiveness have not otherwise been established.

Older adults—Elderly people are especially sensitive to the effects of estrogens. This may increase the chance of side effects during treatment, especially stroke, invasive breast cancer, and memory problems.

Other medicines—Although certain medicines should not be used together at all, in other cases two different medicines may be used together even if an interaction might occur. In these cases, your doctor may want to change the dose, or other precautions may be necessary. Tell your health care professional if you are taking or using any other prescription or nonprescription (over-the-counter [OTC]) medicine.

Other medical problems—The presence of other medical problems may affect the use of estrogens. Make sure you tell your doctor if you have any other medical problems, especially:
- Asthma or
- Epilepsy or
- Heart problems or
- Kidney problems or
- Migraine headaches—Estrogens may worsen these conditions.
- Blood clotting problems—Although worsening of a blood clotting condition is unlikely, some doctors do not prescribe vaginal estrogens for patients with blood clotting problems or a history of these problems

- Certain cancers, including cancers of the breast, bone, or uterus (active or suspected)—Estrogens may interfere with the treatment of breast or bone cancer or worsen cancer of the uterus when these conditions are present
- Diabetes mellitus (sugar diabetes)—Estrogens may alter your body's response to sugar in your diet.
- Endometriosis or
- Fibroid tumors of the uterus—Estrogens may worsen endometriosis or increase the size of fibroid tumors
- Gallbladder problems (gallstones)—Estrogens may increase your chance of getting a gallbladder attack.
- Hepatic hemangioma—Estrogens may worsen this this medical problem.
- Hypercalcemia (too much calcium in your blood)—Estrogens may worsen this this medical problem.
- Hypertriglyceridemia (too much triglycerides in your blood)—Estrogens may increase or chance of getting pancreatitis or other side effects.
- Hypocalcemia (too little calcium in your blood)—Your doctor should treat the low calcium in your blood before starting estrogen therapy.
- Irritation or infection of the vagina—Usually estrogens decrease infections or irritation of the vagina, but sometimes these conditions may become worse
- Liver disease, severe—Estrogens may worsen the condition in some cases; however, many doctors recommend vaginal use of estrogen because it has less effect on the liver than when estrogens are taken by mouth
- Lupus erythematosus, systemic (SLE)—Estrogens may worsen this this medical problem.
- Physical problems within the vagina, such as narrow vagina, vaginal stenosis, or vaginal prolapse—Estradiol vaginal insert may be more likely to slip out of place or cause problems, such as irritation of the vagina
- Porphyria—Estrogens may worsen this medical problem.
- Thyroid problems (underactive thyroid)—Estrogens may alter your body's response to your thyroid medication. Your doctor may alter the amount of thyroid replacement that you take while on estrogen therapy.
- Vision changes, sudden onset including
- Bulging eyes or
- Double vision or
- Migraine headache or
- Vision loss, partial or complete—Estrogens may cause these problems. Tell your doctor if you have had any of these problems.
- Unusual genital or vaginal bleeding of unknown causes—Use of estrogens may delay diagnosis or worsen the condition. The reason for the bleeding should be determined before estrogens are used

Proper Use of This Medicine

Vaginal estrogen products usually come with patient directions. *Read them carefully before using this medicine.*

Wash your hands before and after using the medicine. Also, keep the medicine out of your eyes. If this medicine does get into your eyes, wash them out immediately, but carefully, with large amounts of tap water. If your eyes still burn or are painful, check with your doctor.

Use this medicine only as directed. Do not use more of it and do not use it for a longer time than your doctor ordered. It can take up to 4 months to see the full effect of the estrogens. Your doctor may reconsider continuing your estrogen treatment or may lower your dose several times within the first one or two months, and every 3 to 6 months after that. Sometimes a switch to oral estrogens may be required for added benefits or for higher doses. When using the estradiol vaginal insert, you will need to replace it every 3 months or remove it after 3 months.

For vaginal creams or suppositories Vaginal creams and some vaginal suppositories are inserted with a plastic applicator. Directions for using the applicator are supplied with your medicine. If you do not see your dose marked on the applicator, ask your health care professional for more information.

- *To fill the applicator for cream dosage forms:*
  - Break the metal seal at the opening of the tube by using the point on the top of the cap.
  - Screw the applicator onto the tube.
  - Squeeze the medicine into the applicator slowly until it is measured properly.
  - Remove the applicator from the tube. Replace the cap on the tube.
- *To fill the applicator for suppository dosage form*
  - Place the suppository into the applicator.
- *To place the dose using the applicator for cream and suppository dosage forms:*
  - Relax while lying on your back with your knees bent or stand with one foot on a chair.
  - Hold the full applicator in one hand. Slide the applicator slowly into the vagina. Stop before it becomes uncomfortable.
  - Slowly press the plunger until it stops.
  - Withdraw the applicator. The medicine will be left behind in the vagina.
- *To care for the applicator for cream and suppository dosage forms:*
  - Clean the applicator after use by pulling the plunger out of the applicator and washing both parts completely in warm, soapy water. *Do not use hot or boiling water.*
  - Rinse well.
  - After drying the applicator, replace the plunger.

For vaginal insert dosage form
- *To place the vaginal insert*
  - Relax while lying on your back with your knees bent or stand with one foot on a chair.
  - Pinch or press the sides of the vaginal insert together, between your forefinger and middle finger.
  - With one hand, part the folds of skin around your vagina.
  - Slide the vaginal insert slowly into the upper third of your vagina. Stop before it becomes uncomfortable. The exact location is not too important but it should be comfortable.
  - If it seems uncomfortable, then carefully push the vaginal insert higher into the vagina.

- *To remove the vaginal insert*
  - Stand with one foot on a chair.
  - Slide one finger into the vagina and hook it around the closest part of the vaginal insert.
  - Slowly pull the vaginal insert out.
  - Dispose of the vaginal insert by wrapping it up and throwing it into the trash. *Do not flush it down the toilet.*

Dosing—The dose of vaginal estrogens will be different for different women. *Follow your doctor's orders or the directions on the label.* The following information includes only the average doses of these medicines. *If your dose is different, do not change it* unless your doctor tells you to do so.

For conjugated estrogens
- For *vaginal* dosage form (cream):
  - For treating a genital skin condition (vulvar atrophy) and inflammation of the vagina (atrophic vaginitis):
    - Adults: 0.3 to 1.25 milligrams (mg) of conjugated estrogens (one half to two grams of cream) inserted into the vagina once a day or as directed by your doctor to achieve the lowest dose possible. Usually your doctor will want you to use this medicine for only three weeks of each month (three weeks on and one week off).

For estradiol
- For *vaginal* dosage form (cream):
  - For treating a genital skin condition (vulvar atrophy) and inflammation of the vagina (atrophic vaginitis):
    - Adults: 200 to 400 micrograms (mcg) of estradiol (two to four grams of cream) inserted into the vagina once a day for one to two weeks, decreasing the dose by one half over two and four weeks. After four weeks, your doctor will probably ask you to use the medicine less often, such as 100 mcg (one gram of cream) one to three times a *week* and for only three weeks of each month (three weeks on and one week off).

- For *vaginal* dosage form (insert):
  - For treating a genital skin condition (vulvar atrophy), inflammation of the vagina (atrophic vaginitis) in postmenopausal women, and inflammation of the urethra (urethritis) in postmenopausal women:
    - Adults: 2 milligrams (mg) of estradiol (7.5 mcg released every twenty-four hours with continuous use) and replaced every three months.

For estrone
- For *vaginal* dosage form (cream):
  - For treating a genital skin condition (vulvar atrophy) and inflammation of the vagina (atrophic vaginitis) in postmenopausal women:
    - Adults: 2 to 4 milligrams (mg) of estrone (two to four grams of cream) inserted into the vagina once a day or as directed by your doctor.

- For *vaginal* dosage form (suppository):
  - For treating a genital skin condition (vulvar atrophy) and inflammation of the vagina (atrophic vaginitis) in postmenopausal women:
    - Adults: 250 to 500 micrograms (mcg) inserted into the vagina once a day or as directed by your doctor.

Missed dose—When using the suppository or cream several times a week: If you miss a dose of this medicine and remember it within 1 or 2 days of the missed dose, use the missed dose as soon as possible. However, if it is almost time for your next dose, skip the missed dose and go back to your regular dosing schedule. Do not double doses.

When using the cream or suppositories more than several times a week: If you miss a dose of this medicine, use it as soon as possible if remembered within 12 hours of the missed dose. However, if it is almost time for your next dose, skip the missed dose and go back to your regular dosing schedule. Do not double doses.

Storage—To store this medicine:

- Keep out of the reach of children.
- Store away from heat and direct light.
- Keep the medicine from freezing.
- Do not keep outdated medicine or medicine no longer needed. Be sure that any discarded medicine is out of the reach of children.

Precautions While Using This Medicine

It is very important that your doctor check your progress at regular visits to make sure this medicine does not cause unwanted effects. Plan on going to see your doctor every year, but some doctors require visits more often.

It is not yet known whether the use of vaginal estrogens increases the risk of breast cancer in women. Therefore, it is very important that you regularly check your breasts for any unusual lumps or discharge. Report any problems to your doctor. You should also have a mammogram (x-ray pictures of the breasts) done if your doctor recommends it.

Although the chance is low, use of estrogen may increase your chance of getting cancer of the ovary or uterus (womb). Regular visits to your health professional can help identify these serious side effects early.

If you think that you may be pregnant, stop using the medicine immediately and check with your doctor.

Tell the doctor in charge that you are using this medicine before having any laboratory test, because some test results may be affected.

For vaginal creams

- Avoid using latex condoms, diaphragms, or cervical caps for up to 72 hours after using estrogen vaginal creams. Certain estrogen products may contain oils in the creams that can weaken latex (rubber) products and cause condoms to break or leak, or cervical caps or diaphragms to wear out sooner. Check with your health care professional to make sure the vaginal estrogen product you are using can be used with latex devices.
- This medicine is often used at bedtime to increase effectiveness through better absorption.
- Vaginal creams or suppositories will melt and leak out of the vagina. A minipad or sanitary napkin will protect your clothing. *Do not use tampons* (like those used for menstrual periods) since they may soak up the medicine and make the medicine less effective.
- Avoid exposing your male sexual partner to your vaginal estrogen cream or suppository by not having sexual intercourse right after using these medicines. Your male partner might absorb the medicine through his penis if it comes in contact with the medicine.

For estradiol vaginal insert

- It is not necessary to remove the vaginal insert for sexual intercourse unless desired.
- If you do take it out or if it accidentally slips or comes out of the vagina, you can replace the vaginal insert in the vagina after washing it with lukewarm water. *Never use hot or boiling water.*
- If it slips down, gently push it upwards back into place.
- Replace the vaginal insert every 3 months.

Side Effects of This Medicine

The risk of any serious adverse effect is unlikely for most women using low doses of estrogens vaginally. Even women with special risks have used vaginal estrogens without problems.

Check with your doctor as soon as possible if any of the following side effects occur:

Less common
> Breast pain; enlarged breasts; itching of the vagina or genitals; headache; nausea; stinging or redness of the genital area; thick, white vaginal discharge without odor or with a mild odor

Rare
> Feeling of vaginal pressure (with use of estradiol vaginal insert); vaginal burning or pain (with use of estradiol vaginal insert); unusual or unexpected uterine bleeding or spotting

Other side effects may occur that usually do not need medical attention. These side effects may go away during treatment as your body adjusts to the medicine. However, check with your doctor if any of the following side effects continue or are bothersome:

Less common
> Abdominal or back pain; clear vaginal discharge (usually means the medicine is working)

Also, many women who are using estrogens with a progestin (another female hormone) will start having monthly vaginal bleeding, similar to menstrual periods, again. This effect will continue for as long as the medicine is taken. However, monthly bleeding will not occur in women who have had the uterus removed by surgery (total hysterectomy).

Other side effects not listed above may also occur in some patients. If you notice any other effects, check with your doctor.

ESTROGENS AND PROGESTINS ORAL CONTRACEPTIVES (Systemic)

Some commonly used brand names are:

In the U.S.—

Alesse (3)	Estrostep (4)
Brevicon (5)	Estrostep Fe (4)
Cyclessa (1)	Genora 0.5/35 (5)
Demulen 1/35 (2)	Genora 1/35 (5)
Demulen 1/50 (2)	Genora 1/50 (6)
Desogen (1)	Intercon 0.5/35 (5)

Intercon 1/35 (5)
Intercon 1/50 (6)
Jenest (5)
Levlen (3)
Levlite (3)
Levora 0.15/30 (3)
Loestrin 1/20 (4)
Loestrin Fe 1/20 (4)
Loestrin 1.5/30 (4)
Loestrin Fe 1.5/30 (4)
Lo/Ovral (8)
Mircette (1)
ModiCon (5)
Necon 0.5/35 (5)
Necon 1/35 (5)
Necon 1/50 (6)
Necon 10/11 (5)
N.E.E. 1/35 (5)
N.E.E. 1/50 (5)
Nelova 0.5/35E (5)
Nelova 1/35E (5)
Nelova 1/50M (6)

Nelova 10/11 (5)
Nordette (3)
Norethin 1/35E (5)
Norethin 1/50M (6)
Norinyl 1+35 (5)
Norinyl 1+50 (5)
Ortho-Cept (1)
Ortho-Cyclen (7)
Ortho-Novum 1/35 (5)
Ortho-Novum 1/50 (6)
Ortho-Novum 7/7/7 (5)
Ortho-Novum 10/11 (5)
Ortho Tri-Cyclen (7)
Ovcon-35 (5)
Ovcon-50 (5)
Ovral (8)
Tri-Levlen (3)
Tri-Norinyl (5)
Triphasil (3)
Trivora (3)
Zovia 1/35E (2)
Zovia 1/50E (2)

In Canada—

Brevicon 0.5/35 (5)
Brevicon 1/35 (5)
Cyclen (7)
Demulen 30 (2)
Demulen 50 (2)
Loestrin 1.5/30 (4)
Marvelon (1)
Minestrin 1/20 (4)
Min-Ovral (3)
Norinyl 1/50 (5)
Ortho 0.5/35 (5)

Ortho 1/35 (5)
Ortho 7/7/7 (5)
Ortho 10/11 (5)
Ortho-Cept (1)
Ortho-Novum 1/50 (6)
Ovral (8)
Select 1/35 (5)
Synphasic (5)
Tri-Cyclen (7)
Triphasil (3)
Triquilar (3)

This information applies to the following medicines

1. Desogestrel and Ethinyl Estradiol (des-oh-JES-trel and ETH-in-il es-tra-DYE-ole)
2. Ethynodiol Diacetate and Ethinyl Estradiol (e-thye-noe-DYE-ole dye-AS-e-tate and ETH-in-il es-tra-DYE-ole)
3. Levonorgestrel and Ethinyl Estradiol (LEE-voh-nor-jes-trel and ETH-in-il es-tra-DYE-ole)
4. Norethindrone Acetate and Ethinyl Estradiol (nor-eth-IN-drone AS-e-tate and ETH-in-il es-tra-DYE-ole)
5. Norethindrone and Ethinyl Estradiol (nor-eth-IN-drone and ETH-in-il es-tra-DYE-ole)
6. Norethindrone and Mestranol (nor-eth-IN-drone and MES-tra-nole)
7. Norgestimate and Ethinyl Estradiol (nor-JES-ti-mate and ETH-in-il es-tra-DYE-ole)
8. Norgestrel and Ethinyl Estradiol (nor-JES-trel and ETH-in-il es-tra-DYE-ole)

Category

- **Antiacne agent, systemic**—Norgestimate and Ethinyl Estradiol, triphasic formulation only; Norethindrone and Ethinyl Estradiol, triphasic formulation only

- **Antiendometriotic**—Desogestrel and Ethinyl Estradiol; Ethynodiol Diacetate and Ethinyl Estradiol; Levonorgestrel and Ethinyl Estradiol; Norethindrone and Ethinyl Estradiol; Norethindrone and Mestranol; Norethindrone Acetate and Ethinyl Estradiol; Norgestimate and Ethinyl Estradiol; Norgestrel and Ethinyl Estradiol

- **Contraceptive, postcoital, systemic**—Levonorgestrel and Ethinyl Estradiol; Norgestrel and Ethinyl Estradiol

- **Contraceptive, systemic**—Desogestrel and Ethinyl Estradiol; Ethynodiol Diacetate and Ethinyl Estradiol; Levonorgestrel and Ethinyl Estradiol; Norethindrone and

Ethinyl Estradiol; Norethindrone and Mestranol; Norethindrone Acetate and Ethinyl Estradiol; Norgestimate and Ethinyl Estradiol; Norgestrel and Ethinyl Estradiol

- **Estrogen-progestin**—Desogestrel and Ethinyl Estradiol; Ethynodiol Diacetate and Ethinyl Estradiol; Levonorgestrel and Ethinyl Estradiol; Norethindrone and Ethinyl Estradiol; Norethindrone and Mestranol; Norethindrone Acetate and Ethinyl Estradiol; Norgestimate and Ethinyl Estradiol; Norgestrel and Ethinyl Estradiol

- **Gonadotropin inhibitor, female, noncontraceptive use**—Desogestrel and Ethinyl Estradiol; Ethynodiol Diacetate and Ethinyl Estradiol; Levonorgestrel and Ethinyl Estradiol; Norethindrone and Ethinyl Estradiol; Norethindrone and Mestranol; Norethindrone Acetate and Ethinyl Estradiol; Norgestimate and Ethinyl Estradiol; Norgestrel and Ethinyl Estradiol

Description

Oral contraceptives are known also as the Pill, OCs, BCs, BC tablets, or birth control pills. This medicine usually contains two types of hormones, estrogens (ES-troh-jenz) and progestins (proh-JES-tins) and, when taken properly, prevents pregnancy. It works by stopping a woman's egg from fully developing each month. The egg can no longer accept a sperm and fertilization is prevented. Although oral contraceptives have other effects that help prevent a pregnancy from occurring, this is the main action.

Sometimes a woman's egg can still develop even though the medication is taken once each day, especially when more than 24 hours pass between two doses. In almost all cases when the medicine was taken properly and an egg develops, fertilization can still be stopped by oral contraceptives. This is because oral contraceptives also thicken cervical mucus at the opening of the uterus. This makes it hard for the partner's sperm to reach the egg. In addition, oral contraceptives change the uterus lining just enough so that an egg will not stop in the uterus to develop. All of these effects make it difficult to become pregnant when properly taking an oral contraceptive.

No contraceptive method is 100 percent effective. *Studies show that fewer than one of each one hundred women correctly using oral contraceptives becomes pregnant during the first year of use.* Birth control methods such as having surgery to become sterile or not having sex are more effective. Using condoms, diaphragms, progestin-only oral contraceptives, or spermicides is not as effective as using oral contraceptives containing estrogens and progestins. Discuss with your health care professional your options for birth control.

The triphasic cycle product of norgestimate and ethinyl estradiol (the brand name *Ortho Tri-Cyclen*) and norethindrone acetate and ethinyl estradiol (the brand name *Estrostep*) can be used for the treatment of moderate acne only if the patient is at least 15 years old, has acne that has not improved with topical anti-acne medicines, has gotten approval from her doctor, has begun to have menstrual periods, desires an oral contraceptive for birth control, and plans to stay on it for at least 6 months.

Sometimes these preparations can be used for other conditions as determined by your doctor.

Oral contraceptives are available only with your doctor's prescription, in the following dosage forms:

Oral
- Desogestrel and Ethinyl Estradiol
  - Tablets
- Ethynodiol Diacetate and Ethinyl Estradiol
  - Tablets
- Levonorgestrel and Ethinyl Estradiol
  - Tablets
- Norethindrone Acetate and Ethinyl Estradiol
  - Tablets
- Norethindrone and Ethinyl Estradiol
  - Tablets
- Norethindrone and Mestranol
  - Tablets
- Norgestimate and Ethinyl Estradiol
  - Tablets
- Norgestrel and Ethinyl Estradiol
  - Tablets

Before Using This Medicine

In deciding to use a medicine, the risks of taking the medicine must be weighed against the good it will do. If you are using oral contraceptives for contraception you should understand how their benefits and risks compare to those of other birth control methods. This is a decision you, your sexual partner, and your doctor will make. For oral contraceptives, the following should be considered:

Allergies—Tell your doctor if you have ever had any unusual or allergic reaction to estrogens or progestins. Also tell your health care professional if you are allergic to any other substances, such as foods, preservatives, or dyes.

Diet—Make certain your health care professional knows if you are on any special diet, such as a low-sodium or low-sugar diet.

Pregnancy—Oral contraceptives are not recommended for use during pregnancy and should be discontinued if you become pregnant or think you are pregnant. When oral contraceptives were accidently taken early in pregnancy, problems in the fetus did not occur. Women who are not breast-feeding may begin to take oral contraceptives two weeks after having a baby.

Breast-feeding—Oral contraceptives pass into the breast milk and can change the content or lower the amount of breast milk. Also, they may shorten a woman's ability to breast-feed by about 1 month, especially when the mother is only partially breast-feeding. Because the amount of hormones is so small in low-dose contraceptives, your doctor may allow you to begin using an oral contraceptive after you have been breast-feeding for a while. However, it may be necessary for you to use another method of birth control or to stop breast-feeding while taking oral contraceptives.

Teenagers—This medicine is frequently used for birth control in teenage females and has not been shown to cause different side effects or problems than it does in adults. Some teenagers may need extra information on the importance of taking this medication exactly as prescribed.

Other medicines—Although certain medicines should not be used together at all, in other cases two different medicines may be used together even if an interaction might occur. In these cases, your doctor may want to change the dose, or other precautions may be necessary. When you are taking oral contraceptives, it is especially important that your health care professional know if you are taking any of the following:

- Amiodarone (e.g., Cordarone) or
- Anabolic steroids (nandrolone [e.g., Anabolin], oxandrolone [e.g., Anavar], oxymetholone [e.g., Anadrol], stanozolol [e.g., Winstrol]) or
- Androgens (male hormones) or
- Anti-infectives by mouth or by injection (medicine for infection) or
- Barbiturates or
- Carbamazepine (e.g., Tegretol) or
- Carmustine (e.g., BiCNU) or
- Dantrolene (e.g., Dantrium) or
- Daunorubicin (e.g., Cerubidine) or
- Disulfiram (e.g., Antabuse) or
- Divalproex (e.g., Depakote) or
- Estrogens (female hormones) or
- Etretinate (e.g., Tegison) or
- Gold salts (medicine for arthritis) or
- Griseofulvin (e.g., Fulvicin) or
- Hydroxychloroquine (e.g., Plaquenil) or
- Mercaptopurine (e.g., Purinethol) or
- Methotrexate (e.g., Mexate) or
- Methyldopa (e.g., Aldomet) or
- Naltrexone (e.g., Trexan) (with long-term, high-dose use) or
- Phenothiazines (acetophenazine [e.g., Tindal], chlorpromazine [e.g., Thorazine], fluphenazine [e.g., Prolixin], mesoridazine [e.g., Serentil], perphenazine [e.g., Trilafon], prochlorperazine [e.g., Compazine], promazine [e.g., Sparine], promethazine [e.g., Phenergan], thioridazine [e.g., Mellaril], trifluoperazine [e.g., Stelazine], triflupromazine [e.g., Vesprin], trimeprazine [e.g., Temaril]) or
- Phenylbutazone (e.g., Butazolidin) or
- Phenytoin (e.g., Dilantin) or
- Plicamycin (e.g., Mithracin) or
- Primidone (e.g., Mysoline) or
- Rifabutin (e.g., Mycobutin) or
- Rifampin (e.g., Rifadin) or
- Troleandomycin (e.g., TAO)—These medicines may increase the chance of liver problems if taken with oral contraceptives; also, these medicines may decrease the effect of oral contraceptives and increase your chance of pregnancy. Use of an additional form of birth control is recommended unless directed otherwise by your health care professional
- Corticosteroids (cortisone-like medicine) or
- Theophylline—Oral contraceptives may increase the effects of these medicines and increase the chance of problems occurring
- Cyclosporine—Oral contraceptives increase the effect of cyclosporine and increase the chance of problems occurring

- Ritonavir (e.g., Norvir) or
- Troglitazone (e.g., Rezulin)—These medicines may decrease the effect of oral contraceptives and increase your chance of pregnancy. Use of an additional form of birth control is recommended unless directed otherwise by your health care professional
- Smoking, tobacco—Smoking may decrease the effect of oral contraceptives and increase the chance of causing serious blood clot, vein, or heart problems

Other medical problems—The presence of other medical problems may affect the use of oral contraceptives. Make sure you tell your doctor if you have any other medical problems, especially:

- Abnormal changes in menstrual or uterine bleeding or
- Endometriosis or
- Fibroid tumors of the uterus—Oral contraceptives usually improve these female conditions but sometimes they can make them worse or make the diagnosis of these problems more difficult
- Blood clots (or history of) or
- Heart or circulation disease or
- Stroke (or history of)—If these conditions are already present, oral contraceptives may have a greater chance of causing blood clots or circulation problems, especially in women who smoke tobacco. Otherwise, oral contraceptives may help prevent circulation and heart disease if you are healthy and do not smoke
- Breast disease (not involving cancer)—Oral contraceptives usually protect against certain breast diseases, such as breast cysts or breast lumps; however, your doctor may want to follow your condition more closely
- Cancer, including breast cancer (or history of or family history of)—Oral contraceptives may worsen some cancers, especially when breast, cervical, or uterine cancers already exist. Use of oral contraceptives is not recommended if you have any of these conditions. If you have a family history of breast disease, oral contraceptives may still be a good choice but you may need to be tested more often
- Chorea gravidarum or
- Gallbladder disease or gallstones (or history of) or
- High blood cholesterol or
- Liver disease (or history of, including jaundice during pregnancy or oral contraceptive use) or
- Mental depression (or history of)—Oral contraceptives may make these conditions worse or, rarely, cause them to occur again. Oral contraceptives may still be a good choice but you may need to be tested more often
- Diabetes mellitus (sugar diabetes)—Use of oral contraceptives may cause an increase, usually only a small increase, in your blood sugar and usually does not affect the amount of diabetes medicine that you take. You or your doctor will want to test for any changes in your blood sugar for 12 to 24 months after starting to take oral contraceptives in case the dose of your diabetes medicine needs to be changed
- Epilepsy (seizures) (or history of) or
- Heart or circulation problems or
- High blood pressure (hypertension) or

- Migraine headaches—Oral contraceptives may cause fluid build-up and may cause these conditions to become worse; however, some people have fewer migraine headaches when they use oral contraceptives

Proper Use of This Medicine

To make using oral contraceptives as safe and reliable as possible, you should understand how and when to take them and what effects may be expected.

A paper with information for the patient will be given to you with your filled prescription, and will provide many details concerning the use of oral contraceptives. Read this paper carefully and ask your health care professional if you need additional information or explanation.

Take this medicine with food to help prevent nausea that might occur during the first few weeks. Nausea usually disappears with continued use or if the medicine is taken at bedtime.

When you begin to use oral contraceptives, your body will require at least 7 days to adjust before a pregnancy will be prevented. You will need to use an additional birth control method for at least 7 days. Some doctors recommend using an additional method of birth control for the first cycle (or 3 weeks) to ensure full protection. Follow the advice of your doctor or other health care professional.

Try to take the doses no more than 24 hours apart to reduce the possibility of side effects and to prevent pregnancy. Since one of the most important factors in the proper use of oral contraceptives is taking every dose exactly on schedule, you should never let your tablet supply run out. When possible, try to keep an extra month's supply of tablets on hand and replace it monthly.

It is very important that you keep the tablets in their original container and take the tablets in the same order that they appear in the container. The containers help you keep track of which tablets to take next. Different colored tablets in the same package contain different amounts of hormones or are placebos (tablets that do not contain hormones). *The effectiveness of the medicine is reduced if the tablets are taken out of order.*

- *Monophasic (one-phase) cycle* dosing schedule: Most available dosing schedules are monophasic. If you are taking tablets of one strength (color) for 21 days, you are using a monophasic schedule. For the 28–day monophasic cycle you will also take an additional 7 inactive tablets, which are another color. If you are taking the brand name *Mircette,* the last seven tablets of the 28–day cycle contains two inactive tablets (for Days 22 and 23) and five tablets (for Days 24 through 28) that contain a low dose of estrogen. Taking the last 7 tablets is not required for full protection against pregnancy but they do help to replace estrogen.
- *Biphasic (two-phase) cycle* dosing schedule: If you are using a biphasic twenty-one–day schedule, you are taking tablets of one strength (color) for either seven or ten days, depending on the medication prescribed (the first phase). You then take tablets of a second strength (color) for the next eleven or fourteen days, depending on the medication prescribed (the second phase). At this point, you will have taken a total of twenty-one tablets. For the twenty-eight–day biphasic cycle you will also take an additional seven inactive tablets, which are a third color.

- *Triphasic (three-phase) cycle* dosing schedule: If you are using a triphasic twenty-one– day schedule, you are taking tablets of one strength (color) for five, six or seven days, depending on the medicine prescribed (the first phase). You then take tablets of a second strength (color) for the next five, seven, or nine days, depending on the medicine prescribed (the second phase). After that, you take tablets of a third strength (color) for the next five, seven, nine, or ten days, depending on the medicine prescribed (the third phase). At this point, you will have taken a total of twenty-one tablets. For the twenty-eight– day triphasic cycle you will also take an additional seven inactive tablets, which are a fourth color.

If you are taking one of the brand name products *Estrostep Fe* or *Loestrin Fe* each of the last seven tablets that you will take on Days 21 through 28 of your cycle contains iron. These tablets are also a different color from the other tablets in your package. They help to replace some of the iron you lose when you have a menstrual period.

Dosing—Your health care professional may begin your dose on the first day of your menstrual period (called Day-1 start) or on Sunday (called Sunday start). *When you begin on a certain day it is important that you follow that schedule, even when you miss a dose. Do not change your schedule on your own.* If the schedule that you have been put on is not convenient, check with your health care professional about changing schedules.

- For *oral* dosage forms (monophasic, biphasic, or triphasic tablets):
  - For contraception:
    - Adults and teenagers:
      — For the twenty-one–day cycle: Take 1 tablet a day for twenty-one days. Skip seven days. Then repeat the cycle.
      — For the twenty-eight–day cycle: Take 1 tablet a day for twenty-eight days. Then repeat the cycle.

- For *oral* dosage forms (norethindrone acetate and ethinyl estradiol triphasic tablets and norgestimate and ethinyl estradiol triphasic tablets:
  - To treat acne:
    - Adults and teenagers 15 years of age and over:
      — For the twenty-one–day cycle: Take 1 tablet a day for twenty-one days. Skip seven days. Then repeat the cycle.
      — For the twenty-eight–day cycle: Take 1 tablet a day for twenty-eight days. Then repeat the cycle.
    - Teenagers up to 15 years of age—Use and dose must be determined by your doctor.

Missed dose—*Follow your doctor's orders or the directions on the label* if you miss a dose of this medicine. The following information includes only some of the ways to handle missed doses. Your health care professional may want you to stop taking the medicine and use other birth control methods for the rest of the month until you have your menstrual period. Then your health care professional can tell you how to begin taking your medicine again.

For monophasic, biphasic, or triphasic cycles:

- If you miss the first tablet of a new cycle—Take the missed tablet as soon as you remember and take the next tablet at the usual time. You may take 2 tablets in

one day. Then continue your regular dosing schedule. Also, use another birth control method until you have taken seven days of your tablets after the last missed dose.

- If you miss 1 tablet during the cycle—Take the missed tablet as soon as you remember. Take the next tablet at the usual time. You may take 2 tablets in one day. Then continue your regular dosing schedule.
- If you miss 2 tablets in a row in the first or second week—Take 2 tablets on the day that you remember and 2 tablets the next day. Then continue taking 1 tablet a day. Also use another birth control method until you begin a new cycle.
- If you miss 2 tablets in a row in the third week; or
- If you miss 3 or more tablets in a row at any time during the cycle—
  - Using a Day-1 start: Throw out your current cycle and begin taking a new cycle. Also, use another birth control method until you have taken seven days of your tablets after the last missed dose. You may not have a menstrual period this month. But if you miss two menstrual periods in a row, call your health care professional.
  - Using a Sunday start: Keep taking one tablet a day from your current pack until Sunday. Then, on Sunday, throw out your old pack and begin a new pack. Also use another birth control method until you have taken seven days of your tablets after the last missed dose. You may not have a menstrual period this month. But if you miss two menstrual periods in a row, call your health care professional.

If you miss any of the last seven (inactive) tablets of a twenty-eight– day cycle, there is no danger of pregnancy. However, the first tablet (active) of the next month's cycle must be taken on the regularly scheduled day, in spite of any missed doses, if pregnancy is to be avoided. The active and inactive tablets are colored differently for your convenience.

Storage—To store this medicine:

- Keep out of the reach of children.
- Store away from heat and direct light.
- Do not store in the bathroom, near the kitchen sink, or in other damp places. Heat and moisture may cause the medicine to break down.
- Do not keep outdated medicine or medicine no longer needed. Be sure that any discarded medicine is out of the reach of children.

Precautions While Using This Medicine

It is very important that your doctor check your progress at regular visits to make sure this medicine does not cause unwanted effects. These visits will usually be every 6 to 12 months, but some doctors require them more often.

Tell the medical doctor or dentist in charge that you are taking this medicine before any kind of surgery (including dental surgery) or emergency treatment. Your doctor will decide whether you should continue taking this medicine.

The following medicines may reduce the effectiveness of oral contraceptives. *You should use an additional method of birth control during each cycle in which any of the following medicines are used:*

- Ampicillin
- Barbiturates

- Carbamazepine (e.g., Tegretol)
- Griseofulvin (e.g., Fulvicin)
- Penicillin V
- Phenytoin (e.g., Dilantin)
- Primidone (e.g., Mysoline)
- Rifampin (e.g., Rifadin)
- Ritonavir (e.g., Norvir)
- Tetracyclines (medicine for infection)
- Troglitazone (e.g., Rezulin)

Check with your doctor if you have any questions about this.

Vaginal bleeding of various amounts may occur between your regular menstrual periods during the first 3 months of use. This is sometimes called spotting when slight, or break-through bleeding when heavier. If this should occur:

- Continue on your regular dosing schedule.
- The bleeding usually stops within 1 week.
- Check with your doctor if the bleeding continues for more than 1 week.
- After you have been taking oral contraceptives on schedule and for more than 3 months and bleeding continues, check with your doctor.

Missed menstrual periods may occur:

- If you have not taken the medicine exactly as scheduled. Pregnancy must be considered as a possibility.
- If the medicine is not the right strength or type for your needs.
- If you stop taking oral contraceptives, especially if you have taken oral contraceptives for 2 or more years.

Check with your doctor if you miss any menstrual periods so that the cause may be determined.

In some patients using estrogen-containing oral contraceptives, tenderness, swelling, or bleeding of the gums may occur. Brushing and flossing your teeth carefully and regularly and massaging your gums may help prevent this. See your dentist regularly to have your teeth cleaned. Check with your medical doctor or dentist if you have any questions about how to take care of your teeth and gums, or if you notice any tenderness, swelling, or bleeding of your gums. Also, it has been shown that estrogen-containing oral contraceptives may cause a healing problem called dry socket after a tooth has been removed. If you are going to have a tooth removed, tell your dentist or oral surgeon that you are taking oral contraceptives.

Some people who take oral contraceptives may become more sensitive to sunlight than they are normally. When you begin taking this medicine, avoid too much sun and do not use a sunlamp until you see how you react to the sun, especially if you tend to burn easily. If you have a severe reaction, check with your doctor. Some people may develop brown, blotchy spots on exposed areas. These spots usually disappear gradually when the medicine is stopped.

If you suspect that you may have become pregnant, stop taking this medicine immediately and check with your doctor.

If you are scheduled for any laboratory tests, tell your doctor that you are taking birth control pills.

Check with your doctor before refilling an old prescription, especially after a pregnancy. You will need another physical examination and your doctor may change your prescription.

Side Effects of This Medicine

Healthy women who do not smoke cigarettes have almost no chance of having a severe side effect from taking oral contraceptives. For most women, more problems occur because of pregnancy than will occur from taking oral contraceptives. But for some women who have special health problems, oral contraceptives can cause some unwanted effects. Some of these unwanted effects include benign (not cancerous) liver tumors, liver cancer, or blood clots or related problems, such as a stroke. Although these effects are very rare, they can be serious enough to cause death. You may want to discuss these effects with your doctor.

Smoking cigarettes during the use of oral contraceptives has been found to greatly increase the chances of these serious side effects occurring. *To reduce the risk of serious side effects, do not smoke cigarettes while you are taking oral contraceptives.* Cigarette smoking increases the risk of serious cardiovascular side effects from oral contraceptive use. The risk increases with age and with heavy smoking (15 or more cigarettes per day) and is quite marked in women over 35 years of age.

The following side effects may be caused by blood clots. *Get emergency help immediately* if any of the following side effects occur:

Rare

Abdominal or stomach pain (sudden, severe, or continuing); coughing up blood; headache (severe or sudden); loss of coordination (sudden); loss of vision or change in vision (sudden); pains in chest, groin, or leg (especially in calf of leg); shortness of breath (sudden or unexplained); slurring of speech (sudden); weakness, numbness, or pain in arm or leg (unexplained)

Check with your doctor as soon as possible if any of the following side effects occur:

More common—usually less common after the first 3 months of oral contraceptive use

Changes in the uterine bleeding pattern at menses or between menses, such as decreased bleeding at menses, breakthrough bleeding or spotting between periods, prolonged bleeding at menses, complete stopping of menstrual bleeding that occurs over several months in a row, or stopping of menstrual bleeding that only occurs sometimes

Less common
For women with diabetes mellitus

Mild increase of blood sugar—Faintness, nausea, pale skin, or sweating

Headaches or migraines (although headaches may lessen in many users, in others, they may increase in number or become worse); increased blood pressure; vaginal infection with vaginal itching or irritation, or thick, white, or curd-like discharge

Rare
For women who smoke tobacco

Pains in stomach, side, or abdomen; yellow eyes or skin

For women with a history of breast disease

Lumps in breast

Mental depression; swelling, pain, or tenderness in upper abdominal area

Other side effects may occur that usually do not need medical attention. These side effects may go away during treatment as your body adjusts to the medicine. However, check with your doctor if any of the following side effects continue or are bothersome:

More common
Abdominal cramping or bloating; acne (usually less common after first 3 months and may improve if acne already exists); breast pain, tenderness, or swelling; dizziness; nausea; swelling of ankles and feet; unusual tiredness or weakness; vomiting

Less common
Brown, blotchy spots on exposed skin; gain or loss of body or facial hair; increased or decreased interest in sexual intercourse; increased sensitivity of skin to sunlight; weight gain or loss

Other side effects not listed above may also occur in some patients. If you notice any other effects, check with your doctor.

Additional Information

Once a medicine has been approved for marketing for a certain use, experience may show that it is also useful for other medical problems. Although these uses are not included in product labeling, oral contraceptives are used in certain patients with the following medical conditions:

- Amenorrhea (stopping of menses for several consecutive months)
- Dysfunctional uterine bleeding (abnormal uterine bleeding)
- Dysmenorrhea (painful menstrual bleeding)
- Hypermenorrhea (excessive menstrual bleeding)
- Emergency contraception within 72 hours of unprotected intercourse
- Endometriosis (painful bleeding from uterine-like tissue that can grow in different parts of the female body)
- Hirsutism in females (male-like hair growth)
- Hyperandrogenism, ovarian (excessive production of male hormones)
- Polycystic ovary syndrome (many problems that include amenorrhea, hirsutism, infertility, and many tiny cysts or sacs usually in both ovaries)

For patients taking this medicine for *emergency contraception:*

- Must be taken with food within 72 hours of unprotected sexual intercourse. One single course (2 doses 12 hours apart) is a one-time emergency protection. Using more than one course in a month will reduce the effectiveness.
- Because the hormones are strong, watch for danger signs. Call your doctor if you experience any severe pains in your leg, stomach, or chest; any vision or breathing changes; yellowing of skin; headaches; numbness; or trouble in speaking.
- You may experience nausea so take it with food and call your doctor if you vomit the medicine.
- Your menstrual period may start earlier than usual. If it doesn't start, call your doctor.

For patients taking this medicine for *hirsutism:*

- You may need to use oral contraceptives for 6 to 12 months before you see less new hair growth.

For patients taking this medicine for *endometriosis:*

- Sometimes instead of following the directions on the oral contraceptive's package, your doctor may ask you to follow different directions, such as taking the active tablets in the package each day without stopping for 6 to 9 months. This means that after 21 days you will start a new package of pills. If you are not sure about how to take this medicine, discuss any questions with your health care professional.
- Also, your symptoms of endometriosis may worsen at first but with continued use of the oral contraceptives your symptoms should lessen and your condition improve.

Other than the above information, there is no additional information relating to proper use, precautions, or side effects for these uses.

ESTROGENS AND PROGESTINS
(Ovarian Hormone Therapy)   (Systemic)

Some commonly used brand names are:
In the U.S.—
Activella (3)
femhrt (2)
Ortho-Prefest (1)

This information applies to the following medicines:

1. 17 beta-estradiol and norgestimate (seh-ven-TEEN BAY-tuh estra-DYE-ole and nor-JES-ti-mate)
2. Ethinyl estradiol and norethindrone (ETH-in-il es-tra-DYE-ole and nor-eth-IN-drone)
3. Estradiol and norethindrone (es-tra-DYE-ole and nor-eth-IN-drone)

Category

- **Estrogen-progestin**—17 beta-Estradiol and norgestimate tablets; Ethinyl estradiol and norethindrone tablets; Estradiol and norethindrone tablets
- **Ovarian hormone therapy agent**—17 beta-Estradiol and norgestimate tablets; Ethinyl estradiol and norethindrone tablets; Estradiol and norethindrone tablets
- **Osteoporosis prophylactic**—17 beta-Estradiol and norgestimate tablets; Ethinyl estradiol and norethindrone tablets

Description

Estrogens (ES-troe-jenz) and progestins (pro-GEST-ins) are female hormones. They are produced by the body and are necessary for the normal sexual development of the female and for the regulation of the menstrual cycle during the childbearing years.

The ovaries begin to produce less estrogen after menopause (the change of life). This medicine is prescribed to make up for the lower amount of estrogen. Estrogens help relieve signs of menopause, such as hot flashes and unusual sweating, chills, faintness, or dizziness. Progestins help to regulate the effects of estrogens.

Estrogens are prescribed for several reasons:
- to provide additional hormone when the body does not produce enough of its own, such as during menopause.

They can also help to relieve a genital skin condition called vaginal or vulvar atrophy.

- to help prevent weakening of bones (osteoporosis) in women past menopause.

Estrogens may also be used for other conditions as determined by your doctor.

There is *no* medical evidence to support the belief that the use of estrogens will keep the patient feeling young, keep the skin soft, or delay the appearance of wrinkles. Nor has it been proven that the use of estrogens during menopause will relieve emotional and nervous symptoms, unless these symptoms are caused by other menopausal symptoms, such as hot flashes or hot flushes.

Estrogens and progestins are available only with your doctor's prescription, in the following dosage forms:

Oral
- 17 beta-estradiol and norgestimate
  - Tablets
- Ethinyl estradiol and norethindrone
  - Tablets
- Estradiol and norethindrone
  - Tablets

Before Using This Medicine

In deciding to use a medicine, the risks of taking the medicine must be weighed against the good it will do. This is a decision you and your doctor will make. For estrogens and progestins, the following should be considered:

Allergies—Tell your doctor if you have ever had any unusual or allergic reaction to estrogens or progestins. Also tell your health care professional if you are allergic to any other substances, such as foods, preservatives, or dyes

Pregnancy—Estrogens and progestins are not recommended for use during pregnancy or right after giving birth. Becoming pregnant or maintaining a pregnancy is not likely to occur around the time of menopause.

Breast-feeding—Estrogens and progestins pass into the breast milk and can change the content or lower the amount of breast milk. Use of this medicine is not recommended in nursing mothers.

Older adults—Many medicines have not been studied specifically in older people. Therefore, it may not be known whether they work exactly the same way they do in younger adults or if they cause different side effects or problems in older people. There is no specific information comparing use of estrogens and progestins in the elderly with use in other age groups.

Other medicines—Although certain medicines should not be used together at all, in other cases two different medicines may be used together even if an interaction might occur. In these cases, your doctor may want to change the dose, or other precautions may be necessary. When you are taking estrogens and progestins, it is especially important that your health care professional know if you are taking any of the following:

- Cyclosporine (e.g., Sandimmune)—Estrogens can prevent cyclosporine's removal from the body; this can lead to kidney or liver problems caused by too much cyclosporine

Other medical problems—The presence of other medical problems may affect the use of estrogens and progestins.

Make sure you tell your doctor if you have any other medical problems, especially:

- Asthma or
- Calcium, too much or too little in blood or
- Diabetes mellitus (sugar diabetes)
- Epilepsy (seizures) or
- Heart problems or
- Kidney problems or
- Liver tumors, benign or
- Lupus erythematosus, systemic or
- Migraine headaches or
- Porphyria—Estrogens may worsen these conditions.
- Blood clotting problems (or history of during previous estrogen therapy)—Estrogens usually are not used until blood clotting problems stop; using estrogens is not a problem for most patients without a history of blood clotting problems due to estrogen use
- Breast cancer or
- Bone cancer or
- Cancer of the uterus or
- Fibroid tumors of the uterus—Estrogens may interfere with the treatment of breast or bone cancer or worsen cancer of the uterus when these conditions are present
- Changes in genital or vaginal bleeding of unknown causes—Use of estrogens may delay diagnosis or worsen condition. The reason for the bleeding should be determined before estrogens are used
- Endometriosis or
- Gallbladder disease or gallstones (or history of) or
- High cholesterol or triglycerides (or history of) or
- Liver disease or
- Pancreatitis (inflammation of pancreas)—Estrogens may worsen these conditions; while estrogens can improve blood cholesterol, they may worsen blood triglycerides for some people
- Hypothyroid (too little thyroid hormone)—Dose of thyroid medicine may need to be increased.
- Vision changes, sudden onset including
- Bulging eyes or
- Double vision or
- Migraine headache or
- Vision loss, partial or complete—Estrogens may cause these problems. Tell your doctor if you have had any of these problems, especially while taking estrogen or oral contraceptives ("birth control pills").

Proper Use of This Medicine

Estrogens and progestins usually come with patient information or directions. Read them carefully before taking this medicine.

Take this medicine only as directed by your doctor. Do not take more of it and do not take or use it for a longer time than your doctor ordered. Try to take the medicine at the same time each day to reduce the possibility of side effects and to allow it to work better.

For patients taking estrogens and progestins by mouth:

- Nausea may occur during the first few weeks after you start taking estrogens. This effect usually disappears with continued use. If the nausea is bothersome, it can usually be prevented or reduced by taking each dose with food or immediately after food.

Dosing—The dose of these medicines will be different for different patients. *Follow your doctor's orders or the directions on the label.* The following information includes only the average doses of these medicines. *If your dose is different, do not change it* unless your doctor tells you to do so.

For 17 beta-estradiol and norgestimate
- For *oral* dosage forms (tablets)
  - For treating a genital skin condition (vaginal or vulvar atrophy), or vasomotor symptoms of menopause:
    - Adults—Oral, 1 mg estradiol for three days followed by 1 mg of estradiol combined with 0.09 mg of norgestimate for three days. The regimen is repeated continuously without interruption.
  - To prevent loss of bone (osteoporosis):
    - Adults—Oral, 1 mg estradiol for three days followed by 1mg of estradiol combined with 0.09 mg of norgestimate for three days. The regimen is repeated continuously without interruption.

For ethinyl estradiol and norethindrone
- For *oral* dosage forms (tablets)
  - For treating vasomotor symptoms of menopause:
    - Adults—Oral, 2.5 mcg (0.025 mg) ethinyl estradiol and 0.5 mg norethindrone once daily.
  - To prevent loss of bone (osteoporosis):
    - Adults—Oral, 2.5 mcg (0.025 mg) ethinyl estradiol and 0.5 mg norethindrone once daily.

For estradiol and norethindrone
- For *oral* dosage forms (tablets)
  - For treating vasomotor symptoms of menopause or treatment of vaginal or vulvar atrophy:
    - Adults—Oral, 1 mg estradiol and 0.5 mg norethindrone once daily.
  - To prevent loss of bone (osteoporosis):
    - Adults—Oral, 1 mg estradiol and 0.5 mg norethindrone once daily.

For 17 beta-estradiol and norgestimate
- For *oral* dosage forms (tablets)
  - For treating a genital skin condition (vaginal or vulvar atrophy), or vasomotor symptoms of menopause:
    - Adults—Oral, 1 mg estradiol for three days followed by 1 mg of estradiol combined with 0.09 mg of norgestimate for three days. The regimen is repeated continuously without interruption.
  - To prevent loss of bone (osteoporosis):
    - Adults—Oral, 1 mg estradiol for three days followed by 1mg of estradiol combined with 0.09 mg of norgestimate for three days. The regimen is repeated continuously without interruption.

For ethinyl estradiol and norethindrone
- For *oral* dosage forms (tablets)
  - For treating vasomotor symptoms of menopause:
    - Adults—Oral, 2.5 mcg (0.025 mg) ethinyl estradiol and 0.5 mg norethindrone once daily.
  - To prevent loss of bone (osteoporosis):
    - Adults—Oral, 2.5 mcg (0.025 mg) ethinyl estradiol and 0.5 mg norethindrone once daily.

For estradiol and norethindrone
- For *oral* dosage forms (tablets)
  - For treating vasomotor symptoms of menopause or treatment of vaginal or vulvar atrophy:
    - Adults—Oral, 1 mg estradiol and 0.5 mg norethindrone once daily.
  - To prevent loss of bone (osteoporosis):
    - Adults—Oral, 1 mg estradiol and 0.5 mg norethindrone once daily.

Missed dose—If you miss a dose of this medicine, take it as soon as possible. However, if it is almost time for your next dose, skip the missed dose and take only your next regularly scheduled dose. Do not double doses.

Storage—To store this medicine:
- Keep out of the reach of children.
- Store away from heat and direct light.
- Do not store in the bathroom medicine cabinet because the heat or moisture may cause the medicine to break down.
- Do not keep outdated medicine or medicine no longer needed. Be sure that any discarded medicine is out of the reach of children.

Precautions While Using This Medicine

It is very important that your doctor check your progress at regular visits to make sure this medicine does not cause unwanted effects. These visits will usually be every year, but some doctors require them more often.

It is not yet known whether the use of estrogens increases the risk of breast cancer in women. Therefore, it is very important that you regularly check your breasts for any unusual lumps or discharge. Report any problems to your doctor. You should also have a mammogram (x-ray pictures of the breasts) done if your doctor recommends it. Because breast cancer has occurred in men taking estrogens, regular breast self-exams and exams by your doctor for any unusual lumps or discharge should be done.

Tell the doctor in charge that you are taking this medicine before having any laboratory test because some results may be affected.

Side Effects

Women rarely have severe side effects from taking estrogens to replace estrogen. Discuss these possible effects with your doctor:

- The prolonged use of estrogens has been reported to increase the risk of endometrial cancer (cancer of the lining of the uterus) in women after menopause. This risk seems to increase as the dose and the length of use increase. When estrogens are used in low doses for less than 1 year, there is less risk. The risk is also reduced if a progestin (another female hormone) is added to, or replaces part of, your estrogen dose. If the uterus has been removed by surgery (total hysterectomy), there is no risk of endometrial cancer, and no need to take an estrogen and progestin combination.
- It is not yet known whether the use of estrogens increases the risk of breast cancer in women. Although some large studies show an increased risk, most studies and information gathered to date do not support this idea.

Check with your doctor as soon as possible if any of the following side effects occur:

More common

Breast pain or tenderness; dizziness or light-headedness; headache; swelling of feet and lower legs; rapid weight gain; vaginal bleeding

Rare

Breast lumps; change in vaginal discharge; discharge from nipple; nausea and vomiting; pains in stomach, side, or abdomen; pain or feeling of pressure in pelvis; yellow eyes or skin; severe or sudden headache; sudden loss of coordination; pains in chest, groin, or leg, especially calf; sudden and unexplained shortness of breath; sudden slurred speech; sudden vision changes; weakness or numbness in arm or leg

Other side effects may occur that usually do not need medical attention. These side effects may go away during treatment as your body adjusts to the medicine. However, check with your doctor if any of the following side effects continue or are bothersome:

More common

Back pain; dizziness; general feeling of tiredness; bloating or gas; flu-like symptoms; mental depression; muscle aches; nausea—taking tablet with food may decrease; vaginitis

Other side effects not listed above may also occur in some patients. If you notice any other effects, check with your doctor.

ESZOPICLONE (Oral route) - es-zoe-PIK-lone

Commonly used brand name(s)

In the U.S.—
Lunesta

Available Dosage Forms:

• Tablet

Therapeutic Class: Nonbarbiturate Hypnotic

Uses For This Medicine

Eszopiclone belongs to the group of medicines called central nervous system (CNS) depressants (medicines that make you drowsy or less alert). This medicine is used to treat insomnia (trouble in sleeping). Eszopiclone helps you get to sleep faster and sleep through the night. In general, when sleep medicines are used every night for a long time, they may lose their effectiveness. In most cases, sleep medicines should be used only for short periods of time, such as 7 to 10 days, and generally for no longer than 2 weeks.

This medicine is available only with your doctor's prescription.

Before Using This Medicine

In deciding to use a medicine, the risks of taking the medicine must be weighed against the good it will do. This is a decision you and your doctor will make. For this medicine, the following should be considered:

Allergies—Tell your doctor if you have ever had any unusual or allergic reaction to this medicine or any other medicines. Also tell your health care professional if you have any other types of allergies, such as to foods, dyes, preservatives, or animals. For non-prescription products, read the label or package ingredients carefully.

Pediatric—Studies on this medicine have been done only in adult patients, and there is no specific information comparing use of eszopiclone in children with use in other age groups.

Geriatric—This medicine has been tested and has not been shown to cause different side effects or problems in older adults than it does in younger adults.

Pregnancy—

	Pregnancy Category	Explanation
All Trimesters	C	Animal studies have shown an adverse effect and there are no adequate studies in pregnant women OR no animal studies have been conducted and there are no adequate studies in pregnant women.

Breast Feeding—There are no adequate studies in women for determining infant risk when using this medication during breastfeeding. Weigh the potential benefits against the potential risks before taking this medication while breastfeeding.

Other medicines—

Using this medicine with any of the following medicines may cause an increased risk of certain side effects, but using both drugs may be the best treatment for you. If both medicines are prescribed together, your doctor may change the dose or how often you use one or both of the medicines.

Ketoconazole

Interactions with Food/Tobacco/Alcohol—Certain medicines should not be used at or around the time of eating food or eating certain types of food since interactions may occur. Using alcohol or tobacco with certain medicines may also cause interactions to occur. The following interactions have been selected on the basis of their potential significance and are not necessarily all-inclusive.

Using this medicine with any of the following may cause an increased risk of certain side effects but may be unavoidable in some cases. If used together, your doctor may change the dose or how often you use this medicine, or give you special instructions about the use of food, alcohol, or tobacco.

Ethanol

Other medical problems—The presence of other medical problems may affect the use of this medicine. Make sure you tell your doctor if you have any other medical problems, especially:

• Alcohol abuse (or history of) or

• Drug abuse (or history of) or

• Psychiatric disorders—Dependence on eszopiclone may develop.

• Liver disease (severe)—Higher blood levels of eszopiclone may result, increasing the chance of side effects.

- Mental depression—Eszopiclone may make these conditions worse.

Proper Use of This Medicine

Take this medicine only as directed by your doctor. Do not take more of it, do not take it more often, and do not take it for a longer time than your doctor ordered. If too much is taken, it may become habit-forming (causing mental or physical dependence).

Do not take this medicine when your schedule does not permit you to get a full night's sleep (8 hours). If you must wake up before this, you may continue to feel drowsy and may experience memory problems, because the effects of the medicine have not had time to wear off.

It is important to swallow the tablet whole. Do not chew, crush or break the tablet.

You should not take eszopiclone with or immediately after a high-fat meal or a heavy meal.

Dosing—The dose of this medicine will be different for different patients. Follow your doctor's orders or the directions on the label. The following information includes only the average doses of this medicine. If your dose is different, do not change it unless your doctor tells you to do so.

The amount of medicine that you take depends on the strength of the medicine. Also, the number of doses you take each day, the time allowed between doses, and the length of time you take the medicine depend on the medical problem for which you are using the medicine.

- For oral dosage form (tablets):
  - For the treatment of insomnia (trouble in sleeping):
    - Adults—1 to 2 milligrams (mg) at bedtime.
    - Children—Use and dose must be determined by your doctor.

Precautions While Using This Medicine

This medicine works very quickly. You should take eszopiclone immediately before going to bed.

If you think you need to take eszopiclone for more than 2 weeks, be sure to discuss it with your doctor. Insomnia that lasts longer than this may be a sign of another medical problem.

This medicine will add to the effects of alcohol and other CNS depressants (medicines that cause drowsiness). Some examples of CNS depressants are antihistamines or medicine for hay fever, other allergies, or colds; sedatives, tranquilizers, or sleeping medicine; prescription pain medicine or narcotics; barbiturates; medicine for seizures; muscle relaxants; or anesthetics, including some dental anesthetics. Check with your doctor before taking any of the above while you are using this medicine.

This medicine may cause some people, especially older persons, to become drowsy, dizzy, lightheaded, clumsy or unsteady, or less alert than they are normally. Even though eszopiclone is taken at bedtime, it may cause some people to feel drowsy or less alert on arising. Make sure you know how you react to eszopiclone before you drive, use machines, or do anything else that could be dangerous if you are dizzy, or are not alert or able to see well.

If you develop any unusual and strange thoughts or behavior while you are taking eszopiclone, be sure to discuss it with your doctor. Some changes that have occurred in people taking this medicine are like those seen in people who drink alcohol and then act in a manner that is not normal. Other changes may be more unusual and extreme, such as confusion, worsening of depression, hallucinations (seeing, hearing, or feeling things that are not there), suicidal thoughts, and unusual excitement, nervousness, or irritability.

If you will be taking eszopiclone for a long time, do not stop taking it without first checking with your doctor. Your doctor may want you to gradually reduce the amount you are taking before stopping completely. Stopping this medicine suddenly may cause withdrawal side effects.

After taking eszopiclone for insomnia, you may have difficulty sleeping (rebound insomnia) for the first few nights after you stop taking it.

Side Effects of This Medicine

Along with its needed effects, a medicine may cause some unwanted effects. Although not all of these side effects may occur, if they do occur they may need medical attention.

Check with your doctor immediately if any of the following side effects occur:

Symptoms of overdose

Get emergency help immediately if any of the following symptoms of overdose occur:

Change in consciousness; confusion; loss of consciousness; sleepiness or unusual drowsiness; very drowsy or sleepy

Some side effects may occur that usually do not need medical attention. These side effects may go away during treatment as your body adjusts to the medicine. Also, your health care professional may be able to tell you about ways to prevent or reduce some of these side effects. Check with your health care professional if any of the following side effects continue or are bothersome or if you have any questions about them:

More common

Acid or sour stomach; belching; cough or hoarseness; dizziness; dry mouth; fever or chills; headache; heartburn; indigestion; lower back or side pain; nausea; nervousness; pain; painful or difficult urination; sleepiness or unusual drowsiness; stomach discomfort, upset or pain; unpleasant taste

Less common

Abnormal dreams; accidental injury; bladder pain; bloody or cloudy urine; chills; cold flu-like symptoms; cough or hoarseness; decreased interest in sexual intercourse; diarrhea; difficult, burning, or painful urination; discouragement; fear; feeling sad or empty; frequent urge to urinate; inability to have or keep an erection; irritability; itching skin; lack of appetite; loss in sexual ability, desire, drive, or performance; loss of interest or pleasure; mood or mental changes; nerve pain; nervousness; pain, cramps, heavy bleeding (females); rash; seeing, hearing, or feeling things that are not there; swelling of the breasts or breast soreness (males); tiredness; trouble concentrating; trouble sleeping; vomiting

Frequency not known

Loss of memory; problems with memory

After you stop using this medicine, it may still produce some side effects that need attention. During this period of time, *check with your doctor immediately* if you notice the following side effects:

> Abnormal dreams; fear; nervousness; nausea; upset stomach

Other side effects not listed may also occur in some patients. If you notice any other effects, check with your healthcare professional.

ETANERCEPT (Subcutaneous route) -
et-a-NER-sept

Commonly used brand name(s)

In the U.S.—
Enbrel

Available Dosage Forms:
- Powder for Solution
- Solution

Therapeutic Class: Immune Suppressant
Pharmacologic Class: Tumor Necrosis Factor Inhibitor

Uses For This Medicine

Etanercept is injected under the skin to reduce signs and symptoms of active arthritis or rheumatoid arthritis, such as joint swelling, pain, tiredness, and duration of morning stiffness. This medicine may also slow the progression of damage to the body from active arthritis or rheumatoid arthritis. It may also be used to treat psoriasis or a condition known as ankylosing spondylitis.

This medicine is available only with your doctor's prescription.

Once a medicine has been approved for marketing for a certain use, experience may show that it is also useful for other medical problems. Although this use is not included in the product labeling, etanercept is used in certain patients with the following medical condition:
- Reactive arthritis
- Inflammatory bowel disease arthritis

Before Using This Medicine

In deciding to use a medicine, the risks of taking the medicine must be weighed against the good it will do. This is a decision you and your doctor will make. For this medicine, the following should be considered:

Allergies—Tell your doctor if you have ever had any unusual or allergic reaction to this medicine or any other medicines. Also tell your health care professional if you have any other types of allergies, such as to foods, dyes, preservatives, or animals. For non-prescription products, read the label or package ingredients carefully.

Pediatric—Etanercept has been tested in children 4 to 17 years of age. Studies indicate that etanercept may reduce signs and symptoms in patients with juvenile rheumatoid arthritis. Stomach pain, nausea, headache, and vomiting were seen more often in children than in adults.

Geriatric—Etanercept has been tested in elderly patients and has not been found to cause different side effects or problems in older people than it does in younger adults. Caution should be used in elderly patients who are taking etanercept because they may be more likely to get an infection.

Pregnancy—

	Pregnancy Category	Explanation
All Trimesters	B	Animal studies have revealed no evidence of harm to the fetus, however, there are no adequate studies in pregnant women OR animal studies have shown an adverse effect, but adequate studies in pregnant women have failed to demonstrate a risk to the fetus.

Breast Feeding—There are no adequate studies in women for determining infant risk when using this medication during breastfeeding. Weigh the potential benefits against the potential risks before taking this medication while breastfeeding.

Other medicines—

Using this medicine with any of the following medicines is usually not recommended, but may be required in some cases. If both medicines are prescribed together, your doctor may change the dose or how often you use one or both of the medicines.

Abatacept, Anakinra, Cyclophosphamide

Interactions with Food/Tobacco/Alcohol—Certain medicines should not be used at or around the time of eating food or eating certain types of food since interactions may occur. Using alcohol or tobacco with certain medicines may also cause interactions to occur. Discuss with your healthcare professional the use of your medicine with food, alcohol, or tobacco.

Other medical problems—The presence of other medical problems may affect the use of this medicine. Make sure you tell your doctor if you have any other medical problems, especially:
- Allergy to etanercept or any of its ingredients
- Serious infection that spreads through the bloodstream—You should not use etanercept if you have either of these conditions
- Diseases of the central nervous system, such as multiple sclerosis—Etanercept may make these diseases worse in susceptible patients
- Cancer (or history of) or
- Diabetes mellitus (sugar diabetes) or
- Disease of the immune system (or history of) or
- Infections, serious infections, or continual infections—Etanercept may decrease the body's ability to fight infection
- Blood disorders—Etanercept may make these diseases worse or cause them to appear in susceptible patients
- Heart failure—May make heart conditions worse; use with caution
- Lung problems—May make lung problems worse; use with caution
- Seizure disorder—May make this condition worse; use with caution

Proper Use of This Medicine

If you are injecting this medicine yourself, each package of etanercept will contain a patient instruction sheet. Read this sheet carefully and make sure you understand:

- How to prepare the injection
- How to give the injection
- Proper use and disposal of syringes
- How long the injection is stable
- How to store the medication

Dosing—The dose of this medicine will be different for different patients. Follow your doctor's orders or the directions on the label. The following information includes only the average doses of this medicine. If your dose is different, do not change it unless your doctor tells you to do so.

The amount of medicine that you take depends on the strength of the medicine. Also, the number of doses you take each day, the time allowed between doses, and the length of time you take the medicine depend on the medical problem for which you are using the medicine.

- For prefilled syringe injection dosage form:
  - For the reduction of signs and symptoms of juvenile rheumatoid arthritis
    - Children 4 to 17 years of age and 138 pounds of body weight or more—0.8 milligrams (mg) per kg (0.36 mg per pound) of body weight up to 50 mg, injected under the skin once a week.
    - Children under 4 years of age—Use and dose must be determined by your doctor.
  - For the reduction of signs and symptoms of rheumatoid arthritis or psoriatic arthritis, or to treat ankylosing spondylitis:
    - Adults—50 mg injected under the skin once a week.
    - Children—Use and dose must be determined by your doctor.
  - For plaque psoriasis:
    - Adults—50 mg injected under the skin twice a week for 3 months, then 50 mg injected under the skin once a week.
    - Children up to 18 years—Use and dose must be determined by your doctor.
- For vial injection dosage form:
  - For the reduction of signs and symptoms of juvenile rheumatoid arthritis:
    - Children 4 to 17 years of age and 68 to 136 pounds of body weight—0.4 milligrams (mg) per kg (0.18 mg per pound) of body weight injected under the skin twice a week, or 0.8 mg per kg (0.36 mg per pound) of body weight once a week given as 2 injections under the skin at different sites.
    - Children 4 to 17 years of age and less than 68 pounds of body weight—0.8 mg per kg (0.36 mg per pound) of body weight once a week.
    - Children under 4 years of age—Use and dose must be determined by your doctor.
  - For the reduction of signs and symptoms of rheumatoid arthritis or psoriatic arthritis, or to treat ankylosing spondylitis:
    - Adults—25 mg injected under the skin twice a week.
    - Children—Use and dose must be determined by your doctor.

Missed dose—If you miss a dose of this medicine, take it as soon as possible. However, if it is almost time for your next dose, skip the missed dose and go back to your regular dosing schedule. Do not double doses.

Storage—Store in the refrigerator. Do not freeze.

Keep out of the reach of children.

Do not keep outdated medicine or medicine no longer needed.

Precautions While Using This Medicine

It is important that your doctor check your progress at regular visits to make sure that this medicine is working properly and to check for unwanted effects.

Your body's ability to fight infection may be reduced while you are being treated with etanercept, it is very important that you call your doctor at the first signs of any infection (for example, if you get a fever or chills).

While you are being treated with etanercept, do not have any immunizations (vaccinations) without your doctor's approval. Live virus vaccinations should not be given for 3 months before or while receiving etanercept.

Side Effects of This Medicine

Along with its needed effects, a medicine may cause some unwanted effects. Although not all of these side effects may occur, if they do occur they may need medical attention.

Check with your doctor as soon as possible if any of the following side effects occur:

More common
　　Chills; cough; fever; sneezing; sore throat

Less common
　　Congestion in chest; depression; fast heartbeat; frequent or painful urination; itching, pain, redness, or swelling on the skin; joint or muscle stiffness, tightness, or rigidity; shortness of breath; stomach discomfort and/or pain

Frequency not determined (side effects in adults)
　　Anxiety; blindness; bloating; bloody, black, or tarry stools; blue-yellow color blindness; blurred vision; changes in skin color; chest discomfort or pain; cloudy or bloody urine; confusion; constipation; convulsions; cramping or burning; darkened urine; decreased urine output; decreased vision; difficult, irregular, troubled or labored breathing (or difficulty in breathing gets worse); difficulty in speaking; dilated neck veins; discouragement; double vision; drowsiness; extreme fatigue; eye pain; felling sad or empty; general feeling of discomfort, illness, or weakness; generalized pain; heartburn and/or indigestion; high blood pressure; hives or welts; inability to move arms, legs, or facial muscles; irregular heartbeat; irritability; lack of appetite; large, hive-like swelling on face, eyelids, lips, tongue, throat, hands, legs, feet, or sex organs; lightheadedness; loss of interest or pleasure; lower back or side pain; muscle tenderness; nosebleeds; pain and inflammation at the joints; pain or discomfort in arms, jaw, back or neck; pain, redness, or swelling in arm or leg; pains in stomach, side, or abdomen, possibly radiating to the back; pale skin; problems with bowel or bladder function; severe abdominal pain; severe and continuing nausea; severe numbness, especially on one side of the face or body; skin rash on face, scalp, or stomach; slow speech or inability to speak; sore throat; sores,

ulcers, or white spots on lips or in mouth; swelling of face, fingers, feet, or lower legs; swollen or painful glands; tenderness; tightness in chest; tiredness; trouble concentrating; trouble sleeping; unusual bleeding or bruising; unusual tiredness or weakness; vomiting of blood or material that looks like coffee grounds; weight loss; wheezing; yellow eyes or skin

Incidence not determined (side effects in children)
Accumulation of pus; bladder pain; blisters on skin; burning feeling in chest or stomach; change in personality; difficult or burning urination; difficulty in moving; difficulty in swallowing; dry mouth; fatigue; flushed, dry skin; frequent urge to urinate; fruit-like breath odor; increased hunger; increased thirst; loss of consciousness; sores on the skin; swelling or redness in joints; swollen, red, tender area of infection; tenderness in stomach area; unexplained weight loss

Some side effects may occur that usually do not need medical attention. These side effects may go away during treatment as your body adjusts to the medicine. Also, your health care professional may be able to tell you about ways to prevent or reduce some of these side effects. Check with your health care professional if any of the following side effects continue or are bothersome or if you have any questions about them:

More common
Abdominal pain—more common in children; loss of energy or weakness; nausea and vomiting—more common in children; pain or burning in throat; redness and/or itching, pain, or swelling at the site of injection (under the skin); runny or stuffy nose

Less common
Bumps below the skin; depression; diarrhea; dry eyes; dry mouth; hair loss or thinning; heartburn; irritation or soreness of mouth; itching, redness, or tearing of eye; skin rash

Frequency not determined
Altered sense of taste; burning, crawling, itching, numb, prickling, "pins and needles", or tingling feelings; feeling faint, dizzy, or lightheaded; feeling of warmth or heat; flushing or redness of skin, especially on face and neck; loss of appetite; muscle aches and pains; sweating; weight gain

Other side effects not listed may also occur in some patients. If you notice any other effects, check with your healthcare professional.

ETHAMBUTOL (Oral route) - e-THAM-byoo-tole

Commonly used brand name(s)
In the U.S.—
Myambutol

Available Dosage Forms:
• Tablet

Therapeutic Class: Antitubercular

Uses For This Medicine

Ethambutol is used to treat tuberculosis (TB). It is used with other medicines for TB. This medicine may also be used for other problems as determined by your doctor.

To help clear up your tuberculosis (TB) infection completely, you must keep taking this medicine for the full time of treatment, even if you begin to feel better. This is very important. It is also important that you do not miss any doses.

Ethambutol is available only with your doctor's prescription.

Once a medicine has been approved for marketing for a certain use, experience may show that it is also useful for other medical problems. Although this use is not included in product labeling, ethambutol is used in certain patients with the following medical condition:
• Atypical mycobacterial infections, such as Mycobacterium avium complex (MAC)

Before Using This Medicine

In deciding to use a medicine, the risks of taking the medicine must be weighed against the good it will do. This is a decision you and your doctor will make. For this medicine, the following should be considered:

Allergies—Tell your doctor if you have ever had any unusual or allergic reaction to this medicine or any other medicines. Also tell your health care professional if you have any other types of allergies, such as to foods, dyes, preservatives, or animals. For non-prescription products, read the label or package ingredients carefully.

Pediatric—This medicine has been tested in children 13 years of age or older and has not been shown to cause different side effects or problems than it does in adults. Ethambutol may be used for children with TB when other medicines cannot be used. However, ethambutol is usually not used in children up to 6 years of age because it may be hard to tell if they are having side effects affecting their eyes.

Geriatric—Many medicines have not been studied specifically in older people. Therefore, it may not be known whether they work exactly the same way they do in younger adults. Although there is no specific information comparing use of ethambutol in the elderly with its use in other age groups, this medicine is not expected to cause different side effects or problems in older people than it does in younger adults.

Pregnancy—

	Pregnancy Category	Explanation
All Trimesters	B	Animal studies have revealed no evidence of harm to the fetus, however, there are no adequate studies in pregnant women OR animal studies have shown an adverse effect, but adequate studies in pregnant women have failed to demonstrate a risk to the fetus.

Breast Feeding—There are no adequate studies in women for determining infant risk when using this medication during breastfeeding. Weigh the potential benefits against the potential risks before taking this medication while breastfeeding.

Other medicines—

Using this medicine with any of the following medicines may cause an increased risk of certain side effects, but using both drugs may be the best treatment for you. If both medicines are prescribed together, your doctor may change the dose or how often you use one or both of the medicines.

Aluminum Distearate, Aluminum Hydroxide, Dihydroxyaluminum Aminoacetate, Dihydroxyaluminum Sodium Carbonate, Magaldrate

Interactions with Food/Tobacco/Alcohol—Certain medicines should not be used at or around the time of eating food or eating certain types of food since interactions may occur. Using alcohol or tobacco with certain medicines may also cause interactions to occur. Discuss with your healthcare professional the use of your medicine with food, alcohol, or tobacco.

Other medical problems—The presence of other medical problems may affect the use of this medicine. Make sure you tell your doctor if you have any other medical problems, especially:

- Gouty arthritis—Ethambutol may cause or worsen attacks of gout
- Kidney disease—Patients with kidney disease may be more likely to have side effects
- Optic neuritis (eye nerve damage)—Ethambutol may cause or worsen eye disease

Proper Use of This Medicine

Ethambutol may be taken with food if this medicine upsets your stomach.

To help clear up your tuberculosis (TB) completely, it is very important that you keep taking this medicine for the full time of treatment, even if you begin to feel better after a few weeks. You may have to take it every day for as long as 1 to 2 years or more. It is important that you do not miss any doses.

Dosing—The dose of this medicine will be different for different patients. Follow your doctor's orders or the directions on the label. The following information includes only the average doses of this medicine. If your dose is different, do not change it unless your doctor tells you to do so.

The amount of medicine that you take depends on the strength of the medicine. Also, the number of doses you take each day, the time allowed between doses, and the length of time you take the medicine depend on the medical problem for which you are using the medicine.

- For oral dosage form (tablets):
  - For the treatment of tuberculosis (TB):
    - Adults and children 13 years of age and older— 15 to 25 milligrams (mg) per kilogram (kg) (6.8 to 11.4 mg per pound) of body weight once a day. Instead, your doctor may tell you to take 50 mg per kg (22.8 mg per pound) of body weight, up to a total of 2.5 grams, two times a week. Another dose that your doctor may tell you to take is 25 to 30 mg per kg (11.4 to 13.6 mg per pound) of body weight, up to a total of 2.5 grams, three times a week. Ethambutol must be taken with other medicines to treat tuberculosis.
    - Infants and children up to 13 years of age—Use and dose must be determined by your doctor.

Missed dose—If you miss a dose of this medicine, take it as soon as possible. However, if it is almost time for your next dose, skip the missed dose and go back to your regular dosing schedule. Do not double doses.

Storage—Store the medicine in a closed container at room temperature, away from heat, moisture, and direct light. Keep from freezing.

Keep out of the reach of children.

Do not keep outdated medicine or medicine no longer needed.

Precautions While Using This Medicine

If your symptoms do not improve within 2 to 3 weeks, or if they become worse, check with your doctor.

It is very important that your doctor check your progress at regular visits.

Check with your doctor immediately if blurred vision, eye pain, red-green color blindness, or loss of vision occurs during treatment. Your doctor may want you to have your eyes checked by an ophthalmologist (eye doctor). Also, make sure you know how you react to this medicine before you drive, use machines, or do anything else that could be dangerous if you are not alert or able to see well.

Side Effects of This Medicine

Along with its needed effects, a medicine may cause some unwanted effects. Although not all of these side effects may occur, if they do occur they may need medical attention.

Check with your doctor immediately if any of the following side effects occur:

Less common
Chills; pain and swelling of joints, especially big toe, ankle, or knee; tense, hot skin over affected joints

Rare
Blurred vision, eye pain, red-green color blindness, or any loss of vision (more common with high doses); fever; joint pain; numbness, tingling, burning pain, or weakness in hands or feet; skin rash

Some side effects may occur that usually do not need medical attention. These side effects may go away during treatment as your body adjusts to the medicine. Also, your health care professional may be able to tell you about ways to prevent or reduce some of these side effects. Check with your health care professional if any of the following side effects continue or are bothersome or if you have any questions about them:

Less common
Abdominal pain; confusion; headache; loss of appetite; nausea and vomiting

Other side effects not listed may also occur in some patients. If you notice any other effects, check with your healthcare professional.

ETHINYL ESTRADIOL AND ETONOGESTREL (Vaginal route) - ETH-in-il es-tra-DYE-ole, et-oh-noe-JES-trel

Black Box Warning

Cigarette smoking increases the risk of serious cardiovascular side effects from combination oral contraceptive use. This risk increases with age and with heavy smoking (15 or more cigarettes per day) and is quite marked in women over 35 years of age. Women who use combination hormonal contraceptives, including ethinyl estradiol/etonogestrel, should be strongly advised not to smoke.

Commonly used brand name(s)

In the U.S.—
  Nuvaring

Available Dosage Forms:
- Insert, Extended Release

Therapeutic Class: Contraceptive
Pharmacologic Class: Progestin

Uses For This Medicine

The ethinyl estradiol and etonogestrel vaginal ring is a flexible combination contraceptive vaginal ring. Ethinyl estradiol is a kind of estrogen (ES-troh-jen) and etonogestrel is a kind of progesterone (proe-JES-ter-one). These are both female hormones used for contraception. The etonogestrel and ethinyl estradiol vaginal ring releases these hormones and is used to prevent pregnancy.

Ethinyl estradiol and etonogestrel vaginal ring will not protect a woman from sexually transmitted diseases (STDs), including human immunodeficiency virus (HIV) or acquired immunodeficiency syndrome (AIDS). The use of latex (rubber) condoms or abstinence (not having intercourse) is recommended for protection from these diseases.

Ethinyl estradiol and etonogestrel vaginal ring is available only from your doctor or other authorized health care professional.

Before Using This Medicine

In deciding to use a medicine, the risks of taking the medicine must be weighed against the good it will do. This is a decision you and your doctor will make. For this medicine, the following should be considered:

In deciding whether to use the combined contraceptive vaginal ring as a method of birth control, you need to consider the risks of using it as well as the good it can do. This is a decision you, your sexual partner, and your health care professional will make. For etonogestrel and ethinyl estradiol vaginal ring the following should be considered:

Allergies—Tell your doctor if you have ever had any unusual or allergic reaction to this medicine or any other medicines. Also tell your health care professional if you have any other types of allergies, such as to foods, dyes, preservatives, or animals. For non-prescription products, read the label or package ingredients carefully.

Pediatric—Studies with this contraceptive ring have been done only in adult patients, and it is not expected to cause different side effects in children than it does in adults. The etonogestrel and ethinyl estradiol vaginal ring is not intended for use in children or adolescents who have not yet started menstruating.

Geriatric—Many medicines have not been studied specifically in older people. Therefore, it may not be known if this works the same way in younger adults as it does in older adults. There is no specific information comparing the use of ethinyl estradiol and etonogestrel vaginal ring in the elderly with use in other age groups. The ethinyl estradiol and etonogestrel vaginal ring is not intended for use in women older than child-bearing age.

Other medicines—

Using this medicine with any of the following medicines is usually not recommended, but may be required in some cases. If both medicines are prescribed together, your doctor may change the dose or how often you use one or both of the medicines.

Felbamate, Isotretinoin, Paclitaxel, Paclitaxel Protein-Bound, Theophylline, Tizanidine

Interactions with Food/Tobacco/Alcohol—Certain medicines should not be used at or around the time of eating food or eating certain types of food since interactions may occur. Using alcohol or tobacco with certain medicines may also cause interactions to occur. The following interactions have been selected on the basis of their potential significance and are not necessarily all-inclusive.

Using this medicine with any of the following may cause an increased risk of certain side effects but may be unavoidable in some cases. If used together, your doctor may change the dose or how often you use this medicine, or give you special instructions about the use of food, alcohol, or tobacco.

Caffeine, Grapefruit Juice

Other medical problems—The presence of other medical problems may affect the use of this medicine. Make sure you tell your doctor if you have any other medical problems, especially:

- Abnormal or unusual vaginal bleeding (nonmenstrual)— The use of ethinyl estradiol and etonogestrel vaginal ring may delay diagnosis or worsen this condition. The reason for the bleeding should be determined before etonogestrel and ethinyl estradiol vaginal ring is used.
- Breast cancer (now or in the past or if suspected) or
- Cancer of the lining of the uterus, cervix or vagina (now or in the past) or
- Cancer that worsens when estrogen is present (now or in the past) or
- Confined to bed or inability to move for long period of time or
- Coronary artery disease (now or in the past) or
- Diabetes mellitus with blood vessel problems or
- Headache (severe) with changes in vision, loss of coordination, inability to move, numbness in arms or legs, or fainting or
- High blood pressure, severe or
- Jaundice while using birth control pills or
- Jaundice during pregnancy or
- Liver disease (active) or
- Liver tumors or
- Surgery (major) or
- Problems with circulation or blood clots, now or in the past, such as:
- Blood clots in your brain or
- Blood clots in your legs or
- Blood clots in your lungs or
- Blood clots in your eyes
- Problems with heart valves—These conditions may increase your chance of serious side effects.
- Coronary artery disease risk factors such as:
- Diabetes (sugar diabetes) or
- High blood pressure or
- High cholesterol or
- Obesity—These conditions may increase your chance of serious side effects when using ethinyl estradiol and etonogestrel vaginal ring.

- Depression or
- Diabetes mellitus (sugar diabetes) or
- Headache of type not experience before or
- High blood pressure or
- Kidney disease or
- Migraine headache or
- Problems with too much insulin in your blood or
- Problems with too much sugar in your blood—This medication may make this condition worse.
- Menstrual vaginal bleeding (lack of or heavy)—This problem may occur when contraceptive medicine is stopped, especially if it has happened in the past.
- Smoking cigarettes—Smoking may increase your chance of serious side effects, especially if you are over 35 years of age or smoke 15 cigarettes or more a day.
- Swollen ankles, feet, or hands—This medication may make this condition worse. This medicine may also make other medical problems worse when your body keeps too much water or fluid.

Proper Use of This Medicine

Dosing—The dose of this medicine will be different for different patients. Follow your doctor's orders or the directions on the label. The following information includes only the average doses of this medicine. If your dose is different, do not change it unless your doctor tells you to do so.

The amount of medicine that you take depends on the strength of the medicine. Also, the number of doses you take each day, the time allowed between doses, and the length of time you take the medicine depend on the medical problem for which you are using the medicine.

This ethinyl estradiol and etonogestrel vaginal ring comes with patient information. You must understand this information. You should keep a copy for reference. Be sure you understand possible problems with the ethinyl estradiol and etonogestrel vaginal ring, especially side effects, risks, and signs of a serious problem.

It is important to know how and when to insert, remove, or replace ethinyl estradiol and etonogestrel vaginal ring. If you have any questions about this ask your doctor. It is very important to follow the instructions on when to insert and remove your etonogestrel and ethinyl estradiol vaginal ring.

Pregnancy must be ruled out if there is a problem or change in your regimen. It is important to use additional methods of contraception if there was a problem or change in the regimen. Back-up contraception must be used until the ring has been in place for seven days.

- For vaginal dosage form
  - For preventing pregnancy:
    - Adults—One ring inserted into the vagina for three weeks. The ring is removed for a one week break and the old ring is disposed of. A new ring is inserted one week after the last ring was removed and left in place for three weeks. Note: The ring must be inserted on the appropriate day and left in place for three weeks. This means that the ring is removed three weeks later on the same day of the week it was inserted and at about the same time.

Missed dose—Call your doctor or pharmacist for instructions.

If the ethinyl estradiol and etonogestrel vaginal ring has slipped out of the vagina and it has been out less than three hours, you should still be protected from pregnancy. If the ethinyl estradiol and etonogestrel vaginal ring has been out of the vagina for more than three hours you may not adequately be protected from pregnancy, and you must use an extra method of birth control until the ethinyl estradiol and etonogestrel vaginal ring has been in place for seven days in a row. For additional information changes or problems with your regimen consult your patient information leaflet or ask your doctor.

Storage—Store the medicine in a closed container at room temperature, away from heat, moisture, and direct light. Keep from freezing.

Keep out of the reach of children.

Do not keep outdated medicine or medicine no longer needed.

Precautions While Using This Medicine

It is very important that your doctor check you at regular annual visits. Your doctor may want to see you more often than once a year.

It is very important that you tell your doctor if you think that you might be pregnant or if you miss a period.

This product does not protect against HIV infection (AIDS) and other sexually transmitted diseases.

Side Effects of This Medicine

The risk of serious adverse effects is unlikely for most women using the ethinyl estradiol and etonogestrel vaginal ring. However, oral combination hormonal contraceptives have been associated with unwanted effects which may need medical attention.

Check with your doctor immediately if any of the following side effects occur:

Incidence not determined

Abdominal fullness; abdominal pain or tenderness usually after eating a meal; blurred vision; changes in skin color; chest pain or discomfort; confusion; constipation; diarrhea; dizziness; gaseous abdominal pain; headache; inability to speak; nausea; nervousness; numbness of hands; pain or discomfort in arms, jaw, back or neck; pain; pains in chest, groin, or legs, especially calves of legs; pounding in the ears; prominent superficial veins over affected area with tenderness and warmth; recurrent fever; seizures; severe headaches of sudden onset; shortness of breath; slow or fast heartbeat; sudden loss of coordination; sudden onset of slurred speech; sudden vision changes; sudden and severe weakness in arm and/or leg on one side; sweating; swelling; swelling of foot or leg on one side of the body; temporary blindness; vomiting or vomiting of blood; yellow eyes or skin

Symptoms of overdose

Get emergency help immediately if any of the following symptoms of overdose occur:

Menstrual changes; nausea; vaginal bleeding; vomiting

Some side effects may occur that usually do not need medical attention. These side effects may go away during treatment as your body adjusts to the medicine. Also, your health care professional may be able to tell you about ways to prevent or reduce some of these side effects. Check with your health care professional if any of the following side effects continue or are bothersome or if you have any questions about them:

More common

Cough; fever; headache; itching of the vagina or genital area; pain during sexual intercourse; pain or tenderness around eyes and cheekbones; sore throat; stuffy or runny nose; thick, white vaginal discharge with no odor or with a mild odor; tightness of chest or wheezing; weight gain

Less common

Crying; depersonalization; false or unusual sense of well-being; hoarseness; mental depression; paranoia; quick to react or overreact emotionally; rapidly changing moods, mild feeling of sadness or discouragement that come and go

Incidence not determined

Absent, missed, or irregular menstrual periods; bloody vaginal discharge; brown, blotchy spots on exposed skin; chills; clay-colored stools; contact lenses intolerance; dark urine; decreased amount or quality of milk; dry mouth; dry skin; fatigue; flushed; fruit-like or unpleasant breath odor; increased hunger; increased thirst; increased urination; loss of appetite; medium to heavy, irregular vaginal bleeding between regular monthly periods, which may require the use of a pad or a tampon; rash; soreness, swelling, or discharge from the breast or breasts; trouble getting pregnant; unexplained weight loss; unusual tiredness or weakness

Other side effects not listed may also occur in some patients. If you notice any other effects, check with your healthcare professional.

ETHINYL ESTRADIOL AND NORELGESTROMIN (Transdermal route) - ETH-in-il es-tra-DYE-ole, nor-el-JES-troe-min

Black Box Warning

Cigarette smoking increases the risk of serious cardiovascular side effects from hormonal contraceptive use. This risk increases with age and with heavy smoking (15 or more cigarettes per day) and is quite marked in women over 35 years of age. Women who use hormonal contraceptives, including ethinyl estradiol/norelgestromin, should be strongly advised not to smoke.

Commonly used brand name(s)

In the U.S.—
Ortho Evra

Available Dosage Forms:
• Patch, Extended Release

Therapeutic Class: Monophasic Contraceptive Combination
Pharmacologic Class: Progestin

Uses For This Medicine

Ethinyl Estradiol/Norelgestromin contraceptive skin patch is used to prevent pregnancy. Hormones from the patch are absorbed through your skin into your body. It works by stopping a woman's egg from fully developing each month. The egg can no longer accept a sperm and fertilization is prevented.

This patch allows more estrogen into the blood than oral birth control containing the same amount of estrogen.

No contraceptive method is 100 percent effective. Birth control methods such as having surgery to become sterile or not having sex are more effective. Discuss with your health care professional your options for birth control.

Ethinyl Estradiol/Norelgestromin does not prevent AIDS or other sexually transmitted diseases. It will not prevent, hepatitis B. It will not help as emergency contraception, such as after unprotected sexual contact.

This medicine is available only with your doctor's prescription.

Before Using This Medicine

In deciding to use a medicine, the risks of taking the medicine must be weighed against the good it will do. This is a decision you and your doctor will make. For this medicine, the following should be considered:

Allergies—Tell your doctor if you have ever had any unusual or allergic reaction to this medicine or any other medicines. Also tell your health care professional if you have any other types of allergies, such as to foods, dyes, preservatives, or animals. For non-prescription products, read the label or package ingredients carefully.

Pediatric—Studies on this medicine have been done only in adult patients, and there is no specific information comparing use of ethinyl estradiol/norelgestromin in children with use in other age groups. This medicine should not be used before the start of menstruation. It may be used for birth control in teenage females and has not been shown to cause different side effects or problems than it does in adults. Some teenagers may need extra information on the importance of taking ethinyl estradiol/norelgestromin exactly as prescribed.

Geriatric—Many medicines have not been studied specifically in older people. Therefore, it may not be known whether they work exactly the same way they do in younger adults or if they cause different side effects or problems in older people. There is no specific information comparing use of norelgestromin/ethinyl estradiol in the elderly with use in other age groups.

Pregnancy—

	Pregnancy Category	Explanation
All Trimesters	X	Studies in animals or pregnant women have demonstrated positive evidence of fetal abnormalities. This drug should not be used in women who are or may become pregnant because the risk clearly outweighs any possible benefit.

Breast Feeding—

Ethinyl Estradiol
- Studies suggest that this medication may alter milk production or composition. If an alternative to this medication is not prescribed, you should monitor the infant for side effects and adequate milk intake.

Norelgestromin
- Studies in women breastfeeding have demonstrated harmful infant effects. An alternative to this medication should be prescribed or you should stop breastfeeding while using this medicine.

Other medicines—

Using this medicine with any of the following medicines is usually not recommended, but may be required in some cases. If both medicines are prescribed together, your doctor may change the dose or how often you use one or both of the medicines.

Felbamate, Isotretinoin, Paclitaxel, Paclitaxel Protein-Bound, Theophylline, Tizanidine

Interactions with Food/Tobacco/Alcohol—Certain medicines should not be used at or around the time of eating food or eating certain types of food since interactions may occur. Using alcohol or tobacco with certain medicines may also cause interactions to occur. The following interactions have been selected on the basis of their potential significance and are not necessarily all-inclusive.

Using this medicine with any of the following may cause an increased risk of certain side effects but may be unavoidable in some cases. If used together, your doctor may change the dose or how often you use this medicine, or give you special instructions about the use of food, alcohol, or tobacco.

Caffeine, Grapefruit Juice

Other medical problems—The presence of other medical problems may affect the use of this medicine. Make sure you tell your doctor if you have any other medical problems, especially:
- Breast cancer—Current or suspected diagnosis or
- Breast cancer—Personal history or
- Cancer of the uterus or cervix—Use of hormonal contraceptives may make these conditions worse.
- Jaundice during pregnancy or from using hormonal therapy in the past or
- Liver cancer, disease or tumors—Use of hormonal contraceptives may increase the chance of liver problems or make liver conditions worse.
- Diabetes mellitus (sugar diabetes)—Use of hormonal contraceptives may cause an increase, usually only a small increase, in your blood sugar and usually does not affect the amount of diabetes medicine that you take. You or your doctor will want to test for any changes in your blood sugar.
- Depression or
- Gallbladder disease or
- Heart attack or
- Heart disease, now or in the past or
- High blood pressure or
- Stroke, now or in the past—Use of hormonal contraceptives may cause or worsen these conditions.

- Abnormal or unusual vaginal bleeding—This condition may sometimes be treated with hormone contraceptives, but may make this condition worse.
- Migraine headache, new or worse or a new kind of headache—Use of hormonal contraceptives may cause headaches to be worse.
- Obesity—Use of the transdermal patch may be less effective in women with body weight greater than or equal to 198 pounds (90 kilograms).
- Problems with circulation or blood clots, now or in the past or
- Problems with heart valves or
- Surgery with a long period of inactivity—Use of hormonal contraceptives may increase the chance of blood clots and worsen these conditions.

Proper Use of This Medicine

To make using hormonal contraceptives as safe and reliable as possible, you should understand how and when to use them and what effects may be expected.

A paper with information for the patient will be given to you with your filled prescription, and will provide many details concerning the use of hormonal contraceptives. Read this paper carefully and ask your health care professional if you need additional information or explanation.

When you begin using norelgestromin and ethinyl estradiol, your body will require at least 7 days to adjust before a pregnancy will be prevented. Use a second form of contraception, such as a condom, spermicide, or diaphragm, for the first 7 days of your first cycle.

Keep each patch in the package until you are ready to use it. Apply the patch to clean, dry skin on the abdomen, upper body, the upper outside part of the arm, or the buttocks. Avoid touching the sticky surface of the patch. Make sure there is no lotion, powder, cream, or make-up on the skin. Apply the patch and then press it with the palm of your hand for 10 seconds to make sure it sticks. Change the location of the patch each time you apply a new one. Do not apply a patch to skin that is injured, broken, or cut. Do not apply a patch to your breasts. Check the patch every day to make sure it is in place.

If the patch comes off partly or all the way, try to apply it again or apply a new patch. If it was loose less than 24 hours, no other form of birth control is needed. If the patch has peeled away for more than 24 hours, apply a new patch and start a new cycle. A second form of birth control should be used.

If the patch is not sticky or has stuck to material or itself, remove it and apply a new patch. Do not hold the patch in place with tape or wraps.

If you are switching from a contraceptive pill to using the patch, start the patch on the first day of your period. If you do not start your period after 5 days, you see your health care professional for a pregnancy test. If you start the patch later than the first day of your period, use a second method of birth control with the patch for the first 7 days.

If you have had a baby and are not breast-feeding, you should wait 4 weeks before you start this medicine. If you have not had a period after having your baby, you should make sure you are not pregnant before starting this medicine.

If you have a miscarriage or an abortion in the first trimester of your pregnancy, you may start ethinyl estradiol/norelgestromin right away. You do not need a second form of birth control. If you start this medicine 5 days or more after the miscarriage or abortion, you should use a second form of birth control with the patch for the first 7 days. If you have a miscarriage or abortion after the first trimester, you should wait 4 weeks before starting this medicine

If you have bleeding with the patch in place, continue to use the patches as usual. If the bleeding continues for 2–3 cycles, call your health care professional. If you do not have your period during the time the patch is off stay on your regular schedule and call your health care professional.

If the patch is uncomfortable or causing irritation, change to a new patch in a new location. Change the patch again on your regular schedule. Do not use more than one patch at a time.

When you remove a patch, carefully fold it in half so that it sticks to itself and throw it away. There will still be some hormones on the patch. Do not touch the inside of the patch.

Dosing—The dose of this medicine will be different for different patients. Follow your doctor's orders or the directions on the label. The following information includes only the average doses of this medicine. If your dose is different, do not change it unless your doctor tells you to do so.

The amount of medicine that you take depends on the strength of the medicine. Also, the number of doses you take each day, the time allowed between doses, and the length of time you take the medicine depend on the medical problem for which you are using the medicine.

Your health care professional may begin your patch on the first day of your menstrual period (called Day-1 start) or on Sunday (called Sunday start). When you begin on a certain day it is important that you follow that schedule, even if you forget to change a patch. Do not change your schedule on your own. If the schedule that you have been put on is not convenient, check with your health care professional about changing schedules.

- For transdermal dosage form (skin patch):
  - For contraception (to prevent pregnancy):
    - Adults—Apply 1 patch to the skin and keep it in place for 1 week. Apply a new patch at the beginning of week 2 and again at week 3. Always change the patch on the same day of the week. Do not use a patch during week 4. This is when you will have your period. Start a new patch 7 days after the last patch was removed.
    - Children—Use and dose must be determined by your doctor.

Missed dose—Call your doctor or pharmacist for instructions.

Follow your doctor's orders or the directions on the label if you forget to change your patch. The following information includes only some of the ways to handle this. Your health care professional may want you to stop taking the medicine and use other birth control methods for the rest of the month until you have your menstrual period. Then your health care professional can tell you how to begin taking your medicine again. If you forget to apply your patch during the 1st week, apply it as soon as possible and start a new cycle. Use a second form of birth control for the first week of the new cycle. You will now have a new patch start day. If you forget to change your patch in the 2nd or 3rd week for one or two days, change it as soon as you remember. No other form of birth

control is needed. If you forget to change your patch in the 2nd or 3rd week for more than two days, change to a new patch and start a new cycle. Use a second form of birth control for the first week of the new cycle. If you forget to remove your patch at the end of the 3rd week, remove it as soon as possible and then start a new patch on your regular start day. You should never have the patch off for more than 7 days in a row.

Storage—Store the medicine in a closed container at room temperature, away from heat, moisture, and direct light. Keep from freezing.

Keep out of the reach of children.

Do not keep outdated medicine or medicine no longer needed.

Precautions While Using This Medicine

It is very important that your doctor check your progress at regular visits to make sure this medicine does not cause unwanted effects. These visits will usually be every 6 to 12 months, but some doctors require them more often.

Tell the medical doctor or dentist in charge that you are taking this medicine before any kind of surgery (including dental surgery) or emergency treatment. Your doctor will decide whether you should continue taking this medicine.

Ethinyl estradiol/norelgestromin may not work as well for you if you weigh more than 198 pounds. Talk to your health care professional about the kind of birth control that is best for you.

Vaginal bleeding of various amounts may occur between your regular menstrual periods during the first 3 months of use. This is sometimes called spotting when slight, or breakthrough bleeding when heavier. If this should occur:

- Continue on your regular dosing schedule.
- The bleeding usually stops within 1 week.
- Check with your doctor if the bleeding continues for more than 1 week.
- After you have been taking hormonal contraceptives on schedule and for more than 3 months and bleeding continues, check with your doctor.

Missed menstrual periods may occur:

- If you have not used the patch exactly as scheduled. Pregnancy must be considered as a possibility.
- If the medicine is not the right strength or type for your needs.

Check with your health care professional if you miss any menstrual periods so that the cause may be determined.

If you suspect that you may have become pregnant, stop taking this medicine immediately and check with your doctor.

Check with your doctor before refilling an old prescription, especially after a pregnancy. You will need another physical examination and your doctor may change your prescription.

Side Effects of This Medicine

Healthy women who do not smoke cigarettes have almost no chance of having a severe side effect from using hormonal contraceptives. For most women, more problems occur because of pregnancy than will occur from using hormonal contraceptives. But for some women who have special health problems, hormonal contraceptives can cause some unwanted effects. Some of these unwanted effects include heart disease, heart attack, benign (not cancerous) liver tumors, liver cancer, or blood clots or related problems, such as a stroke. Although these effects are very rare, they can be serious enough to cause death. You may want to discuss these effects with your doctor.

Other health problems that may be affected by using hormonal contraceptives are high blood pressure, high cholesterol, diabetes and being overweight.

Smoking cigarettes during the use of hormonal contraceptives has been found to greatly increase the chances of these serious side effects occurring. This risk increases with heavy smoking (15 or more cigarettes a day) or if you are over 35 years old. To reduce the risk of serious side effects, do not smoke cigarettes while you are taking hormonal contraceptives.

Along with its needed effects, a medicine may cause some unwanted effects. Although not all of these side effects may occur, if they do occur they may need medical attention.

Check with your doctor as soon as possible if any of the following side effects occur:

Use with caution around small children. The contraceptive patch may be a choking hazard if swallowed by a child.

More common
Body aches or pain; chills; cough; difficulty breathing; ear congestion; fever; headache; loss of voice; nasal congestion; runny nose; sneezing; sore throat; unusual tiredness or weakness

Symptoms of overdose

Get emergency help immediately if any of the following symptoms of overdose occur:

Nausea; vomiting; unusual vaginal bleeding in women

Frequency unknown
Anxiety; changes in skin color; chest pain or discomfort; confusion; dark urine; diarrhea; eye pain; dizziness; fainting; inability to speak; itching; lack or loss of appetite; light-colored stools; lightheadedness; nausea; nervousness; numbness in hands; pain in abdomen; pain in chest, groin, or legs, especially the calves; pain, tenderness, or swelling of foot or leg; pain or discomfort in arms, jaw, back or neck; pounding in the ears; rash; seizures; slow or fast heartbeat; slurred speech; sudden headache; sudden loss of coordination; sudden, severe weakness or numbness in arm or leg on one side of the body; sudden, unexplained shortness of breath; sweating; swelling, pain, or tenderness in upper abdominal area; temporary blindness; unpleasant breath odor; vision changes; vomiting of blood; yellow eyes or skin

Some side effects may occur that usually do not need medical attention. These side effects may go away during treatment as your body adjusts to the medicine. Also, your health care professional may be able to tell you about ways to prevent or reduce some of these side effects. Check with your health care professional if any of the following side effects continue or are bothersome or if you have any questions about them:

More common
Burning, itching, or redness of skin; menstrual cramps; pain, soreness, swelling, or discharge from the breast or breasts; swelling or soreness at patch site

Other side effects not listed may also occur in some patients. If you notice any other effects, check with your healthcare professional.

Frequency unknown
Abdominal cramps or bloating; absent, missed, or irregular menstrual periods; bloody vaginal discharge; brown, blotchy spots on exposed skin; change in amount of vaginal discharge; change in menstrual flow; decreased amount of breast milk; discouragement; dry mouth; feeling sad or empty; increased hunger or thirst; increase or decrease in weight; increased urination; irritability; itching of the vagina or outside genitals; light vaginal bleeding between periods and after sexual intercourse; loss of interest or pleasure; pain during sexual intercourse; stopping of menstrual bleeding; swelling; thick, white curd-like vaginal discharge without odor or with mild odor; trouble concentrating; trouble sleeping; unusual vaginal bleeding; vomiting

ETHIONAMIDE   (Oral route) - e-thye-on-AM-ide

Commonly used brand name(s)

In the U.S.—
Trecator
Trecator-SC

Available Dosage Forms:
• Tablet

Therapeutic Class: Antitubercular

Uses For This Medicine

Ethionamide is used with other medicines to treat tuberculosis (TB). Ethionamide may also be used for other problems as determined by your doctor.

To help clear up your tuberculosis (TB) completely, you must keep taking this medicine for the full time of treatment, even if you begin to feel better. This is very important. It is also important that you do not miss any doses.

Ethionamide is available only with your doctor's prescription.

Once a medicine has been approved for marketing for a certain use, experience may show that it is also useful for other medical problems. Although these uses are not included in product labeling, ethionamide is used in certain patients with the following medical conditions:

• Atypical mycobacterial infections, such as Mycobacterium avium complex (MAC)
• Leprosy (Hansen's disease)

Before Using This Medicine

In deciding to use a medicine, the risks of taking the medicine must be weighed against the good it will do. This is a decision you and your doctor will make. For this medicine, the following should be considered:

Allergies—Tell your doctor if you have ever had any unusual or allergic reaction to this medicine or any other medicines. Also tell your health care professional if you have any

other types of allergies, such as to foods, dyes, preservatives, or animals. For non-prescription products, read the label or package ingredients carefully.

Pediatric—Although there is no specific information comparing use of ethionamide in children with use in other age groups, this medicine is not expected to cause different side effects or problems in children than it does in adults.

Geriatric—Many medicines have not been studied specifically in older people. Therefore, it may not be known whether they work exactly the same way they do in younger adults or if they cause different side effects or problems in older people. There is no specific information comparing use of ethionamide in the elderly with use in other age groups.

Pregnancy—

	Pregnancy Category	Explanation
All Trimesters	C	Animal studies have shown an adverse effect and there are no adequate studies in pregnant women OR no animal studies have been conducted and there are no adequate studies in pregnant women.

Breast Feeding—There are no adequate studies in women for determining infant risk when using this medication during breastfeeding. Weigh the potential benefits against the potential risks before taking this medication while breastfeeding.

Other medicines—

Using this medicine with any of the following medicines is usually not recommended, but may be required in some cases. If both medicines are prescribed together, your doctor may change the dose or how often you use one or both of the medicines.

Pyrazinamide, Rifampin

Interactions with Food/Tobacco/Alcohol—Certain medicines should not be used at or around the time of eating food or eating certain types of food since interactions may occur. Using alcohol or tobacco with certain medicines may also cause interactions to occur. Discuss with your healthcare professional the use of your medicine with food, alcohol, or tobacco.

Other medical problems—The presence of other medical problems may affect the use of this medicine. Make sure you tell your doctor if you have any other medical problems, especially:

- Diabetes mellitus (sugar diabetes)—Diabetes may be harder to control in patients taking ethionamide
- Liver disease (severe)—Patients with severe liver disease may have an increased chance of side effects

Proper Use of This Medicine

Ethionamide may be taken with or after meals if it upsets your stomach.

To help clear up your tuberculosis (TB) completely, it is very important that you keep taking this medicine for the full time of treatment, even if you begin to feel better after a few weeks. You may have to take it every day for 1 to 2 years or more. It is important that you do not miss any doses.

Your doctor may also want you to take pyridoxine (e.g., Hexa-Betalin; vitamin B 6) every day to help prevent or lessen some of the side effects of ethionamide. If so, it is very important to take pyridoxine every day along with this medicine. Do not miss any doses.

Dosing—The dose of this medicine will be different for different patients. Follow your doctor's orders or the directions on the label. The following information includes only the average doses of this medicine. If your dose is different, do not change it unless your doctor tells you to do so.

The amount of medicine that you take depends on the strength of the medicine. Also, the number of doses you take each day, the time allowed between doses, and the length of time you take the medicine depend on the medical problem for which you are using the medicine.

- For oral dosage form (tablets):
  - For the treatment of tuberculosis (TB):
    - Adults and teenagers—250 milligrams (mg) every eight to twelve hours. Ethionamide must be taken with other medicines to treat tuberculosis.
    - Children—Dose is based on body weight. The usual dose is 4 to 5 mg per kilogram of body weight every eight hours. Ethionamide must be taken with other medicines to treat tuberculosis.

Missed dose—If you miss a dose of this medicine, take it as soon as possible. However, if it is almost time for your next dose, skip the missed dose and go back to your regular dosing schedule. Do not double doses.

Storage—Store the medicine in a closed container at room temperature, away from heat, moisture, and direct light. Keep from freezing.

Keep out of the reach of children.

Do not keep outdated medicine or medicine no longer needed.

Precautions While Using This Medicine

If your symptoms do not improve within 2 to 3 weeks, or if they become worse, check with your doctor.

It is very important that your doctor check your progress at regular visits. Also, check with your doctor immediately if blurred vision or any loss of vision, with or without eye pain, occurs during treatment. Your doctor may want you to have your eyes checked by an ophthalmologist (eye doctor).

Since this medicine may cause blurred vision or loss of vision, make sure you know how you react to this medicine before you drive, use machines, or do anything else that could be dangerous if you are not able to see well.

If this medicine causes clumsiness; unsteadiness; or numbness, tingling, burning, or pain in the hands and feet, check with your doctor immediately. These may be early warning symptoms of more serious nerve problems that could develop later.

Side Effects of This Medicine

Along with its needed effects, a medicine may cause some unwanted effects. Although not all of these side effects may occur, if they do occur they may need medical attention.

Check with your doctor immediately if any of the following side effects occur:

Less common

Clumsiness or unsteadiness; confusion; mental depression; mood or other mental changes; numbness, tingling, burning, or pain in hands and feet; yellow eyes or skin

Rare

Blurred vision or loss of vision, with or without eye pain; changes in menstrual periods; coldness; decreased sexual ability (in males); difficulty in concentrating; dry, puffy skin; faster heartbeat; increased hunger; nervousness; shakiness; skin rash; swelling of front part of neck; weight gain

Some side effects may occur that usually do not need medical attention. These side effects may go away during treatment as your body adjusts to the medicine. Also, your health care professional may be able to tell you about ways to prevent or reduce some of these side effects. Check with your health care professional if any of the following side effects continue or are bothersome or if you have any questions about them:

More common

Dizziness (especially when getting up from a lying or sitting position); loss of appetite; metallic taste; nausea or vomiting; sore mouth

Less common or rare

Enlargement of the breasts (in males)

Other side effects not listed may also occur in some patients. If you notice any other effects, check with your healthcare professional.

ETIDRONATE (Oral route, Intravenous route) - e-ti-DROE-nate

Commonly used brand name(s)

In the U.S.—
Didronel
Didronel I.V.

Available Dosage Forms:

• Kit
• Solution
• Tablet

Therapeutic Class: Calcium Regulator

Uses For This Medicine

Etidronate is used to treat Paget's disease of bone. It may also be used to treat or prevent a certain type of bone problem that may occur after hip replacement surgery or spinal injury.

Etidronate is also used to treat hypercalcemia (too much calcium in the blood) that may occur with some types of cancer.

This medicine is available only with your doctor's prescription.

Before Using This Medicine

In deciding to use a medicine, the risks of taking the medicine must be weighed against the good it will do. This is a decision you and your doctor will make. For this medicine, the following should be considered:

Allergies—Tell your doctor if you have ever had any unusual or allergic reaction to this medicine or any other medicines. Also tell your health care professional if you have any other types of allergies, such as to foods, dyes, preservatives, or animals. For non-prescription products, read the label or package ingredients carefully.

Pediatric—Some changes in bone growth may occur in children, but will usually go away when the medicine is stopped.

Geriatric—When etidronate is given by injection along with a large amount of fluid, older people tend to retain (keep) the excess fluid.

Pregnancy—

	Pregnancy Category	Explanation
All Trimesters	C	Animal studies have shown an adverse effect and there are no adequate studies in pregnant women OR no animal studies have been conducted and there are no adequate studies in pregnant women.

Breast Feeding—There are no adequate studies in women for determining infant risk when using this medication during breastfeeding. Weigh the potential benefits against the potential risks before taking this medication while breastfeeding.

Other medicines—Although certain medicines should not be used together at all, in other cases two different medicines may be used together even if an interaction might occur. In these cases, your doctor may want to change the dose, or other precautions may be necessary. Tell your healthcare professional if you are taking any other prescription or nonprescription (over-the-counter [OTC]) medicine.

Interactions with Food/Tobacco/Alcohol—Certain medicines should not be used at or around the time of eating food or eating certain types of food since interactions may occur. Using alcohol or tobacco with certain medicines may also cause interactions to occur. The following interactions have been selected on the basis of their potential significance and are not necessarily all-inclusive.

Using this medicine with any of the following may cause an increased risk of certain side effects but may be unavoidable in some cases. If used together, your doctor may change the dose or how often you use this medicine or give you special instructions about the use of food, alcohol, or tobacco.

Dairy Foods

Other medical problems—The presence of other medical problems may affect the use of this medicine. Make sure you tell your doctor if you have any other medical problems, especially:

• Bone fracture, especially of arm or leg—Etidronate may increase the risk of bone fractures.

• Intestinal or bowel disease—Etidronate may increase the risk of diarrhea.

• Kidney disease—High blood levels of etidronate may result, causing serious side effects.

Proper Use of This Medicine

Make certain your health care professional knows if your diet includes large amounts of calcium, such as milk or other dairy products, or if you are on any special diet, such as a low-sodium or low-sugar diet. Calcium in the diet may prevent the absorption of oral etidronate.

Take etidronate with water on an empty stomach at least 2 hours before or after food (mid-morning is best) or at bedtime. Food may decrease the amount of etidronate absorbed by your body.

Take etidronate only as directed. Do not take more of it, do not take it more often, and do not take it for a longer time than your doctor ordered. To do so may increase the chance of side effects.

In some patients, etidronate takes up to 3 months to work. If you feel that the medicine is not working, do not stop taking it on your own. Instead, check with your doctor.

It is important that you eat a well-balanced diet with an adequate amount of calcium and vitamin D (found in milk or other dairy products). Too much or too little of either may increase the chance of side effects while you are taking etidronate. Your doctor can help you choose the meal plan that is best for you. However, do not take any food, especially milk, milk formulas, or other dairy products, or antacids, mineral supplements, or other medicines that are high in calcium or iron (high amounts of these minerals may also be in some vitamin preparations), magnesium, or aluminum within 2 hours of taking etidronate. To do so may keep this medicine from working properly.

Dosing—The dose of this medicine will be different for different patients. Follow your doctor's orders or the directions on the label. The following information includes only the average doses of this medicine. If your dose is different, do not change it unless your doctor tells you to do so.

The amount of medicine that you take depends on the strength of the medicine. Also, the number of doses you take each day, the time allowed between doses, and the length of time you take the medicine depend on the medical problem for which you are using the medicine.

- For oral dosage form (tablets):
  - For treating Paget's disease of bone:
    - Adults—Dose is based on body weight and must be determined by your doctor. The dose to start is 5 milligrams (mg) per kilogram (kg) (2.3 mg per pound) of body weight a day, usually as a single dose, for not more than six months. Some people may need 6 to 10 mg per kg (2.7 to 4.6 mg per pound) of body weight a day for not more than six months. Others may need 11 to 20 mg per kg (5 to 9.1 mg per pound) of body weight a day for not more than three months. Your doctor may change your dose depending on your response to treatment.
    - Children—Dose must be determined by your doctor.
  - For treating or preventing a certain type of bone problem that may occur after hip replacement:
    - Adults—Dose is based on body weight and must be determined by your doctor. The usual dose is 20 mg per kg (9.1 mg per pound) of body weight a day for one month before surgery, and for three months after surgery.
    - Children—Dose must be determined by your doctor.
  - For treating or preventing a certain type of bone problem that may occur after spinal injury:
    - Adults—Dose is based on body weight and must be determined by your doctor. The usual dose is 20 mg per kg (9.1 mg per pound) of body weight a day for two weeks, beginning as soon as possible after your injury. Your doctor may then decrease your dose to 10 mg per kg (4.5 mg per pound) of body weight for an additional ten weeks.
    - Children—Dose must be determined by your doctor.
  - For treating hypercalcemia (too much calcium in the blood):
    - Adults—Dose is based on body weight and must be determined by your doctor. The usual dose is 20 mg per kg (9.1 mg per pound) of body weight

a day for thirty days. Treatment usually does not continue beyond ninety days.
    - Children—Dose must be determined by your doctor.
- For injection dosage form:
  - For treating hypercalcemia (too much calcium in the blood):
    - Adults—Dose is based on body weight and must be determined by your doctor. The usual dose is 7.5 milligrams (mg) per kilogram (kg) (3.4 mg per pound) of body weight, injected slowly into your vein over 2 hours. This dose is repeated for two more days. Your doctor may repeat the treatment after at least seven days.
    - Children—Dose must be determined by your doctor.

Missed dose—If you miss a dose of this medicine, take it as soon as possible. However, if it is almost time for your next dose, skip the missed dose and go back to your regular dosing schedule. Do not double doses.

Storage—Store the medicine in a closed container at room temperature, away from heat, moisture, and direct light. Keep from freezing.

Keep out of the reach of children.

Do not keep outdated medicine or medicine no longer needed.

Precautions While Using This Medicine

It is important that your doctor check your progress at regular visits even if you are between treatments and are not taking this medicine. If your condition has improved and your doctor has told you to stop taking etidronate, your progress must still be checked. The results of laboratory tests or the occurrence of certain symptoms will tell your doctor if more medicine must be taken. Your doctor may want you to begin another course of treatment after you have been off the medicine for at least 3 months.

It is important that you check with your doctor before having any dental procedures or surgeries done while you are receiving etidronate. Tell your doctor right away if you experience jaw tightness, swelling, numbing, or pain or a loose tooth. It could be the sign of a serious jaw disease.

If this medicine causes you to have nausea or diarrhea and it continues, check with your doctor. The dose may need to be changed.

If bone, joint or muscle pain occurs, or worsens during treatment, check with your doctor.

Side Effects of This Medicine

Along with its needed effects, a medicine may cause some unwanted effects. Although not all of these side effects may occur, if they do occur they may need medical attention.

Check with your doctor as soon as possible if any of the following side effects occur:
More common
   Bone pain or tenderness (increased, continuing, or returning—in patients with Paget's disease)
Less common
   Bone fractures, especially of the thigh bone
Rare
   Hives; skin rash or itching; swelling of the arms, legs, face, lips, tongue, and/or throat

Incidence not known
    Bone, joint, or muscle pain that is severe and occasionally disabling; heavy jaw feeling; loosening of a tooth; pain, swelling, or numbness in the mouth or jaw

Some side effects may occur that usually do not need medical attention. These side effects may go away during treatment as your body adjusts to the medicine. Also, your health care professional may be able to tell you about ways to prevent or reduce some of these side effects. Check with your health care professional if any of the following side effects continue or are bothersome or if you have any questions about them:

More common—at higher doses
    Diarrhea; nausea

Less common—with injection
    Loss of taste or metallic or altered taste

Other side effects not listed may also occur in some patients. If you notice any other effects, check with your healthcare professional.

ETOPOSIDE (Oral route, Intravenous route) - e-toe-POE-side

Black Box Warning

Etoposide should be administered under the supervision of a qualified physician experienced in the use of cancer chemotherapeutic agents. Severe myelosuppression with resulting infection or bleeding may occur.

Commonly used brand name(s)

In the U.S.—
    Etopophos
    Vepesid

In Canada—

Dom-Etoposide	Etoposide
Eposin	Pms-Etoposide

Available Dosage Forms:

• Capsule, Liquid Filled	• Solution
• Capsule	• Powder for Solution

Therapeutic Class: Antineoplastic Agent
Pharmacologic Class: Mitotic Inhibitor

Uses For This Medicine

Etoposide belongs to the group of medicines known as antineoplastic agents. It is used to treat cancer of the testicles and certain types of lung cancer. It is also sometimes used to treat some other kinds of cancer in both males and females.

The exact way that etoposide acts against cancer is not known. However, it seems to interfere with the growth of the cancer cells, which are eventually destroyed. Since the growth of normal body cells may also be affected by etoposide, other effects will also occur. Some of these may be serious and must be reported to your doctor. Other effects, like hair loss, may not be serious but may cause concern. Some effects may not occur until months or years after the medicine is used.

Before you begin treatment with etoposide, you and your doctor should talk about the good this medicine will do as well as the risks of using it.

This medicine is available only with your doctor's prescription.

Once a medicine has been approved for marketing for a certain use, experience may show that it is also useful for other medical problems. Although these uses are not included in product labeling, etoposide is used in certain patients with the following medical conditions:

- Autoimmune deficiency syndrome (AIDS)— associated Kaposi's sarcoma (a type of cancer of the skin and mucous membranes that is more common in patients with AIDS)
- Cancer of the adrenal cortex (the outside layer of the adrenal gland)
- Cancers of the blood and lymph system
- Cancer in the bone
- Cancer of the endometrium
- Cancer of the lung (a certain type of lung cancer usually associated with prior smoking, passive smoking, or radon exposure)
- Cancer of the lymph system (a part of the body's immune system) that affects the skin
- Cancer of the stomach
- Cancers of the soft tissues of the body, including the muscles, connective tissues (tendons), vessels that carry blood or lymph, or fat
- Cancer of unknown primary site
- Ewing's sarcoma (a type of cancer found in the bone)
- Gestational trophoblastic tumors (tumors in the uterus or womb)
- Hepatoblastoma (a certain type of liver cancer that occurs in children)
- Multiple myeloma (a certain type of cancer of the blood)
- Myelodysplastic syndromes (MDS)
- Neuroblastoma (a cancer of the nerves that usually occurs in children)
- Retinoblastoma (a cancer of the eye that usually occurs in children)
- Thymoma (a cancer of the thymus, which is a small organ that lies under the breastbone)
- Tumors in the brain
- Wilms' tumor (a cancer of the kidney that usually occurs in children)
- Cancer of the ovaries (a type of cancer found in the egg-making cells)

Before Using This Medicine

In deciding to use a medicine, the risks of taking the medicine must be weighed against the good it will do. This is a decision you and your doctor will make. For this medicine, the following should be considered:

Allergies—Tell your doctor if you have ever had any unusual or allergic reaction to this medicine or any other medicines. Also tell your health care professional if you have any other types of allergies, such as to foods, dyes, preservatives, or animals. For non-prescription products, read the label or package ingredients carefully.

Pediatric—Although this medicine has been used in children, there is no specific information comparing use of etoposide in children with use in other age groups. However, children who receive high doses may be more likely to have a serious allergic reaction to this medicine.

Geriatric—Many medicines have not been studied specifically in older people. Therefore, it may not be known whether they work exactly the same way they do in younger adults or if they cause different side effects or problems in older people. There is no specific information comparing use of etoposide in the elderly with use in other age groups.

Pregnancy—

	Pregnancy Category	Explanation
All Trimesters	D	Studies in pregnant women have demonstrated a risk to the fetus. However, the benefits of therapy in a life threatening situation or a serious disease, may outweigh the potential risk.

Breast Feeding—There are no adequate studies in women for determining infant risk when using this medication during breastfeeding. Weigh the potential benefits against the potential risks before taking this medication while breastfeeding.

Other medicines—

Using this medicine with any of the following medicines is not recommended. Your doctor may decide not to treat you with this medication or change some of the other medicines you take.

Rotavirus Vaccine, Live

Interactions with Food/Tobacco/Alcohol—Certain medicines should not be used at or around the time of eating food or eating certain types of food since interactions may occur. Using alcohol or tobacco with certain medicines may also cause interactions to occur. The following interactions have been selected on the basis of their potential significance and are not necessarily all-inclusive.

Using this medicine with any of the following may cause an increased risk of certain side effects but may be unavoidable in some cases. If used together, your doctor may change the dose or how often you use this medicine, or give you special instructions about the use of food, alcohol, or tobacco.

Grapefruit Juice

Other medical problems—The presence of other medical problems may affect the use of this medicine. Make sure you tell your doctor if you have any other medical problems, especially:

- Chickenpox (including recent exposure) or
- Herpes zoster (shingles)—Risk of severe disease affecting other parts of the body
- Infection—Etoposide can decrease your body's ability to fight infection
- Kidney disease or
- Liver disease—Effects of etoposide may be increased because of slower removal from the body

Proper Use of This Medicine

Take etoposide only as directed by your doctor. Do not use more or less of it, and do not use it more often than your doctor ordered. The exact amount of medicine you need has been carefully worked out. Taking too much may increase the chance of side effects, while taking too little may not improve your condition.

Etoposide is sometimes given together with certain other medicines. If you are using a combination of medicines, make sure that you take each one at the proper time and do not mix them. If you are taking some of these medicines by mouth, ask your health care professional to help you plan a way to remember to take your medicines at the right times.

Etoposide often causes nausea, vomiting, and loss of appetite, which may be severe. However, it is very important that you continue to receive the medicine, even if you begin to feel ill. Ask your health care professional for ways to lessen these effects.

If you vomit shortly after taking a dose of etoposide, check with your doctor. You will be told whether to take the dose again or to wait until the next dose.

Dosing—The dose of this medicine will be different for different patients. Follow your doctor's orders or the directions on the label. The following information includes only the average doses of this medicine. If your dose is different, do not change it unless your doctor tells you to do so.

The amount of medicine that you take depends on the strength of the medicine. Also, the number of doses you take each day, the time allowed between doses, and the length of time you take the medicine depend on the medical problem for which you are using the medicine.

Missed dose—If you miss a dose of this medicine, skip the missed dose and go back to your regular dosing schedule. Do not double doses.

Storage—Store in the refrigerator. Do not freeze.

Keep out of the reach of children.

Do not keep outdated medicine or medicine no longer needed.

Precautions While Using This Medicine

It is very important that your doctor check your progress at regular visits to make sure that etoposide is working properly and to check for unwanted effects.

While you are being treated with etoposide, and after you stop treatment with it, do not have any immunizations (vaccinations) without your doctor's approval. Etoposide may lower your body's resistance and there is a chance you might get the infection the immunization is meant to prevent. In addition, other persons living in your household should not take oral polio vaccine since there is a chance they could pass the polio virus on to you. Also, avoid persons who have taken oral polio vaccine within the last several months. Do not get close to them and do not stay in the same room with them for very long. If you cannot take these precautions, you should consider wearing a protective face mask that covers the nose and mouth.

Etoposide can temporarily lower the number of white blood cells in your blood, increasing the chance of your getting an infection. It can also lower the number of platelets, which are necessary for proper blood clotting. If this occurs, there are certain precautions you can take, especially when your blood count is low, to reduce the risk of infection or bleeding:

- If you can, avoid people with infections. Check with your doctor immediately if you think you are getting an infection or if you get a fever or chills, cough or hoarseness, lower back or side pain, or have painful or difficult urination.

- Check with your doctor immediately if you notice any unusual bleeding or bruising; black, tarry stools; blood in urine or stools; or pinpoint red spots on your skin.

- Be careful when using a regular toothbrush, dental floss, or toothpick. Your medical doctor, dentist, or nurse may recommend other ways to clean your teeth and gums. Check with your medical doctor before having any dental work done.

- Do not touch your eyes or the inside of your nose unless you have just washed your hands and have not touched anything else in the meantime.

- Be careful not to cut yourself when you are using sharp objects such as a safety razor or fingernail or toenail cutters.

- Avoid contact sports or other situations where bruising or injury could occur.

Side Effects of This Medicine

Along with its needed effects, a medicine may cause some unwanted effects. Although not all of these side effects may occur, if they do occur they may need medical attention.

Also, because of the way these medicines act on the body, there is a chance that they might cause other unwanted effects that may not occur until months or years after the medicine is used. These delayed effects may include certain types of cancer, such as leukemia. Discuss these possible effects with your doctor.

Check with your doctor immediately if any of the following side effects occur:

Rare
Fast heartbeat; loss of consciousness; shortness of breath; sweating; swelling of face or tongue; tightness in throat; wheezing

Check with your doctor as soon as possible if any of the following side effects occur:

More common
Unusual tiredness or weakness

Less common
Black, tarry stools; blood in urine or stools; cough or hoarseness, accompanied by fever or chills; fever or chills; lower back or side pain, accompanied by fever or chills; painful or difficult urination, accompanied by fever or chills; pinpoint red spots on skin; sores in mouth or on lips; unusual bleeding or bruising

Rare
Back pain; difficulty in walking; numbness or tingling in fingers and toes; pain at place of injection; skin rash or itching; weakness

Some side effects may occur that usually do not need medical attention. These side effects may go away during treatment as your body adjusts to the medicine. Also, your health care professional may be able to tell you about ways to prevent or reduce some of these side effects. Check with your health care professional if any of the following side effects continue or are bothersome or if you have any questions about them:

More common
Loss of appetite; nausea and vomiting

Less common
Diarrhea

This medicine often causes a temporary loss of hair. After treatment with etoposide has ended, normal hair growth should return.

Other side effects not listed may also occur in some patients. If you notice any other effects, check with your healthcare professional.

EXEMESTANE (Oral route) - ex-e-MES-tane

Commonly used brand name(s)

In the U.S.—
Aromasin

Available Dosage Forms:
- Tablet

Therapeutic Class: Antineoplastic Agent
Pharmacologic Class: Aromatase Inhibitor

Uses For This Medicine

Exemestane is a medicine that is used to treat breast cancer in women whose disease has progressed while they were taking tamoxifen.

Many breast cancer tumors grow in response to estrogen. Exemestane interferes with the production of estrogen in the body. As a result, the amount of estrogen that the tumor is exposed to is reduced, limiting the growth of the tumor. This medicine is meant to be used only by women who have already stopped menstruating.

Before you begin treatment with exemestane, you and your doctor should talk about the good this medicine will do as well as the risks of using it.

Exemestane is available only with your doctor's prescription.

Before Using This Medicine

In deciding to use a medicine, the risks of taking the medicine must be weighed against the good it will do. This is a decision you and your doctor will make. For this medicine, the following should be considered:

Allergies—Tell your doctor if you have ever had any unusual or allergic reaction to this medicine or any other medicines. Also tell your health care professional if you have any other types of allergies, such as to foods, dyes, preservatives, or animals. For non-prescription products, read the label or package ingredients carefully.

Geriatric—Many medicines have not been studied specifically in older people. Therefore, it may not be known whether they work exactly the same way they do in younger adults. Although there is no specific information comparing use of exemestane in the elderly with use in other age groups, this medicine is not expected to cause different side effects or problems in older people than it does in younger adults.

Pregnancy—

	Pregnancy Category	Explanation
All Trimesters	D	Studies in pregnant women have demonstrated a risk to the fetus. However, the benefits of therapy in a life threatening situation or a serious disease, may outweigh the potential risk.

Breast Feeding—There are no adequate studies in women for determining infant risk when using this medication during breastfeeding. Weigh the potential benefits against the potential risks before taking this medication while breastfeeding.

Other medicines—Although certain medicines should not be used together at all, in other cases two different medicines may be used together even if an interaction might occur. In these cases, your doctor may want to change the dose, or other precautions may be necessary. Tell your healthcare professional if you are taking any other prescription or non-prescription (over-the-counter [OTC]) medicine.

Interactions with Food/Tobacco/Alcohol—Certain medicines should not be used at or around the time of eating food or eating certain types of food since interactions may occur. Using alcohol or tobacco with certain medicines may also cause interactions to occur. Discuss with your healthcare professional the use of your medicine with food, alcohol, or tobacco.

Other medical problems—The presence of other medical problems may affect the use of this medicine. Make sure you tell your doctor if you have any other medical problems, especially:

• Kidney disease or

• Liver disease—It is not known whether moderate or severe kidney or liver disease may increase the chance of side effects during treatment

Proper Use of This Medicine

Use this medicine only as directed by your doctor. Do not use more or less of it, and do not use it more often than your doctor ordered. The exact amount of medicine you need has been carefully worked out. Taking too much may increase the chance of side effects, while taking too little may not improve your condition.

Dosing—The dose of this medicine will be different for different patients. Follow your doctor's orders or the directions on the label. The following information includes only the average doses of this medicine. If your dose is different, do not change it unless your doctor tells you to do so.

The amount of medicine that you take depends on the strength of the medicine. Also, the number of doses you take each day, the time allowed between doses, and the length of time you take the medicine depend on the medical problem for which you are using the medicine.

• For oral dosage form (tablets)
  ○ For breast cancer in postmenopausal women:
    ▪ Adults—25 milligrams (mg) once a day after a meal.

Missed dose—If you miss a dose of this medicine, skip the missed dose and go back to your regular dosing schedule. Do not double doses.

Storage—Store the medicine in a closed container at room temperature, away from heat, moisture, and direct light. Keep from freezing.

Keep out of the reach of children.

Do not keep outdated medicine or medicine no longer needed.

Precautions While Using This Medicine

It is very important that your doctor check your progress at regular visits to make sure that this medicine is working properly and to check for unwanted effects.

Side Effects of This Medicine

Along with its needed effects, a medicine may cause some unwanted effects. Although not all of these side effects may occur, if they do occur they may need medical attention.

Check with your doctor as soon as possible if any of the following side effects occur:
More common
Cough or hoarseness; difficult or labored breathing; fever or chills; increased blood pressure; lower back or side pain; mental depression; shortness of breath; swelling of hands, ankles, feet, or lower legs; tightness in chest

Less common
Chest pain; difficult, burning, or painful urination; frequent urge to urinate; headache; sore throat; unexplained broken bones; wheezing

Some side effects may occur that usually do not need medical attention. These side effects may go away during treatment as your body adjusts to the medicine. Also, your health care professional may be able to tell you about ways to prevent or reduce some of these side effects. Check with your health care professional if any of the following side effects continue or are bothersome or if you have any questions about them:
More common
Abdominal or stomach pain; anxiety; constipation; diarrhea; dizziness; general feeling of discomfort or illness; general feeling of tiredness or weakness; hot flashes; increased sweating; loss of appetite; nausea and vomiting; pain; trouble in sleeping

Less common
Back pain; bone pain; burning, tingling or prickly sensations; confusion; decreased sense of touch; increased appetite; itching; joint pain; loss of hair; rash; runny nose; stomach upset; weakness, generalized

Other side effects not listed may also occur in some patients. If you notice any other effects, check with your healthcare professional.

EXENATIDE (Subcutaneous route) -
ex-EN-a-tide

Commonly used brand name(s)

In the U.S.—
Byetta

Available Dosage Forms:
- Solution

Therapeutic Class: Antidiabetic

Uses For This Medicine

Exenatide injection is used to treat high blood sugar levels that are caused by a type of diabetes mellitus or sugar diabetes called type 2 diabetes. Normally, after you eat, your pancreas releases insulin to help your body store excess sugar for later use. This process occurs during normal digestion of food. In type 2 diabetes, your body does not work properly to store the excess sugar and the sugar remains in your bloodstream. Chronic high blood sugar can lead to serious health problems in the future. Proper diet is the first step in managing type 2 diabetes but often medicines are needed to help your body. Exenatide helps your body cope with high blood sugar in several ways. Exenatide helps the cells in the pancreas that produce insulin when there is too much sugar in your blood. Exenatide helps the cells of your liver to decrease the amount of sugar the liver dumps into your blood. Exenatide slows down the passage of food from your stomach and helps to decrease the amount of sugar added to your blood after eating. Exenatide also reduces the amount of food needed because the sugar in the bloodstream is processed more effectively.

This medicine is available only with your doctor's prescription.

Before Using This Medicine

In deciding to use a medicine, the risks of taking the medicine must be weighed against the good it will do. This is a decision you and your doctor will make. For this medicine, the following should be considered:

Allergies—Tell your doctor if you have ever had any unusual or allergic reaction to this medicine or any other medicines. Also tell your health care professional if you have any other types of allergies, such as to foods, dyes, preservatives, or animals. For non-prescription products, read the label or package ingredients carefully.

Pediatric—Studies on this medicine have been done only in adult patients, and there is no specific information comparing use of exenatide in children with use in other age groups.

Geriatric—This medicine has been tested and has not been shown to cause different side effects or problems in older people than it does in younger adults.

Pregnancy—

	Pregnancy Category	Explanation
All Trimesters	C	Animal studies have shown an adverse effect and there are no adequate studies in pregnant women OR no animal studies have been conducted and there are no adequate studies in pregnant women.

Breast Feeding—There are no adequate studies in women for determining infant risk when using this medication during breastfeeding. Weigh the potential benefits against the potential risks before taking this medication while breastfeeding.

Other medicines—Although certain medicines should not be used together at all, in other cases two different medicines may be used together even if an interaction might occur. In these cases, your doctor may want to change the dose, or other precautions may be necessary. Tell your healthcare professional if you are taking any other prescription or non-prescription (over-the-counter [OTC]) medicine.

Interactions with Food/Tobacco/Alcohol—Certain medicines should not be used at or around the time of eating food or eating certain types of food since interactions may occur. Using alcohol or tobacco with certain medicines may also cause interactions to occur. Discuss with your healthcare professional the use of your medicine with food, alcohol, or tobacco.

Other medical problems—The presence of other medical problems may affect the use of this medicine. Make sure you tell your doctor if you have any other medical problems, especially:
- Diabetic ketoacidosis or
- Type 1 diabetes—These conditions should be treated with insulin.
- Gastrointestinal disease, severe or
- Kidney disease, end-stage—May make symptoms such as nausea, diarrhea, and vomiting worse
- Liver disease—Use with caution

Proper Use of This Medicine

Dosing—The dose of this medicine will be different for different patients. Follow your doctor's orders or the directions on the label. The following information includes only the average doses of this medicine. If your dose is different, do not change it unless your doctor tells you to do so.

The amount of medicine that you take depends on the strength of the medicine. Also, the number of doses you take each day, the time allowed between doses, and the length of time you take the medicine depend on the medical problem for which you are using the medicine.
- For subcutaneous dosage form (injection):
  - For type 2 diabetes:
    - Adults—At first, your dose will be an injection to the thigh, upper arm, or stomach of 5 mcg two times a day at any time within the 60–minute period before the morning and evening meals. Your doctor may adjust your dose after the first month of therapy to 10 mcg twice a day.
    - Children—Use and dose must be determined by your doctor.

Missed dose—If you miss a dose of this medicine, skip the missed dose and go back to your regular dosing schedule. Do not double doses.

Storage—Store in the refrigerator. Do not freeze.

Do not keep outdated medicine or medicine no longer needed.

Ask your healthcare professional how you should dispose of any medicine you do not use.

The pen should be discarded 30 days after the first time it is used.

Precautions While Using This Medicine

Your doctor will want to check your progress at regular visits.

It is very important to follow carefully any instructions from your health care team about:

- Alcohol—Drinking alcohol may cause severe low blood sugar. Discuss this with your health care team.
- Other medicines—Do not take other medicines during the time you are taking exenatide unless they have been discussed with your doctor. This especially includes non-prescription medicines such as aspirin, and medicines for appetite control, asthma, colds, cough, hay fever, or sinus problems.
- Counseling—Other family members need to learn how to prevent side effects or help with side effects if they occur. Also, diabetic patients may need special counseling about diabetes medicine dosing changes that might occur because of lifestyle changes, such as changes in exercise and diet. Furthermore, counseling on contraception and pregnancy may be needed because of the problems that can occur in patients with diabetes during pregnancy.
- Travel—Keep a recent prescription and your medical history with you. Be prepared for an emergency as you would normally. Make allowances for changing time zones and keep your meal times as close as possible to your usual meal times.

In case of emergency—There may be a time when you need emergency help for a problem caused by your diabetes. You need to be prepared for these emergencies. It is a good idea to wear a medical identification (ID) bracelet or neck chain at all times. Also, carry an ID card in your wallet or purse that says that you have diabetes and a list of all of your medicines.

This medicine does not cause hypoglycemia (low blood sugar). However, low blood sugar can occur when exenatide is taken with other medicines, such as insulin or sulfonylureas, that can lower blood sugar. Low blood sugar can also occur if you delay or miss a meal or snack, exercise more than usual, drink alcohol, or cannot eat because of nausea or vomiting.

Symptoms of low blood sugar include anxiety; behavior change similar to being drunk; blurred vision; cold sweats; confusion; cool, pale skin; difficulty in thinking; drowsiness; excessive hunger; fast heartbeat; headache (continuing); nausea; nervousness; nightmares; restless sleep; shakiness; slurred speech; or unusual tiredness or weakness.

If symptoms of low blood sugar occur, *eat glucose tablets or gel, corn syrup, honey, or sugar cubes; or drink fruit juice, non-diet soft drink, or sugar dissolved in water to relieve the symptoms.* Also, check your blood for low blood sugar. *Glucagon is used in emergency situations when severe symptoms such as seizures (convulsions) or unconsciousness occur.* Have a glucagon kit available, along with a syringe and needle, and know how to use it. Members of your family should also know how to use it.

Hyperglycemia (high blood sugar) may occur if you do not take enough or skip a dose of your antidiabetic medicine, overeat or do not follow your meal plan, have a fever or infection, or do not exercise as much as usual.

Symptoms of high blood sugar include blurred vision; drowsiness; dry mouth; flushed, dry skin; fruit-like breath odor; increased urination (frequency and amount); ketones in urine; loss of appetite; stomachache, nausea, or vomiting; tiredness; troubled breathing (rapid and deep); unconsciousness; or unusual thirst.

If symptoms of high blood sugar occur, *check your blood sugar level and then call your doctor for instructions.*

Side Effects of This Medicine

Along with its needed effects, a medicine may cause some unwanted effects. Although not all of these side effects may occur, if they do occur they may need medical attention.

Some side effects may occur that usually do not need medical attention. These side effects may go away during treatment as your body adjusts to the medicine. Also, your health care professional may be able to tell you about ways to prevent or reduce some of these side effects. Check with your health care professional if any of the following side effects continue or are bothersome or if you have any questions about them:

More common
> Acid or sour stomach; belching; diarrhea; dizziness; feeling jittery; headache; heartburn; indigestion; nausea; stomach discomfort upset or pain; vomiting

Less common
> Appetite decreased; heartburn; increased sweating; lack or loss of strength

Other side effects not listed may also occur in some patients. If you notice any other effects, check with your healthcare professional.

EZETIMIBE (Oral route) - ez-ET-i-mibe

Commonly used brand name(s)
In the U.S.—
> Zetia

Available Dosage Forms:
- Tablet

Therapeutic Class: Antihyperlipidemic
Pharmacologic Class: Cholesterol Absorption Inhibitor

Uses For This Medicine

Ezetimibe is used to lower cholesterol and triglyceride (fat-like substances) levels in the blood. Using this medicine may help prevent medical problems caused by such substances clogging the blood vessels.

This medicine is available only with your doctor's prescription.

Before Using This Medicine

In deciding to use a medicine, the risks of taking the medicine must be weighed against the good it will do. This is a decision you and your doctor will make. For this medicine, the following should be considered:

Allergies—Tell your doctor if you have ever had any unusual or allergic reaction to this medicine or any other medicines. Also tell your health care professional if you have any other types of allergies, such as to foods, dyes, preservatives, or animals. For non-prescription products, read the label or package ingredients carefully.

Pediatric—This medicine has been tested in children and, in effective doses, has not been shown to cause different side effects or problems than it does in adults. This medicine should only be used in children 10 years of age or older.

Geriatric—Many medicines have not been studied specifically in older people. Therefore, it may not be known whether they work exactly the same way they do in younger adults.

Although there is no specific information comparing use of ezetimibe in the elderly with use in other age groups, this medicine has been used in elderly patients and is not expected to cause different side effects or problems in older people than it does in younger adults.

Pregnancy—

	Pregnancy Category	Explanation
All Trimesters	C	Animal studies have shown an adverse effect and there are no adequate studies in pregnant women OR no animal studies have been conducted and there are no adequate studies in pregnant women.

Breast Feeding—There are no adequate studies in women for determining infant risk when using this medication during breastfeeding. Weigh the potential benefits against the potential risks before taking this medication while breastfeeding.

Other medicines—

Using this medicine with any of the following medicines is usually not recommended, but may be required in some cases. If both medicines are prescribed together, your doctor may change the dose or how often you use one or both of the medicines.

Clofibrate, Gemfibrozil

Interactions with Food/Tobacco/Alcohol—Certain medicines should not be used at or around the time of eating food or eating certain types of food since interactions may occur. Using alcohol or tobacco with certain medicines may also cause interactions to occur. Discuss with your healthcare professional the use of your medicine with food, alcohol, or tobacco.

Other medical problems—The presence of other medical problems may affect the use of this medicine. Make sure you tell your doctor if you have any other medical problems, especially:

- Liver disease (or history of) or
- Liver enzymes, persistently high levels—Use of this medicine may make liver problems worse

Proper Use of This Medicine

Before prescribing medicine for your condition, your doctor will probably try to control your condition by prescribing a personal diet for you. Such a diet may be low in fats, sugars, and/or cholesterol. Many people are able to control their condition by carefully following their doctor's orders for proper diet and exercise. Medicine is prescribed only when additional help is needed and is effective only when a schedule of diet and exercise is properly followed.

Also, this medicine is less effective if you are greatly overweight. It may be very important for you to go on a weight-reducing diet. However, check with your doctor before going on any diet.

Dosing—The dose of this medicine will be different for different patients. Follow your doctor's orders or the directions on the label. The following information includes only the average doses of this medicine. If your dose is different, do not change it unless your doctor tells you to do so.

The amount of medicine that you take depends on the strength of the medicine. Also, the number of doses you take each day, the time allowed between doses, and the length of time you take the medicine depend on the medical problem for which you are using the medicine.

Follow carefully the special diet your doctor gave you. This is the most important part of controlling your condition and is necessary if the medicine is to work properly.

- For tablet dosage form:
  - For high cholesterol:
    - Adults: 10 milligrams (mg) once daily. May take with or without food.
    - Children up to 10 years of age—Use is not recommended.
    - Children 10 years of age and older—10 milligrams (mg) once daily. May take with or without food.

Missed dose—If you miss a dose of this medicine, take it as soon as possible. However, if it is almost time for your next dose, skip the missed dose and go back to your regular dosing schedule. Do not double doses.

Storage—Store the medicine in a closed container at room temperature, away from heat, moisture, and direct light. Keep from freezing.

Keep out of the reach of children.

Do not keep outdated medicine or medicine no longer needed.

Ask your healthcare professional how you should dispose of any medicine you do not use.

Precautions While Using This Medicine

It is very important that your doctor check you at regular visits. This will allow your doctor to see if the medicine is working properly to lower your cholesterol. Your doctor can then decide if you should continue to take it.

Check with your doctor immediately if you think that you may be pregnant. Certain cholesterol medications may cause birth defects or other problems in the baby if taken during pregnancy.

Tell your doctor if you experience any unexplained muscle pain, tenderness, or weakness.

Do not take other medicines unless they have been discussed with your doctor. It is very important that you take all of your medicine. Your doctor will discuss with you any changes in your medicine. Ask your doctor if you have any questions.

Side Effects of This Medicine

Along with its needed effects, a medicine may cause some unwanted effects. Although not all of these side effects may occur, if they do occur they may need medical attention.

Frequency not determined

Abdominal fullness; black tarry stools; bleeding gums; bloating; blood in urine or stools; chills; constipation; darkened urine; fast heartbeat; fever; gaseous abdominal pain; general tiredness or weakness; indigestion; large, hive-like swelling on face, eyelids, lips, tongue, throat, hands, legs, feet, sex organs; loss of appetite; light-colored stools; muscle cramps or spasms; muscular tenderness, wasting or weakness; nausea; pains in stomach, side or abdomen, possibly radiating to the back; pinpoint red spots on skin; recurrent fever; severe nausea; skin rash; unusual bleeding or bruising; upper right abdominal pain; vomiting; yellow eyes or skin

Some side effects may occur that usually do not need medical attention. These side effects may go away during treatment as your body adjusts to the medicine. Also, your health care professional may be able to tell you about ways to prevent or reduce some of these side effects. Check with your health care professional if any of the following side effects continue or are bothersome or if you have any questions about them:

More common
Fever; headache; muscle pain; runny nose; sore throat

Less common
Back pain; body aches or pain; chest pain; chills; cold or flu-like symptoms; congestion; coughing; diarrhea; difficulty in moving; dizziness; dryness or soreness of throat; hoarseness; muscle pain or stiffness; pain in joints; pain or tenderness around eyes and cheek-bones; shortness of breath or troubled breathing; stomach pain; stuffy nose; tender, swollen glands in neck; tightness of chest or wheezing; trouble in swallowing; unusual tiredness or weakness; voice changes

Other side effects not listed may also occur in some patients. If you notice any other effects, check with your healthcare professional.

EZETIMIBE AND SIMVASTATIN
(Oral route) - ez-ET-i-mibe, SIM-va-stat-in

Commonly used brand name(s)

In the U.S.—
Vytorin

Available Dosage Forms:
• Tablet

Therapeutic Class: Antihyperlipidemic
Pharmacologic Class: Cholesterol Absorption Inhibitor

Uses For This Medicine

Ezetimibe and simvastatin is used to lower cholesterol and triglyceride (fat-like substances) levels in the blood. Using this medicine may help prevent medical problems caused by such substances clogging the blood vessels.

This medicine is available only with your doctor's prescription.

Before Using This Medicine

In deciding to use a medicine, the risks of taking the medicine must be weighed against the good it will do. This is a decision you and your doctor will make. For this medicine, the following should be considered:

Allergies—Tell your doctor if you have ever had any unusual or allergic reaction to this medicine or any other medicines. Also tell your health care professional if you have any other types of allergies, such as to foods, dyes, preservatives, or animals. For non-prescription products, read the label or package ingredients carefully.

Pediatric—This medicine has been tested in children and, in effective doses, has not been shown to cause different side effects or problems than it does in adults. This medicine should only be used in children 10 years of age or older.

Geriatric—This medicine has been tested and has not been shown to cause different side effects or problems in older people than it does in younger adults

Other medicines—

Using this medicine with any of the following medicines is not recommended. Your doctor may decide not to treat you with this medication or change some of the other medicines you take.

Itraconazole, Mibefradil

Interactions with Food/Tobacco/Alcohol—Certain medicines should not be used at or around the time of eating food or eating certain types of food since interactions may occur. Using alcohol or tobacco with certain medicines may also cause interactions to occur. The following interactions have been selected on the basis of their potential significance and are not necessarily all-inclusive.

Using this medicine with any of the following is usually not recommended, but may be unavoidable in some cases. If used together, your doctor may change the dose or how often you use this medicine, or give you special instructions about the use of food, alcohol, or tobacco.

Grapefruit Juice

Other medical problems—The presence of other medical problems may affect the use of this medicine. Make sure you tell your doctor if you have any other medical problems, especially:
• Liver disease (or history of) or
• Liver enzymes, persistently high levels—Use of this medicine may make liver problems worse
• Major surgery or serious illness—May increase chance of kidney side effects
• Complicated medical histories or
• Diabetes mellitus (sugar diabetes) or
• Kidney disease—May increase risk of muscle side effects

Proper Use of This Medicine

Before prescribing medicine for your condition, your doctor will probably try to control your condition by prescribing a personal diet for you. Such a diet may be low in fats, sugars, and/or cholesterol. Many people are able to control their condition by carefully following their doctor's orders for proper diet and exercise. Medicine is prescribed only when additional help is needed and is effective only when a schedule of diet and exercise is properly followed.

Also, this medicine is less effective if you are greatly overweight. It may be very important for you to go on a weight-reducing diet. However, check with your doctor before going on any diet.

Dosing—The dose of this medicine will be different for different patients. Follow your doctor's orders or the directions on the label. The following information includes only the average doses of this medicine. If your dose is different, do not change it unless your doctor tells you to do so.

The amount of medicine that you take depends on the strength of the medicine. Also, the number of doses you take each day, the time allowed between doses, and the length of time you take the medicine depend on the medical problem for which you are using the medicine.

Follow carefully the special diet your doctor gave you. This is the most important part of controlling your condition and is necessary if the medicine is to work properly.

- For oral dosage form (tablets):
  - For high cholesterol:
    - Adults—1 tablet a day, tablet strength is determined by your doctor.
    - Children—Use and dose must be determined by your doctor.

Missed dose—If you miss a dose of this medicine, take it as soon as possible. However, if it is almost time for your next dose, skip the missed dose and go back to your regular dosing schedule. Do not double doses.

Storage—Store the medicine in a closed container at room temperature, away from heat, moisture, and direct light. Do not refrigerate. Keep from freezing.

Keep out of the reach of children.

Do not keep outdated medicine or medicine no longer needed.

Ask your healthcare professional how you should dispose of any medicine you do not use.

Precautions While Using This Medicine

It is very important that your doctor check you at regular visits. This will allow your doctor to see if the medicine is working properly to lower your cholesterol. Your doctor can then decide if you should continue to take it.

Check with your doctor immediately if you think that you may be pregnant. Certain cholesterol medications may cause birth defects or other problems in the baby if taken during pregnancy.

Do not take other medicines unless they have been discussed with your doctor. It is very important that you take all of your medicine. Your doctor will discuss with you any changes in your medicine. Ask your doctor if you have any questions.

Check with your doctor immediately if you experience unexplained muscle pain, tenderness, or weakness, especially if it is accompanied by unusual tiredness or fever, because the medicine's adverse effects on muscle can lead to serious kidney problems.

Side Effects of This Medicine

Along with its needed effects, a medicine may cause some unwanted effects. Although not all of these side effects may occur, if they do occur they may need medical attention.

Check with your doctor immediately if any of the following side effects occur:
Incidence not known
  Abdominal fullness; bloating; chills; constipation; darkened urine; fast heartbeat; fever; gaseous abdominal pain; hives; hoarseness; indigestion; irritation; itching; joint pain; large, hive-like swelling on face, eyelids, lips, tongue, throat, hands, legs, feet, sex organs; loss of appetite; nausea; pains in stomach, side, or abdomen, possibly radiating to the back; severe nausea; stomach pain; rash; recurrent fever; redness of skin; shortness of breath; stiffness; swelling of eyelids, face, lips, hands, or feet; tightness in chest; troubled breathing or swallowing; vomiting; wheezing; yellow eyes or skin

Some side effects may occur that usually do not need medical attention. These side effects may go away during treatment as your body adjusts to the medicine. Also, your health care professional may be able to tell you about ways to prevent or reduce some of these side effects. Check with your health care professional if any of the following side effects continue or are bothersome or if you have any questions about them:
Less common
  Body aches or pain; cough; diarrhea; difficulty in breathing; difficulty in moving; ear congestion; general feeling of discomfort or illness; headache; loss of voice; muscle aches and pains or cramping; muscle stiffness; nasal congestion; pain in arms or legs; runny nose; shivering; sneezing; sore throat; sweating; swollen joints; trouble sleeping; unusual tiredness or weakness; vomiting

Other side effects not listed may also occur in some patients. If you notice any other effects, check with your healthcare professional.

FAMCICLOVIR (Oral route) - fam-SYE-kloe-veer

Commonly used brand name(s)

In the U.S.—
  Famvir

Available Dosage Forms:
- Tablet

Therapeutic Class: Antiviral

Uses For This Medicine

Famciclovir is used to treat the symptoms of herpes zoster (also known as shingles), a herpes virus infection of the skin. It is used to treat and suppress herpes labialis (cold sores) and recurrent episodes of genital herpes infection. This medicine is also used to treat recurrent herpes virus infections of the mucous membranes (lips and mouth) and genitals in HIV-infected patients. Although famciclovir will not cure genital herpes or herpes zoster, it does help relieve the pain and discomfort and helps the sores heal faster.

This medicine is available only with your doctor's prescription.

Before Using This Medicine

In deciding to use a medicine, the risks of taking the medicine must be weighed against the good it will do. This is a decision you and your doctor will make. For this medicine, the following should be considered:

Allergies—Tell your doctor if you have ever had any unusual or allergic reaction to this medicine or any other medicines. Also tell your health care professional if you have any other types of allergies, such as to foods, dyes, preservatives, or animals. For non-prescription products, read the label or package ingredients carefully.

Pediatric—No information is available on the relationship of age to the effects of famciclovir in children under 18 years of age. Safety and efficacy have not been established.

Geriatric—Appropriate studies performed to date have not demonstrated geriatrics-specific problems that would limit the usefulness of famciclovir in the elderly. However, elderly patients are more likely to have age-related kidney disease, which may require caution in patients receiving this medicine.

Pregnancy—

	Pregnancy Category	Explanation
All Trimesters	B	Animal studies have revealed no evidence of harm to the fetus, however, there are no adequate studies in pregnant women OR animal studies have shown an adverse effect, but adequate studies in pregnant women have failed to demonstrate a risk to the fetus.

Breast Feeding—There are no adequate studies in women for determining infant risk when using this medication during breastfeeding. Weigh the potential benefits against the potential risks before taking this medication while breastfeeding.

Other medicines—Although certain medicines should not be used together at all, in other cases two different medicines may be used together even if an interaction might occur. In these cases, your doctor may want to change the dose, or other precautions may be necessary. Tell your healthcare professional if you are taking any other prescription or non-prescription (over-the-counter [OTC]) medicine.

Interactions with Food/Tobacco/Alcohol—Certain medicines should not be used at or around the time of eating food or eating certain types of food since interactions may occur. Using alcohol or tobacco with certain medicines may also cause interactions to occur. Discuss with your healthcare professional the use of your medicine with food, alcohol, or tobacco.

Other medical problems—The presence of other medical problems may affect the use of this medicine. Make sure you tell your doctor if you have any other medical problems, especially:

- Galactose intolerance or
- Glucose-galactose malabsorption or
- Severe lactase deficiency—Patients with these condition should not take this medicine.
- Kidney disease—Kidney disease may increase blood levels of this medicine, increasing the chance of side effects. Dosage adjustment may be required.

Proper Use of This Medicine

Famciclovir is best used within 48 hours after the symptoms of shingles (for example, pain, burning, blisters) begin to appear, or within 6 hours after the symptoms of recurrent genital herpes (for example, pain, blisters) begin to appear.

Famciclovir may be taken with or without food

To help clear up your herpes infection, keep taking famciclovir for the full time of treatment, even if your symptoms begin to clear up after a few days. Do not miss any doses. However, do not use this medicine more often or for a longer time than your doctor ordered.

Dosing—The dose of this medicine will be different for different patients. Follow your doctor's orders or the directions on the label. The following information includes only the average doses of this medicine. If your dose is different, do not change it unless your doctor tells you to do so.

The amount of medicine that you take depends on the strength of the medicine. Also, the number of doses you take each day, the time allowed between doses, and the length of time you take the medicine depend on the medical problem for which you are using the medicine.

- For oral dosage form (tablets):
  - For treatment of shingles:
    - Adults—500 milligrams (mg) every eight hours for seven days.
    - Children—Use and dose must be determined by your doctor.
  - For suppression of recurrent genital herpes:
    - Adults—250 mg two times a day for up to one year.
    - Children—Use and dose must be determined by your doctor.
  - For treatment of recurrent genital herpes:
    - Adults—1000 mg two times a day for one day.
    - Children—Use and dose must be determined by your doctor.
  - For treatment of recurrent herpes labialis (cold sores):
    - Adults—1500 mg as a single dose.
    - Children—Use and dose must be determined by your doctor.
  - For treatment of recurrent herpes virus infections of the mucous membranes (lips and mouth) and genitals in HIV-infected patients:
    - Adults—500 mg two times a day for seven days.
    - Children—Use and dose must be determined by your doctor.

Missed dose—If you miss a dose of this medicine, take it as soon as possible. However, if it is almost time for your next dose, skip the missed dose and go back to your regular dosing schedule. Do not double doses.

Storage—Store the medicine in a closed container at room temperature, away from heat, moisture, and direct light. Keep from freezing.

Keep out of the reach of children.

Do not keep outdated medicine or medicine no longer needed.

Precautions While Using This Medicine

If your symptoms do not improve within a few days, or if they become worse, check with your doctor.

The areas affected by herpes should be kept as clean and dry as possible. Also, wear loose-fitting clothing to avoid irritating the sores (blisters).

This medicine may cause some people to become dizzy, drowsy, or less alert than they are normally. If any of these side effects occur, do not drive, use machines, or do anything else that could be dangerous if you are dizzy or are not alert while you are taking famciclovir.

This medicine does not prevent the sexual transmission of genital herpes. You should avoid having sex when lesions are present to avoid infecting your partner.

Side Effects of This Medicine

Along with its needed effects, a medicine may cause some unwanted effects. Although not all of these side effects may occur, if they do occur they may need medical attention.

Check with your doctor immediately if any of the following side effects occur:

Incidence not known

Black, tarry stools; bleeding gums; blistering, peeling, loosening of skin; blood in urine or stools; chills; clay-colored stools; cough; dark urine; dizziness; fever; joint or muscle pain; loss of appetite; pinpoint red spots on skin; red, irritated eyes; sore throat; sores, ulcers, or white spots in mouth or on lips; unpleasant breath odor; unusual bleeding or bruising; vomiting of blood; yellow eyes or skin.

Some side effects may occur that usually do not need medical attention. These side effects may go away during treatment as your body adjusts to the medicine. Also, your health care professional may be able to tell you about ways to prevent or reduce some of these side effects. Check with your health care professional if any of the following side effects continue or are bothersome or if you have any questions about them:

More common

Cramps; diarrhea; headache; heavy bleeding; nausea; stomach pain.

Less common

Bloated full feeling; burning, crawling, itching, numbness, prickling, "pins and needles", or tingling feeling; confusion as to time, place, or person; excess air or gas in stomach or intestines; hives or welts; holding false beliefs that cannot be changed by fact; itching skin; mood or mental changes; passing gas; rash; redness of skin; seeing, hearing, or feeling things that are not there; unusual excitement, nervousness, or restlessness; unusual tiredness or weakness; vomiting.

Incidence not known

Sleepiness or unusual drowsiness.

Other side effects not listed may also occur in some patients. If you notice any other effects, check with your healthcare professional.

FELBAMATE (Oral route) - FEL-ba-mate

Black Box Warning

The use of felbamate is associated with a marked increase in the incidence of aplastic anemia. Accordingly, felbamate should only be used in patients whose epilepsy is so severe that the risk of aplastic anemia is deemed acceptable in light of the benefits conferred by its use. Ordinarily, a patient should not be placed on and/or continued on felbamate without consideration of appropriate expert hematologic consultation.

Among felbamate treated patients, aplastic anemia (pancytopenia in the presence of a bone marrow largely depleted of hematopoietic precursors) occurs at an incidence that may be more than a 100 fold greater than that seen in the untreated population (ie, 2 to 5 per million persons per year).

The risk of death in patients with aplastic anemia generally varies as a function of its severity and etiology; current estimates of the overall case fatality rate are in the range of 20% to 30%, but rates as high as 70% have been reported in the past.

There are too few felbamate associated cases, and too little known about them to provide a reliable estimate of the syndrome's incidence or its case fatality rate or to identify the factors, if any, that might conceivably be used to predict who is at greater or lesser risk.

In managing patients on felbamate, it should be borne in mind that the clinical manifestation of aplastic anemia may not be seen until after a patient has been on felbamate for several months (eg, onset of aplastic anemia among felbamate exposed patients for whom data are available has ranged from 5 weeks to 30 weeks). However, the injury to bone marrow stem cells that is held to be ultimately responsible for the anemia may occur weeks to months earlier. Accordingly, patients who are discontinued from felbamate remain at risk for developing anemia for a variable, and unknown, period afterwards.

It is not known whether or not the risk of developing aplastic anemia changes with duration of exposure. Consequently, it is not safe to assume that a patient who has been on felbamate without signs of hematologic abnormality for long periods of time is without risk.

It is not known whether or not the dose of felbamate affects the incidence of aplastic anemia.

It is not known whether or not concomitant use of antiepileptic drugs and/or other drugs affects the incidence of aplastic anemia.

Aplastic anemia typically develops without premonitory clinical or laboratory signs, the full blown syndrome presenting with signs of infection, bleeding, or anemia. Accordingly, routine blood testing cannot be reliably used to reduce the incidence of aplastic anemia, but, it will, in some cases, allow the detection of the hematologic changes before the syndrome declares itself clinically. Felbamate should be discontinued if any evidence of bone marrow depression occurs.

Evaluation of postmarketing experience suggests that acute liver failure is associated with the use of felbamate. The reported rate in the US has been about 6 cases of liver failure leading to death or transplant per 75,000 patient years of use. This rate is an underestimate because of under reporting, and the true rate could be considerably greater than this. For example, if the reporting rate is 10%, the true rate would be one case per 1,250 patient years of use.

Of the cases reported, about 67% resulted in death or liver transplantation, usually within 5 weeks of the onset of signs and symptoms of liver failure. The earliest onset of severe hepatic dysfunction followed subsequently by liver failure was 3 weeks after initiation of felbamate. Although some reports described dark urine and nonspecific prodromal symptoms (eg, anorexia, malaise, and gastrointestinal symptoms), in other reports it was not clear if any prodromal symptoms preceded the onset of jaundice.

It is not known whether or not the risk of developing hepatic failure changes with duration of exposure.

It is not known whether or not the dosage of felbamate affects the incidence of hepatic failure.

It is not known whether concomitant use of other antiepileptic drugs and/or other drugs affect the incidence of hepatic failure.

Felbamate should not be prescribed for anyone with a history of hepatic dysfunction.

Treatment with felbamate should be initiated only in individuals without active liver disease and with normal baseline serum transaminases. It has not been proved that periodic serum transaminase testing will prevent serious injury but it is generally believed that early detection of drug-induced hepatic injury along with immediate withdrawal of the suspect drug enhances the likelihood for recovery. There is no information available that documents how rapidly patients can progress from normal liver function to liver failure, but other drugs known to be hepatotoxins can cause liver failure rapidly (eg, from normal enzymes to liver failure in 2 weeks to 4 weeks). Accordingly, monitoring of serum transaminase levels (AST and ALT) is recommended at baseline and periodically thereafter. While the more frequent the monitoring the greater the chances of early detection, the precise schedule for monitoring is a matter of clinical judgement.

Felbamate should be discontinued if either serum AST or serum ALT levels become increased greater than or equal to 2 times the upper limit of normal, or if clinical signs and symptoms suggest liver failure. Patients who develop evidence of hepatocellular injury while on felbamate and are withdrawn from the drug for any reason should be presumed to be at increased risk for liver injury if felbamate is reintroduced. Accordingly, such patients should not be considered for re-treatment.

Commonly used brand name(s)

In the U.S.—
    Felbatol

Available Dosage Forms:
- Tablet
- Suspension

Therapeutic Class: Anticonvulsant

Uses For This Medicine

Felbamate is used to control some types of seizures in the treatment of epilepsy. Felbamate acts on the central nervous system (CNS) to make it more difficult for seizures to start or to continue. This medicine cannot cure epilepsy and will only work to control seizures for as long as you continue to use it.

Felbamate is available only with your doctor's prescription.

Before Using This Medicine

In deciding to use a medicine, the risks of taking the medicine must be weighed against the good it will do. This is a decision you and your doctor will make. For this medicine, the following should be considered:

Allergies—Tell your doctor if you have ever had any unusual or allergic reaction to this medicine or any other medicines. Also tell your health care professional if you have any other types of allergies, such as to foods, dyes, preservatives, or animals. For non-prescription products, read the label or package ingredients carefully.

Pediatric—This medicine has some very serious unwanted effects. Children may not be able to tell their parent or guardian or their doctor if they have symptoms of these effects, such as chills or stomach pain. Felbamate should be used in children only if other medicines have not controlled their seizures.

Geriatric—Many medicines have not been studied specifically in older people. Therefore, it may not be known whether they work exactly the same way they do in younger adults or if they cause different side effects or problems in older people. There is no specific information comparing use of felbamate in the elderly with use in other age groups. However, older people are more likely to have other illnesses and to use other medicines that may affect the way felbamate works. Your doctor may start with a lower felbamate dose or may increase the dose more slowly.

Pregnancy—

	Pregnancy Category	Explanation
All Trimesters	C	Animal studies have shown an adverse effect and there are no adequate studies in pregnant women OR no animal studies have been conducted and there are no adequate studies in pregnant women.

Breast Feeding—There are no adequate studies in women for determining infant risk when using this medication during breastfeeding. Weigh the potential benefits against the potential risks before taking this medication while breastfeeding.

Other medicines—

Using this medicine with any of the following medicines is usually not recommended, but may be required in some cases. If both medicines are prescribed together, your doctor may change the dose or how often you use one or both of the medicines.

Ethinyl Estradiol, Gestodene

Interactions with Food/Tobacco/Alcohol—Certain medicines should not be used at or around the time of eating food or eating certain types of food since interactions may occur. Using alcohol or tobacco with certain medicines may also cause interactions to occur. Discuss with your healthcare professional the use of your medicine with food, alcohol, or tobacco.

Other medical problems—The presence of other medical problems may affect the use of this medicine. Make sure you tell your doctor if you have any other medical problems, especially:
- Anemia or other blood problems (or history of) or
- Liver problems (or history of)—Felbamate may make the condition worse

Proper Use of This Medicine

Take this medicine only as directed by your doctor, to benefit your condition as much as possible. Do not take more of it, do not take it more often, and do not take it for a longer time than your doctor ordered.

For patients taking the oral liquid form of this medicine:
- Shake the bottle well before measuring the dose.

- Use a specially marked measuring spoon, a plastic syringe, or a small marked measuring cup to measure each dose accurately. The average household teaspoon may not hold the right amount of liquid.

To lessen stomach upset, felbamate may be taken with food, unless your doctor has told you to take it on an empty stomach.

Dosing—The dose of this medicine will be different for different patients. Follow your doctor's orders or the directions on the label. The following information includes only the average doses of this medicine. If your dose is different, do not change it unless your doctor tells you to do so.

The amount of medicine that you take depends on the strength of the medicine. Also, the number of doses you take each day, the time allowed between doses, and the length of time you take the medicine depend on the medical problem for which you are using the medicine.

- For oral dosage forms (suspension or tablets):
  - For epilepsy:
    - Adults and teenagers 14 years of age and older—At first, usually 1200 milligrams (mg) a day, divided into three or four smaller doses. Your doctor may increase the dose gradually over several weeks if needed. However, the dose is usually not more than 3600 mg a day.
    - Children 2 to 14 years of age—At first, usually 15 mg per kilogram (kg) [6.8 mg per pound] of body weight per day, divided into smaller doses that are given three or four times during the day. Your doctor may increase the dose gradually over a few weeks if needed. However, the dose is usually not more than 45 mg per kg [20.5 mg per pound] or 3600 mg per day, whichever is less.

Missed dose—If you miss a dose of this medicine, take it as soon as possible. However, if it is almost time for your next dose, skip the missed dose and go back to your regular dosing schedule. Do not double doses.

Storage—Store the medicine in a closed container at room temperature, away from heat, moisture, and direct light. Keep from freezing.

Keep out of the reach of children.

Do not keep outdated medicine or medicine no longer needed.

Precautions While Using This Medicine

It is important that your doctor check your progress at regular visits. This is necessary to allow dose adjustments and to test for serious unwanted effects.

Do not stop taking felbamate without first checking with your doctor. Your doctor may want you to gradually reduce the amount you are taking before stopping completely. Stopping the medicine suddenly may cause your seizures to return or to occur more often.

Felbamate may cause blurred vision, double vision, or other changes in vision. It may also cause some people to become dizzy or drowsy. Make sure you know how you react to this medicine before you drive, use machines, or do anything else that could be dangerous if you are not alert or able to see well. If these reactions are especially bothersome, check with your doctor.

Side Effects of This Medicine

Felbamate may cause some serious side effects, including blood problems and liver problems. You and your doctor should discuss the good this medicine will do as well as the risks of receiving it.

Along with its needed effects, a medicine may cause some unwanted effects. Some side effects will have signs or symptoms that you can see or feel. Your doctor may watch for others by doing certain tests. Although not all of these side effects may occur, if they do occur they may need medical attention.

Check with your doctor immediately if any of the following side effects occur:
> *More common*
>> Fever; purple or red spots on skin
>
> *Rare*
>> Black or tarry stools; blood in urine or stools; chills; continuing headache; continuing stomach pain; continuing vomiting; dark-colored urine; general feeling of tiredness or weakness; light-colored stools; nosebleeds or other unusual bruising or bleeding; shortness of breath, trouble in breathing, wheezing, or tightness in chest; sore throat; sores, ulcers, or white spots on lips or in mouth; swelling of face; swollen or painful glands; yellow eyes or skin

Check with your doctor as soon as possible if any of the following side effects occur:
> *More common*
>> Walking in unusual manner
>
> *Less common*
>> Agitation, aggression, or other mood or mental changes; clumsiness or unsteadiness; skin rash; trembling or shaking
>
> *Rare*
>> Chest pain; hives or itching; muscle cramps; nasal congestion; pain; sensitivity of skin to sunlight; swollen lymph nodes

Some side effects may occur that usually do not need medical attention. These side effects may go away during treatment as your body adjusts to the medicine. Also, your health care professional may be able to tell you about ways to prevent or reduce some of these side effects. Check with your health care professional if any of the following side effects continue or are bothersome or if you have any questions about them:
> *More common*
>> Change in your sense of taste; constipation; difficulty in sleeping; dizziness; headache; indigestion; loss of appetite; nausea; stomach pain; vomiting
>
> *Less common*
>> Blurred or double vision; coughing; diarrhea; drowsiness; ear congestion or pain; runny nose; sneezing; weight loss

This medicine may also cause the following side effects that your doctor will watch for:
> *Rare*
>> Blood problems

Other side effects not listed may also occur in some patients. If you notice any other effects, check with your healthcare professional.

FENOFIBRATE (Oral route) - fen-oh-FIB-rate

Commonly used brand name(s)

In the U.S.—

Antara
Lipofen
Lofibra
Tricor
Triglide

Available Dosage Forms:
- Tablet
- Capsule

Therapeutic Class: Antihyperlipidemic

Uses For This Medicine

Fenofibrate is used to lower triglyceride (fat-like substances) levels and cholesterol levels in the blood. This may help prevent the development of pancreatitis (inflammation of the pancreas) caused by high levels of triglycerides in the blood.

This medicine is available only with your doctor's prescription.

Before Using This Medicine

In deciding to use a medicine, the risks of taking the medicine must be weighed against the good it will do. This is a decision you and your doctor will make. For this medicine, the following should be considered:

In addition to its helpful effects in treating your medical problem, this type of medicine may have some harmful effects. Results of large studies using other agents that are similar to fenofibrate seem to suggest that fenofibrate may increase the patient's risk of cancer, pancreatitis (inflammation of the pancreas), gallstones, and problems from gallbladder surgery. Studies with fenofibrate in rats found an increased risk of liver and pancreatic tumors when doses up to 6 times the human dose were given for a long time. Be sure you have discussed this with your doctor before taking this medicine.

Allergies—Tell your doctor if you have ever had any unusual or allergic reaction to this medicine or any other medicines. Also tell your health care professional if you have any other types of allergies, such as to foods, dyes, preservatives, or animals. For non-prescription products, read the label or package ingredients carefully.

Pediatric—Studies on this medicine have been done only in adult patients, and there is no specific information comparing use of fenofibrate in children with use in other age groups.

Geriatric—Although the effects of fenofibrate have not been fully tested in older people, this medicine has been tested in a limited number of patients 77 through 87 years of age and has not been shown to cause problems when given to older people.

Pregnancy—

	Pregnancy Category	Explanation
All Trimesters	C	Animal studies have shown an adverse effect and there are no adequate studies in pregnant women OR no animal studies have been conducted and there are no adequate studies in pregnant women.

Breast Feeding—There are no adequate studies in women for determining infant risk when using this medication during breastfeeding. Weigh the potential benefits against the potential risks before taking this medication while breastfeeding.

Other medicines—

Using this medicine with any of the following medicines is usually not recommended, but may be required in some cases. If both medicines are prescribed together, your doctor may change the dose or how often you use one or both of the medicines.

Acenocoumarol, Anisindione, Atorvastatin, Cerivastatin, Dicumarol, Fluvastatin, Lovastatin, Phenindione, Phenprocoumon, Pravastatin, Simvastatin, Warfarin

Interactions with Food/Tobacco/Alcohol—Certain medicines should not be used at or around the time of eating food or eating certain types of food since interactions may occur. Using alcohol or tobacco with certain medicines may also cause interactions to occur. Discuss with your healthcare professional the use of your medicine with food, alcohol, or tobacco.

Other medical problems—The presence of other medical problems may affect the use of this medicine. Make sure you tell your doctor if you have any other medical problems, especially:
- Gallbladder disease or
- Gallstones or
- Liver disease—Fenofibrate may make these conditions worse. You should NOT use fenofibrate if you have any of these conditions.
- Kidney disease—Higher blood levels of fenofibrate may result, which may increase the chance of side effects or make kidney problems worse. If you have severe kidney problems, you should NOT use fenofibrate.

Proper Use of This Medicine

Before prescribing medicine for your condition, your doctor will probably try to control your condition by prescribing a personal diet for you. Such a diet may be low in fats, sugars, and/or cholesterol. Many people are able to control their condition by carefully following their doctor's orders for proper diet and exercise. *Medicine is prescribed only when additional help is needed* and is effective only when a schedule of diet and exercise is properly followed.

Use this medicine only as directed by your doctor. Take the medication at the same time each day to maintain the medication's effect. Do not use more or less of it, and do not use it more often than your doctor ordered.

Follow carefully the special diet your doctor gave you. This is the most important part of controlling your condition and is necessary if the medicine is to work properly.

This medicine is usually taken once a day. Lipofen®, and Lofibra® should be taken with a meal. Antara®, Tricor®, and Triglide® can be taken with or without a meal.

Dosing—The dose of this medicine will be different for different patients. Follow your doctor's orders or the directions on the label. The following information includes only the average doses of this medicine. If your dose is different, do not change it unless your doctor tells you to do so.

The amount of medicine that you take depends on the strength of the medicine. Also, the number of doses you take

each day, the time allowed between doses, and the length of time you take the medicine depend on the medical problem for which you are using the medicine.

- For oral dosage form (capsules):
  - For hypertriglyceridemia (to lower triglycerides):
    - Adults—
      — Antara®—At first, 43 milligrams (mg) once a day with a meal. Your doctor may increase your dose as needed.
      — Lipofen®—At first, 50 to 150 milligrams (mg) once a day with a meal. Your doctor may increase your dose as needed.
      — Lofibra®—At first, 67 milligrams (mg) once a day with a meal. Your doctor may increase your dose as needed.
  - For hypercholesteremia (to lower cholesterol):
    - Adults—
      — Antara®—130 milligrams (mg) once a day with a meal.
      — Lipofen®—150 milligrams (mg) once a day with a meal.
      — Lofibra®—200 milligrams (mg) once a day with a meal.

- For oral dosage form (tablets):
  - For hypertriglyceridemia (to lower triglycerides):
    - Adults—
      — Tricor®—At first, 48 to 145 milligrams (mg) once daily. Your doctor may increase your dose as needed.
      — Triglide®—At first, 50 to 160 milligrams (mg) once daily. Your doctor may increase your dose as needed.
  - For hypercholesteremia (to lower cholesterol):
    - Adults
      — Tricor®—145 milligrams (mg) once daily.
      — Triglide®—160 milligrams (mg) once daily.

Missed dose—If you miss a dose of this medicine, take it as soon as possible. However, if it is almost time for your next dose, skip the missed dose and go back to your regular dosing schedule. Do not double doses.

Storage—Store the medicine in a closed container at room temperature, away from heat, moisture, and direct light. Keep from freezing.

Keep out of the reach of children.

Do not keep outdated medicine or medicine no longer needed.

Precautions While Using This Medicine

It is very important that your doctor check your progress at regular visits. This will allow your doctor to see if the medicine is working properly to lower your triglyceride levels and to decide if you should continue to take it.

Check with your doctor right away if you experience unexplained muscle pain, tenderness, or weakness, especially if accompanied by unusual tiredness or fever.

Check with your doctor right away if you think that you may be pregnant. Fenofibrate may cause birth defects or other problems in the baby if taken during pregnancy.

Check with your doctor right away if you have signs of an infection, such as a fever, sore throat, or chills.

Side Effects of This Medicine

Along with its needed effects, a medicine may cause some unwanted effects. Although not all of these side effects may occur, if they do occur they may need medical attention.

Check with your doctor immediately if any of the following side effects occur:
  Rare
    Chills, fever, or sore throat

Check with your doctor as soon as possible if any of the following side effects occur:
  Less common
    Chills, fever, muscle aches and pains, or nausea and/or vomiting; hives; infections; itching (generalized); skin rash
  Rare
    Bloating or pain of the stomach; chronic indigestion; cough and shortness of breath or troubled breathing; dark urine; general ill feeling; loss of appetite; muscle cramps, pain, stiffness, swelling, or weakness; nausea; unusual bleeding or bruising; unusual tiredness; vomiting; yellow eyes or skin

Some side effects may occur that usually do not need medical attention. These side effects may go away during treatment as your body adjusts to the medicine. Also, your health care professional may be able to tell you about ways to prevent or reduce some of these side effects. Check with your health care professional if any of the following side effects continue or are bothersome or if you have any questions about them:
  More common
    Chest congestion; difficulty breathing
  Less common
    Back pain; belching; constipation; decreased sexual drive; diarrhea; dizziness; eye irritation; gas; headache; increased sensitivity of the skin to sunlight; lack or loss of strength; stomach pain; stuffy nose

Other side effects not listed may also occur in some patients. If you notice any other effects, check with your healthcare professional.

FENTANYL (Buccal route) - FEN-ta-nil

Black Box Warning

Physicians and other healthcare providers must become familiar with the important warnings in this label.

Fentanyl citrate is indicated only for the management of breakthrough cancer pain in patients with malignancies who are already receiving and who are tolerant to opioid therapy for their underlying persistent cancer pain. Patients considered opioid tolerant are those who are taking at least 60 mg morphine/day, 50 mcg transdermal fentanyl/hour, or an equianalgesic dose of another opioid for a week or longer.

Because life-threatening hypoventilation could occur at any dose in patients not taking chronic opiates, fentanyl citrate is contraindicated in the management of acute or postoperative pain. This product must not be used in opioid non-tolerant patients.

Fentanyl citrate is intended to be used only in the care of cancer patients and only by oncologists and pain specialists who are knowledgeable of and skilled in the use of Schedule II opioids to treat cancer pain.

Patients and their caregivers must be instructed that fentanyl citrate contains a medicine in an amount which can be fatal to a child. Patients and their caregivers must be instructed to keep all units out of the reach of children and to discard opened units properly.

Commonly used brand name(s)

In the U.S.—
   Actiq

Available Dosage Forms:
• Lozenge/Troche

Therapeutic Class: Analgesic

Uses For This Medicine

Fentanyl belongs to the group of medicines called narcotic analgesics (nar-KOT-ik an-al-GEE-ziks). Narcotic analgesics are used to relieve pain. The transmucosal form of fentanyl is used to treat breakthrough cancer pain. Breakthrough episodes of cancer pain are the flares of pain which "breakthrough" the medication used to control the persistent pain. Transmucosal fentanyl is only used in patients who are already taking narcotic analgesics.

Fentanyl acts in the central nervous system (CNS) to relieve pain. Some of its side effects are also caused by actions in the CNS. When a narcotic is used for a long time, it may become habit-forming (causing mental or physical dependence). However, people who have continuing pain should not let the fear of dependence keep them from using narcotics to relieve their pain. Mental dependence (addiction) is not likely to occur when narcotics are used for this purpose. Physical dependence may lead to withdrawal side effects if treatment is stopped suddenly. However, severe withdrawal side effects can usually be prevented by reducing the dose gradually over a period of time before treatment is stopped completely. Your health care professional will take this into consideration when deciding on the amount of transmucosal fentanyl you should receive.

This medicine is available only with your doctor's prescription.

Before Using This Medicine

In deciding to use a medicine, the risks of taking the medicine must be weighed against the good it will do. This is a decision you and your doctor will make. For this medicine, the following should be considered:

Allergies—Tell your doctor if you have ever had any unusual or allergic reaction to this medicine or any other medicines. Also tell your health care professional if you have any other types of allergies, such as to foods, dyes, preservatives, or animals. For non-prescription products, read the label or package ingredients carefully.

Pediatric—Studies with transmucosal fentanyl have been done only in adult patients, and there is no specific information comparing use of transmucosal fentanyl in children with use in other age groups. It contains a medicine in an amount which can be fatal to a child. Patients and their caregivers should keep transmucosal fentanyl out of the reach of children and discard open units properly.

Geriatric—Elderly people may be especially sensitive to the effects of narcotic analgesics. This may increase the chance of side effects during treatment. Your health care professional will take this into consideration when deciding on the amount of transmucosal fentanyl you should receive.

Pregnancy—

	Pregnancy Category	Explanation
All Trimesters	C	Animal studies have shown an adverse effect and there are no adequate studies in pregnant women OR no animal studies have been conducted and there are no adequate studies in pregnant women.

Breast Feeding—Studies in women suggest that this medication poses minimal risk to the infant when used during breastfeeding.

Other medicines—

Using this medicine with any of the following medicines is not recommended. Your doctor may decide not to treat you with this medication or change some of the other medicines you take.

Naltrexone

Interactions with Food/Tobacco/Alcohol—Certain medicines should not be used at or around the time of eating food or eating certain types of food since interactions may occur. Using alcohol or tobacco with certain medicines may also cause interactions to occur. Discuss with your healthcare professional the use of your medicine with food, alcohol, or tobacco.

Other medical problems—The presence of other medical problems may affect the use of this medicine. Make sure you tell your doctor if you have any other medical problems, especially:

• Alcohol abuse or history of or

• Drug dependence, especially narcotic abuse or dependence, history of or

• Kidney disease or

• Liver disease—The chance of side effects may be increased

• Emphysema or other chronic lung disease or

• Head injuries—Some of the side effects of transmucosal fentanyl can cause serious problems in people who have these medical problems

• Slow heartbeat—Transmucosal fentanyl can make this condition worse

---

Proper Use of This Medicine

Transmucosal fentanyl contains a medicine in an amount which can be fatal to a child. Patients and their caregivers should keep transmucosal fentanyl out of the reach of children and discard open units properly.

Transmucosal fentanyl comes with patient instructions. Read them carefully before using the product.

How to use transmucosal fentanyl:
• Keep medication in sealed pouch until ready to use.
• The foil package should be opened with scissors immediately prior to product use.

- Place the medicine in mouth between the cheek and lower gum, occasionally moving the medicine from one side to the other using the handle.
- The medicine should be sucked, not chewed.
- Suck the medicine over a 15–minute period.

Dosing—The dose of this medicine will be different for different patients. Follow your doctor's orders or the directions on the label. The following information includes only the average doses of this medicine. If your dose is different, do not change it unless your doctor tells you to do so.

The amount of medicine that you take depends on the strength of the medicine. Also, the number of doses you take each day, the time allowed between doses, and the length of time you take the medicine depend on the medical problem for which you are using the medicine.

- For oral transmucosal dosage form:
  - For cancer pain:
    - Adults—The initial dose to treat episodes of breakthrough cancer pain in patients who are already receiving and who are tolerant to opioid therapy for their underlying persistent cancer pain is 200 micrograms. Redosing may start 15 minutes after the previous dose has been completed (30 minutes after the start of the previous dose). Patients should not use more than 2 units per episode of breakthrough pain. Patients should record their use over several episodes of breakthrough cancer pain and review their experience with their physicians to determine if a dosage adjustment is warranted.
    - Children—Use and dose must be determined by the doctor.

Missed dose—If you miss a dose of this medicine, take it as soon as possible. However, if it is almost time for your next dose, skip the missed dose and go back to your regular dosing schedule. Do not double doses.

Storage—Store the medicine in a closed container at room temperature, away from heat, moisture, and direct light. Keep from freezing.

Keep out of the reach of children.

Do not keep outdated medicine or medicine no longer needed.

Do not use if the foil pouch has been opened. A temporary storage bottle is provided as part of the Actiq [reg] Welcome Kit. This container is to be used by patients or their caregivers in the event that a partially consumed unit cannot be disposed of promptly. If additional assistance is required, refer to 1–800–615–0187.

Precautions While Using This Medicine

Transmucosal fentanyl contains a medicine in an amount which can be fatal to a child. Patients and their caregivers should keep transmucosal fentanyl out of the reach of children and discard open units properly.

Check with your health care professional at regular times while using fentanyl. Be sure to report any side effects.

Transmucosal fentanyl comes with patient instructions. Read them carefully before using the product.

This medicine will add to the effects of alcohol and other CNS depressants (medicines that can make you drowsy or less alert). Some examples of CNS depressants are antihistamines or medicine for hay fever, other allergies, or colds; sedatives, tranquilizers, or sleeping medicine; other prescription pain medicine or narcotics; barbiturates; medicine for seizures; muscle relaxants; or anesthetics, including some dental anesthetics. Check with your health care professional before taking any of the other medicines listed above while you are using this medicine.

Transmucosal fentanyl may cause some people to become drowsy, dizzy, or lightheaded, or to feel a false sense of well-being. Make sure you know how you react to this medicine before you drive, use machines, or do anything else that could be dangerous if you are dizzy or not alert and clear-headed. These effects usually go away after a few days of treatment, when your body gets used to the medicine. However, check with your health care professional if drowsiness that is severe enough to interfere with your activities continues for more than a few days.

Dizziness, lightheadedness, or even fainting may occur when you get up suddenly from a lying or sitting position. Getting up slowly may help lessen this problem. Also, lying down for a while may relieve dizziness or lightheadedness.

Using narcotics for a long time can cause severe constipation. To prevent this, your health care professional may direct you to take laxatives, drink a lot of fluids, or increase the amount of fiber in your diet. Be sure to follow the directions carefully, because continuing constipation can lead to more serious problems.

Before having any kind of surgery (including dental surgery) or emergency treatment, tell the medical doctor or dentist in charge that you are using this medicine. Serious side effects can occur if your medical doctor or dentist gives you certain other medicines without knowing that you are using transmucosal fentanyl.

If you have been using this medicine regularly for several weeks or more, do not suddenly stop using it without first checking with your health care professional. You may be directed to reduce gradually the amount you are using before stopping treatment completely to lessen the chance of withdrawal side effects.

Using too much transmucosal fentanyl, or taking too much of another narcotic while using transmucosal fentanyl, may cause an overdose. If this occurs, get emergency help right away. An overdose can cause severe breathing problems (breathing may even stop), unconsciousness, and death. Serious signs of an overdose include very slow breathing (fewer than 8 breaths a minute) and drowsiness that is so severe that you are not able to answer when spoken to or, if asleep, cannot be awakened. Other signs of an overdose may include cold, clammy skin; low blood pressure; pinpoint pupils of eyes; and slow heartbeat. It may be best to have a family member or a friend check on you several times a day when you start using a narcotic regularly, and whenever your dose is increased, so that he or she can get help for you if you cannot do so yourself.

Check with your dentist at regular times while using fentanyl. This medicine contains sugar and may increase your chance for tooth decay or other trouble with your teeth or gums.

Side Effects of This Medicine

Along with its needed effects, a medicine may cause some unwanted effects. Although not all of these side effects may occur, if they do occur they may need medical attention.

Check with your doctor as soon as possible if any of the following side effects occur:

More common

Dizziness, feeling faint, lightheadedness, unusual tiredness or weakness; shortness of breath

Less common

Anxiety; confusion; decrease in urine volume; decreased frequency of urination; drowsiness; false sense of well-being; nervousness; seeing, hearing, or feeling things that are not there

Incidence not known

tooth pain; trouble with gums; trouble with teeth

Symptoms of overdose

Cold, clammy skin; convulsions (seizures); feeling faint; pinpoint pupils of the eyes; severe dizziness, drowsiness, nervousness, restlessness, or weakness; slow or troubled breathing

Some side effects may occur that usually do not need medical attention. These side effects may go away during treatment as your body adjusts to the medicine. Also, your health care professional may be able to tell you about ways to prevent or reduce some of these side effects. Check with your health care professional if any of the following side effects continue or are bothersome or if you have any questions about them:

More common

Constipation; dry mouth; nausea and/or vomiting

After you stop using this medicine, it may still produce some side effects that need attention. During this period of time, *check with your doctor immediately* if you notice the following side effects:

Diarrhea; nausea and/or vomiting; restlessness or irritability; speech disorder; stomach cramps; trouble in sleeping; weakness

Other side effects not listed may also occur in some patients. If you notice any other effects, check with your healthcare professional.

FENTANYL (Transdermal route) - FEN-ta-nil

Black Box Warning

- **FENTANYL PATCH, DEVICE ASSISTED**
  - IONSYS(TM) should only be used for the treatment of hospitalized patients. Treatment with IONSYS(TM) should be discontinued before patients are discharged from the hospital.
  - Treatment with fentanyl, the active component of IONSYS(TM), may result in potentially life-threatening respiratory depression and death. To avoid potential overdosing, only the patient should activate IONSYS(TM) dosing.
  - Inappropriate use of IONSYS(TM), leading to ingestion or contact with mucous membranes or unintended exposure to the fentanyl hydrogel could lead to the absorption of a potentially fatal dose of fentanyl. Therefore, the hydrogels should not come into contact with fingers or mouth.
  - IONSYS(TM) contains fentanyl, a potent opioid agonist and a Schedule II controlled substance with high potential for abuse similar to hydromorphone, methadone, morphine, and oxycodone. Fentanyl can be abused in a manner similar to other opioid agonists, legal or illicit. This should be considered when prescribing or dispensing IONSYS(TM) in situations where the Health Care Professional is concerned about an increased risk of misuse, abuse, or diversion. After the maximum dosage administration, a significant amount of fentanyl remains in the device.
  - IONSYS(TM) should always be kept out of reach of children.
  - Prior to discharge from the hospital, medical personnel must remove the IONSYS(TM) system and dispose of it properly. After the maximum dosage administration, a significant amount of fentanyl remains in the device.

- **FENTANYL TRANSDERMAL SYSTEMS**
  - Because serious or life-threatening hypoventilation could occur, fentanyl is contraindicated: 1) in the management of acute or post-operative pain, including use in out-patient surgeries, 2) in the management of mild or intermittent pain responsive to as needed basis or non-opioid therapy and 3) in doses exceeding 25 mcg/hour at the initiation of opioid therapy.
  - Safety of fentanyl has not been established in children under 2 years of age. Fentanyl should be administered to children only if they are opioid tolerant and age 2 years or older.
  - Fentanyl is indicated for treatment of chronic pain (such as that of malignancy) that: 1) cannot be managed by lesser means such as acetaminophen-opioid combinations, non-steroidal analgesics, or as needed basis dosing with short-acting opioids and 2) requires continuous opioid administration.
  - The 50 mcg/hr, 75 mcg/hr, and 100 mcg/hr dosages should only be used in patients who are already on and are tolerant to opioid therapy.

- **FENTANYL TRANSDERMAL SYSTEMS - DURAGESIC®**
  - DURAGESIC® contains a high concentration of a potent Schedule II opioid agonist, fentanyl. Schedule II opioid substances which include fentanyl, hydromorphone, methadone, morphine, oxycodone, and oxymorphone have the highest potential for abuse and associated risk of fatal overdose due to respiratory depression. Fentanyl can be abused and is subject to criminal diversion. The high content of fentanyl in the patches may be a particular target for abuse and diversion.
  - Fentanyl should only be used in patients who are already receiving opioid therapy, who have demonstrated opioid tolerance, and who require a total daily dose at least equivalent to fentanyl 25 mcg/hour. Patients who are considered opioid-tolerant are those who have been taking, for a week or longer, at least 60 mg of morphine daily, or at least 30 mg of oral oxycodone daily, or at least 8 mg of oral hydromorphone daily or an equianalgesic dose of another opioid.
  - Since the peak fentanyl levels occur between 24 hours and 72 hours of treatment, prescribers should be aware that serious or life-threatening hypoventilation may occur, even in opioid-tolerant patients, during the initial application period.

○ The concomitant use of fentanyl with potent cytochrome P450 3A4 (CYP3A4) inhibitors (ritonavir, ketoconazole, itraconazole, troleandomycin, clarithromycin, nelfinavir, and nefazodone) may result in an increase in fentanyl plasma concentrations, which could increase or prolong adverse drug effects and may cause potentially fatal respiratory depression. Patients receiving fentanyl and potent CYP3A4 inhibitors should be carefully monitored for an extended period of time and dosage adjustments should be made if warranted.

○ Fentanyl is only for use in patients who are already tolerant to opioid therapy of comparable potency. Use in non-opioid tolerant patients may lead to fatal respiratory depression. Overestimating the fentanyl dose when converting patients from another opioid medication can result in fatal overdose with the first dose. Due to the mean elimination half-life of 17 hours of fentanyl, patients who are thought to have had a serious adverse event, including overdose, will require monitoring and treatment for at least 24 hours.

○ Fentanyl can be abused in a manner similar to other opioid agonists, legal or illicit. This risk should be considered when administering, prescribing, or dispensing fentanyl in situations where the healthcare professional is concerned about increased risk of misuse, abuse or diversion.

○ Persons at increased risk for opioid abuse include those with a personal or family history of substance abuse (including drug or alcohol abuse or addiction) or mental illness (eg, major depression). Patients should be assessed for their clinical risks for opioid abuse or addiction prior to being prescribed opioids. All patients receiving opioids should be routinely monitored for signs of misuse, abuse and addiction. Patients at increased risk of opioid abuse may still be appropriately treated with modified-release opioid formulations; however, these patients will require intensive monitoring for signs of misuse, abuse, or addiction.

○ Fentanyl patches are intended for transdermal use (on intact skin) only. Using damaged or cut fentanyl patches can lead to the rapid release of the contents of the fentanyl patch and absorption of a potentially fatal dose of fentanyl.

Commonly used brand name(s)

In the U.S.—
Duragesic
Ionsys

Available Dosage Forms:
- Patch, Extended Release
- Patch, Device Assisted

Therapeutic Class: Analgesic

Uses For This Medicine

Fentanyl belongs to the group of medicines called narcotic analgesics. Narcotic analgesics are used to relieve pain. The transdermal system (skin patch) form of fentanyl is used to treat chronic pain (pain that continues for a long time). There is another kind of transdermal system, called iontophoretic, that allows the patient to activate a dosing button on the patch. This is used to treat short-term pain that occurs after an operation, and only while the patient is still in the hospital.

Fentanyl acts in the central nervous system (CNS) to relieve pain. Some of its side effects are also caused by actions in the CNS.

When a narcotic is used for a long time, it may become habit-forming (causing mental or physical dependence). However, people who have continuing pain should not let the fear of dependence keep them from using narcotics to relieve their pain. Mental dependence (addiction) is not likely to occur when narcotics are used for this purpose. Physical dependence may lead to withdrawal side effects if treatment is stopped suddenly. However, severe withdrawal side effects can usually be prevented by reducing the dose gradually over a period of time before treatment is stopped completely.

This medicine is available only with your doctor's prescription.

Before Using This Medicine

In deciding to use a medicine, the risks of taking the medicine must be weighed against the good it will do. This is a decision you and your doctor will make. For this medicine, the following should be considered:

Allergies—Tell your doctor if you have ever had any unusual or allergic reaction to this medicine or any other medicines. Also tell your health care professional if you have any other types of allergies, such as to foods, dyes, preservatives, or animals. For non-prescription products, read the label or package ingredients carefully.

Pediatric—Iontophoretic transdermal patches—Safety and efficacy have not been established in children less than 18 years of age. This dosage form is not for use in children.

Transdermal patches—This medicine has been tested in children 2 years of age and older. In effective doses, the medicine has not been shown to cause different side effects or problems than it does in adults. The child or teenager *must be opioid-tolerant in order to take fentanyl.* If you are unsure if your child or teenager is opioid-tolerant, talk to your doctor.

Geriatric—Elderly people are especially sensitive to the effects of narcotic analgesics. This may increase the chance of side effects, especially breathing problems, during treatment. Your health care professional will take this into consideration when deciding on the amount of transdermal fentanyl you should receive.

Pregnancy—

	Pregnancy Category	Explanation
All Trimesters	C	Animal studies have shown an adverse effect and there are no adequate studies in pregnant women OR no animal studies have been conducted and there are no adequate studies in pregnant women.

Breast Feeding—Studies in women suggest that this medication poses minimal risk to the infant when used during breastfeeding.

Other medicines—

Using this medicine with any of the following medicines is not recommended. Your doctor may decide not to treat you with this medication or change some of the other medicines you take.

Naltrexone

Interactions with Food/Tobacco/Alcohol—Certain medicines should not be used at or around the time of eating food or eating certain types of food since interactions may occur. Using alcohol or tobacco with certain medicines may also cause interactions to occur. Discuss with your healthcare professional the use of your medicine with food, alcohol, or tobacco.

Other medical problems—The presence of other medical problems may affect the use of this medicine. Make sure you tell your doctor if you have any other medical problems, especially:

- Alcohol abuse, or history of, or
- Drug dependence, especially narcotic abuse or dependence, or history of, or
- Emotional problems or
- Kidney disease or
- Liver disease or
- Mental illness (such as major depression) or
- Underactive thyroid—The chance of side effects may be increased.
- Brain tumor or
- Diarrhea caused by antibiotic treatment or poisoning or
- Enlarged prostate or problems with urination or
- Gallbladder disease or gallstones or
- Intestinal problems such as colitis or Crohn's disease or
- Pancreatitis, acute—Some of the side effects of fentanyl can cause serious problems in people who have these medical problems.
- Bronchial asthma, acute or severe or
- Not opioid-tolerant (if you are NOT taking a certain amount of morphine, oxycodone, hydromorphone or other opioid medicine) or
- Ongoing breathing problems—Fentanyl patches should NOT be used in these patients. It could cause very serious breathing problems.
- Paralytic ileus (intestinal blockage)—Fentanyl patches should NOT be used in patients with this condition.
- Slow or irregular heartbeat—Fentanyl can make this condition worse.

Proper Use of This Medicine

Iontophoretic transdermal patches—*Iontophoretic transdermal patches are for hospital use only.* These patches are not for use at home and should be removed before you are discharged from the hospital.

The iontophoretic fentanyl patch comes with patient instructions. Read them carefully before using the product. If you do not receive any printed instructions with the medicine, or do not understand the instructions, check with your nurse or doctor.

Only one iontophoretic transdermal patch should be put on your skin at a time. A doctor or nurse will put the patch on your skin.

Each dose is delivered over a 10–minute period. The fentanyl dose is activated when you press the button firmly two times within 3 seconds. The tone or beep indicates the start of the dose. The red light next to the dosing button will stay on during the 10 minute dosing period.

Transdermal patches—Transdermal fentanyl comes with patient instructions. Read them carefully before using the product. If you do not receive any printed instructions with the medicine, check with your pharmacist.

Fentanyl skin patches are for use in opioid-tolerant patients ONLY. If you are uncertain whether or not you are opioid-tolerant, check with your doctor before using this medicine.

To use the **transdermal fentanyl patch:**

- Use this medicine exactly as directed by your doctor. It will work only if it has been applied correctly.
- Fentanyl skin patches are packaged in sealed pouches. Do not remove the patch from the sealed pouch until you are ready to apply it.
- When handling the skin patch, be careful not to touch the adhesive (sticky) surface with your hand. The adhesive part of the system contains some fentanyl, which can be absorbed into your body too fast through the skin of your hand. If any of the medicine does get on your hand, rinse the area right away with a lot of clear water. Do not use soap or other cleansers.
- Be careful not to tear the patch or make any holes in it. Damage to a patch may allow fentanyl to pass into your skin too quickly. This can cause an overdose.
- Apply the patch to a dry, flat skin area on your upper arm, chest, or back. Choose a place where the skin is not very oily and is free of scars, cuts, burns, or any other skin irritations. Also, do not apply this medicine to areas that have received radiation (x-ray) treatment.
- The patch will stay in place better if it is applied to an area with little or no hair. If you need to apply the patch to a hairy area, you may first clip the hair with scissors, but do not shave it off.
- If you need to clean the area before applying the medicine, use only plain water. Do not use soaps, other cleansers, lotions, or anything that contains oils or alcohol. Be sure that the skin is completely dry before applying the medicine.
- Remove the liner covering the sticky side of the skin patch. Then press the patch firmly in place, using the palm of your hand, for a minimum of 30 seconds. Make sure that the entire adhesive surface is attached to your skin, especially around the edges.
- If the patch becomes loose, tape the edges with first aid tape.
- If the patch falls off after applying it, throw it away and apply a new patch in a different area.
- If you need to apply more than 1 patch at a time, place the patches far enough apart so that the edges do not touch or overlap each other.
- Wash your hands with a lot of clear water after applying the medicine. Do not use soap or other cleansers.

- Remove the patch after 72 hours (3 days), or as directed by your doctor. Choose a different place on your skin to apply the next patch. If possible, use a place on the other side of your body. Wait at least 3 days before using the first area again.

After a patch is applied, the fentanyl it contains passes into the skin a little at a time. A certain amount of the medicine must build up in the skin before it is absorbed into the body. Therefore, up to a day may pass before the first dose begins to work. Your health care professional may need to change the dose during the first several applications (each kept in place for 3 days) before finding the amount that works best for you. Even if you feel that the medicine is not working, do not increase the amount of transdermal fentanyl that you apply. Instead, check with your health care professional.

You will probably need to take a faster-acting narcotic to relieve pain during the first few days of transdermal fentanyl treatment. You may continue to need another narcotic while your dose of fentanyl is being adjusted, and also to relieve any "breakthrough" pain that occurs later on. Be sure that you do not take more of the other narcotic, and do not take it more often, than directed. Taking other narcotics together with fentanyl can increase the chance of an overdose.

Dosing—The dose of this medicine will be different for different patients. Follow your doctor's orders or the directions on the label. The following information includes only the average doses of this medicine. If your dose is different, do not change it unless your doctor tells you to do so.

The amount of medicine that you take depends on the strength of the medicine. Also, the number of doses you take each day, the time allowed between doses, and the length of time you take the medicine depend on the medical problem for which you are using the medicine.

- For transdermal dosage form (stick-on patch):
  - For relief of severe, continuing pain:
    - Adults—If you have not already been using other narcotics regularly, your doctor will determine use and dose. If you have already been using other narcotics regularly, your first dose will depend on the amount of other narcotic you have been taking every day. If necessary, your health care professional will change the dose after 3 days, when the first patch is replaced. The size of the new dose will depend on how well the medicine is working and on whether you had any side effects during the first 3-day application. Other changes in dose may be needed later on. Some people may need to use more than one patch at a time.
    - Children—Use and dose must be determined by the doctor.
- For iontophoretic transdermal dosage form (self-dosing stick-on patch):
  - For relief of short-term pain following an operation:
    - Adults— a 40 microgram (mcg) dose will be delivered over a 10–minute period after the patch is activated.
    - Children—Use and dose must be determined by the doctor.

Missed dose—If you miss a dose of this medicine, apply it as soon as possible. However, if it is almost time for your next dose, skip the missed dose and go back to your regular dosing schedule.

Iontophoretic transdermal patches—The doctor or nurse will replace the patch when necessary until you are discharged from the hospital.

Transdermal patches—Remove the new patch 3 days after applying it.

Storage—Store the medicine in a closed container at room temperature, away from heat, moisture, and direct light. Keep from freezing.

Keep out of the reach of children.

Do not keep outdated medicine or medicine no longer needed.

To dispose of this medicine, first fold the patch in half, with the sticky side inside. If the patch has not been used, take it out of the pouch and remove the liner that covers the sticky side of the patch before folding it in half. Then flush it down the toilet right away.

Precautions While Using This Medicine

Iontophoretic transdermal patches—To avoid an overdose of fentanyl, you should not allow anyone else to activate your transdermal patch. You should activate your medicine as needed to relieve your pain.

You should never give your medicine to other people.

Do not touch the sticky side of the patch or the gel. Fentanyl can be quickly absorbed through the eyes and mouth and can be extremely dangerous. If you do touch the sticky side of the patch or gel, let your nurse or doctor know right away and rinse the area with large amounts of water. Do not use soaps or other cleansers.

Transdermal patches—Check with your health care professional at regular times while using fentanyl. Be sure to report any side effects.

After you have been using this medicine for awhile, "breakthrough" pain may occur more often than usual, and it may not be relieved by your regular dose of medicine. If this occurs, do not increase the amount of transdermal fentanyl or other narcotic that you are taking without first checking with your health care professional.

This medicine will add to the effects of alcohol and other CNS depressants (medicines that can make you drowsy or less alert). Some examples of CNS depressants are antihistamines or medicine for hay fever, other allergies, or colds; sedatives, tranquilizers, or sleeping medicine; other prescription pain medicine or narcotics; barbiturates; medicine for seizures; muscle relaxants; or anesthetics, including some dental anesthetics. You will probably be directed to take other pain relievers if you still have pain while using transdermal fentanyl. However, check with your health care professional before taking any of the other medicines listed above while you are using this medicine.

Fentanyl may cause some people to become drowsy, dizzy, or lightheaded, or to feel a false sense of well-being. Make sure you know how you react to this medicine before you drive, use machines, or do anything else that could be dangerous if you are dizzy or not alert and clearheaded. These effects usually go away after a few days of treatment, when your body gets used to the medicine. However, check with your health care professional if drowsiness that is severe enough to interfere with your activities continues for more than a few days.

Dizziness, lightheadedness, or even fainting may occur when you get up suddenly from a lying or sitting position. Getting up slowly may help lessen this problem. Also, lying down for a while may relieve dizziness or lightheadedness.

Nausea or vomiting may occur, especially during the first several days of treatment. Lying down for a while may relieve these effects. However, if they are especially bothersome or if they continue for more than a few days, check with your health care professional. You may be able to take another medicine to help prevent these problems.

Using narcotics for a long time can cause severe constipation. To prevent this, your health care professional may direct you to take laxatives, drink a lot of fluids, or increase the amount of fiber in your diet. Be sure to follow the directions carefully, because continuing constipation can lead to more serious problems.

Heat can cause the fentanyl in the patch to be absorbed into your body faster. This may increase the chance of serious side effects or an overdose. While you are using this medicine, do not use a heating pad, a sunlamp, or a heated water bed, and do not take sunbaths or long baths or showers in hot water. Also, check with your health care professional if you get a fever.

Before having any kind of surgery (including dental surgery) or emergency treatment, tell the medical doctor or dentist in charge that you are using this medicine. Serious side effects can occur if your medical doctor or dentist gives you certain other medicines without knowing that you are using fentanyl.

You may bathe, shower, or swim while wearing a fentanyl skin patch. However, be careful to wash and dry the area around the patch gently. Rubbing may cause the patch to get loose or come off. If this does occur, throw away the patch and apply a new one in a different place. Make sure the area is completely dry before applying the new patch.

If you have been using this medicine regularly for several weeks or more, do not suddenly stop using it without first checking with your health care professional. You may be directed to reduce gradually the amount you are using before stopping treatment completely, or to take another narcotic for a while, to lessen the chance of withdrawal side effects.

In young children or persons with decreased mental alertness, the patch should be put on the upper back to decrease the chance that the patch will be removed and placed in the mouth.

If the patch comes off and accidentally sticks to the skin of another person, they should take the patch off immediately and wash the exposed area with water. The exposed person should then seek medical attention.

Using too much transdermal fentanyl, or taking too much of another narcotic while using transdermal fentanyl, may cause an overdose. If this occurs, get emergency help right away. An overdose can cause severe breathing problems (breathing may even stop), unconsciousness, and death. Serious signs of an overdose include very slow breathing (fewer than 8 breaths a minute) and drowsiness that is so severe that you are not able to answer when spoken to or, if asleep, cannot be awakened. Other signs of an overdose may include cold, clammy skin; low blood pressure; pinpoint pupils of eyes; and slow heartbeat. It may be best to have a family member or a friend check on you several times a day when you start using a narcotic regularly, and whenever your dose is increased, so that he or she can get help for you if you cannot do so yourself.

Side Effects of This Medicine

Along with its needed effects, a medicine may cause some unwanted effects. Although not all of these side effects may occur, if they do occur they may need medical attention.

Get emergency help immediately if any of the following symptoms of overdose occur:

> Cold, clammy skin; convulsions (seizures); drowsiness that is so severe that you are not able to answer when spoken to or, if asleep, cannot be awakened; low blood pressure; pinpoint pupils of eyes; slow heartbeat; very slow (fewer than 8 breaths a minute) or troubled breathing

Check with your doctor as soon as possible if any of the following side effects occur:

More common
> Decrease in amount of urine or in the frequency of urination; hallucinations (seeing, hearing, or feeling things that are not there)

Less common
> Chest pain; difficulty in speaking; fainting; irregular heartbeat; mood or mental changes; problems with walking; redness, swelling, itching, or bumps on the skin at place of application; spitting blood

Rare
> Any change in vision; bladder pain; difficulty in speaking; fever with or without chills; fluid-filled blisters on skin; frequent urge to urinate; noisy breathing, shortness of breath, tightness in chest, or wheezing; red, thickened, or scaly skin; swelling of abdomen or stomach area; swollen and/or painful glands; unusual bruising

Incidence not known
> Bloating or swelling of face, hands, lower legs and/or feet; fast or pounding heartbeat or pulse; rapid weight gain

Some side effects may occur that usually do not need medical attention. These side effects may go away during treatment as your body adjusts to the medicine. Also, your health care professional may be able to tell you about ways to prevent or reduce some of these side effects. Check with your health care professional if any of the following side effects continue or are bothersome or if you have any questions about them:

More common
> Abdominal or stomach pain that was not present before treatment; confusion; constipation; diarrhea; dizziness, drowsiness, or lightheadedness; false sense of well-being; feeling anxious; headache; indigestion; loss of appetite; nausea or vomiting; nervousness; sweating; weakness

Less common
> Bloated feeling or gas; feeling anxious and restless at the same time; feeling of crawling, tingling, or burning of the skin; memory loss; unusual dreams

Incidence not known
> Decreased interest in sexual intercourse; ejaculatory difficulty; inability to have or keep an erection; loss in sexual ability, desire, drive, or performance; not able to have an orgasm; weight loss

After you stop using this medicine, it may still produce some side effects that need attention. During this period of time, *check with your doctor immediately* if you notice the following side effects:

> Anxiety; body aches; diarrhea; fast heartbeat; fever, runny nose, or sneezing; gooseflesh; increased sweating; increased yawning; loss of appetite; nausea or vomiting; nervousness, restlessness, or irritability; shivering or trembling; stomach cramps; trouble in sleeping; unusually large pupils in eyes; weakness

Other side effects not listed may also occur in some patients. If you notice any other effects, check with your healthcare professional.

FEXOFENADINE (Oral route) - fex-oh-FEN-a-deen

Commonly used brand name(s)

In the U.S.—
Allegra

Available Dosage Forms:
- Tablet
- Capsule

Therapeutic Class: Respiratory Agent
Pharmacologic Class: Antihistamine, Less-Sedating

Uses For This Medicine

Fexofenadine is an antihistamine. It is used to relieve the symptoms of hay fever and hives of the skin.

Antihistamines work by preventing the effects of a substance called histamine, which is produced by the body. Histamine can cause itching, sneezing, runny nose, and watery eyes. Also, in some persons histamine can close up the bronchial tubes (air passages of the lungs) and make breathing difficult. Histamine can also cause some persons to have hives, with severe itching of the skin.

This medicine is available only with your doctor's prescription.

Before Using This Medicine

In deciding to use a medicine, the risks of taking the medicine must be weighed against the good it will do. This is a decision you and your doctor will make. For this medicine, the following should be considered:

Allergies—Tell your doctor if you have ever had any unusual or allergic reaction to this medicine or any other medicines. Also tell your health care professional if you have any other types of allergies, such as to foods, dyes, preservatives, or animals. For non-prescription products, read the label or package ingredients carefully.

Pediatric—This medicine has been tested in children 6 years of age and older and, in effective doses, has not been shown to cause different side effects or problems than it does in adults. There is no specific information comparing use of fexofenadine in children up to 6 years of age.

Geriatric—Fexofenadine has been tested in patients 65 years of age and older and has not been shown to cause different side effects or problems in older people than it does in younger adults.

Pregnancy—

	Pregnancy Category	Explanation
All Trimesters	C	Animal studies have shown an adverse effect and there are no adequate studies in pregnant women OR no animal studies have been conducted and there are no adequate studies in pregnant women.

Breast Feeding—There are no adequate studies in women for determining infant risk when using this medication during breastfeeding. Weigh the potential benefits against the potential risks before taking this medication while breastfeeding.

Other medicines—

Using this medicine with any of the following medicines is usually not recommended, but may be required in some cases. If both medicines are prescribed together, your doctor may change the dose or how often you use one or both of the medicines.

Droperidol

Interactions with Food/Tobacco/Alcohol—Certain medicines should not be used at or around the time of eating food or eating certain types of food since interactions may occur. Using alcohol or tobacco with certain medicines may also cause interactions to occur. The following interactions have been selected on the basis of their potential significance and are not necessarily all-inclusive.

Using this medicine with any of the following may cause an increased risk of certain side effects but may be unavoidable in some cases. If used together, your doctor may change the dose or how often you use this medicine, or give you special instructions about the use of food, alcohol, or tobacco.

Apple Juice, Grapefruit Juice, Orange Juice

Other medical problems—The presence of other medical problems may affect the use of this medicine. Make sure you tell your doctor if you have any other medical problems, especially:
- Kidney disease—Effects of fexofenadine may be increased because of slower removal from the body

Proper Use of This Medicine

You should always take this medicine with water. Do not take it with juice such as grape, orange or apple juice.

You should NOT take antacids that contain aluminum or magnesium hydroxide within 15 minutes of taking this medicine. If you are uncertain about this, ask your doctor or pharmacist.

Dosing—The dose of this medicine will be different for different patients. Follow your doctor's orders or the directions on the label. The following information includes only the average doses of this medicine. If your dose is different, do not change it unless your doctor tells you to do so.

The amount of medicine that you take depends on the strength of the medicine. Also, the number of doses you take each day, the time allowed between doses, and the length of time you take the medicine depend on the medical problem for which you are using the medicine.

- For oral dosage form (capsules, tablets):
  - For symptoms of hay fever:
    - Adults and children 12 years of age and older—60 milligrams (mg) two times a day, or 180 mg once a day.
    - Children 6 to 11 years of age—30 mg two times a day
    - Children younger than 6 years of age—Use and dose must be determined by your doctor.
  - For symptoms of chronic hives:
    - Adults and children 12 years of age and older—60 mg two times a day, or 180 mg once a day.
    - Children 6 to 11 years of age—30 mg two times a day.
    - Children younger than 6 years of age—Use and dose must be determined by your doctor.

Missed dose—If you miss a dose of this medicine, take it as soon as possible. However, if it is almost time for your next dose, skip the missed dose and go back to your regular dosing schedule. Do not double doses.

Storage—Store the medicine in a closed container at room temperature, away from heat, moisture, and direct light. Keep from freezing.

Keep out of the reach of children.

Do not keep outdated medicine or medicine no longer needed.

Side Effects of This Medicine

Along with its needed effects, a medicine may cause some unwanted effects. Although not all of these side effects may occur, if they do occur they may need medical attention.

Check with your doctor immediately if any of the following side effects occur:

Incidence rare
> Chest tightness; feeling of warmth, redness of the face, neck, arms and occasionally, upper chest; large, hive-like swelling on face, eyelids, lips, tongue, throat, hands, legs, feet, sex organs; shortness of breath, difficult or labored breathing

Some side effects may occur that usually do not need medical attention. These side effects may go away during treatment as your body adjusts to the medicine. Also, your health care professional may be able to tell you about ways to prevent or reduce some of these side effects. Check with your health care professional if any of the following side effects continue or are bothersome or if you have any questions about them:

Less common
> Back pain; body aches or pain; chills; coughing; difficulty in moving; dizziness; drowsiness; ear congestion; earache; fever; headache; joint pain; loss of voice; muscle aching or cramping; muscle pains or stiffness; nasal congestion; nausea; pain in arms or legs; pain or tenderness around eyes or cheekbones; painful menstrual bleeding; ringing or buzzing in ears; runny or stuffy nose; sneezing; sore throat; stomach upset; swollen joints; unusual feeling of tiredness or weakness; viral infection (such as cold and flu)

Incidence rare
> Nervousness; rash; sleeplessness; terrifying dreams; trouble sleeping

Other side effects not listed may also occur in some patients. If you notice any other effects, check with your healthcare professional.

FEXOFENADINE AND PSEUDOEPHEDRINE (Oral route) -
fex-oh-FEN-a-deen, soo-doe-e-FED-rin

Commonly used brand name(s)

In the U.S.—
> Allegra-D

Available Dosage Forms:

- Tablet, Extended Release
- Tablet, Extended Release, 24 HR

Therapeutic Class: Antihistamine, Less-Sedating/Decongestant Combination
Pharmacologic Class: Fexofenadine

Uses For This Medicine

Fexofenadine is an antihistamine and pseudoephedrine is a decongestant. The combination of these two medicines is used to treat the nasal congestion (stuffy nose), sneezing, and runny nose caused by hay fever.

This medicine is available only with your doctor's prescription.

Before Using This Medicine

In deciding to use a medicine, the risks of taking the medicine must be weighed against the good it will do. This is a decision you and your doctor will make. For this medicine, the following should be considered:

Allergies—Tell your doctor if you have ever had any unusual or allergic reaction to this medicine or any other medicines. Also tell your health care professional if you have any other types of allergies, such as to foods, dyes, preservatives, or animals. For non-prescription products, read the label or package ingredients carefully.

Pediatric—Use is not recommended in infants and children up to 12 years of age. In children 12 years of age and older, this medicine is not expected to cause different side effects or problems than it does in adults.

Geriatric—Some side effects may be more likely to occur in elderly patients, who are usually more sensitive to the effects of this medicine.

Other medicines—

Using this medicine with any of the following medicines is not recommended. Your doctor may decide not to treat you with this medication or change some of the other medicines you take.

Clorgyline, Dihydroergotamine, Furazolidone, Iproniazid, Isocarboxazid, Moclobemide, Nialamide, Pargyline, Phenelzine, Procarbazine, Rasagiline, Selegiline, Toloxatone, Tranylcypromine

Interactions with Food/Tobacco/Alcohol—Certain medicines should not be used at or around the time of eating food or eating certain types of food since interactions may occur. Using alcohol or tobacco with certain medicines may also cause interactions to occur. The following interactions have been selected on the basis of their potential significance and are not necessarily all-inclusive.

Using this medicine with any of the following may cause an increased risk of certain side effects but may be unavoidable in some cases. If used together, your doctor may change the dose or how often you use this medicine, or give you special instructions about the use of food, alcohol, or tobacco.

Apple Juice, Grapefruit Juice, Orange Juice

Other medical problems—The presence of other medical problems may affect the use of this medicine. Make sure you tell your doctor if you have any other medical problems, especially:

- Diabetes mellitus (sugar diabetes)—Use of this medicine may cause an increase in blood glucose levels
- Enlarged prostate or
- Urinary tract blockage or difficult urination—Use of this medicine may cause urination to be more difficult. You should not take this medicine if you have these conditions.
- Glaucoma or
- Increased pressure in the eye—Use of this medicine may make the condition worse. You should not take this medicine if you have these conditions.
- Heart or blood vessel disease or
- High blood pressure—Use of this medicine may make the condition worse. You should not take this medicine if you have high blood pressure, especially if it is severe.
- Kidney disease—Effects may be increased because of slower removal of the medicine from the body. The 24-hour extended-release tablet should not be used if you have kidney problems.
- Overactive thyroid—Serious effects on the heart may occur

Proper Use of This Medicine

Swallow the extended-release tablet whole. Do not crush, break, or chew it before swallowing.

This medicine is best taken on an empty stomach (either one hour before or two hours after a meal).

This medicine should be taken with water. Do not take with fruit juices or antacids.

Dosing—The dose of this medicine will be different for different patients. Follow your doctor's orders or the directions on the label. The following information includes only the average doses of this medicine. If your dose is different, do not change it unless your doctor tells you to do so.

The amount of medicine that you take depends on the strength of the medicine. Also, the number of doses you take each day, the time allowed between doses, and the length of time you take the medicine depend on the medical problem for which you are using the medicine.

- For oral dosage form (extended-release tablets [12 hour]):
  - For symptoms of hay fever:
    - Adults and teenagers—1 tablet two times a day.
    - Children—Use and dose must be determined by your doctor.

- For oral dosage form (extended-release tablets [24 hour]):
  - For symptoms of hay fever:
    - Adults and teenagers—1 tablet one time a day.
    - Children—Use and dose must be determined by your doctor.

Missed dose—If you miss a dose of this medicine, take it as soon as possible. However, if it is almost time for your next dose, skip the missed dose and go back to your regular dosing schedule. Do not double doses.

Storage—Store the medicine in a closed container at room temperature, away from heat, moisture, and direct light. Keep from freezing.

Keep out of the reach of children.

Do not keep outdated medicine or medicine no longer needed.

Side Effects of This Medicine

Along with its needed effects, a medicine may cause some unwanted effects. Although not all of these side effects may occur, if they do occur they may need medical attention.

Check with your doctor as soon as possible if any of the following side effects occur:

More common
Trouble in sleeping

Less common
Cough; dizziness; irregular heartbeat; nervousness; sore throat

Incidence not known
Difficult or labored breathing; difficulty swallowing; dizziness; fast heartbeat; feeling of warmth; fever; hives or welts; itching skin; itching, puffiness or swelling of the eyelids or around the eyes, face, lips or tongue; large, hive-like swelling on face, eyelids, lips, tongue, throat, hands, legs, feet, sex organs; reddening of the skin, especially around ears; redness of the face, neck, arms and occasionally, upper chest; shortness of breath; skin rash; tightness in chest; swelling of eyes, face, or inside of nose; unusual tiredness or weakness; wheezing

Some side effects may occur that usually do not need medical attention. These side effects may go away during treatment as your body adjusts to the medicine. Also, your health care professional may be able to tell you about ways to prevent or reduce some of these side effects. Check with your health care professional if any of the following side effects continue or are bothersome or if you have any questions about them:

More common
Headache; nausea

Less common
Abdominal or stomach pain; agitation; anxiety; back pain; dry mouth; heartburn

Incidence not known
Terrifying dreams causing sleep disturbances

Other side effects not listed may also occur in some patients. If you notice any other effects, check with your healthcare professional.

FINASTERIDE (Oral route) - fi-NAS-teer-ide

Commonly used brand name(s)

In the U.S.—
Propecia
Proscar

Available Dosage Forms:
- Tablet

Therapeutic Class: Alopecia Agent
Pharmacologic Class: 5–Alpha Reductase Inhibitor

Uses For This Medicine

Note: Women of childbearing potential should not use or handle crushed finasteride tablets. Finasteride can cause birth defects in male fetuses.

Finasteride belongs to the group of medicines called enzyme inhibitors. It is used to treat urinary problems caused by enlargement of the prostate (benign prostatic hyperplasia or BPH). In men with very enlarged prostates and mild to moderate symptoms (difficulty urinating, decreased flow of urination, hesitation at the beginning of urination, getting up at night to urinate), finasteride may decrease the severity of symptoms. Finasteride may also reduce the chance that surgery on the prostate will be needed.

Finasteride blocks an enzyme called 5–alpha-reductase, which is necessary to change testosterone to another hormone that causes the prostate to grow. As a result, the size of the prostate is decreased. The effect of finasteride on the prostate lasts only as long as the medicine is taken. If it is stopped, the prostate begins to grow again.

Finasteride also is used by some balding men to stimulate hair growth. If hair growth is going to occur with the use of finasteride, it usually occurs after the medicine has been used for about 3 months and lasts only as long as the medicine continues to be used. The new hair will be lost within 1 year after finasteride treatment is stopped.

Finasteride is available only with your doctor's prescription.

Before Using This Medicine

In deciding to use a medicine, the risks of taking the medicine must be weighed against the good it will do. This is a decision you and your doctor will make. For this medicine, the following should be considered:

Allergies—Tell your doctor if you have ever had any unusual or allergic reaction to this medicine or any other medicines. Also tell your health care professional if you have any other types of allergies, such as to foods, dyes, preservatives, or animals. For non-prescription products, read the label or package ingredients carefully.

Geriatric—This medicine has been tested and has not been shown to cause different side effects or problems in older people than it does in younger adults.

Pregnancy—

	Pregnancy Category	Explanation
All Trimesters	X	Studies in animals or pregnant women have demonstrated positive evidence of fetal abnormalities. This drug should not be used in women who are or may become pregnant because the risk clearly outweighs any possible benefit.

Breast Feeding—There are no adequate studies in women for determining infant risk when using this medication during breastfeeding. Weigh the potential benefits against the potential risks before taking this medication while breastfeeding.

Other medicines—Although certain medicines should not be used together at all, in other cases two different medicines may be used together even if an interaction might occur. In these cases, your doctor may want to change the dose, or other precautions may be necessary. Tell your healthcare professional if you are taking any other prescription or non-prescription (over-the-counter [OTC]) medicine.

Interactions with Food/Tobacco/Alcohol—Certain medicines should not be used at or around the time of eating food or eating certain types of food since interactions may occur. Using alcohol or tobacco with certain medicines may also cause interactions to occur. Discuss with your healthcare professional the use of your medicine with food, alcohol, or tobacco.

Proper Use of This Medicine

Finasteride tablets may be crushed to make them easier to swallow. However, women who are or may become pregnant should not handle crushed finasteride tablets.

For patients taking this medicine for benign prostatic hyperplasia (BPH):

- To help you remember to take your medicine, try to get into the habit of taking it at the same time each day.

- Remember that this medicine does not cure BPH but it does help reduce the size of the prostate. Therefore, you must continue to take it if you expect to keep the size of your prostate down. You may have to take this medicine for at least 6 months to see the full effect. You may have to take this medicine for the rest of your life. Do not stop taking this medicine without first discussing it with your doctor.

- This medicine helps to reduce urinary problems in men with BPH. In general, it is best to avoid drinking fluids, especially coffee or alcohol, in the evening. Then your sleep will not be disturbed by your need to urinate during the night.

For individuals taking this medicine for hair growth:

- You may have to take this medicine for at least 3 months to see an effect. The effect will last only as long as the medicine continues to be used. The new hair will be lost within 1 year after finasteride is stopped.

Dosing—The dose of this medicine will be different for different patients. Follow your doctor's orders or the directions on the label. The following information includes only the av-

erage doses of this medicine. If your dose is different, do not change it unless your doctor tells you to do so.

The amount of medicine that you take depends on the strength of the medicine. Also, the number of doses you take each day, the time allowed between doses, and the length of time you take the medicine depend on the medical problem for which you are using the medicine.

- For oral dosage form (tablets):
  - For treatment of benign prostatic hyperplasia (BPH):
    - Adults—5 milligrams (mg) once a day.
  - For hair growth:
    - Adults—1 mg once a day.

Missed dose—If you miss a dose of this medicine, take it as soon as possible. However, if it is almost time for your next dose, skip the missed dose and go back to your regular dosing schedule. Do not double doses.

Storage—Store the medicine in a closed container at room temperature, away from heat, moisture, and direct light. Keep from freezing.

Keep out of the reach of children.

Do not keep outdated medicine or medicine no longer needed.

Precautions While Using This Medicine

Women who are or who may become pregnant should not handle crushed finasteride tablets. There is a risk that the medicine could get into the pregnant woman's body and cause birth defects in a male fetus.

Side Effects of This Medicine

Along with its needed effects, a medicine may cause some unwanted effects. Although not all of these side effects may occur, if they do occur they may need medical attention.

Check with your doctor as soon as possible if any of the following side effects occur:

Less common
> Breast enlargement and tenderness; skin rash; swelling of lipsNote: Breast enlargement and tenderness, skin rash and swelling of lips are more likely to occur with the 5–mg dose.

Some side effects may occur that usually do not need medical attention. These side effects may go away during treatment as your body adjusts to the medicine. Also, your health care professional may be able to tell you about ways to prevent or reduce some of these side effects. Check with your health care professional if any of the following side effects continue or are bothersome or if you have any questions about them:

Less common or rare
> Abdominal pain; back pain; decreased libido (decreased interest in sex); decreased volume of ejaculate (decreased amount of semen); diarrhea; dizziness; headache; impotence (inability to have or keep an erection)

Incidence Unknown
> Testicular pain

Note: A decrease in the amount of semen during ejaculation should not affect your sexual performance and is not a sign of any change in fertility.

Other side effects not listed may also occur in some patients. If you notice any other effects, check with your healthcare professional.

FLAVOCOXID (Oral route) - flay-voe-COX-id

Commonly used brand name(s)
In the U.S.—
> Limbrel

Available Dosage Forms:
- Capsule

Therapeutic Class: Nutriceutical

Uses For This Medicine

Flavocoxid is used to treat moderate to severe symptoms of osteoarthritis. This medicine is used in patients 18 years of age or older. Flavocoxid will not cure the disease, but will help with the symptoms as long as you continue to take it.

Before Using This Medicine

In deciding to use a medicine, the risks of taking the medicine must be weighed against the good it will do. This is a decision you and your doctor will make. For this medicine, the following should be considered:

Allergies—Tell your doctor if you have ever had any unusual or allergic reaction to this medicine or any other medicines. Also tell your health care professional if you have any other types of allergies, such as to foods, dyes, preservatives, or animals. For non-prescription products, read the label or package ingredients carefully.

Pediatric—Studies on flavocoxid have been done only in adult patients, and there is no specific information comparing the use flavocoxid in children with use in other age groups.

Geriatric—Many medicines have not been studied specifically in older people. Therefore, it may not be known whether they work exactly the same way they do in younger adults. Although there is no specific information comparing use of flavocoxid in the elderly with use in other age groups, this medicine is not expected to cause different side effects or problems than it does in younger adults.

Breast Feeding—There are no adequate studies in women for determining infant risk when using this medication during breastfeeding. Weigh the potential benefits against the potential risks before taking this medication while breastfeeding.

Other medicines—Although certain medicines should not be used together at all, in other cases two different medicines may be used together even if an interaction might occur. In these cases, your doctor may want to change the dose, or other precautions may be necessary. Tell your healthcare professional if you are taking any other prescription or non-prescription (over-the-counter [OTC]) medicine.

Interactions with Food/Tobacco/Alcohol—Certain medicines should not be used at or around the time of eating food or eating certain types of food since interactions may occur. Using alcohol or tobacco with certain medicines may also cause interactions to occur. Discuss with your healthcare professional the use of your medicine with food, alcohol, or tobacco.

Other medical problems—The presence of other medical problems may affect the use of this medicine. Make sure you tell your doctor if you have any other medical problems, especially:

- Stomach ulcers—May be worsened by flavocoxid

Proper Use of This Medicine

You should take flavocoxid one hour before or after the consumption of food.

Dosing—The dose of this medicine will be different for different patients. Follow your doctor's orders or the directions on the label. The following information includes only the average doses of this medicine. If your dose is different, do not change it unless your doctor tells you to do so.

The amount of medicine that you take depends on the strength of the medicine. Also, the number of doses you take each day, the time allowed between doses, and the length of time you take the medicine depend on the medical problem for which you are using the medicine.

- For oral dosage form (capsules)
  - For rheumatoid arthritis:
    - Adults—250 milligrams (mg) every 12 hours.
    - Children—Use and dose must be determined by your doctor.

Missed dose—If you miss a dose of this medicine, take it as soon as possible. However, if it is almost time for your next dose, skip the missed dose and go back to your regular dosing schedule. Do not double doses.

Storage—Keep out of the reach of children.

Store the medicine in a closed container at room temperature, away from heat, moisture, and direct light. Keep from freezing.

Do not keep outdated medicine or medicine no longer needed.

Side Effects of This Medicine

Some side effects may occur that usually do not need medical attention. These side effects may go away during treatment as your body adjusts to the medicine. Also, your health care professional may be able to tell you about ways to prevent or reduce some of these side effects. Check with your health care professional if any of the following side effects continue or are bothersome or if you have any questions about them:

More common

Blurred vision; dizziness; dull ache or feeling of pressure or heaviness in legs; fluid accumulation in the knee; headache; itching skin near damaged veins; nervousness; pounding in the ears; red, scaling, or cursed skin; slow or fast heartbeat; swollen feet and ankles

FLAVOXATE (Oral route) - fla-VOX-ate

Commonly used brand name(s)

In the U.S.—
  Urispas

Available Dosage Forms:
- Tablet

Therapeutic Class: Urinary Antispasmodic
Pharmacologic Class: Antimuscarinic

Uses For This Medicine

Flavoxate belongs to the group of medicines called antispasmodics. It is taken by mouth to help decrease muscle spasms of the bladder and relieve difficult urination.

Flavoxate is available only with your doctor's prescription.

Before Using This Medicine

In deciding to use a medicine, the risks of taking the medicine must be weighed against the good it will do. This is a decision you and your doctor will make. For this medicine, the following should be considered:

Allergies—Tell your doctor if you have ever had any unusual or allergic reaction to this medicine or any other medicines. Also tell your health care professional if you have any other types of allergies, such as to foods, dyes, preservatives, or animals. For non-prescription products, read the label or package ingredients carefully.

Pediatric—Studies on this medicine have been done only in adult patients and in children over 12 years of age. Flavoxate is not recommended for children younger than 12 years of age because safety and efficacy have not been established.

Geriatric—Confusion may be especially likely to occur in elderly patients, who are usually more sensitive than younger adults to the effects of flavoxate.

Pregnancy—

	Pregnancy Category	Explanation
All Trimesters	B	Animal studies have revealed no evidence of harm to the fetus, however, there are no adequate studies in pregnant women OR animal studies have shown an adverse effect, but adequate studies in pregnant women have failed to demonstrate a risk to the fetus.

Breast Feeding—There are no adequate studies in women for determining infant risk when using this medication during breastfeeding. Weigh the potential benefits against the potential risks before taking this medication while breastfeeding.

Other medicines—Although certain medicines should not be used together at all, in other cases two different medicines may be used together even if an interaction might occur. In these cases, your doctor may want to change the dose, or other precautions may be necessary. Tell your healthcare professional if you are taking any other prescription or non-prescription (over-the-counter [OTC]) medicine.

Interactions with Food/Tobacco/Alcohol—Certain medicines should not be used at or around the time of eating food or eating certain types of food since interactions may occur. Using alcohol or tobacco with certain medicines may also cause interactions to occur. Discuss with your healthcare professional the use of your medicine with food, alcohol, or tobacco.

Other medical problems—The presence of other medical problems may affect the use of this medicine. Make sure you tell your doctor if you have any other medical problems, especially:

- Bleeding (severe) or
- Glaucoma or
- Intestinal blockage or other intestinal or stomach problems or
- Urinary tract blockage—Use of flavoxate may make these conditions worse
- Enlarged prostate—Use of flavoxate may cause difficult urination

Proper Use of This Medicine

This medicine is usually taken with water on an empty stomach. However, your doctor may want you to take it with food or milk to lessen stomach upset.

Take this medicine only as directed. Do not take more of it, do not take it more often, and do not take it for a longer time than your doctor ordered. To do so may increase the chance of side effects.

Dosing—The dose of this medicine will be different for different patients. Follow your doctor's orders or the directions on the label. The following information includes only the average doses of this medicine. If your dose is different, do not change it unless your doctor tells you to do so.

The amount of medicine that you take depends on the strength of the medicine. Also, the number of doses you take each day, the time allowed between doses, and the length of time you take the medicine depend on the medical problem for which you are using the medicine.

- Adults and children 12 years of age and older: 100 to 200 milligrams three or four times a day.
- Children up to 12 years of age: Use and dose must be determined by the doctor.

Missed dose—If you miss a dose of this medicine, take it as soon as possible. However, if it is almost time for your next dose, skip the missed dose and go back to your regular dosing schedule. Do not double doses.

Storage—Store the medicine in a closed container at room temperature, away from heat, moisture, and direct light. Keep from freezing.

Keep out of the reach of children.

Do not keep outdated medicine or medicine no longer needed.

Precautions While Using This Medicine

This medicine may cause your eyes to become more sensitive to light than they are normally. Wearing sunglasses may help lessen the discomfort from bright light.

This medicine may cause some people to become drowsy or have blurred vision. Make sure you know how you react to this medicine before you drive, use machines, or do anything else that could be dangerous if you are not alert or able to see well.

Flavoxate may make you sweat less, causing your body temperature to increase. Use extra care not to become overheated during exercise or hot weather while you are taking this medicine, since overheating may result in heat stroke. Also, hot baths or saunas may make you feel dizzy or faint while you are taking this medicine.

Your mouth and throat may feel very dry while you are taking this medicine. For temporary relief of mouth dryness, use sugarless candy or gum, melt bits of ice in your mouth, or use a saliva substitute. However, if your mouth continues to feel dry for more than 2 weeks, check with your medical doctor or dentist. Continuing dryness of the mouth may increase the chance of dental disease, including tooth decay, gum disease, and fungus infections.

Side Effects of This Medicine

Along with its needed effects, a medicine may cause some unwanted effects. Although not all of these side effects may occur, if they do occur they may need medical attention.

Check with your doctor as soon as possible if any of the following side effects occur:
Rare
Confusion; eye pain; skin rash or hives; sore throat and fever
Symptoms of overdose
Clumsiness or unsteadiness; dizziness (severe); drowsiness (severe); fever; flushing or redness of face; hallucinations (seeing, hearing, or feeling things that are not there); shortness of breath or troubled breathing; unusual excitement, nervousness, restlessness, or irritability

Some side effects may occur that usually do not need medical attention. These side effects may go away during treatment as your body adjusts to the medicine. Also, your health care professional may be able to tell you about ways to prevent or reduce some of these side effects. Check with your health care professional if any of the following side effects continue or are bothersome or if you have any questions about them:
More common
Drowsiness; dryness of mouth and throat
Less common or rare
Blurred vision; constipation; difficult urination; difficulty concentrating; dizziness; fast heartbeat; headache; increased sensitivity of eyes to light; increased sweating; nausea or vomiting; nervousness; stomach pain

Other side effects not listed may also occur in some patients. If you notice any other effects, check with your healthcare professional.

FLECAINIDE (Oral route) - fle-KAY-nide

Black Box Warning

Flecainide acetate was included in the National Heart Lung and Blood Institute's Cardiac Arrhythmia Suppression Trial (CAST), a long-term, multicenter, randomized, double-blind study in patients with asymptomatic non-life threatening ventricular arrhythmias who had a myocardial infarction more than six days but less than two years previously. An excessive mortality or non-fatal cardiac arrest rate was seen in patients treated with flecainide acetate compared with that seen in patients assigned to a carefully matched placebo-treated group. This rate was 16/315 (5.1%) for flecainide acetate and 7/309 (2.3%) for the matched placebo. The average duration of treatment with flecainide acetate in this study was ten months.

The applicability of the CAST results to other populations (eg, those without recent myocardial infarction) is uncertain, but at present, it is prudent to consider the risks of Class IC agents (including flecainide acetate), coupled with the lack of any evidence of improved survival, generally unacceptable in patients without life-threatening ventricular arrhythmias, even if the patients are experiencing unpleasant, but not life-threatening, symptoms or signs.

A review of the world literature revealed reports of 568 patients treated with oral flecainide acetate for paroxysmal atrial fibrillation/flutter (PAF). Ventricular tachycardia was experienced in 0.4% (2/568) of these patients. Of 19 patients in the literature with chronic atrial fibrillation (CAF), 10.5% (2) experienced VT or VF. Flecainide is not recommended for use in patients with chronic atrial fibrillation. Case reports of ventricular proarrhythmic effects in patients treated with flecainide for atrial fibrillation/flutter have included increased PVCs, VT, ventricular fibrillation (VF), and death.

As with other Class I agents, patients treated with flecainide acetate for atrial flutter have been reported with 1:1 atrioventricular conduction due to slowing the atrial rate. A paradoxical increase in the ventricular rate also may occur in patients with atrial fibrillation who receive flecainide acetate. Concomitant negative chronotropic therapy such as digoxin or beta-blockers may lower the risk of this complication.

Commonly used brand name(s)

In the U.S.—
   Tambocor

Available Dosage Forms:
 • Tablet
 • Capsule, Extended Release

Therapeutic Class: Antiarrhythmic, Group IC

Uses For This Medicine

Flecainide belongs to the group of medicines known as antiarrhythmics. It is used to correct irregular heartbeats to a normal rhythm.

Flecainide produces its helpful effects by slowing nerve impulses in the heart and making the heart tissue less sensitive.

There is a chance that flecainide may cause new or make worse existing heart rhythm problems when it is used. Since it has been shown to cause severe problems in some patients, it is only used to treat serious heart rhythm problems. Discuss this possible effect with your doctor.

This medicine is available only with your doctor's prescription.

Before Using This Medicine

In deciding to use a medicine, the risks of taking the medicine must be weighed against the good it will do. This is a decision you and your doctor will make. For this medicine, the following should be considered:

Allergies—Tell your doctor if you have ever had any unusual or allergic reaction to this medicine or any other medicines. Also tell your health care professional if you have any other types of allergies, such as to foods, dyes, preservatives, or animals. For non-prescription products, read the label or package ingredients carefully.

Pediatric—Studies on this medicine have been done only in adult patients, and there is no specific information comparing use of flecainide in children with use in other age groups.

Geriatric—Elderly people are especially sensitive to the effects of flecainide. Flecainide may be more likely to cause irregular heartbeat in the elderly.

Pregnancy—

	Pregnancy Category	Explanation
All Trimesters	C	Animal studies have shown an adverse effect and there are no adequate studies in pregnant women OR no animal studies have been conducted and there are no adequate studies in pregnant women.

Breast Feeding—There are no adequate studies in women for determining infant risk when using this medication during breastfeeding. Weigh the potential benefits against the potential risks before taking this medication while breastfeeding.

Other medicines—

Using this medicine with any of the following medicines is not recommended. Your doctor may decide not to treat you with this medication or change some of the other medicines you take.

Bepridil, Cisapride, Levomethadyl, Mesoridazine, Pimozide, Ritonavir, Saquinavir, Terfenadine, Thioridazine, Tipranavir, Ziprasidone

Interactions with Food/Tobacco/Alcohol—Certain medicines should not be used at or around the time of eating food or eating certain types of food since interactions may occur. Using alcohol or tobacco with certain medicines may also cause interactions to occur. Discuss with your healthcare professional the use of your medicine with food, alcohol, or tobacco.

Other medical problems—The presence of other medical problems may affect the use of this medicine. Make sure you tell your doctor if you have any other medical problems, especially:
 • Congestive heart failure—Flecainide may make this condition worse
 • Kidney disease or
 • Liver disease—Effects of flecainide may be increased because of slower removal from the body
 • Recent heart attack—Risk of irregular heartbeats may be increased
 • If you have a pacemaker—Flecainide may interfere with the pacemaker and require more careful follow-up by the doctor

Proper Use of This Medicine

Take flecainide exactly as directed by your doctor, even though you may feel well. Do not take more medicine than ordered.

This medicine works best when there is a constant amount in the blood. To help keep this amount constant, do not miss any doses. Also, it is best to take the doses 12 hours apart, in the morning and at night, unless otherwise directed by your doctor. If you need help in planning the best times to take your medicine, check with your health care professional.

Dosing—The dose of this medicine will be different for different patients. Follow your doctor's orders or the directions on the label. The following information includes only the average doses of this medicine. If your dose is different, do not change it unless your doctor tells you to do so.

The amount of medicine that you take depends on the strength of the medicine. Also, the number of doses you take each day, the time allowed between doses, and the length of time you take the medicine depend on the medical problem for which you are using the medicine.

- For oral dosage form (tablets):
  - For correcting irregular heartbeat:
    - Adults—50 to 150 milligrams (mg) every twelve hours.
    - Children—Use and dose must be determined by your doctor.

Missed dose—If you miss a dose of this medicine, take it as soon as possible. However, if it is almost time for your next dose, skip the missed dose and go back to your regular dosing schedule. Do not double doses.

Storage—Store the medicine in a closed container at room temperature, away from heat, moisture, and direct light. Keep from freezing.

Keep out of the reach of children.

Do not keep outdated medicine or medicine no longer needed.

Precautions While Using This Medicine

It is important that your doctor check your progress at regular visits to make sure the medicine is working properly. This will allow for changes to be made in the amount of medicine you are taking, if necessary.

Your doctor may want you to carry a medical identification card or bracelet stating that you are using this medicine.

Before having any kind of surgery (including dental surgery) or emergency treatment, tell the medical doctor or dentist in charge that you are taking this medicine.

Flecainide may cause some people to become dizzy, light-headed, or less alert than they are normally. Make sure you know how you react to this medicine before you drive, use machines, or do anything else that could be dangerous if you are dizzy or are not alert.

If you have been using this medicine regularly for several weeks, do not suddenly stop using it. Check with your doctor for the best way to reduce gradually the amount you are taking before stopping completely.

Side Effects of This Medicine

Along with its needed effects, a medicine may cause some unwanted effects. Although not all of these side effects may occur, if they do occur they may need medical attention.

Check with your doctor as soon as possible if any of the following side effects occur:
Less common
    Chest pain; irregular heartbeat; shortness of breath; swelling of feet or lower legs; trembling or shaking
Rare
    Yellow eyes or skin

Some side effects may occur that usually do not need medical attention. These side effects may go away during treatment as your body adjusts to the medicine. Also, your health care professional may be able to tell you about ways to prevent or reduce some of these side effects. Check with your health care professional if any of the following side effects continue or are bothersome or if you have any questions about them:
More common
    Blurred vision or seeing spots; dizziness or lightheadedness
Less common
    Anxiety or mental depression; constipation; headache; nausea or vomiting; skin rash; stomach pain or loss of appetite; unusual tiredness or weakness

Other side effects not listed may also occur in some patients. If you notice any other effects, check with your healthcare professional.

FLOXURIDINE   (Injection route) - flox-YOOR-i-deen

Black Box Warning

It is recommended that floxuridine be given only by or under the supervision of a qualified physician who is experienced in cancer chemotherapy and intra-arterial drug therapy and is well versed in the use of potent antimetabolites.

Because of the possibility of severe toxic reactions, all patients should be hospitalized for initiation of the first course of therapy.

Commonly used brand name(s)
In the U.S.—
    FUDR

Available Dosage Forms:
- Powder for Solution

Therapeutic Class: Antineoplastic Agent
Pharmacologic Class: Antimetabolite

Uses For This Medicine

Floxuridine belongs to the group of medicines known as antimetabolites. It is used to treat some kinds of cancer.

Floxuridine interferes with the growth of cancer cells, which are eventually destroyed. Since the growth of normal body cells may also be affected by floxuridine, other effects will also occur. Some of these may be serious and must be reported to your doctor. Other effects, like hair loss, may not be serious but may cause concern. Some effects may not occur for months or years after the medicine is used.

Before you begin treatment with floxuridine, you and your doctor should talk about the good this medicine will do as well as the risks of using it.

Floxuridine is to be administered only by or under the immediate supervision of your doctor.

Before Using This Medicine

In deciding to use a medicine, the risks of taking the medicine must be weighed against the good it will do. This is a decision you and your doctor will make. For this medicine, the following should be considered:

Allergies—Tell your doctor if you have ever had any unusual or allergic reaction to this medicine or any other medicines. Also tell your health care professional if you have any other types of allergies, such as to foods, dyes, preservatives, or animals. For non-prescription products, read the label or package ingredients carefully.

Pediatric—There is no specific information comparing use of floxuridine in children with use in other age groups.

Geriatric—Many medicines have not been studied specifically in older people. Therefore, it may not be known whether they work exactly the same way they do in younger adults or if they cause different side effects or problems in older people. Although there is no specific information comparing use of floxuridine in the elderly with use in other age groups, this medicine is not expected to cause different side effects or problems in older people than it does in younger adults.

Pregnancy—

	Pregnancy Category	Explanation
All Trimesters	D	Studies in pregnant women have demonstrated a risk to the fetus. However, the benefits of therapy in a life threatening situation or a serious disease, may outweigh the potential risk.

Breast Feeding—There are no adequate studies in women for determining infant risk when using this medication during breastfeeding. Weigh the potential benefits against the potential risks before taking this medication while breastfeeding.

Other medicines—

Using this medicine with any of the following medicines is not recommended. Your doctor may decide not to treat you with this medication or change some of the other medicines you take.

Rotavirus Vaccine, Live

Interactions with Food/Tobacco/Alcohol—Certain medicines should not be used at or around the time of eating food or eating certain types of food since interactions may occur. Using alcohol or tobacco with certain medicines may also cause interactions to occur. Discuss with your healthcare professional the use of your medicine with food, alcohol, or tobacco.

Other medical problems—The presence of other medical problems may affect the use of this medicine. Make sure you tell your doctor if you have any other medical problems, especially:

- Chickenpox (including recent exposure) or
- Herpes zoster (shingles)—Risk of severe disease affecting other parts of the body
- Hepatitis (history of)—Increased risk of hepatitis
- Kidney disease or
- Liver disease (other)—Effects of floxuridine may be increased because of slower removal from the body
- Infection—Floxuridine can decrease your body's ability to fight infection

Proper Use of This Medicine

Floxuridine sometimes causes nausea and vomiting. Tell your doctor if this occurs, especially if you have stomach pain.

Dosing—The dose of this medicine will be different for different patients. Follow your doctor's orders or the directions on the label. The following information includes only the average doses of this medicine. If your dose is different, do not change it unless your doctor tells you to do so.

The amount of medicine that you take depends on the strength of the medicine. Also, the number of doses you take each day, the time allowed between doses, and the length of time you take the medicine depend on the medical problem for which you are using the medicine.

Precautions While Using This Medicine

It is very important that your doctor check your progress at regular visits to make sure that this medicine is working properly and to check for unwanted effects.

While you are being treated with floxuridine, and after you stop treatment with it, do not have any immunizations (vaccinations) without your doctor's approval. Floxuridine may lower your body's resistance and there is a chance you might get the infection the immunization is meant to prevent. In addition, other persons living in your household should not take oral polio vaccine since there is a chance they could pass the polio virus on to you. Also, avoid persons who have recently taken oral polio vaccine. Do not get close to them and do not stay in the same room with them for very long. If you cannot take these precautions, you should consider wearing a protective face mask that covers the nose and mouth.

Side Effects of This Medicine

Along with its needed effects, a medicine may cause some unwanted effects. Although not all of these side effects may occur, if they do occur they may need medical attention.

Also, because of the way these medicines act on the body, there is a chance that they might cause other unwanted effects that may not occur until months or years after the medicine is used. These delayed effects may include certain types of cancer, such as leukemia. Discuss these possible effects with your doctor.

Check with your doctor immediately if any of the following side effects occur:

More common

Diarrhea; sores in mouth and on lips; stomach pain or cramps

Less common

Black, tarry stools; heartburn; nausea and vomiting; scaling or redness of hands or feet; swelling or soreness of the tongue

Rare

Blood in urine or stools; cough or hoarseness; fever or chills; lower back or side pain; painful or difficult urination; pinpoint red spots on skin; trouble in walking; unusual bleeding or bruising; yellow eyes or skin

Some side effects may occur that usually do not need medical attention. These side effects may go away during treatment as your body adjusts to the medicine. Also, your health care professional may be able to tell you about ways to prevent or reduce some of these side effects. Check with your health care professional if any of the following side effects continue or are bothersome or if you have any questions about them:

Less common or rare

Loss of appetite; skin rash or itching

This medicine sometimes causes temporary thinning of hair. After treatment with floxuridine has ended, normal hair growth should return.

Other side effects not listed may also occur in some patients. If you notice any other effects, check with your healthcare professional.

FLUCYTOSINE   (Oral route) - floo-SYE-toe-seen

Black Box Warning

Use with extreme caution in patients with impaired renal function. Close monitoring of hematologic, renal and hepatic status of all patients is essential. These instructions should be thoroughly reviewed before administration of flucytosine.

Commonly used brand name(s)

In the U.S.—

Ancobon

Available Dosage Forms:

- Capsule
- Tablet

Therapeutic Class: Antifungal

Uses For This Medicine

Flucytosine belongs to the group of medicines called antifungals. It is used to treat certain fungus infections.

Flucytosine is available only with your doctor's prescription.

Before Using This Medicine

In deciding to use a medicine, the risks of taking the medicine must be weighed against the good it will do. This is a decision you and your doctor will make. For this medicine, the following should be considered:

Allergies—Tell your doctor if you have ever had any unusual or allergic reaction to this medicine or any other medicines. Also tell your health care professional if you have any other types of allergies, such as to foods, dyes, preservatives, or animals. For non-prescription products, read the label or package ingredients carefully.

Pediatric—Although there is no specific information comparing use of flucytosine in children with use in other age groups, this medicine is not expected to cause different side effects or problems in children than it does in adults.

Geriatric—Many medicines have not been studied specifically in older people. Therefore, it may not be known whether they work exactly the same way they do in younger adults. Although there is no specific information comparing use of flucytosine in the elderly with use in other age groups, this medicine is not expected to cause different side effects or problems in older people than it does in younger adults.

Pregnancy—

	Pregnancy Category	Explanation
All Trimesters	C	Animal studies have shown an adverse effect and there are no adequate studies in pregnant women OR no animal studies have been conducted and there are no adequate studies in pregnant women.

Breast Feeding—There are no adequate studies in women for determining infant risk when using this medication during breastfeeding. Weigh the potential benefits against the potential risks before taking this medication while breastfeeding.

Other medicines—

Using this medicine with any of the following medicines is not recommended. Your doctor may decide not to treat you with this medication or change some of the other medicines you take.

Levomethadyl

Interactions with Food/Tobacco/Alcohol—Certain medicines should not be used at or around the time of eating food or eating certain types of food since interactions may occur. Using alcohol or tobacco with certain medicines may also cause interactions to occur. Discuss with your healthcare professional the use of your medicine with food, alcohol, or tobacco.

Other medical problems—The presence of other medical problems may affect the use of this medicine. Make sure you tell your doctor if you have any other medical problems, especially:

- Blood disease—Flucytosine may cause blood problems
- Kidney disease—Patients with kidney disease may have an increased chance of side effects
- Liver disease—Flucytosine may cause liver side effects

Proper Use of This Medicine

In some patients this medicine may cause nausea or vomiting. If you are taking more than 1 capsule for each dose, you may space them out over a period of 15 minutes to help lessen the nausea or vomiting. If this does not help or if you have any questions, check with your doctor.

To help clear up your infection completely, keep taking this medicine for the full time of treatment, even if you begin to feel better after a few days. Do not miss any doses.

Dosing—The dose of this medicine will be different for different patients. Follow your doctor's orders or the directions on the label. The following information includes only the average doses of this medicine. If your dose is different, do not change it unless your doctor tells you to do so.

The amount of medicine that you take depends on the strength of the medicine. Also, the number of doses you take each day, the time allowed between doses, and the length of time you take the medicine depend on the medical problem for which you are using the medicine.

- For oral dosage form (capsules):
  - For fungus infections:
    - Adults and children—Dose is based on body weight. The usual dose is 12.5 to 37.5 milligrams (mg) per kilogram (kg) (5.7 to 17 mg per pound) of body weight every six hours.

Missed dose—If you miss a dose of this medicine, take it as soon as possible. However, if it is almost time for your next dose, skip the missed dose and go back to your regular dosing schedule. Do not double doses.

Storage—Store the medicine in a closed container at room temperature, away from heat, moisture, and direct light. Keep from freezing.

Keep out of the reach of children.

Do not keep outdated medicine or medicine no longer needed.

Precautions While Using This Medicine

Your doctor should check your progress at regular visits to make sure that this medicine does not cause unwanted effects.

Flucytosine may cause blood problems. These problems may result in a greater chance of infection, slow healing, and bleeding of the gums. Therefore, you should be careful when using regular toothbrushes, dental floss, and toothpicks. Dental work, whenever possible, should be done before you begin taking this medicine or delayed until your blood counts have returned to normal. Check with your medical doctor or dentist if you have any questions about proper oral hygiene (mouth care) during treatment.

Flucytosine may cause your skin to be more sensitive to sunlight than it is normally. Exposure to sunlight, even for brief periods of time, may cause skin rash, itching, redness, or other discoloration of the skin, or a severe sunburn. When you begin taking this medicine:

- Stay out of direct sunlight, especially between the hours of 10:00 a.m. and 3:00 p.m., if possible.
- Wear protective clothing, including a hat. Also, wear sunglasses.
- Apply a sun block product that has a skin protection factor (SPF) of at least 15. Some patients may require a product with a higher SPF number, especially if they have a fair complexion. If you have any questions about this, check with your health care professional.
- Apply a sun block lipstick that has an SPF of at least 15 to protect your lips.
- Do not use a sunlamp or tanning bed or booth.

If you have a severe reaction from the sun, check with your doctor.

This medicine may also cause some people to become dizzy, lightheaded, drowsy, or less alert than they are normally. Make sure you know how you react to this medicine before you drive, use machines, or do anything else that could be dangerous if you are dizzy or are not alert. If these reactions are especially bothersome, check with your doctor.

Side Effects of This Medicine

Along with its needed effects, a medicine may cause some unwanted effects. Although not all of these side effects may occur, if they do occur they may need medical attention.

Check with your doctor immediately if any of the following side effects occur:
> *More common*
>> Skin rash, redness, or itching; sore throat and fever; unusual bleeding or bruising; unusual tiredness or weakness; yellow eyes or skin
> *Less common*
>> Confusion; hallucinations (seeing, hearing, or feeling things that are not there); increased sensitivity of skin to sunlight

Some side effects may occur that usually do not need medical attention. These side effects may go away during treatment as your body adjusts to the medicine. Also, your health care professional may be able to tell you about ways to prevent or reduce some of these side effects. Check with your health care professional if any of the following side effects continue or are bothersome or if you have any questions about them:
> *More common*
>> Abdominal pain; diarrhea; loss of appetite; nausea or vomiting
> *Less common*
>> Dizziness or lightheadedness; drowsiness; headache

Other side effects not listed may also occur in some patients. If you notice any other effects, check with your healthcare professional.

FLUDARABINE   (Oral route) - floo-DARE-a-been

Uses For This Medicine

Fludarabine belongs to the group of medicines called antimetabolites. It is used to treat chronic lymphocytic leukemia (CLL), a type of cancer.

Fludarabine interferes with the growth of cancer cells, which are eventually destroyed. Since the growth of normal body cells may also be affected by fludarabine, other effects will also occur. Some of these may be serious and must be reported to your doctor. Other effects may not be serious but may cause concern. Some effects may not occur for months or years after the medicine is used.

Before you begin treatment with fludarabine, you and your doctor should talk about the good this medicine will do as well as the risks of using it.

Fludarabine is to be administered only by or under the immediate supervision of your doctor.

Before Using This Medicine

In deciding to use a medicine, the risks of taking the medicine must be weighed against the good it will do. This is a decision you and your doctor will make. For this medicine, the following should be considered:

Allergies—Tell your doctor if you have ever had any unusual or allergic reaction to this medicine or any other medicines. Also tell your health care professional if you have any other types of allergies, such as to foods, dyes, preservatives, or animals. For non-prescription products, read the label or package ingredients carefully.

Pediatric—There is no specific information comparing use of fludarabine in children with use in other age groups.

Geriatric—Many medicines have not been studied specifically in older people. Therefore, it may not be known whether they work exactly the same way they do in younger adults. Although there is no specific information comparing use of fludarabine in the elderly with use in other age groups, it is not expected to cause different side effects or problems in older people than it does in younger adults.

Pregnancy—

	Pregnancy Category	Explanation
All Trimesters	D	Studies in pregnant women have demonstrated a risk to the fetus. However, the benefits of therapy in a life threatening situation or a serious disease, may outweigh the potential risk.

Breast Feeding—There are no adequate studies in women for determining infant risk when using this medication during breastfeeding. Weigh the potential benefits against the potential risks before taking this medication while breastfeeding.

Other medicines—

Using this medicine with any of the following medicines is not recommended. Your doctor may decide not to treat you with this medication or change some of the other medicines you take.

Rotavirus Vaccine, Live

Interactions with Food/Tobacco/Alcohol—Certain medicines should not be used at or around the time of eating food or eating certain types of food since interactions may occur. Using alcohol or tobacco with certain medicines may also cause interactions to occur. Discuss with your healthcare professional the use of your medicine with food, alcohol, or tobacco.

Other medical problems—The presence of other medical problems may affect the use of this medicine. Make sure you tell your doctor if you have any other medical problems, especially:

- Anemia or
- Immune deficiency condition—may increase the risk of side effects of fludarabine
- Chickenpox (including recent exposure) or
- Herpes zoster (shingles)—Risk of severe disease affecting other parts of the body
- Gout (history of) or
- Kidney stones (history of)—Fludarabine may increase levels of uric acid in the body, which can cause gout or kidney stones
- Infection—Fludarabine may decrease your body's ability to fight infection
- Kidney disease—Effects of fludarabine may be increased because of slower removal from the body
- Transfusions—non-irradiated blood transfusion may increase the risk of side effects of fludarabine

Proper Use of This Medicine

This medicine may cause nausea and vomiting. However, it is very important that you continue to receive the medicine even if you begin to feel ill. Ask your health care professional for ways to lessen these effects.

Dosing—The dose of this medicine will be different for different patients. Follow your doctor's orders or the directions on the label. The following information includes only the average doses of this medicine. If your dose is different, do not change it unless your doctor tells you to do so.

The amount of medicine that you take depends on the strength of the medicine. Also, the number of doses you take each day, the time allowed between doses, and the length of time you take the medicine depend on the medical problem for which you are using the medicine.

Precautions While Using This Medicine

It is very important that your doctor check your progress at regular visits to make sure that this medicine is working properly and to check for unwanted effects.

While you are being treated with fludarabine, and after you stop treatment with it, do not have any immunizations (vaccinations) without your doctor's approval. Fludarabine may lower your body's resistance and there is a chance you might get the infection the immunization is meant to prevent. In addition, other persons living in your household should not take oral polio vaccine since there is a chance they could pass the polio virus on to you. Also, avoid persons who have recently taken oral polio vaccine. Do not get close to them and do not stay in the same room with them for very long. If you cannot take these precautions, you should consider wearing a protective face mask that covers the nose and mouth.

Fludarabine can temporarily lower the number of white blood cells in your blood, increasing the chance of getting an infection. It can also lower the number of platelets, which are necessary for proper blood clotting. If this occurs, there are certain precautions you can take, especially when your blood count is low, to reduce the risk of infection or bleeding:

- If you can, avoid people with infections. Check with your doctor immediately if you think you are getting an infection or if you get a fever or chills, cough or hoarseness, lower back or side pain, or painful or difficult urination.

- Check with your doctor immediately if you notice any unusual bleeding or bruising; black, tarry stools; blood in urine or stools; or pinpoint red spots on your skin.
- Be careful when using a regular toothbrush, dental floss, or toothpick. Your medical doctor, dentist, or nurse may recommend other ways to clean your teeth and gums. Check with your medical doctor before having any dental work done.
- Do not touch your eyes or the inside of your nose unless you have just washed your hands and have not touched anything else in the meantime.
- Be careful not to cut yourself when you are using sharp objects such as a safety razor or fingernail or toenail cutters.
- Avoid contact sports or other situations where bruising or injury could occur.

Side Effects of This Medicine

Along with its needed effects, a medicine may cause some unwanted effects. Although not all of these side effects may occur, if they do occur they may need medical attention.

Also, because of the way cancer medicines act on the body, there is a chance that they might cause other unwanted effects that may not occur until months or years after the medicine is used. These delayed effects may include certain types of cancer. Discuss these possible effects with your doctor.

Check with your doctor immediately if any of the following side effects occur:

More common
Arm, back or jaw pain; black, tarry stools; blood in urine or stools; chest pain or discomfort; chest tightness or heaviness; constipation; cough or hoarseness; coughing or spitting up blood; fast or irregular heartbeat; fever or chills; general feeling of discomfort or illness; lower back or side pain; nausea; pain; painful, burning, or difficult urination; pale skin; pinpoint red spots on skin; shortness of breath; sneezing; sore throat; sores, ulcers, or white spots on lips or in mouth; stomach pain, severe; sweating; swelling; tender, swollen glands in neck; thickening of bronchial secretions; troubled breathing; unusual bleeding or bruising; unusual tiredness or weakness; vomiting of blood or material that looks like coffee grounds; wheezing

Less common
Agitation; aneurysm; bleeding gums; blurred vision; confusion; decreased urine output; difficulty in breathing or swallowing; dilated neck veins; dizziness; extreme fatigue; fainting; fast, pounding, or irregular heartbeat, or pulse; headache; increased menstrual flow or vaginal bleeding; irregular breathing; loss of hearing; nosebleeds; numbness or tingling in fingers, toes, or face; pain, redness, or swelling in arm or leg; paralysis; prolonged bleeding from cuts; seizures; slurred speech; sudden and severe inability to speak; temporary blindness; weakness in arm and/or leg on one side of the body, sudden and severe; weight gain

Rare
Blindness; continuing vomiting; dark-colored urine; drowsiness; frequent urination; hives; itching; light-colored stools; loss of appetite; loss of consciousness; lower abdominal cramping; muscle tremors; puffiness or swelling of the eyelids or around the eyes, face, lips or tongue; rapid, deep breathing; restlessness; skin rash; stomach pain; trouble speaking, thinking or

walking; unusual tiredness or weakness; yellow eyes or skin

Some side effects may occur that usually do not need medical attention. These side effects may go away during treatment as your body adjusts to the medicine. Also, your health care professional may be able to tell you about ways to prevent or reduce some of these side effects. Check with your health care professional if any of the following side effects continue or are bothersome or if you have any questions about them:

More common
Abdominal pain; bladder pain; body aches or pain; burning, crawling, itching, numbness, prickling, "pins and needles", or tingling feelings; cloudy urine; congestion; diarrhea; difficulty in moving; dry mouth or throat; flushed, dry skin; frequent urge to urinate; fruit-like breath odor; increased hunger; increased thirst; increased urination; joint pain; muscle aching or cramping; muscle pains or stiffness; runny nose; swollen joints; trouble in swallowing; voice changes; weight loss

Less common
Abdominal fullness; bluish color of skin; changes in skin color; cracked lips; dandruff; decreased urination; decrease in height; difficulty in sleeping; discouragement; feeling sad or empty; gaseous abdominal pain; heartburn; irritability; loss of interest or pleasure; lightheadedness; oily skin; pain or tenderness around eyes and cheekbones; rapid breathing; recurrent fever; stuffy nose; sunken eye; trouble concentrating; wrinkled skin

This medicine may rarely cause a temporary loss of hair in some people. After treatment with fludarabine has ended, normal hair growth should return.

After you stop using this medicine, it may still produce some side effects that need attention. During this period of time, *check with your doctor immediately* if you notice the following side effects:

Rare
Cough or hoarseness; fever or chills; loss of vision; lower back or side pain; painful or difficult urination

Other side effects not listed may also occur in some patients. If you notice any other effects, check with your healthcare professional.

FLUDROCORTISONE (Oral route) -
floo-droe-KOR-ti-sone

Commonly used brand name(s)
In the U.S.—
Florinef Acetate

Available Dosage Forms:
- Tablet

Therapeutic Class: Endocrine-Metabolic Agent
Pharmacologic Class: Adrenal Mineralocorticoid

Uses For This Medicine

Fludrocortisone is a corticosteroid (cortisone-like medicine). It belongs to the family of medicines called steroids. Your body naturally produces similar corticosteroids, which are necessary to maintain the balance of certain minerals and water for good health. If your body does not produce enough corticosteroids, your doctor may have prescribed this medicine to help make up the difference.

Fludrocortisone may also be used to treat other medical conditions as determined by your doctor.

Fludrocortisone is available only with your doctor's prescription.

Once a medicine has been approved for marketing for a certain use, experience may show that it is also useful for other medical problems. Although these uses are not included in product labeling, fludrocortisone is used in certain patients with the following medical conditions:

- Idiopathic orthostatic hypotension (a certain type of low blood pressure)
- Too much acid in the blood, caused by kidney disease

Before Using This Medicine

In deciding to use a medicine, the risks of taking the medicine must be weighed against the good it will do. This is a decision you and your doctor will make. For this medicine, the following should be considered:

Allergies—Tell your doctor if you have ever had any unusual or allergic reaction to this medicine or any other medicines. Also tell your health care professional if you have any other types of allergies, such as to foods, dyes, preservatives, or animals. For non-prescription products, read the label or package ingredients carefully.

Pediatric—Fludrocortisone may slow or stop growth in children or growing adolescents when used for a long time. The natural production of corticosteroids by the body may also be decreased by the use of this medicine. Before this medicine is given to a child or adolescent, you and your child's doctor should talk about the good this medicine will do as well as the risks of using it. Follow the doctor's directions very carefully to lessen the chance that these unwanted effects will occur.

Geriatric—Many medicines have not been studied specifically in older people. Therefore, it may not be known whether they work exactly the same way they do in younger adults or if they cause different side effects or problems in older people. There is no specific information comparing the use of fludrocortisone in the elderly with its use in other age groups.

Pregnancy—

	Pregnancy Category	Explanation
All Trimesters	C	Animal studies have shown an adverse effect and there are no adequate studies in pregnant women OR no animal studies have been conducted and there are no adequate studies in pregnant women.

Breast Feeding—There are no adequate studies in women for determining infant risk when using this medication during breastfeeding. Weigh the potential benefits against the potential risks before taking this medication while breastfeeding.

Other medicines—

Using this medicine with any of the following medicines is not recommended. Your doctor may decide not to treat you with this medication or change some of the other medicines you take.

Bupropion, Rotavirus Vaccine, Live

Interactions with Food/Tobacco/Alcohol—Certain medicines should not be used at or around the time of eating food or eating certain types of food since interactions may occur. Using alcohol or tobacco with certain medicines may also cause interactions to occur. Discuss with your healthcare professional the use of your medicine with food, alcohol, or tobacco.

Other medical problems—The presence of other medical problems may affect the use of this medicine. Make sure you tell your doctor if you have any other medical problems, especially:

- Bleeding problems—Using fludrocortisone and also using aspirin may cause bleeding problems to become worse.
- Bone disease—Fludrocortisone may make bone disease worse because it causes more calcium to pass into the urine
- Edema (swelling of feet or lower legs) or
- Heart disease or
- High blood pressure or
- Kidney disease—Fludrocortisone causes the body to retain (keep) more salt and water. These conditions may be made worse by this extra body water
- Herpes infection of the eye—may cause a hole in the cornea of the eye.
- Liver disease or
- Abdominal surgery (fresh) or
- Diseases of the intestines or
- Myasthenia gravis or
- Tuberculosis or
- Ulcers in the stomach or intestines—Fludrocortisone suppresses the immune system. Infections with these conditions may be made worse by this suppression.
- Thyroid disease—The body may not get fludrocortisone out of the bloodstream at the usual rate, which may increase the effect of fludrocortisone or cause more side effects

Proper Use of This Medicine

Your doctor may want you to control the amount of sodium in your diet. When fludrocortisone is used to treat certain types of kidney diseases, too much sodium may cause high blood sodium, high blood pressure, and excess body water.

Take this medicine only as directed by your doctor. Do not take more or less of it, do not take it more often, and do not take it for a longer time than your doctor ordered. To do so may increase the chance of side effects.

Dosing—The dose of this medicine will be different for different patients. Follow your doctor's orders or the directions on the label. The following information includes only the average doses of this medicine. If your dose is different, do not change it unless your doctor tells you to do so.

The amount of medicine that you take depends on the strength of the medicine. Also, the number of doses you take each day, the time allowed between doses, and the length of time you take the medicine depend on the medical problem for which you are using the medicine.

- For oral dosage forms (tablets):
  - Adults
    - For adrenal gland deficiency: 50 to 200 micrograms a day.
    - For adrenogenital syndrome: 100 to 200 micrograms a day.
  - Children: For adrenal gland deficiency: 50 to 100 micrograms a day.

Missed dose—If you miss a dose of this medicine, take it as soon as possible. However, if it is almost time for your next dose, skip the missed dose and go back to your regular dosing schedule. Do not double doses.

Storage—Store the medicine in a closed container at room temperature, away from heat, moisture, and direct light. Keep from freezing.

Keep out of the reach of children.

Do not keep outdated medicine or medicine no longer needed.

Precautions While Using This Medicine

Your doctor should check your progress at regular visits to make sure this medicine does not cause unwanted effects.

If you will be using this medicine for a long time, your doctor may want you to carry a medical identification card stating that you are using this medicine.

While you are taking fludrocortisone, be careful to limit the amount of alcohol you drink.

Side Effects of This Medicine

Along with its needed effects, a medicine may cause some unwanted effects. Although not all of these side effects may occur, if they do occur they may need medical attention.

Check with your doctor immediately if any of the following side effects occur:

Less common or rare

Abdominal pain; agitation or combativeness; anxiety; back or rib pain; blindness; bloating; bloody or black, sticky stools; blurred vision; burning in stomach; changes in skin color; chest pain or tightness; chills; confusion; constipation; convulsions; cough; coughing up blood; darkened urine; decrease in height; decreased range of motion; decreased urine output; decreased vision; depression; difficulty swallowing; dry mouth; expressed fear of impending death; eye pain; eyeballs bulge out of eye sockets; fainting or lightheadedness when getting up from a lying or sitting position; fast or slow heartbeat; fever; flushed dry skin; fractures in arms or legs without any injury; fractures in the neck or back; fruit-like breath odor; hallucinations; headache; heartburn; hives; increased fat deposits on face, neck, and trunk; increased hunger; increased thirst; increased urination; indigestion; irregular breathing or shortness of breath; irregular heartbeat; joint pain; lack or slowing of normal growth in children; walking with a limp; loss of appetite; loss of consciousness; muscle cramps or pain; nausea or vomiting; nervousness; pain, tenderness, or swelling of foot or leg; pains in stomach or side, possibly radiating to the back; patients taking oral medicines or insulin for diabetes may need to increase the amount they take; pounding in the ears; problems with wound healing; redness and itching of skin; redness of eyes; redness of face; severe or continuing dizziness; severe weakness of arms and legs; skin rash; sweating; swelling of face, fingers, feet, or lower legs; swelling of nasal passages, face, or eyelids; swollen neck veins; tearing of eyes; unexplained weight loss; unusual tiredness or weakness; vision changes; weight gain; wheezing; yellow eyes or skin

Some side effects may occur that usually do not need medical attention. These side effects may go away during treatment as your body adjusts to the medicine. Also, your health care professional may be able to tell you about ways to prevent or reduce some of these side effects. Check with your health care professional if any of the following side effects continue or are bothersome or if you have any questions about them:

Less common or rare

Acne, pimples; bruising, large, flat, blue or purplish patches in the skin; change in color of skin or nails; increased sweating; loss of muscle mass; menstrual changes; muscle weakness; reddish purple lines on arms, face, legs, trunk, or groin; sleeplessness, trouble sleeping, unable to sleep; small, red, or purple spots on skin; swelling of abdominal or stomach area, full or bloated feeling or pressure in the stomach; thin, fragile skin; unusual increase in hair growth

Other side effects not listed may also occur in some patients. If you notice any other effects, check with your healthcare professional.

FLUOROQUINOLONE   (Oral route, Injection route, Intravenous route)

Commonly used brand name(s)

In the U.S.—

Avelox	Maxaquin
Avelox I.V.	Noroxin
Ciloxan	Ocuflox
Cipro	Quixin
Cipro IV	Tequin
Factive	Tequin Teq-Paqs
Floxin	Zagam
Levaquin	

In Canada—

Ciprofloxacin
Cipro Iv Minibags
Trovan

Available Dosage Forms:

- Powder for Suspension
- Solution
- Tablet
- Injectable

Uses For This Medicine

Fluoroquinolones are used to treat bacterial infections in many different parts of the body. They work by killing bacteria or preventing their growth. However, these medicines will not work for colds, flu, or other virus infections. Fluoroquinolones may also be used for other problems as determined by your doctor.

Once a medicine has been approved for marketing for a certain use, experience may show that it is also useful for other medical problems. Although these uses are not included in product labeling, fluoroquinolones are used in certain patients with the following medical conditions:

- Chancroid
- Pulmonary exacerbations (airway infections) in cystic fibrosis

Before Using This Medicine

Allergies—Tell your doctor if you have ever had any unusual or allergic reaction to medicines in this group or any other medicines. Also tell your health care professional if you have any other types of allergies, such as to foods dyes, preservatives, or animals. For non-prescription products, read the label or package ingredients carefully.

Pediatric—Use is not recommended for infants or children younger than 18 years of age since fluoroquinolones have been shown to cause bone development problems in young animals. However, your doctor may choose to use one of these medicines if other medicines cannot be used.

Geriatric—These medicines have been tested and, in effective doses, have not been shown to cause different side effects or problems in older people than they do in younger adults.

Pregnancy—Studies have not been done in humans. However, use is not recommended during pregnancy since fluoroquinolones have been reported to cause bone development problems in young animals. Before taking a fluoroquinolone, make sure your doctor knows if you are pregnant or if you may become pregnant.

Breast Feeding—Some of the fluoroquinolones are known to pass into human breast milk. Since fluoroquinolones have been reported to cause bone development problems in young animals, breast-feeding is not recommended during treatment with these medicines. Be sure you have discussed the risks and benefits of the medicine with your doctor.

Other medicines—

Using medicines in this class with any of the following medicines is not recommended. Your doctor may decide not to treat you with a medication in this class or change some of the other medicines you take.

Acecainide, Acetophenazine, Amiodarone, Amitriptyline, Amoxapine, Astemizole, Bepridil, Bretylium, Chlorpromazine, Cisapride, Clomipramine, Desipramine, Disopyramide, Dofetilide, Dothiepin, Doxepin, Erythromycin, Ethopropazine, Fluphenazine, Haloperidol, Ibutilide, Imipramine, Lofepramine, Mesoridazine, Methotrimeprazine, Moricizine, Nortriptyline, Opipramol, Pentamidine, Perphenazine, Pimozide, Pipotiazine, Pirmenol, Prajmaline, Probucol, Procainamide, Prochlorperazine, Promazine, Promethazine, Propiomazine, Protriptyline, Quinidine, Recainam, Sotalol, Terfenadine, Thiethylperazine, Thioridazine, Tizanidine, Trifluoperazine, Triflupromazine, Trimeprazine, Trimipramine, Ziprasidone

Using medicines in this class with any of the following medicines is usually not recommended, but may be required in some cases. If both medicines are prescribed together, your doctor may change the dose or how often you use one or both of the medicines.

Acarbose, Acecainide, Acetohexamide, Acetophenazine, Ajmaline, Alosetron, Amiodarone, Amisulpride, Amitriptyline, Amoxapine, Arsenic Trioxide, Astemizole, Azimilide, Benfluorex, Bretylium, Chloral Hydrate, Chloroquine, Chlorpromazine, Chlorpropamide, Clarithromycin, Clomipramine, Desipramine, Dibenzepin, Disopyramide, Dofetilide, Dolasetron,

Dothiepin, Doxepin, Droperidol, Encainide, Erythromycin, Ethopropazine, Flecainide, Fluconazole, Fluoxetine, Fluphenazine, Foscarnet, Gliclazide, Glimepiride, Glipizide, Gliquidone, Glyburide, Guar Gum, Halofantrine, Haloperidol, Hydroquinidine, Ibutilide, Imipramine, Insulin, Insulin Aspart, Recombinant, Insulin Glulisine, Insulin Lispro, Recombinant, Isradipine, Levomethadyl, Lidocaine, Lidoflazine, Lofepramine, Mefloquine, Metformin, Methotrimeprazine, Mexiletine, Miglitol, Moricizine, Nortriptyline, Octreotide, Opipramol, Pentamidine, Perphenazine, Pipotiazine, Pirmenol, Prajmaline, Prednisone, Probucol, Procainamide, Prochlorperazine, Promazine, Promethazine, Propafenone, Propiomazine, Protriptyline, Quetiapine, Quinidine, Recainam, Risperidone, Sematilide, Sertindole, Sotalol, Spiramycin, Sucralfate, Sulfamethizole, Sultopride, Tedisamil, Theophylline, Thiethylperazine, Tizanidine, Tocainide, Tolazamide, Tolbutamide, Trifluoperazine, Triflupromazine, Trimeprazine, Trimethoprim, Trimipramine, Troglitazone, Vasopressin, Venlafaxine, Ziprasidone, Zolmitriptan, Zotepine

Using this medicine with any of the following may cause an increased risk of certain side effects but using both medicines may be the best treatment for you. If both medicines are prescribed together, your doctor may change the dose or how often you use one or both of the medicines.

Aceclofenac, Acemetacin, Alclofenac, Aluminum Carbonate, Basic, Aluminum Hydroxide, Aluminum Phosphate, Apazone, Benoxaprofen, Betamethasone, Bromfenac, Bufexamac, Calcium, Calcium Carbonate, Carprofen, Clometacin, Clonixin, Corticotropin, Cortisone, Cosyntropin, Cyclosporine, Deflazacort, Dexamethasone, Dexketoprofen, Diclofenac, Didanosine, Diflunisal, Digoxin, Dihydroxyaluminum Aminoacetate, Dihydroxyaluminum Sodium Carbonate, Dipyrone, Droxicam, Duloxetine, Dutasteride, Etodolac, Etofenamate, Felbinac, Fenbufen, Fenoprofen, Fentiazac, Floctafenine, Fludrocortisone, Flufenamic Acid, Fluocortolone, Flurbiprofen, Fosphenytoin, Hydrocortisone, Ibuprofen, Indomethacin, Indoprofen, Iron, Isoxicam, Ketoprofen, Ketorolac, Lornoxicam, Magaldrate, Magnesium Carbonate, Magnesium Hydroxide, Magnesium Oxide, Magnesium Trisilicate, Meclofenamate, Mefenamic Acid, Meloxicam, Methylprednisolone, Nabumetone, Naproxen, Niflumic Acid, Nimesulide, Olanzapine, Oxaprozin, Oxyphenbutazone, Paramethasone, Phenylbutazone, Phenytoin, Pirazolac, Piroxicam, Pirprofen, Prednisolone, Prednisone, Probenecid, Propyphenazone, Proquazone, Ranitidine, Rasagiline, Rifapentine, Ropinirole, Ropivacaine, Sevelamer, Sucralfate, Sulindac, Suprofen, Tenidap, Tenoxicam, Tiaprofenic Acid, Tolmetin, Triamcinolone, Warfarin, Zinc, Zomepirac

Interactions with Food/Tobacco/Alcohol—Certain medicines should not be used at or around the time of eating food or eating certain types of food since interactions may occur. Using alcohol or tobacco with certain medicines may also cause interactions to occur. The following interactions have been selected on the basis of their potential significance and are not necessarily all-inclusive.

Using this medicine with any of the following may cause an increased risk of certain side effects but may be unavoidable in some cases. If used together, your doctor may change the dose or how often you use this medicine or give you special instructions about the use of food, alcohol, or tobacco.

Caffeine, Dairy Food, Milk

Other medical problems—The presence of other medical problems may affect the use of medicines in this class. Make sure you tell your doctor if you have any other medical problems, especially:

- Brain or spinal cord disease, including hardening of the arteries in the brain or epilepsy or other seizures—Fluoroquinolones may cause nervous system side effects

- Diabetes mellitus (sugar diabetes)—Levofloxacin may cause changes in blood sugar, which could lead to problems in controlling blood sugar
- Diarrhea—May be a sign of colon problems and taking fluoroquinolones could make this problem worse. Your doctor will want to check you before you begin taking your medicine.
- Glucose-6–phosphate dehydrogenase activity defect (problem with an enzyme that your body makes)—If you have this condition and you take a fluoroquinolone, you could have problems with anemia.
- Heart disease—Gatifloxacin, gemifloxacin, lomefloxacin, moxifloxacin or sparfloxacin may make this problem worse
- Kidney disease or
- Liver disease—Patients with kidney disease or liver disease may have an increased chance of side effects with any of the fluoroquinolones
- Myasthenia gravis (muscle disease)—This condition may become worse when taking a fluoroquinolone and cause your respiratory muscles to become weak which is life-threatening. Be sure and tell your doctor if you have this condition.
- Sensitivity of the skin to sunlight (previous)—Patients taking sparfloxacin or any of the other fluoroquinolones may have an increased risk of severe reactions to sunlight
- Tendinitis (previous)—Fluoroquinolones may increase the risk of tendon injury

Proper Use of This Medicine

Do not take fluoroquinolones if you are pregnant. Do not give fluoroquinolones to infants, children, or teenagers unless otherwise directed by your doctor. These medicines have been shown to cause bone development problems in young animals.

Fluoroquinolones should be used only to treat bacterial infections and not viral infections like the common cold. To help clear up your infection completely, keep taking your medicine for the full time of treatment, even if you begin to feel better after a few days. If you stop taking this medicine too soon, your symptoms may return.

Fluoroquinolones are best taken with a full glass (8 ounces) of water. Several additional glasses of water should be taken every day, unless you are otherwise directed by your doctor. Drinking extra water will help to prevent some unwanted effects of ciprofloxacin and norfloxacin.

Enoxacin or norfloxacin should be taken on an empty stomach

Ciprofloxacin, gatifloxacin, levofloxacin, lomefloxacin, moxifloxacin, ofloxacin, or sparfloxacin may be taken with meals or on an empty stomach. Ciprofloxacin should NOT be taken with dairy products or calcium-fortified juices alone, but may be taken with a meal that contains these products

This medicine works best when there is a constant amount in the blood or urine. To help keep the amount constant, do not miss any doses. Also, it is best to take the doses at evenly spaced times, day and night. For example, if you are to take two doses a day, the doses should be spaced about 12 hours apart. If this interferes with your sleep or other daily activities, or if you need help in planning the best times to take your medicine, check with your health care professional.

If you need to take this medicine for anthrax, your doctor will want you to begin taking it as soon as possible after you are exposed to anthrax.

Dosing—The dose medicines in this class will be different for different patients. Follow your doctor's orders or the directions on the label. The following information includes only the average doses of these medicines. If your dose is different, do not change it unless your doctor tells you to do so.

The amount of medicine that you take depends on the strength of the medicine. Also, the number of doses you take each day, the time allowed between doses, and the length of time you take the medicine depend on the medical problem for which you are using the medicine.

- For ciprofloxacin:
  - For long-acting oral dosage form (extended-release tablets):
    - Adults: 500 to 1000 milligrams (mg) every twenty-four hours for three to fourteen days, depending on the medical problem being treated.
    - Children up to 18 years of age: This medicine is not recommended for use in infants, children, or teenagers.
  - —For regular (short-acting) oral dosage form (oral suspension or tablets):
    - Adults: 100 to 750 milligrams (mg) every twelve hours for three to twenty-eight days, depending on the medical problem being treated. Bone and joint infections are usually treated for at least four to six weeks. Gonorrhea is usually treated with a single oral dose of 250 mg. Inhalational anthrax is usually treated for sixty days with 500 mg every twelve hours.
  - Children up to 18 years of age: This medicine is not recommended for use in infants, children, or teenagers, except in the case of inhalational anthrax. Inhalational anthrax is usually treated for sixty days with 15 mg per kilogram (kg) (6.8 mg per pound) of body weight every twelve hours.
    - For injection dosage form:
      - Adults: 200 to 400 mg every eight to twelve hours.
      - Children up to 18 years of age: This medicine is not recommended for use in infants, children, or teenagers, except in the case of inhalational anthrax. Inhalational anthrax is usually treated for sixty days with 10 mg per kg (4.5 mg per pound) of body weight every twelve hours.
- For enoxacin:
  - For oral dosage form (tablets):
    - Adults: 200 to 400 mg every twelve hours for seven to fourteen days, depending on the medical problem being treated. Gonorrhea is usually treated with a single oral dose of 400 mg.
    - Children up to 18 years of age: This medicine is not recommended for use in infants, children, or teenagers.
- For gatifloxacin:
  - For oral dosage form (oral suspension or tablets):
    - Adults: 200 to 400 mg every twenty four hours for seven to fourteen days, depending on the medical

problems being treated. Gonorrhea and certain bladder infection are usually treated with a single oral dose of 400 mg.

- Children up to 18 years of age: This medicine is not recommended for use in infants, children, or teenagers.

—For injection dosage form:

- Adults: 200 to 400 mg every twenty four hours for seven to fourteen days, depending on the medical problems being treated. Gonorrhea and certain bladder infection are usually treated with a single oral dose of 400 mg.
- Children up to 18 years of age: This medicine is not recommended for use in infants, children, or teenagers.

- For gemifloxacin:
  ○ For oral dosage form (tablets):
    - Adults: 320 mg once a day for 5 to 7 days, depending on the medical problem being treated.
    - Children up to 18 years of age: This medicine is not recommended for use in infants, children, or teenagers.

- For levofloxacin:
  ○ For oral dosage form (tablets):
    - Adults: 250 to 750 mg once a day for three to twenty-eight days, depending on the medical problem being treated.
    - Children up to 18 years of age: This medicine is not recommended for use in infants, children, or teenagers.
      —For injection dosage form:
      - Adults: 250 to 750 mg, injected slowly into a vein, once a day for three to twenty-eight days, depending on the medical problem being treated.
      - Children up to 18 years of age: This medicine is not recommended for use in infants, children, or teenagers.

- For lomefloxacin:
  ○ For oral dosage form (tablets):
    - Adults: 400 mg once a day for three to fourteen days, depending on the medical problem being treated.
    - Children up to 18 years of age: This medicine is not recommended for use in infants, children, or teenagers.

- For moxifloxacin:
  ○ For oral dosage form (tablets):
    - Adult: 400 mg once a day for five to fourteen days, depending on the medical problem being treated.
    - Children up to 18 years of age: This medicine is not recommended for use in infants, children, or teenagers.
      —For injection dosage form:
      - Adult: 400 mg injected in a vein once a day for five to fourteen days, depending on the medical problem being treated.
      - Children up to 18 years of age: This medicine is not recommended for use in infants, children, or teenagers.

- For norfloxacin:
  ○ For oral dosage form (tablets):
    - Adults: 400 mg every twelve hours for three to twenty-eight days, depending on the medical problem being treated. Gonorrhea is usually treated with a single oral dose of 800 mg.
    - Children up to 18 years of age: This medicine is not recommended for use in infants, children, or teenagers.

- For ofloxacin:
  ○ For oral dosage form (tablets):
    - Adults: 200 to 400 mg every twelve hours for three to fourteen days, depending on the medical problem being treated. Prostatitis is usually treated for six weeks. Gonorrhea is usually treated with a single oral dose of 400 mg.
    - Children up to 18 years of age: This medicine is not recommended for use in infants, children, or teenagers.
      —For injection dosage form:
      - Adults: 200 to 400 mg, injected slowly into a vein, every twelve hours for three to fourteen days, depending on the medical problem being treated. Prostatitis is usually treated for six weeks. Gonorrhea is usually treated with a single dose of 400 mg.
      - Children up to 18 years of age: This medicine is not recommended for use in infants, children, or teenagers.

- For sparfloxacin:
  ○ For oral dosage form (tablet):
    - Adults: 400 mg on the first day, then 200 mg once a day for an additional nine days.
    - Children up to 18 years of age: This medicine is not recommended for use in infants, children, or teenagers.

Missed dose—If you miss a dose of this medicine, take it as soon as possible. However, if it is almost time for your next dose, skip the missed dose and go back to your regular dosing schedule. Do not double doses.

Storage—Store the medicine in a closed container at room temperature, away from heat, moisture, and direct light. Keep from freezing.

Keep out of the reach of children.

Do not keep outdated medicine or medicine no longer needed.

Ciprofloxacin oral suspension may be refrigerated. However, keep this medicine from freezing.

Gatifloxacin oral suspension may be stored in the tightly closed bottle in a refrigerator for 14 days. Shake thoroughly prior to each use.

Precautions While Using This Medicine

If your symptoms do not improve within a few days, or if they become worse, check with your doctor.

If you are taking aluminum- or magnesium-containing antacids, didanosine, or sucralfate, do not take them at the same time that you take this medicine. It is best to take these medicines at least 6 hours before or 2 hours after taking ciprofloxacin; at least 8 hours before or 2 hours after taking enoxacin; at least 4 hours after taking gatifloxacin; at least

4 hours before or 4 hours after taking sparfloxacin; at least 2 hours before or 2 hours after taking levofloxacin, norfloxacin, or ofloxacin; at least 4 hours before or 2 hours after taking lomefloxacin, and at least 8 hours before and 4 hours after taking moxifloxacin. These medicines may keep fluoroquinolones from working properly.

If you are taking metal cations such as iron, and multivitamin preparations with zinc, or didanosine (Videx) chewable/buffered tablets or the pediatric powder for oral solution take moxifloxacin at least 4 hours before or 8 hours after and take ciprofloxacin at least 2 hours before or 6 hours after taking these medicines.

If you are taking levofloxacin or lomefloxacin, you should not take certain medications which correct a fast, slow or irregular heartbeat. Check with your physician to determine whether you are taking one of these medications.

If you are taking enoxacin, you should not take any caffeine-containing products (e.g., coffee, tea, chocolate, certain carbonated beverages). Taking any of these caffeine-containing products while you are taking enoxacin may increase the effects of caffeine.

Some people who take fluoroquinolones, especially sparfloxacin, may become more sensitive to sunlight than they are normally. Exposure to sunlight, even for brief periods of time, may cause severe sunburn, or skin rash, redness, itching, or discoloration. When you begin taking this medicine:

- Stay out of direct sunlight, especially between the hours of 10:00 a.m. and 3:00 p.m., if possible.
- Wear protective clothing, including a hat and sunglasses.
- Apply a sun block product that has a skin protection factor (SPF) of at least 15. Some patients may require a product with a higher SPF number, especially if they have a fair complexion. If you have any questions about this, check with your health care professional.
- Do not use a sunlamp or tanning bed or booth.
- Stay out of direct sunlight and artificial light (e.g., sunlamp, tanning bed or booth) for the next 5 days or until the reaction has stopped.
- If you get a skin rash or other signs of an allergic reaction, stop taking the fluoroquinolone and check with your doctor

Fluoroquinolones may also cause some people to become dizzy, lightheaded, drowsy, or less alert than they are normally. Make sure you know how you react to this medicine before you drive, use machines, or do anything else that can be dangerous if you are dizzy or are not alert. If these reactions are especially bothersome, check with your doctor.

Fluoroquinolones may rarely cause inflammation or even tearing of a tendon (the cord that attaches muscles to bones). If you get sudden pain in a tendon after exercise (for example, in your ankle, back of the knee or leg, shoulder, elbow, or wrist), stop taking the fluoroquinolone and check with your doctor. Rest and do not exercise until the doctor has made sure that you have not injured or torn the tendon.

If you have pain, burning, tingling, numbness and/or weakness, stop taking the fluoroquinolone and check with your doctor.

For patients with diabetes taking insulin or diabetes medicine by mouth: Levofloxacin may cause hypoglycemia (low blood sugar) in some patients. Symptoms of low blood sugar must be treated before they lead to unconsciousness (passing out). Different people may feel different symptoms of low blood sugar. If you experience symptoms of low blood sugar, stop taking levofloxacin and check with your doctor right away:

- Symptoms of low blood sugar can include: Anxious feeling, behavior change similar to being drunk, blurred vision, cold sweats, confusion, cool pale skin, difficulty in concentrating, drowsiness, excessive hunger, headache, nausea, nervousness, rapid heartbeat, shakiness, unusual tiredness or weakness.

For patients with low potassium levels: levofloxacin may increase your risk of experiencing a fast, slow or irregular heartbeat.

Side Effects of This Medicine

Along with its needed effects, a medicine may cause some unwanted effects. Although not all of these side effects may occur, if they do occur they may need medical attention.

Check with your doctor immediately if any of the following side effects occur:

More common—Less common for moxifloxacin; rare for lomefloxacin
   Fainting; irregular or slow heart rate

Less common—More common for lomefloxacin and sparfloxacin
   Bloating or swelling of face, arms, hands, lower legs, or feet; blistering of skin; blurred vision; dizziness; headache; nervousness; pounding in the ears; rapid weight gain; sensation of skin burning; slow or fast heartbeat; skin itching, rash, redness, or swelling; tingling of hands or feet; unusual weight gain or loss

Rare
   Abdominal or stomach cramps and pain (severe); abdominal pain; abdominal tenderness; agitation; area rash; black, tarry stools; bleeding; blisters on mucous membranes, with fever; blistering, itching, loosening, peeling, or redness of skin; bloody or cloudy urine; coldness; burning, crawling, itching, numbness, prickling, "pins and needles", or tingling feelings; chills; chest pain; clay-colored stools; confusion; cough; dark or amber urine; diarrhea (watery and severe, which may also be bloody); difficulty breathing; difficulty swallowing; discoloration of skin; dizziness; dry mouth; excessive muscle tone; fainting; faintness, dizziness, or lightheadedness when getting up from a lying or sitting position suddenly; fast, pounding, or irregular heartbeat or pulse; fatigue; flushed, dry skin; feeling of pressure; feeling of unreality; feeling of warmth or heat; fever; flushing or redness of skin especially on face and neck; fruit-like breath odor; hallucinations (seeing, hearing, or feeling things that are not there); hives or welts; incoordination; increased hunger; increased thirst; increased urination; inflammation; infection; irregular or fast heart rate; itching; joint pain; lack or loss of strength; large amount of fat in the blood; loss of appetite; loss of memory; lower back, side, or stomach pain; lumps; muscle stiffness; muscle tension or tightness; nausea; noisy breathing; numbness; pain; pain at site of injection— for ciprofloxacin or ofloxacin injection; pain in calves, radiating to heels; pain, warmth, or burning in fingers, toes and legs; painful or difficult urination; pale stools; palpitations; peeling of the skin; problems with memory; problems with speech or speaking; problems with vision or hearing; rash; rash with flat lesions or small raised lesions on the skin; redness; redness of skin; redness, swelling, or soreness

of tongue; scarring; seizures; sense of detachment from self or body; shakiness or tremors; shortness of breath skin rash; sore throat; sores, ulcers, or white spots on lips or in mouth; soreness; stomach pain; stinging; sweating; swelling; swelling of face or neck; swelling of calves, feet, or lower legs; swelling or inflammation of the mouth; swelling or puffiness of face; tenderness; tightness in chest; tingling; troubled breathing; ulceration; unpleasant breath odor; unusual tiredness or weakness; vomiting; vomiting of blood; warmth; wheezing; yellow eyes or skin

Incidence not known

Abnormal brain wave patterns; black, tarry stools; bleeding gums; blurred vision; coma; confusion; difficult breathing; failure of the heart, lungs, kidneys and/or liver; fatigue; general body swelling; hives; inability to move arms and legs; increased bleeding time; irregular reading on a electrocardiogram (heart test); joint or muscle pain; sharp drop in blood pressure; sore throat; sudden numbness and weakness in the arms and legs; swollen glands; unsteadiness or awkwardness; unusual bleeding or bruising; weakness in arms, hands, legs, or feet

Some side effects may occur that usually do not need medical attention. These side effects may go away during treatment as your body adjusts to the medicine. Also, your health care professional may be able to tell you about ways to prevent or reduce some of these side effects. Check with your health care professional if any of the following side effects continue or are bothersome or if you have any questions about them:

More common

Abdominal or stomach pain or discomfort (mild); diarrhea (mild); drowsiness; lightheadedness; nervousness; trouble in sleeping; vaginal pain and discharge

Less frequent or rare

Abnormal dream; acid or sour stomach; back pain; bad, unusual or unpleasant (after) taste; belching; bloated full feeling; burning, crawling, itching, numbness, prickling, "pins and needles", or tingling feelings; burning feeling in chest or stomach; change in sense of taste; change in sense of smell; change in taste; change in vision; constipation; continuing ringing or buzzing or other unexplained noise in ears; crying; depersonalization; depression; difficulty in sleeping; difficulty in speaking; difficulty in urination; dysphoria; euphoria; excess air or gas in stomach or intestines; fear; feeling of constant movement of self or surroundings; general feeling of discomfort or illness; hearing loss; heartburn; impaired vision; increased sensitivity of skin to sunlight; indigestion; mental depression; pain, swelling, or redness in joints; paranoia; passing gas; pelvic pain; pinpoint red or purple spots on skin; puffiness or swelling of the eyelids or around the eyes, face, lips or tongue; quick to react or overreact emotionally; rapidly changing moods; sensation of spinning; shortness of breath; sleeplessness; sleepiness or unusual drowsiness; sore mouth or tongue, or white patches in mouth and/or on tongue; spots on skin resembling a blister or pimple; stomach discomfort, upset or pain; tenderness in stomach area; thinking, abnormal; tongue discoloration; unable to sleep; vaginal yeast infection; vision problems; weight loss

Other side effects not listed may also occur in some patients. If you notice any other effects, check with your healthcare professional.

FLUOROURACIL (Intravenous route, Injection route) - flure-oh-YOOR-a-sil

Black Box Warning

It is recommended that fluorouracil be given only by or under the supervision of a qualified physician who is experienced in cancer chemotherapy and who is well versed in the use of potent antimetabolites. Because of the possibility of severe toxic reactions, it is recommended that patients be hospitalized at least during the initial course of therapy.

These instructions should be thoroughly reviewed before administration of fluorouracil.

Commonly used brand name(s)

In the U.S.—
   Adrucil

Available Dosage Forms:
* Solution
* Injectable

Therapeutic Class: Antineoplastic Agent
Pharmacologic Class: Antimetabolite

Uses For This Medicine

Fluorouracil belongs to the group of medicines known as antimetabolites. It is used to treat cancer of the colon, rectum, breast, stomach, and pancreas. It may also be used to treat other kinds of cancer, as determined by your doctor.

Fluorouracil interferes with the growth of cancer cells, which are eventually destroyed. Since the growth of normal body cells may also be affected by fluorouracil, other effects will also occur. Some of these may be serious and must be reported to your doctor. Other effects, like hair loss, may not be serious but may cause concern. Some effects may not occur for months or years after the medicine is used.

Before you begin treatment with fluorouracil, you and your doctor should talk about the good this medicine will do as well as the risks of using it.

Fluorouracil is to be administered only by or under the immediate supervision of your doctor.

Once a medicine has been approved for marketing for a certain use, experience may show that it is also useful for other medical problems. Although these uses are not included in product labeling, fluorouracil is used in certain patients with the following medical conditions:
* Cancer of the outside layer of the adrenal gland
* Cancer of the anus
* Cancer of the bladder
* Cancer of the cervix
* Cancer of the endometrium
* Cancer of the ovaries
* Cancer of the esophagus
* Cancer of the head and neck
* Cancer of the penis
* Cancer of the liver
* Cancer of the prostate
* Cancer of the skin
* Cancer of the vulva
* Carcinoid tumors

- Hepatoblastoma (a certain type of liver cancer that occurs in children)
- Glaucoma, during and after certain surgery (trabeculectomy)

Before Using This Medicine

In deciding to use a medicine, the risks of taking the medicine must be weighed against the good it will do. This is a decision you and your doctor will make. For this medicine, the following should be considered:

Allergies—Tell your doctor if you have ever had any unusual or allergic reaction to this medicine or any other medicines. Also tell your health care professional if you have any other types of allergies, such as to foods, dyes, preservatives, or animals. For non-prescription products, read the label or package ingredients carefully.

Pediatric—Although there is no specific information comparing use of fluorouracil in children with use in other age groups, it is not expected to cause different side effects or problems in children than it does in adults.

Geriatric—Many medicines have not been studied specifically in older people. Therefore, it may not be known whether they work exactly the same way they do in younger adults. Although there is no specific information comparing use of fluorouracil in the elderly with use in other age groups, it is not expected to cause different side effects or problems in older people than it does in younger adults.

Pregnancy—

	Pregnancy Category	Explanation
All Trimesters	X	Studies in animals or pregnant women have demonstrated positive evidence of fetal abnormalities. This drug should not be used in women who are or may become pregnant because the risk clearly outweighs any possible benefit.

Breast Feeding—There are no adequate studies in women for determining infant risk when using this medication during breastfeeding. Weigh the potential benefits against the potential risks before taking this medication while breastfeeding.

Other medicines—

Using this medicine with any of the following medicines is not recommended. Your doctor may decide not to treat you with this medication or change some of the other medicines you take.

Rotavirus Vaccine, Live

Interactions with Food/Tobacco/Alcohol—Certain medicines should not be used at or around the time of eating food or eating certain types of food since interactions may occur. Using alcohol or tobacco with certain medicines may also cause interactions to occur. Discuss with your healthcare professional the use of your medicine with food, alcohol, or tobacco.

Other medical problems—The presence of other medical problems may affect the use of this medicine. Make sure you tell your doctor if you have any other medical problems, especially:
- Chickenpox (including recent exposure) or

- Herpes zoster (shingles)—Risk of severe disease affecting other parts of the body
- Infection—Fluorouracil can decrease your body's ability to fight infection
- Kidney disease or
- Liver disease—Effects of fluorouracil may be increased because of slower removal from the body

Proper Use of This Medicine

This medicine is sometimes given together with certain other medicines. If you are using a combination of medicines, it is important that you receive each one at the proper time. If you are taking some of these medicines by mouth, ask your health care professional to help you plan a way to remember to take them at the right times.

Fluorouracil often causes nausea and vomiting. However, it is very important that you continue to receive the medicine, even if your stomach is upset. Ask your health care professional for ways to lessen these effects.

Dosing—The dose of this medicine will be different for different patients. Follow your doctor's orders or the directions on the label. The following information includes only the average doses of this medicine. If your dose is different, do not change it unless your doctor tells you to do so.

The amount of medicine that you take depends on the strength of the medicine. Also, the number of doses you take each day, the time allowed between doses, and the length of time you take the medicine depend on the medical problem for which you are using the medicine.

Precautions While Using This Medicine

It is very important that your doctor check your progress at regular visits to make sure that this medicine is working properly and to check for unwanted effects.

While you are being treated with fluorouracil, and after you stop treatment with it, do not have any immunizations (vaccinations) without your doctor's approval. Fluorouracil may lower your body's resistance and there is a chance you might get the infection the immunization is meant to prevent. In addition, other persons living in your household should not take oral polio vaccine since there is a chance they could pass the polio virus on to you. Also, avoid persons who have taken oral polio vaccine within the last several months. Do not get close to them and do not stay in the same room with them for very long. If you cannot take these precautions, you should consider wearing a protective face mask that covers the nose and mouth.

Fluorouracil can temporarily lower the number of white blood cells in your blood, increasing the chance of getting an infection. It can also lower the number of platelets, which are necessary for proper blood clotting. If this occurs, there are certain precautions you can take, especially when your blood count is low, to reduce the risk of infection or bleeding:
- If you can, avoid people with infections. Check with your doctor immediately if you think you are getting an infection or if you get a fever or chills, cough or hoarseness, lower back or side pain, or painful or difficult urination.
- Check with your doctor immediately if you notice any unusual bleeding or bruising; black, tarry stools; blood in urine or stools; or pinpoint red spots on your skin.

- Be careful when using a regular toothbrush, dental floss, or toothpick. Your medical doctor, dentist, or nurse may recommend other ways to clean your teeth and gums. Check with your medical doctor before having any dental work done.
- Do not touch your eyes or the inside of your nose unless you have just washed your hands and have not touched anything else in the meantime.
- Be careful not to cut yourself when you are using sharp objects such as a safety razor or fingernail or toenail cutters.
- Avoid contact sports or other situations where bruising or injury could occur.

Side Effects of This Medicine

Along with its needed effects, a medicine may cause some unwanted effects. Although not all of these side effects may occur, if they do occur they may need medical attention.

Also, because of the way these medicines act on the body, there is a chance that they might cause other unwanted effects that may not occur until months or years after the medicine is used. These delayed effects may include certain types of cancer, such as leukemia. Discuss these possible effects with your doctor.

Check with your doctor immediately if any of the following side effects occur:

More common
Diarrhea; heartburn; sores in mouth and on lips

Less common
Black, tarry stools; cough or hoarseness, accompanied by fever or chills; fever or chills; lower back or side pain, accompanied by fever or chills; nausea and vomiting (severe); painful or difficult urination, accompanied by fever or chills; stomach cramps

Rare
Blood in urine or stools; pinpoint red spots on skin; unusual bleeding or bruising

Check with your doctor as soon as possible if any of the following side effects occur:

Rare
Chest pain; cough; shortness of breath; tingling of hands and feet, followed by pain, redness, and swelling; trouble with balance

Some side effects may occur that usually do not need medical attention. These side effects may go away during treatment as your body adjusts to the medicine. Also, your health care professional may be able to tell you about ways to prevent or reduce some of these side effects. Check with your health care professional if any of the following side effects continue or are bothersome or if you have any questions about them:

More common
Loss of appetite; nausea and vomiting; skin rash and itching; weakness

Less common
Dry or cracked skin

This medicine often causes a temporary loss of hair. After treatment with fluorouracil has ended, normal hair growth should return.

After you stop using this medicine, it may still produce some side effects that need attention. During this period of time, *check with your doctor immediately* if you notice the following side effects:

Black, tarry stools; blood in urine or stools; cough or hoarseness, accompanied by fever or chills; fever or chills; lower back or side pain, accompanied by fever or chills; painful or difficult urination, accompanied by fever or chills; pinpoint red spots on skin; unusual bleeding or bruising

Other side effects not listed may also occur in some patients. If you notice any other effects, check with your healthcare professional.

FLUOROURACIL (Topical route) -
flure-oh-YOOR-a-sil

Commonly used brand name(s)

In the U.S.—
Carac
Efudex
Fluoroplex

Available Dosage Forms:
- Solution
- Cream

Therapeutic Class: Antineoplastic, Dermatological
Pharmacologic Class: Antimetabolite

Uses For This Medicine

Fluorouracil belongs to the group of medicines known as antimetabolites. When applied to the skin, it is used to treat certain skin problems, including cancer or conditions that could become cancerous if not treated.

Fluorouracil interferes with the growth of abnormal cells, which are eventually destroyed.

Fluorouracil is available only with your doctor's prescription.

Before Using This Medicine

In deciding to use a medicine, the risks of taking the medicine must be weighed against the good it will do. This is a decision you and your doctor will make. For this medicine, the following should be considered:

Allergies—Tell your doctor if you have ever had any unusual or allergic reaction to this medicine or any other medicines. Also tell your health care professional if you have any other types of allergies, such as to foods, dyes, preservatives, or animals. For non-prescription products, read the label or package ingredients carefully.

Pediatric—There is no specific information comparing use of fluorouracil on the skin in children with use in other age groups.

Geriatric—Many medicines have not been studied specifically in older people. Therefore, it may not be known whether they work exactly the same way they do in younger adults or if they cause different side effects or problems in older people. Although there is no specific information comparing use of fluorouracil on the skin in the elderly with use in other age groups, this medicine is not expected to cause different side effects or problems in older people than it does in younger adults.

Pregnancy—

	Pregnancy Category	Explanation
All Trimesters	X	Studies in animals or pregnant women have demonstrated positive evidence of fetal abnormalities. This drug should not be used in women who are or may become pregnant because the risk clearly outweighs any possible benefit.

Breast Feeding—There are no adequate studies in women for determining infant risk when using this medication during breastfeeding. Weigh the potential benefits against the potential risks before taking this medication while breastfeeding.

Other medicines—

Using this medicine with any of the following medicines is not recommended. Your doctor may decide not to treat you with this medication or change some of the other medicines you take.

Rotavirus Vaccine, Live

Interactions with Food/Tobacco/Alcohol—Certain medicines should not be used at or around the time of eating food or eating certain types of food since interactions may occur. Using alcohol or tobacco with certain medicines may also cause interactions to occur. Discuss with your healthcare professional the use of your medicine with food, alcohol, or tobacco.

Other medical problems—The presence of other medical problems may affect the use of this medicine. Make sure you tell your doctor if you have any other medical problems, especially:

- Dihydropyrimidine dehydrogenase (DPD) enzyme deficiency—May increase your chance of getting serious side effects.
- Other skin problems—May be aggravated

Proper Use of This Medicine

Keep using this medicine for the full time of treatment. However, do not use this medicine more often or for a longer time than your doctor ordered. Apply enough medicine each time to cover the entire affected area with a thin layer.

After washing the area with soap and water and drying carefully, use a cotton-tipped applicator or your fingertips to apply the medicine in a thin layer to your skin.

If you apply this medicine with your fingertips, make sure you wash your hands immediately afterwards, to prevent any of the medicine from accidentally getting in your eyes or mouth.

Fluorouracil may cause redness, soreness, scaling, and peeling of affected skin after 1 or 2 weeks of use. This effect may last for several weeks after you stop using the medicine and is to be expected. Sometimes a pink, smooth area is left when the skin treated with this medicine heals. This area will usually fade after 1 to 2 months. Do not stop using this medicine without first checking with your doctor. If the reaction is very uncomfortable, check with your doctor.

Dosing—The dose of this medicine will be different for different patients. Follow your doctor's orders or the directions on the label. The following information includes only the average doses of this medicine. If your dose is different, do not change it unless your doctor tells you to do so.

The amount of medicine that you take depends on the strength of the medicine. Also, the number of doses you take each day, the time allowed between doses, and the length of time you take the medicine depend on the medical problem for which you are using the medicine.

- For cream dosage form:
  - For precancerous skin condition caused by the sun:
    - Adults—Use the 0.5% or 1% cream on the affected areas of skin one or two times a day. The 5% cream is sometimes used on the hands.
    - Children—Use and dose must be determined by your doctor.
  - For skin cancer:
    - Adults—Use the 5% cream on the affected areas of skin two times a day. Treatment may continue for several weeks.
    - Children—Use and dose must be determined by your doctor.
- For topical solution dosage form:
  - For precancerous skin condition caused by the sun:
    - Adults—Use the 1% solution on the affected areas of skin one or two times a day. The 2% or 5% solution is sometimes used on the hands.
    - Children—Use and dose must be determined by your doctor.
  - For skin cancer:
    - Adults—Use the 5% solution on the affected areas of skin two times a day. Treatment may continue for several weeks.
    - Children—Use and dose must be determined by your doctor.

Missed dose—If you miss a dose of this medicine, take it as soon as possible. However, if it is almost time for your next dose, skip the missed dose and go back to your regular dosing schedule. Do not double doses.

Storage—Store the medicine in a closed container at room temperature, away from heat, moisture, and direct light. Keep from freezing.

Keep out of the reach of children.

Do not keep outdated medicine or medicine no longer needed.

Precautions While Using This Medicine

It is very important that your doctor check your progress at regular visits to make sure that this medicine is working properly and to check for unwanted effects.

Apply this medicine very carefully when using it on your face. Avoid getting any in your eyes, nose, or mouth.

While using this medicine, and for 1 or 2 months after you stop using it, your skin may become more sensitive to sunlight than usual and too much sunlight may increase the effect of the drug. During this period of time:

- Stay out of direct sunlight, especially between the hours of 10:00 a.m. and 3:00 p.m., if possible.
- Wear protective clothing, including a hat and sunglasses.
- Apply a sun block product that has a skin protection factor (SPF) of at least 15. Some patients may require a product with a higher SPF number, especially if they

have a fair complexion. If you have any questions about this, check with your health care professional.

- Do not use a sunlamp or tanning bed or booth.

If you have a severe reaction from the sun, check with your doctor.

Side Effects of This Medicine

Along with its needed effects, a medicine may cause some unwanted effects. Although not all of these side effects may occur, if they do occur they may need medical attention.

Check with your doctor immediately if any of the following side effects occur:

Redness and swelling of normal skin

Some side effects may occur that usually do not need medical attention. These side effects may go away during treatment as your body adjusts to the medicine. Also, your health care professional may be able to tell you about ways to prevent or reduce some of these side effects. Check with your health care professional if any of the following side effects continue or are bothersome or if you have any questions about them:

More common
Burning feeling where medicine is applied; increased sensitivity of skin to sunlight; itching; oozing; skin rash; soreness or tenderness of skin

Less common or rare
Darkening of skin; scaling; watery eyes

Other side effects not listed may also occur in some patients. If you notice any other effects, check with your healthcare professional.

FLUOXETINE   (Oral route) - floo-OX-e-teen

Black Box Warning

Suicidality in Children and Adolescents - Antidepressants increased the risk of suicidal thinking and behavior (suicidality) in short-term studies in children and adolescents with major depressive disorder (MDD) and other psychiatric disorders. Anyone considering the use of fluoxetine hydrochloride or any other antidepressant in a child or adolescent must balance this risk with the clinical need. Patients who are started on therapy should be observed closely for clinical worsening, suicidality, or unusual changes in behavior. Families and caregivers should be advised of the need for close observation and communication with the prescriber. Fluoxetine hydrochloride is approved for use in pediatric patients with MDD and obsessive compulsive disorder (OCD).

Pooled analyses of short-term (4 to 16 weeks) placebo-controlled trials of 9 antidepressant drugs (SSRIs and others) in children and adolescents with MDD, OCD, or other psychiatric disorders (a total of 24 trials involving over 4,400 patients) have revealed a greater risk of adverse events representing suicidal thinking or behavior (suicidality) during the first few months of treatment in those receiving antidepressants. The average risk of such events in patients receiving antidepressants was 4%, twice the placebo risk of 2%. No suicides occurred in these trials.

Commonly used brand name(s)

In the U.S.—

Prozac	Rapiflux
Prozac Weekly	Sarafem

In Canada—
Phl-Fluoxetine

Available Dosage Forms:
- Capsule, Delayed Release
- Solution
- Tablet
- Capsule

Therapeutic Class: Antidepressant
Pharmacologic Class: Serotonin Reuptake Inhibitor

Uses For This Medicine

Fluoxetine is used to treat mental depression. It is also used to treat obsessive-compulsive disorder, bulimia nervosa, and premenstrual dysphoric disorder (PMDD).

Fluoxetine also may be used for other conditions as determined by your doctor.

Fluoxetine belongs to a group of medicines known as selective serotonin reuptake inhibitors (SSRIs). These medicines are thought to work by increasing the activity of a chemical called serotonin in the brain.

This medicine is available only with your doctor's prescription.

Once a medicine has been approved for marketing for a certain use, experience may show that it is also useful for other medical problems. Although these uses are not included in product labeling, fluoxetine is used in certain patients with the following medical conditions:
- Premature ejaculation

Before Using This Medicine

In deciding to use a medicine, the risks of taking the medicine must be weighed against the good it will do. This is a decision you and your doctor will make. For this medicine, the following should be considered:

Allergies—Tell your doctor if you have ever had any unusual or allergic reaction to this medicine or any other medicines. Also tell your health care professional if you have any other types of allergies, such as to foods, dyes, preservatives, or animals. For non-prescription products, read the label or package ingredients carefully.

Pediatric—This medicine has been tested in a limited number of children 7 to 18 years of age. These studies indicate that fluoxetine may help to treat depression and obsessive-compulsive disorder in children. However, unusual excitement, restlessness, irritability, and trouble in sleeping may be especially likely to occur in children, who seem to be more sensitive than adults to the effects of fluoxetine. Fluoxetine must be used with caution in children with depression. Studies have shown occurrences of children thinking about suicide or attempting suicide in clinical trials for this medicine. More study is needed to be sure fluoxetine is safe and effective in children.

Geriatric—Many medicines have not been tested in older people. Therefore, it may not be known whether they work exactly the same way they do in younger adults or if they cause different side effects or problems in older people. In studies done to date that included elderly people, fluoxetine did not cause different side effects or problems in older people than it did in younger adults.

Pregnancy—

	Pregnancy Category	Explanation
All Trimesters	C	Animal studies have shown an adverse effect and there are no adequate studies in pregnant women OR no animal studies have been conducted and there are no adequate studies in pregnant women.

Breast Feeding—There are no adequate studies in women for determining infant risk when using this medication during breastfeeding. Weigh the potential benefits against the potential risks before taking this medication while breastfeeding.

Other medicines—

Using this medicine with any of the following medicines is not recommended. Your doctor may decide not to treat you with this medication or change some of the other medicines you take.

Bepridil, Clorgyline, Dihydroergotamine, Ergoloid Mesylates, Ergonovine, Ergotamine, Furazolidone, Iproniazid, Isocarboxazid, Levomethadyl, Mesoridazine, Methylergonovine, Methysergide, Moclobemide, Nialamide, Pargyline, Phenelzine, Pimozide, Procarbazine, Selegiline, Terfenadine, Thioridazine, Toloxatone, Tranylcypromine

Interactions with Food/Tobacco/Alcohol—Certain medicines should not be used at or around the time of eating food or eating certain types of food since interactions may occur. Using alcohol or tobacco with certain medicines may also cause interactions to occur. Discuss with your healthcare professional the use of your medicine with food, alcohol, or tobacco.

Other medical problems—The presence of other medical problems may affect the use of this medicine. Make sure you tell your doctor if you have any other medical problems, especially:

- Bipolar disorder (mood disorder with alternating episodes of mania and depression) or risk of—May make condition worse. Your doctor will check you for this condition.
- Brain disease or mental retardation or
- Seizures, history of—The chance of having seizures may be increased
- Diabetes—The amount of insulin or oral antidiabetic medicine that you need to take may change
- Diseases that affect your body's metabolism—Caution should be used
- Kidney disease or
- Liver disease—Higher blood levels of fluoxetine may occur, increasing the chance of side effects
- Parkinson's disease—May become worse
- Weight loss—Fluoxetine may cause weight loss. This weight loss is usually small, but if a large weight loss occurs, it may be harmful in some patients

Proper Use of This Medicine

Take this medicine only as directed by your doctor, to benefit your condition as much as possible. Do not take more of it, do not take it more often, and do not take it for a longer time than your doctor ordered.

If this medicine upsets your stomach, it may be taken with food.

If you are taking fluoxetine for depression, it may take 4 weeks or longer before you begin to feel better. Also, you may need to keep taking this medicine for 6 months or longer to stop the depression from returning. If you are taking fluoxetine for obsessive-compulsive disorder, it may take 5 weeks or longer before you begin to get better. Your doctor should check your progress at regular visits during this time.

If you are taking fluoxetine for bulimia nervosa, you may begin to get better after 1 week. However, it may take 4 weeks or longer before you get better.

Dosing—The dose of this medicine will be different for different patients. Follow your doctor's orders or the directions on the label. The following information includes only the average doses of this medicine. If your dose is different, do not change it unless your doctor tells you to do so.

The amount of medicine that you take depends on the strength of the medicine. Also, the number of doses you take each day, the time allowed between doses, and the length of time you take the medicine depend on the medical problem for which you are using the medicine.

- For oral dosage forms (capsules or solution):
  - For depression or obsessive-compulsive disorder:
    - Adults—At first, usually 20 milligrams (mg) a day, taken as a single dose in the morning. Your doctor may increase the dose if needed. However, the dose usually is not more than 80 mg a day. Once your depression is under control, your doctor may wish to change you to a weekly dose. In this case, you will usually take a 90–mg capsule as a single dose one day per week.
    - Children—Use and dose must be determined by your doctor.
  - For bulimia nervosa:
    - Adults—Usually 60 milligrams (mg) a day, taken as a single dose in the morning. Your doctor may start with a lower dose and increase it gradually. The dose usually is not more than 80 mg a day.
    - Children—Use and dose must be determined by your doctor.
  - For premenstrual dysphoric disorder:
    - Adults—At first, usually 20 milligrams (mg) a day, taken as a single dose in the morning. Your doctor may have you take 20 mg every day of your menstrual cycle or for only 14 days out of your cycle. Your doctor will determine the use and dose that is right for you. Your doctor may increase the dose if needed. However, the dose usually is not more than 80 mg a day.
    - Children—Use and dose must be determined by your doctor.

Missed dose—If you miss a dose of this medicine, skip the missed dose and go back to your regular dosing schedule. Do not double doses.

Storage—Store the medicine in a closed container at room temperature, away from heat, moisture, and direct light. Keep from freezing.

Keep out of the reach of children.

Do not keep outdated medicine or medicine no longer needed.

Precautions While Using This Medicine

It is important that your doctor check your progress at regular visits, to allow dosage adjustments and help reduce any side effects.

If you develop a skin rash or hives, stop taking fluoxetine and check with your doctor as soon as possible.

Fluoxetine may cause some people to be agitated, irritable or display other abnormal behaviors. It may also cause some people to have suicidal thoughts and tendencies or to become more depressed. If you or your caregiver notice any of these unwanted effects, tell your doctor right away.

Do not suddenly stop taking your fluoxetine. If you have been instructed to stop taking fluoxetine, ask you healthcare professional how to slowly decrease the dose. This is to decrease the chance of having symptoms such as agitation, breathing problems, chest pain, confusion, diarrhea, dizziness or light-headedness, fast heartbeat, headache, increased sweating, muscle pain, nausea, restlessness, runny nose, trouble in sleeping, trembling or shaking, unusual tiredness or weakness, vision changes, or vomiting.

Do not take fluoxetine within 2 weeks of taking a monoamine oxidase (MAO) inhibitor activity (isocarboxazid [e.g., Marplan], phenelzine [e.g., Nardil], procarbazine [e.g., Matulane], selegiline [e.g., Eldepryl], tranylcypromine [e.g., Parnate]) and do not take an MAO inhibitor for at least 5 weeks after taking fluoxetine. If you do, you may develop extremely high blood pressure or convulsions.

Do not take thioridazine (e.g., Mellaril) while you are taking fluoxetine or less than 5 weeks after you have stopped taking fluoxetine. Using these medicines together can cause very serious heart problems.

Avoid drinking alcohol while you are taking fluoxetine.

For diabetic patients:

- This medicine may affect blood sugar levels. If you notice a change in the results of your blood or urine sugar tests or if you have any questions, check with your doctor.

This medicine may cause some people to become drowsy or less able to think clearly, or to have poor muscle control. Make sure you know how you react to fluoxetine before you drive, use machines, or do anything else that could be dangerous if you are not alert and well able to control your movements.

Side Effects of This Medicine

Along with its needed effects, a medicine may cause some unwanted effects. Although not all of these side effects may occur, if they do occur they may need medical attention.

Check with your doctor as soon as possible if any of the following side effects occur:

More common
　Decreased sexual drive or ability; inability to sit still; restlessness; skin rash, hives, or itching

Less common
　Chills or fever; joint or muscle pain
Rare
　Breast enlargement or pain; convulsions (seizures); fast or irregular heartbeat; purple or red spots on skin; symptoms of hypoglycemia (low blood sugar), including anxiety or nervousness, chills, cold sweats, confusion, cool pale skin, difficulty in concentration, drowsiness, excessive hunger, fast heartbeat, headache, shakiness or unsteady walk, or unusual tiredness or weakness; symptoms of hyponatremia (low blood sodium), including confusion, convulsions (seizures), drowsiness, dryness of mouth, increased thirst, lack of energy; symptoms of serotonin syndrome, including diarrhea, fever, increased sweating, mood or behavior changes, overactive reflexes, racing heartbeat, restlessness, shivering or shaking; talking, feeling, and acting with excitement and activity you cannot control; trouble in breathing; unusual or incomplete body or facial movements; unusual secretion of milk, in females

Incidence not known
　Abdominal or stomach pain; agitation; back or leg pains; bleeding gums; blindness; blistering, peeling, loosening of skin; bloating; blood in urine or stools; bloody, black, or tarry stools; blue-yellow color blindness; blurred vision; changes in behavior; chest pain or discomfort; clay-colored stools; coma; constipation; continuing vomiting; cough/dry cough; dark urine; decreased urine output; decreased vision; depression; difficulty breathing; difficulty swallowing; dizziness or lightheadedness; eye pain; fainting; fainting, fast, pounding, or irregular heartbeat or pulse; fatigue; general body swelling; high fever; high or low blood pressure; hives or welts; hives, itching, puffiness or swelling of the eyelids or around the eyes, face, lips or tongue; hostility; increased hunger; indigestion; irregular or slow heart rate; irritability; itching; joint or muscle pain; large, hive-like swelling on face, eyelids, lips, tongue, throat, hands, legs, feet, sex organs; lethargy; light-colored stools; loss of appetite; loss of bladder control; muscle twitching; nausea; nightmares; no blood pressure or pulse; noisy breathing; nosebleeds; pain in ankles or knees; painful, red lumps under the skin, mostly on the legs; pains in stomach, side, or abdomen, possibly radiating to the back; palpitations; pinpoint red spots on skin; pounding heartbeat; rapid weight gain; red or irritated eyes; red skin lesions, often with a purple center; redness, tenderness, itching, burning, or peeling of skin; severe muscle stiffness; shortness of breath; skin rash; slurred speech; sore throat; sores, ulcers, or white spots on lips or in mouth; stopping of heart; stupor; sudden, severe chest pain; sudden shortness of breath or troubled breathing; sudden weakness in arms or legs; swelling of face, ankles, or hands; swollen or painful glands; thoughts of killing oneself; tightness in chest; tiredness; twitching, twisting, uncontrolled repetitive movements of tongue, lips, face, arms, or legs; unconsciousness; unpleasant breath odor; unusual bleeding or bruising; unusually pale skin; use of extreme physical or emotional force; vomiting of blood; wheezing; yellow eyes or skin

Symptoms of overdose—May be more severe than side effects that may occur from regular doses, or several symptoms may occur together

Agitation and restlessness; convulsions (seizures); drowsiness; fast heartbeat; nausea and vomiting; talking, feeling, and acting with excitement and activity you cannot control; trembling or shaking

Some side effects may occur that usually do not need medical attention. These side effects may go away during treatment as your body adjusts to the medicine. Also, your health care professional may be able to tell you about ways to prevent or reduce some of these side effects. Check with your health care professional if any of the following side effects continue or are bothersome or if you have any questions about them:

More common

Anxiety or nervousness; decreased appetite; diarrhea; drowsiness; headache; increased sweating; nausea; tiredness or weakness; trembling or shaking; trouble in sleeping

Less common or rare

Abnormal dreams; change in sense of taste; changes in vision; chest pain; constipation; dizziness or light-headedness; dryness of mouth; feeling of warmth or heat; flushing or redness of skin, especially on face and neck; frequent urination; hair loss; increased appetite; increased sensitivity of skin to sunlight; menstrual pain; stomach cramps, gas, or pain; vomiting; weight loss; yawning

Incidence not known

Cracks in the skin; loss of heat from the body; painful or prolonged erections of penis; red, swollen skin; scaly skin

After you stop using this medicine, it may still produce some side effects that need attention. During this period of time, *check with your doctor immediately* if you notice the following side effects:

Anxiety; dizziness; feeling that body or surroundings are turning; general feeling of discomfort or illness; headache; nausea; sweating; unusual tiredness or weakness

Incidence not known

Cracks in skin; loss of heat from the body; painful or prolonged erection of the penis; red, swollen skin; scaly skin; swelling of the breasts or breast soreness in both females and males; unusual milk production

After you stop using this medicine, it may still produce some side effects that need attention. During this period of time, *check with your doctor immediately* if you notice the following side effects:

Actions that are out of control; agitation; anxiety; burning, crawling, itching, numbness, prickling, "pins and needles", or tingling feeling; crying; depersonalization; euphoria; feeling of distress; feeling that body or surroundings are turning; general feeling of discomfort or illness; headache; irritability; mental depression; mood or mental changes; nervousness; nausea; paranoia; quick to react or over-react emotionally; rapidly changing moods; sleeplessness; sweating; talking, feeling, and acting with excitement; trouble sleeping; unable to sleep; unusual drowsiness, dullness, tiredness, weakness, or feeling of sluggishness; unusual tiredness or weakness; vaginal bleeding

Other side effects not listed may also occur in some patients. If you notice any other effects, check with your healthcare professional.

FLUTICASONE (Inhalation, oral/ nebulization route) - floo-TIK-a-sone

Commonly used brand name(s)

In the U.S.—

Flovent
Flovent HFA
Flovent Rotadisk

Available Dosage Forms:

- Aerosol Powder
- Powder
- Disk

Therapeutic Class: Anti-Inflammatory
Pharmacologic Class: Adrenal Glucocorticoid

Uses For This Medicine

Fluticasone belongs to the family of medicines known as corticosteroids (cortisone-like medicines). It is used to help prevent the symptoms of asthma. When used regularly every day, inhaled fluticasone decreases the number and severity of asthma attacks. However, it will not relieve an asthma attack that has already started.

Inhaled fluticasone works by preventing certain cells in the lungs and breathing passages from releasing substances that cause asthma symptoms.

This medicine may be used with other asthma medicines, such as bronchodilators (medicines that open up narrowed breathing passages) or other corticosteroids taken by mouth.

This medicine is available only with your doctor's prescription.

Once a medicine has been approved for marketing for a certain use, experience may show that it is also useful for other medical problems. Although these uses are not included in the product labeling, fluticasone propionate is used in certain patients with the following medical conditions:

- Pulmonary disease, chronic obstructive

Before Using This Medicine

In deciding to use a medicine, the risks of taking the medicine must be weighed against the good it will do. This is a decision you and your doctor will make. For this medicine, the following should be considered:

Allergies—Tell your doctor if you have ever had any unusual or allergic reaction to this medicine or any other medicines. Also tell your health care professional if you have any other types of allergies, such as to foods, dyes, preservatives, or animals. For non-prescription products, read the label or package ingredients carefully.

Pediatric—Corticosteroids taken by mouth or injection have been shown to slow or stop growth in children and cause reduced adrenal gland function. If enough fluticasone is absorbed following inhalation, it is possible it also could cause these effects. Your doctor will want you to use the lowest possible dose of fluticasone that controls asthma. This will lessen the chance of an effect on growth or adrenal gland function. It is also important that children taking fluticasone visit their doctors regularly so that their growth rates may be monitored. Children who are taking this medicine may be more susceptible to infections, such as chickenpox or measles. Care should be taken to avoid exposure to chickenpox or measles. If the child is exposed or the disease develops, the doctor should be contacted and his or her directions should be followed carefully. Before this medicine is given to a child, you and your child's doctor should talk about the good this medicine will do as well as the risks of using it.

Geriatric—Inhaled fluticasone has been studied in elderly patients and has not been found to cause different side effects or other problems than it does in younger adults.

Pregnancy—

	Pregnancy Category	Explanation
All Trimesters	C	Animal studies have shown an adverse effect and there are no adequate studies in pregnant women OR no animal studies have been conducted and there are no adequate studies in pregnant women.

Breast Feeding—There are no adequate studies in women for determining infant risk when using this medication during breastfeeding. Weigh the potential benefits against the potential risks before taking this medication while breastfeeding.

Other medicines—

Using this medicine with any of the following medicines is not recommended. Your doctor may decide not to treat you with this medication or change some of the other medicines you take.

Bupropion

Interactions with Food/Tobacco/Alcohol—Certain medicines should not be used at or around the time of eating food or eating certain types of food since interactions may occur. Using alcohol or tobacco with certain medicines may also cause interactions to occur. Discuss with your healthcare professional the use of your medicine with food, alcohol, or tobacco.

Other medical problems—The presence of other medical problems may affect the use of this medicine. Make sure you tell your doctor if you have any other medical problems, especially:

- Herpes simplex (virus) infection of the eye or
- Infections (virus, bacteria, or fungus)—Inhaled fluticasone may make these infections worse.
- Tuberculosis (active or history of)—Inhaled fluticasone may cause this infection to start up again.

Proper Use of This Medicine

Inhaled fluticasone is used to prevent asthma attacks. It is not used to relieve an attack that has already started. For relief of an asthma attack that has already started, you should use another medicine. If you do not have another medicine to use for an attack or if you have any questions about this, check with your health care professional.

Use this medicine only as directed. Do not use more of it and do not use it more often than your doctor ordered. To do so may increase the chance of side effects. The full benefit of this medicine may take 1 to 2 weeks or longer to achieve.

In order for this medicine to help prevent asthma attacks, it must be used every day in regularly spaced doses, as ordered by your doctor.

Gargling and rinsing your mouth with water after each dose may help prevent hoarseness, throat irritation, and infection in the mouth. However, do not swallow the water after rinsing.

Inhaled fluticasone is used with a special inhaler and usually comes with patient directions. Read the directions carefully before using this medicine. If you do not understand the directions or you are not sure how to use the inhaler, ask your health care professional to show you what to do. Also, ask your health care professional to check regularly how you use the inhaler to make sure you are using it properly.

For patients using the inhalation aerosol:

- When you use the inhaler for the first time, or if you have not used it for 4 weeks or longer, it may not deliver the right amount of medicine with the first puff. Therefore, before using the inhaler, prime it by spraying the medicine into the air four times. (Spray the inhaler once into the air if it has not been used in 1 to 3 weeks.) The inhaler will now be ready to give the right amount of medicine when you use it.
- To use the inhaler:
  - Shake the inhaler well for 15 seconds immediately before each use.
  - Take the cap off the mouthpiece (the strap will stay attached to the actuator). Check the mouthpiece and remove any foreign objects. Make sure the canister is fully and firmly inserted into the actuator.
  - Hold the mouthpiece away from your mouth and breathe out slowly and completely.
  - Use the inhalation method recommended by your doctor.
    - Open-mouth method—Place the mouthpiece about 1 or 2 inches (two fingerwidths) in front of your widely opened mouth. Make sure the inhaler is aimed into your mouth so that the spray does not hit the roof of your mouth or your tongue.
    - Closed-mouth method—Place the mouthpiece in your mouth between your teeth and over your tongue, with your lips closed tightly around it. Do not block the mouthpiece with your teeth or tongue.
  - Tilt your head back a little. Start to breathe in slowly and deeply through your mouth and, at the same time, press the top of the canister one time to get one puff of the medicine. Continue to breathe in slowly for 5 to 10 seconds. Count the seconds while inhaling. It is important to press the top of the canister and breathe in slowly at the same time so the medicine is pulled into your lungs. This step may be difficult at first. If you are using the closed-mouth method and you see a fine mist coming from your mouth or nose, the inhaler is not being used correctly.
  - Hold your breath as long as you can up to 10 seconds. This gives the medicine time to settle in your airways and lungs. Take the mouthpiece away from your mouth and breathe out slowly.
  - If your doctor has told you to inhale more than one puff of medicine at each dose, wait about 30 seconds and then gently shake the inhaler again, and take the second puff following exactly the same steps you used for the first puff.
  - When you are finished, wipe off the mouthpiece and replace the cover to keep the mouthpiece clean and free of foreign objects.

- Clean the inhaler and mouthpiece at least once a day to prevent buildup of medicine and blockage of the mouthpiece.
  - To clean the inhaler:
    - Remove the metal canister from the inhaler and set it aside.
    - Rinse the mouthpiece and cover and plastic case in warm, running water.
    - Shake off the excess water and let the inhaler parts air dry completely before replacing the metal canister and cover.

For patients using the powder for inhalation:

- To load the inhaler:
  - Make sure your hands are clean and dry.
  - Do not insert the disk until just before you are ready to use the medicine.
  - Take off the mouthpiece cover and make sure that the mouthpiece is clean.
  - Hold the corners of the white tray and pull out gently until you can see all of the plastic ridges on the sides of the tray.
  - Put your finger and thumb on the ridges, squeeze inward, and gently pull the tray out of the body of the inhaler.
  - Place a disk on the wheel with the numbers facing up, and then slide the tray back into the inhaler.
  - Hold the corners of the tray and slide the tray out and in. This will rotate the disk.
  - Continue to turn the disk in this way until the number 4 appears in the small window. Each disk has four blisters containing the medicine. The window will display how many inhalations you have left after you use it each time. For example, when you see the number 1, you have one inhalation left.
  - To replace the empty disk with a full disk, follow the same steps you used to load the inhaler. Do not throw away the wheel when you discard the empty disk.
- To use the inhaler:
  - Hold the inhaler flat in your hand. Lift the rear edge of the lid until it is fully upright.
  - The plastic needle on the front of the lid will break the blister containing one inhalation of medicine. When the lid is raised as far as it will go, both the upper and the lower surfaces of the blister will be pierced. Do not lift the lid if the cartridge is not in the inhaler. Doing this will break the needle and you will need a new inhaler.
  - After the blister is broken open, close the lid. Keeping the inhaler flat and well away from your mouth, breathe out to the end of a normal breath.
  - Raise the inhaler to your mouth, and place the mouthpiece in your mouth.
  - Close your lips around the mouthpiece and tilt your head slightly back. Do not bite down on the mouthpiece. Do not block the mouthpiece with your teeth or tongue. Do not cover the air holes on the side of the mouthpiece.
  - Breathe in through your mouth as steadily and as deeply as you can until you have taken a full deep breath.
  - Hold your breath and remove the mouthpiece from your mouth. Continue holding your breath as long as you can up to 10 seconds before breathing out. This

gives the medicine time to settle in your airways and lungs.
  - Hold the inhaler well away from your mouth and breathe out to the end of a normal breath.
  - Prepare the cartridge for your next inhalation. Pull the cartridge out once and push it in once. The disk will turn to the next numbered dose as seen in the indicator window. Do not pierce the blister until just before the inhalation.
  - If your doctor has told you to inhale more than one puff of medicine at each dose, take the second puff following exactly the same steps you used for the first puff.
  - When you are finished, wipe off the mouthpiece and replace the cover to keep the mouthpiece clean and free of foreign objects.
- To clean the inhaler:
  - Remove the tray from the body of the inhaler.
  - Hold the wheel between your forefinger and thumb and pull upward to separate it from the tray.
  - Use the brush that is stored in the rear of the body of the inhaler to brush away any powder left behind on the parts of the inhaler.
  - Replace the wheel and push it down firmly until it snaps back into place.
  - Replace the tray and mouthpiece cover.
  - Separate the parts of the inhaler using the steps outlined above.
  - Rinse the parts of the inhaler with warm water and let them air dry before reassembling them as described above.

The inhaler should be cleaned once a week.

Dosing—The dose of this medicine will be different for different patients. Follow your doctor's orders or the directions on the label. The following information includes only the average doses of this medicine. If your dose is different, do not change it unless your doctor tells you to do so.

The amount of medicine that you take depends on the strength of the medicine. Also, the number of doses you take each day, the time allowed between doses, and the length of time you take the medicine depend on the medical problem for which you are using the medicine.

- For bronchial asthma
  - For inhalation aerosol:
    - Adults and children 12 years of age and older— 88 to 880 micrograms (mcg) two times a day, morning and evening.
    - Canadian labeling recommends—For adults and children 16 and older: 100 to 1000 mcg two times a day.
    - Children younger than 12 years of age—Use and dose must be determined by your doctor.
    - Canadian labeling recommends—For children 4 to 16 years of age: 50 to 100 mcg two times a day; For children up to 4 years of age: Use and dose must be determined by your doctor.
  - For powder for inhalation:
    - Adults and children older than 11 years of age— 100 to 1000 mcg two times a day.
    - Children 4 to 11 years of age—50 to 100 mcg two times a day.
    - Canadian labeling recommends—For children 4 to 16 years of age: 50 to 100 mcg two times a day.

- Children younger than 4 years of age—Use and dose must be determined by your doctor.

Missed dose—If you miss a dose of this medicine, take it as soon as possible. However, if it is almost time for your next dose, skip the missed dose and go back to your regular dosing schedule. Do not double doses.

Storage—Store the medicine in a closed container at room temperature, away from heat, moisture, and direct light. Keep from freezing.

Store the canister at room temperature, away from heat and direct light. Do not freeze. Do not keep this medicine inside a car where it could be exposed to extreme heat or cold. Do not poke holes in the canister or throw it into a fire, even if the canister is empty.

Keep out of the reach of children.

Do not keep outdated medicine or medicine no longer needed.

Precautions While Using This Medicine

Check with your doctor if:
- You go through a period of unusual stress to your body, such as surgery, injury, or infection.
- You have an asthma attack that does not improve after you take a bronchodilator medicine.
- Your asthma symptoms do not improve or your condition worsens.
- You are exposed to the chickenpox or measles.

Your doctor may want you to carry a medical identification card stating that you are using this medicine and that you may need additional medicine during times of emergency, a severe asthma attack or other illness, or unusual stress.

Before you have any kind of surgery (including dental surgery) or emergency treatment, tell the medical doctor or dentist in charge that you are using this medicine.

Side Effects of This Medicine

Along with its needed effects, a medicine may cause some unwanted effects. Although not all of these side effects may occur, if they do occur they may need medical attention.

Check with your doctor immediately if any of the following side effects occur:

More common
White patches in mouth and throat

Less common
Diarrhea; ear ache; fever; lower abdominal pain; nausea; pain on passing urine; redness or discharge of the eye, eyelid, or lining of the eye; shortness of breath; sore throat; trouble in swallowing; vaginal discharge (creamy white) and itching; vomiting

Rare
Blindness, blurred vision, eye pain; large hives; bone fractures; diabetes mellitus [increased hunger, thirst, or urination]; excess facial hair in women; fullness or roundness of face, neck, and trunk; growth reduction in children or adolescents; heart problems; high blood pressure; hives and skin rash; impotence in males; lack of menstrual periods; muscle wasting; numbness and weakness of hands and feet; weakness; swelling of face, lips, or eyelids; tightness in chest, troubled breathing, or wheezing

Incidence not known
Difficulty breathing; difficulty swallowing; dizziness; fast heartbeat; growth rate decreased in children and teenagers; itching, puffiness, or swelling of the eyelids or around the eyes, face, lips, or tongue; noisy breathing; swelling of the mouth or throat

Some side effects may occur that usually do not need medical attention. These side effects may go away during treatment as your body adjusts to the medicine. Also, your health care professional may be able to tell you about ways to prevent or reduce some of these side effects. Check with your health care professional if any of the following side effects continue or are bothersome or if you have any questions about them:

More common
Cough; general aches and pains or general feeling of illness; greenish-yellow mucus in nose; headache; hoarseness or other voice changes; loss of appetite; runny, sore, or stuffy nose; unusual tiredness; weakness

Less common
Bloody mucus or unexplained nosebleeds; dizziness; eye irritation; feeling 'faint'; giddiness; irregular or painful menstrual periods; irritation due to inhalant; joint pain; migraines; mouth irritation; muscle soreness, sprain, or strain; sneezing; stomach pain or burning

Rare
Aggression; agitation; bruising; depression; itching; restlessness; weight gain

Incidence not known
Abdominal pain; blurred vision; decrease in height; dry mouth; fatigue; flushed, dry skin; fruit-like breath odor; increased hunger; increased thirst; increased urination; loss of voice; pain in back, ribs, arms or legs; sweating; trouble sitting still; unexplained weight loss

Other side effects not listed may also occur in some patients. If you notice any other effects, check with your healthcare professional.

FLUTICASONE AND SALMETEROL
(Inhalation, oral/nebulization route) - floo-TIK-a-sone, sal-ME-te-role

Black Box Warning

Long-acting beta 2–adrenergic agonists, such as salmeterol, one of the active ingredients in the fluticasone proprionate/salmeterol inhalation powder, may increase the risk of asthma-related death. Therefore, when treating patients with asthma, physicians should only prescribe fluticasone proprionate/salmeterol for patients not adequately controlled on other asthma-controller medications (e.g., low- to medium-dose inhaled corticosteroids) or whose disease severity clearly warrants initiation of treatment with 2 maintenance therapies. Data from a large placebo-controlled US study that compared the safety of salmeterol or placebo added to usual asthma therapy showed an increase in asthma-related deaths in patients receiving salmeterol (13 deaths out of 13,176 patients treated for 28 weeks on salmeterol versus 3 deaths out of 13,179 patients on placebo).

Commonly used brand name(s)

In the U.S.—

Advair Diskus 100/50	Advair Diskus 500/50
Advair Diskus 250/50	Advair HFA

Available Dosage Forms:

- Aerosol Liquid
- Disk
- Aerosol Powder

Therapeutic Class: Antiasthma, Anti-Inflammatory/Bronchodilator Combination

Pharmacologic Class: Fluticasone

Uses For This Medicine

Fluticasone and salmeterol is a combination of two medicines that are used to help control the symptoms of asthma and improve lung function. It is used when a patient's asthma has not been controlled sufficiently on other asthma medicines or when a patient's condition is so severe that more than one maintenance medicine is needed. However, this medicine will not relieve an asthma attack that has already started.

Inhaled fluticasone belongs to the family of medicines known as corticosteroids (cortisone-like medicines). It works by preventing certain cells in the lungs and breathing passages from releasing substances that cause asthma symptoms.

Inhaled salmeterol is a long-acting bronchodilator and it belongs to the family of medicines known as bronchodilators. Bronchodilators are medicines that are breathed in through the mouth to open up the bronchial tubes (air passages) of the lungs. Salmeterol is different than other bronchodilators because it does not act quickly enough to relieve an asthma attack that has already started.

This medicine must be used with a short-acting beta-2 agonist (e.g. albuterol) for the treatment of an asthma attack or asthma symptoms that need immediate attention.

This medicine is available only with your doctor's prescription.

Once a medicine has been approved for marketing for a certain use, experience may show that it is also useful for other medical problems. Although these uses are not included in the product labeling, fluticasone and salmeterol combination is used in certain patients with the following medical conditions:

- Emphysema

Before Using This Medicine

In deciding to use a medicine, the risks of taking the medicine must be weighed against the good it will do. This is a decision you and your doctor will make. For this medicine, the following should be considered:

Allergies—Tell your doctor if you have ever had any unusual or allergic reaction to this medicine or any other medicines. Also tell your health care professional if you have any other types of allergies, such as to foods, dyes, preservatives, or animals. For non-prescription products, read the label or package ingredients carefully.

Pediatric—Corticosteroids taken by mouth or injection have been shown to slow or stop growth in children and cause reduced adrenal gland function. If enough fluticasone is absorbed following inhalation, it is possible it also could cause these effects. Your doctor will want you to use the lowest possible dose of fluticasone that controls asthma. This will lessen the chance of an effect on growth or adrenal gland function. It is also important that children taking fluticasone visit their doctors regularly so that their growth rates may be monitored. Children who are taking this medicine may be more susceptible to infections, such as chickenpox or measles. Care should be taken to avoid exposure to chickenpox or measles. If the child is exposed or the disease develops, the doctor should be contacted and his or her directions should be followed carefully. Before this medicine is given to a child, you and your child's doctor should talk about the good this medicine will do as well as the risks of using it.

Geriatric—Many medicines have not been studied specifically in older people. Therefore, it may not be known whether they work exactly the same way they do in younger adults. Although there is no specific information comparing the use of fluticasone and salmeterol in the elderly with other age groups, this medicine has been used in elderly patients and is not expected to cause different side effects or problems in older people than it does in younger adults. Elderly people who have cardiovascular disease may have increased chances of side effects from this medicine.

Other medicines—

Using this medicine with any of the following medicines is not recommended. Your doctor may decide not to treat you with this medication or change some of the other medicines you take.

Bupropion

Interactions with Food/Tobacco/Alcohol—Certain medicines should not be used at or around the time of eating food or eating certain types of food since interactions may occur. Using alcohol or tobacco with certain medicines may also cause interactions to occur. Discuss with your healthcare professional the use of your medicine with food, alcohol, or tobacco.

Other medical problems—The presence of other medical problems may affect the use of this medicine. Make sure you tell your doctor if you have any other medical problems, especially:

- Asthma attack, severe or
- Infection or
- Stress or
- Surgery or
- Trauma—Supplementary oral corticosteroids may be needed. Check with your doctor.
- Chickenpox (including recent exposure) or
- Measles or
- Herpes simplex (virus) infection of the eye or
- Infections (virus, bacteria, or fungus) or
- Tuberculosis (active or history of)—Inhaled fluticasone can reduce the body's ability to fight off these infections
- Diabetes mellitus or
- Ketoacidosis—Blood sugar levels may increase

- Heart or blood vessel disease or
- High blood pressure or
- Overactive thyroid or
- Seizures—This medicine may worsen these conditions
- Eosinophilic conditions—Fluticasone may make these conditions worse
- Osteoporosis (bone disease)—Inhaled corticosteroids in high doses may make this condition worse.

Proper Use of This Medicine

Inhaled fluticasone and salmeterol is used to prevent asthma attacks. It is not used to relieve an asthma attack that has already started. For relief of an asthma attack that has already started, you should use another medicine. If you do not have another medicine to use for an attack or if you have any questions about this, check with your health care professional.

Use this medicine only as directed. Do not use more of it and do not use it more often than your doctor ordered. Also, do not stop taking this medicine without telling your doctor. To do so may increase the chance of side effects.

In order for this medicine to help prevent asthma attacks, it must be used every day in regularly spaced doses, as ordered by your doctor.

Do not stop using this medicine or other asthma medicines that your doctor has prescribed for you unless you have discussed this with your doctor.

Rinsing your mouth with water after each dose may help prevent hoarseness, throat irritation, and infection in the mouth. However, do not swallow the water after rinsing.

Inhaled fluticasone and salmeterol is used with a special inhaler that comes with patient directions. Read the directions carefully before using this medicine. If you do not understand the directions or you are not sure how to use the inhaler, ask your health care professional to show you what to do. Also, ask your health care professional to check regularly how you use the inhaler to make sure you are using it properly.

To use the disposable inhaler for inhalation powder:

- To open the inhaler, push the thumbgrip away from you as far as it will go. You will hear a click and feel a snap. When open, the mouthpiece will appear.
- Slide the mouthpiece lever away from you as far as it will go until it clicks. The inhaler is now ready to use. If you close the inhaler or push the lever again, you will lose medicine.
- Turn your head away from the inhaler, and breathe out to the end of a normal breath. Do not breathe into the inhaler.
- Holding the inhaler level, put the mouthpiece between your lips and teeth, and close your lips around the mouthpiece. Do not bite down on the mouthpiece. Do not block the mouthpiece with your teeth or tongue.
- Breathe in through your mouth as deeply as you can until you have taken a full deep breath. Do not breathe through your nose.
- Hold your breath and remove the mouthpiece from your mouth. Continue holding your breath as long as you can up to 10 seconds before breathing out slowly. This gives the medicine time to settle in your airways and lungs.

- Turn your head away from the inhaler, and breathe out slowly to the end of a normal breath. Do not breathe into the inhaler.
- If your doctor has told you to inhale more than one puff of medicine at each dose, take the second puff following exactly the same steps you used for the first puff.
- When you are finished, close the inhaler. Place your thumb on the thumbgrip, and slide it back toward you as far as it will go. You will hear it click shut.
- Keep the inhaler dry. Do not wash the mouthpiece, or any other part of the inhaler. You may use a dry cloth to wipe it clean.
- The inhaler has a window that shows the number of doses remaining. This tells you when you are getting low on medicine. The doses counting down from 5 to 0 will show up in red to remind you to refill your prescription.

Dosing—The dose of this medicine will be different for different patients. Follow your doctor's orders or the directions on the label. The following information includes only the average doses of this medicine. If your dose is different, do not change it unless your doctor tells you to do so.

The amount of medicine that you take depends on the strength of the medicine. Also, the number of doses you take each day, the time allowed between doses, and the length of time you take the medicine depend on the medical problem for which you are using the medicine.

- For powder for inhalation
  - For bronchial asthma
    - Adults and children 4 years of age and older: One inhalation twice a day, about 12 hours apart.
    - Children up to 4 years of age: Use and dose must be determined by your doctor.

  - For chronic obstructive pulmonary disease with chronic bronchitis
    - Adults: One inhalation (250/50) twice a day, about 12 hour apart.
    - Children: Use and dose must be determined by your doctor.

Missed dose—If you miss a dose of this medicine, skip the missed dose and go back to your regular dosing schedule. Do not double doses.

Storage—Store the medicine in a closed container at room temperature, away from heat, moisture, and direct light. Keep from freezing.

Keep the medicine in the foil pouch until you are ready to use it. Store at room temperature, away from heat and direct light. Do not freeze.

Keep out of the reach of children.

Do not keep outdated medicine or medicine no longer needed.

Precautions While Using This Medicine

Check with your doctor if your asthma symptoms do not improve or your condition worsens. Check with your doctor if you notice:

- Your short-acting inhaler does not seem to work as well as it used to

- You need to use your short-acting inhaler more often
- You have a significant decrease in your peak flow when measured as directed by your doctor

Do not use this medicine to treat wheezing that is getting worse. Call your doctor right away if wheezing worsens while using this medicine.

Although this medicine decreases the number of asthma episodes, these medicines may increase the chances of a severe asthma episode when they do occur. Be sure to read about these risks in the Medication Guide and talk to your doctor or pharmacist about any questions or concerns that you have.

Side Effects of This Medicine

Along with its needed effects, a medicine may cause some unwanted effects. Although not all of these side effects may occur, if they do occur they may need medical attention.

Check with your doctor as soon as possible if any of the following side effects occur:

Black, tarry stools; blindness; blurred vision; burning, tingling, numbness or pain in the hands, arms, feet, or legs; chills; cough; decreased vision; difficulty breathing or swallowing; eye pain; fast heartbeat; fever; headache; hives or welts; large, hive-like swelling on face, eyelids, lips, tongue, throat, hands, legs, feet, sex organs; nausea or vomiting; noisy breathing; painful or difficult urination; sensation of pins and needles; shortness of breath; skin itching, rash, or redness; sore throat; sores, ulcers or white spots on lips or in mouth; stabbing pain in extremities; swelling of face, throat, or tongue; swollen glands; tearing; unusual bleeding or bruising; wheezing

Symptoms of overdose

Get emergency help immediately if any of the following symptoms of overdose occur:

Blurred vision; chest pain or tightness; confusion; convulsions (seizures); darkening of skin; decreased urine output; diarrhea; dizziness; dry mouth; fainting, faintness, or light-headedness when getting up from a lying or sitting position; fast, pounding, or irregular heartbeat or pulse; fatigue; flushed, dry skin; fruit-like breath odor; general feeling of discomfort or illness; headache; high blood pressure; increased hunger; increased thirst; loss of appetite; mental depression; mood changes; muscle pain or cramps; nausea; nervousness; numbness or tingling in hands, feet, or lips; palpitations; shortness of breath; skin rash; sudden sweating; tremors; trouble in sleeping; unusual tiredness or weakness; vomiting

Some side effects may occur that usually do not need medical attention. These side effects may go away during treatment as your body adjusts to the medicine. Also, your health care professional may be able to tell you about ways to prevent or reduce some of these side effects. Check with your health care professional if any of the following side effects continue or are bothersome or if you have any questions about them:

More common

Body aches or pain; choking; congestion; dryness of throat; high-pitched noise when breathing; hoarseness; runny nose; sneezing; trouble in swallowing; voice changes

Less common

Abdominal or stomach pain; cough-producing mucus; flu-like symptoms; irritation or inflammation of eye; muscle pain; pain or tenderness around eyes and cheekbones; sleep disorders; stuffy nose; tremors; white patches in the mouth or throat or on the tongue

Other side effects not listed may also occur in some patients. If you notice any other effects, check with your healthcare professional.

FLUVOXAMINE   (Oral route) - floo-VOX-a-meen

Commonly used brand name(s)

In the U.S.—
Luvox

Available Dosage Forms:
- Tablet

Therapeutic Class: Antidepressant
Pharmacologic Class: Serotonin Reuptake Inhibitor

Uses For This Medicine

Fluvoxamine is used to treat obsessive-compulsive disorder.

This medicine may also be used for other conditions as determined by your doctor.

Fluvoxamine belongs to a group of medicines known as selective serotonin reuptake inhibitors (SSRIs). These medicines are thought to work by increasing the activity of a chemical called serotonin in the brain.

This medicine is available only with your doctor's prescription.

Once a medicine has been approved for marketing for a certain use, experience may show that it is also useful for other medical problems. Although this use is not included in product labeling, fluvoxamine is used in certain patients with the following medical condition:
- Mental depression

If you are taking fluvoxamine for mental depression, you may have to take it for 3 weeks or longer before you begin to feel better. Your doctor should check your progress at regular visits during this time.

Before Using This Medicine

In deciding to use a medicine, the risks of taking the medicine must be weighed against the good it will do. This is a decision you and your doctor will make. For this medicine, the following should be considered:

Allergies—Tell your doctor if you have ever had any unusual or allergic reaction to this medicine or any other medicines. Also tell your health care professional if you have any other types of allergies, such as to foods, dyes, preservatives, or animals. For non-prescription products, read the label or package ingredients carefully.

Pediatric—This medicine has been tested in children and, in effective doses, has not been shown to cause different side effects or problems than it does in adults. Because fluvoxamine may cause weight loss or a decrease in appetite, children who will be taking fluvoxamine for a long time should have their weight and growth measured by the doctor regularly.

Fluvoxamine must be used with caution in children with depression. Studies have shown occurrences of children thinking about suicide or attempting suicide in clinical trials for this medicine. More study is needed to be sure fluvoxamine is safe and effective in children.

Geriatric—Fluvoxamine has been tested in a limited number of older adults and has not been shown to cause different side effects or problems in older people than it does in younger adults. However, fluvoxamine may be removed from the body more slowly in older adults and an older adult may receive a lower dose than a younger adult.

Pregnancy—

	Pregnancy Category	Explanation
All Trimesters	C	Animal studies have shown an adverse effect and there are no adequate studies in pregnant women OR no animal studies have been conducted and there are no adequate studies in pregnant women.

Breast Feeding—There are no adequate studies in women for determining infant risk when using this medication during breastfeeding. Weigh the potential benefits against the potential risks before taking this medication while breastfeeding.

Other medicines—

Using this medicine with any of the following medicines is not recommended. Your doctor may decide not to treat you with this medication or change some of the other medicines you take.

Alosetron, Astemizole, Cisapride, Dihydroergotamine, Ergoloid Mesylates, Ergonovine, Ergotamine, Furazolidone, Isocarboxazid, Levomethadyl, Methylergonovine, Phenelzine, Rasagiline, Terfenadine, Thioridazine, Tizanidine

Interactions with Food/Tobacco/Alcohol—Certain medicines should not be used at or around the time of eating food or eating certain types of food since interactions may occur. Using alcohol or tobacco with certain medicines may also cause interactions to occur. Discuss with your healthcare professional the use of your medicine with food, alcohol, or tobacco.

Other medical problems—The presence of other medical problems may affect the use of this medicine. Make sure you tell your doctor if you have any other medical problems, especially:

- Brain disease or mental retardation or
- Seizures, history of—The risk of seizures may be increased
- Liver disease—Higher blood levels of fluvoxamine may occur, increasing the chance of side effects
- Mania or hypomania, history of—The condition may be activated

Proper Use of This Medicine

Take this medicine only as directed by your doctor to benefit your condition as much as possible. Do not take more of it, do not take it more often, and do not take it for a longer time than your doctor ordered.

Fluvoxamine may be taken with or without food or on a full or empty stomach. However, if your doctor tells you to take the medicine a certain way, take it exactly as directed.

If you are taking fluvoxamine for obsessive-compulsive disorder, you may have to take it for up to 10 or 12 weeks before you begin to feel better. Your doctor should check your progress at regular visits during this time.

Dosing—The dose of this medicine will be different for different patients. Follow your doctor's orders or the directions on the label. The following information includes only the average doses of this medicine. If your dose is different, do not change it unless your doctor tells you to do so.

The amount of medicine that you take depends on the strength of the medicine. Also, the number of doses you take each day, the time allowed between doses, and the length of time you take the medicine depend on the medical problem for which you are using the medicine.

- For oral dosage form (tablets):
  - For treatment of obsessive-compulsive disorder:
    - Adults—At first, 50 milligrams (mg) once a day at bedtime. Your doctor may increase your dose if needed. However, the dose usually is not more than 300 mg a day. If your daily dose is higher than 100 mg, your doctor may want you to take it in two divided doses.
    - Children younger than 8 years of age—Use and dose must be determined by your doctor.
    - Children 8 to 17 years of age—At first, 25 mg once a day at bedtime. Your doctor may increase your dose if needed. However, the dose usually is not more than 200 mg a day. If your daily dose is higher than 50 mg, your doctor may want you to take it in two divided doses.

Missed dose—If you miss a dose of this medicine, take it as soon as possible. However, if it is almost time for your next dose, skip the missed dose and go back to your regular dosing schedule. Do not double doses.

For twice-a-day dosing: Skip the missed dose and go back to your regular dosing schedule. Do not double doses.

Storage—Store the medicine in a closed container at room temperature, away from heat, moisture, and direct light. Keep from freezing.

Keep out of the reach of children.

Do not keep outdated medicine or medicine no longer needed.

Precautions While Using This Medicine

It is important that your doctor check your progress at regular visits, to allow for changes in your dose and to help reduce any side effects.

Do not take alosetron or tizanidine while you are taking fluvoxamine. If you do, it could increase the amounts of these medicines in your body which may cause serious unwanted effects.

Do not take astemizole, cisapride, or terfenadine while you are taking fluvoxamine. If you do, you may develop a very serious heart problem.

Do not take fluvoxamine if you have taken a monoamine oxidase (MAO) inhibitor in the past 14 days. Do not start taking an MAO inhibitor within 14 days of stopping fluvoxamine. If you do, you may develop agitation, coma, extreme muscle stiffness, sudden high body temperature, or other severe unwanted effects.

Avoid drinking alcohol while taking fluvoxamine.

Check with your doctor as soon as possible if you develop a skin rash, hives, or itching while you are taking fluvoxamine.

Fluvoxamine may cause some people to be agitated, irritable or display other abnormal behaviors. It may also cause some people to have suicidal thoughts and tendencies or to become more depressed. If you or your caregiver notice any of these adverse effects, tell your doctor right away.

Fluvoxamine may cause some people to become drowsy or less able to think clearly, or to have blurred vision or poor muscle control. Make sure you know how you react to this medicine before you drive, use machines, or do anything else that could be dangerous if you are not alert, able to see clearly, or able to control your movements well.

Do not stop taking this medicine without first checking with your doctor. Your doctor may want you to reduce gradually the amount you are taking before stopping completely. This is to decrease the chance of having discontinuation symptoms.

Side Effects of This Medicine

Along with its needed effects, a medicine may cause some unwanted effects. Although not all of these side effects may occur, if they do occur they may need medical attention.

Check with your doctor as soon as possible if any of the following side effects occur:

More common
Change in sexual performance or desire

Less common
Behavior, mood, or mental changes; trouble in breathing; trouble in urinating; twitching

Rare
Absence of or decrease in body movements; blurred vision; clumsiness or unsteadiness; convulsions (seizures); inability to move eyes; increase in body movements; menstrual changes; nose bleeds; red or irritated eyes; redness, tenderness, itching, burning or peeling of skin; skin rash; sore throat, fever, and chills; unusual bruising; unusual, incomplete, or sudden body or facial movements; unusual secretion of milk, in females; weakness

Rare—Symptoms of serotonin syndrome (usually three or more occur together)
Agitation; confusion; diarrhea; fever; overactive reflexes; poor coordination; restlessness; shivering; sweating; talking or acting with excitement you cannot control; trembling or shaking; twitching

Symptoms of overdose—may be more severe than usual side effects, or two or more may occur together
Coma; convulsions (seizures); diarrhea; dizziness; drowsiness; dryness of mouth; fast or slow heartbeat; large pupils; low blood pressure; nausea; trembling or shaking; trouble in urinating; twitching; vomiting

Some side effects may occur that usually do not need medical attention. These side effects may go away during treatment as your body adjusts to the medicine. Also, your health care professional may be able to tell you about ways to prevent or reduce some of these side effects. Check with your health care professional if any of the following side effects

continue or are bothersome or if you have any questions about them:

More common
Constipation; dizziness; drowsiness; headache; nausea; trouble in sleeping; unusual tiredness; vomiting

Less common
Abdominal pain; change in sense of taste; decreased appetite; diarrhea; dryness of mouth; feeling of constant movement of self or surroundings; feeling of fast or irregular heartbeat; frequent urination; heartburn; increased sweating; trembling or shaking; unusual weight gain or loss

After you stop using this medicine, it may still produce some side effects that need attention. During this period of time, *check with your doctor immediately* if you notice the following side effects:

Confusion; decreased energy; dizziness; headache; irritability; nausea; problems with memory; weakness

Other side effects not listed may also occur in some patients. If you notice any other effects, check with your healthcare professional.

FOLIC ACID (Oral route, Injection route) - FOE-lik As-id

Commonly used brand name(s)

In the U.S.—
FA-8
Folacin-800
Nature's Blend Folic Acid

Available Dosage Forms:
- Solution
- Tablet
- Injectable

Therapeutic Class: Nutritive Agent
Pharmacologic Class: Vitamin B

Uses For This Dietary Supplement

Vitamins are compounds that you must have for growth and health. They are needed in small amounts only and are usually available in the foods that you eat. Folic acid (vitamin B 9) is necessary for strong blood.

Lack of folic acid may lead to anemia (weak blood). Your health care professional may treat this by prescribing folic acid for you.

Some conditions may increase your need for folic acid. These include:
- Alcoholism
- Anemia, hemolytic
- Diarrhea (continuing)
- Fever (prolonged)
- Hemodialysis

- Illness (prolonged)
- Intestinal diseases
- Liver disease
- Stress (continuing)
- Surgical removal of stomach

In addition, infants smaller than normal, breast-fed infants, or those receiving unfortified formulas (such as evaporated milk or goat's milk) may need additional folic acid.

Increased need for folic acid should be determined by your health care professional.

Some studies have found that folic acid taken by women before they become pregnant and during early pregnancy may reduce the chances of certain birth defects (neural tube defects).

Claims that folic acid and other B vitamins are effective for preventing mental problems have not been proven. Many of these treatments involve large and expensive amounts of vitamins.

Injectable folic acid is given by or under the direction of your health care professional. Another form of folic acid is available without a prescription.

Importance of Diet—For good health, it is important that you eat a balanced and varied diet. Follow carefully any diet program your health care professional may recommend. For your specific dietary vitamin and/or mineral needs, ask your health care professional for a list of appropriate foods. If you think that you are not getting enough vitamins and/or minerals in your diet, you may choose to take a dietary supplement.

Folic acid is found in various foods, including vegetables, especially green vegetables; potatoes; cereal and cereal products; fruits; and organ meats (for example, liver or kidney). It is best to eat fresh fruits and vegetables whenever possible since they contain the most vitamins. Food processing may destroy some of the vitamins. For example, heat may reduce the amount of folic acid in foods.

Vitamins alone will not take the place of a good diet and will not provide energy. Your body also needs other substances found in food such as protein, minerals, carbohydrates, and fat. Vitamins themselves often cannot work without the presence of other foods.

The daily amount of folic acid needed is defined in several different ways.

For U.S.—
- Recommended Dietary Allowances (RDAs) are the amount of vitamins and minerals needed to provide for adequate nutrition in most healthy persons. RDAs for a given nutrient may vary depending on a person's age, sex, and physical condition (e.g., pregnancy).
- Daily Values (DVs) are used on food and dietary supplement labels to indicate the percent of the recommended daily amount of each nutrient that a serving provides. DV replaces the previous designation of United States Recommended Daily Allowances (USRDAs).

For Canada—
- Recommended Nutrient Intakes (RNIs) are used to determine the amounts of vitamins, minerals, and protein needed to provide adequate nutrition and lessen the risk of chronic disease.

Normal daily recommended intakes in micrograms (mcg) for folic acid are generally defined as follows:

Persons	U.S. (mcg)	Canada (mcg)
Infants and children		
Birth to 3 years of age	25–100	50–80
4 to 6 years of age	75–400	90
7 to 10 years of age	100–400	125–180
Adolescent and adult males	150–400	150–220
Adolescent and adult females	150–400	145–190
Pregnant females	400–800	445–475
Breast-feeding females	260–800	245–275

Before Using This Dietary Supplement

If you are taking this dietary supplement without a prescription, carefully read and follow any precautions on the label. For this supplement, the following should be considered:

In deciding to use folic acid, the risks of taking it must be weighed against the good it will do. This is a decision you and your health care professional will make. For folic acid, the following should be considered:

Allergies—Tell your doctor if you have ever had any unusual or allergic reaction to this medicine or any other medicines. Also tell your health care professional if you have any other types of allergies, such as to foods, dyes, preservatives, or animals. For non-prescription products, read the label or package ingredients carefully.

Pediatric—Problems in children have not been reported with intake of normal daily recommended amounts.

Geriatric—Problems in older adults have not been reported with intake of normal daily recommended amounts.

Breast Feeding—There are no adequate studies in women for determining infant risk when using this medication during breastfeeding. Weigh the potential benefits against the potential risks before taking this medication while breastfeeding.

Other medicines—

Using this dietary supplement with any of the following medicines may cause an increased risk of certain side effects, but using both drugs may be the best treatment for you. If both medicines are prescribed together, your doctor may change the dose or how often you use one or both of the medicines.

Phenytoin

Interactions with Food/Tobacco/Alcohol—Certain medicines should not be used at or around the time of eating food or eating certain types of food since interactions may occur. Using alcohol or tobacco with certain medicines may also cause interactions to occur. Discuss with your healthcare professional the use of your medicine with food, alcohol, or tobacco.

Other medical problems—The presence of other medical problems may affect the use of this dietary supplement. Make sure you tell your doctor if you have any other medical problems, especially:

- Pernicious anemia (a type of blood problem)—Taking folic acid while you have pernicious anemia may cause serious side effects. You should be sure that you do not have pernicious anemia before beginning folic acid supplementation

Proper Use of This Dietary Supplement

Dosing—The dose of this medicine will be different for different patients. Follow your doctor's orders or the directions on the label. The following information includes only the average doses of this medicine. If your dose is different, do not change it unless your doctor tells you to do so.

The amount of medicine that you take depends on the strength of the medicine. Also, the number of doses you take each day, the time allowed between doses, and the length of time you take the medicine depend on the medical problem for which you are using the medicine.

- For oral dosage form (tablets):
  - To prevent deficiency, the amount taken by mouth is based on normal daily recommended intakes:

  For the U.S.
  - Adult and teenage males—150 to 400 micrograms (mcg) per day.
  - Adult and teenage females—150 to 400 mcg per day.
  - Pregnant females—400 to 800 mcg per day.
  - Breast-feeding females—260 to 800 mcg per day.
  - Children 7 to 10 years of age—100 to 400 mcg per day.
  - Children 4 to 6 years of age—75 to 400 mcg per day.
  - Children birth to 3 years of age—25 to 100 mcg per day.

  For Canada
  - Adult and teenage males—150 to 220 mcg per day.
  - Adult and teenage females—145 to 190 mcg per day.
  - Pregnant females—445 to 475 mcg per day.
  - Breast-feeding females—245 to 275 mcg per day.
  - Children 7 to 10 years of age—125 to 180 mcg per day.
  - Children 4 to 6 years of age—90 mcg per day.
  - Children birth to 3 years of age—50 to 80 mcg per day.
  - To treat deficiency:
    - Adults, teenagers, and children—Treatment dose is determined by prescriber for each individual based on the severity of deficiency.

Missed dose—If you miss a dose of this medicine, skip the missed dose and go back to your regular dosing schedule. Do not double doses.

Storage—Store the dietary supplement in a closed container at room temperature, away from heat, moisture, and direct light. Keep from freezing.

Keep out of the reach of children.

Do not keep outdated medicine or medicine no longer needed.

Side Effects of This Dietary Supplement

Along with its needed effects, a medicine may cause some unwanted effects. Although not all of these side effects may occur, if they do occur they may need medical attention.

Check with your doctor as soon as possible if any of the following side effects occur:
> *Rare*
>> Fever; general weakness or discomfort; reddened skin; shortness of breath; skin rash or itching; tightness in chest; troubled breathing; wheezing

Other side effects not listed may also occur in some patients. If you notice any other effects, check with your healthcare professional.

FOLLICLE STIMULATING HORMONE AND LUTEINIZING HORMONE   (Intramuscular route, Subcutaneous route) - FOL-i-kul STIM-yoo-lay-ting HOR-mone, LOO-ten-eye-zing HOR-mone

Commonly used brand name(s)

In the U.S.—
   Menopur
   Pergonal
   Repronex

Available Dosage Forms:
- Powder for Solution

Therapeutic Class: Endocrine-Metabolic Agent
Pharmacologic Class: Human Luteinizing Hormone

Uses For This Medicine

Menotropins are a mixture of follicle-stimulating hormone (FSH) and luteinizing hormone (LH) that are naturally produced by the pituitary gland.

Use in females—FSH is primarily responsible for stimulating growth of the ovarian follicle, which includes the developing egg, the cells surrounding the egg that produce the hormones needed to support a pregnancy, and the fluid around the egg. As the follicle grows, an increasing amount of the hormone estrogen is produced by the cells in the follicle and released into the bloodstream. Estrogen causes the endometrium (lining of the uterus) to thicken before ovulation occurs. The higher blood levels of estrogen will also tell the hypothalamus and pituitary gland to slow the production and release of FSH.

LH also helps to increase the amount of estrogen produced by the follicle cells. However, its main function is to cause ovulation. The sharp rise in the blood level of LH that triggers ovulation is called the LH surge. After ovulation, the group of hormone-producing follicle cells become the corpus luteum, which will produce estrogen and large amounts of another hormone, progesterone. Progesterone causes the endometrium to mature so that it can support implantation of the fertilized egg or embryo. If implantation of a fertilized egg does not occur, the levels of estrogen and progesterone decrease, the endometrium sloughs off, and menstruation occurs.

Menotropins are usually given in combination with human chorionic gonadotropin (hCG). The actions of hCG are almost the same as those of LH. It is given to simulate the natural LH surge. This results in ovulation at an expected time.

Many women choosing treatment with menotropins have already tried clomiphene (e.g., Serophene) and have not been able to conceive yet. Menotropins may also be used to cause the ovary to produce several follicles, which can then be harvested for use in gamete intrafallopian transfer (GIFT) or *in vitro* fertilization (IVF).

Use in males—Menotropins are used to stimulate the production of sperm in some forms of male infertility.

Once a medicine has been approved for marketing for a certain use, experience may show that it is also useful for other medical problems. Although these uses are not included in product labeling, menotropins are used in certain patients with the following medical conditions:
- For causing ovulation in women to help them become pregnant
- For producing sperm in men

Before Using This Medicine

In deciding to use a medicine, the risks of taking the medicine must be weighed against the good it will do. This is a decision you and your doctor will make. For this medicine, the following should be considered:

Allergies—Tell your doctor if you have ever had any unusual or allergic reaction to this medicine or any other medicines. Also tell your health care professional if you have any other types of allergies, such as to foods, dyes, preservatives, or animals. For non-prescription products, read the label or package ingredients carefully.

Pediatric—Studies on this medicine have been done only in adult patients, and there is no specific information comparing use of menotropins in children with use in other age groups.

Geriatric—Many medicines have not been studied specifically in older people. Therefore, it may not be known whether they work exactly the same way they do in younger adults or if they cause different side effects or problems in older people. There is no specific information comparing use of menotropins in the elderly with use in other age groups.

Other medicines—Although certain medicines should not be used together at all, in other cases two different medicines may be used together even if an interaction might occur. In these cases, your doctor may want to change the dose, or other precautions may be necessary. Tell your healthcare professional if you are taking any other prescription or non-prescription (over-the-counter [OTC]) medicine.

Interactions with Food/Tobacco/Alcohol—Certain medicines should not be used at or around the time of eating food or eating certain types of food since interactions may occur. Using alcohol or tobacco with certain medicines may also cause interactions to occur. Discuss with your healthcare professional the use of your medicine with food, alcohol, or tobacco.

Other medical problems—The presence of other medical problems may affect the use of this medicine. Make sure you tell your doctor if you have any other medical problems, especially:
- Adrenal gland or thyroid disease (not controlled) or
- Tumor, brain or
- Tumor, sex hormone-dependent—Menotropins should not be used in patients with these medical problems.
- Cyst on ovary—Menotropins can cause further growth of cysts on the ovary
- Primary ovarian failure—Menotropins will not work in patients whose ovaries no longer develop eggs.
- Unusual vaginal bleeding—Some irregular vaginal bleeding is a sign that the endometrium is growing too rapidly, possibly of endometrial cancer, or some hormone imbalances; the increases in estrogen production caused by menotropins can make these problems worse. If a hormonal imbalance is present, it should be treated before beginning menotropins therapy

Proper Use of This Medicine

Dosing—The dose of this medicine will be different for different patients. Follow your doctor's orders or the directions on the label. The following information includes only the average doses of this medicine. If your dose is different, do not change it unless your doctor tells you to do so.

The amount of medicine that you take depends on the strength of the medicine. Also, the number of doses you take each day, the time allowed between doses, and the length of time you take the medicine depend on the medical problem for which you are using the medicine.
- For injection dosage form:
  - For help in becoming pregnant while using other pregnancy-promoting methods (assisted reproductive technology [ART]):
    - Adults—225 Units of FSH and 225 Units of LH injected under the skin below your belly button. Your doctor will adjust your daily dose after checking your blood and your ovaries. Usually your doctor will give you another medicine called human chorionic gonadotropin (hCG) the day after the last dose of menotropins.

Precautions While Using This Medicine

It is very important that your doctor check your progress at regular visits to make sure that the medicine is working properly and to check for unwanted effects. Your doctor will likely want to watch the development of the ovarian follicle(s) by measuring the amount of estrogen in your bloodstream and by checking the size of the follicle(s) with ultrasound examinations.

For females only:
- If your doctor has asked you to record your basal body temperatures (BBTs) daily, make sure that you do this every day. It is important that intercourse take place around the time of ovulation to give you the best chance of becoming pregnant. Follow your doctor's instructions carefully.
- If you become pregnant as a result of using this medicine, there is an increased chance of a multiple pregnancy.

Side Effects of This Medicine

Along with its needed effects, a medicine may cause some unwanted effects. Although not all of these side effects may occur, if they do occur they may need medical attention.

Check with your doctor as soon as possible if any of the following side effects occur:

For females only
More common
Bloating (mild); pain, swelling, or irritation at place of injection; rash at place of injection or on body; stomach or pelvic pain

Less common or rare
Abdominal or stomach pain (severe); bloating (moderate to severe); decreased amount of urine; feeling of indigestion; nausea, vomiting, or diarrhea (continuing or severe); pelvic pain (severe); shortness of breath; swelling of the lower legs; weight gain (rapid)

For males only
More common
Dizziness; fainting; headache; irregular heartbeat; loss of appetite; more frequent nosebleeds; shortness of breath

For females only
More common
Coughing; headache; mild nausea; sneezing; sore throat; stuffy or runny nose

Less common
Back pain; breast tenderness; chills; difficulty having a bowel movement (stool); dizziness; feeling of warmth, redness of the face, neck, arms and occasionally, upper chest; fever; general feeling of discomfort or illness; headache, severe and throbbing; joint pain; loss of appetite; menstrual changes; mild diarrhea; mild vomiting; muscle aches and pains; pain; severe cramping of the uterus; shivering; sweating; trouble sleeping; unusual tiredness or weakness

Some side effects may occur that usually do not need medical attention. These side effects may go away during treatment as your body adjusts to the medicine. Also, your health care professional may be able to tell you about ways to prevent or reduce some of these side effects. Check with your health care professional if any of the following side effects continue or are bothersome or if you have any questions about them:

For males only
Less common
Enlargement of breasts

After you stop using this medicine, it may still produce some side effects that need attention. During this period of time, *check with your doctor immediately* if you notice the following side effects:

For females only
Abdominal or stomach pain (severe); bloating (moderate to severe); decreased amount of urine; feeling of indigestion; nausea, vomiting, or diarrhea (continuing or severe); pelvic pain (severe); shortness of breath; weight gain (rapid)

Other side effects not listed may also occur in some patients. If you notice any other effects, check with your healthcare professional.

FOLLITROPIN ALFA (Subcutaneous route) - fol-i-TROE-pin AL-fa

Commonly used brand name(s)
In the U.S.—
Gonal-F
Gonal-F RFF

Available Dosage Forms:
- Powder for Solution
- Solution

Therapeutic Class: Female Reproductive Agent
Pharmacologic Class: Human Follicle Stimulating Hormone

Uses For This Medicine

Follitropin alfa is a hormone identical to follicle-stimulating hormone (FSH) produced by the pituitary gland. FSH helps to develop eggs in the ovaries.

Follitropin alfa is used as a fertility medicine to develop eggs in women who have not been able to become pregnant because of problems in ovulation. Also, many women wanting to become pregnant will use this medicine while enrolled in a fertility program (assisted reproductive technology [ART]) that uses procedures such as in vitro fertilization (IVF) or embryo transfer (ET). Follitropin alfa may be used with other medicines for these purposes.

Follitropin alfa is also used as a fertility medicine to help men with low sperm counts produce more sperms. Treatment with human chorionic gonadotropin should come before treatment with follitropin alfa. This pretreatment elevates the amount of testosterone to the correct level. Treatment with human chorionic gonadotropin should continue as long as follitropin alfa is being used.

Some patients may be treated with another hormone called gonadotropin-releasing hormone agonist (GnRHa) before starting treatment with follitropin alfa. GnRHa reduces the amount of FSH released from the pituitary gland. This is done so that the doctor can replace their FSH with follitropin alfa in the proper amounts each day to achieve fertility.

This medicine is available only with your doctor's prescription.

Before Using This Medicine

In deciding to use a medicine, the risks of taking the medicine must be weighed against the good it will do. This is a decision you and your doctor will make. For this medicine, the following should be considered:

Allergies—Tell your doctor if you have ever had any unusual or allergic reaction to this medicine or any other medicines. Also tell your health care professional if you have any other types of allergies, such as to foods, dyes, preservatives, or animals. For non-prescription products, read the label or package ingredients carefully.

Pregnancy—

	Pregnancy Category	Explanation
All Trimesters	X	Studies in animals or pregnant women have demonstrated positive evidence of fetal abnormalities. This drug should not be used in women who are or may become pregnant because the risk clearly outweighs any possible benefit.

Breast Feeding—There are no adequate studies in women for determining infant risk when using this medication during breastfeeding. Weigh the potential benefits against the potential risks before taking this medication while breastfeeding.

Other medicines—Although certain medicines should not be used together at all, in other cases two different medicines may be used together even if an interaction might occur. In these cases, your doctor may want to change the dose, or other precautions may be necessary. Tell your healthcare professional if you are taking any other prescription or non-prescription (over-the-counter [OTC]) medicine.

Interactions with Food/Tobacco/Alcohol—Certain medicines should not be used at or around the time of eating food or eating certain types of food since interactions may occur. Using alcohol or tobacco with certain medicines may also cause interactions to occur. Discuss with your healthcare professional the use of your medicine with food, alcohol, or tobacco.

Other medical problems—The presence of other medical problems may affect the use of this medicine. Make sure you tell your doctor if you have any other medical problems, especially:

- Abnormal bleeding of genitals or uterus (unknown cause)—Use of follitropin alfa may make the diagnosis of this problem more difficult
- Adrenal gland or thyroid disease (not controlled) or
- Asthma or
- Tumor, brain or
- Tumor, sex hormone-dependent—Use of follitropin alfa may make these conditions worse
- Ovarian cyst or enlarged ovaries—Use of follitropin alfa may increase the size of a cyst on an ovary or increase the size of enlarged ovaries
- Primary testicular failure—Follitropin alfa will not work in patients who no longer are able to produce sperms
- Primary ovarian failure—Follitropin alfa will not work in patients whose ovaries no longer develop eggs

Proper Use of This Medicine

To make using follitropin alfa as safe and reliable as possible, you should understand how and when to use this medicine and what effects may be expected. A paper with information for the patient will be given to you with your filled prescription and will provide many details concerning the use of follitropin alfa. Read this paper carefully and ask your health care professional for any additional information or explanation.

Sometimes follitropin alfa can be given by injection at home. If you are using this medicine at home:

- Understand and use the proper method of safely preparing the medicine if you are going to prepare your own medicine.
- Wash yours hands with soap and water and use a clean work area to prepare your injection.
- Make sure you clearly understand and carefully follow your doctor's instructions on how to give yourself an injection, including using the proper needle and syringe.
- Do not inject more or less of the medicine than your doctor ordered.
- Remember to move the site of injection to different areas to prevent skin problems from developing.
- Throw away needles, syringes, bottles, and unused medicine after the injection in a safe manner.

Tell your doctor when you use the last dose of follitropin alfa. Follitropin alfa often requires that another hormone called human chorionic gonadotropin (hCG) be given as a single dose the day after the last dose of follitropin alfa is given. Your doctor will give you this medicine or arrange for you to get this medicine at the right time.

Dosing—The dose of this medicine will be different for different patients. Follow your doctor's orders or the directions on the label. The following information includes only the average doses of this medicine. If your dose is different, do not change it unless your doctor tells you to do so.

The amount of medicine that you take depends on the strength of the medicine. Also, the number of doses you take each day, the time allowed between doses, and the length of time you take the medicine depend on the medical problem for which you are using the medicine.

- For injection dosage form:
  - For treatment of female infertility:
    - Adults—75 international units (IU) injected under the skin once a day for approximately fourteen days. The dose may be increased at weekly intervals by 37.5 IU, up to a total dose of 300 IU once a day. Using follitropin alfa for longer than fourteen days may be needed, but only if directed by your doctor. Report when you receive your last dose of follitropin alfa because you may be given an injection of hCG twenty-four hours later. If abdominal pain occurs with the use of follitropin alfa, report it to your doctor immediately, discontinue treatment, do not receive the dose of hCG, and avoid sexual intercourse.
  - For use with assisted reproductive technology (ART) procedures:
    - Adults—150 international units (IU) injected under the skin once a day for five days beginning on Day 2 or Day 3 of your menstrual cycle. After five days, your dose may be increased by 75 to 150 IU every three to five days, up to a total dose of 450 IU once a day, for up to five more days. Some patients may start treatment at a dose of 225 IU once a day. Using follitropin alfa for longer than ten days may be needed, but only if directed by your doctor. Report when you receive your last dose of follitropin alfa because you may be given an injection of hCG twenty-four hours later.

○ For treatment of male infertility
- Adults—150 international units (IU) injected under the skin three times a week in conjunction with 1000 USP Units of human chorionic gonadotropin (hCG) three times a week. Your dose may be increased up to 300 IU three times a week, and the treatment may last up to eighteen months.

Missed dose—Call your doctor or pharmacist for instructions.

Storage—Store the medicine in a closed container at room temperature, away from heat, moisture, and direct light. Keep from freezing.

Keep out of the reach of children.

Do not keep outdated medicine or medicine no longer needed.

Precautions While Using This Medicine

It is very important that your doctor check your progress often at regular visits to make sure that the medicine is working properly and to check for unwanted effects. Your doctor will probably want to follow the developing eggs inside the ovaries by doing an ultrasound examination and measuring hormones in your blood stream. After you no longer receive follitropin alfa, your progress still must be checked for at least 2 weeks.

If your doctor has asked you to record your basal body temperatures (BBTs) daily, make sure that you do this every day. Using a BBT record or some other method, your doctor will help you decide when you are most fertile and when ovulation occurs. It is important that sexual intercourse take place around the time when you are most fertile to give you the best chance of becoming pregnant. Follow your doctor's directions carefully.

If abdominal pain occurs with use of follitropin alfa, discontinue treatment and report the problem to your doctor immediately. Do not receive the injection of human chorionic gonadotropin (hCG) and avoid sexual intercourse.

This medicine may cause some people to become dizzy. If this side effect occurs, do not drive, use machines, or do anything else that could be dangerous if you are not alert while you are using follitropin alfa and for 24 hours after you stop using it.

Side Effects of This Medicine

Along with its needed effects, a medicine may cause some unwanted effects. Although not all of these side effects may occur, if they do occur they may need medical attention.

Stop taking this medicine and get emergency help immediately if any of the following effects occur:

Abdominal pain (severe), nausea, vomiting, and weight gain (rapid)

Check with your doctor as soon as possible if any of the following side effects occur:
More common
For patients treated for female infertility or patients pretreated with a gonadotropin-releasing hormone agonist (GnRHa) undergoing assisted reproduction technologies (ART)
Abdominal bloating; diarrhea; flu or cold-like symptoms, such as body aches or pain, coughing, fever, headache, loss of voice, runny nose, and unusual tired-

ness or weakness; nausea; passing of gas; vaginal bleeding between menstrual periods
For patients treated for female infertility
Acne; breast pain or tenderness; mood swings
Less common
For patients treated for female infertility or patients pretreated with GnRHa undergoing ART
Dizziness; painful menstrual periods; redness, pain, or swelling at injection site; sleepiness; vaginal bleeding unrelated to menstrual periods (heavy); white vaginal discharge
For patients treated for female infertility
Fainting; light-headedness; migraine headache; nervousness; stomach discomfort
For patients treated pretreated with a GnRHa undergoing ART
Fast, racing heartbeat; itching of skin; loss of appetite; thirst (unusual)

After you stop using this medicine, it may still produce some side effects that need attention. During this period of time, *check with your doctor immediately* if you notice the following side effects:

Abdominal pain (severe), nausea, vomiting, and weight gain (rapid)

Other side effects not listed may also occur in some patients. If you notice any other effects, check with your healthcare professional.

FOLLITROPIN BETA (Subcutaneous route) - fol-i-TROE-pin BAY-ta

Commonly used brand name(s)
In the U.S.—
Follistim
Follistim AQ
Gonal-f RFF

Available Dosage Forms:
- Kit
- Solution
- Powder for Solution

Therapeutic Class: Human Follicle Stimulating Hormone Combination
Pharmacologic Class: Human Follicle Stimulating Hormone

Uses For This Medicine

Follitropin beta is a hormone identical to follicle-stimulating hormone (FSH) produced by the pituitary gland. FSH helps to develop eggs in the ovaries.

Follitropin beta is used as a fertility medicine to develop eggs in women who have not been able to become pregnant because of problems in ovulation. Also, many women wanting to become pregnant will use this medicine while enrolled in a fertility program that uses procedures such as in vitro fertilization (IVF) or embryo transfer (ET). Follitropin beta may be used with other medicines for these purposes.

Some patients may be treated with another hormone called gonadotropin-releasing hormone agonist (GnRHa) before starting treatment with follitropin beta. GnRHa reduces the amount of FSH released from the pituitary gland. This is done so that the doctor can replace their FSH by using follitropin beta in the proper amounts each day to achieve fertility.

Follitropin beta is available only with your doctor's prescription.

Before Using This Medicine

In deciding to use a medicine, the risks of taking the medicine must be weighed against the good it will do. This is a decision you and your doctor will make. For this medicine, the following should be considered:

Allergies—Tell your doctor if you have ever had any unusual or allergic reaction to this medicine or any other medicines. Also tell your health care professional if you have any other types of allergies, such as to foods, dyes, preservatives, or animals. For non-prescription products, read the label or package ingredients carefully.

Pregnancy—

	Pregnancy Category	Explanation
All Trimesters	X	Studies in animals or pregnant women have demonstrated positive evidence of fetal abnormalities. This drug should not be used in women who are or may become pregnant because the risk clearly outweighs any possible benefit.

Breast Feeding—There are no adequate studies in women for determining infant risk when using this medication during breastfeeding. Weigh the potential benefits against the potential risks before taking this medication while breastfeeding.

Other medicines—Although certain medicines should not be used together at all, in other cases two different medicines may be used together even if an interaction might occur. In these cases, your doctor may want to change the dose, or other precautions may be necessary. Tell your healthcare professional if you are taking any other prescription or non-prescription (over-the-counter [OTC]) medicine.

Interactions with Food/Tobacco/Alcohol—Certain medicines should not be used at or around the time of eating food or eating certain types of food since interactions may occur. Using alcohol or tobacco with certain medicines may also cause interactions to occur. Discuss with your healthcare professional the use of your medicine with food, alcohol, or tobacco.

Other medical problems—The presence of other medical problems may affect the use of this medicine. Make sure you tell your doctor if you have any other medical problems, especially:

- Abnormal bleeding of genitals or uterus (unknown cause)—Use of follitropin beta may make the diagnosis of this problem more difficult
- Adrenal gland or thyroid disease (not controlled) or
- Asthma or
- Tumors, brain or
- Tumors, sex hormone-dependent—Use of follitropin beta may make these conditions worse
- Ovarian cyst or enlarged ovaries—Use of follitropin beta may increase the size of a cyst on an ovary or increase the size of enlarged ovaries

- Primary ovarian failure—Follitropin will not work in patients whose ovaries no longer develop eggs

Proper Use of This Medicine

To make using follitropin beta as safe and reliable as possible, you should understand how and when to use this medicine and what effects may be expected. A paper with information for the patient will be given to you with your filled prescription, and will provide many details concerning the use of follitropin beta. Read this paper carefully and ask your health care professional for any additional information or explanation.

Sometimes follitropin beta can be given by injection at home. If you are using this medicine at home:

- Understand and use the proper method of safely preparing the medicine if you are going to prepare your own medicine.
- Wash your hands with soap and water and use a good, clean work area to prepare your injection.
- Make sure you clearly understand and carefully follow your doctor's instructions on how to give yourself an injection, including using the proper needle and syringe.
- Do not inject more or less of the medicine than your doctor ordered.
- Remember to move the site of injection to different areas to prevent skin problems from developing.
- Throw away needles, syringes, bottles, and unused medicine after the injection in a safe manner.

Tell your doctor when you use your last dose of follitropin beta. Follitropin beta often requires that another hormone called human chorionic gonadotropin (hCG) be given as a single dose the day after the last dose of follitropin beta is given. Your doctor will give you this medicine or arrange for you to get this medicine at the right time.

Dosing—The dose of this medicine will be different for different patients. Follow your doctor's orders or the directions on the label. The following information includes only the average doses of this medicine. If your dose is different, do not change it unless your doctor tells you to do so.

The amount of medicine that you take depends on the strength of the medicine. Also, the number of doses you take each day, the time allowed between doses, and the length of time you take the medicine depend on the medical problem for which you are using the medicine.

- For injection dosage form:
  - For treatment of female infertility:
    - Adults—75 international units (IU) injected under the skin or into a muscle once a day for up to fourteen days. The dose may be increased at weekly intervals by 37.5 IU, up to a total dose of 300 IU a day. Tell your doctor when you receive your last dose of follitropin beta. If abdominal pain occurs with the use of follitropin beta, report it to your doctor immediately, discontinue treatment, do not receive the dose of hCG, and avoid sexual intercourse.
  - For use with assisted reproductive technology (ART) procedures:
    - Adults—150 international units (IU) injected under the skin or into a muscle once a day for four days beginning on Day 2 or Day 3 of your menstrual cycle. Then your dose may be increased by 75 to 150 IU up to a total daily dose of 600 IU. Some

patients may start at 375 IU. Tell your doctor when you receive your last dose of follitropin beta.

Missed dose—Call your doctor or pharmacist for instructions.

Storage—Store the medicine in a closed container at room temperature, away from heat, moisture, and direct light. Keep from freezing.

Keep out of the reach of children.

Do not keep outdated medicine or medicine no longer needed.

Precautions While Using This Medicine

It is very important that your doctor check your progress often at regular visits, such as every other day, to make sure that the medicine is working properly and to check for unwanted effects. Your doctor will probably want to follow the developing eggs inside the ovaries by doing an ultrasound examination and measuring hormones in your blood stream. After you no longer receive follitropin beta, your progress still must be checked every other day for at least 2 weeks.

If your doctor has asked you to record your basal body temperature (BBT) daily, make sure that you do this every day. Using a BBT record or some other method, your doctor will help you decide when you are most fertile and when ovulation occurs. It is important that sexual intercourse take place around the time when you are most fertile to give you the best chance of becoming pregnant. Follow your doctor's directions carefully.

If abdominal pain occurs with use of follitropin beta, discontinue treatment and report the problem to your doctor immediately. Do not receive the injection of hCG and avoid sexual intercourse.

This medicine may cause some people to become dizzy. If this side effect occurs, do not drive, use machines, or do anything else that could be dangerous if you are not alert while you are using follitropin beta and for 24 hours after you stop using it.

Side Effects of This Medicine

Along with its needed effects, a medicine may cause some unwanted effects. Although not all of these side effects may occur, if they do occur they may need medical attention.

There is a rare chance that serious lung and blood problems can occur with use of follitropin beta. Discuss these possible effects with your doctor.

Stop taking this medicine and get emergency help immediately if any of the following effects occur:

    Abdominal pain (severe), nausea, vomiting, and weight gain (rapid)

Check with your doctor as soon as possible if any of the following side effects occur:
    Less common
    For patients treated for female infertility or patients pretreated with a gonadotropin-releasing hormone agonist (GnRHa) undergoing assisted reproduction technologies (ART)
      Abdominal pain

For patients pretreated with a GnRHa undergoing ART
    Redness, pain, or swelling at injection site

Some side effects may occur that usually do not need medical attention. These side effects may go away during treatment as your body adjusts to the medicine. Also, your health care professional may be able to tell you about ways to prevent or reduce some of these side effects. Check with your health care professional if any of the following side effects continue or are bothersome or if you have any questions about them:

    Body aches or pain; breast tenderness; chills; difficulty in breathing; dizziness; dry skin; fast, racing heart; fever; hair loss; headache; hives; nausea; quick, shallow breathing; skin rash; unusual tiredness

After you stop using this medicine, it may still produce some side effects that need attention. During this period of time, *check with your doctor immediately* if you notice the following side effects:
    Abdominal pain (severe), nausea, vomiting, and weight gain (rapid)

Other side effects not listed may also occur in some patients. If you notice any other effects, check with your healthcare professional.

FONDAPARINUX (Subcutaneous route) - fon-da-PAR-in-ux

Black Box Warning

When neuraxial anesthesia (epidural/spinal anesthesia) or spinal puncture is employed, patients anticoagulated or scheduled to be anticoagulated with low molecular weight heparins, heparinoids, or fondaparinux sodium for prevention of thromboembolic complications are at risk of developing an epidural or spinal hematoma which can result in long-term or permanent paralysis.

The risk of these events is increased by the use of indwelling epidural catheters for administration of analgesia or by the concomitant use of drugs affecting hemostasis such as non-steroidal anti-inflammatory drugs (NSAIDs), platelet inhibitors, or other anticoagulants. The risk also appears to be increased by traumatic or repeated epidural or spinal puncture.

Patients should be frequently monitored for signs and symptoms of neurologic impairment. If neurologic compromise is noted, urgent treatment is necessary.

The physician should consider the potential benefit versus risk before neuraxial intervention in patients anticoagulated or to be anticoagulated for thromboprophylaxis.

Commonly used brand name(s)

In the U.S.—
    Arixtra

Available Dosage Forms:
- Solution

Therapeutic Class: Anticoagulant
Pharmacologic Class: Factor Xa Inhibitor

Uses For This Medicine

Fondaparinux is used to prevent deep vein thrombosis, a condition in which harmful blood clots form in the blood vessels of the legs. These blood clots can travel to the lungs and can become lodged in the blood vessels of the lungs, causing a condition called pulmonary embolism. This medicine is used for several days after hip fracture surgery, hip replacement surgery or knee replacement surgery. It is also used in patients who are having abdominal surgery who are at risk for blood clots. Blood clots are more likely to form after surgery when you are unable to walk. Fondaparinux is also used to treat deep vein thrombosis and a condition called pulmonary embolism together with warfarin (e.g., Coumadin). Pulmonary embolism occurs when harmful blood clots form in the blood vessels in the lungs and is a very serious and sometimes fatal condition. Fondaparinux also may be used for other conditions as determined by your doctor.

This medicine is available only with your doctor's prescription.

Before Using This Medicine

In deciding to use a medicine, the risks of taking the medicine must be weighed against the good it will do. This is a decision you and your doctor will make. For this medicine, the following should be considered:

Allergies—Tell your doctor if you have ever had any unusual or allergic reaction to this medicine or any other medicines. Also tell your health care professional if you have any other types of allergies, such as to foods, dyes, preservatives, or animals. For non-prescription products, read the label or package ingredients carefully.

Pediatric—Studies on this medicine have been done only in adult patients, and there is no specific information comparing use of fondaparinux in children with use in other age groups.

Geriatric—Bleeding problems may be especially likely to occur in elderly patients, who are usually more sensitive than younger adults to the effects of fondaparinux.

Pregnancy—

	Pregnancy Category	Explanation
All Trimesters	B	Animal studies have revealed no evidence of harm to the fetus, however, there are no adequate studies in pregnant women OR animal studies have shown an adverse effect, but adequate studies in pregnant women have failed to demonstrate a risk to the fetus.

Breast Feeding—There are no adequate studies in women for determining infant risk when using this medication during breastfeeding. Weigh the potential benefits against the potential risks before taking this medication while breastfeeding.

Other medicines—

Using this medicine with any of the following medicines is usually not recommended, but may be required in some cases. If both medicines are prescribed together, your doctor may change the dose or how often you use one or both of the medicines.

Abciximab, Acenocoumarol, Alteplase, Recombinant, Anisindione, Anistreplase, Ardeparin, Argatroban, Bivalirudin, Certoparin, Cilostazol, Clopidogrel, Dalteparin, Danaparoid, Defibrotide, Dermatan Sulfate, Desirudin, Dicumarol, Enoxaparin, Eptifibatide, Fondaparinux, Garlic, Ginkgo, Heparin, Lamifiban, Nadroparin, Papaya, Parnaparin, Phenindione, Phenprocoumon, Reteplase, Recombinant, Reviparin, Sibrafiban, St John's Wort, Streptokinase, Tan-Shen, Tenecteplase, Tinzaparin, Tirofiban, Urokinase, Warfarin, Xemilofiban

Interactions with Food/Tobacco/Alcohol—Certain medicines should not be used at or around the time of eating food or eating certain types of food since interactions may occur. Using alcohol or tobacco with certain medicines may also cause interactions to occur. Discuss with your healthcare professional the use of your medicine with food, alcohol, or tobacco.

Other medical problems—The presence of other medical problems may affect the use of this medicine. Make sure you tell your doctor if you have any other medical problems, especially:

- Blood disease or bleeding problems or
- Eye problems caused by diabetes or high blood pressure or
- Heart infection or
- High blood pressure (hypertension) or
- If you weigh less than 110 pounds or
- Kidney disease or
- Stomach or intestinal ulcer (active) or
- Stroke—The risk of bleeding may be increased

Also, tell your doctor if you have received fondaparinux or heparin before and had a reaction to either of them called thrombocytopenia (a low platelet count in the blood), or if new blood clots formed while you were receiving the medicine.

In addition, tell your doctor if you have recently had medical surgery or spinal anesthesia. This may increase the risk of serious bleeding when you are taking fondaparinux.

Proper Use of This Medicine

If you are using fondaparinux at home, your health care professional will teach you how to inject yourself with the medicine. Be sure to follow the directions carefully. Check with your health care professional if you have any problems using the medicine.

Put used syringes in a puncture-resistant, disposable container, or dispose of them as directed by your health care professional.

Dosing—The dose of this medicine will be different for different patients. Follow your doctor's orders or the directions on the label. The following information includes only the average doses of this medicine. If your dose is different, do not change it unless your doctor tells you to do so.

The amount of medicine that you take depends on the strength of the medicine. Also, the number of doses you take each day, the time allowed between doses, and the length of time you take the medicine depend on the medical problem for which you are using the medicine.

- For injection dosage form:
  - For prevention of deep vein thrombosis (leg clots):
    - Adults—2.5 milligrams (mg) injected under the skin once a day for five to nine days. The first dose is given six to eight hours after surgery.

- Children—Use and dose must be determined by your doctor.
  - For treatment of deep vein thrombosis (leg clots) and pulmonary embolism (blood clots in the lungs):
    - Adults—5 mg (if body weight is less than 110 lbs), 7.5 mg (for 110 lbs to 220 lbs), or 10 mg (for greater 220 lbs) injected under the skin once a day for five to nine days. The first dose is given six to eight hours after surgery.
    - Children—Use and dose must be determined by your doctor.

Missed dose—Call your doctor or pharmacist for instructions.

Storage—Store the medicine in a closed container at room temperature, away from heat, moisture, and direct light. Keep from freezing.

Keep out of the reach of children.

Do not keep outdated medicine or medicine no longer needed.

Precautions While Using This Medicine

Tell all your medical doctors and dentists that you are using this medicine.

Check with your doctor immediately if you notice any of the following side effects:
- Bruising or bleeding, especially bleeding that is hard to stop. (Bleeding inside the body sometimes appears as bloody or black, tarry stools. Feeling faint or vomiting blood are other signs of bleeding.)

Side Effects of This Medicine

Along with its needed effects, a medicine may cause some unwanted effects. Although not all of these side effects may occur, if they do occur they may need medical attention.

Check with your doctor immediately if any of the following side effects occur:

More common
Pale skin; troubled breathing with exertion; unusual bleeding or bruising; unusual tiredness or weakness

Less common
Black, tarry stools; bladder pain; bleeding; bleeding gums; blood in urine or stools; blurred vision; chest pain; chills; collection of blood under skin; confusion; convulsions; cough; decreased or cloudy urine; deep, dark purple bruise; difficult, burning, or painful urination; dizziness; dry mouth; fainting or lightheadedness when getting up from a lying or sitting position; fever; frequent urge to urinate; increased thirst; irregular heartbeat; itching, pain, redness, or swelling at place of injection; loss of appetite; lower back or side pain; mood changes; muscle pain or cramps; nausea or vomiting; numbness or tingling in hands, feet, or lips; painful or difficult urination; pinpoint red spots on skin; red, tender, or oozing skin at incision; shortness of breath; sore throat; sores, ulcers, or white spots on lips or in mouth; sudden sweating

Symptoms of overdose

Get emergency help immediately if any of the following symptoms of overdose occur:
Abdominal pain or swelling; back pain; black, tarry stools; bruising or purple areas on skin; coughing up

blood; decreased alertness; dizziness; headache; joint pain or swelling; nosebleeds

Some side effects may occur that usually do not need medical attention. These side effects may go away during treatment as your body adjusts to the medicine. Also, your health care professional may be able to tell you about ways to prevent or reduce some of these side effects. Check with your health care professional if any of the following side effects continue or are bothersome or if you have any questions about them:

More common
Difficulty having a bowel movement; fever; rash; sleeplessness; swelling; trouble sleeping

Less common
Acid or sour stomach; belching; diarrhea; headache; heartburn; indigestion; pain; pinpoint red or purple spots on skin; skin blisters; stomach discomfort, upset or pain; tightness in chest; unusual changes to site of surgery; wheezing; wound drainage, increased

FORMOTEROL (Inhalation, oral/nebulization route) - for-MOH-te-rol

Commonly used brand name(s)
In the U.S.—
Foradil Aerolizer

Available Dosage Forms:
- Aerosol Powder
- Capsule

Therapeutic Class: Bronchodilator
Pharmacologic Class: Sympathomimetic

Uses For This Medicine

Formoterol belongs to the family of medicines known as beta 2-agonists. It is used to help prevent the symptoms of asthma. When used regularly every day, inhaled formoterol decreases the number and severity of asthma attacks. However, it will not relieve an asthma attack that has already started.

Inhaled formoterol works by preventing certain cells in the lungs and breathing passages from releasing substances that cause asthma symptoms.

This medicine may be taken with other asthma medicines known as corticosteroids.

Formoterol is also used for patients with COPD (Chronic Obstructive Pulmonary Disease). These are diseases such as chronic bronchitis and emphysema.

This medicine is available only with your doctor's prescription.

Before Using This Medicine

In deciding to use a medicine, the risks of taking the medicine must be weighed against the good it will do. This is a decision you and your doctor will make. For this medicine, the following should be considered:

Allergies—Tell your doctor if you have ever had any unusual or allergic reaction to this medicine or any other medi-

cines. Also tell your health care professional if you have any other types of allergies, such as to foods, dyes, preservatives, or animals. For non-prescription products, read the label or package ingredients carefully.

Pediatric—Studies on this medicine been done only in patients 5 years of age and older, and there is no specific information comparing use of formoterol in children less than 5 years of age with use in other age groups.

Geriatric—This medicine has been tested and has not been shown to cause different side effects or problems in older people than it does in younger adults.

Pregnancy—

	Pregnancy Category	Explanation
All Trimesters	C	Animal studies have shown an adverse effect and there are no adequate studies in pregnant women OR no animal studies have been conducted and there are no adequate studies in pregnant women.

Breast Feeding—There are no adequate studies in women for determining infant risk when using this medication during breastfeeding. Weigh the potential benefits against the potential risks before taking this medication while breastfeeding.

Other medicines—

Using this medicine with any of the following medicines is usually not recommended, but may be required in some cases. If both medicines are prescribed together, your doctor may change the dose or how often you use one or both of the medicines.

Clorgyline, Iproniazid, Isocarboxazid, Moclobemide, Nialamide, Pargyline, Phenelzine, Procarbazine, Selegiline, Toloxatone, Tranylcypromine

Interactions with Food/Tobacco/Alcohol—Certain medicines should not be used at or around the time of eating food or eating certain types of food since interactions may occur. Using alcohol or tobacco with certain medicines may also cause interactions to occur. Discuss with your healthcare professional the use of your medicine with food, alcohol, or tobacco.

Other medical problems—The presence of other medical problems may affect the use of this medicine. Make sure you tell your doctor if you have any other medical problems, especially:

- Acutely deteriorating asthma
- Blocked heart or
- High blood pressure or
- Irregular heartbeat or
- Structural problems with the heart or
- Weak heart, unable to circulate blood effectively—Risk of increased side effects
- Diabetes—Risk of increased side effects
- Overactive thyroid
- Seizures or
- Strong response to this kind of medicine—Risk of increased side effects

Proper Use of This Medicine

Dosing—The dose of this medicine will be different for different patients. Follow your doctor's orders or the directions on the label. The following information includes only the average doses of this medicine. If your dose is different, do not change it unless your doctor tells you to do so.

The amount of medicine that you take depends on the strength of the medicine. Also, the number of doses you take each day, the time allowed between doses, and the length of time you take the medicine depend on the medical problem for which you are using the medicine.

Inhaled formoterol is used to prevent asthma attacks. It is not used to relieve an attack that has already started. For relief of an asthma attack that has already started, you should use another medicine. If you do not have another medicine to use for an attack or if you have any questions about this, check with your health care professional.

In order for this medicine to help prevent asthma attacks, it must be used every day in regularly spaced doses, as ordered by your doctor.

Do not stop using this medicine or other asthma medicines that your doctor has prescribed for you unless you have discussed this with your doctor.

Inhaled formoterol is used with a special inhaler and usually comes with patient directions. Read the directions carefully before using this medicine. If you do not understand the directions or you are not sure how to use the inhaler, ask your health care professional to show you what to do. Also, ask your health care professional to check regularly how you use the inhaler to make sure you are using it properly.

Do not wash and reuse your inhaler. Use a new inhaler with each refill of your medicine.

Do not use a spacer with this medicine.

Do not exhale into your inhaler.

Do not use the inhaler for this medicine with any other medicine.

Dry your hands before handling this medicine.

- For inhalation:
  - Adults and children 5 years of age and older— 12 mcg by oral inhalation every 12 hours
  - Children younger than 6 years of age— use and dose must be determined by your doctor

Missed dose—If you miss a dose of this medicine, take it as soon as possible. However, if it is almost time for your next dose, skip the missed dose and go back to your regular dosing schedule. Do not double doses.

Storage—Store the medicine in a closed container at room temperature, away from heat, moisture, and direct light. Keep from freezing.

Keep out of the reach of children.

Do not keep outdated medicine or medicine no longer needed.

Ask your healthcare professional how you should dispose of any medicine you do not use.

Precautions While Using This Medicine

If you will be taking this medicine for a long time, it is very important that your doctor check you at regular visits for any blood or heart problems that may be caused by this medicine.

If your symptoms do not improve within a few days or if they become worse, check with your doctor.

Do not use this medicine to treat wheezing that is getting worse. Call your doctor right away if wheezing worsens while using formoterol.

You may also be taking an anti-inflammatory medicine along with this medicine. *Do not stop taking the anti-inflammatory medicine even if your asthma seems better, unless you are told to do so by your doctor.*

Although this medicine decreases the number of asthma episodes, this medicine may increase the chances of a severe asthma episode when they do occur. Be sure to read about these risks in the Medication Guide and talk to your doctor or pharmacist about any questions or concerns that you have.

Side Effects of This Medicine

Along with its needed effects, a medicine may cause some unwanted effects. Although not all of these side effects may occur, if they do occur they may need medical attention.

Check with your doctor immediately if any of the following side effects occur:

More common
Chills; cold or flu-like symptoms; cough or hoarseness; fever; sneezing; sore throat

Less common
Body aches or pain; chest pain or discomfort; congestion; cough producing mucous; difficulty breathing; dry throat; headache; labored breathing; pain or tenderness around eyes and cheekbones; runny nose; shortness of breath; tender, swollen glands in neck; tightness in chest; trauma; trouble swallowing; voice changes; wheezing

Rare
Convulsions; decreased urine; dry mouth; fainting; fast pounding, or irregular heartbeat or pulse palpitations; increased thirst; irregular heartbeat; loss of appetite; noisy breathing

Symptoms of overdose

Get emergency help immediately if any of the following symptoms of overdose occur:

Arm, back or jaw pain; blurred vision; chest tightness or heaviness; convulsions; decreased urine; dizziness or light-headedness; dry mouth; fainting; fast or irregular heartbeat; fatigue; general feeling or discomfort or illness; headache; increased hunger or thirst; increased urination; loss of appetite; mood changes; muscle pain or cramps; muscle spasm or jerking of all extremities; nausea; nervousness; no blood pressure or pulse; numbness or tingling in hands, feet or lips; palpitations or pounding in the ears; pounding or racing heartbeat or pulse; shortness of breath; sleeplessness; slow heartbeat; stopping of heart; sudden loss of consciousness; sweating; troubled breathing; trouble sleeping; unable to sleep; unconsciousness; unusual tiredness or weakness; vomiting

Some side effects may occur that usually do not need medical attention. These side effects may go away during treatment as your body adjusts to the medicine. Also, your health care professional may be able to tell you about ways to prevent or reduce some of these side effects. Check with your health care professional if any of the following side effects continue or are bothersome or if you have any questions about them:

More common
Headache

Less common
Agitation; anxiety; back pain; cramps; dizziness; hives or welts; increased mucous in throat and lungs; itching; redness of skin; restlessness; shakiness in legs, arms, hands, feet; skin rash; sleeplessness; trembling or shaking of hands or feet; trouble sleeping; unable to sleep

FOSAMPRENAVIR (Oral route) - FOS-am-pren-a-veer

Commonly used brand name(s)

In the U.S.—
Lexiva

Available Dosage Forms:
• Tablet

Therapeutic Class: Antiretroviral Agent
Pharmacologic Class: Protease Inhibitor

Uses For This Medicine

Fosamprenavir is a protease inhibitor. It is used in combination with other medicines to treat patients who are infected with the human immunodeficiency virus (HIV).

HIV is the virus that causes acquired immune deficiency syndrome (AIDS). Fosamprenavir may slow down the destruction of the immune system caused by HIV. This may help delay the development of problems usually related to AIDS or HIV disease. However, this medicine will not cure or prevent HIV infection, and it will not keep you from spreading the virus to other people. Patients who are taking this medicine may continue to have the problems usually related to AIDS or HIV disease.

This medicine is available only with your doctor's prescription.

Before Using This Medicine

In deciding to use a medicine, the risks of taking the medicine must be weighed against the good it will do. This is a decision you and your doctor will make. For this medicine, the following should be considered:

Allergies—Tell your doctor if you have ever had any unusual or allergic reaction to this medicine or any other medicines. Also tell your health care professional if you have any other types of allergies, such as to foods, dyes, preservatives, or animals. For non-prescription products, read the label or package ingredients carefully.

Pediatric—Studies on this medicine have been done only in adult patients, and there is no specific information comparing use of fosamprenavir in children with use in other age groups.

Geriatric—Many medicines have not been studied specifically in older people. Therefore, it may not be known whether

they work exactly the same way they do in younger adults or if they cause different side effects or problems in older people. There is not specific information comparing use of fosamprenavir in the elderly with use in other age groups.

Pregnancy—

	Pregnancy Category	Explanation
All Trimesters	C	Animal studies have shown an adverse effect and there are no adequate studies in pregnant women OR no animal studies have been conducted and there are no adequate studies in pregnant women.

Breast Feeding—There are no adequate studies in women for determining infant risk when using this medication during breastfeeding. Weigh the potential benefits against the potential risks before taking this medication while breastfeeding.

Other medicines—

Using this medicine with any of the following medicines is not recommended. Your doctor may decide not to treat you with this medication or change some of the other medicines you take.

Cisapride, Dihydroergotamine, Ergoloid Mesylates, Ergonovine, Ergotamine, Methylergonovine, Midazolam, Pimozide, Ranolazine, St John's Wort, Triazolam

Interactions with Food/Tobacco/Alcohol—Certain medicines should not be used at or around the time of eating food or eating certain types of food since interactions may occur. Using alcohol or tobacco with certain medicines may also cause interactions to occur. Discuss with your healthcare professional the use of your medicine with food, alcohol, or tobacco.

Other medical problems—The presence of other medical problems may affect the use of this medicine. Make sure you tell your doctor if you have any other medical problems, especially:

- Bleeding problems—May be worsened by recombinant interferon alfa-2b
- Diabetes mellitus (sugar diabetes)
- Hemophilia—Fosamprenavir may make this condition worse.
- Liver disease—Effects of fosamprenavir may be increased because of slower removal of fosamprenavir from the body. Your doctor may need to lower your dose of fosamprenavir.
- Hepatitis B or
- Hepatitis C—May increase certain concentrations of liver enzymes. Your doctor should monitor you closely.

Proper Use of This Medicine

Fosamprenavir suspension should be taken without food on an empty stomach.

Fosamprenavir tablets may be taken with or without food. However, it should not be taken with a high-fat meal. Taking fosamprenavir with a high-fat meal may decrease the amount of fosamprenavir that is absorbed by the body and prevent the medicine from working properly.

It is important to take fosamprenavir as part of a combination treatment. Your dose of medicine will be based on what other medicines you are taking, as well as your weight. Be sure to take all the medicines your doctor has prescribed for you, including fosamprenavir.

Take this medicine exactly as directed by your doctor. Do not take more of it, do not take it more often, and do not take it for a longer time than your doctor ordered. Also, do not stop taking this medicine without checking with your doctor first.

Keep taking fosamprenavir for the full time of treatment, even if you begin to feel better.

This medicine works best when there is a constant amount in the blood. To help keep the amount constant, do not miss any doses. Also, it is best to take the doses at evenly spaced times, day and night. For example, if you are to take two doses a day, the doses should be spaced about 12 hours apart. If you need help in planning the best times to take your medicine, check with your health care professional.

Only take medicine that your doctor has prescribed especially for you. Do not share your medicine with others.

Dosing—The dose of this medicine will be different for different patients. Follow your doctor's orders or the directions on the label. The following information includes only the average doses of this medicine. If your dose is different, do not change it unless your doctor tells you to do so.

The amount of medicine that you take depends on the strength of the medicine. Also, the number of doses you take each day, the time allowed between doses, and the length of time you take the medicine depend on the medical problem for which you are using the medicine.

- For oral dosage form (suspension and tablets):
  - For treatment of HIV infection:
    - Adults who have not taken HIV medicines called protease inhibitors in the past (fosamprenavir alone)—1400 mg two times a day.
    - Adults who have not taken HIV medicines called protease inhibitors in the past (fosamprenavir together with ritonavir)—1400 mg fosamprenavir with 200 mg ritonavir one time per day or 700 mg fosamprenavir with 100 mg ritonavir two times a day.
    - Adults who have taken HIV medicines called protease inhibitors in the past (fosamprenavir together with ritonavir)—700 mg fosamprenavir with 100 mg ritonavir two times a day. Adults who have taken HIV medicines called protease inhibitors in the past should not take the combination of fosamprenavir with ritonavir only one time a day. Check with your doctor if you are unsure of what amounts and how many times a day you should be taking your medicines. If you are taking fosamprenavir with ritonavir and efavirenz, check with your doctor for the correct doses.
    - Children—Use and dose must be determined by your doctor.

Missed dose—If you miss a dose of this medicine, take it as soon as possible. However, if it is almost time for your next dose, skip the missed dose and go back to your regular dosing schedule. Do not double doses.

Storage—Store the medicine in a closed container at room temperature, away from heat, moisture, and direct light. Do not refrigerate. Keep from freezing.

Keep out of the reach of children.

Do not keep outdated medicine or medicine no longer needed.

Ask your healthcare professional how you should dispose of any medicine you do not use.

Precautions While Using This Medicine

Do not take any other medicines without checking with your doctor first. This includes prescription and nonprescription medicines. This also includes food supplements, herbs and vitamins. To do so may increase the chance of side effects from fosamprenavir or other medicines.

This medicine may decrease the effects of some oral contraceptives (birth control pills). To avoid unwanted pregnancy, it is a good idea to use some additional contraceptive measures while being treated with fosamprenavir.

For patients with diabetes: Amprenavir may affect blood sugar levels. If you notice a change in the results of your blood or urine sugar tests or if you have any questions, check with your doctor.

It is very important that your doctor check your progress at regular visits to make sure this medicine is working properly and to check for unwanted effects, especially increases in blood sugar.

Fosamprenavir does not decrease the risk of transmitting the HIV infection to others through sexual contact or by contamination through blood. HIV may be acquired from or spread to others through infected body fluids, including blood, vaginal fluid, or semen. If you are infected, it is best to avoid any sexual activity involving an exchange of body fluids with other people. If you do have sex, always wear (or have your partner wear) a condom ("rubber"). Only use condoms made of latex, and use them every time you have vaginal, anal, or oral sex. The use of a spermicide (such as nonoxynol-9) may also help prevent the spread of HIV if it is not irritating to the vagina, rectum, or mouth. Spermicides have been shown to kill HIV in lab tests. Do not use oil-based jelly, cold cream, baby oil, or shortening as a lubricant— these products can cause the condom to break. Lubricants without oil, such as K-Y Jelly, are recommended. Women may wish to carry their own condoms. Birth control pills and diaphragms will help protect against pregnancy, but they will not prevent someone from giving or getting the AIDS virus. If you inject drugs, get help to stop. Do not share needles or equipment with anyone. In some cities, more than half of the drug users are infected, and sharing even 1 needle or syringe can spread the virus. If you have any questions about this, check with your health care professional.

Side Effects of This Medicine

Along with its needed effects, a medicine may cause some unwanted effects. Although not all of these side effects may occur, if they do occur they may need medical attention.

Check with your doctor immediately if any of the following side effects occur:

More common
  Large amount of triglyceride in the blood; severe skin rash

Less common
  Abdominal pain; blurred vision; depression mood or mental changes; dry mouth; fatigue; flushed, dry skin; fruit-like breath odor; increased hunger; increased thirst; increased urination; nausea; sweating; troubled breathing; unexplained weight loss; vomiting

Rare
  Back, leg, or stomach pains; bleeding gums; blistering, peeling, loosening of skin; chills; cough; dark urine; diarrhea; difficulty breathing; fever; general body swelling; itching; joint or muscle pain; loss of appetite; nosebleeds; pale skin; red irritated eyes; red skin lesions often with a purple center; sore throat; sores, ulcers, or white spots in mouth or on lips; unusual tiredness or weakness; yellowing of the eyes or skin

Some side effects may occur that usually do not need medical attention. These side effects may go away during treatment as your body adjusts to the medicine. Also, your health care professional may be able to tell you about ways to prevent or reduce some of these side effects. Check with your health care professional if any of the following side effects continue or are bothersome or if you have any questions about them:

More common
  Itching skin; mild or moderate rash

Less common
  Burning or prickling sensation around the mouth; headache

Frequency not known
  Breast enlargement; obesity; increased fat deposits on face, neck, and truck; buffalo hump; fat redistribution

Other side effects not listed may also occur in some patients. If you notice any other effects, check with your healthcare professional.

FOSCARNET (Intravenous route) - fos-KAR-net

Black Box Warning

Renal impairment is the major toxicity of foscarnet sodium. Frequent monitoring of serum creatinine, with dose adjustment for changes in renal function, and adequate hydration with administration of foscarnet sodium, is imperative.

Seizures, related to alterations in plasma minerals and electrolytes, have been associated with foscarnet sodium treatment. Therefore, patients must be carefully monitored for such changes and their potential sequelae. Mineral and electrolyte supplementation may be required.

Foscarnet sodium is indicated for use only in immunocompromised patients with CMV retinitis and mucocutaneous acyclovir-resistant HSV infections.

Commonly used brand name(s)

In the U.S.—
  Foscavir

Available Dosage Forms:
• Solution

Therapeutic Class: Antiviral
Pharmacologic Class: Viral DNA Polymerase Inhibitor

Uses For This Medicine

Foscarnet is used to treat the symptoms of cytomegalovirus (CMV) infection of the eyes in patients with acquired immune deficiency syndrome (AIDS). Foscarnet will not cure this eye infection, but it may help to control worsening of the symptoms. It is also used to treat herpes simplex virus (HSV) infections of the skin and mucous membranes in people who are immunocompromised and whose infections did not improve with other therapy. Foscarnet may also be used for other serious viral infections as determined by your doctor. However, it does not work in treating certain viruses, such as the common cold or the flu.

Foscarnet is administered only by or under the supervision of your doctor.

Once a medicine has been approved for marketing for a certain use, experience may show that it is also useful for other medical problems. Although these uses are not included in product labeling, foscarnet is used in certain patients with the following medical conditions:

- Cytomegalovirus infections in places other than the eyes, such as the lungs, esophagus, or intestines
- Varicella-zoster infection (shingles) that does not respond to treatment with acyclovir in patients with HIV infection

Before Using This Medicine

In deciding to use a medicine, the risks of taking the medicine must be weighed against the good it will do. This is a decision you and your doctor will make. For this medicine, the following should be considered:

Allergies—Tell your doctor if you have ever had any unusual or allergic reaction to this medicine or any other medicines. Also tell your health care professional if you have any other types of allergies, such as to foods, dyes, preservatives, or animals. For non-prescription products, read the label or package ingredients carefully.

Pediatric—There is no specific information comparing use of foscarnet in children with use in other age groups. Foscarnet can cause serious side effects in any patient. Therefore, it is especially important that you discuss with the child's doctor the good that this medicine may do as well as the risks of using it.

Geriatric—Many medicines have not been studied specifically in older people. Therefore, it may not be known whether they work exactly the same way they do in younger adults or if they cause different side effects or problems in older people. There is no specific information comparing use of foscarnet in the elderly with use in other age groups.

Pregnancy—

	Pregnancy Category	Explanation
All Trimesters	C	Animal studies have shown an adverse effect and there are no adequate studies in pregnant women OR no animal studies have been conducted and there are no adequate studies in pregnant women.

Breast Feeding—There are no adequate studies in women for determining infant risk when using this medication during breastfeeding. Weigh the potential benefits against the potential risks before taking this medication while breastfeeding.

Other medicines—

Using this medicine with any of the following medicines is not recommended. Your doctor may decide not to treat you with this medication or change some of the other medicines you take.

Arsenic Trioxide, Bepridil, Cisapride, Levomethadyl, Mesoridazine, Pimozide, Probucol, Terfenadine, Thioridazine, Ziprasidone

Interactions with Food/Tobacco/Alcohol—Certain medicines should not be used at or around the time of eating food or eating certain types of food since interactions may occur. Using alcohol or tobacco with certain medicines may also cause interactions to occur. Discuss with your healthcare professional the use of your medicine with food, alcohol, or tobacco.

Other medical problems—The presence of other medical problems may affect the use of this medicine. Make sure you tell your doctor if you have any other medical problems, especially:

- Anemia—Foscarnet may cause or worsen anemia
- Dehydration or
- Kidney disease—Patients who are dehydrated or have kidney disease may have an increased chance of side effects

Proper Use of This Medicine

To ensure the best response, foscarnet must be given for the full time of treatment. Also, this medicine works best when there is a constant amount in the blood. To help keep the amount constant, foscarnet must be given on a regular schedule.

Several glasses of water should be taken every day, unless otherwise directed by your doctor. Drinking extra water will help to prevent some unwanted effects foscarnet has on the kidneys.

This medicine may cause sores on the genitals (sex organs). Washing your genitals after urination may decrease the chance of your developing this problem.

Dosing—The dose of this medicine will be different for different patients. Follow your doctor's orders or the directions on the label. The following information includes only the average doses of this medicine. If your dose is different, do not change it unless your doctor tells you to do so.

The amount of medicine that you take depends on the strength of the medicine. Also, the number of doses you take each day, the time allowed between doses, and the length of time you take the medicine depend on the medical problem for which you are using the medicine.

- For injection dosage form:
  - For cytomegalovirus (CMV) retinitis induction (first stage of dosing):
    - Adults and children—The usual dose is 60 milligrams (mg) per kilogram (kg) (27.3 mg per pound) of body weight every eight hours for fourteen to twenty-one days. Each dose is injected slowly into a vein by an infusion pump over at least one hour.

○ For CMV retinitis maintenance (second stage of dosing):

- Adults and children—The usual dose is 90 to 120 mg per kg (41 to 54.5 mg per pound) of body weight once a day. This dose is injected slowly into a vein by an infusion pump over at least two hours.

○ For herpes simplex infections:

- Adults and children—The usual dose is 40 mg per kg (18.2 mg per pound) of body weight given either every eight or every twelve hours. This dose is injected slowly into a vein by an infusion pump over at least one hour. Treatment is usually continued for two to three weeks or until the infection in healed.

Precautions While Using This Medicine

It is very important that your doctor check your progress at regular visits. This will allow your doctor to check for possible unwanted effects.

It is also very important that your ophthalmologist (eye doctor) check your eyes at regular visits since you may have some loss of eyesight due to retinitis even while you are receiving foscarnet.

Side Effects of This Medicine

Along with their needed effects, medicines like foscarnet can sometimes cause serious side effects such as kidney problems; these are described below. Foscarnet may also decrease the amount of calcium in your blood, causing you to have a tingling sensation around your mouth, and pain or numbness in your hands and feet. If this occurs, especially while you are receiving the medicine, notify your health care professional immediately.

Along with its needed effects, a medicine may cause some unwanted effects. Although not all of these side effects may occur, if they do occur they may need medical attention.

Check with your doctor immediately if any of the following side effects occur:

More common

Increased or decreased frequency of urination or amount of urine; increased thirst

Less common

Convulsions (seizures); fever, chills, and sore throat; muscle twitching; pain at place of injection; pain or numbness in hands or feet; tingling sensation around mouth; tremor; unusual tiredness and weakness

Rare

Sores or ulcers on the mouth or throat, penis, or vulva

Some side effects may occur that usually do not need medical attention. These side effects may go away during treatment as your body adjusts to the medicine. Also, your health care professional may be able to tell you about ways to prevent or reduce some of these side effects. Check with your health care professional if any of the following side effects continue or are bothersome or if you have any questions about them:

More common

Abdominal or stomach pain; anxious feeling; confusion; dizziness; headache; loss of appetite; nausea and vomiting; unusual tiredness or weakness

Other side effects not listed may also occur in some patients. If you notice any other effects, check with your healthcare professional.

FOSFOMYCIN (Oral route) - fos-foe-MYE-sin

Commonly used brand name(s)

In the U.S.—
Monurol

Available Dosage Forms:
- Powder for Solution

Therapeutic Class: Antibiotic

Uses For This Medicine

Fosfomycin is an antibiotic. It is used to treat urinary tract infection and cystitis (bladder infection) in women.

This medicine is available only with your doctor's prescription.

Before Using This Medicine

In deciding to use a medicine, the risks of taking the medicine must be weighed against the good it will do. This is a decision you and your doctor will make. For this medicine, the following should be considered:

Allergies—Tell your doctor if you have ever had any unusual or allergic reaction to this medicine or any other medicines. Also tell your health care professional if you have any other types of allergies, such as to foods, dyes, preservatives, or animals. For non-prescription products, read the label or package ingredients carefully.

Pregnancy—

	Pregnancy Category	Explanation
All Trimesters	B	Animal studies have revealed no evidence of harm to the fetus, however, there are no adequate studies in pregnant women OR animal studies have shown an adverse effect, but adequate studies in pregnant women have failed to demonstrate a risk to the fetus.

Breast Feeding—There are no adequate studies in women for determining infant risk when using this medication during breastfeeding. Weigh the potential benefits against the potential risks before taking this medication while breastfeeding.

Other medicines—Although certain medicines should not be used together at all, in other cases two different medicines may be used together even if an interaction might occur. In these cases, your doctor may want to change the dose, or other precautions may be necessary. Tell your healthcare professional if you are taking any other prescription or non-prescription (over-the-counter [OTC]) medicine.

Interactions with Food/Tobacco/Alcohol—Certain medicines should not be used at or around the time of eating food or eating certain types of food since interactions may occur. Using alcohol or tobacco with certain medicines may also cause interactions to occur. Discuss with your healthcare professional the use of your medicine with food, alcohol, or tobacco.

Other medical problems—The presence of other medical problems may affect the use of this medicine. Make sure you

tell your doctor if you have any other medical problems, especially:
- Kidney disease—Effects of fosfomycin may be increased because of slower removal from the body

Proper Use of This Medicine

Fosfomycin powder must be dissolved in water before it is taken. Take the medicine as soon as it has dissolved.

This medicine can be taken with or without food.

Dosing—The dose of this medicine will be different for different patients. Follow your doctor's orders or the directions on the label. The following information includes only the average doses of this medicine. If your dose is different, do not change it unless your doctor tells you to do so.

The amount of medicine that you take depends on the strength of the medicine. Also, the number of doses you take each day, the time allowed between doses, and the length of time you take the medicine depend on the medical problem for which you are using the medicine.
- For oral dosage form (powder for solution):
  - For treatment of bladder infection:
    - Adults—3 grams (one packet) dissolved in water taken one time.
    - Children—Use and dose must be determined by your doctor.

Storage—Store the medicine in a closed container at room temperature, away from heat, moisture, and direct light. Keep from freezing.

Keep out of the reach of children.

Do not keep outdated medicine or medicine no longer needed.

Precautions While Using This Medicine

Check with your doctor if your symptoms do not improve within 2 or 3 days or if they become worse.

Side Effects of This Medicine

Along with its needed effects, a medicine may cause some unwanted effects. Although not all of these side effects may occur, if they do occur they may need medical attention.

Check with your doctor as soon as possible if any of the following side effects occur:
More common
  Vaginal discharge and pain

Some side effects may occur that usually do not need medical attention. These side effects may go away during treatment as your body adjusts to the medicine. Also, your health care professional may be able to tell you about ways to prevent or reduce some of these side effects. Check with your health care professional if any of the following side effects continue or are bothersome or if you have any questions about them:
More common
  Diarrhea; headache; nausea
Less common
  Abdominal or stomach pain; back pain; dizziness; heartburn; indigestion; pain; painful menstruation; runny or stuffy nose; skin rash; sore throat; weakness

Other side effects not listed may also occur in some patients. If you notice any other effects, check with your healthcare professional.

FROVATRIPTAN (Oral route) - froe-va-TRIP-tan

Commonly used brand name(s)
In the U.S.—
  Frova

Available Dosage Forms:
- Tablet

Therapeutic Class: Antimigraine
Pharmacologic Class: Serotonin Receptor Agonist, 5–HT1

Uses For This Medicine

Frovatriptan is used to treat severe migraine headaches. Many people find that their headaches go away completely after they take frovatriptan. Other people find that their headaches are much less painful, and that they are able to go back to their normal activities even though their headaches are not completely gone. Frovatriptan often relieves other symptoms that occur together with a migraine headache, such as nausea, vomiting, sensitivity to light, and sensitivity to sound.

Frovatriptan is not an ordinary pain reliever. It will not relieve any kind of pain other than migraine headaches. This medicine is usually used for people whose headaches are not relieved by acetaminophen, aspirin, or other pain relievers.

Frovatriptan has caused serious side effects in some people, especially people who have heart or blood vessel disease. Be sure that you discuss with your doctor the risks of using this medicine as well as the good that it can do.

Frovatriptan is available only with your doctor's prescription.

Before Using This Medicine

In deciding to use a medicine, the risks of taking the medicine must be weighed against the good it will do. This is a decision you and your doctor will make. For this medicine, the following should be considered:

Allergies—Tell your doctor if you have ever had any unusual or allergic reaction to this medicine or any other medicines. Also tell your health care professional if you have any other types of allergies, such as to foods, dyes, preservatives, or animals. For non-prescription products, read the label or package ingredients carefully.

Pediatric—Studies on this medicine have been done only in adult patients, and there is no specific information comparing use of frovatriptan in children with use in other age groups. However, frovatriptan is not recommended for use in patients younger than 18 years of age.

Geriatric—Many medicines have not been studied specifically in older people. Therefore, it may not be known whether they work exactly the same way they do in younger adults or if they cause different side effects or problems in older people.

There is no specific information comparing use of frovatriptan in the elderly with use in other age groups.

Pregnancy—

	Pregnancy Category	Explanation
All Trimesters	C	Animal studies have shown an adverse effect and there are no adequate studies in pregnant women OR no animal studies have been conducted and there are no adequate studies in pregnant women.

Breast Feeding—There are no adequate studies in women for determining infant risk when using this medication during breastfeeding. Weigh the potential benefits against the potential risks before taking this medication while breastfeeding.

Other medicines—

Using this medicine with any of the following medicines is not recommended. Your doctor may decide not to treat you with this medication or change some of the other medicines you take.

Almotriptan, Avitriptan, Dihydroergotamine, Eletriptan, Ergoloid Mesylates, Ergonovine, Ergotamine, Metergoline, Methylergonovine, Methysergide, Naratriptan, Pergolide, Rizatriptan, Sumatriptan, Zolmitriptan

Interactions with Food/Tobacco/Alcohol—Certain medicines should not be used at or around the time of eating food or eating certain types of food since interactions may occur. Using alcohol or tobacco with certain medicines may also cause interactions to occur. Discuss with your healthcare professional the use of your medicine with food, alcohol, or tobacco.

Other medical problems—The presence of other medical problems may affect the use of this medicine. Make sure you tell your doctor if you have any other medical problems, especially:

- Uncontrolled high blood pressure—Use of frovatriptan may cause this condition to become worse.

- Coronary artery disease or

- Heart attack (recent) or

- Heart disease

- Risk factors for coronary artery disease such as high cholesterol, family history, diabetes, obesity, women after menopause and men over 40 years of age—Use of frovatriptan may cause problems in patients with these risk factors.

- Blood vessel disease, especially in the intestines and fingers—Use of frovatriptan may cause these conditions to become worse.

- Bleeding in the brain or

- Stroke (or history of)—Use of frovatriptan may increase the chance of having a stroke

Proper Use of This Medicine

Dosing—The dose of this medicine will be different for different patients. Follow your doctor's orders or the directions on the label. The following information includes only the average doses of this medicine. If your dose is different, do not change it unless your doctor tells you to do so.

The amount of medicine that you take depends on the strength of the medicine. Also, the number of doses you take each day, the time allowed between doses, and the length of time you take the medicine depend on the medical problem for which you are using the medicine.

Do not use frovatriptan for a headache that is different from your usual migraines. Instead, check with your doctor.

To relieve your migraine as soon as possible, use frovatriptan as soon as the headache pain begins. Even if you get warning signals of a coming migraine (an aura), you should wait until the headache pain starts before using frovatriptan. Using frovatriptan during the aura probably will not prevent the headache from occurring. However, even if you do not use frovatriptan until your migraine has been present for several hours, the medicine will still work.

Lying down in a quiet, dark room for a while after you use this medicine may help relieve your migraine.

If you are not much better 2 hours after a tablet is taken follow your health care provider's instructions concerning taking one additional dose. A migraine that is not relieved by the first dose of frovatriptan probably will not be relieved by a second dose, either. Ask your doctor ahead of time about other medicine to be taken if frovatriptan does not work. After taking the other medicine, check with your doctor as soon as possible. Headaches that are not relieved by frovatriptan are sometimes caused by conditions that need other treatment. However, even if frovatriptan does not relieve one migraine, it may still relieve the next one.

If you feel much better after a dose of frovatriptan, but your headache comes back or gets worse after a while, you may use one more tablet of frovatriptan. However, use this medicine only as directed by your doctor. Do not use more of it, and do not use it more often, than directed. Using too much frovatriptan may increase the chance of side effects.

Your doctor may direct you to take another medicine to help prevent headaches. It is important that you follow your doctor's directions, even if your headaches continue to occur. Headache-preventing medicines may take several weeks to start working. Even after they do start working, your headaches may not go away completely. However, your headaches should occur less often, and they should be less severe and easier to relieve. This may reduce the amount of frovatriptan or pain relievers that you need. If you do not notice any improvement after several weeks of headache-preventing treatment, check with your doctor.

- For oral dosage form (tablets):
  - For migraine headaches:
    - Adults—Take one tablet (2.5 mg (milligrams) anytime after the start of your migraine headache. You may take a second tablet if your headache comes back after relief from the 1st dose. You should wait at least 2 hours between doses. Do not take more than 3 tablets in a 24 hour period.
    - Children—Use and dose must be determined by your doctor.

Storage—Store the medicine in a closed container at room temperature, away from heat, moisture, and direct light. Keep from freezing.

Keep out of the reach of children.

Do not keep outdated medicine or medicine no longer needed.

Ask your healthcare professional how you should dispose of any medicine you do not use.

Precautions While Using This Medicine

Check with your doctor if you have used frovatriptan for three headaches, and have not had good relief. Also, check with your doctor if your migraine headaches are worse, or if they are occurring more often, than before you started using frovatriptan.

Drinking alcoholic beverages can make headaches worse or cause new headaches to occur. People who suffer from severe headaches should probably avoid alcoholic beverages, especially during a headache.

Some people feel drowsy or dizzy during or after a migraine, or after taking frovatriptan to relieve a migraine. As long as you are feeling drowsy or dizzy, do not drive, use machines, or do anything else that could be dangerous if you are dizzy or are not alert.

Side Effects of This Medicine

Along with its needed effects, a medicine may cause some unwanted effects. Although not all of these side effects may occur, if they do occur they may need medical attention.

Check with your doctor immediately if any of the following side effects occur:
> *Less common*
>> Chest pain

Some side effects may occur that usually do not need medical attention. These side effects may go away during treatment as your body adjusts to the medicine. Also, your health care professional may be able to tell you about ways to prevent or reduce some of these side effects. Check with your health care professional if any of the following side effects continue or are bothersome or if you have any questions about them:
> *More common*
>> Dizziness
> *Less common*
>> Acid or sour stomach, belching, heartburn, indigestion, stomach discomfort, upset or pain; dry mouth; fatigue, such as unusual tiredness or weakness; flushing, such as feeling of warmth, redness of the face, neck, arms and occasionally upper chest; headache; hot or cold sensation; nausea; skeletal pain, such as pain in bones; tingling, burning, or prickly sensations; sleepiness or unusual drowsiness.

Other side effects not listed may also occur in some patients. If you notice any other effects, check with your healthcare professional.

FULVESTRANT (Intramuscular route)
- fool-VES-trant

Commonly used brand name(s)
In the U.S.—
> Faslodex

Available Dosage Forms:
- Solution

Therapeutic Class: Antineoplastic Agent

Uses For This Medicine

Fulvestrant is a medicine that is used to treat breast cancer.

Many breast cancer tumors grow in response to estrogen. This medicine blocks the effects of the estrogen hormone in the body. As a result, the amount of estrogen that the tumor is exposed to is reduced, limiting the growth of the tumor.

This medicine is available only with your doctor's prescription.

Before Using This Medicine

In deciding to use a medicine, the risks of taking the medicine must be weighed against the good it will do. This is a decision you and your doctor will make. For this medicine, the following should be considered:

Allergies—Tell your doctor if you have ever had any unusual or allergic reaction to this medicine or any other medicines. Also tell your health care professional if you have any other types of allergies, such as to foods, dyes, preservatives, or animals. For non-prescription products, read the label or package ingredients carefully.

Geriatric—Many medicines have not been studied specifically in older people. Therefore, it may not be known whether they work exactly the same way they do in younger adults or if they cause different side effects or problems in older people.

Pregnancy—

	Pregnancy Category	Explanation
All Trimesters	D	Studies in pregnant women have demonstrated a risk to the fetus. However, the benefits of therapy in a life threatening situation or a serious disease, may outweigh the potential risk.

Breast Feeding—There are no adequate studies in women for determining infant risk when using this medication during breastfeeding. Weigh the potential benefits against the potential risks before taking this medication while breastfeeding.

Other medicines—Although certain medicines should not be used together at all, in other cases two different medicines may be used together even if an interaction might occur. In these cases, your doctor may want to change the dose, or other precautions may be necessary. Tell your healthcare professional if you are taking any other prescription or nonprescription (over-the-counter [OTC]) medicine.

Interactions with Food/Tobacco/Alcohol—Certain medicines should not be used at or around the time of eating food or eating certain types of food since interactions may occur. Using alcohol or tobacco with certain medicines may also cause interactions to occur. Discuss with your healthcare

professional the use of your medicine with food, alcohol, or tobacco.

Other medical problems—The presence of other medical problems may affect the use of this medicine. Make sure you tell your doctor if you have any other medical problems, especially:

- Bleeding problems—May be worsened by fulvestrant

- Liver disease—Effects of fulvestrant may be increased because of slower removal from the body

Proper Use of This Medicine

Fulvestrant is usually given by a health care professional. However, medicines given by injection are sometimes used at home. If you will be using fulvestrant at home, your health care professional will teach you how the injections are to be given. Be certain that you understand exactly how the medicine is to be injected. Do not reuse needles and syringes.

Put used needles and syringes in a puncture-resistant disposable container, or dispose of them as directed by your health care professional.

Dosing—The dose of this medicine will be different for different patients. Follow your doctor's orders or the directions on the label. The following information includes only the average doses of this medicine. If your dose is different, do not change it unless your doctor tells you to do so.

The amount of medicine that you take depends on the strength of the medicine. Also, the number of doses you take each day, the time allowed between doses, and the length of time you take the medicine depend on the medical problem for which you are using the medicine.

- For parenteral dosage form (injection):
  - For cancer of the breast:
    - Adults—250 milligrams (mg), injected into the muscle of the buttocks on the same day of every month (e.g., the first day of every month). The dose can be given as a single 5 mL (milliliter) injection, or as two 2.5 mL (milliliter) injections, immediately following each other.

Missed dose—Call your doctor or pharmacist for instructions.

If you miss a dose of this medicine, take it as soon as possible and schedule the next dose 30 days later. Do not double doses or use more often than one dose every 30 days. If you have any questions about this, check with your doctor.

Storage—Store in the refrigerator. Do not freeze.

Keep out of the reach of children.

Do not keep outdated medicine or medicine no longer needed.

Ask your healthcare professional how you should dispose of any medicine you do not use.

Precautions While Using This Medicine

Your doctor will want to check your progress at regular visits. This will allow your doctor to see if the medicine is working properly and to check for unwanted effects.

For women of childbearing age—It is very important that you do not become pregnant while taking fulvestrant.

Side Effects of This Medicine

Along with its needed effects, a medicine may cause some unwanted effects. Although not all of these side effects may occur, if they do occur they may need medical attention.

Check with your doctor immediately if any of the following side effects occur:

More common

Bloating or swelling of face, arms, hands, lower legs, or feet; rapid weight gain; tingling of hands or feet; unusual weight gain or loss

Some side effects may occur that usually do not need medical attention. These side effects may go away during treatment as your body adjusts to the medicine. Also, your health care professional may be able to tell you about ways to prevent or reduce some of these side effects. Check with your health care professional if any of the following side effects continue or are bothersome or if you have any questions about them:

More common

Back pain; bladder pain; bloody or cloudy urine; body aches or pain; bone pain; burning, crawling, itching, numbness, prickling, "pins and needles", or tingling feelings; chest pain; chills; congestion; cough, increased; diarrhea; difficult, burning, or painful urination; difficult or labored breathing; difficulty having a bowel movement (stool); discouragement; dizziness; dryness or soreness of throat; feeling faint, dizzy, or light-headedness; feeling of warmth or heat; feeling sad or empty; fever; flushing or redness of skin, especially on face and neck; frequent urge to urinate; general feeling of discomfort or illness; headache; hoarseness; injection site pain; irritability; joint pain; lack or loss of appetite; lack or loss of strength; loss of interest or pleasure; lower back or side pain; muscle aches and pains; nausea; pain; pelvic pain; runny nose; shivering; shortness of breath; skin rash; sleeplessness; sore throat; stomach pain; sweating; tender, swollen glands in neck; tightness in chest; trouble concentrating; trouble in swallowing; trouble sleeping; unable to sleep; unusual tiredness or weakness; voice changes; vomiting; wheezing

Less common

Difficulty in moving; fear; muscle pain or stiffness; nervousness; pain, swelling, or redness in joints; pale skin; troubled breathing with exertion; unusual bleeding or bruising

Rare

Black, tarry stools; feeling of constant movement of self or surroundings; muscle aching or cramping; muscle pains or stiffness; pain in chest, groin, or legs, especially the calves; sensation of spinning; severe, sudden headache; slurred speech; sores, ulcers, or white spots on lips or in mouth; sudden, unexplained shortness of breath; sudden loss of coordination; sudden, severe weakness or numbness in arm or leg; swollen joints; vaginal bleeding; vision changes

Other side effects not listed may also occur in some patients. If you notice any other effects, check with your healthcare professional.

GABAPENTIN   (Oral route) - GA-ba-pen-tin

Commonly used brand name(s)

In the U.S.—
Gabarone
Neurontin

Available Dosage Forms:

- Tablet
- Capsule
- Solution

Therapeutic Class: Anticonvulsant

Uses For This Medicine

Gabapentin is used to help control some types of seizures in the treatment of epilepsy. This medicine cannot cure epilepsy and will only work to control seizures for as long as you continue to take it.

This medicine is also used to manage a condition called postherpetic neuralgia (pain after "shingles").

Gabapentin is available only with your doctor's prescription.

Once a medicine has been approved for marketing for a certain use, experience may show that it is also useful for other medical problems. Although this use is not included in product labeling, gabapentin is used in certain patients:
- To treat diabetic peripheral neuropathic pain.

Before Using This Medicine

In deciding to use a medicine, the risks of taking the medicine must be weighed against the good it will do. This is a decision you and your doctor will make. For this medicine, the following should be considered:

Allergies—Tell your doctor if you have ever had any unusual or allergic reaction to this medicine or any other medicines. Also tell your health care professional if you have any other types of allergies, such as to foods, dyes, preservatives, or animals. For non-prescription products, read the label or package ingredients carefully.

Pediatric—This medicine has been tested in children 3 years to 12 years of age. Children may be sensitive to the effects of gabapentin. This may increase the chance of side effects during treatment. Certain side effects may be especially likely to occur in children. It is especially important that you discuss with the child's doctor the good that this medicine may do as well as the risks of using it

This medicine has been tested in a small number of patients 12 to 18 years of age. In effective doses, gabapentin has not been shown to cause different side effects or problems than it does in adults.

Geriatric—Gabapentin is removed from the body more slowly in elderly people than in younger people. Higher blood levels may occur, which may increase the chance of unwanted effects. Your doctor may give you a different gabapentin dose than a younger person would receive.

Pregnancy—

	Pregnancy Category	Explanation
All Trimesters	C	Animal studies have shown an adverse effect and there are no adequate studies in pregnant women OR no animal studies have been conducted and there are no adequate studies in pregnant women.

Breast Feeding—There are no adequate studies in women for determining infant risk when using this medication during breastfeeding. Weigh the potential benefits against the potential risks before taking this medication while breastfeeding.

Other medicines—

Using this medicine with any of the following medicines may cause an increased risk of certain side effects, but using both drugs may be the best treatment for you. If both medicines are prescribed together, your doctor may change the dose or how often you use one or both of the medicines.

Aluminum Carbonate, Basic, Aluminum Hydroxide, Aluminum Phosphate, Dihydroxyaluminum Aminoacetate, Dihydroxyaluminum Sodium Carbonate, Ginkgo, Magaldrate, Magnesium Carbonate, Magnesium Hydroxide, Magnesium Oxide, Magnesium Trisilicate

Interactions with Food/Tobacco/Alcohol—Certain medicines should not be used at or around the time of eating food or eating certain types of food since interactions may occur. Using alcohol or tobacco with certain medicines may also cause interactions to occur. Discuss with your healthcare professional the use of your medicine with food, alcohol, or tobacco.

Other medical problems—The presence of other medical problems may affect the use of this medicine. Make sure you tell your doctor if you have any other medical problems, especially:
- Kidney disease—Higher blood levels of gabapentin may occur, which may increase the chance of unwanted effects; your doctor may need to change your dose

Proper Use of This Medicine

Take this medicine only as directed by your doctor, to help your condition as much as possible. Do not take more or less of it, and do not take it more or less often than your doctor ordered.

Gabapentin may be taken with or without food or on a full or empty stomach. However, if your doctor tells you to take the medicine a certain way, take it exactly as directed.

When taking gabapentin 3 times a day, do not allow more than 12 hours to pass between any 2 doses.

If you have trouble swallowing capsules, you may open the gabapentin capsule and mix the medicine with applesauce or juice. Mix only one dose at a time just before taking it. Do not mix any doses to save for later, because the medicine may change over time and may not work properly.

Dosing—The dose of this medicine will be different for different patients. Follow your doctor's orders or the directions on the label. The following information includes only the average doses of this medicine. If your dose is different, do not change it unless your doctor tells you to do so.

The amount of medicine that you take depends on the strength of the medicine. Also, the number of doses you take each day, the time allowed between doses, and the length of time you take the medicine depend on the medical problem for which you are using the medicine.

- For oral dosage form (capsules):
  - For epilepsy:
    - Adults and teenagers 12 years of age and older—At first, 300 milligrams (mg) three times a day. Your doctor may increase the dose gradually if needed. However, the dose is usually not more than 1800 mg a day.
    - Children 3 to 12 years of age—Dose is based on body weight. To start, 10 to 15 mg per kilogram (4.5 to 6.8 mg per pound) of body weight a day, divided into three doses. Your doctor may increase your dose as needed. The usual dose for children 5 years of age and older is 25 to 35 mg per kilogram (11.3 to 15.9 mg per pound) of body weight a day, divided into three doses. The usual dose for children 3 to 5 years of age is 40 mg per kilogram (18.1 mg per pound) of body weight a day, divided into three doses.
    - Children less than 3 years of age—Use and dose must be determined by your doctor.
    - Older adults—Dose must be determined by your doctor, but it is usually not more than 600 mg three times a day.
  - For postherpetic neuralgia
    - Adults and teenagers—At first, 300 milligrams (mg) on day 1. On day 2, 300 milligrams (mg) two times a day. On day 3, 300 milligrams (mg) three times a day. Your doctor may want to increase your dose to a maximum daily dose of 1800 milligrams (600 milligrams three times a day).
- For oral dosage form (oral solution):
  - For epilepsy:
    - Adults and teenagers 12 years of age and older—At first, 300 milligrams (mg) three times a day. Your doctor may increase the dose gradually if needed. However, the dose is usually not more than 1800 mg a day.
    - Children 3 to 12 years of age—Dose is based on body weight. To start, 10 to 15 mg per kilogram (4.5 to 6.8 mg per pound) of body weight a day, divided into three doses. Your doctor may increase your dose as needed. The usual dose for children 5 years of age and older is 25 to 35 mg per kilogram (11.3 to 15.9 mg per pound) of body weight a day, divided into three doses. The usual dose for children 3 to 5 years of age is 40 mg per kilogram (18.1 mg per pound) of body weight a day, divided into three doses.
    - Children less than 3 years of age—Use and dose must be determined by your doctor.
    - Older adults—Dose must be determined by your doctor, but it is usually not more than 600 mg three times a day.
  - For postherpetic neuralgia
    - Adults and teenagers—At first, 300 milligrams (mg) on day 1. On day 2, 300 milligrams (mg) two times a day. On day 3, 300 milligrams (mg) three times a day. Your doctor may want to increase your dose to a maximum daily dose of 1800 milligrams (600 milligrams three times a day).
- For oral dosage form (tablets):
  - For epilepsy:
    - Adults and teenagers 12 years of age and older—At first, 300 milligrams (mg) three times a day. Your doctor may increase the dose gradually if needed. However, the dose is usually not more than 1800 mg a day.
    - Children 3 to 12 years of age—Dose is based on body weight. To start, 10 to 15 mg per kilogram (4.5 to 6.8 mg per pound) of body weight a day, divided into three doses. Your doctor may increase your dose as needed. The usual dose for children 5 years of age and older is 25 to 35 mg per kilogram (11.3 to 15.9 mg per pound) of body weight a day, divided into three doses. The usual dose for children 3 to 5 years of age is 40 mg per kilogram (18.1 mg per pound) of body weight a day, divided into three doses.
    - Children less than 3 years of age—Use and dose must be determined by your doctor.
    - Older adults—Dose must be determined by your doctor, but it is usually not more than 600 mg three times a day.
  - For postherpetic neuralgia
    - Adults and teenagers—At first, 300 milligrams (mg) on day 1. On day 2, 300 milligrams (mg) two times a day. On day 3, 300 milligrams (mg) three times a day. Your doctor may want to increase your dose to a maximum daily dose of 1800 milligrams (600 milligrams three times a day).

Note: This medicine may be given as a combination of any of the forms it comes in.

Missed dose—If you miss a dose of this medicine, take it as soon as possible. However, if it is almost time for your next dose, skip the missed dose and go back to your regular dosing schedule. Do not double doses.

Do not allow more than 12 hours to go by between doses. If this happens, call your doctor right away.

Storage—Store the medicine in a closed container at room temperature, away from heat, moisture, and direct light. Keep from freezing.

Keep out of the reach of children.

Do not keep outdated medicine or medicine no longer needed.

Store the liquid form of this medicine in the refrigerator.

Precautions While Using This Medicine

It is important that your doctor check your progress at regular visits, especially for the first few months you take gabapentin. This is necessary to allow dose adjustments and to reduce any unwanted effects.

This medicine will add to the effects of alcohol and other CNS depressants (medicines that make you drowsy or less alert). Some examples of CNS depressants are antihistamines or medicine for hay fever, other allergies, or colds; sedatives, tranquilizers, or sleeping medicine; prescription pain medicine or narcotics; barbiturates; other medicines for seizures; muscle relaxants; or anesthetics, including some dental anesthetics. Check with your medical doctor or dentist before taking any of the above while you are taking gabapentin.

Gabapentin may cause blurred vision, double vision, clumsiness, unsteadiness, dizziness, drowsiness, or trouble in thinking. Make sure you know how you react to this medicine before you drive, use machines, or do anything else that could be dangerous if you are not alert, well-coordinated, or able to think or see well. If these reactions are especially bothersome, check with your doctor.

Before you have any medical tests, tell the doctor in charge that you are taking gabapentin. The results of dipstick tests for protein in the urine may be affected by this medicine.

Do not stop taking gabapentin without first checking with your doctor. Stopping the medicine suddenly may cause your seizures to return or to occur more often. Your doctor may want you to gradually reduce the amount you are taking before stopping completely.

Side Effects of This Medicine

Along with its needed effects, a medicine may cause some unwanted effects. Although not all of these side effects may occur, if they do occur they may need medical attention.

Check with your doctor as soon as possible if any of the following side effects occur:

More common
Clumsiness or unsteadiness; continuous, uncontrolled, back-and-forth and/or rolling eye movements

More common in patients 3 to 12 years of age
Aggressive behaviors or other behavior problems; anxiety; concentration problems and change in school performance; crying; false sense of well-being; hyperactivity or increase in body movements; mental depression; reacting too quickly, too emotionally, or overreacting; rapidly changing moods; restlessness; suspiciousness or distrust

Less common
Black, tarry stools; chills; chest pain; cough; depression, irritability, or other mood or mental changes; fever; loss of memory; pain or swelling in arms or legs; painful or difficult urination; shortness of breath; sore throat; sores, ulcers, or white spots on lips or in mouth; swollen glands; unusual bleeding or bruising; unusual tiredness or weakness

Frequency not determined
abdominal or stomach pain; blistering, peeling, loosening of skin; clay-colored stools; coma; confusion; convulsions; dark urine; decreased urine output; diarrhea; dizziness; fast or irregular heartbeat; headache; increased thirst; itching; joint pain; large, hive-like swelling on face, eyelids, lips, tongue, throat, hands, legs, feet, sex organs; loss of appetite; muscle ache or pain; nausea; red irritated eyes; red skin lesions, often with a purple center; skin rash; sores, ulcers, or white spots in mouth or on lips; unpleasant breath odor; unusual tiredness or weakness; vomiting of blood; yellow eyes or skin

Symptoms of overdose
Diarrhea; double vision; drowsiness; sluggishness; slurred speech

Some side effects may occur that usually do not need medical attention. These side effects may go away during treatment as your body adjusts to the medicine. Also, your health care professional may be able to tell you about ways to prevent or reduce some of these side effects. Check with your health care professional if any of the following side effects continue or are bothersome or if you have any questions about them:

More common
Blurred or double vision; cold or flu-like symptoms; delusions; dementia; drowsiness; hoarseness; lack or loss of strength; lower back or side pain; swelling of hands, feet, or lower legs; trembling or shaking

Less common or rare
Accidental injury; appetite increased; back pain; bloated full feeling; body aches or pain; burning, dry or itching eyes; change in vision; change in walking and balance; clumsiness, or unsteadiness; congestion; constipation; cough producing mucus; decrease in sexual desire or ability; dementia; difficulty breathing; dryness of mouth or throat; earache; excess air or gas in stomach or intestines; excessive tearing; eye discharge; feeling faint, dizzy, or lightheadedness; feeling of warmth or heat; flushing or redness of skin, especially on face and neck; flushed, dry skin; frequent urination; fruit-like breath odor; impaired vision; increased hunger; increased sensitivity to pain; increased sensitivity to touch; increased thirst; incoordination; indigestion; low blood pressure; nervousness; noise in ears; pain, redness, rash, swelling, or bleeding where the skin is rubbed off; passing gas; redness, pain, swelling of eye, eyelid, or inner lining of eyelid; redness or swelling in ear; runny nose; shortness of breath; slurred speech; sneezing; sweating; tender, swollen glands in neck; tightness in chest; tingling in the hands and feet; troubled breathing; trouble in sleeping; trouble in swallowing; trouble in thinking; twitching; unexplained weight loss; voice changes; vomiting; weakness or loss of strength; weight gain; wheezing

Other side effects not listed may also occur in some patients. If you notice any other effects, check with your healthcare professional.

GALANTAMINE (Oral route) - ga-LAN-ta-meen

Commonly used brand name(s)

In the U.S.—

Razadyne	Razadyne IR
Razadyne ER	Reminyl

Available Dosage Forms:
• Capsule, Extended Release
• Tablet
• Solution

Therapeutic Class: Central Nervous System Agent
Pharmacologic Class: Cholinesterase Inhibitor, Centrally/Peripherally Acting

Uses For This Medicine

Galantamine is used to treat the symptoms of mild to moderate Alzheimer's disease. Galantamine will not cure Alzheimer's disease, and it will not stop the disease from getting worse. However, galantamine can improve thinking ability in some patients with Alzheimer's disease

In Alzheimer's disease, many chemical changes take place in the brain. One of the earliest and biggest changes is that there is less of a chemical called acetylcholine (ACh). ACh helps the brain to work properly. Galantamine slows the breakdown of ACh, so it can build up and have a greater effect. However, as Alzheimer's disease gets worse, there will be less and less ACh, so galantamine may not work as well.

This medicine is available only with your doctor's prescription.

Before Using This Medicine

In deciding to use a medicine, the risks of taking the medicine must be weighed against the good it will do. This is a decision you and your doctor will make. For this medicine, the following should be considered:

Allergies—Tell your doctor if you have ever had any unusual or allergic reaction to this medicine or any other medicines. Also tell your health care professional if you have any other types of allergies, such as to foods, dyes, preservatives, or animals. For non-prescription products, read the label or package ingredients carefully.

Pediatric—Studies on this medicine have been done only in adult patients, and there is no specific information comparing use of galantamine in children with use in other age groups. Use in children is not recommended.

Geriatric—Galantamine levels are higher in older adults than in healthy young subjects.

Pregnancy—

	Pregnancy Category	Explanation
All Trimesters	B	Animal studies have revealed no evidence of harm to the fetus, however, there are no adequate studies in pregnant women OR animal studies have shown an adverse effect, but adequate studies in pregnant women have failed to demonstrate a risk to the fetus.

Breast Feeding—There are no adequate studies in women for determining infant risk when using this medication during breastfeeding. Weigh the potential benefits against the potential risks before taking this medication while breastfeeding.

Other medicines—

Using this medicine with any of the following medicines may cause an increased risk of certain side effects, but using both drugs may be the best treatment for you. If both medicines are prescribed together, your doctor may change the dose or how often you use one or both of the medicines.

Amitriptyline, Fluoxetine, Fluvoxamine, Ketoconazole, Paroxetine, Quinidine

Interactions with Food/Tobacco/Alcohol—Certain medicines should not be used at or around the time of eating food or eating certain types of food since interactions may occur. Using alcohol or tobacco with certain medicines may also cause interactions to occur. Discuss with your healthcare professional the use of your medicine with food, alcohol, or tobacco.

Other medical problems—The presence of other medical problems may affect the use of this medicine. Make sure you tell your doctor if you have any other medical problems, especially:

- Asthma (or history of) or
- Lung disease—May make breathing problems worse
- Epilepsy or history of seizures—Galantamine may cause seizures
- Heart problems, including slow heartbeat or heart block (slow and irregular heartbeat)—May make condition worse
- Kidney problems or
- Liver problems—Your doctor may need to adjust your dose. If the problems are severe, you should not take galantamine.
- Mild cognitive impairment (memory problems)—Galantamine should not be used for this condition.
- Stomach ulcer (or history of) or
- Urinary tract blockage or difficult urination—Galantamine may make these conditions worse

Proper Use of This Medicine

Dosing—The dose of this medicine will be different for different patients. Follow your doctor's orders or the directions on the label. The following information includes only the average doses of this medicine. If your dose is different, do not change it unless your doctor tells you to do so.

The amount of medicine that you take depends on the strength of the medicine. Also, the number of doses you take each day, the time allowed between doses, and the length of time you take the medicine depend on the medical problem for which you are using the medicine.

If you are taking the tablets or oral solution: Take this medicine with your morning and evening meals.

If you are taking the extended-release capsules: Take this medicine with your morning meal.

Follow the instruction sheet for the proper dosing of the oral solution and ask your doctor or pharmacist if you have any questions.

Make sure that you are drinking plenty of fluids while you are taking this medicine.

- For oral dosage forms (oral solution and tablets):
  - For treatment of Alzheimer's disease:
    - Adults—To start, take 4 mg (milligrams) two times a day. Your doctor may increase your dose gradually if you are doing well on this medicine.
- For long acting oral dosage forms (extended-release capsules):
  - For treatment of Alzheimer's disease:
    - Adults—To start, take 8 mg one time a day. Your doctor may increase your dose gradually if you are doing well on this medicine.

Missed dose—If you miss a dose of this medicine, take it as soon as possible. However, if it is almost time for your next dose, skip the missed dose and go back to your regular dosing schedule. Do not double doses.

Do not take your morning and evening doses close together.

Storage—Store the medicine in a closed container at room temperature, away from heat, moisture, and direct light. Keep from freezing.

Keep out of the reach of children.

Do not keep outdated medicine or medicine no longer needed.

Ask your healthcare professional how you should dispose of any medicine you do not use.

Precautions While Using This Medicine

It is very important that your doctor check you at regular visits.

Tell your doctor if your symptoms get worse, or if you notice any new symptoms.

Do not take other medicines unless they have been discussed with your doctor. This especially includes nonprescription medicines, such as aspirin, and medicines for appetite control, asthma, colds, cough, hay fever, or sinus problems.

Galantamine causes a large number of patients to have problems with their stomachs and intestines. Tell your doctor about any nausea, vomiting, diarrhea, stomach pain or loss of appetite.

If you think you or someone else may have taken an overdose of galantamine, get emergency help at once. Taking an overdose of galantamine may lead to convulsions (seizures) or shock. Some signs of shock are large pupils, irregular breathing, and fast weak pulse. Other signs of an overdose are severe nausea and vomiting, increasing muscle weakness, greatly increased sweating, and greatly increased watering of the mouth.

Side Effects of This Medicine

Along with its needed effects, a medicine may cause some unwanted effects. Although not all of these side effects may occur, if they do occur they may need medical attention.

Check with your doctor as soon as possible if any of the following side effects occur:

Less common
Chest pain or discomfort; Shortness of breath

Incidence not known
Attack, assault, force; bloody or black, tarry stools; confusion; constipation; convulsions; decreased urination; dry mouth; increase in heart rate; increased thirst; irregular heartbeat; mood changes; muscle pain or cramps; numbness or tingling in hands, feet, or lips; rapid breathing; severe stomach pain; sunken eyes; vomiting of blood or material that looks like coffee grounds; wrinkled skin

Symptoms of overdose
Cramping; defecation or urination, uncontrolled; dizziness; drooling; fainting; increased sweating; low blood pressure; muscle weakness; seizures; slow heart beat; severe nausea or vomiting; slow or troubled breathing; tearing of the eyes; watering of the mouth

Some side effects may occur that usually do not need medical attention. These side effects may go away during treatment as your body adjusts to the medicine. Also, your health care professional may be able to tell you about ways to prevent or reduce some of these side effects. Check with your health care professional if any of the following side effects continue or are bothersome or if you have any questions about them:

More common
Bladder pain; bloody or cloudy urine; diarrhea; difficult, burning, or painful urination; discouragement; feeling sad or empty; frequent urge to urinate; irritability; loss of appetite; loss of interest or pleasure; lower back or side pain; nausea; tiredness; trouble concentrating; vomiting; weight loss

Less common
Abdominal pain; pale skin; troubled breathing with activity; slow or irregular heartbeat (less than 50 beats per minute); light-headedness; dizziness or fainting; unusual tiredness or weakness; indigestion; headache; blood in urine; lower back pain; pain or burning while urinating; trouble sleeping; unable to sleep; sleepiness; sleeplessness; stuffy nose; unusual bleeding or bruising; unusual drowsiness; high or low blood pressure; tremor

Other side effects not listed may also occur in some patients. If you notice any other effects, check with your healthcare professional.

GALSULFASE   (Injection route) - gal-SUL-face

Uses For This Medicine

Galsulfase is used to treat mucopolysaccharidosis (MPS VI) disease caused by the lack of a certain enzyme called N-acetylgalactosamine 4–sulfatase in the body.

Before Using This Medicine

In deciding to use a medicine, the risks of taking the medicine must be weighed against the good it will do. This is a decision you and your doctor will make. For this medicine, the following should be considered:

Allergies—Tell your doctor if you have ever had any unusual or allergic reaction to this medicine or any other medicines. Also tell your health care professional if you have any other types of allergies, such as to foods, dyes, preservatives, or animals. For non-prescription products, read the label or package ingredients carefully.

Pediatric—This medicine has been tested in children 5 years of age and older and has not been shown to cause different side effects or problems than is does in adults. It is not known if children under 5 respond differently from older children.

Geriatric—Many medicines have not been studied specifically in older people. Therefore, it may not be known whether they work exactly the same way they do in younger adults or if they cause different side effects or problems in older people. There is no specific information comparing use of galsulfase in the elderly with use in other age groups.

Other medicines—Although certain medicines should not be used together at all, in other cases two different medicines may be used together even if an interaction might occur. In these cases, your doctor may want to change the dose, or other precautions may be necessary. Tell your healthcare professional if you are taking any other prescription or nonprescription (over-the-counter [OTC]) medicine.

Interactions with Food/Tobacco/Alcohol—Certain medicines should not be used at or around the time of eating food or eating certain types of food since interactions may occur. Using alcohol or tobacco with certain medicines may also cause interactions to occur. Discuss with your healthcare

professional the use of your medicine with food, alcohol, or tobacco.

Proper Use of This Medicine

Dosing—The dose of this medicine will be different for different patients. Follow your doctor's orders or the directions on the label. The following information includes only the average doses of this medicine. If your dose is different, do not change it unless your doctor tells you to do so.

The amount of medicine that you take depends on the strength of the medicine. Also, the number of doses you take each day, the time allowed between doses, and the length of time you take the medicine depend on the medical problem for which you are using the medicine.

- For Mycopolysaccharidosis VI:
  - For injection dosage form:
    - Adults and children—The dose is based on body weight and must be determined by your doctor. The usual dose is 1 milligram (mg) per kilogram (kg), given once weekly. It is injected slowly into a vein over at least four hours.

Precautions While Using This Medicine

Regular visits: If you will be taking this medicine for a long time, *it is very important that your doctor check you at regular visits*

Side Effects of This Medicine

Check with your doctor immediately if any of the following side effects occur:

Less common
Blindness; blurred vision; chest pain; decreased vision; difficult or labored breathing; dizziness; headache; hernia of the naval; nervousness; pounding in the ears; shortness of breath; slow or fast heartbeat; swelling of the face; tightness in chest; wheezing

Frequency unknown
Bluish lips or skin; confusion; cough; dizziness, faintness, or lightheadedness when getting up from a lying or sitting position suddenly; facial swelling; fever or chills; hives or welts; itching; joint pain; large, hive-like swelling on face, eyelids, lips, tongue, throat, hands, legs, feet, sex organs; nausea; noisy breathing; not breathing; pain behind the sternum; redness of skin; skin rash; stomach pain; sweating; troubled breathing; vomiting

Some side effects may occur that usually do not need medical attention. These side effects may go away during treatment as your body adjusts to the medicine. Also, your health care professional may be able to tell you about ways to prevent or reduce some of these side effects. Check with your health care professional if any of the following side effects continue or are bothersome or if you have any questions about them:

More common
Body produces substance that can bind to drug making it less effective or cause side effects; ear pain; stomach pain; diarrhea; loss of appetite; pain

Less common
Body aches or pain; burning, dry, or itching eyes; congestion; discharge; dryness or soreness of throat; excessive tearing; general feeling of discomfort or illness; hoarseness; loss of or increase in reflexes; redness,

pain, swelling of eye, eyelid, or inner lining of eyelid; runny nose; stuffy nose; tender, swollen glands in neck; trouble in swallowing; unusual tiredness or weakness; voice changes

Observed during clinical trials
Difficulty in moving; ear congestion; loss of voice; muscle pain or stiffness; nasal congestion; redness or swelling in ear; sneezing or sore throat

Other side effects not listed may also occur in some patients. If you notice any other effects, check with your healthcare professional.

GANCICLOVIR   (Intraocular route) -
gan-SYE-kloe-veer

Commonly used brand name(s)
In the U.S.—
  Vitrasert

Available Dosage Forms:
- Implant

Therapeutic Class: Antiviral
Pharmacologic Class: Viral DNA Polymerase Inhibitor

Uses For This Medicine

Ganciclovir is an antiviral medicine that is used in an implant that is inserted into the eye during surgery. The ganciclovir implant is used to treat a serious condition called cytomegalovirus (CMV) retinitis in persons who have acquired immune deficiency syndrome (AIDS). Ganciclovir will not cure this eye infection, but it may help to keep the symptoms from becoming worse.

After your eye has used up all the medicine in the implant (generally within 5 to 8 months), the implant is removed by surgery and, at the same time, another implant can be inserted.

The surgery, the implant containing this medicine, or the medicine itself may cause some serious side effects, including detachment of the retina, formation of a cataract, and eye infections. Before you receive this implant, you and your doctor should talk about the good this medicine and surgery will do as well as the risks involved.

This medicine is available only with your doctor's prescription.

Before Receiving This Medicine

In deciding to use a medicine, the risks of taking the medicine must be weighed against the good it will do. This is a decision you and your doctor will make. For this medicine, the following should be considered:

Allergies—Tell your doctor if you have ever had any unusual or allergic reaction to this medicine or any other medicines. Also tell your health care professional if you have any other types of allergies, such as to foods, dyes, preservatives, or animals. For non-prescription products, read the label or package ingredients carefully.

Pediatric—There is no specific information comparing use of ganciclovir eye implants in children younger than 9 years of age with use in other age groups.

Geriatric—Many medicines have not been studied specifically in older people. Therefore, it may not be known whether they work exactly the same way they do in younger adults or if they cause different side effects or problems in older people. There is no specific information comparing use of ganciclovir eye implants in the elderly with use in other age groups.

Other medicines—Although certain medicines should not be used together at all, in other cases two different medicines may be used together even if an interaction might occur. In these cases, your doctor may want to change the dose, or other precautions may be necessary. Tell your healthcare professional if you are taking any other prescription or non-prescription (over-the-counter [OTC]) medicine.

Interactions with Food/Tobacco/Alcohol—Certain medicines should not be used at or around the time of eating food or eating certain types of food since interactions may occur. Using alcohol or tobacco with certain medicines may also cause interactions to occur. Discuss with your healthcare professional the use of your medicine with food, alcohol, or tobacco.

Other medical problems—The presence of other medical problems may affect the use of this medicine. Make sure you tell your doctor if you have any other medical problems, especially:
- Blood problems or
- Eye infection—Surgery on the eye is not recommended

Proper Use of This Medicine

Dosing—The dose of this medicine will be different for different patients. Follow your doctor's orders or the directions on the label. The following information includes only the average doses of this medicine. If your dose is different, do not change it unless your doctor tells you to do so.

The amount of medicine that you take depends on the strength of the medicine. Also, the number of doses you take each day, the time allowed between doses, and the length of time you take the medicine depend on the medical problem for which you are using the medicine.

Precautions After Receiving This Medicine

It is very important that your doctor check your progress at regular visits. This is to make sure the medicine is working properly and to check for any problems from the surgery, implant, or medicine. This will also help the doctor determine when all of the medicine in the implant has been used up, so it can be removed.

You may notice blurred or decreased vision in the eye where the implant has been placed. This is to be expected and will last for 2 to 4 weeks after the surgery to insert the implant into the eye. Tell your doctor if the blurred or decreased vision gets worse, lasts for more than 4 weeks, or gets better for a while and then gets worse again. Also, tell your doctor right away if any other changes in your vision occur. These may be signs of complications from the surgery.

Side Effects of This Medicine

Along with its needed effects, a medicine may cause some unwanted effects. Although not all of these side effects may occur, if they do occur they may need medical attention.

Also, ganciclovir has been found to cause cancerous tumors in animals. Discuss these possible effects with your doctor.

Check with your doctor as soon as possible if any of the following side effects occur:
More common—Usually occur within the first 2 months after the surgery
Decrease in vision (severe); seeing flashes or sparks of light; seeing floating spots before the eyes, or a veil or curtain appearing across part of vision
Less common—Usually occur within the first 2 months after the surgery
Blurred vision or other change in vision; decreased vision or other change in vision; eye pain or tearing; red or bloodshot eye; sensitivity of eye to light
Rare—Usually occur within the first 2 months after the surgery
Eye irritation; swelling of the membrane covering the white part of the eye

Some side effects may occur that usually do not need medical attention. These side effects may go away during treatment as your body adjusts to the medicine. Also, your health care professional may be able to tell you about ways to prevent or reduce some of these side effects. Check with your health care professional if any of the following side effects continue or are bothersome or if you have any questions about them:
More common
Decrease in vision lasting approximately 2 to 4 weeks

Other side effects not listed may also occur in some patients. If you notice any other effects, check with your healthcare professional.

GANCICLOVIR (Oral route, Intravenous route) - gan-SYE-kloe-veer

Black Box Warning

The clinical toxicity of ganciclovir and ganciclovir sodium for injection includes granulocytopenia, anemia, and thrombocytopenia. In animal studies ganciclovir was carcinogenic, teratogenic and caused aspermatogenesis.

Ganciclovir is indicated only for prevention of CMV disease in patients with advanced HIV infection at risk for CMV disease, for maintenance treatment of CMV retinitis in immunocompromised patients, and for prevention of CMV disease in solid organ transplant recipients.

Because ganciclovir is associated with a risk of more rapid rate of CMV retinitis progression, they should be used as maintenance treatment only in those patients for whom this risk is balanced by the benefit associated with avoiding daily intravenous infusions.

Commonly used brand name(s)

In the U.S.—
Cytovene
Cytovene IV

Available Dosage Forms:
- Capsule
- Powder for Solution

Therapeutic Class: Antiviral
Pharmacologic Class: Viral DNA Polymerase Inhibitor

Uses For This Medicine

Ganciclovir is an antiviral. It is used to treat infections caused by viruses.

Ganciclovir is used to treat the symptoms of cytomegalovirus (CMV) infection of the eyes in people whose immune system is not working fully. This includes patients with acquired immune deficiency syndrome (AIDS). Ganciclovir will not cure this eye infection, but it may help to keep the symptoms from becoming worse. It is also used to help prevent CMV infection in patients who receive organ or bone marrow transplants, as well as in patients with advanced human immunodeficiency virus (HIV) infection. Ganciclovir may be used for other serious CMV infections as determined by your doctor. However, it does not work in treating certain viruses, such as the common cold or the flu.

This medicine may cause some serious side effects, including anemia and other blood problems. Before you begin treatment with ganciclovir, you and your doctor should talk about the good this medicine will do as well as the risks of using it.

Ganciclovir is to be administered only by or under the supervision of your doctor.

Before Receiving This Medicine

In deciding to use a medicine, the risks of taking the medicine must be weighed against the good it will do. This is a decision you and your doctor will make. For this medicine, the following should be considered:

Allergies—Tell your doctor if you have ever had any unusual or allergic reaction to this medicine or any other medicines. Also tell your health care professional if you have any other types of allergies, such as to foods, dyes, preservatives, or animals. For non-prescription products, read the label or package ingredients carefully.

Pediatric—Ganciclovir can cause serious side effects in any patient. Therefore, it is especially important that you discuss with the child's doctor the good that this medicine may do as well as the risks of using it.

Geriatric—Many medicines have not been studied specifically in older people. Therefore, it may not be known whether they work exactly the same way they do in younger adults or if they cause different side effects or problems in older people. There is no specific information comparing use of ganciclovir in the elderly with use in other age groups.

Pregnancy—

	Pregnancy Category	Explanation
All Trimesters	C	Animal studies have shown an adverse effect and there are no adequate studies in pregnant women OR no animal studies have been conducted and there are no adequate studies in pregnant women.

Breast Feeding—There are no adequate studies in women for determining infant risk when using this medication during breastfeeding. Weigh the potential benefits against the potential risks before taking this medication while breastfeeding.

Other medicines—

Using this medicine with any of the following medicines is usually not recommended, but may be required in some

cases. If both medicines are prescribed together, your doctor may change the dose or how often you use one or both of the medicines.

Imipenem, Zidovudine

Interactions with Food/Tobacco/Alcohol—Certain medicines should not be used at or around the time of eating food or eating certain types of food since interactions may occur. Using alcohol or tobacco with certain medicines may also cause interactions to occur. Discuss with your healthcare professional the use of your medicine with food, alcohol, or tobacco.

Other medical problems—The presence of other medical problems may affect the use of this medicine. Make sure you tell your doctor if you have any other medical problems, especially:

- Kidney disease—Ganciclovir may build up in the blood in patients with kidney disease, increasing the chance of side effects
- Low platelet count or
- Low white blood cell count—Ganciclovir may make these blood diseases worse

Proper Use of This Medicine

It is important that you take ganciclovir capsules with food. This is to make sure the medicine is fully absorbed into the body and will work properly.

To get the best results, ganciclovir must be given for the full time of treatment. Also, this medicine works best when there is a constant amount in the blood. To help keep the amount constant, ganciclovir must be given on a regular schedule.

Dosing—The dose of this medicine will be different for different patients. Follow your doctor's orders or the directions on the label. The following information includes only the average doses of this medicine. If your dose is different, do not change it unless your doctor tells you to do so.

The amount of medicine that you take depends on the strength of the medicine. Also, the number of doses you take each day, the time allowed between doses, and the length of time you take the medicine depend on the medical problem for which you are using the medicine.

- For oral dosage form (capsules):
  - For treatment of CMV retinitis after you have received ganciclovir injection for at least fourteen to twenty-one days:
    - Adults and teenagers—1000 milligrams (mg) three times a day with food; or 500 mg six times a day, every three hours with food, during waking hours.
    - Children—Use and dose must be determined by your doctor.
  - For prevention of CMV disease in transplant patients and patients with advanced HIV infection:
    - Adults and teenagers—1000 mg three times a day with food.
    - Children—Use and dose must be determined by your doctor.
- For injection dosage form:
  - For treatment of CMV retinitis:
    - Adults and teenagers—Dose is based on body weight and must be determined by your doctor. At first, 5 mg per kilogram (2.3 mg per pound) of body weight is injected into a vein every twelve hours for fourteen to twenty-one days. Then, 5 mg per

kilogram (2.3 mg per pound) of body weight is injected into a vein once a day for seven days of the week; or 6 mg per kilogram (2.7 mg per pound) of body weight is injected into a vein once a day for five days of the week.

- Children—Use and dose must be determined by your doctor.

○ For prevention of CMV in transplant patients:

- Adults and teenagers—Dose is based on body weight and must be determined by your doctor. At first, 5 mg per kilogram (2.3 mg per pound) of body weight is injected into a vein every twelve hours for seven to fourteen days. Then the dose is reduced to 5 mg per kilogram (2.3 mg per pound) of body weight once a day for seven days of the week; or 6 mg per kilogram (2.7 mg per pound) of body weight is injected into a vein once a day for five days of the week.
- Children—Use and dose must be determined by your doctor.

Precautions After Receiving This Medicine

Ganciclovir can lower the number of white blood cells in your blood, increasing the chance of getting an infection. It can also lower the number of platelets, which are necessary for proper blood clotting. If this occurs, there are certain precautions you can take to reduce the risk of infection or bleeding:

- Check with your doctor immediately if you think you are getting an infection or if you get a fever or chills.
- Check with your doctor immediately if you notice any unusual bleeding or bruising; black, tarry stools; blood in urine or stools; or pinpoint red spots on your skin.
- Be careful when using a regular toothbrush, dental floss, or toothpick. Your medical doctor, dentist, or nurse may recommend other ways to clean your teeth and gums. Check with your medical doctor before having any dental work done.
- Be careful not to cut yourself when you are using sharp objects such as a safety razor or fingernail or toenail cutters.

The use of birth control is recommended for both men and women. Women should use effective birth control methods while receiving this medicine. Men should use a condom during treatment with this medicine and for at least 90 days after treatment has been completed.

It is very important that your doctor check you at regular visits for any blood problems that may be caused by this medicine.

If you have CMV retinitis: It is also very important that your ophthalmologist (eye doctor) check your eyes at regular visits since it is still possible that you may have some loss of eyesight during ganciclovir treatment.

Side Effects of This Medicine

Along with its needed effects, a medicine may cause some unwanted effects. Although not all of these side effects may occur, if they do occur they may need medical attention.

Medicines like ganciclovir can sometimes cause serious side effects such as blood problems; these are described below. Discuss these possible effects with your doctor.

Check with your doctor immediately if any of the following side effects occur:

More common
   For oral capsules and injection into the vein only
      Sore throat and fever; unusual bleeding or bruising

Less common
   For oral capsules and injection into the vein only
      Mood or other mental changes; nervousness; pain at place of injection; skin rash; tremor; unusual tiredness and weakness

   For injection into the eye only
      Decreased vision or any change in vision

Some side effects may occur that usually do not need medical attention. These side effects may go away during treatment as your body adjusts to the medicine. Also, your health care professional may be able to tell you about ways to prevent or reduce some of these side effects. Check with your health care professional if any of the following side effects continue or are bothersome or if you have any questions about them:

Less common
      Abdominal or stomach pain; loss of appetite; nausea and vomiting

Other side effects not listed may also occur in some patients. If you notice any other effects, check with your healthcare professional.

GANIRELIX   (Subcutaneous route) - ga-ni-REL-ix

Commonly used brand name(s)
In the U.S.—
   Antagon

Available Dosage Forms:
   • Solution

Therapeutic Class: Endocrine-Metabolic Agent
Pharmacologic Class: Luteinizing Hormone Releasing Hormone Antagonist

Uses For This Medicine

Ganirelixis used as a fertility medicine to prevent premature luteinizing hormone (LH) surges in women undergoing the fertility procedure of controlled ovarian hyperstimulation. LH is involved in ovulation, which is the development of eggs in the ovaries. Ganirelix may help reduce the need for follicle-stimulating hormone (FSH), which is also involved in ovulation.

Ganirelix is available only with your doctor's prescription.

Before Using This Medicine

In deciding to use a medicine, the risks of taking the medicine must be weighed against the good it will do. This is a decision you and your doctor will make. For this medicine, the following should be considered:

Allergies—Tell your doctor if you have ever had any unusual or allergic reaction to this medicine or any other medicines. Also tell your health care professional if you have any other types of allergies, such as to foods, dyes, preservatives,

or animals. For non-prescription products, read the label or package ingredients carefully.

Pregnancy—

	Pregnancy Category	Explanation
All Trimesters	X	Studies in animals or pregnant women have demonstrated positive evidence of fetal abnormalities. This drug should not be used in women who are or may become pregnant because the risk clearly outweighs any possible benefit.

Breast Feeding—There are no adequate studies in women for determining infant risk when using this medication during breastfeeding. Weigh the potential benefits against the potential risks before taking this medication while breastfeeding.

Other medicines—Although certain medicines should not be used together at all, in other cases two different medicines may be used together even if an interaction might occur. In these cases, your doctor may want to change the dose, or other precautions may be necessary. Tell your healthcare professional if you are taking any other prescription or non-prescription (over-the-counter [OTC]) medicine.

Interactions with Food/Tobacco/Alcohol—Certain medicines should not be used at or around the time of eating food or eating certain types of food since interactions may occur. Using alcohol or tobacco with certain medicines may also cause interactions to occur. Discuss with your healthcare professional the use of your medicine with food, alcohol, or tobacco.

Other medical problems—The presence of other medical problems may affect the use of ganirelix. Make sure you tell your doctor if you have any other medical problems.

Proper Use of This Medicine

To make using ganirelix as safe and reliable as possible, you should understand how and when to use this medicine and what effects may be expected. A paper with information for the patient will be given to you with your filled prescription and will provide many details concerning the use of ganirelix. Read this paper carefully and ask your health care professional for any additional information or explanation.

Sometimes ganirelix can be given by injection at home. If you are using this medicine at home:

- Understand and use the proper method of safely preparing the medicine if you are going to prepare your own medicine.
- Wash your hands with soap and water and use a clean work area to prepare your injection.
- Make sure you clearly understand and carefully follow your doctor's instructions on how to give yourself an injection, including using the proper needle and syringe.
- Do not inject more or less of the medicine than your doctor ordered.
- Remember to move the site of injection to different areas to prevent skin problems from developing.
- Throw away needles, syringes, bottles, and unused medicine after the injection in a safe manner.

- Tell your doctor when you use your last dose of ganirelix. Your doctor will give you another medicine called human chorionic gonadotrophin (hCG) or arrange for you to get this medicine at the right time.

Dosing—The dose of this medicine will be different for different patients. Follow your doctor's orders or the directions on the label. The following information includes only the average doses of this medicine. If your dose is different, do not change it unless your doctor tells you to do so.

The amount of medicine that you take depends on the strength of the medicine. Also, the number of doses you take each day, the time allowed between doses, and the length of time you take the medicine depend on the medical problem for which you are using the medicine.

- For injection dosage form:
  - For treatment of female infertility:
    - Adults—After receiving FSH treatment on Day 2 or 3 of your menstrual cycle, 250 micrograms (mcg) of ganirelix is injected under the skin once a day during the early to midfollicular phase (about Day 7 or Day 8 of your menstrual cycle).

Missed dose—Call your doctor or pharmacist for instructions.

Storage—Store the medicine in a closed container at room temperature, away from heat, moisture, and direct light. Keep from freezing.

Keep out of the reach of children.

Do not keep outdated medicine or medicine no longer needed.

Precautions While Using This Medicine

It is very important that your doctor check your progress often at regular visits to make sure that the medicine is working properly and to check for unwanted effects. Your doctor will probably want to follow the developing eggs inside the ovaries by doing an ultrasound examination and measuring hormones in your blood stream.

If your doctor has asked you to record your basal body temperatures (BBTs) daily, make sure that you do this every day. Using a BBT record or some other method, your doctor will help you decide when you are most fertile and when ovulation occurs. It is important that sexual intercourse take place around the time when you are most fertile to give you the best chance of becoming pregnant. Follow your doctor's directions carefully.

If severe abdominal pain occurs with use of ganirelix, discontinue treatment and report the problem to your doctor immediately. Do not receive the injection of human chorionic gonadotropin (hCG) and avoid sexual intercourse.

Side Effects of This Medicine

Along with its needed effects, a medicine may cause some unwanted effects. Although not all of these side effects may occur, if they do occur they may need medical attention.

Stop taking this medicine and get emergency help immediately if any of the following effects occur:

Less common

Abdominal pain (severe); nausea and vomiting; weight gain (rapid)

Check with your doctor as soon as possible if any of the following side effects occur:

Less common
Nausea; vaginal bleeding

Some side effects may occur that usually do not need medical attention. These side effects may go away during treatment as your body adjusts to the medicine. Also, your health care professional may be able to tell you about ways to prevent or reduce some of these side effects. Check with your health care professional if any of the following side effects continue or are bothersome or if you have any questions about them:

Less common
Headache; redness, pain or swelling at injection site

Other side effects not listed may also occur in some patients. If you notice any other effects, check with your healthcare professional.

GATIFLOXACIN (Ophthalmic route) -
ga-ti-FLOKS-a-sin

Commonly used brand name(s)

In the U.S.—
Zymar

Available Dosage Forms:
• Solution

Therapeutic Class: Antibiotic

Uses For This Medicine

Ophthalmic gatifloxacin is used in the eye to treat bacterial infections of the eye. Ophthalmic gatifloxacin works by killing bacteria.

This medicine is available only with your doctor's prescription.

Before Using This Medicine

In deciding to use a medicine, the risks of taking the medicine must be weighed against the good it will do. This is a decision you and your doctor will make. For this medicine, the following should be considered:

Allergies—Tell your doctor if you have ever had any unusual or allergic reaction to this medicine or any other medicines. Also tell your health care professional if you have any other types of allergies, such as to foods, dyes, preservatives, or animals. For non-prescription products, read the label or package ingredients carefully.

Pediatric—Use is not recommended in infants and children under 1 year of age. In children older than 1 year of age, this medicine is not expected to cause different side effects or problems than it does in adults.

Geriatric—Many medicines have not been studied specifically in older people. Therefore, it may not be known whether they work exactly the same way they do in younger adults. Although there is no specific information comparing use of gatifloxacin in the elderly with use in other age groups, this medicine is not expected to cause different side effects or problems in older people than it does in younger adults.

Pregnancy—

	Pregnancy Category	Explanation
All Trimesters	C	Animal studies have shown an adverse effect and there are no adequate studies in pregnant women OR no animal studies have been conducted and there are no adequate studies in pregnant women.

Breast Feeding—There are no adequate studies in women for determining infant risk when using this medication during breastfeeding. Weigh the potential benefits against the potential risks before taking this medication while breastfeeding.

Other medicines—

Using this medicine with any of the following medicines is not recommended. Your doctor may decide not to treat you with this medication or change some of the other medicines you take.

Cisapride, Mesoridazine, Thioridazine, Ziprasidone

Interactions with Food/Tobacco/Alcohol—Certain medicines should not be used at or around the time of eating food or eating certain types of food since interactions may occur. Using alcohol or tobacco with certain medicines may also cause interactions to occur. Discuss with your healthcare professional the use of your medicine with food, alcohol, or tobacco.

Other medical problems—The presence of other medical problems may affect the use of this medicine. Make sure you tell your doctor if you have any other medical problems, especially:

• Allergy to gatifloxacin or
• Allergy to any part of the medicine—Serious allergic reactions can occur

---

Proper Use of This Medicine

To use gatifloxacin ophthalmic solution (eye drops):

• First, wash your hands. Then tilt the head back and pull the lower eyelid away from the eye to form a pouch. Drop the medicine into the pouch and gently close the eyes. Do not blink. Keep the eyes closed for 1 or 2 minutes to allow the medicine to come into contact with the infection.
• If you think you did not get the drop of medicine into your eyes properly, use another drop.
• To keep the medicine as germ-free as possible, do not touch the applicator tip to any surface (including the eye). Also, keep the container tightly closed.

To help clear up your eye infection completely, keep using ophthalmic gatifloxacin for the full time of treatment, even if your symptoms have disappeared. If you stop using this medicine to soon your symptoms may return. Do not miss any doses.

Dosing—The dose of this medicine will be different for different patients. Follow your doctor's orders or the directions on the label. The following information includes only the average doses of this medicine. If your dose is different, do not change it unless your doctor tells you to do so.

The amount of medicine that you take depends on the strength of the medicine. Also, the number of doses you take each day, the time allowed between doses, and the length of

time you take the medicine depend on the medical problem for which you are using the medicine.

- For ophthalmic solution dosage form:
  - For bacterial conjunctivitis:
    - Adults and children 1 year of age and older— Days 1 and 2: Put one drop in the affected eye(s) every two hours while awake. Do not put drops in more than 8 times a day. Days 3 through 7: Put one drop in the affected eye(s) every 4 hours while awake. Do not put drops in more than 4 times a day.
    - Infants and children up to 1 year of age—Use and dose must be determined by your doctor.

Missed dose—If you miss a dose of this medicine, apply it as soon as possible. However, if it is almost time for your next dose, skip the missed dose and go back to your regular dosing schedule.

Storage—Store the medicine in a closed container at room temperature, away from heat, moisture, and direct light. Keep from freezing.

Keep out of the reach of children.

Do not keep outdated medicine or medicine no longer needed.

Ask your healthcare professional how you should dispose of any medicine you do not use.

Precautions While Using This Medicine

If your eye infection does not improve within a few days, or if it becomes worse, check with your doctor.

Stop using these eye drops and contact your doctor at the first sign of a rash or an allergic reaction.

Side Effects of This Medicine

Along with its needed effects, a medicine may cause some unwanted effects. Although not all of these side effects may occur, if they do occur they may need medical attention.

Check with your doctor immediately if any of the following side effects occur:

More common
  Eye irritation; eye pain; eye redness

Less common
  Bloody eye; decrease in vision; swelling of the membrane covering the white part of the eye

Some side effects may occur that usually do not need medical attention. These side effects may go away during treatment as your body adjusts to the medicine. Also, your health care professional may be able to tell you about ways to prevent or reduce some of these side effects. Check with your health care professional if any of the following side effects continue or are bothersome or if you have any questions about them:

More common
  Blurry vision; discharge from eyes; itching eyes; stringy mucus secretions; swelling of eye, eyelid, or inner lining of eyelid; watering eyes

Less common
  Bad, unusual or unpleasant (after) taste; change in taste; dry eye; headache

Other side effects not listed may also occur in some patients. If you notice any other effects, check with your healthcare professional.

GEFITINIB (Oral route) - ge-FI-tye-nib

Commonly used brand name(s)

In the U.S.—
  Iressa

Available Dosage Forms:
- Tablet

Therapeutic Class: Antineoplastic Agent
Pharmacologic Class: Tyrosine Kinase Inhibitor

Uses For This Medicine

Gefitinib belongs to the group of medicines called antineoplastics. It is used to treat non-small cell lung cancer after the failure of other chemotherapy treatment.

Before you begin treatment with gefitinib, you and your doctor should talk about the good this medicine will do as well as the risks of using it.

This medicine is available only with your doctor's prescription.

Before Using This Medicine

In deciding to use a medicine, the risks of taking the medicine must be weighed against the good it will do. This is a decision you and your doctor will make. For this medicine, the following should be considered:

Allergies—Tell your doctor if you have ever had any unusual or allergic reaction to this medicine or any other medicines. Also tell your health care professional if you have any other types of allergies, such as to foods, dyes, preservatives, or animals. For non-prescription products, read the label or package ingredients carefully.

Pediatric—Studies on this medicine have been done only in adult patients, and there is no specific information comparing use of gefitinib in children with use in other age groups.

Geriatric—This medicine has been tested in elderly patients and has not been shown to cause different side effects or problems in older people than it does in younger adults.

Pregnancy—

	Pregnancy Category	Explanation
All Trimesters	D	Studies in pregnant women have demonstrated a risk to the fetus. However, the benefits of therapy in a life threatening situation or a serious disease, may outweigh the potential risk.

Breast Feeding—There are no adequate studies in women for determining infant risk when using this medication during breastfeeding. Weigh the potential benefits against the potential risks before taking this medication while breastfeeding.

Other medicines—

Using this medicine with any of the following medicines is usually not recommended, but may be required in some cases. If both medicines are prescribed together, your doctor may change the dose or how often you use one or both of the medicines.

Vinorelbine

Interactions with Food/Tobacco/Alcohol—Certain medicines should not be used at or around the time of eating food or eating certain types of food since interactions may occur. Using alcohol or tobacco with certain medicines may also cause interactions to occur. Discuss with your healthcare professional the use of your medicine with food, alcohol, or tobacco.

Other medical problems—The presence of other medical problems may affect the use of this medicine. Make sure you tell your doctor if you have any other medical problems, especially:

- Idiopathic pulmonary fibrosis—Condition may worsen while receiving gefitinib therapy
- Kidney disease or
- Liver disease—The chance of serious side effects is greatly increased.

Proper Use of This Medicine

Dosing—The dose of this medicine will be different for different patients. Follow your doctor's orders or the directions on the label. The following information includes only the average doses of this medicine. If your dose is different, do not change it unless your doctor tells you to do so.

The amount of medicine that you take depends on the strength of the medicine. Also, the number of doses you take each day, the time allowed between doses, and the length of time you take the medicine depend on the medical problem for which you are using the medicine.

- For oral dosage form:
  - For lung cancer, non-small cell:
    - Adults—250 milligrams (mg) daily.
    - Children—Use and dose must be determined by your doctor.

Missed dose—If you miss a dose of this medicine, take it as soon as possible. However, if it is almost time for your next dose, skip the missed dose and go back to your regular dosing schedule. Do not double doses.

Precautions While Using This Medicine

It is very important that your doctor check your progress at regular visits to make sure that this medicine is working properly and to check for unwanted effects.

It is very important to check with your doctor if you have diarrhea, nausea or anorexia.

It is very important to check with your doctor if you have problems breathing.

It is very important to check with your doctor if you have any new eye problems.

Side Effects of This Medicine

Along with its needed effects, a medicine may cause some unwanted effects. Although not all of these side effects may occur, if they do occur they may need medical attention.

Check with your doctor immediately if any of the following side effects occur:
Less common
bloating or swelling of face, arms, hands, lower legs, or feet; burning, dry or itching eyes; change in vision; difficult or labored breathing; eye discharge or excessive tearing; redness, pain, swelling of eye, eyelid, or inner lining of eyelid; shortness of breath; tightness in chest;

tingling of hands or feet; unusual weight gain or loss; wheezing
Incidence unknown
abnormal eyelash growth; blistering, peeling, loosening of skin; bloating of stomach; blood in urine; bloody nose; chills; constipation; cough; darkened urine; diarrhea; fainting or loss of consciousness; fast heartbeat; fast or irregular breathing; fever; indigestion; joint or muscle pain; large, hive-like swelling on face, eyelids, lips, tongue, throat, hands, legs, feet, sex organs; loss of appetite; nausea; pains in stomach, side, or abdomen, possibly radiating to the back; redness, tenderness, itching, or burning of skin; seeing floating spots before the eyes; severe stinging of the eye; skin rash; sore throat; sores, ulcers, or white spots in mouth or on lips; unusual tiredness or weakness; vomiting; yellow eyes or skin
Symptoms of overdose
Get emergency help immediately if any of the following symptoms of overdose occur:
Diarrhea; skin rash

Some side effects may occur that usually do not need medical attention. These side effects may go away during treatment as your body adjusts to the medicine. Also, your health care professional may be able to tell you about ways to prevent or reduce some of these side effects. Check with your health care professional if any of the following side effects continue or are bothersome or if you have any questions about them:
More common
blemishes on the skin, pimples; lack or loss of strength; dry skin
Less common
irritation or soreness of mouth; blisters under the skin, large, hard skin blisters

Other side effects not listed may also occur in some patients. If you notice any other effects, check with your healthcare professional.

GEMCITABINE (Intravenous route) - jem-SITE-a-been

Commonly used brand name(s)
In the U.S.—
Gemzar

Available Dosage Forms:
- Powder for Solution

Therapeutic Class: Antineoplastic Agent
Pharmacologic Class: Antimetabolite

Uses For This Medicine

Gemcitabine belongs to the group of medicines called antimetabolites. It is used alone or in combination with other medicines to treat cancer of the breast, ovary, pancreas, and lung. It may also be used to treat other kinds of cancer, as determined by your doctor.

Gemcitabine interferes with the growth of cancer cells, which are eventually destroyed. Since the growth of normal cells may also be affected by the medicine, other effects will also occur. Some of these may be serious and must be reported to your doctor. Other effects, like hair loss, may not be serious but may cause concern. Some effects may occur after treatment with gemcitabine has been stopped.

This medicine is available only with your doctor's prescription.

Once a medicine has been approved for marketing for a certain use, experience may show that it is also useful for other medical problems. Although this use is not included in product labeling, gemcitabine is used in certain patients with the following medical conditions:

- Bladder cancer
- Cancer of the lymph system
- Epithelial ovarian cancer
- Cancer of the bile ducts
- Cancer of the gallbladder
- Germ cell tumors of the ovaries and testes (cancer of the egg- and sperm-producing cells)

Before Using This Medicine

In deciding to use a medicine, the risks of taking the medicine must be weighed against the good it will do. This is a decision you and your doctor will make. For this medicine, the following should be considered:

Allergies—Tell your doctor if you have ever had any unusual or allergic reaction to this medicine or any other medicines. Also tell your health care professional if you have any other types of allergies, such as to foods, dyes, preservatives, or animals. For non-prescription products, read the label or package ingredients carefully.

Pediatric—Gemcitabine has been tested in a limited number of children and was not found to cause different side effects in children than it does in adults. However, side effects specific to children can not be ruled out because appropriate studies have not been done.

Geriatric—Gemcitabine has been tested in elderly patients and has not been shown to cause different side effects or problems in older people than it does in younger adults. However, seriously low blood counts tend to occur more often in elderly patients.

Pregnancy—

	Pregnancy Category	Explanation
All Trimesters	D	Studies in pregnant women have demonstrated a risk to the fetus. However, the benefits of therapy in a life threatening situation or a serious disease, may outweigh the potential risk.

Breast Feeding—There are no adequate studies in women for determining infant risk when using this medication during breastfeeding. Weigh the potential benefits against the potential risks before taking this medication while breastfeeding.

Other medicines—

Using this medicine with any of the following medicines is not recommended. Your doctor may decide not to treat you with this medication or change some of the other medicines you take.

Rotavirus Vaccine, Live

Interactions with Food/Tobacco/Alcohol—Certain medicines should not be used at or around the time of eating food or eating certain types of food since interactions may occur. Using alcohol or tobacco with certain medicines may also cause interactions to occur. Discuss with your healthcare professional the use of your medicine with food, alcohol, or tobacco.

Other medical problems—The presence of other medical problems may affect the use of this medicine. Make sure you tell your doctor if you have any other medical problems, especially:

- Chickenpox (including recent exposure) or
- Herpes zoster (shingles)—Risk of severe disease spreading to other parts of the body
- Infection—Gemcitabine can decrease your body's ability to fight infection
- Kidney disease or
- Liver disease, severe—These conditions sometimes increase the effects of medicines by causing them to be removed from the body more slowly.

Proper Use of This Medicine

Your doctor will prescribe your exact dose and tell you how often it should be given. This medicine is given through a needle placed into one of your veins.

Gemcitabine often causes nausea and vomiting. It can also cause flu-like symptoms such as chills, fever, general feeling of illness, headache, muscle pain, and weakness. It is very important that you continue to receive the medicine even if it makes you feel ill. Ask your health care professional for ways to lessen these effects.

Dosing—The dose of this medicine will be different for different patients. Follow your doctor's orders or the directions on the label. The following information includes only the average doses of this medicine. If your dose is different, do not change it unless your doctor tells you to do so.

The amount of medicine that you take depends on the strength of the medicine. Also, the number of doses you take each day, the time allowed between doses, and the length of time you take the medicine depend on the medical problem for which you are using the medicine.

Precautions While Using This Medicine

It is very important that your doctor check your progress at regular visits to make sure that this medicine is working properly. Blood tests will be needed to check for unwanted effects.

While you are being treated with gemcitabine, and after you stop treatment with it, do not have any immunizations (vaccinations) without your doctor's approval. Gemcitabine may lower your body's resistance, and there is a chance you might get the infection that the immunization is meant to prevent. In addition, other persons living in your household should not take oral polio vaccine, since there is a chance they could pass the polio virus on to you. Also, avoid persons who have taken oral polio vaccine within the past several months. Do not get close to them and do not stay in the same room with them for very long. If you cannot take these precautions, you should consider wearing a protective face mask that covers the nose and mouth.

Check with your doctor immediately if shortness of breath occurs or worsens while you are being treated with gemcitabine.

Gemcitabine can temporarily lower the number of white blood cells in your blood, increasing the chance of getting an infection. It can also lower the number of platelets, which are needed for proper blood clotting. If this occurs, there are certain precautions you can take, especially when your blood count is low, to reduce the risk of infection or bleeding:

- If you can, avoid people with infections. Check with your doctor immediately if you think you are getting an infection or if you get a fever or chills, cough or hoarseness, lower back or side pain, or painful or difficult urination.

- Check with your doctor immediately if you notice any unusual bleeding or bruising; black, tarry stools; blood in urine or stools; or pinpoint red spots on your skin.

- Be careful when using a regular toothbrush, dental floss, or toothpick. Your medical doctor, dentist, or nurse may recommend other ways to clean your teeth and gums. Also, check with your medical doctor before having any dental work done.

- Do not touch your eyes or the inside of your nose unless you have just washed your hands and have not touched anything else in the meantime.

- Be careful not to cut yourself when you are using sharp objects such as a safety razor or fingernail or toenail cutters.

- Avoid contact sports or other situations where bruising or injury could occur.

- This medicine can cause harm to your unborn baby. Make sure your doctor knows if you are pregnant before taking this medicine. If you think you have become pregnant while using the medicine, tell your doctor right away.

Side Effects of This Medicine

Along with its needed effects, a medicine may cause some unwanted effects. Although not all of these side effects may occur, if they do occur they may need medical attention.

Check with your doctor immediately if any of the following side effects occur:

More common

Bleeding gums; blood in urine or stools; burning, crawling, itching, numbness, prickling, "pins and needles", or tingling feelings; chest pain; cloudy urine; coughing up blood; cough or hoarseness; diarrhea; difficult or labored breathing; difficulty in moving; difficulty in swallowing; dizziness; fever or chills; general feeling of discomfort or illness; headache; increased menstrual flow or vaginal bleeding; joint pain; lack or loss of strength; loss of appetite; lower back or side pain; muscle aching or cramping; muscle pains or stiffness; nausea; nosebleeds; painful or difficult urination; pale skin; paralysis; pinpoint red spots on skin; prolonged bleeding from cuts; red or black, tarry stools; red or dark brown urine; runny nose; shivering; shortness of breath; sores, ulcers, or white spots on lips or in mouth; sore throat; sweating; swelling of hands, ankles, feet, or lower legs; swollen glands; swollen joints; tightness in chest; troubled breathing with exertion; trouble sleeping; unusual bleeding or bruising; unusual tiredness or weakness; vomiting; weight loss; wheezing

Less common

Blurred vision; chest discomfort; fainting; fast, slow, or irregular heartbeat; headache (sudden and severe); inability to speak; nervousness; noisy breathing; pain or discomfort in arms, jaw, back or neck; pounding in the ears; seizures; slurred speech; temporary blindness; weakness in arm and/or leg on one side of the body (sudden and severe)

Rare

Confusion; lightheadedness; rapid, shallow breathing

Incidence not determined

Hives; itching; puffiness or swelling of the eyelids or around the eyes, face, lips or tongue; skin rash

Some side effects may occur that usually do not need medical attention. These side effects may go away during treatment as your body adjusts to the medicine. Also, your health care professional may be able to tell you about ways to prevent or reduce some of these side effects. Check with your health care professional if any of the following side effects continue or are bothersome or if you have any questions about them:

More common

Difficulty having a bowel movement (stool); hair loss; pain; sleepiness or unusual drowsiness; swelling or inflammation of the mouth; thinning of hair

Less common

Bleeding, blistering, burning, coldness, discoloration of skin, feeling of pressure, hives, infection, inflammation, itching, lumps, numbness, pain, rash, redness, scarring, soreness, stinging, swelling, tenderness, tingling, ulceration, or warmth at site

Other side effects not listed may also occur in some patients. If you notice any other effects, check with your healthcare professional.

GEMFIBROZIL (Oral route) - jem-FI-broe-zil

Commonly used brand name(s)

In the U.S.—
Lopid

Available Dosage Forms:

- Tablet
- Capsule

Therapeutic Class: Antihyperlipidemic

Uses For This Medicine

Gemfibrozil is used to lower cholesterol and triglyceride (fat-like substances) levels in the blood. This may help prevent medical problems caused by such substances clogging the blood vessels.

Gemfibrozil is available only with your doctor's prescription.

Before Using This Medicine

In deciding to use a medicine, the risks of taking the medicine must be weighed against the good it will do. This is a decision you and your doctor will make. For this medicine, the following should be considered:

In addition to its helpful effects in treating your medical problem, this type of medicine may have some harmful effects.Results of a large study using gemfibrozil seem to show that it may cause a higher rate of some cancers in humans. In addition, the action of gemfibrozil is similar to that of another medicine called clofibrate. Studies with clofibrate have suggested that it may increase the patient's risk of cancer, liver disease, pancreatitis (inflammation of the pancreas), gallstones and problems from gallbladder surgery, although it may also decrease the risk of heart attacks. Other studies have not found all of these effects.Studies with gemfibrozil in rats found an increased risk of liver tumors when doses up to 10 times the human dose were given for a long time.Be sure you have discussed this with your doctor before taking this medicine.

Allergies—Tell your doctor if you have ever had any unusual or allergic reaction to this medicine or any other medicines. Also tell your health care professional if you have any other types of allergies, such as to foods, dyes, preservatives, or animals. For non-prescription products, read the label or package ingredients carefully.

Pediatric—There is no specific information about the use of gemfibrozil in children. However, use is not recommended in children under 2 years of age since cholesterol is needed for normal development.

Geriatric—Many medicines have not been studied specifically in older people. Therefore, it may not be known whether they work exactly the same way they do in younger adults or if they cause different side effects or problems in older people. There is no specific information comparing use of gemfibrozil in the elderly with use in other age groups.

Pregnancy—

	Pregnancy Category	Explanation
All Trimesters	C	Animal studies have shown an adverse effect and there are no adequate studies in pregnant women OR no animal studies have been conducted and there are no adequate studies in pregnant women.

Breast Feeding—There are no adequate studies in women for determining infant risk when using this medication during breastfeeding. Weigh the potential benefits against the potential risks before taking this medication while breastfeeding.

Other medicines—

Using this medicine with any of the following medicines is not recommended. Your doctor may decide not to treat you with this medication or change some of the other medicines you take.

Repaglinide

Interactions with Food/Tobacco/Alcohol—Certain medicines should not be used at or around the time of eating food or eating certain types of food since interactions may occur. Using alcohol or tobacco with certain medicines may also cause interactions to occur. Discuss with your healthcare professional the use of your medicine with food, alcohol, or tobacco.

Other medical problems—The presence of other medical problems may affect the use of this medicine. Make sure you tell your doctor if you have any other medical problems, especially:

- Gallbladder disease or
- Gallstones—Gemfibrozil may make these conditions worse
- Kidney disease or
- Liver disease—Higher blood levels of gemfibrozil may result, which may increase the chance of side effects; a decrease in the dose of gemfibrozil may be needed

Proper Use of This Medicine

Before prescribing medicine for your condition, your doctor will probably try to control your condition by prescribing a personal diet for you. Such a diet may be low in fats, sugars, and/or cholesterol. Many people are able to control their condition by carefully following their doctor's orders for proper diet and exercise. Medicine is prescribed only when additional help is needed and is effective only when a schedule of diet and exercise is properly followed.

Also, this medicine is less effective if you are greatly overweight. It may be very important for you to go on a reducing diet. However, check with your doctor before going on any diet.

Make certain your health care professional knows if you are on a low-sodium, low-sugar, or any other special diet. Most medicines contain more than their active ingredient.

Use this medicine only as directed by your doctor. Do not use more or less of it, and do not use it more often or for a longer time than your doctor ordered.

This medicine is usually taken twice a day. If you are taking 2 doses a day, it is best to take the medicine 30 minutes before your breakfast and evening meal.

Follow carefully the special diet your doctor gave you. This is the most important part of controlling your condition and is necessary if the medicine is to work properly.

Dosing—The dose of this medicine will be different for different patients. Follow your doctor's orders or the directions on the label. The following information includes only the average doses of this medicine. If your dose is different, do not change it unless your doctor tells you to do so.

The amount of medicine that you take depends on the strength of the medicine. Also, the number of doses you take each day, the time allowed between doses, and the length of time you take the medicine depend on the medical problem for which you are using the medicine.

- For oral dosage forms (tablets):
  - Adults: 600 milligrams two times a day to be taken thirty minutes before the morning and evening meals.

Missed dose—If you miss a dose of this medicine, take it as soon as possible. However, if it is almost time for your next dose, skip the missed dose and go back to your regular dosing schedule. Do not double doses.

Storage—Store the medicine in a closed container at room temperature, away from heat, moisture, and direct light. Keep from freezing.

Keep out of the reach of children.

Do not keep outdated medicine or medicine no longer needed.

Precautions While Using This Medicine

It is very important that your doctor check your progress at regular visits. This will allow your doctor to see if the medicine is working properly to lower your cholesterol and triglyceride levels and to decide if you should continue to take it.

Do not stop taking this medication without first checking with your doctor. When you stop taking this medicine, your blood cholesterol levels may increase again. Your doctor may want you to follow a special diet to help prevent this from happening.

Side Effects of This Medicine

Along with its needed effects, a medicine may cause some unwanted effects. Although not all of these side effects may occur, if they do occur they may need medical attention.

Check with your doctor immediately if any of the following side effects occur:
> *Rare*
>> Cough or hoarseness; fever or chills; lower back or side pain; painful or difficult urination; stomach pain (severe) with nausea and vomiting

Check with your doctor as soon as possible if any of the following side effects occur:
> *Rare*
>> Muscle pain; unusual tiredness or weakness

Some side effects may occur that usually do not need medical attention. These side effects may go away during treatment as your body adjusts to the medicine. Also, your health care professional may be able to tell you about ways to prevent or reduce some of these side effects. Check with your health care professional if any of the following side effects continue or are bothersome or if you have any questions about them:
> *More common*
>> Stomach pain, gas, or heartburn
> *Less common*
>> Diarrhea; nausea or vomiting; skin rash

Other side effects not listed may also occur in some patients. If you notice any other effects, check with your healthcare professional.

GEMIFLOXACIN (Oral route) - je-mi-FLOX-a-sin

Commonly used brand name(s)

In the U.S.—
> Factive

Available Dosage Forms:
- Tablet

Therapeutic Class: Antibiotic

Uses For This Medicine

Gemifloxacin belongs to the class of medicines known as antibiotics. It is used to treat bronchitis and pneumonia caused by bacterial infections.

Gemifloxacin works by killing bacteria or preventing their growth. However, this medicine will not work for colds, flu, or other virus infections.

This medicine is available only with your doctor's prescription.

Before Using This Medicine

In deciding to use a medicine, the risks of taking the medicine must be weighed against the good it will do. This is a decision you and your doctor will make. For this medicine, the following should be considered:

Allergies—Tell your doctor if you have ever had any unusual or allergic reaction to this medicine or any other medicines. Also tell your health care professional if you have any other types of allergies, such as to foods, dyes, preservatives, or animals. For non-prescription products, read the label or package ingredients carefully.

Pediatric—Studies on this medicine have only been done in adult patients and there is no specific information comparing the use of gemifloxacin in children with use in other age groups. It is not recommended to use gemifloxacin in children up to 18 years of age because this medicine has been shown to cause bone development problems in young animals.

Geriatric—There is no specific information comparing use of gemifloxacin in the elderly with use in other age groups. However, it has been used in older people and has not been found to cause different side effects or other problems than it does in younger adults.

Pregnancy—

	Pregnancy Category	Explanation
All Trimesters	C	Animal studies have shown an adverse effect and there are no adequate studies in pregnant women OR no animal studies have been conducted and there are no adequate studies in pregnant women.

Breast Feeding—Studies in women breastfeeding have demonstrated harmful infant effects. An alternative to this medication should be prescribed or you should stop breastfeeding while using this medicine.

Other medicines—

Using this medicine with any of the following medicines is not recommended. Your doctor may decide not to treat you with this medication or change some of the other medicines you take.

Bepridil, Cisapride, Mesoridazine, Pimozide, Terfenadine, Thioridazine, Ziprasidone

Interactions with Food/Tobacco/Alcohol—Certain medicines should not be used at or around the time of eating food or eating certain types of food since interactions may occur. Using alcohol or tobacco with certain medicines may also cause interactions to occur. Discuss with your healthcare

professional the use of your medicine with food, alcohol, or tobacco.

Other medical problems—The presence of other medical problems may affect the use of this medicine. Make sure you tell your doctor if you have any other medical problems, especially:

- Brain or spinal cord disease, epilepsy or other seizures—Gemifloxacin may increase the chance of making these problems worse.

- Heart rhythm problems—Gemifloxacin should be used with caution in patients with these conditions.

- Hypokalemia (not enough potassium in your blood) or

- Hypomagnesemia (not enough magnesium in your blood)—These conditions can increase your risk of having a fast, slow or irregular heartbeat when you are taking gemifloxacin.

- QTc prolongation (rare heart rhythm problem)—Gemifloxacin may cause this condition to become worse, especially with higher doses of gemifloxacin.

Proper Use of This Medicine

Gemifloxacin may be taken with or without food. Tablet must be swallowed whole. Do not chew the tablet.

Drink plenty of fluids while you are being treated with this medicine. Drinking extra water will help to prevent some unwanted effects of gemifloxacin.

This medicine works best when there is a constant amount in the blood or urine. To help keep the amount constant, do not miss any doses. Also, it is best to take the doses at evenly spaced times, day and night. For example, if you are to take one dose a day, try to take it at the same time each day.

It is important that you take this medicine exactly as prescribed by your doctor. It is important for you to take this medicine for as long as the doctor tells you to, even if you begin to feel better after a few days.

Dosing—The dose of this medicine will be different for different patients. Follow your doctor's orders or the directions on the label. The following information includes only the average doses of this medicine. If your dose is different, do not change it unless your doctor tells you to do so.

The amount of medicine that you take depends on the strength of the medicine. Also, the number of doses you take each day, the time allowed between doses, and the length of time you take the medicine depend on the medical problem for which you are using the medicine.

- For oral dosage form (tablets):
  - For treatment of infection
    - Adults—320 milligrams (mg) once a day for five to seven days.
    - Children—Use and dose must be determined by your doctor.

Missed dose—If you miss a dose of this medicine, take it as soon as possible. However, if it is almost time for your next dose, skip the missed dose and go back to your regular dosing schedule. Do not double doses.

Storage—Store the medicine in a closed container at room temperature, away from heat, moisture, and direct light. Keep from freezing.

Keep out of the reach of children.

Do not keep outdated medicine or medicine no longer needed.

Ask your healthcare professional how you should dispose of any medicine you do not use.

Precautions While Using This Medicine

If your symptoms do not improve within a few days, or if they become worse, check with your doctor.

Make sure your doctor knows if you recently had an episode of chest pain.

Tell your doctor right away if you have palpitations (pounding heartbeat) or fainting spells while taking this medicine.

Some people who take gemifloxacin may become more sensitive to sunlight than they are normally. Exposure to sunlight, even for brief periods of time, may cause severe sunburn; skin rash, redness, itching, or discoloration; or vision changes. When you begin taking this medicine use caution when you are in the sun and do not use a tanning bed, booth or sunlamp. If you have a severe reaction from the sun, check with your doctor.

If you get a skin rash or other signs of an allergic reaction, stop taking gemifloxacin and check with your doctor immediately.

Gemifloxacin may cause some people to become dizzy, light-headed, drowsy, or less alert than they are normally. Make sure you know how you react to this medicine before you drive, use machines, or do anything else that could be dangerous if you are dizzy or are not alert. If these reactions are especially bothersome, check with your doctor.

This medicine may rarely cause inflammation or even tearing of a tendon (the cord that attaches muscles to bones). If you get sudden pain in a tendon after exercise (for example, in your ankle, back of the knee or leg, shoulder, elbow, or wrist), stop taking gemifloxacin and check with your doctor. Rest and do not exercise until the doctor has made sure that you have not injured or torn the tendon.

Tell your doctor if you have severe diarrhea that does not go away while taking this medicine or after you finish taking this medicine.

Side Effects of This Medicine

Along with its needed effects, a medicine may cause some unwanted effects. Although not all of these side effects may occur, if they do occur they may need medical attention.

Check with your doctor immediately if any of the following side effects occur:

Less common
    Rash

Rare
    Black, tarry stools; bleeding gums; blood in urine or stools; body aches or pain; burning, numbness, tingling, or painful sensations; chest pain; chills; congestion; cough; fever; hives or welts; hoarseness; itching skin; pale skin; painful or difficult urination; pinpoint red spots on skin; redness of skin; runny nose; shortness of breath; skin rash; sneezing; sore throat; sores, ulcers, or white spots on lips or in mouth; swollen glands; tightness in chest; trouble in swallowing; troubled breathing; unsteadiness or awkwardness; unusual bleeding or bruising; unusual tiredness or weakness; voice changes; weakness in arms, hands, legs, or feet; wheezing; yellow eyes or skin

Some side effects may occur that usually do not need medical attention. These side effects may go away during treat-

ment as your body adjusts to the medicine. Also, your health care professional may be able to tell you about ways to prevent or reduce some of these side effects. Check with your health care professional if any of the following side effects continue or are bothersome or if you have any questions about them:

Less common

Diarrhea; headache; nausea

Rare

Abnormal urine; acid or sour stomach; back pain; bad unusual or unpleasant taste; belching; blistering, crusting, irritation, itching, or reddening of skin; blurred vision; change in taste; change in vision; cracked, dry, scaly skin; difficulty having a bowel movement (stool); difficulty in moving; dizziness or light-headedness; dry mouth; dryness or soreness of throat; feeling of constant movement of self or surroundings; feeling of warmth; fruit like breath odor; heartburn; hoarseness; increased hunger and thirst; increased sensitivity of skin to sunlight; increased urination; indigestion; lack or loss of strength; leg cramps; loss of appetite; muscle aching or cramping; muscle pain or stiffness; nervousness; pain; pain in joints; redness of the face, neck, arms and occasionally, upper chest; sensation of spinning; shakiness in legs, arms, hands, feet; sleepiness or drowsiness; sleeplessness; stomach discomfort, upset or pain; sudden sweating; swelling; swollen joints; trembling or shaking of hands or feet; trouble in swallowing; voice changes; vomiting; weight loss

Other side effects not listed may also occur in some patients. If you notice any other effects, check with your healthcare professional.

GEMTUZUMAB OZOGAMICIN
(Intravenous route) - gem-TOO-zoo-mab oh-zoh-ga-MYE-sin

Black Box Warning

Gemtuzumab ozogamicin should be administered under the supervision of physicians experienced in the treatment of acute leukemia and in facilities equipped to monitor and treat leukemia patients.

There are no controlled trials demonstrating efficacy and safety using gemtuzumab ozogamicin in combination with other chemotherapeutic agents. Therefore, gemtuzumab ozogamicin should only be used as single agent chemotherapy and not in combination chemotherapy regimens outside clinical trials.

Severe myelosuppression occurs when gemtuzumab ozogamicin is used at recommended doses.

Gemtuzumab ozogamicin administration can result in severe hypersensitivity reactions (including anaphylaxis), and other infusion-related reactions which may include severe pulmonary events. Infrequently, hypersensitivity reactions and pulmonary events have been fatal. In most cases, infusion-related symptoms occurred during the infusion or within 24 hours of administration of gemtuzumab ozogamicin and resolved. Gemtuzumab ozogamicin infusion should be interrupted for patients experiencing dyspnea or clinically significant hypotension. Patients should be monitored until signs and symptoms completely resolve. Discontinuation of gemtuzumab ozogamicin treatment should be strongly considered for patients who develop anaphylaxis, pulmonary edema, or acute respiratory distress syndrome. Since patients with high peripheral blast counts may be at greater risk for pulmonary events and tumor lysis syndrome, physicians should consider leukoreduction with hydroxyurea or leukapheresis to reduce the peripheral white count to below 30,000/ microliters prior to administration of gemtuzumab ozogamicin.

Hepatotoxicity, including severe hepatic veno-occlusive disease (VOD), has been reported in association with the use of gemtuzumab ozogamicin as a single agent, as part of a combination chemotherapy regimen, and in patients without a history of liver disease or hematopoietic stem-cell transplant (HSCT). Patients who receive gemtuzumab ozogamicin either before or after HSCT, patients with underlying hepatic disease or abnormal liver function, and patients receiving gemtuzumab ozogamicin in combinations with other chemotherapy are at increased risk for developing VOD, including severe VOD. Death from liver failure and from VOD has been reported in patients who received gemtuzumab ozogamicin. Physicians should monitor their patients carefully for symptoms of hepatotoxicity, particularly VOD. These symptoms can include: rapid weight gain, right upper quadrant pain, hepatomegaly, ascites, elevations in bilirubin and/or liver enzymes. However, careful monitoring may not identify all patients at risk or prevent the complications of hepatotoxicity.

Commonly used brand name(s)

In the U.S.—

Mylotarg

Available Dosage Forms:

• Powder for Solution

Therapeutic Class: Antineoplastic Agent
Pharmacologic Class: Monoclonal Antibody

Uses For This Medicine

Gemtuzumab ozogamicin is a monoclonal antibody. It is used to treat a certain type of leukemia which has recurred in patients who are 60 years of age or older. Gemtuzumab ozogamicin is an alternative to chemotherapy for these patients.

This medicine is to be administered only by or under the immediate supervision of your doctor.

Before Using This Medicine

In deciding to use a medicine, the risks of taking the medicine must be weighed against the good it will do. This is a decision you and your doctor will make. For this medicine, the following should be considered:

Allergies—Tell your doctor if you have ever had any unusual or allergic reaction to this medicine or any other medicines. Also tell your health care professional if you have any other types of allergies, such as to foods, dyes, preservatives, or animals. For non-prescription products, read the label or package ingredients carefully.

Pediatric—Studies on this medicine have been done only in adult patients, and there is no specific information comparing use of gemtuzumab ozogamicin in children with use in other age groups.

Geriatric—Many medicines have not been studied specifically in older people. Therefore, it may not be known whether they work exactly the same way they do in younger adults or if they cause different side effects or problems in older people. There is no specific information comparing use of gemtuzumab ozogamicin in the elderly with use in other age groups. However, laboratory values associated with liver problems were observed more often in patients 60 years old or older.

Pregnancy—

	Pregnancy Category	Explanation
All Trimesters	D	Studies in pregnant women have demonstrated a risk to the fetus. However, the benefits of therapy in a life threatening situation or a serious disease, may outweigh the potential risk.

Breast Feeding—There are no adequate studies in women for determining infant risk when using this medication during breastfeeding. Weigh the potential benefits against the potential risks before taking this medication while breastfeeding.

Other medicines—Although certain medicines should not be used together at all, in other cases two different medicines may be used together even if an interaction might occur. In these cases, your doctor may want to change the dose, or other precautions may be necessary. Tell your healthcare professional if you are taking any other prescription or non-prescription (over-the-counter [OTC]) medicine.

Interactions with Food/Tobacco/Alcohol—Certain medicines should not be used at or around the time of eating food or eating certain types of food since interactions may occur. Using alcohol or tobacco with certain medicines may also cause interactions to occur. Discuss with your healthcare professional the use of your medicine with food, alcohol, or tobacco.

Other medical problems—The presence of other medical problems may affect the use of this medicine. Make sure you tell your doctor if you have any other medical problems, especially:

- Chickenpox (including recent exposure) or
- Herpes zoster (shingles)—Risk of severe disease affecting other parts of the body
- High blood cell counts (peripheral blasts)—Risk of side effects increased by gemtuzumab ozogamicin
- Infection—Risk increased by gemtuzumab ozogamicin
- Liver disease—May be worsened by gemtuzumab ozogamicin
- Stem-cell transplant—Risk of side effects increased by gemtuzumab ozogamicin

Proper Use of This Medicine

Dosing—The dose of this medicine will be different for different patients. Follow your doctor's orders or the directions on the label. The following information includes only the average doses of this medicine. If your dose is different, do not change it unless your doctor tells you to do so.

The amount of medicine that you take depends on the strength of the medicine. Also, the number of doses you take each day, the time allowed between doses, and the length of time you take the medicine depend on the medical problem for which you are using the medicine.

Precautions While Using This Medicine

It is very important that your doctor check you at regular visits to make sure this medication is working properly and to check for any unwanted effects.

While you are being treated with gemtuzumab ozogamicin, and after you stop treatment with it, *do not have any immunizations (vaccinations) without your doctor's approval*. Gemtuzumab ozogamicin may lower your body's resistance and there is a chance you might get the infection the immunization is meant to prevent. In addition, other persons living in your household should not take oral polio vaccine since there is a chance they could pass the polio virus on to you. Also, avoid persons who have taken oral polio vaccine within the last several months. Do not get close to them, and do not stay in the same room with them for very long. If you cannot take these precautions, you should consider wearing a protective face mask that covers the nose and mouth.

Gemtuzumab ozogamicin can temporarily lower the number of white blood cells in your blood, increasing the chance of getting an infection. It can also lower the number of platelets, which are necessary for proper blood clotting. If this occurs, there are certain precautions you can take, especially when your blood count is low, to reduce the risk of infection or bleeding:

- If you can, avoid people with infections. Check with your doctor immediately if you think you are getting an infection or if you get a fever or chills, cough or hoarseness, lower back or side pain, or painful or difficult urination.
- Check with your doctor immediately if you notice any unusual bleeding or bruising; black, tarry stools; blood in urine or stools; or pinpoint red spots on your skin.
- Be careful when using a regular toothbrush, dental floss, or toothpick. Your medical doctor, dentist, or nurse may recommend other ways to clean your teeth and gums. Check with your medical doctor before having any dental work done.
- Do not touch your eyes or the inside of your nose unless you have just washed your hands and have not touched anything else in the meantime.
- Be careful not to cut yourself when you are using sharp objects such as a safety razor or fingernail or toenail cutters.
- Avoid contact sports or other situations where bruising or injury could occur.

Side Effects of This Medicine

Along with its needed effects, a medicine may cause some unwanted effects. Although not all of these side effects may occur, if they do occur they may need medical attention.

More common

Black, tarry stools; bloating or swelling of face, arms, hands, lower legs, or feet; blood in stools or urine; bluish color of fingernails, lips, skin, palms, or nail beds; blurred vision; burning or stinging of skin; chest pain; chills; confusion; convulsions (seizures); cough or hoarseness; cracked lips; decrease or increase in urine; diarrhea; difficulty in swallowing; dizziness; dry mouth; excessive sweating; fainting; fast or slow heartbeat; fatigue; fever; flushed, dry skin; fruit-like breath odor; headache, sudden and severe; heavy, nonmenstrual vaginal bleeding; inability to speak; increased thirst or hunger; irregular heartbeat; large, flat, blue or purplish patches in the skin; light-headedness; lower back, joint, or side pain; loss of appetite; mood changes; muscle pain or cramps; muscle trembling or twitching; nausea or vomiting; numbness or tingling in hands, feet, or lips; pain, difficulty, or burning while urinating; painful cold sores or blisters on lips, nose, eyes, or genitals; pale skin; persistent bleeding or oozing from puncture sites, mouth, or nose; palpitations; pinpoint red spots on skin; pounding in the ears; red or purplish patches or spots on skin; rapid, shallow breathing; rapid weight gain; severe or continuing dull nervousness; shortness of breath; slurred speech; small red or purple spots on skin; sneezing; sore throat; sores, ulcers, or white spots on lips, tongue, or inside mouth; stomachache; sweating; swelling or inflammation of the mouth, face, fingers, feet, or lower legs; swollen glands; temporary blindness; tightness in chest; tingling of hands or feet; troubled breathing, exertional; unexplained nosebleeds; unusual bleeding or bruising; unusual tiredness or weakness; unusual weight gain or loss; weakness in arm and/or leg on one side of the body, sudden and severe; wheezing; yellow eyes or skin

Some side effects may occur that usually do not need medical attention. These side effects may go away during treatment as your body adjusts to the medicine. Also, your health care professional may be able to tell you about ways to prevent or reduce some of these side effects. Check with your health care professional if any of the following side effects continue or are bothersome or if you have any questions about them:

More common
Acid or sour stomach; belching; difficulty in moving; dry, red, hot, or irritated skin; full or bloated feeling or pressure in the stomach; heartburn; indigestion; lack or loss of strength; muscle pain or stiffness; pain, swelling, or redness in joints; runny, stuffy nose; stomach discomfort upset; swelling of abdominal or stomach area; trouble in sleeping

Other side effects not listed may also occur in some patients. If you notice any other effects, check with your healthcare professional.

GENTAMICIN (Ophthalmic route) - jen-ta-MYE-sin

Commonly used brand name(s)

In the U.S.—

Garamycin	Gentafair
Genoptic	Gentak
Genoptic S.O.P.	Gentasol
Gentacidin	Ocu-Mycin

Available Dosage Forms:
- Solution
- Ointment

Therapeutic Class: Antibiotic

Uses For This Medicine

Gentamicin belongs to the family of medicines called antibiotics. Gentamicin ophthalmic preparations are used to treat infections of the eye.

Gentamicin is available only with your doctor's prescription.

Before Using This Medicine

In deciding to use a medicine, the risks of taking the medicine must be weighed against the good it will do. This is a decision you and your doctor will make. For this medicine, the following should be considered:

Allergies—Tell your doctor if you have ever had any unusual or allergic reaction to this medicine or any other medicines. Also tell your health care professional if you have any other types of allergies, such as to foods, dyes, preservatives, or animals. For non-prescription products, read the label or package ingredients carefully.

Pediatric—There is no specific information comparing use of this medicine in babies up to one month of age with use in other age groups.

Geriatric—Many medicines have not been studied specifically in older people. Therefore, it may not be known whether they work exactly the same way they do in younger adults or if they cause different side effects or problems in older people. There is no specific information comparing use of this medicine in the elderly with use in other age groups.

Pregnancy—

	Pregnancy Category	Explanation
All Trimesters	D	Studies in pregnant women have demonstrated a risk to the fetus. However, the benefits of therapy in a life threatening situation or a serious disease, may outweigh the potential risk.

Breast Feeding—Studies in women suggest that this medication poses minimal risk to the infant when used during breastfeeding.

Other medicines—

Using this medicine with any of the following medicines is usually not recommended, but may be required in some cases. If both medicines are prescribed together, your doctor may change the dose or how often you use one or both of the medicines.

Alcuronium, Atracurium, Cidofovir, Cisatracurium, Decamethonium, Doxacurium, Fazadinium, Gallamine, Hexafluorenium, Lysine, Metocurine, Mivacurium, Pancuronium, Pipecuronium, Rapacuronium, Rocuronium, Succinylcholine, Tacrolimus, Tubocurarine, Vancomycin, Vecuronium

Interactions with Food/Tobacco/Alcohol—Certain medicines should not be used at or around the time of eating food or eating certain types of food since interactions may occur. Using alcohol or tobacco with certain medicines may also cause interactions to occur. Discuss with your healthcare professional the use of your medicine with food, alcohol, or tobacco.

Proper Use of This Medicine

For patients using the eye drop form of this medicine:

- The bottle is only partially full to provide proper drop control.
- To use:
  - First, wash your hands. Tilt the head back and with the index finger of one hand, press gently on the skin just beneath the lower eyelid and pull the lower eyelid away from the eye to make a space. Drop the medicine into this space. Let go of the eyelid and gently close the eyes. Do not blink. Keep the eyes closed for 1 or 2 minutes, to allow the medicine to come into contact with the infection.
- If you think you did not get the drop of medicine into your eye properly, use another drop.
- Avoid wearing contact lenses during treatment
- To keep the medicine as germ-free as possible, do not touch the applicator tip to any surface (including the eye). Also, keep the container tightly closed.

For patients using the eye ointment form of this medicine:

- First, wash your hands. Tilt the head back and with the index finger of one hand, press gently on the skin just beneath the lower eyelid and pull the lower eyelid away from the eye to make a space. Squeeze a thin strip of ointment into this space. A 1–cm (approximately ⅓-inch) strip of ointment is usually enough unless otherwise directed by your doctor. Let go of the eyelid and gently close the eyes and keep them closed for 1 or 2 minutes, to allow the medicine to come into contact with the infection.
- To keep the medicine as germ-free as possible, do not touch the applicator tip to any surface (including the eye). After using gentamicin eye ointment, wipe the tip of the ointment tube with a clean tissue and keep the tube tightly closed.

To help clear up your infection completely, keep using this medicine for the full time of treatment, even if your symptoms have disappeared. Do not miss any doses.

Dosing—The dose of this medicine will be different for different patients. Follow your doctor's orders or the directions on the label. The following information includes only the average doses of this medicine. If your dose is different, do not change it unless your doctor tells you to do so.

The amount of medicine that you take depends on the strength of the medicine. Also, the number of doses you take each day, the time allowed between doses, and the length of time you take the medicine depend on the medical problem for which you are using the medicine.

- For ophthalmic ointment dosage form:
  - For eye infections:
    - Adults and children—Use every eight to twelve hours.
- For ophthalmic solution (eye drops) dosage form:
  - For mild to moderate eye infections:
    - Adults and children—One to two drops every four hours.
  - For severe eye infections:
    - Adults and children—One to two drops as often as once every hour as directed by your doctor.

Missed dose—If you miss a dose of this medicine, apply it as soon as possible. However, if it is almost time for your next dose, skip the missed dose and go back to your regular dosing schedule.

Storage—Store the medicine in a closed container at room temperature, away from heat, moisture, and direct light. Keep from freezing.

Keep out of the reach of children.

Do not keep outdated medicine or medicine no longer needed.

Precautions While Using This Medicine

If your symptoms do not improve within a few days, or if they become worse, check with your doctor.

Side Effects of This Medicine

Along with its needed effects, a medicine may cause some unwanted effects. Although not all of these side effects may occur, if they do occur they may need medical attention.

Check with your doctor immediately if any of the following side effects occur:

> *Less common*
> Itching, redness, swelling, or other sign of irritation not present before use of this medicine; redness of eye, eyelid, or inner lining of eyelid
>
> *Rare*
> Black, tarry stools; blood in urine or stools; or unusual bleeding or swelling; blurred vision, eye pain, sensitivity to light, and/or tearing; seeing, hearing, or feeling things that are not there
> hallucinations

Some side effects may occur that usually do not need medical attention. These side effects may go away during treatment as your body adjusts to the medicine. Also, your health care professional may be able to tell you about ways to prevent or reduce some of these side effects. Check with your health care professional if any of the following side effects continue or are bothersome or if you have any questions about them:

> *Less common*
> Burning or stinging

After application, eye ointments usually cause your vision to blur for a few minutes.

Other side effects not listed may also occur in some patients. If you notice any other effects, check with your healthcare professional.

GENTAMICIN (Otic route) - jen-ta-MYE-sin

Uses For This Medicine

Gentamicin belongs to the family of medicines called antibiotics. Gentamicin otic preparations are used to treat infections of the ear canal.

Gentamicin is available only with your doctor's prescription.

Before Using This Medicine

In deciding to use a medicine, the risks of taking the medicine must be weighed against the good it will do. This is a decision you and your doctor will make. For this medicine, the following should be considered:

Allergies—Tell your doctor if you have ever had any unusual or allergic reaction to this medicine or any other medicines. Also tell your health care professional if you have any other types of allergies, such as to foods, dyes, preservatives, or animals. For non-prescription products, read the label or package ingredients carefully.

Pediatric—There is no specific information comparing use of gentamicin otic solution in children up to 6 years of age with use in other age groups.

Geriatric—Many medicines have not been studied specifically in older people. Therefore, it may not be known whether they work exactly the same way they do in younger adults. Although there is no specific information comparing use of this medicine in the elderly with use in other age groups, this medicine is not expected to cause different side effects or problems in older people than it does in younger adults.

Other medicines—Although certain medicines should not be used together at all, in other cases two different medicines may be used together even if an interaction might occur. In these cases, your doctor may want to change the dose, or other precautions may be necessary. Tell your healthcare professional if you are taking any other prescription or non-prescription (over-the-counter [OTC]) medicine.

Interactions with Food/Tobacco/Alcohol—Certain medicines should not be used at or around the time of eating food or eating certain types of food since interactions may occur. Using alcohol or tobacco with certain medicines may also cause interactions to occur. Discuss with your healthcare professional the use of your medicine with food, alcohol, or tobacco.

Other medical problems—The presence of other medical problems may affect the use of this medicine. Make sure you tell your doctor if you have any other medical problems, especially:

- Any other ear infection or problem (including punctured or absent eardrum)—Use of gentamicin otic preparations in persons with this condition may lead to systemic absorption, and increase the chance of side effects

Proper Use of This Medicine

To use:

- Lie down or tilt the head so that the infected ear faces up. Gently pull the earlobe up and back for adults (down and back for children) to straighten the ear canal. Drop the medicine into the ear canal. Keep the ear facing up for about 1 or 2 minutes to allow the medicine to come into contact with the infection. A sterile cotton plug may be gently inserted into the ear opening to prevent the medicine from leaking out.
- To keep the medicine as germ-free as possible, do not touch the applicator tip to any surface (including the ear). Also, keep the container tightly closed.

To help clear up your infection completely, keep using this medicine for the full time of treatment, even if your symptoms have disappeared. Do not miss any doses.

Dosing—The dose of this medicine will be different for different patients. Follow your doctor's orders or the directions on the label. The following information includes only the average doses of this medicine. If your dose is different, do not change it unless your doctor tells you to do so.

The amount of medicine that you take depends on the strength of the medicine. Also, the number of doses you take each day, the time allowed between doses, and the length of time you take the medicine depend on the medical problem for which you are using the medicine.

- For ear drops dosage form:
  - For ear infections:
    - Adults and children 6 years of age and older—Place three or four drops in the infected ear three times a day.
    - Children younger than 6 years of age—Use and dose must be determined by your doctor.

Missed dose—If you miss a dose of this medicine, apply it as soon as possible. However, if it is almost time for your next dose, skip the missed dose and go back to your regular dosing schedule.

Storage—Store the medicine in a closed container at room temperature, away from heat, moisture, and direct light. Keep from freezing.

Keep out of the reach of children.

Do not keep outdated medicine or medicine no longer needed.

Precautions While Using This Medicine

If your symptoms do not improve within a few days, or if they become worse, check with your doctor.

Side Effects of This Medicine

Along with its needed effects, a medicine may cause some unwanted effects. Although not all of these side effects may occur, if they do occur they may need medical attention.

Check with your doctor immediately if any of the following side effects occur:
 Less common
  Itching, redness, swelling, or other sign of irritation not present before use of this medicine

Some side effects may occur that usually do not need medical attention. These side effects may go away during treatment as your body adjusts to the medicine. Also, your health care professional may be able to tell you about ways to prevent or reduce some of these side effects. Check with your health care professional if any of the following side effects continue or are bothersome or if you have any questions about them:
 Less common
  Burning or stinging in the ear

Other side effects not listed may also occur in some patients. If you notice any other effects, check with your healthcare professional.

GLIPIZIDE AND METFORMIN (Oral route) - GLIP-i-zide, met-FOR-min

Commonly used brand name(s)

In the U.S.—
Metaglip

Available Dosage Forms:
• Tablet

Therapeutic Class: Antidiabetic

Uses For This Medicine

Glipizide and metformin combination is used to treat high blood sugar levels that are caused by a type of diabetes mellitus or sugar diabetes called type 2 diabetes. Normally, after you eat, your pancreas releases insulin to help your body store excess sugar for later use. This process occurs during normal digestion of food. In type 2 diabetes, your body does not work properly to store the excess sugar and the sugar remains in your bloodstream. Chronic high blood sugar can lead to serious health problems in the future. Proper diet is the first step in managing type 2 diabetes but often medicines are needed to help your body. With two actions, the combination of glipizide and metformin helps your body cope with high blood sugar. Glipizide stimulates the release of insulin from the pancreas, directing your body to store blood sugar. Metformin has three different actions: it slows the absorption of sugar in your small intestine; it also stops your liver from converting stored sugar into blood sugar; and it helps your body use your natural insulin more efficiently.

This medicine is available only with your doctor's prescription.

Before Using This Medicine

In deciding to use a medicine, the risks of taking the medicine must be weighed against the good it will do. This is a decision you and your doctor will make. For this medicine, the following should be considered:

Allergies—Tell your doctor if you have ever had any unusual or allergic reaction to this medicine or any other medicines. Also tell your health care professional if you have any other types of allergies, such as to foods, dyes, preservatives, or animals. For non-prescription products, read the label or package ingredients carefully.

Pediatric—Studies on this medicine have been done only in adult patients, and there is no specific information comparing use of glipizide and metformin in children with use in other age groups.

Geriatric—Some older adults may be more sensitive than younger adults to the effects of these medicines. The first signs of low or high blood sugar are not easily seen or do not occur at all in older adults. This may increase the chance of low blood sugar developing during treatment. Older adults are more likely to have age-related problems and glipizide and metformin should be used carefully as age increases. This medicine should not be started in adults over 80 years of age unless kidney function is not reduced.

Pregnancy—

	Pregnancy Category	Explanation
All Trimesters	C	Animal studies have shown an adverse effect and there are no adequate studies in pregnant women OR no animal studies have been conducted and there are no adequate studies in pregnant women.

Breast Feeding—There are no adequate studies in women for determining infant risk when using this medication during breastfeeding. Weigh the potential benefits against the potential risks before taking this medication while breastfeeding.

Other medicines—

Using this medicine with any of the following medicines is not recommended. Your doctor may decide not to treat you with this medication or change some of the other medicines you take.

Acetrizoic Acid, Diatrizoate, Ethiodized Oil, Iobenzamic Acid, Iobitridol, Iocarmic Acid, Iocetamic Acid, Iodamide, Iodipamide, Iodixanol, Iodohippuric Acid, Iodopyracet, Iodoxamic Acid, Ioglicic Acid, Ioglycamic Acid, Iohexol, Iomeprol, Iopamidol, Iopanoic Acid, Iopentol, Iophendylate, Iopromide, Iopronic Acid, Ioseric Acid, Iosimide, Iotasul, Iothalamate, Iotrolan, Iotroxic Acid, Ioversol, Ioxaglate, Ioxitalamic Acid, Ipodate, Metrizamide, Metrizoic Acid, Tyropanoate Sodium

Interactions with Food/Tobacco/Alcohol—Certain medicines should not be used at or around the time of eating food or eating certain types of food since interactions may occur. Using alcohol or tobacco with certain medicines may also cause interactions to occur. The following interactions have been selected on the basis of their potential significance and are not necessarily all-inclusive.

Using this medicine with any of the following is usually not recommended, but may be unavoidable in some cases. If used together, your doctor may change the dose or how often you use this medicine, or give you special instructions about the use of food, alcohol, or tobacco.

Ethanol

Other medical problems—The presence of other medical problems may affect the use of this medicine. Make sure you tell your doctor if you have any other medical problems, especially:
• Acid in the blood (acidosis or ketoacidosis) or
• Surgery (major)—Use of insulin is best to help control diabetes in patients with these conditions.
• Blood poisoning or
• Dehydration (severe) or
• Heart or blood vessel disorders or
• Kidney disease or
• Liver disease—Lactic acidosis can occur in these conditions and chances of it occurring are even greater with a medicine that contains metformin.

- Congestive heart failure—Glipizide and metformin should not be used in patients who have this medical condition.
- Kidney, heart, or other problems that require medical tests or examinations that use certain medicines called contrast agents, with x-ray exams—Because this medicine contains metformin, your doctor should advise you to stop taking it before you have any medical exams or diagnostic tests that might cause less urine output than usual; you may be advised to start taking the medicine again 48 hours after the exams or tests if your kidney function is tested and found to be normal.
- Alcohol intoxication or
- Strenuous exercise not accompanied by adequate intake of food or
- Underactive adrenal gland, not properly controlled or
- Underactive pituitary gland, not properly controlled or
- Undernourished condition or
- Weakened physical condition or
- Any other condition that causes low blood sugar—Patients with these conditions may be more likely to develop low blood sugar while taking a medication that contains glipizide and metformin.
- Vitamin B12 deficiency—This condition may be made worse by this medication.

Proper Use of This Medicine

Follow carefully the special meal plan your doctor gave you. This is the most important part of controlling your condition, and is necessary if the medicine is to work properly. Also, exercise regularly and test for sugar in your blood or urine as directed.

Glipizide and metformin combination should be taken with meals to help reduce the gastrointestinal side effects that may occur during treatment.

Dosing—The dose of this medicine will be different for different patients. Follow your doctor's orders or the directions on the label. The following information includes only the average doses of this medicine. If your dose is different, do not change it unless your doctor tells you to do so.

The amount of medicine that you take depends on the strength of the medicine. Also, the number of doses you take each day, the time allowed between doses, and the length of time you take the medicine depend on the medical problem for which you are using the medicine.

- For oral dosage form (tablets):
  - For type 2 diabetes:
    - For first-time treatment:
      - Adults: At first, 2.5 milligrams (mg) of glipizide and 250 milligrams (mg) of metformin once a day with a meal. Then, your doctor may increase your dose a little at a time every two weeks until your blood sugar is controlled.
      - Children: Use and dose must be determined by your doctor.
    - As second-line therapy:
      - Oral, 2.5 milligrams (mg) of glipizide and 500 milligrams (mg) of metformin or 5 milligrams (mg) of glipizide and 500 milligrams (mg) of metformin two times a day, with the morning and evening meals. Then, your doctor may increase your dose a little at a time until your blood sugar is controlled. The starting dose should not exceed the daily dose of glipizide or metformin already being taken.
      - Children: Use and dose must be determined by your doctor.
  - For patients previously treated with a sulfonylurea antidiabetic agent and/or metformin:
    - Adults: When switching patients from a sulfonylurea plus metformin to the glipizide and metformin combination, the initial dose should not exceed the daily dose of glipizide (or equivalent dose of another sulfonylurea) and metformin that was being taken.
    - Children: Use and dose must be determined by your doctor.

Missed dose—If you miss a dose of this medicine, take it as soon as possible. However, if it is almost time for your next dose, skip the missed dose and go back to your regular dosing schedule. Do not double doses.

Storage—Store the medicine in a closed container at room temperature, away from heat, moisture, and direct light. Keep from freezing.

Keep out of the reach of children.

Do not keep outdated medicine or medicine no longer needed.

Ask your healthcare professional how you should dispose of any medicine you do not use.

Precautions While Using This Medicine

Your doctor will want to check your progress at regular visits, especially during the first few weeks that you take this medicine.

Under certain conditions, too much glipizide and metformin can cause lactic acidosis. Symptoms of lactic acidosis are severe and quick to appear and usually occur when other health problems not related to the medicine are present and are very severe, such as a heart attack or kidney failure. Symptoms of lactic acidosis include abdominal or stomach discomfort; decreased appetite; diarrhea; fast, shallow breathing; general feeling of discomfort; muscle pain or cramping; and unusual sleepiness, tiredness, or weakness.

If symptoms of lactic acidosis occur, you should get immediate emergency medical help.

It is very important to follow carefully any instructions from your health care team about:

- Alcohol—Drinking alcohol may cause severe low blood sugar. Discuss this with your health care team.
- Other medicines—Do not take other medicines unless they have been discussed with your doctor.
- Counseling—Other family members need to learn how to prevent side effects or help with side effects if they occur. Also, patients with diabetes may need special counseling about diabetes medicine dosing changes that might occur because of lifestyle changes, such as changes in exercise and diet. Furthermore, counseling on contraception and pregnancy may be needed be-

cause of the problems that can occur in patients with diabetes during pregnancy.

- Travel—Keep a recent prescription and your medical history with you. Be prepared for an emergency as you would normally. Make allowances for changing time zones and keep your meal times as close as possible to your usual meal times.

In case of emergency—There may be a time when you need emergency help for a problem caused by your diabetes. You need to be prepared for these emergencies. It is a good idea to wear a medical identification (ID) bracelet or neck chain at all times. Also, carry an ID card in your wallet or purse that says that you have diabetes and a list of all your medicines.

Symptoms of hypoglycemia (low blood sugar) include anxiety; behavior change similar to being drunk; blurred vision; cold sweats; confusion; cool, pale skin; difficulty in thinking; drowsiness; excessive hunger; fast heartbeat; headache (continuing); nausea; nervousness; nightmares; restless sleep; shakiness; slurred speech; or unusual tiredness or weakness.

Glipizide and metformin combination can cause low blood sugar. However, it also can occur if you delay or miss a meal or snack, drink alcohol, exercise more than usual, cannot eat because of nausea or vomiting, take certain medicines, or take glipizide and metformin with another type of diabetes medicine. Symptoms of low blood sugar must be treated before they lead to unconsciousness (passing out). Different people feel different symptoms of low blood sugar. It is important that you learn which symptoms of low blood sugar you usually have so that you can treat it quickly.

If symptoms of low blood sugar occur, eat glucose tablets or gel, corn syrup, honey, or sugar cubes; or drink fruit juice, nondiet soft drink, or sugar dissolved in water. Also, check your blood for low blood sugar. Glucagon is used in emergency situations when severe symptoms such as seizures (convulsions) or unconsciousness occur. Have a glucagon kit available, along with a syringe or needle, and know how to use it. Members of your household also should know how to use it.

Symptoms of hyperglycemia (high blood sugar) include blurred vision; drowsiness; dry mouth; flushed, dry skin; fruit-like breath odor; increased urination (frequency and volume); ketones in urine; loss of appetite; sleepiness; stomachache, nausea, or vomiting; tiredness; troubled breathing (rapid and deep); unconsciousness; or unusual thirst.

High blood sugar may occur if you do not exercise as much as usual, have a fever or infection, do not take enough or skip a dose of your diabetes medicine, or overeat or do not follow your meal plan.

If symptoms of high blood sugar occur, check your blood sugar level and then call your health care professional for instructions.

Side Effects of This Medicine

Along with its needed effects, a medicine may cause some unwanted effects. Although not all of these side effects may occur, if they do occur they may need medical attention.

Check with your doctor immediately if any of the following side effects occur:
  More common
    Anxiety; blurred vision; chills; cold sweats; coma; confusion; cool pale skin; cough; depression; dizziness;

fast heartbeat; fever; headache; increased hunger; nausea; nervousness; nightmares; seizures; shakiness; slurred speech; sneezing; sore throat; unusual tiredness or weakness
  Less common
    Bladder pain; bloody or cloudy urine; difficult, burning, or painful urination; frequent urge to urinate; lower back or side pain; pounding in the ears; slow heartbeat
  Rare
    Abdominal discomfort; decreased appetite; diarrhea; fainting spells; fast, shallow breathing; general feeling of discomfort; muscle pain or cramping; shortness of breath; sleepiness
  Symptoms of overdose
    Get emergency help immediately if any of the following symptoms of overdose occur:
      Abdominal discomfort; anxiety; behavior change, similar to drunkenness; blurred vision; cold sweats; coma; confusion; cool, pale skin; decreased appetite; diarrhea; difficulty in concentrating; drowsiness; excessive hunger; fast heartbeat; fast, shallow breathing; general feeling of discomfort; headache; muscle pain or cramping; nausea; nervousness; nightmares; restless sleep; seizures; shakiness; slurred speech; unusual sleepiness; unusual tiredness or weakness

Some side effects may occur that usually do not need medical attention. These side effects may go away during treatment as your body adjusts to the medicine. Also, your health care professional may be able to tell you about ways to prevent or reduce some of these side effects. Check with your health care professional if any of the following side effects continue or are bothersome or if you have any questions about them:
  More common
    Muscle or bone pain; stomach pain; vomiting

Other side effects not listed may also occur in some patients. If you notice any other effects, check with your healthcare professional.

GLUCAGON   (Injection route) - GLOO-ka-gon

Commonly used brand name(s)
In the U.S.—
  Glucagen   Glucagon Diagnostic Kit
  Glucagen Diagnostic Kit   Glucagon Emergency Kit
  Glucagon

Available Dosage Forms:
- Powder for Solution

Therapeutic Class: Glucose Regulation, Antihypoglycemic

Uses For This Medicine

Glucagon belongs to the group of medicines called hormones. It is an emergency medicine used to treat severe hypoglycemia (low blood sugar) in patients with diabetes who have passed out or cannot take some form of sugar by mouth.

Glucagon is also used during x-ray tests of the stomach and bowels to improve test results by relaxing the muscles of the stomach and bowels. This also makes the testing more comfortable for the patient.

Glucagon also may be used for other conditions as determined by your doctor.

Glucagon is available only with your doctor's prescription.

Once a medicine has been approved for marketing for a certain use, experience may show that it is also useful for other medical problems. Although these uses are not included in product labeling, glucagon is used in certain patients with the following medical conditions or undergoing certain medical procedures:

- Overdose of beta-adrenergic blocking medicines
- Overdose of calcium channel blocking medicines
- Removing food or an object stuck in the esophagus
- Hysterosalpingography (x-ray examination of the uterus and fallopian tubes)

Before Using This Medicine

In deciding to use a medicine, the risks of taking the medicine must be weighed against the good it will do. This is a decision you and your doctor will make. For this medicine, the following should be considered:

Allergies—Tell your doctor if you have ever had any unusual or allergic reaction to this medicine or any other medicines. Also tell your health care professional if you have any other types of allergies, such as to foods, dyes, preservatives, or animals. For non-prescription products, read the label or package ingredients carefully.

Pediatric—This medicine has been tested in children and, in effective doses, has not been shown to cause different side effects or problems than it does in adults.

Geriatric—Many medicines have not been studied specifically in older people. Therefore, it may not be known whether they work exactly the same way they do in younger adults. Although there is no specific information comparing use of glucagon in the elderly with use in other age groups, it is not expected to cause different side effects or problems in older people than it does in younger adults.

Pregnancy—

	Pregnancy Category	Explanation
All Trimesters	B	Animal studies have revealed no evidence of harm to the fetus, however, there are no adequate studies in pregnant women OR animal studies have shown an adverse effect, but adequate studies in pregnant women have failed to demonstrate a risk to the fetus.

Breast Feeding—There are no adequate studies in women for determining infant risk when using this medication during breastfeeding. Weigh the potential benefits against the potential risks before taking this medication while breastfeeding.

Other medicines—

Using this medicine with any of the following medicines may cause an increased risk of certain side effects, but using both drugs may be the best treatment for you. If both medicines

are prescribed together, your doctor may change the dose or how often you use one or both of the medicines.

Acenocoumarol, Anisindione, Dicumarol, Phenindione, Phenprocoumon, Warfarin

Interactions with Food/Tobacco/Alcohol—Certain medicines should not be used at or around the time of eating food or eating certain types of food since interactions may occur. Using alcohol or tobacco with certain medicines may also cause interactions to occur. Discuss with your healthcare professional the use of your medicine with food, alcohol, or tobacco.

Other medical problems—The presence of other medical problems may affect the use of this medicine. Make sure you tell your doctor if you have any other medical problems, especially:

- Diabetes mellitus—When glucagon is used for test or x-ray procedures in patients with diabetes that is well-controlled, a rise in blood sugar may occur; otherwise, glucagon is an important part of the management of diabetes because it is used to treat hypoglycemia (low blood sugar)
- Insulinoma (tumors of the pancreas gland that make too much insulin) (or history of)—Blood sugar concentrations may decrease
- Pheochromocytoma—Glucagon can cause high blood pressure

Proper Use of This Medicine

Glucagon is an emergency medicine and must be used only as directed by your doctor. Make sure that you and a member of your family or a friend understand exactly when and how to use this medicine before it is needed.

Glucagon is packaged in a kit with a vial of powder containing the medicine and a syringe filled with liquid to mix with the medicine. Directions for mixing and injecting the medicine are in the package. Read the directions carefully and ask your health care professional for additional explanation, if necessary.

Glucagon should not be mixed after the expiration date printed on the kit and on one vial. Check the date regularly and replace the medicine before it expires. The printed expiration date does not apply after mixing, when any unused portion must be discarded.

Dosing—The dose of this medicine will be different for different patients. Follow your doctor's orders or the directions on the label. The following information includes only the average doses of this medicine. If your dose is different, do not change it unless your doctor tells you to do so.

The amount of medicine that you take depends on the strength of the medicine. Also, the number of doses you take each day, the time allowed between doses, and the length of time you take the medicine depend on the medical problem for which you are using the medicine.

- As an emergency treatment for hypoglycemia:
  - Adults and children weighing 20 kilograms (kg) (44 pounds) or more: 1 milligram (mg). The dose may be repeated after fifteen minutes if necessary.
  - Children weighing up to 20 kg (44 pounds): 0.5 mg or 20 to 30 micrograms (mcg) per kg (9.1 to 13.6 mcg per pound) of body weight. The dose may be repeated after fifteen minutes if necessary.

Storage—Store the medicine in a closed container at room temperature, away from heat, moisture, and direct light. Keep from freezing.

Keep out of the reach of children.

Do not keep outdated medicine or medicine no longer needed.

Precautions While Using This Medicine

Patients with diabetes should be aware of the symptoms of hypoglycemia (low blood sugar). These symptoms may develop in a very short time and may result from:

- using too much insulin ("insulin reaction") or as a side effect from oral antidiabetic medicines.
- delaying or missing a scheduled snack or meal.
- sickness (especially with vomiting or diarrhea).
- exercising more than usual.

Unless corrected, hypoglycemia will lead to unconsciousness, convulsions (seizures), and possibly death. Early symptoms of hypoglycemia include: anxious feeling, behavior change similar to being drunk, blurred vision, cold sweats, confusion, cool pale skin, difficulty in concentrating, drowsiness, excessive hunger, fast heartbeat, headache, nausea, nervousness, nightmares, restless sleep, shakiness, slurred speech, and unusual tiredness or weakness.

Symptoms of hypoglycemia can differ from person to person. It is important that you learn your own signs of low blood sugar so that you can treat it quickly. It is a good idea also to check your blood sugar to confirm that it is low.

You should know what to do if symptoms of low blood sugar occur. Eating or drinking something containing sugar when symptoms of low blood sugar first appear will usually prevent them from getting worse, and will probably make the use of glucagon unnecessary. Good sources of sugar include glucose tablets or gel, corn syrup, honey, sugar cubes or table sugar (dissolved in water), fruit juice, or nondiet soft drinks. If a meal is not scheduled soon (1 hour or less), you should also eat a light snack, such as crackers and cheese or half a sandwich or drink a glass of milk to keep your blood sugar from going down again. You should not eat hard candy or mints because the sugar will not get into your blood stream quickly enough. You also should not eat foods high in fat such as chocolate because the fat slows down the sugar entering the blood stream. After 10 to 20 minutes, check your blood sugar again to make sure it is not still too low.

Tell someone to take you to your doctor or to a hospital right away if the symptoms do not improve after eating or drinking a sweet food. Do not try to drive yourself.

If severe symptoms such as convulsions (seizures) or unconsciousness occur, the patient with diabetes should not be given anything to eat or drink. There is a chance that he or she could choke from not swallowing correctly. Glucagon should be administered and the patient's doctor should be called at once.

If it becomes necessary to inject glucagon, a family member or friend should know the following:

- After the injection, turn the patient on his or her left side. Glucagon may cause some patients to vomit and this position will reduce the possibility of choking.
- The patient should become conscious in less than 15 minutes after glucagon is injected, but if not, a second dose may be given. Get the patient to a doctor or to hospital emergency care as soon as possible because being unconscious too long can be harmful.
- When the patient is conscious and can swallow, give him or her some form of sugar. Glucagon is not effective for much longer than 1½ hours and is used only until the patient is able to swallow. Fruit juice, corn syrup, honey, and sugar cubes or table sugar (dissolved in water) all work quickly. Then, if a snack or meal is not scheduled for an hour or more, the patient should also eat some crackers and cheese or half a sandwich, or drink a glass of milk. This will prevent hypoglycemia from occurring again before the next meal or snack.
- The patient or caregiver should continue to monitor the patient's blood sugar. For about 3 to 4 hours after the patient regains consciousness, the blood sugar should be checked every hour.
- If nausea and vomiting prevent the patient from swallowing some form of sugar for an hour after glucagon is given, medical help should be obtained.

Keep your doctor informed of any hypoglycemic episodes or use of glucagon even if the symptoms are successfully controlled and there seem to be no continuing problems. Complete information is necessary for the doctor to provide the best possible treatment of any condition.

Replace your supply of glucagon as soon as possible, in case another hypoglycemic episode occurs.

You should wear a medical identification (I.D.) bracelet or chain at all times. In addition, you should carry an I.D. card that lists your medical condition and medicines.

Side Effects of This Medicine

Along with its needed effects, a medicine may cause some unwanted effects. Although not all of these side effects may occur, if they do occur they may need medical attention.

Check with your doctor immediately if any of the following side effects occur:

Less common
    Dizziness; lightheadedness; trouble in breathing

Symptoms of overdose
    Diarrhea; irregular heartbeat; loss of appetite; muscle cramps or pain; nausea (continuing); vomiting (continuing); weakness of arms, legs, and trunk (severe)

Check with your doctor as soon as possible if any of the following side effects occur:

Less common
    Skin rash

Some side effects may occur that usually do not need medical attention. These side effects may go away during treatment as your body adjusts to the medicine. Also, your health care professional may be able to tell you about ways to prevent or reduce some of these side effects. Check with your health care professional if any of the following side effects continue or are bothersome or if you have any questions about them:

Less common or rare
    Fast heartbeat; nausea; vomiting

Other side effects not listed may also occur in some patients. If you notice any other effects, check with your healthcare professional.

GLUTAMINE (Oral route) - GLOO-ta-meen

Commonly used brand name(s)

In the U.S.—
Enterex Glutapak-10	Sympt-X
Resource Glutasolve	Sympt-X G.I.

Available Dosage Forms:

- Capsule
- Powder
- Powder for Solution
- Tablet
- Powder for Suspension
- Packet

Therapeutic Class: Amino Acid Supplement

Uses For This Medicine

Glutamine is a substance naturally produced in the body to help regulate cell growth and function. There may also be man-made versions of these substances. Glutamine is used along with human growth hormone and a specialized diet to treat short bowel syndrome

This medicine is available only with your doctor's prescription.

Importance of Diet—For good health, it is important that you eat a balanced and varied diet. Follow carefully any diet program your health care professional may recommend. For your specific dietary vitamin and/or mineral needs, ask your health care professional for a list of appropriate foods. If you think that you are not getting enough vitamins and/or minerals in your diet, you may choose to take a dietary supplement.

Before Using This Medicine

In deciding to use a medicine, the risks of taking the medicine must be weighed against the good it will do. This is a decision you and your doctor will make. For this medicine, the following should be considered:

In deciding to use glutamine, the risks of taking it must be weighed against the good it will do. This is a decision you and your doctor will make. For glutamine, the following should be considered:

Allergies—Tell your doctor if you have ever had any unusual or allergic reaction to this medicine or any other medicines. Also tell your health care professional if you have any other types of allergies, such as to foods, dyes, preservatives, or animals. For non-prescription products, read the label or package ingredients carefully.

Pediatric—Studies on this medicine have been done only in adult patients, and there is no specific information comparing use of glutamine in children with use in other age groups.

Geriatric—Many medicines have not been studied specifically in older people. Therefore, it may not be known whether they work exactly the same way they do in younger adults or if they cause different side effects or problems in older people. There is no specific information comparing use of glutamine in the elderly with use in other age groups. However, elderly patients are more likely to be sensitive requiring the need for dosage adjustment.

Pregnancy—

	Pregnancy Category	Explanation
All Trimesters	C	Animal studies have shown an adverse effect and there are no adequate studies in pregnant women OR no animal studies have been conducted and there are no adequate studies in pregnant women.

Breast Feeding—There are no adequate studies in women for determining infant risk when using this medication during breastfeeding. Weigh the potential benefits against the potential risks before taking this medication while breastfeeding.

Other medicines—Although certain medicines should not be used together at all, in other cases two different medicines may be used together even if an interaction might occur. In these cases, your doctor may want to change the dose, or other precautions may be necessary. Tell your healthcare professional if you are taking any other prescription or nonprescription (over-the-counter [OTC]) medicine.

Interactions with Food/Tobacco/Alcohol—Certain medicines should not be used at or around the time of eating food or eating certain types of food since interactions may occur. Using alcohol or tobacco with certain medicines may also cause interactions to occur. Discuss with your healthcare professional the use of your medicine with food, alcohol, or tobacco.

Other medical problems—The presence of other medical problems may affect the use of this medicine. Make sure you tell your doctor if you have any other medical problems, especially:

- Liver disease—May be worsened by glutamine.

Proper Use of This Medicine

Dosing—The dose of this medicine will be different for different patients. Follow your doctor's orders or the directions on the label. The following information includes only the average doses of this medicine. If your dose is different, do not change it unless your doctor tells you to do so.

The amount of medicine that you take depends on the strength of the medicine. Also, the number of doses you take each day, the time allowed between doses, and the length of time you take the medicine depend on the medical problem for which you are using the medicine.

- For oral dosage form (powder for oral solution):
  - For short bowel syndrome
    - Adults—30 grams per day in divided doses (5 grams taken 6 times a day) for up to 16 weeks. Taken with meals or snacks, 2 to 3 hours apart while awake.
    - Children—Use and dose must be determined by your doctor.

Missed dose—If you miss a dose of this medicine, take it as soon as possible. However, if it is almost time for your next dose, skip the missed dose and go back to your regular dosing schedule. Do not double doses.

Storage—Store the medicine in a closed container at room temperature, away from heat, moisture, and direct light. Keep from freezing.

Keep out of the reach of children.

Do not keep outdated medicine or medicine no longer needed.

Ask your healthcare professional how you should dispose of any medicine you do not use.

Precautions While Using This Medicine

It is very important that your doctor check you at regular visits.

Side Effects of This Medicine

Along with its needed effects, a medicine may cause some unwanted effects. Although not all of these side effects may occur, if they do occur they may need medical attention.

Check with your doctor immediately if any of the following side effects occur:

Less common

Blood in urine; changes in skin color; chills; cold hands and feet; confusion; cough; difficulty swallowing; dizziness; fainting; fast heartbeat; fever; frequent and painful urination; headache; hives; itching; lightheadedness; lower back or side pain; pain, redness, or swelling in arm or leg; puffiness or swelling of the eyelids or around the eyes, face, lips or tongue; rapid, shallow breathing; shortness of breath; skin rash; stomach pain; sudden decrease in amount of urine; tightness in chest; unusual tiredness or weakness; wheezing

Some side effects may occur that usually do not need medical attention. These side effects may go away during treatment as your body adjusts to the medicine. Also, your health care professional may be able to tell you about ways to prevent or reduce some of these side effects. Check with your health care professional if any of the following side effects continue or are bothersome or if you have any questions about them:

More common

Cough or hoarseness; frequent urge to defecate; straining while passing stool

Less common

Abnormal or decreased touch sensation; back pain; bacterial infection; bleeding after defecation; bleeding, blistering, burning, coldness, discoloration of skin, feeling of pressure, hives, infection, inflammation, itching, lumps, numbness, pain, rash, redness, scarring, soreness, stinging, swelling, tenderness, tingling, ulceration, or warmth at site; bloated full feeling; body aches or pain; breast pain, female; chest pain; change in the color, amount, or odor of vaginal discharge; congestion; constipation; Crohn's disease, aggravated; dark urine; decreased urination; diarrhea; difficulty having a bowel movement (stool); difficulty in moving; discoloration of fingernails or toenails; discouragement; dry mouth; dryness or soreness of throat; ear or hearing symptoms; excess air or gas in stomach or intestines; feeling sad or empty; feeling unusually cold shivering; flatulence; full or bloated feeling; general feeling of discomfort or illness; increase in heart rate; indigestion; irritability; joint pain; lack of appetite; light-colored stools; loss of appetite; loss of interest or pleasure; muscle aches and pains; muscle pain or stiffness; nausea; pain in joints; pain or burning while urinating; pains in stomach, side, or abdomen, possibly radiating to the back; passing gas; pressure in the stomach; rash; rectal bleeding; runny nose; shivering; sleepless-

ness; sneezing; sore throat; stomach bloating, burning, cramping, or pain; stuffy nose; sunken eyes; sweating; swelling of abdominal or stomach area; swelling of face; swelling of hands, ankles, feet, or lower legs; swollen joints; tender, swollen glands in neck; thirst; trouble concentrating; trouble sleeping; trouble in swallowing; unable to sleep; uncomfortable swelling around anus; unpleasant breath odor; unusual tiredness or weakness; voice changes; vomiting; vomiting of blood; weight loss; wrinkled skin; yellow eyes or skin

Other side effects not listed may also occur in some patients. If you notice any other effects, check with your healthcare professional.

GLYBURIDE AND METFORMIN
(Oral route) - GLYE-byoo-ride, met-FOR-min

Black Box Warning

Lactic acidosis is a rare, but serious, metabolic complication that can occur due to metformin accumulation during treatment with glyburide/metformin hydrochloride; when it occurs, it is fatal in approximately 50% of cases. Lactic acidosis may also occur in association with a number of pathophysiologic conditions, including diabetes mellitus, and whenever there is significant tissue hypoperfusion and hypoxemia. Lactic acidosis is characterized by elevated blood lactate levels (greater than 5 mmol/L), decreased blood pH, electrolyte disturbances with an increased anion gap, and an increased lactate/pyruvate ratio. When metformin is implicated as the cause of lactic acidosis, metformin plasma levels greater than 5 mcg/mL are generally found.

The reported incidence of lactic acidosis in patients receiving metformin hydrochloride is very low (approximately 0.03 cases/1,000 patient-years, with approximately 0.015 fatal cases/1,000 patient-years). Reported cases have occurred primarily in diabetic patients with significant renal insufficiency, including both intrinsic renal disease and renal hypoperfusion, often in the setting of multiple concomitant medical/surgical problems and multiple concomitant medications. Patients with congestive heart failure requiring pharmacologic management, in particular those with unstable or acute congestive heart failure who are at risk of hypoperfusion and hypoxemia, are at increased risk of lactic acidosis. The risk of lactic acidosis increases with the degree of renal dysfunction and the patient's age. The risk of lactic acidosis may, therefore, be significantly decreased by regular monitoring of renal function in patients taking metformin and by use of the minimum effective dose of metformin. In particular, treatment of the elderly should be accompanied by careful monitoring of renal function. Glyburide/metformin hydrochloride treatment should not be initiated in patients greater than or equal to 80 years of age unless measurement of creatinine clearance demonstrates that renal function is not reduced, as these patients are more susceptible to developing lactic acidosis. In addition, glyburide/metformin hydrochloride should be promptly withheld in the presence of any condition associated with hypoxemia, dehydration, or sepsis. Because impaired hepatic function may significantly limit the ability to clear lactate, glyburide/metformin hydrochloride should generally be avoided in patients with clinical or laboratory evidence of hepatic disease. Patients should be cautioned against excessive alcohol intake, either acute or chronic, when taking glyburide/metformin hydrochloride, since alcohol potentiates the effects of metformin hydrochloride on lactate metabolism. In addition, glyburide/metformin hydrochloride should be temporarily discontinued prior to any intravascular radiocontrast study and for any surgical procedure.

The onset of lactic acidosis often is subtle, and accompanied only by nonspecific symptoms such as malaise, myalgias, respiratory distress, increasing somnolence, and nonspecific abdominal distress. There may be associated hypothermia, hypotension, and resistant bradyarrhythmias with more marked acidosis. The patient and the patient's physician must be aware of the possible importance of such symptoms and the patient should be instructed to notify the physician immediately if they occur. Glyburide/metformin hydrochloride should be withdrawn until the situation is clarified. Serum electrolytes, ketones, blood glucose, and, if indicated, blood pH, lactate levels, and even blood metformin levels may be useful. Once a patient is stabilized on any dose level of glyburide/metformin hydrochloride, gastrointestinal symptoms, which are common during initiation of therapy with metformin, are unlikely to be drug related. Later occurrence of gastrointestinal symptoms could be due to lactic acidosis or other serious disease.

Levels of fasting venous plasma lactate above the upper limit of normal but less than 5 mmol/L in patients taking glyburide/metformin hydrochloride do not necessarily indicate impending lactic acidosis and may be explainable by other mechanisms, such as poorly controlled diabetes or obesity, vigorous physical activity, or technical problems in sample handling.

Lactic acidosis should be suspected in any diabetic patient with metabolic acidosis lacking evidence of ketoacidosis (ketonuria and ketonemia).

Lactic acidosis is a medical emergency that must be treated in a hospital setting. In a patient with lactic acidosis who is taking glyburide/metformin hydrochloride, the drug should be discontinued immediately and general supportive measures promptly instituted. Because metformin hydrochloride is dialyzable (with a clearance of up to 170 mL/min under good hemodynamic conditions), prompt hemodialysis is recommended to correct the acidosis and remove the accumulated metformin. Such management often results in prompt reversal of symptoms and recovery.

Commonly used brand name(s)

In the U.S.—
Glucovance

Available Dosage Forms:
• Tablet

Therapeutic Class: Hypoglycemic, Biguanide/Sulfonylurea Combination

Uses For This Medicine

Glyburide and metformin combination is used to treat high blood sugar levels that are caused by a type of diabetes mellitus or sugar diabetes called type 2 diabetes. Normally, after you eat, your pancreas releases insulin to help your body store excess sugar for later use. This process occurs during normal digestion of food. In type 2 diabetes, your body does not work properly to store the excess sugar and the sugar remains in your bloodstream. Chronic high blood sugar can lead to serious health problems in the future. Proper diet is the first step in managing type 2 diabetes but often medicines are needed to help your body. With two actions, the combination of glyburide and metformin helps your body cope with high blood sugar. Glyburide stimulates the release of insulin from the pancreas, directing your body to store blood sugar. Metformin has three different actions: it slows the absorption of sugar in your small intestine; it also stops your liver from converting stored sugar into blood sugar; and it helps your body use your natural insulin more efficiently.

This medicine is available only with your doctor's prescription.

Before Using This Medicine

In deciding to use a medicine, the risks of taking the medicine must be weighed against the good it will do. This is a decision you and your doctor will make. For this medicine, the following should be considered:

Allergies—Tell your doctor if you have ever had any unusual or allergic reaction to this medicine or any other medicines. Also tell your health care professional if you have any other types of allergies, such as to foods, dyes, preservatives, or animals. For non-prescription products, read the label or package ingredients carefully.

Pediatric—Studies on this medicine have been done only in adult patients, and there is no specific information comparing use of glyburide and metformin in children with use in other age groups.

Geriatric—This medicine has been tested and has not been shown to cause different side effects or problems in older people than it does in younger adults.

Pregnancy—

	Pregnancy Category	Explanation
All Trimesters	B	Animal studies have revealed no evidence of harm to the fetus, however, there are no adequate studies in pregnant women OR animal studies have shown an adverse effect, but adequate studies in pregnant women have failed to demonstrate a risk to the fetus.

Breast Feeding—There are no adequate studies in women for determining infant risk when using this medication during breastfeeding. Weigh the potential benefits against the potential risks before taking this medication while breastfeeding.

Other medicines—

Using this medicine with any of the following medicines is not recommended. Your doctor may decide not to treat you with this medication or change some of the other medicines you take.

Acetrizoic Acid, Bosentan, Diatrizoate, Ethiodized Oil, Iobenzamic Acid, Iobitridol, Iocarmic Acid, Iocetamic Acid, Iodamide, Iodipamide, Iodixanol, Iodohippuric Acid, Iodopyracet, Iodoxamic Acid, Ioglicic Acid, Ioglycamic Acid, Iohexol, Iomeprol, Iopamidol, Iopanoic Acid, Iopentol, Iophendylate, Iopromide, Iopronic Acid, Ioseric Acid, Iosimide, Iotasul, Iothalamate, Iotrolan, Iotroxic Acid, Ioversol, Ioxaglate, Ioxita-

Iamic Acid, Ipodate, Metrizamide, Metrizoic Acid, Tyropanoate Sodium

Interactions with Food/Tobacco/Alcohol—Certain medicines should not be used at or around the time of eating food or eating certain types of food since interactions may occur. Using alcohol or tobacco with certain medicines may also cause interactions to occur. The following interactions have been selected on the basis of their potential significance and are not necessarily all-inclusive.

Using this medicine with any of the following is usually not recommended, but may be unavoidable in some cases. If used together, your doctor may change the dose or how often you use this medicine, or give you special instructions about the use of food, alcohol, or tobacco.

Ethanol

Other medical problems—The presence of other medical problems may affect the use of this medicine. Make sure you tell your doctor if you have any other medical problems, especially:

- Acid in the blood (acidosis or ketoacidosis) or
- Surgery (major)—Use of insulin is best to help control diabetes in patients with these conditions.
- Blood poisoning or
- Dehydration (severe) or
- Heart or blood vessel disorders or
- Kidney disease or
- Liver disease—Lactic acidosis can occur in these conditions and chances of it occurring are even greater with a medicine that contains metformin.
- Kidney, heart, or other problems that require medical tests or examinations that use certain medicines called contrast agents, with x-ray exams—Because this medicine contains metformin, your doctor should advise you to stop taking it before you have any medical exams or diagnostic tests that might cause less urine output than usual; you may be advised to start taking the medicine again 48 hours after the exams or tests if your kidney function is tested and found to be normal.

Proper Use of This Medicine

Follow carefully the special meal plan your doctor gave you. This is the most important part of controlling your condition, and is necessary if the medicine is to work properly. Also, exercise regularly and test for sugar in your blood or urine as directed.

Glyburide and metformin combination should be taken with meals to help reduce the gastrointestinal side effects that may occur during the first few weeks of treatment.

Dosing—The dose of this medicine will be different for different patients. Follow your doctor's orders or the directions on the label. The following information includes only the average doses of this medicine. If your dose is different, do not change it unless your doctor tells you to do so.

The amount of medicine that you take depends on the strength of the medicine. Also, the number of doses you take each day, the time allowed between doses, and the length of time you take the medicine depend on the medical problem for which you are using the medicine.

- For oral dosage form (tablets):
  - For type 2 diabetes:
    - For first-time treatment:
      — Adults: At first, 1.25 milligrams (mg) of glyburide and 250 mg of metformin one or two times a day with meals. Then, your doctor may increase your dose a little at a time every two weeks until your blood sugar is controlled.
      — Children: Use and dose must be determined by your doctor.
    - For patients previously treated with a sulfonylurea antidiabetic agent and/or metformin:
      — Adults: At first, 2.5 mg of glyburide and 500 mg of metformin or 5 mg of glyburide and 500 mg of metformin two times a day, with the morning and evening meals. Then, your doctor may increase your dose a little at a time until your blood sugar is controlled.
      — Children: Use and dose must be determined by your doctor.

Storage—Store the medicine in a closed container at room temperature, away from heat, moisture, and direct light. Keep from freezing.

Keep out of the reach of children.

Do not keep outdated medicine or medicine no longer needed.

Ask your healthcare professional how you should dispose of any medicine you do not use.

Precautions While Using This Medicine

Your doctor will want to check your progress at regular visits, especially during the first few weeks that you take this medicine.

Under certain conditions, too much metformin can cause lactic acidosis. Symptoms of lactic acidosis are severe and quick to appear and usually occur when other health problems not related to the medicine are present and are very severe, such as a heart attack or kidney failure. Symptoms of lactic acidosis include abdominal or stomach discomfort; decreased appetite; diarrhea; fast, shallow breathing; general feeling of discomfort; muscle pain or cramping; and unusual sleepiness, tiredness, or weakness.

If symptoms of lactic acidosis occur, you should get immediate emergency medical help.

It is very important to follow carefully any instructions from your health care team about:

- Alcohol—Drinking alcohol may cause severe low blood sugar. Discuss this with your health care team.
- Other medicines—Do not take other medicines unless they have been discussed with your doctor. This especially includes nonprescription medicines such as aspirin, and medicines for appetite control, asthma, colds, cough, hay fever, or sinus problems.
- Counseling—Other family members need to learn how to prevent side effects or help with side effects if they occur. Also, patients with diabetes may need special counseling about diabetes medicine dosing changes that might occur because of lifestyle changes, such as changes in exercise and diet. Furthermore, counseling on contraception and pregnancy may be needed be-

cause of the problems that can occur in patients with diabetes during pregnancy.

- Travel—Keep a recent prescription and your medical history with you. Be prepared for an emergency as you would normally. Make allowances for changing time zones and keep your meal times as close as possible to your usual meal times.

In case of emergency—There may be a time when you need emergency help for a problem caused by your diabetes. You need to be prepared for these emergencies. It is a good idea to wear a medical identification (ID) bracelet or neck chain at all times. Also, carry an ID card in your wallet or purse that says that you have diabetes and a list of all your medicines.

Symptoms of hypoglycemia (low blood sugar) include anxiety; behavior change similar to being drunk; blurred vision; cold sweats; confusion; cool, pale skin; difficulty in thinking; drowsiness; excessive hunger; fast heartbeat; headache (continuing); nausea; nervousness; nightmares; restless sleep; shakiness; slurred speech; or unusual tiredness or weakness.

Glyburide and metformin combination can cause low blood sugar. However, it also can occur if you delay or miss a meal or snack, drink alcohol, exercise more than usual, cannot eat because of nausea or vomiting, take certain medicines, or take glyburide and metformin with another type of diabetes medicine. Symptoms of low blood sugar must be treated before they lead to unconsciousness (passing out). Different people feel different symptoms of low blood sugar. It is important that you learn which symptoms of low blood sugar you usually have so that you can treat it quickly.

If symptoms of low blood sugar occur, eat glucose tablets or gel, corn syrup, honey, or sugar cubes; or drink fruit juice, nondiet soft drink, or sugar dissolved in water. Also, check your blood for low blood sugar. Glucagon is used in emergency situations when severe symptoms such as seizures (convulsions) or unconsciousness occur. Have a glucagon kit available, along with a syringe or needle, and know how to use it. Members of your household also should know how to use it.

Symptoms of hyperglycemia (high blood sugar) include blurred vision; drowsiness; dry mouth; flushed, dry skin; fruit-like breath odor; increased urination (frequency and volume); ketones in urine; loss of appetite; sleepiness; stomachache, nausea, or vomiting; tiredness; troubled breathing (rapid and deep); unconsciousness; or unusual thirst.

High blood sugar may occur if you do not exercise as much as usual, have a fever or infection, do not take enough or skip a dose of your diabetes medicine, or overeat or do not follow your meal plan.

If symptoms of high blood sugar occur, check your blood sugar level and then call your health care professional for instructions.

Side Effects of This Medicine

Along with its needed effects, a medicine may cause some unwanted effects. Although not all of these side effects may occur, if they do occur they may need medical attention.

Check with your doctor immediately if any of the following side effects occur:
More common
Convulsions (seizures); unconsciousness

Rare
Lactic acidosis, including abdominal discomfort, decreased appetite, diarrhea, fast shallow breathing, general feeling of discomfort, muscle pain or cramping, unusual sleepiness, or unusual tiredness or weakness

Check with your doctor as soon as possible if any of the following side effects occur:
More common
Cough; fever; hypoglycemia (low blood sugar), including anxious feeling, behavior change similar to being drunk, blurred vision, cold sweats, confusion, cool pale skin, difficulty in concentrating, drowsiness, excessive hunger, fast heartbeat, headache (continuing), nausea, nervousness, nightmares, restless sleep, shakiness, slurred speech, or unusual tiredness or weakness; sneezing; sore throat

Some side effects may occur that usually do not need medical attention. These side effects may go away during treatment as your body adjusts to the medicine. Also, your health care professional may be able to tell you about ways to prevent or reduce some of these side effects. Check with your health care professional if any of the following side effects continue or are bothersome or if you have any questions about them:
More common
Dizziness; headache; vomiting

Other side effects not listed may also occur in some patients. If you notice any other effects, check with your healthcare professional.

GONADORELIN (Intravenous route, Injection route) - goe-nad-oh-RELL-in

Commonly used brand name(s)
In the U.S.—
Factrel

Available Dosage Forms:
- Powder for Solution
- Kit

Therapeutic Class: Endocrine-Metabolic Agent
Pharmacologic Class: Gonadotropin Releasing Hormone Agonist

Uses For This Medicine

Gonadorelin is a medicine that is the same as gonadotropin-releasing hormone (GnRH) that is naturally released from the hypothalamus gland. GnRH causes the pituitary gland to release other hormones (luteinizing hormone [LH] and follicle-stimulating hormone [FSH]). LH and FSH control development in children and fertility in adults.

Gonadorelin is used to test how well the hypothalamus and the pituitary glands are working. It is also used to cause ovulation (release of an egg from the ovary) in women who do not have regular ovulation and menstrual periods because the hypothalamus gland does not release enough GnRH.

Gonadorelin may also be used for other conditions as determined by your doctor.

Once a medicine has been approved for marketing for a certain use, experience may show that it is also useful for other medical problems. Although not specifically included in product labeling, gonadorelin is used in certain patients with the following medical conditions:

- Delayed puberty
- Infertility in males caused by pituitary or hypothalamus problems

Before Using This Medicine

In deciding to use a medicine, the risks of taking the medicine must be weighed against the good it will do. This is a decision you and your doctor will make. For this medicine, the following should be considered:

Allergies—Tell your doctor if you have ever had any unusual or allergic reaction to this medicine or any other medicines. Also tell your health care professional if you have any other types of allergies, such as to foods, dyes, preservatives, or animals. For non-prescription products, read the label or package ingredients carefully.

Pediatric—Gonadorelin, used as a test, has been studied only in children 12 years of age and older. The medicine has not caused different side effects or problems in children 12 years of age and older than it does in adults. Children up to 12 years of age may not be sensitive to the effects of gonadorelin. Infants may be very sensitive to the effects of gonadorelin and use in infants is not recommended.

Pregnancy—

	Pregnancy Category	Explanation
All Trimesters	B	Animal studies have revealed no evidence of harm to the fetus, however, there are no adequate studies in pregnant women OR animal studies have shown an adverse effect, but adequate studies in pregnant women have failed to demonstrate a risk to the fetus.

Breast Feeding—There are no adequate studies in women for determining infant risk when using this medication during breastfeeding. Weigh the potential benefits against the potential risks before taking this medication while breastfeeding.

Other medicines—Although certain medicines should not be used together at all, in other cases two different medicines may be used together even if an interaction might occur. In these cases, your doctor may want to change the dose, or other precautions may be necessary. Tell your healthcare professional if you are taking any other prescription or non-prescription (over-the-counter [OTC]) medicine.

Interactions with Food/Tobacco/Alcohol—Certain medicines should not be used at or around the time of eating food or eating certain types of food since interactions may occur. Using alcohol or tobacco with certain medicines may also cause interactions to occur. Discuss with your healthcare professional the use of your medicine with food, alcohol, or tobacco.

Other medical problems—The presence of other medical problems may affect the use of this medicine. Make sure you tell your doctor if you have any other medical problems, especially:

- Gonadotropin-releasing hormone adenoma—Although this condition is rare, use of gonadorelin when this condition exists may cause problems in the pituitary gland and could result in sudden blindness
- Any condition that may be made worse by estrogens, progestins, or androgens, such as a hormone-dependent tumor—The increase of estrogens and progestins in women or androgens in men that can result from use of multiple doses of gonadorelin may make a tumor worse if the tumor depends on estrogens, progestins, or androgens for growth

Proper Use of This Medicine

If you are having a test done with gonadorelin, one or more samples of your blood will be taken. Then gonadorelin is given by an intravenous (into a vein) or a subcutaneous (under the skin) injection. At regular times after the medicine is given, more blood samples will be taken. Then the results of the test will be studied.

Some medicines given by injection or by injection pump may sometimes be given at home to patients who do not need to be in the hospital. If you are using this medicine at home, make sure you clearly understand and carefully follow your doctor's instructions.

Dosing—The dose of this medicine will be different for different patients. Follow your doctor's orders or the directions on the label. The following information includes only the average doses of this medicine. If your dose is different, do not change it unless your doctor tells you to do so.

The amount of medicine that you take depends on the strength of the medicine. Also, the number of doses you take each day, the time allowed between doses, and the length of time you take the medicine depend on the medical problem for which you are using the medicine.

- For injection dosage form (for Lutrepulse pump):
  - For treating amenorrhea or infertility in women caused by pituitary or hypothalamus problems:
    - Adults—5 microgram (mcg) injected by the pump into a vein or under the skin slowly over 1 minute, every ninety minutes for twenty-one days. As determined by doctor, dose may be changed slowly, decreased to 1 mcg or increased to 20 mcg if needed.
    - Children up to 18 years of age—Use and dose must be determined by the doctor.
- For injection dosage form (single-dose injection):
  - For testing the hypothalamus and pituitary glands:
    - Adults—0.1 milligram (mg) injected once as a single dose under the skin or into a vein.
    - Children 12 years of age and older—2 micrograms (mcg) per kilogram (kg) (0.9 mcg per pound) of body weight, not to exceed a single dose of 100 mcg, injected once under the skin or into vein.
    - Children up to 12 years of age—Use and dose must be determined by doctor.

Precautions While Using This Medicine

For *Lutrepulse* pump—*It is very important that your doctor check your progress at regular visits.* This will allow the doctor to see if the medicine is working properly and to decide if you should continue to use it.

If you are using gonadorelin to help you become pregnant, *closely follow your doctor's advice on the best times to have sexual intercourse.* Your doctor can help you decide when having sexual intercourse will not result in a pregnancy with twins or triplets.

Tell your doctor when you suspect your are pregnant.

Side Effects of This Medicine

Along with its needed effects, a medicine may cause some unwanted effects. Although not all of these side effects may occur, if they do occur they may need medical attention.

Check with your doctor immediately if any of the following side effects occur:

With repeated doses
  Difficulty in breathing; flushing (continuing); rapid heartbeat

Check with your doctor as soon as possible if any of the following side effects occur:

With repeated doses
  Hardening of skin at place of injection; hives

With single or repeated doses
  Itching, pain, redness or swelling of skin at place of injection; skin rash (at place of injection or over entire body)

Some side effects may occur that usually do not need medical attention. These side effects may go away during treatment as your body adjusts to the medicine. Also, your health care professional may be able to tell you about ways to prevent or reduce some of these side effects. Check with your health care professional if any of the following side effects continue or are bothersome or if you have any questions about them:

Less common
With single dose
  Abdominal or stomach discomfort; flushing (lasting only a short time); headaches; lightheadedness; nausea

Other side effects not listed may also occur in some patients. If you notice any other effects, check with your healthcare professional.

GOSERELIN (Subcutaneous route) -
GOE-se-rel-in

Commonly used brand name(s)

In the U.S.—
  Zoladex

Available Dosage Forms:
  • Implant

Therapeutic Class: Antineoplastic Agent
Pharmacologic Class: Luteinizing Hormone Releasing Hormone Agonist

Uses For This Medicine

Goserelin is a hormone similar to the one normally released from the hypothalamus gland in the brain. It is used to treat a number of medical problems. These include:

  • Cancer of the prostate in men
  • Cancer of the breast in women if it develops before or around the time of menopause
  • Endometriosis, a painful condition caused by extra tissue growing inside or outside of the uterus and
  • Thinning of the lining of the uterus before surgery on the uterus

When given regularly as an implant, goserelin works every day to decrease the amount of estrogen and testosterone in the blood.

Reducing the amount of estrogen in the body is one way of treating endometriosis and cancer of the breast, and can help thin the uterus lining before surgery. Goserelin prevents the growth of tissue associated with endometriosis in adult women during treatment and for up to 6 months after treatment is discontinued.

Reducing the amount of testosterone in the body is one way of treating cancer of the prostate.

Suppressing estrogen can thin the bones or slow their growth. This is a problem for adult women whose bones are no longer growing like the bones of children. This is why goserelin is used only for up to 6 months in adult women treated for endometriosis.

Goserelin is to be given only by or under the supervision of your doctor. It is injected under the skin.

Before Using This Medicine

In deciding to use a medicine, the risks of taking the medicine must be weighed against the good it will do. This is a decision you and your doctor will make. For this medicine, the following should be considered:

Allergies—Tell your doctor if you have ever had any unusual or allergic reaction to this medicine or any other medicines. Also tell your health care professional if you have any other types of allergies, such as to foods, dyes, preservatives, or animals. For non-prescription products, read the label or package ingredients carefully.

Pediatric—Studies of this medicine have been done only in adult patients, and there is no specific information comparing use of goserelin in children younger than 18 years of age with use in other age groups. Endometriosis is not likely to occur before puberty.

Geriatric—Many medicines have not been tested in older people. Therefore, it may not be known whether they work exactly the same way they do in younger adults. Although there is no specific information comparing use of goserelin in the elderly to use in other age groups, it has been used mostly in elderly patients and is not expected to cause different side effects or problems in older people than it does in younger adults.

Pregnancy—

	Pregnancy Category	Explanation
All Trimesters	X	Studies in animals or pregnant women have demonstrated positive evidence of fetal abnormalities. This drug should not be used in women who are or may become pregnant because the risk clearly outweighs any possible benefit.

Breast Feeding—There are no adequate studies in women for determining infant risk when using this medication during breastfeeding. Weigh the potential benefits against the potential risks before taking this medication while breastfeeding.

Other medicines—Although certain medicines should not be used together at all, in other cases two different medicines may be used together even if an interaction might occur. In these cases, your doctor may want to change the dose, or other precautions may be necessary. Tell your healthcare professional if you are taking any other prescription or nonprescription (over-the-counter [OTC]) medicine.

Interactions with Food/Tobacco/Alcohol—Certain medicines should not be used at or around the time of eating food or eating certain types of food since interactions may occur. Using alcohol or tobacco with certain medicines may also cause interactions to occur. Discuss with your healthcare professional the use of your medicine with food, alcohol, or tobacco.

Other medical problems—The presence of other medical problems may affect the use of this medicine. Make sure you tell your doctor if you have any other medical problems, especially:

- Changes in vaginal bleeding from an unknown cause—Gonadorelin may delay diagnosis or worsen condition. The reason for the bleeding should be determined before goserelin is used
- Conditions that increase the chances of developing thinning bones or
- Osteoporosis (brittle bones), history of, or family history of—It is important that your doctor know if you already have an increased risk of osteoporosis. Some things that can increase your risk for having osteoporosis include cigarette smoking, alcohol abuse, and a family history of osteoporosis or easily broken bones. Some medicines, such as corticosteroids (cortisone-like medicines) or anticonvulsants (seizure medicine), can also cause thinning of the bones when used for a long time
- Nerve problems caused by bone lesions in the spine (in treatment of cancer of the prostate) or
- Problems in passing urine (in treatment of cancer of the prostate)—Conditions may get worse for a short time after goserelin treatment is started

Proper Use of This Medicine

Goserelin sometimes causes unwanted effects such as hot flashes or decreased sexual ability. However, it is very important that you continue to receive the medicine, even after you begin to feel better. Do not stop treatment with this medicine without first checking with your doctor.

Dosing—The dose of this medicine will be different for different patients. Follow your doctor's orders or the directions on the label. The following information includes only the average doses of this medicine. If your dose is different, do not change it unless your doctor tells you to do so.

The amount of medicine that you take depends on the strength of the medicine. Also, the number of doses you take each day, the time allowed between doses, and the length of time you take the medicine depend on the medical problem for which you are using the medicine.

- For implants dosage form:
  - For treating cancer of the breast:
    - Adults—3.6 milligrams (mg) (one implant) injected under the skin of the upper abdomen every twenty-eight days.
    - Children up to 18 years of age—Use and dose must be determined by the doctor.
  - For treating cancer of the prostate:
    - Adults—3.6 milligrams (mg) (one implant) injected under the skin of the upper abdomen every twenty-eight days or 10.8 mg (one implant) injected under the skin of the upper abdomen every twelve weeks.
    - Children up to 18 years of age—Use and dose must be determined by the doctor.
  - For treating endometriosis:
    - Adults—3.6 milligrams (mg) (one implant) injected under the skin of the upper abdomen every twenty-eight days for six months.
    - Children up to 18 years of age—Use must be determined by the doctor.
  - For thinning the uterus before surgery of the uterus:
    - Adults—3.6 milligrams (mg) (one implant) injected under the skin of the upper abdomen every twenty-eight days for two doses.
    - Children up to 18 years of age—Use and dose must be determined by the doctor.

Missed dose—Call your doctor or pharmacist for instructions.

If you miss getting a dose of this medicine, receive it as soon as possible.

Precautions While Using This Medicine

It is very important that your doctor check your progress at regular visits to make sure that this medicine is working properly and to check for unwanted effects.

For women—

- During the time you are receiving goserelin, your menstrual period may not be regular or you may not have a menstrual period at all. This is to be expected when being treated with this medicine. If regular menstrual periods continue during treatment or do not begin within 2 to 3 months after you stop using this medicine, check with your health care professional.
- To prevent pregnancy if you are sexually active and able to become pregnant, you should use birth control methods that do not contain hormones, such as vaginal spermicides with condoms, a diaphragm, or a cervical cap. If you have any questions about this, check with your health care professional.
- If you suspect you are pregnant, check with your doctor immediately. There is a chance goserelin could cause problems to the unborn baby if taken during a pregnancy.

During use of goserelin, and usually for a short time after discontinuing it, the medicine decreases fertility in men by reducing sperm counts and in many women by suppressing egg development. Be sure you have discussed this with your doctor before receiving the medicine.

Side Effects of This Medicine

Along with its needed effects, a medicine may cause some unwanted effects. Although not all of these side effects may occur, if they do occur they may need medical attention.

Check with your doctor immediately if any of the following side effects occur:

> *For adults*
>> *Less common*
>>> Fast or irregular heartbeat
>>
>> *Rare*
>>> Bone, muscle, or joint pain; changes in skin color of face; fainting; fast or irregular breathing; numbness or tingling of hands or feet; puffiness or swelling of the eyelids or around the eyes; shortness of breath; skin rash, hives, and/or itching; sudden, severe decrease in blood pressure and collapse; tightness in chest or wheezing; troubled breathing
>
> *For males only*
>> *Rare*
>>> Pains in chest; pain in groin or legs (especially in calves of legs)

Check with your doctor as soon as possible if any of the following side effects occur:

> *For females only*
>> *Rare*
>>> Anxiety; deepening of voice; increased hair growth; mental depression; mood changes; nervousness

Some side effects may occur that usually do not need medical attention. These side effects may go away during treatment as your body adjusts to the medicine. Also, your health care professional may be able to tell you about ways to prevent or reduce some of these side effects. Check with your health care professional if any of the following side effects continue or are bothersome or if you have any questions about them:

> *For females and males*
>> *More common*
>>> Sudden sweating and feelings of warmth (also called hot flashes)
>>
>> *Less common*
>>> Blurred vision; burning, itching, redness, or swelling at place of injection; decreased interest in sexual intercourse; dizziness; headache; nausea or vomiting; swelling and increased tenderness of breasts; swelling of feet or lower legs; trouble in sleeping; weight gain
>
> *For females only*
>> *More common*
>>> Light, irregular vaginal bleeding; stopping of menstrual periods
>>
>> *Less common*
>>> Burning, dryness, or itching of vagina; pelvic pain
>
> *For males only*
>> *Less common*
>>> Bone pain; constipation; decreased size of testicles; inability to have or keep an erection

Other side effects not listed may also occur in some patients. If you notice any other effects, check with your healthcare professional.

GRANISETRON (Oral route, Intravenous route) - gra-NI-se-tron

Commonly used brand name(s)

In the U.S.—
  Kytril

Available Dosage Forms:
  • Solution
  • Tablet

Therapeutic Class: Antiemetic
Pharmacologic Class: Serotonin Receptor Antagonist, 5–HT3

Uses For This Medicine

Granisetron is used to prevent the nausea and vomiting that may occur after treatment with anticancer medicines (chemotherapy) or with radiation therapy.

Granisetron is to be given only by or under the immediate supervision of your doctor.

Once a medicine has been approved for marketing for a certain use, experience may show that it is also useful for other medical problems. Although this use is not included in product labeling, granisetron injection is used in certain patients:

  • To prevent the nausea and vomiting that may occur after cancer radiation treatment in patients undergoing bone marrow transplantation.

Before Receiving This Medicine

In deciding to use a medicine, the risks of taking the medicine must be weighed against the good it will do. This is a decision you and your doctor will make. For this medicine, the following should be considered:

Allergies—Tell your doctor if you have ever had any unusual or allergic reaction to this medicine or any other medicines. Also tell your health care professional if you have any other types of allergies, such as to foods, dyes, preservatives, or animals. For non-prescription products, read the label or package ingredients carefully.

Pediatric—This medicine has been tested in children 2 years of age and older and, in effective doses, has not been shown to cause different side effects or problems than it does in adults.

Geriatric—This medicine has been tested in a limited number of patients 65 years of age or older and has not been shown to cause different side effects or problems in older people than it does in younger adults.

Pregnancy—

	Pregnancy Category	Explanation
All Trimesters	B	Animal studies have revealed no evidence of harm to the fetus, however, there are no adequate studies in pregnant women OR animal studies have shown an adverse effect, but adequate studies in pregnant women have failed to demonstrate a risk to the fetus.

Breast Feeding—There are no adequate studies in women for determining infant risk when using this medication during

breastfeeding. Weigh the potential benefits against the potential risks before taking this medication while breastfeeding.

Other medicines—

Using this medicine with any of the following medicines is not recommended. Your doctor may decide not to treat you with this medication or change some of the other medicines you take.

Apomorphine

Interactions with Food/Tobacco/Alcohol—Certain medicines should not be used at or around the time of eating food or eating certain types of food since interactions may occur. Using alcohol or tobacco with certain medicines may also cause interactions to occur. Discuss with your healthcare professional the use of your medicine with food, alcohol, or tobacco.

Other medical problems—The presence of other medical problems may affect the use of this medicine. Make sure you tell your doctor if you have any other medical problems, especially:

The presence of other medical problems may affect the use of granisetron. Make sure you tell your doctor if you have any other medical problems, especially:

- Abdominal (stomach) surgery, very recent or

- Nausea and vomiting from the chemotherapy—If granisetron is taken when these medical problems exist, it may mask very serious stomach problems.

Proper Use of This Medicine

Dosing—The dose of this medicine will be different for different patients. Follow your doctor's orders or the directions on the label. The following information includes only the average doses of this medicine. If your dose is different, do not change it unless your doctor tells you to do so.

The amount of medicine that you take depends on the strength of the medicine. Also, the number of doses you take each day, the time allowed between doses, and the length of time you take the medicine depend on the medical problem for which you are using the medicine.

- For prevention of nausea and vomiting caused by anticancer medicine:
  - For oral dosage form (tablets):
    - Adults and teenagers—Dose is usually 1 milligram (mg) taken up to one hour before the anticancer medicine. The 1–mg dose is taken again twelve hours after the first dose. Alternatively, 2 mg may be taken as one dose, up to one hour before the anticancer medicine.
    - Children—Dose must be determined by your doctor.
  - For injection dosage form:
    - Adults and children 2 years of age or older—Dose is based on body weight and must be determined by your doctor. It is usually 10 micrograms (mcg) per kilogram (kg) (4.5 mcg per pound) of body weight. It is injected into a vein over a period of five minutes, beginning within thirty minutes before the anticancer medicine is given.
    - Children up to 2 years of age—Dose must be determined by your doctor.

- For prevention of nausea and vomiting caused by radiation therapy:
  - For oral dosage form (tablets):
    - Adults and teenagers—Dose is 2 milligrams (two 1 milligram tablets) taken within 1 hour of radiation.
    - Children—Dose must be determined by your doctor.

Precautions After Receiving This Medicine

Check with your doctor if severe nausea and vomiting occur after receiving the anticancer medicine.

Side Effects of This Medicine

Along with its needed effects, a medicine may cause some unwanted effects. Although not all of these side effects may occur, if they do occur they may need medical attention.

Check with your doctor as soon as possible if any of the following side effects occur:

Less common
   Blurred vision; fever; nervousness; pounding in the ears; slow or fast heartbeat

Rare
   Arm, back or jaw pain; chest pain or discomfort; chest tightness or heaviness; confusion; dizziness, faintness, or lightheadedness when getting up from a lying or sitting position suddenly; fainting; irregular heartbeat; nausea; shortness of breath; skin rash, hives, and itching; sweating

Some side effects may occur that usually do not need medical attention. These side effects may go away during treatment as your body adjusts to the medicine. Also, your health care professional may be able to tell you about ways to prevent or reduce some of these side effects. Check with your health care professional if any of the following side effects continue or are bothersome or if you have any questions about them:

More common
   Abdominal pain; constipation; diarrhea; headache; lack or loss of strength; unusual tiredness or weakness; vomiting

Less common
   Agitation; dizziness; drowsiness; fear; heartburn; indigestion; nervousness; sleepiness or unusual drowsiness; sour stomach; trouble in sleeping; unusual taste in mouth

GRISEOFULVIN (Oral route) - gri-see-oh-FUL-vin

Commonly used brand name(s)

In the U.S.—
   Fulvicin P/G   Grifulvin V
   Fulvicin-U/F   Gris-PEG

Available Dosage Forms:
- Capsule
- Tablet
- Suspension

Therapeutic Class: Antifungal

Uses For This Medicine

Griseofulvin belongs to the group of medicines called antifungals. It is used to treat fungus infections of the skin, hair, fingernails, and toenails. This medicine may be taken alone or used along with medicines that are applied to the skin for fungus infections.

Griseofulvin is available only with your doctor's prescription.

Before Using This Medicine

In deciding to use a medicine, the risks of taking the medicine must be weighed against the good it will do. This is a decision you and your doctor will make. For this medicine, the following should be considered:

Allergies—Tell your doctor if you have ever had any unusual or allergic reaction to this medicine or any other medicines. Also tell your health care professional if you have any other types of allergies, such as to foods, dyes, preservatives, or animals. For non-prescription products, read the label or package ingredients carefully.

Pediatric—This medicine has been tested in a limited number of children 2 years of age or older. In effective doses, the medicine has not been shown to cause different side effects or problems than it does in adults.

Geriatric—Many medicines have not been studied specifically in older people. Therefore, it may not be known whether they work exactly the same way they do in younger adults. Although there is no specific information comparing use of griseofulvin in the elderly with use in other age groups, this medicine is not expected to cause different side effects or problems in older people than it does in younger adults.

Breast Feeding—There are no adequate studies in women for determining infant risk when using this medication during breastfeeding. Weigh the potential benefits against the potential risks before taking this medication while breastfeeding.

Other medicines—

Using this medicine with any of the following medicines may cause an increased risk of certain side effects, but using both drugs may be the best treatment for you. If both medicines are prescribed together, your doctor may change the dose or how often you use one or both of the medicines.

Ethinyl Estradiol, Etonogestrel, Levonorgestrel, Mestranol, Norelgestromin, Norethindrone, Norgestrel, Phenobarbital, Warfarin

Interactions with Food/Tobacco/Alcohol—Certain medicines should not be used at or around the time of eating food or eating certain types of food since interactions may occur. Using alcohol or tobacco with certain medicines may also cause interactions to occur. The following interactions have been selected on the basis of their potential significance and are not necessarily all-inclusive.

Using this medicine with any of the following is usually not recommended, but may be unavoidable in some cases. If used together, your doctor may change the dose or how often you use this medicine, or give you special instructions about the use of food, alcohol, or tobacco.

Ethanol

Other medical problems—The presence of other medical problems may affect the use of this medicine. Make sure you tell your doctor if you have any other medical problems, especially:

- Liver disease—Griseofulvin may on rare occasion cause side effects affecting the liver

- Lupus erythematosus or lupus-like diseases—Griseofulvin may worsen lupus symptoms in patients who have lupus erythematosus or lupus-like diseases

- Porphyria—Griseofulvin may increase attacks of porphyria in patients with acute intermittent porphyria

Proper Use of This Medicine

Griseofulvin is absorbed best when it is taken with a high fat meal, such as a cheeseburger, whole milk, or ice cream. Tell your doctor if you are on a low-fat diet.

Griseofulvin is best taken with or after meals, especially fatty ones (for example, whole milk or ice cream). This lessens possible stomach upset and helps to clear up the infection by helping your body absorb the medicine better. However, if you are on a low-fat diet, check with your doctor.

For patients taking the oral liquid form of griseofulvin:

- Use a specially marked measuring spoon or other device to measure each dose accurately. The average household teaspoon may not hold the right amount of liquid.

To help clear up your infection completely, keep taking this medicine for the full time of treatment, even if you begin to feel better after a few days. Do not miss any doses.

Dosing—The dose of this medicine will be different for different patients. Follow your doctor's orders or the directions on the label. The following information includes only the average doses of this medicine. If your dose is different, do not change it unless your doctor tells you to do so.

The amount of medicine that you take depends on the strength of the medicine. Also, the number of doses you take each day, the time allowed between doses, and the length of time you take the medicine depend on the medical problem for which you are using the medicine.

- For microsize capsules, tablets, and suspension:
  - Adults and teenagers:
    - Treatment of fungus infections of the feet and nails—500 milligrams (mg) every twelve hours.
    - Treatment of fungus infections of the scalp, skin, and groin—250 mg every twelve hours; or 500 mg once a day.
  - Children:
    - Treatment of fungus infections—Dose is based on body weight. The usual dose is 5 mg per kilogram (kg) (2.3 mg per pound) of body weight every twelve hours; or 10 mg per kg (4.6 mg per pound) of body weight once a day.

- For ultramicrosize tablets:
  - Adults and teenagers:
    - Treatment of fungus infections of the feet and nails—250 to 375 mg every twelve hours.
    - Treatment of fungus infections of the scalp, skin, and groin—125 to 187.5 mg every twelve hours; or 250 to 375 mg once a day.
  - Infants and children up to 2 years of age:
    - Treatment of fungus infections—Use and dose must be determined by your doctor.
  - Children 2 years of age and over:
    - Treatment of fungus infections—Dose is based on body weight. The usual dose is 2.75 to 3.65 mg per kg (1.25 to 1.7 mg per pound) of body weight every twelve hours; or 5.5 to 7.3 mg per kg (2.5 to 3.3 mg per pound) of body weight once a day.

Missed dose—If you miss a dose of this medicine, take it as soon as possible. However, if it is almost time for your next dose, skip the missed dose and go back to your regular dosing schedule. Do not double doses.

Storage—Store the medicine in a closed container at room temperature, away from heat, moisture, and direct light. Keep from freezing.

Keep out of the reach of children.

Do not keep outdated medicine or medicine no longer needed.

Precautions While Using This Medicine

Your doctor should check your progress at regular visits to make sure that griseofulvin does not cause unwanted effects.

Oral contraceptives (birth control pills) containing estrogen may not work properly if you take them while you are taking griseofulvin. Unplanned pregnancies may occur. You should use a different or additional means of birth control while you are taking griseofulvin and for one month after stopping griseofulvin. If you have any questions about this, check with your health care professional.

Griseofulvin may increase the effects of alcohol. If taken with alcohol it may also cause fast heartbeat, flushing, increased sweating, or redness of the face. Therefore, if you have this reaction, do not drink alcoholic beverages while you are taking this medicine, unless you have first checked with your doctor.

This medicine may cause some people to become dizzy or less alert than they are normally. Make sure you know how you react to this medicine before you drive, use machines, or do other things that could be dangerous if you are dizzy or are not alert. If these reactions are especially bothersome, check with your doctor.

Griseofulvin may cause your skin to be more sensitive to sunlight than it is normally. Exposure to sunlight, even for brief periods of time, may cause a skin rash, itching, redness or other discoloration of the skin, or a severe sunburn. When you begin taking this medicine:

- Stay out of direct sunlight, especially between the hours of 10:00 a.m. and 3:00 p.m., if possible.
- Wear protective clothing, including a hat. Also, wear sunglasses.
- Apply a sun block product that has a skin protection factor (SPF) of at least 15. Some patients may require a product with a higher SPF number, especially if they have a fair complexion. If you have any questions about this, check with your health care professional.

- Apply a sun block lipstick that has an SPF of at least 15 to protect your lips.
- Do not use a sunlamp or tanning bed or booth.

If you have a severe reaction from the sun, check with your doctor.

Side Effects of This Medicine

Griseofulvin has been shown to cause liver and thyroid tumors in some animals. You and your doctor should discuss the good this medicine will do, as well as the risks of taking it.

Along with its needed effects, a medicine may cause some unwanted effects. Although not all of these side effects may occur, if they do occur they may need medical attention.

Check with your doctor as soon as possible if any of the following side effects occur:

Less common
> Confusion; increased sensitivity of skin to sunlight; skin rash, hives, or itching; soreness or irritation of mouth or tongue

Rare
> Numbness, tingling, pain, or weakness in hands or feet; sore throat and fever; yellow eyes or skin

Some side effects may occur that usually do not need medical attention. These side effects may go away during treatment as your body adjusts to the medicine. Also, your health care professional may be able to tell you about ways to prevent or reduce some of these side effects. Check with your health care professional if any of the following side effects continue or are bothersome or if you have any questions about them:

More common
> Headache

Less common
> Diarrhea; dizziness; nausea or vomiting; stomach pain; trouble in sleeping; unusual tiredness

Other side effects not listed may also occur in some patients. If you notice any other effects, check with your healthcare professional.

GROWTH HORMONE   (Systemic)

Some commonly used brand names are:

In the U.S.—

Genotropin (2)	Nutropin (2)
Genotropin Miniquick (2)	Nutropin AQ (2)
Humatrope (2)	Protropin (1)
Norditropin cartridges (2)	Saizen (2)
Norditropin NordiFlex (2)	Serostim (2)

In Canada—

Humatrope (2)	Protropin (1)
Nutropin (2)	Saizen (2)
Nutropin AQ (2)	Serostim (2)

This information applies to the following medicines:

1. Somatrem (SOE-ma-trem)
2. Somatropin, Recombinant (soe-ma-TROE-pin, re-KOM-bi-nant)

Category

- **Growth hormone**—Somatrem; Somatropin

Description

Somatrem and somatropin are man-made versions of human growth hormone. Growth hormone is naturally produced by the pituitary gland and is necessary to stimulate growth in children. Man-made growth hormone may be used in children who have certain conditions that cause failure to grow normally. These conditions include growth hormone deficiency (inability to produce enough growth hormone), kidney disease, Prader-Willi Syndrome (PWS), and Turner's syndrome. Growth hormone is also used in adults to treat growth failure and to treat weight loss caused by acquired immunodeficiency syndrome (AIDS).

This medicine is available only with your doctor's prescription, in the following dosage forms:

Parenteral
- Somatrem
  - Injection
- Somatropin, Recombinant
  - Injection

Before Using This Medicine

In deciding to use a medicine, the risks of taking the medicine must be weighed against the good it will do. This is a decision you and your doctor will make. For growth hormone, the following should be considered:

Allergies—Tell your doctor if you have ever had any unusual or allergic reaction to growth hormone. Also tell your health care professional if you are allergic to any other substances, such as foods, preservatives (especially benzyl alcohol), or dyes.

Pregnancy—Growth hormone has not been studied in pregnant women. However, in animal studies, growth hormone has not been shown to cause birth defects or other problems. This drug should be used during pregnancy only if clearly needed. Tell your doctor if you are pregnant or plan on becoming pregnant.

Breast-feeding—It is not known whether growth hormone passes into breast milk. However, you should tell your doctor if you are nursing.

Children—There is no specific information comparing use of growth hormone in children with acquired immunodeficiency syndrome (AIDS) with use in other age groups.

Older adults—Many medicines have not been studied specifically in older people. Therefore, it may not be known whether they work exactly the same way they do in younger adults. Although there is no specific information comparing use of growth hormone in the elderly with use in other age groups, it is not expected to cause different side effects or problems in older people than it does in younger adults. However, elderly patients may be more sensitive to the action of growth hormone drugs and may be more at risk to develop adverse reactions.

Other medicines—Although certain medicines should not be used together at all, in other cases two different medicines may be used together even if an interaction might occur. In these cases, your doctor may want to change the dose, or other precautions may be necessary. When you are taking growth hormone, it is especially important that your health care professional know if you are taking any of the following:

- Corticosteroids (cortisone-like medicines)—These medicines can interfere with the effects of growth hormone

Other medical problems—The presence of other medical problems may affect the use of growth hormone. Make sure you tell your doctor if you have any other medical problems, especially:

- Acute critical illnesses (e.g., complications following open heart or abdominal surgery, accidental trauma, or respiratory failure)—Growth hormone use has not been studied in patients with these serious illnesses. Your doctor will weigh the benefits and risks before starting you on this medicine.
- Brain tumor—Growth hormone should not be used in patients who have a brain tumor that is still growing
- Diabetes mellitus (sugar diabetes) or a family history of diabetes mellitus—Growth hormone may prevent insulin from working as well as it should; your doctor may have to change your dose of insulin
- Diabetic retinopathy (inflammation of the retina in diabetic patients)—Growth hormone should not be used in these patients.
- Prader-Willi syndrome [a rare genetic disorder]—Certain patients with this rare genetic disorder may be at increased risk for side effects from growth hormone therapy. You and your doctor will decide if growth hormone is right for you.
- Tumors—If you already have a tumor, your doctor should treat you for it before beginning this medicine. If the tumor comes back, growth hormone medicine should be stopped.
- Underactive thyroid—This condition can interfere with the effects of growth hormone

Proper Use of This Medicine

Some medicines given by injection may sometimes be given at home to patients who do not need to be in the hospital. If you are using this medicine at home, your health care professional will teach you how to prepare and inject the medicine. You will have a chance to practice preparing and injecting it. *Be certain that you understand exactly how the medicine is to be prepared and injected.*

It is important to read the patient information and instructions for use, if provided with your medicine, each time your prescription is filled.

It is important to follow any instructions from your doctor about the careful selection and rotation of injection sites on your body. This will help to prevent skin problems.

Put used needles and syringes in a puncture-resistant disposable container or dispose of them as directed by your health care professional. *Do not reuse needles and syringes.*

Dosing—The dose of these medicines will be different for different patients. *Follow your doctor's orders or the directions on the label.* The following information includes only the average doses of these medicines. *If your dose is different, do not change it* unless your doctor tells you to do so.

For somatrem
- For *injection* dosage form:
  - For treatment of growth failure caused by growth hormone deficiency:
    - Children—Dose is based on body weight and must be determined by your doctor. The usual total weekly dose is 0.3 milligram (mg) per kilogram

(kg) (0.136 mg per pound) of body weight. This is divided into smaller doses and usually is injected under the skin, but may be injected into a muscle as determined by your doctor.

For somatropin

- For *injection* dosage form:
  - For treatment of growth failure caused by growth hormone deficiency:
    - Adults—Dose is based on body weight and must be determined by your doctor. At first, it is usually 0.005 milligram (mg) per kilogram (kg) (0.0023 mg per pound) of body weight injected under the skin once a day. Your doctor may then increase the dose if needed.
    - Adults using Norditropin Cartridges or Norditropin NordiFlex—Dose is based on body weight and must be determined by your doctor. At first, it is usually 0.004 milligram (mg) per kilogram (kg) (0.0002 mg per pound) of body weight injected under the skin once a day. Your doctor may then increase the dose if needed. The dose is given using a NordiPen injection device for Norditropin cartridges and a prefilled pen for Norditropin NordiFlex.
    - Children—Dose is based on body weight and must be determined by your doctor. The usual total weekly dose is 0.16 to 0.3 mg per kg (0.073 to 0.136 mg per pound) of body weight. This is divided into smaller doses and usually is injected under the skin, but may be injected into a muscle as determined by your doctor.
    - Children using Norditropin Cartridges or Norditropin NordiFlex—Dose is based on body weight and must be determined by your doctor. The usual dose is 0.024 to 0.034 mg per kg (0.011 to 0.015 mg per pound of body weight) injected under the skin, on 6 to 7 days a week. The dose is given using a NordiPen injection device for Norditropin cartridges and a prefilled pen for Norditropin NordiFlex.
  - For treatment of growth failure caused by kidney disease:
    - Children—Dose is based on body weight and must be determined by your doctor. The usual total weekly dose is 0.35 mg per kg (0.16 mg per pound) of body weight. This is divided into smaller daily doses and is injected under the skin or into a muscle.
  - For treatment of growth failure caused by Turner's syndrome:
    - Children—Dose is based on body weight and must be determined by your doctor. The usual total weekly dose is 0.375 mg per kg (0.17 mg per pound) of body weight. This is divided into smaller doses and is injected under the skin.
  - For treatment of growth failure caused by Prader-Willi syndrome:
    - Children—Dose is based on body weight and must be determined by your doctor. The usual total weekly dose is 0.24 mg per kg (0.11 mg per pound) of body weight. This is divided into 6 or 7 smaller doses over the course of the week and is injected under the skin.
  - For treatment of weight loss caused by acquired immunodeficiency disease (AIDS):
    - Adults weighing more than 121 pounds (55 kg)—6 mg injected under the skin once a day at bedtime.
    - Adults weighing 99 to 121 pounds (45 to 55 kg)—5 mg injected under the skin once a day at bedtime.
    - Adults weighing 77 to 98 pounds (35 to 44 kg)—4 mg injected under the skin once a day at bedtime.
    - Adults weighing less than 77 pounds (35 kg)—Dose is based on body weight and must be determined by your doctor. It is usually 0.1 mg per kg (0.045 mg per pound) of body weight injected under the skin once a day at bedtime.
    - Children—Use and dose must be determined by your doctor.

Storage—To store this medicine:

- Keep out of the reach of children.
- Store away from heat and direct light.
- Store at temperature directed by your health care professional or the manufacturer.
- Do not keep outdated medicine or medicine no longer needed. Be sure that any discarded medicine is out of the reach of children.

Precautions While Using This Medicine

It is important that your doctor check your progress at regular visits.

Side Effects of This Medicine

Leukemia has been reported in a few patients after treatment with growth hormone. However, it is not definitely known whether the leukemia was caused by the growth hormone. Leukemia has also been reported in patients whose bodies do not make enough growth hormone and who have not yet been treated with man-made growth hormone. However, discuss this possible effect with your doctor.

If growth hormone is given to children or adults with normal growth, who do not need growth hormone, serious unwanted effects may occur because levels in the body become too high. These effects include the development of diabetes; abnormal growth of bones and internal organs such as the heart, kidneys, and liver; atherosclerosis (hardening of the arteries); and hypertension (high blood pressure).

Side Effects of This Medicine
  More common
  Abnormal or decreased touch sensation; blurred vision; burning, crawling, itching, numbness, prickling, "pins and needles", or tingling feelings; dizziness; ear infection or other ear problems (in patients with Turner's syndrome); nervousness; pounding in the ears; severe headache; slow or fast heartbeat

Less common
  Chest pain

Rare
  Abdominal pain or bloating; changes in vision; depression of skin at place of injection; headache; limp; nausea and vomiting; pain and swelling at place of injection; pain in hip or knee; skin rash or itching

Other side effects may occur that usually do not need medical attention. These side effects may go away during treatment as your body adjusts to the medicine. However, check with your doctor if any of the following side effects continue or are bothersome:

More common

Back pain; chills; cough or cough producing mucus; constipation; depressed mood; diarrhea; difficulty in breathing; difficulty in moving; dizziness; dry skin and hair; ear congestion; feeling cold; fever; general feeling of discomfort or illness; hair loss; hoarseness or husky voice; loss of appetite; loss of voice; runny nose; shivering; shortness of breath; sore throat; slowed heartbeat; sneezing; stuffy nose; sweating; swollen joints; tightness in chest; trouble sleeping; weight gain; wheezing

Less common or rare

Carpal tunnel syndrome; discouragement; enlargement of breasts; feeling sad or empty; increased growth of birthmarks; irritability; joint pain; loss of interest or pleasure; muscle pain, cramps, or stiffness; skeletal pain; sleepiness; swelling of hands, feet, or lower legs; trouble concentrating; unable to sleep; unusual tiredness or weakness

Other side effects not listed above may also occur in some patients. If you notice any other effects, check with your doctor.

GUAIFENESIN (Oral route) - gwye-FEN-e-sin

Commonly used brand name(s)

In the U.S.—

Allfen	Diabetic Tussin EX
Altarussin	Drituss G
Amibid LA	Guaifenex G
Antitussin	Guaifenex LA
Bidex 400	Mucinex
Diabetic Siltussin DAS-Na	Robitussin

In Canada—

Benylin-E	Broncho-Grippex Expectorant
Benylin E Extra Strength Chest Congestion	Robitussin Extra Strength

Available Dosage Forms:

- Liquid
- Tablet
- Elixir
- Capsule, Extended Release
- Tablet, Extended Release
- Syrup
- Capsule
- Solution

Therapeutic Class: Expectorant

Uses For This Medicine

Guaifenesin is used to help coughs caused by colds or similar illnesses clear mucus or phlegm (pronounced flem) from the chest. It works by thinning the mucus or phlegm in the lungs.

Some guaifenesin preparations are available only with your doctor's prescription.

Before Using This Medicine

In deciding to use a medicine, the risks of taking the medicine must be weighed against the good it will do. This is a decision you and your doctor will make. For this medicine, the following should be considered:

Allergies—Tell your doctor if you have ever had any unusual or allergic reaction to this medicine or any other medicines. Also tell your health care professional if you have any other types of allergies, such as to foods, dyes, preservatives, or animals. For non-prescription products, read the label or package ingredients carefully.

Pediatric—Although there is no specific information comparing use of guaifenesin in children with use in other age groups, this medicine is not expected to cause different side effects or problems in children than it does in adults. However, check with your doctor before using this medicine in children who have a chronic cough, such as occurs with asthma, or who have an unusually large amount of mucus or phlegm with the cough. Children with these conditions may need a different kind of medicine. Also, guaifenesin should not be given to children younger than 2 years of age unless you are directed to do so by your doctor.

Geriatric—Many medicines have not been studied specifically in older people. Therefore, it may not be known whether they work exactly the same way they do in younger adults. Although there is no specific information comparing use of guaifenesin in the elderly with use in other age groups, this medicine is not expected to cause different side effects or problems in older people than it does in younger adults.

Pregnancy—

	Pregnancy Category	Explanation
All Trimesters	C	Animal studies have shown an adverse effect and there are no adequate studies in pregnant women OR no animal studies have been conducted and there are no adequate studies in pregnant women.

Breast Feeding—There are no adequate studies in women for determining infant risk when using this medication during breastfeeding. Weigh the potential benefits against the potential risks before taking this medication while breastfeeding.

Other medicines—Although certain medicines should not be used together at all, in other cases two different medicines may be used together even if an interaction might occur. In these cases, your doctor may want to change the dose, or other precautions may be necessary. Tell your healthcare professional if you are taking any other prescription or non-prescription (over-the-counter [OTC]) medicine.

Interactions with Food/Tobacco/Alcohol—Certain medicines should not be used at or around the time of eating food or eating certain types of food since interactions may occur. Using alcohol or tobacco with certain medicines may also cause interactions to occur. Discuss with your healthcare professional the use of your medicine with food, alcohol, or tobacco.

Proper Use of This Medicine

Drinking plenty of water while taking guaifenesin may help loosen mucus or phlegm in the lungs.

For patients taking the extended-release capsule form of this medicine:

- Swallow the capsule whole, or open the capsule and sprinkle the contents on soft food such as applesauce, jelly, or pudding and swallow without crushing or chewing.

For patients taking the extended-release tablet form of this medicine:

- If the tablet has a groove in it, you may carefully break it into two pieces along the groove. Then swallow the pieces whole, without crushing or chewing them.
- If the tablet does not have a groove in it, it must be swallowed whole. Do not break, crush, or chew it before swallowing.

Dosing—The dose of this medicine will be different for different patients. Follow your doctor's orders or the directions on the label. The following information includes only the average doses of this medicine. If your dose is different, do not change it unless your doctor tells you to do so.

The amount of medicine that you take depends on the strength of the medicine. Also, the number of doses you take each day, the time allowed between doses, and the length of time you take the medicine depend on the medical problem for which you are using the medicine.

- For regular (short-acting) oral dosage forms (capsules, oral solution, syrup, or tablets):
  - For cough:
    - Adults—200 to 400 milligrams (mg) every four hours.
    - Children younger than 2 years of age—Use and dose must be determined by your doctor.
    - Children 2 to 6 years of age—50 to 100 mg every four hours.
    - Children 6 to 12 years of age—100 to 200 mg every four hours.
- For long-acting oral dosage forms (extended-release capsules or tablets):
  - For cough:
    - Adults—600 to 1200 mg every twelve hours.
    - Children younger than 2 years of age—Use is not recommended.
    - Children 2 to 6 years of age—300 mg every twelve hours.
    - Children 6 to 12 years of age—600 mg every twelve hours.

Missed dose—If you miss a dose of this medicine, take it as soon as possible. However, if it is almost time for your next dose, skip the missed dose and go back to your regular dosing schedule. Do not double doses.

Storage—Store the medicine in a closed container at room temperature, away from heat, moisture, and direct light. Keep from freezing.

Keep out of the reach of children.

Do not keep outdated medicine or medicine no longer needed.

Precautions While Using This Medicine

If your cough has not improved after 7 days or if you have a fever, skin rash, continuing headache, or sore throat with the cough, check with your doctor. These signs may mean that you have other medical problems.

Side Effects of This Medicine

Along with its needed effects, a medicine may cause some unwanted effects. Although not all of these side effects may occur, if they do occur they may need medical attention.

Some side effects may occur that usually do not need medical attention. These side effects may go away during treatment as your body adjusts to the medicine. Also, your health care professional may be able to tell you about ways to prevent or reduce some of these side effects. Check with your health care professional if any of the following side effects continue or are bothersome or if you have any questions about them:

Less common or rare
  Diarrhea; dizziness; headache; hives; nausea or vomiting; skin rash; stomach pain

Other side effects not listed may also occur in some patients. If you notice any other effects, check with your healthcare professional.

HAEMOPHILUS B CONJUGATE VACCINE   (Systemic)

Some commonly used brand names are:

In the U.S.—

Act-Hib (4)	Pedvaxhib (3)
Hibtiter (1)	Prohibit (2)

In Canada—

Act-Hib (4)	Pedvaxhib (3)
Hibtiter (1)	Prohibit (2)

This information applies to the following medicines:

1. Haemophilus b Conjugate Vaccine (HbOC—Diphtheria CRM 197 Protein Conjugate)
2. Haemophilus b Conjugate Vaccine (PRP-D—Diphtheria Toxoid Conjugate)
3. Haemophilus b Conjugate Vaccine (PRP-OMP—Meningococcal Protein Conjugate)
4. Haemophilus b Conjugate Vaccine (PRP-T—Tetanus Protein Conjugate)

Category

- **Immunizing agent, active—**

Description

Haemophilus b conjugate (hem-OFF-fil-us BEE KON-ja-gat) vaccine is an active immunizing agent used to prevent infection by Haemophilus influenza type b (Hib) bacteria. The vaccine works by causing your body to produce its own protection (antibodies) against the disease.

Haemophilus b conjugate vaccine is an haemophilus b vaccine that has been prepared by adding a diphtheria-, meningococcal-, or tetanus-related substance. However, this vaccine does *not* take the place of the regular diphtheria or tetanus toxoid injections (for example, DTP, DT, or T) that children should receive, the regular tetanus toxoid or diphtheria and tetanus toxoid injections (for example T or Td) that adults should receive, or the meningococcal vaccine injection that some children and adults should receive.

Infection by Haemophilus influenza type b (Hib) bacteria can cause life-threatening illnesses, such as meningitis, which affects the brain; epiglottitis, which can cause death by suffocation; pericarditis, which affects the heart; pneumonia, which affects the lungs; and septic arthritis, which affects the bones and joints. Hib meningitis causes death in 5 to 10% of children who are infected. Also, approximately 30% of children who survive Hib meningitis are left with some type of serious permanent damage, such as mental retardation, deafness, epilepsy, or partial blindness.

Immunization against Hib is recommended for all children 2 months up to 5 years of age (i.e., up to the 5th birthday).

Immunization against Hib may also be recommended for adults and children over 5 years of age with certain medical problems.

This vaccine is to be administered only by or under the supervision of your doctor or other authorized health care professional. It is available in the following dosage form:

Parenteral
- Injection

Before Receiving This Vaccine

In deciding to use a medicine, the risks of taking the medicine must be weighed against the good it will do. This is a decision you and your doctor will make. For haemophilus b conjugate vaccine, the following should be considered:

Allergies—Tell your doctor if you have ever had any unusual or allergic reaction to haemophilus b conjugate vaccine, haemophilus b polysaccharide vaccine, diphtheria or tetanus toxoid, or meningococcal vaccine. Also tell your health care professional if you are allergic to any other substances, such as preservatives.

Pregnancy—Studies on effects in pregnancy have not been done in either humans or animals.

Breast-feeding—This vaccine has not been reported to cause problems in nursing babies.

Children—This vaccine is not recommended for children less than 2 months of age.

Older adults—Many medicines have not been studied specifically in older people. Therefore, it may not be known whether they work exactly the same way they do in younger adults. Although there is no specific information comparing use of this vaccine in the elderly with use in other age groups, this vaccine is not expected to cause different side effects or problems in older people than it does in younger adults.

Other medicines—Although certain medicines should not be used together at all, in other cases two different medicines may be used together even if an interaction might occur. In these cases, your doctor may want to change the dose, or other precautions may be necessary. Tell your health care professional if you are using any other prescription or nonprescription (over-the-counter [OTC]) medicine.

Other medical problems—The presence of other medical problems may affect the use of haemophilus b conjugate vac-

cine. Make sure you tell your doctor if you have any other medical problems, especially:
- Fever or
- Serious illness—The symptoms of the condition may be confused with some of the possible side effects of the vaccine

Proper Use of This Vaccine

Dosing—Haemophilus b conjugate vaccine is an haemophilus b vaccine that has been prepared by adding a diphtheria-, meningococcal-, or tetanus-related substance to it. If the vaccine was prepared using a diphtheria-related substance, it is called either HbOC or PRP-D. If the vaccine was prepared using a meningococcal-related substance, it is called PRP-OMP. If the vaccine was prepared using a tetanus-related substance, it is called PRP-T. *All of these subtypes of haemophilus b conjugate vaccine work the same way*, but may be given at different ages or times.

The dose of haemophilus b conjugate vaccine will be different for different patients. The following information includes only the average doses of haemophilus b conjugate vaccine.
- For prevention of *Haemophilus influenzae* type b infection:
  - For *HbOC or PRP-T injection* dosage form:
    - Adults and children 5 years of age and older—Use and dose must be determined by your doctor.
    - Infants 2 to 6 months of age at the first dose—Three doses, two months apart, then a booster dose at fifteen months of age. The doses are injected into a muscle.
    - Children 7 to 11 months of age at the first dose—Two doses, two months apart, then a booster dose at fifteen months of age. The doses are injected into a muscle.
    - Children 12 to 14 months of age at the first dose—One dose, then a booster dose at fifteen months of age. The doses are injected into a muscle.
    - Children 15 to 59 months of age at the first dose—One dose injected into a muscle.
  - For *PRP-D injection* dosage form:
    - Adults and children 5 years of age and older—Use and dose must be determined by your doctor.
    - Infants and children up to 15 months of age—Use is not recommended.
    - Children 15 to 59 months of age at the first dose—One dose injected into a muscle.
  - For *PRP-OMP injection* dosage form:
    - Adults and children 5 years of age and older—Use and dose must be determined by your doctor.
    - Infants 2 to 6 months of age at the first dose—Two doses, two months apart, then a booster dose at twelve months of age. The doses are injected into a muscle.
    - Children 7 to 11 months of age at the first dose—Two doses, two months apart, then a booster dose at fifteen months of age. The doses are injected into a muscle.
    - Children 12 to 14 months of age at the first dose—One dose, then a booster dose at fifteen months of age. The doses are injected into a muscle.
    - Children 15 to 59 months of age at the first dose—One dose injected into a muscle.

After Receiving This Vaccine

This vaccine may interfere with laboratory tests that check for Hib disease. Make sure your doctor knows that you have received Hib vaccine if you are treated for a severe infection during the 2 weeks after you receive this vaccine.

Side Effects of This Vaccine

Along with its needed effects, a vaccine may cause some unwanted effects. Although not all of these side effects may occur, if they do occur they may need medical attention.

Get emergency help immediately if any of the following side effects occur:

Symptoms of allergic reactions
Difficulty in breathing or swallowing; hives; itching (especially of feet or hands); reddening of skin (especially around ears); swelling of eyes, face, or inside of nose; unusual tiredness or weakness (sudden and severe)

Check with your doctor immediately if the following side effect occurs:

Rare
Convulsions (seizures)

Other side effects may occur that usually do not need medical attention. However, check with your doctor if any of the following side effects continue or are bothersome:

More common
Fever of up to 102 °F (39 °C) (usually lasts less than 48 hours); irritability; loss of appetite; lack of interest; redness at place of injection; reduced physical activity; tenderness at place of injection; tiredness

Less common
Diarrhea; fever over 102 °F (39 °C) (usually lasts less than 48 hours); hard lump, swelling, or warm feeling at place of injection; skin rash; vomiting

Other side effects not listed above may also occur in some patients. If you notice any other effects, check with your doctor.

HAEMOPHILUS B POLYSACCHARIDE VACCINE
(Intramuscular route, Injection route) - hem-OFF-i-lus B pol-ee-sak-a-ride vak-SEEN

Uses For This Vaccine

Haemophilus b polysaccharide vaccine is an active immunizing agent used to prevent infection by Haemophilus influenzae type b (Hib) bacteria. The vaccine works by causing your body to produce its own protection (antibodies) against the disease.

The following information applies only to the Haemophilus b polysaccharide vaccine.

Infection by Haemophilus influenzae type b (Hib) bacteria can cause life-threatening illnesses, such as meningitis, which affects the brain; epiglottitis, which can cause death by suffocation; pericarditis, which affects the heart; pneumonia, which affects the lungs; and septic arthritis, which affects the bones

and joints. Hib meningitis causes death in 5 to 10% of children who are infected. Also, approximately 30% of children who survive Hib meningitis are left with some type of serious permanent damage, such as mental retardation, deafness, epilepsy, or partial blindness.

Immunization against Hib is recommended for all children 24 months up to 5 years of age (i.e., up to the 5th birthday). In addition, immunization is recommended for children 18 to 24 months of age, especially:

- Children attending day-care facilities.
- Children with chronic illnesses associated with increased risk of Hib disease. These illnesses include asplenia, sickle cell disease, antibody deficiency syndromes, immunosuppression, and Hodgkin's disease.
- Children 18 to 24 months of age who have already had Hib disease. These children may get the disease again if they are not immunized. Children who developed Hib disease when 24 months of age or older do not need to be immunized, since most children in this age group will develop antibodies against the disease.
- Children with human immunodeficiency virus (HIV) infection or acquired immunodeficiency syndrome (AIDS).
- Children of certain racial groups, such as American Indian and Alaskan Eskimo. Children in these groups seem to be at increased risk of Hib disease.
- Children living close together with groups of other persons. Close living conditions increase a child's risk of being exposed to persons who have Hib infection or who carry the bacteria.

It is recommended that children immunized when they were 18 to 24 months of age receive a second dose of vaccine, since these children may not produce enough antibodies to fully protect them from Hib disease. Children who were first immunized when they were 24 months of age or older do not need to be reimmunized.

This vaccine is available only from your doctor or other authorized health care professional.

Before Receiving This Vaccine

In deciding to use a vaccine, the risks of taking the vaccine must be weighed against the good it will do. This is a decision you and your doctor will make. For this vaccine, the following should be considered:

Allergies—Tell your doctor if you have ever had any unusual or allergic reaction to this medicine or any other medicines. Also tell your health care professional if you have any other types of allergies, such as to foods, dyes, preservatives, or animals. For non-prescription products, read the label or package ingredients carefully.

Pediatric—This vaccine is not recommended for children less than 18 months of age.

Pregnancy—

	Pregnancy Category	Explanation
All Trimesters	C	Animal studies have shown an adverse effect and there are no adequate studies in pregnant women OR no animal studies have been conducted and there are no adequate studies in pregnant women.

Breast Feeding—Studies in women suggest that this medication poses minimal risk to the infant when used during breastfeeding.

Other medicines—Although certain medicines should not be used together at all, in other cases two different medicines may be used together even if an interaction might occur. In these cases, your doctor may want to change the dose, or other precautions may be necessary. Tell your healthcare professional if you are taking any other prescription or non-prescription (over-the-counter [OTC]) medicine.

Interactions with Food/Tobacco/Alcohol—Certain medicines should not be used at or around the time of eating food or eating certain types of food since interactions may occur. Using alcohol or tobacco with certain medicines may also cause interactions to occur. Discuss with your healthcare professional the use of your medicine with food, alcohol, or tobacco.

Other medical problems—The presence of other medical problems may affect the use of this vaccine. Make sure you tell your doctor if you have any other medical problems, especially:

- Fever or
- Serious illness—The symptoms of the condition may be confused with the possible side effects of the vaccine

Proper Use of This Vaccine

Dosing—The dose of this medicine will be different for different patients. Follow your doctor's orders or the directions on the label. The following information includes only the average doses of this medicine. If your dose is different, do not change it unless your doctor tells you to do so.

The amount of medicine that you take depends on the strength of the medicine. Also, the number of doses you take each day, the time allowed between doses, and the length of time you take the medicine depend on the medical problem for which you are using the medicine.

- For injection dosage form:
  - For prevention of Haemophilus influenzae type b infection:
    - Adults and children 5 years of age and older— Use is not recommended.
    - Children up to 18 months of age—Use is not recommended.
    - Children 18 to 24 months of age—Use and dose must be determined by your doctor.
    - Children 24 months to 5 years of age—One dose injected under the skin or into a muscle.

Side Effects of This Vaccine

Along with its needed effects, a medicine may cause some unwanted effects. Although not all of these side effects may occur, if they do occur they may need medical attention.

Check with your doctor immediately if any of the following side effects occur:
Symptoms of allergic reaction
Difficulty in breathing or swallowing; hives; itching (especially of feet or hands); reddening of skin (especially around ears); swelling of eyes, face, or inside of nose; unusual tiredness or weakness (sudden and severe)

Check with your doctor immediately if any of the following side effects occur:
Rare
Convulsions (seizures)

Some side effects may occur that usually do not need medical attention. These side effects may go away during treatment as your body adjusts to the medicine. Also, your health care professional may be able to tell you about ways to prevent or reduce some of these side effects. Check with your health care professional if any of the following side effects continue or are bothersome or if you have any questions about them:
More common
Diarrhea; fever up to 102 °F (39 °C) (usually lasts less than 48 hours); irritability; lack of appetite; lack of interest; redness at place of injection; reduced physical activity; tenderness at place of injection
Less common
Fever over 102 °F (39 °C) (usually lasts less than 48 hours); hard lump at place of injection; itching; joint aches or pains; skin rash; swelling at place of injection; trouble in sleeping; vomiting

Other side effects not listed may also occur in some patients. If you notice any other effects, check with your healthcare professional.

HALOPERIDOL (Oral route, Intramuscular route, Injection route) - ha-loe-PER-i-dole

Commonly used brand name(s)
In the U.S.—
Haldol
Haldol Decanoate

In Canada—

Alti-Haloperidol	Peridol
Apo-Haloperidol	Pms-Haloperidol
Novo-Peridol	Ratio-Haloperidol

Available Dosage Forms:
- Solution
- Tablet
- Injectable
- Suspension
- Oil

Therapeutic Class: Antipsychotic
Pharmacologic Class: Dopamine Antagonist

Uses For This Medicine

Haloperidol is used to treat nervous, mental, and emotional conditions. It is also used to control the symptoms of Tourette's disorder. Haloperidol may also be used for other conditions as determined by your doctor.

Haloperidol is available only with your doctor's prescription.

Once a medicine has been approved for marketing for a certain use, experience may show that it is also useful for other medical problems. Although these uses are not included in product labeling, haloperidol is used in certain patients with the following medical conditions:

- Huntington's chorea (an hereditary movement disorder)
- Infantile autism
- Nausea and vomiting caused by cancer chemotherapy

Before Using This Medicine

In deciding to use a medicine, the risks of taking the medicine must be weighed against the good it will do. This is a decision you and your doctor will make. For this medicine, the following should be considered:

Allergies—Tell your doctor if you have ever had any unusual or allergic reaction to this medicine or any other medicines. Also tell your health care professional if you have any other types of allergies, such as to foods, dyes, preservatives, or animals. For non-prescription products, read the label or package ingredients carefully.

Pediatric—Side effects, especially muscle spasms of the neck and back, twisting movements of the body, trembling of fingers and hands, and inability to move the eyes are more likely to occur in children, who usually are more sensitive than adults to the effects of haloperidol.

Geriatric—Constipation, dizziness or fainting, drowsiness, dryness of mouth, trembling of the hands and fingers, and symptoms of tardive dyskinesia (such as rapid, worm-like movements of the tongue or any other uncontrolled movements of the mouth, tongue, or jaw, and/or arms and legs) are especially likely to occur in elderly patients, who are usually more sensitive than younger adults to the effects of haloperidol.

Pregnancy—

	Pregnancy Category	Explanation
All Trimesters	C	Animal studies have shown an adverse effect and there are no adequate studies in pregnant women OR no animal studies have been conducted and there are no adequate studies in pregnant women.

Breast Feeding—There are no adequate studies in women for determining infant risk when using this medication during breastfeeding. Weigh the potential benefits against the potential risks before taking this medication while breastfeeding.

Other medicines—

Using this medicine with any of the following medicines is not recommended. Your doctor may decide not to treat you with this medication or change some of the other medicines you take.

Bepridil, Cisapride, Levomethadyl, Mesoridazine, Pimozide, Sparfloxacin, Terfenadine, Thioridazine, Ziprasidone

Interactions with Food/Tobacco/Alcohol—Certain medicines should not be used at or around the time of eating food or eating certain types of food since interactions may occur. Using alcohol or tobacco with certain medicines may also cause interactions to occur. Discuss with your healthcare professional the use of your medicine with food, alcohol, or tobacco.

Other medical problems—The presence of other medical problems may affect the use of this medicine. Make sure you

tell your doctor if you have any other medical problems, especially:

- Alcohol abuse—The risk of heat stroke may be increased
- Difficult urination or
- Glaucoma or
- Heart or blood vessel disease or
- Lung disease or
- Parkinson's disease—Haloperidol may make the condition worse
- Epilepsy—The risk of seizures may be increased
- Kidney disease or
- Liver disease—Higher blood levels of haloperidol may occur, increasing the chance of side effects
- Overactive thyroid—Serious unwanted effects may occur

Proper Use of This Medicine

If this medicine upsets your stomach, it may be taken with food or milk to lessen stomach irritation.

For patients taking the liquid form of this medicine:

- This medicine is to be taken by mouth even if it comes in a dropper bottle. Each dose is to be measured with the specially marked dropper provided with your prescription. Do not use other droppers since they may not deliver the correct amount of medicine.
- This medicine should be mixed with water or a beverage such as orange juice, apple juice, tomato juice, or cola and taken immediately after mixing. Haloperidol should not be mixed with tea or coffee, since they cause the medicine to separate out of solution.

Take this medicine only as directed by your doctor. Do not take more of it, do not take it more often, and do not take it for a longer time than your doctor ordered. This is particularly important for children or elderly patients, since they may react very strongly to this medicine.

Continue taking this medicine for the full time of treatment. Sometimes haloperidol must be taken for several days to several weeks before its full effect is reached.

Dosing—The dose of this medicine will be different for different patients. Follow your doctor's orders or the directions on the label. The following information includes only the average doses of this medicine. If your dose is different, do not change it unless your doctor tells you to do so.

The amount of medicine that you take depends on the strength of the medicine. Also, the number of doses you take each day, the time allowed between doses, and the length of time you take the medicine depend on the medical problem for which you are using the medicine.

- For oral dosage forms (solution and tablets):
  - Adults and adolescents: To start, 500 micrograms to 5 milligrams two or three times a day. Your doctor may increase your dose if needed. However, the dose is usually not more than 100 milligrams a day.
  - Children 3 to 12 years of age or weighing 15 to 40 kilograms (33 to 88 pounds): Dose is based on body weight. The usual dose is 25 to 150 micrograms per kilogram (11 to 68 micrograms per pound) a day, taken in smaller doses two or three times a day.

- ○ Children up to 3 years of age: Dose must be determined by the doctor.
- ○ Older adults: To start, 500 micrograms to 2 milligrams two or three times a day. The doctor may increase your dose if needed.
- For short-acting injection dosage form:
  - ○ Adults and adolescents: To start, 2 to 5 milligrams, usually injected into a muscle. The dose may be repeated every one to eight hours, depending on your condition.
  - ○ Children: Dose must be determined by the doctor.
- For long-acting or depot injection dosage form:
  - ○ Adults and adolescents: To start, the dose is usually 10 to 15 times the daily oral dose you were taking, injected into a muscle once a month. The doctor may adjust how much of this medicine you need and how often you will need it, depending on your condition.
  - ○ Children: Dose must be determined by the doctor.

Missed dose—If you miss a dose of this medicine, take it as soon as possible. However, if it is almost time for your next dose, skip the missed dose and go back to your regular dosing schedule. Do not double doses.

Storage—Store the medicine in a closed container at room temperature, away from heat, moisture, and direct light. Keep from freezing.

Keep out of the reach of children.

Do not keep outdated medicine or medicine no longer needed.

Precautions While Using This Medicine

Your doctor should check your progress at regular visits, especially during the first few months of treatment with this medicine. The amount of haloperidol you take may be changed often to meet the needs of your condition. This also helps prevent side effects.

Do not stop taking this medicine without first checking with your doctor. Your doctor may want you to reduce gradually the amount you are taking before stopping completely. This will allow your body time to adjust and help avoid a worsening of your medical condition.

This medicine will add to the effects of alcohol and other CNS depressants (medicines that slow down the nervous system, possibly causing drowsiness). Some examples of CNS depressants are antihistamines or medicine for hay fever, other allergies, or colds; sedatives, tranquilizers, or sleeping medicine; prescription pain medicine or narcotics; barbiturates; medicine for seizures; muscle relaxants; or anesthetics, including some dental anesthetics. Check with your doctor before taking any of the above while you are taking this medicine.

This medicine may cause some people to become dizzy, drowsy, or less alert than they are normally, especially as the amount of medicine is increased. Even if you take haloperidol at bedtime, you may feel drowsy or less alert on arising. Make sure you know how you react to this medicine before you drive, use machines, or do anything else that could be dangerous if you are dizzy or are not alert.

Although not a problem for many patients, dizziness, lightheadedness, or fainting may occur, especially when you get up from a lying or sitting position. Getting up slowly may help.

However, if the problem continues or gets worse, check with your doctor.

This medicine will often make you sweat less, causing your body temperature to increase. Use extra care not to become overheated during exercise or hot weather while you are taking this medicine, since overheating may result in heat stroke. Also, hot baths or saunas may make you feel dizzy or faint while you are taking this medicine.

Before using any prescription or over-the-counter (OTC) medicine for colds or allergies, check with your doctor. These medicines may increase the chance of heat stroke or other unwanted effects, such as dizziness, dry mouth, blurred vision, and constipation, while you are taking haloperidol.

Before having any kind of surgery, dental treatment, or emergency treatment, tell the medical doctor or dentist in charge that you are using this medicine. Taking haloperidol together with medicines that are used during surgery or dental or emergency treatments may increase the CNS depressant effects.

Haloperidol may cause your skin to be more sensitive to sunlight than it is normally. Exposure to sunlight, even for brief periods of time, may cause a skin rash, itching, redness or other discoloration of the skin, or a severe sunburn. When you begin taking this medicine:

- Stay out of direct sunlight, especially between the hours of 10:00 a.m. and 3:00 p.m., if possible.
- Wear protective clothing, including a hat. Also, wear sunglasses.
- Apply a sun block product that has a skin protection factor (SPF) of at least 15. Some patients may require a product with a higher SPF number, especially if they have a fair complexion. If you have any questions about this, check with your health care professional.
- Apply a sun block lipstick that has an SPF of at least 15 to protect your lips.
- Do not use a sunlamp or tanning bed or booth.

If you have a severe reaction from the sun, check with your doctor.

Haloperidol may cause dryness of the mouth. For temporary relief, use sugarless candy or gum, melt bits of ice in your mouth, or use a saliva substitute. However, if your mouth continues to feel dry for more than 2 weeks, check with your medical doctor or dentist. Continuing dryness of the mouth may increase the chance of dental disease, including tooth decay, gum disease, and fungus infections.

If you are taking the liquid form of this medicine, avoid getting it on your skin because it may cause a skin rash or other irritation.

If you are receiving this medicine by injection:

- The effects of the long-acting injection form of this medicine may last for up to 6 weeks. The precautions and side effects information for this medicine applies during this time.

Side Effects of This Medicine

Along with its needed effects, haloperidol can sometimes cause serious side effects. Tardive dyskinesia (a movement disorder) may occur and may not go away after you stop using the medicine. Signs of tardive dyskinesia include fine, worm-like movements of the tongue, or other uncontrolled movements of the mouth, tongue, cheeks, jaw, or arms and legs. Other serious but rare side effects may also occur. These include severe muscle stiffness, fever, unusual tiredness or weakness, fast heartbeat, difficult breathing, increased sweating, loss of bladder control, and seizures (neuroleptic malignant syndrome). You and your doctor should discuss the good this medicine will do as well as the risks of taking it.

Stop taking this medicine and get emergency help immediately if any of the following effects occur:

Rare
Convulsions (seizures); difficult or fast breathing; fast heartbeat or irregular pulse; fever (high); high or low blood pressure; increased sweating; loss of bladder control; muscle stiffness (severe); unusually pale skin; unusual tiredness or weakness

Check with your doctor as soon as possible if any of the following side effects occur:

More common
Difficulty in speaking or swallowing; inability to move eyes; loss of balance control; mask-like face; muscle spasms, especially of the neck and back; restlessness or need to keep moving (severe); shuffling walk; stiffness of arms and legs; trembling and shaking of fingers and hands; twisting movements of body; weakness of arms and legs

Less common
Decreased thirst; difficulty in urination; dizziness, lightheadedness, or fainting; hallucinations (seeing or hearing things that are not there); lip smacking or puckering; puffing of cheeks; rapid or worm-like movements of tongue; skin rash; uncontrolled chewing movements; uncontrolled movements of arms and legs

Rare
Confusion; hot, dry skin, or lack of sweating; increased blinking or spasms of eyelid; muscle weakness; sore throat and fever; uncontrolled twisting movements of neck, trunk, arms, or legs; unusual bleeding or bruising; unusual facial expressions or body positions; yellow eyes or skin

Symptoms of overdose
Difficulty in breathing (severe); dizziness (severe); drowsiness (severe); muscle trembling, jerking, stiffness, or uncontrolled movements (severe); unusual tiredness or weakness (severe)

Some side effects may occur that usually do not need medical attention. These side effects may go away during treatment as your body adjusts to the medicine. Also, your health care professional may be able to tell you about ways to prevent or reduce some of these side effects. Check with your health care professional if any of the following side effects continue or are bothersome or if you have any questions about them:

More common
Blurred vision; changes in menstrual period; constipation; dryness of mouth; swelling or pain in breasts (in females); unusual secretion of milk; weight gain

Less common
Decreased sexual ability; drowsiness; increased sensitivity of skin to sun (skin rash, itching, redness or other discoloration of skin, or severe sunburn); nausea or vomiting

Some side effects, such as trembling of fingers and hands, or uncontrolled movements of the mouth, tongue, and jaw,

may occur after you have stopped taking this medicine. If you notice any of these effects, check with your doctor as soon as possible.

Other side effects not listed may also occur in some patients. If you notice any other effects, check with your healthcare professional.

HEADACHE MEDICINES, ERGOT DERIVATIVE-CONTAINING (Systemic)

Some commonly used brand names are:

In the U.S.—

Belcomp-PB (5)	Ergomar (2)
Cafergot (3)	Migergot (3)
D.H.E. 45 (1)	Migracet-PB (5)
Ergocaff-PB (5)	Wigraine (3)

In Canada—

Cafergot (3)	Ergodryl (8)
D.H.E. (1)	Gravergol (7)

This information applies to the following medicines:

1. Dihydroergotamine (dye-hye-droe-er-GOT-a-meen)
2. Ergotamine (er-GOT-a-meen)
3. Ergotamine and Caffeine (er-GOT-a-meen and kaf-EEN)
4. Ergotamine, Caffeine, and Belladonna Alkaloids (er-GOT-a-meen, kaf-EEN, and bell-a-DON-a AL-ka-loids)
5. Ergotamine, Caffeine, Belladonna Alkaloids, and Pentobarbital (er-GOT-a-meen, kaf-EEN, bell-a-DON-a AL-ka-loids, and pentoe-BAR-bi-tal)
6. Ergotamine, Caffeine, and Cyclizine (er-GOT-a-meen, kaf-EEN, and SYE-kli-zeen)
7. Ergotamine, Caffeine, and Dimenhydrinate (er-GOT-a-meen, kaf-EEN, and dye-men-HYE-dri-nate)
8. Ergotamine, Caffeine, and Diphenhydramine (er-GOT-a-meen, kaf-EEN, and dye-fen-HYE-dra-mine)

Category

- **Antihypotensive—**
- **Thrombosis prophylaxis adjunct—**
- **Vascular headache suppressant—**

Description

Dihydroergotamine and ergotamine belong to the group of medicines known as ergot alkaloids. They are used to treat severe, throbbing headaches, such as migraine and cluster headaches. Dihydroergotamine and ergotamine are not ordinary pain relievers. They will not relieve any kind of pain other than throbbing headaches. Because these medicines can cause serious side effects, they are usually used for patients whose headaches are not relieved by acetaminophen, aspirin, or other pain relievers.

Dihydroergotamine and ergotamine may cause blood vessels in the body to constrict (become narrower). This effect can lead to serious side effects that are caused by a decrease in the flow of blood (blood circulation) to many parts of the body.

The caffeine present in many ergotamine-containing combinations helps ergotamine work better and faster by causing more of it to be quickly absorbed into the body. The belladonna alkaloids, dimenhydrinate, and diphenhydramine in some combinations help to relieve nausea and vomiting, which often occur together with the headaches. Dimenhydrinate, diphenhydramine, and pentobarbital also help the patient relax and even sleep. This also helps relieve headaches.

Dihydroergotamine is also used for other conditions, as determined by your doctor.

These medicines are available only with your doctor's prescription, in the following dosage forms:

  Oral
  - Ergotamine
    ○ Sublingual tablets
  - Ergotamine and Caffeine
    ○ Tablets
  - Ergotamine, Caffeine, and Dimenhydrinate
    ○ Capsules
  - Ergotamine, Caffeine, and Diphenhydramine
    ○ Capsules
  Parenteral
  - Dihydroergotamine
    ○ Injection
  Rectal
  - Ergotamine and Caffeine
    ○ Suppositories
  - Ergotamine, Caffeine, Belladonna Alkaloids, and Pentobarbital
    ○ Suppositories

Before Using This Medicine

In deciding to use a medicine, the risks of taking the medicine must be weighed against the good it will do. This is a decision you and your doctor will make. For these headache medicines, the following should be considered:

Allergies—Tell your doctor if you have ever had any unusual or allergic reaction to atropine, belladonna, pentobarbital or other barbiturates, caffeine, dimenhydrinate, diphenhydramine, or an ergot medicine. Also tell your health care professional if you are allergic to any other substances, such as foods, preservatives, or dyes.

Pregnancy—Use of dihydroergotamine or ergotamine by pregnant women may cause serious harm, including death of the fetus and miscarriage. Therefore, *these medicines should not be used during pregnancy.*

Breast-feeding—Be sure that you discuss these possible problems with your doctor before taking any of these medicines.
  - *For dihydroergotamine and ergotamine:* These medicines pass into the breast milk and may cause unwanted effects, such as vomiting, diarrhea, weak pulse, changes in blood pressure, or convulsions (seizures) in nursing babies. Large amounts of these medicines may also decrease the flow of breast milk.
  - *For caffeine:* Caffeine passes into the breast milk. Large amounts of it may cause the baby to appear jittery or to have trouble in sleeping.
  - *For belladonna alkaloids, dimenhydrinate, and diphenhydramine:* These medicines have drying effects. Therefore, it is possible that they may reduce the amount of breast milk in some people. Dimenhydrinate passes into the breast milk.

  - *For pentobarbital:* Pentobarbital passes into the breast milk. Large amounts of it may cause unwanted effects such as drowsiness in nursing babies.

Be sure that you discuss these possible problems with your doctor before taking any of these medicines.

Children—
  - *For dihydroergotamine and ergotamine:* These medicines are used to relieve severe, throbbing headaches in children 6 years of age or older. They have not been shown to cause different side effects or problems in children than they do in adults. However, these medicines can cause serious side effects in any patient. Therefore, it is especially important that you discuss with the child's doctor the good that this medicine may do as well as the risks of using it.
  - *For belladonna alkaloids:* Young children, especially children with spastic paralysis or brain damage, may be especially sensitive to the effects of belladonna alkaloids. This may increase the chance of side effects during treatment.
  - *For dimenhydrinate, diphenhydramine, and pentobarbital:* Although these medicines often cause drowsiness, some children become excited after taking them.

Older adults—
  - *For dihydroergotamine and ergotamine:* The chance of serious side effects caused by decreases in blood flow is increased in elderly people receiving these medicines.
  - *For belladonna alkaloids, dimenhydrinate, diphenhydramine, and pentobarbital:* Elderly people are more sensitive than younger adults to the effects of these medicines. This may increase the chance of side effects such as excitement, depression, dizziness, drowsiness, and confusion.

Other medicines—Although certain medicines should not be used together at all, in other cases two different medicines may be used together even if an interaction might occur. In these cases, your doctor may want to change the dose, or other precautions may be necessary. Many medicines can add to or decrease the effects of the belladonna alkaloids, caffeine, dimenhydrinate, diphenhydramine, or pentobarbital present in some of these headache medicines. Therefore, you should tell your health care professional if you are taking *any* other prescription or nonprescription (over-the-counter [OTC]) medicine. This is especially important if any medicine you take causes excitement, trouble in sleeping, dryness of the mouth, dizziness, or drowsiness.

When you are taking dihydroergotamine or ergotamine, it is especially important that your health care professional know if you are taking any of the following:
  - Cocaine or
  - Epinephrine by injection [e.g., Epi-Pen] or
  - Other ergot medicines (ergoloid mesylates [e.g., Hydergine], ergonovine [e.g., Ergotrate], methylergonovine [e.g., Methergine], methysergide [e.g., Sansert])—The chance of serious side effects caused by dihydroergotamine or ergotamine may be increased
  - Itraconazole (e.g., Sporanox) or
  - Ketoconazole (e.g., Nizoral) or
  - Macrolide antibiotics (clarithromycin [e.g., Biaxin], erythromycin [e.g., Ery-Tab], troleandomycin [e.g., TAO]) or

- Protease inhibitors (indinavir [e.g., Crixivan], nelfinavir [e.g., Viracept], ritonavir [e.g., Norvir])—Use of any of these medicines with ergotamine can cause serious or life-threatening problems with blood circulation. **These medicines should not be used with ergotamine.**

- 5–HT$_1$ agonists (almotriptan [e.g., Axert], eletriptan [e.g., Relpax], frovatriptan [e.g., Frova], naratriptan [e.g., Amerge], rizatriptan [e.g., Maxalt], sumatriptan [e.g., Imitrex], zolmitriptan [e.g., Zomig])—Use of these medicines may cause serious side effects if taken within 24 hours of an ergot-containing medicine.

Other medical problems—The presence of other medical problems may affect the use of these headache medicines. Make sure you tell your doctor if you have any other medical problems, especially:

- Agoraphobia (fear of open or public places) or
- Panic attacks or
- Stomach ulcer or
- Trouble in sleeping (insomnia)—Caffeine can make your condition worse
- Diarrhea—Rectal dosage forms (suppositories) will not be effective if you have diarrhea
- Difficult urination or
- Enlarged prostate or
- Glaucoma (not well controlled) or
- Heart or blood vessel disease or
- High blood pressure (not well controlled) or
- Infection or
- Intestinal blockage or other intestinal problems or
- Itching (severe) or
- Kidney disease or
- Liver disease or
- Mental depression or
- Overactive thyroid or
- Trauma from an accident (broken arm or leg) or
- Urinary tract blockage—The chance of side effects may be increased

Also, tell your doctor if you need, or if you have recently had, an angioplasty (a procedure done to improve the flow of blood in a blocked blood vessel) or surgery on a blood vessel. The chance of serious side effects caused by dihydroergotamine or ergotamine may be increased.

Proper Use of This Medicine

Use this medicine only as directed by your doctor. Do not use more of it, and do not use it more often, than directed. If the amount you are to use does not relieve your headache, check with your doctor. Taking too much dihydroergotamine or ergotamine, or taking it too often, may cause serious effects, especially in elderly patients. Also, if a headache medicine (especially ergotamine) is used too often for migraines, it may lose its effectiveness or even cause a type of physical dependence. If this occurs, your headaches may actually get worse.

This medicine works best if you:

- *Use it at the first sign of headache or migraine attack. If you get warning signals of a coming migraine, take it before the headache actually starts.*

- *Lie down in a quiet, dark room until you are feeling better.*

Your doctor may direct you to take another medicine to help prevent headaches. *It is important that you follow your doctor's directions, even if your headaches continue to occur.* Headache-preventing medicines may take several weeks to start working. Even after they do start working, your headaches may not go away completely. However, your headaches should occur less often, and they should be less severe and easier to relieve. This can reduce the amount of dihydroergotamine, ergotamine, or pain relievers that you need. If you do not notice any improvement after several weeks of headache-preventing treatment, check with your doctor.

For patients using *dihydroergotamine:*

- Dihydroergotamine is given only by injection. Your health care professional will teach you how to inject yourself with the medicine. Be sure to follow the directions carefully. Check with your health care professional if you have any problems using the medicine.

For patients using the *sublingual (under-the-tongue) tablets of ergotamine:*

- To use—Place the tablet under your tongue and let it remain there until it disappears. The sublingual tablet should not be chewed or swallowed, because it works faster when it is absorbed into the body through the lining of the mouth. Do not eat, drink, or smoke while the tablet is under your tongue.

For patients using *rectal suppository forms of a headache medicine:*

- If the suppository is too soft to use, chill it in the refrigerator for 30 minutes or run cold water over it before removing the foil wrapper.

- If you have been directed to use part of a suppository, you should divide the suppository into pieces that all contain the same amount of medicine. To do this, use a sharp knife and carefully cut the suppository lengthwise (from top to bottom) into pieces that are the same size. The suppository will be easier to cut if it has been kept in the refrigerator.

- To insert the suppository—First remove the foil wrapper and moisten the suppository with cold water. Lie down on your side and use your finger to push the suppository well up into the rectum.

Dosing—The dose of these headache medicines will be different for different patients. *Follow your doctor's orders or the directions on the label.* The following information includes only the average doses of these medicines. *If your dose is different, do not change it* unless your doctor tells you to do so.

For dihydroergotamine

- Adults: For relieving a migraine or cluster headache—1 mg. If your headache is not better, and no side effects are occurring, a second 1–mg dose may be used at least one hour later.

- Children 6 years of age and older: For relieving a migraine headache—It is not likely that a child will be receiving dihydroergotamine at home. If a child needs the medicine, the dose will have to be determined by the doctor.

For ergotamine
- Some headache medicines contain only ergotamine. Some of them contain other medicines along with the ergotamine. The number of tablets, capsules, or suppositories that you need for each dose depends on the amount of ergotamine in them. The size of each dose, and the number of doses that you take, also depends on the reason you are taking the medicine and on how you react to the medicine.
- For *oral* (capsule or tablet) and *sublingual* (under-the-tongue tablet) dosage forms:
  - Adults:
    - For relieving a migraine or cluster headache—1 or 2 mg of ergotamine. If your headache is not better, and no side effects are occurring, a second dose and even a third dose may be taken; however the doses should be taken at least 30 minutes apart. People who usually need more than one dose of the medicine, and who do not get side effects from it, may be able to take a larger first dose of not more than 3 mg of ergotamine. This may provide better relief of the headache with only one dose. *The medicine should not be taken more often than 2 times a week, at least five days apart.*
    - For preventing cluster headaches—The dose of ergotamine, and the number of doses you need every day, will depend on how many headaches you usually get each day. For some people, 1 or 2 mg of ergotamine once a day may be enough. Other people may need to take 1 or 2 mg of ergotamine 2 or 3 times a day.
    - For all uses—*Do not take more than 6 mg of ergotamine a day in the form of capsules or tablets.*
  - Children 6 years of age and older: For relieving migraine headaches—1 mg of ergotamine. If the headache is not better, and no side effects are occurring, a second dose and even a third dose may be taken; however, the doses should be taken at least 30 minutes apart. *Children should not take more than 3 mg of ergotamine a day in the form of capsules or tablets. Also, this medicine should not be taken more often than 2 times a week, at least five days apart.*
- For *rectal suppository* dosage forms:
  - Adults: For relieving migraine or cluster headaches— Usually 1 mg of ergotamine, but the dose may range from half of this amount to up to 2 mg. If your headache is not better, and no side effects are occurring, a second dose and even a third dose may be used; however the doses should be taken at least 30 minutes apart. People who usually need more than one dose of the medicine, and who do not get side effects from it, may be able to use a larger first dose of not more than 3 mg. This may provide better relief of the headache with only one dose. *Adults should not use more than 4 mg of ergotamine a day in suppository form. Also, this medicine should not be used more often than 2 times a week, at least five days apart.*
  - Children 6 years of age and older: For relieving migraine headaches—One-half or 1 mg of ergotamine. *Children should not receive more than 1 mg a day of ergotamine in suppository form. Also, this med-*

icine should not be used more often than 2 times a week, at least five days apart.

Storage—To store this medicine:
- Keep out of the reach of children since overdose is especially dangerous in children.
- Store away from heat and direct light.
- Do not store in the bathroom, near the kitchen sink, or in other damp places. Heat or moisture may cause the medicine to break down.
- Suppositories should be stored in a cool place, but not allowed to freeze. Some manufacturers recommend keeping them in a refrigerator; others do not. Follow the directions on the package. However, cutting the suppository into smaller pieces, if you need to do so, will be easier if the suppository is kept in the refrigerator.
- Do not keep outdated medicine or medicine no longer needed. Be sure that any discarded medicine is out of the reach of children.

Precautions While Using This Medicine

Check with your doctor:
- If your migraine headaches are worse than they were before you started using this medicine, or your headache medicine stops working as well as it did when you first started using it. This may mean that you are in danger of becoming dependent on the headache medicine. *Do not try to get better relief by increasing the dose.*
- If your migraine headaches are occurring more often than they did before you started using this medicine. This is especially important if a new headache occurs within 1 day after you took your last dose of headache medicine, or if you are having headaches every day. This may mean that you are dependent on the headache medicine. *Continuing to take this medicine will cause even more headaches later on.* Your doctor can give you advice on how to relieve the headaches.

Drinking alcoholic beverages can make headaches worse or cause new headaches to occur. People who suffer from severe headaches should probably avoid alcoholic beverages, especially during a headache.

Smoking or nicotine replacement therapy products may increase some of the harmful effects of dihydroergotamine or ergotamine. It is best to avoid smoking or the use of nicotine replacement therapy products for several hours after taking these medicines.

Dihydroergotamine and ergotamine may make you more sensitive to cold temperatures, especially if you have blood circulation problems. They tend to decrease blood flow in the skin, fingers, and toes. Dress warmly during cold weather and be careful during prolonged exposure to cold temperatures. This is especially important for older patients, who are more likely than younger adults to already have problems with their circulation.

If you have a serious infection or illness of any kind, check with your doctor before using this medicine, since you may be more sensitive to its effects.

For patients taking one of the combination medicines that contains *caffeine:*
- Caffeine may interfere with the results of a test that uses dipyridamole (e.g., Persantine) to help find out how well your blood is flowing through certain blood vessels. You

should not have any caffeine for at least 12 hours before the test.

Caffeine may also interfere with some other laboratory tests. Before having any other laboratory tests, tell the person in charge if you have taken a medicine that contains caffeine.

For patients taking one of the combination medicines that contains *belladonna alkaloids, dimenhydrinate, diphenhydramine, or pentobarbital:*

- These medicines may cause some people to have blurred vision or to become drowsy, dizzy, lightheaded, or less alert than they are normally. These effects may be especially severe if you also take CNS depressants (medicines that slow down the nervous system, possibly causing drowsiness) together with one of these combination medicines. Some examples of CNS depressants are antihistamines or medicine for hay fever, other allergies, or colds; sedatives, tranquilizers, or sleeping medicine; prescription pain medicine or narcotics; barbiturates; medicine for seizures; muscle relaxants; and antiemetics (medicines that prevent or relieve nausea or vomiting). If you are not able to lie down for a while, *make sure you know how you react to this medicine or combination of medicines before you drive, use machines, or do anything else that could be dangerous if you are dizzy or are not alert and able to see well.*
- Belladonna alkaloids, dimenhydrinate, and diphenhydramine may cause dryness of the mouth, nose, and throat. For temporary relief of mouth dryness, use sugarless candy or gum, melt bits of ice in your mouth, or use a saliva substitute.
- Belladonna alkaloids may interfere with certain laboratory tests that check the amount of acid in your stomach. They should not be taken for 24 hours before the test.
- Dimenhydrinate and diphenhydramine may interfere with skin tests that show whether you are allergic to certain substances. They should not be taken for 3 days before the test.

Side Effects of This Medicine

Along with its needed effects, a medicine may cause some unwanted effects. Although not all of these side effects may occur, if they do occur they may need medical attention.

Check with your doctor immediately if the following side effects occur, because they may mean that you are developing a problem with blood circulation:

Less common or rare
Anxiety or confusion (severe); change in vision; chest pain; increase in blood pressure; muscle pain; pain in arms, legs, or lower back, especially if pain occurs in your calves or heels while you are walking; pale, bluish-colored, or cold hands or feet (not caused by cold temperatures and occurring together with other side effects listed in this section); red or violet-colored blisters on the skin of the hands or feet

Also check with your doctor immediately if any of the following side effects occur, because they may mean that you have taken an overdose of the medicine:

Less common or rare
Convulsions (seizures); diarrhea, nausea, vomiting, or stomach pain or bloating (severe) occurring together with other signs of overdose or of problems with blood circulation; dizziness, drowsiness, or weakness (severe), occurring together with other signs of overdose or of problems with blood circulation; fast or slow heart-

beat; diarrhea; headaches, more often and/or more severe than before; problems with moving bowels, occurring together with pain or discomfort in the rectum (with rectal suppositories only); shortness of breath; unusual excitement

The following side effects may go away after a little while. *Do not take any more medicine while they are present.* If any of them occur together with other signs of problems with blood circulation, *check with your doctor right away.* Even if any of the following side effects occur without other signs of problems with blood circulation, *check with your doctor if any of them continue for more than one hour:*

More common
Itching of skin; coldness, numbness, or tingling in fingers, toes, or face; weakness in legs

Also, check with your doctor as soon as possible if you notice any of the following side effects:

More common
Swelling of face, fingers, feet, or lower legs

Less common or rare
Absence of pulse; blurred vision; decrease in blood pressure; lightheadedness; fainting; fever; general feeling of illness; loss of appetite; lower abdominal pain; lower back pain; pounding in the ears; rapid, weak pulse; slow or irregular heartbeat; unusual tiredness

Other side effects may occur that usually do not need medical attention. These side effects may go away after a little while. However, check with your doctor if any of the following side effects continue or are bothersome:

More common
Diarrhea, nausea, or vomiting (occurring without other signs of overdose or problems with blood circulation); dizziness or drowsiness (occurring without other signs of overdose or problems with blood circulation, especially with combinations containing dimenhydrinate, diphenhydramine, or pentobarbital); nervousness or restlessness; dryness of mouth (especially with combinations containing belladonna alkaloids, dimenhydrinate, or diphenhydramine)

Rare
Abdominal pain; difficulty in moving bowels; irregular bowel movements; rectal discomfort

After you stop taking this medicine, your body may need time to adjust. The length of time this takes depends on the amount of medicine you were taking and how long you took it. During this time check with your doctor if your headaches begin again or worsen.

Other side effects not listed above may also occur in some patients. If you notice any other effects, check with your doctor.

Additional Information

Once a medicine has been approved for marketing for a certain use, experience may show that it is also useful for other medical problems. Although this use is not specifically included in product labeling, dihydroergotamine is sometimes used together with another medicine (heparin) to help prevent blood clots that may occur after certain kinds of surgery. It is also used to prevent or treat low blood pressure in some patients.

For patients receiving this medicine for *preventing blood clots:*

- You may need to receive this medicine two or three times a day for several days in a row. This may increase the chance of problems caused by decreased blood flow. Your health care professional will be following your progress, to make sure that this medicine is not causing problems with blood circulation.

For patients using this medicine to *prevent or treat low blood pressure:*

- Take this medicine every day as directed by your doctor.
- The dose of dihydroergotamine will depend on whether the medicine is going to be injected under the skin or into a muscle, and, sometimes, on the weight of the patient. For these reasons, the dose will have to be determined by your doctor.
- Your doctor will need to check your progress at regular visits, to make sure that the medicine is working properly without causing side effects.
- This medicine is less likely to cause problems with blood circulation in patients with low blood pressure than it is in patients with normal or high blood pressure.
- In patients being treated for low blood pressure, an increase in blood pressure is the wanted effect, not a side effect that may need medical attention.

Other than the above information, there is no additional information relating to proper use, precautions, or side effects for these uses.

HEPATITIS A VACCINE INACTIVATED AND HEPATITIS B VACCINE RECOMBINANT

(Intramuscular route) - hep-a-TYE-tis A vak-seen, in-AK-ti-vay-ted, hep-ah-TY-tiss B vak-seen re-KOM-bin-ant

Commonly used brand name(s)

In the U.S.—
  Twinrix

Available Dosage Forms:

- Suspension

Therapeutic Class: Vaccine

Uses For This Vaccine

Hepatitis A virus vaccine inactivated and hepatitis B virus vaccine recombinant is used to prevent infection caused by Hepatitis A and Hepatitis B in patients 18 years of age or older. The vaccine works by causing your body to produce its own protection (antibodies) against the disease. Hepatitis A and Hepatitis B are highly contagious, serious diseases of the liver.

The hepatitis A virus (HAV) is spread most often through infected food or water. Hepatitis A may also be spread by close person-to-person contact with infected persons (such as between persons living in the same household). Although some infected persons do not appear to be sick, they are still able to spread the virus to others.

Hepatitis A is less common in the U.S. and other areas of the world that have a higher level of sanitation and good water

and sewage (waste) systems. However, it is a significant health problem in parts of the world that do not have such systems. If you are traveling to certain countries or remote (out-of-the-way) areas, hepatitis A vaccine will help protect you from hepatitis A disease.

Hepatitis B (HBV) is spread by contact with body fluids, such as blood, saliva, semen, or vaginal fluids; by needle sticks or sharing needles; or from mother to child.

Hepatitis A and Hepatitis B combination vaccine is recommended for all persons 18 years of age or older who are at risk from infection from their jobs or some behaviors, or from traveling to the following parts of the world:

- Africa.
- the Caribbean.
- Central and South America.
- Eastern and southern Europe.
- the Middle East.
- South and southeast Asia (except Japan).
- the Soviet Union (former).

Hepatitis A and Hepatitis B combination vaccine is also recommended for:

- Military personnel.
- Persons living in or moving to areas that have a high rate of HAV infection and who are at a high risk of HBV infection.
- Persons engaging in high-risk sexual activity, such as homosexual and bisexual males.
- Persons who use illegal injectable drugs.
- Persons at risk through their work, such as laboratory workers who handle live hepatitis A and hepatitis B virus, police and those who give first aid or medical help, and workers who come in contact with stool or sewage.
- People who work in child day-care centers and correctional facilities, residents of drug and alcohol treatment centers, and patients and staff in hemodialysis units.
- Patients who frequently receive blood and blood products, including those people who have problems with clotting, such as hemophiliacs.
- Persons with chronic liver disease.
- Healthcare workers who give first aid or emergency medical care.
- People who are at increased risk for HBV infection and who are in close contact with patients that have hepatitis A or B.

This medicine is available only with your doctor's prescription.

Before Receiving This Vaccine

In deciding to use a vaccine, the risks of taking the vaccine must be weighed against the good it will do. This is a decision you and your doctor will make. For this vaccine, the following should be considered:

Allergies—Tell your doctor if you have ever had any unusual or allergic reaction to this medicine or any other medicines. Also tell your health care professional if you have any other types of allergies, such as to foods, dyes, preservatives, or animals. For non-prescription products, read the label or package ingredients carefully.

Pediatric—Studies on this vaccine have been done only in adult patients, and there is no specific information comparing use of hepatitis A and hepatitis B combination vaccine in children with use in other age groups.

Geriatric—Many medicines have not been studied specifically in older people. Therefore, it may not be known whether they work exactly the same way they do in younger adults. Although there is no specific information comparing use of hepatitis A and hepatitis B combination vaccine in the elderly with use in other age groups, this vaccine is not expected to cause different side effects or problems in older people than it does in younger adults.

Pregnancy—

	Pregnancy Category	Explanation
All Trimesters	C	Animal studies have shown an adverse effect and there are no adequate studies in pregnant women OR no animal studies have been conducted and there are no adequate studies in pregnant women.

Breast Feeding—Studies in women suggest that this medication poses minimal risk to the infant when used during breastfeeding.

Other medicines—Although certain medicines should not be used together at all, in other cases two different medicines may be used together even if an interaction might occur. In these cases, your doctor may want to change the dose, or other precautions may be necessary. Tell your healthcare professional if you are taking any other prescription or non-prescription (over-the-counter [OTC]) medicine.

Interactions with Food/Tobacco/Alcohol—Certain medicines should not be used at or around the time of eating food or eating certain types of food since interactions may occur. Using alcohol or tobacco with certain medicines may also cause interactions to occur. Discuss with your healthcare professional the use of your medicine with food, alcohol, or tobacco.

Other medical problems—The presence of other medical problems may affect the use of this vaccine. Make sure you tell your doctor if you have any other medical problems, especially:

- Allergy to yeast—Hepatitis A and hepatitis B combination vaccine is made with yeast
- Bleeding problems or
- Low blood platelet count—Because hepatitis A and hepatitis B combination vaccine must be injected into a muscle, it may cause bleeding
- Hepatitis A or
- Hepatitis B—The vaccine will not work in patients who already have the disease
- Illness, moderate or severe, with or without fever—The vaccine should not be given until after the illness has cleared up
- Immune system problems—The vaccine may not work properly in patients with this condition

Proper Use of This Vaccine

Dosing—The dose of this medicine will be different for different patients. Follow your doctor's orders or the directions on the label. The following information includes only the average doses of this medicine. If your dose is different, do not change it unless your doctor tells you to do so.

The amount of medicine that you take depends on the strength of the medicine. Also, the number of doses you take each day, the time allowed between doses, and the length of time you take the medicine depend on the medical problem for which you are using the medicine.

- For injection dosage form:
  - For prevention of hepatitis A and hepatitis B:
    - Adults—One milliliter (mL) injected into the arm muscle during the first office visit, then at one month and six months after the first dose, for a total of three doses.
    - Children—Use and dose must be determined by your doctor.

Side Effects of This Vaccine

Along with its needed effects, a medicine may cause some unwanted effects. Although not all of these side effects may occur, if they do occur they may need medical attention.

Check with your doctor immediately if any of the following side effects occur:

Symptoms of allergic reaction—Rare
> Difficulty in breathing or swallowing; hives; itching, especially of feet or hands; reddening of skin, especially around ears; swelling of eyes, face, or inside of nose; unusual tiredness or weakness (sudden and severe)

Some side effects may occur that usually do not need medical attention. These side effects may go away during treatment as your body adjusts to the medicine. Also, your health care professional may be able to tell you about ways to prevent or reduce some of these side effects. Check with your health care professional if any of the following side effects continue or are bothersome or if you have any questions about them:

More common
> Soreness at the place of injection

Less common
> Cough; fever; hardening or thickening of skin at the place of injection; sneezing; sore throat

Rare
> Abdominal or stomach pain; back pain; bruising at the place of injection; difficulty in moving; dizziness; fainting or lightheadedness when getting up from a lying or sitting position; feeling of constant movement of self or surroundings; feeling of warmth; headache, may be severe; irritability and agitation; itching, redness, or swelling at the place of injection; large, flat, blue or purplish patches in the skin at the place of injection; loss of appetite; muscle pain; nausea; pain, swelling, or redness in joints; palpitations; rash; runny nose; sensation of spinning; sleepiness; sleeplessness; small, red or purple spots on skin; sweating; tingling, burning, or prickly sensations; trouble sleeping; unusual drowsiness; unusually fast heartbeat; unusually warm skin; vomiting; weakness; weight loss

Other side effects not listed may also occur in some patients. If you notice any other effects, check with your healthcare professional.

HEPATITIS A VACCINE, INACTIVATED   (Intramuscular route) -
hep-a-TYE-tis A vak-seen, in-AK-ti-vay-ted

Commonly used brand name(s)

In the U.S.—
Havrix	Vaqta
Havrix Pediatric	Vaqta Pediatric

Available Dosage Forms:
- Suspension
- Solution
- Injectable

Therapeutic Class: Vaccine

Uses For This Vaccine

Hepatitis A is a serious disease of the liver that can cause death. It is caused by the hepatitis A virus (HAV), and is spread most often through infected food or water. Hepatitis A may also be spread by close person-to-person contact with infected persons (such as between persons living in the same household). Although some infected persons do not appear to be sick, they are still able to spread the virus to others.

Hepatitis A is less common in the U.S. and other areas of the world that have a higher level of sanitation and good water and sewage (waste) systems. However, it is a significant health problem in parts of the world that do not have such systems. If you are traveling to certain countries or remote (out-of-the-way) areas, hepatitis A vaccine will help protect you from hepatitis A disease.

It is recommended that persons 12 months of age or 2 years of age and older (depending on which brand of the vaccine is given) be vaccinated with hepatitis A vaccine when traveling to the following parts of the world:
- Africa
- Asia (except Japan)
- Parts of the Caribbean
- Central and South America
- Eastern Europe
- The Mediterranean basin
- The Middle East
- Mexico

Hepatitis A vaccine is also recommended for all persons 12 months or 2 years of age and older (depending on which brand of the vaccine is given) who live in areas that have frequent outbreaks of hepatitis A disease or who may be at increased risk of infection from hepatitis A virus. These persons include:
- Military personnel
- Persons living in or moving to areas that have a high rate of HAV infection
- Persons who may be exposed to the hepatitis A virus repeatedly due to a high rate of hepatitis A disease, such as Alaskan Eskimos and Native Americans
- Persons engaging in high-risk sexual activity, such as homosexual and bisexual males
- Persons who use illegal injectable drugs
- Persons living in a community experiencing an outbreak of hepatitis A

- Persons working in facilities for the mentally retarded
- Employees of child day-care centers.
- Persons who work with hepatitis A virus in the laboratory
- Persons who handle primate animals
- Persons with hemophilia
- Food handlers
- Persons with chronic liver disease

Hepatitis A vaccine is to be used only by or under the supervision of a doctor.

Before Receiving This Vaccine

In deciding to use a vaccine, the risks of taking the vaccine must be weighed against the good it will do. This is a decision you and your doctor will make. For this vaccine, the following should be considered:

Allergies—Tell your doctor if you have ever had any unusual or allergic reaction to this medicine or any other medicines. Also tell your health care professional if you have any other types of allergies, such as to foods, dyes, preservatives, or animals. For non-prescription products, read the label or package ingredients carefully.

Pediatric—*Havrix* brand hepatitis A vaccine is not recommended for infants and children younger than 2 years of age. For children 2 years of age and older, this vaccine is not expected to cause different side effects or problems than it does in adults.

Vaqta brand hepatitis A vaccine is not recommended for infants and children younger than 12 months of age. For infants 12 months of age and older, this vaccine is not expected to cause different side effects or problems than it dose in adults.

Geriatric—This vaccine has been tested and has not been shown to cause different side effects or problems in older people than it does in younger adults. Elderly people may be more sensitive than younger adults to the effects of hepatitis A vaccine.

Pregnancy—

	Pregnancy Category	Explanation
All Trimesters	C	Animal studies have shown an adverse effect and there are no adequate studies in pregnant women OR no animal studies have been conducted and there are no adequate studies in pregnant women.

Breast Feeding—Studies in women suggest that this medication poses minimal risk to the infant when used during breastfeeding.

Other medicines—Although certain medicines should not be used together at all, in other cases two different medicines may be used together even if an interaction might occur. In these cases, your doctor may want to change the dose, or other precautions may be necessary. Tell your healthcare professional if you are taking any other prescription or non-prescription (over-the-counter [OTC]) medicine.

Interactions with Food/Tobacco/Alcohol—Certain medicines should not be used at or around the time of eating food or eating certain types of food since interactions may occur. Using alcohol or tobacco with certain medicines may also cause interactions to occur. Discuss with your healthcare

professional the use of your medicine with food, alcohol, or tobacco.

Other medical problems—The presence of other medical problems may affect the use of this vaccine. Make sure you tell your doctor if you have any other medical problems, especially:

- Bleeding problems such as hemophilia or abnormal bleeding—Hepatitis A vaccine injection should be given with caution to avoid increased risks.

- Illness with fever or

- Severe infection—May need to delay receiving vaccine until patient is feeling better

- Patients with unsatisfactory immune response—May cause the vaccine to not work as well

Proper Use of This Vaccine

Dosing—The dose of this medicine will be different for different patients. Follow your doctor's orders or the directions on the label. The following information includes only the average doses of this medicine. If your dose is different, do not change it unless your doctor tells you to do so.

The amount of medicine that you take depends on the strength of the medicine. Also, the number of doses you take each day, the time allowed between doses, and the length of time you take the medicine depend on the medical problem for which you are using the medicine.

- For injection dosage form:
  - For prevention of hepatitis A disease:
    - Adults—One adult dose injected into a muscle. A booster (repeat) dose may be needed six to eighteen months after the first dose.
    - Havrix brand: Children 2 to 18 years of age—One or two pediatric doses injected into a muscle. A booster (repeat) dose may be needed six to twelve months after the first dose.
    - Children up to 2 years of age—Use is not recommended.
    - Vaqta brand: Children 12 months to 18 years of age—One or two pediatric doses injected into a muscle. A booster (repeat) dose may be needed six to eighteen months after the first dose.
    - Infants up to 12 months of age—Use is not recommended.

Side Effects of This Vaccine

Along with its needed effects, a vaccine may cause some unwanted effects. Although not all of these side effects may occur, if they do occur they may need medical attention. It is very important that you tell your doctor about any side effects that occur after a dose of hepatitis A vaccine, even though the side effect may have gone away without treatment. Some types of side effects may mean that you should not receive any more doses of hepatitis A vaccine.

Check with your doctor immediately if any of the following side effects occur:

Rare

Difficulty in breathing or swallowing; hives; itching, especially of feet or hands; reddening of skin, especially around ears; swelling of eyes, face, or inside of nose; unusual tiredness or weakness (sudden and severe)

Incidence not known

Black, tarry stools; bleeding gums; blood in urine or stools; confusion; inability to move arms and legs; irritability; pinpoint red spots on skin; seizures; shakiness and unsteady walk; stiff neck; sudden numbness and weakness in the arms and legs; unsteadiness, trembling, or other problems with muscle control or coordination; unusual bleeding or bruising

Some side effects may occur that usually do not need medical attention. These side effects may go away during treatment as your body adjusts to the medicine. Also, your health care professional may be able to tell you about ways to prevent or reduce some of these side effects. Check with your health care professional if any of the following side effects continue or are bothersome or if you have any questions about them:

More common

Soreness at place of injection

Less common

Arm or back pain; bleeding between periods; body aches or pain; change in amount of bleeding during periods; change in pattern of monthly periods; congestion; cough; dryness of throat; fever of 37.7 °C (100 °F) or higher; general feeling of discomfort or illness; headache; hoarseness; lack of appetite; lack or loss of strength; nausea; pain, soreness; runny nose; sneezing; sore throat; stiffness; stuffy nose; tender, swollen glands in neck; tenderness or warmth at injection site; trouble in swallowing; unusual stopping of menstrual bleeding; voice changes

Rare

Aches or pain in joints or muscles; diarrhea or stomach cramps or pain; itching; swelling of glands in armpits or neck; vomiting; welts

Other side effects not listed may also occur in some patients. If you notice any other effects, check with your healthcare professional.

HEPATITIS B IMMUNE GLOBULIN
(Intramuscular route) - hep-a-TYE-tis B im-MYOON GLOB-yoo-lin

Commonly used brand name(s)

In the U.S.—

Bayhep B	Nabi-HB
HepaGam B	Nabi-HB NovaPlus
HyperHEP B	

Available Dosage Forms:

- Solution

Therapeutic Class: Vaccine

Uses For This Medicine

Hepatitis B Immune Globulin (Human) is used to prevent hepatitis B.

Hepatitis B Immune Globulin (Human) may be used for the following patients:

- Sexual partners of persons with hepatitis B.

- Persons who may be exposed to the virus by means of blood, blood products, or human bites, such as health care workers, employees in medical facilities, patients and staff of live-in facilities and day-care programs for the developmentally disabled, morticians and embalmers, police and fire department personnel, and military personnel.
- Those who have household exposure to persons with acute hepatitis B and babies less than 12 months old whose caregiver tests positive for hepatitis B.
- Babies born to mothers who test positive for hepatitis B.

This medicine is available only from your doctor or other authorized health care professional.

Once a medicine has been approved for marketing for a certain use, experience may show that it is also useful for other medical problems. Although this use is not included in product labeling, hepatitis B immune globulin (human) is used to prevent infection by the hepatitis B virus in patients who have had liver transplants.

Before Using This Medicine

In deciding to use a medicine, the risks of taking the medicine must be weighed against the good it will do. This is a decision you and your doctor will make. For this medicine, the following should be considered:

Allergies—Tell your doctor if you have ever had any unusual or allergic reaction to this medicine or any other medicines. Also tell your health care professional if you have any other types of allergies, such as to foods, dyes, preservatives, or animals. For non-prescription products, read the label or package ingredients carefully.

Pediatric—Although there is no specific information comparing use of hepatitis B immune globulin (human) in children with use in other age groups, this medicine is not expected to cause different side effects or problems in children than it does in adults.

Geriatric—Many medicines have not been studied specifically in older people. Therefore, it may not be known whether they work exactly the same way they do in younger adults or if they cause different side effects or problems in older people. There is no specific information comparing use of hepatitis B immune globulin in the elderly with use in other age groups.

Pregnancy—

	Pregnancy Category	Explanation
All Trimesters	C	Animal studies have shown an adverse effect and there are no adequate studies in pregnant women OR no animal studies have been conducted and there are no adequate studies in pregnant women.

Breast Feeding—There are no adequate studies in women for determining infant risk when using this medication during breastfeeding. Weigh the potential benefits against the potential risks before taking this medication while breastfeeding.

Other medicines—Although certain medicines should not be used together at all, in other cases two different medicines may be used together even if an interaction might occur. In these cases, your doctor may want to change the dose, or

other precautions may be necessary. Tell your healthcare professional if you are taking any other prescription or non-prescription (over-the-counter [OTC]) medicine.

Interactions with Food/Tobacco/Alcohol—Certain medicines should not be used at or around the time of eating food or eating certain types of food since interactions may occur. Using alcohol or tobacco with certain medicines may also cause interactions to occur. Discuss with your healthcare professional the use of your medicine with food, alcohol, or tobacco.

Other medical problems—The presence of other medical problems may affect the use of this medicine. Make sure you tell your doctor if you have any other medical problems, especially:

- Bleeding problems—Because hepatitis B immune globulin (human) is given as a shot into a muscle, it may cause more bleeding
- Immune system problems—Hepatitis B immune globulin (human) may cause severe allergic reactions

Proper Use of This Medicine

Hepatitis B immune globulin (human) is given as a shot into the muscle of the upper arm, upper thigh, or outer area of the buttocks.

Dosing—The dose of this medicine will be different for different patients. Follow your doctor's orders or the directions on the label. The following information includes only the average doses of this medicine. If your dose is different, do not change it unless your doctor tells you to do so.

The amount of medicine that you take depends on the strength of the medicine. Also, the number of doses you take each day, the time allowed between doses, and the length of time you take the medicine depend on the medical problem for which you are using the medicine.

- For injectable dosage form:
  - For prevention of hepatitis B following nonsexual exposure:
    - Adults—Dose is based on weight and will be determined by your doctor. If you have never been vaccinated with hepatitis B virus vaccine, your doctor may start the vaccination series. If you have been vaccinated, you may need a booster.
    - Infants with mothers who test positive for hepatitis B—Dose is usually 0.5 milliliters (mL) injected into a muscle in the thigh.
  - For prevention of hepatitis B following sexual exposure:
    - Adults—Dose is based on weight and will be determined by your doctor. Your doctor may start the hepatitis B virus vaccination series if the exposure has been within the last 14 days or if sexual contact is likely to continue.
  - For prevention of hepatitis B following household exposure:
    - Infants less than 12 months of age—Dose is usually 0.5 mL injected into a muscle in the thigh.

Side Effects of This Medicine

Some side effects may occur that usually do not need medical attention. These side effects may go away during treatment as your body adjusts to the medicine. Also, your health care

professional may be able to tell you about ways to prevent or reduce some of these side effects. Check with your health care professional if any of the following side effects continue or are bothersome or if you have any questions about them:

More common
Back pain; general feeling of discomfort; headache; muscle aches or pain; nausea; pain at the injection site

Less common
Abdominal or stomach cramping; burning, heat, and redness at the injection site; chills; diarrhea; feeling as if you are going to vomit; joint pain; lightheadedness; skin rash; unusual tiredness or weakness

Other side effects not listed may also occur in some patients. If you notice any other effects, check with your healthcare professional.

HEPATITIS B VACCINE RECOMBINANT   (Intramuscular route)
- hep-ah-TY-tiss B vak-seen re-KOM-bin-ant

Commonly used brand name(s)
In the U.S.—

Engerix-B	Recombivax HB Pediatric/
Engerix-B Pediatric	Adolescent
Recombivax HB	

Available Dosage Forms:
• Suspension

Therapeutic Class: Vaccine

Uses For This Vaccine

Hepatitis B vaccine recombinant is used to prevent infection by the hepatitis B virus. The vaccine works by causing your body to produce its own protection (antibodies) against the disease.

Hepatitis B vaccine recombinant is made without any human blood or blood products or any other substances of human origin and cannot give you the hepatitis B virus (HBV) or the human immunodeficiency virus (HIV).

HBV infection is a major cause of serious liver diseases, such as virus hepatitis and cirrhosis, and a type of liver cancer called primary hepatocellular carcinoma.

Pregnant women who have hepatitis B infection or are carriers of hepatitis B virus can give the disease to their babies when they are born. These babies often suffer serious long-term illnesses from the disease.

Immunization against hepatitis B disease is recommended for all newborn babies, infants, children, and adolescents up to 19 years old. It is also recommended for adults who live in areas that have a high rate of hepatitis B disease or who may be at increased risk of infection from hepatitis B virus. These adults include:
• Sexually active homosexual and bisexual males, including those with HIV infection.
• Sexually active heterosexual persons with multiple partners.
• Persons who may be exposed to the virus by means of blood, blood products, or human bites, such as health care workers, employees in medical facilities, patients and staff of live-in facilities and day-care programs for the developmentally disabled, morticians and embalmers, police and fire department personnel, and military personnel.
• Persons who have kidney disease or who undergo blood dialysis for kidney disease.
• Persons with blood clotting disorders who receive transfusions of clotting-factor concentrates.
• Household and sexual contacts of HBV carriers.
• Persons in areas with high risk of HBV infection [in the population], such as Alaskan Eskimos, Pacific Islanders, Haitian and Indochinese immigrants, and refugees from areas that have a high rate of hepatitis B disease; persons accepting orphans or adoptees from these areas; and travelers to these areas.
• Persons who use illegal injection drugs.
• Prisoners.

This vaccine is available only from your doctor or other authorized health care professional.

Before Receiving This Vaccine

In deciding to use a vaccine, the risks of taking the vaccine must be weighed against the good it will do. This is a decision you and your doctor will make. For this vaccine, the following should be considered:

Allergies—Tell your doctor if you have ever had any unusual or allergic reaction to this medicine or any other medicines. Also tell your health care professional if you have any other types of allergies, such as to foods, dyes, preservatives, or animals. For non-prescription products, read the label or package ingredients carefully.

Pediatric—Hepatitis B vaccine has been tested in newborns, infants, and children and, in effective doses, has not been shown to cause different side effects or problems than it does in adults. The vaccine strength for use in dialysis patients has been studied only in adult patients, and there is no specific information about its use in children receiving dialysis.

Hepatitis B vaccine is very effective when administered to adolescents and young adults. It is recommended that all adolescents who have not previously received three doses of hepatitis B vaccine should start or complete the vaccine series at 11 to 12 years of age. Hepatitis B vaccine has not been shown to cause different side effects or problems in adolescents and young adults than it does in other age groups.

Geriatric—This vaccine is not expected to cause different side effects or problems in older people than it does in younger adults. However, persons over 50 years of age may not become as immune to the virus as do younger adults.

Pregnancy—

	Pregnancy Category	Explanation
All Trimesters	C	Animal studies have shown an adverse effect and there are no adequate studies in pregnant women OR no animal studies have been conducted and there are no adequate studies in pregnant women.

Breast Feeding—Studies in women suggest that this medication poses minimal risk to the infant when used during breastfeeding.

Other medicines—Although certain medicines should not be used together at all, in other cases two different medicines may be used together even if an interaction might occur. In these cases, your doctor may want to change the dose, or other precautions may be necessary. Tell your healthcare professional if you are taking any other prescription or non-prescription (over-the-counter [OTC]) medicine.

Interactions with Food/Tobacco/Alcohol—Certain medicines should not be used at or around the time of eating food or eating certain types of food since interactions may occur. Using alcohol or tobacco with certain medicines may also cause interactions to occur. Discuss with your healthcare professional the use of your medicine with food, alcohol, or tobacco.

Other medical problems—The presence of other medical problems may affect the use of this vaccine. Make sure you tell your doctor if you have any other medical problems, especially:

- Allergic reaction to hepatitis B vaccine, history of—Use of hepatitis B vaccine is not recommended

Proper Use of This Vaccine

Dosing—The dose of this medicine will be different for different patients. Follow your doctor's orders or the directions on the label. The following information includes only the average doses of this medicine. If your dose is different, do not change it unless your doctor tells you to do so.

The amount of medicine that you take depends on the strength of the medicine. Also, the number of doses you take each day, the time allowed between doses, and the length of time you take the medicine depend on the medical problem for which you are using the medicine.

- For injection dosage form:
  - For prevention of hepatitis B infection:
    - Adults, adolescents, and older children—2.5 to 20 micrograms (mcg) injected into the arm muscle during the first office visit, then one month and six months after the first dose, for a total of three doses.
    - Adults who also receive or will receive blood dialysis—40 mcg injected into the arm muscle during the first office visit, then one month and six months after the first dose, for a total of three doses; or 40 mcg injected into the arm muscle during the first office visit, then one month, two months, and six months after the first dose, for a total of four doses.
    - Infants and young children—2.5 to 20 mcg injected into the thigh muscle during the first office visit, then one month and six months after the first dose, for a total of three doses.
    - Newborn babies—2.5 to 20 mcg injected into the thigh muscle at birth or within seven days of birth, then one month and six months after the first dose, for a total of three doses; or 10 or 20 mcg injected into the thigh muscle at birth or within seven days of birth, then one month, two months, and twelve months after the first dose, for a total of four doses.

Side Effects of This Vaccine

Along with its needed effects, a medicine may cause some unwanted effects. Although not all of these side effects may occur, if they do occur they may need medical attention.

Check with your doctor immediately if any of the following side effects occur:

Symptoms of allergic reaction—Rare
> Difficulty in breathing or swallowing; hives; itching, especially of feet or hands; reddening of skin, especially around ears; swelling of eyes, face, or inside of nose; unusual tiredness or weakness (sudden and severe)

Check with your doctor as soon as possible if any of the following side effects occur:

Rare
> Aches or pain in joints, fever, or skin rash or welts (may occur days or weeks after receiving the vaccine); blurred vision or other vision changes; muscle weakness or numbness or tingling of arms and legs

Some side effects may occur that usually do not need medical attention. These side effects may go away during treatment as your body adjusts to the medicine. Also, your health care professional may be able to tell you about ways to prevent or reduce some of these side effects. Check with your health care professional if any of the following side effects continue or are bothersome or if you have any questions about them:

More common
> Soreness at the place of injection

Less common
> Dizziness; fever of 37.7 °C (100 °F) or higher; hard lump, redness, swelling, pain, itching, purple spot, tenderness, or warmth at place of injection; headache; unusual tiredness or weakness

Rare
> Aches or pain in muscles; back pain or stiffness or pain in neck or shoulder; chills; diarrhea or stomach cramps or pain; general feeling of discomfort or illness; increased sweating; headache (mild), sore throat, runny nose, or fever (mild); itching; lack of appetite or decreased appetite; nausea or vomiting; sudden redness of skin; swelling of glands in armpit or neck; trouble in sleeping; welts

Other side effects not listed may also occur in some patients. If you notice any other effects, check with your healthcare professional.

HISTAMINE H₂ ANTAGONIST (Oral route, Injection route, Intravenous route)

Commonly used brand name(s)
In the U.S.—

Axid	Tagamet
Axid AR	Tagamet HB
Axid Pulvules	Zantac
Heartburn Relief	Zantac 150
Pepcid	Zantac 150 Efferdose
Pepcid AC	Zantac 25

In Canada—

Alti-Ranitidine	Apo-Famotidine
Apo-Cimetidine	Famotidine

Available Dosage Forms:
- Powder for Suspension
- Tablet
- Solution
- Tablet, Chewable
- Capsule
- Syrup
- Tablet, Effervescent
- Powder for Solution
- Tablet, Disintegrating
- Injectable
- Capsule, Liquid Filled
- Granule
- Packet
- Suspension

Uses For This Medicine

Histamine H$_2$–receptor antagonists, also known as H$_2$–blockers, are used to treat duodenal ulcers and prevent their return. They are also used to treat gastric ulcers and for some conditions, such as Zollinger-Ellison disease, in which the stomach produces too much acid. In over-the-counter (OTC) strengths, these medicines are used to relieve and/or prevent heartburn, acid indigestion, and sour stomach. H$_2$–blockers may also be used for other conditions as determined by your doctor.

H$_2$–blockers work by decreasing the amount of acid produced by the stomach.

Once a medicine has been approved for marketing for a certain use, experience may show that it is also useful for other medical problems. Although these uses are not included in product labeling, H$_2$–blockers are used in certain patients with the following medical conditions:
- Damage to the stomach and/or intestines due to stress or trauma
- Hives
- Pancreatic problems
- Stomach or intestinal ulcers (sores) resulting from damage caused by medication used to treat rheumatoid arthritis

Before Using This Medicine

Allergies—Tell your doctor if you have ever had any unusual or allergic reaction to medicines in this group or any other medicines. Also tell your health care professional if you have any other types of allergies, such as to foods dyes, preservatives, or animals. For non-prescription products, read the label or package ingredients carefully.

Pediatric—This medicine has been tested in children and, in effective doses, has not been shown to cause different side effects or problems than it does in adults when used for short periods of time.

Geriatric—Confusion and dizziness may be especially likely to occur in elderly patients, who are usually more sensitive than younger adults to the effects of H$_2$–blockers.

Pregnancy—H$_2$–blockers have not been studied in pregnant women. In animal studies, famotidine and ranitidine have not been shown to cause birth defects or other problems. However, one study in rats suggested that cimetidine may affect male sexual development. More studies are needed to confirm this. Also, studies in rabbits with very high doses have shown that nizatidine causes miscarriages and low birth weights. Make sure your doctor knows if you are pregnant or if you may become pregnant before taking H$_2$–blockers.

Breast Feeding—Cimetidine, famotidine, nizatidine, and ranitidine pass into the breast milk and may cause unwanted effects, such as decreased amounts of stomach acid and increased excitement, in the nursing baby. It may be necessary for you to take another medicine or to stop breast-feeding during treatment. Be sure you have discussed the risks and benefits of the medicine with your doctor.

Other medicines—

Using medicines in this class with any of the following medicines is not recommended. Your doctor may decide not to treat you with a medication in this class or change some of the other medicines you take.

Dofetilide

Using medicines in this class with any of the following medicines is usually not recommended, but may be required in some cases. If both medicines are prescribed together, your doctor may change the dose or how often you use one or both of the medicines.

Alosetron, Carmustine, Chloroquine, Delavirdine, Meperidine, Metformin, Morphine, Morphine Sulfate Liposome, Theophylline, Tizanidine, Tolazoline, Zalcitabine

Using this medicine with any of the following may cause an increased risk of certain side effects but using both medicines may be the best treatment for you. If both medicines are prescribed together, your doctor may change the dose or how often you use one or both of the medicines.

Alprazolam, Amitriptyline, Atazanavir, Azelastine, Carvedilol, Cefditoren Pivoxil, Cefpodoxime Proxetil, Clozapine, Cyclosporine, Desipramine, Dicumarol, Dilevalol, Diltiazem, Doxepin, Dutasteride, Enoxacin, Epirubicin, Escitalopram, Flecainide, Fluconazole, Fosamprenavir, Fosphenytoin, Gefitinib, Glipizide, Imipramine, Itraconazole, Labetalol, Levomethadyl, Lidocaine, Lornoxicam, Metoprolol, Midazolam, Nifedipine, Nisoldipine, Nortriptyline, Paroxetine, Pentoxifylline, Phenindione, Phenytoin, Pramipexole, Procainamide, Propranolol, Quinidine, Saquinavir, Sertraline, Tamsulosin, Timolol, Tocainide, Triazolam, Trimetrexate, Warfarin, Zaleplon, Zolmitriptan

Interactions with Food/Tobacco/Alcohol—Certain medicines should not be used at or around the time of eating food or eating certain types of food since interactions may occur. Using alcohol or tobacco with certain medicines may also cause interactions to occur. The following interactions have been selected on the basis of their potential significance and are not necessarily all-inclusive.

Using this medicine with any of the following may cause an increased risk of certain side effects but may be unavoidable in some cases. If used together, your doctor may change the dose or how often you use this medicine or give you special instructions about the use of food, alcohol, or tobacco.

Grapefruit Juice

Other medical problems—The presence of other medical problems may affect the use of medicines in this class. Make sure you tell your doctor if you have any other medical problems, especially:
- Kidney disease or
- Liver disease—The H$_2$–blocker may build up in the bloodstream, which may increase the risk of side effects.
- Phenylketonuria (PKU)—Some H$_2$–blockers contain aspartame. Aspartame is converted to phenylalanine in the body and must be used with caution in patients with PKU. The Pepcid AC brand of famotidine chewable tablets contains 1.4 mg of phenylalanine per 10–mg dose. The Pepcid RPD brand of famotidine oral dispersible tablets contains 1.05 mg of phenylalanine per 20–mg dose. The Zantac brand of ranitidine EFFERdose tablets contains 2.81 mg of phenylalanine per 25–mg dose and 16.84 mg of phenylalanine per 150–mg dose.

- Porphyria (rare family disease that affects the way your body digests food)—May make condition worse in patients who have acute porphyria
- Weakened immune system (difficulty fighting infection)—Decrease in stomach acid caused by H₂–blockers may increase the possibility of a certain type of infection

Proper Use of This Medicine

For patients taking the nonprescription strengths of these medicines for heartburn, acid indigestion, and sour stomach:

- Do not take the maximum daily dosage continuously for more than 2 weeks, unless directed to do so by your doctor.
- If you have trouble in swallowing, or persistent abdominal pain, see your doctor promptly. These may be signs of a serious condition that may need different treatment.

For patients taking the prescription strengths of these medicines for more serious problems:

- One dose a day—Take it at bedtime, unless otherwise directed.
- Two doses a day—Take one in the morning and one at bedtime.
- Several doses a day—Take them with meals and at bedtime for best results.

It may take several days before this medicine begins to relieve stomach pain. To help relieve this pain, antacids may be taken with the H₂–blocker, unless your doctor has told you not to use them. However, you should wait one-half to one hour between taking the antacid and the H₂–blocker. Take this medicine for the full time of treatment, even if you begin to feel better. Also, it is important that you keep your appointments with your doctor for check-ups so that your doctor will be better able to tell you when to stop taking this medicine.

For patients taking famotidine chewable tablets:

- Chew the tablets well before swallowing.

For patients taking famotidine oral disintegrating tablets:

- Make sure your hands are dry.
- Leave tablets in unopened package until the time of use, then open the pack and remove the tablet.
- Immediately place the tablet on the tongue.
- The tablet will dissolve in seconds, and you may swallow it with your saliva. You do not need to drink water or other liquid to swallow the tablet.

For patients taking ranitidine effervescent tablets:

- Do not chew, swallow whole or dissolve on the tongue.
- Remove the foil wrapping and dissolve the 150–mg tablet in 6 to 8 ounces of water before drinking.
- For infants and children: Dissolve the 25–mg tablet in no less than 5 mL (1 teaspoonful) of water in a dosing cup. Wait until the tablet is completely dissolved before administering the solution to the infant or child. You may give the medicine to your infant by dropper or oral syringe. Ask your doctor if you are unsure how much medicine to give your infant.

Dosing—The dose medicines in this class will be different for different patients. Follow your doctor's orders or the directions on the label. The following information includes only the average doses of these medicines. If your dose is different, do not change it unless your doctor tells you to do so.

The amount of medicine that you take depends on the strength of the medicine. Also, the number of doses you take each day, the time allowed between doses, and the length of time you take the medicine depend on the medical problem for which you are using the medicine.

- For cimetidine:
  - For oral dosage forms (solution and tablets):
    - To treat duodenal or gastric ulcers:
      — Older adults, adults, and teenagers— 300 milligrams (mg) four times a day, with meals and at bedtime. Some people may take 400 or 600 mg two times a day, on waking up and at bedtime. Others may take 800 mg at bedtime.
      — Children—20 to 40 mg per kilogram (kg) (9.1 to 18.2 mg per pound) of body weight a day, divided into four doses, taken with meals and at bedtime.
    - To prevent duodenal ulcers:
      — Older adults, adults, and teenagers— 300 mg two times a day, on waking up and at bedtime. Instead some people may take 400 mg at bedtime.
      — Children—Dose must be determined by your doctor.
    - To treat heartburn, acid indigestion, and sour stomach:
      — Adults and teenagers—100 to 200 mg with water when symptoms start. The dose may be repeated once in twenty-four hours. Do not take more than 400 mg in twenty-four hours.
      — Children—Dose must be determined by your doctor.
    - To prevent heartburn, acid indigestion, and sour stomach:
      — Adults and teenagers—100 to 200 mg with water up to one hour before eating food or drinking beverages you expect to cause symptoms. Do not take more than 400 mg in twenty-four hours.
      — Children—Dose must be determined by your doctor.
    - To treat conditions in which the stomach produces too much acid:
      — Adults—300 mg four times a day, with meals and at bedtime. Your doctor may change the dose if needed.
      — Children—Dose must be determined by your doctor.
    - To treat gastroesophageal reflux disease:
      — Adults—800 to 1600 mg a day, divided into smaller doses. Treatment usually lasts for 12 weeks.
      — Children—Dose must be determined by your doctor.
  - For injection dosage form:
    - To treat duodenal ulcers, gastric ulcers or conditions in which the stomach produces too much acid:
      — Older adults, adults, and teenagers— 300 mg injected into muscle, every six to eight hours. Or, 300 mg injected slowly into a vein every six to eight hours. Instead, 900 mg may be injected slowly into a vein around the clock at the rate of 37.5 mg per hour. Some

people may need 150 mg at first, before beginning the around-the-clock treatment.
— Children—5 to 10 mg per kg (2.3 to 4.5 mg per pound) of body weight injected into a vein or muscle, every six to eight hours.
- To prevent stress-related bleeding:
— Older adults, adults, and teenagers—50 mg per hour injected slowly into a vein around the clock for up to 7 days.
— Children—Dose must be determined by your doctor.

- For famotidine:
  ○ For oral dosage forms (suspension, tablets, chewable tablets, and oral disintegrating tablets):
    - To treat duodenal ulcers:
      — Older adults, adults, and teenagers—40 milligrams (mg) once a day at bedtime. Some people may take 20 mg two times a day.
      — Children—Dose must be determined by your doctor.
    - To prevent duodenal ulcers:
      — Older adults, adults, and teenagers—20 mg once a day at bedtime.
      — Children—Dose must be determined by your doctor.
    - To treat gastric ulcers:
      — Older adults, adults, and teenagers—40 mg once a day at bedtime.
      — Children—Dose must be determined by your doctor.
    - To treat heartburn, acid indigestion, and sour stomach:
      — Adults and teenagers—10 mg with water when symptoms start. The dose may be repeated once in twenty-four hours. Do not take more than 20 mg in twenty-four hours.
      — Children—Dose must be determined by your doctor.
    - To prevent heartburn, acid indigestion, and sour stomach:
      — Adults and teenagers—10 mg taken one hour before eating a meal you expect to cause symptoms. The dose may be repeated once in twenty-four hours. Do not take more than 20 mg in twenty-four hours.
      — Children—Dose must be determined by your doctor.
    - To treat conditions in which the stomach produces too much acid:
      — Older adults, adults, and children—20 mg every six hours. Your doctor may change the dose if needed.
      — Children—Dose must be determined by your doctor.
    - To treat gastroesophageal reflux disease:
      — Older adults, adults, and teenagers—20 mg two times a day, usually for up to 6 weeks.
      — Children weighing more than 10 kg (22 pounds)—1 to 2 mg per kilogram (kg) (0.5 to 0.9 mg per pound) of body weight a day, divided into two doses.
      — Children weighing less than 10 kg (22 pounds)—1 to 2 mg per kg (0.5 to 0.9 mg

per pound) of body weight a day, divided into three doses.
  ○ For injection dosage form:
    - To treat duodenal ulcers, gastric ulcers, or conditions in which the stomach produces too much acid:
      — Older adults, adults, and teenagers—20 mg injected into a vein, every twelve hours.
      — Children—Dose must be determined by your doctor.

- For nizatidine:
  ○ For oral dosage forms (capsules and oral solution):
    - To treat duodenal or gastric ulcers:
      — Older adults, adults, and teenagers—300 milligrams (mg) once a day at bedtime. Some people may take 150 mg two times a day.
      — Children—Dose must be determined by your doctor.
    - To prevent duodenal ulcers:
      — Adults and teenagers—150 mg once a day at bedtime.
      — Children—Dose must be determined by your doctor.
    - To prevent heartburn, acid indigestion, and sour stomach:
      — Adults and teenagers—75 mg taken thirty to sixty minutes before eating a meal you expect to cause symptoms. The dose may be repeated once in twenty-four hours.
      — Children—Dose must be determined by your doctor.
    - To treat gastroesophageal reflux disease:
      — Adults and teenagers—150 mg two times a day.
      — Children—Dose must be determined by your doctor.

- For ranitidine:
  ○ For oral dosage forms (syrup, tablets, effervescent tablets):
    - To treat active duodenal ulcers:
      — Older adults, adults, and teenagers—150 milligrams (mg) two times a day. Some people may take 300 mg once a day at bedtime.
      — Children and infants—2 to 4 mg per kilogram (kg) (1 to 2 mg per pound) of body weight twice a day. However, the total dose will not be more than 300 mg a day.
    - To maintain healing of duodenal ulcers:
      — Older adults, adults, and teenagers—150 mg once a day at bedtime.
      — Children and infants—2 to 4 mg per kg (1 to 2 mg per pound) of body weight once a day. However, the total dose will not be more than 150 mg a day.
    - To treat erosive esophagitis:
      — Older adults, adults, and teenagers—150 mg four times a day
      — Children and infants—5 to 10 mg per kg (2.3 to 4.6 mg per pound) of body weight per day, usually divided and given in two doses during the day.

- To maintain healing of erosive esophagitis:
  - — Older adults, adults, and teenagers— 150 mg twice a day
  - — Children and infants—Dose must be determined by your doctor.
- To treat benign gastric ulcers:
  - — Older adults, adults, and teenagers— 150 mg two times a day.
  - — Children and infants—2 to 4 mg per kg (1 to 2 mg per pound) of body weight twice a day. However, the total dose will not be more than 300 mg a day.
- To maintain healing of gastric ulcers:
  - — Older adults, adults, and teenagers— 150 mg once a day at bedtime.
  - — Children and infants—2 to 4 mg per kg (1 to 2 mg per pound) of body weight once a day. However, the total dose will not be more than 150 mg a day.
- To treat heartburn, acid indigestion, and sour stomach:
  - — Adults and teenagers—150 mg with water when symptoms start. The dose may be repeated once in twenty-four hours. Do not take more than 300 mg in twenty-four hours.
  - — Children—Dose must be determined by your doctor.
- To prevent heartburn, acid indigestion, and sour stomach:
  - — Adults and teenagers—150 mg with water taken thirty to sixty minutes before eating a meal or drinking beverages you expect to cause symptoms. Do not take more than 300 mg in twenty-four hours.
  - — Children—Dose must be determined by your doctor.
- To treat some conditions in which the stomach produces too much acid:
  - — Older adults, adults, and teenagers— 150 mg two times a day. Your doctor may change the dose if needed.
  - — Children—Dose must be determined by your doctor.
- To treat gastroesophageal reflux disease:
  - — Older adults, adults, and teenagers— 150 mg two times a day. Your dose may be increased if needed.
  - — Children and infants—5 to 10 mg per kg (2.3 to 4.6 mg per pound) of body weight per day, usually divided and given in two doses during the day.
  - For injection dosage form:
    - To treat duodenal ulcers, gastric ulcers, or conditions in which the stomach produces too much acid:
      - — Older adults, adults, and teenagers— 50 milligrams (mg) injected into a muscle every six to eight hours. Or, 50 mg injected slowly into a vein every six to eight hours. Instead, you may receive 6.25 mg per hour injected slowly into a vein around the clock. However, most people will usually not need more than 400 mg a day.

- To treat duodenal or gastric ulcers:
  - — Children—2 to 4 mg per kilogram (kg) (1 to 2 mg per pound) of body weight per day, usually divided and injected slowly into a vein every six to eight hours. However the total dose will not be more than 50 mg every six to eight hours.

Missed dose—If you miss a dose of this medicine, take it as soon as possible. However, if it is almost time for your next dose, skip the missed dose and go back to your regular dosing schedule. Do not double doses.

Storage—Store the medicine in a closed container at room temperature, away from heat, moisture, and direct light. Keep from freezing.

Keep out of the reach of children.

Do not keep outdated medicine or medicine no longer needed.

Precautions While Using This Medicine

Some tests may be affected by this medicine. Tell the doctor in charge that you are taking this medicine before:
- You have any skin tests for allergies.
- You have any tests to determine how much acid your stomach produces.

Remember that certain medicines, such as aspirin, and certain foods and drinks (e.g., citrus products, carbonated drinks) irritate the stomach and may make your problem worse.

Cigarette smoking tends to decrease the effect of H$_2$–blockers by increasing the amount of acid produced by the stomach. This is more likely to affect the stomach's night-time production of acid. While taking H$_2$–blockers, stop smoking completely, or at least do not smoke after taking the last dose of the day.

Drinking alcoholic beverages while taking an H$_2$–receptor antagonist has been reported to increase the blood levels of alcohol. You should consult your health care professional for guidance.

Check with your doctor if your ulcer pain continues or gets worse.

Side Effects of This Medicine

Along with its needed effects, a medicine may cause some unwanted effects. Although not all of these side effects may occur, if they do occur they may need medical attention.

Check with your doctor as soon as possible if any of the following side effects occur:

Rare

Abdominal pain; back, leg, or stomach pain; bleeding or crusting sores on lips; blistering, burning, redness, scaling, or tenderness of skin; blisters on palms of hands and soles of feet; changes in vision or blurred vision; confusion; coughing or difficulty in swallowing; dark-colored urine; dizziness; fainting; fast, pounding, or irregular heartbeat; fever and/or chills; flu-like symptoms; general feeling of discomfort or illness; hives; inflammation of blood vessels; joint pain; light-colored stools; mood or mental changes, including anxiety, agitation, confusion, hallucinations (seeing, hearing, or feeling things that are not there), mental depression, nervousness, or severe mental illness; muscle cramps or aches; nausea, vomiting, or loss of appetite; pain; peeling or sloughing of skin; red or irritated eyes; shortness of breath; skin rash or itching; slow heartbeat; sore throat; sores, ulcers, or white spots on lips, in mouth, or on genitals; sudden difficult breathing; swelling of face, lips, mouth, tongue, or eyelids; swelling of hands or feet; swollen or painful glands; tightness in chest; troubled breathing; unusual bleeding or bruising; unusual tiredness or weakness; unusually slow or irregular breathing; wheezing; yellow eyes or skin

Some side effects may occur that usually do not need medical attention. These side effects may go away during treatment as your body adjusts to the medicine. Also, your health care professional may be able to tell you about ways to prevent or reduce some of these side effects. Check with your health care professional if any of the following side effects continue or are bothersome or if you have any questions about them:

Less common or rare

Constipation; decrease in sexual desire; decreased sexual ability (especially in patients with Zollinger-Ellison disease who have received high doses of cimetidine for at least 1 year); diarrhea; difficult urination; dizziness; drowsiness; dryness of mouth or skin; headache; increased or decreased urination; increased sweating; loss of hair; ringing or buzzing in ears; runny nose; swelling of breasts or breast soreness in females and males; trouble in sleeping

Not all of the side effects listed above have been reported for each of these medicines, but they have been reported for at least one of them. All of the H2–blockers are similar, so any of the above side effects may occur with any of these medicines.

Other side effects not listed may also occur in some patients. If you notice any other effects, check with your healthcare professional.

HMG-COA REDUCTASE INHIBITOR (Oral route)

Commonly used brand name(s)

In the U.S.—

Altoprev	Lipitor
Crestor	Mevacor
Lescol	Pravachol
Lescol XL	Zocor

Available Dosage Forms:

• Capsule

• Tablet, Extended Release

• Tablet

Uses For This Medicine

Atorvastatin, cerivastatin, fluvastatin, lovastatin, pravastatin, and simvastatin are used to lower levels of cholesterol and other fats in the blood. This may help prevent medical problems caused by cholesterol clogging the blood vessels.

These medicines belong to the group of medicines called 3–hydroxy-3–methylglutaryl coenzyme A (HMG-CoA) reduc-

tase inhibitors. They work by blocking an enzyme that is needed by the body to make cholesterol. Thus, less cholesterol is made.

Cerivastatin was removed from the market by Bayer in August 2001.

Importance of Diet—Before prescribing medicines to lower your cholesterol, your doctor will probably try to control your condition by prescribing a personal diet for you. Such a diet will be lower in total fat, particularly saturated fat, and dietary cholesterol. Many people are able to control their condition by carefully following their doctor's orders for proper diet and exercise. Medicine is prescribed only when additional help is needed and is effective only when a schedule of diet and exercise is properly followed.

Also, this medicine is less effective if you are greatly overweight. It may be very important for you to go on a reducing diet. However, check with your doctor before going on any diet.

Before Using This Medicine

Allergies—Tell your doctor if you have ever had any unusual or allergic reaction to medicines in this group or any other medicines. Also tell your health care professional if you have any other types of allergies, such as to foods dyes, preservatives, or animals. For non-prescription products, read the label or package ingredients carefully.

Pediatric—Studies on this medicine have been done only in adult patients, and there is no specific information comparing use of HMG-CoA reductase inhibitors in children with use in other age groups. However, atorvastatin, lovastatin, and simvastatin have been used in a limited number of children under 18 years of age. Early information seems to show that these medicines may be effective in children, but their long-term safety has not been studied.

Geriatric—This medicine has been tested in a limited number of patients 65 years of age or older and has not been shown to cause different side effects or problems in older people than it does in younger adults.

Pregnancy—HMG-CoA reductase inhibitors should not be used during pregnancy or by women who plan to become pregnant in the near future. These medicines block formation of cholesterol, which is necessary for the fetus to develop properly. HMG-CoA reductase inhibitors may cause birth defects or other problems in the baby if taken during pregnancy. An effective form of birth control should be used during treatment with these medicines. Check with your doctor immediately if you think you have become pregnant while taking this medicine. Be sure you have discussed this with your doctor.

Breast Feeding—These medicines should not be used during breast-feeding because they may cause unwanted effects in nursing babies.

Other medicines—

Using medicines in this class with any of the following medicines is not recommended. Your doctor may decide not to treat you with a medication in this class or change some of the other medicines you take.

Itraconazole, Mibefradil

Using medicines in this class with any of the following medicines is usually not recommended, but may be required in some cases. If both medicines are prescribed together, your doctor may change the dose or how often you use one or both of the medicines.

Amiodarone, Amprenavir, Atazanavir, Bezafibrate, Ciprofibrate, Clarithromycin, Clofibrate, Cyclosporine, Dalfopristin, Danazol, Darunavir, Delavirdine, Diltiazem, Erythromycin, Fenofibrate, Fluconazole, Fosamprenavir, Fusidic Acid, Gemfibrozil, Indinavir, Itraconazole, Ketoconazole, Lopinavir, Mibefradil, Nefazodone, Nelfinavir, Niacin, Quinupristin, Risperidone, Ritonavir, Saquinavir, Telithromycin, Tipranavir, Troleandomycin, Verapamil

Using this medicine with any of the following may cause an increased risk of certain side effects but using both medicines may be the best treatment for you. If both medicines are prescribed together, your doctor may change the dose or how often you use one or both of the medicines.

Amprenavir, Bosentan, Carbamazepine, Cholestyramine, Conivaptan, Cyclosporine, Darunavir, Delavirdine, Desogestrel, Digoxin, Diltiazem, Efavirenz, Ethinyl Estradiol, Ethynodiol, Etonogestrel, Fluconazole, Fosphenytoin, Imatinib, Itraconazole, Levonorgestrel, Mestranol, Nefazodone, Nelfinavir, Norelgestromin, Norethindrone, Norgestimate, Norgestrel, Oat Bran, Oxcarbazepine, Pectin, Phenytoin, Pioglitazone, Rifampin, Ritonavir, Saquinavir, St John's Wort, Voriconazole, Warfarin

Interactions with Food/Tobacco/Alcohol—Certain medicines should not be used at or around the time of eating food or eating certain types of food since interactions may occur. Using alcohol or tobacco with certain medicines may also cause interactions to occur. The following interactions have been selected on the basis of their potential significance and are not necessarily all-inclusive.

Using medicines in this class with any of the following is usually not recommended, but may be unavoidable in some cases. If used together, your doctor may change the dose or how often you use your medicine, or give you special instructions about the use of food, alcohol, or tobacco.

Grapefruit Juice

Other medical problems—The presence of other medical problems may affect the use of medicines in this class. Make sure you tell your doctor if you have any other medical problems, especially:

- Alcohol abuse (or history of) or
- Liver disease—Use of this medicine may make liver problems worse
- Convulsions (seizures), not well-controlled, or
- Organ transplant with therapy to prevent transplant rejection or
- If you have recently had major surgery—Patients with these conditions may be at risk of developing problems that may lead to kidney failure

Proper Use of This Medicine

Use this medicine only as directed by your doctor. Do not use more or less of it, and do not use it more often or for a longer time than your doctor ordered.

Remember that this medicine will not cure your condition but it does help control it. Therefore, you must continue to take it as directed if you expect to keep your cholesterol levels down.

Follow carefully the special diet your doctor gave you. This is the most important part of controlling your condition, and is necessary if the medicine is to work properly.

For patients taking atorvastatin and simvastatin:
- Do not take these medicines with large amounts of grapefruit juice

For patients taking fluvastatin:
- For extended-release tablets: The extended-release tablets should be swallowed whole. They should not be chewed, crushed, or cut.

For patients taking lovastatin:
- For extended-release tablets: This medicine works better when it is taken at bedtime. The extended-release tablets should be swallowed whole. They should not be chewed, crushed, or cut.
- For tablets: This medicine works better when it is taken with food. If you are taking this medicine once a day, take it with the evening meal. If you are taking more than one dose a day, take each dose with a meal or snack

Dosing—The dose medicines in this class will be different for different patients. Follow your doctor's orders or the directions on the label. The following information includes only the average doses of these medicines. If your dose is different, do not change it unless your doctor tells you to do so.

The amount of medicine that you take depends on the strength of the medicine. Also, the number of doses you take each day, the time allowed between doses, and the length of time you take the medicine depend on the medical problem for which you are using the medicine.

- For atorvastatin:
  - For high cholesterol:
    - Adults—10 to 80 milligrams (mg) once a day.
    - Children 10 to 17 years of age—10 to 20 milligrams (mg) once a day.
    - Children younger than 10 years of age—Use and dose must be determined by your doctor.

- For cerivastatin:
  - For oral dosage form:
    - Removed from the market by Bayer in August 2001

- For fluvastatin:
  - For high cholesterol:
    - For oral dosage form (capsules):
      — Adults—20 to 80 milligrams (mg) once a day in the evening.
      — Children—Use and dose must be determined by your doctor.
    - For long-acting oral dosage form (extended-release tablets):
      ○ Adults—80 mg once a day in the evening.
      ○ Children—Use and dose must be determined by your doctor.

- For lovastatin:
  - For high cholesterol:
    - For oral dosage form (extended-release tablets):
      — Adults—10 to 60 milligrams (mg) once a day at bedtime.
      — Children—Use and dose must be determined by your doctor.
    - For oral dosage form (tablets):
      ○ Adults—20 to 80 milligrams (mg) a day taken as a single dose or divided into smaller doses. Take with evening meals.
      ○ Children—Use and dose must be determined by your doctor.

- For pravastatin:
  - For high cholesterol:
    - For oral dosage form (tablets):
      — Adults—10 to 40 mg once a day at bedtime.
      — Children—Use and dose must be determined by your doctor.

- For rosuvastatin:
  - For high cholesterol:
    - For oral dosage form (tablets):
      — Adults—5 to 40 mg once a day
      — Children—Use and dose must be determined by your doctor.

- For simvastatin:
  - For high cholesterol:
    - For oral dosage form (tablets):
      — Adults—5 to 80 mg a day.
      — Children—Use and dose must be determined by your doctor.

Missed dose—If you miss a dose of this medicine, take it as soon as possible. However, if it is almost time for your next dose, skip the missed dose and go back to your regular dosing schedule. Do not double doses.

Storage—Store the medicine in a closed container at room temperature, away from heat, moisture, and direct light. Do not refrigerate. Keep from freezing.

Keep out of the reach of children.

Do not keep outdated medicine or medicine no longer needed.

Precautions While Using This Medicine

It is very important that your doctor check your progress at regular visits. This will allow your doctor to see if the medicine is working properly to lower your cholesterol levels and that it does not cause unwanted effects.

Check with your doctor immediately if you think that you may be pregnant. HMG-CoA reductase inhibitors may cause birth defects or other problems in the baby if taken during pregnancy. Your doctor may recommend an appropriate method of birth control to prevent adolescent girls and women of child bearing potential from getting pregnant.

Do not stop taking this medicine without first checking with your doctor. When you stop taking this medicine, your blood cholesterol levels may increase again. Your doctor may want you to follow a special diet to help prevent this from happening.

Before having any kind of surgery (including dental surgery) or emergency treatment, tell the medical doctor or dentist in charge that you are taking this medicine.

Check with your doctor immediately if you have unexplained muscle pain, tenderness, or weakness.

Side Effects of This Medicine

Along with its needed effects, a medicine may cause some unwanted effects. Although not all of these side effects may occur, if they do occur they may need medical attention.

Check with your doctor as soon as possible if any of the following side effects occur:
  Less common or rare
    Fever; muscle aches or cramps; severe stomach pain; unusual tiredness or weakness

Some side effects may occur that usually do not need medical attention. These side effects may go away during treatment as your body adjusts to the medicine. Also, your health care professional may be able to tell you about ways to prevent or reduce some of these side effects. Check with your health care professional if any of the following side effects continue or are bothersome or if you have any questions about them:
  More common
    Constipation; diarrhea; dizziness; gas; headache; heartburn; nausea; skin rash; stomach pain
  Rare
    Decreased sexual ability; trouble in sleeping

Other side effects not listed may also occur in some patients. If you notice any other effects, check with your healthcare professional.

HYDRALAZINE   (Oral route, Injection route, Intravenous route) - hye-DRAL-a-zeen

Commonly used brand name(s)
In the U.S.—
  Apresoline

Available Dosage Forms:
- Powder for Solution
- Solution
- Tablet

Therapeutic Class: Peripheral Vasodilator

Uses For This Medicine

Hydralazine belongs to the general class of medicines called antihypertensives. It is used to treat high blood pressure (hypertension). It is also used to control high blood pressure in the mother during pregnancy (pre-eclampsia or eclampsia) or in emergency situations when blood pressure is extremely high (hypertensive crisis).

High blood pressure adds to the workload of the heart and arteries. If it continues for a long time, the heart and arteries may not function properly. This can damage the blood vessels of the brain, heart, and kidneys, resulting in a stroke, heart failure, or kidney failure. High blood pressure may also increase the risk of heart attacks. These problems may be less likely to occur if blood pressure is controlled.

Hydralazine works by relaxing blood vessels and increasing the supply of blood and oxygen to the heart while reducing its workload.

Hydralazine may also be used for other conditions as determined by your doctor.

Hydralazine is available only with your doctor's prescription.

Once a medicine has been approved for marketing for a certain use, experience may show that it is also useful for other medical problems. Although this use is not specifically included in product labeling, hydralazine is used in certain patients with the following medical condition:
- Congestive heart failure

Before Using This Medicine

In deciding to use a medicine, the risks of taking the medicine must be weighed against the good it will do. This is a decision you and your doctor will make. For this medicine, the following should be considered:

Allergies—Tell your doctor if you have ever had any unusual or allergic reaction to this medicine or any other medicines. Also tell your health care professional if you have any other types of allergies, such as to foods, dyes, preservatives, or animals. For non-prescription products, read the label or package ingredients carefully.

Pediatric—Although there is no specific information comparing use of hydralazine in children with use in other age groups, this medicine is not expected to cause different side effects or problems in children than it does in adults. However, the oral solution contains aspartame, which is converted to phenylalanine in the body. Children with phenylketonuria cannot process phenylalanine and high levels of this substance in body fluids may cause brain damage.

Geriatric—Many medicines have not been studied specifically in older people. Therefore, it may not be known whether they work exactly the same way they do in younger adults. Although there is no specific information comparing use of hydralazine in the elderly with use in other age groups, this medicine is not expected to cause different side effects or problems in older people than it does in younger adults.

Pregnancy—

	Pregnancy Category	Explanation
All Trimesters	C	Animal studies have shown an adverse effect and there are no adequate studies in pregnant women OR no animal studies have been conducted and there are no adequate studies in pregnant women.

Breast Feeding—There are no adequate studies in women for determining infant risk when using this medication during breastfeeding. Weigh the potential benefits against the potential risks before taking this medication while breastfeeding.

Other medicines—

Using this medicine with any of the following medicines may cause an increased risk of certain side effects, but using both drugs may be the best treatment for you. If both medicines are prescribed together, your doctor may change the dose or how often you use one or both of the medicines.

Metoprolol

Interactions with Food/Tobacco/Alcohol—Certain medicines should not be used at or around the time of eating food or eating certain types of food since interactions may occur. Using alcohol or tobacco with certain medicines may also cause interactions to occur. The following interactions have been selected on the basis of their potential significance and are not necessarily all-inclusive.

Using this medicine with any of the following may cause an increased risk of certain side effects but may be unavoidable in some cases. If used together, your doctor may change the dose or how often you use this medicine, or give you special instructions about the use of food, alcohol, or tobacco.

Enteral Nutrition

Other medical problems—The presence of other medical problems may affect the use of this medicine. Make sure you tell your doctor if you have any other medical problems, especially:

- Heart or blood vessel disease or
- Stroke—Lowering blood pressure may make problems resulting from these conditions worse
- Kidney disease—Effects may be increased because of slower removal of hydralazine from the body
- Phenylketonuria—The oral solution of hydralazine contains aspartame, which is converted to phenylalanine in the body. Patients with phenylketonuria cannot process phenylalanine and high levels of this substance in body fluids may cause brain damage

Proper Use of This Medicine

For patients taking this medicine for high blood pressure:

- In addition to the use of the medicine your doctor has prescribed, treatment for your high blood pressure may include weight control and care in the types of foods you eat, especially foods high in sodium. Your doctor will tell you which of these are most important for you. You should check with your doctor before changing your diet.
- Many patients who have high blood pressure will not notice any signs of the problem. In fact, many may feel normal. It is very important that you take your medicine exactly as directed and that you keep your appointments with your doctor even if you feel well.
- Remember that hydralazine will not cure your high blood pressure but it does help control it. Therefore, you must continue to take it as directed if you expect to lower your blood pressure and keep it down. You may have to take high blood pressure medicine for the rest of your life. If high blood pressure is not treated, it can cause serious problems such as heart failure, blood vessel disease, stroke, or kidney disease.

For patients taking the oral solution form of hydralazine:

- The oral solution may be mixed with fruit juice or applesauce. If mixed with fruit juice or applesauce, take immediately after mixing. Be sure to take all of the mixture to get the full dose of the medicine.

This medicine works best if there is a constant amount in the blood. To help keep this amount constant, do not miss any doses and take the medicine at the same times each day.

Dosing—The dose of this medicine will be different for different patients. Follow your doctor's orders or the directions on the label. The following information includes only the average doses of this medicine. If your dose is different, do not change it unless your doctor tells you to do so.

The amount of medicine that you take depends on the strength of the medicine. Also, the number of doses you take each day, the time allowed between doses, and the length of time you take the medicine depend on the medical problem for which you are using the medicine.

- For oral dosage forms (oral solution and tablets):
  - For high blood pressure:
    - Adults—40 to 200 milligrams (mg) per day divided into two or four doses
    - Children—Dose is based on body weight. The usual dose is 0.75 to 7.5 mg per kilogram (kg) (0.34 to 3.4 mg per pound) of body weight a day. This is divided into two or four doses.

- For injection dosage form:
  - For high blood pressure:
    - Adults—5 to 40 mg injected into a muscle or a vein. Your doctor may repeat the dose as needed.
    - Children—Dose is based on body weight. The usual dose is 1.7 to 3.5 mg per kg (0.77 to 1.6 mg per pound) of body weight a day. This is divided into four to six doses and injected into a muscle or a vein.
  - For high blood pressure during pregnancy:
    - Adults—5 mg injected into a vein every fifteen to twenty minutes.

Missed dose—If you miss a dose of this medicine, take it as soon as possible. However, if it is almost time for your next dose, skip the missed dose and go back to your regular dosing schedule. Do not double doses.

Storage—Keep the bottle closed when you are not using it. Keep it in the refrigerator. Do not freeze.

Keep out of the reach of children.

Do not keep outdated medicine or medicine no longer needed.

Precautions While Using This Medicine

It is important that your doctor check your progress at regular visits to make sure that this medicine is working properly.

Hydralazine may cause some people to have headaches or to feel dizzy. Make sure you know how you react to this medicine before you drive, use machines, or do anything else that could be dangerous if you are dizzy or are not alert.

The oral solution contains 1.4 milligrams (mg) of phenylalanine per teaspoonful (5 mL). Patients with phenylketonuria cannot process phenylalanine and high levels of this substance in body fluids may cause brain damage.

For patients taking this medicine for high blood pressure:

- Do not take other medicines unless they have been discussed with your doctor. This especially includes over-the-counter (nonprescription) medicines for appetite control, asthma, colds, cough, hay fever, or sinus problems, since they may tend to increase your blood pressure.

Side Effects of This Medicine

Along with its needed effects, a medicine may cause some unwanted effects. Although not all of these side effects may occur, if they do occur they may need medical attention.

Check with your doctor as soon as possible if any of the following side effects occur:

Less common

Blisters on skin; chest pain; general feeling of discomfort or illness or weakness; joint pain; muscle pain; numbness, tingling, pain, or weakness in hands or feet; skin rash or itching; sore throat and fever; swelling of feet or lower legs; swelling of lymph glands

Rare

Fever; general feeling of discomfort or illness; sore throat; weakness

Some side effects may occur that usually do not need medical attention. These side effects may go away during treatment as your body adjusts to the medicine. Also, your health care professional may be able to tell you about ways to pre-

vent or reduce some of these side effects. Check with your health care professional if any of the following side effects continue or are bothersome or if you have any questions about them:

More common

Diarrhea; fast heartbeat; headache; loss of appetite; nausea or vomiting; pounding heartbeat

Less common

Constipation; dizziness or lightheadedness; redness or flushing of face; shortness of breath; stuffy nose; watery eyes

Other side effects not listed may also occur in some patients. If you notice any other effects, check with your healthcare professional.

HYDROCODONE AND IBUPROFEN
(Oral route) - hye-droe-KOE-done, eye-byoo-PROE-fen

Black Box Warning

- CARDIOVASCULAR RISK
  - NSAIDs may cause an increased risk of serious cardiovascular thrombotic events, myocardial infarction, and stroke, which can be fatal. This risk may increase with duration of use. Patients with cardiovascular disease or risk factors for cardiovascular disease may be at greater risk
- Ibuprofen is contraindicated for the treatment of peri-operative pain in the setting of coronary artery bypass graft (CABG) surgery.
- GASTROINTESTINAL RISK
  - NSAIDs cause an increased risk of serious gastrointestinal adverse events including bleeding, ulceration, and perforation of the stomach or intestines, which can be fatal. These events can occur at any time during use and without warning symptoms. Elderly patients are at greater risk for serious gastrointestinal events.

Commonly used brand name(s)

In the U.S.—
Reprexain
Vicoprofen

Available Dosage Forms:

- Tablet

Therapeutic Class: Opioid/NSAID Combination
Pharmacologic Class: NSAID

Uses For This Medicine

Hydrocodone and ibuprofen combination is used to relieve pain.

The hydrocodone is a narcotic analgesic that acts in the central nervous system to relieve pain. If hydrocodone is used for a long time, it may become habit-forming (causing mental or physical dependence). Physical dependence may lead to withdrawal side effects when you stop taking the medicine. Since hydrocodone and ibuprofen combination is only used for short-term (10 days or less) relief of pain, physical dependence will probably not occur.

Ibuprofen is a nonsteroidal anti-inflammatory drug (NSAID) used in this combination to relieve inflammation, swelling, and pain.

This medicine is available only with your doctor's prescription.

Before Using This Medicine

In deciding to use a medicine, the risks of taking the medicine must be weighed against the good it will do. This is a decision you and your doctor will make. For this medicine, the following should be considered:

Allergies—Tell your doctor if you have ever had any unusual or allergic reaction to this medicine or any other medicines. Also tell your health care professional if you have any other types of allergies, such as to foods, dyes, preservatives, or animals. For non-prescription products, read the label or package ingredients carefully.

Pediatric—Studies on this medicine have been done only in adult patients, and there is no specific information comparing use of hydrocodone and ibuprofen combination in children with its use in other age groups.

Geriatric—Elderly people are especially sensitive to the effects of hydrocodone and ibuprofen combination. This may increase the chance of side effects during treatment. Constipation may be especially likely to occur in elderly patients.

Other medicines—

Using this medicine with any of the following medicines is not recommended. Your doctor may decide not to treat you with this medication or change some of the other medicines you take.

Ketorolac, Naltrexone

Interactions with Food/Tobacco/Alcohol—Certain medicines should not be used at or around the time of eating food or eating certain types of food since interactions may occur. Using alcohol or tobacco with certain medicines may also cause interactions to occur. The following interactions have been selected on the basis of their potential significance and are not necessarily all-inclusive.

Using this medicine with any of the following may cause an increased risk of certain side effects but may be unavoidable in some cases. If used together, your doctor may change the dose or how often you use this medicine or give you special instructions about the use of food, alcohol, or tobacco.

Ethanol

Other medical problems—The presence of other medical problems may affect the use of this medicine. Make sure you tell your doctor if you have any other medical problems, especially:

- Asthma or other chronic lung disease or
- Brain disease or head injury or
- Enlarged prostate or problems with urination—Side effects of hydrocodone and ibuprofen combination may be dangerous with these conditions
- Abdominal conditions or
- Anemia or
- Alcohol abuse, or history of, or
- Bleeding problems or
- Dehydration or

- Drug dependence, especially narcotic abuse, or history of or
- Heart disease or
- Kidney disease or
- Liver disease or
- Stomach ulcer or
- Tobacco use or
- Underactive thyroid—The chance of side effects may be increased

Proper Use of This Medicine

For safe and effective use of this medicine, do not take more of it, do not take it more often, and do not take it for a longer time than ordered by your health care professional. Taking too much of this medicine may increase the chance of unwanted effects.

Dosing—The dose of this medicine will be different for different patients. Follow your doctor's orders or the directions on the label. The following information includes only the average doses of this medicine. If your dose is different, do not change it unless your doctor tells you to do so.

The amount of medicine that you take depends on the strength of the medicine. Also, the number of doses you take each day, the time allowed between doses, and the length of time you take the medicine depend on the medical problem for which you are using the medicine.

- For oral dosage form (tablets):
  - For pain:
    - Adults—1 tablet of Vicoprofen every four to six hours as needed.
    - Children—Use and dose must be determined by your doctor.

Missed dose—If you miss a dose of this medicine, take it as soon as possible. However, if it is almost time for your next dose, skip the missed dose and go back to your regular dosing schedule. Do not double doses.

Storage—Store the medicine in a closed container at room temperature, away from heat, moisture, and direct light. Keep from freezing.

Keep out of the reach of children.

Do not keep outdated medicine or medicine no longer needed.

Precautions While Using This Medicine

Hydrocodone and ibuprofen combination will add to the effects of alcohol and other central nervous system (CNS) depressants (medicines that slow down the nervous system, possibly causing drowsiness). Some examples of CNS depressants are antihistamines or medicine for hay fever, other allergies, or colds; sedatives, tranquilizers, sleeping medicine, or other prescription pain medication. Do not drink alcoholic beverages, and check with your medical doctor or dentist before taking any of the medicines listed above, while you are using this medicine.

This medicine may cause some people to become drowsy, dizzy, or lightheaded, or to feel a false sense of well-being. Make sure you know how you react to this medicine before you drive, use machines, or do anything else that could be dangerous if you are dizzy or are not alert and clearheaded.

If these reactions are especially bothersome, check with your doctor.

Dizziness, lightheadedness, or fainting may occur, especially when getting up suddenly from a lying or sitting position. Getting up slowly may lessen this problem.

Serious side effects can occur during treatment with this medicine. Sometimes serious side effects can occur without any warning. However, possible warning signs often occur, including swelling of the face, fingers, feet, and/or lower legs; severe stomach pain, black, tarry stools, and/or vomiting of blood or material that looks like coffee grounds; unusual weight gain; and/or skin rash. Also, signs of serious heart problems could occur such as chest pain, tightness in chest, fast or irregular heartbeat, or unusual flushing or warmth of skin. *Stop taking this medicine and check with your doctor immediately if you notice any of these warning signs.*

Before having any kind of surgery (including dental surgery) or emergency treatment, tell the medical doctor or dentist in charge that you are taking this medicine.

Hydrocodone and ibuprofen combination may cause dryness of the mouth. For temporary relief, use sugarless candy or gum, melt bits of ice in your mouth, or use a saliva substitute. However, if dry mouth continues for more than 2 weeks, check with your dentist. Continuing dryness of the mouth may increase the chance of dental disease, including tooth decay, gum disease, and fungus infections.

Side Effects of This Medicine

Along with its needed effects, a medicine may cause some unwanted effects. Although not all of these side effects may occur, if they do occur they may need medical attention.

Check with your doctor as soon as possible if any of the following side effects occur:

Less common or rare
Bloody stools; burning feeling in chest or stomach; congestion in chest; changes in facial skin color; cough; diarrhea; difficulty in swallowing; fast or irregular breathing; fever; frequent urge to urinate; heartburn; inability to urinate; irregular heartbeat; lightheadedness or dizziness; loss of bladder control; puffiness or swelling of the eyelids or around the eyes; ringing or buzzing in the ears; shortness of breath, troubled breathing, tightness in chest and/or wheezing; skin rash, hives, and/or itching; stomach pain; tenderness in stomach

Symptoms of overdose
Blurred vision; cold or clammy skin; confusion; difficulty hearing or ringing or buzzing in ears; dizziness; general feeling of illness; headache; mood or mental changes; nausea and/or vomiting; severe drowsiness; severe stomach pain; skin rash; slow heartbeat; slow or troubled breathing; stiff neck and/or back; swelling of the face, fingers, feet, or lower legs

Some side effects may occur that usually do not need medical attention. These side effects may go away during treatment as your body adjusts to the medicine. Also, your health care professional may be able to tell you about ways to prevent or reduce some of these side effects. Check with your health care professional if any of the following side effects continue or are bothersome or if you have any questions about them:

More common
Anxiety; constipation; dry mouth; gas; increased sweating; nausea and/or vomiting; nervousness;

pounding heartbeat; sleepiness; swelling of feet or lower legs; trouble in sleeping; unusual tiredness or weakness

Less common or rare
Confusion; decreased appetite; decrease in sexual ability; depression; headache; heartburn; increased thirst; irritability; mood or mental changes; mouth ulcers; pain or burning in throat; runny nose; sensation of burning, warmth, heat, numbness, tightness, or tingling; slurred speech; stomach upset; thinking abnormalities; trembling or shaking of hands or feet; unexplained weight loss; unusual feeling of well-being; visual disturbances

Other side effects not listed may also occur in some patients. If you notice any other effects, check with your healthcare professional.

HYDROCORTISONE AND ACETIC ACID (Otic route) - hye-droe-KOR-ti-sone, a-SEE-tik AS-id

Commonly used brand name(s)
In the U.S.—
Acetasol HC

Available Dosage Forms:
• Solution

Therapeutic Class: Anti-Infective/Anti-Inflammatory Combination
Pharmacologic Class: Adrenal Glucocorticoid

Uses For This Medicine

Corticosteroid and acetic acid combinations are used to treat certain problems of the ear canal. They also help relieve the redness, itching, and swelling that may accompany these conditions.

These medicines may also be used for other conditions as determined by your doctor.

Corticosteroid and acetic acid combinations are available only with your doctor's prescription.

Before Using This Medicine

In deciding to use a medicine, the risks of taking the medicine must be weighed against the good it will do. This is a decision you and your doctor will make. For this medicine, the following should be considered:

Allergies—Tell your doctor if you have ever had any unusual or allergic reaction to this medicine or any other medicines. Also tell your health care professional if you have any other types of allergies, such as to foods, dyes, preservatives, or animals. For non-prescription products, read the label or package ingredients carefully.

Pediatric—There is no specific information comparing the use of otic corticosteroids in children under 3 years of age with use in other age groups.

Geriatric—Although there is no specific information comparing the use of otic corticosteroids in the elderly with use in other age groups, they are not expected to cause different side effects or problems in older people than they do in younger adults.

Pregnancy—

	Pregnancy Category	Explanation
All Trimesters	C	Animal studies have shown an adverse effect and there are no adequate studies in pregnant women OR no animal studies have been conducted and there are no adequate studies in pregnant women.

Breast Feeding—There are no adequate studies in women for determining infant risk when using this medication during breastfeeding. Weigh the potential benefits against the potential risks before taking this medication while breastfeeding.

Other medicines—

Using this medicine with any of the following medicines is not recommended. Your doctor may decide not to treat you with this medication or change some of the other medicines you take.

Bupropion, Rotavirus Vaccine, Live

Interactions with Food/Tobacco/Alcohol—Certain medicines should not be used at or around the time of eating food or eating certain types of food since interactions may occur. Using alcohol or tobacco with certain medicines may also cause interactions to occur. Discuss with your healthcare professional the use of your medicine with food, alcohol, or tobacco.

Other medical problems—The presence of other medical problems may affect the use of this medicine. Make sure you tell your doctor if you have any other medical problems, especially:

- Any other ear infection or condition—Otic corticosteroids may worsen existing infections or cause new infections
- Punctured ear drum—Using otic corticosteroids when you have a punctured ear drum may damage the ear

Proper Use of This Medicine

To use:

- Lie down or tilt the head so that the affected ear faces up. Gently pull the ear lobe up and back for adults (down and back for children) to straighten the ear canal. Drop the medicine into the ear canal. Keep the ear facing up for several (about 5) minutes to allow the medicine to run to the bottom of the ear canal. A sterile cotton plug may be gently inserted into the ear opening to prevent the medicine from leaking out. At first, your doctor may want you to put more medicine on the cotton plug during the day to keep it moist.

To keep the medicine as germ-free as possible, avoid touching the dropper or applicator tip to any surface as much as possible (including the ear). Also, always keep the container tightly closed.

For patients using hydrocortisone and acetic acid ear drops:

- Do not wash the dropper or applicator tip, because water may get into the medicine and make it weaker. If necessary, you may wipe the dropper or applicator tip with a clean tissue.

Do not use corticosteroids more often or for a longer time than your doctor ordered. To do so may increase the chance of side effects.

Do not use any leftover medicine for future ear problems without first checking with your doctor. This medicine should not be used if certain kinds of infections are present. To do so may make the infection worse.

Dosing—The dose of this medicine will be different for different patients. Follow your doctor's orders or the directions on the label. The following information includes only the average doses of this medicine. If your dose is different, do not change it unless your doctor tells you to do so.

The amount of medicine that you take depends on the strength of the medicine. Also, the number of doses you take each day, the time allowed between doses, and the length of time you take the medicine depend on the medical problem for which you are using the medicine.

For hydrocortisone and acetic acid
- For ear drops dosage form:
  - For ear infections:
    - Adults and children over 3 years of age—Use 3 to 5 drops in the affected ear every four to six hours for the first twenty-four hours, then 5 drops three to four times daily.
    - Children under 3 years of age—Use and dose must be determined by your doctor.

Missed dose—If you miss a dose of this medicine, apply it as soon as possible. However, if it is almost time for your next dose, skip the missed dose and go back to your regular dosing schedule.

Do not stop treatment abruptly.

Storage—Store the medicine in a closed container at room temperature, away from heat, moisture, and direct light. Keep from freezing.

Keep out of the reach of children.

Do not keep outdated medicine or medicine no longer needed.

Precautions While Using This Medicine

If your condition does not improve within 5 to 7 days, or if it becomes worse, check with your doctor.

Side Effects of This Medicine

Along with its needed effects, a medicine may cause some unwanted effects. Although not all of these side effects may occur, if they do occur they may need medical attention.

Some side effects may occur that usually do not need medical attention. These side effects may go away during treatment as your body adjusts to the medicine. Also, your health care professional may be able to tell you about ways to prevent or reduce some of these side effects. Check with your health care professional if any of the following side effects continue or are bothersome or if you have any questions about them:

Less common
Anorexia, weakness, weight loss (in children); stinging, itching, irritation, or burning of the ear

There have not been any other side effects reported with this medicine. However, if you notice any other effects, check with your doctor.

HYDROXYCHLOROQUINE (Oral route) - hye-drox-ee-KLOR-oh-kwin

Commonly used brand name(s)

In the U.S.—
Plaquenil

Available Dosage Forms:
- Tablet

Therapeutic Class: Antimalarial

Uses For This Medicine

Hydroxychloroquine belongs to the family of medicines called antiprotozoals. Protozoa are tiny, one-celled animals. Some are parasites that can cause many different kinds of infections in the body.

This medicine is used to prevent and to treat malaria and to treat some conditions such as liver disease caused by protozoa. It is also used in the treatment of arthritis to help relieve inflammation, swelling, stiffness, and joint pain and to help control the symptoms of lupus erythematosus (lupus; SLE).

This medicine may be given alone or with one or more other medicines. It may also be used for other conditions as determined by your doctor.

Hydroxychloroquine is available only with your doctor's prescription.

Once a medicine has been approved for marketing for a certain use, experience may show that it is also useful for other medical problems. Although these uses are not included in product labeling, hydroxychloroquine is used in certain patients with the following medical conditions:
- Arthritis, juvenile
- Hypercalcemia, sarcoid-associated
- Polymorphous light eruption
- Porphyria cutanea tarda
- Urticaria, solar
- Vasculitis, chronic cutaneous

Before Using This Medicine

In deciding to use a medicine, the risks of taking the medicine must be weighed against the good it will do. This is a decision you and your doctor will make. For this medicine, the following should be considered:

Allergies—Tell your doctor if you have ever had any unusual or allergic reaction to this medicine or any other medicines. Also tell your health care professional if you have any other types of allergies, such as to foods, dyes, preservatives, or animals. For non-prescription products, read the label or package ingredients carefully.

Pediatric—Children are especially sensitive to the effects of hydroxychloroquine. This may increase the chance of side effects during treatment. Overdose is especially dangerous in children. Taking as few as 3 or 4 tablets (250–milligrams [mg] strength) of chloroquine has resulted in death in small children. Because hydroxychloroquine is so similar to chloroquine, it is probably just as toxic.

Geriatric—Many medicines have not been studied specifically in older people. Therefore, it may not be known whether they work exactly the same way they do in younger adults or if they cause different side effects or problems in older people.

There is no specific information comparing use of hydroxychloroquine in the elderly with use in other age groups.

Breast Feeding—There are no adequate studies in women for determining infant risk when using this medication during breastfeeding. Weigh the potential benefits against the potential risks before taking this medication while breastfeeding.

Other medicines—

Using this medicine with any of the following medicines is not recommended. Your doctor may decide not to treat you with this medication or change some of the other medicines you take.

Aurothioglucose

Interactions with Food/Tobacco/Alcohol—Certain medicines should not be used at or around the time of eating food or eating certain types of food since interactions may occur. Using alcohol or tobacco with certain medicines may also cause interactions to occur. Discuss with your healthcare professional the use of your medicine with food, alcohol, or tobacco.

Other medical problems—The presence of other medical problems may affect the use of this medicine. Make sure you tell your doctor if you have any other medical problems, especially:
- Blood disease (severe)—Hydroxychloroquine may cause blood disorders
- Eye or vision problems—Hydroxychloroquine may cause serious eye side effects, especially in high doses
- Glucose-6–phosphate dehydrogenase (G6PD) deficiency—Hydroxychloroquine may cause serious blood side effects in patients with this deficiency
- Kidney disease—There may be an increased chance of side effects in patients with kidney disease
- Liver disease—May decrease the removal of hydroxychloroquine from the blood, increasing the chance of side effects
- Nerve or brain disease (severe), including convulsions (seizures)—Hydroxychloroquine may cause muscle weakness and, in high doses, seizures
- Porphyria—Hydroxychloroquine may worsen the symptoms of porphyria
- Psoriasis—Hydroxychloroquine may bring on severe attacks of psoriasis
- Stomach or intestinal disease (severe)—Hydroxychloroquine may cause stomach irritation

Proper Use of This Medicine

Take this medicine with meals or milk to lessen possible stomach upset, unless otherwise directed by your doctor.

Keep this medicine out of the reach of children. Children are especially sensitive to the effects of hydroxychloroquine and overdose is especially dangerous in children. Taking as few as 3 or 4 tablets (250–mg strength) of chloroquine has resulted in death in small children. Hydroxychloroquine is probably just as dangerous.

It is very important that you take this medicine only as directed. Do not take more of it, do not take it more often, and do not take it for a longer time than your doctor ordered. To do so may increase the chance of serious side effects.

If you are taking this medicine to help keep you from getting malaria, keep taking it for the full time of treatment. If you already have malaria, you should still keep taking this medicine for the full time of treatment even if you begin to feel better after a few days. This will help to clear up your infection completely. If you stop taking this medicine too soon, your symptoms may return.

Hydroxychloroquine works best when you take it on a regular schedule. For example, if you are to take it once a week to prevent malaria, it is best to take it on the same day each week. Or if you are to take 2 doses a day, 1 dose may be taken with breakfast and the other with the evening meal. Make sure that you do not miss any doses. If you have any questions about this, check with your health care professional.

For patients taking hydroxychloroquine to prevent malaria:

- Your doctor may want you to start taking this medicine 1 to 2 weeks before you travel to an area where there is a chance of getting malaria. This will help you to see how you react to the medicine. Also, it will allow time for your doctor to change to another medicine if you have a reaction to this medicine.
- Also, you should keep taking this medicine while you are in the area and for 4 to 6 weeks after you leave the area. No medicine will protect you completely from malaria. However, to protect you as completely as possible, it is important to keep taking this medicine for the full time your doctor ordered. Also, if fever develops during your travels or within 2 months after you leave the area, check with your doctor immediately.

For patients taking hydroxychloroquine for arthritis or lupus:

- This medicine must be taken regularly as ordered by your doctor in order for it to help you. It may take up to several weeks before you begin to feel better. It may take up to 6 months before you feel the full benefit of this medicine.

For patients unable to swallow hydroxychloroquine tablets:

- Your pharmacist can crush the tablets and put each dose in a capsule. Contents of the capsules may then be mixed with a teaspoonful of jam, jelly, or jello. Be sure you take all the food in order to get the full dose of medicine.

Dosing—The dose of this medicine will be different for different patients. Follow your doctor's orders or the directions on the label. The following information includes only the average doses of this medicine. If your dose is different, do not change it unless your doctor tells you to do so.

The amount of medicine that you take depends on the strength of the medicine. Also, the number of doses you take each day, the time allowed between doses, and the length of time you take the medicine depend on the medical problem for which you are using the medicine.

- For tablets dosage form:
  - For prevention of malaria:
    - Adults—400 milligrams (mg) once every seven days.
    - Children—Dose is based on body weight and must be determined by your doctor. The usual dose is 6.4 mg per kilogram (kg) (2.9 mg per pound) of body weight once every seven days.
  - For treatment of malaria:
    - Adults—800 mg as a single dose. This may sometimes be followed by a dose of 400 mg six to eight hours after the first dose, then 400 mg once a day on the second and third days.
    - Children—Dose is based on body weight and must be determined by your doctor. The usual

dose is 32 mg per kg (14.5 mg per pound) of body weight taken over a period of three days.
  - For treatment of arthritis:
    - Adults—Dose is based on body weight and must be determined by your doctor. The usual dose is 6.5 mg per kg (2.9 mg per pound) of body weight per day.

Missed dose—If you miss a dose of this medicine, take it as soon as possible. However, if it is almost time for your next dose, skip the missed dose and go back to your regular dosing schedule. Do not double doses.

Storage—Store the medicine in a closed container at room temperature, away from heat, moisture, and direct light. Keep from freezing.

Keep out of the reach of children.

Do not keep outdated medicine or medicine no longer needed.

Precautions While Using This Medicine

Check with your doctor immediately if blurred vision, difficulty in reading, or any other change in vision occurs during or after long-term treatment. Your doctor may want you to have your eyes checked by an ophthalmologist (eye doctor).

If your symptoms do not improve within a few days (or a few weeks or months for arthritis), or if they become worse, check with your doctor.

Hydroxychloroquine may cause blurred vision, difficulty in reading, or other change in vision. It may also cause some people to become dizzy or lightheaded. Make sure you know how you react to this medicine before you drive, use machines, or do anything else that could be dangerous if you are dizzy or are not alert or able to see well. If these reactions are especially bothersome, check with your doctor.

Malaria is spread by mosquitoes. If you are living in, or will be traveling to, an area where there is a chance of getting malaria, the following mosquito-control measures will help to prevent infection:

- If possible, sleep under mosquito netting to avoid being bitten by malaria-carrying mosquitoes.
- Wear long-sleeved shirts or blouses and long trousers to protect your arms and legs, especially from dusk through dawn when mosquitoes are out.
- Apply mosquito repellent to uncovered areas of the skin from dusk through dawn when mosquitoes are out.

Side Effects of This Medicine

Along with its needed effects, a medicine may cause some unwanted effects. Although not all of these side effects may occur, if they do occur they may need medical attention. When this medicine is used for short periods of time, side effects usually are rare. However, when it is used for a long time and/or in high doses, side effects are more likely to occur and may be serious.

Check with your doctor immediately if any of the following side effects occur:

Less common

  Blurred vision or any other change in vision— this side effect may also occur or get worse after you stop taking this medicine

Rare

  Convulsions (seizures); increased muscle weakness; mood or other mental changes; ringing or buzzing in ears or any loss of hearing; sore throat and fever; unusual bleeding or bruising; unusual tiredness; weakness

Symptoms of overdose

Drowsiness; headache; increased excitability

Some side effects may occur that usually do not need medical attention. These side effects may go away during treatment as your body adjusts to the medicine. Also, your health care professional may be able to tell you about ways to prevent or reduce some of these side effects. Check with your health care professional if any of the following side effects continue or are bothersome or if you have any questions about them:

More common

Diarrhea; difficulty in seeing to read; headache; itching (more common in black patients); loss of appetite; nausea or vomiting; stomach cramps or pain

Less common

Bleaching of hair or increased hair loss; blue-black discoloration of skin, fingernails, or inside of mouth; dizziness or lightheadedness; nervousness or restlessness; skin rash

Other side effects not listed may also occur in some patients. If you notice any other effects, check with your healthcare professional.

HYDROXYPROPYL CELLULOSE
(Ophthalmic route) - hye-drox-ee-PROE-pil SELL-yoo-lose

Commonly used brand name(s)

In the U.S.—
Lacrisert

Available Dosage Forms:
• Device

Therapeutic Class: Lubricant, Ocular

Uses For This Medicine

Hydroxypropyl cellulose belongs to the group of medicines known as artificial tears. It is inserted in the eye to relieve dryness and irritation caused by reduced tear flow that occurs in certain eye diseases.

This medicine is available only with your doctor's prescription.

Before Using This Medicine

In deciding to use a medicine, the risks of taking the medicine must be weighed against the good it will do. This is a decision you and your doctor will make. For this medicine, the following should be considered:

Allergies—Tell your doctor if you have ever had any unusual or allergic reaction to this medicine or any other medicines. Also tell your health care professional if you have any other types of allergies, such as to foods, dyes, preservatives, or animals. For non-prescription products, read the label or package ingredients carefully.

Pediatric—Although there is no specific information comparing use of this medicine in children with use in other age groups, this medicine is not expected to cause different side effects or problems in children than it does in adults.

Geriatric—Many medicines have not been studied specifically in older people. Therefore, it may not be known whether they work exactly the same way they do in younger adults. Although there is no specific information comparing use of this medicine in the elderly with use in other age groups, this medicine is not expected to cause different side effects or problems in older people than it does in younger adults.

Other medicines—Although certain medicines should not be used together at all, in other cases two different medicines may be used together even if an interaction might occur. In these cases, your doctor may want to change the dose, or other precautions may be necessary. Tell your healthcare professional if you are taking any other prescription or non-prescription (over-the-counter [OTC]) medicine.

Interactions with Food/Tobacco/Alcohol—Certain medicines should not be used at or around the time of eating food or eating certain types of food since interactions may occur. Using alcohol or tobacco with certain medicines may also cause interactions to occur. Discuss with your healthcare professional the use of your medicine with food, alcohol, or tobacco.

Proper Use of This Medicine

To use:

• This medicine usually comes with patient directions. Read them carefully before using this medicine. It is very important that you understand how to insert this eye system properly. If you have any questions about this, check with your doctor.

• Before opening the package containing this medicine, wash your hands thoroughly with soap and water.

• If the eye system accidentally comes out of your eye, as sometimes occurs when the eye is rubbed, do not put it back in the eye, since it may be contaminated. Instead, insert another eye system if needed.

• You may have to use this medicine for several weeks before your eye symptoms get better.

Dosing—The dose of this medicine will be different for different patients. Follow your doctor's orders or the directions on the label. The following information includes only the average doses of this medicine. If your dose is different, do not change it unless your doctor tells you to do so.

The amount of medicine that you take depends on the strength of the medicine. Also, the number of doses you take each day, the time allowed between doses, and the length of time you take the medicine depend on the medical problem for which you are using the medicine.

• For eye system dosage form:
  ○ For dry eyes or eye irritation:
    ▪ Adults and children—Place one insert in the eye each day.

Missed dose—If you miss a dose of this medicine, take it as soon as possible. However, if it is almost time for your next dose, skip the missed dose and go back to your regular dosing schedule. Do not double doses.

Storage—Store the medicine in a closed container at room temperature, away from heat, moisture, and direct light. Keep from freezing.

Keep out of the reach of children.

Do not keep outdated medicine or medicine no longer needed.

Precautions While Using This Medicine

This medicine may cause blurred vision for a short time after each dose is applied. Make sure your vision is clear before you drive, use machines, or do anything else that could be dangerous if you are not able to see well.

This medicine may also cause your eyes to become more sensitive to light than they are normally. Wearing sunglasses and avoiding too much exposure to bright light may help lessen the discomfort.

If your eye symptoms get worse or if you get new eye symptoms, remove the eye system and check with your doctor as soon as possible.

Side Effects of This Medicine

Along with its needed effects, a medicine may cause some unwanted effects. Although not all of these side effects may occur, if they do occur they may need medical attention.

Some side effects may occur that usually do not need medical attention. These side effects may go away during treatment as your body adjusts to the medicine. Also, your health care professional may be able to tell you about ways to prevent or reduce some of these side effects. Check with your health care professional if any of the following side effects continue or are bothersome or if you have any questions about them:

    Less common

        Blurred vision; eye redness or discomfort or other irritation not present before use of this medicine; increased sensitivity of eyes to light; matting or stickiness of eyelashes; swelling of eyelids; watering of eyes

Other side effects not listed may also occur in some patients. If you notice any other effects, check with your healthcare professional.

HYDROXYUREA (Oral route) - hye-drox-ee-yoor-EE-a

Black Box Warning

Treatment of patients with hydroxyurea may be complicated by severe, sometimes life-threatening, adverse effects. Hydroxyurea should be administered under the supervision of a physician experienced in the use of this medication for the treatment of sickle cell anemia.

Hydroxyurea is mutagenic and clastogenic, and causes cellular transformation to a tumorigenic phenotype. Hydroxyurea is thus unequivocally genotoxic and a presumed transspecies carcinogen which implies a carcinogenic risk to humans. In patients receiving long-term hydroxyurea for myeloproliferative disorders, such as polycythemia vera and thrombocythemia, secondary leukemias have been reported. It is unknown whether this leukemogenic effect is secondary to hydroxyurea or is associated with the patients' underlying disease. The physician and patient must very carefully consider the potential benefits of hydroxyurea relative to the undefined risk of developing secondary malignancies.

Commonly used brand name(s)

In the U.S.—
    Droxia
    Hydrea

Available Dosage Forms:
- Tablet
- Capsule

Therapeutic Class: Antineoplastic Agent
Pharmacologic Class: Antimetabolite

Uses For This Medicine

Hydroxyurea belongs to the group of medicines called antimetabolites. It is used to treat some kinds of cancer and to prevent painful episodes associated with sickle cell anemia.

Hydroxyurea seems to interfere with the growth of cancer cells, which are eventually destroyed. Since the growth of normal body cells may also be affected by hydroxyurea, other effects will also occur. Some of these may be serious and must be reported to your doctor. Other effects may not be serious but may cause concern. Some effects may not occur for months or years after the medicine is used.

When used in sickle cell anemia, hydroxyurea appears to increase the flexibility of sickled cells.

Before you begin treatment with hydroxyurea, you and your doctor should talk about the good this medicine will do as well as the risks of using it.

Hydroxyurea is available only with your doctor's prescription.

Before Using This Medicine

In deciding to use a medicine, the risks of taking the medicine must be weighed against the good it will do. This is a decision you and your doctor will make. For this medicine, the following should be considered:

Allergies—Tell your doctor if you have ever had any unusual or allergic reaction to this medicine or any other medicines. Also tell your health care professional if you have any other types of allergies, such as to foods, dyes, preservatives, or animals. For non-prescription products, read the label or package ingredients carefully.

Pediatric—Side effects may be likely to occur in children, who may be more sensitive to the effects of hydroxyurea.

Geriatric—Side effects may be more likely to occur in the elderly, who may be more sensitive to the effects of hydroxyurea. And, because elderly people are more likely to have kidney problems, the doctor may want to adjust the dose and monitor kidney function.

Pregnancy—

	Pregnancy Category	Explanation
All Trimesters	D	Studies in pregnant women have demonstrated a risk to the fetus. However, the benefits of therapy in a life threatening situation or a serious disease, may outweigh the potential risk.

Breast Feeding—There are no adequate studies in women for determining infant risk when using this medication during breastfeeding. Weigh the potential benefits against the potential risks before taking this medication while breastfeeding.

Other medicines—

Using this medicine with any of the following medicines is not recommended. Your doctor may decide not to treat you with this medication or change some of the other medicines you take.

Rotavirus Vaccine, Live

Interactions with Food/Tobacco/Alcohol—Certain medicines should not be used at or around the time of eating food or eating certain types of food since interactions may occur. Using alcohol or tobacco with certain medicines may also cause interactions to occur. Discuss with your healthcare professional the use of your medicine with food, alcohol, or tobacco.

Other medical problems—The presence of other medical problems may affect the use of this medicine. Make sure you tell your doctor if you have any other medical problems, especially:

- Anemia or
- Leukopenia or
- Neutropenia or
- Thrombocytopenia—May worsen and affect the decision to continue therapy
- Chickenpox (including recent exposure) or
- Herpes zoster (shingles)—Risk of severe disease affecting other parts of the body
- Gout or
- Kidney stones—Hydroxyurea may increase levels of uric acid in the body, which can cause gout or kidney stones.
- History of interferon (e.g., Intron A, Roferon-A) use—If you have received interferon treatment in the past, you may have a greater chance of getting severe unwanted effects of the skin.
- Infection (especially AIDS or HIV)—Hydroxyurea may decrease your body's ability to fight infection or cause serious liver, pancreas, or peripheral nerve reactions with certain specific HIV treatments
- Kidney disease—Effects may be increased because of slower removal of hydroxyurea from the body

Proper Use of This Medicine

Take hydroxyurea only as directed by your doctor. Do not use more or less of it, and do not use it more often than your doctor ordered. The exact amount of medicine you need has been carefully worked out. Taking too much may increase the chance of side effects, while taking too little may not improve your condition.

Hydroxyurea should be handled with care and people who are not taking this medicine should take proper precautions to avoid it. To decrease the chances of coming into contact with hydroxyurea:

- Wear disposable gloves when handling hydroxyurea or bottles containing hydroxyurea.
- Wash your hands before and after contact with the bottle or capsules.
- If powder from the capsule is spilled, you should wipe it up immediately with a damp disposable towel and discard it in a closed container, such as a plastic bag.
- You should keep medicine away from children and pets.
- You should contact your doctor for instructions on how to dispose of capsules that are past their expiration date.

For patients who cannot swallow the capsules:

- The contents of the capsule may be emptied into a glass of water and then taken immediately. Some powder may float on the surface of the water, but that is just filler from the capsule.

This medicine is sometimes given together with certain other medicines. If you are using a combination of medicines, make sure that you take each one at the right time and do not mix them. Ask your health care professional to help you plan a way to take your medicine at the right times.

While you are using this medicine, your doctor may want you to drink extra fluids so that you will pass more urine. This will help prevent kidney problems and keep your kidneys working well.

This medicine commonly causes nausea, vomiting, and diarrhea. However, it is very important that you continue to use the medicine, even if you begin to feel ill. Ask your health care professional for ways to lessen these effects.

If you vomit shortly after taking a dose of hydroxyurea, check with your doctor. You will be told whether to take the dose again or to wait until the next scheduled dose.

Dosing—The dose of this medicine will be different for different patients. Follow your doctor's orders or the directions on the label. The following information includes only the average doses of this medicine. If your dose is different, do not change it unless your doctor tells you to do so.

The amount of medicine that you take depends on the strength of the medicine. Also, the number of doses you take each day, the time allowed between doses, and the length of time you take the medicine depend on the medical problem for which you are using the medicine.

Missed dose—If you miss a dose of this medicine, skip the missed dose and go back to your regular dosing schedule. Do not double doses.

Storage—Store the medicine in a closed container at room temperature, away from heat, moisture, and direct light. Keep from freezing.

Keep out of the reach of children.

Do not keep outdated medicine or medicine no longer needed.

Precautions While Using This Medicine

It is very important that your doctor check your progress at regular visits to make sure that this medicine is working properly and to check for unwanted effects.

While you are being treated with hydroxyurea, and after you stop treatment with it, do not have any immunizations (vaccinations) without your doctor's approval. Hydroxyurea may lower your body's resistance and there is a chance you might get the infection the immunization is meant to prevent. In addition, other persons living in your household should not take oral polio vaccine since there is a chance they could pass the polio virus on to you. Also, avoid persons who have recently taken oral polio vaccine. Do not get close to them and do not stay in the same room with them for very long. If you cannot take these precautions, you should consider wearing a protective face mask that covers the nose and mouth.

Hydroxyurea can temporarily lower the number of white blood cells in your blood, increasing the chance of getting an infection. It can also lower the number of platelets, which are necessary for proper blood clotting. If this occurs, there are certain precautions you can take, especially when your blood count is low, to reduce the risk of infection or bleeding:

- If you can, avoid people with infections. Check with your doctor immediately if you think you are getting an infection or if you get a fever or chills, cough or hoarseness, lower back or side pain, or painful or difficult urination.
- Check with your doctor immediately if you notice any unusual bleeding or bruising; black, tarry stools; blood in urine or stools; or pinpoint red spots on your skin.
- Be careful when using a regular toothbrush, dental floss, or toothpick. Your medical doctor, dentist, or nurse may recommend other ways to clean your teeth and gums. Check with your medical doctor before having any dental work done.
- Do not touch your eyes or the inside of your nose unless you have just washed your hands and have not touched anything else in the meantime.
- Be careful not to cut yourself when you are using sharp objects such as a safety razor or fingernail or toenail cutters.
- Avoid contact sports or other situations where bruising or injury could occur.

Side Effects of This Medicine

Along with their needed effects, medicines like hydroxyurea can sometimes cause unwanted effects such as blood problems and other side effects. These and others are described below. Also, because of the way these medicines act on the body, there is a chance that they might cause other unwanted effects that may not occur until months or years after the medicine is used. These delayed effects may include certain types of cancer, such as leukemia. Ask your health care professional for ways to lessen these effects.

Although not all of these side effects may occur, if they do occur they may need medical attention.

Check with your doctor immediately if any of the following side effects occur:

More common
Cough or hoarseness; fever or chills; lower back or side pain; painful or difficult urination

Less common
Black, tarry stools; blood in urine or stools; pinpoint red spots on skin; unusual bleeding or bruising

Check with your doctor as soon as possible if any of the following side effects occur:

Less common
Blackening of fingernails and toenails; sores in mouth and on lips

Rare
Confusion; convulsions (seizures); difficulty in urination; dizziness; hallucinations (seeing, hearing, or feeling things that are not there); headache; joint pain; swelling of feet or lower legs

Incidence not known
Bleeding under skin; blisters on skin; cold, pale or a bluish color skin of the fingers or toes; crater-like lesions; fatigue; itching skin; numbness or tingling of the fingers or toes; pain in the fingers or toes; weight loss

Symptoms of overdose
Scaling of skin on hands and feet; severe darkening of skin color; soreness; sores in mouth and on lips; swelling of palms and soles of feet; violet flushing of the skin

Some side effects may occur that usually do not need medical attention. These side effects may go away during treatment as your body adjusts to the medicine. Also, your health care professional may be able to tell you about ways to prevent or reduce some of these side effects. Check with your health care professional if any of the following side effects continue or are bothersome or if you have any questions about them:

More common
Diarrhea; drowsiness; loss of appetite; nausea or vomiting

Less common
Constipation; redness of skin at place of irradiation; skin rash and itching

Hydroxyurea may cause temporary loss of hair in some people. After treatment has ended, normal hair growth should return, although the new hair may be a slightly different color or texture.

After you stop using this medicine, it may still produce some side effects that need attention. During this period of time, *check with your doctor immediately* if you notice the following side effects:

Black, tarry stools; blood in urine; cough or hoarseness; fever or chills; lower back or side pain; painful or difficult urination; pinpoint red spots on skin; unusual bleeding or bruising

Other side effects not listed may also occur in some patients. If you notice any other effects, check with your healthcare professional.

HYPROMELLOSE (Ophthalmic route)
- hye-PROE-me-lose

Commonly used brand name(s)

In the U.S.—

Genteal	Isopto Tears
Genteal Mild	Nature's Tears
Gonak	Tearisol
Goniosoft	Tears Again Mc

Available Dosage Forms:

- Gel/Jelly
- Solution

Therapeutic Class: Surgical Aid, Ocular

Uses For This Medicine

Hydroxypropyl methylcellulose belongs to the group of medicines known as artificial tears. It is used to relieve dryness and irritation caused by reduced tear flow. It helps prevent damage to the eye in certain eye diseases. Hydroxypropyl methylcellulose may also be used to moisten hard contact lenses and artificial eyes. In addition, it may be used in certain eye examinations.

Some of these preparations are available only with your doctor's prescription.

Before Using This Medicine

In deciding to use a medicine, the risks of taking the medicine must be weighed against the good it will do. This is a decision you and your doctor will make. For this medicine, the following should be considered:

Allergies—Tell your doctor if you have ever had any unusual or allergic reaction to this medicine or any other medicines. Also tell your health care professional if you have any other types of allergies, such as to foods, dyes, preservatives, or animals. For non-prescription products, read the label or package ingredients carefully.

Pediatric—Although there is no specific information comparing use of hydroxypropyl methylcellulose in children with use in other age groups, this medicine is not expected to cause different side effects or problems in children than it does in adults.

Geriatric—Many medicine have not been studied specifically in older people. Therefore, it may not be known whether they work exactly the same way they do in younger adults. Although there is no specific information comparing use of hydroxypropyl methylcellulose in the elderly with use in other age groups, this medicine is not expected to cause different side effects or problems in older people than it does in younger adults.

Other medicines—Although certain medicines should not be used together at all, in other cases two different medicines may be used together even if an interaction might occur. In these cases, your doctor may want to change the dose, or other precautions may be necessary. Tell your healthcare professional if you are taking any other prescription or non-prescription (over-the-counter [OTC]) medicine.

Interactions with Food/Tobacco/Alcohol—Certain medicines should not be used at or around the time of eating food or eating certain types of food since interactions may occur. Using alcohol or tobacco with certain medicines may also cause interactions to occur. Discuss with your healthcare professional the use of your medicine with food, alcohol, or tobacco.

Proper Use of This Medicine

To use:

- First, wash your hands. Then tilt the head back and pull the lower eyelid away from the eye to form a pouch. Drop the medicine into the pouch and gently close the eyes. Do not blink. Keep the eyes closed for 1 or 2 minutes to allow the medicine to be absorbed.
- To keep the medicine as germ-free as possible, do not touch the applicator tip to any surface (including the eye). Also, keep the container tightly closed.

For patients wearing hard contact lenses:

- Take care not to float the lens from your eye when applying this medicine. If you have any questions about this, check with your health care professional.

Dosing—The dose of this medicine will be different for different patients. Follow your doctor's orders or the directions on the label. The following information includes only the average doses of this medicine. If your dose is different, do not change it unless your doctor tells you to do so.

The amount of medicine that you take depends on the strength of the medicine. Also, the number of doses you take each day, the time allowed between doses, and the length of time you take the medicine depend on the medical problem for which you are using the medicine.

- For dry eyes:
  - For ophthalmic solution (eye drops) dosage form:
    - Adults and children—Use 1 drop three or four times a day.

Storage—Store the medicine in a closed container at room temperature, away from heat, moisture, and direct light. Keep from freezing.

Keep out of the reach of children.

Do not keep outdated medicine or medicine no longer needed.

Precautions While Using This Medicine

If you experience eye pain, changes in vision, continued redness or irritation of the eye, or if your symptoms continue for more than 3 days or become worse, check with your doctor.

Side Effects of This Medicine

Along with its needed effects, a medicine may cause some unwanted effects. Although not all of these side effects may occur, if they do occur they may need medical attention.

Check with your doctor as soon as possible if any of the following side effects occur:

Eye irritation not present before use of this medicine

Some side effects may occur that usually do not need medical attention. These side effects may go away during treatment as your body adjusts to the medicine. Also, your health care professional may be able to tell you about ways to prevent or reduce some of these side effects. Check with your health care professional if any of the following side effects continue or are bothersome or if you have any questions about them:

Less common—more common with 1% solution
    Blurred vision; matting or stickiness of eyelashes

Other side effects not listed may also occur in some patients. If you notice any other effects, check with your healthcare professional.

IBANDRONATE (Oral route, Injection route) - i-BAN-droh-nate

Commonly used brand name(s)
In the U.S.—
  Boniva

Available Dosage Forms:
  • Tablet

Therapeutic Class: Calcium Regulator

Uses For This Medicine

Ibandronate is used to treat or prevent osteoporosis (thinning of the bone) in women after menopause.

This medicine is available only with your doctor's prescription.

Before Using This Medicine

In deciding to use a medicine, the risks of taking the medicine must be weighed against the good it will do. This is a decision you and your doctor will make. For this medicine, the following should be considered:

Allergies—Tell your doctor if you have ever had any unusual or allergic reaction to this medicine or any other medicines. Also tell your health care professional if you have any other types of allergies, such as to foods, dyes, preservatives, or animals. For non-prescription products, read the label or package ingredients carefully.

Pediatric—Studies on this medicine have been done only in adult patients and there is no specific information comparing use of ibandronate in children with use in other age groups.

Geriatric—This medicine has been tested and has not been shown to cause different side effects or problems in older people than it does in younger adults.

Pregnancy—

	Pregnancy Category	Explanation
All Trimesters	C	Animal studies have shown an adverse effect and there are no adequate studies in pregnant women OR no animal studies have been conducted and there are no adequate studies in pregnant women.

Breast Feeding—There are no adequate studies in women for determining infant risk when using this medication during breastfeeding. Weigh the potential benefits against the potential risks before taking this medication while breastfeeding.

Other medicines—Although certain medicines should not be used together at all, in other cases two different medicines may be used together even if an interaction might occur. In these cases, your doctor may want to change the dose, or other precautions may be necessary. Tell your healthcare professional if you are taking any other prescription or non-prescription (over-the-counter [OTC]) medicine.

Interactions with Food/Tobacco/Alcohol—Certain medicines should not be used at or around the time of eating food or eating certain types of food since interactions may occur. Using alcohol or tobacco with certain medicines may also cause interactions to occur. The following interactions have been selected on the basis of their potential significance and are not necessarily all-inclusive.

Using this medicine with any of the following may cause an increased risk of certain side effects but may be unavoidable in some cases. If used together, your doctor may change the dose or how often you use this medicine, or give you special instructions about the use of food, alcohol, or tobacco.

Dairy Food

Other medical problems—The presence of other medical problems may affect the use of this medicine. Make sure you tell your doctor if you have any other medical problems, especially:

  • Hypocalcemia (low calcium levels in the blood)—Must be treated first, before beginning treatment with ibandronate
  • Inability to stand or sit upright for at least 60 minutes—You should not take this medicine because it could cause serious problems to your esophagus and stomach.
  • Anemia or
  • Blood clotting problems or
  • Cancer or
  • Cancer treatment or
  • Dental or oral disease or
  • Infection—May put you at risk for a serious jaw problem
  • Asian or Caucasian race or
  • Family history of osteoporosis or
  • Other bone problems or
  • Previous broken bone or
  • Smoking or
  • Thin body frame—These conditions may make it more difficult for this medicine to prevent osteoporosis.
  • Digestion problems—Taking ibandronate may be harmful to the esophagus, intestine, or stomach
  • Esophagus problems or
  • Intestine problems or
  • Stomach problems—Ibandronate may make these conditions worse
  • Kidney problems—The effects of ibandronate may be increased

Proper Use of This Medicine

Make certain your health care professional knows if you are on any special diet, such as a low-sodium or low-sugar diet. Your doctor may recommend that you eat a balanced diet with an adequate amount of calcium and vitamin D (found in milk or other dairy products).

Take ibandronate with a full glass (6 to 8 ounces) of plain water on an empty stomach. It should be taken in the morning at least 60 minutes before any food, beverage, or other medicines. Food and beverages, such as mineral water, coffee, tea, or juice, will decrease the amount of ibandronate absorbed by the body. Waiting longer than 60 minutes will allow more of the drug to be absorbed. Medicines such as antacids, calcium or vitamin supplements will also decrease the absorption of ibandronate.

Do not lie down for 60 minutes after taking ibandronate. This will help ibandronate reach your stomach faster. It will also help prevent irritation to your esophagus.

Your doctor may recommend that you eat a balanced diet with an adequate amount of calcium and vitamin D (found in milk or other dairy products). However, do not take any food, beverages, or calcium or vitamin supplements within 60 minutes or longer of taking ibandronate. To do so may keep this medicine from working properly.

For the *injection:* You will receive this medicine from a healthcare professional every 3 months. You should not receive this injection more often than every 3 months.

Dosing—The dose of this medicine will be different for different patients. Follow your doctor's orders or the directions on the label. The following information includes only the average doses of this medicine. If your dose is different, do not change it unless your doctor tells you to do so.

The amount of medicine that you take depends on the strength of the medicine. Also, the number of doses you take each day, the time allowed between doses, and the length of time you take the medicine depend on the medical problem for which you are using the medicine.

- For oral dosage form (tablets):
  - For treatment of postmenopausal osteoporosis (thinning of bone)
    - Adults—2.5 mg once a day in the morning or 150 mg once a month on the same date each month, taken at least 60 minutes before the first food, beverage, or medication. You should take ibandronate with six to eight ounces of plain water.
    - Children—Use and dose must be determined by your doctor.
  - For prevention of postmenopausal osteoporosis (thinning of bone)
    - Adults—2.5 mg once a day in the morning or 150 mg once a month on the same date each month (if directed by your doctor), taken at least 60 minutes before the first food, beverage, or medication. You should take ibandronate with six to eight ounces of plain water.
    - Children—Use and dose must be determined by your doctor.

Missed dose—If you miss a dose of this medicine, skip the missed dose and go back to your regular dosing schedule. Do not double doses.

Call your doctor or pharmacist for instructions.

Storage—Store the medicine in a closed container at room temperature, away from heat, moisture, and direct light. Keep from freezing.

Keep out of the reach of children.

Do not keep outdated medicine or medicine no longer needed.

Ask your healthcare professional how you should dispose of any medicine you do not use.

Precautions While Using This Medicine

It is important that your doctor check your progress at regular visits to make sure this medicine is working properly and watch for unwanted effects.

Tell your doctor right away if you develop symptoms of your esophagus being irritated such as new or worsening difficulty swallowing, pain on swallowing, pain behind your breast bone, or heartburn.

Importance of not lying down for at least 60 minutes after taking ibandronate.

Importance of taking ibandronate at least 60 minutes before first food, beverage, or medication of the day.

Importance of taking antacids, calcium supplements, or other products containing aluminum, iron, or magnesium at least 60 minutes after ibandronate.

Use of aspirin or nonsteroidal anti-inflammatory drugs (e.g. Aleve, Motrin) may increase your risk for stomach problems.

Do not chew or suck on the tablet. Swallow whole with 6 to 8 ounces of plain water.

Side Effects of This Medicine

Along with its needed effects, a medicine may cause some unwanted effects. Although not all of these side effects may occur, if they do occur they may need medical attention.

Check with your doctor immediately if any of the following side effects occur:
  More common
  Bladder pain; bloody or cloudy urine; chest pain; cough producing mucus; difficulty breathing; difficult, burning, or painful urination; fever or chills; frequent urge to urinate; lower back or side pain; nervousness; pounding in the ears; shortness of breath; slow or fast heartbeat; sneezing; sore throat; tightness in chest; wheezing

  Less common
  Bloody or cloudy urine; body aches or pain; congestion; difficult, burning, or painful urination; difficulty swallowing; dizziness; dryness of throat; fast heartbeat; frequent urge to urinate; hives; hoarseness; itching; large amount of cholesterol in the blood; numbness; puffiness or swelling of the eyelids or around the eyes, face, lips or tongue; runny nose; skin rash; tender, swollen glands in neck; tingling; trouble in swallowing; unusual tiredness or weakness; voice changes

  Incidence unknown
  Blurred vision or other change in vision; bone, joint, and/or muscle pain, severe and occasionally incapacitating; eye redness; eye tenderness; heavy jaw feeling; loosening of a tooth; pain, swelling, or numbness in the mouth or jaw; sensitivity to light; severe eye pain; tearing

Symptoms of overdose

Get emergency help immediately if any of the following symptoms of overdose occur:

  Abdominal cramps; acid or sour stomach; belching; bone pain; burning feeling in chest or stomach; chest pain; confusion; convulsions; difficulty in breathing; difficulty in swallowing; heartburn; indigestion; irregular heartbeats; loss of appetite; mood or mental changes; muscle cramps in hands, arms, feet, legs, or face; numbness and tingling around the mouth, fingertips, or feet; pain or burning in throat; shortness of breath; stomach discomfort upset or pain; sores, ulcers; tenderness in stomach area; tremor; ulcer; unusual tiredness or weakness; upset stomach; vomiting; white spots on lips or tongue or inside the mouth

Some side effects may occur that usually do not need medical attention. These side effects may go away during treatment as your body adjusts to the medicine. Also, your health care professional may be able to tell you about ways to prevent or reduce some of these side effects. Check with your health care professional if any of the following side effects continue or are bothersome or if you have any questions about them:

More common

Acid or sour stomach; belching; diarrhea; ear congestion; headache; heartburn; indigestion; loss of voice; pain in extremity (arms and legs); stomach discomfort, upset or pain

Less common

Abdominal or stomach pain; bleeding, blistering, burning, coldness, discoloration of skin, feeling of pressure, hives, infection, inflammation, itching, lumps, numbness, pain, rash, redness, scarring, soreness, stinging, swelling, tenderness, tingling, ulceration, or warmth at site; cough; difficulty having a bowel movement [stool] difficulty in moving; discouragement; feeling of constant movement of self or surroundings; feeling sad or empty; general feeling of discomfort or illness; irritability; joint pain; lack of appetite; lack or loss of strength; lightheadedness; loss of interest or pleasure; muscle aches and pain; muscle pain or stiffness; nausea; pain, swelling, or redness in joints; sensation of spinning; shivering; sore throat; stuffy or runny nose; sweating; tiredness; tooth disorder; trouble concentrating; trouble sleeping; vomiting; weakness

Rare

Sleeplessness; unable to sleep

Other side effects not listed may also occur in some patients. If you notice any other effects, check with your healthcare professional.

IDARUBICIN   (Intravenous route) - eye-da-ROO-bi-sin

Black Box Warning

Idarubicin hydrochloride injection should be given slowly into a freely flowing intravenous infusion. It must never be given intramuscularly or subcutaneously. Severe local tissue necrosis can occur if there is extravasation during administration.

As is the case with other anthracyclines the use of idarubicin hydrochloride injection can cause myocardial toxicity leading to congestive heart failure. Cardiac toxicity is more common in patients who have received prior anthracyclines or who have pre-existing cardiac disease.

It is recommended that idarubicin hydrochloride injection be administered only under the supervision of a physician who is experienced in leukemia chemotherapy and in facilities with laboratory and supportive resources adequate to monitor drug tolerance and protect and maintain a patient compromised by drug toxicity. The physician and institution must be capable of responding rapidly and completely to severe hemorrhagic conditions and/or overwhelming infection.

Dosage should be reduced in patients with impaired hepatic or renal function.

Commonly used brand name(s)

In the U.S.—
Idamycin PFS

Available Dosage Forms:

• Solution
• Powder for Solution

Therapeutic Class: Antineoplastic Agent

Uses For This Medicine

Idarubicin belongs to the general group of medicines known as antineoplastics. It is used to treat some kinds of cancer, including leukemia.

Idarubicin seems to interfere with the growth of cancer cells, which are eventually destroyed. Since the growth of normal body cells may also be affected by idarubicin, other effects will also occur. Some of these may be serious and must be reported to your doctor. Other effects, like hair loss, may not be serious but may cause concern. Some effects may not occur for months or years after the medicine is used.

Before you begin treatment with idarubicin, you and your doctor should talk about the good this medicine will do as well as the risks of using it.

Idarubicin is to be administered only by or under the supervision of your doctor.

Before Using This Medicine

In deciding to use a medicine, the risks of taking the medicine must be weighed against the good it will do. This is a decision you and your doctor will make. For this medicine, the following should be considered:

Allergies—Tell your doctor if you have ever had any unusual or allergic reaction to this medicine or any other medicines. Also tell your health care professional if you have any other types of allergies, such as to foods, dyes, preservatives, or animals. For non-prescription products, read the label or package ingredients carefully.

Pediatric—There is no specific information comparing use of idarubicin in children with use in other age groups.

Geriatric—Heart problems are more likely to occur in the elderly, who are usually more sensitive to the effects of idarubicin.

Pregnancy—

	Pregnancy Category	Explanation
All Trimesters	D	Studies in pregnant women have demonstrated a risk to the fetus. However, the benefits of therapy in a life threatening situation or a serious disease, may outweigh the potential risk.

Breast Feeding—There are no adequate studies in women for determining infant risk when using this medication during breastfeeding. Weigh the potential benefits against the potential risks before taking this medication while breastfeeding.

Other medicines—

Using this medicine with any of the following medicines is not recommended. Your doctor may decide not to treat you with this medication or change some of the other medicines you take.

Rotavirus Vaccine, Live

Interactions with Food/Tobacco/Alcohol—Certain medicines should not be used at or around the time of eating food or eating certain types of food since interactions may occur. Using alcohol or tobacco with certain medicines may also cause interactions to occur. Discuss with your healthcare professional the use of your medicine with food, alcohol, or tobacco.

Other medical problems—The presence of other medical problems may affect the use of this medicine. Make sure you tell your doctor if you have any other medical problems, especially:

- Chickenpox (including recent exposure) or
- Herpes zoster (shingles)—Risk of severe disease affecting other parts of the body
- Gout or
- Kidney stones—Idarubicin may increase levels of a chemical called uric acid in the body, which can cause gout or kidney stones
- Heart disease—Risk of heart problems caused by idarubicin may be increased
- Kidney disease or
- Liver disease—Effects may be increased because of slower removal of idarubicin from the body

Proper Use of This Medicine

Idarubicin is sometimes given together with certain other medicines. If you are receiving a combination of medicines, it is important that you receive each one at the proper time. If you are taking some of these medicines by mouth, ask your health care professional to help you plan a way to take them at the right times.

While you are receiving this medicine, your doctor may want you to drink extra fluids so that you will pass more urine. This will help prevent kidney problems and keep your kidneys working well.

Idarubicin often causes nausea and vomiting. However, it is very important that you continue to receive it, even if you begin to feel ill. Ask your health care professional for ways to lessen these effects.

Dosing—The dose of this medicine will be different for different patients. Follow your doctor's orders or the directions on the label. The following information includes only the average doses of this medicine. If your dose is different, do not change it unless your doctor tells you to do so.

The amount of medicine that you take depends on the strength of the medicine. Also, the number of doses you take each day, the time allowed between doses, and the length of time you take the medicine depend on the medical problem for which you are using the medicine.

Precautions While Using This Medicine

It is very important that your doctor check your progress at regular visits to make sure that this medicine is working properly and to check for unwanted effects.

While you are being treated with idarubicin, and after you stop treatment with it, do not have any immunizations (vaccinations) without your doctor's approval. Idarubicin may lower your body's resistance, and there is a chance you might get the infection the immunization is meant to prevent. In addition, other persons living in your household should not take oral polio vaccine since there is a chance they could pass the polio virus on to you. Also, avoid persons who have taken oral polio vaccine. Do not get close to them, and do not stay in the same room with them for very long. If you cannot take these precautions, you should consider wearing a protective face mask that covers the nose and mouth.

Idarubicin can temporarily lower the number of white blood cells in your blood, increasing the chance of getting an infection. It can also lower the number of platelets, which are necessary for proper blood clotting. If this occurs, there are certain precautions you can take, especially when your blood count is low, to reduce the risk of infection or bleeding:

- If you can, avoid people with infections. Check with your doctor immediately if you think you are getting an infection or if you get a fever or chills, cough or hoarseness, lower back or side pain, or painful or difficult urination.
- Check with your doctor immediately if you notice any unusual bleeding or bruising; black, tarry stools; blood in urine or stools; or pinpoint red spots on your skin.
- Be careful when using a regular toothbrush, dental floss, or toothpick. Your medical doctor, dentist, or nurse may recommend other ways to clean your teeth and gums. Check with your medical doctor before having any dental work done.
- Do not touch your eyes or the inside of your nose unless you have just washed your hands and have not touched anything else in the meantime.
- Be careful not to cut yourself when you are using sharp objects such as a safety razor or fingernail or toenail cutters.
- Avoid contact sports or other situations where bruising or injury could occur.

If idarubicin accidentally seeps out of the vein into which it is injected, it may damage some tissues and cause scarring. Tell the health care professional right away if you notice redness, pain, or swelling at the place of injection.

Side Effects of This Medicine

Along with its needed effects, a medicine may cause some unwanted effects. Although not all of these side effects may occur, if they do occur they may need medical attention.

Also, because of the way cancer medicines act on the body, there is a chance that they might cause other unwanted effects that may not occur until months or years after the medicine is used. These delayed effects may include certain types of cancer. Discuss these possible effects with your doctor.

Check with your doctor immediately if any of the following side effects occur:

More common

Black, tarry stools; blood in urine or stools; cough or hoarseness; fever or chills; lower back or side pain; painful or difficult urination; pinpoint red spots on skin; unusual bleeding or bruising

Less common

Fast or irregular heartbeat; pain at place of injection; shortness of breath; swelling of feet and lower legs

Rare
Stomach pain (severe)

Check with your doctor as soon as possible if any of the following side effects occur:

More common
Sores in mouth and on lips

Less common
Joint pain

Rare
Skin rash or hives

Some side effects may occur that usually do not need medical attention. These side effects may go away during treatment as your body adjusts to the medicine. Also, your health care professional may be able to tell you about ways to prevent or reduce some of these side effects. Check with your health care professional if any of the following side effects continue or are bothersome or if you have any questions about them:

More common
Diarrhea or stomach cramps; headache; nausea and vomiting

Less common
Darkening or redness of skin (after x-ray treatment); numbness or tingling of fingers, toes, or face

Idarubicin causes the urine to turn reddish in color, which may stain clothes. This is not blood. It is perfectly normal and lasts for only a day or two after each dose is given.

This medicine often causes a temporary and total loss of hair. After treatment with idarubicin has ended, normal hair growth should return.

After you stop using this medicine, it may still produce some side effects that need attention. During this period of time, *check with your doctor immediately* if you notice the following side effects:

Fast or irregular heartbeat; shortness of breath; swelling of feet and lower legs

Other side effects not listed may also occur in some patients. If you notice any other effects, check with your healthcare professional.

IDOXURIDINE (Ophthalmic route) - eye-dox-YOOR-i-deen

Commonly used brand name(s)

In Canada—
Herplex

Available Dosage Forms:
• Solution
• Ointment

Therapeutic Class: Antiviral

Uses For This Medicine

Idoxuridine belongs to the family of medicines called antivirals. Idoxuridine is used to treat virus infections of the eye.

Idoxuridine is available only with your doctor's prescription.

Before Using This Medicine

In deciding to use a medicine, the risks of taking the medicine must be weighed against the good it will do. This is a decision you and your doctor will make. For this medicine, the following should be considered:

Allergies—Tell your doctor if you have ever had any unusual or allergic reaction to this medicine or any other medicines. Also tell your health care professional if you have any other types of allergies, such as to foods, dyes, preservatives, or animals. For non-prescription products, read the label or package ingredients carefully.

Pediatric—Studies on this medicine have been done only in adult patients, and there is no specific information comparing use of this medicine in children with use in other age groups.

Geriatric—Many medicines have not been studied specifically in older people. Therefore, it may not be known whether they work exactly the same way they do in younger adults or if they cause different side effects or problems in older people. There is no specific information comparing use of idoxuridine in the elderly with use in other age groups.

Other medicines—

Using this medicine with any of the following medicines is usually not recommended, but may be required in some cases. If both medicines are prescribed together, your doctor may change the dose or how often you use one or both of the medicines.

Boric Acid

Interactions with Food/Tobacco/Alcohol—Certain medicines should not be used at or around the time of eating food or eating certain types of food since interactions may occur. Using alcohol or tobacco with certain medicines may also cause interactions to occur. Discuss with your healthcare professional the use of your medicine with food, alcohol, or tobacco.

Proper Use of This Medicine

For patients using the eye drop form of idoxuridine:

• The bottle is only partially full to provide proper drop control.
• To use:
  ◦ First, wash your hands. Then tilt the head back and pull the lower eyelid away from the eye to form a pouch. Drop the medicine into the pouch and gently close the eyes. Do not blink. Keep the eyes closed for 1 or 2 minutes to allow the medicine to come into contact with the infection.
  ◦ If you think you did not get the drop of medicine into your eye properly, use another drop.
  ◦ To keep the medicine as germ-free as possible, do not touch the applicator tip to any surface (including the eye). Also, keep the container tightly closed.

For patients using the eye ointment form of idoxuridine:

• To use:
  ◦ First, wash your hands. Then pull the lower eyelid away from the eye to form a pouch. Squeeze a thin strip of ointment into the pouch. A 1–cm (approximately ⅓-inch) strip of ointment is usually enough unless otherwise directed by your doctor. Gently close the eyes and keep them closed for 1 or 2 minutes to

allow the medicine to come into contact with the infection.

- To keep the medicine as germ-free as possible, do not touch the applicator tip to any surface (including the eye). After using idoxuridine eye ointment, wipe the tip of the ointment tube with a clean tissue and keep the tube tightly closed.

Do not use this medicine more often or for a longer time than your doctor ordered. To do so may cause problems in the eyes. If you have any questions about this, check with your doctor.

To help clear up your infection completely, keep using this medicine for the full time of treatment, even though your symptoms may have disappeared. Do not miss any doses.

Dosing—The dose of this medicine will be different for different patients. Follow your doctor's orders or the directions on the label. The following information includes only the average doses of this medicine. If your dose is different, do not change it unless your doctor tells you to do so.

The amount of medicine that you take depends on the strength of the medicine. Also, the number of doses you take each day, the time allowed between doses, and the length of time you take the medicine depend on the medical problem for which you are using the medicine.

- For virus infections of the eye:
  - For eye ointment dosage form:
    - Adults and children—Use every four hours during the day (five times a day).
  - For eye solution (eye drops) dosage form:
    - Adults and children—Use every hour during the day and every two hours during the night. After the eye condition gets better, use every two hours during the day and every four hours during the night.

Missed dose—If you miss a dose of this medicine, apply it as soon as possible. However, if it is almost time for your next dose, skip the missed dose and go back to your regular dosing schedule.

Storage—Store in the refrigerator. Do not freeze.

Keep out of the reach of children.

Do not keep outdated medicine or medicine no longer needed.

Precautions While Using This Medicine

It is very important that your doctor check your progress at regular visits.

If your symptoms do not improve within a week, or if they become worse, check with your doctor.

This medicine may cause your eyes to become more sensitive to light than they are normally. Wearing sunglasses and avoiding too much exposure to bright light may help lessen the discomfort.

Side Effects of This Medicine

Along with its needed effects, a medicine may cause some unwanted effects. Although not all of these side effects may occur, if they do occur they may need medical attention.

Check with your doctor as soon as possible if any of the following side effects occur:

Less common
    Increased sensitivity of eyes to light; itching, redness, swelling, pain, or other sign of irritation not present before use of this medicine

Rare
    Blurring, dimming, or haziness of vision

Some side effects may occur that usually do not need medical attention. These side effects may go away during treatment as your body adjusts to the medicine. Also, your health care professional may be able to tell you about ways to prevent or reduce some of these side effects. Check with your health care professional if any of the following side effects continue or are bothersome or if you have any questions about them:

Less common
    Excess flow of tears

After application, eye ointments usually cause your vision to blur for a few minutes.

Other side effects not listed may also occur in some patients. If you notice any other effects, check with your healthcare professional.

IFOSFAMIDE   (Intravenous route) -
eye-FOS-fa-mide

Black Box Warning

Ifosfamide should be administered under the supervision of a qualified physician experienced in the use of cancer chemotherapeutic agents. Urotoxic side effects, especially hemorrhagic cystitis, as well as CNS toxicities such as confusion and coma have been associated with the use of ifosfamide. When they occur, they may require cessation of ifosfamide therapy. Severe myelosuppression has been reported.

Commonly used brand name(s)

In the U.S.—
    Ifex

Available Dosage Forms:
- Powder for Solution

Therapeutic Class: Antineoplastic Agent
Pharmacologic Class: Alkylating Agent

Uses For This Medicine

Ifosfamide belongs to the group of medicines called alkylating agents. It is used to treat cancer of the testicles as well as some other kinds of cancer. Another medicine, called mesna, is usually given along with ifosfamide to prevent bladder problems that can be caused by ifosfamide.

Ifosfamide interferes with the growth of cancer cells, which are eventually destroyed. Since the growth of normal body cells may also be affected by ifosfamide, other effects will also occur. Some of these may be serious and must be reported to your doctor. Other effects, like hair loss, may not be serious but may cause concern. Some effects may not occur until months or years after the medicine is used.

Before you begin treatment with ifosfamide, you and your doctor should talk about the good this medicine will do as well as the risks of using it.

Ifosfamide is to be administered only by or under the immediate supervision of your doctor.

Once a medicine has been approved for marketing for a certain use, experience may show that it is also useful for other medical problems. Although these uses are not included in product labeling, ifosfamide is used in certain patients with the following medical conditions:

- Acute lymphocytic leukemia (a type of cancer of the blood)
- Cancer of the bladder
- Cancer of the bone (including Ewing's sarcoma)
- Cancer of the breast
- Cancer of the cervix
- Cancer of the endometrium
- Cancers of the head and neck
- Cancer of the lung
- Cancer of the ovaries
- Lymphomas
- Neuroblastoma (a certain type of brain cancer)
- Thymoma and other cancer of the thymus (a small organ beneath the breastbone)
- Tumors in the ovaries
- Wilms' tumor (a cancer of the kidneys occurring mainly in children)

Before Using This Medicine

In deciding to use a medicine, the risks of taking the medicine must be weighed against the good it will do. This is a decision you and your doctor will make. For this medicine, the following should be considered:

Allergies—Tell your doctor if you have ever had any unusual or allergic reaction to this medicine or any other medicines. Also tell your health care professional if you have any other types of allergies, such as to foods, dyes, preservatives, or animals. For non-prescription products, read the label or package ingredients carefully.

Pediatric—Although there is no specific information comparing use of ifosfamide in children with use in other age groups, this medicine is not expected to cause different side effects or problems in children than it does in adults.

Geriatric—Many medicines have not been studied specifically in older people. Therefore, it may not be known whether they work exactly the same way they do in younger adults or if they cause different side effects or problems in older people. There is no specific information comparing use of ifosfamide in the elderly with use in other age groups.

Pregnancy—

	Pregnancy Category	Explanation
All Trimesters	D	Studies in pregnant women have demonstrated a risk to the fetus. However, the benefits of therapy in a life threatening situation or a serious disease, may outweigh the potential risk.

Breast Feeding—There are no adequate studies in women for determining infant risk when using this medication during breastfeeding. Weigh the potential benefits against the potential risks before taking this medication while breastfeeding.

Other medicines—

Using this medicine with any of the following medicines is not recommended. Your doctor may decide not to treat you with this medication or change some of the other medicines you take.

Rotavirus Vaccine, Live

Interactions with Food/Tobacco/Alcohol—Certain medicines should not be used at or around the time of eating food or eating certain types of food since interactions may occur. Using alcohol or tobacco with certain medicines may also cause interactions to occur. Discuss with your healthcare professional the use of your medicine with food, alcohol, or tobacco.

Other medical problems—The presence of other medical problems may affect the use of this medicine. Make sure you tell your doctor if you have any other medical problems, especially:

- Chickenpox (including recent exposure) or
- Herpes zoster (shingles)—Risk of severe disease affecting other parts of the body
- Infection—Ifosfamide can decrease your body's ability to fight infection
- Kidney disease—Effects may be increased because of slower removal of ifosfamide from the body
- Liver disease—Effects may be increased or decreased because the liver both makes ifosfamide work and removes it from the body

Proper Use of This Medicine

Ifosfamide is sometimes given together with certain other medicines. If you are using a combination of medicines, make sure that you take each one at the proper time and do not mix them. Ask your health care professional to help you plan a way to remember to take your medicines at the right times.

While you are receiving ifosfamide, it is important that you drink extra fluids so that you will pass more urine. Also, empty your bladder frequently, including at least once during the night. This will help prevent kidney and bladder problems and keep your kidneys working well. Ifosfamide passes from the body in the urine. If too much of it appears in the urine or if the urine stays in the bladder too long, it can cause dangerous irritation. Follow your doctor's instructions carefully about how much fluid to drink every day. Some patients may have to drink up to 7 to 12 cups (3 quarts) of fluid a day.

Ifosfamide often causes nausea and vomiting. However, it is very important that you continue to receive the medicine even if you begin to feel ill. Ask your health care professional for ways to lessen these effects.

Dosing—The dose of this medicine will be different for different patients. Follow your doctor's orders or the directions on the label. The following information includes only the average doses of this medicine. If your dose is different, do not change it unless your doctor tells you to do so.

The amount of medicine that you take depends on the strength of the medicine. Also, the number of doses you take each day, the time allowed between doses, and the length of

time you take the medicine depend on the medical problem for which you are using the medicine.

Precautions While Using This Medicine

It is very important that your doctor check your progress at regular visits to make sure that this medicine is working properly and to check for unwanted effects.

While you are being treated with ifosfamide, and after you stop treatment with it, do not have any immunizations (vaccinations) without your doctor's approval. Ifosfamide may lower your body's resistance and there is a chance you might get the infection the immunization is meant to prevent. In addition, other persons living in your house should not take oral polio vaccine since there is a chance they could pass the polio virus on to you. Also, avoid persons who have taken oral polio vaccine within the past several months. Do not get close to them, and do not stay in the same room with them for very long. If you cannot take these precautions, you should consider wearing a protective face mask that covers the nose and mouth.

Ifosfamide can temporarily lower the number of white blood cells in your blood, increasing the chance of getting an infection. It can also lower the number of platelets, which are necessary for proper blood clotting. If this occurs, there are certain precautions you can take to reduce the risk of infection or bleeding:

- If you can, avoid people with infections. Check with your doctor immediately if you think you are getting an infection or if you get a fever or chills, cough or hoarseness, lower back or side pain, or have painful or difficult urination.
- Check with your doctor immediately if you notice any unusual bleeding or bruising; black, tarry stools; blood in urine or stools; or pinpoint red spots on your skin.
- Be careful when using a regular toothbrush, dental floss, or toothpick. Your medical doctor, dentist, or nurse may recommend other ways to clean your teeth and gums. Check with your medical doctor before having any dental work done.
- Do not touch your eyes or the inside of your nose unless you have just washed your hands and have not touched anything else in the meantime.
- Be careful not to cut yourself when you are using sharp objects such as a safety razor or fingernail or toenail cutters.
- Avoid contact sports or other situations where bruising or injury could occur.

Side Effects of This Medicine

Along with their needed effects, medicines like ifosfamide can sometimes cause unwanted effects such as blood problems, loss of hair, and problems with the bladder. These and others are described below. Also, because of the way these medicines act on the body, there is a chance that they might cause other unwanted effects that may not occur until months or years after the medicine is used. These may include certain types of cancer, such as leukemia. Discuss these possible effects with your doctor.

Although not all of these side effects may occur, if they do occur they may need medical attention.

Check with your doctor immediately if any of the following side effects occur:

More common
Blood in urine; frequent urination; painful urination

Less common
Cough or hoarseness accompanied by fever or chills; fever or chills; lower back or side pain accompanied by fever or chills

Rare
Black, tarry stools; blood in stools; pinpoint red spots on skin; unusual bleeding or bruising

Check with your doctor as soon as possible if any of the following side effects occur:

More common
Agitation; confusion; hallucinations (seeing, hearing, or feeling things that are not there); unusual tiredness

Less common
Dizziness; redness, swelling, or pain at place of injection

Rare
Convulsions (seizures); cough or shortness of breath; sores in mouth and on lips

Some side effects may occur that usually do not need medical attention. These side effects may go away during treatment as your body adjusts to the medicine. Also, your health care professional may be able to tell you about ways to prevent or reduce some of these side effects. Check with your health care professional if any of the following side effects continue or are bothersome or if you have any questions about them:

More common
Nausea and vomiting

Ifosfamide often causes a temporary loss of hair. After treatment has ended, normal hair growth should return.

After you stop using this medicine, it may still produce some side effects that need attention. During this period of time, *check with your doctor immediately* if you notice the following side effects:

Blood in urine

Other side effects not listed may also occur in some patients. If you notice any other effects, check with your healthcare professional.

ILOPROST (Inhalation, oral/ nebulization route) - EYE-loe-prost

Commonly used brand name(s)

In the U.S.—
Ventavis

Available Dosage Forms:
- Solution

Therapeutic Class: Vasodilator
Pharmacologic Class: Prostaglandin

Uses For This Medicine

Iloprost is used to treat the symptoms of pulmonary arterial hypertension. This is the high blood pressure that occurs in the main artery that carries blood from the right side of the heart (the ventricle) to the lungs. When the smaller blood vessels in the lungs become more resistant to blood flow, the right ventricle must work harder to pump enough blood through the lungs. Iloprost works by blocking a hormone (a naturally occurring substance), that is found in the blood and lungs in large quantities of the people with pulmonary arterial hypertension. Iloprost helps by increasing the supply of blood to the lungs and reducing the workload of the heart.

This medicine is available only with your doctor's prescription.

Before Using This Medicine

In deciding to use a medicine, the risks of taking the medicine must be weighed against the good it will do. This is a decision you and your doctor will make. For this medicine, the following should be considered:

Allergies—Tell your doctor if you have ever had any unusual or allergic reaction to this medicine or any other medicines. Also tell your health care professional if you have any other types of allergies, such as to foods, dyes, preservatives, or animals. For non-prescription products, read the label or package ingredients carefully.

Pediatric—Studies on this medicine have been done only in adult patients, and there is no specific information comparing use of iloprost in children with use in other age groups.

Geriatric—Many medicines have not been studied specifically in older people. Therefore, it may not be known whether they work exactly the same way they do in younger adults. Although there is no specific information comparing use of iloprost in the elderly with use in other age groups, elderly patients may be more sensitive to the effects of this medicine.

Pregnancy—

	Pregnancy Category	Explanation
All Trimesters	C	Animal studies have shown an adverse effect and there are no adequate studies in pregnant women OR no animal studies have been conducted and there are no adequate studies in pregnant women.

Breast Feeding—There are no adequate studies in women for determining infant risk when using this medication during breastfeeding. Weigh the potential benefits against the potential risks before taking this medication while breastfeeding.

Other medicines—

Using this medicine with any of the following medicines is usually not recommended, but may be required in some cases. If both medicines are prescribed together, your doctor may change the dose or how often you use one or both of the medicines.

Ginkgo

Interactions with Food/Tobacco/Alcohol—Certain medicines should not be used at or around the time of eating food or eating certain types of food since interactions may occur. Using alcohol or tobacco with certain medicines may also cause interactions to occur. Discuss with your healthcare professional the use of your medicine with food, alcohol, or tobacco.

Other medical problems—The presence of other medical problems may affect the use of this medicine. Make sure you tell your doctor if you have any other medical problems, especially:

- Asthma or
- Chronic obstructive pulmonary disease or
- Lung infection—Caution, iloprost has not been studied in patients these conditions
- Kidney disease or
- Liver disease—May increase the amount of iloprost in your blood
- Low blood pressure—Iloprost therapy should not be started in patients with low blood pressure

Proper Use of This Medicine

The importance of proper administration techniques including dosing frequency, ampule dispensing, Prodose AAD System operation, and equipment cleaning.

The importance of proper dosing intervals of not less than 2 hours apart

The importance of a back-up Prodose AAD System, to avoid potential interruptions in drug delivery due to equipment malfunctions.

Discarding any remaining solution in the medication chamber after each inhalation session

Dosing—The dose of this medicine will be different for different patients. Follow your doctor's orders or the directions on the label. The following information includes only the average doses of this medicine. If your dose is different, do not change it unless your doctor tells you to do so.

The amount of medicine that you take depends on the strength of the medicine. Also, the number of doses you take each day, the time allowed between doses, and the length of time you take the medicine depend on the medical problem for which you are using the medicine.

- For inhalation dosage form (solutions):
  - For pulmonary arterial hypertension:
    - Adults—2.5 micrograms (mcg) for the first dose; if well tolerated, dosing may be increased to 5 mcg and maintained at that dose, taken 6 to 9 times per day (no more than every 2 hours) during waking hours.
    - Children—Use and dose must be determined by your doctor.

Missed dose—If you miss a dose of this medicine, take it as soon as possible. However, if it is almost time for your next dose, skip the missed dose and go back to your regular dosing schedule. Do not double doses.

Storage—Store the medicine in a closed container at room temperature, away from heat, moisture, and direct light. Keep from freezing.

Keep out of the reach of children.

Do not keep outdated medicine or medicine no longer needed.

Ask your healthcare professional how you should dispose of any medicine you do not use.

Precautions While Using This Medicine

Regular visits: If you will be taking this medicine for a long time, it is very important that your doctor check you at regular visits.

Patients may have a drop in blood pressure, and may become dizzy or faint. Make sure you know how you react to this medicine before you drive, use machines, or do anything else that could be dangerous if you are dizzy.

Side Effects of This Medicine

Along with its needed effects, a medicine may cause some unwanted effects. Although not all of these side effects may occur, if they do occur they may need medical attention.

Check with your doctor immediately if any of the following side effects occur:

Frequency unknown

Chest pain; decreased urine output; difficult or labored breathing; dilated neck veins; extreme fatigue; fainting; fast, pounding, or irregular heartbeat or pulse; irregular breathing; irregular heartbeat; kidney failure; palpitations; shortness of breath; swelling of face, fingers, feet, or lower legs; tightness in chest; troubled breathing; tingling of hands or feet; unusual weight gain or loss; weight gain; wheezing

Symptoms of overdose

Get emergency help immediately if any of the following symptoms of overdose occur:

Blurred vision; confusion; diarrhea; dizziness, faintness, or lightheadedness when getting up from a lying or sitting position suddenly; feeling of warmth; headache; nausea; redness of the face, neck, arms and occasionally, upper chest; sweating; unusual tiredness or weakness; vomiting

Some side effects may occur that usually do not need medical attention. These side effects may go away during treatment as your body adjusts to the medicine. Also, your health care professional may be able to tell you about ways to prevent or reduce some of these side effects. Check with your health care professional if any of the following side effects continue or are bothersome or if you have any questions about them:

More common

Abnormal lab test; back pain; blurred vision, confusion, dizziness, faintness, or lightheadedness when getting up from a lying or sitting position suddenly; chills; cough increased; coughing or spitting up blood; diarrhea; difficulty opening the mouth; feeling of warmth; fever; general feeling of discomfort or illness; headache; joint pain; lockjaw; loss of appetite; muscle aches and pains; muscle cramps; muscle spasms, especially of neck and back; nausea; redness of the face, neck, arms and occasionally, upper chest; runny nose; shivering; sore throat; sweating; trouble sleeping; sleeplessness; unable to sleep; unusual tiredness or weakness; vomiting

Less common

Sneezing; tongue pain; troubled breathing

Other side effects not listed may also occur in some patients. If you notice any other effects, check with your healthcare professional.

IMATINIB   (Oral route) - i-ma-TIN-ib

Commonly used brand name(s)

In the U.S.—
   Gleevec

Available Dosage Forms:

- Tablet
- Capsule

Therapeutic Class: Antineoplastic Agent
Pharmacologic Class: Tyrosine Kinase Inhibitor

Uses For This Medicine

Imatinib is a new type of medication that prevents and stops the growth of cancer cells. It helps your body fight against a type of cancer called chronic myeloid leukemia (CML) or gastrointestinal stromal tumor (GIST). CML is a disease in which your body makes too many abnormal white blood cells which can cause you to become sick more often and also to feel weak or tired. Imatinib helps your body to stop making these abnormal white blood cells. GIST is a group of cancer cells that started growing in the wall of the stomach, intestines, or rectum. Imatinib helps your body to stop making these abnormal cells.

Before you begin treatment with imatinib, you and your doctor should talk about the good this medicine will do as well as the risks of using it.

This medicine is available only with your doctor's prescription.

Once a medicine has been approved for marketing for a certain use, experience may show that it is also useful for other medical problems. Although this use is not included in product labeling, imatinib is used in certain patients with the following medical condition:

- Acute lymphoblastic leukemia, Philadelphia chromosome-positive, newly diagnosed, as part of combination chemotherapy

Before Using This Medicine

In deciding to use a medicine, the risks of taking the medicine must be weighed against the good it will do. This is a decision you and your doctor will make. For this medicine, the following should be considered:

Allergies—Tell your doctor if you have ever had any unusual or allergic reaction to this medicine or any other medicines. Also tell your health care professional if you have any other types of allergies, such as to foods, dyes, preservatives, or animals. For non-prescription products, read the label or package ingredients carefully.

Pediatric—Studies on this medicine have been done only in children over 3 years of age with Ph+ chronic phase CML and adult patients, and there is no specific information comparing use of imatinib to treat other conditions in children with use in other age groups. Safety and effectiveness have not been established in these children.

Geriatric—This medicine has been tested and has not been shown to cause different side effects or problems in older people than it does in younger adults. Fluid retention may be more likely to occur in elderly patients, who may be more sensitive than younger adults to the effects of imatinib.

Pregnancy—

	Pregnancy Category	Explanation
All Trimesters	D	Studies in pregnant women have demonstrated a risk to the fetus. However, the benefits of therapy in a life threatening situation or a serious disease, may outweigh the potential risk.

Breast Feeding—There are no adequate studies in women for determining infant risk when using this medication during breastfeeding. Weigh the potential benefits against the potential risks before taking this medication while breastfeeding.

Other medicines—

Using this medicine with any of the following medicines is usually not recommended, but may be required in some cases. If both medicines are prescribed together, your doctor may change the dose or how often you use one or both of the medicines.

Aprepitant, Carbamazepine, Dexamethasone, Phenobarbital, Phenytoin, Rifampin, St John's Wort, Warfarin

Interactions with Food/Tobacco/Alcohol—Certain medicines should not be used at or around the time of eating food or eating certain types of food since interactions may occur. Using alcohol or tobacco with certain medicines may also cause interactions to occur. Discuss with your healthcare professional the use of your medicine with food, alcohol, or tobacco.

Other medical problems—The presence of other medical problems may affect the use of this medicine. Make sure you tell your doctor if you have any other medical problems, especially:

- Anemia or
- Platelet problems or
- White blood cell problems—May worsen and affect the decision to continue therapy.
- Chickenpox (including recent exposure) or
- Herpes zoster (shingles)—Risk of severe disease affecting other parts of the body.
- Liver disease—Effects may be increased because of slower removal of imatinib from the body.
- Infection—Imatinib may decrease your body's ability to fight infection.

Proper Use of This Medicine

Take imatinib only as directed by your doctor. Do not use more or less of it, and do not use it more often than your doctor ordered. The exact amount of medicine you need has been carefully worked out. Taking too much may increase the chance of side effects, while taking too little may not improve your condition.

This medicine should be taken with a tall glass of water and a meal.

Do not take imatinib with grapefruit, grapefruit juice, or grapefruit-containing foods or supplements.

Dosing—The dose of this medicine will be different for different patients. Follow your doctor's orders or the directions on the label. The following information includes only the average doses of this medicine. If your dose is different, do not change it unless your doctor tells you to do so.

The amount of medicine that you take depends on the strength of the medicine. Also, the number of doses you take each day, the time allowed between doses, and the length of time you take the medicine depend on the medical problem for which you are using the medicine.

Missed dose—If you miss a dose of this medicine, skip the missed dose and go back to your regular dosing schedule. Do not double doses.

Storage—Store the medicine in a closed container at room temperature, away from heat, moisture, and direct light. Keep from freezing.

Keep out of the reach of children.

Do not keep outdated medicine or medicine no longer needed.

Precautions While Using This Medicine

It is very important that your doctor check your progress at regular visits to make sure that this medicine is working properly and to check for unwanted effects.

While you are being treated with imatinib, and after you stop treatment with it, do not have any immunizations (vaccinations) without your doctor's approval. Imatinib may lower your body's resistance and there is a chance you might get the infection the immunization is meant to prevent. In addition, other persons living in your household should not take oral polio vaccine since there is a chance they could pass the polio virus on to you. Also, avoid persons who have recently taken oral polio vaccine. Do not get close to them and do not stay in the same room with them for very long. If you cannot take these precautions, you should consider wearing a protective face mask that covers the nose and mouth.

Imatinib can temporarily lower the number of white blood cells in your blood, increasing the chance of getting an infection. It can also lower the number of platelets, which are necessary for proper blood clotting. If this occurs, there are certain precautions you can take, especially when your blood count is low, to reduce the risk of infection or bleeding:

- If you can, avoid people with infections. Check with your doctor immediately if you think you are getting an infection or if you get a fever or chills, cough or hoarseness, lower back or side pain, or painful or difficult urination.
- Check with your doctor immediately if you notice any unusual bleeding or bruising; black, tarry stools; blood in urine or stools; or pinpoint red spots on your skin.
- Be careful when using a regular toothbrush, dental floss, or toothpick. Your medical doctor, dentist, or nurse may recommend other ways to clean your teeth and gums. Check with your medical doctor before having any dental work done.
- Do not touch your eyes or the inside of your nose unless you have just washed your hands and have not touched anything else in the meantime.

- Be careful not to cut yourself when you are using sharp objects such as a safety razor or fingernail or toenail cutters.
- Avoid contact sports or other situations where bruising or injury could occur.

Side Effects of This Medicine

Along with its needed effects, a medicine may cause some unwanted effects. Although not all of these side effects may occur, if they do occur they may need medical attention.

Check with your doctor as soon as possible if any of the following side effects occur:

More common
Black, tarry stools; bleeding problems; bloating or swelling of face, hands, lower legs, and/or feet; chest pain; chills; cough; decreased urination; fever; painful or difficult urination; pale skin; rapid weight gain; shortness of breath; sore throat; sores, ulcers, or white spots on lips or in mouth; swollen glands; trouble breathing, exertional; unusual bleeding or bruising; unusual tiredness or weakness

Less common
Body aches or pain; convulsions (seizures); dry mouth; ear congestion; general feeling of discomfort or illness; headache, sudden and severe; increased thirst; irregular heartbeat; loss of appetite; loss of voice; mood changes; muscle pain or cramps; nausea and vomiting; numbness or tingling in hands, feet, or lips; runny nose; shivering; small red or purple spots on skin; sneezing; stuffy nose; sweating; tightness in chest; wheezing

Rare
Bloody stools; blurred vision; inability to speak; slurred speech; temporary blindness; vomiting of blood or material that looks like coffee grounds; weakness in arm and/or leg on one side of the body, sudden and severe

Some side effects may occur that usually do not need medical attention. These side effects may go away during treatment as your body adjusts to the medicine. Also, your health care professional may be able to tell you about ways to prevent or reduce some of these side effects. Check with your health care professional if any of the following side effects continue or are bothersome or if you have any questions about them:

More common
Bone pain; increased bowel movements; joint pain; loose stools; skin rash; stomach pain

Less common
Acid indigestion; back pain; bad, unusual or unpleasant (after) taste; bloated full feeling; bloody nose; change in taste; difficulty having a bowel movement (stool); dizziness; excess air or gas in stomach or intestines; headache; itching skin; lack or loss of strength; large, flat, blue or purplish patches in the skin; loss of appetite; night sweats; passing gas; sleeplessness; trouble sleeping; unable to sleep; upset stomach; watering of eyes; weight loss

Other side effects not listed may also occur in some patients. If you notice any other effects, check with your healthcare professional.

IMIPENEM AND CILASTATIN
(Intravenous route, Intramuscular route) -
i-mi-PEN-em, sye-la-STAT-in

Commonly used brand name(s)

In the U.S.—
Primaxin IM
Primaxin IV

Available Dosage Forms:
- Powder for Solution

Therapeutic Class: Antibiotic
Pharmacologic Class: Beta-Lactam

Uses For This Medicine

Imipenem and cilastatin combination is used in the treatment of infections caused by bacteria. It works by killing bacteria or preventing their growth. This medicine will not work for colds, flu, or other virus infections.

Imipenem and cilastatin combination is used to treat infections in many different parts of the body. It is sometimes given with other antibiotics.

This medicine is available only with your doctor's prescription.

Once a medicine has been approved for marketing for a certain use, experience may show that it is also useful for other medical problems. Although these uses are not included in product labeling, imipenem and cilastatin combination is used in certain patients with the following medical conditions:

- Febrile neutropenia (treatment)
- Melioidosis (treatment)

Before Receiving This Medicine

In deciding to use a medicine, the risks of taking the medicine must be weighed against the good it will do. This is a decision you and your doctor will make. For this medicine, the following should be considered:

Allergies—Tell your doctor if you have ever had any unusual or allergic reaction to this medicine or any other medicines. Also tell your health care professional if you have any other types of allergies, such as to foods, dyes, preservatives, or animals. For non-prescription products, read the label or package ingredients carefully.

Pediatric—This medicine has been tested in a limited number of children 12 years of age and older and, in effective doses, has not been reported to cause different side effects or problems in children than it does in adults.

Geriatric—Many medicines have not been studied specifically in older people. Therefore, it may not be known whether they work exactly the same way they do in younger adults. Although there is no specific information comparing use of imipenem and cilastatin in the elderly with use in other age groups, this medicine is not expected to cause different side effects or problems in older people than it does in younger adults.

Pregnancy—

	Pregnancy Category	Explanation
All Trimesters	C	Animal studies have shown an adverse effect and there are no adequate studies in pregnant women OR no animal studies have been conducted and there are no adequate studies in pregnant women.

Breast Feeding—There are no adequate studies in women for determining infant risk when using this medication during breastfeeding. Weigh the potential benefits against the potential risks before taking this medication while breastfeeding.

Other medicines—

Using this medicine with any of the following medicines is usually not recommended, but may be required in some cases. If both medicines are prescribed together, your doctor may change the dose or how often you use one or both of the medicines.

Ganciclovir, Theophylline

Interactions with Food/Tobacco/Alcohol—Certain medicines should not be used at or around the time of eating food or eating certain types of food since interactions may occur. Using alcohol or tobacco with certain medicines may also cause interactions to occur. Discuss with your healthcare professional the use of your medicine with food, alcohol, or tobacco.

Other medical problems—The presence of other medical problems may affect the use of this medicine. Make sure you tell your doctor if you have any other medical problems, especially:

- Central nervous system (CNS) disorders (for example, brain disease or history of seizures)—Patients with nervous system disorders, including seizures, may be more likely to have side effects
- Kidney disease—Patients with kidney disease may be more likely to have side effects

Proper Use of This Medicine

To help clear up your infection completely, imipenem and cilastatin combination must be given for the full time of treatment, even if you begin to feel better after a few days. Also, this medicine works best when there is a constant amount in the blood or urine. To help keep the amount constant, it must be given on a regular schedule.

Dosing—The dose of this medicine will be different for different patients. Follow your doctor's orders or the directions on the label. The following information includes only the average doses of this medicine. If your dose is different, do not change it unless your doctor tells you to do so.

The amount of medicine that you take depends on the strength of the medicine. Also, the number of doses you take each day, the time allowed between doses, and the length of time you take the medicine depend on the medical problem for which you are using the medicine.

- For injection dosage form:
  - For bacterial infections:
    - Adults and children 12 years of age and over—250 milligrams (mg) to 1 gram injected into a vein

every six to eight hours; or 500 to 750 mg injected into a muscle every twelve hours, depending on how severe your infection is.
    - Children up to 12 years of age—Use and dose must be determined by your doctor.

Precautions After Receiving This Medicine

Some patients may develop tremors or seizures while receiving this medicine. If you already have a history of seizures and you are taking anticonvulsants, you should continue to take them unless otherwise directed by your doctor.

In some patients, imipenem and cilastatin combination may cause diarrhea.

- Severe diarrhea may be a sign of a serious side effect. Do not take any diarrhea medicine without first checking with your doctor. Diarrhea medicines may make your diarrhea worse or make it last longer.
- For mild diarrhea, diarrhea medicine containing kaolin (e.g., Kaopectate liquid) or attapulgite (e.g., Kaopectate tablets, Diasorb) may be taken. However, other kinds of diarrhea medicine should not be taken. They may make your diarrhea worse or make it last longer.
- If you have any questions about this or if mild diarrhea continues or gets worse, check with your health care professional.

Side Effects of This Medicine

Along with its needed effects, a medicine may cause some unwanted effects. Although not all of these side effects may occur, if they do occur they may need medical attention.

Check with your doctor immediately if any of the following side effects occur:

More common

Confusion; convulsions (seizures); dizziness; pain at place of injection; skin rash, hives, itching, fever, or wheezing; tremors

Less common

Dizziness; increased sweating; nausea or vomiting; unusual tiredness or weakness

Rare

Fever; severe abdominal or stomach cramps and pain; watery and severe diarrhea, which may also be bloody (these side effects may also occur up to several weeks after you stop receiving this medicine)

Some side effects may occur that usually do not need medical attention. These side effects may go away during treatment as your body adjusts to the medicine. Also, your health care professional may be able to tell you about ways to prevent or reduce some of these side effects. Check with your health care professional if any of the following side effects continue or are bothersome or if you have any questions about them:

More common

Diarrhea; nausea and vomiting

Other side effects not listed may also occur in some patients. If you notice any other effects, check with your healthcare professional.

IMIQUIMOD (Topical route) - i-mi-KWI-mod

Commonly used brand name(s)

In the U.S.—
Aldara

Available Dosage Forms:
- Kit
- Cream

Therapeutic Class: Immune Modulator

Uses For This Medicine

Imiquimod is used to treat external warts around the genital and rectal areas called condyloma acuminatum. It is not used on warts inside the vagina, penis, or rectum. Imiquimod is also used to treat a skin condition of the face and scalp called actinic keratoses. Imiquimod can also be used to treat certain types of skin cancer called superficial basal cell carcinoma (sBCC).

It works by aiding the immune system to help protect the body from viruses that cause warts. The medicine does not fight the viruses that cause warts directly. It does help to relieve and control wart production. It is not known how imiquimod helps actinic keratoses or skin cancer.

This medicine is available only with your doctor's prescription.

Before Using This Medicine

In deciding to use a medicine, the risks of taking the medicine must be weighed against the good it will do. This is a decision you and your doctor will make. For this medicine, the following should be considered:

Allergies—Tell your doctor if you have ever had any unusual or allergic reaction to this medicine or any other medicines. Also tell your health care professional if you have any other types of allergies, such as to foods, dyes, preservatives, or animals. For non-prescription products, read the label or package ingredients carefully.

Pediatric—Studies of this medicine have been done only in adult patients, and there is no specific information comparing use of imiquimod in children up to 12 years of age with use in other age groups. Actinic keratosis and basal cell carcinoma usually do not occur in children.

Geriatric—Many medicines have not been studied specifically in older people. Therefore, it may not be known whether they work exactly the same way they do in younger adults or if they cause different side effects or problems in older people. There is no specific information comparing use of imiquimod in the elderly with use in other age groups. However, older adults may be more sensitive to the effects of imiquimod.

Pregnancy—

	Pregnancy Category	Explanation
All Trimesters	C	Animal studies have shown an adverse effect and there are no adequate studies in pregnant women OR no animal studies have been conducted and there are no adequate studies in pregnant women.

Breast Feeding—There are no adequate studies in women for determining infant risk when using this medication during breastfeeding. Weigh the potential benefits against the potential risks before taking this medication while breastfeeding.

Other medicines—Although certain medicines should not be used together at all, in other cases two different medicines may be used together even if an interaction might occur. In these cases, your doctor may want to change the dose, or other precautions may be necessary. Tell your healthcare professional if you are taking any other prescription or non-prescription (over-the-counter [OTC]) medicine.

Interactions with Food/Tobacco/Alcohol—Certain medicines should not be used at or around the time of eating food or eating certain types of food since interactions may occur. Using alcohol or tobacco with certain medicines may also cause interactions to occur. Discuss with your healthcare professional the use of your medicine with food, alcohol, or tobacco.

Other medical problems—The presence of other medical problems may affect the use of this medicine. Make sure you tell your doctor if you have any other medical problems, especially:
- Allergy to imiquimod, parabens, or any ingredients in the product—This drug should not be used
- Autoimmune disorders—Tell your doctor if you have this condition; you and your doctor will decide if this medicine is right for you.
- Inflamed skin—May make condition worse
- Lower immune response (your body is not able to fight infections as well)—It is not known if imiquimod is safe to use with this condition
- Medicine that you have taken recently for the same skin problem or
- Surgery (recent)—Imiquimod should not be used until the skin is completely healed from any previous treatments that you have had with medicine or surgery
- Sensitive to sunlight—Use caution as you may have a higher risk of getting a sunburn
- Sunburn—Should not use until sunburn is gone

Proper Use of This Medicine

To apply the medicine:
- Wash your hands before and after using the medicine. Avoid getting the medicine into your eyes, lips, or nostrils or in vagina or anus.
- Use the medicine only as directed by your doctor. Do not use more of it, do not use it more often, and do not use it longer than directed.
- Allow medicine to stay on skin for 8 hours if you are using it for actinic keratoses or basal cell carcinoma, and 6 to 10 hours for genital warts, then wash area thoroughly with soap and water.
- Men not circumcised treating genital warts under the foreskin should retract the foreskin and clean the area daily.
- Throw out any unused cream from the single-dose packet.
- Do not apply an occlusive dressing (airtight covering, such as kitchen plastic wrap) over the medicine, unless told to do so by your doctor. To do so may cause irritation

of the skin. Other materials that are not airtight, such as cotton gauze or cotton underclothes, may be used.

Dosing—The dose of this medicine will be different for different patients. Follow your doctor's orders or the directions on the label. The following information includes only the average doses of this medicine. If your dose is different, do not change it unless your doctor tells you to do so.

The amount of medicine that you take depends on the strength of the medicine. Also, the number of doses you take each day, the time allowed between doses, and the length of time you take the medicine depend on the medical problem for which you are using the medicine.

- For topical dosage form (cream):
  - For skin condition on face and scalp called actinic keratoses:
    - Adults—Apply a thin film to the treatment area two times a week before normal sleeping hours Monday and Thursday or Tuesday and Friday. Rub in well and leave on for about 8 hours. Remove medicine from skin by washing with mild soap and water. Continue treatment until skin condition is gone or for up to sixteen weeks.
    - Children—Use and dose must be determined by doctor.
  - For skin cancer called basal cell carcinoma:
    - Adults—Apply a thin film to the treatment area five times a week before normal sleeping hours Monday through Friday. Rub in well and leave on for about 8 hours. Remove medicine from skin by washing with mild soap and water. Continue treatment until skin condition is gone or for up to six weeks.
    - Children—Use and dose must be determined by doctor.
  - For warts on the skin outside of the genital or rectal areas (condyloma acuminatum):
    - Adults—Apply a thin film to wart once every other day (three times a week) before normal sleeping hours. Rub in well and leave on for six to ten hours. Remove medicine from wart by washing with mild soap and water. Continue treatment until wart is gone or for up to sixteen weeks.
    - Children—Use and dose must be determined by doctor.

Missed dose—If you miss a dose of this medicine, skip the missed dose and go back to your regular dosing schedule. Do not double doses.

Storage—Store the medicine in a closed container at room temperature, away from heat, moisture, and direct light. Do not refrigerate. Keep from freezing.

Keep out of the reach of children.

Do not keep outdated medicine or medicine no longer needed.

Precautions While Using This Medicine

If you notice severe skin irritation or flu-like symptoms (diarrhea, fatigue, fever, headache, or muscle pain), check with your doctor. It may be necessary for you to reduce the number of times a week that you use the medicine or to stop using the medicine for a short time until your skin is less irritated or your flu-like symptoms disappear.

For treatment of warts on the skin outside of the genital or rectal areas (condyloma acuminatum), avoid having genital, oral, or anal sex while the medicine is on your skin. Make sure you wash the cream off your skin before you engage in any sexual activity. Also, the medicine contains oils that can weaken latex (rubber) condoms, diaphragms, or cervical caps causing them not to work properly to prevent pregnancy.

Imiquimod is not a cure for genital warts. New warts may develop during treatment with imiquimod.

Imiquimod will not keep your from spreading genital warts to other people.

Do not use any other skin product on the same skin area on which you use this medicine, unless directed otherwise by your doctor.

Do not share your medicine with others, even if you think that they have the same condition you have.

Side Effects of This Medicine

Along with its needed effects, a medicine may cause some unwanted effects. Although not all of these side effects may occur, if they do occur they may need medical attention.

Check with your doctor as soon as possible if any of the following side effects occur:

More common

Blisters on skin; body aches or pain; chills; cough; difficulty in breathing; ear congestion; itching in genital or other skin areas; loss of voice; nasal congestion; open sores or scabs on skin; pain or tenderness around eyes and cheekbones; redness of skin (severe); scaling; shortness of breath or troubled breathing; skin rash; sneezing; sore throat; stuffy or runny nose; tightness of chest or wheezing; unusual tiredness or weakness

Less common

Abdominal pain; ankle, knee, or great toe joint pain; blurred vision; chest pain; dizziness; bladder pain; bloody or cloudy urine; cold flu-like symptoms; difficult, burning, or painful urination; fainting; fast or irregular heartbeat; frequent urge to urinate; joint stiffness or swelling; high amount of cholesterol in the blood; hoarseness; lower back or side pain; lump in abdomen; nervousness; persistent non-healing sore; pink growth on skin; pounding in the ears; reddish patch or irritated area; severe headache; shiny bump on skin; slow or fast heartbeat; swollen, painful, or tender lymph glands in neck, armpit, or groin; white, yellow or waxy scar-like area

Incidence unknown—Observed during clinical practice, estimates of frequency can not be determined

Blurred vision; blue lips and fingernails; convulsions; coughing that sometimes produces a pink frothy sputum; difficulty breathing; dilated neck veins; dizziness; extreme fatigue; faintness; fast, irregular or pounding heartbeat; headache; irregular breathing; irregular heartbeat; nausea or vomiting; pain in the shoulders, arms, jaw or neck; seizures; shortness of breath; slurred speech; sudden and severe inability to speak; suicide; sweating; swelling of face, fingers, feet, or lower legs; temporary blindness; weakness in arm and/or leg on one side of the body; weight gain; wheezing

Symptoms of overdose

Flu-like symptoms, including diarrhea, fatigue, fever, headache, or muscle pain

Some side effects may occur that usually do not need medical attention. These side effects may go away during treatment as your body adjusts to the medicine. Also, your health care professional may be able to tell you about ways to prevent or reduce some of these side effects. Check with your health care professional if any of the following side effects continue or are bothersome or if you have any questions about them:

More common

Burning or stinging of skin (mild); flaking of skin; mild headache; pain, soreness, or tenderness of skin (mild); rash; redness of skin (mild); swelling at place of application

Less common

Back pain; fever; lightening of the treated skin; nausea

Other side effects not listed may also occur in some patients. If you notice any other effects, check with your healthcare professional.

IMMUNE GLOBULIN (Intramuscular route, Intravenous route, Injection route) - im-MYOON GLOB-yoo-lin

Black Box Warning

Immune globulin intravenous (human) products have been reported to be associated with renal dysfunction, acute renal failure, osmotic nephrosis, and death. Patients predisposed to acute renal failure include patients with any degree of pre-existing renal insufficiency, diabetes mellitus, age greater than 65, volume depletion, sepsis, paraproteinemia, or patients receiving known nephrotoxic drugs. Especially in such patients, IGIV products should be administered at the minimum concentration available and the minimum rate of infusion practicable. While these reports of renal dysfunction and acute renal failure have been associated with the use of many of the licensed IGIV products, those containing sucrose as a stabilizer accounted for a disproportionate share of the total number.

- GAMMAGARD S/D
  - GAMMAGARD S/D does not contain sucrose.

Commonly used brand name(s)

In the U.S.—

Baygam	Gamunex
Carimune	Iveegam EN
Carimune NF	Octagam
Gamimune N 10 %	Panglobulin NF
Gammagard S/D	Polygam S/D
Gammar-P I.V.	Sandoglobulin

In Canada—
Iveegam
Iveegam Immuno

Available Dosage Forms:

- Solution
- Powder for Solution
- Injectable

Therapeutic Class: Immune Serum

Uses For This Medicine

Immune globulin intravenous (IGIV) belongs to a group of medicines known as immunizing agents. IGIV is used to prevent or treat some illnesses that can occur when your body does not produce enough of its own immunity to prevent those diseases.

IGIV should be administered only by or under the supervision of your doctor or other health care professional.

Once a medicine has been approved for marketing for a certain use, experience may show that it is also useful for other medical problems. Although these uses are not included in product labeling, IGIV is used in certain patients with the following medical conditions:

- Chronic parvovirus B19 infection (treatment)
- Chronic inflammatory demyelinating polyneuropathies (treatment)
- Dermatomyositis (treatment)
- Guillain-BarrÃ(C syndrome (treatment)
- Hyperimmunoglobulinemia E syndrome (treatment)
- Infections in low-birth-weight preterm high-risk neonates (prophylaxis and treatment adjunct)
- Lambert-Eaton myasthenic syndrome (treatment)
- Multifocal motor neuropathy (treatment)
- Relapsing-remitting multiple sclerosis (treatment)

Before Using This Medicine

In deciding to use a medicine, the risks of taking the medicine must be weighed against the good it will do. This is a decision you and your doctor will make. For this medicine, the following should be considered:

Allergies—Tell your doctor if you have ever had any unusual or allergic reaction to this medicine or any other medicines. Also tell your health care professional if you have any other types of allergies, such as to foods, dyes, preservatives, or animals. For non-prescription products, read the label or package ingredients carefully.

Pediatric—Although there is no specific information comparing use of IGIV in children with use in other age groups, this medicine is not expected to cause different side effects or problems in children than it does in adults.

Geriatric—Many medicines have not been studied specifically in older people. Therefore, it may not be known whether they work exactly the same way they do in younger adults. Although there is no specific information comparing use of IGIV in the elderly with use in other age groups, this medicine is not expected to cause different side effects or problems in older people than it does in younger adults.

Pregnancy—

	Pregnancy Category	Explanation
All Trimesters	C	Animal studies have shown an adverse effect and there are no adequate studies in pregnant women OR no animal studies have been conducted and there are no adequate studies in pregnant women.

Breast Feeding—There are no adequate studies in women for determining infant risk when using this medication during breastfeeding. Weigh the potential benefits against the potential risks before taking this medication while breastfeeding.

Other medicines—

Using this medicine with any of the following medicines may cause an increased risk of certain side effects, but using both drugs may be the best treatment for you. If both medicines are prescribed together, your doctor may change the dose or how often you use one or both of the medicines.

Measles Virus Vaccine, Live, Mumps Virus Vaccine, Live, Rotavirus Vaccine, Live, Rubella Virus Vaccine, Live, Smallpox Vaccine, Varicella Virus Vaccine

Interactions with Food/Tobacco/Alcohol—Certain medicines should not be used at or around the time of eating food or eating certain types of food since interactions may occur. Using alcohol or tobacco with certain medicines may also cause interactions to occur. Discuss with your healthcare professional the use of your medicine with food, alcohol, or tobacco.

Other medical problems—The presence of other medical problems may affect the use of this medicine. Make sure you tell your doctor if you have any other medical problems, especially:

• Allergy to maltose or sucrose—May be in some IGIV products
• Blood clotting problems (or history of) or
• Diabetes mellitus (sugar diabetes) or
• Heart disease (or history of) or
• Heart problems or
• Immunoglobulin A (IgA) deficiencies or
• Kidney problems or
• Severe allergic reaction to IGIV—IGIV may make these conditions worse.
• Kidney problems or
• Conditions that make a person susceptible or more likely to have kidney problems such as:
    ◦ Abnormal kidney function or
    ◦ Being older than 65 years of age or
    ◦ Diabetes mellitus (sugar diabetes) or
    ◦ Paraproteinemia (having abnormal proteins called paraproteins in the blood) or
    ◦ Sepsis (serious infection in the body) or
    ◦ Volume depletion (loss of body fluids)—May cause kidney dysfunction, failure, and can be fatal

Proper Use of This Medicine

Make certain your health care professional knows if you are on any special diet, such as a low-sodium or low-sugar diet.

Waiting at least 2 to 3 weeks after receiving live virus vaccines before receiving IGIV, depending on the vaccine received.

Waiting at least 5 to 11 months after receiving IGIV before receiving live virus vaccines, depending on the vaccine to be received.

Dosing—The dose of this medicine will be different for different patients. Follow your doctor's orders or the directions on the label. The following information includes only the average doses of this medicine. If your dose is different, do not change it unless your doctor tells you to do so.

The amount of medicine that you take depends on the strength of the medicine. Also, the number of doses you take each day, the time allowed between doses, and the length of time you take the medicine depend on the medical problem for which you are using the medicine.

Side Effects of This Medicine

Along with its needed effects, a medicine may cause some unwanted effects. Although not all of these side effects may occur, if they do occur they may need medical attention.

Check with your doctor as soon as possible if any of the following side effects occur:

More common
    Fast or pounding heartbeat; troubled breathing

Less common
    Bluish coloring of lips or nailbeds; burning sensation in head; faintness or lightheadedness; unusual tiredness or weakness; wheezing

Rare
    Difficulty in breathing or swallowing; hives or welts; itching, especially of feet or hands; reddening of skin, especially around ears; swelling of eyes, face, or inside of nose; unusual tiredness or weakness (sudden and severe)

Incidence not determined
    Blistering, peeling, loosening of skin; bloody, black, or tarry stools; change in consciousness; cloudy urine; convulsions; coughing that sometimes produces a pink frothy sputum; dark urine; decrease in urine output or decrease in urine-concentrating ability; diarrhea; difficult, fast, noisy breathing, sometimes with wheezing; feeling unusually cold; high fever; increased sweating; loss of bladder control; loss of consciousness; muscle spasm or jerking of all extremities; no blood pressure or pulse; noisy breathing; not breathing; painful or difficult urination; pains in chest, groin, or legs, especially calves of legs; pale skin; red, irritated eyes; red skin lesions, often with a purple center; severe headaches that occur suddenly; shakiness in legs, arms, hands, feet; shivering; shortness of breath; shortness of breath that occurs suddenly for no apparent reason; skin blisters; slurred speech that occurs suddenly; sore throat; sores, ulcers, or white spots in mouth or on lips; stomach pain; stopping of heart; sudden loss of consciousness; sudden loss of coordination; sudden vision changes; swelling in legs and ankles; swollen glands; tightness in chest; tiredness; trembling or shaking of hands or feet; unconsciousness; unexplained or unusual bleeding or bruising; yellow eyes or skin

Some side effects may occur that usually do not need medical attention. These side effects may go away during treatment as your body adjusts to the medicine. Also, your health care professional may be able to tell you about ways to prevent or reduce some of these side effects. Check with your health care professional if any of the following side effects continue or are bothersome or if you have any questions about them:

More common
    Backache or pain; general feeling of discomfort or illness; headache; joint pain; muscle pain; nausea; vomiting

Less common

Chest or hip pain; leg cramps; redness, rash, or pain at place of injection

Incidence not determined

Blurred vision, confusion, dizziness, faintness, or light-headedness when getting up from a lying or sitting position suddenly; chills; confusion; dizziness; fever; feeling of warmth; high blood pressure; lightheadedness; redness of the face, neck, arms and occasionally, upper chest; skin rash; sweating

Other side effects not listed may also occur in some patients. If you notice any other effects, check with your healthcare professional.

INAMRINONE (Intravenous route) - eye-NAM-ri-none

Commonly used brand name(s)

In the U.S.—
Inocor

Available Dosage Forms:
• Solution

Therapeutic Class: Vasodilator
Pharmacologic Class: Inotropic Agent

Uses For This Medicine

Inamrinone is used to treat heart failure. Inamrinone helps your heart to work better. This medicine may be used only if other treatments have not worked for you.

This medicine is available only with your doctor's prescription.

Before Using This Medicine

In deciding to use a medicine, the risks of taking the medicine must be weighed against the good it will do. This is a decision you and your doctor will make. For this medicine, the following should be considered:

Allergies—Tell your doctor if you have ever had any unusual or allergic reaction to this medicine or any other medicines. Also tell your health care professional if you have any other types of allergies, such as to foods, dyes, preservatives, or animals. For non-prescription products, read the label or package ingredients carefully.

Pediatric—This medicine has been tested in children and, in effective doses, has not been shown to cause specific problems.

Geriatric—Many medicines have not been studied specifically in older people. Therefore, it may not be known whether they work exactly the same way they do in younger adults or if they cause different side effects or problems in older people. There is no specific information comparing use of inamrinone in the elderly with use in other age groups.

Pregnancy—

	Pregnancy Category	Explanation
All Trimesters	C	Animal studies have shown an adverse effect and there are no adequate studies in pregnant women OR no animal studies have been conducted and there are no adequate studies in pregnant women.

Breast Feeding—There are no adequate studies in women for determining infant risk when using this medication during breastfeeding. Weigh the potential benefits against the potential risks before taking this medication while breastfeeding.

Other medicines—Although certain medicines should not be used together at all, in other cases two different medicines may be used together even if an interaction might occur. In these cases, your doctor may want to change the dose, or other precautions may be necessary. Tell your healthcare professional if you are taking any other prescription or non-prescription (over-the-counter [OTC]) medicine.

Interactions with Food/Tobacco/Alcohol—Certain medicines should not be used at or around the time of eating food or eating certain types of food since interactions may occur. Using alcohol or tobacco with certain medicines may also cause interactions to occur. Discuss with your healthcare professional the use of your medicine with food, alcohol, or tobacco.

Other medical problems—The presence of other medical problems may affect the use of this medicine. Make sure you tell your doctor if you have any other medical problems, especially:

• Blood vessel disease or

• Heart disease—Inamrinone may make these conditions worse

• Kidney disease or

• Liver disease—Inamrinone may make liver problems worse; your doctor may need to change your dose

Proper Use of This Medicine

Dosing—The dose of this medicine will be different for different patients. Follow your doctor's orders or the directions on the label. The following information includes only the average doses of this medicine. If your dose is different, do not change it unless your doctor tells you to do so.

The amount of medicine that you take depends on the strength of the medicine. Also, the number of doses you take each day, the time allowed between doses, and the length of time you take the medicine depend on the medical problem for which you are using the medicine.

• For injection dosage form:
  ○ For congestive heart failure:
    ▪ Adults—Dose is based on your weight and must be determined by your doctor.
    ▪ Children—Use and dose must be determined by your doctor.

Side Effects of This Medicine

Along with its needed effects, a medicine may cause some unwanted effects. Although not all of these side effects may occur, if they do occur they may need medical attention.

Check with your doctor immediately if any of the following side effects occur:

Less common
 Dizziness; irregular heartbeat; low blood pressure

Rare
 Black, sticky stools; blood in urine or stools; burning at site of injection; chest pain or discomfort; loss of appetite; pinpoint red spots on skin; unusual bleeding or bruising; weight loss; yellow eyes or skin

Some side effects may occur that usually do not need medical attention. These side effects may go away during treatment as your body adjusts to the medicine. Also, your health care professional may be able to tell you about ways to prevent or reduce some of these side effects. Check with your health care professional if any of the following side effects continue or are bothersome or if you have any questions about them:

Less common
 Fever; nausea or vomiting; stomach pain

Other side effects not listed may also occur in some patients. If you notice any other effects, check with your healthcare professional.

INDAPAMIDE (Oral route) - in-DAP-a-mide

Commonly used brand name(s)

In the U.S.—
 Lozol

Available Dosage Forms:
• Tablet

Therapeutic Class: Cardiovascular Agent
Pharmacologic Class: Diuretic

Uses For This Medicine

Indapamide belongs to the group of medicines known as diuretics. It is commonly used to treat high blood pressure (hypertension).

High blood pressure adds to the workload of the heart and arteries. If it continues for a long time, the heart and arteries may not function properly. This can damage the blood vessels of the brain, heart, and kidneys resulting in a stroke, heart failure, or kidney failure. High blood pressure may also increase the risk of heart attacks. These problems may be less likely to occur if blood pressure is controlled.

Indapamide is also used to help reduce the amount of water in the body by increasing the flow of urine.

Indapamide is available only with your doctor's prescription.

Before Using This Medicine

In deciding to use a medicine, the risks of taking the medicine must be weighed against the good it will do. This is a decision you and your doctor will make. For this medicine, the following should be considered:

Allergies—Tell your doctor if you have ever had any unusual or allergic reaction to this medicine or any other medicines. Also tell your health care professional if you have any other types of allergies, such as to foods, dyes, preservatives, or animals. For non-prescription products, read the label or package ingredients carefully.

Pediatric—Studies on this medicine have been done only in adult patients, and there is no specific information comparing use of indapamide in children with use in other age groups.

Geriatric—Dizziness or lightheadedness and signs and symptoms of too much potassium loss are more likely to occur in the elderly, who are usually more sensitive than younger adults to the effects of indapamide.

Pregnancy—

	Pregnancy Category	Explanation
All Trimesters	B	Animal studies have revealed no evidence of harm to the fetus, however, there are no adequate studies in pregnant women OR animal studies have shown an adverse effect, but adequate studies in pregnant women have failed to demonstrate a risk to the fetus.

Breast Feeding—There are no adequate studies in women for determining infant risk when using this medication during breastfeeding. Weigh the potential benefits against the potential risks before taking this medication while breastfeeding.

Other medicines—

Using this medicine with any of the following medicines is usually not recommended, but may be required in some cases. If both medicines are prescribed together, your doctor may change the dose or how often you use one or both of the medicines.

Acetyldigoxin, Arsenic Trioxide, Deslanoside, Digitalis, Digitoxin, Digoxin, Dofetilide, Droperidol, Ketanserin, Levomethadyl, Lithium, Metildigoxin, Sotalol

Interactions with Food/Tobacco/Alcohol—Certain medicines should not be used at or around the time of eating food or eating certain types of food since interactions may occur. Using alcohol or tobacco with certain medicines may also cause interactions to occur. Discuss with your healthcare professional the use of your medicine with food, alcohol, or tobacco.

Other medical problems—The presence of other medical problems may affect the use of this medicine. Make sure you tell your doctor if you have any other medical problems, especially:
• Diabetes mellitus (sugar diabetes) or
• Gout (history of)—Indapamide may make these conditions worse

- Kidney disease—May prevent indapamide from working properly
- Liver disease—Higher blood levels of indapamide may occur, which may increase the chance of side effects

Proper Use of This Medicine

Indapamide may cause you to have an unusual feeling of tiredness when you begin to take it. You may also notice an increase in the amount of urine or in your frequency of urination. After taking the medicine for a while, these effects should lessen. In general, to keep the increase in urine from affecting your sleep:

- If you are to take a single dose a day, take it in the morning after breakfast.
- If you are to take more than one dose a day, take the last dose no later than 6 p.m., unless otherwise directed by your doctor.

However, it is best to plan your dose or doses according to a schedule that will least affect your personal activities and sleep. Ask your health care professional to help you plan the best time to take this medicine.

To help you remember to take indapamide, try to get into the habit of taking it at the same time each day.

For patients taking indapamide for high blood pressure:

- In addition to the use of the medicine your doctor has prescribed, treatment for your high blood pressure may include weight control and care in the types of foods you eat, especially foods high in sodium. Your doctor will tell you which of these are most important for you. You should check with your doctor before changing your diet.
- Many patients who have high blood pressure will not notice any signs of the problem. In fact, many may feel normal. It is very important that you take your medicine exactly as directed and that you keep your appointments with your doctor even if you feel well.
- Remember that this medicine will not cure your high blood pressure but it does help control it. Therefore, you must continue to take it as directed if you expect to lower your blood pressure and keep it down. You may have to take high blood pressure medicine for the rest of your life. If high blood pressure is not treated, it can cause serious problems such as heart failure, blood vessel disease, stroke, or kidney disease.

Dosing—The dose of this medicine will be different for different patients. Follow your doctor's orders or the directions on the label. The following information includes only the average doses of this medicine. If your dose is different, do not change it unless your doctor tells you to do so.

The amount of medicine that you take depends on the strength of the medicine. Also, the number of doses you take each day, the time allowed between doses, and the length of time you take the medicine depend on the medical problem for which you are using the medicine.

- For oral dosage forms (tablets):
  - Adults: 2.5 to 5 milligrams once a day.

Missed dose—If you miss a dose of this medicine, take it as soon as possible. However, if it is almost time for your next dose, skip the missed dose and go back to your regular dosing schedule. Do not double doses.

Storage—Store the medicine in a closed container at room temperature, away from heat, moisture, and direct light. Keep from freezing.

Keep out of the reach of children.

Do not keep outdated medicine or medicine no longer needed.

Precautions While Using This Medicine

It is important that your doctor check your progress at regular visits to make sure that indapamide is working properly.

This medicine may cause a loss of potassium from your body:

- To help prevent this, your doctor may want you to:
  - eat or drink foods that have a high potassium content (for example, orange or other citrus fruit juices), or
  - take a potassium supplement, or
  - take another medication to help prevent the loss of the potassium in the first place.
- It is very important to follow these directions. Also, it is important not to change your diet on your own. This is more important if you are already on a special diet (as for diabetes), or if you are taking a potassium supplement or a medicine to reduce potassium loss. Extra potassium may not be necessary and, in some cases, too much potassium could be harmful.

Check with your doctor if you become sick and have severe or continuing vomiting or diarrhea. These problems may cause you to lose additional water and potassium.

For patients taking this medicine for high blood pressure:

- Do not take other medicines unless they have been discussed with your doctor. This especially includes over-the-counter (nonprescription) medicines for appetite control, asthma, colds, hay fever, or sinus problems, since they may tend to increase your blood pressure.

Side Effects of This Medicine

Along with its needed effects, a medicine may cause some unwanted effects. Although not all of these side effects may occur, if they do occur they may need medical attention.

Check with your doctor as soon as possible if any of the following side effects occur:

Signs and symptoms of an imbalance of water or potassium in the body
  Dryness of mouth; increased thirst; irregular heartbeat; mood or mental changes; muscle cramps or pain; nausea or vomiting; unusual tiredness or weakness; weak pulse

Rare
  Skin rash, itching, or hives

Some side effects may occur that usually do not need medical attention. These side effects may go away during treatment as your body adjusts to the medicine. Also, your health care professional may be able to tell you about ways to prevent or reduce some of these side effects. Check with your health care professional if any of the following side effects continue or are bothersome or if you have any questions about them:

Less common or rare
  Diarrhea; dizziness or lightheadedness, especially when getting up from a lying or sitting position; head-

ache; loss of appetite; trouble in sleeping; stomach upset

Other side effects not listed may also occur in some patients. If you notice any other effects, check with your healthcare professional.

INDINAVIR (Oral route) - in-DIN-a-veer

Commonly used brand name(s)

In the U.S.—
Crixivan

Available Dosage Forms:
• Capsule

Therapeutic Class: Antiretroviral Agent
Pharmacologic Class: Protease Inhibitor

Uses For This Medicine

Indinavir is used, alone or in combination with other medicines, in the treatment of the infection caused by the human immunodeficiency virus (HIV). HIV is the virus that causes acquired immune deficiency syndrome (AIDS).

Indinavir will not cure or prevent HIV infection or AIDS; however, it helps keep HIV from reproducing and appears to slow down the destruction of the immune system. This may help delay the development of problems usually related to AIDS or HIV disease. Indinavir will not keep you from spreading HIV to other people. People who receive this medicine may continue to have other problems usually related to AIDS or HIV disease.

This medicine is available only with your doctor's prescription.

Before Using This Medicine

In deciding to use a medicine, the risks of taking the medicine must be weighed against the good it will do. This is a decision you and your doctor will make. For this medicine, the following should be considered:

Allergies—Tell your doctor if you have ever had any unusual or allergic reaction to this medicine or any other medicines. Also tell your health care professional if you have any other types of allergies, such as to foods, dyes, preservatives, or animals. For non-prescription products, read the label or package ingredients carefully.

Pediatric—Studies on this medicine have been done only in adult patients, and there is limited recommendations comparing the use of indinavir in children with use in other age groups.

Geriatric—Indinavir has not been studied specifically in older people. Therefore, it is not known whether it causes different side effects or problems in the elderly than it does in younger adults.

Pregnancy—

	Pregnancy Category	Explanation
All Trimesters	C	Animal studies have shown an adverse effect and there are no adequate studies in pregnant women OR no animal studies have been conducted and there are no adequate studies in pregnant women.

Breast Feeding—There are no adequate studies in women for determining infant risk when using this medication during breastfeeding. Weigh the potential benefits against the potential risks before taking this medication while breastfeeding.

Other medicines—

Using this medicine with any of the following medicines is not recommended. Your doctor may decide not to treat you with this medication or change some of the other medicines you take.

Amiodarone, Astemizole, Cisapride, Conivaptan, Dihydroergotamine, Ergoloid Mesylates, Ergonovine, Ergotamine, Methylergonovine, Midazolam, Pimozide, Ranolazine, St John's Wort, Terfenadine, Triazolam

Interactions with Food/Tobacco/Alcohol—Certain medicines should not be used at or around the time of eating food or eating certain types of food since interactions may occur. Using alcohol or tobacco with certain medicines may also cause interactions to occur. Discuss with your healthcare professional the use of your medicine with food, alcohol, or tobacco.

Other medical problems—The presence of other medical problems may affect the use of this medicine. Make sure you tell your doctor if you have any other medical problems, especially:

• Hemophilia—Increased effects of hemophilia may occur when using indinavir

• Hepatitis—Increased effects of hepatitis and hepatic failure may happen when using indinavir

• Hyperbilirubinemia— may make these effects greater in newborn babies

• Liver disease—Effects of indinavir may be increased because of slower removal from the body

Proper Use of This Medicine

This medicine should be taken with water on an empty stomach (1 hour before or 2 hours after a meal) or with a light meal Indinavir may also be taken with other liquids (skim milk, juice, coffee, or tea) or with a light meal (dry toast with jelly, juice, coffee with skim milk and sugar, or corn flakes with skim milk and sugar).

While you are taking indinavir, it is important that you drink extra fluids so that you will pass more urine. This will help prevent possible kidney stones. Follow your doctor's instructions carefully about how much fluid to drink. Usually you will need to drink at least 48 ounces (1.5 liters) of fluids every day during your treatment.

Take this medicine exactly as directed by your doctor. Do not take it more often, and do not take it for a longer time than your doctor ordered. Also, do not stop taking this medicine without checking with your doctor first.

Keep taking indinavir for the full time of treatment, even if you begin to feel better.

This medicine works best when there is a constant amount in the blood. To help keep the amount constant, do not miss any doses. Also, it is best to take the doses at evenly spaced times, day and night. For example, if you are to take three doses a day, the doses should be spaced about 8 hours apart. If you need help in planning the best times to take your medicine, check with your health care professional.

Only take medicine that your doctor has prescribed specially for you. Do not share your medicine with others.

Dosing—The dose of this medicine will be different for different patients. Follow your doctor's orders or the directions on the label. The following information includes only the average doses of this medicine. If your dose is different, do not change it unless your doctor tells you to do so.

The amount of medicine that you take depends on the strength of the medicine. Also, the number of doses you take each day, the time allowed between doses, and the length of time you take the medicine depend on the medical problem for which you are using the medicine.

- For oral dosage form (capsules):
  - For treatment of HIV infection:
    - Adults—800 mg every eight hours.
    - Children—Use and dose must be determined by your doctor.

Note: This medicine may be taken in combination with other medicines that are used to treat HIV infection. Check with your health care professional for information and dose amounts.

Missed dose—If you miss a dose of this medicine, take it as soon as possible. However, if it is almost time for your next dose, skip the missed dose and go back to your regular dosing schedule. Do not double doses.

Storage—Store the medicine in a closed container at room temperature, away from heat, moisture, and direct light. Keep from freezing.

Keep out of the reach of children.

Do not keep outdated medicine or medicine no longer needed.

Indinavir capsules are very sensitive to moisture. Keep them in their original container and leave the drying packet in the container.

Precautions While Using This Medicine

Do not take any other medicines without checking with your doctor first. To do so may increase the chance of side effects from indinavir.

It is very important that your doctor check your progress at regular visits to make sure this medicine is working properly and to check for unwanted effects.

Side Effects of This Medicine

Along with its needed effects, a medicine may cause some unwanted effects. Although not all of these side effects may occur, if they do occur they may need medical attention.

Check with your doctor immediately if any of the following side effects occur:
More common
Blood in urine; sharp back pain just below ribs

Check with your doctor as soon as possible if any of the following side effects occur:
Less common
Abdominal or stomach pain; chills; clay-colored stools; dark urine; dizziness; fever; headache; itching; loss of appetite; nausea; rash; unpleasant breath odor; unusual tiredness or weakness; vomiting of blood; yellow eyes or skin
Rare
Confusion; dehydration; dry or itchy skin; fatigue; fruity mouth odor; increased hunger; increased thirst; increased urination; pale skin; troubled breathing with exertion; unusual bleeding or bruising; unusual tiredness or weakness; vomiting; weight loss

Some side effects may occur that usually do not need medical attention. These side effects may go away during treatment as your body adjusts to the medicine. Also, your health care professional may be able to tell you about ways to prevent or reduce some of these side effects. Check with your health care professional if any of the following side effects continue or are bothersome or if you have any questions about them:
More common
Change in sense of taste; diarrhea; difficulty in sleeping; generalized weakness
Less common
Acid regurgitation; acid or sour stomach; appetite increase; belching; cough; general feeling of discomfort or illness; heartburn; indigestion; sleepiness

Note: Other side effects not listed above have occurred since indinavir was released on the market and these side effects may also occur in some patients. How often these side effects occur is unknown. If you notice any other effects, check with your doctor.

INFLIXIMAB (Injection route, Intravenous route) - in-FLIX-i-mab

Black Box Warning

- RISK OF INFECTIONS
  - Tuberculosis (frequently disseminated or extrapulmonary at clinical presentation), invasive fungal infections, and other opportunistic infections, have been observed in patients receiving infliximab. Some of these infections have been fatal. Anti-tuberculosis treatment of patients with a reactive tuberculin skin test reduces the risk of TB reactivation in patients receiving treatment with infliximab. However, active tuberculosis has developed in patients receiving infliximab who were tuberculin skin test negative prior to receiving infliximab.
  - Patients should be evaluated for latent tuberculosis infection with a tuberculin skin test. Treatment of latent tuberculosis infection should be initiated prior to therapy with infliximab. Physicians should monitor

patients receiving infliximab for signs and symptoms of active tuberculosis, including patients who are tuberculin skin test negative.

- HEPATOSPLENIC T-CELL LYMPHOMAS
  - ◦ Rare postmarketing cases of hepatosplenic t-cell lymphoma have been reported in adolescent and young adult patients with Crohn's disease treated with infliximab. This rare type of t-cell lymphoma has a very aggressive disease course and is usually fatal. All of these hepatosplenic t-cell lymphomas with infliximab have occurred in patients on concomitant treatment with azathioprine or 6–mercaptopurine.

Commonly used brand name(s)

In the U.S.—
  Remicade

Available Dosage Forms:

- Powder for Solution

Therapeutic Class: Immunological Agent
Pharmacologic Class: Tumor Necrosis Factor Inhibitor

Uses For This Medicine

Infliximab is a monoclonal antibody. It is used to treat Crohn's disease in children 6 years of age and older and adults who have not been helped by other medicines and also in patients who have a type of Crohn's disease in which fistulas form. It is also used to treat rheumatoid arthritis and ankylosing spondylitis which is a type of arthritis that affects the joints in the spine. In addition, it is used to treat psoriatic arthritis which is a type of arthritis that causes pain and swelling of the joints and patches of scaly skin on some areas of the body. Psoriatic arthritis is related to the skin condition, psoriasis.

Infliximab is also used to treat ulcerative colitis.

This medicine is available only with your doctor's prescription.

Once a medicine has been approved for marketing for a certain use, experience may show that it is also useful for other medical problems. Although this use is not included in the product labeling, infliximab is used in certain patients with the following medical conditions:

- Psoriasis
- Reactive arthritis
- Inflammatory bowel disease arthritis

Before Using This Medicine

In deciding to use a medicine, the risks of taking the medicine must be weighed against the good it will do. This is a decision you and your doctor will make. For this medicine, the following should be considered:

Allergies—Tell your doctor if you have ever had any unusual or allergic reaction to this medicine or any other medicines. Also tell your health care professional if you have any other types of allergies, such as to foods, dyes, preservatives, or animals. For non-prescription products, read the label or package ingredients carefully.

Pediatric—Studies of this medicine for treatment of Crohn's with fistulas, ankylosing spondylitis, rheumatoid arthritis, psoriatic arthritis, and ulcerative colitis have been done only in adult patients, and there is no specific information comparing use of infliximab in children for these conditions with use in other age groups.

Appropriate studies performed to date have not demonstrated pediatric-specific problems that would limit the usefulness of infliximab for the treatment of Crohn's disease in children 6 years of age and older.

Your child's vaccinations need to be current before he/she begins taking infliximab. Be sure to ask your child's doctor if you have any questions about this.

A very serious kind of cancer called hepatosplenic T-cell lymphoma has been reported in some teenagers and young adults who were taking this medicine. They were also taking azathioprine or 6–mercaptopurine. The connection between infliximab and this cancer is unclear.

Geriatric—Many medicines have not been studied specifically in older people. Therefore, it may not be known whether they work exactly the same way they do in younger adults or if they cause different side effects or problems in older people. There is no specific information comparing use of infliximab in the elderly with use in other age groups. However, older adults generally get more infections than do younger adults, and it is not known if infliximab may affect the number of infections that older people get.

Pregnancy—

	Pregnancy Category	Explanation
All Trimesters	B	Animal studies have revealed no evidence of harm to the fetus, however, there are no adequate studies in pregnant women OR animal studies have shown an adverse effect, but adequate studies in pregnant women have failed to demonstrate a risk to the fetus.

Breast Feeding—There are no adequate studies in women for determining infant risk when using this medication during breastfeeding. Weigh the potential benefits against the potential risks before taking this medication while breastfeeding.

Other medicines—

Using this medicine with any of the following medicines is usually not recommended, but may be required in some cases. If both medicines are prescribed together, your doctor may change the dose or how often you use one or both of the medicines.

Abatacept, Anakinra

Interactions with Food/Tobacco/Alcohol—Certain medicines should not be used at or around the time of eating food or eating certain types of food since interactions may occur. Using alcohol or tobacco with certain medicines may also cause interactions to occur. Discuss with your healthcare professional the use of your medicine with food, alcohol, or tobacco.

Other medical problems—The presence of other medical problems may affect the use of this medicine. Make sure you tell your doctor if you have any other medical problems, especially:

- Blood problems, ongoing or in the past—Caution should be used.
- Cancer, history—This medicine should be used with caution. If you have a history of cancer, you may be more susceptible to lymphoma (a type of blood cancer).

- Heart disease—Infliximab is not recommended for patients with a certain type of heart disease called congestive heart failure.
- Hepatitis B—Infliximab could cause your hepatitis B to become active again if you have a history of hepatitis B.
- Infection—Infliximab is not recommended for patients with an active infection. Caution should be used if you have a chronic infection or history of a recurring infection.
- Inactive tuberculosis infection—Should be treated before starting infliximab therapy.
- Nervous system problems or
- Seizures—Caution should be used; your doctor will consider discontinuing this medicine if you develop serious CNS reactions.

Proper Use of This Medicine

You will be given a Patient Information Sheet prior to each treatment. Make sure you read it each time you are scheduled for an infliximab treatment.

Dosing—The dose of this medicine will be different for different patients. Follow your doctor's orders or the directions on the label. The following information includes only the average doses of this medicine. If your dose is different, do not change it unless your doctor tells you to do so.

The amount of medicine that you take depends on the strength of the medicine. Also, the number of doses you take each day, the time allowed between doses, and the length of time you take the medicine depend on the medical problem for which you are using the medicine.

- For treatment of Crohn's with fistulas, ankylosing spondylitis, psoriatic arthritis, or ulcerative colitis:
  - Adults—5 milligrams (mg) per kilogram (kg) (2.27 mg per pound) of body weight, injected into a vein.
  - Children—Use and dose must be determined by your doctor.
- For treatment of rheumatoid arthritis:
  - Adults—3 milligrams (mg) per kilogram (kg) (1.36 mg per pound) of body weight, injected into a vein
  - Children—Use and dose must be determined by your doctor.
- For treatment of Crohn's disease:
  - Adults—5 milligrams (mg) per kilogram (kg) (2.27 mg per pound) of body weight, injected into a vein
  - Children—5 mg per kg (2.27 mg per pound) of body weight, injected into a vein.

Storage—Store in the refrigerator. Do not freeze.

Keep out of the reach of children.

Do not keep outdated medicine or medicine no longer needed.

Precautions While Using This Medicine

Infliximab may cause chest pain, fever, chills, itching, hives, flushing of face, or troubled breathing within a few hours after you receive it. Check with your doctor or nurse immediately if you have any of these symptoms.

Check with your doctor immediately if you have any symptoms of liver problems including skin and eyes turning yellow, dark brown-colored urine, right sided abdominal pain, fever or severe tiredness.

It is important to have a tuberculin skin test to make sure that you do not have an inactive tuberculosis infection, which could worsen while you are on infliximab therapy.

It is important to have your heart closely checked if you take infliximab, and have existing heart disease, which could worsen while you are on infliximab therapy

Your doctor will check you for active infections before each infliximab treatment. Tell your doctor if you are not feeling well or if you have symptoms of a cold or other type of infection.

Side Effects of This Medicine

Along with its needed effects, a medicine may cause some unwanted effects. Although not all of these side effects may occur, if they do occur they may need medical attention.

Check with your doctor immediately if any of the following side effects occur:
  More common
    Chest pain; chills; fever; flushing of face; hives; itching; troubled breathing

Check with your doctor as soon as possible if any of the following side effects occur:
  More common
    Abdominal pain; cough; dizziness; fainting; headache; muscle pain; nasal congestion; nausea; runny nose; shortness of breath; sneezing; sore throat; tightness in chest; unusual tiredness or weakness; vomiting; wheezing
  Less common
    Back pain; bloody or cloudy urine; cracks in skin at the corners of mouth; diarrhea; difficult or painful urination; frequent urge to urinate; high blood pressure; low blood pressure; pain; pain or tenderness around eyes and cheekbones; skin rash; soreness or irritation of mouth or tongue; soreness or redness around fingernails or toenails; vaginal burning or itching and discharge; white patches in mouth and/or on tongue
  Rare
    Abscess (swollen, red, tender area of infection containing pus); back or side pain; black, tarry stools; blood in urine or stools; bone or joint pain; constipation; falls; feeling of fullness; general feeling of illness; hernia (bulge of tissue through the wall of the abdomen); infection; irregular or pounding heartbeat; pain in rectum; pain spreading from the abdomen to the left shoulder; pinpoint red spots on skin; stomach pain (severe); swollen or painful glands; tendon injury; unusual bleeding or bruising; weight loss (unusual); yellow skin and eyes
  Incidence not known— occurred during clinical practice
    Area rash; bloody nose; burning, tingling, numbness or pain in the hands, arms, feet or legs; change in mental status; clay-colored stools; continuing vomiting; convulsions; dark or bloody urine; difficulty breathing; difficulty speaking; difficulty swallowing; fast heartbeat; general feeling of tiredness or weakness; heavier menstrual periods; hives; hoarseness; inability to move arms and legs; itching, puffiness, or swelling of the eyelids or around the eyes, face, lips or tongue; light colored stools; loss of appetite; loss of bladder control; lower back or side pain; muscle spasm or jerking of all extremities; noisy breathing; painful or difficult urination; painless swelling in neck, armpits or groin; pale skin; redness, soreness or itching skin; seizures; sen-

sation of pins and needles; severe abdominal pain; severe muscle weakness, sudden and progressing; slow or irregular breathing; sore throat; sores, welting, or blisters; stabbing pain; stomach pain; sudden loss of consciousness; sudden numbness and weakness in the arms and legs; ulcers, sore, or white spots in mouth; unpleasant breath odor; upper right abdominal pain; vomiting of blood

INFLUENZA VIRUS VACCINE
(Intramuscular route, Nasal route) - in-floo-EN-za VYE-rus vak-SEEN

Commonly used brand name(s)
In the U.S.—

Fluarix	Fluzone
FluMist	Fluzone Pediatric
Fluvirin	

Available Dosage Forms:
- Solution

Therapeutic Class: Vaccine

Uses For This Vaccine

Influenza virus vaccine is used to prevent infection by the influenza viruses. The vaccine works by causing your body to produce its own protection (antibodies) against the disease. It is also known as a "flu shot." New for the 2003–2004 flu season, influenza virus vaccine is also available as a nasal spray.

There are many kinds of influenza viruses, but not all will cause problems in any given year. Therefore, before the influenza vaccine for each year is produced, the World Health Organization (WHO) and the U.S. and Canadian Public Health Services decide which influenza viruses will be most likely to cause influenza infection that year. Then they include the antigens (substances that cause protective antibodies to be formed) to these viruses in the influenza vaccine made available. Usually, the U.S. and Canada use the same influenza vaccine; however, they are not required to do so.

It is necessary to receive an influenza vaccine injection each year, since influenza infections are usually caused by different kinds of influenza viruses each year and because the protection gained by the vaccine lasts less than a year.

Influenza is a virus infection of the throat, bronchial tubes, and lungs. Influenza infection causes fever, chills, cough, headache, and muscle aches and pains in your back, arms, and legs. In addition, adults and children weakened by other diseases or medical conditions and persons 50 years of age and over, even if they are healthy, may get a much more serious illness and may have to be treated in a hospital. Each year thousands of people die as a result of an influenza infection.

The best way to help prevent influenza infection is to get an influenza vaccination each year, usually in early November.

Immunization (administration of vaccine) against influenza is approved for infants 6 months of age and over, all children, and all adults.

Influenza virus vaccine may not protect all persons given the vaccine.

This vaccine is to be administered only by or under the supervision of your doctor or other health care professional.

Before Receiving This Vaccine

In deciding to use a vaccine, the risks of taking the vaccine must be weighed against the good it will do. This is a decision you and your doctor will make. For this vaccine, the following should be considered:

Allergies—Tell your doctor if you have ever had any unusual or allergic reaction to this medicine or any other medicines. Also tell your health care professional if you have any other types of allergies, such as to foods, dyes, preservatives, or animals. For non-prescription products, read the label or package ingredients carefully.

Pediatric—Use is not recommended for infants up to 6 months of age. In addition, only a split-virus influenza vaccine ("shot") should be given to children 6 months to 12 years of age. Some side effects of the vaccine, such as fever, unusual tiredness or weakness, or aches or pains in muscles, are more likely to occur in infants and children, who are usually more sensitive than adults to the effects of influenza vaccine.

The nasal mist vaccine should not be used in children less than 5 years of age.

Geriatric—This vaccine ("shot") is not expected to cause different side effects or problems in older persons than it does in younger adults. However, elderly persons may not become as immune to head and upper chest influenza infections as younger adults, although the vaccine may still be effective in preventing lower chest influenza infections and other complications of influenza.

The nasal mist vaccine should not be used in adults 50 years of age and older.

Pregnancy—

	Pregnancy Category	Explanation
All Trimesters	C	Animal studies have shown an adverse effect and there are no adequate studies in pregnant women OR no animal studies have been conducted and there are no adequate studies in pregnant women.

Breast Feeding—Studies in women suggest that this medication poses minimal risk to the infant when used during breastfeeding.

Other medicines—

Receiving this vaccine with any of the following medicines may cause an increased risk of certain side effects, but using both drugs may be the best treatment for you. If both medicines are prescribed together, your doctor may change the dose or how often you use one or both of the medicines.

Carbamazepine, Vaccinia Immune Globulin, Human

Interactions with Food/Tobacco/Alcohol—Certain medicines should not be used at or around the time of eating food or eating certain types of food since interactions may occur. Using alcohol or tobacco with certain medicines may also cause interactions to occur. Discuss with your healthcare professional the use of your medicine with food, alcohol, or tobacco.

Other medical problems—The presence of other medical problems may affect the use of this vaccine. Make sure you tell your doctor if you have any other medical problems, especially:

- Asthma, bronchitis, pneumonia, or other illness involving lungs or bronchial tubes—Use of influenza vaccine (nasal mist or "shot") may make the condition worse

- Immune deficiency diseases such as:
  - Agammaglobulinemia or
  - Cancer or
  - Human immunodeficiency virus infection (HIV) or
  - Immunodeficiency or
  - Leukemia or
  - Lymphoma or
  - Thymus gland problems—Use of live virus vaccines like nasal mist influenza vaccine is not recommended for patients with these medical problems.

- Guillain Barré syndrome, history of—Use of influenza vaccine (nasal mist or "shot") may cause a recurrence of the symptoms of the condition

- Medical conditions that may make influenza infection more severe, such as:
  - Blood problems (hemoglobinopathies) or
  - Diabetes Mellitus (sugar diabetes) or
  - Heart disease (history of) or
  - Immunosuppression (inability of body to fight an infection) or
  - Kidney disease (history of) or
  - Lung disease (history of) or
  - Metabolic problems (history of)—Use of nasal mist influenza virus vaccine is not recommended. Your doctor will decide if use of inactivated influenza virus vaccine ("shot") is right for you.

- Severe illness with fever—Influenza virus vaccine should not be given when a fever is present. Your doctor will decide when you are well enough to get your influenza virus vaccine.

Proper Use of This Vaccine

Dosing—The dose of this medicine will be different for different patients. Follow your doctor's orders or the directions on the label. The following information includes only the average doses of this medicine. If your dose is different, do not change it unless your doctor tells you to do so.

The amount of medicine that you take depends on the strength of the medicine. Also, the number of doses you take each day, the time allowed between doses, and the length of time you take the medicine depend on the medical problem for which you are using the medicine.

- For nasal dosage form:
  - To help prevent influenza infection:
    - Adults and children age 9 through 49 years—One dose (0.5 mL) each year.

- Children 5 through 8 years of age—One or two doses (0.5 mL), depending on whether the child has received nasal mist influenza vaccine in the past. The dose is given each year. If two doses are needed, they should be spaced 6 weeks apart.

- For injection dosage form:
  - To help prevent influenza infection:
    - Adults and children 9 years of age and older—One injection each year.
    - Children 6 months to 9 years of age—One or two injections, depending on whether the child has received influenza vaccine in the past. The dose is given each year. If two doses are needed, they should be spaced 4 weeks apart.

Side Effects of This Vaccine

In 1976, a number of persons who received the "swine flu" influenza vaccine developed Guillain-Barré syndrome (GBS). Most of these persons were over 25 years of age. Although only 10 out of one million persons receiving the vaccine actually developed GBS, this number was 6 times more than would normally have been expected. Most of the persons who got GBS recovered completely from the paralysis it caused.

It is assumed that the "swine flu" virus included in the 1976 vaccine caused the problem, but this has not been proven. Since that time, the "swine flu" virus has not been used in influenza vaccines, and there has been no recurrence of GBS associated with influenza vaccinations.

Along with its needed effects, a medicine may cause some unwanted effects. Although not all of these side effects may occur, if they do occur they may need medical attention.

Check with your doctor immediately if any of the following side effects occur:
  Symptoms of allergic reaction
    Difficulty in breathing or swallowing; hives; itching, especially of feet or hands; reddening of skin, especially around ears; swelling of eyes, face, or inside of nose; unusual tiredness or weakness (sudden and severe)

Some side effects may occur that usually do not need medical attention. These side effects may go away during treatment as your body adjusts to the medicine. Also, your health care professional may be able to tell you about ways to prevent or reduce some of these side effects. Check with your health care professional if any of the following side effects continue or are bothersome or if you have any questions about them:
  More common
    Headache (nasal mist); nasal congestion (nasal mist); runny nose (nasal mist); tenderness, redness, or hard lump at place of injection ("shot")

  Less common
    Abdominal pain (nasal mist); aches or pains in muscles; cough (nasal mist); diarrhea (nasal mist); earache (nasal mist); fever; or general feeling of discomfort or illness; pain or tenderness around eyes and cheekbones (nasal mist); redness or swelling in ear (nasal mist)

Other side effects not listed may also occur in some patients. If you notice any other effects, check with your healthcare professional.

INSULIN (Systemic)

Some commonly used brand names are:

In the U.S.—

Humulin 50/50 (14)
Humulin 70/30 (14)
Humulin 70/30 Pen (14)
Humulin L (10)
Humulin N (13)
Humulin N Pen (13)
Humulin R (7)
Humulin R, Regular U-500 (Concentrated) (7)
Humulin U (5)
Lente Iletin II (8)
Lente (8)
Novolin L (10)
Novolin 70/30 (14)
Novolin N (13)

Novolin N PenFill (13)
Novolin N Prefilled (13)
Novolin 70/30 PenFill (14)
Novolin 70/30 Prefilled (14)
Novolin R (7)
Novolin R PenFill (7)
Novolin R Prefilled (7)
NPH Iletin II (11)
NPH Purified Insulin (11)
Regular (Concentrated) Iletin II, U-500 (6)
Regular Iletin II (6)
Regular Insulin (6)
Velosulin BR (1)

In Canada—

Humulin 10/90 (14)
Humulin 20/80 (14)
Humulin 30/70 (14)
Humulin 40/60 (14)
Humulin 50/50 (14)
Humulin-L (10)
Humulin-N (13)
Humulin-R (7)
Humulin-U (5)
Lente Iletin (8)
Lente Iletin II (8)
Novolin ge 30/70 (14)
Novolin ge Lente (10)
Novolin ge NPH (13)

Novolin ge NPH Penfill (13)
Novolin ge 10/90 Penfill (14)
Novolin ge 20/80 Penfill (14)
Novolin ge 30/70 Penfill (14)
Novolin ge 40/60 Penfill (14)
Novolin ge 50/50 Penfill (14)
Novolin ge Toronto (7)
Novolin ge Toronto Penfill (7)
Novolin ge Ultralente (5)
NPH Iletin (11)
NPH Iletin II (11)
Regular Iletin II (6)
Velosulin Human (1)

This information applies to the following medicines:

1. Buffered Insulin Human (R) (IN-su-lin)
2. Buffered Insulin Human (R) or Insulin (R) or Insulin Human (R)
3. Extended Insulin Zinc (U)
4. Extended Insulin Zinc (U) or Extended Insulin Human Zinc (U)
5. Extended Insulin Human Zinc (U)
6. Insulin (R)
7. Insulin Human (R)
8. Insulin Zinc (L)
9. Insulin Zinc (L) or Insulin Human Zinc (L)
10. Insulin Human Zinc (L)
11. Isophane Insulin (NPH) (EYE-so-fayn)
12. Isophane Insulin (NPH) or Isophane Insulin Human (NPH)
13. Isophane Insulin Human (NPH)
14. Isophane Insulin Human and Insulin Human (NPH and R)
15. Prompt Insulin Zinc (S)

Category

- **Antidiabetic agent**—Buffered Insulin Human; Extended Insulin Zinc; Extended Insulin Human Zinc; Insulin; Insulin Human; Insulin Zinc; Insulin Human Zinc; Isophane Insulin; Isophane Insulin Human; Isophane Insulin and Insulin Human; Prompt Insulin Zinc; Buffered Insulin Human; Insulin; Insulin Human

- **Diagnostic aid, pituitary growth hormone reserve—**

Description

Insulin IN-su-lin is one of many hormones that helps the body turn the food we eat into energy. Also, insulin helps us store energy that we can use later. After we eat, insulin works by causing sugar (glucose) to go from the blood into our body's

cells to make fat, sugar, and protein. When we need more energy between meals, insulin will help us use the fat, sugar, and protein that we have stored. This occurs whether we make our own insulin in the pancreas gland or take it by injection.

Diabetes mellitus (sugar diabetes) is a condition in which the body does not make enough insulin to meet its needs or does not properly use the insulin it makes. Without insulin, glucose cannot get into the body's cells. Without glucose, the cells will not work properly.

To work properly, the amount of insulin you use must be balanced against the amount and type of food you eat and the amount of exercise you do. If you change your diet, your exercise, or both without changing your insulin dose, your blood glucose level can drop too low or rise too high. A prescription is not necessary to purchase most insulin. However, your doctor must first determine your insulin needs and provide you with special instructions for control of your diabetes.

Insulin can be obtained from beef or pork pancreas glands. Another type of insulin that you may use is called human insulin. It is just like the insulin made by humans but it is made by methods called semi-synthetic or recombinant DNA. All types of insulin must be injected because, if taken by mouth, insulin is destroyed in the stomach.

Insulin is available in the following dosage forms:

Parenteral

- Buffered Insulin Human (a regular insulin)
  - Injection
- Extended Insulin Zinc (an ultralente insulin)
  - Injection
- Extended Insulin Human Zinc (an ultralente insulin)
  - Injection
- Insulin (a regular insulin)
  - Injection
- Insulin Human (a regular insulin)
  - Injection
- Insulin Zinc (a lente insulin)
  - Injection
- Insulin Human Zinc (a lente insulin)
  - Injection
- Isophane Insulin (an NPH insulin)
  - Injection
- Isophane Insulin Human (an NPH insulin)
  - Injection
- Isophane Insulin Human and Insulin Human (an NPH and a regular insulin)
  - Injection
- Prompt Insulin Zinc (a semilente insulin)
  - Injection

Before Using This Medicine

In deciding to use a medicine, the risks of taking the medicine must be weighed against the good it will do. This is a decision you and your doctor will make. For insulin, the following should be considered:

Allergies—Tell your doctor if you have ever had any reactions to insulin, especially in the skin area where you injected the insulin. Also, tell your health care professional if you are allergic to any other substances, such as foods, preservatives, or dyes.

Pregnancy—The amount of insulin you need changes during and after pregnancy. It is especially important for your health and your baby's health that your blood sugar be closely controlled. Close control of your blood sugar can reduce the chance of your baby gaining too much weight, having birth defects, or having high or low blood sugar. Be sure to tell your doctor if you plan to become pregnant or if you think you are pregnant.

Breast-feeding—Insulin does not pass into breast milk and will not affect the nursing infant. However, most women need less insulin while breast-feeding than they needed before. You will need to test your blood sugar often for several months in case your insulin dose needs to be changed.

Children—Children are especially sensitive to the effects of insulin before puberty (the time when sexual changes occur). Therefore, low blood sugar may be especially likely to occur.

Use in teenagers is similar to use in older age groups. The insulin need may be higher during puberty and lower after puberty.

Older adults—Use in older adults is similar to use in other age groups. However, sometimes the first signs of low or high blood sugar are missing or not easily seen in older patients. This may increase the chance of low blood sugar during treatment. Also, some older people may have vision problems or other medical problems that make it harder for them to measure and inject the medicine. Special training and equipment may be needed.

Other medicines—Although certain medicines should not be used together at all, in other cases two different medicines may be used together even if an interaction might occur. In these cases, your doctor may want to change the dose, or other precautions may be necessary. *Do not take any other medicine, unless prescribed or approved by your doctor.* When you are using insulin, it is especially important that your health care professional know if you are taking any of the following:

- Alcohol—Small amounts of alcohol taken with meals do not usually cause a problem; however, larger amounts of alcohol taken for a long time or in one sitting without food can increase the effect of insulin to lower the blood sugar level. This can keep the blood sugar low for a longer period of time than normal

- Beta-adrenergic blocking agents (acebutolol [e.g., Sectral], atenolol [e.g., Tenormin], betaxolol [e.g., Kerlone], bisoprolol [e.g., Zebeta], carteolol [e.g., Cartrol], labetalol [e.g., Normodyne], metoprolol [e.g., Lopressor], nadolol [e.g., Corgard], oxprenolol [e.g., Trasicor], penbutolol [e.g., Levatol], pindolol [e.g., Visken], propranolol [e.g., Inderal], sotalol [e.g., Sotacor], timolol [e.g., Blocadren])—Beta-adrenergic blocking agents may increase the chance of developing either high or low blood sugar levels. Also, they can cover up symptoms of low blood sugar (such as fast heartbeat). Because of this, a person with diabetes might not recognize that he or she has low blood sugar and might not take immediate steps to treat it. Beta-adrenergic blocking agents can also cause a low blood sugar level to last longer than normal

- Corticosteroids (e.g., prednisone or other cortisone-like medicines)—Corticosteroids taken over several weeks, applied to the skin over a long period of time, or injected into a joint may increase the blood sugar level. Higher doses of insulin may be needed during corticosteroid

treatment and for a period of time after corticosteroid treatment ends

- Pentamidine (e.g., NebuPent)—Your dose of pentamidine or insulin or both may need to be adjusted if your pancreas can still make some insulin because pentamidine may cause your pancreas to release its insulin too fast. This effect at first lowers the blood sugar but then causes high blood sugar

Other medical problems—The presence of other medical problems may affect the dose of insulin you need. Be sure to tell your doctor if you have any other medical problems, especially:

- Changes in female hormones for some women (e.g., during puberty, pregnancy, or menstruation) or

- High fever or

- Infection, severe or

- Mental stress or

- Overactive adrenal gland, not properly controlled or

- Other conditions that cause high blood sugar—These conditions increase blood sugar and may increase the amount of insulin you need to take, make it necessary to change the time when you inject the insulin dose, and increase the need to take blood sugar tests

- Diarrhea or

- Gastroparesis (slow stomach emptying) or

- Intestinal blockage or

- Vomiting or

- Other conditions that delay food absorption or stomach emptying—These conditions may slow the time it takes to break down and absorb your meal from your stomach or intestines, which may change the amount of insulin you need, make it necessary to change the time when you inject the insulin dose, and increase the need to take blood sugar tests

- Injury or

- Surgery—Effects of insulin may be increased or decreased; the amount and type of insulin you need may change rapidly

- Kidney disease or

- Liver disease—Effects of insulin may be increased or decreased, partly because of slower removal of insulin from the body; this may change the amount of insulin you need

- Overactive thyroid, not properly controlled—Effects of insulin may be increased or decreased, partly because of faster removal of insulin from the body. Until your thyroid condition is controlled, the amount of insulin you need may change, make it necessary to change the time when you inject the insulin dose, and increase the need to take blood sugar tests

- Underactive adrenal gland, not properly controlled or

- Underactive pituitary gland, not properly controlled or

- Other conditions that cause low blood sugar—These conditions lower blood sugar and may lower the amount of insulin you need, make it necessary for you to change the time when you inject the insulin dose, and increase the need to take blood sugar tests

Proper Use of This Medicine

Make sure you have the type (beef and pork, pork, or human) and the strength of insulin that your doctor ordered for you. You may find that keeping an insulin label with you is helpful when buying insulin supplies.

The concentration (strength) of insulin is measured in USP Insulin Units and USP Insulin Human Units and is usually expressed in terms such as U-100 insulin. Insulin doses are measured and injected with specially marked insulin syringes. *The appropriate syringe is chosen based on your insulin dose to make measuring the dose easy to read. This helps you measure your dose accurately.* These syringes come in three sizes: 3/10 cubic centimeters (cc) measuring up to 30 USP Units of insulin, ½ cc measuring up to 50 USP Units of insulin, and 1 cc measuring up to 100 USP Units of insulin.

It is important to follow any instructions from your doctor about the careful selection and rotation of injection sites on your body.

There are several important steps that will help you successfully prepare your insulin injection. To draw the insulin up into the syringe correctly, you need to follow these steps:

- Wash your hands with soap and water.
- If your insulin contains zinc or isophane (normally cloudy), be sure that it is completely mixed. Mix the insulin by slowly rolling the bottle between your hands or gently tipping the bottle over a few times.
- Never shake the bottle vigorously (hard).
- Do not use the insulin if it looks lumpy or grainy, seems unusually thick, sticks to the bottle, or seems to be even a little discolored. Do not use the insulin if it contains crystals or if the bottle looks frosted. Regular insulin (short-acting) should be used only if it is clear and colorless.
- Remove the colored protective cap on the bottle. Do *not* remove the rubber stopper.
- Wipe the top of the bottle with an alcohol swab.
- Remove the needle cover from the insulin syringe.

How to prepare your insulin dose if you are using one type of insulin:

- Draw air into the syringe by pulling back on the plunger. The amount of air should be equal to your insulin dose.
- Gently push the needle through the top of the rubber stopper with the bottle standing upright.
- Push plunger in all the way to inject air into the bottle.
- Turn the bottle with syringe upside down in one hand. Be sure the tip of the needle is covered by the insulin. With your other hand, draw the plunger back slowly to draw the correct dose of insulin into the syringe.
- Check your dose. Hold the syringe with the scale at eye level to see that the proper dose is withdrawn and to check for air bubbles. Tap gently on the measuring scale of the syringe to move any bubbles to the top of the syringe near the needle. Then, push the insulin slowly back into the bottle and draw up your dose again.
- If your dose measures too low in the syringe, withdraw more solution from the bottle. If there is too much insulin in the syringe, put some back into the bottle. Then check your dose again.

- Remove the needle from the bottle and re-cover the needle.

How to prepare your insulin dose if you are using two types of insulin:

- When you mix regular insulin with another type of insulin, *always* draw the regular insulin into the syringe first. When you mix two types of insulins other than regular insulin, it does not matter in what order you draw them into the syringe.
- After you decide on a certain order for drawing up your insulin, you should use the same order each time.
- Some mixtures of insulins have to be injected immediately. Others may be stable for longer periods of time, which means that you can wait before you inject the mixture. Check with your health care professional to find out which type you have.
- Draw air into the syringe by pulling back on the plunger. The amount of air in the syringe should be equal to the part of the dose that you will be taking from the first bottle. Inject the air into the first bottle. *Do not draw the insulin yet.* Next, draw into the syringe an amount of air equal to the part of the dose that you will be taking from the *second* bottle. Inject the air into the second bottle.
- Return to the first bottle of the combination. With the plunger at zero, draw the first insulin dose of the combination (usually regular insulin) into the syringe.
- Check your dose. Hold the syringe with the scale at eye level to help you see that the proper dose is withdrawn and to check for air bubbles. Tap gently on the measuring scale of the syringe to move any bubbles to the top of the syringe near the needle.
- At this point, if the first part of the dose measures too low in the syringe, you can withdraw more solution from the bottle. If there is too much insulin in your syringe, put some back into the bottle. Then check your dose again.
- Then, without moving the plunger, insert the needle into the second bottle of insulin and withdraw the dose. Sometimes withdrawing a little bit more insulin from the second bottle than needed will help you correct the second dose more easily when you remove the air bubbles.
- Again, check that the proper dose is withdrawn. The syringe will now contain two types of insulin. It is important *not* to squirt *any* extra solution from the syringe back into the bottle. Doing so might change the insulin in the bottle. Throw away any extra insulin in the syringe.
- *If you are not sure that you have done this correctly,* throw away the dose into the sink and begin the steps again. *Do not place any of the solutions back into either bottle.* You can use the same syringe to begin the procedure again.
- If you prepared your mixture ahead of time, gently turn the filled syringe back and forth to remix the insulins before you inject them. Do not shake the syringe.

How to inject your insulin dose:

- After you have prepared your syringe and chosen the area of your body to inject, you are ready to inject the insulin into the fatty skin.
  - Clean the area where the injection is to be given with an alcohol swab or with soap and water. Let the area dry.

○ Pinch up a large area of skin and hold it firmly. With your other hand, hold the syringe like a pencil. Push the needle straight into the pinched-up skin at a 90–degree angle for an adult or at a 45–degree angle for a child. Be sure the needle is all the way in. It is not necessary to draw back on the syringe each time to check for blood (also called routine aspiration).

○ Push the plunger all the way down, using less than 5 seconds to inject the dose. Let go of the skin. Hold an alcohol swab near the needle and pull the needle straight out of the skin.

○ Press the swab against the injection area for several seconds. Do not rub.

○ If you are either thin or greatly overweight, you may be given special instructions for giving yourself insulin injections.

How to use special injection devices:

• It is important to follow the information that comes with your insulin and with the device you use for injecting your insulin. This will ensure proper use and proper insulin dosing. If you need more information about this, ask your health care professional.

For patients using an *automatic injector* (with a disposable syringe):

• After the dose is drawn, the disposable syringe is placed inside the automatic injector. Pressing a button on the device quickly plunges the needle into the skin, releasing the insulin dose.

For patients using *a continuous subcutaneous infusion insulin pump:*

• Buffered regular human insulin, when available, is the recommended insulin for insulin pumps. Otherwise non-buffered regular insulin can be used.

• The pump consists of a tube, with a needle on the end of it that is taped to the abdomen, and a computerized device that is worn at the waist. Insulin is received continuously from the pump. A button is pressed at mealtime to release an extra insulin dose.

• It is important to follow the pump manufacturer's directions on how to load the syringe and/or pump reservoir. If you do not load the syringe and/or pump properly, you may not get the correct insulin dose.

• Check the infusion tubing and infusion-site dressing as often as your health care professional recommends to make sure the pump is working properly.

For patients using *disposable syringes:*

• Manufacturers of disposable syringes recommend that they be used only once, because the sterility of a reused syringe cannot be guaranteed. However, some patients prefer to reuse a syringe until its needle becomes dull. Most insulins have chemicals added that keep them from growing the bacteria that are usually found on the skin. However, the syringe should be thrown away when the needle becomes dull, has been bent, or has come into contact with any surface other than the cleaned and swabbed area of skin. If you plan to reuse a syringe, the needle must be recapped after each use. Check with your health care professional to find out the best way to reuse syringes.

For patients using an *insulin pen device* (cartridge and disposable needles):

• Change the dose by rotating the head of the pen. Put the pen next to your skin and press the plunger to inject the medicine. Some pen devices can only inject certain doses of insulin with each injection. Injection amounts can be different for different pen devices. To receive the right dose, you might have to count the number of times you press the plunger. Also, these devices use special cartridges of isophane insulin (NPH), regular insulin (R), or a mixture of these two types.

For patients using *nondisposable syringes* (glass syringe and metal needle):

• These types of syringes and needles may be used repeatedly if they are sterilized after each use. You should get an instruction sheet that tells you how to do this. If you need more information about this, ask your health care professional.

For patients using *a spray injector* (device without needles):

• The dose is measured by rotating part of the device. Insulin is drawn up into the spray device from an insulin bottle. Pressing a button forcefully sprays the insulin dose into the skin. This involves a wider area of skin than an injection would.

Laws in some states require that used insulin syringes and needles be destroyed. Be careful when you recap, bend, or break a needle, because these actions increase the chances of a needle-stick injury. It is best to put used syringes and needles in a disposable container that is puncture-resistant (such as an empty plastic liquid laundry detergent or bleach bottle) or to use a needle-clipping device. The chance of a syringe being reused by someone else is smaller if the plunger is taken out of the barrel and broken in half when you dispose of a syringe.

Use this medicine only as directed. Do not use more or less insulin than recommended by your doctor. To do so may increase the chance of serious side effects.

Your doctor will give you instructions about diet, exercise, how to test your blood sugar levels, and how to adjust your dose when you are sick.

• Diet—The daily number of calories in the meal plan should be adjusted by your doctor or a registered dietitian to help you reach and maintain a healthy body weight. In addition, regular meals and snacks are arranged to meet the energy needs of your body at different times of the day. *It is very important that you carefully follow your meal plan.*

• Exercise—Ask your doctor what kind of exercise to do, the best time to do it, and how much you should do each day.

• Blood tests—This is the best way to tell whether your diabetes is being controlled properly. Blood sugar testing helps you and your health care team adjust your insulin dose, meal plan, and exercise schedule.

• Changes in dose—Your doctor may change the first dose of the day. A change in the first dose of the day might change your blood sugar later in the day or change the amount of insulin you should use in other doses later that day. *That is why your doctor should know any time your dose changes, even temporarily, unless you have been told otherwise.*

• On sick days—When you become sick with a cold, fever, or the flu, you need to take your usual insulin dose, even if you feel too ill to eat. This is especially true if you have nausea, vomiting, or diarrhea. Infection usually increases your need for insulin. Call your doctor for specific instructions. Continue taking your insulin and try to stay on your regular meal plan. However, if you have trouble eating solid food, drink fruit juices, nondiet soft drinks, or clear soups, or eat small amounts of bland foods. A dietitian or your doctor can give you a list of foods and the amounts to use for sick days.Test your blood sugar level at least every 4 hours while you are awake and check your urine for ketones. If ketones are present, call your doctor at once. If you have severe or prolonged vomiting, check with your doctor. Even when you start feeling better, let your doctor know how you are doing.

Dosing—The dose of these medicines will be different for different patients. *Follow your doctor's orders or the directions on the label.* The following information applies to the average doses of these medicines. *If your dose is different, do not change it* unless your doctor tells you to do so.

The number of injections that you receive each day depends on the strength or type of the medicine. Also, *the number of doses you receive each day, the time allowed between doses, and the length of time you receive the medicine depend on the amount of sugar in your blood or urine.*

For regular insulin (R)—Crystalline zinc, human buffered, and human regular insulins
- For *injection* dosage form:
  ○ For treating sugar diabetes (diabetes mellitus):
    ▪ Adults and teenagers—The dose is based on your blood sugar and must be determined by your doctor. The medicine is injected under the skin fifteen or thirty minutes before meals and/or a bedtime snack. Also, your doctor may want you to use more than one type of insulin.
    ▪ Children—Dose is based on your blood sugar and body weight and must be determined by your doctor.

For isophane insulin (NPH)—Isophane and human isophane insulins
- For *injection* dosage form:
  ○ For treating sugar diabetes (diabetes mellitus):
    ▪ Adults and teenagers—The dose is based on your blood sugar and must be determined by your doctor. The medicine is injected under the skin thirty to sixty minutes before a meal and/or a bedtime snack. Also, your doctor may want you to use more than one type of insulin.
    ▪ Children—Dose is based on your blood sugar and body weight and must be determined by your doctor.

For isophane insulin human/insulin human (NPH/R)—Human isophane/human regular insulin
- For *injection* dosage form:
  ○ For treating sugar diabetes (diabetes mellitus):
    ▪ Adults and teenagers—The dose is based on your blood sugar and must be determined by your doctor. The medicine is injected under the skin fifteen to thirty minutes before breakfast. You may need a dose before another meal or at bedtime. Also, your doctor may want you to use more than one type of insulin.
    ▪ Children—Dose is based on your blood sugar and body weight and must be determined by your doctor.

For insulin zinc (L)—Lente and human lente insulins
- For *injection* dosage form:
  ○ For treating sugar diabetes (diabetes mellitus):
    ▪ Adults and teenagers—The dose is based on your blood sugar and must be determined by your doctor. The medicine is injected under the skin thirty minutes before breakfast. You may need a dose before another meal and/or a bedtime snack. Also, your doctor may want you to use more than one type of insulin.
    ▪ Children—Dose is based on your blood sugar and body weight and must be determined by your doctor.

For insulin zinc extended (U)—Ultralente and human ultralente insulins
- For *injection* dosage form:
  ○ For treating sugar diabetes (diabetes mellitus):
    ▪ Adults and teenagers—The dose is based on your blood sugar and must be determined by your doctor. The medicine is injected under the skin thirty to sixty minutes before a meal and/or a bedtime snack. Your doctor may want you to use more than one type of insulin.
    ▪ Children—Dose is based on your blood sugar and body weight and must be determined by your doctor.

For prompt insulin zinc (S)—Semilente insulin
- For *injection* dosage form:
  ○ For treating sugar diabetes (diabetes mellitus):
    ▪ Adults and teenagers—The dose is based on your blood sugar and must be determined by your doctor. The medicine is injected under the skin thirty to sixty minutes before breakfast. You may need a dose thirty minutes before another meal and/or a bedtime snack. Your doctor may want you to use more than one type of insulin.
    ▪ Children—Dose is based on your blood sugar and body weight and must be determined by your doctor.

Storage—To store this medicine:
- Unopened bottles of insulin should be refrigerated until needed and may be used until the printed expiration date on the label. Insulin should never be frozen. Remove the insulin from the refrigerator and allow it to reach room temperature before injecting it.
- An insulin bottle in use may be kept at room temperature for up to 1 month. Insulin that has been kept at room temperature for longer than a month should be thrown away.
- Storing prefilled syringes in the refrigerator with the needle pointed up reduces problems that can occur, such as crystals forming in the needle and blocking it up.
- Do not expose insulin to extremely hot temperatures or to sunlight. Extreme heat will cause insulin to become less effective much more quickly.

Precautions While Using This Medicine

It is very important that your doctor check your progress at regular visits, especially during the first few weeks of insulin treatment.

It is very important to follow carefully any instructions from your health care team about:

- Alcohol—Drinking alcohol may cause severe low blood sugar. Discuss this with your health care team.
- Tobacco—If you have been smoking for a long time and suddenly stop, your dosage of insulin may need to be reduced. If you decide to quit, tell your doctor first.
- Other medicines—Do not take other medicines unless they have been discussed with your doctor. This especially includes nonprescription medicines such as aspirin, and medicines for appetite control, asthma, colds, cough, hay fever, or sinus problems.
- Counseling—Other family members need to learn how to prevent side effects or help with side effects if they occur. Also, patients with diabetes, especially teenagers, may need special counseling about insulin dosing changes that might occur because of lifestyle changes, such as changes in exercise and diet. Furthermore, counseling on contraception and pregnancy may be needed because of the problems that can occur in women with diabetes who become pregnant.
- Travel—Keep a recent prescription and your medical history with you. Be prepared for an emergency as you would normally. Make allowances for changing time zones, keep your meal times as close as possible to your usual meal times, and store insulin properly.

In case of emergency—There may be a time when you need emergency help for a problem caused by your diabetes. You need to be prepared for these emergencies. It is a good idea to:

- Wear a medical identification (ID) bracelet or neck chain at all times. Also, carry an ID card in your wallet or purse that says that you have diabetes and lists all of your medicines.
- Keep an extra supply of insulin and syringes with needles on hand in case high blood sugar occurs.
- Keep some kind of quick-acting sugar handy to treat low blood sugar.
- Have a glucagon kit available in case severe low blood sugar occurs. Check and replace any expired kits regularly.

Too much insulin can cause low blood sugar (also called hypoglycemia or insulin reaction). *Symptoms of low blood sugar must be treated before they lead to unconsciousness (passing out).* Different people may feel different symptoms of low blood sugar. *It is important that you learn what symptoms of low blood sugar you usually have so that you can treat it quickly.*

- Symptoms of low blood sugar can include: anxious feeling, behavior change similar to being drunk, blurred vision, cold sweats, confusion, cool pale skin, difficulty in concentrating, drowsiness, excessive hunger, fast heartbeat, headache, nausea, nervousness, nightmares, restless sleep, shakiness, slurred speech, and unusual tiredness or weakness.
- The symptoms of low blood sugar may develop quickly and may result from:
  - delaying or missing a scheduled meal or snack.
  - exercising more than usual.
  - drinking a significant amount of alcohol.
  - taking certain medicines.
  - using too much insulin.
  - sickness (especially with vomiting or diarrhea).

- Know what to do if symptoms of low blood sugar occur. Eating some form of quick-acting sugar when symptoms of low blood sugar first appear will usually prevent them from getting worse. Good sources of sugar include:
  - Glucose tablets or gel, fruit juice or nondiet soft drink (4 to 6 ounces [one-half cup]), corn syrup or honey (1 tablespoon), sugar cubes (six one-half inch size), or table sugar (dissolved in water).
    - If a snack is not scheduled for an hour or more you should also eat a light snack, such as cheese and crackers, half a sandwich, or drink an 8-ounce glass of milk.
    - Do not use chocolate because its fat slows down the sugar entering into the blood stream.
  - Glucagon is used in emergency situations such as unconsciousness. Have a glucagon kit available and know how to prepare and use it. Members of your household also should know how and when to use it.

High blood sugar (hyperglycemia) is another problem related to uncontrolled diabetes. *If you have any symptoms of high blood sugar, contact your health care team right away.* If high blood sugar is not treated, severe hyperglycemia can occur, leading to ketoacidosis (diabetic coma) and death.

- The symptoms of mild high blood sugar appear more slowly than those of low blood sugar. Symptoms can include: blurred vision; drowsiness; dry mouth; flushed and dry skin; fruit-like breath odor; increased urination (frequency and volume); loss of appetite; stomachache, nausea, or vomiting; tiredness; troubled breathing (rapid and deep); and unusual thirst.
- Symptoms of severe high blood sugar (called ketoacidosis or diabetic coma) that need immediate hospitalization include: flushed and dry skin, fruit-like breath odor, ketones in urine, passing out, and troubled breathing (rapid and deep).
- High blood sugar symptoms may occur if you:
  - have diarrhea, a fever, or an infection.
  - do not take enough insulin or skip a dose of insulin.
  - do not exercise as much as usual.
  - overeat or do not follow your meal plan.
- Know what to do if high blood sugar occurs. Your doctor may recommend changes in your insulin dose or meal plan to avoid high blood sugar. Symptoms of high blood sugar must be corrected before they progress to more serious conditions. Check with your doctor often to make sure you are controlling your blood sugar. Your doctor might discuss the following with you:
  - Increasing your insulin dose when you plan to eat an unusually large dinner, such as on holidays. This type of increase is called an anticipatory dose.
  - Decreasing your dose for a short time for special needs, such as when you cannot exercise as you normally do. Changing only one type of insulin dose (usually the first dose) and anticipating how the change may affect other doses during the day. Contacting your doctor if you need a permanent change in dose.
  - Delaying a meal if your blood glucose is over 200 mg/dL to allow time for your blood sugar to go down. An extra insulin dose may be needed if your blood sugar does not come down shortly.
  - Not exercising if your blood glucose is over 240 mg/dL and reporting this to your doctor immediately.
  - Being hospitalized if ketoacidosis or diabetic coma occurs.

Side Effects

Along with its needed effects, a medicine may cause some unwanted effects. Although not all of these side effects may occur, if they do occur they may need medical attention.

Check with your doctor immediately if any of the following side effects occur:

More common
> Convulsions (seizures); unconsciousness

Also, check with your doctor as soon as possible if any of the following side effects occur:

More common
> Low blood sugar (mild), including anxious feeling, behavior change similar to being drunk, blurred vision, cold sweats, confusion, cool pale skin, difficulty in concentrating, drowsiness, excessive hunger, fast heartbeat, headache, nausea, nervousness, nightmares, restless sleep, shakiness, slurred speech, unusual tiredness or weakness; weight gain

Rare
> Depressed skin at the place of injection; swelling of face, fingers, feet, or ankles; thickening of the skin at the place of injection

Not all of the side effects listed above have been reported for each of these medicines, but they have been reported for at least one of them. All of the insulins are similar, so any of the above side effects may occur with any of these medicines.

Other side effects not listed above may also occur in some patients. If you notice any other effects, check with your doctor.

Additional Information

Once a medicine has been approved for marketing for a certain use, experience may show that it is also useful for other medical problems. Although this use is not included in product labeling, regular insulin is used in certain patients:

- To treat high blood sugar (hyperglycemia) in low birth weight infants.
- To test for growth hormone deficiency
- To prevent complications of diabetes, including eye problems (retinopathy), kidney disease (nephropathy), and nerve damage (neuropathy)

Other than the above information, there is no additional information relating to proper use, precautions, or side effects for this use.

INSULIN ASPART, RECOMBINANT
(Subcutaneous route) - IN-su-lin AS-part, re-KOM-bi-nant

Commonly used brand name(s)
In the U.S.—
> Novolog
> Novolog FlexPen

Available Dosage Forms:
- Solution

Therapeutic Class: Antidiabetic
Pharmacologic Class: Insulin, Ultra Rapid Acting

Uses For This Medicine

Insulin aspart is a fast-acting type of human insulin. Insulin is used by people with type 2 diabetes to help keep blood sugar levels under control. If you have type 2 diabetes, your body cannot make enough or does not use insulin properly. So, you must take additional insulin to regulate your blood sugar and keep your body healthy. This is very important as too much sugar in your blood can be harmful to your health. Since insulin aspart acts faster than regular human insulin, you normally should use insulin aspart with a longer-acting insulin.

This medicine is available only with your doctor's prescription.

Before Using This Medicine

In deciding to use a medicine, the risks of taking the medicine must be weighed against the good it will do. This is a decision you and your doctor will make. For this medicine, the following should be considered:

Allergies—Tell your doctor if you have ever had any unusual or allergic reaction to this medicine or any other medicines. Also tell your health care professional if you have any other types of allergies, such as to foods, dyes, preservatives, or animals. For non-prescription products, read the label or package ingredients carefully.

Pediatric—Studies on this medicine have been done only in adult patients, and there is no specific information comparing use of insulin aspart in children with use in other age groups.

Geriatric—This medicine has been tested in a limited number of patients 65 years of age or older and has not been shown to cause different side effects or problems in older people than it does in younger adults.

Pregnancy—

	Pregnancy Category	Explanation
All Trimesters	C	Animal studies have shown an adverse effect and there are no adequate studies in pregnant women OR no animal studies have been conducted and there are no adequate studies in pregnant women.

Breast Feeding—There are no adequate studies in women for determining infant risk when using this medication during breastfeeding. Weigh the potential benefits against the potential risks before taking this medication while breastfeeding.

Other medicines—

Using this medicine with any of the following medicines is usually not recommended, but may be required in some cases. If both medicines are prescribed together, your doctor may change the dose or how often you use one or both of the medicines.

Alatrofloxacin, Balofloxacin, Ciprofloxacin, Clinafloxacin, Enoxacin, Fleroxacin, Flumequine, Gatifloxacin, Gemifloxacin, Grepafloxacin, Levofloxacin, Lomefloxacin, Moxifloxacin, Norfloxacin, Ofloxacin, Pefloxacin, Prulifloxacin, Rufloxacin, Sparfloxacin, Temafloxacin, Tosufloxacin, Trovafloxacin Mesylate

Interactions with Food/Tobacco/Alcohol—Certain medicines should not be used at or around the time of eating food or eating certain types of food since interactions may occur. Using alcohol or tobacco with certain medicines may also cause interactions to occur. Discuss with your healthcare professional the use of your medicine with food, alcohol, or tobacco.

Other medical problems—The presence of other medical problems may affect the use of this medicine. Make sure you tell your doctor if you have any other medical problems, especially:

- Hypoglycemia (low blood sugar)—If you have low blood sugar and take insulin, your blood sugar may reach dangerously low levels
- Kidney disease or
- Liver disease—Effects of insulin aspart may be increased or decreased; your doctor may need to change your insulin dose

Proper Use of This Medicine

It is best to use a different place on the body for each injection (e.g., abdomen, thigh, or upper arm). If you have questions about this, contact a member of your health care team.

When used as a mealtime insulin, insulin aspart should be taken within 5–10 minutes before the meal or immediately before the meal.

Follow carefully the special meal plan your doctor gave you. This is the most important part of controlling your condition, and is necessary if the medicine is to work properly. Also, exercise regularly and test for sugar in your blood or urine as directed.

Dosing—The dose of this medicine will be different for different patients. Follow your doctor's orders or the directions on the label. The following information includes only the average doses of this medicine. If your dose is different, do not change it unless your doctor tells you to do so.

The amount of medicine that you take depends on the strength of the medicine. Also, the number of doses you take each day, the time allowed between doses, and the length of time you take the medicine depend on the medical problem for which you are using the medicine.

- For injection dosage form:
  - For type 2 diabetes mellitus:
    - Adults—The dose is based on your blood sugar and must be determined by your doctor.
    - Children—Use and dose must be determined by your doctor.

Storage—Store in the refrigerator. Do not freeze.

Keep out of the reach of children.

Do not keep outdated medicine or medicine no longer needed.

After a cartridge has been inserted into a pen, store the cartridge and pen at room temperature, not in the refrigerator.

Precautions While Using This Medicine

Your doctor will want to check your progress at regular visits, especially during the first few weeks you take this medicine.

It is very important to follow carefully any instructions from your health care team about:

- Alcohol—Drinking alcohol may cause severe low blood sugar. Discuss this with your health care team.
- Other medicines—Do not take other medicines during the time you are taking insulin aspart unless they have been discussed with your doctor. This especially includes nonprescription medicines such as aspirin, and medicines for appetite control, asthma, colds, cough, hay fever, or sinus problems.
- Counseling—Other family members need to learn how to prevent side effects or help with side effects if they occur. Also, patients with diabetes may need special counseling about diabetes medicine dosing changes that might occur because of lifestyle changes, such as changes in exercise and diet. Furthermore, counseling on contraception and pregnancy may be needed because of the problems that can occur in patients with diabetes during pregnancy.
- Travel—Keep a recent prescription and your medical history with you. Be prepared for an emergency as you would normally. Make allowances for changing time zones and keep your meal times as close as possible to your usual meal times.

In case of emergency—There may be a time when you need emergency help for a problem caused by your diabetes. You need to be prepared for these emergencies. It is a good idea to:

- Wear a medical identification (ID) bracelet or neck chain at all times. Also, carry an ID card in your wallet or purse that says that you have diabetes and a list of all of your medicines.

Too much insulin aspart can cause hypoglycemia (low blood sugar). Symptoms of low blood sugar include anxiety; behavior change similar to being drunk; blurred vision; cold sweats; confusion; depression; difficulty in thinking; dizziness or light-headedness; drowsiness; excessive hunger; fast heartbeat; headache; irritability or abnormal behavior; nervousness; nightmares; restless sleep; shakiness; slurred speech; and tingling in the hands, feet, lips, or tongue.

Low blood sugar also can occur if you use insulin aspart with another antidiabetic medicine, delay or miss a meal or snack, exercise more than usual, drink alcohol, or cannot eat because of nausea or vomiting or have diarrhea.

If symptoms of low blood sugar occur, eat glucose tablets or gel to relieve the symptoms. Also, check your blood for low blood sugar. Get to a doctor or a hospital right away if the symptoms do not improve. Someone should call for emergency help immediately if severe symptoms such as convulsions (seizures) or unconsciousness occur. Have a glucagon kit available, along with a syringe and needle, and know how to use it. Members of your household also should know how to use it.

Symptoms of high blood sugar include blurred vision; drowsiness; dry mouth; flushed, dry skin; fruit-like breath odor; increased urination; ketones in urine; loss of appetite; stomachache, nausea, or vomiting; tiredness; troubled breathing (rapid and deep); unconsciousness; and unusual thirst.

Hyperglycemia (high blood sugar) may occur if you do not take enough or skip a dose of your antidiabetic medicine, overeat or do not follow your meal plan, have a fever or infection, or do not exercise as much as usual.

If symptoms of high blood sugar occur, check your blood sugar level and then call your doctor for instructions.

Side Effects of This Medicine

Along with its needed effects, a medicine may cause some unwanted effects. Although not all of these side effects may occur, if they do occur they may need medical attention.

Check with your doctor immediately if any of the following side effects occur:

More common

Convulsions (seizures); unconsciousness

Check with your doctor as soon as possible if any of the following side effects occur:

More common

Low blood sugar; anxious feeling; behavior change similar to being drunk; blurred vision; cold sweats; confusion; depression; difficulty in thinking; dizziness or light-headedness; drowsiness; excessive hunger; fast heartbeat; headache; irritability or abnormal behavior; nervousness; nightmares; restless sleep; shakiness; slurred speech; tingling in the hands, feet, lips, or tongue

Less common or rare

Depression of the skin at place of injection; thickening of the skin at place of injection; dryness of mouth; irregular heartbeat; increased thirst; loss of appetite; mood or mental changes; muscle cramps or pain; nausea or vomiting; shortness of breath; unusual tiredness or weakness; fast or weak pulse; sweating; skin rash or itching over the whole body; wheezing; feeling of pressure, itching, redness, soreness, stinging; swelling, or tingling at place of injection

Other side effects not listed may also occur in some patients. If you notice any other effects, check with your healthcare professional.

INSULIN DETEMIR   (Injection route)

Uses For This Medicine

Insulin is one of many hormones that help the body turn the food we eat into energy. This is done by using the glucose (sugar) in the blood as quick energy. Also, insulin helps us store energy that we can use later. When you have diabetes mellitus, your body does not produce enough insulin, or the insulin produced is not used properly. This causes you to have too much sugar in your blood. Like other types of insulin, insulin detemir is used to keep your blood sugar level close to normal. Insulin detemir is a long-acting insulin that works slowly over about 24 hours. You may have to use insulin detemir in combination with another type of insulin or with a type of oral diabetes medicine to keep your blood sugar under control.

This medicine is available only with your doctor's prescription

Before Using This Medicine

In deciding to use a medicine, the risks of taking the medicine must be weighed against the good it will do. This is a decision you and your doctor will make. For this medicine, the following should be considered:

Allergies—Tell your doctor if you have ever had any unusual or allergic reaction to this medicine or any other medicines. Also tell your health care professional if you have any other types of allergies, such as to foods, dyes, preservatives, or animals. For non-prescription products, read the label or package ingredients carefully.

Pediatric—Studies on this medicine have been done only in adult patients, and there is no specific information comparing use of insulin detemir in children with use in other age groups.

Geriatric—This medicine has been tested in a limited number of patients 65 years of age or older and has not been shown to cause different side effects or problems in older people than it does in younger adults.

Pregnancy—

	Pregnancy Category	Explanation
All Trimesters	C	Animal studies have shown an adverse effect and there are no adequate studies in pregnant women OR no animal studies have been conducted and there are no adequate studies in pregnant women.

Breast Feeding—There are no adequate studies in women for determining infant risk when using this medication during breastfeeding. Weigh the potential benefits against the potential risks before taking this medication while breastfeeding.

Other medicines—Although certain medicines should not be used together at all, in other cases two different medicines may be used together even if an interaction might occur. In these cases, your doctor may want to change the dose, or other precautions may be necessary. Tell your healthcare professional if you are taking any other prescription or non-prescription (over-the-counter [OTC]) medicine.

Interactions with Food/Tobacco/Alcohol—Certain medicines should not be used at or around the time of eating food or eating certain types of food since interactions may occur. Using alcohol or tobacco with certain medicines may also cause interactions to occur. Discuss with your healthcare professional the use of your medicine with food, alcohol, or tobacco.

Other medical problems—The presence of other medical problems may affect the use of this medicine. Make sure you tell your doctor if you have any other medical problems, especially:

• Emotional disturbances or

• Stress—These conditions increase blood sugar and may increase the amount of insulin or insulin detemir you need.

• Hypoglycemia (low blood sugar)—If you have low blood sugar and take insulin, your blood sugar may reach dangerously low levels.

• Kidney disease or

• Liver disease—Effects of insulin detemir may be increased or decreased; your doctor may need to change your insulin dose.

Proper Use of This Medicine

Each package of insulin detemir contains a patient information sheet. Read this sheet carefully before beginning treatment and each time you refill for any new information, and make sure you understand:

- How to prepare the medicine.
- How to inject the medicine.
- How to dispose of syringes, needles, and injection devices.

It is best to use a different place on the body for each injection (e.g., abdomen, thigh, or upper arm). If you have questions about this, contact a member of your health care team.

Follow carefully special instructions your doctor gave you. This is the most important part of controlling your condition, and is necessary if the medicine is to work properly. Also, exercise regularly and test for sugar in your blood or urine as directed.

Do not dilute or mix insulin detemir with any other insulins or solutions. This may cause the medicine to not work properly.

Dosing—The dose of this medicine will be different for different patients. Follow your doctor's orders or the directions on the label. The following information includes only the average doses of this medicine. If your dose is different, do not change it unless your doctor tells you to do so.

The amount of medicine that you take depends on the strength of the medicine. Also, the number of doses you take each day, the time allowed between doses, and the length of time you take the medicine depend on the medical problem for which you are using the medicine.

- For injection dosage form:
  - For diabetes mellitus:
    - Adults—The dose is based on your blood sugar and must be determined by your doctor.
    - Children—Use and dose must be determined by your doctor.

Storage—Keep out of the reach of children.

Store in the refrigerator. Do not freeze.

Do not keep outdated medicine or medicine no longer needed.

Precautions While Using This Medicine

Your doctor will want to check your progress at regular visits, especially during the first few weeks you take this medicine.

Avoid drinking alcohol while using this medicine. It is very important to follow carefully any instructions from your health care team about:

- Alcohol—Drinking alcohol may cause severe low blood sugar. Discuss this with your health care team.
- Other medicines—Do not take other medicines during the time you are taking insulin detemir unless they have been discussed with your doctor. This especially includes nonprescription medicines such as aspirin, and medicines for appetite control, asthma, colds, cough, hay fever, or sinus problems.
- Counseling—Other family members need to learn how to prevent side effects or help with side effects if they occur. Also, patients with diabetes may need special counseling about diabetes medicine dosing changes that might occur because of lifestyle changes, such as changes in exercise and diet. Furthermore, counseling on contraception and pregnancy is needed because of the problems that can occur in patients with diabetes during pregnancy.
- Travel—Keep a recent prescription and your medical history with you. Be prepared for an emergency as you would normally. Make allowances for changing time zones and keep your meal times as close as possible to your usual meal times.

In case of emergency—There may be a time when you need emergency help for a problem caused by your diabetes. You need to be prepared for these emergencies. It is a good idea to:

- Wear a medical identification (ID) bracelet or neck chain at all times. Also, carry an ID card in your wallet or purse that says that you have diabetes and a list of all of your medicines.
- Keep an extra supply of insulin detemir and syringes with needles or injection devices on hand in case high blood sugar occurs.
- Keep some kind of quick-acting sugar handy to treat low blood sugar.
- Have a glucagon kit and a syringe and needle available in case severe low blood sugar occurs. Check and replace any expired kits regularly.

Too much insulin detemir can cause hypoglycemia (low blood sugar). Low blood sugar also can occur if you use insulin detemir with another antidiabetic medicine, delay or miss a meal or snack, exercise more than usual, or drink alcohol. *Symptoms of low blood sugar must be treated before they lead to unconsciousness (passing out).* Different people may feel different symptoms of low blood sugar. *It is important that you learn which symptoms of low blood sugar you usually have so that you can treat it quickly.*

Symptoms of low blood sugar include: anxiety; behavior change similar to being drunk; blurred vision; cold sweats; confusion; difficulty in thinking; dizziness or lightheadedness; drowsiness; excessive hunger; fast heartbeat; headache; irritability or abnormal behavior; nervousness; nightmares; restless sleep; shakiness; slurred speech; and tingling in the hands, feet, lips, or tongue.

If symptoms of low blood sugar occur, *eat glucose tablets or gel, corn syrup, honey, or sugar cubes; or drink fruit juice, nondiet soft drink, or sugar dissolved in water to relieve the symptoms.* Also, check your blood for low blood sugar. *Get to a doctor or a hospital right away if the symptoms do not improve. Someone should call for emergency help immediately if severe symptoms such as convulsions (seizures) or unconsciousness occur.* Have a glucagon kit available, along with a syringe and needle, and know how to use it. Members of your household also should know how to use it.

Hyperglycemia (high blood sugar) may occur if you do not take enough or skip a dose of your antidiabetic medicine, overeat or do not follow your meal plan, have emotional stress or infection, or do not exercise as much as usual.

Symptoms of high blood sugar include: blurred vision; drowsiness; dry mouth; flushed, dry skin; fruit-like breath odor; increased urination; ketones in urine; loss of appetite; stomachache, nausea, or vomiting; tiredness; troubled breathing (rapid and deep); unconsciousness; and unusual thirst.

Side Effects of This Medicine

Along with its needed effects, a medicine may cause some unwanted effects. Although not all of these side effects may occur, if they do occur they may need medical attention.

Check with your doctor immediately if any of the following side effects occur:
> *Incidence unknown*
>> Anxiety; blurred vision; chills; cold sweats; coma; confusion; cool pale skin; cough; depression; difficulty swallowing; dizziness; fast heartbeat; fever; headache; hives; hoarseness; increased hunger; irritation; itching; joint pain; nausea; nervousness; nightmares; puffiness or swelling of the eyelids or around the eyes, face, lips or tongue; redness of skin; seizures; shakiness; shortness of breath; skin rash; slurred speech; stiffness or swelling; swelling of eyelids, face, lips, hands, or feet; tightness in chest; troubled breathing or swallowing; unusual tiredness or weakness; wheezing

Get emergency help immediately if any of the following symptoms of overdose occur:
> *Symptoms of overdose*
>> Anxiety; blurred vision; chills; cold sweats; coma; confusion; cool pale skin; depression; dizziness; fast heartbeat; headache; increased hunger; nausea; nervousness; nightmares; seizures; shakiness; slurred speech; unusual tiredness or weakness

Some side effects may occur that usually do not need medical attention. These side effects may go away during treatment as your body adjusts to the medicine. Also, your health care professional may be able to tell you about ways to prevent or reduce some of these side effects. Check with your health care professional if any of the following side effects continue or are bothersome or if you have any questions about them:
> *Incidence unknown*
>> Bleeding, blistering, burning, coldness, discoloration of skin; feeling of pressure, hives, infection, inflammation, itching, lumps, numbness, pain, rash, redness, scarring, soreness, stinging, swelling, tenderness, tingling, ulceration, or warmth at injection site; decrease in amount of urine; noisy, rattling breathing; redistribution or accumulation of body fat; swelling of fingers, hands, feet, or lower legs; swelling; troubled breathing at rest; weight gain

Other side effects not listed may also occur in some patients. If you notice any other effects, check with your healthcare professional.

INSULIN GLARGINE, RECOMBINANT (Subcutaneous route)
- IN-su-lin GLAR-jeen, re-KOM-bi-nant

Commonly used brand name(s)

In the U.S.—
> Lantus

Available Dosage Forms:
- Solution

Therapeutic Class: Antidiabetic
Pharmacologic Class: Insulin, Long Acting

Uses For This Medicine

Insulin glargine is a type of insulin. Insulin is one of many hormones that help the body turn the food we eat into energy. This is done by using the glucose (sugar) in the blood as quick energy. Also, insulin helps us store energy that we can use later. When you have type 2 diabetes mellitus, your body does not produce enough insulin, or the insulin produced is not used properly. This causes you to have too much sugar in your blood. Like other types of insulin, insulin glargine is used to keep your blood sugar level close to normal. Insulin glargine is a long-acting insulin that works slowly over about 24 hours. You may have to use insulin glargine in combination with another type of insulin or with a type of oral diabetes medicine to keep your blood sugar under control.

This medicine is available only with your doctor's prescription.

Before Using This Medicine

In deciding to use a medicine, the risks of taking the medicine must be weighed against the good it will do. This is a decision you and your doctor will make. For this medicine, the following should be considered:

Allergies—Tell your doctor if you have ever had any unusual or allergic reaction to this medicine or any other medicines. Also tell your health care professional if you have any other types of allergies, such as to foods, dyes, preservatives, or animals. For non-prescription products, read the label or package ingredients carefully.

Pediatric—This medicine has been tested in a limited number of children 6 years of age or older. In effective doses, the medicine has not been shown to cause different side effects or problems than it does in adults.

Geriatric—This medicine has been tested in a limited number of patients 65 years of age or older and has not been shown to cause different side effects or problems in older people than it does in younger adults.

Pregnancy—

	Pregnancy Category	Explanation
All Trimesters	C	Animal studies have shown an adverse effect and there are no adequate studies in pregnant women OR no animal studies have been conducted and there are no adequate studies in pregnant women.

Other medicines—Although certain medicines should not be used together at all, in other cases two different medicines may be used together even if an interaction might occur. In these cases, your doctor may want to change the dose, or other precautions may be necessary. Tell your healthcare professional if you are taking any other prescription or non-prescription (over-the-counter [OTC]) medicine.

Interactions with Food/Tobacco/Alcohol—Certain medicines should not be used at or around the time of eating

food or eating certain types of food since interactions may occur. Using alcohol or tobacco with certain medicines may also cause interactions to occur. Discuss with your healthcare professional the use of your medicine with food, alcohol, or tobacco.

Other medical problems—The presence of other medical problems may affect the use of this medicine. Make sure you tell your doctor if you have any other medical problems, especially:

- Emotional disturbances or
- Infection or
- Stress—These conditions increase blood sugar and may increase the amount of insulin or insulin glargine you need
- Kidney disease or
- Liver disease—Effects of insulin glargine may be increased; this may change the amount of insulin glargine you need

Proper Use of This Medicine

Dosing—The dose of this medicine will be different for different patients. Follow your doctor's orders or the directions on the label. The following information includes only the average doses of this medicine. If your dose is different, do not change it unless your doctor tells you to do so.

The amount of medicine that you take depends on the strength of the medicine. Also, the number of doses you take each day, the time allowed between doses, and the length of time you take the medicine depend on the medical problem for which you are using the medicine.

Each package of insulin glargine contains a patient information sheet. Read this sheet carefully and make sure you understand:

- How to prepare the medicine.
- How to inject the medicine.
- How to dispose of syringes, needles, and injection devices.

It is best to use a different place on the body for each injection (e.g., abdomen, thigh, or upper arm). If you have questions about this, contact a member of your health care team.

Since insulin glargine lowers the blood glucose over 24 hours, it should be taken once daily at bedtime

Follow carefully the special meal plan your doctor gave you. This is the most important part of controlling your condition, and is necessary if the medicine is to work properly. Also, exercise regularly and test for sugar in your blood or urine as directed.

- For injection dosage form:
  ○ For type 2 diabetes mellitus:
    ▪ Adults, teenagers, and children 6 years of age or older—The dose is based on your blood sugar and must be determined by your doctor.
    ▪ Children up to 6 years of age—Use and dose must be determined by your doctor.

Storage—Store in the refrigerator. Do not freeze.

Keep out of the reach of children.

Do not keep outdated medicine or medicine no longer needed.

After a cartridge has been inserted into a pen, store the cartridge and pen at room temperature, not in the refrigerator.

Precautions While Using This Medicine

Your doctor will want to check your progress at regular visits, especially during the first few weeks you take this medicine.

It is very important to follow carefully any instructions from your health care team about:

- Alcohol—Drinking alcohol may cause severe low blood sugar. Discuss this with your health care team.
- Other medicines—Do not take other medicines during the time you are taking insulin glargine unless they have been discussed with your doctor. This especially includes nonprescription medicines such as aspirin, and medicines for appetite control, asthma, colds, cough, hay fever, or sinus problems.
- Counseling—Other family members need to learn how to prevent side effects or help with side effects if they occur. Also, patients with diabetes may need special counseling about diabetes medicine dosing changes that might occur because of lifestyle changes, such as changes in exercise and diet. Furthermore, counseling on contraception and pregnancy is needed because of the problems that can occur in patients with diabetes during pregnancy.
- Travel—Keep a recent prescription and your medical history with you. Be prepared for an emergency as you would normally. Make allowances for changing time zones and keep your meal times as close as possible to your usual meal times.

In case of emergency—There may be a time when you need emergency help for a problem caused by your diabetes. You need to be prepared for these emergencies. It is a good idea to:

- Wear a medical identification (ID) bracelet or neck chain at all times. Also, carry an ID card in your wallet or purse that says that you have diabetes and a list of all of your medicines.
- Keep an extra supply of insulin glargine and syringes with needles or injection devices on hand in case high blood sugar occurs.
- Keep some kind of quick-acting sugar handy to treat low blood sugar.
- Have a glucagon kit and a syringe and needle available in case severe low blood sugar occurs. Check and replace any expired kits regularly.

Too much insulin glargine can cause hypoglycemia (low blood sugar). Low blood sugar also can occur if you use insulin glargine with another antidiabetic medicine, delay or miss a meal or snack, exercise more than usual, or drink alcohol. Symptoms of low blood sugar must be treated before they lead to unconsciousness (passing out). Different people may feel different symptoms of low blood sugar. It is important that you learn which symptoms of low blood sugar you usually have so that you can treat it quickly.

Symptoms of low blood sugar include anxiety; behavior change similar to being drunk; blurred vision; cold sweats; confusion; difficulty in thinking; dizziness or lightheadedness; drowsiness; excessive hunger; fast heartbeat; headache; irritability or abnormal behavior; nervousness; nightmares; restless sleep; shakiness; slurred speech; and tingling in the hands, feet, lips, or tongue.

If symptoms of low blood sugar occur, eat glucose tablets or gel, corn syrup, honey, or sugar cubes; or drink fruit juice, nondiet soft drink, or sugar dissolved in water to relieve the symptoms. Also, check your blood for low blood sugar. Get to a doctor or a hospital right away if the symptoms do not improve. Someone should call for emergency help immediately if severe symptoms such as convulsions (seizures) or unconsciousness occur. Have a glucagon kit available, along with a syringe and needle, and know how to use it. Members of your household also should know how to use it.

Hyperglycemia (high blood sugar) may occur if you do not take enough or skip a dose of your antidiabetic medicine, overeat or do not follow your meal plan, have emotional stress or infection, or do not exercise as much as usual.

Symptoms of high blood sugar include blurred vision; drowsiness; dry mouth; flushed, dry skin; fruit-like breath odor; increased urination; ketones in urine; loss of appetite; stomachache, nausea, or vomiting; tiredness; troubled breathing (rapid and deep); unconsciousness; and unusual thirst.

If symptoms of high blood sugar occur, check your blood sugar level and then call your doctor for instructions.

Side Effects of This Medicine

Along with its needed effects, a medicine may cause some unwanted effects. Although not all of these side effects may occur, if they do occur they may need medical attention.

Check with your doctor immediately if any of the following side effects occur:

More common

Convulsions (seizures); unconsciousness

Check with your doctor as soon as possible if any of the following side effects occur:

More common

Low blood sugar, including anxious feeling; behavior change similar to being drunk; blurred vision; cold sweats; confusion; cool, pale skin; difficulty in thinking; dizziness or lightheadedness; drowsiness; excessive hunger; fast heartbeat; headache; nausea; nervousness; nightmares; restless sleep; shakiness; slurred speech; and tingling in the hands, feet, lips, or tongue

Less common or rare

Allergic reaction, including fast pulse, shortness of breath, skin rash or itching over the entire body, sweating, and wheezing

Some side effects may occur that usually do not need medical attention. These side effects may go away during treatment as your body adjusts to the medicine. Also, your health care professional may be able to tell you about ways to prevent or reduce some of these side effects. Check with your health care professional if any of the following side effects continue or are bothersome or if you have any questions about them:

Less common or rare

Bloating or swelling of face, hands, lower legs, and/or feet; depression of skin at injection site; injection site pain; local allergy, including itching, redness, or swelling at injection site; thickening of skin at injection site

Other side effects not listed may also occur in some patients. If you notice any other effects, check with your healthcare professional.

INSULIN GLULISINE (Subcutaneous route) - IN-su-lin gloo-LYE-seen

Commonly used brand name(s)

In the U.S.—
Apidra

Available Dosage Forms:
• Solution

Therapeutic Class: Antidiabetic
Pharmacologic Class: Insulin, Ultra Rapid Acting

Uses For This Medicine

Insulin glulisine is a fast-acting type of human insulin. Insulin is used by people with sugar diabetes to help keep blood sugar levels under control. If you have sugar diabetes, your body cannot make enough or does not use insulin properly. So, you must take additional insulin to regulate your blood sugar and keep your body healthy. This is very important as too much sugar in your blood can be harmful to your health. Since insulin glulisine acts faster than regular human insulin, you normally should use insulin glulisine with a longer-acting insulin.

This medicine is available only with your doctor's prescription.

Before Using This Medicine

In deciding to use a medicine, the risks of taking the medicine must be weighed against the good it will do. This is a decision you and your doctor will make. For this medicine, the following should be considered:

Allergies—Tell your doctor if you have ever had any unusual or allergic reaction to this medicine or any other medicines. Also tell your health care professional if you have any other types of allergies, such as to foods, dyes, preservatives, or animals. For non-prescription products, read the label or package ingredients carefully.

Pediatric—Studies on this medicine have been done only in adult patients, and there is no specific information comparing use of insulin glulisine in children with use in other age groups.

Geriatric—This medicine has been tested in a limited number of patients 65 years of age or older and has not been shown to cause different side effects or problems in older people than it does in younger adults.

Pregnancy—

	Pregnancy Category	Explanation
All Trimesters	C	Animal studies have shown an adverse effect and there are no adequate studies in pregnant women OR no animal studies have been conducted and there are no adequate studies in pregnant women.

Breast Feeding—There are no adequate studies in women for determining infant risk when using this medication during breastfeeding. Weigh the potential benefits against the potential risks before taking this medication while breastfeeding.

Other medicines—

Using this medicine with any of the following medicines is usually not recommended, but may be required in some cases. If both medicines are prescribed together, your doctor may change the dose or how often you use one or both of the medicines.

Alatrofloxacin, Balofloxacin, Ciprofloxacin, Clinafloxacin, Enoxacin, Fleroxacin, Flumequine, Gatifloxacin, Gemifloxacin, Grepafloxacin, Levofloxacin, Lomefloxacin, Moxifloxacin, Norfloxacin, Ofloxacin, Pefloxacin, Prulifloxacin, Rufloxacin, Sparfloxacin, Temafloxacin, Tosufloxacin, Trovafloxacin Mesylate

Interactions with Food/Tobacco/Alcohol—Certain medicines should not be used at or around the time of eating food or eating certain types of food since interactions may occur. Using alcohol or tobacco with certain medicines may also cause interactions to occur. Discuss with your healthcare professional the use of your medicine with food, alcohol, or tobacco.

Other medical problems—The presence of other medical problems may affect the use of this medicine. Make sure you tell your doctor if you have any other medical problems, especially:

- Hypoglycemia (low blood sugar)—If you have low blood sugar and take insulin, your blood sugar may reach dangerously low levels
- Kidney disease or
- Liver disease—Effects of insulin glulisine may be increased or decreased; your doctor may need to change your insulin dose

Proper Use of This Medicine

It is best to use a different place on the body for each injection (e.g., abdomen, thigh, or upper arm). If you have questions about this, contact a member of your health care team.

When used as a mealtime insulin, insulin glulisine should be taken within 15 minutes before the meal or within 20 minutes after starting a meal.

Follow carefully the special meal plan your doctor gave you. This is the most important part of controlling your condition, and is necessary if the medicine is to work properly. Also, exercise regularly and test for sugar in your blood or urine as directed.

The dose of insulin glulisine will be different for different patients. Follow your doctor's orders.

- For injection dosage form:
  - For diabetes mellitus (sugar diabetes):
    - Adults—The dose is based on your blood sugar and must be determined by your doctor.
    - Children—Use and dose must be determined by your doctor.

Dosing—The dose of this medicine will be different for different patients. Follow your doctor's orders or the directions on the label. The following information includes only the average doses of this medicine. If your dose is different, do not change it unless your doctor tells you to do so.

The amount of medicine that you take depends on the strength of the medicine. Also, the number of doses you take each day, the time allowed between doses, and the length of time you take the medicine depend on the medical problem for which you are using the medicine.

Storage—Store in the refrigerator. Do not freeze.

Keep out of the reach of children.

Do not keep outdated medicine or medicine no longer needed.

Ask your healthcare professional how you should dispose of any medicine you do not use.

Precautions While Using This Medicine

Your doctor will want to check your progress at regular visits, especially during the first few weeks you take this medicine.

It is very important to follow carefully any instructions from your health care team about:

- Alcohol—Drinking alcohol may cause severe low blood sugar. Discuss this with your health care team.
- Other medicines—Do not take other medicines during the time you are taking insulin glulisine unless they have been discussed with your doctor. This especially includes nonprescription medicines such as aspirin, and medicines for appetite control, asthma, colds, cough, hay fever, or sinus problems.
- Counseling—Other family members need to learn how to prevent side effects or help with side effects if they occur. Also, patients with diabetes may need special counseling about diabetes medicine dosing changes that might occur because of lifestyle changes, such as changes in exercise and diet. Furthermore, counseling on contraception and pregnancy may be needed because of the problems that can occur in patients with diabetes during pregnancy.
- Travel—Keep a recent prescription and your medical history with you. Be prepared for an emergency as you would normally. Make allowances for changing time zones and keep your meal times as close as possible to your usual meal times.

In case of emergency—There may be a time when you need emergency help for a problem caused by your diabetes. You need to be prepared for these emergencies. It is a good idea to:

- Wear a medical identification (ID) bracelet or neck chain at all times. Also, carry an ID card in your wallet or purse that says that you have diabetes and a list of all of your medicines.

Too much insulin glulisine can cause hypoglycemia (low blood sugar). Symptoms of low blood sugar include anxiety; behavior change similar to being drunk; blurred vision; cold sweats; confusion; depression; difficulty in thinking; dizziness or light-headedness; drowsiness; excessive hunger; fast heartbeat; headache; irritability or abnormal behavior; nervousness; nightmares; restless sleep; shakiness; slurred speech; and tingling in the hands, feet, lips, or tongue.

Low blood sugar also can occur if you use insulin glulisine with another antidiabetic medicine, delay or miss a meal or snack, exercise more than usual, drink alcohol, or cannot eat because of nausea or vomiting or have diarrhea.

If symptoms of low blood sugar occur, eat glucose tablets or gel to relieve the symptoms. Also, check your blood for low blood sugar. Get to a doctor or a hospital right away if the symptoms do not improve. Someone should call for emergency help immediately if severe symptoms such as convulsions (seizures) or unconsciousness occur. Have a glucagon kit available, along with a syringe and needle, and know how to use it. Members of your household also should know how to use it.

Symptoms of high blood sugar include blurred vision; drowsiness; dry mouth; flushed, dry skin; fruit-like breath odor; increased urination; ketones in urine; loss of appetite; stomachache, nausea, or vomiting; tiredness; troubled breathing (rapid and deep); unconsciousness; and unusual thirst.

Hyperglycemia (high blood sugar) may occur if you do not take enough or skip a dose of your antidiabetic medicine, overeat or do not follow your meal plan, have a fever or infection, or do not exercise as much as usual.

If symptoms of high blood sugar occur, check your blood sugar level and then call your doctor for instructions.

Side Effects of This Medicine

Along with its needed effects, a medicine may cause some unwanted effects. Although not all of these side effects may occur, if they do occur they may need medical attention.

Check with your doctor immediately if any of the following side effects occur:

More common
  Convulsions (seizures); unconsciousness

Check with your doctor as soon as possible if any of the following side effects occur:

More common
  Low blood sugar, including anxiety; blurred vision; chills; cold sweats; confusion; cool pale skin; depression; dizziness; fast heartbeat; headache; increased hunger; nervousness; nightmares; shakiness; slurred speech; and unusual tiredness or weakness

Less common
  Accumulation of body fat; bleeding, blistering, burning, coldness, discoloration of skin; decrease in blood pressure; depression of the skin at place of injection; feeling of pressure; hives; infection, inflammation, itching, lumps, numbness, pain, rash, redness, scarring, soreness, stinging, swelling, tenderness, tingling, ulceration, or warmth at site of injection; rapid pulse; shortness of breath; skin rash or itching over the entire body; sweating; wheezing

Other side effects not listed may also occur in some patients. If you notice any other effects, check with your healthcare professional.

INSULIN LISPRO, RECOMBINANT
(Subcutaneous route) - IN-su-lin LYE-sproe, re-KOM-bi-nant

Commonly used brand name(s)

In the U.S.—
  Humalog
  Lispro-PFC

Available Dosage Forms:
  • Suspension

Therapeutic Class: Antidiabetic
Pharmacologic Class: Insulin, Ultra Rapid Acting

Uses For This Medicine

Insulin lispro is a type of insulin. Insulin is one of many hormones that help the body turn the food we eat into energy. This is done by using the glucose (sugar) in the blood as quick energy. Also, insulin helps us store energy that we can use later. When you have diabetes mellitus (sugar diabetes), your body does not produce enough insulin, or the insulin produced is not used properly. This causes you to have too much sugar in your blood. Like other types of insulin, insulin lispro is used to keep your blood sugar level close to normal. Insulin lispro works faster than other types of insulin; therefore, you may have to use insulin lispro in combination with another type of insulin or with a type of oral diabetes medicine called a sulfonylurea to keep your blood sugar under control.

This medicine is available only with your doctor's prescription.

Before Using This Medicine

In deciding to use a medicine, the risks of taking the medicine must be weighed against the good it will do. This is a decision you and your doctor will make. For this medicine, the following should be considered:

Allergies—Tell your doctor if you have ever had any unusual or allergic reaction to this medicine or any other medicines. Also tell your health care professional if you have any other types of allergies, such as to foods, dyes, preservatives, or animals. For non-prescription products, read the label or package ingredients carefully.

Pediatric—This medicine has been tested in a limited number of children 3 years of age or older. In effective doses, the medicine has not been shown to cause different side effects or problems than it does in adults.

Geriatric—This medicine has been tested in a limited number of patients 65 years of age or older and has not been shown to cause different side effects or problems in older people than it does in younger adults.

Pregnancy—

	Pregnancy Category	Explanation
All Trimesters	B	Animal studies have revealed no evidence of harm to the fetus, however, there are no adequate studies in pregnant women OR animal studies have shown an adverse effect, but adequate studies in pregnant women have failed to demonstrate a risk to the fetus.

Breast Feeding—There are no adequate studies in women for determining infant risk when using this medication during breastfeeding. Weigh the potential benefits against the potential risks before taking this medication while breastfeeding.

Other medicines—

Using this medicine with any of the following medicines is usually not recommended, but may be required in some cases. If both medicines are prescribed together, your doctor may change the dose or how often you use one or both of the medicines.

Alatrofloxacin, Balofloxacin, Ciprofloxacin, Clinafloxacin, Enoxacin, Fleroxacin, Flumequine, Gatifloxacin, Gemifloxacin, Grepafloxacin, Levofloxacin, Lomefloxacin, Moxifloxacin,

Norfloxacin, Ofloxacin, Pefloxacin, Prulifloxacin, Rufloxacin, Sparfloxacin, Temafloxacin, Tosufloxacin, Trovafloxacin Mesylate

Interactions with Food/Tobacco/Alcohol—Certain medicines should not be used at or around the time of eating food or eating certain types of food since interactions may occur. Using alcohol or tobacco with certain medicines may also cause interactions to occur. The following interactions have been selected on the basis of their potential significance and are not necessarily all-inclusive.

Using this medicine with any of the following may cause an increased risk of certain side effects but may be unavoidable in some cases. If used together, your doctor may change the dose or how often you use this medicine or give you special instructions about the use of food, alcohol, or tobacco.

Ethanol

Other medical problems—The presence of other medical problems may affect the use of this medicine. Make sure you tell your doctor if you have any other medical problems, especially:

- Diarrhea or
- Underactive adrenal gland or
- Underactive pituitary gland or
- Vomiting—These conditions lower blood sugar and may lower the amount of insulin or insulin lispro you need
- Fever or
- Infection—These conditions increase blood sugar and may increase the amount of insulin or insulin lispro you need
- Kidney disease or
- Liver disease—Effects of insulin lispro may be increased or decreased; this may change the amount of insulin lispro you need

Proper Use of This Medicine

Each package of insulin lispro contains a patient information sheet. Read this sheet carefully and make sure you understand:

- How to prepare the medicine.
- How to inject the medicine.
- How to use disposable insulin delivery device.
- How to use external insulin pump. How and when to change the infusion set, cartridge adapter, and insulin in the external insulin pump reservoir. How and when to change the insulin lispro 3–mL cartridge.
- How to dispose of syringes, needles, and injection devices.

It is best to use a different place on the body for each injection (e.g., abdomen, thigh, or upper arm). If you have questions about this, contact a member of your health care team.

When used as a mealtime insulin, insulin lispro should be taken within 15 minutes before the meal or immediately after the meal.

When used in an insulin pump: Carefully read and follow the external insulin pump instructions. This insulin should not be mixed with any other insulin or diluted when used in an insulin pump. If you do not understand how you are to use the insulin pump, contact your health care professional.

Follow carefully the special meal plan your doctor gave you. This is the most important part of controlling your condition, and is necessary if the medicine is to work properly. Also, exercise regularly and test for sugar in your blood or urine as directed.

Dosing—The dose of this medicine will be different for different patients. Follow your doctor's orders or the directions on the label. The following information includes only the average doses of this medicine. If your dose is different, do not change it unless your doctor tells you to do so.

The amount of medicine that you take depends on the strength of the medicine. Also, the number of doses you take each day, the time allowed between doses, and the length of time you take the medicine depend on the medical problem for which you are using the medicine.

- For injection dosage form:
  - For diabetes mellitus (sugar diabetes):
    - Adults and teenagers—The dose is based on your blood sugar and must be determined by your doctor.
    - Children—Use and dose must be determined by your doctor.

Storage—Store in the refrigerator. Do not freeze.

Keep out of the reach of children.

Do not keep outdated medicine or medicine no longer needed.

After a cartridge has been inserted into a pen, store the cartridge and pen at room temperature, not in the refrigerator.

Precautions While Using This Medicine

Your doctor will want to check your progress at regular visits, especially during the first few weeks you take this medicine.

It is very important to follow carefully any instructions from your health care team about:

- Alcohol—Drinking alcohol may cause severe low blood sugar. Discuss this with your health care team.
- Other medicines—Do not take other medicines during the time you are taking insulin lispro unless they have been discussed with your doctor. This especially includes nonprescription medicines such as aspirin, and medicines for appetite control, asthma, colds, cough, hay fever, or sinus problems.
- Counseling—Other family members need to learn how to prevent side effects or help with side effects if they occur. Also, patients with diabetes may need special counseling about diabetes medicine dosing changes that might occur because of lifestyle changes, such as changes in exercise and diet. Furthermore, counseling on contraception and pregnancy may be needed because of the problems that can occur in patients with diabetes during pregnancy.
- Travel—Keep a recent prescription and your medical history with you. Be prepared for an emergency as you would normally. Make allowances for changing time zones and keep your meal times as close as possible to your usual meal times.

In case of emergency—There may be a time when you need emergency help for a problem caused by your diabetes. You need to be prepared for these emergencies. It is a good idea to:

- Wear a medical identification (ID) bracelet or neck chain at all times. Also, carry an ID card in your wallet or purse that says that you have diabetes and a list of all of your medicines.
- Keep an extra supply of insulin lispro and syringes with needles or injection devices on hand in case high blood sugar occurs.

- Keep some kind of quick-acting sugar handy to treat low blood sugar.
- Have a glucagon kit and a syringe and needle available in case severe low blood sugar occurs. Check and replace any expired kits regularly.

Too much insulin lispro can cause hypoglycemia (low blood sugar). Low blood sugar also can occur if you use insulin lispro with another antidiabetic medicine, delay or miss a meal or snack, exercise more than usual, drink alcohol, or cannot eat because of nausea or vomiting or have diarrhea. Symptoms of low blood sugar must be treated before they lead to unconsciousness (passing out). Different people may feel different symptoms of low blood sugar. It is important that you learn which symptoms of low blood sugar you usually have so that you can treat it quickly.

Symptoms of low blood sugar include anxiety; behavior change similar to being drunk; blurred vision; cold sweats; confusion; depression; difficulty in thinking; dizziness or lightheadedness; drowsiness; excessive hunger; fast heartbeat; headache; irritability or abnormal behavior; nervousness; nightmares; restless sleep; shakiness; slurred speech; and tingling in the hands, feet, lips, or tongue.

If symptoms of low blood sugar occur, eat glucose tablets or gel, corn syrup, honey, or sugar cubes; or drink fruit juice, nondiet soft drink, or sugar dissolved in water to relieve the symptoms. Also, check your blood for low blood sugar. Get to a doctor or a hospital right away if the symptoms do not improve. Someone should call for emergency help immediately if severe symptoms such as convulsions (seizures) or unconsciousness occur. Have a glucagon kit available, along with a syringe and needle, and know how to use it. Members of your household also should know how to use it.

Hyperglycemia (high blood sugar) may occur if you do not take enough or skip a dose of your antidiabetic medicine, overeat or do not follow your meal plan, have a fever or infection, or do not exercise as much as usual.

Symptoms of high blood sugar include blurred vision; drowsiness; dry mouth; flushed, dry skin; fruit-like breath odor; increased urination; ketones in urine; loss of appetite; stomachache, nausea, or vomiting; tiredness; troubled breathing (rapid and deep); unconsciousness; and unusual thirst.

If symptoms of high blood sugar occur, check your blood sugar level and then call your doctor for instructions.

Side Effects of This Medicine

Along with its needed effects, a medicine may cause some unwanted effects. Although not all of these side effects may occur, if they do occur they may need medical attention.

Check with your doctor immediately if any of the following side effects occur:

> *More common*
> Convulsions (seizures); unconsciousness

Check with your doctor as soon as possible if any of the following side effects occur:

> *More common*
> Low blood sugar, including anxious feeling; behavior change similar to being drunk; blurred vision; cold sweats; confusion; depression; difficulty in thinking; dizziness or lightheadedness; drowsiness; excessive hunger; fast heartbeat; headache; irritability or abnormal behavior; nervousness; nightmares; restless

sleep; shakiness; slurred speech; and tingling in the hands, feet, lips, or tongue

> *Less common or rare*
> Depression of the skin at place of injection; dryness of mouth; fast or weak pulse; increased thirst; irregular heartbeat; itching, redness, or swelling at place of injection; mood or mental changes; muscle cramps or pain; nausea or vomiting; shortness of breath; skin rash or itching over the whole body; sweating; thickening of the skin at place of injection; unusual tiredness or weakness; wheezing

Other side effects not listed may also occur in some patients. If you notice any other effects, check with your healthcare professional.

INTERFERON ALFACON-1
(Subcutaneous route) - in-ter-FEER-on AL-fa-kon-1

Black Box Warning

Alpha interferons, including interferon alfacon-1, cause or aggravate fatal or life-threatening neuropsychiatric, autoimmune, ischemic, and infectious disorders.

Patients should be monitored closely with periodic clinical and laboratory evaluations. Patients with persistently severe or worsening symptoms of these conditions should be withdrawn from therapy. In many but not all cases, these disorders resolve after stopping interferon alfacon-1 therapy.

Commonly used brand name(s)

In the U.S.—
 Infergen

Available Dosage Forms:
- Solution

Therapeutic Class: Immunological Agent
Pharmacologic Class: Interferon, Alfa (class)

Uses For This Medicine

Interferon is a substance naturally produced in cells in the body to help fight infections. There also are synthetic (manmade) versions of this substance, such as interferon alfacon-1. Interferon alfacon-1 is used to treat hepatitis C, a type of infection of the liver, in adults who also have other types of liver disease.

This medicine is available only with your doctor's prescription.

Before Using This Medicine

In deciding to use a medicine, the risks of taking the medicine must be weighed against the good it will do. This is a decision you and your doctor will make. For this medicine, the following should be considered:

Allergies—Tell your doctor if you have ever had any unusual or allergic reaction to this medicine or any other medicines. Also tell your health care professional if you have any other types of allergies, such as to foods, dyes, preservatives,

or animals. For non-prescription products, read the label or package ingredients carefully.

Pediatric—Studies on this medicine have been done only in adult patients, and there is no specific information comparing use of interferon alfacon-1 in children with use in other age groups. However, use in children less than 18 years of age is not recommended.

Geriatric—Many medicines have not been studied specifically in older people. Therefore, it may not be known whether they work exactly the same way they do in younger adults or if they cause different side effects or problems in older people. There is no specific information comparing use of interferon alfacon-1 in the elderly with use in other age groups.

Pregnancy—

	Pregnancy Category	Explanation
All Trimesters	C	Animal studies have shown an adverse effect and there are no adequate studies in pregnant women OR no animal studies have been conducted and there are no adequate studies in pregnant women.

Breast Feeding—There are no adequate studies in women for determining infant risk when using this medication during breastfeeding. Weigh the potential benefits against the potential risks before taking this medication while breastfeeding.

Other medicines—

Using this medicine with any of the following medicines is not recommended. Your doctor may decide not to treat you with this medication or change some of the other medicines you take.

Rotavirus Vaccine, Live

Interactions with Food/Tobacco/Alcohol—Certain medicines should not be used at or around the time of eating food or eating certain types of food since interactions may occur. Using alcohol or tobacco with certain medicines may also cause interactions to occur. Discuss with your healthcare professional the use of your medicine with food, alcohol, or tobacco.

Other medical problems—The presence of other medical problems may affect the use of this medicine. Make sure you tell your doctor if you have any other medical problems, especially:

- Decreased bone marrow production or other blood problems or
- Heart disease or
- Liver disease or
- Mental problems (or history of) or
- Thyroid disease—Interferon alfacon-1 may make these conditions worse
- Problems with an overactive immune system—Interferon alfacon-1 may make the immune system even more active

Proper Use of This Medicine

If you are injecting this medicine yourself, use it exactly as directed by your doctor. Do not use more or less of it, and do not use it more often than your doctor ordered. The exact amount of medicine you need has been carefully worked out. Using too much will increase the risk of side effects, while using too little may not improve your condition.

To help clear up your infection completely, interferon alfacon-1 must be used for the full time of treatment, even if you begin to feel better after a few days or weeks. It is also very important that you receive your injection at the same time for each day of treatment.

Each package of interferon alfacon-1 contains a patient instruction sheet. Read this sheet carefully and make sure you understand:

- How to prepare the injection.
- Proper use of disposable syringes.
- How to give the injection.
- How long the injection is stable.

If you have any questions about any of this, check with your health care professional.

Dosing—The dose of this medicine will be different for different patients. Follow your doctor's orders or the directions on the label. The following information includes only the average doses of this medicine. If your dose is different, do not change it unless your doctor tells you to do so.

The amount of medicine that you take depends on the strength of the medicine. Also, the number of doses you take each day, the time allowed between doses, and the length of time you take the medicine depend on the medical problem for which you are using the medicine.

- For injection dosage form:
  - For hepatitis C:
    - Adults—9 micrograms per dose, injected under the skin, three times per week at intervals of at least forty-eight hours, for twenty-four weeks.
    - Children—Use is not recommended.

Missed dose—If you miss a dose of this medicine, skip the missed dose and go back to your regular dosing schedule. Do not double doses.

Call your doctor or pharmacist for instructions.

Storage—Store in the refrigerator. Do not freeze.

Keep out of the reach of children.

Do not keep outdated medicine or medicine no longer needed.

Ask your healthcare professional how you should dispose of any medicine you do not use.

Precautions While Using This Medicine

It is very important that your doctor check your progress at regular visits to make sure that this medicine is working properly and to check for unwanted effects. It is also important that you tell your doctor if you notice any changes in your ability to see clearly.

Do not change to another brand of alpha interferon without checking with your physician. Different kinds of alpha interferon have different doses. If you refill your medicine and it looks different, check with your pharmacist.

This medicine commonly causes a flu-like reaction, with aching muscles, fever and chills, and headache. To prevent problems from your temperature going too high, your doctor may ask you to take acetaminophen before each dose of interferon alfacon-1. You may also need to take acetaminophen after a dose of interferon alfacon-1 to bring your temperature down. Follow your doctor's instructions carefully about taking your temperature, and how much and when to take the acetaminophen.

In some patients, this medicine may cause mental depression. Tell your doctor right away:

- if you or anyone else notices unusual changes in your mood.
- if you start having early-morning sleeplessness or unusually vivid dreams or nightmares.

Interferon alfacon-1 can lower the number of white blood cells in your blood temporarily, increasing the chance of getting an infection. It can also lower the number of platelets, which are necessary for proper blood clotting. If this occurs, there are certain precautions you can take, especially when your blood count is low, to reduce the risk of infection or bleeding:

- If you can, avoid people with infections. Check with your doctor immediately if you think you are getting an infection or if you get a fever or chills, cough or hoarseness, lower back or side pain, or painful or difficult urination.
- Check with your doctor immediately if you notice any unusual bleeding or bruising; black, tarry stools; blood in urine or stools; or pinpoint red spots on your skin.
- Be careful when using a regular toothbrush, dental floss, or toothpick. Your medical doctor, dentist, or nurse may recommend other ways to clean your teeth and gums. Check with your medical doctor before having any dental work done.
- Do not touch your eyes or the inside of your nose unless you have just washed your hands and have not touched anything else in the meantime.
- Be careful not to cut yourself when you are using sharp objects, such as a safety razor or fingernail or toenail cutters.
- Avoid contact sports or other situations where bruising or injury could occur.

Interferon alfacon-1 may cause some people to become unusually tired or dizzy, or less alert than they are normally. Make sure you know how you react to this medicine before you drive, use machines, or do anything else that could be dangerous if you are dizzy or if you are not alert.

Side Effects of This Medicine

Along with its needed effects, a medicine may cause some unwanted effects. Although not all of these side effects may occur, if they do occur they may need medical attention.

Check with your doctor as soon as possible if any of the following side effects occur:

More common
    Anxiety; black, tarry stools; blood in urine or stools; confusion; cough or hoarseness; fever or chills; lower back or side pain; mental depression; nervousness; painful or difficult urination; pinpoint red spots on skin; redness at place of injection; trouble in sleeping; trouble in thinking or concentrating; unusual bleeding or bruising

Less common
    Chest pain; irregular heartbeat; numbness or tingling of fingers, toes, or face

Rare
    Blurred vision or loss of vision; skin rash, hives, or itching

Some side effects may occur that usually do not need medical attention. These side effects may go away during treatment as your body adjusts to the medicine. Also, your health care professional may be able to tell you about ways to prevent or reduce some of these side effects. Check with your health care professional if any of the following side effects continue or are bothersome or if you have any questions about them:

More common
    Abdominal pain; aching muscles; decreased appetite; diarrhea; dizziness; general feeling of discomfort or illness; headache; heartburn or indigestion; nausea or vomiting; pain in back or joints; sore throat; unusual tiredness or weakness

Interferon alfacon-1 may cause a temporary loss of some hair. After treatment has ended, normal hair growth should return.

Other side effects not listed may also occur in some patients. If you notice any other effects, check with your healthcare professional.

INTERFERON BETA-1A
(Intramuscular route, Subcutaneous route, Injection route) - in-ter-FEER-on BAY-ta-1a

Commonly used brand name(s)

In the U.S.—
    Avonex
    Rebif

Available Dosage Forms:

- Solution
- Kit

Therapeutic Class: Immunological Agent
Pharmacologic Class: Interferon, Beta (class)

Uses For This Medicine

Interferon beta-1a is used to treat the relapsing forms of multiple sclerosis (MS). This medicine will not cure MS, but it may slow some disabling effects and decrease the number of relapses of the disease.

Interferon beta-1a is also used to treat genital warts.

This medicine is available only with your doctor's prescription.

Before Using This Medicine

In deciding to use a medicine, the risks of taking the medicine must be weighed against the good it will do. This is a decision you and your doctor will make. For this medicine, the following should be considered:

Allergies—Tell your doctor if you have ever had any unusual or allergic reaction to this medicine or any other medicines. Also tell your health care professional if you have any other types of allergies, such as to foods, dyes, preservatives, or animals. For non-prescription products, read the label or package ingredients carefully.

Pediatric—Studies on this medicine have been done only in adult patients, and there is no specific information comparing use of interferon beta-1a in children with use in other age groups.

Geriatric—Many medicines have not been studied specifically in older people. Therefore, it may not be known whether they work exactly the same way they do in younger adults. Although there is no specific information comparing use of interferon beta-1a in the elderly with use in other age groups, this medicine is not expected to cause different side effects or problems in older people than it does in younger adults.

Pregnancy—

	Pregnancy Category	Explanation
All Trimesters	C	Animal studies have shown an adverse effect and there are no adequate studies in pregnant women OR no animal studies have been conducted and there are no adequate studies in pregnant women.

Breast Feeding—Studies in women suggest that this medication poses minimal risk to the infant when used during breastfeeding.

Other medicines—

Using this medicine with any of the following medicines is not recommended. Your doctor may decide not to treat you with this medication or change some of the other medicines you take.

Rotavirus Vaccine, Live

Interactions with Food/Tobacco/Alcohol—Certain medicines should not be used at or around the time of eating food or eating certain types of food since interactions may occur. Using alcohol or tobacco with certain medicines may also cause interactions to occur. Discuss with your healthcare professional the use of your medicine with food, alcohol, or tobacco.

Other medical problems—The presence of other medical problems may affect the use of this medicine. Make sure you tell your doctor if you have any other medical problems, especially:

- Alcohol abuse or
- Higher concentration of a liver enzyme called SGPT
- Liver disease, active or in the past—This medicine should be used cautiously. You should tell your doctor if you have any of these conditions. If you start having symptoms of liver problems such as jaundice (yellow skin and eyes), tell your doctor right away; your medicine may need to be stopped.
- Heart disease—Some side effects of this medicine may be harmful to patients with serious heart problems
- Mental depression or thoughts of suicide or
- Psychiatric disorders or
- Other mood disorders—This medicine may make the condition worse
- Seizure disorder—The risk of seizures may be increased

Proper Use of This Medicine

If you are injecting this medicine yourself, use it exactly as directed by your doctor.

Special patient directions come with interferon beta-1a injection. Read the directions carefully before using the medicine. Make sure you understand:

- How to prepare the injection.
- Proper use of disposable syringes.
- How to give the injection.
- How long the injection is stable.

If you have any questions about any of this, check with your health care professional.

Dosing—The dose of this medicine will be different for different patients. Follow your doctor's orders or the directions on the label. The following information includes only the average doses of this medicine. If your dose is different, do not change it unless your doctor tells you to do so.

The amount of medicine that you take depends on the strength of the medicine. Also, the number of doses you take each day, the time allowed between doses, and the length of time you take the medicine depend on the medical problem for which you are using the medicine.

- For injection dosage form:
  - For multiple sclerosis (MS):
    - Adults
      — For Avonex
        - 30 micrograms (mcg) once a week, injected into a muscle.
      — For Rebif
        - 22 micrograms (mcg) or 44 mcg 3 times a week, injected under the skin; your doctor may start you at a lower dose at first.
    - Children—Use and dose must be determined by the physician.
  - For genital warts:
    - Adults
      — For Rebif
        - 3.67 micrograms (mcg) per lesion 3 times a week for 3 weeks

Missed dose—If you miss a dose of this medicine, take it as soon as possible. However, if it is almost time for your next dose, skip the missed dose and go back to your regular dosing schedule. Do not double doses.

The next injection should be scheduled at least 48 hours later.

Storage—Keep out of the reach of children.

Do not keep outdated medicine or medicine no longer needed.

Store prefilled syringes or vials of interferon beta-1a in the refrigerator. Do not freeze. If refrigeration is not available, the vials that have not been mixed with diluent may be kept for up to 30 days at room temperature, as long as the temperature does not go above 77 °F.

Precautions While Using This Medicine

It is very important that your doctor check your progress at regular visits to make sure that this medicine is working properly and to check for unwanted effects.

Importance of caretaker and/or patient informing doctor of any signs or symptoms of depression or other mental or mood disturbances.

Check with your doctor right away if you experience dark urine, persistent loss of appetite, yellow eyes or skin, influenza (flu)-like symptoms, right upper quadrant tenderness, headache, stomach pain, continuing vomiting, general feeling of tiredness or weakness, or light-colored stools. These could be symptoms of serious liver problems.

You should avoid alcohol while you are taking this medicine. It can cause serious liver problems.

This medicine commonly causes a flu-like reaction, with aching muscles, chills, fever, headache, joint pain, and nausea. Your doctor may ask you to take acetaminophen to help control these effects. Follow your doctor's instructions carefully about how much and when to take acetaminophen.

Side Effects of This Medicine

Along with its needed effects, a medicine may cause some unwanted effects. Although not all of these side effects may occur, if they do occur they may need medical attention.

Check with your doctor as soon as possible if any of the following side effects occur:

More common
Black, tarry stools; chest pain; chills; cough; diarrhea; fever; flu-like symptoms including headache, joint pain, muscle aches, and nausea; pain; painful or difficult urination; shortness of breath; sores, ulcers, or white spots on lips or in mouth; swollen glands; unusual bleeding or bruising; unusual tiredness or weakness

Less common
Abdominal pain; chest pain; clumsiness or unsteadiness; convulsions (seizures); coughing; decreased hearing; difficulty in swallowing; dizziness; fainting; flushing; hives or itching; mood changes, especially with thoughts of suicide; muscle spasms; pain or discharge from the vagina; pelvic discomfort, aching, or heaviness; redness, swelling, or tenderness at place of injection; runny or stuffy nose; skin lesions; sneezing; sore throat; speech problems; swelling of face, lips, or eyelids; troubled breathing; wheezing

Rare
Earache; general feeling of discomfort or illness; loss of appetite; painful blisters on trunk of body— also known as shingles; painful cold sores or blisters on lips, nose, eyes, or genitals

Incidence not known
Bleeding gums; blood in urine or stools; bloody nose; chest discomfort; confusion; constipation; continuing vomiting; convulsions; dark urine; decreased urine output; depressed mood; dilated neck veins; dry skin and hair; extreme fatigue; faintness; fast, irregular, or pounding heartbeat; feeling cold; general tiredness and weakness; hair loss; heavier menstrual periods; high fever; hoarseness or husky voice; irregular breathing; light-colored stools; loss of bladder control; mental depression; mood or other mental changes; muscle cramps and stiffness; muscle spasm or jerking of all extremities; nausea and vomiting; nervousness; pale skin; persistent anorexia; pinpoint red spots on skin; pruritus; puffiness or swelling of the eyelids, or around the eyes, face, lips, or tongue; redness, blistering, peeling, or loosening of the skin; right upper quadrant tenderness; sensitivity to heat; shortness of breath; skin rash; slowed heartbeat; stomach pain; sudden loss of consciousness; sweating; swelling of face, fingers, feet, or lower legs; swelling of the mouth or throat; tightness in chest; tightness in throat; upper right abdominal pain; vesicular rash; weight gain; weight loss; yellow eyes and skin

Some side effects may occur that usually do not need medical attention. These side effects may go away during treatment as your body adjusts to the medicine. Also, your health care professional may be able to tell you about ways to prevent or reduce some of these side effects. Check with your health care professional if any of the following side effects continue or are bothersome or if you have any questions about them:

More common
Heartburn; indigestion; sour stomach

Less common
Hair loss; trouble in sleeping

Other side effects not listed may also occur in some patients. If you notice any other effects, check with your healthcare professional.

INTERFERON BETA-1B
(Subcutaneous route) - in-ter-FEER-on BAY-ta-1b

Commonly used brand name(s)
In the U.S.—
Betaseron

Available Dosage Forms:
• Powder for Solution

Therapeutic Class: Immunological Agent
Pharmacologic Class: Interferon, Beta (class)

Uses For This Medicine

Interferon beta-1b is used to treat the relapsing-remitting form of multiple sclerosis (MS). This medicine will not cure MS, but may decrease the number of relapses of the disease.

This medicine is available only with your doctor's prescription.

Before Using This Medicine

In deciding to use a medicine, the risks of taking the medicine must be weighed against the good it will do. This is a decision you and your doctor will make. For this medicine, the following should be considered:

Allergies—Tell your doctor if you have ever had any unusual or allergic reaction to this medicine or any other medicines. Also tell your health care professional if you have any other types of allergies, such as to foods, dyes, preservatives, or animals. For non-prescription products, read the label or package ingredients carefully.

Pediatric—Studies on this medicine have been done only in adult patients, and there is no specific information com-

paring use of interferon beta-1b in children with use in other age groups.

Geriatric—Many medicines have not been studied specifically in older people. Therefore, it may not be known whether they work exactly the same way they do in younger adults. Although there is no specific information comparing use of interferon beta-1b in the elderly with use in other age groups, this medicine is not expected to cause different side effects or problems in older people than it does in younger adults.

Pregnancy—

	Pregnancy Category	Explanation
All Trimesters	C	Animal studies have shown an adverse effect and there are no adequate studies in pregnant women OR no animal studies have been conducted and there are no adequate studies in pregnant women.

Breast Feeding—There are no adequate studies in women for determining infant risk when using this medication during breastfeeding. Weigh the potential benefits against the potential risks before taking this medication while breastfeeding.

Other medicines—

Using this medicine with any of the following medicines is not recommended. Your doctor may decide not to treat you with this medication or change some of the other medicines you take.

Rotavirus Vaccine, Live

Interactions with Food/Tobacco/Alcohol—Certain medicines should not be used at or around the time of eating food or eating certain types of food since interactions may occur. Using alcohol or tobacco with certain medicines may also cause interactions to occur. Discuss with your healthcare professional the use of your medicine with food, alcohol, or tobacco.

Other medical problems—The presence of other medical problems may affect the use of this medicine. Make sure you tell your doctor if you have any other medical problems, especially:

- Mental depression or thoughts of suicide—This medicine may make the condition worse

---

Proper Use of This Medicine

Use this medicine exactly as directed by your doctor in order to help your condition as much as possible.

Taking interferon beta-1b at bedtime may help lessen the flu-like symptoms.

Special patient directions come with interferon beta-1b. Read the directions carefully before using this medicine.

It is important to follow several steps to prepare your interferon beta-1b injection correctly. Before injecting the medication, you need to:

- Collect the items you will need before you begin.
- Wash your hands thoroughly with soap and water. Do not touch your hair or skin afterwards.
- Make sure the needle guards are on the needles tightly.

- Remove the plastic cap from the interferon beta-1b and the diluent vial. Use an alcohol wipe to clean the tops of the vials. Move the alcohol wipe in one direction and use one wipe per vial. Leave the alcohol wipe on top of each vial until you are ready to use it.

In order to keep everything sterile, it is important that you do not touch the tops of the vials or the needles. If you do touch a stopper, clean it with a fresh alcohol wipe. If you touch a needle, or if the needle touches any surface, throw away the entire syringe and start over with a new syringe. Also, use only the diluent (sodium chloride 0.54%) provided with the interferon beta-1b to dilute the medicine for injection.

To mix the contents of one vial:

- Resting your hands on a stable surface, remove the needle cover on the 3–mL syringe by pulling the cover straight off the needle. Do not touch the needle itself.
- Pull back the plunger of the syringe back to the 1.2–mL mark.
- Holding the vial of diluent for interferon beta-1b on a stable surface, slowly insert the needle straight through the stopper into the top of the vial.
- Push in the plunger all the way to gently inject 1.2 mL of air into the vial. Leave the needle in the vial of diluent.
- Turn the vial upside down using one hand and make sure the tip of the needle is covered by solution. With your other hand, slowly pull back the plunger of the syringe to withdraw 1.2 mL of diluent into the syringe.
- Keeping the vial upside down, gently tap the syringe until any air bubbles that formed rise to the top of the barrel of the syringe.
- Carefully push in the plunger to eject only the air through the needle. Remove the needle/syringe from the vial of diluent.
- Holding the interferon beta-1b vial on a stable surface, slowly insert the needle of the syringe (containing 1.2 mL of diluent) all the way through the stopper of the vial.
- Push the plunger down slowly, directing the needle toward the side of the vial to allow the diluent to run down the inside wall. Injecting the diluent directly onto the white cake of medicine will cause excess foaming.
- Remove the needle/syringe from the vial of interferon beta-1b.
- Roll the vial between your hands gently to completely dissolve the white cake of medicine.
- Check the solution to make sure it is clear. If you can see anything solid in the solution or if the solution is discolored, discard it and start again.

To prepare the injection syringe:

- Remove the needle guard from the 1–mL syringe and pull back the plunger to the 1–mL mark.
- Insert the needle of the 1–mL syringe through the stopper of the vial of interferon beta-1b solution.
- Gently push the plunger all the way down to inject air into the vial.
- Turn the vial of interferon beta-1b solution upside down, keeping the needle tip in the liquid.
- Pull back the plunger of the syringe to withdraw 1 mL of liquid into the syringe.

- Hold the syringe with the needle pointing upward. Tap the syringe gently until any air bubbles that formed rise to the top of the barrel of the syringe.
- Carefully push in the plunger to eject only the air through the needle.
- Remove the needle/syringe from the vial. Replace the needle guard on the syringe.
- Throw away the unused portion of the solution remaining in the vial.

The injection should be administered immediately after mixing. If the injection is delayed, refrigerate the solution and inject it within 3 hours.

To give yourself the injection:

Before you self-inject the interferon beta-1b dose, decide where you will inject yourself. There are eight areas for injection, and each area has an upper, a middle, and a lower injection site. To help prevent injection site reactions, select a site in an area different from the area where you last injected yourself. You should not choose the same area for two injections in a row. Keeping a record of your injections will help make sure you rotate areas.

Do not self-inject into any area in which you feel lumps, bumps, firm knots, or pain. Do not use any area in which the skin is discolored, depressed, red, scabbed, tender, or has broken open. Talk to your doctor or other health care professional about these or any other unusual conditions that you find. If you experience a break in the skin or drainage of fluid from the injection site, contact your doctor before continuing injections with interferon beta-1b.

- Clean the injection site with a fresh alcohol wipe, and let it air dry.
- Pick up the 1–mL syringe you already filled with interferon beta-1b. Hold the syringe as you would a pencil or dart. Remove the needle guard from the needle, but do not touch the needle itself.
- Gently pinch the skin together around the site, to lift it up a bit.
- Resting your wrist on the skin near the site, stick the needle straight into the skin at a 90° angle with a quick, firm motion.
- Using a slow steady push, inject the medicine by pushing the plunger all the way in until the syringe is empty.
- Hold a swab on the injection site. Remove the needle by pulling straight out.
- Gently massage the injection site with a dry cotton ball or gauze.

To dispose of needles and syringes:

Needles, syringes, and vials should be used for only one injection. Place all used syringes, needles, and vials in a syringe disposal unit or in a hard-walled plastic container, such as a liquid laundry detergent container. Keep the cover closed tightly, and keep the container out of the reach of children. When the container is full, check with your physician or nurse about proper disposal, as laws vary from state to state.

Dosing—The dose of this medicine will be different for different patients. Follow your doctor's orders or the directions on the label. The following information includes only the average doses of this medicine. If your dose is different, do not change it unless your doctor tells you to do so.

The amount of medicine that you take depends on the strength of the medicine. Also, the number of doses you take each day, the time allowed between doses, and the length of time you take the medicine depend on the medical problem for which you are using the medicine.

- For injection dosage form:
  - For multiple sclerosis (MS):
    - Adults—0.25 milligrams (mg) every other day.
    - Children—Use and dose must be determined by your doctor.

Missed dose—If you miss a dose of this medicine, take it as soon as possible. However, if it is almost time for your next dose, skip the missed dose and go back to your regular dosing schedule. Do not double doses.

The next injection should be scheduled about 48 hours later.

Storage—Store in the refrigerator. Do not freeze.

Keep out of the reach of children.

Do not keep outdated medicine or medicine no longer needed.

If refrigeration is not available, vials may be kept for up to 7 days at room temperature, as long as the temperature does not go above 86 °F.

Side Effects of This Medicine

Along with its needed effects, a medicine may cause some unwanted effects. Although not all of these side effects may occur, if they do occur they may need medical attention.

Check with your doctor as soon as possible if any of the following side effects occur:

More common
Abdominal pain; break in the skin at place of injection, with blue-black discoloration, swelling, or drainage of fluid; flu-like symptoms including chills, fever, generalized feeling of discomfort or illness, increased sweating, and muscle pain; headache or migraine; hives, itching, or swelling at place of injection; hypertension (high blood pressure); irregular or pounding heartbeat; pain at place of injection; redness or feeling of heat at place of injection; stuffy nose

Less common
Breast pain; bloody or cloudy urine; changes in vision; cold hands and feet; difficult, burning, or painful urination; fast or racing heartbeat; frequent urge to urinate; pain; pelvic pain; swollen glands; troubled breathing; unusual weight gain

Rare
Abnormal growth in breast; benign lumps in breast; bleeding problems; bloating or swelling; changes in menstrual periods; confusion; convulsions (seizures); cyst (abnormal growth filled with fluid or semisolid material); decreased sexual ability in males; dry, puffy skin; feeling cold; hyperactivity; increased muscle tone; increased urge to urinate; loss of memory; mental depression with thoughts of suicide; problems in speaking; red, itching, or swollen eyes; swelling of front part of neck; unusual weight loss

Some side effects may occur that usually do not need medical attention. These side effects may go away during treatment as your body adjusts to the medicine. Also, your health care professional may be able to tell you about ways to prevent or reduce some of these side effects. Check with your health care professional if any of the following side effects continue or are bothersome or if you have any questions about them:

More common

Constipation; diarrhea; dizziness; laryngitis (loss of voice); menstrual pain or other changes; unusual tiredness or weakness

Less common

Anxiety; drowsiness; hair loss; nervousness; vomiting

Other side effects not listed may also occur in some patients. If you notice any other effects, check with your healthcare professional.

INTERFERON GAMMA

(Subcutaneous route, Injection route) - inter-FEER-on GAM-ma

Commonly used brand name(s)
In the U.S.—
    Actimmune

Available Dosage Forms:
  • Solution

Therapeutic Class: Immunological Agent
Pharmacologic Class: Interferon, Gamma (class)

Uses For This Medicine

Gamma interferon is a synthetic (man-made) version of a substance naturally produced by cells in the body to help fight infections and tumors. Gamma interferon is used to treat chronic granulomatous disease and osteopetrosis.

Gamma interferon is available only with your doctor's prescription.

Before Using This Medicine

In deciding to use a medicine, the risks of taking the medicine must be weighed against the good it will do. This is a decision you and your doctor will make. For this medicine, the following should be considered:

Allergies—Tell your doctor if you have ever had any unusual or allergic reaction to this medicine or any other medicines. Also tell your health care professional if you have any other types of allergies, such as to foods, dyes, preservatives, or animals. For non-prescription products, read the label or package ingredients carefully.

Pediatric—Studies on this medicine have been done mostly in children and it is not expected to cause different side effects or problems than it does in adults.

Geriatric—Many medicines have not been studied specifically in older people. Therefore, it may not be known whether they work exactly the same way they do in younger adults or if they cause different side effects or problems in older people. There is no specific information comparing use of gamma interferon in the elderly with use in other age groups.

Pregnancy—

	Pregnancy Category	Explanation
All Trimesters	C	Animal studies have shown an adverse effect and there are no adequate studies in pregnant women OR no animal studies have been conducted and there are no adequate studies in pregnant women.

Breast Feeding—There are no adequate studies in women for determining infant risk when using this medication during breastfeeding. Weigh the potential benefits against the potential risks before taking this medication while breastfeeding.

Other medicines—

Using this medicine with any of the following medicines is not recommended. Your doctor may decide not to treat you with this medication or change some of the other medicines you take.

Rotavirus Vaccine, Live

Interactions with Food/Tobacco/Alcohol—Certain medicines should not be used at or around the time of eating food or eating certain types of food since interactions may occur. Using alcohol or tobacco with certain medicines may also cause interactions to occur. Discuss with your healthcare professional the use of your medicine with food, alcohol, or tobacco.

Other medical problems—The presence of other medical problems may affect the use of this medicine. Make sure you tell your doctor if you have any other medical problems, especially:

  • Convulsions (seizures) or
  • Mental problems (or history of)—Risk of problems affecting the central nervous system may be increased
  • Heart disease or
  • Multiple sclerosis or
  • Systemic lupus erythematosus—May be worsened by gamma interferon

Proper Use of This Medicine

If you are injecting this medicine yourself, use it exactly as directed by your doctor. Do not use more or less of it, and do not use it more often than your doctor ordered. The exact amount of medicine you need has been carefully worked out. Using too much will increase the risk of side effects, while using too little may not improve your condition.

Each package of gamma interferon contains a patient instruction sheet. Read this sheet carefully and make sure you understand:

  • How to prepare the injection.
  • Proper use of disposable syringes.
  • How to give the injection.
  • How long the injection is stable.

If you have any questions about any of this, check with your health care professional.

While you are using gamma interferon, your doctor may want you to drink extra fluids. This will help prevent low blood pressure due to loss of too much water.

Gamma interferon often causes flu-like symptoms, which can be severe. This effect is less likely to cause problems if you inject your gamma interferon at bedtime.

Dosing—The dose of this medicine will be different for different patients. Follow your doctor's orders or the directions on the label. The following information includes only the average doses of this medicine. If your dose is different, do not change it unless your doctor tells you to do so.

The amount of medicine that you take depends on the strength of the medicine. Also, the number of doses you take each day, the time allowed between doses, and the length of time you take the medicine depend on the medical problem for which you are using the medicine.

Missed dose—If you miss a dose of this medicine, skip the missed dose and go back to your regular dosing schedule. Do not double doses.

Call your doctor or pharmacist for instructions.

Storage—Store in the refrigerator. Do not freeze.

Keep out of the reach of children.

Do not keep outdated medicine or medicine no longer needed.

Discard any unopened vials that are left at room temperature for more than 12 hours.

Precautions While Using This Medicine

It is very important that your doctor check your progress at regular visits to make sure that this medicine is working properly and to check for unwanted effects.

This medicine commonly causes a flu-like reaction, with aching muscles, fever and chills, and headache. To prevent problems from your temperature going too high, your doctor may ask you to take acetaminophen before each dose of gamma interferon. You may also need to take it after a dose to bring your temperature down. Follow your doctor's instructions carefully about taking your temperature, and how much and when to take the acetaminophen.

Side Effects of This Medicine

Along with its needed effects, a medicine may cause some unwanted effects. Although not all of these side effects may occur, if they do occur they may need medical attention.

Check with your doctor as soon as possible if any of the following side effects occur:
Rare
    Black, tarry stools; blood in urine or stools; confusion; cough or hoarseness; loss of balance control; lower back or side pain; mask-like face; painful or difficult urination; pinpoint red spots on skin; shuffling walk; stiffness of arms or legs; trembling and shaking of hands and fingers; trouble in speaking or swallowing; trouble in thinking or concentrating; trouble in walking; unusual bleeding or bruising

Some side effects may occur that usually do not need medical attention. These side effects may go away during treatment as your body adjusts to the medicine. Also, your health care professional may be able to tell you about ways to prevent or reduce some of these side effects. Check with your health care professional if any of the following side effects

continue or are bothersome or if you have any questions about them:
More common
    Aching muscles; diarrhea; fever and chills; general feeling of discomfort or illness; headache; nausea or vomiting; skin rash; unusual tiredness
Less common
    Back pain; dizziness; joint pain; loss of appetite; weight loss

Other side effects not listed may also occur in some patients. If you notice any other effects, check with your healthcare professional.

INTERFERON, ALFA (Injection route, Intravenous route, Subcutaneous route)

Commonly used brand name(s)
In the U.S.—

Alferon N	PEG-Intron
Infergen	Peg Intron RP
Intron A	Roferon-A
Pegasys	

In Canada—
    Unitron Peg

Available Dosage Forms:
- Solution
- Kit
- Powder for Solution
- Injectable

Uses For This Medicine

Interferons are substances naturally produced by cells in the body to help fight infections and tumors. They may also be synthetic (man-made) versions of these substances. Alpha interferons are used to treat hairy cell leukemia, malignant melanoma, and AIDS-related Kaposi's sarcoma. They are also used to treat laryngeal papillomatosis (growths in the respiratory tract) in children, genital warts, and some kinds of hepatitis.

Alpha interferons may also be used for other conditions as determined by your doctor.

Alpha interferons are available only with your doctor's prescription.

Once a medicine has been approved for marketing for a certain use, experience may show that it is also useful for other medical problems. Although these uses are not included in product labeling, alpha interferons are used in certain patients with the following medical conditions:
- Bladder cancer
- Carcinoid tumors
- Chronic myelocytic leukemia
- Kidney cancer
- Laryngeal papillomatosis (growths on larynx)
- Lymphomas, non-Hodgkin's
- Multiple myeloma
- Mycosis fungoides
- Ovarian cancer
- Polycythemia vera (a type of cancer of the blood)

- Skin cancer
- Thrombocytosis

Before Receiving This Medicine

Allergies—Tell your doctor if you have ever had any unusual or allergic reaction to medicines in this group or any other medicines. Also tell your health care professional if you have any other types of allergies, such as to foods dyes, preservatives, or animals. For non-prescription products, read the label or package ingredients carefully.

Pediatric—There is no specific information comparing use of alpha interferon for cancer or genital warts in children with use in other age groups.

Alpha interferons may cause changes in the menstrual cycle. Discuss this possible effect with your doctor.

Geriatric—Some side effects of alpha interferons (chest pain, irregular heartbeat, unusual tiredness, confusion, mental depression, trouble in thinking or concentrating) may be more likely to occur in the elderly, who are usually more sensitive to the effects of alpha interferons.

Pregnancy—Alpha interferons have not been shown to cause birth defects or other problems in humans. However, in monkeys given 20 to 500 times the human dose of recombinant interferon alfa-2a or given 90 to 180 times the usual dose of recombinant interferon alfa-2b, there was an increase in death of the fetuses.

Breast Feeding—It is not known whether alpha interferons pass into breast milk. However, because this medicine may cause serious side effects, breast-feeding may not be recommended while you are receiving it. Discuss with your doctor whether or not you should breast-feed while you are receiving alpha interferon.

Other medicines—

Using medicines in this class with any of the following medicines is not recommended. Your doctor may decide not to treat you with a medication in this class or change some of the other medicines you take.

Rotavirus Vaccine, Live

Using medicines in this class with any of the following medicines is usually not recommended, but may be required in some cases. If both medicines are prescribed together, your doctor may change the dose or how often you use one or both of the medicines.

Autumn Crocus, Bacillus of Calmette and Guerin Vaccine, Live, Captopril, Colchicine, Enalaprilat, Enalapril Maleate, Lamivudine, Measles Virus Vaccine, Live, Mumps Virus Vaccine, Live, Poliovirus Vaccine, Live, Rubella Virus Vaccine, Live, Smallpox Vaccine, Theophylline, Typhoid Vaccine, Varicella Virus Vaccine, Yellow Fever Vaccine, Zidovudine

Using this medicine with any of the following may cause an increased risk of certain side effects but using both medicines may be the best treatment for you. If both medicines are prescribed together, your doctor may change the dose or how often you use one or both of the medicines.

Aldesleukin, Ribavirin, Theophylline

Interactions with Food/Tobacco/Alcohol—Certain medicines should not be used at or around the time of eating food or eating certain types of food since interactions may occur. Using alcohol or tobacco with certain medicines may also cause interactions to occur. Discuss with your healthcare professional the use of your medicine with food, alcohol, or tobacco.

Other medical problems—The presence of other medical problems may affect the use of medicines in this class. Make sure you tell your doctor if you have any other medical problems, especially:

- Bleeding problems—May be worsened by recombinant interferon alfa-2b
- Chickenpox (including recent exposure) or
- Herpes zoster (shingles)—Risk of severe disease affecting other parts of the body
- Convulsions (seizures) or
- Mental problems (or history of)—Risk of problems affecting the central nervous system may be increased
- Eye problems—May be worsened by interferon alphas; your doctor will want you to have periodic eye exams while you are receiving this medicine.
- Diabetes mellitus (sugar diabetes) or
- Heart attack (recent) or
- Heart disease or
- Infections or
- Kidney disease or
- Lack of blood supply to any part of the body or
- Liver disease or
- Lung disease—May be worsened by alpha interferons
- Problems with overactive immune system—Alpha interferons make the immune system even more active
- Thyroid disease—Recombinant interferon alfa-2b can cause thyroid problems when it is used to treat hepatitis

Proper Use of This Medicine

If you are injecting this medicine yourself, use it exactly as directed by your doctor. Do not use more or less of it, and do not use it more often than your doctor ordered. The exact amount of medicine you need has been carefully worked out. Using too much will increase the risk of side effects, while using too little may not improve your condition.

Each package of alpha interferon contains a patient instruction sheet. Read this sheet carefully and make sure you understand:

- How to prepare the injection.
- Proper use of disposable syringes.
- How to give the injection.
- How long the injection is stable.

If you have any questions about any of this, check with your health care professional.

While you are using alpha interferon, your doctor may want you to drink extra fluids. This will help prevent low blood pressure due to loss of too much water.

Alpha interferons often cause unusual tiredness, which can be severe. This effect is less likely to cause problems if you inject your interferon at bedtime.

Dosing—The dose medicines in this class will be different for different patients. Follow your doctor's orders or the directions on the label. The following information includes only the average doses of these medicines. If your dose is different, do not change it unless your doctor tells you to do so.

The amount of medicine that you take depends on the strength of the medicine. Also, the number of doses you take

each day, the time allowed between doses, and the length of time you take the medicine depend on the medical problem for which you are using the medicine.

Missed dose—If you miss a dose of this medicine, take it as soon as possible. However, if it is almost time for your next dose, skip the missed dose and go back to your regular dosing schedule. Do not double doses.

Storage—Keep out of the reach of children.

Store in the refrigerator. Do not freeze.

Do not keep outdated medicine or medicine no longer needed.

Ask your healthcare professional how you should dispose of any medicine you do not use.

Precautions After Receiving This Medicine

It is very important that your doctor check your progress at regular visits to make sure that this medicine is working properly and to check for unwanted effects.

Do not change to another brand of alpha interferon without checking with your physician. Different kinds of alpha interferon have different doses. If you refill your medicine and it looks different, check with your pharmacist.

This medicine will add to the effects of alcohol and other CNS depressants (medicines that slow down the nervous system, possibly causing drowsiness). Some examples of CNS depressants are antihistamines or medicine for hay fever, other allergies, or colds; sedatives, tranquilizers, or sleeping medicine; prescription pain medicine or narcotics; barbiturates; medicine for seizures; muscle relaxants; or anesthetics, including some dental anesthetics. Check with your doctor before drinking alcohol or taking any of the above while you are using this medicine.

Alpha interferon may cause some people to become unusually tired or dizzy, or less alert than they are normally. Make sure you know how you react to this medicine before you drive, use machines, or do anything else that could be dangerous if you are dizzy or if you are not alert.

This medicine commonly causes a flu-like reaction, with aching muscles, fever and chills, and headache. To prevent problems from your temperature going too high, your doctor may ask you to take acetaminophen (e.g., Tylenol) before each dose of interferon. You may also need to take it after a dose to bring your temperature down. Follow your doctor's instructions carefully about taking your temperature, and how much and when to take the acetaminophen.

Alpha interferon can lower the number of white blood cells in your blood temporarily, increasing the chance of getting an infection. It can also lower the number of platelets, which are necessary for proper blood clotting. If this occurs, there are certain precautions you can take, especially when your blood count is low, to reduce the risk of infection or bleeding:

- If you can, avoid being close to people with infections. Check with your doctor immediately if you think you are getting an infection or if you get a fever or chills, cough or hoarseness, lower back or side pain, or have painful or difficult urination.
- Check with your doctor immediately if you notice any unusual bleeding or bruising; black, tarry stools; blood in urine or stools; or pinpoint red spots on your skin.

- Be careful when using a regular toothbrush, dental floss, or toothpick. Your medical doctor, dentist, or nurse may recommend other ways to clean your teeth and gums. Check with your medical doctor before having any dental work done.
- Do not touch your eyes or the inside of your nose unless you have just washed your hands and have not touched anything else in the meantime.
- Be careful not to cut yourself when you are using sharp objects such as a safety razor or fingernail or toenail cutters.
- Avoid contact sports or other situations where bruising or injury could occur.

If you experience vision problems while receiving an interferon alpha, you should contact your doctor for an eye examination.

Side Effects of This Medicine

Along with its needed effects, a medicine may cause some unwanted effects. Although not all of these side effects may occur, if they do occur they may need medical attention.

Because this medicine is used for many different conditions and in many different doses, the actual frequency of side effects may vary. In general, side effects are less common with low doses than with high doses. Also, when alpha interferon is used for genital warts, very little of it gets into the rest of the body, so side effects are generally less common than in other conditions.

Check with your doctor as soon as possible if any of the following side effects occur:
Less common
Confusion; mental depression; nervousness; numbness or tingling of fingers, toes, and face; trouble in sleeping; trouble in thinking or concentrating

Rare
Black, tarry stools; blood in urine or stools; chest pain; cough or hoarseness accompanied by fever or chills; fever or chills (beginning after 3 weeks of treatment); headache; irregular heartbeat; lower back or side pain accompanied by fever or chills; muscle pain; numbness or tingling in the legs; pain, swelling or redness in the joints; painful or difficult urination accompanied by fever or chills; pinpoint red spots on skin; trouble speaking; unusual bleeding or bruising

Some side effects may occur that usually do not need medical attention. These side effects may go away during treatment as your body adjusts to the medicine. Also, your health care professional may be able to tell you about ways to prevent or reduce some of these side effects. Check with your health care professional if any of the following side effects continue or are bothersome or if you have any questions about them:
More common
Aching muscles; change in taste or metallic taste; fever and chills (should lessen after the first 1 or 2 weeks of treatment); general feeling of discomfort or illness; headache; loss of appetite; nausea and vomiting; skin rash; unusual tiredness

Less common or rare
Back pain; blurred vision; diarrhea; dizziness; dry skin or itching; dryness of mouth; increased sweating; joint

pain; leg cramps; sores in mouth and on lips; weight loss

Alpha interferon may cause a temporary loss of some hair. After treatment has ended, normal hair growth should return.

Other side effects not listed may also occur in some patients. If you notice any other effects, check with your healthcare professional.

IPECAC (Oral route) - IP-e-kak

Uses For This Medicine

Ipecac is used in the emergency treatment of certain kinds of poisoning. It is used to cause vomiting of the poison.

Only the syrup form of ipecac should be used. A bottle of ipecac labeled as being Ipecac Fluidextract or Ipecac Tincture should not be used. These dosage forms are too strong and may cause serious side effects or death. Only ipecac syrup contains the proper strength of ipecac for treating poisonings.

Ordinarily, this medicine should not be used if strychnine, corrosives such as alkalies (lye) and strong acids, or petroleum distillates such as kerosene, gasoline, coal oil, fuel oil, paint thinner, or cleaning fluid have been swallowed. It may cause seizures, additional injury to the throat, or pneumonia.

Ipecac should not be used to cause vomiting as a means of losing weight. If used regularly for this purpose, serious heart problems or even death may occur.

This medicine in amounts of more than 1 ounce is available only with your doctor's prescription. It is available in ½- and 1-ounce bottles without a prescription. However, before using ipecac syrup, call a poison control center, your doctor, or an emergency room for advice.

Before Using This Medicine

In deciding to use a medicine, the risks of taking the medicine must be weighed against the good it will do. This is a decision you and your doctor will make. For this medicine, the following should be considered:

Allergies—Tell your doctor if you have ever had any unusual or allergic reaction to this medicine or any other medicines. Also tell your health care professional if you have any other types of allergies, such as to foods, dyes, preservatives, or animals. For non-prescription products, read the label or package ingredients carefully.

Pediatric—Infants and very young children are at a greater risk of choking with their own vomit (or getting vomit in their lungs). Therefore, it is especially important to call a poison control center, your doctor, or an emergency room for instructions before giving ipecac to an infant or young child.

Geriatric—This medicine has been tested and has not been shown to cause different side effects or problems in older people than it does in younger adults.

Breast Feeding—There are no adequate studies in women for determining infant risk when using this medication during breastfeeding. Weigh the potential benefits against the potential risks before taking this medication while breastfeeding.

Other medicines—Although certain medicines should not be used together at all, in other cases two different medicines may be used together even if an interaction might occur. In these cases, your doctor may want to change the dose, or other precautions may be necessary. Tell your healthcare professional if you are taking any other prescription or nonprescription (over-the-counter [OTC]) medicine.

Interactions with Food/Tobacco/Alcohol—Certain medicines should not be used at or around the time of eating food or eating certain types of food since interactions may occur. Using alcohol or tobacco with certain medicines may also cause interactions to occur. Discuss with your healthcare professional the use of your medicine with food, alcohol, or tobacco.

Other medical problems—The presence of other medical problems may affect the use of this medicine. Make sure you tell your doctor if you have any other medical problems, especially:

- Heart disease—There is an increased risk of heart problems, such as unusually fast heartbeat, if the ipecac is not vomited

Proper Use of This Medicine

It is very important that you take this medicine only as directed. Do not take more of it and do not take it more often than recommended on the label, unless otherwise directed. When too much ipecac is used, it can cause damage to the heart and other muscles, and may even cause death.

Do not give this medicine to unconscious or very drowsy persons, since the vomited material may enter the lungs and cause pneumonia.

To help this medicine cause vomiting of the poison, adults should drink 1 full glass (8 ounces) of water and children should drink ½ to 1 full glass (4 to 8 ounces) of water immediately after taking this medicine. Water may be given first in the case of a small or scared child.

Do not take this medicine with milk, milk products, or with carbonated beverages. Milk or milk products may prevent this medicine from working properly, and carbonated beverages may cause swelling of the stomach.

If vomiting does not occur within 20 to 30 minutes after you have taken the first dose of this medicine, take a second dose. If vomiting does not occur after you have taken the second dose, you must immediately see your doctor or go to an emergency room.

If you have been told to take both this medicine and activated charcoal to treat the poisoning, do not take the activated charcoal until after you have taken this medicine to cause vomiting and vomiting has stopped. This takes usually about 30 minutes.

Dosing—The dose of this medicine will be different for different patients. Follow your doctor's orders or the directions on the label. The following information includes only the average doses of this medicine. If your dose is different, do not change it unless your doctor tells you to do so.

The amount of medicine that you take depends on the strength of the medicine. Also, the number of doses you take each day, the time allowed between doses, and the length of time you take the medicine depend on the medical problem for which you are using the medicine.

- For oral dosage form (syrup):
  - For treatment of poisoning:
    - Adults and teenagers—The usual dose is 15 to 30 milliliters (mL) (1 to 2 tablespoonfuls), followed immediately by one full glass (240 mL) of water. The dose may be repeated one time after twenty to thirty minutes if vomiting does not occur.
    - Children 1 to 12 years of age—The usual dose is 15 mL (1 tablespoonful). One-half to one full glass (120 to 240 mL) of water should be taken right before or right after the dose. The dose may be repeated one time after twenty to thirty minutes if vomiting does not occur.
    - Children 6 months to 1 year of age—The usual dose is 5 to 10 mL (1 to 2 teaspoonfuls). One-half to one full glass (120 to 240 mL) of water should be taken right before or right after the dose. The dose may be repeated one time after twenty to thirty minutes if vomiting does not occur.
    - Children up to 6 months of age—Ipecac must be given only under the direction of your doctor.

Storage—Store the medicine in a closed container at room temperature, away from heat, moisture, and direct light. Keep from freezing.

Keep out of the reach of children.

Do not keep outdated medicine or medicine no longer needed.

Do not keep a bottle of ipecac that has been opened. Ipecac may evaporate over a period of time. It is best to replace it with a new one.

Side Effects of This Medicine

Along with its needed effects, a medicine may cause some unwanted effects. Although not all of these side effects may occur, if they do occur they may need medical attention.

Check with your doctor as soon as possible if any of the following side effects occur:

Symptoms of overdose (may also occur if ipecac is taken regularly)

Diarrhea; fast or irregular heartbeat; nausea or vomiting (continuing more than 30 minutes); stomach cramps or pain; troubled breathing; unusual tiredness or weakness; weakness, aching, and stiffness of muscles, especially those of the neck, arms, and legs

Other side effects not listed may also occur in some patients. If you notice any other effects, check with your healthcare professional.

IPRATROPIUM (Inhalation, oral/ nebulization route) - i-pra-TROE-pee-um

Commonly used brand name(s)
In the U.S.—
Atrovent

Available Dosage Forms:
- Solution
- Aerosol Powder

Therapeutic Class: Bronchodilator
Pharmacologic Class: Anticholinergic

Uses For This Medicine

Ipratropium is a bronchodilator (medicine that opens up narrowed breathing passages). It is taken by inhalation to help control the symptoms of lung diseases, such as asthma, chronic bronchitis, and emphysema. Ipratropium helps decrease coughing, wheezing, shortness of breath, and troubled breathing by increasing the flow of air into the lungs.

When ipratropium inhalation is used to treat acute, severe attacks of asthma, bronchitis, or emphysema, it is used only in combination with other bronchodilators.

Ipratropium is available only with your doctor's prescription.

Before Using This Medicine

In deciding to use a medicine, the risks of taking the medicine must be weighed against the good it will do. This is a decision you and your doctor will make. For this medicine, the following should be considered:

Allergies—Tell your doctor if you have ever had any unusual or allergic reaction to this medicine or any other medicines. Also tell your health care professional if you have any other types of allergies, such as to foods, dyes, preservatives, or animals. For non-prescription products, read the label or package ingredients carefully.

Pediatric—This medicine has been tested in children and, in effective doses, has not been shown to cause different side effects or problems in children than it does in adults.

Geriatric—Ipratropium inhalation has been tested in patients 65 years of age or older. This medicine is not expected to cause different side effects or problems in older people than it does in younger adults.

Pregnancy—

	Pregnancy Category	Explanation
All Trimesters	B	Animal studies have revealed no evidence of harm to the fetus, however, there are no adequate studies in pregnant women OR animal studies have shown an adverse effect, but adequate studies in pregnant women have failed to demonstrate a risk to the fetus.

Breast Feeding—There are no adequate studies in women for determining infant risk when using this medication during breastfeeding. Weigh the potential benefits against the potential risks before taking this medication while breastfeeding.

Other medicines—

Using this medicine with any of the following medicines may cause an increased risk of certain side effects, but using both drugs may be the best treatment for you. If both medicines are prescribed together, your doctor may change the dose or how often you use one or both of the medicines.

Betel Nut

Interactions with Food/Tobacco/Alcohol—Certain medicines should not be used at or around the time of eating food or eating certain types of food since interactions may occur. Using alcohol or tobacco with certain medicines may also cause interactions to occur. Discuss with your healthcare

professional the use of your medicine with food, alcohol, or tobacco.

Other medical problems—The presence of other medical problems may affect the use of this medicine. Make sure you tell your doctor if you have any other medical problems, especially:

The presence of other medical problems may affect the use of ipratropium. Make sure you tell your doctor if you have any other medical problem, especially:

- Difficult urination or
- Enlarged prostate or
- Urinary bladder blockage—Ipratropium may make the condition worse.
- Glaucoma—Ipratropium may make the condition worse if it gets into the eyes

Proper Use of This Medicine

Ipratropium is used to help control the symptoms of lung diseases, such as chronic bronchitis, emphysema, and asthma. However, for treatment of bronchospasm or asthma attacks that have already started, ipratropium is used only in combination with other bronchodilators.

It is very important that you use ipratropium only as directed. Do not use more of it and do not use it more often than your doctor ordered. To do so may increase the chance of side effects.

Keep the spray or solution away from the eyes because this medicine may cause irritation or blurred vision. Closing your eyes while you are inhaling ipratropium may keep the medicine from getting into your eyes. Rinsing your eyes with cool water may help if any medicine does get into your eyes.

Ipratropium usually comes with patient directions. Read them carefully before using this medicine.

If you are taking this medicine every day to help control your symptoms, it must be taken at regularly spaced times as ordered by your doctor.

Contact your doctor before using other inhaled medicines.

For patients using *ipratropium inhalation aerosol:*

- If you do not understand the directions or you are not sure how to use the inhaler, ask your health care professional to show you how to use it. Also, ask your health care professional to check regularly how you use the inhaler to make sure you are using it properly.
- There are two formulas of the inhaled aerosol. One contains chlorofluorocarbons and the other contains HFA as the propellant. The taste and inhalation of these may seem different, but the safety and effectiveness of both formulas are similar.
- The ipratropium aerosol canister provides about 200 inhalations, depending on the size of the canister your doctor ordered. You should try to keep a record of the number of inhalations you use so you will know when the canister is almost empty. This canister, unlike some other aerosol canisters, cannot be floated in water to test its fullness.
- When you use the inhaler for the first time, or if you have not used it for a while, the inhaler may not give the right amount of medicine with the first puff. Therefore, before using the inhaler, test or prime it.

- To test or prime the inhaler:
  ◦ Insert the canister firmly into the clean mouthpiece according to the manufacturer's instructions. Check to make sure it is placed properly into the mouthpiece.
  ◦ Take the cap off the mouthpiece and shake the inhaler three or four times.
  ◦ Hold the inhaler away from you at arm's length and press the top of the canister, spraying the medicine once into the air. The inhaler will now be ready to give the right amount of medicine when you use it.
- To use the inhaler:
  ◦ Using your thumb and one or two fingers, hold the inhaler upright, with the mouthpiece end down and pointing toward you.
  ◦ Take the cap off the mouthpiece. Check the mouthpiece to make sure it is clear. Then, gently shake the inhaler three or four times.
  ◦ Breathe out slowly to the end of a normal breath.
  ◦ Use the inhalation method recommended by your doctor:
    ▪ Open-mouth method—Place the mouthpiece about 1 or 2 inches (2 fingerwidths) in front of your widely opened mouth. Make sure the inhaler is aimed into your mouth so the spray does not hit the roof of your mouth or your tongue.
    ▪ Closed-mouth method—Place the mouthpiece in your mouth between your teeth and over your tongue with your lips closed tightly around it. Make sure your tongue or teeth are not blocking the opening.
  ◦ Start to breathe in slowly and deeply through your mouth. At the same time, press the top of the canister once to get one puff of medicine. Continue to breathe in slowly for 5 to 10 seconds. Count the seconds while breathing in. It is important to press the canister and breathe in slowly at the same time so the medicine gets into your lungs. This step may be difficult at first. If you are using the closed-mouth method and you see a fine mist coming from your mouth or nose, the inhaler is not being used correctly.
  ◦ Hold your breath as long as you can up to 10 seconds. This gives the medicine time to settle into your airways and lungs.
  ◦ Take the mouthpiece away from your mouth and breathe out slowly.
  ◦ If your doctor has told you to inhale more than one puff of medicine at each dose, gently shake the inhaler again, and take the second puff following exactly the same steps you used for the first puff. Press the canister one time for each puff of medicine.
  ◦ When you are finished, wipe off the mouthpiece and replace the cap.
- Your doctor may want you to use a spacer device or holding chamber with the inhaler. A spacer helps get the medicine into the lungs and reduces the amount of medicine that stays in your mouth and throat.
  ◦ To use a spacer device with the inhaler:
    ▪ Attach the spacer to the inhaler according to the manufacturer's directions. There are different types of spacers available, but the method of breathing remains the same with most spacers.
    ▪ Gently shake the inhaler and spacer three or four times.

- Hold the mouthpiece of the spacer away from your mouth and breathe out slowly to the end of a normal breath.
- Place the mouthpiece into your mouth between your teeth and over your tongue with your lips closed around it.
- Press the top of the canister once to release one puff of medicine into the spacer. Within 1 or 2 seconds, start to breathe in slowly and deeply through your mouth for 5 to 10 seconds. Count the seconds while inhaling. Do not breathe in through your nose.
- Hold your breath as long as you can up to 10 seconds.
- Take the mouthpiece away from your mouth and breathe out slowly.
- If your doctor has told you to take more than one puff of medicine at each dose, gently shake the inhaler and spacer again and take the next puff, following exactly the same steps you used for the first puff. Do not put more than one puff of medicine into the spacer at a time.
- When you are finished, remove the spacer device from the inhaler and replace the cap.
- Clean the inhaler, mouthpiece, and spacer at least twice a week.
  - To clean the inhaler:
    - Remove the canister from the inhaler and set aside.
    - Wash the mouthpiece, cap, and the spacer with warm, soapy water. Then, rinse well with warm, running water.
    - Shake off the excess water and let the inhaler parts air dry completely before putting the inhaler back together.

For patients using ipratropium inhalation solution:

- Use this medicine only in a power-operated nebulizer with an adequate flow rate and equipped with a face mask or mouthpiece. Your doctor will tell you which nebulizer to use. Make sure you understand exactly how to use it. If you have any questions about this, check with your doctor.
- To prepare the medicine for use in the nebulizer:
  - If you are using the single-dose vial of ipratropium:
    - Break away one vial by pulling it firmly from the strip.
    - Twist off the top to open the vial. Use the contents of the vial as soon as possible after opening it.
    - Squeeze the contents of the vial into the cup of the nebulizer. If your doctor has told you to use less than a full vial of solution, use a syringe to withdraw the correct amount of solution from the vial and add it to the nebulizer cup. Be sure to throw away the syringe after one use.
  - If you are using the multiple-dose bottle of ipratropium:
    - Use a syringe to withdraw the correct amount of solution from the bottle and add it to the nebulizer cup. Do not use the same syringe more than once.
- If you have been told to dilute the ipratropium inhalation solution in the nebulizer cup with the sodium chloride solution provided, use a new syringe to add the sodium chloride solution to the cup as directed by your health care professional.

- If your doctor told you to use another inhalation solution with the ipratropium inhalation solution, add that solution also to the nebulizer cup.
- To use the nebulizer:
  - Gently shake the nebulizer cup to mix the solutions well.
  - Connect the nebulizer tube to the air or oxygen pump and begin the treatment. Adjust the mask, if you are using one, to prevent mist from getting into your eyes.
  - Use the method of breathing your doctor told you to use to take the treatment. One way is to breathe slowly and deeply through the mask or mouthpiece. Another way is to breathe in and out normally with the mouthpiece in your mouth, taking a deep breath every 1 or 2 minutes. Continue to breathe in the medicine as instructed until no more mist is formed in the nebulizer cup or until you hear a sputtering (spitting or popping) sound.
  - When you have finished, replace the caps on the solutions. Store the bottles of solution in the refrigerator until the next treatment.
  - Clean the nebulizer according to the manufacturer's directions.

Dosing—The dose of this medicine will be different for different patients. Follow your doctor's orders or the directions on the label. The following information includes only the average doses of this medicine. If your dose is different, do not change it unless your doctor tells you to do so.

The amount of medicine that you take depends on the strength of the medicine. Also, the number of doses you take each day, the time allowed between doses, and the length of time you take the medicine depend on the medical problem for which you are using the medicine.

- For symptoms of chronic obstructive pulmonary disease, such as chronic bronchitis or emphysema:
  - For inhalation aerosol dosage form:
    - Adults and children 12 years of age and older—2 to 4 inhalations (puffs) three or four times a day, at regularly spaced times. Some patients may need up to 6 to 8 puffs three times a day.
  - For inhalation solution dosage form:
    - Adults and children 12 years of age and older—250 to 500 mcg used in a nebulizer three or four times a day, every six to eight hours.
- For symptoms of asthma:
  - For inhalation aerosol dosage form:
    - Adults and children 12 years of age and older—1 to 4 inhalations (puffs) four times a day, at regularly spaced times, as needed.
    - Children up to 12 years of age—1 or 2 inhalations (puffs) three or four times a day, at regularly spaced times, as needed.
  - For inhalation solution dosage form:
    - Adults and children 12 years of age and older—500 mcg used in a nebulizer three or four times a day, every six to eight hours, as needed.
    - Children 5 to 12 years of age—125 to 250 mcg used in a nebulizer three or four times a day, every four to six hours as needed.
    - Children up to 5 years of age—Use and dose must be determined by your doctor.

Missed dose—If you miss a dose of this medicine, take it as soon as possible. However, if it is almost time for your next

dose, skip the missed dose and go back to your regular dosing schedule. Do not double doses.

Storage—Store in the refrigerator. Do not freeze.

Store the canister at room temperature, away from heat and direct light. Do not freeze. Do not keep this medicine inside a car where it could be exposed to extreme heat or cold. Do not poke holes in the canister or throw it into a fire, even if the canister is empty.

Keep out of the reach of children.

Do not keep outdated medicine or medicine no longer needed.

Precautions While Using This Medicine

Check with your doctor at once if your symptoms do not improve within 30 minutes after using a dose of this medicine or if your condition gets worse.

If symptoms of an allergic reaction such as abdominal or stomach pain, diarrhea, fever, joint or muscle pain, nausea, numbness or tingling of face, hands, or feet, redness and soreness of eyes, skin rash, shortness of breath, sores in mouth, swelling of feet or lower legs, or vomiting occur, contact your doctor right away.

For patients using ipratropium inhalation solution:

- If you are also using cromolyn inhalation solution, do not mix that solution with the ipratropium inhalation solution containing the preservative benzalkonium chloride for use in a nebulizer. To do so will cause the solution to become cloudy. However, if your condition requires you to use cromolyn inhalation solution with ipratropium inhalation solution, it may be mixed with ipratropium inhalation solution that is preservative-free.

Side Effects of This Medicine

Along with its needed effects, a medicine may cause some unwanted effects. Although not all of these side effects may occur, if they do occur they may need medical attention.

Check with your doctor as soon as possible if any of the following side effects occur:

Rare

Constipation (continuing) or lower abdominal pain or bloating; fainting; fast, pounding, or irregular heartbeat or pulse; increased wheezing, tightness in chest, or difficulty in breathing; palpitations; severe eye pain; skin rash or hives; swelling of face, lips, or eyelids

Some side effects may occur that usually do not need medical attention. These side effects may go away during treatment as your body adjusts to the medicine. Also, your health care professional may be able to tell you about ways to prevent or reduce some of these side effects. Check with your health care professional if any of the following side effects continue or are bothersome or if you have any questions about them:

More common

Cough; dryness of mouth; unpleasant taste

Less common or rare

Acid or sour stomach; belching; bladder pain; bloody or cloudy urine; blurred vision or other changes in vision; body aches or pain; burning eyes; chills; cough producing mucus; diarrhea; difficult, burning, or painful urination; difficulty breathing; dizziness; ear congestion; fever; frequent urge to urinate; general feeling of dis-

comfort or illness; headache; heartburn; indigestion; joint pain; loss of appetite; loss of voice; lower back or side pain; muscle aches and pains; nasal congestion; nausea; nervousness; pain or tenderness around eyes and cheekbones; pounding heartbeat; runny nose; shivering; shortness of breath or troubled breathing; sneezing; sore throat; stomach discomfort, upset, or pain; stuffy or runny nose; sweating; tightness in chest; trembling; trouble sleeping; unusual tiredness or weakness; vomiting; wheezing

Other side effects not listed may also occur in some patients. If you notice any other effects, check with your healthcare professional.

IPRATROPIUM (Nasal route) - i-pra-TROE-pee-um

Commonly used brand name(s)

In the U.S.—

Atrovent

Available Dosage Forms:

- Spray

Therapeutic Class: Nasal Agent
Pharmacologic Class: Anticholinergic

Uses For This Medicine

Ipratropium nasal spray is used to relieve runny nose (rhinorrhea).

The 0.03% nasal solution is used to relieve a runny nose associated with allergic and nonallergic perennial rhinitis. However, it does not relieve the nasal congestion, sneezing, or postnasal drip associated with allergic or nonallergic perennial rhinitis.

The 0.06% nasal solution is used for 4 days to relieve a runny nose associated with the common cold. However, it does not relieve the nasal congestion or sneezing associated with the common cold.

When this medicine is sprayed into your nose, it works by preventing the glands in your nose from producing large amounts of fluid.

Ipratropium is available only with your doctor's prescription.

Before Using This Medicine

In deciding to use a medicine, the risks of taking the medicine must be weighed against the good it will do. This is a decision you and your doctor will make. For this medicine, the following should be considered:

Allergies—Tell your doctor if you have ever had any unusual or allergic reaction to this medicine or any other medicines. Also tell your health care professional if you have any other types of allergies, such as to foods, dyes, preservatives, or animals. For non-prescription products, read the label or package ingredients carefully.

Pediatric—Although there is no specific information comparing the use of ipratropium nasal spray in children with use in other age groups, this medicine is not expected to cause different side effects or problems in children than it does in adults.

Geriatric—Many medicines have not been studied specifically in older people. Therefore, it may not be known whether they work exactly the same way they do in younger adults. Although there is no specific information comparing the use of ipratropium nasal spray in the elderly with use in other age groups, this medicine is not expected to cause different side effects in older people than it does in younger adults.

Pregnancy—

	Pregnancy Category	Explanation
All Trimesters	B	Animal studies have revealed no evidence of harm to the fetus, however, there are no adequate studies in pregnant women OR animal studies have shown an adverse effect, but adequate studies in pregnant women have failed to demonstrate a risk to the fetus.

Breast Feeding—There are no adequate studies in women for determining infant risk when using this medication during breastfeeding. Weigh the potential benefits against the potential risks before taking this medication while breastfeeding.

Other medicines—

Using this medicine with any of the following medicines may cause an increased risk of certain side effects, but using both drugs may be the best treatment for you. If both medicines are prescribed together, your doctor may change the dose or how often you use one or both of the medicines.

Betel Nut

Interactions with Food/Tobacco/Alcohol—Certain medicines should not be used at or around the time of eating food or eating certain types of food since interactions may occur. Using alcohol or tobacco with certain medicines may also cause interactions to occur. Discuss with your healthcare professional the use of your medicine with food, alcohol, or tobacco.

Other medical problems—The presence of other medical problems may affect the use of this medicine. Make sure you tell your doctor if you have any other medical problems, especially:

The presence of other medical problems may affect the use of ipratropium nasal spray. Make sure you tell your doctor if you have any other medical problem, especially:
- Bladder neck obstruction or
- Enlarged prostate—Ipratropium nasal may make the condition worse
- Glaucoma, angle-closure—If ipratropium nasal is sprayed into the eyes, it may make the condition worse

Proper Use of This Medicine

It is very important that you use ipratropium nasal spray only as directed. Do not use more of it and do not use it more often than your doctor ordered. To do so may increase the chance of side effects.

Keep the nasal spray away from your eyes. If the nasal spray gets in your eyes, immediately flush your eyes with cool tap water for several minutes. If you get the nasal spray in your

eyes, you may experience an increased sensitivity to light (which may last a few hours), blurring of vision, or eye pain. If eye pain or blurred vision occurs, check with your doctor as soon as possible.

Ipratropium nasal spray usually comes with patient directions. Read them carefully before using this medicine.

If you do not understand the directions or if you are not sure how to use the ipratropium nasal spray, ask your health care professional to show you how to use it.

When you use the nasal spray for the first time or if you have not used it for a while, the spray device may not deliver the right amount of medicine with the first spray. Therefore, before using the nasal spray, prime the device to make sure it works properly.

To prime the nasal spray device:
- The nasal spray pump must be primed before the nasal spray is used for the first time.
- To prime the pump, hold the bottle with your thumb at the base and your index and middle fingers on the white shoulder area. Make sure the bottle points upright and away from your eyes.
- Press your thumb firmly and quickly against the bottle seven times. The pump is now primed and can be used.
- Your pump should not have to be reprimed unless you have not used the medication for more than 24 hours. Repriming the pump will only require two sprays. However, if you have not used your nasal spray for more than seven days, repriming the pump will require seven sprays.

To use the nasal spray:
- Before using the nasal spray, blow your nose gently to clear your nostrils.
- Remove the clear plastic dust cap and the green safety clip from the nasal spray pump. The safety clip prevents the accidental discharge of the spray when you are not using it.
- Close one nostril by gently placing your finger against the side of your nose, tilt your head slightly forward and, keeping the bottle upright, insert the nasal tip into the other nostril. Point the tip toward the back and outer side of the nose.
- Press firmly and quickly upwards with the thumb at the base while holding the white shoulder portion of the pump between your index and middle fingers. Do not breathe in while spraying.
- After spraying the nostril and removing the unit, sniff deeply and breathe out through the nose. Tilt your head backwards for a few seconds to let the spray spread over the back of the nose.
- Repeat these steps for the second spray in the first nostril and for the two sprays in the other nostril.
- Replace the clear plastic dust cap and the green safety clip.
- You should not take extra doses of the nasal spray without checking with your doctor.

To clean the nasal spray device:
- If the nasal tip becomes clogged, remove the clear plastic dust cap and the green safety clip.
- Hold the nasal tip under running warm tap water for about a minute.

- Dry the nasal tip, reprime the nasal spray pump (see above, To prime the nasal spray device), and replace the clear plastic dust cap and green safety clip.

Dosing—The dose of this medicine will be different for different patients. Follow your doctor's orders or the directions on the label. The following information includes only the average doses of this medicine. If your dose is different, do not change it unless your doctor tells you to do so.

The amount of medicine that you take depends on the strength of the medicine. Also, the number of doses you take each day, the time allowed between doses, and the length of time you take the medicine depend on the medical problem for which you are using the medicine.

- For the 0.03% nasal spray:
  - For runny nose associated with allergic and nonallergic perennial rhinitis:
    - Adults and children 6 years of age and older— 2 sprays of the 0.03% nasal solution into each nostril two or three times a day.
    - Children up to 6 years of age—Use and dose must be determined by your doctor.
- For the 0.06% nasal spray:
  - For runny nose associated with the common cold:
    - Adults and children 5 years of age and older— 2 sprays of the 0.06% nasal solution into each nostril three or four times a day. Do not use the medicine for more than 4 days.
    - Children up to 5 years of age—Use and dose must be determined by your doctor.

Missed dose—If you miss a dose of this medicine, take it as soon as possible. However, if it is almost time for your next dose, skip the missed dose and go back to your regular dosing schedule. Do not double doses.

Storage—Store the medicine in a closed container at room temperature, away from heat, moisture, and direct light. Keep from freezing.

Keep out of the reach of children.

Do not keep outdated medicine or medicine no longer needed.

Precautions While Using This Medicine

Some improvement in your runny nose is usually seen during the first full day of treatment. However:

- If you are using the 0.03% nasal spray for runny nose associated with allergic and nonallergic perennial rhinitis, and your symptoms do not improve within one or two weeks or if your condition becomes worse, check with your doctor.
- If you are using the 0.06% nasal spray for runny nose associated with the common cold, and your condition becomes worse, check with your doctor.

Ipratropium nasal spray may cause dryness of the mouth or throat. For temporary relief, use sugarless candy or gum, melt bits of ice in your mouth, or use a saliva substitute. However, if your mouth continues to feel dry for more than 2 weeks, check with your medical doctor or dentist. Continuing dryness of the mouth may increase the chance of dental disease, including tooth decay, gum disease, and fungus infections.

Side Effects of This Medicine

Along with its needed effects, a medicine may cause some unwanted effects. Although not all of these side effects may occur, if they do occur they may need medical attention.

Check with your doctor as soon as possible if any of the following side effects occur:

For the 0.03% nasal spray
Less common
  Nasal dryness; nosebleeds; sore throat
Rare
  Blurred vision; dizziness; eye redness, irritation, or pain; pain or cramping in abdomen; painful or difficult urination
For the 0.06% nasal spray used for 4 days
Less common
  Nasal dryness; nosebleeds
Rare
  Blurred vision; dizziness; eye redness or pain; fast, slow, or irregular heartbeat; pain or cramping in abdomen; painful or difficult urination; ringing or buzzing in ears; sore throat

Some side effects may occur that usually do not need medical attention. These side effects may go away during treatment as your body adjusts to the medicine. Also, your health care professional may be able to tell you about ways to prevent or reduce some of these side effects. Check with your health care professional if any of the following side effects continue or are bothersome or if you have any questions about them:

For the 0.03% nasal spray
Less common or rare
  Dry mouth or throat; increased nasal congestion or runny nose; nasal itching, burning, or irritation; nausea
For the 0.06% nasal spray
Less common or rare
  Dry mouth or throat; increased nasal congestion

Other side effects not listed may also occur in some patients. If you notice any other effects, check with your healthcare professional.

IRBESARTAN (Oral route) - ir-be-SAR-tan

Black Box Warning

When used in pregnancy during the second and third trimesters, drugs that act directly on the renin-angiotensin system can cause injury and even death to the developing fetus. When pregnancy is detected, irbesartan should be discontinued as soon as possible.

Commonly used brand name(s)
In the U.S.—
  Avapro

Available Dosage Forms:
- Tablet

Therapeutic Class: Cardiovascular Agent
Pharmacologic Class: Angiotensin II Receptor Antagonist

Uses For This Medicine

Irbesartan belongs to the class of medicines called angiotensin II inhibitor antihypertensives. It is used to treat high blood pressure (hypertension).

High blood pressure adds to the workload of the heart and arteries. If it continues for a long time, the heart and arteries may not function properly. This can damage the blood vessels of the brain, heart, and kidneys, resulting in a stroke, heart failure, or kidney failure. High blood pressure also may increase the risk of heart attacks. These problems may be less likely to occur if blood pressure is controlled.

Irbesartan works by blocking the action of a substance in the body that causes blood vessels to tighten. As a result, irbesartan relaxes blood vessels. This lowers blood pressure.

This medicine is available only with your doctor's prescription.

Before Using This Medicine

In deciding to use a medicine, the risks of taking the medicine must be weighed against the good it will do. This is a decision you and your doctor will make. For this medicine, the following should be considered:

Allergies—Tell your doctor if you have ever had any unusual or allergic reaction to this medicine or any other medicines. Also tell your health care professional if you have any other types of allergies, such as to foods, dyes, preservatives, or animals. For non-prescription products, read the label or package ingredients carefully.

Pediatric—This medicine has been tested in children over 6 years of age and has not been shown to cause different side effects or problems than it does in adults.

Geriatric—This medicine has been tested in patients 65 years of age or older and has not been shown to cause different side effects or problems in older people than it does in younger adults. However, blood levels of irbesartan may be increased in the elderly and elderly patients may be more sensitive to the effects of irbesartan.

Pregnancy—

	Pregnancy Category	Explanation
1st Trimester	C	Animal studies have shown an adverse effect and there are no adequate studies in pregnant women OR no animal studies have been conducted and there are no adequate studies in pregnant women.
2nd Trimester	D	Studies in pregnant women have demonstrated a risk to the fetus. However, the benefits of therapy in a life threatening situation or a serious disease, may outweigh the potential risk.
3rd Trimester	D	Studies in pregnant women have demonstrated a risk to the fetus. However, the benefits of therapy in a life threatening situation or a serious disease, may outweigh the potential risk.

Breast Feeding—There are no adequate studies in women for determining infant risk when using this medication during breastfeeding. Weigh the potential benefits against the potential risks before taking this medication while breastfeeding.

Other medicines—Although certain medicines should not be used together at all, in other cases two different medicines may be used together even if an interaction might occur. In these cases, your doctor may want to change the dose, or other precautions may be necessary. Tell your healthcare professional if you are taking any other prescription or non-prescription (over-the-counter [OTC]) medicine.

Interactions with Food/Tobacco/Alcohol—Certain medicines should not be used at or around the time of eating food or eating certain types of food since interactions may occur. Using alcohol or tobacco with certain medicines may also cause interactions to occur. Discuss with your healthcare professional the use of your medicine with food, alcohol, or tobacco.

Other medical problems—The presence of other medical problems may affect the use of this medicine. Make sure you tell your doctor if you have any other medical problems, especially:

- Congestive heart failure, severe—Lowering of blood pressure by irbesartan may make this condition worse
- Dehydration—Blood pressure-lowering effects of irbesartan may be increased.
- Kidney disease—Effects of irbesartan may be increased because of slower removal of medicine from the body.

Proper Use of This Medicine

Take this medicine only as directed by your doctor. Do not take more of it and do not take it more often than your doctor ordered. This medicine works best when there is a constant amount in the blood. To help keep the amount constant, do not miss any doses. Also, it is best to take the doses at the same time each day.

Dosing—The dose of this medicine will be different for different patients. Follow your doctor's orders or the directions on the label. The following information includes only the average doses of this medicine. If your dose is different, do not change it unless your doctor tells you to do so.

The amount of medicine that you take depends on the strength of the medicine. Also, the number of doses you take each day, the time allowed between doses, and the length of time you take the medicine depend on the medical problem for which you are using the medicine.

- For oral dosage form (tablets):
  - For high blood pressure:
    - Adults and adolescents over 13 years of age— 150 milligrams (mg) once a day. Your doctor may increase your dose if needed.
    - Children 6 to 12 years of age—75 mg once a day. Your doctor may increase your dose if needed.
    - Children under 6 years of age—Use and dose must be determined by your doctor.

Missed dose—If you miss a dose of this medicine, take it as soon as possible. However, if it is almost time for your next dose, skip the missed dose and go back to your regular dosing schedule. Do not double doses.

Storage—Store the medicine in a closed container at room temperature, away from heat, moisture, and direct light. Keep from freezing.

Keep out of the reach of children.

Do not keep outdated medicine or medicine no longer needed.

Precautions While Using This Medicine

It is important that your doctor check your progress at regular visits to make sure that this medicine is working properly and to check for unwanted effects.

Check with your doctor immediately if you think that you may be pregnant. Irbesartan may cause birth defects or other problems in the baby if taken during pregnancy.

Do not take other medicines unless they have been discussed with your doctor. This especially includes over-the-counter (nonprescription) medicines for appetite control, asthma, colds, cough, hay fever, or sinus problems, since they may tend to increase your blood pressure.

Dizziness or light-headedness may occur, especially if you have been taking a diuretic (water pill). Make sure you know how you react to this medicine before you drive, use machines, or do anything else that could be dangerous if you experience these effects.

Check with your doctor right away if you become sick while taking this medicine, especially with severe or continuing nausea and vomiting or diarrhea. These conditions may cause you to lose too much water and lead to low blood pressure.

Dizziness, lightheadedness, or fainting may also occur if you exercise or if the weather is hot. Heavy sweating can cause loss of too much water and result in low blood pressure. Use extra care during exercise or hot weather.

Side Effects of This Medicine

Along with its needed effects, a medicine may cause some unwanted effects. Although not all of these side effects may occur, if they do occur they may need medical attention.

Check with your doctor as soon as possible if any of the following side effects occur:

Rare
Dizziness, lightheadedness, or fainting

Frequency not determined
Confusion, irregular heartbeat, numbness or tingling in hands, feet, or lips, shortness of breath, difficult breathing, or weakness or heaviness of legs; clay-colored stools, dark urine, itching, loss of appetite, stomach pain, or yellow eyes or skin; large, hive-like swelling on face, eyelids, lips, tongue, throat, hands, legs, feet or sex organsSome side effects may occur that usually do not need medical attention. These side effects may go away during treatment as your body adjusts to the medicine. Also, your health care professional may be able to tell you about ways to prevent or reduce some of these side effects. Check with your health care professional if any of the following side effects continue or are bothersome or if you have any questions about them:

Less common
Anxiety and/or nervousness; cold-like symptoms; belching, heartburn, and stomach discomfort; cold symptoms; diarrhea; headache; muscle or bone pain; unusual tiredness

Frequency not determined
Hives or welts, itching, redness of skin, or skin rash

Other side effects not listed may also occur in some patients. If you notice any other effects, check with your healthcare professional.

IRINOTECAN (Intravenous route) -
eye-ri-noe-TEE-kan

Black Box Warning

Irinotecan hydrochloride should be administered only under the supervision of a physician who is experienced in the use of cancer chemotherapeutic agents. Appropriate management of complications is possible only when adequate diagnostic and treatment facilities are readily available. Irinotecan hydrochloride can induce both early and late forms of diarrhea that appear to be mediated by different mechanisms. Both forms of diarrhea may be severe. Early diarrhea (occurring during or shortly after infusion of irinotecan hydrochloride) may be accompanied by cholinergic symptoms of rhinitis, increased salivation, miosis, lacrimation, diaphoresis, flushing, and intestinal hyperperistalsis that can cause abdominal cramping. Early diarrhea and other cholinergic symptoms may be prevented or ameliorated by atropine. Late diarrhea (generally occurring more than 24 hours after administration of irinotecan hydrochloride) can be life threatening since it may be prolonged and may lead to dehydration, electrolyte imbalance, or sepsis. Late diarrhea should be treated promptly with loperamide. Patients with diarrhea should be carefully monitored and given fluid and electrolyte replacement if they become dehydrated or antibiotic therapy if they develop ileus, fever, or severe neutropenia. Administration of irinotecan hydrochloride should be interrupted and subsequent doses reduced if severe diarrhea occurs.

Severe myelosuppression may occur.

Commonly used brand name(s)

In the U.S.—
Camptosar

Available Dosage Forms:
• Solution

Therapeutic Class: Antineoplastic Agent
Pharmacologic Class: Topoisomerase I Inhibitor

Uses For This Medicine

Irinotecan belongs to the group of medicines called antineoplastics. It is used to treat cancer of the colon or rectum.

Irinotecan interferes with the growth of cancer cells, which are eventually destroyed. Since the growth of normal cells may also be affected by the medicine, other effects may also occur. Some of these may be serious and must be reported to your doctor. Other effects, like hair loss, may not be serious but may cause concern. Some effects may occur after treatment with irinotecan has been stopped. Be sure that you have discussed with your doctor the possible side effects of this medicine as well as the good it can do.

This medicine is available only with your doctor's prescription.

Once a medicine has been approved for marketing for a certain use, experience may show that it is also useful for other medical problems. Although these uses are not included in

product labeling, irinotecan is used in certain patients with the following medical conditions:

- Carcinoma, lung, non-small cell (treatment) (cancer of the lung [non-small cell]
- Extensive-stage small-cell lung cancer, first-line treatment, in combination with cisplatin (to treat lung cancer; used together with cisplatin [e.g., Platinol])

Before Receiving This Medicine

In deciding to use a medicine, the risks of taking the medicine must be weighed against the good it will do. This is a decision you and your doctor will make. For this medicine, the following should be considered:

Allergies—Tell your doctor if you have ever had any unusual or allergic reaction to this medicine or any other medicines. Also tell your health care professional if you have any other types of allergies, such as to foods, dyes, preservatives, or animals. For non-prescription products, read the label or package ingredients carefully.

Pediatric—There is no specific information comparing use of irinotecan in children with use in other age groups. However, one study had to be discontinued due to serious unwanted effects in children.

Geriatric—Patients greater than 65 years of age may be at an increased risk for severe diarrhea.

Pregnancy—

	Pregnancy Category	Explanation
All Trimesters	D	Studies in pregnant women have demonstrated a risk to the fetus. However, the benefits of therapy in a life threatening situation or a serious disease, may outweigh the potential risk.

Breast Feeding—There are no adequate studies in women for determining infant risk when using this medication during breastfeeding. Weigh the potential benefits against the potential risks before taking this medication while breastfeeding.

Other medicines—

Using this medicine with any of the following medicines is not recommended. Your doctor may decide not to treat you with this medication or change some of the other medicines you take.

Rotavirus Vaccine, Live, St John's Wort

Interactions with Food/Tobacco/Alcohol—Certain medicines should not be used at or around the time of eating food or eating certain types of food since interactions may occur. Using alcohol or tobacco with certain medicines may also cause interactions to occur. Discuss with your healthcare professional the use of your medicine with food, alcohol, or tobacco.

Other medical problems—The presence of other medical problems may affect the use of this medicine. Make sure you tell your doctor if you have any other medical problems, especially:

- Bowel obstruction—This medicine should NOT be used until this condition is treated.
- Chickenpox (including recent exposure) or

- Herpes zoster (shingles)—Irinotecan may cause these conditions to get worse and spread to other parts of your body.
- Hereditary fructose intolerance—The risk of having severe diarrhea as a side effect of this medicine may be increased.
- Infection—Irinotecan may decrease your body's ability to fight an infection
- Kidney disease—Irinotecan may worsen condition, usually due to dehydration from severe vomiting or diarrhea.
- Liver disease or
- Severe bone marrow disease—The risk of dangerously low white blood cell counts may be increased.
- Lung disease—An unusual side effect consisting of fever and of shortness of breath and other problems with the lungs has occurred, very rarely, in some people with lung disease who received irinotecan.

Proper Use of This Medicine

Irinotecan often causes nausea and vomiting. It is very important that you continue to receive the medicine even if it makes you feel ill. Ask your health care professional about ways to lessen these effects.

Dosing—The dose of this medicine will be different for different patients. Follow your doctor's orders or the directions on the label. The following information includes only the average doses of this medicine. If your dose is different, do not change it unless your doctor tells you to do so.

The amount of medicine that you take depends on the strength of the medicine. Also, the number of doses you take each day, the time allowed between doses, and the length of time you take the medicine depend on the medical problem for which you are using the medicine.

Precautions After Receiving This Medicine

It is very important that your doctor check your progress at regular visits to make sure that this medicine is working properly and to check for unwanted effects. Some of the side effects of this medicine do not have any symptoms and must be found with a blood test.

While you are being treated with irinotecan, and after you stop treatment with it, do not have any immunizations (vaccinations) without your doctor's approval. Irinotecan may lower your body's resistance, and there is a chance you might get the infection the immunization is meant to prevent. In addition, other persons living in your household should not get live vaccines (e.g., oral poliovirus vaccine, nasal influenza [flu] virus vaccine). Try to avoid persons who have taken live vaccines. Do not get close to them and do not stay in the same room with them for very long. If you cannot take these precautions, you should wear a protective face mask that covers the nose and mouth.

Irinotecan may cause diarrhea, which can last long enough and be severe enough to cause serious medical problems. If diarrhea occurs while you are being treated with irinotecan:

- Check with your doctor immediately. Be sure to let your doctor know if the diarrhea started during an irinotecan injection or less than 24 hours afterwards. Also, be sure to tell your doctor if you had any other symptoms, such as stomach cramps or sweating, before the diarrhea started. This means that you are having a certain kind of diarrhea that may need to be treated by your doctor.

- If diarrhea first occurs more than 24 hours after a dose of irinotecan, start taking loperamide (e.g., Imodium A-D) as soon as you notice that your bowel movements are occurring more often, or are more loose than usual. Loperamide is available without a prescription. Buy some of it ahead of time, so that you will have it on hand in case it is needed. Unless otherwise directed by your doctor, take 4 milligrams (mg) of loperamide (2 capsules or tablets, or 4 teaspoonfuls of the oral solution dosage form) for the first dose, then 2 mg (1 capsule or tablet, or 2 teaspoonfuls of the oral solution dosage form) every two hours. To interrupt your sleep less often, you may take 4 mg of loperamide every four hours during the night. Continue taking loperamide, day and night, until you have not had any diarrhea for twelve hours. It is very important that you follow these (or your doctor's) directions, even though they are different from the directions on the nonprescription (over-the-counter [OTC]) loperamide package label. The largest amount of loperamide recommended on the package label for use in a twenty-four-hour period (8 mg) is not enough for treating diarrhea caused by irinotecan. Notify your doctor if the diarrhea is not controlled within 24 hours.

- Diarrhea causes loss of body fluid, which can lead to dehydration, a serious medical problem. To prevent this, it is very important that you replace the lost fluid. While you have diarrhea, and for a day or two after the diarrhea has stopped, drink plenty of clear liquids, such as ginger ale, caffeine-free cola, decaffeinated tea, and broth. Ask your doctor about the amount of liquid you should be drinking every day. Also, ask your doctor whether you should use a sports drink (e.g., Gatorade), which contains other substances, such as sodium and potassium, that may be lost along with body fluid. Follow your doctor's directions very carefully.

- Because alcohol and caffeine can increase fluid loss, you should not drink beverages or take any medicines that contain them while you have diarrhea. Also, avoid eating foods that may make diarrhea worse, such as bran, raw fruits or vegetables, or fatty, fried, or spicy foods.

- Vomiting can also increase the amount of fluid lost by the body and increase the risk of dehydration. If vomiting occurs at the same time as diarrhea, check with your doctor right away.

- Signs of too much fluid loss (dehydration) include decreased urination, dizziness or light-headedness, dryness of the mouth, fainting, increased thirst, and wrinkled skin. If any of these occur, check with your doctor immediately.

Irinotecan can temporarily lower the number of white blood cells in your blood, increasing the chance of getting an infection. It can also lower the number of platelets, which are needed for proper blood clotting. If this occurs, there are certain precautions you can take, especially when your blood count is low, to reduce the risk of infection or bleeding:

- If you can, avoid people with infections. Check with your doctor immediately if you think you are getting an infection or if you get a fever or chills, cough or hoarseness, lower back or side pain, or painful or difficult urination.

- Check with your doctor immediately if you notice any unusual bleeding or bruising; black, tarry stools; blood in urine or stools; or pinpoint red spots on your skin.

- Be careful when using a regular toothbrush, dental floss, or toothpick. Your medical doctor, dentist, or nurse may recommend other ways to clean your teeth and gums. Also, check with your medical doctor before having any dental work done.

- Do not touch your eyes or the inside of your nose unless you have just washed your hands and have not touched anything else in the meantime.

- Be careful not to cut yourself when you are using sharp objects such as a safety razor or fingernail or toenail cutters.

- Avoid contact sports or other situations where bruising or injury could occur.

This medicine may cause some people to become dizzy, drowsy, or less alert than they are normally. This medicine may also cause blurred vision or other vision problems. If any of these side effects occur, do not drive, use machines, or do anything else that could be dangerous if you are not alert or not able to see well. If these reactions are especially bothersome, check with your doctor.

Using this medicine while you are pregnant can harm your unborn baby. If you think you have become pregnant while using the medicine, tell your doctor right away.

St. John's Wort or ketoconazole (Nizoral®) should not be used during irinotecan therapy. If you are using St. John's Wort, it should be discontinued at least 2 weeks before the first cycle of irinotecan.

Side Effects of This Medicine

Along with its needed effects, a medicine may cause some unwanted effects. Although not all of these side effects may occur, if they do occur they may need medical attention.

Check with your doctor immediately if any of the following side effects occur:
    More common
        Anxiety; black, tarry stools; blood in urine or stools; blurred vision; changes in skin color; chest pain or discomfort; chest tightness or heaviness; chills; clay colored stools; cold hands and feet; confusion; constricted pupils; cough or hoarseness; diarrhea with or without stomach cramps or sweating; dark urine; dizziness; fainting; fast, slow, or irregular heartbeat; fever; full or bloated feeling or pressure in the stomach; headache; increased production of saliva; increased tear production; itching; lightheadedness when getting up from a lying or sitting position suddenly; loss of appetite; lower back or side pain; nausea or vomiting; no blood pressure or pulse; no breathing; numbness or tingling in face, arms, legs; pain; painful or difficult urination; pain in chest, groin, or legs, especially calves of legs; pain in the shoulders, arms, jaw, or neck; pale skin; pinpoint red spots on skin; redness or swelling of leg; runny nose; seizures; severe headache of sudden onset; shortness of breath or troubled breathing; skin rash; slurred speech; sore throat; stomach pain; stopping of heart; sudden and severe weakness in arm and/or leg on one side of the body; sudden loss of coordination; sudden vision changes; sweating; swelling; swelling of abdominal or stomach area; temporary blindness; ten-

derness, pain, or swelling of arm, foot, or leg; trouble speaking or walking; ulcers, sores, or white spots on lips or in mouth; unconsciousness; unpleasant breath odor; unusual bleeding or bruising; unusual tiredness or weakness; vomiting of blood; warm, red feeling over body; yellow eyes or skin

Less common

Bleeding gums; coughing up blood; decreased urination; difficulty in swallowing; dryness of mouth; increased menstrual flow or vaginal bleeding; increased thirst; nosebleeds; paralysis; prolonged bleeding from cuts; sneezing; wheezing; wrinkled skin

Rare

Decreased amount of urine; decreased frequency of urination; fast, irregular, or troubled breathing; hives; increased blood pressure; puffiness or swelling of the eyelids or around the eyes, face, lips or tongue; rapid weight gain

Incidence not known

Abdominal pain and tenderness; agitation; bloating, full feeling; burning, crawling, itching, numbness, prickling, "pins and needles", or tingling feelings; coma; constipation; convulsions; depression; heartburn or indigestion; hostility; increased thirst; irritability; lethargy; muscle pain and cramps; muscle twitching; pain in stomach, side, or abdomen, possibly radiating to the back; rectal bleeding; severe abdominal cramping or burning; severe and continuing nausea; stupor; swelling of face, lower legs, ankles, fingers or hands; tightness in chest; unusual tiredness or weakness; vomiting of material that looks like coffee grounds

Some side effects may occur that usually do not need medical attention. These side effects may go away during treatment as your body adjusts to the medicine. Also, your health care professional may be able to tell you about ways to prevent or reduce some of these side effects. Check with your health care professional if any of the following side effects continue or are bothersome or if you have any questions about them:

More common

Accidental injury; acid or sour stomach; belching; blistering, peeling, redness, and/or swelling of palms of hands or bottoms of feet; cracked lips; excess air or gas in stomach or intestines; feeling of constant movement of self or surroundings; numbness, pain, tingling, or unusual sensations in palms of hands or bottoms of feet; passing gas; right upper abdominal pain and fullness; sensation of spinning; sleepiness or unusual drowsiness; sleeplessness; stomach discomfort, upset, or pain; trouble sleeping; unable to sleep; weight loss

The side effects listed above may occur, or continue to occur, after treatment with irinotecan has ended. Check with your doctor if you notice any of them after you stop receiving the medicine.

Irinotecan may also cause a temporary loss of hair in some people. After treatment with irinotecan has ended, normal hair growth should return.

Irinotecan sometimes causes flushing of the face. This effect is harmless and does not need medical treatment.

Other side effects not listed may also occur in some patients. If you notice any other effects, check with your healthcare professional.

IRON SUPPLEMENTS (Systemic)

Some commonly used brand names are:

In the U.S.—

DexFerrum (4)	Ferretts (1)
Femiron (1)	Ferrlecit (8)
Feosol Caplets (3)	Fumasorb (1)
Feosol Tablets (3)	Fumerin (1)
Feostat (1)	Hemocyte (1)
Feostat Drops (1)	Hytinic (5)
Feratab (3)	InFeD (4)
Fer-gen-sol (3)	Ircon (1)
Fergon (2)	Mol-Iron (3)
Fer-In-Sol Drops (3)	Nephro-Fer (1)
Fer-In-Sol Syrup (3)	Niferex (5)
Fer-Iron Drops (3)	Niferex-150 (5)
Fero-Gradumet (3)	Nu-Iron (5)
Ferospace (3)	Nu-Iron 150 (5)
Ferralet (2)	Simron (2)
Ferralet Slow Release (2)	Slow Fe (3)
Ferralyn Lanacaps (3)	Span-FF (1)
Ferra-TD (3)	Venofer (7)

In Canada—

Apo-Ferrous Gluconate (2)	Fertinic (2)
Apo-Ferrous Sulfate (3)	Jectofer (6)
DexIron (4)	Neo-Fer (1)
Fer-In-Sol Drops (3)	Novofumar (1)
Fer-In-Sol Syrup (3)	Palafer (1)
Ferodan Infant Drops (3)	Slow Fe (3)
Ferodan Syrup (3)	

This information applies to the following:

1. Ferrous Fumarate (FER-us FYOO-ma-rate)
2. Ferrous Gluconate (FER-us GLOO-koe-nate)
3. Ferrous Sulfate (FER-us SUL-fate)
4. Iron Dextran (DEX-tran)
5. Iron-Polysaccharide (pol-i-SAK-a-ride)
6. Iron Sorbitol (SOR-bi-tole)
7. Iron Sucrose (SU-crose)
8. Sodium Ferric Gluconate (SO-dee-um FAIR-ic GLU-con-ate)

Category

- **Antianemic**—Ferrous Fumarate; Ferrous Gluconate; Ferrous Sulfate; Iron Dextran; Iron-Polysaccharide; Iron Sorbitol; Iron Sucrose; Sodium Ferric Gluconate
- **Nutritional supplement, mineral**—Ferrous Fumarate; Ferrous Gluconate; Ferrous Sulfate; Iron Dextran; Iron Sorbitol; Iron-Polysaccharide

Description

Iron is a mineral that the body needs to produce red blood cells. When the body does not get enough iron, it cannot produce the number of normal red blood cells needed to keep you in good health. This condition is called iron deficiency (iron shortage) or iron deficiency anemia.

Although many people in the U.S. get enough iron from their diet, some must take additional amounts to meet their needs. For example, iron is sometimes lost with slow or small amounts of bleeding in the body that you would not be aware of and which can only be detected by your doctor. Your doctor can determine if you have an iron deficiency, what is causing the deficiency, and if an iron supplement is necessary.

Lack of iron may lead to unusual tiredness, shortness of breath, a decrease in physical performance, and learning problems in children and adults, and may increase your chance of getting an infection.

Some conditions may increase your need for iron. These include:

- Bleeding problems
- Burns
- Hemodialysis
- Intestinal diseases
- Stomach problems
- Stomach removal
- Use of medicines to increase your red blood cell count

In addition, infants, especially those receiving breast milk or low-iron formulas, may need additional iron.

Increased need for iron supplements should be determined by your health care professional.

Injectable iron is administered only by or under the supervision of your health care professional. Other forms of iron are available without a prescription; however, your health care professional may have special instructions on the proper use and dose for your condition.

Iron supplements are available in the following dosage forms:

Oral
- Ferrous Fumarate
  - Capsules
  - Extended-release capsules
  - Oral solution
  - Oral suspension
  - Tablets
  - Chewable tablets
- Ferrous Gluconate
  - Capsules
  - Elixir
  - Syrup
  - Tablets
  - Extended-release tablets
- Ferrous Sulfate
  - Capsules
  - Extended-release capsules
  - Oral solution
  - Syrup
  - Tablets
  - Delayed-release tablets
  - Extended-release tablets
- Iron-Polysaccharide
  - Capsules
  - Oral solution
  - Tablets

Parenteral
- Iron Dextran
  - Injection
- Iron Sorbitol
  - Injection
- Iron Sucrose
  - Injection
- Sodium Ferric Gluconate Complex
  - Injection

Importance of Diet

For good health, it is important that you eat a balanced and varied diet. Follow carefully any diet program your health care professional may recommend. For your specific dietary vitamin and/or mineral needs, ask your health care professional for a list of appropriate foods. If you think that you are not getting enough vitamins and/or minerals in your diet, you may choose to take a dietary supplement.

Iron is found in the diet in two forms— heme iron, which is well absorbed, and nonheme iron, which is poorly absorbed. The best dietary source of absorbable (heme) iron is lean red meat. Chicken, turkey, and fish are also sources of iron, but they contain less than red meat. Cereals, beans, and some vegetables contain poorly absorbed (nonheme) iron. Foods rich in vitamin C (e.g., citrus fruits and fresh vegetables), eaten with small amounts of heme iron-containing foods, such as meat, may increase the amount of nonheme iron absorbed from cereals, beans, and other vegetables. Some foods (e.g., milk, eggs, spinach, fiber-containing, coffee, tea) may decrease the amount of nonheme iron absorbed from foods. Additional iron may be added to food from cooking in iron pots.

The daily amount of iron needed is defined in several different ways.

For U.S.—
- Recommended Dietary Allowances (RDAs) are the amount of vitamins and minerals needed to provide for adequate nutrition in most healthy persons. RDAs for a given nutrient may vary depending on a person's age, sex, and physical condition (e.g., pregnancy).
- Daily Values (DVs) are used on food and dietary supplement labels to indicate the percent of the recommended daily amount of each nutrient that a serving provides. DV replaces the previous designation of United States Recommended Daily Allowances (USRDAs).

For Canada—
- Recommended Nutrient Intakes (RNIs) are used to determine the amounts of vitamins, minerals, and protein needed to provide adequate nutrition and lessen the risk of chronic disease.

Normal daily recommended intakes in milligrams (mg) for iron are generally defined as follows (Note that the RDA and RNI are expressed as an actual amount of iron, which is referred to as "elemental"' iron. The product form [e.g., ferrous fumarate, ferrous gluconate, ferrous sulfate] has a different strength):

Persons	U.S. (mg)	Canada (mg)
Infants and children	6–10	0.3–6
Birth to 3 years of age		
4 to 6 years of age	10	8
7 to 10 years of age	10	8–10
Adolescent and adult males	10	8–10
Adolescent and adult females	10–15	8–13
Pregnant females	30	17–22
Breast-feeding females	15	8–13

Before Using This Dietary Supplement

If you are taking this dietary supplement without a prescription, carefully read and follow any precautions on the label. For iron supplements, the following should be considered:

Allergies—Tell your health care professional if you have ever had any unusual or allergic reaction to iron medicine.

Also tell your health care professional if you are allergic to any other substances, such as foods, preservatives, or dyes.

Pregnancy—It is especially important that you are receiving enough vitamins and minerals when you become pregnant and that you continue to receive the right amount of vitamins and minerals throughout your pregnancy. Healthy fetal growth and development depend on a steady supply of nutrients from mother to fetus. During the first 3 months of pregnancy, a proper diet usually provides enough iron. However, during the last 6 months, in order to meet the increased needs of the developing baby, an iron supplement may be recommended by your health care professional.

However, taking large amounts of a dietary supplement in pregnancy may be harmful to the mother and/or fetus and should be avoided.

Breast-feeding—It is especially important that you receive the right amounts of vitamins and minerals so that your baby will also get the vitamins and minerals needed to grow properly. Iron normally is present in breast milk in small amounts. When prescribed by a health care professional, iron preparations are not known to cause problems during breast-feeding. However, nursing mothers are advised to check with their health care professional before taking iron supplements or any other medication. Taking large amounts of a dietary supplement while breast-feeding may be harmful to the mother and/or infant and should be avoided.

Children—Problems in children have not been reported with intake of normal daily recommended amounts. Iron supplements, when prescribed by your health care professional, are not expected to cause different side effects in children than they do in adults. However, it is important to follow the directions carefully, since iron overdose in children is especially dangerous.

Studies on sodium ferric gluconate have shown that this supplement is safe to use in children ages 6 to 15 years. The safety of sodium ferric gluconate has not been determined in patients who are younger than 6 years of age.

Older adults—Problems in older adults have not been reported with intake of normal daily recommended amounts. Elderly people sometimes do not absorb iron as easily as younger adults and may need a larger dose. If you think you need to take an iron supplement, check with your health care professional first. Only your health care professional can decide if you need an iron supplement and how much you should take.

Medicines or other dietary supplements—Although certain medicines or dietary supplements should not be used together at all, in other cases they may be used together even if an interaction might occur. In these cases, your health care professional may want to change the dose, or other precautions may be necessary. When you are taking iron supplements, it is especially important that your health care professional know if you are taking any of the following:

- Acetohydroxamic acid (e.g., Lithostat)—Use with iron supplements may cause either medicine to be less effective

- Antacids—Use with iron supplements may make the iron supplements less effective; iron supplements should be taken 1 or 2 hours before or after antacids

- Dimercaprol—Iron supplements and dimercaprol may combine in the body to form a harmful chemical

- Etidronate or

- Fluoroquinolones (e.g., ciprofloxacin, enoxacin, lomefloxacin, norfloxacin, ofloxacin) or

- Tetracyclines (taken by mouth) (medicine for infection)—Use with iron supplements may make these medicines less effective; iron supplements should be taken 2 hours before or after these medicines

Other medical problems—The presence of other medical problems may affect the use of iron supplements. Make sure you tell your health care professional if you have any other medical problems, especially:

- Alcohol abuse (or history of) or

- Blood transfusions (with high red blood cell iron content) or

- Kidney infection or

- Liver disease or

- Porphyria cutaneous tarda—Higher blood levels of the iron supplement may occur, which may increase the chance of side effects

- Arthritis (rheumatoid) or

- Asthma or allergies or

- Heart disease—The injected form of iron may make these conditions worse

- Colitis or other intestinal problems or

- Iron overload conditions (e.g., hemochromatosis, hemosiderosis, hemoglobinopathies) or

- Stomach ulcer—Iron supplements may make these conditions worse

- Other anemias—Iron supplements may increase iron to toxic levels in anemias not associated with iron deficiency

---

Proper Use of This Dietary Supplement

Dosing—The amount of iron needed to meet normal daily recommended intakes will be different for different individuals. The following information includes only the average amounts of iron.

- For *oral* dosage forms (capsules, tablets, oral solution):
  - To prevent deficiency, the amount taken by mouth is based on normal daily recommended intakes:

  For the U.S.
  - Adult and teenage males—10 milligrams (mg) per day.
  - Adult and teenage females—10 to 15 mg per day.
  - Pregnant females—30 mg per day.
  - Breast-feeding females—15 mg per day.
  - Children 7 to 10 years of age—10 mg per day.
  - Children 4 to 6 years of age—10 mg per day.
  - Children birth to 3 years of age—6 to 10 mg per day.

For Canada
- Adult and teenage males—8 to 10 mg per day.
- Adult and teenage females—8 to 13 mg per day.
- Pregnant females—17 to 22 mg per day.
- Breast-feeding females—8 to 13 mg per day.
- Children 7 to 10 years of age—8 to 10 mg per day.
- Children 4 to 6 years of age—8 mg per day.
- Children birth to 3 years of age—0.3 to 6 mg per day.
  - To treat deficiency:
    - Adults, teenagers, and children—The dose will be determined by your doctor, based on your condition.
- For injection dosage forms:
  - Adults, teenagers, and children—The dose will be determined by your doctor, based on your condition.

After you start using this dietary supplement, continue to return to your health care professional to see if you are benefiting from the iron. Some blood tests may be necessary for this.

Iron is best absorbed when taken on an empty stomach, with water or fruit juice (adults: full glass or 8 ounces; children: ½ glass or 4 ounces), about 1 hour before or 2 hours after meals. However, to lessen the possibility of stomach upset, iron may be taken with food or immediately after meals.

For safe and effective use of iron supplements:

- Follow your health care professional's instructions if this dietary supplement was prescribed.

- Follow the manufacturer's package directions if you are treating yourself. If you think you still need iron after taking it for 1 or 2 months, check with your health care professional.

Liquid forms of iron supplement tend to stain the teeth. To prevent, reduce, or remove these stains:

- Mix each dose in water, fruit juice, or tomato juice. You may use a drinking tube or straw to help keep the iron supplement from getting on the teeth.

- When doses of liquid iron supplement are to be given by dropper, the dose may be placed well back on the tongue and followed with water or juice.

- Iron stains on teeth can usually be removed by brushing with baking soda (sodium bicarbonate) or medicinal peroxide (hydrogen peroxide 3%).

Missed dose—If you miss a dose of this dietary supplement, skip the missed dose and go back to your regular dosing schedule. Do not double doses.

Storage—To store this dietary supplement:

- Keep out of the reach of children because iron overdose is especially dangerous in children. As few as 3 or 4 adult iron tablets can cause serious poisoning in small children. Vitamin-iron products for use during pregnancy and flavored vitamins with iron often cause iron overdose in small children.

- Store away from heat and direct light.

- Do not store in the bathroom, near the kitchen sink, or in other damp places. Heat or moisture may cause the dietary supplement to break down.

- Keep the liquid form of this dietary supplement from freezing.

- Do not keep outdated dietary supplements or those no longer needed. Be sure that any discarded dietary supplement is out of the reach of children.

Precautions While Using This Dietary Supplement

When iron is combined with certain foods it may lose much of its value. If you are taking iron, the following foods should be avoided, or only taken in very small amounts, for at least 1 hour before or 2 hours after you take iron:

- Cheese and yogurt
- Eggs
- Milk
- Spinach
- Tea or coffee
- Whole-grain breads and cereals and bran

Do not take iron supplements and antacids or calcium supplements at the same time. It is best to space doses of these 2 products 1 to 2 hours apart, to get the full benefit from each medicine or dietary supplement.

If you are taking iron supplements *without a prescription:*

- Do not take iron supplements by mouth if you are receiving iron injections. To do so may result in iron poisoning.

- Do not regularly take large amounts of iron for longer than 6 months without checking with your health care professional. People differ in their need for iron, and those with certain medical conditions can gradually become poisoned by taking too much iron over a period of time. Also, unabsorbed iron can mask the presence of blood in the stool, which may delay discovery of a serious condition.

If you have been taking a long-acting or coated iron tablet and your stools have *not* become black, check with your health care professional. The tablets may not be breaking down properly in your stomach, and you may not be receiving enough iron.

It is important to keep iron preparations out of the reach of children. Keep a 1-ounce bottle of *syrup* of ipecac available at home to be taken in case of an iron overdose emergency when a doctor, poison control center, or emergency room orders its use.

If you think you or anyone else has taken an overdose of iron medicine:
- *Immediate medical attention is very important.*
- *Call your doctor, a poison control center, or the nearest hospital emergency room at once.* Always keep these phone numbers readily available.
- *Follow any instructions given to you.* If syrup of ipecac has been ordered and given, do not delay going to the emergency room while waiting for the ipecac syrup to empty the stomach, since it may require 20 to 30 minutes to show results.
- *Go to the emergency room without delay.*
- *Take the container of iron with you.*

Early signs of iron overdose may not appear for up to 60 minutes or more. Do not delay going to the emergency room while waiting for signs to appear.

Side Effects of This Dietary Supplement

Along with its needed effects, a dietary supplement may cause some unwanted effects. Although not all of these effects may occur, if they do occur they may need medical attention.

Check with your health care professional if any of the following side effects occur:

More common—with injection only
Backache, groin, side, or muscle pain; chest pain; chills; dizziness; fainting; fast heartbeat; fever with increased sweating; flushing; headache; metallic taste; nausea or vomiting; numbness, pain, or tingling of hands or feet; pain or redness at injection site; redness of skin; skin rash or hives; swelling of mouth or throat; troubled breathing

More common—when taken by mouth only
Abdominal or stomach pain; cramping (continuing) or soreness

Less common or rare—with injection only
Double vision; general unwell feeling; weakness without feeling dizzy or faint

Less common or rare—when taken by mouth only
Chest or throat pain, especially when swallowing; stools with signs of blood (red or black color)

Early symptoms of iron overdose
Diarrhea (may contain blood); fever; nausea; stomach pain or cramping (sharp); vomiting, severe (may contain blood)

Late symptoms of iron overdose
Bluish-colored lips, fingernails, and palms of hands; convulsions (seizures); drowsiness; pale, clammy skin; shallow and rapid breathing; unusual tiredness or weakness; weak and fast heartbeat

Other side effects may occur that usually do not need medical attention. These side effects may go away during treatment as your body adjusts to the dietary supplement. However, check with your health care professional if any of the following side effects continue or are bothersome:

More common
Constipation; diarrhea; leg cramps; nausea; vomiting

Less common
Darkened urine; heartburn; stained teeth

Stools commonly become dark green or black when iron preparations are taken by mouth. This is caused by unabsorbed iron and is harmless. However, in rare cases, black stools of a sticky consistency may occur along with other side effects such as red streaks in the stool, cramping, soreness, or sharp pains in the stomach or abdominal area. Check with your health care professional immediately if these side effects appear.

If you have been receiving injections of iron, you may notice a brown discoloration of your skin. This color usually fades within several weeks or months.

Other side effects not listed above may also occur in some individuals. If you notice any other effects, check with your health care professional.

ISOMETHEPTENE, DICHLORALPHENAZONE, AND ACETAMINOPHEN (Oral route) - eye-soe-me-THEP-teen, dye-klor-al-FEN-a-zone, a-seet-a-MIN-oh-fen

Commonly used brand name(s)

In the U.S.—

Amidrine	Migquin
Duradrin	Migratine
Epidrin	Migrazone
Iso-Acetazone	Migrin-A
Midrin	Va-Zone

Available Dosage Forms:

• Capsule

Therapeutic Class: Acetaminophen Combination
Pharmacologic Class: Isometheptene

Uses For This Medicine

Isometheptene, dichloralphenazone, and acetaminophen combination is used to treat certain kinds of headaches, such as "tension" headaches and migraine headaches. This combination is not used regularly (for example, every day) to prevent headaches. It should be taken only after headache pain begins, or after a warning sign that a migraine is coming appears. Isometheptene helps to relieve throbbing headaches, but it is not an ordinary pain reliever. Dichloralphenazone helps you to relax, and acetaminophen relieves pain.

This medicine is available only with your doctor's prescription.

Before Using This Medicine

In deciding to use a medicine, the risks of taking the medicine must be weighed against the good it will do. This is a decision you and your doctor will make. For this medicine, the following should be considered:

Allergies—Tell your doctor if you have ever had any unusual or allergic reaction to this medicine or any other medicines. Also tell your health care professional if you have any other types of allergies, such as to foods, dyes, preservatives, or animals. For non-prescription products, read the label or package ingredients carefully.

Pediatric—Studies with this medicine have been done only in adult patients, and there is no specific information about its use in children.

Geriatric—Many medicines have not been tested in older people. Therefore, it may not be known whether they work exactly the same way they do in younger adults or if they cause different side effects or problems in older people. There is no specific information comparing use of this combination medicine in the elderly with use in other age groups.

Other medicines—

Using this medicine with any of the following medicines is not recommended. Your doctor may decide not to treat you with

this medication or change some of the other medicines you take.

Clorgyline, Iproniazid, Isocarboxazid, Moclobemide, Nialamide, Pargyline, Phenelzine, Procarbazine, Selegiline, Toloxatone, Tranylcypromine

Interactions with Food/Tobacco/Alcohol—Certain medicines should not be used at or around the time of eating food or eating certain types of food since interactions may occur. Using alcohol or tobacco with certain medicines may also cause interactions to occur. The following interactions have been selected on the basis of their potential significance and are not necessarily all-inclusive.

Using this medicine with any of the following is usually not recommended, but may be unavoidable in some cases. If used together, your doctor may change the dose or how often you use this medicine, or give you special instructions about the use of food, alcohol, or tobacco.

Ethanol

Using this medicine with any of the following may cause an increased risk of certain side effects but may be unavoidable in some cases. If used together, your doctor may change the dose or how often you use this medicine, or give you special instructions about the use of food, alcohol, or tobacco.

Cabbage

Other medical problems—The presence of other medical problems may affect the use of this medicine. Make sure you tell your doctor if you have any other medical problems, especially:

- Alcohol abuse or
- Heart attack (recent) or
- Heart or blood vessel disease or
- Kidney disease or
- Liver disease or
- Stroke (recent) or
- Virus infection of the liver (viral hepatitis)—The chance of side effects may be increased
- Glaucoma, not well controlled, or
- High blood pressure (hypertension), not well controlled—The isometheptene in this combination medicine may make these conditions worse

Proper Use of This Medicine

Take this medicine only as directed by your doctor. Do not take more of it, do not take it more often than directed, and do not take it every day for several days in a row. If the amount you are to take does not relieve your headache, check with your doctor. If a headache medicine is used too often, it may lose its effectiveness or even cause a type of physical dependence. If this occurs, your headaches may actually get worse. Also, taking too much acetaminophen can cause liver damage.

This medicine works best if you:

- Take it as soon as the headache begins. If you get warning signals of a migraine, take this medicine as soon

as you are sure that the migraine is coming. This may even stop the headache pain from occurring.

- Lie down in a quiet, dark room until you are feeling better.

People who get a lot of headaches may need to take a different medicine to help prevent headaches. It is important that you follow your doctor's directions, even if your headaches continue to occur. Headache-preventing medicines may take several weeks to start working. Even after they do start working, your headaches may not go away completely. However, your headaches should occur less often, and they should be less severe and easier to relieve, than before. This will reduce the amount of headache relievers that you need. If you do not notice any improvement after several weeks of headache-preventing treatment, check with your doctor.

Dosing—The dose of this medicine will be different for different patients. Follow your doctor's orders or the directions on the label. The following information includes only the average doses of this medicine. If your dose is different, do not change it unless your doctor tells you to do so.

The amount of medicine that you take depends on the strength of the medicine. Also, the number of doses you take each day, the time allowed between doses, and the length of time you take the medicine depend on the medical problem for which you are using the medicine.

- For "tension" headaches:
  - Adults: 1 or 2 capsules every 4 hours, as needed. Not more than 8 capsules a day.
  - Children: Dose must be determined by the doctor.

- For migraine headaches:
  - Adults: 2 capsules for the first dose, then 1 capsule every hour, as needed. Not more than 5 capsules in 12 hours.
  - Children: Dose must be determined by the doctor.

Precautions While Using This Medicine

Check with your doctor:

- If the medicine stops working as well as it did when you first started using it. This may mean that you are in danger of becoming dependent on the medicine. Do not try to get better relief by increasing the dose.

- If you are having headaches more often than you did before you started using this medicine. This is especially important if a new headache occurs within 1 day after you took your last dose of headache medicine, headaches begin to occur every day, or a headache continues for several days in a row. This may mean that you are dependent on the medicine. Continuing to take this medicine will cause even more headaches later on. Your doctor can give you advice on how to relieve the headaches.

Check the labels of all nonprescription (over-the-counter [OTC]) and prescription medicines you now take. Taking other medicines that contain acetaminophen together with this medicine may lead to an overdose. If you have any questions about this, check with your health care professional.

This medicine may cause some people to become drowsy, dizzy, or less alert than they are normally. These effects may be especially severe if you also take CNS depressants (medicines that slow down the nervous system, possibly causing drowsiness) together with this medicine. Some examples of CNS depressants are antihistamines or medicine for hay fever, other allergies, or colds; sedatives, tranquilizers, or sleeping medicine; prescription pain medicine or narcotics; barbiturates; medicine for seizures; muscle relaxants; antiemetics (medicines that prevent or relieve nausea or vomiting), and anesthetics. If you are not able to lie down for a while, make sure you know how you react to this medicine or combination of medicines before you drive, use machines, or do anything else that could be dangerous if you are drowsy or dizzy or are not alert.

Do not drink alcoholic beverages while taking this medicine. To do so may increase the chance of liver damage caused by acetaminophen, especially if you drink large amounts of alcoholic beverages regularly. Also, because drinking alcoholic beverages may make your headaches worse or cause new headaches to occur, people who often get headaches should probably avoid alcohol.

Side Effects of This Medicine

Along with its needed effects, a medicine may cause some unwanted effects. Although not all of these side effects may occur, if they do occur they may need medical attention.

Check with your doctor as soon as possible if any of the following side effects occur:
Less common
Unusual tiredness or weakness

Rare
Black, tarry stools; blood in urine or stools; pinpoint red spots on skin; skin rash, hives, or itching; sore throat and fever; unusual bleeding or bruising; yellow eyes or skin

Symptoms of dependence on this medicine
Headaches, more severe and/or more frequent than before

Symptoms of acetaminophen overdose
Diarrhea; increased sweating; loss of appetite; nausea or vomiting; pain, tenderness, and/or swelling in the upper abdominal (stomach) area; stomach cramps or pain

Some side effects may occur that usually do not need medical attention. These side effects may go away during treatment as your body adjusts to the medicine. Also, your health care professional may be able to tell you about ways to prevent or reduce some of these side effects. Check with your health care professional if any of the following side effects continue or are bothersome or if you have any questions about them:
More common
Drowsiness

Rare
Dizziness; fast or irregular heartbeat

Other side effects not listed may also occur in some patients. If you notice any other effects, check with your healthcare professional.

ISONIAZID (Oral route, Intramuscular route) - eye-soe-NYE-a-zid

Black Box Warning

Severe and sometimes fatal hepatitis associated with isoniazid therapy has been reported and may occur or may develop even after many months of treatment. The risk of developing hepatitis is age related. Approximate case rates by age are: less than 1 per 1,000 for persons under 20 years of age, 3 per 1,000 for persons in the 20 year to 34 year age group, 12 per 1,000 for persons in the 35 year to 49 year age group, 23 per 1,000 for persons in the 50 year to 64 year age group, and 8 per 1,000 for persons over 65 years of age. The risk of hepatitis is increased with daily consumption of alcohol. Precise data to provide fatality rate for isoniazid related hepatitis is not available; however, in a U.S. Public Health Service Surveillance Study involving 13,838 persons taking isoniazid, there were 8 deaths among the 174 cases of hepatitis.

Therefore, patients given isoniazid should be carefully monitored and interviewed at monthly intervals. For persons 35 and older, in addition to monthly symptom reviews, hepatic enzymes (specifically, AST and ALT (formerly SGOT and SGPT, respectively) should be measured prior to starting isoniazid therapy and periodically throughout treatment. Isoniazid-associated hepatitis usually occurs during the first three months of treatment. Usually, enzyme levels return to normal despite continuance of drug, but in some cases progressive liver dysfunction occurs. Other factors associated with an increased risk of hepatitis include daily use of alcohol, chronic liver disease and injection drug use. A recent report suggests an increased risk of fatal hepatitis associated with isoniazid among women, particularly black and Hispanic women. The risk may also be increased during the post partum period. More careful monitoring should be considered in these groups, possibly including more frequent laboratory monitoring. If abnormalities of liver function exceed three to five times the upper limit of normal, discontinuation of isoniazid should be strongly considered. Liver function tests are not a substitute for a clinical evaluation at monthly intervals or for the prompt assessment of signs or symptoms of adverse reactions occurring between regularly scheduled evaluations. Patients should be instructed to immediately report signs or symptoms consistent with liver damage or other adverse effects. These include any of the following: unexplained anorexia, nausea, vomiting, dark urine, icterus, rash, persistent paresthesias of the hands and feet, persistent fatigue, weakness or fever of greater than 3 days duration and/or abdominal tenderness, especially right upper quadrant discomfort. If these symptoms appear or if signs suggestive of hepatic damage are detected, isoniazid should be discontinued promptly, since continued use of the drug in these cases has been reported to cause a more severe form of liver damage.

Patients with tuberculosis who have hepatitis attributed to isoniazid should be given appropriate treatment with alternative drugs. If isoniazid must be reinstituted, it should be reinstituted only after symptoms and laboratory abnormalities have cleared. The drug should be restarted in very small and gradually increasing doses and should be withdrawn immediately if there is any indication of recurrent liver involvement.

Preventive treatment should be deferred in persons with acute hepatic disease.

Commonly used brand name(s)
In the U.S.—
Nydrazid

In Canada—
Pms-Isoniazid

Available Dosage Forms:
- Tablet
- Solution
- Syrup

Therapeutic Class: Antitubercular

Uses For This Medicine

Isoniazid is used to treat tuberculosis (TB) or prevent its return (reactivation). It may be given alone, or in combination with other medicines, to treat TB or to prevent its return (reactivation). This medicine may also be used for other problems as determined by your doctor.

This medicine may cause some serious side effects, including damage to the liver. Liver damage is more likely to occur in patients over 50 years of age. You and your doctor should talk about the good this medicine will do, as well as the risks of taking it.

If you are being treated for active tuberculosis (TB): To help clear up your TB infection completely, you must keep taking this medicine for the full time of treatment, even if you begin to feel better. This is very important. It is also important that you do not miss any doses.

Isoniazid is available only with your doctor's prescription.

Before Using This Medicine

In deciding to use a medicine, the risks of taking the medicine must be weighed against the good it will do. This is a decision you and your doctor will make. For this medicine, the following should be considered:

Allergies—Tell your doctor if you have ever had any unusual or allergic reaction to this medicine or any other medicines. Also tell your health care professional if you have any other types of allergies, such as to foods, dyes, preservatives, or animals. For non-prescription products, read the label or package ingredients carefully.

Pediatric—Isoniazid can cause serious side effects in any patient. Therefore, it is especially important that you discuss with the child's doctor the good that this medicine may do as well as the risks of using it.

Geriatric—Hepatitis may be especially likely to occur in patients over 50 years of age, who are usually more sensitive than younger adults to the effects of isoniazid.

Breast Feeding—There are no adequate studies in women for determining infant risk when using this medication during breastfeeding. Weigh the potential benefits against the potential risks before taking this medication while breastfeeding.

Other medicines—

Using this medicine with any of the following medicines is usually not recommended, but may be required in some cases. If both medicines are prescribed together, your doctor may change the dose or how often you use one or both of the medicines.

Itraconazole, Levodopa, Rifampin

Interactions with Food/Tobacco/Alcohol—Certain medicines should not be used at or around the time of eating food or eating certain types of food since interactions may occur. Using alcohol or tobacco with certain medicines may also cause interactions to occur. The following interactions have been selected on the basis of their potential significance and are not necessarily all-inclusive.

Using this medicine with any of the following is usually not recommended, but may be unavoidable in some cases. If used together, your doctor may change the dose or how often you use this medicine, or give you special instructions about the use of food, alcohol, or tobacco.

Ethanol

Using this medicine with any of the following may cause an increased risk of certain side effects but may be unavoidable in some cases. If used together, your doctor may change the dose or how often you use this medicine, or give you special instructions about the use of food, alcohol, or tobacco.

Tyramine Containing Food

Other medical problems—The presence of other medical problems may affect the use of this medicine. Make sure you tell your doctor if you have any other medical problems, especially:
- Alcohol abuse (or history of) or
- Liver disease—There may be an increased chance of hepatitis with daily drinking of alcohol or in patients with liver disease
- Kidney disease (severe)—There may be an increased chance of side effects in patients with severe kidney disease
- Seizure disorders such as epilepsy—There may be an increased chance of seizures (convulsions) in some patients

Proper Use of This Medicine

Make certain your health care professional knows if you are on a low-sodium, low-sugar, or any other special diet. Most medicines contain more than just the active ingredient, and many liquid medicines contain alcohol.

If you are taking isoniazid by mouth and it upsets your stomach, take it with food. Antacids may also help. However, do not take aluminum-containing antacids within 1 hour of taking isoniazid. They may keep this medicine from working properly.

For patients taking the oral liquid form of isoniazid:
- Use a specially marked measuring spoon or other device to measure each dose accurately. The average household teaspoon may not hold the right amount of liquid.

To help clear up your tuberculosis (TB) completely, it is very important that you keep taking this medicine for the full time of treatment, even if you begin to feel better after a few weeks. You may have to take it every day for as long as 6 months to 2 years. It is important that you do not miss any doses.

Your doctor may also want you to take pyridoxine (e.g., Hexa-Betalin, vitamin B_6) every day to help prevent or lessen some of the side effects of isoniazid. This is not usually needed in children, who receive enough pyridoxine in their diet. If it is needed, it is very important to take pyridoxine every day along with this medicine. Do not miss any doses.

Dosing—The dose of this medicine will be different for different patients. Follow your doctor's orders or the directions on the label. The following information includes only the average doses of this medicine. If your dose is different, do not change it unless your doctor tells you to do so.

The amount of medicine that you take depends on the strength of the medicine. Also, the number of doses you take each day, the time allowed between doses, and the length of time you take the medicine depend on the medical problem for which you are using the medicine.

- For oral dosage forms (tablets, syrup):
  - For preventing the return (reactivation) of tuberculosis:
    - Adults and teenagers—300 milligrams (mg) once a day.
    - Children—Dose is based on body weight. The usual dose is 10 mg per kilogram (kg) (4.5 mg per pound) of body weight, up to 300 mg, once a day.
  - For treatment of tuberculosis:
    - Adults and teenagers—300 mg once a day; or 15 mg per kg (6.8 mg per pound) of body weight, up to 900 mg, two times a week or three times a week, depending on the schedule your doctor chooses for you.
    - Children—Dose is based on body weight. The usual dose is 10 to 20 mg per kg (4.5 to 9.1 mg per pound) of body weight, up to 300 mg, once a day; or 20 to 40 mg per kg (9.1 to 18.2 mg per pound) of body weight, up to 900 mg, two times a week or three times a week, depending on the schedule your doctor chooses for you.
- For injection dosage form:
  - For preventing the return (reactivation) of tuberculosis:
    - Adults and teenagers—300 mg once a day.
    - Children—Dose is based on body weight. The usual dose is 10 mg per kg (4.5 mg per pound) of body weight, up to 300 mg, once a day.
  - For treatment of tuberculosis:
    - Adults and teenagers—300 mg once a day; or 15 mg per kg (6.8 mg per pound) of body weight, up to 900 mg, two times a week or three times a week, depending on the schedule your doctor chooses for you.
    - Children—Dose is based on body weight. The usual dose is 10 to 20 mg per kg (4.5 to 9.1 mg per pound) of body weight, up to 300 mg, once a day; or 20 to 40 mg per kg (9.1 to 18.2 mg per pound) of body weight, up to 900 mg, two times a week or three times a week, depending on the schedule your doctor chooses for you.

Missed dose—If you miss a dose of this medicine, take it as soon as possible. However, if it is almost time for your next dose, skip the missed dose and go back to your regular dosing schedule. Do not double doses.

Storage—Store the medicine in a closed container at room temperature, away from heat, moisture, and direct light. Keep from freezing.

Keep out of the reach of children.

Do not keep outdated medicine or medicine no longer needed.

Precautions While Using This Medicine

It is very important that your doctor check your progress at regular visits. Also, check with your doctor immediately if blurred vision or loss of vision, with or without eye pain, occurs during treatment. Your doctor may want you to have your eyes checked by an ophthalmologist (eye doctor).

If your symptoms do not improve within 2 to 3 weeks, or if they become worse, check with your doctor.

Certain foods such as cheese (Swiss or Cheshire) or fish (tuna, skipjack, or Sardinella) may rarely cause reactions in some patients taking isoniazid. Check with your doctor if redness or itching of the skin, hot feeling, fast or pounding heartbeat, sweating, chills or clammy feeling, headache, or lightheadedness occurs while you are taking this medicine.

Liver problems may be more likely to occur if you drink alcoholic beverages regularly while you are taking this medicine. Also, the regular use of alcohol may keep this medicine from working properly. Therefore, you should strictly limit the amount of alcoholic beverages you drink while you are taking this medicine.

If this medicine causes you to feel very tired or very weak; or causes clumsiness; unsteadiness; a loss of appetite; nausea; numbness, tingling, burning, or pain in the hands and feet; or vomiting, check with your doctor immediately. These may be early warning signs of more serious liver or nerve problems that could develop later.

For diabetic patients:
- This medicine may cause false test results with some urine sugar tests. Check with your doctor before changing your diet or the dosage of your diabetes medicine.

Side Effects of This Medicine

Along with its needed effects, a medicine may cause some unwanted effects. Although not all of these side effects may occur, if they do occur they may need medical attention.

Check with your doctor immediately if any of the following side effects occur:

More common
  Clumsiness or unsteadiness; dark urine; loss of appetite; nausea or vomiting; numbness, tingling, burning, or pain in hands and feet; unusual tiredness or weakness; yellow eyes or skin

Rare
  Blurred vision or loss of vision, with or without eye pain; convulsions (seizures); fever and sore throat; joint pain; mental depression; mood or other mental changes; skin rash; unusual bleeding or bruising

Some side effects may occur that usually do not need medical attention. These side effects may go away during treatment as your body adjusts to the medicine. Also, your health care professional may be able to tell you about ways to prevent or reduce some of these side effects. Check with your health care professional if any of the following side effects continue or are bothersome or if you have any questions about them:

More common
  Diarrhea; stomach pain

For injection form
  Irritation at the place of injection

Dark urine and yellowing of the eyes or skin (signs of liver problems) are more likely to occur in patients over 50 years of age.

Other side effects not listed may also occur in some patients. If you notice any other effects, check with your healthcare professional.

ISOTRETINOIN   (Oral route) - eye-soe-TRET-i-noyn

Black Box Warning

Isotretinoin must not be used by female patients who are or may become pregnant. There is an extremely high risk that severe birth defects will result if pregnancy occurs while taking isotretinoin in any amount, even for short periods of time. Potentially any fetus exposed during pregnancy can be affected. There are no accurate means of determining whether an exposed fetus has been affected.

Birth defects which have been documented following isotretinoin exposure include abnormalities of the face, eyes, ears, skull, central nervous system, cardiovascular system, and thymus and parathyroid glands. Cases of IQ scores less than 85 with or without other abnormalities have been reported. There is an increased risk of spontaneous abortion, and premature births have been reported.

Documented external abnormalities include: skull abnormality; ear abnormalities (including anotia, micropinna, small or absent external auditory canals); eye abnormalities (including microphthalmia); facial dysmorphia; cleft palate. Documented internal abnormalities include: CNS abnormalities (including cerebral abnormalities, cerebellar malformation, hydrocephalus, microcephaly, cranial nerve deficit); cardiovascular abnormalities; thymus gland abnormality; parathyroid hormone deficiency. In some cases death has occurred with certain of the abnormalities previously noted.

If pregnancy does occur during treatment of a female patient who is taking isotretinoin, isotretinoin must be discontinued immediately and she should be referred to an Obstetrician-Gynecologist experienced in reproductive toxicity for further evaluation and counseling.

Special Prescribing Requirements:

Because of isotretinoin's teratogenicity and to minimize fetal exposure, isotretinoin is approved for marketing only under a special restricted distribution program approved by the Food and Drug Administration. This program is called iPLEDGE. Isotretinoin must only be prescribed by prescribers who are registered and activated with the iPLEDGE program. Isotretinoin must only be dispensed by a pharmacy registered and activated with iPLEDGE, and must only be dispensed to patients who are registered and meet all the requirements of iPLEDGE.

Commonly used brand name(s)

In the U.S.—
Accutane	Claravis
Amnesteem	Sotret

Available Dosage Forms:
- Capsule, Liquid Filled

Therapeutic Class: Antiacne

Uses For This Medicine

Isotretinoin is used to treat severe, disfiguring nodular acne. It should be used only after other acne medicines have been tried and have failed to help the acne. Isotretinoin may also be used to treat other skin diseases as determined by your doctor.

Isotretinoin must not be used to treat women who are able to bear children unless other forms of treatment have been tried first and have failed. Isotretinoin must not be taken during pregnancy because it causes birth defects in humans. If you are able to bear children, it is very important that you read, understand, and follow the pregnancy warnings for isotretinoin.

This medicine is available only with your doctor's prescription.

Once a medicine has been approved for marketing for a certain use, experience may show that it is also useful for other medical problems. Although these uses are not included in product labeling, isotretinoin is used in certain patients with the following medical conditions:
- Folliculitis, gram-negative (bacterial infection of skin on face beginning near the nose)
- Hidradenitis suppurativa (sweat gland problem)
- Rosacea (red skin disorder of the face, usually of the nose and cheeks)
- Thickened or patchy skin disorders, such as keratosis follicularis, palmoplantar keratoderma, lamellar ichthyosis, or pityriasis rubra pilaris

Before Using This Medicine

In deciding to use a medicine, the risks of taking the medicine must be weighed against the good it will do. This is a decision you and your doctor will make. For this medicine, the following should be considered:

Allergies—Tell your doctor if you have ever had any unusual or allergic reaction to this medicine or any other medicines. Also tell your health care professional if you have any other types of allergies, such as to foods, dyes, preservatives, or animals. For non-prescription products, read the label or package ingredients carefully.

Pediatric—Children may be especially sensitive to the effects of isotretinoin. This may increase the chance of side effects during treatment. Children may have the side effects of back, joint, or muscle pain more often than adults.

This medicine should be used with caution in teenagers, especially those with bone problems or diseases.

Geriatric—Many medicines have not been studied specifically in older people. Therefore, it may not be known whether they work exactly the same way they do in younger adults or if they cause different side effects or problems in older people. There is no specific information comparing use of isotretinoin in the elderly with use in other age groups. However, older people may have a greater risk of problems and adverse effects when taking isotretinoin.

Pregnancy—

	Pregnancy Category	Explanation
All Trimesters	X	Studies in animals or pregnant women have demonstrated positive evidence of fetal abnormalities. This drug should not be used in women who are or may become pregnant because the risk clearly outweighs any possible benefit.

Breast Feeding—There are no adequate studies in women for determining infant risk when using this medication during

breastfeeding. Weigh the potential benefits against the potential risks before taking this medication while breastfeeding.

Other medicines—

Using this medicine with any of the following medicines is usually not recommended, but may be required in some cases. If both medicines are prescribed together, your doctor may change the dose or how often you use one or both of the medicines.

Desogestrel, Doxycycline, Ethinyl Estradiol, Ethynodiol, Etonogestrel, Levonorgestrel, Mestranol, Minocycline, Norelgestromin, Norethindrone, Norgestimate, Norgestrel, Tetracycline

Interactions with Food/Tobacco/Alcohol—Certain medicines should not be used at or around the time of eating food or eating certain types of food since interactions may occur. Using alcohol or tobacco with certain medicines may also cause interactions to occur. The following interactions have been selected on the basis of their potential significance and are not necessarily all-inclusive.

Using this medicine with any of the following is usually not recommended, but may be unavoidable in some cases. If used together, your doctor may change the dose or how often you use this medicine, or give you special instructions about the use of food, alcohol, or tobacco.

Ethanol

Other medical problems—The presence of other medical problems may affect the use of this medicine. Make sure you tell your doctor if you have any other medical problems, especially:

- Alcoholism or excess use of alcohol (or history of) or

- Diabetes mellitus (sugar diabetes) (or a family history of) or

- Family history of high triglyceride (a fat-like substance) levels in the blood or

- Severe weight problems—Use of isotretinoin may increase blood levels of triglyceride (a fat-like substance), which may increase the chance of heart or blood vessel problems in patients who have a family history of high triglycerides, are greatly overweight, are diabetic, or use a lot of alcohol. For persons with diabetes mellitus, use of isotretinoin also may change blood sugar levels

- Anorexia (eating disorder) or

- Osteoporosis (brittle bones), childhood or family history of or

- Osteomalacia (softening of the bones) or

- Other bone disorders or diseases—Isotretinoin should be used with caution. It is not known whether this medicine effects bone loss.

- Kidney disease or

- Lipids in blood, sudden and large increase or

- Liver disease or

- Vitamin A overdose (too much vitamin A in your body)—Isotretinoin should not be used in patients with these medical problems.

- Mental disorders such as mental depression or psychosis—Isotretinoin may make these problems worse.

Proper Use of This Medicine

Isotretinoin comes with patient information. It is very important that you read and understand this information. Be sure to ask your doctor about anything you do not understand.

Women of reproductive age are required to sign up for a pregnancy risk program called iPLEDGE in order to receive their isotretinoin prescription each month. You can sign up on the internet (www.ipledge.com) or by telephone (1–866–495–0654). Be sure to ask your doctor if you have any questions about this program. It is very important that you understand and follow all of its requirements.

Isotretinoin must not be taken by women of reproductive age unless two effective forms of contraception (birth control) have been used for at least 1 month before the beginning of treatment. Contraception must be continued during the period of treatment, which is up to 20 weeks, and for 1 month after isotretinoin is stopped. Be sure you have discussed this information with your doctor.

If you are a woman who is able to have children, you must have a pregnancy blood test within 1 week before beginning treatment with isotretinoin to make sure you are not pregnant. Treatment with isotretinoin will then be started within the week, on the second or third day of your next normal menstrual period. In addition, you must have a pregnancy blood test each month while you are taking this medicine and one month after treatment is completed.

Take isotretinoin with food and a full glass of liquid, like water. Taking with food is important for getting the right amount of medicine out of your stomach. Taking with a full glass of liquid will reduce chest or stomach discomfort that may occur from isotretinoin.

It is very important that you take isotretinoin only as directed. Do not take more of it, do not take it more often, and do not take it for a longer time than your doctor ordered. To do so may increase the chance of side effects.

Importance of not sharing medication with anyone else because of the risk of birth defects and other serious side effects.

Dosing—The dose of this medicine will be different for different patients. Follow your doctor's orders or the directions on the label. The following information includes only the average doses of this medicine. If your dose is different, do not change it unless your doctor tells you to do so.

The amount of medicine that you take depends on the strength of the medicine. Also, the number of doses you take each day, the time allowed between doses, and the length of time you take the medicine depend on the medical problem for which you are using the medicine.

- For oral dosage form (capsules):
  - For acne:
    - Adults and teenagers—Dose is based on body weight and must be determined by your doctor. The usual dose is 0.5 to 1 milligram (mg) per kilogram (kg) (0.23 to 0.45 mg per pound) of body weight a day. It is recommended that the dose per day be divided and not taken all at one time. For adult patients with severe acne, dosage adjust-

ments may be needed and must be determined by your doctor.

- Children—Use is usually not recommended.

Missed dose—If you miss a dose of this medicine, take it as soon as possible. However, if it is almost time for your next dose, skip the missed dose and go back to your regular dosing schedule. Do not double doses.

Storage—Store the medicine in a closed container at room temperature, away from heat, moisture, and direct light. Keep from freezing.

Keep out of the reach of children.

Do not keep outdated medicine or medicine no longer needed.

Precautions While Using This Medicine

Your doctor should check your progress at regular visits to make sure this medicine does not cause unwanted effects.

Isotretinoin causes birth defects in humans if taken during pregnancy. Therefore, if you suspect that you may have become pregnant, stop taking this medicine immediately and check with your doctor.

Importance of checking with your doctor before taking any medications including vitamins, herbal products, or over-the-counter (OTC) medicines. Some of these medicines or nutritional supplements (e.g., St. John's wort) may make your birth control pills not work.

During the first 3 weeks you are taking isotretinoin, your skin may become irritated. Also, your acne may seem to get worse before it gets better. Check with your doctor if your skin condition does not improve within 1 to 2 months after starting this medicine or at any time your skin irritation becomes severe. Full improvement continues after you stop taking isotretinoin and may take up to 6 months. Your health care professional can help you choose the right skin products to reduce skin dryness and irritation.

Do not donate blood to a blood bank while you are taking isotretinoin or for 30 days after you stop taking it. This is to prevent the possibility of a pregnant patient receiving the blood containing the medicine.

In some patients, isotretinoin may cause a decrease in night vision. This decrease may occur suddenly. If it does occur, do not drive, use machines, or do anything else that could be dangerous if you are not able to see well. Also, check with your doctor.

Isotretinoin may cause dryness of the eyes. Therefore, if you wear contact lenses, your eyes may be more sensitive to them during the time you are taking isotretinoin and for up to about 2 weeks after you stop taking it. To help relieve dryness of the eyes, check with your doctor about using an eye-lubricating solution, such as artificial tears. If eye inflammation occurs, check with your doctor.

Isotretinoin may cause dryness of the mouth and nose. For temporary relief of mouth dryness, use sugarless candy or gum, melt bits of ice in your mouth, or use a saliva substitute. However, if dry mouth continues for more than 2 weeks, check with your medical doctor or dentist. Continuing dryness of the mouth may increase the chance of dental disease, including tooth decay, gum disease, and fungus infections.

Avoid overexposing your skin to sunlight, wind, or cold weather. Your skin will be more prone to sunburn, dryness,

or irritation, especially during the first 2 or 3 weeks of treatment. However, you should not stop taking this medicine unless the skin irritation becomes too severe. Do not use a sunlamp.

To help isotretinoin work properly, regularly use sunscreen or sunblocking lotions with a sun protection factor (SPF) of at least 15. Also, wear protective clothing and hats.

Isotretinoin may cause mood or behavior problems, including having thoughts about hurting themselves; check with you doctor right away if unusual mood or behavior problems occur.

Isotretinoin may cause bone or muscle problems, including joint pain, muscle pain or stiffness, or difficulty moving. Check with your doctor if these problems are bothersome.

Do not take vitamin A or any vitamin supplement containing vitamin A while taking this medicine, unless otherwise directed by your doctor. To do so may increase the chance of side effects.

Importance of not removing hair by wax epilation while taking isotretinoin and for 6 months after stopping isotretinoin. Isotretinoin can increase your chance of scarring from wax epilation.

Importance of not having any cosmetic procedures to smooth your skin (e.g., dermabrasion, laser) while taking isotretinoin and for 6 months after stopping isotretinoin. Isotretinoin can increase your chance of scarring from these cosmetic procedures.

For diabetic patients:

- This medicine may affect blood sugar levels. If you notice a change in the results of your blood or urine sugar tests or if you have any questions, check with your doctor.

Side Effects of This Medicine

Along with its needed effects, a medicine may cause some unwanted effects. Although not all of these side effects may occur, if they do occur they may need medical attention.

Check with your doctor as soon as possible if any of the following side effects occur:

More common

Bone or joint pain; burning, redness, itching, or other signs of eye inflammation; difficulty in moving; nosebleeds; scaling, redness, burning, pain, or other signs of inflammation of lips; skin infection or rash

Rare

Abdominal or stomach pain (severe); attempts at suicide or thoughts of suicide (usually stops after medicine is stopped); back pain; bleeding or inflammation of gums; blurred vision or other changes in vision; changes in behavior; decreased vision after sunset or before sunrise (sudden or may continue after medicine is stopped); diarrhea (severe); headache (severe or continuing); mental depression; nausea and vomiting; pain or tenderness of eyes; pain, tenderness, or stiffness in muscles (long-term treatment); rectal bleeding; yellow eyes or skin

Incidence not determined

Attack, assault, or use of force; black, tarry stools; bleeding from sore in mouth; bloating; bloody cough; bloody or cloudy urine; bone pain, tenderness, or aching; burning or stinging of skin; chest pain; chills;

confusion; constipation; convulsions; cough or hoarse-ness; dark-colored urine; decrease in height; difficulty breathing; difficulty in speaking; difficulty in swallowing; discharge from eye; dizziness; double vision; ear pain; excessive tearing; fainting; fast, irregular, pounding, or racing heartbeat or pulse; fever with or without chills; fractures and/or delayed healing; general feeling of dis-comfort or illness; heartburn; high blood pressure; hives; inability to move arms, legs, or facial muscles; inability to speak; indigestion; inflamed tissue from in-fection; irregular yellow patch or lump on skin; irritation; joint pain, redness, stiffness, or swelling; killing oneself; lack or slowing of normal growth in children; loosening of the fingernails; loss of appetite; loss of bladder con-trol; loss or change in hearing; muscle cramps or spasms; muscle spasm or jerking of all extremities; muscle weakness; noisy breathing; pain in ribs, arms, or legs; pain or burning in throat; pain or tenderness around eyes and cheekbones; painful cold sores or blisters on lips, nose, eyes, or genitals; painful or diffi-cult urination; pains in chest, groin, or legs, especially calves of legs; pains in stomach, side, or abdomen, possibly radiating to the back; pale skin; pinpoint red spots on skin; redness or soreness around fingernails; redness, soreness or itching skin; sensitivity of eyes to sunlight; shortness of breath; skin rash; slow speech; sneezing; sore throat; sores, ulcers, or white spots on lips or tongue or inside the mouth; sores, welting or blisters; stuffy or runny nose; sudden loss of conscious-ness; sudden loss of coordination; sudden onset of se-vere acne on chest and trunk; sudden onset of short-ness of breath for no apparent reason; sudden onset of slurred speech; swelling of eyelids, face, lips, hands, lower legs, or feet; swollen, painful or tender lymph glands in neck, armpit, or groin; tightness in chest; un-usual bleeding or bruising; unusual tiredness or weak-ness; unusual weight gain or loss; use of extreme phys-ical or emotional force; watery or bloody diarrhea; wheezing

Some side effects may occur that usually do not need med-ical attention. These side effects may go away during treat-ment as your body adjusts to the medicine. Also, your health care professional may be able to tell you about ways to pre-vent or reduce some of these side effects. Check with your health care professional if any of the following side effects continue or are bothersome or if you have any questions about them:

More common
Crusting of skin; difficulty in wearing contact lenses (may continue after medicine is stopped); dryness of eyes (may continue after treatment is stopped); dry-ness of mouth or nose; dryness or itching of skin; head-ache (mild); increased sensitivity of skin to sunlight; peeling of skin on palms of hands or soles of feet; stomach upset; thinning of hair (may continue after treatment is stopped)

Incidence not determined
Abnormal menstruation; burning, crawling, itching, numbness, prickling, "pins and needles" or tingling feeling; changes in fingernails or toenails; continuing ringing or buzzing, or other unexplained noise in ears; dandruff; darkening of skin; fatigue; flushing; hair ab-normalities; hair loss; increased hair growth, especially on the face; large amount of triglyceride in the blood;

lightening of normal skin color; lightening of treated areas of dark skin; nervousness; oily skin; redness of face; severe sunburn; skin rash, encrusted, scaly and oozing; sleeplessness; stomach burning; sweating; trouble sleeping; unable to sleep; unusual drowsiness, dullness, tiredness, weakness or feeling of sluggish-ness; unusually warm skin of face; voice changes

Other side effects not listed may also occur in some patients. If you notice any other effects, check with your healthcare professional.

KETOCONAZOLE (Topical route) - kee-toe-KOE-na-zole

Commonly used brand name(s)

In the U.S.—
Nizoral
Nizoral A-D
Xolegel

In Canada—
Ketoderm

Available Dosage Forms:

- Cream
- Shampoo
- Solution
- Gel/Jelly

Therapeutic Class: Antifungal

Uses For This Medicine

Ketoconazole is used to treat infections caused by a fungus or yeast. It works by killing the fungus or yeast or preventing its growth.

Ketoconazole cream is used to treat:
- Athlete's foot (tinea pedis; ringworm of the foot);
- Ringworm of the body (tinea corporis);
- Ringworm of the groin (tinea cruris; jock itch);
- Seborrheic dermatitis;
- "Sun fungus" (tinea versicolor; pityriasis versicolor); and
- Yeast infection of the skin (cutaneous candidiasis).

Ketoconazole 1% shampoo is used to treat dandruff.

Ketoconazole 2% shampoo is used to treat "sun fungus" (tinea versicolor; pityriasis versicolor).

This medicine may also be used for other fungus infections of the skin as determined by your doctor.

Ketoconazole is available without a doctor's prescription.

Before Using This Medicine

In deciding to use a medicine, the risks of taking the medicine must be weighed against the good it will do. This is a decision you and your doctor will make. For this medicine, the following should be considered:

Allergies—Tell your doctor if you have ever had any un-usual or allergic reaction to this medicine or any other medi-cines. Also tell your health care professional if you have any other types of allergies, such as to foods, dyes, preservatives,

or animals. For non-prescription products, read the label or package ingredients carefully.

Pediatric—Studies on this medicine have been done only in adult patients, and there is no specific information comparing use of this medicine in children with use in other age groups.

Geriatric—Many medicines have not been studied specifically in older people. Therefore, it may not be known whether they work exactly the same way they do in younger adults or if they cause different side effects or problems in older people. There is no specific information comparing use of topical ketoconazole in the elderly with use in other age groups.

Other medicines—Although certain medicines should not be used together at all, in other cases two different medicines may be used together even if an interaction might occur. In these cases, your doctor may want to change the dose, or other precautions may be necessary. Tell your healthcare professional if you are taking any other prescription or nonprescription (over-the-counter [OTC]) medicine.

Interactions with Food/Tobacco/Alcohol—Certain medicines should not be used at or around the time of eating food or eating certain types of food since interactions may occur. Using alcohol or tobacco with certain medicines may also cause interactions to occur. Discuss with your healthcare professional the use of your medicine with food, alcohol, or tobacco.

Proper Use of This Medicine

Keep this medicine away from the eyes.

For patients using the cream form of this medicine:

- Apply enough ketoconazole cream to cover the affected and surrounding skin areas, and rub in gently.
- To help clear up your infection completely, it is very important that you keep using ketoconazole cream for the full time of treatment, even if your symptoms begin to clear up after a few days. Since fungus or yeast infections may be very slow to clear up, you may have to continue using this medicine every day for up to several weeks. If you stop using this medicine too soon, your symptoms may return. Do not miss any doses.

For patients using the 1% shampoo form of this medicine:

- Wet your hair and scalp well with water.
- Apply enough shampoo to work up a good lather and gently massage it over your entire scalp.
- Rinse your hair and scalp with warm water.
- Repeat application.
- Rinse your hair and scalp well with warm water, and dry your hair.

For patients using the 2% shampoo form of this medicine:

- Wet your hair and scalp well with water.
- Apply the shampoo to the skin of the affected area and a wide margin surrounding this area.
- Work up a good lather and leave it in place for 5 minutes.
- Rinse your hair and scalp well with warm water, and dry your hair.

Dosing—The dose of this medicine will be different for different patients. Follow your doctor's orders or the directions on the label. The following information includes only the average doses of this medicine. If your dose is different, do not change it unless your doctor tells you to do so.

The amount of medicine that you take depends on the strength of the medicine. Also, the number of doses you take each day, the time allowed between doses, and the length of time you take the medicine depend on the medical problem for which you are using the medicine.

- For cream dosage form:
  - For cutaneous candidiasis, tinea corporis, tinea cruris, tinea pedis, or pityriasis versicolor:
    - Adults—Apply once a day to the affected skin and surrounding area.
    - Children—Use and dose must be determined by your doctor.
  - For seborrheic dermatitis:
    - Adults—Apply two times a day to the affected skin and surrounding area.
    - Children—Use and dose must be determined by your doctor.
- For 1% shampoo dosage form:
  - For dandruff:
    - Adults—Use every 3 or 4 days for up to 8 weeks. Then use only as needed to keep dandruff under control.
    - Children—Use and dose must be determined by your doctor.
- For 2% shampoo dosage form:
  - For pityriasis versicolor:
    - Adults—Use once.
    - Children—Use and dose must be determined by your doctor.

Missed dose—If you miss a dose of this medicine, apply it as soon as possible. However, if it is almost time for your next dose, skip the missed dose and go back to your regular dosing schedule.

Storage—Store the medicine in a closed container at room temperature, away from heat, moisture, and direct light. Keep from freezing.

Keep out of the reach of children.

Do not keep outdated medicine or medicine no longer needed.

Precautions While Using This Medicine

If your skin problem does not improve within:

- 2 weeks for cutaneous candidiasis, pityriasis versicolor, tinea corporis, or tinea cruris;
- 4 weeks for seborrheic dermatitis; or
- 4 to 6 weeks for tinea pedis;

or if it becomes worse, check with your doctor.

For patients using the cream form of this medicine:

- To help clear up your infection completely and to help make sure it does not return, good health habits are also required.
- For patients using ketoconazole cream for athlete's foot (tinea pedis; ringworm of the foot), the following instructions will help keep the feet cool and dry.
  - Avoid wearing socks made from wool or synthetic materials (for example, rayon or nylon). Instead, wear clean, cotton socks and change them daily or more often if your feet sweat a lot.
  - Wear sandals or well-ventilated shoes (for examples, shoes with holes).

- ○ Use a bland, absorbent powder (for example, talcum powder) or an antifungal powder between the toes, on the feet, and in socks and shoes one or two times a day. It is best to use the powder between the times you use ketoconazole cream.
- ○ If you have any questions about these instructions, check with your health care professional.
- For patients using ketoconazole cream for ringworm of the groin (tinea cruris; jock itch), the following instructions will help reduce chafing and irritation and will also help keep the groin area cool and dry.
  - ○ Avoid wearing underwear that is tight-fitting or made from synthetic materials (for example, rayon or nylon). Instead, wear loose-fitting, cotton underwear.
  - ○ Use a bland, absorbent powder (for example, talcum powder) or an antifungal powder on the skin. It is best to use the powder between the times you use ketoconazole cream.
  - ○ If you have any questions about these instructions, check with your health care professional.

Side Effects of This Medicine

Along with its needed effects, a medicine may cause some unwanted effects. Although not all of these side effects may occur, if they do occur they may need medical attention.

Check with your doctor as soon as possible if any of the following side effects occur:

Less common—For cream or shampoo
Itching, stinging, or irritation not present before use of this medicine

Rare—For cream
Skin rash

Some side effects may occur that usually do not need medical attention. These side effects may go away during treatment as your body adjusts to the medicine. Also, your health care professional may be able to tell you about ways to prevent or reduce some of these side effects. Check with your health care professional if any of the following side effects continue or are bothersome or if you have any questions about them:

Less common—For shampoo
Dry skin; dryness or oiliness of the hair and scalp

Other side effects not listed may also occur in some patients. If you notice any other effects, check with your healthcare professional.

KETOROLAC (Ophthalmic route) -
kee-toe-ROLE-ak

Commonly used brand name(s)

In the U.S.—
Acular
Acular LS
Acular PF

Available Dosage Forms:
- Solution

Therapeutic Class: Ophthalmologic Agent
Pharmacologic Class: NSAID

Uses For This Medicine

Ophthalmic ketorolac is an anti-inflammatory medicine. It is used in the eye to treat itching caused by seasonal allergic conjunctivitis (an allergy that occurs at only certain times of the year). Ophthalmic ketorolac is also used to treat inflammation of the eye following cataract surgery.

This medicine may also be used to prevent or treat other conditions, as determined by your ophthalmologist (eye doctor).

Before Using This Medicine

In deciding to use a medicine, the risks of taking the medicine must be weighed against the good it will do. This is a decision you and your doctor will make. For this medicine, the following should be considered:

Allergies—Tell your doctor if you have ever had any unusual or allergic reaction to this medicine or any other medicines. Also tell your health care professional if you have any other types of allergies, such as to foods, dyes, preservatives, or animals. For non-prescription products, read the label or package ingredients carefully.

Pediatric—Studies on this medicine have been done only in adult patients, and there is no specific information comparing use of ophthalmic ketorolac in children with use in other age groups.

Geriatric—Many medicines have not been studied specifically in older people. Therefore, it may not be known whether they work exactly the same way they do in younger adults. Although there is no specific information comparing use of ophthalmic ketorolac in the elderly with use in other age groups, this medicine is not expected to cause different side effects or problems in older people than it does in younger adults.

Other medicines—Although certain medicines should not be used together at all, in other cases two different medicines may be used together even if an interaction might occur. In these cases, your doctor may want to change the dose, or other precautions may be necessary. Tell your healthcare professional if you are taking any other prescription or non-prescription (over-the-counter [OTC]) medicine.

Interactions with Food/Tobacco/Alcohol—Certain medicines should not be used at or around the time of eating food or eating certain types of food since interactions may occur. Using alcohol or tobacco with certain medicines may also cause interactions to occur. Discuss with your healthcare professional the use of your medicine with food, alcohol, or tobacco.

Other medical problems—The presence of other medical problems may affect the use of this medicine. Make sure you tell your doctor if you have any other medical problems, especially:
- Hemophilia or
- Other bleeding problems—The possibility of bleeding may be increased during eye surgery

Proper Use of This Medicine

To use:

- First, wash your hands. Tilt the head back and, pressing your finger gently on the skin just beneath the lower eyelid, pull the lower eyelid away from the eye to make a space. Drop the medicine into this space. Let go of the eyelid and gently close the eyes. Do not blink. Keep the eyes closed for 1 or 2 minutes to allow the medicine to be absorbed by the eye.
- If you think you did not get the drop of medicine into your eye properly, use another drop.
- To keep the medicine as germ-free as possible, do not touch the applicator tip to any surface (including the eye). Also, keep the container tightly closed.

Dosing—The dose of this medicine will be different for different patients. Follow your doctor's orders or the directions on the label. The following information includes only the average doses of this medicine. If your dose is different, do not change it unless your doctor tells you to do so.

The amount of medicine that you take depends on the strength of the medicine. Also, the number of doses you take each day, the time allowed between doses, and the length of time you take the medicine depend on the medical problem for which you are using the medicine.

- For ophthalmic solution (eye drops) dosage form:
  - For itching of the eye
    - Adults—Use one drop in each eye four times a day for up to one week or as directed by your doctor.
    - Children—Use and dose must be determined by your doctor.
  - For inflammation of the eye following cataract surgery
    - Adults—Use one drop in the affected eye(s) four times a day beginning twenty-four hours after surgery and continuing for two weeks.
    - Children—Use and dose must be determined by your doctor.

Missed dose—If you miss a dose of this medicine, take it as soon as possible. However, if it is almost time for your next dose, skip the missed dose and go back to your regular dosing schedule. Do not double doses.

Storage—Store the medicine in a closed container at room temperature, away from heat, moisture, and direct light. Keep from freezing.

Keep out of the reach of children.

Do not keep outdated medicine or medicine no longer needed.

Precautions While Using This Medicine

If your symptoms do not improve within a few days, or if they become worse, check with your doctor.

While applying this medicine, your eyes will probably sting or burn for a short time. This is to be expected.

Side Effects of This Medicine

Along with its needed effects, a medicine may cause some unwanted effects. Although not all of these side effects may occur, if they do occur they may need medical attention.

Check with your doctor as soon as possible if any of the following side effects occur:

Less common or rare

Burning, itching, redness, swelling, tearing, or other sign of eye irritation not present before therapy or becoming worse during therapy; skin rash around eye

Some side effects may occur that usually do not need medical attention. These side effects may go away during treatment as your body adjusts to the medicine. Also, your health care professional may be able to tell you about ways to prevent or reduce some of these side effects. Check with your health care professional if any of the following side effects continue or are bothersome or if you have any questions about them:

More common

Stinging or burning of eye when medicine is applied

Other side effects not listed may also occur in some patients. If you notice any other effects, check with your healthcare professional.

KETOROLAC (Oral route, Intravenous route, Injection route, Intramuscular route) - kee-toe-ROLE-ak

Black Box Warning

- Ketorolac tromethamine, a nonsteroidal anti-inflammatory drug (NSAID), is indicated for the short-term (up to 5 days in adults) management of moderately severe acute pain that requires analgesia at the opioid level. It is not indicated for minor or chronic painful conditions. Ketorolac tromethamine is a potent NSAID analgesic, and its administration carries many risks. The resulting NSAID-related adverse events can be serious in certain patients for whom ketorolac tromethamine is indicated, especially when the drug is used inappropriately. Increasing the dose of ketorolac tromethamine beyond the label recommendations will not provide better efficacy but will result in increasing the risk of developing serious adverse events.

- Gastrointestinal effects
  - Ketorolac tromethamine can cause peptic ulcers, gastrointestinal bleeding and/or perforation. Therefore, ketorolac tromethamine is contraindicated in patients with active peptic ulcer disease, in patients with recent gastrointestinal bleeding or perforation, and in patients with a history of peptic ulcer disease or gastrointestinal bleeding.

- Renal effects
  - Ketorolac tromethamine is contraindicated in patients with advanced renal impairment and in patients at risk for renal failure due to volume depletion.

- Risk of bleeding
  - Ketorolac tromethamine inhibits platelet function and is, therefore, contraindicated in patients with suspected or confirmed cerebrovascular bleeding, pa-

tients with hemorrhagic diathesis, incomplete hemostasis and those at high risk of bleeding.
  ○ Ketorolac tromethamine is contraindicated as prophylactic analgesic before any major surgery and is contraindicated intraoperatively when hemostasis is critical because of the increased risk of bleeding.
- Hypersensitivity
  ○ Hypersensitivity reactions, ranging from bronchospasm to anaphylactic shock, have occurred and appropriate counteractive measures must be available when administering the first dose of ketorolac tromethamine IV/IM. Ketorolac tromethamine is contraindicated in patients with previously demonstrated hypersensitivity to ketorolac tromethamine or allergic manifestations to aspirin or other nonsteroidal anti-inflammatory drugs (NSAIDs).
- Intrathecal or epidural administration
  ○ Ketorolac tromethamine is contraindicated for intrathecal or epidural administration due to its alcohol content.
- Labor, delivery and nursing
  ○ The use of ketorolac tromethamine in labor and delivery is contraindicated because it may adversely affect fetal circulation and inhibit uterine contractions.
  ○ The use of ketorolac tromethamine is contraindicated in nursing mothers because of the potential adverse effects of prostaglandin-inhibiting drugs on neonates.
- Concomitant use with NSAIDs
  ○ Ketorolac tromethamine is contraindicated in patients currently receiving ASA or NSAIDs because of the cumulative risk of inducing serious NSAID-related side effects.
- Dosage and administration
  ○ Ketorolac tromethamine oral is indicated only as continuation therapy to ketorolac tromethamine IV/IM, and the combined duration of use of ketorolac tromethamine IV/IM and ketorolac tromethamine oral is not to exceed 5 days because of the increased risk of serious adverse events.
  ○ The recommended total daily dose of ketorolac tromethamine oral (maximum 40 mg) is significantly lower than for ketorolac tromethamine IV/IM (maximum 120 mg).
- Special populations
  ○ Dosage should be adjusted for patients 65 years or older, for patients under 50 kg (110 lbs) of body weight and for patients with moderately elevated serum creatinine. Doses of ketorolac tromethamine IV/IM are not to exceed 60 mg (total dose per day) in these patients. Ketorolac tromethamine IV/IM is indicated as a single dose therapy in pediatric patients; not to exceed 30 mg for IM administration and 15 mg for IV administration.

Commonly used brand name(s)

In the U.S.—
  Toradol
  Toradol IV/IM

Available Dosage Forms:
- Solution
- Tablet
- Injectable

Therapeutic Class: Analgesic
Pharmacologic Class: NSAID

Uses For This Medicine

Ketorolac is used to relieve moderately severe pain, usually pain that occurs after an operation or other painful procedure. It belongs to the group of medicines called nonsteroidal anti-inflammatory drugs (NSAIDs). Ketorolac is not a narcotic and is not habit-forming. It will not cause physical or mental dependence, as narcotics can. However, ketorolac is sometimes used together with a narcotic to provide better pain relief than either medicine used alone.

Ketorolac has side effects that can be very dangerous. The risk of having a serious side effect increases with the dose of ketorolac and with the length of treatment. Therefore, ketorolac should not be used for more than 5 days. Before using this medicine, you should discuss with your doctor the good that this medicine can do as well as the risks of using it.

Ketorolac is available only with your doctor's prescription.

Once a medicine has been approved for marketing for a certain use, experience may show that it is also useful for other medical problems. Although these uses are not included in product labeling, ketorolac is used in certain patients with the following medical conditions:
- Pain after surgery in children

Before Using This Medicine

In deciding to use a medicine, the risks of taking the medicine must be weighed against the good it will do. This is a decision you and your doctor will make. For this medicine, the following should be considered:

Allergies—Tell your doctor if you have ever had any unusual or allergic reaction to this medicine or any other medicines. Also tell your health care professional if you have any other types of allergies, such as to foods, dyes, preservatives, or animals. For non-prescription products, read the label or package ingredients carefully.

Pediatric—Studies on this medicine have been done only in adult patients, and there is no specific information comparing use of ketorolac in children up to 16 years of age with use in other age groups.

Geriatric—Stomach or intestinal problems, swelling of the face, feet, or lower legs, or sudden decrease in the amount of urine may be especially likely to occur in elderly patients, who are usually more sensitive than younger adults to the effects of ketorolac. Also, elderly people are more likely than younger adults to get very sick if the medicine causes stomach problems. Studies in older adults have shown that ketorolac stays in the body longer than it does in younger people. Your doctor will consider this when deciding on how much ketorolac should be given for each dose and how often it should be given.

Pregnancy—

	Pregnancy Category	Explanation
All Trimesters	C	Animal studies have shown an adverse effect and there are no adequate studies in pregnant women OR no animal studies have been conducted and there are no adequate studies in pregnant women.

Breast Feeding—There are no adequate studies in women for determining infant risk when using this medication during breastfeeding. Weigh the potential benefits against the potential risks before taking this medication while breastfeeding.

Other medicines—

Using this medicine with any of the following medicines is not recommended. Your doctor may decide not to treat you with this medication or change some of the other medicines you take.

Aceclofenac, Acemetacin, Alclofenac, Apazone, Aspirin, Benoxaprofen, Bufexamac, Carprofen, Clometacin, Clonixin, Dexketoprofen, Diclofenac, Diflunisal, Dipyrone, Droxicam, Etodolac, Etofenamate, Felbinac, Fenbufen, Fenoprofen, Fentiazac, Floctafenine, Flufenamic Acid, Flurbiprofen, Ibuprofen, Indomethacin, Indoprofen, Isoxicam, Ketoprofen, Lornoxicam, Meclofenamate, Mefenamic Acid, Meloxicam, Nabumetone, Naproxen, Niflumic Acid, Nimesulide, Oxaprozin, Oxyphenbutazone, Phenylbutazone, Pirazolac, Piroxicam, Pirprofen, Propyphenazone, Proquazone, Sulindac, Suprofen, Tenidap, Tenoxicam, Tiaprofenic Acid, Tolmetin, Zomepirac

Interactions with Food/Tobacco/Alcohol—Certain medicines should not be used at or around the time of eating food or eating certain types of food since interactions may occur. Using alcohol or tobacco with certain medicines may also cause interactions to occur. Discuss with your healthcare professional the use of your medicine with food, alcohol, or tobacco.

Other medical problems—The presence of other medical problems may affect the use of this medicine. Make sure you tell your doctor if you have any other medical problems, especially:

- Alcohol abuse or
- Diabetes mellitus (sugar diabetes) or
- Edema (swelling of face, fingers, feet or lower legs caused by too much fluid in the body) or
- Kidney disease or
- Liver disease (severe) or
- Systemic lupus erythematosus (SLE)—The chance of serious side effects may be increased
- Asthma or
- Heart disease or
- High blood pressure—Ketorolac may make your condition worse.
- Bleeding in the brain (history of) or
- Hemophilia or other bleeding problems—Ketorolac may increase the chance of serious bleeding

- Bleeding from the stomach or intestines (history of) or
- Colitis, stomach ulcer, or other stomach or intestinal problems (or history of)—Ketorolac may make stomach or intestinal problems worse. Also, bleeding from the stomach or intestines is more likely to occur during ketorolac treatment in people with these conditions

Proper Use of This Medicine

For patients taking ketorolac tablets:

- To lessen stomach upset, ketorolac tablets should be taken with food (a meal or a snack) or with an antacid.
- Take this medicine with a full glass of water. Also, do not lie down for about 15 to 30 minutes after taking it. This helps to prevent irritation that may lead to trouble in swallowing.

For patients using ketorolac injection:

- Medicines given by injection are sometimes used at home. If you will be using ketorolac at home, your health care professional will teach you how the injections are to be given. You will also have a chance to practice giving injections. Be certain that you understand exactly how the medicine is to be injected.

For safe and effective use of this medicine, do not use more of it, do not use it more often, and do not use it for more than 5 days. Using too much of this medicine increases the chance of unwanted effects, especially in elderly patients.

Ketorolac should be used only when it is ordered by your doctor for treating certain kinds of pain. Because of the risk of serious side effects, do not save any leftover ketorolac for use in the future, and do not share it with other people.

Dosing—The dose of this medicine will be different for different patients. Follow your doctor's orders or the directions on the label. The following information includes only the average doses of this medicine. If your dose is different, do not change it unless your doctor tells you to do so.

The amount of medicine that you take depends on the strength of the medicine. Also, the number of doses you take each day, the time allowed between doses, and the length of time you take the medicine depend on the medical problem for which you are using the medicine.

- For oral dosage form (tablets):
  - For pain:
    - Adults (patients 16 years of age and older)—One 10–milligram (mg) tablet four times a day, four to six hours apart. Some people may be directed to take two tablets for the first dose only.
    - Children up to 16 years of age—Use and dose must be determined by your doctor.
- For injection dosage form:
  - For pain:
    - Adults (patients 16 years of age and older)—15 or 30 mg, injected into a muscle or a vein four times a day, at least 6 hours apart. This amount of medicine may be contained in 1 mL or in one-half (0.5) mL of the injection, depending on the strength. Some people who do not need more than one injection may receive one dose of 60 mg, injected into a muscle.
    - Children up to 16 years of age—Use and dose must be determined by your doctor.

Missed dose—If you miss a dose of this medicine, take it as soon as possible. However, if it is almost time for your next dose, skip the missed dose and go back to your regular dosing schedule. Do not double doses.

Storage—Store the medicine in a closed container at room temperature, away from heat, moisture, and direct light. Do not refrigerate. Keep from freezing.

Keep out of the reach of children.

Do not keep outdated medicine or medicine no longer needed.

Precautions While Using This Medicine

Taking certain other medicines together with ketorolac may increase the chance of unwanted effects. The risk will depend on how much of each medicine you take every day, and on how long you take the medicines together. Therefore, do not take acetaminophen (e.g., Tylenol) together with ketorolac for more than a few days, unless otherwise directed by your medical doctor or dentist. Also, do not take any of the following medicines together with ketorolac, unless your medical doctor or dentist has directed you to do so and is following your progress:

- Aspirin or other salicylates
- Diclofenac (e.g., Voltaren)
- Diflunisal (e.g., Dolobid)
- Etodolac (e.g., Lodine)
- Fenoprofen (e.g., Nalfon)
- Floctafenine (e.g., Idarac)
- Flurbiprofen (e.g., Ansaid)
- Ibuprofen (e.g., Motrin)
- Indomethacin (e.g., Indocin)
- Ketoprofen (e.g., Orudis)
- Meclofenamate (e.g., Meclomen)
- Mefenamic acid (e.g., Ponstel)
- Nabumetone (e.g., Relafen)
- Naproxen (e.g., Naprosyn)
- Oxaprozin (e.g., Daypro)
- Phenylbutazone (e.g., Butazolidin)
- Piroxicam (e.g., Feldene)
- Sulindac (e.g., Clinoril)
- Tenoxicam (e.g., Mobiflex)
- Tiaprofenic acid (e.g., Surgam)
- Tolmetin (e.g., Tolectin)
- Zomepirac (e.g., Zomax)

Ketorolac may cause some people to become dizzy or drowsy. If either of these side effects occurs, *do not drive, use machines, or do anything else that could be dangerous if you are not alert.*

Serious side effects can occur during treatment with this medicine. Sometimes serious side effects can occur without any warning. However, possible warning signs often occur, including swelling of the face, fingers, feet, and/or lower legs; severe stomach pain, black, tarry stools, and/or vomiting of blood or material that looks like coffee grounds; unusual weight gain; and/or skin rash. Also, signs of serious heart problems could occur such as chest pain, tightness in chest, fast or irregular heartbeat, or unusual flushing or warmth of skin. *Stop taking this medicine and check with your doctor immediately if you notice any of these warning signs.*

Side Effects of This Medicine

Along with its needed effects, a medicine may cause some unwanted effects. Although not all of these side effects may occur, if they do occur they may need medical attention.

Stop taking this medicine and get emergency help immediately if any of the following effects occur:
Rare
Bleeding from the rectum or bloody or black, tarry stools; bleeding or crusting sores on lips; blue lips and fingernails; chest pain; convulsions; fainting; shortness of breath, fast, irregular, noisy, or troubled breathing, tightness in chest, and/or wheezing; vomiting of blood or material that looks like coffee grounds

Check with your doctor as soon as possible if any of the following side effects occur:
More common
Swelling of face, fingers, lower legs, ankles, and/or feet; weight gain (unusual)

Less common
Bruising (not at place of injection); high blood pressure; skin rash or itching; small, red spots on skin; sores, ulcers, or white spots on lips or in mouth

Rare
Abdominal or stomach pain, cramping, or burning (severe); bloody or cloudy urine; blurred vision of other vision change; burning, red, tender, thick, scaly, or peeling skin; cough or hoarseness; dark urine; decrease in amount of urine (sudden); fever with severe headache, drowsiness, confusion, and stiff neck or back; fever with or without chills or sore throat; general feeling of illness; hallucinations (seeing, hearing, or feeling things that are not there); hearing loss; hives; increase in amount of urine or urinating often; light-colored stools; loss of appetite; low blood pressure; mood changes or unusual behavior; muscle cramps or pain; nausea, heartburn, and/or indigestion (severe and continuing); nosebleeds; pain in lower back and/or side; pain, tenderness, and/or swelling in the upper abdominal area; painful or difficult urination; pale skin; puffiness or swelling of the eyelids or around the eyes; ringing or buzzing in ears; runny nose; severe restlessness; swollen and/or painful glands; swollen tongue; thirst (continuing); unusual tiredness or weakness; yellow eyes or skin

Some side effects may occur that usually do not need medical attention. These side effects may go away during treatment as your body adjusts to the medicine. Also, your health care professional may be able to tell you about ways to prevent or reduce some of these side effects. Check with your health care professional if any of the following side effects continue or are bothersome or if you have any questions about them:
More common
Abdominal or stomach pain (mild or moderate); bruising at place of injection; diarrhea; dizziness; drowsiness; headache; indigestion; nausea

Less common or rare

> Bloating or gas; burning or pain at place of injection; constipation; feeling of fullness in abdominal or stomach area; increased sweating; vomiting

Other side effects not listed may also occur in some patients. If you notice any other effects, check with your healthcare professional.

KETOTIFEN (Ophthalmic route) - kee-toe-TYE-fen

Commonly used brand name(s)

In the U.S.—
> Zaditor

Available Dosage Forms:
- Solution

Therapeutic Class: Ophthalmologic Agent
Pharmacologic Class: Mast Cell Stabilizer

Uses For This Medicine

Ketotifen ophthalmic (eye) solution is used to temporarily prevent itching of the eye caused by a condition known as allergic conjunctivitis. It works by acting on certain cells, called mast cells, to prevent them from releasing substances that cause the allergic reaction.

This medicine is available only with your doctor's prescription.

Before Using This Medicine

In deciding to use a medicine, the risks of taking the medicine must be weighed against the good it will do. This is a decision you and your doctor will make. For this medicine, the following should be considered:

Allergies—Tell your doctor if you have ever had any unusual or allergic reaction to this medicine or any other medicines. Also tell your health care professional if you have any other types of allergies, such as to foods, dyes, preservatives, or animals. For non-prescription products, read the label or package ingredients carefully.

Pediatric—Studies on this medicine have been done only in adult patients, and there is no specific information comparing use of ketotifen in children younger than 3 years of age with use in other age groups.

Geriatric—Many medicines have not been studied specifically in older people. Therefore, it may not be known whether they work exactly the same way they do in younger adults or if they cause different side effects or problems in older people. There is no specific information comparing use of ophthalmic ketotifen in the elderly with use in other age groups.

Pregnancy—

	Pregnancy Category	Explanation
All Trimesters	C	Animal studies have shown an adverse effect and there are no adequate studies in pregnant women OR no animal studies have been conducted and there are no adequate studies in pregnant women.

Breast Feeding—There are no adequate studies in women for determining infant risk when using this medication during breastfeeding. Weigh the potential benefits against the potential risks before taking this medication while breastfeeding.

Other medicines—Although certain medicines should not be used together at all, in other cases two different medicines may be used together even if an interaction might occur. In these cases, your doctor may want to change the dose, or other precautions may be necessary. Tell your healthcare professional if you are taking any other prescription or non-prescription (over-the-counter [OTC]) medicine.

Interactions with Food/Tobacco/Alcohol—Certain medicines should not be used at or around the time of eating food or eating certain types of food since interactions may occur. Using alcohol or tobacco with certain medicines may also cause interactions to occur. Discuss with your healthcare professional the use of your medicine with food, alcohol, or tobacco.

Proper Use of This Medicine

Do not wear contact lenses if your eyes are red. Also, do not use this medicine to treat irritation related to contact lens use. If you wear contact lenses: Take out your contact lenses before using ketotifen eye drops. Wait at least 10 minutes after putting the eye drops in before putting the contact lenses back in.

To use the eye drops:

- First, wash your hands. Tilt the head back and, pressing your finger gently on the skin just beneath the lower eyelid, pull the lower eyelid away from the eye to make a space. Drop the medicine into this space. Let go of the eyelid and gently close the eyes. Do not blink. Keep the eyes closed for 1 to 2 minutes to allow the medicine to be absorbed by the eye.

- If you think you did not get the drop of medicine into your eye properly, use another drop.

- To keep the medicine as germ-free as possible, do not touch the applicator tip to any surface (including the eye). Also, keep the container tightly closed.

Dosing—The dose of this medicine will be different for different patients. Follow your doctor's orders or the directions on the label. The following information includes only the average doses of this medicine. If your dose is different, do not change it unless your doctor tells you to do so.

The amount of medicine that you take depends on the strength of the medicine. Also, the number of doses you take each day, the time allowed between doses, and the length of

time you take the medicine depend on the medical problem for which you are using the medicine.

- For ophthalmic dosage form (eye drops):
  - For prevention of itching of the eye due to allergic conjunctivitis (eye allergy):
    - Adults and children 3 years of age and older— Use one drop in each affected eye every 8 to 12 hours.
    - Children up to 3 years of age—Use and dose must be determined by your doctor.

Missed dose—If you miss a dose of this medicine, take it as soon as possible. However, if it is almost time for your next dose, skip the missed dose and go back to your regular dosing schedule. Do not double doses.

Storage—Store the medicine in a closed container at room temperature, away from heat, moisture, and direct light. Keep from freezing.

Keep out of the reach of children.

Do not keep outdated medicine or medicine no longer needed.

Ask your healthcare professional how you should dispose of any medicine you do not use.

Precautions While Using This Medicine

If your symptoms do not improve or if your condition becomes worse, check with your doctor.

Side Effects of This Medicine

Along with its needed effects, a medicine may cause some unwanted effects. Although not all of these side effects may occur, if they do occur they may need medical attention.

Check with your doctor as soon as possible if any of the following side effects occur:
More common
  Eye redness and swelling

Less common
  Eye discharge; eye discomfort; eye pain; hives; increased itching of eyes; rash.

Some side effects may occur that usually do not need medical attention. These side effects may go away during treatment as your body adjusts to the medicine. Also, your health care professional may be able to tell you about ways to prevent or reduce some of these side effects. Check with your health care professional if any of the following side effects continue or are bothersome or if you have any questions about them:
More common
  Headaches; stuffy or runny nose

Less common
  Burning or stinging of eyes; dry eyes; eyelid disorder; eye sensitivity to light; fever, tiredness, achiness, and sore throat; increase in size of pupils; sore throat; tearing.

Other side effects not listed may also occur in some patients. If you notice any other effects, check with your healthcare professional.

KETOTIFEN (Oral route) - kee-toe-TYE-fen

Uses For This Medicine

Ketotifen is a type of asthma medication which, when taken every day and used along with other antiasthma medications, may reduce the frequency, severity, and duration of asthma symptoms or attacks in children. It may also lead to a reduction in daily requirements of other antiasthma medications. Ketotifen is not effective for the prevention or treatment of acute asthma attacks. Ketotifen works by inhibiting certain substances in the body that are known to cause inflammation and symptoms of asthma.

This medicine is available only with your doctor's prescription.

Before Using This Medicine

In deciding to use a medicine, the risks of taking the medicine must be weighed against the good it will do. This is a decision you and your doctor will make. For this medicine, the following should be considered:

Allergies—Tell your doctor if you have ever had any unusual or allergic reaction to this medicine or any other medicines. Also tell your health care professional if you have any other types of allergies, such as to foods, dyes, preservatives, or animals. For non-prescription products, read the label or package ingredients carefully.

Pediatric—This medicine has been tested in children and, in effective doses, has not been shown to cause different side effects or problems than it does in adults.

Geriatric—Many medicines have not been studied specifically in older people. Therefore, it may not be known whether they work exactly the same way they do in younger adults or if they cause different side effects or problems in older people. There is no specific information comparing use of ketotifen in the elderly with use in other age groups.

Other medicines—Although certain medicines should not be used together at all, in other cases two different medicines may be used together even if an interaction might occur. In these cases, your doctor may want to change the dose, or other precautions may be necessary. Tell your healthcare professional if you are taking any other prescription or non-prescription (over-the-counter [OTC]) medicine.

Interactions with Food/Tobacco/Alcohol—Certain medicines should not be used at or around the time of eating food or eating certain types of food since interactions may occur. Using alcohol or tobacco with certain medicines may also cause interactions to occur. Discuss with your healthcare professional the use of your medicine with food, alcohol, or tobacco.

Other medical problems—The presence of other medical problems may affect the use of this medicine. Make sure you tell your doctor if you have any other medical problems, especially:

- Diabetes mellitus (sugar diabetes)—May alter low-sugar diet (syrup contains carbohydrates)
- Epilepsy—May increase risk of convulsions (seizures)

Proper Use of This Medicine

Make certain your health care professional knows if you are on any special diet, such as a low-sugar diet. The syrup contains carbohydrates.

Ketotifen is used to help prevent asthma attacks. It will not relieve an asthma attack that has already started.

Ketotifen must be taken continuously in order to be effective.

Continue taking your current asthma medications until instructed otherwise by your doctor.

Ketotifen may be taken with or without food.

Dosing—The dose of this medicine will be different for different patients. Follow your doctor's orders or the directions on the label. The following information includes only the average doses of this medicine. If your dose is different, do not change it unless your doctor tells you to do so.

The amount of medicine that you take depends on the strength of the medicine. Also, the number of doses you take each day, the time allowed between doses, and the length of time you take the medicine depend on the medical problem for which you are using the medicine.

- For oral dosage form (tablets and syrup):
  - For asthma:
    - Adults and children 3 years of age and older—The usual dose is 1 milligram (mg) (1 tablet or 5 milliliters [mL] of syrup) twice daily, once in the morning and once in the evening.
    - Infants and children from 6 months to 3 years of age—Dose is based on body weight and must be determined by the doctor. It is usually 0.25 mL (50 mcg or 0.05 mg) of syrup per kilogram (kg) (110 micrograms [mcg] or 0.110 mg per pound) of body weight twice daily, once in the morning and once in the evening.

Missed dose—If you miss a dose of this medicine, take it as soon as possible. However, if it is almost time for your next dose, skip the missed dose and go back to your regular dosing schedule. Do not double doses.

Storage—Store the medicine in a closed container at room temperature, away from heat, moisture, and direct light. Keep from freezing.

Keep out of the reach of children.

Do not keep outdated medicine or medicine no longer needed.

Precautions While Using This Medicine

It is very important that your doctor check your progress at regular visits. This will allow your doctor to see if the medicine is working properly and to decide if you should continue to take it. If your symptoms worsen, you should check with your doctor.

This medicine may cause some people to become drowsy, dizzy, or less alert than they are normally. Make sure you know how you react to this medicine before you drive, use machines, or do anything else that could be dangerous if you are dizzy or are not alert.

This medicine may cause some people to become excited, irritable, or nervous or to have trouble in sleeping. These are symptoms of central nervous system stimulation and are especially likely to occur in children.

For patients with diabetes:
- The syrup form of this medicine may affect blood sugar levels. If you notice a change in the results of your blood or urine sugar tests or if you have any questions, check with your doctor.

Side Effects of This Medicine

Along with its needed effects, a medicine may cause some unwanted effects. Although not all of these side effects may occur, if they do occur they may need medical attention.

Check with your doctor as soon as possible if any of the following side effects occur:

Less common
Chills; cough; diarrhea; fever; general feeling of discomfort or illness; headache; joint pain; loss of appetite; muscle aches and pains; nausea; runny nose; shivering; sore throat; sweating; trouble sleeping; unusual tiredness or weakness; vomiting

Rare
Abdominal or stomach pain; blistering, itching, peeling, or redness of skin; bloody or cloudy urine; clay-colored stools; convulsions; dark urine; difficult, burning, or painful urination; dizziness; frequent urge to urinate; muscle spasm or jerking of all extremities; rash; sudden loss of consciousness; unpleasant breath odor; vomiting of blood; yellow eyes or skin

Symptoms of overdose

Get emergency help immediately if any of the following symptoms of overdose occur:

Blurred vision; confusion; convulsions; disorientation; dizziness; drowsiness (severe); faintness or lightheadedness when getting up from a lying or sitting position; fast, pounding, or irregular heartbeat or pulse; hyperexcitability; loss of consciousness; palpitations; sweating; unusual tiredness or weakness

Some side effects may occur that usually do not need medical attention. These side effects may go away during treatment as your body adjusts to the medicine. Also, your health care professional may be able to tell you about ways to prevent or reduce some of these side effects. Check with your health care professional if any of the following side effects continue or are bothersome or if you have any questions about them:

More common
Weight gain

Less common or rare
Bloody nose; drowsiness; dryness of mouth; excitation; increased appetite; irritability; nervousness; swelling of eyelids; unexplained nosebleeds

Other side effects not listed may also occur in some patients. If you notice any other effects, check with your healthcare professional.

LAMIVUDINE   (Oral route) - la-MI-vyoo-deen

Black Box Warning

Lactic acidosis and severe hepatomegaly with steatosis, including fatal cases, have been reported with the use of nucleoside analogues alone or in combination, including lamivudine and other antiretrovirals.

- EPIVIR®
  - EPIVIR® tablets and oral solution (used to treat HIV infection) contain a higher dose of the active ingredient (lamivudine) than EPIVIR-HBV® tablets and oral solution (used to treat chronic hepatitis B). Patients with HIV infection should receive only dosing forms appropriate for treatment of HIV.
  - Severe acute exacerbations of hepatitis B have been reported in patients who are co-infected with hepatitis B virus (HBV) and HIV and have discontinued lamivudine. Hepatic function should be monitored closely with both clinical and laboratory follow-up for at least several months in patients who discontinue lamivudine and are co-infected with HIV and HBV. If appropriate, initiation of anti-hepatitis B therapy may be warranted.
- EPIVIR-HBV®
  - Human immunodeficiency virus (HIV) counseling and testing should be offered to all patients before beginning EPIVIR-HBV® and periodically during treatment, because EPIVIR-HBV® tablets and oral solution contain a lower dose of the same active ingredient (lamivudine) as EPIVIR® tablets and oral solution used to treat HIV infection. If treatment with EPIVIR-HBV® is prescribed for chronic hepatitis B for a patient with unrecognized or untreated HIV infection, rapid emergence of HIV resistance is likely because of subtherapeutic dose and inappropriate monotherapy.
  - Severe acute exacerbations of hepatitis B have been reported in patients who have discontinued anti-hepatitis B therapy (including EPIVIR-HBV®). Hepatic function should be monitored closely with both clinical and laboratory follow-up for at least several months in patients who discontinue anti-hepatitis B therapy. If appropriate, initiation of anti-hepatitis B therapy may be warranted.

Commonly used brand name(s)

In the U.S.—
Epivir
Epivir HBV

In Canada—
3tc
Heptovir

Available Dosage Forms:
- Tablet
- Solution

Therapeutic Class: Antiretroviral Agent
Pharmacologic Class: Nucleoside Reverse Transcriptase Inhibitor

Uses For This Medicine

Lamivudine is used in the treatment of the infection caused by the human immunodeficiency virus (HIV) or hepatitis B virus. HIV is the virus that causes acquired immune deficiency syndrome (AIDS). Lamivudine is taken together with zidovudine (AZT) or other medications used to treat HIV.

Lamivudine will not cure or prevent HIV infection or AIDS; however, it helps keep HIV from reproducing and appears to slow down the destruction of the immune system. This may help delay the development of problems usually related to AIDS or HIV disease. Lamivudine will not keep you from spreading HIV to other people. People who receive this medicine may continue to have other problems usually related to AIDS or HIV disease. Lamivudine is not a cure for the hepatitis B virus; the long-term effects of the drug on the infection and the liver are unknown at this time.

Lamivudine is available only with your doctor's prescription.

Once a medicine has been approved for marketing for a certain use, experience may show that it is also useful for other medical problems. Although this use is not included in product labeling, lamivudine is used in certain patients with the following medical condition:

- Human immunodeficiency virus (HIV) infection due to occupational exposure (possible prevention of)

Before Using This Medicine

In deciding to use a medicine, the risks of taking the medicine must be weighed against the good it will do. This is a decision you and your doctor will make. For this medicine, the following should be considered:

Allergies—Tell your doctor if you have ever had any unusual or allergic reaction to this medicine or any other medicines. Also tell your health care professional if you have any other types of allergies, such as to foods, dyes, preservatives, or animals. For non-prescription products, read the label or package ingredients carefully.

Pediatric—Lamivudine can cause serious side effects. In one study, children with advanced AIDS were more likely than children who were less ill to develop pancreatitis (inflammation of the pancreas) and peripheral neuropathy (a problem involving the nerves). Therefore, it is especially important that you discuss with your child's doctor the good that this medicine may do as well as the risks of using it. Your child must be seen frequently and your child's progress carefully followed by the doctor while the child is taking lamivudine.

Geriatric—Lamivudine has not been studied specifically in older people. Therefore, it is not known whether it causes different side effects or problems in the elderly than it does in younger adults. Talk to your doctor first if you have liver, kidney, heart problems or other diseases. Your doctor may need to adjust your dose.

Pregnancy—

	Pregnancy Category	Explanation
All Trimesters	C	Animal studies have shown an adverse effect and there are no adequate studies in pregnant women OR no animal studies have been conducted and there are no adequate studies in pregnant women.

Breast Feeding—There are no adequate studies in women for determining infant risk when using this medication during

breastfeeding. Weigh the potential benefits against the potential risks before taking this medication while breastfeeding.

Other medicines—

Using this medicine with any of the following medicines is usually not recommended, but may be required in some cases. If both medicines are prescribed together, your doctor may change the dose or how often you use one or both of the medicines.

Interferon Alfa, Ribavirin, Zalcitabine

Interactions with Food/Tobacco/Alcohol—Certain medicines should not be used at or around the time of eating food or eating certain types of food since interactions may occur. Using alcohol or tobacco with certain medicines may also cause interactions to occur. Discuss with your healthcare professional the use of your medicine with food, alcohol, or tobacco.

Other medical problems—The presence of other medical problems may affect the use of this medicine. Make sure you tell your doctor if you have any other medical problems, especially:

- Combined infection of HIV and hepatitis B—May make the condition of either of these infections worse
- Diabetes mellitus (sugar diabetes)—Lamivudine oral solution contains sucrose
- Hepatitis C or
- Hepatitis delta—Caution should be used; lamivudine safety has not been determined in patients who have hepatitis infections
- Human immunodeficiency virus—For patients with hepatitis B virus, your physician will talk to you about HIV before you begin taking lamivudine. You may be tested for HIV. Lamivudine tablets and oral solution for hepatitis B virus contain lower amounts of the drug than the tablets and solution for HIV. If you start on the lower-dose medication and later learn that you have HIV, the higher-dose lamivudine may not then be effective against the infection caused by HIV.
- Inflamed pancreas or
- Problems with inflamed pancreas in the past or
- Other risk factors for developing an inflamed pancreas or
- Nerve damage—These conditions may occur or worsen when taking lamivudine
- Kidney disease—Patients with kidney disease may have an increased chance of side effects
- Liver disease or
- Risk factors for liver disease or
- Obesity (being overweight)—This medicine may make liver disease worse in patients with liver disease, obesity and other HIV medicine use.
- Organ transplant—Caution should be used; lamivudine safety has not been determined in patients who have received an organ transplant

Proper Use of This Medicine

Take this medicine exactly as directed by your doctor. Do not take more of it, do not take it more often, and do not take it for a longer time than your doctor ordered. Also, do not stop taking lamivudine or zidovudine without checking with your doctor first.

Keep taking lamivudine for the full time of treatment, even if you begin to feel better.

This medicine works best when there is a constant amount in the blood. To help keep the amount constant, do not miss any doses. If you need help in planning the best times to take your medicine, check with your health care professional.

If you are using lamivudine oral suspension, use a specially marked measuring spoon or other device to measure each dose accurately. The average household teaspoon may not hold the right amount of liquid. The lamivudine oral suspension contains sucrose. Tell your doctor if you are diabetic before you start taking this medicine.

Only take medicine that your doctor has prescribed specifically for you. Do not share your medicine with others.

Dosing—The dose of this medicine will be different for different patients. Follow your doctor's orders or the directions on the label. The following information includes only the average doses of this medicine. If your dose is different, do not change it unless your doctor tells you to do so.

The amount of medicine that you take depends on the strength of the medicine. Also, the number of doses you take each day, the time allowed between doses, and the length of time you take the medicine depend on the medical problem for which you are using the medicine.

- For oral dosage forms (oral solution and tablets):
  - For treatment of hepatitis B infection:
    - Adults—100 milligrams (mg) once a day.
    - Children younger than 16 years of age—Use and dose must be determined by your doctor.
  - For treatment of HIV infection or AIDS:
    - Adults weighing 50 kilograms (kg) (110 pounds) or more—150 milligrams (mg) twice a day together with other HIV medications.
    - Adults weighing less than 50 kg (110 pounds)—2 mg per kg of body weight twice a day together with other HIV medications.
    - Children 3 months to 16 years of age—4 mg per kg of body weight, up to 150 mg per dose, twice a day together with other HIV medications.
    - Children younger than 3 months of age—Use and dose must be determined by your doctor.

Note: Patients that require treatment for both hepatitis B and either AIDS or HIV should follow the dosing schedule for HIV or AIDS

Missed dose—If you miss a dose of this medicine, take it as soon as possible. However, if it is almost time for your next dose, skip the missed dose and go back to your regular dosing schedule. Do not double doses.

Storage—Store the medicine in a closed container at room temperature, away from heat, moisture, and direct light. Keep from freezing.

Keep out of the reach of children.

Do not keep outdated medicine or medicine no longer needed.

Precautions While Using This Medicine

It is very important that your doctor check your progress at regular visits.

Do not take any other medicines without checking with your doctor first. To do so may increase the chance of side effects from lamivudine.

If you have both HIV and hepatitis B virus (HBV) infections, deterioration of liver disease has occurred when lamivudine treatment is stopped. Discuss any changes in your treatment and medicines with your doctor.

HIV may be acquired from or spread to other people through infected body fluids, including blood, vaginal fluid, or semen. If you are infected, it is best to avoid any sexual activity involving an exchange of body fluids with other people. If you do have sex, always wear (or have your partner wear) a condom ("rubber"). Only use condoms made of latex, and use them every time you have vaginal, anal, or oral sex. The use of a spermicide (such as nonoxynol-9) may also help prevent transmission of HIV if it is not irritating to the vagina, rectum, or mouth. Spermicides have been shown to kill HIV in lab tests. Do not use oil-based jelly, cold cream, baby oil, or short-ening as a lubricant— these products can cause the condom to break. Lubricants without oil, such as K-Y Jelly, are recommended. Women may wish to carry their own condoms. Birth control pills and diaphragms will help protect against pregnancy, but they will not prevent someone from giving or getting the AIDS virus. If you inject drugs, get help to stop. Do not share needles or equipment with anyone. In some cities, more than half of the drug users are infected, and sharing even 1 needle or syringe can spread the virus. If you have any questions about this, check with your health care professional.

Side Effects of This Medicine

Along with its needed effects, a medicine may cause some unwanted effects. Although not all of these side effects may occur, if they do occur they may need medical attention.

Check with your doctor immediately if any of the following side effects occur:

More common— especially in children
Abdominal or stomach pain (severe); feeling of fullness; nausea; sensation or pins and needles; skin rash; stabbing pain; tingling, burning, numbness, or pain in the hands, arms, feet, or legs; unsteadiness or awkward-ness; vomiting

Rare
Abdominal discomfort; decreased appetite; diarrhea; fast, shallow breathing; feeling of fullness; fever, chills, or sore throat; general feeling of discomfort; muscle pain or cramping; nausea; shortness of breath; sleepi-ness; unusual tiredness or weakness

Incidence not determined
Cough; dark urine; difficulty swallowing; dizziness; fast heartbeat; fever; hives or welts; itching; light-colored stools; puffiness or swelling of the eyelids or around the eyes, face, lips, or tongue; redness of skin; tightness in chest; upper right abdominal pain; wheezing; yellow eyes and skin

Some side effects may occur that usually do not need medical attention. These side effects may go away during treatment as your body adjusts to the medicine. Also, your health care professional may be able to tell you about ways to prevent or reduce some of these side effects. Check with your health care professional if any of the following side effects continue or are bothersome or if you have any questions about them:

More common
Canker sores; difficulty in moving; discouragement; ear discharge; ear swelling; feeling sad or empty; general

feeling of discomfort or illness; irritability; loss of ap-petite; loss of interest or pleasure; nasal discharge or congestion; pain in joints; sores, ulcers, or white spots on lips or tongue or inside the mouth; stomach pain or cramps; swollen and painful spots on neck, armpit, or groin; swollen joints; trouble concentrating; trouble sleeping; unusually warm skin; weight loss

Less common
Acid or sour stomach; belching; cough; heartburn; in-digestion; stomach discomfort or upset

Other side effects not listed may also occur in some patients. If you notice any other effects, check with your healthcare professional.

Incidence not determined
Body fat redistribution or accumulation; blurred vision; dry mouth; flushed, dry skin; fruit-like breath odor; hair loss; increased hunger or thirst; increased urination; sweating; thinning of hair

LAMIVUDINE AND ZIDOVUDINE
(Oral route) - la-MI-vyoo-deen, zye-DOE-vyoo-deen

Black Box Warning

Zidovudine, one of the two active ingredients in lamivudine/zidovudine, has been associated with hematologic toxicity including neutropenia and severe anemia, particularly in patients with advanced HIV disease. Prolonged use of zidovudine has been associated with symptomatic myopathy.

Lactic acidosis and severe hepatomegaly with steatosis, including fatal cases, have been reported with the use of nucleoside analogues alone or in combination, including lamivudine, zidovudine, and other antiretrovirals.

Severe acute exacerbations of hepatitis B have been reported in patients who are co-infected with hepatitis B virus (HBV) and HIV and have discontinued lamivudine, which is one component of lamivudine/zidovudine. Hepatic function should be monitored closely with both clinical and laboratory follow-up for at least several months in patients who discontinue lamivudine/zidovudine and are co-infected with HIV and HBV. If appropriate, initiation of anti-hepatitis B therapy may be warranted.

Commonly used brand name(s)

In the U.S.—
Combivir

Available Dosage Forms:

• Tablet

Therapeutic Class: Antiretroviral Agent
Pharmacologic Class: Nucleoside Reverse Transcriptase Inhibitor

Uses For This Medicine

Lamivudine and zidovudine combination is used in the treatment of human immunodeficiency virus (HIV) infection. HIV is the virus that causes acquired immune deficiency syndrome (AIDS).

Lamivudine and zidovudine combination will not cure or prevent HIV infection or the symptoms of AIDS; however, it helps keep HIV from reproducing, and appears to slow down the destruction of the immune system. This may help delay the development of serious health problems usually related to AIDS or HIV infection. Lamivudine and zidovudine combination will not keep you from spreading HIV to other people. People who receive this medicine may continue to have other problems usually related to AIDS or HIV infection.

The zidovudine component of this combination medicine may cause some serious side effects, including bone marrow problems. Symptoms of bone marrow problems include fever, chills, sore throat, pale skin, and unusual tiredness or weakness. These problems may require blood transfusion or temporarily stopping treatment with lamivudine and zidovudine combination. Check with your doctor if any new health problems or symptoms occur while you are taking lamivudine and zidovudine combination.

This medicine is available only with your doctor's prescription.

Before Using This Medicine

In deciding to use a medicine, the risks of taking the medicine must be weighed against the good it will do. This is a decision you and your doctor will make. For this medicine, the following should be considered:

Allergies—Tell your doctor if you have ever had any unusual or allergic reaction to this medicine or any other medicines. Also tell your health care professional if you have any other types of allergies, such as to foods, dyes, preservatives, or animals. For non-prescription products, read the label or package ingredients carefully.

Pediatric—Either lamivudine or zidovudine used alone may cause serious side effects, and children should receive less of these medicines than adults. However, lamivudine and zidovudine combination contains a fixed amount of each medicine that cannot be decreased. Therefore, lamivudine and zidovudine combination is not recommended for children less than 12 years of age, or children who weigh less than 50 kilograms (110 pounds) because the amounts of lamivudine and zidovudine in this product cannot be adjusted for smaller body sizes.

Geriatric—Many medicines have not been studied specifically in older people. Therefore, it may not be known whether they work exactly the same way they do in younger adults or if they cause different side effects or problems in older people. Many older people have problems with their liver, heart and kidneys. Your doctor may change the amount of medicine you take because of other health problems.

Other medicines—

Using this medicine with any of the following medicines is usually not recommended, but may be required in some cases. If both medicines are prescribed together, your doctor may change the dose or how often you use one or both of the medicines.

Dapsone, Doxorubicin Hydrochloride, Flucytosine, Ganciclovir, Interferon Alfa, Pyrazinamide, Pyrimethamine, Ribavirin, Stavudine, Vinblastine, Vincristine, Vincristine Liposome, Zalcitabine

Interactions with Food/Tobacco/Alcohol—Certain medicines should not be used at or around the time of eating food or eating certain types of food since interactions may occur. Using alcohol or tobacco with certain medicines may also cause interactions to occur. Discuss with your healthcare professional the use of your medicine with food, alcohol, or tobacco.

Other medical problems—The presence of other medical problems may affect the use of this medicine. Make sure you tell your doctor if you have any other medical problems, especially:

- Blood problems, including decreased bone marrow production—Lamivudine and zidovudine combination may make these conditions worse

- Infection of human immunodeficiency virus (HIV) and hepatitis B virus (HBV) at the same time—This medicine could make your hepatitis worse or prevent the medicine from working properly.

- Kidney disease—Patients with kidney disease may experience an increase in side effects

- Liver disease or

- Risk factors for liver disease or

- Obesity (being overweight) or

- Use of other HIV medicines over a long period of time—This medicine may make liver disease worse in patients with liver disease, obesity or other HIV medicine use.

Proper Use of This Medicine

Lamivudine and zidovudine combination may be taken with food or on an empty stomach.

Take this medicine exactly as directed by your doctor. Do not take more of it, do not take it more often, and do not take it for a longer time than your doctor ordered. Also, do not stop taking lamivudine and zidovudine combination without checking with your doctor first.

Keep taking lamivudine and zidovudine combination for the full time of treatment, even if you begin to feel better.

This medicine works best when there is a constant amount in the blood. To help keep the amount constant, do not miss any doses. If you need help in planning the best times to take your medicine, check with your health care professional.

Only take medicine that your doctor has prescribed specifically for you. Do not share your medicine with others.

Dosing—The dose of this medicine will be different for different patients. Follow your doctor's orders or the directions on the label. The following information includes only the average doses of this medicine. If your dose is different, do not change it unless your doctor tells you to do so.

The amount of medicine that you take depends on the strength of the medicine. Also, the number of doses you take each day, the time allowed between doses, and the length of time you take the medicine depend on the medical problem for which you are using the medicine.

Lamivudine and zidovudine combination contains a fixed amount of each medicine.

- For oral dosage form (tablets):
  - For human immunodeficiency virus (HIV) infection:
    - Adults and teenagers who weigh more than 50 kilograms (kg) (110 pounds)—150 milligrams (mg) of lamivudine and 300 mg of zidovudine (equivalent to one tablet) two times a day.

- Adults and teenagers who weigh 50 kg (110 pounds) or less—Use is not recommended.
- Children—Use is not recommended.

Missed dose—If you miss a dose of this medicine, take it as soon as possible. However, if it is almost time for your next dose, skip the missed dose and go back to your regular dosing schedule. Do not double doses.

Storage—Store the medicine in a closed container at room temperature, away from heat, moisture, and direct light. Keep from freezing.

Keep out of the reach of children.

Do not keep outdated medicine or medicine no longer needed.

Precautions While Using This Medicine

It is very important that your doctor check your progress at regular visits. Lamivudine and zidovudine combination may cause blood problems, and your doctor will want to test your blood regularly.

Do not take any other medicines without checking with your doctor first. To do so may increase the chance of side effects from lamivudine and zidovudine combination.

If you have both HIV and hepatitis B virus (HBV) infections, deterioration of liver disease has occurred when lamivudine and zidovudine treatment is stopped. Discuss any changes in your treatment and medicines with your doctor.

HIV may be acquired from or spread to other people through infected body fluids, including blood, vaginal fluid, or semen. If you are infected, it is best to avoid any sexual activity involving an exchange of body fluids with other people. If you do have sex, always wear (or have your partner wear) a condom ("rubber"). Only use condoms made of latex, and use them every time you have vaginal, anal, or oral sex. The use of a spermicide (such as nonoxynol-9) may also help prevent transmission of HIV if it is not irritating to the vagina, rectum, or mouth. Spermicides have been shown to kill HIV in lab tests. Do not use oil-based jelly, cold cream, baby oil, or shortening as a lubricant— these products can cause the condom to break. Lubricants without oil, such as K-Y Jelly, are recommended. Women may wish to carry their own condoms. Birth control pills and diaphragms will help protect against pregnancy, but they will not prevent someone from giving or getting the AIDS virus. If you inject drugs, get help to stop. Do not share needles or equipment with anyone. In some cities, more than half of the drug users are infected, and sharing even 1 needle or syringe can spread the virus. If you have any questions about this, check with your health care professional.

Side Effects of This Medicine

Along with its needed effects, a medicine may cause some unwanted effects. Although not all of these side effects may occur, if they do occur they may need medical attention.

Check with your doctor as soon as possible if any of the following side effects occur:

More common
Chills; fever; pale skin; sore throat; unusual tiredness or weakness

Less common
Abdominal pain (severe); burning, tingling, numbness, or pain in the hands, arms, feet, or legs; muscle tenderness and weakness; nausea; skin rash; vomiting; yellow eyes or skin

Incidence unknown
Blistering, peeling, loosening of skin; canker sores; chest discomfort or pain; chills; convulsions; dark urine; decreased appetite; difficulty breathing; difficulty swallowing; dizziness; faintness; fast, irregular, or pounding heartbeat; fast shallow breathing; feeling of fullness; general feeling of discomfort; general tiredness and weakness; hives or welts; itching; itching, puffiness or selling of the eyelids or around the eyes, face, lips, or tongue; jerking of all extremities; joint or muscle pain; light-colored stools; loss of bladder control; muscle pain, spasms, stiffness, or cramping; red, irritated eyes; red skin lesions often with a purple center; redness, soreness, or itching skin; sensation of pins and needles; shortness of breath; sleepiness; sores, ulcers, or white spots in mouth or on lips or tongue; sores, welting or blisters; stabbing pain; sudden loss of consciousness; swelling of feet or lower legs; tingling, burning, numbness, or pain the hands, arms, feet, or legs; tightness in chest; troubled breathing; unsteadiness or awkwardness; wheezing

Some side effects may occur that usually do not need medical attention. These side effects may go away during treatment as your body adjusts to the medicine. Also, your health care professional may be able to tell you about ways to prevent or reduce some of these side effects. Check with your health care professional if any of the following side effects continue or are bothersome or if you have any questions about them:

More common
Headache

Less common
Abdominal pain (mild); coughing; decreased appetite; diarrhea; dizziness; trouble in sleeping

Incidence unknown
Abnormal breathing; blurred vision; body fat redistribution/accumulation; darkening of skin and mucous membranes; dry mouth; fatigue; flushed, dry skin; fruit-like breath odor; hair loss; increased hunger; increased thirst; increased urination; sweating; swelling of the breasts or breast soreness in both females and males; swollen, painful, or tender lymph glands in neck, armpit, or groin; thinning of hair; troubled breathing, unexplained

Other side effects not listed may also occur in some patients. If you notice any other effects, check with your healthcare professional.

LAMOTRIGINE (Oral route) - la-MOE-tri-jeen

Black Box Warning

Serious rashes requiring hospitalization and discontinuation of treatment have been reported in association with the use of lamotrigine. The incidence of these rashes, which have included Stevens-Johnson syndrome, is approximately 0.8% (8 per 1,000) in pediatric patients (age less than 16 years) receiving lamotrigine as adjunctive therapy for epilepsy and 0.3% (3 per 1,000) in adults on adjunctive therapy for epilepsy. In clinical trials of bipolar and other mood disorders, the rate of serious rash was 0.08% (0.8 per 1,000) in adult patients receiving lamotrigine as initial monotherapy and 0.13% (1.3 per 1,000) in adult patients receiving lamotrigine as adjunctive therapy. In a prospectively followed cohort of 1,983 pediatric patients with epilepsy taking adjunctive lamotrigine, there was 1 rash-related death. In worldwide post-marketing experience, rare cases of toxic epidermal necrolysis and/or rash-related death have been reported in adult and pediatric patients, but their numbers are too few to permit a precise estimate of the rate.

Because the rate of serious rash is greater in pediatric patients than in adults, it bears emphasis that lamotrigine is approved only for use in pediatric patients below the age of 16 years who have seizures associated with the Lennox-Gastaut syndrome or in patients with partial seizures.

Other than age, there are as yet no factors identified that are known to predict the risk of occurrence or the severity of rash associated with lamotrigine. There are suggestions, yet to be proven, that the risk of rash may also be increased by coadministration of lamotrigine with valproate (includes valproic acid and divalproex sodium), exceeding the recommended initial dose of lamotrigine, or exceeding the recommended dose escalation for lamictal. However, cases have been reported in the absence of these factors.

Nearly all cases of life-threatening rashes associated with lamotrigine have occurred within 2 to 8 weeks of treatment initiation. However, isolated cases have been reported after prolonged treatment (eg, 6 months). Accordingly, duration of therapy cannot be relied upon as a means to predict the potential risk heralded by the first appearance of a rash.

Although benign rashes also occur with lamotrigine, it is not possible to predict reliably which rashes will prove to be serious or life threatening. Accordingly, lamotrigine should ordinarily be discontinued at the first sign of rash, unless the rash is clearly not drug related. Discontinuation of treatment may not prevent a rash from becoming life threatening or permanently disabling or disfiguring.

Commonly used brand name(s)

In the U.S.—
Lamictal
Lamictal CD

Available Dosage Forms:
- Tablet
- Tablet, Chewable

Therapeutic Class: Anticonvulsant

Uses For This Medicine

Lamotrigine is used to help control some types of seizures in the treatment of epilepsy. This medicine cannot cure epilepsy and will only work to control seizures for as long as you continue to take it. It can also be used in the treatment of bipolar disorder (manic-depressive illness) in adults older than 18 years of age.

Lamotrigine is available only with your doctor's prescription.

Before Using This Medicine

In deciding to use a medicine, the risks of taking the medicine must be weighed against the good it will do. This is a decision you and your doctor will make. For this medicine, the following should be considered:

Allergies—Tell your doctor if you have ever had any unusual or allergic reaction to this medicine or any other medicines. Also tell your health care professional if you have any other types of allergies, such as to foods, dyes, preservatives, or animals. For non-prescription products, read the label or package ingredients carefully.

Pediatric—Skin rashes may be more likely to occur in children younger than 16 years of age than in adults. Some of these rashes may be serious and life-threatening. It is especially important that you discuss with the child's doctor the good that this medicine may do as well as the risks of using it. Lamotrigine is not indicated for bipolar disorder in children under 18 years of age.

Geriatric—Lamotrigine is removed from the body more slowly in elderly people than in younger people. Higher blood levels of the medicine may occur, which may increase the chance of unwanted effects. Your doctor may give you a different lamotrigine dose than a younger person would receive.

Pregnancy—

	Pregnancy Category	Explanation
All Trimesters	C	Animal studies have shown an adverse effect and there are no adequate studies in pregnant women OR no animal studies have been conducted and there are no adequate studies in pregnant women.

Breast Feeding—There are no adequate studies in women for determining infant risk when using this medication during breastfeeding. Weigh the potential benefits against the potential risks before taking this medication while breastfeeding.

Other medicines—

Using this medicine with any of the following medicines is usually not recommended, but may be required in some cases. If both medicines are prescribed together, your doctor may change the dose or how often you use one or both of the medicines.

Valproic Acid

Interactions with Food/Tobacco/Alcohol—Certain medicines should not be used at or around the time of eating food or eating certain types of food since interactions may occur. Using alcohol or tobacco with certain medicines may also cause interactions to occur. Discuss with your healthcare professional the use of your medicine with food, alcohol, or tobacco.

Other medical problems—The presence of other medical problems may affect the use of this medicine. Make sure you tell your doctor if you have any other medical problems, especially:
- Heart disease—It is not clear if patients who have problems with heart rhythms will have increased problems while taking lamotrigine
- Kidney disease or

- Liver disease—Higher blood levels of lamotrigine may occur, which may increase the chance of unwanted effects; your doctor may need to change your dose
- Thalassemia—Lamotrigine may cause your body to stop making or to make fewer red blood cells

Proper Use of This Medicine

Take lamotrigine only as directed by your doctor to help your condition as much as possible and to decrease the chance of unwanted effects. Do not take more or less of this medicine, and do not take it more or less often than your doctor ordered.

Lamotrigine may be taken with or without food or on a full or empty stomach. However, if your doctor tells you to take the medicine a certain way, take it exactly as directed.

If you are taking the chewable/dispersible tablets: These tablets may be swallowed whole, chewed and swallowed, or dispersed in a small amount of liquid and swallowed. If the tablets are chewed, they should be followed with a small amount of water or diluted fruit juice to aid in swallowing. If tablets are to be dispersed: Place tablets in enough water or diluted fruit juice to cover the tablets (about a teaspoonful), wait until the tablets are completely dispersed (about 1 minute), then swirl the solution and swallow it immediately.

Dosing—The dose of this medicine will be different for different patients. Follow your doctor's orders or the directions on the label. The following information includes only the average doses of this medicine. If your dose is different, do not change it unless your doctor tells you to do so.

The amount of medicine that you take depends on the strength of the medicine. Also, the number of doses you take each day, the time allowed between doses, and the length of time you take the medicine depend on the medical problem for which you are using the medicine.

- For oral dosage forms (tablets):
  - For treatment of bipolar disorder:
    - Adults not taking valproic acid (e.g., Depakote) and not taking carbamazepine (e.g., Tegretol), phenobarbital (e.g., Luminal), phenytoin (e.g., Dilantin), and/or primidone (e.g., Mysoline)—At first, 25 milligrams (mg) of lamotrigine once a day for two weeks, then a total of 50 mg divided into two smaller doses each day for two weeks. After this, your doctor may increase the dose gradually if needed. However, the dose is usually not more than 200 mg a day.
    - Adults taking valproic acid (e.g., Depakote)—At first, 25 mg of lamotrigine once every other day for two weeks, then 25 mg once every day for two weeks. After this, your doctor may increase the dose gradually if needed. However, the dose is usually not more than 100 mg a day.
    - Adults not taking valproic acid (e.g., Depakote) but taking carbamazepine (e.g., Tegretol), phenobarbital (e.g., Luminal), phenytoin (e.g., Dilantin), and/or primidone (e.g., Mysoline)—At first, 50 mg of lamotrigine once a day for two weeks, then a total of 100 mg divided into two smaller doses each day for two weeks. After this, your doctor may increase the dose gradually if needed. However, the dose is usually not more than 400 mg a day.
    - Adults who are discontinuing valproic acid (e.g., Depakote) or discontinuing carbamazepine (e.g.,

Tegretol), phenobarbital (e.g., Luminal), phenytoin (e.g., Dilantin), and/or primidone (e.g., Mysoline)—Dose will be determined by your doctor.
    - Children under 18 years of age—Use and dose must be determined by your doctor.
  - For treatment of epilepsy:
    - Adults not taking valproic acid (e.g., Depakote) but taking carbamazepine (e.g., Tegretol), phenobarbital (e.g., Luminal), phenytoin (e.g., Dilantin), and/or primidone (e.g., Mysoline)—At first, 50 milligrams (mg) of lamotrigine once a day for two weeks, then a total of 100 mg divided into two smaller doses each day for two weeks. After this, your doctor may increase the dose gradually if needed. However, the dose is usually not more than 500 mg a day.
    - Adults taking valproic acid (e.g., Depakote) and also taking carbamazepine (e.g., Tegretol), phenobarbital (e.g., Luminal), phenytoin (e.g., Dilantin), and/or primidone (e.g., Mysoline)—At first, 25 mg of lamotrigine once every other day for two weeks, then 25 mg once every day for two weeks. After this, your doctor may increase the dose gradually if needed. However, the dose is usually not more than 400 mg a day.
    - Children 2 to 12 years of age:
      — Children not taking valproic acid (e.g., Depakote) but taking carbamazepine (e.g., Tegretol), phenobarbital (e.g., Luminal), phenytoin (e.g., Dilantin), and/or primidone (e.g., Mysoline): At first, 0.6 milligrams (mg) per kilogram (kg) (0.27 mg per pound) of body weight of lamotrigine once a day for two weeks, then 1.2 mg/kg (0.54 mg per pound) of body weight divided into two smaller doses each day for two weeks. After this, your doctor may increase the dose gradually if needed. However, the dose is usually not more than 400 mg a day.
      — Children taking valproic acid (e.g., Depakote) and also taking carbamazepine (e.g., Tegretol), phenobarbital (e.g., Luminal), phenytoin (e.g., Dilantin), and/or primidone (e.g., Mysoline): At first, 0.15 mg per kg (0.07 mg per pound) of body weight of lamotrigine given in one dose or two smaller doses each day for two weeks, then 0.3 mg/kg (0.136 mg per pound) of body weight given in one dose or two smaller doses each day for two weeks. After this, your doctor may increase the dose gradually if needed. However, the dose is usually not more than 200 mg a day.
    - Children older than 12 years of age usually receive the adult dose.

Missed dose—If you miss a dose of this medicine, take it as soon as possible. However, if it is almost time for your next dose, skip the missed dose and go back to your regular dosing schedule. Do not double doses.

Storage—Store the medicine in a closed container at room temperature, away from heat, moisture, and direct light. Keep from freezing.

Keep out of the reach of children.

Do not keep outdated medicine or medicine no longer needed.

Precautions While Using This Medicine

It is important that your doctor check your progress at regular visits, especially during the first few months of your treatment with lamotrigine. This will allow your doctor to change your dose, if necessary, and will help reduce any unwanted effects.

You should not start or stop using birth control pills or other female hormonal products while you are taking this medicine until you have consulted your doctor.

Tell your doctor right away if you experience unusual changes in your menstrual cycle such as breakthrough bleeding while taking lamotrigine and birth control pills or other female hormonal products.

This medicine may increase the effects of alcohol and other central nervous system (CNS) depressants (medicines that make you drowsy or less alert). Some examples of CNS depressants are antihistamines or medicine for hay fever, other allergies, or colds; sedatives, tranquilizers, or sleeping medicine; prescription pain medicine or narcotics; barbiturates; medicine for seizures; muscle relaxants; or anesthetics, including some dental anesthetics. *Check with your doctor before taking any of the above while you are using this medicine.*

Lamotrigine may cause blurred vision, double vision, clumsiness, unsteadiness, dizziness, or drowsiness. *Make sure you know how you react to this medicine before you drive, use machines, or do anything else that could be dangerous if you are not alert, well-coordinated, or able to see well.* If these reactions are especially bothersome, check with your doctor.

Skin rash may be a sign of a serious unwanted effect. *Check with your doctor immediately if you develop a rash, fever, flu-like symptoms, or swollen glands, or if your seizures increase.*

If suicidal thoughts or behavior occur, especially if you are taking this medicine to treat bipolar disorder, contact your doctor right away.

Do not stop taking lamotrigine without first checking with your doctor. Stopping this medicine suddenly may cause your seizures to return or to occur more often. Your doctor may want you to gradually reduce the amount you are taking before stopping completely.

Side Effects of This Medicine

Along with its needed effects, a medicine may cause some unwanted effects. Although not all of these side effects may occur, if they do occur they may need medical attention.

Check with your doctor immediately if any of the following side effects occur:
More common
   Skin rash
Less common
   Increase in seizures
Rare
   Blistering, peeling, or loosening of skin; dark-colored urine; fever, chills, and/or sore throat; flu-like symptoms; itching; muscle cramps, pain, or weakness; red or irritated eyes; small red or purple spots on skin; sores, ulcers, or white spots on lips or in mouth;

swelling of face, mouth, hands, or feet; swollen lymph nodes; trouble in breathing; unusual bleeding or bruising; unusual tiredness or weakness; yellow eyes or skin

Symptoms of overdose
   Clumsiness or unsteadiness (severe); coma; continuous, uncontrolled back and forth and/or rolling eye movements (severe); dizziness (severe); drowsiness (severe); dryness of mouth (severe); headache (severe); increased heart rate; slurred speech (severe)

Check with your doctor as soon as possible if any of the following side effects occur:
More common
   Blurred or double vision or other changes in vision; clumsiness or unsteadiness; poor coordination
Less common
   Anxiety, confusion, depression, irritability, or other mood or mental changes; chest pain; continuous, uncontrolled back and forth and/or rolling eye movements; infection
Rare
   Memory loss
Incidence not known
   Back, leg, or stomach pains; bleeding gums; bloating; blood in urine; bloody, black or tarry stools; bluish lips or skin; bruising; chills; confusion; constipation; cough or hoarseness; coughing or vomiting blood; dark urine; difficulty breathing; difficulty swallowing; fainting; fast heartbeat; fatigue; fever; general body swelling; general feeling of discomfort or illness or weakness; general feeling of tiredness or weakness; heartburn; high fever; lightheadedness; loss of appetite; loss of balance control; lower back or side pain; mask-like face; muscle spasms; muscle stiffness; nosebleeds; not breathing; pain or burning in throat; painful or difficult urination; pains in stomach, side, or abdomen, possibly radiating to the back; pale skin; persistent bleeding or oozing from puncture sites, mouth, or nose; rapid, shallow breathing; redness, soreness or itching skin; shortness of breath; shuffling walk; slowed movement; slurred speech; sores, welting or blisters; stiffness of arms and legs; swollen or painful glands; tic-like [jerky] movements; tightness in chest; unexplained bleeding or bruising; wheezing

Some side effects may occur that usually do not need medical attention. These side effects may go away during treatment as your body adjusts to the medicine. Also, your health care professional may be able to tell you about ways to prevent or reduce some of these side effects. Check with your health care professional if any of the following side effects continue or are bothersome or if you have any questions about them:
More common
   Dizziness (more common in women); drowsiness; headache; nausea; vomiting
Less common
   Constipation; diarrhea; dryness of mouth; indigestion; loss of strength; menstrual pain; pain; runny nose; slurred speech; trembling or shaking; trouble in sleeping; unusual weight loss

Other side effects not listed may also occur in some patients. If you notice any other effects, check with your healthcare professional.

LANSOPRAZOLE (Oral route) - lan-SOE-pra-zole

Commonly used brand name(s)

In the U.S.—
Prevacid
Prevacid SoluTab

Available Dosage Forms:

- Packet
- Capsule, Delayed Release
- Tablet Disintegrating, Delayed Release

Therapeutic Class: Antiulcer
Pharmacologic Class: Proton Pump Inhibitor

Uses For This Medicine

Lansoprazole is used to treat certain conditions in which there is too much acid in the stomach. It is used to treat duodenal and gastric ulcers and gastroesophageal reflux disease (GERD), a condition in which the acid in the stomach washes back up into the esophagus. Sometimes lansoprazole is used in combination with antibiotics to treat ulcers associated with infection caused by the H. pylori bacteria (germ).

Lansoprazole is also used to treat Zollinger-Ellison disease, a condition in which the stomach produces too much acid.

Lansoprazole works by decreasing the amount of acid produced by the stomach.

This medicine is available only with your doctor's prescription.

Before Using This Medicine

In deciding to use a medicine, the risks of taking the medicine must be weighed against the good it will do. This is a decision you and your doctor will make. For this medicine, the following should be considered:

Allergies—Tell your doctor if you have ever had any unusual or allergic reaction to this medicine or any other medicines. Also tell your health care professional if you have any other types of allergies, such as to foods, dyes, preservatives, or animals. For non-prescription products, read the label or package ingredients carefully.

Pediatric—There is no specific information comparing the use of oral lansoprazole in children less than 1 year of age with use in other age groups. It is safe to use oral lansoprazole to treat heartburn and erosive esophagitis in people between 1 and 17 years of age.

Studies on lansoprazole for injection have been done only in adult patients, and there is no specific information comparing use of lansoprazole for injection in children with use in other age groups.

Geriatric—In studies done to date that have included older adults, lansoprazole did not cause different side effects or problems than it did in younger adults.

Pregnancy—

	Pregnancy Category	Explanation
All Trimesters	B	Animal studies have revealed no evidence of harm to the fetus, however, there are no adequate studies in pregnant women OR animal studies have shown an adverse effect, but adequate studies in pregnant women have failed to demonstrate a risk to the fetus.

Breast Feeding—There are no adequate studies in women for determining infant risk when using this medication during breastfeeding. Weigh the potential benefits against the potential risks before taking this medication while breastfeeding.

Other medicines—

Using this medicine with any of the following medicines is usually not recommended, but may be required in some cases. If both medicines are prescribed together, your doctor may change the dose or how often you use one or both of the medicines.

Atazanavir, Delavirdine

Interactions with Food/Tobacco/Alcohol—Certain medicines should not be used at or around the time of eating food or eating certain types of food since interactions may occur. Using alcohol or tobacco with certain medicines may also cause interactions to occur. Discuss with your healthcare professional the use of your medicine with food, alcohol, or tobacco.

Proper Use of This Medicine

Take oral lansoprazole before a meal, preferably in the morning.

For Delayed-Release Capsules: Swallow the capsule whole. Do not crush, break, or chew the capsule. If you cannot swallow the capsule whole, you may open it and sprinkle the granules contained in the capsule on one tablespoonful of applesauce and swallow it immediately; or you may mix the granules in some fruit or vegetable juice and drink it immediately. Juices you may use include apple, cranberry, grape, orange, pineapple, prune, tomato, and V-8 vegetable juice. Do not chew or crush the granules.

For Delayed-Release Oral Suspension: Empty the packet contents into a container containing 2 tablespoons of water. Stir well and drink immediately. If any of the content remains after drinking, add more water and drink immediately. If you have enteral administration tubes, do not take this medicine through them.

For Delayed-Release Orally Disintegrating Tablets: Do not chew. Place on tongue and allow to disintegrate, with or without water, until particles can be swallowed

- If you are using this medicine with an Oral Syringe:
  - Place a 15 mg tablet in oral syringe and fill with 4 mL of water, or place a 30 mg tablet in oral syringe and fill with 10 mL of water
  - Shake gently
  - After medicine mixes completely with the water, take the mixture within 15 minutes
  - Refill the syringe with 2 mL (5 mL for the 30 mg tablet) of water, shake gently and take any remaining contents
- If you are using this medicine with a Nasogastric Tube:
  - Place a 15 mg tablet in oral syringe and fill with 4 mL of water, or place a 30 mg tablet in oral syringe and fill with 10 mL of water
  - Shake gently
  - After tablet has dispersed, inject through the nasogastric tube into the stomach within 15 minutes
  - Refill the syringe with approximately 5 mL of water, shake gently and administer any remaining contents

Take this medicine for the full time of treatment, even if you begin to feel better. Also, keep your appointments with your doctor for check-ups so that your doctor will be better able to tell you when to stop taking this medicine.

Dosing—The dose of this medicine will be different for different patients. Follow your doctor's orders or the directions on the label. The following information includes only the average doses of this medicine. If your dose is different, do not change it unless your doctor tells you to do so.

The amount of medicine that you take depends on the strength of the medicine. Also, the number of doses you take each day, the time allowed between doses, and the length of time you take the medicine depend on the medical problem for which you are using the medicine.

- For oral dosage form (delayed-release capsule, delayed-release oral suspension, or delayed-release orally disintegrating tablet):
  - To treat gastroesophageal reflux disease (GERD):
    - Adults—15 to 30 mg once a day, preferably taken in the morning before a meal.
    - Children less than 1 year of age—Use and dose must be determined by your doctor
    - Children 1 to 18 years of age—15 to 30 mg once daily for 8 to 12 weeks
  - To treat duodenal ulcers:
    - Adults—At first, 15 milligrams (mg) once a day, preferably taken in the morning before a meal. Your doctor may increase your dose if needed.
    - Children up to 18 years of age—Use and dose must be determined by your doctor.
  - To treat duodenal ulcers related to infection with H. pylori:
    - Adults—30 mg plus amoxicillin 1000 mg (1 gram) plus clarithromycin 500 mg, taken together before meals twice a day for ten to fourteen days. Alternatively, your doctor may want you to take lansoprazole 30 mg plus amoxicillin 1000 mg (1 gram) before meals three times a day for fourteen days.
    - Children up to 18 years of age—Use and dose must be determined by your doctor.
  - To treat gastric ulcers:
    - Adults—15 to 30 mg once a day, preferably taken in the morning before a meal.
    - Children up to 18 years of age—Use and dose must be determined by your doctor.
  - To treat conditions in which the stomach produces too much acid:
    - Adults—At first, 60 mg once a day, preferably taken in the morning before a meal. Your doctor may increase your dose if needed.
    - Children up to 18 years of age—Use and dose must be determined by your doctor.
- For injection dosage form:
  - To treat erosive esophagitis in patients who cannot take oral lansoprazole:
    - Adults—30 mg once a day injected into a vein.
    - Children—Use and dose must be determined by your doctor.

Missed dose—If you miss a dose of this medicine, take it as soon as possible. However, if it is almost time for your next dose, skip the missed dose and go back to your regular dosing schedule. Do not double doses.

Storage—Store the medicine in a closed container at room temperature, away from heat, moisture, and direct light. Keep from freezing.

Keep out of the reach of children.

Do not keep outdated medicine or medicine no longer needed.

Precautions While Using This Medicine

It is important that your doctor check your progress at regular intervals. If your condition does not improve, or if it becomes worse, discuss this with your doctor.

Side Effects of This Medicine

Along with its needed effects, a medicine may cause some unwanted effects. Although not all of these side effects may occur, if they do occur they may need medical attention.

Check with your doctor as soon as possible if any of the following side effects occur:

More common
    Diarrhea; skin rash or itching

Less common
    Abdominal or stomach pain; increased or decreased appetite; joint pain; nausea; vomiting

Rare
    Anxiety; cold or flu-like symptoms; constipation; increased cough; mental depression; muscle pain; rectal bleeding; unusual bleeding or bruising

Incidence not known
    Abdominal tenderness; back, leg or stomach pains; bleeding gums; blistering, peeling, loosening of skin; bloating; bloody, black, or tarry stools; change in mental status; chest pain; chills; clay colored stools; constipation; cough or hoarseness; dark or bloody urine; difficulty swallowing; fast heartbeat; fatigue; fever; general body swelling; high fever; hives; indigestion; loss of appetite; lower back or side pain; nosebleeds; painful or difficult urination; pains in stomach, side or abdomen, possibly radiating to the back; pale skin; puffiness or swelling of the eyelids or around the eyes, face, lips or tongue; red irritated eyes; pinpoint red spots on skin; red skin lesions, often with a purple center; seizures; shortness of breath; sore throat; sores, ulcers or white spots on lips or in mouth; swelling of feet or lower legs; swollen or painful glands; tightness in chest; un-

usual tiredness or weakness; wheezing; yellowing of the eyes or skin

Some side effects may occur that usually do not need medical attention. These side effects may go away during treatment as your body adjusts to the medicine. Also, your health care professional may be able to tell you about ways to prevent or reduce some of these side effects. Check with your health care professional if any of the following side effects continue or are bothersome or if you have any questions about them:

More common
Dizziness; headache

Less common
Bleeding, blistering, burning, coldness, discoloration of skin; feeling of pressure, hives, infection, inflammation, itching, lumps, numbness, pain, rash, redness, scarring, soreness, stinging, swelling, tenderness, tingling, ulceration, or warmth at injection site; mild nausea

Rare
Acid or sour stomach; bad, unusual or unpleasant (after)taste; belching; burning, crawling, itching, numbness, prickling, "pins and needles", or tingling feelings; change in taste; feeling faint, dizzy, or light-headedness; feeling of heat or warmth; flushing or redness of skin, especially on face and neck; heartburn; indigestion; mild diarrhea; mild headache; mild vomiting; stomach discomfort, upset or pain; sweating

Incidence not known
Difficulty in speaking; decrease in frequency of urination; decrease in urine volume; decrease in passing urine [dribbling]

Other side effects not listed may also occur in some patients. If you notice any other effects, check with your healthcare professional.

LANTHANUM CARBONATE (Oral route) - LAN-tha-num KAR-boh-nate

Commonly used brand name(s)

In the U.S.—
Fosrenol

Available Dosage Forms:
• Tablet, Chewable

Therapeutic Class: Phosphate Binder

Uses For This Medicine

Lanthanum is used to treat hyperphosphatemia (too much phosphate in the blood) in patients with kidney disease who are on dialysis.

This medicine is available only with your doctor's prescription.

Before Using This Medicine

In deciding to use a medicine, the risks of taking the medicine must be weighed against the good it will do. This is a decision you and your doctor will make. For this medicine, the following should be considered:

Allergies—Tell your doctor if you have ever had any unusual or allergic reaction to this medicine or any other medicines. Also tell your health care professional if you have any other types of allergies, such as to foods, dyes, preservatives, or animals. For non-prescription products, read the label or package ingredients carefully.

Pediatric—Studies on this medicine have been done only in adult patients, and there is no specific information comparing use of lanthanum in children with use in other age groups.

Geriatric—This medicine has been tested and has not been been shown to cause different side effects or problems in older people than it does in younger adults.

Pregnancy—

	Pregnancy Category	Explanation
All Trimesters	C	Animal studies have shown an adverse effect and there are no adequate studies in pregnant women OR no animal studies have been conducted and there are no adequate studies in pregnant women.

Breast Feeding—There are no adequate studies in women for determining infant risk when using this medication during breastfeeding. Weigh the potential benefits against the potential risks before taking this medication while breastfeeding.

Other medicines—Although certain medicines should not be used together at all, in other cases two different medicines may be used together even if an interaction might occur. In these cases, your doctor may want to change the dose, or other precautions may be necessary. Tell your healthcare professional if you are taking any other prescription or non-prescription (over-the-counter [OTC]) medicine.

Interactions with Food/Tobacco/Alcohol—Certain medicines should not be used at or around the time of eating food or eating certain types of food since interactions may occur. Using alcohol or tobacco with certain medicines may also cause interactions to occur. Discuss with your healthcare professional the use of your medicine with food, alcohol, or tobacco.

Other medical problems—The presence of other medical problems may affect the use of this medicine. Make sure you tell your doctor if you have any other medical problems, especially:

• Bowel obstruction (blockage) or other disorders affecting the gastrointestinal tract or

• Crohn's disease or

• Peptic ulcer (an ulcer in the wall of the stomach) or

• Ulcerative colitis (inflammatory disease of the colon)—Use of lanthanum has not been studied in patients with these medical problems.

Proper Use of This Medicine

Take this medicine with meals.

Take this medicine only as directed by your doctor. Do not take more or less of it, and do not take it more often than your doctor ordered.

Chew the tablet before swallowing. Do not swallow the tablet whole.

Follow carefully any diet program your doctor may recommend.

Dosing—The dose of this medicine will be different for different patients. Follow your doctor's orders or the directions on the label. The following information includes only the average doses of this medicine. If your dose is different, do not change it unless your doctor tells you to do so.

The amount of medicine that you take depends on the strength of the medicine. Also, the number of doses you take each day, the time allowed between doses, and the length of time you take the medicine depend on the medical problem for which you are using the medicine.

- For oral dosage form (chewable tablets):
  ○ For high phosphorus levels in the blood:
    ▪ Adults—Your dose will be determined by your doctor depending on how high your blood phosphorus level is.
    ▪ Children—Use and dose must be determined by your doctor.

Missed dose—If you miss a dose of this medicine, take it as soon as possible. However, if it is almost time for your next dose, skip the missed dose and go back to your regular dosing schedule. Do not double doses.

Storage—Store the medicine in a closed container at room temperature, away from heat, moisture, and direct light. Keep from freezing.

Keep out of the reach of children.

Do not keep outdated medicine or medicine no longer needed.

Precautions While Using This Medicine

Regular visits: If you will be taking this medicine for a long time, it is very important that your doctor check you at regular visits.

Side Effects of This Medicine

Along with its needed effects, a medicine may cause some unwanted effects. Although not all of these side effects may occur, if they do occur they may need medical attention.

Check with your doctor immediately if any of the following side effects occur:

More common
  Dialysis graft blockage

Along with its needed effects, a medicine may cause some unwanted effects. Although not all of these side effects may occur, if they do occur they may need medical attention.

Some side effects may occur that usually do not need medical attention. These side effects may go away during treatment as your body adjusts to the medicine. Also, your health care professional may be able to tell you about ways to prevent or reduce some of these side effects. Check with your health care professional if any of the following side effects continue or are bothersome or if you have any questions about them:

More common
  Diarrhea; difficulty having a bowel movement (stool); nausea; runny nose; sneezing; stomach pain; stuffy nose; vomiting

Other side effects not listed may also occur in some patients. If you notice any other effects, check with your healthcare professional.

LARONIDASE   (Intravenous route) -
lair-OH-ni-days

Commonly used brand name(s)
In the U.S.—
  Aldurazyme

Available Dosage Forms:
- Solution

Therapeutic Class: Endocrine-Metabolic Agent
Pharmacologic Class: Enzyme

Uses For This Medicine

Laronidase is used to treat Hurler and Hurler-Schele syndrome forms of mucopolysaccharidosis (MPS I) disease caused by the lack of a certain enzyme called α-Liduronidasein the body.

Laronidase is available only with your doctor's prescription.

Before Using This Medicine

In deciding to use a medicine, the risks of taking the medicine must be weighed against the good it will do. This is a decision you and your doctor will make. For this medicine, the following should be considered:

Allergies—Tell your doctor if you have ever had any unusual or allergic reaction to this medicine or any other medicines. Also tell your health care professional if you have any other types of allergies, such as to foods, dyes, preservatives, or animals. For non-prescription products, read the label or package ingredients carefully.

Pediatric—This medicine has been tested in children 5 years of age and older, and has not been shown to cause different side effects or problems than is does in adults. It is not know if children under 5 respond differently from older children.

Geriatric—Many medicines have not been studied specifically in older people. Therefore, it may not be known whether they work exactly the same way they do in younger adults or if they cause different side effects or problems in older people. There is no specific information comparing use of laronidase in the elderly with use in other age groups.

Pregnancy—

	Pregnancy Category	Explanation
All Trimesters	B	Animal studies have revealed no evidence of harm to the fetus, however, there are no adequate studies in pregnant women OR animal studies have shown an adverse effect, but adequate studies in pregnant women have failed to demonstrate a risk to the fetus.

Breast Feeding—There are no adequate studies in women for determining infant risk when using this medication during breastfeeding. Weigh the potential benefits against the potential risks before taking this medication while breastfeeding.

Other medicines—Although certain medicines should not be used together at all, in other cases two different medicines may be used together even if an interaction might occur. In these cases, your doctor may want to change the dose, or other precautions may be necessary. Tell your healthcare professional if you are taking any other prescription or non-prescription (over-the-counter [OTC]) medicine.

Interactions with Food/Tobacco/Alcohol—Certain medicines should not be used at or around the time of eating food or eating certain types of food since interactions may occur. Using alcohol or tobacco with certain medicines may also cause interactions to occur. Discuss with your healthcare professional the use of your medicine with food, alcohol, or tobacco.

Proper Use of This Medicine

Dosing—The dose of this medicine will be different for different patients. Follow your doctor's orders or the directions on the label. The following information includes only the average doses of this medicine. If your dose is different, do not change it unless your doctor tells you to do so.

The amount of medicine that you take depends on the strength of the medicine. Also, the number of doses you take each day, the time allowed between doses, and the length of time you take the medicine depend on the medical problem for which you are using the medicine.

- For Mycopolysaccharidosis I:
  - For injection dosage form:
    - Adults and children—The dose is based on body weight and must be determined by your doctor. The usual dose is 0.58 milligrams (mg) per kilogram (kg), (0.26 mg per pound) given once weekly. It is injected slowly into a vein over three to four hours.

Precautions While Using This Medicine

Regular visits: If you will be taking this medicine for a long time, it is very important that your doctor check you at regular visits

Side Effects of This Medicine

Along with its needed effects, a medicine may cause some unwanted effects. Although not all of these side effects may occur, if they do occur they may need medical attention.

Check with your doctor immediately if any of the following side effects occur:

More common
Abdominal or stomach pain; accumulation of pus; black, tarry stools; bleeding gums; blood in urine or stools; blurred vision; chest pain; chills; clay-colored stools; confusion; dark urine; dizziness; facial swelling; faintness; fever; headache; itching; lightheadedness when getting up from a lying or sitting position suddenly; loss of appetite; nausea or vomiting; pinpoint red spots on skin; shortness of breath; skin rash; sweating; swollen, red, tender area of infection; unpleasant breath odor; unusual bleeding or bruising; unusual tiredness or weakness; vomiting of blood; yellow eyes or skin

Less common
Cough; difficulty breathing; itching skin; large, hive-like swelling on face, eyelids, lips, tongue, throat, hands, legs, feet, sex organs; noisy breathing; redness of skin; shortness of breath; tightness in chest; wheezing

Some side effects may occur that usually do not need medical attention. These side effects may go away during treatment as your body adjusts to the medicine. Also, your health care professional may be able to tell you about ways to prevent or reduce some of these side effects. Check with your health care professional if any of the following side effects continue or are bothersome or if you have any questions about them:

More common
Bleeding, blistering, burning, coldness, discoloration of skin; blindness; body aches or pain; body produces substance that can bind to drug making it less effective or cause side effects; burning, crawling, itching, numbness, prickling, "pins and needles", or tingling feelings; decreased vision; ear congestion; feeling of pressure; hives, infection, inflammation, itching, lumps, numbness, pain, rash, redness, scarring, soreness, stinging, swelling, tenderness, tingling, ulceration, or warmth at injection site; loss of voice; nasal congestion; overactive reflexes; runny nose; sneezing; sore throat; swelling of legs and feet; swelling or puffiness of face; varicose or spider veins

Other side effects not listed may also occur in some patients. If you notice any other effects, check with your healthcare professional.

LATANOPROST (Ophthalmic route) -
la-TA-noe-prost

Commonly used brand name(s)

In the U.S.—
    Xalatan

Available Dosage Forms:
- Solution

Therapeutic Class: Antiglaucoma
Pharmacologic Class: Prostaglandin

Uses For This Medicine

Latanoprost is used to treat certain kinds of glaucoma. It is also used to treat a condition called hypertension of the eye. Latanoprost appears to work by increasing the outflow of fluid from the eye. This lowers the pressure in the eye.

This medicine is available only with your doctor's prescription.

Before Using This Medicine

In deciding to use a medicine, the risks of taking the medicine must be weighed against the good it will do. This is a decision you and your doctor will make. For this medicine, the following should be considered:

Allergies—Tell your doctor if you have ever had any unusual or allergic reaction to this medicine or any other medicines. Also tell your health care professional if you have any other types of allergies, such as to foods, dyes, preservatives, or animals. For non-prescription products, read the label or package ingredients carefully.

Pediatric—Studies on this medicine have been done only in adult patients, and there is no specific information com-

paring use of latanoprost in children with use in other age groups.

Geriatric—Many medicines have not been studied specifically in older people. Therefore, it may not be known whether they work exactly the same way they do in younger adults. Although there is no specific information comparing use of latanoprost in the elderly with use in other age groups, this medicine has been used mostly in elderly patients and is not expected to cause different side effects or problems in older people than it does in younger adults.

Other medicines—Although certain medicines should not be used together at all, in other cases two different medicines may be used together even if an interaction might occur. In these cases, your doctor may want to change the dose, or other precautions may be necessary. Tell your healthcare professional if you are taking any other prescription or non-prescription (over-the-counter [OTC]) medicine.

Interactions with Food/Tobacco/Alcohol—Certain medicines should not be used at or around the time of eating food or eating certain types of food since interactions may occur. Using alcohol or tobacco with certain medicines may also cause interactions to occur. Discuss with your healthcare professional the use of your medicine with food, alcohol, or tobacco.

Other medical problems—The presence of other medical problems may affect the use of this medicine. Make sure you tell your doctor if you have any other medical problems, especially:

- Eye disease, such as iritis or uveitis—Use of latanoprost may make the condition worse
- Eye problems, such as loss of the lens of the eye or
- Intraocular lens (IOL) replacement—May be more prone to an adverse reaction called macular edema
- Kidney disease or
- Liver disease—Higher blood levels of latanoprost may result, which may lead to increased side effects

Proper Use of This Medicine

Use this medicine only as directed. Do not use more of it and do not use it more often than your doctor ordered. To do so may increase the chance of too much medicine being absorbed into the body and the chance of side effects.

If your doctor ordered two different eye drops to be used together, wait at least 5 minutes between the times you apply the medicines. This will help to keep the second medicine from "washing out" the first one.

It is important that your doctor check your eye pressure at regular visits to make certain that your glaucoma is being controlled.

Contact lenses should be removed before you use this medicine. You should wait at least 15 minutes after using the eye drops before reinserting them.

To use the eye drops:

- First, wash your hands. Tilt the head back and, pressing your finger gently on the skin just beneath the lower eyelid, pull the lower eyelid away from the eye to make a space. Drop the medicine into this space. Let go of the eyelid and gently close the eyes. Do not blink. Keep the eyes closed and apply pressure to the inner corner of the eye with your finger for 1 or 2 minutes to allow the medicine to be absorbed by the eye.

- Immediately after using the eye drops, wash your hands to remove any medicine that may be on them.
- To keep the medicine as germ-free as possible, do not touch the applicator tip to any surface (including the eye). Also, keep the container tightly closed.

Dosing—The dose of this medicine will be different for different patients. Follow your doctor's orders or the directions on the label. The following information includes only the average doses of this medicine. If your dose is different, do not change it unless your doctor tells you to do so.

The amount of medicine that you take depends on the strength of the medicine. Also, the number of doses you take each day, the time allowed between doses, and the length of time you take the medicine depend on the medical problem for which you are using the medicine.

- For ophthalmic solution (eye drops) dosage form:
  - For glaucoma or hypertension of the eye:
    - Adults—Use one drop in the affected eye(s) once a day in the evening.
    - Children—Use and dose must be determined by your doctor.

Missed dose—If you miss a dose of this medicine, take it as soon as possible. However, if it is almost time for your next dose, skip the missed dose and go back to your regular dosing schedule. Do not double doses.

Storage—Keep out of the reach of children.

Do not keep outdated medicine or medicine no longer needed.

Before the bottle has been opened for the first time, store in the refrigerator. After the bottle has been opened, store at room temperature (up to 25 °C [77 °F]) for up to 6 weeks, or in the refrigerator.

Precautions While Using This Medicine

While you are using latanoprost, the iris (colored part) of your treated eye(s) may slowly become more brown in color. This is more likely to happen if you have blue-brown, gray-brown, green-brown, or yellow-brown eyes. The change in color of the iris is noticeable usually within several months or years from the start of treatment with latanoprost. In addition, there may be a darkening of eyelid skin color. Also, your eyelashes may become longer, thicker, and darker. These changes to the iris, eyelid, and lashes may be permanent even if you stop using latanoprost. Also, these changes to the iris, eyelid, and lashes will affect only the eye being treated with latanoprost. Therefore, if only one eye is being treated, only that eye may develop darker iris, eyelid, and eyelashes and other changes to the eyelashes, and you may have differently appearing eyes. Check with your doctor if you have any questions about this.

Latanoprost may cause your eyes to become more sensitive to light than they are normally. Wearing sunglasses and avoiding too much exposure to bright light may help lessen the discomfort.

Side Effects of This Medicine

Along with its needed effects, a medicine may cause some unwanted effects. Although not all of these side effects may occur, if they do occur they may need medical attention.

Check with your doctor immediately if any of the following side effects occur:

Less common

Eyelid crusting, redness, swelling, discomfort, or pain

Rare

Cough; difficulty breathing; noisy breathing; redness of eye or inside of eyelid; shortness of breath; swelling of the eye; tightness in chest; wheezing

Check with your doctor as soon as possible if any of the following side effects occur:

More common

Blurred vision, eye irritation, or tearing; darkening of eyelid skin color; increase in brown color in colored part of eye; longer, thicker, and darker eyelashes

Less common

Angina pectoris or other chest pain; cold or flu symptoms; eye pain; pain in muscles, joints, or back; skin rash

Rare

Discharge from the eye; double vision or other change in vision; fever; sensitivity of eye to light; sore throat

Some side effects may occur that usually do not need medical attention. These side effects may go away during treatment as your body adjusts to the medicine. Also, your health care professional may be able to tell you about ways to prevent or reduce some of these side effects. Check with your health care professional if any of the following side effects continue or are bothersome or if you have any questions about them:

More common

Burning of eye; feeling of something in eye; itching of eye; stinging of eye

Less common

Dryness of eye

Other side effects not listed may also occur in some patients. If you notice any other effects, check with your healthcare professional.

LAXATIVES (Oral)

Some commonly used brand names are:

In the U.S.—

Agoral 350
Alophen 25
Alphamul 30
Alramucil Orange 7
Alramucil Regular 7
Bisac-Evac 25
Black-Draught 26
Black-Draught Lax-Senna 32
Carter's Little Pills 25
Cholac 14
Citroma 16
Citrucel Orange Flavor 3
Citrucel Sugar-Free Orange Flavor 3
Colace 39
Constilac 14
Constulose 14
Correctol 25
Correctol Caplets 25
Correctol Herbal Tea 32
Correctol Stool Softener Soft Gels 39
DC Softgels 39
Diocto 39
Diocto-C 35
Dioeze 39
Diosuccin 39
Docu-K Plus 35
DOK 39
DOK Softgels 39
D.O.S. Softgels 39
Dr. Caldwell Senna Laxative 32
D-S-S 39
D-S-S plus 35
Dulcolax 25
Emulsoil 30
Enulose 14
Epsom salts 19
Equalactin 4
Evac-U-Gen 33

Ex-Lax 33iV
Ex-Lax Chocolate 33
FemiLax 25
Fiberall 7
Fibercon Caplets 4
Fiber-Lax 4
FiberNorm 4
Fleet Laxative 25
Fleet Mineral Oil 24
Fleet Phospho-Soda 20
Fleet Soflax Gelcaps 39
Fleet Soflax Overnight Gelcaps 35
Fletcher's Castoria 32
Genasoft Plus Softgels 35
Gentle Laxative 25
Haley's M-O 21
Herbal Laxative 33
Hydrocil Instant 7
Kondremul Plain 24
Konsyl 6
Konsyl-D 7
Konsyl Easy Mix 7
Konsyl-Orange 7
Konsyl-Orange Sugar Free 7
Laxinate 100 39
Liqui-Doss 24
Mag-Ox 400 18
Maltsupex 1
Metamucil 7
Metamucil Apple Crisp Fiber Wafers 7
Metamucil Cinnamon Spice Fiber Wafers 7
Metamucil Orange Flavor 7
Metamucil Smooth, Citrus Flavor 7
Metamucil Smooth, Orange Flavor 7
Metamucil Smooth Sugar-Free, Citrus Flavor 7
Metamucil Smooth Sugar-Free, Orange Flavor 7
Metamucil Smooth Sugar-Free, Regular Flavor 7
Metamucil Sugar-Free, Lemon-Lime Flavor 7

Metamucil Orange Flavor 7
Metamucil Sugar-Free, Orange Flavor 7
MiraLax 15
Modane 25
Modane Bulk 7
Mylanta Natural Fiber Supplement 7
Mylanta Sugar Free Natural Fiber Supplement 7
Nature's Remedy 33
Neoloid 30
Perdiem 9
Perdiem Fiber 6
Peri-Colace 35
Peri-Dos Softgels 35
Phillips' Chewable 17
Phillips' Concentrated 17
Phillips' Stool Softner Laxative Softgels 39
Phillips' Milk of Magnesia 17
Prompt 11
Purge 30
Reguloid Natural 7
Reguloid Natural Sugar Free 7
Reguloid Orange 7
Reguloid Orange Sugar Free 7
Senexon 32
Senna-Gen 32
Senokot 33
Senokot Children's Syrup 33
Senokot-S 38
SenokotXTRA 33
Senolax 32
Serutan 7
Serutan Toasted Granules 8
Silace 39
Silace-C 35
Sulfolax 39
Surfak 39
Syllact 6
Veracolate 25
V-Lax 7
X-Prep Liquid 32

In Canada—
Acilac 14
Apo-Bisacodyl 25
Bicholate Lilas 29
Bisacolax 25

Carter's Little Pills 25
Citro-Mag 16
Colace 39
Correctol 25
Correctol Stool Softener Soft Gels 39
Dulcolax 25
Ex-Lax 33
Ex-Lax Chocolate 33
Ex-Lax Extra Strength 33
Ex-Lax Gentle Strength 38
Feen-a-Mint 25
Fletcher's Castoria 33
Glysennid 33
Herbal Laxative 32
Kondremul 24
Lansol 24
Lansol Sugar Free 24
Magnolax 21
Metamucil 7
Metamucil Orange Flavor 7
Metamucil Sugar Free 7
Metamucil Sugar-Free, Orange Flavor 7
Natural Source Fibre Laxative 7
Nature's Remedy 33
Nujol 24
Peri-Colace 35
Phillips' Magnesia Tablets 17
Phillips' Milk of Magnesia 17
PMS-Bisacodyl 25
PMS-Docusate Calcium 39
PMS-Docusate Sodium 39
PMS-Lactulose 14
PMS-Sennosides 33
Prodiem Plain 7
Prodiem Plus 10
Pro-Lax 15
Senokot 33
Senokot-S 38
SenoKot XTRA 33
Silace 39
Soflax 39
Surfak 39
Vitalax Super Smooth Sugar Free Orange Flavor 7
Vitalax Unflavored 7

Note: For quick reference the following laxatives are numbered to match the corresponding brand names.

Bulk-forming laxatives—

1. Malt Soup Extract (malt soup EX-tract)
2. Malt Soup Extract and Psyllium (malt soup EX-tract and SILL-i-yum)
3. Methylcellulose (meth-ill-SELL-yoo-lose)
4. Polycarbophil (pol-i-KAR-boe-fil)

5. Polycarbophil and Psyllium (pol-i-KAR-boe-fil and SILL-i-yum)
6. Psyllium (SILL-i-yum)
7. Psyllium Hydrophilic Mucilloid (SILL-i-yumhye-droe-FILL-ik MYOO-sill-oid)
8. Psyllium Hydrophilic Mucilloid and Carboxymethylcellulose (SILL-i-yum hye-droe-FILL-ik MYOO-sill-oid and kar-box-ee-meth-ill-SELL-yoo-lose)

Bulk-forming and stimulant combinations—
9. Psyllium and Senna (SILL-i-yum and SEN-na)
10. Psyllium Hydrophilic Mucilloid and Senna (SILL-i-yum hye-droe-FILL-ik MYOO-sill-oid and SEN-na)
11. Psyllium Hydrophilic Mucilloid and Sennosides (SILL-i-yum hye-droe-FILL-ik MYOO-sill-oid and SEN-no-sydes)

Bulk-forming, stimulant, and stool softener (emollient) combinations—
12. Product not available

Bulk-forming and stool softener (emollient) combinations—
13. Product not available

Hyperosmotic laxatives—Lactulose—
14. Lactulose (LAC-tu-los)

Hyperosmotic laxatives—Polymer—
15. Polyethylene glycol 3350 (pol-ee-ETH-ill-een GLYE-cal)

Hyperosmotic laxatives—Saline—
16. Magnesium Citrate (mag-NEE-zhum SI-trate)
17. Magnesium Hydroxide (mag-NEE-zhumhye-DROX-ide)
18. Magnesium Oxide (mag-NEE-zhum OX-ide)
19. Magnesium Sulfate (mag-NEE-zhum SUL-fate)
20. Sodium Phosphate (SOE-dee-um FOS-fate)

Hyperosmotic and lubricant combinations—
21. Milk of Magnesia and Mineral Oil (milk of mag-NEE-zha and MIN-er-al oil)
22. Mineral Oil and Glycerin (MIN-er-aloil and GLIH-ser-in)*

Hyperosmotic and stimulant combinations—
23. Milk of Magnesia and Cascara Sagrada (milk of mag-NEE-zha and kas-KAR-a sa-GRA-da)

Lubricant laxatives—
24. Mineral Oil (MIN-er-al oil)

Stimulant laxatives—
25. Bisacodyl (bis-a-KOE-dill)
26. Casanthranol (cas-SAN-thrah-nole)
27. Cascara Sagrada (kas-KAR-a sa-GRA-da)
28. Cascara Sagrada and Aloe (kas-KAR-a sa-GRA-da and AL-owe)
29. Cascara Sagrada and Bisacodyl (kas-KAR-a sa-GRA-da and bis-a-KOE-dill)
30. Castor Oil (KAS-tor)
31. Dehydrocholic Acid (dee-hye-droe-KOE-likacid)
32. Senna (SEN-na)
33. Sennosides (SEN-no-sides)

Stimulant and stool softener (emollient) combinations—
34. Bisacodyl and Docusate (bis-a-KOE-dilland doc-CUE-sayt)*
35. Casanthranol and Docusate (cas-SAN-thrah-nole and doc-CUE-sayt)
36. Danthron and Docusate (DAN-thron and doc-CUE-sayt)*
37. Dehydrocholic Acid and Docusate (dee-hye-droe-KOE-lik acid and doc-CUE-sayt)
38. Sennosides and Docusate (SEN-no-sides and doc-CUE-sayt)

Stool softener (emollient) laxatives—
39. Docusate (doc-CUE-sayt)
40. Poloxamer 188 (pol-OX-a-mer 188)

Category

• **Antacid**—Magnesium Hydroxide; Magnesium Oxide

• **Antidiarrheal**—Polycarbophil; Psyllium Hydrophilic Mucilloid

• **Antihyperammonemic**—Lactulose

• **Antihyperlipidemic**—Psyllium Hydrophilic Mucilloid

• **Hydrocholeretic**—Dehydrocholic Acid

• **Laxative, bulk-forming**—Malt Soup Extract; Malt Soup Extract and Psyllium; Methylcellulose; Polycarbophil; Psyllium; Psyllium Hydrophilic Mucilloid; Psyllium Hydrophilic Mucilloid and Carboxymethylcellulose

• **Laxative, bulk-forming and stimulant**—Psyllium and Senna; Psyllium Hydrophilic Mucilloid and Senna; Psyllium Hydrophilic Mucilloid and Sennosides

• **Laxative, carbon dioxide-releasing**—Potassium Bitartrate and Sodium Bicarbonate

• **Laxative, hyperosmotic**—Glycerin; Lactulose; Polyethylene Glycol

• **Laxative, hyperosmotic and lubricant**—Magnesium Hydroxide and Mineral Oil; Mineral Oil and Glycerin

• **Laxative, hyperosmotic and stimulant**—Magnesium Hydroxide and Cascara Sagrada

• **Laxative, hyperosmotic, saline**—Magnesium Citrate; Magnesium Hydroxide; Magnesium Oxide; Magnesium Sulfate; Sodium Phosphate

• **Laxative, lubricant**—Mineral Oil

• **Laxative, stimulant and stool softener (emollient)**—Bisacodyl and Docusate; Casanthranol and Docusate; Danthron and Docusate; Dehydrocholic Acid and Docusate; Sennosides and Docusate

• **Laxative, stimulant or contact**—Bisacodyl; Casanthranol; Cascara Sagrada and Bisacodyl; Cascara Sagrada; Cascara Sagrada and Aloe; Castor Oil; Dehydrocholic Acid; Senna; Sennosides

• **Laxative, stool softener (emollient)**—Docusate; Poloxamer 188

Description

Oral laxatives are medicines taken by mouth to encourage bowel movements to relieve constipation.

There are several different types of oral laxatives and they work in different ways. Since directions for use are different for each type, it is important to know which one you are taking. The different types of oral laxatives include:

Bulk-formers—Bulk-forming laxatives are not digested but absorb liquid in the intestines and swell to form a soft, bulky stool. The bowel is then stimulated normally by the presence of the bulky mass. Some bulk-forming laxatives, like psyllium and polycarbophil, may be prescribed by your doctor to treat diarrhea.

Hyperosmotics—Hyperosmotic laxatives encourage bowel movements by drawing water into the bowel from surrounding body tissues. This provides a soft stool mass and increased bowel action.

There are three types of hyperosmotic laxatives taken by mouth— the saline, the lactulose, and the polymer types. The *saline type* is often called "salts." They are used for rapid emptying of the lower intestine and bowel. They are not used for long-term or repeated correction of constipation. With smaller doses than those used for the laxative effect, some saline laxatives are used as antacids. The information that follows applies only to their use as laxatives. Sodium phosphate may also be prescribed for other conditions as determined by your doctor.

The *lactulose type* is a special sugar-like laxative that works the same way as the saline type. However, it produces results much more slowly and is often used for long-term treatment of chronic constipation. Lactulose may sometimes be used in the treatment of certain medical conditions to reduce the amount of ammonia in the blood. It is available only with your doctor's prescription.

The *polymer type* is a polyglycol (polyethylene glycol), a large molecule that causes water to be retained in the stool; this will soften the stool and increase the number of bowel movements. It is used for short periods of time to treat constipation.

Lubricants—Lubricant laxatives, such as mineral oil, taken by mouth encourage bowel movements by coating the bowel and the stool mass with a waterproof film. This keeps moisture in the stool. The stool remains soft and its passage is made easier.

Stimulants—Stimulant laxatives, also known as contact laxatives, encourage bowel movements by acting on the intestinal wall. They increase the muscle contractions that move along the stool mass. Stimulant laxatives are a popular type of laxative for self-treatment. However, they also are more likely to cause side effects. One of the stimulant laxatives, dehydrocholic acid, may also be used for treating certain conditions of the biliary tract.

Stool softeners (emollients)—Stool softeners encourage bowel movements by helping liquids mix into the stool and prevent dry, hard stool masses. This type of laxative has been said not to *cause* a bowel movement but instead *allows* the patient to have a bowel movement without straining.

Combinations—There are many products that you can buy for constipation that contain more than one type of laxative. For example, a product may contain both a stool softener and a stimulant laxative. In general, combination products may be more likely to cause side effects because of the multiple ingredients. In addition, they may not offer any advantage over products containing only one type of laxative. *If you are taking a combination laxative, make certain you know the proper use and precautions for each of the different ingredients.*

Most laxatives (except saline laxatives) may be used to provide relief:

- during pregnancy.
- for a few days after giving birth.
- during preparation for examination or surgery.
- for constipation of bedfast patients.
- for constipation caused by other medicines.
- following surgery when straining should be avoided.
- following a period of poor eating habits or a lack of physical exercise in order to develop normal bowel function (bulk-forming laxatives only).
- for some medical conditions that may be made worse by straining, for example:
  - Heart disease
  - Hemorrhoids
  - Hernia (rupture)
  - High blood pressure (hypertension)
  - History of stroke

Saline laxatives have more limited uses and may be used to provide rapid results:

- during preparation for examination or surgery.
- for elimination of food or drugs from the body in cases of poisoning or overdose.

- for simple constipation that happens on occasion (although another type of laxative may be preferred).
- in supplying a fresh stool sample for diagnosis.

Most laxatives are available without a prescription; however, your doctor may have special instructions for the proper use and dose for your medical condition. They are available in the following dosage forms:

Oral

- **Bulk-forming laxatives—**
  - Malt Soup Extract
    - Powder
    - Oral solution
    - Tablets
  - Malt Soup Extract and Psyllium
    - Powder
  - Methylcellulose
    - Capsules
    - Granules
    - Powder
    - Oral solution
    - Tablets
  - Polycarbophil
    - Tablets
    - Chewable tablets
  - Psyllium
    - Caramels
    - Granules
    - Powder
  - Psyllium Hydrophilic Mucilloid
    - Granules
    - Powder
    - Effervescent powder
    - For oral suspension
    - Wafers
  - Psyllium Hydrophilic Mucilloid and Carboxymethylcellulose
    - Granules
- **Bulk-forming and stimulant combinations—**
  - Psyllium and Senna
    - Granules
  - Psyllium Hydrophilic Mucilloid and Senna
    - Granules
  - Psyllium Hydrophilic Mucilloid and Sennosides
    - Powder
- **Hyperosmotic laxative—Lactulose:**
  - Lactulose
    - Solution
- **Hyperosmotic laxative—Polyethylene Glycol:**
  - Polyethylene glycol 3350
    - Powder
- **Hyperosmotic laxatives—Saline:**
  - Magnesium Citrate
    - Oral solution
  - Magnesium Hydroxide
    - Milk of magnesia
    - Tablets
  - Magnesium Oxide
    - Tablets
  - Magnesium Sulfate
    - Crystals
    - Tablets
  - Sodium Phosphate
    - Effervescent powder
    - Oral solution

- **Hyperosmotic and lubricant combinations—**
  - Milk of Magnesia and Mineral Oil
    - Emulsion
  - Mineral Oil and Glycerin
    - Emulsion
- **Hyperosmotic and stimulant combination—**
  - Milk of Magnesia and Cascara Sagrada
    - Oral Suspension
- **Lubricant laxatives—**
  - Mineral Oil
    - Oil
    - Emulsion
    - Gel
    - Oral suspension
- **Stimulant laxatives—**
  - Bisacodyl
    - Tablets
  - Casanthranol
    - Syrup
  - Cascara Sagrada
    - Fluid extract
    - Tablets
  - Cascara Sagrada and Aloe
    - Tablets
  - Cascara Sagrada and Bisacodyl
    - Tablets
  - Castor Oil
    - Oil
    - Emulsion
  - Dehydrocholic Acid
    - Tablets
  - Senna
    - Granules
    - Oral solution
    - For oral solution
    - Syrup
    - Tablets
  - Sennosides
    - Granules
    - Oral solution
    - Syrup
    - Tablets
- **Stimulant and stool softener (emollient) combinations—**
  - Bisacodyl and Docusate
    - Tablets
  - Casanthranol and Docusate
    - Capsules
    - Syrup
    - Tablets
  - Danthron and Docusate
    - Capsules
    - Tablets
  - Dehydrocholic Acid and Docusate
    - Capsules
    - Tablets
  - Sennosides and Docusate
    - Tablets
- **Stool softener (emollient) laxatives—**
  - Docusate
    - Capsules
    - Oral solution
    - Syrup
    - Tablets
  - Poloxamer 188
    - Capsules

Before Using This Medicine

Importance of diet, fluids, and exercise to prevent constipation—Laxatives are to be used to provide short-term relief only, unless otherwise directed by a doctor. A proper diet containing roughage (whole grain breads and cereals, bran, fruit, and green, leafy vegetables), with 6 to 8 full glasses (8 ounces each) of liquids each day, and daily exercise are most important in maintaining healthy bowel function. Also, for individuals who have problems with constipation, foods such as pastries, puddings, sugar, candy, cake, and cheese may make the constipation worse.

If you are taking this medicine without a prescription, carefully read and follow any precautions on the label. For oral laxatives, the following should be considered:

Allergies—Tell your doctor if you have ever had any unusual or allergic reaction to laxatives. Also tell your health care professional if you are allergic to any other substances, such as foods, preservatives, or dyes.

Diet—Make certain your health care professional knows if you are on any special diet, such as a low-sodium or low-sugar diet. Some laxatives have large amounts of sodium or sugars in them.

Pregnancy—Although laxatives are often used during pregnancy, some types are better than others. Stool softeners (emollient) laxatives and bulk-forming laxatives are probably used most often. If you are using a laxative during pregnancy, remember that:

- Some laxatives (in particular, the bulk-formers) contain a large amount of sodium or sugars, which may have possible unwanted effects such as increasing blood pressure or causing water to be held in the body.
- Saline laxatives containing magnesium, potassium, or phosphates may have to be avoided if your kidney function is not normal.
- Mineral oil is usually not used during pregnancy because of possible unwanted effects on the mother or infant. Mineral oil may interfere with the absorption of nutrients and vitamins in the mother. Also, if taken for a long time during pregnancy, mineral oil may cause severe bleeding in the newborn infant.
- Stimulant laxatives may cause unwanted effects in the expectant mother if improperly used. Castor oil in particular should not be used as it may cause contractions of the womb.

Breast-feeding—Laxatives containing cascara and danthron may pass into the breast milk. Although the amount of laxative in the milk is generally thought to be too small to cause problems in the baby, your doctor should be told if you plan to use such laxatives. Some reports claim that diarrhea has been caused in the infant.

Children—*Laxatives should not be given to young children (up to 6 years of age) unless prescribed by their doctor.* Since children usually cannot describe their symptoms very well, they should be checked by a doctor before being given a laxative. The child may have a condition that needs other treatment. If so, laxatives will not help, and may even cause unwanted effects or make the condition worse.

Mineral oil should not be given to young children (up to 6 years of age) because a form of pneumonia may be caused by the inhalation of oil droplets into the lungs.

Also, bisacodyl tablets should not be given to children up to 6 years of age because if chewed they may cause stomach irritation.

Older adults—Mineral oil should not be taken by bedridden elderly persons because a form of pneumonia may be caused by the inhalation of oil droplets into the lungs. Also, stimulant laxatives (e.g., bisacodyl or casanthranol), if taken too often, may worsen weakness, lack of coordination, or dizziness and light-headedness.

Polyethylene glycol 3350 should be discontinued if diarrhea occurs, especially in elderly persons in nursing homes.

Other medicines—Although certain medicines should not be used together at all, in other cases two different medicines may be used together even if an interaction might occur. In these cases, your doctor may want to change the dose, or other precautions may be necessary. When you are taking oral laxatives, it is especially important that your health care professional know if you are taking any of the following:

- Anticoagulants, oral (blood thinners you take by mouth) or
- Digitalis glycosides (heart medicine)—The use of magnesium-containing laxatives may reduce the effects of these medicines
- Ciprofloxacin (e.g., Cipro) or
- Etidronate (e.g., Didronel) or
- Sodium polystyrene sulfonate—Use of magnesium-containing laxatives will keep these medicines from working
- Tetracyclines taken by mouth (medicine for infection)—Use of bulk-forming or magnesium-containing laxatives will keep the tetracycline medicine from working

Other medical problems—The presence of other medical problems may affect the use of oral laxatives. Make sure you tell your doctor if you have any other medical problems, especially:

- Appendicitis (or signs of) or
- Rectal bleeding of unknown cause—These conditions need immediate attention by a doctor
- Colostomy or
- Intestinal blockage or
- Ileostomy—The use of laxatives may create other problems if these conditions are present
- Diabetes mellitus (sugar diabetes)—Diabetic patients should be careful since some laxatives contain large amounts of sugars, such as dextrose, galactose, and/or sucrose
- Heart disease or
- High blood pressure—Some laxatives contain large amounts of sodium, which may make these conditions worse
- Kidney disease—Magnesium and potassium (contained in some laxatives) may build up in the body if kidney disease is present; a serious condition may develop
- Swallowing difficulty—Mineral oil should not be used since it may get into the lungs by accident and cause pneumonia; also, bulk-forming laxatives may get lodged in the esophagus of patients who have difficulty in swallowing

Proper Use of This Medicine

For safe and effective use of your laxative:
- Follow your doctor's instructions if this laxative was prescribed.
- Follow the manufacturer's package directions if you are treating yourself.

With all kinds of laxatives, at least 6 to 8 glasses (8 ounces each) of liquids should be taken each day. This will help make the stool softer.

For *patients taking laxatives containing a bulk-forming ingredient:*
- Do not try to swallow in the dry form. Take with liquid.
- To allow bulk-forming laxatives to work properly and to prevent intestinal blockage, it is necessary to drink plenty of fluids during their use. Each dose should be taken in or with a full glass (8 ounces) or more of cold water or fruit juice. This will provide enough liquid for the laxative to work properly. A second glass of water or juice by itself is often recommended with each dose for best effect and to avoid side effects.
- When taking a product that contains only a bulk-forming ingredient, results often may be obtained in 12 hours. However, this may not occur for some individuals until after 2 or 3 days.

For *patients taking laxatives containing a stool softener (emollient):*
- Liquid forms may be taken in milk or fruit juice to improve flavor.
- When taking a product that contains only a stool softener, results usually occur 1 to 2 days after the first dose. However, this may not occur for some individuals until after 3 to 5 days.

For *patients taking laxatives containing a hyperosmotic ingredient:*
- Each dose should be taken in or with a full glass (8 ounces) or more of cold water or fruit juice. This will provide enough liquid for the laxative to work properly. A second glass of water or juice by itself is often recommended with each dose for best effect and, in the case of saline laxatives, to prevent you from becoming dehydrated.
- The unpleasant taste produced by some hyperosmotic laxatives may be improved by following each dose with citrus fruit juice or citrus-flavored carbonated beverage.
- Lactulose may not produce laxative results for 24 to 48 hours.
- Polyethylene glycol may not produce laxative results for 2 to 4 days.
- Saline laxatives usually produce results within ½ to 3 hours following a dose. When a larger dose is taken on an empty stomach, the results are quicker. When a smaller dose is taken with food, the results are delayed. Therefore, large doses of saline laxatives are usually not taken late in the day on an empty stomach.

For *patients taking laxatives containing mineral oil:*
- Mineral oil should not be taken within 2 hours of meals because of possible interference with food digestion and absorption of nutrients and vitamins.
- Mineral oil is usually taken at bedtime (but not while lying down) for convenience and because it requires about 6 to 8 hours to produce results.

For *patients taking laxatives containing a stimulant ingredient:*
- Stimulant laxatives are usually taken on an empty stomach for rapid effect. Results are slowed if taken with food.
- Many stimulant laxatives (but not castor oil) are often taken at bedtime to produce results the next morning (although some may require 24 hours or more).

- *Castor oil* is not usually taken late in the day because its results occur within 2 to 6 hours.
- The unpleasant taste of *castor oil* may be improved by chilling in the refrigerator for at least an hour and then stirring the dose into a full glass of cold orange juice just before it is taken. Also, flavored preparations of castor oil are available.
- *Bisacodyl tablets* are specially coated to allow them to work properly without causing irritation and/or nausea. To protect this coating, do not chew, crush, or take the tablets within an hour of milk or antacids.

Dosing—There are a large number of laxative products on the market. The dose of laxatives will be different for different products. The number of capsules or tablets or teaspoonfuls of crystals, gel, granules, liquid, or powder that you use; the number of caramels or wafers that you eat; or the number of pieces of gum that you chew depends on the strength of the medicine. *Follow your doctor's orders if this medicine was prescribed, or follow the directions on the box if you are buying this medicine without a prescription.*

Storage—To store this medicine:
- Keep out of the reach of children.
- Store away from heat and direct light.
- Do not store the capsule, tablet, granules, or powder form of this medicine in the bathroom, near the kitchen sink, or in other damp places. Heat or moisture may cause the medicine to break down.
- Keep the liquid form of this medicine from freezing.
- Do not keep outdated medicine or medicine no longer needed. Be sure that any discarded medicine is out of the reach of children.

Precautions While Using This Medicine

Do not take any type of laxative:
- *if you have signs of appendicitis or inflamed bowel* (such as stomach or lower abdominal pain, cramping, bloating, soreness, nausea, or vomiting). Instead, check with your doctor as soon as possible.
- *for more than 1 week* unless your doctor has prescribed or ordered a special schedule for you. This is true even when you have had no results from the laxative.
- *within 2 hours of taking other medicine* because the desired effect of the other medicine may be reduced.
- *if you do not need it,* as for the common cold," to clean out your system" or as a" tonic to make you feel better."
- *if you miss a bowel movement for a day or two.*
- *if you develop a skin rash* while taking a laxative or if you had a rash the last time you took it. Instead, check with your doctor.

If you notice a sudden change in bowel habits or function that lasts longer than 2 weeks, or that keeps returning off and on, check with your doctor before using a laxative. This will allow the cause of your problem to be determined before it may become more serious.

The "laxative habit"—Laxative products are overused by many people. Such a practice often leads to dependence on the laxative action to produce a bowel movement. In severe cases, overuse of some laxatives has caused damage to the nerves, muscles, and tissues of the intestines and bowel. If you have any questions about the use of laxatives, check with your health care professional.

Many laxatives often contain large amounts of sugars, carbohydrates, and sodium. If you are on a low-sugar, low-caloric, or low-sodium diet, check with your health care professional before using a laxative.

For *patients taking laxatives containing mineral oil:*
- Mineral oil should not be taken often or for long periods of time because:
  ○ gradual build-up in body tissues may create additional problems.
  ○ the use of mineral oil may interfere with the body's ability to absorb certain food nutrients and vitamins A, D, E, and K.
- Large doses of mineral oil may cause some leakage from the rectum. The use of absorbent pads or a decrease in dose may be necessary to prevent the soiling of clothing.
- Do not take mineral oil within 2 hours of a stool softener (emollient laxative). The stool softener may increase the amount of mineral oil absorbed.

For *patients taking laxatives containing a stimulant ingredient:*
- Stimulant laxatives are most often associated with:
  ○ overuse and the laxative habit.
  ○ skin rashes.
  ○ intestinal cramping after dosing (especially if taken on an empty stomach).
  ○ potassium loss.

Side Effects of This Medicine

Along with its needed effects, a medicine may cause some unwanted effects. Although not all of these side effects may occur, if they do occur they may need medical attention.

Check with your doctor as soon as possible if any of the following side effects occur:
For bulk-forming-containing
  Difficulty in breathing; intestinal blockage; skin rash or itching; swallowing difficulty (feeling of lump in throat)
For hyperosmotic-containing
  Confusion; dizziness or light-headedness; irregular heartbeat; muscle cramps; unusual tiredness or weakness
For stimulant-containing
  Confusion; irregular heartbeat; muscle cramps; pink to red, red to violet, or red to brown coloration of alkaline urine (for cascara, danthron, and/or senna only); skin rash; unusual tiredness or weakness; yellow to brown coloration of acid urine (for cascara, and/or senna only)
For stool softener (emollient)-containing
  Skin rash

Other side effects may occur that usually do not need medical attention. These side effects are less common and may go away during treatment as your body adjusts to the medicine. However, check with your doctor if any of the following side effects continue or are bothersome:
For hyperosmotic-containing
  Bloating; cramping; diarrhea; nausea; gas; increased thirst

For lubricant-containing
  Skin irritation surrounding rectal area
For stimulant-containing
  Belching; cramping; diarrhea; nausea
For stool softener (emollient)-containing
  Stomach and/or intestinal cramping; throat irritation
  (liquid forms only)

Other side effects not listed above may also occur in some patients. If you notice any other effects, check with your doctor.

Additional Information

Once a medicine has been approved for marketing for a certain use, experience may show that it is also useful for other medical problems. Although this use is not included in product labeling, psyllium hydrophilic mucilloid is used in certain patients with high cholesterol (hypercholesterolemia).

For patients taking psyllium hydrophilic mucilloid for *high cholesterol:*

• Importance of diet—Before prescribing medicine for your condition, your doctor will probably try to control your condition by prescribing a personal diet for you. Such a diet may be low in fats, sugars, and/or cholesterol. Many people are able to control their condition by carefully following their doctor's orders for proper diet and exercise. Medicine is prescribed only when additional help is needed. *Follow carefully the special diet your doctor gave you*, since the medicine is effective only when a schedule of diet and exercise is properly followed.

• Do not try to swallow the powder form of this medicine in the dry form. Mix with liquid following the directions in the package.

• Remember that this medicine will not cure your cholesterol problem but it will help control it. Therefore, you must continue to take it as directed by your doctor if you expect to lower your cholesterol level.

Other than the above information, there is no additional information relating to proper use, precautions, or side effects for this use.

LAXATIVES (Rectal)

Some commonly used brand names are:

In the U.S.—

Bisco-Lax (1)	Fleet Enema Mineral Oil (4)
Ceo-Two (5)	Fleet Glycerin Laxative (3)
Dacodyl (1)	Fleet Laxative (1)
Deficol (1)	Sani-Supp (3)
Dulcolax (1)	Senokot (6)
Fleet Babylax (3)	Theralax (1)
Fleet Bisacodyl (1)	Therevac Plus (2)
Fleet Enema (7)	Therevac-SB (2)
Fleet Enema for Children (7)	

In Canada—

Apo-Bisacodyl (1)	Fleet Pediatric Enema (7)
Bisacolax (1)	Gent-L-Tip (7)
Dulcolax (1)	Laxit (1)
Enemol (7)	PMS-Bisacodyl (1)
Fleet Enema (7)	Senokot (6)
Fleet Enema Mineral Oil (4)	

This information applies to the following medicines:

1. Bisacodyl (bis-a-KOE-dill)
2. Docusate (DOK-yoo-sate)
3. Glycerin (GLI-ser-in)
4. Mineral Oil
5. Potassium Bitartrate and Sodium Bicarbonate (pot-TAS-ee-um bye-TAR-trayte and SOE-dee-um bye-KAR-boe-nate)
6. Senna
7. Sodium Phosphates (SOE-dee-um FOS-fates)

Category

• **Laxative, carbon dioxide–releasing**—Potassium Bitartrate and Sodium Bicarbonate
• **Laxative, hyperosmotic**—Glycerin
• **Laxative, hyperosmotic, saline**—Sodium Phosphates
• **Laxative, lubricant**—Mineral Oil
• **Laxative, stimulant (contact)**—Bisacodyl; Senna
• **Laxative, stool softener (emollient)**—Docusate

Description

Rectal laxatives are used as enemas or suppositories to produce bowel movements in a short time.

There are several different types of rectal laxatives and they work in different ways. Since directions for use are different for each type, it is important to know which one you are taking. The different types of rectal laxatives include:

Carbon dioxide-releasing—Carbon dioxide-releasing laxatives (e.g., potassium bitartrate and sodium bicarbonate) are suppositories that encourage bowel movements by forming carbon dioxide, a gas. This gas pushes against the intestinal wall, causing contractions that move along the stool mass.

Hyperosmotic—Hyperosmotic laxatives (e.g., glycerin; sodium phosphates) draw water into the bowel from surrounding body tissues. This provides a soft stool mass and increased bowel action.

Lubricant—Mineral oil coats the bowel and the stool mass with a waterproof film. This keeps moisture in the stool. The stool remains soft and its passage is made easier.

Stimulants—Stimulant laxatives (e.g., bisacodyl; senna), also known as contact laxatives, act on the intestinal wall. They increase the muscle contractions that move along the stool mass.

Stool softeners (emollients)—Stool softeners (emollient laxatives— e.g., docusate) encourage bowel movements by helping liquids mix into the stool and prevent dry, hard stool masses. This type of laxative has been said not to *cause* a bowel movement but instead *allows* the patient to have a bowel movement without straining.

Rectal laxatives may provide relief in a number of situations such as:

- before giving birth.
- for a few days after giving birth.
- preparation for examination or surgery.
- to aid in developing normal bowel function following a period of poor eating habits or a lack of physical exercise (glycerin suppositories only).
- following surgery when straining should be avoided.
- constipation caused by other medicines.

Some of these laxatives are available only with your doctor's prescription. Others are available without a prescription; however, your doctor may have special instructions for the proper use and dose for your medical condition. They are available in the following dosage forms:

Rectal
- Bisacodyl
  - Rectal solution
  - Suppositories
- Docusate
  - Rectal solution
- Glycerin
  - Rectal solution
  - Suppositories
- Mineral Oil
  - Enema
- Potassium Bitartrate and Sodium Bicarbonate
  - Suppositories
- Senna
  - Suppositories
- Sodium Phosphates
  - Enema

Before Using This Medicine

Importance of diet, fluids, and exercise to prevent constipation—Laxatives are to be used to provide short-term relief only, unless otherwise directed by your doctor. A proper diet containing roughage (whole grain breads and cereals, bran, fruit, and green, leafy vegetables), with 6 to 8 full glasses (8 ounces each) of liquids each day, and daily exercise are most important in maintaining healthy bowel function. Also, for individuals who have problems with constipation, foods such as pastries, puddings, sugar, candy, cake, and cheese may make the constipation worse.

If you are using this medicine without a prescription, carefully read and follow any precautions on the label. For rectal laxatives, the following should be considered:

Allergies—Tell your doctor if you have ever had any unusual or allergic reaction to rectal laxatives. Also tell your health care professional if you are allergic to any other substances, such as preservatives or dyes.

Children—*Laxatives should not be given to young children (up to 6 years of age) unless prescribed by their doctor.* Since children cannot usually describe their symptoms very well, they should be checked by a doctor before being given a laxative. The child may have a condition that needs other treatment. If so, laxatives will not help and may even cause unwanted effects or make the condition worse.

Also, weakness, increased sweating, and convulsions (seizures) may be especially likely to occur in children receiving enemas or rectal solutions, since they may be more sensitive than adults to their effects.

Older adults—Weakness, increased sweating, and convulsions (seizures) may be especially likely to occur in elderly patients, since they may be more sensitive than younger adults to the effects of rectal laxatives.

Other medical problems—The presence of other medical problems may affect the use of rectal laxatives. Make sure you tell your doctor if you have any other medical problems, especially:

- Appendicitis (or signs of) or
- Rectal bleeding of unknown cause—These conditions need immediate attention by a doctor
- Intestinal blockage—The use of laxatives may create other problems if this condition is present

Proper Use of This Medicine

For safe and effective use of laxatives:

- Follow your doctor's orders if this laxative was prescribed.
- Follow the manufacturer's package directions if you are treating yourself.

For patients using *the enema or rectal solution form* of this medicine:

- This medicine usually comes with patient directions. Read them carefully before using this medicine.
- Lubricate anus with petroleum jelly before inserting the enema applicator.
- Gently insert the rectal tip of the enema applicator to prevent damage to the rectal wall.
- Results often may be obtained with:
  - bisacodyl enema in 15 minutes to 1 hour.
  - docusate enema in 2 to 15 minutes.
  - glycerin enema in 15 minutes to 1 hour.
  - mineral oil enema in 2 to 15 minutes.
  - senna enema in 30 minutes, but may not occur for some individuals for up to 2 hours.
  - sodium phosphates enema in 2 to 5 minutes.

For patients using *the suppository form* of this medicine:

- If the suppository is too soft to insert, chill the suppository in the refrigerator for 30 minutes or run cold water over it, before removing the foil wrapper.
- To insert suppository: First remove the foil wrapper and moisten the suppository with cold water. Lie down on your side and use your finger to push the suppository well up into the rectum.
- Results often may be obtained with:
  - bisacodyl suppositories in 15 minutes to 1 hour.
  - carbon dioxide– releasing suppositories in 5 to 30 minutes.
  - glycerin suppositories in 15 minutes to 1 hour.
  - senna suppositories in 30 minutes, but may not occur for some individuals for up to 2 hours.

Dosing—There are a large number of laxative products on the market. The dose of laxatives will be different for different products. The amount of enema or the number of suppositories that you use depends on the strength of the medicine. *Follow your doctor's orders if this medicine was prescribed, or follow the directions on the box if you are buying this medicine without a prescription.*

Storage—To store this medicine:
- Keep out of the reach of children.
- Store away from heat and direct light.
- Do not store in the bathroom, near the kitchen sink, or in other damp places. Heat or moisture may cause the medicine to break down.
- Do not keep outdated medicine or medicine no longer needed. Be sure that any discarded medicine is out of the reach of children.

Precautions While Using This Medicine

Do not use any type of laxative:
- *if you have signs of appendicitis or inflamed bowel* (such as stomach or lower abdominal pain, cramping, bloating, soreness, nausea, or vomiting). Instead, check with your doctor as soon as possible.
- *more often than your doctor prescribed. This is true even when you have had no results from the laxative.*
- *if you do not need it,* as for the common cold, "to clean out your system," or as a "tonic to make you feel better."
- *if you miss a bowel movement for a day or two.*

If you notice a sudden change in bowel habits or function that lasts longer than 2 weeks, or keeps returning off and on, check with your doctor before using a laxative. This will allow the cause of your problem to be determined before it becomes more serious.

The "laxative habit"—Laxative products are overused by many people. Such a practice often leads to dependence on the laxative action to produce a bowel movement. In severe cases, overuse of some laxatives has caused damage to the nerves, muscles, and tissues of the intestines and bowel. If you have any questions about the use of laxatives, check with your health care professional.

For patients using *the enema or rectal solution form* of this medicine:
- *Check with your doctor if you notice rectal bleeding, blistering, pain, burning, itching, or other sign of irritation not present before you started using this medicine.*

For patients using *the suppository form* of this medicine:
- Do not lubricate the suppository with mineral oil or petroleum jelly before inserting into the rectum. To do so may affect the way the suppository works. Moisten only with water.

Side Effects

Along with its needed effects, a medicine may cause some unwanted effects. Although not all of these side effects may occur, if they do occur they may need medical attention.

Check with your doctor as soon as possible if any of the following side effects occur:
Less common
 Rectal bleeding, blistering, burning, itching, or pain (with enemas only)

Other side effects may occur that usually do not need medical attention. These side effects may go away during treatment as your body adjusts to the medicine. However, check with your doctor if the following side effect continues or is bothersome:
Less common
 Skin irritation surrounding rectal area

Other side effects not listed above may also occur in some patients. If you notice any other effects, check with your doctor.

LEFLUNOMIDE (Oral route) - le-FLOO-noh-mide

Black Box Warning

Pregnancy must be excluded before the start of treatment with leflunomide. Leflunomide is contraindicated in pregnant women, or women of childbearing potential who are not using reliable contraception. Pregnancy must be avoided during leflunomide treatment or prior to the completion of the drug elimination procedure after leflunomide treatment.

Commonly used brand name(s)

In the U.S.—
 Arava

Available Dosage Forms:
- Tablet

Therapeutic Class: Immune Suppressant
Pharmacologic Class: Dihydroorotate Dehydrogenase Inhibitor

Uses For This Medicine

Leflunomide is used to relieve some symptoms caused by rheumatoid arthritis, such as inflammation, swelling, stiffness, and joint pain. This medicine works by stopping the body from producing too many of the immune cells that are responsible for the swelling and inflammation.

This medicine is available only with your doctor's prescription.

Before Using This Medicine

In deciding to use a medicine, the risks of taking the medicine must be weighed against the good it will do. This is a decision you and your doctor will make. For this medicine, the following should be considered:

Allergies—Tell your doctor if you have ever had any unusual or allergic reaction to this medicine or any other medicines. Also tell your health care professional if you have any other types of allergies, such as to foods, dyes, preservatives, or animals. For non-prescription products, read the label or package ingredients carefully.

Pediatric—Although there is no specific information comparing use of leflunomide in children with use in any other age group, use is not recommended in children up to 18 years of age.

Geriatric—Many medicines have not been studied specifically in older people. Therefore, it may not be known whether they work exactly the same way as they do in younger adults or if they cause different side effects or problems in older people. There is no specific information comparing use of leflunomide in the elderly with use in other age groups. However, elderly people may be more sensitive to the effects of leflunomide. This may increase the chance of side effects during treatment.

Pregnancy—

	Pregnancy Category	Explanation
All Trimesters	X	Studies in animals or pregnant women have demonstrated positive evidence of fetal abnormalities. This drug should not be used in women who are or may become pregnant because the risk clearly outweighs any possible benefit.

Breast Feeding—There are no adequate studies in women for determining infant risk when using this medication during breastfeeding. Weigh the potential benefits against the potential risks before taking this medication while breastfeeding.

Other medicines—

Using this medicine with any of the following medicines is usually not recommended, but may be required in some cases. If both medicines are prescribed together, your doctor may change the dose or how often you use one or both of the medicines.

Methotrexate, Warfarin

Interactions with Food/Tobacco/Alcohol—Certain medicines should not be used at or around the time of eating food or eating certain types of food since interactions may occur. Using alcohol or tobacco with certain medicines may also cause interactions to occur. Discuss with your healthcare professional the use of your medicine with food, alcohol, or tobacco.

Other medical problems—The presence of other medical problems may affect the use of this medicine. Make sure you tell your doctor if you have any other medical problems, especially:

- Blood problems, history—May make side effects worse
- Disease of the immune system or
- Infections, severe—Leflunomide may decrease the body's ability to fight infection
- Liver disease, including hepatitis B or C or
- Renal disease—The chance of side effects may be increased

Proper Use of This Medicine

Take this medicine only as directed by your doctor. Do not take more or less of it, and do not take it more often than your doctor ordered.

Dosing—The dose of this medicine will be different for different patients. Follow your doctor's orders or the directions on the label. The following information includes only the average doses of this medicine. If your dose is different, do not change it unless your doctor tells you to do so.

The amount of medicine that you take depends on the strength of the medicine. Also, the number of doses you take each day, the time allowed between doses, and the length of time you take the medicine depend on the medical problem for which you are using the medicine.

- For oral dosage form (tablets):
  - For rheumatoid arthritis:
    - Adults—At first, 100 mg once a day for three days, then 20 mg once a day. Your doctor may decrease the dose as needed.
    - Children—Use and dose must be determined by your doctor.

Missed dose—If you miss a dose of this medicine, take it as soon as possible. However, if it is almost time for your next dose, skip the missed dose and go back to your regular dosing schedule. Do not double doses.

Storage—Store the medicine in a closed container at room temperature, away from heat, moisture, and direct light. Keep from freezing.

Keep out of the reach of children.

Do not keep outdated medicine or medicine no longer needed.

Precautions While Using This Medicine

It is important that your doctor check your progress at regular visits to make sure that this medicine is working properly and to check for unwanted effects.

Leflunomide may cause birth defects in humans if taken during pregnancy. Therefore, if you suspect that you may have become pregnant, stop taking this medicine immediately and check with your doctor.

Leflunomide may cause birth defects in the children of the men taking it during the time of conception. Therefore, men taking leflunomide should use condoms as a form of birth control during sexual intercourse. A man intending to father a child should stop taking this medicine and check with his doctors.

Studies have not been done in animals or humans to determine if leflunomide will cause birth defects in the children of men taking leflunomide at the time of conception. However, it is recommended that men taking this medicine use condoms as a form of birth control during sexual intercourse. Men taking leflunomide who intend to father a child, should stop taking the medicine and tell their doctor immediately.

Check with your doctor right away if you begin having symptoms of lung problems such as cough or shortness of breath with or without a fever

Do not drink alcohol while using this medicine. Alcohol can increase the chance of liver problems.

While you are being treated with leflunomide, and after you stop treatment with it, do not have any immunizations (vaccinations) without your doctor's approval.

Side Effects of This Medicine

Along with its needed effects, a medicine may cause some unwanted effects. Although not all of these side effects may occur, if they do occur they may need medical attention.

Check with your doctor as soon as possible if any of the following side effects occur:

More common

Bloody or cloudy urine; congestion in chest; cough; difficult, burning, or painful urination; difficult or painful breathing; dizziness; fever; frequent urge to urinate; headache; loss of appetite; nausea and/or vomiting; sneezing; sore throat; yellow eyes and/or skin

Less common

Burning feeling in chest or stomach; burning, prickling, or tingling sensation in fingers and/or toes; chest pain; diarrhea; fast heartbeat; indigestion; joint or muscle pain or stiffness; pounding heartbeat; severe stomach pain; shortness of breath; tenderness in stomach area; unusual tiredness or weakness

Incidence not known

Area rash; black or tarry stools; bleeding gums; blistering, peeling, loosening of skin; bloating; blood in stools; burning, numbness, tingling, or painful sensations; chest pain; chills; clay-colored stools; confusion; constipation; continuing vomiting; cough or hoarseness; dark urine; fainting; fast heartbeat; fever with or without chills; general feeling of tiredness or weakness; high fever; large, hive-like swelling on face, eyelids, lips, tongue, throat, hands, legs, feet, sex organs; light-colored stools; lightheadedness; loss of appetite; lower back or side pain; painful or difficult urination; pains in stomach, side, or abdomen, possibly radiating to the back; pale skin; pinpoint red spots on skin; rapid, shallow breathing; red, irritated eyes; red skin lesions, often with a purple center; sores, ulcers, or white spots in mouth or on lips; swollen glands; unexplained bleeding or bruising; unpleasant breath odor; unsteadiness or awkwardness; unusual bleeding or bruising; upper right abdominal pain; vomiting of blood; weakness in arms, hands, legs, or feet

Some side effects may occur that usually do not need medical attention. These side effects may go away during treatment as your body adjusts to the medicine. Also, your health care professional may be able to tell you about ways to prevent or reduce some of these side effects. Check with your health care professional if any of the following side effects continue or are bothersome or if you have any questions about them:

More common

Back pain; hair loss; heartburn; skin rash; stomach pain; weight loss (unexplained)

Less common

Acne; anxiety; constipation; decreased appetite; dry mouth; gas; irritation or soreness of mouth; itching of the skin; pain or burning in throat; red or irritated eyes; runny nose

Other side effects not listed may also occur in some patients. If you notice any other effects, check with your healthcare professional.

LENALIDOMIDE (Oral route) - le-na-LID-oh-mide

Black Box Warning

- POTENTIAL FOR HUMAN BIRTH DEFECTS
  - Lenalidomide is an analogue of thalidomide. Thalidomide is a known human teratogen that causes severe life-threatening human birth defects. If lenalidomide is taken during pregnancy, it may cause birth defects or death to an unborn baby. Females should be advised to avoid pregnancy while taking lenalidomide.
  - SPECIAL PRESCRIBING REQUIREMENTS: Because of this potential toxicity and to avoid fetal exposure to lenalidomide, lenalidomide is only available under a special restricted distribution program. This program is called RevAssist(SM). Under this program, only prescribers and pharmacists registered with the program are able to prescribe and dispense the product. In addition, lenalidomide must only be dispensed to patients who are registered and meet all the conditions of the the RevAssist(SM) program. Please see the following information for prescribers, female patients, and male patients about this restricted distribution program.
  - REVASSIST(SM) PROGRAM DESCRIPTION
  - PRESCRIBERS: Lenalidomide can be prescribed only by licensed prescribers who are registered in the RevAssist(SM) program and understand the potential risk of teratogenicity if lenalidomide is used during pregnancy. Effective contraception must be used by female patients of childbearing potential for at least 4 weeks before beginning lenalidomide therapy, during lenalidomide therapy, during dose interruptions and for 4 weeks following discontinuation of lenalidomide therapy. Reliable contraception is indicated even where there has been a history of infertility, unless due to hysterectomy or because the patient has been postmenopausal naturally for at least 24 consecutive months. Two reliable forms of contraception must be used simultaneously unless continuous abstinence from heterosexual sexual contact is the chosen method. Females of childbearing potential should be referred to a qualified provider of contraceptive methods, if needed. Sexually mature females who have not undergone a hysterectomy, have not had a bilateral oophorectomy, or who have not been postmenopausal naturally for at least 24 consecutive months (ie, who have had menses at some time in the preceding 24 consecutive months) are considered to be females of childbearing potential.
  - Before prescribing lenalidomide, FEMALES of childbearing potential should have 2 negative pregnancy tests (sensitivity of at least 50 mIU/mL). The first test should be performed within 10 to 14 days, and the second test within 24 hours prior to prescribing lenalidomide. A prescription for lenalidomide for a female of childbearing potential must not be issued by the prescriber until negative pregnancy tests have been verified by the prescriber.
  - For MALE patients, it is not known whether lenalidomide is present in the semen of patients receiving

the drug. Therefore, males receiving lenalidomide must always use a latex condom during any sexual contact with females of childbearing potential even if they have undergone a successful vasectomy.

○ Once treatment has started and during dose interruptions, pregnancy testing for females of childbearing potential should occur weekly during the first 4 weeks of use, then pregnancy testing should be repeated every 4 weeks in females with regular menstrual cycles. If menstrual cycles are irregular, the pregnancy testing should occur every 2 weeks. Pregnancy testing and counseling should be performed if a patient misses her period or if there is any abnormality in ther pregnancy test or in her menstrual bleeding. Lenalidomide treatment must be discontinued during this evaluation.

○ Pregnancy test results should be verified by the prescriber and the pharmacist prior to dispensing any prescription.

○ If pregnancy does occur during lenalidomide treatment, lenalidomide must be discontinued immediately.

○ Any suspected fetal exposure to lenalidomide should be reported to the FDA via the MedWatch number at 1–800–FDA-1088 and also to Celgene Corporation at 1–888–423–5436. The patient should be referred to an obstetrician/gynecologist experienced in reproductive toxicity for further evaluation and counseling.

○ FEMALE PATIENTS: Lenalidomide should be used in females of childbearing potential only when the patient meets all of the following conditions (ie, she is unable to become pregnant while on lenalidomide therapy):

○ she understands and can reliably carry out instructions.

○ she is capable of complying with the mandatory contraceptive measures, pregnancy testing, patient registration, and patient survey as described in the RevAssist(SM) program.

○ she has received and understands both oral and written warnings of the potential risks of taking lenalidomide during pregnancy and of exposing a fetus to the drug.

○ she has received both oral and written warnings of the risk of possible contraception failure and of the need to use two reliable forms of contraception simultaneously, unless continuous abstinence from heterosexual sexual contact is the chosen method. Sexually mature females who have not undergone a hysterectomy or who have not been postmenopausal for at least 24 consecutive months (ie, who have had menses at some time in the preceding 24 consecutive months) are considered to be females of childbearing potential.

○ she acknowledges, in writing, her understanding of these warnings and of the need for using two reliable methods of contraception for 4 weeks prior to beginning lenalidomide therapy, during lenalidomide therapy, during dose interruptions and for 4 weeks after discontinuation of lenalidomide therapy.

○ she has had two negative pregnancy tests with a sensitivity of at least 50 mIU/mL, within 10 to 14 days and 24 hours prior to beginning therapy.

○ if the patient is between 12 and 18 years of age, her parent or legal guardian must have read the educa-

tional materials and agreed to ensure compliance with the above.

○ MALE PATIENTS: Lenalidomide should be used in sexually active males when the PATIENT MEETS ALL OF THE FOLLOWING CONDITIONS:

○ he understands and can reliably carry out instructions.

○ he is capable of complying with the mandatory contraceptive measures that are appropriate for men, patient registration, and patient survey as described in the RevAssist(SM) program.

○ he has received and understands both oral and written warnings of the potential risks of taking lenalidomide and exposing a fetus to the drug.

○ he has received both oral and written warnings of the risk of possible contraception failure and that it is unknown whether lenalidomide is present in semen. He has been instructed that he must always use a latex condom during any sexual contact with females of childbearing potential, even if he has undergone a successful vasectomy.

○ he acknowledges, in writing, his understanding of these warnings and of the need to use a latex condom during any sexual contact with females of childbearing potential, even if he has undergone a successful vasectomy. Females of childbearing potential are considered to be sexually mature females who have not undergone a hysterectomy, have not had a bilateral oophorectomy, or who have not been postmenopausal for at least 24 consecutive months (ie, who have had menses at any time in the preceding 24 consecutive months).

○ if the patient is between 12 and 18 years of age, his parent or legal guardian must have read the educational material and agreed to ensure compliance with the above.

• HEMATOLOGIC TOXICITY (NEUTROPENIA AND THROMBOCYTOPENIA)

○ This drug is associated with significant neutropenia and thrombocytopenia. Eighty percent of patients with del 5q myelodysplastic syndromes had to have a dose delay/reduction during the major study. Thirty-four percent of patients had to have a second dose delay/reduction. Grade 3 or 4 hematologic toxicity was seen in 80% of patients enrolled in the study. Patients on therapy for del 5q myelodysplastic syndromes should have their complete blood counts monitored weekly for the first 8 weeks of therapy and at least monthly thereafter. Patients may require dose interruption and/or reduction. Patients may require use of blood product support and/or growth factors.

• DEEP VENOUS THROMBOSIS AND PULMONARY EMBOLISM

○ This drug has demonstrated a significantly increased risk of deep venous thrombosis (DVT) and pulmonary embolism (PE) in patients with multiple myeloma who were treated with lenalidomide combination therapy. Patients and physicians are advised to be observant for the signs and symptoms of thromboembolism. Patients should be instructed to seek medical care if they develop symptoms such as shortness of breath, chest pain, or arm or leg swelling. It is not known whether prophylactic anticoagulation or antiplatelet therapy prescribed in conjunction with lenalidomide may lessen the potential for venous thromboembolic events. The decision to take prophylactic measures should be done carefully after an assessment of an individual patient's underlying risk factors

- You can get the information about lenalidomide and the RevAssist(SM) program on the internet at www.revlimid.com or by calling the manufacturer's toll free number 1–888–423–5436.

Commonly used brand name(s)

In the U.S.—
Revlimid

Available Dosage Forms:
- Capsule

Therapeutic Class: Immune Modulator

Uses For This Medicine

Lenalidomide is a medicine used to treat anemia in patients with a certain type of myelodysplastic syndrome (MDS) called 5q MDS. Patients with this type of MDS may have low red blood cell counts that require blood transfusions.

This medicine is available only with your doctor's prescription.

Before Using This Medicine

In deciding to use a medicine, the risks of taking the medicine must be weighed against the good it will do. This is a decision you and your doctor will make. For this medicine, the following should be considered:

Allergies—Tell your doctor if you have ever had any unusual or allergic reaction to this medicine or any other medicines. Also tell your health care professional if you have any other types of allergies, such as to foods, dyes, preservatives, or animals. For non-prescription products, read the label or package ingredients carefully.

Pediatric—Studies on this medicine have been done only in adult patients, and there is no specific information comparing use of lenalidomide in children with use in other age groups.

Geriatric—This medicine has been tested and has not been shown to cause different side effects or problems in older people than it does in younger adults.

Pregnancy—

	Pregnancy Category	Explanation
All Trimesters	X	Studies in animals or pregnant women have demonstrated positive evidence of fetal abnormalities. This drug should not be used in women who are or may become pregnant because the risk clearly outweighs any possible benefit.

Breast Feeding—There are no adequate studies in women for determining infant risk when using this medication during breastfeeding. Weigh the potential benefits against the potential risks before taking this medication while breastfeeding.

Other medicines—

Using this medicine with any of the following medicines may cause an increased risk of certain side effects, but using both drugs may be the best treatment for you. If both medicines are prescribed together, your doctor may change the dose or how often you use one or both of the medicines.

Digoxin

Interactions with Food/Tobacco/Alcohol—Certain medicines should not be used at or around the time of eating food or eating certain types of food since interactions may occur. Using alcohol or tobacco with certain medicines may also cause interactions to occur. Discuss with your healthcare professional the use of your medicine with food, alcohol, or tobacco.

Other medical problems—The presence of other medical problems may affect the use of this medicine. Make sure you tell your doctor if you have any other medical problems, especially:

- Kidney disease—May increase the amount of lenalidomide in your body and increase the risk of side effects.

- Liver disease—Use caution as studies have not been done.

- Multiple myeloma—May increase your risk for serious side effects.

Proper Use of This Medicine

It is very important that you become educated and counseled on the requirements of the RevAssist program, and become familiar with the RevAssist educational materials, and Patient Medication Guide. Direct any questions to a physician or pharmacist prior to starting lenalidomide therapy.

You should take the necessary precautions to avoid pregnancy while taking lenalidomide. Use one highly effective form of birth control plus an additional effective form of birth control at the same time, if abstinence is not the chosen method. Begin this 4 weeks before starting lenalidomide and continue it for 4 weeks after stopping the medication.

There is a telephone survey and patient registry that you must participate in while taking lenalidomide. Ask your doctor or pharmacist if you have any questions about what you need to do.

Swallow whole, do not break, chew, or open the capsule.

It is important that you have laboratory blood tests at regular intervals.

It is important that you have pregnancy tests at regular intervals.

Male patients, even those who have had a vasectomy, must use a latex condom during sexual contact with a female patient.

Do not donate blood while taking lenalidomide.

You should not share this medication with anyone, even someone with similar symptoms.

For male patients: *Do not donate semen or sperm while taking lenalidomide.*

Dosing—The dose of this medicine will be different for different patients. Follow your doctor's orders or the directions on the label. The following information includes only the average doses of this medicine. If your dose is different, do not change it unless your doctor tells you to do so.

The amount of medicine that you take depends on the strength of the medicine. Also, the number of doses you take each day, the time allowed between doses, and the length of time you take the medicine depend on the medical problem for which you are using the medicine.

- For oral dosage form (capsules):
  - For treating anemia in patients with myelodysplastic syndrome:
    - Adults—10 milligrams daily, taken with water. Your doctor may adjust your dose.
    - Children—Use and dose must be determined by your doctor.

Missed dose—If you miss a dose of this medicine, take it as soon as possible. However, if it is almost time for your next dose, skip the missed dose and go back to your regular dosing schedule. Do not double doses.

Storage—Keep out of the reach of children.

Store the medicine in a closed container at room temperature, away from heat, moisture, and direct light. Keep from freezing.

Do not keep outdated medicine or medicine no longer needed.

Precautions While Using This Medicine

Your doctor will want to see you every 4 weeks for pregnancy testing if you have a regular menstrual cycle and every 2 weeks if you have an irregular cycle.

Call your doctor or 1–888–688–2528 for emergency contraception information if you for any reason think you are pregnant or, for males, if you think that your sexual partner may be pregnant.

Seek medical attention if you develop any shortness of breath, chest pain, or arm or leg swelling.

Side Effects of This Medicine

Along with its needed effects, a medicine may cause some unwanted effects. Although not all of these side effects may occur, if they do occur they may need medical attention.

Check with your doctor immediately if any of the following side effects occur:

More common
    Black, tarry stools; bleeding gums; blood in urine or stools; chest pain; chills; convulsions; cough; decreased urine; difficult or labored breathing; dry mouth; fever; increased thirst; irregular heartbeat; loss of appetite; lower back or side pain; mood changes; muscle pain or cramps; nausea or vomiting; numbness or tingling in hands, feet, or lips; painful or difficult urination; pale skin; pinpoint red spots on skin; shortness of breath; sore throat; sores, ulcers, or white spots on lips or in mouth; swollen glands; tightness in chest; unusual bleeding or bruising; unusual tiredness or weakness; wheezing

Frequency not known
    Anxiety; dizziness or light-headedness; fainting; fast heartbeat; pain, redness, or swelling in arm or leg; sudden shortness of breath or troubled breathing

Some side effects may occur that usually do not need medical attention. These side effects may go away during treatment as your body adjusts to the medicine. Also, your health care professional may be able to tell you about ways to prevent or reduce some of these side effects. Check with your health care professional if any of the following side effects continue or are bothersome or if you have any questions about them:

More common
    Abnormal or decreased touch sensation; back pain; bloody nose; blurred vision; body aches or pain;

bruising; burning, numbness, tingling, or painful sensations; burning while urinating; change in taste; constipation; contusion; cough producing mucus; depressed mood; diarrhea; difficulty having a bowel movement (stool); difficulty in moving; discouragement; drowsiness; dry skin and hair; dryness or soreness of throat; ear congestion; fast, irregular, pounding, or racing heartbeat or pulse; feeling sad or empty; feeling unusually cold; flushing, redness of skin; hair loss; headache; hoarseness or husky voice; irritability; itching, pain, redness, swelling, tenderness, warmth on skin; itching skin; lack or loss of strength; large, flat, blue or purplish patches in the skin; loose stools; loss of appetite; loss of interest or pleasure; loss of taste; loss of voice; muscle aching; muscle pain or stiffness; muscle spasms; nasal congestion; nervousness; night sweats; pain; pain in arms or legs; pain in joints; pain or tenderness around eyes and cheekbones; pounding in the ears; rash; runny nose; seizures; shivering; sleeplessness; slow or fast heartbeat; sneezing; stomach pain; stuffy or runny nose; sweating increased; swelling of hands, ankles, feet or lower legs; swollen joints; tender, swollen glands in neck; [tetany] or twitching; tiredness; trembling; trouble concentrating; trouble sleeping; trouble swallowing; troubled breathing with exertion; unable to sleep; unsteadiness or awkwardness; unusually warm skin; upper abdominal pain; voice changes; vomiting; weakness in arms, hands, legs, or feet; weight gain; weight loss

Other side effects not listed may also occur in some patients. If you notice any other effects, check with your healthcare professional.

LETROZOLE   (Oral route) - LET-roe-zole

Commonly used brand name(s)

In the U.S.—
    Femara

Available Dosage Forms:
- Tablet

Therapeutic Class: Antineoplastic Agent
Pharmacologic Class: Aromatase Inhibitor

Uses For This Medicine

Letrozole is used to treat certain types of breast cancer in women. Female hormones that occur naturally in the body can increase the growth of some breast cancers. Letrozole works by decreasing the amounts of these hormones in the body. This medicine is meant to be used only by women who have already stopped menstruating.

This medicine is available only with your doctor's prescription.

Before Using This Medicine

In deciding to use a medicine, the risks of taking the medicine must be weighed against the good it will do. This is a decision

you and your doctor will make. For this medicine, the following should be considered:

Allergies—Tell your doctor if you have ever had any unusual or allergic reaction to this medicine or any other medicines. Also tell your health care professional if you have any other types of allergies, such as to foods, dyes, preservatives, or animals. For non-prescription products, read the label or package ingredients carefully.

Geriatric—This medicine has been tested and has not been shown to cause different effects in older women than in younger adults.

Pregnancy—

	Pregnancy Category	Explanation
All Trimesters	D	Studies in pregnant women have demonstrated a risk to the fetus. However, the benefits of therapy in a life threatening situation or a serious disease, may outweigh the potential risk.

Breast Feeding—There are no adequate studies in women for determining infant risk when using this medication during breastfeeding. Weigh the potential benefits against the potential risks before taking this medication while breastfeeding.

Other medicines—

Using this medicine with any of the following medicines may cause an increased risk of certain side effects, but using both drugs may be the best treatment for you. If both medicines are prescribed together, your doctor may change the dose or how often you use one or both of the medicines.

Tamoxifen

Interactions with Food/Tobacco/Alcohol—Certain medicines should not be used at or around the time of eating food or eating certain types of food since interactions may occur. Using alcohol or tobacco with certain medicines may also cause interactions to occur. Discuss with your healthcare professional the use of your medicine with food, alcohol, or tobacco.

Other medical problems—The presence of other medical problems may affect the use of this medicine. Make sure you tell your doctor if you have any other medical problems, especially:

- Cirrhosis or
- Kidney disease or
- Liver disease or
- Severe liver disease—Problems are not likely to occur in people with mild kidney or liver disease. However, the dose of letrozole should be reduced in patients with cirrhosis and severe liver disease.

Proper Use of This Medicine

Take this medicine only as directed by your doctor. Do not take more of it, and do not take it more often than your doctor ordered.

Dosing—The dose of this medicine will be different for different patients. Follow your doctor's orders or the directions on the label. The following information includes only the average doses of this medicine. If your dose is different, do not change it unless your doctor tells you to do so.

The amount of medicine that you take depends on the strength of the medicine. Also, the number of doses you take each day, the time allowed between doses, and the length of time you take the medicine depend on the medical problem for which you are using the medicine.

- For oral dosage form (tablets):
  - For breast cancer:
    - Adults—One 2.5–milligram tablet a day.

Missed dose—If you miss a dose of this medicine, take it as soon as possible. However, if it is almost time for your next dose, skip the missed dose and go back to your regular dosing schedule. Do not double doses.

Storage—Store the medicine in a closed container at room temperature, away from heat, moisture, and direct light. Keep from freezing.

Keep out of the reach of children.

Do not keep outdated medicine or medicine no longer needed.

Precautions While Using This Medicine

It is very important that your doctor check your progress at regular visits to make sure that the medicine is working properly and does not cause unwanted effects.

This medicine may cause you to become dizzy or drowsy; use caution if you are driving an automobile or using machinery.

Side Effects of This Medicine

Along with its needed effects, a medicine may cause some unwanted effects. Although not all of these side effects may occur, if they do occur they may need medical attention.

Stop taking this medicine and get emergency help immediately if any of the following effects occur:
More common
　Shortness of breath

Less common
　Chest pain

Rare
　Continuing or severe nervousness; cough; dizziness or lightheadedness; fainting; fast heartbeat; heart attack; increased sweating; nausea; pain in chest, groin, or legs, especially the calves; severe, sudden headache; slurred speech; severe and sudden, unexplained shortness of breath; sudden loss of coordination; sudden, severe weakness or numbness in arm or leg; vision changes

Check with your doctor as soon as possible if any of the following side effects occur:
Less common
　Bone fracture; breast pain; chills, fever, or flu-like symptoms; mental depression; swelling of feet or lower legs

Rare
　Vaginal bleeding

Some side effects may occur that usually do not need medical attention. These side effects may go away during treatment as your body adjusts to the medicine. Also, your health care professional may be able to tell you about ways to prevent or reduce some of these side effects. Check with your health care professional if any of the following side effects continue or are bothersome or if you have any questions about them:

More common
Back pain; bone pain; hot flashes (sudden sweating and feeling of warmth); joint pain; muscle pain

Less common
Anxiety; confusion; constipation; diarrhea; dry mouth; headache; increased thirst and urination; loss of appetite or weight loss; metallic taste; skin rash or itching; sleepiness; spinning or whirling sensation causing loss of balance; stomach pain or upset; trouble sleeping; unusual tiredness; vomiting; weakness; weight gain

Incidence not known
Blurred vision

Letrozole sometimes causes a loss of hair.

Other side effects not listed may also occur in some patients. If you notice any other effects, check with your healthcare professional.

LEUCOVORIN   (Oral route, Intravenous route, Injection route) - loo-koe-VOR-in

Uses For This Medicine

Leucovorin is used as an antidote to the harmful effects of methotrexate (a cancer medicine) that is given in high doses. It is used also to prevent or treat certain kinds of anemia. Leucovorin acts the same way in the body as folic acid, which may be low in these patients.

Leucovorin is also used along with fluorouracil (a cancer medicine) to treat cancer of the colon (bowel).

Leucovorin is available only with a prescription.

Once a medicine has been approved for marketing for a certain use, experience may show that it is also useful for other medical problems. Although these uses are not included in the product labeling, leucovorin is used in certain patients with the following medical conditions:

* Ewing's sarcoma (type of cancer found in the bone)
* Gestational trophoblastic tumors (tumors in the uterus or womb)
* Head and neck cancer
* Non-Hodgkin's lymphoma (cancer of the lymph system)

Before Using This Medicine

In deciding to use a medicine, the risks of taking the medicine must be weighed against the good it will do. This is a decision you and your doctor will make. For this medicine, the following should be considered:

Allergies—Tell your doctor if you have ever had any unusual or allergic reaction to this medicine or any other medicines. Also tell your health care professional if you have any other types of allergies, such as to foods, dyes, preservatives, or animals. For non-prescription products, read the label or package ingredients carefully.

Pediatric—In children with seizures, leucovorin may increase the number of seizures that occur.

Geriatric—Many medicines have not been studied specifically in older people. Therefore, it may not be known whether they work exactly the same way they do in younger adults or

if they cause different side effects or problems in older people. There is no specific information comparing use of leucovorin in the elderly with use in other age groups.

Pregnancy—

	Pregnancy Category	Explanation
All Trimesters	C	Animal studies have shown an adverse effect and there are no adequate studies in pregnant women OR no animal studies have been conducted and there are no adequate studies in pregnant women.

Breast Feeding—There are no adequate studies in women for determining infant risk when using this medication during breastfeeding. Weigh the potential benefits against the potential risks before taking this medication while breastfeeding.

Other medicines—

Using this medicine with any of the following medicines may cause an increased risk of certain side effects, but using both drugs may be the best treatment for you. If both medicines are prescribed together, your doctor may change the dose or how often you use one or both of the medicines.

Capecitabine, Fluorouracil, Phenobarbital, Primidone

Interactions   with   Food/Tobacco/Alcohol—Certain medicines should not be used at or around the time of eating food or eating certain types of food since interactions may occur. Using alcohol or tobacco with certain medicines may also cause interactions to occur. Discuss with your healthcare professional the use of your medicine with food, alcohol, or tobacco.

Other medical problems—The presence of other medical problems may affect the use of this medicine. Make sure you tell your doctor if you have any other medical problems, especially:

* Kidney disease—Levels of methotrexate may be increased because of its slower removal from the body, so the dose of leucovorin may not be enough to block the unwanted effects of methotrexate

* Nausea and vomiting—Not enough leucovorin may be absorbed into the body to block the unwanted effects of methotrexate

Proper Use of This Medicine

It is very important that you take leucovorin exactly as directed, especially when it is being taken to counteract the harmful effects of cancer medicine. Do not miss any doses. Also, it is best to take the doses at evenly spaced times day and night. For example, if you are to take 4 doses a day, the doses should be spaced about 6 hours apart. If this interferes with your sleep or other daily activities, or if you need help in planning the best times to take your medicine, check with your health care professional.

Do not stop taking leucovorin without checking with your doctor. It is very important that you get exactly the right amount.

Dosing—The dose of this medicine will be different for different patients. Follow your doctor's orders or the directions on the label. The following information includes only the average doses of this medicine. If your dose is different, do not change it unless your doctor tells you to do so.

The amount of medicine that you take depends on the strength of the medicine. Also, the number of doses you take each day, the time allowed between doses, and the length of time you take the medicine depend on the medical problem for which you are using the medicine.

- For use as an antidote to methotrexate:
  - For oral (tablets) or injection dosage forms:
    - Adults, teenagers, and children—Dose is based on body size and must be determined by your doctor.
- For use as an antidote to other medicines:
  - For oral (tablets) or injection dosage forms:
    - Adults, teenagers, and children—Dose may range from 0.4 milligrams (mg) to 15 mg a day and must be determined by your doctor.
- For certain kinds of anemia:
  - For oral (tablets) or injection dosage forms:
    - Adults, teenagers, and children—Up to 1 mg a day.
- For colon cancer:
  - For injection dosage forms:
    - Adults and teenagers—Dose is based on body size and must be determined by your doctor.
    - Children—Dose must be determined by your doctor.

Missed dose—Call your doctor or pharmacist for instructions.

Storage—Store the medicine in a closed container at room temperature, away from heat, moisture, and direct light. Keep from freezing.

Keep out of the reach of children.

Do not keep outdated medicine or medicine no longer needed.

Side Effects of This Medicine

Along with its needed effects, a medicine may cause some unwanted effects. Although not all of these side effects may occur, if they do occur they may need medical attention.

Check with your doctor immediately if any of the following side effects occur:
  Rare
    Skin rash, hives, or itching; wheezing

Check with your doctor as soon as possible if any of the following side effects occur:
  Rare—reported with use in treatment of cancer
    Convulsions (seizures)

Other side effects not listed may also occur in some patients. If you notice any other effects, check with your healthcare professional.

LEUPROLIDE (Intramuscular route, Subcutaneous route, Intradermal route, Injection route) - loo-PROE-lide

Commonly used brand name(s)
In the U.S.—
  Eligard   Lupron Depot-Ped
  Lupron   Viadur
  Lupron Depot

Available Dosage Forms:

- Powder for Solution
- Solution
- Powder for Suspension, 1 Month
- Powder for Suspension, 3 Month
- Powder for Suspension
- Powder for Suspension, 4 Month
- Kit
- Powder for Suspension, 6 Month

Therapeutic Class: Endocrine-Metabolic Agent
Pharmacologic Class: Luteinizing Hormone Releasing Hormone Agonist

Uses For This Medicine

Leuprolide may be used for a number of different medical problems. These include treatment of:
- anemia caused by bleeding of uterine leiomyomas (tumors in the uterus);
- cancer of the prostate gland in men;
- central precocious puberty (CPP), a condition that causes early puberty in boys (before 9 years of age) and in girls (before 8 years of age);
- pain due to endometriosis in women.

Leuprolide is similar to a hormone normally released from the hypothalamus gland.

When given regularly to men and boys, leuprolide decreases testosterone levels. Reducing the amount of testosterone in the body is one way of treating cancer of the prostate.

When given regularly to women and girls, leuprolide decreases estrogen levels. Reducing the amount of estrogen in the body is one way of treating endometriosis. By shrinking tumors in the uterus, leuprolide helps stop anemia by decreasing the vaginal bleeding from these tumors. Iron supplements should be used to help treat the anemia.

When given to boys and girls experiencing early puberty, leuprolide slows down the development of the genital areas in both sexes and breast development in girls. This medicine delays puberty in a child only as long as the child continues to receive it.

Suppressing estrogen can cause thinning of the bones or slowing of their growth. This is a problem for adult women whose bones are no longer growing like the bones of children. Slowing the growth of bones is a positive effect in girls and boys whose bones grow too fast when puberty begins too early. Boys and girls may benefit by adding inches to their adult height when leuprolide helps their bones grow at the proper and expected rate for children.

Leuprolide is available only with your doctor's prescription.

Once a medicine has been approved for marketing for a certain use, experience may show that it is also useful for other medical problems. Although this use is not included in product labeling, leuprolide is used in certain patients with the following medical condition:
- Cancer of the breast

Before Using This Medicine

In deciding to use a medicine, the risks of taking the medicine must be weighed against the good it will do. This is a decision you and your doctor will make. For this medicine, the following should be considered:

Allergies—Tell your doctor if you have ever had any unusual or allergic reaction to this medicine or any other medicines. Also tell your health care professional if you have any other types of allergies, such as to foods, dyes, preservatives,

or animals. For non-prescription products, read the label or package ingredients carefully.

Pediatric—Leuprolide will stop having an effect on a child treated for central precocious puberty soon after the child stops using it, and puberty will advance normally. It is not known if using leuprolide around the time of puberty causes changes in boys' and girls' future abilities to have babies. Their chances of having children later are thought to be normal. It is especially important that you discuss with the child's doctor the good that this medicine may do as well as the risks of using it.

Geriatric—Many medicines have not been studied specifically in older people. Therefore, it may not be known whether they work exactly the same way they do in younger adults. Although there is no specific information comparing use of leuprolide in the elderly to use in other age groups, it is not expected to cause different side effects or problems in older people than it does in younger adults.

Pregnancy—

	Pregnancy Category	Explanation
All Trimesters	X	Studies in animals or pregnant women have demonstrated positive evidence of fetal abnormalities. This drug should not be used in women who are or may become pregnant because the risk clearly outweighs any possible benefit.

Breast Feeding—There are no adequate studies in women for determining infant risk when using this medication during breastfeeding. Weigh the potential benefits against the potential risks before taking this medication while breastfeeding.

Other medicines—Although certain medicines should not be used together at all, in other cases two different medicines may be used together even if an interaction might occur. In these cases, your doctor may want to change the dose, or other precautions may be necessary. Tell your healthcare professional if you are taking any other prescription or non-prescription (over-the-counter [OTC]) medicine.

Interactions with Food/Tobacco/Alcohol—Certain medicines should not be used at or around the time of eating food or eating certain types of food since interactions may occur. Using alcohol or tobacco with certain medicines may also cause interactions to occur. Discuss with your healthcare professional the use of your medicine with food, alcohol, or tobacco.

Other medical problems—The presence of other medical problems may affect the use of this medicine. Make sure you tell your doctor if you have any other medical problems, especially:

- Changes in vaginal bleeding from an unknown cause (for use for endometriosis or anemia due to tumors of the uterus)—Leuprolide may delay diagnosis or worsen condition. The reason for the bleeding should be determined before leuprolide is used
- Conditions that increase the chances of developing thinning bones or
- Osteoporosis (brittle bones), history of, or family history of—It is important that your doctor know if you already have an increased risk of osteoporosis. Some things that can increase your risk for having osteoporosis include

cigarette smoking, alcohol abuse, and a family history of osteoporosis or easily broken bones. Some medicines, such as corticosteroids (cortisone-like medicines) or anticonvulsants (seizure medicine), can also cause thinning of the bones when used for a long time

- Nerve problems caused by bone lesions in spine (for use for cancer of the prostate) and
- Problems in passing urine (for use for cancer of the prostate)—Conditions may get worse for a short time after leuprolide treatment is started

---

Proper Use of This Medicine

Leuprolide comes with patient directions. Read these instructions carefully.

Use the syringes provided in the kit. Other syringes may not provide the correct dose. These disposable syringes and needles are already sterilized and are designed to be used one time only and then discarded. If you have any questions about the use of disposable syringes, check with your health care professional.

Use this medicine only as directed by your doctor. Do not use more or less of it, and do not use it more often than your doctor ordered. The exact amount of medicine you need has been carefully worked out. Using too much may increase the chance of side effects, while using too little may not improve your condition.

For adult patients receiving leuprolide for anemia caused by tumors of the uterus or for endometriosis:

- Leuprolide sometimes causes unwanted effects such as hot flashes or decreased interest in sex. It may also cause a temporary increase in pain when you first begin to use it. However, it is very important that you continue to use the medicine, even after you begin to feel better. Do not stop using this medicine without first checking with your doctor.

For adult patients receiving leuprolide for cancer of the prostate:

- Leuprolide sometimes causes unwanted effects such as hot flashes or decreased sexual ability. It may also cause a temporary increase in pain or difficulty in urinating, as well as temporary numbness or tingling of hands or feet or weakness when you first begin to use it. However, it is very important that you continue to use the medicine, even after you begin to feel better. Do not stop using this medicine without first checking with your doctor.

Dosing—The dose of this medicine will be different for different patients. Follow your doctor's orders or the directions on the label. The following information includes only the average doses of this medicine. If your dose is different, do not change it unless your doctor tells you to do so.

The amount of medicine that you take depends on the strength of the medicine. Also, the number of doses you take each day, the time allowed between doses, and the length of time you take the medicine depend on the medical problem for which you are using the medicine.

- For short-acting (daily) injection dosage forms:
  - For cancer of the prostate:
    - Adults—1 milligram (mg) injected under the skin once a day.
  - For central precocious puberty:
    - Children—Dose is based on body weight and must be determined by your doctor. It is injected

under the skin once a day. The dose should be changed over time as weight changes.

- For long-acting (1–month) injection dosage forms:
  - For anemia caused by tumors of the uterus:
    - Adults—3.75 milligrams (mg) injected into a muscle once a month for up to three months.
  - For cancer of the prostate:
    - Adults—7.5 milligrams (mg) injected into a muscle or under the skin (depending on the specific product used) once a month.
  - For central precocious puberty:
    - Children—Dose is based on body weight and must be determined by the doctor. It is injected into a muscle once a month. The dose should be changed over time as weight changes.
  - For endometriosis:
    - Adults—3.75 milligrams (mg) injected into a muscle once a month for up to six months.

- For long-acting (3–month) injection dosage forms:
  - For anemia caused by tumors of the uterus:
    - Adults—11.25 milligrams (mg) injected into a muscle as a single injection to last for three months.
  - For cancer of the prostate:
    - Adults—22.5 milligrams (mg) injected into a muscle or under the skin (depending on the specific product used) once every three months.
  - For endometriosis:
    - Adults—11.25 milligrams (mg) injected into a muscle once every three months for up to six months.

- For long-acting (4–month) injection dosage form:
  - For cancer of the prostate:
    - Adults—30 milligrams (mg) injected into a muscle or under the skin (depending on the specific product used) once every four months.

- For long-acting (12–month) implant dosage form:
  - For cancer of the prostate:
    - Adults— one implant every 12 months.

Missed dose—If you miss a dose of this medicine, take it as soon as possible. However, if it is almost time for your next dose, skip the missed dose and go back to your regular dosing schedule. Do not double doses.

Storage—Store the medicine in a closed container at room temperature, away from heat, moisture, and direct light. Keep from freezing.

Keep out of the reach of children.

Do not keep outdated medicine or medicine no longer needed.

Dispose of used syringes properly in the container provided.

Precautions While Using This Medicine

It is very important that your doctor check your progress at regular visits to make sure that this medicine is working properly and to check for unwanted effects.

For patients receiving leuprolide for endometriosis or for anemia caused by tumors of the uterus:

- During the time you are receiving leuprolide, your menstrual period may not be regular or you may not have a menstrual period at all. This is to be expected when being treated with this medicine. If regular menstruation

does not begin within 60 to 90 days after you stop receiving this medicine, check with your doctor.

- During the time you are receiving leuprolide, you should use birth control methods that do not contain hormones. If you have any questions about this, check with your health care professional.
- If you suspect you may have become pregnant, stop using this medicine and check with your doctor. There is a chance that continued use of leuprolide during pregnancy could cause birth defects or a miscarriage.

Side Effects of This Medicine

Along with its needed effects, a medicine may cause some unwanted effects. Although not all of these side effects may occur, if they do occur they may need medical attention.

Check with your doctor immediately if any of the following side effects occur:
> For adults
> Less common
>> Fast or irregular heartbeat
>
> Rare
>> Bone, muscle, or joint pain; fainting; fast or irregular breathing; numbness or tingling of hands or feet; puffiness or swelling of the eyelids or around the eyes; shortness of breath; skin rash, hives, and/or itching; sudden, severe decrease in blood pressure and collapse; tightness in chest or wheezing; troubled breathing
>
> For males only (adults)
> Rare
>> Pains in chest; pain in groin or legs (especially in calves of legs)
>
> Unknown—Observed during clinical practice, estimates of frequency can not be determined
>> Altered mental status; cardiovascular collapse; double vision; visual changes; vomiting

Check with your doctor as soon as possible if any of the following side effects occur:
> For females only (adults)
> Rare
>> Anxiety; deepening of voice; increased hair growth; mental depression; mood changes; nervousness
>
> For children
> Rare
>> Body pain; burning, itching, redness, or swelling at place of injection; skin rash
>
> For females only (children)— expected in first few weeks
> Rare
>> Vaginal bleeding (continuing); white vaginal discharge (continuing)

Some side effects may occur that usually do not need medical attention. These side effects may go away during treatment as your body adjusts to the medicine. Also, your health care professional may be able to tell you about ways to prevent or reduce some of these side effects. Check with your health care professional if any of the following side effects continue or are bothersome or if you have any questions about them:
> For adults
> More common
>> Sudden sweating and feelings of warmth (also called hot flashes)

Less common

Blurred vision; bleeding, bruising, burning, itching, pain, redness, or swelling at place of injection; decreased interest in sexual intercourse; dizziness; headache; nausea; swelling of feet or lower legs; swelling or increased tenderness of breasts; trouble in sleeping; weight gain

For females only (adults)

More common

Light, irregular vaginal bleeding; stopping of menstrual periods

Less common

Burning, dryness, or itching of vagina; pelvic pain

For males only (adults)

Less common

Bone pain; constipation; decreased size of testicles; inability to have or keep an erection

Other side effects not listed may also occur in some patients. If you notice any other effects, check with your healthcare professional.

LEVALBUTEROL (Inhalation, oral/ nebulization route) - lev-al-BYOO-ter-ol

Commonly used brand name(s)

In the U.S.—

Xopenex

Xopenex HFA

Xopenex Pediatric

Available Dosage Forms:

• Solution

• Aerosol Powder

Therapeutic Class: Bronchodilator

Pharmacologic Class: Sympathomimetic

Uses For This Medicine

Levalbuterol belongs to the family of adrenergic bronchodilators. Levalbuterol is used to prevent or treat chest tightness, shortness of breath, troubled breathing and wheezing associated with bronchospasm.

This medicine is breathed in through the mouth by using a nebulizer and compressor or by using an inhaler. Levalbuterol opens up the bronchial tubes (air passages) of the lungs.

This medicine is available only with your doctor's prescription.

Before Using This Medicine

In deciding to use a medicine, the risks of taking the medicine must be weighed against the good it will do. This is a decision you and your doctor will make. For this medicine, the following should be considered:

Allergies—Tell your doctor if you have ever had any unusual or allergic reaction to this medicine or any other medicines. Also tell your health care professional if you have any other types of allergies, such as to foods, dyes, preservatives, or animals. For non-prescription products, read the label or package ingredients carefully.

Pediatric—The inhalation solution has been tested in children 12 years of age and older. The inhalation aerosol has

been tested in children 4 years of age and older. In effective doses, this medicine has not been shown to cause different side effects or problems than it does in other age groups.

Geriatric—Many medicines have not been studied specifically in older people. Therefore, it may not be known whether they work exactly the same as they do in young adults. Although there is limited information comparing the use of levalbuterol in the elderly with use in other age groups, this medicine is not expected to cause different side effects or problems in older people than it does in younger adults. Your doctor may want to begin with a lesser dose and increase the dosage as tolerated.

Pregnancy—

	Pregnancy Category	Explanation
All Trimesters	C	Animal studies have shown an adverse effect and there are no adequate studies in pregnant women OR no animal studies have been conducted and there are no adequate studies in pregnant women.

Breast Feeding—There are no adequate studies in women for determining infant risk when using this medication during breastfeeding. Weigh the potential benefits against the potential risks before taking this medication while breastfeeding.

Other medicines—

Using this medicine with any of the following medicines is usually not recommended, but may be required in some cases. If both medicines are prescribed together, your doctor may change the dose or how often you use one or both of the medicines.

Clorgyline, Iproniazid, Isocarboxazid, Moclobemide, Nialamide, Pargyline, Phenelzine, Procarbazine, Selegiline, Toloxatone, Tranylcypromine

Interactions with Food/Tobacco/Alcohol—Certain medicines should not be used at or around the time of eating food or eating certain types of food since interactions may occur. Using alcohol or tobacco with certain medicines may also cause interactions to occur. Discuss with your healthcare professional the use of your medicine with food, alcohol, or tobacco.

Other medical problems—The presence of other medical problems may affect the use of this medicine. Make sure you tell your doctor if you have any other medical problems, especially:

• Heart disease (irregular heartbeat or decreased blood flow through the heart) or

• High blood pressure—Use of levalbuterol may worsen these conditions

• Diabetes mellitus (sugar diabetes)—Levalbuterol may worsen blood glucose control

• Hyperthyroidism (overactive thyroid)

• Seizures—Concurrent use may worsen this condition

Proper Use of This Medicine

These medicines come with patient directions. Read them carefully before using the medicine. If you do not understand the directions or if you are not sure how to use the medicine, ask your health care professional to show you what to do.

Also, ask your health care professional to check regularly how you use the medicine to make sure you are using it properly.

Use this medicine only as directed. Do not use more of it and do not use it more often than recommended on the label, unless otherwise directed by your doctor. Using the medicine more often may increase the chance of serious unwanted effects. Deaths have occurred when too much of an inhalation bronchodilator medicine was used.

For patients using levalbuterol inhalation aerosol:

- The levalbuterol aerosol canister provides about 200 inhalations, depending on the size of the canister your doctor ordered. You should try to keep a record of the number of inhalations you use so you will know when the canister is almost empty. This canister, unlike some other aerosol canisters, cannot be floated in water to test its fullness.
- When you use the inhaler for the first time, or if you have not used it in a while, the inhaler may not deliver the right amount of medicine with the first puff. Therefore, before using the inhaler, test or prime it.
- To test or prime the inhaler:
  - Shake the inhaler well immediately before each use.
  - Take the cap off the actuator (or mouthpiece). Inspect the actuator for the presence of foreign objects and make sure that the canister is seated in the actuator before each use.
  - Prime the inhaler by releasing 4 test sprays in the air, away from your face. The inhaler will now be ready to provide the right amount of medicine when you use it.
- To use the inhaler:
  - Shake the inhaler well
  - Breathe out fully through your mouth, expelling as much air from your lungs as possible. Place the mouthpiece fully into your mouth, holding the inhaler in the mouthpiece-down position and closing your lips around it.
  - While breathing in deeply and slowly through your mouth, fully depress the top of the metal canister with your middle finger. Immediately after the puff is delivered, release your finger from the canister and remove the inhaler from your mouth.
  - Hold your breath for 10 seconds, if possible.
  - If your doctor has prescribed more than a single inhalation/puff, wait 1 minute between inhalations. Then, shake the inhaler well and repeat.
  - Replace the cap on the mouthpiece after each use
  - Clean the actuator or mouthpiece at least once a week.
- To clean the inhaler:
  - To clean the blue plastic actuator (or mouthpiece), remove the canister and red mouthpiece cap.
  - Wash the actuator through the top and bottom with warm running water for 30 seconds at least once a week
  - Shake off the excess water and let the inhaler parts air dry completely before putting the inhaler back together.
  - Do not clean the metal canister or allow the metal canister to become wet. Never immerse the metal canister in water.
  - To dry, shake off excess water and let the actuator air dry thoroughly, such as overnight.

- When the actuator is dry, replace the canister and the mouthpiece cap. Make sure the canister is fully and firmly inserted into the actuator. Blockage from medicine build-up is more likely to occur if the actuator is not allowed to air dry thoroughly.

If your actuator becomes blocked (little or no medicine coming out of the mouthpiece), wash your actuator and air dry thoroughly. If you need your inhaler before the plastic actuator is completely dry, shake excess water off the actuator, replace canister, shake well, and test spray twice into the air away from your face, to remove most of the water remaining in the actuator. Then take your dose as prescribed. After such use, rewash and air dry the actuator thoroughly.

For patients using levalbuterol inhalation solution dosage form:

- If you are using this medicine in a nebulizer, make sure you understand exactly how to use it. If you have any questions about this, check with your health care professional.
- Do not use if solution becomes cloudy.
- Do not mix another inhalation medicine with levalbuterol in the nebulizer unless told to do so by your health care professional.

Dosing—The dose of this medicine will be different for different patients. Follow your doctor's orders or the directions on the label. The following information includes only the average doses of this medicine. If your dose is different, do not change it unless your doctor tells you to do so.

The amount of medicine that you take depends on the strength of the medicine. Also, the number of doses you take each day, the time allowed between doses, and the length of time you take the medicine depend on the medical problem for which you are using the medicine.

- For inhalation aerosol dosage form:
  - For preventing or treating bronchospasm:
    - Adults and children 4 years of age and older— This medicine is used in an aerosol inhaler The usual dose is 2 inhalations (puffs) every 4 to 6 hours. In some patients 1 inhalation (puff) every 4 hours may be enough.
    - Children up to 4 years of age—Use and dose must be determined by your doctor.

- For inhalation solution dosage form:
  - For preventing or treating bronchospasm:
    - Adults and children 12 years of age and older— This medicine is used in a nebulizer and is taken by inhalation over a period of five to fifteen minutes. The usual dose is 0.63 milligrams (mg) to 1.25 mg three times a day, every six to eight hours.
    - Children up to 12 years of age—Use and dose must be determined by your doctor.

Missed dose—If you miss a dose of this medicine, take it as soon as possible. However, if it is almost time for your next dose, skip the missed dose and go back to your regular dosing schedule. Do not double doses.

If your dosing schedule is different from all of the above and you miss a dose of this medicine, or if you have any questions about this, check with your doctor.

Storage—Store the medicine in a closed container at room temperature, away from heat, moisture, and direct light. Keep from freezing.

Keep out of the reach of children.

Do not keep outdated medicine or medicine no longer needed.

Precautions While Using This Medicine

It is important that your doctor check your progress at regular intervals to make sure that your medicine is working properly.

If you still have trouble breathing after using this medicine, if your condition becomes worse, or if you are using more medicine than the amount prescribed, check with your doctor at once.

Do not add or stop taking inhaled or other asthma medicines without first checking with your doctor.

Side Effects of This Medicine

Along with its needed effects, a medicine may cause some unwanted effects. Although not all of these side effects may occur, if they do occur they may need medical attention.

Check with your doctor as soon as possible if any of the following side effects occur:

More common
    Fast heartbeat

Less common or rare
    Chest pain or tightness; dizziness; feeling "faint” high or low blood pressure; hives; light-headedness; shortness of breath; troubled breathing; wheezing

Incidence not known
    Cough; Difficult or labored breathing; difficulty swallowing; extra heartbeats; fainting; fast, pounding, slow, or irregular heartbeat or pulse; hives or welts; itching; large, hive-like swelling on face, eyelids, lips, tongue, throat, hands, legs, feet, sex organs; noisy breathing; palpitations; puffiness or swelling of the eyelids or around the eyes, face, lips, or tongue; rash; redness of skin; tightness in chest; unusual tiredness or weakness

Symptoms of overdose
    Chest pain; dizziness; dry mouth; fatigue; general feeling of discomfort or illness; headache; high blood pressure; impaired consciousness; irregular or fast heartbeat; light-headedness; nausea; nervousness; seizures; sleeplessness; sweating; tremor

Some side effects may occur that usually do not need medical attention. These side effects may go away during treatment as your body adjusts to the medicine. Also, your health care professional may be able to tell you about ways to prevent or reduce some of these side effects. Check with your health care professional if any of the following side effects continue or are bothersome or if you have any questions about them:

More common
    Accidental injury (in children 4 to 11 years of age); anxiety; body aches or pain; chills; congestion; cough or hoarseness; dryness or soreness of throat; fever; general aches and pains; headache; hoarseness; increased cough; leg cramps; loss of appetite; migraines or other headaches; muscle tightness; nervousness; runny or stuffy nose

Less common or rare
    Abdominal or stomach pain; abnormal growth filled with fluid or semisolid material; blemishes on the skin; blood

in urine; bloody nose; burning, dry or itching eyes; burning or stinging of skin; cough producing mucus; cramps; diarrhea; difficulty breathing; difficulty having a bowel movement (stool); discharge from the eye; dry mouth or throat; ear pain; excessive tearing; eye itch; heavy menstrual bleeding; muscle pain; nausea; night sweats; numbness or decreased sensitivity of the hand; pain; painful cold sores or blisters on lips, nose, eyes, or genitals; pimples; redness, pain, swelling of eye, eyelid, or inner lining of eyelid; sleeplessness; tingling sensation in extremities; vaginal yeast infection; weight loss

Other side effects not listed may also occur in some patients. If you notice any other effects, check with your healthcare professional.

LEVETIRACETAM (Oral route) - lee-ve-tye-RA-se-tam

Commonly used brand name(s)
In the U.S.—
    Keppra

Available Dosage Forms:
- Tablet
- Solution

Therapeutic Class: Anticonvulsant

Uses For This Medicine

Levetiracetam is used to help control some types of seizures in the treatment of epilepsy. This medicine cannot cure epilepsy and will only work to control seizures for as long as you continue to take it.

This medicine is available only with your doctor's prescription.

Before Using This Medicine

In deciding to use a medicine, the risks of taking the medicine must be weighed against the good it will do. This is a decision you and your doctor will make. For this medicine, the following should be considered:

Allergies—Tell your doctor if you have ever had any unusual or allergic reaction to this medicine or any other medicines. Also tell your health care professional if you have any other types of allergies, such as to foods, dyes, preservatives, or animals. For non-prescription products, read the label or package ingredients carefully.

Pediatric—Studies on this medicine have been done only in adult patients, and there is no specific information comparing use of levetiracetam in children with use in other age groups.

Geriatric—This medicine has been tested in a limited number of patients 65 years of age and older and has not been shown to cause different side effects or problems in older people than it does in younger adults.

Pregnancy—

	Pregnancy Category	Explanation
All Trimesters	C	Animal studies have shown an adverse effect and there are no adequate studies in pregnant women OR no animal studies have been conducted and there are no adequate studies in pregnant women.

Breast Feeding—There are no adequate studies in women for determining infant risk when using this medication during breastfeeding. Weigh the potential benefits against the potential risks before taking this medication while breastfeeding.

Other medicines—

Using this medicine with any of the following medicines may cause an increased risk of certain side effects, but using both drugs may be the best treatment for you. If both medicines are prescribed together, your doctor may change the dose or how often you use one or both of the medicines.

Ginkgo

Interactions with Food/Tobacco/Alcohol—Certain medicines should not be used at or around the time of eating food or eating certain types of food since interactions may occur. Using alcohol or tobacco with certain medicines may also cause interactions to occur. Discuss with your healthcare professional the use of your medicine with food, alcohol, or tobacco.

Other medical problems—The presence of other medical problems may affect the use of this medicine. Make sure you tell your doctor if you have any other medical problems, especially:

- Kidney problems—Higher blood levels of levetiracetam may occur, which may increase the chance of unwanted effects; your doctor may need to change your dose.

Proper Use of This Medicine

Take this medicine only as directed by your doctor, to help your condition as much as possible. Do not take it more or less often than your doctor ordered.

Swallow the tablet form of this medicine whole

Levetiracetam may be taken with or without food or on a full or empty stomach. However, if your doctor tells you to take the medicine a certain way, take it exactly as directed.

This medicine is to be taken by mouth even if it comes in a dropper bottle. The amount you should take is to be measured with the special dropper provided with your prescription.

Dosing—The dose of this medicine will be different for different patients. Follow your doctor's orders or the directions on the label. The following information includes only the average doses of this medicine. If your dose is different, do not change it unless your doctor tells you to do so.

The amount of medicine that you take depends on the strength of the medicine. Also, the number of doses you take each day, the time allowed between doses, and the length of time you take the medicine depend on the medical problem for which you are using the medicine.

- For oral dosage form (tablets):
  - For epilepsy:
    - Adults—At first, 500 milligrams (mg) two times a day. Your doctor may increase the dose gradually if needed. However, the dose is usually not more than 3000 mg a day.
    - Children—Use and dose must be determined by your doctor.
- For oral dosage form (solution):
  - For epilepsy:
    - Adults—At first, 500 milligrams (mg) two times a day. Your doctor may increase the dose gradually if needed. However, the dose is usually not more than 3000 mg a day.
    - Children—Use and dose must be determined by your doctor.

Missed dose—Call your doctor or pharmacist for instructions.

Storage—Store the medicine in a closed container at room temperature, away from heat, moisture, and direct light. Keep from freezing.

Keep out of the reach of children.

Do not keep outdated medicine or medicine no longer needed.

Ask your healthcare professional how you should dispose of any medicine you do not use.

Precautions While Using This Medicine

It is important that your doctor check your progress at regular visits, especially for the first few months you take levetiracetam. This is necessary to allow dose adjustments and to reduce any unwanted effects.

This medicine may cause some people to become drowsy, dizzy, or less alert than they are normally. Make sure you know how you react to this medicine before you drive, use machines, or do anything else that could be dangerous if you are dizzy or are not alert

Do not stop taking levetiracetam without first checking with your doctor. Stopping the medicine suddenly may cause your seizures to return or to occur more often. Your doctor may want you to gradually reduce the amount you are taking before stopping completely.

Side Effects of This Medicine

Along with its needed effects, a medicine may cause some unwanted effects. Although not all of these side effects may occur, if they do occur they may need medical attention.

Check with your doctor as soon as possible if any of the following side effects occur:

Less common

Clumsiness or unsteadiness; cough or hoarseness; crying; depersonalization; depression; double vision; fever or chills; headache; loss of memory or problems with memory; lower back or side pain; mood or mental changes; nervousness; outburst of anger; pain or tenderness around eyes and cheekbones; painful or difficult urination; paranoia; problems with muscle control or coordination; quick to react or overreact; rapidly changing emotional moods; shortness of breath or troubled breathing,; stuffy or runny nose; tightness of chest or wheezing

Incidence not determined—Observed during clinical practice with levetiracetam; estimates of frequency cannot be determined

 Black, tarry stools; bloating; constipation; dark urine; indigestion; painful or difficult urination; pinpoint red spots on skin; shortness of breath; sores, ulcers, or white spots on lips or in mouth; unusual bleeding or bruising; unusual tiredness or weakness

Some side effects may occur that usually do not need medical attention. These side effects may go away during treatment as your body adjusts to the medicine. Also, your health care professional may be able to tell you about ways to prevent or reduce some of these side effects. Check with your health care professional if any of the following side effects continue or are bothersome or if you have any questions about them:

More common

 Cough; dizziness; dryness or soreness of throat; fever; hoarseness; loss of strength or energy; muscle pain or weakness; pain; runny nose; sleepiness or unusual drowsiness; tender, swollen glands in neck; trouble in swallowing; unusual weak feeling; voice changes

Less common

 Burning, crawling, itching, numbness, prickling, "pins and needles," or tingling feelings; cough increased; dizziness or light-headedness; feeling of constant movement of self or surroundings; loss of appetite; sensation of spinning; weight loss

Incidence not determined—Observed during clinical practice with levetiracetam; estimates of frequency cannot be determined

 Hair loss

Other side effects not listed may also occur in some patients. If you notice any other effects, check with your healthcare professional.

LEVODOPA (Oral route) - lee-voe-DOE-pa

Uses For This Medicine

Levodopa is used alone or in combination with carbidopa to treat Parkinson's disease, sometimes referred to as shaking palsy. Some patients require the combination of medicine, while others benefit from levodopa alone. By improving muscle control, this medicine allows more normal movements of the body.

Levodopa alone or in combination is available only with your doctor's prescription.

Before Using This Medicine

In deciding to use a medicine, the risks of taking the medicine must be weighed against the good it will do. This is a decision you and your doctor will make. For this medicine, the following should be considered:

Allergies—Tell your doctor if you have ever had any unusual or allergic reaction to this medicine or any other medicines. Also tell your health care professional if you have any other types of allergies, such as to foods, dyes, preservatives,

or animals. For non-prescription products, read the label or package ingredients carefully.

Pediatric—Studies on this medicine have been done only in adult patients, and there is no specific information comparing use of levodopa or carbidopa in children with use in other age groups.

Geriatric—Elderly people are especially sensitive to the effects of levodopa. This may increase the chance of side effects during treatment.

Pregnancy—

	Pregnancy Category	Explanation
All Trimesters	C	Animal studies have shown an adverse effect and there are no adequate studies in pregnant women OR no animal studies have been conducted and there are no adequate studies in pregnant women.

Breast Feeding—Studies suggest that this medication may alter milk production or composition. If an alternative to this medication is not prescribed, you should monitor the infant for side effects and adequate milk intake.

Other medicines—

Using this medicine with any of the following medicines is not recommended. Your doctor may decide not to treat you with this medication or change some of the other medicines you take.

Clorgyline, Iproniazid, Isocarboxazid, Nialamide, Pargyline, Phenelzine, Procarbazine, Selegiline, Toloxatone, Tranylcypromine

Interactions with Food/Tobacco/Alcohol—Certain medicines should not be used at or around the time of eating food or eating certain types of food since interactions may occur. Using alcohol or tobacco with certain medicines may also cause interactions to occur. Discuss with your healthcare professional the use of your medicine with food, alcohol, or tobacco.

Other medical problems—The presence of other medical problems may affect the use of this medicine. Make sure you tell your doctor if you have any other medical problems, especially:

- Diabetes mellitus (sugar diabetes)—The amount of insulin or antidiabetic medicine that you need to take may change

- Emphysema, asthma, bronchitis, or other chronic lung disease or

- Glaucoma or

- Heart or blood vessel disease or

- Hormone problems or

- Melanoma (a type of skin cancer) (or history of) or

- Mental illness—Levodopa may make the condition worse

- Kidney disease or
- Liver disease—Higher blood levels of levodopa may occur, increasing the chance of side effects
- Seizure disorders, such as epilepsy (history of)—The risk of seizures may be increased
- Stomach ulcer (history of)—The ulcer may occur again

Proper Use of This Medicine

Since protein may interfere with the body's response to levodopa, high protein diets should be avoided. Intake of normal amounts of protein should be spaced equally throughout the day, or taken as directed by your doctor.

For patients taking levodopa by itself:

- Pyridoxine (vitamin B 6) has been found to reduce the effects of levodopa when levodopa is taken by itself. This does not happen with the combination of carbidopa and levodopa. If you are taking levodopa by itself, do not take vitamin products containing vitamin B 6 during treatment, unless prescribed by your doctor.
- Large amounts of pyridoxine are also contained in some foods such as bananas, egg yolks, lima beans, meats, peanuts, and whole grain cereals. Check with your doctor about how much of these foods you may have in your diet while you are taking levodopa. Also, ask your health care professional for help when selecting vitamin products.

At first, levodopa may be taken with a meal or a snack, so that any effects like stomach upset will be lessened. Later, as your body becomes accustomed to the medicine, it should be taken on an empty stomach so that it works better. Be sure to talk to your doctor about the best time for you to take this medicine.

Take this medicine only as directed. Do not take more or less of it, and do not take it more often than your doctor ordered.

For patients taking carbidopa and levodopa extended-release tablets:

- Swallow the tablet whole without crushing or chewing, unless your doctor tells you not to. If your doctor tells you to, you may break the tablet in half.

Some people must take this medicine for several weeks or months before full benefit is received. Do not stop taking it even if you do not think it is working. Instead, check with your doctor.

Dosing—The dose of this medicine will be different for different patients. Follow your doctor's orders or the directions on the label. The following information includes only the average doses of this medicine. If your dose is different, do not change it unless your doctor tells you to do so.

The amount of medicine that you take depends on the strength of the medicine. Also, the number of doses you take each day, the time allowed between doses, and the length of time you take the medicine depend on the medical problem for which you are using the medicine.

For levodopa
- For Parkinson's disease:
  - For oral dosage form (tablets):
    - Adults and teenagers—At first, 250 milligrams (mg) two to four times a day. Your doctor may increase your dose if needed. However, the dose is usually not more than 8000 mg (8 grams) a day.
    - Children up to 12 years of age—Use and dose must be determined by your doctor.

For levodopa and carbidopa combination
- For Parkinson's disease:
  - For oral tablet dosage form:
    - Adults—At first, 1 tablet three or four times a day. Your doctor may need to change your dose, depending on how you respond to this combination medicine.
    - Children and teenagers—Use and dose must be determined by your doctor.
  - For oral extended-release tablet dosage form:
    - Adults—At first, 1 tablet two times a day. However, you may need to take more than this. Your doctor will decide the right dose for you, depending on your condition and the other medicines you may be taking for Parkinson's disease.
    - Children and teenagers—Use and dose must be determined by your doctor.

Missed dose—If you miss a dose of this medicine, take it as soon as possible. However, if it is almost time for your next dose, skip the missed dose and go back to your regular dosing schedule. Do not double doses.

Storage—Store the medicine in a closed container at room temperature, away from heat, moisture, and direct light. Keep from freezing.

Keep out of the reach of children.

Do not keep outdated medicine or medicine no longer needed.

Precautions While Using This Medicine

Before having any kind of surgery (including dental surgery) or emergency treatment, tell the medical doctor or dentist in charge that you are taking this medicine.

For patients with diabetes:

- This medicine may cause test results for urine sugar or ketones to be wrong. Check with your doctor before depending on home tests using the paper-strip or tablet method.

This medicine may cause some people to become dizzy, confused, or have blurred or double vision. Make sure you know how you react to this medicine before you drive, use machines, or do anything else that could be dangerous if you are not alert or not able to see well.

Dizziness, lightheadedness, or fainting may occur, especially when you get up from a lying or sitting position. Getting up slowly may help. If the problem continues or gets worse, check with your doctor.

For patients taking levodopa by itself:

- Pyridoxine (vitamin B 6) has been found to reduce the effects of levodopa when levodopa is taken by itself. This does not happen with the combination of carbidopa and levodopa. If you are taking levodopa by itself, do not take vitamin products containing vitamin B 6 during treatment, unless prescribed by your doctor.
- Large amounts of pyridoxine are also contained in some foods such as bananas, egg yolks, lima beans, meats, peanuts, and whole grain cereals. Check with your doctor about how much of these foods you may have in your diet while you are taking levodopa. Also, ask your health care professional for help when selecting vitamin products.

As your condition improves and your body movements become easier, be careful not to overdo physical activities. Injuries resulting from falls may occur. Physical activities must be increased gradually to allow your body to adjust to changing balance, circulation, and coordination. This is especially important in the elderly.

Side Effects of This Medicine

Along with its needed effects, a medicine may cause some unwanted effects. Although not all of these side effects may occur, if they do occur they may need medical attention.

Check with your doctor as soon as possible if any of the following side effects occur:

More common

Abnormal thinking: holding false beliefs that cannot be changed by fact; agitation; anxiety; clenching or grinding of teeth; clumsiness or unsteadiness; confusion; difficulty swallowing; dizziness; excessive watering of mouth; false sense of well being; feeling faint; general feeling of discomfort or illness; hallucinations (seeing, hearing, or feeling things that are not there); hand tremor, increased; nausea or vomiting; numbness; unusual and uncontrolled movements of the body, including the face, tongue, arms, hands, head, and upper body; unusual tiredness or weakness

Less common

Blurred vision; difficult urination; difficulty opening mouth; dilated (large) pupils; dizziness or lightheadedness when getting up from a lying or sitting position; double vision; fast, irregular, or pounding heartbeat; hot flashes; increased blinking or spasm of eyelids; loss of bladder control; mental depression; other mood or mental changes; skin rash; unusual weight gain or loss

Rare

Back or leg pain; bloody or black tarry stools; chills; convulsions (seizures); fever; high blood pressure; inability to move eyes; loss of appetite; pain, tenderness, or swelling of foot or leg; pale skin; prolonged, painful, inappropriate penile erection; sore throat; stomach pain; swelling of face; swelling of feet or lower legs; vomiting of blood or material that looks like coffee grounds

Some side effects may occur that usually do not need medical attention. These side effects may go away during treatment as your body adjusts to the medicine. Also, your health care professional may be able to tell you about ways to prevent or reduce some of these side effects. Check with your health care professional if any of the following side effects continue or are bothersome or if you have any questions about them:

More common

Abdominal pain; dryness of mouth; loss of appetite; nightmares; passing gas

Less common

Constipation; diarrhea; flushing of skin; headache; hiccups; increased sweating; muscle twitching; trouble in sleeping

This medicine may sometimes cause the urine, saliva, and sweat to be darker in color than usual. The urine may at first be reddish, then turn to nearly black after being exposed to air. Some bathroom cleaning products will produce a similar effect when in contact with urine containing this medicine. This is to be expected during treatment with this medicine. Also, this medicine may cause a bitter taste, or a burning sensation of the tongue.

Other side effects not listed may also occur in some patients. If you notice any other effects, check with your healthcare professional.

LEVOFLOXACIN (Ophthalmic route) -
lee-voe-FLOX-a-sin

Commonly used brand name(s)

In the U.S.—
Quixin

Available Dosage Forms:

• Solution

Therapeutic Class: Antibiotic

Uses For This Medicine

Ophthalmic levofloxacin is used in the eye to treat bacterial infections of the eye. Ophthalmic levofloxacin works by killing bacteria.

This medicine is available only with your doctor's prescription.

Before Using This Medicine

In deciding to use a medicine, the risks of taking the medicine must be weighed against the good it will do. This is a decision you and your doctor will make. For this medicine, the following should be considered:

Allergies—Tell your doctor if you have ever had any unusual or allergic reaction to this medicine or any other medicines. Also tell your health care professional if you have any other types of allergies, such as to foods, dyes, preservatives, or animals. For non-prescription products, read the label or package ingredients carefully.

Pediatric—Use is not recommended in infants under 1 year of age. In children older than 1 year, this medicine is not expected to cause different side effects or problems than it does in adults.

Geriatric—Many medicines have not been studied specifically in older people. Therefore, it may not be known whether they work exactly the same way they do in younger adults. Although there is no specific information comparing use of levofloxacin in the elderly with use in other age groups, this medicine is not expected to cause different side effects or problems in older people than it does in younger adults.

Pregnancy—

	Pregnancy Category	Explanation
All Trimesters	C	Animal studies have shown an adverse effect and there are no adequate studies in pregnant women OR no animal studies have been conducted and there are no adequate studies in pregnant women.

Breast Feeding—There are no adequate studies in women for determining infant risk when using this medication during breastfeeding. Weigh the potential benefits against the potential risks before taking this medication while breastfeeding.

Other medicines—

Using this medicine with any of the following medicines is not recommended. Your doctor may decide not to treat you with this medication or change some of the other medicines you take.

Mesoridazine, Thioridazine

Interactions with Food/Tobacco/Alcohol—Certain medicines should not be used at or around the time of eating food or eating certain types of food since interactions may occur. Using alcohol or tobacco with certain medicines may also cause interactions to occur. Discuss with your healthcare professional the use of your medicine with food, alcohol, or tobacco.

Proper Use of This Medicine

Dosing—The dose of this medicine will be different for different patients. Follow your doctor's orders or the directions on the label. The following information includes only the average doses of this medicine. If your dose is different, do not change it unless your doctor tells you to do so.

The amount of medicine that you take depends on the strength of the medicine. Also, the number of doses you take each day, the time allowed between doses, and the length of time you take the medicine depend on the medical problem for which you are using the medicine.

To use levofloxacin ophthalmic solution (eye drops):

- First, wash your hands. Then tilt the head back and pull the lower eyelid away from the eye to form a pouch. Drop the medicine into the pouch and gently close the eyes. Do not blink. Keep the eyes closed for 1 or 2 minutes to allow the medicine to come into contact with the infection.

- If you think you did not get the drop of medicine into your eyes properly, use another drop.

- To keep the medicine as germ-free as possible, do not touch the applicator tip to any surface (including the eye). Also, keep the container tightly closed.

- For ophthalmic solution dosage form:
  - For bacterial conjunctivitis:
    - Adults and children 1 year of age and older— Days 1 and 2: Put one to two drops in the affected eye(s) every two hours while awake. Do not put drops in more than 8 times a day. Days 3 through 7: Put one to two drops in the affected eye(s) every 4 hours while awake. Do not put drops in more than 4 times a day.
    - Infants and children up to 1 year of age—Use and dose must be determined by your doctor.

Missed dose—If you miss a dose of this medicine, take it as soon as possible. However, if it is almost time for your next dose, skip the missed dose and go back to your regular dosing schedule. Do not double doses.

Storage—Store the medicine in a closed container at room temperature, away from heat, moisture, and direct light. Keep from freezing.

Keep out of the reach of children.

Do not keep outdated medicine or medicine no longer needed.

Ask your healthcare professional how you should dispose of any medicine you do not use.

Precautions While Using This Medicine

If your eye infection does not improve within a few days, or if it becomes worse, check with your doctor.

This medicine may cause your eyes to become more sensitive to light than they are normally. Wearing sunglasses and avoiding too much exposure to bright light may help lessen the discomfort.

Side Effects of This Medicine

Along with its needed effects, a medicine may cause some unwanted effects. Although not all of these side effects may occur, if they do occur they may need medical attention.

Some side effects may occur that usually do not need medical attention. These side effects may go away during treatment as your body adjusts to the medicine. Also, your health care professional may be able to tell you about ways to prevent or reduce some of these side effects. Check with your health care professional if any of the following side effects continue or are bothersome or if you have any questions about them:
> *Less common*
> Itching, pain, redness or swelling of eye or eyelid; watering of eyes; decreased vision; fever; feeling of having something in the eye; headache; hoarseness; eye burning, dryness, itching, or pain; increased sensitivity of eyes to lightbody aches or pain; congestion; dryness or soreness of throat; runny nose; swelling of the eyelid; tender, swollen glands in neck; trouble in swallowingvoice changes

Other side effects not listed may also occur in some patients. If you notice any other effects, check with your healthcare professional.

LEVOFLOXACIN (Oral route, Intravenous route) - lee-voe-FLOX-a-sin

Commonly used brand name(s)

In the U.S.—
Levaquin

Available Dosage Forms:

- Tablet
- Solution

Therapeutic Class: Antibiotic

Uses For This Medicine

Levofloxacin belongs to the class of medicines known as antibiotics. It is used to treat bacterial infections in many different parts of the body. Levofloxacin is also used to treat anthrax.

Levofloxacin works by killing bacteria or preventing their growth. However, this medicine will not work for colds, flu, or other virus infections.

This medicine is available only with your doctor's prescription.

Before Using This Medicine

In deciding to use a medicine, the risks of taking the medicine must be weighed against the good it will do. This is a decision you and your doctor will make. For this medicine, the following should be considered:

Allergies—Tell your doctor if you have ever had any unusual or allergic reaction to this medicine or any other medi-

cines. Also tell your health care professional if you have any other types of allergies, such as to foods, dyes, preservatives, or animals. For non-prescription products, read the label or package ingredients carefully.

Pediatric—Caution is recommended in using levofloxacin in children up to 18 years of age because this medicine has been shown to cause bone development problems in young animals. However, your doctor may choose to use this medicine if other medicines cannot be used.

Geriatric—There is no specific information comparing use of levofloxacin in the elderly with use in other age groups. However, it has been used in older people and has not been found to cause different side effects or other problems than it does in younger adults.

Pregnancy—

	Pregnancy Category	Explanation
All Trimesters	C	Animal studies have shown an adverse effect and there are no adequate studies in pregnant women OR no animal studies have been conducted and there are no adequate studies in pregnant women.

Breast Feeding—There are no adequate studies in women for determining infant risk when using this medication during breastfeeding. Weigh the potential benefits against the potential risks before taking this medication while breastfeeding.

Other medicines—

Using this medicine with any of the following medicines is not recommended. Your doctor may decide not to treat you with this medication or change some of the other medicines you take.

Mesoridazine, Thioridazine

Interactions with Food/Tobacco/Alcohol—Certain medicines should not be used at or around the time of eating food or eating certain types of food since interactions may occur. Using alcohol or tobacco with certain medicines may also cause interactions to occur. Discuss with your healthcare professional the use of your medicine with food, alcohol, or tobacco.

Other medical problems—The presence of other medical problems may affect the use of this medicine. Make sure you tell your doctor if you have any other medical problems, especially:

- Brain or spinal cord disease, including hardening of the arteries in the brain, or epilepsy or other seizures—Levofloxacin may increase the chance of convulsions (seizures) occurring
- Diabetes mellitus (sugar diabetes)—Levofloxacin may cause changes in blood sugar, which could lead to problems in controlling blood sugar
- Kidney disease—Effects may be increased because of slower removal of levofloxacin from the body

Proper Use of This Medicine

Levofloxacin oral solution should be taken 1 hour before eating or 2 hours after eating.

Levofloxacin tablets may be taken with meals or on an empty stomach.

This medicine is best taken with a full glass (8 ounces) of water. Several additional glasses of water should be taken every day, unless you are otherwise directed by your doctor. Drinking extra water will help to prevent some unwanted effects of levofloxacin.

This medicine works best when there is a constant amount in the blood or urine. To help keep the amount constant, do not miss any doses. Also, it is best to take the doses at evenly spaced times, day and night. For example, if you are to take one dose a day, try to take it at the same time each day.

If you need to take this medicine for anthrax, your doctor will want you to begin taking it as soon as possible after you are exposed to anthrax.

Dosing—The dose of this medicine will be different for different patients. Follow your doctor's orders or the directions on the label. The following information includes only the average doses of this medicine. If your dose is different, do not change it unless your doctor tells you to do so.

The amount of medicine that you take depends on the strength of the medicine. Also, the number of doses you take each day, the time allowed between doses, and the length of time you take the medicine depend on the medical problem for which you are using the medicine.

- For oral dosage form (oral solution or tablets):
  - For treatment of infection:
    - Adults—250 to 750 milligrams (mg) once a day.
    - Children younger than 18 years of age—Use and dose must be determined by your doctor
- For parenteral dosage form (injection):
  - For treatment of infection:
    - Adults—250 to 750 mg once a day.
    - Children younger than 18 years of age—Use and dose must be determined by your doctor.

Missed dose—If you miss a dose of this medicine, take it as soon as possible. However, if it is almost time for your next dose, skip the missed dose and go back to your regular dosing schedule. Do not double doses.

Storage—Store the medicine in a closed container at room temperature, away from heat, moisture, and direct light. Keep from freezing.

Keep out of the reach of children.

Do not keep outdated medicine or medicine no longer needed.

Ask your healthcare professional how you should dispose of any medicine you do not use.

Precautions While Using This Medicine

If your symptoms do not improve within a few days, or if they become worse, check with your doctor.

For patients with an abnormally slow heartbeat: Levofloxacin may increase your risk of experiencing a fast, slow or irregular heartbeat

If you are taking aluminum-, calcium-, or magnesium-containing antacids, didanosine, iron supplements, sucralfate, or zinc, do not take them at the same time that you take this medicine. It is best to take these medicines at least 2 hours before or 2 hours after taking levofloxacin. These medicines may keep levofloxacin from working properly.

Some people who take levofloxacin may become more sensitive to sunlight than they are normally. Exposure to sunlight, even for brief periods of time, may cause severe sunburn or skin rash, redness, itching, or discoloration. When you begin taking this medicine:

- Stay out of direct sunlight, especially between the hours of 10:00 a.m. and 3:00 p.m., if possible.
- Wear protective clothing, including a hat and sunglasses.
- Apply a sun block product that has a skin protection factor (SPF) of at least 15. Some patients may require a product with a higher SPF number, especially if they have a fair complexion. If you have any questions about this, check with your health care professional.
- Do not use a sun lamp or tanning bed or booth.

If you have a severe reaction from the sun, check with your doctor.

If you get a skin rash or other signs of an allergic reaction, stop taking levofloxacin and check with your doctor.

Levofloxacin may cause some people to become dizzy, lightheaded, drowsy, or less alert than they are normally. Make sure you know how you react to this medicine before you drive, use machines, or do anything else that could be dangerous if you are dizzy or are not alert. If these reactions are especially bothersome, check with your doctor.

Levofloxacin may cause pain, inflammation, or rupture of a tendon. If you experience these symptoms in your hands, shoulders, or calves, stop taking levofloxacin and check with your doctor right away. Refrain from exercise until your doctor says otherwise.

For diabetic patients taking insulin or diabetes medicine by mouth: Levofloxacin may cause hypoglycemia (low blood sugar) in some patients. Symptoms of low blood sugar must be treated before they lead to unconsciousness (passing out). Different people may feel different symptoms of low blood sugar. If you experience symptoms of low blood sugar, stop taking levofloxacin and check with your doctor right away:

- Symptoms of low blood sugar can include: Anxious feeling, behavior change similar to being drunk, blurred vision, cold sweats, confusion, cool pale skin, difficulty in concentrating, drowsiness, excessive hunger, headache, nausea, nervousness, rapid heartbeat, shakiness, unusual tiredness or weakness.

For patients with low potassium levels: Levofloxacin may increase your risk of experiencing a fast, slow or irregular heartbeat

Side Effects of This Medicine

Along with its needed effects, a medicine may cause some unwanted effects. Although not all of these side effects may occur, if they do occur they may need medical attention.

Check with your doctor immediately if any of the following side effects occur:

  Rare
    Skin rash, itching, or redness

Check with your doctor as soon as possible if any of the following side effects occur:

  Rare
    Abdominal or stomach cramps or pain (severe); abdominal tenderness; agitation; blisters; confusion; diarrhea (watery and severe) which may also be bloody; fever; hallucinations (seeing, hearing, or feeling things that are not there); pain, inflammation, or swelling in

calves of legs, shoulders, or hands; psychosis; sensation of skin burning; redness and swelling of skin; trembling

  Incidence not determined—Observed during clinical practice; estimates of frequency cannot be determined
    Abnormal brain wave patterns; black, tarry stools; bleeding gums; blurred vision; burning, numbness, tingling, or painful sensations; coma; confusion; cough; dark-colored urine; difficult breathing; difficulty swallowing; failure of the heart, lungs, kidneys and/or liver; fast or irregular heartbeat; fatigue; general body swelling; hives; hoarseness; increased bleeding time; joint or muscle pain; muscle cramps or spasms; muscle pain or stiffness; peeling, loosening of skin; puffiness or swelling of the eyelids or around the eyes, face, lips or tongue; severe dizziness; sharp drop in blood pressure; shortness of breath; sore throat; swollen glands; tightness in chest; unsteadiness or awkwardness; unusual bleeding or bruising; unusual tiredness or weakness; voice changes; weakness in arms, hands, legs, or feet; wheezing

Some side effects may occur that usually do not need medical attention. These side effects may go away during treatment as your body adjusts to the medicine. Also, your health care professional may be able to tell you about ways to prevent or reduce some of these side effects. Check with your health care professional if any of the following side effects continue or are bothersome or if you have any questions about them:

  Less common
    Abdominal or stomach pain or discomfort; change in sense of taste; constipation; diarrhea; dizziness; drowsiness; headache; lightheadedness; nausea; nervousness; trouble in sleeping; vaginal itching and discharge; vomiting

  Incidence not determined—Observed during clinical practice; estimates of frequency cannot be determined
    feeling of warmth or heat; flushing or redness of skin, especially on face and neck; feeling faint; sweating

After you stop using this medicine, it may still produce some side effects that need attention. During this period of time, *check with your doctor immediately* if you notice the following side effects:
    Abdominal or stomach cramps and pain (severe); abdominal tenderness; diarrhea (watery and severe) which may also be bloody; fever

Other side effects not listed may also occur in some patients. If you notice any other effects, check with your healthcare professional.

LINDANE (Topical route) - LIN-dane

Black Box Warning

Lindane should only be used in patients who cannot tolerate or have failed first-line treatment with safer medications for the treatment of scabies.

Seizures and deaths have been reported following lindane use with repeat or prolonged application, but also in rare cases following a single application used according to directions. Lindane should be used with caution for infants, children, the elderly, and individuals with other skin conditions (eg, atopic dermatitis, psoriasis) and in those who weigh less than 110 lbs (50 kg) as they may be at risk of serious neurotoxicity.

Lindane is contraindicated in premature infants and individuals with known uncontrolled seizure disorders.

Instruct patients on the proper use of lindane, the amount to apply, how long to leave it on, and avoiding retreatment. Inform patients that itching occurs after the successful killing of scabies and is not necessarily an indication for retreatment with lindane.

Commonly used brand name(s)

In the U.S.—
 Kwell
 Thionex

In Canada—
 Kwellada Lotion 1%
 Lindane
 Pms-Lindane

Available Dosage Forms:

- Lotion
- Cream
- Shampoo

Therapeutic Class: Scabicide

Uses For This Medicine

Lindane, formerly known as gamma benzene hexachloride, is an insecticide and is used to treat scabies and lice infestations.

Lindane cream and lotion are usually used to treat only scabies infestation. Lindane shampoo is used to treat only lice infestations.

Lindane is available only with your doctor's prescription.

Before Using This Medicine

In deciding to use a medicine, the risks of taking the medicine must be weighed against the good it will do. This is a decision you and your doctor will make. For this medicine, the following should be considered:

Allergies—Tell your doctor if you have ever had any unusual or allergic reaction to this medicine or any other medicines. Also tell your health care professional if you have any other types of allergies, such as to foods, dyes, preservatives, or animals. For non-prescription products, read the label or package ingredients carefully.

Pediatric—Infants and children or people who weigh less than 110 pounds (50 kilograms) are especially sensitive to the effects of lindane. This may increase the chance of serious side effects during treatment. Be sure you have discussed the risks and benefits of using this medicine with your doctor. In addition, use of lindane is not to be used in premature infants.

Geriatric—Elderly people or people who weigh less than 110 pounds (50 kilograms) are especially sensitive to the effects of lindane. This may increase the chance of serious side effects during treatment. Be sure you have discussed the risks and benefits of this medicine with your doctor.

Pregnancy—

	Pregnancy Category	Explanation
All Trimesters	C	Animal studies have shown an adverse effect and there are no adequate studies in pregnant women OR no animal studies have been conducted and there are no adequate studies in pregnant women.

Breast Feeding—There are no adequate studies in women for determining infant risk when using this medication during breastfeeding. Weigh the potential benefits against the potential risks before taking this medication while breastfeeding.

Other medicines—Although certain medicines should not be used together at all, in other cases two different medicines may be used together even if an interaction might occur. In these cases, your doctor may want to change the dose, or other precautions may be necessary. Tell your healthcare professional if you are taking any other prescription or non-prescription (over-the-counter [OTC]) medicine.

Interactions with Food/Tobacco/Alcohol—Certain medicines should not be used at or around the time of eating food or eating certain types of food since interactions may occur. Using alcohol or tobacco with certain medicines may also cause interactions to occur. Discuss with your healthcare professional the use of your medicine with food, alcohol, or tobacco.

Other medical problems—The presence of other medical problems may affect the use of this medicine. Make sure you tell your doctor if you have any other medical problems, especially:

- Alcohol use that is excessive, or
- Brain tumor or
- Head injuries, history of, or
- HIV Infection or
- Liver disease, or
- Seizures, history of
- Suddenly stopping the regular use of alcohol or sedatives—Patients with these conditions should use lindane carefully because these patients have a greater risk of having a seizure
- Hypersensitivity to lindane
- Seizure disorder—This medicine should not be used in patients with seizure disorders
- Skin conditions—This medicine should not be used in people with crusted scabies, atopic dermatitis, or psoriasis. These problems of the skin could cause more lindane to be absorbed in your body and result in serious side effects.

Proper Use of This Medicine

Lindane is poisonous. Keep it away from the mouth because it is harmful and may be fatal if swallowed.

Use lindane only as directed by your doctor. Do not use more of it, do not use it more often, and do not use it for a longer time than your doctor ordered. To do so may increase the chance of absorption through the skin and the chance of lindane poisoning.

Keep lindane away from the eyes. If you should accidentally get some in your eyes, flush them thoroughly with water at once and contact your doctor.

Do not use lindane on open wounds, such as cuts or sores on the skin or scalp. To do so may increase the chance of lindane poisoning.

When applying lindane to another person, you should wear plastic disposable or rubber gloves made of latex or vinyl, especially if you are pregnant or are breast-feeding. Do not use natural latex gloves because lindane can go through those gloves and be absorbed by your skin. Wash hands very well after applying the lotion. This will prevent lindane from being absorbed through your skin. If you have any questions about this, check with your healthcare professional.

Put lindane lotion under fingernails, and trim fingernails short. Use a toothbrush to get the lindane lotion under fingernails, and throw out the toothbrush when finished.

Do not cover the area completely. Use a light clothing.

Lindane comes with patient directions. Be sure that you read them very carefully before using lindane. If you have any questions check with your healthcare professional.

Your sexual partner or partners, especially, and all members of your household may need to be treated also, since the infestation may spread to persons in close contact. If these persons have not been checked for an infestation or if you have any questions about this, check with your healthcare professional

To use the cream or lotion form of lindane for scabies:

- If your skin has any cream, lotion, ointment, or oil on it, wash, rinse, and dry your skin well before applying lindane.
- If you take a warm bath or shower before using lindane, dry the skin well before applying it.
- Apply enough lindane to your dry skin to cover the entire skin surface from the neck down, including the soles of your feet, and rub in well.
- Leave lindane on for 8 to 12 hours, then remove by washing thoroughly.

To use the shampoo form of lindane for lice:

- If your hair has any cream, lotion, ointment, or oil-based product on it, shampoo, rinse, and dry your hair and scalp well before applying lindane.
- If you apply this shampoo in the shower or in the bathtub, make sure the shampoo is not allowed to run down on other parts of your body. Also, do not apply this shampoo in a bathtub where the shampoo may run into the bath water in which you are sitting. To do so may increase the chance of absorption through the skin. When you rinse out the shampoo, be sure to thoroughly rinse your entire body also to remove any shampoo that may have gotten on it.
- Apply enough shampoo to your dry hair (1 ounce or less for short hair, 1½ ounces for medium length hair, and 2 ounces or less for long hair) to thoroughly wet the hair and skin or scalp of the affected and surrounding hairy areas.
- Thoroughly rub the shampoo into the hair and skin or scalp and allow to remain in place for 4 minutes. Then, use just enough water to work up a good lather.
- Rinse thoroughly and dry with a clean towel.
- When the hair is dry, comb with a fine-toothed comb to remove any remaining nits (eggs) or nit shells.
- Do not use as a regular shampoo.

Dosing—The dose of this medicine will be different for different patients. Follow your doctor's orders or the directions on the label. The following information includes only the average doses of this medicine. If your dose is different, do not change it unless your doctor tells you to do so.

The amount of medicine that you take depends on the strength of the medicine. Also, the number of doses you take each day, the time allowed between doses, and the length of time you take the medicine depend on the medical problem for which you are using the medicine.

- For cream and lotion dosage forms:
  - For scabies:
    - Adults and children—Apply to the affected area(s) of the skin one time.
    - Premature infants—Use is not recommended.
- For shampoo dosage form:
  - For lice:
    - Adults and children—Apply to the scalp or the affected area(s) of the skin one time.
    - Premature infants—Use is not recommended.

Storage—Store the medicine in a closed container at room temperature, away from heat, moisture, and direct light. Keep from freezing.

Keep out of the reach of children.

Do not keep outdated medicine or medicine no longer needed.

Precautions While Using This Medicine

To help prevent reinfestation or spreading of the infestation to other persons:

- For scabies—All recently worn underwear and pajamas and used sheets, pillowcases, and towels should be washed in very hot water or dry-cleaned.
- For lice—All recently worn clothing and used bed linens and towels should be washed in very hot water or dry-cleaned.

Side Effects of This Medicine

Along with its needed effects, a medicine may cause some unwanted effects. Although not all of these side effects may occur, if they do occur they may need medical attention.

Check with your doctor as soon as possible if any of the following side effects occur:

Rare

Convulsions (seizures); dizziness, clumsiness, or unsteadiness; fast heartbeat; muscle cramps; nervousness, restlessness, or irritability; vomiting; skin irritation not present before use of lindane; skin rash

After you stop using this medicine, it may still produce some side effects that need attention. During this period of time, *check with your doctor immediately* if you notice the following side effects:

Serious side effects have resulted in patients using lindane. Sometime it has occurred even when used according to the labeled directions. Serious side effects have been reported following lindane use with repeat or prolonged use, but also in rare cases following a single application. You should discuss these possible effects with your doctor.

Other side effects not listed may also occur in some patients. If you notice any other effects, check with your healthcare professional.

LINEZOLID (Intravenous route, Oral route) - li-NE-zoh-lid

Commonly used brand name(s)
In the U.S.—
  Zyvox

Available Dosage Forms:
- Solution
- Powder for Suspension
- Tablet

Therapeutic Class: Antibiotic

Uses For This Medicine

Linezolid belongs to the family of medicines called antibiotics. Antibiotics are medicines used in the treatment of infections caused by bacteria. They work by killing bacteria or preventing their growth. Linezolid will not work for colds, flu, or other virus infections.

Linezolid is used to treat infections of the blood, lungs, and skin. It may also be used for other conditions as determined by your doctor. It is given by injection or orally. It is used mainly for serious infection for which other medicines may not work.

This medicine is available only with your doctor's prescription.

Before Using This Medicine

In deciding to use a medicine, the risks of taking the medicine must be weighed against the good it will do. This is a decision you and your doctor will make. For this medicine, the following should be considered:

Allergies—Tell your doctor if you have ever had any unusual or allergic reaction to this medicine or any other medicines. Also tell your health care professional if you have any other types of allergies, such as to foods, dyes, preservatives, or animals. For non-prescription products, read the label or package ingredients carefully.

Pediatric—
This medicine has been tested in children and, in effective doses, has not been shown to cause different side effects or problems than it does in adults

Geriatric—This medicine has been tested and has not been shown to cause different side effects or problems in older people than it does in younger adults.

Pregnancy—

	Pregnancy Category	Explanation
All Trimesters	C	Animal studies have shown an adverse effect and there are no adequate studies in pregnant women OR no animal studies have been conducted and there are no adequate studies in pregnant women.

Breast Feeding—There are no adequate studies in women for determining infant risk when using this medication during breastfeeding. Weigh the potential benefits against the potential risks before taking this medication while breastfeeding.

Other medicines—
Using this medicine with any of the following medicines is usually not recommended, but may be required in some cases. If both medicines are prescribed together, your doctor may change the dose or how often you use one or both of the medicines.

Amitriptyline, Bupropion, Carbidopa, Citalopram, Clovoxamine, Dextromethorphan, Dopamine, Duloxetine, Epinephrine, Escitalopram, Femoxetine, Flesinoxan, Fluoxetine, Fluvoxamine, Levodopa, Lithium, Metoclopramide, Mirtazapine, Nefazodone, Paroxetine, Phenylpropanolamine, Pseudoephedrine, Risperidone, Sertraline, Sibutramine, St John's Wort, Tramadol, Trazodone, Venlafaxine, Zimeldine

Interactions with Food/Tobacco/Alcohol—Certain medicines should not be used at or around the time of eating food or eating certain types of food since interactions may occur. Using alcohol or tobacco with certain medicines may also cause interactions to occur. The following interactions have been selected on the basis of their potential significance and are not necessarily all-inclusive.

Using this medicine with any of the following may cause an increased risk of certain side effects but may be unavoidable in some cases. If used together, your doctor may change the dose or how often you use this medicine, or give you special instructions about the use of food, alcohol, or tobacco.

Tyramine Containing Food

Other medical problems—The presence of other medical problems may affect the use of this medicine. Make sure you tell your doctor if you have any other medical problems, especially:
- Diarrhea—May be a sign of a serious condition that your doctor will want to check before you start taking this medicine.
- Phenylketonuria—The oral suspension contains phenylalanine, which may cause side effects; however, the other dosage forms do not contain phenylalanine

Proper Use of This Medicine

- The liquid form of linezolid should be gently mixed by turning the bottle upside down 3 to 5 times before each dose. Do not shake this product.
- Do not use after the expiration date on the label. The medicine may not work properly after that date. If you have any questions about this, check with your pharmacist.

To help clear up your infection completely, keep taking this medicine for the full time of treatment, even if you begin to feel better after a few days. Also, it works best when there is a constant amount in the blood. To help keep the amount constant, linezolid must be given on a regular schedule.

Dosing—The dose of this medicine will be different for different patients. Follow your doctor's orders or the directions on the label. The following information includes only the average doses of this medicine. If your dose is different, do not change it unless your doctor tells you to do so.

The amount of medicine that you take depends on the strength of the medicine. Also, the number of doses you take each day, the time allowed between doses, and the length of time you take the medicine depend on the medical problem for which you are using the medicine.

- For oral dosage forms:
  - Adults—400 or 600 mg every 12 hours.
  - Children—10 mg per kg (2.2 lbs.) every 8 or 12 hours as determined by your doctor
- For parenteral dosage form (injection):
  - Adults—600 mg every 12 hours.
  - Children—10 mg per kg (2.2 lbs.) every 8 hours as determined by your doctor

Missed dose—If you miss a dose of this medicine, take it as soon as possible. However, if it is almost time for your next dose, skip the missed dose and go back to your regular dosing schedule. Do not double doses.

Storage—Store the medicine in a closed container at room temperature, away from heat, moisture, and direct light. Keep from freezing.

Keep out of the reach of children.

Do not keep outdated medicine or medicine no longer needed.

Ask your healthcare professional how you should dispose of any medicine you do not use.

Precautions While Using This Medicine

If your symptoms do not improve within a few days or if they become worse, check with your doctor.

Contact your doctor right away if you develop abdominal discomfort, decreased appetite, diarrhea, fast, shallow breathing, general feeling of discomfort, muscle pain or cramping, nausea, shortness of breath, sleepiness, unusual tiredness or weakness or vomiting. These could be symptoms of a serious condition.

If you begin to have visual impairment problems such as changes in color vision, blurred vision, or visual field defect, make an appointment with an eye doctor as soon as possible.

Linezolid can lower the number of white blood cells in your blood temporarily, increasing the chance of getting an infection. It can also lower the number of platelets, which are necessary for proper blood clotting. If this occurs, there are certain precautions your doctor may ask you to take, especially when your blood count is low, to reduce the risk of infection or bleeding:

- If you can, avoid people with infections. Check with your doctor immediately if you think you are getting an infection or if you get a fever or chills.
- Check with your doctor immediately if you notice any unusual bleeding or bruising.
- Do not touch your eyes or the inside of your nose unless you have just washed your hands and have not touched anything else in the meantime.
- Be careful not to cut yourself when you are using sharp objects such as a safety razor or fingernail or toenail cutters.
- Avoid contact sports or other situations where bruising or injury could occur.

When taken with certain foods or drinks, linezolid can cause an increase in blood pressure. To avoid this, do not eat large amounts of foods or drink beverages that have a high tyramine content (most common in foods that are aged, fermented, pickled, or smoked to increase their flavor, such as aged cheeses; air-dried, fermented, or smoked fish, meat, or poultry; sauerkraut; soy sauce; red wine; or tap beer. If a list of these foods and beverages is not given to you, ask your health care professional to provide one.

Side Effects of This Medicine

Along with its needed effects, a medicine may cause some unwanted effects. Although not all of these side effects may occur, if they do occur they may need medical attention.

More common
　Diarrhea

Less common or rare
　Abdominal or stomach cramps or pain (severe); black, tarry stools; blood in urine or stools; chills; cough; diarrhea (severe and watery, may also be bloody); discharge from the vagina; fever; headache; hoarseness; itching of the vagina; lower back or side pain; painful or difficult urination; pinpoint red spots on skin; shortness of breath; sore mouth or tongue; unusual bleeding or bruising; unusual tiredness or weakness; white patches in mouth, tongue, or throat

Incidence not known
　Abdominal discomfort; blindness; blurred vision; burning, numbness, tingling, or painful sensations; decreased appetite; decreased vision; eye pain; fast, shallow breathing; general feeling of discomfort; muscle pain or cramping; sleepiness; unsteadiness or awkwardness; weakness in arms, hands, legs, or feet

Some side effects may occur that usually do not need medical attention. These side effects may go away during treatment as your body adjusts to the medicine. Also, your health care professional may be able to tell you about ways to prevent or reduce some of these side effects. Check with your health care professional if any of the following side effects continue or are bothersome or if you have any questions about them:

More common
　Nausea

Less common or rare
　Bad taste in the mouth; change in sense of taste; change in color of tongue; dizziness; loss of taste; vomiting

Other side effects not listed may also occur in some patients. If you notice any other effects, check with your healthcare professional.

LITHIUM　(Oral route) - LITH-ee-um

Black Box Warning

Lithium toxicity is closely related to serum lithium levels, and can occur at doses close to therapeutic levels. Facilities for prompt and accurate serum lithium determinations should be available before initiating therapy.

Commonly used brand name(s)

In the U.S.—
　Eskalith
　Eskalith-CR
　Lithobid

Available Dosage Forms:
- Solution
- Syrup
- Capsule
- Tablet, Extended Release
- Tablet

Therapeutic Class: Antimanic

Uses For This Medicine

Lithium is used to treat the manic stage of bipolar disorder (manic-depressive illness). Manic-depressive patients experience severe mood changes, ranging from an excited or manic state (for example, unusual anger or irritability or a false sense of well-being) to depression or sadness. Lithium is used to reduce the frequency and severity of manic states. Lithium may also reduce the frequency and severity of depression in bipolar disorder.

It is not known how lithium works to stabilize a person's mood. However, it does act on the central nervous system. It helps you to have more control over your emotions and helps you cope better with the problems of living.

It is important that you and your family understand all the effects of lithium. These effects depend on your individual condition and response and the amount of lithium you use. You also must know when to contact your doctor if there are problems with the medicine's use. Lithium may also be used for other conditions as determined by your doctor.

This medicine is available only with your doctor's prescription.

Once a medicine has been approved for marketing for a certain use, experience may show that it is also useful for other medical problems. Although these uses are not included in product labeling, lithium is used in certain patients with the following medical conditions:
- Cluster headaches
- Mental depression
- Neutropenia (a blood condition in which there is a decreased number of a certain type of white blood cells)

Before Using This Medicine

In deciding to use a medicine, the risks of taking the medicine must be weighed against the good it will do. This is a decision you and your doctor will make. For this medicine, the following should be considered:

Allergies—Tell your doctor if you have ever had any unusual or allergic reaction to this medicine or any other medicines. Also tell your health care professional if you have any other types of allergies, such as to foods, dyes, preservatives, or animals. For non-prescription products, read the label or package ingredients carefully.

Pediatric—Lithium may cause weakened bones in children during treatment.

Geriatric—Unusual thirst, an increase in amount of urine, diarrhea, drowsiness, loss of appetite, muscle weakness, trembling, slurred speech, nausea or vomiting, goiter, or symptoms of underactive thyroid are especially likely to occur

in elderly patients, who are often more sensitive than younger adults to the effects of lithium.

Pregnancy—

	Pregnancy Category	Explanation
All Trimesters	D	Studies in pregnant women have demonstrated a risk to the fetus. However, the benefits of therapy in a life threatening situation or a serious disease, may outweigh the potential risk.

Breast Feeding—There are no adequate studies in women for determining infant risk when using this medication during breastfeeding. Weigh the potential benefits against the potential risks before taking this medication while breastfeeding.

Other medicines—

Using this medicine with any of the following medicines is usually not recommended, but may be required in some cases. If both medicines are prescribed together, your doctor may change the dose or how often you use one or both of the medicines.

Acetophenazine, Azosemide, Bemetizide, Bendroflumethiazide, Benzthiazide, Bromperidol, Bumetanide, Buthiazide, Candesartan Cilexetil, Canrenoate, Chlorothiazide, Chlorpromazine, Chlorprothixene, Chlorthalidone, Clozapine, Cyclothiazide, Domperidone, Droperidol, Ethacrynic Acid, Ethopropazine, Flupentixol, Fluphenazine, Furosemide, Haloperidol, Hydrochlorothiazide, Hydroflumethiazide, Indapamide, Linezolid, Losartan, Loxapine, Melperone, Mesoridazine, Methotrimeprazine, Methyclothiazide, Metolazone, Molindone, Olanzapine, Penfluridol, Periciazine, Perphenazine, Phenelzine, Pimozide, Pipamperone, Pipotiazine, Piretanide, Polythiazide, Prochlorperazine, Promazine, Promethazine, Quinethazone, Remoxipride, Risperidone, Sertindole, Sibutramine, Spironolactone, Sulpiride, Thiopropazate, Thioproperazine, Thioridazine, Thiothixene, Tiapride, Torsemide, Trichlormethiazide, Trifluoperazine, Triflupromazine, Trimeprazine, Valsartan, Xipamide, Zotepine, Zuclopenthixol

Interactions with Food/Tobacco/Alcohol—Certain medicines should not be used at or around the time of eating food or eating certain types of food since interactions may occur. Using alcohol or tobacco with certain medicines may also cause interactions to occur. Discuss with your healthcare professional the use of your medicine with food, alcohol, or tobacco.

Other medical problems—The presence of other medical problems may affect the use of this medicine. Make sure you tell your doctor if you have any other medical problems, especially:
- Brain disease or
- Schizophrenia—You may be especially sensitive to lithium, and mental effects (such as increased confusion) may occur
- Diabetes mellitus (sugar diabetes)—Lithium may increase the blood levels of insulin; the dose of insulin you need to take may change

- Difficult urination or
- Infection (severe, occurring with fever, prolonged sweating, diarrhea, or vomiting) or
- Kidney disease—Higher blood levels of lithium may occur, increasing the chance of serious side effects
- Epilepsy or
- Goiter or other thyroid disease, or
- Heart disease or
- Parkinson's disease or
- Psoriasis—Lithium may make the condition worse
- Leukemia (history of)—Lithium may cause the leukemia to occur again

Proper Use of This Medicine

Make certain your health care professional knows if you are on a low-sodium or low-salt diet. Too little salt in your diet could lead to serious side effects.

Take this medicine after a meal or snack. Doing so will reduce stomach upset, tremors, or weakness and may also prevent a laxative effect.

For patients taking the long-acting or slow-release form of lithium:

- Swallow the tablet or capsule whole.
- Do not break, crush, or chew before swallowing.

For patients taking the syrup form of lithium:

- Dilute the syrup in fruit juice or another flavored beverage before taking.

During treatment with lithium, drink 2 or 3 quarts of water or other fluids each day, and use a normal amount of salt in your food, unless otherwise directed by your doctor.

Take this medicine exactly as directed. Do not take more or less of it, do not take it more or less often, and do not take it for a longer time than your doctor ordered. To do so may increase the chance of unwanted effects.

Sometimes lithium must be taken for 1 to several weeks before you begin to feel better.

In order for lithium to work properly, it must be taken every day in regularly spaced doses as ordered by your doctor. This is necessary to keep a constant amount of lithium in your blood. To help keep the amount constant, do not miss any doses and do not stop taking the medicine even if you feel better.

Dosing—The dose of this medicine will be different for different patients. Follow your doctor's orders or the directions on the label. The following information includes only the average doses of this medicine. If your dose is different, do not change it unless your doctor tells you to do so.

The amount of medicine that you take depends on the strength of the medicine. Also, the number of doses you take each day, the time allowed between doses, and the length of time you take the medicine depend on the medical problem for which you are using the medicine.

- For short-acting oral dosage forms (capsules, tablets, syrup):
  - Adults and adolescents: To start, 300 to 600 milligrams three times a day.
  - Children up to 12 years of age: The dose is based on body weight. To start, the usual dose is 15 to 20 mil

ligrams per kilogram of body weight (6.8 to 9 milligrams per pound) a day, given in smaller doses two or three times during the day.

- For long-acting oral dosage forms (slow-release capsules, extended-release tablets):
  - Adults and adolescents: 300 to 600 milligrams three times a day, or 450 to 900 milligrams two times a day.
  - Children up to 12 years of age: Dose must be determined by the doctor.

Missed dose—If you miss a dose of this medicine, take it as soon as possible. However, if it is almost time for your next dose, skip the missed dose and go back to your regular dosing schedule. Do not double doses.

Storage—Store the medicine in a closed container at room temperature, away from heat, moisture, and direct light. Keep from freezing.

Keep out of the reach of children.

Do not keep outdated medicine or medicine no longer needed.

Precautions While Using This Medicine

Your doctor should check your progress at regular visits to make sure that the medicine is working properly and that possible side effects are avoided. Laboratory tests may be necessary.

Lithium may not work properly if you drink large amounts of caffeine-containing coffee, tea, or colas.

This medicine may cause some people to become dizzy, drowsy, or less alert than they are normally. Make sure you know how you react to this medicine before you drive, use machines, or do anything else that could be dangerous if you are dizzy or are not alert.

Use extra care in hot weather and during activities that cause you to sweat heavily, such as hot baths, saunas, or exercising. The loss of too much water and salt from your body could lead to serious side effects from this medicine.

If you have an infection or illness that causes heavy sweating, vomiting, or diarrhea, check with your doctor. The loss of too much water and salt from your body could lead to serious side effects from lithium.

Do not go on a diet to lose weight and do not make a major change in your diet without first checking with your doctor. Improper dieting could cause the loss of too much water and salt from your body and could lead to serious side effects from this medicine.

For patients taking the slow-release capsules or the extended-release tablets:

- Do not use this medicine interchangeably with other lithium products.

It is important that you and your family know the early symptoms of lithium overdose or toxicity and when to call the doctor.

Side Effects of This Medicine

Along with its needed effects, a medicine may cause some unwanted effects. Although not all of these side effects may occur, if they do occur they may need medical attention.

Check with your doctor immediately if any of the following side effects occur:

Early symptoms of overdose or toxicity

Diarrhea; drowsiness; lack of coordination; loss of appetite; muscle weakness; nausea or vomiting; slurred speech; trembling

Late symptoms of overdose or toxicity
Blurred vision; clumsiness or unsteadiness; confusion; convulsions (seizures); dizziness; increase in amount of urine; ringing in the ears; trembling (severe)

Check with your doctor as soon as possible if any of the following side effects occur:
Less common
Confusion, poor memory or lack of awareness; fainting; fast or slow heartbeat; frequent urination; irregular pulse; increased thirst; stiffness of arms or legs; troubled breathing (especially during hard work or exercise); slurred speech; unusual tiredness or weakness; weight gain
Rare
Blue color and pain in fingers and toes; coldness of arms and legs; dizziness; eye pain; headache; noises in the ears; vision problems
Signs of low thyroid function
Dry, rough skin; hair loss; hoarseness; mental depression; sensitivity to cold; swelling of feet or lower legs; swelling of neck; unusual excitement

Some side effects may occur that usually do not need medical attention. These side effects may go away during treatment as your body adjusts to the medicine. Also, your health care professional may be able to tell you about ways to prevent or reduce some of these side effects. Check with your health care professional if any of the following side effects continue or are bothersome or if you have any questions about them:
More common
Increased frequency of urination or loss of bladder control— more common in women than in men, usually beginning 2 to 7 years after start of treatment; increased thirst; nausea (mild); trembling of hands (slight)
Less common
Acne or skin rash; bloated feeling or pressure in the stomach; muscle twitching (slight)

Other side effects not listed may also occur in some patients. If you notice any other effects, check with your healthcare professional.

LOPERAMIDE (Oral route) - loe-PER-a-mide

Commonly used brand name(s)
In the U.S.—
Diamode / Imotil
Imodium / Imperim
Imodium A-D / Kaodene A-D
Imogen / Kao-Paverin Caps

Available Dosage Forms:
• Capsule   • Tablet
• Liquid   • Solution

Therapeutic Class: Antidiarrheal

Uses For This Medicine

Loperamide is a medicine used along with other measures to treat diarrhea. Loperamide helps stop diarrhea by slowing down the movements of the intestines.

In the U.S., loperamide capsules are available only with your doctor's prescription.

Before Using This Medicine

In deciding to use a medicine, the risks of taking the medicine must be weighed against the good it will do. This is a decision you and your doctor will make. For this medicine, the following should be considered:

Allergies—Tell your doctor if you have ever had any unusual or allergic reaction to this medicine or any other medicines. Also tell your health care professional if you have any other types of allergies, such as to foods, dyes, preservatives, or animals. For non-prescription products, read the label or package ingredients carefully.

Pediatric—This medicine should not be used in children under 6 years of age unless directed by a doctor. Children, especially very young children, are very sensitive to the effects of loperamide. This may increase the chance of side effects during treatment. Also, the fluid loss caused by diarrhea may result in a serious health problem (dehydration). Loperamide may hide the symptoms of dehydration. For these reasons, do not give medicine for diarrhea to children without first checking with their doctor. If you have any questions about this, check with your health care professional.

Geriatric—The fluid loss caused by diarrhea may result in a serious health problem (dehydration). Loperamide may hide the symptoms of dehydration. For this reason, elderly persons with diarrhea, in addition to using medicine for diarrhea, must receive a sufficient amount of liquids to replace the fluid lost by the body. If you have any questions about this, check with your health care professional.

Pregnancy—

	Pregnancy Category	Explanation
All Trimesters	C	Animal studies have shown an adverse effect and there are no adequate studies in pregnant women OR no animal studies have been conducted and there are no adequate studies in pregnant women.

Breast Feeding—There are no adequate studies in women for determining infant risk when using this medication during breastfeeding. Weigh the potential benefits against the potential risks before taking this medication while breastfeeding.

Other medicines—Although certain medicines should not be used together at all, in other cases two different medicines may be used together even if an interaction might occur. In these cases, your doctor may want to change the dose, or other precautions may be necessary. Tell your healthcare professional if you are taking any other prescription or non-prescription (over-the-counter [OTC]) medicine.

Interactions with Food/Tobacco/Alcohol—Certain medicines should not be used at or around the time of eating food or eating certain types of food since interactions may occur. Using alcohol or tobacco with certain medicines may also cause interactions to occur. Discuss with your healthcare professional the use of your medicine with food, alcohol, or tobacco.

Other medical problems—The presence of other medical problems may affect the use of this medicine. Make sure you

tell your doctor if you have any other medical problems, especially:

- Colitis (severe)—A more serious problem of the colon may develop if you use loperamide
- Dysentery—This condition may get worse; a different kind of treatment may be needed
- Liver disease—The chance of severe central nervous system (CNS) side effects may be greater in patients with liver disease

Proper Use of This Medicine

Do not use loperamide to treat your diarrhea if you have a fever or if there is blood or mucus in your stools. Contact your doctor.

For safe and effective use of this medicine:

- Follow your doctor's instructions if this medicine was prescribed.
- Follow the manufacturer's package directions if you are treating yourself.

Use a specially marked measuring spoon or other device to measure each dose accurately. The average household teaspoon may not hold the right amount of liquid.

Importance of diet and fluid intake while treating diarrhea:

- In addition to using medicine for diarrhea, it is very important that you replace the fluid lost by the body and follow a proper diet. For the first 24 hours, you should eat gelatin, and drink plenty of caffeine-free clear liquids, such as ginger ale, decaffeinated cola, decaffeinated tea, and broth. During the next 24 hours you may eat bland foods, such as cooked cereals, bread, crackers, and applesauce. Fruits, vegetables, fried or spicy foods, bran, candy, caffeine, and alcoholic beverages may make the condition worse.
- If too much fluid has been lost by the body due to the diarrhea, a serious condition (dehydration) may develop. Check with your doctor as soon as possible if any of the following signs or symptoms of too much fluid loss occur:
  - Decreased urination
  - Dizziness and lightheadedness
  - Dryness of mouth
  - Increased thirst
  - Wrinkled skin

Dosing—The dose of this medicine will be different for different patients. Follow your doctor's orders or the directions on the label. The following information includes only the average doses of this medicine. If your dose is different, do not change it unless your doctor tells you to do so.

The amount of medicine that you take depends on the strength of the medicine. Also, the number of doses you take each day, the time allowed between doses, and the length of time you take the medicine depend on the medical problem for which you are using the medicine.

- For diarrhea:
  - For oral dosage form (capsules):
    - Adults and teenagers—The usual dose is 4 milligrams (mg) (2 capsules) after the first loose bowel movement, and 2 mg (1 capsule) after each loose bowel movement after the first dose has been taken. No more than 16 mg (8 capsules) should be taken in any twenty-four-hour period.
    - Children 8 to 12 years of age—The usual dose is 2 mg (1 capsule) three times a day.

- Children 6 to 8 years of age—The usual dose is 2 mg (1 capsule) two times a day.
- Children up to 6 years of age—Use is not recommended unless directed by your doctor.
  - For oral dosage form (oral solution):
    - Adults and teenagers—The usual dose is 4 teaspoonfuls (4 mg) after the first loose bowel movement, and 2 teaspoonfuls (2 mg) after each loose bowel movement after the first dose has been taken. No more than 8 teaspoonfuls (8 mg) should be taken in any twenty-four-hour period.
    - Children 9 to 11 years of age—The usual dose is 2 teaspoonfuls (2 mg) after the first loose bowel movement, and 1 teaspoonful (1 mg) after each loose bowel movement after the first dose has been taken. No more than 6 teaspoonfuls (6 mg) should be taken in any twenty-four-hour period.
    - Children 6 to 8 years of age—The usual dose is 2 teaspoonfuls (2 mg) after the first loose bowel movement, and 1 teaspoonful (1 mg) after each loose bowel movement after the first dose has been taken. No more than 4 teaspoonfuls (4 mg) should be taken in any twenty-four-hour period.
    - Children up to 6 years of age—Use is not recommended unless directed by your doctor.
  - For oral dosage form (tablets):
    - Adults and teenagers—The usual dose is 4 mg (2 tablets) after the first loose bowel movement, and 2 mg (1 tablet) after each loose bowel movement after the first dose has been taken. No more than 8 mg (4 tablets) should be taken in any twenty-four-hour period.
    - Children 9 to 11 years of age—The usual dose is 2 mg (1 tablet) after the first loose bowel movement, and 1 mg (½ tablet) after each loose bowel movement after the first dose has been taken. No more than 6 mg (3 tablets) should be taken in any twenty-four-hour period.
    - Children 6 to 8 years of age—The usual dose is 2 mg (1 tablet) after the first loose bowel movement, and 1 mg (½ tablet) after each loose bowel movement after the first dose has been taken. No more than 4 mg (2 tablets) should be taken in any twenty-four-hour period.
    - Children up to 6 years of age—Use is not recommended unless directed by your doctor.

Missed dose—If you miss a dose of this medicine, take it as soon as possible. However, if it is almost time for your next dose, skip the missed dose and go back to your regular dosing schedule. Do not double doses.

Storage—Store the medicine in a closed container at room temperature, away from heat, moisture, and direct light. Keep from freezing.

Keep out of the reach of children.

Do not keep outdated medicine or medicine no longer needed.

Precautions While Using This Medicine

Loperamide should not be used for more than 2 days, unless directed by your doctor. If you will be taking this medicine regularly for a long time, your doctor should check your progress at regular visits.

Check with your doctor if your diarrhea does not stop after two days or if you develop a fever.

Side Effects of This Medicine

Along with its needed effects, a medicine may cause some unwanted effects. Although not all of these side effects may occur, if they do occur they may need medical attention.

Check with your doctor immediately if any of the following side effects occur:

> *Rare*
>> Bloating; constipation; loss of appetite; stomach pain (severe) with nausea and vomiting

Check with your doctor as soon as possible if any of the following side effects occur:

> *Rare*
>> Skin rash

Some side effects may occur that usually do not need medical attention. These side effects may go away during treatment as your body adjusts to the medicine. Also, your health care professional may be able to tell you about ways to prevent or reduce some of these side effects. Check with your health care professional if any of the following side effects continue or are bothersome or if you have any questions about them:

> *Rare*
>> Dizziness or drowsiness; dryness of mouth

Other side effects not listed may also occur in some patients. If you notice any other effects, check with your healthcare professional.

LOPINAVIR AND RITONAVIR (Oral route) - loe-PIN-a-veer, ri-TOE-na-veer

Commonly used brand name(s)

In the U.S.—
   Kaletra

Available Dosage Forms:

• Capsule, Liquid Filled
• Tablet
• Solution

Therapeutic Class: Antiretroviral Agent
Pharmacologic Class: Protease Inhibitor

Uses For This Medicine

The combination of lopinavir and ritonavir is used in the treatment of the infection caused by the human immuno-deficiency virus (HIV). HIV is the virus responsible for acquired immune deficiency syndrome (AIDS). It is used to slow the progression of disease in patients infected with HIV who have advanced symptoms, early symptoms, or no symptoms at all.

Lopinavir and ritonavir will not cure or prevent HIV infection or AIDS; however, it helps keep HIV from reproducing and appears to slow down the destruction of the immune system.

This may help delay the development of problems usually related to AIDS or HIV disease. Lopinavir and ritonavir will not keep you from spreading HIV to other people. People who receive this medicine may continue to have other problems usually related to AIDS or HIV disease.

This medicine is available only with your doctor's prescription.

Before Using This Medicine

In deciding to use a medicine, the risks of taking the medicine must be weighed against the good it will do. This is a decision you and your doctor will make. For this medicine, the following should be considered:

Allergies—Tell your doctor if you have ever had any unusual or allergic reaction to this medicine or any other medicines. Also tell your health care professional if you have any other types of allergies, such as to foods, dyes, preservatives, or animals. For non-prescription products, read the label or package ingredients carefully.

Pediatric—The twice-daily dose of this medicine has been tested in children 6 months of age and older and, in effective doses, has not been shown to cause different side effects or problems than it does in adults.

The once-daily dose of this medicine has been tested only in adult patients and there is no specific information comparing use in children with use in other age groups.

Geriatric—Many medicines have not been studied specifically in older people. Therefore, it may not be known whether they work exactly the same way they do in younger adults or if they cause different side effects or problems in older people. There is no specific information comparing use of lopinavir and ritonavir in the elderly with use in other age groups.

Other medicines—

Using this medicine with any of the following medicines is not recommended. Your doctor may decide not to treat you with this medication or change some of the other medicines you take.

Alfuzosin, Amiodarone, Astemizole, Bepridil, Cisapride, Conivaptan, Dihydroergotamine, Encainide, Eplerenone, Ergoloid Mesylates, Ergonovine, Ergotamine, Flecainide, Methylergonovine, Methysergide, Midazolam, Pimozide, Propafenone, Quinidine, Ranolazine, St John's Wort, Terfenadine, Triazolam, Voriconazole

Interactions with Food/Tobacco/Alcohol—Certain medicines should not be used at or around the time of eating food or eating certain types of food since interactions may occur. Using alcohol or tobacco with certain medicines may also cause interactions to occur. Discuss with your healthcare professional the use of your medicine with food, alcohol, or tobacco.

Other medical problems—The presence of other medical problems may affect the use of this medicine. Make sure you tell your doctor if you have any other medical problems, especially:

• Diabetes mellitus (sugar diabetes)—Lopinavir and ritonavir may increase blood sugar; it may be necessary to adjust your dose of insulin or oral diabetes medicine

• Hemophilia—Lopinavir and ritonavir may increase the risk of major bleeding.

- Liver problems or
- Hepatitis B or
- Hepatitis C—Effects of lopinavir and ritonavir may be increased because of slower removal of the medicines from the body
- Pancreatitis (history of)—The chance that this condition will return is increased

Proper Use of This Medicine

A paper with information about lopinavir and ritonavir will be given to you with your filled prescription. Read this paper carefully and ask your health care professional if you need additional information or explanation.

It is important that lopinavir and ritonavir capsules and oral solution be taken with food.

Lopinavir and ritonavir tablets may be taken with or without food.

For oral solution dosage form, use calibrated dosing syringe to measure dose.

For tablet dosage form, swallow whole and do not crush or chew.

Take this medicine exactly as directed by your doctor. Do not take it more often and do not take it for a longer time than your doctor ordered. Also, do not stop taking this medicine without checking with your doctor first.

Dosing—The dose of this medicine will be different for different patients. Follow your doctor's orders or the directions on the label. The following information includes only the average doses of this medicine. If your dose is different, do not change it unless your doctor tells you to do so.

The amount of medicine that you take depends on the strength of the medicine. Also, the number of doses you take each day, the time allowed between doses, and the length of time you take the medicine depend on the medical problem for which you are using the medicine.

- For oral dosage form (capsules):
  - For treatment of HIV infection:
    - Adults: 400 milligrams (mg) of lopinavir and 100 mg of ritonavir (3 capsules) twice a day with food or 800 mg of lopinavir and 200 mg of ritonavir (6 capsules) one time a day with food.
    - Children: This dosage form is usually not used for children. Please refer to the oral solution dosage form.
- For oral dosage form (oral solution):
  - For treatment of HIV infection:
    - Adults and adolescents: 400 mg of lopinavir and 100 mg of ritonavir (5 milliliters [mL]) twice a day with food or 800 mg of lopinavir and 200 mg of ritonavir (10 mL) one time a day with food.
    - Children 6 months to 12 years of age: Dose is based on body weight and must be determined by your doctor.
    - Children less than 6 months of age: Use and dose must be determined by your doctor.
    - Use and dose must be determined by a doctor for all children receiving the once-daily dose.
  - For oral dosage form (tablets):
    - For treatment of HIV infection:

- Adults: 400 milligrams (mg) of lopinavir and 100 mg of ritonavir (2 tablets) twice a day with food or 800 mg of lopinavir and 200 mg of ritonavir (4 tablets) one time a day with or without food.
- Children: This dosage form is usually not used for children. Please refer to the oral solution dosage form.

Missed dose—If you miss a dose of this medicine, take it as soon as possible. However, if it is almost time for your next dose, skip the missed dose and go back to your regular dosing schedule. Do not double doses.

Storage—Store in the refrigerator. Do not freeze.

Keep out of the reach of children.

Do not keep outdated medicine or medicine no longer needed.

Ask your healthcare professional how you should dispose of any medicine you do not use.

Precautions While Using This Medicine

It is very important that your doctor check your progress at regular visits to make sure this medicine is working properly and to check for unwanted effects.

If you are taking the oral solution form of this medicine, you should limit the amount of alcohol you drink. The oral solution contains 42% alcohol.

It is very important that you use a second type of birth control if you are currently using an estrogen-containing form of birth control.

If you are taking sildenafil, tadalafil, or vardenafil, it is very important to report any side effects, especially dizziness, fainting, or changes in your vision.

Side Effects of This Medicine

Along with its needed effects, a medicine may cause some unwanted effects. Although not all of these side effects may occur, if they do occur they may need medical attention.

Less common
Bloating; blurred vision; chills; constipation; darkened urine; dry mouth; fast heart beat; fatigue; fever; flushed, dry skin; fruit-like breath odor; increased hunger; increased thirst; increased urination; indigestion; loss of appetite; loss of consciousness; nausea; pains in stomach, side, or abdomen, possibly moving to the back; sweating; troubled breathing; unexplained weight loss; vomiting; yellow eyes or skin

Frequency not determined
chest pain or discomfort; lightheadedness, dizziness or fainting; shortness of breath; slow or irregular heartbeat; unusual tiredness

Some side effects may occur that usually do not need medical attention. These side effects may go away during treatment as your body adjusts to the medicine. Also, your health care professional may be able to tell you about ways to prevent or reduce some of these side effects. Check with your health care professional if any of the following side effects continue or are bothersome or if you have any questions about them:

More common
Diarrhea

Less common
> Abnormal stools; acid or sour stomach; belching; headache; heartburn; lack or loss of strength; pain; skin rash; stomach discomfort, upset, or pain; trouble in sleeping

Other side effects not listed may also occur in some patients. If you notice any other effects, check with your healthcare professional.

Frequency not determined
> Redistribution of body fat

Other side effects not listed may also occur in some patients. If you notice any other effects, check with your healthcare professional.

LORACARBEF (Oral route) - lor-a-KAR-bef

Commonly used brand name(s)

In the U.S.—
> Lorabid
> Lorabid Pulvules

Available Dosage Forms:

- Capsule
- Powder for Suspension

Therapeutic Class: Antibiotic
Pharmacologic Class: 2nd Generation Cephalosporin

Uses For This Medicine

Loracarbef is used to treat bacterial infections in many different parts of the body. It works by killing bacteria or preventing their growth. This medicine will not work for colds, flu, or other virus infections.

Loracarbef is available only with your doctor's prescription.

Before Using This Medicine

In deciding to use a medicine, the risks of taking the medicine must be weighed against the good it will do. This is a decision you and your doctor will make. For this medicine, the following should be considered:

Allergies—Tell your doctor if you have ever had any unusual or allergic reaction to this medicine or any other medicines. Also tell your health care professional if you have any other types of allergies, such as to foods, dyes, preservatives, or animals. For non-prescription products, read the label or package ingredients carefully.

Pediatric—This medicine has been tested in a limited number of children 6 months of age and older. In effective doses, the medicine has not been shown to cause different side effects or problems than it does in adults.

Geriatric—This medicine has been tested in a limited number of elderly patients and has not been shown to cause different side effects or problems in older people than it does in younger adults.

Pregnancy—

	Pregnancy Category	Explanation
All Trimesters	B	Animal studies have revealed no evidence of harm to the fetus, however, there are no adequate studies in pregnant women OR animal studies have shown an adverse effect, but adequate studies in pregnant women have failed to demonstrate a risk to the fetus.

Breast Feeding—There are no adequate studies in women for determining infant risk when using this medication during breastfeeding. Weigh the potential benefits against the potential risks before taking this medication while breastfeeding.

Other medicines—Although certain medicines should not be used together at all, in other cases two different medicines may be used together even if an interaction might occur. In these cases, your doctor may want to change the dose, or other precautions may be necessary. Tell your healthcare professional if you are taking any other prescription or non-prescription (over-the-counter [OTC]) medicine.

Interactions with Food/Tobacco/Alcohol—Certain medicines should not be used at or around the time of eating food or eating certain types of food since interactions may occur. Using alcohol or tobacco with certain medicines may also cause interactions to occur. The following interactions have been selected on the basis of their potential significance and are not necessarily all-inclusive.

Using this medicine with any of the following may cause an increased risk of certain side effects but may be unavoidable in some cases. If used together, your doctor may change the dose or how often you use this medicine, or give you special instructions about the use of food, alcohol, or tobacco.

Other medical problems—The presence of other medical problems may affect the use of this medicine. Make sure you tell your doctor if you have any other medical problems, especially:

- Kidney disease—Kidney disease may increase the blood level of loracarbef, increasing the chance of side effects

Proper Use of This Medicine

Loracarbef should be taken at least 1 hour before or at least 2 hours after meals.

To help clear up your infection completely, keep taking loracarbef for the full time of treatment, even if you begin to feel better after a few days. If you have a "strep" infection, you should keep taking this medicine for at least 10 days. This is especially important in "strep" infections. Serious heart problems could develop later if your infection is not cleared up completely. Also, if you stop taking this medicine too soon, your symptoms may return.

This medicine works best when there is a constant amount in the blood or urine. To help keep the amount constant, do not miss any doses. Also, it is best to take the doses at evenly spaced times, day and night. If this interferes with your sleep or other daily activities, or if you need help in planning the best times to take your medicine, check with your health care professional.

Dosing—The dose of this medicine will be different for different patients. Follow your doctor's orders or the directions on the label. The following information includes only the average doses of this medicine. If your dose is different, do not change it unless your doctor tells you to do so.

The amount of medicine that you take depends on the strength of the medicine. Also, the number of doses you take each day, the time allowed between doses, and the length of time you take the medicine depend on the medical problem for which you are using the medicine.

- For oral dosage forms (capsules or oral suspension):
  - For bronchitis:
    - Adults and children 13 years of age and older—200 to 400 milligrams (mg) every twelve hours for seven days.
    - Children 6 months to 12 years of age—Use and dose to be determined by your doctor.
  - For otitis media (ear infection):
    - Children 6 months to 12 years of age—Dose is based on body weight and must be determined by your doctor.
  - For pneumonia:
    - Adults and children 13 years of age and older—400 mg every twelve hours for fourteen days.
    - Children 6 months to 12 years of age—Use and dose to be determined by your doctor.
  - For sinusitis:
    - Adults and children 13 years of age and older—400 mg every twelve hours for ten days.
    - Children 6 months to 12 years of age—Use and dose to be determined by your doctor.
  - For skin and soft tissue infections:
    - Adults and children 13 years of age and older—200 mg every twelve hours for seven days.
    - Children 6 months to 12 years of age—Dose is based on body weight and must be determined by your doctor.
  - For streptococcal pharyngitis ("strep throat"):
    - Adults and children 13 years of age and older—200 mg every twelve hours for ten days.
    - Children 6 months to 12 years of age—Dose is based on body weight and must be determined by your doctor.
  - For urinary tract infections:
    - Adults and children 13 years of age and older—200 to 400 mg every twelve to twenty-four hours for seven to fourteen days.
    - Children 6 months to 12 years of age—Use and dose to be determined by your doctor.

Missed dose—If you miss a dose of this medicine, take it as soon as possible. However, if it is almost time for your next dose, skip the missed dose and go back to your regular dosing schedule. Do not double doses.

Storage—Store the medicine in a closed container at room temperature, away from heat, moisture, and direct light. Keep from freezing.

Keep out of the reach of children.

Do not keep outdated medicine or medicine no longer needed.

Precautions While Using This Medicine

If your symptoms do not improve within a few days, or if they become worse, check with your doctor.

In some patients, loracarbef may cause diarrhea.

- Severe diarrhea may be a sign of a serious side effect. Do not take any diarrhea medicine without first checking with your doctor. Diarrhea medicines may make your diarrhea worse or last longer.
- For mild diarrhea, diarrhea medicine containing kaolin or attapulgite (e.g., Kaopectate tablets, Diasorb) may be taken. However, other kinds of diarrhea medicine should not be taken. They may make your diarrhea worse or last longer.
- If you have any questions about this or if mild diarrhea continues or gets worse, check with your health care professional.

Side Effects of This Medicine

Along with its needed effects, a medicine may cause some unwanted effects. Although not all of these side effects may occur, if they do occur they may need medical attention.

Check with your doctor as soon as possible if any of the following side effects occur:
> *More common*
> Itching; skin rash

Some side effects may occur that usually do not need medical attention. These side effects may go away during treatment as your body adjusts to the medicine. Also, your health care professional may be able to tell you about ways to prevent or reduce some of these side effects. Check with your health care professional if any of the following side effects continue or are bothersome or if you have any questions about them:
> *More common*
> Diarrhea; loss of appetite; nausea and vomiting; stomach pain
> *Rare*
> Dizziness; drowsiness; headache; itching or discharge from the vagina; nervousness; trouble in sleeping

Other side effects not listed may also occur in some patients. If you notice any other effects, check with your healthcare professional.

LOSARTAN   (Oral route) - loe-SAR-tan

Black Box Warning

When used in pregnancy during the second and third trimesters, drugs that act directly on the renin-angiotensin system can cause injury and even death to the developing fetus. When pregnancy is detected, losartan potassium should be discontinued as soon as possible.

Commonly used brand name(s)
In the U.S.—
   Cozaar

Available Dosage Forms:
- Tablet

Therapeutic Class: Cardiovascular Agent
Pharmacologic Class: Angiotensin II Receptor Antagonist

Uses For This Medicine

Losartan is used to treat high blood pressure (hypertension). High blood pressure adds to the work load of the heart and arteries. If it continues for a long time, the heart and arteries may not function properly. This can damage the blood vessels of the brain, heart, and kidneys, resulting in a stroke, heart failure, or kidney failure. High blood pressure may also increase the risk of heart attacks. These problems may be less likely to occur if blood pressure is controlled.

Losartan works by blocking the action of a substance in the body that causes blood vessels to tighten. As a result, losartan relaxes blood vessels. This lowers blood pressure.

Losartan is also used to decrease the risk of stroke in patients with high blood pressure and a condition called left ventricular hypertrophy (LVH). LVH is an enlargement of the left pumping chamber of the heart and can cause problems with the way the heart pumps blood.

Losartan is also used to treat a condition called diabetic nephropathy. Diabetic nephropathy is a complication of type 2 diabetes which causes the kidneys to not work properly.

Losartan is available only with your doctor's prescription.

Before Using This Medicine

In deciding to use a medicine, the risks of taking the medicine must be weighed against the good it will do. This is a decision you and your doctor will make. For this medicine, the following should be considered:

Allergies—Tell your doctor if you have ever had any unusual or allergic reaction to this medicine or any other medicines. Also tell your health care professional if you have any other types of allergies, such as to foods, dyes, preservatives, or animals. For non-prescription products, read the label or package ingredients carefully.

Pediatric—Studies on this medicine have been done only in adult patients, and there is no specific information comparing use of losartan in children younger than 6 years of age with use in other age groups.

Geriatric—This medicine has been tested in a limited number of patients 65 years of age or older and has not been shown to cause different side effects or problems in older people than it does in younger adults.

Pregnancy—

	Pregnancy Category	Explanation
1st Trimester	C	Animal studies have shown an adverse effect and there are no adequate studies in pregnant women OR no animal studies have been conducted and there are no adequate studies in pregnant women.
2nd Trimester	D	Studies in pregnant women have demonstrated a risk to the fetus. However, the benefits of therapy in a life threatening situation or a serious disease, may outweigh the potential risk.
3rd Trimester	D	Studies in pregnant women have demonstrated a risk to the fetus. However, the benefits of therapy in a life threatening situation or a serious disease, may outweigh the potential risk.

Breast Feeding—There are no adequate studies in women for determining infant risk when using this medication during breastfeeding. Weigh the potential benefits against the potential risks before taking this medication while breastfeeding.

Other medicines—

Using this medicine with any of the following medicines is usually not recommended, but may be required in some cases. If both medicines are prescribed together, your doctor may change the dose or how often you use one or both of the medicines.

Lithium

Interactions with Food/Tobacco/Alcohol—Certain medicines should not be used at or around the time of eating food or eating certain types of food since interactions may occur. Using alcohol or tobacco with certain medicines may also cause interactions to occur. Discuss with your healthcare professional the use of your medicine with food, alcohol, or tobacco.

Other medical problems—The presence of other medical problems may affect the use of this medicine. Make sure you tell your doctor if you have any other medical problems, especially:

- Kidney disease or
- Liver disease—Effects may be increased because of slower removal of losartan from the body

Proper Use of This Medicine

Make certain your health care professional knows if you are on any special diet, such as a low-sodium diet.

To help you remember to take your medicine, try to get into the habit of taking it at the same time each day.

In addition to the use of the medicine your doctor has prescribed, treatment for your high blood pressure may include weight control and care in the types of foods you eat, especially foods high in sodium. Your doctor will tell you which of these are most important for you. You should check with your doctor before changing your diet.

Many patients who have high blood pressure will not notice any signs of the problem. In fact, many may feel normal. It is very important that you take your medicine exactly as directed and that you keep your appointments with your doctor even if you feel well.

Remember that this medicine will not cure your high blood pressure but it does help control it. Therefore, you must continue to take it as directed if you expect to lower your blood pressure and keep it down. You may have to take high blood pressure medicine for the rest of your life. If high blood pressure is not treated, it can cause serious problems such as heart failure, blood vessel disease, stroke, or kidney disease.

This medicine may be taken with or without food.

If you are unable to swallow tablets, ask your pharmacist about preparing an oral suspension for you.

Dosing—The dose of this medicine will be different for different patients. Follow your doctor's orders or the directions on the label. The following information includes only the average doses of this medicine. If your dose is different, do not change it unless your doctor tells you to do so.

The amount of medicine that you take depends on the strength of the medicine. Also, the number of doses you take each day, the time allowed between doses, and the length of time you take the medicine depend on the medical problem for which you are using the medicine.

- For oral dosage form (tablets):
  - For high blood pressure:
    - Adults—25 to 100 milligrams (mg) a day. The dose may be taken once a day or divided into two doses.
    - Children 6 years of age and older—Use and dose must be determined by your doctor.
    - Children younger than 6 years of age—Use and dose must be determined by your doctor.
  - For high blood pressure with left ventricular hypertrophy:
    - Adults—50 to 100 milligrams (mg) once a day. Your doctor may adjust your dose and add another medicine based on your blood pressure response.
    - Children 6 years of age and older—Use and dose must be determined by your doctor.
    - Children younger than 6 years of age—Use and dose must be determined by your doctor.
  - For diabetic neuropathy:
    - Adults—50 to 100 milligrams (mg) once a day. Your doctor may adjust your dose based on your blood pressure response.
    - Children 6 years of age and older—Use and dose must be determined by your doctor.
    - Children younger than 6 years of age—Use and dose must be determined by your doctor.

Missed dose—If you miss a dose of this medicine, take it as soon as possible. However, if it is almost time for your next dose, skip the missed dose and go back to your regular dosing schedule. Do not double doses.

Storage—Store the medicine in a closed container at room temperature, away from heat, moisture, and direct light. Keep from freezing.

Keep out of the reach of children.

Do not keep outdated medicine or medicine no longer needed.

Precautions While Using This Medicine

Check with your doctor immediately if you think that you may be pregnant. Losartan may cause birth defects or other problems in the baby if taken during pregnancy.

It is important that your doctor check your progress at regular visits to make sure that this medicine is working properly and to check for unwanted effects.

Do not take other medicines unless they have been discussed with your doctor. This especially includes over-the-counter (nonprescription) medicines for appetite control, asthma, colds, cough, hay fever, or sinus problems, since they may tend to increase your blood pressure.

Dizziness or lightheadedness may occur after the first dose of this medicine, especially if you have been taking a diuretic (water pill). Make sure you know how you react to this medicine before you drive, use machines, or do anything else that could be dangerous if you are dizzy.

Check with your doctor right away if you become sick while taking this medicine, especially with severe or continuing nausea and vomiting or diarrhea. These conditions may cause you to lose too much water and lead to low blood pressure.

Dizziness, lightheadedness, or fainting may also occur if you exercise or if the weather is hot. Heavy sweating can cause loss of too much water and result in low blood pressure. Use extra care during exercise or hot weather.

Avoid alcoholic beverages until you have discussed their use with your doctor. Alcohol may make the low blood pressure effect worse and/or increase the possibility of dizziness or fainting.

Side Effects of This Medicine

Along with its needed effects, a medicine may cause some unwanted effects. Although not all of these side effects may occur, if they do occur they may need medical attention.

Check with your doctor immediately if any of the following side effects occur:
Rare
Hoarseness; swelling of face, mouth, hands, or feet; trouble in swallowing or breathing (sudden)

Incidence not known
Abdominal pain; black, tarry stools; bleeding gums; blood in urine or stools; coma; confusion; convulsions; decreased urine output; difficult breathing; fast or irregular breathing; headache; increased thirst; irregular heartbeat; large, flat, bluish patches on the skin; muscle pain or cramps; nausea or vomiting; painful knees and ankles; pinpoint red spots on skin; unusual bleeding or bruising; unusual tiredness or weakness; upper right abdominal pain; weakness or heaviness of legs; yellow eyes and skin

Check with your doctor as soon as possible if any of the following side effects occur:
Less common
Cough, fever or sore throat; dizziness

Some side effects may occur that usually do not need medical attention. These side effects may go away during treatment as your body adjusts to the medicine. Also, your health care professional may be able to tell you about ways to prevent or reduce some of these side effects. Check with your health care professional if any of the following side effects continue or are bothersome or if you have any questions about them:
More common
Headache
Less common
Back pain; diarrhea; fatigue; nasal congestion
Rare
Cough, dry; leg pain; muscle cramps or pain; sinus problems; trouble in sleeping

Other side effects not listed may also occur in some patients. If you notice any other effects, check with your healthcare professional.

LOTEPREDNOL (Ophthalmic route) - loe-te-PRED-nol

Commonly used brand name(s)
In the U.S.—
Alrex
Lotemax

Available Dosage Forms:
- Suspension

Therapeutic Class: Ophthalmologic Agent
Pharmacologic Class: Adrenal Glucocorticoid

Uses For This Medicine

Loteprednol belongs to the group of medicines known as corticosteroids (cortisone-like medicines). It is used to treat inflammation (redness) of the eye, which may occur with certain eye problems or following eye surgery. This medicine is also used to temporarily treat the symptoms of the eye caused by a condition known as seasonal allergic conjunctivitis (seasonal eye allergy).

This medicine is available only with your doctor's prescription.

Before Using This Medicine

In deciding to use a medicine, the risks of taking the medicine must be weighed against the good it will do. This is a decision you and your doctor will make. For this medicine, the following should be considered:

Allergies—Tell your doctor if you have ever had any unusual or allergic reaction to this medicine or any other medicines. Also tell your health care professional if you have any other types of allergies, such as to foods, dyes, preservatives, or animals. For non-prescription products, read the label or package ingredients carefully.

Pediatric—There is no specific information comparing use of ophthalmic loteprednol in children with use in other age groups.

Geriatric—Many medicines have not been studied specifically in older people. Therefore, it may not be known whether they work exactly the same way they do in younger adults or if they cause different side effects or problems in older people. There is no specific information comparing use of ophthalmic loteprednol in the elderly with use in other age groups.

Other medicines—Although certain medicines should not be used together at all, in other cases two different medicines may be used together even if an interaction might occur. In these cases, your doctor may want to change the dose, or other precautions may be necessary. Tell your healthcare professional if you are taking any other prescription or non-prescription (over-the-counter [OTC]) medicine.

Interactions with Food/Tobacco/Alcohol—Certain medicines should not be used at or around the time of eating food or eating certain types of food since interactions may occur. Using alcohol or tobacco with certain medicines may also cause interactions to occur. Discuss with your healthcare professional the use of your medicine with food, alcohol, or tobacco.

Other medical problems—The presence of other medical problems may affect the use of this medicine. Make sure you tell your doctor if you have any other medical problems, especially:

- Certain eye diseases that cause the cornea to get thin—Use of ophthalmic loteprednol could cause a hole to form (perforation)
- Fungus infection of the eye or
- Herpes infection of the eye or
- Virus infection of the eye or
- Yeast infection of the eye or
- Any other eye infection—Ophthalmic loteprednol may make existing infections worse or cause new infections

- Glaucoma—Prolonged use of corticosteroids may result in glaucoma; caution should be used when corticosteroids are used in patients who have glaucoma

Proper Use of This Medicine

Shake the container very well before applying the eye drops.

If you are using the 0.5% strength of this medicine: Do not wear soft contact lenses while you are using this medicine.

If you are using the 0.2% strength of this medicine: If your eyes are red, you should not wear contact lenses. If your eyes are not red, soft contact lenses should be removed before you use this medicine. You should wait at least 10 minutes after using the eye drops before reinserting the contact lenses.

To use:

- First, wash your hands. Tilt your head back and, pressing your finger gently on the skin just beneath the lower eyelid, pull the lower eyelid away from the eye to make a space. Drop the medicine into this space. Let go of the eyelid and gently close the eyes. Do not blink. Keep the eyes closed and apply pressure to the inner corner of the eye with your finger for 1 or 2 minutes to allow the medicine to be absorbed by the eye.
- If you think you did not get the drop of medicine into your eye properly, use another drop.
- To keep the medicine as germ-free as possible, do not touch the applicator tip to any surface (including the eye). Also, keep the container tightly closed.

Dosing—The dose of this medicine will be different for different patients. Follow your doctor's orders or the directions on the label. The following information includes only the average doses of this medicine. If your dose is different, do not change it unless your doctor tells you to do so.

The amount of medicine that you take depends on the strength of the medicine. Also, the number of doses you take each day, the time allowed between doses, and the length of time you take the medicine depend on the medical problem for which you are using the medicine.

- For ophthalmic suspension dosage form (eye drops):
  - For seasonal allergic conjunctivitis:
    - Adults—Use one drop of the 0.2% eye suspension in the affected eye four times a day.
    - Children—Use and dose must be determined by your doctor.
  - For inflammation after surgery:
    - Adults—Use one or two drops of the 0.5% eye suspension in the affected eye four times a day beginning twenty-four hours after surgery and continuing throughout the first two weeks after surgery.
    - Children—Use and dose must be determined by your doctor.
  - For other eye problems as determined by your doctor:
    - Adults—Use one or two drops of the 0.5% eye suspension in the affected eye four times a day. During the first week your doctor may want you to use the eye drops more often.
    - Children—Use and dose must be determined by your doctor.

Missed dose—If you miss a dose of this medicine, take it as soon as possible. However, if it is almost time for your next

dose, skip the missed dose and go back to your regular dosing schedule. Do not double doses.

Storage—Store the medicine in a closed container at room temperature, away from heat, moisture, and direct light. Keep from freezing.

Keep out of the reach of children.

Do not keep outdated medicine or medicine no longer needed.

Precautions While Using This Medicine

If you will be using this medicine for more than few weeks, an ophthalmologist (eye doctor) should examine your eyes at regular visits to make sure it does not cause unwanted effects.

If your symptoms do not improve or if your condition becomes worse, check with your doctor.

Side Effects of This Medicine

Along with its needed effects, a medicine may cause some unwanted effects. Although not all of these side effects may occur, if they do occur they may need medical attention.

Check with your doctor as soon as possible if any of the following side effects occur:

More common
Blurred vision or other change in vision; redness or swelling of the eye; swelling of the membrane covering the white part of the eye

Less common
Discharge from the eye; eye discomfort, irritation, or pain; increased sensitivity of eye to light; redness of eyelid or inner lining of eyelid; tiny bumps on the inner lining of eyelid

Some side effects may occur that usually do not need medical attention. These side effects may go away during treatment as your body adjusts to the medicine. Also, your health care professional may be able to tell you about ways to prevent or reduce some of these side effects. Check with your health care professional if any of the following side effects continue or are bothersome or if you have any questions about them:

More common
Burning when medicine is applied; dry eye; feeling of something in the eye; headache; itching; runny nose; sore throat; tearing or watery eye

Other side effects not listed may also occur in some patients. If you notice any other effects, check with your healthcare professional.

LOTEPREDNOL ETABONATE AND TOBRAMYCIN (Ophthalmic route) -
loe-te-PRED-nol e-TA-boh-nate, toe-bra-MYE-sin

Commonly used brand name(s)

In the U.S.—
Zylet

Available Dosage Forms:
• Suspension

Therapeutic Class: Aminoglycoside/Corticosteroid Combination
Pharmacologic Class: Loteprednol

Uses For This Medicine

Loteprednol and tobramycin is a combination of an antibiotic and a corticosteroid. It is used in the eye to prevent permanent damage, which may occur with certain eye problems.

This medicine is available only with your doctor's prescription.

Before Using This Medicine

In deciding to use a medicine, the risks of taking the medicine must be weighed against the good it will do. This is a decision you and your doctor will make. For this medicine, the following should be considered:

Allergies—Tell your doctor if you have ever had any unusual or allergic reaction to this medicine or any other medicines. Also tell your health care professional if you have any other types of allergies, such as to foods, dyes, preservatives, or animals. For non-prescription products, read the label or package ingredients carefully.

Pediatric—Studies on this medicine have been done only in adult patients, and there is no specific information comparing use of loteprednol and tobramycin in children with use in other age groups.

Geriatric—This medicine has been tested and has not been shown to cause different side effects or problems in older people than it does in younger adults.

Other medicines—

Using this medicine with any of the following medicines is usually not recommended, but may be required in some cases. If both medicines are prescribed together, your doctor may change the dose or how often you use one or both of the medicines.

Alcuronium, Atracurium, Cidofovir, Cisatracurium, Decamethonium, Doxacurium, Fazadinium, Gallamine, Hexafluorenium, Lysine, Metocurine, Mivacurium, Pancuronium, Pipecuronium, Rapacuronium, Rocuronium, Succinylcholine, Tacrolimus, Tubocurarine, Vecuronium

Interactions with Food/Tobacco/Alcohol—Certain medicines should not be used at or around the time of eating food or eating certain types of food since interactions may occur. Using alcohol or tobacco with certain medicines may also cause interactions to occur. Discuss with your healthcare professional the use of your medicine with food, alcohol, or tobacco.

Other medical problems—The presence of other medical problems may affect the use of this medicine. Make sure you tell your doctor if you have any other medical problems, especially:

• Cataract surgery—Use of loteprednol after cataract surgery may delay healing and increase the chance of side effects

• Certain eye diseases that cause the cornea to get thin—Use of ophthalmic loteprednol could cause a hole to form (perforation)

- Fungus infection of the eye or
- Herpes infection of the eye or
- Pussy conditions of the eye or
- Virus infection of the eye or
- Yeast infection of the eye—Ophthalmic loteprednol and tobramycin may mask or make existing infections worse.
- Glaucoma—Prolonged use of corticosteroids may result in glaucoma; caution should be used when corticosteroids are used in patients who have glaucoma

Proper Use of This Medicine

Shake the container very well before applying the eye drops.

Using only if the imprinted neckband is intact.

Do not wear soft contact lenses while you are using this medicine

Decrease use gradually as symptoms improve.

To help clear up your eye infection completely, keep using loteprednol and tobramycin for the full time of treatment, even if your symptoms have disappeared.

To use:

- First, wash your hands. Tilt your head back and, pressing your finger gently on the skin just beneath the lower eyelid, pull the lower eyelid away from the eye to make a space. Drop the medicine into this space. Let go of the eyelid and gently close the eyes. Do not blink. Keep the eyes closed and apply pressure to the inner corner of the eye with your finger for 1 or 2 minutes to allow the medicine to be absorbed by the eye.
- If you think you did not get the drop of medicine into your eye properly, use another drop.
- To keep the medicine as germ-free as possible, do not touch the applicator tip to any surface (including the eye). Also, keep the container tightly closed.

Dosing—The dose of this medicine will be different for different patients. Follow your doctor's orders or the directions on the label. The following information includes only the average doses of this medicine. If your dose is different, do not change it unless your doctor tells you to do so.

The amount of medicine that you take depends on the strength of the medicine. Also, the number of doses you take each day, the time allowed between doses, and the length of time you take the medicine depend on the medical problem for which you are using the medicine.

- For ophthalmic suspension dosage form (eye drops):
  - For eye disorders:
    - Adults—Use one or two drops into the affected eye every four to six hours. Your doctor may have you use the drops more frequently during the first day or two and will probably have you space the doses further apart as the eye gets better.
    - Children—Use and dose must be determined by your doctor.

Missed dose—If you miss a dose of this medicine, take it as soon as possible. However, if it is almost time for your next dose, skip the missed dose and go back to your regular dosing schedule. Do not double doses.

Storage—Store the medicine in a closed container at room temperature, away from heat, moisture, and direct light. Keep from freezing.

Keep out of the reach of children.

Do not keep outdated medicine or medicine no longer needed.

Ask your healthcare professional how you should dispose of any medicine you do not use.

Store upright.

Precautions While Using This Medicine

If you will be using this medicine for more than a few weeks, an ophthalmologist (eye doctor) should examine your eyes at regular visits to make sure it does not cause unwanted effects.

If your eye infection does not improve or if your condition becomes worse, check with your doctor.

Side Effects of This Medicine

Along with its needed effects, a medicine may cause some unwanted effects. Although not all of these side effects may occur, if they do occur they may need medical attention.

Check with your doctor immediately if any of the following side effects occur:

> *More common*
> Increased intraocular pressure; painful irritation of the clear front part of the eye
>
> *Less common*
> Blurred vision or blue-green halos seen around objects; blurred vision or other changes in vision; decreased vision; discharge from the eye; dry eyes; eyelid burning, redness, itching, pain, or tenderness; fast heartbeat; fever; hives; hoarseness; irritation and swelling of the eye; itching; joint pain; lid itching and swelling; pain in eye; rash; redness of skin; redness of eyelid; sensitivity of eyes to light; shortness of breath; stiffness or swelling; swelling of eyelids, face, lips, hands, or feet; tightness in chest; troubled breathing or swallowing; wheezing
>
> *Incidence not known*
> Redness of eye; tearing

Some side effects may occur that usually do not need medical attention. These side effects may go away during treatment as your body adjusts to the medicine. Also, your health care professional may be able to tell you about ways to prevent or reduce some of these side effects. Check with your health care professional if any of the following side effects continue or are bothersome or if you have any questions about them:

> *More common*
> Burning; dry eyes; headache; increased sensitivity of eyes to light; itching; stinging

Other side effects not listed may also occur in some patients. If you notice any other effects, check with your healthcare professional.

LOVASTATIN AND NIACIN (Oral route) - LOE-va-sta-tin, NYE-a-sin

Commonly used brand name(s)

In the U.S.—
  Advicor

Available Dosage Forms:
- Tablet, Extended Release
- Tablet

Therapeutic Class: Antihyperlipidemic
Pharmacologic Class: Vitamin B

Uses For This Medicine

Lovastatin and niacin extended-release combination medicine is used to help lower high cholesterol and fat levels in the blood. This may help prevent medical problems caused by cholesterol and fat clogging the blood vessels.

Lovastatin and niacin extended-release combination medicine combines two drugs that work together to treat cholesterol and lipid (fat) disorders. Lovastatin belongs to the group of medicines called 3–hydroxy-3–methylglutaryl coenzyme A (HMG-CoA) reductase inhibitors. It works by blocking an enzyme that is needed by the body to make cholesterol, thereby reducing the amount of cholesterol in the blood. Niacin is a B-complex vitamin that reduces the amount of cholesterol in the blood.

This medicine is available only with your doctor's prescription.

Before Using This Medicine

In deciding to use a medicine, the risks of taking the medicine must be weighed against the good it will do. This is a decision you and your doctor will make. For this medicine, the following should be considered:

This combination medicine should not be used until after your body has adjusted to each of the individual medicines. Be sure to check with your doctor about this.

Allergies—Tell your doctor if you have ever had any unusual or allergic reaction to this medicine or any other medicines. Also tell your health care professional if you have any other types of allergies, such as to foods, dyes, preservatives, or animals. For non-prescription products, read the label or package ingredients carefully.

Pediatric—Studies on this medicine have been done only in adult patients, and there is no specific information comparing use of niacin extended-release and lovastatin combination in children with use in other age groups.

Geriatric—This medicine has been tested in a limited number of patients 65 years of age or older and has not been shown to cause different side effects or problems in older people than it does in younger adults.

Other medicines—

Using this medicine with any of the following medicines is not recommended. Your doctor may decide not to treat you with this medication or change some of the other medicines you take.

Itraconazole, Mibefradil

Interactions with Food/Tobacco/Alcohol—Certain medicines should not be used at or around the time of eating food or eating certain types of food since interactions may occur. Using alcohol or tobacco with certain medicines may also cause interactions to occur. The following interactions have been selected on the basis of their potential significance and are not necessarily all-inclusive.

Using this medicine with any of the following may cause an increased risk of certain side effects but may be unavoidable in some cases. If used together, your doctor may change the dose or how often you use this medicine, or give you special instructions about the use of food, alcohol, or tobacco.

Grapefruit Juice

Other medical problems—The presence of other medical problems may affect the use of this medicine. Make sure you tell your doctor if you have any other medical problems, especially:
- Bleeding problems or
- Diabetes mellitus (sugar diabetes) or
- Endocrine problems or
- Gout or
- Heart disease or
- Liver disease or
- Low blood pressure or
- Stomach ulcer—Lovastatin and niacin extended-release combination may make these conditions worse.
- Kidney disease—Effects of lovastatin and niacin extended-release combination may be increased because of slower removal of medicine from the body.

Proper Use of This Medicine

Before prescribing medicine for your condition, your doctor will probably try to control your condition by prescribing a personal diet for you. Such a diet may be low in fats, particularly saturated fat, sugars, and/or cholesterol. Many people are able to control their condition by carefully following their doctor's orders for proper diet and exercise. Medicine is prescribed only when additional help is needed and is effective only when a schedule of diet and exercise is properly followed.

Make certain your doctor knows if you are on any special diet, such as a low-sodium or low-sugar diet.

Use this medicine only as directed by your doctor. Do not use more or less of it, and do not use it more often or for a longer time than your doctor ordered. Also, this medicine works best if there is a constant amount in the blood. To help keep this amount constant, do not miss any doses and take the medicine at the same time each day.

Remember that this medicine will not cure your condition but it does help control it. Therefore, you must continue to take it as directed to keep your cholesterol levels down.

Follow carefully the special diet your doctor gave you. This is an important part of controlling your condition, and is necessary if the medicine is to work properly.

Do not drink any grapefruit juice around the time you take this medicine. It may be best to drink any grapefruit juice approximately 12 hours before or after you take your medicine. In addition, do not drink grapefruit juice in large quantities (more than one quart per day) while you are being treated with lovastatin and niacin extended-release combination. To do so may increase the risk of developing muscle problems. Check with your doctor if you have any questions.

Take this medicine at bedtime after eating a low fat snack. Swallow the tablet whole. Do not crush, break, or chew the tablet before you swallow it.

This medicine may cause you to have skin flushing which makes your face, neck, arms and occasionally, your upper chest to feel warm and look red. Flushing usually starts about two to four hours after you take your medicine, and may last up to several hours. Flushing can also cause itching and/or a tingling sensation. A more intense episode of flushing may include dizziness or faintness. If you take your medicine at bedtime, you may sleep through any flushing that occurs. If awakened by flushing, rise slowly to minimize the potential for dizziness or fainting. Avoiding alcohol or hot drinks may reduce the flushing. This effect should lessen after several weeks as your body gets used to the medicine. However, if the problem continues or gets worse, check with your doctor.

Dosing—The dose of this medicine will be different for different patients. Follow your doctor's orders or the directions on the label. The following information includes only the average doses of this medicine. If your dose is different, do not change it unless your doctor tells you to do so.

The amount of medicine that you take depends on the strength of the medicine. Also, the number of doses you take each day, the time allowed between doses, and the length of time you take the medicine depend on the medical problem for which you are using the medicine.

- For oral dosage form (tablets):
  ○ Adults—The starting dose is usually, 500 milligrams (mg) of niacin extended-release and 20 mg of lovastatin (combined in one tablet) one time a day, at bedtime with a low fat snack. Then your doctor may increase your dose a little at a time every 4 weeks, as your body gets used to the medicine, until your cholesterol is controlled.
  ○ Children—Use and dose must be determined by your doctor.

Missed dose—If you miss a dose of this medicine, take it as soon as possible. However, if it is almost time for your next dose, skip the missed dose and go back to your regular dosing schedule. Do not double doses.

If you have not taken this medicine for more than 7 days, check with your doctor. You may need to have your dose reduced before you can start taking this medicine again.

Storage—Store the medicine in a closed container at room temperature, away from heat, moisture, and direct light. Keep from freezing.

Keep out of the reach of children.

Do not keep outdated medicine or medicine no longer needed.

Ask your healthcare professional how you should dispose of any medicine you do not use.

Precautions While Using This Medicine

Check with your doctor immediately if you have dark-colored urine, a fever, muscle cramps or spasms, muscle pain or stiffness, or feel very tired or weak. Niacin extended-release and lovastatin combination may cause a serious, but rare, problem called rhabdomyolysis. It is important to call your doctor right away if you have any of these symptoms.

It is very important that your doctor check your progress at regular visits. This will allow your doctor to see if the medicine is working properly to lower your cholesterol and triglyceride (fat) levels and that it does not cause unwanted side effects. At regular intervals, your doctor will want to do routine blood tests.

For diabetic patients: This medicine may affect blood sugar levels. If you notice a change in the results of your blood or urine sugar tests or if you have any questions, check with your doctor.

Do not stop taking lovastatin and niacin extended-release combination without first checking with your doctor. When you stop taking this medicine, your blood cholesterol levels may increase again.

Check with your doctor immediately if you think that you may be pregnant. Lovastatin and niacin extended-release combination may cause birth defects or other problems in the baby if taken during pregnancy.

Before having any kind of surgery (including dental surgery) or emergency treatment, tell the medical doctor or dentist in charge that you are taking this medicine.

Side Effects of This Medicine

Along with its needed effects, a medicine may cause some unwanted effects. Although not all of these side effects may occur, if they do occur they may need medical attention.

Check with your doctor immediately if any of the following side effects occur:

More common
 Asthenia, such as, lack or loss of strength; infection, such as, cough or hoarseness, fever or chills, lower back or side pain, painful or difficult urination; pain

Less common
 Abdominal pain, such as, stomach pain; hyperglycemia, such as, abdominal pain, blurred vision, dry mouth, fatigue, dry skin, fruit-like breath odor, increased hunger, increased thirst, increased urination, nausea, unexplained weight loss, vomiting; myalgia, such as, difficulty in moving, joint pain, muscle aching, cramping pain or stiffness, swollen joints; myopathy, such as, muscle aches, weakness, tenderness, or pain; stomach pain

Rare
 Rhabdomyolysis, such as, dark-colored urine, fever, muscle cramps, pain, spasm, or stiffness, unusual tiredness or weakness

Symptoms of overdose

Get emergency help immediately if any of the following symptoms of overdose occur:

 Cardiac arrhythmia, such as, chest pain or discomfort, dizziness, fainting, fast, slow or irregular heartbeat, lightheadedness, pounding or rapid pulse; diarrhea; dizziness; flushing, severe, such as, feeling of warmth, redness, itching, and/or tingling of the face, neck, arms, and occasionally, upper chest, dizziness, fainting; hypotension, such as, blurred vision, confusion, dizziness, faintness, lightheadedness when getting up from a lying or sitting position, sudden sweating, unusual tiredness or weakness; nausea and vomiting; syncope, such as, fainting

Some side effects may occur that usually do not need medical attention. These side effects may go away during treatment as your body adjusts to the medicine. Also, your health care professional may be able to tell you about ways to prevent or reduce some of these side effects. Check with your health care professional if any of the following side effects continue or are bothersome or if you have any questions about them:

More common
Chills; diarrhea; flu syndrome, such as, chills, diarrhea, fever, general feeling of discomfort or illness, headache, joint pain, loss of appetite, muscle aches and pains, nausea, runny nose, shivering, sore throat, sweating, trouble sleeping, unusual tiredness or weakness, vomiting; flushing, such as, feeling of warmth, redness, itching, and/or tingling of the face, neck, arms, and occasionally, upper chest; edema, such as, swelling; headache; nausea; pruritus, such as, itching skin; rash; shortness of breath; sweating; syncope, such as, feeling faint or fainting; tachycardia, such as, fast, pounding, or irregular heartbeat or pulse

Less common
dyspepsia, such as, acid or sour stomach, belching, heartburn, indigestion, stomach discomfort, upset or pain

Other side effects not listed may also occur in some patients. If you notice any other effects, check with your healthcare professional.

LOXAPINE (Oral route, Intramuscular route) - LOX-a-peen

Commonly used brand name(s)

In the U.S.—
Loxitane

Available Dosage Forms:
- Solution
- Capsule
- Tablet

Therapeutic Class: Antipsychotic

Uses For This Medicine

Loxapine is used to treat nervous, mental, and emotional conditions.

Loxapine is available only with your doctor's prescription.

Once a medicine has been approved for marketing for a certain use, experience may show that it is also useful for other medical problems. Although this use is not included in product labeling, loxapine is used in certain patients with the following medical condition:

- Anxiety associated with mental depression

Before Using This Medicine

In deciding to use a medicine, the risks of taking the medicine must be weighed against the good it will do. This is a decision you and your doctor will make. For this medicine, the following should be considered:

Allergies—Tell your doctor if you have ever had any unusual or allergic reaction to this medicine or any other medicines. Also tell your health care professional if you have any other types of allergies, such as to foods, dyes, preservatives, or animals. For non-prescription products, read the label or package ingredients carefully.

Pediatric—Studies on this medicine have been done only in adult patients, and there is no specific information comparing use of loxapine in children with use in other age groups.

Geriatric—Elderly patients are usually more sensitive than younger adults to the effects of loxapine. Constipation, dizziness or fainting, drowsiness, dry mouth, trembling of the hands and fingers, and symptoms of tardive dyskinesia (such as rapid, worm-like movements of the tongue or any other uncontrolled movements of the mouth, tongue, or jaw, and/or arms and legs) are especially likely to occur in elderly patients.

Pregnancy—

	Pregnancy Category	Explanation
All Trimesters	C	Animal studies have shown an adverse effect and there are no adequate studies in pregnant women OR no animal studies have been conducted and there are no adequate studies in pregnant women.

Breast Feeding—There are no adequate studies in women for determining infant risk when using this medication during breastfeeding. Weigh the potential benefits against the potential risks before taking this medication while breastfeeding.

Other medicines—

Using this medicine with any of the following medicines is usually not recommended, but may be required in some cases. If both medicines are prescribed together, your doctor may change the dose or how often you use one or both of the medicines.

Lithium, Tramadol, Zotepine

Interactions with Food/Tobacco/Alcohol—Certain medicines should not be used at or around the time of eating food or eating certain types of food since interactions may occur. Using alcohol or tobacco with certain medicines may also cause interactions to occur. Discuss with your healthcare professional the use of your medicine with food, alcohol, or tobacco.

Other medical problems—The presence of other medical problems may affect the use of this medicine. Make sure you tell your doctor if you have any other medical problems, especially:

- Alcohol abuse—CNS depressant effects may be increased
- Difficult urination or
- Enlarged prostate or
- Glaucoma (or predisposition to) or
- Parkinson's disease—Loxapine may make the condition worse
- Heart or blood vessel disease—An increased risk of low blood pressure (hypotension) or changes in the rhythm of your heart may occur
- Liver disease—Higher blood levels of loxapine may occur, increasing the chance of side effects
- Seizure disorders—Loxapine may increase the risk of seizures

Proper Use of This Medicine

This medicine may be taken with food or a full glass (8 ounces) of water or milk to reduce stomach irritation.

For patients taking the oral solution:

- Measure the solution only with the dropper provided by the manufacturer. This will give a more accurate dose.

The liquid medicine must be mixed with orange juice or grape-fruit juice just before you take it to make it easier to take.

Do not take more of this medicine, do not take it more often, and do not take it for a longer time than your doctor ordered. To do so may increase the chance of unwanted effects.

Dosing—The dose of this medicine will be different for different patients. Follow your doctor's orders or the directions on the label. The following information includes only the average doses of this medicine. If your dose is different, do not change it unless your doctor tells you to do so.

The amount of medicine that you take depends on the strength of the medicine. Also, the number of doses you take each day, the time allowed between doses, and the length of time you take the medicine depend on the medical problem for which you are using the medicine.

- For oral dosage forms (capsules, oral solution, or tablets):
    - Adults: To start, 10 milligrams taken two times a day. Your doctor may increase your dose if needed.
    - Children up to 16 years of age: The dose must be determined by the doctor.
- For injection dosage form:
    - Adults: 12.5 to 50 milligrams every four to six hours, injected into a muscle.
    - Children up to 16 years of age: The dose must be determined by the doctor.

Missed dose—If you miss a dose of this medicine, take it as soon as possible. However, if it is almost time for your next dose, skip the missed dose and go back to your regular dosing schedule. Do not double doses.

Storage—Store the medicine in a closed container at room temperature, away from heat, moisture, and direct light. Keep from freezing.

Keep out of the reach of children.

Do not keep outdated medicine or medicine no longer needed.

Precautions While Using This Medicine

Your doctor should check your progress at regular visits, especially during the first few months of treatment with this medicine. The amount of loxapine you take may be changed often to meet the needs of your condition and to help avoid side effects.

Do not stop taking this medicine without first checking with your doctor. Your doctor may want you to reduce gradually the amount you are taking before stopping completely. This will allow your body time to adjust and to keep your condition from becoming worse.

This medicine will add to the effects of alcohol and other CNS depressants (medicines that slow down the nervous system, possibly causing drowsiness). Some examples of CNS depressants are antihistamines or medicine for hay fever, other allergies, or colds; sedatives, tranquilizers, or sleeping medicine; prescription pain medicine or narcotics; barbiturates; medicine for seizures; or anesthetics, including some dental anesthetics. Check with your doctor before taking any of the above while you are taking this medicine.

Do not take this medicine within two hours of taking antacids or medicine for diarrhea. Taking loxapine and antacids or medicine for diarrhea too close together may make this medicine less effective.

This medicine may cause some people to become drowsy or less alert than they are normally, especially as the amount of medicine is increased. Even if you take this medicine at bedtime, you may feel drowsy or less alert on arising. Make sure you know how you react to this medicine before you drive, use machines, or do anything else that could be dangerous if you are not alert.

Although it is not a problem for most patients, dizziness, light-headedness, or fainting may occur, especially when you get up from a lying or sitting position. Getting up slowly may help. However, if the problem continues or gets worse, check with your doctor.

Loxapine may cause your skin to be more sensitive to sunlight than it is normally. Exposure to sunlight, even for brief periods of time, may cause a skin rash, itching, redness or other discoloration of the skin, or a severe sunburn. When you begin taking this medicine:

- Stay out of direct sunlight, especially between the hours of 10:00 a.m. and 3:00 p.m., if possible.
- Wear protective clothing, including a hat. Also, wear sunglasses.
- Apply a sun block product that has a skin protection factor (SPF) of at least 15. Some patients may require a product with a higher SPF number, especially if they have a fair complexion. If you have any questions about this, check with your health care professional.
- Apply a sun block lipstick that has an SPF of at least 15 to protect your lips.
- Do not use a sunlamp or tanning bed or booth.

If you have a severe reaction from the sun, check with your doctor.

Loxapine may cause dryness of the mouth. For temporary relief, use sugarless candy or gum, melt bits of ice in your mouth, or use a saliva substitute. However, if your mouth continues to feel dry for more than 2 weeks, check with your medical doctor or dentist. Continuing dryness of the mouth may increase the chance of dental disease, including tooth decay, gum disease, and fungus infections.

Before having any kind of surgery, dental treatment, or emergency treatment, tell the medical doctor or dentist in charge that you are taking this medicine. Taking loxapine together with medicines that are used during surgery or dental or emergency treatments may increase the CNS depressant effects.

Side Effects of This Medicine

Along with its needed effects, loxapine can sometimes cause serious side effects. Tardive dyskinesia (a movement disorder) may occur and may not go away after you stop using the medicine. Signs of tardive dyskinesia include fine, worm-like movements of the tongue, or other uncontrolled movements of the mouth, tongue, cheeks, jaw, or arms and legs. Other serious but rare side effects may also occur. These include severe muscle stiffness, fever, unusual tiredness or weakness, fast heartbeat, difficult breathing, increased sweating, loss of bladder control, and seizures (neuroleptic malignant syndrome). You and your doctor should discuss the good this medicine will do as well as the risks of taking it.

Stop taking this medicine and get emergency help immediately if any of the following effects occur:

Rare
Convulsions (seizures); difficult or fast breathing; fast heartbeat or irregular pulse; fever (high); high or low blood pressure; increased sweating; loss of bladder control; muscle stiffness (severe); unusually pale skin; unusual tiredness or weakness

Check with your doctor immediately if any of the following side effects occur:

More common
Lip smacking or puckering; puffing of cheeks; rapid or fine, worm-like movements of tongue; uncontrolled chewing movements; uncontrolled movements of arms or legs

Check with your doctor as soon as possible if any of the following side effects occur:

More common (occurring with increase of dosage)
Difficulty in speaking or swallowing; loss of balance control; mask-like face; restlessness or desire to keep moving; shuffling walk; slowed movements; stiffness of arms and legs; trembling and shaking of fingers and hands

Less common
Constipation (severe); difficult urination; inability to move eyes; muscle spasms, especially of the neck and back; skin rash; twisting movements of the body

Rare
Sore throat and fever; increased blinking or spasms of eyelid; uncontrolled twisting movements of neck, trunk, arms, or legs; unusual bleeding or bruising; unusual facial expressions or body positions; yellow eyes or skin

Symptoms of overdose
Dizziness (severe); drowsiness (severe); muscle trembling, jerking, stiffness, or uncontrolled movements (severe); troubled breathing (severe); unusual tiredness or weakness (severe)

Some side effects may occur that usually do not need medical attention. These side effects may go away during treatment as your body adjusts to the medicine. Also, your health care professional may be able to tell you about ways to prevent or reduce some of these side effects. Check with your health care professional if any of the following side effects continue or are bothersome or if you have any questions about them:

More common
Blurred vision; confusion; dizziness, lightheadedness, or fainting; drowsiness; dryness of mouth

Less common
Constipation (mild); decreased sexual ability; enlargement of breasts (males and females); headache; increased sensitivity of skin to sun; missing menstrual periods; nausea or vomiting; trouble in sleeping; unusual secretion of milk; weight gain

After you stop using this medicine, it may still produce some side effects that need attention. During this period of time, *check with your doctor immediately* if you notice the following side effects:

Dizziness; nausea and vomiting; rapid or worm-like movements of the tongue; stomach upset or pain; trembling of fingers and hands; uncontrolled chewing movements

Other side effects not listed may also occur in some patients. If you notice any other effects, check with your healthcare professional.

LUTROPIN ALFA (Subcutaneous route) - LOO-troe-pin alfa

Commonly used brand name(s)

In the U.S.—
Luveris

Available Dosage Forms:
• Powder for Solution

Therapeutic Class: Endocrine-Metabolic Agent
Pharmacologic Class: Human Luteinizing Hormone

Uses For This Medicine

Lutropin alfa is a drug whose actions are almost the same as those of luteinizing hormone (LH), which is produced by the pituitary gland. It is a hormone also normally produced by the placenta in pregnancy.

Lutropin alfa is used to help conception occur. It is usually given in combination with follitropin alfa. Many women being treated with these drugs usually have not been able to conceive yet.

This medicine is available only with your doctor's prescription.

Before Using This Medicine

In deciding to use a medicine, the risks of taking the medicine must be weighed against the good it will do. This is a decision

you and your doctor will make. For this medicine, the following should be considered:

Allergies—Tell your doctor if you have ever had any unusual or allergic reaction to this medicine or any other medicines. Also tell your health care professional if you have any other types of allergies, such as to foods, dyes, preservatives, or animals. For non-prescription products, read the label or package ingredients carefully.

Pregnancy—

	Pregnancy Category	Explanation
All Trimesters	X	Studies in animals or pregnant women have demonstrated positive evidence of fetal abnormalities. This drug should not be used in women who are or may become pregnant because the risk clearly outweighs any possible benefit.

Breast Feeding—There are no adequate studies in women for determining infant risk when using this medication during breastfeeding. Weigh the potential benefits against the potential risks before taking this medication while breastfeeding.

Other medicines—Although certain medicines should not be used together at all, in other cases two different medicines may be used together even if an interaction might occur. In these cases, your doctor may want to change the dose, or other precautions may be necessary. Tell your healthcare professional if you are taking any other prescription or non-prescription (over-the-counter [OTC]) medicine.

Interactions with Food/Tobacco/Alcohol—Certain medicines should not be used at or around the time of eating food or eating certain types of food since interactions may occur. Using alcohol or tobacco with certain medicines may also cause interactions to occur. Discuss with your healthcare professional the use of your medicine with food, alcohol, or tobacco.

Other medical problems—The presence of other medical problems may affect the use of this medicine. Make sure you tell your doctor if you have any other medical problems, especially:

- Abnormal bleeding of genitals or uterus (unknown cause)—Use of lutropin alfa may make the diagnosis of this problem more difficult
- Adrenal gland or thyroid disease (not controlled) or
- Tumor, brain or
- Tumor, sex hormone-dependent—Use of lutropin alfa may make these conditions worse
- Ovarian cyst or enlarged ovaries—Use of lutropin alfa may increase the size of a cyst on an ovary or increase the size of enlarged ovaries
- Primary ovarian failure—Lutropin alfa will not work in patients whose ovaries no longer develop eggs
- Thrombophlebitis, active—Lutropin alfa may increase the risk of side effects

Proper Use of This Medicine

To make using lutropin alfa as safe and reliable as possible, you should understand how and when to use this medicine and what effects may be expected. A paper with information for the patient will be given to you with your filled prescription and will provide many details concerning the use of lutropin alfa. Read this paper carefully and ask your health care professional for any additional information or explanation.

Sometimes lutropin alfa can be given by injection at home. If you are using this medicine at home:

- Understand and use the proper method of safely preparing the medicine if you are going to prepare your own medicine.
- Wash your hands with soap and water and use a clean work area to prepare your injection.
- Make sure you clearly understand and carefully follow your doctor's instructions on how to give yourself an injection, including using the proper needle and syringe.
- Do not inject more or less of the medicine than your doctor ordered.
- Remember to move the site of injection to different areas to prevent skin problems from developing.
- Throw away needles, syringes, bottles, and unused medicine after the injection in a safe manner.

Tell your doctor when you use the last dose of lutropin alfa. Follitropin alfa often requires that another hormone called human chorionic gonadotropin (hCG) be given as a single dose the day after the last dose of lutropin alfa is given. Your doctor will give you this medicine or arrange for you to get this medicine at the right time.

Dosing—The dose of this medicine will be different for different patients. Follow your doctor's orders or the directions on the label. The following information includes only the average doses of this medicine. If your dose is different, do not change it unless your doctor tells you to do so.

The amount of medicine that you take depends on the strength of the medicine. Also, the number of doses you take each day, the time allowed between doses, and the length of time you take the medicine depend on the medical problem for which you are using the medicine.

- For injection dosage form
  - For treatment of female infertility:
    - Adults—75 international units (IU) injected under the skin once a day for approximately fourteen days. Lutropin alfa is administered together with 75 to 150 IU of follitropin alfa as two separate injections. Using lutropin alfa for longer than fourteen days may be needed, but only if directed by your doctor. Report when you receive your last dose of lutropin alfa because you may be given an injection of hCG twenty-four hours later. If abdominal pain occurs with the use of lutropin alfa, report it to your doctor immediately, discontinue treatment, do not receive the dose of hCG, and avoid sexual intercourse.
    - Children—Not for use in children.

Missed dose—Call your doctor or pharmacist for instructions.

Storage—Store the medicine in a closed container at room temperature, away from heat, moisture, and direct light. Keep from freezing.

Keep out of the reach of children.

Do not keep outdated medicine or medicine no longer needed.

Precautions While Using This Medicine

It is very important that your doctor check your progress often at regular visits to make sure that the medicine is working properly and to check for unwanted effects. Your doctor will probably want to follow the developing eggs inside the ovaries by doing an ultrasound examination and measuring hormones in your blood stream. After you no longer receive lutropin alfa and follitropin alfa therapy, your progress still must be checked for at least 2 weeks.

If your doctor has asked you to record your basal body temperatures (BBTs) daily, make sure that you do this every day. Using a BBT record or some other method, your doctor will help you decide when you are most fertile and when ovulation occurs. It is important that sexual intercourse take place around the time when you are most fertile to give you the best chance of becoming pregnant. Follow your doctor's directions carefully.

If abdominal pain occurs with use of lutropin alfa, discontinue treatment and report the problem to your doctor immediately. Do not receive the injection of human chorionic gonadotropin (hCG) and avoid sexual intercourse.

Side Effects of This Medicine

Along with its needed effects, a medicine may cause some unwanted effects. Although not all of these side effects may occur, if they do occur they may need medical attention.

Stop taking this medicine and get emergency help immediately if any of the following effects occur:

Abdominal pain (severe), nausea, vomiting, and weight gain (rapid)

Check with your doctor as soon as possible if any of the following side effects occur:

More common
Bleeding, blistering, burning, coldness, discoloration of skin, feeling of pressure, hives, infection, inflammation, itching, lumps, numbness, pain, rash, redness, scarring, soreness, stinging, swelling, tenderness, tingling, ulceration, or warmth at injection site; bloating; stomach or pelvic discomfort, aching, or heaviness; diarrhea

Observed after pregnancy, frequency unknown
Congenital abnormalities; ectopic pregnancy; postpartum fever; premature labor; spontaneous abortion

Observed during menotropin therapy, frequency unknown
Adnexal torsion as a complication of ovarian enlargement; changes in skin color; cold hands and feet; blood in the peritoneal cavity; ovarian enlargement mild to moderate; pain, redness, or swelling in arm or leg; shortness of breath or troubled breathing

Symptoms of overdose
Get emergency help immediately if any of the following symptoms of overdose occur:
Abdominal pain; bloating; diarrhea; multiple gestation; rapid weight gain; severe nausea; vomiting

Some side effects may occur that usually do not need medical attention. These side effects may go away during treatment as your body adjusts to the medicine. Also, your health care professional may be able to tell you about ways to prevent or reduce some of these side effects. Check with your health care professional if any of the following side effects continue or are bothersome or if you have any questions about them:

More common
Breast pain; bloated full feeling; excess air or gas in stomach or intestines; headache; pain; passing gas; unusual tiredness or weakness

Less common
Body aches or pain; chills; cough; cramps; difficulty in breathing; difficulty having a bowel movement (stool); ear congestion; fever; heavy bleeding; loss of voice; nasal congestion; ovarian disorder; pain; runny nose; sneezing, or sore throat

---

MAFENIDE (Topical route) - MA-fe-nide

Commonly used brand name(s)

In the U.S.—
Sulfamylon

Available Dosage Forms:
- Powder for Solution
- Powder for Suspension
- Cream

Therapeutic Class: Antibacterial

Uses For This Medicine

Mafenide, a sulfa medicine, is used to prevent and treat bacterial or fungus infections. It works by preventing growth of the fungus or bacteria.

Mafenide cream is applied to the skin and/or burned area(s) to prevent and treat bacterial or fungus infections that may occur in burns.

Other medicines are used along with this medicine for burns. Patients with severe burns or burns over a large area of the body must be treated in a hospital.

This medicine is available only with your doctor's prescription.

Before Using This Medicine

In deciding to use a medicine, the risks of taking the medicine must be weighed against the good it will do. This is a decision you and your doctor will make. For this medicine, the following should be considered:

Allergies—Tell your doctor if you have ever had any unusual or allergic reaction to this medicine or any other medicines. Also tell your health care professional if you have any other types of allergies, such as to foods, dyes, preservatives, or animals. For non-prescription products, read the label or package ingredients carefully.

Pediatric—Use of mafenide is not recommended in premature or newborn infants up to 2 months of age. Sulfa medicines may cause liver problems in these infants.

Geriatric—Many medicines have not been tested in older people. Therefore, it may not be known whether they work exactly the same way they do in younger adults or if they cause different side effects or problems in older people. There is no specific information comparing use of mafenide in the elderly with use in other age groups.

Pregnancy—

	Pregnancy Category	Explanation
All Trimesters	C	Animal studies have shown an adverse effect and there are no adequate studies in pregnant women OR no animal studies have been conducted and there are no adequate studies in pregnant women.

Breast Feeding—There are no adequate studies in women for determining infant risk when using this medication during breastfeeding. Weigh the potential benefits against the potential risks before taking this medication while breastfeeding.

Other medicines—Although certain medicines should not be used together at all, in other cases two different medicines may be used together even if an interaction might occur. In these cases, your doctor may want to change the dose, or other precautions may be necessary. Tell your healthcare professional if you are taking any other prescription or non-prescription (over-the-counter [OTC]) medicine.

Interactions with Food/Tobacco/Alcohol—Certain medicines should not be used at or around the time of eating food or eating certain types of food since interactions may occur. Using alcohol or tobacco with certain medicines may also cause interactions to occur. Discuss with your healthcare professional the use of your medicine with food, alcohol, or tobacco.

Other medical problems—The presence of other medical problems may affect the use of this medicine. Make sure you tell your doctor if you have any other medical problems, especially:

- Blood problems—Use of mafenide may make the condition worse.
- Glucose-6–phosphate dehydrogenase deficiency (lack of G6PD enzyme)—Use of mafenide in persons with this condition may result in hemolytic anemia.
- Kidney problems or
- Lung problems or
- Metabolic acidosis—Use of mafenide in persons with any of these conditions may increase the risk of a side effect called metabolic acidosis.

Proper Use of This Medicine

To use:
- Before applying this medicine, cleanse the affected area(s). Remove dead or burned skin and other debris.
- Wear a sterile glove to apply this medicine. For the topical creak, apply a thin layer (about 1/16 inch) of mafenide to the affected area(s). For the topical solution, the solution is applied to the dressing covering the affected area(s). Keep the affected area(s) covered with the medicine at all times.
- If this medicine is rubbed off the affected area(s) by moving around or if it is washed off during bathing, showering, or the use of a whirlpool bath, reapply the medicine.
- After this medicine has been applied, the treated area(s) may be covered with a dressing or left uncovered as desired.

To help clear up your skin and/or burn infection completely, keep using mafenide for the full time of treatment. You should keep using this medicine until the burn area has healed or is ready for skin grafting. Do not miss any doses.

Dosing—The dose of this medicine will be different for different patients. Follow your doctor's orders or the directions on the label. The following information includes only the average doses of this medicine. If your dose is different, do not change it unless your doctor tells you to do so.

The amount of medicine that you take depends on the strength of the medicine. Also, the number of doses you take each day, the time allowed between doses, and the length of time you take the medicine depend on the medical problem for which you are using the medicine.

- For topical dosage form (cream):
  - For bacterial or fungus infection:
    - Adults and children 2 months of age and over— Use one or two times a day.
    - Infants and children up to 2 months of age—Use is not recommended.
- For topical dosage form (solution):
  - For bacterial or fungus infection:
    - Adults and children 3 months of age and over— Use every 4 to 8 hours each day as needed to keep the dressing wet.
    - Infants and children up to 3 months of age—Use is not recommended.

Missed dose—If you miss a dose of this medicine, apply it as soon as possible. However, if it is almost time for your next dose, skip the missed dose and go back to your regular dosing schedule.

Storage—Store the medicine in a closed container at room temperature, away from heat, moisture, and direct light. Keep from freezing.

Keep out of the reach of children.

Do not keep outdated medicine or medicine no longer needed.

Precautions While Using This Medicine

It is important that your doctor check your progress at regular visits.

If your skin infection or burn does not improve within a few days or if your more serious burns or burns over larger areas do not improve within a few weeks, or if they become worse, check with your doctor.

Side Effects of This Medicine

Along with its needed effects, a medicine may cause some unwanted effects. Although not all of these side effects may occur, if they do occur they may need medical attention.

Check with your doctor immediately if any of the following side effects occur:
Less common
   Itching; skin rash or redness; swelling of face or skin; wheezing or troubled breathing
Rare
   Bleeding or oozing of skin; drowsiness; fast, deep breathing; nausea
Incidence unknown
   Black, tarry stools; chest pain; chills; cough or hoarseness; dark urine; dizziness; fever; fluid-filled skin blis-

ters; light-colored stools; lower back or side pain; numbness to feet, hands and around mouth; painful or difficult urination; rapid shallow breathing; sensitivity to the sun; shortness of breath; skin thinness; sore throat; sores, ulcers, or white spots on lips or in mouth; swollen glands; unusual bleeding or bruising; unusual tiredness or weakness; yellow eyes or skin

Some side effects may occur that usually do not need medical attention. These side effects may go away during treatment as your body adjusts to the medicine. Also, your health care professional may be able to tell you about ways to prevent or reduce some of these side effects. Check with your health care professional if any of the following side effects continue or are bothersome or if you have any questions about them:

More common
   Pain or burning feeling on treated area(s)
Incidence unknown
   Blisters; flushing; raised red swellings on the skin, lips, tongue, or in the throat; redness of skin; skin rash; softening of the skin; swelling; unusually warm skin

Other side effects not listed may also occur in some patients. If you notice any other effects, check with your healthcare professional.

MAPROTILINE (Oral route) - ma-PROE-ti-leen

Commonly used brand name(s)

In the U.S.—
   Ludiomil

Available Dosage Forms:
   • Tablet

Therapeutic Class: Antidepressant
Pharmacologic Class: Antidepressant, Tetracyclic

Uses For This Medicine

Maprotiline is used to relieve mental depression, including anxiety that sometimes occurs with depression.

Maprotiline is available only with your doctor's prescription.

Once a medicine has been approved for marketing for a certain use, experience may show that it is also useful for other medical problems. Although this use is not included in product labeling, maprotiline is used in certain patients with the following medical condition:
   • Chronic neurogenic pain (a certain type of pain that is continuing)

Before Using This Medicine

In deciding to use a medicine, the risks of taking the medicine must be weighed against the good it will do. This is a decision you and your doctor will make. For this medicine, the following should be considered:

Allergies—Tell your doctor if you have ever had any unusual or allergic reaction to this medicine or any other medicines. Also tell your health care professional if you have any other types of allergies, such as to foods, dyes, preservatives,

or animals. For non-prescription products, read the label or package ingredients carefully.

Pediatric—Maprotiline must be used with caution in children with depression. Studies have shown occurrences of children thinking about suicide or attempting suicide in clinical trials for this medicine. More study is needed to be sure maprotiline is safe and effective in children

Geriatric—Drowsiness, dizziness or lightheadedness; confusion; vision problems; dryness of mouth; constipation; and difficulty in urinating may be especially likely to occur in elderly patients, who are usually more sensitive than younger adults to the effects of maprotiline.

Pregnancy—

	Pregnancy Category	Explanation
All Trimesters	B	Animal studies have revealed no evidence of harm to the fetus, however, there are no adequate studies in pregnant women OR animal studies have shown an adverse effect, but adequate studies in pregnant women have failed to demonstrate a risk to the fetus.

Breast Feeding—There are no adequate studies in women for determining infant risk when using this medication during breastfeeding. Weigh the potential benefits against the potential risks before taking this medication while breastfeeding.

Other medicines—

Using this medicine with any of the following medicines is not recommended. Your doctor may decide not to treat you with this medication or change some of the other medicines you take.

Cisapride, Clorgyline, Iproniazid, Isocarboxazid, Moclobemide, Nialamide, Pargyline, Phenelzine, Procarbazine, Selegiline, Toloxatone, Tranylcypromine

Interactions with Food/Tobacco/Alcohol—Certain medicines should not be used at or around the time of eating food or eating certain types of food since interactions may occur. Using alcohol or tobacco with certain medicines may also cause interactions to occur. Discuss with your healthcare professional the use of your medicine with food, alcohol, or tobacco.

Other medical problems—The presence of other medical problems may affect the use of this medicine. Make sure you tell your doctor if you have any other medical problems, especially:
   • Alcohol abuse or
   • Seizure disorders (including epilepsy)—The risk of seizures may be increased
   • Asthma or
   • Difficult urination or
   • Enlarged prostate or
   • Glaucoma or
   • Mental illness (severe) or
   • Stomach or intestinal problems—Maprotiline may make the condition worse
   • Heart or blood vessel disease or

- Overactive thyroid—Serious effects on your heart may occur
- Liver disease—Higher blood levels of maprotiline may occur, increasing the chance of side effects

Proper Use of This Medicine

Take this medicine only as directed by your doctor to benefit your condition as much as possible. Do not take more of it, do not take it more often, and do not take it for a longer time than your doctor ordered.

Sometimes this medicine must be taken for up to two or three weeks before you begin to feel better. Your doctor should check your progress at regular visits.

Dosing—The dose of this medicine will be different for different patients. Follow your doctor's orders or the directions on the label. The following information includes only the average doses of this medicine. If your dose is different, do not change it unless your doctor tells you to do so.

The amount of medicine that you take depends on the strength of the medicine. Also, the number of doses you take each day, the time allowed between doses, and the length of time you take the medicine depend on the medical problem for which you are using the medicine.

- For oral dosage form (tablets):
  - For depression:
    - Adults—At first, 25 milligrams (mg) taken one to three times a day. Your doctor may increase your dose as needed. However, the dose is usually not more than 150 mg a day, unless you are in the hospital. Some hospitalized patients may need higher doses.
    - Children—Use and dose must be determined by your doctor.

Missed dose—If you miss a dose of this medicine, take it as soon as possible. However, if it is almost time for your next dose, skip the missed dose and go back to your regular dosing schedule. Do not double doses.

For once daily dosing at bedtime: Do not take the missed dose in the morning since it may cause disturbing side effects during waking hours. Instead, check with your doctor.

Storage—Store the medicine in a closed container at room temperature, away from heat, moisture, and direct light. Keep from freezing.

Keep out of the reach of children.

Do not keep outdated medicine or medicine no longer needed.

Precautions While Using This Medicine

It is very important that your doctor check your progress at regular visits. This will allow your dosage to be changed if necessary and will help to reduce side effects.

This medicine will add to the effects of alcohol and other CNS depressants (medicines that slow down the nervous system, possibly causing drowsiness). Some examples of CNS depressants are antihistamines or medicine for hay fever, other allergies, or colds; sedatives, tranquilizers, or sleeping medicine; prescription pain medicine or narcotics; barbiturates; medicine for seizures; or anesthetics, including some dental anesthetics. Check with your doctor before taking any of the above while you are using this medicine.

Maprotiline may cause some people to be agitated, irritable or display other abnormal behaviors. It may also cause some people to have suicidal thoughts and tendencies or to become more depressed. If you or your caregiver notice any of these adverse effects, tell your doctor right away.

This medicine may cause blurred vision, especially during the first few weeks of treatment. It may also cause some people to become drowsy or less alert than they are normally. If these effects occur, do not drive, use machines, or do anything else that could be dangerous if you are not alert or able to see well.

Dizziness, lightheadedness, or fainting may occur, especially when you get up from a lying or sitting position. Getting up slowly may help. If this problem continues or gets worse, check with your doctor.

Maprotiline may cause dryness of the mouth. For temporary relief, use sugarless gum or candy, melt bits of ice in your mouth, or use a saliva substitute. However, if your mouth continues to feel dry for more than 2 weeks, check with your medical doctor or dentist. Continuing dryness of the mouth may increase the chance of dental disease, including tooth decay, gum disease, and fungus infections.

Before having any kind of surgery, dental treatment, or emergency treatment, tell the medical doctor or dentist in charge that you are using this medicine. Taking maprotiline together with medicines that are used during surgery or dental or emergency treatments may increase the CNS depressant effects.

Do not stop taking this medicine without first checking with your doctor. Your doctor may want you to reduce gradually the amount you are taking before stopping completely. This will allow your body to adjust properly and will reduce the possibility of unwanted effects.

Side Effects of This Medicine

Along with its needed effects, a medicine may cause some unwanted effects. Although not all of these side effects may occur, if they do occur they may need medical attention.

Check with your doctor as soon as possible if any of the following side effects occur:

More common
  Skin rash, redness, swelling, or itching
Less common
  Constipation (severe); nausea or vomiting; shakiness or trembling; seizures (convulsions); unusual excitement; weight loss
Rare
  Breast enlargement— in males and females; confusion (especially in the elderly); difficulty in urinating; fainting; hallucinations (seeing, hearing, or feeling things that are not there); inappropriate secretion of milk— in females; irregular heartbeat (pounding, racing, skipping); sore throat and fever; swelling of testicles; yellow eyes or skin
Symptoms of overdose
  Convulsions (seizures); dizziness (severe); drowsiness (severe); fast or irregular heartbeat; fever; muscle stiffness or weakness (severe); restlessness or agitation; trouble in breathing; vomiting

Some side effects may occur that usually do not need medical attention. These side effects may go away during treat-

ment as your body adjusts to the medicine. Also, your health care professional may be able to tell you about ways to prevent or reduce some of these side effects. Check with your health care professional if any of the following side effects continue or are bothersome or if you have any questions about them:

More common
Blurred vision; decreased sexual ability; dizziness or lightheadedness (especially in the elderly); drowsiness; dryness of mouth; headache; increased or decreased sexual drive; tiredness or weakness

Less common
Constipation (mild); diarrhea; heartburn; increased appetite and weight gain; increased sensitivity of skin to sunlight; increased sweating; trouble in sleeping; weight loss

After you stop using this medicine, it may still produce some side effects that need attention. During this period of time, *check with your doctor immediately* if you notice the following side effects:

Other side effects not listed may also occur in some patients. If you notice any other effects, check with your healthcare professional.

MEASLES VIRUS VACCINE, LIVE
(Subcutaneous route) - MEE-zuls VYE-rus vak-SEEN, lyve

Commonly used brand name(s)
In the U.S.—
Attenuvax

Available Dosage Forms:
• Powder for Solution

Therapeutic Class: Vaccine

Uses For This Vaccine

Measles Virus Vaccine Live is an immunizing agent used to prevent infection by the measles virus. It works by causing your body to produce its own protection (antibodies) against the virus. This vaccine does not protect you against German measles (Rubella). A separate immunization is needed for that type of measles.

Measles (also known as coughing measles, hard measles, morbilli, red measles, rubeola, and ten-day measles) is an infection that is easily spread from one person to another. Infection with measles can lead to serious problems, such as pneumonia, ear infections, sinus problems, convulsions (seizures), brain damage, and possibly death. The risk of serious complications and death is greater for adults and infants than for children and teenagers.

Immunization against measles is recommended for everyone 12 to 15 months of age and older. In addition, there may be special reasons why children from 6 months of age up to 12 months of age may also require measles vaccine.

Immunization against measles is usually not recommended for infants up to 12 months of age, unless the risk of their getting a measles infection is high. This is because antibodies they received from their mothers before birth may interfere with the effectiveness of the vaccine. Children who were immunized against measles before 12 months of age should be immunized twice again.

You can be considered to be immune to measles only if you received two doses of measles vaccine starting on or after your first birthday and have the medical record to prove it, if you have a doctor's diagnosis of a previous measles infection, or if you have had a blood test showing immunity to measles.

This vaccine is to be administered only by or under the supervision of your doctor or other health care professional.

Before Receiving This Vaccine

In deciding to use a vaccine, the risks of taking the vaccine must be weighed against the good it will do. This is a decision you and your doctor will make. For this vaccine, the following should be considered:

Allergies—Tell your doctor if you have ever had any unusual or allergic reaction to this medicine or any other medicines. Also tell your health care professional if you have any other types of allergies, such as to foods, dyes, preservatives, or animals. For non-prescription products, read the label or package ingredients carefully.

Pediatric—Measles vaccine usually is not recommended for infants up to 12 months of age. In special cases, such as children traveling outside the U.S. or children living in high-risk areas, measles vaccine may be given to children as young as 6 months of age.

Pregnancy—

	Pregnancy Category	Explanation
All Trimesters	C	Animal studies have shown an adverse effect and there are no adequate studies in pregnant women OR no animal studies have been conducted and there are no adequate studies in pregnant women.

Breast Feeding—Studies in women suggest that this medication poses minimal risk to the infant when used during breastfeeding.

Other medicines—

Receiving this vaccine with any of the following medicines is usually not recommended, but may be required in some cases. If both medicines are prescribed together, your doctor may change the dose or how often you use one or both of the medicines.

Aclarubicin, Aldesleukin, Alemtuzumab, Altretamine, Amonafide, Amsacrine, Asparaginase, Azacitidine, Azathioprine, Bleomycin, Broxuridine, Busulfan, Capecitabine, Carboplatin, Carmustine, Chlorambucil, Cisplatin, Cladribine, Cyclophosphamide, Cytarabine, Cytarabine Liposome, Dacarbazine, Dactinomycin, Daunorubicin, Daunorubicin Citrate Liposome, Decitabine, Docetaxel, Doxifluridine, Doxorubicin Hydrochloride, Doxorubicin Hydrochloride Liposome, Edatrexate, Eflornithine, Epirubicin, Estramustine, Etoposide, Floxuridine, Fludarabine, Fluorouracil, Fotemustine, Gallium Nitrate, Gemcitabine, Hydroxyurea, Idarubicin, Ifosfamide, Interferon Alfa,

Interferon Alfacon-1, Interferon Beta, Interferon Beta-1a, Interferon Beta-1b, Interferon Gamma, Irinotecan, Lomustine, Mechlorethamine, Melphalan, Meningococcal Polysaccharide Vaccine, Mercaptopurine, Methotrexate, Mitolactol, Mitomycin, Mitotane, Mitoxantrone, Oxaliplatin, Paclitaxel, Pegaspargase, Pentostatin, Pipobroman, Pirarubicin, Plicamycin, Procarbazine, Raltitrexed, Rituximab, Sirolimus, Streptozocin, Tacrolimus, Teceleukin, Tegafur, Teniposide, Thioguanine, Thiotepa, Topotecan, Treosulfan, Trimetrexate, Trofosfamide, Uracil Mustard, Vinblastine, Vincristine, Vincristine Liposome, Vindesine, Vinorelbine

Interactions with Food/Tobacco/Alcohol—Certain medicines should not be used at or around the time of eating food or eating certain types of food since interactions may occur. Using alcohol or tobacco with certain medicines may also cause interactions to occur. Discuss with your healthcare professional the use of your medicine with food, alcohol, or tobacco.

Other medical problems—The presence of other medical problems may affect the use of this vaccine. Make sure you tell your doctor if you have any other medical problems, especially:

- Immune deficiency condition (or family history of)—Condition may increase the chance and severity of side effects of the vaccine and/or may decrease the useful effects of the vaccine

- Severe illness with fever—The symptoms of the condition may be confused with the possible side effects of the vaccine

Proper Use of This Vaccine

Dosing—The dose of this medicine will be different for different patients. Follow your doctor's orders or the directions on the label. The following information includes only the average doses of this medicine. If your dose is different, do not change it unless your doctor tells you to do so.

The amount of medicine that you take depends on the strength of the medicine. Also, the number of doses you take each day, the time allowed between doses, and the length of time you take the medicine depend on the medical problem for which you are using the medicine.

- For injection dosage form:
  - For prevention of measles:
    - Adults and children 12 months of age and older— One dose injected under the skin, followed by a second dose at least one month later.

Precautions While Using This Vaccine

Do not become pregnant for 3 months after receiving measles vaccine without first checking with your doctor.

Tell your doctor that you have received this vaccine:

- If you are to receive a tuberculin skin test within 4 to 6 weeks after receiving this vaccine. The results of the test may be affected by this vaccine.

- If you are to receive this vaccine within 2 weeks before or 3 to 11 months after receiving blood transfusions or other blood products.

- If you are to receive this vaccine 2 weeks before or 3 to 11 months after receiving gamma globulin or other immune globulins.

Side Effects of This Vaccine

Along with its needed effects, a medicine may cause some unwanted effects. Although not all of these side effects may occur, if they do occur they may need medical attention.

Check with your doctor immediately if any of the following side effects occur:
> *Symptoms of allergic reaction*
>> Difficulty in breathing or swallowing; hives; itching, especially of feet or hands; reddening of skin, especially around ears; swelling of eyes, face, or inside of nose; unusual tiredness or weakness (sudden and severe)

Check with your doctor as soon as possible if any of the following side effects occur:
> *More common*
>> Fever over 103 °F (39.4 °C)
> *Rare*
>> Bruising or purple spots on skin; confusion; double vision; headache (severe or continuing); irritability; stiff neck; swelling, blistering or pain at place of injection; swelling of glands in neck; vomiting

Some side effects may occur that usually do not need medical attention. These side effects may go away during treatment as your body adjusts to the medicine. Also, your health care professional may be able to tell you about ways to prevent or reduce some of these side effects. Check with your health care professional if any of the following side effects continue or are bothersome or if you have any questions about them:
> *More common*
>> Burning or stinging at place of injection; fever of 100 °F (37.7 °C) or less
> *Less common*
>> Fever between 100 and 103 °F (37.7 and 39.4 °C); itching, swelling, redness, tenderness, or hard lump at place of injection; skin rash

Fever or skin rash may occur from 5 to 12 days after vaccination and usually lasts several days.

Other side effects not listed may also occur in some patients. If you notice any other effects, check with your healthcare professional.

MEASLES, MUMPS, AND RUBELLA VIRUS VACCINE LIVE
(Subcutaneous route, Intramuscular route) - MEE-zuls, mumps, roo-BELL-a VYE-rus vak-SEEN lyve

Commonly used brand name(s)
In the U.S.—
M-M-R II

Available Dosage Forms:
- Powder for Solution

Therapeutic Class: Vaccine

Uses For This Vaccine

Measles, mumps, and rubella virus vaccine live is an active immunizing agent used to prevent infection by the measles, mumps, and rubella viruses. It works by causing your body to produce its own protection (antibodies) against the virus.

Measles (also known as coughing measles, hard measles, morbilli, red measles, rubeola, and 10–day measles) is an infection that is easily spread from one person to another. Infection with measles can cause serious problems, such as stomach problems, pneumonia, ear infections, sinus problems, convulsions (seizures), brain damage, and possibly death. The risk of serious complications and death is greater for adults and infants than for children and teenagers.

Mumps is an infection that can cause serious problems, such as encephalitis and meningitis, which affect the brain. In addition, adolescent boys and men are very susceptible to a condition called orchitis, which causes pain and swelling in the testicles and scrotum and, in rare cases, sterility. Also, mumps infection can cause spontaneous abortion (miscarriage) in women during the first 3 months of pregnancy.

Rubella (also known as German measles) is a serious infection that causes miscarriages, stillbirths, or birth defects in unborn babies when pregnant women get the disease.

While immunization against measles, mumps, and rubella is recommended for all persons 12 months of age and older, it is especially important for women of childbearing age and persons traveling outside the U.S.

If measles, mumps, and rubella vaccine is to be given to a child, the child should be at least 12 months of age. This is to make sure the measles vaccine is effective. In a younger child, antibodies from the mother may interfere with the effectiveness of the vaccine.

This vaccine should be administered only by or under the supervision of your doctor or other health care professional.

Before Receiving This Vaccine

In deciding to use a vaccine, the risks of taking the vaccine must be weighed against the good it will do. This is a decision you and your doctor will make. For this vaccine, the following should be considered:

Allergies—Tell your doctor if you have ever had any unusual or allergic reaction to this medicine or any other medicines. Also tell your health care professional if you have any other types of allergies, such as to foods, dyes, preservatives, or animals. For non-prescription products, read the label or package ingredients carefully.

Pediatric—Use is not recommended for infants younger than 12 months of age, unless the risk of measles infection is high. Waiting until children are at least 12 months of age is important because antibodies that infants receive from their mothers before birth may interfere with the effectiveness of the vaccine. There may be special reasons why children between 6 months and 12 months of age also may require measles vaccination.

Pregnancy—

	Pregnancy Category	Explanation
All Trimesters	C	Animal studies have shown an adverse effect and there are no adequate studies in pregnant women OR no animal studies have been conducted and there are no adequate studies in pregnant women.

Breast Feeding—

Measles Virus Vaccine, Live
- Studies in women suggest that this medication poses minimal risk to the infant when used during breastfeeding.

Mumps Virus Vaccine, Live
- Studies in women suggest that this medication poses minimal risk to the infant when used during breastfeeding.

Rubella Virus Vaccine, Live
- There are no adequate studies in women for determining infant risk when using this medication during breastfeeding. Weigh the potential benefits against the potential risks before taking this medication while breastfeeding.

Other medicines—

Receiving this vaccine with any of the following medicines is usually not recommended, but may be required in some cases. If both medicines are prescribed together, your doctor may change the dose or how often you use one or both of the medicines.

Aclarubicin, Aldesleukin, Alemtuzumab, Altretamine, Amonafide, Amsacrine, Asparaginase, Azacitidine, Azathioprine, Bleomycin, Broxuridine, Busulfan, Capecitabine, Carboplatin, Carmustine, Chlorambucil, Cisplatin, Cladribine, Cyclophosphamide, Cytarabine, Cytarabine Liposome, Dacarbazine, Dactinomycin, Daunorubicin, Daunorubicin Citrate Liposome, Decitabine, Docetaxel, Doxifluridine, Doxorubicin Hydrochloride, Doxorubicin Hydrochloride Liposome, Edatrexate, Eflornithine, Epirubicin, Estramustine, Etoposide, Floxuridine, Fludarabine, Fluorouracil, Fotemustine, Gallium Nitrate, Gemcitabine, Hydroxyurea, Idarubicin, Ifosfamide, Interferon Alfa, Interferon Alfacon-1, Interferon Beta, Interferon Beta-1a, Interferon Beta-1b, Interferon Gamma, Irinotecan, Lomustine, Mechlorethamine, Melphalan, Meningococcal Polysaccharide Vaccine, Mercaptopurine, Methotrexate, Mitolactol, Mitomycin, Mitotane, Mitoxantrone, Oxaliplatin, Paclitaxel, Pegaspargase, Pentostatin, Pipobroman, Pirarubicin, Plicamycin, Procarbazine, Raltitrexed, Rituximab, Sirolimus, Streptozocin, Tacrolimus, Teceleukin, Tegafur, Teniposide, Thioguanine, Thiotepa, Topotecan, Treosulfan, Trimetrexate, Trofosfamide, Uracil Mustard, Vinblastine, Vincristine, Vincristine Liposome, Vindesine, Vinorelbine

Interactions with Food/Tobacco/Alcohol—Certain medicines should not be used at or around the time of eating food or eating certain types of food since interactions may occur. Using alcohol or tobacco with certain medicines may also cause interactions to occur. Discuss with your healthcare professional the use of your medicine with food, alcohol, or tobacco.

Other medical problems—The presence of other medical problems may affect the use of this vaccine. Make sure you

tell your doctor if you have any other medical problems, especially:

- Immune deficiency condition (or family history of)—Condition may increase the chance of developing side effects and the severity of side effects of the vaccine and/or may decrease the useful effects of the vaccine
- Severe illness with fever—The symptoms of the condition may be confused with the possible side effects of the vaccine

Proper Use of This Vaccine

Dosing—The dose of this medicine will be different for different patients. Follow your doctor's orders or the directions on the label. The following information includes only the average doses of this medicine. If your dose is different, do not change it unless your doctor tells you to do so.

The amount of medicine that you take depends on the strength of the medicine. Also, the number of doses you take each day, the time allowed between doses, and the length of time you take the medicine depend on the medical problem for which you are using the medicine.

- For injection dosage form:
  - For prevention of measles, mumps, and rubella:
    - Adults and children 12 months of age and older—One dose injected under the skin.
    - Children up to 12 months of age—Use is not recommended.

Precautions While Using This Vaccine

Do not become pregnant for 3 months after receiving measles, mumps, and rubella vaccine. There is a chance that this vaccine may cause birth defects.

Tell your doctor that you have received this vaccine:

- If you are to receive a tuberculin skin test within 8 weeks after receiving this vaccine. The results of the test may be affected by this vaccine.
- If you are to receive any other live virus vaccines within 1 month after receiving this vaccine.
- If you are to receive blood transfusions or other blood products within 2 weeks after receiving this vaccine.
- If you are to receive gamma globulin or other globulins within 2 weeks after receiving this vaccine.

Side Effects of This Vaccine

Along with its needed effects, a medicine may cause some unwanted effects. Although not all of these side effects may occur, if they do occur they may need medical attention.

Check with your doctor immediately if any of the following side effects occur:

Symptoms of allergic reaction
  Difficulty in breathing or swallowing; hives; itching, especially of feet or hands; reddening of skin, especially around ears; swelling of eyes, face, or inside of nose; unusual tiredness or weakness (sudden and severe)

Check with your doctor as soon as possible if any of the following side effects occur:

More common
  Fever higher than 103 °F (39.4 °C)

Less common
  Pain or tenderness of eyes

Rare
  Bruising or purple spots on skin; confusion; convulsions (seizures); double vision; headache (severe or continuing); irritability; pain, numbness, or tingling of hands, arms, legs, or feet; pain, tenderness, or swelling in testicles and scrotum; stiff neck; vomiting

Some side effects may occur that usually do not need medical attention. These side effects may go away during treatment as your body adjusts to the medicine. Also, your health care professional may be able to tell you about ways to prevent or reduce some of these side effects. Check with your health care professional if any of the following side effects continue or are bothersome or if you have any questions about them:

More common
  Burning or stinging at place of injection; fever between 100 and 103 °F (37.7 and 39.4 °C); skin rash; swelling of glands in neck

Less common
  Aches or pain in joints; headache (mild); itching, swelling, redness, tenderness, or hard lump at place of injection; nausea; runny nose; sore throat; vague feeling of bodily discomfort

The above side effects (especially aches or pain in joints) are more likely to occur in adults, particularly women.

Other side effects not listed may also occur in some patients. If you notice any other effects, check with your healthcare professional.

MEBENDAZOLE (Oral route) - me-BEN-da-zole

Commonly used brand name(s)
In the U.S.—
  Vermox

Available Dosage Forms:
- Tablet, Chewable
- Suspension

Therapeutic Class: Anthelmintic

Uses For This Medicine

Mebendazole belongs to the family of medicines called anthelmintics. Anthelmintics are medicines used in the treatment of worm infections.

Mebendazole is used to treat:
- Common roundworms (ascariasis);
- Hookworm infections (uncinariasis);
- Pinworms (enterobiasis; oxyuriasis);
- Whipworms (trichuriasis); and
- More than one worm infection at a time.

This medicine may also be used for other worm infections as determined by your doctor.

Mebendazole works by keeping the worm from absorbing sugar (glucose). This gradually causes loss of energy and death of the worm.

Mebendazole is available only with your doctor's prescription.

Before Using This Medicine

In deciding to use a medicine, the risks of taking the medicine must be weighed against the good it will do. This is a decision you and your doctor will make. For this medicine, the following should be considered:

Allergies—Tell your doctor if you have ever had any unusual or allergic reaction to this medicine or any other medicines. Also tell your health care professional if you have any other types of allergies, such as to foods, dyes, preservatives, or animals. For non-prescription products, read the label or package ingredients carefully.

Pediatric—This medicine has been tested in a limited number of children 2 years of age or older and, in effective doses, has not been shown to cause different side effects or problems in children than it does in adults.

Geriatric—Many medicines have not been studied specifically in older people. Therefore, it may not be known whether they work exactly the same way they do in younger adults or if they cause different side effects or problems in older people. There is no specific information comparing use of mebendazole in the elderly with use in other age groups.

Pregnancy—

	Pregnancy Category	Explanation
All Trimesters	C	Animal studies have shown an adverse effect and there are no adequate studies in pregnant women OR no animal studies have been conducted and there are no adequate studies in pregnant women.

Breast Feeding—There are no adequate studies in women for determining infant risk when using this medication during breastfeeding. Weigh the potential benefits against the potential risks before taking this medication while breastfeeding.

Other medicines—Although certain medicines should not be used together at all, in other cases two different medicines may be used together even if an interaction might occur. In these cases, your doctor may want to change the dose, or other precautions may be necessary. Tell your healthcare professional if you are taking any other prescription or non-prescription (over-the-counter [OTC]) medicine.

Interactions with Food/Tobacco/Alcohol—Certain medicines should not be used at or around the time of eating food or eating certain types of food since interactions may occur. Using alcohol or tobacco with certain medicines may also cause interactions to occur. Discuss with your healthcare professional the use of your medicine with food, alcohol, or tobacco.

Other medical problems—The presence of other medical problems may affect the use of this medicine. Make sure you tell your doctor if you have any other medical problems, especially:

- Crohn's disease or
- Liver disease or
- Ulcerative colitis—Patients with these diseases may have an increased chance of side effects from mebendazole

Proper Use of This Medicine

Mebendazole usually comes with patient directions. Read them carefully before using this medicine.

No special preparations or other steps (for example, special diets, fasting, other medicines, laxatives, or enemas) are necessary before, during, or immediately after taking mebendazole.

Mebendazole tablets may be chewed, swallowed whole, or crushed and mixed with food.

For patients taking mebendazole for hookworms, roundworms, or whipworms:

- To help clear up your infection completely, take this medicine exactly as directed by your doctor for the full time of treatment. In some patients a second course of this medicine may be required to clear up the infection completely. Do not miss any doses.

For patients taking mebendazole for pinworms:

- To help clear up your infection completely, take this medicine exactly as directed by your doctor. A second course of this medicine is usually required to clear up the infection completely.
- Pinworms may be easily passed from one person to another, especially in a household. Therefore, all household members may have to be treated at the same time. This helps to prevent infection or reinfection of other household members. Also, all household members may have to be treated again in 2 to 3 weeks to clear up the infection completely.

For patients taking mebendazole for infections in which high doses are needed:

- Mebendazole is best taken with meals, especially fatty ones (for example, meals that include whole milk or ice cream). This helps to clear up the infection by helping your body absorb the medicine better. However, if you are on a low-fat diet, check with your doctor.

Dosing—The dose of this medicine will be different for different patients. Follow your doctor's orders or the directions on the label. The following information includes only the average doses of this medicine. If your dose is different, do not change it unless your doctor tells you to do so.

The amount of medicine that you take depends on the strength of the medicine. Also, the number of doses you take each day, the time allowed between doses, and the length of time you take the medicine depend on the medical problem for which you are using the medicine.

- For oral dosage form (chewable tablets):
  - For common roundworms, hookworms, and whipworms:
    - Adults and children 2 years of age and over—100 milligrams (mg) two times a day, morning and evening, for three days. Treatment may need to be repeated in two to three weeks.
    - Children up to 2 years of age—Use and dose must be determined by your doctor.
  - For pinworms:
    - Adults and children 2 years of age and over—100 mg once a day for one day. Treatment may need to be repeated in two to three weeks.
    - Children up to 2 years of age—Use and dose must be determined by your doctor.

◦ For more than one worm infection at a time:
  ▪ Adults and children 2 years of age and over— 100 mg two times a day, morning and evening, for three days.
  ▪ Children up to 2 years of age—Use and dose must be determined by your doctor.

Missed dose—If you miss a dose of this medicine, take it as soon as possible. However, if it is almost time for your next dose, skip the missed dose and go back to your regular dosing schedule. Do not double doses.

Storage—Store the medicine in a closed container at room temperature, away from heat, moisture, and direct light. Keep from freezing.

Keep out of the reach of children.

Do not keep outdated medicine or medicine no longer needed.

Precautions While Using This Medicine

It is important that your doctor check your progress at regular visits, especially in infections in which high doses are needed. This is to make sure that the infection is cleared up completely and to allow your doctor to check for any unwanted effects.

If your symptoms do not improve within a few days, or if they become worse, check with your doctor.

For patients taking mebendazole for pinworms:
- In some patients, pinworms may return after treatment with mebendazole. Washing (not shaking) all bedding and nightclothes (pajamas) after treatment may help to prevent this.
- Some doctors may also recommend other measures to help keep your infection from returning. If you have any questions about this, check with your doctor.

For patients taking mebendazole for hookworms or whipworms:
- In hookworm and whipworm infections anemia may occur. Therefore, your doctor may want you to take iron supplements to help clear up the anemia. If so, it is important to take iron every day while you are being treated for hookworms or whipworms; do not miss any doses. Your doctor may also want you to keep taking iron supplements for up to 6 months after you stop taking mebendazole. If you have any questions about this, check with your doctor.

Side Effects of This Medicine

Along with its needed effects, a medicine may cause some unwanted effects. Although not all of these side effects may occur, if they do occur they may need medical attention.

Check with your doctor as soon as possible if any of the following side effects occur:
  Rare
    Fever; skin rash or itching; sore throat and fever; unusual tiredness and weakness

Some side effects may occur that usually do not need medical attention. These side effects may go away during treatment as your body adjusts to the medicine. Also, your health care professional may be able to tell you about ways to prevent or reduce some of these side effects. Check with your health care professional if any of the following side effects continue or are bothersome or if you have any questions about them:

  Less common
    Abdominal or stomach pain or upset; diarrhea; nausea or vomiting
  Rare
    Dizziness; hair loss; headache

Other side effects not listed may also occur in some patients. If you notice any other effects, check with your healthcare professional.

MECASERMIN (Subcutaneous route) - mek-a-SER-min

Commonly used brand name(s)

In the U.S.—
  Increlex
  Iplex

Available Dosage Forms:
- Solution

Therapeutic Class: Endocrine-Metabolic Agent

Uses For This Medicine

Mecasermin is a synthetic (man-made) version of insulin-like growth factor-1 (IGF-1) hormone. IGF-1 is produced in the liver and plays an important role in childhood growth. Mecasermin is used to replace IGF-1 in children who are severely lacking it in their bodies.

This medicine is available only with your doctor's prescription.

Before Using This Medicine

In deciding to use a medicine, the risks of taking the medicine must be weighed against the good it will do. This is a decision you and your doctor will make. For this medicine, the following should be considered:

Allergies—Tell your doctor if you have ever had any unusual or allergic reaction to this medicine or any other medicines. Also tell your health care professional if you have any other types of allergies, such as to foods, dyes, preservatives, or animals. For non-prescription products, read the label or package ingredients carefully.

Pediatric—Studies on this medicine have not been done in children under 2 years of age.

Geriatric—This medicine is not used in adults or older adults.

Pregnancy—

	Pregnancy Category	Explanation
All Trimesters	C	Animal studies have shown an adverse effect and there are no adequate studies in pregnant women OR no animal studies have been conducted and there are no adequate studies in pregnant women.

Breast Feeding—There are no adequate studies in women for determining infant risk when using this medication during

breastfeeding. Weigh the potential benefits against the potential risks before taking this medication while breastfeeding.

Other medicines—Although certain medicines should not be used together at all, in other cases two different medicines may be used together even if an interaction might occur. In these cases, your doctor may want to change the dose, or other precautions may be necessary. Tell your healthcare professional if you are taking any other prescription or non-prescription (over-the-counter [OTC]) medicine.

Interactions with Food/Tobacco/Alcohol—Certain medicines should not be used at or around the time of eating food or eating certain types of food since interactions may occur. Using alcohol or tobacco with certain medicines may also cause interactions to occur. Discuss with your healthcare professional the use of your medicine with food, alcohol, or tobacco.

Other medical problems—The presence of other medical problems may affect the use of this medicine. Make sure you tell your doctor if you have any other medical problems, especially:

- Closed epiphyses (e.g., growth centers in the bones show no more growth potential)—Mecasermin should NOT be used in these patients.

- Hypothyroidism (e.g., underactive thyroid) or

- Nutrition deficiencies—These problems should be corrected before starting treatment with mecasermin.

- Neoplasia, active or suspected (e.g., cancerous or non-cancerous tumor)—Mecasermin should NOT be used. It should be discontinued if signs of neoplasia occur.

Proper Use of This Medicine

Some medicines given by injection may sometimes be given at home to patients who do not need to be in the hospital. If you are using this medicine at home, your health care professional will teach you how to prepare and inject the medicine. You will have a chance to practice preparing and injecting it. *Be certain that you understand exactly how the medicine is to be prepared and injected.*

It is important to read the patient information and instructions for use, if provided with your medicine, each time your prescription is filled.

This medicine must be taken 20 minutes before or 20 minutes after a snack or meal.

If a meal or snack is not given, then the dose should not be given.

It is important to follow any instructions from your doctor about the careful selection and rotation of injection sites on your body. This will help to prevent skin problems.

This medicine should NEVER be injected into a vein or muscle. It should always be injected under the skin.

Put used needles and syringes in a puncture-resistant disposable container or dispose of them as directed by your health care professional. *Do not reuse needles and syringes.*

Dosing—The dose of this medicine will be different for different patients. Follow your doctor's orders or the directions on the label. The following information includes only the average doses of this medicine. If your dose is different, do not change it unless your doctor tells you to do so.

The amount of medicine that you take depends on the strength of the medicine. Also, the number of doses you take each day, the time allowed between doses, and the length of time you take the medicine depend on the medical problem for which you are using the medicine.

- For injection
  - For treatment of growth failure caused by IGF-1 deficiency:
    - Children—At first, 0.04 to 0.08 milligrams (mg) per kg (0.018 to 0.036 mg per lb) under the skin two times a day. Your doctor may then increase the dose, if necessary.

Missed dose—Call your doctor or pharmacist for instructions. Do not double doses.

Storage—Keep out of the reach of children.

Store in the refrigerator. Do not freeze.

Ask your healthcare professional how you should dispose of any medicine you do not use.

Be sure that any discarded medicine is out of the reach of children.

Precautions While Using This Medicine

It is very important that your doctor check you at regular visits.

This medicine may cause low blood sugar with the following symptoms that you should be aware of: anxiety; blurred vision; chills; cold sweats; coma; confusion; cool pale skin; depression; dizziness; fast heartbeat; headache; increased hunger; nausea; nervousness; nightmares; seizures; shakiness; slurred speech; unusual tiredness or weakness. It is important to have a source of sugar such as orange juice, candy, soda, glucose gel, or milk, if these symptoms occur.

You should avoid participating in high risk activities such as driving within 2 to 3 hours after your mecasermin injection, especially at the beginning of mecasermin treatment.

Side Effects of This Medicine

Along with its needed effects, a medicine may cause some unwanted effects. Although not all of these side effects may occur, if they do occur they may need medical attention.

Check with your doctor immediately if any of the following side effects occur:

More common
Anxiety; bluish skin color of fingertips; blurred vision; breathlessness; chest pain; chills; cold sweats; coma; confusion; cool pale skin; depression; dizziness; fast heartbeat; fatigue; headache; increased hunger; loss of hearing; nausea; nervousness; nightmares; rapid growth of normal cells of thymus (no symptoms); seizures; shakiness; slurred speech; thickening of the skin; unusual tiredness or weakness

Incidence not known
Change in ability to see colors, especially blue or yellow; limp; pain in hip or knee; vomiting

Symptoms of overdose

Get emergency help immediately if any of the following symptoms of overdose occur:

Anxiety; backache; blurred vision; changes in vision; chills; cold sweats; coma; confusion; cool pale skin; depression; dizziness; excessive sweating; extreme weakness; fast heartbeat; frequent urination; headache; increase in hands and feet size; increased hunger; increased thirst; increased volume of pale diluted urine; joint pain; nausea; nervousness; nightmares; pain in extremities; seizures; shakiness;

slurred speech; stop in menstruation; unusual tired-ness or weakness

Some side effects may occur that usually do not need medical attention. These side effects may go away during treatment as your body adjusts to the medicine. Also, your health care professional may be able to tell you about ways to prevent or reduce some of these side effects. Check with your health care professional if any of the following side effects continue or are bothersome or if you have any questions about them:

More common
  Abnormal response of tympanic membrane to air pres-sure; difficulty in moving; difficulty swallowing; dizzi-ness; ear pain; earache; large, flat, blue or purplish patches in the skin; muffled hearing; muscle pain or stiffness; pain in arms or legs; pain in joints; redness or swelling in ear; sense of fullness in the ear; snoring; sore throat; voice changing

Other side effects not listed may also occur in some patients. If you notice any other effects, check with your healthcare professional.

MECHLORETHAMINE (Intravenous route) - me-klor-ETH-a-meen

Black Box Warning

Mechlorethamine hydrochloride should be administered only under the supervision of a physician who is experienced in the use of cancer chemotherapeutic agents.

This drug is highly toxic and both powder and solution must be handled and administered with care. Inhalation of dust or vapors and contact with skin or mucous membranes, espe-cially those of the eyes, must be avoided. Avoid exposure during pregnancy. Due to the toxic properties of mechloreth-amine (eg, corrosivity, carcinogenicity, mutagenicity, terato-genicity), special handling procedures should be reviewed prior to handling and followed diligently.

Extravasation of the drug into subcutaneous tissues results in a painful inflammation. The area usually becomes indu-rated and sloughing may occur. If leakage of drug is obvious, prompt infiltration of the area with sterile isotonic sodium thi-osulfate (1/6 molar) and application of an ice compress for 6 hours to 12 hours may minimize the local reaction. For a 1/6 molar solution of sodium thiosulfate, use 4.14 g of sodium thiosulfate per 100 mL of sterile water for injection or 2.64 g of anhydrous sodium thiosulfate per 100 mL or dilute 4 ml of sodium thiosulfate injection (10%) with 6 mL of Sterile Water for Injection.

Commonly used brand name(s)

In the U.S.—
  Mustargen

Available Dosage Forms:
  • Powder for Solution

Therapeutic Class: Antineoplastic Agent
Pharmacologic Class: Alkylating Agent

Uses For This Medicine

Mechlorethamine belongs to the group of medicines called alkylating agents. It is used to treat some kinds of cancer as well as some noncancerous conditions.

Mechlorethamine interferes with the growth of cancer cells, which are eventually destroyed. Since the growth of normal body cells may also be affected by mechlorethamine, other effects will also occur. Some of these may be serious and must be reported to your doctor. Other effects, like hair loss, may not be serious but may cause concern. Some effects may not occur for months or years after the medicine is used.

Before you begin treatment with mechlorethamine, you and your doctor should talk about the good this medicine will do as well as the risks of using it.

Mechlorethamine is to be administered only by or under the immediate supervision of your doctor.

Once a medicine has been approved for marketing for a cer-tain use, experience may show that it is also useful for other medical problems. Although these uses are not included in product labeling, mechlorethamine is used in certain patients with the following medical conditions:
  • Cancer of the lymph system (part of the immune system) that affects the skin

Before Using This Medicine

In deciding to use a medicine, the risks of taking the medicine must be weighed against the good it will do. This is a decision you and your doctor will make. For this medicine, the following should be considered:

Allergies—Tell your doctor if you have ever had any un-usual or allergic reaction to this medicine or any other medi-cines. Also tell your health care professional if you have any other types of allergies, such as to foods, dyes, preservatives, or animals. For non-prescription products, read the label or package ingredients carefully.

Pediatric—Although there is no specific information com-paring use of mechlorethamine in children with use in other age groups, it is not expected to cause different side effects or problems in children than it does in adults.

Geriatric—Many medicines have not been studied specifi-cally in older people. Therefore, it may not be known whether they work exactly the same way they do in younger adults or if they cause different side effects or problems in older people. There is no specific information comparing use of mechlor-ethamine in the elderly with use in other age groups.

Pregnancy—

	Pregnancy Category	Explanation
All Trimesters	D	Studies in pregnant women have demonstrated a risk to the fetus. However, the bene-fits of therapy in a life threat-ening situation or a serious disease, may outweigh the po-tential risk.

Breast Feeding—There are no adequate studies in women for determining infant risk when using this medication during breastfeeding. Weigh the potential benefits against the po-tential risks before taking this medication while breastfeeding.

Other medicines—

Using this medicine with any of the following medicines is not recommended. Your doctor may decide not to treat you with this medication or change some of the other medicines you take.

Rotavirus Vaccine, Live

Interactions with Food/Tobacco/Alcohol—Certain medicines should not be used at or around the time of eating food or eating certain types of food since interactions may occur. Using alcohol or tobacco with certain medicines may also cause interactions to occur. Discuss with your healthcare professional the use of your medicine with food, alcohol, or tobacco.

Other medical problems—The presence of other medical problems may affect the use of this medicine. Make sure you tell your doctor if you have any other medical problems, especially:

- Chickenpox (including recent exposure) or
- Herpes zoster (shingles)—Risk of severe disease affecting other parts of the body
- Gout or
- Kidney stones—Mechlorethamine may increase levels of uric acid in the body, which can cause gout and kidney stones
- Infection—Mechlorethamine may decrease your body's ability to fight infection

Proper Use of This Medicine

Mechlorethamine is sometimes given together with certain other medicines. If you are using a combination of medicines, it is important that you receive each one at the proper time. If you are taking some of these medicines by mouth, ask your health care professional to help you plan a way to take them at the right times.

While you are using this medicine, your doctor may want you to drink extra fluids so that you will pass more urine. This will help prevent kidney problems and keep your kidneys working well.

Mechlorethamine often causes nausea and vomiting, which usually last only 8 to 24 hours. It is very important that you continue to receive the medicine, even if you begin to feel ill. Ask your health care professional for ways to lessen these effects.

Dosing—The dose of this medicine will be different for different patients. Follow your doctor's orders or the directions on the label. The following information includes only the average doses of this medicine. If your dose is different, do not change it unless your doctor tells you to do so.

The amount of medicine that you take depends on the strength of the medicine. Also, the number of doses you take each day, the time allowed between doses, and the length of time you take the medicine depend on the medical problem for which you are using the medicine.

Precautions While Using This Medicine

It is very important that your doctor check your progress at regular visits to make sure that this medicine is working properly and to check for unwanted effects.

While you are being treated with mechlorethamine, and after you stop treatment with it, do not have any immunizations (vaccinations) without your doctor's approval. Mechlorethamine may lower your body's resistance and there is a chance you might get the infection the immunization is meant to prevent. In addition, other persons living in your household should not take oral polio vaccine since there is a chance they could pass the polio virus on to you. Also, avoid persons who have taken oral polio vaccine. Do not get close to them, and do not stay in the same room with them for very long. If you cannot take these precautions, you should consider wearing a protective face mask that covers the nose and mouth.

Mechlorethamine can temporarily lower the number of white blood cells in your blood, increasing the chance of getting an infection. It can also lower the number of platelets, which are necessary for proper blood clotting. If this occurs, there are certain precautions you can take, especially when your blood count is low, to reduce the risk of infection or bleeding:

- If you can, avoid people with infections. Check with your doctor immediately if you think you are getting an infection or if you get a fever or chills, cough or hoarseness, lower back or side pain, or painful or difficult urination.
- Check with your doctor immediately if you notice any unusual bleeding or bruising; black, tarry stools; blood in urine or stools; or pinpoint red spots on your skin.
- Be careful when using a regular toothbrush, dental floss, or toothpick. Your medical doctor, dentist, or nurse may recommend other ways to clean your teeth and gums. Check with your medical doctor before having any dental work done.
- Do not touch your eyes or the inside of your nose unless you have just washed your hands and have not touched anything else in the meantime.
- Be careful not to cut yourself when you are using sharp objects such as a safety razor or fingernail or toenail cutters.
- Avoid contact sports or other situations where bruising or injury could occur.

If mechlorethamine accidentally seeps out of the vein into which it is injected, it may damage some tissues and cause scarring. Tell the health care professional right away if you notice redness, pain, or swelling at the place of injection.

Side Effects of This Medicine

Along with its needed effects, a medicine may cause some unwanted effects. Although not all of these side effects may occur, if they do occur they may need medical attention.

Also, because of the way cancer medicines act on the body, there is a chance that they might cause other effects that may not occur until months or years after these medicines are used. These delayed effects may include certain types of cancer. Discuss these possible effects with your doctor.

Check with your doctor immediately if any of the following side effects occur:

Less common

Black, tarry stools; blood in urine or stools; cough or hoarseness; fever or chills; lower back or side pain; pain or redness at place of injection; painful or difficult urination; pinpoint red spots on skin; unusual bleeding or bruising

Rare

Shortness of breath, itching, or wheezing

Check with your doctor as soon as possible if any of the following side effects occur:

More common

Missing menstrual periods; painful rash

Less common

Dizziness; joint pain; loss of hearing; ringing in ears; swelling of feet or lower legs

Rare

Numbness, tingling, or burning of fingers, toes, or face; sores in mouth and on lips; yellow eyes or skin

Some side effects may occur that usually do not need medical attention. These side effects may go away during treatment as your body adjusts to the medicine. Also, your health care professional may be able to tell you about ways to prevent or reduce some of these side effects. Check with your health care professional if any of the following side effects continue or are bothersome or if you have any questions about them:

More common

Nausea and vomiting (usually lasts only 8 to 24 hours)

Less common

Confusion; diarrhea; drowsiness; headache; loss of appetite; metallic taste; weakness

This medicine may cause a temporary loss of hair in some people. After treatment with mechlorethamine has ended, normal hair growth should return.

After you stop using this medicine, it may still produce some side effects that need attention. During this period of time, *check with your doctor immediately* if you notice the following side effects:

Black, tarry stools; blood in urine or stools; cough or hoarseness; fever or chills; lower back or side pain; painful or difficult urination; pinpoint red spots on skin; unusual bleeding or bruising

Other side effects not listed may also occur in some patients. If you notice any other effects, check with your healthcare professional.

MEFLOQUINE (Oral route) - ME-floe-kwin

Commonly used brand name(s)

In the U.S.—

Lariam

Available Dosage Forms:

• Tablet

Therapeutic Class: Antimalarial

Uses For This Medicine

Mefloquine belongs to a group of medicines called antimalarials. It is used to prevent or treat malaria, a red blood cell infection transmitted by the bite of a mosquito.

Malaria transmission occurs in large areas of Central and South America, Hispaniola, sub-Saharan Africa, the Indian subcontinent, Southeast Asia, the Middle East, and Oceania. Country-specific information on malaria can be obtained from the Centers for Disease Control and Prevention (CDC), or from the CDC's web site at http://www.cdc.gov/travel.

This medicine may cause some serious side effects. Therefore, it is usually used only to prevent the symptoms of malaria or to treat serious malaria infections in areas where it is known that other medicines may not work.

Mefloquine is available only with your doctor's prescription.

Before Using This Medicine

In deciding to use a medicine, the risks of taking the medicine must be weighed against the good it will do. This is a decision you and your doctor will make. For this medicine, the following should be considered:

Allergies—Tell your doctor if you have ever had any unusual or allergic reaction to this medicine or any other medicines. Also tell your health care professional if you have any other types of allergies, such as to foods, dyes, preservatives, or animals. For non-prescription products, read the label or package ingredients carefully.

Pediatric—Children should avoid traveling to areas where there is a chance of getting malaria, unless they can take effective antimalarial medicines such as mefloquine. Studies on this medicine have not been done in infants below the age of 6 months old.

Geriatric—Many medicines have not been studied specifically in older people. Therefore, it may not be known whether they work exactly the same way they do in younger adults or if they cause different side effects or problems in older people. There is no specific information comparing use of mefloquine in the elderly with use in other age groups. However, elderly people may be more sensitive to the adverse effects of mefloquine which may require caution.

Pregnancy—

	Pregnancy Category	Explanation
All Trimesters	C	Animal studies have shown an adverse effect and there are no adequate studies in pregnant women OR no animal studies have been conducted and there are no adequate studies in pregnant women.

Breast Feeding—There are no adequate studies in women for determining infant risk when using this medication during breastfeeding. Weigh the potential benefits against the potential risks before taking this medication while breastfeeding.

Other medicines—

Using this medicine with any of the following medicines is not recommended. Your doctor may decide not to treat you with this medication or change some of the other medicines you take.

Aurothioglucose, Bepridil, Cisapride, Halofantrine, Isradipine, Levomethadyl, Mesoridazine, Pimozide, Terfenadine, Thioridazine, Ziprasidone

Interactions with Food/Tobacco/Alcohol—Certain medicines should not be used at or around the time of eating food or eating certain types of food since interactions may occur. Using alcohol or tobacco with certain medicines may also cause interactions to occur. Discuss with your healthcare

professional the use of your medicine with food, alcohol, or tobacco.

Other medical problems—The presence of other medical problems may affect the use of this medicine. Make sure you tell your doctor if you have any other medical problems, especially:

- Allergy to mefloquine or similar medicines such as quinine and quinidine or
- Psychiatric conditions such as
  - Active depression or recent history of depression or
  - Generalized anxiety disorder or
  - Psychosis or
  - Schizophrenia or
  - Other major psychiatric disorders or
- Convulsions, history of—Mefloquine should not be taken if you have any of these conditions.
- Depression previous history of—Mefloquine should be used with caution.
- Epilepsy or
- Seizure disorder—Mefloquine may make these conditions worse.
- Heart conditions or
- Liver problems—Mefloquine should be used with caution.

Proper Use of This Medicine

Mefloquine is best taken with a full glass (8 ounces) of water and with food, unless otherwise directed by your doctor.

Mefloquine may be crushed and put in water, milk, or juice to make it easier to take.

For patients taking mefloquine to prevent the symptoms of malaria:

- Your doctor will want you to start taking this medicine one week before you travel to an area where there is a chance of getting malaria.
- Also, you should keep taking this medicine while you are in the area where malaria is present and for 4 weeks after you leave the area. No medicine will protect you completely from malaria. However, to protect you as completely as possible, it is important that you keep taking this medicine for the full time your doctor ordered. Also, if fever or "flu-like" symptoms develop during your travels or within 2 to 3 months after you leave the area, check with your doctor immediately.
- This medicine works best when you take it on a regular schedule. For example, if you are to take it once a week, it is best to take it on the same day each week. Do not miss any doses. If you have any questions about this, check with your health care professional.

For patients taking mefloquine to treat malaria:

- To help clear up your infection completely, take this medicine exactly as directed by your doctor.

Children taking mefloquine to treat malaria may vomit after taking this medicine. Your child may vomit some of the dose of medicine. Contact your child's doctor if vomiting occurs. The doctor may need for you to give your child more medicine.

Dosing—The dose of this medicine will be different for different patients. Follow your doctor's orders or the directions on the label. The following information includes only the average doses of this medicine. If your dose is different, do not change it unless your doctor tells you to do so.

The amount of medicine that you take depends on the strength of the medicine. Also, the number of doses you take each day, the time allowed between doses, and the length of time you take the medicine depend on the medical problem for which you are using the medicine.

The number of doses you take each day, the time allowed between doses, and the length of time you take the medicine depend on whether you are using mefloquine to prevent or to treat malaria.

- For oral dosage form (tablets):
  - For prevention of malaria:
    - Adults and children weighing over 45 kilograms (kg) (99 pounds)—250 milligrams (mg) (1 tablet) one week before traveling to an area where malaria occurs. Then 250 mg once a week on the same day of each week and preferably after your main meal while staying in the area and every week for four weeks after leaving the area.
    - Children—Dose is based on body weight and must be determined by your doctor.
      — Children weighing 5 to 9 kg (11 to 20 pounds): 5 mg per kg of body weight one week before traveling to an area where malaria occurs.
      — Children weighing 10 to 19 kg (21 to 43 pounds): 62.5 mg (¼ tablet) one week before traveling to an area where malaria occurs. Then 62.5 mg once a week while staying in the area where malaria occurs and every week for four weeks after leaving the area.
      — Children weighing 20 to 30 kg (44 to 66 pounds): 125 mg (½ tablet) one week before traveling to an area where malaria occurs. Then 125 mg once a week while staying in the area and every week for four weeks after leaving the area.
      — Children weighing 31 to 45 kg (67 to 99 pounds): 187.5 mg (¾ tablet) one week before traveling to an area where malaria occurs. Then 187.5 mg once a week while staying in the area and every week for four weeks after leaving the area.
  - For treatment of malaria:
    - Adults—1250 mg as a single dose, or 750 mg as one dose, then a 500 mg dose 8 hours later, or may be determined by your doctor based on body weight
    - Children—Dose is based on body weight and must be determined by your doctor. The usual dose is 20 to 25 mg per kg (9 to 11 mg per pound) of body weight as a single dose or two doses (divide the single dose by two) taken 6 to 8 hours apart. Taking two doses may decrease the occurrence of unwanted side effects.

Missed dose—If you miss a dose of this medicine, take it as soon as possible. However, if it is almost time for your next dose, skip the missed dose and go back to your regular dosing schedule. Do not double doses.

Storage—Store the medicine in a closed container at room temperature, away from heat, moisture, and direct light. Keep from freezing.

Keep out of the reach of children.

Do not keep outdated medicine or medicine no longer needed.

Precautions While Using This Medicine

Mefloquine may cause vision problems. It may also cause some people to become dizzy or lightheaded or to have hallucinations (seeing, hearing, or feeling things that are not there). Make sure you know how you react to this medicine before you drive, use machines, or do anything else that could be dangerous if you are dizzy or are not alert or able to see well. This is especially important for people whose jobs require fine coordination. If these reactions are especially bothersome, check with your doctor.

Malaria is spread by the bite of certain kinds of infected female mosquitoes. If you are living in, or will be traveling to, an area where there is a chance of getting malaria, the following mosquito-control measures will help to prevent infection:

- If possible, sleep under mosquito netting, preferably netting coated or soaked with pyrethrum, to avoid being bitten by malaria-carrying mosquitoes.
- Remain in air-conditioned rooms to reduce contact with mosquitoes
- Wear long-sleeved shirts or blouses and long trousers to protect your arms and legs, especially from dusk through dawn when mosquitoes are out.
- Apply mosquito repellant, preferably one containing DEET, to uncovered areas of the skin from dusk through dawn when mosquitoes are out.
- Using a pyrethrum-containing flying insect spray to kill mosquitoes in living and sleeping quarters during evening and nighttime hours.

If you are taking quinidine (e.g., Quinidex) or quinine, talk to your doctor before you take mefloquine. While you are taking mefloquine, take mefloquine at least 12 hours after the last dose of quinidine or quinine. Taking mefloquine and either of these medicines at the same time may result in a greater chance of serious side effects.

If you are taking anticonvulsants (e.g., Tegetrol, Dilantin), halofantrine (e.g., Halfan), or typhoid vaccine, talk to your doctor before you take mefloquine. Taking mefloquine and any of these medicines at the same time may result in a greater chance of serious side effects.

For patients taking mefloquine to treat malaria:
- If your symptoms do not improve within a few days, or if they become worse, check with your doctor.

Side Effects of This Medicine

Along with its needed effects, a medicine may cause some unwanted effects. Although not all of these side effects may occur, if they do occur they may need medical attention.

Check with your doctor immediately if any of the following side effects occur:
  Rare
    Aching joints and muscles; anxiety; blistering, loosening, peeling, or redness of the skin; chest pain or discomfort; chills, fever, and/or sore throat; confusion; convulsions (seizures); dizziness; cough or hoarseness; depression; fainting; hallucinations (seeing, hearing, or feeling things that are not there); irregular, pounding, slow, or fast heartbeat or pulse; irritability;

lightheadedness; lower back or side pain; nervousness; painful or difficult urination; pinpoint red spots on skin; mood or mental changes, mental depression, and/or restlessness; red or irritated eye; sores, ulcers, and/or white spots in mouth or on lips; stiff neck; swelling of ankles, feet, and/or lower legs; unusual bleeding or bruising; unusual tiredness or weakness; vomiting

  Incidence not determined
    Blurred or loss of vision; convulsions; disturbed color perception; dizziness; double vision; halos around lights; hearing problems; loss of bladder control; muscle spasm or jerking of all extremities; night blindness; overbright appearance of lights; severe or continuing headache; shortness of breath and or wheezing; sudden loss of consciousness; troubled breathing; tunnel vision

Some side effects may occur that usually do not need medical attention. These side effects may go away during treatment as your body adjusts to the medicine. Also, your health care professional may be able to tell you about ways to prevent or reduce some of these side effects. Check with your health care professional if any of the following side effects continue or are bothersome or if you have any questions about them:
  More common
    Chills; continuing ringing or buzzing or other unexplained noise in ears or hearing loss; diarrhea; emotional problems; loss of balance; nausea; stomach pain
  Less common
    Abnormal dreams; loss of appetite; skin rash; trouble in sleeping; unusual tiredness or weakness; vertigo
  Rare
    Loss of hair

Mefloquine very rarely may cause partial loss of hair. After treatment with mefloquine has ended, normal hair growth should return.
  Incidence not determined
    Acid or sour stomach; belching; flushing, redness of skin; heartburn; indigestion; skin rash with a general disease; stomach discomfort, upset or pain; swelling; unusually warm skin

Other side effects not listed may also occur in some patients. If you notice any other effects, check with your healthcare professional.

MELOXICAM   (Oral route) - mel-OKS-i-kam

Black Box Warning

NSAIDs may cause an increased risk of serious cardiovascular thrombotic events, myocardial infarction, and stroke, which can be fatal. This risk may increase with duration of use. Patients with cardiovascular disease or risk factors for cardiovascular disease may be at greater risk.

Meloxicam is contraindicated for the treatment of peri-operative pain in the setting of coronary artery bypass graft (CABG) surgery.

NSAIDs cause an increased risk of serious gastrointestinal adverse events including bleeding, ulceration, and perforation of the stomach or intestines, which can be fatal. These events can occur at any time during use and without warning symptoms. Elderly patients are at greater risk for serious gastrointestinal events.

Commonly used brand name(s)

In the U.S.—
  Mobic

Available Dosage Forms:
  • Tablet
  • Suspension

Therapeutic Class: Analgesic
Pharmacologic Class: NSAID

Uses For This Medicine

Meloxicam is a nonsteroidal anti-inflammatory drug (NSAID) used to relieve some symptoms of arthritis and rheumatoid arthritis, such as inflammation, swelling, stiffness, and joint pain. However, this medicine does not cure arthritis and will help you only as long as you continue to take it.

This medicine is available only with your doctor's prescription.

Before Using This Medicine

In deciding to use a medicine, the risks of taking the medicine must be weighed against the good it will do. This is a decision you and your doctor will make. For this medicine, the following should be considered:

Allergies—Tell your doctor if you have ever had any unusual or allergic reaction to this medicine or any other medicines. Also tell your health care professional if you have any other types of allergies, such as to foods, dyes, preservatives, or animals. For non-prescription products, read the label or package ingredients carefully.

Pediatric—Meloxicam has been tested in children 2 to 17 years of age. Studies show that meloxicam may reduce signs and symptoms in patients with juvenile rheumatoid arthritis.

Geriatric—This medicine has been tested and has not been shown to cause different side effects or problems in older people than it does in younger adults. Caution should be used in elderly patients who are taking this medicine because they may be at greater risk for serious gastrointestinal (GI) problems.

Pregnancy—

	Pregnancy Category	Explanation
All Trimesters	C	Animal studies have shown an adverse effect and there are no adequate studies in pregnant women OR no animal studies have been conducted and there are no adequate studies in pregnant women.

Breast Feeding—There are no adequate studies in women for determining infant risk when using this medication during breastfeeding. Weigh the potential benefits against the potential risks before taking this medication while breastfeeding.

Other medicines—

Using this medicine with any of the following medicines is not recommended. Your doctor may decide not to treat you with this medication or change some of the other medicines you take.

Ketorolac

Interactions with Food/Tobacco/Alcohol—Certain medicines should not be used at or around the time of eating food or eating certain types of food since interactions may occur. Using alcohol or tobacco with certain medicines may also cause interactions to occur. Discuss with your healthcare professional the use of your medicine with food, alcohol, or tobacco.

Other medical problems—The presence of other medical problems may affect the use of this medicine. Make sure you tell your doctor if you have any other medical problems, especially:

  • Alcohol abuse or
  • Bleeding problems or
  • Stomach ulcer or other stomach problems or
  • Tobacco (or recent history of)—The chance of side effects may be increased
  • Anemia or
  • Asthma or
  • Dehydration or
  • Fluid retention (swelling of feet or lower legs) or
  • High blood pressure or
  • Kidney disease or
  • Liver disease—Meloxicam may make these conditions worse
  • Aspirin triad (asthma, nasal polyps, and aspirin intolerance) or
  • Previous allergic or anaphylactic response to aspirin or other nonsteroidal anti-inflammatory drugs—Use of meloxicam may cause a serious allergic reaction
  • Coronary artery bypass graft (CABG) surgery—Meloxicam should NOT be used for pain during this surgery.
  • Heart disease or
  • Risk factors for heart disease—This medicine may cause you to be at greater risk for serious problems with blood clots.

Proper Use of This Medicine

For oral suspension: Shake gently before using.

For safe and effective use of this medicine, do not take more of it, do not take it more often, and do not take it for a longer time than ordered by your health care professional. Taking too much of this medicine may increase the chance of unwanted side effects.

Dosing—The dose of this medicine will be different for different patients. Follow your doctor's orders or the directions on the label. The following information includes only the average doses of this medicine. If your dose is different, do not change it unless your doctor tells you to do so.

The amount of medicine that you take depends on the strength of the medicine. Also, the number of doses you take each day, the time allowed between doses, and the length of time you take the medicine depend on the medical problem for which you are using the medicine.

  • For oral dosage form (suspension or tablets):
    ○ For symptoms of osteoarthritis or rheumatoid arthritis:
      ▪ Adults—7.5 milligrams (mg) once a day
      ▪ Children—Use must be determined by your doctor
      ▪ For symptoms of juvenile rheumatoid arthritis:
        — Children—Dose is based on weight and must be determined by your doctor.

Missed dose—If you miss a dose of this medicine, take it as soon as possible. However, if it is almost time for your next dose, skip the missed dose and go back to your regular dosing schedule. Do not double doses.

Storage—Store the medicine in a closed container at room temperature, away from heat, moisture, and direct light. Keep from freezing.

Keep out of the reach of children.

Do not keep outdated medicine or medicine no longer needed.

Ask your healthcare professional how you should dispose of any medicine you do not use.

Precautions While Using This Medicine

If you will be taking this medicine for a long time, it is very important that your doctor check you at regular visits for any blood problems that may be caused by this medicine.

Stomach problems may be more likely to occur if you drink alcoholic beverages while being treated with this medicine. Therefore, do not regularly drink alcoholic beverages while taking this medicine, unless otherwise directed by your doctor.

Taking two or more of the nonsteroidal anti-inflammatory drugs together on a regular basis may increase the chance of unwanted effects. Also, taking acetaminophen, aspirin or other salicylates, or ketorolac (e.g., Toradol) regularly while you are taking a nonsteroidal anti-inflammatory drug may increase the chance of unwanted effects. The risk will depend on how much of each medicine you take every day, and on how long you take the medicines together. If your health care professional directs you to take these medicines together on a regular basis, follow his or her directions carefully. However, do not take acetaminophen or aspirin or other salicylates together with this medicine for more than a few days, and do not take any ketorolac (e.g., Toradol) while taking this medicine, unless your doctor has directed you to do so and is following your progress.

Serious side effects can occur during treatment with this medicine. Sometimes serious side effects can occur without warning. However, possible warning signs often occur, including severe stomach pain, black tarry stools, and/or vomiting of blood or material that looks like coffee grounds; skin rash; swelling of face, fingers, feet and/or lower legs. Also, signs of serious heart problems could occur such as chest pain, tightness in chest, fast or irregular heartbeat, or unusual flushing or warmth of skin. *Stop taking this medicine and check with your doctor immediately if you notice any of these warning signs.*

If you notice signs of liver toxicity including nausea, unusual tiredness, itching of the skin, stomach pain or fever,

Stop taking this medicine and check with your doctor immediately if you notice any of these warning signs.

Meloxicam may cause a serious type of allergic reaction called anaphylaxis. Although this is rare, it may occur often in patients who are allergic to aspirin or other nonsteroidal anti-inflammatory drugs. Anaphylaxis requires immediate medical attention. The most serious signs of this reaction are very fast or irregular breathing, gasping for breath, wheezing, or fainting. Other signs may include changes in skin color of face; very fast but irregular heartbeat or pulse; hive-like swellings on the skin; puffiness or swelling of the eyelids or around the eyes. If these effects occur, get emergency help at once.

Ask someone to drive you to the nearest hospital emergency room. Call an ambulance, lie down, cover yourself to keep warm, and prop your feet higher than your head. Stay in that position until help arrives.

Side Effects of This Medicine

Along with its needed effects, a medicine may cause some unwanted effects. Although not all of these side effects may occur, if they do occur they may need medical attention.

Check with your doctor immediately if any of the following side effects occur:

Less common

Arm, back, or jaw pain; bleeding gums; bloating; blood in urine; blurred vision; burning upper abdominal pain; canker sores; chest tightness or heaviness; chills; cloudy urine; cough; cramping; dark urine; decreased frequency/amount of urine; difficult or labored breathing; dilated neck veins; dizziness; dizziness, faintness, or lightheadedness when getting up from a lying or sitting position suddenly; extreme fatigue; general tiredness and weakness; headache; hives or welts; increased blood pressure; increased sensitivity of skin to sunlight; increased thirst; irregular breathing; itching, redness or other discoloration of skin; large, hive-like swelling on face, eyelids, lips, tongue, throat, hands, legs, feet, sex organs; light-colored stools; loss of appetite; lower side/back pain; noisy breathing; pain or discomfort in arms, jaw, back or neck; painful or difficult urination; pains in stomach, side, or abdomen, possibly radiating to the back; pinpoint red or purple spots on skin; pounding in the ears; redness, soreness, or itching skin; seizures; severe and continuing nausea; severe sunburn; shakiness in legs, arms, hands, feet; skin blisters; sore throat; sores, ulcers, or white spots on lips or tongue or inside the mouth; sores, welting or blisters; stomach bloating, burning, cramping, tenderness, or pain; sweating; swelling or puffiness of face; swollen glands; trembling or shaking of hands or feet; trouble breathing; unusual bleeding or bruising; upper right abdominal pain; watery or bloody diarrhea; weight gain or loss; yellow eyes or skin

Rare

Area rash; blistering, peeling, loosening of skin; bloody or black, tarry stools; clay-colored stools; cold, clammy skin; continuing vomiting; cough or hoarseness; cracks in the skin; difficulty swallowing; fast, weak pulse; fever with or without chills; greatly decreased frequency of urination or amount of urine; joint or muscle pain; lightheadedness; loss of heat from the body; puffiness or swelling of the eyelids or around the eyes, face, lips or tongue; red irritated eyes; red skin lesions, often with a purple center; red, swollen skin; scaly skin; severe stomach pain; shortness of breath; tightness in chest; unpleasant breath odor; unusual tiredness or weakness; vomiting of blood or material that looks like coffee grounds; wheezing

Incidence not known

Difficulty in speaking; double vision; inability to move arms, legs, or facial muscles; inability to speak; pains in chest, groin or legs, especially calves; severe headaches of sudden onset; slow speech; sudden loss of coordination; sudden onset of shortness of breath for no apparent reason; sudden onset of slurred speech; sudden vision changes

Symptoms of overdose

Get emergency help immediately if any of the following symptoms of overdose occur:

Bloody or black tarry stools; blue lips, fingernails or skin; blurred vision; confusion; convulsions (seizures); dark urine; decreased urine output; difficulty breathing; difficulty swallowing; dizziness; fever with or without chills; pain in chest, upper stomach, or throat; pounding in ears; skin rash; slow or fast heartbeat; swelling around eyes, face, lips, or tongue; shortness of breath; severe stomach pain; unusual tiredness or weakness; tightness in chest; vomiting of blood or material that looks like coffee grounds; weight gain (rapid); wheezing; yellow eyes or skin

Some side effects may occur that usually do not need medical attention. These side effects may go away during treatment as your body adjusts to the medicine. Also, your health care professional may be able to tell you about ways to prevent or reduce some of these side effects. Check with your health care professional if any of the following side effects continue or are bothersome or if you have any questions about them:

More common

Diarrhea; gas; heartburn; indigestion

Less common or rare

Abdominal pain; abnormal dreaming; anxiety; appetite increased; bad, unusual, or unpleasant aftertaste; belching; bloated full feeling; burning feeling in chest or stomach; burning, crawling, itching, numbness, prickling, "pins and needles", or tingling feelings; burning, dry, or itching eyes; change in taste; changes in vision; confusion; constipation; continuing ringing or buzzing or other unexplained noise in ears; decreased urination; discharge; discouragement; dry mouth; excess air or gas in stomach; excessive tearing; feeling sad or empty; feeling of constant movement of self or surroundings; general feeling of discomfort or illness; hair loss; hearing loss; hot flushes; increase in heart rate; irritability; loss of interest or pleasure; nausea and/or vomiting; nervousness; pain or burning in throat; rapid breathing; redness, pain, swelling of eye, eyelid, or inner lining of eyelid; sensation of spinning; sleepiness; stomach upset; sunken eyes; tenderness in stomach area; thinning of hair; thirst; tiredness; trouble concentrating; trouble sleeping; wrinkled skin

Other side effects not listed may also occur in some patients. If you notice any other effects, check with your healthcare professional.

MELPHALAN (Oral route, Intravenous route) - MEL-fa-lan

Black Box Warning

Melphalan should be administered under the supervision of a qualified physician experienced in the use of cancer chemotherapeutic agents. Severe bone marrow suppression with resulting infection or bleeding may occur. Melphalan is leukemogenic in humans.

Melphalan produces chromosomal aberrations in vitro and in vivo and, therefore, should be considered potentially mutagenic in humans.

Commonly used brand name(s)

In the U.S.—
Alkeran
Alkeran IV

Available Dosage Forms:
- Tablet
- Powder for Solution

Therapeutic Class: Antineoplastic Agent
Pharmacologic Class: Alkylating Agent

Uses For This Medicine

Melphalan belongs to the group of medicines called alkylating agents. It is used to treat cancer of the ovaries and a certain type of cancer in the bone marrow.

Melphalan interferes with the growth of cancer cells, which are eventually destroyed. Since the growth of normal body cells may also be affected by melphalan, other effects will also occur. Some of these may be serious and must be reported to your doctor. Other effects may not be serious but may cause concern. Some effects may not occur for months or years after the medicine is used.

Before you begin treatment with melphalan, you and your doctor should talk about the good this medicine will do as well as the risks of using it.

Melphalan is available only with your doctor's prescription.

Once a medicine has been approved for marketing for a certain use, experience may show that it is also useful for other medical problems. Although these uses are not included in product labeling, melphalan is used in certain patients with the following conditions:
- Cancer of the breast
- Waldenström's macroglobulinemia (a certain type of cancer of the blood)
- Cancer of the blood and lymph system
- Cancer of the endometrium
- Malignant melanoma (a type of skin cancer that has spread to other parts of the body)

Before Using This Medicine

In deciding to use a medicine, the risks of taking the medicine must be weighed against the good it will do. This is a decision you and your doctor will make. For this medicine, the following should be considered:

Allergies—Tell your doctor if you have ever had any unusual or allergic reaction to this medicine or any other medicines. Also tell your health care professional if you have any other types of allergies, such as to foods, dyes, preservatives, or animals. For non-prescription products, read the label or package ingredients carefully.

Pediatric—Although there is no specific information comparing use of melphalan in children with use in other age groups, this medicine is not expected to cause different side effects or problems in children than it does in adults.

Geriatric—Many medicines have not been studied specifically in older people. Therefore, it may not be known whether they work exactly the same way they do in younger adults or if they cause different side effects or problems in older people. There is no specific information comparing the use of melphalan in the elderly with use in other age groups.

Pregnancy—

	Pregnancy Category	Explanation
All Trimesters	D	Studies in pregnant women have demonstrated a risk to the fetus. However, the benefits of therapy in a life threatening situation or a serious disease, may outweigh the potential risk.

Breast Feeding—There are no adequate studies in women for determining infant risk when using this medication during breastfeeding. Weigh the potential benefits against the potential risks before taking this medication while breastfeeding.

Other medicines—

Using this medicine with any of the following medicines is not recommended. Your doctor may decide not to treat you with this medication or change some of the other medicines you take.

Rotavirus Vaccine, Live

Interactions with Food/Tobacco/Alcohol—Certain medicines should not be used at or around the time of eating food or eating certain types of food since interactions may occur. Using alcohol or tobacco with certain medicines may also cause interactions to occur. Discuss with your healthcare professional the use of your medicine with food, alcohol, or tobacco.

Other medical problems—The presence of other medical problems may affect the use of this medicine. Make sure you tell your doctor if you have any other medical problems, especially:

- Chickenpox (including recent exposure) or
- Herpes zoster (shingles)—Risk of severe disease affecting other parts of the body
- Gout (history of) or
- Kidney stones (history of)—Melphalan may increase levels of a chemical called uric acid in the body, which can cause gout or kidney stones
- Infection—Melphalan decreases your body's ability to fight infection
- Kidney disease—Risk of toxic effects on the blood may be increased

---

Proper Use of This Medicine

Take melphalan only as directed by your doctor. Do not take more or less of it, do not take it more often, and do not take it for a longer time than your doctor ordered. The exact amount of medicine you need has been carefully worked out. Taking too much may increase the chance of side effects, while taking too little may not improve your condition.

Melphalan is sometimes given together with certain other medicines. If you are using a combination of medicines, it is important that you receive each one at the proper time. If you are taking some of these medicines by mouth, ask your health care professional to help you plan a way to remember to take your medicine at the right times.

While you are using melphalan, your doctor may want you to drink extra fluids so that you will pass more urine. This will help prevent kidney problems and keep your kidneys working well.

This medicine may cause nausea, vomiting, and loss of appetite. However, it is very important that you continue to receive the medicine, even if you begin to feel ill. Ask your health care professional for ways to lessen these effects.

If you vomit shortly after taking a dose of melphalan, check with your doctor. You will be told whether to take the dose again or to wait until the next scheduled dose.

Dosing—The dose of this medicine will be different for different patients. Follow your doctor's orders or the directions on the label. The following information includes only the average doses of this medicine. If your dose is different, do not change it unless your doctor tells you to do so.

The amount of medicine that you take depends on the strength of the medicine. Also, the number of doses you take each day, the time allowed between doses, and the length of time you take the medicine depend on the medical problem for which you are using the medicine.

Missed dose—If you miss a dose of this medicine, skip the missed dose and go back to your regular dosing schedule. Do not double doses.

Call your doctor or pharmacist for instructions.

Storage—Store the medicine in a closed container at room temperature, away from heat, moisture, and direct light. Keep from freezing.

Keep out of the reach of children.

Do not keep outdated medicine or medicine no longer needed.

Precautions While Using This Medicine

It is very important that your doctor check your progress at regular visits to make sure that this medicine is working properly and to check for unwanted effects.

While you are being treated with melphalan, and after you stop treatment with it, do not have any immunizations (vaccinations) without your doctor's approval. Melphalan may lower your body's resistance and there is a chance you might get the infection the immunization is meant to prevent. In addition, other persons living in your household should not take or should not have taken oral polio vaccine within the last several months since there is a chance they could pass the polio virus on to you. Also, avoid other persons who have taken oral polio vaccine. Do not get close to them and do not stay in the same room with them for very long. If you cannot take these precautions, you should consider wearing a protective face mask that covers the nose and mouth.

Melphalan can lower the number of white blood cells in your blood temporarily, increasing the chance of getting an infection. It can also lower the number of platelets, which are necessary for proper blood clotting. If this occurs, there are certain precautions you can take, especially when your blood count is low, to reduce the risk of infection or bleeding:

- If you can, avoid people with infections. Check with your doctor immediately if you think you are getting an infection or if you get a fever or chills, cough or hoarseness, lower back or side pain, or painful or difficult urination.
- Check with your doctor immediately if you notice any unusual bleeding or bruising; black, tarry stools; blood in urine or stools; or pinpoint red spots on your skin.

- Be careful when using a regular toothbrush, dental floss, or toothpick. Your medical doctor, dentist, or nurse may recommend other ways to clean your teeth and gums. Check with your medical doctor before having any dental work done.
- Do not touch your eyes or the inside of your nose unless you have just washed your hands and have not touched anything else in the meantime.
- Be careful not to cut yourself when you are using sharp objects such as a safety razor or fingernail or toenail cutters.
- Avoid contact sports or other situations where bruising or injury could occur.

Side Effects of This Medicine

Along with their needed effects, medicines like melphalan can sometimes cause unwanted effects such as blood problems and other side effects. These and others are described below. Also, because of the way these medicines act on the body, there is a chance that they might cause other unwanted effects that may not occur until months or years after the medicine is used. These delayed effects may include certain types of cancer, such as leukemia. Discuss these possible effects with your doctor.

Although not all of these side effects may occur, if they do occur they may need medical attention.

Check with your doctor immediately if any of the following side effects occur:
Less common
Black, tarry stools; blood in urine or stools; cough or hoarseness, accompanied by fever or chills; fast or irregular heart beat; fever or chills; lower back or side pain, accompanied by fever or chills; painful or difficult urination, accompanied by fever or chills; pinpoint red spots on skin; redness and/or soreness at the infusion site; shortness of breath; skin rash or itching (sudden); troubled breathing; unusual bleeding or bruising

Check with your doctor as soon as possible if any of the following side effects occur:
Less common or rare
Diarrhea; difficulty swallowing; joint pain; redness and/or soreness in arm or leg; sores in mouth and on lips; swelling of feet or lower legs

Some side effects may occur that usually do not need medical attention. These side effects may go away during treatment as your body adjusts to the medicine. Also, your health care professional may be able to tell you about ways to prevent or reduce some of these side effects. Check with your health care professional if any of the following side effects continue or are bothersome or if you have any questions about them:
Less common
Nausea and vomiting

After you stop using this medicine, it may still produce some side effects that need attention. During this period of time, *check with your doctor immediately* if you notice the following side effects:

Black, tarry stools; blood in urine or stools; cough or hoarseness, accompanied by fever or chills; fever or chills; lower back or side pain, accompanied by fever or chills; painful or difficult urination, accompanied by fever or chills; pinpoint red spots on skin; unusual bleeding or bruising

Other side effects not listed may also occur in some patients. If you notice any other effects, check with your healthcare professional.

MEMANTINE   (Oral route) - me-MAN-teen

Commonly used brand name(s)
In the U.S.—
Namenda

Available Dosage Forms:
- Tablet
- Solution

Therapeutic Class: Central Nervous System Agent
Pharmacologic Class: N-Methyl-D-Aspartate Receptor Antagonist

Uses For This Medicine

Memantine is used to treat moderate to severe Alzheimer's disease. Memantine is not a cure for Alzheimer's disease but it can help people with the disease. Memantine will not cure Alzheimer's disease, and it will not stop the disease from getting worse.

This medicine is available only with your doctor's prescription.

Before Using This Medicine

In deciding to use a medicine, the risks of taking the medicine must be weighed against the good it will do. This is a decision you and your doctor will make. For this medicine, the following should be considered:

Allergies—Tell your doctor if you have ever had any unusual or allergic reaction to this medicine or any other medicines. Also tell your health care professional if you have any other types of allergies, such as to foods, dyes, preservatives, or animals. For non-prescription products, read the label or package ingredients carefully.

Pediatric—Studies on this medicine have only been done in adult patients, and there is no specific information comparing the use of memantine in children with use in other age groups. This medicine is generally not used in children.

Geriatric—This medicine has been studied in older adults and has not been shown to cause different side effects or problems in older people than it does in younger adults.

Pregnancy—

	Pregnancy Category	Explanation
All Trimesters	B	Animal studies have revealed no evidence of harm to the fetus, however, there are no adequate studies in pregnant women OR animal studies have shown an adverse effect, but adequate studies in pregnant women have failed to demonstrate a risk to the fetus.

Breast Feeding—There are no adequate studies in women for determining infant risk when using this medication during

breastfeeding. Weigh the potential benefits against the potential risks before taking this medication while breastfeeding.

Other medicines—Although certain medicines should not be used together at all, in other cases two different medicines may be used together even if an interaction might occur. In these cases, your doctor may want to change the dose, or other precautions may be necessary. Tell your healthcare professional if you are taking any other prescription or non-prescription (over-the-counter [OTC]) medicine.

Interactions with Food/Tobacco/Alcohol—Certain medicines should not be used at or around the time of eating food or eating certain types of food since interactions may occur. Using alcohol or tobacco with certain medicines may also cause interactions to occur. Discuss with your healthcare professional the use of your medicine with food, alcohol, or tobacco.

Other medical problems—The presence of other medical problems may affect the use of this medicine. Make sure you tell your doctor if you have any other medical problems, especially:

- Kidney disease—Memantine may make this condition worse. Patients with severe kidney disease may need to take a smaller amount of memantine.

- Difficult urination

- Urinary tract problems

- Urinary tract blockage—Memantine may make these conditions worse

- Epilepsy or history of seizures—Memantine may make this medical condition worse

Proper Use of This Medicine

For patients taking the *oral solution form* of this medicine:

- Remove oral dosing syringe along with the cap and plastic tube from the bag and attach to tube to the cap.

- Open the child-resistant cap on the bottle by pushing down on the cap while turning the cap counter-clockwise (to the left) and remove the cap and seal from the bottle.

- Insert the plastic tube fully into the bottle and screw the cap tightly onto the bottle by turning the cap clockwise (to the right).

- Keeping the bottle upright on the table, remove the lid to uncover the opening on the top of the cap. With the plunger fully depressed, insert the tip of the syringe firmly into the opening of the cap.

- While holding the syringe, gently pull the plunger of the syringe up to draw medicine into the syringe.

- Remove the syringe from the cap opening. Invert the syringe (point tip upwards) and slowly press the plunger to a level that pushed out any large air bubbles that may be present. Keep the plunger in this position.

- Re-insert the tip of the syringe into the cap opening. While holding the syringe, continue to gently pull out the plunger until the bottom of the black ring of the plunger reaches the appropriate mark on the syringe that corresponds to the dose prescribed.

- Remove the syringe from the bottle and swallow the oral solution directly from the syringe. Do not mix with any other liquid.

- After use, reseal the bottle by snapping the attached lid closed.

- Rinse the empty syringe by inserting the open end of the syringe into a glass of water, pulling the plunger out to draw in water, and pushing the plunger in to remove the water. Repeat several times. Allow the syringe to air dry.

Dosing—The dose of this medicine will be different for different patients. Follow your doctor's orders or the directions on the label. The following information includes only the average doses of this medicine. If your dose is different, do not change it unless your doctor tells you to do so.

The amount of medicine that you take depends on the strength of the medicine. Also, the number of doses you take each day, the time allowed between doses, and the length of time you take the medicine depend on the medical problem for which you are using the medicine.

- For oral dosage form (oral solution and tablets)
  - For treatment of Alzheimer's disease
    - Adults—To start, take 5 mg (milligrams) once a day. Your doctor may increase your dose gradually up to 10 mg (milligrams) twice a day.
    - Children—This medicine is not used in children.

Missed dose—If you miss a dose of this medicine, take it as soon as possible. However, if it is almost time for your next dose, skip the missed dose and go back to your regular dosing schedule. Do not double doses.

Storage—Store the medicine in a closed container at room temperature, away from heat, moisture, and direct light. Keep from freezing.

Keep out of the reach of children.

Do not keep outdated medicine or medicine no longer needed.

Ask your healthcare professional how you should dispose of any medicine you do not use.

Precautions While Using This Medicine

It is very important that your healthcare professional check your progress at regular visits to make sure that this medicine is working properly and to check for unwanted effects.

Side Effects of This Medicine

Along with its needed effects, a medicine may cause some unwanted effects. Although not all of these side effects may occur, if they do occur they may need medical attention.

Check with your doctor immediately if any of the following side effects occur:

Less common

Bloating or swelling of face, arms, hands, lower legs, or feet; blurred vision; dizziness; headache; nervousness; pounding in the ears; rapid weight gain; slow or fast heartbeat; tingling of hands or feet; unusual weight gain or loss

Incidence not known

Abdominal pain; agitation; black, tarry stools; bleeding gums; blistering, peeling, loosening of skin; bloating; blood in urine or stools; chest pain; coma; constipation; continuing vomiting; convulsions; dark-colored urine; decreased urine output; depression; fainting; fast, pounding, or irregular heartbeat or pulse; general feeling of tiredness or weakness; high fever; high or low blood pressure; hostility; increased sweating; indigestion; infection from breathing foreign substances into the lungs; itching; lethargy; light-colored stools; lip smacking or puckering; loss of consciousness; muscle twitching; no blood pressure; no breathing; no pulse; numbness or tingling in face, arms, legs; pain or swelling in arms or legs without any injury; pain, tension, and weakness upon walking that subsides during periods of rest; pain in stomach, side, or abdomen, possibly radiating to the back; palpitations; pinpoint red spots on skin; pounding, slow heartbeat; puffing of cheeks; rapid or worm-like movements of tongue; rapid weight gain; recurrent fainting; red irritated eyes; red skin lesions, often with a purple center; seizures; severe constipation; severe headache; severe muscle stiffness; severe vomiting; sores, ulcers, or white spots in mouth or on lips; stomach pain; stupor; sudden severe weakness; swelling of face, ankles, or hands; total body jerking; trouble speaking or walking; troubled breathing; twitching, twisting, uncontrolled repetitive movements of tongue, lips, face, arms, or legs; uncontrolled chewing movements; uncontrolled movements of arms and legs; unusual bleeding or bruising; unusually pale skin; vomiting; yellow eyes and skin

Some side effects may occur that usually do not need medical attention. These side effects may go away during treatment as your body adjusts to the medicine. Also, your health care professional may be able to tell you about ways to prevent or reduce some of these side effects. Check with your health care professional if any of the following side effects continue or are bothersome or if you have any questions about them:

More common
Confusion

Less common
Anxiety; back pain; bladder pain; bloody or cloudy urine; change in walking and balance; chills; clumsiness or unsteadiness; cough producing mucus; coughing; difficult, burning, or painful urination; difficulty breathing; difficulty moving; difficulty having a bowel movement (stool); diarrhea; discouragement; dry mouth; fear; feeling sad or empty; fever; frequent urge to urinate; general feeling of discomfort or illness; hyperventilation; insomnia; irregular heartbeats; irritability; joint pain; loss of appetite; loss of bladder control; loss of interest or pleasure; lower back or side pain; muscle pain or stiffness; nausea; nervousness; pain; pain in joints; restlessness; seeing, hearing, or feeling things that are not there; shortness of breath; sleepiness or unusual drowsiness; sore throat; tightness in chest; tiredness; trouble concentrating; trouble sleeping; unusual tiredness or weakness; vomiting; wheezing

Incidence not known
Burning feeling in chest or stomach; burning, numbness, pain, or tingling in all fingers except smallest finger; cold sweats; cool pale skin; decreased interest in sexual intercourse; difficulty swallowing; general feeling of discomfort or illness; heartburn; inability to have or keep an erection; increased hunger; large amounts of fat in the blood; loss in sexual ability, desire, drive, or performance; nightmares; shakiness; slurred speech; stomach cramps; stomach upset; tenderness in stomach area; watery or bloody diarrhea

Other side effects not listed may also occur in some patients. If you notice any other effects, check with your healthcare professional.

MENINGOCOCCAL POLYSACCHARIDE VACCINE
(Subcutaneous route) - me-NINJ-oh-kok-kal pol-ee-SAK-a-ride vak-SEEN

Commonly used brand name(s)
In the U.S.—
Menomune-A/C/Y/W-135

Available Dosage Forms:
• Powder for Solution
• Injectable

Therapeutic Class: Vaccine

Uses For This Vaccine

Meningococcal polysaccharide vaccine is an active immunizing agent used to prevent infection by certain groups of meningococcal bacteria. The vaccine works by causing your body to produce its own protection (antibodies) against the disease.

The following information applies only to the meningococcal vaccine used for meningococcal bacteria Groups A, C, Y, and W-135. These groups cause approximately 50% of meningococcal meningitis cases in the U.S. The vaccine will not protect against infection caused by other meningococcal bacteria groups, such as Group B.

Meningococcal infection can cause life-threatening illnesses, such as meningococcal meningitis, which affects the brain, and meningococcemia, which affects the blood. Some persons with meningococcal meningitis and/or meningococcemia also may die. These diseases are more likely to occur in young children and in persons with certain diseases or conditions that make them more susceptible to a meningococcal infection or more likely to develop serious problems from a meningococcal infection.

Immunization against meningococcal disease is recommended for persons 2 years of age or older who are at risk of getting the disease because:
• they have certain diseases or conditions that make them more susceptible to a meningococcal infection or more likely to develop serious problems from a meningococcal infection.
• they are living in, working in, or visiting an area where there is a strong possibility of contracting meningococcal disease.

Usually a person needs to receive meningococcal vaccine only once. However, additional injections may be needed for young children who remain at high risk for meningococcal disease.

Meningococcal polysaccharide vaccine is to be administered only by or under the supervision of your doctor or other health care professional.

Before Receiving This Vaccine

In deciding to use a vaccine, the risks of taking the vaccine must be weighed against the good it will do. This is a decision you and your doctor will make. For this vaccine, the following should be considered:

Allergies—Tell your doctor if you have ever had any unusual or allergic reaction to this medicine or any other medi-

cines. Also tell your health care professional if you have any other types of allergies, such as to foods, dyes, preservatives, or animals. For non-prescription products, read the label or package ingredients carefully.

Pediatric—In general the use of meningococcal vaccine is restricted to persons 2 years of age and older; however, in some cases children as young as 3 months of age may be vaccinated. This vaccine has been tested in older children and, in effective doses, has not been shown to cause different side effects or problems than it does in adults.

Geriatric—Many medicines have not been studied specifically in older people. Therefore, it may not be known whether they work exactly the same way they do in younger adults. Although there is no specific information comparing use of this vaccine in the elderly with use in other age groups, this vaccine is not expected to cause different side effects or problems in older people than it does in younger adults.

Pregnancy—

	Pregnancy Category	Explanation
All Trimesters	C	Animal studies have shown an adverse effect and there are no adequate studies in pregnant women OR no animal studies have been conducted and there are no adequate studies in pregnant women.

Breast Feeding—Studies in women suggest that this medication poses minimal risk to the infant when used during breastfeeding.

Other medicines—

Receiving this vaccine with any of the following medicines is usually not recommended, but may be required in some cases. If both medicines are prescribed together, your doctor may change the dose or how often you use one or both of the medicines.

Measles Virus Vaccine, Live

Interactions with Food/Tobacco/Alcohol—Certain medicines should not be used at or around the time of eating food or eating certain types of food since interactions may occur. Using alcohol or tobacco with certain medicines may also cause interactions to occur. Discuss with your healthcare professional the use of your medicine with food, alcohol, or tobacco.

Other medical problems—The presence of other medical problems may affect the use of this vaccine. Make sure you tell your doctor if you have any other medical problems, especially:
- Severe illness with fever—The symptoms of the condition may be confused with the possible side effects of the vaccine

Proper Use of This Vaccine

Dosing—The dose of this medicine will be different for different patients. Follow your doctor's orders or the directions on the label. The following information includes only the average doses of this medicine. If your dose is different, do not change it unless your doctor tells you to do so.

The amount of medicine that you take depends on the strength of the medicine. Also, the number of doses you take each day, the time allowed between doses, and the length of time you take the medicine depend on the medical problem for which you are using the medicine.
- For injection dosage form:
  - For prevention of meningococcal meningitis:
    - Adults and children—One dose injected under the skin.

Side Effects of This Vaccine

Along with its needed effects, a medicine may cause some unwanted effects. Although not all of these side effects may occur, if they do occur they may need medical attention.

Check with your doctor immediately if any of the following side effects occur:
Symptoms of allergic reaction
    Difficulty in breathing or swallowing; hives; itching, especially of feet or hands; reddening of skin, especially around ears; swelling of eyes, face, or inside of nose; unusual tiredness or weakness (sudden and severe)

Some side effects may occur that usually do not need medical attention. These side effects may go away during treatment as your body adjusts to the medicine. Also, your health care professional may be able to tell you about ways to prevent or reduce some of these side effects. Check with your health care professional if any of the following side effects continue or are bothersome or if you have any questions about them:
More common
    Redness at place of injection—may last 1 or 2 days; tenderness, soreness, or pain at place of injection
Less common
    Chills; fever over 100 °F (37.8 °C); general feeling of discomfort or illness; hard lump at place of injection; headache; tiredness or weakness

Other side effects not listed may also occur in some patients. If you notice any other effects, check with your healthcare professional.

MENINGOCOCCAL VACCINE, DIPHTHERIA CONJUGATE
(Intramuscular route) - me-NINJ-oh-kok-kal vak-SEEN, dif-THEER-ee-a KON-joo-gate

Commonly used brand name(s)
In the U.S.—
    Menactra

Available Dosage Forms:
- Suspension
- Powder for Suspension

Therapeutic Class: Vaccine

Uses For This Vaccine

Meningococcal diphtheria conjugate vaccine is an active immunizing agent used to prevent infection by certain groups of meningococcal bacteria. The vaccine works by causing your body to produce its own protection (antibodies) against the disease.

The following information applies only to the meningococcal vaccine used for meningococcal bacteria Groups A, C, Y, and W-135. These groups cause nearly all of the meningococcal meningitis cases in the U.S. The vaccine will not protect against infection caused by other meningococcal bacteria groups, such as Group B.

Meningococcal infection can cause life-threatening illnesses, such as meningococcal meningitis, which affects the brain, and meningococcemia, which affects the blood. Some persons with meningococcal meningitis and/or meningococcemia also may die. The rate of these diseases peak in adolescence and early adulthood and are more likely to occur in persons with certain diseases or conditions that make them more susceptible to a meningococcal infection or more likely to develop serious problems from a meningococcal infection.

Immunization against meningococcal disease is recommended for persons 11 to 55 years of age who are at risk of getting the disease because:

- They have certain diseases or conditions that make them more susceptible to a meningococcal infection or more likely to develop serious problems from a meningococcal infection.
- They are living in, working in, or visiting an area where there is a strong possibility of contracting meningococcal disease.

Usually a person needs to receive meningococcal vaccine only once.

Meningococcal polysaccharide vaccine is to be administered only by or under the supervision of your doctor or other health care professional.

Before Receiving This Vaccine

In deciding to use a vaccine, the risks of taking the vaccine must be weighed against the good it will do. This is a decision you and your doctor will make. For this vaccine, the following should be considered:

Allergies—Tell your doctor if you have ever had any unusual or allergic reaction to this medicine or any other medicines. Also tell your health care professional if you have any other types of allergies, such as to foods, dyes, preservatives, or animals. For non-prescription products, read the label or package ingredients carefully.

Pediatric—Studies on this vaccine have been done only in patients older than 11 years of age, and there is no specific information comparing use of meningococcal diphtheria conjugate vaccine in children with use in other age groups. This vaccine has been tested in children 11 and 12 years of age and teenagers and, in effective doses, has not been shown to cause different side effects or problems than it does in adults.

Geriatric—Studies on this vaccine have been done only in patients younger than 55 years of age, and there is no specific information comparing use of meningococcal diphtheria conjugate vaccine in the elderly with use in other age groups.

Pregnancy—

	Pregnancy Category	Explanation
All Trimesters	C	Animal studies have shown an adverse effect and there are no adequate studies in pregnant women OR no animal studies have been conducted and there are no adequate studies in pregnant women.

Breast Feeding—Studies in women suggest that this medication poses minimal risk to the infant when used during breastfeeding.

Other medicines—Although certain medicines should not be used together at all, in other cases two different medicines may be used together even if an interaction might occur. In these cases, your doctor may want to change the dose, or other precautions may be necessary. Tell your healthcare professional if you are taking any other prescription or non-prescription (over-the-counter [OTC]) medicine.

Interactions with Food/Tobacco/Alcohol—Certain medicines should not be used at or around the time of eating food or eating certain types of food since interactions may occur. Using alcohol or tobacco with certain medicines may also cause interactions to occur. Discuss with your healthcare professional the use of your medicine with food, alcohol, or tobacco.

Other medical problems—The presence of other medical problems may affect the use of this vaccine. Make sure you tell your doctor if you have any other medical problems, especially:

- Guillain-Barré syndrome (GBS), history of—This vaccine should not be used if you have this condition.
- Hemophilia (blood disorder with tendency to bleed uncontrollably) or
- Other bleeding problems—May be worsened by meningococcal diphtheria conjugate vaccine
- Illness, recent or critical—May make your condition worse
- Lower immune system response (body's ability to fight infection is suppressed)—This vaccine has not been studied in patients with this problem.

Proper Use of This Vaccine

Dosing—The dose of this medicine will be different for different patients. Follow your doctor's orders or the directions on the label. The following information includes only the average doses of this medicine. If your dose is different, do not change it unless your doctor tells you to do so.

The amount of medicine that you take depends on the strength of the medicine. Also, the number of doses you take each day, the time allowed between doses, and the length of time you take the medicine depend on the medical problem for which you are using the medicine.

- For injection dosage form:
  - For prevention of meningococcal meningitis:
    - Adults and teenagers—One dose injected into the shoulder muscle

- Children 11 to 12 years of age—One dose injected into the shoulder muscle—
- Children younger than 11 years of age—Use and dose must be determined by your doctor.

Precautions While Using This Vaccine

It is very important to tell your doctor if you are allergic to rubber. The stopper of the vial contains dry natural rubber latex, which may cause an allergic reaction if you have a latex allergy.

Check with your doctor right away if you experience a cough, difficulty swallowing, dizziness, fast heartbeat, hives, itching, puffiness or swelling of the eyelids or around the eyes, face, lips or tongue, shortness of breath, skin rash, tightness in chest, unusual tiredness or weakness, and/or wheezing. These could be symptoms of an allergic reaction to the vaccine.

Contact your doctor immediately if you have sudden weakness or are not able to move your arms or legs. This could be a sign of a serious condition called Guillain-Barré syndrome.

Side Effects of This Vaccine

Along with its needed effects, a medicine may cause some unwanted effects. Although not all of these side effects may occur, if they do occur they may need medical attention.

Check with your doctor immediately if any of the following side effects occur:

Rare

Cough; difficulty swallowing; dizziness; fast heartbeat; hives; itching; puffiness or swelling of the eyelids or around the eyes, face, lips, or tongue; shortness of breath; skin rash; tightness in chest; unusual tiredness or weakness; wheezing

Incidence not known

Inability to move arms and legs; sudden and progressing muscle weakness; sudden and severe back pain; sudden numbness and weakness in the arms and legs

Some side effects may occur that usually do not need medical attention. These side effects may go away during treatment as your body adjusts to the medicine. Also, your health care professional may be able to tell you about ways to prevent or reduce some of these side effects. Check with your health care professional if any of the following side effects continue or are bothersome or if you have any questions about them:

More common

Chills; diarrhea; difficulty in moving; fever; general feeling of discomfort or illness; hard lump at injection site; headache; loss of appetite; muscle pain or stiffness; pain in joints; pain, redness or swelling at injection site; weight loss

Less common

Vomiting

Other side effects not listed may also occur in some patients. If you notice any other effects, check with your healthcare professional.

MEPROBAMATE AND ASPIRIN
(Oral route) - me-proe-BA-mate, AS-pir-in

Commonly used brand name(s)

In the U.S.—
Equagesic
Micrainin

Available Dosage Forms:
- Tablet

Therapeutic Class: Salicylate, Aspirin Combination
Pharmacologic Class: NSAID

Uses For This Medicine

Meprobamate and aspirin combination is used to relieve pain, anxiety, and tension in certain disorders or diseases.

This medicine is available only with your doctor's prescription.

Before Using This Medicine

In deciding to use a medicine, the risks of taking the medicine must be weighed against the good it will do. This is a decision you and your doctor will make. For this medicine, the following should be considered:

Allergies—Tell your doctor if you have ever had any unusual or allergic reaction to this medicine or any other medicines. Also tell your health care professional if you have any other types of allergies, such as to foods, dyes, preservatives, or animals. For non-prescription products, read the label or package ingredients carefully.

Pediatric—Do not give a medicine containing aspirin to a child or teenager with a fever or other symptoms of a virus infection, especially flu or chickenpox, without first discussing this with your child's doctor. This is very important because aspirin may cause a serious illness called Reye's syndrome in children or teenagers with fever caused by a virus infection, especially flu or chickenpox. Children who do not have a virus infection may also be more sensitive to the effects of aspirin (contained in this combination medicine), especially if they have a fever or have lost large amounts of body fluid because of vomiting, diarrhea, or sweating. This may increase the chance of side effects during treatment.

Geriatric—Elderly people may be especially sensitive to the effects of meprobamate and aspirin. This may increase the chance of side effects during treatment.

Pregnancy—

	Pregnancy Category	Explanation
All Trimesters	D	Studies in pregnant women have demonstrated a risk to the fetus. However, the benefits of therapy in a life threatening situation or a serious disease, may outweigh the potential risk.

Breast Feeding—There are no adequate studies in women for determining infant risk when using this medication during breastfeeding. Weigh the potential benefits against the potential risks before taking this medication while breastfeeding.

Other medicines—

Using this medicine with any of the following medicines is not recommended. Your doctor may decide not to treat you with this medication or change some of the other medicines you take.

Ketorolac

Interactions with Food/Tobacco/Alcohol—Certain medicines should not be used at or around the time of eating food or eating certain types of food since interactions may occur. Using alcohol or tobacco with certain medicines may also cause interactions to occur. The following interactions have been selected on the basis of their potential significance and are not necessarily all-inclusive.

Using this medicine with any of the following may cause an increased risk of certain side effects but may be unavoidable in some cases. If used together, your doctor may change the dose or how often you use this medicine, or give you special instructions about the use of food, alcohol, or tobacco.

Ethanol

Other medical problems—The presence of other medical problems may affect the use of this medicine. Make sure you tell your doctor if you have any other medical problems, especially:

- Alcohol abuse (or history of) or
- Drug abuse or dependence (or history of)—Dependence on meprobamate may develop
- Anemia or
- Stomach ulcer or other stomach problems—Aspirin may make your condition worse
- Asthma, allergies, and nasal polyps (history of) or
- Kidney disease or
- Liver disease—The chance of side effects may be increased.
- Epilepsy—The risk of seizures may be increased
- Gout—Aspirin may make this condition worse and may also lessen the effects of some medicines used to treat gout
- Hemophilia or other bleeding problems—The chance of bleeding may be increased by aspirin
- Porphyria—Meprobamate may make the condition worse

Proper Use of This Medicine

Take this medicine with food or a full glass (8 ounces) of water to lessen stomach irritation.

Do not take this medicine if it has a strong vinegar-like odor. This odor means the aspirin in it is breaking down. If you have any questions about this, check with your health care professional.

Take this medicine only as directed by your doctor. Do not take more of it, do not take it more often, and do not take it for a longer time than your doctor ordered. If too much meprobamate is taken, it may become habit-forming. Also, taking too much aspirin may cause stomach problems or lead to medical problems because of an overdose.

Dosing—The dose of this medicine will be different for different patients. Follow your doctor's orders or the directions on the label. The following information includes only the av-

erage doses of this medicine. If your dose is different, do not change it unless your doctor tells you to do so.

The amount of medicine that you take depends on the strength of the medicine. Also, the number of doses you take each day, the time allowed between doses, and the length of time you take the medicine depend on the medical problem for which you are using the medicine.

- Adults—Oral, 1 or 2 tablets three or four times a day, as needed.
- Children up to 12 years of age: Use is not recommended.

Storage—Store the medicine in a closed container at room temperature, away from heat, moisture, and direct light. Keep from freezing.

Keep out of the reach of children.

Do not keep outdated medicine or medicine no longer needed.

Precautions While Using This Medicine

If you will be taking this medicine regularly for a long time:
- Your doctor should check your progress at regular visits.
- Check with your doctor at least every 4 months to make sure you need to continue taking this medicine.

If you will be taking this medicine in large doses or for a long time, do not stop taking it without first checking with your doctor. Your doctor may want you to reduce gradually the amount you are taking before stopping completely.

Check the labels of all nonprescription (over-the-counter [OTC]) and prescription medicines you now take. If any contain aspirin or other salicylates (including bismuth subsalicylate [e.g., Pepto-Bismol]), be especially careful. Taking or using any of these medicines while taking this combination medicine containing aspirin may lead to overdose. If you have any questions about this, check with your health care professional.

This medicine will add to the effects of alcohol and other CNS depressants (medicines that slow down the nervous system, possibly causing drowsiness). Some examples of CNS depressants are antihistamines or medicine for hay fever, other allergies, or colds; sedatives, tranquilizers, or sleeping medicine; prescription pain medicine or narcotics; barbiturates; medicine for seizures; muscle relaxants; or anesthetics, including some dental anesthetics. Check with your doctor before taking any of the above while you are taking this medicine.

Stomach problems may be more likely to occur if you drink alcoholic beverages while being treated with this medicine, especially if you are taking the medicine in high doses or for a long time. Check with your doctor if you have any questions about this.

Too much use of this medicine together with certain other medicines may increase the chance of stomach problems. Therefore, do not regularly take this medicine together with any of the following medicines, unless directed to do so by your medical doctor or dentist:
- Acetaminophen (e.g., Tylenol)
- Diclofenac (e.g., Voltaren)
- Diflunisal (e.g., Dolobid)
- Etodolac (e.g., Lodine)

- Fenoprofen (e.g., Nalfon)
- Floctafenine (e.g., Idarac)
- Flurbiprofen (oral) (e.g., Ansaid)
- Ibuprofen (e.g., Motrin)
- Indomethacin (e.g., Indocin)
- Ketoprofen (e.g., Orudis)
- Ketorolac (e.g., Toradol)
- Meclofenamate (e.g., Meclomen)
- Mefenamic acid (e.g., Ponstel)
- Naproxen (e.g., Naprosyn)
- Phenylbutazone (e.g., Butazolidin)
- Piroxicam (e.g., Feldene)
- Sulindac (e.g., Clinoril)
- Tiaprofenic acid (e.g., Surgam)
- Tolmetin (e.g., Tolectin)

If you are taking a laxative containing cellulose, do not take it within 2 hours of taking this medicine. Taking these medicines close together may make this medicine less effective by preventing the aspirin (contained in this combination medicine) from being absorbed by your body.

For diabetic patients:
- False urine sugar test results may occur if you take 8 or more 325-mg (5-grain) doses of aspirin (contained in this combination medicine) every day for several days in a row. Smaller doses or occasional use of aspirin usually will not affect urine sugar tests. If you have any questions about this, check with your doctor, especially if your diabetes is not well controlled.

Before you have any medical tests, tell the medical doctor in charge that you are taking this medicine. The results of some tests, such as the metyrapone test and the phentolamine test, may be affected by this medicine.

If you plan to have surgery, including dental surgery, do not take aspirin (contained in this combination medicine) for 5 days before the surgery, unless otherwise directed by your medical doctor or dentist. Taking aspirin during this time may cause bleeding problems.

If you think you or someone else may have taken an overdose of this medicine, get emergency help at once. Taking an overdose of this medicine or taking alcohol or other CNS depressants with it may lead to unconsciousness and possibly death. Some signs of an overdose are continuing ringing or buzzing in ears; any hearing loss; severe confusion, drowsiness, or weakness; shortness of breath or slow or troubled breathing; staggering; and slow heartbeat.

This medicine may cause some people to become dizzy, lightheaded, drowsy, or less alert than they are normally. Make sure you know how you react to this medicine before you drive, use machines, or do anything else that could be dangerous if you are dizzy or are not alert.

Meprobamate (contained in this combination medicine) may cause dryness of the mouth. For temporary relief, use sugarless candy or gum, melt bits of ice in your mouth, or use a saliva substitute. However, if your mouth continues to feel dry for more than 2 weeks, check with your medical doctor or dentist. Continuing dryness of the mouth may increase the chance of dental disease, including tooth decay, gum disease, and fungus infections.

Side Effects of This Medicine

Along with its needed effects, a medicine may cause some unwanted effects. Although not all of these side effects may occur, if they do occur they may need medical attention.

Check with your doctor immediately if any of the following side effects occur:

Rare
Wheezing, shortness of breath, troubled breathing, or tightness in chest

Symptoms of overdose
Any loss of hearing; bloody urine; confusion (severe); convulsions (seizures); diarrhea (severe or continuing); dizziness or lightheadedness (continuing); drowsiness (severe); fast or deep breathing; hallucinations (seeing, hearing, or feeling things that are not there); headache (severe or continuing); increased sweating; nausea or vomiting (continuing); nervousness or excitement (severe); ringing or buzzing in ears (continuing); slow heartbeat; slurred speech; staggering; stomach pain (severe or continuing); unexplained fever; unusual or uncontrolled flapping movements of the hands, especially in elderly patients; unusual thirst; vision problems; weakness (severe)

Symptoms of overdose in children
Changes in behavior; drowsiness or tiredness (severe); fast or deep breathing

Check with your doctor as soon as possible if any of the following side effects occur:

Rare
Bloody or black, tarry stools; confusion; skin rash, hives, or itching; sore throat and fever; unusual bleeding or bruising; unusual excitement; unusual tiredness or weakness; vomiting of blood or material that looks like coffee grounds

Some side effects may occur that usually do not need medical attention. These side effects may go away during treatment as your body adjusts to the medicine. Also, your health care professional may be able to tell you about ways to prevent or reduce some of these side effects. Check with your health care professional if any of the following side effects continue or are bothersome or if you have any questions about them:

More common
Drowsiness; heartburn or indigestion; nausea with or without vomiting; stomach pain (mild)

Less common
Blurred vision or change in near or distant vision; dizziness or lightheadedness; headache

After you stop using this medicine, it may still produce some side effects that need attention. During this period of time, *check with your doctor immediately* if you notice the following side effects:

Clumsiness or unsteadiness; confusion; convulsions (seizures); hallucinations (seeing, hearing, or feeling things that are not there); increased dreaming; muscle twitching; nausea or vomiting; nervousness or restlessness; nightmares; trembling; trouble in sleeping

Other side effects not listed may also occur in some patients. If you notice any other effects, check with your healthcare professional.

MEQUINOL AND TRETINOIN
(Topical route) - ME-kwi-nole, TRET-i noyn

Commonly used brand name(s)

In the U.S.—
   Solage

Available Dosage Forms:
- Solution

Therapeutic Class: Hypopigmentation Agent

Uses For This Medicine

Mequinol and Tretinoin is used to treat areas of the skin that have become darker after repeated exposure to the sun. These areas are called solar lentigines, or age or liver spots.

Mequinol and tretinoin is available only with your doctor's prescription.

Before Using This Medicine

In deciding to use a medicine, the risks of taking the medicine must be weighed against the good it will do. This is a decision you and your doctor will make. For this medicine, the following should be considered:

Allergies—Tell your doctor if you have ever had any unusual or allergic reaction to this medicine or any other medicines. Also tell your health care professional if you have any other types of allergies, such as to foods, dyes, preservatives, or animals. For non-prescription products, read the label or package ingredients carefully.

Pediatric—Studies on this medicine have been done only in adult patients, and there is no specific information comparing use of this medicine in children with use in other age groups. Mequinol and tretinoin should not be used in children.

Geriatric—This medicine has been tested and has not been shown to cause different side effects or problems in older people than it does in younger adults.

Other medicines—

Using this medicine with any of the following medicines is usually not recommended, but may be required in some cases. If both medicines are prescribed together, your doctor may change the dose or how often you use one or both of the medicines.

Aminocaproic Acid, Aprotinin, Tetracycline, Tranexamic Acid

Interactions with Food/Tobacco/Alcohol—Certain medicines should not be used at or around the time of eating food or eating certain types of food since interactions may occur. Using alcohol or tobacco with certain medicines may also cause interactions to occur. Discuss with your healthcare professional the use of your medicine with food, alcohol, or tobacco.

Other medical problems—The presence of other medical problems may affect the use of this medicine. Make sure you tell your doctor if you have any other medical problems, especially:
- Eczema or
- Frequent exposure to sunlight or sunlamps or
- Sunburn—Use of this medicine may cause or increase the irritation associated with these conditions
- Vitiligo (or a family history of this condition)—Use of this medicine may cause lightening of areas of the skin that have not been treated

Proper Use of This Medicine

It is very important that you use this medicine only as directed. Do not use more of it, do not use it more often, and do not use it for a longer time than your doctor ordered. To do so may cause irritation of the skin.

Do not apply this medicine to windburned or sunburned skin or on open wounds.

Do not use this medicine in or around the eyes or lips, or inside of the nose. Spread the medicine away from these areas when applying. If the medicine accidentally gets on these areas, wash with water at once.

This medicine usually comes with patient directions. Read them carefully before using the medicine.

To use this medicine:
- Using the applicator tip, apply enough mequinol and tretinoin solution to cover the affected areas. Apply only enough medicine to make the lesion appear moist. Avoid areas of normally colored skin.
- You should not shower or bathe for at least 6 hours after applying the medicine.
- Cosmetics may be applied 30 minutes after application of the medicine.

Dosing—The dose of this medicine will be different for different patients. Follow your doctor's orders or the directions on the label. The following information includes only the average doses of this medicine. If your dose is different, do not change it unless your doctor tells you to do so.

The amount of medicine that you take depends on the strength of the medicine. Also, the number of doses you take each day, the time allowed between doses, and the length of time you take the medicine depend on the medical problem for which you are using the medicine.

- For topical dosage form (solution):
  - For age or liver spots:
    - Adults—Apply to the affected areas of the skin twice daily, morning and evening, at least 8 hours apart.
    - Children—Use is not recommended.

Missed dose—If you miss a dose of this medicine, skip the missed dose and go back to your regular dosing schedule. Do not double doses.

Storage—Store the medicine in a closed container at room temperature, away from heat, moisture, and direct light. Keep from freezing.

Keep out of the reach of children.

Do not keep outdated medicine or medicine no longer needed.

The product is flammable and should be kept away from fire or excessive heat.

Precautions While Using This Medicine

You may notice redness, stinging, burning or irritation when you first start using this medicine. It may take up to 6 months before you notice full beneficial effects, even if you use the medicine every day. Check with your health care professional at any time skin irritation becomes severe or if your age spots get darker in color.

Unless your doctor tells you otherwise, it is especially important to avoid using the following skin products on the same area as mequinol and tretinoin topical solution:

- Hair products that are irritating, such as permanents or hair removal products
- Skin products that cause sensitivity to the sun, such as those containing spices or limes
- Skin products containing a large amount of alcohol, such as astringents, shaving creams, or after-shave lotions
- Skin products that are too drying or abrasive, such as some cosmetics, soaps, or skin cleansers

Using these products along with mequinol and tretinoin may cause mild to severe irritation of the skin. Check with your doctor before using other topical medicines.

Avoid overexposing the treated areas to sunlight, wind, or cold weather. The skin will be more prone to sunburn, dryness, or irritation. Do not use a sunlamp.

Regularly use sunscreen or sunblocking lotions with a sun protection factor (SPF) of at least 15. Also, wear protective clothing and hats, and apply creams, lotions, or moisturizers often.

Check with your doctor any time your skin becomes too dry and irritated. Your health care professional can help you choose the right skin products for you to reduce skin dryness and irritation and may include:

- Taking part in an ongoing program to avoid further damage to your skin from the sun. The program should stress staying out of the sun when possible and wearing proper clothing or hats to protect your skin from sunlight.
- Regular use of oil-based creams or lotions to help to reduce skin irritation or dryness caused by the use of mequinol and tretinoin topical solution.

Side Effects of This Medicine

In some animal studies, mequinol and tretinoin has been shown to cause skin tumors to develop faster when the treated area is exposed to ultraviolet light (sunlight or artificial sunlight from a sunlamp). Other studies have not shown the same result and more studies need to be done. It is not known if mequinol and tretinoin topical solution causes skin tumors to develop faster in humans.

Along with its needed effects, a medicine may cause some unwanted effects. Although not all of these side effects may occur, if they do occur they may need medical attention.

Check with your doctor as soon as possible if any of the following side effects occur:

More common
> Burning feeling or stinging skin (severe); itching (severe); peeling of skin (severe); redness of skin (severe)

Less common
> Allergic reaction; large blisters on the skin

Some side effects may occur that usually do not need medical attention. These side effects may go away during treat-

ment as your body adjusts to the medicine. Also, your health care professional may be able to tell you about ways to prevent or reduce some of these side effects. Check with your health care professional if any of the following side effects continue or are bothersome or if you have any questions about them:

More common
> Burning feeling, stinging, or tingling of skin (mild)— lasting for a short time after first applying the medicine; itching (mild); chapping or slight peeling of skin (mild); lightening of skin around treated area; lightening of skin on treated area; redness of skin (mild); skin irritation; unusually warm skin (mild)

Less common
> Crusting of skin; dry skin; skin rash

Other side effects not listed may also occur in some patients. If you notice any other effects, check with your healthcare professional.

MERCAPTOPURINE (Oral route) - mer-kap-toe-PYOOR-een

Commonly used brand name(s)

In the U.S.—
> Purinethol

Available Dosage Forms:
- Tablet

Therapeutic Class: Antineoplastic Agent
Pharmacologic Class: Antimetabolite

Uses For This Medicine

Mercaptopurine belongs to the group of medicines known as antimetabolites. It is used to treat some kinds of cancer.

Mercaptopurine interferes with the growth of cancer cells, which are eventually destroyed. Since the growth of normal body cells may also be affected by mercaptopurine, other effects will also occur. Some of these may be serious and must be reported to your doctor. Other effects may not be serious but may cause concern. Some effects may not occur for months or years after the medicine is used.

Before you begin treatment with mercaptopurine, you and your doctor should talk about the good this medicine will do as well as the risks of using it.

Mercaptopurine may also be used for other conditions as determined by your doctor.

Mercaptopurine is available only with your doctor's prescription.

Before Using This Medicine

In deciding to use a medicine, the risks of taking the medicine must be weighed against the good it will do. This is a decision you and your doctor will make. For this medicine, the following should be considered:

Allergies—Tell your doctor if you have ever had any unusual or allergic reaction to this medicine or any other medicines. Also tell your health care professional if you have any other types of allergies, such as to foods, dyes, preservatives,

or animals. For non-prescription products, read the label or package ingredients carefully.

Pediatric—Although there is no specific information comparing use of mercaptopurine in children with use in other age groups, it is not expected to cause different side effects or problems in children than it does in adults.

Geriatric—Many medicines have not been studied specifically in older people. Therefore, it may not be known whether they work exactly the same way they do in younger adults or if they cause different side effects or problems in older people. There is no specific information comparing use of mercaptopurine in the elderly with use in other age groups.

Pregnancy—

	Pregnancy Category	Explanation
All Trimesters	D	Studies in pregnant women have demonstrated a risk to the fetus. However, the benefits of therapy in a life threatening situation or a serious disease, may outweigh the potential risk.

Breast Feeding—There are no adequate studies in women for determining infant risk when using this medication during breastfeeding. Weigh the potential benefits against the potential risks before taking this medication while breastfeeding.

Other medicines—

Using this medicine with any of the following medicines is not recommended. Your doctor may decide not to treat you with this medication or change some of the other medicines you take.

Rotavirus Vaccine, Live

Interactions with Food/Tobacco/Alcohol—Certain medicines should not be used at or around the time of eating food or eating certain types of food since interactions may occur. Using alcohol or tobacco with certain medicines may also cause interactions to occur. Discuss with your healthcare professional the use of your medicine with food, alcohol, or tobacco.

Other medical problems—The presence of other medical problems may affect the use of this medicine. Make sure you tell your doctor if you have any other medical problems, especially:

- Chickenpox (including recent exposure) or
- Herpes zoster (shingles)—Risk of severe disease affecting other parts of the body
- Gout (history of) or
- Kidney stones (history of)—Mercaptopurine may increase levels of uric acid in the body, which can cause gout or kidney stones
- Infection—Mercaptopurine may decrease your body's ability to fight infection
- Kidney disease or
- Liver disease—Effects of mercaptopurine may be increased because of slower removal from the body

Proper Use of This Medicine

Use this medicine only as directed by your doctor. Do not use more or less of it, and do not use it more often than your doctor ordered. The exact amount of medicine you need has been carefully worked out. Taking too much may increase the chance of side effects, while taking too little may not improve your condition.

Mercaptopurine is often given together with certain other medicines. If you are using a combination of medicines, make sure that you take each one at the right time and do not mix them. Ask your health care professional to help you plan a way to remember to take your medicines at the right times.

While you are using mercaptopurine, your doctor may want you to drink extra fluids so that you will pass more urine. This will help prevent kidney problems and keep your kidneys working well.

If you vomit shortly after taking a dose of mercaptopurine, check with your doctor. You will be told whether to take the dose again or to wait until the next scheduled dose.

Dosing—The dose of this medicine will be different for different patients. Follow your doctor's orders or the directions on the label. The following information includes only the average doses of this medicine. If your dose is different, do not change it unless your doctor tells you to do so.

The amount of medicine that you take depends on the strength of the medicine. Also, the number of doses you take each day, the time allowed between doses, and the length of time you take the medicine depend on the medical problem for which you are using the medicine.

Missed dose—If you miss a dose of this medicine, skip the missed dose and go back to your regular dosing schedule. Do not double doses.

Call your doctor or pharmacist for instructions.

Storage—Store the medicine in a closed container at room temperature, away from heat, moisture, and direct light. Keep from freezing.

Keep out of the reach of children.

Do not keep outdated medicine or medicine no longer needed.

Precautions While Using This Medicine

It is very important that your doctor check your progress at regular visits to make sure that this medicine is working properly and to check for unwanted effects.

Avoid alcoholic beverages until you have discussed their use with your doctor. Alcohol may increase the harmful effects of this medicine.

While you are being treated with mercaptopurine, and after you stop treatment with it, do not have any immunizations (vaccinations) without your doctor's approval. Mercaptopurine may lower your body's resistance and there is a chance you might get the infection the immunization is meant to prevent. In addition, other persons living in your household should not take oral polio vaccine since there is a chance they could pass the polio virus on to you. Also, avoid persons who have taken oral polio vaccine. Do not get close to them and do not stay in the same room with them for very long. If you cannot take these precautions, you should consider wearing a protective face mask that covers the nose and mouth.

Mercaptopurine can temporarily lower the number of white blood cells in your blood, increasing the chance of getting an infection. It can also lower the number of platelets, which are necessary for proper blood clotting. If this occurs, there are certain precautions you can take, especially when your blood count is low, to reduce the risk of infection or bleeding:

- If you can, avoid people with infections. Check with your doctor immediately if you think you are getting an infection or if you get a fever or chills, cough or hoarseness, lower back or side pain, or painful or difficult urination.
- Check with your doctor immediately if you notice any unusual bleeding or bruising; black, tarry stools; blood in urine or stools; or pinpoint red spots on your skin.
- Be careful when using a regular toothbrush, dental floss, or toothpick. Your medical doctor, dentist, or nurse may recommend other ways to clean your teeth and gums. Check with your medical doctor before having any dental work done.
- Do not touch your eyes or the inside of your nose unless you have just washed your hands and have not touched anything else in the meantime.
- Be careful not to cut yourself when you are using sharp objects such as a safety razor or fingernail or toenail cutters.
- Avoid contact sports or other situations where bruising or injury could occur.

Tell the doctor in charge that you are taking this medicine before you have any medical tests. The results of tests for the amount of sugar or uric acid in the blood measured by a machine called a sequential multiple analyzer (SMA) may be affected by this medicine.

Side Effects of This Medicine

Along with its needed effects, a medicine may cause some unwanted effects. Although not all of these side effects may occur, if they do occur they may need medical attention.

Also, because of the way cancer medicines act on the body, there is a chance that they might cause other unwanted effects that may not occur until months or years after the medicine is used. These delayed effects may include certain types of cancer. Discuss these possible effects with your doctor.

Check with your doctor immediately if any of the following side effects occur:
Less common
   Black, tarry stools; blood in urine or stools; cough or hoarseness; fever or chills; lower back or side pain; painful or difficult urination; pinpoint red spots on skin; unusual bleeding or bruising

Check with your doctor as soon as possible if any of the following side effects occur:
More common
   Unusual tiredness or weakness; yellow eyes or skin

Less common
   Joint pain; loss of appetite; nausea and vomiting; swelling of feet or lower legs

Rare
   Sores in mouth and on lips

Some side effects may occur that usually do not need medical attention. These side effects may go away during treatment as your body adjusts to the medicine. Also, your health care professional may be able to tell you about ways to prevent or reduce some of these side effects. Check with your health care professional if any of the following side effects

continue or are bothersome or if you have any questions about them:
Less common
   Darkening of skin; diarrhea; headache; skin rash and itching; weakness

After you stop using this medicine, it may still produce some side effects that need attention. During this period of time, *check with your doctor immediately* if you notice the following side effects:

   Black, tarry stools; blood in urine or stools; cough or hoarseness; fever or chills; lower back or side pain; painful or difficult urination; pinpoint red spots on skin; unusual bleeding or bruising; yellow eyes or skin

Other side effects not listed may also occur in some patients. If you notice any other effects, check with your healthcare professional.

MESALAMINE (Oral route) - me-SAL-a-meen

Commonly used brand name(s)
In the U.S.—
   Asacol
   Pentasa

In Canada—
   Asacol 800

Available Dosage Forms:
- Tablet, Delayed Release
- Tablet, Enteric Coated
- Capsule, Extended Release
- Tablet

Therapeutic Class: Gastrointestinal Agent

Uses For This Medicine

Mesalamine is used to treat inflammatory bowel disease, such as ulcerative colitis. It works inside the bowel by helping to reduce the inflammation and other symptoms of the disease.

Mesalamine is available only with your doctor's prescription.

Once a medicine has been approved for marketing for a certain use, experience may show that it is also useful for other medical problems. Although this use is not included in product labeling, mesalamine may be used to treat mild or moderate Crohn's disease and help prevent it from occurring again.

Before Using This Medicine

In deciding to use a medicine, the risks of taking the medicine must be weighed against the good it will do. This is a decision you and your doctor will make. For this medicine, the following should be considered:

Allergies—Tell your doctor if you have ever had any unusual or allergic reaction to this medicine or any other medicines. Also tell your health care professional if you have any other types of allergies, such as to foods, dyes, preservatives, or animals. For non-prescription products, read the label or package ingredients carefully.

Pediatric—Studies on this medicine have been done only in adult patients, and there is no specific information comparing use of mesalamine in children with use in other age groups.

Geriatric—Many medicines have not been studied specifically in older people. Therefore, it may not be known whether they work exactly the same way they do in younger adults or if they cause different side effects or problems in older people. There is no information comparing use of mesalamine in the elderly with use in other age groups.

Pregnancy—

	Pregnancy Category	Explanation
All Trimesters	B	Animal studies have revealed no evidence of harm to the fetus, however, there are no adequate studies in pregnant women OR animal studies have shown an adverse effect, but adequate studies in pregnant women have failed to demonstrate a risk to the fetus.

Breast Feeding—There are no adequate studies in women for determining infant risk when using this medication during breastfeeding. Weigh the potential benefits against the potential risks before taking this medication while breastfeeding.

Other medicines—

Using this medicine with any of the following medicines is usually not recommended, but may be required in some cases. If both medicines are prescribed together, your doctor may change the dose or how often you use one or both of the medicines.

Varicella Virus Vaccine

Interactions with Food/Tobacco/Alcohol—Certain medicines should not be used at or around the time of eating food or eating certain types of food since interactions may occur. Using alcohol or tobacco with certain medicines may also cause interactions to occur. Discuss with your healthcare professional the use of your medicine with food, alcohol, or tobacco.

Other medical problems—The presence of other medical problems may affect the use of this medicine. Make sure you tell your doctor if you have any other medical problems, especially:

- Kidney disease—The use of mesalamine may cause further damage to the kidneys
- Narrowing of the tube where food passes out of the stomach—May delay release of mesalamine into the body

Proper Use of This Medicine

Swallow the capsule or tablet whole. Do not break, crush, or chew it before swallowing.

Take this medicine before meals and at bedtime with a full glass (8 ounces) of water, unless otherwise directed by your doctor.

Keep taking this medicine for the full time of treatment, even if you begin to feel better after a few days. Do not miss any doses.

Do not change to another brand without checking with your doctor. The doses are different for different brands. If you refill your medicine and it looks different, check with your pharmacist.

Dosing—The dose of this medicine will be different for different patients. Follow your doctor's orders or the directions on the label. The following information includes only the average doses of this medicine. If your dose is different, do not change it unless your doctor tells you to do so.

The amount of medicine that you take depends on the strength of the medicine. Also, the number of doses you take each day, the time allowed between doses, and the length of time you take the medicine depend on the medical problem for which you are using the medicine.

The number of capsules or tablets that you take depends on the brand and strength of the medicine.

- For inflammatory bowel disease:
  - For long-acting oral dosage form (extended-release capsules or tablets):
    - Adults—1 gram four times a day for up to eight weeks.
    - Children—Use and dose must be determined by your doctor.
  - For long-acting oral dosage form (delayed-release tablets):
    - Adults—
      - For Asacol: 800 milligrams (mg) three times a day for six weeks. For maintenance treatment of ulcerative colitis, 1600 mg a day, divided into smaller doses that are taken at separate times.
      - For Mesasal: A total of 1.5 to 3 grams a day, divided into smaller doses that are taken at separate times.
      - For Salofalk: 1 gram three or four times a day.
    - Children—Use and dose must be determined by your doctor.

Missed dose—If you miss a dose of this medicine, take it as soon as possible. However, if it is almost time for your next dose, skip the missed dose and go back to your regular dosing schedule. Do not double doses.

Storage—Store the medicine in a closed container at room temperature, away from heat, moisture, and direct light. Keep from freezing.

Keep out of the reach of children.

Do not keep outdated medicine or medicine no longer needed.

Precautions While Using This Medicine

It is important that your doctor check your progress at regular visits.

For patients taking the capsule form of this medicine:
- You may sometimes notice what looks like small beads in your stool. These are just the empty shells that are left after the medicine has been absorbed into your body.

For patients taking the tablet form of this medicine:
- You may sometimes notice what looks like a tablet in your stool. This is just the empty shell that is left after the medicine has been absorbed into your body.

Side Effects of This Medicine

Along with its needed effects, a medicine may cause some unwanted effects. Although not all of these side effects may occur, if they do occur they may need medical attention.

Stop taking this medicine and get emergency help immediately if any of the following effects occur:

Less common

Abdominal or stomach cramps or pain (severe); bloody diarrhea; fever; headache (severe); skin rash and itching

Rare

Anxiety; back or stomach pain (severe); blue or pale skin; chest pain, possibly moving to the left arm, neck, or shoulder; chills; fast heartbeat; nausea or vomiting; shortness of breath; swelling of the stomach; unusual tiredness or weakness; yellow eyes or skin

Symptoms of overdose

Confusion; diarrhea (severe or continuing); dizziness or lightheadedness; drowsiness (severe); fast or deep breathing; headache (severe or continuing); hearing loss or ringing or buzzing in ears (continuing); nausea or vomiting (continuing)

Some side effects may occur that usually do not need medical attention. These side effects may go away during treatment as your body adjusts to the medicine. Also, your health care professional may be able to tell you about ways to prevent or reduce some of these side effects. Check with your health care professional if any of the following side effects continue or are bothersome or if you have any questions about them:

More common

Abdominal or stomach cramps or pain (mild); diarrhea (mild); dizziness; headache (mild); runny or stuffy nose or sneezing

Less common

Acne; back or joint pain; gas or flatulence; indigestion; loss of appetite; loss of hair

Other side effects not listed may also occur in some patients. If you notice any other effects, check with your healthcare professional.

METFORMIN   (Oral route) - met-FOR-min

Black Box Warning

Lactic acidosis is a rare, but serious, metabolic complication that can occur due to metformin accumulation during treatment with metformin hydrochloride; when it occurs, it is fatal in approximately 50% of cases. Lactic acidosis may also occur in association with a number of pathophysiologic conditions, including diabetes mellitus, and whenever there is significant tissue hypoperfusion and hypoxemia. Lactic acidosis is characterized by elevated blood lactate levels (greater than 5 mmol/L), decreased blood pH, electrolyte disturbances with an increased anion gap, and an increased lactate/pyruvate ratio. When metformin is implicated as the cause of lactic acidosis, metformin plasma levels greater than 5 mcg/mL are generally found.

The reported incidence of lactic acidosis in patients receiving metformin hydrochloride is very low (approximately 0.03 cases/1000 patient-years, with approximately 0.015 fatal cases/1000 patient-years). In more than 20,000 patient-years exposure to metformin in clinical trials, there were no reports of lactic acidosis. Reported cases have occurred primarily in diabetic patients with significant renal insufficiency, including both intrinsic renal disease and renal hypoperfusion, often in the setting of multiple concomitant medical/surgical problems and multiple concomitant medications. Patients with congestive heart failure requiring pharmacologic management, in particular those with unstable or acute congestive heart failure who are at risk of lactic acidosis. The risk of lactic acidosis increases with the degree of renal dysfunction and the patient's age. The risk of lactic acidosis may, therefore, be significantly decreased by regular monitoring of renal function in patients taking metformin hydrochloride and by use of the minimum effective dose of metformin hydrochloride. In particular, treatment of the elderly should be accompanied by careful monitoring of renal function. Metformin hydrochloride treatment should not be initiated in patients greater than or equal to 80 years of age unless measurement of creatinine clearance demonstrates that renal function is not reduced, as these patients are more susceptible to developing lactic acidosis. In addition, metformin hydrochloride should be promptly withheld in the presence of any condition associated with hypoxemia, dehydration, or sepsis. Because impaired hepatic function may significantly limit the ability to clear lactate, metformin hydrochloride should generally be avoided in patients with clinical or laboratory evidence of hepatic disease. Patients should be cautioned against excessive alcohol intake, either acute or chronic, when taking metformin hydrochloride, since alcohol potentiates the effects of metformin hydrochloride on lactate metabolism. In addition, metformin hydrochloride should be temporarily discontinued prior to any intravascular radiocontrast study and for any surgical procedure.

The onset of lactic acidosis often is subtle, and accompanied only by nonspecific symptoms such as malaise, myalgias, respiratory distress, increasing somnolence, and nonspecific abdominal distress. There may be associated hypothermia, hypotension, and resistant bradyarrhythmias with more marked acidosis. The patient and the patient's physician must be aware of the possible importance of such symptoms and the patient should be instructed to notify the physician immediately if they occur. Metformin hydrochloride should be withdrawn until the situation is clarified. Serum electrolytes, ketones, blood glucose and, if indicated, blood pH, lactate levels, and even blood metformin levels may be useful. Once a patient is stabilized on any dose level of metformin hydrochloride, gastrointestinal symptoms, which are common during initiation of therapy, are unlikely to be drug related. Later occurrence of gastrointestinal symptoms could be due to lactic acidosis or other serious disease.

Levels of fasting venous plasma lactate above the upper limit of normal but less than 5 mmol/L in patients taking metformin hydrochloride do not necessarily indicate impending lactic acidosis and may be explainable by other mechanisms, such as poorly controlled diabetes or obesity, vigorous physical activity, or technical problems in sample handling.

Lactic acidosis should be suspected in any diabetic patient with metabolic acidosis lacking evidence of ketoacidosis (ketonuria and ketonemia).

Lactic acidosis is a medical emergency that must be treated in a hospital setting. In a patient with lactic acidosis who is taking metformin hydrochloride, the drug should be discontinued immediately and general supportive measures promptly instituted. Because metformin hydrochloride is dialyzable (with a clearance of up to 170 mL/min under good hemodynamic conditions), prompt hemodialysis is recommended to correct the acidosis and remove the accumulated metformin. Such management often results in prompt reversal of symptoms and recovery.

Commonly used brand name(s)
In the U.S.—

Fortamet	Glucophage XR
Glucophage	Riomet

Available Dosage Forms:
- Solution
- Tablet
- Tablet, Extended Release

Therapeutic Class: Hypoglycemic

Uses For This Medicine

Metformin is used to treat a type of diabetes mellitus (sugar diabetes) called type 2 diabetes. With this type of diabetes, insulin produced by the pancreas is not able to get sugar into the cells of the body where it can work properly. Using metformin alone, with a type of oral antidiabetic medicine called a sulfonylurea, or with insulin will help to lower blood sugar when it is too high and help restore the way you use food to make energy.

Many people can control type 2 diabetes with diet alone or diet and exercise. Following a specially planned diet and exercising will always be important when you have diabetes, even when you are taking medicines. To work properly, the amount of metformin you take must be balanced against the amount and type of food you eat and the amount of exercise you do. If you change your diet, your exercise, or both, you will want to test your blood sugar to find out if it is too low. Your health care professional will teach you what to do if this happens.

At some point, this medicine may stop working as well and your blood glucose will increase. You will need to know if this happens and what to do. Instead of taking more of this medicine, your doctor may want you to change to another antidiabetic medicine. If that does not lower your blood sugar, your doctor may have you stop taking the medicine and begin receiving insulin injections instead.

Metformin does not help patients who have insulin-dependent or type 1 diabetes because they cannot produce insulin from their pancreas gland. Their blood glucose is best controlled by insulin injections.

Metformin is available only with your doctor's prescription.

Once a medicine has been approved for marketing for a certain use, experience may show that it is also useful for other medical problems. Although this use is not included in product labeling, metformin is used in certain patients with the following medical conditions:
- Polycystic ovary syndrome

Before Using This Medicine

In deciding to use a medicine, the risks of taking the medicine must be weighed against the good it will do. This is a decision you and your doctor will make. For this medicine, the following should be considered:

Allergies—Tell your doctor if you have ever had any unusual or allergic reaction to this medicine or any other medicines. Also tell your health care professional if you have any other types of allergies, such as to foods, dyes, preservatives, or animals. For non-prescription products, read the label or package ingredients carefully.

Pediatric—Metformin tablets have been tested in children older than 10 years old and, in effective doses, have not been shown to cause different side effects or problems than it does in adults.

Studies with metformin extended-release tablets have been done only in adult patients, and there is no specific information comparing use of this medicine in children with use in other age groups.

Geriatric—Use in older adults is similar to use in adults of younger age. However, if you have blood vessel disorders or kidney problems, your health care professional may adjust your dose or tell you to stop taking this medicine, if necessary.

Pregnancy—

	Pregnancy Category	Explanation
All Trimesters	B	Animal studies have revealed no evidence of harm to the fetus, however, there are no adequate studies in pregnant women OR animal studies have shown an adverse effect, but adequate studies in pregnant women have failed to demonstrate a risk to the fetus.

Breast Feeding—Studies in women suggest that this medication poses minimal risk to the infant when used during breastfeeding.

Other medicines—

Using this medicine with any of the following medicines is not recommended. Your doctor may decide not to treat you with this medication or change some of the other medicines you take.

Acetrizoic Acid, Diatrizoate, Ethiodized Oil, Iobenzamic Acid, Iobitridol, Iocarmic Acid, Iocetamic Acid, Iodamide, Iodipamide, Iodixanol, Iodohippuric Acid, Iodopyracet, Iodoxamic Acid, Ioglicic Acid, Ioglycamic Acid, Iohexol, Iomeprol, Iopamidol, Iopanoic Acid, Iopentol, Iophendylate, Iopromide, Iopronic Acid, Ioseric Acid, Iosimide, Iotasul, Iothalamate, Iotrolan, Iotroxic Acid, Ioversol, Ioxaglate, Ioxitalamic Acid, Ipodate, Metrizamide, Metrizoic Acid, Tyropanoate Sodium

Interactions with Food/Tobacco/Alcohol—Certain medicines should not be used at or around the time of eating food or eating certain types of food since interactions may occur. Using alcohol or tobacco with certain medicines may also cause interactions to occur. Discuss with your healthcare professional the use of your medicine with food, alcohol, or tobacco.

Other medical problems—The presence of other medical problems may affect the use of this medicine. Make sure you tell your doctor if you have any other medical problems, especially:
- Acid in the blood (ketoacidosis or lactic acidosis) or
- Burns (severe) or

- Dehydration or
- Diarrhea (severe) or
- Female hormone changes for some women (e.g., during puberty, pregnancy, or menstruation) or
- Fever, high or
- Infection (severe) or
- Injury (severe) or
- Ketones in the urine or
- Mental stress (severe) or
- Overactive adrenal gland (not properly controlled) or
- Problems with intestines (severe) or
- Slow stomach emptying or
- Surgery (major) or
- Vomiting or
- Any other condition that causes problems with eating or absorbing food or
- Any other condition in which blood sugar changes rapidly—Metformin in many cases will be replaced with insulin by your doctor, possibly only for a short time. Use of insulin is best to help control diabetes mellitus in patients with these conditions that without warning cause quick changes in the blood sugar.
- Heart or blood vessel disorders or
- Kidney disease or kidney problems or
- Liver disease (or history of)—Lactic acidosis can occur in these conditions and chances of it occurring are even greater with use of metformin
- Kidney, heart, or other problems that require medical tests or examinations that use certain medicines called contrast agents, with x-rays—Metformin should be stopped before medical exams or diagnostic tests that might cause less urine output than usual. Passing unusually low amounts of urine may increase the chance of a build up of metformin and unwanted effects. Metformin may be restarted 48 hours after the exams or tests if kidney function is tested and found to be normal
- Overactive thyroid (not properly controlled) or
- Underactive thyroid (not properly controlled)—Until the thyroid condition is controlled, it may change the amount or type of antidiabetic medicine you need
- Underactive adrenal gland (not properly controlled) or
- Underactive pituitary gland (not properly controlled) or
- Undernourished condition or
- Weakened physical condition or
- Any other condition that causes low blood sugar—Patients who have any of these conditions may be more likely to develop low blood sugar, which can affect the dose of metformin you need and increase the need for blood sugar testing

Proper Use of This Medicine

Use this medicine as directed even if you feel well and do not notice any signs of high blood sugar. Do not take more of this medicine and do not take it more often than your doctor ordered. To do so may increase the chance of serious side effects. Remember that this medicine will not cure your dia-

betes, but it does help control it. Therefore, you must continue to take it as directed if you expect to lower your blood sugar and keep it low. You may have to take an antidiabetic medicine for the rest of your life. If high blood sugar is not treated, it can cause serious problems, such as heart failure, blood vessel disease, eye disease, or kidney disease.

Your doctor will give you instructions about diet, exercise, how to test your blood sugar, and how to adjust your dose when you are sick.

- Blood sugar tests: Testing for blood sugar is the best way to tell whether your diabetes is being controlled properly. Blood sugar testing helps you and your health care team adjust your antidiabetic medicine dose, meal plan, and exercise schedule.
- Diet: The daily number of calories in your meal plan should be adjusted by your doctor or a registered dietitian to help you reach and maintain a healthy body weight. In addition, regular meals and snacks are arranged to meet the energy needs of your body at different times of the day. It is very important that you carefully follow your meal plan.
- Exercise: Ask your doctor what kind of exercise to do, the best time to do it, and how much you should do each day.
- Fluid (water) replacement: It is important to replace the water or fluid that your body uses. Tell your doctor if you have less urine output than usual or severe diarrhea that lasts for more than 1 day.
- On sick days:
  - When you become sick with a cold, fever, or the flu, you need to take your usual dose of metformin, even if you feel too ill to eat. This is especially true if you have nausea, vomiting, or diarrhea. Infection usually increases your need to produce more insulin. Sometimes you may need to be switched from metformin to insulin for a short period of time while you are sick to properly control blood sugar. Call your doctor for specific instructions, especially if severe or prolonged vomiting occurs.
  - Continue taking your metformin and try to stay on your regular meal plan. If you have trouble eating solid food, drink fruit juices, non-diet soft drinks, or clear soups, or eat small amounts of bland foods. A dietitian or your health care professional can give you a list of foods and the amounts to use for sick days.
  - Test your blood sugar and check your urine for ketones. If ketones are present, call your doctor at once. Even when you start feeling better, let your doctor know how you are doing.
- For patients taking a long-acting form of this medicine
  - Swallow the tablets whole. Do not crush or chew before swallowing.

Dosing—The dose of this medicine will be different for different patients. Follow your doctor's orders or the directions on the label. The following information includes only the average doses of this medicine. If your dose is different, do not change it unless your doctor tells you to do so.

The amount of medicine that you take depends on the strength of the medicine. Also, the number of doses you take each day, the time allowed between doses, and the length of time you take the medicine depend on the medical problem for which you are using the medicine.

- For oral dosage form (tablets):
  - For type 2 diabetes:
    - For patients taking metformin tablets
    - Adults:
      — Metformin alone: At first, 500 milligrams (mg) two times a day taken with the morning and evening meals. Or, 850 mg a day taken with the morning meal. Then, your doctor may increase your dose a little at a time every week or every other week if needed. Later, your doctor may want you to take 500 or 850 mg two to three times a day with meals.
      — Metformin with a sulfonylurea: Your doctor will determine the dose of each medicine.
      — Metformin with insulin: At first, 500 mg a day. Then, your doctor may increase your dose by 500 mg every week if needed.
    - Children up to 10 years of age—Use and dose must be determined by your doctor.
    - Children 10 years of age and over—At first, 500 milligrams (mg) with your morning meal and 500 mg with your evening meal. Then, your doctor may increase your dose a little at a time every week if needed.
    - For patients taking metformin extended-release tablets
    - Adults and teenagers:
      — Metformin alone (Glucophage® ER): At first, 500 milligrams (mg) once daily with the evening meal. Then, your doctor may increase your dose a little at a time every week if needed. If you need more medicine, your doctor may tell you to take more than one dose a day.
      — Metformin alone (Glumetza®): At first, 1000 milligrams (mg) once daily with the evening meal. Then, your doctor may increase your dose a little at a time every week if needed. If you need more medicine, your doctor may tell you to take more than one dose a day.
      — Metformin with a sulfonylurea: Your doctor will determine the dose of each medicine.
      — Metformin with insulin: At first, 500 mg a day. Then, your doctor may increase your dose by 500 mg every week if needed.
    - Children up to 17 years of age—Use and dose must be determined by your doctor.

Missed dose—If you miss a dose of this medicine, take it as soon as possible. However, if it is almost time for your next dose, skip the missed dose and go back to your regular dosing schedule. Do not double doses.

Storage—Store the medicine in a closed container at room temperature, away from heat, moisture, and direct light. Keep from freezing.

Keep out of the reach of children.

Do not keep outdated medicine or medicine no longer needed.

Precautions While Using This Medicine

Your doctor will want to check your progress at regular visits, especially during the first few weeks that you take this medicine.

It is very important to follow carefully any instructions from your health care team about:

- Alcohol—Drinking alcohol may cause very low blood sugar. Discuss this with your health care team.
- Other medicines—Do not take other medicines unless they have been discussed with your doctor. This especially includes nonprescription medicines such as aspirin, and medicines for appetite control, asthma, colds, cough, hay fever, or sinus problems.
- Counseling—Other family members need to learn how to prevent side effects or help with side effects if they occur. Counseling on birth control and pregnancy may be needed because of the problems that can occur in pregnancy for patients with diabetes.
- Travel—Carry a recent prescription and your medical history. Be prepared for an emergency as you would normally. Make allowances for changing time zones, but keep your meal times as close as possible to your usual meal times.

In case of emergency—There may be a time when you need emergency help for a problem caused by your diabetes. You need to be prepared for these emergencies. It is a good idea to:

- Wear a medical identification (I.D.) bracelet or neck chain at all times. Also, carry an I.D. card in your wallet or purse that says that you have diabetes and a list of all of your medicines.
- Have a glucagon kit available in case severe low blood sugar occurs. Check and replace any expired kits regularly.
- Keep some kind of quick-acting sugar handy to treat low blood sugar.

If you are scheduled to have surgery or medical tests that involve x-rays, you should tell your doctor that you are taking metformin. Your doctor will instruct you to stop taking metformin until at least 2 days after the surgery or medical tests. During this time, if your blood sugar cannot be controlled by diet and exercise, you may be advised to take insulin.

Too much metformin, under certain conditions, can cause lactic acidosis. Symptoms of lactic acidosis are severe and quick to appear and usually occur when other health problems not related to the medicine are present and are very severe, such as a heart attack or kidney failure. Symptoms include diarrhea, fast and shallow breathing, severe muscle pain or cramping, unusual sleepiness, and unusual tiredness or weakness.

If symptoms of lactic acidosis occur, you should check your blood sugar and get immediate emergency medical help. Also, tell your doctor if severe vomiting occurs.

Too much metformin also can cause low blood sugar (hypoglycemia) when it is used under certain conditions. Symptoms of low blood sugar must be treated before they lead to unconsciousness (passing out). Different people may feel different symptoms of low blood sugar. It is important that you learn which symptoms of low blood sugar you usually have so that you can treat it quickly and call someone on your health care team right away when you need advice.

- Symptoms of low blood sugar can include: anxious feeling, behavior change similar to being drunk, blurred vision, cold sweats, confusion, cool pale skin, difficulty in concentrating, drowsiness, excessive hunger, fast heartbeat, headache, nausea, nervousness, nightmares, restless sleep, shakiness, slurred speech, and unusual tiredness or weakness.

- The symptoms of low blood sugar may develop quickly and may result from:
  - delaying or missing a scheduled meal or snack.
  - exercising more than usual.
  - drinking a large amount of alcohol.
  - taking certain medicines.
  - if also using insulin or a sulfonylurea, using too much of these medicines.
  - sickness (especially with vomiting or diarrhea).

- Know what to do if symptoms of low blood sugar occur. Eating some form of quick-acting sugar when symptoms of low blood sugar first appear will usually prevent them from getting worse.

- Good ways to increase your blood sugar include:
  - Using glucagon injections in emergency situations such as unconsciousness. Have a glucagon kit available and know how to prepare and use it. Members of your household also should know how and when to use it.
  - Eating glucose tablets or gel or sugar cubes (6 one-half–inch size). Or drinking fruit juice or nondiet soft drink (4 to 6 ounces [one-half cup]), corn syrup or honey (1 tablespoon), or table sugar (dissolved in water).
    - Do not use chocolate. The sugar in chocolate may not enter into your blood stream fast enough. This is because the fat in chocolate slows down the sugar entering into the blood stream.
    - If a meal is not scheduled for an hour or more, you should also eat a light snack, such as crackers or half a sandwich.

High blood sugar (hyperglycemia) is another problem related to uncontrolled diabetes. Symptoms of mild high blood sugar appear more slowly than those of low blood sugar.

- Check with your health care team as soon as possible if you notice any of the following symptoms: Blurred vision, drowsiness, dry mouth, increased frequency and volume of urination, loss of appetite, nausea or vomiting, stomachache, tiredness, or unusual thirst.

- Get emergency help right away if you notice any of the following symptoms: Flushed dry skin, fruit-like breath odor, ketones in urine, passing out, or troubled breathing (rapid and deep). If high blood sugar is not treated, severe hyperglycemia can occur, leading to ketoacidosis (diabetic coma) and death.

- It is important to recognize what can cause the loss of blood glucose control. Calling your doctor early may be important to prevent problems from developing when the following occur. High blood sugar symptoms may occur if you:
  - have a fever or an infection.
  - are using insulin, sulfonylurea, or metformin and do not take enough of these medicines or skip a dose.
  - do not exercise as much as usual.
  - take certain medicines to treat conditions other than diabetes that change the amount of sugar in your blood.
  - overeat or do not follow your meal plan.

- Know what to do if high blood sugar occurs. Your doctor may recommend changes in your antidiabetic medicine dose(s) or meal plan to avoid high blood sugar. Symptoms of high blood sugar must be corrected before they progress to more serious conditions. Check with your doctor often to make sure you are controlling your blood sugar, but do not change your dose without checking with your doctor. Your doctor might discuss the following with you:
  - Delaying a meal if your blood glucose is over 200 mg/dL to allow time for your blood sugar to go down. An extra dose of metformin or an injection of insulin may be needed if your blood sugar does not come down shortly.
  - Not exercising if your blood glucose is over 240 mg/dL and reporting this to your doctor immediately.
  - Being hospitalized if ketoacidosis or diabetic coma occurs.

Side Effects of This Medicine

Along with its needed effects, a medicine may cause some unwanted effects. Although not all of these side effects may occur, if they do occur they may need medical attention.

Check with your doctor immediately if any of the following side effects occur:

   Rare
   Lactic acidosis (quick and severe), including diarrhea, fast shallow breathing, muscle pain or cramping, unusual sleepiness, unusual tiredness or weakness

Check with your doctor as soon as possible if any of the following side effects occur:

   Rare
   Low blood sugar (mild), including anxious feeling, behavior change similar to being drunk, blurred vision, cold sweats, confusion, cool pale skin, difficulty in concentrating, drowsiness, excessive hunger, fast heartbeat, headache, nausea, nervousness, nightmares, restless sleep, shakiness, slurred speech

Some side effects may occur that usually do not need medical attention. These side effects may go away during treatment as your body adjusts to the medicine. Also, your health care professional may be able to tell you about ways to prevent or reduce some of these side effects. Check with your health care professional if any of the following side effects continue or are bothersome or if you have any questions about them:

   More common
   Loss of appetite; metallic taste in mouth; passing of gas; stomachache; vomiting; weight loss

Other side effects not listed may also occur in some patients. If you notice any other effects, check with your healthcare professional.

METFORMIN AND PIOGLITAZONE
(Oral route) - met-FOR-min, pye-oh-GLI-ta-zone

Uses For This Medicine

Metformin and pioglitazone is a combination medicine used to treat a type of diabetes mellitus (sugar diabetes) called type 2 diabetes. With this type of diabetes, insulin produced by the pancreas is not able to get sugar into the cells of the body where it can work properly. Using metformin and pioglitazone will help to lower blood sugar when it is too high and help restore the way you use food to make energy.

Many people can control type 2 diabetes with diet alone or diet and exercise. Following a specially planned diet and exercising will always be important when you have diabetes, even when you are taking medicines. To work properly, the amount of metformin/pioglitazone you take must be balanced against the amount and type of food you eat and the amount of exercise you do. If you change your diet, your exercise, or both, you will want to test your blood sugar to find out if it is too low. Your health care professional will teach you what to do if this happens.

This medicine is available only with your doctor's prescription.

Before Using This Medicine

In deciding to use a medicine, the risks of taking the medicine must be weighed against the good it will do. This is a decision you and your doctor will make. For this medicine, the following should be considered:

Allergies—Tell your doctor if you have ever had any unusual or allergic reaction to this medicine or any other medicines. Also tell your health care professional if you have any other types of allergies, such as to foods, dyes, preservatives, or animals. For non-prescription products, read the label or package ingredients carefully.

Pediatric—Studies with this medicine have been done only in adult patients, and there is no specific information comparing use of metformin/pioglitazone in children with use in other age groups.

Geriatric—Use in older adults is similar to use in adults of younger age. However, if you have kidney problems, your health care professional may adjust your dose or tell you to stop taking this medicine, if necessary.

Pregnancy—

	Pregnancy Category	Explanation
All Trimesters	C	Animal studies have shown an adverse effect and there are no adequate studies in pregnant women OR no animal studies have been conducted and there are no adequate studies in pregnant women.

Breast Feeding—
Metformin
• Studies in women suggest that this medication poses minimal risk to the infant when used during breastfeeding.
Pioglitazone
• There are no adequate studies in women for determining infant risk when using this medication during breastfeeding. Weigh the potential benefits against the potential risks before taking this medication while breastfeeding.

Other medicines—

Using this medicine with any of the following medicines is not recommended. Your doctor may decide not to treat you with this medication or change some of the other medicines you take.

Acetrizoic Acid, Diatrizoate, Ethiodized Oil, Iobenzamic Acid, Iobitridol, Iocarmic Acid, Iocetamic Acid, Iodamide, Iodi-

pamide, Iodixanol, Iodohippuric Acid, Iodopyracet, Iodoxamic Acid, Ioglicic Acid, Ioglycamic Acid, Iohexol, Iomeprol, Iopamidol, Iopanoic Acid, Iopentol, Iophendylate, Iopromide, Iopronic Acid, Ioseric Acid, Iosimide, Iotasul, Iothalamate, Iotrolan, Iotroxic Acid, Ioversol, Ioxaglate, Ioxitalamic Acid, Ipodate, Metrizamide, Metrizoic Acid, Tyropanoate Sodium

Interactions with Food/Tobacco/Alcohol—Certain medicines should not be used at or around the time of eating food or eating certain types of food since interactions may occur. Using alcohol or tobacco with certain medicines may also cause interactions to occur. Discuss with your healthcare professional the use of your medicine with food, alcohol, or tobacco.

Other medical problems—The presence of other medical problems may affect the use of this medicine. Make sure you tell your doctor if you have any other medical problems, especially:
• Acid in the blood (acidosis or ketoacidosis)—This medicine should NOT be used in these patients.
• Blood poisoning or
• Dehydration (severe) or
• Heart or blood vessel disorders or
• Kidney disease or
• Liver disease—Lactic acidosis can occur with these conditions and chances of it occurring are even greater with a medicine that contains metformin.
• Adrenal gland problems or
• Debilitation (severe weakness and loss of energy) or
• Malnourishment (e.g., not having enough food or calorie intake) or
• Older age or
• Pituitary gland problems—These conditions could make you more vulnerable to the effects of low blood sugar.
• Edema (e.g., swelling or retaining fluids)—Metformin/pioglitazone may cause this condition to become worse.
• Kidney, heart, or other problems that require medical tests, or examinations that use certain medicines called contrast agents with x-ray exams or
• Major surgery—Because this medicine contains metformin, your doctor should advise you to stop taking it before you have any medical exams, diagnostic tests, or major surgeries that might cause less urine output than usual; you may be advised to start taking the medicine again 48 hours after the exam or test if your kidney function is tested and found to be normal.

Proper Use of This Medicine

Follow carefully the special meal plan your doctor gave you. This is a very important part of controlling your condition, and is necessary if the medicine is to work properly. Also, exercise regularly and test for sugar in your blood or urine as directed.

Metformin/pioglitazone should be taken with meals to help reduce the gastrointestinal side effects that may occur during the first few weeks of treatment.

Dosing—The dose of this medicine will be different for different patients. Follow your doctor's orders or the directions on the label. The following information includes only the average doses of this medicine. If your dose is different, do not change it unless your doctor tells you to do so.

The amount of medicine that you take depends on the strength of the medicine. Also, the number of doses you take each day, the time allowed between doses, and the length of time you take the medicine depend on the medical problem for which you are using the medicine.

- For oral dosage form (tablets):
  - For type 2 diabetes:
    - For patients already taking metformin alone:
      — Adults: At first, either the 15 milligrams (mg) pioglitazone/500 mg metformin tablet or the 15 mg pioglitazone/850 mg metformin tablet once or twice a day, as instructed by your doctor. Then, your doctor may increase your dose a little at a time until your blood sugar is controlled.
      — Children: Use and dose must be determined by your doctor.
    - For patients already taking pioglitazone alone:
      — Adults: At first, either the 15 milligrams (mg) pioglitazone/500 mg metformin tablet twice a day or the 15 mg pioglitazone/850 mg metformin tablet once a day, as instructed by your doctor. Then, your doctor may increase your dose a little at a time until your blood sugar is controlled.
      — Children: Use and dose must be determined by your doctor.
    - For patients switching from a combination of metformin and pioglitazone as separate tablets:
      — Adults: At first, either the 15 milligrams (mg) pioglitazone/500 mg metformin tablet or the 15 mg pioglitazone/850 mg metformin tablet, based on the doses of pioglitazone and metformin already being taken, as instructed by your doctor. Then, your doctor may increase your dose a little at a time until your blood sugar is controlled.
      — Children: Use and dose must be determined by your doctor.

Missed dose—Call your doctor or pharmacist for instructions.

Storage—Keep out of the reach of children.

Keep the bottle closed when you are not using it. Store it at room temperature, away from light and heat. Do not freeze.

Ask your healthcare professional how you should dispose of any medicine you do not use.

Precautions While Using This Medicine

Your doctor will want to check your progress at regular visits, especially during the first few weeks that you take this medicine.

Under certain conditions, too much metformin can cause lactic acidosis. *The symptoms of lactic acidosis are severe and quick to appear,* and usually occur when other health problems not related to the medicine are present and are very severe, such as a heart attack or kidney failure. Symptoms of lactic acidosis include: abdominal or stomach discomfort; decreased appetite; diarrhea; fast or shallow breathing; a general feeling of discomfort; muscle pain or cramping; and unusual sleepiness, tiredness, or weakness.

If symptoms of lactic acidosis occur, you should get immediate emergency medical help.

It is very important to carefully follow any instructions from your health care team about:

- Alcohol—Drinking alcohol may cause severe low blood sugar. Discuss this with your health care team.
- Other medicines—Do not take other medicines unless they have been discussed with your doctor. This especially includes nonprescription medicines such as aspirin, and medicines for appetite control, asthma, colds, cough, hay fever, or sinus problems.
- Counseling—Other family members need to learn how to prevent side effects or help with side effects if they occur. Also, patients with diabetes may need special counseling about diabetes medicine dosing changes that might occur with life-style changes, such as changes in exercise or diet. Furthermore, counseling on contraception and pregnancy may be needed, because of the problems that can occur in patients with diabetes during pregnancy.
- Travel—Keep a recent prescription and your medical history with you. Be prepared for an emergency as you would normally. Make allowances for changing time zones and keep your meal times as close as possible to your usual meal times.

In case of emergency—There may be a time when you need emergency help for a problem caused by your diabetes. You need to be prepared for these emergencies. It is a good idea to wear a medical identification (ID) bracelet or neck chain at all times. Also, carry an ID card in your wallet or purse that says you have diabetes and that lists all of your medicines.

Symptoms of hypoglycemia (low blood sugar) include: anxiety; behavior changes similar to being drunk; blurred vision; cold sweats; confusion; cool, pale skin; difficulty in thinking; drowsiness; excessive hunger; fast heartbeat; headache (continuing); nausea; nervousness; nightmares; restless sleep; shakiness; slurred speech; or unusual tiredness or weakness.

Metformin/pioglitazone can cause low blood sugar. However, this can also occur if you delay or miss a meal or snack, drink alcohol, exercise more than usual, cannot eat because of nausea or vomiting, take certain medicines, or take metformin/pioglitazone with another type of diabetes medicine. *The symptoms of low blood sugar must be treated before they lead to unconsciousness (passing out).* Different people feel different symptoms of low blood sugar. *It is important that you learn which symptoms of low blood sugar you usually have so you can treat it quickly.*

If symptoms of low blood sugar occur, *eat glucose tablets or gel, corn syrup, honey, or sugar cubes; or drink fruit juice, non-diet soft drink, or sugar dissolved in water.* Also, check your blood for low blood sugar. *Glucagon is used in emergency situations when severe symptoms such as seizures (convulsions) or unconsciousness occur.* Have a glucagon kit available, along with a syringe and needle, and know how to use it. The members of your household should also know how to use it.

Symptoms of hyperglycemia (high blood sugar) include: blurred vision; drowsiness; dry mouth; flushed, dry skin; fruit-like breath odor; increased urination (frequency and volume); ketones in the urine; loss of appetite; sleepiness; stomachache, nausea, or vomiting; tiredness; troubled breathing (rapid and deep); unconsciousness; or unusual thirst.

High blood sugar may occur if you do not exercise as much as usual, have a fever or infection, do not take enough or skip a dose of your diabetes medicine, or overeat or do not follow your meal plan.

If symptoms of high blood sugar occur, *check your blood sugar level and then call your health care professional for instructions.*

Side Effects of This Medicine

Along with its needed effects, a medicine may cause some unwanted effects. Although not all of these side effects may occur, if they do occur they may need medical attention.

Also, because of the way these medicines act on the body, there is a chance that they might cause other unwanted effects that may not occur until months or years after the medicine is used. These may include certain types of cancer, such as leukemia or bladder cancer. Discuss these possible effects with your doctor.

Check with your doctor immediately if any of the following side effects occur:

More common
Bladder pain; bloody or cloudy urine; difficult, burning, or painful urination; frequent urge to urinate; lower back or side pain

Less common
Pale skin; troubled breathing with exertion; unusual bleeding or bruising; unusual tiredness or weakness

Rare
Abdominal discomfort; anxiety; blurred vision; chills; cold sweats; coma; confusion; cool pale skin; decreased appetite; depression; diarrhea; dizziness; fast heartbeat; fast, shallow breathing; general feeling of discomfort; headache; increased hunger; muscle pain or cramping; nausea; nervousness; nightmares; seizures; shakiness; shortness of breath; sleepiness; slurred speech

Some side effects may occur that usually do not need medical attention. These side effects may go away during treatment as your body adjusts to the medicine. Also, your health care professional may be able to tell you about ways to prevent or reduce some of these side effects. Check with your health care professional if any of the following side effects continue or are bothersome or if you have any questions about them:

More common
Body aches or pain; cough; difficulty in breathing; ear congestion; fever, sneezing or sore throat; loss of voice; nasal congestion; runny nose

Other side effects not listed may also occur in some patients. If you notice any other effects, check with your healthcare professional.

METHOTREXATE (Oral route, Injection route) - meth-oh-TREX-ate

Black Box Warning

- INJECTION
  - ○ The use of methotrexate high dose regimens recommended for osteosarcoma requires meticulous care. High dose regimens for other neoplastic diseases are investigational and a therapeutic advantage has not been established.
  - ○ Methotrexate formulations and diluents containing preservatives must not be used for intrathecal or high dose methotrexate therapy.
- ORAL AND INJECTION
  - ○ Methotrexate should be used only by physicians whose knowledge and experience include the use of antimetabolite therapy.
  - ○ Because of the possibility of serious toxic reactions (which can be fatal):
    - ▪ Methotrexate should be used only in life threatening neoplastic diseases, or in patients with psoriasis or rheumatoid arthritis with severe, recalcitrant, disabling disease which is not adequately responsive to other forms of therapy.
    - ▪ Deaths have been reported with the use of methotrexate in the treatment of malignancy, psoriasis, and rheumatoid arthritis.
    - ▪ Patients should be closely monitored for bone marrow, liver, lung and kidney toxicities.
    - ▪ Patients should be informed by their physician of the risks involved and be under physician's care throughout therapy.
  - ○ Methotrexate has been reported to cause fetal death and/or congenital anomalies. Therefore, it is not recommended for women of childbearing potential unless there is clear medical evidence that the benefits can be expected to outweigh the considered risks. Pregnant women with psoriasis or rheumatoid arthritis should not receive methotrexate.
  - ○ Methotrexate elimination is reduced in patients with impaired renal functions, ascites, or pleural effusions. Such patients require especially careful monitoring for toxicity, and require dose reduction or, in some cases, discontinuation of methotrexate administration.
  - ○ Unexpectedly severe (sometimes fatal) bone marrow suppression, aplastic anemia, and gastrointestinal toxicity have been reported with concomitant administration of methotrexate (usually in high dosage) along with some nonsteroidal anti-inflammatory drugs (NSAIDs).
  - ○ Methotrexate causes hepatotoxicity, fibrosis and cirrhosis, but generally only after prolonged use. Acutely, liver enzyme elevations are frequently seen. These are usually transient and asymptomatic, and also do not appear predictive of subsequent hepatic disease. Liver biopsy after sustained use often shows histologic changes, and fibrosis and cirrhosis have been reported; these latter lesions may not be preceded by symptoms or abnormal liver function tests in the psoriasis population. For this reason, periodic liver biopsies are usually recommended for psoriatic patients who are under long-term treatment. Persistent abnormalities in liver function tests may precede appearance of fibrosis or cirrhosis in the rheumatoid arthritis population.
  - ○ Methotrexate-induced lung disease, including acute or chronic interstitial pneumonitis, is a potentially dangerous lesion, which may occur acutely at any time during therapy and has been reported at oral doses as low as 7.5 mg/week. It is not always fully reversible and fatalities have been reported. Pulmonary symp-

toms (especially a dry, nonproductive cough) may require interruption of treatment and careful investigation.

○ Diarrhea and ulcerative stomatitis require interruption of therapy; otherwise, hemorrhagic enteritis and death from intestinal perforation may occur.

○ Malignant lymphomas, which may regress following withdrawal of methotrexate, may occur in patients receiving low-dose methotrexate and, thus, may not require cytotoxic treatment. Discontinue methotrexate first and, if the lymphoma does not regress, appropriate treatment should be instituted.

○ Like other cytotoxic drugs, methotrexate may induce "tumor lysis syndrome" in patients with rapidly growing tumors. Appropriate supportive and pharmacologic measures may prevent or alleviate this complication.

○ Severe, occasionally fatal, skin reactions have been reported following single or multiple doses of methotrexate. Reactions have occurred within days of oral, intramuscular, intravenous, or intrathecal methotrexate administration. Recovery has been reported with discontinuation of therapy.

○ Potentially fatal opportunistic infections, especially Pneumocystis carinii pneumonia, may occur with methotrexate therapy.

○ Methotrexate given concomitantly with radiotherapy may increase the risk of soft tissue necrosis and osteonecrosis.

Commonly used brand name(s)

In the U.S.—
Rheumatrex Dose Pack
Trexall

Available Dosage Forms:

- Tablet
- Solution
- Powder for Solution
- Injectable

Therapeutic Class: Antineoplastic Agent
Pharmacologic Class: Antimetabolite

Uses For This Medicine

Methotrexate belongs to the group of medicines known as antimetabolites. It is used to treat cancer of the breast, head and neck, lung, blood, bone, and lymph, and tumors in the uterus. It may also be used to treat other kinds of cancer, as determined by your doctor.

Methotrexate blocks an enzyme needed by the cell to live. This interferes with the growth of cancer cells, which are eventually destroyed. Since the growth of normal body cells may also be affected by methotrexate, other effects will also occur. Some of these may be serious and must be reported to your doctor. Other effects, like hair loss, may not be serious but may cause concern. Some effects may not occur for months or years after the medicine is used.

Before you begin treatment with methotrexate, you and your doctor should talk about the good this medicine will do as well as the risks of using it.

Methotrexate is available only with your doctor's prescription.

Once a medicine has been approved for marketing for a certain use, experience may show that it is also useful for other medical problems. Although these uses are not included in

product labeling, methotrexate is used in certain patients with the following medical conditions:

- Acute nonlymphocytic leukemia (a type of cancer of the blood and lymph system)
- Cancer in the membranes that cover and protect the brain and spinal cord (the meninges)
- Cancer of the bladder
- Cancer of the brain (lymphoma)
- Cancer of the cervix
- Cancer of colon and rectum
- Cancer of the esophagus
- Cancer of the ovaries
- Cancer of the pancreas
- Cancer of the penis
- Cancers of the soft tissues of the body, including the muscles, connective tissues (tendons), vessels that carry blood or lymph, or fat
- Cancer of the stomach
- Hodgkin's lymphoma (a cancer of the lymph system, a part of the body's immune system)

Before Using This Medicine

In deciding to use a medicine, the risks of taking the medicine must be weighed against the good it will do. This is a decision you and your doctor will make. For this medicine, the following should be considered:

Allergies—Tell your doctor if you have ever had any unusual or allergic reaction to this medicine or any other medicines. Also tell your health care professional if you have any other types of allergies, such as to foods, dyes, preservatives, or animals. For non-prescription products, read the label or package ingredients carefully.

Pediatric—Newborns and other infants may be more sensitive to the effects of methotrexate. However, in other children it is not expected to cause different side effects or problems than it does in adults.

Geriatric—Side effects may be more likely to occur in the elderly, who are usually more sensitive to the effects of methotrexate.

Pregnancy—

	Pregnancy Category	Explanation
All Trimesters	X	Studies in animals or pregnant women have demonstrated positive evidence of fetal abnormalities. This drug should not be used in women who are or may become pregnant because the risk clearly outweighs any possible benefit.

Breast Feeding—Studies in women breastfeeding have demonstrated harmful infant effects. An alternative to this medication should be prescribed or you should stop breastfeeding while using this medicine.

Other medicines—

Using this medicine with any of the following medicines is not recommended. Your doctor may decide not to treat you with this medication or change some of the other medicines you take.

Rotavirus Vaccine, Live

Interactions with Food/Tobacco/Alcohol—Certain medicines should not be used at or around the time of eating food or eating certain types of food since interactions may occur. Using alcohol or tobacco with certain medicines may also cause interactions to occur. Discuss with your healthcare professional the use of your medicine with food, alcohol, or tobacco.

Other medical problems—The presence of other medical problems may affect the use of this medicine. Make sure you tell your doctor if you have any other medical problems, especially:

- Alcohol abuse (or history of)—Increased risk of unwanted effects on the liver
- Chickenpox (including recent exposure) or
- Herpes zoster (shingles)—Risk of severe disease affecting other parts of the body
- Colitis
- Disease of the immune system
- Gout (history of) or
- Kidney stones (or history of)—Methotrexate may increase levels of a chemical called uric acid in the body, which can cause gout or kidney stones
- Infection—Methotrexate can reduce immunity to infection
- Intestine blockage or
- Kidney disease or
- Liver disease—Effects may be increased because of slower removal of methotrexate from the body
- Mouth sores or inflammation or
- Stomach ulcer—May be worsened

Proper Use of This Medicine

Take this medicine only as directed by your doctor. Do not take more or less of it, and do not take it more often than your doctor ordered. The exact amount of medicine you need has been carefully worked out. Taking too much may increase the chance of side effects, while taking too little may not improve your condition.

Methotrexate is often given together with certain other medicines. If you are using a combination of medicines, make sure that you take each one at the proper time and do not mix them. Ask your health care professional to help you plan a way to remember to take your medicines at the right times.

While you are using methotrexate, your doctor may want you to drink extra fluids so that you will pass more urine. This will help the drug to pass from the body, and will prevent kidney problems and keep your kidneys working well.

Methotrexate commonly causes nausea and vomiting. Even if you begin to feel ill, do not stop using this medicine without first checking with your doctor. Ask your health care professional for ways to lessen these effects.

If you vomit shortly after taking a dose of methotrexate, check with your doctor. You will be told whether to take the dose again or to wait until the next scheduled dose.

Dosing—The dose of this medicine will be different for different patients. Follow your doctor's orders or the directions on the label. The following information includes only the average doses of this medicine. If your dose is different, do not change it unless your doctor tells you to do so.

The amount of medicine that you take depends on the strength of the medicine. Also, the number of doses you take each day, the time allowed between doses, and the length of time you take the medicine depend on the medical problem for which you are using the medicine.

Missed dose—If you miss a dose of this medicine, skip the missed dose and go back to your regular dosing schedule. Do not double doses.

Call your doctor or pharmacist for instructions.

Storage—Store the medicine in a closed container at room temperature, away from heat, moisture, and direct light. Keep from freezing.

Keep out of the reach of children.

Do not keep outdated medicine or medicine no longer needed.

Precautions While Using This Medicine

It is very important that your doctor check your progress at regular visits to make sure that this medicine is working properly and to check for unwanted effects.

Do not drink alcohol while using this medicine. Alcohol can increase the chance of liver problems.

Some patients who take methotrexate may become more sensitive to sunlight than they are normally. When you first begin taking methotrexate, avoid too much sun and do not use a sunlamp until you see how you react to the sun, especially if you tend to burn easily. In case of a severe burn, check with your doctor.

Do not take medicine for inflammation or pain (aspirin or other salicylates, diclofenac, diflunisal, fenoprofen, ibuprofen, indomethacin, ketoprofen, meclofenamate, mefenamic acid, naproxen, phenylbutazone, piroxicam, sulindac, suprofen, tolmetin) without first checking with your doctor. These medicines may increase the effects of methotrexate, which could be harmful.

While you are being treated with methotrexate, and after you stop treatment with it, do not have any immunizations (vaccinations) without your doctor's approval. Methotrexate may lower your body's resistance and there is a chance you might get the infection the immunization is meant to prevent. In addition, other persons living in your household should not take oral polio vaccine since there is a chance they could pass the polio virus on to you. Also, avoid other persons who have taken oral polio vaccine within the last several months. Do not get close to them, and do not stay in the same room with them for very long. If you cannot take these precautions, you should consider wearing a protective face mask that covers the nose and mouth.

Methotrexate can lower the number of white blood cells in your blood temporarily, increasing the chance of getting an infection. It can also lower the number of platelets, which are necessary for proper blood clotting. If this occurs, there are certain precautions you can take, especially when your blood count is low, to reduce the risk of infection or bleeding:

- If you can, avoid people with infections. Check with your doctor immediately if you think you are getting an infection or if you get a fever or chills, cough or hoarseness, lower back or side pain, or painful or difficult urination.

- Check with your doctor immediately if you notice any unusual bleeding or bruising; black, tarry stools; blood in urine or stools; or pinpoint red spots on your skin.
- Be careful when using a regular toothbrush, dental floss, or toothpick. Your medical doctor, dentist, or nurse may recommend other ways to clean your teeth and gums. Check with your medical doctor before having any dental work done.
- Do not touch your eyes or the inside of your nose unless you have just washed your hands and have not touched anything else in the meantime.
- Be careful not to cut yourself when you are using sharp objects such as a safety razor or fingernail or toenail cutters.
- Avoid contact sports or other situations where bruising or injury could occur.

Side Effects of This Medicine

Along with their needed effects, medicines like methotrexate can sometimes cause unwanted effects such as blood problems, kidney problems, stomach or liver problems, loss of hair, and other side effects. These and others are described below. Also, because of the way these medicines act on the body, there is a chance that they might cause other unwanted effects that may not occur until months or years after the medicine is used. These delayed effects may include certain types of cancer, such as leukemia. Discuss these possible effects with your doctor.

Although not all of these side effects may occur, if they do occur they may need medical attention.

Check with your doctor immediately if any of the following side effects occur:

More common
Black, tarry stools; blood in urine or stools; bloody vomit; diarrhea; joint pain; reddening of skin; stomach pain; swelling of feet or lower legs

Less common
Blurred vision; confusion; convulsions (seizures); cough; pinpoint red spots on skin; shortness of breath; unusual bleeding or bruising

Check with your doctor as soon as possible if any of the following side effects occur:

More common
Sores in mouth and on lips

Less common
Back pain; cough or hoarseness accompanied by fever or chills; dark urine; dizziness; drowsiness; fever or chills; headache; lower back or side pain accompanied by fever or chills; painful or difficult urination accompanied by fever or chills; unusual tiredness or weakness; yellow eyes or skin

Some side effects may occur that usually do not need medical attention. These side effects may go away during treatment as your body adjusts to the medicine. Also, your health care professional may be able to tell you about ways to prevent or reduce some of these side effects. Check with your health care professional if any of the following side effects continue or are bothersome or if you have any questions about them:

More common
Loss of appetite; nausea or vomiting

Less common
Acne; boils; pale skin; skin rash or itching

This medicine may cause a temporary loss of hair in some people. After treatment with methotrexate has ended, normal hair growth should return.

After you stop using this medicine, it may still produce some side effects that need attention. During this period of time, *check with your doctor immediately* if you notice the following side effects:

Back pain; blurred vision; confusion; convulsions (seizures); dizziness; drowsiness; fever; headache; unusual tiredness or weakness

Other side effects not listed may also occur in some patients. If you notice any other effects, check with your healthcare professional.

METHOXSALEN   (Injection route) -
meth-OX-a-len

Black Box Warning

- CAPSULE
  - Methoxsalen with UV radiation should be used only by physicians who have special competence in diagnosis and treatment of psoriasis and who have special training and experience in photochemotherapy. The use of psoralen and ultraviolet radiation therapy should be under constant supervision of such a physician. For the treatment of patients with psoriasis, photochemotherapy should be restricted to patients with severe, recalcitrant, disabling psoriasis which is not adequately responsive to other forms of therapy, and only when the diagnosis has been supported by biopsy. Because of the possibilities of ocular damage, aging of the skin, and skin cancer (including melanoma), the patient should be fully informed by the physician of the risks inherent in this therapy.
  - Methoxsalen soft gelatin capsules should not be used interchangeably with regular Methoxsalen hard gelatin capsules. This new dosage form of methoxsalen exhibits significantly greater bioavailability and earlier photosensitization onset time than previous methoxsalen dosage forms. Patients should be treated in accordance with the dosimetry specifically recommended for this product. The minimum phototoxic dose (MPD) and phototoxic peak time after drug administration prior to onset of photochemotherapy with this dosage form should be determined.
- INJECTION
  - Read the UVAR photophoresis system operator's manual prior to prescribing or dispensing this medication. Methoxsalen sterile solution should be used only by physicians who have special competence in the diagnosis and treatment of cutaneous T-cell lymphoma and who have special training and experience in the UVAR® or UVAR® XTS® Photopheresis System. Please consult the appropriate Operator's Manual before using this product.

Commonly used brand name(s)

In the U.S.—
  Uvadex

Available Dosage Forms:
  • Solution
  • Injectable

Therapeutic Class: Antipsoriatic

Uses For This Medicine

Methoxsalen belongs to the group of medicines called psoralens. It is used along with ultraviolet light (found in sunlight and some special lamps) to treat the white blood cells from your blood in a process called photopheresis. The treated white blood cells are returned to your body to control skin problems associated with cutaneous T-cell lymphoma, a cancer of the lymph system.

Methoxsalen is to be administered only by or under the supervision of your doctor or other health care professional.

Before Using This Medicine

In deciding to use a medicine, the risks of taking the medicine must be weighed against the good it will do. This is a decision you and your doctor will make. For this medicine, the following should be considered:

Allergies—Tell your doctor if you have ever had any unusual or allergic reaction to this medicine or any other medicines. Also tell your health care professional if you have any other types of allergies, such as to foods, dyes, preservatives, or animals. For non-prescription products, read the label or package ingredients carefully.

Pediatric—Studies on this medicine have been done only in adult patients, and there is no specific information comparing use of methoxsalen in children with use in other age groups.

Geriatric—Many medicines have not been studied specifically in older people. Therefore, it may not be known whether they work exactly the same way they do in younger adults or if they cause different side effects or problems in older people. There is no specific information comparing use of methoxsalen in the elderly with use in other age groups.

Pregnancy—

	Pregnancy Category	Explanation
All Trimesters	C	Animal studies have shown an adverse effect and there are no adequate studies in pregnant women OR no animal studies have been conducted and there are no adequate studies in pregnant women.

Breast Feeding—There are no adequate studies in women for determining infant risk when using this medication during breastfeeding. Weigh the potential benefits against the potential risks before taking this medication while breastfeeding.

Other medicines—

Using this medicine with any of the following medicines may cause an increased risk of certain side effects, but using both drugs may be the best treatment for you. If both medicines are prescribed together, your doctor may change the dose or how often you use one or both of the medicines.

Phenytoin

Interactions with Food/Tobacco/Alcohol—Certain medicines should not be used at or around the time of eating food or eating certain types of food since interactions may occur. Using alcohol or tobacco with certain medicines may also cause interactions to occur. Discuss with your healthcare professional the use of your medicine with food, alcohol, or tobacco.

Other medical problems—The presence of other medical problems may affect the use of this medicine. Make sure you tell your doctor if you have any other medical problems, especially:
  • Albinism (pigment lacking in the skin, hair, and eyes, or eyes only) or
  • Erythropoietic protoporphyria or
  • Lupus erythematosus or
  • Porphyria cutanea tarda or
  • Skin cancer or
  • Variegate porphyria or
  • Xeroderma pigmentosum—Methoxsalen treatment may make condition worse
  • Eye problems, such as cataracts or loss of the lens of the eye—Methoxsalen and light treatment may make these conditions worse or may cause damage to the eye

Proper Use of This Medicine

Dosing—The dose of this medicine will be different for different patients. Follow your doctor's orders or the directions on the label. The following information includes only the average doses of this medicine. If your dose is different, do not change it unless your doctor tells you to do so.

The amount of medicine that you take depends on the strength of the medicine. Also, the number of doses you take each day, the time allowed between doses, and the length of time you take the medicine depend on the medical problem for which you are using the medicine.

Precautions While Using This Medicine

Eating certain foods while you are receiving methoxsalen treatment may increase your skin's sensitivity to sunlight. To help prevent this, avoid eating limes, figs, parsley, parsnips, mustard, carrots, and celery while you are being treated with this medicine.

Your doctor should check your progress at regular visits to make sure this treatment is working and that it does not cause unwanted effects. You also should have regular eye examinations.

This medicine increases the sensitivity of your skin to sunlight and also may cause premature aging of the skin. Therefore, exposure to the sun, even through window glass or on a cloudy day, could cause a serious burn. If you must go out during the daylight hours:
  • After each treatment, cover your skin with protective clothing for at least 24 hours. In addition, use a sun block product that has a skin protection factor (SPF) of at least 15 on those areas of your body that cannot be covered. If you have any questions about this, check with your health care professional.

For 24 hours after your methoxsalen treatment, your eyes should be protected during daylight hours with special wrap-around sunglasses that totally block or absorb ultraviolet light (ordinary sunglasses are not adequate). This is to prevent cataracts. Your doctor will tell you what kind of sunglasses to use. These glasses should be worn even in indirect light, such as light coming through a window, or on a cloudy day.

Side Effects of This Medicine

Along with its needed effects, a medicine may cause some unwanted effects. Although not all of these side effects may occur, if they do occur they may need medical attention.

Check with your doctor immediately if any of the following side effects occur:

Rare
Fever; irregular heartbeat; redness or pain at catheter site

Symptoms of overdose
Blistering and peeling of skin; reddened, sore skin

Some side effects may occur that usually do not need medical attention. These side effects may go away during treatment as your body adjusts to the medicine. Also, your health care professional may be able to tell you about ways to prevent or reduce some of these side effects. Check with your health care professional if any of the following side effects continue or are bothersome or if you have any questions about them:

Reddening of skin, slight

Treatment with this medicine usually causes a slight reddening of your skin 24 to 48 hours after the treatment. This is an expected effect and is no cause for concern. However, check with your doctor right away if your skin becomes sore and red or blistered.

There is an increased risk of developing skin cancer after use of methoxsalen. You should check your body regularly and show your doctor any skin sores that do not heal, new skin growths, or skin growths that have changed in the way they look or feel.

Premature aging of the skin may occur as a result of prolonged methoxsalen therapy. This effect is permanent and is similar to what happens when a person sunbathes for long periods of time.

Other side effects not listed may also occur in some patients. If you notice any other effects, check with your healthcare professional.

METHOXSALEN (Oral route) - meth-OX-a-len

Black Box Warning

- CAPSULE
  ○ Methoxsalen with UV radiation should be used only by physicians who have special competence in diagnosis and treatment of psoriasis and who have special training and experience in photochemotherapy. The use of psoralen and ultraviolet radiation

therapy should be under constant supervision of such a physician. For the treatment of patients with psoriasis, photochemotherapy should be restricted to patients with severe, recalcitrant, disabling psoriasis which is not adequately responsive to other forms of therapy, and only when the diagnosis has been supported by biopsy. Because of the possibilities of ocular damage, aging of the skin, and skin cancer (including melanoma), the patient should be fully informed by the physician of the risks inherent in this therapy.
  ○ Methoxsalen soft gelatin capsules should not be used interchangeably with regular Methoxsalen hard gelatin capsules. This new dosage form of methoxsalen exhibits significantly greater bioavailability and earlier photosensitization onset time than previous methoxsalen dosage forms. Patients should be treated in accordance with the dosimetry specifically recommended for this product. The minimum phototoxic dose (MPD) and phototoxic peak time after drug administration prior to onset of photochemotherapy with this dosage form should be determined.

- INJECTION
  ○ Read the UVAR photophoresis system operator's manual prior to prescribing or dispensing this medication. Methoxsalen sterile solution should be used only by physicians who have special competence in the diagnosis and treatment of cutaneous T-cell lymphoma and who have special training and experience in the UVAR® or UVAR® XTS® Photopheresis System. Please consult the appropriate Operator's Manual before using this product.

Commonly used brand name(s)

In the U.S.—
8–Mop
Oxsoralen-Ultra

Available Dosage Forms:
- Capsule

Therapeutic Class: Antipsoriatic

Uses For This Medicine

Methoxsalen belongs to the group of medicines called psoralens. It is used along with ultraviolet light (found in sunlight and some special lamps) in a treatment called PUVA to treat vitiligo, a disease in which skin color is lost, and psoriasis, a skin condition associated with red and scaly patches.

Methoxsalen is also used with ultraviolet light in the treatment of white blood cells. This treatment is called photopheresis and is used to treat the skin problems associated with mycosis fungoides, which is a type of lymphoma.

Methoxsalen may also be used for other conditions as determined by your doctor.

This medicine is available only with your doctor's prescription.

Once a medicine has been approved for marketing for a certain use, experience may show that it is also useful for other medical problems. Although these uses are not included in the product labeling, methoxsalen is used in certain patients with the following medical conditions:
- Alopecia areata
- Atopic dermatitis

- Eczema
- Lichen planus
- Skin that is abnormally sensitive to sunlight

Before Using This Medicine

In deciding to use a medicine, the risks of taking the medicine must be weighed against the good it will do. This is a decision you and your doctor will make. For this medicine, the following should be considered:

Methoxsalen is a very strong medicine that increases the skin's sensitivity to sunlight. In addition to causing serious sunburns if not properly used, it has been reported to increase the chance of skin cancer and cataracts. Also, like too much sunlight, PUVA can cause premature aging of the skin. Therefore, methoxsalen should be used only as directed and it should not be used simply for suntanning. Before using this medicine, be sure that you have discussed its use with your doctor.

Allergies—Tell your doctor if you have ever had any unusual or allergic reaction to this medicine or any other medicines. Also tell your health care professional if you have any other types of allergies, such as to foods, dyes, preservatives, or animals. For non-prescription products, read the label or package ingredients carefully.

Pediatric—Some of the side effects are more likely to occur in children up to 12 years of age, since these children may be more sensitive to the effects of methoxsalen.

Geriatric—Many medicines have not been studied specifically in older people. Therefore, it may not be known whether they work exactly the same way they do in younger adults or if they cause different side effects or problems in older people. There is no specific information comparing use of methoxsalen in the elderly with use in other age groups.

Pregnancy—

	Pregnancy Category	Explanation
All Trimesters	C	Animal studies have shown an adverse effect and there are no adequate studies in pregnant women OR no animal studies have been conducted and there are no adequate studies in pregnant women.

Breast Feeding—There are no adequate studies in women for determining infant risk when using this medication during breastfeeding. Weigh the potential benefits against the potential risks before taking this medication while breastfeeding.

Other medicines—

Using this medicine with any of the following medicines may cause an increased risk of certain side effects, but using both drugs may be the best treatment for you. If both medicines are prescribed together, your doctor may change the dose or how often you use one or both of the medicines.

Phenytoin

Interactions with Food/Tobacco/Alcohol—Certain medicines should not be used at or around the time of eating food or eating certain types of food since interactions may occur. Using alcohol or tobacco with certain medicines may also cause interactions to occur. Discuss with your healthcare professional the use of your medicine with food, alcohol, or tobacco.

Other medical problems—The presence of other medical problems may affect the use of this medicine. Make sure you tell your doctor if you have any other medical problems, especially:

- Allergy to sunlight (or family history of) or
- Infection or
- Lupus erythematosus or
- Porphyria or
- Skin cancer (history of) or
- Skin conditions (other) or
- Stomach problems—Use of PUVA may make the condition worse
- Eye problems, such as cataracts or loss of the lens of the eye—The light treatment may make the condition worse or may cause damage to the eye
- Heart or blood vessel disease (severe)—The heat or prolonged standing associated with each light treatment may make the condition worse
- Liver disease—Condition may cause increased blood levels of the medicine and cause an increase in side effects

Proper Use of This Medicine

Eating certain foods while you are taking methoxsalen may increase your skin's sensitivity to sunlight. To help prevent this, avoid eating limes, figs, parsley, parsnips, mustard, carrots, and celery while you are being treated with this medicine.

Methoxsalen usually comes with patient directions. Read them carefully before using this medicine.

This medicine may take 6 to 8 weeks to really help your condition. Do not increase the amount of methoxsalen you are taking or spend extra time in the sunlight or under an ultraviolet lamp. This will not make the medicine act any more quickly and may result in a serious burn.

If this medicine upsets your stomach:

- Patients taking the hard gelatin capsules may take them with food or milk.
- Patients taking the soft gelatin capsules may take them with low-fat food or low-fat milk.

Dosing—The dose of this medicine will be different for different patients. Follow your doctor's orders or the directions on the label. The following information includes only the average doses of this medicine. If your dose is different, do not change it unless your doctor tells you to do so.

The amount of medicine that you take depends on the strength of the medicine. Also, the number of doses you take each day, the time allowed between doses, and the length of time you take the medicine depend on the medical problem for which you are using the medicine.

- For oral dosage form (hard gelatin capsule):
  - For treating mycosis fungoides and psoriasis:
    - Adults and children 12 years of age and over—Dose is based on body weight and must be determined by your doctor. However, the usual dose is 0.6 mg per kilogram (kg) (0.27 mg per pound) of

body weight taken two hours before UVA exposure. This treatment (methoxsalen and UVA) is given two or three times a week with the treatment spaced at least forty-eight hours apart.
- Children up to 12 years of age—Dose must be determined by your doctor.
  ○ For vitiligo:
    - Adults and children 12 years of age and over—20 milligrams (mg) per day taken two to four hours before ultraviolet light A (UVA) exposure. This treatment (methoxsalen and UVA) is given two or three times a week with the treatment spaced at least forty-eight hours apart.
    - Children up to 12 years of age—Dose must be determined by your doctor.
- For oral dosage form (soft gelatin capsule):
  ○ For psoriasis:
    - Adults and children 12 years of age and over—Dose is based on body weight and must be determined by your doctor. The usual dose is 0.4 mg per kg (0.18 mg per pound) of body weight taken one and one-half to two hours before UVA exposure. This treatment (methoxsalen and UVA) is given two or three times a week, with the treatment spaced at least forty-eight hours apart.
    - Children up to 12 years of age—Dose must be determined by your doctor.

Missed dose—Call your doctor or pharmacist for instructions.

If you are late in taking, or miss taking, a dose of this medicine, notify your doctor so your light treatment can be rescheduled. Remember that exposure to sunlight or ultraviolet light must take place a certain number of hours after you take the medicine or it will not work. For patients taking the hard gelatin capsules, this is 2 to 4 hours. For patients taking the soft gelatin capsules, this is 1½ to 2 hours. If you have any questions about this, check with your doctor.

Storage—Store the medicine in a closed container at room temperature, away from heat, moisture, and direct light. Keep from freezing.

Keep out of the reach of children.

Do not keep outdated medicine or medicine no longer needed.

Precautions While Using This Medicine

Your doctor should check your progress at regular visits to make sure this medicine is working and that it does not cause unwanted effects. Eye examinations should be included.

This medicine increases the sensitivity of your skin and lips to sunlight. Therefore, exposure to the sun, even through window glass or on a cloudy day, could cause a serious burn. If you must go out during the daylight hours:
- Before each treatment, cover your skin for at least 24 hours by wearing protective clothing, such as long-sleeved shirts, full-length slacks, wide-brimmed hat, and gloves. In addition, protect your lips with a special sun block lipstick that has a skin protection factor (SPF) of at least 15. Check with your doctor before using sun block products on other parts of your body before a treatment, since sun block products should not be used on the areas of your skin that are to be treated.
- After each treatment, cover your skin for at least 8 hours by wearing protective clothing. In addition, use a sun

block product that has a skin protection factor (SPF) of at least 15 on your lips and on those areas of your body that cannot be covered.

If you have any questions about this, check with your health care professional.

Your skin may continue to be sensitive to sunlight for some time after treatment with this medicine. Use extra caution for at least 48 hours following each treatment if you plan to spend any time in the sun. In addition, do not sunbathe anytime during your course of treatment with methoxsalen.

For 24 hours after you take each dose of methoxsalen, your eyes should be protected during daylight hours with special wraparound sunglasses that totally block or absorb ultraviolet light (ordinary sunglasses are not adequate). This is to prevent cataracts. Your doctor will tell you what kind of sunglasses to use. These glasses should be worn even in indirect light, such as light coming through window glass or on a cloudy day.

This medicine may cause your skin to become dry or itchy. However, check with your doctor before applying anything to your skin to treat this problem.

Side Effects of This Medicine

Along with its needed effects, a medicine may cause some unwanted effects. Although not all of these side effects may occur, if they do occur they may need medical attention.

Check with your doctor immediately if any of the following side effects occur:

Blistering and peeling of skin; reddened, sore skin; swelling (especially of feet or lower legs)

Some side effects may occur that usually do not need medical attention. These side effects may go away during treatment as your body adjusts to the medicine. Also, your health care professional may be able to tell you about ways to prevent or reduce some of these side effects. Check with your health care professional if any of the following side effects continue or are bothersome or if you have any questions about them:

More common
Itching of skin; nausea

Less common
Dizziness; headache; mental depression; nervousness; trouble in sleeping

Treatment with this medicine usually causes a slight reddening of your skin 24 to 48 hours after the treatment. This is an expected effect and is no cause for concern. However, check with your doctor right away if your skin becomes sore and red or blistered.

There is an increased risk of developing skin cancer after use of methoxsalen. You should check your body regularly and show your doctor any skin sores that do not heal, new skin growths, and skin growths that have changed in the way they look or feel.

Premature aging of the skin may occur as a result of prolonged methoxsalen therapy. This effect is permanent and is similar to what happens when a person sunbathes for long periods of time.

Other side effects not listed may also occur in some patients. If you notice any other effects, check with your healthcare professional.

METHOXSALEN   (Topical route) -
meth-OX-a-len

Commonly used brand name(s)

In the U.S.—
Oxsoralen

In Canada—
Ultramop

Available Dosage Forms:
- Lotion

Therapeutic Class: Hypopigmentation Agent

Uses For This Medicine

Methoxsalen belongs to the group of medicines called psoralens. It is used along with ultraviolet light (found in sunlight and some special lamps) in a treatment called psoralen plus ultraviolet light A (PUVA) to treat vitiligo, a disease in which skin color is lost. Methoxsalen may also be used for other conditions as determined by your doctor.

Methoxsalen is available only with a prescription and is to be administered by or under the direct supervision of your doctor.

Once a medicine has been approved for marketing for a certain use, experience may show that it is also useful for other medical problems. Although these uses are not included in product labeling, topical methoxsalen is used in certain patients with the following medical conditions:

- Alopecia areata
- Eczema
- Inflammatory dermatoses
- Lichen planus
- Mycosis fungoides
- Need to increase tolerance of skin to sunlight
- Psoriasis

Before Using This Medicine

In deciding to use a medicine, the risks of taking the medicine must be weighed against the good it will do. This is a decision you and your doctor will make. For this medicine, the following should be considered:

Methoxsalen is a very strong medicine that increases the skin's sensitivity to sunlight. In addition to causing serious sunburns if not properly used, it has been reported to increase the chance of skin cancer. Also, like too much sunlight, PUVA can cause premature aging of the skin. Therefore, methoxsalen should be used only as directed and should not be used simply for suntanning. Before using this medicine, be sure that you have discussed its use with your doctor.

Allergies—Tell your doctor if you have ever had any unusual or allergic reaction to this medicine or any other medicines. Also tell your health care professional if you have any other types of allergies, such as to foods, dyes, preservatives, or animals. For non-prescription products, read the label or package ingredients carefully.

Pediatric—Studies on this medicine have been done only in adult patients, and there is no specific information comparing use of methoxsalen in children up to 12 years of age with use in other age groups.

Geriatric—Many medicines have not been studied specifically in older people. Therefore, it may not be known whether they work exactly the same way they do in younger adults or if they cause different side effects or problems in older people. There is no specific information comparing use of topical methoxsalen in the elderly with use in other age groups.

Pregnancy—

	Pregnancy Category	Explanation
All Trimesters	C	Animal studies have shown an adverse effect and there are no adequate studies in pregnant women OR no animal studies have been conducted and there are no adequate studies in pregnant women.

Breast Feeding—There are no adequate studies in women for determining infant risk when using this medication during breastfeeding. Weigh the potential benefits against the potential risks before taking this medication while breastfeeding.

Other medicines—

Using this medicine with any of the following medicines may cause an increased risk of certain side effects, but using both drugs may be the best treatment for you. If both medicines are prescribed together, your doctor may change the dose or how often you use one or both of the medicines.

Phenytoin

Interactions with Food/Tobacco/Alcohol—Certain medicines should not be used at or around the time of eating food or eating certain types of food since interactions may occur. Using alcohol or tobacco with certain medicines may also cause interactions to occur. Discuss with your healthcare professional the use of your medicine with food, alcohol, or tobacco.

Other medical problems—The presence of other medical problems may affect the use of this medicine. Make sure you tell your doctor if you have any other medical problems, especially:

- Allergy to sunlight (or family history of) or
- Infection or
- Lupus erythematosus or
- Porphyria or
- Skin cancer (history of) or
- Skin conditions (other)—Use of PUVA may make the condition worse
- Heart or blood vessel disease (severe)—The heat or prolonged standing associated with each light treatment may make the condition worse

Proper Use of This Medicine

Eating certain foods while you are using methoxsalen may increase your skin's sensitivity to sunlight. To help prevent this, avoid eating limes, figs, parsley, parsnips, mustard, carrots, and celery while you are being treated with this medicine.

Use this medicine only under the direct supervision of your doctor.

After UVA exposure, wash the treated area of skin with soap and water. Then use a sunscreen or wear protective clothing to protect the area.

Dosing—The dose of this medicine will be different for different patients. Follow your doctor's orders or the directions on the label. The following information includes only the average doses of this medicine. If your dose is different, do not change it unless your doctor tells you to do so.

The amount of medicine that you take depends on the strength of the medicine. Also, the number of doses you take each day, the time allowed between doses, and the length of time you take the medicine depend on the medical problem for which you are using the medicine.

- For topical solution dosage form:
  - For vitiligo:
    - Adults and children 12 years of age and over— Apply to the affected area of the skin and allow to dry for one to two minutes, then apply again within two to two and one-half hours before UVA exposure.
    - Children under 12 years of age—Use and dose must be determined by your doctor.

Precautions While Using This Medicine

It is important that you visit your doctor as directed for treatments and to have your progress checked.

This medicine increases the sensitivity of the treated areas of your skin to sunlight. Therefore, exposure to the sun, even through window glass or on a cloudy day, could cause a serious burn. After each light treatment, thoroughly wash the treated areas of your skin. Also, if you must go out during daylight hours, cover the treated areas of your skin for at least 12 to 48 hours following treatment by wearing protective clothing or a sun block product that has a skin protection factor (SPF) of at least 15. Some patients may require a product with a higher SPF number, especially if they have a fair complexion. If you have any questions about this, check with your health care professional.

The treated areas of your skin may continue to be sensitive to sunlight for some time after treatment with this medicine. Use extra caution for at least 72 hours following each treatment if you plan to spend any time in the sun. In addition, do not sunbathe anytime during your course of treatment with methoxsalen.

This medicine may cause your skin to become dry or itchy. However, check with your doctor before applying anything to your skin to treat this problem.

Side Effects of This Medicine

Along with its needed effects, a medicine may cause some unwanted effects. Although not all of these side effects may occur, if they do occur they may need medical attention.

Check with your doctor immediately if any of the following side effects occur:

Blistering and peeling of skin; reddened, sore skin; swelling, especially of the feet or lower legs

There is an increased risk of developing skin cancer after use of methoxsalen. You should check the treated areas of your body regularly and show your doctor any skin sores that do not heal, new skin growths, and skin growths that have changed in the way they look or feel.

Premature aging of the skin may occur as a result of prolonged methoxsalen therapy. This effect is permanent and is similar to the result of sunbathing for long periods of time.

Other side effects not listed may also occur in some patients. If you notice any other effects, check with your healthcare professional.

METHYLDOPA   (Oral route, Intravenous route) - meth-il-DOE-pa

Commonly used brand name(s)

In the U.S.—
   Aldomet

Available Dosage Forms:
- Tablet
- Suspension
- Solution

Therapeutic Class: Antihypertensive
Pharmacologic Class: Alpha-Adrenergic Agonist

Uses For This Medicine

Methyldopa belongs to the general class of medicines called antihypertensives. It is used to treat high blood pressure (hypertension).

High blood pressure adds to the work load of the heart and arteries. If it continues for a long time, the heart and arteries may not function properly. This can damage the blood vessels of the brain, heart, and kidneys, resulting in a stroke, heart failure, or kidney failure. High blood pressure may also increase the risk of heart attacks. These problems may be less likely to occur if blood pressure is controlled.

Methyldopa works by controlling impulses along certain nerve pathways. As a result, it relaxes blood vessels so that blood passes through them more easily. This helps to lower blood pressure.

Methyldopa is available only with your doctor's prescription.

Before Using This Medicine

In deciding to use a medicine, the risks of taking the medicine must be weighed against the good it will do. This is a decision you and your doctor will make. For this medicine, the following should be considered:

Allergies—Tell your doctor if you have ever had any unusual or allergic reaction to this medicine or any other medicines. Also tell your health care professional if you have any other types of allergies, such as to foods, dyes, preservatives, or animals. For non-prescription products, read the label or package ingredients carefully.

Pediatric—Although there is no specific information comparing use of methyldopa in children with use in other age groups, this medicine is not expected to cause different side effects or problems in children than it does in adults.

Geriatric—Dizziness or lightheadedness and drowsiness may be more likely to occur in the elderly, who are more sensitive to the effects of methyldopa.

Pregnancy—

	Pregnancy Category	Explanation
All Trimesters	B	Animal studies have revealed no evidence of harm to the fetus, however, there are no adequate studies in pregnant women OR animal studies have shown an adverse effect, but adequate studies in pregnant women have failed to demonstrate a risk to the fetus.

Breast Feeding—Studies in women suggest that this medication poses minimal risk to the infant when used during breastfeeding.

Other medicines—

Using this medicine with any of the following medicines is not recommended. Your doctor may decide not to treat you with this medication or change some of the other medicines you take.

Clorgyline, Iproniazid, Isocarboxazid, Moclobemide, Nialamide, Pargyline, Phenelzine, Procarbazine, Selegiline, Toloxatone, Tranylcypromine

Interactions with Food/Tobacco/Alcohol—Certain medicines should not be used at or around the time of eating food or eating certain types of food since interactions may occur. Using alcohol or tobacco with certain medicines may also cause interactions to occur. Discuss with your healthcare professional the use of your medicine with food, alcohol, or tobacco.

Other medical problems—The presence of other medical problems may affect the use of this medicine. Make sure you tell your doctor if you have any other medical problems, especially:

- Angina (chest pain) or
- Parkinson's disease—Methyldopa may make these conditions worse
- Kidney disease or
- Liver disease—Effects of methyldopa may be increased because of slower removal from the body
- Mental depression (history of)—Methyldopa can cause mental depression
- Pheochromocytoma—Methyldopa may interfere with tests for the condition; in addition, there have been reports of increased blood pressure
- If you have taken methyldopa in the past and developed liver problems

Proper Use of This Medicine

In addition to the use of the medicine your doctor has prescribed, treatment for your high blood pressure may include weight control and care in the types of foods you eat, especially foods high in sodium. Your doctor will tell you which of these are most important for you. You should check with your doctor before changing your diet.

Many patients who have high blood pressure will not notice any signs of the problem. In fact, many may feel normal. It is very important that you take your medicine exactly as directed and that you keep your appointments with your doctor even if you feel well.

Remember that methyldopa will not cure your high blood pressure but it does help control it. Therefore, you must continue to take it as directed if you expect to lower your blood pressure and keep it down. You may have to take high blood pressure medicine for the rest of your life. If high blood pressure is not treated, it can cause serious problems such as heart failure, blood vessel disease, stroke, or kidney disease.

To help you remember to take your medicine, try to get into the habit of taking it at the same time each day.

Dosing—The dose of this medicine will be different for different patients. Follow your doctor's orders or the directions on the label. The following information includes only the average doses of this medicine. If your dose is different, do not change it unless your doctor tells you to do so.

The amount of medicine that you take depends on the strength of the medicine. Also, the number of doses you take each day, the time allowed between doses, and the length of time you take the medicine depend on the medical problem for which you are using the medicine.

- For oral dosage form (suspension or tablets):
  - For high blood pressure:
    - Adults—250 milligrams (mg) to 2 grams a day. This is divided into two to four doses.
    - Children—Dose is based on body weight or size and must be determined by your doctor. The usual dose is 10 mg per kilogram (kg) (4.5 mg per pound) of body weight a day. This is divided into two to four doses. Your doctor may increase the dose as needed.

- For injection dosage form:
  - For high blood pressure:
    - Adults—250 to 500 mg mixed in 100 milliliters (mL) of solution (5% dextrose) and slowly injected into a vein every six hours as needed.
    - Children—Dose is based on body weight and must be determined by your doctor. The usual dose is 20 to 40 mg per kg (9.1 to 18.2 mg per pound) of body weight. This is mixed in a solution (5% dextrose) and slowly injected into a vein every six hours as needed.

Missed dose—If you miss a dose of this medicine, take it as soon as possible. However, if it is almost time for your next dose, skip the missed dose and go back to your regular dosing schedule. Do not double doses.

Storage—Store the medicine in a closed container at room temperature, away from heat, moisture, and direct light. Keep from freezing.

Keep out of the reach of children.

Do not keep outdated medicine or medicine no longer needed.

Precautions While Using This Medicine

It is important that your doctor check your progress at regular visits to make sure that this medicine is working properly.

Do not take other medicines unless they have been discussed with your doctor. This especially includes over-the-counter (nonprescription) medicines for appetite control, asthma, colds, cough, hay fever, or sinus problems, since they may tend to increase your blood pressure.

If you have a fever and there seems to be no reason for it, check with your doctor. This is especially important during the first few weeks you take methyldopa, since fever may be a sign of a serious reaction to this medicine.

Before having any kind of surgery (including dental surgery) or emergency treatment, make sure the medical doctor or dentist in charge knows that you are taking this medicine.

Methyldopa may cause some people to become drowsy or less alert than they are normally. This is more likely to happen when you begin to take it or when you increase the amount of medicine you are taking. Make sure you know how you react to this medicine before you drive, use machines, or do anything else that could be dangerous if you are not alert.

Dizziness, lightheadedness, or fainting may occur, especially when you get up from a lying or sitting position. Getting up slowly may help, but if the problem continues or gets worse, check with your doctor.

Methyldopa may cause dryness of the mouth. For temporary relief, use sugarless candy or gum, melt bits of ice in your mouth, or use a saliva substitute. However, if your mouth continues to feel dry for more than 2 weeks, check with your medical doctor or dentist. Continuing dryness of the mouth may increase the chance of dental disease, including tooth decay, gum disease, and fungus infections.

Tell the doctor in charge that you are taking this medicine before you have any medical tests. The results of some tests may be affected by this medicine.

Side Effects of This Medicine

Along with its needed effects, a medicine may cause some unwanted effects. Although not all of these side effects may occur, if they do occur they may need medical attention.

Check with your doctor immediately if any of the following side effects occur:

Less common
> Fever, shortly after starting to take this medicine

Check with your doctor as soon as possible if any of the following side effects occur:

More common
> Swelling of feet or lower legs

Less common
> Mental depression or anxiety; nightmares or unusually vivid dreams

Rare
> Dark or amber urine; diarrhea or stomach cramps (severe or continuing); fever, chills, troubled breathing, and fast heartbeat; general feeling of discomfort or illness or weakness; joint pain; pale stools; skin rash or itching; stomach pain (severe) with nausea and vom-

iting; tiredness or weakness after having taken this medicine for several weeks (continuing); yellow eyes or skin

Some side effects may occur that usually do not need medical attention. These side effects may go away during treatment as your body adjusts to the medicine. Also, your health care professional may be able to tell you about ways to prevent or reduce some of these side effects. Check with your health care professional if any of the following side effects continue or are bothersome or if you have any questions about them:

More common
> Drowsiness; dryness of mouth; headache

Less common
> Decreased sexual ability or interest in sex; diarrhea; dizziness or lightheadedness when getting up from a lying or sitting position; nausea or vomiting; numbness, tingling, pain, or weakness in hands or feet; slow heartbeat; stuffy nose; swelling of breasts or unusual milk production

Other side effects not listed may also occur in some patients. If you notice any other effects, check with your healthcare professional.

METHYLPHENIDATE   (Oral route) -
meth-il-FEN-i-date

Black Box Warning

- ORAL
  - Methylphenidate hydrochloride should be given cautiously to emotionally unstable patients, such as those with a history of drug dependence or alcoholism, because such patients may increase dosage on their own initiative.
  - Chronically abusive use can lead to marked tolerance and psychic dependence with varying degrees of abnormal behavior. Frank psychotic episodes can occur, especially with parenteral abuse. Careful supervision is required during drug withdrawal, since severe depression as well as the effects of chronic overactivity can be unmasked. Long term follow-up may be required because of the patient's basic personality disturbances

- TRANSDERMAL
  - Methylphenidate patch should be given cautiously to patients with a history of drug dependence or alcoholism. Chronic abusive use can lead to marked tolerance and psychological dependence with varying degrees of abnormal behavior. Frank psychotic episodes can occur, especially with parenteral abuse. Careful supervision is required during withdrawal from abusive use, since severe depression may occur. Withdrawal following chronic therapeutic use may unmask symptoms of the underlying disorder that may require follow-up

Commonly used brand name(s)

In the U.S.—

Concerta	Methylin ER
Metadate CD	Ritalin
Metadate ER	Ritalin LA
Methylin	Ritalin-SR

Available Dosage Forms:

- Tablet, Extended Release
- Capsule, Extended Release
- Solution
- Tablet, Chewable
- Tablet

Therapeutic Class: CNS Stimulant

Uses For This Medicine

Methylphenidate belongs to the group of medicines called central nervous system (CNS) stimulants. It is used to treat attention-deficit hyperactivity disorder (ADHD), narcolepsy (uncontrollable desire for sleep or sudden attacks of deep sleep), and other conditions as determined by the doctor.

Methylphenidate works in the treatment of ADHD by increasing attention and decreasing restlessness in children and adults who are overactive, cannot concentrate for very long or are easily distracted, and are impulsive. This medicine is used as part of a total treatment program that also includes social, educational, and psychological treatment.

This medicine is available only with a doctor's prescription.

Once a medicine has been approved for marketing for a certain use, experience may show that it is also useful for other medical problems. Although not specifically included in product labeling, methylphenidate may be used in certain patients with the following condition:

- Depressive disorder secondary to physical illness in patients who cannot take antidepressant medicines.

Before Using This Medicine

In deciding to use a medicine, the risks of taking the medicine must be weighed against the good it will do. This is a decision you and your doctor will make. For this medicine, the following should be considered:

Allergies—Tell your doctor if you have ever had any unusual or allergic reaction to this medicine or any other medicines. Also tell your health care professional if you have any other types of allergies, such as to foods, dyes, preservatives, or animals. For non-prescription products, read the label or package ingredients carefully.

Pediatric—Loss of appetite, trouble in sleeping, stomach pain, fast heartbeat, and weight loss may be especially likely to occur in children, who are usually more sensitive than adults to the effects of methylphenidate. Some children who used medicines like methylphenidate for a long time grew more slowly than expected. It is not known whether long-term use of methylphenidate causes slowed growth. The doctor should regularly measure the height and weight of children who are taking methylphenidate. Some doctors recommend stopping treatment with methylphenidate during times when the child is not under stress, such as on weekends.

This medicine should not be used in children under 6 years of age.

Geriatric—Many medicines have not been studied specifically in older people. Therefore, it may not be known whether they work exactly the same way they do in younger adults or if they cause different side effects or problems in older people. There is no specific information comparing use of methylphenidate in the elderly with use in other age groups.

Pregnancy—

	Pregnancy Category	Explanation
All Trimesters	C	Animal studies have shown an adverse effect and there are no adequate studies in pregnant women OR no animal studies have been conducted and there are no adequate studies in pregnant women.

Breast Feeding—There are no adequate studies in women for determining infant risk when using this medication during breastfeeding. Weigh the potential benefits against the potential risks before taking this medication while breastfeeding.

Other medicines—

Using this medicine with any of the following medicines is not recommended. Your doctor may decide not to treat you with this medication or change some of the other medicines you take.

Clorgyline, Iproniazid, Isocarboxazid, Lazabemide, Moclobemide, Nialamide, Pargyline, Phenelzine, Procarbazine, Selegiline, Toloxatone, Tranylcypromine

Interactions with Food/Tobacco/Alcohol—Certain medicines should not be used at or around the time of eating food or eating certain types of food since interactions may occur. Using alcohol or tobacco with certain medicines may also cause interactions to occur. Discuss with your healthcare professional the use of your medicine with food, alcohol, or tobacco.

Other medical problems—The presence of other medical problems may affect the use of this medicine. Make sure you tell your doctor if you have any other medical problems, especially:

- Alcohol abuse (or history of) or
- Drug abuse or dependence (or history of)—Dependence on methylphenidate may be more likely to develop.
- Epilepsy or other seizure disorders—The risk of having convulsions (seizures) may be increased.
- Gilles de la Tourette's disorder (or family history of) or
- Glaucoma or
- Heart failure or
- High blood pressure or
- Psychosis or
- Severe anxiety, agitation, tension, or depression or
- Thyroid (overactive) or
- Tics (other than Tourette's disorder)—Methylphenidate may make the condition worse.
- Heart problems or
- Family history of heart problems—May make the condition worse and cause serious problems.

Proper Use of This Medicine

Take this medicine only as directed by your doctor. Do not take more of it, do not take it more often, and do not take it for a longer time than your doctor ordered. If too much is taken, it may become habit-forming.

This medicine may be taken with or without food, depending on which brand is used.

To help prevent trouble in sleeping, take the last dose of the short-acting tablets before 6 p.m., unless otherwise directed by your doctor.

If you think this medicine is not working properly after you have taken it for several weeks, do not increase the dose. Instead, check with your doctor.

If you are taking the long-acting form of this medicine:

- These tablets or capsules are to be swallowed whole. Do not break, open, crush, or chew before swallowing.
- If you are taking the Concerta® brand of methylphenidate extended-release tablets, you may sometimes notice what looks like a tablet in your stool. This is just the empty shell that is left after the medicine has been absorbed into your body.

For patients using the *transdermal system (skin patch):*

- Methylphenidate patches come with patient instructions. Read them carefully before using this medicine. Methylphenidate patches will work only if applied correctly.
- Do not remove the patch from its sealed pouch until you are ready to put it on your skin. The patch may not work as well if it is unwrapped too soon.
- Apply the patch 2 hours before the desired effect.
- Do not try to trim or cut the adhesive patch to adjust the dosage. Check with your healthcare professional if you think the medicine is not working as it should.
- Apply the patch to a clean, dry area of skin on your hip. Choose an area that is not very oily, has little or no hair, and is free of scars, cuts, burns, or any other skin irritations. A different place on either hip should be chosen each day. The patch should not be applied to the waistline, or where tight clothing may rub it.
- Press the patch firmly in place with the palm of your hand for about 10 seconds. Make sure there is good contact with your skin, especially around the edges of the patch.
- The patch should stay in place even when you are showering, bathing, or swimming. Apply a new patch if one falls off. However, the total time of wearing a patch for that day should not exceed the total amount of time in one day that your doctor prescribed for you to wear the patch.
- Remove the patch approximately 9 hours after it has been applied, as directed by your doctor.
- After removing a used patch, fold the patch in half with the sticky sides together. Place the folded, used patch in its protective pouch or in aluminum foil. Make sure to dispose of it out of the reach of children and pets.

Dosing—The dose of this medicine will be different for different patients. Follow your doctor's orders or the directions on the label. The following information includes only the average doses of this medicine. If your dose is different, do not change it unless your doctor tells you to do so.

The amount of medicine that you take depends on the strength of the medicine. Also, the number of doses you take each day, the time allowed between doses, and the length of time you take the medicine depend on the medical problem for which you are using the medicine.

- For attention-deficit hyperactivity disorder:
  - For short-acting oral dosage form (tablets):
    - Adults and teenagers—5 to 20 milligrams (mg) two or three times a day, taken with or after meals.
    - Children 6 years of age and older—To start, 5 mg two times a day, taken with or after breakfast and

lunch. If needed, your doctor may increase the dose once a week by 5 to 10 mg a day until symptoms improve or a maximum dose is reached.
    - Children up to 6 years of age—The dose must be determined by the doctor.
  - For long-acting oral dosage form (extended-release tablets):
    - Adults, teenagers, and children—The dose must be determined by the doctor.
  - For long-acting oral dosage form (extended-release capsules):
    - Adults, teenagers, and children over 6 years of age—The recommended starting dose is 20 milligrams (mg) a day, taken in the morning before breakfast. Your doctor may increase the dose once a week as needed up to 60 mg a day.
    - Children up to 6 years of age—The dose must be determined by the doctor.
  - For the transdermal (stick-on) skin patch:
    - Adults, teenagers, and children over 6 years of age—The dose you receive will be determined by your doctor on an individual basis.
    - Children up to 6 years of age—The dose must be determined by the doctor.
- For narcolepsy:
  - For short-acting oral dosage form (tablets):
    - Adults and teenagers—5 to 20 milligrams (mg) two or three times a day, taken with or after meals.
  - For long-acting oral dosage form (extended-release tablets):
    - Adults and teenagers—The dose must be determined by the doctor.

Missed dose—Call your doctor or pharmacist for instructions.

Storage—Store the medicine in a closed container at room temperature, away from heat, moisture, and direct light. Keep from freezing.

Keep out of the reach of children.

Do not keep outdated medicine or medicine no longer needed.

Precautions While Using This Medicine

Your doctor should check your progress at regular visits and make sure that this medicine does not cause unwanted effects, such as high blood pressure.

Methylphenidate may cause dizziness, drowsiness, or changes in vision. Do not drive a car, ride a bicycle, operate machinery, or do other things that might be dangerous until you know how this medicine affects you.

If you take this medicine in large doses and/or for a long time, do not stop taking it without first checking with your doctor. Your doctor may want you to reduce gradually the amount you are taking before you stop completely. This is to help reduce unwanted effects.

If you think you may have become mentally or physically dependent on this medicine, check with your doctor. Some signs of dependence on methylphenidate are:

- A strong desire or need to continue taking the medicine.
- A need to increase the dose to receive the effects of the medicine.

- Withdrawal side effects (for example, mental depression, unusual behavior, or unusual tiredness or weakness) occurring after the medicine is stopped.

If you are using the methylphenidate transdermal patches and you experience any swelling or blistering where the patch has been, you should be seen by your doctor.

Side Effects of This Medicine

Along with its needed effects, a medicine may cause some unwanted effects. Although not all of these side effects may occur, if they do occur they may need medical attention.

Check with your doctor as soon as possible if any of the following side effects occur:

More common
Fast heartbeat; increased blood pressure

Less common
Chest pain; fever; joint pain; skin rash or hives; uncontrolled movements of the body

Rare
Black, tarry stools; blistering, burning, itching, peeling, skin rash, redness, or other signs of irritation; blood in urine or stools; blurred vision or other changes in vision; convulsions (seizures); crusting, dryness, flaking of skin; muscle cramps; pinpoint red spots on skin; scaling, severe redness, soreness, swelling of skin; uncontrolled vocal outbursts and/or tics (uncontrolled and repeated body movements); unusual bleeding or bruising

Incidence unknown
Abnormal liver function; confusion; cracks in the skin; hives or welts; loss of heat from the body; numbness of hands; painful or difficult urination; pale skin; red, irritated eyes; red, swollen, scaly skin; severe or sudden headache; shortness of breath; sore throat; sores, ulcers, or white spots on lips or in mouth; sudden loss of coordination; sudden slurring of speech; swollen glands; troubled breathing with exertion; unusual bleeding or bruising; unusual tiredness or weakness

With long-term use or at high doses
Changes in mood; confusion; delusions (false beliefs); depersonalization (feeling that self or surroundings are not real); hallucinations (seeing, hearing, or feeling things that are not there); weight loss

Symptoms of overdose
Agitation; confusion (severe); convulsions (seizures); dryness of mouth or mucous membranes; false sense of well-being; fast, pounding, or irregular heartbeat; fever; flushing; hallucinations (seeing, hearing, or feeling things that are not there); headache (severe); increased blood pressure; increased sweating; large pupils; muscle twitching; overactive reflexes; sweating; trembling or shaking; vomiting

Some side effects may occur that usually do not need medical attention. These side effects may go away during treatment as your body adjusts to the medicine. Also, your health care professional may be able to tell you about ways to prevent or reduce some of these side effects. Check with your health care professional if any of the following side effects continue or are bothersome or if you have any questions about them:

More common
Blisters under the skin; flushing, redness of skin; loss of appetite; nervousness; small, rounded bumps rising

from the skin; stuffy nose; swelling at site of patch application; trouble in sleeping; unusually warm skin

Less common
Anger; dizziness; drowsiness; fear; headache; irritability; muscle aches; nausea; nervousness; runny nose; scalp hair loss; sleeplessness; stomach pain; talking, feeling, and acting with excitement; trouble sleeping; unable to sleep

After you stop using this medicine, it may still produce some side effects that need attention. During this period of time, *check with your doctor immediately* if you notice the following side effects:

Mental depression (severe); unusual behavior; unusual tiredness or weakness

Other side effects not listed may also occur in some patients. If you notice any other effects, check with your healthcare professional.

METOCLOPRAMIDE (Oral route, Intravenous route) - met-oh-kloe-PRA-mide

Commonly used brand name(s)

In the U.S.—
Reglan

Available Dosage Forms:

- Solution
- Syrup
- Tablet

Therapeutic Class: Antiemetic
Pharmacologic Class: Dopamine Antagonist

Uses For This Medicine

Metoclopramide is a medicine that increases the movements or contractions of the stomach and intestines. When given by injection, it is used to help diagnose certain problems of the stomach and/or intestines. It is also used by injection to prevent the nausea and vomiting that may occur after treatment with anticancer medicines. Another medicine may be used with metoclopramide to prevent side effects that may occur when metoclopramide is used with anticancer medicines.

When taken by mouth, metoclopramide is used to treat the symptoms of a certain type of stomach problem called diabetic gastroparesis. It relieves symptoms such as nausea, vomiting, continued feeling of fullness after meals, and loss of appetite. Metoclopramide is also used, for a short time, to treat symptoms such as heartburn in patients who suffer esophageal injury from a backward flow of gastric acid into the esophagus.

Metoclopramide may also be used for other conditions as determined by your doctor.

Metoclopramide is available only with your doctor's prescription.

Once a medicine has been approved for marketing for a certain use, experience may show that it is also useful for other medical problems. Although these uses are not included in

product labeling, metoclopramide is used in certain patients with the following medical conditions:

- Failure of the stomach to empty its contents
- Nausea and vomiting caused by other medicines
- Persistent hiccups
- Prevention of aspirating fluid into the lungs during surgery
- Vascular headaches

Before Using This Medicine

In deciding to use a medicine, the risks of taking the medicine must be weighed against the good it will do. This is a decision you and your doctor will make. For this medicine, the following should be considered:

Allergies—Tell your doctor if you have ever had any unusual or allergic reaction to this medicine or any other medicines. Also tell your health care professional if you have any other types of allergies, such as to foods, dyes, preservatives, or animals. For non-prescription products, read the label or package ingredients carefully.

Pediatric—Muscle spasms, especially of jaw, neck, and back, and tic-like (jerky) movements of head and face may be especially likely to occur in children, who are usually more sensitive than adults to the effects of metoclopramide. Premature and full-term infants may develop blood problems if given high doses of metoclopramide.

Geriatric—Shuffling walk and trembling and shaking of hands may be especially likely to occur in elderly patients after they have taken metoclopramide over a long time.

Pregnancy—

	Pregnancy Category	Explanation
All Trimesters	B	Animal studies have revealed no evidence of harm to the fetus, however, there are no adequate studies in pregnant women OR animal studies have shown an adverse effect, but adequate studies in pregnant women have failed to demonstrate a risk to the fetus.

Breast Feeding—There are no adequate studies in women for determining infant risk when using this medication during breastfeeding. Weigh the potential benefits against the potential risks before taking this medication while breastfeeding.

Other medicines—

Using this medicine with any of the following medicines is usually not recommended, but may be required in some cases. If both medicines are prescribed together, your doctor may change the dose or how often you use one or both of the medicines.

Linezolid

Interactions with Food/Tobacco/Alcohol—Certain medicines should not be used at or around the time of eating food or eating certain types of food since interactions may occur. Using alcohol or tobacco with certain medicines may also cause interactions to occur. Discuss with your healthcare professional the use of your medicine with food, alcohol, or tobacco.

Other medical problems—The presence of other medical problems may affect the use of this medicine. Make sure you tell your doctor if you have any other medical problems, especially:

- Abdominal or stomach bleeding or
- Asthma or
- Cirrhosis (liver disease) or
- Congestive heart failure or
- High blood pressure or
- Intestinal blockage or
- Mental depression or
- Parkinson's disease or
- Pheochromocytoma (catecholamine-producing tumor)—Metoclopramide may make these conditions worse
- Epilepsy—Metoclopramide may increase the risk of having a seizure
- Kidney disease (severe)—Higher blood levels of metoclopramide may result, possibly increasing the chance of side effects
- Nicotinamide adenine dinucleotide (NADH) methemoglobin reductase deficiency—Metoclopramide may increase your chance of side effects affecting the blood.

Proper Use of This Medicine

Take this medicine 30 minutes before meals and at bedtime, unless otherwise directed by your doctor.

Take metoclopramide only as directed. Do not take more of it, do not take it more often, and do not take it for a longer time than your doctor ordered. To do so may increase the chance of side effects.

To take metoclopramide oral concentrate: This medicine should be mixed with another liquid, such as water, juices, soda or soda-like beverages, or with a semi-solid food, such as applesauce or pudding.

Dosing—The dose of this medicine will be different for different patients. Follow your doctor's orders or the directions on the label. The following information includes only the average doses of this medicine. If your dose is different, do not change it unless your doctor tells you to do so.

The amount of medicine that you take depends on the strength of the medicine. Also, the number of doses you take each day, the time allowed between doses, and the length of time you take the medicine depend on the medical problem for which you are using the medicine.

- For oral dosage forms (concentrate, solution, or tablets):
  - To treat the symptoms of a stomach problem called diabetic gastroparesis:
    - Adults and teenagers—10 milligrams (mg) thirty minutes before symptoms are likely to begin or before each meal and at bedtime. The dose may be taken up to four times a day. However, most people usually will not take more than 500 micrograms (mcg) per kilogram (kg) (227 mcg per pound) of body weight a day.
    - Children—Dose must be determined by your doctor.
  - For heartburn:
    - Adults and teenagers—10 to 15 mg thirty minutes before symptoms are likely to begin or before each

meal and at bedtime. The dose may be taken up to four times a day. However, most people usually will not take more than 500 mcg per kg (227 mcg per pound) of body weight a day.

- Children—Dose must be determined by your doctor.

○ To increase movements or contractions of the stomach and intestines:

- Children 5 to 14 years of age—2.5 to 5 mg three times a day, thirty minutes before meals.

• For injection dosage form:

○ To increase movements or contractions of the stomach and intestine:

- Adults and teenagers—10 mg injected into a vein.
- Children—Dose is based on body weight and must be determined by your doctor. The usual dose is 1 mg per kilogram (kg) (0.45 mg per pound) of body weight injected into a vein. Your doctor may repeat this dose after sixty minutes if needed.

○ To prevent nausea and vomiting caused by anti-cancer medicines:

- Adults and teenagers—Dose is based on body weight and must be determined by your doctor. The usual dose is 1 to 2 mg per kg (0.45 to 0.9 mg per pound) of body weight, injected slowly into a vein, thirty minutes before you take your anti-cancer medicine. Your doctor may repeat this dose every two or three hours if needed. Some people may need a larger dose to start.
- Children—1 mg per kg (0.45 mg per pound) of body weight injected into a vein. Your doctor may repeat this dose after sixty minutes if needed.

○ To prevent vomiting after surgery:

- Adults and teenagers—10 to 20 mg injected into a muscle near the end of surgery.
- Children—Dose must be determined by your doctor.

Missed dose—If you miss a dose of this medicine, take it as soon as possible. However, if it is almost time for your next dose, skip the missed dose and go back to your regular dosing schedule. Do not double doses.

Storage—Store the medicine in a closed container at room temperature, away from heat, moisture, and direct light. Keep from freezing.

Keep out of the reach of children.

Do not keep outdated medicine or medicine no longer needed.

Precautions While Using This Medicine

This medicine will add to the effects of alcohol and other CNS depressants (medicines that cause drowsiness). Some examples of CNS depressants are antihistamines or medicine for hay fever, other allergies, or colds; sedatives, tranquilizers, or sleeping medicine; prescription pain medicine or narcotics; barbiturates; medicine for seizures; muscle relaxants; or anesthetics, including some dental anesthetics. Check with your doctor before taking any of the above while you are using this medicine.

This medicine may cause some people to become dizzy, lightheaded, drowsy, or less alert than they are normally. Make sure you know how you react to this medicine before

you drive, use machines, or do anything else that could be dangerous if you are dizzy or are not alert.

Side Effects of This Medicine

Along with its needed effects, a medicine may cause some unwanted effects. Although not all of these side effects may occur, if they do occur they may need medical attention.

Check with your doctor as soon as possible if any of the following side effects occur:

Rare

Abdominal pain or tenderness; chills; clay colored stools; convulsions; dark urine; difficulty in breathing; difficulty in speaking or swallowing; dizziness or fainting; fast or irregular heartbeat; fever; general feeling of tiredness or weakness; headache (severe or continuing); inability to move eyes; increase in blood pressure; increased sweating; itching; lip smacking or puckering; loss of appetite; loss of balance control; loss of bladder control; mask-like face; muscle spasms of face, neck, and back; nausea and vomiting; puffing of cheeks; rapid or worm-like movements of tongue; shuffling walk; skin rash; sore throat; stiffness of arms or legs; swelling of feet or lower legs; trembling and shaking of hands and fingers; tic-like or twitching movements; twisting movements of body; uncontrolled chewing movements; uncontrolled movements of arms and legs; unusually pale skin; weakness of arms and legs; yellow eyes or skin

With high doses—may occur within minutes of receiving a dose of metoclopramide and last for 2 to 24 hours

Aching or discomfort in lower legs; panic-like sensation; sensation of crawling in legs; unusual nervousness, restlessness, or irritability

Symptoms of overdose—may also occur rarely with usual doses, especially in children and young adults, and with high doses used to treat the nausea and vomiting caused by anticancer medicines

Confusion; convulsions (seizures); drowsiness (severe)

Some side effects may occur that usually do not need medical attention. These side effects may go away during treatment as your body adjusts to the medicine. Also, your health care professional may be able to tell you about ways to prevent or reduce some of these side effects. Check with your health care professional if any of the following side effects continue or are bothersome or if you have any questions about them:

More common

Diarrhea— with high doses; drowsiness; restlessness

Less common or rare

Breast tenderness and swelling; changes in menstruation; constipation; decreased interest in sexual intercourse; inability to have or keep an erection; increased flow of breast milk; increased need to urinate; loss in sexual ability, desire, drive, or performance; mental depression; nausea; passing urine more often; skin rash; trouble in sleeping; unusual dryness of mouth; unusual irritability

Other side effects not listed may also occur in some patients. If you notice any other effects, check with your healthcare professional.

METRONIDAZOLE (Oral route, Intravenous route) - me-troe-NI-da-zole

Black Box Warning

Metronidazole has been shown to be carcinogenic in mice and rats. Unnecessary use of the drug should be avoided

Commonly used brand name(s)

In the U.S.—

Flagyl	Flagyl I.V.
Flagyl ER	Flagyl I.V. RTU

Available Dosage Forms:

- Tablet, Extended Release
- Capsule
- Solution
- Powder for Solution
- Tablet
- Suspension

Therapeutic Class: Antibiotic

Uses For This Medicine

Metronidazole is used to treat infections. It may also be used for other problems as determined by your doctor. It will not work for colds, flu, or other virus infections.

Metronidazole is available only with your doctor's prescription.

Once a medicine has been approved for marketing for a certain use, experience may show that it is also useful for other medical problems. Although these uses are not included in product labeling, metronidazole is used in certain patients with the following medical conditions:

- Antibiotic-associated colitis
- Balantidiasis
- Dental infections
- Gastritis or ulcer due to Helicobacter pylori
- Giardiasis
- Inflammatory bowel disease

For patients taking this medicine for giardiasis:

- After treatment, it is important that your doctor check whether or not the infection in your intestinal tract has been cleared up completely.

Before Using This Medicine

In deciding to use a medicine, the risks of taking the medicine must be weighed against the good it will do. This is a decision you and your doctor will make. For this medicine, the following should be considered:

Allergies—Tell your doctor if you have ever had any unusual or allergic reaction to this medicine or any other medicines. Also tell your health care professional if you have any other types of allergies, such as to foods, dyes, preservatives, or animals. For non-prescription products, read the label or package ingredients carefully.

Pediatric—Metronidazole has been used in children and, in effective doses, has not been shown to cause different side effects or problems in children than it does in adults.

Geriatric—Many medicines have not been studied specifically in older people. Therefore, it may not be known whether they work exactly the same way they do in younger adults or if they cause different side effects or problems in older people.

There is no specific information comparing use of metronidazole in the elderly with use in other age groups.

Pregnancy—

	Pregnancy Category	Explanation
All Trimesters	B	Animal studies have revealed no evidence of harm to the fetus, however, there are no adequate studies in pregnant women OR animal studies have shown an adverse effect, but adequate studies in pregnant women have failed to demonstrate a risk to the fetus.

Breast Feeding—Studies in women suggest that this medication poses minimal risk to the infant when used during breastfeeding.

Other medicines—

Using this medicine with any of the following medicines is not recommended. Your doctor may decide not to treat you with this medication or change some of the other medicines you take.

Amprenavir, Dihydroergotamine, Disulfiram, Ergoloid Mesylates, Ergonovine, Ergotamine, Methylergonovine

Interactions with Food/Tobacco/Alcohol—Certain medicines should not be used at or around the time of eating food or eating certain types of food since interactions may occur. Using alcohol or tobacco with certain medicines may also cause interactions to occur. The following interactions have been selected on the basis of their potential significance and are not necessarily all-inclusive.

Using this medicine with any of the following is usually not recommended, but may be unavoidable in some cases. If used together, your doctor may change the dose or how often you use this medicine, or give you special instructions about the use of food, alcohol, or tobacco.

Ethanol

Other medical problems—The presence of other medical problems may affect the use of this medicine. Make sure you tell your doctor if you have any other medical problems, especially:

- Blood disease or a history of blood disease—Metronidazole may make the condition worse
- Central nervous system (CNS) disease, including epilepsy—Metronidazole may increase the chance of seizures (convulsions) or other CNS side effects
- Heart disease—Metronidazole by injection may make heart disease worse
- Liver disease, severe—Patients with severe liver disease may have an increase in side effects
- Oral thrush or vaginal yeast infection—Metronidazole may make yeast infections worse.

Proper Use of This Medicine

If this medicine upsets your stomach, it may be taken with meals or a snack. If stomach upset (nausea, vomiting, stomach pain, or diarrhea) continues, check with your doctor. If you are taking the extended- release formulation, you should try to take it an hour before or two hours after your meal.

To help clear up your infection completely, keep taking this medicine for the full time of treatment, even if you begin to feel better after a few days. If you stop taking this medicine too soon, your symptoms may return.

In some kinds of infections, this medicine works best when there is a constant amount in the blood. To help keep the amount constant, do not miss any doses. Also, it is best to take the doses at evenly spaced times, day and night. For example, if you are to take 4 doses a day, the doses should be spaced about 6 hours apart. If this interferes with your sleep or other daily activities, or if you need help in planning the best times to take your medicine, check with your health care professional.

Dosing—The dose of this medicine will be different for different patients. Follow your doctor's orders or the directions on the label. The following information includes only the average doses of this medicine. If your dose is different, do not change it unless your doctor tells you to do so.

The amount of medicine that you take depends on the strength of the medicine. Also, the number of doses you take each day, the time allowed between doses, and the length of time you take the medicine depend on the medical problem for which you are using the medicine.

- For oral dosage forms (capsules, tablets):
  - For bacterial infections:
    - Adults and teenagers—Dose is based on body weight. The usual dose is 7.5 milligrams (mg) per kilogram (kg) (3.4 mg per pound) of body weight, up to a maximum dose of 1 gram, every six hours for at least seven days.
    - Children—Dose is based on body weight. The usual dose is 7.5 mg per kg (3.4 mg per pound) of body weight every six hours; or 10 mg per kg (4.5 mg per pound) every eight hours.
  - For amebiasis infections:
    - Adults and teenagers—500 to 750 mg three times a day for five to ten days.
    - Children—Dose is based on body weight. The usual dose is 11.6 to 16.7 mg per kg (5.3 to 7.6 mg per pound) of body weight three times a day for ten days.
  - For trichomoniasis infections:
    - Adults and teenagers—A single dose of 2 grams; or 1 gram two times a day for one day; or 250 mg three times a day for seven days.
    - Children—Dose is based on body weight. The usual dose is 5 mg per kg (2.3 mg per pound) of body weight three times a day for seven days.
- For oral dosage form (extended release tablets):
  - For bacterial vaginosis:
    - Adults and teenagers—750 mg once a day for seven days.
    - Children—Use and dose must be determined by your doctor.
- For injection dosage form:
  - For bacterial infections:
    - Adults and children over 1 week of age—Dose is based on body weight. The usual dose is 15 mg per kg (6.8 mg per pound) of body weight one time to start, then 7.5 mg per kg (3.4 mg per pound) of

body weight injected into a vein every six hours for at least seven days.
  - Preterm infants—Dose is based on body weight. The usual dose is 15 mg per kg (6.8 mg per pound) of body weight one time to start, then 7.5 mg per kg (3.4 mg per pound) of body weight, injected into a vein, every twelve hours starting forty-eight hours after the first dose.
  - Full-term infants—Dose is based on body weight. The usual dose is 15 mg per kg (6.8 mg per pound) of body weight one time to start, then 7.5 mg per kg (3.4 mg per pound) of body weight, injected into a vein, every twelve hours starting twenty-four hours after the first dose.
  - For treatment before and during bowel surgery:
    - Adults and teenagers—Dose is based on body weight. The usual dose is 15 mg per kg (6.8 mg per pound), injected into a vein, one hour before surgery, then 7.5 mg per kg (3.4 mg per pound) of body weight, injected into a vein, six hours and twelve hours after the first dose.
    - Children—Use and dose must be determined by your doctor.

Missed dose—If you miss a dose of this medicine, take it as soon as possible. However, if it is almost time for your next dose, skip the missed dose and go back to your regular dosing schedule. Do not double doses.

Storage—Store the medicine in a closed container at room temperature, away from heat, moisture, and direct light. Keep from freezing.

Keep out of the reach of children.

Do not keep outdated medicine or medicine no longer needed.

Precautions While Using This Medicine

If your symptoms do not improve within a few days, or if they become worse, check with your doctor.

Drinking alcoholic beverages while taking this medicine may cause stomach pain, nausea, vomiting, headache, or flushing or redness of the face. Other alcohol-containing preparations (for example, elixirs, cough syrups, tonics) may also cause problems. These problems may last for at least a day after you stop taking metronidazole. Also, this medicine may cause alcoholic beverages to taste different. Therefore, you should not drink alcoholic beverages or take other alcohol-containing preparations while you are taking this medicine and for at least 3 days after stopping it.

Metronidazole may cause dryness of the mouth, an unpleasant or sharp metallic taste, and a change in taste sensation. For temporary relief of dry mouth, use sugarless candy or gum, melt bits of ice in your mouth, or use a saliva substitute. However, if your mouth continues to feel dry for more than 2 weeks, check with your medical doctor or dentist. Continuing dryness of the mouth may increase the chance of dental disease, including tooth decay, gum disease, and fungus infections.

This medicine may also cause some people to become dizzy or lightheaded. Make sure you know how you react to this medicine before you drive, use machines, or do anything else that could be dangerous if you are dizzy or are not alert. If these reactions are especially bothersome, check with your doctor.

If you are taking this medicine for trichomoniasis (an infection of the sex organs in males and females), your doctor may want to treat your sexual partner at the same time you are being treated, even if he or she has no symptoms. Also, it may be desirable to use a condom (prophylactic) during intercourse. These measures will help keep you from getting the infection back again from your partner. If you have any questions about this, check with your doctor.

Side Effects of This Medicine

Along with its needed effects, a medicine may cause some unwanted effects. Although not all of these side effects may occur, if they do occur they may need medical attention.

Check with your doctor immediately if any of the following side effects occur:

Less common
    Numbness, tingling, pain, or weakness in hands or feet

Rare
    Convulsions (seizures)

Check with your doctor as soon as possible if any of the following side effects occur:

Less common
    Any vaginal irritation, discharge, or dryness not present before use of this medicine; black, tarry stools; blood in urine or stools; clumsiness or unsteadiness; frequent or painful urination; inability to control urine flow; mood or other mental changes; nausea and vomiting; pinpoint red spots on skin; sense of pelvic pressure; skin rash, hives, redness, or itching; sore throat and fever; stomach and back pain (severe); unusual bleeding or bruising

For injection form
    Pain, tenderness, redness, or swelling over vein in which the medicine is given

Some side effects may occur that usually do not need medical attention. These side effects may go away during treatment as your body adjusts to the medicine. Also, your health care professional may be able to tell you about ways to prevent or reduce some of these side effects. Check with your health care professional if any of the following side effects continue or are bothersome or if you have any questions about them:

More common
    Diarrhea; dizziness or light– headedness; headache; loss of appetite; nausea or vomiting; stomach pain or cramps

Less common or rare
    Change in taste sensation; dryness of mouth; unpleasant or sharp metallic taste

In some patients metronidazole may cause dark urine. This is only temporary and will go away when you stop taking this medicine.

Other side effects not listed may also occur in some patients. If you notice any other effects, check with your healthcare professional.

METRONIDAZOLE   (Topical route) -
me-troe-NI-da-zole

Commonly used brand name(s)

In the U.S.—
Metrocream	Noritate
Metrogel	Rozex
Metrolotion	

Available Dosage Forms:

• Emulsion	• Gel/Jelly
• Cream	• Lotion

Therapeutic Class: Antiacne Antibacterial

Uses For This Medicine

Topical metronidazole is applied to the skin in adults to help control rosacea, also known as acne rosacea and "adult acne." This medicine helps to reduce the redness of the skin and the number of pimples, usually found on the face, in patients with rosacea.

Topical metronidazole is available only with your doctor's prescription.

Before Using This Medicine

In deciding to use a medicine, the risks of taking the medicine must be weighed against the good it will do. This is a decision you and your doctor will make. For this medicine, the following should be considered:

Allergies—Tell your doctor if you have ever had any unusual or allergic reaction to this medicine or any other medicines. Also tell your health care professional if you have any other types of allergies, such as to foods, dyes, preservatives, or animals. For non-prescription products, read the label or package ingredients carefully.

Pediatric—Rosacea is usually considered an adult disease. Therefore, topical metronidazole is not generally used in children.

Geriatric—Many medicines have not been studied specifically in older people. Therefore, it may not be known whether they work exactly the same way they do in younger adults or if they cause different side effects or problems in older people. There is no specific information comparing use of topical metronidazole in the elderly with use in other age groups.

Other medicines—Although certain medicines should not be used together at all, in other cases two different medicines may be used together even if an interaction might occur. In these cases, your doctor may want to change the dose, or other precautions may be necessary. Tell your healthcare professional if you are taking any other prescription or non-prescription (over-the-counter [OTC]) medicine.

Interactions with Food/Tobacco/Alcohol—Certain medicines should not be used at or around the time of eating food or eating certain types of food since interactions may occur. Using alcohol or tobacco with certain medicines may also cause interactions to occur. Discuss with your healthcare professional the use of your medicine with food, alcohol, or tobacco.

Other medical problems—The presence of other medical problems may affect the use of this medicine. Make sure you

tell your doctor if you have any other medical problems, especially:

- Blood disease or a history of blood disease—Metronidazole may make the condition worse

Proper Use of This Medicine

Do not use this medicine in or near the eyes. Watering of the eyes may occur when the medicine is used too close to the eyes.

If this medicine does get into your eyes, wash them out immediately, but carefully, with large amounts of cool tap water. If your eyes still burn or are painful, check with your doctor.

Before applying this medicine, thoroughly wash the affected area(s) with a mild, nonirritating cleanser, rinse well, and gently pat dry.

To use:

- After washing the affected area(s), apply this medicine with your fingertips.
- Apply and rub in a thin film of medicine, using enough to cover the affected area(s) lightly. You should apply the medicine to the whole area usually affected by rosacea, not just to the pimples themselves.
- Wash the medicine off your hands.

To help keep your rosacea under control, keep using this medicine for the full time of treatment. You may have to continue using this medicine every day for 9 weeks or longer. Do not miss any doses.

Dosing—The dose of this medicine will be different for different patients. Follow your doctor's orders or the directions on the label. The following information includes only the average doses of this medicine. If your dose is different, do not change it unless your doctor tells you to do so.

The amount of medicine that you take depends on the strength of the medicine. Also, the number of doses you take each day, the time allowed between doses, and the length of time you take the medicine depend on the medical problem for which you are using the medicine.

- For topical dosage forms (cream, gel, and lotion):
  - For rosacea:
    - Adults—Apply to the affected area(s) of skin two times a day, morning and evening, for nine weeks.
    - Children—Use and dose must be determined by your doctor.

Missed dose—If you miss a dose of this medicine, apply it as soon as possible. However, if it is almost time for your next dose, skip the missed dose and go back to your regular dosing schedule.

Storage—Store the medicine in a closed container at room temperature, away from heat, moisture, and direct light. Keep from freezing.

Keep out of the reach of children.

Do not keep outdated medicine or medicine no longer needed.

Precautions While Using This Medicine

If your rosacea does not improve within 3 weeks, or if it becomes worse, check with your doctor. However, treatment of rosacea may take up to 9 weeks or longer before you see full improvement.

Stinging or burning of the skin may be expected after this medicine is applied. These effects may last up to a few minutes or more. If irritation continues, check with your doctor. You may have to use the medicine less often or stop using it altogether. Follow your doctor's directions.

You may continue to use cosmetics (make-up) while you are using this medicine for rosacea. However, it is best to use only "oil-free" cosmetics. Also, it is best not to use cosmetics too heavily or too often. They may make your rosacea worse. If you have any questions about this, check with your doctor.

Side Effects of This Medicine

Along with its needed effects, a medicine may cause some unwanted effects. Although not all of these side effects may occur, if they do occur they may need medical attention.

Some side effects may occur that usually do not need medical attention. These side effects may go away during treatment as your body adjusts to the medicine. Also, your health care professional may be able to tell you about ways to prevent or reduce some of these side effects. Check with your health care professional if any of the following side effects continue or are bothersome or if you have any questions about them:

Less common
  Dry skin; redness or other signs of skin irritation not present before use of this medicine; stinging or burning of the skin; watering of eyes

Rare
  Metallic taste in the mouth; nausea; tingling or numbness of arms, legs, hands, or feet

Other side effects not listed may also occur in some patients. If you notice any other effects, check with your healthcare professional.

METRONIDAZOLE (Vaginal route) -
me-troe-NI-da-zole

Commonly used brand name(s)

In the U.S.—
  Metrogel-Vaginal

In Canada—
  Flagyl
  Neo-Metric
  Nidagel

Available Dosage Forms:

- Suppository
- Gel/Jelly
- Cream

Therapeutic Class: Antibacterial

Uses For This Medicine

Metronidazole is used to treat certain vaginal infections. It works by killing bacteria. This medicine will not work for vaginal fungus or yeast infections.

Metronidazole is available only with your doctor's prescription.

Before Using This Medicine

In deciding to use a medicine, the risks of taking the medicine must be weighed against the good it will do. This is a decision you and your doctor will make. For this medicine, the following should be considered:

In deciding whether to use a medicine, the risks of using the medicine must be weighed against the good it will do. This is a decision you and your doctor will make. For vaginal metronidazole, the following should be considered:

Allergies—Tell your doctor if you have ever had any unusual or allergic reaction to this medicine or any other medicines. Also tell your health care professional if you have any other types of allergies, such as to foods, dyes, preservatives, or animals. For non-prescription products, read the label or package ingredients carefully.

Pediatric—Studies on these medicines have been done only in adult patients, and there is no specific information comparing use of vaginal metronidazole in children with use in other age groups.

Geriatric—Many medicines have not been studied specifically in older people. Therefore, it may not be known whether they work exactly the same way they do in younger adults or if they cause different side effects or problems in older people. There is no specific information comparing use of metronidazole in the elderly with use in other age groups.

Pregnancy—

	Pregnancy Category	Explanation
All Trimesters	B	Animal studies have revealed no evidence of harm to the fetus, however, there are no adequate studies in pregnant women OR animal studies have shown an adverse effect, but adequate studies in pregnant women have failed to demonstrate a risk to the fetus.

Breast Feeding—Studies in women suggest that this medication poses minimal risk to the infant when used during breastfeeding.

Other medicines—

Using this medicine with any of the following medicines is not recommended. Your doctor may decide not to treat you with this medication or change some of the other medicines you take.

Amprenavir, Dihydroergotamine, Disulfiram, Ergoloid Mesylates, Ergonovine, Ergotamine, Methylergonovine

Interactions with Food/Tobacco/Alcohol—Certain medicines should not be used at or around the time of eating food or eating certain types of food since interactions may occur. Using alcohol or tobacco with certain medicines may also cause interactions to occur. The following interactions have been selected on the basis of their potential significance and are not necessarily all-inclusive.

Using this medicine with any of the following is usually not recommended, but may be unavoidable in some cases. If used together, your doctor may change the dose or how often you use this medicine, or give you special instructions about the use of food, alcohol, or tobacco.

Ethanol

Other medical problems—The presence of other medical problems may affect the use of this medicine. Make sure you tell your doctor if you have any other medical problems, especially:

- Central nervous system (CNS) disease, including epilepsy—Metronidazole may increase the chance of seizures (convulsions) or other side effects
- Liver disease, severe—Patients with severe liver disease may have an increase in side effects
- Low white blood cell count (or history of)—Metronidazole may make the condition worse

Proper Use of This Medicine

Wash your hands before and after using the medicine. Also, keep the medicine out of your eyes.

If this medicine does get into your eyes, wash them out immediately, but carefully, with large amounts of tap water. If your eyes still burn or are painful, check with your doctor.

Vaginal metronidazole products usually come with patient directions. Read them carefully before using this medicine.

Use vaginal metronidazole exactly as directed by your doctor.

- To fill the applicator
  - For cream or gel dosage forms:
    - Break the metal seal at the opening of the tube by using the point on the top of the cap.
    - Screw the applicator onto the tube.
    - Squeeze the medicine into the applicator slowly until it is full.
    - Remove the applicator from the tube. Replace the cap on the tube.
  - For vaginal tablet dosage form:
    - Place the vaginal tablet into the applicator. Wet the vaginal tablet with water for a few seconds.
- To insert vaginal metronidazole using the applicator
  - For all dosage forms:
    - Relax while lying on your back with your knees bent.
    - Hold the full applicator in one hand. Insert it slowly into the vagina. Stop before it becomes uncomfortable.
    - Slowly press the plunger until it stops.
    - Withdraw the applicator. The medicine will be left behind in the vagina.
- To care for the applicator
  - For all dosage forms:
    - Clean the applicator after use by pulling the plunger out of the applicator and washing both parts completely in warm soapy water.
    - Rinse well.
    - After drying the applicator, replace the plunger.

To help clear up your infection completely, it is very important that you keep using this medicine for the full time of treatment, even if your symptoms begin to clear up after a few days. If you stop using this medicine too soon, your symptoms may return. Do not miss any doses. Also, continue using this medicine even if your menstrual period starts during the time of treatment.

Dosing—The dose of this medicine will be different for different patients. Follow your doctor's orders or the directions on the label. The following information includes only the average doses of this medicine. If your dose is different, do not change it unless your doctor tells you to do so.

The amount of medicine that you take depends on the strength of the medicine. Also, the number of doses you take each day, the time allowed between doses, and the length of time you take the medicine depend on the medical problem for which you are using the medicine.

- Forvaginal cream dosage form:
  - For bacterial vaginosis or trichomoniasis:
    - Adults and teenagers—One applicatorful (500 milligrams [mg]), inserted into the vagina. Use the medicine one or two times a day for ten or twenty days.
    - Children—Use and dose must be determined by your doctor.
- Forvaginal gel dosage form:
  - For bacterial vaginosis:
    - Adults and teenagers—One applicatorful (37.5 mg), inserted into the vagina one or two times a day for five days.
    - Children—Use and dose must be determined by your doctor.
- Forvaginal tablets dosage form:
  - For bacterial vaginosis or trichomoniasis:
    - Adults and teenagers—One 500–mg tablet, inserted high into the vagina. Use the medicine once a day in the evening for ten or twenty days.
    - Children—Use and dose must be determined by your doctor.

Missed dose—If you miss a dose of this medicine, take it as soon as possible. However, if it is almost time for your next dose, skip the missed dose and go back to your regular dosing schedule. Do not double doses.

Storage—Store the medicine in a closed container at room temperature, away from heat, moisture, and direct light. Keep from freezing.

Keep out of the reach of children.

Do not keep outdated medicine or medicine no longer needed.

Precautions While Using This Medicine

If your symptoms do not improve within a few days, or if they become worse, check with your doctor.

It is important that you visit your doctor after you have used all your medicine to make sure that the infection is gone.

Drinking alcoholic beverages while using this medicine may cause stomach pain, nausea, vomiting, headache, or flushing or redness of the face. Alcohol-containing medicines (for example, elixirs, cough syrups, tonics) may also cause problems. The chance of these problems occurring may continue for at least a day after you stop using metronidazole. Therefore, you should not drink alcoholic beverages or take other alcohol-containing medicines while you are using this medicine and for at least a day after stopping it.

This medicine may cause some people to become dizzy or lightheaded. Make sure you know how you react to this medicine before you drive, use machines, or do anything else that could be dangerous if you are dizzy or are not alert. If these reactions are especially bothersome, check with your doctor.

Vaginal medicines usually leak out of the vagina during treatment. To keep the medicine from getting on your clothing, wear a minipad or sanitary napkin. Do not use tampons (like those used for menstrual periods) since they may soak up the medicine.

To help clear up your infection completely and to help make sure it does not return, good health habits are also required.

- Wear cotton panties (or panties or pantyhose with cotton crotches) instead of synthetic (for example, nylon or rayon) panties.
- Wear only freshly washed panties daily.

Do not have sexual intercourse while you are using this medicine. Having sexual intercourse may reduce the strength of the medicine. This may cause the medicine to not work as well. Also, oils in the cream and vaginal tablets (but not the vaginal gel) may damage latex (rubber) contraceptive devices, such as cervical caps, condoms, or diaphragms, causing them to leak, wear out sooner, or not work properly.

Many vaginal infections (for example, trichomoniasis) are spread by having sexual intercourse. You can give the infection to your sexual partner, and the infection could be given back to you. Your partner may also need to be treated for some infections. Until you are sure that the infection is completely cleared up after your treatment with this medicine, your partner should wear a condom during sexual intercourse. If you have any questions about this, check with your health care professional.

Side Effects of This Medicine

Along with its needed effects, a medicine may cause some unwanted effects. Although not all of these side effects may occur, if they do occur they may need medical attention.

Check with your doctor as soon as possible if any of the following side effects occur:

More common
> Itching in the vagina; pain during sexual intercourse; thick, white vaginal discharge with no odor or with a mild odor

Less common
> Abdominal or stomach cramping or pain; burning or irritation of penis of sexual partner; burning on urination or need to urinate more often; itching, stinging or redness of the genital area

Some side effects may occur that usually do not need medical attention. These side effects may go away during treatment as your body adjusts to the medicine. Also, your health care professional may be able to tell you about ways to prevent or reduce some of these side effects. Check with your health care professional if any of the following side effects continue or are bothersome or if you have any questions about them:

Less common
> Diarrhea; dizziness or lightheadedness; dryness of mouth; headache; feeling of a furry tongue; loss of appetite; metallic taste or other change in taste sensation; nausea; vomiting

Metronidazole may cause your urine to become dark. This is harmless and will go away when you stop using this medicine.

After you stop using this medicine, it may still produce some side effects that need attention. During this period of time, *check with your doctor immediately* if you notice the following side effects:

> Any vaginal or genital irritation or itching; pain during sexual intercourse; thick, white vaginal discharge not present before treatment, with no odor or with a mild odor

Other side effects not listed may also occur in some patients. If you notice any other effects, check with your healthcare professional.

METYROSINE (Oral route) - me-TYE-roe-seen

Commonly used brand name(s)

In the U.S.—
> Demser

Available Dosage Forms:
- Capsule

Therapeutic Class: Antihypertensive
Pharmacologic Class: Tyrosine Hydroxylase Inhibitor

Uses For This Medicine

Metyrosine belongs to the general class of medicines called antihypertensives. It is used to treat high blood pressure (hypertension) caused by a disease called pheochromocytoma (a noncancerous tumor of the adrenal gland).

Metyrosine reduces the amount of certain chemicals in the body. When these chemicals are present in large amounts, they cause high blood pressure.

Metyrosine is available only with your doctor's prescription.

Before Using This Medicine

In deciding to use a medicine, the risks of taking the medicine must be weighed against the good it will do. This is a decision you and your doctor will make. For this medicine, the following should be considered:

Allergies—Tell your doctor if you have ever had any unusual or allergic reaction to this medicine or any other medicines. Also tell your health care professional if you have any other types of allergies, such as to foods, dyes, preservatives, or animals. For non-prescription products, read the label or package ingredients carefully.

Pediatric—Studies on this medicine have been done only in adult patients, and there is no specific information comparing use of metyrosine in children with use in other age groups.

Geriatric—Many medicines have not been studied specifically in older people. Therefore, it may not be known whether they work exactly the same way they do in younger adults or if they cause different side effects or problems in older people. There is no specific information comparing use of metyrosine in the elderly with use in other age groups.

Pregnancy—

	Pregnancy Category	Explanation
All Trimesters	C	Animal studies have shown an adverse effect and there are no adequate studies in pregnant women OR no animal studies have been conducted and there are no adequate studies in pregnant women.

Breast Feeding—There are no adequate studies in women for determining infant risk when using this medication during breastfeeding. Weigh the potential benefits against the potential risks before taking this medication while breastfeeding.

Other medicines—Although certain medicines should not be used together at all, in other cases two different medicines may be used together even if an interaction might occur. In these cases, your doctor may want to change the dose, or other precautions may be necessary. Tell your healthcare professional if you are taking any other prescription or non-prescription (over-the-counter [OTC]) medicine.

Interactions with Food/Tobacco/Alcohol—Certain medicines should not be used at or around the time of eating food or eating certain types of food since interactions may occur. Using alcohol or tobacco with certain medicines may also cause interactions to occur. Discuss with your healthcare professional the use of your medicine with food, alcohol, or tobacco.

Other medical problems—The presence of other medical problems may affect the use of this medicine. Make sure you tell your doctor if you have any other medical problems, especially:
- Kidney disease or
- Liver disease—Effects of metyrosine may be increased because of slower removal from the body
- Mental depression (or history of) or
- Parkinson's disease—Metyrosine may make these conditions worse

Proper Use of This Medicine

Take this medicine only as directed by your doctor. Do not take more or less of it than your doctor ordered.

To help you remember to take your medicine, try to get into the habit of taking it at the same times each day.

Dosing—The dose of this medicine will be different for different patients. Follow your doctor's orders or the directions on the label. The following information includes only the average doses of this medicine. If your dose is different, do not change it unless your doctor tells you to do so.

The amount of medicine that you take depends on the strength of the medicine. Also, the number of doses you take each day, the time allowed between doses, and the length of time you take the medicine depend on the medical problem for which you are using the medicine.

- For oral dosage forms (capsules):
  - Adults and children 12 years of age and older: 1000 milligrams to 3000 milligrams (1 to 3 grams) a day, divided into four doses.

Missed dose—If you miss a dose of this medicine, take it as soon as possible. However, if it is almost time for your next dose, skip the missed dose and go back to your regular dosing schedule. Do not double doses.

Storage—Store the medicine in a closed container at room temperature, away from heat, moisture, and direct light. Keep from freezing.

Keep out of the reach of children.

Do not keep outdated medicine or medicine no longer needed.

Precautions While Using This Medicine

It is important that your doctor check your progress at regular visits to make sure that this medicine is working properly and to check for unwanted effects.

While taking this medicine, it is important that you drink plenty of fluids and urinate often. This will help prevent kidney problems and keep your kidneys working well. If you have any questions about how much you should drink, check with your doctor.

This medicine will add to the effects of alcohol and other CNS depressants (medicines that slow down the nervous system, possibly causing drowsiness). Some examples of CNS depressants are antihistamines or medicine for hay fever, other allergies, or colds; sedatives, tranquilizers, or sleeping medicine; prescription pain medicine or narcotics; barbiturates; medicine for seizures; tricyclic antidepressants (medicine for depression); muscle relaxants; or anesthetics, including some dental anesthetics. Check with your doctor before taking any of the above while you are taking this medicine.

Before having any kind of surgery (including dental surgery), tell the medical doctor or dentist in charge that you are taking this medicine.

This medicine may cause most people to become drowsy or less alert than they are normally. Make sure you know how you react to this medicine before you drive, use machines, or do anything else that could be dangerous if you are not alert.

Side Effects of This Medicine

Along with its needed effects, a medicine may cause some unwanted effects. Although not all of these side effects may occur, if they do occur they may need medical attention.

Check with your doctor as soon as possible if any of the following side effects occur:

More common
 Diarrhea; drooling; trembling and shaking of hands and fingers; trouble in speaking

Less common
 Anxiety; confusion; hallucinations (seeing, hearing, or feeling things that are not there); mental depression

Rare
 Black, tarry stools; blood in urine or stools; unusual bleeding or bruising; muscle spasms, especially of neck and back; painful urination; pinpoint red spots on skin; restlessness; shortness of breath; shuffling walk; skin rash and itching; swelling of feet or lower legs; tic-like (jerky) movements of head, face, mouth, and neck; unusual tiredness or weakness

Some side effects may occur that usually do not need medical attention. These side effects may go away during treatment as your body adjusts to the medicine. Also, your health care professional may be able to tell you about ways to prevent or reduce some of these side effects. Check with your health care professional if any of the following side effects continue or are bothersome or if you have any questions about them:

More common
 Drowsiness

Less common
 Decreased sexual ability in men; dryness of mouth; nausea, vomiting, or stomach pain; stuffy nose; swelling of breasts or unusual milk production

After you stop using this medicine, it may still produce some side effects that need attention. During this period of time, *check with your doctor immediately* if you notice the following side effects:

More common
 Diarrhea

Also, after you stop taking this medicine, you may have feelings of increased energy or you may have trouble sleeping. However, these effects should last only for two or three days.

Other side effects not listed may also occur in some patients. If you notice any other effects, check with your healthcare professional.

MEXILETINE (Oral route) - MEX-i-le-teen

Black Box Warning

Mortality: In the National Heart, Lung and Blood Institute's Cardiac Arrhythmia Suppression Trial (CAST), a long-term, multicentered, randomized, double-blind study in patients with asymptomatic non-life-threatening ventricular arrhythmias who had a myocardial infarction more than six days but less than two years previously, an excessive mortality or non-fatal cardiac arrest rate (7.7%) was seen in patients treated with encainide or flecainide compared with that seen in patients assigned to carefully matched placebo-treated groups (3%). The average duration of treatment with encainide or flecainide in this study was ten months.

The applicability of the CAST results to other populations (eg, those without recent myocardial infarction) is uncertain. Considering the known proarrhythmic properties of mexiletine hydrochloride and the lack of evidence of improved survival for any antiarrhythmic drug in patients without life-threatening arrhythmias, the use of mexiletine hydrochloride as well as other antiarrhythmic agents should be reserved for patients with life-threatening ventricular arrhythmia.

Commonly used brand name(s)

In the U.S.—
 Mexitil

Available Dosage Forms:
- Capsule
- Capsule, Extended Release

Therapeutic Class: Antiarrhythmic, Group IB

Uses For This Medicine

Mexiletine belongs to the group of medicines known as antiarrhythmics. It is used to correct irregular heartbeats to a normal rhythm.

Mexiletine produces its helpful effects by slowing nerve impulses in the heart and making the heart tissue less sensitive.

Mexiletine is available only with your doctor's prescription.

Before Using This Medicine

In deciding to use a medicine, the risks of taking the medicine must be weighed against the good it will do. This is a decision

you and your doctor will make. For this medicine, the following should be considered:

Allergies—Tell your doctor if you have ever had any unusual or allergic reaction to this medicine or any other medicines. Also tell your health care professional if you have any other types of allergies, such as to foods, dyes, preservatives, or animals. For non-prescription products, read the label or package ingredients carefully.

Pediatric—Studies on this medicine have been done only in adult patients, and there is no specific information comparing use of mexiletine in children with use in other age groups.

Geriatric—Many medicines have not been studied specifically in older people. Therefore, it may not be known whether they work exactly the same way they do in younger adults or if they cause different side effects or problems in older people. There is no specific information comparing use of mexiletine in the elderly with use in other age groups.

Pregnancy—

	Pregnancy Category	Explanation
All Trimesters	C	Animal studies have shown an adverse effect and there are no adequate studies in pregnant women OR no animal studies have been conducted and there are no adequate studies in pregnant women.

Breast Feeding—There are no adequate studies in women for determining infant risk when using this medication during breastfeeding. Weigh the potential benefits against the potential risks before taking this medication while breastfeeding.

Other medicines—

Using this medicine with any of the following medicines is not recommended. Your doctor may decide not to treat you with this medication or change some of the other medicines you take.

Levomethadyl

Interactions with Food/Tobacco/Alcohol—Certain medicines should not be used at or around the time of eating food or eating certain types of food since interactions may occur. Using alcohol or tobacco with certain medicines may also cause interactions to occur. Discuss with your healthcare professional the use of your medicine with food, alcohol, or tobacco.

Other medical problems—The presence of other medical problems may affect the use of this medicine. Make sure you tell your doctor if you have any other medical problems, especially:

- Congestive heart failure or
- Low blood pressure—Mexiletine may make these conditions worse
- Heart attack (severe) or
- Liver disease—Effects may last longer because of slower removal of mexiletine from the body
- Seizures (history of)—Mexiletine can cause seizures

Proper Use of This Medicine

Take mexiletine exactly as directed by your doctor, even though you may feel well. Do not take more medicine than ordered.

To lessen the possibility of stomach upset, mexiletine should be taken with food or immediately after meals or with milk or an antacid.

This medicine works best when there is a constant amount in the blood. To help keep this amount constant, do not miss any doses. Also it is best to take the doses at evenly spaced times day and night. For example, if you are to take 3 doses a day, the doses should be spaced about 8 hours apart. If this interferes with your sleep or other daily activities, or if you need help in planning the best times to take your medicine, check with your health care professional.

Dosing—The dose of this medicine will be different for different patients. Follow your doctor's orders or the directions on the label. The following information includes only the average doses of this medicine. If your dose is different, do not change it unless your doctor tells you to do so.

The amount of medicine that you take depends on the strength of the medicine. Also, the number of doses you take each day, the time allowed between doses, and the length of time you take the medicine depend on the medical problem for which you are using the medicine.

- For oral dosage form (capsules):
  - For irregular heartbeat (arrhythmias):
    - Adults—At first, 200 milligrams (mg) every eight hours. Then, your doctor may raise or lower your dose as needed.
    - Children—Use and dose must be determined by your doctor.

Missed dose—If you miss a dose of this medicine, take it as soon as possible. However, if it is almost time for your next dose, skip the missed dose and go back to your regular dosing schedule. Do not double doses.

Storage—Store the medicine in a closed container at room temperature, away from heat, moisture, and direct light. Keep from freezing.

Keep out of the reach of children.

Do not keep outdated medicine or medicine no longer needed.

Precautions While Using This Medicine

It is important that your doctor check your progress at regular visits to make sure the medicine is working properly. This will allow for changes to be made in the amount of medicine you are taking, if necessary.

Your doctor may want you to carry a medical identification card or bracelet stating that you are using this medicine.

Before having any kind of surgery (including dental surgery) or emergency treatment, tell the medical doctor or dentist in charge that you are taking this medicine.

Mexiletine may cause some people to become dizzy, lightheaded, or less alert than they are normally. Make sure you know how you react to this medicine before you drive, use machines, or do anything else that could be dangerous if you are dizzy or are not alert.

Side Effects of This Medicine

Along with its needed effects, a medicine may cause some unwanted effects. Although not all of these side effects may occur, if they do occur they may need medical attention.

Check with your doctor as soon as possible if any of the following side effects occur:

Less common
   Chest pain; fast or irregular heartbeat; shortness of breath

Rare
   Convulsions (seizures); fever or chills; unusual bleeding or bruising

Some side effects may occur that usually do not need medical attention. These side effects may go away during treatment as your body adjusts to the medicine. Also, your health care professional may be able to tell you about ways to prevent or reduce some of these side effects. Check with your health care professional if any of the following side effects continue or are bothersome or if you have any questions about them:

More common
   Dizziness or lightheadedness; heartburn; nausea and vomiting; nervousness; trembling or shaking of the hands; unsteadiness or difficulty in walking

Less common
   Blurred vision; confusion; constipation or diarrhea; headache; numbness or tingling of fingers and toes; ringing in the ears; skin rash; slurred speech; trouble in sleeping; unusual tiredness or weakness

Other side effects not listed may also occur in some patients. If you notice any other effects, check with your healthcare professional.

MICONAZOLE (Topical route) - mi-KON-a-zole

Commonly used brand name(s)

In the U.S.—

Aloe Vesta 2–N-1 Antifungal	Monistat 1
Baza Antifungal	Monistat Derm
Carrington Antifungal	Neosporin AF
Derma Gran AF	QC Miconazole Nitrate
DiabetAid Antifungal Foot Bath	Secura Antifungal
	Soothe & Cool Inzo Antifungal
Fungoid	Tetterine
Lotrimin AF	Therasoft Antifungal
Micatin	Triple Care Antifungal
Micro-Guard	Triple Care EPC
Mitrazol	Zeasorb-AF

Available Dosage Forms:

- Cream
- Ointment
- Tincture
- Powder
- Tablet, Effervescent
- Spray
- Kit
- Lotion

Therapeutic Class: Antifungal

Uses For This Medicine

Miconazole belongs to the group of medicines called antifungals. Topical miconazole is used to treat some types of fungus infections.

Some of these preparations may be available without a prescription.

Before Using This Medicine

In deciding to use a medicine, the risks of taking the medicine must be weighed against the good it will do. This is a decision you and your doctor will make. For this medicine, the following should be considered:

Allergies—Tell your doctor if you have ever had any unusual or allergic reaction to this medicine or any other medicines. Also tell your health care professional if you have any other types of allergies, such as to foods, dyes, preservatives, or animals. For non-prescription products, read the label or package ingredients carefully.

Pediatric—Although there is no specific information comparing use of topical miconazole in children with use in other age groups, this medicine is not expected to cause different side effects or problems in children than it does in adults.

Geriatric—Many medicines have not been studied specifically in older people. Therefore, it may not be known whether they work exactly the same way they do in younger adults. Although there is no specific information comparing use of topical miconazole in the elderly with use in other age groups, this medicine is not expected to cause different side effects or problems in older people than it does in younger adults.

Other medicines—Although certain medicines should not be used together at all, in other cases two different medicines may be used together even if an interaction might occur. In these cases, your doctor may want to change the dose, or other precautions may be necessary. Tell your healthcare professional if you are taking any other prescription or non-prescription (over-the-counter [OTC]) medicine.

Interactions with Food/Tobacco/Alcohol—Certain medicines should not be used at or around the time of eating food or eating certain types of food since interactions may occur. Using alcohol or tobacco with certain medicines may also cause interactions to occur. Discuss with your healthcare professional the use of your medicine with food, alcohol, or tobacco.

Proper Use of This Medicine

Keep this medicine away from the eyes.

Apply enough miconazole to cover the affected area, and rub in gently.

To use the aerosol powder form of miconazole:

- Shake well before using.
- From a distance of 6 to 10 inches, spray the powder on the affected areas. If it is used on the feet, spray it between the toes, on the feet, and in the socks and shoes.
- Do not inhale the powder.
- Do not use near heat, near open flame, or while smoking.

To use the aerosol solution form of miconazole:

- Shake well before using.

- From a distance of 4 to 6 inches, spray the solution on the affected areas. If it is used on the feet, spray it between the toes and on the feet.
- Do not inhale the vapors from the spray.
- Do not use near heat, near open flame, or while smoking.

To use the powder form of miconazole:

- If the powder is used on the feet, sprinkle it between the toes, on the feet, and in the socks and shoes.

When miconazole is used to treat certain types of fungus infections of the skin, an occlusive dressing (airtight covering, such as kitchen plastic wrap) should not be applied over this medicine. To do so may cause irritation of the skin. Do not apply an occlusive dressing over this medicine unless you have been directed to do so by your doctor.

To help clear up your infection completely, keep using this medicine for the full time of treatment, even if your condition has improved. Do not miss any doses.

Dosing—The dose of this medicine will be different for different patients. Follow your doctor's orders or the directions on the label. The following information includes only the average doses of this medicine. If your dose is different, do not change it unless your doctor tells you to do so.

The amount of medicine that you take depends on the strength of the medicine. Also, the number of doses you take each day, the time allowed between doses, and the length of time you take the medicine depend on the medical problem for which you are using the medicine.

- For aerosol powder, aerosol solution, cream, and powder dosage forms:
  - For fungus infections:
    - Adults and children—Apply to the affected area(s) of the skin two times a day, morning and evening.
- For cream and lotion dosage forms:
  - For sun fungus:
    - Adults and children—Apply to the affected area(s) of the skin once a day.

Missed dose—If you miss a dose of this medicine, apply it as soon as possible. However, if it is almost time for your next dose, skip the missed dose and go back to your regular dosing schedule.

Storage—Store the medicine in a closed container at room temperature, away from heat, moisture, and direct light. Keep from freezing.

Store the canister at room temperature, away from heat and direct light. Do not freeze. Do not keep this medicine inside a car where it could be exposed to extreme heat or cold. Do not poke holes in the canister or throw it into a fire, even if the canister is empty.

Keep out of the reach of children.

Do not keep outdated medicine or medicine no longer needed.

Precautions While Using This Medicine

If your skin problem does not improve within 4 weeks, or if it becomes worse, check with your health care professional.

Side Effects of This Medicine

Along with its needed effects, a medicine may cause some unwanted effects. Although not all of these side effects may occur, if they do occur they may need medical attention.

Check with your doctor as soon as possible if any of the following side effects occur:

Blistering, burning, redness, skin rash, or other sign of skin irritation not present before use of this medicine

Other side effects not listed may also occur in some patients. If you notice any other effects, check with your healthcare professional.

MIDODRINE   (Oral route) - MI-doe-dreen

Black Box Warning

Because midodrine hydrochloride can cause marked elevation of supine blood pressure, it should be used in patients whose lives are considerably impaired despite standard clinical care. The indication for use of midodrine hydrochloride in the treatment of symptomatic orthostatic hypotension is based primarily on a change in a surrogate marker of effectiveness, an increase in systolic blood pressure measured one minute after standing, a surrogate marker considered likely to correspond to a clinical benefit. At present, however, clinical benefits of midodrine hydrochloride, principally improved ability to carry out activities of daily living, have not been verified.

Commonly used brand name(s)

In the U.S.—
Orvaten
Proamatine

Available Dosage Forms:

- Tablet

Therapeutic Class: Vasopressor
Pharmacologic Class: Sympathomimetic

Uses For This Medicine

Midodrine is a medicine used to treat low blood pressure (hypotension). It works by stimulating nerve endings in blood vessels, causing the blood vessels to tighten. As a result, blood pressure is increased.

This medicine is available only with your doctor's prescription.

Once a medicine has been approved for marketing for a certain use, experience may show that it is also useful for other medical problems. Although not specifically included in product labeling, midodrine is used in certain patients with the following medical conditions:

- Low blood pressure (hypotension) caused by kidney dialysis
- Low blood pressure caused by certain medicines used to treat mental illness
- Low blood pressure in children with an infection

Before Using This Medicine

In deciding to use a medicine, the risks of taking the medicine must be weighed against the good it will do. This is a decision you and your doctor will make. For this medicine, the following should be considered:

Allergies—Tell your doctor if you have ever had any unusual or allergic reaction to this medicine or any other medi-

cines. Also tell your health care professional if you have any other types of allergies, such as to foods, dyes, preservatives, or animals. For non-prescription products, read the label or package ingredients carefully.

Pediatric—This medicine has been tested in a limited number of children 6 months to 12 years of age. In effective doses, the medicine has not been shown to cause different side effects or problems than it does in adults.

Geriatric—This medicine has been tested and has not been shown to cause different side effects or problems in older people than it dose in younger adults.

Pregnancy—

	Pregnancy Category	Explanation
All Trimesters	C	Animal studies have shown an adverse effect and there are no adequate studies in pregnant women OR no animal studies have been conducted and there are no adequate studies in pregnant women.

Breast Feeding—There are no adequate studies in women for determining infant risk when using this medication during breastfeeding. Weigh the potential benefits against the potential risks before taking this medication while breastfeeding.

Other medicines—

Using this medicine with any of the following medicines is not recommended. Your doctor may decide not to treat you with this medication or change some of the other medicines you take.

Dihydroergotamine

Interactions with Food/Tobacco/Alcohol—Certain medicines should not be used at or around the time of eating food or eating certain types of food since interactions may occur. Using alcohol or tobacco with certain medicines may also cause interactions to occur. Discuss with your healthcare professional the use of your medicine with food, alcohol, or tobacco.

Other medical problems—The presence of other medical problems may affect the use of this medicine. Make sure you tell your doctor if you have any other medical problems, especially:

- Heart disease, severe or
- Hypertension (high blood pressure) or
- Overactive thyroid or
- Visual problems—Effects of midodrine on blood pressure may aggravate these problems
- Kidney disease or
- Liver disease—Effects of midodrine may be increased because of slower removal of the medicine from the body
- Urinary retention—Effects of midodrine on the bladder may aggravate this condition

Proper Use of This Medicine

The last dose of midodrine should not be taken after the evening meal or less than 3 to 4 hours before bedtime because high blood pressure upon lying down (supine hypertension) can occur, which can cause blurred vision, headaches, and

pounding in the ears while lying down after taking this medicine.

Also, midodrine should not be taken if you will be lying down for any length of time.

Dosing—The dose of this medicine will be different for different patients. Follow your doctor's orders or the directions on the label. The following information includes only the average doses of this medicine. If your dose is different, do not change it unless your doctor tells you to do so.

The amount of medicine that you take depends on the strength of the medicine. Also, the number of doses you take each day, the time allowed between doses, and the length of time you take the medicine depend on the medical problem for which you are using the medicine.

- For oral dosage form (tablets):
  - Low blood pressure (hypotension):
    - Adults—10 milligrams (mg) three times a day in approximately four-hour intervals during the daytime hours: shortly before or upon rising in the morning, at midday, and in the late afternoon (not later than six p.m.). Your doctor may increase your dose if needed.
    - Children—Use and dose must be determined by your doctor.

Missed dose—If you miss a dose of this medicine, take it as soon as possible. However, if it is almost time for your next dose, skip the missed dose and go back to your regular dosing schedule. Do not double doses.

Storage—Store the medicine in a closed container at room temperature, away from heat, moisture, and direct light. Keep from freezing.

Keep out of the reach of children.

Do not keep outdated medicine or medicine no longer needed.

Precautions While Using This Medicine

Do not take other medicines unless they have been discussed with your doctor. This especially includes over-the-counter (nonprescription) medicines for appetite control, asthma, colds, cough, hayfever, or sinus problems, since they may tend to increase your blood pressure.

Side Effects of This Medicine

Along with its needed effects, a medicine may cause some unwanted effects. Although not all of these side effects may occur, if they do occur they may need medical attention.

Check with your doctor as soon as possible if any of the following side effects occur:
More common
    Blurred vision, cardiac awareness, headache, and/or pounding in the ears
Rare
    Fainting; increased dizziness; slow pulse

Some side effects may occur that usually do not need medical attention. These side effects may go away during treatment as your body adjusts to the medicine. Also, your health care professional may be able to tell you about ways to prevent or reduce some of these side effects. Check with your health care professional if any of the following side effects

continue or are bothersome or if you have any questions about them:

More common

Burning, itching, or prickling of the scalp; chills; goosebumps; urinary frequency, retention, or urgency

Less common

Anxiety or nervousness; confusion; dry mouth; flushing; headache or feeling of pressure in the head; skin rash

Rare

Backache; canker sores; dizziness; drowsiness; dry skin; leg cramps; pain or sensitivity of skin to touch; stomach problems such as gas, heartburn, or nausea; trouble in sleeping; trouble seeing; weakness

Other side effects not listed may also occur in some patients. If you notice any other effects, check with your healthcare professional.

MIFEPRISTONE   (Oral route) - mi-FE-pri-stone

Black Box Warning

Serious and sometimes fatal infections and bleeding occur very rarely following spontaneous, surgical, and medical abortions, including following mifepristone use. No causal relationship between the use of mifepristone and misoprostol and these events has been established. Before prescribing mifepristone, inform the patient about the risk of these serious events and discuss the medication guide and the patient agreement. Ensure that the patient knows whom to call and what to do, including going to an emergency room if none of the provided contacts are reachable, if she experiences sustained fever, severe abdominal pain, prolonged heavy bleeding, or syncope,or if she experiences abdominal pain or discomfort or general malaise (including weakness, nausea, vomiting or diarrhea) more than 24 hours after taking misoprostol.

Atypical Presentation of Infection. Patients with serious bacterial infections (e.g. Clostridium sordellii) and sepsis can present without fever, bacteremia or significant findings on pelvic examination following an abortion. Very rarely, deaths have been reported in patients who presented without fever, with or without abdominal pain, but with leukocytosis with a marked left shift, tachycardia, hemoconcentration, and general malaise. A high index of suspicion is needed to rule out serious infection and sepsis.

Bleeding. Prolonged heavy bleeding may be a sign of incomplete abortion or other complications and prompt medical or surgical intervention may be needed. Advise patients to seek immediate medical attention if they experience prolonged heavy vaginal bleeding.

Patients should be advised to take their medication guide with them if they visit an emergency room or another health care provider who did not prescribe mifepristone, so that provider will be aware that the patient is undergoing a medical abortion.

Commonly used brand name(s)

In the U.S.—
Mifeprex

Available Dosage Forms:

• Tablet

Therapeutic Class: Antiprogesterone

Uses For This Medicine

Mifepristone is used to end a pregnancy that is less than 49 days in duration. It works by stopping the supply of hormones that maintains the interior of the uterus. Without these hormones, the uterus cannot support the pregnancy and the contents of the uterus are expelled.

This medicine is available only with your doctor's prescription.

Before Using This Medicine

In deciding to use a medicine, the risks of taking the medicine must be weighed against the good it will do. This is a decision you and your doctor will make. For this medicine, the following should be considered:

Allergies—Tell your doctor if you have ever had any unusual or allergic reaction to this medicine or any other medicines. Also tell your health care professional if you have any other types of allergies, such as to foods, dyes, preservatives, or animals. For non-prescription products, read the label or package ingredients carefully.

Pregnancy—

	Pregnancy Category	Explanation
All Trimesters	X	Studies in animals or pregnant women have demonstrated positive evidence of fetal abnormalities. This drug should not be used in women who are or may become pregnant because the risk clearly outweighs any possible benefit.

Breast Feeding—There are no adequate studies in women for determining infant risk when using this medication during breastfeeding. Weigh the potential benefits against the potential risks before taking this medication while breastfeeding.

Other medicines—Although certain medicines should not be used together at all, in other cases two different medicines may be used together even if an interaction might occur. In these cases, your doctor may want to change the dose, or other precautions may be necessary. Tell your healthcare professional if you are taking any other prescription or nonprescription (over-the-counter [OTC]) medicine.

Interactions with   Food/Tobacco/Alcohol—Certain medicines should not be used at or around the time of eating food or eating certain types of food since interactions may occur. Using alcohol or tobacco with certain medicines may also cause interactions to occur. Discuss with your healthcare professional the use of your medicine with food, alcohol, or tobacco.

Other medical problems—The presence of other medical problems may affect the use of this medicine. Make sure you tell your doctor if you have any other medical problems, especially:

• Adrenal failure—Mifepristone may not work appropriately

• Bleeding   problems—May cause excessive vaginal bleeding

- Diabetes or
- Heart disease or
- High blood pressure or
- Kidney disease or
- Liver disease or
- Lung disease
- Women older than 35 years of age who smoke cigarettes (10 or more a day)—You should use caution if you have any of these chronic conditions and let your doctor know before beginning treatment with this medicine.
- Ectopic pregnancy (e.g., a pregnancy that develops in fallopian tubes instead of the uterus) or
- Lower abdominal mass—Mifepristone will not terminate an ectopic pregnancy
- An intrauterine device (IUD) that is still in the uterus— Must be removed before mifepristone therapy is started
- Porphyria, inherited
- Anemia, severe or
- Poor blood circulation or
- Inability of blood to clot properly—Mifepristone causes heavy bleeding in a small portion of users, this may be intensified in patients with bleeding disorders

Proper Use of This Medicine

Dosing—The dose of this medicine will be different for different patients. Follow your doctor's orders or the directions on the label. The following information includes only the average doses of this medicine. If your dose is different, do not change it unless your doctor tells you to do so.

The amount of medicine that you take depends on the strength of the medicine. Also, the number of doses you take each day, the time allowed between doses, and the length of time you take the medicine depend on the medical problem for which you are using the medicine.

- To terminate a pregnancy of 49 days or less duration:
  - For oral dosage form (tablets):
    - Adults—600 milligrams (mg) (three 200 mg tablets) as a single oral dose followed two days later by 400 micrograms (mcg) (two 200 mcg tablets) of misoprostol as a single oral dose as needed.

Precautions While Using This Medicine

You must have 3 visits to your physicians office during the treatment procedure. It is extremely important that you attend all three visits.

Check with your physician if the vaginal bleeding becomes severe or seems to last longer than expected (i.e., soaking through two thick full-size sanitary pads per hour for two consecutive hours).

You may need to have a surgical procedure to stop excessive vaginal bleeding or to terminate a pregnancy that was not terminated with the medical treatment procedure.

You should check with your physician immediately if signs or symptoms of serious infection (i.e., continuing fever ≥ 100.4 °F, severe stomach pain, pelvic tenderness, weakness, nausea, vomiting, diarrhea or abnormally fast heartbeat) occur.

Side Effects of This Medicine

Along with its needed effects, a medicine may cause some unwanted effects. Although not all of these side effects may occur, if they do occur they may need medical attention.

Check with your doctor as soon as possible if any of the following side effects occur:

Less common
 Excessively heavy vaginal bleeding; unusual tiredness or weakness

Incidence not known
 Chest pain or discomfort; confusion; cough or hoarseness; fast, weak pulse; fever or chills; lower back or side pain; pain or discomfort in arms, jaw, back or neck; painful or difficult urination; pale, cold, clammy skin; shortness of breath; sudden increase in abdominal or shoulder pain; sweating; unusual or large amount of vaginal bleeding

Some side effects may occur that usually do not need medical attention. These side effects may go away during treatment as your body adjusts to the medicine. Also, your health care professional may be able to tell you about ways to prevent or reduce some of these side effects. Check with your health care professional if any of the following side effects continue or are bothersome or if you have any questions about them:

More common
 Abdominal pain or uterine cramping; back pain; diarrhea; dizziness; headache; nausea or vomiting

Less common
 Acid or sour stomach; anxiety; belching; cough; fainting or light-headedness when getting up from a lying or sitting position; fever; flu-like symptoms; headache; heartburn; increased clear or white vaginal discharge; indigestion; itching of the vagina or genital area; lack or loss of strength; pain during sexual intercourse; pain or tenderness around eyes and cheekbones; pale skin; shaking chills; shortness of breath or troubled breathing; sleeplessness or trouble sleeping; stomach discomfort, upset, or pain; tightness of chest or wheezing; troubled breathing, exertional; unusual bleeding or bruising; stuffy or runny nose

Other side effects not listed may also occur in some patients. If you notice any other effects, check with your healthcare professional.

MIGLITOL (Oral route) - MIG-li-tol

Commonly used brand name(s)

In the U.S.—
 Glyset

Available Dosage Forms:
- Tablet

Therapeutic Class: Antidiabetic
Pharmacologic Class: Alpha-Glucosidase Inhibitor

Uses For This Medicine

Miglitol is used to treat high blood sugar levels that are caused by type 2 diabetes. Normally, after you eat, your pancreas releases insulin to help your body store excess sugar for later use. This process occurs during normal digestion of food. In type 2 diabetes, your body does not work properly to store the excess sugar and the sugar remains in your bloodstream. Having high blood sugar can lead to serious health problems in the future. Proper diet is the first step in managing type 2 diabetes but often medicines are needed to help your body. Miglitol is a medicine that slows the digestion of sugars so your body has time to store extra sugar. Sometimes another medicine called sulfonylurea can be used in combination with miglitol to help your body store more sugar.

This medicine is available only with your doctor's prescription.

Before Using This Medicine

In deciding to use a medicine, the risks of taking the medicine must be weighed against the good it will do. This is a decision you and your doctor will make. For this medicine, the following should be considered:

Allergies—Tell your doctor if you have ever had any unusual or allergic reaction to this medicine or any other medicines. Also tell your health care professional if you have any other types of allergies, such as to foods, dyes, preservatives, or animals. For non-prescription products, read the label or package ingredients carefully.

Pediatric—Studies on this medicine have been done only in adult patients, and there is no specific information comparing use of miglitol in children with use in other age groups.

Geriatric—This medicine has been tested and has not been shown to cause different side effects or problems in older people than it does in younger adults.

Pregnancy—

	Pregnancy Category	Explanation
All Trimesters	B	Animal studies have revealed no evidence of harm to the fetus, however, there are no adequate studies in pregnant women OR animal studies have shown an adverse effect, but adequate studies in pregnant women have failed to demonstrate a risk to the fetus.

Breast Feeding—There are no adequate studies in women for determining infant risk when using this medication during breastfeeding. Weigh the potential benefits against the potential risks before taking this medication while breastfeeding.

Other medicines—

Using this medicine with any of the following medicines is usually not recommended, but may be required in some cases. If both medicines are prescribed together, your doctor may change the dose or how often you use one or both of the medicines.

Alatrofloxacin, Balofloxacin, Ciprofloxacin, Clinafloxacin, Enoxacin, Fleroxacin, Flumequine, Gatifloxacin, Gemifloxacin, Grepafloxacin, Levofloxacin, Lomefloxacin, Moxifloxacin, Norfloxacin, Ofloxacin, Pefloxacin, Prulifloxacin, Rufloxacin,

Sparfloxacin, Temafloxacin, Tosufloxacin, Trovafloxacin Mesylate

Interactions with Food/Tobacco/Alcohol—Certain medicines should not be used at or around the time of eating food or eating certain types of food since interactions may occur. Using alcohol or tobacco with certain medicines may also cause interactions to occur. Discuss with your healthcare professional the use of your medicine with food, alcohol, or tobacco.

Other medical problems—The presence of other medical problems may affect the use of this medicine. Make sure you tell your doctor if you have any other medical problems, especially:

- Digestion problems or
- Inflammatory bowel disease or
- Intestinal blockage or
- Other intestinal problems—Miglitol should not be used
- Kidney disease—Higher levels of miglitol may result and a smaller dose may be needed

Proper Use of This Medicine

Follow carefully the special meal plan you doctor gave you. This is the most important part of controlling your condition, and is necessary if the medicine is to work properly. Also, exercise regularly and test for sugar in your blood or urine as directed.

For this medicine to work properly it should be taken with the first bite of each main meal.

Dosing—The dose of this medicine will be different for different patients. Follow your doctor's orders or the directions on the label. The following information includes only the average doses of this medicine. If your dose is different, do not change it unless your doctor tells you to do so.

The amount of medicine that you take depends on the strength of the medicine. Also, the number of doses you take each day, the time allowed between doses, and the length of time you take the medicine depend on the medical problem for which you are using the medicine.

- For oral dosage form (tablets):
  - For type 2 diabetes:
    - Adults—At first the dose is 25 milligrams (mg) three times a day, at the start (with the first bite) of each main meal. After four to eight weeks, your doctor may increase your dose to 50 mg three times a day. Then, after an additional twelve weeks, if necessary, your doctor may increase your dose to 100 mg three times a day.
    - Children—Use and dose must be determined by your doctor.

Missed dose—If you miss a dose of this medicine, skip the missed dose and go back to your regular dosing schedule. Do not double doses.

Storage—Store the medicine in a closed container at room temperature, away from heat, moisture, and direct light. Keep from freezing.

Keep out of the reach of children.

Do not keep outdated medicine or medicine no longer needed.

Ask your healthcare professional how you should dispose of any medicine you do not use.

Precautions While Using This Medicine

Your doctor will want to check your progress at regular visits, especially during the first few weeks that you take this medicine.

It is very important to follow carefully any instructions from your health care team about:

- Alcohol—Drinking alcohol may cause severe low blood sugar. Discuss this with your health care team.
- Other medicines—Do not take other medicines during the time you are taking miglitol unless they have been discussed with your doctor. This especially includes non-prescription medicines such as aspirin, and medicines for appetite control, asthma, colds, cough, hay fever, or sinus problems.
- Counseling—Other family members need to learn how to prevent side effects or help with side effects if they occur. Also, patients with diabetes may need special counseling about diabetes medicine dosing changes that might occur because of lifestyle changes, such as changes in exercise and diet. Furthermore, counseling on contraception and pregnancy may be needed because of the problems that can occur in patients with diabetes during pregnancy.
- Travel—Keep a recent prescription and your medical history with you. Be prepared for an emergency as you would normally. Make allowances for changing time zones and keep your meal times as close as possible to your usual meal times.

In case of emergency—There may be a time when you need emergency help for a problem caused by your diabetes. You need to be prepared for these emergencies. It is a good idea to wear a medical identification (ID) bracelet or neck chain at all times. Also, carry an ID card in your wallet or purse that says that you have diabetes and a list of all your medicines.

Symptoms of hypoglycemia (low blood sugar) include anxiety; behavior change similar to being drunk; blurred vision; cold sweats; confusion; cool, pale skin; difficulty in thinking; drowsiness; excessive hunger; fast heartbeat; headache (continuing); nausea; nervousness; nightmares; restless sleep; shakiness; slurred speech; or unusual tiredness or weakness.

Miglitol does not cause low blood sugar. However, it can occur if you delay or miss a meal or snack, drink alcohol, exercise more than usual, cannot eat because of nausea or vomiting, or take miglitol with another type of diabetes medicine. Symptoms of low blood sugar must be treated before they lead to unconsciousness (passing out). Different people feel different symptoms of low blood sugar. It is important that you learn which symptoms of low blood sugar you usually have so that you can treat it quickly.

If symptoms of low blood sugar occur, eat glucose tablets or gel or honey, or drink fruit juice to relieve the symptoms. Table sugar (sucrose) or regular (nondiet) soft drinks will not work. Also, check your blood for low blood sugar. Glucagon is used in emergency situations when severe symptoms such as seizures (convulsions) or unconsciousness occur. Have a glucagon kit available, along with a syringe or needle, and know how to use it. Members of your household also should know how to use it.

Symptoms of hyperglycemia (high blood sugar) include blurred vision; drowsiness; dry mouth; flushed, dry skin; fruit-like breath odor; increased urination; ketones in urine; loss of appetite; stomachache, nausea, or vomiting; tiredness; troubled breathing (rapid and deep); unconsciousness; or unusual thirst.

High blood sugar may occur if you do not exercise as much as usual, have a fever or infection, do not take enough or skip a dose of your diabetes medicine, or overeat or do not follow your meal plan.

If symptoms of high blood sugar occur, check your blood sugar level and then call your health care professional for instructions.

Side Effects of This Medicine

Some side effects may occur that usually do not need medical attention. These side effects may go away during treatment as your body adjusts to the medicine. Also, your health care professional may be able to tell you about ways to prevent or reduce some of these side effects. Check with your health care professional if any of the following side effects continue or are bothersome or if you have any questions about them:

More common
Bloated full feeling; excess air or gas in stomach or intestines; increase in bowel movements; loose stools; passing gas; soft stools; stomach or abdomen pain

Less common
Skin rash

Other side effects not listed may also occur in some patients. If you notice any other effects, check with your healthcare professional.

MIGLUSTAT   (Oral route) - MIG-loo-stat

Commonly used brand name(s)
In the U.S.—
Zavesca

Available Dosage Forms:
- Capsule

Therapeutic Class: Endocrine-Metabolic Agent
Pharmacologic Class: Glucosylceramide Synthase Inhibitor

Uses For This Medicine

Miglustat is used to treat adults with mild to moderate type 1 Gaucher disease. Miglustat is only used in people who cannot be treated with enzyme replacement therapy. Type 1 Gaucher disease is a disease you get from both your parents. People with type 1 Gaucher disease are missing an enzyme (naturally occurring substance in your body) that breaks down a chemical in your body called glucosylceramide. Too much glucosylceramide causes liver and spleen enlargement, changes in the blood, and bone disease. Miglustat works by stopping the body from making glucosylceramide.

This medicine is available only with your doctor's prescription.

Before Using This Medicine

In deciding to use a medicine, the risks of taking the medicine must be weighed against the good it will do. This is a decision

you and your doctor will make. For this medicine, the following should be considered:

Allergies—Tell your doctor if you have ever had any unusual or allergic reaction to this medicine or any other medicines. Also tell your health care professional if you have any other types of allergies, such as to foods, dyes, preservatives, or animals. For non-prescription products, read the label or package ingredients carefully.

Pediatric—This medicine is not used in children under 18 years of age.

Geriatric—Many medicines have not been specifically studied in older people. Therefore, it may not be known whether they work the same way the do in younger adults. This medicine is not expected to cause different side effects or problems in older people than it does in younger adults.

Pregnancy—

	Pregnancy Category	Explanation
All Trimesters	X	Studies in animals or pregnant women have demonstrated positive evidence of fetal abnormalities. This drug should not be used in women who are or may become pregnant because the risk clearly outweighs any possible benefit.

Breast Feeding—There are no adequate studies in women for determining infant risk when using this medication during breastfeeding. Weigh the potential benefits against the potential risks before taking this medication while breastfeeding.

Other medicines—Although certain medicines should not be used together at all, in other cases two different medicines may be used together even if an interaction might occur. In these cases, your doctor may want to change the dose, or other precautions may be necessary. Tell your healthcare professional if you are taking any other prescription or non-prescription (over-the-counter [OTC]) medicine.

Interactions with Food/Tobacco/Alcohol—Certain medicines should not be used at or around the time of eating food or eating certain types of food since interactions may occur. Using alcohol or tobacco with certain medicines may also cause interactions to occur. Discuss with your healthcare professional the use of your medicine with food, alcohol, or tobacco.

Other medical problems—The presence of other medical problems may affect the use of this medicine. Make sure you tell your doctor if you have any other medical problems, especially:

- Gaucher disease, Type 1, severe—This medicine is not currently being used in patients with severe Type 1 Gaucher disease
- Kidney disease—This condition may cause you to have more miglustat in your body; your doctor may want to change the amount of miglustat that you take

Proper Use of This Medicine

It is important to take miglustat exactly as your doctor prescribed. You should take your medicine at the same time or at the same times each day.

The capsules should be swallowed whole with water and may be taken with or without food. Check with your doctor or pharmacist if you have any questions.

Your doctor may recommend changes to your diet to help with some side effects. It is important that you follow these changes.

Dosing—The dose of this medicine will be different for different patients. Follow your doctor's orders or the directions on the label. The following information includes only the average doses of this medicine. If your dose is different, do not change it unless your doctor tells you to do so.

The amount of medicine that you take depends on the strength of the medicine. Also, the number of doses you take each day, the time allowed between doses, and the length of time you take the medicine depend on the medical problem for which you are using the medicine.

- For oral dosage form (capsules):
  - For Mild to Moderate Type 1 Gaucher disease
    - Adults—One 100 milligram (mg) capsule given three times a day; your doctor may change this dose as needed.
    - Children—Use is not recommended in children under the age of 18.

Missed dose—If you miss a dose of this medicine, take it as soon as possible. However, if it is almost time for your next dose, skip the missed dose and go back to your regular dosing schedule. Do not double doses.

Storage—Store the medicine in a closed container at room temperature, away from heat, moisture, and direct light. Keep from freezing.

Keep out of the reach of children.

Do not keep outdated medicine or medicine no longer needed.

Ask your healthcare professional how you should dispose of any medicine you do not use.

Precautions While Using This Medicine

Miglustat can cause problems affecting your nerves. If you have hand tremors (shaky movements) or if miglustat worsens a hand tremor you already have call your doctor. Your doctor might want to change your dose of miglustat.

If you experience numbness and tingling in your hands, arms, legs, or feet (peripheral neuropathy) call your doctor right away.

It is very important that your doctor check you at regular visits. Your doctor will also want to test your nerves (neurological exam) before you start taking miglustat and may repeat this test at a later time.

Diarrhea is the most common side effect for people taking miglustat. Your doctor may give you another medicine (antidiarrheal) to help treat diarrhea if it is a problem for you. Your doctor may also recommend changes to your diet. You may also lose weight when you start treatment with miglustat.

It is very important to discuss with your doctor if you are pregnant or plan to become pregnant before starting miglustat. You should use effective birth control while taking miglustat. Miglustat may also harm a man's sperm. All men should use effective birth control during treatment and for three months after stopping treatment.

Side Effects of This Medicine

Along with its needed effects, a medicine may cause some unwanted effects. Although not all of these side effects may occur, if they do occur they may need medical attention.

Check with your doctor immediately if any of the following side effects occur:

More common

Black, tarry stools; bleeding gums; blood in urine or stools; burning, crawling, itching, numbness, prickling, "pins and needles", or tingling feelings; pinpoint red spots on skin; unusual bleeding or bruising

Unknown

Painful sensations; shakiness in legs, arms, hands, feet; trembling or shaking of hands or feet; unsteadiness or awkwardness; weakness in arms, hands, legs, or feet

Some side effects may occur that usually do not need medical attention. These side effects may go away during treatment as your body adjusts to the medicine. Also, your health care professional may be able to tell you about ways to prevent or reduce some of these side effects. Check with your health care professional if any of the following side effects continue or are bothersome or if you have any questions about them:

More common

Acid or sour stomach; back pain; belching; bloated, full feeling; change in vision; cramps; diarrhea; difficulty having a bowel movement (stool); dizziness; dry mouth; excess air or gas in stomach or intestines; full or bloated feeling or pressure in the stomach; headache; heartburn; heaviness in limbs; indigestion; leg cramps; loss of appetite; memory loss; menstrual changes; nausea; pain or discomfort in chest, upper stomach, or throat; passing gas; stomach discomfort, upset or pain; swelling; swelling of abdominal or stomach area; unsteady walk; vomiting; weakness; weight loss

Other side effects not listed may also occur in some patients. If you notice any other effects, check with your healthcare professional.

MINOCYCLINE (Subgingival route) -
mi-noe-SYE-kleen

Uses For This Medicine

Minocycline is used to help treat periodontal disease (a disease of your gums). Periodontal disease is caused by bacteria growing beneath the gum line. Minocycline works by keeping the number of bacteria from growing. Lowering the amount of bacteria helps to reduce inflammation and swelling in your mouth, and the amount of bleeding around the teeth. Minocycline is placed in deep gum pockets next to your teeth in order to reduce the depth of the pockets.

This medicine will be applied by your dentist or other oral health care professional,.

Before Receiving This Medicine

In deciding to use a medicine, the risks of taking the medicine must be weighed against the good it will do. This is a decision you and your doctor will make. For this medicine, the following should be considered:

Allergies—Tell your doctor if you have ever had any unusual or allergic reaction to this medicine or any other medicines. Also tell your health care professional if you have any other types of allergies, such as to foods, dyes, preservatives,

or animals. For non-prescription products, read the label or package ingredients carefully.

Pediatric—Use is not recommended in infants and children up to 8 years of age. Tetracyclines, such as minocycline, may cause permanent discoloration of teeth and slow down the growth of bones. The safety and effectiveness of minocycline have not been determined in children 8 years of age or older.

Geriatric—Many medicines have not been studied specifically in older people. Therefore, it may not be known whether they work exactly the same way they do in younger adults or if they cause different side effects or problems in older people. There is no specific information comparing use of minocycline in the elderly with use in other age groups.

Pregnancy—

	Pregnancy Category	Explanation
All Trimesters	D	Studies in pregnant women have demonstrated a risk to the fetus. However, the benefits of therapy in a life threatening situation or a serious disease, may outweigh the potential risk.

Breast Feeding—Studies suggest that this medication may alter milk production or composition. If an alternative to this medication is not prescribed, you should monitor the infant for side effects and adequate milk intake.

Other medicines—

Using this medicine with any of the following medicines is not recommended. Your doctor may decide not to treat you with this medication or change some of the other medicines you take.

Acitretin

Interactions with Food/Tobacco/Alcohol—Certain medicines should not be used at or around the time of eating food or eating certain types of food since interactions may occur. Using alcohol or tobacco with certain medicines may also cause interactions to occur. Discuss with your healthcare professional the use of your medicine with food, alcohol, or tobacco.

Proper Use of This Medicine

After minocycline is placed in your mouth try to avoid any actions that may cause the medicine to come out. For example:

- Do not chew hard, crunchy, or sticky foods for 1 week after treatment.
- Do not brush near any treated areas. Wait 12 hours after the procedure before brushing the other teeth.
- Do not use dental floss or any other cleaning tools that go between the teeth for 10 days after treatment.
- Do not probe or pick at the treated areas with your tongue, toothpicks, or fingers.

Dosing—The dose of this medicine will be different for different patients. Follow your doctor's orders or the directions on the label. The following information includes only the average doses of this medicine. If your dose is different, do not change it unless your doctor tells you to do so.

The amount of medicine that you take depends on the strength of the medicine. Also, the number of doses you take each day, the time allowed between doses, and the length of time you take the medicine depend on the medical problem for which you are using the medicine.

The amount of minocycline that will be put into your gum pockets will be determined by your dentist. The number of teeth that need treatment and the depth of the pockets will determine the amount of medicine that is used.

Precautions After Receiving This Medicine

Check with your dentist as soon as possible if you have pain or swelling or other problems in the treated areas.

It is very important that your dentist check your progress. Do not miss any dental appointments.

Tetracyclines, such as minocycline, may cause your skin to be more sensitive to sunlight than it is normally. Exposure to sunlight, even for brief periods of time, may cause a skin rash, itching, redness or other discoloration of the skin, or a severe sunburn. After receiving minocycline:

- Stay out of direct sunlight, especially between the hours of 10:00 a.m. and 3:00 p.m., if possible.
- Wear protective clothing, including a hat. Also, wear sunglasses.
- Apply a sun block product that has a skin protection factor (SPF) of at least 15. Some patients may require a product with a higher SPF number, especially if they have a fair complexion. If you have any questions about this, check with your health care professional.
- Apply a sun block lip balm or lipstick that has an SPF of at least 15 to protect your lips.
- Do not use a sunlamp or tanning bed or booth.

If you have a severe reaction from the sun, check with your dentist or doctor.

Side Effects of This Medicine

Along with its needed effects, a medicine may cause some unwanted effects. Although not all of these side effects may occur, if they do occur they may need medical attention.

Check with your doctor as soon as possible if any of the following side effects occur:

More common
Bleeding from gums; chills; dental pain; fever; pain, redness, and swelling in the mouth; problems with teeth; redness or swelling of gums; toothache

Less common
Bad taste in mouth; discharge from gums; foul breath odor; painful sores in the mouth; problems in the lining of the mouth

Some side effects may occur that usually do not need medical attention. These side effects may go away during treatment as your body adjusts to the medicine. Also, your health care professional may be able to tell you about ways to prevent or reduce some of these side effects. Check with your health care professional if any of the following side effects continue or are bothersome or if you have any questions about them:

More common
Headache

Less common
Acid or sour stomach; belching; cough; heartburn; increased sensitivity to sunlight; indigestion; pain, general; pain in joints or muscles; runny nose; sneezing; sore throat; stomach discomfort, upset, or pain

Other side effects not listed may also occur in some patients. If you notice any other effects, check with your healthcare professional.

MINOXIDIL   (Oral route) - mi-NOX-i-dil

Black Box Warning

Minoxidil tablets contain the powerful antihypertensive agent, minoxidil, which may produce serious adverse effects. It can cause pericardial effusion, occasionally progressing to tamponade, and angina pectoris may be exacerbated. Minoxidil should be reserved for hypertensive patients who do not respond adequately to maximum therapeutic doses of a diuretic and two other antihypertensive agents.

In experimental animals, minoxidil caused several kinds of myocardial lesions as well as other adverse cardiac effects.

Minoxidil must be administered under close supervision, usually concomitantly with therapeutic doses of a beta-adrenergic blocking agent to prevent tachycardia and increased myocardial workload. It must also usually be given with a diuretic, frequently one acting in the ascending limb of the loop of Henle, to prevent serious fluid accumulation. Patients with malignant hypertension and those already receiving guanethidine should be hospitalized when minoxidil is first administered so that they can be monitored to avoid too rapid, or large orthostatic, decreases in blood pressure.

Commonly used brand name(s)
In the U.S.—
    Loniten

Available Dosage Forms:
- Tablet

Therapeutic Class: Antihypertensive, Peripheral Vasodilator

Uses For This Medicine

Minoxidil belongs to the general class of medicines called antihypertensives. It is used to treat high blood pressure (hypertension).

High blood pressure adds to the workload of the heart and arteries. If it continues for a long time, the heart and arteries may not function properly. This can damage the blood vessels of the brain, heart, and kidneys, resulting in a stroke, heart failure, or kidney failure. High blood pressure may also increase the risk of heart attacks. These problems may be less likely to occur if blood pressure is controlled.

Minoxidil works by relaxing blood vessels so that blood passes through them more easily. This helps to lower blood pressure.

Minoxidil has other effects that could be bothersome for some patients. These include increased hair growth, weight gain, fast heartbeat, and chest pain. Before you take this medicine, be sure that you have discussed the use of it with your doctor.

Minoxidil is being applied to the scalp in liquid form by some balding men to stimulate hair growth. However, improper use of liquids made from minoxidil tablets can result in minoxidil being absorbed into the body, where it may cause unwanted effects on the heart and blood vessels.

Minoxidil is available only with your doctor's prescription.

Before Using This Medicine

In deciding to use a medicine, the risks of taking the medicine must be weighed against the good it will do. This is a decision you and your doctor will make. For this medicine, the following should be considered:

Allergies—Tell your doctor if you have ever had any unusual or allergic reaction to this medicine or any other medicines. Also tell your health care professional if you have any other types of allergies, such as to foods, dyes, preservatives, or animals. For non-prescription products, read the label or package ingredients carefully.

Pediatric—Although there is no specific information comparing use of minoxidil in children with use in other age groups, this medicine is not expected to cause different side effects or problems in children than it does in adults.

Geriatric—Elderly patients may be more sensitive to the effects of minoxidil. In addition, minoxidil may reduce tolerance to cold temperatures in elderly patients.

Pregnancy—

	Pregnancy Category	Explanation
All Trimesters	C	Animal studies have shown an adverse effect and there are no adequate studies in pregnant women OR no animal studies have been conducted and there are no adequate studies in pregnant women.

Breast Feeding—There are no adequate studies in women for determining infant risk when using this medication during breastfeeding. Weigh the potential benefits against the potential risks before taking this medication while breastfeeding.

Other medicines—Although certain medicines should not be used together at all, in other cases two different medicines may be used together even if an interaction might occur. In these cases, your doctor may want to change the dose, or other precautions may be necessary. Tell your healthcare professional if you are taking any other prescription or non-prescription (over-the-counter [OTC]) medicine.

Interactions with Food/Tobacco/Alcohol—Certain medicines should not be used at or around the time of eating food or eating certain types of food since interactions may occur. Using alcohol or tobacco with certain medicines may also cause interactions to occur. Discuss with your healthcare professional the use of your medicine with food, alcohol, or tobacco.

Other medical problems—The presence of other medical problems may affect the use of this medicine. Make sure you tell your doctor if you have any other medical problems, especially:

- Angina (chest pain)—Minoxidil may make this condition worse
- Heart attack or stroke (recent)—Lowering blood pressure may make problems resulting from heart attack or stroke worse
- Heart or blood vessel disease—Minoxidil can cause fluid buildup, which can cause problems
- Kidney disease—Effects may be increased because of slower removal of minoxidil from the body
- Pheochromocytoma—Minoxidil may cause the tumor to be more active

Proper Use of This Medicine

In addition to the use of the medicine your doctor has prescribed, treatment for your high blood pressure may include weight control and care in the types of foods you eat, especially foods high in sodium. Your doctor will tell you which of these are most important for you. You should check with your doctor before changing your diet.

Many patients who have high blood pressure will not notice any signs of the problem. In fact, many may feel normal. It is very important that you take your medicine exactly as directed and that you keep your appointments with your doctor even if you feel well.

Remember that minoxidil will not cure your high blood pressure but it does help control it. Therefore, you must continue to take it as directed if you expect to lower your blood pressure and keep it down. You may have to take high blood pressure medicine for the rest of your life. If high blood pressure is not treated, it can cause serious problems such as heart failure, blood vessel disease, stroke, or kidney disease.

To help you remember to take your medicine, try to get into the habit of taking it at the same time each day.

This medicine is usually given together with certain other medicines. If you are using a combination of drugs, make sure that you take each medicine at the proper time and do not mix them. Ask your health care professional to help you plan a way to remember to take your medicines at the right time.

Dosing—The dose of this medicine will be different for different patients. Follow your doctor's orders or the directions on the label. The following information includes only the average doses of this medicine. If your dose is different, do not change it unless your doctor tells you to do so.

The amount of medicine that you take depends on the strength of the medicine. Also, the number of doses you take each day, the time allowed between doses, and the length of time you take the medicine depend on the medical problem for which you are using the medicine.

- For oral dosage forms (tablets):
  - Adults and children over 12 years of age: 5 to 40 milligrams taken as a single dose or in divided doses.
  - Children up to 12 years of age: 200 micrograms to 1 milligram per kilogram of body weight a day to be taken as a single dose or in divided doses.

Missed dose—If you miss a dose of this medicine, take it as soon as possible. However, if it is almost time for your next dose, skip the missed dose and go back to your regular dosing schedule. Do not double doses.

Storage—Store the medicine in a closed container at room temperature, away from heat, moisture, and direct light. Keep from freezing.

Keep out of the reach of children.

Do not keep outdated medicine or medicine no longer needed.

Precautions While Using This Medicine

It is important that your doctor check your progress at regular visits to make sure that this medicine is working properly.

Ask your doctor about checking your pulse rate before and after taking minoxidil. Then, while you are taking this medicine, check your pulse regularly while you are resting. If it increases by 20 beats or more a minute, check with your doctor right away.

While you are taking minoxidil, weigh yourself every day. A weight gain of 2 to 3 pounds (about 1 kg) in an adult is normal and should be lost with continued treatment. However, if you suddenly gain 5 pounds (2 kg) or more (for a child, 2 pounds [1 kg] or more) or if you notice swelling of your feet or lower legs, check with your doctor right away.

Do not take other medicines unless they have been discussed with your doctor. This especially includes over-the-counter (nonprescription) medicines for appetite control, asthma, colds, cough, hay fever, or sinus problems, since they may tend to increase your blood pressure.

Side Effects of This Medicine

Along with its needed effects, a medicine may cause some unwanted effects. Although not all of these side effects may occur, if they do occur they may need medical attention.

Check with your doctor immediately if any of the following side effects occur:

More common
  Fast or irregular heartbeat; weight gain (rapid) of more than 5 pounds (2 pounds in children)

Less common
  Chest pain; shortness of breath

Check with your doctor as soon as possible if any of the following side effects occur:

More common
  Bloating; flushing or redness of skin; swelling of feet or lower legs

Less common
  Numbness or tingling of hands, feet, or face

Rare
  Skin rash and itching

Some side effects may occur that usually do not need medical attention. These side effects may go away during treatment as your body adjusts to the medicine. Also, your health care professional may be able to tell you about ways to prevent or reduce some of these side effects. Check with your health care professional if any of the following side effects continue or are bothersome or if you have any questions about them:

More common
  Increase in hair growth, usually on face, arms, and back

Less common or rare
  Breast tenderness in males and females; headache

This medicine causes a temporary increase in hair growth in most people. Hair may grow longer and darker in both men and women. This may first be noticed on the face several weeks after you start taking minoxidil. Later, new hair growth may be noticed on the back, arms, legs, and scalp. Talk to your doctor about shaving or using a hair remover during this time. After treatment with minoxidil has ended, the hair will stop growing, although it may take several months for the new hair growth to go away.

Other side effects not listed may also occur in some patients. If you notice any other effects, check with your healthcare professional.

MINOXIDIL (Topical route) - mi-NOX-i-dil

Commonly used brand name(s)

In the U.S.—
  Rogaine
  Rogaine For Men Extra
  Strength

In Canada—

Apo-Gain	Hair Regrowth Treatment
Gen-Minoxidol	Med Minoxidil
Hairgro	Minox

Available Dosage Forms:
  • Solution

Therapeutic Class: Alopecia Agent

Uses For This Medicine

Minoxidil applied to the scalp is used to stimulate hair growth in adult men and women with a certain type of baldness. The exact way that this medicine works is not known.

If hair growth is going to occur with the use of minoxidil, it usually occurs after the medicine has been used for several months and lasts only as long as the medicine continues to be used. Hair loss will begin again within a few months after minoxidil treatment is stopped.

In the U.S., this medicine is available without a prescription.

Before Using This Medicine

In deciding to use a medicine, the risks of taking the medicine must be weighed against the good it will do. This is a decision you and your doctor will make. For this medicine, the following should be considered:

Allergies—Tell your doctor if you have ever had any unusual or allergic reaction to this medicine or any other medicines. Also tell your health care professional if you have any other types of allergies, such as to foods, dyes, preservatives, or animals. For non-prescription products, read the label or package ingredients carefully.

Pediatric—Studies of this medicine have been done only in adult patients, and there is no specific information comparing use of topical minoxidil in children up to 18 years of age with use in other age groups. Use in infants and children is not recommended. If you think your child has hair loss, discuss it with the doctor.

Geriatric—This medicine has been tested in a limited number of older patients up to 65 years of age and has not been shown to cause different side effects or problems in this age group than it does in younger adults. However, studies have shown that the medicine works best in younger patients who have a short history of hair loss. Minoxidil has not been studied in patients older than 65 years of age.

Pregnancy—

	Pregnancy Category	Explanation
All Trimesters	C	Animal studies have shown an adverse effect and there are no adequate studies in pregnant women OR no animal studies have been conducted and there are no adequate studies in pregnant women.

Breast Feeding—There are no adequate studies in women for determining infant risk when using this medication during breastfeeding. Weigh the potential benefits against the potential risks before taking this medication while breastfeeding.

Other medicines—Although certain medicines should not be used together at all, in other cases two different medicines may be used together even if an interaction might occur. In these cases, your doctor may want to change the dose, or other precautions may be necessary. Tell your healthcare professional if you are taking any other prescription or non-prescription (over-the-counter [OTC]) medicine.

Interactions with Food/Tobacco/Alcohol—Certain medicines should not be used at or around the time of eating food or eating certain types of food since interactions may occur. Using alcohol or tobacco with certain medicines may also cause interactions to occur. Discuss with your healthcare professional the use of your medicine with food, alcohol, or tobacco.

Other medical problems—The presence of other medical problems may affect the use of this medicine. Make sure you tell your doctor if you have any other medical problems, especially:

- Any other skin problems or an irritation or a sunburn on the scalp—The condition may cause too much topical minoxidil to be absorbed into the body and may increase the chance of side effects
- Heart disease or
- Hypertension (high blood pressure)—Topical minoxidil has not been studied in patients who have these conditions, but more serious problems may develop for these patients if they use more medicine than is recommended over a large area and too much minoxidil is absorbed into the body

Proper Use of This Medicine

This medicine usually comes with patient instructions. It is important that you read the instructions carefully.

It is very important that you use this medicine only as directed. Do not use more of it and do not use it more often than your doctor ordered. To do so may increase the chance of it being absorbed through the skin. For the same reason, do not apply minoxidil to other parts of your body. Absorption into the body may affect the heart and blood vessels and cause unwanted effects.

Do not use any other skin products on the same skin area on which you use minoxidil. Hair coloring, hair permanents, and hair relaxers may be used during minoxidil therapy as long as the scalp is washed just before applying the hair coloring, permanent, or relaxer. Minoxidil should not be used 24 hours before and after the hair treatment procedure. Be sure to not double your doses of minoxidil to make up for any missed doses.

To apply minoxidil solution:

- Make sure your hair and scalp are completely dry before applying this medicine.
- Apply the amount prescribed to the area of the scalp being treated, beginning in the center of the area. Follow your doctor's instructions on how to apply the solution, using the applicator provided.
- Do not shampoo your hair for 4 hours after applying minoxidil.
- Immediately after using this medicine, wash your hands to remove any medicine that may be on them.
- Do not use a hairdryer to dry the scalp after you apply minoxidil solution. Blowing with a hairdryer on the scalp may make the treatment less effective.
- Allow the minoxidil to completely dry for 2 to 4 hours after applying it, including before going to bed. Minoxidil can stain clothing, hats, or bed linen if your hair or scalp is not fully dry after using the medicine.
- Avoid transferring the medicine while wet to other parts of the body. This can occur if the medicine gets on your pillowcase or bed linens or if your hands are not washed after applying minoxidil.

If your scalp becomes abraded, irritated, or sunburned, check with your doctor before applying minoxidil.

Keep this medicine away from the eyes, nose, and mouth. If you should accidentally get some in your eyes, nose, or mouth, flush the area thoroughly with cool tap water. If you are using the pump spray, be careful not to breathe in the spray.

Dosing—The dose of this medicine will be different for different patients. Follow your doctor's orders or the directions on the label. The following information includes only the average doses of this medicine. If your dose is different, do not change it unless your doctor tells you to do so.

The amount of medicine that you take depends on the strength of the medicine. Also, the number of doses you take each day, the time allowed between doses, and the length of time you take the medicine depend on the medical problem for which you are using the medicine.

- For topical solution dosage form:
  - For hair growth:
    - Adults up to 65 years of age—Apply 1 milliliter to the scalp two times a day.
    - Adults 65 years of age and older—Use and dose must be determined by the doctor.
    - Infants—Use is not recommended.
    - Children up to 18 years of age—Use and dose must be determined by the doctor.

Missed dose—If you miss a dose of this medicine, skip the missed dose and go back to your regular dosing schedule. Do not double doses.

Storage—Store the medicine in a closed container at room temperature, away from heat, moisture, and direct light. Keep from freezing.

Keep out of the reach of children.

Do not keep outdated medicine or medicine no longer needed.

Flammable: Keep away from fire or flame.

Precautions While Using This Medicine

It is important that your doctor check your progress at regular visits to make sure that this medicine is working properly and to check for unwanted effects.

Tell your doctor if you notice continued itching, redness, or burning of your scalp after you apply minoxidil. If the itching, redness, or burning is severe, wash the medicine off and check with your doctor before using it again.

Hair loss may continue for 2 weeks after you start using minoxidil. Tell your doctor if your hair loss continues after

2 weeks. Also, tell your doctor if your hair growth does not increase after using minoxidil for 4 months.

Side Effects of This Medicine

Along with its needed effects, a medicine may cause some unwanted effects. Although not all of these side effects may occur, if they do occur they may need medical attention.

Check with your doctor as soon as possible if any of the following side effects occur:

Less common
    Itching or skin rash (continued)

Rare
    Acne at site of application; burning of scalp; increased hair loss; inflammation or soreness at root of hair; reddened skin; swelling of face

Signs and symptoms of too much medicine being absorbed into the body—Rare
    Blurred vision or other changes in vision; chest pain; decrease of sexual ability or desire; fast or irregular heartbeat; flushing; headache; lightheadedness; numbness or tingling of hands, feet, or face; swelling of face, hands, feet, or lower legs; weight gain (rapid)

Other side effects not listed may also occur in some patients. If you notice any other effects, check with your healthcare professional.

MIRTAZAPINE   (Oral route) - mir-TAZ-a-peen

Black Box Warning

Antidepressants increased the risk of suicidal thinking and behavior (suicidality) in short-term studies in children and adolescents with Major Depressive Disorder (MDD) and other psychiatric disorders. Anyone considering the use of mirtazapine or any other antidepressant in a child or adolescent must balance this risk with the clinical need. Patients who are started on therapy should be observed closely for clinical worsening, suicidality, or unusual changes in behavior. Families and caregivers should be advised of the need for close observation and communication with the prescriber. Mirtazapine is not approved for use in pediatric patients.

Pooled analyses of short-term (4 to 16 weeks) placebo-controlled trials of 9 antidepressant drugs (SSRIs and others) in children and adolescents with MDD, obsessive compulsive disorder (OCD), or other psychiatric disorders (a total of 24 trials involving over 4,400 patients) have revealed a greater risk of adverse events representing suicidal thinking or behavior (suicidality) during the first few months of treatment in those receiving antidepressants. The average risk of such events in patients receiving antidepressants was 4%, twice the placebo risk of 2%. No suicides occurred in these trials.

Commonly used brand name(s)

In the U.S.—
Remeron
Remeron Soltab

In Canada—
Remeron RD

Available Dosage Forms:

- Tablet

- Tablet, Disintegrating

Therapeutic Class: Antidepressant
Pharmacologic Class: Antidepressant, Tetracyclic

Uses For This Medicine

Mirtazapine is used to treat mental depression.

This medicine is available only with your doctor's prescription.

Before Using This Medicine

In deciding to use a medicine, the risks of taking the medicine must be weighed against the good it will do. This is a decision you and your doctor will make. For this medicine, the following should be considered:

Allergies—Tell your doctor if you have ever had any unusual or allergic reaction to this medicine or any other medicines. Also tell your health care professional if you have any other types of allergies, such as to foods, dyes, preservatives, or animals. For non-prescription products, read the label or package ingredients carefully.

Pediatric—Mirtazapine must be used with caution in children with depression. Studies have shown occurrences of children thinking about suicide or attempting suicide in clinical trials for this medicine. More study is needed to be sure mirtazapine is safe and effective in children.

Geriatric—This medicine has been tested and has not been shown to cause different side effects or problems in older people than it does in younger adults. However, it is removed from the body more slowly in older people.

Pregnancy—

	Pregnancy Category	Explanation
All Trimesters	C	Animal studies have shown an adverse effect and there are no adequate studies in pregnant women OR no animal studies have been conducted and there are no adequate studies in pregnant women.

Breast Feeding—There are no adequate studies in women for determining infant risk when using this medication during breastfeeding. Weigh the potential benefits against the potential risks before taking this medication while breastfeeding.

Other medicines—

Using this medicine with any of the following medicines is not recommended. Your doctor may decide not to treat you with this medication or change some of the other medicines you take.

Clorgyline, Iproniazid, Isocarboxazid, Moclobemide, Nialamide, Pargyline, Phenelzine, Procarbazine, Rasagiline, Selegiline, Toloxatone, Tranylcypromine

Interactions with Food/Tobacco/Alcohol—Certain medicines should not be used at or around the time of eating food or eating certain types of food since interactions may occur. Using alcohol or tobacco with certain medicines may also cause interactions to occur. The following interactions have been selected on the basis of their potential significance and are not necessarily all-inclusive.

Using this medicine with any of the following may cause an increased risk of certain side effects but may be unavoidable in some cases. If used together, your doctor may change the dose or how often you use this medicine, or give you special instructions about the use of food, alcohol, or tobacco.

Other medical problems—The presence of other medical problems may affect the use of this medicine. Make sure you tell your doctor if you have any other medical problems, especially:

- Convulsions (seizures) (history of)—Mirtazapine has been reported to cause seizures rarely
- Dehydration or
- Heart disease or
- Stroke (history of)—Mirtazapine may make the condition worse by causing low blood pressure (hypotension)
- Kidney disease—Effects of mirtazapine may be increased because of slower removal from the body
- Liver disease—Mirtazapine may cause liver problems; also, effects of mirtazapine may be increased because of slower removal from the body
- Mania (a type of mental illness) (or history of)—Mirtazapine may cause this problem to recur
- Phenylketonuria (PKU)—The oral disintegrating tablets may contain aspartame, which can make your condition worse

Proper Use of This Medicine

Take this medicine only as directed by your doctor in order to improve your condition as much as possible. Do not take more of it and do not take it more often than your doctor ordered.

Mirtazapine may be taken with or without food, on a full or empty stomach. If your doctor tells you to take it a certain way, follow your doctor's instructions.

For patients using the oral disintegrating tablet form of this medicine:

- Make sure your hands are dry.
- Do not push the tablet through the foil backing of the package. Instead, gently peel back the foil backing and remove the tablet.
- Immediately place the tablet on top of the tongue.
- The tablet will dissolve in seconds, and you may swallow it with your saliva. You do not need to drink water or other liquid to swallow the tablet.

Dosing—The dose of this medicine will be different for different patients. Follow your doctor's orders or the directions on the label. The following information includes only the av-

erage doses of this medicine. If your dose is different, do not change it unless your doctor tells you to do so.

The amount of medicine that you take depends on the strength of the medicine. Also, the number of doses you take each day, the time allowed between doses, and the length of time you take the medicine depend on the medical problem for which you are using the medicine.

- For oral dosage form (tablets and oral disintegrating tablets):
  - For mental depression:
    - Adults—At first, 15 milligrams (mg) once a day, preferably in the evening just before you go to sleep. Your doctor may increase the dose if necessary. However, the dose usually is not more than 45 mg a day.
    - Children—Use and dose must be determined by your doctor.

Missed dose—If you miss a dose of this medicine, take it as soon as possible. However, if it is almost time for your next dose, skip the missed dose and go back to your regular dosing schedule. Do not double doses.

Storage—Store the medicine in a closed container at room temperature, away from heat, moisture, and direct light. Keep from freezing.

Keep out of the reach of children.

Do not keep outdated medicine or medicine no longer needed.

Precautions While Using This Medicine

It is important that your doctor check your progress at regular visits, to allow for changes in your dose and to help reduce any side effects.

Do not take mirtazapine with monoamine oxidase (MAO) inhibitors (e.g., furazolidone, phenelzine, procarbazine, selegiline, or tranylcypromine) or sooner than 14 days after stopping an MAO inhibitor. Do not take an MAO inhibitor sooner than 14 days after stopping mirtazapine. To do so may increase the chance of serious side effects.

Mirtazapine may cause some people to be agitated, irritable or display other abnormal behaviors. It may also cause some people to have suicidal thoughts and tendencies or to become more depressed. If you or your caregiver notice any of these adverse effects, tell your doctor right away.

This medicine may add to the effects of alcohol and other CNS depressants (medicines that make you drowsy or less alert). Some examples of CNS depressants are antihistamines or medicine for hay fever, other allergies, or colds; sedatives, tranquilizers, or sleeping medicine; prescription pain medicine or narcotics; barbiturates; medicine for seizures; muscle relaxants; or anesthetics, including some dental anesthetics. Check with your doctor before taking any of the above while you are taking this medicine.

Check with your doctor immediately if you develop fever, chills, sore throat, or sores in the mouth. These may be signs of a very serious blood problem that has occurred rarely in patients taking mirtazapine.

Mirtazapine may cause drowsiness or trouble in thinking. Make sure you know how you react to this medicine before you drive, use machines, or do other jobs that require you to be alert and clearheaded.

Dizziness, light-headedness, or fainting may occur, especially when you get up from a lying or sitting position. Getting up slowly may help. If this problem continues or gets worse, check with your doctor.

This medicine may cause dryness of the mouth. For temporary relief, use sugarless gum or candy, melt bits of ice in your mouth, or use a saliva substitute. However, if your mouth feels dry for more than 2 weeks, check with your medical doctor or dentist. Continuing dryness of the mouth may increase the chance of dental disease, including tooth decay, gum disease, and fungus infections.

Side Effects of This Medicine

Along with its needed effects, a medicine may cause some unwanted effects. Although not all of these side effects may occur, if they do occur they may need medical attention.

Check with your doctor immediately if any of the following side effects occur:

Rare
Convulsions (seizures); mouth sores; sore throat, chills, or fever

Check with your doctor as soon as possible if any of the following side effects occur:

Less common
Decreased or increased movement; mood or mental changes, including abnormal thinking, agitation, anxiety, confusion, and feelings of not caring; shortness of breath; skin rash; swelling

Rare
Decreased sexual ability; menstrual pain; missing periods; mood or mental changes, including anger, feelings of being outside the body, hallucinations (seeing, hearing, or feeling things that are not there), mood swings, and unusual excitement

Some side effects may occur that usually do not need medical attention. These side effects may go away during treatment as your body adjusts to the medicine. Also, your health care professional may be able to tell you about ways to prevent or reduce some of these side effects. Check with your health care professional if any of the following side effects continue or are bothersome or if you have any questions about them:

More common
Constipation; dizziness; drowsiness; dryness of mouth; increased appetite; weight gain

Less common
Abdominal pain; abnormal dreams; back pain; dizziness or fainting when getting up suddenly from a lying or sitting position; increased need to urinate; increased sensitivity to touch; increased thirst; low blood pressure; muscle pain; nausea; sense of constant movement of self or surroundings; trembling or shaking; vomiting; weakness

Other side effects not listed may also occur in some patients. If you notice any other effects, check with your healthcare professional.

MISOPROSTOL (Oral route) - mye-soe-PROST-ole

Black Box Warning

Misoprostol administration to women who are pregnant can cause abortion, premature birth, or birth defects. Uterine rupture has been reported when misoprostol was administered in pregnant women to induce labor or to induce abortion beyond the eight week of pregnancy. Misoprostol should not be taken by pregnant women to reduce the risk of ulcers induced by nonsteroidal anti-inflammatory drugs (NSAIDs).

Patients must be advised of the abortifacient property and warned not to give the drug to others.

Misoprostol should not be used for reducing the risk of NSAID-induced ulcers in women of childbearing potential unless the patient is at high risk of complications from gastric ulcers associated with use of the NSAID, or is at high risk of developing gastric ulceration. In such patients, misoprostol may be prescribed if the patient

- has had a negative serum pregnancy test within 2 weeks prior to beginning therapy.
- is capable of complying with effective contraceptive measures.
- has received both oral and written warnings of the hazards of misoprostol, the risk of possible contraception failure, and the danger to other women of childbearing potential should the drug be taken by mistake.
- will begin misoprostol on the second or third day of the next menstrual period

Commonly used brand name(s)

In the U.S.—
Cytotec

Available Dosage Forms:
- Tablet

Therapeutic Class: Endocrine-Metabolic Agent
Pharmacologic Class: Prostaglandin

Uses For This Medicine

Misoprostol is taken to prevent stomach ulcers in patients taking anti-inflammatory drugs, including aspirin. Misoprostol may also be used for other conditions as determined by your doctor.

Misoprostol helps the stomach protect itself against acid damage. It also decreases the amount of acid produced by the stomach.

This medicine is available only with your doctor's prescription.

Once a medicine has been approved for marketing for a certain use, experience may show that it is also useful for other medical problems. Although these uses are not included in product labeling, misoprostol may be used in certain patients with the following medical conditions:
- Abortion, first trimester
- Abortion, second trimester
- Cervical ripening
- Induction of labor
- Postpartum hemorrhage

Before Using This Medicine

In deciding to use a medicine, the risks of taking the medicine must be weighed against the good it will do. This is a decision you and your doctor will make. For this medicine, the following should be considered:

Allergies—Tell your doctor if you have ever had any unusual or allergic reaction to this medicine or any other medicines. Also tell your health care professional if you have any other types of allergies, such as to foods, dyes, preservatives, or animals. For non-prescription products, read the label or package ingredients carefully.

Pediatric—Studies on this medicine have been done only in adult patients, and there is no specific information comparing use of misoprostol in children with use in other age groups.

Geriatric—This medicine has been tested and has not been shown to cause different side effects or problems in older people than it does in younger adults.

Pregnancy—

	Pregnancy Category	Explanation
All Trimesters	X	Studies in animals or pregnant women have demonstrated positive evidence of fetal abnormalities. This drug should not be used in women who are or may become pregnant because the risk clearly outweighs any possible benefit.

Breast Feeding—There are no adequate studies in women for determining infant risk when using this medication during breastfeeding. Weigh the potential benefits against the potential risks before taking this medication while breastfeeding.

Other medicines—

Using this medicine with any of the following medicines may cause an increased risk of certain side effects, but using both drugs may be the best treatment for you. If both medicines are prescribed together, your doctor may change the dose or how often you use one or both of the medicines.

Phenylbutazone

Interactions with Food/Tobacco/Alcohol—Certain medicines should not be used at or around the time of eating food or eating certain types of food since interactions may occur. Using alcohol or tobacco with certain medicines may also cause interactions to occur. Discuss with your healthcare professional the use of your medicine with food, alcohol, or tobacco.

Other medical problems—The presence of other medical problems may affect the use of this medicine. Make sure you tell your doctor if you have any other medical problems, especially:

- Blood vessel disease—Medicines similar to misoprostol have been shown to make this condition worse
- Epilepsy (uncontrolled)—Medicines similar to misoprostol have been shown to cause convulsions (seizures)
- Inflammatory bowel disease—Misoprostol may worsen diarrhea, which could lead to dehydration

Proper Use of This Medicine

Misoprostol is best taken with or after meals and at bedtime, unless otherwise directed by your doctor. To help prevent loose stools, diarrhea, and abdominal cramping, always take this medicine with food or milk.

Dosing—The dose of this medicine will be different for different patients. Follow your doctor's orders or the directions on the label. The following information includes only the average doses of this medicine. If your dose is different, do not change it unless your doctor tells you to do so.

The amount of medicine that you take depends on the strength of the medicine. Also, the number of doses you take each day, the time allowed between doses, and the length of time you take the medicine depend on the medical problem for which you are using the medicine.

- To prevent stomach ulcers in patients taking anti-inflammatory medicines including aspirin:
  - For oral dosage form (tablets):
    - Adults—200 micrograms (mcg) four times a day, with or after meals and at bedtime. Or, your dose may be 400 mcg two times a day with the last dose taken at bedtime. Your doctor may reduce the dose to 100 mcg if you are sensitive to high doses.
    - Children and teenagers—Dose must be determined by your doctor.

Missed dose—If you miss a dose of this medicine, take it as soon as possible. However, if it is almost time for your next dose, skip the missed dose and go back to your regular dosing schedule. Do not double doses.

Storage—Store the medicine in a closed container at room temperature, away from heat, moisture, and direct light. Keep from freezing.

Keep out of the reach of children.

Do not keep outdated medicine or medicine no longer needed.

Precautions While Using This Medicine

Misoprostol may cause miscarriage if taken during pregnancy. Therefore, if you suspect that you may have become pregnant, stop taking this medicine immediately and check with your doctor.

This medicine may cause diarrhea, stomach cramps, or nausea in some people. These effects will usually disappear within a few days as your body adjusts to the medicine. However, check with your doctor if the diarrhea, cramps, or nausea is severe and/or does not stop after a week. Your doctor may have to lower the dose of misoprostol you are taking.

Side Effects of This Medicine

Along with its needed effects, a medicine may cause some unwanted effects. Although not all of these side effects may occur, if they do occur they may need medical attention.

Some side effects may occur that usually do not need medical attention. These side effects may go away during treatment as your body adjusts to the medicine. Also, your health care professional may be able to tell you about ways to prevent or reduce some of these side effects. Check with your health

care professional if any of the following side effects continue or are bothersome or if you have any questions about them:

More common
　　Abdominal or stomach pain (mild); diarrhea

Less common or rare
　　Bleeding from vagina; constipation; cramps in lower abdomen or stomach area; gas; headache; heartburn, indigestion, or acid stomach; nausea and/or vomiting

Symptoms of overdose
　　Abdominal pain; convulsions (seizures); diarrhea; drowsiness; fast or pounding heartbeat; fever; low blood pressure; slow heartbeat; tremor; troubled breathing

Other side effects not listed may also occur in some patients. If you notice any other effects, check with your healthcare professional.

MITOMYCIN (Intravenous route) - mye-toe-MYE-sin

Black Box Warning

Mitomycin for injection should be administered under the supervision of a qualified physician experienced in the use of cancer chemotherapeutic agents. Appropriate management of therapy and complications is possible only when adequate diagnostic and treatment facilities are readily available.

Bone marrow suppression, notably thrombocytopenia and leukopenia, which may contribute to overwhelming infections in an already compromised patient, is the most common and severe of the toxic effects of mitomycin.

Hemolytic Uremic Syndrome (HUS) a serious complication of chemotherapy, consisting primarily of microangiopathic hemolytic anemia, thrombocytopenia, and irreversible renal failure has been reported in patients receiving systemic mitomycin. The syndrome may occur at any time during systemic therapy with mitomycin as a single agent or in combination with other cytotoxic drugs, however, most cases occur at doses greater than or equal to 60 mg of mitomycin. Blood product transfusion may exacerbate the symptoms associated with this syndrome.

The incidence of the syndrome has not been defined.

Commonly used brand name(s)

In the U.S.—
　　Mutamycin

Available Dosage Forms:
　　• Powder for Solution

Therapeutic Class: Antineoplastic Agent

Uses For This Medicine

Mitomycin belongs to the group of medicines known as antineoplastics. It is used to treat some kinds of cancer.

Mitomycin interferes with the growth of cancer cells, which are eventually destroyed. Since the growth of normal body cells may also be affected by mitomycin, other effects will also occur. Some of these may be serious and must be reported to your doctor. Other effects, like hair loss, may not be serious but may cause concern. Some effects may not occur for months or years after the medicine is used.

Before you begin treatment with mitomycin, you and your doctor should talk about the good this medicine will do as well as the risks of using it.

Mitomycin is to be administered only by or under the immediate supervision of your doctor.

Before Using This Medicine

In deciding to use a medicine, the risks of taking the medicine must be weighed against the good it will do. This is a decision you and your doctor will make. For this medicine, the following should be considered:

Allergies—Tell your doctor if you have ever had any unusual or allergic reaction to this medicine or any other medicines. Also tell your health care professional if you have any other types of allergies, such as to foods, dyes, preservatives, or animals. For non-prescription products, read the label or package ingredients carefully.

Pediatric—Although there is no specific information comparing use of mitomycin in children with use in other age groups, it is not expected to cause different side effects or problems in children than it does in adults.

Geriatric—Many medicines have not been studied specifically in older people. Therefore, it may not be known whether they work exactly the same way they do in younger adults or if they cause different side effects or problems in older people. There is no specific information comparing use of mitomycin in the elderly with use in other age groups.

Breast Feeding—There are no adequate studies in women for determining infant risk when using this medication during breastfeeding. Weigh the potential benefits against the potential risks before taking this medication while breastfeeding.

Other medicines—

Using this medicine with any of the following medicines is not recommended. Your doctor may decide not to treat you with this medication or change some of the other medicines you take.

Rotavirus Vaccine, Live

Interactions with Food/Tobacco/Alcohol—Certain medicines should not be used at or around the time of eating food or eating certain types of food since interactions may occur. Using alcohol or tobacco with certain medicines may also cause interactions to occur. Discuss with your healthcare professional the use of your medicine with food, alcohol, or tobacco.

Other medical problems—The presence of other medical problems may affect the use of this medicine. Make sure you tell your doctor if you have any other medical problems, especially:
　　• Bleeding problems
　　• Chickenpox (including recent exposure) or
　　• Herpes zoster (shingles)—Risk of severe disease affecting other parts of the body
　　• Infection—Mitomycin may decrease your body's ability to fight infection
　　• Kidney disease—May be worsened

Proper Use of This Medicine

Mitomycin is usually given together with certain other medicines. If you are using a combination of medicines, it is important that you receive each one at the proper time. If you are taking some of these medicines by mouth, ask your health care professional to help you plan a way to remember to take them at the right times.

This medicine often causes nausea, vomiting, and loss of appetite. However, it is very important that you continue to receive the medicine, even if you begin to feel ill. Ask your health care professional for ways to lessen these effects.

Dosing—The dose of this medicine will be different for different patients. Follow your doctor's orders or the directions on the label. The following information includes only the average doses of this medicine. If your dose is different, do not change it unless your doctor tells you to do so.

The amount of medicine that you take depends on the strength of the medicine. Also, the number of doses you take each day, the time allowed between doses, and the length of time you take the medicine depend on the medical problem for which you are using the medicine.

Precautions While Using This Medicine

It is very important that your doctor check your progress at regular visits to make sure that this medicine is working properly and to check for unwanted effects.

While you are being treated with mitomycin, and after you stop treatment with it, do not have any immunizations (vaccinations) without your doctor's approval. Mitomycin may lower your body's resistance and there is a chance you might get the infection the immunization is meant to prevent. In addition, other persons living in your household should not take oral polio vaccine since there is a chance they could pass the polio virus on to you. Also, avoid persons who have taken oral polio vaccine. Do not get close to them, and do not stay in the same room with them for very long. If you cannot take these precautions, you should consider wearing a protective face mask that covers the nose and mouth.

Mitomycin can temporarily lower the number of white blood cells in your blood, increasing the chance of getting an infection. It can also lower the number of platelets, which are necessary for proper blood clotting. If this occurs, there are certain precautions you can take, especially when your blood count is low, to reduce the risk of infection or bleeding:

- If you can, avoid people with infections. Check with your doctor immediately if you think you are getting an infection or if you get a fever or chills, cough or hoarseness, lower back or side pain, or painful or difficult urination.
- Check with your doctor immediately if you notice any unusual bleeding or bruising; black, tarry stools; blood in urine or stools; or pinpoint red spots on your skin.
- Be careful when using a regular toothbrush, dental floss, or toothpick. Your medical doctor, dentist, or nurse may recommend other ways to clean your teeth and gums. Check with your medical doctor before having any dental work done.
- Do not touch your eyes or the inside of your nose unless you have just washed your hands and have not touched anything else in the meantime.

- Be careful not to cut yourself when you are using sharp objects such as a safety razor or fingernail or toenail cutters.
- Avoid contact sports or other situations where bruising or injury could occur.

If mitomycin accidentally seeps out of the vein into which it is injected, it may damage the skin and cause scarring. In some patients, this may occur weeks or even months after this medicine is given. Tell the doctor or nurse right away if you notice redness, pain, or swelling at the place of injection or anywhere else on your skin.

Side Effects of This Medicine

Along with its needed effects, a medicine may cause some unwanted effects. Although not all of these side effects may occur, if they do occur they may need medical attention.

Also, because of the way cancer medicines act on the body, there is a chance that they might cause other unwanted effects that may not occur until months or years after the medicine is used. These delayed effects may include certain types of cancer. Discuss these possible effects with your doctor.

Check with your doctor immediately if any of the following side effects occur:

Less common
Black, tarry stools; blood in urine or stools; cough or hoarseness; fever or chills; lower back or side pain; painful or difficult urination; pinpoint red spots on skin; unusual bleeding or bruising

Rare
Redness or pain, especially at place of injection

Check with your doctor as soon as possible if any of the following side effects occur:

Less common
Cough; decreased urination; shortness of breath; sores in mouth and on lips; swelling of feet or lower legs

Rare
Bloody vomit

Some side effects may occur that usually do not need medical attention. These side effects may go away during treatment as your body adjusts to the medicine. Also, your health care professional may be able to tell you about ways to prevent or reduce some of these side effects. Check with your health care professional if any of the following side effects continue or are bothersome or if you have any questions about them:

More common
Loss of appetite; nausea and vomiting

Less common
Numbness or tingling in fingers and toes; purple-colored bands on nails; skin rash; unusual tiredness or weakness

Mitomycin sometimes causes a temporary loss of hair. After treatment has ended, normal hair growth should return.

After you stop using this medicine, it may still produce some side effects that need attention. During this period of time, *check with your doctor immediately* if you notice the following side effects:

Blood in urine

Also, check with your doctor if you notice any of the following:

Black, tarry stools; blood in stools; cough or hoarseness; decreased urination; fever or chills; lower back or side pain; painful or difficult urination; pinpoint red spots on skin; red or painful skin; shortness of breath; swelling of feet or lower legs; unusual bleeding or bruising

Other side effects not listed may also occur in some patients. If you notice any other effects, check with your healthcare professional.

MITOTANE   (Oral route) - MYE-toe-tane

Black Box Warning

Mitotane should be administered under the supervision of a qualified physician experienced in the uses of cancer chemotherapeutic agents. Mitotane should be temporarily discontinued immediately following shock or severe trauma since adrenal suppression is its prime action. Exogenous steroids should be administered in such circumstances, since the depressed adrenal may not immediately start to secrete steroids.

Commonly used brand name(s)

In the U.S.—
Lysodren

Available Dosage Forms:
• Tablet

Therapeutic Class: Adrenocortical Suppressant

Uses For This Medicine

Mitotane is a medicine that acts on a part of the body called the adrenal cortex. It is used to treat some kinds of cancer that affect the adrenal cortex. Also, it is sometimes used when the adrenal cortex is overactive without being cancerous.

Mitotane reduces the amounts of adrenocorticoids (cortisone-like hormones) produced by the adrenal cortex. These steroids are important for various functions of the body, including growth. However, too much of these steroids can cause problems.

Mitotane is available only with your doctor's prescription.

Before Using This Medicine

In deciding to use a medicine, the risks of taking the medicine must be weighed against the good it will do. This is a decision you and your doctor will make. For this medicine, the following should be considered:

Allergies—Tell your doctor if you have ever had any unusual or allergic reaction to this medicine or any other medicines. Also tell your health care professional if you have any other types of allergies, such as to foods, dyes, preservatives, or animals. For non-prescription products, read the label or package ingredients carefully.

Pediatric—Although there is no specific information about the use of mitotane in children, it is not expected to cause different side effects or problems in children than it does in adults.

Geriatric—Many medicines have not been tested in older people. Therefore, it may not be known whether they work exactly the same way they do in younger adults or if they cause different side effects or problems in older people. There is no specific information about the use of mitotane in the elderly.

Pregnancy—

	Pregnancy Category	Explanation
All Trimesters	C	Animal studies have shown an adverse effect and there are no adequate studies in pregnant women OR no animal studies have been conducted and there are no adequate studies in pregnant women.

Breast Feeding—There are no adequate studies in women for determining infant risk when using this medication during breastfeeding. Weigh the potential benefits against the potential risks before taking this medication while breastfeeding.

Other medicines—

Using this medicine with any of the following medicines is not recommended. Your doctor may decide not to treat you with this medication or change some of the other medicines you take.

Rotavirus Vaccine, Live

Interactions with Food/Tobacco/Alcohol—Certain medicines should not be used at or around the time of eating food or eating certain types of food since interactions may occur. Using alcohol or tobacco with certain medicines may also cause interactions to occur. Discuss with your healthcare professional the use of your medicine with food, alcohol, or tobacco.

Other medical problems—The presence of other medical problems may affect the use of this medicine. Make sure you tell your doctor if you have any other medical problems, especially:

• Infection

• Liver disease—Effects may be increased because of slower removal of mitotane from the body

Proper Use of This Medicine

Take mitotane only as directed by your doctor. Do not take more or less of it, and do not take it more often than your doctor ordered.

Do not stop taking this medicine without first checking with your doctor. To do so may increase the chance of unwanted effects.

Dosing—The dose of this medicine will be different for different patients. Follow your doctor's orders or the directions on the label. The following information includes only the average doses of this medicine. If your dose is different, do not change it unless your doctor tells you to do so.

The amount of medicine that you take depends on the strength of the medicine. Also, the number of doses you take each day, the time allowed between doses, and the length of time you take the medicine depend on the medical problem for which you are using the medicine.

Missed dose—If you miss a dose of this medicine, take it as soon as possible. However, if it is almost time for your next dose, skip the missed dose and go back to your regular dosing schedule. Do not double doses.

Storage—Store the medicine in a closed container at room temperature, away from heat, moisture, and direct light. Keep from freezing.

Keep out of the reach of children.

Do not keep outdated medicine or medicine no longer needed.

Precautions While Using This Medicine

It is very important that your doctor check your progress at regular visits to make sure this medicine is working properly and to check for unwanted effects.

Your doctor may want you to carry an identification card stating that you are taking this medicine.

This medicine will add to the effects of alcohol and other CNS depressants (medicines that slow down the nervous system, possibly causing drowsiness). Some examples of CNS depressants are antihistamines or medicine for hay fever, other allergies, or colds; sedatives, tranquilizers, or sleeping medicine; prescription pain medicine or narcotics; barbiturates; medicine for seizures; tricyclic antidepressants (medicine for depression); muscle relaxants; or anesthetics, including some dental anesthetics. Check with your doctor before taking any of the above while you are using this medicine.

This medicine may cause some people to become dizzy, drowsy, or less alert than they are normally. Make sure you know how you react to this medicine before you drive, use machines, or do anything else that could be dangerous if you are dizzy or are not alert.

Check with your doctor right away if you get an injury, infection, or illness of any kind. This medicine may weaken your body's defenses against infection or inflammation.

Side Effects of This Medicine

Along with its needed effects, a medicine may cause some unwanted effects. Although not all of these side effects may occur, if they do occur they may need medical attention.

Check with your doctor as soon as possible if any of the following side effects occur:
More common
  Darkening of skin; diarrhea; dizziness; drowsiness; loss of appetite; mental depression; nausea and vomiting; skin rash; unusual tiredness

Less common
  Blood in urine; blurred vision; double vision

Rare
  Shortness of breath; wheezing

Some side effects may occur that usually do not need medical attention. These side effects may go away during treatment as your body adjusts to the medicine. Also, your health care professional may be able to tell you about ways to prevent or reduce some of these side effects. Check with your health care professional if any of the following side effects continue or are bothersome or if you have any questions about them:
Less common
  Aching muscles; dizziness or lightheadedness when getting up from a lying or sitting position; fever; flushing or redness of skin; muscle twitching

Other side effects not listed may also occur in some patients. If you notice any other effects, check with your healthcare professional.

MITOXANTRONE (Intravenous route, Injection route) - mye-toe-ZAN-trone

Black Box Warning

Mitoxantrone for injection concentrate should be administered under the supervision of a physician experienced in the use of cytotoxic chemotherapy agents.

Mitoxantrone should be given slowly into a freely flowing intravenous infusion. It must never be given subcutaneously, intramuscularly, or intra-arterially. Severe local tissue damage may occur if there is extravasation during administration.

Not for intrathecal use. Severe injury with permanent sequelae can result from intrathecal administration.

Except for the treatment of acute nonlymphocytic leukemia, mitoxantrone therapy generally should not be given to patients with baseline neutrophil counts of less than 1,500 cells/mm(3). In order to monitor the occurrence of bone marrow suppression, primarily neutropenia, which may be severe and result in infection, it is recommended that frequent peripheral blood cell counts be performed on all patients receiving mitoxantrone.

Use of mitoxantrone has been associated with cardiotoxicity. Cardiotoxicity can occur at any time during mitoxantrone therapy, and the risk increases with cumulative dose. Congestive heart failure (CHF), potentially fatal, may occur either during therapy with mitoxantrone or months to years after termination of therapy. All patients should be carefully assessed for cardiac signs and symptoms by history and physical examination prior to start of mitoxantrone therapy. Baseline evaluation of left ventricular ejection fraction (LVEF) by echocardiogram or multi-gated radionuclide angiography (MUGA) should be performed. Multiple sclerosis patients with a baseline LVEF less than 50% should not be treated with mitoxantrone. LVEF should be reevaluated by echocardiogram or MUGA prior to each dose administered to patients with multiple sclerosis. Additional doses of mitoxantrone should not be administered to multiple sclerosis patients who have experienced either a drop in LVEF to below 50% or a clinically significant reduction in LVEF during mitoxantrone therapy. Patients with multiple sclerosis should not receive a cumulative dose greater than 140 mg/m(2). In cancer patients, the risk of symptomatic CHF was estimated to be 2.6% for patients receiving up to a cumulative dose of 140 mg/m(2). Presence or history of cardiovascular disease, prior or concomitant radiotherapy to the mediastinal/pericardial area, previous therapy with other anthracyclines or anthracenediones, or concomitant use of other cardiotoxic drugs may increase the risk of cardiac toxicity. Cardiac toxicity with mitoxantrone may occur whether or not cardiac risk factors are present.

Secondary acute myelogenous leukemia (AML) has been reported in multiple sclerosis and cancer patients treated with mitoxantrone. In a cohort of mitoxantrone treated MS patients followed for varying periods of time, an elevated leukemia risk of 0.25% (2/802) has been observed. Postmarketing cases of secondary AML have also been reported. In 1,774 patients with breast cancer who received mitoxantrone concomitantly with other cytotoxic agents and radiotherapy, the cumulative risk of developing treatment-related AML, was estimated as 1.1% and 1.6% at 5 and 10 years, respectively. Secondary acute myelogenous leukemia (AML) has been reported in cancer patients treated with anthracyclines. Mitoxantrone is an anthracenedione, a related drug.

The occurrence of refractory secondary leukemia is more common when anthracyclines are given in combination with DNA-damaging antineoplastic agents, when patients have been heavily pretreated with cytotoxic drugs, or when doses of anthracyclines have been escalated.

Commonly used brand name(s)

In the U.S.—
Novantrone

Available Dosage Forms:
- Liquid
- Solution

Uses For This Medicine

Mitoxantrone belongs to the general group of medicines known as antineoplastics. It is used to treat some kinds of cancer. It is also used to treat some forms of multiple sclerosis (MS). This medicine will not cure MS, but may extend the time between relapses.

Mitoxantrone seems to interfere with the growth of cancer cells, which are eventually destroyed. Since the growth of normal body cells may also be affected by mitoxantrone, other effects will also occur. Some of these may be serious and must be reported to your doctor. Other effects, like hair loss, may not be serious but may cause concern. Some effects may not occur for months or years after the medicine is used.

Before you begin treatment with mitoxantrone, you and your doctor should talk about the good this medicine will do as well as the risks of using it.

Mitoxantrone is to be administered only by or under the immediate supervision of your doctor.

Before Using This Medicine

In deciding to use a medicine, the risks of taking the medicine must be weighed against the good it will do. This is a decision you and your doctor will make. For this medicine, the following should be considered:

Allergies—Tell your doctor if you have ever had any unusual or allergic reaction to this medicine or any other medicines. Also tell your health care professional if you have any other types of allergies, such as to foods, dyes, preservatives, or animals. For non-prescription products, read the label or package ingredients carefully.

Pediatric—There is no specific information comparing use of mitoxantrone in children with use in other age groups.

Geriatric—Many medicines have not been studied specifically in older people. Therefore, it may not be known whether they work exactly the same way they do in younger adults or if they cause different side effects or problems in older people. There is no specific information comparing use of mitoxantrone in the elderly with use in other age groups.

Pregnancy—

	Pregnancy Category	Explanation
All Trimesters	D	Studies in pregnant women have demonstrated a risk to the fetus. However, the benefits of therapy in a life threatening situation or a serious disease, may outweigh the potential risk.

Breast Feeding—There are no adequate studies in women for determining infant risk when using this medication during breastfeeding. Weigh the potential benefits against the potential risks before taking this medication while breastfeeding.

Other medicines—

Using this medicine with any of the following medicines is not recommended. Your doctor may decide not to treat you with this medication or change some of the other medicines you take.

Rotavirus Vaccine, Live

Interactions with Food/Tobacco/Alcohol—Certain medicines should not be used at or around the time of eating food or eating certain types of food since interactions may occur. Using alcohol or tobacco with certain medicines may also cause interactions to occur. Discuss with your healthcare professional the use of your medicine with food, alcohol, or tobacco.

Other medical problems—The presence of other medical problems may affect the use of this medicine. Make sure you tell your doctor if you have any other medical problems, especially:
- Chickenpox (including recent exposure) or
- Herpes zoster (shingles)—Risk of severe disease affecting other parts of the body
- Gout (history of) or
- Kidney stones—Mitoxantrone may increase levels of uric acid in the body, which can cause gout or kidney stones
- Heart disease—Risk of heart problems caused by mitoxantrone may be increased
- Infection—Mitoxantrone may decrease your body's ability to fight infection
- Liver disease—Effects of mitoxantrone may be increased because of slower removal from the body

Proper Use of This Medicine

Mitoxantrone is sometimes given together with certain other medicines. If you are using a combination of medicines, it is important that you receive each one at the proper time. If you are taking some of these medicines by mouth, ask your health care professional to help you plan a way to take them at the right times.

While you are receiving mitoxantrone, your doctor may want you to drink extra fluids so that you will pass more urine. This will help prevent kidney problems and keep your kidneys working well.

Mitoxantrone often causes nausea and vomiting. However, it is very important that you continue to receive the medicine, even if your stomach is upset. Ask your health care professional for ways to lessen these effects.

Dosing—The dose of this medicine will be different for different patients. Follow your doctor's orders or the directions

on the label. The following information includes only the average doses of this medicine. If your dose is different, do not change it unless your doctor tells you to do so.

The amount of medicine that you take depends on the strength of the medicine. Also, the number of doses you take each day, the time allowed between doses, and the length of time you take the medicine depend on the medical problem for which you are using the medicine.

Precautions While Using This Medicine

It is very important that your doctor check your progress at regular visits to make sure that this medicine is working properly and to check for unwanted effects.

While you are being treated with mitoxantrone, and after you stop treatment with it, do not have any immunizations (vaccinations) without your doctor's approval. Mitoxantrone may lower your body's resistance and there is a chance you might get the infection the immunization is meant to prevent. In addition, other persons living in your household should not take oral polio vaccine since there is a chance they could pass the polio virus on to you. Also, avoid persons who have taken oral polio vaccine. Do not get close to them and do not stay in the same room with them for very long. If you cannot take these precautions, you should consider wearing a protective face mask that covers the nose and mouth.

Mitoxantrone can temporarily lower the number of white blood cells in your blood, increasing the chance of getting an infection. It can also lower the number of platelets, which are necessary for proper blood clotting. If this occurs, there are certain precautions you can take, especially when your blood count is low, to reduce the risk of infection or bleeding:

- If you can, avoid people with infections. Check with your doctor immediately if you think you are getting an infection or if you get a fever or chills, cough or hoarseness, lower back or side pain, or painful or difficult urination.
- Check with your doctor immediately if you notice any unusual bleeding or bruising; black, tarry stools; blood in urine or stools; or pinpoint red spots on your skin.
- Be careful when using a regular toothbrush, dental floss, or toothpick. Your medical doctor, dentist, or nurse may recommend other ways to clean your teeth and gums. Check with your medical doctor before having any dental work done.
- Do not touch your eyes or the inside of your nose unless you have just washed your hands and have not touched anything else in the meantime.
- Be careful not to cut yourself when you are using sharp objects such as a safety razor or fingernail or toenail cutters.
- Avoid contact sports or other situations where bruising or injury could occur.

Side Effects of This Medicine

Along with its needed effects, a medicine may cause some unwanted effects. Although not all of these side effects may occur, if they do occur they may need medical attention.

Also, because of the way cancer medicines act on the body, there is a chance that they might cause other unwanted effects that may not occur until months or years after the medicine is used. These delayed effects may include certain types of cancer, such as leukemia. Discuss these possible effects with your doctor.

Check with your doctor immediately if any of the following side effects occur:
More common
Black, tarry stools; cough or shortness of breath
Less common
Blood in urine or stools; fast or irregular heartbeat; fever or chills; lower back or side pain; painful or difficult urination; pinpoint red spots on skin; swelling of feet and lower legs; unusual bleeding or bruising

Check with your doctor as soon as possible if any of the following side effects occur:
More common
Sores in mouth and on lips; stomach pain
Less common
Decrease in urination; seizures; sore, red eyes; yellow eyes or skin
Rare
Blue skin at place of injection; pain or redness at place of injection; skin rash

Some side effects may occur that usually do not need medical attention. These side effects may go away during treatment as your body adjusts to the medicine. Also, your health care professional may be able to tell you about ways to prevent or reduce some of these side effects. Check with your health care professional if any of the following side effects continue or are bothersome or if you have any questions about them:
More common
Body aches or pains; congestion; constipation; diarrhea; dryness or soreness of throat; headache; irregular menstrual periods; longer or heavier menstrual periods; nausea and vomiting; oral bleeding; runny nose; sneezing; stuffy nose; tender, swollen glands in neck

Mitoxantrone may cause the urine to turn a blue-green color. It may also cause the whites of the eyes to turn a blue color. These effects are normal and last for only 1 or 2 days after each dose is given.

This medicine often causes a temporary loss of hair. After treatment with mitoxantrone has ended, normal hair growth should return.

Other side effects not listed may also occur in some patients. If you notice any other effects, check with your healthcare professional.

MODAFINIL (Oral route) - moe-DAF-i-nil

Commonly used brand name(s)
In the U.S.—
Provigil

Available Dosage Forms:
- Tablet

Therapeutic Class: CNS Stimulant

Uses For This Medicine

Modafinil is used to help people who have narcolepsy, obstructive sleep apnea/hyponea, or shift work sleep disorder to stay awake during the day. Modafinil does not cure these conditions and will only work as long as you continue to take it.

This medicine is available only with your doctor's prescription.

Before Using This Medicine

In deciding to use a medicine, the risks of taking the medicine must be weighed against the good it will do. This is a decision you and your doctor will make. For this medicine, the following should be considered:

Allergies—Tell your doctor if you have ever had any unusual or allergic reaction to this medicine or any other medicines. Also tell your health care professional if you have any other types of allergies, such as to foods, dyes, preservatives, or animals. For non-prescription products, read the label or package ingredients carefully.

Pediatric—Studies on this medicine have been done only in adult patients, and there is no specific information comparing use of modafinil in children with use in other age groups.

Geriatric—Many medicines have not been studied specifically in older people. Therefore, it may not be known whether they work exactly the same way they do in younger adults. Although there is no specific information comparing use of modafinil in the elderly with use in other age groups, this medicine has been used in a few elderly patients and was not shown to cause different side effects or problems in older people than it does in younger adults.

Pregnancy—

	Pregnancy Category	Explanation
All Trimesters	C	Animal studies have shown an adverse effect and there are no adequate studies in pregnant women OR no animal studies have been conducted and there are no adequate studies in pregnant women.

Breast Feeding—There are no adequate studies in women for determining infant risk when using this medication during breastfeeding. Weigh the potential benefits against the potential risks before taking this medication while breastfeeding.

Other medicines—

Using this medicine with any of the following medicines may cause an increased risk of certain side effects, but using both drugs may be the best treatment for you. If both medicines are prescribed together, your doctor may change the dose or how often you use one or both of the medicines.

Clomipramine, Cyclosporine, Desogestrel, Ethinyl Estradiol, Ethynodiol, Etonogestrel, Levonorgestrel, Mestranol, Norelgestromin, Norethindrone, Norgestimate, Norgestrel, Triazolam

Interactions with Food/Tobacco/Alcohol—Certain medicines should not be used at or around the time of eating food or eating certain types of food since interactions may occur. Using alcohol or tobacco with certain medicines may also cause interactions to occur. Discuss with your healthcare professional the use of your medicine with food, alcohol, or tobacco.

Other medical problems—The presence of other medical problems may affect the use of this medicine. Make sure you tell your doctor if you have any other medical problems, especially:

- Heart disease or
- Heart attack, recent or
- High blood pressure—It is not known how modafinil will affect these conditions
- Heart problems during the use of other central nervous system (CNS) stimulating medicines, history of—Similar problems may occur when you use modafinil
- Kidney disease, severe—Higher blood levels of a breakdown product of modafinil may occur. It is not known if this will cause any problems
- Liver disease, severe—Higher blood levels of modafinil may occur, increasing the chance of having unwanted effects. You will probably receive a lower dose than a patient without liver disease
- Severe mental illness, history of—Modafinil may cause the illness to return

Proper Use of This Medicine

Take this medicine only as directed by your doctor. Do not take more of it, do not take it more often, and do not take it for a longer time than your doctor ordered. If too much is taken, it may become habit-forming.

Dosing—The dose of this medicine will be different for different patients. Follow your doctor's orders or the directions on the label. The following information includes only the average doses of this medicine. If your dose is different, do not change it unless your doctor tells you to do so.

The amount of medicine that you take depends on the strength of the medicine. Also, the number of doses you take each day, the time allowed between doses, and the length of time you take the medicine depend on the medical problem for which you are using the medicine.

- For oral dosage form (tablets):
  - For narcolepsy:
    - Adults—Usually 200 milligrams (mg) a day, taken as a single dose; dose should be taken in the morning if you also have obstructive sleep apnea/hyponea syndrome; dose should be taken 1 hour prior to the start of work if you have shift work sleep disorder.
    - Children—Use and dose must be determined by your doctor.

Missed dose—If you miss a dose of this medicine, skip the missed dose and go back to your regular dosing schedule. Do not double doses.

If you miss a dose of modafinil and you remember it before 12:00 noon the same day, take the missed dose as soon as possible.

Storage—Store the medicine in a closed container at room temperature, away from heat, moisture, and direct light. Keep from freezing.

Keep out of the reach of children.

Do not keep outdated medicine or medicine no longer needed.

Precautions While Using This Medicine

Your doctor should check your progress at regular visits to make sure that this medicine is working properly.

If you think modafinil is not working properly after you have taken it for a few weeks, do not increase the dose. Instead, check with your doctor.

If you are using a medicine for birth control, such as birth control pills or implants, it may not work properly while you are taking modafinil and for 1 month after stopping modafinil. Another form of birth control should be used during this time.

Modafinil may cause some people to feel dizzy, to have changes in thinking, to have difficulty controlling movements, or to have blurred vision. Make sure you know how you react to this medicine before you drive, use machines, or do anything else that could be dangerous.

If you have been taking this medicine for a long time or in large doses and you think you may have become mentally or physically dependent on it, check with your doctor. Some signs of dependence on modafinil are:

- a strong desire or need to continue taking the medicine.
- a need to increase the dose to receive the effects of the medicine.
- withdrawal side effects when you stop taking the medicine.

If you have been taking this medicine in large doses or for a long time, do not stop taking it without first checking with your doctor. Your doctor may want you to reduce gradually the amount you are taking before you stop completely.

Side Effects of This Medicine

Along with its needed effects, a medicine may cause some unwanted effects. Although not all of these side effects may occur, if they do occur they may need medical attention.

Check with your doctor as soon as possible if any of the following side effects occur:

Less common
Blurred vision or other vision changes; chest pain; chills or fever; clumsiness or unsteadiness; confusion; dizziness or fainting; increased thirst and increased urination; mental depression; problems with memory; rapidly changing moods; shortness of breath; sore throat; trouble in urinating; uncontrolled movements of the face, mouth, or tongue

Symptoms of overdose—may be more severe than side effects seen with regular doses or several symptoms may occur together
Agitation or excitement; fast or pounding heartbeat; increased blood pressure; trouble in sleeping

Some side effects may occur that usually do not need medical attention. These side effects may go away during treatment as your body adjusts to the medicine. Also, your health care professional may be able to tell you about ways to prevent or reduce some of these side effects. Check with your health care professional if any of the following side effects continue or are bothersome or if you have any questions about them:

More common
Anxiety; headache; nausea; nervousness; trouble in sleeping

Less common
Back pain; belching; black, tarry stools; decrease in appetite; diarrhea; difficulty having a bowel movement; dryness of mouth; dryness of skin; feeling of constant movement of self or surroundings; flushing or redness of skin; heartburn; indigestion; muscle stiffness; sores;

ulcers or white spots on lips or in mouth; sour stomach; stomach discomfort upset or pain; stuffy or runny nose; swelling; tingling, burning, or prickling sensations in the skin; trembling or shaking; unusual bleeding or bruising; unusual tiredness or weakness; vomiting

After you stop using this medicine, it may still produce some side effects that need attention. During this period of time, *check with your doctor immediately* if you notice the following side effects:

Other side effects not listed may also occur in some patients. If you notice any other effects, check with your healthcare professional.

MOLINDONE   (Oral route) - moe-LIN-done

Commonly used brand name(s)

In the U.S.—
Moban

Available Dosage Forms:

- Tablet
- Syrup

Therapeutic Class: Antipsychotic

Uses For This Medicine

Molindone is used to treat nervous, mental, and emotional conditions.

Molindone is available only with your doctor's prescription.

Before Using This Medicine

In deciding to use a medicine, the risks of taking the medicine must be weighed against the good it will do. This is a decision you and your doctor will make. For this medicine, the following should be considered:

Allergies—Tell your doctor if you have ever had any unusual or allergic reaction to this medicine or any other medicines. Also tell your health care professional if you have any other types of allergies, such as to foods, dyes, preservatives, or animals. For non-prescription products, read the label or package ingredients carefully.

Pediatric—Studies on this medicine have been done only in adult patients, and there is no specific information comparing use of molindone in children with use in other age groups.

Geriatric—Elderly patients are usually more sensitive than younger adults to the effects of molindone. Constipation, dizziness or lightheadedness, drowsiness, dryness of mouth, trembling of the hands and fingers, and symptoms of tardive dyskinesia (such as rapid, worm-like movements of the tongue or any other uncontrolled movements of the mouth, tongue, or jaw, and/or arms and legs) are especially likely to occur in elderly patients.

Pregnancy—

	Pregnancy Category	Explanation
All Trimesters	C	Animal studies have shown an adverse effect and there are no adequate studies in pregnant women OR no animal studies have been conducted and there are no adequate studies in pregnant women.

Breast Feeding—There are no adequate studies in women for determining infant risk when using this medication during breastfeeding. Weigh the potential benefits against the potential risks before taking this medication while breastfeeding.

Other medicines—

Using this medicine with any of the following medicines is not recommended. Your doctor may decide not to treat you with this medication or change some of the other medicines you take.

Droperidol

Interactions with Food/Tobacco/Alcohol—Certain medicines should not be used at or around the time of eating food or eating certain types of food since interactions may occur. Using alcohol or tobacco with certain medicines may also cause interactions to occur. Discuss with your healthcare professional the use of your medicine with food, alcohol, or tobacco.

Other medical problems—The presence of other medical problems may affect the use of this medicine. Make sure you tell your doctor if you have any other medical problems, especially:

- Brain tumor or
- Intestinal blockage—Molindone may interfere with the diagnosis of these conditions
- Difficult urination or
- Enlarged prostate or
- Glaucoma or
- Liver disease or
- Parkinson's disease—Molindone may make the condition worse

Proper Use of This Medicine

Molindone should be taken with food or a full glass (8 ounces) of water or milk to reduce stomach irritation.

The liquid form of molindone may be taken undiluted or mixed with milk, water, fruit juice, or carbonated beverages.

Take this medicine only as directed by your doctor. Do not take more of it, do not take it more often, and do not take it for a longer time than your doctor ordered. To do so may increase the chance of side effects.

Sometimes this medicine must be taken for several weeks before its full effect is reached in the treatment of certain mental and emotional conditions.

Dosing—The dose of this medicine will be different for different patients. Follow your doctor's orders or the directions on the label. The following information includes only the average doses of this medicine. If your dose is different, do not change it unless your doctor tells you to do so.

The amount of medicine that you take depends on the strength of the medicine. Also, the number of doses you take each day, the time allowed between doses, and the length of time you take the medicine depend on the medical problem for which you are using the medicine.

- For oral dosage forms (solution or tablets):
  - Adults: To start, 50 to 75 milligrams a day, taken in smaller doses three or four times during the day. For maintenance, the dose you take will depend on your condition and may be from 15 to 225 milligrams a day, taken in smaller doses three or four times during the day.
  - Children up to 12 years of age: The dose must be determined by the doctor.

Missed dose—If you miss a dose of this medicine, take it as soon as possible. However, if it is almost time for your next dose, skip the missed dose and go back to your regular dosing schedule. Do not double doses.

Storage—Store the medicine in a closed container at room temperature, away from heat, moisture, and direct light. Keep from freezing.

Keep out of the reach of children.

Do not keep outdated medicine or medicine no longer needed.

Precautions While Using This Medicine

Your doctor should check your progress at regular visits. This will allow the dosage of the medicine to be adjusted when necessary and also will reduce the possibility of side effects.

Do not stop taking this medicine without first checking with your doctor. Your doctor may want you to reduce gradually the amount you are taking before stopping completely.

Do not take molindone within 1 or 2 hours of taking antacids or medicine for diarrhea. Taking them too close together may make molindone less effective.

This medicine will add to the effects of alcohol and other CNS depressants (medicines that slow down the nervous system, possibly causing drowsiness). Some examples of CNS depressants are antihistamines or medicine for hay fever, other allergies, or colds; sedatives, tranquilizers, or sleeping medicine; prescription pain medicine or narcotics; barbiturates; medicine for seizures; muscle relaxants; or anesthetics, including some dental anesthetics. Check with your doctor before taking any of the above while you are using this medicine.

Molindone may cause some people to become drowsy or less alert than they are normally, especially during the first few weeks the medicine is being taken. Even if you take this medicine only at bedtime, you may feel drowsy or less alert on arising. Make sure you know how you react to this medicine before you drive, use machines, or do anything else that could be dangerous if you are not alert.

Dizziness or lightheadedness may occur, especially when you get up from a lying or sitting position. Getting up slowly may help. If the problem continues or gets worse, check with your doctor.

These medicines may make you sweat less, causing your body temperature to increase. Use extra care not to become overheated during exercise or hot weather while you are taking this medicine, since overheating may result in heat stroke. Also, hot baths or saunas may make you feel dizzy or faint while you are taking this medicine.

Molindone may cause dryness of the mouth. For temporary relief, use sugarless candy or gum, melt bits of ice in your mouth, or use a saliva substitute. However, if your mouth continues to feel dry for more than 2 weeks, check with your medical doctor or dentist. Continuing dryness of the mouth may increase the chance of dental disease, including tooth decay, gum disease, and fungus infection.

Side Effects of This Medicine

Along with its needed effects, molindone can sometimes cause serious side effects. Tardive dyskinesia (a movement disorder) may occur and may not go away after you stop using the medicine. Symptoms of tardive dyskinesia include fine, worm-like movements of the tongue, or other uncontrolled movements of the mouth, tongue, cheeks, jaw, or arms and legs. Other serious but rare side effects may also occur. These include severe muscle stiffness, fever, unusual tiredness or weakness, fast heartbeat, difficult breathing, increased sweating, loss of bladder control, and seizures (neuroleptic malignant syndrome). You and your doctor should discuss the good this medicine will do as well as the risks of taking it.

Stop taking this medicine and get emergency help immediately if any of the following effects occur:
Rare
   Convulsions (seizures); difficult or fast breathing; fast heartbeat or irregular pulse; fever (high); high or low (irregular) blood pressure; increased sweating; loss of bladder control; muscle stiffness (severe); unusually pale skin; unusual tiredness or weakness

Check with your doctor as soon as possible if any of the following side effects occur:
More common
   Difficulty in talking or swallowing; inability to move eyes; lip smacking or puckering; loss of balance control; mask-like face; muscle spasms, especially of the neck and back; puffing of cheeks; rapid or worm-like movements of tongue; restlessness or need to keep moving (severe); shuffling walk; stiffness of arms and legs; trembling and shaking of hands; twisting movements of body; uncontrolled movements of arms and legs; unusual chewing movements

Less common
   Mental depression
Rare
   Confusion; hot, dry skin, or lack of sweating; muscle weakness; skin rash; yellow eyes or skin

Some side effects may occur that usually do not need medical attention. These side effects may go away during treatment as your body adjusts to the medicine. Also, your health care professional may be able to tell you about ways to prevent or reduce some of these side effects. Check with your health care professional if any of the following side effects continue or are bothersome or if you have any questions about them:
More common
   Blurred vision; constipation; decreased sweating; difficult urination; dizziness or lightheadedness, especially when getting up suddenly from a lying or sitting position; drowsiness; dryness of mouth; headache; nausea; stuffy nose

Less common
   Changes in menstrual periods; decreased sexual ability; false sense of well-being; swelling of breasts; unusual secretion of milk

After you stop using this medicine, it may still produce some side effects that need attention. During this period of time, *check with your doctor immediately* if you notice the following side effects:
   Lip smacking or puckering; puffing of cheeks; rapid or worm-like movements of tongue; uncontrolled chewing movements; uncontrolled movements of arms and legs

Other side effects not listed may also occur in some patients. If you notice any other effects, check with your healthcare professional.

MOMETASONE (Inhalation, oral/nebulization route) - moe-MET-a-sone

Commonly used brand name(s)
In the U.S.—
   Asmanex Twist

Available Dosage Forms:
 • Powder

Therapeutic Class: Anti-Inflammatory
Pharmacologic Class: Adrenal Glucocorticoid

Uses For This Medicine

Mometasone belongs to the family of medicines known as corticosteroids (cortisone-like medicines). It is used to help prevent the symptoms of asthma. When used regularly every day, inhaled mometasone decreases the number and severity of asthma attacks. However, it will not relieve an asthma attack that has already started.

Inhaled mometasone works by preventing certain cells in the lungs and breathing passages from releasing substances that cause asthma symptoms.

This medicine is available only with your doctor's prescription.

Before Using This Medicine

In deciding to use a medicine, the risks of taking the medicine must be weighed against the good it will do. This is a decision you and your doctor will make. For this medicine, the following should be considered:

Allergies—Tell your doctor if you have ever had any unusual or allergic reaction to this medicine or any other medicines. Also tell your health care professional if you have any other types of allergies, such as to foods, dyes, preservatives, or animals. For non-prescription products, read the label or package ingredients carefully.

Pediatric—This medicine has only been tested in children 12 years of age or older. Mometasone powder for inhalation may adversely effect the adrenal gland and stunt growth in pediatric patients. Before this medicine is given to a child, you and your child's doctor should talk about the good this medicine will do as well as the risks of using it.

Geriatric—Many medicines have not been studied specifically in older people. Therefore, it may not be known whether they work exactly the same way they do in younger adults or if they cause different side effects or problems in older people. There is no specific information comparing use of mometasone inhalation powder in the elderly with use in other age groups.

Pregnancy—

	Pregnancy Category	Explanation
All Trimesters	C	Animal studies have shown an adverse effect and there are no adequate studies in pregnant women OR no animal studies have been conducted and there are no adequate studies in pregnant women.

Breast Feeding—There are no adequate studies in women for determining infant risk when using this medication during breastfeeding. Weigh the potential benefits against the potential risks before taking this medication while breastfeeding.

Other medicines—

Using this medicine with any of the following medicines may cause an increased risk of certain side effects, but using both drugs may be the best treatment for you. If both medicines are prescribed together, your doctor may change the dose or how often you use one or both of the medicines.

Ketoconazole

Interactions with Food/Tobacco/Alcohol—Certain medicines should not be used at or around the time of eating food or eating certain types of food since interactions may occur. Using alcohol or tobacco with certain medicines may also cause interactions to occur. Discuss with your healthcare professional the use of your medicine with food, alcohol, or tobacco.

Other medical problems—The presence of other medical problems may affect the use of this medicine. Make sure you tell your doctor if you have any other medical problems, especially:

- Eye problems such as:
- Cataracts or
- Glaucoma or
- Intraocular pressure increased—Mometasone may make these conditions worse
- Liver problems—May increase the amount of mometasone that stays in the body
- Immobilization for long periods of time or
- Osteoporosis, family history—Mometasone may make your bones weaker and increase the chance of a broken bone after a minor fall or injury.
- Infections—Mometasone may make infections like chickenpox and measles more dangerous; it might also hide the effects of certain infections
- Tuberculosis of the respiratory tract—Mometasone may either hide the effects of this disease or make it worse

Proper Use of This Medicine

Dosing—The dose of this medicine will be different for different patients. Follow your doctor's orders or the directions on the label. The following information includes only the average doses of this medicine. If your dose is different, do not change it unless your doctor tells you to do so.

The amount of medicine that you take depends on the strength of the medicine. Also, the number of doses you take each day, the time allowed between doses, and the length of time you take the medicine depend on the medical problem for which you are using the medicine.

- For asthma (treatment)
  - If you have had previous asthma therapy with bronchodilators alone:
    - Adults—220 mcg once daily in the evening
    - Children—Use and dose must be determined by your doctor.
  - If you have had previous asthma therapy with inhaled corticosteroids alone:
    - Adults—220 mcg once daily in the evening
    - Children—Use and dose must be determined by your doctor.
  - If you have had previous asthma therapy with oral corticosteroids:
    - Adults—440 mcg twice daily
    - Children—Use and dose must be determined by your doctor.

Storage—Store the medicine in a closed container at room temperature, away from heat, moisture, and direct light. Keep from freezing.

Keep out of the reach of children.

Do not keep outdated medicine or medicine no longer needed.

Ask your healthcare professional how you should dispose of any medicine you do not use.

Precautions While Using This Medicine

Check with your doctor if:
- You go through a period of unusual stress to your body, such as surgery, injury, or infection.
- You have an asthma attack that does not improve after you take a bronchodilator medicine.
- Your asthma symptoms do not improve or your condition worsens.
- You are exposed to the chickenpox or measles.

Your doctor may want you to carry a medical identification card stating that you are using this medicine and that you may need additional medicine during times of emergency, a severe asthma attack or other illness, or unusual stress.

Side Effects of This Medicine

Along with its needed effects, a medicine may cause some unwanted effects. Although not all of these side effects may occur, if they do occur they may need medical attention.

Check with your doctor immediately if any of the following side effects occur:
More common
  Body aches or pain; cold or flu-like symptoms; congestion; cough; dryness or soreness of throat
Less common
  Abdominal or stomach pain; diarrhea; fever or chills; loss of appetite; lower back or side pain; nausea
Rare
  White patches inside nose or mouth

Some side effects may occur that usually do not need medical attention. These side effects may go away during treatment as your body adjusts to the medicine. Also, your health care professional may be able to tell you about ways to prevent or reduce some of these side effects. Check with your health care professional if any of the following side effects continue or are bothersome or if you have any questions about them:

More common

Difficulty in moving; discouragement; fatigue; feeling sad or empty; increased abdominal pain and cramping during menstrual periods; irritability; lack of appetite; loss of interest or pleasure; muscle pain or stiffness; musculoskeletal pain; nasal burning and irritation; pain in joints; stomach discomfort following meals; stuffy or runny nose or headache; tiredness; trouble concentrating; trouble sleeping; unexplained runny nose or sneezing; upset stomach

Less common

Accidental injury; bladder pain; bloody or cloudy urine; bloody mucus or unexplained nosebleeds; chest congestion; chills; cough; diarrhea; difficult, burning, or painful urination; flatulence; frequent urge to urinate; general feeling of discomfort or illness; lower back or side pain; menstrual changes; nausea; post-procedure pain; shivering; sore throat; sweating; unusual tiredness or weakness; vomiting

Other side effects not listed may also occur in some patients. If you notice any other effects, check with your healthcare professional.

MONTELUKAST   (Oral route) - mon-te-LOO-kast

Commonly used brand name(s)

In the U.S.—
   Singulair

Available Dosage Forms:

- Tablet
- Tablet, Chewable
- Packet

Therapeutic Class: Anti-Inflammatory
Pharmacologic Class: Leukotriene Pathway Inhibitor

Uses For This Medicine

Montelukast is used in mild to moderate asthma to decrease the symptoms of asthma and the number of acute asthma attacks. However, this medicine should not be used to relieve an asthma attack that has already started. This medicine is also used to treat the symptoms (sneezing, runny nose, itching, wheezing) of seasonal (short-term) allergies.

This medicine is available only with your doctor's prescription.

Before Using This Medicine

In deciding to use a medicine, the risks of taking the medicine must be weighed against the good it will do. This is a decision you and your doctor will make. For this medicine, the following should be considered:

Allergies—Tell your doctor if you have ever had any unusual or allergic reaction to this medicine or any other medicines. Also tell your health care professional if you have any other types of allergies, such as to foods, dyes, preservatives, or animals. For non-prescription products, read the label or package ingredients carefully.

Pediatric—No information is available regarding use of montelukast in infants younger than 12 months of age.

Geriatric—Many medicines have not been studied specifically in older people. Therefore, it may not be known whether they work exactly the same way they do in younger adults. There is no specific information comparing use of montelukast in the elderly with its use in other age groups. However, it has been used in some elderly patients and no differences in effectiveness or side effects were seen from those that occurred in younger adults.

Pregnancy—

	Pregnancy Category	Explanation
All Trimesters	B	Animal studies have revealed no evidence of harm to the fetus, however, there are no adequate studies in pregnant women OR animal studies have shown an adverse effect, but adequate studies in pregnant women have failed to demonstrate a risk to the fetus.

Breast Feeding—There are no adequate studies in women for determining infant risk when using this medication during breastfeeding. Weigh the potential benefits against the potential risks before taking this medication while breastfeeding.

Other medicines—

Using this medicine with any of the following medicines may cause an increased risk of certain side effects, but using both drugs may be the best treatment for you. If both medicines are prescribed together, your doctor may change the dose or how often you use one or both of the medicines.

Prednisone

Interactions with Food/Tobacco/Alcohol—Certain medicines should not be used at or around the time of eating food or eating certain types of food since interactions may occur. Using alcohol or tobacco with certain medicines may also cause interactions to occur. Discuss with your healthcare professional the use of your medicine with food, alcohol, or tobacco.

Other medical problems—The presence of other medical problems may affect the use of this medicine. Make sure you tell your doctor if you have any other medical problems, especially:

- Allergy to aspirin or non-steroidal anti-inflammatory agents (NSAIDs) (etodolac [e.g., Lodine], ibuprofen [e.g., Advil, Motrin], ketoprofen [e.g., Orudis], naproxen [e.g., Aleve])—Patients should continue to avoid aspirin or NSAIDs while taking montelukast.

- Liver disease—Effects of montelukast may be increased because of slower removal from the body
- Phenylketonuria (PKU)—The chewable tablets may contain aspartame, which can make your condition worse.

Proper Use of This Medicine

Montelukast is used to prevent asthma attacks. It is not used to relieve an attack that has already started. For relief of an asthma attack that has already started, you should use another medicine. If you do not have another medicine to use for an attack or if you have any questions about this, check with your health care professional.

For patients taking the oral granule form of this medicine— May be taken on a full or empty stomach. Packet of oral granules may either be swallowed whole or mixed with a spoonful of soft food such as applesauce, carrots, rice or ice cream. The oral granules should not be chewed.

Dosing—The dose of this medicine will be different for different patients. Follow your doctor's orders or the directions on the label. The following information includes only the average doses of this medicine. If your dose is different, do not change it unless your doctor tells you to do so.

The amount of medicine that you take depends on the strength of the medicine. Also, the number of doses you take each day, the time allowed between doses, and the length of time you take the medicine depend on the medical problem for which you are using the medicine.

- For asthma or seasonal allergies:
  - For tablets dosage form:
    - Adults and children 15 years of age and over— 10 milligrams (mg) once a day.
  - For chewable tablets dosage form:
    - Children 6 to 14 years of age—5 mg once a day.
    - Children 2 to 5 years of age—4 mg once a day.
  - For oral granules dosage form:
    - Children 2 to 5 years of age—4 mg (one packet) once a day.
    - Infants 12 to 23 months of age—4 mg (one packet) once a day.
    - Infants younger than 12 months of age—Use and dose must be determined by your doctor.

Missed dose—If you miss a dose of this medicine, take it as soon as possible. However, if it is almost time for your next dose, skip the missed dose and go back to your regular dosing schedule. Do not double doses.

Storage—Store the medicine in a closed container at room temperature, away from heat, moisture, and direct light. Keep from freezing.

Keep out of the reach of children.

Do not keep outdated medicine or medicine no longer needed.

Precautions While Using This Medicine

To work properly, montelukast must be taken every day at the same time, even if your asthma seems better.

Do not stop taking montelukast, even if your asthma seems better, unless you are told to do so by your doctor.

Check with your doctor if your symptoms do not improve or if your asthma gets worse.

You may be taking other medicines for asthma along with montelukast. Do not stop taking or reduce the dose of the other medicines, even if your asthma seems better, unless you are told to do so by your doctor.

Side Effects of This Medicine

Along with its needed effects, a medicine may cause some unwanted effects. Although not all of these side effects may occur, if they do occur they may need medical attention.

Check with your doctor as soon as possible if any of the following side effects occur:
Rare
  Pus in the urine

Incidence not determined
  Abdominal or stomach pain; anxiety; assault; attack; bloating; chills; clay-colored stools; constipation; convulsions; darkened urine; diarrhea; difficulty swallowing; dry mouth; fast, irregular, pounding, or racing heartbeat or pulse; force; general tiredness and weakness; hives or welts; hyperventilation; indigestion; irregular heartbeats; irritability; itching; itching, puffiness, or swelling of the eyelids or around the eyes, face, lips or tongue; itching skin; large, hive-like swelling on face, eyelids, lips, tongue, throat, hands, legs, feet, sex organs; light-colored stools; loss of appetite; loss of bladder control; muscle spasm or jerking of all extremities; nausea; nervousness; pains in stomach, side, or abdomen, possibly radiating to the back; redness of skin; restlessness; seeing, hearing, or feeling things that are not there; shaking; shortness of breath; sudden loss of consciousness; tightness in chest; trouble sleeping; unpleasant breath odor; upper right abdominal pain; unusual tiredness or weakness; vomiting; vomiting of blood; wheezing; yellow eyes or skin

Some side effects may occur that usually do not need medical attention. These side effects may go away during treatment as your body adjusts to the medicine. Also, your health care professional may be able to tell you about ways to prevent or reduce some of these side effects. Check with your health care professional if any of the following side effects continue or are bothersome or if you have any questions about them:
More common
  Headache

Less common
  Abdominal or stomach pain; cough; dental pain; dizziness; fever; heartburn; skin rash; stuffy nose; weakness or unusual tiredness

Incidence not determined
  Burning, crawling, itching, numbness, prickling, "pins and needles", or tingling feelings; difficulty in moving; dream abnormalities; increased bleeding tendency; irritability; joint pain; large, flat, blue or purplish patches in the skin; muscle aching or cramping; muscle pain or stiffness; sleepiness; sleeplessness; swelling; swollen joints; trouble sleeping; unable to sleep

Other side effects not listed may also occur in some patients. If you notice any other effects, check with your healthcare professional.

MOXIFLOXACIN   (Ophthalmic route) -
mox-i-FLOX-a-sin

Commonly used brand name(s)

In the U.S.—
Vigamox

Available Dosage Forms:
• Solution

Therapeutic Class: Antibiotic

Uses For This Medicine

Moxifloxacin belongs to the family of medicines called antibiotics. Moxifloxacin ophthalmic solution (eye drops) is used to treat infections of the eye, such as bacterial conjunctivitis. Ophthalmic moxifloxacin works by killing the bacteria in your eye.

This medicine is available only with your doctor's prescription.

Before Using This Medicine

In deciding to use a medicine, the risks of taking the medicine must be weighed against the good it will do. This is a decision you and your doctor will make. For this medicine, the following should be considered:

Allergies—Tell your doctor if you have ever had any unusual or allergic reaction to this medicine or any other medicines. Also tell your health care professional if you have any other types of allergies, such as to foods, dyes, preservatives, or animals. For non-prescription products, read the label or package ingredients carefully.

Pediatric—Although there is no specific information comparing use of moxifloxacin eye drops in children with use in other age groups, this medicine is not expected to cause different side effects or problems in children than it does in older adults. This medicine should not be used in children younger than one year old.

Geriatric—Many medicines have not been studied specifically in older people. Therefore, it may not be known whether they work exactly the same way they do in younger adults or if they cause different side effects or problems in older people. Moxifloxacin eye drops are not expected to cause different side effects or problems in older people than they do in younger adults.

Pregnancy—

	Pregnancy Category	Explanation
All Trimesters	C	Animal studies have shown an adverse effect and there are no adequate studies in pregnant women OR no animal studies have been conducted and there are no adequate studies in pregnant women.

Breast Feeding—There are no adequate studies in women for determining infant risk when using this medication during breastfeeding. Weigh the potential benefits against the potential risks before taking this medication while breastfeeding.

Other medicines—
Using this medicine with any of the following medicines is not recommended. Your doctor may decide not to treat you with this medication or change some of the other medicines you take.

Cisapride, Mesoridazine, Thioridazine, Ziprasidone

Interactions with Food/Tobacco/Alcohol—Certain medicines should not be used at or around the time of eating food or eating certain types of food since interactions may occur. Using alcohol or tobacco with certain medicines may also cause interactions to occur. Discuss with your healthcare professional the use of your medicine with food, alcohol, or tobacco.

Proper Use of This Medicine

To use:
• First, wash your hands. Tilt the head back and pressing your finger gently on the skin just beneath the lower eyelid, pull the lower eyelid away from the eye to make a space. Drop the medicine into this space. Let go of the eyelid and gently close the eyes. Do not blink.
• If you think you did not get the drop of medicine into your eye properly, use another drop.
• Immediately after using the eye drops, wash your hands to remove any medicine that may be on them.
• To keep the medicine as germ free as possible, do not touch the applicator tip to any surface (including the eye).

Dosing—The dose of this medicine will be different for different patients. Follow your doctor's orders or the directions on the label. The following information includes only the average doses of this medicine. If your dose is different, do not change it unless your doctor tells you to do so.

The amount of medicine that you take depends on the strength of the medicine. Also, the number of doses you take each day, the time allowed between doses, and the length of time you take the medicine depend on the medical problem for which you are using the medicine.

To keep the medicine as germ free as possible, do not touch the applicator tip to any surface (including your eye).

You should not wear your contact lenses if you have any signs or symptoms of an eye infection.

For ophthalmic solution (eye drops) dosage form:
• For bacterial conjunctivitis (eye infections)
  ◦ Adults and children 1 year of age and older—One drop in your infected eye(s) three times a day for 7 days.
  ◦ Children up to 1 year of age—Use and dose must be determined by your doctor.

Missed dose—If you miss a dose of this medicine, take it as soon as possible. However, if it is almost time for your next dose, skip the missed dose and go back to your regular dosing schedule. Do not double doses.

Storage—Keep out of the reach of children.

Do not keep outdated medicine or medicine no longer needed.

Ask your healthcare professional how you should dispose of any medicine you do not use.

Precautions While Using This Medicine

If your symptoms do not improve within a few days or if they become worse, check with your doctor.

Check with your doctor right away if you have any of the following symptoms: cough, difficulty swallowing, dizziness, fast heartbeat, hives, itching, puffiness or swelling of the eyelids or around the eyes, face, lips or tongue, shortness of breath, skin rash, tightness in chest, unusual tiredness or weakness or wheezing. These could be symptoms of an allergic reaction.

Side Effects of This Medicine

Along with its needed effects, a medicine may cause some unwanted effects. Although not all of these side effects may occur, if they do occur they may need medical attention.

Check with your doctor immediately if any of the following side effects occur:

Incidence unknown
>   Fainting or loss of consciousness; fast or irregular breathing; itching; skin rash; swelling of eyes or eyelids; tightness in chest, and/or wheezing; trouble in breathing

Some side effects may occur that usually do not need medical attention. These side effects may go away during treatment as your body adjusts to the medicine. Also, your health care professional may be able to tell you about ways to prevent or reduce some of these side effects. Check with your health care professional if any of the following side effects continue or are bothersome or if you have any questions about them:

More common
>   Burning, dry or itching eyes; change in vision; decreased vision; dry eye; eye discharge; itching of eye; pain in eye; redness of eye; swelling of eye, eyelid, or inner lining of eyelid; tearing

Less common
>   Body aches or pain; congestion; cough or hoarseness; decreased hearing; dryness or soreness of throat; fever or chills; general body discomfort; lower back or side pain; painful or difficult urination; rash; rubbing or pulling of the ears (in children); runny nose; sore throat; tender, swollen glands in neck; trouble in swallowing; voice changes; vomiting and diarrhea (in infants)

Other side effects not listed may also occur in some patients. If you notice any other effects, check with your healthcare professional.

MUPIROCIN (Topical route) - myoo-PEER-oh-sin

Commonly used brand name(s)

In the U.S.—
>   Bactroban
>   Centany

Available Dosage Forms:
- Ointment
- Cream

Therapeutic Class: Antibacterial

Uses For This Medicine

Mupirocin is used to treat bacterial infections. It works by killing bacteria or preventing their growth.

Mupirocin ointment is applied to the skin to treat impetigo. It may also be used for other bacterial skin infections as determined by your doctor.

Mupirocin cream is applied to the skin to treat secondarily infected traumatic skin lesions.

Mupirocin is available in the U.S. only with your doctor's prescription.

Before Using This Medicine

In deciding to use a medicine, the risks of taking the medicine must be weighed against the good it will do. This is a decision you and your doctor will make. For this medicine, the following should be considered:

Allergies—Tell your doctor if you have ever had any unusual or allergic reaction to this medicine or any other medicines. Also tell your health care professional if you have any other types of allergies, such as to foods, dyes, preservatives, or animals. For non-prescription products, read the label or package ingredients carefully.

Pediatric—Safety and effectiveness of mupirocin cream have not been established in children up to 3 months of age.

Safety and effectiveness of mupirocin ointment have not been established in children up to 2 months of age.

Geriatric—No overall difference in safety and efficacy were observed in patients over 65 years of age.

Pregnancy—

	Pregnancy Category	Explanation
All Trimesters	B	Animal studies have revealed no evidence of harm to the fetus, however, there are no adequate studies in pregnant women OR animal studies have shown an adverse effect, but adequate studies in pregnant women have failed to demonstrate a risk to the fetus.

Breast Feeding—There are no adequate studies in women for determining infant risk when using this medication during breastfeeding. Weigh the potential benefits against the potential risks before taking this medication while breastfeeding.

Other medicines—Although certain medicines should not be used together at all, in other cases two different medicines may be used together even if an interaction might occur. In these cases, your doctor may want to change the dose, or other precautions may be necessary. Tell your healthcare professional if you are taking any other prescription or non-prescription (over-the-counter [OTC]) medicine.

Interactions with Food/Tobacco/Alcohol—Certain medicines should not be used at or around the time of eating

food or eating certain types of food since interactions may occur. Using alcohol or tobacco with certain medicines may also cause interactions to occur. Discuss with your healthcare professional the use of your medicine with food, alcohol, or tobacco.

Proper Use of This Medicine

Do not use this medicine in the eyes.

To use:

- Before applying this medicine, wash the affected area(s) with soap and water, and dry thoroughly. Then apply a small amount to the affected area(s) and rub in gently.
- After applying this medicine, the treated area(s) may be covered with a gauze dressing if desired.

To help clear up your skin infection completely, keep using mupirocin for the full time of treatment, even if your symptoms have disappeared. Do not miss any doses.

Dosing—The dose of this medicine will be different for different patients. Follow your doctor's orders or the directions on the label. The following information includes only the average doses of this medicine. If your dose is different, do not change it unless your doctor tells you to do so.

The amount of medicine that you take depends on the strength of the medicine. Also, the number of doses you take each day, the time allowed between doses, and the length of time you take the medicine depend on the medical problem for which you are using the medicine.

- For ointment dosage form:
  - Impetigo:
    - Adults and children 2 months of age and older—Apply three times a day.
    - Children under 2 months of age—Use and dose must be determined by your doctor.
- For cream dosage form:
  - Secondarily infected traumatic skin lesions
    - Adults and children 3 months of age and older—Apply three times a day, for 10 days.
    - Children under 3 months of age—Use and dose must be determined by your doctor.

Missed dose—If you miss a dose of this medicine, apply it as soon as possible. However, if it is almost time for your next dose, skip the missed dose and go back to your regular dosing schedule.

Storage—Store the medicine in a closed container at room temperature, away from heat, moisture, and direct light. Keep from freezing.

Keep out of the reach of children.

Do not keep outdated medicine or medicine no longer needed.

Precautions While Using This Medicine

If your skin infection does not improve within 3 to 5 days, or if it becomes worse, check with your health care professional.

Side Effects of This Medicine

Along with its needed effects, a medicine may cause some unwanted effects. Although not all of these side effects may occur, if they do occur they may need medical attention.

Some side effects may occur that usually do not need medical attention. These side effects may go away during treatment as your body adjusts to the medicine. Also, your health care professional may be able to tell you about ways to prevent or reduce some of these side effects. Check with your health care professional if any of the following side effects continue or are bothersome or if you have any questions about them:

Less common
  Dry skin; skin burning, itching, pain, rash, redness, stinging, or swelling; headache; nausea

Rare
  Abdominal pain; dizziness; secondary wound infection; sores on mouth and on lips

Other side effects not listed may also occur in some patients. If you notice any other effects, check with your healthcare professional.

MYCOPHENOLATE MOFETIL (Oral route, Intravenous route) - mye-koe-FEN-oh-late MOE-fe-til

Black Box Warning

Increased susceptibility to infection and the possible development of lymphoma may result from immunosuppression. Only physicians experienced in immunosuppressive therapy and management of renal, cardiac or hepatic transplant patients should use mycophenolate mofetil. Patients receiving the drug should be managed in facilities equipped and staffed with adequate laboratory and supportive medical resources. The physician responsible for maintenance therapy should have complete information requisite for the follow-up of the patient.

Commonly used brand name(s)

In the U.S.—
  Cellcept

Available Dosage Forms:

- Capsule
- Powder for Suspension
- Tablet

Therapeutic Class: Immune Suppressant

Uses For This Medicine

Mycophenolate belongs to a group of medicines known as immunosuppressive agents. It is used to lower the body's natural immunity in patients who receive organ transplants.

When a patient receives an organ transplant, the body's white blood cells will try to get rid of (reject) the transplanted organ. Mycophenolate works by preventing the white blood cells from getting rid of the transplanted organ.

This medicine is available only with your doctor's prescription.

Once a medicine has been approved for marketing for a certain use, experience may show that it is also useful for other medical problems. Although this use is not included in product labeling, mycophenolate is used in certain patients with the following medical condition:

• Lupus nephritis

Before Using This Medicine

In deciding to use a medicine, the risks of taking the medicine must be weighed against the good it will do. This is a decision you and your doctor will make. For this medicine, the following should be considered:

Allergies—Tell your doctor if you have ever had any unusual or allergic reaction to this medicine or any other medicines. Also tell your health care professional if you have any other types of allergies, such as to foods, dyes, preservatives, or animals. For non-prescription products, read the label or package ingredients carefully.

Pediatric—For kidney transplants—This medicine has been tested in children 3 months and older and, in effective doses, has not been shown to cause different side effects or problems than it does in adults.

For heart or liver transplants—Studies of this medicine have been done only in adult patients, and there is no specific information comparing use of mycophenolate in children with use in other age groups.

Geriatric—Many medicines have not been studied specifically in older people. Therefore, it may not be known whether they work exactly the same way they do in younger adults or if they cause different side effects or problems in older people. There is no specific information comparing use of mycophenolate in the elderly with use in other age groups. However, elderly people may be especially sensitive to the effects of mycophenolate.

Pregnancy—

	Pregnancy Category	Explanation
All Trimesters	C	Animal studies have shown an adverse effect and there are no adequate studies in pregnant women OR no animal studies have been conducted and there are no adequate studies in pregnant women.

Breast Feeding—There are no adequate studies in women for determining infant risk when using this medication during breastfeeding. Weigh the potential benefits against the potential risks before taking this medication while breastfeeding.

Other medicines—

Using this medicine with any of the following medicines is usually not recommended, but may be required in some cases. If both medicines are prescribed together, your doctor may change the dose or how often you use one or both of the medicines.

Activated Charcoal, Aluminum Carbonate, Basic, Aluminum Hydroxide, Aluminum Phosphate, Cholestyramine, Colesevelam, Colestipol, Dihydroxyaluminum Aminoacetate, Dihydroxyaluminum Sodium Carbonate, Magaldrate, Magnesium Carbonate, Magnesium Hydroxide, Magnesium Oxide, Magnesium Trisilicate

Interactions with Food/Tobacco/Alcohol—Certain medicines should not be used at or around the time of eating food or eating certain types of food since interactions may occur. Using alcohol or tobacco with certain medicines may also cause interactions to occur. Discuss with your healthcare professional the use of your medicine with food, alcohol, or tobacco.

Other medical problems—The presence of other medical problems may affect the use of this medicine. Make sure you tell your doctor if you have any other medical problems, especially:

• Delayed kidney function following kidney transplantation or

• Kidney problems, severe—Reduced elimination of mycophenolate and increased chance of developing fever and chills, cough or hoarseness, lower back or side pain, painful or difficult urination.

• Digestive system disease, active—Risk of bleeding from the stomach

• Phenylketonuria (PKU)—The oral suspension may contain aspartame, which can make your condition worse.

Proper Use of This Medicine

This medicine should be taken on an empty stomach.

Take this medicine only as directed by your doctor. Do not take more or less of it and do not take it more often than your doctor ordered. Taking too much may increase the chance of side effects, while taking too little may lead to rejection of your transplanted organ.

To help you remember to take your medicine, try to get into the habit of taking it at the same time each day.

Do not stop taking this medicine without first checking with your doctor. Your physician will use the results of tests and your physical examination to decide how long you should take this medicine.

The capsules or tablets of mycophenolate should be swallowed whole. The tablets should not be crushed and the capsules should not be opened because it is important that other people not be exposed to mycophenolate powder. You should not inhale the powder or allow the powder or oral suspension liquid to touch your skin.

You should use the dispenser that was given to you by your pharmacist to measure out the correct amount of oral suspension. If you have any questions about this, ask your doctor or pharmacist.

Dosing—The dose of this medicine will be different for different patients. Follow your doctor's orders or the directions on the label. The following information includes only the average doses of this medicine. If your dose is different, do not change it unless your doctor tells you to do so.

The amount of medicine that you take depends on the strength of the medicine. Also, the number of doses you take each day, the time allowed between doses, and the length of time you take the medicine depend on the medical problem for which you are using the medicine.

• For oral dosage form (capsules or tablets):
  ○ For prevention of rejection of transplanted heart:
    ▪ Adults—1.5 grams (six capsules or three tablets) two times a day.
  ○ For prevention of rejection of transplanted kidney:
    ▪ Adults—1 gram (four capsules or two tablets) two times a day.
    ▪ Children 3 months and older—Dose is based on child's size as instructed by the doctor.

○ For prevention of rejection of transplanted liver:
  ▪ Adults—1.5 grams (six capsules or three tablets) two times a day.

• For oral dosage form (suspension):
  ○ For prevention of rejection of transplanted heart:
    ▪ Adults—1.5 grams two times a day.
  ○ For prevention of rejection of transplanted kidney:
    ▪ Adults—1 gram two times a day.
    ▪ Children 3 months and older—Dose is based on child's size as instructed by the doctor.
  ○ For prevention of rejection of transplanted liver:
    ▪ Adults—1.5 grams two times a day.

• For injection dosage form:
  ○ For prevention of rejection of transplanted heart:
    ▪ Adults—1.5 grams two times a day.
  ○ For prevention of rejection of transplanted kidney:
    ▪ Adults—1 gram two times a day.
  ○ For prevention of rejection of transplanted liver:
    ▪ Adults—1 gram two times a day.

Missed dose—If you miss a dose of this medicine, take it as soon as possible. However, if it is almost time for your next dose, skip the missed dose and go back to your regular dosing schedule. Do not double doses.

Call your doctor or pharmacist for instructions.

Storage—Store the medicine in a closed container at room temperature, away from heat, moisture, and direct light. Keep from freezing.

Keep out of the reach of children.

Do not keep outdated medicine or medicine no longer needed.

Precautions While Using This Medicine

It is very important that your doctor check your progress at regular visits. Your doctor will want to do laboratory tests to make sure that mycophenolate is working properly and to check for unwanted effects.

While you are taking mycophenolate, it is important to maintain good dental hygiene and see a dentist regularly for teeth cleaning.

Treatment with mycophenolate may increase the chance of getting other infections. If you can, avoid contact with people with colds or other infections. The effects of mycophenolate may cause increased infections and delayed healing. Dental work, whenever possible, should be completed prior to beginning this medicine. If you think you are getting a cold or other infection, check with your doctor.

It is important that you handle mycophenolate with care. If the medicine gets on your skin, wash thoroughly with soap and water, and if it gets in your eyes, rinse with water. Should a spill occur, wipe it up using paper towels wetted with water to remove the powder or liquid.

The oral suspension expires and should be discarded at 60 days.

Side Effects of This Medicine

Along with its needed effects, a medicine may cause some unwanted effects. Although not all of these side effects may occur, if they do occur they may need medical attention.

Check with your doctor as soon as possible if any of the following side effects occur:
More common
  Blood in the urine; chest pain or discomfort; cough or hoarseness; fever or chills; increased cough; lower back or side pain; painful or difficult urination; shortness of breath; swelling of feet or lower legs
Less common
  Abdominal pain; black, tarry stools; bloody vomit; enlarged gums; irregular heartbeat; joint pain; muscle aches or pain; pinpoint red spots on the skin; red, inflamed, bleeding gums; sores inside mouth; trembling or shaking of hands or feet; unusual bleeding or bruising; white patches on the mouth, tongue, or throat
Incidence not known
  Abdominal distention; blue lips, fingernails, or skin; chronic or occasional diarrhea; confusion; coughing or spitting up blood; difficult or troubled breathing; drowsiness; general feeling of illness or nausea; heart murmur; irregular, fast or slow, or shallow breathing; night sweats; severe headache; sore throat; stiff neck and/or back; stools that float, are foul smelling or "fatty"; sudden high fever or low-grade fever for months; unusual tiredness

Some side effects may occur that usually do not need medical attention. These side effects may go away during treatment as your body adjusts to the medicine. Also, your health care professional may be able to tell you about ways to prevent or reduce some of these side effects. Check with your health care professional if any of the following side effects continue or are bothersome or if you have any questions about them:
More common
  Constipation; diarrhea; headache; heartburn; nausea; stomach pain; vomiting; weakness
Less common
  Acne; dizziness; skin rash; trouble in sleeping

Other side effects not listed may also occur in some patients. If you notice any other effects, check with your healthcare professional.

NADROPARIN (Subcutaneous route) - na-droe-PARE-in

Uses For This Medicine

Nadroparin is used to prevent and treat deep vein thrombosis, a condition in which harmful blood clots form in the blood vessels of the legs. These blood clots can travel to the lungs and can become lodged in the blood vessels of the lungs, causing a condition called pulmonary embolism. Nadroparin is used for several days after surgery, while you are unable to walk. Nadroparin also is used to prevent blood clots from forming during hemodialysis.

This medicine is available only with your doctor's prescription.

Before Using This Medicine

In deciding to use a medicine, the risks of taking the medicine must be weighed against the good it will do. This is a decision

you and your doctor will make. For this medicine, the following should be considered:

Allergies—Tell your doctor if you have ever had any unusual or allergic reaction to this medicine or any other medicines. Also tell your health care professional if you have any other types of allergies, such as to foods, dyes, preservatives, or animals. For non-prescription products, read the label or package ingredients carefully.

Pediatric—Studies on this medicine have been done only in adult patients and there is no specific information comparing use of nadroparin in children with use in other age groups.

Geriatric—This medicine has been tested and has not been shown to cause different side effects or problems in older people than it does in younger adults.

Other medicines—

Using this medicine with any of the following medicines is usually not recommended, but may be required in some cases. If both medicines are prescribed together, your doctor may change the dose or how often you use one or both of the medicines.

Abciximab, Aceclofenac, Acemetacin, Acenocoumarol, Alclofenac, Alteplase, Recombinant, Ancrod, Anisindione, Anistreplase, Antithrombin III Human, Apazone, Ardeparin, Argatroban, Benoxaprofen, Bivalirudin, Bromfenac, Bufexamac, Carprofen, Certoparin, Clometacin, Clonixin, Clopidogrel, Dalteparin, Danaparoid, Defibrotide, Dermatan Sulfate, Desirudin, Dexketoprofen, Diclofenac, Dicumarol, Diflunisal, Dipyrone, Droxicam, Enoxaparin, Eptifibatide, Etodolac, Etofenamate, Felbinac, Fenbufen, Fenoprofen, Fentiazac, Floctafenine, Flufenamic Acid, Flurbiprofen, Fondaparinux, Heparin, Ibuprofen, Indomethacin, Indoprofen, Isoxicam, Ketoprofen, Ketorolac, Lamifiban, Lornoxicam, Meclofenamate, Mefenamic Acid, Meloxicam, Nabumetone, Nadroparin, Naproxen, Niflumic Acid, Nimesulide, Oxaprozin, Oxyphenbutazone, Parnaparin, Pentosan Polysulfate Sodium, Phenindione, Phenprocoumon, Phenylbutazone, Pirazolac, Piroxicam, Pirprofen, Propyphenazone, Proquazone, Reteplase, Recombinant, Reviparin, Sibrafiban, Streptokinase, Sulindac, Suprofen, Tenecteplase, Tenidap, Tenoxicam, Tiaprofenic Acid, Tinzaparin, Tirofiban, Tolmetin, Urokinase, Warfarin, Xemilofiban, Zomepirac

Interactions with Food/Tobacco/Alcohol—Certain medicines should not be used at or around the time of eating food or eating certain types of food since interactions may occur. Using alcohol or tobacco with certain medicines may also cause interactions to occur. Discuss with your healthcare professional the use of your medicine with food, alcohol, or tobacco.

Other medical problems—The presence of other medical problems may affect the use of this medicine. Make sure you tell your doctor if you have any other medical problems, especially:

- Abortion (risk of) or
- Bleeding problems or
- Eye problems caused by diabetes or high blood pressure or
- Heart infection or
- High blood pressure or

- Injury or surgery involving the brain, ears, eyes, or spinal cord or
- Liver disease or
- Low blood platelet count or
- Stomach or intestinal ulcer or
- Stroke—The risk of bleeding may be increased
- Kidney disease—Nadroparin is removed from the body by the kidneys; patients with kidney disease may need to receive a lower dose of nadroparin

Proper Use of This Medicine

If you are using nadroparin at home, your health care professional will teach you how to inject yourself with the medicine. Be sure to follow the directions carefully. Check with your health care professional if you have any problems using the medicine.

Put used syringes in a puncture-resistant, disposable container or dispose of them as directed by your health care professional.

Dosing—The dose of this medicine will be different for different patients. Follow your doctor's orders or the directions on the label. The following information includes only the average doses of this medicine. If your dose is different, do not change it unless your doctor tells you to do so.

The amount of medicine that you take depends on the strength of the medicine. Also, the number of doses you take each day, the time allowed between doses, and the length of time you take the medicine depend on the medical problem for which you are using the medicine.

- For injection dosage form:
  - For unstable angina or certain types of heart attacks:
    - Adults: The dose is based on body weight. It is usually 86 anti-factor Xa International Units (IU) per kilogram (kg) (39.1 anti-factor Xa IU per pound) of body weight injected under the skin every twelve hours for six days.
    - Children: Use and dose must be determined by your doctor.
  - For prevention of deep vein thrombosis (blood clots in the legs) or pulmonary embolism (blood clots in the lungs) after general surgery:
    - Adults: The dose is usually 2850 anti-factor Xa IU injected under the skin once a day beginning two to four hours before surgery and continuing for at least seven days.
    - Children: Use and dose must be determined by your doctor.
  - For prevention of deep vein thrombosis or pulmonary embolism after hip replacement surgery:
    - Adults: The dose is usually 38 anti-factor Xa IU per kg (17.3 anti-factor Xa IU per pound) of body weight injected under the skin twelve hours before surgery, twelve hours after surgery, and once a day for the first three days after surgery. Then, the dose is 57 anti-factor Xa IU per kg (26 anti-factor Xa IU per pound) of body weight injected under the skin once a day from the fourth through the tenth days after surgery.
    - Children: Use and dose must be determined by your doctor.

○ For treatment of deep vein thrombosis:
  ▪ Adults:
    — Patients weighing less than 40 kg (88 pounds) or more than 100 kg (220 pounds): Dose must be determined by your doctor.
    — Patients weighing 40 to 100 kg (88 to 220 pounds): The dose is usually 171 anti-factor Xa IU per kg (77.7 anti-factor Xa IU per pound) of body weight injected under the skin once a day. Or, the dose may be 86 anti-factor Xa IU per kg (39.1 anti-factor Xa IU per pound) of body weight injected under the skin two times a day.
  ▪ Children: Use and dose must be determined by your doctor.
○ For prevention of blood clots during hemodialysis (kidney dialysis):
  ▪ Adults: The dose is usually 65 anti-factor Xa IU per kg (29.5 anti-factor Xa IU per pound) of body weight injected into an artery at the start of each dialysis session.
  ▪ Children: Use and dose must be determined by your doctor.

Storage—Store the medicine in a closed container at room temperature, away from heat, moisture, and direct light. Keep from freezing.

Keep out of the reach of children.

Do not keep outdated medicine or medicine no longer needed.

Ask your healthcare professional how you should dispose of any medicine you do not use.

Precautions While Using This Medicine

Tell all of your medical doctors and dentists that you are using this medicine.

Side Effects of This Medicine

Along with its needed effects, a medicine may cause some unwanted effects. Although not all of these side effects may occur, if they do occur they may need medical attention.

Stop taking this medicine and get emergency help immediately if any of the following effects occur:
More common
Deep, dark purple bruise, pain, or swelling at place of injection
Rare
Back pain; black, tarry stools; bleeding from the mouth or gums; blood in the urine; blue-green to black skin discoloration; bluish discoloration, flushing, or redness of skin; burning, pricking, tickling, or tingling sensation; coughing; difficulty in swallowing; dizziness or feeling faint; fever; hives; itching; leg weakness; nosebleed; numbness; paralysis; problems with bladder or bowel function; redness or sloughing of skin at place of injection; skin rash; small purple or red spots in the mouth, on the gums, or on the skin; swelling of eyelids, face, or lips; tightness in chest, troubled breathing, and/or wheezing; vomiting of blood or coffee ground-like material

Other side effects not listed may also occur in some patients. If you notice any other effects, check with your healthcare professional.

NAFARELIN (Nasal route) - NAF-a-re-lin

Commonly used brand name(s)
In the U.S.—
  Synarel

Available Dosage Forms:
  • Spray

Therapeutic Class: Endocrine-Metabolic Agent
Pharmacologic Class: Luteinizing Hormone Releasing Hormone Agonist

Uses For This Medicine

Nafarelin is a hormone similar to the one normally released from the hypothalamus gland in the brain. It is used in the treatment of:
  • Endometriosis, a painful condition caused by extra tissue similar to the lining of the uterus growing inside and outside of the uterus.
  • Central precocious puberty (CPP), puberty developing too early in boys and girls.

Nafarelin works by decreasing the amount of estrogen and testosterone in the blood.

When given regularly to boys and girls, this medicine helps to prevent them from continuing to develop the sexual features associated with puberty, slowing down the development of breasts in girls and the development of genital areas in boys and girls. This medicine delays puberty in a child only as long as the child continues to take it.

Nafarelin prevents the growth of tissue associated with endometriosis in adult women during treatment and for 6 months after treatment is discontinued. Reducing the amount of estrogen in the body is one way of treating endometriosis.

Suppressing estrogen can thin the bones or slow their growth. This is a problem for adult women whose bones are no longer growing like the bones of children. Slowing the growth of bones is a positive effect for girls and boys whose bones grow too fast when puberty begins too early. This is why nafarelin is used only for up to 6 months in adult women treated for endometriosis, but often is used for a longer time in girls and boys with pubertal problems. Boys and girls may benefit by adding inches to their adult height when nafarelin causes their bones to grow at a proper rate.

Nafarelin is available only with your doctor's prescription.

Before Using This Medicine

In deciding to use a medicine, the risks of taking the medicine must be weighed against the good it will do. This is a decision you and your doctor will make. For this medicine, the following should be considered:

Allergies—Tell your doctor if you have ever had any unusual or allergic reaction to this medicine or any other medicines. Also tell your health care professional if you have any other types of allergies, such as to foods, dyes, preservatives, or animals. For non-prescription products, read the label or package ingredients carefully.

Pediatric—Studies of this medicine for treatment of endometriosis have been done only in adult patients, and there is no specific information comparing use of nafarelin to treat this condition in children younger than 18 years of age with use in other age groups. Endometriosis is not likely to occur before puberty.

When used to treat a child for central precocious puberty, nafarelin will stop having an effect soon after the child stops using it, and puberty will advance normally. It is not known if nafarelin causes:

- Changes in boys' and girls' future abilities to have babies after having used nafarelin around the time of puberty. Their chances of having children later are thought to be normal.
- Problems in the ovaries, such as cysts or a larger than normal ovary. Nafarelin stimulates the ovaries in adult women and has caused these problems in the ovary. It is not known whether nafarelin can also have these effects in younger girls treated for central precocious puberty.

It is especially important that you discuss with the child's doctor the good that this medicine may do as well as the risks of using it.

Pregnancy—

	Pregnancy Category	Explanation
All Trimesters	X	Studies in animals or pregnant women have demonstrated positive evidence of fetal abnormalities. This drug should not be used in women who are or may become pregnant because the risk clearly outweighs any possible benefit.

Breast Feeding—There are no adequate studies in women for determining infant risk when using this medication during breastfeeding. Weigh the potential benefits against the potential risks before taking this medication while breastfeeding.

Other medicines—Although certain medicines should not be used together at all, in other cases two different medicines may be used together even if an interaction might occur. In these cases, your doctor may want to change the dose, or other precautions may be necessary. Tell your healthcare professional if you are taking any other prescription or nonprescription (over-the-counter [OTC]) medicine.

Interactions with Food/Tobacco/Alcohol—Certain medicines should not be used at or around the time of eating food or eating certain types of food since interactions may occur. Using alcohol or tobacco with certain medicines may also cause interactions to occur. Discuss with your healthcare professional the use of your medicine with food, alcohol, or tobacco.

Other medical problems—The presence of other medical problems may affect the use of this medicine. Make sure you tell your doctor if you have any other medical problems, especially:

- Bleeding from the vagina (abnormal or of unknown cause)—For adult women treated for endometriosis or girls treated for central precocious puberty, using nafarelin when the reason for vaginal bleeding is not known may make it harder for the doctor to find the cause of the problem, and may cause a delay in treatment of the condition

- Other conditions that increase the chances of developing thinning bones or osteoporosis (brittle bones)—If you are an adult female being treated for endometriosis, it is important that your doctor knows if you already have an increased risk of osteoporosis. Some things that can increase your risk for having osteoporosis include cigarette smoking, alcohol abuse, and a family history of osteoporosis or easily broken bones. Some medicines, such as corticosteroids (cortisone-like medicines) or anticonvulsants (seizure medicine), can also cause thinning of the bones when used for a long time

Proper Use of This Medicine

You will be given a fact sheet with your prescription for nafarelin that explains how to use the pump spray bottle. If you have any questions about using the pump spray, ask your health care professional.

To use nafarelin spray:

- Before you use each new bottle of nafarelin, the spray pump needs to be started. To do this, point the bottle away from you and pump the bottle firmly about seven times. A spray should come out by the seventh time you pump the spray bottle. This only needs to be done once for each new bottle of nafarelin. Be careful not to breathe in this spray. You could inhale extra doses of nafarelin, since the medicine is dissolved in the spray.
- Before you take your daily doses of nafarelin, blow your nose gently. Hold your head forward a little. Put the spray tip into one nostril. Aim the tip toward the back and outside of your nostril. You do not need to put the tip too far into your nose.
- Close your other nostril off by pressing on the outside of your nose with a finger. Then, sniff in the spray as you pump the bottle once.
- Take the spray bottle out of your nose. Tilt your head back for 30 seconds, to let the spray get onto the back of your nose.
- Repeat these steps for each dose of medicine.
- Each time you use the spray bottle, wipe off the tip with a clean tissue or cloth. Keep the blue safety clip and plastic cap on the bottle when you are not using it.
- Every 3 or 4 days you should clean the tip of the spray bottle. To do this, hold the bottle sideways. Rinse the tip with warm water, while wiping the tip with your finger or a soft cloth for about 15 seconds. Dry the tip with a soft cloth or tissue. Replace the cap right after use. Be careful not to get water into the bottle, since this could dilute the medicine.

It is important to avoid sneezing when spraying and immediately after using the medicine. If you sneeze, the medicine may not be absorbed as well.

Use this medicine only as directed by your doctor. Do not use more or less of it, and do not use it more often than your doctor ordered. The exact amount of medicine you need has been carefully worked out. Using too much may increase the chance of side effects, while using too little may not improve your condition.

Many boys and girls who have central precocious puberty will not feel sick or will not understand the importance of taking the medicine regularly. It is very important that the medicine is used exactly as directed and that the proper amount is used at the proper time. It works best when there is a constant amount in the blood. To help keep the amount constant, nafarelin must be given on a regular schedule.

Dosing—The dose of this medicine will be different for different patients. Follow your doctor's orders or the directions on the label. The following information includes only the average doses of this medicine. If your dose is different, do not change it unless your doctor tells you to do so.

The amount of medicine that you take depends on the strength of the medicine. Also, the number of doses you take each day, the time allowed between doses, and the length of time you take the medicine depend on the medical problem for which you are using the medicine.

- For nasal solution dosage form:
  - For treating central precocious puberty:
    - Children—800 micrograms (mcg) (two sprays into each nostril) two times a day, once in the morning and once in the evening. This provides a total daily dose of eight sprays or 1600 mcg a day. Sometimes a larger dose may be needed. 1800 mcg a day is provided by using three sprays in alternating nostrils three times a day to provide a total of nine sprays a day.
  - For treating endometriosis:
    - Adults—200 mcg (one spray) inhaled into one nostril in the morning and one spray inhaled into the other nostril in the evening, for six months. Begin your treatment on Day 2, 3, or 4 of your menstrual period.

Missed dose—If you miss a dose of this medicine, take it as soon as possible. However, if it is almost time for your next dose, skip the missed dose and go back to your regular dosing schedule. Do not double doses.

Storage—Store the medicine in a closed container at room temperature, away from heat, moisture, and direct light. Keep from freezing.

Keep out of the reach of children.

Do not keep outdated medicine or medicine no longer needed.

The bottle should be stored standing upright, with the tip up.

Precautions While Using This Medicine

All scheduled visits to the doctor should be kept, even if the medicine seems to be working properly and you feel well. This is especially important for children using the medicine for treatment of central precocious puberty, even if their condition improves. Their progress still must be checked by the doctor when they are no longer using the medicine.

For children treated for central precocious puberty—Tell the doctor if nafarelin does not stop puberty from progressing within 6 to 8 weeks. You may notice puberty progressing in your child for the first few weeks of therapy, but you should see signs that puberty is stopping within 4 weeks after your child begins nafarelin therapy.

For adult women treated for endometriosis—
- During the time you are receiving nafarelin, your menstrual period may not be regular or you may not have a menstrual period at all. This is to be expected when being treated with this medicine. If regular menstrual periods do not begin within 2 to 3 months after you stop using this medicine, check with your health care professional.

- To prevent pregnancy if you are sexually active during the time you are using nafarelin, you should use birth control methods that do not contain hormones, such as condoms or a diaphragm or a cervical cap with a spermicide. If you have any questions about this, check with your health care professional.

- Use a water-based vaginal lubricant product if dryness of the vagina causes problems, such as pain during sexual intercourse. Make sure the lubricant you choose can be used with a latex birth control device if you are using one. Some lubricants contain oils, which can break down the latex rubber of condoms, a cervical cap, or a diaphragm, and cause them to rip or tear.

- If you suspect you are pregnant, stop using this medicine and check with your doctor immediately. There is a chance that nafarelin could cause problems to the unborn baby if taken during a pregnancy.

Side Effects of This Medicine

In the first few weeks of therapy, you may notice puberty progressing in your child, including vaginal bleeding and breast enlargement in girls. Within 4 weeks after nafarelin has had time to begin working properly, you should see signs in boys and girls that puberty is stopping. However, pubic hair may continue to show or grow in either boys or girls.

Along with its needed effects, a medicine may cause some unwanted effects. Although not all of these side effects may occur, if they do occur they may need medical attention.

Check with your doctor as soon as possible if any of the following side effects occur:

More common
  For adults (female)
    Breast enlargement; light vaginal bleeding between regular menstrual periods called spotting; longer or heavier menstrual periods; vaginal bleeding between regular menstrual periods called breakthrough bleeding

  For children (male)
    Body odor; growth of pubic hair

  For children (female)
    Body odor; breast enlargement; growth of pubic hair; light vaginal bleeding between regular menstrual periods called spotting; longer or heavier menstrual periods; vaginal bleeding between regular menstrual periods called breakthrough bleeding

Less common or rare
  For adults (female)
    Allergic reaction (shortness of breath, chest pain, hives); fast or irregular heartbeat; numbness or tingling of hands or feet; pain in eyes or joints; patchy brown or dark brown discoloration of skin; pelvic bloating or tenderness; unexpected or excess milk flow from breasts; unusual tiredness or weakness

  For children (male and female)
    Allergic reaction (shortness of breath, chest pain, hives)

Some side effects may occur that usually do not need medical attention. These side effects may go away during treatment as your body adjusts to the medicine. Also, your health care professional may be able to tell you about ways to prevent or reduce some of these side effects. Check with your health care professional if any of the following side effects continue or are bothersome or if you have any questions about them:

More common
For adults (female)
Acne; dandruff; hot flashes; increase or decrease in sexual desire; increased hair growth, often abnormally distributed; mood swings; muscle pain; oily skin; pain during sexual intercourse; rapid weight gain; reduced breast size; stopping of menstrual periods; swelling of feet or lower legs; vaginal dryness

For children (male)
Acne; dandruff; mood swings; oily skin

For children (female)
Acne; dandruff; hot flashes; mood swings; oily skin

Less common or rare
For adults (female)
Breast pain; headache (mild and transient); irritated or runny nose; mental depression (mild and transient); skin rash

For children (male)
Irritated or runny nose

For children (female)
Irritated or runny nose; white or brownish vaginal discharge

Other side effects not listed may also occur in some patients. If you notice any other effects, check with your healthcare professional.

NAPHAZOLINE (Ophthalmic route) -
naf-AZ-oh-leen

Commonly used brand name(s)

In the U.S.—

AK-Con	Naphcon
Albalon	Ocu-Zoline
Allersol	Vasoclear
Clear Eyes	

Available Dosage Forms:

• Gel/Jelly

• Solution

Therapeutic Class: Decongestant
Pharmacologic Class: Alpha-Adrenergic Agonist

Uses For This Medicine

Naphazoline is used to relieve redness due to minor eye irritations, such as those caused by colds, dust, wind, smog, pollen, swimming, or wearing contact lenses.

Some of these preparations are available only with your doctor's prescription.

Before Using This Medicine

In deciding to use a medicine, the risks of taking the medicine must be weighed against the good it will do. This is a decision you and your doctor will make. For this medicine, the following should be considered:

Allergies—Tell your doctor if you have ever had any unusual or allergic reaction to this medicine or any other medicines. Also tell your health care professional if you have any other types of allergies, such as to foods, dyes, preservatives, or animals. For non-prescription products, read the label or package ingredients carefully.

Pediatric—Use by infants and children is not recommended, since they are especially sensitive to the effects of naphazoline.

Geriatric—Many medicines have not been studied specifically in older people. Therefore, it may not be known whether they work exactly the same way they do in younger adults or if they cause different side effects or problems in older people. There is no specific information comparing use of naphazoline in the elderly with use in other age groups.

Pregnancy—

	Pregnancy Category	Explanation
All Trimesters	C	Animal studies have shown an adverse effect and there are no adequate studies in pregnant women OR no animal studies have been conducted and there are no adequate studies in pregnant women.

Breast Feeding—There are no adequate studies in women for determining infant risk when using this medication during breastfeeding. Weigh the potential benefits against the potential risks before taking this medication while breastfeeding.

Other medicines—Although certain medicines should not be used together at all, in other cases two different medicines may be used together even if an interaction might occur. In these cases, your doctor may want to change the dose, or other precautions may be necessary. Tell your healthcare professional if you are taking any other prescription or non-prescription (over-the-counter [OTC]) medicine.

Interactions with Food/Tobacco/Alcohol—Certain medicines should not be used at or around the time of eating food or eating certain types of food since interactions may occur. Using alcohol or tobacco with certain medicines may also cause interactions to occur. Discuss with your healthcare professional the use of your medicine with food, alcohol, or tobacco.

Other medical problems—The presence of other medical problems may affect the use of this medicine. Make sure you tell your doctor if you have any other medical problems, especially:

• Type 2 diabetes mellitus or

• Heart disease or

• High blood pressure or

• Overactive thyroid—Use of ophthalmic naphazoline may make the condition worse

• Eye disease, infection, or injury—The symptoms of the condition may be confused with possible side effects of ophthalmic naphazoline

Proper Use of This Medicine

Do not use naphazoline ophthalmic solution if it becomes cloudy or changes color.

Naphazoline should not be used in infants and children. It may cause severe slowing down of the central nervous system (CNS), which may lead to unconsciousness. It may also cause a severe decrease in body temperature.

Use this medicine only as directed. Do not use more of it, do not use it more often, and do not use it for more than 72 hours, unless otherwise directed by your doctor. To do so may make your eye redness and irritation worse and may also increase the chance of side effects.

To use:

- First, wash your hands. With the middle finger, apply pressure to the inside corner of the eye (and continue to apply pressure for 1 or 2 minutes after the medicine has been placed in the eye). Tilt the head back and with the index finger of the same hand, pull the lower eyelid away from the eye to form a pouch. Drop the medicine into the pouch and gently close the eyes. Do not blink. Keep the eyes closed for 1 or 2 minutes to allow the medicine to be absorbed.
- To keep the medicine as germ-free as possible, do not touch the applicator tip to any surface (including the eye). Also, keep the container tightly closed.

Dosing—The dose of this medicine will be different for different patients. Follow your doctor's orders or the directions on the label. The following information includes only the average doses of this medicine. If your dose is different, do not change it unless your doctor tells you to do so.

The amount of medicine that you take depends on the strength of the medicine. Also, the number of doses you take each day, the time allowed between doses, and the length of time you take the medicine depend on the medical problem for which you are using the medicine.

- For ophthalmic solution (eye drop) dosage form:
  ○ For eye redness:
    - Adults—Use one drop not more often than every four hours.
    - Children—Use is not recommended.

Storage—Store the medicine in a closed container at room temperature, away from heat, moisture, and direct light. Keep from freezing.

Keep out of the reach of children.

Do not keep outdated medicine or medicine no longer needed.

Precautions While Using This Medicine

If eye pain or change in vision occurs or if redness or irritation of the eye continues, gets worse, or lasts for more than 72 hours, stop using the medicine and check with your doctor.

Side Effects of This Medicine

Along with its needed effects, a medicine may cause some unwanted effects. Although not all of these side effects may occur, if they do occur they may need medical attention.

Check with your doctor as soon as possible if any of the following side effects occur:

With overuse or long-term use
  Increase in eye irritation

Symptoms of too much medicine being absorbed into the body
  Dizziness; headache; increased sweating; nausea; nervousness; weakness

Symptoms of overdose
  Decrease in body temperature; drowsiness; slow heartbeat; weakness (severe)

Some side effects may occur that usually do not need medical attention. These side effects may go away during treatment as your body adjusts to the medicine. Also, your health care professional may be able to tell you about ways to prevent or reduce some of these side effects. Check with your health care professional if any of the following side effects continue or are bothersome or if you have any questions about them:

Less common or rare
  Blurred vision; large pupils

Other side effects not listed may also occur in some patients. If you notice any other effects, check with your healthcare professional.

NARATRIPTAN   (Oral route) - NAR-a-trip-tan

Commonly used brand name(s)

In the U.S.—
  Amerge

Available Dosage Forms:
- Tablet

Therapeutic Class: Antimigraine
Pharmacologic Class: Serotonin Receptor Agonist, 5–HT1

Uses For This Medicine

Naratriptan is used to treat severe migraine headaches. Many people find that their headaches go away completely after they take naratriptan. Other people find that their headaches are much less painful, and that they are able to go back to their normal activities even though their headaches are not completely gone. Naratriptan often relieves symptoms that occur together with a migraine headache, such as nausea, vomiting, sensitivity to light, and sensitivity to sound.

Naratriptan is not an ordinary pain reliever. It should not be used to relieve any kind of pain other than migraine headaches.

Naratriptan may cause serious side effects in some people, especially people who have heart or blood vessel disease. Be sure that you discuss with your doctor the risks of using this medicine as well as the good that it can do.

Naratriptan is available only with your doctor's prescription.

Before Using This Medicine

In deciding to use a medicine, the risks of taking the medicine must be weighed against the good it will do. This is a decision you and your doctor will make. For this medicine, the following should be considered:

Allergies—Tell your doctor if you have ever had any unusual or allergic reaction to this medicine or any other medicines. Also tell your health care professional if you have any other types of allergies, such as to foods, dyes, preservatives, or animals. For non-prescription products, read the label or package ingredients carefully.

Pediatric—This medicine has been tested in a limited number of children 12 years of age or older. In effective doses, the medicine has not been shown to cause different side effects or problems than it does in adults.

Geriatric—Although there is no specific information comparing the use of naratriptan in the elderly with use in other age groups, use of this medicine is not recommended in older adults.

Pregnancy—

	Pregnancy Category	Explanation
All Trimesters	C	Animal studies have shown an adverse effect and there are no adequate studies in pregnant women OR no animal studies have been conducted and there are no adequate studies in pregnant women.

Breast Feeding—There are no adequate studies in women for determining infant risk when using this medication during breastfeeding. Weigh the potential benefits against the potential risks before taking this medication while breastfeeding.

Other medicines—

Using this medicine with any of the following medicines is not recommended. Your doctor may decide not to treat you with this medication or change some of the other medicines you take.

Almotriptan, Dihydroergotamine, Ergoloid Mesylates, Ergonovine, Ergotamine, Frovatriptan, Methylergonovine, Methysergide, Rizatriptan, Sumatriptan, Zolmitriptan

Interactions with Food/Tobacco/Alcohol—Certain medicines should not be used at or around the time of eating food or eating certain types of food since interactions may occur. Using alcohol or tobacco with certain medicines may also cause interactions to occur. Discuss with your healthcare professional the use of your medicine with food, alcohol, or tobacco.

Other medical problems—The presence of other medical problems may affect the use of this medicine. Make sure you tell your doctor if you have any other medical problems, especially:

- Angina (chest pain) or
- Heart or blood vessel disease or
- High blood pressure or
- Kidney disease or
- Liver disease or
- Stroke (history of)—The chance of side effects may be increased. Heart or blood vessel disease and high blood pressure sometimes do not cause any symptoms, so some people do not know that they have these problems. Before deciding whether you should use naratriptan, your doctor may need to do some tests to make sure that you do not have any of these conditions.

Proper Use of This Medicine

Do not use naratriptan for a headache that is different from your usual migraines. Instead, check with your doctor.

To relieve your migraine as soon as possible, use naratriptan as soon as the headache pain begins. Even if you get warning signals of a coming migraine (an aura), you should wait until the headache pain starts before using naratriptan.

Lying down in a quiet, dark room for a while after you use this medicine may help relieve your migraine.

Ask your doctor ahead of time about any other medicine you may take if naratriptan does not work. After you take the other medicine, check with your doctor as soon as possible. Headaches that are not relieved by naratriptan are sometimes caused by conditions that need other treatment.

If you feel much better after a dose of naratriptan, but your headache comes back or gets worse after a while, you may use more naratriptan. However, use this medicine only as directed by your doctor. Do not use more of it, and do not use it more often, than directed. Using too much naratriptan may increase the chance of side effects.

Your doctor may direct you to take another medicine to help prevent headaches. It is important that you follow your doctor's directions, even if your headaches continue to occur. Headache-preventing medicines may take several weeks to start working. Even after they do start working, your headaches may not go away completely. However, your headaches should occur less often, and they should be less severe and easier to relieve. This can reduce the amount of naratriptan or other pain medicines that you need. If you do not notice any improvement after several weeks of headache-preventing treatment, check with your doctor.

Dosing—The dose of this medicine will be different for different patients. Follow your doctor's orders or the directions on the label. The following information includes only the average doses of this medicine. If your dose is different, do not change it unless your doctor tells you to do so.

The amount of medicine that you take depends on the strength of the medicine. Also, the number of doses you take each day, the time allowed between doses, and the length of time you take the medicine depend on the medical problem for which you are using the medicine.

- For oral dosage form (tablets):
  - For migraine headaches:
    - Adults—1 or 2.5 mg as a single dose. If the migraine comes back after being relieved, another dose may be taken four hours after the last dose. Do not take more than 5 mg in any twenty-four-hour period (one day). Patients with kidney or liver disease should take less than 2.5 mg as a single

dose once daily and should not exceed 2.5 mg in a twenty-four-hour period.

- Children—Use and dose must be determined by your doctor.

Storage—Store the medicine in a closed container at room temperature, away from heat, moisture, and direct light. Keep from freezing.

Keep out of the reach of children.

Do not keep outdated medicine or medicine no longer needed.

Precautions While Using This Medicine

Drinking alcoholic beverages can make headaches worse or cause new headaches to occur. People who suffer from severe headaches should probably avoid alcoholic beverages, especially during a headache.

Some people feel drowsy or dizzy during or after a migraine, or after taking naratriptan to relieve a migraine. As long as you are feeling drowsy or dizzy, do not drive, use machines, or do anything else that could be dangerous if you are dizzy or are not alert.

Side Effects of This Medicine

Along with its needed effects, a medicine may cause some unwanted effects. Although not all of these side effects may occur, if they do occur they may need medical attention.

Stop taking this medicine and get emergency help immediately if any of the following effects occur:

More common
Chest pain (severe); heaviness, tightness, or pressure in chest, throat, and/or neck; sensation of burning, warmth, heat, numbness, tightness, or tingling

Less common or rare
Convulsions (seizures); irregular heartbeat; slow heartbeat

Other side effects may occur that usually do not need medical attention. Some of the following effects, such as nausea, vomiting, drowsiness, dizziness, and general feeling of illness or tiredness, often occur during or after a migraine, even when naratriptan has not been used. However, check with your doctor if any of the following side effects continue or are bothersome:

More common
Dizziness; drowsiness; increased tiredness; nausea and/or vomiting

Less common or rare
Acne; anxiety; blurred vision; bone or skeletal pain; change in taste sensation; chills and/or fever; confusion; constipation; diarrhea; difficulty sleeping; eye problems; fainting; fluid imbalance; increased thirst; itching of the skin; joint pain; mood or mental changes; muscle or joint stiffness, tightness, or rigidity; muscle pain or spasms; pounding heartbeat; restlessness; skin rash; stomach discomfort and/or pain; sudden large increase in frequency and amount of urine; trembling or shaking of hands or feet; unusual tiredness or weakness

Other side effects not listed may also occur in some patients. If you notice any other effects, check with your healthcare professional.

NARCOTIC ANALGESICS—FOR PAIN RELIEF (Systemic)

Some commonly used brand names are:

In the U.S.—

Astramorph PF (10)	MS/L Concentrate (10)
AVINZA (10)	MS/S (10)
Buprenex (2)	Nubain (11)
Cotanal-65 (16)	Numorphan (14)
Darvon (16)	OMS Concentrate (10)
Darvon-N (16)	Oramorph SR (10)
Demerol (8)	OxyContin (13)
Dilaudid (6)	PP-Cap (16)
Dilaudid-5 (6)	Rescudose (10)
Dilaudid-HP (6)	RMS Uniserts (10)
Dolophine (9)	Roxanol (10)
Duramorph (10)	Roxanol 100 (10)
Hydrostat IR (6)	Roxanol UD (10)
Kadian (10)	Roxicodone (13)
Levo-Dromoran (7)	Roxicodone Intensol (13)
Methadose (9)	Stadol (3)
M S Contin (10)	Talwin (15)
MSIR (10)	Talwin-Nx (15)
MS/L (10)	

In Canada—

Darvon-N (16)	MS´IR (10)
Demerol (8)	Nubain (11)
Dilaudid (6)	Numorphan (14)
Dilaudid-HP (6)	Oramorph SR (10)
Epimorph (10)	OxyContin (13)
Hycodan (5)	Pantopon (12)
Kadian (10)	Paveral (4)
Leritine (1)	PMS-Hydromorphone (6)
Levo-Dromoran (7)	PMS-Hydromorphone Syrup
M-Eslon (10)	(6)
Morphine Extra-Forte (10)	Robidone (5)
Morphine Forte (10)	642 (16)
Morphine H.P. (10)	Statex (10)
Morphitec (10)	Statex Drops (10)
M.O.S. (10)	Supeudol (13)
M.O.S.-S.R. (10)	Talwin (15)
M S Contin (10)	

This information applies to the following medicines:

1. Anileridine (an-i-LER-i-deen))
2. Buprenorphine (byoo-pre-NOR-feen)
3. Butorphanol (byoo-TOR-fa-nole)
4. Codeine (KOE-deen)
5. Hydrocodone (hye-droe-KOE-done)
6. Hydromorphone (hye-droe-MOR-fone)
7. Levorphanol (lee-VOR-fa-nole)
8. Meperidine (me-PER-i-deen)
9. Methadone (METH-a-done)
10. Morphine (MOR-feen)
11. Nalbuphine (NAL-byoo-feen)
12. Opium Injection (OH-pee-um)
13. Oxycodone (ox-i-KOE-done)
14. Oxymorphone (ox-i-MOR-fone)
15. Pentazocine (pen-TAZ-oh-seen)
16. Propoxyphene (proe-POX-i-feen)

Category

- **Analgesic**—Anileridine; Buprenorphine; Butorphanol; Codeine; Hydrocodone; Hydromorphone; Levorphanol; Meperidine; Methadone; Morphine; Nalbuphine; Opium Injection; Oxycodone; Oxymorphone; Pentazocine; Propoxyphene

- **Anesthesia adjunct**—Anileridine; Buprenorphine

- **Anesthesia adjunct, opioid analgesic**—Butorphanol; Hydromorphone; Levorphanol; Meperidine; Morphine; Nalbuphine; Oxymorphone; Pentazocine
- **Antidiarrheal**—Codeine; Morphine
- **Antitussive**—Codeine; Hydrocodone; Hydromorphone; Methadone; Morphine
- **Pulmonary edema therapy adjunct**—Morphine
- **Suppressant, narcotic abstinence syndrome**—Methadone

Description

Narcotic (nar-KOT-ik) analgesics (an-al-JEE-zicks) are used to relieve pain. Some of these medicines are also used just before or during an operation to help the anesthetic work better. Codeine and hydrocodone are also used to relieve coughing. Methadone is also used to help some people control their dependence on heroin or other narcotics. Narcotic analgesics may also be used for other conditions as determined by your doctor.

Narcotic analgesics act in the central nervous system (CNS) to relieve pain. Some of their side effects are also caused by actions in the CNS.

If a narcotic is used for a long time, it may become habit-forming (causing mental or physical dependence). Physical dependence may lead to withdrawal side effects when you stop taking the medicine.

These medicines are available only with your medical doctor's or dentist's prescription. For some of them, prescriptions cannot be refilled and you must obtain a new prescription from your medical doctor or dentist each time you need the medicine. In addition, other rules and regulations may apply when methadone is used to treat narcotic dependence.

These medicines are available in the following dosage forms:

Oral
- Anileridine
  - Tablets
- Codeine
  - Oral solution
  - Tablets
- Hydrocodone
  - Syrup
  - Tablets
- Hydromorphone
  - Extended-release capsule
  - Oral solution
  - Tablets
- Levorphanol
  - Tablets
- Meperidine
  - Syrup
  - Tablets
- Methadone
  - Oral concentrate
  - Oral solution
  - Tablets
  - Dispersible tablets
- Morphine
  - Capsules
  - Extended-release capsules
  - Oral solution
  - Syrup

- Tablets
  - Extended-release tablets
- Oxycodone
  - Oral solution
  - Tablets
  - Extended-release tablets
- Pentazocine
  - Tablets
- Pentazocine and Naloxone
  - Tablets
- Propoxyphene
  - Capsules
  - Oral suspension
  - Tablets

Parenteral
- Buprenorphine
  - Injection
- Butorphanol
  - Injection
- Codeine
  - Injection
- Hydromorphone
  - Injection
- Levorphanol
  - Injection
- Meperidine
  - Injection
- Methadone
  - Injection
- Morphine
  - Injection
- Nalbuphine
  - Injection
- Opium
  - Injection
- Oxymorphone
  - Injection
- Pentazocine
  - Injection

Rectal
- Hydromorphone
  - Suppositories
- Morphine
  - Suppositories
- Oxycodone
  - Suppositories
- Oxymorphone
  - Suppositories

Before Using This Medicine

In deciding to use a medicine, the risks of taking the medicine must be weighed against the good it will do. This is a decision you and your doctor will make. For narcotic analgesics, the following should be considered:

Allergies—Tell your doctor if you have ever had any unusual or allergic reaction to any of the narcotic analgesics. Also tell your health care professional if you are allergic to any other substances, such as foods, preservatives, or dyes.

Pregnancy—Although studies on birth defects with narcotic analgesics have not been done in pregnant women, these medicines have not been reported to cause birth defects. However, hydrocodone, hydromorphone, and morphine caused birth defects in animals when given in very large doses. Buprenorphine and codeine did not cause birth defects in animal studies, but they caused other unwanted effects. Butorphanol, nalbuphine, pentazocine, and propoxyphene did not cause birth defects in animals. There is no information about whether other narcotic analgesics cause birth defects in animals.

Too much use of a narcotic during pregnancy may cause the baby to become dependent on the medicine. This may lead to withdrawal side effects after birth. Also, some of these medicines may cause breathing problems in the newborn infant if taken just before delivery.

Breast-feeding—Most narcotic analgesics have not been reported to cause problems in nursing babies. However, when the mother is taking large amounts of methadone (in a methadone maintenance program), the nursing baby may become dependent on the medicine. Also, butorphanol, codeine, meperidine, morphine, opium, and propoxyphene pass into the breast milk.

Children—Breathing problems may be especially likely to occur in children younger than 2 years of age. These children are usually more sensitive than adults to the effects of narcotic analgesics. Also, unusual excitement or restlessness may be more likely to occur in children receiving these medicines. Hydromorphone extended-release capsules should not be used in children younger than 18 years of age.

Older adults—Elderly people are especially sensitive to the effects of narcotic analgesics. This may increase the chance of side effects, especially breathing problems, during treatment.

Other medicines—Although certain medicines should not be used together at all, in other cases two different medicines may be used together even if an interaction might occur. In these cases, your doctor may want to change the dose, or other precautions may be necessary. When you are taking a narcotic analgesic, it is especially important that your health care professional know if you are taking any of the following:

- Carbamazepine (e.g., Tegretol)—Propoxyphene may increase the blood levels of carbamazepine, which increases the chance of serious side effects
- Central nervous system (CNS) depressants or
- Monoamine oxidase (MAO) inhibitor activity (isocarboxazid [e.g., Marplan], phenelzine [e.g., Nardil], procarbazine [e.g., Matulane], tranylcypromine [e.g., Parnate] (taken currently or within the past 2 weeks) or
- Tricyclic antidepressants (amitriptyline [e.g., Elavil], amoxapine [e.g., Asendin], clomipramine [e.g., Anafranil], desipramine [e.g., Pertofrane], doxepin [e.g., Sinequan], imipramine [e.g., Tofranil], nortriptyline [e.g., Aventyl], protriptyline [e.g., Vivactil], trimipramine [e.g., Surmontil])—The chance of side effects may be increased; the combination of meperidine (e.g., Demerol) and MAO inhibitors is especially dangerous
- Naltrexone (e.g., Trexan)—Narcotics will not be effective in people taking naltrexone
- Rifampin (e.g., Rifadin)—Rifampin decreases the effects of methadone and may cause withdrawal symptoms in people who are dependent on methadone

- Zidovudine (e.g., AZT, Retrovir)—Morphine may increase the blood levels of zidovudine and increase the chance of serious side effects

Other medical problems—The presence of other medical problems may affect the use of narcotic analgesics. Make sure you tell your doctor if you have any other medical problems, especially:

- Alcohol abuse, or history of, or
- Drug dependence, especially narcotic abuse, or history of, or
- Emotional problems—The chance of side effects may be increased; also, withdrawal symptoms may occur if a narcotic you are dependent on is replaced by buprenorphine, butorphanol, nalbuphine, or pentazocine
- Brain disease or head injury or
- Emphysema, asthma, or other chronic lung disease or
- Enlarged prostate or problems with urination or
- Gallbladder disease or gallstones—Some of the side effects of narcotic analgesics can be dangerous if these conditions are present
- Colitis or
- Heart disease or
- Kidney disease or
- Liver disease or
- Underactive thyroid—The chance of side effects may be increased
- Convulsions (seizures), history of—Some of the narcotic analgesics can cause convulsions

Proper Use of This Medicine

Some narcotic analgesics given by injection may be given at home to patients who do not need to be in the hospital. If you are using an injection form of this medicine at home, *make sure you clearly understand and carefully follow your doctor's instructions.*

To take *long-acting hydromorphone capsules:*

- *These capsules must be swallowed whole.* Do not chew, crush or dissolve.
- If the capsules is not swallowed whole, you could overdose on this medicine.
- Check with your doctor right away if you are not sure how to take extended-release hydromorphone capsules.

To take the *syrup form of meperidine:*

- Unless otherwise directed by your medical doctor or dentist, *take this medicine mixed with a half glass (4 ounces) of water* to lessen the numbing effect of the medicine on your mouth and throat.

To take the *oral liquid forms of methadone:*

- *This medicine may have to be mixed with water or another liquid before you take it.* Read the label carefully for directions. If you have any questions about this, check with your health care professional.

To take the *dispersible tablet form of methadone:*

- *These tablets must be stirred into water or fruit juice just before each dose is taken. Read the label carefully for directions.* If you have any questions about this, check with your health care professional.

To take *oral liquid forms of morphine:*

- This medicine may be mixed with a glass of fruit juice just before you take it, if desired, to improve the taste.

To take *long-acting morphine and oxycodone tablets:*

- *These tablets must be swallowed whole.* Do not break, crush, or chew them before swallowing.

To take *long-acting morphine capsules:*

- *These capsules must be swallowed whole.* Do not chew, crush or dissolve.
- Or, the capsule can be opened and all of the beads inside sprinkled over applesauce and used right away. *The beads must not be chewed, crushed, or dissolved.*
- If capsules or beads from the capsules are not swallowed whole, you could overdose on this medicine.
- Check with your doctor right away if you are not sure how to take long-acting morphine capsules.

To use *suppositories:*

- If the suppository is too soft to insert, chill it in the refrigerator for 30 minutes or run cold water over it before removing the foil wrapper.
- To insert the suppository: First remove the foil wrapper and moisten the suppository with cold water. Lie down on your side and use your finger to push the suppository well up into the rectum.

Take this medicine only as directed by your medical doctor or dentist. Do not take more of it, do not take it more often, and do not take it for a longer time than your medical doctor or dentist ordered. This is especially important for young children and elderly patients, who are especially sensitive to the effects of narcotic analgesics. If too much is taken, the medicine may become habit-forming (causing mental or physical dependence) or lead to medical problems because of an overdose.

If you think this medicine is not working properly after you have been taking it for a few weeks, *do not increase the dose.* Instead, check with your doctor.

Dosing—The dose of these medicines will be different for different patients. *Follow your doctor's orders or the directions on the label.* The following information includes only the average doses of these medicines. *If your dose is different, do not change it* unless your doctor tells you to do so.

The number of capsules or tablets or teaspoonfuls of oral solution or syrup that you take, or the amount of injection that you are directed to use, depends on the strength of the medicine. Also, *the number of doses you take each day, the time allowed between doses, and the length of time you take the medicine depend on the narcotic you are taking, whether or not you are taking a long-acting form of the medicine, and the reason you are taking the medicine.*

For anileridine
- For *oral* dosage form:
  - For pain
    - Adults and teenagers—25 to 50 milligrams (mg) every 6 hours as needed.
    - Children up to 13 years of age—Dose must be determined by your doctor.

For buprenorphine
- For *injection* dosage form:
  - For pain:
    - Adults and teenagers—0.3 milligrams (mg), injected into a muscle or a vein every six hours as needed.
    - Children up to 2 years of age—Dose must be determined by your doctor.
    - Children 2 to 12 years of age—0.002 to 0.006 mg per kilogram (kg) (0.0008 to 0.0024 mg per pound) of body weight, injected into a muscle or a vein every four to six hours as needed.

For butorphanol
- For *injection* dosage form:
  - For pain:
    - Adults—1 to 4 milligrams (mg) (usually 2 mg), injected into a muscle every three or four hours as needed. Some people may receive 0.5 to 2 mg (usually 1 mg) injected into a vein every three or four hours as needed.
    - Children and teenagers—Dose must be determined by your doctor.

For codeine
- For *oral* dosage forms (oral solution or tablets):
  - For pain:
    - Adults—15 to 60 milligrams (mg) (usually 30 mg) every three to six hours as needed.
    - Children—0.5 mg per kilogram (kg) (0.2 mg per pound) of body weight every four to six hours as needed. Young children will probably take the oral solution, rather than tablets. Small doses may need to be measured by a special dropper instead of a teaspoon.
  - For cough:
    - Adults—10 to 20 mg every four to six hours.
    - Children up to 2 years of age—Use is not recommended.
    - Children 2 years of age—3 mg every four to six hours, up to a maximum of 12 mg a day. Children this young will probably take the oral solution, rather than tablets. Small doses may need to be measured by a special dropper instead of a teaspoon.
    - Children 3 years of age—3.5 mg every four to six hours, up to a maximum of 14 mg a day. Children this young will probably take the oral solution, rather than tablets. Small doses may need to be measured by a special dropper instead of a teaspoon.
    - Children 4 years of age—4 mg every four to six hours, up to a maximum of 16 mg a day. Children this young will probably take the oral solution, rather than tablets. Small doses may need to be measured by a special dropper instead of a teaspoon.
    - Children 5 years of age—4.5 mg every four to six hours, up to a maximum of 18 mg a day. Children this young will probably take the oral solution, rather than tablets. Small doses may need to be measured by a special dropper instead of a teaspoon.
    - Children 6 to 12 years of age—5 to 10 mg every four to six hours, up to a maximum of 60 mg a day.

- For *injection* dosage form:
  - For pain:
    - Adults—15 to 60 mg (usually 30 mg), injected into a muscle or a vein or under the skin every four to six hours as needed.
    - Children—0.5 mg per kg (0.2 mg per pound) of body weight, injected into a muscle or under the skin every four to six hours as needed.

For hydrocodone
- For *oral* dosage form (syrup or tablets):
  - For pain:
    - Adults—5 to 10 milligrams (mg) every four to six hours as needed.
    - Children—0.15 mg per kilogram (kg) (0.06 mg per pound) of body weight every six hours as needed.
  - For cough:
    - Adults—5 mg every four to six hours as needed.
    - Children—Dose must be determined by your doctor.

For hydromorphone
- For *short-acting oral* dosage form (oral solution or tablets):
  - For pain:
    - Adults—2 or 2.5 milligrams (mg) every three to six hours as needed.
    - Children—Dose must be determined by your doctor.
- For *long-acting oral* dosage forms (extended-release capsules):
  - For severe, chronic pain (severe pain that lasts a long time):
    - Adults—Long-acting forms of hydromorphone are usually used for patients who have already been receiving narcotics to relieve pain. The starting dose will depend on the amount of narcotic you have been receiving every day. Your doctor will then adjust the dose according to your individual needs. To be helpful, these medicines need to be taken at regularly scheduled times according to your doctor's instructions. It is important that you take the dose at the time and as often as your doctor tells you.
    - Children—Dose must be determined by your doctor.
- For *injection* dosage form:
  - For pain:
    - Adults—1 or 2 mg, injected into a muscle or under the skin every three to six hours as needed. Some people may receive 0.5 mg, injected slowly into a vein every three hours as needed.
    - Children—Dose must be determined by your doctor.
- For *rectal suppository* dosage form:
  - For pain:
    - Adults—3 mg every four to eight hours as needed.
    - Children—Dose must be determined by your doctor.

For levorphanol
- For *oral* dosage form (tablets):
  - For pain:
    - Adults—2 milligrams (mg). Some people with severe pain may need 3 or 4 mg.

- Children—Dose must be determined by your doctor.
- For *injection* dosage form:
  - For pain:
    - Adults—2 mg, injected under the skin or into a vein. Some people may need 3 mg.
    - Children—Dose must be determined by your doctor.

For meperidine
- For *oral* dosage form (syrup or tablets):
  - For pain:
    - Adults—50 to 150 milligrams (mg) (usually 100 mg) every three or four hours as needed.
    - Children—1.1 to 1.76 mg per kilogram (kg) (0.44 to 0.8 mg per pound) of body weight, up to a maximum of 100 mg, every three or four hours as needed. Young children will probably take the syrup, rather than tablets. Small doses may need to be measured by a special dropper instead of a teaspoon.
- For *injection* dosage form:
  - For pain:
    - Adults—50 to 150 milligrams (mg) (usually 100 mg), injected into a muscle or under the skin every three or four hours as needed. The medicine may also be injected continuously into a vein at a rate of 15 to 35 mg an hour.
    - Children—1.1 to 1.76 mg per kg (0.44 to 0.8 mg per pound) of body weight, up to a maximum of 100 mg, injected into a muscle or under the skin every three or four hours as needed.

For methadone
- For *oral solution* dosage form:
  - For pain:
    - Adults—5 to 20 mg every four to eight hours.
    - Children—Dose must be determined by your doctor.
  - For narcotic addiction:
    - Adults 18 years of age or older—
      - For detoxification: At first, 15 to 40 mg once a day. Your doctor will gradually decrease the dose you take every day until you do not need the medicine any more.
      - For maintenance: Dose must be determined by the needs of the individual patient, up to a maximum of 120 mg a day.
    - Children up to 18 years of age—Special conditions must be met before methadone can be used for narcotic addiction in patients younger than 18 years of age. Use and dose must be determined by your doctor.
- For *oral tablet* dosage form:
  - For pain:
    - Adults—2.5 to 10 mg every three or four hours as needed.
    - Children—Dose must be determined by your doctor.
  - For narcotic addiction:
    - Adults 18 years of age or older—
      - For detoxification: At first, 15 to 40 mg once a day. Your doctor will gradually decrease the dose you take every day until you do not need the medicine any more.

— For maintenance: Dose must be determined by the needs of the individual patient, up to a maximum of 120 mg a day.

- Children up to 18 years of age—Special conditions must be met before methadone can be used for narcotic addiction in patients younger than 18 years of age. Use and dose must be determined by your doctor.

- For *injection* dosage form:
  ○ For pain:
    ▪ Adults—2.5 to 10 mg, injected into a muscle or under the skin, every three or four hours as needed.
    ▪ Children—Dose must be determined by your doctor.
  ○ For narcotic addiction:
    ▪ Adults 18 years of age and older—For detoxification only, in patients unable to take medicine by mouth: At first, 15 to 40 mg a day. Your doctor will gradually decrease the dose you receive every day until you do not need the medicine any more.
    ▪ Children younger than 18 years of age—Use and dose must be determined by your doctor.

For morphine
- For *short-acting oral* dosage forms (capsules, oral solution, syrup, or tablets):
  ○ For severe, chronic pain (severe pain that lasts a long time):
    ▪ Adults—At first, 10 to 30 milligrams (mg) every four hours. Your doctor will then adjust the dose according to your individual needs. If you have already been taking other narcotics to relieve severe, chronic pain, your starting dose will depend on the amount of other narcotic you were taking every day.
    ▪ Children—Dose must be determined by your doctor.
- For *long-acting oral* dosage forms (extended-release capsules or tablets):
  ○ For severe, chronic pain (severe pain that lasts a long time):
    ▪ Adults—Long-acting forms of morphine are usually used for patients who have already been receiving narcotics to relieve pain. The starting dose will depend on the amount of narcotic you have been receiving every day. Your doctor will then adjust the dose according to your individual needs. To be helpful, these medicines need to be taken at regularly scheduled times according to your doctor's instructions. It is important that you take the dose at the time and as often as your doctor tells you. Some people may need to take a short-acting form of morphine if breakthrough pain occurs between doses of the long-acting medicine.
    ▪ Children—Dose must be determined by your doctor.
- For once daily *long-acting oral* dosage forms (extended-release capsules):
  ○ For severe, chronic pain (severe pain that lasts a long time):
    ▪ Adults—Long-acting forms of morphine are usually used for patients who have already been receiving narcotics to relieve pain. The starting dose will depend on the amount of narcotic you have

been receiving every day. Your doctor will then adjust the dose according to your individual needs. To be helpful, these medicines need to be taken once a day at regularly scheduled times according to your doctor's instructions. It is important that you take the dose at the time and as often as your doctor tells you. Some people may need to take a short-acting form of morphine if breakthrough pain occurs between doses of the long-acting medicine.
    ▪ Children—Dose must be determined by your doctor.
- For *injection* dosage form:
  ○ For pain:
    ▪ Adults—5 to 20 mg (usually 10 mg), injected into a muscle or under the skin every four hours as needed. Some people may receive 4 to 10 mg, injected slowly into a vein. Morphine may also be injected continuously into a vein or under the skin at a rate that depends on the needs of the patient. This medicine may also be injected into the spinal area. The dose will depend on where and how the medicine is injected into the spinal area and on the needs of the patient.
    ▪ Children—0.1 to 0.2 mg per kg (0.04 or 0.09 mg per pound) of body weight, up to a maximum of 15 mg, injected under the skin every four hours as needed. Some patients may receive 0.05 to 0.1 mg per kg (0.02 to 0.04 mg per pound) of body weight, injected slowly into a vein.
- For *rectal suppository* dosage form:
  ○ For pain:
    ▪ Adults—10 to 30 mg every four to six hours as needed.
    ▪ Children—Dose must be determined by your doctor.

For nalbuphine
- For *injection* dosage form:
  ○ For pain:
    ▪ Adults—10 milligrams (mg) every three to six hours as needed, injected into a muscle or a vein or under the skin.
    ▪ Children—Dose must be determined by your doctor.

For opium
- For *injection* dosage form:
  ○ For pain:
    ▪ Adults—5 to 20 milligrams (mg), injected into a muscle or under the skin every four to five hours as needed.
    ▪ Children—Dose must be determined by your doctor.

For oxycodone
- For *oral* dosage form (oral solution or tablets):
  ○ For pain:
    ▪ Adults—5–15 milligrams (mg) every 4–6 hours as needed.
    ▪ Children—Dose must be determined by your doctor. Children up to 6 years of age will probably take the oral solution, rather than tablets. Small doses may need to be measured by a special dropper instead of a teaspoon.

- For *long-acting oral* dosage form (extended-release tablets):
  - For pain (continuous and lasts a long time):
    - Adults—Your doctor will determine the dose according to your individual needs. To be helpful, these medicines need to be taken two times a day at regularly scheduled times.
    - Children—Use and dose must be determined by your doctor.
- For *rectal suppository* dosage form:
  - For pain:
    - Adults—10 to 40 mg three or four times a day.
    - Children—Dose must be determined by your doctor.

For oxymorphone
- For *injection* dosage form:
  - For pain:
    - Adults—1 to 1.5 milligrams (mg), injected into a muscle or under the skin every three to six hours as needed. Some patients may receive 0.5 mg, injected into a vein.
    - Children—Dose must be determined by your doctor.
- For *rectal suppository* dosage form:
  - For pain:
    - Adults—5 mg every four to six hours as needed.
    - Children—Dose must be determined by your doctor.

For pentazocine
- For *oral* dosage form (tablets):
  - For pain:
    - Adults—50 mg every three to four hours as needed. Some patients may need 100 mg every three to four hours. The usual maximum dose is 600 mg a day.
    - Children—Dose must be determined by your doctor.
- For *injection* dosage form:
  - For pain:
    - Adults—30 mg, injected into a muscle or a vein or under the skin every three to four hours as needed.
    - Children—Dose must be determined by your doctor.

For propoxyphene
- For *oral* dosage form (capsules, oral suspension, or tablets):
  - For pain:
    - Adults—Propoxyphene comes in two different forms, propoxyphene hydrochloride and propoxyphene napsylate. 100 mg of propoxyphene napsylate provides the same amount of pain relief as 65 mg of propoxyphene hydrochloride. The dose of propoxyphene hydrochloride is 65 milligrams (mg) every four hours as needed, up to a maximum of 390 mg a day. The dose of propoxyphene napsylate is 100 mg every four hours as needed, up to a maximum of 600 mg a day.
    - Children—Dose must be determined by your doctor.

Missed dose—If your medical doctor or dentist has ordered you to take this medicine according to a regular schedule and you miss a dose, take it as soon as you remember. However, if it is almost time for your next dose, skip the missed dose and go back to your regular dosing schedule. *Do not double doses.*

Storage—To store this medicine:
- Keep out of the reach of children. Overdose is very dangerous in young children.
- Store away from heat and direct light.
- Do not store tablets or capsules in the bathroom, near the kitchen sink, or in other damp places. Heat or moisture may cause the medicine to break down.
- Store hydromorphone, oxycodone, or oxymorphone suppositories in the refrigerator.
- Keep liquid (including injections) and suppository forms of the medicine from freezing.
- Do not keep outdated medicine or medicine no longer needed. Be sure that any discarded medicine is out of the reach of children.

Precautions While Using This Medicine

If you will be taking this medicine for a long time (for example, for several months at a time), your doctor should check your progress at regular visits.

Narcotic analgesics will add to the effects of alcohol and other CNS depressants (medicines that slow down the nervous system, possibly causing drowsiness). Some examples of CNS depressants are antihistamines or medicine for hay fever, other allergies, or colds; sedatives, tranquilizers, or sleeping medicine; other prescription pain medicines including other narcotics; barbiturates; medicine for seizures; muscle relaxants; or anesthetics, including some dental anesthetics. *Do not drink alcoholic beverages, and check with your medical doctor or dentist before taking any of the medicines listed above, while you are using this medicine.*

This medicine may cause some people to become drowsy, dizzy, or lightheaded, or to feel a false sense of well-being. *Make sure you know how you react to this medicine before you drive, use machines, or do anything else that could be dangerous if you are dizzy or are not alert and clearheaded.*

Dizziness, light-headedness, or fainting may occur, especially when you get up suddenly from a lying or sitting position. Getting up slowly may help lessen this problem.

Nausea or vomiting may occur, especially after the first couple of doses. This effect may go away if you lie down for a while. However, if nausea or vomiting continues, check with your medical doctor or dentist. Lying down for a while may also help relieve some other side effects, such as dizziness or light-headedness, that may occur.

Before having any kind of surgery (including dental surgery) or emergency treatment, tell the medical doctor or dentist in charge that you are taking this medicine.

Narcotic analgesics may cause dryness of the mouth. For temporary relief, use sugarless candy or gum, melt bits of ice in your mouth, or use a saliva substitute. However, if dry mouth continues for more than 2 weeks, check with your dentist. Continuing dryness of the mouth may increase the chance of dental disease, including tooth decay, gum disease, and fungus infections.

If you have been taking this medicine regularly for several weeks or more, *do not suddenly stop using it without first checking with your doctor.* Your doctor may want you to reduce gradually the amount you are taking before stopping completely, in order to lessen the chance of withdrawal side effects.

If you think you or someone else may have taken an overdose, get emergency help at once. Taking an overdose of this medicine or taking alcohol or CNS depressants with this medicine may lead to unconsciousness or death. Signs of overdose include convulsions (seizures), confusion, severe nervousness or restlessness, severe dizziness, severe drowsiness, slow or troubled breathing, and severe weakness.

Side Effects of This Medicine

Along with its needed effects, a medicine may cause some unwanted effects. Although not all of these side effects may occur, if they do occur they may need medical attention.

Get emergency help immediately if any of the following symptoms of overdose occur:

Cold, clammy skin; confusion; convulsions (seizures); dizziness (severe); drowsiness (severe); low blood pressure; nervousness or restlessness (severe); pinpoint pupils of eyes; slow heartbeat; slow or troubled breathing; weakness (severe)

Also, check with your doctor as soon as possible if any of the following side effects occur:

Less common or rare

Dark urine (for propoxyphene only); fast, slow, or pounding heartbeat; feelings of unreality; hallucinations (seeing, hearing, or feeling things that are not there); hives, itching, or skin rash; increased sweating (more common with hydrocodone, meperidine, and methadone); irregular breathing; mental depression or other mood or mental changes; pale stools (for propoxyphene only); redness or flushing of face (more common with hydrocodone, meperidine, and methadone); ringing or buzzing in the ears; shortness of breath, wheezing, or troubled breathing; swelling of face; trembling or uncontrolled muscle movements; unusual excitement or restlessness (especially in children); yellow eyes or skin (for propoxyphene only)

Other side effects may occur that usually do not need medical attention. These side effects may go away during treatment as your body adjusts to the medicine. However, check with your doctor if any of the following side effects continue or are bothersome:

More common

Dizziness, light-headedness, or feeling faint; drowsiness; nausea or vomiting

Less common or rare

Blurred or double vision or other changes in vision; constipation (more common with long-term use and with codeine); decrease in amount of urine; difficult or painful urination; dry mouth; false sense of well-being; frequent urge to urinate; general feeling of discomfort or illness; headache; loss of appetite; nervousness or restlessness; nightmares or unusual dreams; redness, swelling, pain, or burning at place of injection; stomach cramps or pain; trouble in sleeping; unusual tiredness or weakness

After you stop using this medicine, your body may need time to adjust. The length of time this takes depends on the amount of medicine you were using and how long you used it. During this period of time check with your doctor if you notice any of the following side effects:

Body aches; diarrhea; fast heartbeat; fever, runny nose, or sneezing; gooseflesh; increased sweating; increased yawning; loss of appetite; nausea or vomiting; nervousness, restlessness, or irritability; shivering or trembling; stomach cramps; trouble in sleeping; unusually large pupils of eyes; weakness

Other side effects not listed above may also occur in some patients. If you notice any other effects, check with your doctor.

Additional Information

Once a medicine has been approved for marketing for a certain use, experience may show that it is also useful for other medical problems. Although not specifically included in product labeling, morphine by injection is used in certain pediatric patients with the following medical conditions:

• Pain, during mechanical ventilation, neonatal

• Pain, postoperative, neonatal

Other than the above information, there is no additional information relating to proper use, precautions, or side effects for these uses.

NARCOTIC ANALGESICS—FOR SURGERY AND OBSTETRICS (Systemic)

Some commonly used brand names are:

In the U.S.—

Alfenta (1)	Nubain (7)
Astramorph (6)	Stadol (3)
Astramorph PF (6)	Sublimaze (4)
Buprenex (2)	Sufenta (9)
Demerol (5)	Ultiva (8)
Duramorph (6)	

In Canada—

Alfenta (1)	Stadol (3)
Demerol (5)	Sufenta (9)
Epimorph (6)	Ultiva (8)
Nubain (7)	

This information applies to the following medicines:

1. Alfentanil (al-FEN-ta-nil)
2. Buprenorphine (byoo-pre-NOR-feen)
3. Butorphanol (byoo-TOR-fa-nole)
4. Fentanyl (FEN-ta-nil)
5. Meperidine (me-PER-i-deen)
6. Morphine (MOR-feen)
7. Nalbuphine (NAL-byoo-feen)
8. Remifentanil (rem-i-FEN-ta-nil)
9. Sufentanil (soo-FEN-ta-nil)

Category

- **Analgesic—**
- **Anesthesia adjunct—**
- **Anesthesia adjunct, opioid analgesic—**

Description

Narcotic analgesics (nar-KOT-ik an-al-JEE-zicks) are given to relieve pain before and during surgery (including dental surgery) or during labor and delivery. These medicines may also be given before or together with an anesthetic (either a general anesthetic or a local anesthetic), even when the patient is not in pain, to help the anesthetic work better.

When a narcotic analgesic is used for surgery or obstetrics (labor and delivery), it will be given by or under the immediate supervision of a medical doctor or dentist, or by a specially trained nurse, in the doctor's office or in a hospital.

The following information applies only to these special uses of narcotic analgesics. If you are taking or receiving a narcotic analgesic to relieve pain after surgery, or for any other reason, ask your health care professional for additional information about the medicine and its use.

These medicines are available in the following dosage forms:

Parenteral
- Alfentanil
  - Injection
- Buprenorphine
  - Injection
- Butorphanol
  - Injection
- Fentanyl
  - Injection
- Meperidine
  - Injection
- Morphine
  - Injection
- Nalbuphine
  - Injection
- Remifentanil
  - Injection
- Sufentanil
  - Injection

Before Receiving This Medicine

In deciding to use a medicine, the risks of using the medicine must be weighed against the good it will do. This is a decision you and your doctor will make. For narcotic analgesics, the following should be considered:

Allergies—Tell your doctor if you have ever had any unusual or allergic reaction to a narcotic analgesic. Also tell your health care professional if you are allergic to any other substances, such as foods, preservatives, or dyes.

Pregnancy—Although studies on birth defects have not been done in pregnant women, these medicines have not been reported to cause birth defects. However, in animal studies, many narcotics have caused birth defects or other unwanted effects when they were given for a long time in amounts that were large enough to cause harmful effects in the mother.

Use of a narcotic during labor and delivery sometimes causes drowsiness or breathing problems in the newborn baby. If this happens, your health care professional can give the baby another medicine that will overcome these effects. Narcotics are usually not used during the delivery of a premature baby.

Breast-feeding—Some narcotics have been shown to pass into the breast milk. However, these medicines have not been reported to cause problems in nursing babies.

Children—Children younger than 2 years of age may be especially sensitive to the effects of narcotic analgesics. This may increase the chance of side effects.

Older adults—Elderly people are especially sensitive to the effects of narcotic analgesics. This may increase the chance of side effects.

Other medicines—Although certain medicines should not be used together at all, in other cases two different medicines may be used together even if an interaction might occur. In these cases, it may be necessary to change the dose, or other precautions may be necessary. It is very important that you tell the person in charge if you are taking:
- Any other medicine, prescription or nonprescription (over-the-counter [OTC]), or
- "Street" drugs, such as amphetamines ("uppers"), barbiturates ("downers"), cocaine (including "crack"), marijuana, phencyclidine (PCP, "angel dust"), and heroin or other narcotics—Serious side effects may occur if anyone gives you an anesthetic without knowing that you have taken another medicine
- Benzodiazepines or
- Central nervous system (CNS) depressants (medicine that causes drowsiness)—The CNS depressant and other effects of either these medicines or the narcotic analgesics may be increased
- Buprenorphine or similar medicines—The narcotic analgesics may not work if you are taking buprenorphine or other similar medicines
- Cimetidine or
- Erythromycin—Increased chance of side effects with some narcotic analgesics
- Naltrexone—The narcotic analgesics will not work if you are taking naltrexone

Other medical problems—The presence of other medical problems may affect the use of narcotic analgesics. Make sure you tell your doctor if you have *any* other medical problems, especially:
- Abdominal problems or
- Brain tumor or
- Head injury or
- Gallbladder disease or
- Heart disease or
- Kidney disease or
- Liver disease or
- Lung disease or
- Prostate disease or
- Thyroid disease or
- Urinary tract disease—Narcotic analgesics may make these conditions or the symptoms of these conditions worse

Proper Use of This Medicine

Dosing—The dose of narcotic analgesic will be different for different patients. Your health care professional will decide on the right amount for you, depending on:

- Your age;
- Your general physical condition;
- The reason you are receiving the narcotic analgesic; and
- Other medicines you are taking or will receive before or after the narcotic analgesic is given.

Precautions After Receiving This Medicine

For patients going home within a few hours after surgery:

- Narcotic analgesics and other medicines that may be given with them during surgery may cause some people to feel drowsy, tired, or weak for up to a few days after they have been given. Therefore, for at least 24 hours (or longer if necessary) after receiving this medicine, *do not drive, use machines, or do anything else that could be dangerous if you are dizzy or are not alert.*
- Unless otherwise directed by your medical doctor or dentist, *do not drink alcoholic beverages or take other CNS depressants (medicines that slow down the nervous system, possibly causing drowsiness) for about 24 hours after you have received this medicine.* To do so may add to the effects of the narcotic analgesic. Some examples of CNS depressants are antihistamines or medicine for hay fever, other allergies, or colds; sedatives, tranquilizers, or sleeping medicine; prescription pain medicine or narcotics; barbiturates; medicine for seizures; and muscle relaxants.

Side Effects

Along with its needed effects, a medicine may cause some unwanted effects. Before you leave the hospital or doctor's office, your health care professional will closely follow the effects of this medicine. However, some effects may continue, or may not be noticed until later.

Check with your medical doctor or dentist as soon as possible if any of the following side effects occur:

More common
Dizziness, light-headedness, or feeling faint; drowsiness; nausea or vomiting; unusual tiredness or weakness

Less common or rare
Blurred or double vision or other vision problems; confusion; constipation; convulsions (seizures); difficult or painful urination; mental depression; shortness of breath, trouble in breathing, tightness in the chest, or wheezing; skin rash, hives, or itching; unusual excitement

Other side effects not listed above may also occur in some patients. If you notice any other effects, check with your doctor.

Additional Information

Once a medicine has been approved for marketing for a certain use, experience may show that it is also useful for other medical problems. Although not specifically included in

product labeling, fentanyl by injection is used in certain pediatric patients with the following medical conditions:

- Pain, during surgery, neonatal

Other than the above information, there is no additional information relating to proper use, precautions, or side effects for these uses.

NARCOTIC ANALGESICS AND ACETAMINOPHEN (Systemic)

Some commonly used brand names are:

In the U.S.—

Allay (4)	Panacet 5/500 (4)
Anexsia 5/500 (4)	Panlor (4)
Anexsia 7.5/650 (4)	Percocet 2.5/325 (5)
Anolor DH 5 (4)	Percocet 5/325 (5)
Bancap-HC (4)	Percocet 7.5/500 (5)
Capital with Codeine (1)	Percocet 10/650 (5)
Co-Gesic (4)	Phenaphen with Codeine
Darvocet-N 50 (7)	No.3 (1)
Darvocet-N 100 (7)	Phenaphen with Codeine
DHCplus (3)	No.4 (1)
Dolacet (4)	Polygesic (4)
Dolagesic (4)	Propacet 100 (7)
Duocet (4)	Pyregesic-C (1)
E-Lor (7)	Roxicet (5)
Endocet (5)	Roxicet 5/500 (5)
EZ III (1)	Roxilox (5)
Hycomed (4)	Stagesic (4)
Hyco-Pap (4)	Talacen (6)
Hydrocet (4)	T-Gesic (4)
Hydrogesic (4)	Tylenol with Codeine Elixir (1)
HY-PHEN (4)	Tylenol with Codeine No.2 (1)
Lorcet 10/650 (4)	Tylenol with Codeine No.3 (1)
Lorcet-HD (4)	Tylenol with Codeine No.4 (1)
Lorcet Plus (4)	Tylox (5)
Lortab (4)	Ugesic (4)
Lortab 2.5/500 (4)	Vanacet (4)
Lortab 5/500 (4)	Vendone (4)
Lortab 7.5/500 (4)	Vicodin (4)
Lortab 10/500 (4)	Vicodin ES (4)
Margesic #3 (1)	Wygesic (7)
Margesic-H (4)	Zydone (4)
Oncet (4)	

In Canada—

Acet-2 (2)	Lenoltec with Codeine
Acet-3 (2)	No.4 (1)
Acet Codeine 30 (1)	Novo-Gesic C8 (2)
Acet Codeine 60 (1)	Novo-Gesic C15 (2)
Atasol-8 (2)	Novo-Gesic C30 (2)
Atasol-15 (2)	Oxycocet (5)
Atasol-30 (2)	Percocet (5)
Cetaphen with Codeine (2)	Percocet-Demi (5)
Cetaphen Extra-Strength with	PMS-Acetaminophen with
Codeine (2)	Codeine (1)
Cotabs (2)	Roxicet (5)
Empracet-30 (1)	Triatec-8 (2)
Empracet-60 (1)	Triatec-30 (1)
Emtec-30 (1)	Triatec-8 Strong (2)
Endocet (5)	Tylenol with Codeine Elixir (1)
Exdol-8 (2)	Tylenol with Codeine No.1 (2)
Lenoltec with Codeine	Tylenol with Codeine No.2 (2)
No.1 (2)	Tylenol with Codeine No.3 (2)
Lenoltec with Codeine	Tylenol with Codeine No.4 (1)
No.2 (2)	Tylenol with Codeine
Lenoltec with Codeine	No.1 Forte (2)
No.3 (2)	

This information applies to the following medicines:

1. Acetaminophen and Codeine (a-seat-a-MIN-oh-fen and KOE-deen)
2. Acetaminophen, Codeine, and Caffeine (a-seat-a-MIN-oh-fen, KOE-deen, and kaf-EEN)
3. Dihydrocodeine, Acetaminophen, and Caffeine (dye-hye-droe-KOE-deen, a-seat-a-MIN-oh-fen, and kaf-EEN)
4. Hydrocodone and Acetaminophen (hye-droe-KOE-done and a-seat-a-MIN-oh-fen)
5. Oxycodone and Acetaminophen (ox-i-KOE-done and a-seat-a-MIN-oh-fen)
6. Pentazocine and Acetaminophen (pen-TAZ-oh-seen and a-seat-a-MIN-oh-fen)
7. Propoxyphene and Acetaminophen (proe-POX-i-feen and a-seat-a-MIN-oh-fen)

Category

• **Analgesic—**

Description

Combination medicines containing narcotic analgesics (nar-KOT-ik an-al-JEE-zicks) and acetaminophen (a-seat-a-MIN-oh-fen) are used to relieve pain. A narcotic analgesic and acetaminophen used together may provide better pain relief than either medicine used alone. In some cases, relief of pain may come at lower doses of each medicine.

Narcotic analgesics act in the central nervous system (CNS) to relieve pain. Many of their side effects are also caused by actions in the CNS. When narcotics are used for a long time, your body may get used to them so that larger amounts are needed to relieve pain. This is called tolerance to the medicine. Also, when narcotics are used for a long time or in large doses, they may become habit-forming (causing mental or physical dependence). Physical dependence may lead to withdrawal symptoms when you stop taking the medicine.

Acetaminophen does not become habit-forming when taken for a long time or in large doses, but it may cause other unwanted effects, including liver damage, if too much is taken.

In the U.S., these medicines are available only with your medical doctor's or dentist's prescription. In Canada, some acetaminophen, codeine, and caffeine combinations are available without a prescription.

These medicines are available in the following dosage forms:

Oral
- Acetaminophen and Codeine
  - Capsules
  - Oral solution
  - Oral suspension
  - Tablets
- Acetaminophen, Codeine, and Caffeine
  - Tablets
- Dihydrocodeine, Acetaminophen, and Caffeine
  - Capsules
- Hydrocodone and Acetaminophen
  - Capsules
  - Oral solution
  - Tablets
- Oxycodone and Acetaminophen
  - Capsules
  - Oral solution
  - Tablets
- Pentazocine and Acetaminophen
  - Tablets
- Propoxyphene and Acetaminophen
  - Tablets

Before Using This Medicine

In deciding to use a medicine, the risks of taking the medicine must be weighed against the good it will do. This is a decision you and your doctor will make. For narcotic analgesic and acetaminophen combinations, the following should be considered:

Allergies—Tell your doctor if you have ever had any unusual or allergic reaction to acetaminophen or to a narcotic analgesic. Also tell your health care professional if you are allergic to any other substances, such as foods, preservatives, or dyes.

Pregnancy—
- *For acetaminophen:* Although studies on birth defects with acetaminophen have not been done in pregnant women, it has not been reported to cause birth defects or other problems.
- *For narcotic analgesics:* Although studies on birth defects with narcotic analgesics have not been done in pregnant women, they have not been reported to cause birth defects. However, hydrocodone caused birth defects in animal studies when very large doses were used. Codeine did not cause birth defects in animals, but it caused slower development of bones and other toxic or harmful effects in the fetus. Pentazocine and propoxyphene did not cause birth defects in animals. There is no information about whether dihydrocodeine or oxycodone causes birth defects in animals.Too much use of a narcotic during pregnancy may cause the fetus to become dependent on the medicine. This may lead to withdrawal side effects in the newborn baby. Also, some of these medicines may cause breathing problems in the newborn baby if taken just before or during delivery.
- *For caffeine:* Studies in humans have not shown that caffeine (contained in some of these combination medicines) causes birth defects. However, studies in animals have shown that caffeine causes birth defects when given in very large doses (amounts equal to those present in 12 to 24 cups of coffee a day).

Breast-feeding—Acetaminophen, codeine, and propoxyphene pass into the breast milk. It is not known whether other narcotic analgesics pass into the breast milk. However, these medicines have not been reported to cause problems in nursing babies.

Children—Breathing problems may be especially likely to occur when narcotic analgesics are given to children younger than 2 years of age. These children are usually more sensitive than adults to the effects of narcotic analgesics. Also, unusual excitement or restlessness may be more likely to occur in children receiving these medicines.

Acetaminophen has been tested in children and has not been shown to cause different side effects or problems in children than it does in adults.

Older adults—Elderly people are especially sensitive to the effects of narcotic analgesics. This may increase the chance of side effects, especially breathing problems, during treatment.

Acetaminophen has been tested and has not been shown to cause different side effects or problems in older people than it does in younger adults.

Other medicines—Although certain medicines should not be used together at all, in other cases two different medicines may be used together even if an interaction might occur. In these cases, your doctor may want to change the dose, or other precautions may be necessary. When you are taking a narcotic analgesic and acetaminophen combination, it is especially important that your health care professional know if you are taking any of the following:

- Carbamazepine (e.g., Tegretol)—Propoxyphene may increase the blood levels of carbamazepine, which increases the chance of serious side effects
- Central nervous system (CNS) depressants or
- Monoamine oxidase (MAO) inhibitor activity (isocarboxazid [e.g., Marplan], phenelzine [e.g., Nardil], procarbazine [e.g., Matulane], selegiline [e.g., Eldepryl], tranylcypromine [e.g., Parnate]) (taken currently or within the past 2 weeks) or
- Tricyclic antidepressants (amitriptyline [e.g., Elavil], amoxapine [e.g., Asendin], clomipramine [e.g., Anafranil], desipramine [e.g., Pertofrane], doxepin [e.g., Sinequan], imipramine [e.g., Tofranil], nortriptyline [e.g., Aventyl], protriptyline [e.g., Vivactil], trimipramine [e.g., Surmontil])—Taking these medicines together with a narcotic analgesic may increase the chance of serious side effects
- Naltrexone (e.g., Trexan)—Naltrexone keeps narcotic analgesics from working to relieve pain; people taking naltrexone should take pain relievers that do not contain a narcotic
- Zidovudine (e.g., AZT, Retrovir)—Acetaminophen may increase the blood levels of zidovudine, which increases the chance of serious side effects

Other medical problems—The presence of other medical problems may affect the use of narcotic analgesic and acetaminophen combinations. Make sure you tell your doctor if you have any other medical problems, especially:

- Alcohol and/or other drug abuse, or history of, or
- Brain disease or head injury or
- Colitis or
- Convulsions (seizures), history of, or
- Emotional problems or mental illness or
- Emphysema, asthma, or other chronic lung disease or
- Hepatitis or other liver disease or
- Kidney disease or
- Underactive thyroid—The chance of serious side effects may be increased
- Enlarged prostate or problems with urination or
- Gallbladder disease or gallstones—Some of the effects of narcotic analgesics may be especially serious in people with these medical problems
- Heart disease—Caffeine (present in some of these combination medicines) can make some kinds of heart disease worse

Proper Use of This Medicine

Take this medicine only as directed by your medical doctor or dentist. Do not take more of it, do not take it more often, and do not take it for a longer time than your medical doctor or dentist ordered. This is especially important for young children and elderly patients, who may be more sensitive than other people to the effects of narcotic analgesics. If too much of a narcotic analgesic is taken, it may become habit-forming (causing mental or physical dependence) or lead to medical problems because of an overdose. Taking too much acetaminophen may cause liver damage.

If you think that this medicine is not working properly after you have been taking it for a few weeks, *do not increase the dose.* Instead, check with your medical doctor or dentist.

Dosing—The dose of these medicines will be different for different patients. *Follow your doctor's orders or the directions on the label.* The following information includes only the average doses of these medicines. *If your dose is different, do not change it* unless your doctor tells you to do so.

The number of capsules or tablets or teaspoonfuls of solution or suspension that you take depends on the strength of the medicine.

For acetaminophen and codeine
- For *oral capsule or tablet* dosage form:
  - For pain:
    - Adults—1 or 2 capsules or tablets containing acetaminophen with 15 or 30 milligrams (mg) of codeine, or 1 capsule or tablet containing acetaminophen with 60 mg of codeine, every four hours as needed.
    - Children—Dose must be determined by the doctor, depending on the age of the child. Most young children will receive the oral solution or suspension, rather than tablets or capsules.
- For *oral solution or suspension* dosage form:
  - For pain:
    - Adults—1 tablespoonful (3 teaspoonfuls) every four hours as needed.
    - Children younger than 3 years of age—Dose must be determined by your doctor.
    - Children 3 to 7 years of age—1 teaspoonful three or four times a day as needed.
    - Children 7 to 12 years of age—2 teaspoonfuls three or four times a day as needed.

For acetaminophen, codeine, and caffeine
- For *oral tablet* dosage form:
  - For pain:
    - Adults—1 or 2 tablets every four hours as needed.
    - Children—Dose must be determined by your doctor.

For dihydrocodeine, acetaminophen, and caffeine
- For *oral capsule* dosage form:
  - For pain:
    - Adults—2 capsules every four hours.
    - Children—Dose must be determined by your doctor.

For hydrocodone and acetaminophen
- For *oral capsule* dosage form:
  - For pain:
    - Adults—1 capsule every four to six hours as needed.
    - Children—Dose must be determined by your doctor.

- For *oral solution* dosage form:
  - For pain:
    - Adults—1 to 3 teaspoonfuls every four to six hours as needed.
    - Children—Dose must be determined by your doctor.
- For *oral tablet* dosage form:
  - For pain:
    - Adults—1 or 2 tablets containing acetaminophen with 2.5 milligrams (mg) of hydrocodone, or 1 tablet containing acetaminophen with 5, 7.5, or 10 mg of hydrocodone, every four to six hours as needed.
    - Children—Dose must be determined by your doctor.

For oxycodone and acetaminophen
- For *oral capsule or tablet* dosage form:
  - For pain:
    - Adults—1 to 2 capsules or tablets every four to six hours as needed.
    - Children—Dose must be determined by your doctor.
- For *oral solution* dosage form:
  - For pain:
    - Adults—1 teaspoonful every four to six hours as needed.
    - Children—Dose must be determined by your doctor.

For pentazocine and acetaminophen
- For *oral tablet* dosage form:
  - For pain:
    - Adults—1 tablet every four hours.
    - Children—Dose must be determined by your doctor.

For propoxyphene and acetaminophen
- For *oral tablet* dosage form:
  - For pain:
    - Adults—1 or 2 tablets, depending on the strength, every four hours as needed.
    - Children—Dose must be determined by your doctor.

Missed dose—If your medical doctor or dentist has ordered you to take this medicine according to a regular schedule and you miss a dose, take it as soon as you remember. However, if it is almost time for your next dose, skip the missed dose and go back to your regular dosing schedule. *Do not double doses.*

Storage—To store this medicine:
- Keep out of the reach of children. Overdose is very dangerous in young children.
- Store away from heat and direct light.
- Do not store tablets or capsules in the bathroom, near the kitchen sink, or in other damp places. Heat or moisture may cause the medicine to break down.
- Keep the liquid forms of this medicine from freezing.
- Do not keep outdated medicine or medicine no longer needed. Be sure that any discarded medicine is out of the reach of children.

Precautions While Using This Medicine

If you will be taking this medicine for a long time (for example, for several months at a time), or in high doses, your doctor should check your progress at regular visits.

Check the labels of all nonprescription (over-the-counter [OTC]) and prescription medicines you now take. If any contain acetaminophen or a narcotic be especially careful, since taking them while taking this medicine may lead to overdose. If you have any questions about this, check with your medical doctor, dentist, or pharmacist.

The narcotic analgesic in this medicine will add to the effects of alcohol and other CNS depressants (medicines that slow down the nervous system, possibly causing drowsiness). Some examples of CNS depressants are antihistamines or medicine for hay fever, other allergies, or colds; sedatives, tranquilizers, or sleeping medicine; other prescription pain medicine or narcotics; barbiturates; medicine for seizures; muscle relaxants; or anesthetics, including some dental anesthetics. Also, there may be a greater risk of liver damage if you drink three or more alcoholic beverages while you are taking acetaminophen. *Do not drink alcoholic beverages, and check with your medical doctor or dentist before taking any of the medicines listed above, while you are using this medicine.*

Too much use of the acetaminophen in this combination medicine together with certain other medicines may increase the chance of unwanted effects. The risk will depend on how much of each medicine you take every day, and on how long you take the medicines together. If your doctor directs you to take these medicines together on a regular basis, follow his or her directions carefully. However, do not take this medicine together with any of the following medicines for more than a few days, unless your doctor has directed you to do so and is following your progress:
- Aspirin or other salicylates
- Diclofenac (e.g., Voltaren)
- Diflunisal (e.g., Dolobid)
- Etodolac (e.g., Lodine)
- Fenoprofen (e.g., Nalfon)
- Floctafenine (e.g., Idarac)
- Flurbiprofen, oral (e.g., Ansaid)
- Ibuprofen (e.g., Motrin)
- Indomethacin (e.g., Indocin)
- Ketoprofen (e.g., Orudis)
- Ketorolac (e.g., Toradol)
- Meclofenamate (e.g., Meclomen)
- Mefenamic acid (e.g., Ponstel)
- Nabumetone (e.g., Relafen)
- Naproxen (e.g., Naprosyn)
- Oxaprozin (e.g., Daypro)
- Phenylbutazone (e.g., Butazolidin)
- Piroxicam (e.g., Feldene)
- Sulindac (e.g., Clinoril)
- Tenoxicam (e.g., Mobiflex)
- Tiaprofenic acid (e.g., Surgam)
- Tolmetin (e.g., Tolectin)

This medicine may cause some people to become drowsy, dizzy, or lightheaded, or to feel a false sense of well-being. *Make sure you know how you react to this medicine be-*

fore you drive, use machines, or do anything else that could be dangerous if you are dizzy or are not alert and clearheaded.

Dizziness, lightheadedness, or fainting may occur, especially when you get up suddenly from a lying or sitting position. Getting up slowly may help lessen this problem.

Nausea or vomiting may occur, especially after the first couple of doses. This effect may go away if you lie down for a while. However, if nausea or vomiting continues, check with your medical doctor or dentist. Lying down for a while may also help relieve some other side effects, such as dizziness or lightheadedness, that may occur.

Before having any kind of surgery (including dental surgery) or emergency treatment, tell the medical doctor or dentist in charge that you are taking this medicine.

Narcotic analgesics may cause dryness of the mouth. For temporary relief, use sugarless candy or gum, melt bits of ice in your mouth, or use a saliva substitute. However, if dry mouth continues for more than 2 weeks, check with your dentist. Continuing dryness of the mouth may increase the chance of dental disease, including tooth decay, gum disease, and fungus infections.

If you have been taking this medicine regularly for several weeks or more, *do not suddenly stop taking it without first checking with your doctor.* Your doctor may want you to reduce gradually the amount you are taking before stopping completely, to lessen the chance of withdrawal side effects. This will depend on which of these medicines you have been taking, and the amount you have been taking every day.

If you think you or someone else may have taken an overdose of this medicine, get emergency help at once. Taking an overdose of this medicine or taking alcohol or CNS depressants with this medicine may lead to unconsciousness or death. Signs of overdose of narcotics include convulsions (seizures), confusion, severe nervousness or restlessness, severe dizziness, severe drowsiness, shortness of breath or troubled breathing, and severe weakness. Signs of severe acetaminophen overdose may not occur until several days after the overdose is taken.

Side Effects

Along with its needed effects, a medicine may cause some unwanted effects. Although not all of these side effects may occur, if they do occur they may need medical attention.

Get emergency help immediately if any of the following symptoms of overdose occur:
> Cold, clammy skin; confusion (severe); convulsions (seizures); diarrhea; dizziness (severe); drowsiness (severe); increased sweating; low blood pressure; nausea or vomiting (continuing); nervousness or restlessness (severe); pinpoint pupils of eyes; shortness of breath or unusually slow or troubled breathing; slow heartbeat; stomach cramps or pain; weakness (severe)

Also, check with your doctor as soon as possible if any of the following side effects occur:
Less common or rare
> Black, tarry stools; bloody or cloudy urine; confusion; dark urine; difficult or painful urination; fast, slow, or pounding heartbeat; frequent urge to urinate; hallucinations (seeing, hearing, or feeling things that are not there); increased sweating; irregular breathing or

wheezing; mental depression; pain in lower back and/or side (severe and/or sharp); pale stools; pinpoint red spots on skin; redness or flushing of face; ringing or buzzing in ears; skin rash, hives, or itching; sore throat and fever; sudden decrease in amount of urine; swelling of face; trembling or uncontrolled muscle movements; unusual bleeding or bruising; unusual excitement (especially in children); yellow eyes or skin

Other side effects may occur that usually do not need medical attention. These side effects may go away during treatment as your body adjusts to the medicine. However, check with your medical doctor or dentist if any of the following side effects continue or are bothersome:
More common
> Dizziness, lightheadedness, or feeling faint; drowsiness; nausea or vomiting; unusual tiredness or weakness

Less common or rare
> Blurred or double vision or other changes in vision; constipation (more common with long-term use and with codeine or meperidine); dry mouth; false sense of well-being; general feeling of discomfort or illness; headache; loss of appetite; nervousness or restlessness; nightmares or unusual dreams; trouble in sleeping

Although not all of the side effects listed above have been reported for all of these combination medicines, they have been reported for at least one of them. However, since all of the narcotic analgesics are very similar, any of the above side effects may occur with any of these medicines.

After you stop using this medicine, your body may need time to adjust. The length of time this takes depends on which of these medicines you were taking, the amount of medicine you were using, and how long you used it. During this time check with your doctor if you notice any of the following side effects:
> Body aches; diarrhea; fast heartbeat; fever, runny nose, or sneezing; gooseflesh; increased sweating; increased yawning; loss of appetite; nausea or vomiting; nervousness, restlessness, or irritability; shivering or trembling; stomach cramps; trouble in sleeping; weakness

Other side effects not listed above may also occur in some patients. If you notice any other effects, check with your doctor.

NARCOTIC ANALGESICS AND ASPIRIN (Systemic)

Some commonly used brand names are:

In the U.S.—

Damason-P (5)	Percodan (6)
Darvon Compound-65 (9)	Percodan-Demi (6)
Empirin with Codeine No.3 (2)	Propoxyphene Compound-
Empirin with Codeine No.4 (2)	65 (9)
Endodan (6)	Roxiprin (6)
Lortab ASA (5)	Synalgos-DC (1)
Panasal 5/500 (5)	Talwin Compound (7)
PC-Cap (9)	

In Canada—

Anacin with Codeine (3)	Oxycodan (6)
C2 Buffered with Codeine (4)	Percodan (6)
C2 with Codeine (3)	Percodan-Demi (6)
Darvon-N Compound (9)	692 (9)
Darvon-N with A.S.A. (8)	222 (3)
Endodan (6)	282 (3)
Novo-AC and C (3)	292 (3)

This information applies to the following medicines:

1. Aspirin, Caffeine, and Dihydrocodeine (AS-pir-in kaf-EEN and dye-hye-droe-KOE-deen)
2. Aspirin and Codeine (AS-pir-in and KOE-deen)
3. Aspirin, Codeine, and Caffeine (AS-pir-in KOE-deen and kaf-EEN)
4. Aspirin, Codeine, and Caffeine, Buffered
5. Hydrocodone and Aspirin (hye-droe-KOE-done and AS-pir-in)
6. Oxycodone and Aspirin (ox-i-KOE-done and AS-pir-in)
7. Pentazocine and Aspirin (pen-TAZ-oh-seen and AS-pir-in)
8. Propoxyphene and Aspirin (proe-POX-i-feen and AS-pir-in)
9. Propoxyphene, Aspirin, and Caffeine (proe-POX-i-feen AS-pir-in and kaf-EEN)

Category

- **Analgesic—**

Description

Combination medicines containing narcotic analgesics (nar-KOT-ik an-al-JEE-zicks) and aspirin (AS-pir-in) are used to relieve pain. A narcotic analgesic and aspirin used together may provide better pain relief than either medicine used alone. In some cases, relief of pain may come at lower doses of each medicine.

Narcotic analgesics act in the central nervous system (CNS) to relieve pain. Many of their side effects are also caused by actions in the CNS. When narcotics are used for a long time, your body may get used to them so that larger amounts are needed to relieve pain. This is called tolerance to the medicine. Also, when narcotics are used for a long time or in large doses, they may become habit-forming (causing mental or physical dependence). Physical dependence may lead to withdrawal symptoms when you stop taking the medicine.

Aspirin does not become habit-forming when taken for a long time or in large doses, but it may cause other unwanted effects if too much is taken.

In the U.S., these medicines are available only with your medical doctor's or dentist's prescription. In Canada, some strengths of aspirin, codeine, and caffeine combination are available without a prescription.

These medicines are available in the following dosage forms:

Oral

- Aspirin, Caffeine, and Dihydrocodeine
  - Capsules
- Aspirin and Codeine
  - Tablets
- Aspirin, Codeine, and Caffeine
  - Tablets
- Aspirin, Codeine, and Caffeine, Buffered
  - Tablets
- Hydrocodone and Aspirin
  - Tablets
- Oxycodone and Aspirin
  - Tablets
- Pentazocine and Aspirin
  - Tablets
- Propoxyphene and Aspirin
  - Capsules
- Propoxyphene, Aspirin, and Caffeine
  - Capsules
  - Tablets

Before Using This Medicine

In deciding to use a medicine, the risks of taking the medicine must be weighed against the good it will do. This is a decision you and your doctor will make. For narcotic analgesic and aspirin combinations, the following should be considered:

Allergies—Tell your doctor if you have ever had any unusual or allergic reaction to a narcotic analgesic, aspirin or other salicylates, including methyl salicylate (oil of wintergreen), or any of the following medicines:

- Diclofenac (e.g., Voltaren)
- Diflunisal (e.g., Dolobid)
- Etodolac (e.g., Lodine)
- Fenoprofen (e.g., Nalfon)
- Floctafenine (e.g., Idarac)
- Flurbiprofen, oral (e.g., Ansaid)
- Ibuprofen (e.g., Motrin)
- Indomethacin (e.g., Indocin)
- Ketoprofen (e.g., Orudis)
- Ketorolac (e.g., Toradol)
- Meclofenamate (e.g., Meclomen)
- Mefenamic acid (e.g., Ponstel)
- Nabumetone (e.g., Relafen)
- Naproxen (e.g., Naprosyn)
- Oxaprozin (e.g., Daypro)
- Oxyphenbutazone (e.g., Tandearil)
- Phenylbutazone (e.g., Butazolidin)
- Piroxicam (e.g., Feldene)
- Sulindac (e.g., Clinoril)
- Suprofen (e.g., Suprol)
- Tenoxicam (e.g., Mobiflex)
- Tiaprofenic acid (e.g., Surgam)
- Tolmetin (e.g., Tolectin)
- Zomepirac (e.g., Zomax)

Also tell your health care professional if you are allergic to any other substances, such as foods, preservatives, or dyes.

Pregnancy—

- *For aspirin:* Studies in humans have not shown that aspirin causes birth defects. However, studies in animals have shown that aspirin causes birth defects.Some reports have suggested that too much use of aspirin late in pregnancy may cause a decrease in the newborn's weight and possible death of the fetus or newborn baby. However, the mothers in these reports had been taking much larger amounts of aspirin than are usually recommended. Studies of mothers taking aspirin in the doses that are usually recommended did not show these effects. However, regular use of aspirin late in pregnancy may cause unwanted effects on the heart or blood flow in the fetus or in the newborn baby. Also, use of aspirin during the last 2 weeks of pregnancy may cause bleeding problems in the fetus before or during delivery or in the newborn baby. Too much use of aspirin during the last 3 months of pregnancy may increase the length of pregnancy, prolong labor, cause other problems during delivery, or cause severe bleeding in the mother before, during, or after delivery. *Do not take aspirin during the last 3 months of pregnancy unless it has been ordered by your doctor.*

• *For narcotic analgesics:* Although studies on birth defects with narcotic analgesics have not been done in pregnant women, they have not been reported to cause birth defects. However, hydrocodone caused birth defects in animal studies when given in very large doses. Codeine did not cause birth defects in animals, but it caused slower development of bones and other toxic or harmful effects on the fetus. Pentazocine and propoxyphene did not cause birth defects in animals. There is no information about whether dihydrocodeine or oxycodone causes birth defects in animals. Too much use of a narcotic during pregnancy may cause the fetus to become dependent on the medicine. This may lead to withdrawal side effects in the newborn baby. Also, some of these medicines may cause breathing problems in the newborn baby if taken just before or during delivery.

• *For caffeine:* Studies in humans have not shown that caffeine (contained in some of these combination medicines) causes birth defects. However, studies in animals have shown that caffeine causes birth defects when given in very large doses (amounts equal to those present in 12 to 24 cups of coffee a day).

Breast-feeding—These combination medicines have not been reported to cause problems in nursing babies. However, aspirin, caffeine, codeine, and propoxyphene pass into the breast milk. It is not known whether dihydrocodeine, hydrocodone, oxycodone, or pentazocine passes into the breast milk.

Children—*Do not give a medicine containing aspirin to a child or a teenager with a fever or other symptoms of a virus infection, especially flu or chickenpox, without first discussing its use with your child's doctor.* This is very important because aspirin may cause a serious illness called Reye's syndrome in children with fever caused by a virus infection, especially flu or chickenpox. Children who do not have a virus infection may also be more sensitive to the effects of aspirin, especially if they have a fever or have lost large amounts of body fluid because of vomiting, diarrhea, or sweating. This may increase the chance of side effects during treatment.

The narcotic analgesic in this combination medicine can cause breathing problems, especially in children younger than 2 years of age. These children are usually more sensitive than adults to the effects of narcotic analgesics. Also, unusual excitement or restlessness may be more likely to occur in children receiving these medicines.

Older adults—Elderly people are especially sensitive to the effects of aspirin and of narcotic analgesics. This may increase the chance of side effects, especially breathing problems caused by narcotic analgesics, during treatment.

Other medicines—Although certain medicines should not be used together at all, in other cases two different medicines may be used together even if an interaction might occur. In these cases, your doctor may want to change the dose, or other precautions may be necessary. When you are taking a narcotic analgesic and aspirin combination, it is especially important that your health care professional know if you are taking any of the following:

• Anticoagulants (blood thinners) or
• Carbenicillin by injection (e.g., Geopen) or
• Cefamandole (e.g., Mandol) or
• Cefoperazone (e.g., Cefobid) or
• Cefotetan (e.g., Cefotan) or
• Dipyridamole (e.g., Persantine) or
• Divalproex (e.g., Depakote) or
• Heparin or
• Medicine for inflammation or pain, except narcotics, or
• Pentoxifylline (e.g., Trental) or
• Plicamycin (e.g., Mithracin) or
• Ticarcillin (e.g., Ticar) or
• Valproic acid (e.g., Depakene)—Taking these medicines together with aspirin may increase the chance of bleeding
• Antidiabetics, oral (diabetes medicine you take by mouth)—Aspirin may increase the effects of the antidiabetic medicine; a change in the dose of the antidiabetic medicine may be needed if aspirin is taken regularly
• Carbamazepine (e.g., Tegretol)—Propoxyphene can increase the blood levels of carbamazepine, which increases the chance of serious side effects
• Central nervous system (CNS) depressants or
• Diarrhea medicine or
• Methotrexate (e.g., Mexate) or
• Tricyclic antidepressants (amitriptyline [e.g., Elavil], amoxapine [e.g., Asendin], clomipramine [e.g., Anafranil], desipramine [e.g., Pertofrane], doxepin [e.g., Sinequan], imipramine [e.g., Tofranil], nortriptyline [e.g., Aventyl], protriptyline [e.g., Vivactil], trimipramine [e.g., Surmontil]) or
• Vancomycin (e.g., Vancocin)—The chance of side effects may be increased
• Naltrexone (e.g., Trexan)—Naltrexone keeps narcotic analgesics from working to relieve pain; people taking naltrexone should use pain relievers that do not contain a narcotic
• Probenecid (e.g., Benemid) or
• Sulfinpyrazone (e.g., Anturane)—Aspirin can keep these medicines from working as well for treating gout; also, use of sulfinpyrazone and aspirin together may increase the chance of bleeding
• Urinary alkalizers (medicine that makes the urine less acid, such as acetazolamide [e.g., Diamox], calcium- and/or magnesium-containing antacids, dichlorphenamide [e.g., Daranide], methazolamide [e.g., Neptazane], potassium or sodium citrate and/or citric acid, sodium bicarbonate [baking soda])—These medicines may make aspirin less effective by causing it to be removed from the body more quickly
• Zidovudine (e.g., AZT, Retrovir)—Higher blood levels of zidovudine and an increased chance of serious side effects may occur

Other medical problems—The presence of other medical problems may affect the use of narcotic analgesic and aspirin combinations. Make sure you tell your doctor if you have any other medical problems, especially:

- Alcohol and/or other drug abuse, or history of, or
- Asthma, allergies, and nasal polyps (history of) or
- Brain disease or head injury or
- Colitis or
- Convulsions (seizures), history of, or
- Emotional problems or mental illness or
- Emphysema or other chronic lung disease or
- Kidney disease or
- Liver disease or
- Underactive thyroid—The chance of serious side effects may be increased
- Anemia or
- Overactive thyroid or
- Stomach ulcer or other stomach problems—Aspirin may make these conditions worse
- Enlarged prostate or problems with urination or
- Gallbladder disease or gallstones—Narcotic analgesics have side effects that may be dangerous if these medical problems are present
- Gout—Aspirin can make this condition worse and can also lessen the effects of some medicines used to treat gout
- Heart disease—Large amounts of aspirin and caffeine (present in some of these combination medicines) can make some kinds of heart disease worse
- Hemophilia or other bleeding problems or
- Vitamin K deficiency—Aspirin increases the chance of serious bleeding

Proper Use of This Medicine

Take this medicine with food or a full glass (8 ounces) of water to lessen stomach irritation.

Do not take this medicine if it has a strong vinegar-like odor. This odor means the aspirin in it is breaking down. If you have any questions about this, check with your health care professional.

Take this medicine only as directed by your medical doctor or dentist. Do not take more of it, do not take it more often, and do not take it for a longer time than your medical doctor or dentist ordered. This is especially important for children and elderly patients, who are usually more sensitive to the effects of these medicines. If too much of a narcotic analgesic is taken, it may become habit-forming (causing mental or physical dependence) or lead to medical problems because of an overdose. Also, taking too much aspirin may cause stomach problems or lead to medical problems because of an overdose.

If you think that this medicine is not working as well after you have been taking it for a few weeks, *do not increase the dose.* Instead, check with your medical doctor or dentist.

Dosing—The dose of these medicines will be different for different patients. *Follow your doctor's orders or the directions on the label.* The following information includes only the average doses of these medicines. *If your dose is dif-*

ferent, do not change it unless your doctor tells you to do so.

The number of capsules or tablets that you take depends on the strength of the medicine and on the amount of pain you are having.

For aspirin, caffeine, and dihydrocodeine
- For *oral* dosage form (capsules):
  - For pain:
    - Adults—2 capsules every four hours as needed.
    - Children—Dose must be determined by your doctor.

For aspirin and codeine
- For *oral* dosage form (tablets):
  - For pain:
    - Adults—1 or 2 tablets every four hours as needed.
    - Children—Dose must be determined by your doctor.

For aspirin, codeine, and caffeine
- For *oral* dosage form (tablets):
  - For pain:
    - Adults—1 or 2 tablets every four hours as needed.
    - Children—Dose must be determined by your doctor.

For buffered aspirin, codeine, and caffeine
- For *oral* dosage form (tablets):
  - For pain:
    - Adults—1 or 2 tablets every four hours as needed.
    - Children—Dose must be determined by your doctor.

For hydrocodone and aspirin
- For *oral* dosage form (tablets):
  - For pain:
    - Adults—1 or 2 tablets every four to six hours as needed.
    - Children—Dose must be determined by your doctor.

For oxycodone and aspirin
- For *oral* dosage form (tablets):
  - For pain:
    - Adults—1 or 2 half-strength tablets, or 1 full-strength tablet, every four to six hours as needed.
    - Children up to 6 years of age—Use is not recommended.
    - Children 6 to 12 years of age—One-quarter of a half-strength tablet every six hours as needed.
    - Children 12 years of age and older—One-half of a half-strength tablet every six hours as needed.

For pentazocine and aspirin
- For *oral* dosage form (tablets):
  - For pain:
    - Adults—2 tablets three or four times a day as needed.
    - Children—Dose must be determined by your doctor.

For propoxyphene and aspirin
- For *oral* dosage form (capsules):
  - For pain:
    - Adults—1 capsule every four hours as needed.
    - Children—Dose must be determined by your doctor.

For propoxyphene, aspirin, and caffeine
- For *oral* dosage form (capsules or tablets):
  - For pain:
    - Adults—1 capsule or tablet every four hours as needed.
    - Children—Dose must be determined by your doctor.

Missed dose—If your medical doctor or dentist has ordered you to take this medicine according to a regular schedule and you miss a dose, take it as soon as you remember. However, if it is almost time for your next dose, skip the missed dose and go back to your regular dosing schedule. *Do not double doses.*

Storage—To store this medicine:
- Keep out of the reach of children. Overdose is very dangerous in young children.
- Store away from heat and direct light.
- Do not store this medicine in the bathroom, near the kitchen sink, or in other damp places. Heat or moisture may cause the medicine to break down.
- Do not keep outdated medicine or medicine no longer needed. Be sure that any discarded medicine is out of the reach of children.

Precautions While Using This Medicine

If you will be taking this medicine for a long time (for example, for several months at a time), your doctor should check your progress at regular visits.

Check the labels of all nonprescription (over-the-counter [OTC]) and prescription medicines you now take. If any contain a narcotic, aspirin, or other salicylates, check with your health care professional. Taking them together with this medicine may cause an overdose.

This medicine will add to the effects of alcohol and other CNS depressants (medicines that slow down the nervous system, possibly causing drowsiness). Some examples of CNS depressants are antihistamines or medicine for hay fever, other allergies, or colds; sedatives, tranquilizers, or sleeping medicine; other prescription pain medicine or narcotics; barbiturates; medicine for seizures; muscle relaxants; or anesthetics, including some dental anesthetics. Also, stomach problems may be more likely to occur if you drink alcoholic beverages while you are taking aspirin. *Do not drink alcoholic beverages, and check with your medical doctor or dentist before taking any of the medicines listed above, while you are using this medicine.*

Taking acetaminophen or certain other medicines together with the aspirin in this combination medicine may increase the chance of unwanted effects. The risk will depend on how much of each medicine you take every day, and on how long you take the medicines together. If your medical doctor or dentist directs you to take these medicines together on a regular basis, follow his or her directions carefully. However, do not take acetaminophen or any of the following medicines together with this combination medicine for more than a few days, unless your medical doctor or dentist has directed you to do so and is following your progress:
- Diclofenac (e.g., Voltaren)
- Diflunisal (e.g., Dolobid)
- Etodolac (e.g., Lodine)
- Fenoprofen (e.g., Nalfon)
- Floctafenine (e.g., Idarac)
- Flurbiprofen, oral (e.g., Ansaid)
- Ibuprofen (e.g., Motrin)
- Indomethacin (e.g., Indocin)
- Ketoprofen (e.g., Orudis)
- Ketorolac (e.g., Toradol)
- Meclofenamate (e.g., Meclomen)
- Mefenamic acid (e.g., Ponstel)
- Nabumetone (e.g., Relafen)
- Naproxen (e.g., Naprosyn)
- Oxaprozin (e.g., Daypro)
- Phenylbutazone (e.g., Butazolidin)
- Piroxicam (e.g., Feldene)
- Sulindac (e.g., Clinoril)
- Tenoxicam (e.g., Mobiflex)
- Tiaprofenic acid (e.g., Surgam)
- Tolmetin (e.g., Tolectin)

This medicine may cause some people to become drowsy, dizzy, or lightheaded, or to feel a false sense of well-being. *Make sure you know how you react to this medicine before you drive, use machines, or do anything else that could be dangerous if you are dizzy or are not alert and clearheaded.*

Dizziness, lightheadedness, or fainting may occur, especially when you get up suddenly from a lying or sitting position. Getting up slowly may help lessen this problem.

Nausea or vomiting may occur, especially after the first couple of doses. This effect may go away if you lie down for a while. However, if nausea or vomiting continues, check with your doctor. Lying down for a while may also help some other side effects, such as dizziness or lightheadedness.

Before having any kind of surgery (including dental surgery) or emergency treatment, tell the medical doctor or dentist in charge that you are taking this medicine.

Do not take this medicine for 5 days before any surgery, including dental surgery, unless otherwise directed by your medical doctor or dentist. Taking aspirin during this time may cause bleeding problems.

For patients taking the *buffered aspirin, codeine, and caffeine* combination (C2 Buffered with Codeine):
- This product contains antacids that can keep many other medicines, especially some medicines used to treat infections, from working properly. This problem can be prevented by not taking the 2 medicines too close together. Ask your pharmacist how long you should wait between taking any other medicine and the buffered aspirin, codeine, and caffeine combination.

For *diabetic patients:*
- False urine sugar test results may occur if you are regularly taking 8 or more 325–mg (5–grain) or 5 or more 500–mg doses of aspirin a day. Smaller amounts or occasional use of aspirin usually will not affect urine sugar tests. If you have any questions about this, check with your health care professional, especially if your diabetes is not well controlled.

Narcotic analgesics may cause dryness of the mouth. For temporary relief, use sugarless candy or gum, melt bits of ice in your mouth, or use a saliva substitute. However, if dry mouth continues for more than 2 weeks, check with your dentist. Continuing dryness of the mouth may increase the chance of dental disease, including tooth decay, gum disease, and fungus infections.

If you have been taking this medicine regularly for several weeks or more, *do not suddenly stop using it without first checking with your doctor.* Depending on which of these medicines you have been taking, and the amount you have been taking every day, your doctor may want you to reduce gradually the amount you are taking before stopping completely, to lessen the chance of withdrawal side effects.

If you think you or someone else may have taken an overdose of this medicine, get emergency help at once. Taking an overdose of this medicine or taking alcohol or CNS depressants with this medicine may lead to unconsciousness or death. Signs of overdose of this medicine include convulsions (seizures); hearing loss; confusion; ringing or buzzing in the ears; severe excitement, nervousness, or restlessness; severe dizziness, severe drowsiness, shortness of breath or troubled breathing, and severe weakness.

Side Effects of This Medicine

Along with its needed effects, a medicine may cause some unwanted effects. Although not all of these side effects may occur, if they do occur they may need medical attention.

Get emergency help immediately if any of the following symptoms of overdose occur:

Any loss of hearing; bloody urine; cold, clammy skin; confusion (severe); convulsions (seizures); diarrhea (severe or continuing); dizziness or lightheadedness (severe); drowsiness (severe); excitement, nervousness, or restlessness (severe); fever; hallucinations (seeing, hearing, or feeling things that are not there); headache (severe or continuing); increased sweating; increased thirst; low blood pressure; nausea or vomiting (severe or continuing); pinpoint pupils of eyes; ringing or buzzing in the ears; shortness of breath or unusually slow or troubled breathing; slow heartbeat; stomach pain (severe or continuing); uncontrollable flapping movements of the hands (especially in elderly patients); vision problems; weakness (severe)

Also, check with your doctor as soon as possible if any of the following side effects occur:

Less common or rare

Bloody or black, tarry stools; confusion; dark urine; fast, slow, or pounding heartbeat; increased sweating (more common with hydrocodone); irregular breathing; mental depression; pale stools; redness or flushing of face (more common with hydrocodone); skin rash, hives, or itching; stomach pain (severe); swelling of face; tightness in chest or wheezing; trembling or uncontrolled muscle movements; unusual excitement (especially in children); unusual tiredness or weakness; vomiting of blood or material that looks like coffee grounds; yellow eyes or skin

Other side effects may occur that usually do not need medical attention. These side effects may go away during treatment as your body adjusts to the medicine. However, check with your doctor if any of the following side effects continue or are bothersome:

More common

Dizziness, lightheadedness, or feeling faint; drowsiness; heartburn or indigestion; nausea or vomiting; stomach pain (mild)

Less common or rare

Blurred or double vision or other changes in vision; constipation (more common with long-term use and with

codeine); difficult, painful, or decreased urination; dryness of mouth; false sense of well-being; frequent urge to urinate; general feeling of discomfort or illness; headache; loss of appetite; nervousness or restlessness; nightmares or unusual dreams; trouble in sleeping; unusual tiredness; unusual weakness

Although not all of the side effects listed above have been reported for all of these medicines, they have been reported for at least one of them. However, since all of the narcotic analgesics are very similar, any of the above side effects may occur with any of these medicines.

After you stop using this medicine, your body may need time to adjust. The length of time this takes depends on which of these medicines you were taking, the amount of medicine you were using, and how long you used it. During this period of time check with your doctor if you notice any of the following side effects:

Body aches; diarrhea; fever, runny nose, or sneezing; gooseflesh; increased sweating; increased yawning; loss of appetite; nausea or vomiting; nervousness, restlessness, or irritability; shivering or trembling; stomach cramps; trouble in sleeping; weakness

Other side effects not listed above may also occur in some patients. If you notice any other effects, check with your medical doctor or dentist.

NATALIZUMAB (Intravenous route) -
na-ta-LYE-zoo-mab

Black Box Warning

- Natalizumab increases the risk of progressive multifocal leukoencephalopathy (PML), an opportunistic viral infection of the brain that usually leads to death or severe disability. Although the cases of PML were limited to patients with recent or concomitant exposure to immunomodulators or immunosuppressants, there were too few cases to rule out the possibility that PML may occur with natalizumab monotherapy.
  - Because of the risk of PML, natalizumab is available only through a special restricted distribution program called the TOUCH® Prescribing Program. Under the TOUCH® Prescribing Program, only prescribers, infusion centers, and pharmacies associated with infusion centers registered with the program are able to prescribe, distribute, or infuse the product. In addition, natalizumab must be administered only to patients who are enrolled in and meet all the conditions of the TOUCH® Prescribing Program.
  - Healthcare professionals should monitor patients on natalizumab for any new sign or symptoms that may be suggestive of PML. Natalizumab dosing should be withheld immediately at the first sign or symptoms suggestive of PML. For diagnosis, an evaluation that includes a gadolinium-enhanced magnetic resonance imaging scan of the brain and, when indicated, cerebrospinal fluid analysis for JC viral DNA are recommended.

Commonly used brand name(s)

In the U.S.—
  Tysabri

Available Dosage Forms:
  • Solution

Therapeutic Class: Immune Suppressant
Pharmacologic Class: Monoclonal Antibody

Uses For This Medicine

Natalizumab is used to treat patients with relapsing forms of multiple sclerosis (MS). This medicine will not cure MS, but may delay physical disability and extend the time between relapses.

This medicine is only available with your doctor's prescription.

Before Receiving This Medicine

In deciding to use a medicine, the risks of taking the medicine must be weighed against the good it will do. This is a decision you and your doctor will make. For this medicine, the following should be considered:

Allergies—Tell your doctor if you have ever had any unusual or allergic reaction to this medicine or any other medicines. Also tell your health care professional if you have any other types of allergies, such as to foods, dyes, preservatives, or animals. For non-prescription products, read the label or package ingredients carefully.

Pediatric—Studies with this medicine have only been done in adult patients, and there is no specific information comparing use of natalizumab in children with use in other age groups. This medicine is not indicated for use in children under 18 years of age.

Geriatric—Many medicines have not been studied specifically in older people. Therefore, it may not be known whether they work exactly the same way they do in younger adults or if they cause different side effects or problems in older people. There is no specific information comparing use of natalizumab in the elderly with use in other age groups.

Pregnancy—

	Pregnancy Category	Explanation
All Trimesters	C	Animal studies have shown an adverse effect and there are no adequate studies in pregnant women OR no animal studies have been conducted and there are no adequate studies in pregnant women.

Breast Feeding—There are no adequate studies in women for determining infant risk when using this medication during breastfeeding. Weigh the potential benefits against the potential risks before taking this medication while breastfeeding.

Other medicines—Although certain medicines should not be used together at all, in other cases two different medicines may be used together even if an interaction might occur. In these cases, your doctor may want to change the dose, or other precautions may be necessary. Tell your healthcare professional if you are taking any other prescription or non-prescription (over-the-counter [OTC]) medicine.

Interactions with Food/Tobacco/Alcohol—Certain medicines should not be used at or around the time of eating food or eating certain types of food since interactions may occur. Using alcohol or tobacco with certain medicines may also cause interactions to occur. Discuss with your healthcare professional the use of your medicine with food, alcohol, or tobacco.

Other medical problems—The presence of other medical problems may affect the use of this medicine. Make sure you tell your doctor if you have any other medical problems, especially:
  • Kidney problems or
  • Liver disease—Use with caution; natalizumab has not been studied in patients with these conditions.
  • Progressive multifocal leukoencephalopathy (PML; a rare viral infection of the brain that causes severe muscle disability)—People who have PML or who have ever had PML should not receive this medicine.
  • Weakened immune system (e.g., HIV infection, AIDS, leukemia, lymphoma, or organ transplant recipient)—This medicine is not recommended, because people with these conditions may be more likely to get infections.

Proper Use of This Medicine

Natalizumab comes with a medication guide. It is very important that you read and understand this information. Be sure to ask your doctor about anything you do not understand.

You must enroll in a prescribing program called TOUCH in order to begin receiving natalizumab. Your doctor will explain the program and have you sign an enrollment form. Be sure to ask your doctor if you have any questions about the TOUCH prescribing program. It is very important that you understand and follow all of the instructions.

Dosing—The dose of this medicine will be different for different patients. Follow your doctor's orders or the directions on the label. The following information includes only the average doses of this medicine. If your dose is different, do not change it unless your doctor tells you to do so.

The amount of medicine that you take depends on the strength of the medicine. Also, the number of doses you take each day, the time allowed between doses, and the length of time you take the medicine depend on the medical problem for which you are using the medicine.

Missed dose—Call your doctor or pharmacist for instructions.

Storage—Store in the refrigerator. Do not freeze.

Keep out of the reach of children.

Do not keep outdated medicine or medicine no longer needed.

Ask your healthcare professional how you should dispose of any medicine you do not use.

Precautions After Receiving This Medicine

Your doctor will want to check your progress 3 months after the first injection, 6 months after the first injection, and every 6 months after that.

If you are taking interferon beta (e.g., Avonex, Betaseron, Rebif) or azathioprine (e.g., Imuran), you should not take natalizumab.

Other medicines—Do not take other medicines unless they have been discussed with your doctor. This includes prescription or non-prescription (over-the-counter [OTC]) medicines and herbal or vitamin supplements.

If your symptoms do not improve within a few days or if they become worse, check with your doctor.

Avoid getting any immunizations (vaccines) unless they are approved by your doctor.

Side Effects of This Medicine

Along with its needed effects, a medicine may cause some unwanted effects. Although not all of these side effects may occur, if they do occur they may need medical attention.

Check with your doctor immediately if any of the following side effects occur:

More common
> Body produces substance that can bind to drug making it less effective or cause side effects; cough; difficulty swallowing; dizziness; fast heartbeat; hives; itching; puffiness or swelling of the eyelids or around the eyes, face, lips or tongue; shortness of breath; skin rash; tightness in chest; unusual tiredness or weakness; wheezing

Rare
> Abdominal fullness; blurred vision; changes in behavior; chest pain; confusion; difficult or labored breathing; faintness, or lightheadedness when getting up from a lying or sitting position suddenly; feeling of warmth; feeling unusually cold; fever; gaseous abdominal pain; nausea; redness of the face, neck, arms and occasionally, upper chest; shivering; sneezing; sore throat; sweating; thoughts of killing oneself; troubled breathing; yellow eyes or skin

Frequency unknown
> Back pain; convulsions; drowsiness; headache

Some side effects may occur that usually do not need medical attention. These side effects may go away during treatment as your body adjusts to the medicine. Also, your health care professional may be able to tell you about ways to prevent or reduce some of these side effects. Check with your health care professional if any of the following side effects continue or are bothersome or if you have any questions about them:

More common
> Bladder pain; blistering, crusting, irritation, itching, or reddening of skin; bloody or cloudy urine; cracked, dry, scaly skin; diarrhea; difficult, burning, or painful urination; difficulty in moving; discouragement; feeling sad or empty; frequent, strong or increased urge to urinate; headache; irregular menstruation; irritability; itching of the vagina or genital area; lack of appetite; loss of appetite; loss of interest or pleasure; lower back or side pain; muscle pain or stiffness; nausea; pain, cramps, heavy bleeding; pain during sexual intercourse; pain in joints; passing urine more often; stomach pain; stomach soreness or discomfort; swelling; swollen glands; thick, white vaginal discharge with no odor or with a mild odor; trouble concentrating; trouble sleeping

Less common
> Absent, missed, or irregular menstrual periods; chest discomfort; fainting; local bleeding; shakiness in legs, arms, hands, or feet; stopping of menstrual bleeding; trembling or shaking of hands or feet

Other side effects not listed may also occur in some patients. If you notice any other effects, check with your healthcare professional.

NATEGLINIDE   (Oral route) - na-te-GLYE-nide

Commonly used brand name(s)
In the U.S.—
> Starlix

Available Dosage Forms:
- Tablet

Therapeutic Class: Hypoglycemic

Uses For This Medicine

Nateglinide is used to treat a type of diabetes mellitus (sugar diabetes) called type 2 diabetes. With this type of diabetes, insulin produced by the pancreas is not able to get sugar into the cells of the body where it can work properly. Using nateglinide alone, or with metformin or a thiazolidinedione (other types of oral antidiabetic medicines), will help to lower blood sugar when it is too high and help restore the way you use food to make energy.

Many people can control type 2 diabetes with diet alone or with diet and exercise. Following a specially planned diet and exercising will always be important when you have diabetes, even when you are taking medicines. To work properly, the amount of nateglinide you take must be balanced against the amount and type of food you eat and the amount of exercise you do. If you change your diet, your exercise, or both, you will want to test your blood sugar to find out if it is too low. Your health care professional will teach you what to do if this happens.

Nateglinide does not help patients who have insulin-dependent or type 1 diabetes because they cannot produce insulin from their pancreas gland. Their blood glucose is best controlled by insulin injections.

Nateglinide does not help patients who have already been treated with other antidiabetic medicines for a long time.

Nateglinide may be used together with metformin or a thiazolidinedione, but should not take the place of these medicines.

Nateglinide is available only with your doctor's prescription.

Before Using This Medicine

In deciding to use a medicine, the risks of taking the medicine must be weighed against the good it will do. This is a decision you and your doctor will make. For this medicine, the following should be considered:

Allergies—Tell your doctor if you have ever had any unusual or allergic reaction to this medicine or any other medi-

cines. Also tell your health care professional if you have any other types of allergies, such as to foods, dyes, preservatives, or animals. For non-prescription products, read the label or package ingredients carefully.

Pediatric—Studies on this medicine have been done only in adult patients, and there is no specific information comparing use of nateglinide in children with use in other age groups.

Geriatric—This medicine has been tested and has not been shown to cause different side effects or problems in older people than it does in younger adults. However, older patients may be more likely to develop low blood sugar.

Pregnancy—

	Pregnancy Category	Explanation
All Trimesters	C	Animal studies have shown an adverse effect and there are no adequate studies in pregnant women OR no animal studies have been conducted and there are no adequate studies in pregnant women.

Breast Feeding—There are no adequate studies in women for determining infant risk when using this medication during breastfeeding. Weigh the potential benefits against the potential risks before taking this medication while breastfeeding.

Other medicines—

Using this medicine with any of the following medicines may cause an increased risk of certain side effects, but using both drugs may be the best treatment for you. If both medicines are prescribed together, your doctor may change the dose or how often you use one or both of the medicines.

Bitter Melon, Glucomannan, Guar Gum, Psyllium, St John's Wort

Interactions with Food/Tobacco/Alcohol—Certain medicines should not be used at or around the time of eating food or eating certain types of food since interactions may occur. Using alcohol or tobacco with certain medicines may also cause interactions to occur. Discuss with your healthcare professional the use of your medicine with food, alcohol, or tobacco.

Other medical problems—The presence of other medical problems may affect the use of this medicine. Make sure you tell your doctor if you have any other medical problems, especially:

- Adrenal gland or pituitary gland not producing enough hormones or
- Malnourishment (not getting enough nutrients in your diet) or
- Severe kidney problems—These conditions can make patients on nateglinide be more at risk for having low blood sugar.
- Alcohol use or
- Not eating enough or
- Strenuous physical exercise—May increase risk of low blood sugar
- Fever or
- Infection or
- Surgery or

- Trauma—Temporary loss of blood sugar control may occur in patients with these conditions. Insulin therapy may be needed.
- Ketones in the blood (diabetic ketoacidosis) or
- Type 1 (insulin-dependent) diabetes—Insulin is needed to control diabetes in patients with these conditions
- Liver disease, moderate to severe—Use of nateglinide in patients with this condition have not been studied. Caution should be used.
- Nervous system disorder (autonomic neuropathy)—Patients with this condition might not be able to detect the symptoms of low blood sugar and might not take immediate steps to treat it

Proper Use of This Medicine

Follow carefully the special meal plan that your doctor gave you. This is the most important part of controlling your condition and is necessary if the medicine is to work properly. Also, exercise regularly and test for sugar in your blood or urine as directed.

This medicine is usually taken between 1 and 30 minutes before a meal. If you skip the meal, also skip the scheduled dose of nateglinide.

Use this medicine as directed even if you feel well and do not notice any signs of high blood sugar. Remember that this medicine will not cure your diabetes, but it does help to control it. You must to continue to take it as directed if you expect to lower your blood sugar and keep it low. You may have to take an antidiabetic medicine for the rest of your life. If high blood sugar is not treated, it can cause serious problems, such as blood vessel disease, eye disease, heart failure, or kidney disease.

Dosing—The dose of this medicine will be different for different patients. Follow your doctor's orders or the directions on the label. The following information includes only the average doses of this medicine. If your dose is different, do not change it unless your doctor tells you to do so.

The amount of medicine that you take depends on the strength of the medicine. Also, the number of doses you take each day, the time allowed between doses, and the length of time you take the medicine depend on the medical problem for which you are using the medicine.

- For oral dosage form (tablets):
  - For type 2 diabetes:
    - Adults—60 to 120 mg three times a day taken between one and thirty minutes before meals.
    - Children—Use and dose must be determined by your doctor.

Missed dose—If you miss a dose of this medicine, take it as soon as possible. However, if it is almost time for your next dose, skip the missed dose and go back to your regular dosing schedule. Do not double doses.

Take it before your next main meal.

Storage—Store the medicine in a closed container at room temperature, away from heat, moisture, and direct light. Keep from freezing.

Keep out of the reach of children.

Do not keep outdated medicine or medicine no longer needed.

Ask your healthcare professional how you should dispose of any medicine you do not use.

Precautions While Using This Medicine

Your doctor will want to check your progress at regular visits, especially during the first few weeks that you take this medicine.

It is very important to follow carefully any instructions from your health care team about:

- Alcohol—Drinking alcohol may cause severe low blood sugar. Discuss this with your health care team.

- Other medicines—Do not take other medicines during the time you are taking nateglinide unless they have been discussed with your doctor. This especially includes nonprescription medicines for appetite control, asthma, colds, cough, hay fever, pain relief, or sinus problems.

- Counseling—Other family members need to learn how to prevent side effects or help with side effects if they occur. Also, patients with diabetes may need special counseling about diabetes medicine dosing changes that might occur because of lifestyle changes, such as changes in exercise and diet. Furthermore, counseling on contraception and pregnancy may be needed because of the problems that can occur in patients with diabetes during pregnancy.

- Travel—Keep a recent prescription and your medical history with you. Be prepared for an emergency as you would normally. Make allowances for changing time zones and keep your meal times as close as possible to your usual meal times.

In case of emergency—There may be a time when you need emergency help for a problem caused by your diabetes. You need to be prepared for these emergencies. It is a good idea to wear a medical identification (ID) bracelet or neck chain at all times. Also, carry an ID card in your wallet or purse that says that you have diabetes and a list of all of your medicines.

Nateglinide can cause low blood sugar (hypoglycemia). Low blood sugar also can occur if you use nateglinide with another antidiabetic medicine, delay or miss a meal or snack, exercise more than usual, drink alcohol, or cannot eat because of nausea or vomiting. Symptoms of low blood sugar must be treated before they lead to unconsciousness (passing out). Different people may feel different symptoms of low blood sugar. It is important that you learn which symptoms of low blood sugar you usually have so that you can treat it quickly.

Symptoms of low blood sugar include anxiety; behavior change similar to being drunk; blurred vision; cold sweats; confusion; cool, pale skin; difficulty in thinking; drowsiness; excessive hunger; fast heartbeat; headache (continuing); nausea; nervousness; nightmares; restless sleep; shakiness; slurred speech; or unusual tiredness or weakness.

If symptoms of low blood sugar occur, eat glucose tablets or gel, corn syrup, honey, or sugar cubes; or drink fruit juice, nondiet soft drink, or sugar dissolved in water to relieve the symptoms. Also, check your blood for low blood sugar. Get to a doctor or a hospital right away if the symptoms do not improve. Someone should call for emergency help immediately if severe symptoms such as convulsions (seizures) or unconsciousness occur. Food or drink should not be forced because the patient could choke from not swallowing correctly.

Hyperglycemia (high blood sugar) may occur if you do not take enough or skip a dose of your antidiabetic medicine, overeat or do not follow your meal plan, have a fever or infection, or do not exercise as much as usual.

Symptoms of high blood sugar include blurred vision; drowsiness; dry mouth; flushed, dry skin; fruit-like breath odor; increased urination; ketones in urine; loss of appetite; stomachache, nausea, or vomiting; tiredness; troubled breathing (rapid and deep); unconsciousness; or unusual thirst.

If symptoms of high blood sugar occur, check your blood sugar level and then call your doctor for instructions.

Side Effects of This Medicine

Along with its needed effects, a medicine may cause some unwanted effects. Although not all of these side effects may occur, if they do occur they may need medical attention.

Check with your doctor immediately if any of the following side effects occur:

Less common

Convulsions (seizures); unconsciousness

Check with your doctor as soon as possible if any of the following side effects occur:

Less common

Low blood sugar, including anxious feeling, behavior change similar to being drunk, blurred vision, cold sweats, confusion, cool pale skin, difficulty in thinking, drowsiness, excessive hunger, fast heartbeat, headache, nausea, nervousness, nightmares, restless sleep, shakiness, slurred speech, or unusual tiredness or weakness

Incidence not known-occurred during clinical practice

Hives or welts; itching; redness of skin; skin rash

Some side effects may occur that usually do not need medical attention. These side effects may go away during treatment as your body adjusts to the medicine. Also, your health care professional may be able to tell you about ways to prevent or reduce some of these side effects. Check with your health care professional if any of the following side effects continue or are bothersome or if you have any questions about them:

More common

Cough; runny or stuffy nose; sore throat

Less common

Abdominal or stomach pain; back pain; chills; dizziness; pain in joints or muscles; sneezing; swelling in joints

Other side effects not listed may also occur in some patients. If you notice any other effects, check with your healthcare professional.

NEDOCROMIL (Inhalation, oral/ nebulization route) - ne-doe-KROE-mil

Commonly used brand name(s)

In the U.S.—

Tilade

Available Dosage Forms:

- Aerosol Powder

Therapeutic Class: Antiasthma
Pharmacologic Class: Mast Cell Stabilizer

Uses For This Medicine

Nedocromil is used to prevent the symptoms of asthma. When it is used regularly, nedocromil lessens the number and severity of asthma attacks by reducing inflammation in the lungs. Nedocromil is also used just before exposure to conditions or substances (for example, allergens, chemicals, cold air, or air pollutants) that cause reactions, to prevent bronchospasm (wheezing or difficulty in breathing). In addition, nedocromil is used to prevent bronchospasm following exercise. This medicine will not help an asthma or bronchospasm attack that has already started.

Nedocromil may be used alone or with other asthma medicines, such as bronchodilators (medicines that open up narrowed breathing passages) and corticosteroids (cortisone-like medicines).

Nedocromil works by acting on certain inflammatory cells in the lungs to prevent them from releasing substances that cause asthma symptoms and/or bronchospasm.

This medicine is available only with your doctor's prescription.

Before Using This Medicine

In deciding to use a medicine, the risks of taking the medicine must be weighed against the good it will do. This is a decision you and your doctor will make. For this medicine, the following should be considered:

Allergies—Tell your doctor if you have ever had any unusual or allergic reaction to this medicine or any other medicines. Also tell your health care professional if you have any other types of allergies, such as to foods, dyes, preservatives, or animals. For non-prescription products, read the label or package ingredients carefully.

Pediatric—Nedocromil has been tested in children 6 years of age and older. In effective doses, it is not expected to cause different side effects or problems in children than it does in adults.

Geriatric—Many medicines have not been studied specifically in older people. Therefore, it may not be known whether they work the same way they do in younger adults. Although there is no specific information comparing use of nedocromil in the elderly with use in other age groups, it is not expected to cause different side effects or problems in older people than it does in younger adults.

Pregnancy—

	Pregnancy Category	Explanation
All Trimesters	B	Animal studies have revealed no evidence of harm to the fetus, however, there are no adequate studies in pregnant women OR animal studies have shown an adverse effect, but adequate studies in pregnant women have failed to demonstrate a risk to the fetus.

Breast Feeding—There are no adequate studies in women for determining infant risk when using this medication during breastfeeding. Weigh the potential benefits against the potential risks before taking this medication while breastfeeding.

Other medicines—Although certain medicines should not be used together at all, in other cases two different medicines may be used together even if an interaction might occur. In these cases, your doctor may want to change the dose, or other precautions may be necessary. Tell your healthcare professional if you are taking any other prescription or non-prescription (over-the-counter [OTC]) medicine.

Interactions with Food/Tobacco/Alcohol—Certain medicines should not be used at or around the time of eating food or eating certain types of food since interactions may occur. Using alcohol or tobacco with certain medicines may also cause interactions to occur. Discuss with your healthcare professional the use of your medicine with food, alcohol, or tobacco.

Proper Use of This Medicine

Nedocromil is used to help prevent symptoms of asthma or bronchospasm (wheezing or difficulty in breathing). When this medicine is used regularly, it decreases the number and severity of asthma attacks. Nedocromil will not relieve an asthma or bronchospasm attack that has already started.

Nedocromil inhalation aerosol usually comes with patient directions. Read them carefully before using this medicine. If you do not understand the directions or if you are not sure how to use the inhaler, ask your health care professional to show you what to do. Also, ask your health care professional to check regularly how you use the inhaler to make sure you are using it properly.

The nedocromil aerosol canister provides 104 inhalations for the inhaler that is available in the U.S. or 112 inhalations for the Canadian inhaler. You should keep a record of the number of inhalations you use so you will know when the canister is almost empty. This canister, unlike other aerosol canisters, cannot be floated in water to test its fullness.

When you use the inhaler for the first time, or if you have not used it for more than seven days, the inhaler may not deliver the right amount of medicine with the first puff. Therefore, before using the inhaler, prime it to make sure it provides the correct dose.

To prime the inhaler:

- Insert the metal canister firmly into the clean mouthpiece according to the manufacturer's instructions. Check to make sure the canister is placed properly into the mouthpiece.
- Take the cover off the mouthpiece and shake the inhaler well.
- Hold the canister well away from you against a light background, and press the top of the canister, spraying the medicine one time into the air. Repeat this two more times for a total of three sprays. If the inhaler is working properly, a fine mist will be sprayed from the mouthpiece.

To use the inhaler:

- Using your thumb and one or two fingers, hold the inhaler upright with the mouthpiece end down and pointing toward you.
- Take the cover off the mouthpiece. Check the mouthpiece for any foreign objects. Do not use the inhaler with any other mouthpieces.
- Gently shake the inhaler three or four times.
- Hold the mouthpiece away from your mouth and breathe out slowly and completely to the end of a normal breath.

- Use the inhalation method recommended by your doctor.
  - Open-mouth method: Place the mouthpiece about 1 to 2 inches (2 fingerwidths) in front of your widely opened mouth. Make sure the inhaler is aimed into your mouth so the spray does not hit the roof of your mouth or your tongue. Close your eyes just before spraying to keep the spray out of your eyes.
  - Closed-mouth method: Place the mouthpiece in your mouth between your teeth and over your tongue with your lips closed tightly around it. Make sure your tongue or teeth are not blocking the opening.
- Tilt your head back a little. Start to breathe in slowly and deeply through your mouth and, at the same time, press the top of the canister once to get one puff of medicine. Continue to breathe in slowly for 3 to 4 seconds until you have taken a full breath. It is important to press down on the canister and breathe in slowly at the same time so the medicine is pulled into your lungs. This step may be difficult at first. If you are using the closed-mouth method and you see a fine mist coming from your mouth or nose, the inhaler is not being used correctly.
- Hold your breath as long as you can for up to 10 seconds (count slowly to 10). This gives the medicine time to get into your airways and lungs.
- Take the mouthpiece away from your mouth and breathe out slowly.
- If your doctor has told you to inhale more than one puff of medicine at each dose, wait 1 minute between puffs. Then, gently shake the inhaler again, and take the second puff following exactly the same steps you used for the first puff. Breathe in only one puff at a time.
- If your doctor has told you to use an inhaled bronchodilator before using nedocromil, you should wait at least 2 minutes after using the bronchodilator before using nedocromil. This allows the nedocromil to get deeper into your lungs.
- When you are finished, wipe off the mouthpiece and replace the cover to keep the mouthpiece clean and free of foreign objects.
- Keep track of the number of sprays you have used by noting each one on the chart provided with the inhaler. The inhaler should be discarded once 104 sprays have been used. Even though the inhaler may not be empty after 104 sprays, the dose may be inaccurate so you may not receive the correct amount of medicine.

Your doctor may want you to use a spacer device with the inhaler. A spacer makes the inhaler easier to use. It allows more of the medicine to reach your lungs and helps make sure that less of it stays in your mouth and throat.

To use a spacer device with the inhaler:

- Attach the spacer to the inhaler according to the manufacturer's directions. There are different types of spacers available, but the method of breathing remains the same with most spacers.
- Gently shake the inhaler and spacer three or four times.
- Hold the mouthpiece of the spacer away from your mouth and breathe out slowly to the end of a normal breath.
- Place the mouthpiece into your mouth between your teeth and over your tongue with your lips closed around it.

- Press down on the canister top once to release one puff of medicine into the spacer. Then, within one or two seconds, begin to breathe in slowly and deeply through your mouth for 5 to 10 seconds. Count the seconds while inhaling. Do not breathe in through your nose.
- Hold your breath as long as you can for up to 10 seconds (count slowly to ten).
- Breathe out slowly. Do not remove the mouthpiece from your mouth. Breathe in and out slowly two or three times to make sure the spacer device is emptied.
- If your doctor has told you to take more than one puff of medicine at each dose, wait a minute between puffs. Then, gently shake the inhaler and spacer again and take the second puff, following exactly the same steps you used for the first puff.
- When you have finished, remove the spacer device from the inhaler and replace the cover of the mouthpiece.

To clean the inhaler:

- Clean the inhaler often to prevent build-up of medicine and blocking of the mouthpiece. The mouthpiece can be washed every day and should be washed at least twice a week.
- Remove the metal canister from the inhaler and set it aside. Do not get the canister wet.
- Wash the mouthpiece in hot water.
- Shake off the excess water and let the mouthpiece air dry completely before replacing the metal canister and cover.

For patients using nedocromil regularly (for example, every day):

- In order for nedocromil to work properly, it must be inhaled every day in regularly spaced doses as ordered by your doctor.
- Usually about 2 to 4 weeks may pass before you begin to feel the full effects of this medicine.

Dosing—The dose of this medicine will be different for different patients. Follow your doctor's orders or the directions on the label. The following information includes only the average doses of this medicine. If your dose is different, do not change it unless your doctor tells you to do so.

The amount of medicine that you take depends on the strength of the medicine. Also, the number of doses you take each day, the time allowed between doses, and the length of time you take the medicine depend on the medical problem for which you are using the medicine.

- For inhalation dosage form (inhalation aerosol):
  - For prevention of asthma symptoms:
    - Adults and children 6 years of age or older— 3.5 or 4 milligrams (mg) (2 puffs) two to four times a day at regularly spaced times.
    - Children up to 6 years of age—Use and dose must be determined by the doctor.
  - For prevention of bronchospasm caused by exercise or a substance:
    - Adults and children 12 years of age or older— 4 mg (2 puffs) as a single dose up to thirty minutes before exercise or exposure to any condition or substance that may cause an attack.
    - Children up to 12 years of age—Use and dose must be determined by the doctor.

Missed dose—If you miss a dose of this medicine, take it as soon as possible. However, if it is almost time for your next

dose, skip the missed dose and go back to your regular dosing schedule. Do not double doses.

Storage—Store the medicine in a closed container at room temperature, away from heat, moisture, and direct light. Keep from freezing.

Store the canister at room temperature, away from heat and direct light. Do not freeze. Do not keep this medicine inside a car where it could be exposed to extreme heat or cold. Do not poke holes in the canister or throw it into a fire, even if the canister is empty.

Keep out of the reach of children.

Do not keep outdated medicine or medicine no longer needed.

Precautions While Using This Medicine

If your symptoms do not improve within 2 to 4 weeks, check with your doctor. Also, check with your doctor if your condition becomes worse.

You may also be taking a corticosteroid or a bronchodilator for asthma along with this medicine. Do not stop taking the corticosteroid or bronchodilator even if your asthma seems better, unless you are told to do so by your doctor.

Throat irritation and/or an unpleasant taste may occur after you use this medicine. Gargling and rinsing the mouth after each dose may help prevent these effects.

Side Effects of This Medicine

Along with its needed effects, a medicine may cause some unwanted effects. Although not all of these side effects may occur, if they do occur they may need medical attention.

Check with your doctor as soon as possible if any of the following side effects occur:

Less common
 Abdominal pain; increased wheezing, tightness in chest, or difficulty in breathing

Rare
 Pain, stiffness, or swelling of joints; signs of infection, such as fever, sore throat, body aches, or chills

Some side effects may occur that usually do not need medical attention. These side effects may go away during treatment as your body adjusts to the medicine. Also, your health care professional may be able to tell you about ways to prevent or reduce some of these side effects. Check with your health care professional if any of the following side effects continue or are bothersome or if you have any questions about them:

Less common or rare
 Cough; headache; nausea or vomiting; runny or stuffy nose; sensation of warmth; throat irritation; tremor

After you use nedocromil inhalation aerosol, you may notice an unpleasant taste. This may be expected and will usually go away after a while.

Other side effects not listed may also occur in some patients. If you notice any other effects, check with your healthcare professional.

NEDOCROMIL (Ophthalmic route) -
ne-doe-KROE-mil

Commonly used brand name(s)
In the U.S.—
 Alocril

Available Dosage Forms:
 • Solution

Therapeutic Class: Ophthalmologic Agent
Pharmacologic Class: Mast Cell Stabilizer

Uses For This Medicine

Nedocromil is used to treat the itching in your eyes that happens with allergies.

Nedocromil works by acting on certain inflammatory cells to prevent them from releasing substances that cause allergic symptom.

This medicine is available only with your doctor's prescription.

Before Using This Medicine

In deciding to use a medicine, the risks of taking the medicine must be weighed against the good it will do. This is a decision you and your doctor will make. For this medicine, the following should be considered:

Allergies—Tell your doctor if you have ever had any unusual or allergic reaction to this medicine or any other medicines. Also tell your health care professional if you have any other types of allergies, such as to foods, dyes, preservatives, or animals. For non-prescription products, read the label or package ingredients carefully.

Pediatric—Nedocromil has been tested in children 3 years of age and older. In effective doses, it is not expected to cause different side effects or problems in children than it does in adults.

Geriatric—No differences in safety or effectiveness have been observed between elderly and younger patients.

Pregnancy—

	Pregnancy Category	Explanation
All Trimesters	B	Animal studies have revealed no evidence of harm to the fetus, however, there are no adequate studies in pregnant women OR animal studies have shown an adverse effect, but adequate studies in pregnant women have failed to demonstrate a risk to the fetus.

Breast Feeding—There are no adequate studies in women for determining infant risk when using this medication during breastfeeding. Weigh the potential benefits against the potential risks before taking this medication while breastfeeding.

Other medicines—Although certain medicines should not be used together at all, in other cases two different medicines may be used together even if an interaction might occur. In these cases, your doctor may want to change the dose, or other precautions may be necessary. Tell your healthcare

professional if you are taking any other prescription or non-prescription (over-the-counter [OTC]) medicine.

Interactions with Food/Tobacco/Alcohol—Certain medicines should not be used at or around the time of eating food or eating certain types of food since interactions may occur. Using alcohol or tobacco with certain medicines may also cause interactions to occur. Discuss with your healthcare professional the use of your medicine with food, alcohol, or tobacco.

Proper Use of This Medicine

Dosing—The dose of this medicine will be different for different patients. Follow your doctor's orders or the directions on the label. The following information includes only the average doses of this medicine. If your dose is different, do not change it unless your doctor tells you to do so.

The amount of medicine that you take depends on the strength of the medicine. Also, the number of doses you take each day, the time allowed between doses, and the length of time you take the medicine depend on the medical problem for which you are using the medicine.

Nedocromil is used to help treat the itching that occurs with allergic conjunctivitis. To use the ophthalmic solution (eye drops)form of this medicine:

- First, wash your hands. Tilt the head back and, pressing your finger gently on the skin just beneath the lower eyelid, pull the lower eyelid away from the eye to make a space. Drop the medicine into this space. Let go of the eyelid and gently close the eyes. Blink a few times to make sure the eye is covered with the medicine.
- To keep the medicine as germ-free as possible, do not touch the applicator tip to any surface (including the eye). Also, keep the container tightly closed.

Missed dose—If you miss a dose of this medicine, take it as soon as possible. However, if it is almost time for your next dose, skip the missed dose and go back to your regular dosing schedule. Do not double doses.

Storage—Keep out of the reach of children.

Do not keep outdated medicine or medicine no longer needed.

Ask your healthcare professional how you should dispose of any medicine you do not use.

Precautions While Using This Medicine

You should avoid wearing your contact lenses while your eyes are itching from your allergies.

Side Effects of This Medicine

Some side effects may occur that usually do not need medical attention. These side effects may go away during treatment as your body adjusts to the medicine. Also, your health care professional may be able to tell you about ways to prevent or reduce some of these side effects. Check with your health care professional if any of the following side effects continue or are bothersome or if you have any questions about them:

More common

Blurred vision; change in color vision; cough; difficulty breathing; noisy breathing; shortness of breath, tightness in chest, or wheezing; difficulty seeing at night;

dry or itching eyes; headache; increased sensitivity of eyes to sunlight; redness, pain, or swelling of eye, eyelid, or inner lining of the eye; runny or stuffy nose; sneezing; stinging, irritation or burning of your eyes; unpleasant taste; unusual watering of eyes or discharge

Other side effects not listed may also occur in some patients. If you notice any other effects, check with your healthcare professional.

NEFAZODONE (Oral route) - nef-AY-zoe-done

Black Box Warning

Cases of life-threatening hepatic failure have been reported in patients treated with nefazodone hydrochloride.

The reported rate in the United States is about 1 case of liver failure resulting in death or transplant per 250,000 patient-years to 300,000 patient-years of nefazodone hydrochloride treatment. The total patient-years is a summation of each patient's duration of exposure expressed in years. For example, 1 patient-year is equal to 2 patients each treated for 6 months, 3 patients each treated for 4 months, etc.

Ordinarily, treatment with nefazodone hydrochloride should not be initiated in individuals with active liver disease or with elevated baseline serum transaminases. There is no evidence that pre-existing liver disease increases the likelihood of developing liver failure, however, baseline abnormalities can complicate patient monitoring.

Patients should be advised to be alert for signs and symptoms of liver dysfunction (jaundice, anorexia, gastrointestinal complaints, malaise, etc) and to report them to their doctor immediately if they occur.

Nefazodone hydrochloride should be discontinued if clinical signs or symptoms suggest liver failure. Patients who develop evidence of hepatocellular injury such as increased serum AST or serum ALT levels greater or equal to 3 times the upper limit of normal, while on nefazodone hydrochloride should be withdrawn from the drug. These patients should be presumed to be at increased risk for liver injury if nefazodone hydrochloride is reintroduced. Accordingly, such patients should not be considered for re-treatment.

Commonly used brand name(s)

In the U.S.—
Serzone

Available Dosage Forms:
- Tablet

Therapeutic Class: Antidepressant
Pharmacologic Class: Serotonin/Norepinephrine Reuptake Inhibitor

Uses For This Medicine

Nefazodone is used to treat mental depression.

This medicine is available only with your doctor's prescription.

Before Using This Medicine

In deciding to use a medicine, the risks of taking the medicine must be weighed against the good it will do. This is a decision you and your doctor will make. For this medicine, the following should be considered:

Allergies—Tell your doctor if you have ever had any unusual or allergic reaction to this medicine or any other medicines. Also tell your health care professional if you have any other types of allergies, such as to foods, dyes, preservatives, or animals. For non-prescription products, read the label or package ingredients carefully.

Pediatric—Studies on nefazodone have been done only in adult patients, and there is no specific information comparing use of this medicine in children up to 18 years of age with use in other age groups.

Nefazodone must be used with caution in children with depression. Studies have shown occurrences of children thinking about suicide or attempting suicide in clinical trials for this medicine. More study is needed to be sure nefazodone is safe and effective in children.

Geriatric—The relationship of age to the effects of nefazodone has not been systematically studied in older people. However, blood levels of nefazodone have been found to be higher in older patients. An older adult may require a lower dose of nefazodone than a younger adult.

Pregnancy—

	Pregnancy Category	Explanation
All Trimesters	C	Animal studies have shown an adverse effect and there are no adequate studies in pregnant women OR no animal studies have been conducted and there are no adequate studies in pregnant women.

Breast Feeding—Studies in women breastfeeding have demonstrated harmful infant effects. An alternative to this medication should be prescribed or you should stop breast-feeding while using this medicine.

Other medicines—

Using this medicine with any of the following medicines is not recommended. Your doctor may decide not to treat you with this medication or change some of the other medicines you take.

Astemizole, Cisapride, Dihydroergotamine, Eplerenone, Ergoloid Mesylates, Ergonovine, Ergotamine, Furazolidone, Isocarboxazid, Methylergonovine, Phenelzine, Pimozide, Terfenadine

Interactions with Food/Tobacco/Alcohol—Certain medicines should not be used at or around the time of eating food or eating certain types of food since interactions may occur. Using alcohol or tobacco with certain medicines may also cause interactions to occur. Discuss with your healthcare professional the use of your medicine with food, alcohol, or tobacco.

Other medical problems—The presence of other medical problems may affect the use of this medicine. Make sure you

tell your doctor if you have any other medical problems, especially:

- Convulsions (seizures) (history of)—The risk of seizures may be increased

- Dehydration or

- Hypovolemia (low blood volume)—May increase the chance that low blood pressure (hypotension) will occur

- Heart disease or

- Stroke (or history of)—Nefazodone may make these conditions worse by causing low blood pressure (hypotension)

- Liver function problems—If your liver does not function well, due to liver problems or liver disease and you take nefazodone, the amount of nefazodone in your blood may be too high. This may cause serious disease or damage in your liver.

- Liver function problems when taking this medicine before and you had to stop taking it—You may have a greater chance of having liver problems if you take nefazodone again. Tell your doctor immediately if you have taken this medicine before.

- Mania (a type of mental illness) (history of)—Nefazodone may cause this problem to recur

Proper Use of This Medicine

Take this medicine only as directed by your doctor. Do not take more or less of it and do not take it more or less often than your doctor ordered.

Sometimes this medicine must be taken for several weeks before you begin to feel better.

Dosing—The dose of this medicine will be different for different patients. Follow your doctor's orders or the directions on the label. The following information includes only the average doses of this medicine. If your dose is different, do not change it unless your doctor tells you to do so.

The amount of medicine that you take depends on the strength of the medicine. Also, the number of doses you take each day, the time allowed between doses, and the length of time you take the medicine depend on the medical problem for which you are using the medicine.

- For oral dosage form (tablets):
  - For mental depression:
    - Adults (18 years of age and older)—To start, 200 milligrams (mg) a day, divided into two doses. Your doctor may increase the dose if needed.
    - Older adults—To start, 100 mg a day, divided into two doses. Your doctor may increase the dose if needed.
    - Children up to 18 years of age—Use and dose must be determined by the doctor.

Missed dose—If you miss a dose of this medicine, take it as soon as possible. However, if it is almost time for your next dose, skip the missed dose and go back to your regular dosing schedule. Do not double doses.

Storage—Store the medicine in a closed container at room temperature, away from heat, moisture, and direct light. Keep from freezing.

Keep out of the reach of children.

Do not keep outdated medicine or medicine no longer needed.

Precautions While Using This Medicine

It is important that your doctor check your progress at regular visits to allow dosage adjustments and to help reduce side effects.

Do not take astemizole, cisapride, pimozide, or terfenadine while you are taking nefazodone. If you do, you may develop a very serious change in the rhythm of your heartbeat.

Do not take carbamazepine while you are taking nefazodone. It may cause the medicine to not work or to not work as well.

This medicine may cause serious problems with your liver. Call your doctor right away for any of the following problems. Abdominal pain, nausea, vomiting, yellow eyes or skin, dark colored urine, light-colored stools, feeling very tired or weak

Do not take a monoamine oxidase (MAO) inhibitor (furazolidone, phenelzine, procarbazine, selegiline, tranylcypromine) while you are taking or less than 7 days after taking nefazodone. Do not take nefazodone less than 14 days after taking an MAO inhibitor. If you do, you may develop convulsions (seizures), extremely high fever, or other serious unwanted effects.

Nefazodone may cause some people to be agitated, irritable or display other abnormal behaviors. It may also cause some people to have suicidal thoughts and tendencies or to become more depressed. If you or your caregiver notice any of these adverse effects, tell your doctor right away.

This medicine may add to the effects of alcohol and other central nervous system (CNS) depressants (medicines that make you drowsy or less alert). Some examples of CNS depressants are antihistamines or medicine for hay fever, other allergies, or colds; sedatives, tranquilizers, or sleeping medicine; prescription pain medicine or narcotics; barbiturates; medicine for seizures; muscle relaxants; or anesthetics, including some dental anesthetics. Check with your doctor before taking any of the above while you are using this medicine.

This medicine may cause some people to become dizzy or drowsy, or to have blurred vision or other vision changes. Make sure you know how you react to this medicine before you drive, use machines, or do other jobs that require you to be alert and able to see well.

Dizziness, lightheadedness, or fainting may occur, especially when you get up from a lying or sitting position. Getting up slowly may help. If this problem continues or gets worse, check with your doctor.

This medicine may cause dryness of the mouth. For temporary relief, use sugarless gum or candy, melt bits of ice in your mouth, or use a saliva substitute. However, if your mouth feels dry for more than 2 weeks, check with your medical doctor or dentist. Continuing dryness of the mouth may increase the chance of dental disease, including tooth decay, gum disease, and fungus infections.

Side Effects of This Medicine

Along with its needed effects, a medicine may cause some unwanted effects. Although not all of these side effects may occur, if they do occur they may need medical attention.

Check with your doctor as soon as possible if any of the following side effects occur:

More common
   Blurred vision or other changes in vision; clumsiness or unsteadiness; lightheadedness or fainting; ringing in the ears; skin rash or itching

Less common
   Bladder pain; bloody or cloudy; cough or hoarseness; diarrhea; excessive muscle tone; eye pain; feeling dizzy; frequent urge to urinate; itching of the vagina or genital area; muscle stiffness; muscle tension or tightness; nausea; pain during sexual intercourse; painful, burning, or difficult urination; shortness of breath, tightness in chest, or wheezing; stomach pain; thick, white vaginal discharge with no odor or with a mild odor; troubled breathing

Rare
   Asthma; bleeding from the rectum; bloody or black, tarry stools; change in sexual desire or performance; chest pain; double vision; dryness of eye; ear pain; fainting; fast heartbeat; fever, chills, or sore throat; hallucinations (seeing, hearing, or feeling things that are not there); hives; increased sense of hearing; increased sensitivity to sun; irritation or soreness of mouth; joint or muscle pain or stiffness; kidney stones; large pupils of eyes; lower back, side, or stomach pain; menstrual changes; mood or mental changes; nerve pain or twitching; pelvic pain; problems in speaking; problems with urination; prolonged, painful, inappropriate penile erection; red or irritated eyes; sensitivity of eyes to light; swelling of face; swollen glands; talking, feeling, and acting with excitement and activity you cannot control; unusual bleeding or bruising; unusual feeling of well-being; unusual tiredness or weakness; vomiting of blood or material that looks like coffee grounds

Incidence not known
   Blistering, peeling, or loosening of skin; light-colored stools; confusion; dark urine; decreased urine output; fever; increased thirst; itching; lack of appetite; large, hive-like swelling on face, eyelids, lips, tongue, throat, hands, legs, feet, or sex organs; muscle pain or cramps; muscle spasm or jerking of all extremities; muscle stiffness; pain, warmth, or burning in fingers, toes, and legs; red skin lesions, often with a purple center; sore throat; sudden loss of consciousness; sweating; vomiting

Some side effects may occur that usually do not need medical attention. These side effects may go away during treatment as your body adjusts to the medicine. Also, your health care professional may be able to tell you about ways to prevent or reduce some of these side effects. Check with your health care professional if any of the following side effects continue or are bothersome or if you have any questions about them:

More common
   Abnormal dreams; agitation; confusion; constipation; diarrhea; dizziness; drowsiness; dryness of mouth; flushing or feeling of warmth; headache; heartburn; increased appetite; increased cough; memory problems; nausea; swelling of arms or legs; tingling, burning, or prickly sensations; tremor; trouble in sleeping; vomiting

Less common or rare
    Breast pain; generalized slowing of mental and physical activity; increased thirst; loss of strength or energy; muscle weakness

Incidence not known
    Unexpected or excess milk flow from breasts; swelling of the breasts or breast soreness in males

Other side effects not listed may also occur in some patients. If you notice any other effects, check with your healthcare professional.

NELFINAVIR (Oral route) - nel-FIN-a-veer

Commonly used brand name(s)

In the U.S.—
    Viracept

Available Dosage Forms:
- Powder for Suspension
- Tablet

Therapeutic Class: Antiretroviral Agent
Pharmacologic Class: Protease Inhibitor

Uses For This Medicine

Nelfinavir is used, usually in combination with other medicines, in the treatment of the infection caused by the human immunodeficiency virus (HIV). HIV is the virus that causes acquired immune deficiency syndrome (AIDS).

Nelfinavir will not cure or prevent HIV infection or AIDS; however, it helps keep HIV from reproducing and appears to slow down the destruction of the immune system. This may help delay the development of problems usually related to AIDS or HIV disease. Nelfinavir will not keep you from spreading HIV to other people. People who receive this medicine may continue to have other problems usually related to AIDS or HIV disease.

This medicine is available only with your doctor's prescription.

Before Using This Medicine

In deciding to use a medicine, the risks of taking the medicine must be weighed against the good it will do. This is a decision you and your doctor will make. For this medicine, the following should be considered:

Allergies—Tell your doctor if you have ever had any unusual or allergic reaction to this medicine or any other medicines. Also tell your health care professional if you have any other types of allergies, such as to foods, dyes, preservatives, or animals. For non-prescription products, read the label or package ingredients carefully.

Pediatric—This medicine has not been reported to cause different side effects or problems in children between 2 and 13 years of age than it does in adults.

This medicine does not work as well in patients less than 2 years of age as it does in others.

Geriatric—Many medicines have not been studied specifically in older people. Therefore, it may not be known whether they work exactly the same way they do in younger adults.

There is no specific information comparing use of nelfinavir in the elderly with use in other age groups.

Pregnancy—

	Pregnancy Category	Explanation
All Trimesters	B	Animal studies have revealed no evidence of harm to the fetus, however, there are no adequate studies in pregnant women OR animal studies have shown an adverse effect, but adequate studies in pregnant women have failed to demonstrate a risk to the fetus.

Breast Feeding—There are no adequate studies in women for determining infant risk when using this medication during breastfeeding. Weigh the potential benefits against the potential risks before taking this medication while breastfeeding.

Other medicines—

Using this medicine with any of the following medicines is not recommended. Your doctor may decide not to treat you with this medication or change some of the other medicines you take.

Amiodarone, Astemizole, Cisapride, Dihydroergotamine, Eplerenone, Ergoloid Mesylates, Ergonovine, Ergotamine, Methylergonovine, Midazolam, Pimozide, Quinidine, Ranolazine, St John's Wort, Triazolam

Interactions with Food/Tobacco/Alcohol—Certain medicines should not be used at or around the time of eating food or eating certain types of food since interactions may occur. Using alcohol or tobacco with certain medicines may also cause interactions to occur. Discuss with your healthcare professional the use of your medicine with food, alcohol, or tobacco.

Other medical problems—The presence of other medical problems may affect the use of this medicine. Make sure you tell your doctor if you have any other medical problems, especially:
- Diabetes or
- Hyperglycemia—Nelfinavir may make the effects of these conditions worse
- Hemophilia—May increase the possibility of bleeding
- Liver disease—Effects of nelfinavir may be increased because of slower removal from the body
- Phenylketonuria (a metabolic problem)—The oral powder form of nelfinavir contains phenylalanine, which may not be broken down properly in people with this condition

Proper Use of This Medicine

Nelfinavir works best if it is taken with food.

Take this medicine exactly as directed by your doctor. Do not take it more often, and do not take it for a longer time than your doctor ordered. Also, do not stop taking this medicine without checking with your doctor first.

Keep taking nelfinavir for the full time of treatment, even if you begin to feel better.

This medicine works best when there is a constant amount in the blood. To help keep the amount constant, do not miss any doses. Also, it is best to take the doses at evenly spaced times, day and night. For example, if you are to take three doses a day, the doses should be spaced about 8 hours apart. If you need help in planning the best times to take your medicine, check with your health care professional.

Only take medicine that your doctor has prescribed specially for you. Do not share your medicine with others.

Dosing—The dose of this medicine will be different for different patients. Follow your doctor's orders or the directions on the label. The following information includes only the average doses of this medicine. If your dose is different, do not change it unless your doctor tells you to do so.

The amount of medicine that you take depends on the strength of the medicine. Also, the number of doses you take each day, the time allowed between doses, and the length of time you take the medicine depend on the medical problem for which you are using the medicine.

- For oral dosage form (oral powder):
  - For treatment of HIV infection:
    - Children 2 to 13 years of age—Dose is based on body weight and must be determined by your doctor. The usual dose is 25 to 35 milligrams (mg) per kilogram (kg) (11.36 to 15.9 mg per pound) of body weight three times a day or 45 to 55 milligrams (mg) per kilogram (kg) (20.45 to 25 mg per pound) two times a day with food
    - Children less than 2 years of age—Use and dose must be determined by your doctor.
- For oral dosage form (tablets):
  - For treatment of HIV infection:
    - Adults and teenagers—750 mg three times a day or 1250 mg two times a day with food.
    - Children 2 to 13 years of age—Dose is based on body weight and must be determined by your doctor. The usual dose is 25 to 35 milligrams (mg) per kilogram (kg) (11.36 to 15.9 mg per pound) of body weight three times a day or 45 to 55 milligrams (mg) per kilogram (kg) (20.45 to 25 mg per pound) two times a day with food
    - Children less than 2 years of age—Use and dose must be determined by your doctor.

Missed dose—If you miss a dose of this medicine, take it as soon as possible. However, if it is almost time for your next dose, skip the missed dose and go back to your regular dosing schedule. Do not double doses.

Storage—Store the medicine in a closed container at room temperature, away from heat, moisture, and direct light. Keep from freezing.

Keep out of the reach of children.

Do not keep outdated medicine or medicine no longer needed.

Precautions While Using This Medicine

Do not take any other medicines without checking with your doctor first. To do so may increase the chance of side effects from nelfinavir.

Nelfinavir should be taken at least 2 hours before or 1 hour after taking didanosine.

This medicine may decrease the effects of some oral contraceptives (birth control pills). To avoid unwanted pregnancy, it is a good idea to use some additional contraceptive measures while being treated with nelfinavir.

It is very important that your doctor check your progress at regular visits to make sure this medicine is working properly and check for unwanted effects, especially increases in blood sugar.

Side Effects of This Medicine

Along with its needed effects, a medicine may cause some unwanted effects. Although not all of these side effects may occur, if they do occur they may need medical attention.

Check with your doctor as soon as possible if any of the following side effects occur:

Confusion; dehydration; dry or itchy skin; fatigue; fruity mouth odor; increased hunger; increased thirst; increased urination; nausea; vomiting; weight loss

Incidence not determined—Observed during clinical practice with levofloxacin; estimates of frequency cannot be determined

cough; difficulty breathing; noisy breathing; shortness of breath; tightness in chest; wheezing; chills; clay-colored stools; dark urine; dizziness; fever; headache; loss of appetite; abdominal or stomach pain; area rash; unpleasant breath odor; unusual tiredness or weakness; vomiting of blood; yellow eyes or skin; drowsiness; muscle tremors; rapid, deep breathing; restlessness; stomach cramps; irregular heartbeat; recurrent fainting

Some side effects may occur that usually do not need medical attention. These side effects may go away during treatment as your body adjusts to the medicine. Also, your health care professional may be able to tell you about ways to prevent or reduce some of these side effects. Check with your health care professional if any of the following side effects continue or are bothersome or if you have any questions about them:

More common
Diarrhea

Less common
Intestinal gas

Other side effects not listed may also occur in some patients. If you notice any other effects, check with your healthcare professional.

NEOMYCIN (Oral route) - nee-oh-MEY-sin

Black Box Warning

Systemic absorption of neomycin occurs following oral administration and toxic reactions may occur. Patients treated with neomycin should be under close clinical observation because of the potential toxicity associated with their use.

Neurotoxicity (including ototoxicity) and nephrotoxicity following the oral use of neomycin sulfate have been reported, even when used in recommended doses. The potential for nephrotoxicity, permanent bilateral auditory ototoxicity and sometimes vestibular toxicity is present in patients with normal renal function when treated with higher doses of neomycin and/or for longer periods that recommended. Serial, vestibular, and audiometric tests, as well as tests of renal function, should be performed (especially in high risk patients).

The risk of nephrotoxicity and ototoxicity is greater in patients with impaired renal function. Ototoxicity is often delayed in onset and patients developing cochlear damage will not have symptoms during therapy to warn them of developing eighth nerve destruction and total or partial deafness may occur long after neomycin has been discontinued.

Neuromuscular blockage and respiratory paralysis have been reported following the oral use of neomycin. The possibility of the occurrence of neuromuscular blockage and respiratory paralysis should be considered if neomycin is administered, especially to patients receiving anesthetics, neuromuscular blocking agents such as tubocurarine, succinylcholine, decamethonium, or in patients receiving massive transfusions of citrate anticoagulated blood. If blockage occurs, calcium salts may reverse these phenomena but mechanical respiratory assistance may be necessary.

Concurrent and/or sequential systemic, oral, or topical use of other aminoglycosides including paromomycin and other potentially nephrotoxic and/or neurotoxic drugs such as bacitracin, cisplatin, vancomycin, amphotericin B, polymyxin B, colistin, and viomycin should be avoided because the toxicity may be additive.

Other factors which increase the risk of toxicity are advanced age and dehydration.

The concurrent use of neomycin with potent diuretics such as ethacrynic acid or furosemide should be avoided since certain diuretics by themselves may cause ototoxicity. In addition, when administered intravenously, diuretics may enhance neomycin toxicity by altering the antibiotic concentration in serum and tissue.

Commonly used brand name(s)

In the U.S.—
Neo-Fradin

Available Dosage Forms:
- Solution
- Tablet

Therapeutic Class: Antibiotic

Uses For This Medicine

Oral neomycin is used to help lessen the symptoms of hepatic coma, a complication of liver disease. In addition, it may be used with another medicine before any surgery affecting the bowels to help prevent infection during surgery.

Neomycin is available only with your doctor's prescription.

Before Using This Medicine

In deciding to use a medicine, the risks of taking the medicine must be weighed against the good it will do. This is a decision you and your doctor will make. For this medicine, the following should be considered:

Allergies—Tell your doctor if you have ever had any unusual or allergic reaction to this medicine or any other medicines. Also tell your health care professional if you have any other types of allergies, such as to foods, dyes, preservatives,

or animals. For non-prescription products, read the label or package ingredients carefully.

Pediatric—Damage to hearing, sense of balance, and kidneys is more likely to occur in premature infants and neonates, who are more sensitive than adults to the effects of neomycin.

Geriatric—Serious side effects, such as damage to hearing, sense of balance, and kidneys may occur in elderly patients, who are usually more sensitive than younger adults to the effects of neomycin.

Pregnancy—

	Pregnancy Category	Explanation
All Trimesters	D	Studies in pregnant women have demonstrated a risk to the fetus. However, the benefits of therapy in a life threatening situation or a serious disease, may outweigh the potential risk.

Breast Feeding—There are no adequate studies in women for determining infant risk when using this medication during breastfeeding. Weigh the potential benefits against the potential risks before taking this medication while breastfeeding.

Other medicines—

Using this medicine with any of the following medicines is usually not recommended, but may be required in some cases. If both medicines are prescribed together, your doctor may change the dose or how often you use one or both of the medicines.

Alcuronium, Atracurium, Cidofovir, Cisatracurium, Decamethonium, Doxacurium, Fazadinium, Gallamine, Hexafluorenium, Metocurine, Mivacurium, Pancuronium, Pipecuronium, Rapacuronium, Rocuronium, Tacrolimus, Tubocurarine, Vecuronium

Interactions with Food/Tobacco/Alcohol—Certain medicines should not be used at or around the time of eating food or eating certain types of food since interactions may occur. Using alcohol or tobacco with certain medicines may also cause interactions to occur. Discuss with your healthcare professional the use of your medicine with food, alcohol, or tobacco.

Other medical problems—The presence of other medical problems may affect the use of this medicine. Make sure you tell your doctor if you have any other medical problems, especially:
- Blockage of the bowel
- Eighth-cranial-nerve disease (loss of hearing and/or balance)—Oral neomycin may increase the chance of hearing loss and/or balance problems
- Kidney disease—Patients with kidney disease may have an increased chance of side effects
- Myasthenia gravis or
- Parkinson's disease—Patients with myasthenia gravis or Parkinson's disease may have an increased chance of developing muscular weakness
- Ulcers of the bowel—Patients with ulcers of the bowel may have an increased chance of side effects since more neomycin may be absorbed by the body

Proper Use of This Medicine

This medicine may be taken on a full or empty stomach.

For patients taking the oral liquid form of neomycin:

- Use a specially marked measuring spoon or other device to measure each dose accurately. The average household teaspoon may not hold the right amount of liquid.

Keep taking this medicine for the full time of treatment. Do not miss any doses.

Dosing—The dose of this medicine will be different for different patients. Follow your doctor's orders or the directions on the label. The following information includes only the average doses of this medicine. If your dose is different, do not change it unless your doctor tells you to do so.

The amount of medicine that you take depends on the strength of the medicine. Also, the number of doses you take each day, the time allowed between doses, and the length of time you take the medicine depend on the medical problem for which you are using the medicine.

- For oral dosage forms (solution, tablets):
  - For patients in a coma from liver disease:
    - Adults and teenagers—1 to 3 grams every six hours for five or six days.
    - Children—Dose is based on body size (not weight) and must be determined by your doctor. That dose is given every six hours for five or six days.
  - For cleaning the bowel before surgery:
    - Adults and teenagers—1 gram every hour for four hours, then 1 gram every four hours for the rest of a twenty-four hour period; or 1 gram nineteen hours before surgery, 1 gram eighteen hours before surgery, and 1 gram nine hours before surgery.
    - Children—Dose is based on body weight. The usual dose is 14.7 milligrams (mg) per kilogram (kg) (6.7 mg per pound) of body weight every four hours for three days.

Missed dose—If you miss a dose of this medicine, take it as soon as possible. However, if it is almost time for your next dose, skip the missed dose and go back to your regular dosing schedule. Do not double doses.

Storage—Store the medicine in a closed container at room temperature, away from heat, moisture, and direct light. Keep from freezing.

Keep out of the reach of children.

Do not keep outdated medicine or medicine no longer needed.

Side Effects of This Medicine

Along with its needed effects, a medicine may cause some unwanted effects. Although not all of these side effects may occur, if they do occur they may need medical attention.

Check with your doctor immediately if any of the following side effects occur:

Rare

Any loss of hearing; clumsiness; diarrhea; difficulty in breathing; dizziness; drowsiness; greatly decreased frequency of urination or amount of urine; increased amount of gas; increased thirst; light-colored, frothy, fatty-appearing stools; ringing or buzzing or a feeling of fullness in the ears; skin rash; unsteadiness; weakness

Some side effects may occur that usually do not need medical attention. These side effects may go away during treatment as your body adjusts to the medicine. Also, your health care professional may be able to tell you about ways to prevent or reduce some of these side effects. Check with your health care professional if any of the following side effects continue or are bothersome or if you have any questions about them:

More common

Irritation or soreness of the mouth or rectal area; nausea or vomiting

Other side effects not listed may also occur in some patients. If you notice any other effects, check with your healthcare professional.

NEOMYCIN (Topical route) - nee-oh-MEY-sin

Uses For This Medicine

Neomycin belongs to the family of medicines called antibiotics. Neomycin topical preparations are used to help prevent infections of the skin. This medicine may be used for other problems as determined by your doctor.

Neomycin topical preparations are available without a prescription.

Before Using This Medicine

In deciding to use a medicine, the risks of taking the medicine must be weighed against the good it will do. This is a decision you and your doctor will make. For this medicine, the following should be considered:

Allergies—Tell your doctor if you have ever had any unusual or allergic reaction to this medicine or any other medicines. Also tell your health care professional if you have any other types of allergies, such as to foods, dyes, preservatives, or animals. For non-prescription products, read the label or package ingredients carefully.

Pediatric—Studies on this medicine have been done only in adult patients, and there is no specific information comparing use of topical neomycin in children with use in other age groups.

Geriatric—Many medicines have not been studied specifically in older people. Therefore, it may not be known whether they work exactly the same way they do in younger adults or if they cause different side effects or problems in older people. There is no specific information comparing use of topical neomycin in the elderly with use in other age groups.

Pregnancy—

	Pregnancy Category	Explanation
All Trimesters	D	Studies in pregnant women have demonstrated a risk to the fetus. However, the benefits of therapy in a life threatening situation or a serious disease, may outweigh the potential risk.

Breast Feeding—There are no adequate studies in women for determining infant risk when using this medication during breastfeeding. Weigh the potential benefits against the potential risks before taking this medication while breastfeeding.

Other medicines—

Using this medicine with any of the following medicines is usually not recommended, but may be required in some cases. If both medicines are prescribed together, your doctor may change the dose or how often you use one or both of the medicines.

Alcuronium, Atracurium, Cidofovir, Cisatracurium, Decamethonium, Doxacurium, Fazadinium, Gallamine, Hexafluorenium, Metocurine, Mivacurium, Pancuronium, Pipecuronium, Rapacuronium, Rocuronium, Tacrolimus, Tubocurarine, Vecuronium

Interactions with Food/Tobacco/Alcohol—Certain medicines should not be used at or around the time of eating food or eating certain types of food since interactions may occur. Using alcohol or tobacco with certain medicines may also cause interactions to occur. Discuss with your healthcare professional the use of your medicine with food, alcohol, or tobacco.

Proper Use of This Medicine

If you are using this medicine without a prescription, do not use it to treat deep wounds, puncture wounds, serious burns, or raw areas without first checking with your health care professional.

Do not use this medicine in the eyes.

Before applying this medicine, wash the affected area with soap and water, and dry thoroughly.

For patients using the cream form of this medicine:

- Apply a generous amount of cream to the affected area, and rub in gently until the cream disappears.

For patients using the ointment form of this medicine:

- Apply a generous amount of ointment to the affected area, and rub in gently.

After this medicine is applied, the treated area may be covered with a gauze dressing if desired.

To help clear up your infection completely, keep using this medicine for the full time of treatment, even if your symptoms have disappeared. Do not miss any doses.

Dosing—The dose of this medicine will be different for different patients. Follow your doctor's orders or the directions on the label. The following information includes only the average doses of this medicine. If your dose is different, do not change it unless your doctor tells you to do so.

The amount of medicine that you take depends on the strength of the medicine. Also, the number of doses you take each day, the time allowed between doses, and the length of time you take the medicine depend on the medical problem for which you are using the medicine.

- For topical dosage forms (cream or ointment):
  - For minor bacterial skin infections:
    - Adults and children—Apply to the affected area(s) of the skin one to three times a day.

Missed dose—If you miss a dose of this medicine, apply it as soon as possible. However, if it is almost time for your next dose, skip the missed dose and go back to your regular dosing schedule.

Storage—Store the medicine in a closed container at room temperature, away from heat, moisture, and direct light. Keep from freezing.

Keep out of the reach of children.

Do not keep outdated medicine or medicine no longer needed.

Precautions While Using This Medicine

If your skin problem does not improve within 1 week, or if it becomes worse, check with your health care professional.

Side Effects of This Medicine

Along with its needed effects, a medicine may cause some unwanted effects. Although not all of these side effects may occur, if they do occur they may need medical attention.

Check with your doctor immediately if any of the following side effects occur:

  More common
    Itching, rash, redness, swelling, or other sign of skin irritation not present before use of this medicine

  Rare
    Any loss of hearing

Other side effects not listed may also occur in some patients. If you notice any other effects, check with your healthcare professional.

NEOMYCIN AND POLYMYXIN B
(Topical route) - nee-oh-MEY-sin, pol-i-MIX-in B

Available Dosage Forms:

- Cream
- Powder

Therapeutic Class: Antibacterial Combination

Uses For This Medicine

Neomycin and polymyxin B combination is used to prevent bacterial infections. It works by killing bacteria.

Neomycin and polymyxin B cream is applied to the skin to prevent minor bacterial skin infections. It may also be used for other problems as determined by your doctor.

This medicine is available without a prescription.

Before Using This Medicine

In deciding to use a medicine, the risks of taking the medicine must be weighed against the good it will do. This is a decision you and your doctor will make. For this medicine, the following should be considered:

Allergies—Tell your doctor if you have ever had any unusual or allergic reaction to this medicine or any other medicines. Also tell your health care professional if you have any other types of allergies, such as to foods, dyes, preservatives, or animals. For non-prescription products, read the label or package ingredients carefully.

Pediatric—Although there is no specific information comparing use of neomycin and polymyxin B combination in children with use in other age groups, this medicine is not expected to cause different side effects or problems in children than it does in adults.

Geriatric—Many medicines have not been studied specifically in older people. Therefore, it may not be known whether they work exactly the same way they do in younger adults or if they cause different side effects or problems in older people. There is no specific information comparing use of neomycin and polymyxin B combination in the elderly with use in other age groups.

Pregnancy—

	Pregnancy Category	Explanation
All Trimesters	D	Studies in pregnant women have demonstrated a risk to the fetus. However, the benefits of therapy in a life threatening situation or a serious disease, may outweigh the potential risk.

Breast Feeding—There are no adequate studies in women for determining infant risk when using this medication during breastfeeding. Weigh the potential benefits against the potential risks before taking this medication while breastfeeding.

Other medicines—

Using this medicine with any of the following medicines is usually not recommended, but may be required in some cases. If both medicines are prescribed together, your doctor may change the dose or how often you use one or both of the medicines.

Alcuronium, Atracurium, Cidofovir, Cisatracurium, Decamethonium, Doxacurium, Fazadinium, Gallamine, Hexaflurorenium, Metocurine, Mivacurium, Pancuronium, Pipecuronium, Rapacuronium, Rocuronium, Tacrolimus, Tubocurarine, Vecuronium

Interactions with Food/Tobacco/Alcohol—Certain medicines should not be used at or around the time of eating food or eating certain types of food since interactions may occur. Using alcohol or tobacco with certain medicines may also cause interactions to occur. Discuss with your healthcare professional the use of your medicine with food, alcohol, or tobacco.

Proper Use of This Medicine

If you are using this medicine without a prescription, do not use it to treat deep wounds, puncture wounds, animal bites, serious burns, or raw areas without first checking with your health care professional.

Do not use this medicine in the eyes.

To use:

- Before applying this medicine, wash the affected area(s) with soap and water, and dry thoroughly.
- Apply a small amount of this medicine to the affected area(s) and rub in gently.
- After applying this medicine, the treated area(s) may be covered with a gauze dressing if desired.

Do not use this medicine for longer than 1 week or on large areas of the skin, unless otherwise directed by your doctor. To do so may increase the chance of side effects.

To help clear up your skin infection completely, keep using this medicine for the full time of treatment, even if your symptoms have disappeared. Do not miss any doses.

Dosing—The dose of this medicine will be different for different patients. Follow your doctor's orders or the directions on the label. The following information includes only the average doses of this medicine. If your dose is different, do not change it unless your doctor tells you to do so.

The amount of medicine that you take depends on the strength of the medicine. Also, the number of doses you take each day, the time allowed between doses, and the length of time you take the medicine depend on the medical problem for which you are using the medicine.

- For topical dosage form (cream):
  - For prevention of minor bacterial infections:
    - Adults and children 2 years of age and older— Apply to the affected area(s) of the skin one to three times a day.
    - Children up to 2 years of age—Use and dose must be determined by your doctor.

Missed dose—If you miss a dose of this medicine, apply it as soon as possible. However, if it is almost time for your next dose, skip the missed dose and go back to your regular dosing schedule.

Storage—Store the medicine in a closed container at room temperature, away from heat, moisture, and direct light. Keep from freezing.

Keep out of the reach of children.

Do not keep outdated medicine or medicine no longer needed.

Precautions While Using This Medicine

If your skin infection does not improve within 1 week, or if it becomes worse, check with your health care professional.

Side Effects of This Medicine

Along with its needed effects, a medicine may cause some unwanted effects. Although not all of these side effects may occur, if they do occur they may need medical attention.

Check with your doctor immediately if any of the following side effects occur:

> **More common**
>> Itching, pain, skin rash, swelling, redness, or other sign of skin irritation not present before use of this medicine
>
> *Rare*
>> Loss of hearing

Other side effects not listed may also occur in some patients. If you notice any other effects, check with your healthcare professional.

NEOMYCIN, POLYMYXIN B, AND BACITRACIN (Ophthalmic route) -
nee-oh-MEY-sin, pol-i-MIX-in B, bas-i-TRAY-sin

Uses For This Medicine

Neomycin, polymyxin B, and bacitracin combination antibiotic medicine is used to treat infections of the eye.

Neomycin, polymyxin B, and bacitracin combination is available only with your doctor's prescription.

Before Using This Medicine

In deciding to use a medicine, the risks of taking the medicine must be weighed against the good it will do. This is a decision you and your doctor will make. For this medicine, the following should be considered:

Allergies—Tell your doctor if you have ever had any unusual or allergic reaction to this medicine or any other medicines. Also tell your health care professional if you have any other types of allergies, such as to foods, dyes, preservatives, or animals. For non-prescription products, read the label or package ingredients carefully.

Pediatric—Studies on this medicine have been done only in adult patients, and there is no specific information comparing use of neomycin, polymyxin B, and bacitracin combination in children with use in other age groups.

Geriatric—Many medicines have not been studied specifically in older people. Therefore, it may not be known whether they work exactly the same way they do in younger adults or if they cause different side effects or problems in older people. There is no specific information comparing use of neomycin, polymyxin B, and bacitracin combination in the elderly with use in other age groups.

Breast Feeding—There are no adequate studies in women for determining infant risk when using this medication during breastfeeding. Weigh the potential benefits against the potential risks before taking this medication while breastfeeding.

Other medicines—Although certain medicines should not be used together at all, in other cases two different medicines may be used together even if an interaction might occur. In these cases, your doctor may want to change the dose, or other precautions may be necessary. Tell your healthcare professional if you are taking any other prescription or non-prescription (over-the-counter [OTC]) medicine.

Interactions with Food/Tobacco/Alcohol—Certain medicines should not be used at or around the time of eating food or eating certain types of food since interactions may occur. Using alcohol or tobacco with certain medicines may also cause interactions to occur. Discuss with your healthcare professional the use of your medicine with food, alcohol, or tobacco.

Proper Use of This Medicine

To use:

- First, wash your hands. Tilt the head back and, pressing your finger gently on the skin just beneath the lower eyelid, pull the lower eyelid away from the eye to make a space. Squeeze a thin strip of ointment into this space. A 1–cm (approximately ⅓-inch) strip of ointment is usually enough, unless you have been told by your doctor to use a different amount. Let go of the eyelid and gently close the eyes. Keep the eyes closed for 1 or 2 minutes to allow the medicine to come into contact with the infection.
- To keep the medicine as germ-free as possible, do not touch the applicator tip to any surface (including the eye). After using neomycin, polymyxin B, and bacitracin eye ointment, wipe the tip of the ointment tube with a clean tissue and keep the tube tightly closed.

To help clear up your infection completely, keep using this medicine for the full time of treatment, even if your symptoms have disappeared. Do not miss any doses.

Dosing—The dose of this medicine will be different for different patients. Follow your doctor's orders or the directions on the label. The following information includes only the average doses of this medicine. If your dose is different, do not change it unless your doctor tells you to do so.

The amount of medicine that you take depends on the strength of the medicine. Also, the number of doses you take each day, the time allowed between doses, and the length of time you take the medicine depend on the medical problem for which you are using the medicine.

- For eye infections:
  - For eye ointment dosage forms:
    - Adults and children—Use a thin strip of ointment in the eyes every three or four hours for seven to ten days.

Missed dose—If you miss a dose of this medicine, apply it as soon as possible. However, if it is almost time for your next dose, skip the missed dose and go back to your regular dosing schedule.

Storage—Store the medicine in a closed container at room temperature, away from heat, moisture, and direct light. Keep from freezing.

Keep out of the reach of children.

Do not keep outdated medicine or medicine no longer needed.

Precautions While Using This Medicine

If your symptoms do not improve within a few days, or if they become worse, check with your doctor.

Side Effects of This Medicine

Along with its needed effects, a medicine may cause some unwanted effects. Although not all of these side effects may occur, if they do occur they may need medical attention.

Check with your doctor immediately if any of the following side effects occur:

   More common
      Itching, rash, redness, swelling, or other sign of irritation not present before use of this medicine

After application, eye ointments usually cause your vision to blur for a few minutes.

Other side effects not listed may also occur in some patients. If you notice any other effects, check with your healthcare professional.

NEOMYCIN, POLYMYXIN B, AND BACITRACIN (Topical route) - nee-oh-MEY-sin, pol-i-MIX-in B, bas-i-TRAY-sin

Uses For This Medicine

Neomycin, polymyxin B, and bacitracin is a combination antibiotic medicine used to help prevent infections of the skin.

Neomycin, polymyxin B, and bacitracin combination is available without a prescription.

Before Using This Medicine

In deciding to use a medicine, the risks of taking the medicine must be weighed against the good it will do. This is a decision you and your doctor will make. For this medicine, the following should be considered:

Allergies—Tell your doctor if you have ever had any unusual or allergic reaction to this medicine or any other medicines. Also tell your health care professional if you have any other types of allergies, such as to foods, dyes, preservatives, or animals. For non-prescription products, read the label or package ingredients carefully.

Pediatric—Studies on this medicine have been done only in adult patients, and there is no specific information comparing use of topical neomycin, polymyxin B, and bacitracin combination in children with use in other age groups.

Geriatric—Many medicines have not been studied specifically in older people. Therefore, it may not be known whether they work exactly the same way they do in younger adults or if they cause different side effects or problems in older people. There is no specific information comparing use of topical neomycin, polymyxin B, and bacitracin combination in the elderly with use in other age groups.

Pregnancy—

	Pregnancy Category	Explanation
All Trimesters	D	Studies in pregnant women have demonstrated a risk to the fetus. However, the benefits of therapy in a life threatening situation or a serious disease, may outweigh the potential risk.

Breast Feeding—There are no adequate studies in women for determining infant risk when using this medication during breastfeeding. Weigh the potential benefits against the potential risks before taking this medication while breastfeeding.

Other medicines—

Using this medicine with any of the following medicines is usually not recommended, but may be required in some cases. If both medicines are prescribed together, your doctor may change the dose or how often you use one or both of the medicines.

Alcuronium, Atracurium, Cidofovir, Cisatracurium, Decamethonium, Doxacurium, Fazadinium, Gallamine, Hexafluorenium, Metocurine, Mivacurium, Pancuronium, Pipecuronium, Rapacuronium, Rocuronium, Tacrolimus, Tubocurarine, Vecuronium

Interactions with Food/Tobacco/Alcohol—Certain medicines should not be used at or around the time of eating food or eating certain types of food since interactions may occur. Using alcohol or tobacco with certain medicines may also cause interactions to occur. Discuss with your healthcare professional the use of your medicine with food, alcohol, or tobacco.

Proper Use of This Medicine

If you are using this medicine without a prescription, do not use it to treat deep wounds, puncture wounds, serious burns, or raw areas without first checking with your health care professional.

Do not use this medicine in the eyes.

Before applying this medicine, wash the affected area with soap and water, and dry thoroughly.

After applying this medicine, the treated area may be covered with a gauze dressing if desired.

To help clear up your infection completely, keep using this medicine for the full time of treatment, even if your symptoms have disappeared. Do not miss any doses.

Dosing—The dose of this medicine will be different for different patients. Follow your doctor's orders or the directions on the label. The following information includes only the average doses of this medicine. If your dose is different, do not change it unless your doctor tells you to do so.

The amount of medicine that you take depends on the strength of the medicine. Also, the number of doses you take each day, the time allowed between doses, and the length of time you take the medicine depend on the medical problem for which you are using the medicine.

- For topical dosage form (ointment):
  - For prevention of minor bacterial infections:
    - Adults and children—Apply to the affected area(s) of the skin two to five times a day.

Missed dose—If you miss a dose of this medicine, apply it as soon as possible. However, if it is almost time for your next dose, skip the missed dose and go back to your regular dosing schedule.

Storage—Store the medicine in a closed container at room temperature, away from heat, moisture, and direct light. Keep from freezing.

Keep out of the reach of children.

Do not keep outdated medicine or medicine no longer needed.

Precautions While Using This Medicine

If your skin problem does not improve within 1 week, or if it becomes worse, check with your health care professional.

Side Effects of This Medicine

Along with its needed effects, a medicine may cause some unwanted effects. Although not all of these side effects may occur, if they do occur they may need medical attention.

Check with your doctor immediately if any of the following side effects occur:

More common
Itching, skin rash, redness, swelling, or other sign of irritation not present before use of this medicine

Rare
Any loss of hearing

Other side effects not listed may also occur in some patients. If you notice any other effects, check with your healthcare professional.

NEOMYCIN, POLYMYXIN B, AND GRAMICIDIN (Ophthalmic route) - nee-oh-MEY-sin, pol-i-MIX-in B, gram-i-SI-din

Commonly used brand name(s)

In the U.S.—
Neosporin
Ocu-Spor-G

Available Dosage Forms:
- Solution

Therapeutic Class: Antibiotic Combination

Uses For This Medicine

Neomycin, polymyxin B, and gramicidin is a combination antibiotic medicine used to treat infections of the eye.

Neomycin, polymyxin B, and gramicidin combination is available only with your doctor's prescription.

Before Using This Medicine

In deciding to use a medicine, the risks of taking the medicine must be weighed against the good it will do. This is a decision you and your doctor will make. For this medicine, the following should be considered:

Allergies—Tell your doctor if you have ever had any unusual or allergic reaction to this medicine or any other medicines. Also tell your health care professional if you have any other types of allergies, such as to foods, dyes, preservatives, or animals. For non-prescription products, read the label or package ingredients carefully.

Pediatric—Studies on this medicine have been done only in adult patients, and there is no specific information comparing use of this combination in children with use in other age groups.

Geriatric—Many medicines have not been studied specifically in older people. Therefore, it may not be known whether they work exactly the same way they do in younger adults or if they cause different side effects or problems in older people. There is no specific information comparing use of neomycin, polymyxin B, and gramicidin combination in the elderly with use in other age groups.

Breast Feeding—There are no adequate studies in women for determining infant risk when using this medication during breastfeeding. Weigh the potential benefits against the potential risks before taking this medication while breastfeeding.

Other medicines—Although certain medicines should not be used together at all, in other cases two different medicines may be used together even if an interaction might occur. In these cases, your doctor may want to change the dose, or other precautions may be necessary. Tell your healthcare professional if you are taking any other prescription or nonprescription (over-the-counter [OTC]) medicine.

Interactions with Food/Tobacco/Alcohol—Certain medicines should not be used at or around the time of eating food or eating certain types of food since interactions may occur. Using alcohol or tobacco with certain medicines may also cause interactions to occur. Discuss with your healthcare professional the use of your medicine with food, alcohol, or tobacco.

Proper Use of This Medicine

The bottle is only partially full to provide proper drop control.

To use:

- First, wash your hands. Tilt the head back and, pressing your finger gently on the skin just beneath the lower eyelid, pull the lower eyelid away from the eye to make a space. Drop the medicine into this space. Let go of the eyelid and gently close the eyes. Do not blink. Keep the eyes closed for 1 or 2 minutes to allow the medicine to come into contact with the infection.

- If you think you did not get the drop of medicine into your eye properly, use another drop.

- To keep the medicine as germ-free as possible, do not touch the applicator tip or dropper to any surface (including the eye). Also, keep the container tightly closed.

To help clear up your infection completely, keep using this medicine for the full time of treatment, even if your symptoms have disappeared. Do not miss any doses.

Dosing—The dose of this medicine will be different for different patients. Follow your doctor's orders or the directions on the label. The following information includes only the average doses of this medicine. If your dose is different, do not change it unless your doctor tells you to do so.

The amount of medicine that you take depends on the strength of the medicine. Also, the number of doses you take each day, the time allowed between doses, and the length of time you take the medicine depend on the medical problem for which you are using the medicine.

- For eye infections:
  - For eye drops dosage form:
    - Adults and children—Use one drop in the eye two to four times a day for seven to ten days. If you have a more serious infection, your doctor may want you to use one drop in the eye every fifteen to thirty minutes at first. Then your doctor may have you use the medicine less often.

Missed dose—If you miss a dose of this medicine, apply it as soon as possible. However, if it is almost time for your next dose, skip the missed dose and go back to your regular dosing schedule.

Storage—Store the medicine in a closed container at room temperature, away from heat, moisture, and direct light. Keep from freezing.

Keep out of the reach of children.

Do not keep outdated medicine or medicine no longer needed.

Precautions While Using This Medicine

If your symptoms do not improve within a few days, or if they become worse, check with your doctor.

Side Effects of This Medicine

Along with its needed effects, a medicine may cause some unwanted effects. Although not all of these side effects may occur, if they do occur they may need medical attention.

Check with your doctor immediately if any of the following side effects occur:
  More common
    Itching, rash, redness, swelling, or other sign of irritation in or around the eye not present before use of this medicine

Some side effects may occur that usually do not need medical attention. These side effects may go away during treatment as your body adjusts to the medicine. Also, your health care professional may be able to tell you about ways to prevent or reduce some of these side effects. Check with your health care professional if any of the following side effects continue or are bothersome or if you have any questions about them:

Less common
  Burning or stinging sensation in the eye

Other side effects not listed may also occur in some patients. If you notice any other effects, check with your healthcare professional.

NEOMYCIN, POLYMYXIN B, AND HYDROCORTISONE (Ophthalmic route) - nee-oh-MEY-sin, pol-i-MIX-in B, hye-droe-KOR-ti-sone

Commonly used brand name(s)

In the U.S.—
  Cortisporin

Available Dosage Forms:
- Suspension

Therapeutic Class: Aminoglycoside/Corticosteroid Combination
Pharmacologic Class: Adrenal Glucocorticoid

Uses For This Medicine

Neomycin, polymyxin B, and hydrocortisone is a combination antibiotic and cortisone-like medicine. It is used to treat infections of the eye and to help provide relief from redness, irritation, and discomfort of certain eye problems. It is also used to help prevent permanent damage of certain eye problems.

Neomycin, polymyxin B, and hydrocortisone combination is available only with your doctor's prescription.

Before Using This Medicine

In deciding to use a medicine, the risks of taking the medicine must be weighed against the good it will do. This is a decision you and your doctor will make. For this medicine, the following should be considered:

Allergies—Tell your doctor if you have ever had any unusual or allergic reaction to this medicine or any other medicines. Also tell your health care professional if you have any other types of allergies, such as to foods, dyes, preservatives, or animals. For non-prescription products, read the label or package ingredients carefully.

Pediatric—Studies on this medicine have been done only in adult patients, and there is no specific information comparing use in children with use in other age groups.

Geriatric—Many medicines have not been studied specifically in older people. Therefore, it may not be known whether they work exactly the same way they do in younger adults or if they cause different side effects or problems in older people. There is no specific information comparing use of ophthalmic neomycin, polymyxin B, and hydrocortisone combination in the elderly with use in other age groups.

Other medicines—

Using this medicine with any of the following medicines is not recommended. Your doctor may decide not to treat you with this medication or change some of the other medicines you take.

Bupropion, Rotavirus Vaccine, Live

Interactions with Food/Tobacco/Alcohol—Certain medicines should not be used at or around the time of eating food or eating certain types of food since interactions may occur. Using alcohol or tobacco with certain medicines may also cause interactions to occur. Discuss with your healthcare professional the use of your medicine with food, alcohol, or tobacco.

Other medical problems—The presence of other medical problems may affect the use of this medicine. Make sure you tell your doctor if you have any other medical problems, especially:

- Any other eye infection or condition or

- Glaucoma—Use of neomycin, polymyxin B, and hydrocortisone ophthalmic drops may make the condition worse

- Cataract surgery, recent—Use of neomycin, polymyxin B, and hydrocortisone ophthalmic drops may delay healing or cause other problems

Proper Use of This Medicine

The bottle is only partially full to provide proper drop control.

To use:

- First, wash your hands. Then tilt the head back and pull the lower eyelid away from the eye to form a pouch. Drop the medicine into the pouch and gently close the eyes. Do not blink. Keep the eyes closed for 1 or 2 minutes to allow the medicine to come into contact with the infection.

- If you think you did not get the drop of medicine into your eye properly, use another drop.

- To keep the medicine as germ-free as possible, do not touch the applicator tip to any surface (including the eye). Also, keep the container tightly closed.

To help clear up your infection completely, keep using this medicine for the full time of treatment, even if your symptoms have disappeared. Do not miss any doses.

Dosing—The dose of this medicine will be different for different patients. Follow your doctor's orders or the directions on the label. The following information includes only the average doses of this medicine. If your dose is different, do not change it unless your doctor tells you to do so.

The amount of medicine that you take depends on the strength of the medicine. Also, the number of doses you take each day, the time allowed between doses, and the length of time you take the medicine depend on the medical problem for which you are using the medicine.

- For eye infection:
  - For ophthalmic suspension dosage forms:
    - Adults—One or two drops every three or four hours.
    - Children—Use and dose must be determined by your doctor.

Missed dose—If you miss a dose of this medicine, apply it as soon as possible. However, if it is almost time for your next dose, skip the missed dose and go back to your regular dosing schedule.

Storage—Store the medicine in a closed container at room temperature, away from heat, moisture, and direct light. Keep from freezing.

Keep out of the reach of children.

Do not keep outdated medicine or medicine no longer needed.

Precautions While Using This Medicine

If you will be using this medicine for more than 10 days, your doctor should check your eyes at regular visits.

If your symptoms do not improve within a few days, or if they become worse, check with your doctor.

If a rash or allergic reaction develops, you should check with your doctor right away.

You should not let anyone else use your medicine. It could cause infection to spread.

Do not use any leftover medicine for future eye problems without checking with your doctor first. This medicine should not be used on many different kinds of infection.

Side Effects of This Medicine

Along with its needed effects, a medicine may cause some unwanted effects. Although not all of these side effects may occur, if they do occur they may need medical attention.

Stop taking this medicine and get emergency help immediately if any of the following effects occur:
Rare
    Fainting; lightheadedness (sudden and severe); shortness of breath or trouble breathing (severe); swelling around face

Check with your doctor immediately if any of the following side effects occur:
More common
    Itching, rash, redness, swelling, or other sign of irritation not present before use of this medicine

Rare
    Blurred vision or other change in vision; delayed healing of eye infection

Some side effects may occur that usually do not need medical attention. These side effects may go away during treatment as your body adjusts to the medicine. Also, your health care professional may be able to tell you about ways to prevent or reduce some of these side effects. Check with your health care professional if any of the following side effects continue or are bothersome or if you have any questions about them:
Less common
    Burning or stinging when applying medicine

Other side effects not listed may also occur in some patients. If you notice any other effects, check with your healthcare professional.

NEOMYCIN, POLYMYXIN B, AND HYDROCORTISONE (Otic route) -

nee-oh-MEY-sin, pol-i-MIX-in B, hye-droe-KOR-ti-sone

Commonly used brand name(s)

In the U.S.—

Antibiotic Otic	Cortomycin
Cort-Biotic	Oti-Sone
Cortisporin	Pediotic

Available Dosage Forms:

- Suspension
- Solution

Therapeutic Class: Anti-Infective/Anti-Inflammatory Combination
Pharmacologic Class: Adrenal Glucocorticoid

Uses For This Medicine

Neomycin, polymyxin B, and hydrocortisone is a combination antibiotic and cortisone-like medicine. It is used to treat infections of the ear canal and to help provide relief from redness, irritation, and discomfort of certain ear problems.

Neomycin, polymyxin B, and hydrocortisone preparation is available only with your doctor's prescription.

Before Using This Medicine

In deciding to use a medicine, the risks of taking the medicine must be weighed against the good it will do. This is a decision you and your doctor will make. For this medicine, the following should be considered:

Allergies—Tell your doctor if you have ever had any unusual or allergic reaction to this medicine or any other medicines. Also tell your health care professional if you have any other types of allergies, such as to foods, dyes, preservatives, or animals. For non-prescription products, read the label or package ingredients carefully.

Pediatric—Although there is no specific information comparing use of otic neomycin, polymyxin B, and hydrocortisone preparation in children with use in other age groups, this preparation is not expected to cause different side effects or problems in children than it does in adults.

Geriatric—Many medicines have not been studied specifically in older people. Therefore, it may not be known whether they work exactly the same way they do in younger adults. Although there is no specific information comparing use of otic neomycin, polymyxin B, and hydrocortisone preparation in the elderly with use in other age groups, this preparation is not expected to cause different side effects or problems in older people than it does in younger adults.

Other medicines—Although certain medicines should not be used together at all, in other cases two different medicines may be used together even if an interaction might occur. In these cases, your doctor may want to change the dose, or other precautions may be necessary. Tell your healthcare professional if you are taking any other prescription or non-prescription (over-the-counter [OTC]) medicine.

Interactions with Food/Tobacco/Alcohol—Certain medicines should not be used at or around the time of eating food or eating certain types of food since interactions may occur. Using alcohol or tobacco with certain medicines may also cause interactions to occur. Discuss with your healthcare professional the use of your medicine with food, alcohol, or tobacco.

Other medical problems—The presence of other medical problems may affect the use of this medicine. Make sure you tell your doctor if you have any other medical problems, especially:

- Any other ear infection or condition (including punctured eardrum)—Use of neomycin, polymyxin B, and hydrocortisone otic preparations may make the condition worse

Proper Use of This Medicine

You may warm the ear drops to body temperature (37 °C or 98.6 °F), but no higher, by holding the bottle in your hand for a few minutes before using the medicine. If the medicine gets too warm, it may break down and not work at all.

To use:

- Lie down or tilt the head so that the infected ear faces up. Gently pull the earlobe up and back for adults (down and back for children) to straighten the ear canal. Drop the medicine into the ear canal. Keep the ear facing up for about 5 minutes to allow the medicine to coat the ear canal. (For young children and other patients who cannot stay still for 5 minutes, try to keep the ear facing up for at least 1 or 2 minutes.) Your doctor may have inserted a gauze or cotton wick into your ear and may want you to keep the wick moistened with this medicine. Your doctor also may have other directions for you, such as how long you should keep the wick in your ear or when you should return to your doctor to have the wick replaced. If you have any questions about this, check with your doctor.
- To keep the medicine as germ-free as possible, do not touch the dropper to any surface (including the ear). Also, keep the container tightly closed.

To help clear up your infection completely, keep using this medicine for the full time of treatment, even if your symptoms have disappeared. Do not miss any doses.

Dosing—The dose of this medicine will be different for different patients. Follow your doctor's orders or the directions on the label. The following information includes only the average doses of this medicine. If your dose is different, do not change it unless your doctor tells you to do so.

The amount of medicine that you take depends on the strength of the medicine. Also, the number of doses you take each day, the time allowed between doses, and the length of time you take the medicine depend on the medical problem for which you are using the medicine.

- For otic (ear drops) dosage forms:
  - For ear canal infection:
    - Adults—Use four drops in the ear three or four times a day.
    - Children—Use three drops in the ear three or four times a day.
  - For mastoid cavity infection:
    - Adults—Use four to ten drops in the ear every six to eight hours.
    - Children—Use four or five drops in the ear every six to eight hours.

Missed dose—If you miss a dose of this medicine, apply it as soon as possible. However, if it is almost time for your next dose, skip the missed dose and go back to your regular dosing schedule.

Storage—Store the medicine in a closed container at room temperature, away from heat, moisture, and direct light. Keep from freezing.

Keep out of the reach of children.

Do not keep outdated medicine or medicine no longer needed.

Precautions While Using This Medicine

If your symptoms do not improve within 1 week, or if they become worse, check with your doctor.

Do not use this medicine for more than 10 days unless otherwise directed by your doctor.

Side Effects of This Medicine

Along with its needed effects, a medicine may cause some unwanted effects. Although not all of these side effects may occur, if they do occur they may need medical attention.

Check with your doctor immediately if any of the following side effects occur:

> *More common*
> Itching, skin rash, redness, swelling, or other sign of irritation in or around the ear not present before use of this medicine

Other side effects not listed may also occur in some patients. If you notice any other effects, check with your healthcare professional.

NEPAFENAC (Ophthalmic route) - ne-pa-FEN-ak

Commonly used brand name(s)
In the U.S.—
> Nevanac

Available Dosage Forms:
- Suspension

Therapeutic Class: Anti-Inflammatory
Pharmacologic Class: NSAID

Uses For This Medicine

Nepafenac is an ophthalmic anti-inflammatory medicine used in the eye to relieve pain and inflammation or edema (too much fluid in the eye) that can occur during or after some kinds of eye surgery.

Before Using This Medicine

In deciding to use a medicine, the risks of taking the medicine must be weighed against the good it will do. This is a decision you and your doctor will make. For this medicine, the following should be considered:

Allergies—Tell your doctor if you have ever had any unusual or allergic reaction to this medicine or any other medicines. Also tell your health care professional if you have any other types of allergies, such as to foods, dyes, preservatives, or animals. For non-prescription products, read the label or package ingredients carefully.

Pediatric—Nepafenac eye drops have only been studied in children age 10 years and older. Discuss with your child's doctor the good that this medicine may do as well as the risks of using it.

Pregnancy—

	Pregnancy Category	Explanation
All Trimesters	C	Animal studies have shown an adverse effect and there are no adequate studies in pregnant women OR no animal studies have been conducted and there are no adequate studies in pregnant women.

Breast Feeding—There are no adequate studies in women for determining infant risk when using this medication during breastfeeding. Weigh the potential benefits against the potential risks before taking this medication while breastfeeding.

Other medicines—Although certain medicines should not be used together at all, in other cases two different medicines may be used together even if an interaction might occur. In these cases, your doctor may want to change the dose, or other precautions may be necessary. Tell your healthcare professional if you are taking any other prescription or non-prescription (over-the-counter [OTC]) medicine.

Interactions with Food/Tobacco/Alcohol—Certain medicines should not be used at or around the time of eating food or eating certain types of food since interactions may occur. Using alcohol or tobacco with certain medicines may also cause interactions to occur. Discuss with your healthcare professional the use of your medicine with food, alcohol, or tobacco.

Other medical problems—The presence of other medical problems may affect the use of this medicine. Make sure you tell your doctor if you have any other medical problems, especially:
- Bleeding problems—The possibility of bleeding may be increased
- Use of soft contact lenses—Eye irritation, such as redness and burning of the eyes, may occur
- Vision problems—The possibility of increased side effects and loss of vision

Proper Use of This Medicine

- First, wash your hands. Tilt the head back and, pressing your finger gently on the skin just beneath the lower eyelid, pull the lower eyelid away from the eye to make a space. Drop the medicine into this space. Let go of the eyelid and gently close the eyes. Do not blink. Keep the eyes closed and apply pressure to the inner corner of the eye with your finger for 1 or 2 minutes to allow the medicine to be absorbed by the eye.
- Immediately after using the eye drops, wash your hands to remove any medicine that may be on them.
- To keep the medicine as germ-free as possible, do not touch the applicator tip to any surface (including the eye). Also, always keep the container tightly closed.

Dosing—The dose of this medicine will be different for different patients. Follow your doctor's orders or the directions on the label. The following information includes only the av-

erage doses of this medicine. If your dose is different, do not change it unless your doctor tells you to do so.

The amount of medicine that you take depends on the strength of the medicine. Also, the number of doses you take each day, the time allowed between doses, and the length of time you take the medicine depend on the medical problem for which you are using the medicine.

- For ophthalmic solution (eye drops) dosage form:
  - Inflammation in the eye following cataract surgery:
    - Adults—1 drop in the eye three times a day beginning 1 day before cataract surgery and on the day of surgery and throughout the first two weeks following surgery.
    - Children—Use and dose must be determined by your doctor.

Missed dose—If you miss a dose of this medicine, take it as soon as possible. However, if it is almost time for your next dose, skip the missed dose and go back to your regular dosing schedule. Do not double doses.

Storage—Keep out of the reach of children.

Do not keep outdated medicine or medicine no longer needed.

Precautions While Using This Medicine

Wearing soft contact lenses during treatment with nepafenac has caused severe irritation (redness and itching) in some people. Therefore, *do not wear soft contact lenses during the time that you are being treated with nepafenac.*

Side Effects of This Medicine

Check with your doctor immediately if any of the following side effects occur:
> *Less common*
>> Seeing flashes or sparks of light; seeing floating spots before the eyes, or a veil or curtain appearing across part of vision

Some side effects may occur that usually do not need medical attention. These side effects may go away during treatment as your body adjusts to the medicine. Also, your health care professional may be able to tell you about ways to prevent or reduce some of these side effects. Check with your health care professional if any of the following side effects continue or are bothersome or if you have any questions about them:
> *More common*
>> Blurred vision; change in vision; decrease in vision; feeling of having something in the eye; loss of vision; sticky sensation of eyelids
>
> *Less common*
>> Change in color vision; cough; crusting in corner of eye; difficulty seeing at night; dry eye; eye itching; eye pain; fever; headache; increased sensitivity of eyes to sunlight; nausea; nervousness; pain in eye; pounding in the ears; redness of eye; shortness of breath or troubled breathing; slow or fast heartbeat; stuffy or runny nose; swelling and/or redness of eye and lining of eyelid; tenderness around eyes and cheekbone; tightness of chest or wheezing

Other side effects not listed may also occur in some patients. If you notice any other effects, check with your healthcare professional.

NESIRITIDE　(Intravenous route) - ni-SIR-i-tide

Commonly used brand name(s)

In the U.S.—
　Natrecor

Available Dosage Forms:
- Powder for Solution

Therapeutic Class: Cardiovascular Agent
Pharmacologic Class: Natriuretic Peptide

Uses For This Medicine

Nesiritide is used for patients who have severe congestive heart failure that has recently become worse. Nesiritide is for patients who are short of breath while at rest or with minimal activity.

Before Using This Medicine

In deciding to use a medicine, the risks of taking the medicine must be weighed against the good it will do. This is a decision you and your doctor will make. For this medicine, the following should be considered:

Allergies—Tell your doctor if you have ever had any unusual or allergic reaction to this medicine or any other medicines. Also tell your health care professional if you have any other types of allergies, such as to foods, dyes, preservatives, or animals. For non-prescription products, read the label or package ingredients carefully.

Pediatric—Studies on this medicine have been done only in adult patients, and there is no specific information comparing use of nesiritide in children with use in other age groups.

Geriatric—This medicine has been tested and has not been shown to cause different side effects or problems in older people than it does in younger adults.

Pregnancy—

	Pregnancy Category	Explanation
All Trimesters	C	Animal studies have shown an adverse effect and there are no adequate studies in pregnant women OR no animal studies have been conducted and there are no adequate studies in pregnant women.

Breast Feeding—There are no adequate studies in women for determining infant risk when using this medication during breastfeeding. Weigh the potential benefits against the potential risks before taking this medication while breastfeeding.

Other medicines—

Using this medicine with any of the following medicines is usually not recommended, but may be required in some cases. If both medicines are prescribed together, your doctor may change the dose or how often you use one or both of the medicines.

Arsenic Trioxide

Interactions with Food/Tobacco/Alcohol—Certain medicines should not be used at or around the time of eating food or eating certain types of food since interactions may

occur. Using alcohol or tobacco with certain medicines may also cause interactions to occur. Discuss with your healthcare professional the use of your medicine with food, alcohol, or tobacco.

Other medical problems—The presence of other medical problems may affect the use of this medicine. Make sure you tell your doctor if you have any other medical problems, especially:

- Heart disease (other than congestive heart failure)—Nesiritide may make heart problems worse.
- Low blood pressure—Nesiritide may make this condition worse.

Proper Use of This Medicine

Dosing—The dose of this medicine will be different for different patients. Follow your doctor's orders or the directions on the label. The following information includes only the average doses of this medicine. If your dose is different, do not change it unless your doctor tells you to do so.

The amount of medicine that you take depends on the strength of the medicine. Also, the number of doses you take each day, the time allowed between doses, and the length of time you take the medicine depend on the medical problem for which you are using the medicine.

- For injection dosage form:
  - For congestive heart failure:
    - Adults—Dose is based on your weight and must be determined by your doctor.
    - Children—Use and dose must be determined by your doctor.

Side Effects of This Medicine

Along with its needed effects, a medicine may cause some unwanted effects. Although not all of these side effects may occur, if they do occur they may need medical attention.

Check with your doctor immediately if any of the following side effects occur:

More common

Low blood pressure

Less common

Bluish lips or skin; chest pain, tightness, or discomfort; cool, clammy skin; difficulty in breathing or shortness of breath; dizziness; fainting; lightheadedness; fast, slow, or irregular heartbeat; unusual tiredness or weakness

Some side effects may occur that usually do not need medical attention. These side effects may go away during treatment as your body adjusts to the medicine. Also, your health care professional may be able to tell you about ways to prevent or reduce some of these side effects. Check with your health care professional if any of the following side effects continue or are bothersome or if you have any questions about them:

More common

Headache

Less common

Abdominal or stomach pain; anxiety; back pain; burning, crawling, itching, numbness, prickling, "pins and needles", or tingling feelings on the skin; change in vision; confusion; coughing or spitting up blood; fever; increased cough; itching skin; leg cramps; nausea; pain or irritation at the injection site; pale skin;

unusual bleeding or bruising; rash; sleepiness or unusual drowsiness; sleeplessness; sweating; trembling or shakiness; vomiting

Other side effects not listed may also occur in some patients. If you notice any other effects, check with your healthcare professional.

NEVIRAPINE (Oral route) - ne-VYE-ra-peen

Black Box Warning

Severe, life-threatening, and in some cases fatal hepatotoxicity, particularly in the first 18 weeks, has been reported in patients treated with nevirapine. In some cases, patients presented with non-specific prodromal signs or symptoms of hepatitis and progressed to hepatic failure. These events are often associated with rash. Female gender and higher CD4 counts at initiation of therapy place patients at increased risk; women with CD4 counts greater than 250 cells/mm(3), including pregnant women receiving nevirapine in combination with other antiretrovirals for the treatment of HIV infection, are at the greatest risk. However, hepatotoxicity associated with nevirapine use can occur in both genders, all CD4 counts and at any time during treatment. Patients with signs or symptoms of hepatitis, or with increased transaminases combined with rash or other systemic symptoms, must discontinue nevirapine and seek medical evaluation immediately.

Severe, life-threatening skin reactions, including fatal cases, have occurred in patients treated with nevirapine. These have included cases of Stevens-Johnson syndrome, toxic epidermal necrolysis, and hypersensitivity reactions characterized by rash, constitutional findings, and organ dysfunction. Patients developing signs or symptoms of severe skin reactions or hypersensitivity reactions must discontinue nevirapine and seek medical evaluation immediately.

It is essential that patients be monitored intensively during the first 18 weeks of therapy with nevirapine to detect potentially life-threatening hepatotoxicity or skin reactions. Extra vigilance is warranted during the first 6 weeks of therapy, which is the period of greatest risk of these events. Do not restart nevirapine following severe hepatic, skin or hypersensitivity reactions. In some cases, hepatic injury has progressed despite discontinuation of treatment. In addition, the 14–day lead-in period with nevirapine 200 mg daily dosing must be strictly followed.

Commonly used brand name(s)

In the U.S.—

Viramune

Available Dosage Forms:

- Suspension
- Tablet
- Elixir

Therapeutic Class: Antiretroviral Agent
Pharmacologic Class: Non-Nucleoside Reverse Transcriptase Inhibitor

Uses For This Medicine

Nevirapine is used, with other medicines, in the treatment of the infection caused by the human immunodeficiency virus (HIV).

Nevirapine will not cure HIV infection or AIDS; however, it helps keep HIV from reproducing and appears to slow down the destruction of the immune system. This may help delay the development of problems usually related to AIDS or HIV disease. Nevirapine will not keep you from spreading HIV to other people. People who receive this medicine may continue to have other problems usually related to AIDS or HIV disease.

This medicine is available only with your doctor's prescription.

Once a medicine has been approved for marketing for a certain use, experience may show that it is also useful for other medical problems. Although this use is not included in product labeling, nevirapine is used in certain patients with the following medical condition:

- Mother-to-child transmission of HIV during labor and at birth (prevention)

Before Using This Medicine

In deciding to use a medicine, the risks of taking the medicine must be weighed against the good it will do. This is a decision you and your doctor will make. For this medicine, the following should be considered:

Allergies—Tell your doctor if you have ever had any unusual or allergic reaction to this medicine or any other medicines. Also tell your health care professional if you have any other types of allergies, such as to foods, dyes, preservatives, or animals. For non-prescription products, read the label or package ingredients carefully.

Pediatric—Granulocytopenia may be more likely to occur in children, who are usually more sensitive than adults to this effect of nevirapine.

Geriatric—Many medicines have not been studied specifically in older people. Therefore, it may not be known whether they work exactly the same way they do in younger adults. There is no specific information comparing use of nevirapine in the elderly with use in other age groups.

Pregnancy—

	Pregnancy Category	Explanation
All Trimesters	C	Animal studies have shown an adverse effect and there are no adequate studies in pregnant women OR no animal studies have been conducted and there are no adequate studies in pregnant women.

Breast Feeding—There are no adequate studies in women for determining infant risk when using this medication during breastfeeding. Weigh the potential benefits against the potential risks before taking this medication while breastfeeding.

Other medicines—

Using this medicine with any of the following medicines is not recommended. Your doctor may decide not to treat you with this medication or change some of the other medicines you take.

St John's Wort

Interactions with Food/Tobacco/Alcohol—Certain medicines should not be used at or around the time of eating food or eating certain types of food since interactions may occur. Using alcohol or tobacco with certain medicines may also cause interactions to occur. Discuss with your healthcare professional the use of your medicine with food, alcohol, or tobacco.

Other medical problems—The presence of other medical problems may affect the use of this medicine. Make sure you tell your doctor if you have any other medical problems, especially:

- Kidney disease—Nevirapine may be removed more slowly from the body
- Liver disease—Nevirapine has been reported to cause unwanted and sometimes serious effects in the liver

Proper Use of This Medicine

Nevirapine may be taken with or without food.

Take this medicine exactly as directed by your doctor. Do not take it more often, and do not take it for a longer time than your doctor ordered. Also, do not stop taking this medicine without checking with your doctor first.

Keep taking nevirapine for the full time of treatment, even if you begin to feel better.

This medicine works best when there is a constant amount in the blood. To help keep the amount constant, do not miss any doses. Also, it is best to take the doses at evenly spaced times, day and night. For example, if you are to take one dose a day, try to take it at the same time each day. If you are taking two doses a day, the doses should be spaced about 12 hours apart. If you need help in planning the best times to take your medicine, check with your health care professional.

If you are taking the oral solution shake it gently before use. Use an oral dosing syringe or dosing cup to measure the right dose. After drinking the medicine, rinse the dosing cup with water and drink the rinse to make sure you get all of the medicine. If your dose is less than 5 ml (one teaspoon) use the syringe.

It is important that you read the patient information package insert before you start taking this medicine. Read it again each time you refill your prescription. There may be new information. Reading the patient information leaflet does not take the place of talking to your doctor. You and your doctor should discuss nevirapine when you start taking your medicine and at regular checkups.

Only take medicine that your doctor has prescribed specially for you. Do not share your medicine with others.

Dosing—The dose of this medicine will be different for different patients. Follow your doctor's orders or the directions on the label. The following information includes only the average doses of this medicine. If your dose is different, do not change it unless your doctor tells you to do so.

The amount of medicine that you take depends on the strength of the medicine. Also, the number of doses you take each day, the time allowed between doses, and the length of time you take the medicine depend on the medical problem for which you are using the medicine.

- For oral dosage form (suspension or tablets):
  - For treatment of HIV infection:
    - Adults—200 milligrams (mg) once a day for two weeks, followed by 200 mg two times a day, in combination with other medicines.

- Children 8 years of age and older—Dose is based on body weight and must be determined by your doctor. The usual dose is 4 mg per kilogram (kg) (1.8 mg per pound) of body weight once a day for two weeks, followed by 4 mg per kg (1.8 mg per pound) of body weight two times a day, in combination with other medicines.
- Infants 2 months old and children up to 8 years of age—Dose is based on body weight and must be determined by your doctor. The usual dose is 4 mg per kilogram (kg) (1.8 mg per pound) of body weight once a day for two weeks, followed by 7 mg per kg (3.2 mg per pound) of body weight two times a day, in combination with other medicines.

Missed dose—If you miss a dose of this medicine, take it as soon as possible. However, if it is almost time for your next dose, skip the missed dose and go back to your regular dosing schedule. Do not double doses.

Storage—Store the medicine in a closed container at room temperature, away from heat, moisture, and direct light. Keep from freezing.

Keep out of the reach of children.

Do not keep outdated medicine or medicine no longer needed.

Precautions While Using This Medicine

Do not take any other medicines without checking with your doctor first. To do so may increase the chance of side effects from nevirapine or other medicines.

Patients taking nevirapine may develop severe liver disease or severe skin reactions that could cause serious side effects. Your doctor will want to check you and do liver function tests in the first 18 weeks of therapy. The risk of serious reactions is greatest during the first 18 weeks of treatment. Checks for liver problems should continue regularly during your therapy. Patients with higher liver function tests and patients with hepatitis B or C have a greater chance of liver damage while taking nevirapine. Women and patients with higher CD4 counts (blood counts) seem to have a greater chance of developing liver damage, often accompanied by a rash, while taking nevirapine.

It is very important that your doctor check your progress at regular visits to make sure this medicine is working properly and check for unwanted effects such as serious skin reactions or rashes. Your health care professional may also want to check certain things such as your blood levels, your liver functions, and your response to this medicine.

This medicine may decrease the effects of some contraceptives (birth control). To avoid unwanted pregnancy, it is a good idea to use additional contraceptive measures while being treated with nevirapine.

Side Effects of This Medicine

Along with its needed effects, a medicine may cause some unwanted effects. Although not all of these side effects may occur, if they do occur they may need medical attention.

Check with your doctor as soon as possible if any of the following side effects occur:

More common

Blistering, peeling, loosening of skin; chills; fever; skin rash; cough; dark urine; diarrhea; fever; general tired-

ness and weakness; itching; joint or muscle pain; light-colored stools; nausea and vomiting; red irritated eyes; red skin lesions, often with a purple center; sore throat; sores, ulcers, or white spots in mouth or on lips; upper right abdominal pain; unusual tiredness or weakness; yellow eyes and skin

Less common

Hives; loss of appetite

Rare

Pain, numbness, or tingling of hands, arms, legs, or feet; tingling, burning, or prickly sensations; sleepiness or unusual drowsiness

Note: Chills, fever, and sore throat are more commonly seen in children.

Some side effects may occur that usually do not need medical attention. These side effects may go away during treatment as your body adjusts to the medicine. Also, your health care professional may be able to tell you about ways to prevent or reduce some of these side effects. Check with your health care professional if any of the following side effects continue or are bothersome or if you have any questions about them:

More common

Abdominal or stomach pain; diarrhea; headache

Other side effects not listed may also occur in some patients. If you notice any other effects, check with your healthcare professional.

It is possible that the fat on your body may distribute itself differently or you may accumulate more body fat while you are taking this medicine. If you have concerns about this, check with your doctor.

NIACIN   (Oral route) - NYE-a-sin

Commonly used brand name(s)

In the U.S.—

Niacinol	Nicotinex
Niacor	Slo-Niacin
Niaspan	

Available Dosage Forms:

- Tablet, Extended Release
- Capsule
- Capsule, Extended Release
- Elixir
- Tablet

Therapeutic Class: Antihyperlipidemic
Pharmacologic Class: Vitamin B

Uses For This Medicine

Niacin is used to help lower high cholesterol and fat levels in the blood. This may help prevent medical problems caused by cholesterol and fat clogging the blood vessels.

Some strengths of niacin are available only with your doctor's prescription.

Importance of Diet—Before prescribing medicine for your condition, your doctor will probably try to control your condition by prescribing a personal diet for you. Such a diet may be low in fats, sugars, and/or cholesterol. Many people are able to control their condition by carefully following their doctor's orders for proper diet and exercise. Medicine is prescribed only when additional help is needed and is effective only when a schedule of diet and exercise is properly followed.

Also, this medicine is less effective if you are greatly overweight. It may be very important for you to go on a reducing diet. However, check with your doctor before going on any diet.

Make certain your health care professional knows if you are on any special diet, such as a low-sodium or low-sugar diet.

Before Using This Medicine

In deciding to use a medicine, the risks of taking the medicine must be weighed against the good it will do. This is a decision you and your doctor will make. For this medicine, the following should be considered:

Allergies—Tell your doctor if you have ever had any unusual or allergic reaction to this medicine or any other medicines. Also tell your health care professional if you have any other types of allergies, such as to foods, dyes, preservatives, or animals. For non-prescription products, read the label or package ingredients carefully.

Pediatric—There is no specific information comparing the use of niacin for high cholesterol in children with use in other age groups. However, use is not recommended in children under 2 years of age since cholesterol is needed for normal development.

Geriatric—Many medicines have not been studied specifically in older people. Therefore, it may not be known whether they work exactly the same way they do in younger adults or if they cause different side effects or problems in older people. Although there is no specific information comparing the use of niacin for high cholesterol in the elderly with use in other age groups, it is not expected to cause different side effects or problems in older people than in younger adults.

Pregnancy—

	Pregnancy Category	Explanation
All Trimesters	C	Animal studies have shown an adverse effect and there are no adequate studies in pregnant women OR no animal studies have been conducted and there are no adequate studies in pregnant women.

Breast Feeding—There are no adequate studies in women for determining infant risk when using this medication during breastfeeding. Weigh the potential benefits against the potential risks before taking this medication while breastfeeding.

Other medicines—

Using this medicine with any of the following medicines is usually not recommended, but may be required in some cases. If both medicines are prescribed together, your doctor may change the dose or how often you use one or both of the medicines.

Atorvastatin, Cerivastatin, Lovastatin, Rosuvastatin, Simvastatin

Interactions with Food/Tobacco/Alcohol—Certain medicines should not be used at or around the time of eating food or eating certain types of food since interactions may

occur. Using alcohol or tobacco with certain medicines may also cause interactions to occur. The following interactions have been selected on the basis of their potential significance and are not necessarily all-inclusive.

Using this medicine with any of the following may cause an increased risk of certain side effects but may be unavoidable in some cases. If used together, your doctor may change the dose or how often you use this medicine, or give you special instructions about the use of food, alcohol, or tobacco.

Ethanol

Other medical problems—The presence of other medical problems may affect the use of this medicine. Make sure you tell your doctor if you have any other medical problems, especially:

- Bleeding problems or
- Diabetes mellitus (sugar diabetes) or
- Glaucoma or
- Gout or
- Liver disease or history of jaundice
- Low blood pressure or
- Stomach ulcer—Niacin may make these conditions worse
- Kidney problems—Niacin (extended release tablets) may make your kidney problems worse.

Proper Use of This Medicine

Use this medicine only as directed by your doctor. Do not use more or less of it, do not use it more often, and do not use it for a longer time than your doctor ordered. To do so may increase the chance of unwanted effects.

Remember that niacin will not cure your condition but it does help control it. Therefore, you must continue to take it as directed if you expect to keep your cholesterol levels down.

Follow carefully the special diet your doctor gave you. This is the most important part of controlling your condition, and is necessary if the medicine is to work properly.

If this medicine upsets your stomach, it may be taken with meals or milk. If stomach upset (nausea or diarrhea) continues, check with your doctor.

For patients taking the extended-release capsule form of this medicine:

- Swallow the capsule whole. Do not crush, break, or chew before swallowing. However, if the capsule is too large to swallow, you may mix the contents of the capsule with jam or jelly and swallow without chewing.

For patients taking the extended-release tablet form of this medicine:

- Swallow the tablet whole. If the tablet is scored, it may be broken, but not crushed or chewed, before being swallowed.
- Tablet (Niaspan) should be taken at bedtime after a low-fat snack.
- To decrease flushing of your face (redness), take aspirin or ibuprofen (e.g., Advil, Motrin) 30 minutes before taking tablet (Niaspan).
- Avoid drinking alcohol or hot drinks around the time you take your tablet (Niaspan). This helps decrease flushing of your face (redness).
- Take this medication exactly as your doctor ordered. If you stop taking this medication for any period of time, contact your doctor prior to restarting taking niacin.

Dosing—The dose of this medicine will be different for different patients. Follow your doctor's orders or the directions on the label. The following information includes only the average doses of this medicine. If your dose is different, do not change it unless your doctor tells you to do so.

The amount of medicine that you take depends on the strength of the medicine. Also, the number of doses you take each day, the time allowed between doses, and the length of time you take the medicine depend on the medical problem for which you are using the medicine.

- For oral dosage form (extended-release capsules, extended-release tablets, oral solution, or regular tablets):
  - For treatment of high cholesterol:
    - Adults and teenagers—500 milligrams to 2 grams one to three times a day: use and dose will be determined by your doctor. Do not exceed the amount the doctor prescribes.
    - Children—Use and dose must be determined by your doctor.

Missed dose—If you miss a dose of this medicine, take it as soon as possible. However, if it is almost time for your next dose, skip the missed dose and go back to your regular dosing schedule. Do not double doses.

Storage—Store the medicine in a closed container at room temperature, away from heat, moisture, and direct light. Keep from freezing.

Keep out of the reach of children.

Do not keep outdated medicine or medicine no longer needed.

Precautions While Using This Medicine

It is very important that your doctor check your progress at regular visits. This will allow your doctor to see if the medicine is working properly to lower your cholesterol and triglyceride (fat) levels and if you should continue to take it.

Do not stop taking niacin without first checking with your doctor. When you stop taking this medicine, your blood cholesterol levels may increase again. Your doctor may want you to follow a special diet to help prevent this from happening.

Do not take vitamins or other dietary supplements unless they have been discussed with your doctor. This especially includes vitamins or dietary supplements that contain niacin or similar ingredients.

This medicine may affect blood sugar levels. If you notice a change in the results of your blood or urine sugar tests or if you have any questions, check with your doctor.

This medicine may cause you to feel dizzy or faint, especially when you get up from a lying or sitting position. Getting up slowly may help. This effect should lessen after a week or two as your body gets used to the medicine. However, if the problem continues or gets worse, check with your doctor.

Side Effects of This Medicine

Along with its needed effects, a medicine may cause some unwanted effects. Although not all of these side effects may occur, if they do occur they may need medical attention.

Check with your doctor immediately if any of the following side effects occur:
> *Less common*
> *With prolonged use of extended-release niacin*
>> Darkening of urine; light gray-colored stools; loss of appetite; severe stomach pain; yellow eyes or skin

Some side effects may occur that usually do not need medical attention. These side effects may go away during treatment as your body adjusts to the medicine. Also, your health care professional may be able to tell you about ways to prevent or reduce some of these side effects. Check with your health care professional if any of the following side effects continue or are bothersome or if you have any questions about them:
> *Less common*
>> Abdominal pain; feeling of warmth; flushing or redness of skin, especially on face and neck; headache; rash; runny nose; sneezing; stuffy nose
> *With high doses*
>> Diarrhea; dizziness or faintness; dryness of skin; fever; frequent urination; itching of skin; joint pain; muscle aching or cramping; nausea or vomiting; side, lower back, or stomach pain; swelling of feet or lower legs; unusual thirst; unusual tiredness or weakness; unusually fast, slow, or irregular heartbeat

Other side effects not listed may also occur in some patients. If you notice any other effects, check with your healthcare professional.

NIACIN   (Vitamin B 3)   (Systemic)

Some commonly used brand names are:

In the U.S.—
Niacor (1)   Nicotinex Elixir (1)
Nicolar (1)   Slo-Niacin (1)

In Canada—
Novo-Niacin (1)

This information applies to the following products:

1. Niacin (nye-a-SIN)
2. Niacinamide (nye-a-SIN-a-mide)

Category

- **Nutritional supplement, vitamin—**

Description

Vitamins (VYE-ta-mins) are compounds that you *must* have for growth and health. They are needed in small amounts only and are usually available in the foods that you eat. Niacin and niacinamide are necessary for many normal functions of the body, including normal tissue metabolism. They may have other effects as well.

Lack of niacin may lead to a condition called pellagra. Pellagra causes diarrhea, stomach problems, skin problems, sores in the mouth, anemia (weak blood), and mental problems. Your health care professional may treat this by prescribing niacin for you.

Some conditions may increase your need for niacin. These include:
- Cancer
- Diabetes mellitus (sugar diabetes)
- Diarrhea (prolonged)
- Fever (prolonged)

- Hartnup disease
- Infection (prolonged)
- Intestinal problems
- Liver disease
- Mouth or throat sores
- Overactive thyroid
- Pancreas disease
- Stomach ulcer
- Stress (prolonged)
- Surgical removal of stomach

Increased need for niacin should be determined by your health care professional.

Claims that niacin is effective for treatment of acne, alcoholism, unwanted effects of drug abuse, leprosy, motion sickness, muscle problems, poor circulation, and mental problems, and for prevention of heart attacks, have not been proven. Many of these treatments involve large and expensive amounts of vitamins.

Injectable niacin and niacinamide are given by or under the supervision of a health care professional. Other forms of niacin and niacinamide are available without a prescription.

Niacin and niacinamide are available in the following dosage forms:

Oral
- Niacin
  - Extended-release capsules
  - Solution
  - Tablets
  - Extended-release tablets
- Niacinamide
  - Tablets

Parenteral
- Niacin
  - Injection
- Niacinamide
  - Injection

Before Using This Dietary Supplement

If you are taking this dietary supplement without a prescription, carefully read and follow any precautions on the label. For niacin or niacinamide, the following should be considered:

Allergies—Tell your health care professional if you have ever had any unusual or allergic reaction to niacin or niacinamide. Also tell your health care professional if you are allergic to any other substances, such as foods, preservatives, or dyes.

Pregnancy—It is especially important that you are receiving enough vitamins when you become pregnant and that you continue to receive the right amount of vitamins throughout your pregnancy. The healthy growth and development of the fetus depend on a steady supply of nutrients from the mother. However, taking large amounts of a dietary supplement in pregnancy may be harmful to the mother and/or fetus and should be avoided.

Breast-feeding—It is especially important that you receive the right amounts of vitamins so that your baby will also get the vitamins needed to grow properly. However, taking large amounts of a dietary supplement while breast-feeding may be harmful to the mother and/or baby and should be avoided.

Children—Problems in children have not been reported with intake of normal daily recommended amounts.

Older adults—Problems in older adults have not been reported with intake of normal daily recommended amounts.

Medicines or other dietary supplements—Although certain medicines or dietary supplements should not be used together at all, in other cases they may be used together even if an interaction might occur. In these cases, your health care professional may want to change the dose, or other precautions may be necessary. Tell your health care professional if you are using any other dietary supplement or any prescription or nonprescription (over-the-counter [OTC]) medicine.

Other medical problems—The presence of other medical problems may affect the use of niacin or niacinamide. Make sure you tell your health care professional if you have any other medical problems, especially:
- Bleeding problems or
- Diabetes mellitus (sugar diabetes) or
- Glaucoma or
- Gout or
- Liver disease or
- Low blood pressure or
- Stomach ulcer—Niacin or niacinamide may make these conditions worse

Proper Use of This Dietary Supplement

For good health, it is important that you eat a balanced and varied diet. Follow carefully any diet program your health care professional may recommend. For your specific dietary vitamin and/or mineral needs, ask your health care professional for a list of appropriate foods. If you think that you are not getting enough vitamins and/or minerals in your diet, you may choose to take a dietary supplement.

Niacin is found in meats, eggs, and milk and dairy products. Little niacin is lost from foods during ordinary cooking.

Vitamins alone will not take the place of a good diet and will not provide energy. Your body also needs other substances found in food such as protein, minerals, carbohydrates, and fat. Vitamins themselves often cannot work without the presence of other foods.

The daily amount of niacin needed is defined in several different ways.

For U.S.—
- Recommended Dietary Allowances (RDAs) are the amount of vitamins and minerals needed to provide for adequate nutrition in most healthy persons. RDAs for a given nutrient may vary depending on a person's age, sex, and physical condition (e.g., pregnancy).
- Daily Values (DVs) are used on food and dietary supplement labels to indicate the percent of the recommended daily amount of each nutrient that a serving provides. DV replaces the previous designation of United States Recommended Daily Allowances (USRDAs).

For Canada—
- Recommended Nutrient Intakes (RNIs) are used to determine the amounts of vitamins, minerals, and protein needed to provide adequate nutrition and lessen the risk of chronic disease.

Normal daily recommended intakes in milligrams (mg) for niacin are generally defined as follows:

Persons	U.S. (mg)	Canada (mg)
Infants and children	5–9	4–9
Birth to 3 years of age		
4 to 6 years of age	12	13
7 to 10 years of age	13	14–18
Adolescent and adult males	15–20	14–23
Adolescent and adult females	13–15	14–16
Pregnant females	17	14–16
Breast-feeding females	20	14–16

Dosing—The amount of niacin and niacinamide needed to meet normal daily recommended intakes will be different for different individuals. The following information includes only the average amounts of niacin and niacinamide.

For niacin
- For *oral* dosage form (capsules, extended-release capsules and tablets, tablets, oral solution):
  - To prevent deficiency, the amount taken by mouth is based on normal daily recommended intakes:

  For the U.S.
  - Adult and teenage males—15 to 20 milligrams (mg) per day.
  - Adult and teenage females—13 to 15 mg per day.
  - Pregnant females—17 mg per day.
  - Breast-feeding females—20 mg per day.
  - Children 7 to 10 years of age—13 mg per day.
  - Children 4 to 6 years of age—12 mg per day.
  - Children birth to 3 years of age—5 to 9 mg per day.

  For Canada
  - Adult and teenage males—14 to 23 mg per day.
  - Adult and teenage females—14 to 16 mg per day.
  - Pregnant females—14 to 16 mg per day.
  - Breast-feeding females—14 to 16 mg per day.
  - Children 7 to 10 years of age—14 to 18 mg per day.
  - Children 4 to 6 years of age—13 mg per day.
  - Children birth to 3 years of age—4 to 9 mg per day.
  - To treat deficiency:
    - Adults, teenagers, and children—Treatment dose is determined by prescriber for each individual based on the severity of deficiency.

For niacinamide
- For *oral* dosage form (tablets):
  - To prevent deficiency, the amount taken by mouth is based on normal daily recommended intakes:

  For the U.S.
  - Adult and teenage males—15 to 20 milligrams (mg) per day.
  - Adult and teenage females—13 to 15 mg per day.
  - Pregnant females—17 mg per day.
  - Breast-feeding females—20 mg per day.
  - Children 7 to 10 years of age—13 mg per day.
  - Children 4 to 6 years of age—12 mg per day.
  - Children birth to 3 years of age—5 to 9 mg per day.

  For Canada
  - Adult and teenage males—14 to 23 mg per day.
  - Adult and teenage females—14 to 16 mg per day.
  - Pregnant females—14 to 16 mg per day.

- Breast-feeding females—14 to 16 mg per day.
- Children 7 to 10 years of age—14 to 18 mg per day.
- Children 4 to 6 years of age—13 mg per day.
- Children birth to 3 years of age—4 to 9 mg per day.
  - To treat deficiency:
    - Adults, teenagers, and children—Treatment dose is determined by prescriber for each individual based on the severity of deficiency.

If this dietary supplement upsets your stomach, it may be taken with meals or milk. If stomach upset (nausea or diarrhea) continues, check with your health care professional.

For individuals taking the *extended-release capsule form* of this dietary supplement:

- Swallow the capsule whole. Do not crush, break, or chew before swallowing. However, if the capsule is too large to swallow, you may mix the contents of the capsule with jam or jelly and swallow without chewing.

For individuals taking the *extended-release tablet form* of this dietary supplement:

- Swallow the tablet whole. If the tablet is scored, it may be broken, but not crushed or chewed, before being swallowed.

Missed dose—If you miss taking a vitamin for one or more days there is no cause for concern, since it takes some time for your body to become seriously low in vitamins. However, if your health care professional has recommended that you take this vitamin, try to remember to take it as directed every day.

Storage—To store this dietary supplement:

- Keep out of the reach of children.
- Store away from heat and direct light.
- Do not store in the bathroom, near the kitchen sink, or in other damp places. Heat or moisture may cause the dietary supplement to break down.
- Keep the liquid form of this dietary supplement from freezing.
- Do not keep outdated dietary supplements or those no longer needed. Be sure that any discarded dietary supplement is out of the reach of children.

Precautions While Using This Dietary Supplement

This dietary supplement may cause you to feel dizzy or faint, especially when you get up from a lying or sitting position. Getting up slowly may help. This effect should lessen after a week or two as your body gets used to the dietary supplement. However, if the problem continues or gets worse, check with your health care professional.

Side Effects of This Dietary Supplement

Along with its needed effects, a dietary supplement may cause some unwanted effects. Although not all of these side effects may occur, if they do occur they may need medical attention.

Check with your health care professional immediately if any of the following side effects occur:

With injection only

Skin rash or itching; wheezing

With prolonged use of extended-release niacin

Darkening of urine; light gray-colored stools; loss of appetite; severe stomach pain; yellow eyes or skin

Other side effects may occur that usually do not need medical attention. These side effects may go away during treatment as your body adjusts to the dietary supplement. However, check with your health care professional if any of the following side effects continue or are bothersome:

Less common—with niacin only

Feeling of warmth; flushing or redness of skin, especially on face and neck; headache

With high doses

Diarrhea; dizziness or faintness; dryness of skin; fever; frequent urination; itching of skin; joint pain; muscle aching or cramping; nausea or vomiting; side, lower back, or stomach pain; swelling of feet or lower legs; unusual thirst; unusual tiredness or weakness; unusually fast, slow, or irregular heartbeat

Other side effects not listed above may also occur in some individuals. If you notice any other effects, check with your health care professional.

NICOTINE   (Inhalation, oral/nebulization route) - NIK-oh-teen

Commonly used brand name(s)

In the U.S.—

Nicotrol

In Canada—

Nicorette Inhaler

Available Dosage Forms:

- Aerosol Liquid
- Aerosol Powder
- Device

Therapeutic Class: Smoking Cessation Agent
Pharmacologic Class: Cholinergic

Uses For This Medicine

Nicotine, in an inhaler, is used to help you stop smoking. It is used for up to 6 months as part of a stop-smoking program. This program may include counseling, education, specific behavior change techniques, or support groups.

With the inhaler, nicotine is inhaled through the mouth and is absorbed in the mouth and throat, but not in the lungs. Eight to ten puffs on the inhaler provide about the same amount of nicotine as one puff on an average cigarette. This nicotine takes the place of the nicotine that you would otherwise get from smoking. In this way, the withdrawal effects of not smoking are less severe. Then, as your body adjusts to not smoking, the use of the nicotine inhaler is decreased gradually over several weeks. Finally, use is stopped altogether.

This medicine is available only with your doctor's prescription.

Before Using This Medicine

In deciding to use a medicine, the risks of taking the medicine must be weighed against the good it will do. This is a decision you and your doctor will make. For this medicine, the following should be considered:

Allergies—Tell your doctor if you have ever had any unusual or allergic reaction to this medicine or any other medicines. Also tell your health care professional if you have any other types of allergies, such as to foods, dyes, preservatives, or animals. For non-prescription products, read the label or package ingredients carefully.

Pediatric—Small amounts of nicotine can cause poisoning in children. Even used nicotine inhaler cartridges contain enough nicotine to cause serious harm in children. Also, the cartridges are small enough that they can cause choking if they are swallowed.

Geriatric—This medicine has been tested in a limited number of patients 60 years of age or older and has not been shown to cause different side effects or problems in older people than it does in younger adults.

Pregnancy—

	Pregnancy Category	Explanation
All Trimesters	D	Studies in pregnant women have demonstrated a risk to the fetus. However, the benefits of therapy in a life threatening situation or a serious disease, may outweigh the potential risk.

Breast Feeding—Studies in women breastfeeding have demonstrated harmful infant effects. An alternative to this medication should be prescribed or you should stop breast-feeding while using this medicine.

Other medicines—

Using this medicine with any of the following medicines may cause an increased risk of certain side effects, but using both drugs may be the best treatment for you. If both medicines are prescribed together, your doctor may change the dose or how often you use one or both of the medicines.

Clozapine

Interactions with Food/Tobacco/Alcohol—Certain medicines should not be used at or around the time of eating food or eating certain types of food since interactions may occur. Using alcohol or tobacco with certain medicines may also cause interactions to occur. Discuss with your healthcare professional the use of your medicine with food, alcohol, or tobacco.

Other medical problems—The presence of other medical problems may affect the use of this medicine. Make sure you tell your doctor if you have any other medical problems, especially:

- Asthma or other breathing problems or
- Heart or blood vessel disease or
- High blood pressure or
- Liver disease or
- Overactive thyroid or
- Pheochromocytoma or

- Stomach ulcer or
- Type 1 diabetes mellitus (sugar diabetes)—Nicotine may make the condition worse

Proper Use of This Medicine

The nicotine inhaler usually comes with patient directions. Read the directions carefully before using this medicine.

The nicotine inhaler should be used at or above room temperature (60 °F [16 °C]). Cold temperatures decrease the amount of nicotine you inhale.

It is important to participate in a stop-smoking program during treatment. This may make it easier for you to stop smoking.

To decrease the risk of becoming dependent on the nicotine inhaler, your doctor may instruct you to stop treatment gradually. This may be done by keeping track of, and steadily reducing, use of the nicotine inhaler or by setting a planned date for stopping use of the inhaler.

Dosing—The dose of this medicine will be different for different patients. Follow your doctor's orders or the directions on the label. The following information includes only the average doses of this medicine. If your dose is different, do not change it unless your doctor tells you to do so.

The amount of medicine that you take depends on the strength of the medicine. Also, the number of doses you take each day, the time allowed between doses, and the length of time you take the medicine depend on the medical problem for which you are using the medicine.

- For cartridge for inhalation dosage form:
  - To help you stop smoking:
    - Adults and older teenagers—At first, the dose is 6 to 16 cartridges per day for up to twelve weeks. Then the dose is gradually reduced over a period of up to twelve weeks.
    - Children—Use and dose must be determined by your doctor.

Storage—Store the medicine in a closed container at room temperature, away from heat, moisture, and direct light. Keep from freezing.

Keep out of the reach of children.

Do not keep outdated medicine or medicine no longer needed.

Precautions While Using This Medicine

Do not smoke during treatment with the nicotine inhaler because of the risk of nicotine overdose.

Do not use the nicotine inhaler for longer than 6 months if you have stopped smoking because continuing use of nicotine in any form can be harmful and addictive.

Nicotine should not be used in pregnancy. If there is a possibility you might become pregnant, you may want to use some type of birth control. If you think you may have become pregnant, stop taking this medicine immediately and check with your doctor.

Nicotine products must be kept out of the reach of children and pets. Even used nicotine inhaler cartridges contain enough nicotine to cause serious harm in children. If a child chews on or swallows a cartridge, contact your doctor or poison control center at once.

Side Effects of This Medicine

Along with its needed effects, a medicine may cause some unwanted effects. Although not all of these side effects may occur, if they do occur they may need medical attention.

Check with your doctor as soon as possible if any of the following side effects occur:

Less common
   Fast or irregular heartbeat; fever with or without chills; headache; nausea with or without vomiting; runny nose; shortness of breath, tightness in chest, trouble in breathing, or wheezing; skin rash, itching, or hives; tearing of eyes

Symptoms of overdose
   Abdominal or stomach pain; cold sweat; confusion; convulsions (seizures); disturbed hearing and vision; drooling; extreme exhaustion; pale skin; slow heartbeat; tremors

Some side effects may occur that usually do not need medical attention. These side effects may go away during treatment as your body adjusts to the medicine. Also, your health care professional may be able to tell you about ways to prevent or reduce some of these side effects. Check with your health care professional if any of the following side effects continue or are bothersome or if you have any questions about them:

More common
   Coughing; indigestion; mouth and throat irritation; stuffy nose

Less common
   Anxiety; back pain; change in taste; diarrhea; dizziness; feeling of burning, numbness, tightness, tingling, warmth or heat; feelings of drug dependence; flu-like symptoms; general pain; hiccups; mental depression; pain in jaw and neck; pain in muscles; passing of gas; problems with teeth; trouble in sleeping; unusual tiredness or weakness

Other side effects not listed may also occur in some patients. If you notice any other effects, check with your healthcare professional.

NICOTINE   (Nasal route) - NIK-oh-teen

Commonly used brand name(s)

In the U.S.—
   Nicotrol NS

Available Dosage Forms:
- Spray

Therapeutic Class: Smoking Cessation Agent
Pharmacologic Class: Cholinergic

Uses For This Medicine

Nicotine in a nasal spray is used to help you stop smoking. It is used for up to 3 months as part of a stop-smoking program. This program may include counseling, education, or psychological support.

With the nasal spray, nicotine is inhaled through your nose and passes into your blood stream. This nicotine takes the place of the nicotine you would otherwise get from smoking. In this way, the withdrawal effects of not smoking are less severe. Then, as your body adjusts to not smoking, the use of nicotine nasal spray is decreased gradually over several weeks. Finally, use is stopped altogether.

This medicine is available only with your doctor's prescription.

Before Using This Medicine

In deciding to use a medicine, the risks of taking the medicine must be weighed against the good it will do. This is a decision you and your doctor will make. For this medicine, the following should be considered:

Allergies—Tell your doctor if you have ever had any unusual or allergic reaction to this medicine or any other medicines. Also tell your health care professional if you have any other types of allergies, such as to foods, dyes, preservatives, or animals. For non-prescription products, read the label or package ingredients carefully.

Pediatric—Small amounts of nicotine can cause poisoning in children.

Geriatric—This medicine has been tested in a limited number of patients 60 years of age or older and has not been shown to cause different side effects or problems in older people than it does in younger adults.

Pregnancy—

	Pregnancy Category	Explanation
All Trimesters	D	Studies in pregnant women have demonstrated a risk to the fetus. However, the benefits of therapy in a life threatening situation or a serious disease, may outweigh the potential risk.

Breast Feeding—Studies in women breastfeeding have demonstrated harmful infant effects. An alternative to this medication should be prescribed or you should stop breastfeeding while using this medicine.

Other medicines—

Using this medicine with any of the following medicines may cause an increased risk of certain side effects, but using both drugs may be the best treatment for you. If both medicines are prescribed together, your doctor may change the dose or how often you use one or both of the medicines.

Clozapine

Interactions with Food/Tobacco/Alcohol—Certain medicines should not be used at or around the time of eating food or eating certain types of food since interactions may occur. Using alcohol or tobacco with certain medicines may also cause interactions to occur. Discuss with your healthcare professional the use of your medicine with food, alcohol, or tobacco.

Other medical problems—The presence of other medical problems may affect the use of this medicine. Make sure you tell your doctor if you have any other medical problems, especially:
* Allergies or

* Heart or blood vessel disease or
* High blood pressure or
* Liver disease or
* Nose polyps or
* Overactive thyroid or
* Pheochromocytoma or
* Sinus problems or
* Stomach ulcer or
* Type 1 diabetes (sugar diabetes)—Nicotine may make the condition worse
* Common cold or
* Stuffy nose—Nicotine nasal spray may not work properly

Proper Use of This Medicine

Nicotine nasal spray usually comes with patient directions. Read the directions carefully before using this medicine.

It is important to participate in a stop-smoking program during treatment. To do so may make it easier for you to stop smoking.

Use of nicotine nasal spray may be gradually reduced by using only one half of a dose at a time or skipping doses by not using the spray every hour. You may also keep track of the number of doses and use fewer each day, or set a date to stop using nicotine nasal spray.

Dosing—The dose of this medicine will be different for different patients. Follow your doctor's orders or the directions on the label. The following information includes only the average doses of this medicine. If your dose is different, do not change it unless your doctor tells you to do so.

The amount of medicine that you take depends on the strength of the medicine. Also, the number of doses you take each day, the time allowed between doses, and the length of time you take the medicine depend on the medical problem for which you are using the medicine.

* For the nasal spray dosage form:
  ○ To help you stop smoking:
    ▪ Adults—At first, the dose is 1 or 2 sprays into each nostril every hour. The dose should then be adjusted based on the number of cigarettes you smoked each day before beginning treatment with the nasal spray and the side effects the nasal spray causes.
    ▪ Children—Use and dose must be determined by your doctor.

Storage—Store the medicine in a closed container at room temperature, away from heat, moisture, and direct light. Keep from freezing.

Keep out of the reach of children.

Do not keep outdated medicine or medicine no longer needed.

Precautions While Using This Medicine

Nicotine nasal spray should not be used by people who do not smoke because they can become addicted to nicotine.

During the first week of use, you may have a hot, peppery feeling in the back of your throat or nose; coughing; runny nose; sneezing; or watery eyes. Do not stop using this medicine. If you continue to use nicotine nasal spray regularly, you should adjust to these effects. If these effects do not lessen after 1 week, check with your doctor.

Avoid contact with the skin, mouth, eyes, and ears. If even a small amount of nicotine nasal spray comes into contact with the skin, mouth, eyes, or ears, the affected area should be immediately rinsed with water only.

Do not use nicotine nasal spray for longer than 3 months. To do so may result in physical dependence on the nicotine.

Nicotine should not be used in pregnancy. If there is a possibility you might become pregnant, you may want to use some type of birth control. If you think you may have become pregnant, stop using this medicine immediately and check with your doctor.

Nicotine products must be kept out of the reach of children and pets. Even very small amounts of nicotine may cause poisoning in children. If a child uses nicotine nasal spray, contact your doctor or poison control center at once.

Side Effects of This Medicine

Along with its needed effects, a medicine may cause some unwanted effects. Although not all of these side effects may occur, if they do occur they may need medical attention.

Check with your doctor as soon as possible if any of the following side effects occur:

More common
Feelings of dependence; joint pain; shortness of breath; swelling of gums, mouth, or tongue; tightness in chest; tingling in arms, legs, hands, or feet

Less common
Burning, tingling, or prickly sensations in nose, mouth, or head; confusion; difficulty in swallowing; dryness or pain in throat; fast or irregular heartbeat; muscle pain; nasal blister or sore; numbness of nose or mouth

Rare
Blood-containing blisters on skin; difficulty in speaking; loss of memory; migraine headache; skin rash; swelling of feet or lower legs; wheezing

Symptoms of overdose
Cold sweat; convulsions (seizures); disturbed hearing and vision; dizziness; drooling; pale skin; slow heartbeat; tremors; vomiting; unusual tiredness or weakness

Some side effects may occur that usually do not need medical attention. These side effects may go away during treatment as your body adjusts to the medicine. Also, your health care professional may be able to tell you about ways to prevent or reduce some of these side effects. Check with your health care professional if any of the following side effects continue or are bothersome or if you have any questions about them:

More common
Back pain; constipation; cough; headache; hot, peppery feeling in the back of the throat or nose; indigestion; nausea; runny nose; sneezing; watery eyes

Less common
Abdominal or stomach pain; acne; change in sense of smell or taste; dryness, burning, itching, or irritation of the eyes; earache; flushing of face; passing of gas; hoarseness; itching; menstrual problems; nosebleed;

sinus problems; soreness of teeth and gums; stuffy nose

Rare
Changes in vision; diarrhea; dryness of mouth; hiccups; increased amount of sputum

Other side effects not listed may also occur in some patients. If you notice any other effects, check with your healthcare professional.

NICOTINE (Oral route, Transdermal route) - NIK-oh-teen

Commonly used brand name(s)

In the U.S.—
Habitrol
Nicoderm CQ
Nicotrol

In Canada—
Nicoderm

Available Dosage Forms:
• Patch, Extended Release

Therapeutic Class: Smoking Cessation Agent
Pharmacologic Class: Cholinergic

Uses For This Medicine

Nicotine, in a flavored chewing gum, a lozenge, or a skin patch, is used to help you stop smoking. It is used for up to 12 weeks as part of a stop-smoking program. This program may include education, counseling, and psychological support.

As you chew nicotine gum or suck on the nicotine lozenge, nicotine passes through the lining of your mouth and into your blood stream. When you wear a nicotine patch, nicotine passes through your skin into your blood stream. This nicotine takes the place of nicotine that you would otherwise get from smoking. In this way, the withdrawal effects of not smoking are less severe. Then, as your body adjusts to not smoking, the use of the nicotine gum is decreased gradually until use is stopped altogether. For most brands of patches, the strength of the patch you use will be decreased over a few weeks until use is stopped. If you are using the brand of patch that is available in only one strength, use is stopped after the treatment period indicated on the label.

Children, pregnant women, and nonsmokers should not use nicotine gum or patches because of harmful effects.

Nicotine gum or lozenge is available without a prescription.

Before Using This Medicine

In deciding to use a medicine, the risks of taking the medicine must be weighed against the good it will do. This is a decision you and your doctor will make. For this medicine, the following should be considered:

Allergies—Tell your doctor if you have ever had any unusual or allergic reaction to this medicine or any other medicines. Also tell your health care professional if you have any other types of allergies, such as to foods, dyes, preservatives,

or animals. For non-prescription products, read the label or package ingredients carefully.

Pediatric—Small amounts of nicotine can cause serious harm in children. Even nicotine patches that have been used still contain enough nicotine to cause problems in children. Although there is no specific information comparing use of nicotine in teenagers with use in other age groups, this medicine is not expected to cause different side effects or problems in nicotine-dependent teenagers than it does in adults.

Geriatric—Nicotine gum, lozenges, and patches have been used in a limited number of patients 60 years of age or older, and have not been shown to cause different side effects or problems in older people than in younger adults.

Pregnancy—

	Pregnancy Category	Explanation
All Trimesters	D	Studies in pregnant women have demonstrated a risk to the fetus. However, the benefits of therapy in a life threatening situation or a serious disease, may outweigh the potential risk.

Breast Feeding—Studies in women breastfeeding have demonstrated harmful infant effects. An alternative to this medication should be prescribed or you should stop breast-feeding while using this medicine.

Other medicines—

Using this medicine with any of the following medicines may cause an increased risk of certain side effects, but using both drugs may be the best treatment for you. If both medicines are prescribed together, your doctor may change the dose or how often you use one or both of the medicines.

Clozapine

Interactions with Food/Tobacco/Alcohol—Certain medicines should not be used at or around the time of eating food or eating certain types of food since interactions may occur. Using alcohol or tobacco with certain medicines may also cause interactions to occur. Discuss with your healthcare professional the use of your medicine with food, alcohol, or tobacco.

Other medical problems—The presence of other medical problems may affect the use of this medicine. Make sure you tell your doctor if you have any other medical problems, especially:

- Dental problems (with gum only) or
- Diabetes, type 1 (sugar diabetes) or
- Heart or blood vessel disease or
- High blood pressure or
- Inflammation of mouth or throat (with gum only) or
- Irritated skin (with patches only) or
- Overactive thyroid or
- Pheochromocytoma (PCC) or
- Stomach ulcer or
- Stroke, recent or
- Temporomandibular (jaw) joint disorder (TMJ) (with gum only)—Nicotine may make the condition worse

Proper Use of This Medicine

For patients using the chewing gum:

- Nicotine gum usually comes with patient directions. Read the directions carefully before using this medicine.
- Use nicotine gum exactly as directed on the label. Remember that it is also important to participate in a stop-smoking program during treatment. This may make it easier for you to stop smoking.
- When you feel the urge to smoke, chew one piece of gum very slowly until you taste it or feel a slight tingling in your mouth. Stop chewing, and place ("park") the chewing gum between your cheek and gum until the taste or tingling is almost gone. Then chew slowly until you taste it again. Continue chewing and stopping ("parking") in this way for about 30 minutes in order to get the full dose of nicotine.
- Do not chew too fast, do not chew more than one piece at a time, and do not chew more than one piece of gum within an hour. To do so may cause unpleasant side effects or an overdose. Also, slower chewing will reduce the possibility of belching.
- You should not drink acidic beverages, such as citrus fruit juices, coffee, soft drinks, or tea within 15 minutes before or while chewing a piece of gum. The acid will prevent the nicotine from being released from the gum.
- As your urge to smoke becomes less frequent, gradually reduce the number of pieces of gum you chew each day until you are chewing three to six pieces a day. This may be possible within 2 to 3 months.
- Remember to carry nicotine gum with you at all times in case you feel the sudden urge to smoke. One cigarette may be enough to start you on the smoking habit again.
- Using hard sugarless candy between doses of gum may help to relieve any nicotine cravings you may have between doses of gum.

For patients using the lozenge:

- Nicotine lozenges usually come with patient directions. Read the directions carefully before using this medicine.
- Use nicotine lozenges exactly as directed on the label. Remember that it is also important to participate in a stop-smoking program during treatment. This may make it easier for you to stop smoking.
- Do not eat or drink for 15 minutes before using a nicotine lozenge.
- When you feel the urge to smoke, suck one lozenge slowly until it dissolves. Do not bite or chew the lozenge like a hard candy. Do not swallow the lozenge.
- As your urge to smoke becomes less frequent, gradually reduce the number of lozenges you use each day until you are using three to six lozenges a day. This should be possible within 12 weeks.
- Remember to carry nicotine lozenges with you at all times in case you feel the sudden urge to smoke. One cigarette may be enough to start you on the smoking habit again.

For patients using the transdermal system (skin patch):

- Nicotine patches usually come with patient instructions. Read them carefully before using this medicine. Nicotine patches will work only if applied correctly.

- Remember that it is also important to participate in a stop-smoking program during treatment. This may make it easier for you to stop smoking.
- Do not remove the patch from its sealed pouch until you are ready to put it on your skin. The patch may not work as well if it is unwrapped too soon.
- Do not try to trim or cut the adhesive patch to adjust the dosage. Check with your healthcare professional if you think the medicine is not working as it should.
- Apply the patch to a clean, dry area of skin on your upper arm, chest, or back. Choose an area that is not very oily, has little or no hair, and is free of scars, cuts, burns, or any other skin irritations.
- Press the patch firmly in place with the palm of your hand for about 10 seconds. Make sure there is good contact with your skin, especially around the edges of the patch.
- The patch should stay in place even when you are showering, bathing, or swimming. Apply a new patch if one falls off.
- Rinse your hands with plain water after you have finished applying the patch to your skin. Nicotine on your hands could get into your eyes and nose and cause stinging, redness, or more serious problems. Using soap to wash your hands will increase the amount of nicotine that passes through your skin.
- After 16 or 24 hours, depending on which product you are using, remove the patch. Choose a different place on your skin to apply the next patch. Do not put a new patch in the same place for at least 1 week. Do not leave the patch on for more than 24 hours. It will not work as well after that time and it may irritate your skin.
- After removing a used patch, fold the patch in half with the sticky sides together. Place the folded, used patch in its protective pouch or in aluminum foil. Make sure to dispose of it out of the reach of children and pets.
- Try to change the patch at the same time each day. If you want to change the time when you put on your patch, just remove the patch you are wearing and put on a new patch. After that, apply a fresh patch at the new time each day.
- Nicotine patches should be removed from the skin during strenuous exercise. If a patch is left on, too much nicotine may pass through your skin into your blood stream.
- If you are using a 24–hour patch and begin having unusual dreams or disturbed sleep, you may take the patch off before going to bed and put a new one on after you wake up the next morning.

Dosing—The dose of this medicine will be different for different patients. Follow your doctor's orders or the directions on the label. The following information includes only the average doses of this medicine. If your dose is different, do not change it unless your doctor tells you to do so.

The amount of medicine that you take depends on the strength of the medicine. Also, the number of doses you take each day, the time allowed between doses, and the length of time you take the medicine depend on the medical problem for which you are using the medicine.

- For the oral dosage form (chewing gum):
  - To help you stop smoking:
    - Adults and teenagers—The usual dose is one piece of chewing gum every one to two hours for six weeks, one piece of chewing gum every two to four hours for three weeks, then one piece of chewing gum every four to eight hours for three weeks. You should not chew more than 24 pieces of gum a day.
    - Children—Use and dose must be determined by your healthcare professional.
- For the oral dosage form (lozenge):
  - To help you stop smoking:
    - Adults and teenagers—The usual dose is suck slowly one lozenge until it dissolves every one to two hours for six weeks, suck one lozenge every two to four hours for three weeks, then suck one lozenge every four to eight hours for three weeks. You should not use more than 20 lozenges a day.
    - Children—Use and dose must be determined by your healthcare professional.
- For the transdermal (stick-on) skin patch:
  - To help you stop smoking:
    - Adults and teenagers—The dose you receive will be based on your body weight, how often you have the urge to smoke, and the brand and strength of the patch you use. This dose will be provided on the package label.
    - Children—Use and dose must be determined by your healthcare professional.

Storage—Store the medicine in a closed container at room temperature, away from heat, moisture, and direct light. Keep from freezing.

Keep out of the reach of children.

Do not keep outdated medicine or medicine no longer needed.

Precautions While Using This Medicine

Do not smoke during treatment with nicotine gum, lozenges, or patches because of the risk of nicotine overdose.

Nicotine should not be used in pregnancy. If there is a possibility you might become pregnant, you may want to use some type of birth control. If you think you may have become pregnant, stop using this medicine immediately and check with your healthcare professional.

Nicotine products must be kept out of the reach of children and pets. Even nicotine patches that have been used still contain enough nicotine to cause problems in children. If a child chews or swallows one or more pieces of nicotine gum or lozenges, contact your healthcare professional or poison control center at once. If a child puts on a nicotine patch or plays with a patch that is out of the sealed pouch, take it away from the child and contact your healthcare professional or poison control center at once.

For patients using the chewing gum:

- Do not chew more than 24 pieces of gum a day. Chewing too many pieces may be harmful because of the risk of overdose.
- Do not use nicotine gum for longer than 12 weeks. To do so may result in physical dependence on the nicotine. If you feel the need to continue using the gum after 12 weeks, contact your healthcare professional.
- If the gum sticks to your dental work, stop using it and check with your medical healthcare professional or dentist. Dentures or other dental work may be damaged be-

cause nicotine gum is stickier and harder to chew than ordinary gum.

For patients using the lozenges:
- Do not use more than 20 lozenges a day. Sucking too many pieces may be harmful because of the risk of overdose.
- Do not use nicotine lozenges for longer than 12 weeks. If you feel the need to continue using the lozenges after 12 weeks, contact your healthcare professional.

For patients using the transdermal system (skin patch):
- Mild itching, burning, or tingling may occur when the patch is first applied, and should go away within 24 hours. After a patch is removed, the skin underneath it may be red. It should not remain red for more than a day. If you get a skin rash from the patch, or if the skin becomes swollen or very red, call your healthcare professional. Do not put on a new patch. If you become allergic to the nicotine in the patch, you could get sick from using cigarettes or other products that contain nicotine.
- Do not use nicotine patches for longer than 12 weeks if you have stopped smoking. If you feel the need to continue using nicotine patches after 12 weeks, contact your healthcare professional.

Side Effects of This Medicine

Along with its needed effects, a medicine may cause some unwanted effects. Although not all of these side effects may occur, if they do occur they may need medical attention.

Check with your doctor as soon as possible if any of the following side effects occur:

More common
Injury or irritation to mouth, teeth, or dental work—with chewing gum only

Less common
High blood pressure

Rare
Fast or irregular heartbeat; hives, itching, rash, redness, or swelling of skin

Symptoms of overdose (may occur in the following order)
Nausea and/or vomiting; increased watering of mouth (severe); abdominal or stomach pain (severe); diarrhea (severe); pale skin; cold sweat; headache (severe); dizziness (severe); disturbed hearing and vision; tremor; confusion; weakness (severe); extreme exhaustion; fainting; low blood pressure; difficulty in breathing (severe); fast, weak, or irregular heartbeat; convulsions (seizures)

Some side effects may occur that usually do not need medical attention. These side effects may go away during treatment as your body adjusts to the medicine. Also, your health care professional may be able to tell you about ways to prevent or reduce some of these side effects. Check with your health care professional if any of the following side effects continue or are bothersome or if you have any questions about them:

More common
Belching—with chewing gum and lozenges; headache (mild); increased appetite; increased watering of mouth (mild)—with chewing gum only; jaw muscle ache—with chewing gum only; redness, itching, and/or burning

at site of application of patch—usually stops within 24 hours; sore mouth or throat—with chewing gum only

Less common or rare
Abdominal or stomach pain (mild); change in sense of taste; constipation; coughing (increased); diarrhea; dizziness or lightheadedness (mild); drowsiness; dryness of mouth; hiccups—with chewing gum and lozenges; hoarseness—with chewing gum only; indigestion (mild); loss of appetite; menstrual pain; muscle or joint pain; nausea or vomiting (mild); passing of gas; sweating (increased); trouble in sleeping or unusual dreams; unusual irritability or nervousness

Other side effects not listed may also occur in some patients. If you notice any other effects, check with your healthcare professional.

NISOLDIPINE (Oral route) - NYE-sole-di-peen

Commonly used brand name(s)

In the U.S.—
Sular

Available Dosage Forms:
- Tablet, Extended Release

Therapeutic Class: Cardiovascular Agent
Pharmacologic Class: Calcium Channel Blocker

Uses For This Medicine

Nisoldipine is a calcium channel blocking agent used to treat high blood pressure. Nisoldipine affects the movement of calcium into the cells of the heart and blood vessels. It relaxes blood vessels and increases the supply of blood and oxygen to the heart while reducing the heart's workload.

High blood pressure adds to the workload of the heart and arteries. If it continues for a long time, the heart and arteries may not function properly. This can damage the blood vessels of the brain, heart, and kidneys, resulting in a stroke, heart failure, or kidney failure. High blood pressure may also increase the risk of heart attacks. These problems may be less likely to occur if blood pressure is controlled.

This medicine is available only with your doctor's prescription.

Before Using This Medicine

In deciding to use a medicine, the risks of taking the medicine must be weighed against the good it will do. This is a decision you and your doctor will make. For this medicine, the following should be considered:

Allergies—Tell your doctor if you have ever had any unusual or allergic reaction to this medicine or any other medicines. Also tell your health care professional if you have any other types of allergies, such as to foods, dyes, preservatives, or animals. For non-prescription products, read the label or package ingredients carefully.

Pediatric—Studies on this medicine have been done only in adult patients, and there is no specific information com-

paring use of nisoldipine in children with use in other age groups.

Geriatric—Elderly people may have higher blood levels of nisoldipine, which may increase the chance of side effects during treatment.

Pregnancy—

	Pregnancy Category	Explanation
All Trimesters	C	Animal studies have shown an adverse effect and there are no adequate studies in pregnant women OR no animal studies have been conducted and there are no adequate studies in pregnant women.

Breast Feeding—There are no adequate studies in women for determining infant risk when using this medication during breastfeeding. Weigh the potential benefits against the potential risks before taking this medication while breastfeeding.

Other medicines—

Using this medicine with any of the following medicines is usually not recommended, but may be required in some cases. If both medicines are prescribed together, your doctor may change the dose or how often you use one or both of the medicines.

Amiodarone, Fentanyl, Mibefradil

Interactions with Food/Tobacco/Alcohol—Certain medicines should not be used at or around the time of eating food or eating certain types of food since interactions may occur. Using alcohol or tobacco with certain medicines may also cause interactions to occur. The following interactions have been selected on the basis of their potential significance and are not necessarily all-inclusive.

Using this medicine with any of the following may cause an increased risk of certain side effects but may be unavoidable in some cases. If used together, your doctor may change the dose or how often you use this medicine, or give you special instructions about the use of food, alcohol, or tobacco.

Grapefruit Juice

Other medical problems—The presence of other medical problems may affect the use of this medicine. Make sure you tell your doctor if you have any other medical problems, especially:

- Blood vessel disease (coronary artery disease)—Nisoldipine may cause chest pain or a heart attack
- Congestive heart failure—Nisoldipine may make this condition worse
- Liver disease—Higher blood levels of nisoldipine may result and a smaller dose may be needed

Proper Use of This Medicine

Take this medicine exactly as directed even if you feel well. Do not take more of this medicine and do not take it more often than your doctor ordered. This medicine works best if there is a constant amount in the blood. To keep blood levels constant, take this medicine at the same time each day and do not miss any doses.

Swallow the tablet whole, without breaking, crushing, or chewing it.

Nisoldipine should not be taken with a high-fat meal or with grapefruit juice or other grapefruit products because these may increase the levels of nisoldipine in the body.

Dosing—The dose of this medicine will be different for different patients. Follow your doctor's orders or the directions on the label. The following information includes only the average doses of this medicine. If your dose is different, do not change it unless your doctor tells you to do so.

The amount of medicine that you take depends on the strength of the medicine. Also, the number of doses you take each day, the time allowed between doses, and the length of time you take the medicine depend on the medical problem for which you are using the medicine.

- For oral dosage form (tablets):
  - For high blood pressure:
    - Adults—10 to 20 mg once a day. Your doctor may increase your dose if needed.
    - Children—Use and dose must be determined by your doctor.

Missed dose—If you miss a dose of this medicine, take it as soon as possible. However, if it is almost time for your next dose, skip the missed dose and go back to your regular dosing schedule. Do not double doses.

Storage—Store the medicine in a closed container at room temperature, away from heat, moisture, and direct light. Keep from freezing.

Keep out of the reach of children.

Do not keep outdated medicine or medicine no longer needed.

Precautions While Using This Medicine

It is important that your doctor check your progress at regular visits. This will allow your doctor to make sure the medicine is working properly and to change the dosage if needed.

This medicine may cause dizziness, lightheadedness, or fainting. Make sure you know how you react to this medicine before you drive, use machines, or do anything else that could be dangerous if you experience these effects.

Side Effects of This Medicine

Along with its needed effects, a medicine may cause some unwanted effects. Although not all of these side effects may occur, if they do occur they may need medical attention.

Check with your doctor as soon as possible if any of the following side effects occur:

More common
Swelling of ankles, feet, or lower legs

Less common
Chest pain; dizziness, lightheadedness, or fainting; rash

Rare
A reaction which may include swelling of the arms, face, legs, lips, tongue, and/or throat; shortness of breath; fast heart rate; chest tightness; dizziness, lightheadedness, or fainting; and/or skin rash

Some side effects may occur that usually do not need medical attention. These side effects may go away during treatment as your body adjusts to the medicine. Also, your health care professional may be able to tell you about ways to prevent or reduce some of these side effects. Check with your health care professional if any of the following side effects

continue or are bothersome or if you have any questions about them:

More common

Headache

Less common

Dizziness; hoarseness and/or sore throat; heartbeat sensations; stuffy nose

Other side effects not listed may also occur in some patients. If you notice any other effects, check with your healthcare professional.

NITAZOXANIDE (Oral route) - nye-ta-ZOX-a-nide

Commonly used brand name(s)

In the U.S.—

Alinia

Available Dosage Forms:

* Powder for Suspension
* Tablet

Therapeutic Class: Antiprotozoal

Uses For This Medicine

Nitazoxanide belongs to a group of medicines called antiprotozoals. It is used to treat diarrhea that is caused by certain types of protozoa (tiny, one-celled animals).

This medicine is available only with your healthcare professional's prescription.

Once a medicine has been approved for marketing for a certain use, experience may show that it is also useful for other medical problems. Although this use is not included in product labeling, nitazoxanide is used in certain patients with the following medical condition:

* Intestinal parasitic infections

Before Using This Medicine

In deciding to use a medicine, the risks of taking the medicine must be weighed against the good it will do. This is a decision you and your doctor will make. For this medicine, the following should be considered:

Allergies—Tell your doctor if you have ever had any unusual or allergic reaction to this medicine or any other medicines. Also tell your health care professional if you have any other types of allergies, such as to foods, dyes, preservatives, or animals. For non-prescription products, read the label or package ingredients carefully.

Pediatric—This medicine has been tested in children and it is not expected to cause different problems in children than it does in other age groups.

Geriatric—Many medicines have not been specifically studied in older people. Therefore it may not be known whether they work the same way they do in younger adults or if they cause different side effects or problems in older people. There is no specific information comparing the use of nitazoxanide in the elderly with use in other age groups.

Pregnancy—

	Pregnancy Category	Explanation
All Trimesters	B	Animal studies have revealed no evidence of harm to the fetus, however, there are no adequate studies in pregnant women OR animal studies have shown an adverse effect, but adequate studies in pregnant women have failed to demonstrate a risk to the fetus.

Breast Feeding—There are no adequate studies in women for determining infant risk when using this medication during breastfeeding. Weigh the potential benefits against the potential risks before taking this medication while breastfeeding.

Other medicines—Although certain medicines should not be used together at all, in other cases two different medicines may be used together even if an interaction might occur. In these cases, your doctor may want to change the dose, or other precautions may be necessary. Tell your healthcare professional if you are taking any other prescription or non-prescription (over-the-counter [OTC]) medicine.

Interactions with Food/Tobacco/Alcohol—Certain medicines should not be used at or around the time of eating food or eating certain types of food since interactions may occur. Using alcohol or tobacco with certain medicines may also cause interactions to occur. Discuss with your healthcare professional the use of your medicine with food, alcohol, or tobacco.

Other medical problems—The presence of other medical problems may affect the use of this medicine. Make sure you tell your doctor if you have any other medical problems, especially:

* Biliary (gallbladder) disease or
* Immune deficiency condition, including HIV or AIDS or
* Kidney disease or
* Liver disease—It is not known how this medicine will effect these conditions and it should be used with caution
* Diabetes mellitus (sugar diabetes)—The oral suspension of nitazoxanide contains 1.48 grams of sucrose per 5 milliliters (mL).

Proper Use of This Medicine

Dosing—The dose of this medicine will be different for different patients. Follow your doctor's orders or the directions on the label. The following information includes only the average doses of this medicine. If your dose is different, do not change it unless your doctor tells you to do so.

The amount of medicine that you take depends on the strength of the medicine. Also, the number of doses you take each day, the time allowed between doses, and the length of time you take the medicine depend on the medical problem for which you are using the medicine.

It is important to take nitazoxanide with food.

It is very important to shake the oral suspension for of the medicine well before measuring each dose.

For the oral suspension dosage form: Use a specially marked measuring syringe or spoon to measure each dose accurately. The average household teaspoon may not hold the right amount of liquid.

- For oral dosage form (oral suspension):
  - For treatment of diarrhea caused by protozoal infections
    - Adults and adolescents—Ages 12 years or older: 25 milliliters (mL) every 12 hours for 3 days.
    - Children—Ages 12 to 47 months: 5 milliliters (mL) every 12 hours for 3 days.
    - Children—Ages 4 to 11 years: 10 milliliters (mL) every 12 hours for 3 days.
- For oral dosage form (tablets):
  - For treatment of diarrhea caused by protozoal infections
    - Adults and adolescents—Ages 12 years or older: 500 milligrams (mg) every 12 hours for 3 days.
    - Children—Ages 11 months or younger: Tablet dosage form is not for use in children.

Missed dose—If you miss a dose of this medicine, take it as soon as possible. However, if it is almost time for your next dose, skip the missed dose and go back to your regular dosing schedule. Do not double doses.

Storage—Store the medicine in a closed container at room temperature, away from heat, moisture, and direct light. Keep from freezing.

Keep out of the reach of children.

Do not keep outdated medicine or medicine no longer needed.

Ask your healthcare professional how you should dispose of any medicine you do not use.

The suspension may be stored for 7 days. Any unused suspension must be disposed of after 7 days.

Precautions While Using This Medicine

It is very important that your healthcare professional check you at regular visits

If your symptoms do not improve within a few days or if they become worse, check with your healthcare professional.

Side Effects of This Medicine

Some side effects may occur that usually do not need medical attention. These side effects may go away during treatment as your body adjusts to the medicine. Also, your health care professional may be able to tell you about ways to prevent or reduce some of these side effects. Check with your health care professional if any of the following side effects continue or are bothersome or if you have any questions about them:

More common
  Stomach pain
Less common
  Diarrhea; headache; vomiting
Rare
  Appetite increase; bloated full feeling; discolored urine; dizziness; enlarged salivary glands; excess air or gas in stomach or intestines; eye discoloration, pale yellow; fever; general feeling of discomfort or illness; infection; itching skin; loss of appetite; nausea; passing gas; runny nose; sneezing; stuffy nose; sweating; unusual tiredness or weakness; weight loss

Other side effects not listed may also occur in some patients. If you notice any other effects, check with your healthcare professional.

NITISINONE   (Oral route) - nye-TIS-i-none

Commonly used brand name(s)

In the U.S.—
  Orfadin

Available Dosage Forms:

- Capsule

Therapeutic Class: Gastrointestinal Agent

Uses For This Medicine

Nitisinone is given along with a special diet to treat hereditary tyrosinemia, type 1. This disease is caused by too much tyrosine in the blood. It may cause damage to the liver, kidneys, eyes, skin, and nervous system. Treatment with nitisinone and diet may slow the disease, but it will not cure it.

This medicine is available only with your or your child's doctor's prescription.

Before Using This Medicine

In deciding to use a medicine, the risks of taking the medicine must be weighed against the good it will do. This is a decision you and your doctor will make. For this medicine, the following should be considered:

Allergies—Tell your doctor if you have ever had any unusual or allergic reaction to this medicine or any other medicines. Also tell your health care professional if you have any other types of allergies, such as to foods, dyes, preservatives, or animals. For non-prescription products, read the label or package ingredients carefully.

Pediatric—This medicine has been tested in children and, in effective doses, has not been shown to cause specific problems.

Geriatric—Many medicines have not been studied specifically in older people. Therefore, it may not be known whether they work exactly the same way they do in younger adults or if they cause different side effects or problems in older people. There is no specific information comparing use of nitisinone in the elderly with use in other age groups.

Pregnancy—

	Pregnancy Category	Explanation
All Trimesters	C	Animal studies have shown an adverse effect and there are no adequate studies in pregnant women OR no animal studies have been conducted and there are no adequate studies in pregnant women.

Breast Feeding—There are no adequate studies in women for determining infant risk when using this medication during breastfeeding. Weigh the potential benefits against the potential risks before taking this medication while breastfeeding.

Other medicines—Although certain medicines should not be used together at all, in other cases two different medicines may be used together even if an interaction might occur. In these cases, your doctor may want to change the dose, or other precautions may be necessary. Tell your healthcare

professional if you are taking any other prescription or non-prescription (over-the-counter [OTC]) medicine.

Interactions with Food/Tobacco/Alcohol—Certain medicines should not be used at or around the time of eating food or eating certain types of food since interactions may occur. Using alcohol or tobacco with certain medicines may also cause interactions to occur. Discuss with your healthcare professional the use of your medicine with food, alcohol, or tobacco.

Proper Use of This Medicine

To use:
- It is not known how nitisinone reacts with food. It is best to take it at least 1 hour before a meal.
- For small children, you may open the capsule and put the medicine in a small amount of water, formula, or applesauce. Give the medicine as soon as it is mixed.

Dosing—The dose of this medicine will be different for different patients. Follow your doctor's orders or the directions on the label. The following information includes only the average doses of this medicine. If your dose is different, do not change it unless your doctor tells you to do so.

The amount of medicine that you take depends on the strength of the medicine. Also, the number of doses you take each day, the time allowed between doses, and the length of time you take the medicine depend on the medical problem for which you are using the medicine.

- For oral dosage form (capsules):
  - For hereditary tyrosinemia, type 1:
    - Adults—The dose is based on body weight and will be determined by your doctor. Your doctor may increase the dose as needed.
    - Children—The dose is based on body weight and will be determined by your child's doctor. Your child's doctor may increase the dose as needed.

Missed dose—If you miss a dose of this medicine, take it as soon as possible. However, if it is almost time for your next dose, skip the missed dose and go back to your regular dosing schedule. Do not double doses.

Storage—Store the medicine in a closed container at room temperature, away from heat, moisture, and direct light. Keep from freezing.

Keep out of the reach of children.

Do not keep outdated medicine or medicine no longer needed.

Ask your healthcare professional how you should dispose of any medicine you do not use.

Precautions While Using This Medicine

While taking this medicine, it is important that you or your child maintain a diet with restricted amounts of tyrosine and phenylalanine A nutritionist may be able to help you with the special diet needed to treat you. A nutritionist that has special training with children may help with a diet for your child.

Call your doctor right away for any redness, swelling, or burning of your or your child's eyes, an unusual rash, bleeding, or if your or your child's skin is yellow.

It is very important that the doctor check you or your child at regular visits to see how the medicine is working and increase the dose if needed. The doctor may test your your child's blood often.

A special examination of your or your child's eyes should be done before this medicine is started.

Wearing sunglasses that block ultraviolet light is recommended. Nitisinone may cause sensitivity of the eyes to the sunlight.

Side Effects of This Medicine

Along with its needed effects, a medicine may cause some unwanted effects. Although not all of these side effects may occur, if they do occur they may need medical attention.

Check with your doctor immediately if any of the following side effects occur:
More common
Bloated abdomen; dark-colored urine; dull, achy upper abdominal pain; general feeling of tiredness or weakness; headache; light-colored stools; loss of appetite; unexplained weight loss; vomiting; yellow eyes or skin

Less common
Black, tarry stools
blindness; blood in urine or stools; blisters on skin; bloody nose; blurred vision; change in color vision; chest pain or discomfort; chills; cough; darkening of urine; decreased vision; difficulty seeing at night; dry or itching eyes; dry skin; excessive tearing from eyes; eye pain; fever; fluid-filled skin blisters; general feeling of discomfort or illness; increased sensitivity of eyes to sunlight; irritation or inflammation of the eye; itching of the skin; painful or difficult urination; pinpoint red spots on skin; rash with flat lesions or small raised lesions on the skin; red, thickened, or scaly skin; redness, pain, swelling of eye, eyelid, or inner lining of eyelid burning; sensitivity to the sun; shortness of breath; skin thinness; sore throat; sores, ulcers, or white spots on lips or in mouth; swollen and/or painful glands; unusual bleeding or bruising; unexplained nosebleed

Rare
Agitation; anxiety; back pain; bloody stools; bluish color of fingernails, lips, skin, palms, or nail beds; change in personality; change in vision; cold sweats; coma; confusion; cool, pale skin; cough producing mucus; decreased urination; diarrhea; difficulty breathing; dizziness; drowsiness; dry mouth; earache; fainting; fast heartbeat; feeling full in upper abdomen; increase in heart rate; increase in body movements; increased hunger; infection; irregular, fast or slow, or shallow breathing; irritability; lightheadedness; mood or mental changes; nausea; nervousness; pain or swelling in arms or legs without any injury; pale skin; problems with walking or talking; rapid breathing; redness or swelling in ear; seeing things that are not there; shakiness; skin rash found mostly on mucous membranes such as eyes and mouth; stiff neck; sunken eyes; thirst; tightness in chest; vomiting of blood or material that looks like coffee grounds; wheezing; wrinkled skin

Some side effects may occur that usually do not need medical attention. These side effects may go away during treatment as your body adjusts to the medicine. Also, your health care professional may be able to tell you about ways to prevent or reduce some of these side effects. Check with your health care professional if any of the following side effects continue or are bothersome or if you have any questions about them:
Less common or rare
Absent, missed, or irregular menstrual periods; burning feeling in chest or stomach; hair loss; indigestion;

sleepiness; stomach upset; stopping of menstrual bleeding; tenderness in stomach area; thinning of hair; tooth discoloration

Other side effects not listed may also occur in some patients. If you notice any other effects, check with your healthcare professional.

NITRATES—ORAL (Systemic)

Some commonly used brand names are:

In the U.S.—

Dilatrate-SR (1)	Nitrocot (3)
IMDUR (2)	Nitroglyn E-R (3)
ISDN (1)	Nitro-par (3)
ISMO (2)	Nitro-time (3)
Isordil Tembids (1)	Nitrong (3)
Isordil Titradose (1)	Sorbitrate (1)
Monoket (2)	

In Canada—

Apo-ISDN (1)	IMDUR (2)
Cedocard-SR (1)	ISMO (2)
Coradur (1)	Isordil Titradose (1)
Coronex (1)	Nitrong SR (3)

This information applies to the following medicines:

1. Isosorbide Dinitrate (eye-soe-SOR-bide dye-NYE-trate)
2. Isosorbide Mononitrate (eye-soe-SOR-bide mon-oh-NYE-trate)
3. Nitroglycerin (nye-troe-GLI-ser-in)

Category

- **Antianginal**—Isosorbide Dinitrate; Isosorbide Mononitrate; Nitroglycerin
- **Vasodilator, congestive heart failure**—Isosorbide Dinitrate; Nitroglycerin

Description

Nitrates (NYE-trates) are used to treat the symptoms of angina (chest pain). Depending on the type of dosage form and how it is taken, nitrates are used to treat angina in three ways:

- to relieve an attack that is occurring by using the medicine when the attack begins;
- to prevent attacks from occurring by using the medicine just before an attack is expected to occur; or
- to reduce the number of attacks that occur by using the medicine regularly on a long-term basis.

When taken orally and swallowed, nitrates are used to reduce the number of angina attacks that occur. They do not act fast enough to relieve the pain of an angina attack.

Nitrates work by relaxing blood vessels and increasing the supply of blood and oxygen to the heart while reducing its work load.

Nitrates may also be used for other conditions as determined by your doctor.

The nitrates discussed here are available only with your doctor's prescription, in the following dosage forms:

Oral

- Isosorbide dinitrate
  - Extended-release capsules
  - Tablets
  - Chewable tablets
  - Extended-release tablets
- Isosorbide mononitrate
  - Extended-release tablets
  - Tablets
- Nitroglycerin
  - Extended-release capsules
  - Extended-release tablets

Before Using This Medicine

In deciding to use a medicine, the risks of taking the medicine must be weighed against the good it will do. This is a decision you and your doctor will make. For nitrates, the following should be considered:

Allergies—Tell your doctor if you have ever had any unusual or allergic reaction to nitrates or nitrites. Also tell your health care professional if you are allergic to any other substances, such as certain foods, preservatives, or dyes.

Pregnancy—Nitrates have not been studied in pregnant women. However, studies in rabbits given large doses of isosorbide dinitrate have shown adverse effects on the fetus. Before taking these medicines, make sure your doctor knows if you are pregnant or if you may become pregnant.

Breast-feeding—It is not known whether these medicines pass into breast milk. Although most medicines pass into breast milk in small amounts, many of them may be used safely while breast-feeding. Mothers who are taking these medicines and who wish to breast-feed should discuss this with their doctor.

Children—Studies on these medicines have been done only in adult patients, and there is no specific information comparing use of nitrates in children with use in other age groups.

Older adults—Dizziness or lightheadedness may be more likely to occur in the elderly, who may be more sensitive to the effects of nitrates.

Other medicines—Although certain medicines should not be used together at all, in other cases two different medicines may be used together even if an interaction might occur. In these cases, your doctor may want to change the dose, or other precautions may be necessary. When you are taking nitrates, it is especially important that your health care professional know if you are taking any of the following:

- Antihypertensives (high blood pressure medicine) or
- Other heart medicine—May increase the effects of nitrates on blood pressure
- Sildenafil (e.g., Viagra) or
- Tadalafil (e.g., Cialis) or
- Vardenafil (e.g., Levitra)—These medicines which treat sexual impotence **should not** be used together with nitrates. You should tell your doctor right away if you are taking one of these drugs.

Other medical problems—The presence of other medical problems may affect the use of nitrates. Make sure you tell your doctor if you have any other medical problems, especially:

- Anemia (severe)
- Glaucoma—May be worsened by nitrates
- Head injury (recent) or

- Stroke (recent)—Nitrates may increase pressure in the brain, which can make problems worse
- Heart attack (recent)—Nitrates may lower blood pressure, which can aggravate problems associated with heart attack
- Kidney disease or
- Liver disease—Effects may be increased because of slower removal of nitroglycerin from the body
- Overactive thyroid

Proper Use of This Medicine

Take this medicine exactly as directed by your doctor. It will work only if taken correctly.

This form of nitrate is used to reduce the number of angina attacks. In most cases, it will not relieve an attack that has already started because it works too slowly (the extended-release form releases medicine gradually over a 6–hour period to provide its effect for 8 to 10 hours). Check with your doctor if you need a fast-acting medicine to relieve the pain of an angina attack.

Take this medicine with a full glass (8 ounces) of water on an empty stomach. If taken either 1 hour before or 2 hours after meals, it will start working sooner.

Extended-release capsules and tablets are not to be broken, crushed, or chewed before they are swallowed. If broken up, they will not release the medicine properly.

Dosing—The dose of nitrates will be different for different patients. *Follow your doctor's orders or the directions on the label.* The following information includes only the average doses of nitrates. *If your dose is different, do not change it* unless your doctor tells you to do so.

The number of capsules or tablets that you take depends on the strength of the medicine. Also, *the number of doses you take each day, the time allowed between doses, and the length of time you take the medicine depend on the medical problem for which you are taking nitrates.*

For isosorbide dinitrate
- For angina (chest pain):
  - For *regular (short-acting) oral* dosage forms (capsules or tablets):
    - Adults—5 to 40 mg four times a day.
    - Children—Dose must be determined by your doctor.
  - For *long-acting oral* dosage forms (extended-release capsules or tablets):
    - Adults—20 to 80 mg every eight to twelve hours.
    - Children—Dose must be determined by your doctor.

For isosorbide mononitrate
- For angina (chest pain):
  - For *regular (short-acting) oral* dosage form (tablets):
    - Adults—20 mg two times a day. The two doses should be taken seven hours apart.
    - Children—Use and dose must be determined by your doctor.
  - For *long-acting oral* dosage forms (extended-release tablets):
    - Adults—30 to 240 mg once a day.
    - Children—Use and dose must be determined by your doctor.

For nitroglycerin
- For angina (chest pain):
  - For *long-acting oral* dosage forms (capsules or tablets):
    - Adults—2.5 to 9 mg every eight to twelve hours.
    - Children—Dose must be determined by your doctor.

Missed dose—If you are taking this medicine regularly and you miss a dose, take it as soon as possible. However, if the next scheduled dose is within 2 hours (or within 6 hours for extended-release capsules or tablets), skip the missed dose and go back to your regular dosing schedule. Do not double doses.

Storage—To store this medicine:
- Keep out of the reach of children.
- Store away from heat and direct light.
- Do not store in the bathroom, near the kitchen sink, or in other damp places. Heat or moisture may cause the medicine to break down.
- Do not keep outdated medicine or medicine no longer needed. Be sure that any discarded medicine is out of the reach of children.

Precautions While Using This Medicine

Do not take sildenafil (e.g., Viagra), tadalafil (e.g., Cialis), or vardenafil (e.g., Levitra) if you are taking this medicine. When sildenafil, tadalafil, or vardenafil are taken with nitrates, the combination can lower blood pressure and cause dizziness, lightheadedness, or fainting. *In some cases, sildenafil, tadalafil, or vardenafil taken with nitrates has caused death.* If you are taking sildenafil, tadalafil, or vardenafil and you experience an angina attack, you must go to the hospital right away.

If you have been taking this medicine regularly for several weeks or more, do not suddenly stop using it. Stopping suddenly may bring on attacks of angina. Check with your doctor for the best way to reduce gradually the amount you are taking before stopping completely.

Dizziness, lightheadedness, or faintness may occur, especially when you get up quickly from a lying or sitting position. Getting up slowly may help. If you feel dizzy, sit or lie down.

The dizziness, lightheadedness, or fainting is also more likely to occur if you drink alcohol, stand for long periods of time, exercise, or if the weather is hot. *While you are taking this medicine, be careful to limit the amount of alcohol you drink. Also, use extra care during exercise or hot weather or if you must stand for long periods of time.*

After taking a dose of this medicine you may get a headache that lasts for a short time. This is a common side effect, which should become less noticeable after you have taken the medicine for a while. If this effect continues, or if the headaches are severe, check with your doctor.

For patients taking the *extended-release dosage forms of isosorbide dinitrate:*
- Partially dissolved tablets have been found in the stools of a few patients taking the extended-release tablets. Be alert to this possibility, especially if you have frequent bowel movements, diarrhea, or digestive problems. Notify your doctor if any such tablets are discovered. The

tablets must be properly digested to provide the correct dose of medicine.

Side Effects

Along with its needed effects, a medicine may cause some unwanted effects. Although not all of these side effects may occur, if they do occur they may need medical attention.

Check with your doctor as soon as possible if any of the following side effects occur:

Rare
   Blurred vision; dryness of mouth; headache (severe or prolonged); skin rash

Signs and symptoms of overdose (in the order in which they may occur)
   Bluish-colored lips, fingernails, or palms of hands; dizziness (extreme) or fainting; feeling of extreme pressure in head; shortness of breath; unusual tiredness or weakness; weak and fast heartbeat; fever; convulsions (seizures)

Other side effects may occur that usually do not need medical attention. These side effects may go away during treatment as your body adjusts to the medicine. However, check with your doctor if any of the following side effects continue or are bothersome:

More common
   Dizziness or lightheadedness, especially when getting up from a lying or sitting position; fast pulse; flushing of face and neck; headache; nausea or vomiting; restlessness

Other side effects not listed above may also occur in some patients. If you notice any other effects, check with your doctor.

NITRATES—SUBLINGUAL, CHEWABLE, BUCCAL (Systemic)

Some commonly used brand names are:

In the U.S.—
   Isordil (1)   Nitrostat (2)
   Nitrogard (2)   Sorbitrate (1)
In Canada—
   Apo-ISDN (1)   Isordil (1)
   Coronex (1)   Nitrostat (2)

This information applies to the following medicines:

1. Isosorbide Dinitrate (eye-soe-SOR-bide dye-NYE-trate)
2. Nitroglycerin (nye-troe-GLI-ser-in)

Category

- **Antianginal—**
- **Vasodilator, congestive heart failure—**

Description

Nitrates (NYE-trates) are used to treat the symptoms of angina (chest pain). Depending on the type of dosage form and how it is taken, nitrates are used to treat angina in three ways:

- to relieve an attack that is occurring by using the medicine when the attack begins;

- to prevent attacks from occurring by using the medicine just before an attack is expected to occur; or
- to reduce the number of attacks that occur by using the medicine regularly on a long-term basis.

Nitrates are available in different forms. Sublingual nitrates are generally placed under the tongue where they dissolve and are absorbed through the lining of the mouth. Some can also be used buccally, being placed under the lip or in the cheek. The chewable dosage forms, after being chewed and held in the mouth before swallowing, are absorbed in the same way. *It is important to remember that each dosage form is different and that the specific directions for each type must be followed if the medicine is to work properly.*

Nitrates that are used *to relieve the pain* of an angina attack include:

- sublingual nitroglycerin;
- buccal nitroglycerin;
- sublingual isosorbide dinitrate; and
- chewable isosorbide dinitrate.

Those that can be used *to prevent expected attacks* of angina include:

- sublingual nitroglycerin;
- buccal nitroglycerin;
- sublingual isosorbide dinitrate; and
- chewable isosorbide dinitrate.

Products that are used regularly on a long-term basis *to reduce the number of attacks* that occur include:

- buccal nitroglycerin;
- chewable isosorbide dinitrate; and
- sublingual isosorbide dinitrate.

Nitrates work by relaxing blood vessels and increasing the supply of blood and oxygen to the heart while reducing its work load.

Nitrates may also be used for other conditions as determined by your doctor.

The nitrates discussed here are available only with your doctor's prescription, in the following dosage forms:

Buccal
- Nitroglycerin
   - Extended-release tablets
Chewable
- Isosorbide dinitrate
   - Tablets
Sublingual
- Isosorbide dinitrate
   - Tablets
- Nitroglycerin
   - Tablets

Before Using This Medicine

In deciding to use a medicine, the risks of taking the medicine must be weighed against the good it will do. This is a decision you and your doctor will make. For nitrates, the following should be considered:

Allergies—Tell your doctor if you have ever had any unusual or allergic reaction to nitrates or nitrites. Also tell your health care professional if you are allergic to any other substances, such as certain foods, preservatives, or dyes.

Pregnancy—Nitrates have not been studied in pregnant women. However, studies in rabbits given large doses of isosorbide dinitrate have shown adverse effects on the fetus. Before taking these medicines, make sure your doctor knows if you are pregnant or if you may become pregnant.

Breast-feeding—It is not known whether these medicines pass into breast milk. Although most medicines pass into breast milk in small amounts, many of them may be used safely while breast-feeding. Mothers who are taking these medicines and who wish to breast-feed should discuss this with their doctor.

Children—Studies on these medicines have been done only in adult patients, and there is no specific information comparing use of nitrates in children with use in other age groups.

Older adults—Dizziness or lightheadedness may be more likely to occur in the elderly, who may be more sensitive to the effects of nitrates.

Other medicines—Although certain medicines should not be used together at all, in other cases two different medicines may be used together even if an interaction might occur. In these cases, your doctor may want to change the dose, or other precautions may be necessary. When you are taking nitrates, it is especially important that your health care professional know if you are taking any of the following:

- Antihypertensives (high blood pressure medicine) or
- Other heart medicine—May increase the effects of nitrates on blood pressure
- Sildenafil (e.g., Viagra) or
- Tadalafil (e.g., Cialis) or
- Vardenafil (e.g., Levitra)—These medicines which treat sexual impotence **should not** be used together with nitrates. You should tell your doctor right away if you are taking one of these drugs.

Other medical problems—The presence of other medical problems may affect the use of nitrates. Make sure you tell your doctor if you have any other medical problems, especially:

- Anemia (severe)
- Glaucoma—May be worsened by nitrates
- Head injury (recent) or
- Stroke (recent)—Nitrates may increase pressure in the brain, which can make problems worse
- Heart attack (recent)—Nitrates may lower blood pressure, which can aggravate problems associated with heart attack
- Kidney disease or
- Liver disease—Effects may be increased because of slower removal of nitroglycerin from the body
- Overactive thyroid

Proper Use of This Medicine

Take this medicine exactly as directed by your doctor. It will work only if taken correctly.

Sublingual tablets should not be chewed, crushed, or swallowed. They work much faster when absorbed through the lining of the mouth. Place the tablet under the tongue, between the lip and gum, or between the cheek and gum and let it dissolve there. Do not eat, drink, smoke, or use chewing tobacco while a tablet is dissolving.

Buccal extended-release tablets should not be chewed, crushed, or swallowed. They are designed to release a dose of nitroglycerin over a period of hours, not all at once.

- Allow the tablet to dissolve slowly in place between the upper lip and gum (above the front teeth), or between the cheek and upper gum. If food or drink is to be taken during the 3 to 5 hours when the tablet is dissolving, place the tablet between the *upper* lip and gum, above the front teeth. If you have dentures, you may place the tablet anywhere between the cheek and gum.
- Touching the tablet with your tongue or drinking hot liquids may cause the tablet to dissolve faster.
- Do not go to sleep while a tablet is dissolving because it could slip down your throat and cause choking.
- If you accidentally swallow the tablet, replace it with another one.
- Do not use chewing tobacco while a tablet is in place.

Chewable tablets must be chewed well and held in the mouth for about 2 minutes before you swallow them. This will allow the medicine to be absorbed through the lining of the mouth.

For patients using *nitroglycerin or isosorbide dinitrate to relieve the pain of an angina attack:*

- *When you begin to feel an attack of angina starting (chest pains or a tightness or squeezing in the chest), sit down. Then place a tablet in your mouth, either sublingually or buccally, or chew a chewable tablet.* This medicine works best when you are standing or sitting. However, since you may become dizzy, lightheaded, or faint soon after using a tablet, it is safer to sit rather than stand while the medicine is working. If you become dizzy or faint while sitting, take several deep breaths and bend forward with your head between your knees.
- Remain calm and you should feel better in a few minutes.
- *This medicine usually gives relief in 1 to 5 minutes.* However, if the pain is not relieved, and you are using:
  - Sublingual tablets, either sublingually or buccally: Use a second tablet. If the pain continues for another 5 minutes, a third tablet may be used. *If you still have the chest pains after a total of 3 tablets in a 15–minute period, contact your doctor or go to a hospital emergency room immediately.*
  - Buccal extended-release tablets: *Use a sublingual (under the tongue) nitroglycerin tablet and check with your doctor.* Do not use another buccal tablet since the effects of a buccal tablet last for several hours.

For patients using *nitroglycerin or isosorbide dinitrate to prevent an expected angina attack:*

- You may prevent anginal chest pains for up to 1 hour (6 hours for the extended-release nitroglycerin tablet) by using a buccal or sublingual tablet or chewing a chewable tablet 5 to 10 minutes before expected emotional stress or physical exertion that in the past seemed to bring on an attack.

For patients using *isosorbide dinitrate or extended-release buccal nitroglycerin regularly on a long-term basis to reduce the number of angina attacks that occur:*

- Chewable or sublingual isosorbide dinitrate and buccal extended-release nitroglycerin tablets can be used either to prevent angina attacks or to help relieve an attack that has already started.

Dosing—The dose of nitrates will be different for different patients. *Follow your doctor's orders or the directions on the label.* The following information includes only the average doses of nitrates. *If your dose is different, do not change it* unless your doctor tells you to do so.

For isosorbide dinitrate
- For angina (chest pain):
  - For *chewable* dosage form (tablets):
    - Adults—5 mg every two to three hours, chewed well and held in mouth for one or two minutes.
    - Children—Dose must be determined by your doctor.
  - For *sublingual* dosage form (tablets):
    - Adults—2.5 to 5 mg every two to three hours.
    - Children—Dose must be determined by your doctor.

For nitroglycerin
- For angina (chest pain):
  - For *buccal* dosage form (extended-release tablets):
    - Adults—1 mg every five hours while awake. Your doctor may increase your dose.
    - Children—Dose must be determined by your doctor.
  - For *sublingual* dosage form (tablets):
    - Adults—300 to 600 micrograms (mcg) (0.3 to 0.6 mg) every five minutes. If you still have chest pain after a total of three tablets in fifteen minutes, call your doctor or go to the emergency room right away.
    - Children—Dose must be determined by your doctor.

Missed dose—For patients using isosorbide dinitrate or extended-release buccal nitroglycerin regularly on a long-term basis to reduce the number of angina attacks that occur:

- If you miss a dose of this medicine, use it as soon as possible. However, if the next scheduled dose is within 2 hours, skip the missed dose and go back to your regular dosing schedule. Do not double doses.

Stability and proper storage—

For sublingual nitroglycerin
- Sublingual nitroglycerin tablets may lose some of their strength if they are exposed to air, heat, or moisture for long periods of time. However, if you screw the cap on tightly after each use and you properly store the bottle, the tablets should retain their strength until the expiration date on the bottle.
- Some people think they should test the strength of their sublingual nitroglycerin tablets by looking for a tingling or burning sensation, a feeling of warmth or flushing, or a headache after a tablet has been dissolved under the tongue. This kind of testing is not completely reliable since some patients may be unable to detect these effects. In addition, newer, stabilized sublingual nitroglycerin tablets are less likely to produce these detectable effects.
- To help keep the nitroglycerin tablets at full strength:
  - keep the medicine in the original glass, screw-cap bottle. For patients who wish to carry a small number of tablets with them for emergency use, a specially

designed container is available. However, only containers specifically labeled as suitable for use with nitroglycerin sublingual tablets should be used.
  - remove the cotton plug that comes in the bottle and *do not* put it back.
  - *put the cap on the bottle quickly and tightly after each use.*
  - to select a tablet for use, pour several into the bottle cap, take one, and pour the others back into the bottle. Try not to hold them in the palm of your hand because they may pick up moisture and crumble.
  - do not keep other medicines in the same bottle with the nitroglycerin since they will weaken the nitroglycerin effect.
  - keep the medicine handy at all times but try not to carry the bottle close to the body. Medicine may lose strength because of body warmth. Instead, carry the tightly closed bottle in your purse or the pocket of a jacket or other loose-fitting clothing whenever possible.
  - store the bottle of nitroglycerin tablets in a cool, dry place. Storage at average room temperature away from direct heat or direct sunlight is best. Do not store in the refrigerator or in a bathroom medicine cabinet because the moisture usually present in these areas may cause the tablets to crumble if the container is not tightly closed. Do not keep the tablets in your automobile glove compartment.
- Keep out of the reach of children.
- Do not keep outdated medicine or medicine no longer needed. Be sure that any discarded medicine is out of the reach of children.

For isosorbide dinitrate and buccal extended-release nitroglycerin
- These forms of nitrates are more stable than sublingual nitroglycerin.
- Keep out of the reach of children.
- Store away from heat and direct light.
- Do not store in the bathroom, near the kitchen sink, or in other damp places. Heat or moisture may cause the medicine to break down.
- Do not keep outdated medicine or medicine no longer needed. Be sure that any discarded medicine is out of the reach of children.

Precautions While Using This Medicine

Do not take sildenafil (e.g., Viagra), tadalafil (e.g., Cialis), or vardenafil (e.g., Levitra) if you are taking this medicine. When sildenafil, tadalafil, or vardenafil are taken with nitrates, the combination can lower blood pressure and cause dizziness, lightheadedness, or fainting. *In some cases, sildenafil, tadalafil, or vardenafil taken with nitrates has caused death.*

If you have been taking this medicine regularly for several weeks, do not suddenly stop using it. If you are taking sildenafil, tadalafil, or vardenafil and you experience an angina attack, you must go to the hospital right away. Stopping suddenly may bring on attacks of angina. Check with your doctor for the best way to reduce gradually the amount you are taking before stopping completely.

Dizziness, lightheadedness, or faintness may occur, especially when you get up quickly from a lying or sitting position. Getting up slowly may help. If you feel dizzy, sit or lie down.

The dizziness, lightheadedness, or fainting is also more likely to occur if you drink alcohol, stand for long periods of time, exercise, or if the weather is hot. *While you are taking this medicine, be careful to limit the amount of alcohol you drink. Also, use extra care during exercise or hot weather or if you must stand for long periods of time.*

After taking a dose of this medicine you may get a headache that lasts for a short time. This is a common side effect, which should become less noticeable after you have taken the medicine for a while. If this effect continues or if the headaches are severe, check with your doctor.

Side Effects

Along with its needed effects, a medicine may cause some unwanted effects. Although not all of these side effects may occur, if they do occur they may need medical attention.

Check with your doctor as soon as possible if any of the following side effects occur:

Rare
Blurred vision; dryness of mouth; headache (severe or prolonged); skin rash

Signs and symptoms of overdose (in the order in which they may occur)
Bluish-colored lips, fingernails, or palms of hands; dizziness (extreme) or fainting; feeling of extreme pressure in head; shortness of breath; unusual tiredness or weakness; weak and fast heartbeat; fever; convulsions (seizures)

Other side effects may occur that usually do not need medical attention. These side effects may go away during treatment as your body adjusts to the medicine. However, check with your doctor if any of the following side effects continue or are bothersome:

More common
Dizziness or lightheadedness, especially when getting up from a lying or sitting position; fast pulse; flushing of face and neck; headache; nausea or vomiting; restlessness

Other side effects not listed above may also occur in some patients. If you notice any other effects, check with your doctor.

NITRATES—TOPICAL (Systemic)

Some commonly used brand names are:

In the U.S.—

Deponit (2)	Nitro-Dur (2)
Minitran (2)	Nitrol (1)
Nitro-Bid (1)	Transderm-Nitro (2)
Nitrodisc (2)	

In Canada—

Minitran (2)	Nitrol (1)
Nitro-Dur (2)	Transderm-Nitro (2)

This information applies to the following medicines:

1. Nitroglycerin Ointment
2. Nitroglycerin Transdermal Patches

Category

- **Antianginal—**
- **Vasodilator, congestive heart failure—**

Description

Nitrates (NYE-trates) are used to treat the symptoms of angina (chest pain). Depending on the type of dosage form and how it is taken, nitrates are used to treat angina in three ways:

- to relieve an attack that is occurring by using the medicine when the attack begins;
- to prevent attacks from occurring by using the medicine just before an attack is expected to occur; or
- to reduce the number of attacks that occur by using the medicine regularly on a long-term basis.

When applied to the skin, nitrates are used to reduce the number of angina attacks that occur. The only nitrate available for this purpose is topical nitroglycerin nye-troe-GLI-ser-in.

Topical nitroglycerin is absorbed through the skin. It works by relaxing blood vessels and increasing the supply of blood and oxygen to the heart while reducing its work load. This helps prevent future angina attacks from occurring.

Topical nitroglycerin may also be used for other conditions as determined by your doctor.

Nitroglycerin as discussed here is available only with your doctor's prescription, in the following dosage forms:

Topical
- Ointment
- Transdermal (stick-on) patch

Before Using This Medicine

In deciding to use a medicine, the risks of taking the medicine must be weighed against the good it will do. This is a decision you and your doctor will make. For nitroglycerin applied to the skin, the following should be considered:

Allergies—Tell your doctor if you have ever had any unusual or allergic reaction to nitrates or nitrites. Also tell your health care professional if you are allergic to any other substances, such as certain foods, preservatives, or dyes.

Pregnancy—Nitrates have not been studied in pregnant women. Before taking these medicines, make sure your doctor knows if you are pregnant or if you may become pregnant.

Breast-feeding—It is not known whether this medicine passes into breast milk. Although most medicines pass into breast milk in small amounts, many of them may be used safely while breast-feeding. Mothers who are taking these medicines and who wish to breast-feed should discuss this with their doctor.

Children—Studies on these medicines have been done only in adult patients, and there is no specific information comparing use of nitrates in children with use in other age groups.

Older adults—Dizziness or lightheadedness may be more likely to occur in the elderly, who may be more sensitive to the effects of nitrates.

Other medicines—Although certain medicines should not be used together at all, in other cases two different medicines may be used together even if an interaction might occur. In these cases, your doctor may want to change the dose, or other precautions may be necessary. When you are using nitroglycerin, it is especially important that your health care professional know if you are taking any of the following:

- Antihypertensives (high blood pressure medicine) or

- Other heart medicine—May increase the effects of nitroglycerin on blood pressure

- Sildenafil (e.g., Viagra) or

- Tadalafil (e.g., Cialis) or

- Vardenafil (e.g., Levitra)—These medicines which treat sexual impotence **should not** be used together with nitrates. You should tell your doctor right away if you are taking one of these drugs.

Other medical problems—The presence of other medical problems may affect the use of nitroglycerin. Make sure you tell your doctor if you have any other medical problems, especially:

- Anemia (severe)

- Glaucoma—May be worsened by nitroglycerin

- Head injury (recent) or

- Stroke (recent)—Nitroglycerin may increase pressure in the brain, which can make problems worse

- Heart attack (recent)—Nitroglycerin may lower blood pressure, which can aggravate problems associated with heart attack

- Kidney disease or

- Liver disease—Effects may be increased because of slower removal of nitroglycerin from the body

- Overactive thyroid

Proper Use of This Medicine

Use nitroglycerin exactly as directed by your doctor. It will work only if applied correctly.

The ointment and transdermal forms of nitroglycerin are used to reduce the number of angina attacks. They will not relieve an attack that has already started because they work too slowly. Check with your doctor if you need a fast-acting medicine to relieve the pain of an angina attack.

This medicine usually comes with patient instructions. Read them carefully before using this medicine.

For patients using the *ointment* form of this medicine:

- Before applying a new dose of ointment, remove any ointment remaining on the skin from a previous dose. This will allow the fresh ointment to release the nitroglycerin properly.

- This medicine comes with dose-measuring papers. Use them to measure the length of ointment squeezed from the tube and to apply the ointment to the skin. *Do not rub or massage the ointment into the skin; just spread in a thin, even layer, covering an area of the same size each time it is applied.*

- Apply the ointment to skin that has little or no hair.

- Apply each dose of ointment to a different area of skin to prevent irritation or other skin problems.

- If your doctor has ordered an occlusive dressing (airtight covering, such as kitchen plastic wrap) to be applied over this medicine, make sure you know how to apply it. Since occlusive dressings increase the amount of med-

icine absorbed through the skin and the possibility of side effects, use them only as directed. If you have any questions about this, check with your health care professional.

For patients using the *transdermal (stick-on patch) system:*

- Do not try to trim or cut the adhesive patch to adjust the dosage. Check with your doctor if you think the medicine is not working as it should.

- Apply the patch to a clean, dry skin area with little or no hair and free of scars, cuts, or irritation. Remove the previous patch before applying a new one.

- Apply a new patch if the first one becomes loose or falls off.

- Apply each dose to a different area of skin to prevent skin irritation or other problems.

Dosing—The dose of nitroglycerin will be different for different patients. *Follow your doctor's orders or the directions on the label.* The following information includes only the average doses of nitrates. *If your dose is different, do not change it* unless your doctor tells you to do so.

For nitroglycerin
- For angina (chest pain):
  - For *ointment* dosage form:
    - Adults—15 to 30 milligrams (mg) (about one to two inches of ointment squeezed from tube) every six to eight hours.
    - Children—Use and dose must be determined by your doctor.
  - For *transdermal system (skin patch)* dosage form:
    - Adults—Apply one transdermal dosage system (skin patch) to intact skin once a day. The patch is usually left on for 12 to 14 hours a day and then taken off. Follow your doctor's instructions for when to put on and take off the skin patch.
    - Children—Use and dose must be determined by your doctor.

Missed dose—

- For patients using the *ointment* form of this medicine: If you miss a dose of this medicine, apply it as soon as possible unless the next scheduled dose is within 2 hours. Then go back to your regular dosing schedule. Do not increase the amount used.

- For patients using the *transdermal (stick-on patch) system:* If you miss a dose of this medicine, apply it as soon as possible. Then go back to your regular dosing schedule.

Storage—

- To store the *ointment* form of this medicine:
  - Keep out of the reach of children.
  - Store the tube of nitroglycerin ointment in a cool place and keep it tightly closed.
  - Do not keep outdated medicine or medicine no longer needed. Be sure that any discarded medicine is out of the reach of children.

- To store the *transdermal (stick-on patch) system:*
  - Keep out of the reach of children.
  - Store away from heat and direct light.
  - Do not store in the bathroom, near the kitchen sink, or in other damp places. Heat or moisture may cause the medicine to break down.

○ Do not keep outdated medicine or medicine no longer needed. Be sure that any discarded medicine is out of the reach of children.

Precautions While Using This Medicine

Do not take sildenafil (e.g., Viagra), tadalafil (e.g., Cialis), or vardenafil (e.g., Levitra) if you are taking this medicine. When sildenafil, tadalafil, or vardenafil are taken with nitrates, the combination can lower blood pressure and cause dizziness, lightheadedness, or fainting. *In some cases, sildenafil, tadalafil, or vardenafil taken with nitrates has caused death.* If you are taking sildenafil, tadalafil, or vardenafil and you experience an angina attack, you must go to the hospital right away.

If you have been using nitroglycerin regularly for several weeks or more, do not suddenly stop using it. Stopping suddenly may bring on attacks of angina. Check with your doctor for the best way to reduce gradually the amount you are using before stopping completely.

Dizziness, lightheadedness, or faintness may occur, especially when you get up quickly from a lying or sitting position. Getting up slowly may help. If you feel dizzy, sit or lie down.

The dizziness, lightheadedness, or fainting is also more likely to occur if you drink alcohol, stand for long periods of time, exercise, or if the weather is hot. *While you are taking this medicine, be careful to limit the amount of alcohol you drink. Also, use extra care during exercise or hot weather or if you must stand for long periods of time.*

After using a dose of this medicine you may get a headache that lasts for a short time. This is a common side effect, which should become less noticeable after you have used the medicine for a while. If this effect continues, or if the headaches are severe, check with your doctor.

Side Effects

Along with its needed effects, a medicine may cause some unwanted effects. Although not all of these side effects may occur, if they do occur they may need medical attention.

Check with your doctor as soon as possible if any of the following side effects occur:
Rare
Blurred vision; dryness of mouth; headache (severe or prolonged)

Signs and symptoms of overdose (in the order in which they may occur)
Bluish-colored lips, fingernails, or palms of hands; dizziness (extreme) or fainting; feeling of extreme pressure in head; shortness of breath; unusual tiredness or weakness; weak and fast heartbeat; fever; convulsions (seizures)

Other side effects may occur that usually do not need medical attention. These side effects may go away during treatment as your body adjusts to the medicine. However, check with your doctor if any of the following side effects continue or are bothersome:
More common
Dizziness or lightheadedness, especially when getting up from a lying or sitting position; fast pulse; flushing of face and neck; headache; nausea or vomiting; restlessness

Less common
Sore, reddened skin

Other side effects not listed above may also occur in some patients. If you notice any other effects, check with your doctor.

Additional Information

Once a medicine has been approved for marketing for a certain use, experience may show that it is also useful for other medical problems. Although this use is not included in the product labeling, topical nitroglycerin is used in certain patients with the following medical conditions:

• Chronic anal fissures

Other than the above information, there is no additional information relating to proper use, precautions, or side effects for this use.

NITROFURANTOIN   (Oral route) - nye-troe-fyoor-AN-toyn

Commonly used brand name(s)

In the U.S.—
Furadantin
Macrodantin

In Canada—
Novo-Furan Suspension

Available Dosage Forms:
• Tablet
• Suspension
• Capsule

Therapeutic Class: Antibiotic

Uses For This Medicine

Nitrofurantoin belongs to the family of medicines called anti-infectives. It is used to treat infections of the urinary tract. It may also be used for other conditions as determined by your doctor.

Nitrofurantoin is available only with your doctor's prescription.

Before Using This Medicine

In deciding to use a medicine, the risks of taking the medicine must be weighed against the good it will do. This is a decision you and your doctor will make. For this medicine, the following should be considered:

Allergies—Tell your doctor if you have ever had any unusual or allergic reaction to this medicine or any other medicines. Also tell your health care professional if you have any other types of allergies, such as to foods, dyes, preservatives, or animals. For non-prescription products, read the label or package ingredients carefully.

Pediatric—This medicine has been tested in children 1 month of age and older and, in effective doses, has not been shown to cause different side effects or problems in children than it does in adults. However, infants up to 1 month of age should not be given this medicine because they are especially sensitive to the effects of nitrofurantoin.

Geriatric—Elderly people may be more sensitive to the effects of nitrofurantoin. This may increase the chance of side effects during treatment.

Pregnancy—

	Pregnancy Category	Explanation
All Trimesters	B	Animal studies have revealed no evidence of harm to the fetus, however, there are no adequate studies in pregnant women OR animal studies have shown an adverse effect, but adequate studies in pregnant women have failed to demonstrate a risk to the fetus.

Breast Feeding—There are no adequate studies in women for determining infant risk when using this medication during breastfeeding. Weigh the potential benefits against the potential risks before taking this medication while breastfeeding.

Other medicines—

Using this medicine with any of the following medicines is usually not recommended, but may be required in some cases. If both medicines are prescribed together, your doctor may change the dose or how often you use one or both of the medicines.

Fluconazole

Interactions with Food/Tobacco/Alcohol—Certain medicines should not be used at or around the time of eating food or eating certain types of food since interactions may occur. Using alcohol or tobacco with certain medicines may also cause interactions to occur. Discuss with your healthcare professional the use of your medicine with food, alcohol, or tobacco.

Other medical problems—The presence of other medical problems may affect the use of this medicine. Make sure you tell your doctor if you have any other medical problems, especially:

- Anemia or
- Diabetes mellitus or
- Lung disease or
- Nerve damage or
- Other serious illness or
- Vitamin B deficiency—These conditions may increase the chance for side effects
- Glucose-6–phosphate dehydrogenase (G6PD) deficiency—Nitrofurantoin may cause anemia in patients with G6PD deficiency
- Kidney disease (other than infection)—The chance of side effects of this medicine may be increased and the medicine may be less effective in patients with kidney disease

Proper Use of This Medicine

Do not give this medicine to infants up to 1 month of age.

Nitrofurantoin is best taken with food or milk. This may lessen stomach upset and help your body to better absorb the medicine.

For patients taking the oral liquid form of this medicine:

- Shake the oral liquid forcefully before each dose to help make it pour more smoothly and to be sure the medicine is evenly mixed.
- Use a specially marked measuring spoon or other device to measure each dose accurately. The average household teaspoon may not hold the right amount of liquid.
- Nitrofurantoin may be mixed with water, milk, fruit juices, or infants' formulas. If it is mixed with any of these liquids, take the medicine immediately after mixing. Be sure to drink all the liquid in order to get the full dose of medicine.

For patients taking the extended-release capsule form of this medicine:

- Swallow the capsules whole.
- Do not open, crush, or chew the capsules before swallowing them.

To help clear up your infection completely, keep taking this medicine for the full time of treatment, even if you begin to feel better after a few days. Do not miss any doses.

Dosing—The dose of this medicine will be different for different patients. Follow your doctor's orders or the directions on the label. The following information includes only the average doses of this medicine. If your dose is different, do not change it unless your doctor tells you to do so.

The amount of medicine that you take depends on the strength of the medicine. Also, the number of doses you take each day, the time allowed between doses, and the length of time you take the medicine depend on the medical problem for which you are using the medicine.

- For the capsule, oral suspension, and tablet dosage forms:
  - For the prevention of urinary tract infection:
    - Adults and adolescents—50 to 100 mg once a day at bedtime.
    - Children 1 month of age and older—Dose is based on body weight and must be determined by your doctor.
    - Children up to 1 month of age—Use is not recommended.
  - For the treatment of urinary tract infection:
    - Adults and adolescents—50 to 100 mg every six hours.
    - Children 1 month of age and older—Dose is based on body weight and must be determined by your doctor.
    - Children up to 1 month of age—Use is not recommended.
- For the extended-release capsule dosage form:
  - Adults and children 12 years of age and older: 100 mg every twelve hours for seven days.
  - Children up to 12 years of age: Dose must be determined by the doctor.

Missed dose—If you miss a dose of this medicine, take it as soon as possible. However, if it is almost time for your next dose, skip the missed dose and go back to your regular dosing schedule. Do not double doses.

Storage—Store the medicine in a closed container at room temperature, away from heat, moisture, and direct light. Keep from freezing.

Keep out of the reach of children.

Do not keep outdated medicine or medicine no longer needed.

Precautions While Using This Medicine

It is important that your doctor check your progress at regular visits if you will be taking this medicine for a long time.

If your symptoms do not improve within a few days, or if they become worse, check with your doctor.

For diabetic patients:
- This medicine may cause false test results with some urine sugar tests. Check with your doctor before changing your diet or the dosage of your diabetes medicine.

Side Effects of This Medicine

Along with its needed effects, a medicine may cause some unwanted effects. Although not all of these side effects may occur, if they do occur they may need medical attention.

Check with your doctor immediately if any of the following side effects occur:

More common
Changes in facial skin color; chest pain; chills; cough; fever; general feeling of discomfort or illness; hives; hoarseness; itching; joint or muscle pain; shortness of breath; skin rash; sudden trouble in swallowing or breathing; swelling of face, mouth, hands, or feet; troubled breathing

Less common
Black, tarry stools; blood in urine or stools; burning, numbness, tingling, or painful sensations; dizziness; drowsiness; headache; pinpoint red spots on skin; sore throat; unusual bleeding or bruising; unusual tiredness or weakness; weakness in arms, hands, legs, or feet

Rare
Abdominal or stomach pain; blistering, peeling, or loosening of skin and mucous membranes; bluish color of skin; blurred vision or loss of vision, with or without eye pain; bulging fontanel in infants; confusion; darkening of urine; diarrhea, watery and severe, which may also be bloody; loss of appetite; mental depression; mood or mental changes; nausea or vomiting; pale skin; pale stools; red skin lesions, often with a purple center; red, thickened, or scaly skin; skin rash; sores, ulcers, or white spots on lips or in mouth; swollen or painful glands; unpleasant breath odor; visual changes; vomiting of blood; wheezing or tightness in chest; yellow eyes or skin

Some side effects may occur that usually do not need medical attention. These side effects may go away during treatment as your body adjusts to the medicine. Also, your health care professional may be able to tell you about ways to prevent or reduce some of these side effects. Check with your health care professional if any of the following side effects continue or are bothersome or if you have any questions about them:

More common
Diarrhea; gas

After you stop using this medicine, it may still produce some side effects that need attention. During this period of time, *check with your doctor immediately* if you notice the following side effects:
Abdominal or stomach cramps or pain, severe; diarrhea, watery and severe, which may also be bloody; fever

This medicine may cause the urine to become rust-yellow to brown. This side effect does not require medical attention.

Nitrofurantoin may cause a temporary loss of hair in some people.

Other side effects not listed may also occur in some patients. If you notice any other effects, check with your healthcare professional.

NORFLOXACIN (Ophthalmic route) -
nor-FLOX-a-sin

Commonly used brand name(s)

In Canada—
Noroxin

Available Dosage Forms:
- Solution

Therapeutic Class: Antibiotic

Uses For This Medicine

Norfloxacin is an antibiotic. The ophthalmic preparation is used to treat infections of the eye.

Norfloxacin is available only with your doctor's prescription.

Before Using This Medicine

In deciding to use a medicine, the risks of taking the medicine must be weighed against the good it will do. This is a decision you and your doctor will make. For this medicine, the following should be considered:

Allergies—Tell your doctor if you have ever had any unusual or allergic reaction to this medicine or any other medicines. Also tell your health care professional if you have any other types of allergies, such as to foods, dyes, preservatives, or animals. For non-prescription products, read the label or package ingredients carefully.

Pediatric—Use is not recommended in infants and children up to 1 year of age. Norfloxacin taken by mouth has been shown to cause bone problems in young animals. It is not known whether ophthalmic norfloxacin can cause bone problems in infants. In children 1 year of age and older, this medicine is not expected to cause different side effects or problems than it does in adults.

Geriatric—Many medicines have not been studied specifically in older people. Therefore, it may not be known whether they work exactly the same way they do in younger adults. Although there is no specific information comparing use of ophthalmic norfloxacin in the elderly with use in other age groups, this medicine is not expected to cause different side effects or problems in older people than it does in younger adults.

Other medicines—Although certain medicines should not be used together at all, in other cases two different medicines may be used together even if an interaction might occur. In these cases, your doctor may want to change the dose, or other precautions may be necessary. Tell your healthcare professional if you are taking any other prescription or non-prescription (over-the-counter [OTC]) medicine.

Interactions with Food/Tobacco/Alcohol—Certain medicines should not be used at or around the time of eating food or eating certain types of food since interactions may occur. Using alcohol or tobacco with certain medicines may also cause interactions to occur. Discuss with your healthcare professional the use of your medicine with food, alcohol, or tobacco.

Proper Use of This Medicine

To use:

- First, wash your hands. Tilt the head back and with the index finger of one hand, press gently on the skin just beneath the lower eyelid and pull the lower eyelid away from the eye to make a space. Drop the medicine into this space. Let go of the eyelid and gently close the eyes. Do not blink. Keep the eyes closed for 1 or 2 minutes, to allow the medicine to come into contact with the infection.

- If you think you did not get the drop of medicine into your eye properly, use another drop.

- To keep the medicine as germ-free as possible, do not touch the applicator tip to any surface (including the eye). Also, keep the container tightly closed.

Dosing—The dose of this medicine will be different for different patients. Follow your doctor's orders or the directions on the label. The following information includes only the average doses of this medicine. If your dose is different, do not change it unless your doctor tells you to do so.

The amount of medicine that you take depends on the strength of the medicine. Also, the number of doses you take each day, the time allowed between doses, and the length of time you take the medicine depend on the medical problem for which you are using the medicine.

- For infants and children up to 1 year of age: Use is not recommended.

- For adults and children 1 year of age and over: Place 1 drop in each eye four times a day for 7 days.

To help clear up your infection completely, keep using this medicine for the full time of treatment, even if your symptoms begin to clear up after a few days. If you stop using this medicine too soon, your symptoms may return. Do not miss any doses.

Missed dose—If you miss a dose of this medicine, apply it as soon as possible. However, if it is almost time for your next dose, skip the missed dose and go back to your regular dosing schedule.

Storage—Store the medicine in a closed container at room temperature, away from heat, moisture, and direct light. Keep from freezing.

Keep out of the reach of children.

Do not keep outdated medicine or medicine no longer needed.

Precautions While Using This Medicine

If your symptoms do not improve within a few days, or if they become worse, check with your doctor.

This medicine may cause your eyes to become more sensitive to light than they are normally. Wearing sunglasses and avoiding too much exposure to bright light may help lessen the discomfort.

Side Effects of This Medicine

Along with its needed effects, a medicine may cause some unwanted effects. Although not all of these side effects may occur, if they do occur they may need medical attention.

Check with your doctor immediately if any of the following side effects occur:
  Rare
    Skin rash or other sign of allergic reaction

Some side effects may occur that usually do not need medical attention. These side effects may go away during treatment as your body adjusts to the medicine. Also, your health care professional may be able to tell you about ways to prevent or reduce some of these side effects. Check with your health care professional if any of the following side effects continue or are bothersome or if you have any questions about them:
  More common
    Burning or other eye discomfort
  Less common
    Bitter taste following use in the eye; increased sensitivity of eye to light; redness of the lining of the eyelids; swelling of the membrane covering the white part of the eye

Other side effects not listed may also occur in some patients. If you notice any other effects, check with your healthcare professional.

NYSTATIN (Oral route) - nye-STA-tin

Commonly used brand name(s)

In the U.S.—
    Bio-Statin

In Canada—

Mycostatin Suspension	Nilstat Powder
Nadostine	Nyaderm
Nadostine Sucrose-Free	Pms-Nystatin
Nilstat Drops	

Available Dosage Forms:

- Suspension
- Tablet
- Capsule

Therapeutic Class: Antifungal

Uses For This Medicine

Nystatin belongs to the group of medicines called antifungals. The dry powder, lozenge (pastille), and liquid forms of this medicine are used to treat fungus infections in the mouth.

Nystatin is available only with your doctor's prescription.

Once a medicine has been approved for marketing for a certain use, experience may show that it is also useful for other medical problems. Although this use is not included in product labeling, nystatin is used in certain patients with the following medical condition:

- Candidiasis, oral (fungus infection of the mouth) (prevention)

Before Using This Medicine

In deciding to use a medicine, the risks of taking the medicine must be weighed against the good it will do. This is a decision you and your doctor will make. For this medicine, the following should be considered:

Allergies—Tell your doctor if you have ever had any unusual or allergic reaction to this medicine or any other medicines. Also tell your health care professional if you have any other types of allergies, such as to foods, dyes, preservatives, or animals. For non-prescription products, read the label or package ingredients carefully.

Pediatric—This medicine has been tested in children and has not been reported to cause different side effects or problems in children than it does in adults. However, since children up to 5 years of age may be too young to use the lozenges (pastilles) or tablets safely, the oral suspension dosage form is best for this age group.

Geriatric—Many medicines have not been studied specifically in older people. Therefore, it may not be known whether they work exactly the same way they do in younger adults or if they cause different side effects or problems in older people. There is no specific information comparing use of oral nystatin in the elderly with use in other age groups.

Other medicines—Although certain medicines should not be used together at all, in other cases two different medicines may be used together even if an interaction might occur. In these cases, your doctor may want to change the dose, or other precautions may be necessary. Tell your healthcare professional if you are taking any other prescription or non-prescription (over-the-counter [OTC]) medicine.

Interactions with Food/Tobacco/Alcohol—Certain medicines should not be used at or around the time of eating food or eating certain types of food since interactions may occur. Using alcohol or tobacco with certain medicines may also cause interactions to occur. Discuss with your healthcare professional the use of your medicine with food, alcohol, or tobacco.

Proper Use of This Medicine

For patients taking the dry powder form of nystatin:

- Add about ⅛ teaspoonful of dry powder to about 4 ounces of water immediately before taking. Stir well.
- After it is mixed, take this medicine by dividing the whole amount (4 ounces) into several portions. Hold each portion of the medicine in your mouth or swish it around in your mouth for as long as possible, gargle, and swallow. Be sure to use all the liquid to get the full dose of medicine.

For patients taking the lozenge (pastille) form of nystatin:

- Nystatin lozenges (pastilles) should be held in the mouth and allowed to dissolve slowly and completely. This may take 15 to 30 minutes. Also, the saliva should be swallowed during this time. Do not chew or swallow the lozenges whole.
- Do not give nystatin lozenges (pastilles) to infants or children up to 5 years of age. They may be too young to use the lozenges safely.

For patients taking the oral liquid form of nystatin:

- This medicine is to be taken by mouth even if it comes in a dropper bottle. If it does come in a dropper bottle, use the specially marked dropper to measure each dose accurately.

- Take this medicine by placing one-half of the dose in each side of your mouth. Hold the medicine in your mouth or swish it around in your mouth for as long as possible, then gargle and swallow.

Patients with full or partial dentures may need to soak their dentures nightly in nystatin for oral suspension to eliminate the fungus from the dentures. In rare cases when this does not eliminate the fungus, it may be necessary to have new dentures made.

To help clear up your infection completely, keep taking this medicine for the full time of treatment, even if your condition has improved. Do not miss any doses.

Dosing—The dose of this medicine will be different for different patients. Follow your doctor's orders or the directions on the label. The following information includes only the average doses of this medicine. If your dose is different, do not change it unless your doctor tells you to do so.

The amount of medicine that you take depends on the strength of the medicine. Also, the number of doses you take each day, the time allowed between doses, and the length of time you take the medicine depend on the medical problem for which you are using the medicine.

- For the lozenge (pastille) and tablet dosage forms:
  - Adults and children 5 years of age and older: 1 or 2 lozenges or tablets three to five times a day for up to fourteen days.
  - Children up to 5 years of age: Children this young may not be able to use the lozenges or tablets safely. The oral suspension is better for this age group.
- For the suspension dosage form:
  - Adults and children 5 years of age and older: 4 to 6 milliliters (mL) (about 1 teaspoonful) four times a day.
  - For older infants: 2 mL four times a day.
  - For premature and low-birth-weight infants: 1 mL four times a day.

Missed dose—If you miss a dose of this medicine, take it as soon as possible. However, if it is almost time for your next dose, skip the missed dose and go back to your regular dosing schedule. Do not double doses.

Storage—Store the medicine in a closed container at room temperature, away from heat, moisture, and direct light. Keep from freezing.

Keep out of the reach of children.

Do not keep outdated medicine or medicine no longer needed.

Store the lozenge (pastille) form in the refrigerator.

Side Effects of This Medicine

Along with its needed effects, a medicine may cause some unwanted effects. Although not all of these side effects may occur, if they do occur they may need medical attention.

Some side effects may occur that usually do not need medical attention. These side effects may go away during treatment as your body adjusts to the medicine. Also, your health care professional may be able to tell you about ways to prevent or reduce some of these side effects. Check with your health care professional if any of the following side effects continue or are bothersome or if you have any questions about them:

Less common

Diarrhea; nausea or vomiting; stomach pain

Other side effects not listed may also occur in some patients. If you notice any other effects, check with your healthcare professional.

NYSTATIN (Topical route) - nye-STA-tin

Commonly used brand name(s)

In the U.S.—
Mycostatin
Nystop

Pedi-Dri

In Canada—
Mycostatin Cream
Mycostatin Ointment
Mycostatin Powder
Nadostine

Nilstat Topical Cream
Nilstat Topical Ointment
Nyaderm Cream
Nyaderm Ointment

Available Dosage Forms:
- Powder
- Ointment
- Cream

Therapeutic Class: Antifungal

Uses For This Medicine

Nystatin belongs to the group of medicines called antifungals. Topical nystatin is used to treat some types of fungus infections of the skin.

Nystatin is available in the U.S. only with your doctor's prescription.

Before Using This Medicine

In deciding to use a medicine, the risks of taking the medicine must be weighed against the good it will do. This is a decision you and your doctor will make. For this medicine, the following should be considered:

Allergies—Tell your doctor if you have ever had any unusual or allergic reaction to this medicine or any other medicines. Also tell your health care professional if you have any other types of allergies, such as to foods, dyes, preservatives, or animals. For non-prescription products, read the label or package ingredients carefully.

Pediatric—Although there is no specific information comparing use of topical nystatin in children with use in other age groups, this medicine is not expected to cause different side effects or problems in children than it does in adults.

Geriatric—Many medicines have not been studied specifically in older people. Therefore, it may not be known whether they work exactly the same way they do in younger adults or if they cause different side effects or problems in older people. There is no specific information comparing use of topical nystatin in the elderly with use in other age groups.

Other medicines—Although certain medicines should not be used together at all, in other cases two different medicines may be used together even if an interaction might occur. In these cases, your doctor may want to change the dose, or other precautions may be necessary. Tell your healthcare professional if you are taking any other prescription or non-prescription (over-the-counter [OTC]) medicine.

Interactions with Food/Tobacco/Alcohol—Certain medicines should not be used at or around the time of eating food or eating certain types of food since interactions may occur. Using alcohol or tobacco with certain medicines may also cause interactions to occur. Discuss with your healthcare professional the use of your medicine with food, alcohol, or tobacco.

Proper Use of This Medicine

Topical nystatin should not be used in the eyes.

Apply enough nystatin to cover the affected area.

For patients using the powder form of this medicine on the feet:

- Sprinkle the powder between the toes, on the feet, and in socks and shoes.

The use of any kind of occlusive dressing (airtight covering, such as kitchen plastic wrap) over this medicine may increase the chance of irritation. Therefore, do not bandage, wrap, or apply any occlusive dressing over this medicine unless directed to do so by your doctor. When using this medicine on the diaper area of children, avoid tight-fitting diapers and plastic pants.

To help clear up your infection completely, keep using this medicine for the full time of treatment, even if your condition has improved. Do not miss any doses.

Dosing—The dose of this medicine will be different for different patients. Follow your doctor's orders or the directions on the label. The following information includes only the average doses of this medicine. If your dose is different, do not change it unless your doctor tells you to do so.

The amount of medicine that you take depends on the strength of the medicine. Also, the number of doses you take each day, the time allowed between doses, and the length of time you take the medicine depend on the medical problem for which you are using the medicine.

- For topical dosage forms (cream or ointment):
  - For fungus infections:
    - Adults and children—Apply to the affected area(s) of the skin two times a day.
- For topical dosage form (powder):
  - For fungus infections:
    - Adults and children—Apply to the affected area(s) of the skin two or three times a day.

Missed dose—If you miss a dose of this medicine, take it as soon as possible. However, if it is almost time for your next dose, skip the missed dose and go back to your regular dosing schedule. Do not double doses.

Storage—Store the medicine in a closed container at room temperature, away from heat, moisture, and direct light. Keep from freezing.

Keep out of the reach of children.

Do not keep outdated medicine or medicine no longer needed.

Side Effects of This Medicine

Along with its needed effects, a medicine may cause some unwanted effects. Although not all of these side effects may occur, if they do occur they may need medical attention.

Check with your doctor as soon as possible if any of the following side effects occur:

Skin irritation not present before use of this medicine

Other side effects not listed may also occur in some patients. If you notice any other effects, check with your healthcare professional.

NYSTATIN (Vaginal route) - nye-STA-tin

Commonly used brand name(s)

In Canada—

Mycostatin

Mycostatin Vaginal Cream

Nadostine

Nilstat Vaginal Cream

Nilstat Vaginal Tablet

Nyaderm Vaginal Cream

Available Dosage Forms:

• Cream

• Tablet

Therapeutic Class: Antifungal

Uses For This Medicine

Nystatin belongs to the group of medicines called antifungals. Vaginal nystatin is used to treat fungus infections of the vagina. Nystatin vaginal cream or tablets may also be used for other problems as determined by your doctor.

Nystatin is available only with your doctor's prescription.

Before Using This Medicine

In deciding to use a medicine, the risks of taking the medicine must be weighed against the good it will do. This is a decision you and your doctor will make. For this medicine, the following should be considered:

Allergies—Tell your doctor if you have ever had any unusual or allergic reaction to this medicine or any other medicines. Also tell your health care professional if you have any other types of allergies, such as to foods, dyes, preservatives, or animals. For non-prescription products, read the label or package ingredients carefully.

Pediatric—Studies on this medicine have been done only in adults, and there is no specific information comparing use of vaginal nystatin in children with use in other age groups.

Geriatric—Many medicines have not been studied specifically in older people. Therefore, it may not be known whether they work exactly the same way they do in younger adults or if they cause different side effects or problems in older people. There is no specific information comparing the use of vaginal nystatin in the elderly with use in other age groups.

Other medicines—Although certain medicines should not be used together at all, in other cases two different medicines may be used together even if an interaction might occur. In these cases, your doctor may want to change the dose, or other precautions may be necessary. Tell your healthcare professional if you are taking any other prescription or non-prescription (over-the-counter [OTC]) medicine.

Interactions with Food/Tobacco/Alcohol—Certain medicines should not be used at or around the time of eating food or eating certain types of food since interactions may occur. Using alcohol or tobacco with certain medicines may also cause interactions to occur. Discuss with your healthcare professional the use of your medicine with food, alcohol, or tobacco.

Proper Use of This Medicine

Nystatin usually comes with patient directions. Read them carefully before using this medicine.

This medicine is usually inserted into the vagina with an applicator. However, if you are pregnant, check with your doctor before using the applicator to insert the vaginal tablet.

To help clear up your infection completely, keep using this medicine for the full time of treatment, even if your condition has improved. Also, keep using this medicine even if you begin to menstruate during the time of treatment. Do not miss any doses.

Dosing—The dose of this medicine will be different for different patients. Follow your doctor's orders or the directions on the label. The following information includes only the average doses of this medicine. If your dose is different, do not change it unless your doctor tells you to do so.

The amount of medicine that you take depends on the strength of the medicine. Also, the number of doses you take each day, the time allowed between doses, and the length of time you take the medicine depend on the medical problem for which you are using the medicine.

- For treating fungus (yeast) infections:
  - For vaginal cream dosage form:
    - Adults and teenagers—One 100,000–unit applicatorful inserted into the vagina one or two times a day for two weeks. Or, your doctor may want you to insert one 500,000–unit applicatorful into the vagina once a day.
    - Children—Dose must be determined by your doctor.
  - For vaginal tablet dosage form:
    - Adults and teenagers—One 100,000–unit tablet inserted into the vagina one or two times a day for two weeks.
    - Children—Dose must be determined by your doctor.

Missed dose—If you miss a dose of this medicine, take it as soon as possible. However, if it is almost time for your next dose, skip the missed dose and go back to your regular dosing schedule. Do not double doses.

Storage—Store the medicine in a closed container at room temperature, away from heat, moisture, and direct light. Keep from freezing.

Keep out of the reach of children.

Do not keep outdated medicine or medicine no longer needed.

Precautions While Using This Medicine

To help cure the infection and to help prevent reinfection, good health habits are required.

- Wear cotton panties (or panties or pantyhose with cotton crotches) instead of synthetic (for example, nylon, rayon) underclothes.
- Wear freshly laundered underclothes.

If you have any questions about this, check with your health care professional.

If you have any questions about douching or intercourse during the time of treatment with nystatin, check with your doctor.

Since there may be some vaginal drainage while you are using this medicine, a sanitary napkin may be worn to protect your clothing.

Side Effects of This Medicine

Along with its needed effects, a medicine may cause some unwanted effects. Although not all of these side effects may occur, if they do occur they may need medical attention.

Check with your doctor as soon as possible if any of the following side effects occur:

Rare

Vaginal burning or itching not present before use of this medicine

Other side effects not listed may also occur in some patients. If you notice any other effects, check with your healthcare professional.

OCTREOTIDE (Injection route, Intramuscular route) - ok-TREE-oh-tide

Commonly used brand name(s)

In the U.S.—
Sandostatin
Sandostatin LAR Depot

Available Dosage Forms:
- Solution
- Powder for Solution
- Powder for Suspension

Therapeutic Class: Endocrine-Metabolic Agent
Pharmacologic Class: Somatostatin (class)

Uses For This Medicine

Octreotide is used to treat the severe diarrhea and other symptoms that occur with certain intestinal tumors. It does not cure the tumor but it helps the patient live a more normal life.

Also, this medicine is used to treat a condition called acromegaly, which is caused by too much growth hormone in the body. Too much growth hormone produced in adults causes the hands, feet, and parts of the face to become large, thick, and bulky. Other problems such as arthritis also can develop. Octreotide works by reducing the amount of growth hormone that the body produces.

Octreotide may also be used for other medical conditions as determined by your doctor.

Octreotide is available only with your doctor's prescription.

Once a medicine has been approved for marketing for a certain use, experience may show that it is also useful for other medical problems. Although these uses are not included in product labeling, octreotide is used in certain patients with the following medical conditions:

- Acquired immunodeficiency syndrome (AIDS)-related diarrhea.
- Chemotherapy-induced diarrhea.
- Insulin-producing tumors of the pancreas.

Before Using This Medicine

In deciding to use a medicine, the risks of taking the medicine must be weighed against the good it will do. This is a decision you and your doctor will make. For this medicine, the following should be considered:

Allergies—Tell your doctor if you have ever had any unusual or allergic reaction to this medicine or any other medicines. Also tell your health care professional if you have any other types of allergies, such as to foods, dyes, preservatives, or animals. For non-prescription products, read the label or package ingredients carefully.

Pediatric—The short-acting form of this medicine has been tested in a limited number of children as young as 1 month of age and has not been shown to cause different side effects or problems than it does in adults.

Studies on the long-acting form of this medicine have been done in children 6 to 17 years and have not demonstrated pediatrics-specific problems that would limit the usefulness of octreotide in children.

Geriatric—Although appropriate studies on the relationship of age to the effects of octreotide have not been performed in the geriatric population, geriatrics-specific problems are not expected to limit the usefulness of octreotide in the elderly. However, elderly patients are more likely to have age-related kidney or heart problems, which may require caution and dosage adjustment in patients receiving octreotide.

Pregnancy—

	Pregnancy Category	Explanation
All Trimesters	B	Animal studies have revealed no evidence of harm to the fetus, however, there are no adequate studies in pregnant women OR animal studies have shown an adverse effect, but adequate studies in pregnant women have failed to demonstrate a risk to the fetus.

Breast Feeding—There are no adequate studies in women for determining infant risk when using this medication during breastfeeding. Weigh the potential benefits against the potential risks before taking this medication while breastfeeding.

Other medicines—

Using this medicine with any of the following medicines is not recommended. Your doctor may decide not to treat you with this medication or change some of the other medicines you take.

Bepridil, Cisapride, Levomethadyl, Mesoridazine, Pimozide, Terfenadine, Thioridazine, Ziprasidone

Interactions   with   Food/Tobacco/Alcohol—Certain medicines should not be used at or around the time of eating food or eating certain types of food since interactions may occur. Using alcohol or tobacco with certain medicines may also cause interactions to occur. Discuss with your healthcare professional the use of your medicine with food, alcohol, or tobacco.

Other medical problems—The presence of other medical problems may affect the use of this medicine. Make sure you tell your doctor if you have any other medical problems, especially:

- Type 1 and type 2 diabetes mellitus—Octreotide may cause high or low blood sugar; your doctor may need to change the dose of your diabetes medicine.
- Heart disease or heart rhythm problem—Your doctor may need to change the dose of your heart medicines.
- Gallbladder disease or gallstones (or history of)—This medicine may increase the chance of having gallstones.
- Kidney disease (severe)—If you have this condition, octreotide may remain in the body longer than normal; your doctor may need to change the dose of your medicine.

Proper Use of This Medicine

To control the symptoms of your medical problem, this medicine must be taken as ordered by your doctor. Make sure that you understand exactly how to take this medicine.

Octreotide is packaged in a kit containing an ampule opener, alcohol swabs, ampules of the medicine, and, in some kits, a vial of diluent to mix with the medicine. Directions on how to prepare and inject the medicine are in the package. Read the directions carefully and ask your health care professional for additional explanation, if necessary.

It is important to follow any instructions from your doctor about the careful selection and rotation of injection sites on your body. This will help to prevent skin problems, such as irritation.

Some patients may feel pain, stinging, tingling, or burning sensations at the place where they inject the medicine. These sensations usually last only a few moments and may be eased by rubbing the spot after the injection. Injecting the medicine after it has been warmed to room temperature rather than cold from the refrigerator may reduce the discomfort. The medicine should be taken from the refrigerator 20 to 60 minutes before it is to be used. However, do not use heat to warm it faster because heat can destroy the medicine.

Put used needles and syringes in a puncture-resistant disposable container or dispose of them as directed by your health care professional. Do not reuse needles and syringes.

Dosing—The dose of this medicine will be different for different patients. Follow your doctor's orders or the directions on the label. The following information includes only the average doses of this medicine. If your dose is different, do not change it unless your doctor tells you to do so.

The amount of medicine that you take depends on the strength of the medicine. Also, the number of doses you take each day, the time allowed between doses, and the length of time you take the medicine depend on the medical problem for which you are using the medicine.

- For long-acting injection dosage form:
  - For treating the severe diarrhea that occurs with certain types of intestinal tumors:
    - Adults and teenagers—At first, 20 milligrams (mg) injected into the gluteal muscle once every four weeks for two months. Then, the dose will be adjusted by your doctor, based on your response to the medicine.
    - Children—Use and dose must be determined by your doctor.

- For treating acromegaly:
  - Adults—At first, 20 mg injected into the gluteal muscle once every four weeks for three months. Then, the dose will be adjusted by your doctor, based on your response to the medicine.

- For short-acting injection dosage form:
  - For treating the severe diarrhea that occurs with certain types of intestinal tumors:
    - Adults and teenagers—At first, 50 micrograms (mcg) injected under the skin two or three times a day. Then, the dose is slowly increased. Some people may need doses as high as 600 mcg a day for the first two weeks. Thereafter, the dose is usually between 50 and 1500 mcg per day.
    - Children—The dose is based on body weight and must be determined by your doctor. The usual dose is 1 to 10 mcg per kilogram (kg) (0.45 to 4.5 mcg per pound) of body weight a day, injected under the skin.
  - For treating acromegaly:
    - Adults—At first, 50 mcg injected under the skin or into a vein three times a day. Then, the dose is slowly increased to 100 to 200 mcg three times a day. Higher doses may be needed, as determined by your doctor.

Missed dose—If you miss a dose of this medicine, take it as soon as possible. However, if it is almost time for your next dose, skip the missed dose and go back to your regular dosing schedule. Do not double doses.

If you miss a dose of the long-acting form of this medicine, contact your doctor.

Storage—Store in the refrigerator. Do not freeze.

Keep out of the reach of children.

Do not keep outdated medicine or medicine no longer needed.

Ampules of the short-acting form of octreotide may be kept at room temperature for 14 days when they are protected from light. If the ampuls are not protected from light, problems with the solution can develop much sooner.

Precautions While Using This Medicine

It is very important that your doctor check your progress at regular visits to make sure that this medicine is working properly and to check for unwanted effects.

Side Effects of This Medicine

Along with its needed effects, a medicine may cause some unwanted effects. Although not all of these side effects may occur, if they do occur they may need medical attention.

Check with your doctor immediately if any of the following side effects occur:

Less common or rare

Changes in menstrual periods; convulsions (seizures); decreased sexual ability in males; depressed mood; dry skin and hair; dry, puffy skin; feeling cold; hoarseness or husky voice; muscle cramps and stiffness; slowed heartbeat; swelling of front part of neck; unconsciousness; unusual tiredness or weakness; weight gain

Check with your doctor as soon as possible if any of the following side effects occur:

More common

Irregular heartbeat; slow heartbeat

Less common or rare

Hyperglycemia (high blood sugar), including blurred vision, drowsiness, dry mouth, flushed dry skin, fruit-like breath odor, increased urination (frequency and volume), ketones in urine, loss of appetite, nausea, stomachache, tiredness, troubled breathing (rapid and deep), unusual thirst, or vomiting; hypoglycemia (low blood sugar), including anxious feeling, behavior change similar to drunkenness, blurred vision, cold sweats, confusion, cool pale skin, difficulty in concentrating, drowsiness, excessive hunger, fast heartbeat, headache, nausea, nervousness, nightmares, restless sleep, shakiness, slurred speech, or unusual tiredness or weakness; inflammation of the pancreas gland, including abdominal or stomach pain or bloating, nausea, or vomiting

Some side effects may occur that usually do not need medical attention. These side effects may go away during treatment as your body adjusts to the medicine. Also, your health care professional may be able to tell you about ways to prevent or reduce some of these side effects. Check with your health care professional if any of the following side effects continue or are bothersome or if you have any questions about them:

More common

Constipation; diarrhea; headache; pain, stinging, tingling, or burning sensation at place of injection, with redness and swelling; passing of gas

Less common or rare

Backache; bladder pain; bloody or cloudy urine; blurred or loss of vision; chills; cough; difficult, burning, or painful urination; discouragement; disturbed color perception; dizziness or light-headedness; double vision; feeling sad or empty; fever; frequent urge to urinate; frequent urination usually with very small amounts of urine; general feeling of discomfort or illness; hair loss; halos around lights; irritability; itching skin; joint pain; lack or loss of appetite; loss of interest or pleasure; lower back or side pain; muscle aches and pains; nausea; night blindness; overbright appearance of lights; redness or flushing of face; runny nose; shivering; sore throat; stools that float, are foul smelling, and fatty in appearance; sweating; swelling of feet or lower legs; tiredness; trouble concentrating; trouble sleeping; tunnel vision; vomiting

Other side effects not listed may also occur in some patients. If you notice any other effects, check with your healthcare professional.

OFLOXACIN (Ophthalmic route) - oh-FLOX-a-sin

Commonly used brand name(s)

In the U.S.—

Ocuflox

In Canada—

Ofloxacin
Ophtho-Flox

Available Dosage Forms:

• Solution

Therapeutic Class: Antibiotic

Uses For This Medicine

Ofloxacin is an antibiotic used to treat bacterial infections of the eye, such as conjunctivitis and corneal ulcers.

Ofloxacin is available only with your doctor's prescription.

Before Using This Medicine

In deciding to use a medicine, the risks of taking the medicine must be weighed against the good it will do. This is a decision you and your doctor will make. For this medicine, the following should be considered:

Allergies—Tell your doctor if you have ever had any unusual or allergic reaction to this medicine or any other medicines. Also tell your health care professional if you have any other types of allergies, such as to foods, dyes, preservatives, or animals. For non-prescription products, read the label or package ingredients carefully.

Pediatric—Use is not recommended in infants up to 1 year of age. In children 1 year of age and older, this medicine is not expected to cause different side effects or problems than it does in adults.

Geriatric—Many medicines have not been studied specifically in older people. Therefore, it may not be known whether they work exactly the same way they do in younger adults or if they cause different side effects or problems in older people. There is no specific information comparing use of ophthalmic ofloxacin in the elderly with use in other age groups.

Pregnancy—

	Pregnancy Category	Explanation
All Trimesters	C	Animal studies have shown an adverse effect and there are no adequate studies in pregnant women OR no animal studies have been conducted and there are no adequate studies in pregnant women.

Breast Feeding—There are no adequate studies in women for determining infant risk when using this medication during breastfeeding. Weigh the potential benefits against the potential risks before taking this medication while breastfeeding.

Other medicines—

Using this medicine with any of the following medicines is usually not recommended, but may be required in some cases. If both medicines are prescribed together, your doctor may change the dose or how often you use one or both of the medicines.

Acarbose, Acetohexamide, Alosetron, Benfluorex, Chlorpropamide, Disopyramide, Droperidol, Encainide, Flecainide, Gliclazide, Glimepiride, Glipizide, Gliquidone, Glyburide, Guar Gum, Insulin, Insulin Aspart, Recombinant, Insulin Glulisine, Insulin Lispro, Recombinant, Lidocaine, Metformin, Mexiletine, Miglitol, Moricizine, Procainamide, Propafenone, Quinidine, Tocainide, Tolazamide, Tolbutamide, Troglitazone

Interactions with Food/Tobacco/Alcohol—Certain medicines should not be used at or around the time of eating

food or eating certain types of food since interactions may occur. Using alcohol or tobacco with certain medicines may also cause interactions to occur. Discuss with your healthcare professional the use of your medicine with food, alcohol, or tobacco.

Proper Use of This Medicine

To use:

- First, wash your hands. Tilt the head back and with the index finger of one hand, press gently on the skin just beneath the lower eyelid and pull the lower eyelid away from the eye to make a space. Drop the medicine into this space. Let go of the eyelid and gently close the eyes. Do not blink. Keep the eyes closed for 1 to 2 minutes, to allow the medicine to come into contact with the infection.
- If you think you did not get the drop of medicine into your eyes properly, use another drop.
- To keep the medicine as germ-free as possible, do not touch the applicator tip to any surface (including the eye). Also, keep the container tightly closed.

To help clear up your eye infection completely, keep using ophthalmic ofloxacin for the full time of treatment, even if your symptoms have disappeared. Do not miss any doses.

Dosing—The dose of this medicine will be different for different patients. Follow your doctor's orders or the directions on the label. The following information includes only the average doses of this medicine. If your dose is different, do not change it unless your doctor tells you to do so.

The amount of medicine that you take depends on the strength of the medicine. Also, the number of doses you take each day, the time allowed between doses, and the length of time you take the medicine depend on the medical problem for which you are using the medicine.

- For ophthalmic (eye drops) dosage form:
  - For conjunctivitis:
    - Adults and children 1 year of age and older—Use 1 drop in the affected eye every two to four hours, while you are awake, for two days. Then, use 1 drop in each eye four times a day for up to five more days.
    - Infants up to 1 year of age—Use and dose must be determined by your doctor.
  - For bacterial corneal ulcers:
    - Adults and children 1 year of age and older—Use 1 drop in the affected eye every thirty minutes while you are awake and 1 drop four to six hours after you go to bed, for two days. Then use 1 drop every hour while you are awake for up to seven more days. After the seventh, eighth, or ninth day, as instructed by your doctor, use 1 drop four times a day until your doctor determines that the treatment is complete.
    - Infants up to 1 year of age—Use and dose must be determined by your doctor.

Missed dose—If you miss a dose of this medicine, take it as soon as possible. However, if it is almost time for your next dose, skip the missed dose and go back to your regular dosing schedule. Do not double doses.

Storage—Store the medicine in a closed container at room temperature, away from heat, moisture, and direct light. Keep from freezing.

Keep out of the reach of children.

Do not keep outdated medicine or medicine no longer needed.

Precautions While Using This Medicine

If your eye infection does not improve within 7 days, or if it becomes worse, check with your doctor.

Discontinue using these eye drops immediately and contact your physician at the first sign of a rash or an allergic reaction.

This medicine may cause your eyes to become more sensitive to light than they are normally. Wearing sunglasses and avoiding too much exposure to bright light may help lessen the discomfort.

Side Effects of This Medicine

Along with its needed effects, a medicine may cause some unwanted effects. Although not all of these side effects may occur, if they do occur they may need medical attention.

Check with your doctor immediately if any of the following side effects occur:

> *Rare*
> > Puffiness or swelling of eyes; signs of an allergic reaction, such as hives, itching, rash, swelling of face or lips, tightness in chest, troubled breathing, or wheezing

Check with your doctor as soon as possible if any of the following side effects occur:

> *Rare*
> > Dizziness

Some side effects may occur that usually do not need medical attention. These side effects may go away during treatment as your body adjusts to the medicine. Also, your health care professional may be able to tell you about ways to prevent or reduce some of these side effects. Check with your health care professional if any of the following side effects continue or are bothersome or if you have any questions about them:

> *More common*
> > Burning of eye

> *Less common*
> > Blurred vision; eye pain; feeling of something in the eye; increased sensitivity of eye to light; redness, irritation, or itching of eye, eyelid, or inner lining of eyelid; stinging, tearing, or dryness of eye

Other side effects not listed may also occur in some patients. If you notice any other effects, check with your healthcare professional.

OFLOXACIN   (Otic route) - oh-FLOX-a-sin

Commonly used brand name(s)
In the U.S.—
>   Floxin

Available Dosage Forms:
- Solution

Therapeutic Class: Antibacterial

Uses For This Medicine

Ofloxacin belongs to the family of medicines called antibiotics. Ofloxacin otic solution is used to treat infections of the ear canal. It also is used to treat infections of the middle ear in patients with nonintact tympanic membranes (holes or tubes in the eardrums).

This medicine is available only with your doctor's prescription.

Before Using This Medicine

In deciding to use a medicine, the risks of taking the medicine must be weighed against the good it will do. This is a decision you and your doctor will make. For this medicine, the following should be considered:

Allergies—Tell your doctor if you have ever had any unusual or allergic reaction to this medicine or any other medicines. Also tell your health care professional if you have any other types of allergies, such as to foods, dyes, preservatives, or animals. For non-prescription products, read the label or package ingredients carefully.

Pediatric—Use is not recommended in infants younger than 1 year of age.

Geriatric—Many medicines have not been studied specifically in older people. Therefore, it may not be known whether they work exactly the same way they do in younger adults or if they cause different side effects or problems in older people. There is no specific information comparing use of otic ofloxacin in the elderly with use in other age groups.

Pregnancy—

	Pregnancy Category	Explanation
All Trimesters	C	Animal studies have shown an adverse effect and there are no adequate studies in pregnant women OR no animal studies have been conducted and there are no adequate studies in pregnant women.

Breast Feeding—There are no adequate studies in women for determining infant risk when using this medication during breastfeeding. Weigh the potential benefits against the potential risks before taking this medication while breastfeeding.

Other medicines—

Using this medicine with any of the following medicines is usually not recommended, but may be required in some cases. If both medicines are prescribed together, your doctor may change the dose or how often you use one or both of the medicines.

Acarbose, Acetohexamide, Alosetron, Benfluorex, Chlorpropamide, Disopyramide, Droperidol, Encainide, Flecainide, Gliclazide, Glimepiride, Glipizide, Gliquidone, Glyburide, Guar Gum, Insulin, Insulin Aspart, Recombinant, Insulin Glulisine, Insulin Lispro, Recombinant, Lidocaine, Metformin, Mexiletine, Miglitol, Moricizine, Procainamide, Propafenone, Quinidine, Tocainide, Tolazamide, Tolbutamide, Troglitazone

Interactions with Food/Tobacco/Alcohol—Certain medicines should not be used at or around the time of eating food or eating certain types of food since interactions may occur. Using alcohol or tobacco with certain medicines may also cause interactions to occur. Discuss with your healthcare professional the use of your medicine with food, alcohol, or tobacco.

Proper Use of This Medicine

Ofloxacin eardrops comes with patient information and instructions (Medication Guide). Be sure to read these instructions before using the eardrops. If you have any questions, check with your doctor or health care professional.

To use:

- Hold the bottle in your hands for 1 or 2 minutes to warm up the solution before putting it in your ear. Otherwise, putting cold solution in your ear could cause you to become dizzy.
- Wash your hands with soap and water.
- Gently clean any discharge that can be removed easily from the outer ear, but do not insert any object or swab into the ear canal.
- If you are using the eardrops for a middle ear infection— Drop the medicine into the ear canal. Then, gently press the tragus of the ear (see the diagram in the Medication Guide) four times in a pumping motion. This will allow the drops to pass through the hole or tube in the eardrum and into the middle ear.
- If you are using the eardrops for an ear canal infection— Gently pull the outer ear up and back for adults (down and back for children) to straighten the ear canal. This will allow the eardrops to flow down into the ear canal.
- Keep the ear facing up for about 5 minutes to allow the medicine to come into contact with the infection.
- If both ears are being treated, turn over after 5 minutes, and repeat the application for the other ear.
- To keep the medicine as germ-free as possible, do not touch the applicator tip to any surface (including the ear). Also, keep the container tightly closed.

To help clear up your infection completely, keep using this medicine for the full time of treatment, even if your symptoms have disappeared. Do not miss any doses.

Dosing—The dose of this medicine will be different for different patients. Follow your doctor's orders or the directions on the label. The following information includes only the average doses of this medicine. If your dose is different, do not change it unless your doctor tells you to do so.

The amount of medicine that you take depends on the strength of the medicine. Also, the number of doses you take each day, the time allowed between doses, and the length of time you take the medicine depend on the medical problem for which you are using the medicine.

- For eardrops dosage form:
  - For ear infections:
    - Adults and teenagers (12 years of age and older)—Place 10 drops in each affected ear two times a day for ten to fourteen days, depending on the infection.
    - Children 1 to 12 years of age—Place 5 drops in each affected ear two times a day for ten days.
    - Children younger than 1 year of age—Use and dose must be determined by your doctor.

Missed dose—If you miss a dose of this medicine, take it as soon as possible. However, if it is almost time for your next

dose, skip the missed dose and go back to your regular dosing schedule. Do not double doses.

Storage—Store the medicine in a closed container at room temperature, away from heat, moisture, and direct light. Keep from freezing.

Keep out of the reach of children.

Do not keep outdated medicine or medicine no longer needed.

Precautions While Using This Medicine

If your symptoms do not improve within a few days, or if they become worse, check with your doctor.

Oral and systemic ofloxacin and other similar antibiotics have sometimes caused a severe allergic reaction. It is not known if otic ofloxacin may cause this reaction. However, stop using this medicine and check with your doctor immediately if you notice skin rash or itching, shortness of breath, or swelling of the face or neck.

Side Effects of This Medicine

Along with its needed effects, a medicine may cause some unwanted effects. Although not all of these side effects may occur, if they do occur they may need medical attention.

Check with your doctor immediately if any of the following side effects occur:

> *Less common*
>> Burning, itching, redness, skin rash, swelling, or other sign of irritation not present before use of this medicine

Check with your doctor as soon as possible if any of the following side effects occur:

> *Less common*
>> Dizziness

> *Rare*
>> Bleeding from the ear; fast heartbeat; fever; headache; ringing in the ear; runny or stuffy nose; sore throat

Some side effects may occur that usually do not need medical attention. These side effects may go away during treatment as your body adjusts to the medicine. Also, your health care professional may be able to tell you about ways to prevent or reduce some of these side effects. Check with your health care professional if any of the following side effects continue or are bothersome or if you have any questions about them:

> *Less common*
>> Change in taste; earache; numbness or tingling

Other side effects not listed may also occur in some patients. If you notice any other effects, check with your healthcare professional.

OLANZAPINE (Intramuscular route) - oh-LAN-za-peen

Black Box Warning

Elderly patients with dementia-related psychosis treated with atypical antipsychotic drugs are at an increased risk of death compared to placebo. Analyses of seventeen placebo-controlled trials (modal duration of 10 weeks) in these patients revealed a risk of death in the drug-treated patients of between 1.6 times to 1.7 times that seen in placebo-treated patients. Over the course of a typical 10–week controlled trial, the rate of death in drug-treated patients was about 4.5%, compared to a rate of about 2.6% in the placebo group. Although the causes of death were varied, most of the deaths appeared to be either cardiovascular (eg, heart failure, sudden death) or infectious (eg, pneumonia) in nature. Olanzapine is not approved for the treatment of patients with dementia-related psychosis.

Commonly used brand name(s)

In the U.S.—
> Zyprexa IntraMuscular

Available Dosage Forms:
- Powder for Solution

Therapeutic Class: Antipsychotic

Uses For This Medicine

Olanzapine is used to treat psychotic mental disorders, such as schizophrenia, bipolar disorder, and agitation that occurs with schizophrenia and bipolar mania. This medicine should NOT be used to treat behavioral problems in older adult patients who have dementia.

This medicine is available only with your doctor's prescription.

Before Using This Medicine

In deciding to use a medicine, the risks of taking the medicine must be weighed against the good it will do. This is a decision you and your doctor will make. For this medicine, the following should be considered:

Allergies—Tell your doctor if you have ever had any unusual or allergic reaction to this medicine or any other medicines. Also tell your health care professional if you have any other types of allergies, such as to foods, dyes, preservatives, or animals. For non-prescription products, read the label or package ingredients carefully.

Pediatric—Studies on this medicine have been done only in adult patients, and there is no specific information comparing use of olanzapine in children up to 18 years of age with use in other age groups.

Geriatric—This medicine has been tested and has not been shown to cause different side effects or problems in older people than it does in younger adults. However, it is removed from the body more slowly in older people and they may need a lower dose of this medicine. This medicine should not be used for behavioral problems in older adults with dementia.

Pregnancy—

	Pregnancy Category	Explanation
All Trimesters	C	Animal studies have shown an adverse effect and there are no adequate studies in pregnant women OR no animal studies have been conducted and there are no adequate studies in pregnant women.

Breast Feeding—There are no adequate studies in women for determining infant risk when using this medication during breastfeeding. Weigh the potential benefits against the potential risks before taking this medication while breastfeeding.

Other medicines—

Using this medicine with any of the following medicines is not recommended. Your doctor may decide not to treat you with this medication or change some of the other medicines you take.

Levomethadyl

Interactions with Food/Tobacco/Alcohol—Certain medicines should not be used at or around the time of eating food or eating certain types of food since interactions may occur. Using alcohol or tobacco with certain medicines may also cause interactions to occur. Discuss with your healthcare professional the use of your medicine with food, alcohol, or tobacco.

Other medical problems—The presence of other medical problems may affect the use of this medicine. Make sure you tell your doctor if you have any other medical problems, especially:

- Alzheimer's disease—Risk of aspiration pneumonia and convulsions (seizures) may be increased
- Aspiration pneumonia, risk or history of— may increase risk of adverse events
- Breast cancer (or history of)—Certain types of breast cancer may be worsened
- Convulsions (seizures) (existing or history of)—Olanzapine has been reported to cause seizures rarely
- Dehydration or
- Exposure to extreme heat or
- Strenuous exercise—Increased risk of heat stroke because olanzapine affects the body's ability to cool itself
- Diabetes or family history of diabetes—May make condition worse and cause serious side effects
- Enlarged prostate or
- Glaucoma, narrow-angle or
- Paralytic ileus (severe intestinal problem) (history of)— May be worsened
- Heart or blood vessel disease, including previous heart attack or
- Poor circulation to the brain—Low blood pressure may be worsened or may make these conditions worse
- Liver disease—Olanzapine can cause liver problems

Proper Use of This Medicine

Take this medicine only as directed by your doctor in order to improve your condition as much as possible. Do not take more of it and do not take it more often than your doctor ordered.

Olanzapine may be taken with or without food, on a full or an empty stomach. If your doctor tells you to take it a certain way, follow your doctor's instructions.

Dosing—The dose of this medicine will be different for different patients. Follow your doctor's orders or the directions on the label. The following information includes only the average doses of this medicine. If your dose is different, do not change it unless your doctor tells you to do so.

The amount of medicine that you take depends on the strength of the medicine. Also, the number of doses you take each day, the time allowed between doses, and the length of time you take the medicine depend on the medical problem for which you are using the medicine.

- For oral dosage form (orally disintegrating tablets and tablets):
  - For treatment of psychotic disorders, including bipolar disorder and schizophrenia:
    - Adults—At first, 5 to 10 milligrams (mg) once a day. This dose may be changed to a higher or lower dose by your doctor as needed.
    - Children up to 18 years of age—Use and dose must be determined by your doctor.

- For parenteral dosage form (intramuscular injection)
  - For treatment of agitation that occurs with schizophrenia or bipolar mania:
    - Adults—At first, 10 mg per dose. This dose may be changed to a higher or lower dose by your doctor as needed.
    - Children—Use and dose must be determined by your doctor.

Missed dose—If you miss a dose of this medicine, take it as soon as possible. However, if it is almost time for your next dose, skip the missed dose and go back to your regular dosing schedule. Do not double doses.

Storage—Store the medicine in a closed container at room temperature, away from heat, moisture, and direct light. Keep from freezing.

Keep out of the reach of children.

Do not keep outdated medicine or medicine no longer needed.

Precautions While Using This Medicine

It is important that your doctor check your progress at regular visits, to allow for changes in your dose and help reduce any side effects.

This medicine may add to the effects of alcohol and other central nervous system (CNS) depressants (medicines that make you drowsy or less alert). Some examples of CNS depressants are antihistamines or medicine for hay fever, other allergies, or colds; sedatives, tranquilizers, or sleeping medicine; prescription pain medicine or narcotics; barbiturates; medicine for seizures; muscle relaxants; or anesthetics, including some dental anesthetics. Check with your doctor before taking any CNS depressants while you are taking this medicine.

Olanzapine may cause drowsiness, trouble in thinking, trouble in controlling movements, or trouble in seeing clearly. Make sure you know how you react to this medicine before you drive, use machines, or do other jobs that require you to be alert, well-coordinated, or able to think or see well.

Dizziness, lightheadedness, or fainting may occur, especially when you get up from a lying or sitting position. Getting up slowly may help. If this problem continues or gets worse, check with your doctor.

This medicine may make it more difficult for your body to cool itself down. Use care not to become overheated during exercise or hot weather since overheating may result in heat stroke.

Olanzapine may cause dryness of the mouth. For temporary relief, use sugarless gum or candy, melt bits of ice in your mouth, or use a saliva substitute. However, if your mouth feels dry for more than 2 weeks, check with your medical doctor or dentist. Continuing dryness of the mouth may increase the chance of dental disease, including tooth decay, gum disease, and fungus infections.

Side Effects of This Medicine

Along with its needed effects, a medicine may cause some unwanted effects. Although not all of these side effects may occur, if they do occur they may need medical attention.

Check with your doctor as soon as possible if any of the following side effects occur:

More common
> Agitation; behavior problems; difficulty in speaking or swallowing; restlessness or need to keep moving; stiffness of arms or legs; trembling or shaking of hands and fingers

Less common
> Blurred vision; chest pain; fever; flu-like symptoms; headache; inability to move eyes; itching of the vagina or genital area; lip smacking or puckering; mood or mental changes, such as anger, anxiety, giddiness, loss of memory, or nervousness; muscle spasms of face, neck, and back; muscle twitching or jerking; nervousness; pain during sexual intercourse; pounding in the ears; puffing of cheeks; rapid or worm-like movements of tongue; rhythmic movement of muscles; slow or fast heartbeat; swelling of feet or ankles; thick, white vaginal discharge with no odor or with a mild odor; twitching movements; twitching, twisting, uncontrolled repetitive movements of tongue, lips, face, arms, or legs; uncontrolled chewing movements; uncontrolled jerking or twisting movements of hands, arms and legs; uncontrolled movements of lips, tongue, or cheeks; unusual or incomplete body or facial movements

Rare
> Changes in menstrual period; confusion; extra heartbeat; mental or physical sluggishness; skin rash; swelling of face; trouble in breathing

Incidence not known
> Bloating; cough; constipation; darkened urine; diabetic coma; difficulty swallowing; hives; indigestion; itching skin; itching, puffiness or swelling of the eyelids or around the eyes, face, lips, or tongue; large, hive-like swelling on face, eyelids, lips, tongue, throat, hands, legs, feet, sex organs; loss of appetite; nausea; pain in stomach, side, or abdomen, possibly radiating to the back; painful or prolonged erection of the penis; redness of skin; shortness of breath; skin rash; tightness in chest; unusual tiredness or weakness; vomiting; wheezing; yellow eyes or skin

Some side effects may occur that usually do not need medical attention. These side effects may go away during treatment as your body adjusts to the medicine. Also, your health care professional may be able to tell you about ways to prevent or reduce some of these side effects. Check with your health care professional if any of the following side effects

continue or are bothersome or if you have any questions about them:

More common
> Acid or sour stomach; belching; change in walking and balance; clumsiness; constipation; difficulty in speaking; dizziness; dizziness or fainting when getting up suddenly from a lying or sitting position; drowsiness; dryness of mouth; headache; heartburn; runny nose; sleepiness or unusual drowsiness; stomach discomfort, upset, or pain; unsteadiness; vision problems; weakness; weight gain

Less common or rare
> Abdominal pain; awareness of heartbeat; blemishes on the skin; burning, crawling, itching, numbness, prickling, "pins and needles", or tingling feelings; changes in vision; cramps; decrease in sexual desire; double vision; fast heartbeat; heavy bleeding; increased appetite; increased cough; increased sensitivity of skin to sunlight; joint pain; lack of feeling or emotion; low blood pressure; nausea; pain in arms or legs; pimples; sore throat; stuttering; sweating; thirst; tightness of muscles; trouble in controlling urine; trouble in sleeping; uncaring; vomiting; watering of mouth; weight loss

Other side effects not listed may also occur in some patients. If you notice any other effects, check with your healthcare professional.

OLMESARTAN AND HYDROCHLOROTHIAZIDE (Oral route) - ol-me-SAR-tan, hye-droe-klor-oh-THYE-a-zide

Black Box Warning

When used in pregnancy during the second and third trimesters, drugs that act directly on the renin-angiotensin system can cause injury and even death to the developing fetus. When pregnancy is detected, hydrochlorothiazide/olmesartan medoxomil should be discontinued as soon as possible.

Commonly used brand name(s)

In the U.S.—
> Benicar HCT

Available Dosage Forms:

- Tablet

Therapeutic Class: Angiotensin II Receptor Antagonist/Thiazide Combination

Pharmacologic Class: Angiotensin II Receptor Antagonist

Uses For This Medicine

Olmesartan and hydrochlorothiazide is a combination medicine that belongs to the class of medicines called high blood pressure medicines (antihypertensives). It is used to treat high blood pressure (hypertension).

High blood pressure adds to the workload of the heart and arteries. If it continues for a long time, the heart and arteries may not function properly. This can damage the blood vessels of the brain, heart, and kidneys, resulting in a stroke, heart failure, or kidney failure. High blood pressure may also increase the risk of heart attacks. These problems may be less likely to occur if blood pressure is controlled.

Olmesartan works by blocking a substance in the body that causes blood vessels to tighten. As a result, olmesartan relaxes blood vessels. This lowers blood pressure and increases the supply of blood and oxygen to the heart. Hydrochlorothiazide helps reduce the amount of salt and water in the body by acting on the kidneys to increase the flow of urine; this also helps to lower blood pressure.

This combination also may be used for other conditions as determined by your doctor.

This medicine is available only with your doctor's prescription.

Before Using This Medicine

In deciding to use a medicine, the risks of taking the medicine must be weighed against the good it will do. This is a decision you and your doctor will make. For this medicine, the following should be considered:

Allergies—Tell your doctor if you have ever had any unusual or allergic reaction to this medicine or any other medicines. Also tell your health care professional if you have any other types of allergies, such as to foods, dyes, preservatives, or animals. For non-prescription products, read the label or package ingredients carefully.

Pediatric—Studies on this medicine have been done only in adult patients, and there is no specific information comparing use of olmesartan and hydrochlorothiazide combination in children with use in other age groups.

Geriatric—This medicine has been tested and has not been shown to cause different side effects or problems in older people than it does in younger adults. However, older adults may be more sensitive to the effects of olmesartan and hydrochlorothiazide and should be monitored by the doctor.

Other medicines—

Using this medicine with any of the following medicines is not recommended. Your doctor may decide not to treat you with this medication or change some of the other medicines you take.

Dofetilide

Interactions with Food/Tobacco/Alcohol—Certain medicines should not be used at or around the time of eating food or eating certain types of food since interactions may occur. Using alcohol or tobacco with certain medicines may also cause interactions to occur. Discuss with your healthcare professional the use of your medicine with food, alcohol, or tobacco.

Other medical problems—The presence of other medical problems may affect the use of this medicine. Make sure you tell your doctor if you have any other medical problems, especially:

- Fluid or electrolyte (e.g., potassium, chloride, sodium) imbalance (due to excessive perspiration, vomiting, diarrhea, etc.)—The side effects of olmesartan and hydrochlorothiazide may be increased.

- Diabetes mellitus (sugar diabetes) or
- Gout or
- Hyperglycemia or
- Hyperuricemia—These conditions may be made worse by hydrochlorothiazide.
- Hypersensitivity to olmesartan, hydrochlorothiazide, sulfa drugs or any of its components
- Kidney disease or
- Liver disease—These conditions may be aggravated by olmesartan and hydrochlorothiazide.
- Sympathectomy—Blood pressure-lowering effects may be increased.
- Systemic lupus erythematosus (SLE)—Symptoms of this condition may be made worse with use of hydrochlorothiazide.

Proper Use of This Medicine

Dosing—The dose of this medicine will be different for different patients. Follow your doctor's orders or the directions on the label. The following information includes only the average doses of this medicine. If your dose is different, do not change it unless your doctor tells you to do so.

The amount of medicine that you take depends on the strength of the medicine. Also, the number of doses you take each day, the time allowed between doses, and the length of time you take the medicine depend on the medical problem for which you are using the medicine.

- For oral dosage form (tablets):
  - For high blood pressure:
    - Adults—1 tablet (20 mg/12.5 mg) once a day. Your doctor may increase your dose if needed.
    - Children—Use and dose must be determined by your doctor.

Precautions While Using This Medicine

Check with your doctor immediately if you think that you may be pregnant. Olmesartan and hydrochlorothiazide may cause birth defects or other problems in the baby if taken during pregnancy.

It is important that your doctor check your progress at regular visits to make sure that this medicine is working properly and to check for unwanted effects.

Do not take other medicines unless they have been discussed with your doctor. This especially includes potassium supplements or salt substitutes that contain potassium, since they may change your blood potassium levels, or over-the-counter (nonprescription) medicines for appetite control, asthma, colds, cough, hay fever, or sinus problems, since they may tend to increase your blood pressure.

Dizziness, lightheadedness, or fainting may occur with this medicine. Make sure you know how you react to this medicine before you drive, use machines, or do anything else that could be dangerous if you experience these effects.

Use extra care during exercise or hot weather. Heavy sweating can cause loss of too much water and result in low blood pressure.

Check with your doctor right away if you become sick while taking this medicine, especially with severe or continuing nausea and vomiting or diarrhea. These conditions may cause you to lose too much water and lead to low blood pressure.

Avoid alcoholic beverages until you have discussed their use with your doctor. Alcohol may make the low blood pressure effect worse and/or increase the possibility of dizziness or fainting.

For diabetic patients:

- Hydrochlorothiazide may raise blood sugar levels. Check with your doctor if any changes in your blood sugar levels occur.

Side Effects of This Medicine

Along with its needed effects, a medicine may cause some unwanted effects. Although not all of these side effects may occur, if they do occur they may need medical attention.

Also, because of the way these medicines act on the body, there is a chance that they might cause other unwanted effects that may not occur until months or years after the medicine is used. These may include certain types of cancer, such as leukemia or bladder cancer. Discuss these possible effects with your doctor.

Symptoms of fluid and electrolyte imbalance
Dry mouth; increased thirst; weak and/or irregular heartbeat; muscle cramps or pain; nausea or vomiting; unusual tiredness or weakness

Some side effects may occur that usually do not need medical attention. These side effects may go away during treatment as your body adjusts to the medicine. Also, your health care professional may be able to tell you about ways to prevent or reduce some of these side effects. Check with your health care professional if any of the following side effects continue or are bothersome or if you have any questions about them:

More common
Chest pain; chills; cough; dizziness; ear congestion or pain; fever; head congestion; hoarseness or other voice changes; nasal congestion; runny nose; sneezing; sore throat

Less common
Joint pain stiffness, or swelling; lower back, side, or stomach pain; swelling of face, feet or lower legs

Incidence unknown
Acid or sour stomach; belching; blood in urine; convulsions; decrease in amount of urine; diarrhea; difficult breathing; difficulty in moving; dizziness; dizziness, faintness, or lightheadedness when getting up from lying or sitting position; fainting; feeling of constant movement of self or surroundings; fruit-like breath odor; heartburn; increased hunger; indigestion; joint pain; large amount of fat in the blood; loss of appetite; mood changes; muscle pain or stiffness; nervousness; numbness or tingling in hands, feet, or lips; numbness, tingling, pain, or weakness in hands or feet; pain in lower back or side; rash; redness in joints; seizures; sensation of spinning; shortness of breath; stomach discomfort upset or pain; swelling or puffiness of face; thirst; tingling of hands or feet; trembling; weakness or heaviness of legs

OLMESARTAN MEDOXOMIL (Oral route) - ol-me-SAR-tan me-DOX-oh-mil

Black Box Warning

When used in pregnancy during the second and third trimesters, drugs that act directly on the renin-angiotensin system can cause injury and even death to the developing fetus. When pregnancy is detected, olmesartan medoxomil should be discontinued as soon as possible.

Commonly used brand name(s)

In the U.S.—
Benicar

Available Dosage Forms:

- Tablet

Therapeutic Class: Cardiovascular Agent
Pharmacologic Class: Angiotensin II Receptor Antagonist

Uses For This Medicine

Olmesartan belongs to the class of medicines called angiotensin II inhibitor antihypertensives. It is used to treat high blood pressure (hypertension).

High blood pressure adds to the workload of the heart and arteries. If it continues for a long time, the heart and arteries may not function properly. This can damage the blood vessels of the brain, heart, and kidneys, resulting in a stroke, heart failure, or kidney failure. High blood pressure also may increase the risk of heart attacks. These problems may be less likely to occur if blood pressure is controlled.

Olmesartan works by blocking the action of a substance in the body that causes blood vessels to tighten. As a result, olmesartan relaxes blood vessels. This lowers blood pressure.

This medicine is available only with your doctor's prescription.

Before Using This Medicine

In deciding to use a medicine, the risks of taking the medicine must be weighed against the good it will do. This is a decision you and your doctor will make. For this medicine, the following should be considered:

Allergies—Tell your doctor if you have ever had any unusual or allergic reaction to this medicine or any other medicines. Also tell your health care professional if you have any other types of allergies, such as to foods, dyes, preservatives, or animals. For non-prescription products, read the label or package ingredients carefully.

Pediatric—Studies on this medicine have only been done in adult patients, and there is no specific information comparing the use of olmesartan in children with use in other age groups.

Geriatric—This medicine has been tested in patients 65 years of age or older and has not been shown to cause different side effects or problems in older people than it does in younger adults. Elderly patients may have a greater sensitivity to olmesartan than younger adults.

Pregnancy—

	Pregnancy Category	Explanation
1st Trimester	C	Animal studies have shown an adverse effect and there are no adequate studies in pregnant women OR no animal studies have been conducted and there are no adequate studies in pregnant women.
2nd Trimester	D	Studies in pregnant women have demonstrated a risk to the fetus. However, the benefits of therapy in a life threatening situation or a serious disease, may outweigh the potential risk.
3rd Trimester	D	Studies in pregnant women have demonstrated a risk to the fetus. However, the benefits of therapy in a life threatening situation or a serious disease, may outweigh the potential risk.

Breast Feeding—There are no adequate studies in women for determining infant risk when using this medication during breastfeeding. Weigh the potential benefits against the potential risks before taking this medication while breastfeeding.

Other medicines—Although certain medicines should not be used together at all, in other cases two different medicines may be used together even if an interaction might occur. In these cases, your doctor may want to change the dose, or other precautions may be necessary. Tell your healthcare professional if you are taking any other prescription or non-prescription (over-the-counter [OTC]) medicine.

Interactions with Food/Tobacco/Alcohol—Certain medicines should not be used at or around the time of eating food or eating certain types of food since interactions may occur. Using alcohol or tobacco with certain medicines may also cause interactions to occur. Discuss with your healthcare professional the use of your medicine with food, alcohol, or tobacco.

Other medical problems—The presence of other medical problems may affect the use of this medicine. Make sure you tell your doctor if you have any other medical problems, especially:

- Congestive heart failure, severe—Lowering of blood pressure by olmesartan may make this condition worse
- Dehydration—Blood pressure-lowering effects of olmesartan may be increased
- Kidney disease or
- Liver disease—Effects of olmesartan may be increased because of slower removal of medicine from the body.

Proper Use of This Medicine

Make certain your health care professional knows if you are on any special diet, such as a low-sodium diet.

To help you remember to take your medicine, try to get into the habit of taking it at the same time each day.

In addition to the use of the medicine your doctor has prescribed, treatment for your high blood pressure may include weight control and care in the types of foods you eat, especially foods high in sodium. Your doctor will tell you which of these are most important for you. You should check with your doctor before changing your diet.

Many patients who have high blood pressure will not notice any signs of the problem. In fact, many may feel normal. It is very important that you take your medicine exactly as directed and that you keep your appointments with your doctor even if you feel well.

Remember that this medicine will not cure your high blood pressure but it does help control it. Therefore, you must continue to take it as directed if you expect to lower your blood pressure and keep it down. You may have to take high blood pressure medicine for the rest of your life. If high blood pressure is not treated, it can cause serious problems such as heart failure, blood vessel disease, stroke, or kidney disease.

This medicine may be taken with or without food.

Dosing—The dose of this medicine will be different for different patients. Follow your doctor's orders or the directions on the label. The following information includes only the average doses of this medicine. If your dose is different, do not change it unless your doctor tells you to do so.

The amount of medicine that you take depends on the strength of the medicine. Also, the number of doses you take each day, the time allowed between doses, and the length of time you take the medicine depend on the medical problem for which you are using the medicine.

- For oral dosage form (tablets):
  - For high blood pressure:
    - Adults—20 milligrams (mg) once a day. Your doctor may increase your dose to 40 milligrams (mg) once a day if needed.

Missed dose—If you miss a dose of this medicine, take it as soon as possible. However, if it is almost time for your next dose, skip the missed dose and go back to your regular dosing schedule. Do not double doses.

Storage—Store the medicine in a closed container at room temperature, away from heat, moisture, and direct light. Keep from freezing.

Keep out of the reach of children.

Do not keep outdated medicine or medicine no longer needed.

Precautions While Using This Medicine

It is important that your doctor checks your progress at regular visits to make sure that this medicine is working properly and to check for unwanted effects.

Check with your doctor immediately if you think that you may be pregnant. Olmesartan may cause birth defects or other problems in the baby if taken during pregnancy.

Do not take other medicines unless they have been discussed with your doctor. This especially includes over-the-counter (nonprescription) medicines for appetite control, asthma, colds, cough, hay fever, or sinus problems, since they may tend to increase your blood pressure.

Dizziness or lightheadedness may occur after the first dose of this medicine, especially if you have been taking a diuretic (water pill). Make sure you know how you react to this medicine before you drive, use machines, or do anything else that could be dangerous if you are dizzy.

Check with your doctor right away if you become sick while taking this medicine, especially with severe or continuing nausea and vomiting or diarrhea. These conditions may cause you to lose too much water and lead to low blood pressure.

Dizziness, lightheadedness, or fainting may also occur if you exercise or if the weather is hot. Heavy sweating can cause loss of too much water and result in low blood pressure. Use extra care during exercise or hot weather.

Avoid alcoholic beverages until you have discussed their use with your doctor. Alcohol may make the low blood pressure effect worse and/or increase the possibility of dizziness or fainting.

Side Effects of This Medicine

Along with its needed effects, a medicine may cause some unwanted effects. Although not all of these side effects may occur, if they do occur they may need medical attention.

Check with your doctor immediately if any of the following side effects occur:

Less common
Body aches or pain; blood in urine; chills; cough or cough producing mucus; difficulty breathing; ear congestion; fever; headache; loss of voice; nasal congestion; runny nose; shortness of breath; sneezing; sore throat; tightness in chest; unusual tiredness or weakness; wheezing

Rare
Bladder pain; bloody or cloudy urine; difficult, burning, or painful urination; fast, pounding, or irregular heartbeat or pulse; frequent urge to urinate; joint pain, stiffness, or swelling; large amount of fat in the blood; lower back, side, or stomach pain; swelling of feet or lower legs

Frequency not known
Dark-colored urine; large, hive-like swelling on face, eyelids, lips, tongue, throat, hands, legs, feet, sex organs; muscle cramps or spasms; muscle pain or stiffness

Symptoms of overdose
Get emergency help immediately if any of the following symptoms of overdose occur:

Blurred vision; chest pain or discomfort; confusion; dizziness, faintness, or lightheadedness; fast, pounding, slow, or irregular heartbeat or pulse; shortness of breath; sweating; unusual tiredness or weakness

Some side effects may occur that usually do not need medical attention. These side effects may go away during treatment as your body adjusts to the medicine. Also, your health care professional may be able to tell you about ways to prevent or reduce some of these side effects. Check with your health care professional if any of the following side effects continue or are bothersome or if you have any questions about them:

Less common
Abdominal pain; back pain; blurred vision; body aches or pain; diarrhea; dizziness; dry mouth; fatigue; flushed,

dry skin; fruit-like breath odor; general feeling of discomfort or illness; increased hunger; increased thirst; increased urination; loss of appetite; muscle aches and pains; nausea; pain or tenderness around eyes and cheekbones; shivering; sweating; tender, swollen glands in neck; troubled breathing; trouble sleeping; trouble in swallowing; unexplained weight loss; vomiting

Rare
Acid or sour stomach; belching; bloating or swelling of face, arms, hands, lower legs, or feet; chest pain; difficulty in moving; feeling of constant movement of self or surroundings; heartburn; indigestion; muscle pains or stiffness; nausea; rash; rapid weight gain; sensation of spinning; skeletal pain; sleeplessness; stomach pain; swelling or puffiness of face; tingling of hands or feet; unusual weight gain or loss

Other side effects not listed may also occur in some patients. If you notice any other effects, check with your healthcare professional.

OLOPATADINE (Ophthalmic route) -
oh-loe-pa-TA-deen

Commonly used brand name(s)

In the U.S.—
Patanol

Available Dosage Forms:
• Solution

Therapeutic Class: Ophthalmologic Agent
Pharmacologic Class: Antihistamine

Uses For This Medicine

Olopatadine ophthalmic (eye) solution is used to temporarily prevent itching of the eye caused by a condition known as allergic conjunctivitis. It works by acting on certain cells, called mast cells, to prevent them from releasing substances that cause the allergic reaction.

This medicine is available only with your doctor's prescription.

Before Using This Medicine

In deciding to use a medicine, the risks of taking the medicine must be weighed against the good it will do. This is a decision you and your doctor will make. For this medicine, the following should be considered:

Allergies—Tell your doctor if you have ever had any unusual or allergic reaction to this medicine or any other medicines. Also tell your health care professional if you have any other types of allergies, such as to foods, dyes, preservatives, or animals. For non-prescription products, read the label or package ingredients carefully.

Pediatric—Studies on this medicine have been done only in adult patients, and there is no specific information comparing use of olopatadine in children up to 3 years of age with use in other age groups.

Geriatric—Many medicines have not been studied specifically in older people. Therefore, it may not be known whether

they work exactly the same way they do in younger adults or if they cause different side effects or problems in older people. There is no specific information comparing use of olopatadine in the elderly with use in other age groups.

Pregnancy—

	Pregnancy Category	Explanation
All Trimesters	C	Animal studies have shown an adverse effect and there are no adequate studies in pregnant women OR no animal studies have been conducted and there are no adequate studies in pregnant women.

Breast Feeding—There are no adequate studies in women for determining infant risk when using this medication during breastfeeding. Weigh the potential benefits against the potential risks before taking this medication while breastfeeding.

Other medicines—Although certain medicines should not be used together at all, in other cases two different medicines may be used together even if an interaction might occur. In these cases, your doctor may want to change the dose, or other precautions may be necessary. Tell your healthcare professional if you are taking any other prescription or non-prescription (over-the-counter [OTC]) medicine.

Interactions with Food/Tobacco/Alcohol—Certain medicines should not be used at or around the time of eating food or eating certain types of food since interactions may occur. Using alcohol or tobacco with certain medicines may also cause interactions to occur. Discuss with your healthcare professional the use of your medicine with food, alcohol, or tobacco.

Proper Use of This Medicine

This medicine should not be used for irritation caused by contact lenses.

If your eye is red, do not wear your contact lens.

If you wear contact lenses: Take out your contact lenses before using olopatadine eye drops. Wait at least 10 minutes after putting the eye drops in before you put your contact lenses back in only if your eye is not red.

To use the eye drops:

- First, wash your hands. Tilt your head back and, pressing your finger gently on the skin just beneath the lower eyelid, pull the lower eyelid away from the eye to make a space. Drop the medicine into this space. Let go of the eyelid and gently close the eyes. Do not blink. Keep the eyes closed for 1 or 2 minutes to allow the medicine to be absorbed by the eye.
- If you think you did not get the drop of medicine into your eye properly, use another drop.
- To keep the medicine as germ-free as possible, do not touch the applicator tip to any surface (including the eye). Also, keep the container tightly closed.

Dosing—The dose of this medicine will be different for different patients. Follow your doctor's orders or the directions on the label. The following information includes only the av-

erage doses of this medicine. If your dose is different, do not change it unless your doctor tells you to do so.

The amount of medicine that you take depends on the strength of the medicine. Also, the number of doses you take each day, the time allowed between doses, and the length of time you take the medicine depend on the medical problem for which you are using the medicine.

- For ophthalmic dosage form (eye drops):
  - For treatment of allergic conjunctivitis:
    - Adults and children 3 years of age and older—Use one drop (0.1% solution) in each affected eye two times a day, with each dose being at least six to eight hours apart. Or, use one drop (0.2% solution) in each affected eye one time a day.
    - Children up to 3 years of age—Use and dose must be determined by your doctor.

Missed dose—If you miss a dose of this medicine, take it as soon as possible. However, if it is almost time for your next dose, skip the missed dose and go back to your regular dosing schedule. Do not double doses.

Storage—Store the medicine in a closed container at room temperature, away from heat, moisture, and direct light. Keep from freezing.

Keep out of the reach of children.

Do not keep outdated medicine or medicine no longer needed.

Precautions While Using This Medicine

If your symptoms do not improve or if your condition becomes worse, check with your doctor.

Side Effects of This Medicine

Along with its needed effects, a medicine may cause some unwanted effects. Although not all of these side effects may occur, if they do occur they may need medical attention.

Some side effects may occur that usually do not need medical attention. These side effects may go away during treatment as your body adjusts to the medicine. Also, your health care professional may be able to tell you about ways to prevent or reduce some of these side effects. Check with your health care professional if any of the following side effects continue or are bothersome or if you have any questions about them:

More common
Headache; runny or stuffy nose; sore throat

Less common
Back pain; burning, dryness, itching, or stinging of the eye; change in taste; chills; diarrhea; eye irritation or pain; feeling of something in the eye; general feeling of discomfort or illness; increased cough; loss of appetite; muscle aches and pains; nausea; pain; redness of eye or inside of eyelid; shivering; sweating; swelling of eyelid; trouble sleeping; unusual tiredness or weakness; vomiting

Other side effects not listed may also occur in some patients. If you notice any other effects, check with your healthcare professional.

OLSALAZINE   (Oral route) - ole-SAL-a-zeen

Commonly used brand name(s)

In the U.S.—
Dipentum

Available Dosage Forms:
• Capsule

Therapeutic Class: Gastrointestinal Agent

Uses For This Medicine

Olsalazine is used in patients who have had ulcerative colitis to prevent the condition from occurring again. It works inside the bowel by helping to reduce inflammation and other symptoms of the disease.

Olsalazine is available only with your doctor's prescription.

Once a medicine has been approved for marketing for a certain use, experience may show that it is also useful for other medical problems. Although this use is not included in product labeling, olsalazine may be used in certain patients to treat mild or moderate ulcerative colitis.

Before Using This Medicine

In deciding to use a medicine, the risks of taking the medicine must be weighed against the good it will do. This is a decision you and your doctor will make. For this medicine, the following should be considered:

Allergies—Tell your doctor if you have ever had any unusual or allergic reaction to this medicine or any other medicines. Also tell your health care professional if you have any other types of allergies, such as to foods, dyes, preservatives, or animals. For non-prescription products, read the label or package ingredients carefully.

Pediatric—Studies on this medicine have been done only in adult patients, and there is no specific information comparing use of olsalazine in children with use in other age groups.

Geriatric—Many medicines have not been studied specifically in older people. Therefore, it may not be known whether they work exactly the same way they do in younger adults. Although there is no specific information comparing use of olsalazine in the elderly with use in other age groups, this medicine is not expected to cause different side effects or problems in older people than it does in younger adults.

Pregnancy—

	Pregnancy Category	Explanation
All Trimesters	C	Animal studies have shown an adverse effect and there are no adequate studies in pregnant women OR no animal studies have been conducted and there are no adequate studies in pregnant women.

Breast Feeding—Studies in women breastfeeding have demonstrated harmful infant effects. An alternative to this medication should be prescribed or you should stop breast-feeding while using this medicine.

Other medicines—

Using this medicine with any of the following medicines is usually not recommended, but may be required in some cases. If both medicines are prescribed together, your doctor may change the dose or how often you use one or both of the medicines.

Varicella Virus Vaccine

Interactions with Food/Tobacco/Alcohol—Certain medicines should not be used at or around the time of eating food or eating certain types of food since interactions may occur. Using alcohol or tobacco with certain medicines may also cause interactions to occur. Discuss with your healthcare professional the use of your medicine with food, alcohol, or tobacco.

Other medical problems—The presence of other medical problems may affect the use of this medicine. Make sure you tell your doctor if you have any other medical problems, especially:
• Kidney disease—The use of olsalazine may cause further damage to the kidneys

Proper Use of This Medicine

Olsalazine is best taken with food, to lessen stomach upset. If stomach or intestinal problems continue or are bothersome, check with your doctor.

Keep taking this medicine for the full time of treatment, even if you begin to feel better after a few days. Do not miss any doses.

Dosing—The dose of this medicine will be different for different patients. Follow your doctor's orders or the directions on the label. The following information includes only the average doses of this medicine. If your dose is different, do not change it unless your doctor tells you to do so.

The amount of medicine that you take depends on the strength of the medicine. Also, the number of doses you take each day, the time allowed between doses, and the length of time you take the medicine depend on the medical problem for which you are using the medicine.

• For oral dosage form (capsules):
  ○ To prevent ulcerative colitis from occurring again:
    ▪ Adults and teenagers—500 milligrams (mg) two times a day.
    ▪ Children—Use and dose must be determined by your doctor.

Missed dose—If you miss a dose of this medicine, take it as soon as possible. However, if it is almost time for your next dose, skip the missed dose and go back to your regular dosing schedule. Do not double doses.

Storage—Store the medicine in a closed container at room temperature, away from heat, moisture, and direct light. Keep from freezing.

Keep out of the reach of children.

Do not keep outdated medicine or medicine no longer needed.

Precautions While Using This Medicine

It is very important that your doctor check your progress at regular visits, especially if you will be taking olsalazine for a long time.

Side Effects of This Medicine

Along with its needed effects, a medicine may cause some unwanted effects. Although not all of these side effects may occur, if they do occur they may need medical attention.

Check with your doctor as soon as possible if any of the following side effects occur:

Rare
> Back or stomach pain (severe); bloody diarrhea; fast heartbeat; fever; nausea or vomiting; skin rash; swelling of the stomach; yellow eyes or skin

Some side effects may occur that usually do not need medical attention. These side effects may go away during treatment as your body adjusts to the medicine. Also, your health care professional may be able to tell you about ways to prevent or reduce some of these side effects. Check with your health care professional if any of the following side effects continue or are bothersome or if you have any questions about them:

More common
> Abdominal or stomach pain or upset; diarrhea; loss of appetite

Less common
> Aching joints and muscles; acne; anxiety or depression; dizziness or drowsiness; headache; trouble in sleeping

Other side effects not listed may also occur in some patients. If you notice any other effects, check with your healthcare professional.

OMALIZUMAB (Subcutaneous route) -
oh-mah-LYE-zoo-mab

Commonly used brand name(s)

In the U.S.—
> Xolair

Available Dosage Forms:
- Powder for Solution

Therapeutic Class: Antiasthma
Pharmacologic Class: Monoclonal Antibody

Uses For This Medicine

Omalizumab is used to treat moderate to severe persistent allergic asthma. Omalizumab is a shot (injection) given under the skin (subcutaneous) The shot is given every 2 or 4 weeks. For many patients who still have asthma symptoms even though they are taking inhaled steroids, omalizumab helps to reduce the number of asthma attacks.

Omalizumab is a medicine called an IgE blocker. IgE is short for immunoglobulin E. IgE is a substance that occurs naturally in the body in small amounts. This substance plays an important role in allergic asthma. When people with allergic asthma breathe in a year-round allergen, such as cat or dog dander, their bodies make more IgE. This may cause a series of reactions in your body that can lead to asthma attacks and symptoms. Omalizumab works by helping to block IgE.

This medicine is available only with your doctor's prescription.

Before Using This Medicine

In deciding to use a medicine, the risks of taking the medicine must be weighed against the good it will do. This is a decision you and your doctor will make. For this medicine, the following should be considered:

Allergies—Tell your doctor if you have ever had any unusual or allergic reaction to this medicine or any other medicines. Also tell your health care professional if you have any other types of allergies, such as to foods, dyes, preservatives, or animals. For non-prescription products, read the label or package ingredients carefully.

Pediatric—Although there is no specific information comparing the use of omalizumab in children with other age groups, this medicine is not expected to cause different side effects or problems in children than it does in older adults. This medicine can be used in children 12 years of age and older.

Geriatric—Many medicines have not been specifically studied in older people. Therefore, it may not be known whether they work exactly the same way they do in younger adults or if they cause different side effects or problems in older people. There is no specific information comparing the use of omalizumab in the elderly with use in other age groups.

Pregnancy—

	Pregnancy Category	Explanation
All Trimesters	B	Animal studies have revealed no evidence of harm to the fetus, however, there are no adequate studies in pregnant women OR animal studies have shown an adverse effect, but adequate studies in pregnant women have failed to demonstrate a risk to the fetus.

Breast Feeding—There are no adequate studies in women for determining infant risk when using this medication during breastfeeding. Weigh the potential benefits against the potential risks before taking this medication while breastfeeding.

Other medicines—Although certain medicines should not be used together at all, in other cases two different medicines may be used together even if an interaction might occur. In these cases, your doctor may want to change the dose, or other precautions may be necessary. Tell your healthcare professional if you are taking any other prescription or nonprescription (over-the-counter [OTC]) medicine.

Interactions with Food/Tobacco/Alcohol—Certain medicines should not be used at or around the time of eating food or eating certain types of food since interactions may occur. Using alcohol or tobacco with certain medicines may also cause interactions to occur. Discuss with your healthcare professional the use of your medicine with food, alcohol, or tobacco.

Proper Use of This Medicine

Dosing—The dose of this medicine will be different for different patients. Follow your doctor's orders or the directions on the label. The following information includes only the average doses of this medicine. If your dose is different, do not change it unless your doctor tells you to do so.

The amount of medicine that you take depends on the strength of the medicine. Also, the number of doses you take each day, the time allowed between doses, and the length of time you take the medicine depend on the medical problem for which you are using the medicine.

You will receive omalizumab once every 2 or 4 weeks. Your dose will be determined by your IgE level, which your doctor will measure with a simple blood test before treatment begins, and your body weight. Based on your dose, your doctor will also tell you if you will need 1, 2, or 3 injections per dose. If you need more than 1 injection, each will be given in a different place on your body.

Omalizumab is not a rescue medication and should not be used to treat sudden asthma attacks. It is not a substitute for the medicines you are already taking. Never suddenly stop taking, or change the dose of, your inhaled steroids or any other asthma medicine you are taking unless your doctor tells you to do so.

- For parenteral dosage form (injection):
  - For allergic asthma:
    - Adults—150 to 375 milligrams (mg) is administered by a shot (injection) under the skin every 2 or 4 weeks.
    - Children—Use and dose for children under 12 years of age must be determined by your doctor.

Precautions While Using This Medicine

If you stop receiving omalizumab injections, your symptoms can be expected to return.

You may not see immediate improvement in your asthma after omalizumab treatment begins. It takes time for the medicine to work. So if you don't feel a difference right away, it doesn't mean omalizumab is not working. It is important to continue your omalizumab injections until your doctor tells you otherwise.

It is important to know the signs of an allergic reaction to this medicine and to know what to do. Get medical help immediately if you have any symptoms such as rash, itching, and swelling of the tongue and throat.

Your doctor will ask you to remain at the healthcare facility or clinic for a period of time after each injection to watch for immediate side effects that can be serious.

Side Effects of This Medicine

Along with its needed effects, a medicine may cause some unwanted effects. Although not all of these side effects may occur, if they do occur they may need medical attention.

Check with your doctor immediately if any of the following side effects occur:
  Rare
    Cough; difficulty swallowing; dizziness; fast heartbeat; hives; itching; malignant tumor; puffiness or swelling of the eyelids or around the eyes, face, lips or tongue; shortness of breath; skin rash; tightness in chest; unusual tiredness or weakness; wheezing

Some side effects may occur that usually do not need medical attention. These side effects may go away during treatment as your body adjusts to the medicine. Also, your health care professional may be able to tell you about ways to prevent or reduce some of these side effects. Check with your health care professional if any of the following side effects continue or are bothersome or if you have any questions about them:
  More common
    Bleeding; blistering; body aches or pain; burning; chills; cold or flu-like symptoms; coldness; congestion; discoloration of skin; dryness or soreness of throat; feeling of pressure; fever; headache; hoarseness; infection; inflammation; itching; leg pain; lumps; muscle or joint pain; numbness; pain; pain or tenderness around eyes and cheekbones; redness; runny nose; scarring; shortness of breath or troubled breathing; sore throat; soreness; stinging; stuffy or runny nose; swelling; tender, swollen glands in neck; tenderness; tingling; trouble in swallowing; ulceration; voice changes; warmth
  Less common or uncommon
    Arm pain; blistering, crusting, irritation, itching, or reddening of skim; body produces substance that can bind to drug making it less effective or cause side effects; cracked, dry, scaly skin; earache; itching skin

Other side effects not listed may also occur in some patients. If you notice any other effects, check with your healthcare professional.

OMEGA-3 ACID ETHYL ESTERS
(Oral route) - oh-ME-ga 3 AS-id ETH-il ES-ters

Commonly used brand name(s)

In the U.S.—
  Omacor

Available Dosage Forms:
- Capsule, Liquid Filled

Therapeutic Class: Antihyperlipidemic

Uses For This Medicine

Omega-3–acid ethyl esters are used to lower very high triglyceride (fat-like substance) levels in the blood. This may help prevent medical problems caused by this substance clogging the blood vessels.

This medicine is available only with your doctor's prescription.

Before Using This Medicine

In deciding to use a medicine, the risks of taking the medicine must be weighed against the good it will do. This is a decision

you and your doctor will make. For this medicine, the following should be considered:

Allergies—Tell your doctor if you have ever had any unusual or allergic reaction to this medicine or any other medicines. Also tell your health care professional if you have any other types of allergies, such as to foods, dyes, preservatives, or animals. For non-prescription products, read the label or package ingredients carefully.

Pediatric—Studies on omega-3–acid ethyl esters have been done only in adult patients and there is no specific information comparing use of omega-3–acid ethyl esters in children with use in other age groups.

Geriatric—This medicine has been tested in a limited number of patients 65 years of age or older and has not been shown to cause different problems in older people than it does in younger adults.

Pregnancy—

	Pregnancy Category	Explanation
All Trimesters	C	Animal studies have shown an adverse effect and there are no adequate studies in pregnant women OR no animal studies have been conducted and there are no adequate studies in pregnant women.

Breast Feeding—There are no adequate studies in women for determining infant risk when using this medication during breastfeeding. Weigh the potential benefits against the potential risks before taking this medication while breastfeeding.

Other medicines—Although certain medicines should not be used together at all, in other cases two different medicines may be used together even if an interaction might occur. In these cases, your doctor may want to change the dose, or other precautions may be necessary. Tell your healthcare professional if you are taking any other prescription or non-prescription (over-the-counter [OTC]) medicine.

Interactions with Food/Tobacco/Alcohol—Certain medicines should not be used at or around the time of eating food or eating certain types of food since interactions may occur. Using alcohol or tobacco with certain medicines may also cause interactions to occur. Discuss with your healthcare professional the use of your medicine with food, alcohol, or tobacco.

Proper Use of This Medicine

Use this medicine only as directed by your doctor. Do not use more or less of it, and do not use it more often or for a longer time than your doctor ordered.

Remember that this medicine will not cure your condition but it does help control it. Therefore, you must continue to take it as directed if you expect to keep your triglyceride levels down.

Before prescribing medicine for your condition your doctor will probably try to control your condition prescribing a personal diet for you. Follow carefullly the special diet your doctor gave you. Such a diet may be low in fats, sugars, and/or cholesterol. Many people are able to control their condition by carefully following their doctor's orders for proper diet and exercise. Medicine is prescribed only when additional help is needed and is effective only when a schedule of diet and

exercise is properly followed. Also, this medicine is less effective if you are greatly overweight. It may be very important for you to go on a weight-reducing diet. However, check with your doctor before going on any diet.

This medicine may be taken with meals.

Dosing—The dose of this medicine will be different for different patients. Follow your doctor's orders or the directions on the label. The following information includes only the average doses of this medicine. If your dose is different, do not change it unless your doctor tells you to do so.

The amount of medicine that you take depends on the strength of the medicine. Also, the number of doses you take each day, the time allowed between doses, and the length of time you take the medicine depend on the medical problem for which you are using the medicine.

- For oral dosage form (capsules):
  - For high triglycerides:
    - Adults—4 grams (g) daily.
    - Children—Use and dose must be determined by your doctor.

Missed dose—If you miss a dose of this medicine, take it as soon as possible. However, if it is almost time for your next dose, skip the missed dose and go back to your regular dosing schedule. Do not double doses.

Storage—Store the medicine in a closed container at room temperature, away from heat, moisture, and direct light. Do not refrigerate. Keep from freezing.

Keep out of the reach of children.

Do not keep outdated medicine or medicine no longer needed.

Ask your healthcare professional how you should dispose of any medicine you do not use.

Precautions While Using This Medicine

It is very important that your doctor check your progress at regular visits. This will allow your doctor to see if the medicine is working properly to lower triglyceride levels and to decide if you should continue to take it.

Compliance with prescribed diet during treatment.

Side Effects of This Medicine

Along with its needed effects, a medicine may cause some unwanted effects. Although not all of these side effects may occur, if they do occur they may need medical attention.

Check with your doctor immediately if any of the following side effects occur:

More common

Arm, back or jaw pain; chest pain or discomfort; chest tightness or heaviness; difficult or labored breathing; fast or irregular heartbeat; nausea; shortness of breath; sweating; tightness in chest; wheezing

Some side effects may occur that usually do not need medical attention. These side effects may go away during treatment as your body adjusts to the medicine. Also, your health care professional may be able to tell you about ways to prevent or reduce some of these side effects. Check with your health care professional if any of the following side effects

continue or are bothersome or if you have any questions about them:

Less common

> Back pain; bad unusual or unpleasant (after)taste; belching; bloated full feeling; change in taste; chills; cough; diarrhea; excess air or gas in stomach; fever; general feeling of discomfort or illness; headache; hoarseness; joint pain; loss of appetite; lower back or side pain; muscle aches and pains; pain; painful or difficult urination; rash; runny nose; shivering; sore throat; sweating; trouble sleeping; unusual tiredness or weakness; vomiting

Other side effects not listed may also occur in some patients. If you notice any other effects, check with your healthcare professional.

OMEPRAZOLE   (Oral route) - oh-ME-pray-zol

Commonly used brand name(s)

In the U.S.—
> Prilosec
> Prilosec OTC

Available Dosage Forms:

- Capsule, Delayed Release
- Tablet, Delayed Release

Therapeutic Class: Antiulcer
Pharmacologic Class: Proton Pump Inhibitor

Uses For This Medicine

Omeprazole is used to treat certain conditions in which there is too much acid in the stomach. It is used to treat gastric and duodenal ulcers and gastroesophageal reflux disease, a condition in which the acid in the stomach washes back up into the esophagus. Sometimes omeprazole is used in combination with antibiotics to treat ulcers associated with infection caused by the H. pylori bacteria (germ).

Omeprazole is also used to treat Zollinger-Ellison disease, a condition in which the stomach produces too much acid.

Omeprazole is also used to treat dyspepsia, a condition that causes sour stomach, belching, heart burn, or indigestion.

In addition, omeprazole is used to prevent upper gastrointestinal tract bleeding in seriously ill patients.

Omeprazole works by decreasing the amount of acid produced by the stomach.

This medicine is available only with your doctor's prescription.

Before Using This Medicine

In deciding to use a medicine, the risks of taking the medicine must be weighed against the good it will do. This is a decision you and your doctor will make. For this medicine, the following should be considered:

Allergies—Tell your doctor if you have ever had any unusual or allergic reaction to this medicine or any other medicines. Also tell your health care professional if you have any other types of allergies, such as to foods, dyes, preservatives, or animals. For non-prescription products, read the label or package ingredients carefully.

Pediatric—There is no specific information comparing the use of omeprazole in children with use in other age groups.

Geriatric—Many medicines have not been studied specifically in older people. Therefore, it may not be known whether they work exactly the same way they do in younger adults or if they cause different side effects or problems in older people. There is no specific information comparing use of omeprazole in the elderly with use in other age groups.

Pregnancy—

	Pregnancy Category	Explanation
All Trimesters	C	Animal studies have shown an adverse effect and there are no adequate studies in pregnant women OR no animal studies have been conducted and there are no adequate studies in pregnant women.

Breast Feeding—There are no adequate studies in women for determining infant risk when using this medication during breastfeeding. Weigh the potential benefits against the potential risks before taking this medication while breastfeeding.

Other medicines—

Using this medicine with any of the following medicines is usually not recommended, but may be required in some cases. If both medicines are prescribed together, your doctor may change the dose or how often you use one or both of the medicines.

Atazanavir, Clorazepate, Delavirdine, Methotrexate

Interactions with Food/Tobacco/Alcohol—Certain medicines should not be used at or around the time of eating food or eating certain types of food since interactions may occur. Using alcohol or tobacco with certain medicines may also cause interactions to occur. Discuss with your healthcare professional the use of your medicine with food, alcohol, or tobacco.

Other medical problems—The presence of other medical problems may affect the use of this medicine. Make sure you tell your doctor if you have any other medical problems, especially:

- Liver disease or a history of liver disease—This condition may cause omeprazole to build up in the body

Proper Use of This Medicine

Take omeprazole *capsules* immediately before a meal, preferably in the morning. Omeprazole *tablets* may be taken with food or on an empty stomach. Take omeprazole *powder for oral suspension* on an empty stomach at least 1 hour before a meal. For patients receiving continuous feeding through a tube, feeding should be temporarily stopped about 3 hours before and 1 hour after administration of omeprazole *powder for oral suspension.*

It may take several days before this medicine begins to relieve stomach pain. To help relieve this pain, antacids may be taken with omeprazole, unless your doctor has told you not to use them.

Swallow the capsule and tablet forms of omeprazole whole. Do not open the capsule. Do not crush, break, or chew the capsule or the tablet.

To use the powder for oral suspension:

- Empty packet of powder into a small cup containing 2 tablespoons of water
- Do not use other liquids or foods
- Stir well and drink immediately
- Refill cup with water and drink

Take this medicine for the full time of treatment, even if you begin to feel better. Also, keep your appointments with your doctor for check-ups so that your doctor will be better able to tell you when to stop taking this medicine.

Dosing—The dose of this medicine will be different for different patients. Follow your doctor's orders or the directions on the label. The following information includes only the average doses of this medicine. If your dose is different, do not change it unless your doctor tells you to do so.

The amount of medicine that you take depends on the strength of the medicine. Also, the number of doses you take each day, the time allowed between doses, and the length of time you take the medicine depend on the medical problem for which you are using the medicine.

- For oral dosage forms (capsules, tablets):
  - To treat dyspepsia:
    - Adults—20 milligrams (mg) taken once a day for four weeks. Patients may respond adequately to 10 mg once daily, so individual dose adjustment may be considered.
    - Children—Use and dose must be determined by your doctor.
  - To treat gastroesophageal reflux disease (GERD):
    - Adults—20 milligrams (mg) taken once a day for four to eight weeks. Or your doctor may tell you to take 40 mg a day for certain conditions. Also, your doctor may want you to take omeprazole for more than eight weeks for certain conditions.
    - Children—Use and dose must be determined by your doctor.
  - To treat conditions in which the stomach produces too much acid:
    - Adults—60 mg taken once a day. Your doctor may change the dose as needed. Your treatment may be continued for as long as it is needed.
    - Children—Use and dose must be determined by your doctor.
  - To treat duodenal ulcers:
    - Adults—20 mg taken once a day. Or your doctor may tell you to take 40 mg a day for certain conditions.
    - Children—Use and dose must be determined by your doctor.
  - To treat gastric ulcers:
    - Adults—40 mg taken once a day for four to eight weeks.
    - Children—Use and dose must be determined by your doctor.
  - To treat ulcers related to infection with H. pylori:
    - Adults—40 mg once a day, taken along with clarithromycin 500 mg three times a day, for the first fourteen days. For days 15 through 28, omeprazole 20 mg taken once a day.

- Children—Use and dose must be determined by your doctor.
- For oral dosage form (powder for suspension):
  - To prevent upper gastrointestinal tract bleeding in seriously ill patients:
    - Adults—The first day: 40 milligrams (mg) for the first dose; then after 6 to 8 hours, a second 40 mg dose. After the first day: 40 mg once a day for up to 14 days.
    - Children—Use and dose must be determined by your doctor.
  - To treat duodenal ulcer:
    - Adults—20 milligrams (mg) taken once a day for four to eight weeks.
    - Children—Use and dose must be determined by your doctor.
  - To treat gastric ulcers:
    - Adults—40 mg taken once a day for four to eight weeks.
    - Children—Use and dose must be determined by your doctor.
  - To treat gastroesophageal reflux disease (GERD) for erosive esophagitis:
    - Adults—20 mg taken once a day for four to eight weeks.
    - Children—Use and dose must be determined by your doctor.

Missed dose—If you miss a dose of this medicine, take it as soon as possible. However, if it is almost time for your next dose, skip the missed dose and go back to your regular dosing schedule. Do not double doses.

Storage—Store the medicine in a closed container at room temperature, away from heat, moisture, and direct light. Keep from freezing.

Keep out of the reach of children.

Do not keep outdated medicine or medicine no longer needed.

Precautions While Using This Medicine

It is important that your doctor check your progress at regular visits. If your condition does not improve, or if it becomes worse, check with your doctor.

Side Effects of This Medicine

Along with its needed effects, a medicine may cause some unwanted effects. Although not all of these side effects may occur, if they do occur they may need medical attention.

Check with your doctor as soon as possible if any of the following side effects occur:

Rare

Back, leg, or stomach pain; bleeding or crusting sores on lips; blisters; bloody or cloudy urine; chills; continuing ulcers or sores in mouth; difficult, burning, or painful urination; fever; frequent urge to urinate; general feeling of discomfort or illness; joint pain; loss of appetite; muscle aches or cramps; pain; red or irritated eyes; redness, tenderness, itching, burning, or peeling of skin; skin rash or itching; sore throat; sores, ulcers, or white spots on lips, in mouth, or on genitals; unusual bleeding or bruising; unusual tiredness or weakness

Symptoms of overdose

Blurred vision; confusion; drowsiness; dryness of mouth; fast or irregular heartbeat; flushing; general feeling of discomfort or illness; headache; increased sweating; nausea; vomiting

Some side effects may occur that usually do not need medical attention. These side effects may go away during treatment as your body adjusts to the medicine. Also, your health care professional may be able to tell you about ways to prevent or reduce some of these side effects. Check with your health care professional if any of the following side effects continue or are bothersome or if you have any questions about them:

More common

Abdominal or stomach pain

Less common

Back pain; body aches or pain; chest pain; constipation; cough; diarrhea or loose stools; difficulty in breathing; dizziness; ear congestion; gas; headache; heartburn; loss of voice; muscle pain; nasal congestion; nausea and vomiting; runny nose; skin rash or itching; sneezing; unusual drowsiness; unusual tiredness

Other side effects not listed may also occur in some patients. If you notice any other effects, check with your healthcare professional.

ONDANSETRON (Oral route, Injection route, Intravenous route) - on-DAN-se-tron

Commonly used brand name(s)

In the U.S.—

Zofran

Zofran ODT

Available Dosage Forms:

- Tablet, Disintegrating
- Solution
- Tablet

Therapeutic Class: Antiemetic

Pharmacologic Class: Serotonin Receptor Antagonist, 5–HT3

Uses For This Medicine

Ondansetron is used to prevent the nausea and vomiting that may occur after therapy with anticancer medicines (chemotherapy) or radiation, or after surgery.

Ondansetron is available only with your doctor's prescription.

Before Using This Medicine

In deciding to use a medicine, the risks of taking the medicine must be weighed against the good it will do. This is a decision you and your doctor will make. For this medicine, the following should be considered:

Allergies—Tell your doctor if you have ever had any unusual or allergic reaction to this medicine or any other medicines. Also tell your health care professional if you have any other types of allergies, such as to foods, dyes, preservatives, or animals. For non-prescription products, read the label or package ingredients carefully.

Pediatric—This medicine has been tested in a limited number of children with cancer 6 months of age or older and after surgery in children 1 month to 12 years of age. In effective doses, the medicine has not been shown to cause different side effects or problems than it does in adults.

Geriatric—This medicine has been tested in a limited number of cancer patients 65 years of age or older and has not been shown to cause different side effects or problems in older people than it does in younger adults.

Pregnancy—

	Pregnancy Category	Explanation
All Trimesters	B	Animal studies have revealed no evidence of harm to the fetus, however, there are no adequate studies in pregnant women OR animal studies have shown an adverse effect, but adequate studies in pregnant women have failed to demonstrate a risk to the fetus.

Breast Feeding—There are no adequate studies in women for determining infant risk when using this medication during breastfeeding. Weigh the potential benefits against the potential risks before taking this medication while breastfeeding.

Other medicines—

Using this medicine with any of the following medicines is not recommended. Your doctor may decide not to treat you with this medication or change some of the other medicines you take.

Apomorphine, Mesoridazine, Pimozide, Thioridazine

Interactions with Food/Tobacco/Alcohol—Certain medicines should not be used at or around the time of eating food or eating certain types of food since interactions may occur. Using alcohol or tobacco with certain medicines may also cause interactions to occur. Discuss with your healthcare professional the use of your medicine with food, alcohol, or tobacco.

Other medical problems—The presence of other medical problems may affect the use of this medicine. Make sure you tell your doctor if you have any other medical problems, especially:

- Abdominal surgery—Use of ondansetron may cover up stomach problems

- Allergy to selective 5–HT3 receptor antagonists (alosetron [e.g., Lotronex], dolasetron [e.g., Anzemet], granisetron [e.g., Kytril], palonosetron [e.g., Aloxi])—If you are allergic to one of these, you may be allergic to ondansetron because they are in the same group of medicines.

- Liver disease—Patients with liver disease may have an increased chance of side effects

- Phenylketonuria (PKU)—The oral disintegrating tablets may contain aspartame, which can make your condition worse.

Proper Use of This Medicine

If you vomit within 30 minutes after taking this medicine, take the same amount of medicine again. If vomiting continues, check with your doctor.

For patients using the oral disintegrating tablet form of this medicine:

- Make sure your hands are dry.
- Do not push the tablet through the foil backing of the package. Instead, gently peel back the foil backing and remove the tablet.
- Immediately place the tablet on top of the tongue.
- The tablet will dissolve in seconds, and you may swallow it with your saliva. You do not need to drink water or other liquid to swallow the tablet.

Dosing—The dose of this medicine will be different for different patients. Follow your doctor's orders or the directions on the label. The following information includes only the average doses of this medicine. If your dose is different, do not change it unless your doctor tells you to do so.

The amount of medicine that you take depends on the strength of the medicine. Also, the number of doses you take each day, the time allowed between doses, and the length of time you take the medicine depend on the medical problem for which you are using the medicine.

- For oral dosage forms (solution, oral disintegrating tablets, and tablets):
  - For prevention of moderate nausea and vomiting after anticancer medicine:
    - Adults and children 12 years of age and older—At first, the dose is 8 milligrams (mg) taken thirty minutes before the anticancer medicine is given. The 8–mg dose is taken again eight hours after the first dose. Then, the dose is 8 mg every twelve hours for one to two days.
    - Children 4 to 11 years of age—At first, the dose is 4 mg taken thirty minutes before the anticancer medicine is given. The 4–mg dose is taken again four and eight hours after the first dose. Then, the dose is 4 mg every eight hours for one to two days.
    - Children up to 4 years of age—Dose must be determined by your doctor.
  - For prevention of more severe nausea and vomiting after anticancer medicine:
    - Adults and children 12 years of age and older—One 24–milligram (mg) tablet taken thirty minutes before the anticancer medicine is given.
    - Children up to 12 years of age—Use and dose must be determined by your doctor.
  - For prevention of nausea and vomiting after surgery:
    - Adults—Dose is usually 16 mg one hour before anesthesia (medicine to put you to sleep before surgery).
    - Children—Dose must be determined by your doctor.
  - For prevention of nausea and vomiting after radiation treatment:
    - Adults—At first, the dose is 8 mg taken one to two hours before radiation treatment. Then, the dose is 8 mg every eight hours.
    - Children—Dose must be determined by your doctor.
- For injection dosage form:
  - For prevention of nausea and vomiting after anticancer medicine:
    - Adults—Dose is usually 32 mg injected into a vein, over a period of fifteen minutes, beginning thirty minutes before the anticancer medicine is given. Or, if the dose is based on body weight, it

is usually 150 micrograms (mcg) per kilogram (kg) (68 mcg per pound) of body weight. This dose is injected into a vein over a period of fifteen minutes, beginning thirty minutes before the anticancer medicine is given. It is injected again four and eight hours after the first dose.

- Children 6 months to 18 years of age—Dose is based on body weight and must be determined by your doctor. It is usually 150 mcg per kg (68 mcg per pound) of body weight, injected into a vein over a period of fifteen minutes, beginning thirty minutes before the anticancer medicine is given. The dose is given again four and eight hours after the first dose.
- Children up to 6 months of age—Dose must be determined by your doctor.
  - For prevention of nausea and vomiting after surgery:
- Adults—Dose is usually 4 mg injected into a vein over a period of thirty seconds to five minutes. It is given just before anesthesia (medicine to put you to sleep before surgery) or right after surgery if nausea and vomiting begin.
- Children 1 month to 12 years of age—Dose is based on body weight and must be determined by your doctor. It is usually 100 mcg per kg (45.5 mcg per pound) of body weight for children weighing 40 kg or less (88 pounds or less), or 4 mg for children weighing over 40 kg (over 88 pounds). The dose is injected into a vein over a period of thirty seconds to five minutes. It is given just before anesthesia or after surgery if nausea and vomiting begin.
- Children up to 1 month of age—Dose must be determined by your doctor.

Missed dose—If you miss a dose of this medicine, skip the missed dose and go back to your regular dosing schedule. Do not double doses.

If you miss a dose of this medicine, and you feel nauseated or you vomit, take the missed dose as soon as possible.

Storage—Store the medicine in a closed container at room temperature, away from heat, moisture, and direct light. Keep from freezing.

Keep out of the reach of children.

Do not keep outdated medicine or medicine no longer needed.

Side Effects of This Medicine

Along with its needed effects, a medicine may cause some unwanted effects. Although not all of these side effects may occur, if they do occur they may need medical attention.

Check with your doctor immediately if any of the following side effects occur:
Rare

Chest pain or discomfort; pain, redness, or burning at place of injection; shortness of breath; skin rash, hives, redness, and/or itching; tightness in chest; troubled breathing; wheezing

Incidence not known

Blurred vision; cold, clammy skin; confusion; coughing; decreased or irregular heartbeat; difficulty in breathing or swallowing; dizziness or fainting; dizziness, faintness, or lightheadedness when getting up from a lying position; fast, pounding, slow, or irregular heartbeat or pulse; fast, weak pulse; fixed position of eye; heart stops; hives or welts; hoarseness; inability to move eyes; increased blinking or spasms of eyelid; lab results that show problems with liver; large, hive-like swelling on face, eyelids, lips, tongue, throat, hands, legs, feet, sex organs; lightheadedness; no breathing; no pulse or blood pressure; noisy breathing; pain in neck, back, or jaw; palpitations; shortness of breath; slow or irregular breathing; sticking out of tongue; sweating; swelling of face, throat, or tongue; trouble in breathing, speaking, or swallowing; unconscious; uncontrolled twisting movements of neck, trunk, arms, or legs; unusual facial expressions; weakness; weakness of arms and legs

Some side effects may occur that usually do not need medical attention. These side effects may go away during treatment as your body adjusts to the medicine. Also, your health care professional may be able to tell you about ways to prevent or reduce some of these side effects. Check with your health care professional if any of the following side effects continue or are bothersome or if you have any questions about them:

More common
Constipation; diarrhea; fever; headache

Less common
Abdominal pain or stomach cramps; burning, tingling, or prickling sensations; dizziness or lightheadedness; drowsiness; dryness of mouth; feeling cold; itching; unusual tiredness or weakness

Other side effects not listed may also occur in some patients. If you notice any other effects, check with your healthcare professional.

ORLISTAT (Oral route) - OR-li-stat

Commonly used brand name(s)
In the U.S.—
Xenical

Available Dosage Forms:
- Capsule

Therapeutic Class: Dietary Fat Absorption Inhibitor
Pharmacologic Class: Lipase Inhibitor

Uses For This Medicine

Orlistat is used as an aid to help you lose weight. The medicine prevents the digestion of some of the fat you eat. Fats that are not digested cannot be absorbed and therefore do not contribute calories. To give the greatest weight loss, orlistat must be used with a weight-reduction diet.

Orlistat is available only with your doctor's prescription.

Before Using This Medicine

In deciding to use a medicine, the risks of taking the medicine must be weighed against the good it will do. This is a decision you and your doctor will make. For this medicine, the following should be considered:

Allergies—Tell your doctor if you have ever had any unusual or allergic reaction to this medicine or any other medicines. Also tell your health care professional if you have any other types of allergies, such as to foods, dyes, preservatives, or animals. For non-prescription products, read the label or package ingredients carefully.

Pediatric—Studies on this medicine have been done only in adult patients, and there is no specific information comparing use of orlistat in children with use in other age groups.

Geriatric—There is no specific information comparing use of orlistat in the elderly with use in younger adults. However, this medicine is not expected to cause different side effects or problems in older people than it does in younger adults.

Pregnancy—

	Pregnancy Category	Explanation
All Trimesters	B	Animal studies have revealed no evidence of harm to the fetus, however, there are no adequate studies in pregnant women OR animal studies have shown an adverse effect, but adequate studies in pregnant women have failed to demonstrate a risk to the fetus.

Breast Feeding—There are no adequate studies in women for determining infant risk when using this medication during breastfeeding. Weigh the potential benefits against the potential risks before taking this medication while breastfeeding.

Other medicines—

Using this medicine with any of the following medicines is usually not recommended, but may be required in some cases. If both medicines are prescribed together, your doctor may change the dose or how often you use one or both of the medicines.

Cyclosporine

Interactions with Food/Tobacco/Alcohol—Certain medicines should not be used at or around the time of eating food or eating certain types of food since interactions may occur. Using alcohol or tobacco with certain medicines may also cause interactions to occur. Discuss with your healthcare professional the use of your medicine with food, alcohol, or tobacco.

Other medical problems—The presence of other medical problems may affect the use of this medicine. Make sure you tell your doctor if you have any other medical problems, especially:
- Kidney stones or
- Gallbladder problems—Orlistat may make the condition worse

Proper Use of This Medicine

Orlistat prevents the absorption of some of the fat you eat. Therefore, you should take it during the meal or within 1 hour of eating. If you occasionally miss a meal or eat a meal that contains no fat, you should skip the dose of orlistat.

Because orlistat may decrease the amount of some vitamins that your body can absorb from food, you will need to take a multivitamin supplement once a day. Take the vitamin supplement at least 2 hours before or after taking orlistat.

When using orlistat, your diet should contain no more than 30% of calories as fat. More fat in your diet will increase the side effects of this medicine. Your diet should be nutritionally balanced, and your daily intake of fat, carbohydrates, and protein should be distributed over three main meals.

Dosing—The dose of this medicine will be different for different patients. Follow your doctor's orders or the directions on the label. The following information includes only the average doses of this medicine. If your dose is different, do not change it unless your doctor tells you to do so.

The amount of medicine that you take depends on the strength of the medicine. Also, the number of doses you take each day, the time allowed between doses, and the length of time you take the medicine depend on the medical problem for which you are using the medicine.

- For oral dosage form (capsules):
  - For treatment of obesity:
    - Adults—120 milligrams (mg) three times a day with meals containing fat.
    - Children—Use and dose must be determined by your doctor.

Missed dose—If you miss a dose of this medicine, skip the missed dose and go back to your regular dosing schedule. Do not double doses.

Storage—Store the medicine in a closed container at room temperature, away from heat, moisture, and direct light. Keep from freezing.

Keep out of the reach of children.

Do not keep outdated medicine or medicine no longer needed.

Precautions While Using This Medicine

It is very important that your doctor check your progress at regular visits to make sure that this medicine is working properly and to check for unwanted effects.

For patients with diabetes: Weight loss may result in an improvement in your condition, and your doctor may need to change your dose of oral diabetes medicine or insulin.

Side Effects of This Medicine

Along with its needed effects, a medicine may cause some unwanted effects. Although not all of these side effects may occur, if they do occur they may need medical attention.

Check with your doctor as soon as possible if any of the following side effects occur:

More common
Bodyache; chills; cough; fever; headache; nasal congestion; runny nose; sneezing; sore throat

Less common
Tightness in chest; tooth or gum problems; troubled breathing; wheezing

Rare
Bloody or cloudy urine; change in hearing; contagious diarrhea; difficult or painful urination; earache; frequent urge to urinate; pain in ear

Other side effects may occur that usually do not need medical attention. These side effects may go away during treatment as your body adjusts to the medicine. However, check with your doctor if any of the following side effects continue or are bothersome:

More common
Gas with leaky bowel movements; inability to hold bowel movement; increases in bowel movements; oily bowel movements; oily spotting of underclothes

Less common
Anxiety; back pain; menstrual changes; rectal pain or discomfort

After you stop using this medicine, your body may need time to adjust. Side effects caused by orlistat usually disappear within 2 to 3 days after stopping it.

Other side effects not listed may also occur in some patients. If you notice any other effects, check with your healthcare professional.

ORPHENADRINE (Oral route, Injection route) - or-FEN-a-dreen

Commonly used brand name(s)

In the U.S.—

Antiflex	Orfro
Mio-Rel	Orphenate
Norflex	

Available Dosage Forms:

- Tablet
- Tablet, Extended Release
- Solution

Therapeutic Class: Skeletal Muscle Relaxant, Centrally Acting
Pharmacologic Class: Antimuscarinic

Uses For This Medicine

Orphenadrine is used to help relax certain muscles in your body and relieve the stiffness, pain, and discomfort caused by strains, sprains, or other injury to your muscles. One form of orphenadrine is also used to relieve trembling caused by Parkinson's disease. However, this medicine does not take the place of rest, exercise or physical therapy, or other treatment that your doctor may recommend for your medical problem.

Orphenadrine acts in the central nervous system (CNS) to produce its muscle relaxant effects. Orphenadrine also has other actions (anticholinergic) that produce its helpful effects in Parkinson's disease. Orphenadrine's CNS and anticholinergic actions may also be responsible for some of its side effects.

In the U.S., this medicine is available only with your doctor's prescription.

Before Using This Medicine

In deciding to use a medicine, the risks of taking the medicine must be weighed against the good it will do. This is a decision you and your doctor will make. For this medicine, the following should be considered:

Allergies—Tell your doctor if you have ever had any unusual or allergic reaction to this medicine or any other medicines. Also tell your health care professional if you have any other types of allergies, such as to foods, dyes, preservatives, or animals. For non-prescription products, read the label or package ingredients carefully.

Pediatric—Studies on this medicine have been done only in adult patients, and there is no specific information com-

paring use of orphenadrine in children with use in other age groups.

Geriatric—Many medicines have not been tested in older people. Therefore, it may not be known whether they work exactly the same way they do in younger adults or if they cause different side effects or problems in older people. There is no specific information about the use of orphenadrine in the elderly.

Pregnancy—

	Pregnancy Category	Explanation
All Trimesters	C	Animal studies have shown an adverse effect and there are no adequate studies in pregnant women OR no animal studies have been conducted and there are no adequate studies in pregnant women.

Breast Feeding—There are no adequate studies in women for determining infant risk when using this medication during breastfeeding. Weigh the potential benefits against the potential risks before taking this medication while breastfeeding.

Other medicines—

Using this medicine with any of the following medicines may cause an increased risk of certain side effects, but using both drugs may be the best treatment for you. If both medicines are prescribed together, your doctor may change the dose or how often you use one or both of the medicines.

Perphenazine

Interactions with Food/Tobacco/Alcohol—Certain medicines should not be used at or around the time of eating food or eating certain types of food since interactions may occur. Using alcohol or tobacco with certain medicines may also cause interactions to occur. Discuss with your healthcare professional the use of your medicine with food, alcohol, or tobacco.

Other medical problems—The presence of other medical problems may affect the use of this medicine. Make sure you tell your doctor if you have any other medical problems, especially:

- Disease of the digestive tract, especially esophagus disease, stomach ulcer, or intestinal blockage, or
- Enlarged prostate or
- Fast or irregular heartbeat or
- Glaucoma or
- Myasthenia gravis or
- Urinary tract blockage—Orphenadrine has side effects that may be harmful to people with these conditions
- Heart disease or
- Kidney disease or
- Liver disease—The chance of side effects may be increased

Proper Use of This Medicine

Dosing—The dose of this medicine will be different for different patients. Follow your doctor's orders or the directions on the label. The following information includes only the av-

erage doses of this medicine. If your dose is different, do not change it unless your doctor tells you to do so.

The amount of medicine that you take depends on the strength of the medicine. Also, the number of doses you take each day, the time allowed between doses, and the length of time you take the medicine depend on the medical problem for which you are using the medicine.

- For extended-release tablet dosage form:
  - For relaxing stiff, sore muscles:
    - Adults and teenagers—100 milligrams (mg) two times a day, in the morning and evening.
    - Children—Use and dose must be determined by your doctor.
- For oral tablet dosage form:
  - For relaxing stiff, sore muscles and for Parkinson's disease:
    - Adults—50 mg three times a day.
    - Children—Dose must be determined by your doctor.
- For injection dosage form:
  - For relaxing stiff, sore muscles:
    - Adults—60 mg, injected into a muscle or a vein, every twelve hours as needed.
    - Children—Use and dose must be determined by your doctor.

Missed dose—If you miss a dose of this medicine, take it as soon as possible. However, if it is almost time for your next dose, skip the missed dose and go back to your regular dosing schedule. Do not double doses.

Storage—Store the medicine in a closed container at room temperature, away from heat, moisture, and direct light. Keep from freezing.

Keep out of the reach of children.

Do not keep outdated medicine or medicine no longer needed.

Precautions While Using This Medicine

If you will be taking this medicine for a long time (for example, more than a few weeks), your doctor should check your progress at regular visits.

This medicine may add to the effects of alcohol and other CNS depressants (medicines that slow down the nervous system, possibly causing drowsiness). Some examples of CNS depressants are antihistamines or medicine for hay fever, other allergies, or colds; sedatives, tranquilizers, or sleeping medicine; prescription pain medicine or narcotics; barbiturates; medicine for seizures; other muscle relaxants; or anesthetics, including some dental anesthetics. Do not drink alcoholic beverages, and check with your doctor before taking any of the medicines listed above, while you are using this medicine.

This medicine may cause some people to have blurred vision or to become drowsy, dizzy, lightheaded, faint, or less alert than they are normally. It may also cause muscle weakness in some people. Make sure you know how you react to this medicine before you drive, use machines, or do anything else that could be dangerous if you are dizzy or are not alert and able to see well.

Orphenadrine may cause dryness of the mouth. For temporary relief, use sugarless candy or gum, melt bits of ice in your mouth, or use a saliva substitute. However, if dry mouth continues for more than 2 weeks, check with your dentist.

Continuing dryness of the mouth may increase the chance of dental disease, including tooth decay, gum disease, and fungus infections.

Side Effects of This Medicine

Along with its needed effects, a medicine may cause some unwanted effects. Although not all of these side effects may occur, if they do occur they may need medical attention.

Check with your doctor as soon as possible if any of the following side effects occur:

Less common
Decreased urination; eye pain; fainting; fast or pounding heartbeat

Rare
Hallucinations (seeing, hearing, or feeling things that are not there); shortness of breath, troubled breathing, tightness in chest, and/or wheezing; skin rash, hives, itching, or redness; sores, ulcers, or white spots on lips or in mouth; swollen and/or painful glands; unusual bruising or bleeding; unusual tiredness or weakness

Some side effects may occur that usually do not need medical attention. These side effects may go away during treatment as your body adjusts to the medicine. Also, your health care professional may be able to tell you about ways to prevent or reduce some of these side effects. Check with your health care professional if any of the following side effects continue or are bothersome or if you have any questions about them:

More common
Dryness of mouth

Less common or rare
Abdominal or stomach cramps or pain; blurred or double vision or other vision problems; confusion; constipation; difficult urination; dizziness or lightheadedness; drowsiness; excitement, irritability, nervousness, or restlessness; headache; muscle weakness; nausea or vomiting; trembling; unusually large pupils of eyes

Other side effects not listed may also occur in some patients. If you notice any other effects, check with your healthcare professional.

ORPHENADRINE, ASPIRIN, AND CAFFEINE (Oral route) - or-FEN-a-dreen SIT-rate, AS-pir-in, kaf-EEN

Uses For This Medicine

Orphenadrine and aspirin combination is used to help relax certain muscles in your body and relieve the pain and discomfort caused by strains, sprains, or other injury to your muscles. However, this medicine does not take the place of rest, exercise, or other treatment that your doctor may recommend for your medical problem.

Orphenadrine acts in the central nervous system (CNS) to produce its muscle relaxant effects. Actions in the CNS may also be responsible for some of its side effects. Orphenadrine also has other actions (antimuscarinic) that may be responsible for some of its side effects.

This combination medicine also contains caffeine.

In the U.S., this combination medicine is available only with your doctor's prescription.

Before Using This Medicine

In deciding to use a medicine, the risks of taking the medicine must be weighed against the good it will do. This is a decision you and your doctor will make. For this medicine, the following should be considered:

Allergies—Tell your doctor if you have ever had any unusual or allergic reaction to this medicine or any other medicines. Also tell your health care professional if you have any other types of allergies, such as to foods, dyes, preservatives, or animals. For non-prescription products, read the label or package ingredients carefully.

Pediatric—Do not give a medicine containing aspirin to a child or a teenager with a fever or other symptoms of a virus infection, especially flu or chickenpox, without first discussing its use with your child's doctor. This is very important because aspirin may cause a serious illness called Reye's syndrome in children with fever caused by a virus infection, especially flu or chickenpox. Children who do not have a virus infection may also be more sensitive to the effects of aspirin, especially if they have a fever or have lost large amounts of body fluid because of vomiting, diarrhea, or sweating. This may increase the chance of side effects during treatment.

There is no specific information about the use of orphenadrine in children.

Geriatric—Elderly people are especially sensitive to the effects of aspirin. This may increase the chance of side effects during treatment.

There is no specific information about the use of orphenadrine in the elderly.

Pregnancy—

	Pregnancy Category	Explanation
All Trimesters	D	Studies in pregnant women have demonstrated a risk to the fetus. However, the benefits of therapy in a life threatening situation or a serious disease, may outweigh the potential risk.

Breast Feeding—There are no adequate studies in women for determining infant risk when using this medication during breastfeeding. Weigh the potential benefits against the potential risks before taking this medication while breastfeeding.

Other medicines—

Using this medicine with any of the following medicines is not recommended. Your doctor may decide not to treat you with this medication or change some of the other medicines you take.

Ketorolac

Interactions with Food/Tobacco/Alcohol—Certain medicines should not be used at or around the time of eating food or eating certain types of food since interactions may occur. Using alcohol or tobacco with certain medicines may also cause interactions to occur. The following interactions have been selected on the basis of their potential significance and are not necessarily all-inclusive.

Using this medicine with any of the following may cause an increased risk of certain side effects but may be unavoidable in some cases. If used together, your doctor may change the dose or how often you use this medicine, or give you special instructions about the use of food, alcohol, or tobacco.

Ethanol

Other medical problems—The presence of other medical problems may affect the use of this medicine. Make sure you tell your doctor if you have any other medical problems, especially:

- Anemia or
- Overactive thyroid or
- Stomach ulcer or other stomach problems—Aspirin may make your condition worse
- Asthma, allergies, and nasal polyps, history of or
- Glucose-6–phosphate dehydrogenase (G6PD) deficiency or
- Kidney disease or
- Liver disease—The chance of side effects may be increased
- Disease of the digestive tract, especially esophagus disease or intestinal blockage, or
- Enlarged prostate or
- Fast or irregular heartbeat or
- Glaucoma or
- Myasthenia gravis or
- Urinary tract blockage—Orphenadrine has side effects that may be harmful to people with these conditions
- Gout—Aspirin can make this condition worse and can also lessen the effects of some medicines used to treat gout
- Heart disease—The chance of some side effects may be increased. Also, the caffeine present in this combination medicine can make your condition worse
- Hemophilia or other bleeding problems or
- Vitamin K deficiency—Aspirin may increase the chance of bleeding

Proper Use of This Medicine

Take this medicine with food or a full glass (8 ounces) of water to lessen stomach irritation.

Do not take this medicine if it has a strong vinegar-like odor. This odor means the aspirin in it is breaking down. If you have any questions about this, check with your health care professional.

Do not take more of this medicine than your doctor ordered to lessen the chance of side effects or overdose.

Dosing—The dose of this medicine will be different for different patients. Follow your doctor's orders or the directions on the label. The following information includes only the average doses of this medicine. If your dose is different, do not change it unless your doctor tells you to do so.

The amount of medicine that you take depends on the strength of the medicine. Also, the number of doses you take each day, the time allowed between doses, and the length of time you take the medicine depend on the medical problem for which you are using the medicine.

- For oral dosage forms (tablets):
  - For muscle pain and stiffness:
    - Adults and teenagers—One or two tablets containing 25 milligrams (mg) of orphenadrine and 385 mg of aspirin, or one-half or one tablet containing 50 mg of orphenadrine and 770 mg of aspirin, three or four times a day.
    - Children—Dose must be determined by your doctor.

Missed dose—If you miss a dose of this medicine, take it as soon as possible. However, if it is almost time for your next dose, skip the missed dose and go back to your regular dosing schedule. Do not double doses.

Storage—Store the medicine in a closed container at room temperature, away from heat, moisture, and direct light. Keep from freezing.

Keep out of the reach of children.

Do not keep outdated medicine or medicine no longer needed.

Precautions While Using This Medicine

If you will be taking this medicine for a long time (for example, more than a few weeks), your doctor should check your progress at regular visits.

Check the labels of all nonprescription (over-the-counter [OTC]) and prescription medicines you now take. If any contain orphenadrine or aspirin or other salicylates be especially careful, since taking them while taking this medicine may lead to overdose. If you have any questions about this, check with your health care professional.

Too much use of acetaminophen or certain other medicines together with the aspirin in this combination medicine may increase the chance of unwanted effects. The risk depends on how much of each medicine you take every day, and on how long you take the medicines together. If your doctor directs you to take these medicines together on a regular basis, follow his or her directions carefully. However, do not take acetaminophen or any of the following medicines together with this combination medicine for more than a few days, unless your doctor has directed you to do so and is following your progress:

- Diclofenac (e.g., Voltaren)
- Diflunisal (e.g., Dolobid)
- Etodolac (e.g., Lodine)
- Fenoprofen (e.g., Nalfon)
- Floctafenine (e.g., Idarac)
- Flurbiprofen, oral (e.g., Ansaid)
- Ibuprofen (e.g., Motrin)
- Indomethacin (e.g., Indocin)
- Ketoprofen (e.g., Orudis)
- Ketorolac (e.g., Toradol)
- Meclofenamate (e.g., Meclomen)
- Mefenamic acid (e.g., Ponstel)
- Nabumetone (e.g., Relafen)
- Naproxen (e.g., Naprosyn)
- Oxaprozin (e.g., Daypro)
- Phenylbutazone (e.g., Butazolidin)
- Piroxicam (e.g., Feldene)
- Sulindac (e.g., Clinoril)
- Tenoxicam (e.g., Mobiflex)
- Tiaprofenic acid (e.g., Surgam)
- Tolmetin (e.g., Tolectin)

For diabetic patients:
- The aspirin in this combination medicine may cause false urine sugar test results if you are regularly taking

6 or more of the regular-strength tablets or 3 or more of the double-strength tablets of this medicine a day. Smaller doses or occasional use of aspirin usually will not affect urine sugar tests. If you have any questions about this, check with your health care professional especially if your diabetes is not well controlled.

Do not take this medicine for 5 days before any surgery, including dental surgery, unless otherwise directed by your medical doctor or dentist. Taking aspirin during this time may cause bleeding problems.

The orphenadrine in this combination medicine may add to the effects of alcohol and other CNS depressants (medicines that slow down the nervous system, possibly causing drowsiness). Some examples of CNS depressants are antihistamines or medicine for hay fever, other allergies, or colds; sedatives, tranquilizers, or sleeping medicine; prescription pain medicine or narcotics; barbiturates; medicine for seizures; other muscle relaxants; or anesthetics, including some dental anesthetics. Also, stomach problems may be more likely to occur if you drink alcoholic beverages while you are taking aspirin. Do not drink alcoholic beverages, and check with your doctor before taking any of the medicines listed above, while you are using this medicine.

This medicine may cause some people to have blurred vision or to become drowsy, dizzy, lightheaded, faint, or less alert than they are normally. Make sure you know how you react to this medicine before you drive, use machines, or do anything else that could be dangerous if you are dizzy or are not alert.

Dryness of the mouth may occur while you are taking this medicine. For temporary relief, use sugarless candy or gum, melt bits of ice in your mouth, or use a saliva substitute. However, if dry mouth continues for more than 2 weeks, check with your dentist. Continuing dryness of the mouth may increase the chance of dental disease, including tooth decay, gum disease, and fungus infections.

If you think that you or someone else may have taken an overdose of this medicine, get emergency help at once. Taking an overdose of this medicine may cause unconsciousness or death. Signs of overdose include convulsions (seizures), hearing loss, confusion, ringing or buzzing in the ears, severe drowsiness or tiredness, severe excitement or nervousness, and fast or deep breathing.

Side Effects of This Medicine

Along with its needed effects, a medicine may cause some unwanted effects. Although not all of these side effects may occur, if they do occur they may need medical attention.

Get emergency help immediately if any of the following symptoms of overdose occur:

Any loss of hearing; bloody urine; confusion; convulsions (seizures); diarrhea; dizziness or lightheadedness (severe); drowsiness (severe); excitement or nervousness (severe); fast or deep breathing; hallucinations (seeing, hearing, or feeling things that are not there); headache (severe or continuing); increased sweating; nausea or vomiting (severe or continuing); ringing or buzzing in the ears (continuing); uncontrollable flapping movements of the hands, especially in elderly patients; unexplained fever; unusual thirst; vision problems

Symptoms of overdose in children

Changes in behavior; drowsiness or tiredness (severe); fast or deep breathing

Check with your doctor as soon as possible if any of the following side effects occur:

Less common or rare

Abdominal or stomach pain, cramping, or burning (severe); bloody or black, tarry stools; decreased urination; eye pain; fainting; fast or pounding heartbeat; shortness of breath, troubled breathing, tightness in chest, or wheezing; skin rash, hives, itching, or redness; sores, ulcers, or white spots on lips or in mouth; swollen and/or painful glands; unusual bleeding or bruising; unusual tiredness or weakness; vomiting of blood or material that looks like coffee grounds

Some side effects may occur that usually do not need medical attention. These side effects may go away during treatment as your body adjusts to the medicine. Also, your health care professional may be able to tell you about ways to prevent or reduce some of these side effects. Check with your health care professional if any of the following side effects continue or are bothersome or if you have any questions about them:

More common

Abdominal or stomach cramps, pain, or discomfort (mild to moderate); dryness of mouth; heartburn or indigestion; nausea or vomiting (mild)

Less common

Blurred or double vision or other vision problems; confusion; constipation; difficult urination; dizziness or lightheadedness; drowsiness; excitement, nervousness, or restlessness; headache; muscle weakness; trembling; unusually large pupils of eyes

Other side effects not listed may also occur in some patients. If you notice any other effects, check with your healthcare professional.

OSELTAMIVIR   (Oral route) - oh-sel-TAM-i-vir

Commonly used brand name(s)

In the U.S.—

Tamiflu

Available Dosage Forms:

- Powder for Suspension
- Capsule

Therapeutic Class: Antiviral
Pharmacologic Class: Neuraminidase Inhibitor, Influenza A&B Virus

Uses For This Medicine

Oseltamivir belongs to the family of medicines called antivirals, which are used to treat infections caused by viruses. Oseltamivir is used in the treatment of the infection caused by the flu virus (influenza A and influenza B). Oseltamivir may reduce flu symptoms (weakness, headache, fever, cough, and sore throat) by 1 day. Oseltamivir is also used to prevent influenza infection if you have come into close contact with someone who has the flu.

If you receive the flu vaccine every year, continue to do so. Oseltamivir is not a substitute for your yearly flu shot.

Oseltamivir is available only with your doctor's prescription.

Before Using This Medicine

In deciding to use a medicine, the risks of taking the medicine must be weighed against the good it will do. This is a decision you and your doctor will make. For this medicine, the following should be considered:

Allergies—Tell your doctor if you have ever had any unusual or allergic reaction to this medicine or any other medicines. Also tell your health care professional if you have any other types of allergies, such as to foods, dyes, preservatives, or animals. For non-prescription products, read the label or package ingredients carefully.

Pediatric—This medicine has not been tested in children younger than 1 year of age.

Geriatric—This medicine has been tested in older adults and has not been shown to cause different side effects or problems in older adults than it does in younger adults.

Pregnancy—

	Pregnancy Category	Explanation
All Trimesters	C	Animal studies have shown an adverse effect and there are no adequate studies in pregnant women OR no animal studies have been conducted and there are no adequate studies in pregnant women.

Breast Feeding—There are no adequate studies in women for determining infant risk when using this medication during breastfeeding. Weigh the potential benefits against the potential risks before taking this medication while breastfeeding.

Other medicines—Although certain medicines should not be used together at all, in other cases two different medicines may be used together even if an interaction might occur. In these cases, your doctor may want to change the dose, or other precautions may be necessary. Tell your healthcare professional if you are taking any other prescription or non-prescription (over-the-counter [OTC]) medicine.

Interactions with Food/Tobacco/Alcohol—Certain medicines should not be used at or around the time of eating food or eating certain types of food since interactions may occur. Using alcohol or tobacco with certain medicines may also cause interactions to occur. Discuss with your healthcare professional the use of your medicine with food, alcohol, or tobacco.

Other medical problems—The presence of other medical problems may affect the use of this medicine. Make sure you tell your doctor if you have any other medical problems, especially:
- Kidney disease or
- Heart disease or
- Illnesses caused by viruses other than influenza Type A or B or
- Liver disease or
- Lung disease or
- Serious medical problems that may need admission to a hospital—Safety of this medicine for people with these conditions is not established.

Proper Use of This Medicine

Talk to your doctor about the possibility of getting a flu shot if you have not had one yet. Patient information about oseltamivir is available. Read this information carefully.

For patients taking oseltamivir for treatment of the flu: This medicine works best if taken within 2 days of having flu symptoms (weakness, headache, fever, cough, and sore throat). Oseltamivir capsules may be taken with meals or on an empty stomach. Taking oseltamivir with food may lessen the possibility of stomach upset. This medicine should be taken for 5 days. Continue taking this medicine for the full time of treatment even if you begin to feel better after a few days. This will help to clear up your infection completely. If you stop taking this medicine too soon, your symptoms may return.

For patients taking oseltamivir for prevention of the flu after exposure: The medicine should be taken within 2 days of being exposed to the flu. Oseltamivir capsules may be taken with meals or on an empty stomach. Taking oseltamivir with food may lessen the possibility of stomach upset. This medicine should be taken for at least 10 days.

For patients taking the oral suspension form of this medicine:
- This medicine is to be taken only by mouth. Use the specially marked measuring device that is given to you with the medicine to measure each dose accurately. The average household spoon may not hold the right amount of liquid. If the measuring device provided with the medicine is lost or damaged, contact your pharmacist or doctor to find out the appropriate doses.
- Do not use after the expiration date on the label. The medicine may not work properly after that date. If you have any questions about this, check with your pharmacist.

Dosing—The dose of this medicine will be different for different patients. Follow your doctor's orders or the directions on the label. The following information includes only the average doses of this medicine. If your dose is different, do not change it unless your doctor tells you to do so.

The amount of medicine that you take depends on the strength of the medicine. Also, the number of doses you take each day, the time allowed between doses, and the length of time you take the medicine depend on the medical problem for which you are using the medicine.

- For oral dosage forms (capsules and oral suspension):
  - For treatment of the flu:
    - Adults and teenagers: 75 milligrams (mg) two times a day for five days.
    - Children 1 year of age or older: Dose is based on body weight and must be determined by your doctor. It is usually between 30 and 75 mg two times a day for five days.
    - Children up to 1 year of age: Use and dose must be determined by your doctor.
  - For prevention of the flu:
    - Adults and teenagers: 75 mg once a day for at least ten days.
    - Children 1 year of age or older: Dose is based on body weight and must be determined by your doctor. It is usually between 30 and 75 mg one time a day for ten days.
    - Children up to 1 year of age: Use and dose must be determined by your doctor.

Missed dose—If you miss a dose of this medicine, take it as soon as possible. However, if it is almost time for your next dose, skip the missed dose and go back to your regular dosing schedule. Do not double doses.

Storage—Store the medicine in a closed container at room temperature, away from heat, moisture, and direct light. Keep from freezing.

Keep out of the reach of children.

Do not keep outdated medicine or medicine no longer needed.

Precautions While Using This Medicine

If your symptoms do not improve after you finish taking the medicine, or if they become worse, check with your doctor.

Side Effects of This Medicine

Side Effects of This Medicine

Along with its needed effects, a medicine may cause some unwanted effects. Although not all of these side effects may occur, if they do occur they may need medical attention.

Stop taking this medicine and get emergency help immediately if any of the following effects occur:

Less common
> Phlegm producing cough; wheezing

Rare
> Abdominal or stomach cramps or tenderness; arm, back or jaw pain; bloating; chest pain or discomfort; chest tightness or heaviness; diarrhea, watery and severe, which may also be bloody; drooling; facial swelling; fast or irregular heartbeat; fever; hoarseness; humerus fracture (broken forearm); increased thirst; pain; shortness of breath; tender glands of jaw and throat; unusual tiredness or weakness; unusual weight loss

Incidence not known
> Blistering, peeling, loosening of skin; chills; convulsions; dark urine; difficulty swallowing; fainting; fast, slow or irregular heartbeat; general tiredness and weakness; hives or welts; itching; itching, puffiness or swelling of the eyelids or around the eyes, face, lips or tongue; joint or muscle pain; light-colored stools; loss of bladder control; loss of consciousness; muscle spasm or jerking of all extremities; red irritated eyes; red skin lesions, often with a purple center; redness of skin; shortness of breath; skin rash; skin rash or itching over the entire body; sore throat; sores, ulcers, or white spots in mouth or on lips; sudden loss of consciousness; sweating; swelling of the face or tongue; tightness in chest; unusual tiredness or weakness; upper right abdominal pain; weakness; yellow eyes and skin

Some side effects may occur that usually do not need medical attention. These side effects may go away during treatment as your body adjusts to the medicine. Also, your health care professional may be able to tell you about ways to prevent or reduce some of these side effects. Check with your health care professional if any of the following side effects continue or are bothersome or if you have any questions about them:

More common
> Diarrhea; nausea; vomiting

Less common
> Abdominal or stomach pain; bloody nose or unexplained nosebleeds (occurs mainly in children); burning, dry or itching eyes, redness, pain, swelling of eye or eyelid, or excessive tearing (occurs mainly in children); cough; dizziness; ear disorder (occurs mainly in children); fatigue; headache; trouble in sleeping

Rare
> Pale skin; sneezing; tightness in chest; troubled breathing; troubled breathing with exertion; unusual bleeding or bruising

Incidence not known
> Blistering, crusting, irritation, itching, or reddening of skin; blurred vision; cracked, dry, scaly skin; dry mouth; flushed, dry skin; fruit-like breath odor; increased hunger; increased urination; mood or mental changes; skin rash encrusted, scaly and oozing; stomachache; swelling; unexplained weight loss

Other side effects not listed may also occur in some patients. If you notice any other effects, check with your healthcare professional.

OXALIPLATIN   (Intravenous route) - ox-AL-i-pla-tin

Black Box Warning

Oxaliplatin should be administered under the supervision of a qualified physician experienced in the use of cancer chemotherapeutic agents. Appropriate management of therapy and complications is possible only when adequate diagnostic and treatment facilities are readily available.

Anaphylactic-like reactions to oxaliplatin have been reported, and may occur within minutes of oxaliplatin administration. Epinephrine, corticosteroids, and antihistamines have been employed to alleviate symptoms.

Commonly used brand name(s)

In the U.S.—
> Eloxatin

Available Dosage Forms:
- Powder for Solution
- Solution

Therapeutic Class: Antineoplastic Agent
Pharmacologic Class: Platinum Coordination Complex

Uses For This Medicine

Oxaliplatin belongs to the group of medicines called antineoplastics. It is used to treat cancer of the colon or rectum. Oxaliplatin is usually given along with other medicines to treat cancer.

Oxaliplatin interferes with the growth of cancer cells, which are eventually destroyed. Since the growth of normal cells may also be affected by the medicine, other effects may also occur. Some of these may be serious and must be reported to your healthcare professional. Other effects may not be serious but may cause concern. Some effects may occur after treatment with oxaliplatin has been stopped. Be sure that you have discussed with your healthcare professional the possible side effects of this medicine as well as the good it can do.

This medicine is available only with your healthcare professional's prescription.

Once a medicine has been approved for marketing for a certain use, experience may show that it is also useful for other medical problems. Although these uses are not included in product labeling, oxaliplatin is used in certain patients with the following medical conditions:

- Colon cancer, stage II, adjuvant treatment in combination with 5–fluorouracil/leucovorin
- Gastric carcinoma, advanced/metastatic

Before Using This Medicine

In deciding to use a medicine, the risks of taking the medicine must be weighed against the good it will do. This is a decision you and your doctor will make. For this medicine, the following should be considered:

Allergies—Tell your doctor if you have ever had any unusual or allergic reaction to this medicine or any other medicines. Also tell your health care professional if you have any other types of allergies, such as to foods, dyes, preservatives, or animals. For non-prescription products, read the label or package ingredients carefully.

Pediatric—Studies of this medicine have been done only in adult patients, and there is no specific information comparing the use of oxaliplatin in children with use in other age groups.

Geriatric—This medicine may increase your chance of getting certain side effects, such as diarrhea or dizziness, if you are 65 years of age or older.

Pregnancy—

	Pregnancy Category	Explanation
All Trimesters	D	Studies in pregnant women have demonstrated a risk to the fetus. However, the benefits of therapy in a life threatening situation or a serious disease, may outweigh the potential risk.

Breast Feeding—There are no adequate studies in women for determining infant risk when using this medication during breastfeeding. Weigh the potential benefits against the potential risks before taking this medication while breastfeeding.

Other medicines—

Using this medicine with any of the following medicines is not recommended. Your doctor may decide not to treat you with this medication or change some of the other medicines you take.

Rotavirus Vaccine, Live

Interactions with Food/Tobacco/Alcohol—Certain medicines should not be used at or around the time of eating food or eating certain types of food since interactions may occur. Using alcohol or tobacco with certain medicines may also cause interactions to occur. Discuss with your healthcare professional the use of your medicine with food, alcohol, or tobacco.

Other medical problems—The presence of other medical problems may affect the use of this medicine. Make sure you tell your doctor if you have any other medical problems, especially:

- Kidney disease—Effects of oxaliplatin may be increased because of slower removal from the body

Proper Use of This Medicine

Dosing—The dose of this medicine will be different for different patients. Follow your doctor's orders or the directions on the label. The following information includes only the average doses of this medicine. If your dose is different, do not change it unless your doctor tells you to do so.

The amount of medicine that you take depends on the strength of the medicine. Also, the number of doses you take each day, the time allowed between doses, and the length of time you take the medicine depend on the medical problem for which you are using the medicine.

This medicine often causes nausea and vomiting. However, it is very important that you continue to receive the medicine even if you begin to feel ill. Other medicines may be given to you to help with the nausea and vomiting. Ask your health care professional for other ways to lessen these effects.

Precautions While Using This Medicine

It is very important that your healthcare professional check your progress at regular visits to make sure that this medicine is working properly and to check for unwanted effects.

While you are being treated with oxaliplatin, and after you stop treatment with it, do not have any immunizations (vaccinations) without your healthcare professional's approval. Oxaliplatin may lower your body's resistance and there is a chance you might get the infection the immunization is meant to prevent. In addition, other persons living in your household should not take oral polio vaccine since there is a chance they could pass the polio virus on to you. Also, avoid persons who have taken oral polio vaccine within the last several months. Do not get close to them and do not stay in the same room with them for very long. If you cannot take these precautions, you should consider wearing a protective face mask that covers the nose and mouth.

Oxaliplatin can temporarily lower the number of white blood cells in your blood, increasing the chance of getting an infection. It can also lower the number of platelets, which are necessary for proper blood clotting. If this occurs, there are certain precautions you can take, especially when your blood count is low, to reduce the risk of infection or bleeding:

- If you can, avoid people with infections. Check with your healthcare professional immediately if you think you are getting an infection or if you get a fever or chills, cough or hoarseness, lower back or side pain, or painful or difficult urination and persistent diarrhea.
- Check with your healthcare professional immediately if you have persistent vomiting, diarrhea, dehydration, cough or difficulty breathing
- Check with your healthcare professional immediately if you notice any unusual bleeding or bruising; black, tarry stools; blood in urine or stools; or pinpoint red spots on your skin.
- Check with your healthcare professional immediately if you notice any redness, pain, or swelling in the area you are receiving your medicine.
- Avoid cold drinks, and the use of ice cubes in drinks. Avoid cold temperatures and cold objects. Cover your

skin if you must go outside in cold temperatures. Do not put ice or ice packs on your body. Do not breathe deeply when exposed to cold air. Do not take things from the freezer or refrigerator without wearing gloves. Do not run the air conditioner at high levels in the house or in the car in hot weather.

- Be careful when using a regular toothbrush, dental floss, or toothpick. Your medical healthcare professional, dentist, or nurse may recommend other ways to clean your teeth and gums. Check with your medical healthcare professional before having any dental work done.

- Do not touch your eyes or the inside of your nose unless you have just washed your hands and have not touched anything else in the meantime.

- Be careful not to cut yourself when you are using sharp objects such as a safety razor or fingernail or toenail cutters.

- Avoid contact sports or other situations where bruising or injury could occur.

Side Effects of This Medicine

Along with its needed effects, a medicine may cause some unwanted effects. Although not all of these side effects may occur, if they do occur they may need medical attention.

More common
Abnormal tongue sensation; black, tarry stools; bleeding gums; blistering, peeling, redness, and/or swelling of palms of hands or bottoms of feet; blood in urine or stools; burning, prickling, itching, or tingling of skin; chest pain; chills; confusion; cough; decreased feeling, or pain in the hands, feet, around mouth, or throat; decreased urination; difficult breathing; difficulty in articulating words; difficulty in moving; difficulty performing daily activities such as writing, buttoning, swallowing or walking; difficulty swallowing; dizziness; dry mouth; eye pain; fainting; fever; increase in heart rate; jaw spasm; lightheadedness; muscle pain or stiffness; numbness; numbness, pain, tingling, or unusual sensations in palms of hands or bottoms of feet; pain in chest, groin, or legs, especially the calves; pain in joints; painful or difficult urination; pale skin; pinpoint red spots on skin; rapid breathing; sensation of pins and needles; severe, sudden headache; shortness of breath; slurred speech; sore throat; sores, ulcers, or white spots on lips or in mouth; stabbing pain; sudden loss of coordination; sudden, severe weakness or numbness in arm or leg; sudden, unexplained shortness of breath; sunken eyes; swelling; swelling or inflammation of the mouth; swollen glands; thirst; troubled breathing with exertion; unusual bleeding or bruising; unusual tiredness or weakness; vision changes; wrinkled skin

Less common
Convulsions; fast heartbeat; hives; increased thirst; irregular heartbeat; itching; loss of appetite; mood changes; nausea or vomiting; numbness or tingling in hands, feet, or lips; puffiness or swelling of the eyelids or around the eyes, face, lips or tongue; skin rash; tightness in chest; wheezing

Incidence not known
Back, leg, or stomach pains; blindness; bloated abdomen; blue-yellow color blindness; blurred vision; changes in patterns and rhythms of speech; dark urine;

deafness; decreased vision; deep breathing; drowsiness; electric shock-like sensation that moves down the back and into the legs following a bending movement of the neck; fatigue; general body swelling; increased urination; large, hive-like swelling on face, eyelids, lips, tongue, throat, hands, legs, feet, sex organs; loss of deep tendon reflexes; muscle tremors; pain and fullness in right upper abdomen; restlessness; severe constipation; severe diarrhea; severe nosebleeds; severe stomach cramps or tenderness; severe vomiting; swelling of face, fingers, feet, or lower legs; trouble in speaking; twitches of the muscle visible under the skin; weakness of the muscles in your face; weight gain; yellow eyes or skin

Symptoms of overdose

Get emergency help immediately if any of the following symptoms of overdose occur:

Agitation; black, tarry stools; bleeding gums; blood in urine or stools; burning, prickling, itching, or tingling of skin; chest pain or discomfort; coma; confusion; cough or hoarseness; diarrhea; difficult urination; disorientation; dizziness or fainting; fever or chills; involuntary, rapid, rhythmic movement of the eyes; lack of coordination; lack of sensation; lethargy; lightheadedness; lower back or side pain; muscle twitching; paralysis; pinpoint red spots on skin; respiratory failure; seizures; severe weakness; shortness of breath; slow or irregular heartbeat; slurred speech; tremors; unusual tiredness; unusual bleeding or bruising; vomiting, profuse; wheezing

Some side effects may occur that usually do not need medical attention. These side effects may go away during treatment as your body adjusts to the medicine. Also, your health care professional may be able to tell you about ways to prevent or reduce some of these side effects. Check with your health care professional if any of the following side effects continue or are bothersome or if you have any questions about them:

More common
Abdominal pain; acid or sour stomach; back pain; belching; body aches or pain; diarrhea; ear congestion; feeling unusually cold, shivering; headache; heartburn; indigestion; loss of appetite; loss of voice; nasal congestion; nausea; runny nose; sleeplessness; sneezing; sore throat; stomach discomfort, upset or pain; stuffy nose; trouble sleeping; unable to sleep; weight loss

Less common
Bad, unusual or unpleasant (after) taste; bloated, full feeling; bloating or swelling of face, arms, hands, lower legs, or feet; bloody nose; burning while urinating; change in taste; congestion; cracked lips; dryness or soreness of throat; excess air or gas in stomach or intestines; feeling of warmth; hoarseness; passing gas; rapid weight gain; redness of the face, neck, arms and occasionally upper chest; tender, swollen glands in neck; tingling of hands or feet; trouble in swallowing; unusual tearing of eyes; voice changes; vomiting

Some side effects may occur that usually do not need medical attention. These side effects may go away during treatment as your body adjusts to the medicine. Also, your health care professional may be able to tell you about ways to prevent or reduce some of these side effects. Check with your health care professional if any of the following side effects

continue or are bothersome or if you have any questions about them:

Less common
Hair loss; thinning of hair

Other side effects not listed may also occur in some patients. If you notice any other effects, check with your healthcare professional.

OXCARBAZEPINE (Oral route) - OX-kar-BAZ-e-peen

Commonly used brand name(s)
In the U.S.—
Trileptal

Available Dosage Forms:
• Tablet
• Suspension

Therapeutic Class: Anticonvulsant

Uses For This Medicine

Oxcarbazepine is used to control some types of seizures in the treatment of epilepsy. This medicine cannot cure epilepsy and will only work to control seizures for as long as you continue to take it.

Oxcarbazepine is available only with your doctor's prescription.

Before Using This Medicine

In deciding to use a medicine, the risks of taking the medicine must be weighed against the good it will do. This is a decision you and your doctor will make. For this medicine, the following should be considered:

Allergies—Tell your doctor if you have ever had any unusual or allergic reaction to this medicine or any other medicines. Also tell your health care professional if you have any other types of allergies, such as to foods, dyes, preservatives, or animals. For non-prescription products, read the label or package ingredients carefully.

Pediatric—This medicine has been tested in children 4 years of age and older, and in effective doses, has not been shown to cause different side effects or problems than in adults.

Pregnancy—

	Pregnancy Category	Explanation
All Trimesters	C	Animal studies have shown an adverse effect and there are no adequate studies in pregnant women OR no animal studies have been conducted and there are no adequate studies in pregnant women.

Breast Feeding—There are no adequate studies in women for determining infant risk when using this medication during breastfeeding. Weigh the potential benefits against the potential risks before taking this medication while breastfeeding.

Other medicines—

Using this medicine with any of the following medicines may cause an increased risk of certain side effects, but using both drugs may be the best treatment for you. If both medicines are prescribed together, your doctor may change the dose or how often you use one or both of the medicines.

Carbamazepine, Ethinyl Estradiol, Etonogestrel, Felodipine, Fosphenytoin, Ginkgo, Lamotrigine, Levonorgestrel, Mestranol, Norelgestromin, Norethindrone, Norgestrel, Phenobarbital, Phenytoin, Simvastatin, Valproic Acid, Verapamil

Interactions with Food/Tobacco/Alcohol—Certain medicines should not be used at or around the time of eating food or eating certain types of food since interactions may occur. Using alcohol or tobacco with certain medicines may also cause interactions to occur. Discuss with your healthcare professional the use of your medicine with food, alcohol, or tobacco.

Other medical problems—The presence of other medical problems may affect the use of this medicine. Make sure you tell your doctor if you have any other medical problems, especially:

• Kidney disease or

• Prior hypersensitivity reaction to carbamazepine or

• Hyponatremia (condition in which your body has too little sodium)—May make these conditions worse

---

Proper Use of This Medicine

Take this medicine only as directed by your doctor. Do not take more or less of it, and do not take more or less often than your doctor ordered.

For patients taking the *oral suspension form* of this medicine:

• Shake the bottle well before measuring the dose.

• Use the oral dosing syringe supplied to measure each dose accurately.

• The dose of medicine can be mixed in a small glass of water just before taking it or you may swallow it directly from the syringe.

• After each use, close the bottle and rinse the syringe with warm water and allow it to dry completely before the next use.

Do not suddenly stop taking this medicine without first checking with your doctor. To keep your seizures under control, it is usually best to gradually reduce the amount of oxcarbazepine you are taking before stopping completely.

Dosing—The dose of this medicine will be different for different patients. Follow your doctor's orders or the directions on the label. The following information includes only the average doses of this medicine. If your dose is different, do not change it unless your doctor tells you to do so.

The amount of medicine that you take depends on the strength of the medicine. Also, the number of doses you take each day, the time allowed between doses, and the length of time you take the medicine depend on the medical problem for which you are using the medicine.

• For oral dosage form (oral suspension and tablets):
  ○ For epilepsy:
    ▪ Adults and teenagers 17 years of age and older—At first, 300 milligrams (mg) two times a day. Your doctor may increase your dose as needed. How-

ever, the dose is usually not more than 2400 mg a day.

- Children 4 to 16 years of age—Dose is based on body weight. The usual dose is 8 to 10 mg per kg (3.7 to 4.5 mg per pound) of body weight. The doctor may need to adjust the dose based on your response to the medicine.
- Children up to 4 years of age—Use and dose must be determined by your doctor.

Missed dose—If you miss a dose of this medicine, take it as soon as possible. However, if it is almost time for your next dose, skip the missed dose and go back to your regular dosing schedule. Do not double doses.

Storage—Store the medicine in a closed container at room temperature, away from heat, moisture, and direct light. Keep from freezing.

Keep out of the reach of children.

Do not keep outdated medicine or medicine no longer needed.

Ask your healthcare professional how you should dispose of any medicine you do not use.

Precautions While Using This Medicine

Your doctor should check your progress at regular visits. This is to make sure the medicine is working for you and to allow the dosage to be changed if needed.

If your symptoms do not improve within a few days or if they become worse, check with your doctor.

Do not take other medicines unless they have been discussed with your doctor. This medicine will add to the effects of alcohol and other CNS depressants (medicines that make you drowsy or less alert). Some examples of CNS depressants are antihistamines or medicines for hay fever, other allergies or colds; sedatives, tranquilizers, or sleeping medicine; prescription pain medicine or narcotics; and other medicines for seizures.

Tell your doctor right away if a skin reaction occurs while you are taking this medicine. There have been serious skin reactions associated with oxcarbazepine.

If you develop a fever along with a rash or swollen glands, contact your doctor right away.

This medicine may cause some people to become drowsy, dizzy, or less alert than they are normally. Make sure you know how you react to this medicine before you drive, use machines, or do anything else that could be dangerous if you are dizzy or are not alert.

Oral contraceptives (birth control pills) containing estrogen or progestin, contraceptive progestin injections (e.g., Depo-Provera), and implant contraceptive forms of progestin (e.g., Norplant) may not work properly if you take them while you are taking oxcarbazepine. Unplanned pregnancies may occur. You should use a different or additional means of birth control while you are taking oxcarbazepine. If you have any questions about this, check with your health care professional.

Dizziness, lightheadedness, or fainting may occur, especially when you get up from a lying or sitting position. Getting up slowly may help. If the problem continues or gets worse, check with your doctor.

Do not stop taking this medicine without first checking with your doctor. Stopping the medicine suddenly may cause your seizures to return or to occur more often. Your doctor may

want you to gradually reduce the amount of oxcarbazepine you are taking before stopping completely.

Side Effects of This Medicine

Along with its needed effects, a medicine may cause some unwanted effects. Although not all of these side effects may occur, if they do occur they may need medical attention.

Check with your doctor as soon as possible if any of the following side effects occur:

More common

Change in vision; change in walking or balance; clumsiness or unsteadiness; cough, fever, sneezing, or sore throat; crying; dizziness; double vision; false sense of well-being; feeling of constant movement of self or surroundings; mental depression; sensation of spinning; uncontrolled back-and-forth and/or rolling eye movements

Less common

Agitation; awkwardness; bloody or cloudy urine; blurred vision; bruising; confusion; congestion; convulsions (seizures); decreased urination; difficulty in focusing eyes; disorientation; faintness or light-headedness when getting up from a lying or sitting position; fast or irregular heartbeat; frequent falls; frequent urge to urinate; general feeling of illness; headache; hoarseness; increased thirst; itching of the vagina, with or without white vaginal discharge; loss of consciousness; memory loss; muscle cramps; pain or burning while urinating; pain or tenderness around eyes or cheekbones; poor control in body movements—for example, when reaching or stepping; problems with coordination; shaking or trembling of arms, legs, hands, and feet; shortness of breath; skin rash; stuffy or runny nose; tightness in chest; trouble in walking; troubled breathing; unusual feelings; unusual tiredness or weakness; wheezing

Rare

Anxiety; bleeding or crusting sores on lips; burning feeling in chest or stomach; chest pain; chills; decreased response to stimulation; hives or itching; irritability; joint pain; muscle pain or weakness; nervousness; purple spots on skin; rectal bleeding; redness, blistering, peeling, or loosening of skin; restlessness; sores, ulcers, or white spots in mouth or on lips; stomach upset; swelling of legs; swollen glands

Some side effects may occur that usually do not need medical attention. These side effects may go away during treatment as your body adjusts to the medicine. Also, your health care professional may be able to tell you about ways to prevent or reduce some of these side effects. Check with your health care professional if any of the following side effects continue or are bothersome or if you have any questions about them:

More common

Abdominal pain; burning feeling in chest or stomach; nausea and vomiting; runny or stuffy nose; sleepiness or unusual drowsiness

Less common

Acid or sour stomach; acne; back pain; belching; bloody nose; blurred vision; change in your sense of taste; constipation; diarrhea; difficulty in speaking; dryness of mouth; feeling of warmth and redness of face, neck, arms, and occasionally chest; heartburn; increased sweating; increased urination; nervousness; trouble in sleeping

Other side effects not listed may also occur in some patients. If you notice any other effects, check with your healthcare professional.

OXYBUTYNIN (Oral route) - ox-i-BYOO-ti-nin

Commonly used brand name(s)

In the U.S.—
Ditropan
Ditropan XL

Available Dosage Forms:
- Tablet, Extended Release
- Syrup
- Tablet

Therapeutic Class: Urinary Antispasmodic
Pharmacologic Class: Antimuscarinic

Uses For This Medicine

Oxybutynin belongs to the group of medicines called antispasmodics. It helps decrease muscle spasms of the bladder and the frequent urge to urinate caused by these spasms.

Oxybutynin is available only with your doctor's prescription.

Before Using This Medicine

In deciding to use a medicine, the risks of taking the medicine must be weighed against the good it will do. This is a decision you and your doctor will make. For this medicine, the following should be considered:

Allergies—Tell your doctor if you have ever had any unusual or allergic reaction to this medicine or any other medicines. Also tell your health care professional if you have any other types of allergies, such as to foods, dyes, preservatives, or animals. For non-prescription products, read the label or package ingredients carefully.

Pediatric—There is no specific information about the use of oxybutynin in children under 5 years of age. In older children, oxybutynin is not expected to cause different side effects or problems than it does in adults.

Geriatric—Elderly people are especially sensitive to the effects of oxybutynin. This may increase the chance of side effects during treatment.

Pregnancy—

	Pregnancy Category	Explanation
All Trimesters	B	Animal studies have revealed no evidence of harm to the fetus, however, there are no adequate studies in pregnant women OR animal studies have shown an adverse effect, but adequate studies in pregnant women have failed to demonstrate a risk to the fetus.

Breast Feeding—Studies suggest that this medication may alter milk production or composition. If an alternative to this medication is not prescribed, you should monitor the infant for side effects and adequate milk intake.

Other medicines—Although certain medicines should not be used together at all, in other cases two different medicines may be used together even if an interaction might occur. In these cases, your doctor may want to change the dose, or other precautions may be necessary. Tell your healthcare professional if you are taking any other prescription or non-prescription (over-the-counter [OTC]) medicine.

Interactions with Food/Tobacco/Alcohol—Certain medicines should not be used at or around the time of eating food or eating certain types of food since interactions may occur. Using alcohol or tobacco with certain medicines may also cause interactions to occur. Discuss with your healthcare professional the use of your medicine with food, alcohol, or tobacco.

Other medical problems—The presence of other medical problems may affect the use of this medicine. Make sure you tell your doctor if you have any other medical problems, especially:
- Bleeding (severe)—Oxybutynin may increase heart rate, which may make this condition worse
- Colitis (severe) or
- Dryness of mouth (severe and continuing) or
- Enlarged prostate or
- Glaucoma or
- Heart disease or
- Hiatal hernia or
- High blood pressure (hypertension) or
- Intestinal blockage or other intestinal or stomach problems or
- Myasthenia gravis or
- Toxemia of pregnancy or
- Urinary tract blockage or problems with urination—Oxybutynin may make these conditions worse
- Kidney disease or
- Liver disease—Higher blood levels of oxybutynin may occur, which increases the chance of side effects
- Overactive thyroid—Oxybutynin may further increase heart rate

Proper Use of This Medicine

This medicine is usually taken with water on an empty stomach. However, your doctor may want you to take it with food or milk to lessen stomach upset.

For extended release tablets—Swallow this medicine whole. Do not chew it or crush it up.

Take this medicine only as directed. Do not take more of it, do not take it more often, and do not take it for a longer time than your doctor ordered. To do so may increase the chance of side effects.

Dosing—The dose of this medicine will be different for different patients. Follow your doctor's orders or the directions on the label. The following information includes only the av-

erage doses of this medicine. If your dose is different, do not change it unless your doctor tells you to do so.

The amount of medicine that you take depends on the strength of the medicine. Also, the number of doses you take each day, the time allowed between doses, and the length of time you take the medicine depend on the medical problem for which you are using the medicine.

- For oral dosage forms (syrup or tablets):
  - For treatment of bladder problems:
    - Adults and children 12 years of age and over—5 milligrams (mg) two or three times a day.
    - Children up to 5 years of age—Use and dose have not been determined.
    - Children 5 to 12 years of age—5 mg two or three times a day. The dose is usually not more than 15 mg a day.
- For oral dosage form (extended release tablets):
  - For treatment of bladder problems:
    - Adults and children 12 years of age and over—5 mg to 10 mg once daily
    - Children up to 6 years of age—Use and dose have not been determined.
    - Children 6 to 12 years of age—5 mg once daily. The dose is usually not more than 20 mg per day.

Missed dose—If you miss a dose of this medicine, take it as soon as possible. However, if it is almost time for your next dose, skip the missed dose and go back to your regular dosing schedule. Do not double doses.

Storage—Store the medicine in a closed container at room temperature, away from heat, moisture, and direct light. Keep from freezing.

Keep out of the reach of children.

Do not keep outdated medicine or medicine no longer needed.

Precautions While Using This Medicine

This medicine will add to the effects of alcohol and other CNS depressants (medicines that slow down the nervous system, possibly causing drowsiness). Some examples of CNS depressants are antihistamines or medicine for hay fever, other allergies, or colds; sedatives, tranquilizers, or sleeping medicine; prescription pain medicine or narcotics; barbiturates; medicine for seizures; muscle relaxants; or anesthetics, including some dental anesthetics. Check with your doctor before taking any of the above while you are using this medicine.

This medicine may cause your eyes to become more sensitive to light than they are normally. Wearing sunglasses and avoiding too much exposure to bright light may help lessen the discomfort.

This medicine may cause some people to become drowsy or have blurred vision. Make sure you know how you react to this medicine before you drive, use machines, or do anything else that could be dangerous if you are not alert or able to see well.

Oxybutynin may make you sweat less, causing your body temperature to increase. Use extra care not to become overheated during exercise or hot weather while you are taking this medicine, since overheating may result in heat stroke. Also, hot baths or saunas may make you feel dizzy or faint while you are taking this medicine.

Your mouth, nose, and throat may feel very dry while you are taking this medicine. For temporary relief of mouth dryness, use sugarless candy or gum, melt bits of ice in your mouth, or use a saliva substitute. However, if your mouth continues to feel dry for more than 2 weeks, check with your medical doctor or dentist. Continuing dryness of the mouth may increase the chance of dental disease, including tooth decay, gum disease, and fungus infections.

The extended release tablet shell may be removed from your body and visible in your stool.

Side Effects of This Medicine

Along with its needed effects, a medicine may cause some unwanted effects. Although not all of these side effects may occur, if they do occur they may need medical attention.

Check with your doctor as soon as possible if any of the following side effects occur:

Rare
  Eye pain; skin rash or hives

Symptoms of overdose
  Clumsiness or unsteadiness; confusion; convulsions; dizziness; drowsiness (severe); fainting; fast, slow, or irregular heartbeat; fever; flushing or redness of face; hallucinations (seeing, hearing, or feeling things that are not there); shortness of breath or troubled breathing; unusual excitement, nervousness, restlessness, or irritability

Some side effects may occur that usually do not need medical attention. These side effects may go away during treatment as your body adjusts to the medicine. Also, your health care professional may be able to tell you about ways to prevent or reduce some of these side effects. Check with your health care professional if any of the following side effects continue or are bothersome or if you have any questions about them:

More common
  Acid or sour stomach; belching; constipation; decreased sweating; diarrhea; dizziness; drowsiness; dryness of eyes, mouth, nose, and throat; heartburn; indigestion; stomach discomfort, upset or pain; decreased sweating; runny nose

Less common or rare
  Blurred vision; decreased flow of breast milk; decreased sexual ability; difficult urination; difficulty in swallowing; feeling of warmth or heat; flushing or redness of skin, especially on face and neck; headache; increased sensitivity of eyes to light; nausea or vomiting; trouble in sleeping; unusual tiredness or weakness

Other side effects not listed may also occur in some patients. If you notice any other effects, check with your healthcare professional.

Incidence not determined—Observed during clinical practice with levofloxacin; estimates of frequency cannot be determined
  Bloating or swelling of face, arms, hands, lower legs, or feet; decreased interest in sexual intercourse; inability to have or keep an erection; loss in sexual ability, desire, drive, or performance; rapid weight gain; seeing, hearing, or feeling things that are not there; tingling of hands or feet; unusual weight gain or loss

---

OXYCODONE AND IBUPROFEN

(Oral route) - oks-ee-KOE-done, eye-byoo-PROE-fen

Black Box Warning

- CARDIOVASCULAR RISK
  - NSAIDs may cause an increased risk of serious cardiovascular thrombotic events, myocardial infarction, and stroke, which can be fatal. This risk may increase with duration of use. Patients with cardiovascular disease or risk factors for cardiovascular disease may be at greater risk.
  - Ibuprofen/oxycodone hydrochloride is contraindicated for the treatment of peri-operative pain in the setting of coronary artery bypass graft (CABG) surgery.
- GASTROINTESTINAL RISK
  - NSAIDs cause an increased risk of serious gastrointestinal adverse events including bleeding, ulceration, and perforation of the stomach or intestines, which can be fatal. These events can occur at any time during use and without warning symptoms. Elderly patients are at greater risk for serious gastrointestinal events.

Commonly used brand name(s)

In the U.S.—
   Combunox

Available Dosage Forms:

- Tablet

Therapeutic Class: Opioid/NSAID Combination
Pharmacologic Class: NSAID

Uses For This Medicine

Ibuprofen and oxycodone combination is used to relieve pain.

Ibuprofen is a nonsteroidal anti-inflammatory drug (NSAID) used in this combination to relieve inflammation, swelling, and pain.

The oxycodone is a narcotic analgesic that acts in the central nervous system to relieve pain. If oxycodone is used for a long time, it may become habit-forming (causing mental or physical dependence). Physical dependence may lead to withdrawal side effects when you stop taking the medicine. Since ibuprofen and oxycodone combination is only used for short-term (7 days or less) relief of pain, physical dependence probably will not occur.

This medicine is available only with your doctor's prescription.

Before Using This Medicine

In deciding to use a medicine, the risks of taking the medicine must be weighed against the good it will do. This is a decision you and your doctor will make. For this medicine, the following should be considered:

Allergies—Tell your doctor if you have ever had any unusual or allergic reaction to this medicine or any other medicines. Also tell your health care professional if you have any other types of allergies, such as to foods, dyes, preservatives, or animals. For non-prescription products, read the label or package ingredients carefully.

Pediatric—Appropriate studies have not been performed on the relationship of age to the effects of ibuprofen and oxycodone combination in children under 14 years of age. Safety and efficacy have not been established in children below the age of 14 years.

Geriatric—Respiratory problems, kidney problems, or gastrointestinal (GI) tract problems may be more likely to occur in elderly patients, who may be more sensitive than younger adults to the effects of ibuprofen and oxycodone combination. Special care should be taken when treating these patients.

Pregnancy—

	Pregnancy Category	Explanation
All Trimesters	C	Animal studies have shown an adverse effect and there are no adequate studies in pregnant women OR no animal studies have been conducted and there are no adequate studies in pregnant women.

Breast Feeding—Studies in women breastfeeding have demonstrated harmful infant effects. An alternative to this medication should be prescribed or you should stop breastfeeding while using this medicine.

Other medicines—

Using this medicine with any of the following medicines is not recommended. Your doctor may decide not to treat you with this medication or change some of the other medicines you take.

Ketorolac, Naltrexone

Interactions with Food/Tobacco/Alcohol—Certain medicines should not be used at or around the time of eating food or eating certain types of food since interactions may occur. Using alcohol or tobacco with certain medicines may also cause interactions to occur. Discuss with your healthcare professional the use of your medicine with food, alcohol, or tobacco.

Other medical problems—The presence of other medical problems may affect the use of this medicine. Make sure you tell your doctor if you have any other medical problems, especially:

- Addison's disease (rare hormonal disease causing fatigue, low blood pressure) or
- Anemia or
- Alcohol abuse, or history of, or
- Bleeding problems or
- Dehydration or
- Drug dependence, especially narcotic abuse, or history of or
- Enlarged prostate or

- High blood pressure or
- Kidney disease or
- Kyphoscoliosis (curvature of spine that can cause breathing problems) or
- Liver disease or
- Seizure disorders or
- Tobacco use or
- Toxic psychosis (hallucinations, paranoia) or
- Tremors or
- Underactive thyroid—The chance of side effects may be increased.
- Brain disease or head injury or
- Enlarged prostate or problems with urination—The side effects of ibuprofen and oxycodone combination may be dangerous with these conditions.
- Bronchial asthma, acute or severe, or other chronic lung disease or
- Hypercarbia (large amount of carbon dioxide in the blood) or
- Paralytic ileus (blockage in the intestines) or
- Respiratory depression (troubled breathing)—Ibuprofen and oxycodone combination should NOT be taken by patients with these conditions.
- Coronary artery bypass graft (CABG) surgery (routes blood around blocked or hardened arteries in the heart)—Ibuprofen and oxycodone combination should NOT be used to relieve pain during this operation.
- Gallstone problems or
- Pancreatitis (inflammation of the pancreas)—May make these conditions worse.
- Heart disease or
- Heart failure or
- Risk factors for heart disease—May increase the risk of serious heart problems, heart attacks, or strokes which could be fatal.
- Lupus (disease affecting immune system)—May cause severe unwanted effects in patients taking ibuprofen.
- Postoperative period (after a major surgery)—Oxycodone may cause problems if taken right after surgery.
- Stomach or intestinal bleeding or ulcers—This medicine should be prescribed with extreme caution in these patients.

Proper Use of This Medicine

Dosing—The dose of this medicine will be different for different patients. Follow your doctor's orders or the directions on the label. The following information includes only the average doses of this medicine. If your dose is different, do not change it unless your doctor tells you to do so.

The amount of medicine that you take depends on the strength of the medicine. Also, the number of doses you take each day, the time allowed between doses, and the length of time you take the medicine depend on the medical problem for which you are using the medicine.

For safe and effective use of this medicine, do not take more of it, do not take it more often, and do not take it for a longer time than ordered by your health care professional. Taking too much of this medicine may increase the chance of unwanted effects and the chances of abuse.

- For oral dosage form (tablets):
  - For pain
    - Adults and teenagers (14 years of age and older)—1 tablet (400 milligrams (mg) ibuprofen and 5 mg oxycodone). You should not use more than 4 tablets per day, and this medicine should not be used for longer than 7 days, unless directed by your doctor.
    - Children—Use and dose must be determined by your doctor.

Missed dose—If you miss a dose of this medicine, take it as soon as possible. However, if it is almost time for your next dose, skip the missed dose and go back to your regular dosing schedule. Do not double doses.

Storage—Store the medicine in a closed container at room temperature, away from heat, moisture, and direct light. Keep from freezing.

Keep out of the reach of children.

Do not keep outdated medicine or medicine no longer needed.

Ask your healthcare professional how you should dispose of any medicine you do not use.

Precautions While Using This Medicine

Your doctor will want to check your blood pressure at the beginning of treatment and monitor it throughout treatment with this medicine. If high blood pressure occurs or worsens while taking this medicine, it may lead to serious heart problems.

Ibuprofen and oxycodone combination will add to the effects of alcohol and other central nervous system (CNS) depressants (medicines that slow down the nervous system, possibly causing drowsiness). Some examples of CNS depressants are antihistamines or medicines for hay fever, other allergies, or colds; sedatives, tranquilizers, sleeping medicine, or other prescription pain medication. Do not drink alcoholic beverages, and check with your medical doctor or dentist before taking any of the medicines listed above, while you are using this medicine.

You should tell your doctor if you are taking corticosteroids or anticoagulants (medicines that prevent blood clots). These medicines could increase your chances of stomach or intestinal bleeding when taken with ibuprofen.

Ibuprofen is an NSAID (nonsteroidal antiinflammatory drug) and NSAIDs can cause serious gastrointestinal (GI) problems including inflammation, bleeding ulcers or tearing of the stomach, small intestine or large intestine. These problems can occur at any time with or without warning, and can be fatal. *You should contact your doctor immediately* if any of the following symptoms occur including black, tarry stools; bloody stools; vomiting of blood or material that looks like coffee grounds; severe or continuing stomach pain, cramping, or burning; trouble breathing; severe or continuing nausea, heartburn and/or indigestion.

Your chances of having GI bleeding could be greater if you are on this medicine for a long period of time, if you smoke or use alcohol, if you are older, or if you are in poor health.

This medicine may cause some people to become drowsy, dizzy, light-headed, or to feel a false sense of well-being. Make sure you know how you react to this medicine before you drive, use machines, or do anything else that could be dangerous if you are dizzy or are not alert and clearheaded. If these reactions are especially bothersome, check with your doctor.

Dizziness, light-headedness, or fainting may occur, especially when getting up suddenly from a lying or sitting position. Getting up slowly may lessen this problem.

Before having any kind of surgery (including dental surgery) or emergency treatment, tell the medical doctor or dentist in charge that you are taking this medicine.

Ibuprofen and oxycodone combination may cause dryness of the mouth. For temporary relief, use sugarless candy or gum, melt bits of ice in your mouth, or use a saliva substitute. However, if dry mouth continues for more than 2 weeks, check with your dentist. Continuing dryness of the mouth may increase the chance of dental disease, including tooth decay, gum disease, and fungus infections.

Side Effects of This Medicine

Along with its needed effects, a medicine may cause some unwanted effects. Although not all of these side effects may occur, if they do occur they may need medical attention.

Check with your doctor immediately if any of the following side effects occur:

Less common

Feeling faint, dizzy, or light-headed; feeling of warmth or heat; flushing or redness of skin, especially on face and neck; headache; sweating

Rare

Abdominal pain; blurred vision; changes in skin color; chest pain; confusion; convulsions; decrease in frequency of urination; decreased urine; difficulty in breathing; difficulty in passing urine (dribbling); dizziness; dizziness, faintness, or light-headedness when getting up from a lying position; dry mouth; excessive muscle tone; fainting; fast heartbeat; fast, pounding, or irregular heartbeat or pulse; increased need to urinate; increased thirst; irregular heartbeat; loss of appetite; mood changes; muscle pain or cramps; muscle stiffness; muscle tension or tightness; nausea or vomiting; numbness or tingling in hands, feet, or lips; pain, tenderness, swelling of foot or leg; painful urination; pale skin; passing urine more often; severe constipation; severe vomiting; shortness of breath; troubled breathing with exertion; unusual bleeding or bruising; unusual tiredness or weakness; weakness

Symptoms of overdose

Get emergency help immediately if any of the following symptoms of overdose occur:

Blurred vision; change in consciousness; chest pain or discomfort; cold and clammy skin; confusion; constricted pupils; continuing ringing or buzzing or other unexplained noise in ears; convulsions; decreased awareness or responsiveness; difficult or troubled breathing; difficulty sleeping; disorientation; dizziness; dizziness, faintness, or light-headedness when getting up from a lying position; drowsiness to profound coma; fainting; fast or irregular heartbeat; fast, pounding, or irregular heartbeat or pulse; hallucination; headache; hearing loss; irregular, fast or slow, or shallow breathing; lethargy; light-headedness, dizziness, or fainting; loss of bladder control; loss of consciousness; mood or other mental changes; muscle spasm or jerking of all extremities; nausea; pale or blue lips, fingernails, or skin; severe sleepiness; shortness of breath; skeletal muscle flaccidity; sleepiness or unusual drowsiness; slow or irregular heartbeat; stomach pain; sudden fainting; sudden loss of consciousness; sweating; trouble breathing; unusual tiredness or weakness; vomiting

Some side effects may occur that usually do not need medical attention. These side effects may go away during treatment as your body adjusts to the medicine. Also, your health care professional may be able to tell you about ways to prevent or reduce some of these side effects. Check with your health care professional if any of the following side effects continue or are bothersome or if you have any questions about them:

More common

Headache; sleepiness or unusual drowsiness

Less common

Acid or sour stomach; belching; bloated full feeling; diarrhea; difficulty having a bowel movement (stool); excess air or gas in stomach or intestines; fever; heartburn; indigestion; lack or loss of strength; passing gas; stomach discomfort, upset, or pain

Rare

Back pain; body aches or pain; bruising, large, flat, blue or purplish patches in the skin; changes in vision; chills; congestion; cough or hoarseness; delusions; dementia; difficult urination; difficulty in moving; dryness or soreness of throat; enlarged abdomen; false or unusual sense of well-being; fear; hoarseness; impaired vision; increase in body movements; lower back or side pain; nervousness; pain, swelling, or redness in joints; rash; runny nose; sleeplessness; stomach pain; swelling; taste perversion; tender, swollen glands in neck; trouble in swallowing; trouble sleeping; unable to sleep; voice changes

Other side effects not listed may also occur in some patients. If you notice any other effects, check with your healthcare professional.

OXYMETAZOLINE (Nasal route) - ox-i-met-AZ-oh-leen

Commonly used brand name(s)

In the U.S.—

4–Way Long Lasting	Nasin
Afrin	Neo-Synephrine 12 Hour
Duramist Plus	Nostrilla
Duration	NRS-Nasal Relief
Genasal	Sinarest Nasal
Nasacon	Vicks Sinex 12 Hour

Available Dosage Forms:
- Spray
- Solution

Therapeutic Class: Decongestant

Uses For This Medicine

Oxymetazoline is used for the temporary relief of nasal (of the nose) congestion or stuffiness caused by hay fever or other allergies, colds, or sinus trouble.

This medicine may also be used for other conditions as determined by your doctor.

This medicine is available without a prescription.

Before Using This Medicine

In deciding to use a medicine, the risks of taking the medicine must be weighed against the good it will do. This is a decision you and your doctor will make. For this medicine, the following should be considered:

Allergies—Tell your doctor if you have ever had any unusual or allergic reaction to this medicine or any other medicines. Also tell your health care professional if you have any other types of allergies, such as to foods, dyes, preservatives, or animals. For non-prescription products, read the label or package ingredients carefully.

Pediatric—Children may be especially sensitive to the effects of oxymetazoline. This may increase the chance of side effects during treatment.

Geriatric—Many medicines have not been tested in older people. Therefore, it may not be known whether they work exactly the same way they do in younger adults or if they cause different side effects or problems in older people. There is no specific information about the use of oxymetazoline in the elderly.

Breast Feeding—There are no adequate studies in women for determining infant risk when using this medication during breastfeeding. Weigh the potential benefits against the potential risks before taking this medication while breastfeeding.

Other medicines—Although certain medicines should not be used together at all, in other cases two different medicines may be used together even if an interaction might occur. In these cases, your doctor may want to change the dose, or other precautions may be necessary. Tell your healthcare professional if you are taking any other prescription or non-prescription (over-the-counter [OTC]) medicine.

Interactions with Food/Tobacco/Alcohol—Certain medicines should not be used at or around the time of eating food or eating certain types of food since interactions may occur. Using alcohol or tobacco with certain medicines may also cause interactions to occur. Discuss with your healthcare professional the use of your medicine with food, alcohol, or tobacco.

Other medical problems—The presence of other medical problems may affect the use of this medicine. Make sure you tell your doctor if you have any other medical problems, especially:

- Type 2 diabetes mellitus
- Dry membranes in nose
- Enlarged prostate—Difficulty urinating may worsen
- Glaucoma
- Heart or blood vessel disease or
- High blood pressure—Oxymetazoline may make the condition worse
- Overactive thyroid

Proper Use of This Medicine

To use the nose drops:
- Blow your nose gently. Tilt the head back while standing or sitting up, or lie down on a bed and hang the head over the side. Place the drops into each nostril and keep the head tilted back for a few minutes to allow the medicine to spread throughout the nose.
- Rinse the dropper with hot water and dry with a clean tissue. Replace the cap right after use.
- To avoid spreading the infection, do not use the container for more than one person.

To use the nose spray:
- Blow your nose gently. With the head upright, spray the medicine into each nostril. Sniff briskly while squeezing the bottle quickly and firmly. For best results, spray once into each nostril, wait 3 to 5 minutes to allow the medicine to work, then blow the nose gently and thoroughly. Repeat until the complete dose is used.
- Rinse the tip of the spray bottle with hot water, taking care not to suck water into the bottle, and dry with a clean tissue. Replace the cap right after use.
- To avoid spreading the infection, do not use the container for more than one person.

Use this medicine only as directed. Do not use more of it, do not use it more often, and do not use it for longer than 3 days without first checking with your doctor. To do so may make your runny or stuffy nose worse and may also increase the chance of side effects.

Dosing—The dose of this medicine will be different for different patients. Follow your doctor's orders or the directions on the label. The following information includes only the average doses of this medicine. If your dose is different, do not change it unless your doctor tells you to do so.

The amount of medicine that you take depends on the strength of the medicine. Also, the number of doses you take each day, the time allowed between doses, and the length of time you take the medicine depend on the medical problem for which you are using the medicine.

- For nasal dosage form (nose drops or spray):
  - For nasal congestion or stuffiness:
    - Adults and children 6 years of age and older—Use 2 or 3 drops or sprays of 0.05% solution in each nostril every ten to twelve hours. Do not use more than two times in twenty four hours.
    - Children up to 6 years of age—Use and dose must be determined by your doctor.

Missed dose—If you miss a dose of this medicine, take it as soon as possible. However, if it is almost time for your next dose, skip the missed dose and go back to your regular dosing schedule. Do not double doses.

Storage—Store the medicine in a closed container at room temperature, away from heat, moisture, and direct light. Keep from freezing.

Keep out of the reach of children.

Do not keep outdated medicine or medicine no longer needed.

Side Effects of This Medicine

Along with its needed effects, a medicine may cause some unwanted effects. Although not all of these side effects may occur, if they do occur they may need medical attention.

Check with your doctor as soon as possible if any of the following side effects occur:

> Increase in runny or stuffy nose

Symptoms of too much medicine being absorbed into the body

> Blurred vision; fast, irregular, or pounding heartbeat; headache, dizziness, drowsiness, or lightheadedness; high blood pressure; nervousness; trembling; trouble in sleeping; weakness.

The above side effects are more likely to occur in children because there is a greater chance in children that too much of this medicine may be absorbed into the body.

Some side effects may occur that usually do not need medical attention. These side effects may go away during treatment as your body adjusts to the medicine. Also, your health care professional may be able to tell you about ways to prevent or reduce some of these side effects. Check with your health care professional if any of the following side effects continue or are bothersome or if you have any questions about them:

> Burning, dryness, or stinging inside of nose; increase in nasal discharge; sneezing

Other side effects not listed may also occur in some patients. If you notice any other effects, check with your healthcare professional.

OXYMETAZOLINE (Ophthalmic route)
- ox-i-met-AZ-oh-leen

Commonly used brand name(s)

In the U.S.—
> Ocuclear
> Visine L.R.

Available Dosage Forms:
- Solution

Therapeutic Class: Decongestant

Uses For This Medicine

Oxymetazoline is used to relieve redness due to minor eye irritations, such as those caused by colds, dust, wind, smog, pollen, swimming, or wearing contact lenses.

Oxymetazoline is available without a prescription.

Before Using This Medicine

In deciding to use a medicine, the risks of taking the medicine must be weighed against the good it will do. This is a decision you and your doctor will make. For this medicine, the following should be considered:

Allergies—Tell your doctor if you have ever had any unusual or allergic reaction to this medicine or any other medicines. Also tell your health care professional if you have any other types of allergies, such as to foods, dyes, preservatives, or animals. For non-prescription products, read the label or package ingredients carefully.

Pediatric—Check with your doctor before using oxymetazoline eye drops in children up to 6 years of age. Eye redness in children can occur with illnesses, such as allergies, fevers, colds, and measles, that may require medical attention.

Geriatric—Many medicines have not been studied specifically in older people. Therefore, it may not be known whether they work exactly the same way they do in younger adults or if they cause different side effects or problems in older people. There is no specific information comparing use of oxymetazoline in the elderly with use in other age groups.

Breast Feeding—There are no adequate studies in women for determining infant risk when using this medication during breastfeeding. Weigh the potential benefits against the potential risks before taking this medication while breastfeeding.

Other medicines—Although certain medicines should not be used together at all, in other cases two different medicines may be used together even if an interaction might occur. In these cases, your doctor may want to change the dose, or other precautions may be necessary. Tell your healthcare professional if you are taking any other prescription or non-prescription (over-the-counter [OTC]) medicine.

Interactions with Food/Tobacco/Alcohol—Certain medicines should not be used at or around the time of eating food or eating certain types of food since interactions may occur. Using alcohol or tobacco with certain medicines may also cause interactions to occur. Discuss with your healthcare professional the use of your medicine with food, alcohol, or tobacco.

Other medical problems—The presence of other medical problems may affect the use of this medicine. Make sure you tell your doctor if you have any other medical problems, especially:
- Eye disease, infection, or injury—This medicine may mask the symptoms of these conditions
- Heart or blood vessel disease or
- High blood pressure or
- Overactive thyroid—If absorbed into the body, this medicine may cause side effects that may make the medical problem worse
- Use of soft contact lenses—Because of the preservative in this medicine, some eye conditions may get worse if this medicine is used on top of soft contact lenses

Proper Use of This Medicine

Do not use oxymetazoline ophthalmic solution if it becomes cloudy or changes color.

To use:

- First, wash your hands. With the middle finger, apply pressure to the inside corner of the eye (and continue to apply pressure for 1 or 2 minutes after the medicine has been placed in the eye). Tilt the head back and with the index finger of the same hand, pull the lower eyelid away from the eye to form a pouch. Drop the medicine into the pouch and gently close the eyes. Do not blink. Keep the eyes closed for 1 or 2 minutes to allow the medicine to be absorbed.
- To keep the medicine as germ-free as possible, do not touch the applicator tip to any surface (including the eye). Also, keep the container tightly closed.

Use this medicine only as directed. Do not use more of it, do not use it more often, and do not use it for more than 72 hours, unless otherwise directed by your doctor. To do so may make your eye irritation worse and may also increase the chance of side effects.

Dosing—The dose of this medicine will be different for different patients. Follow your doctor's orders or the directions on the label. The following information includes only the average doses of this medicine. If your dose is different, do not change it unless your doctor tells you to do so.

The amount of medicine that you take depends on the strength of the medicine. Also, the number of doses you take each day, the time allowed between doses, and the length of time you take the medicine depend on the medical problem for which you are using the medicine.

- For ophthalmic solution (eye drops) dosage form:
  - For eye redness:
    - Adults and children 6 years of age and older— Use 1 drop in the eye every six hours.
    - Children up to 6 years of age—Use and dose must be determined by your doctor.

Storage—Store the medicine in a closed container at room temperature, away from heat, moisture, and direct light. Keep from freezing.

Keep out of the reach of children.

Do not keep outdated medicine or medicine no longer needed.

Precautions While Using This Medicine

If eye pain or change in vision occurs or if redness or irritation of the eye continues, gets worse, or lasts for more than 72 hours, stop using the medicine and check with your doctor.

Side Effects of This Medicine

Along with its needed effects, a medicine may cause some unwanted effects. Although not all of these side effects may occur, if they do occur they may need medical attention.

When this medicine is used for short periods of time at low doses, side effects usually are rare.

Check with your doctor as soon as possible if any of the following side effects occur:

With overuse or long-term use
Increase in irritation or redness of eyes

Symptoms of too much medicine being absorbed into the body

Fast, irregular, or pounding heartbeat; headache or lightheadedness; nervousness; trembling; trouble in sleeping

Other side effects not listed may also occur in some patients. If you notice any other effects, check with your healthcare professional.

OXYTOCIN (Nasal route, Intravenous route, Injection route) - ox-i-TOE-sin

Black Box Warning

Elective induction of labor is defined as the initiation of labor in a pregnant individual who has no medical indications for induction. Since the available data are inadequate to evaluate the benefits-to-risks considerations, oxytocin is not indicated for elective induction of labor.

Commonly used brand name(s)

In the U.S.—
Pitocin

In Canada—
Syntocinon

Available Dosage Forms:

- Solution
- Injectable
- Spray

Therapeutic Class: Uterine Stimulant
Pharmacologic Class: Pituitary Hormone, Posterior

Uses For This Medicine

Oxytocin is a hormone used to help start or continue labor and to control bleeding after delivery. It is also sometimes used to help milk secretion in breast-feeding.

Oxytocin may also be used for other conditions as determined by your doctor.

In general, oxytocin should not be used to start labor unless there are specific medical reasons. Be sure you have discussed this with your doctor before receiving this medicine.

Oxytocin is available only with your doctor's prescription.

Once a medicine has been approved for marketing for a certain use, experience may show that it is also useful for other medical problems. Although this use is not included in product labeling, oxytocin is used in certain patients for the following:

- Testing the ability of the placenta to support a pregnancy

Before Using This Medicine

In deciding to use a medicine, the risks of taking the medicine must be weighed against the good it will do. This is a decision

you and your doctor will make. For this medicine, the following should be considered:

Allergies—Tell your doctor if you have ever had any unusual or allergic reaction to this medicine or any other medicines. Also tell your health care professional if you have any other types of allergies, such as to foods, dyes, preservatives, or animals. For non-prescription products, read the label or package ingredients carefully.

Breast Feeding—Studies suggest that this medication may alter milk production or composition. If an alternative to this medication is not prescribed, you should monitor the infant for side effects and adequate milk intake.

Other medicines—

Using this medicine with any of the following medicines is not recommended. Your doctor may decide not to treat you with this medication or change some of the other medicines you take.

Dinoprostone

Interactions with Food/Tobacco/Alcohol—Certain medicines should not be used at or around the time of eating food or eating certain types of food since interactions may occur. Using alcohol or tobacco with certain medicines may also cause interactions to occur. Discuss with your healthcare professional the use of your medicine with food, alcohol, or tobacco.

Other medical problems—The presence of other medical problems may affect the use of this medicine. Make sure you tell your doctor if you have any other medical problems, especially:

* Heart disease
* Hypertension
* Kidney disease

Proper Use of This Medicine

For patients using the nasal spray form of this medicine:

* This medicine usually comes with directions for use. Read them carefully before using.

Dosing—The dose of this medicine will be different for different patients. Follow your doctor's orders or the directions on the label. The following information includes only the average doses of this medicine. If your dose is different, do not change it unless your doctor tells you to do so.

The amount of medicine that you take depends on the strength of the medicine. Also, the number of doses you take each day, the time allowed between doses, and the length of time you take the medicine depend on the medical problem for which you are using the medicine.

* For nasal dosage form:
  * For increasing milk production in breast feeding:
    * Adults—One spray into one or both nostrils two or three minutes before nursing or pumping milk from breasts.
* For injection dosage form:
  * For helping to start or continue labor:
    * Adults—At first, 0.5 to 2 milliunits per minute slowly injected into a vein. Then, your doctor may increase the dose every fifteen to sixty minutes as needed.

* For treating incomplete abortion, causing abortion, or controlling bleeding after an abortion:
  * Adults—10 units injected slowly into a vein.
* For helping to control bleeding after delivery:
  * Adults—10 units injected into a muscle or slowly into a vein.

Storage—Store the medicine in a closed container at room temperature, away from heat, moisture, and direct light. Keep from freezing.

Keep out of the reach of children.

Do not keep outdated medicine or medicine no longer needed.

Precautions While Using This Medicine

Oxytocin nasal spray may not help milk secretion in some breast-feeding women. Call your doctor if this medicine is not working.

Side Effects of This Medicine

Oxytocin can be very useful for helping labor. However, there are certain risks with using it. Oxytocin causes contractions of the uterus. In women who are unusually sensitive to its effects, these contractions may become too strong. In rare cases, this may lead to tearing of the uterus. Also, if contractions are too strong, the supply of blood and oxygen to the fetus may be decreased.

Oxytocin has been reported to cause irregular heartbeat and increase bleeding after delivery in some women. It has also been reported to cause jaundice in some newborn infants.

Along with its needed effects, a medicine may cause some unwanted effects. Although not all of these side effects may occur, if they do occur they may need medical attention.

Rare (with use of injection)
  Confusion; convulsions (seizures); difficulty in breathing; dizziness; fast or irregular heartbeat; headache (continuing or severe); hives; pelvic or abdominal pain (severe); skin rash or itching; vaginal bleeding (increased or continuing); weakness; weight gain (rapid)

Rare (with use of nasal spray)
  Convulsions (seizures); mental disturbances; unexpected bleeding or contractions of the uterus

Some side effects may occur that usually do not need medical attention. These side effects may go away during treatment as your body adjusts to the medicine. Also, your health care professional may be able to tell you about ways to prevent or reduce some of these side effects. Check with your health care professional if any of the following side effects continue or are bothersome or if you have any questions about them:

Rare (with use of injection)
  Nausea; vomiting

Rare (with use of nasal spray)
  Nasal irritation; runny nose; tearing of the eyes

Other side effects not listed may also occur in some patients. If you notice any other effects, check with your healthcare professional.

PACLITAXEL   (Intravenous route) -
PAK-li-tax-el

Commonly used brand name(s)

In the U.S.—

Nov-Onxol	Paclitaxel Novaplus
Onxol	Taxol

Available Dosage Forms:

- Solution

Therapeutic Class: Antineoplastic Agent
Pharmacologic Class: Mitotic Inhibitor

Uses For This Medicine

Paclitaxel belongs to the group of medicines called antineoplastics. It is used to treat cancer of the ovaries, breast, certain types of lung cancer, and a cancer of the skin and mucous membranes more commonly found in patients with acquired immunodeficiency syndrome (AIDS). It may also be used to treat other kinds of cancer, as determined by your doctor.

Paclitaxel interferes with the growth of cancer cells, which are eventually destroyed. Since the growth of normal body cells may also be affected by paclitaxel, other effects will also occur. Some of these may be serious and must be reported to your doctor. Other effects may not be serious but may cause concern. Some effects may not occur until months or years after the medicine is used.

Before you begin treatment with paclitaxel, you and your doctor should talk about the good this medicine will do as well as the risks of using it.

Paclitaxel is to be administered only by or under the immediate supervision of your doctor.

Once a medicine has been approved for marketing for a certain use, experience may show that it is also useful for other medical problems. Although these uses are not included in product labeling, paclitaxel is used in certain patients with the following medical conditions:

- Cancer of the bladder
- Cancer of the cervix
- Cancer of the endometrium
- Cancer of the fallopian tube or lining of the abdomen (spreading from the ovary)
- Cancer of the esophagus
- Cancers of the head and neck
- Small cell lung cancer (a certain type found in the tissues of the lungs)
- Cancer of the stomach
- Cancer of the prostate
- Cancer of the testes
- Cancer of unknown primary site

Before Using This Medicine

In deciding to use a medicine, the risks of taking the medicine must be weighed against the good it will do. This is a decision you and your doctor will make. For this medicine, the following should be considered:

Allergies—Tell your doctor if you have ever had any unusual or allergic reaction to this medicine or any other medicines. Also tell your health care professional if you have any

other types of allergies, such as to foods, dyes, preservatives, or animals. For non-prescription products, read the label or package ingredients carefully.

Pediatric—There is no specific information comparing use of paclitaxel in children with use in other age groups.

Geriatric—This medicine has been tested in a limited number of patients and has not been shown to cause different side effects or problems in older people than it does in younger adults.

Pregnancy—

	Pregnancy Category	Explanation
All Trimesters	D	Studies in pregnant women have demonstrated a risk to the fetus. However, the benefits of therapy in a life threatening situation or a serious disease, may outweigh the potential risk.

Breast Feeding—There are no adequate studies in women for determining infant risk when using this medication during breastfeeding. Weigh the potential benefits against the potential risks before taking this medication while breastfeeding.

Other medicines—

Using this medicine with any of the following medicines is not recommended. Your doctor may decide not to treat you with this medication or change some of the other medicines you take.

Rotavirus Vaccine, Live

Interactions with Food/Tobacco/Alcohol—Certain medicines should not be used at or around the time of eating food or eating certain types of food since interactions may occur. Using alcohol or tobacco with certain medicines may also cause interactions to occur. Discuss with your healthcare professional the use of your medicine with food, alcohol, or tobacco.

Other medical problems—The presence of other medical problems may affect the use of this medicine. Make sure you tell your doctor if you have any other medical problems, especially:

- Chickenpox (including recent exposure) or
- Herpes zoster (shingles)—Risk of severe disease affecting other parts of the body
- Heart rhythm problems—May be made worse by paclitaxel
- Infection—Paclitaxel may decrease your body's ability to fight infection

Proper Use of This Medicine

This medicine often causes nausea and vomiting, which is usually mild. However, it is very important that you continue to receive the medicine even if you begin to feel ill. Ask your health care professional for ways to lessen these effects.

Dosing—The dose of this medicine will be different for different patients. Follow your doctor's orders or the directions on the label. The following information includes only the average doses of this medicine. If your dose is different, do not change it unless your doctor tells you to do so.

The amount of medicine that you take depends on the strength of the medicine. Also, the number of doses you take

each day, the time allowed between doses, and the length of time you take the medicine depend on the medical problem for which you are using the medicine.

Precautions While Using This Medicine

It is very important that your doctor check your progress at regular visits to make sure that this medicine is working properly and to check for unwanted effects.

While you are being treated with paclitaxel, and after you stop treatment with it, do not have any immunizations (vaccinations) without your doctor's approval. Paclitaxel may lower your body's resistance and there is a chance you might get the infection the immunization is meant to prevent. In addition, other persons living in your household should not take oral polio vaccine since there is a chance they could pass the polio virus on to you. Also, avoid persons who have taken oral polio vaccine within the last several months. Do not get close to them and do not stay in the same room with them for very long. If you cannot take these precautions, you should consider wearing a protective face mask that covers the nose and mouth.

Paclitaxel can temporarily lower the number of white blood cells in your blood, increasing the chance of getting an infection. It can also lower the number of platelets, which are necessary for proper blood clotting. If this occurs, there are certain precautions you can take, especially when your blood count is low, to reduce the risk of infection or bleeding:

- If you can, avoid people with infections. Check with your doctor immediately if you think you are getting an infection or if you get a fever or chills, cough or hoarseness, lower back or side pain, or painful or difficult urination.
- Check with your doctor immediately if you notice any unusual bleeding or bruising; black, tarry stools; blood in urine or stools; or pinpoint red spots on your skin.
- Be careful when using a regular toothbrush, dental floss, or toothpick. Your medical doctor, dentist, or nurse may recommend other ways to clean your teeth and gums. Check with your medical doctor before having any dental work done.
- Do not touch your eyes or the inside of your nose unless you have just washed your hands and have not touched anything else in the meantime.
- Be careful not to cut yourself when you are using sharp objects such as a safety razor or fingernail or toenail cutters.
- Avoid contact sports or other situations where bruising or injury could occur.

Side Effects of This Medicine

Along with its needed effects, a medicine may cause some unwanted effects. Some side effects will have signs or symptoms that you can see or feel. Your doctor may watch for others by doing certain tests.

Also, because of the way these medicines act on the body, there is a chance that they might cause other unwanted effects that may not occur until months or years after the medicine is used. These delayed effects may include certain types of cancer. Discuss these possible effects with your doctor.

Check with your doctor immediately if any of the following side effects occur:
Less common
Black, tarry stools; blood in urine or stools; pinpoint red spots on skin; unusual bleeding or bruising

Rare
Shortness of breath (severe); skin reaction (severe)

Check with your doctor as soon as possible if any of the following side effects occur:
More common
Cough or hoarseness accompanied by fever or chills; fever or chills; flushing of face; lower back or side pain accompanied by fever or chills; painful or difficult urination accompanied by fever or chills; shortness of breath; skin rash or itching
Rare
Pain or redness at place of injection; sores in mouth and on lips (usually get better within 7 days after treatment)

This medicine may also cause the following side effects that your doctor will watch out for:
More common
Anemia; low platelet count in blood; low white blood cell count
Less common
Effects on liver; low blood pressure; slow heartbeat

Some side effects may occur that usually do not need medical attention. These side effects may go away during treatment as your body adjusts to the medicine. Also, your health care professional may be able to tell you about ways to prevent or reduce some of these side effects. Check with your health care professional if any of the following side effects continue or are bothersome or if you have any questions about them:
More common
Diarrhea; nausea and vomiting; numbness, burning, or tingling in hands or feet; pain in joints or muscles, especially in arms or legs (begins 2 to 3 days after treatment and may last up to 5 days)

This medicine usually causes a temporary and total loss of hair (including eyebrows, eyelashes, and pubic hair) about 2 to 3 weeks after treatment begins. After treatment with paclitaxel has ended, normal hair growth should return.

Other side effects not listed may also occur in some patients. If you notice any other effects, check with your healthcare professional.

PACLITAXEL PROTEIN-BOUND
(Injection route)

Uses For This Medicine

Paclitaxel protein-bound belongs to the group of medicines called antineoplastics. It is used to treat cancer of the breast after other treatments have failed.

Paclitaxel interferes with the growth of cancer cells, which are eventually destroyed. Since the growth of normal body cells may also be affected by paclitaxel protein bound, other effects will also occur. Some of these may be serious and must be reported to your doctor. Other effects may not be serious but may cause concern. Some effects may not occur until months or years after the medicine is used.

Before you begin treatment with paclitaxel protein-bound, you and your doctor should talk about the good this medicine will do as well as the risks of using it.

Paclitaxel protein-bound is to be administered only by or under the immediate supervision of your doctor.

Before Receiving This Medicine

In deciding to use a medicine, the risks of taking the medicine must be weighed against the good it will do. This is a decision you and your doctor will make. For this medicine, the following should be considered:

Allergies—Tell your doctor if you have ever had any unusual or allergic reaction to this medicine or any other medicines. Also tell your health care professional if you have any other types of allergies, such as to foods, dyes, preservatives, or animals. For non-prescription products, read the label or package ingredients carefully.

Pediatric—There is no specific information comparing use of paclitaxel protein-bound in children with use in other age groups.

Geriatric—This medicine has been tested in a limited number of patients and has not been shown to cause different side effects or problems in older people than it does in younger adults.

Pregnancy—

	Pregnancy Category	Explanation
All Trimesters	D	Studies in pregnant women have demonstrated a risk to the fetus. However, the benefits of therapy in a life threatening situation or a serious disease, may outweigh the potential risk.

Breast Feeding—There are no adequate studies in women for determining infant risk when using this medication during breastfeeding. Weigh the potential benefits against the potential risks before taking this medication while breastfeeding.

Other medicines—

Using this medicine with any of the following medicines is usually not recommended, but may be required in some cases. If both medicines are prescribed together, your doctor may change the dose or how often you use one or both of the medicines.

Ethinyl Estradiol, Testosterone, Tretinoin

Interactions with Food/Tobacco/Alcohol—Certain medicines should not be used at or around the time of eating food or eating certain types of food since interactions may occur. Using alcohol or tobacco with certain medicines may also cause interactions to occur. Discuss with your healthcare professional the use of your medicine with food, alcohol, or tobacco.

Other medical problems—The presence of other medical problems may affect the use of this medicine. Make sure you tell your doctor if you have any other medical problems, especially:

- Infection—Paclitaxel may decrease your body's ability to fight infection.
- Kidney problems or
- Liver problems or
- Neuropathy, grade 3—May require a break in treatment or a decrease in the dose

Proper Use of This Medicine

If you are receiving paclitaxel protein-bound at home, follow your doctor's orders or the directions on the label. If you have any questions about the proper dose of paclitaxel protein-bound, ask your doctor.

Dosing—The dose of this medicine will be different for different patients. Follow your doctor's orders or the directions on the label. The following information includes only the average doses of this medicine. If your dose is different, do not change it unless your doctor tells you to do so.

The amount of medicine that you take depends on the strength of the medicine. Also, the number of doses you take each day, the time allowed between doses, and the length of time you take the medicine depend on the medical problem for which you are using the medicine.

- For parenteral dosage form:
  - For advanced breast cancer:
    - Adults—260 milligrams per m² of body surface area, injected into the vein over 30 minutes once every 3 weeks.
    - Children—Use and dose must be determined by your doctor.

Precautions After Receiving This Medicine

It is very important that your doctor check your progress at regular visits to make sure that this medicine is working properly and to check for unwanted effects.

Men receiving paclitaxel protein-bound should not father a child.

Paclitaxel can temporarily lower the number of white blood cells in your blood, increasing the chance of getting an infection. It can also lower the number of platelets, which are necessary for proper blood clotting. If this occurs, there are certain precautions you can take, especially when your blood count is low, to reduce the risk of infection or bleeding:

- If you can, avoid people with infections. Check with your doctor immediately if you think you are getting an infection or if you get a fever or chills, cough or hoarseness, lower back or side pain, or painful or difficult urination.
- Check with your doctor immediately if you notice any unusual bleeding or bruising; black, tarry stools; blood in urine or stools; or pinpoint red spots on your skin.
- Be careful when using a regular toothbrush, dental floss, or toothpick. Your medical doctor, dentist, or nurse may recommend other ways to clean your teeth and gums. Check with your medical doctor before having any dental work done.
- Do not touch your eyes or the inside of your nose unless you have just washed your hands and have not touched anything else in the meantime.
- Be careful not to cut yourself when you are using sharp objects such as a safety razor or fingernail or toenail cutters.
- Avoid contact sports or other situations where bruising or injury could occur.

Side Effects of This Medicine

Along with its needed effects, a medicine may cause some unwanted effects. Although not all of these side effects may occur, if they do occur they may need medical attention.

Also, because of the way these medicines act on the body, there is a chance that they might cause other unwanted effects that may not occur until months or years after the medicine is used. These may include certain types of cancer, such as leukemia or bladder cancer. Discuss these possible effects with your doctor.

Check with your doctor immediately if any of the following side effects occur:

More common

Black, tarry stools; blurred or double vision; chest pain; chills; cough; fever; loss of taste; lower back or side pain; painful or difficult urination; pale skin; shortness of breath; sneezing; sore mouth or tongue; sore throat; troubled breathing with exertion; tightness in chest; ulcers, sores, or white spots in mouth; unusual bleeding or bruising; unusual tiredness or weakness; wheezing; white patches in mouth and/or on tongue

Less common

Abnormal electrocardiogram (ECG); anxiety; bleeding; bleeding gums; blood in urine or stools; burning, tingling, numbness or pain in the hands, arms, feet, or legs; confusion; difficulty breathing; difficulty in swallowing; dizziness, faintness, or lightheadedness when getting up from a lying or sitting position suddenly; dizziness or lightheadedness; fainting; fast, pounding, or irregular heartbeat or pulse; no blood pressure or pulse; pain in chest, groin, or legs, especially the calves; painful or difficult urination; palpitations; pinpoint red spots on skin; sensation of pins and needles; severe, sudden headache; slow or irregular heartbeat; slurred speech; stabbing pain; skin itching, rash, or redness; stopping of heart; sudden loss of coordination; sudden, severe weakness or numbness in arm or leg; sudden, unexplained shortness of breath; sweating; swelling of face, throat, or tongue; tenderness, pain, swelling, warmth, skin discoloration, and prominent superficial veins over affected area; unconsciousness; vision changes

Rare

Difficulty in speaking; headache; inability to move arms, legs, or facial muscles; inability to speak; numbness or tingling in face, arms or legs; severe pain in chest; slow speech; sudden onset of severe breathing difficulty; trouble speaking, thinking or walking

Get emergency help immediately if any of the following symptoms of overdose occur:

Symptoms of overdose

Blurred or double vision; chest pain; chills; cough or hoarseness; cracked lips; diarrhea; difficulty in swallowing; fever; loss of taste; lower back or side pain; painful or difficult urination; shortness of breath; sores, ulcers, or white spots on lips, tongue, or inside mouth; swollen glands; unusual bleeding or bruising; unusual tiredness or weakness

Some side effects may occur that usually do not need medical attention. These side effects may go away during treatment as your body adjusts to the medicine. Also, your health care professional may be able to tell you about ways to prevent or reduce some of these side effects. Check with your health care professional if any of the following side effects continue or are bothersome or if you have any questions about them:

More common

Cracked lips; diarrhea; difficulty in moving; difficulty in swallowing; lack or loss of strength; loss of hair; muscle pain or stiffness; nausea; pain in joints; swelling; vomiting

Less common

Bleeding, blistering, burning, coldness, discoloration of skin, feeling of pressure, hives, infection, inflammation, itching, lumps, numbness, pain, rash, redness, scarring, soreness, stinging, swelling, tenderness, tingling, ulceration, or warmth at site of injection

Rare

Nail changes

Observed during clinical trials

Disturbed color perception; halos around lights; loss of vision; night blindness; overbright appearance of lights; tunnel vision

Other side effects not listed may also occur in some patients. If you notice any other effects, check with your healthcare professional.

PALIFERMIN (Intravenous route) - pal-ee-FER-min

Commonly used brand name(s)

In the U.S.—
Kepivance

Available Dosage Forms:
• Powder for Solution

Therapeutic Class: Protectant, Dental
Pharmacologic Class: Keratinocyte Growth Factor

Uses For This Medicine

Palifermin is used to help prevent or lessen some side effects caused by other medicines or radiation therapy that are used to treat cancer.

This medicine is available only with your doctor's prescription.

Before Using This Medicine

In deciding to use a medicine, the risks of taking the medicine must be weighed against the good it will do. This is a decision you and your doctor will make. For this medicine, the following should be considered:

Allergies—Tell your doctor if you have ever had any unusual or allergic reaction to this medicine or any other medicines. Also tell your health care professional if you have any other types of allergies, such as to foods, dyes, preservatives, or animals. For non-prescription products, read the label or package ingredients carefully.

Pediatric—Studies on this medicine have been done only in adult patients, and there is no specific information comparing use of palifermin in children with use in other age groups.

Geriatric—Many medicines have not been studied specifically in older people. Therefore, it may not be known whether they work exactly the same way they do in younger adults or if they cause different side effects or problems in older people. There is no specific information comparing use of palifermin in the elderly with use in other age groups.

Pregnancy—

	Pregnancy Category	Explanation
All Trimesters	C	Animal studies have shown an adverse effect and there are no adequate studies in pregnant women OR no animal studies have been conducted and there are no adequate studies in pregnant women.

Breast Feeding—There are no adequate studies in women for determining infant risk when using this medication during breastfeeding. Weigh the potential benefits against the potential risks before taking this medication while breastfeeding.

Other medicines—Although certain medicines should not be used together at all, in other cases two different medicines may be used together even if an interaction might occur. In these cases, your doctor may want to change the dose, or other precautions may be necessary. Tell your healthcare professional if you are taking any other prescription or non-prescription (over-the-counter [OTC]) medicine.

Interactions with Food/Tobacco/Alcohol—Certain medicines should not be used at or around the time of eating food or eating certain types of food since interactions may occur. Using alcohol or tobacco with certain medicines may also cause interactions to occur. Discuss with your healthcare professional the use of your medicine with food, alcohol, or tobacco.

Other medical problems—The presence of other medical problems may affect the use of this medicine. Make sure you tell your doctor if you have any other medical problems, especially:

- Non-hematologic malignancies (e.g., other cancerous tumors)—May be worsened by palifermin

Proper Use of This Medicine

Dosing—The dose of this medicine will be different for different patients. Follow your doctor's orders or the directions on the label. The following information includes only the average doses of this medicine. If your dose is different, do not change it unless your doctor tells you to do so.

The amount of medicine that you take depends on the strength of the medicine. Also, the number of doses you take each day, the time allowed between doses, and the length of time you take the medicine depend on the medical problem for which you are using the medicine.

- For parenteral dosage form (injection):
  - For preventing or lessening side effects caused by medicines used to treat cancer:
    - Adults—60 milligrams (mg) per square meter of body surface area, injected into a vein for 3 consecutive days before and 3 consecutive days after myelotoxic therapy for a total of 6 doses.
    - Children—Use and dose must be determined by your doctor.

Storage—Store in the refrigerator. Do not freeze.

Keep out of the reach of children.

Do not keep outdated medicine or medicine no longer needed.

Ask your healthcare professional how you should dispose of any medicine you do not use.

Precautions While Using This Medicine

Your doctor will want to check your progress at regular visits.

This medicine may cause some other tumors (not bone marrow tumors) to grow in animal models. Make sure your doctor knows if you have had any other type of tumor or cancer.

The importance of reporting any side effects to your doctor

Side Effects of This Medicine

Along with its needed effects, a medicine may cause some unwanted effects. Although not all of these side effects may occur, if they do occur they may need medical attention.

Check with your doctor immediately if any of the following side effects occur:

Rare
> Skin rash, severe

Some side effects may occur that usually do not need medical attention. These side effects may go away during treatment as your body adjusts to the medicine. Also, your health care professional may be able to tell you about ways to prevent or reduce some of these side effects. Check with your health care professional if any of the following side effects continue or are bothersome or if you have any questions about them:

More common
> Bad unusual or unpleasant (after) taste; blurred vision; burning, crawling, itching, numbness, prickling, "pins and needles" or tingling feelings; change in taste; difficulty in moving; dizziness; elevated serum amylase; elevated serum lipase; fever; flushing, redness of skin; headache; increased sensitivity to pain; increased sensitivity to touch; itching skin; muscle pain or stiffness; nervousness; pain; pain in joints; pounding in the ears; rash; slow or fast heartbeat; swelling; tingling in the hands and feet; tongue discoloration; tongue thickening; unusually warm skin

Frequency unknown
> Body produces substance that can bind to drug making it less effective or cause side effects

Other side effects not listed may also occur in some patients. If you notice any other effects, check with your healthcare professional.

PALIVIZUMAB   (Intramuscular route) -
pal-i-VIZ-yoo-mab

Commonly used brand name(s)

In the U.S.—
> Synagis

Available Dosage Forms:
- Powder for Solution
- Solution

Therapeutic Class: Immunological Agent
Pharmacologic Class: Monoclonal Antibody

Uses For This Medicine

Palivizumab belongs to a group of medicines known as immunizing agents. Palivizumab is used to prevent infection in children and babies caused by respiratory syncytial virus (RSV). This medicine works by giving your body the antibodies it needs to protect it against RSV infection.

RSV infection can cause serious problems that affect the lungs, such as pneumonia and bronchitis, and in severe cases even can cause death. These problems are more likely to occur in infants and children younger than 6 months of age with chronic lung disease and breathing problems and in babies who were premature, and babies who were born with heart disease.

Palivizumab is used to prevent serious lower respiratory tract infection caused by the RSV.

Onset of RSV activity usually occurs in November and continues through April, but it may begin earlier or continue later in certain communities. A good way to help prevent RSV infection is to receive palivizumab before the start of the RSV season.

Palivizumab is to be administered only by or under the supervision of your doctor or other health care professional.

Before Using This Medicine

In deciding to use a medicine, the risks of taking the medicine must be weighed against the good it will do. This is a decision you and your doctor will make. For this medicine, the following should be considered:

Allergies—Tell your doctor if you have ever had any unusual or allergic reaction to this medicine or any other medicines. Also tell your health care professional if you have any other types of allergies, such as to foods, dyes, preservatives, or animals. For non-prescription products, read the label or package ingredients carefully.

Pediatric—Studies on this medicine have been done only in children, and it has been shown to be effective in children with breathing problems and those with a history of premature birth.

Geriatric—Studies on this medicine have been done only in infants and children, and there is no specific information about its use in older patients.

Pregnancy—

	Pregnancy Category	Explanation
All Trimesters	C	Animal studies have shown an adverse effect and there are no adequate studies in pregnant women OR no animal studies have been conducted and there are no adequate studies in pregnant women.

Breast Feeding—There are no adequate studies in women for determining infant risk when using this medication during breastfeeding. Weigh the potential benefits against the potential risks before taking this medication while breastfeeding.

Other medicines—Although certain medicines should not be used together at all, in other cases two different medicines may be used together even if an interaction might occur. In these cases, your doctor may want to change the dose, or

other precautions may be necessary. Tell your healthcare professional if you are taking any other prescription or non-prescription (over-the-counter [OTC]) medicine.

Interactions with Food/Tobacco/Alcohol—Certain medicines should not be used at or around the time of eating food or eating certain types of food since interactions may occur. Using alcohol or tobacco with certain medicines may also cause interactions to occur. Discuss with your healthcare professional the use of your medicine with food, alcohol, or tobacco.

Other medical problems—The presence of other medical problems may affect the use of this medicine. Make sure you tell your doctor if you have any other medical problems, especially:
- Allergy to palivizumab

Proper Use of This Medicine

Dosing—The dose of this medicine will be different for different patients. Follow your doctor's orders or the directions on the label. The following information includes only the average doses of this medicine. If your dose is different, do not change it unless your doctor tells you to do so.

The amount of medicine that you take depends on the strength of the medicine. Also, the number of doses you take each day, the time allowed between doses, and the length of time you take the medicine depend on the medical problem for which you are using the medicine.

Side Effects of This Medicine

Along with its needed effects, a medicine may cause some unwanted effects. Although not all of these side effects may occur, if they do occur they may need medical attention.

Check with your doctor as soon as possible if any of the following side effects occur:
More common
  bluish color of fingernails, lips, skin, palms, or nail beds (in patients with heart disease); Difficulty in breathing; ringing or buzzing in the ears; skin rash

Less common or rare
  Abdominal pain; diarrhea; dizziness; fainting; fast, slow, or irregular heartbeat; loss of appetite; lump in abdomen; nausea; weakness

Incidence not known
  Difficult or troubled breathing; hives or welts; irregular, fast or slow, or shallow breathing; itching skin; large, hive-like swelling on face, eyelids, lips, tongue, throat, hands, feet, legs, sex organs; loss of strength or energy; muscle pain or weakness; redness of skin; shortness of breath; tightness in chest; unresponsiveness; unusual weak feeling; wheezing

Some side effects may occur that usually do not need medical attention. These side effects may go away during treatment as your body adjusts to the medicine. Also, your health care professional may be able to tell you about ways to prevent or reduce some of these side effects. Check with your health care professional if any of the following side effects continue or are bothersome or if you have any questions about them:
Less common or rare
  Cough; runny nose; sneezing; stuffy nose; vomiting

Other side effects not listed may also occur in some patients. If you notice any other effects, check with your healthcare professional.

PALONOSETRON (Intravenous route)
- pal-oh-NOE-se-tron

Commonly used brand name(s)

In the U.S.—
  Aloxi

Available Dosage Forms:
  • Solution

Therapeutic Class: Antiemetic
Pharmacologic Class: Serotonin Receptor Antagonist, 5–HT3

Uses For This Medicine

Palonosetron is a substance that is used to treat the nausea and vomiting that is sometimes associated with cancer therapy.

This medicine is available only with your doctor's prescription.

Before Using This Medicine

In deciding to use a medicine, the risks of taking the medicine must be weighed against the good it will do. This is a decision you and your doctor will make. For this medicine, the following should be considered:

Allergies—Tell your doctor if you have ever had any unusual or allergic reaction to this medicine or any other medicines. Also tell your health care professional if you have any other types of allergies, such as to foods, dyes, preservatives, or animals. For non-prescription products, read the label or package ingredients carefully.

Pediatric—Studies on this medicine have only been done in adult patients, and there is no specific information comparing use of palonosetron in children with use in other age groups.

Geriatric—This medicine has been tested in a limited number of patients 65 years of age or older and has not been shown to cause different side effects or problems in older people than it does in younger adults.

Pregnancy—

	Pregnancy Category	Explanation
All Trimesters	B	Animal studies have revealed no evidence of harm to the fetus, however, there are no adequate studies in pregnant women OR animal studies have shown an adverse effect, but adequate studies in pregnant women have failed to demonstrate a risk to the fetus.

Breast Feeding—There are no adequate studies in women for determining infant risk when using this medication during breastfeeding. Weigh the potential benefits against the potential risks before taking this medication while breastfeeding.

Other medicines—

Using this medicine with any of the following medicines is not recommended. Your doctor may decide not to treat you with this medication or change some of the other medicines you take.

Apomorphine

Interactions with Food/Tobacco/Alcohol—Certain medicines should not be used at or around the time of eating food or eating certain types of food since interactions may occur. Using alcohol or tobacco with certain medicines may also cause interactions to occur. Discuss with your healthcare professional the use of your medicine with food, alcohol, or tobacco.

Other medical problems—The presence of other medical problems may affect the use of this medicine. Make sure you tell your doctor if you have any other medical problems, especially:

  • Irregular heartbeats—May increase the risk of certain side effects
  • Kidney problems—May increase the amount of palonosetron in the body

Proper Use of This Medicine

Dosing—The dose of this medicine will be different for different patients. Follow your doctor's orders or the directions on the label. The following information includes only the average doses of this medicine. If your dose is different, do not change it unless your doctor tells you to do so.

The amount of medicine that you take depends on the strength of the medicine. Also, the number of doses you take each day, the time allowed between doses, and the length of time you take the medicine depend on the medical problem for which you are using the medicine.

  • For parenteral dosage form (injection):
    ○ For prevention of nausea and vomiting after anti-cancer medicine:
      ▪ Adults and adolescents 18 years of age or older—0.25 mg as a single dose injected into a vein, over a period of thirty seconds, beginning approximately 30 minutes before the start of chemotherapy. Dose should not be repeated within seven consecutive days.
      ▪ Children up to 18 years of age—Use and dose must be determined by your doctor.

Storage—Store the medicine in a closed container at room temperature, away from heat, moisture, and direct light. Keep from freezing.

Keep out of the reach of children.

Do not keep outdated medicine or medicine no longer needed.

Precautions While Using This Medicine

Check with your doctor if severe nausea and vomiting occur after receiving the anticancer medicine.

Side Effects of This Medicine

Along with its needed effects, a medicine may cause some unwanted effects. Although not all of these side effects may occur, if they do occur they may need medical attention.

Symptoms of overdose

Get emergency help immediately if any of the following symptoms of overdose occur:

bluish color of fingernails, lips, skin, palms, or nail beds; collapse; gasping to breathe; paleness of skin; seizures

Some side effects may occur that usually do not need medical attention. These side effects may go away during treatment as your body adjusts to the medicine. Also, your health care professional may be able to tell you about ways to prevent or reduce some of these side effects. Check with your health care professional if any of the following side effects continue or are bothersome or if you have any questions about them:

More common

Difficulty having a bowel movement (stool); headache

Less common

abdominal pain; acid or sour stomach; belching; bloated full feeling; blood in urine; bloody or black, tarry stools; blurred vision; burning, crawling, itching, numbness, prickling, "pins and needles", or tingling feelings; change in vision; chest pain or discomfort; chills; confusion; continuing ringing or buzzing; cough; decrease in frequency of urination; decrease in urine volume; deep breathing; diarrhea; difficult breathing; difficulty in passing urine; dizziness; dizziness, faintness, or light-headedness when getting up from a lying or sitting position suddenly; [dribbling] painful urination; drowsiness; dry mouth; excess air or gas in stomach or intestines; excessive sleeping; eye irritation; fainting; fast, pounding heartbeat or pulse; fear; feeling of warmth; fever; flushed dry skin; fruit-like breath odor; general feeling of discomfort or illness; happy; heartburn; hearing loss; hiccups; impaired vision; increased hunger; increased thirst; increased urination; indigestion; irregular heartbeat; joint pain; large, flat, blue or purplish patches in the skin; light-headedness; loss of appetite; muscle aches and pains; muscle tremors; nausea or vomiting; nervousness; numbness or tingling in hands, feet, or lips; painful knees and ankles; pain or discomfort in arms, jaw, back or neck; passing gas; pounding in the ears; raised red swellings on the skin, the buttocks, legs or ankles; rash; red, sore eyes; redness of the face, neck, arms and occasionally, upper chest; restlessness; runny nose; seizures; shivering; shortness of breath; slow heartbeat; sore throat; stomach discomfort, upset, or pain; sugar in the urine; sweating; swelling or protruding veins; trembling; troubled breathing; trouble sleeping; unexplained noise in ears; unexplained weight loss; unusual tiredness; unusually deep sleep; unusually long duration of sleep; vein discoloration; weakness or heaviness of legs

Other side effects not listed may also occur in some patients. If you notice any other effects, check with your healthcare professional.

PAMIDRONATE (Intravenous route) -
pa-mi-DROE-nate

Commonly used brand name(s)

In the U.S.—
Aredia

Available Dosage Forms:
- Powder for Solution
- Solution

Therapeutic Class: Calcium Regulator

Uses For This Medicine

Pamidronate is used to treat hypercalcemia (too much calcium in the blood) that may occur with some types of cancer. It is also used to treat Paget's disease of bone and to treat bone metastases (spread of cancer).

This medicine is to be administered only by or under the supervision of your doctor.

Once a medicine has been approved for marketing for a certain use, experience may show that it is also useful for other medical problems. Although these uses are not included in product labeling, pamidronate is used in certain patients with the following medical conditions:
- Osteogenesis imperfecta

Before Receiving This Medicine

In deciding to use a medicine, the risks of taking the medicine must be weighed against the good it will do. This is a decision you and your doctor will make. For this medicine, the following should be considered:

Allergies—Tell your doctor if you have ever had any unusual or allergic reaction to this medicine or any other medicines. Also tell your health care professional if you have any other types of allergies, such as to foods, dyes, preservatives, or animals. For non-prescription products, read the label or package ingredients carefully.

Pediatric—Studies on this medicine have been done only in adult patients, and there is no specific information comparing use of pamidronate in children with use in other age groups.

Geriatric—When pamidronate is given along with a large amount of fluids, older people tend to retain (keep) the excess fluid.

Pregnancy—

	Pregnancy Category	Explanation
All Trimesters	D	Studies in pregnant women have demonstrated a risk to the fetus. However, the benefits of therapy in a life threatening situation or a serious disease, may outweigh the potential risk.

Breast Feeding—There are no adequate studies in women for determining infant risk when using this medication during breastfeeding. Weigh the potential benefits against the potential risks before taking this medication while breastfeeding.

Other medicines—Although certain medicines should not be used together at all, in other cases two different medicines may be used together even if an interaction might occur. In these cases, your doctor may want to change the dose, or other precautions may be necessary. Tell your healthcare professional if you are taking any other prescription or non-prescription (over-the-counter [OTC]) medicine.

Interactions with Food/Tobacco/Alcohol—Certain medicines should not be used at or around the time of eating food or eating certain types of food since interactions may occur. Using alcohol or tobacco with certain medicines may also cause interactions to occur. Discuss with your healthcare professional the use of your medicine with food, alcohol, or tobacco.

Other medical problems—The presence of other medical problems may affect the use of this medicine. Make sure you tell your doctor if you have any other medical problems, especially:
- Blood problems, such as
- Anemia or
- Leukopenia or
- Thrombocytopenia—Your healthcare professional will watch your progress closely for two weeks after treatment.
- Heart problems—The increased amount of fluid may make this condition worse.
- Kidney problems—Pamidronate may build up in the bloodstream, which may increase the chance of unwanted effects.

Proper Use of This Medicine

Dosing—The dose of this medicine will be different for different patients. Follow your doctor's orders or the directions on the label. The following information includes only the average doses of this medicine. If your dose is different, do not change it unless your doctor tells you to do so.

The amount of medicine that you take depends on the strength of the medicine. Also, the number of doses you take each day, the time allowed between doses, and the length of time you take the medicine depend on the medical problem for which you are using the medicine.
- For injection dosage form:
  - For treating hypercalcemia (too much calcium in the blood):
    - Adults: 60 to 90 milligrams (mg) in a solution to be injected over 2 to 24 hours into a vein.
    - Children: Use and dose must be determined by your doctor.
  - For treating Paget's disease of bone:
    - Adults: Dose and frequency must be determined by your doctor. The usual dose range is 30 mg in a solution injected into a vein. Your doctor may repeat this dose each day for a total of 3 days of treatment.
    - Children: Use and dose must be determined by your doctor.
  - For treating bone metastases:
    - Adults—90 mg in a solution to be injected over 2 to 4 hours into a vein. Your dose may be given every three to four weeks or once a month.
      - Children—Use and dose must be determined by your doctor.

Precautions After Receiving This Medicine

It is important that your doctor check your progress at regular visits after you have received pamidronate. If your condition has improved, your progress must still be checked. The results of laboratory tests or the occurrence of certain symptoms will tell your doctor if your condition is coming back and a second treatment is needed.

For patients using this medicine for hypercalcemia (too much calcium in the blood):
- Your doctor may want you to follow a low-calcium diet. If you have any questions about this, check with your doctor.

Side Effects of This Medicine

Along with its needed effects, a medicine may cause some unwanted effects. Although not all of these side effects may occur, if they do occur they may need medical attention.

Check with your doctor as soon as possible if any of the following side effects occur:
More common
Abdominal cramps; black, tarry stools; bleeding gums; bloody in urine or stools; blurred vision; chest pain; chills; confusion; convulsions (seizures); decrease in amount of urine; dizziness; drowsiness; dry mouth; fainting; fast or irregular heartbeat; fever; headache; increased thirst; loss of appetite; mood or mental changes; muscle pain or cramps; muscle spasms; muscle twitching; nausea; nervousness; noisy, rattling breathing; numbness or tingling in hands, feet, or lips; pinpoint red spots on skin; pounding in the ears; shortness of breath; slow or fast heartbeat; spread of cancer; sore throat; swelling of fingers, hands, feet, or lower legs; trembling; troubled breathing at rest; unusual bleeding or bruising; unusual tiredness or weakness; vomiting; vomiting of blood or material that looks like coffee grounds; weight gain

Less common
Cough; dilated neck veins; extreme fatigue; irregular breathing; lower back or side pain; painful or difficult urination; pale skin; swelling; ulcers, sores, or white spots in mouth; wheezing

Rare
Decreased vision; difficulty swallowing; eye pain or tenderness; eye redness; hives; itching; large, hive-like swelling on face, eyelids, lips, tongue, throat, hands, legs, feet, sex organs; sensitivity of eye to light; skin rash; sweating; tearing of eye; tightness in chest

Frequency not determined
Faintness, or light-headedness when getting up from a lying or sitting position suddenly; hives; itching of the skin; large, hive-like swelling on face, eyelids, lips, tongue, throat, hands, legs, feet, sex organs; skin rash; tightness in chest

Note: Abdominal cramps, confusion, and muscle spasms are less common when pamidronate is given in doses of 60 mg or less.

Some side effects may occur that usually do not need medical attention. These side effects may go away during treatment as your body adjusts to the medicine. Also, your health care professional may be able to tell you about ways to prevent or reduce some of these side effects. Check with your health care professional if any of the following side effects continue or are bothersome or if you have any questions about them:

More common

Abdominal pain; acid or sour stomach; belching; bladder pain; bloody or cloudy urine; body aches or pain; bone pain; cracks in skin at the corners of mouth; constipation; degenerative disease of the joint; diarrhea; difficult, burning, or painful urination; difficult or labored breathing; difficulty in moving; ear congestion; fear; frequent urge to urinate; general feeling of body discomfort or illness; heartburn; indigestion; joint pain; lack or loss of strength; loss of voice; lower back or side pain; muscle aching or cramping; muscle pains or stiffness; nasal congestion; nervousness; pain and swelling at place of injection; pain or tenderness around eyes and cheekbones; runny nose; sensitivity to heat; shivering; skin rash; sleeplessness; small clicking, bubbling, or rattling sounds in the lung when listening with a stethoscope; sneezing; soreness or redness around fingernails and toenails; stomach discomfort, upset or pain; stuffy nose; sweating; swollen joints; trouble sleeping; ulcers, sores, or white spots in mouth; unable to sleep; weight loss

Less common

Ammonia-like breath odor; feeling that others are watching you or controlling your behavior; feeling that others can hear your thoughts; feeling, seeing, or hearing things that are not there; feeling unusually cold; swelling or inflammation of the mouth; unusual behavior

Other side effects not listed may also occur in some patients. If you notice any other effects, check with your healthcare professional.

PANCRELIPASE (Oral route) - pan-kre-LI-pase

Commonly used brand name(s)

In the U.S.—

Pancote
Pancreatin

Panokase
Ultrase

Available Dosage Forms:

- Tablet
- Capsule
- Capsule, Extended Release
- Tablet, Enteric Coated
- Capsule, Delayed Release
- Powder

Therapeutic Class: Digestant
Pharmacologic Class: Enzyme

Uses For This Medicine

Pancrelipase is used to help digestion in certain conditions in which the pancreas is not working properly. It may also be used for other conditions as determined by your doctor.

Pancrelipase contains the enzymes needed for the digestion of proteins, starches, and fats.

Pancrelipase is available only with your doctor's prescription.

Before Using This Medicine

In deciding to use a medicine, the risks of taking the medicine must be weighed against the good it will do. This is a decision you and your doctor will make. For this medicine, the following should be considered:

Allergies—Tell your doctor if you have ever had any unusual or allergic reaction to this medicine or any other medicines. Also tell your health care professional if you have any other types of allergies, such as to foods, dyes, preservatives, or animals. For non-prescription products, read the label or package ingredients carefully.

Pediatric—This medicine has been tested in children 6 months of age or older and has not been shown to cause different side effects or problems than it does in adults.

Geriatric—Many medicines have not been studied specifically in older people. Therefore, it may not be known whether they work exactly the same way they do in younger adults. Although there is no specific information comparing use of pancrelipase in the elderly with use in other age groups, this medicine is not expected to cause different side effects or problems in older people than it does in younger adults.

Pregnancy—

	Pregnancy Category	Explanation
All Trimesters	B	Animal studies have revealed no evidence of harm to the fetus, however, there are no adequate studies in pregnant women OR animal studies have shown an adverse effect, but adequate studies in pregnant women have failed to demonstrate a risk to the fetus.

Breast Feeding—There are no adequate studies in women for determining infant risk when using this medication during breastfeeding. Weigh the potential benefits against the potential risks before taking this medication while breastfeeding.

Other medicines—Although certain medicines should not be used together at all, in other cases two different medicines may be used together even if an interaction might occur. In these cases, your doctor may want to change the dose, or other precautions may be necessary. Tell your healthcare professional if you are taking any other prescription or non-prescription (over-the-counter [OTC]) medicine.

Interactions with Food/Tobacco/Alcohol—Certain medicines should not be used at or around the time of eating food or eating certain types of food since interactions may occur. Using alcohol or tobacco with certain medicines may also cause interactions to occur. Discuss with your healthcare professional the use of your medicine with food, alcohol, or tobacco.

Other medical problems—The presence of other medical problems may affect the use of this medicine. Make sure you

tell your doctor if you have any other medical problems, especially:

- Pancreatitis (sudden, severe inflammation of the pancreas)—Pancrelipase may make this condition worse

Proper Use of This Medicine

Take this medicine before or with meals and snacks, unless otherwise directed by your doctor.

When prescribing this medicine for your condition, your doctor may also prescribe a personal diet for you. Follow carefully the special diet your doctor gave you. This is most important and necessary for the medicine to work properly and to avoid indigestion. It is important to drink plenty of water while you are on this medicine.

For patients taking the tablet form of this medicine:

- Swallow the tablets quickly with some liquid, without chewing, to avoid mouth irritation.

For patients taking the capsules containing the enteric-coated spheres:

- Swallow the capsule whole.
- Do not crush, break, or chew before swallowing.
- When given to children, the capsule may be opened and sprinkled on a small amount of liquid or soft food that can be swallowed without chewing, such as applesauce or gelatin. However, it should not be mixed with alkaline foods, such as milk and ice cream, which may reduce its effect.

Dosing—The dose of this medicine will be different for different patients. Follow your doctor's orders or the directions on the label. The following information includes only the average doses of this medicine. If your dose is different, do not change it unless your doctor tells you to do so.

The amount of medicine that you take depends on the strength of the medicine. Also, the number of doses you take each day, the time allowed between doses, and the length of time you take the medicine depend on the medical problem for which you are using the medicine.

- To help digestion:
  - For oral dosage form (capsules):
    - Older adults, adults, and teenagers—One to three capsules before or with meals and snacks. Your doctor may change your dose if needed.
    - Children—The contents of one to three capsules sprinkled on food at each meal. Your doctor may change your dose if needed.
  - For oral dosage form (delayed-release capsules):
    - Older adults, adults, and teenagers—One to four capsules (4000 to 20000 units) before or with meals and snacks. Your doctor will decide what your dose should be at first. Your doctor may change your dose if needed.
    - Children over 6 years old—The contents of one to four capsules (4000 to 12,000 units) with meals. Your doctor will decide what dose to start with. Your doctor may change your dose if needed. You should take the contents of the capsules with a liquid or a small amount of a soft food that you do not have to chew. You should eat the food with the medicine in it right away and follow that with a glass of water or juice.

- Children 1 to 6 years old—The contents of one to two capsules (4000 to 8000 units) with meals. Your doctor will decide what dose to start with. Your doctor may change your dose if needed. You should take the contents of the capsules with a liquid or a small amount of a soft food that you do not have to chew. You should eat the food with the medicine in it right away and follow that with a glass of water or juice.
- Infants 6 months to 1 year old—The contents of half a capsule (2000 units) per meal. Your baby's doctor may change the dose if needed.
- Infants under 6 months—Use and dose should be determined by your baby's doctor.
  - For oral dosage form (powder):
    - Older adults, adults, and teenagers—¼ teaspoonful (0.7 gram) with meals and snacks. Your doctor may change your dose if needed.
    - Children—¼ teaspoonful with meals. Your doctor may change your dose if needed.
  - For oral dosage form (tablets):
    - Older adults, adults, and teenagers—One to three tablets before or with meals and snacks. Your doctor may change your dose if needed.
    - Children—One to two tablets with meals.

Missed dose—If you miss a dose of this medicine, take it as soon as possible. However, if it is almost time for your next dose, skip the missed dose and go back to your regular dosing schedule. Do not double doses.

Storage—Store the medicine in a closed container at room temperature, away from heat, moisture, and direct light. Keep from freezing.

Keep out of the reach of children.

Do not keep outdated medicine or medicine no longer needed.

Precautions While Using This Medicine

Your doctor may recommend that you take pancrelipase with another medicine, such as certain antacids or anti-ulcer medicines. However, antacids that contain calcium carbonate and/or magnesium hydroxate may not let the pancrelipase work properly and should be avoided.

Do not change brands or dosage forms of pancrelipase without first checking with your doctor. Different products may not work in the same way. If you refill your medicine and it looks different, check with your pharmacist.

For patients taking the capsules containing the powder:

- If the capsules are opened to mix with food, be careful not to breathe in the powder. To do so may cause harmful effects such as stuffy nose, shortness of breath, troubled breathing, wheezing, or tightness in chest.

For patients taking the capsule form containing delayed-release microspheres:

- Swallow whole. Do not crush or chew.
- If you are unable to swallow the capsule whole, the capsule may be opened and the microspheres shaken into a small quantity of a soft food (e.g., applesauce, gelatin, etc.) which does not require chewing, and swallowed immediately.
- Some foods can dissolve the protective coating of the microspheres and change the effects of this medicine. If

you are unsure which foods you can put the microspheres in, check with your doctor.

For patients taking the powder form of this medicine:
- Avoid breathing in the powder. To do so may cause harmful effects such as stuffy nose, shortness of breath, troubled breathing, wheezing, or tightness in chest.

Side Effects of This Medicine

Along with its needed effects, a medicine may cause some unwanted effects. Although not all of these side effects may occur, if they do occur they may need medical attention.

Check with your doctor as soon as possible if any of the following side effects occur:

Rare
Skin rash or hives

With high doses
Diarrhea; intestinal blockage; nausea; stomach cramps or pain

With very high doses
Blood in urine; joint pain; swelling of feet or lower legs

With powder dosage form or powder from opened capsules—if breathed in
Shortness of breath; stuffy nose; tightness in chest; troubled breathing; wheezing

With tablets—if held in mouth
Irritation of the mouth

Other side effects not listed may also occur in some patients. If you notice any other effects, check with your healthcare professional.

PANTOPRAZOLE (Intravenous route)
- pan-TOE-pra-zole

Commonly used brand name(s)

In the U.S.—
Protonix

Available Dosage Forms:
- Powder for Solution

Therapeutic Class: Antiulcer
Pharmacologic Class: Proton Pump Inhibitor

Uses For This Medicine

Pantoprazole is used to treat certain conditions in which there is too much acid in the stomach. It is used to treat duodenal and gastric ulcers and gastroesophageal reflux disease (GERD), a condition in which the acid in the stomach washes back up into the esophagus.

Pantoprazole works by decreasing the amount of acid produced by the stomach.

This medicine is available only with your doctor's prescription.

Before Using This Medicine

In deciding to use a medicine, the risks of taking the medicine must be weighed against the good it will do. This is a decision you and your doctor will make. For this medicine, the following should be considered:

Allergies—Tell your doctor if you have ever had any unusual or allergic reaction to this medicine or any other medicines. Also tell your health care professional if you have any other types of allergies, such as to foods, dyes, preservatives, or animals. For non-prescription products, read the label or package ingredients carefully.

Pediatric—Studies on this medicine have been done only in adult patients, and there is no specific information comparing the use of pantoprazole in children with use in other age groups.

Geriatric—This medicine has been tested and has not been shown to cause different side effects or problems in older people than it does in younger adults.

Pregnancy—

	Pregnancy Category	Explanation
All Trimesters	B	Animal studies have revealed no evidence of harm to the fetus, however, there are no adequate studies in pregnant women OR animal studies have shown an adverse effect, but adequate studies in pregnant women have failed to demonstrate a risk to the fetus.

Breast Feeding—There are no adequate studies in women for determining infant risk when using this medication during breastfeeding. Weigh the potential benefits against the potential risks before taking this medication while breastfeeding.

Other medicines—

Using this medicine with any of the following medicines is usually not recommended, but may be required in some cases. If both medicines are prescribed together, your doctor may change the dose or how often you use one or both of the medicines.

Atazanavir

Interactions with Food/Tobacco/Alcohol—Certain medicines should not be used at or around the time of eating food or eating certain types of food since interactions may occur. Using alcohol or tobacco with certain medicines may also cause interactions to occur. Discuss with your healthcare professional the use of your medicine with food, alcohol, or tobacco.

Other medical problems—The presence of other medical problems may affect the use of this medicine. Make sure you tell your doctor if you have any other medical problems, especially:
- Liver disease—This condition may cause pantoprazole to build up in the body
- Zinc deficiency, or prone to—May make your condition worse.

Proper Use of This Medicine

Take pantoprazole tablets immediately before a meal, preferably in the morning. Pantoprazole tablets may be taken with food or on an empty stomach.

Swallow the tablet whole. Do not crush, break, or chew the tablet.

It may take several days before this medicine begins to relieve stomach pain. To help relieve this pain, antacids may be taken with pantoprazole, unless your doctor has told you not to use them.

Tell your doctor if you have ever had problems with a lack of zinc in your body. Your doctor may have you take zinc supplements.

Take this medicine for the full time of treatment, even if you begin to feel better. Also, keep your appointments with your doctor for check-ups so that your doctor will be better able to tell you when to stop taking this medicine.

Dosing—The dose of this medicine will be different for different patients. Follow your doctor's orders or the directions on the label. The following information includes only the average doses of this medicine. If your dose is different, do not change it unless your doctor tells you to do so.

The amount of medicine that you take depends on the strength of the medicine. Also, the number of doses you take each day, the time allowed between doses, and the length of time you take the medicine depend on the medical problem for which you are using the medicine.

- For oral dosage form (delayed-release tablets):
  - To treat gastroesophageal reflux disease (GERD):
    - Adults—40 milligrams (mg) once a day, preferably in the morning for up to eight weeks. Your doctor may advise you to continue taking the medicine for an additional eight weeks if your condition does not improve after the first eight weeks.
    - Children—Use and dose must be determined by your doctor.
  - To treat gastric ulcers:
    - Adults—40 mg once a day, preferably in the morning for four weeks.
    - Children—Use and dose must be determined by your doctor.
  - To treat duodenal ulcers:
    - Adults—40 mg once a day, preferably in the morning for two weeks.
    - Children—Use and dose must be determined by your doctor.
- For injection dosage form:
  - To treat GERD:
    - Adults—40 mg injected into a vein once a day for seven to ten days.
    - Children—Use and dose must be determined by your doctor.
- For injection dosage form:
  - To treat conditions in which the stomach produces too much acid:
    - Adults—80 mg injected into a vein twice a day. Your doctor may adjust your dose.
    - Children—Use and dose must be determined by your doctor.

Missed dose—If you miss a dose of this medicine, take it as soon as possible. However, if it is almost time for your next dose, skip the missed dose and go back to your regular dosing schedule. Do not double doses.

Storage—Store the medicine in a closed container at room temperature, away from heat, moisture, and direct light. Keep from freezing.

Keep out of the reach of children.

Do not keep outdated medicine or medicine no longer needed.

Precautions While Using This Medicine

It is important that your doctor check your progress at regular visits. If your condition does not improve, or if it becomes worse, check with your doctor.

Side Effects of This Medicine

Along with its needed effects, a medicine may cause some unwanted effects. Although not all of these side effects may occur, if they do occur they may need medical attention.

Check with your doctor as soon as possible if any of the following side effects occur:

Less common or rare

Abdominal or stomach pain; blistering, loosening, peeling, or redness of skin; bull's eye-like rash on skin; changes in facial skin color; chest pain; diarrhea; difficulty in speaking; difficulty in urinating; discoloration, itching, numbness, pain, or redness at place of injection; fast or irregular breathing; increased frequency and volume of urination; infection; large, hive-like swellings on eyelids, face, lips, mouth, and/or tongue; loosening and/or stripping off of top layer of skin; loss of appetite; loss of vision (sudden); nausea; painful urination; pain in joints or muscles; puffiness or swelling of the eyelids or around the eyes; shortness of breath, troubled breathing, tightness in chest, and/or wheezing; skin rash, hives, and itching; skin tenderness with burning; unusual tiredness or weakness; unusual thirst; vomiting; yellow eyes or skin

Incidence not known

Blindness; bloody or cloudy urine; bloody, black or tarry stools; continuing vomiting; dark-colored urine; decreased vision; fever; general feeling of tiredness or weakness; greatly decreased frequency of urination or amount of urine; high fever; light-colored stools; muscle cramps or spasms; muscle pain or stiffness; pale skin; sores, ulcers, or white spots on lips or in mouth; stomach pain; swelling of feet or lower legs; swollen glands; unexplained bleeding or bruising

Get emergency help immediately if any of the following symptoms of overdose occur:

Symptoms of overdose

Abdominal pain; blurred vision; confusion; fast, pounding, or irregular heartbeat or pulse; feeling faint, dizzy, or lightheaded; feeling of warmth or heat; flushing or redness of skin, especially on face and neck; headache; nausea and vomiting; sleepiness or unusual drowsiness; sweating

Some side effects may occur that usually do not need medical attention. These side effects may go away during treatment as your body adjusts to the medicine. Also, your health care professional may be able to tell you about ways to prevent or reduce some of these side effects. Check with your health care professional if any of the following side effects continue or are bothersome or if you have any questions about them:

More common

Headache

Less common or rare

Aching, fullness, or tension in sinuses; anxiety; back pain; belching; blurred vision; chills; confusion; constipation; cough; difficulty in moving; dizziness; drooling; feeling of constant movement of self or surroundings; flatulence; hoarseness; indigestion; loss of energy or strength; migraine headache; muscle rigidity or stiffness; neck pain; pain; rectal problems; ringing or buzzing in the ears; runny or stuffy nose; sensation of spinning; sneezing; sore throat; trouble in sleeping

Other side effects not listed may also occur in some patients. If you notice any other effects, check with your healthcare professional.

PAROXETINE (Oral route) - pa-ROX-e-teen

Black Box Warning

Antidepressants increased the risk of suicidal thinking and behavior (suicidality) in short-term studies in children and adolescents with Major Depressive Disorder (MDD) and other psychiatric disorders. Anyone considering the use of paroxetine hydrochloride or any other antidepressant in a child or adolescent must balance this risk with the clinical need. Patients who are started on therapy should be observed closely for clinical worsening, suicidality, or unusual changes in behavior. Families and caregivers should be advised of the need for close observation and communication with the prescriber. Paroxetine hydrochloride is not approved for use in pediatric patients.

Pooled analyses of short-term (4 weeks to 16 weeks) placebo-controlled trials of 9 antidepressant drugs (SSRIs and others) in children and adolescents with MDD, obsessive compulsive disorder (OCD), or other psychiatric disorders (a total of 24 trials involving over 4,400 patients) have revealed a greater risk of adverse events representing suicidal thinking or behavior (suicidality) during the first few months of treatment in those receiving antidepressants. The average risk of such events in patients receiving antidepressants was 4%, twice the placebo risk of 2%. No suicides occurred in these trials.

Commonly used brand name(s)

In the U.S.—
Paxil   Pexeva
Paxil CR

Available Dosage Forms:
- Tablet   • Suspension
- Tablet, Extended Release

Therapeutic Class: Antidepressant
Pharmacologic Class: Serotonin Reuptake Inhibitor

Uses For This Medicine

Paroxetine is used to treat mental depression, obsessive-compulsive disorder, panic disorder, generalized anxiety disorder, social anxiety disorder (also known as social phobia), premenstrual dysphoric disorder (PMDD), and posttraumatic stress disorder (PTSD).

Paroxetine belongs to a group of medicines known as selective serotonin reuptake inhibitors (SSRIs). These medicines are thought to work by increasing the activity of the chemical serotonin in the brain.

This medicine is available only with your doctor's prescription.

Before Using This Medicine

In deciding to use a medicine, the risks of taking the medicine must be weighed against the good it will do. This is a decision you and your doctor will make. For this medicine, the following should be considered:

Allergies—Tell your doctor if you have ever had any unusual or allergic reaction to this medicine or any other medicines. Also tell your health care professional if you have any other types of allergies, such as to foods, dyes, preservatives, or animals. For non-prescription products, read the label or package ingredients carefully.

Pediatric—Paroxetine must be used with caution in children with depression. Studies have shown occurrences of children thinking about suicide or attempting suicide in clinical trials for this medicine. More study is needed to be sure paroxetine is safe and effective in children.

Geriatric—In studies that have included elderly people, paroxetine did not cause different side effects or problems in older people than it did in younger adults. However, paroxetine may be removed from the body more slowly in elderly people. An older adult may need a lower dose than a younger adult.

Pregnancy—

	Pregnancy Category	Explanation
All Trimesters	D	Studies in pregnant women have demonstrated a risk to the fetus. However, the benefits of therapy in a life threatening situation or a serious disease, may outweigh the potential risk.

Breast Feeding—Studies in women suggest that this medication poses minimal risk to the infant when used during breastfeeding.

Other medicines—

Using this medicine with any of the following medicines is not recommended. Your doctor may decide not to treat you with this medication or change some of the other medicines you take.

Clorgyline, Furazolidone, Iproniazid, Isocarboxazid, Moclobemide, Nialamide, Pargyline, Phenelzine, Pimozide, Procarbazine, Selegiline, Thioridazine, Toloxatone, Tranylcypromine

Interactions with Food/Tobacco/Alcohol—Certain medicines should not be used at or around the time of eating food or eating certain types of food since interactions may occur. Using alcohol or tobacco with certain medicines may also cause interactions to occur. Discuss with your healthcare professional the use of your medicine with food, alcohol, or tobacco.

Other medical problems—The presence of other medical problems may affect the use of this medicine. Make sure you

tell your doctor if you have any other medical problems, especially:

- Bipolar disorder (mood disorder with alternating episodes of mania and depression) or risk of—May make condition worse. Your doctor will check you for this condition.
- Brain disease or damage or
- Mental retardation or
- Epilepsy or seizures (history of)—The risk of seizures may be increased.
- Glaucoma, narrow angle—Patients with this condition should use paroxetine with caution.
- Heart disease or
- Heart attack, recent—Use must be determined by your doctor.
- Kidney disease, severe, or
- Liver disease, severe—Higher blood levels of paroxetine may occur, increasing the chance of side effects.
- Mania (history of)—The condition may be activated.

Proper Use of This Medicine

Take this medicine only as directed by your doctor to benefit your condition as much as possible. Do not take more of it, do not take it more often, and do not take it for a longer time than your doctor ordered.

Paroxetine may be taken with or without food or on a full or empty stomach. However, if your doctor tells you to take the medicine a certain way, take it exactly as directed.

You may have to take paroxetine for several weeks before you begin to feel better. Your doctor should check your progress at regular visits during this time. Also, if you are taking paroxetine for depression, you will probably need to continue taking it for at least 6 months to help prevent the depression from returning.

If you are taking the oral suspension form of paroxetine, shake the bottle well before measuring each dose. Use a small measuring cup or a measuring spoon to measure each dose. The teaspoons and tablespoons that are used for serving and eating food do not measure exact amounts.

If you are taking the extended-release tablet form of this medicine, swallow the tablet whole. Do not crush, break, or chew before swallowing.

Dosing—The dose of this medicine will be different for different patients. Follow your doctor's orders or the directions on the label. The following information includes only the average doses of this medicine. If your dose is different, do not change it unless your doctor tells you to do so.

The amount of medicine that you take depends on the strength of the medicine. Also, the number of doses you take each day, the time allowed between doses, and the length of time you take the medicine depend on the medical problem for which you are using the medicine.

- For oral suspension dosage form:
  - For treatment of depression:
    - Adults—At first, 20 milligrams (mg) (10 milliliters [mL]) once a day, usually taken in the morning. Your doctor may increase your dose if needed. However, the dose usually is not more than 50 mg (25 mL) a day.
    - Children—Use and dose must be determined by your doctor.
    - Older adults—At first, 10 mg (5 mL) once a day, usually taken in the morning. Your doctor may increase your dose if needed. However, the dose usually is not more than 40 mg (20 mL) a day.
  - For treatment of generalized anxiety disorder:
    - Adults—At first, 20 milligrams (mg) (10 milliliters [mL]) once a day, usually taken in the morning. Your doctor may increase your dose if needed. However, the dose usually is not more than 50 mg (25 mL) a day.
    - Children—Use and dose must be determined by your doctor.
    - Older adults—At first, 10 mg (5 mL) once a day, usually taken in the morning. Your doctor may increase your dose if needed. However, the dose usually is not more than 40 mg (20 mL) a day.
  - For treatment of obsessive-compulsive disorder:
    - Adults—At first, 20 milligrams (mg) (10 milliliters [mL]) once a day, usually taken in the morning. Your doctor may increase your dose if needed. However, the dose usually is not more than 60 mg (30 mL) a day.
    - Children—Use and dose must be determined by your doctor.
    - Older adults—At first, 10 mg (5 mL) once a day, usually taken in the morning. Your doctor may increase your dose if needed. However, the dose usually is not more than 40 mg (20 mL) a day.
  - For treatment of panic disorder:
    - Adults—At first, 10 milligrams (mg) (5 milliliters [mL]) once a day, usually taken in the morning. Your doctor may increase your dose if needed. However, the dose usually is not more than 60 mg (30 mL) a day.
    - Children—Use and dose must be determined by your doctor.
    - Older adults—At first, 10 mg (5 mL) once a day, usually taken in the morning. Your doctor may increase your dose if needed. However, the dose usually is not more than 40 mg (20 mL) a day.
  - For treatment of posttraumatic stress disorder:
    - Adults—At first, 20 milligrams (mg) (10 milliliters [mL]) once a day, usually taken in the morning. Your doctor may increase your dose if needed. However, the dose usually is not more than 50 mg (25 mL) a day.
    - Children—Use and dose must be determined by your doctor.
    - Older adults—At first, 10 mg (5 mL) once a day, usually taken in the morning. Your doctor may increase your dose if needed. However, the dose usually is not more than 40 mg (20 mL) a day.
  - For treatment of social anxiety disorder:
    - Adults—At first, 20 milligrams (mg) (10 milliliters [mL]) once a day, usually taken in the morning.
    - Children—Use and dose must be determined by your doctor.
    - Older adults—At first, 10 mg (5 mL) once a day, usually taken in the morning. Your doctor may increase your dose if needed. However, the dose usually is not more than 20 mg (10 mL) a day.

- For oral tablet dosage form:
  - For treatment of depression:
    - Adults—At first, 20 milligrams (mg) once a day, usually taken in the morning. Your doctor may increase your dose if needed. However, the dose usually is not more than 50 mg a day.
    - Children—Use and dose must be determined by your doctor.
    - Older adults—At first, 10 mg once a day, usually taken in the morning. Your doctor may increase your dose if needed. However, the dose usually is not more than 40 mg a day.
  - For treatment of generalized anxiety disorder:
    - Adults—At first, 20 milligrams (mg) once a day, usually taken in the morning. Your doctor may increase your dose if needed. However, the dose usually is not more than 50 mg a day.
    - Children—Use and dose must be determined by your doctor.
    - Older adults—At first, 10 mg once a day, usually taken in the morning. Your doctor may increase your dose if needed. However, the dose usually is not more than 40 mg a day.
  - For treatment of obsessive-compulsive disorder:
    - Adults—At first, 20 milligrams (mg) once a day, usually taken in the morning. Your doctor may increase your dose if needed. However, the dose usually is not more than 60 mg a day.
    - Children—Use and dose must be determined by your doctor.
    - Older adults—At first, 10 mg once a day, usually taken in the morning. Your doctor may increase your dose if needed. However, the dose usually is not more than 40 mg a day.
  - For treatment of panic disorder:
    - Adults—At first, 10 milligrams (mg) once a day, usually taken in the morning. Your doctor may increase your dose if needed. However, the dose usually is not more than 60 mg a day.
    - Children—Use and dose must be determined by your doctor.
    - Older adults—At first, 10 mg once a day, usually taken in the morning. Your doctor may increase your dose if needed. However, the dose usually is not more than 40 mg a day.
  - For treatment of posttraumatic stress disorder:
    - Adults—At first, 20 milligrams (mg) once a day, usually taken in the morning. Your doctor may increase your dose if needed. However, the dose usually is not more than 50 mg a day.
    - Children—Use and dose must be determined by your doctor.
    - Older adults—At first, 10 mg once a day, usually taken in the morning. Your doctor may increase your dose if needed. However, the dose usually is not more than 40 mg a day.
  - For treatment of social anxiety disorder:
    - Adults—At first, 20 milligrams (mg) once a day, usually taken in the morning.
    - Children—Use and dose must be determined by your doctor.
    - Older adults—At first, 10 mg once a day, usually taken in the morning. Your doctor may increase

your dose if needed. However, the dose usually is not more than 20 mg a day.

- For oral extended-release tablet dosage form:
  - For treatment of depression:
    - Adults—At first, 25 milligrams (mg) once a day, usually taken in the morning. Your doctor may increase your dose if needed. However, the dose usually is not more than 62.5 mg a day.
    - Children—Use and dose must be determined by your doctor.
    - Older adults—At first, 12.5 mg once a day, usually taken in the morning. Your doctor may increase your dose if needed. However, the dose usually is not more than 50 mg a day.
  - For treatment of panic disorder:
    - Adults—At first, 12.5 milligrams (mg) once a day, usually taken in the morning. Your doctor may increase your dose if needed. However, the dose usually is not more than 75 mg a day.
    - Children—Use and dose must be determined by your doctor.
    - Older adults—At first, 12.5 mg once a day, usually taken in the morning. Your doctor may increase your dose if needed. However, the dose usually is not more than 50 mg a day.
  - For treatment of social anxiety disorder:
    - Adults—At first, 12.5 milligrams (mg) once a day, usually taken in the morning. Your doctor may increase your dose if needed. However, the dose usually is not more than 37.5 mg a day.
    - Children—Use and dose must be determined by your doctor.
    - Older adults—At first, 12.5 mg once a day, usually taken in the morning. Your doctor may increase your dose if needed. However, the dose usually is not more than 37.5 mg a day.
  - For treatment of premenstrual dysphoric disorder:
    - Adults—At first, 12.5 milligrams (mg) once a day, usually taken in the morning. Your doctor may increase your dose if needed. However, the dose usually is not more than 25 mg a day.
    - Children—Use and dose must be determined by your doctor.
    - Older adults—Use and dose must be determined by your doctor.

Missed dose—If you miss a dose of this medicine, take it as soon as possible. However, if it is almost time for your next dose, skip the missed dose and go back to your regular dosing schedule. Do not double doses.

Storage—Store the medicine in a closed container at room temperature, away from heat, moisture, and direct light. Keep from freezing.

Keep out of the reach of children.

Do not keep outdated medicine or medicine no longer needed.

Precautions While Using This Medicine

It is important that your doctor check your progress at regular visits, to allow for changes in your dose and to help reduce any side effects.

Tell your doctor right away if you develop any allergic reactions, such as skin rash or hives, while taking paroxetine.

Paroxetine may cause some people to be agitated, irritable or display other abnormal behaviors. It may also cause some people to have suicidal thoughts and tendencies or to become more depressed. If you or your caregiver notice any of these adverse effects, tell your doctor right away.

Paroxetine may cause some people to be agitated, irritable or display other abnormal behaviors. It may also cause some people to have suicidal thoughts and tendencies or to become more depressed. If you or your caregiver notice any of these adverse effects, tell your doctor right away.

Do not suddenly stop taking your paroxetine. If you have been instructed to stop taking paroxetine, ask your healthcare professional how to slowly decrease the dose. This is to decrease the chance of having discontinuation symptoms such as agitation, breathing problems, chest pain, confusion, diarrhea, dizziness or light-headedness, fast heartbeat, headache, increased sweating, muscle pain, nausea, restlessness, runny nose, trouble in sleeping, trembling or shaking, unusual tiredness or weakness, vision changes, or vomiting.

Do not take paroxetine if you have taken a monoamine oxidase (MAO) inhibitor (furazolidone, phenelzine, procarbazine, selegiline, tranylcypromine) in the past 2 weeks. Do not start taking an MAO inhibitor within 2 weeks of stopping paroxetine. If you do, you may develop confusion, agitation, restlessness, stomach or intestinal symptoms, sudden high body temperature, extremely high blood pressure, severe convulsions, or the serotonin syndrome.

Paroxetine has not been shown to add to the effects of alcohol. However, use of alcohol is not recommended in patients who are taking paroxetine.

Paroxetine may cause some people to become drowsy or have blurred vision. Make sure you know how you react to this medicine before you drive, use machines, or do anything else that could be dangerous if you are not alert or able to see clearly.

Side Effects of This Medicine

Along with its needed effects, a medicine may cause some unwanted effects. One rare but serious unwanted effect that may occur with paroxetine use is the serotonin syndrome. This syndrome (group of symptoms) is more likely to occur shortly after the dose of paroxetine is increased.

Although not all of these side effects may occur, if they do occur they may need medical attention.

Check with your doctor as soon as possible if any of the following side effects occur:

Less common

Agitation; chest congestion; chest pain; chills; cold sweats; confusion; difficulty breathing; dizziness, faintness, or lightheadedness when getting up from a lying or sitting position; fast, pounding, or irregular heartbeat or pulse; muscle pain or weakness; skin rash

Rare

Absence of or decrease in body movements; bigger, dilated, or enlarged pupils [black part of eye] difficulty in speaking; inability to move eyes; incomplete, sudden, or unusual body or facial movements; increased sensitivity of eyes to light; low blood sodium (confusion, convulsions [seizures], drowsiness, dryness of mouth, increased thirst, lack of energy); red or purple patches on skin; serotonin syndrome (confusion, diarrhea, fever, poor coordination, restlessness, shiv-

ering, sweating, talking and acting with excitement you cannot control, trembling or shaking, twitching); talking, feeling, and acting with excitement and activity you cannot control

Incidence not determined

Back, leg, or stomach pains; bleeding gums; blindness; blistering, peeling, loosening of skin; bloated, full feeling; bloody or black, tarry stools; bloody urine; blue-yellow color blindness; blurred vision; coma; constipation; cough or hoarseness; dark urine; decreased frequency or amount of urine; decreased vision; depression; difficulty opening the mouth; difficulty swallowing; electric shock sensations; epileptic seizure that will not stop; excessive muscle tone; eye pain; fainting; fixed position of eye; fluid-filled skin blisters; general body swelling; general feeling of tiredness or weakness; headache; high fever; hives; inability to move arms and legs; inability to sit still; increased blood pressure; increased sweating; increased thirst; incremental or ratchet-like movement of muscle; indigestion; itching skin; joint pain; lab results that show problems with liver; light-colored stools; lockjaw; loss of appetite; loss of bladder control; low blood pressure; lower back or side pain; muscle spasm, especially of neck and back; muscle tension or tightness; nausea; need to keep moving; nosebleeds; painful knees and ankles; painful or difficult urination; painful or prolonged erection of the penis; pale skin; puffiness or swelling of the eyelids or around the eyes, face, lips, or tongue; raised red swellings on the skin, the buttocks, legs, or ankles; red irritated eyes; rigid muscles; seizure or coma late in pregnancy; sensitivity to the sun; skin redness or soreness; skin sores, welts or blisters; skin thinness; sore throat; sores, ulcers, or white spots on lips or in mouth; swelling of breasts; swollen or painful glands; shortness of breath; slow heart rate; slow movement; slow reflexes; spasms of throat; stiff muscles; stomach pain; sudden numbness and weakness in the arms and legs; swelling of face, fingers, lower legs; tightness in chest; unexpected or excess milk flow from breasts; unusual bleeding or bruising; unusual or decreased blood cell production; unusual tiredness or weakness; vomiting; weight gain; wheezing; yellowing of the eyes or skin

Symptoms of overdose

Dizziness; drowsiness; dryness of mouth; flushing of face; irritability; large pupils; nausea; racing heartbeat; trembling or shaking; vomiting

Some side effects may occur that usually do not need medical attention. These side effects may go away during treatment as your body adjusts to the medicine. Also, your health care professional may be able to tell you about ways to prevent or reduce some of these side effects. Check with your health care professional if any of the following side effects continue or are bothersome or if you have any questions about them:

More common

Acid or sour stomach; belching; decreased appetite; decreased sexual ability or desire; excess air or gas in stomach or intestines; heartburn; nervousness; pain or tenderness around eyes and cheekbones; passing gas; problems in urinating; runny or stuffy nose; sexual problems, especially ejaculatory disturbances; sleepiness or unusual drowsiness; stomach discomfort, upset, or pain; sweating; trauma; trembling or shaking; trouble in sleeping

Less common

Abnormal dreams; anxiety; bladder pain; body aches or pain; change in sense of taste; changes in vision; cloudy urine; confusion; congestion; difficulty in focusing eyes; difficulty in moving; discouragement, feeling sad or empty; drugged feeling; dryness of throat; excessive muscle tone; fainting or loss of consciousness; fast or irregular breathing; feeling of unreality; feeling of warmth or heat; flushing or redness of skin, especially on face and neck; frequent urge to urinate; headache, severe and throbbing; heavy bleeding; increase in body movements; increased appetite; irritability; itching, pain, redness, or swelling of eye or eyelid; itching of the vagina or genital area; lack of emotion; loss of interest or pleasure; loss of memory; lump in throat; menstrual changes; menstrual pain or cramps; muscle twitching or jerking; pain during sexual intercourse; problems with memory; problems with tooth; rhythmic movement of muscles; sense of detachment from self or body; severe sunburn; slow heartbeat; sneezing; thick, white vaginal discharge with no odor or with a mild odor; tightness in throat; tingling, burning, or prickling sensations; trouble concentrating; voice changes; watering of eyes; weight loss; yawn

After you stop using this medicine, it may still produce some side effects that need attention. During this period of time, *check with your doctor immediately* if you notice the following side effects:

Abnormal dreams; actions that are out of control; agitation, confusion, or restlessness; burning, crawling, itching, numbness, prickling, "pins and needles", or tingling feelings; crying; depersonalization; diarrhea; dizziness or light-headedness; dysphoria; electric shock sensations; euphoria; fear; feeling unwell or unhappy; headache; increased sweating; irritability; mental depression; muscle pain; nausea or vomiting; nervousness; paranoia; quick to react or overreact emotionally; rapidly changing moods; runny nose; talking, feeling, and acting with excitement; trembling or shaking; trouble in sleeping; unusual drowsiness, dullness or feeling of sluggishness; unusual tiredness or weakness; vision changes

Other side effects not listed may also occur in some patients. If you notice any other effects, check with your healthcare professional.

PEGASPARGASE (Intramuscular route, Intravenous route) - peg-AS-par-jase

Commonly used brand name(s)

In the U.S.—
Oncaspar

Available Dosage Forms:
• Solution

Therapeutic Class: Antineoplastic Agent
Pharmacologic Class: Asparaginase (class)

Uses For This Medicine

Pegaspargase belongs to the general group of medicines known as antineoplastics. It is used with other cancer medicines as a first-line treatment to a certain type of blood cancer called acute lymphoblastic leukemia (ALL). This medicine also treats ALL in patients who have had serious allergic reactions to L-asparaginase.

Pegaspargase seems to interfere with the growth of cancer cells, which are eventually destroyed. Since the growth of normal body cells also may be affected by pegaspargase, other effects also occur. Some of these effects may be serious and must be reported to your doctor.

Before you begin treatment with pegaspargase, you and your doctor should talk about the good this medicine will do as well as the risks of using it.

Pegaspargase is to be administered only by or under the immediate supervision of your doctor.

This medicine is available only with your doctor's prescription.

Before Receiving This Medicine

In deciding to use a medicine, the risks of taking the medicine must be weighed against the good it will do. This is a decision you and your doctor will make. For this medicine, the following should be considered:

Allergies—Tell your doctor if you have ever had any unusual or allergic reaction to this medicine or any other medicines. Also tell your health care professional if you have any other types of allergies, such as to foods, dyes, preservatives, or animals. For non-prescription products, read the label or package ingredients carefully.

Pediatric—Infants up to 1 year of age—Safety and efficacy have not been established.

Children 1 year of age and older—This medicine has been studied in children 1 year of age and older and has not been shown to cause different side effects or problems than it does in adults. In fact, the side effects of this medicine seem to be less severe in children than in adults.

Geriatric—There is no specific information comparing the use of pegaspargase in the elderly with use in other age groups. Safety and efficacy of pegaspargase in the elderly have not been established.

Pregnancy—

	Pregnancy Category	Explanation
All Trimesters	C	Animal studies have shown an adverse effect and there are no adequate studies in pregnant women OR no animal studies have been conducted and there are no adequate studies in pregnant women.

Breast Feeding—There are no adequate studies in women for determining infant risk when using this medication during breastfeeding. Weigh the potential benefits against the potential risks before taking this medication while breastfeeding.

Other medicines—

Using this medicine with any of the following medicines is not recommended. Your doctor may decide not to treat you with this medication or change some of the other medicines you take.

Rotavirus Vaccine, Live

Interactions with Food/Tobacco/Alcohol—Certain medicines should not be used at or around the time of eating food or eating certain types of food since interactions may occur. Using alcohol or tobacco with certain medicines may also cause interactions to occur. Discuss with your healthcare professional the use of your medicine with food, alcohol, or tobacco.

Other medical problems—The presence of other medical problems may affect the use of this medicine. Make sure you tell your doctor if you have any other medical problems, especially:

- Anticoagulant therapy (treatment with blood thinners) or
- Bleeding problems—The chance of bleeding may be increased
- Blood clots
- Chickenpox (including recent exposure) or
- Herpes zoster (shingles)—Risk of severe disease affecting other parts of the body
- Type 2 diabetes mellitus—The chance of side effects may be increased
- Infection—Pegaspargase can decrease your body's ability to fight infection
- Liver disease—Effects of pegaspargase may be increased because of slower removal of this medicine from the body
- Pancreatitis—The chance of side effects may be increased

Proper Use of This Medicine

Pegaspargase sometimes is given together with certain other medicines. If you are using a combination of medicines, it is important that you receive each one at the proper time. If you are taking some of these medicines by mouth, ask your doctor to help you plan a way to take them at the right times.

While you are receiving pegaspargase, your doctor may want you to drink extra fluids so that you will pass more urine. This will help prevent kidney problems and keep your kidneys working well.

This medicine often causes nausea and vomiting. However, it is very important that you continue to receive the medicine, even if you begin to feel ill. Ask your health care professional for ways to lessen these effects, especially if they are severe.

Dosing—The dose of this medicine will be different for different patients. Follow your doctor's orders or the directions on the label.

The amount of medicine that you take depends on the strength of the medicine. Also, the number of doses you take each day, the time allowed between doses, and the length of time you take the medicine depend on the medical problem for which you are using the medicine.

Precautions After Receiving This Medicine

It is very important that your doctor check your progress at regular visits to make sure that this medicine is working properly and to check for unwanted effects.

While you are being treated with pegaspargase, and after you stop treatment with it, do not have any immunizations (vaccinations) without your doctor's approval. Pegaspargase may lower your body's resistance and there is a chance you might get the infection the immunization is meant to prevent. In addition, other persons living in your household should not take oral poliovirus vaccine, since there is a chance they could pass the poliovirus on to you. Also, avoid persons who have taken oral poliovirus vaccine. Do not get close to them, and do not stay in the same room with them for long. If you cannot take these precautions, you should consider wearing a protective face mask that covers the nose and the mouth.

Pegaspargase can temporarily lower the number of white blood cells in your blood, increasing the chance of getting infection. It can also lower the number of platelets, which are necessary for proper blood clotting. If this occurs, there are certain precautions you can take, especially when your blood count is low, to reduce the risk of infection or bleeding:

- If you can, avoid people with infection. Check with your doctor immediately if you think you are getting an infection or if you get a fever or chills, cough or hoarseness, lower back or side pain, or have painful or difficult urination.
- Check with your doctor immediately if you notice any unusual bleeding or bruising; black tarry stools; blood in urine or stools; or pinpoint red spots on your skin.
- Be careful when using a regular toothbrush, dental floss, or toothpick. Your medical doctor, dentist, or nurse may recommend other ways to clean your teeth and gums. Check with your medical doctor before having any dental work done.
- Do not touch your eyes or the inside of your nose unless you have just washed your hands and have not touched anything else in the meantime.
- Be careful not to cut yourself when you are using sharp objects such as safety razor or fingernail or toenail cutters.
- Avoid contact sports or other situations where bruising or injury can occur.

If pegaspargase accidentally seeps out of the vein into which it is injected, it may damage some tissue and cause scarring. Tell the doctor or nurse right away if you notice redness, pain, or swelling at the place of injection.

This medicine may cause serious allergic reaction. Tell your doctor immediately if you start having trouble breathing, chest tightness, skin rash, or itching while you are receiving this medicine.

Some people who have received this medicine developed pancreatitis (inflammation of the pancreas). Check with your doctor if you experience sudden and severe stomach pain, nausea, vomiting, fever, or chills while on this medicine.

Check with your doctor immediately if you start having increased thirst or hunger, increased urination, pale skin, nausea, sweating, or faintness. This may be signs that you are having problems with the amount of blood sugar in your body.

This medicine may increase your risk of developing serious blood clots. Tell your doctor right away if you develop any sudden and severe headache, arm or leg swelling, shortness of breath, or chest pain.

Side Effects of This Medicine

Along with its needed effects, a medicine may cause some unwanted effects. Although not all of these side effects may occur, if they do occur they may need medical attention.

Check with your doctor as soon as possible if any of the following side effects occur:

More common

Abdominal or stomach pain; blurry vision; constipation; dry mouth and skin; faintness; fatigue; fruit-like breath odor; increased hunger or thirst; increased need to urinate; nausea; skin paleness; skin rash; sweating; troubled breathing; unexplained weight loss; unusual bleeding or bruising; vomiting

Less common

Bloating; chest pain; confusion; cough; darkened urine; difficulty in breathing or swallowing; dizziness; fast heartbeat; fever or chills; headache; hives or itching; indigestion; itching, especially of hands and feet; loss of appetite; numbness, tingling, or swelling in arms or legs; pains in stomach, side, or abdomen, possibly radiating to the back; puffiness or swelling of the eyelids or around the eyes, face, lips or tongue; reddening of the skin, especially around ears; shortness of breath; swelling of eyes, face, or inside of nose; tightness in chest; unusual tiredness or weakness (sudden and severe); wheezing; yellow eyes or skin

Rare

Black, tarry stools; blood in urine; hoarseness; lower back or side pain; painful or difficult urination; pinpoint red spots on skin

Some side effects may occur that usually do not need medical attention. These side effects may go away during treatment as your body adjusts to the medicine. Also, your health care professional may be able to tell you about ways to prevent or reduce some of these side effects. Check with your health care professional if any of the following side effects continue or are bothersome or if you have any questions about them:

More common

General feeling of discomfort or illness

Less common

Anxiety; behavior change similar to drunkenness; blurred vision; cold sweats; convulsions (seizures); cool pale skin; difficulty in concentrating; drowsiness; lack of appetite; nervousness; nightmares; pain at place of injection; pain in joints or muscles; restless sleep; shakiness; slurred speech

PEGFILGRASTIM (Subcutaneous route) - peg-fil-GRA-stim

Commonly used brand name(s)

In the U.S.—
Neulasta

Available Dosage Forms:
• Solution

Therapeutic Class: Hematopoietic
Pharmacologic Class: Colony Stimulating Factor

Uses For This Medicine

Pegfilgrastim is a substance called a Colony Stimulating Factor. These substances, are synthetic (man-made) versions of substances naturally produced in your body which help the bone marrow to make new white blood cells.

Certain medicines affect those white blood cells in your body that fight infection. To help prevent infections when these medicines are used, colony stimulating factors may be given.

This medicine is available only with your doctor's prescription.

Before Using This Medicine

In deciding to use a medicine, the risks of taking the medicine must be weighed against the good it will do. This is a decision you and your doctor will make. For this medicine, the following should be considered:

Allergies—Tell your doctor if you have ever had any unusual or allergic reaction to this medicine or any other medicines. Also tell your health care professional if you have any other types of allergies, such as to foods, dyes, preservatives, or animals. For non-prescription products, read the label or package ingredients carefully.

Pediatric—Studies on this medicine have been done only in adult patients and there is no specific information comparing use of pegfilgrastim in children with use in other age groups. The 6–mg syringe should not be used in infants, children, and smaller adolescents weighing less than 45 kilograms (99 lbs) of body weight.

Geriatric—This medicine has been tested in a limited number of patients 65 years of age or older and has not been shown to cause different side effects or problems in older people than it does in younger adults.

Pregnancy—

	Pregnancy Category	Explanation
All Trimesters	C	Animal studies have shown an adverse effect and there are no adequate studies in pregnant women OR no animal studies have been conducted and there are no adequate studies in pregnant women.

Breast Feeding—There are no adequate studies in women for determining infant risk when using this medication during breastfeeding. Weigh the potential benefits against the potential risks before taking this medication while breastfeeding.

Other medicines—Although certain medicines should not be used together at all, in other cases two different medicines may be used together even if an interaction might occur. In these cases, your doctor may want to change the dose, or other precautions may be necessary. Tell your healthcare professional if you are taking any other prescription or nonprescription (over-the-counter [OTC]) medicine.

Interactions with Food/Tobacco/Alcohol—Certain medicines should not be used at or around the time of eating food or eating certain types of food since interactions may occur. Using alcohol or tobacco with certain medicines may also cause interactions to occur. Discuss with your healthcare professional the use of your medicine with food, alcohol, or tobacco.

Other medical problems—The presence of other medical problems may affect the use of this medicine. Make sure you tell your doctor if you have any other medical problems, especially:

• Bone marrow cancer or other bone marrow problems— Pegfilgrastim may make cancer or other problems worse.

- Liver problems—Safety of this medicine in patients with liver problems has not been studied.
- Peripheral blood progenitor cell (PBPC) mobilization—Use of pegfilgrastim is not recommended for PBPC mobilization.
- Sepsis (serious infection)—There have been reports of adult respiratory distress syndrome (ARDS) in patients who had a serious infection and were receiving a similar medicine called filgrastim.
- Sickle cell disease—Pegfilgrastim may increase the risk of unwanted effects.

Proper Use of This Medicine

Dosing—The dose of this medicine will be different for different patients. Follow your doctor's orders or the directions on the label. The following information includes only the average doses of this medicine. If your dose is different, do not change it unless your doctor tells you to do so.

The amount of medicine that you take depends on the strength of the medicine. Also, the number of doses you take each day, the time allowed between doses, and the length of time you take the medicine depend on the medical problem for which you are using the medicine.

- For injectable dosage form:
  - To increase white blood cell count:
    - Adults—6 mg as an injection one time every chemotherapy cycle
    - Children—Use and dose must be determined by your doctor.

Storage—Store in the refrigerator. Do not freeze.

Keep out of the reach of children.

Do not keep outdated medicine or medicine no longer needed.

Ask your healthcare professional how you should dispose of any medicine you do not use.

Precautions While Using This Medicine

It is very important that your doctor check your progress at regular visits for any problems that may be caused by this medicine and to make sure that this medicine is working properly.

If you experience upper stomach pain or shoulder tip pain, *contact your doctor right away.*

Side Effects of This Medicine

Along with its needed effects, a medicine may cause some unwanted effects. Although not all of these side effects may occur, if they do occur they may need medical attention.

Some of the side effects listed below may be caused by your cancer or by the cancer medicines that you are also receiving.

Check with your doctor immediately if any of the following side effects occur:

More common
> Fever; granulocytopenia, including chills; cough; fever; sore throat; ulcers; sores, or white spots in mouth

Rare
> Shortness of breath; tightness in chest; troubled breathing; or wheezing; bluish lips or skin; pain, left upper abdomen or shoulder

Incidence not known
> Cough; difficulty swallowing; fast heartbeat; hives or welts; itching, puffiness or swelling of the eyelids or around the eyes, face, lips or tongue; redness of skin; skin rash; unusual tiredness or weakness

Some side effects may occur that usually do not need medical attention. These side effects may go away during treatment as your body adjusts to the medicine. Also, your health care professional may be able to tell you about ways to prevent or reduce some of these side effects. Check with your health care professional if any of the following side effects continue or are bothersome or if you have any questions about them:

More common
> Abdominal pain; acid or sour stomach; belching; heartburn; indigestion; or stomach discomfort, upset, or pain; bone pain; change in sense of taste; constipation; diarrhea; dizziness; hair loss or thinning of hair; lack or loss of strength; loss of appetite or weight loss; fatigue; headache; joint pain; mucositis, including cracked lips; diarrhea; difficulty in swallowing; or sores, ulcers, or white spots on lips, tongue, or inside mouth; muscle soreness; nausea; swelling of hands, ankles, feet, or lower legs; swelling or inflammation of the mouth; trouble sleeping; vomiting; weakness, generalized

Incidence not known
> Body produces substance that can bind to drug making it less effective or cause side effects

Other side effects not listed may also occur in some patients. If you notice any other effects, check with your healthcare professional.

PEGINTERFERON ALFA-2A
(Subcutaneous route) - peg-in-ter-FEER-on AL-fa-2a

Black Box Warning

Alpha interferons, including peginterferon alfa-2a, may cause or aggravate fatal or life-threatening neuropsychiatric, autoimmune, ischemic, and infectious disorders. Patients should be monitored closely with periodic clinical and laboratory evaluations. Therapy should be withdrawn in patients with persistently severe or worsening signs or symptoms of these conditions. In many, but not all cases, these disorders resolve after stopping peginterferon alfa-2a therapy.

Usage with ribavirin: Ribavirin, may cause birth defects and/or death of the fetus. Extreme care must be taken to avoid pregnancy in female patients and in female partners of male patients. Ribavirin causes hemolytic anemia. The anemia associated with ribavirin therapy may result in a worsening of cardiac disease. Ribavirin is genotoxic and mutagenic and should be considered a potential carcinogen.

Commonly used brand name(s)

In the U.S.—
> Pegasys

Available Dosage Forms:
• Solution

Therapeutic Class: Antineoplastic Agent
Pharmacologic Class: Interferon, Alfa (class)

Uses For This Medicine

Peginterferon alfa-2a is a synthetic (man-made) version of substances normally produced in the body to fight infection. Peginterferon alfa-2a is used to treat chronic hepatitis C. It is used for patients who have never been treated by alpha interferons. Peginterferon alfa-2a is also used to treat adult patients with HBeAg negative chronic hepatitis B. It is used in patients who have liver disease and evidence of viral replication and liver inflammation.

This medicine is available only with your doctor's prescription.

Before Using This Medicine

In deciding to use a medicine, the risks of taking the medicine must be weighed against the good it will do. This is a decision you and your doctor will make. For this medicine, the following should be considered:

Allergies—Tell your doctor if you have ever had any unusual or allergic reaction to this medicine or any other medicines. Also tell your health care professional if you have any other types of allergies, such as to foods, dyes, preservatives, or animals. For non-prescription products, read the label or package ingredients carefully.

Pediatric—Studies of this medicine have been done only in adult patients and there is no specific information comparing use of peginterferon alfa–2a in children with use in other age groups. However, this medicine should not be used in newborns and infants because it has a substance that is harmful to newborns and infants.

Geriatric—Many medicines have not been studied specifically in older people. Therefore, it may not be known whether they work exactly the same way they do in younger adults or if they cause different side effects or problems in older people. There is no specific information comparing use of peginterferon alfa–2a in the elderly with use in other age groups. However, specific side effects may be especially likely to occur in elderly patients who may be more sensitive than younger adults to the effects of this medicine.

Pregnancy—

	Pregnancy Category	Explanation
All Trimesters	C	Animal studies have shown an adverse effect and there are no adequate studies in pregnant women OR no animal studies have been conducted and there are no adequate studies in pregnant women.

Breast Feeding—There are no adequate studies in women for determining infant risk when using this medication during breastfeeding. Weigh the potential benefits against the potential risks before taking this medication while breastfeeding.

Other medicines—

Using this medicine with any of the following medicines is usually not recommended, but may be required in some cases. If both medicines are prescribed together, your doctor

may change the dose or how often you use one or both of the medicines.

Theophylline

Interactions with Food/Tobacco/Alcohol—Certain medicines should not be used at or around the time of eating food or eating certain types of food since interactions may occur. Using alcohol or tobacco with certain medicines may also cause interactions to occur. Discuss with your healthcare professional the use of your medicine with food, alcohol, or tobacco.

Other medical problems—The presence of other medical problems may affect the use of this medicine. Make sure you tell your doctor if you have any other medical problems, especially:

• Autoimmune hepatitis (serious liver disease)—Peginterferon alfa-2a should not be used if you have this disease.

• Anemia (blood disease) or

• Blood problems—Peginterferon alfa-2a may make these conditions worse and your doctor may have you take a lower dose of this medicine.

• Bone marrow illness—Peginterferon alfa-2a may make these conditions worse.

• Lung or breathing problems—Peginterferon alfa-2a may make these conditions worse.

• Diabetes mellitus (sugar diabetes) or

• Hyperglycemia (high blood sugar) or

• Hypoglycemia (low blood sugar) or

• Hyperthyroidism (overactive thyroid gland) or

• Hypothyroidism (underactive thyroid gland)—This medicine should be used with caution in patients with these conditions; if your condition is not well controlled with your medicine you should not start using peginterferon alfa-2a.

• Heart problems—Peginterferon alfa-2a should be with caution in people with heart problems.

• HIV (human immunodeficiency virus) or

• Hepatitis B virus (liver disease caused by a virus) or

• Hepatitic C virus—It is unclear how well this medicine works and how safe this medicine is when a patient has these conditions.

• Infections (serious infections caused by bacteria)—Peginterferon alfa-2a therapy should be stopped in patients who have serious infections

• Interstitial nephritis (kidney inflammation) or

• Myositis (muscular pain) or

• Psoriasis (skin disease) or

• Rheumatoid arthritis or

• Systemic Lupus (connective tissue disease) or

• Thyroiditis (thyroid gland problem)—Peginterferon alfa-2a may make these conditions worse and it should be used with caution in patients who have these conditions.

• Kidney failure—The dose of peginterferon alfa-2a may need to be lower for patients who have this condition.

• Depression or

• Mental illness—Peginterferon alfa-2a should be used with caution in patients with these conditions.

• Organ transplants—It is not known if this medicine is safe to use in patients who have recently had organ transplants.

Proper Use of This Medicine

Dosing—The dose of this medicine will be different for different patients. Follow your doctor's orders or the directions on the label. The following information includes only the average doses of this medicine. If your dose is different, do not change it unless your doctor tells you to do so.

The amount of medicine that you take depends on the strength of the medicine. Also, the number of doses you take each day, the time allowed between doses, and the length of time you take the medicine depend on the medical problem for which you are using the medicine.

- For parenteral dosage form (injection):
  - For chronic hepatitis B and hepatitis C:
    - Adults—180 micrograms once weekly for 24 to 48 weeks
    - Children—This medicine is not usually used in children under the age of 18

Missed dose—If you miss a dose of this medicine, take it as soon as possible. However, if it is almost time for your next dose, skip the missed dose and go back to your regular dosing schedule. Do not double doses.

Storage—Store in the refrigerator. Do not freeze.

Keep out of the reach of children.

Do not keep outdated medicine or medicine no longer needed.

Ask your healthcare professional how you should dispose of any medicine you do not use.

Precautions While Using This Medicine

This medicine may cause some people to become drowsy, dizzy, or less alert than they are normally. Make sure you know how you react to this medicine before you drive, use machines, or do anything else that could be dangerous if you are dizzy and not alert.

It is very important that your doctor check your progress at regular visits. This will allow your doctor to see if the medicine is working properly and to check for any problems that this medicine may cause.

Side Effects of This Medicine

Along with its needed effects, a medicine may cause some unwanted effects. Although not all of these side effects may occur, if they do occur they may need medical attention.

Check with your doctor immediately if any of the following side effects occur:

More common
> black, tarry, stools; chills; cough; discouragement; feeling sad or empty; fever; irritability; lack of appetite; loss of interest or pleasure; lower back or side pain; painful or difficult urination; pale skin; shortness of breath; sore throat; tiredness; trouble concentrating; trouble sleeping; ulcers, sores, or white spots in mouth; unusual bleeding or bruising; unusual tiredness or weakness

Less common
> bone pain; chest pain or discomfort; confusion; constipation; depressed mood; difficult urination; dizziness; dry skin and hair; fainting; fast heartbeat; feeling cold; hair loss; headache; heart murmur; hives; hoarseness or husky voice; lightheadedness; muscle cramps and stiffness; pale skin; rapid, shallow breathing; slowed

heartbeat; sneezing; stomach pain; tightness in chest; troubled breathing with exertion; unusual bleeding or bruising; unusual tiredness or weakness; wheezing; weight gain

Some side effects may occur that usually do not need medical attention. These side effects may go away during treatment as your body adjusts to the medicine. Also, your health care professional may be able to tell you about ways to prevent or reduce some of these side effects. Check with your health care professional if any of the following side effects continue or are bothersome or if you have any questions about them:

More common
> back pain; blistering, crusting, irritation, itching, or reddening of skin; cracked, dry, scaly skin; diarrhea; dry mouth; fear; feeling unusually cold, shivering; fever; hair loss or thinning; muscle or joint pain; nervousness; numbness; pain; rash; redness; scarring; soreness; stinging; stomach pain; swelling; tenderness; tingling; ulceration; vomiting; warmth

Less common
> acid or sour stomach; belching; blurred vision; heartburn; indigestion; memory problems; stomach discomfort upset or pain

Incidence not known
> Change of hearing; loss of hearing

Other side effects not listed may also occur in some patients. If you notice any other effects, check with your healthcare professional.

PEGINTERFERON ALFA-2B
(Subcutaneous route) - peg-in-ter-FEER-on AL-fa-2b

Black Box Warning

Alpha interferons, including peginterferon alfa-2b, may cause or aggravate fatal or life-threatening neuropsychiatric, autoimmune, ischemic, and infectious disorders. Patients should be monitored closely with periodic clinical and laboratory evaluations. Patients with persistently severe or worsening signs or symptoms of these conditions should be withdrawn from therapy. In many but not all cases these disorders resolve after stopping peginterferon alfa-2b therapy.

Usage with Ribavirin: Ribavirin, may cause birth defects and/or death of the unborn child. Extreme care must be taken to avoid pregnancy in female patients and in female partners of male patients. Ribavirin causes hemolytic anemia. The anemia associated with ribavirin therapy may result in a worsening of cardiac disease. Ribavirin is genotoxic and mutagenic and should be considered a potential carcinogen.

Commonly used brand name(s)

In the U.S.—
> PEG-Intron
> Peg Intron RP

Available Dosage Forms:
- Kit
- Powder for Solution

Therapeutic Class: Antineoplastic Agent
Pharmacologic Class: Interferon, Alfa (class)

Uses For This Medicine

Peginterferon alfa-2b is a synthetic (man-made) version of substances normally produced in the body to fight infection. Peginterferon alfa-2b is used to treat chronic hepatitis C. It is used for patients who have never been treated by alpha interferons and who do not have symptoms of worsening liver disease.

This medicine is available only with your doctor's prescription.

Before Using This Medicine

In deciding to use a medicine, the risks of taking the medicine must be weighed against the good it will do. This is a decision you and your doctor will make. For this medicine, the following should be considered:

Allergies—Tell your doctor if you have ever had any unusual or allergic reaction to this medicine or any other medicines. Also tell your health care professional if you have any other types of allergies, such as to foods, dyes, preservatives, or animals. For non-prescription products, read the label or package ingredients carefully.

Pediatric—Studies on this medicine have been done only in adult patients, and there is no specific information comparing use of peginterferon alfa-2b in children with use in other age groups.

Geriatric—This medicine has been tested in a limited number of patients 65 years of age or older and has not been shown to cause different side effects or problems in older people than it does in younger adults.

Pregnancy—

	Pregnancy Category	Explanation
All Trimesters	C	Animal studies have shown an adverse effect and there are no adequate studies in pregnant women OR no animal studies have been conducted and there are no adequate studies in pregnant women.

Breast Feeding—There are no adequate studies in women for determining infant risk when using this medication during breastfeeding. Weigh the potential benefits against the potential risks before taking this medication while breastfeeding.

Other medicines—Although certain medicines should not be used together at all, in other cases two different medicines may be used together even if an interaction might occur. In these cases, your doctor may want to change the dose, or other precautions may be necessary. Tell your healthcare professional if you are taking any other prescription or non-prescription (over-the-counter [OTC]) medicine.

Interactions with Food/Tobacco/Alcohol—Certain medicines should not be used at or around the time of eating food or eating certain types of food since interactions may occur. Using alcohol or tobacco with certain medicines may also cause interactions to occur. Discuss with your healthcare professional the use of your medicine with food, alcohol, or tobacco.

Other medical problems—The presence of other medical problems may affect the use of this medicine. Make sure you

tell your doctor if you have any other medical problems, especially:

- Autoimmune hepatitis—May cause severe disease affecting other parts of the body
- Decompensated liver disease—May cause liver disease to become worse
- Type 2 diabetes mellitus or
- Heart or blood vessel disease or
- Hyperglycemia (high blood sugar) or
- Kidney disease or
- Lung disease or
- Psoriasis or
- Psychiatric problems or
- Rheumatoid arthritis or
- Systemic lupus erythematosus or
- Thyroid disease—May be worsened by peginterferon alfa-2b
- Human immunodeficiency virus (HIV) infection or
- Liver or other organ transplant—It is not known if peginterferon alfa-2b will work in patients with these conditions

Proper Use of This Medicine

If you are injecting this medicine yourself, use it exactly as directed by your doctor. Do not use more or less of it, and do not use it more often than your doctor ordered. The exact amount of medicine you need has been carefully worked out. Using too much will increase the risk of side effects, while using too little may not improve your condition.

Each package of peginterferon alfa-2b contains a patient instruction sheet. Read this sheet carefully and make sure you understand:

- How to prepare the injection.
- Proper use of disposable syringes.
- How to give the injection.
- How long the injection is stable.

If you have any questions about any of this, check with your health care professional.

Dosing—The dose of this medicine will be different for different patients. Follow your doctor's orders or the directions on the label. The following information includes only the average doses of this medicine. If your dose is different, do not change it unless your doctor tells you to do so.

The amount of medicine that you take depends on the strength of the medicine. Also, the number of doses you take each day, the time allowed between doses, and the length of time you take the medicine depend on the medical problem for which you are using the medicine.

- For injection dosage form:
  - For treating chronic hepatitis C:
    - Adults—Dose is based on body weight. It is usually between 40 and 150 micrograms (mcg) injected under the skin once a week for one year. The medicine should be taken on the same day each week.
    - Children—Use and dose must be determined by your doctor.

Missed dose—If you miss a dose of this medicine, take it as soon as possible. However, if it is almost time for your next dose, skip the missed dose and go back to your regular dosing schedule. Do not double doses.

Call your doctor or pharmacist for instructions.

Storage—Keep out of the reach of children.

Do not keep outdated medicine or medicine no longer needed.

Ask your healthcare professional how you should dispose of any medicine you do not use.

Store in the refrigerator after you have mixed the powder with the sterile water. You can keep it up to 24 hours. Keep from freezing.

Precautions While Using This Medicine

It is very important that your doctor check your progress at regular visits to make sure that this medicine is working properly and to check for unwanted effects.

You may have feelings of anxiety or depression while taking peginterferon alfa-2b. Call your doctor right away if you have these feelings or if you are thinking about hurting yourself or someone else.

Side Effects of This Medicine

Along with its needed effects, a medicine may cause some unwanted effects. Although not all of these side effects may occur, if they do occur they may need medical attention.

Check with your doctor as soon as possible if any of the following side effects occur:

More common
Abdominal pain; anxiety; black, tarry stools; blood in urine or stools; bloody diarrhea; chills; cough or hoarseness; depression; fever; infection; irritability; lower back or side pain; mood swings; nausea; painful or difficult urination; pinpoint red spots on skin; trouble in sleeping; unusual bleeding or bruising; vomiting

Less common
Changes in menstrual cycle; constipation; drowsiness; dry hair and skin; sensitivity to cold; unusual tiredness or weakness; weight gain

Rare
Aching, pain, and/or stiffness in joints; aggressive behavior; attempt to kill yourself; backache; chest pain (severe); cool, pale skin; decrease in vision; diarrhea; difficulty speaking; dizziness; drug addiction or overdose; eye pain; fast or irregular heartbeat; feeling of constant movement of self or surroundings; headache; hives or skin rash; itching of skin; loss of appetite; muscle weakness; nervousness; numbness or loss of feeling in one or both limbs on the same side of the body; palpitations; paralysis; possible decrease in amount of urine; restlessness; sensation of spinning; sensitivity to heat; sensitivity to sunlight; shortness of breath; sweating (excessive); thoughts of killing someone; thoughts of killing yourself; thick, scaly skin; trouble in sleeping; warm, smooth, moist skin; weight loss

Some side effects may occur that usually do not need medical attention. These side effects may go away during treatment as your body adjusts to the medicine. Also, your health care professional may be able to tell you about ways to prevent or reduce some of these side effects. Check with your health care professional if any of the following side effects continue or are bothersome or if you have any questions about them:

More common
Aching, fullness, or tension in sinuses; bruising, irritation, or itching at place of injection; flushing of skin; hair loss; indigestion; pain in bones or muscles; runny nose; sneezing; sore throat

Less common
Muscle rigidity or stiffness; pain at place of injection

Other side effects not listed may also occur in some patients. If you notice any other effects, check with your healthcare professional.

PEGVISOMANT   (Subcutaneous route)
- peg-VI-soe-mant

Commonly used brand name(s)

In the U.S.—
Somavert

Available Dosage Forms:
• Powder for Solution

Therapeutic Class: Endocrine-Metabolic Agent
Pharmacologic Class: Growth Hormone Receptor Antagonist

Uses For This Medicine

Pegvisomant is used to treat a condition called acromegaly, which is caused by too much growth hormone in the body. Too much growth hormone produced in adults causes the hands, feet, and parts of the face to become large, thick, and bulky. Other problems such as arthritis also can develop. Pegvisomant works by binding to the growth hormone receptor and preventing the actions of too much growth hormone.

This medicine is available only with your doctor's prescription.

Before Using This Medicine

In deciding to use a medicine, the risks of taking the medicine must be weighed against the good it will do. This is a decision you and your doctor will make. For this medicine, the following should be considered:

Allergies—Tell your doctor if you have ever had any unusual or allergic reaction to this medicine or any other medicines. Also tell your health care professional if you have any other types of allergies, such as to foods, dyes, preservatives, or animals. For non-prescription products, read the label or package ingredients carefully.

Pediatric—Studies on this medicine have been done only in adult patients, and there is no specific information comparing use of pegvisomant in children with use in other age groups.

Geriatric—Many medicines have not been studied specifically in older people. Therefore, it may not be known whether they work exactly the same way they do in younger adults or if they cause different side effects or problems in older people. There is no specific information comparing use of pegvisomant in the elderly with use in other age groups.

Pregnancy—

	Pregnancy Category	Explanation
All Trimesters	B	Animal studies have revealed no evidence of harm to the fetus, however, there are no adequate studies in pregnant women OR animal studies have shown an adverse effect, but adequate studies in pregnant women have failed to demonstrate a risk to the fetus.

Breast Feeding—There are no adequate studies in women for determining infant risk when using this medication during breastfeeding. Weigh the potential benefits against the potential risks before taking this medication while breastfeeding.

Other medicines—Although certain medicines should not be used together at all, in other cases two different medicines may be used together even if an interaction might occur. In these cases, your doctor may want to change the dose, or other precautions may be necessary. Tell your healthcare professional if you are taking any other prescription or non-prescription (over-the-counter [OTC]) medicine.

Interactions with Food/Tobacco/Alcohol—Certain medicines should not be used at or around the time of eating food or eating certain types of food since interactions may occur. Using alcohol or tobacco with certain medicines may also cause interactions to occur. Discuss with your healthcare professional the use of your medicine with food, alcohol, or tobacco.

Other medical problems—The presence of other medical problems may affect the use of this medicine. Make sure you tell your doctor if you have any other medical problems, especially:

- Type 2 diabetes mellitus—Pegvisomant may cause low blood sugar; your doctor may need to change the dose of your diabetes medicine
- Kidney disease, or
- Liver disease—If you have this condition, pegvisomant may remain in the body longer than normal; your doctor may need to change the dose of your medicine

Proper Use of This Medicine

To control the symptoms of your medical problem, this medicine must be taken as ordered by your doctor. Make sure that you understand exactly how to take this medicine.

Directions on how to prepare and inject the medicine are in the package. Read the directions carefully and ask your health care professional for additional explanation, if necessary.

Take within six hours of mixing the pegvisomant powder with the diluent

Do not use the solution if it is discolored or cloudy.

Dosing—The dose of this medicine will be different for different patients. Follow your doctor's orders or the directions on the label. The following information includes only the average doses of this medicine. If your dose is different, do not change it unless your doctor tells you to do so.

The amount of medicine that you take depends on the strength of the medicine. Also, the number of doses you take each day, the time allowed between doses, and the length of time you take the medicine depend on the medical problem for which you are using the medicine.

- For injection dosage form
  - For treating acromegaly:
    - Adults—At first, 40 mg injected by the doctor. Then, 10 mg daily injected by the patient. Higher doses may be needed, as determined by your doctor.
    - Children—Use and dose must be determined by your doctor.

Missed dose—If you miss a dose of this medicine, take it as soon as possible. However, if it is almost time for your next dose, skip the missed dose and go back to your regular dosing schedule. Do not double doses.

Storage—Store in the refrigerator. Do not freeze.

Keep out of the reach of children.

Do not keep outdated medicine or medicine no longer needed.

Ask your healthcare professional how you should dispose of any medicine you do not use.

Precautions While Using This Medicine

It is very important that your doctor check your progress at regular visits to make sure that this medicine is working properly and to check for unwanted effects.

It is very important to tell your doctor if a latex allergy exists.

Side Effects of This Medicine

Along with its needed effects, a medicine may cause some unwanted effects. Although not all of these side effects may occur, if they do occur they may need medical attention.

Check with your doctor immediately if any of the following side effects occur:

More common

Bleeding, blistering, burning, coldness, or discoloration of skin at site of injection; chest pain; chills; cough; feeling of pressure; fever; hives; hoarseness; infection, inflammation, itching, or lump at site of injection; lab results that show problems with liver; lower back or side pain; painful or difficult urination

Symptoms of overdose

Get emergency help immediately if any of the following symptoms of overdose occur:

unusual tiredness; weakness

Some side effects may occur that usually do not need medical attention. These side effects may go away during treatment as your body adjusts to the medicine. Also, your health care professional may be able to tell you about ways to prevent or reduce some of these side effects. Check with your health care professional if any of the following side effects continue or are bothersome or if you have any questions about them:

More common

Accidental injury; bloating or swelling of face, arms, hands, lower legs, or feet; blurred vision; burning, crawling, itching, numbness, prickling, "pins and needles", or tingling feelings; diarrhea; dizziness; general feeling of discomfort or illness; headache; joint pain; loss of appetite; muscle aches and pains; nausea;

nervousness; pain; pain or tenderness around eyes and cheekbones; pounding in the ears; runny or stuffy nose; shivering; shortness of breath or troubled breathing; slow or fast heartbeat; sore throat; sweating; tightness of chest or wheezing; trouble sleeping; unusual tiredness; unusual weight gain or loss; vomiting; weakness

Other side effects not listed may also occur in some patients. If you notice any other effects, check with your healthcare professional.

PEMETREXED (Intravenous route) -
pem-e-TREKS-ed

Commonly used brand name(s)

In the U.S.—
Alimta

Available Dosage Forms:
• Powder for Solution

Therapeutic Class: Antineoplastic Agent

Uses For This Medicine

Pemetrexed belongs to the group of medicines called antineoplastics. It is used to treat a type of cancer called malignant pleural mesothelioma (MPM). This cancer affects the inside lining of the chest cavity. Pemetrexed is given with cisplatin, another anti-cancer medicine (chemotherapy). Pemetrexed is also used to treat a type of lung cancer. For this treatment, pemetrexed is given alone, not with cisplatin.

To lower your chances of side effects of pemetrexed, you must also take folic acid and vitamin B$_{12}$ prior to and during your treatment with pemetrexed. Your doctor will prescribe a medicine called a "corticosteroid" to take for 3 days during your treatment with pemetrexed. Corticosteroid medicines lower your chances of getting skin reactions with pemetrexed.

This medicine is available only with your doctor's prescription.

Before Using This Medicine

In deciding to use a medicine, the risks of taking the medicine must be weighed against the good it will do. This is a decision you and your doctor will make. For this medicine, the following should be considered:

Allergies—Tell your doctor if you have ever had any unusual or allergic reaction to this medicine or any other medicines. Also tell your health care professional if you have any other types of allergies, such as to foods, dyes, preservatives, or animals. For non-prescription products, read the label or package ingredients carefully.

Pediatric—Studies on this medicine have only been done in adult patients. There is no specific information comparing the use of pemetrexed in children with use in other age groups.

Geriatric—This medicine has been tested in a limited number of older patients and has not been shown to cause different side effects or problems in older people than it does in younger adults.

Pregnancy—

	Pregnancy Category	Explanation
All Trimesters	D	Studies in pregnant women have demonstrated a risk to the fetus. However, the benefits of therapy in a life threatening situation or a serious disease, may outweigh the potential risk.

Breast Feeding—There are no adequate studies in women for determining infant risk when using this medication during breastfeeding. Weigh the potential benefits against the potential risks before taking this medication while breastfeeding.

Other medicines—Although certain medicines should not be used together at all, in other cases two different medicines may be used together even if an interaction might occur. In these cases, your doctor may want to change the dose, or other precautions may be necessary. Tell your healthcare professional if you are taking any other prescription or non-prescription (over-the-counter [OTC]) medicine.

Interactions with Food/Tobacco/Alcohol—Certain medicines should not be used at or around the time of eating food or eating certain types of food since interactions may occur. Using alcohol or tobacco with certain medicines may also cause interactions to occur. Discuss with your healthcare professional the use of your medicine with food, alcohol, or tobacco.

Other medical problems—The presence of other medical problems may affect the use of this medicine. Make sure you tell your doctor if you have any other medical problems, especially:
• Kidney disease—Patients with kidney disease should not use pemetrexed. Patients with kidney disease may have more pemetrexed in their bodies.
• Third space fluid (extra fluid in your body), such as
• Ascites (extra fluid in your stomach area) or
• Pleural effusion (extra fluid in your lungs and chest)—Pemetrexed should be used carefully in these patients and the effects are not known

Proper Use of This Medicine

It is very important to take folic acid and vitamin B$_{12}$ during your treatment with pemetrexed to lower your chances of harmful side effects. You must start taking 350–1000 micrograms of folic acid every day for at least 5 days out of the 7 days before your first dose of pemetrexed. You must keep taking folic acid every day during the time you are getting treatment with pemetrexed, and for 21 days after your last treatment. You can get folic acid vitamins over-the-counter. Folic acid is also found in many multivitamin pills. Ask your doctor or pharmacist for help if you are not sure how to choose a folic acid product. Your doctor will give you vitamin B$_{12}$ injections while you are getting treatment with pemetrexed. You will get your first vitamin B$_{12}$ injection during the week before your first dose of pemetrexed, and then about every 9 weeks during treatment.

Pemetrexed should be administered under the supervision of a qualified physician experienced in the use of antineoplastic agents.

Pemetrexed is given together with certain other medicines. If you are using a combination of medicines, it is important that you receive each one at the proper time. If you are taking some of these medicines by mouth, ask your health care professional to help you plan a way to take them at the right times.

You will have regular blood tests before and during your treatment with pemetrexed. Your doctor may adjust your dose of pemetrexed or delay treatment based on the results of your blood tests and on your general condition.

Your doctor will prescribe a medicine called a "corticosteroid" to take for 3 days during your treatment with pemetrexed. Corticosteroid medicines lower your chances for getting skin reactions with pemetrexed.

Dosing—The dose of this medicine will be different for different patients. Follow your doctor's orders or the directions on the label. The following information includes only the average doses of this medicine. If your dose is different, do not change it unless your doctor tells you to do so.

The amount of medicine that you take depends on the strength of the medicine. Also, the number of doses you take each day, the time allowed between doses, and the length of time you take the medicine depend on the medical problem for which you are using the medicine.

Storage—Store the medicine in a closed container at room temperature, away from heat, moisture, and direct light. Keep from freezing.

Keep out of the reach of children.

Do not keep outdated medicine or medicine no longer needed.

Ask your healthcare professional how you should dispose of any medicine you do not use.

Precautions While Using This Medicine

It is very important that your doctor check you at regular visits. Your doctor may adjust your dose or delay your treatment based on your general condition.

It is important that you check with your doctor immediately if you have fever or chills, diarrhea, or mouth sores. These may be signs that you have an infection.

You may feel tired or weak for a few days after your pemetrexed treatments. If you have severe weakness or tiredness, call your doctor.

You may get redness or sores in your mouth, throat, or on your lips. These symptoms may happen a few days after pemetrexed treatment.

You may get a rash or itching during treatment. These usually appear between treatments with pemetrexed and usually go away before the next treatment. Call your doctor if you get a severe rash or itching.

Pemetrexed and the other anti-cancer medicine it is given with (cisplatin) can sometimes causes nausea and vomiting. However, it is very important that you continue to receive the medicine, even if you begin to feel ill. You can get medicines to help control some of these symptoms. Talk with your doctor if you get any of these symptoms.

You may lose your appetite and lose weight during your treatment. Talk to your doctor if this is a problem for you.

While you are being treated with pemetrexed, and after you stop treatment with it, do not have any immunizations (vaccinations) without your doctor's approval. Pemetrexed may lower your body's resistance and there is a chance you might get the infection the immunization is meant to prevent. In ad-

dition, other persons living in your household should not take oral polio vaccine since there is a chance they could pass the polio virus on to you. Also, avoid other persons who have taken oral polio vaccine within the last several months. Do not get close to them, and do not stay in the same room with them for very long. If you cannot take these precautions, you should consider wearing a protective face mask that covers the nose and mouth.

Pemetrexed can temporarily affect your blood counts and your doctor will do blood tests to check your blood counts before and during treatment with pemetrexed. Low red blood cells may make you feel tired, get tired easily, appear pale, and become short of breath. Low white blood cells may give you a greater chance for infection. If you have a fever (temperature above 100.4°F) or other signs of infection, call your doctor right away. Low platelets give you a greater chance for bleeding. If this occurs, there are certain precautions you can take, especially when your blood count is low, to reduce the risk of infection or bleeding:

- If you can, avoid people with infections. Check with your doctor immediately if you think you are getting an infection or if you get a fever or chills, cough or hoarseness, diarrhea, lower back or side pain, mouth sores or painful or difficult urination.
- Check with your doctor immediately if you notice any unusual bleeding or bruising; black, tarry stools; blood in urine or stools; or pinpoint red spots on your skin.
- Be careful when using a regular toothbrush, dental floss, or toothpick. Your medical doctor, dentist, or nurse may recommend other ways to clean your teeth and gums. Check with your medical doctor before having any dental work done.
- Do not touch your eyes or the inside of your nose unless you have just washed your hands and have not touched anything else in the meantime.
- Be careful not to cut yourself when you are using sharp objects such as a safety razor or fingernail or toenail cutters.
- Avoid contact sports or other situations where bruising or injury could occur.

Side Effects of This Medicine

Along with its needed effects, a medicine may cause some unwanted effects. Although not all of these side effects may occur, if they do occur they may need medical attention.

Check with your doctor immediately if any of the following side effects occur:
More common
   Black, tarry stools; bleeding gums; chest pain; chills; cough; fever; loss of coordination; lower back or side pain; pains in chest, groin, or legs, especially calves of legs; painful or difficult urination; pale skin; pinpoint red spots on skin; severe headaches of sudden onset sudden; shortness of breath; sore throat; sudden onset of slurred speech; sudden vision changes; swollen glands; troubled breathing; ulcers, sores, or white spots in mouth; unusual bleeding or bruising; unusual tiredness or weakness

Less common
   Bloody urine or bloody stools; decreased frequency/amount of urine; fainting or loss of consciousness; fast or irregular breathing; increased blood pressure; increased thirst; itching; loss of appetite; nausea; skin rash; swelling of eyes or eyelids; swelling of face, fin-

gers, lower legs; tightness in chest, and/or wheezing; vomiting; weight gain

Some side effects may occur that usually do not need medical attention. These side effects may go away during treatment as your body adjusts to the medicine. Also, your health care professional may be able to tell you about ways to prevent or reduce some of these side effects. Check with your health care professional if any of the following side effects continue or are bothersome or if you have any questions about them:

More common

Burning, tingling, numbness or pain in the hands, arms, feet, or legs; confusion; cough or hoarseness; decreased urination; diarrhea (without colostomy); difficulty having a bowel movement (stool); difficulty in moving; difficulty in swallowing; discouragement; dizziness; dry mouth; feeling sad or empty; headache; hair loss; heartburn; increase in heart rate; irritability; lightheadedness; loss of interest or pleasure; mood changes; muscle aches or cramping; muscle pain or stiffness; pain in joints; pain produced by swallowing; pain or burning in throat; peeling of skin; rapid breathing; sensation of pins and needles; stabbing pain; stuffy or runny nose; sunken eyes; swelling; swelling or inflammation of the mouth; swollen joints; thinning of hair; thirst; tiredness; trouble concentrating; trouble sleeping; weight loss; wheezing; wrinkled skin

Other side effects not listed may also occur in some patients. If you notice any other effects, check with your healthcare professional.

PEMIROLAST (Ophthalmic route) - pe-MIR-oh-last

Commonly used brand name(s)
In the U.S.—
   Alamast

Available Dosage Forms:
   • Solution

Therapeutic Class: Ophthalmologic Agent
Pharmacologic Class: Mast Cell Stabilizer

Uses For This Medicine

Pemirolast is used to treat the itching in your eyes that happens with allergies.

Pemirolast works by preventing certain types of inflammatory cells from releasing irritating substances that cause allergic symptoms.

This medicine is available only with your doctor's prescription.

Before Using This Medicine

In deciding to use a medicine, the risks of taking the medicine must be weighed against the good it will do. This is a decision you and your doctor will make. For this medicine, the following should be considered:

Allergies—Tell your doctor if you have ever had any unusual or allergic reaction to this medicine or any other medi-

cines. Also tell your health care professional if you have any other types of allergies, such as to foods, dyes, preservatives, or animals. For non-prescription products, read the label or package ingredients carefully.

Pediatric—This medicine has been tested in children 3 years of age and older and, in effective doses, has not been shown to cause different side effects or problems than it does in adults.

Geriatric—There is no specific information available comparing the use of pemirolast in the elderly with use in other age groups.

Pregnancy—

	Pregnancy Category	Explanation
All Trimesters	C	Animal studies have shown an adverse effect and there are no adequate studies in pregnant women OR no animal studies have been conducted and there are no adequate studies in pregnant women.

Breast Feeding—There are no adequate studies in women for determining infant risk when using this medication during breastfeeding. Weigh the potential benefits against the potential risks before taking this medication while breastfeeding.

Other medicines—Although certain medicines should not be used together at all, in other cases two different medicines may be used together even if an interaction might occur. In these cases, your doctor may want to change the dose, or other precautions may be necessary. Tell your healthcare professional if you are taking any other prescription or nonprescription (over-the-counter [OTC]) medicine.

Interactions with Food/Tobacco/Alcohol—Certain medicines should not be used at or around the time of eating food or eating certain types of food since interactions may occur. Using alcohol or tobacco with certain medicines may also cause interactions to occur. Discuss with your healthcare professional the use of your medicine with food, alcohol, or tobacco.

Other medical problems—The presence of other medical problems may affect the use of this medicine. Make sure you tell your doctor if you have any other medical problems, especially:

• Contact lens–related irritation—Pemirolast should not be used to treat this condition

Proper Use of This Medicine

Pemirolast is used to help treat the itching that often occurs with allergic conjunctivitis.

• To use the eye drops form of this medicine:
   ° First, wash your hands. Then tilt the head back and, pressing your finger gently on the skin just beneath the lower eyelid, pull the lower eyelid away from the eye to make a space. Drop the medicine into this space. Let go of the eyelid and gently close the eyes. Blink a few times to make sure the eye is covered with the medicine.
   ° To keep the medicine as germ-free as possible, do not touch the applicator tip to any surface (including the eye). Also, keep the container tightly closed. Se-

rious damage to the eye and possible loss of vision may result from using contaminated eye drops.

Dosing—The dose of this medicine will be different for different patients. Follow your doctor's orders or the directions on the label. The following information includes only the average doses of this medicine. If your dose is different, do not change it unless your doctor tells you to do so.

The amount of medicine that you take depends on the strength of the medicine. Also, the number of doses you take each day, the time allowed between doses, and the length of time you take the medicine depend on the medical problem for which you are using the medicine.

Use this medicine only as directed. Do not use more of it and do not use it more often than your doctor ordered.

- For ophthalmic dosage form (eye drops):
  - For eye allergies:
    - Adults and children 3 years of age and older— Use one to two drops in each affected eye four times a day.
    - Children up to 3 years of age—Use and dose must be determined by your doctor.

Missed dose—If you miss a dose of this medicine, take it as soon as possible. However, if it is almost time for your next dose, skip the missed dose and go back to your regular dosing schedule. Do not double doses.

Storage—Store the medicine in a closed container at room temperature, away from heat, moisture, and direct light. Keep from freezing.

Keep out of the reach of children.

Do not keep outdated medicine or medicine no longer needed.

Ask your healthcare professional how you should dispose of any medicine you do not use.

Precautions While Using This Medicine

You should avoid wearing contact lenses when your eyes are red and irritated from your allergies.

For patients who continue to wear contact lenses and whose eyes are not red, be certain to wait at least 10 minutes after applying pemirolast to your eyes before replacing any contact lenses normally worn.

Side Effects of This Medicine

Along with its needed effects, a medicine may cause some unwanted effects. Although not all of these side effects may occur, if they do occur they may need medical attention.

Check with your doctor as soon as possible if any of the following side effects occur:
  Less common
    Cough (mucus-producing); headache (severe); stomach pain and cramping; pain and tenderness around eyes and cheekbones; painful menstrual bleeding; runny or stuffy nose; tightness in chest; troubled breathing

Some side effects may occur that usually do not need medical attention. These side effects may go away during treatment as your body adjusts to the medicine. Also, your health care professional may be able to tell you about ways to prevent or reduce some of these side effects. Check with your health care professional if any of the following side effects

continue or are bothersome or if you have any questions about them:
  More common
    Chills; cough; fever; sneezing; sore throat
  Less common
    Back pain; burning feeling in eye; eyelid swelling; eye dryness; foreign body feeling in eye; general feeling of eye discomfort; increased itching of the eye; redness of the eye

Other side effects not listed may also occur in some patients. If you notice any other effects, check with your healthcare professional.

PENCICLOVIR (Topical route) - pen-SYE-kloe-veer

Commonly used brand name(s)

In the U.S.—
  Denavir

Available Dosage Forms:
  - Cream

Therapeutic Class: Antiviral
Pharmacologic Class: Viral DNA Polymerase Inhibitor

Uses For This Medicine

Penciclovir belongs to the family of medicines called antivirals. Antivirals are used to treat infections caused by viruses. Usually they work for only one kind or group of virus infections.

Topical penciclovir is used to treat the symptoms of herpes simplex virus infections around the mouth (cold sores). Although topical penciclovir will not cure herpes simplex, it may help relieve the pain and discomfort and may help the sores heal faster.

This medicine is available only with your doctor's prescription.

Before Using This Medicine

In deciding to use a medicine, the risks of taking the medicine must be weighed against the good it will do. This is a decision you and your doctor will make. For this medicine, the following should be considered:

Allergies—Tell your doctor if you have ever had any unusual or allergic reaction to this medicine or any other medicines. Also tell your health care professional if you have any other types of allergies, such as to foods, dyes, preservatives, or animals. For non-prescription products, read the label or package ingredients carefully.

Pediatric—There is no specific information comparing the use of topical penciclovir in children with use in other age groups.

Geriatric—Many medicines have not been studied specifically in older people. Therefore, it may not be known whether they work exactly the same way they do in younger adults. There is no specific information comparing use of penciclovir in the elderly with use in other age groups. However, this medicine has been used in some older patients and has not been found to cause different side effects or other problems than it does in younger adults.

Pregnancy—

	Pregnancy Category	Explanation
All Trimesters	B	Animal studies have revealed no evidence of harm to the fetus, however, there are no adequate studies in pregnant women OR animal studies have shown an adverse effect, but adequate studies in pregnant women have failed to demonstrate a risk to the fetus.

Breast Feeding—There are no adequate studies in women for determining infant risk when using this medication during breastfeeding. Weigh the potential benefits against the potential risks before taking this medication while breastfeeding.

Other medicines—Although certain medicines should not be used together at all, in other cases two different medicines may be used together even if an interaction might occur. In these cases, your doctor may want to change the dose, or other precautions may be necessary. Tell your healthcare professional if you are taking any other prescription or non-prescription (over-the-counter [OTC]) medicine.

Interactions with Food/Tobacco/Alcohol—Certain medicines should not be used at or around the time of eating food or eating certain types of food since interactions may occur. Using alcohol or tobacco with certain medicines may also cause interactions to occur. Discuss with your healthcare professional the use of your medicine with food, alcohol, or tobacco.

Other medical problems—The presence of other medical problems may affect the use of this medicine. Make sure you tell your doctor if you have any other medical problems, especially:

- Immune system problems—It is not known if this medicine will work properly in patients with these problems

Proper Use of This Medicine

This medicine should only be used on the lips or face.

Penciclovir is best used as soon as possible after the symptoms of herpes infection (for example, pain, burning, or blisters) begin to appear.

Do not use this medicine in or near the eyes.

Do not use this medicine inside the mouth or nose or on other internal parts of the body.

Dosing—The dose of this medicine will be different for different patients. Follow your doctor's orders or the directions on the label. The following information includes only the average doses of this medicine. If your dose is different, do not change it unless your doctor tells you to do so.

The amount of medicine that you take depends on the strength of the medicine. Also, the number of doses you take each day, the time allowed between doses, and the length of time you take the medicine depend on the medical problem for which you are using the medicine.

- For topical dosage form (cream):
  - For herpes simplex infection (cold sores):
    - Adults—Apply to the affected area(s) of the skin every two hours, while awake, for four days.
    - Children—Use and dose must be determined by your doctor.

Missed dose—If you miss a dose of this medicine, take it as soon as possible. However, if it is almost time for your next dose, skip the missed dose and go back to your regular dosing schedule. Do not double doses.

Storage—Store the medicine in a closed container at room temperature, away from heat, moisture, and direct light. Keep from freezing.

Keep out of the reach of children.

Do not keep outdated medicine or medicine no longer needed.

Side Effects of This Medicine

Along with its needed effects, a medicine may cause some unwanted effects. Although not all of these side effects may occur, if they do occur they may need medical attention.

Check with your doctor as soon as possible if any of the following side effects occur:
   Rare
   Mild pain, burning, or stinging

Some side effects may occur that usually do not need medical attention. These side effects may go away during treatment as your body adjusts to the medicine. Also, your health care professional may be able to tell you about ways to prevent or reduce some of these side effects. Check with your health care professional if any of the following side effects continue or are bothersome or if you have any questions about them:
   More common
   Headache

   Less common
   Change in sense of taste; decreased sensitivity of skin, particularly to touch; redness of the skin; skin rash

Other side effects not listed may also occur in some patients. If you notice any other effects, check with your healthcare professional.

PENICILLIN   (Oral route, Injection route, Intravenous route, Intramuscular route)

Commonly used brand name(s)

In the U.S.—

Amoxil	Nafcil
Bactocill	Pfizerpen
Bicillin L-A	Pipracil
Cloxapen	Principen
Crysticillin	Staphcillin
Dynapen	Ticar
Geocillin	Veetids

In Canada—

Amoxil Pediatric	Gen-Amoxicillin
Ampicillin Sodium	Med Amoxicillin
Apo-Amoxi	Nadopen V 200
Apo-Amoxi Sugar-Free	Nadopen V 400
Apo-Cloxi	Novamoxin
Apo-Pen-Vk	

Available Dosage Forms:

- Capsule
- Powder for Solution
- Tablet
- Powder for Suspension
- Suspension
- Tablet, Chewable
- Syrup
- Solution
- Tablet for Suspension

Uses For This Medicine

Penicillins are used to treat infections caused by bacteria. They work by killing the bacteria or preventing their growth.

There are several different kinds of penicillins. Each is used to treat different kinds of infections. One kind of penicillin usually may not be used in place of another. In addition, penicillins are used to treat bacterial infections in many different parts of the body. They are sometimes given with other antibacterial medicines (antibiotics). Some of the penicillins may also be used for other problems as determined by your doctor. However, none of the penicillins will work for colds, flu, or other virus infections.

Penicillins are available only with your doctor's prescription.

Once a medicine has been approved for marketing for a certain use, experience may show that it is also useful for other medical problems. Although these uses are not included in product labeling, penicillins are used in certain patients with the following medical conditions:

- Chlamydia infections in pregnant women—Amoxicillin and ampicillin
- Gas gangrene—Penicillin G
- Helicobacter pylori-associated gastritis or peptic ulcer disease—Amoxicillin
- Leptospirosis—Ampicillin and penicillin G
- Lyme disease—Amoxicillin and penicillin V
- Typhoid fever—Amoxicillin and ampicillin

Before Using This Medicine

Allergies—Tell your doctor if you have ever had any unusual or allergic reaction to medicines in this group or any other medicines. Also tell your health care professional if you have any other types of allergies, such as to foods dyes, preservatives, or animals. For non-prescription products, read the label or package ingredients carefully.

Pediatric—Many penicillins have been used in children and, in effective doses, are not expected to cause different side effects or problems in children than they do in adults.

Some strengths of the chewable tablets of amoxicillin contain aspartame, which is changed by the body to phenylalanine, a substance that is harmful to patients with phenylketonuria.

Geriatric—Penicillins have been used in the elderly and have not been shown to cause different side effects or problems in older people than they do in younger adults.

Pregnancy—Penicillins have not been studied in pregnant women. However, penicillins have been widely used in pregnant women and have not been shown to cause birth defects or other problems in animal studies.

Breast Feeding—Penicillins pass into the breast milk. Even though only small amounts may pass into breast milk, allergic reactions, diarrhea, fungus infections, and skin rash may occur in nursing babies.

Other medicines—

Using medicines in this class with any of the following medicines is usually not recommended, but may be required in some cases. If both medicines are prescribed together, your doctor may change the dose or how often you use one or both of the medicines.

Cyclosporine, Methotrexate, Vecuronium

Using this medicine with any of the following may cause an increased risk of certain side effects but using both medicines may be the best treatment for you. If both medicines are prescribed together, your doctor may change the dose or how often you use one or both of the medicines.

Acenocoumarol, Ethinyl Estradiol, Etonogestrel, Khat, Mestranol, Nifedipine, Norelgestromin, Norethindrone, Norgestrel, Probenecid, Warfarin

Interactions with Food/Tobacco/Alcohol—Certain medicines should not be used at or around the time of eating food or eating certain types of food since interactions may occur. Using alcohol or tobacco with certain medicines may also cause interactions to occur. Discuss with your healthcare professional the use of your medicine with food, alcohol, or tobacco.

Other medical problems—The presence of other medical problems may affect the use of medicines in this class. Make sure you tell your doctor if you have any other medical problems, especially:

- Allergy, general (such as asthma, eczema, hay fever, hives), history of—Patients with a history of general allergies may be more likely to have a severe reaction to penicillins
- Bleeding problems, history of—Patients with a history of bleeding problems may be more likely to have bleeding when receiving carbenicillin, piperacillin, or ticarcillin
- Congestive heart failure (CHF) or
- High blood pressure—Large doses of carbenicillin or ticarcillin may make these conditions worse, because these medicines contain a large amount of salt
- Cystic fibrosis—Patients with cystic fibrosis may have an increased chance of fever and skin rash when receiving piperacillin
- Kidney disease—Patients with kidney disease may have an increased chance of side effects
- Mononucleosis ("mono")—Patients with mononucleosis may have an increased chance of skin rash when receiving ampicillin, bacampicillin, or pivampicillin
- Phenylketonuria—Some strengths of the amoxicillin chewable tablets contain aspartame, which is changed by the body to phenylalanine, a substance that is harmful to patients with phenylketonuria.
- Stomach or intestinal disease, history of (especially colitis, including colitis caused by antibiotics)—Patients with a history of stomach or intestinal disease may be more likely to develop colitis while taking penicillins

Proper Use of This Medicine

Penicillins (except bacampicillin tablets, amoxicillin, penicillin V, pivampicillin, and pivmecillinam) are best taken with a full glass (8 ounces) of water on an empty stomach (either 1 hour before or 2 hours after meals) unless otherwise directed by your doctor.

For patients taking amoxicillin, penicillin V, pivampicillin, and pivmecillinam:

- Amoxicillin, penicillin V, pivampicillin, and pivmecillinam may be taken on a full or empty stomach.
- The liquid form of amoxicillin may also be taken by itself or mixed with formulas, milk, fruit juice, water, ginger ale, or other cold drinks. If mixed with other liquids, take immediately after mixing. Be sure to drink all the liquid to get the full dose of medicine.

For patients taking bacampicillin:

- The liquid form of this medicine is best taken with a full glass (8 ounces) of water on an empty stomach (either 1 hour before or 2 hours after meals) unless otherwise directed by your doctor.
- The tablet form of this medicine may be taken on a full or empty stomach.

For patients taking penicillin G by mouth:

- Do not drink acidic fruit juices (for example, orange or grapefruit juice) or other acidic beverages within 1 hour of taking penicillin G since this may keep the medicine from working properly.

For patients taking the oral liquid form of penicillins:

- This medicine is to be taken by mouth even if it comes in a dropper bottle. If this medicine does not come in a dropper bottle, use a specially marked measuring spoon or other device to measure each dose accurately. The average household teaspoon may not hold the right amount of liquid.
- Do not use after the expiration date on the label. The medicine may not work properly after that date. If you have any questions about this, check with your pharmacist.

For patients taking the chewable tablet form of amoxicillin:

- Tablets should be chewed or crushed before they are swallowed.

To help clear up your infection completely, keep taking this medicine for the full time of treatment, even if you begin to feel better after a few days. If you have a" strep" infection, you should keep taking this medicine for at least 10 days. This is especially important in "strep" infections. Serious heart problems could develop later if your infection is not cleared up completely. Also, if you stop taking this medicine too soon, your symptoms may return.

This medicine works best when there is a constant amount in the blood or urine. To help keep the amount constant, do not miss any doses. Also, it is best to take the doses at evenly spaced times, day and night. For example, if you are to take four doses a day, the doses should be spaced about 6 hours apart. If this interferes with your sleep or other daily activities, or if you need help in planning the best times to take your medicine, check with your health care professional.

Make certain your health care professional knows if you are on a low-sodium (low-salt) diet. Some of these medicines contain enough sodium to cause problems in some people.

Dosing—The dose medicines in this class will be different for different patients. Follow your doctor's orders or the directions on the label. The following information includes only the average doses of these medicines. If your dose is different, do not change it unless your doctor tells you to do so.

The amount of medicine that you take depends on the strength of the medicine. Also, the number of doses you take each day, the time allowed between doses, and the length of time you take the medicine depend on the medical problem for which you are using the medicine.

The number of tablets or teaspoonfuls of suspension that you take depends on the strength of the medicine. Also, the number of doses you take each day, the time allowed between doses, and the length of time you take the medicine depend on the medical problem for which you are taking a penicillin.

- For amoxicillin:
    - For bacterial infections:
        - For oral dosage forms (capsules, oral suspension, tablets, and chewable tablets):
            — Adults, teenagers, and children weighing more than 40 kilograms (kg) (88 pounds)— 250 to 500 milligrams (mg) every eight hours or 500 to 875 mg every twelve hours, depending on the type and severity of the infection.
            — Neonates and infants up to 3 months of age—Dose is based on body weight and must be determined by your doctor. The usual dose is 15 mg per kg (6.8 mg per pound) of body weight or less every twelve hours.
            — Infants 3 months of age and older and children weighing up to 40 kg (88 lbs.)—Dose is based on body weight and must be determined by your doctor. The usual dose is 6.7 to 13.3 mg per kg (3 to 6 mg per pound) of body weight every eight hours or 12.5 to 22.5 mg per kg (5.7 to 10.2 mg per pound) of body weight every twelve hours.
    - For duodenal ulcers (associated with Helicobacter pylori bacterial infection):
        - For oral dosage forms (capsules, oral suspension, tablets, and chewable tablets):
            — Adults: 1000 mg twice a day every twelve hours for fourteen days, along with the two other medicines, clarithromycin and lansoprazole, as directed by your doctor.
            — Teenagers and children: Use and dose must be determined by your doctor.
        - For dual medicine therapy—
            — Adults: 1000 mg three times a day every eight hours for fourteen days, along with the other medicine, lansoprazole, as directed by your doctor.
            — Teenagers and children: Use and dose must be determined by your doctor.
- For ampicillin:
    - For bacterial infections:
        - For oral dosage forms (capsules and oral suspension):
            — Adults, teenagers, and children weighing more than 20 kilograms (kg) (44 pounds)— 250 to 500 milligrams (mg) every six hours.
            — Infants and children weighing up to 20 kg (44 pounds)—Dose is based on body weight and must be determined by your doctor. The usual dose is 12.5 to 25 mg per kg (5.7 to 11.4 mg per pound) of body weight every six

hours; or 16.7 to 33.3 mg per kg (7.6 to 15 mg per pound) of body weight every eight hours.

- For injection dosage form:
  - Adults, teenagers, and children weighing more than 20 kg (44 pounds)—250 to 500 mg, injected into a vein or muscle every three to six hours.
  - Infants and children weighing up to 20 kg (44 pounds)—Dose is based on body weight and must be determined by your doctor. The usual dose is 12.5 mg per kg (5.7 mg per pound) of body weight, injected into a vein or muscle every six hours.

- For bacampicillin:
  - For bacterial infections:
    - For oral dosage forms (oral suspension and tablets):
      - Adults, teenagers, and children weighing more than 25 kilograms (kg) (55 pounds)—400 to 800 milligrams (mg) every twelve hours.
      - Children weighing up to 25 kg (55 pounds)—Bacampicillin tablets are not recommended for use in children weighing up to 25 kg (55 pounds). The dose of the oral suspension is based on body weight and must be determined by your doctor. The usual dose is 12.5 to 25 mg per kg (5.7 to 11.4 mg per pound) of body weight every twelve hours.

- For carbenicillin:
  - For bacterial infections:
    - For oral dosage form (tablets):
      - Adults and teenagers—500 milligrams (mg) to 1 gram every six hours.
      - Children—Dose must be determined by your doctor.
    - For injection dosage form:
      - Adults and teenagers—Dose is based on body weight and must be determined by your doctor. The usual dose is 50 to 83.3 mg per kilogram (kg) (22.8 to 37.9 mg per pound) of body weight, injected into a vein or muscle every four hours.
      - Older infants and children—Dose is based on body weight and must be determined by your doctor. The usual dose is 16.7 to 75 mg per kg (7.6 to 34 mg per pound) of body weight, injected into a vein or muscle every four to six hours.

- For cloxacillin:
  - For bacterial infections:
    - For oral dosage form (capsules and oral solution):
      - Adults, teenagers, and children weighing more than 20 kilograms (kg) (44 pounds)—250 to 500 milligrams (mg) every six hours.
      - Infants and children weighing up to 20 kg (44 pounds)—Dose is based on body weight and must be determined by your doctor. The usual dose is 6.25 to 12.5 mg per kg (2.8 to 5.7 mg per pound) of body weight every six hours.

- For injection dosage form:
  - Adults, teenagers, and children weighing more than 20 kg—250 to 500 mg, injected into a vein every six hours.
  - Infants and children weighing up to 20 kg (44 pounds)—Dose is based on body weight and must be determined by your doctor. The usual dose is 6.25 to 12.5 mg per kg (2.8 to 5.7 mg per pound) of body weight, injected into a vein every six hours.

- For dicloxacillin:
  - For bacterial infections:
    - For oral dosage form (capsules and oral suspension):
      - Adults, teenagers, and children weighing more than 40 kilograms (kg) (88 pounds)—125 to 250 milligrams (mg) every six hours.
      - Infants and children weighing up to 40 kg (88 pounds)—Dose is based on body weight and must be determined by your doctor. The usual dose is 3.1 to 6.2 mg per kg (1.4 to 2.8 mg per pound) of body weight every six hours.

- For flucloxacillin:
  - For bacterial infections:
    - For oral dosage form (capsules and oral suspension):
      - Adults, teenagers, and children more than 12 years of age and weighing more than 40 kilograms (kg) (88 pounds)—250 to 500 milligrams (mg) every six hours.
      - Children less than 12 years of age and weighing up to 40 kg (88 pounds)—125 to 250 mg every six hours; or 6.25 to 12.5 mg per kg (2.8 to 5.7 mg per pound) of body weight every six hours.
      - Infants up to 6 months of age—Dose is based on body weight and must be determined by your doctor. The usual dose is 6.25 mg per kg (2.8 mg per pound) of body weight every six hours.

- For methicillin:
  - For bacterial infections:
    - For injection dosage form:
      - Adults, teenagers, and children weighing more than 40 kilograms (kg) (88 pounds)—1 gram injected into a muscle every four to six hours; or 1 gram injected into a vein every six hours.
      - Children weighing up to 40 kg (88 pounds)—Dose is based on body weight and must be determined by your doctor. The usual dose is 25 milligrams (mg) per kg (11.4 mg per pound) of body weight, injected into a vein or muscle every six hours.

- For mezlocillin:
  - For bacterial infections:
    - For injection dosage form:
      - Adults and teenagers—Dose is based on body weight and must be determined by your doctor. The usual dose is 33.3 to 87.5 milligrams (mg) per kilogram (kg) (15.1 to 39.8 mg per pound) of body weight, injected

into a vein or muscle every four to six hours; or 3 to 4 grams every four to six hours.

— Infants over 1 month of age and children up to 12 years of age—Dose is based on body weight and must be determined by your doctor. The usual dose is 50 mg per kg (22.7 mg per pound) of body weight, injected into a vein or muscle every four hours.

- For nafcillin:
  - For bacterial infections:
    - For oral dosage form (capsules and tablets):
      — Adults and teenagers—250 milligrams (mg) to 1 gram every four to six hours.
      — Older infants and children—Dose is based on body weight and must be determined by your doctor. The usual dose is 6.25 to 12.5 mg per kilogram (kg) (2.8 to 5.7 mg per pound) of body weight every six hours.
      — Newborns—Dose is based on body weight and must be determined by your doctor. The usual dose is 10 mg per kg (4.5 mg per pound) of body weight every six to eight hours.
    - For injection dosage form:
      — Adults and teenagers—500 mg to 2 grams injected into a vein or muscle every four to six hours.
      — Infants and children—Dose is based on body weight and must be determined by your doctor. The usual dose is 10 to 25 mg per kg (4.5 to 11.4 mg per pound) of body weight, injected into a muscle every twelve hours; or 10 to 40 mg per kg (4.5 to 18.2 mg per pound) of body weight, injected into a vein every four to eight hours.

- For oxacillin:
  - For bacterial infections:
    - For oral dosage form (capsules and oral solution):
      — Adults, teenagers, and children weighing more than 40 kilograms (kg) (88 pounds)—500 milligrams (mg) to 1 gram every four to six hours.
      — Children weighing up to 40 kg (88 pounds)—Dose is based on body weight and must be determined by your doctor. The usual dose is 12.5 to 25 mg per kg (5.7 to 11.4 mg per pound) of body weight every six hours.
    - For injection dosage form:
      — Adults, teenagers, and children weighing more than 40 kg (88 pounds)—250 mg to 1 gram injected into a vein or muscle every four to six hours.
      — Children weighing up to 40 kg (88 pounds)—Dose is based on body weight and must be determined by your doctor. The usual dose is 12.5 to 25 mg per kg (5.7 to 11.4 mg per pound) of body weight, injected into a vein or muscle every four to six hours.
      — Premature infants and newborns—Dose is based on body weight and must be determined by your doctor. The usual dose is 6.25 mg per kg (2.8 mg per pound) of body weight, injected into a vein or muscle every six hours.

- For penicillin G:
  - For bacterial infections:
    - For oral dosage form (oral solution, oral suspension, and tablets):
      — Adults and teenagers—200,000 to 500,000 Units (125 to 312 milligrams [mg]) every four to six hours.
      — Infants and children less than 12 years of age—Dose is based on body weight and must be determined by your doctor. The usual dose is 4167 to 30,000 Units per kilogram (kg) (189 to 13,636 Units per pound) of body weight every four to eight hours.
    - For benzathine injection dosage form:
      — Adults and teenagers—1,200,000 to 2,400,000 Units injected into a muscle as a single dose.
      — Infants and children—300,000 to 1,200,000 Units injected into a muscle as a single dose; or 50,000 Units per kg (22,727 Units per pound) of body weight injected into a muscle as a single dose.
    - For injection dosage forms (potassium and sodium salts):
      — Adults and teenagers—1,000,000 to 5,000,000 Units, injected into a vein or muscle every four to six hours.
      — Older infants and children—Dose is based on body weight and must be determined by your doctor. The usual dose is 8333 to 25,000 Units per kg (3788 to 11,363 Units per pound) of body weight, injected into a vein or muscle every four to six hours.
      — Premature infants and newborns—Dose is based on body weight and must be determined by your doctor. The usual dose is 30,000 Units per kg (13,636 Units per pound) of body weight, injected into a vein or muscle every twelve hours.
    - For procaine injection dosage form:
      — Adults and teenagers—600,000 to 1,200,000 Units injected into a muscle once a day.
      — Children—Dose is based on body weight and must be determined by your doctor. The usual dose is 50,000 Units per kg (22,727 Units per pound) of body weight, injected into a muscle once a day.

- For penicillin V:
  - For bacterial infections:
    - For the benzathine salt oral dosage form (oral solution):
      — Adults and teenagers—200,000 to 500,000 Units every six to eight hours.
      — Children—100,000 to 250,000 Units every six to eight hours.
    - For the potassium salt oral dosage forms (oral solution, oral suspension, and tablets):
      — Adults and teenagers—125 to 500 milligrams (mg) every six to eight hours.
      — Children—Dose is based on body weight and must be determined by your doctor. The usual dose is 2.5 to 16.7 mg per kilogram (kg)

(1.1 to 7.6 mg per pound) of body weight every four to eight hours.

- For piperacillin:
  - For bacterial infections:
    - For injection dosage form:
      — Adults and teenagers—3 to 4 grams, injected into a vein or muscle every four to six hours.
      — Infants and children—Dose must be determined by your doctor.

- For pivampicillin:
  - For bacterial infections:
    - For oral dosage form (oral suspension):
      — Adults, teenagers, and children 10 years of age and older—525 to 1050 milligrams (mg) two times a day.
      — Children 7 to 10 years of age—350 mg two times a day.
      — Children 4 to 6 years of age—262.5 mg two times a day.
      — Children 1 to 3 years of age—175 mg two times a day.
      — Infants 3 to 12 months of age—Dose is based on body weight and must be determined by your doctor. The usual dose is 20 to 30 mg per kilogram (kg) (9.1 to 13.6 mg per pound) of body weight two times a day.
    - For oral dosage form (tablets):
      — Adults, teenagers, and children 10 years of age and older—500 mg to 1 gram two times a day.
      — Children up to 10 years of age—Dose must be determined by your doctor.

- For pivmecillinam:
  - For bacterial infections:
    - For oral dosage form (tablets):
      — Adults, teenagers, and children weighing more than 40 kilograms (kg) (88 pounds)—200 milligrams (mg) two to four times a day for three days.
      — Children up to 40 kg (88 pounds)—Dose must be determined by your doctor.

- For ticarcillin:
  - For bacterial infections:
    - For injection dosage form:
      — Adults, teenagers, and children weighing more than 40 kilograms (kg) (88 pounds)—3 grams injected into a vein every four hours; or 4 grams injected into a vein every six hours.
      — Children up to 40 kg (88 pounds)—Dose is based on body weight and must be determined by your doctor. The usual dose is 33.3 to 75 milligrams (mg) per kg (15 to 34 mg per pound) of body weight, injected into a vein every four to six hours.

Missed dose—If you miss a dose of this medicine, take it as soon as possible. However, if it is almost time for your next dose, skip the missed dose and go back to your regular dosing schedule. Do not double doses.

Storage—Store the medicine in a closed container at room temperature, away from heat, moisture, and direct light. Keep from freezing.

Keep out of the reach of children.

Do not keep outdated medicine or medicine no longer needed.

Precautions While Using This Medicine

If your symptoms do not improve within a few days, or if they become worse, check with your doctor.

Penicillins may cause diarrhea in some patients.

- Check with your doctor if severe diarrhea occurs. Severe diarrhea may be a sign of a serious side effect. Do not take any diarrhea medicine without first checking with your doctor. Diarrhea medicines may make your diarrhea worse or make it last longer.
- For mild diarrhea, diarrhea medicine containing kaolin or attapulgite (e.g., Kaopectate tablets, Diasorb) may be taken. However, other kinds of diarrhea medicine should not be taken. They may make your diarrhea worse or make it last longer.
- If you have any questions about this or if mild diarrhea continues or gets worse, check with your health care professional.

Oral contraceptives (birth control pills) containing estrogen may not work properly if you take them while you are taking ampicillin, amoxicillin, or penicillin V. Unplanned pregnancies may occur. You should use a different or additional means of birth control while you are taking any of these penicillins. If you have any questions about this, check with your health care professional.

For diabetic patients:

- Penicillins may cause false test results with some urine sugar tests. Check with your doctor before changing your diet or the dosage of your diabetes medicine.

Before you have any medical tests, tell the doctor in charge that you are taking this medicine. The results of some tests may be affected by this medicine.

Side Effects of This Medicine

Along with its needed effects, a medicine may cause some unwanted effects. Although not all of these side effects may occur, if they do occur they may need medical attention.

Stop taking this medicine and get emergency help immediately if any of the following effects occur:

Less common
Fast or irregular breathing; fever; joint pain; lightheadedness or fainting (sudden); puffiness or swelling around the face; red, scaly skin; shortness of breath; skin rash, hives, itching

Check with your doctor immediately if any of the following side effects occur:

Rare
Abdominal or stomach cramps and pain (severe); abdominal tenderness; convulsions (seizures); decreased amount of urine; diarrhea (watery and severe), which may also be bloody; mental depression; nausea and vomiting; pain at place of injection; sore throat and fever; unusual bleeding or bruising; yellow eyes or skin

Rare—For penicillin G procaine only
Agitation or combativeness; anxiety; confusion; fear of impending death; feeling, hearing, or seeing things that are not real

Some side effects may occur that usually do not need medical attention. These side effects may go away during treatment as your body adjusts to the medicine. Also, your health care professional may be able to tell you about ways to prevent or reduce some of these side effects. Check with your health care professional if any of the following side effects continue or are bothersome or if you have any questions about them:

More common
> Diarrhea (mild); headache; sore mouth or tongue; vaginal itching and discharge; white patches in the mouth and/or on the tongue

Other side effects not listed may also occur in some patients. If you notice any other effects, check with your healthcare professional.

PENICILLINS AND BETA-LACTAMASE INHIBITORS (Systemic)

Some commonly used brand names are:

In the U.S.—

Augmentin (1)	Unasyn (2)
Timentin (4)	Zosyn (3)

In Canada—

Clavulin-250 (1)	Clavulin-500F (1)
Clavulin-125F (1)	Tazocin (3)
Clavulin-250F (1)	Timentin (4)

This information applies to the following medicines:

1. Amoxicillin and Clavulanate (a-mox-i-SILL-in and klav-yoo-LAN-ate)
2. Ampicillin and Sulbactam (am-pi-SILL-in and sul-BAK-tam)
3. Piperacillin and Tazobactam (pi-PER-a-sill-in and ta-zoe-BAK-tam)
4. Ticarcillin and Clavulanate (tye-kar-SILL-in and klav-yoo-LAN-ate)

Category

- **Antibacterial, systemic**—Amoxicillin and Clavulanate; Ampicillin and Sulbactam; Piperacillin and Tazobactam; Ticarcillin and Clavulanate

Description

Penicillins and beta-lactamase inhibitors are used to treat infections caused by bacteria. They work by killing the bacteria or preventing their growth. The beta-lactamase inhibitor is added to the penicillin to protect the penicillin from certain substances (enzymes) that will destroy the penicillin before it can kill the bacteria.

There are several different kinds of penicillins. Each is used to treat different kinds of infections. One kind of penicillin usually may not be used in place of another. In addition, penicillins are used to treat bacterial infections in many different parts of the body. They are sometimes given with other antibacterial medicines. Some of the penicillins may also be used for other problems as determined by your doctor. However, none of the penicillins will work for colds, flu, or other virus infections.

Penicillins are available only with your doctor's prescription, in the following dosage forms:

Oral
- Amoxicillin and Clavulanate
  - Oral suspension
  - Tablets
  - Chewable tablets

Parenteral
- Ampicillin and Sulbactam
  - Injection
- Piperacillin and Tazobactam
  - Injection
- Ticarcillin and Clavulanate
  - Injection

Before Using This Medicine

In deciding to use a medicine, the risks of taking the medicine must be weighed against the good it will do. This is a decision you and your doctor will make. For penicillins, the following should be considered:

Allergies—Tell your doctor if you have ever had any unusual or allergic reaction to any of the penicillins, cephalosporins, or beta-lactamase inhibitors. Also tell your health care professional if you are allergic to any other substances, such as foods, preservatives, or dyes.

Diet—Tell your doctor if you are on a low-sodium (low-salt) diet. Some of these medicines contain enough sodium to cause problems in some people.

Pregnancy—Penicillins and beta-lactamase inhibitors have not been studied in pregnant women. However, penicillins have not been shown to cause birth defects or other problems in animal studies.

Breast-feeding—Penicillins and sulbactam, a beta-lactamase inhibitor, pass into the breast milk. Even though only small amounts may pass into breast milk, allergic reactions, diarrhea, fungus infections, and skin rash may occur in nursing babies.

Children—Penicillins and beta-lactamase inhibitors have been used in children and, in effective doses, are not expected to cause different side effects or problems in children than they do in adults.

Some strengths of the chewable tablets and oral suspensions of amoxicillin and clavulanate combination contain aspartame, which is changed by the body to phenylalanine, a substance that is harmful to patients with phenylketonuria.

Older adults—Penicillins and beta-lactamase inhibitors have been used in the elderly and have not been shown to cause different side effects or problems in older people than they do in younger adults.

Other medicines—Although certain medicines should not be used together at all, in other cases two different medicines may be used together even if an interaction might occur. In these cases, your doctor may want to change the dose, or other precautions may be necessary. When you are taking a penicillin and beta-lactamase inhibitor combination, it is especially important that your health care professional know if you are taking any of the following:

- Anticoagulants (blood thinners) or
- Dipyridamole (e.g., Persantine) or
- Divalproex (e.g., Depakote) or
- Heparin (e.g., Panheprin) or

- Inflammation or pain medicine (except narcotics) or
- Pentoxifylline (e.g., Trental) or
- Plicamycin (e.g., Mithracin) or
- Sulfinpyrazone (e.g., Anturane) or
- Valproic acid (e.g., Depakene)—Use of these medicines with piperacillin and tazobactam combination or with ticarcillin and clavulanate combination may increase the chance of bleeding
- Oral contraceptives (birth control pills)—Use of penicillins and beta-lactamase inhibitors may prevent oral contraceptives from working properly, increasing the chance for pregnancy
- Probenecid (e.g., Benemid)—Probenecid causes penicillins, sulbactam, and tazobactam to build up in the blood. This may increase the chance of side effects. However, your doctor may want to give you probenecid with a penicillin and beta-lactamase inhibitor combination to treat some infections

Other medical problems—The presence of other medical problems may affect the use of penicillin and beta-lactamase inhibitor combinations. Make sure you tell your doctor if you have any other medical problems, especially:

- Allergies or a history of allergies, such as asthma, eczema, hay fever, or hives—Patients with a history of allergies may be more likely to have a severe allergic reaction to a penicillin and beta-lactamase inhibitor combination
- Bleeding problems, history of—Patients with a history of bleeding problems may be more likely to have bleeding when receiving piperacillin and tazobactam combination or ticarcillin and clavulanate combination
- Congestive heart failure (CHF) or
- High blood pressure—Large doses of ticarcillin and clavulanate combination may make these conditions worse, because this medicine contains a large amount of salt
- Cystic fibrosis—Patients with cystic fibrosis may have an increased chance of fever and skin rash when receiving piperacillin and tazobactam combination
- Kidney disease—Patients with kidney disease may have an increased chance of side effects
- Liver disease (active or a history of)—Penicillins and beta-lactamase inhibitor combinations may cause this condition to recur or become worse
- Mononucleosis ("mono")—Patients with mononucleosis may have an increased chance of skin rash when receiving ampicillin and sulbactam combination
- Phenylketonuria—Some strengths of the amoxicillin and clavulanate combination chewable tablets and oral suspension contain aspartame, which is changed by the body to phenylalanine.
- Stomach or intestinal disease, history of (especially colitis, including colitis caused by antibiotics)—Patients with a history of stomach or intestinal disease may be more likely to develop colitis while taking penicillins and beta-lactamase inhibitors

Proper Use of This Medicine

Amoxicillin and clavulanate combination may be taken on a full or empty stomach. Taking amoxicillin and clavulanate combination with food may decrease the chance of diarrhea, nausea, and vomiting.

For patients taking the *oral liquid form of amoxicillin and clavulanate combination:*

- Use a specially marked measuring spoon or other device to measure each dose accurately. The average household teaspoon may not hold the right amount of liquid.
- Do not use after the expiration date on the label. The medicine may not work properly after that date. If you have any questions about this, check with your pharmacist.

For patients taking the *chewable tablet form of amoxicillin and clavulanate combination:*

- Tablets should be chewed or crushed before they are swallowed.

To help clear up your infection completely, *keep taking this medicine for the full time of treatment,* even if you begin to feel better after a few days.

This medicine works best when there is a constant amount in the blood or urine. *To help keep the amount constant, do not miss any doses. Also, it is best to take the doses at evenly spaced times, day and night.* For example, if you are to take four doses a day, the doses should be spaced about 6 hours apart. If this interferes with your sleep or other daily activities, or if you need help in planning the best times to take your medicine, check with your health care professional.

Dosing—The dose of these medicines will be different for different patients. *Follow your doctor's orders or the directions on the label.* The following information includes only the average doses of these medicines. *If your dose is different, do not change it* unless your doctor tells you to do so.

The number of tablets or teaspoonfuls of suspension that you take depends on the strength of the medicine. Also, *the number of doses you take each day, the time allowed between doses, and the length of time you take the medicine depend on the medical problem for which you are taking a penicillin and beta-lactamase inhibitor combination.*

For amoxicillin and clavulanate combination
- For bacterial infections:
  - For *oral* dosage forms (chewable tablets and suspension):
    - Adults, teenagers, and children weighing more than 40 kilograms (kg) (88 pounds)—250 to 500 milligrams (mg) of amoxicillin, in combination with 125 mg of clavulanate, every eight hours or 500 to 875 mg of amoxicillin, in combination with 125 mg of clavulanate, every twelve hours.
    - Neonates and infants up to 12 weeks (3 months) of age—Dose is based on body weight and must be determined by your doctor. The usual dose is 15 mg of amoxicillin per kg (6.8 mg per pound) of body weight every twelve hours.
    - Infants 3 months of age and older and children weighing up to 40 kg (88 pounds)—6.7 to 22.5 mg of amoxicillin per kg (3 to 10.2 mg per pound) of body weight, in combination with 1.7 to 3.2 mg of clavulanate per kg (0.8 to 1.5 mg per pound) of body weight, every eight or twelve hours.
  - For *oral* dosage form (tablets):
    - Adults, teenagers, and children weighing more than 40 kg (88 pounds)—250 to 500 mg of amoxicillin, in combination with 125 mg of clavulanate,

every eight hours or 500 to 875 mg of amoxicillin, in combination with 125 mg of clavulanate, every twelve hours.

- Infants and children weighing up to 40 kg (88 pounds)—The amoxicillin and clavulanate combination tablets are too strong for children weighing less than 40 kg (88 pounds). The chewable tablets or oral suspension are used in these children.

For ampicillin and sulbactam combination
- For bacterial infections:
  - For *injection* dosage form:
    - Adults and teenagers—1 to 2 grams of ampicillin, in combination with 500 milligrams (mg) to 1 gram of sulbactam, injected into a vein or a muscle every six hours.
    - Children 1 to 12 years of age—Dose must be determined by your doctor.
    - Children up to 1 year of age—Use and dose must be determined by your doctor.

For piperacillin and tazobactam combination
- For bacterial infections:
  - For *injection* dosage form:
    - Adults and teenagers—3 to 4 grams of piperacillin, in combination with 0.375 to 0.5 grams of tazobactam, injected into a vein every six to eight hours for seven to ten days.
    - Children up to 12 years of age—Dose must be determined by your doctor.

For ticarcillin and clavulanate combination
- For bacterial infections:
  - For *injection* dosage form:
    - Adults and teenagers weighing 60 kilograms (kg) (132 pounds) or more—3 grams of ticarcillin, in combination with 100 milligrams (mg) of clavulanate, injected into a vein every four to six hours.
    - Adults and teenagers weighing less than 60 kg (132 pounds)—50 mg of ticarcillin per kg (22.7 mg per pound) of body weight, in combination with 1.7 mg of clavulanate per kg (0.8 mg per pound) of body weight, injected into a vein every four to six hours.
    - Infants and children 1 month to 12 years of age—50 mg of ticarcillin per kg (22.7 mg per pound) of body weight, in combination with 1.7 mg of clavulanate per kg (0.8 mg per pound) of body weight, injected into a vein every four to six hours.
    - Infants up to 1 month of age—Use and dose must be determined by your doctor.

Missed dose—If you miss a dose of this medicine, take it as soon as possible. This will help to keep a constant amount of medicine in the blood or urine. However, if it is almost time for your next dose, skip the missed dose and go back to your regular dosing schedule. Do not double doses.

Storage—To store this medicine:
- Keep out of the reach of children.
- Store away from heat and direct light.
- Do not store tablets in the bathroom, near the kitchen sink, or in other damp places. Heat or moisture may cause the medicine to break down.
- Store the oral liquid form of penicillins in the refrigerator because heat will cause this medicine to break down.

However, keep the medicine from freezing. Follow the directions on the label.

- Do not keep outdated medicine or medicine no longer needed. Be sure that any discarded medicine is out of the reach of children.

Precautions While Using This Medicine

If your symptoms do not improve within a few days, or if they become worse, check with your doctor.

Penicillins may cause diarrhea in some patients.

- *Check with your doctor if severe diarrhea occurs.* Severe diarrhea may be a sign of a serious side effect. *Do not take any diarrhea medicine.* Diarrhea medicines may make your diarrhea worse or make it last longer.
- For mild diarrhea, diarrhea medicine containing kaolin or attapulgite (e.g., Kaopectate tablets, Diasorb) may be taken. However, other kinds of diarrhea medicine should not be taken. They may make your diarrhea worse or make it last longer.
- If you have any questions about this or if mild diarrhea continues or gets worse, check with your health care professional.

For *patients with diabetes:*
- *Penicillin and beta-lactamase inhibitor combinations may cause false test results with some urine sugar tests.* Check with your doctor before changing your diet or the dosage of your diabetes medicine.

Before you have any medical tests, tell the doctor in charge that you are taking this medicine. The results of some tests may be affected by this medicine.

Side Effects

Along with its needed effects, a medicine may cause some unwanted effects. Although not all of these side effects may occur, if they do occur they may need medical attention.

Stop taking this medicine and get emergency help immediately if any of the following side effects occur:
> *Less common*
> Cough; fast or irregular breathing; fever; joint pain; lightheadedness or fainting (sudden); pain, redness, or swelling at site of injection; puffiness or swelling around the face; red, irritated eyes; shortness of breath; skin rash, hives, itching; sore mouth or tongue; unusual tiredness or weakness; vaginal itching and discharge; white patches in mouth and/or on tongue

In addition to the side effects mentioned above, *check with your doctor immediately* if any of the following side effects occur:
> *Rare*
> Abdominal or stomach cramps and pain (severe); blistering, peeling, or loosening of skin and mucous membranes; chest pain; cloudy urine; convulsions (seizures); diarrhea (watery and severe), which may also be bloody; general feeling of illness or discomfort; nausea or vomiting; redness, soreness, or swelling of tongue; red skin lesions, often with a purple center; sore throat; swelling of face, fingers, lower legs, or feet; trouble in urinating; unusual bleeding or bruising; weight gain; yellow eyes or skin

Other side effects may occur that usually do not need medical attention. These side effects may go away during treatment as your body adjusts to the medicine. However, check with your doctor if any of the following side effects continue or are bothersome:

More common
 Diarrhea (mild); gas; headache; stomach pain; swelling of abdomen

Less common or rare
 Chills; nosebleed; long-lasting muscle relaxation (with piperacillin and tazobactam combination); unusual tiredness or weakness

Other side effects not listed above may also occur in some patients. If you notice any other effects, check with your doctor.

Additional Information

Once a medicine has been approved for marketing for a certain use, experience may show that it is also useful for other medical problems. Although these uses are not included in product labeling, penicillins and beta-lactamase inhibitor combinations are used in certain patients with the following medical conditions:

Amoxicillin and clavulanate combination

- Bronchitis
- Chancroid

Ampicillin and sulbactam combination

- Gonorrhea

Ticarcillin and clavulanate combination

- Certain surgeries, such as colorectal surgery, abdominal hysterectomy, and high-risk cesarean section: This medicine is sometimes used to prevent infection from these surgical procedures.

Other than the above information, there is no additional information relating to proper use, precautions, or side effects for these uses.

PENTAMIDINE (Inhalation, oral/ nebulization route) - pen-TAM-i-deen

Commonly used brand name(s)

In the U.S.—
 Nebupent

Available Dosage Forms:
- Powder for Solution

Therapeutic Class: Antiprotozoal

Uses For This Medicine

Pentamidine is used to try to prevent Pneumocystis carinii pneumonia (PCP), a very serious type of pneumonia. This type of pneumonia occurs commonly in patients whose immune systems are not working normally, such as patients with acquired immune deficiency syndrome (AIDS). Inhaled pentamidine does not prevent illness in parts of the body outside the lungs. This medicine may also be used for other conditions as determined by your doctor.

Pentamidine is available only with your doctor's prescription.

Before Using This Medicine

In deciding to use a medicine, the risks of taking the medicine must be weighed against the good it will do. This is a decision you and your doctor will make. For this medicine, the following should be considered:

Allergies—Tell your doctor if you have ever had any unusual or allergic reaction to this medicine or any other medicines. Also tell your health care professional if you have any other types of allergies, such as to foods, dyes, preservatives, or animals. For non-prescription products, read the label or package ingredients carefully.

Pediatric—Studies on this medicine have been done only in adult patients, and there is no specific information comparing use of pentamidine inhalation in children with use in other age groups. However, pentamidine inhalation is recommended in children 5 years of age and older who cannot tolerate other medicines.

Geriatric—Many medicines have not been studied specifically in older people. Therefore, it may not be known whether they work exactly the same way they do in younger adults or if they cause different side effects or problems in older people. There is no specific information comparing use of pentamidine inhalation in the elderly with use in other age groups.

Pregnancy—

	Pregnancy Category	Explanation
All Trimesters	C	Animal studies have shown an adverse effect and there are no adequate studies in pregnant women OR no animal studies have been conducted and there are no adequate studies in pregnant women.

Breast Feeding—There are no adequate studies in women for determining infant risk when using this medication during breastfeeding. Weigh the potential benefits against the potential risks before taking this medication while breastfeeding.

Other medicines—

Using this medicine with any of the following medicines is not recommended. Your doctor may decide not to treat you with this medication or change some of the other medicines you take.

Bepridil, Cisapride, Grepafloxacin, Levomethadyl, Mesoridazine, Pimozide, Sparfloxacin, Terfenadine, Thioridazine, Ziprasidone

Interactions with Food/Tobacco/Alcohol—Certain medicines should not be used at or around the time of eating food or eating certain types of food since interactions may occur. Using alcohol or tobacco with certain medicines may also cause interactions to occur. Discuss with your healthcare professional the use of your medicine with food, alcohol, or tobacco.

Other medical problems—The presence of other medical problems may affect the use of this medicine. Make sure you tell your doctor if you have any other medical problems, especially:
- Asthma—Patients with asthma may have an increase in coughing or difficulty in breathing while receiving pentamidine inhalation

Proper Use of This Medicine

To help prevent the development or return of pneumocystis pneumonia, you must receive pentamidine inhalation on a regular basis, even if you are feeling well.

Dosing—The dose of this medicine will be different for different patients. Follow your doctor's orders or the directions on the label. The following information includes only the average doses of this medicine. If your dose is different, do not change it unless your doctor tells you to do so.

The amount of medicine that you take depends on the strength of the medicine. Also, the number of doses you take each day, the time allowed between doses, and the length of time you take the medicine depend on the medical problem for which you are using the medicine.

- For the inhalation dosage form:
  - For the prevention of Pneumocystis carinii pneumonia (PCP):
    - Adults and children 5 years of age and older—300 milligrams (mg) by oral inhalation once every four weeks.
    - Children younger than 5 years of age—Use and dose must be determined by your doctor.

Missed dose—If you miss a dose of this medicine, take it as soon as possible. However, if it is almost time for your next dose, skip the missed dose and go back to your regular dosing schedule. Do not double doses.

Precautions While Using This Medicine

If you are also using the inhalation form of a bronchodilator (medicine used to help relieve breathing problems), use the pentamidine inhalation at least 5 to 10 minutes after the bronchodilator, unless otherwise directed by your doctor. This will help to reduce the possibility of side effects. Do not use the bronchodilator or any medicine other than pentamidine in the nebulizer.

A bitter or metallic taste may occur during use of this medicine. Sucking on a hard candy after each treatment can help reduce this problem.

Cigarette smoking can increase the chance of coughing and difficulty in breathing during pentamidine inhalation therapy.

Side Effects of This Medicine

On rare occasions, pneumocystis infections have occurred in parts of the body outside the lungs in patients receiving pentamidine inhalation therapy. You should discuss this possible problem with your doctor.

Along with its needed effects, a medicine may cause some unwanted effects. Although not all of these side effects may occur, if they do occur they may need medical attention.

Check with your doctor immediately if any of the following side effects occur:
More common
Burning pain, dryness, or sensation of lump in throat; chest pain or congestion; coughing; difficulty in breathing; difficulty in swallowing; skin rash; wheezing
Rare
Nausea and vomiting; pain in upper abdomen, possibly radiating to the back; pain in side of chest (severe); shortness of breath (sudden and severe)

Rare—with daily treatment doses only
Anxiety; chills; cold sweats; cool, pale skin; decreased urination; headache; increased hunger; loss of appetite; nausea and vomiting; nervousness; shakiness; stomach pain; unusual tiredness

Other side effects not listed may also occur in some patients. If you notice any other effects, check with your healthcare professional.

PENTETATE CALCIUM TRISODIUM (Intravenous route, Inhalation, oral/nebulization route) - PEN-te-tate KAL-see-um trye-SOE-dee-um

Uses For This Medicine

Pentetate calcium trisodium is used to remove harmful substances, such as plutonium, americium, or curium from your body.

This medicine is available only with your doctor's prescription.

Before Using This Medicine

In deciding to use a medicine, the risks of taking the medicine must be weighed against the good it will do. This is a decision you and your doctor will make. For this medicine, the following should be considered:

Allergies—Tell your doctor if you have ever had any unusual or allergic reaction to this medicine or any other medicines. Also tell your health care professional if you have any other types of allergies, such as to foods, dyes, preservatives, or animals. For non-prescription products, read the label or package ingredients carefully.

Pediatric—Although there is no specific information comparing use of pentetate calcium trisodium in children with use in other age groups, this medicine when given by injection is not expected to cause different side effects or problems in children than it does in adults.

Geriatric—Many medicines have not been studied specifically in older people. Therefore, it may not be known whether they work exactly the same way they do in younger adults or if they cause different side effects or problems in older people. There is no specific information comparing use of pentetate calcium trisodium in the elderly with use in other age groups.

Pregnancy—

	Pregnancy Category	Explanation
All Trimesters	C	Animal studies have shown an adverse effect and there are no adequate studies in pregnant women OR no animal studies have been conducted and there are no adequate studies in pregnant women.

Breast Feeding—There are no adequate studies in women for determining infant risk when using this medication during

breastfeeding. Weigh the potential benefits against the potential risks before taking this medication while breastfeeding.

Other medicines—Although certain medicines should not be used together at all, in other cases two different medicines may be used together even if an interaction might occur. In these cases, your doctor may want to change the dose, or other precautions may be necessary. Tell your healthcare professional if you are taking any other prescription or non-prescription (over-the-counter [OTC]) medicine.

Interactions with Food/Tobacco/Alcohol—Certain medicines should not be used at or around the time of eating food or eating certain types of food since interactions may occur. Using alcohol or tobacco with certain medicines may also cause interactions to occur. Discuss with your healthcare professional the use of your medicine with food, alcohol, or tobacco.

Other medical problems—The presence of other medical problems may affect the use of this medicine. Make sure you tell your doctor if you have any other medical problems, especially:

- Asthma—May be worsened by pentetate calcium trisodium given by inhalation.
- Hemochromatosis (iron disorder)—May increase the chance for serious side effects.
- Kidney disease—May lower the rate at which the harmful substances can be removed. Dialysis may be needed to increase removal of these harmful substances.

Proper Use of This Medicine

Harmful substances may accumulate in your bladder. Therefore, to increase the flow of urine and decrease the time your bladder contains these harmful substances, your doctor may instruct you to drink plenty of liquids and urinate often while being treated with pentetate calcium trisodium to help eliminate the harmful substances.

Dosing—The dose of this medicine will be different for different patients. Follow your doctor's orders or the directions on the label. The following information includes only the average doses of this medicine. If your dose is different, do not change it unless your doctor tells you to do so.

The amount of medicine that you take depends on the strength of the medicine. Also, the number of doses you take each day, the time allowed between doses, and the length of time you take the medicine depend on the medical problem for which you are using the medicine.

- For inhalation dosage form
  - To help with the removal of harmful substances in individuals breathing in the harmful substances
    - Adults—1 gram once a day.
    - Children—Use and dose must be determined by your doctor.
- For parenteral dosage form
  - To help with the removal of harmful substances in individuals exposed by some other way than breathing in the substances
    - Adults—1 gram once a day.
    - Children—14 milligrams per kilogram (mg/kg) once a day.

Missed dose—Call your doctor or pharmacist for instructions.

Precautions While Using This Medicine

To prevent radiation contamination of other persons or environment:

- Using a normal toilet instead of a urinal
- Flushing toilet several times after each use
- Completely cleaning up any spilled urine with a tissue and flushing it away
- Washing hands thoroughly with soap after urinating or a bowel movement
- Immediately laundering clothes and linens soiled with urine, feces or blood; washing them separately from other clothes

Avoid swallowing any solid substances that may be coughed up. Dispose of solid substances in sink or toilet. Flush several times if put in toilet or flush sink by washing hands thoroughly with soap after disposal.

Extra precaution in handling urine, feces, and substances coughed up by children to avoid additional exposure to the care-giver or to the child.

If you are breast-feeding your baby, talk to your doctor about how long you must formula feed your baby and how to dispose of the breast milk containing harmful substances

Side Effects of This Medicine

Along with its needed effects, a medicine may cause some unwanted effects. Although not all of these side effects may occur, if they do occur they may need medical attention.

Also, because of the way these medicines act on the body, there is a chance that they might cause other unwanted effects that may not occur until months or years after the medicine is used. These may include certain types of cancer, such as leukemia or bladder cancer. Discuss these possible effects with your doctor.

Check with your doctor immediately if any of the following side effects occur:
  Incidence unknown
    Chest pain; cough; difficulty swallowing; dizziness; fast heartbeat; hives; itching; puffiness or swelling of the eyelids or around the eyes, face, lips or tongue; shortness of breath; skin rash; tightness in chest; unusual tiredness or weakness; wheezing

Some side effects may occur that usually do not need medical attention. These side effects may go away during treatment as your body adjusts to the medicine. Also, your health care professional may be able to tell you about ways to prevent or reduce some of these side effects. Check with your health care professional if any of the following side effects continue or are bothersome or if you have any questions about them:
  Incidence unknown
    Bleeding, blistering, burning, coldness, discoloration of skin, feeling of pressure, hives, infection, inflammation, itching, lumps, numbness, pain, rash, redness, scarring, soreness, stinging, swelling, tenderness, tingling, ulceration, or warmth at site; blistering, crusting, irritation, itching, or reddening of skin; cracked, dry, scaly skin; diarrhea; headache; lightheadedness; metallic taste; nausea; swelling

Other side effects not listed may also occur in some patients. If you notice any other effects, check with your healthcare professional.

PENTOSAN POLYSULFATE SODIUM (Oral route) - PEN-toe-san pol-ee-SUL-fate SOE-dee-um

---

Commonly used brand name(s)

In the U.S.—
Elmiron

Available Dosage Forms:
• Capsule

Therapeutic Class: Cystitis Agent

Uses For This Medicine

Pentosan is used to relieve the symptoms of the bladder condition called interstitial cystitis.

This medicine is available only with your doctor's prescription.

Before Using This Medicine

In deciding to use a medicine, the risks of taking the medicine must be weighed against the good it will do. This is a decision you and your doctor will make. For this medicine, the following should be considered:

Allergies—Tell your doctor if you have ever had any unusual or allergic reaction to this medicine or any other medicines. Also tell your health care professional if you have any other types of allergies, such as to foods, dyes, preservatives, or animals. For non-prescription products, read the label or package ingredients carefully.

Pediatric—Studies on this medicine have been done only in adult patients, and there is no specific information comparing use of pentosan in children with use in other age groups.

Geriatric—This medicine has been tested and has not been shown to cause different side effects or problems in older people than it does in younger adults.

Pregnancy—

	Pregnancy Category	Explanation
All Trimesters	B	Animal studies have revealed no evidence of harm to the fetus, however, there are no adequate studies in pregnant women OR animal studies have shown an adverse effect, but adequate studies in pregnant women have failed to demonstrate a risk to the fetus.

Breast Feeding—There are no adequate studies in women for determining infant risk when using this medication during breastfeeding. Weigh the potential benefits against the potential risks before taking this medication while breastfeeding.

Other medicines—

Using this medicine with any of the following medicines is usually not recommended, but may be required in some cases. If both medicines are prescribed together, your doctor may change the dose or how often you use one or both of the medicines.

Alteplase, Recombinant, Anistreplase, Ardeparin, Certoparin, Dalteparin, Enoxaparin, Garlic, Nadroparin, Papaya, Parnaparin, Reteplase, Recombinant, Reviparin, St John's Wort, Streptokinase, Tan-Shen, Tenecteplase, Tinzaparin, Urokinase, Warfarin

Interactions with Food/Tobacco/Alcohol—Certain medicines should not be used at or around the time of eating food or eating certain types of food since interactions may occur. Using alcohol or tobacco with certain medicines may also cause interactions to occur. Discuss with your healthcare professional the use of your medicine with food, alcohol, or tobacco.

Other medical problems—The presence of other medical problems may affect the use of this medicine. Make sure you tell your doctor if you have any other medical problems, especially:

• Blood or blood vessel disease or other blood problems or
• Blockage or obstruction of the intestine or
• Polyps or
• Stomach ulcers—The risk of bleeding may be increased
• Liver disease or
• Spleen problems—Pentosan may not be broken down in the body as fast as it normally would; the chance of side effects may be increased

Proper Use of This Medicine

Take this medicine on an empty stomach (at least 1 hour before or 2 hours after meals) and at least 1 hour before or after any other food, milk, or medicine. Also, always take it with a full glass (8 ounces) of water.

Sometimes pentosan must be taken for up to 3 to 6 months before you begin to feel better. Your doctor should check your progress at regular visits during this time.

It is important that you follow any special instructions from your doctor. Some foods and beverages may aggravate your condition. Also, make certain your health care professional knows if you are on any special diet, such as a low-sodium or low-sugar diet.

Dosing—The dose of this medicine will be different for different patients. Follow your doctor's orders or the directions on the label. The following information includes only the average doses of this medicine. If your dose is different, do not change it unless your doctor tells you to do so.

The amount of medicine that you take depends on the strength of the medicine. Also, the number of doses you take

each day, the time allowed between doses, and the length of time you take the medicine depend on the medical problem for which you are using the medicine.

- For oral dosage form (capsules):
  - To treat interstitial cystitis:
    - Adults—100 milligrams (mg) three times a day for three months. Your doctor may tell you to repeat this dose.
    - Children—Use and dose must be determined by your doctor.

Missed dose—If you miss a dose of this medicine, take it as soon as possible. However, if it is almost time for your next dose, skip the missed dose and go back to your regular dosing schedule. Do not double doses.

Storage—Store the medicine in a closed container at room temperature, away from heat, moisture, and direct light. Keep from freezing.

Keep out of the reach of children.

Do not keep outdated medicine or medicine no longer needed.

Precautions While Using This Medicine

This medicine may increase the risk of serious bleeding. Before having any kind of surgery or dental or emergency treatment, tell the medical doctor or dentist in charge that you are using this medicine.

It is important that you follow any special dietary instructions from your doctor. Some foods and beverages may aggravate your condition.

Side Effects of This Medicine

Along with its needed effects, a medicine may cause some unwanted effects. Although not all of these side effects may occur, if they do occur they may need medical attention.

Check with your doctor as soon as possible if any of the following side effects occur:

Rare
Chills; difficulty in breathing; fever; skin rash or hives; sore throat; unusual bleeding or bruising; unusual tiredness or weakness; vision impairment

Some side effects may occur that usually do not need medical attention. These side effects may go away during treatment as your body adjusts to the medicine. Also, your health care professional may be able to tell you about ways to prevent or reduce some of these side effects. Check with your health care professional if any of the following side effects continue or are bothersome or if you have any questions about them:

Less common or rare
Abdominal pain; bleeding gums; constipation; diarrhea; difficulty or pain upon swallowing; dizziness; dryness of throat; hair loss; headache; heartburn; increased sensitivity of skin to sunlight; irritated or red eyes; itching; loss of appetite; nausea; nosebleed; ringing in the ears; runny nose; sores in mouth; stomach gas; stomach upset; vomiting

Other side effects not listed may also occur in some patients. If you notice any other effects, check with your healthcare professional.

PENTOXIFYLLINE (Oral route) - pen-tox-I-fi-leen

Commonly used brand name(s)
In the U.S.—
Pentopak
Pentoxil
Trental

Available Dosage Forms:
- Tablet, Extended Release

Therapeutic Class: Hemorheologic

Uses For This Medicine

Pentoxifylline improves the flow of blood through blood vessels. It is used to reduce leg pain caused by poor blood circulation. Pentoxifylline makes it possible to walk farther before having to rest because of leg cramps.

Pentoxifylline is available only with your doctor's prescription.

Before Using This Medicine

In deciding to use a medicine, the risks of taking the medicine must be weighed against the good it will do. This is a decision you and your doctor will make. For this medicine, the following should be considered:

Allergies—Tell your doctor if you have ever had any unusual or allergic reaction to this medicine or any other medicines. Also tell your health care professional if you have any other types of allergies, such as to foods, dyes, preservatives, or animals. For non-prescription products, read the label or package ingredients carefully.

Pediatric—Studies on this medicine have been done only in adult patients, and there is no specific information comparing use of pentoxifylline in children with use in other age groups.

Geriatric—Side effects may be more likely to occur in the elderly, who are usually more sensitive than younger adults to the effects of pentoxifylline.

Pregnancy—

	Pregnancy Category	Explanation
All Trimesters	C	Animal studies have shown an adverse effect and there are no adequate studies in pregnant women OR no animal studies have been conducted and there are no adequate studies in pregnant women.

Breast Feeding—There are no adequate studies in women for determining infant risk when using this medication during breastfeeding. Weigh the potential benefits against the potential risks before taking this medication while breastfeeding.

Other medicines—

Using this medicine with any of the following medicines may cause an increased risk of certain side effects, but using both drugs may be the best treatment for you. If both medicines are prescribed together, your doctor may change the dose or how often you use one or both of the medicines.

Cimetidine, Dicumarol, Theophylline

Interactions with Food/Tobacco/Alcohol—Certain medicines should not be used at or around the time of eating food or eating certain types of food since interactions may occur. Using alcohol or tobacco with certain medicines may also cause interactions to occur. Discuss with your healthcare professional the use of your medicine with food, alcohol, or tobacco.

Other medical problems—The presence of other medical problems may affect the use of this medicine. Make sure you tell your doctor if you have any other medical problems, especially:

- Any condition in which there is a risk of bleeding (e.g., recent stroke)—Pentoxifylline may make the condition worse
- Kidney disease or
- Liver disease—The chance of side effects may be increased

Proper Use of This Medicine

Swallow the tablet whole. Do not crush, break, or chew it before swallowing.

Pentoxifylline should be taken with meals to lessen the chance of stomach upset. Taking an antacid with the medicine may also help.

Dosing—The dose of this medicine will be different for different patients. Follow your doctor's orders or the directions on the label. The following information includes only the average doses of this medicine. If your dose is different, do not change it unless your doctor tells you to do so.

The amount of medicine that you take depends on the strength of the medicine. Also, the number of doses you take each day, the time allowed between doses, and the length of time you take the medicine depend on the medical problem for which you are using the medicine.

- For oral dosage form (extended-release tablets):
  - For peripheral vascular disease (circulation problems):
    - Adults—400 milligrams (mg) two to three times a day, taken with meals.
    - Children—Use must be determined by your doctor.

Missed dose—If you miss a dose of this medicine, take it as soon as possible. However, if it is almost time for your next dose, skip the missed dose and go back to your regular dosing schedule. Do not double doses.

Storage—Store the medicine in a closed container at room temperature, away from heat, moisture, and direct light. Keep from freezing.

Keep out of the reach of children.

Do not keep outdated medicine or medicine no longer needed.

Precautions While Using This Medicine

It may take several weeks for this medicine to work. If you feel that pentoxifylline is not working, do not stop taking it on your own. Instead, check with your doctor.

Smoking tobacco may worsen your condition since nicotine may further narrow your blood vessels. Therefore, it is best to avoid smoking.

Side Effects of This Medicine

Along with its needed effects, a medicine may cause some unwanted effects. Although not all of these side effects may occur, if they do occur they may need medical attention.

Check with your doctor as soon as possible if any of the following side effects occur:

Rare

Chest pain; irregular heartbeat

Signs and symptoms of overdose (in the order in which they may occur)

Drowsiness; flushing; faintness; unusual excitement; convulsions (seizures)

Some side effects may occur that usually do not need medical attention. These side effects may go away during treatment as your body adjusts to the medicine. Also, your health care professional may be able to tell you about ways to prevent or reduce some of these side effects. Check with your health care professional if any of the following side effects continue or are bothersome or if you have any questions about them:

Less common

Dizziness; headache; nausea or vomiting; stomach discomfort

Other side effects not listed may also occur in some patients. If you notice any other effects, check with your healthcare professional.

PERFLUTREN LIPID MICROSPHERE   (Intravenous route) -
per-FLOO-tren LIP-id MYE-kroe-sfeers

Commonly used brand name(s)

In the U.S.—
Definity

Available Dosage Forms:
- Suspension

Therapeutic Class: Radiological Non-Ionic Contrast Media

Uses For This Medicine

Perflutren lipid microsphere preparation is an ultrasound contrast agent. Ultrasound contrast agents are used to help provide a clear picture during ultrasound. Ultrasound is a special kind of diagnostic procedure. It uses high-frequency sound waves to create images or "pictures" of certain areas inside the body. The sound waves produced by the ultrasound equipment can be reflected (bounced off) by different parts of the body, like for example, the heart. As the sound waves return they are electronically converted into images on a television screen. Unlike x-rays, ultrasound does not involve ionizing radiation.

The perflutren lipid microspheres preparation contains very small gas-filled lipid microspheres that reflect the sound waves and help create a better picture. The lipid microsphere preparation is given by injection into a vein before ultrasound to help diagnose problems of the heart.

The lipid microsphere preparation is to be given only by or under the direct supervision of a doctor with specialized training in ultrasound procedures.

This medicine is available only with your doctor's prescription.

Before Using This Medicine

In deciding to use a medicine, the risks of taking the medicine must be weighed against the good it will do. This is a decision you and your doctor will make. For this medicine, the following should be considered:

In deciding to use a diagnostic agent, any risks of the test must be weighed against the good it will do. This is a decision you and your doctor will make. Also, test results may be affected by other things. For the perflutren lipid microspheres preparation, the following should be considered:

Allergies—Tell your doctor if you have ever had any unusual or allergic reaction to this medicine or any other medicines. Also tell your health care professional if you have any other types of allergies, such as to foods, dyes, preservatives, or animals. For non-prescription products, read the label or package ingredients carefully.

Pediatric—Studies on this agent have been done only in adult patients, and there is no specific information comparing use of perflutren lipid microspheres in children with use in other age groups.

Geriatric—Many medicines have not been studied specifically in older people. Therefore, it may not be known whether they work exactly the same way they do in younger adults. There is no specific information comparing use of perflutren lipid microspheres in the elderly with use in other age groups.

Other medicines—Although certain medicines should not be used together at all, in other cases two different medicines may be used together even if an interaction might occur. In these cases, your doctor may want to change the dose, or other precautions may be necessary. Tell your healthcare professional if you are taking any other prescription or non-prescription (over-the-counter [OTC]) medicine.

Interactions with Food/Tobacco/Alcohol—Certain medicines should not be used at or around the time of eating food or eating certain types of food since interactions may occur. Using alcohol or tobacco with certain medicines may also cause interactions to occur. Discuss with your healthcare professional the use of your medicine with food, alcohol, or tobacco.

Other medical problems—The presence of other medical problems may affect the use of this medicine. Make sure you tell your doctor if you have any other medical problems, especially:

- Heart shunt— perflutren lipid microspheres can bypass filtering by the lungs and directly enter the blood stream and be trapped in small blood vessels

- Lung disease, especially emphysema, pulmonary vasculitis or any conditions that lower the lung area that comes in contact with the blood or

- Respiratory distress syndrome—May increase the side effects of perflutren lipid microsphere

Proper Use of This Medicine

Your doctor may have special instructions for you in preparation for your test. If you do not understand the instructions you receive or if you have not received such instructions, check with your doctor in advance.

Dosing—The dose of this medicine will be different for different patients. Follow your doctor's orders or the directions on the label.

The amount of medicine that you take depends on the strength of the medicine. Also, the number of doses you take each day, the time allowed between doses, and the length of time you take the medicine depend on the medical problem for which you are using the medicine.

Precautions While Using This Medicine

There are no special precautions to observe after having this test.

Side Effects of This Medicine

Along with its needed effects, a medicine may cause some unwanted effects. Although not all of these side effects may occur, if they do occur they may need medical attention.

Check with your doctor immediately if any of the following side effects occur:
Rare
  Black, tarry stools; blurred vision; chest pain; chills; difficult breathing; dizziness, severe or continuing; fast, pounding, or irregular heartbeat or pulse; hives; itching; lightheadedness when getting up from a lying or sitting position; palpitations; shortness of breath; skin rash; slow or irregular heartbeat; swollen glands; unusual bleeding or bruising

Some side effects may occur that usually do not need medical attention. These side effects may go away during treatment as your body adjusts to the medicine. Also, your health care professional may be able to tell you about ways to prevent or reduce some of these side effects. Check with your health care professional if any of the following side effects continue or are bothersome or if you have any questions about them:
Less common
  Back pain; feeling of warmth on skin; headache; nausea; redness of the face, neck arms and occasionally, upper chest

Rare
  Acid or sour stomach; bruising; diarrhea; difficulty in moving; dizziness; dryness of the mouth; feeling of constant movement of self or surroundings; fever; heartburn; indigestion; leg cramps; muscle stiffness or tension; pain at injection site; pain or swelling in the joints; prickly or tingling sensation; sneezing or runny nose; stomach upset or pain; unusual tiredness or weakness

Other side effects not listed may also occur in some patients. If you notice any other effects, check with your healthcare professional.

PERFLUTREN PROTEIN TYPE A MICROSPHERE (Intravenous route) -
per-FLOO-tren PROE-teen type A MYE-kroe-sfeers

Commonly used brand name(s)
In the U.S.—
    Optison

Available Dosage Forms:
• Suspension

Therapeutic Class: Diagnostic Agent, Cardiac Function

Uses For This Test

The albumin microspheres sonicated preparation is an ultrasound contrast agent. Ultrasound contrast agents are used to help provide a clear picture during ultrasound. Ultrasound is a special kind of diagnostic procedure. It uses high-frequency sound waves to create images or "pictures" of certain areas inside the body. The sound waves produced by the ultrasound equipment can be reflected (bounced off) by different parts of the body, like for example, the heart. As the sound waves return they are electronically converted into images on a television screen. Unlike x-rays, ultrasound does not involve ionizing radiation.

The albumin microspheres sonicated preparation contains very small gas-filled albumin microspheres that reflect the sound waves and help create a better picture. The albumin microspheres sonicated preparation is given by injection into a vein before ultrasound to help diagnose problems of the heart.

The albumin microspheres sonicated preparation is to be given only by or under the direct supervision of a doctor with specialized training in ultrasound procedures.

Before Having This Test

In deciding to use a diagnostic test, any risks of the test must be weighed against the good it will do. This is a decision you and your doctor will make. Also, other things may affect test results. For this test, the following should be considered:

In deciding to use a diagnostic agent, any risks of the test must be weighed against the good it will do. This is a decision you and your doctor will make. Also, test results may be affected by other things. For the albumin microspheres sonicated preparation, the following should be considered:

Allergies—Tell your doctor if you have ever had any unusual or allergic reaction to this medicine or any other medicines. Also tell your health care professional if you have any other types of allergies, such as to foods, dyes, preservatives, or animals. For non-prescription products, read the label or package ingredients carefully.

Pediatric—Studies on this agent have been done only in adult patients, and there is no specific information comparing use of albumin microspheres sonicated in children with use in other age groups.

Geriatric—Many medicines have not been studied specifically in older people. Therefore, it may not be known whether they work exactly the same way they do in younger adults. There is no specific information comparing use of albumin microspheres sonicated in the elderly with use in other age groups.

Pregnancy—

	Pregnancy Category	Explanation
All Trimesters	C	Animal studies have shown an adverse effect and there are no adequate studies in pregnant women OR no animal studies have been conducted and there are no adequate studies in pregnant women.

Breast Feeding—There are no adequate studies in women for determining infant risk when using this medication during breastfeeding. Weigh the potential benefits against the potential risks before taking this medication while breastfeeding.

Other medicines—Although certain medicines should not be used together at all, in other cases two different medicines may be used together even if an interaction might occur. In these cases, your doctor may want to change the dose, or other precautions may be necessary. Tell your healthcare professional if you are taking any other prescription or nonprescription (over-the-counter [OTC]) medicine.

Interactions   with   Food/Tobacco/Alcohol—Certain medicines should not be used at or around the time of eating food or eating certain types of food since interactions may occur. Using alcohol or tobacco with certain medicines may also cause interactions to occur. Discuss with your healthcare professional the use of your medicine with food, alcohol, or tobacco.

Other medical problems—The presence of other medical problems may affect the use of this diagnostic test. Make sure you tell your doctor if you have any other medical problems, especially:
• Congenital heart defects or
• Heart shunt or
• Liver problems—Use of the albumin microspheres sonicated preparation is not recommended because its effect when these conditions are present is not known

Proper Use of This Test

Your doctor may have special instructions for you in preparation for your test. If you do not understand the instructions you receive or if you have not received such instructions, check with your doctor in advance.

Dosing—The dose of this medicine will be different for different patients. Follow your doctor's orders or the directions on the label. The following information includes only the average doses of this medicine. If your dose is different, do not change it unless your doctor tells you to do so.

The amount of medicine that you take depends on the strength of the medicine. Also, the number of doses you take each day, the time allowed between doses, and the length of time you take the medicine depend on the medical problem for which you are using the medicine.

Precautions When Having This Test

There are no special precautions to observe after having this test.

Side Effects of This Test

Along with its needed effects, a medicine may cause some unwanted effects. Although not all of these side effects may occur, if they do occur they may need medical attention.

Check with your doctor immediately if any of the following side effects occur:

Less common or rare
    Chest pain; difficulty breathing or shortness of breath; itching; skin rash

Some side effects may occur that usually do not need medical attention. These side effects may go away during treatment as your body adjusts to the medicine. Also, your health care professional may be able to tell you about ways to prevent or reduce some of these side effects. Check with your health care professional if any of the following side effects continue or are bothersome or if you have any questions about them:

More common
    Dizziness; flushing of skin or sensation of warmth; headache; nausea and/or vomiting

Less common
    Changes in taste; dryness of mouth; fatigue; pain at injection site; weakness

Other side effects not listed may also occur in some patients. If you notice any other effects, check with your healthcare professional.

PERGOLIDE (Oral route) - PER-go-lide

Commonly used brand name(s)

In the U.S.—
    Permax

Available Dosage Forms:
 • Tablet

Therapeutic Class: Antiparkinsonian
Pharmacologic Class: Dopamine Agonist

Uses For This Medicine

Pergolide belongs to the group of medicines known as ergot alkaloids. It is used with levodopa or with carbidopa and levodopa combination to treat people who have Parkinson's disease. It works by stimulating certain parts of the central nervous system (CNS) that are involved in this disease.

Pergolide is available only with your doctor's prescription.

Once a medicine has been approved for marketing for a certain use, experience may show that it is also useful for other medical problems. Although this use is not included in the product labeling, pergolide is used in certain patients with the following medical condition:
 • Restless legs syndrome

Before Using This Medicine

In deciding to use a medicine, the risks of taking the medicine must be weighed against the good it will do. This is a decision you and your doctor will make. For this medicine, the following should be considered:

Allergies—Tell your doctor if you have ever had any unusual or allergic reaction to this medicine or any other medicines. Also tell your health care professional if you have any other types of allergies, such as to foods, dyes, preservatives, or animals. For non-prescription products, read the label or package ingredients carefully.

Pediatric—Studies on this medicine have been done only in adult patients, and there is no specific information about its use in children.

Geriatric—This medicine has been tested and has not been shown to cause different side effects or problems in older people than it does in younger adults.

Pregnancy—

	Pregnancy Category	Explanation
All Trimesters	B	Animal studies have revealed no evidence of harm to the fetus, however, there are no adequate studies in pregnant women OR animal studies have shown an adverse effect, but adequate studies in pregnant women have failed to demonstrate a risk to the fetus.

Breast Feeding—Studies suggest that this medication may alter milk production or composition. If an alternative to this medication is not prescribed, you should monitor the infant for side effects and adequate milk intake.

Other medicines—

Using this medicine with any of the following medicines is not recommended. Your doctor may decide not to treat you with this medication or change some of the other medicines you take.

Frovatriptan

Interactions with Food/Tobacco/Alcohol—Certain medicines should not be used at or around the time of eating food or eating certain types of food since interactions may occur. Using alcohol or tobacco with certain medicines may also cause interactions to occur. Discuss with your healthcare professional the use of your medicine with food, alcohol, or tobacco.

Other medical problems—The presence of other medical problems may affect the use of this medicine. Make sure you tell your doctor if you have any other medical problems, especially:
 • Heart disease or
 • Mental problems (history of)—Pergolide may make the condition worse

Proper Use of This Medicine

If pergolide upsets your stomach, it may be taken with meals. If stomach upset continues, check with your doctor.

Dosing—The dose of this medicine will be different for different patients. Follow your doctor's orders or the directions on the label. The following information includes only the average doses of this medicine. If your dose is different, do not change it unless your doctor tells you to do so.

The amount of medicine that you take depends on the strength of the medicine. Also, the number of doses you take each day, the time allowed between doses, and the length of time you take the medicine depend on the medical problem for which you are using the medicine.

- For oral dosage form (tablets):
  - Adults: 50 micrograms a day for the first two days. The dose may be increased every three days as needed. However, the usual dose is not more than 5000 micrograms.

Missed dose—If you miss a dose of this medicine, take it as soon as possible. However, if it is almost time for your next dose, skip the missed dose and go back to your regular dosing schedule. Do not double doses.

Storage—Store the medicine in a closed container at room temperature, away from heat, moisture, and direct light. Keep from freezing.

Keep out of the reach of children.

Do not keep outdated medicine or medicine no longer needed.

Precautions While Using This Medicine

It is important that your doctor check your progress at regular visits, to make sure that this medicine is working and to check for unwanted effects.

This medicine may cause some people to become drowsy, dizzy, or less alert than they are normally. Make sure you know how you react to this medicine before you drive, use machines, or do anything else that could be dangerous if you are dizzy or are not alert.

Dizziness, light-headedness, or fainting may occur after the first doses of pergolide, especially when you get up from a lying or sitting position. Getting up slowly may help. Taking the first dose at bedtime or when you are able to lie down may also lessen problems. If the problem continues or gets worse, check with your doctor.

Pergolide may cause dryness of the mouth. For temporary relief, use sugarless candy or gum, melt bits of ice in your mouth, or use a saliva substitute. However, if your mouth continues to feel dry for more than 2 weeks, check with your medical doctor or dentist. Continuing dryness of the mouth may increase the chance of dental disease, including tooth decay, gum disease, and fungus infections.

It may take several weeks for pergolide to work. Do not stop taking this medicine or reduce the amount you are taking without first checking with your doctor.

Side Effects of This Medicine

Along with its needed effects, a medicine may cause some unwanted effects. Although not all of these side effects may occur, if they do occur they may need medical attention.

Check with your doctor immediately if any of the following side effects occur:
  Rare
     Chest pain (severe); convulsions (seizures); difficulty in breathing; fainting; fast heartbeat or irregular pulse; headache (severe or continuing); high fever; high or low (irregular) blood pressure; increased sweating; loss of bladder control; nausea and vomiting (continuing or severe); nervousness; severe muscle stiffness; sudden weakness; unexplained shortness of breath; unusual

tiredness or weakness; unusually pale skin; vision changes, such as blurred vision or temporary blindness

Check with your doctor as soon as possible if any of the following side effects occur:
  More common
     Anxiety; bloody or cloudy urine; confusion; difficult or painful urination; frequent urge to urinate; hallucinations (seeing, hearing, or feeling things that are not there); uncontrolled movements of the body, such as the face, tongue, arms, hands, head, and upper body
  Less common
     Dizziness; headache; swelling in hands and legs
  Rare
     Abdominal pain or pressure; chills; cough; decreased flow of urine; fever; pain in side or lower back

Some side effects may occur that usually do not need medical attention. These side effects may go away during treatment as your body adjusts to the medicine. Also, your health care professional may be able to tell you about ways to prevent or reduce some of these side effects. Check with your health care professional if any of the following side effects continue or are bothersome or if you have any questions about them:
  More common
     Chest congestion; constipation; dizziness or light-headedness, especially when getting up from a lying or sitting position; drowsiness; heartburn; lower back pain; muscle pain; nausea; runny or stuffy nose; trouble in sleeping; weakness
  Less common
     Diarrhea; dryness of mouth; loss of appetite; swelling of the face; vomiting

Other side effects not listed may also occur in some patients. If you notice any other effects, check with your healthcare professional.

PERMETHRIN (Topical route) - per-METH-rin

Commonly used brand name(s)

In the U.S.—
    Acticin   Nix Creme Rinse
    Elimite

In Canada—
    Nix
    Nix Dermal Cream

Available Dosage Forms:
- Liquid
- Lotion
- Cream

Therapeutic Class: Pediculicide

Uses For This Medicine

Permethrin 1% lotion is used to treat head lice infections. It acts by destroying both the lice and their eggs. The 5% cream is used to treat scabies infections by destroying the mites which cause scabies.

Before Using This Medicine

In deciding to use a medicine, the risks of taking the medicine must be weighed against the good it will do. This is a decision you and your doctor will make. For this medicine, the following should be considered:

Allergies—Tell your doctor if you have ever had any unusual or allergic reaction to this medicine or any other medicines. Also tell your health care professional if you have any other types of allergies, such as to foods, dyes, preservatives, or animals. For non-prescription products, read the label or package ingredients carefully.

Pediatric—Studies on this medicine have been done only in adult patients, and there is no specific information comparing use of topical permethrin in children with use in other age groups.

Geriatric—Many medicines have not been studied specifically in older people. Therefore, it may not be known whether they work exactly the same way they do in younger adults or if they cause different side effects or problems in older people. There is no specific information comparing use of topical permethrin in the elderly with use in other age groups.

Pregnancy—

	Pregnancy Category	Explanation
All Trimesters	B	Animal studies have revealed no evidence of harm to the fetus, however, there are no adequate studies in pregnant women OR animal studies have shown an adverse effect, but adequate studies in pregnant women have failed to demonstrate a risk to the fetus.

Breast Feeding—There are no adequate studies in women for determining infant risk when using this medication during breastfeeding. Weigh the potential benefits against the potential risks before taking this medication while breastfeeding.

Other medicines—Although certain medicines should not be used together at all, in other cases two different medicines may be used together even if an interaction might occur. In these cases, your doctor may want to change the dose, or other precautions may be necessary. Tell your healthcare professional if you are taking any other prescription or non-prescription (over-the-counter [OTC]) medicine.

Interactions with Food/Tobacco/Alcohol—Certain medicines should not be used at or around the time of eating food or eating certain types of food since interactions may occur. Using alcohol or tobacco with certain medicines may also cause interactions to occur. Discuss with your healthcare professional the use of your medicine with food, alcohol, or tobacco.

Other medical problems—The presence of other medical problems may affect the use of this medicine. Make sure you tell your doctor if you have any other medical problems, especially:

The presence of other medical problems may affect the use of topical permethrin. Make sure you tell your doctor if you have other medical problems, especially:
- Severe inflammation of the scalp—Use of permethrin may make the condition worse

Proper Use of This Medicine

Keep this medicine away from the eyes. If you accidentally get some in your eyes, flush them thoroughly with water at once.

Permethrin lotion which is used to treat lice, comes in a container that holds only one treatment. Use as much of the medicine as you need and discard any remaining lotion properly.

For the treatment of head lice (1% lotion):
- Shampoo the hair and scalp using regular shampoo.
- Thoroughly rinse and towel dry the hair and scalp.
- Allow hair to air dry for a few minutes.
- Shake the permethrin lotion well before applying.
- Thoroughly wet the hair and scalp with the permethrin lotion. Be sure to cover the areas behind the ears and on the back of the neck also. Allow the lotion to remain in place for 10 minutes.
- Then, rinse the hair and scalp thoroughly and dry with a clean towel.
- When the hair is dry, you may want to comb the hair with a fine-toothed comb to remove any remaining nits (eggs) or nit shells.

Head lice can be easily transferred from one person to another by direct contact with clothing, hats, scarves, bedding, towels, washcloths, hairbrushes and combs, or hairs from infected persons. Therefore, all members of your household should be examined for head lice and should receive treatment if they are found to be infected. If you have any questions about this, check with your doctor.

For the treatment of scabies (5% cream):
- Read package directions carefully before using.
- Thoroughly wash and dry skin.
- Massage the cream into the skin from the head to the soles of the feet, paying special attention to creases in the skin, hands, feet, between fingers and toes, underarms, and groin.
- Scabies rarely infests the scalp of adults, although the hairline, neck, side of the head, and forehead may be infested in older people and in infants. Infants should be treated on the scalp, side of the head, and forehead.
- Leave the permethrin cream on the skin for 8 to 14 hours.
- Wash off by taking a shower or bath.
- Change into clean clothes.
- After treatment, itching may continue for up to 4 weeks.

Dosing—The dose of this medicine will be different for different patients. Follow your doctor's orders or the directions on the label. The following information includes only the average doses of this medicine. If your dose is different, do not change it unless your doctor tells you to do so.

The amount of medicine that you take depends on the strength of the medicine. Also, the number of doses you take each day, the time allowed between doses, and the length of

time you take the medicine depend on the medical problem for which you are using the medicine.

- For topical dosage forms (cream and lotion):
    - For head lice:
        - Adults and children 2 years of age and older— Apply to the hair and scalp one time.
        - Children up to 2 years of age—Use and dose must be determined by your doctor.
    - For scabies:
        - Adults and children 2 months of age and older— Apply to the skin one time.
        - Children up to 2 months of age—Use and dose must be determined by your doctor.

Storage—Store the medicine in a closed container at room temperature, away from heat, moisture, and direct light. Keep from freezing.

Keep out of the reach of children.

Do not keep outdated medicine or medicine no longer needed.

Precautions While Using This Medicine

To prevent reinfection or spreading of the infection to other people, good health habits are required. These include the following:

- Machine wash all clothing (including hats, scarves, and coats), bedding, towels, and washcloths in very hot water and dry them by using the hot cycle of a dryer for at least 20 minutes. Clothing or bedding that cannot be washed should be dry cleaned or sealed in an airtight plastic bag for 2 weeks.
- Shampoo all wigs and hairpieces.
- Wash all hairbrushes and combs in very hot soapy water (above 130 °F) for 5 to 10 minutes and do not share them with other people.
- Clean the house or room by thoroughly vacuuming upholstered furniture, rugs, and floors.
- Wash all toys in very hot soapy water (above 130 °F) for 5 to 10 minutes or seal in an airtight plastic bag for 2 weeks. This is especially important for stuffed toys used on the bed.

Side Effects of This Medicine

Along with its needed effects, a medicine may cause some unwanted effects. Although not all of these side effects may occur, if they do occur they may need medical attention.

Some side effects may occur that usually do not need medical attention. These side effects may go away during treatment as your body adjusts to the medicine. Also, your health care professional may be able to tell you about ways to prevent or reduce some of these side effects. Check with your health care professional if any of the following side effects continue or are bothersome or if you have any questions about them:

Less common or rare

Burning, itching, numbness, rash, redness, stinging, swelling, or tingling of the scalp

Other side effects not listed may also occur in some patients. If you notice any other effects, check with your healthcare professional.

PHENAZOPYRIDINE (Oral route) -
fen-az-oh-PEER-i-deen

Commonly used brand name(s)

In the U.S.—

Azo-Gesic	Pyridiate
Azo-Septic	Pyridium
Azo-Standard	RE-Azo
Baridium	Urinary Pain Relief
Phenazo 95	Uristat
Prodium	UTI Relief

Available Dosage Forms:

- Tablet
- Kit

Therapeutic Class: Analgesic

Uses For This Medicine

Phenazopyridine is used to relieve the pain, burning, and discomfort caused by infection or irritation of the urinary tract. It is not an antibiotic and will not cure the infection itself.

In the U.S., phenazopyridine is available only with your doctor's prescription.

Before Using This Medicine

In deciding to use a medicine, the risks of taking the medicine must be weighed against the good it will do. This is a decision you and your doctor will make. For this medicine, the following should be considered:

Allergies—Tell your doctor if you have ever had any unusual or allergic reaction to this medicine or any other medicines. Also tell your health care professional if you have any other types of allergies, such as to foods, dyes, preservatives, or animals. For non-prescription products, read the label or package ingredients carefully.

Pediatric—Although there is no specific information comparing use of phenazopyridine in children with use in other age groups, it is not expected to cause different side effects or problems in children than it does in adults.

Geriatric—Many medicines have not been studied specifically in older people. Therefore, it may not be known whether they work exactly the same way they do in younger adults. Although there is no specific information comparing use of phenazopyridine in the elderly with use in other age groups, this medicine is not expected to cause different side effects or problems in older people than it does in younger adults.

Pregnancy—

	Pregnancy Category	Explanation
All Trimesters	B	Animal studies have revealed no evidence of harm to the fetus, however, there are no adequate studies in pregnant women OR animal studies have shown an adverse effect, but adequate studies in pregnant women have failed to demonstrate a risk to the fetus.

Breast Feeding—There are no adequate studies in women for determining infant risk when using this medication during breastfeeding. Weigh the potential benefits against the potential risks before taking this medication while breastfeeding.

Other medicines—Although certain medicines should not be used together at all, in other cases two different medicines may be used together even if an interaction might occur. In these cases, your doctor may want to change the dose, or other precautions may be necessary. Tell your healthcare professional if you are taking any other prescription or non-prescription (over-the-counter [OTC]) medicine.

Interactions with Food/Tobacco/Alcohol—Certain medicines should not be used at or around the time of eating food or eating certain types of food since interactions may occur. Using alcohol or tobacco with certain medicines may also cause interactions to occur. Discuss with your healthcare professional the use of your medicine with food, alcohol, or tobacco.

Other medical problems—The presence of other medical problems may affect the use of this medicine. Make sure you tell your doctor if you have any other medical problems, especially:

- Glucose-6–phosphate dehydrogenase (G6PD) deficiency or
- Hepatitis or
- Kidney disease—The chance of side effects may be increased.

Proper Use of This Medicine

This medicine is best taken with food or after eating a meal or a snack to lessen stomach upset.

Do not use any leftover medicine for future urinary tract problems without first checking with your doctor. An infection may require additional medicine.

Dosing—The dose of this medicine will be different for different patients. Follow your doctor's orders or the directions on the label. The following information includes only the average doses of this medicine. If your dose is different, do not change it unless your doctor tells you to do so.

The amount of medicine that you take depends on the strength of the medicine. Also, the number of doses you take each day, the time allowed between doses, and the length of time you take the medicine depend on the medical problem for which you are using the medicine.

- For oral dosage form (tablets):
  - For relieving pain, burning, and discomfort in the urinary tract:
    - Adults and teenagers—200 milligrams (mg) three times a day.
    - Children—The dose is based on body weight and must be determined by your doctor. The usual dose is 4 mg per kilogram (kg) (about 1.8 mg per pound) of body weight three times a day.

Missed dose—If you miss a dose of this medicine, take it as soon as possible. However, if it is almost time for your next dose, skip the missed dose and go back to your regular dosing schedule. Do not double doses.

Storage—Store the medicine in a closed container at room temperature, away from heat, moisture, and direct light. Keep from freezing.

Keep out of the reach of children.

Do not keep outdated medicine or medicine no longer needed.

Precautions While Using This Medicine

Check with your doctor if symptoms such as bloody urine, difficult or painful urination, frequent urge to urinate, or sudden decrease in the amount of urine appear or become worse while you are taking this medicine.

Phenazopyridine causes the urine to turn reddish orange. This is to be expected while you are using it. This effect is harmless and will go away after you stop taking the medicine. Also, the medicine may stain clothing.

For patients who wear soft contact lenses:

- It is best not to wear soft contact lenses while being treated with this medicine. Phenazopyridine may cause discoloration or staining of contact lenses. It may not be possible to remove the stain.

For diabetic patients:

- This medicine may cause false test results with urine sugar tests and urine ketone tests. If you have any questions about this, check with your health care professional, especially if your diabetes is not well controlled.

Before you have any medical tests, tell the person in charge that you are taking this medicine. The results of some tests may be affected by this medicine.

Side Effects of This Medicine

Along with its needed effects, a medicine may cause some unwanted effects. Although not all of these side effects may occur, if they do occur they may need medical attention.

Check with your doctor as soon as possible if any of the following side effects occur:

Rare

Blue or blue-purple color of skin; fever and confusion; shortness of breath, tightness in chest, wheezing, or troubled breathing; skin rash; sudden decrease in the amount of urine; swelling of face, fingers, feet, and/or lower legs; unusual tiredness or weakness; weight gain; yellow eyes or skin

Some side effects may occur that usually do not need medical attention. These side effects may go away during treatment as your body adjusts to the medicine. Also, your health care professional may be able to tell you about ways to prevent or reduce some of these side effects. Check with your health care professional if any of the following side effects continue or are bothersome or if you have any questions about them:

Less common or rare

Dizziness; headache; indigestion; itching of the skin; stomach cramps or pain

Other side effects not listed may also occur in some patients. If you notice any other effects, check with your healthcare professional.

PHENOTHIAZINES (Systemic)

Some commonly used brand names are:

In the U.S.—

Chlorpromazine Hydrochloride	Prolixin Decanoate (2)
Intensol (1)	Prolixin Enanthate (2)
Compazine (8)	Serentil (3)
Compazine Spansule (8)	Serentil Concentrate (3)
Mellaril (11)	Stelazine (12)
Mellaril Concentrate (11)	Stelazine Concentrate (12)
Mellaril-S (11)	Thorazine (1)
Permitil (2)	Thorazine Spansule (1)
Permitil Concentrate (2)	Trilafon (6)
Prolixin (2)	Trilafon Concentrate (6)
Prolixin Concentrate (2)	Vesprin (13)

In Canada—

Apo-Fluphenazine (2)	Novo-Trifluzine (12)
Apo-Perphenazine (6)	Novo-Ridazine (11)
Apo-Thioridazine (11)	Nozinan (4)
Apo-Trifluoperazine (12)	Nozinan Liquid (4)
Chlorpromanyl-20 (1)	Nozinan Oral Drops (4)
Chlorpromanyl-40 (1)	Nu-Prochlor (8)
Largactil (1)	Piportil L (7)
Largactil Liquid (1)	PMS Fluphenazine (2)
Largactil Oral Drops (1)	PMS Perphenazine (6)
Majeptil (10)	PMS Prochlorperazine (8)
Mellaril (11)	PMS Thioridazine (11)
Modecate (2)	PMS Trifluoperazine (12)
Modecate Concentrate (2)	Serentil (3)
Moditen Enanthate (2)	Stelazine (12)
Moditen HCl (2)	Stemetil (8)
Neuleptil (5)	Stemetil Liquid (8)
Novo-Chlorpromazine (1)	

This information applies to the following medicines:

1. Chlorpromazine (klor-PROE-ma-zeen)
2. Fluphenazine (floo-FEN-a-zeen)
3. Mesoridazine (mez-oh-RID-a-zeen)
4. Methotrimeprazine (meth-oh-trye-MEP-ra-zeen)
5. Pericyazine (pair-ee-SYE-a-zeen)
6. Perphenazine (per-FEN-a-zeen)
7. Pipotiazine (pip-oh-TYE-a-zeen)
8. Prochlorperazine (proe-klor-PAIR-a-zeen)
9. Promazine (PROE-ma-zeen)
10. Thioproperazine (thye-oh-proe-PAIR-a-zeen)
11. Thioridazine (thye-oh-RID-a-zeen)
12. Trifluoperazine (trye-floo-oh-PAIR-a-zeen)
13. Triflupromazine (trye-floo-PROE-ma-zeen)

Category

- **Analgesic**—Methotrimeprazine

- **Anesthetic adjunct**—Chlorpromazine; Methotrimeprazine, intravenous

- **Antidyskinetic, Huntington's chorea**—Chlorpromazine; Thioridazine

- **Antiemetic**—Chlorpromazine; Methotrimeprazine; Perphenazine; Prochlorperazine; Trifluoperazine; Triflupromazine

- **Antineuralgia adjunct**—Fluphenazine

- **Antipsychotic**—Chlorpromazine; Fluphenazine; Mesoridazine; Methotrimeprazine; Perphenazine; Pipotiazine; Prochlorperazine; Promazine; Thioproperazine; Thioridazine; Trifluoperazine; Triflupromazine

- **Antipsychotic adjunct**—Pericyazine

- **Sedative**—Chlorpromazine; Methotrimeprazine; Thioridazine

Description

Phenothiazines (FEE-noe-THYE-a-zeens) are used to treat serious mental and emotional disorders, including schizophrenia and other psychotic disorders. Some are used also to control agitation in certain patients, severe nausea and vomiting, severe hiccups, and moderate to severe pain in some hospitalized patients. Chlorpromazine is used also in the treatment of certain types of porphyria, and with other medicines in the treatment of tetanus. Phenothiazines may also be used for other conditions as determined by your doctor.

Phenothiazines may cause unwanted, unattractive, and uncontrolled face or body movements that may not go away when you stop taking the medicine. They may also cause other serious unwanted effects. You and your doctor should talk about the good this medicine will do as well as the risks of using it. Also, your doctor should look for early signs of these effects at regular visits. Your doctor may be able to stop or decrease some unwanted effects, if they do occur, by changing your dose or by making other changes in your treatment.

Phenothiazines are available only with your doctor's prescription in the following dosage forms:

Oral

- Chlorpromazine
  - Extended-release capsules
  - Oral concentrate
  - Syrup
  - Tablets
- Fluphenazine
  - Elixir
  - Oral solution
  - Tablets
- Mesoridazine
  - Oral solution
  - Tablets
- Methotrimeprazine
  - Oral solution
  - Tablets
- Pericyazine
  - Capsules
  - Oral solution
- Perphenazine
  - Oral solution
  - Tablets
- Prochlorperazine
  - Extended-release capsules
  - Oral solution
  - Tablets
- Thioproperazine
  - Tablets
- Thioridazine
  - Oral solution
  - Oral suspension
  - Tablets
- Trifluoperazine
  - Syrup
  - Tablets

Parenteral

- Chlorpromazine
  - Injection
- Fluphenazine
  - Injection
- Mesoridazine
  - Injection
- Methotrimeprazine
  - Injection
- Perphenazine
  - Injection
- Pipotiazine
  - Injection
- Prochlorperazine
  - Injection
- Promazine
  - Injection
- Trifluoperazine
  - Injection
- Triflupromazine
  - Injection

Rectal

- Chlorpromazine
  - Suppositories
- Prochlorperazine
  - Suppositories

Before Using This Medicine

In deciding to use a medicine, the risks of taking the medicine must be weighed against the good it will do. This is a decision you and your doctor will make. For phenothiazines, the following should be considered:

Allergies—Tell your doctor if you have ever had any unusual or allergic reaction to phenothiazines. Also tell your health care professional if you are allergic to any other substances, such as foods, preservatives, or dyes. Some of the phenothiazine dosage forms contain parabens, sulfites, or tartrazine.

Pregnancy—Although studies have not been done in pregnant women, some side effects, such as jaundice and movement disorders, have occurred in a few newborns whose mothers received phenothiazines during pregnancy. Studies in animals have shown that, when given to the mother during pregnancy, these medicines can decrease the number of successful pregnancies and cause problems with bone development in the offspring. Before taking this medicine, make sure your doctor knows if you are pregnant or if you may become pregnant.

Breast-feeding—Phenothiazines pass into breast milk and may cause drowsiness or unusual muscle movements in the nursing baby. It may be necessary for you to take a different medicine or to stop breast-feeding during treatment. Be sure you have discussed the risks and benefits of the medicine with your doctor.

Children—Certain side effects, such as muscle spasms of the face, neck, and back, tic-like or twitching movements, inability to move the eyes, twisting of the body, or weakness of the arms and legs, are more likely to occur in children, especially those with severe illness or dehydration. Children are usually more sensitive than adults to the effects of phenothiazines.

Older adults—Constipation, trouble urinating, dryness of mouth, confusion, problems with memory, dizziness or fainting, drowsiness, trembling of the hands and fingers, and problems with muscle movement, such as decreased or unusual movements, are especially likely to occur in elderly patients, who are usually more sensitive than younger adults to the effects of phenothiazines.

Other medicines—Although certain medicines should not be used together at all, in other cases two different medicines may be used together even if an interaction might occur. In these cases, your doctor may want to change the dose, or other precautions may be necessary. When you are taking phenothiazines, it is especially important that your health care professional know if you are taking any of the following:

- Amantadine (e.g., Symmetrel) or
- Antihypertensives (high blood pressure medicine) or
- Bromocriptine (e.g., Parlodel) or
- Deferoxamine (e.g., Desferal) or
- Diuretics (water pills) or
- Levobunolol (e.g., Betagan) or
- Medicine for heart disease or
- Metipranolol (e.g., OptiPranolol) or
- Nabilone (e.g., Cesamet) (with high doses) or
- Narcotic pain medicine or
- Pentamidine (e.g., Pentam)—Severe low blood pressure may occur
- Antidepressants (medicine for depression)—The risk of developing serious side effects, including severe constipation, low blood pressure, severe drowsiness, unusual body or facial movements, and changes in heart rhythm, may be increased
- Antipsychotics, other (medicine for mental illness) or
- Promethazine (e.g., Phenergan) or
- Trimeprazine (e.g., Temaril)—Severe low blood pressure or unusual body or facial movements may occur
- Antithyroid agents (medicine for overactive thyroid)—The risk of developing serious blood problems may be increased
- Astemizole (e.g., Hismanal) or
- Cisapride (e.g., Propulsid) or
- Disopyramide (e.g., Norpace) or
- Erythromycin (e.g., E.E.S., EryPed) or
- Probucol (e.g., Lorelco) or
- Procainamide (e.g., Procan SR) or
- Quinidine (e.g., Duraquin)—Serious changes in heart rhythm may occur
- Central nervous system (CNS) depressants (medicines that cause drowsiness)—Severe drowsiness and trouble in breathing may occur
- Epinephrine (e.g., Adrenalin)—Severe low blood pressure and fast heartbeat may occur
- Levodopa (e.g., Dopar)—Phenothiazines may prevent levodopa from working properly in the treatment of Parkinson's disease

- Lithium (e.g., Lithane, Lithizine, Lithobid)—Some unwanted effects, such as decreased or unusual body or facial movements, may be increased. The blood levels of the phenothiazine and/or lithium may be changed, so the medicines may not work properly. Your doctor may need to change your dose of either or both medicines
- Metoclopramide (e.g., Reglan) or
- Metyrosine (e.g., Demser) or
- Pemoline (e.g., Cylert) or
- Rauwolfia alkaloids (deserpidine [e.g., Harmonyl], rauwolfia serpentina [e.g., Raudixin], reserpine [e.g., Serpasil])—Taking these medicines with phenothiazines may increase the chance of having decreased or unusual body or facial movements or may make the movement problems worse
- Pimozide (e.g., Orap)—Serious changes in heart rhythm, severe low blood pressure, or unusual body or facial movements may occur

Other medical problems—The presence of other medical problems may affect the use of phenothiazines. Make sure you tell your doctor if you have any other medical problems, especially:

- Alcohol abuse—Certain unwanted effects, such as heatstroke and liver disease, may be more likely to occur
- Blood disease or
- Breast cancer or
- Difficult urination or
- Glaucoma or
- Heart or blood vessel disease or
- Parkinson's disease or
- Seizure disorders, or history of or
- Stomach ulcers—Phenothiazines may make the condition worse
- Brain damage or
- Blood vessel disease in the brain—Serious increase in body temperature may occur
- Enlarged prostate—Difficulty in urinating may occur or may become more severe
- Liver disease—Phenothiazines may make the condition worse. Higher blood levels of phenothiazines may occur, increasing the chance of having unwanted effects
- Lung disease—Difficulty in breathing may become more severe. Decrease in cough reflex caused by phenothiazines may increase the risk of developing complications, such as pneumonia
- Pheochromocytoma or
- Kidney disease—Severe low blood pressure may occur
- Reye's syndrome—The risk that the phenothiazine will have unwanted effects on the liver may be increased

Proper Use of This Medicine

For patients taking this medicine *by mouth:*

- This medicine may be taken with food or a full glass (8 ounces) of water or milk to reduce stomach irritation.
- *If your medicine comes in a dropper bottle,* measure each dose with the special dropper provided with your prescription and dilute it in a small glass (4 ounces) of orange or grapefruit juice or water just before taking it.

- If you are taking the *extended-release capsule form* of this medicine, each dose should be swallowed whole. *Do not break, crush, or chew before swallowing.*

For patients using the *suppository form* of this medicine:

- If the suppository is too soft to insert, chill it in the refrigerator for 30 minutes or run cold water over it before removing the foil wrapper.
- To insert the suppository: First remove the foil wrapper and moisten the suppository with cold water. Lie down on your side and use your finger to push the suppository well up into the rectum.

Do not take more or less of this medicine and do not take it more or less often than your doctor ordered. Not taking more than your doctor ordered is particularly important for children or elderly patients, since they may react very strongly to this medicine.

This medicine must be taken for several weeks before its full effect is reached when it is used to treat mental and emotional conditions.

Dosing—The dose of phenothiazines will be different for different patients. *Follow your doctor's orders or the directions on the label.* The following information includes only the average doses of phenothiazines. *If your dose is different, do not change it* unless your doctor tells you to do so.

The number of capsules, tablets, or teaspoonfuls of elixir, solution, suspension, or syrup that you take, or the number of injections you receive or suppositories that you use, depends on the strength of the medicine. Also, *the number of doses you use each day, the time allowed between doses, and the length of time you take the medicine depend on the medical problem for which you are taking phenothiazines.*

For chlorpromazine

- For *oral extended-release capsule* dosage form:
  - For mental or emotional disorders:
    - Adults—30 to 300 milligrams (mg) one to three times a day. Your doctor may increase your dose if needed.
    - Children—This dosage form is not recommended for use in children.
- For *oral concentrate, syrup, or tablet* dosage forms:
  - For mental or emotional disorders:
    - Adults and teenagers—At first, 10 to 25 mg two to four times a day. Your doctor may increase your dose if needed.
    - Children up to 6 months of age—Dose must be determined by your doctor.
    - Children 6 months to 12 years of age—Dose is based on body weight or size, and must be determined by your doctor. The usual dose is 0.55 mg per kilogram (kg) (0.25 mg per pound) of body weight, every four to six hours.
  - For nausea and vomiting:
    - Adults and teenagers—10 to 25 mg every four to six hours as needed.
    - Children up to 6 months of age—Dose must be determined by your doctor.
    - Children 6 months to 12 years of age—Dose is based on body weight or size, and must be determined by your doctor. The usual dose is 0.55 mg per kg (0.25 mg per pound) of body weight, every four to six hours.

- For sedation before surgery:
  - Adults and teenagers—25 to 50 mg two to three hours before surgery.
  - Children—Dose is based on body weight or size, and must be determined by your doctor. The usual dose is 0.55 mg per kg (0.25 mg per pound) of body weight, two to three hours before surgery.
- For treatment of hiccups:
  - Adults and teenagers—25 to 50 mg three or four times a day. If hiccups remain after two to three days of oral treatment, treatment by injection may be needed.
  - Children—Dose must be determined by your doctor.
- For porphyria:
  - Adults and teenagers—25 to 50 mg three or four times a day.
  - Children—Dose must be determined by your doctor.
- For *injection* dosage form:
  - For severe mental or emotional disorders:
    - Adults—At first, 25 to 50 mg, injected into a muscle. The dose may be repeated in one hour, and every three to twelve hours thereafter. Your doctor may increase your dose if needed.
    - Children up to 6 months of age—Dose must be determined by your doctor.
    - Children 6 months to 12 years of age—Dose is based on body weight or size and must be determined by your doctor. The usual dose is 0.55 mg per kg (0.25 mg per pound) of body weight, injected into a muscle every six to eight hours as needed.
  - For nausea and vomiting:
    - Adults—At first, 25 mg injected into a muscle. If needed, doses of 25 to 50 mg may be given every three to four hours.
    - Children up to 6 months of age—Dose must be determined by your doctor.
    - Children 6 months to 12 years of age—Dose is based on body weight or size and must be determined by your doctor. The usual dose is 0.55 mg per kg (0.25 mg per pound) of body weight, injected into a muscle every six to eight hours as needed.
  - For nausea and vomiting during surgery:
    - Adults—At first, 12.5 mg injected into a muscle. The dose may be repeated if needed. Or up to 25 mg may be diluted and injected slowly into a vein.
    - Children up to 6 months of age—Dose must be determined by your doctor.
    - Children 6 months to 12 years of age—Dose is based on body weight or size and must be determined by your doctor. The usual dose is 0.275 mg per kg (0.125 mg per pound) of body weight injected into a muscle or diluted and injected slowly into a vein.
  - For sedation before surgery:
    - Adults—12.5 to 25 mg, injected into a muscle one to two hours before surgery.
    - Children up to 6 months of age—Dose must be determined by your doctor.
    - Children 6 months to 12 years of age—Dose is based on body weight and must be determined by

your doctor. The usual dose is 0.55 mg per kg (0.25 mg per pound) of body weight, injected into a muscle one to two hours before surgery.
  - For treatment of hiccups:
    - Adults—25 to 50 mg, injected into a muscle three or four times a day. If hiccups remain after treatment by injection into muscle, 25 to 50 mg may be diluted and injected slowly into a vein.
    - Children—Dose must be determined by your doctor.
  - For porphyria:
    - Adults—25 mg injected into a muscle every six to eight hours.
    - Children—Dose must be determined by your doctor.
  - For tetanus:
    - Adults—25 to 50 mg, injected into a muscle three or four times a day. Or 25 to 50 mg, diluted and injected slowly into a vein. Your doctor may increase your dose if needed.
    - Children up to 6 months of age—Dose must be determined by your doctor.
    - Children 6 months to 12 years of age—Dose is based on body weight and must be determined by your doctor. The usual dose is 0.55 mg per kg (0.25 mg per pound) of body weight, injected into a muscle every six to eight hours or diluted and injected slowly into a vein.
- For *rectal* dosage form (suppositories):
  - For nausea and vomiting:
    - Adults and teenagers—50 to 100 mg, inserted into the rectum every six to eight hours as needed.
    - Children up to 6 months of age—Dose must be determined by your doctor.
    - Children 6 months to 12 years of age—Dose is based on body weight and must be determined by your doctor. The usual dose is 1 mg per kg (0.45 mg per pound) of body weight, inserted into the rectum every six to eight hours as needed.

For fluphenazine
- For *oral* dosage form (elixir, solution, or tablets):
  - For mental or emotional disorders:
    - Adults—At first, a total of 2.5 to 10 milligrams (mg) a day, taken in smaller doses every six to eight hours during the day. Your doctor may increase your dose if needed. However, the dose usually is not more than 20 mg a day.
    - Children—0.25 to 0.75 mg one to four times a day.
    - Older adults—1 to 2.5 mg a day. Your doctor may increase your dose if needed.
- For *long-acting decanoate injection* dosage form:
  - For mental or emotional disorders:
    - Adults—At first, 12.5 to 25 mg, injected into a muscle or under the skin every one to three weeks. Your doctor may increase your dose if needed. However, the dose usually is not more than 100 mg.
    - Children 5 to 12 years of age—3.125 to 12.5 mg, injected into a muscle or under the skin every one to three weeks.
    - Children 12 years of age and older—At first, 6.25 to 18.75 mg, injected into a muscle or under the skin once a week. Your doctor may increase your

dose if needed. However, the dose usually is not more than 25 mg every one to three weeks.
- For *long-acting enanthate injection* dosage form:
  ○ For mental or emotional disorders:
    ▪ Adults and teenagers—At first, 25 mg, injected into a muscle or under the skin every two weeks. Your doctor may adjust your dose if needed. However, the dose usually is not more than 100 mg.
    ▪ Children up to 12 years of age—Dose must be determined by your doctor.
- For *short-acting hydrochloride injection* dosage form:
  ○ For mental or emotional disorders:
    ▪ Adults and teenagers—At first, 1.25 mg, injected into a muscle. Your doctor may repeat and increase your dose if needed. However, the dose usually is not more than 10 mg a day.
    ▪ Children up to 12 years of age—Dose must be determined by your doctor.
    ▪ Older adults—1 to 2.5 mg a day, injected into a muscle. Your doctor may increase your dose if needed.

For mesoridazine
- For *oral* dosage form (solution or tablets):
  ○ For mental or emotional disorders:
    ▪ Adults and teenagers—At first, 50 milligrams (mg) three times a day. Your doctor may adjust your dose if needed.
    ▪ Children up to 12 years of age—Dose must be determined by your doctor.
- For *injection* dosage form:
  ○ For mental or emotional disorders:
    ▪ Adults and teenagers—25 mg injected into a muscle. The dose may be repeated in thirty to sixty minutes if needed.
    ▪ Children up to 12 years of age—Dose must be determined by your doctor.

For methotrimeprazine
- For *oral* dosage form (solution or tablets):
  ○ For mental or emotional disorders:
    ▪ Adults and teenagers—At first, a total of 50 to 75 milligrams (mg) a day, taken in smaller doses two or three times a day with meals. Your doctor may increase your dose if needed.
    ▪ Children—Dose is based on body weight and must be determined by your doctor. At first, the usual dose is a total of 0.25 mg per kilogram (kg) (0.11 mg per pound) of body weight a day, taken in smaller doses two or three times a day with meals. Your doctor may increase your dose if needed.
  ○ For pain:
    ▪ Adults and teenagers—For moderate pain, at first a total of 6 to 25 mg a day, taken in smaller doses three times a day with meals. For severe pain, at first a total of 50 to 75 mg a day, taken in smaller doses two or three times a day with meals. Your doctor may increase your dose if needed.
    ▪ Children—Dose is based on body weight and must be determined by your doctor. At first, the usual dose is a total of 0.25 mg per kg (0.11 mg per pound) of body weight a day, taken in smaller doses two or three times a day with meals. Your doctor may increase your dose if needed. However, the dose usually is not more than 40 mg a day.

○ For sedation:
  ▪ Adults and teenagers—At first, a total of 6 to 25 mg a day, taken in smaller doses three times a day with meals. Your doctor may increase your dose if needed.
  ▪ Children—Dose is based on body weight and must be determined by your doctor. At first, the usual dose is a total of 0.25 mg per kg (0.11 mg per pound) of body weight a day, taken in smaller doses two or three times a day with meals. Your doctor may increase your dose if needed. However, the dose usually is not more than 40 mg a day.
- For *injection* dosage form:
  ○ For mental or emotional disorders:
    ▪ Adults and teenagers—At first, 10 to 20 mg, injected into a muscle every four to six hours. Your doctor may increase your dose if needed.
    ▪ Children—Dose is based on body weight and must be determined by your doctor. The usual dose is a total of 0.062 to 0.125 mg per kg (0.028 to 0.057 mg per pound) of body weight a day, injected into a muscle in one dose or in a few smaller doses.
  ○ For pain:
    ▪ Adults and teenagers—At first, 2.5 to 20 mg, injected into a muscle. Your doctor may repeat or increase your dose if needed.
    ▪ Children—Dose is based on body weight and must be determined by your doctor. The usual dose is a total of 0.062 to 0.125 mg per kg (0.028 to 0.057 mg per pound) of body weight a day, injected into a muscle in one dose or in a few smaller doses.
    ▪ Older adults—At first, 5 to 10 mg injected into a muscle every four to six hours. Your doctor may increase your dose if needed.
  ○ For sedation before surgery:
    ▪ Adults and teenagers—2 to 20 mg, injected into a muscle forty-five minutes to three hours before surgery.
    ▪ Children—Dose must be determined by your doctor.

For pericyazine
- For *oral* dosage form (capsules or solution):
  ○ For mental or emotional disorders:
    ▪ Adults—At first, 5 milligrams (mg) taken in the morning, and 10 mg taken in the evening. Your doctor may change your dose if needed. However, the dose usually is not more than 20 mg taken in the morning and 40 mg taken in the evening.
    ▪ Children up to 5 years of age—Dose must be determined by your doctor.
    ▪ Children 5 years of age and older—2.5 to 10 mg taken in the morning, and 5 to 30 mg taken in the evening.
    ▪ Older adults—At first, 5 mg a day. Your doctor may increase your dose if needed. However, the dose usually is not more than 30 mg a day.

For perphenazine
- For *oral solution* dosage form:
  ○ For mental or emotional disorders in hospitalized patients:
    ▪ Adults and teenagers—8 to 16 milligrams (mg) two to four times a day.

- Children up to 12 years of age—Dose must be determined by your doctor.

- For *oral tablet* dosage form:
  - For mental or emotional disorders:
    - Adults and teenagers—4 to 16 mg two to four times a day.
    - Children up to 12 years of age—Dose must be determined by your doctor.
  - For nausea and vomiting:
    - Adults and teenagers—A total of 8 to 16 mg a day, taken in smaller doses during the day. Your doctor will lower your dose as soon as possible.
    - Children up to 12 years of age—Dose must be determined by your doctor.

- For *injection* dosage form:
  - For mental or emotional disorders:
    - Adults and teenagers—5 to 10 mg injected into a muscle every six hours.
    - Children up to 12 years of age—Dose must be determined by your doctor.
  - For nausea and vomiting:
    - Adults and teenagers—At first, 5 to 10 mg injected into a muscle, or 5 mg diluted and injected slowly into a vein. Your doctor may adjust your dose if needed.
    - Children up to 12 years of age—Dose must be determined by your doctor.

For pipotiazine
- For *injection* dosage form:
  - For mental or emotional disorders:
    - Adults and teenagers—At first, 50 to 100 milligrams (mg) injected into a muscle every two to three weeks. Your doctor may increase your dose if needed. However, the dose usually is not more than 150 mg every four weeks.
    - Children up to 12 years of age—Dose must be determined by your doctor.

For prochlorperazine
- For *oral extended-release capsule* dosage form:
  - For mental or emotional disorders:
    - Adults and teenagers—Dose must be determined by your doctor.
    - Children—This dosage form is not recommended for use in children.
  - For nausea and vomiting:
    - Adults and teenagers—At first, 15 mg taken once a day in the morning, or 10 mg taken every twelve hours. Your doctor may increase your dose if needed. However, the dose usually is not more than 40 mg a day.
    - Children—This dosage form is not recommended for use in children.
- For *oral* dosage form (solution or tablets):
  - For mental or emotional disorders:
    - Adults and teenagers—At first, 5 to 10 milligrams (mg) three or four times a day. Your doctor may increase your dose if needed. However, the dose usually is not more than 150 mg a day.
    - Children up to 2 years of age—Dose must be determined by your doctor.
    - Children 2 to 12 years of age—2.5 mg two or three times a day. Your doctor may increase your dose if needed. However, for children 2 through

5 years of age, the dose usually is not more than 20 mg a day. For children 6 to 12 years of age, the dose usually is not more than 25 mg a day.
  - For nausea and vomiting:
    - Adults and teenagers—5 to 10 mg three or four times a day.
    - Children—Dose is based on body weight and must be determined by your doctor. The usual dose is 2.5 mg taken one to three times a day.

- For *injection* dosage form:
  - For mental or emotional disorders:
    - Adults and teenagers—At first, 10 to 20 mg injected into a muscle. The dose may be repeated if needed. Later, the dose is usually 10 to 20 mg every four to six hours. However, the dose usually is not more than 200 mg a day.
    - Children up to 2 years of age—Dose must be determined by your doctor.
    - Children 2 to 12 years of age—Dose is based on body weight and must be determined by your doctor. The usual dose is 0.132 mg per kilogram (kg) (0.06 mg per pound) of body weight, injected into a muscle. However, the dose for children 2 through 5 years of age usually is not more than 20 mg a day. The dose for children 6 to 12 years of age usually is not more than 25 mg a day.
  - For nausea and vomiting:
    - Adults and teenagers—5 to 10 mg, injected into a muscle every three to four hours as needed. Or 2.5 to 10 mg injected slowly into a vein. The dose usually is not more than 40 mg a day.
    - Children up to 2 years of age—Dose must be determined by your doctor.
    - Children 2 to 12 years of age—Dose is based on body weight and must be determined by your doctor. The usual dose is 0.132 mg per kg (0.06 mg per pound) of body weight, injected into a muscle. However, the dose for children 2 through 5 years of age usually is not more than 20 mg a day. The dose for children 6 to 12 years of age usually is not more than 25 mg a day.
  - For nausea and vomiting in surgery:
    - Adults and teenagers—5 to 10 mg, injected into a muscle or injected slowly into a vein. The dose may be repeated if needed. However, the total dose usually is not more than 40 mg a day.
    - Children—Dose must be determined by your doctor.

- For *rectal* dosage form (suppositories):
  - For mental or emotional disorders:
    - Adults and teenagers—10 mg inserted into the rectum three or four times a day. Your doctor may increase your dose if needed.
    - Children 2 to 12 years of age—2.5 mg inserted into the rectum two or three times a day. Your doctor may increase your dose if needed. However, for children 2 through 5 years of age, the dose usually is not more than 20 mg a day. For children 6 to 12 years of age, the dose usually is not more than 25 mg a day.
  - For nausea and vomiting:
    - Adults and teenagers—25 mg inserted into the rectum two times a day.
    - Children up to 2 years of age—Dose must be determined by your doctor.

- Children 2 to 12 years of age—Dose is based on body weight and must be determined by your doctor. The usual dose is 2.5 mg inserted into the rectum one to three times a day.

For promazine
- For *injection* dosage form:
  ○ For mental or emotional disorders:
    ▪ Adults—At first, 50 to 150 mg, injected into a muscle or, in hospitalized patients, diluted and injected into a vein. Later, 10 to 200 mg, injected into a muscle every four to six hours.
    ▪ Children up to 12 years of age—Dose must be determined by your doctor.
    ▪ Children 12 years of age and older—10 to 25 mg, injected into a muscle, every four to six hours.

For thioproperazine
- For *oral* dosage form (tablets):
  ○ For mental or emotional disorders:
    ▪ Adults and teenagers—At first, 5 milligrams (mg) a day. Your doctor may increase your dose if needed.
    ▪ Children 3 through 10 years of age—Dose must be determined by your doctor.
    ▪ Children 11 years of age and older—At first, a total of 1 to 3 mg a day taken all at one time in a single dose each day or divided and taken in smaller doses several times during the day. Your doctor may increase your dose if needed.

For thioridazine
- For *oral* dosage form (suspension, solution, or tablets):
  ○ For mental or emotional disorders:
    ▪ Adults and teenagers—At first, 50 to 100 milligrams (mg) one to three times a day. Your doctor may adjust your dose if needed. However, the dose usually is not more than 800 mg a day.
    ▪ Children up to 2 years of age—Dose must be determined by your doctor.
    ▪ Children 2 to 12 years of age—At first, 10 to 25 mg two or three times a day. Your doctor may adjust your dose, if needed, based on body weight or size.

For trifluoperazine
- For *oral* dosage form (syrup or tablets):
  ○ For mental or emotional disorders:
    ▪ Adults and teenagers—At first, 2 to 5 milligrams (mg) one or two times a day. Your doctor may increase your dose if needed. However, the dose usually is not more than 40 mg a day.
    ▪ Children up to 6 years of age—Dose must be determined by your doctor.
    ▪ Children 6 to 12 years of age—At first, 1 mg one or two times a day. Your doctor may increase your dose if needed.
- For *injection* dosage form:
  ○ For mental or emotional disorders:
    ▪ Adults and teenagers—1 to 2 mg, injected into a muscle every four to six hours as needed. However, the dose usually is not more than 10 mg a day.
    ▪ Children up to 6 years of age—Dose must be determined by your doctor.
    ▪ Children 6 to 12 years of age—1 mg injected into a muscle one or two times a day.

For triflupromazine
- For *injection* dosage form:
  ○ For mental or emotional disorders:
    ▪ Adults and teenagers—60 milligrams (mg) injected into a muscle as needed. However, the dose usually is not more than 150 mg a day.
    ▪ Children up to 2½ years of age—Dose must be determined by your doctor.
    ▪ Children 2½ years of age and older—Dose is based on body weight and must be determined by your doctor. The usual dose is 0.2 to 0.25 mg per kilogram (kg) (0.09 to 0.11 mg per pound) of body weight, injected into a muscle. However, the dose usually is not more than 10 mg a day.
  ○ For nausea and vomiting:
    ▪ Adults and teenagers—5 to 15 mg injected into a muscle every four hours, as needed. However, the dose usually is not more than 60 mg a day injected into a muscle. Or 1 mg injected into a vein, the dose being repeated as needed. However, the dose usually is not more than 3 mg a day injected into a vein.
    ▪ Children up to 2½ years of age—Dose must be determined by your doctor.
    ▪ Children 2½ years of age and older—Dose is based on body weight and must be determined by your doctor. The usual dose is 0.2 to 0.25 mg per kg (0.09 to 0.11 mg per pound) of body weight, injected into a muscle. However, the dose usually is not more than 10 mg a day.

Missed dose—If you miss a dose of this medicine and your dosing schedule is:
- One dose a day—Take the missed dose as soon as possible. Then go back to your regular dosing schedule. However, if you do not remember the missed dose until the next day, skip it and go back to your regular dosing schedule. Do not double doses.
- More than one dose a day—If you remember within an hour or so of the missed dose, take it right away. However, if you do not remember until later, skip the missed dose and go back to your regular dosing schedule. Do not double doses.

If you have any questions about this, check with your doctor.

Storage—To store this medicine:
- Keep out of the reach of children.
- Store away from heat and direct light.
- Do not store the capsule or tablet form of this medicine in the bathroom, near the kitchen sink, or in other damp places. Heat or moisture may cause the medicine to break down.
- Keep the liquid form of this medicine from freezing.
- Do not keep outdated medicine or medicine no longer needed. Be sure that any discarded medicine is out of the reach of children.

Precautions While Using This Medicine

Your doctor should check your progress at regular visits, especially during the first few months of treatment with this medicine. This will allow your dosage to be changed if necessary to meet your needs.

Do not stop taking this medicine without first checking with your doctor. Your doctor may want you to reduce gradually the amount you are taking before stopping completely. This is to prevent side effects and to keep your condition from becoming worse.

Do not take this medicine within 2 hours of taking antacids or medicine for diarrhea. Taking these products too close together may make this medicine less effective.

This medicine will add to the effects of alcohol and other central nervous system (CNS) depressants (medicines that slow down the nervous system, possibly causing drowsiness). Some examples of CNS depressants are antihistamines or medicine for hay fever, other allergies, or colds; sedatives, tranquilizers, or sleeping medicine; prescription pain medicine or narcotics; barbiturates; medicine for seizures; muscle relaxants; or anesthetics, including some dental anesthetics. *Check with your doctor before taking any of the above while you are using this medicine.*

Before using any prescription or over-the-counter (OTC) medicine for colds or allergies, check with your doctor. These medicines may increase the chance of developing heatstroke or other unwanted effects, such as dizziness, dry mouth, blurred vision, and constipation, while you are taking a phenothiazine.

Before you have any medical tests, tell the medical doctor in charge that you are taking this medicine. The results of some tests (such as electrocardiogram [ECG or EKG] readings, the gonadorelin test, the metyrapone test, tests for phenylketonurea, and urine bilirubin tests) may be affected by this medicine.

Before having any kind of surgery, dental treatment, or emergency treatment, tell the medical doctor or dentist in charge that you are using this medicine. Taking phenothiazines together with medicines that are used during surgery, dental treatments, or emergency treatments may increase CNS depression or cause low blood pressure.

This medicine may cause some people to become drowsy or less alert than they are normally. Even if this medicine is taken only at bedtime, it may cause some people to feel drowsy or less alert on arising. *Make sure you know how you react to this medicine before you drive, use machines, or do anything else that could be dangerous if you are not alert.*

Phenothiazines may cause blurred vision, difficulty in reading, or other changes in vision, especially during the first few weeks of treatment. Do not drive, use machines, or do anything else that could be dangerous if you are not able to see well. *If the problem continues or gets worse, check with your doctor.*

Dizziness, lightheadedness, or fainting may occur, especially when you get up from a lying or sitting position. Getting up slowly may help. If the problem continues or gets worse, check with your doctor.

This medicine may make you sweat less, causing your body temperature to increase. *Use extra care not to become overheated during exercise or hot weather while you are taking this medicine,* since overheating may result in heatstroke. Also, hot baths or saunas may make you feel dizzy or faint while you are taking this medicine.

This medicine also may make you more sensitive to cold temperatures. Dress warmly during cold weather. Be careful during prolonged exposure to cold, such as in winter sports or swimming in cold water.

Phenothiazines may cause dryness of the mouth. For temporary relief, use sugarless candy or gum, melt bits of ice in your mouth, or use a saliva substitute. However, if your mouth continues to feel dry for more than 2 weeks, check with your medical doctor or dentist. Continuing dryness of the mouth may increase the chance of dental disease, including tooth decay, gum disease, and fungus infections.

Phenothiazines may cause your skin to be more sensitive to sunlight than it is normally. Exposure to sunlight, even for brief periods of time, may cause a skin rash, itching, redness or other discoloration of the skin, or a severe sunburn. When you begin taking this medicine:

- Stay out of direct sunlight, especially between the hours of 10:00 a.m. and 3:00 p.m., if possible.
- Wear protective clothing, including a hat. Also, wear sunglasses.
- Apply a sunblock product that has a skin protection factor (SPF) of at least 15. You may require a product with a higher SPF number, especially if you have a fair complexion. If you have any questions about this, check with your health care professional.
- Apply a sunblock lipstick that has an SPF of at least 15 to protect your lips.
- Do not use a sunlamp or tanning bed or booth.

If you have a severe reaction from the sun, check with your doctor.

Phenothiazines may cause your eyes to be more sensitive to sunlight than they are normally. Exposure to sunlight over a period of time (several months to years) may cause blurred vision, change in color vision, or difficulty in seeing at night. When you go out during the daylight hours, even on cloudy days, wear sunglasses that block ultraviolet (UV) light. Ordinary sunglasses may not protect your eyes. If you have any questions about the kind of sunglasses to wear, check with your medical doctor or eye doctor.

If you are taking a liquid form of this medicine, avoid getting it on your skin or clothing because it may cause a skin rash or other irritation.

If you are receiving this medicine by injection:

- The effects of the long-acting injection form of this medicine may last for 6 to 12 weeks. *The precautions and side effects information for this medicine applies during this time.*

Side Effects of This Medicine

Along with their needed effects, phenothiazines can sometimes cause serious unwanted effects. Tardive dyskinesia or tardive dystonia (muscle movement disorders) may occur and may not go away after you stop using the medicine. Signs of tardive dyskinesia or tardive dystonia include worm-like movements of the tongue, or other uncontrolled movements of the mouth, tongue, cheeks, jaw, body, arms, or legs. Another possible serious unwanted effect is the neuroleptic malignant syndrome (NMS). Signs and symptoms of NMS include severe muscle stiffness, fever, fast heartbeat, difficult breathing, increased sweating, and loss of bladder control. *You and your doctor should discuss the good this medicine will do as well as the risks of taking it.*

Stop taking this medicine and check with your doctor immediately if any of the following side effects occur:

Rare—Symptoms of neuroleptic malignant syndrome
  Confusion (severe) or coma; difficult or fast breathing; drooling; fast heartbeat; fever; high or low (irregular)

blood pressure; increased sweating; loss of bladder control; muscle stiffness (severe); trembling or shaking; trouble in speaking or swallowing

Check with your doctor immediately if any of the following side effects occur:

More common
Inability to move eyes; increased blinking or spasms of eyelid; lip smacking or puckering; muscle spasms of face, neck, body, arms, or legs causing unusual postures or unusual expressions on face; puffing of cheeks; rapid or worm-like movements of tongue; sticking out of tongue; tic-like or twitching movements; trouble in breathing, speaking, or swallowing; uncontrolled chewing movements; uncontrolled movements of arms or legs; uncontrolled twisting movements of neck, trunk, arms, or legs

Rare
irregular or slow heart rate; recurrent fainting

Also, check with your doctor as soon as possible if any of the following side effects occur:

More common
Blurred vision, change in color vision, or difficulty in seeing at night; fainting; loss of balance control; mask-like face; restlessness or need to keep moving; shuffling walk; stiffness of arms or legs; trembling and shaking of hands and fingers

Less common
Difficulty in urinating; skin rash; sunburn (severe)

Rare
Abdominal or stomach pains; aching muscles and joints; agitation, bizarre dreams, excitement, or trouble in sleeping; bleeding or bruising (unusual); chest pain; clumsiness; confusion (mild); constipation (severe); convulsions (seizures); dark urine; fever and chills; hair loss; headaches; hot, dry skin or lack of sweating; itchy skin (severe); muscle weakness; nausea, vomiting, or diarrhea; pain in joints; prolonged, painful, inappropriate erection of the penis; redness of hands; shivering; skin discoloration (tan or blue-gray); sore throat and fever; sores in mouth; unusual bleeding or bruising; unusual tiredness or weakness; yellow eyes or skin

Phenothiazines may cause your urine to be dark. In most cases, this is not a sign of a serious problem. However, if your urine does become dark, discuss it with your doctor.

Other side effects may occur that usually do not need medical attention. These side effects may go away during treatment as your body adjusts to the medicine. However, check with your doctor if any of the following side effects continue or are bothersome:

More common
Constipation (mild); decreased sweating; dizziness; drowsiness; dryness of mouth; nasal congestion

Less common
Changes in menstrual period; decreased sexual ability; increased sensitivity of eyes to light; rough or "fuzzy" tongue; secretion of milk (unusual); swelling or pain in breasts; watering of mouth; weight gain (unusual)

After you stop using this medicine, your body may need time to adjust. The length of time this takes depends on the amount of medicine you were using and how long you used it. During this time, check with your doctor if you notice dizziness, nausea and vomiting, stomach pain, trembling of the

fingers and hands, or any of the following signs of tardive dyskinesia or tardive dystonia:

Inability to move eyes; lip smacking or puckering; muscle spasms of face, neck, body, arms, or legs, causing unusual body positions or unusual expressions on face; puffing of cheeks; rapid or worm-like movements of tongue; sticking out of tongue; tic-like or twitching movements; trouble in breathing, speaking, or swallowing; uncontrolled chewing movements; uncontrolled twisting or other movements of neck, trunk, arms, or legs

Although not all of the side effects listed above have been reported for all of the phenothiazines, they have been reported for at least one of them. However, since all of the phenothiazines are very similar, any of the above side effects may occur with any of these medicines.

Other side effects not listed above may also occur in some patients. If you notice any other effects, check with your doctor.

Additional Information

Once a medicine has been approved for marketing for a certain use, experience may show that it also is useful for other medical problems. Although these uses are not included in product labeling, phenothiazines are used in certain patients with the following medical conditions:

- Chronic neurogenic pain (certain continuing pain conditions)
- Huntington's chorea (hereditary movement disorder)
- Migraine headaches

Other than the above information, there is no additional information relating to proper use, precautions, or side effects for these uses.

PHENOXYBENZAMINE (Oral route) -
fen-ox-ee-BEN-za-meen

Commonly used brand name(s)

In the U.S.—
Dibenzyline

Available Dosage Forms:
- Capsule

Therapeutic Class: Cardiovascular Agent
Pharmacologic Class: Alpha-Adrenergic Blocker

Uses For This Medicine

Phenoxybenzamine belongs to the general class of medicines called antihypertensives. It is used to treat high blood pressure (hypertension) due to a disease called pheochromocytoma.

Phenoxybenzamine blocks the effects of certain chemicals in the body. When these chemicals are present in large amounts, they cause high blood pressure.

Phenoxybenzamine may also be used for other conditions as determined by your doctor.

Phenoxybenzamine is available only with your doctor's prescription.

Once a medicine has been approved for marketing for a certain use, experience may show that it is also useful for other medical problems. Although this use is not included in product labeling, phenoxybenzamine is used in certain patients with the following medical condition:

- Benign prostatic hypertrophy

Before Using This Medicine

In deciding to use a medicine, the risks of taking the medicine must be weighed against the good it will do. This is a decision you and your doctor will make. For this medicine, the following should be considered:

Allergies—Tell your doctor if you have ever had any unusual or allergic reaction to this medicine or any other medicines. Also tell your health care professional if you have any other types of allergies, such as to foods, dyes, preservatives, or animals. For non-prescription products, read the label or package ingredients carefully.

Pediatric—Although there is no specific information about the use of phenoxybenzamine in children, it is not expected to cause different side effects or problems in children than it does in adults.

Geriatric—Dizziness or lightheadedness may be more likely to occur in the elderly, who are more sensitive to the effects of phenoxybenzamine. In addition, phenoxybenzamine may reduce tolerance to cold temperatures in elderly patients.

Pregnancy—

	Pregnancy Category	Explanation
All Trimesters	C	Animal studies have shown an adverse effect and there are no adequate studies in pregnant women OR no animal studies have been conducted and there are no adequate studies in pregnant women.

Breast Feeding—There are no adequate studies in women for determining infant risk when using this medication during breastfeeding. Weigh the potential benefits against the potential risks before taking this medication while breastfeeding.

Other medicines—

Using this medicine with any of the following medicines is usually not recommended, but may be required in some cases. If both medicines are prescribed together, your doctor may change the dose or how often you use one or both of the medicines.

Tadalafil, Vardenafil

Interactions with Food/Tobacco/Alcohol—Certain medicines should not be used at or around the time of eating food or eating certain types of food since interactions may occur. Using alcohol or tobacco with certain medicines may also cause interactions to occur. Discuss with your healthcare professional the use of your medicine with food, alcohol, or tobacco.

Other medical problems—The presence of other medical problems may affect the use of this medicine. Make sure you tell your doctor if you have any other medical problems, especially:

- Angina (chest pain) or
- Heart or blood vessel disease—Some kinds may be worsened by phenoxybenzamine
- Kidney disease—Effects may be increased
- Lung infection—Symptoms such as stuffy nose may be worsened
- Recent heart attack or stroke—Lowering blood pressure may make problems resulting from stroke or heart attack worse

Proper Use of This Medicine

To help you remember to take your medicine, try to get into the habit of taking it at the same time each day.

Dosing—The dose of this medicine will be different for different patients. Follow your doctor's orders or the directions on the label. The following information includes only the average doses of this medicine. If your dose is different, do not change it unless your doctor tells you to do so.

The amount of medicine that you take depends on the strength of the medicine. Also, the number of doses you take each day, the time allowed between doses, and the length of time you take the medicine depend on the medical problem for which you are using the medicine.

- For oral dosage form (capsules):
  - For high blood pressure caused by pheochromocytoma:
    - Adults—At first, 10 milligrams (mg) two times a day. Then, your doctor may increase your dose to 20 to 40 mg two or three times a day.
    - Children—Dose is based on body weight and must be determined by your doctor. The usual starting dose is 0.2 mg per kilogram (kg) (0.09 mg per pound) of body weight taken once a day. Then, your doctor may increase your dose to 0.4 to 1.2 mg per kg (0.18 to 0.55 mg per pound) of body weight a day. This is divided into three or four doses.

Missed dose—If you miss a dose of this medicine, take it as soon as possible. However, if it is almost time for your next dose, skip the missed dose and go back to your regular dosing schedule. Do not double doses.

Storage—Store the medicine in a closed container at room temperature, away from heat, moisture, and direct light. Keep from freezing.

Keep out of the reach of children.

Do not keep outdated medicine or medicine no longer needed.

Precautions While Using This Medicine

It is important that your doctor check your progress at regular visits to make sure that this medicine is working properly and to check for unwanted effects.

Do not take other medicines unless they have been discussed with your doctor. This especially includes over-the-counter (nonprescription) medicines for appetite control, asthma, colds, cough, hay fever, or sinus problems, since they may interfere with the effects of this medicine.

Phenoxybenzamine may cause some people to become dizzy, drowsy, or less alert than they are normally. This is more likely to happen when you begin to take it or when you increase the amount of medicine you are taking. Make sure you know how you react to this medicine before you drive, use machines, or do anything else that could be dangerous if you are dizzy or not alert.

Dizziness, lightheadedness, or fainting may occur, especially when you get up from a lying or sitting position. Getting up slowly may help, but if the problem continues or gets worse, check with your doctor.

The dizziness, lightheadedness, or fainting is also more likely to occur if you drink alcohol, stand for a long time, exercise, or if the weather is hot. While you are taking this medicine, be careful in the amount of alcohol you drink. Also, use extra care during exercise or hot weather or if you must stand for a long time.

Before having any kind of surgery (including dental surgery) or emergency treatment, tell the medical doctor or dentist in charge that you are using this medicine.

Phenoxybenzamine may cause dryness of the mouth, nose, and throat. For temporary relief of mouth dryness, use sugarless candy or gum, melt bits of ice in your mouth, or use a saliva substitute. However, if dry mouth continues for more than 2 weeks, check with your medical doctor or dentist. Continuing dryness of the mouth may increase the chance of dental disease, including tooth decay, gum disease, and fungus infections.

Side Effects of This Medicine

In rats and mice, phenoxybenzamine has been found to increase the risk of development of malignant tumors. It is not known if phenoxybenzamine increases the chance of tumors in humans.

Along with its needed effects, a medicine may cause some unwanted effects. Although not all of these side effects may occur, if they do occur they may need medical attention.

Some side effects may occur that usually do not need medical attention. These side effects may go away during treatment as your body adjusts to the medicine. Also, your health care professional may be able to tell you about ways to prevent or reduce some of these side effects. Check with your health care professional if any of the following side effects continue or are bothersome or if you have any questions about them:

　More common
　　Dizziness or lightheadedness, especially when getting up from a lying or sitting position; fast heartbeat; pinpoint pupils; stuffy nose
　Less common
　　Confusion; drowsiness; dryness of mouth; headache; lack of energy; sexual problems in males; unusual tiredness or weakness

Other side effects not listed may also occur in some patients. If you notice any other effects, check with your healthcare professional.

PHENYLEPHRINE   (Nasal route) - fen-il-EF-rin

Commonly used brand name(s)
In the U.S.—
　Neo-Synephrine　　　　Rhinall
　Nostril　　　　　　　　Tur-Bi-Cal
　Pretz-D　　　　　　　　Vicks Sinex

Available Dosage Forms:
　• Solution
　• Spray
　• Gel/Jelly

Therapeutic Class: Decongestant
Pharmacologic Class: Adrenergic

Uses For This Medicine

Phenylephrine is used for the temporary relief of congestion or stuffiness in the nose caused by hay fever or other allergies, colds, or sinus trouble. It may also be used in ear infections to relieve congestion.

This medicine may also be used for other conditions as determined by your doctor.

This medicine is available without a prescription.

Before Using This Medicine

In deciding to use a medicine, the risks of taking the medicine must be weighed against the good it will do. This is a decision you and your doctor will make. For this medicine, the following should be considered:

Allergies—Tell your doctor if you have ever had any unusual or allergic reaction to this medicine or any other medicines. Also tell your health care professional if you have any other types of allergies, such as to foods, dyes, preservatives, or animals. For non-prescription products, read the label or package ingredients carefully.

Pediatric—Children may be especially sensitive to the effects of nasal phenylephrine. This may increase the chance of side effects during treatment.

Geriatric—Many medicines have not been studied specifically in older people. Therefore, it may not be known whether they work exactly the same way they do in younger adults or if they cause different side effects or problems in older people. There is no specific information comparing use of nasal phenylephrine in the elderly with use in other age groups.

Pregnancy—

	Pregnancy Category	Explanation
All Trimesters	C	Animal studies have shown an adverse effect and there are no adequate studies in pregnant women OR no animal studies have been conducted and there are no adequate studies in pregnant women.

Breast Feeding—There are no adequate studies in women for determining infant risk when using this medication during breastfeeding. Weigh the potential benefits against the potential risks before taking this medication while breastfeeding.

Other medicines—

Using this medicine with any of the following medicines is not recommended. Your doctor may decide not to treat you with this medication or change some of the other medicines you take.

Rasagiline, Selegiline

Interactions with Food/Tobacco/Alcohol—Certain medicines should not be used at or around the time of eating food or eating certain types of food since interactions may occur. Using alcohol or tobacco with certain medicines may also cause interactions to occur. Discuss with your healthcare professional the use of your medicine with food, alcohol, or tobacco.

Other medical problems—The presence of other medical problems may affect the use of this medicine. Make sure you tell your doctor if you have any other medical problems, especially:

- Type 2 diabetes mellitus or
- Heart or blood vessel disease or
- High blood pressure or
- Overactive thyroid—Nasal phenylephrine may make the condition worse

Proper Use of This Medicine

To use the nose drops:

- Blow your nose gently. Tilt the head back while standing or sitting up, or lie down on a bed and hang head over the side. Place the drops into each nostril and keep the head tilted back for a few minutes to allow the medicine to spread throughout the nose.
- Rinse the dropper with hot water and dry with a clean tissue. Replace the cap right after use.
- To avoid spreading the infection, do not use the container for more than one person.

To use the nose spray:

- Blow your nose gently. With the head upright, spray the medicine into each nostril. Sniff briskly while squeezing the bottle quickly and firmly. For best results, spray once or twice into each nostril and wait 3 to 5 minutes to allow the medicine to work. Then, blow your nose gently and thoroughly. Repeat until the complete dose is used.
- Rinse the tip of the spray bottle with hot water, taking care not to suck water into the bottle, and dry with a clean tissue. Replace the cap right after use.
- To avoid spreading the infection, do not use the container for more than one person.

To use the nose jelly:

- Blow your nose gently. Wash your hands before applying the medicine. With your finger, place a small amount of jelly (about the size of a pea) up each nostril. Sniff it well back into the nose.
- Wipe the tip of the tube with a clean, damp tissue and replace the cap right after use.

Use this medicine only as directed. Do not use more of it, do not use it more often, and do not use it for longer than 3 days without first checking with your doctor. To do so may make your runny or stuffy nose worse and may also increase the chance of side effects.

Dosing—The dose of this medicine will be different for different patients. Follow your doctor's orders or the directions on the label. The following information includes only the average doses of this medicine. If your dose is different, do not change it unless your doctor tells you to do so.

The amount of medicine that you take depends on the strength of the medicine. Also, the number of doses you take each day, the time allowed between doses, and the length of time you take the medicine depend on the medical problem for which you are using the medicine.

- For stuffy nose:
  - For nose jelly dosage form:
    - Adults—Use a small amount in the nose every three or four hours as needed.
    - Children—Use is not recommended.
  - For nose drops dosage form:
    - Adults and children 12 years of age and older—Use two or three drops of a 0.25 to 0.5% solution in the nose every four hours as needed.
    - Children 6 to 12 years of age—Use two or three drops of a 0.25% solution in the nose every four hours as needed.
    - Children 2 to 6 years of age—Use two or three drops of a 0.125 or 0.16% solution in the nose every four hours as needed.
    - Children up to 2 years of age—Use and dose must be determined by your doctor.
  - For nose spray dosage form:
    - Adults and children 12 years of age and older—Use two or three sprays of a 0.25 to 0.5% solution in the nose every four hours as needed.
    - Children 6 to 12 years of age—Use two or three sprays of a 0.25% solution in the nose every four hours as needed.
    - Children up to 6 years of age—Use and dose must be determined by your doctor.

Missed dose—If you miss a dose of this medicine, take it as soon as possible. However, if it is almost time for your next dose, skip the missed dose and go back to your regular dosing schedule. Do not double doses.

Storage—Store the medicine in a closed container at room temperature, away from heat, moisture, and direct light. Keep from freezing.

Keep out of the reach of children.

Do not keep outdated medicine or medicine no longer needed.

Side Effects of This Medicine

Along with its needed effects, a medicine may cause some unwanted effects. Although not all of these side effects may occur, if they do occur they may need medical attention.

Check with your doctor as soon as possible if any of the following side effects occur:

Increase in runny or stuffy nose
Symptoms of too much medicine being absorbed into the body

Fast, irregular, or pounding heartbeat; headache or dizziness; increased sweating; nervousness; paleness; trembling; trouble in sleepingNote: The above side effects are more likely to occur in children because there is a greater chance that too much of this medicine may be absorbed into the body.

Some side effects may occur that usually do not need medical attention. These side effects may go away during treatment as your body adjusts to the medicine. Also, your health care professional may be able to tell you about ways to prevent or reduce some of these side effects. Check with your health care professional if any of the following side effects continue or are bothersome or if you have any questions about them:

Burning, dryness, or stinging of inside of nose

Other side effects not listed may also occur in some patients. If you notice any other effects, check with your healthcare professional.

PHOSPHATES (Systemic)

Some commonly used brand names are:

In the U.S.—
K-Phos M. F. (2)	Neutra-Phos (2)
K-Phos Neutral (2)	Neutra-Phos-K (1)
K-Phos No. 2 (2)	Uro-KP-Neutral (2)
K-Phos Original (1)	

In Canada—
Uro-KP-Neutral (2)

This information applies to the following medicines:

1. Potassium Phosphates (poe-TASS-ee-um FOS-fates)
2. Potassium and Sodium Phosphates (poe-TASS-ee-um and SOE-dee-um FOS-fates)
3. Sodium Phosphates (SOE-dee-um FOS-fates)

Category

- **Acidifier, urinary**—Potassium and Sodium Phosphates; Monobasic Potassium Phosphates
- **Antiurolithic, calcium calculi**—Potassium and Sodium Phosphates; Monobasic Potassium Phosphates
- **Electrolyte replenisher**—Potassium and Sodium Phosphates; Potassium Phosphates; Sodium Phosphates

Description

Phosphates are used as dietary supplements for patients who are unable to get enough phosphorus in their regular diet, usually because of certain illnesses or diseases. Phosphate is the drug form (salt) of phosphorus. Some phosphates are used to make the urine more acid, which helps treat certain urinary tract infections. Some phosphates are used to prevent the formation of calcium stones in the urinary tract.

Injectable phosphates are to be administered only by or under the supervision of your health care professional. Some of these oral preparations are available only with a prescription. Others are available without a prescription; however, your health care professional may have special instructions on the proper dose of this medicine for your medical condition. You should take phosphates only under the supervision of your health care professional.

Phosphates are available in the following dosage forms:

Oral
- Potassium Phosphates
  - Capsules for solution
  - Powder for solution
  - Tablets for solution
- Potassium and Sodium Phosphates
  - Capsules for solution
  - Powder for solution
  - Tablets for solution

Parenteral
- Potassium Phosphates
  - Injection
- Sodium Phosphates
  - Injection

Importance of Diet

For good health, it is important that you eat a balanced and varied diet. Follow carefully any diet program your health care professional may recommend. For your specific dietary vitamin and/or mineral needs, ask your health care professional for a list of appropriate foods. If you think that you are not getting enough vitamins and/or minerals in your diet, you may choose to take a dietary supplement.

The best dietary sources of phosphorus include dairy products, meat, poultry, fish, and cereal products.

The daily amount of phosphorus needed is defined in several different ways.

For U.S.—
- Recommended Dietary Allowances (RDAs) are the amount of vitamins and minerals needed to provide for adequate nutrition in most healthy persons. RDAs for a given nutrient may vary depending on a person's age, sex, and physical condition (e.g., pregnancy).
- Daily Values (DVs) are used on food and dietary supplement labels to indicate the percent of the recommended daily amount of each nutrient that a serving provides. DV replaces the previous designation of United States Recommended Daily Allowances (USRDAs).

For Canada—
- Recommended Nutrient Intakes (RNIs) are used to determine the amounts of vitamins, minerals, and protein needed to provide adequate nutrition and lessen the risk of chronic disease.

Normal daily recommended intakes for phosphorus are generally defined as follows:

Persons	U.S. (mg)	Canada (mg)
Infants and children		
Birth to 3 years of age	300–800	150–350
4 to 6 years of age	800	400
7 to 10 years of age	800	500–800
Adolescent and adult males	800–1200	700–1000
Adolescent and adult females	800–1200	800–850
Pregnant females	1200	1050
Breast-feeding females	1200	1050

Before Using This Medicine

In deciding to use a medicine, the risks of taking the medicine must be weighed against the good it will do. This is a decision

you and your health care professional will make. For phosphates the following should be considered:

Allergies—Tell your health care professional if you have ever had any unusual or allergic reaction to potassium, sodium, or phosphates. Also, tell your health care professional if you are allergic to any other substances, such as foods, preservatives, or dyes.

Pregnancy—It is especially important that you are receiving enough vitamins and minerals when you become pregnant and that you continue to receive the right amount of vitamins and minerals throughout your pregnancy. The healthy growth and development of the fetus depend on a steady supply of nutrients from the mother. However, taking large amounts of a dietary supplement in pregnancy may be harmful to the mother and/or fetus and should be avoided.

Breast-feeding—It is especially important that you receive the right amount of vitamins and minerals so that your baby will also get the vitamins and minerals needed to grow properly. However, taking large amounts of a dietary supplement while breast-feeding may be harmful to the mother and/or baby and should be avoided.

Children—Problems in children have not been reported with intake of normal daily recommended amounts. However, use of enemas that contain phosphates in children has resulted in high blood levels of phosphorus.

Older adults—Problems in older adults have not been reported with intake of normal daily recommended amounts.

Other medicines—Although certain medicines should not be used together at all, in other cases two different medicines may be used together even if an interaction might occur. In these cases, your health care professional may want to change the dose, or other precautions may be necessary. When you are taking phosphates, it is especially important that your health care professional know if you are taking any of the following:

- Amiloride (e.g., Midamor) or
- Angiotensin-converting enzyme (ACE) inhibitors (benazepril [e.g., Lotensin], captopril [e.g., Capoten], enalapril [e.g., Vasotec], fosinopril [e.g., Monopril], lisinopril [e.g., Zestril, Prinivil], quinapril [e.g., Accupril], ramipril [e.g., Altace]) or
- Cyclosporine or
- Digitalis glycosides (heart medicine) or
- Heparin (e.g., Panheprin), with long-term use, or
- Medicine for inflammation or pain (except narcotics) or
- Other potassium-containing medicine or
- Salt substitutes, low-salt foods, or milk or
- Spironolactone (e.g., Aldactone) or
- Triamterene (e.g., Dyrenium)—Use with potassium-containing phosphates may increase the risk of hyperkalemia (too much potassium in the blood), possibly leading to serious side effects
- Antacids—Use with phosphates may prevent the phosphate from working properly
- Calcium-containing medicine, including antacids and calcium supplements—Use with phosphates may prevent the phosphate from working properly; calcium deposits may form in tissues

- Corticosteroids (cortisone-like medicine)—Use with sodium-containing phosphates may increase the risk of swelling
- Phosphate-containing medications, other, including phosphate enemas—Use with sodium or potassium phosphates may cause high blood levels of phosphorus which may increase the chance of side effects
- Sodium-containing medicines (other)—Use with sodium phosphates may cause your body to retain (keep) water

Other medical problems—The presence of other medical problems may affect the use of phosphates. Make sure you tell your health care professional if you have any other medical problems, especially:

- Burns, severe or
- Heart disease or
- Pancreatitis (inflammation of the pancreas) or
- Rickets or
- Softening of bones or
- Underactive parathyroid glands—Sodium- or potassium-containing phosphates may make these conditions worse
- Dehydration or
- Underactive adrenal glands—Potassium-containing phosphates may increase the risk of hyperkalemia (too much potassium in the blood)
- Edema (swelling in feet or lower legs or fluid in lungs) or
- High blood pressure or
- Liver disease or
- Toxemia of pregnancy—Sodium-containing phosphates may make these conditions worse
- High blood levels of phosphate (hyperphosphatemia)—Use of phosphates may make this condition worse
- Infected kidney stones—Phosphates may make this condition worse
- Kidney disease—Sodium-containing phosphates may make this condition worse; potassium-containing phosphates may increase the risk of hyperkalemia (too much potassium in the blood)
- Myotonia congenita—Potassium-containing phosphates may increase the risk of hyperkalemia (too much potassium in the blood), and make this condition worse

Proper Use of This Medicine

For patients taking the *tablet form* of this medicine:

- *Do not swallow the tablet*. Before taking, dissolve the tablet in ¾ to 1 glass (6 to 8 ounces) of water. Let the tablet soak in water for 2 to 5 minutes and then stir until completely dissolved.

For patients using the *capsule form* of this medicine:

- *Do not swallow the capsule*. Before taking, mix the contents of 1 capsule in one-third glass (about 2½ ounces) of water or juice or the contents of 2 capsules in two-thirds glass (about 5 ounces) of water and stir well until dissolved.

For patients using the *powder form* of this medicine:

- Add the entire contents of 1 bottle (2¼ ounces) to enough warm water to make 1 gallon of solution *or* the contents of one packet to enough warm water to make

⅓ of a glass (about 2.5 ounces) of solution. Shake the container for 2 or 3 minutes or until all the powder is dissolved.

- Do not dilute solution further.
- This solution may be chilled to improve the flavor; do not allow it to freeze.
- Discard unused solution after 60 days.

Take this medicine immediately after meals or with food to lessen possible stomach upset or laxative action.

To help prevent kidney stones, *drink at least a full glass (8 ounces) of water every hour during waking hours,* unless otherwise directed by your health care professional.

Take this medicine only as directed. Do not take more of it and do not take it more often than recommended on the label, unless otherwise directed by your health care professional.

Dosing—The dose of these single or combination medicines will be different for different patients. *Follow your health care professional's orders or the directions on the label.* The following information includes only the average doses of these medicines. *If your dose is different, do not change it* unless your health care professional tells you to do so.

The number of teaspoonfuls or ounces of prepared solution that you drink depends on the equivalent amount of phosphorus contained in the product. Also, *the number of doses you take each day, the time allowed between doses, and the length of time you take the medicine depend on the medical problem for which you are taking the single or combination medicine.*

For potassium phosphates
- For *tablets for oral solution* dosage form:
  - To replace phosphorus lost by the body or to make the urine more acid or to prevent the formation of kidney stones in the urinary tract:
    - Adults and teenagers—The equivalent of 228 milligrams (mg) of phosphorus (2 tablets) dissolved in six to eight ounces of water four times a day, with meals and at bedtime.
  - To replace phosphorus lost by the body:
    - Children over 4 years of age—The equivalent of 228 mg of phosphorus (2 tablets) dissolved in six to eight ounces of water four times a day, with meals and at bedtime.
    - Children up to 4 years of age—The dose must be determined by your doctor.
- For *capsules for oral solution* dosage form:
  - To replace phosphorus lost by the body:
    - Adults, teenagers, and children over 4 years of age—The equivalent of 250 mg of phosphorus (contents of 1 capsule) dissolved in two and one-half ounces of water or juice four times a day, after meals and at bedtime.
    - Children up to 4 years of age—Dose must be determined by your doctor.
- For *powder for oral solution* dosage form:
  - To replace phosphorus lost by the body:
    - Adults, teenagers, and children over 4 years of age—The equivalent of 250 mg of phosphorus dissolved in two and one-half ounces of water four times a day, after meals and at bedtime.
    - Children up to 4 years of age—Dose must be determined by your doctor.

For potassium and sodium phosphates
- For *tablets for oral solution* dosage form:
  - To replace phosphorus lost by the body or to make the urine more acid or to prevent the formation of kidney stones in the urinary tract:
    - Adults and teenagers—The equivalent of 250 milligrams (mg) of phosphorus dissolved in eight ounces of water four times a day, after meals and at bedtime.
  - To replace phosphorus lost by the body:
    - Children over 4 years of age—The equivalent of 250 mg of phosphorus dissolved in eight ounces of water four times a day, after meals and at bedtime.
    - Children up to 4 years of age—Dose must be determined by your doctor.
- For *capsules for oral solution* dosage form:
  - To replace phosphorus lost by the body:
    - Adults, teenagers, and children over 4 years of age—The equivalent of 250 mg of phosphorus (the contents of 1 capsule) dissolved in two and one-half ounces of water or juice four times a day, after meals and at bedtime.
    - Children up to 4 years of age—Dose must be determined by your doctor.
- For *powder for oral solution* dosage form:
  - To replace phosphorus lost by the body:
    - Adults, teenagers, and children over 4 years of age—The equivalent of 250 mg of phosphorus dissolved in two and one-half ounces of water four times a day, after meals and at bedtime.
    - Children up to 4 years of age—Dose must be determined by your doctor.
- For *tablets for oral solution* dosage form:
  - To replace phosphorus lost by the body:
    - Adults, teenagers, and children over 4 years of age—The equivalent of 250 mg of phosphorus (1 tablet) dissolved in eight ounces of water four times a day.
    - Children up to 4 years of age—Dose must be determined by your doctor.

Missed dose—If you miss a dose of this medicine, take it as soon as possible. However, if it is within 1 or 2 hours of your next dose, skip the missed dose and go back to your regular dosing schedule. Do not double doses.

Storage—To store this medicine:
- Keep out of the reach of children.
- Store away from heat and direct light.
- Do not store the capsule, tablet, or powder form of this medicine in the bathroom, near the kitchen sink, or in other damp places. Heat or moisture may cause the medicine to break down.
- Keep the liquid form of this medicine from freezing.
- Do not keep outdated medicine or medicine no longer needed. Be sure that any discarded medicine is out of the reach of children.

Precautions While Using This Medicine

Your health care professional should check your progress at regular visits to make sure that this medicine does not cause unwanted effects.

Do not take iron supplements within 1 to 2 hours of taking this medicine. To do so may keep the iron from working properly.

For patients taking potassium phosphate-containing medicines:
- Check with your health care professional before starting any strenuous physical exercise, especially if you are out of condition and are taking other medication. Exercise and certain medicines may increase the amount of potassium in the blood.

For patients on a *potassium-restricted diet:*
- This medicine may contain a large amount of potassium. If you have any questions about this, check with your health care professional.
- Do not use salt substitutes and low-salt milk unless told to do so by your health care professional. They may contain potassium.

For patients on a sodium-restricted diet:
- This medicine may contain a large amount of sodium. If you have any questions about this, check with your health care professional.

Side Effects of This Medicine

Along with its needed effects, a medicine may cause some unwanted effects. Although not all of these side effects may occur, if they do occur they may need medical attention.

Check with your health care professional as soon as possible if any of the following side effects occur:
Less common or rare
 Confusion; convulsions (seizures); decrease in amount of urine or in frequency of urination; fast, slow, or irregular heartbeat; headache or dizziness; increased thirst; muscle cramps; numbness, tingling, pain, or weakness in hands or feet; numbness or tingling around lips; shortness of breath or troubled breathing; swelling of feet or lower legs; tremor; unexplained anxiety; unusual tiredness or weakness; weakness or heaviness of legs; weight gain

Other side effects may occur that usually do not need medical attention. These side effects may go away during treatment as your body adjusts to the medicine. However, check with your health care professional if any of the following side effects continue or are bothersome:
 Diarrhea; nausea or vomiting; stomach pain

Other side effects not listed above may also occur in some patients. If you notice any other effects, check with your health care professional.

PILOCARPINE (Ophthalmic route) -
pye-loe-KAR-peen

Commonly used brand name(s)
In the U.S.—
 Isopto Carpine Pilocar
 Ocu-Carpine Pilopine-HS
 Ocusert Pilo

In Canada—
 Minims Pilocarpine 2%
 Minims Pilocarpine 4%

Available Dosage Forms:
- Device
- Suspension
- Solution
- Gel/Jelly

Therapeutic Class: Direct Acting Miotic
Pharmacologic Class: Cholinergic

Uses For This Medicine

Pilocarpine is used to treat glaucoma and other eye conditions.

This medicine is available only with your doctor's prescription.

Before Using This Medicine

In deciding to use a medicine, the risks of taking the medicine must be weighed against the good it will do. This is a decision you and your doctor will make. For this medicine, the following should be considered:

Allergies—Tell your doctor if you have ever had any unusual or allergic reaction to this medicine or any other medicines. Also tell your health care professional if you have any other types of allergies, such as to foods, dyes, preservatives, or animals. For non-prescription products, read the label or package ingredients carefully.

Pediatric—Although there is no specific information comparing use of this medicine in children with use in other age groups, pilocarpine is not expected to cause different side effects or problems in children than it does in adults.

Geriatric—Many medicines have not been studied specifically in older people. Therefore, it may not be known whether they work exactly the same way they do in younger adults or if they cause different side effects or problems in older people. Although there is no specific information comparing use of pilocarpine in the elderly with use in other age groups, this medicine is not expected to cause different side effects or problems in older people than it does in younger adults.

Pregnancy—

	Pregnancy Category	Explanation
All Trimesters	C	Animal studies have shown an adverse effect and there are no adequate studies in pregnant women OR no animal studies have been conducted and there are no adequate studies in pregnant women.

Breast Feeding—There are no adequate studies in women for determining infant risk when using this medication during breastfeeding. Weigh the potential benefits against the potential risks before taking this medication while breastfeeding.

Other medicines—Although certain medicines should not be used together at all, in other cases two different medicines may be used together even if an interaction might occur. In these cases, your doctor may want to change the dose, or other precautions may be necessary. Tell your healthcare professional if you are taking any other prescription or non-prescription (over-the-counter [OTC]) medicine.

Interactions with Food/Tobacco/Alcohol—Certain medicines should not be used at or around the time of eating food or eating certain types of food since interactions may occur. Using alcohol or tobacco with certain medicines may also cause interactions to occur. Discuss with your healthcare

professional the use of your medicine with food, alcohol, or tobacco.

Other medical problems—The presence of other medical problems may affect the use of this medicine. Make sure you tell your doctor if you have any other medical problems, especially:

- Asthma or
- Eye disease or problems (other)—Pilocarpine may make the condition worse

Proper Use of This Medicine

To use the eye drop form of pilocarpine:

- First, wash your hands. Tilt the head back and, pressing your finger gently on the skin just beneath the lower eyelid, pull the lower eyelid away from the eye to make a space. Drop the medicine into this space. Let go of the eyelid and gently close the eyes. Do not blink. Keep the eyes closed and apply pressure to the inner corner of the eye with your finger for 1 or 2 minutes to allow the medicine to be absorbed by the eye.
- Immediately after using the eye drops, wash your hands to remove any medicine that may be on them.
- To keep the medicine as germ-free as possible, do not touch the applicator tip to any surface (including the eye). Also, keep the container tightly closed.

To use the eye gel form of pilocarpine:

- First, wash your hands. Tilt the head back and, pressing your finger gently on the skin just beneath the lower eyelid, pull the lower eyelid away from the eye to make a space. Squeeze a thin strip of gel into this space. A 1½-cm (approximately ½-inch) strip of gel is usually enough, unless you have been told by your doctor to use a different amount. Let go of the eyelid and gently close the eyes. Keep the eyes closed for 1 or 2 minutes to allow the medicine to be absorbed by the eye.
- Immediately after using the eye gel, wash your hands to remove any medicine that may be on them.
- To keep the medicine as germ-free as possible, do not touch the applicator tip to any surface (including the eye). After using the eye gel, wipe the tip of the gel tube with a clean tissue and keep the tube tightly closed.

To use the eye insert form of pilocarpine:

- This medicine usually comes with patient directions. Read them carefully before using this medicine.
- If you think this medicine unit may be damaged, do not use it. If you have any questions about this, check with your health care professional.
- If the unit seems to be releasing too much medicine into your eye, remove it and replace with a new unit. If you have any questions about this, check with your doctor.

Use this medicine only as directed. Do not use more of it and do not use it more often than your doctor ordered. To do so may increase the chance of too much medicine being absorbed into the body and the chance of side effects.

Dosing—The dose of this medicine will be different for different patients. Follow your doctor's orders or the directions on the label. The following information includes only the average doses of this medicine. If your dose is different, do not change it unless your doctor tells you to do so.

The amount of medicine that you take depends on the strength of the medicine. Also, the number of doses you take each day, the time allowed between doses, and the length of time you take the medicine depend on the medical problem for which you are using the medicine.

- For eye drop dosage form:
  - For chronic glaucoma:
    - Adults and children—One drop one to four times a day.
  - For acute angle-closure glaucoma:
    - Adults and children—One drop every five to ten minutes for three to six doses. Then one drop every one to three hours until eye pressure is reduced.
- For eye gel dosage form:
  - For glaucoma:
    - Adults and teenagers—Use once a day at bedtime.
    - Children—Use and dose must be determined by your doctor.
- For eye insert dosage form:
  - For glaucoma:
    - Adults and children—Insert one ocular system every seven days.
    - Infants—Use and dose must be determined by your doctor.

Missed dose—If you miss a dose of this medicine, take it as soon as possible. However, if it is almost time for your next dose, skip the missed dose and go back to your regular dosing schedule. Do not double doses.

Storage—Keep out of the reach of children.

Do not keep outdated medicine or medicine no longer needed.

Store the eye system form of this medicine in the refrigerator. Keep from freezing. Store the 3.5–gram size (of the gel form) at room temperature.

Precautions While Using This Medicine

Your doctor should check your eye pressure at regular visits.

For patients using the eye drop or gel form of this medicine:

- For a short time after you use this medicine, your vision may be blurred or there may be a change in your near or far vision, especially at night. Make sure your vision is clear before you drive, use machines, or do anything else that could be dangerous if you are not able to see well.

For patients using the eye insert form of this medicine:

- For the first several hours after you insert this unit in the eye, your vision may be blurred or there may be a change in your near or far vision, especially at night. Therefore, insert this unit in the eye at bedtime, unless otherwise directed by your doctor. If this unit is inserted in the eye at any other time of the day, make sure your vision is clear before you drive, use machines, or do anything else that could be dangerous if you are not able to see well.

Side Effects of This Medicine

Along with its needed effects, a medicine may cause some unwanted effects. Although not all of these side effects may occur, if they do occur they may need medical attention.

Check with your doctor as soon as possible if any of the following side effects occur:

Symptoms of too much medicine being absorbed into the body

Increased sweating; muscle tremors; nausea, vomiting, or diarrhea; troubled breathing or wheezing; watering of mouth

Less common or rare
Eye pain

Some side effects may occur that usually do not need medical attention. These side effects may go away during treatment as your body adjusts to the medicine. Also, your health care professional may be able to tell you about ways to prevent or reduce some of these side effects. Check with your health care professional if any of the following side effects continue or are bothersome or if you have any questions about them:

More common
Blurred vision or change in near or far vision; decrease in night vision

Less common
Eye irritation; headache or browache

Other side effects not listed may also occur in some patients. If you notice any other effects, check with your healthcare professional.

PIMECROLIMUS   (Topical route) - pim-e-KROE-li-mus

Black Box Warning

Long-term safety of topical calcineurin inhibitors has not been established. Although a causal relationship has not been established, rare cases of malignancy (e.g., skin and lymphoma) have been reported in patients treated with topical calcineurin inhibitors, including pimecrolimus cream. Therefore:

Continuous long-term use of topical calcineurin inhibitors, including pimecrolimus cream, in any age group should be avoided, and application limited to areas of involvement with atopic dermatitis. Pimecrolimus cream is not indicated for use in children less than 2 years of age.

Commonly used brand name(s)

In the U.S.—
Elidel

Available Dosage Forms:
• Cream

Therapeutic Class: Dermatological Agent

Uses For This Medicine

Pimecrolimus cream is used for mild to moderate atopic dermatitis. This is a skin condition where there is itching, redness and inflammation, much like an allergic reaction. Pimecrolimus helps to suppress these symptoms which are a reaction caused by the body's immune system. It can be used for short-term or long-term periodic treatment (not beyond one year). It is often used when other types of treatment are either not working or when you cannot tolerate other types of treatment.

Pimecrolimus is available only with your doctor's prescription.

Once a medicine has been approved for marketing for a certain use, experience may show that it is also useful for other medical problems. Although this use is not included in product labeling, pimecrolimus is used in certain patients with the following medical condition:
• Atopic dermatitis in children less than 2 years of age

Before Using This Medicine

In deciding to use a medicine, the risks of taking the medicine must be weighed against the good it will do. This is a decision you and your doctor will make. For this medicine, the following should be considered:

Allergies—Tell your doctor if you have ever had any unusual or allergic reaction to this medicine or any other medicines. Also tell your health care professional if you have any other types of allergies, such as to foods, dyes, preservatives, or animals. For non-prescription products, read the label or package ingredients carefully.

Pediatric—This medicine is not known to cause different types of side effects or problems in children over the age of two, than it does in adults, although some side effects may occur more often than they do in adult patients. This medicine has not been tested and should not be used in children under 2 years of age.

Geriatric—There is no specific information comparing the use of pimecrolimus in the elderly with the use in other age groups. Pimecrolimus is not expected to cause different side effects or problems in older people than it does in younger adults.

Pregnancy—

	Pregnancy Category	Explanation
All Trimesters	C	Animal studies have shown an adverse effect and there are no adequate studies in pregnant women OR no animal studies have been conducted and there are no adequate studies in pregnant women.

Breast Feeding—There are no adequate studies in women for determining infant risk when using this medication during breastfeeding. Weigh the potential benefits against the potential risks before taking this medication while breastfeeding.

Other medicines—Although certain medicines should not be used together at all, in other cases two different medicines may be used together even if an interaction might occur. In these cases, your doctor may want to change the dose, or other precautions may be necessary. Tell your healthcare professional if you are taking any other prescription or non-prescription (over-the-counter [OTC]) medicine.

Interactions with Food/Tobacco/Alcohol—Certain medicines should not be used at or around the time of eating food or eating certain types of food since interactions may occur. Using alcohol or tobacco with certain medicines may also cause interactions to occur. Discuss with your healthcare professional the use of your medicine with food, alcohol, or tobacco.

Other medical problems—The presence of other medical problems may affect the use of this medicine. Make sure you tell your doctor if you have any other medical problems, especially:
• Eczema herpeticum (Kaposi's varicelliform eruption), or
• Herpes simplex virus infection or

- Varicella zoster virus infection (chicken pox or shingles)—Increases the risk of skin infections
- Erythroderma (exfoliative dermatitis [ED])—The safety of this medicine is not known for patients who have this condition.
- Immunocompromised patients (weakened immune system)—The safety of these patients using pimecrolimus cream has not been established.
- Lymphadenopathy or
- Mononucleosis, acute infectious—May cause enlargement of lymph nodes
- Netherton's syndrome—May cause too much of the pimecrolimus cream to be absorbed into the body
- Precancerous condition of the skin or
- Skin cancer—You should not use this medicine.
- Skin infections—Safety of using pimecrolimus cream for some skin infections is unknown.
- Skin papilloma or
- Warts—May worsen condition

Proper Use of This Medicine

Dosing—The dose of this medicine will be different for different patients. Follow your doctor's orders or the directions on the label. The following information includes only the average doses of this medicine. If your dose is different, do not change it unless your doctor tells you to do so.

The amount of medicine that you take depends on the strength of the medicine. Also, the number of doses you take each day, the time allowed between doses, and the length of time you take the medicine depend on the medical problem for which you are using the medicine.

Infections in the affected areas should be treated before starting treatment with pimecrolimus cream.

Apply a thin layer of pimecrolimus cream and rub it in well to cover the affected areas.

Do not use this medicine in the eyes and do not swallow it.

Wash hands thoroughly after applying pimecrolimus cream, unless your hands are part of the area for treatment.

Use of this medicine may cause reactions at the site of application such as a mild to moderate feeling of warmth and/or sensation of burning. You should contact your doctor if this reaction is severe or persists for more than 1 week.

While using pimecrolimus, if symptoms of your skin condition go away, consult your doctor.

If after your doctor tells you to stop using pimecrolimus, your skin condition reoccurs, consult your doctor.

Do not use any occlusive dressings (a dressing that seals the area that is being treated such as a plastic exercise suit or plastic wraps used to store foods).

Do not bathe, shower or swim right after applying this medicine. This could wash off the cream.

- For cream dosage form
  - For atopic dermatitis
    - Adults—Gently apply cream to skin that is clean and dry two times a day. Stop using when the signs and symptoms of eczema, such as itching, rash, and redness go away, as directed by your doctor.
    - Children over 2 years old—Gently apply cream to skin that is clean and dry two times a day. Stop using when the signs and symptoms of eczema, such as itching, rash, and redness go away, as directed by your doctor.
    - Children under 2 years of age—Use and dose must be determined by your doctor.

Storage—Store the medicine in a closed container at room temperature, away from heat, moisture, and direct light. Keep from freezing.

Keep out of the reach of children.

Do not keep outdated medicine or medicine no longer needed.

Ask your healthcare professional how you should dispose of any medicine you do not use.

Precautions While Using This Medicine

It is very important that your doctor check your progress at regular visits. Your doctor will want to make sure the pimecrolimus cream is working properly and to check for unwanted effects. If your condition has not improved after 6 weeks, your doctor will want to reexamine you.

Report any adverse reactions or side effects to your doctor or if your skin condition seems to be getting worse.

Use this medicine only for the condition for which it was prescribed by your doctor.

You should not use this medicine beyond a year.

Exposure to natural or artificial sunlight should be minimized or avoided.

- Stay out of direct sunlight, especially between the hours of 10:00 a.m. and 3:00 p.m., if possible.
- Wear protective clothing, including a hat. Also, wear sunglasses.
- Apply a sun block product that has a skin protection factor (SPF) of at least 15. Some people may require a product with a higher SPF number, especially if they have a fair complexion. If you have any questions about this, check with your health care professional.
- Apply a sun block lipstick that has an SPF of at least 15 to protect your lips.
- Do not use a sunlamp or tanning bed or booth.

Side Effects of This Medicine

Along with its needed effects, a medicine may cause some unwanted effects. Although not all of these side effects may occur, if they do occur they may need medical attention.

Check with your doctor as soon as possible if any of the following side effects occur:

More common
    Abdominal or stomach pain; body aches or pain; burning, itching, redness, skin rash, swelling, or soreness at site; change in hearing; chills; cold or flu-like symptoms; congestion, ear or nasal; cough producing mucus; diarrhea; difficulty breathing or shortness of breath; dryness or soreness of throat; earache or pain in ear; ear drainage; fever; general feeling of discomfort or illness; headache; hoarseness; itching; joint pain; loss of appetite; loss of voice; muscle aches and pains; nausea; pain; redness; runny nose; shivering; sneezing; sore throat; sweating; swelling; tenderness; tender,

swollen glands in neck; tightness in chest, wheezing; trouble in swallowing; trouble sleeping; unusual tiredness or weakness; voice changes; vomiting; warmth on skin

Less common

Blistering, crusting, irritation, itching, or reddening of skin; blurred vision or other change in vision; eye pain; fast heartbeat; hives; hives or welts, itching, redness of skin; hoarseness; itching; itchy, raised, round, smooth, skin-colored bumps found on just one area of the body that are oozing, thick, white fluid; irritation; joint pain, stiffness or swelling; rash; redness of eye; redness of skin; sensitivity of eye to light; shortness of breath; skin rash on face, scalp, or stomach; swelling of eyelids, face, lips, hands, or feet; tearing; tightness in chest; troubled breathing or swallowing; wheezing

Incidence not known

Black, tarry stools; change in size, shape or color of existing mole; cough; dizziness; itching, puffiness or swelling of the eyelids or around the eyes, face, lips or tongue; large, hive-like swelling on face; mole that leaks fluid or bleeds; new mole; skin rash; small, red skin lesion, growth, or bump usually on face, ears, neck, hands or arms; sores that will not heal; swelling or puffiness of face; unusual tiredness or weakness; weight loss; yellow skin and eyes

Some side effects may occur that usually do not need medical attention. These side effects may go away during treatment as your body adjusts to the medicine. Also, your health care professional may be able to tell you about ways to prevent or reduce some of these side effects. Check with your health care professional if any of the following side effects continue or are bothersome or if you have any questions about them:

More common

Burning, itching, and pain in hairy areas, pus at root of hair

Less common

Blemishes on the skin; pimples; bloody nose; burning or stinging of skin; difficulty having a bowel movement (stool); earache, redness or swelling in ear; flushing; redness of skin; unusually warm skin at site; painful cold sores or blisters on lips, nose, eyes, or genitals; vaginal pain and cramps, heavy bleeding

Incidence not known

Burning, stinging, itching or mild discomfort of the eye (after applying the cream to eyelids or near eyes); feeling of warmth (with alcohol use); redness of the face, neck, arms and occasionally, upper chest (with alcohol use)

PIMOZIDE (Oral route) - PI-moe-zide

Commonly used brand name(s)

In the U.S.—

Orap

Available Dosage Forms:

- Tablet

Therapeutic Class: Antipsychotic
Pharmacologic Class: Dopamine Antagonist

Uses For This Medicine

Pimozide is used to treat the symptoms of Tourette's syndrome. It is meant only for patients with severe symptoms who cannot take or have not been helped by other medicine.

Pimozide works in the central nervous system to help control the vocal outbursts and uncontrolled, repeated movements of the body (tics) that interfere with normal life. It will not completely cure the tics, but will help to reduce their number and severity.

Pimozide may also be used for other conditions as determined by your doctor.

This medicine is available only with your doctor's prescription.

Once a medicine has been approved for marketing for a certain use, experience may show that it is also useful for other medical problems. Although this use is not included in product labeling, pimozide is used in certain patients with the following medical condition:

- Psychotic disorders, such as schizophrenia

Before Using This Medicine

In deciding to use a medicine, the risks of taking the medicine must be weighed against the good it will do. This is a decision you and your doctor will make. For this medicine, the following should be considered:

Allergies—Tell your doctor if you have ever had any unusual or allergic reaction to this medicine or any other medicines. Also tell your health care professional if you have any other types of allergies, such as to foods, dyes, preservatives, or animals. For non-prescription products, read the label or package ingredients carefully.

Pediatric—Children are especially sensitive to the effects of pimozide. This may increase the chance of side effects during treatment. Pimozide usually is not used in children for any condition other than Tourette's syndrome.

Geriatric—Constipation, dizziness or fainting, drowsiness, dryness of mouth, and trembling of the hands and fingers, and symptoms of tardive dyskinesia (such as rapid, worm-like movements of the tongue or any other uncontrolled movements of the mouth, tongue, or jaw, and/or arms and legs) may be especially likely to occur in the elderly, who are usually more sensitive than younger adults to the effects of pimozide.

Pregnancy—

	Pregnancy Category	Explanation
All Trimesters	C	Animal studies have shown an adverse effect and there are no adequate studies in pregnant women OR no animal studies have been conducted and there are no adequate studies in pregnant women.

Breast Feeding—There are no adequate studies in women for determining infant risk when using this medication during breastfeeding. Weigh the potential benefits against the potential risks before taking this medication while breastfeeding.

Other medicines—

Using this medicine with any of the following medicines is not recommended. Your doctor may decide not to treat you with

this medication or change some of the other medicines you take.

Acecainide, Ajmaline, Amiodarone, Amisulpride, Amitriptyline, Amoxapine, Amprenavir, Aprepitant, Aprindine, Arsenic Trioxide, Astemizole, Atazanavir, Azimilide, Azithromycin, Bepridil, Bretylium, Chloral Hydrate, Chloroquine, Chlorpromazine, Cisapride, Clarithromycin, Dalfopristin, Darunavir, Delavirdine, Desipramine, Dibenzepin, Dirithromycin, Disopyramide, Dofetilide, Dolasetron, Doxepin, Droperidol, Encainide, Enflurane, Erythromycin, Flecainide, Fluconazole, Fluoxetine, Fosamprenavir, Foscarnet, Gemifloxacin, Halofantrine, Haloperidol, Halothane, Hydroquinidine, Ibutilide, Imipramine, Indinavir, Isoflurane, Isradipine, Itraconazole, Ketoconazole, Levomethadyl, Lidoflazine, Lorcainide, Mefloquine, Mesoridazine, Miconazole, Nefazodone, Nelfinavir, Nortriptyline, Octreotide, Ondansetron, Paroxetine, Pentamidine, Pirmenol, Prajmaline, Probucol, Procainamide, Prochlorperazine, Propafenone, Protriptyline, Quinidine, Quinupristin, Risperidone, Ritonavir, Roxithromycin, Saquinavir, Sematilide, Sertindole, Sertraline, Sotalol, Spiramycin, Sulfamethoxazole, Sultopride, Tedisamil, Telithromycin, Terfenadine, Thioridazine, Tipranavir, Trifluoperazine, Trimethoprim, Trimipramine, Troleandomycin, Vasopressin, Venlafaxine, Voriconazole, Ziprasidone, Zolmitriptan, Zotepine

Interactions with Food/Tobacco/Alcohol—Certain medicines should not be used at or around the time of eating food or eating certain types of food since interactions may occur. Using alcohol or tobacco with certain medicines may also cause interactions to occur. The following interactions have been selected on the basis of their potential significance and are not necessarily all-inclusive.

Using this medicine with any of the following is usually not recommended, but may be unavoidable in some cases. If used together, your doctor may change the dose or how often you use this medicine, or give you special instructions about the use of food, alcohol, or tobacco.

Grapefruit Juice

Other medical problems—The presence of other medical problems may affect the use of this medicine. Make sure you tell your doctor if you have any other medical problems, especially:

- Breast cancer (history of) or
- Glaucoma, narrow angle or
- Heart disease or
- Intestinal blockage or
- Urinary tract blockage or difficult urination—Pimozide may make the condition worse
- Kidney disease or
- Liver disease—Higher blood levels of pimozide may occur, increasing the chance of side effects
- Low blood potassium—Pimozide may increase the chance of developing serious changes in heart rhythm
- Seizures, history of—Pimozide may increase the chance of having seizures
- Tics other than those caused by Tourette's syndrome—Pimozide should not be used because of the risk of serious side effects

Proper Use of This Medicine

Use pimozide only as directed by your doctor. Do not use more of it, do not use it more often, and do not use it for a longer time than your doctor ordered. To do so may increase the chance of side effects.

It is very important that you do not take pimozide with grapefruit juice. Studies have shown that taking pimozide with grapefruit juice may cause heart rhythm problems.

Dosing—The dose of this medicine will be different for different patients. Follow your doctor's orders or the directions on the label. The following information includes only the average doses of this medicine. If your dose is different, do not change it unless your doctor tells you to do so.

The amount of medicine that you take depends on the strength of the medicine. Also, the number of doses you take each day, the time allowed between doses, and the length of time you take the medicine depend on the medical problem for which you are using the medicine.

- For oral dosage form (tablets):
  - For Tourette's syndrome:
    - Adults—To start, 1 to 2 milligrams (mg) a day. Your doctor may increase your dose if needed. However, the dose is usually not more than 10 mg a day.
    - Children up to 12 years of age—Dose must be determined by the doctor.
    - Children 12 years of age and older—To start, 0.05 mg per kilogram (0.023 mg per pound) of body weight a day. Your doctor may increase your dose if needed. However, the dose is usually not more than 10 mg a day.

Missed dose—If you miss a dose of this medicine, skip the missed dose and go back to your regular dosing schedule. Do not double doses.

Storage—Store the medicine in a closed container at room temperature, away from heat, moisture, and direct light. Keep from freezing.

Keep out of the reach of children.

Do not keep outdated medicine or medicine no longer needed.

Precautions While Using This Medicine

Your doctor should check your progress at regular visits, especially during the first few months of treatment with this medicine. The amount of pimozide you take may be changed often to meet the needs of your condition and to help avoid unwanted effects.

Do not take azithromycin, clarithromycin, dirithromycin, disopyramide, erythromycin, indinavir, itraconazole, ketoconazole, maprotiline, nefazodone, nelfinavir, phenothiazines, probucol, procainamide, quinidine, ritonavir, saquinavir, tricyclic antidepressants, troleandomycin, or zileuton while you are taking pimozide, or you may develop a very serious irregular heartbeat.

Do not suddenly stop taking this medicine without first checking with your doctor. Your doctor may want you to reduce gradually the amount you are taking before stopping completely. This will allow your body time to adjust and help to avoid worsening of your medical condition.

This medicine will add to the effects of alcohol and other CNS depressants (medicines that slow down the nervous system, possibly causing drowsiness). Some examples of CNS depressants are antihistamines or medicine for hay fever, other allergies, or colds; sedatives, tranquilizers, or sleeping medicine; prescription pain medicine or narcotics; barbiturates;

medicine for seizures; muscle relaxants; or anesthetics, including some dental anesthetics. Check with your doctor before taking any of the above while you are using this medicine.

This medicine may cause some people to become drowsy or less alert or to have blurred vision or muscle stiffness, especially as the amount of medicine is increased. Even if you take pimozide at bedtime, you may feel drowsy or less alert on arising. Make sure you know how you react to this medicine before you drive, use machines, or do anything else that could be dangerous if you are not alert or able to see well or if you do not have good muscle control.

Although not a problem for many patients, dizziness, lightheadedness, or fainting may occur when you get up from a sitting or lying position. Getting up slowly may help. If the problem continues or gets worse, check with your doctor.

Before having any kind of surgery, dental treatment, or emergency treatment, tell the medical doctor or dentist in charge that you are using this medicine. Taking pimozide together with medicines that are used during surgery or dental or emergency treatment may increase the CNS depressant effects.

Pimozide may cause dryness of the mouth. For temporary relief, use sugarless gum or candy, melt bits of ice in your mouth, or use a saliva substitute. However, if your mouth continues to feel dry for more than 2 weeks, check with your medical doctor or dentist. Continuing dryness of the mouth may increase the chance of dental disease, including tooth decay, gum disease, and fungus infections.

Side Effects of This Medicine

Along with its needed effects, pimozide can sometimes cause serious unwanted effects. Tardive dyskinesia (a movement disorder) may occur and may not go away after you stop using the medicine. Signs of tardive dyskinesia include fine, worm-like movements of the tongue, or other uncontrolled movements of the mouth, tongue, cheeks, jaw, or arms and legs. Other serious but rare side effects, such as abnormal heart rhythm or the neuroleptic malignant syndrome, may also occur. You and your doctor should discuss the good this medicine will do as well as the risks of taking it.

Stop taking this medicine and get emergency help immediately if any of the following effects occur:
Rare—Signs of the neuroleptic malignant syndrome (usually two or more occur together)
    Convulsions (seizures); difficult or unusually fast breathing; fast heartbeat or irregular pulse; fever (high); high or low (irregular) blood pressure; increased sweating; loss of bladder control; muscle stiffness (severe)
Symptoms of overdose
    Coma; convulsions (seizures); dizziness (severe); muscle trembling, jerking, or stiffness (severe); troubled breathing (severe); uncontrolled movements (severe)

Check with your doctor as soon as possible if any of the following side effects occur:
More common
    Difficulty in speaking; dizziness or fainting; fast or irregular heartbeat; loss of balance control; lack of facial expression; mood or behavior changes; restlessness or need to keep moving; shuffling walk; slowed movements; stiffness of arms and legs; swelling or soreness of breasts (less common in males); trembling and shaking of fingers and hands; unusual secretion of milk (rare in males)
Less common or rare
    Difficulty in swallowing; inability to move eyes; increased blinking or spasms of eyelid; lip smacking or puckering; menstrual changes; muscle spasms, especially of the face, neck, or back; puffing of cheeks; rapid or worm-like movements of tongue; skin rash and itching; sore throat and fever; swelling of face; uncontrolled chewing movements; uncontrolled movements of neck, trunk, arms, or legs, including twisting movements; unusual bleeding or bruising; unusual facial expressions or body positions; yellow eyes or skin

Some side effects may occur that usually do not need medical attention. These side effects may go away during treatment as your body adjusts to the medicine. Also, your health care professional may be able to tell you about ways to prevent or reduce some of these side effects. Check with your health care professional if any of the following side effects continue or are bothersome or if you have any questions about them:
More common
    Blurred vision or other vision problems; constipation; dizziness, lightheadedness, or fainting when getting up from a lying or sitting position; drowsiness; dryness of mouth; skin discoloration
Less common
    Decreased sexual ability; diarrhea; headache; loss of appetite and weight; mental depression; nausea and vomiting; tiredness or weakness

After you stop using this medicine, it may still produce some side effects that need attention. During this period of time, *check with your doctor immediately* if you notice the following side effects:
    Lip smacking or puckering; puffing of cheeks; rapid or worm-like movements of the tongue; uncontrolled chewing movements; uncontrolled movements of the arms and legs

Other side effects not listed may also occur in some patients. If you notice any other effects, check with your healthcare professional.

PIOGLITAZONE   (Oral route) - pye-oh-GLI-ta-zone

Commonly used brand name(s)
In the U.S.—
    Actos

Available Dosage Forms:
  • Tablet

Therapeutic Class: Antidiabetic

Uses For This Medicine

Pioglitazone is used to treat a certain type of diabetes mellitus (sugar diabetes) called type 2 diabetes. It may be used alone, with insulin, or with metformin or another type of oral diabetes medicine called a sulfonylurea. Pioglitazone is to be used when diet and exercise plus another diabetes medicine do not result in good blood sugar control.

This medicine is available only with your doctor's prescription.

Before Using This Medicine

In deciding to use a medicine, the risks of taking the medicine must be weighed against the good it will do. This is a decision you and your doctor will make. For this medicine, the following should be considered:

Allergies—Tell your doctor if you have ever had any unusual or allergic reaction to this medicine or any other medicines. Also tell your health care professional if you have any other types of allergies, such as to foods, dyes, preservatives, or animals. For non-prescription products, read the label or package ingredients carefully.

Pediatric—Studies on this medicine have been done only in adult patients, and there is no specific information comparing use of pioglitazone in children with use in other age groups.

Geriatric—This medicine has been tested in a limited number of patients 65 years of age or older and has not been shown to cause different side effects or problems in older people than it does in younger adults. In a post-marketing safety study, patients over 64 years of age were shown to be more affected by heart failure requiring them to be hospitalized when compared with others in the study.

Pregnancy—

	Pregnancy Category	Explanation
All Trimesters	C	Animal studies have shown an adverse effect and there are no adequate studies in pregnant women OR no animal studies have been conducted and there are no adequate studies in pregnant women.

Breast Feeding—There are no adequate studies in women for determining infant risk when using this medication during breastfeeding. Weigh the potential benefits against the potential risks before taking this medication while breastfeeding.

Other medicines—

Using this medicine with any of the following medicines may cause an increased risk of certain side effects, but using both drugs may be the best treatment for you. If both medicines are prescribed together, your doctor may change the dose or how often you use one or both of the medicines.

Atorvastatin, Bitter Melon, Ethinyl Estradiol, Fenugreek, Glucomannan, Guar Gum, Ketoconazole, Levonorgestrel, Mestranol, Norethindrone, Norgestrel, Psyllium, St John's Wort, Topiramate

Interactions with Food/Tobacco/Alcohol—Certain medicines should not be used at or around the time of eating food or eating certain types of food since interactions may occur. Using alcohol or tobacco with certain medicines may also cause interactions to occur. Discuss with your healthcare professional the use of your medicine with food, alcohol, or tobacco.

Other medical problems—The presence of other medical problems may affect the use of this medicine. Make sure you tell your doctor if you have any other medical problems, especially:

- Heart disease or
- Liver disease—Pioglitazone may make these conditions worse
- Problems with fluid retention or swelling—May make these conditions worse
- Hypersensitivity to pioglitazone or any ingredients in pioglitazone.

Proper Use of This Medicine

Follow carefully the special meal plan your doctor gave you. This is the most important part of controlling your condition, and is necessary if the medicine is to work properly. Also, exercise regularly and test for sugar in your blood or urine as directed.

Pioglitazone may be taken with or without food.

Certain women may be at an increased risk for pregnancy while taking pioglitazone. Adequate contraception is recommended.

Dosing—The dose of this medicine will be different for different patients. Follow your doctor's orders or the directions on the label. The following information includes only the average doses of this medicine. If your dose is different, do not change it unless your doctor tells you to do so.

The amount of medicine that you take depends on the strength of the medicine. Also, the number of doses you take each day, the time allowed between doses, and the length of time you take the medicine depend on the medical problem for which you are using the medicine.

- For oral dosage form (tablets):
  - For type 2 diabetes:
    - Pioglitazone alone:
      — Adults: At first, the dose is 15 or 30 milligrams (mg) once daily with or without meals. Your doctor may later increase your dose up to 45 mg once daily.
      — Children: Use and dose must be determined by your doctor.
    - Pioglitazone with insulin:
      — Adults: At first, the dose is 15 or 30 mg once daily with or without meals.
      — Children: Use and dose must be determined by your doctor.
    - Pioglitazone with metformin:
      — Adults: At first, the dose is 15 or 30 mg once daily with or without meals.
      — Children: Use and dose must be determined by your doctor.
    - Pioglitazone with a sulfonylurea:
      — Adults: At first, the dose is 15 or 30 mg once daily with or without meals.
      — Children: Use and dose must be determined by your doctor.

Missed dose—If you miss a dose of this medicine, take it as soon as possible. However, if it is almost time for your next dose, skip the missed dose and go back to your regular dosing schedule. Do not double doses.

Storage—Store the medicine in a closed container at room temperature, away from heat, moisture, and direct light. Keep from freezing.

Keep out of the reach of children.

Do not keep outdated medicine or medicine no longer needed.

Ask your healthcare professional how you should dispose of any medicine you do not use.

Precautions While Using This Medicine

If you experience abdominal or stomach pain, dark urine, loss of appetite, nausea or vomiting, unusual tiredness or weakness, or yellow eyes or skin, check with your doctor immediately. These may be symptoms of liver problems.

It is very important that your doctor check your progress at regular visits to make sure that this medicine is working properly and to check for unwanted effects

It is very important to follow carefully any instructions from your health care team about

- Alcohol—Drinking alcohol may cause severe low blood sugar. Discuss this with your health care team.

- Other medicines—Do not take other medicines during the time you are taking pioglitazone unless they have been discussed with your doctor. This especially includes nonprescription medicines such as aspirin, and medicines for appetite control, asthma, colds, cough, hay fever, or sinus problems.

- Counseling—Other family members need to learn how to prevent side effects or help with side effects if they occur. Also, diabetic patients may need special counseling about diabetes medicine dosing changes that might occur because of lifestyle changes, such as changes in exercise and diet. Furthermore, counseling on contraception and pregnancy may be needed because of the problems that can occur during pregnancy in patients with diabetes.

- Travel—Keep a recent prescription and your medical history with you. Be prepared for an emergency as you would normally. Make allowances for changing time zones and keep your meal times as close as possible to your usual meal times.

- In case of emergency—There may be a time when you need emergency help for a problem caused by your diabetes. You need to be prepared for these emergencies. It is a good idea to wear a medical identification (ID) bracelet or neck chain at all times. Also, carry an ID card in your wallet or purse that says that you have diabetes and a list of all of your medicines.

- Symptoms of fluid retention—Know what to do if you start to retain fluid. Fluid retention may worsen or lead to heart problems.

- This medicine does not cause hypoglycemia (low blood sugar). However, low blood sugar can occur when you take pioglitazone with other medicines that can lower blood sugar, such as insulin, metformin, or a sulfonylurea. Low blood sugar also can occur if you delay or miss a meal or snack, exercise more than usual, drink alcohol, or cannot eat because of nausea or vomiting.

- Symptoms of low blood sugar include anxiety; behavior change similar to being drunk; blurred vision; cold sweats; confusion; cool, pale skin; difficulty in thinking; drowsiness; excessive hunger; fast heartbeat; headache (continuing); nausea; nervousness; nightmares; restless sleep; shakiness; slurred speech; or unusual tiredness or weakness.

- If symptoms of low blood sugar occur, eat glucose tablets or gel, corn syrup, honey, or sugar cubes; or drink fruit juice, nondiet soft drink, or sugar dissolved in water to relieve the symptoms. Also, check your blood for low blood sugar. Glucagon is used in emergency situations when severe symptoms such as seizures (convulsions) or unconsciousness occur. Have a glucagon kit available, along with a syringe and needle, and know how to use it. Members of your family also should know how to use it.

Hyperglycemia (high blood sugar) may occur if you do not take enough or skip a dose of your antidiabetic medicine, overeat or do not follow your meal plan, have a fever or infection, or do not exercise as much as usual.

Symptoms of high blood sugar include blurred vision; drowsiness; dry mouth; flushed, dry skin; fruit-like breath odor; increased urination (frequency and amount); ketones in urine; loss of appetite; stomachache, nausea, or vomiting; tiredness; troubled breathing (rapid and deep); unconsciousness; or unusual thirst.

If symptoms of high blood sugar occur, check your blood sugar level and then call your doctor for instructions.

Side Effects of This Medicine

Side Effects of This Medicine

Along with its needed effects, a medicine may cause some unwanted effects. Although not all of these side effects may occur, if they do occur they may need medical attention.

Check with your doctor as soon as possible if any of the following side effects occur:

More common
Chest pain; decreased urine output; dilated neck veins; extreme fatigue; irregular breathing; irregular heartbeat; problems with teeth; shortness of breath; swelling of face, fingers, feet, or lower legs; tightness in chest; troubled breathing; weight gain; wheezing

Less common
Swelling

Incidence unknown
Unexplained, rapid weight gain

Some side effects may occur that usually do not need medical attention. These side effects may go away during treatment as your body adjusts to the medicine. Also, your health care professional may be able to tell you about ways to prevent or reduce some of these side effects. Check with your health care professional if any of the following side effects continue or are bothersome or if you have any questions about them:

More common
Blurred vision; cough; dry mouth; fatigue; flushed, dry skin; fruit like breath odor; headache; increased hunger; increased thirst; increased urination; loss of consciousness; muscle soreness; nausea; runny or stuffy nose; sore throat; stomachache; sweating; troubled breathing; unexplained weight loss; vomiting

Less common

> Pale skin; trouble breathing with activity; unusual bleeding or bruising; unusual tiredness or weakness

Other side effects not listed may also occur in some patients. If you notice any other effects, check with your healthcare professional.

PLICAMYCIN (Intravenous route) -
plye-kay-MYE-sin

Uses For This Medicine

Plicamycin belongs to the group of medicines known as antineoplastics. It may be used to treat certain types of cancer. It is also used to treat hypercalcemia or hypercalciuria (too much calcium in the blood or urine) that may occur with some types of cancer.

Plicamycin may also be used for other conditions as determined by your doctor.

Plicamycin is to be administered by or under the immediate care of your doctor. It is available only with a prescription.

Once a medicine has been approved for marketing for a certain use, experience may show that it is also useful for other medical problems. Although this use is not included in product labeling, plicamycin is used in certain patients with the following medical condition:

- Paget's disease of the bone

Before Receiving This Medicine

In deciding to use a medicine, the risks of taking the medicine must be weighed against the good it will do. This is a decision you and your doctor will make. For this medicine, the following should be considered:

Plicamycin is a very strong medicine. In addition to its helpful effects in treating your medical problem, it has side effects that could be very serious. Before you receive this medicine, be sure that you have discussed its use with your doctor.

Allergies—Tell your doctor if you have ever had any unusual or allergic reaction to this medicine or any other medicines. Also tell your health care professional if you have any other types of allergies, such as to foods, dyes, preservatives, or animals. For non-prescription products, read the label or package ingredients carefully.

Pediatric—Studies on this medicine have not been done in children; however, plicamycin can cause serious side effects in any patient. Therefore, it is especially important that you discuss with the child's doctor the good that this medicine may do as well as the risks of using it.

Geriatric—Many medicines have not been studied specifically in older people. Therefore, it may not be known whether they work exactly the same way they do in younger adults or if they cause different side effects or problems in older people.

There is no specific information comparing use of plicamycin in the elderly with use in other age groups.

Pregnancy—

	Pregnancy Category	Explanation
All Trimesters	X	Studies in animals or pregnant women have demonstrated positive evidence of fetal abnormalities. This drug should not be used in women who are or may become pregnant because the risk clearly outweighs any possible benefit.

Breast Feeding—There are no adequate studies in women for determining infant risk when using this medication during breastfeeding. Weigh the potential benefits against the potential risks before taking this medication while breastfeeding.

Other medicines—

Using this medicine with any of the following medicines is not recommended. Your doctor may decide not to treat you with this medication or change some of the other medicines you take.

Rotavirus Vaccine, Live

Interactions with Food/Tobacco/Alcohol—Certain medicines should not be used at or around the time of eating food or eating certain types of food since interactions may occur. Using alcohol or tobacco with certain medicines may also cause interactions to occur. Discuss with your healthcare professional the use of your medicine with food, alcohol, or tobacco.

Other medical problems—The presence of other medical problems may affect the use of this medicine. Make sure you tell your doctor if you have any other medical problems, especially:

- Bleeding problems—Use of plicamycin may increase the risk of bleeding
- Blood disease or
- Kidney disease or
- Liver disease—Use of plicamycin may make these conditions worse
- Chickenpox (including recent exposure) or
- Herpes zoster (shingles)—Use of plicamycin may make your reaction to either of these conditions worse

Proper Use of This Medicine

Plicamycin sometimes causes nausea, vomiting, and loss of appetite. However, it is very important that you continue to receive the medicine, even if you begin to feel ill. If you have any questions about this, check with your doctor.

Dosing—The dose of this medicine will be different for different patients. Follow your doctor's orders or the directions on the label. The following information includes only the average doses of this medicine. If your dose is different, do not change it unless your doctor tells you to do so.

The amount of medicine that you take depends on the strength of the medicine. Also, the number of doses you take each day, the time allowed between doses, and the length of time you take the medicine depend on the medical problem for which you are using the medicine.

- For injection dosage form:
  - To treat cancer:
    - Adults and children—The dose that is used may depend on a number of things, including what the medicine is being used for, the patient's weight, and whether or not other medicines are also being taken. If you are receiving plicamycin at home, follow your doctor's orders or the directions on the label. If you have any questions about the proper dose of plicamycin, ask your doctor.
  - To treat hypercalcemia or hypercalciuria (too much calcium in the blood or urine):
    - Adults—The dose is based on body weight and must be determined by your doctor. At first, the usual dose is 15 to 25 micrograms (mcg) per kg (6.8 to 11.4 mcg per pound) of body weight a day, injected slowly into a vein. The dose is given over a period of four to six hours once a day for three to four days. Your doctor may repeat the treatment if needed.
    - Children—Dose must be determined by your doctor.

Precautions After Receiving This Medicine

It is very important that your doctor check your progress daily while you are receiving plicamycin to make sure that this medicine does not cause unwanted effects.

Your doctor may want you to follow a low-calcium, low–vitamin D diet. If you have any questions about this, check with your doctor.

Do not take aspirin or large amounts of any other preparations containing aspirin, other salicylates, or acetaminophen without first checking with your doctor. These medicines may increase the effects of plicamycin.

While you are being treated with plicamycin, and after you stop treatment with it, do not have any immunizations (vaccinations) without your doctor's approval. Plicamycin may lower your body's resistance and there is a chance you might get the infection the immunization is meant to prevent. In addition, other persons living in your household should not take or have recently taken oral polio vaccine since there is a chance they could pass the polio virus on to you. Also, avoid other persons who have taken oral polio vaccine. Do not get close to them, and do not stay in the same room with them for very long. If you cannot take these precautions, you should consider wearing a protective face mask that covers the nose and mouth.

Plicamycin can lower the number of white blood cells in your blood temporarily, increasing the chance of getting an infection. It can also lower the number of platelets, which are necessary for proper blood clotting. If this occurs, there are certain precautions your doctor may ask you to take, especially when your blood count is low, to reduce the risk of infection or bleeding:

- If you can, avoid people with infections. Check with your doctor immediately if you think you are getting an infection or if you get a fever or chills.
- Check with your doctor immediately if you notice any unusual bleeding or bruising.
- Be careful when using a regular toothbrush, dental floss, or toothpick. Your medical doctor, dentist, or nurse may recommend other ways to clean your teeth and gums. Check with your medical doctor before having any dental work done.
- Do not touch your eyes or the inside of your nose unless you have just washed your hands and have not touched anything else in the meantime.
- Be careful not to cut yourself when you are using sharp objects such as a safety razor or fingernail or toenail cutters.
- Avoid contact sports or other situations where bruising or injury could occur.

Side Effects of This Medicine

Along with its needed effects, a medicine may cause some unwanted effects. Although not all of these side effects may occur, if they do occur they may need medical attention.

Check with your doctor immediately if any of the following side effects occur:

Less common
   Muscle and abdominal cramps

Symptoms of overdose
   Bloody or black, tarry stools; flushing or redness or swelling of face; nosebleed; skin rash or small red spots on skin; sore throat and fever; unusual bleeding or bruising; vomiting of blood; yellow eyes or skin

Some side effects may occur that usually do not need medical attention. These side effects may go away during treatment as your body adjusts to the medicine. Also, your health care professional may be able to tell you about ways to prevent or reduce some of these side effects. Check with your health care professional if any of the following side effects continue or are bothersome or if you have any questions about them:

More common
   Diarrhea; irritation or soreness of mouth; loss of appetite; nausea or vomiting—may occur 1 to 2 hours after the injection is started and continue for 12 to 24 hours

Less common
   Drowsiness; fever; headache; mental depression; pain, redness, soreness, or swelling at place of injection; unusual tiredness or weakness

After you stop using this medicine, it may still produce some side effects that need attention. During this period of time, *check with your doctor immediately* if you notice the following side effects:

   Bloody or black, tarry stools; nosebleed; sore throat and fever; unusual bleeding or bruising; vomiting of blood

Other side effects not listed may also occur in some patients. If you notice any other effects, check with your healthcare professional.

PNEUMOCOCCAL VACCINE POLYVALENT (Intramuscular route) -
NOO-moe-KOK-al vak-seen pol-ee-vay-lent

Commonly used brand name(s)

In the U.S.—
Pneumovax 23
Pnu-Imune 23

In Canada—
Prevnar

Available Dosage Forms:
• Solution

Therapeutic Class: Vaccine

Uses For This Vaccine

Pneumococcal vaccine polyvalent is an active immunizing agent used to prevent infection by pneumococcal bacteria. It works by causing your body to produce its own protection (antibodies) against the disease.

The following information applies only to the polyvalent 23 pneumococcal vaccine. Other polyvalent pneumococcal vaccines may be available in countries other than the U.S.

Pneumococcal infection can cause serious problems, such as pneumonia, which affects the lungs; meningitis, which affects the brain; bacteremia, which is a severe infection in the blood; and possibly death. These problems are more likely to occur in older adults and persons with certain diseases or conditions that make them more susceptible to a pneumococcal infection or more apt to develop serious problems from a pneumococcal infection.

Unless otherwise contraindicated, immunization against pneumococcal disease is recommended for all adults and children 2 years of age and older, especially:
• Older adults, especially those 65 years of age and older.
• Adults and children 2 to 64 years of age with chronic illnesses.
• Adults and children 2 to 64 years of age with sickle cell disease, those with spleen problems or without spleens, and those who are to have their spleens removed.
• Adults and children 2 to 64 years of age who are at increased risk for pneumococcal disease because of other illness (e.g., heart disease, lung disease, diabetes, alcoholism, and liver disease).
• Adults and children 2 to 64 years of age who are living in special environments or social settings (e.g., Alaskan Natives and certain American Indian populations) and residents of nursing homes and other long-term-care facilities.
• Adults and children 2 to 64 years of age with decreased disease-fighting ability (e.g., those with human immunodeficiency virus (HIV) infection, organ or bone marrow transplantations, and cancer).

Immunization against pneumococcal infection is not recommended for infants and children younger than 2 years of age, because these persons cannot produce enough antibodies to the vaccine to protect them against a pneumococcal infection.

Pneumococcal vaccine usually is given only once to each person. Additional injections are not given, except in special cases, because of the possibility of more frequent and more severe side effects.

This vaccine is to be administered only by or under the supervision of your doctor or other health care professional.

Before Receiving This Vaccine

In deciding to use a vaccine, the risks of taking the vaccine must be weighed against the good it will do. This is a decision you and your doctor will make. For this vaccine, the following should be considered:

Allergies—Tell your doctor if you have ever had any unusual or allergic reaction to this medicine or any other medicines. Also tell your health care professional if you have any other types of allergies, such as to foods, dyes, preservatives, or animals. For non-prescription products, read the label or package ingredients carefully.

Pediatric—Use of pneumococcal vaccine is not recommended in infants and children younger than 2 years of age. In children 2 years of age and older, this vaccine is not expected to cause different side effects or problems than it does in adults.

Geriatric—Many medicines have not been studied specifically in older people. Therefore, it may not be known whether they work exactly the same way they do in younger adults. Although there is no specific information comparing use of pneumococcal vaccine in the elderly with use in other age groups, this vaccine is not expected to cause different side effects or problems in older people than it does in younger adults.

Other medicines—Although certain medicines should not be used together at all, in other cases two different medicines may be used together even if an interaction might occur. In these cases, your doctor may want to change the dose, or other precautions may be necessary. Tell your healthcare professional if you are taking any other prescription or non-prescription (over-the-counter [OTC]) medicine.

Interactions with Food/Tobacco/Alcohol—Certain medicines should not be used at or around the time of eating food or eating certain types of food since interactions may occur. Using alcohol or tobacco with certain medicines may also cause interactions to occur. Discuss with your healthcare professional the use of your medicine with food, alcohol, or tobacco.

Other medical problems—The presence of other medical problems may affect the use of this vaccine. Make sure you tell your doctor if you have any other medical problems, especially:
• Severe illness with fever—The symptoms of the illness may be confused with possible side effects of the vaccine
• Previous severe reaction to the vaccine or
• Thrombocytopenic purpura (blood disorder)—Use of pneumococcal vaccine may make the condition worse

Proper Use of This Vaccine

Dosing—The dose of this medicine will be different for different patients. Follow your doctor's orders or the directions

on the label. The following information includes only the average doses of this medicine. If your dose is different, do not change it unless your doctor tells you to do so.

The amount of medicine that you take depends on the strength of the medicine. Also, the number of doses you take each day, the time allowed between doses, and the length of time you take the medicine depend on the medical problem for which you are using the medicine.

- For injection dosage form:
  - For prevention of pneumococcal pneumonia:
    - Adults and children 2 years of age and older— One dose injected under the skin or into a muscle.
    - Children up to 2 years of age—Use is not recommended.

Precautions While Using This Vaccine

If you have more than one doctor, be sure they all know that you have received pneumococcal vaccine polyvalent 23 so that they can put the information into your medical records. This vaccine usually is given only once to each person, except in special cases.

Side Effects of This Vaccine

Along with its needed effects, a medicine may cause some unwanted effects. Although not all of these side effects may occur, if they do occur they may need medical attention.

Check with your doctor immediately if any of the following side effects occur:

Symptoms of allergic reaction
Difficulty in breathing or swallowing; hives; itching, especially of feet or hands; reddening of skin, especially around ears; swelling of eyes, face, or inside of nose; unusual tiredness or weakness (sudden and severe)

Check with your doctor as soon as possible if any of the following side effects occur:

Rare
Fever over 102.2 °F (39 °C)

Some side effects may occur that usually do not need medical attention. These side effects may go away during treatment as your body adjusts to the medicine. Also, your health care professional may be able to tell you about ways to prevent or reduce some of these side effects. Check with your health care professional if any of the following side effects continue or are bothersome or if you have any questions about them:

More common
Redness, soreness, hard lump, swelling, or pain at place of injection

Less common or rare
Aches or pain in joints or muscles; fever of 101 °F (38.3 °C) or less; skin rash; swollen glands; unusual tiredness or weakness; vague feeling of bodily discomfort

Other side effects not listed may also occur in some patients. If you notice any other effects, check with your healthcare professional.

PNEUMOCOCCAL VACCINE, DIPHTHERIA CONJUGATE

(Intramuscular route) - NOO-moe-KOK-al vak-seen dif-THEER-ee-a KON-joo-gate

Commonly used brand name(s)

In the U.S.—
Prevnar

Available Dosage Forms:
- Suspension

Therapeutic Class: Vaccine

Uses For This Vaccine

Pneumococcalconjugate vaccine is an active immunizing agent used to prevent infection by pneumococcal bacteria. It works by causing your body to produce its own protection (antibodies) against the disease.

Pneumococcal infection can cause serious problems, such as pneumonia, which affects the lungs; meningitis, which affects the brain; and bacteremia, which is a severe infection in the blood. Pneumococcal infection is also an important cause of ear infections in children.

Unless otherwise contraindicated, immunization against pneumococcal disease is recommended for infants and young children.

Immunization requires 1 to 4 doses of the vaccine, depending on the age at the first dose. This vaccine can be given at the same time as other routine vaccinations.

This vaccine is to be administered only by or under the supervision of your doctor or other health care professional.

Before Receiving This Vaccine

In deciding to use a vaccine, the risks of taking the vaccine must be weighed against the good it will do. This is a decision you and your doctor will make. For this vaccine, the following should be considered:

Allergies—Tell your doctor if you have ever had any unusual or allergic reaction to this medicine or any other medicines. Also tell your health care professional if you have any other types of allergies, such as to foods, dyes, preservatives, or animals. For non-prescription products, read the label or package ingredients carefully.

Pediatric—This vaccine is generally well tolerated and effective in infants. The safety and effectiveness in infants below 6 weeks of age has not been established.

Geriatric—This vaccine is not recommended for use in adult populations.

Pregnancy—

	Pregnancy Category	Explanation
All Trimesters	C	Animal studies have shown an adverse effect and there are no adequate studies in pregnant women OR no animal studies have been conducted and there are no adequate studies in pregnant women.

Breast Feeding—Studies in women suggest that this medication poses minimal risk to the infant when used during breastfeeding.

Other medicines—Although certain medicines should not be used together at all, in other cases two different medicines may be used together even if an interaction might occur. In these cases, your doctor may want to change the dose, or other precautions may be necessary. Tell your healthcare professional if you are taking any other prescription or non-prescription (over-the-counter [OTC]) medicine.

Interactions with Food/Tobacco/Alcohol—Certain medicines should not be used at or around the time of eating food or eating certain types of food since interactions may occur. Using alcohol or tobacco with certain medicines may also cause interactions to occur. Discuss with your healthcare professional the use of your medicine with food, alcohol, or tobacco.

Proper Use of This Vaccine

Dosing—The dose of this medicine will be different for different patients. Follow your doctor's orders or the directions on the label. The following information includes only the average doses of this medicine. If your dose is different, do not change it unless your doctor tells you to do so.

The amount of medicine that you take depends on the strength of the medicine. Also, the number of doses you take each day, the time allowed between doses, and the length of time you take the medicine depend on the medical problem for which you are using the medicine.

The number of injections your child will receive for protection from pneumococcal infection will depend on your child's age at the first dose:

- Children 6 weeks to 6 months of age—4 doses
- Children 7 to 11 months of age—3 doses
- Children 12 to 23 months of age—2 doses
- Children 2 years through 9 years of age—1 dose
- Children older than 9 years of age—Use of this vaccine is not recommended in this age group.

Your doctor will tell you when your child should receive the next dose.

Precautions While Using This Vaccine

If your child has more than one doctor, be sure they all know that your child has received pneumococcal conjugated vaccine so that they can put the information into your child's medical records.

Side Effects of This Vaccine

Along with its needed effects, a medicine may cause some unwanted effects. Although not all of these side effects may occur, if they do occur they may need medical attention.

Check with your doctor immediately if any of the following side effects occur:

Symptoms of allergic reaction
　Difficulty in breathing or swallowing; hives; itching, especially of feet or hands; reddening of skin, especially around ears; swelling of eyes, face, or inside of nose; unusual tiredness or weakness (sudden and severe)

Check with your doctor as soon as possible if any of the following side effects occur:

Less common
　Fever over 39 °C (102.2 °F)
Rare
　Collapse or shock-like state; convulsions

Some side effects may occur that usually do not need medical attention. These side effects may go away during treatment as your body adjusts to the medicine. Also, your health care professional may be able to tell you about ways to prevent or reduce some of these side effects. Check with your health care professional if any of the following side effects continue or are bothersome or if you have any questions about them:

More common
　Decreased appetite; diarrhea; drowsiness; fever of less than 39 °C (102.2 °F); irritability; redness, soreness, hard lump, swelling, or pain at injection site; restless sleep; vomiting
Less common
　Skin rash or hives

Other side effects not listed may also occur in some patients. If you notice any other effects, check with your healthcare professional.

PODOFILOX (Topical route) - po-do-FIL-ox

Commonly used brand name(s)
In the U.S.—
　Condylox

In Canada—
　Condyline

Available Dosage Forms:
- Gel/Jelly
- Solution

Therapeutic Class: Keratolytic

Uses For This Medicine

Podofilox is used to remove certain types of warts on the outside skin of the genital areas (penis or vulva). The gel is used also to treat warts between the genitals and the rectum, the solution is not. Neither the gel nor the solution is used to treat warts that occur inside the rectum, vagina, or urine passageways inside the penis (male) or the vulva (female). Podofilox works by destroying the skin of the wart.

This medicine is available only with your doctor's prescription.

Before Using This Medicine

In deciding to use a medicine, the risks of taking the medicine must be weighed against the good it will do. This is a decision you and your doctor will make. For this medicine, the following should be considered:

Allergies—Tell your doctor if you have ever had any unusual or allergic reaction to this medicine or any other medicines. Also tell your health care professional if you have any other types of allergies, such as to foods, dyes, preservatives, or animals. For non-prescription products, read the label or package ingredients carefully.

Pediatric—Studies of this medicine have been done only in adult patients, and there is no specific information comparing use of podofilox in children with use in other age groups.

Geriatric—Many medicines have not been studied specifically in older people. Therefore, it may not be known whether they work exactly the same way they do in younger adults or if they cause different side effects or problems in older people. There is no specific information comparing use of podofilox in the elderly with use in other age groups.

Pregnancy—

	Pregnancy Category	Explanation
All Trimesters	C	Animal studies have shown an adverse effect and there are no adequate studies in pregnant women OR no animal studies have been conducted and there are no adequate studies in pregnant women.

Breast Feeding—There are no adequate studies in women for determining infant risk when using this medication during breastfeeding. Weigh the potential benefits against the potential risks before taking this medication while breastfeeding.

Other medicines—Although certain medicines should not be used together at all, in other cases two different medicines may be used together even if an interaction might occur. In these cases, your doctor may want to change the dose, or other precautions may be necessary. Tell your healthcare professional if you are taking any other prescription or nonprescription (over-the-counter [OTC]) medicine.

Interactions with Food/Tobacco/Alcohol—Certain medicines should not be used at or around the time of eating food or eating certain types of food since interactions may occur. Using alcohol or tobacco with certain medicines may also cause interactions to occur. Discuss with your healthcare professional the use of your medicine with food, alcohol, or tobacco.

Proper Use of This Medicine

A paper with information for the patient will be given to you with your filled prescription and will provide many details concerning the use of podofilox. Read this paper carefully and ask your health care professional if you need additional information.

Also, keep podofilox away from the eyes and mucous membranes, such as the inside of the penis, rectum, or vagina. This medicine may cause severe irritation. If you get this medicine in your eyes or on one of these areas, immediately flush the area with water for 15 minutes.

Use podofilox only as directed, no more than 3 days a week and no more than 4 treatment cycles. Do not use more of it,

do not use it more often, and do not use it for a longer time than your doctor ordered. To do so may increase the chances that this medicine is absorbed into the body and that side effects could occur.

Do not apply the medicine to any other wart until you discuss it with your doctor. The total dose of podofilox used on all warts should not exceed that which would cover an area measuring 1.6 square inches (10 square centimeters), about the size of a dollar coin.

To use:

- To apply the solution, use the applicators that come with the solution or a cotton-tipped applicator. To apply the gel, use a cotton-tipped applicator or your finger. Never reuse an applicator or dip a used applicator into the bottle.
- Apply podofilox only to the wart(s) discussed with your doctor.
- Podofilox can cause severe irritation of normal skin. If you get medicine on normal skin, wash it off immediately.
- Make sure the treated area is dry before allowing the treated skin to come in contact with normal, untreated skin.
- Immediately after applying this medicine, wash your hands to remove any medicine. Properly discard used applicator(s).

Dosing—The dose of this medicine will be different for different patients. Follow your doctor's orders or the directions on the label. The following information includes only the average doses of this medicine. If your dose is different, do not change it unless your doctor tells you to do so.

The amount of medicine that you take depends on the strength of the medicine. Also, the number of doses you take each day, the time allowed between doses, and the length of time you take the medicine depend on the medical problem for which you are using the medicine.

- For topical dosage form (gel):
  - For warts on penis or vulva (genitals) or on skin between genitals and rectum:
    - Adults—Apply to the wart(s) two times a day for three days in a row using an applicator tip or finger. Skip four days by not applying any medicine for four days in a row. If the wart can still be seen, this application cycle may be repeated each week for up to four weeks, until the wart is gone. No more than 0.5 grams of gel should be used each day of treatment.
    - Children—Use and dose must be determined by the doctor.
- For topical dosage form (solution):
  - For warts on penis or vulva (genitals) only:
    - Adults—Apply to the wart(s) two times a day (every twelve hours) for three days in a row using applicator tip. Skip four days by not applying any medicine for four days in a row. If the wart can still be seen, this application cycle may be repeated each week for up to four weeks, until the wart is gone. No more than 0.5 milliliters of solution should be used each day of treatment.

- Children—Use and dose must be determined by the doctor.

Missed dose—If you miss a dose of this medicine, take it as soon as possible. However, if it is almost time for your next dose, skip the missed dose and go back to your regular dosing schedule. Do not double doses.

Storage—Store the medicine in a closed container at room temperature, away from heat, moisture, and direct light. Keep from freezing.

Keep out of the reach of children.

Do not keep outdated medicine or medicine no longer needed.

Precautions While Using This Medicine

Podofilox may not be able to prevent previously healed warts from reappearing or stop new warts from growing.

This medicine contains alcohol and therefore may be flammable. Do not use near heat, near open flame, or while smoking.

Side Effects of This Medicine

Along with its needed effects, a medicine may cause some unwanted effects. Although not all of these side effects may occur, if they do occur they may need medical attention.

Check with your doctor as soon as possible if any of the following side effects occur:

More common
Bad odor (solution only); bleeding of treated skin; blistering, crusting, or scabbing of treated skin; bloody urine (solution only); burning feeling of treated skin; dizziness (solution only); headache (gel only); itching of treated skin; pain during sexual intercourse (solution only); pain of treated skin; problems with foreskin of penis (solution only); redness or swelling of treated skin; scarring of treated skin (solution only); skin ulcers of treated skin; vomiting (solution only)

Symptoms of overdose—in order of occurrence
Nausea; vomiting; diarrhea; chills; fever; sore throat; unusual bleeding or bruising; oral ulcers

Some side effects may occur that usually do not need medical attention. These side effects may go away during treatment as your body adjusts to the medicine. Also, your health care professional may be able to tell you about ways to prevent or reduce some of these side effects. Check with your health care professional if any of the following side effects continue or are bothersome or if you have any questions about them:

More common
Dryness of treated skin; peeling of treated skin; soreness or tenderness of treated skin; stinging or tingling of treated skin; trouble in sleeping (solution only)

Less common
Changes in color of treated skin (gel only); skin rash (gel only)

Other side effects not listed may also occur in some patients. If you notice any other effects, check with your healthcare professional.

POLYETHYLENE GLYCOL, POTASSIUM CHLORIDE, SODIUM BICARBONATE, SODIUM CHLORIDE, AND SODIUM SULFATE (Oral route) - pol-ee-ETH-i-leen GLYE-kol, poe-TAS-ee-um KLOR-ide, SOE-dee-um bye-KARB-oh-nate, SOE-dee-um KLOR-ide, SOE-dee-um SUL-fate

Available Dosage Forms:
- Powder for Suspension
- Powder for Solution
- Solution

Therapeutic Class: Laxative, Hyperosmotic

Uses For This Medicine

The polyethylene glycol (PEG) and electrolytes solution is used to clean the colon (large bowel or lower intestine) before certain tests or surgery of the colon. The PEG-electrolyte solution is usually taken by mouth. However, sometimes it is given in the hospital through a nasogastric tube (a tube inserted through the nose).

The PEG-electrolyte solution acts like a laxative. It causes liquid stools or mild diarrhea. In this way, it flushes all solid material from the colon, so the doctor can have a clear view of the colon.

The PEG-electrolyte solution is available only with your doctor's prescription.

Before Using This Medicine

In deciding to use a medicine, the risks of taking the medicine must be weighed against the good it will do. This is a decision you and your doctor will make. For this medicine, the following should be considered:

Allergies—Tell your doctor if you have ever had any unusual or allergic reaction to this medicine or any other medicines. Also tell your health care professional if you have any other types of allergies, such as to foods, dyes, preservatives, or animals. For non-prescription products, read the label or package ingredients carefully.

Pediatric—Although there is no specific information comparing use of PEG-electrolyte solution in children with use in other age groups, this medicine is not expected to cause different side effects or problems in children than it does in adults.

Geriatric—This medicine has been tested and has not been shown to cause different side effects or problems in older people than it does in younger adults.

Pregnancy—

	Pregnancy Category	Explanation
All Trimesters	C	Animal studies have shown an adverse effect and there are no adequate studies in pregnant women OR no animal studies have been conducted and there are no adequate studies in pregnant women.

Breast Feeding—

Polyethylene Glycol

- There are no adequate studies in women for determining infant risk when using this medication during breastfeeding. Weigh the potential benefits against the potential risks before taking this medication while breastfeeding.

Potassium

- There are no adequate studies in women for determining infant risk when using this medication during breastfeeding. Weigh the potential benefits against the potential risks before taking this medication while breastfeeding.

Sodium Bicarbonate

- There are no adequate studies in women for determining infant risk when using this medication during breastfeeding. Weigh the potential benefits against the potential risks before taking this medication while breastfeeding.

Sodium Chloride

- Studies in women suggest that this medication poses minimal risk to the infant when used during breastfeeding.

Other medicines—

Using this medicine with any of the following medicines is usually not recommended, but may be required in some cases. If both medicines are prescribed together, your doctor may change the dose or how often you use one or both of the medicines.

Alacepril, Amiloride, Benazepril, Canrenoate, Captopril, Cilazapril, Delapril, Enalaprilat, Enalapril Maleate, Fosinopril, Imidapril, Indomethacin, Licorice, Lisinopril, Moexipril, Pentopril, Perindopril, Quinapril, Ramipril, Spirapril, Spironolactone, Temocapril, Trandolapril, Triamterene, Zofenopril

Interactions with Food/Tobacco/Alcohol—Certain medicines should not be used at or around the time of eating food or eating certain types of food since interactions may occur. Using alcohol or tobacco with certain medicines may also cause interactions to occur. Discuss with your healthcare professional the use of your medicine with food, alcohol, or tobacco.

Other medical problems—The presence of other medical problems may affect the use of this medicine. Make sure you tell your doctor if you have any other medical problems, especially:

- Blockage or obstruction of the intestine or
- Paralytic ileus or
- Perforated bowel or
- Toxic colitis or
- Toxic megacolon—PEG-electrolyte solution may make these conditions worse; in some cases the colon may rip open or tear

Proper Use of This Medicine

Your doctor may have special instructions for you, depending on the type of test you are going to have. If you have not received such instructions or if you do not understand them, check with your doctor in advance.

Take the PEG-electrolyte solution exactly as directed. Otherwise, the test you are going to have may not work and may have to be done again.

It will take close to 3 hours to drink all of the PEG-electrolyte solution. The first bowel movement may start an hour or so after you start drinking the solution. Continue drinking all the solution to get the best results, unless otherwise directed by your doctor.

Do not eat anything for at least 3 hours before taking the PEG-electrolyte solution. If you do so, the colon may not get completely clean. If you are drinking the PEG-electrolyte solution the evening before the test, you may drink clear liquids (e.g., water, ginger ale, decaffeinated cola, decaffeinated tea, broth, gelatin) up until the time of the test. However, check first with your doctor.

For patients using the powder form of this medicine:

- The powder must be mixed with water before it is used. Add lukewarm water to the fill mark on the bottle.
- Shake well until all the ingredients are dissolved.
- Do not add any other ingredients, such as flavoring, to the solution.
- After you mix the solution, you must use it within 48 hours.

Dosing—The dose of this medicine will be different for different patients. Follow your doctor's orders or the directions on the label. The following information includes only the average doses of this medicine. If your dose is different, do not change it unless your doctor tells you to do so.

The amount of medicine that you take depends on the strength of the medicine. Also, the number of doses you take each day, the time allowed between doses, and the length of time you take the medicine depend on the medical problem for which you are using the medicine.

- For cleaning the colon:
  - For oral dosage forms (oral solution and powder for oral solution):
    - Adults and teenagers—Drink one full glass (8 ounces) of the PEG-electrolyte solution rapidly every ten minutes. If you sip small amounts of the solution, it will not work as well.
    - Children—The amount of PEG-electrolyte solution taken is based on body weight and must be determined by your doctor. It is usually 25 to 40 milliliters (mL) per kilogram (kg) (11.3 to 18.2 mL per pound) of body weight per hour.

Storage—Store in the refrigerator. Do not freeze.

Keep out of the reach of children.

Do not keep outdated medicine or medicine no longer needed.

Side Effects of This Medicine

Along with its needed effects, a medicine may cause some unwanted effects. Although not all of these side effects may occur, if they do occur they may need medical attention.

Check with your doctor as soon as possible if any of the following side effects occur:

Rare

Skin rash

Some side effects may occur that usually do not need medical attention. These side effects may go away during treatment as your body adjusts to the medicine. Also, your health care professional may be able to tell you about ways to prevent or reduce some of these side effects. Check with your health care professional if any of the following side effects continue or are bothersome or if you have any questions about them:

More common
  Bloating; nausea

Less common
  Abdominal or stomach cramps; irritation of the anus; vomiting

Other side effects not listed may also occur in some patients. If you notice any other effects, check with your healthcare professional.

POTASSIUM SUPPLEMENTS
(Systemic)

Some commonly used brand names are:

In the U.S.—

Cena-K (5)	Klor-Con Powder (5)
Effer-K (4)	Klor-Con/25 Powder (5)
Gen-K (5)	Klorvess (3)
Glu-K (6)	Klorvess Effervescent
K-8 (5)	Granules (3)
K+ 10 (5)	Klorvess 10% Liquid (5)
Kaochlor 10% (5)	Klotrix (5)
Kaochlor S-F 10% (5)	K-Lyte (2)
Kaon (6)	K-Lyte/Cl (3)
Kaon-Cl (5)	K-Lyte/Cl 50 (3)
Kaon-Cl-10 (5)	K-Lyte/Cl Powder (5)
Kaon-Cl 20% Liquid (5)	K-Lyte DS (4)
Kato (5)	K-Norm (5)
Kay Ciel (5)	Kolyum (7)
Kaylixir (6)	K-Sol (5)
K+ Care (5)	K-Tab (5)
K+ Care ET (2)	K-Vescent (2)
K-Dur (5)	Micro-K (5)
K-Electrolyte (2)	Micro-K 10 (5)
K-G Elixir (6)	Micro-K LS (5)
K-Ide (3)	Potasalan (5)
K-Lease (5)	Rum-K (5)
K-Lor (5)	Slow-K (5)
Klor-Con 8 (5)	Ten-K (5)
Klor-Con 10 (5)	Tri-K (9)
Klor-Con/EF (2)	Twin-K (8)

In Canada—

Apo-K (5)	K-Lyte (2)
K-10 (5)	K-Lyte/Cl (5)
Kalium Durules (5)	K-Med 900 (5)
Kaochlor-10 (5)	Micro-K (5)
Kaochlor-20 (5)	Micro-K 10 (5)
Kaon (6)	Neo-K (3)
KCL 5% (5)	Potassium-Rougier (6)
K-Dur (5)	Potassium-Sandoz (3)
K-Long (5)	Roychlor-10% (5)
K-Lor (5)	Slow-K (5)

This information applies to the following:

1. Potassium Acetate (poe-TAS-ee-um AS-a-tate)
2. Potassium Bicarbonate (poe-TAS-ee-um bi-KAR-bo-nate)
3. Potassium Bicarbonate and Potassium Chloride (poe-TAS-ee-um bi-KAR-bo-nate and poe-TAS-ee-um KLOR-ide)
4. Potassium Bicarbonate and Potassium Citrate (poe-TAS-ee-um bi-KAR-bo-nate and poe-TAS-ee-um SIH-trayt)
5. Potassium Chloride (poe-TAS-ee-um KLOR-ide)
6. Potassium Gluconate (poe-TAS-ee-um GLOO-ko-nate)
7. Potassium Gluconate and Potassium Chloride (poe-TAS-ee-um GLOO-ko-nate and poe-TAS-ee-um KLOR-ide)
8. Potassium Gluconate and Potassium Citrate (poe-TAS-ee-um GLOO-ko-nate and poe-TAS-ee-um SIH-trayt)
9. Trikates (TRI-kates)

Category

- **Antihypokalemic**—Potassium Acetate; Potassium Bicarbonate; Potassium Bicarbonate and Potassium Chloride; Potassium Bicarbonate and Potassium Citrate; Potassium Chloride; Potassium Gluconate; Potassium Gluconate and Potassium Chloride; Potassium Gluconate and Potassium Citrate; Trikates

- **Electrolyte replenisher**—Potassium Acetate; Potassium Bicarbonate; Potassium Bicarbonate and Potassium Chloride; Potassium Bicarbonate and Potassium Citrate; Potassium Chloride; Potassium Gluconate; Potassium Gluconate and Potassium Chloride; Potassium Gluconate and Potassium Citrate; Trikates

Description

Potassium is needed to maintain good health. Although a balanced diet usually supplies all the potassium a person needs, potassium supplements may be needed by patients who do not have enough potassium in their regular diet or have lost too much potassium because of illness or treatment with certain medicines.

There is no evidence that potassium supplements are useful in the treatment of high blood pressure.

Lack of potassium may cause muscle weakness, irregular heartbeat, mood changes, or nausea and vomiting.

Injectable potassium is administered only by or under the supervision of your doctor. Some forms of oral potassium may be available in stores without a prescription. Since too much potassium may cause health problems, you should take potassium supplements only if directed by your doctor. Potassium supplements are available with your doctor's prescription in the following dosage forms:

Oral
- Potassium Bicarbonate
  - Tablets for solution
- Potassium Bicarbonate and Potassium Chloride
  - Powder for solution
  - Tablets for solution
- Potassium Bicarbonate and Potassium Citrate
  - Tablets for solution
- Potassium Chloride
  - Extended-release capsules
  - Solution
  - Powder for solution
  - Powder for suspension
  - Extended-release tablets
- Potassium Gluconate
  - Elixir
  - Tablets

- Potassium Gluconate and Potassium Chloride
  - Solution
  - Powder for solution
- Potassium Gluconate and Potassium Citrate
  - Solution
- Trikates
  - Solution

Parenteral
- Potassium Acetate
  - Injection
- Potassium Chloride
  - Concentrate for injection

Importance of Diet

For good health, it is important that you eat a balanced and varied diet. Follow carefully any diet program your health care professional may recommend. For your specific dietary vitamin and/or mineral needs, ask your health care professional for a list of appropriate foods.

The following table includes some potassium-rich foods.

Food (amount)	Milligrams of potassium	Milliequivalents of potassium
Acorn squash, cooked (1 cup)	896	23
Potato with skin, baked (1 long)	844	22
Spinach, cooked (1 cup)	838	21
Lentils, cooked (1 cup)	731	19
Kidney beans, cooked (1 cup)	713	18
Split peas, cooked (1 cup)	710	18
White navy beans, cooked (1 cup)	669	17
Butternut squash, cooked (1 cup)	583	15
Watermelon (1/16)	560	14
Raisins (½ cup)	553	14
Yogurt, low-fat, plain (1 cup)	531	14
Orange juice, frozen (1 cup)	503	13
Brussel sprouts, cooked (1 cup)	494	13
Zucchini, cooked, sliced (1 cup)	456	12
Banana (medium)	451	12
Collards, frozen, cooked (1 cup)	427	11
Cantaloupe (¼)	412	11
Milk, low-fat 1% (1 cup)	348	9
Broccoli, frozen, cooked (1 cup)	332	9

The daily amount of potassium needed is defined in several different ways.

For U.S.—
- Recommended Dietary Allowances (RDAs) are the amount of vitamins and minerals needed to provide for adequate nutrition in most healthy persons. RDAs for a given nutrient may vary depending on a person's age, sex, and physical condition (e.g., pregnancy).
- Daily Values (DVs) are used on food and dietary supplement labels to indicate the percent of the recommended daily amount of each nutrient that a serving provides. DV replaces the previous designation of United States Recommended Daily Allowances (USRDAs).

For Canada—
- Recommended Nutrient Intakes (RNIs) are used to determine the amounts of vitamins, minerals, and protein needed to provide adequate nutrition and lessen the risk of chronic disease.

Because lack of potassium is rare, there is no RDA or RNI for this mineral. However, it is thought that 1600 to 2000 mg (40 to 50 milliequivalents [mEq]) per day for adults is adequate.

Remember:
- The total amount of potassium that you get every day includes what you get from food *and* what you may take as a supplement. Read the labels of processed foods. Many foods now have added potassium.
- Your total intake of potassium should not be greater than the recommended amounts, unless ordered by your doctor. In some cases, too much potassium may cause muscle weakness, confusion, irregular heartbeat, or difficult breathing.

Before Using This Medicine

In deciding to use a medicine, the risks of taking the medicine must be weighed against the good it will do. This is a decision you and your doctor will make. For potassium supplements, the following should be considered:

Allergies—Tell your doctor if you have ever had any unusual or allergic reaction to potassium preparations. Also tell your doctor and pharmacist if you are allergic to any other substances, such as foods, preservatives, or dyes.

Pregnancy—Potassium supplements have not been shown to cause problems in humans.

Breast-feeding—Potassium supplements pass into breast milk. However, this medicine has not been reported to cause problems in nursing babies.

Children—Although there is no specific information comparing use of potassium supplements in children with use in other age groups, they are not expected to cause different side effects or problems in children than they do in adults.

Older adults—Many medicines have not been studied specifically in older people. Therefore, it may not be known whether they work exactly the same way they do in younger adults. Although there is no specific information comparing use of potassium supplements in the elderly with use in other age groups, they are not expected to cause different side effects or problems in older people than they do in younger adults.

Older adults may be at a greater risk of developing high blood levels of potassium (hyperkalemia).

Other medicines—Although certain medicines should not be used together at all, in other cases two different medicines may be used together even if an interaction might occur. In these cases, your doctor may want to change the dose, or other precautions may be necessary. When you are taking potassium supplements, it is especially important that your doctor and pharmacist know if you are taking any of the following:
- Amantadine (e.g., Symmetrel) or
- Anticholinergics (medicine for abdominal or stomach spasms or cramps) or
- Antidepressants (medicine for depression) or
- Antidyskinetics (medicine for Parkinson's disease or other conditions affecting control of muscles) or
- Antihistamines or
- Antipsychotic medicine (medicine for mental illness) or
- Buclizine (e.g., Bucladin) or
- Carbamazepine (e.g., Tegretol) or

- Cyclizine (e.g., Marezine) or
- Cyclobenzaprine (e.g., Flexeril) or
- Disopyramide (e.g., Norpace) or
- Flavoxate (e.g., Urispas) or
- Ipratropium (e.g., Atrovent) or
- Meclizine (e.g., Antivert) or
- Methylphenidate (e.g., Ritalin) or
- Orphenadrine (e.g., Norflex) or
- Oxybutynin (e.g., Ditropan) or
- Procainamide (e.g., Pronestyl) or
- Promethazine (e.g., Phenergan) or
- Quinidine (e.g., Quinidex) or
- Trimeprazine (e.g., Temaril)—Use with potassium supplements may cause or worsen certain stomach or intestine problems
- Angiotensin-converting enzyme (ACE) inhibitors (benazepril [e.g., Lotensin], captopril [e.g., Capoten], enalapril [e.g., Vasotec], fosinopril [e.g., Monotril], lisinopril [e.g., Prinivil, Zestril], quinapril [e.g., Accupril], ramipril [e.g., Altace]) or
- Amiloride (e.g., Midamor) or
- Beta-adrenergic blocking agents (acebutolol [e.g., Sectral], atenolol [e.g., Tenormin], betaxolol [e.g., Kerlone], carteolol [e.g., Cartrol], labetalol [e.g., Normodyne], metoprolol [e.g., Lopressor], nadolol [e.g., Corgard], oxprenolol [e.g., Trasicor], penbutolol [e.g., Levatol], pindolol [e.g., Visken], propranolol [e.g., Inderal], sotalol [e.g., Sotacor], timolol [e.g., Blocadren]) or
- Heparin (e.g., Panheprin) or
- Inflammation or pain medicine (except narcotics) or
- Potassium-containing medicines (other) or
- Salt substitutes, low-salt foods, or milk or
- Spironolactone (e.g., Aldactone) or
- Triamterene (e.g., Dyrenium)—Use with potassium supplements may further increase potassium blood levels, which may cause or worsen heart problems
- Digitalis glycosides (heart medicine)—Use with potassium supplements may make heart problems worse
- Thiazide diuretics (water pills)—If you have been taking a potassium supplement and a thiazide diuretic together, stopping the thiazide diuretic may cause hyperkalemia (high blood levels of potassium)

Other medical problems—The presence of other medical problems may affect the use of potassium supplements. Make sure you tell your doctor if you have any other medical problems, especially:

- Addison's disease (underactive adrenal glands) or
- Dehydration (excessive loss of body water, continuing or severe) or
- Diabetes mellitus (sugar diabetes) or
- Kidney disease—Potassium supplements may increase the risk of hyperkalemia (high blood levels of potassium), which may worsen or cause heart problems in patients with these conditions
- Diarrhea (continuing or severe)—The loss of fluid in combination with potassium supplements may cause

kidney problems, which may increase the risk of hyperkalemia (high blood levels of potassium)
- Heart disease—Potassium supplements may make this condition worse
- Intestinal or esophageal blockage—Potassium supplements may damage the intestines
- Stomach ulcer—Potassium supplements may make this condition worse

Proper Use of This Medicine

For patients taking the *liquid form* of this medicine:

- This medicine *must be diluted* in at least one-half glass (4 ounces) of cold water or juice to reduce its possible stomach-irritating or laxative effect.
- If you are on a salt (sodium)-restricted diet, check with your doctor before using tomato juice to dilute your medicine. Tomato juice has a high salt content.

For patients taking the *soluble granule, soluble powder, or soluble tablet form* of this medicine:

- This medicine must be completely dissolved in at least one-half glass (4 ounces) of cold water or juice to reduce its possible stomach-irritating or laxative effect.
- Allow any "fizzing" to stop before taking the dissolved medicine.
- If you are on a salt (sodium)-restricted diet, check with your doctor before using tomato juice to dilute your medicine. Tomato juice has a high salt content.

For patients taking the *extended-release tablet form* of this medicine:

- Swallow the tablets whole with a full (8–ounce) glass of water. Do not chew or suck on the tablet.
- Some tablets may be broken or crushed and sprinkled on applesauce or other soft food. However, check with your doctor or pharmacist first, since this should not be done for most tablets.
- If you have trouble swallowing tablets or if they seem to stick in your throat, check with your doctor. When this medicine is not properly released, it can cause irritation that may lead to ulcers.

For patients taking the *extended-release capsule form* of this medicine:

- Do not crush or chew the capsule. Swallow the capsule whole with a full (8–ounce) glass of water.
- Some capsules may be opened and the contents sprinkled on applesauce or other soft food. However, check with your doctor or pharmacist first, since this should not be done for most capsules.

Take this medicine immediately after meals or with food to lessen possible stomach upset or laxative action.

Take this medicine only as directed by your doctor. Do not take more of it, do not take it more often, and do not take it for a longer time than your doctor ordered. *This is especially important if you are also taking both diuretics (water pills) and digitalis medicines for your heart.*

Dosing—The dose of these single or combination medicines will be different for different patients. *Follow your doctor's orders or the directions on the label.* The following information includes only the average dose of these medicines. *If your dose is different, do not change it* unless your doctor tells you to do so.

The number of ounces of solution that you drink, or the number of tablets or capsules you take, depends on the strength of the medicine. Also, *the number of doses you take each day, the time allowed between doses, and the length of time you take the medicine depend on the medical problem for which you are taking the single or combination medicine.*

For potassium bicarbonate
- For *oral* dosage form (tablets for solution):
  - To prevent potassium loss or replace potassium lost by the body:
    - Adults and teenagers—25 to 50 milliequivalents (mEq) dissolved in one-half to one glass of cold water, taken one or two times a day. Your doctor may change the dose if needed. However, most people will not take more than 100 mEq a day.
    - Children—Dose must be determined by your doctor.

For potassium bicarbonate and potassium chloride
- For *oral* dosage form (granules for solution):
  - To prevent potassium loss or replace potassium lost by the body:
    - Adults and teenagers—20 milliequivalents (mEq) dissolved in one-half to one glass of cold water, taken one or two times a day. Your doctor may change the dose if needed. However, most people will not take more than 100 mEq a day.
    - Children—Dose must be determined by your doctor.
- For *oral* dosage form (tablets for solution):
  - To prevent potassium loss or replace potassium lost by the body:
    - Adults and teenagers—20, 25, or 50 mEq dissolved in one-half to one glass of cold water, taken one or two times a day. Your doctor may change the dose if needed. However, most people will not take more than 100 mEq a day.
    - Children—Dose must be determined by your doctor.

For potassium bicarbonate and potassium citrate
- For *oral* dosage form (tablets for solution):
  - To prevent potassium loss or replace potassium lost by the body:
    - Adults and teenagers—25 or 50 milliequivalents (mEq) dissolved in one-half to one glass of cold water, taken one or two times a day. Your doctor may change the dose if needed. However, most people will not take more than 100 mEq a day.
    - Children—Dose must be determined by your doctor.

For potassium chloride
- For *oral* dosage form (extended-release capsules):
  - To replace potassium lost by the body:
    - Adults and teenagers—40 to 100 milliequivalents (mEq) a day, divided into two or three smaller doses during the day. Your doctor may change the dose if needed. However, most people will not take more than 100 mEq a day.
  - To prevent potassium loss:
    - Adults and teenagers—16 to 24 mEq a day, divided into two or three smaller doses during the day. Your doctor may change the dose if needed. However, most people will not take more than 100 mEq a day.

- Children—Dose must be determined by your doctor.
- For *oral* dosage form (liquid for solution):
  - To prevent potassium loss or replace potassium lost by the body:
    - Adults and teenagers—20 mEq mixed into one-half glass of cold water or juice, taken one to four times a day. Your doctor may change the dose if needed. However, most people will not take more than 100 mEq a day.
    - Children—Dose is based on body weight and must be determined by your doctor. The usual dose is 1 to 3 mEq of potassium per kilogram (kg) (0.45 to 1.36 mEq per pound) of body weight taken in smaller doses during the day. The solution should be well mixed in water or juice.
- For *oral* dosage form (powder for solution):
  - To prevent potassium loss or replace potassium lost by the body:
    - Adults and teenagers—15 to 25 mEq dissolved in four to six ounces of cold water, taken two or four times a day. Your doctor may change the dose if needed. However, most people will not take more than 100 mEq a day.
    - Children—Dose is based on body weight and must be determined by your doctor. The usual dose is 1 to 3 mEq per kg (0.45 to 1.36 mEq per pound) of body weight taken in smaller doses during the day. The solution should be mixed into water or juice.
- For *oral* dosage form (powder for suspension):
  - To prevent potassium loss or replace potassium lost by the body:
    - Adults and teenagers—20 mEq dissolved in two to six ounces of cold water, taken one to five times a day. Your doctor may change the dose if needed. However, most people will not take more than 100 mEq a day.
    - Children—Dose must be determined by your doctor.
- For *oral* dosage form (extended-release tablets):
  - To prevent potassium loss or replace potassium lost by the body:
    - Adults and teenagers—6.7 to 20 mEq taken three times a day. However, most people will not take more than 100 mEq a day.
    - Children—Dose must be determined by your doctor.

For potassium gluconate
- For *oral* dosage form (liquid for solution):
  - To prevent potassium loss or replace potassium lost by the body:
    - Adults and teenagers—20 milliequivalents (mEq) mixed into one-half glass of cold water or juice, taken two to four times a day. Your doctor may change the dose if needed. However, most people will not take more than 100 mEq a day.
    - Children—Dose is based on body weight and must be determined by your doctor. The usual dose is 2 to 3 mEq per kilogram (kg) (0.9 to 1.36 mEq per pound) of body weight a day, taken in smaller doses during the day. The solution should be completely mixed into water or juice.

- For *oral* dosage form (tablets):
  - To prevent potassium loss or replace potassium lost by the body:
    - Adults and teenagers—5 to 10 mEq taken two to four times a day. However, most people will not take more than 100 mEq a day.
    - Children—Dose must be determined by your doctor.

For potassium gluconate and potassium chloride
- For *oral* dosage form (liquid for solution):
  - To prevent potassium loss or replace potassium lost by the body:
    - Adults and teenagers—20 milliequivalents (mEq) diluted in 2 tablespoonfuls or more of cold water or juice, taken two to four times a day. Your doctor may change the dose if needed. However, most people will not take more than 100 mEq a day.
    - Children—Dose is based on body weight and must be determined by your doctor. The usual dose is 2 to 3 mEq per kilogram (kg) (0.9 to 1.36 mEq per pound) of body weight taken in smaller doses during the day. The solution should be well mixed into water or juice.
- For *oral* dosage form (powder for solution):
  - To prevent potassium loss or replace potassium lost by the body:
    - Adults and teenagers—20 mEq mixed in 2 tablespoonfuls or more of cold water or juice taken two to four times a day. Your doctor may change the dose if needed. However, most people will not take more than 100 mEq a day.
    - Children—Dose is base on body weight and must be determined by your doctor. The usual dose is 2 to 3 mEq per kg (0.9 to 1.36 mEq per pound) of body weight taken in smaller doses during the day. The solution should be well mixed into water or juice.

For potassium gluconate and potassium citrate
- For *oral* dosage form (liquid for solution):
  - To prevent potassium loss or replace potassium lost by the body:
    - Adults and teenagers—20 milliequivalents (mEq) mixed into one-half glass of cold water or juice, taken two to four times a day. Your doctor may change the dose if needed. However, most people will not take more than 100 mEq a day.
    - Children—Dose is based on body weight and must be determined by your doctor. The usual dose is 2 to 3 mEq per kg (0.9 to 1.36 mEq per pound) of body weight taken in smaller doses during the day. The solution should be well mixed into water or juice.

For trikates
- For *oral* dosage form (liquid for solution):
  - To prevent potassium loss or replace potassium lost by the body:
    - Adults and teenagers—15 milliequivalents (mEq) mixed into one-half glass of cold water or juice, taken three or four times a day. Your doctor may change the dose if needed. However, most people will not take more than 100 mEq a day.
    - Children—Dose is based on body weight and must be determined by your doctor. The usual dose is 2 to 3 mEq per kilogram (kg) (0.9 to

1.36 mEq per pound) of body weight taken in smaller doses during the day. The solution should be well mixed into water or juice.

Missed dose—If you miss a dose of this medicine and remember within 2 hours, take the missed dose right away with food or liquids. Then go back to your regular dosing schedule. However, if you do not remember until later, skip the missed dose and go back to your regular dosing schedule. Do not double doses.

Storage—To store this medicine:
- Keep out of the reach of children.
- Store away from heat and direct light.
- Do not store in the bathroom, near the kitchen sink, or in other damp places. Heat or moisture may cause the medicine to break down.
- Keep the liquid form of this medicine from freezing.
- Do not keep outdated medicine or medicine no longer needed. Be sure that any discarded medicine is out of the reach of children.

Precautions While Using This Medicine

Your doctor should check your progress at regular visits to make sure the medicine is working properly and that possible side effects are avoided. Laboratory tests may be necessary.

Do not use salt substitutes, eat low-sodium foods, especially some breads and canned foods, or drink low-sodium milk unless you are told to do so by your doctor, since these products may contain potassium. It is important to read the labels carefully on all low-sodium food products.

Check with your doctor before starting any physical exercise program, especially if you are out of condition and are taking any other medicine. Exercise and certain medicines may increase the amount of potassium in the blood.

Check with your doctor at once if you notice blackish stools or other signs of stomach or intestinal bleeding. This medicine may cause such a condition to become worse, especially when taken in tablet form.

Side Effects of This Medicine

Along with its needed effects, a medicine may cause some unwanted effects. Although not all of these side effects may occur, if they do occur they may need medical attention.

Stop taking this medicine and check with your doctor immediately if any of the following side effects occur:
  Less common
    Confusion; irregular or slow heartbeat; numbness or tingling in hands, feet, or lips; shortness of breath or difficult breathing; unexplained anxiety; unusual tiredness or weakness; weakness or heaviness of legs

Also, check with your doctor if any of the following side effects occur:
  Rare
    Abdominal or stomach pain, cramping, or soreness (continuing); chest or throat pain, especially when swallowing; stools with signs of blood (red or black color)

Other side effects may occur that usually do not need medical attention. These side effects may go away during treatment as your body adjusts to the medicine. However, check with your doctor if any of the following side effects continue or are bothersome:

More common

Diarrhea; nausea; stomach pain, discomfort, or gas (mild); vomiting

Sometimes you may see what appears to be a whole tablet in the stool after taking certain extended-release potassium chloride tablets. This is to be expected. Your body has absorbed the potassium from the tablet and the shell is then expelled.

Other side effects not listed above may also occur in some patients. If you notice any other effects, check with your doctor.

PRAMIPEXOLE (Oral route) - pra-mi-PEX-ole

Commonly used brand name(s)

In the U.S.—
Mirapex

Available Dosage Forms:
• Tablet

Therapeutic Class: Antiparkinsonian
Pharmacologic Class: Dopamine Agonist

Uses For This Medicine

Pramipexole is used to treat Parkinson's disease. It may be used alone, or in combination with levodopa or other medicines to treat this disease.

This medicine is available only with your doctor's prescription.

Before Using This Medicine

In deciding to use a medicine, the risks of taking the medicine must be weighed against the good it will do. This is a decision you and your doctor will make. For this medicine, the following should be considered:

Allergies—Tell your doctor if you have ever had any unusual or allergic reaction to this medicine or any other medicines. Also tell your health care professional if you have any other types of allergies, such as to foods, dyes, preservatives, or animals. For non-prescription products, read the label or package ingredients carefully.

Pediatric—Studies on this medicine have been done only in adult patients, and there is no specific information comparing use of pramipexole in children with use in other age groups.

Geriatric—Hallucinations (seeing, hearing, or feeling things that are not there) may be especially likely to occur in elderly patients, who are usually more sensitive than younger adults to the effects of pramipexole.

Pregnancy—

	Pregnancy Category	Explanation
All Trimesters	C	Animal studies have shown an adverse effect and there are no adequate studies in pregnant women OR no animal studies have been conducted and there are no adequate studies in pregnant women.

Breast Feeding—Studies suggest that this medication may alter milk production or composition. If an alternative to this medication is not prescribed, you should monitor the infant for side effects and adequate milk intake.

Other medicines—

Using this medicine with any of the following medicines may cause an increased risk of certain side effects, but using both drugs may be the best treatment for you. If both medicines are prescribed together, your doctor may change the dose or how often you use one or both of the medicines.

Cimetidine, Kava

Interactions with Food/Tobacco/Alcohol—Certain medicines should not be used at or around the time of eating food or eating certain types of food since interactions may occur. Using alcohol or tobacco with certain medicines may also cause interactions to occur. Discuss with your healthcare professional the use of your medicine with food, alcohol, or tobacco.

Other medical problems—The presence of other medical problems may affect the use of this medicine. Make sure you tell your doctor if you have any other medical problems, especially:

• Eye problems, especially with the retina—Animal studies have shown that problems with the retina may occur; it is not certain if this may occur in humans

• Hallucinations (seeing, hearing, or feeling things that are not there) or

• Hypotension (low blood pressure) or

• Postural hypotension (dizziness, lightheadedness, or fainting, especially when getting up from a lying or sitting position)—Pramipexole may make these conditions worse

• Kidney problems—Higher blood levels of pramipexole may result, and cause an increase in side effects

Proper Use of This Medicine

Take this medicine every day exactly as directed by your doctor in order to improve your condition as much as possible. Do not take more of it or less of it, and do not take it more or less often than your doctor ordered.

Dosing—The dose of this medicine will be different for different patients. Follow your doctor's orders or the directions on the label. The following information includes only the average doses of this medicine. If your dose is different, do not change it unless your doctor tells you to do so.

The amount of medicine that you take depends on the strength of the medicine. Also, the number of doses you take each day, the time allowed between doses, and the length of time you take the medicine depend on the medical problem for which you are using the medicine.

- For oral dosage form (tablets):
  - For Parkinson's disease:
    - Adults—At first, 0.125 milligrams (mg) three times a day. Your doctor will increase your dose gradually as needed and tolerated. However, the dose usually is not more than 4.5 mg a day.
    - Children—Use and dose must be determined by your doctor.

Missed dose—If you miss a dose of this medicine, take it as soon as possible. However, if it is almost time for your next dose, skip the missed dose and go back to your regular dosing schedule. Do not double doses.

Storage—Store the medicine in a closed container at room temperature, away from heat, moisture, and direct light. Keep from freezing.

Keep out of the reach of children.

Do not keep outdated medicine or medicine no longer needed.

Precautions While Using This Medicine

It is important that your doctor check your progress at regular visits. This is necessary to allow dose adjustments and to reduce any unwanted effects.

Do not stop taking this medicine without first checking with your doctor. Your doctor may want you to reduce gradually the amount you are taking before stopping completely.

This medicine may cause some people to become drowsy, dizzy or lightheaded, or to have vision problems, weakness, or problems with coordination. Make sure you know how you react to this medicine before you drive, use machines, or do anything else that could be dangerous if you are not alert, well-coordinated, or able to think or see well.

Patients receiving this medicine have reported falling asleep while engaged in daily living activities, including the operation of motor vehicles. Some patients have further reported that they were fully alert just prior to falling asleep and had no warning signs such as excessive drowsiness.

Dizziness, lightheadedness, or fainting may occur, especially when you get up from a lying or sitting position. These symptoms are more likely to occur when you begin taking this medicine, or when the dose is increased. Getting up slowly may help. If you should have this problem, check with your doctor.

Hallucinations (seeing, hearing, or feeling things that are not there) may occur in some patients. This is more common with elderly patients.

Side Effects of This Medicine

Along with its needed effects, a medicine may cause some unwanted effects. Although not all of these side effects may occur, if they do occur they may need medical attention.

Check with your doctor as soon as possible if any of the following side effects occur:

More common
  Dizziness, lightheadedness, or fainting, especially when standing up; drowsiness; hallucinations (seeing, hearing, or feeling things that are not there); nausea; trouble in sleeping; twitching, twisting, or other unusual body movements; unusual tiredness or weakness

Less common
  Confusion; cough; difficulty in swallowing; double vision or other changes in vision; falling asleep without warning; fearfulness, suspiciousness, or other mental changes; fever; frequent urination; memory loss; muscle or joint pain; muscle weakness; restlessness or need to keep moving; shortness of breath; swelling of body; tightness in chest; troubled breathing; wheezing; writhing, twisting, or other unusual body movements

Rare
  Abnormal thinking; anxiety; bloody or cloudy urine; chest pain; difficult, burning, or painful urination; dizziness; frequent urge to urinate; loss of bladder control; mood or mental changes; swelling of arms or legs

Some side effects may occur that usually do not need medical attention. These side effects may go away during treatment as your body adjusts to the medicine. Also, your health care professional may be able to tell you about ways to prevent or reduce some of these side effects. Check with your health care professional if any of the following side effects continue or are bothersome or if you have any questions about them:

More common
  Constipation; dryness of mouth; headache; heartburn, indigestion, or acid stomach

Less common
  Abnormal dreams; decreased sexual drive or ability; general feeling of discomfort or illness; increased cough; increased sweating; itching; joint pain; loss of appetite; runny nose; skin problems, such as rash or itching; weight loss

Other side effects not listed may also occur in some patients. If you notice any other effects, check with your healthcare professional.

PRAMLINTIDE (Subcutaneous route) - PRAM-lin-tide

Black Box Warning

Pramlintide acetate is used with insulin and has been associated with an increased risk of insulin-induced severe hypoglycemia, particularly in patients with type 1 diabetes. When severe hypoglycemia associated with pramlintide acetate use occurs, it is seen within 3 hours following a pramlintide acetate injection. If severe hypoglycemia occurs while operating a motor vehicle, heavy machinery, or while engaging in other high-risk activities, serious injuries may occur. Appropriate patient selection, careful patient instruction, and insulin dose adjustments are critical elements for reducing this risk.

Commonly used brand name(s)

In the U.S.—
  Symlin

Available Dosage Forms:
- Solution

Therapeutic Class: Antidiabetic

Uses For This Medicine

Pramlintide is used to control blood sugar in patients with type 1 and type 2 diabetes. It is always used with insulin.

This medicine is available only with your doctor's prescription.

Before Using This Medicine

In deciding to use a medicine, the risks of taking the medicine must be weighed against the good it will do. This is a decision you and your doctor will make. For this medicine, the following should be considered:

Allergies—Tell your doctor if you have ever had any unusual or allergic reaction to this medicine or any other medicines. Also tell your health care professional if you have any other types of allergies, such as to foods, dyes, preservatives, or animals. For non-prescription products, read the label or package ingredients carefully.

Pediatric—Studies on this medicine have been done only in adult patients, and there is no specific information comparing use of pramlintide in children with use in other age groups.

Geriatric—This medicine has been tested and has not been shown to cause different side effects or problems in older people than it does in younger adults. However, some elderly people may be especially sensitive to the effects of low blood sugar. The doctor should manage pramlintide and insulin treatment to prevent an increased risk of severely low blood sugar.

Pregnancy—

	Pregnancy Category	Explanation
All Trimesters	C	Animal studies have shown an adverse effect and there are no adequate studies in pregnant women OR no animal studies have been conducted and there are no adequate studies in pregnant women.

Breast Feeding—There are no adequate studies in women for determining infant risk when using this medication during breastfeeding. Weigh the potential benefits against the potential risks before taking this medication while breastfeeding.

Other medicines—Although certain medicines should not be used together at all, in other cases two different medicines may be used together even if an interaction might occur. In these cases, your doctor may want to change the dose, or other precautions may be necessary. Tell your healthcare professional if you are taking any other prescription or non-prescription (over-the-counter [OTC]) medicine.

Interactions with Food/Tobacco/Alcohol—Certain medicines should not be used at or around the time of eating food or eating certain types of food since interactions may occur. Using alcohol or tobacco with certain medicines may also cause interactions to occur. Discuss with your healthcare professional the use of your medicine with food, alcohol, or tobacco.

Other medical problems—The presence of other medical problems may affect the use of this medicine. Make sure you tell your doctor if you have any other medical problems, especially:

- Gastroparesis (a condition where the stomach takes too long to empty its contents) or
- HbA1c9% (lab test that shows too high or low amount of sugar in the blood) or

- Hypoglycemia unawareness (unable to recognize symptoms of low blood sugar until it becomes severe) or
- Severe hypoglycemia (severe low blood sugar that comes back and has required assistance from medical personnel in the past 6 months)—If you have any of these conditions, you should NOT take pramlintide.
- Hypoglycemia, insulin-induced, history of (low blood sugar brought on by using insulin in the past)—May increase risk of severe hypoglycemia occurring again

Proper Use of This Medicine

Dosing—The dose of this medicine will be different for different patients. Follow your doctor's orders or the directions on the label. The following information includes only the average doses of this medicine. If your dose is different, do not change it unless your doctor tells you to do so.

The amount of medicine that you take depends on the strength of the medicine. Also, the number of doses you take each day, the time allowed between doses, and the length of time you take the medicine depend on the medical problem for which you are using the medicine.

It is important to follow any instructions from your doctor about the careful selection and rotation of injection sites on your body.

You should never mix your insulin and pramlintide injections. These injections should be done separately. If you have questions about this, ask your doctor or pharmacist.

- For injection dosage form:
  - Diabetes, type 1 or type 2:
    - Adults—The dose is based on your blood sugar and how well your body adjusts to the medicine. This must be determined by your doctor. The medicine is injected under the skin in your abdomen or thigh right before major meals. Also, your doctor will reduce your insulin dose by half before you begin receiving pramlintide.
    - Children—Use and dose must be determined by your doctor.

Missed dose—Call your doctor or pharmacist for instructions.

Storage—Store in the refrigerator. Do not freeze.

A pramlintide vial in use may be kept in the refrigerator or at room temperature for up to 28 days. An open vial of pramlintide that has been kept in the refrigerator or at room temperature for longer than 28 days should be thrown away. Storing prefilled syringes in the refrigerator with the needle pointed up reduces problems that can occur, such as crystals forming in the needle and blocking it up.

Precautions While Using This Medicine

It is very important that your doctor check your progress at regular visits, especially during the first few weeks of pramlintide treatment.

It is very important to follow carefully any instructions from your health care team about:

- Alcohol—Drinking alcohol may cause severe low blood sugar. Discuss this with your health care team.
- Other medicines—Do not take other medicines unless they have been discussed with your doctor. This especially includes nonprescription medicines such as as-

pirin, and medicines for appetite control, asthma, colds, cough, hay fever, or sinus problems.

- Counseling—Other family members need to learn how to prevent side effects or help with side effects if they occur. Also, patients with diabetes, especially teenagers, may need special counseling about pramlintide dosing changes that might occur because of lifestyle changes, such as changes in exercise and diet. Furthermore, counseling on contraception and pregnancy may be needed because of the problems that can occur in women with diabetes who become pregnant.

- Travel—Keep a recent prescription and your medical history with you. Be prepared for an emergency as you would normally. Make allowances for changing time zones, keep your meal times as close as possible to your usual meal times, and store pramlintide properly.

In case of emergency—There may be a time when you need emergency help for a problem caused by your diabetes. You need to be prepared for these emergencies. It is a good idea to:

- Wear a medical identification (ID) bracelet or neck chain at all times. Also, carry an ID card in your wallet or purse that says that you have diabetes and lists all of your medicines.
- Keep an extra supply of insulin and syringes with needles on hand in case high blood sugar occurs.
- Keep some kind of quick-acting sugar handy to treat low blood sugar.
- Have a glucagon kit available in case severe low blood sugar occurs. Check and replace any expired kits regularly.

Too much insulin can cause low blood sugar (also called hypoglycemia or insulin reaction). Symptoms of low blood sugar must be treated before they lead to unconsciousness (passing out). Different people may feel different symptoms of low blood sugar. It is important that you learn what symptoms of low blood sugar you usually have so that you can treat it quickly.

- Symptoms of low blood sugar can include: anxious feeling, behavior change similar to being drunk, blurred vision, cold sweats, confusion, cool pale skin, difficulty in concentrating, drowsiness, excessive hunger, fast heartbeat, headache, nausea, nervousness, nightmares, restless sleep, shakiness, slurred speech, and unusual tiredness or weakness.

- The symptoms of low blood sugar may develop quickly and may result from:
  ◦ delaying or missing a scheduled meal or snack.
  ◦ exercising more than usual.
  ◦ drinking a significant amount of alcohol.
  ◦ taking certain medicines.
  ◦ using too much insulin.
  ◦ sickness (especially with vomiting or diarrhea).

- Know what to do if symptoms of low blood sugar occur. Eating some form of quick-acting sugar when symptoms of low blood sugar first appear will usually prevent them from getting worse. Good sources of sugar include:
  ◦ Glucose tablets or gel, fruit juice or nondiet soft drink (4 to 6 ounces [one-half cup]), corn syrup or honey (1 tablespoon), sugar cubes (six one-half inch size), or table sugar (dissolved in water).
    ▪ If a snack is not scheduled for an hour or more you should also eat a light snack, such as cheese and crackers, half a sandwich, or drink an 8–ounce glass of milk.

- Do not use chocolate because its fat slows down the sugar entering into the blood stream.
  ◦ Glucagon is used in emergency situations such as unconsciousness. Have a glucagon kit available and know how to prepare and use it. Members of your household also should know how and when to use it.

High blood sugar (hyperglycemia) is another problem related to uncontrolled diabetes. If you have any symptoms of high blood sugar, contact your health care team right away. If high blood sugar is not treated, severe hyperglycemia can occur, leading to ketoacidosis (diabetic coma) and death.

- The symptoms of mild high blood sugar appear more slowly than those of low blood sugar. Symptoms can include: blurred vision; drowsiness; dry mouth; flushed and dry skin; fruit-like breath odor; increased urination (frequency and volume); loss of appetite; stomachache, nausea, or vomiting; tiredness; troubled breathing (rapid and deep); and unusual thirst.

- Symptoms of severe high blood sugar (called ketoacidosis or diabetic coma) that need immediate hospitalization include: flushed and dry skin, fruit-like breath odor, ketones in urine, passing out, and troubled breathing (rapid and deep).

- High blood sugar symptoms may occur if you:
  ◦ have diarrhea, a fever, or an infection.
  ◦ do not take enough insulin or skip a dose of insulin.
  ◦ do not exercise as much as usual.
  ◦ overeat or do not follow your meal plan.

- Know what to do if high blood sugar occurs. Your doctor may recommend changes in your pramlintide and/or insulin dose or meal plan to avoid high blood sugar. Symptoms of high blood sugar must be corrected before they progress to more serious conditions. Check with your doctor often to make sure you are controlling your blood sugar. Your doctor might discuss the following with you:

  ◦ Increasing your insulin dose when you plan to eat an unusually large dinner, such as on holidays. This type of increase is called an anticipatory dose.
  ◦ Decreasing your dose for a short time for special needs, such as when you cannot exercise as you normally do. Changing only one type of insulin dose (usually the first dose) and anticipating how the change may affect other doses during the day. Contacting your doctor if you need a permanent change in dose.
  ◦ Delaying a meal if your blood glucose is over 200 mg/dL to allow time for your blood sugar to go down. An extra insulin dose may be needed if your blood sugar does not come down shortly.
  ◦ Not exercising if your blood glucose is over 240 mg/dL and reporting this to your doctor immediately.
  ◦ Being hospitalized if ketoacidosis or diabetic coma occurs.

Side Effects of This Medicine

Along with its needed effects, a medicine may cause some unwanted effects. Although not all of these side effects may occur, if they do occur they may need medical attention.

Check with your doctor immediately if any of the following side effects occur:

More common

   Anxiety; blurred vision; chills; cold sweats; coma; confusion; cool pale skin; cough; depression; difficulty swallowing; dizziness; fast heartbeat; headache; hives; increased hunger; itching; nausea; nervousness; nightmares; puffiness or swelling of the eyelids or around the eyes, face, lips, or tongue; seizures; shakiness; shortness of breath; skin rash; slurred speech; tightness in chest; unusual tiredness or weakness; wheezing

Some side effects may occur that usually do not need medical attention. These side effects may go away during treatment as your body adjusts to the medicine. Also, your health care professional may be able to tell you about ways to prevent or reduce some of these side effects. Check with your health care professional if any of the following side effects continue or are bothersome or if you have any questions about them:

More common

Difficulty in moving; inflicted injury; loss of appetite; muscle pain or stiffness; pain in joints; stomach pain; vomiting; weight loss

Less common

Body aches or pain; congestion; dryness or soreness of throat; fever; hoarseness; runny nose; tender, swollen glands in neck; trouble in swallowing; voice changes

Other side effects not listed may also occur in some patients. If you notice any other effects, check with your healthcare professional.

PRAZOSIN   (Oral route) - PRA-zoe-sin

Commonly used brand name(s)

In the U.S.—
   Minipress

Available Dosage Forms:
   • Capsule
   • Tablet

Therapeutic Class: Cardiovascular Agent
Pharmacologic Class: Alpha-1 Adrenergic Blocker

Uses For This Medicine

Prazosin belongs to the general class of medicines called antihypertensives. It is used to treat high blood pressure (hypertension).

High blood pressure adds to the work load of the heart and arteries. If it continues for a long time, the heart and arteries may not function properly. This can damage the blood vessels of the brain, heart, and kidneys, resulting in a stroke, heart failure, or kidney failure. High blood pressure may also increase the risk of heart attacks. These problems may be less likely to occur if blood pressure is controlled.

Prazosin works by relaxing blood vessels so that blood passes through them more easily. This helps to lower blood pressure.

Prazosin may also be used for other conditions as determined by your doctor.

Prazosin is available only with your doctor's prescription.

Once a medicine has been approved for marketing for a certain use, experience may show that it is also useful for other medical problems. Although these uses are not included in product labeling, prazosin is used in certain patients with the following medical conditions:
   • Congestive heart failure
   • Ergot alkaloid poisoning
   • Pheochromocytoma
   • Raynaud's disease
   • Benign enlargement of the prostate

For patients taking this medicine for benign enlargement of the prostate:
   • Prazosin will not shrink the size of your prostate, but it does help to relieve the symptoms.

Before Using This Medicine

In deciding to use a medicine, the risks of taking the medicine must be weighed against the good it will do. This is a decision you and your doctor will make. For this medicine, the following should be considered:

Allergies—Tell your doctor if you have ever had any unusual or allergic reaction to this medicine or any other medicines. Also tell your health care professional if you have any other types of allergies, such as to foods, dyes, preservatives, or animals. For non-prescription products, read the label or package ingredients carefully.

Pediatric—Studies on this medicine have been done only in adult patients, and there is no specific information comparing use of prazosin in children with use in other age groups.

Geriatric—Dizziness, lightheadedness, or fainting (especially when getting up from a lying or sitting position) may be more likely to occur in the elderly, who are more sensitive to the effects of prazosin. In addition, prazosin may reduce tolerance to cold temperatures in elderly patients.

Pregnancy—

	Pregnancy Category	Explanation
All Trimesters	C	Animal studies have shown an adverse effect and there are no adequate studies in pregnant women OR no animal studies have been conducted and there are no adequate studies in pregnant women.

Breast Feeding—There are no adequate studies in women for determining infant risk when using this medication during breastfeeding. Weigh the potential benefits against the potential risks before taking this medication while breastfeeding.

Other medicines—

Using this medicine with any of the following medicines is usually not recommended, but may be required in some cases. If both medicines are prescribed together, your doctor may change the dose or how often you use one or both of the medicines.

Tadalafil, Vardenafil

Interactions with Food/Tobacco/Alcohol—Certain medicines should not be used at or around the time of eating food or eating certain types of food since interactions may occur. Using alcohol or tobacco with certain medicines may also cause interactions to occur. Discuss with your healthcare professional the use of your medicine with food, alcohol, or tobacco.

Other medical problems—The presence of other medical problems may affect the use of this medicine. Make sure you tell your doctor if you have any other medical problems, especially:

- Angina (chest pain) or
- Heart disease (severe)—Prazosin may make these conditions worse
- Kidney disease—Possible increased sensitivity to the effects of prazosin

Proper Use of This Medicine

For patients taking this medicine for high blood pressure:

- In addition to the use of the medicine your doctor has prescribed, treatment for your high blood pressure may include weight control and care in the types of foods you eat, especially foods high in sodium. Your doctor will tell you which of these are most important for you. You should check with your doctor before changing your diet.
- Many patients who have high blood pressure will not notice any signs of the problem. In fact, many may feel normal. It is very important that you take your medicine exactly as directed and that you keep your appointments with your doctor even if you feel well.
- Remember that prazosin will not cure your high blood pressure but it does help control it. Therefore, you must continue to take it as directed if you expect to lower your blood pressure and keep it down. You may have to take high blood pressure medicine for the rest of your life. If high blood pressure is not treated, it can cause serious problems such as heart failure, blood vessel disease, stroke, or kidney disease.

To help you remember to take your medicine, try to get into the habit of taking it at the same time each day.

Dosing—The dose of this medicine will be different for different patients. Follow your doctor's orders or the directions on the label. The following information includes only the average doses of this medicine. If your dose is different, do not change it unless your doctor tells you to do so.

The amount of medicine that you take depends on the strength of the medicine. Also, the number of doses you take each day, the time allowed between doses, and the length of time you take the medicine depend on the medical problem for which you are using the medicine.

- For oral dosage form (capsules or tablets):
  - For high blood pressure:
    - Adults—At first, 0.5 or 1 milligram (mg) two or three times a day. Then, your doctor will slowly increase your dose to 6 to 15 mg a day. This is divided into two or three doses.
    - Children—Dose is based on body weight and must be determined by your doctor. The usual dose is 50 to 400 micrograms (mcg) (0.05 to 0.4 mg) per kilogram of body weight (22.73 to 181.2 mcg per pound [0.023 to 0.18 mg per pound]) a day. This is divided into two or three doses.

Missed dose—If you miss a dose of this medicine, take it as soon as possible. However, if it is almost time for your next dose, skip the missed dose and go back to your regular dosing schedule. Do not double doses.

Storage—Store the medicine in a closed container at room temperature, away from heat, moisture, and direct light. Keep from freezing.

Keep out of the reach of children.

Do not keep outdated medicine or medicine no longer needed.

Precautions While Using This Medicine

It is important that your doctor check your progress at regular visits to make sure that this medicine is working properly.

For patients taking this medicine for high blood pressure:

- Do not take other medicines unless they have been discussed with your doctor. This especially includes over-the-counter (nonprescription) medicines for appetite control, asthma, colds, cough, hay fever, or sinus problems, since they may tend to make prazosin less effective.

Dizziness, lightheadedness, or sudden fainting may occur after you take this medicine, especially when you get up from a lying or sitting position. These effects are more likely to occur when you take the first dose of this medicine. Taking the first dose at bedtime may prevent problems. However, be especially careful if you need to get up during the night. These effects may also occur with any doses you take after the first dose. Getting up slowly may help lessen this problem. If you feel dizzy, lie down so that you do not faint. Then sit for a few moments before standing to prevent the dizziness from returning.

The dizziness, lightheadedness, or fainting is more likely to occur if you drink alcohol, stand for a long time, exercise, or if the weather is hot. While you are taking this medicine, be careful to limit the amount of alcohol you drink. Also, use extra care during exercise or hot weather or if you must stand for a long time.

Prazosin may cause some people to become drowsy or less alert than they are normally. Make sure you know how you react to this medicine before you drive, use machines, or do anything else that could be dangerous if you are dizzy, drowsy, or are not alert. After you have taken several doses of this medicine, these effects should lessen.

Side Effects of This Medicine

Along with its needed effects, a medicine may cause some unwanted effects. Although not all of these side effects may occur, if they do occur they may need medical attention.

Check with your doctor as soon as possible if any of the following side effects occur:

More common

    Dizziness or lightheadedness, especially when getting up from a lying or sitting position; fainting (sudden)

Less common

    Loss of bladder control; pounding heartbeat; swelling of feet or lower legs

Rare

    Chest pain; painful inappropriate erection of penis (continuing); shortness of breath

Some side effects may occur that usually do not need medical attention. These side effects may go away during treatment as your body adjusts to the medicine. Also, your health care professional may be able to tell you about ways to prevent or reduce some of these side effects. Check with your health care professional if any of the following side effects continue or are bothersome or if you have any questions about them:

More common
 Drowsiness; headache; lack of energy

Less common
 Dryness of mouth; nervousness; unusual tiredness or weakness

Rare
 Frequent urge to urinate; nausea

Other side effects not listed may also occur in some patients. If you notice any other effects, check with your healthcare professional.

PREGABALIN (Oral route) - pre-GAB-a-lin

Commonly used brand name(s)

In the U.S.—
 Lyrica

Available Dosage Forms:

• Capsule

Therapeutic Class: Neuropathic Pain Agent

Uses For This Medicine

Pregabalin is used to help control some types of seizures in the treatment of epilepsy. This medicine cannot cure epilepsy and will only work to control seizures for as long as you continue to take it.

This medicine is also used to manage a condition called postherpetic neuralgia (pain after "shingles"). It is also used for pain caused by nerve damage associated with diabetes.

Pregabalin is available only with your doctor's prescription.

Before Using This Medicine

In deciding to use a medicine, the risks of taking the medicine must be weighed against the good it will do. This is a decision you and your doctor will make. For this medicine, the following should be considered:

Allergies—Tell your doctor if you have ever had any unusual or allergic reaction to this medicine or any other medicines. Also tell your health care professional if you have any other types of allergies, such as to foods, dyes, preservatives, or animals. For non-prescription products, read the label or package ingredients carefully.

Pediatric—Studies on this medicine have been done only in adult patients, and there is no specific information comparing use of pregabalin in children with use in other age groups.

Geriatric—This medicine has been tested and has not been shown to cause different side effects or problems in older people than it does in younger adults. However, elderly patients are more likely to be more sensitive to pregabalin than younger adults and may require a lower dose.

Pregnancy—

	Pregnancy Category	Explanation
All Trimesters	C	Animal studies have shown an adverse effect and there are no adequate studies in pregnant women OR no animal studies have been conducted and there are no adequate studies in pregnant women.

Breast Feeding—There are no adequate studies in women for determining infant risk when using this medication during breastfeeding. Weigh the potential benefits against the potential risks before taking this medication while breastfeeding.

Other medicines—Although certain medicines should not be used together at all, in other cases two different medicines may be used together even if an interaction might occur. In these cases, your doctor may want to change the dose, or other precautions may be necessary. Tell your healthcare professional if you are taking any other prescription or non-prescription (over-the-counter [OTC]) medicine.

Interactions with Food/Tobacco/Alcohol—Certain medicines should not be used at or around the time of eating food or eating certain types of food since interactions may occur. Using alcohol or tobacco with certain medicines may also cause interactions to occur. Discuss with your healthcare professional the use of your medicine with food, alcohol, or tobacco.

Other medical problems—The presence of other medical problems may affect the use of this medicine. Make sure you tell your doctor if you have any other medical problems, especially:

• Diabetes mellitus—May increase your weight and may increase your risk for skin ulcerations

• Heart disease—May increase your chance of side effects

• Kidney disease—Your doctor may lower your dose of pregabalin.

Proper Use of This Medicine

Pregabalin may be taken with or without food or on a full or empty stomach.

Read the patient information leaflet prior to beginning pregabalin therapy.

Dosing—The dose of this medicine will be different for different patients. Follow your doctor's orders or the directions on the label. The following information includes only the average doses of this medicine. If your dose is different, do not change it unless your doctor tells you to do so.

The amount of medicine that you take depends on the strength of the medicine. Also, the number of doses you take each day, the time allowed between doses, and the length of time you take the medicine depend on the medical problem for which you are using the medicine.

• For oral dosage form (capsules):
  ◦ For diabetic nerve pain:
    ▪ Adults—Oral, 150 milligrams per day, divided (50 mg three times a day).

- Children—Dose must be determined by your doctor.
  - For epilepsy:
    - Adults—Oral, 150 to 600 milligrams per day. The total daily dose should be divided and given two or three times a day.
    - Children—Dose must be determined by your doctor.
  - For post-herpetic neuralgia:
    - Adults—Oral, 150 to 300 milligrams per day. The total daily dose should be divided and given two or three times a day.
    - Children—Dose must be determined by your doctor.

Missed dose—If you miss a dose of this medicine, take it as soon as possible. However, if it is almost time for your next dose, skip the missed dose and go back to your regular dosing schedule. Do not double doses.

Storage—Keep out of the reach of children.

Store the medicine in a closed container at room temperature, away from heat, moisture, and direct light. Keep from freezing.

Do not keep outdated medicine or medicine no longer needed.

Precautions While Using This Medicine

It is important that your doctor check your progress at regular visits, especially for the first few months you take pregabalin. This is necessary to allow dose adjustments and to reduce any unwanted effects.

This medicine will add to the effects of alcohol and other CNS depressants (medicines that make you drowsy or less alert). Some examples of CNS depressants are antihistamines or medicine for hay fever, other allergies, or colds; sedatives, tranquilizers, or sleeping medicine; prescription pain medicine or narcotics; barbiturates; other medicines for seizures; muscle relaxants; or anesthetics, including some dental anesthetics. *Check with your medical doctor or dentist before taking any of the above while you are taking pregabalin.*

Pregabalin may cause blurred vision, double vision, clumsiness, unsteadiness, dizziness, drowsiness, or trouble in thinking. *Make sure you know how you react to this medicine before you drive, use machines, or do anything else that could be dangerous if you are not alert, well-coordinated, or able to think or see well.* If these reactions are especially bothersome, check with your doctor.

This medicine *may cause you to keep extra fluid in your body or cause you to gain weight.* If this side effect is bothersome, check with your doctor.

Do not suddenly stop taking your pregabalin. If you have been instructed to stop taking pregabalin, ask your healthcare professional how to slowly decrease the dose. This is to decrease the chance of having discontinuation symptoms such as dizziness, nausea, headache, vomiting, irritability, nightmares, prickling or tingling feelings.

Report any unexplained muscle pain, tenderness, or weakness particularly if accompanied by a fever. For patients with diabetes, *check with your doctor if you notice changes to your skin or skin sores while taking pregabalin.*

Notify your doctor if you become pregnant, if you plan to become pregnant, or if you father a child while taking pregabalin.

Side Effects of This Medicine

Along with its needed effects, a medicine may cause some unwanted effects. Although not all of these side effects may occur, if they do occur they may need medical attention.

Check with your doctor immediately if any of the following side effects occur:

Less common
Difficult or labored breathing; shortness of breath; tightness in chest; wheezing

Rare
Blistering, peeling, loosening of skin; chills; cough; difficulty swallowing; diarrhea; dizziness; fast heartbeat; hives; itching; joint or muscle pain; puffiness or swelling of the eyelids or around the eyes, face, lips or tongue; red, irritated eyes; red skin lesions, often with a purple center; skin rash; sore throat; sores, ulcers, or white spots in mouth or on lips; unusual tiredness or weakness

Some side effects may occur that usually do not need medical attention. These side effects may go away during treatment as your body adjusts to the medicine. Also, your health care professional may be able to tell you about ways to prevent or reduce some of these side effects. Check with your health care professional if any of the following side effects continue or are bothersome or if you have any questions about them:

More common
Accidental injury; bloating or swelling of face, arms, hands, lower legs, or feet; blurry vision; burning, tingling, numbness or pain in the hands, arms, feet or legs; change in walking and balance; clumsiness; confusion; delusions; dementia; difficulty having a bowel movement (stool); difficulty in speaking; double vision; dry mouth; double vision; dry mouth; fever; headache; hoarseness; increased appetite; lack of coordination; loss of memory; lower back or side pain; mood or mental changes; painful or difficult urination; problems with memory; rapid weight gain; seeing double; shakiness and unsteady walk; sensation of pins and needles; sleepiness or unusual drowsiness; stabbing pain; swelling; tingling of hands or feet; trembling, or other problems with muscle control or coordination; unusual weight gain or loss

Less common
Anxiety; bloated full feeling; burning, crawling, itching, numbness, prickling, "pins and needles", or tingling feelings; chest pain; cold sweats; coma; cool pale skin; cough producing mucus; decrease or change in vision; depression; eye disorder; excess air or gas in stomach or intestines; false or unusual sense of well-being; general feeling of discomfort or illness; increased hunger; joint pain; loss of appetite; loss of bladder control; loss of strength or energy; muscle aches and pains; muscle weakness; muscle twitching or jerking; nausea; nervousness; nightmares; noisy breathing; pain; passing gas; rhythmic movement of muscles; runny nose; seizures; shivering; slurred speech; sweating; trouble sleeping; twitching; uncontrolled eye movements; vomiting

Other side effects not listed may also occur in some patients. If you notice any other effects, check with your healthcare professional.

PRIMIDONE (Oral route) - PRI-mi-done

Commonly used brand name(s)

In the U.S.—
Mysoline

Available Dosage Forms:
- Tablet
- Suspension

Therapeutic Class: Anticonvulsant
Pharmacologic Class: Barbiturate, Intermediate Acting

Uses For This Medicine

Primidone belongs to the group of medicines called anticonvulsants. It is used in the treatment of epilepsy to manage certain types of seizures. Primidone may be used alone or in combination with other anticonvulsants. It acts by controlling nerve impulses in the brain.

Primidone is available only with your doctor's prescription.

Once a medicine has been approved for marketing for a certain use, experience may show that it is also useful for other medical problems. Although this use is not included in product labeling, primidone is used in certain patients with the following medical conditions:
- Essential tremor

Before Using This Medicine

In deciding to use a medicine, the risks of taking the medicine must be weighed against the good it will do. This is a decision you and your doctor will make. For this medicine, the following should be considered:

Allergies—Tell your doctor if you have ever had any unusual or allergic reaction to this medicine or any other medicines. Also tell your health care professional if you have any other types of allergies, such as to foods, dyes, preservatives, or animals. For non-prescription products, read the label or package ingredients carefully.

Pediatric—Unusual excitement or restlessness may occur in children, who are usually more sensitive than adults to these effects of primidone.

Geriatric—Unusual excitement or restlessness may occur in elderly patients, who are usually more sensitive than younger adults to these effects of primidone.

Pregnancy—

	Pregnancy Category	Explanation
All Trimesters	D	Studies in pregnant women have demonstrated a risk to the fetus. However, the benefits of therapy in a life threatening situation or a serious disease, may outweigh the potential risk.

Breast Feeding—There are no adequate studies in women for determining infant risk when using this medication during breastfeeding. Weigh the potential benefits against the potential risks before taking this medication while breastfeeding.

Other medicines—

Using this medicine with any of the following medicines is usually not recommended, but may be required in some cases. If both medicines are prescribed together, your doctor may change the dose or how often you use one or both of the medicines.

Adinazolam, Alprazolam, Amobarbital, Anisindione, Aprobarbital, Bromazepam, Brotizolam, Butabarbital, Butalbital, Carisoprodol, Chloral Hydrate, Chlordiazepoxide, Chlorzoxazone, Clobazam, Clonazepam, Clorazepate, Dantrolene, Diazepam, Dicumarol, Estazolam, Ethchlorvynol, Flunitrazepam, Flurazepam, Halazepam, Ketazolam, Lorazepam, Lormetazepam, Medazepam, Mephenesin, Mephobarbital, Meprobamate, Metaxalone, Methocarbamol, Methohexital, Midazolam, Nitrazepam, Nordazepam, Oxazepam, Pentobarbital, Phenindione, Phenobarbital, Phenprocoumon, Prazepam, Primidone, Quazepam, Quetiapine, Secobarbital, Sodium Oxybate, Temazepam, Thiopental, Triazolam, Valproic Acid

Interactions with Food/Tobacco/Alcohol—Certain medicines should not be used at or around the time of eating food or eating certain types of food since interactions may occur. Using alcohol or tobacco with certain medicines may also cause interactions to occur. The following interactions have been selected on the basis of their potential significance and are not necessarily all-inclusive.

Using this medicine with any of the following may cause an increased risk of certain side effects but may be unavoidable in some cases. If used together, your doctor may change the dose or how often you use this medicine, or give you special instructions about the use of food, alcohol, or tobacco.

Ethanol

Other medical problems—The presence of other medical problems may affect the use of this medicine. Make sure you tell your doctor if you have any other medical problems, especially:
- Asthma, emphysema, or chronic lung disease—Primidone may cause serious problems in breathing
- Hyperactivity (in children) or
- Kidney disease or
- Liver disease—Primidone may make the condition worse
- Porphyria—Primidone should not be used when this medical problem exists because it may make the condition worse

Proper Use of This Medicine

Take primidone every day in regularly spaced doses as ordered by your doctor. This will provide the proper amount of medicine needed to prevent seizures.

Dosing—The dose of this medicine will be different for different patients. Follow your doctor's orders or the directions on the label. The following information includes only the average doses of this medicine. If your dose is different, do not change it unless your doctor tells you to do so.

The amount of medicine that you take depends on the strength of the medicine. Also, the number of doses you take each day, the time allowed between doses, and the length of time you take the medicine depend on the medical problem for which you are using the medicine.
- For oral dosage forms (chewable tablets, tablets or suspension):
  - For epilepsy:
    - Adults, teenagers, and children 8 years of age or older—At first, 100 or 125 milligrams (mg) once a day at bedtime. Your doctor may increase your

dose if needed. However, the dose is usually not more than 2000 mg a day.
- Children up to 8 years of age—At first, 50 mg once a day at bedtime. Your doctor may increase your dose if needed.

Missed dose—If you miss a dose of this medicine, take it as soon as possible. However, if it is almost time for your next dose, skip the missed dose and go back to your regular dosing schedule. Do not double doses.

Storage—Store the medicine in a closed container at room temperature, away from heat, moisture, and direct light. Keep from freezing.

Keep out of the reach of children.

Do not keep outdated medicine or medicine no longer needed.

Precautions While Using This Medicine

It is very important that your doctor check your progress at regular visits, especially during the first few months of treatment with primidone. This will allow your doctor to adjust the amount of medicine you are taking to meet your needs.

If you have been taking primidone regularly for several weeks, you should not suddenly stop taking it. Your doctor may want you to reduce gradually the amount you are taking before stopping completely.

Before you have any medical tests, tell the medical doctor in charge that you are taking this medicine. The results of some tests (such as the metyrapone and phentolamine tests) may be affected by this medicine.

Before having any kind of surgery, dental treatment, or emergency treatment, tell the medical doctor or dentist in charge that you are using this medicine.

This medicine will add to the effects of alcohol and other CNS depressants (medicines that cause drowsiness). Some examples of CNS depressants are antihistamines or medicine for hay fever, other allergies, or colds; sedatives, tranquilizers, or sleeping medicine; prescription pain medicine or narcotics; barbiturates; medicine for seizures; muscle relaxants; or anesthetics, including some dental anesthetics. Check with your doctor before taking any of the above while you are using this medicine.

Primidone may cause some people to become dizzy, lightheaded, drowsy, or less alert than they are normally. Even if taken at bedtime, it may cause some people to feel drowsy or less alert on arising. Make sure you know how you react to this medicine before you drive, use machines, or do anything else that could be dangerous if you are dizzy or are not alert.

Oral contraceptives (birth control pills) containing estrogen may not work properly if you take them while you are taking primidone. Unplanned pregnancies may occur. You should use a different or additional means of birth control while you are taking primidone. If you have any questions about this, check with your health care professional.

Side Effects of This Medicine

Along with its needed effects, a medicine may cause some unwanted effects. Although not all of these side effects may occur, if they do occur they may need medical attention.

Check with your doctor as soon as possible if any of the following side effects occur:

Less common
Unusual excitement or restlessness (especially in children and in the elderly)

Rare
Skin rash; unusual tiredness or weakness

Symptoms of overdose
Confusion; continuous, uncontrolled back-and-forth and/or rolling eye movements; double vision; shortness of breath or troubled breathing

Some side effects may occur that usually do not need medical attention. These side effects may go away during treatment as your body adjusts to the medicine. Also, your health care professional may be able to tell you about ways to prevent or reduce some of these side effects. Check with your health care professional if any of the following side effects continue or are bothersome or if you have any questions about them:

More common
Clumsiness or unsteadiness; dizziness

Less common
Decreased sexual ability; drowsiness; loss of appetite; mood or mental changes; nausea or vomiting

Other side effects not listed may also occur in some patients. If you notice any other effects, check with your healthcare professional.

PROBENECID   (Oral route) - proe-BEN-e-sid

Commonly used brand name(s)

In the U.S.—
Benemid
Probalan

Available Dosage Forms:
- Tablet

Therapeutic Class: Antigout

Uses For This Medicine

Probenecid is used in the treatment of chronic gout or gouty arthritis. These conditions are caused by too much uric acid in the blood. The medicine works by removing the extra uric acid from the body. Probenecid does not cure gout, but after you have been taking it for a few months it will help prevent gout attacks. This medicine will help prevent gout attacks only as long as you continue to take it.

Probenecid is also used to prevent or treat other medical problems that may occur if too much uric acid is present in the body.

Probenecid is sometimes used with certain kinds of antibiotics to make them more effective in the treatment of infections.

Probenecid is available only with your doctor's prescription.

Before Using This Medicine

In deciding to use a medicine, the risks of taking the medicine must be weighed against the good it will do. This is a decision you and your doctor will make. For this medicine, the following should be considered:

Allergies—Tell your doctor if you have ever had any unusual or allergic reaction to this medicine or any other medicines. Also tell your health care professional if you have any other types of allergies, such as to foods, dyes, preservatives, or animals. For non-prescription products, read the label or package ingredients carefully.

Pediatric—Probenecid has been tested in children 2 to 14 years of age for use together with antibiotics. It has not been shown to cause different side effects or problems than it does in adults. Studies on the effects of probenecid in patients with gout have been done only in adults. Gout is very rare in children.

Geriatric—Many medicines have not been studied specifically in older people. Therefore, it may not be known whether they work exactly the same way they do in younger adults. There is no specific information comparing use of probenecid in the elderly with use in other age groups.

Pregnancy—

	Pregnancy Category	Explanation
All Trimesters	B	Animal studies have revealed no evidence of harm to the fetus, however, there are no adequate studies in pregnant women OR animal studies have shown an adverse effect, but adequate studies in pregnant women have failed to demonstrate a risk to the fetus.

Breast Feeding—There are no adequate studies in women for determining infant risk when using this medication during breastfeeding. Weigh the potential benefits against the potential risks before taking this medication while breastfeeding.

Other medicines—

Using this medicine with any of the following medicines is usually not recommended, but may be required in some cases. If both medicines are prescribed together, your doctor may change the dose or how often you use one or both of the medicines.

Methotrexate, Zalcitabine

Interactions with Food/Tobacco/Alcohol—Certain medicines should not be used at or around the time of eating food or eating certain types of food since interactions may occur. Using alcohol or tobacco with certain medicines may also cause interactions to occur. Discuss with your healthcare professional the use of your medicine with food, alcohol, or tobacco.

Other medical problems—The presence of other medical problems may affect the use of this medicine. Make sure you tell your doctor if you have any other medical problems, especially:

- Blood disease or
- Cancer being treated by antineoplastics (cancer medicine) or radiation (x-rays) or

- Kidney disease or stones (or history of) or
- Stomach ulcer (history of)—The chance of side effects may be increased

Proper Use of This Medicine

If probenecid upsets your stomach, it may be taken with food. If this does not work, an antacid may be taken. If stomach upset (nausea, vomiting, or loss of appetite) continues, check with your doctor.

For patients taking probenecid for gout:

- After you begin to take probenecid, gout attacks may continue to occur for a while. However, if you take this medicine regularly as directed by your doctor, the attacks will gradually become less frequent and less painful than before. After you have been taking probenecid for several months, they may stop completely.
- This medicine will help prevent gout attacks but it will not relieve an attack that has already started. Even if you take another medicine for gout attacks, continue to take this medicine also. If you have any questions about this, check with your doctor.

For patients taking probenecid for gout or to help remove uric acid from the body:

- When you first begin taking probenecid, the amount of uric acid in the kidneys is greatly increased. This may cause kidney stones or other kidney problems in some people. To help prevent this, your doctor may want you to drink at least 10 to 12 full glasses (8 ounces each) of fluids each day, or to take another medicine to make your urine less acid. It is important that you follow your doctor's instructions very carefully.

Dosing—The dose of this medicine will be different for different patients. Follow your doctor's orders or the directions on the label. The following information includes only the average doses of this medicine. If your dose is different, do not change it unless your doctor tells you to do so.

The amount of medicine that you take depends on the strength of the medicine. Also, the number of doses you take each day, the time allowed between doses, and the length of time you take the medicine depend on the medical problem for which you are using the medicine.

- For treating gout or removing uric acid from the body:
  - Adults: 250 mg (one-half of a 500–mg tablet) two times a day for about one week, then 500 mg (one tablet) two times a day for a few weeks. After this, the dose will depend on the amount of uric acid in your blood or urine. Most people need 2, 3, or 4 tablets a day, but some people may need higher doses.
  - Children: It is not likely that probenecid will be needed to treat gout or to remove uric acid from the body in children. If a child needs this medicine, however, the dose would have to be determined by the doctor.

- For helping antibiotics work better:
  - Adults: The amount of probenecid will depend on the condition being treated. Sometimes, only one dose of 2 tablets is needed. Other times, the dose will be 1 tablet four times a day.
  - Children: The dose will have to be determined by the doctor. It depends on the child's weight, as well as on the condition being treated. Older children and teenagers may need the same amount as adults.

Missed dose—If you miss a dose of this medicine, take it as soon as possible. However, if it is almost time for your next dose, skip the missed dose and go back to your regular dosing schedule. Do not double doses.

Storage—Store the medicine in a closed container at room temperature, away from heat, moisture, and direct light. Keep from freezing.

Keep out of the reach of children.

Do not keep outdated medicine or medicine no longer needed.

Precautions While Using This Medicine

If you will be taking probenecid for more than a few weeks, your doctor should check your progress at regular visits.

Before you have any medical tests, tell the person in charge that you are taking this medicine. The results of some tests may be affected by probenecid.

For diabetic patients:

- Probenecid may cause false test results with copper sulfate urine sugar tests (Clinitest®), but not with glucose enzymatic urine sugar tests (Clinistix®). If you have any questions about this, check with your health care professional.

For patients taking probenecid for gout or to help remove uric acid from the body:

- Taking aspirin or other salicylates may lessen the effects of probenecid. This will depend on the dose of aspirin or other salicylate that you take, and on how often you take it. Also, drinking too much alcohol may increase the amount of uric acid in the blood and lessen the effects of this medicine. Therefore, do not take aspirin or other salicylates or drink alcoholic beverages while taking this medicine, unless you have first checked with your doctor.

Side Effects of This Medicine

Along with its needed effects, a medicine may cause some unwanted effects. Although not all of these side effects may occur, if they do occur they may need medical attention.

Check with your doctor immediately if any of the following side effects occur:

Rare
 Fast or irregular breathing; puffiness or swellings of the eyelids or around the eyes; shortness of breath, troubled breathing, tightness in chest, or wheezing; changes in the skin color of the face occurring together with any of the other side effects listed here; or skin rash, hives, or itching occurring together with any of the other side effects listed here

Check with your doctor as soon as possible if any of the following side effects occur:

Less common
 Bloody urine; difficult or painful urination; lower back or side pain (especially if severe or sharp); skin rash, hives, or itching (occurring without other signs of an allergic reaction)

Rare
 Cloudy urine; cough or hoarseness; fast or irregular breathing; fever; pain in back and/or ribs; sores, ulcers, or white spots on lips or in mouth; sore throat and fever

with or without chills; sudden decrease in the amount of urine; swelling of face, fingers, feet, and/or lower legs; swollen and/or painful glands; unusual bleeding or bruising; unusual tiredness or weakness; yellow eyes or skin; weight gain

Some side effects may occur that usually do not need medical attention. These side effects may go away during treatment as your body adjusts to the medicine. Also, your health care professional may be able to tell you about ways to prevent or reduce some of these side effects. Check with your health care professional if any of the following side effects continue or are bothersome or if you have any questions about them:

More common
 Headache; joint pain, redness, or swelling; loss of appetite; nausea or vomiting (mild)

Less common
 Dizziness; flushing or redness of face (occurring without any signs of an allergic reaction); frequent urge to urinate; sore gums

Other side effects not listed may also occur in some patients. If you notice any other effects, check with your healthcare professional.

PROBENECID AND COLCHICINE
(Oral route) - proe-BEN-e-sid, KOL-chi-seen

Uses For This Medicine

Probenecid and colchicine combination is used to treat gout or gouty arthritis.

The probenecid in this medicine helps to prevent gout attacks by removing extra uric acid from the body. The colchicine in this medicine also helps to prevent gout attacks. Although colchicine may also be used to relieve an attack of gout, this requires more colchicine than this combination medicine contains. Probenecid and colchicine combination does not cure gout. This medicine will help prevent gout attacks only as long as you continue to take it.

Probenecid and colchicine combination is available only with your doctor's prescription.

Before Using This Medicine

In deciding to use a medicine, the risks of taking the medicine must be weighed against the good it will do. This is a decision you and your doctor will make. For this medicine, the following should be considered:

Allergies—Tell your doctor if you have ever had any unusual or allergic reaction to this medicine or any other medicines. Also tell your health care professional if you have any other types of allergies, such as to foods, dyes, preservatives, or animals. For non-prescription products, read the label or package ingredients carefully.

Pediatric—Studies on this combination medicine have been done only in adult patients, and there is no specific information about its use in children.

Geriatric—Elderly people are especially sensitive to the effects of colchicine. This may increase the chance of side effects during treatment.

There is no specific information comparing use of probenecid in the elderly with use in other age groups.

Pregnancy—

	Pregnancy Category	Explanation
All Trimesters	D	Studies in pregnant women have demonstrated a risk to the fetus. However, the benefits of therapy in a life threatening situation or a serious disease, may outweigh the potential risk.

Breast Feeding—
Colchicine
• Studies in women suggest that this medication poses minimal risk to the infant when used during breastfeeding.
Probenecid
• There are no adequate studies in women for determining infant risk when using this medication during breastfeeding. Weigh the potential benefits against the potential risks before taking this medication while breastfeeding.

Other medicines—

Using this medicine with any of the following medicines is usually not recommended, but may be required in some cases. If both medicines are prescribed together, your doctor may change the dose or how often you use one or both of the medicines.

Clarithromycin, Cyclosporine, Erythromycin, Interferon Alfa-2a, Methotrexate, Zalcitabine

Interactions with Food/Tobacco/Alcohol—Certain medicines should not be used at or around the time of eating food or eating certain types of food since interactions may occur. Using alcohol or tobacco with certain medicines may also cause interactions to occur. The following interactions have been selected on the basis of their potential significance and are not necessarily all-inclusive.

Using this medicine with any of the following is usually not recommended, but may be unavoidable in some cases. If used together, your doctor may change the dose or how often you use this medicine, or give you special instructions about the use of food, alcohol, or tobacco.

Grapefruit Juice

Other medical problems—The presence of other medical problems may affect the use of this medicine. Make sure you tell your doctor if you have any other medical problems, especially:
• Alcohol abuse or
• Blood disease or
• Cancer being treated by antineoplastics (cancer medicine) or radiation (x-rays) or
• Heart disease (severe) or
• Intestinal disease (severe) or
• Kidney disease or stones (or history of) or
• Liver disease or

• Stomach ulcer or other stomach problems (or history of)—The chance of serious side effects may be increased

Proper Use of This Medicine

If this medicine upsets your stomach, it may be taken with food. If this does not work, an antacid may be taken. If stomach upset (nausea, vomiting, loss of appetite, or stomach pain) continues, check with your doctor.

Take this medicine only as directed by your doctor. Do not take more of it and do not take it more often than your doctor ordered. The colchicine in this combination medicine may cause serious side effects if too much is taken.

After you begin to take this medicine, gout attacks may continue to occur for a while. However, if you take this medicine regularly as directed by your doctor, the attacks will gradually become less frequent and less painful than before. After you have been taking this medicine for several months, they may stop completely.

This medicine will help prevent gout attacks but it will not relieve an attack that has already started. Even if you take another medicine for gout attacks, continue to take this medicine also.

When you first begin taking this medicine, the amount of uric acid in the kidneys is greatly increased. This may cause kidney stones or other kidney problems in some people. To help prevent this, your doctor may want you to drink at least 10 to 12 full glasses (8 ounces each) of fluids each day, or to take another medicine to make your urine less acid. It is important that you follow your doctor's instructions very carefully.

Dosing—The dose of this medicine will be different for different patients. Follow your doctor's orders or the directions on the label. The following information includes only the average doses of this medicine. If your dose is different, do not change it unless your doctor tells you to do so.

The amount of medicine that you take depends on the strength of the medicine. Also, the number of doses you take each day, the time allowed between doses, and the length of time you take the medicine depend on the medical problem for which you are using the medicine.

• For oral dosage form (tablets):
   ○ For preventing gout attacks:
      ▪ Adults—One tablet a day for one week, then one tablet twice a day. If you are still having a lot of gout attacks a month after you start taking two tablets a day, your doctor may direct you to increase the dose.
      ▪ Children—Dose must be determined by your doctor.

Missed dose—If you miss a dose of this medicine, take it as soon as possible. However, if it is almost time for your next dose, skip the missed dose and go back to your regular dosing schedule. Do not double doses.

Storage—Store the medicine in a closed container at room temperature, away from heat, moisture, and direct light. Keep from freezing.

Keep out of the reach of children.

Do not keep outdated medicine or medicine no longer needed.

Precautions While Using This Medicine

Your doctor should check your progress at regular visits while you are taking this medicine.

Before you have any medical tests, tell the person in charge that you are taking this medicine. The results of some tests may be affected by probenecid or by colchicine.

For diabetic patients:

- The probenecid in this combination medicine may cause false test results with copper sulfate urine sugar tests (e.g., Clinitest®), but not with glucose enzymatic urine sugar tests (e.g., Clinistix®). If you have any questions about this, check with your health care professional.

Taking aspirin or other salicylates may lessen the effects of the probenecid in this combination medicine. This will depend on the dose of aspirin or other salicylate that you take, and on how often you take it. Also, drinking large amounts of alcoholic beverages may increase the chance of stomach problems and may increase the amount of uric acid in your blood. Therefore, do not take aspirin or other salicylates or drink alcoholic beverages while you are taking this medicine, unless you have first checked with your doctor.

For patients taking 4 tablets or more of this medicine a day:

- Stop taking this medicine immediately and check with your doctor as soon as possible if severe diarrhea, nausea or vomiting, or stomach pain occurs while you are taking this medicine.

Side Effects of This Medicine

Along with its needed effects, a medicine may cause some unwanted effects. Although not all of these side effects may occur, if they do occur they may need medical attention.

Check with your doctor immediately if any of the following side effects occur:

Rare

Fast or irregular breathing; puffiness or swelling of the eyelids or around the eyes; shortness of breath, troubled breathing, tightness in chest, or wheezing; changes in the skin color of the face occurring together with any of the other side effects listed here; or skin rash, hives, or itching occurring together with any of the other side effects listed here

Check with your doctor immediately if any of the following side effects occur:

Symptoms of overdose

Bloody urine; burning feeling in stomach, throat, or skin; convulsions (seizures); diarrhea (severe or bloody); fever; mood or mental changes; muscle weakness (severe); nausea or vomiting (severe and continuing); sudden decrease in amount of urine; troubled or difficult breathing

Check with your doctor as soon as possible if any of the following side effects occur:

Less common

Difficult or painful urination; lower back or side pain (especially if severe or sharp); skin rash, hives, or itching (occurring without other signs of an allergic reaction)

Rare

Black or tarry stools; cloudy urine; cough or hoarseness; fast or irregular breathing; numbness, tingling, pain, or weakness in hands or feet; pinpoint red spots on skin; sores, ulcers, or white spots on lips or in mouth; sore throat, fever, and chills; sudden decrease in the amount of urine; swelling of face, fingers, feet, and/or lower legs; swollen and/or painful glands; unusual bleeding or bruising; unusual tiredness or weakness; yellow eyes or skin; weight gain

Some side effects may occur that usually do not need medical attention. These side effects may go away during treatment as your body adjusts to the medicine. Also, your health care professional may be able to tell you about ways to prevent or reduce some of these side effects. Check with your health care professional if any of the following side effects continue or are bothersome or if you have any questions about them:

More common

Diarrhea (mild); headache; loss of appetite; nausea or vomiting (mild); stomach pain

Less common

Dizziness; flushing or redness of face (occurring without any signs of an allergic reaction); frequent urge to urinate; sore gums; unusual loss of hair

Other side effects not listed may also occur in some patients. If you notice any other effects, check with your healthcare professional.

PROBUCOL (Oral route) - PROE-byoo-kole

Uses For This Medicine

Probucol is used to lower levels of cholesterol (a fat-like substance) in the blood. This may help prevent medical problems caused by cholesterol clogging the blood vessels.

Probucol is available only with your doctor's prescription.

Before Using This Medicine

In deciding to use a medicine, the risks of taking the medicine must be weighed against the good it will do. This is a decision you and your doctor will make. For this medicine, the following should be considered:

Allergies—Tell your doctor if you have ever had any unusual or allergic reaction to this medicine or any other medicines. Also tell your health care professional if you have any other types of allergies, such as to foods, dyes, preservatives, or animals. For non-prescription products, read the label or package ingredients carefully.

Pediatric—There is no specific information about the use of probucol in children. However, use is not recommended in children under 2 years of age since cholesterol is needed for normal development.

Geriatric—Many medicines have not been studied specifically in older people. Therefore, it may not be known whether they work exactly the same way they do in younger adults or if they cause different side effects or problems in older people. There is no specific information comparing use of probucol in the elderly with use in other age groups.

Pregnancy—

	Pregnancy Category	Explanation
All Trimesters	B	Animal studies have revealed no evidence of harm to the fetus, however, there are no adequate studies in pregnant women OR animal studies have shown an adverse effect, but adequate studies in pregnant women have failed to demonstrate a risk to the fetus.

Breast Feeding—There are no adequate studies in women for determining infant risk when using this medication during breastfeeding. Weigh the potential benefits against the potential risks before taking this medication while breastfeeding.

Other medicines—

Using this medicine with any of the following medicines is not recommended. Your doctor may decide not to treat you with this medication or change some of the other medicines you take.

Bepridil, Cisapride, Foscarnet, Levomethadyl, Mesoridazine, Pimozide, Sparfloxacin, Terfenadine, Thioridazine, Ziprasidone

Interactions with Food/Tobacco/Alcohol—Certain medicines should not be used at or around the time of eating food or eating certain types of food since interactions may occur. Using alcohol or tobacco with certain medicines may also cause interactions to occur. Discuss with your healthcare professional the use of your medicine with food, alcohol, or tobacco.

Other medical problems—The presence of other medical problems may affect the use of this medicine. Make sure you tell your doctor if you have any other medical problems, especially:

- Gallbladder disease or gallstones or
- Heart disease—Probucol may make these conditions worse
- Liver disease—Higher blood levels of probucol may result, which may increase the chance of side effects

Proper Use of This Medicine

Many patients who have high cholesterol levels will not notice any signs of the problem. In fact, many may feel normal. Take this medicine exactly as directed by your doctor, even though you may feel well. Try not to miss any doses and do not take more medicine than your doctor ordered.

Remember that this medicine will not cure your condition but it does help control it. Therefore, you must continue to take it as directed if you expect to keep your cholesterol levels down.

Follow carefully the special diet your doctor gave you. This is the most important part of controlling your condition, and is necessary if the medicine is to work properly.

This medicine works better when taken with meals.

Before prescribing medicine for your condition, your doctor will probably try to control your condition by prescribing a personal diet for you. Such a diet may be low in fats, sugars, and/or cholesterol. Many people are able to control their condition by carefully following their doctor's orders for proper diet and exercise. Medicine is prescribed only when additional help is needed and is effective only when a schedule of diet and exercise is properly followed.

Also, this medicine is less effective if you are greatly overweight. It may be very important for you to go on a reducing diet. However, check with your doctor before going on any diet.

Make certain your health care professional knows if you are on a low-sodium, low-sugar, or any other special diet.

Dosing—The dose of this medicine will be different for different patients. Follow your doctor's orders or the directions on the label. The following information includes only the average doses of this medicine. If your dose is different, do not change it unless your doctor tells you to do so.

The amount of medicine that you take depends on the strength of the medicine. Also, the number of doses you take each day, the time allowed between doses, and the length of time you take the medicine depend on the medical problem for which you are using the medicine.

- The number of tablets that you take depends on the strength of the medicine.
- For oral dosage form (tablets):
  - Adults: 500 milligrams two times a day taken with the morning and evening meals.
  - Children:
    - Up to 2 years of age—Use is not recommended.
    - 2 years of age and over—Dose must be determined by your doctor.

Missed dose—If you miss a dose of this medicine, take it as soon as possible. However, if it is almost time for your next dose, skip the missed dose and go back to your regular dosing schedule. Do not double doses.

Storage—Store the medicine in a closed container at room temperature, away from heat, moisture, and direct light. Keep from freezing.

Keep out of the reach of children.

Do not keep outdated medicine or medicine no longer needed.

Precautions While Using This Medicine

It is very important that your doctor check your progress at regular visits. This will allow your doctor to see if the medicine is working properly to lower your cholesterol levels and to decide if you should continue to take it.

Do not stop taking this medicine without first checking with your doctor. When you stop taking this medicine, your blood fat levels may increase again. Your doctor may want you to follow a special diet to help prevent this.

Side Effects of This Medicine

Along with its needed effects, a medicine may cause some unwanted effects. Although not all of these side effects may occur, if they do occur they may need medical attention.

Check with your doctor as soon as possible if any of the following side effects occur:
More common
   Dizziness or fainting; fast or irregular heartbeat
Rare
   Swellings on face, hands, or feet, or in mouth; unusual bleeding or bruising; unusual tiredness or weakness

Some side effects may occur that usually do not need medical attention. These side effects may go away during treatment as your body adjusts to the medicine. Also, your health

care professional may be able to tell you about ways to prevent or reduce some of these side effects. Check with your health care professional if any of the following side effects continue or are bothersome or if you have any questions about them:

   More common
      Bloating; diarrhea; nausea and vomiting; stomach pain
   Less common
      Headache; numbness or tingling of fingers, toes, or face

Other side effects not listed may also occur in some patients. If you notice any other effects, check with your healthcare professional.

PROCAINAMIDE (Oral route, Intravenous route) - proe-kane-A-mide

Black Box Warning

Positive Anti-nuclear Antibody (ANA) Titer: The prolonged administration of procainamide often leads to the development of a positive ANA test, with or without symptoms of a lupus erythematosus-like syndrome. If a positive ANA titer develops, the benefit versus risks of continued procainamide therapy should be assessed.

Mortality: In the National Heart, Lung, and Blood Institute's Cardiac Arrhythmia Suppression Trial (CAST), a long-term, muliticentered, randomized, double-blind study in patients with asymptomatic non-life-threatening ventricular arrhythmias who had a myocardial infarction more than six days but less than two years previously, an excessive mortality or non-fatal cardiac arrest rate (7.7%) was seen in patients treated with encainide or flecainide compared with that seen in patients assigned to carefully matched placebo-treated groups (3.0%). The average duration of treatment with encainide or flecainide in this study was 10 months.

The applicability of the CAST results to other populations (eg, those without recent myocardial infarction) is uncertain. Considering the known proarrhythmic properties of procainamide and the lack of evidence of improved survival for any antiarrhythmic drug in patients without life-threatening arrhythmias, the use of procainamide hydrochloride as well as other antiarrhythmic agents should be reserved for patients with life-threatening ventricular arrhythmias.

Blood Dyscrasias: Agranulocytosis, bone marrow depression, neutropenia, hypoplastic anemia and thrombocytopenia in patients receiving procainamide hydrochloride have been reported at a rate of approximately 0.5%. Most of these patients received procainamide hydrochloride within the recommended dosage range. Fatalities have occurred (with approximately 20% to 25 % mortality in reported cases of agranulocytosis). Since most of these events have been noted during the first 12 weeks of therapy, it is recommended that complete blood counts including white cell, differential and platelet counts be performed at weekly intervals for the first three months of therapy, and periodically thereafter. Complete blood counts should be performed promptly if the patient develops any signs of infection (such as fever, chills, sore throat, or stomatitis), bruising or bleeding. If any of these hematologic disorders are identified, procainamide therapy should be discontinued. Blood counts usually return to normal within one month of discontinuation. Caution should be used in patients with pre-existing marrow failure or cytopenia of any type.

Commonly used brand name(s)
In the U.S.—
   Procanbid
   Pronestyl
   Pronestyl-SR

Available Dosage Forms:
   • Solution   • Tablet
   • Tablet, Extended Release   • Capsule

Therapeutic Class: Antiarrhythmic, Group IA

Uses For This Medicine

Procainamide is used to correct irregular heartbeats to a normal rhythm and to slow an overactive heart. This allows the heart to work more efficiently. Procainamide produces its beneficial effects by slowing nerve impulses in the heart and reducing sensitivity of heart tissues.

Procainamide is available only with your doctor's prescription.

Before Using This Medicine

In deciding to use a medicine, the risks of taking the medicine must be weighed against the good it will do. This is a decision you and your doctor will make. For this medicine, the following should be considered:

Allergies—Tell your doctor if you have ever had any unusual or allergic reaction to this medicine or any other medicines. Also tell your health care professional if you have any other types of allergies, such as to foods, dyes, preservatives, or animals. For non-prescription products, read the label or package ingredients carefully.

Pediatric—Procainamide has been used in a limited number of children. In effective doses, the medicine has not been shown to cause different side effects or problems than it does in adults.

Geriatric—Dizziness or lightheadedness is more likely to occur in the elderly, who are usually more sensitive to the effects of this medicine.

Pregnancy—

	Pregnancy Category	Explanation
All Trimesters	C	Animal studies have shown an adverse effect and there are no adequate studies in pregnant women OR no animal studies have been conducted and there are no adequate studies in pregnant women.

Breast Feeding—There are no adequate studies in women for determining infant risk when using this medication during breastfeeding. Weigh the potential benefits against the potential risks before taking this medication while breastfeeding.

Other medicines—

Using this medicine with any of the following medicines is not recommended. Your doctor may decide not to treat you with this medication or change some of the other medicines you take.

Bepridil, Cisapride, Grepafloxacin, Levomethadyl, Mesoridazine, Pimozide, Ranolazine, Sparfloxacin, Terfenadine, Thioridazine, Ziprasidone

Interactions with Food/Tobacco/Alcohol—Certain medicines should not be used at or around the time of eating food or eating certain types of food since interactions may occur. Using alcohol or tobacco with certain medicines may also cause interactions to occur. Discuss with your healthcare professional the use of your medicine with food, alcohol, or tobacco.

Other medical problems—The presence of other medical problems may affect the use of this medicine. Make sure you tell your doctor if you have any other medical problems, especially:

- Asthma—Possible allergic reaction

- Kidney disease or

- Liver disease—Effects may be increased because of slower removal of procainamide from the body

- Lupus erythematosus (history of)—Procainamide may cause the condition to become active

- Myasthenia gravis—Procainamide may increase muscle weakness

Proper Use of This Medicine

Take procainamide exactly as directed by your doctor, even though you may feel well. Do not take more medicine than ordered.

Procainamide should be taken with a glass of water on an empty stomach 1 hour before or 2 hours after meals so that it will be absorbed more quickly. However, to lessen stomach upset, your doctor may want you to take the medicine with food or milk.

For patients taking the extended-release tablets:

- Swallow the tablet whole without breaking, crushing, or chewing it.

This medicine works best when there is a constant amount in the blood. To help keep the amount constant, do not miss any doses. Also, it is best to take the doses at evenly spaced times day and night. For example, if you are to take 6 doses a day, the doses should be spaced about 4 hours apart. If this interferes with your sleep or other daily activities, or if you need help in planning the best times to take your medicine, check with your health care professional.

Dosing—The dose of this medicine will be different for different patients. Follow your doctor's orders or the directions on the label. The following information includes only the average doses of this medicine. If your dose is different, do not change it unless your doctor tells you to do so.

The amount of medicine that you take depends on the strength of the medicine. Also, the number of doses you take each day, the time allowed between doses, and the length of time you take the medicine depend on the medical problem for which you are using the medicine.

- For regular (short-acting) oral dosage forms (capsules or tablets):
  - For atrial arrhythmias (fast or irregular heartbeat):
    - Adults—500 milligrams (mg) to 1000 mg (1 gram) every four to six hours.
    - Children—12.5 mg per kilogram (5.68 mg per pound) of body weight four times a day.

- For ventricular arrhythmias (fast or irregular heartbeat):
    - Adults—50 mg per kilogram (22.73 mg per pound) of body weight per day divided into eight doses taken every three hours.
    - Children—12.5 mg per kilogram (5.68 mg per pound) of body weight four times a day.

- For long-acting oral dosage form (extended-release tablets):
  - For atrial arrhythmias (fast or irregular heartbeat):
    - Adults—1000 mg (1 gram) every six hours.
    - Children—Use is not recommended.
  - For ventricular arrhythmias (fast or irregular heartbeat):
    - Adults—50 mg per kilogram (22.73 mg per pound) of body weight per day divided into four doses taken every six hours.

- For injection dosage form:
  - For arrhythmias (fast or irregular heartbeat):
    - Adults—
      - First few doses: May be given intramuscularly (into the muscle) at 50 mg per kilogram (22.73 mg per pound) of body weight per day in divided doses every three hours; or may be given intravenously (into the vein) by slowly injecting 100 mg (mixed in fluid) every five minutes or infusing 500 to 600 mg (mixed in fluid) over a twenty-five to thirty minute period.
      - Doses after the first few doses: 2 to 6 mg (mixed in fluid) per minute infused into the vein.
    - Children—Dose must be determined by your doctor.

Missed dose—If you miss a dose of this medicine, take it as soon as possible. However, if it is almost time for your next dose, skip the missed dose and go back to your regular dosing schedule. Do not double doses.

Storage—Store the medicine in a closed container at room temperature, away from heat, moisture, and direct light. Keep from freezing.

Keep out of the reach of children.

Do not keep outdated medicine or medicine no longer needed.

Precautions While Using This Medicine

It is important that your doctor check your progress at regular visits to make sure the medicine is working properly. This will allow necessary changes in the amount of medicine you are taking, which also may help reduce side effects.

Do not stop taking this medicine without first checking with your doctor. Stopping it suddenly may cause a serious change in the activity of your heart. Your doctor may want you to reduce gradually the amount you are taking before stopping completely.

Before having any kind of surgery (including dental surgery) or emergency treatment, tell the medical doctor or dentist in charge that you are taking this medicine.

Your doctor may want you to carry a medical identification card or bracelet stating that you are taking this medicine.

Dizziness or lightheadedness may occur, especially in elderly patients and when large doses are used. Elderly patients should use extra care to avoid falling. Make sure you know how you react to this medicine before you drive, use machines, or do anything else that could be dangerous if you are dizzy or are not alert.

Tell the doctor in charge that you are taking this medicine before you have any medical tests. The results of some tests may be affected by this medicine.

Side Effects of This Medicine

Along with its needed effects, a medicine may cause some unwanted effects. Although not all of these side effects may occur, if they do occur they may need medical attention.

Check with your doctor as soon as possible if any of the following side effects occur:

Less common
> Fever and chills; joint pain or swelling; pains with breathing; skin rash or itching

Rare
> Confusion; fever or sore mouth, gums, or throat; hallucinations (seeing, hearing, or feeling things that are not there); mental depression; unusual bleeding or bruising; unusual tiredness or weakness

Signs and symptoms of overdose
> Confusion; decrease in urination; dizziness (severe) or fainting; drowsiness; fast or irregular heartbeat; nausea and vomiting

Some side effects may occur that usually do not need medical attention. These side effects may go away during treatment as your body adjusts to the medicine. Also, your health care professional may be able to tell you about ways to prevent or reduce some of these side effects. Check with your health care professional if any of the following side effects continue or are bothersome or if you have any questions about them:

More common
> Diarrhea; loss of appetite

Less common
> Dizziness or lightheadedness

The medicine in the extended-release tablets is contained in a special wax form (matrix). The medicine is slowly released, after which the wax matrix passes out of the body. Sometimes it may be seen in the stool. This is normal and is no cause for concern.

Other side effects not listed may also occur in some patients. If you notice any other effects, check with your healthcare professional.

PROCARBAZINE (Oral route) - proe-KAR-ba-zeen

Black Box Warning

It is recommended that procarbazine hydrochloride be given only by or under the supervision of a physician experienced in the use of potent antineoplastic drugs. Adequate clinical and laboratory facilities should be available to patients for proper monitoring of treatment.

Commonly used brand name(s)

In the U.S.—
> Matulane

Available Dosage Forms:
• Capsule

Therapeutic Class: Antineoplastic Agent
Pharmacologic Class: Alkylating Agent

Uses For This Medicine

Procarbazine belongs to the group of medicines known as alkylating agents. It is used to treat some kinds of cancer.

Procarbazine is thought to interfere with the growth of cancer cells which are eventually destroyed. It also blocks the action of a chemical substance in the central nervous system called monoamine oxidase (MAO), but this is probably not related to its effect against cancer. Since the growth of normal body cells may also be affected by procarbazine, other effects will also occur. Some of these may be serious and must be reported to your doctor. Other effects, like hair loss, may not be serious but may cause concern. Some effects may not occur for months or years after the medicine is used.

Before you begin treatment with procarbazine, you and your doctor should talk about the good this medicine will do as well as the risks of using it.

Procarbazine is available only with your doctor's prescription.

Before Using This Medicine

In deciding to use a medicine, the risks of taking the medicine must be weighed against the good it will do. This is a decision you and your doctor will make. For this medicine, the following should be considered:

Allergies—Tell your doctor if you have ever had any unusual or allergic reaction to this medicine or any other medicines. Also tell your health care professional if you have any other types of allergies, such as to foods, dyes, preservatives, or animals. For non-prescription products, read the label or package ingredients carefully.

Pediatric—Although there is no specific information about the use of procarbazine in children, it is not expected to cause different side effects or problems in children than it does in adults.

Geriatric—Side effects may be more likely to occur in elderly patients, who are usually more sensitive to the effects of procarbazine.

Pregnancy—

	Pregnancy Category	Explanation
All Trimesters	D	Studies in pregnant women have demonstrated a risk to the fetus. However, the benefits of therapy in a life threatening situation or a serious disease, may outweigh the potential risk.

Breast Feeding—There are no adequate studies in women for determining infant risk when using this medication during breastfeeding. Weigh the potential benefits against the potential risks before taking this medication while breastfeeding.

Other medicines—

Using this medicine with any of the following medicines is not recommended. Your doctor may decide not to treat you with this medication or change some of the other medicines you take.

Amitriptyline, Amphetamine, Apraclonidine, Benzphetamine, Brimonidine, Bupropion, Carbamazepine, Citalopram, Cyclobenzaprine, Cyproheptadine, Dexfenfluramine, Dexmethylphenidate, Dextroamphetamine, Dextromethorphan, Diethylpropion, Fenfluramine, Fluoxetine, Guanadrel, Guanethidine, Isocarboxazid, Isometheptene, Levodopa, Levomethadyl, Maprotiline, Mazindol, Meperidine, Methamphetamine, Methyldopa, Methylphenidate, Mirtazapine, Morphine, Morphine Sulfate Liposome, Nefopam, Opipramol, Paroxetine, Phendimetrazine, Phenelzine, Phenmetrazine, Phentermine, Phenylephrine, Phenylpropanolamine, Pseudoephedrine, Reserpine, Rizatriptan, Rotavirus Vaccine, Live, Sertraline, Sibutramine, Sumatriptan, Tranylcypromine, Venlafaxine, Zolmitriptan

Interactions with Food/Tobacco/Alcohol—Certain medicines should not be used at or around the time of eating food or eating certain types of food since interactions may occur. Using alcohol or tobacco with certain medicines may also cause interactions to occur. The following interactions have been selected on the basis of their potential significance and are not necessarily all-inclusive.

Using this medicine with any of the following is usually not recommended, but may be unavoidable in some cases. If used together, your doctor may change the dose or how often you use this medicine, or give you special instructions about the use of food, alcohol, or tobacco.

Ethanol

Using this medicine with any of the following may cause an increased risk of certain side effects but may be unavoidable in some cases. If used together, your doctor may change the dose or how often you use this medicine, or give you special instructions about the use of food, alcohol, or tobacco.

Tyramine Containing Food

Other medical problems—The presence of other medical problems may affect the use of this medicine. Make sure you tell your doctor if you have any other medical problems, especially:

- Alcoholism
- Angina (chest pain) or
- Heart or blood vessel disease or
- Heart attack or stroke (recent)—Lowered blood pressure caused by procarbazine may make problems associated with some of these conditions worse
- Chickenpox (including recent exposure) or
- Herpes zoster (shingles)—Risk of severe disease affecting other parts of the body
- Type 2 diabetes mellitus—Procarbazine may change the amount of diabetes medicine needed
- Epilepsy—Procarbazine may change the seizures
- Headaches (severe or frequent)—You may not realize when a severe headache is caused by a dangerous reaction to procarbazine
- Infection—Procarbazine can reduce immunity to infection

- Kidney disease—Effects may be increased because of slower removal of procarbazine from the body
- Liver disease—Procarbazine can cause severe liver disease to become much worse
- Mental illness (or history of)—Some cases of mental illness may be worsened
- Overactive thyroid—Increased risk of dangerous reaction to procarbazine
- Parkinson's disease—May be worsened
- Pheochromocytoma—Blood pressure may be affected

Proper Use of This Medicine

Use this medicine only as directed by your doctor. Do not use more or less of it and do not use it more often than your doctor ordered. The exact amount of medicine you need has been carefully worked out. Taking too much may increase the chance of side effects while taking too little may not improve your condition.

Procarbazine is sometimes given together with certain other medicines. If you are using a combination of medicines, make sure that you take each one at the right time and do not mix them. Ask your health care professional to help you plan a way to take your medicines at the right times.

Procarbazine commonly causes nausea and vomiting. Even if you begin to feel ill, do not stop using this medicine without first checking with your doctor. Ask your health care professional for ways to lessen these effects.

If you vomit shortly after taking a dose of procarbazine, check with your doctor. You will be told whether to take the dose again or to wait until the next scheduled dose.

Dosing—The dose of this medicine will be different for different patients. Follow your doctor's orders or the directions on the label. The following information includes only the average doses of this medicine. If your dose is different, do not change it unless your doctor tells you to do so.

The amount of medicine that you take depends on the strength of the medicine. Also, the number of doses you take each day, the time allowed between doses, and the length of time you take the medicine depend on the medical problem for which you are using the medicine.

Missed dose—If you miss a dose of this medicine, take it as soon as possible. However, if it is almost time for your next dose, skip the missed dose and go back to your regular dosing schedule. Do not double doses.

Storage—Store the medicine in a closed container at room temperature, away from heat, moisture, and direct light. Keep from freezing.

Keep out of the reach of children.

Do not keep outdated medicine or medicine no longer needed.

Precautions While Using This Medicine

It is very important that your doctor check your progress at regular visits to make sure that this medicine is working properly and to check for unwanted effects.

Check with your doctor or hospital emergency room immediately if severe headache, stiff neck, chest pains, fast heartbeat, or nausea and vomiting occur while you are taking this medicine. These may be symptoms of a serious high blood pressure reaction that should have a doctor's attention.

When taken with certain foods, drinks, or other medicines, procarbazine can cause very dangerous reactions such as sudden high blood pressure. To avoid such reactions, obey the following rules of caution:

- Do not eat foods that have a high tyramine content (most common in foods that are aged or fermented to increase their flavor), such as cheeses, yeast or meat extracts, fava or broad bean pods, smoked or pickled meat, poultry, or fish, fermented sausage (bologna, pepperoni, salami, and summer sausage) or other unfresh meat, or any overripe fruit. If a list of these foods and beverages is not given to you, ask your health care professional to provide one.
- Do not drink alcoholic beverages or alcohol-free or reduced-alcohol beer or wine.
- Do not eat or drink large amounts of caffeine-containing food or beverages, such as chocolate, coffee, tea, or cola.
- Do not take any other medicine unless approved or prescribed by your doctor. This especially includes over-the-counter (OTC) or nonprescription medicine such as that for colds (including nose drops or sprays), cough, asthma, hay fever, appetite control; "keep awake" products; or products that make you sleepy.

After you stop using this medicine you must continue to obey the rules of caution concerning food, drink, and other medication for at least 2 weeks since procarbazine may continue to react with certain foods or other medicines for up to 14 days after you stop taking it.

This medicine will add to the effects of alcohol and other CNS depressants (medicines that slow down the nervous system, possibly causing drowsiness). Some examples of CNS depressants are antihistamines or medicine for hay fever, other allergies, or colds; sedatives, tranquilizers, or sleeping medicine; prescription pain medicine or narcotics; barbiturates; medicine for seizures; muscle relaxants; or anesthetics, including some dental anesthetics. Check with your doctor before taking any of the above while you are using this medicine.

This medicine may cause some people to become drowsy or less alert than they are normally. Make sure you know how you react to this medicine before you drive, use machines, or do anything else that could be dangerous if you are not alert.

While you are being treated with procarbazine, and after you stop treatment with it, do not have any immunizations (vaccinations) without your doctor's approval. Procarbazine may lower your body's resistance and there is a chance you might get the infection the immunization is meant to prevent. In addition, other persons living in your household should not take or should not have recently taken oral polio vaccine since there is a chance they could pass the polio virus on to you. Also, avoid persons who have taken oral polio vaccine. Do not get close to them and do not stay in the same room with them for very long. If you cannot take these precautions, you should consider wearing a protective face mask that covers the nose and mouth.

Procarbazine can lower the number of white blood cells in your blood temporarily, increasing the chance of getting an infection. It can also lower the number of platelets, which are necessary for proper blood clotting. If this occurs, there are certain precautions you can take, especially when your blood count is low, to reduce the risk of infection or bleeding:

- If you can, avoid people with infections. Check with your doctor immediately if you think you are getting an infection or if you get a fever or chills, cough or hoarseness, lower back or side pain, or painful or difficult urination.
- Check with your doctor immediately if you notice any unusual bleeding or bruising; black, tarry stools; blood in urine or stools; or pinpoint red spots on your skin.
- Be careful when using a regular toothbrush, dental floss, or toothpick. Your medical doctor, dentist, or nurse may recommend other ways to clean your teeth and gums. Check with your medical doctor before having any dental work done.
- Do not touch your eyes or the inside of your nose unless you have just washed your hands and have not touched anything else in the meantime.
- Be careful not to cut yourself when you are using sharp objects such as a safety razor or fingernail or toenail cutters.
- Avoid contact sports or other situations where bruising or injury could occur.

For diabetic patients:
- Procarbazine may affect blood sugar levels. While you are using this medicine, be especially careful in testing for sugar in your blood or urine.

If you are going to have surgery (including dental surgery) or emergency treatment tell the medical doctor or dentist in charge that you are using this medicine or have used it within the past 2 weeks.

Your doctor may want you to carry an identification card stating that you are using this medicine.

Side Effects of This Medicine

Along with their needed effects, medicines like procarbazine can sometimes cause unwanted effects such as blood problems, loss of hair, high blood pressure reactions, and other side effects. These and others are described below. Also, because of the way these medicines act on the body, there is a chance that they might cause other unwanted effects that may not occur until months or years after the medicine is used. These delayed effects may include certain types of cancer, such as leukemia. Discuss these possible effects with your doctor.

Although not all of these side effects may occur, if they do occur they may need medical attention.

Stop taking this medicine and get emergency help immediately if any of the following effects occur:
Rare
   Chest pain (severe); enlarged pupils of eyes; fast or slow heartbeat; headache (severe); increased sensitivity of eyes to light; increased sweating (possibly with fever or cold, clammy skin); stiff or sore neck

Check with your doctor immediately if any of the following side effects occur:
Less common
   Black, tarry stools; blood in urine or stools; bloody vomit; cough or hoarseness; fever or chills; lower back or side pain; painful or difficult urination; pinpoint red spots on skin; unusual bleeding or bruising

Check with your doctor as soon as possible if any of the following side effects occur:

More common

Confusion; convulsions (seizures); cough; hallucinations (seeing, hearing, or feeling things that are not there); missing menstrual periods; shortness of breath; thickening of bronchial secretions; tiredness or weakness (continuing)

Less common

Diarrhea; sores in mouth and on lips; tingling or numbness of fingers or toes; unsteadiness or awkwardness; yellow eyes or skin

Rare

Fainting; skin rash, hives, or itching; wheezing

Some side effects may occur that usually do not need medical attention. These side effects may go away during treatment as your body adjusts to the medicine. Also, your health care professional may be able to tell you about ways to prevent or reduce some of these side effects. Check with your health care professional if any of the following side effects continue or are bothersome or if you have any questions about them:

More common

Drowsiness; muscle or joint pain; muscle twitching; nausea and vomiting; nervousness; nightmares; trouble in sleeping; unusual tiredness or weakness

Less common

Constipation; darkening of skin; difficulty in swallowing; dizziness or lightheadedness when getting up from a lying or sitting position; dry mouth; feeling of warmth and redness in face; headache; loss of appetite; mental depression

This medicine may cause a temporary loss of hair in some people. After treatment with procarbazine has ended, normal hair growth should return.

Other side effects not listed may also occur in some patients. If you notice any other effects, check with your healthcare professional.

PROGESTINS (Systemic)

Some commonly used brand names are:

In the U.S.—

Depo-Provera Contraceptive   NORPLANT System (1)
Injection (2)   Nor-QD (3)
depo-subQ provera 104 (2)   Ovrette (4)
Micronor (3)   Plan B (1)

In Canada—

Depo-Provera (2)   NORPLANT System (1)
Micronor (3)

This information applies to the following medicines

1. Levonorgestrel (LEE-voe-nor-jes-trel)
2. Medroxyprogesterone (me-DROX-ee-proe-JES-te-rone)
3. Norethindrone (nor-eth-IN-drone)
4. Norgestrel (nor-JES-trel)

Category

- **Contraceptive (systemic)—**
- **Progestational agent—**

Description

Progestins (proe-JES-tins) are hormones.

The low-dose progestins for contraception are used to prevent pregnancy. Other names for progestin-only oral contraceptives are minipills and progestin-only pills (POPs). Progestins can prevent fertilization by preventing a woman's egg from fully developing.

Also, progestins cause changes at the opening of the uterus, such as thickening of the cervical mucus. This makes it hard for the partner's sperm to reach the egg. The fertilization of the woman's egg with her partner's sperm is less likely to occur while she is taking, receiving, or using a progestin, but it can occur. Even so, the progestins make it harder for the fertilized egg to become attached to the walls of the uterus, making it difficult to become pregnant.

No contraceptive method is 100 percent effective. *Studies show that fewer than 1 of each 100 women become pregnant during the first year of use when correctly receiving the injection on time or receiving the levonorgestrel implants. Fewer than 10 of each 100 women correctly taking progestins by mouth for contraception become pregnant during the first year of use.* Methods that do not work as well include using condoms, diaphragms, or spermicides. Discuss with your health care professional what your options are for birth control.

Progestins are available only with your doctor's prescription, in the following dosage forms:

Oral

- Levonorgestrel
  ○ Tablets
- Norethindrone
  ○ Tablets
- Norgestrel
  ○ Tablets

Subdermal

- Levonorgestrel
  ○ Implants

Parenteral

- Medroxyprogesterone
  ○ Intramuscular injection
  ○ Subcutaneous injection

Before Using This Medicine

In deciding to use a medicine, the risks of taking the medicine must be weighed against the good it will do. If you are using progestins for contraception you should understand how their benefits and risks compare to those of other birth control methods. This is a decision you, your sexual partner, and your doctor will make. For progestins, the following should be considered:

Allergies—Tell your doctor if you have ever had any unusual or allergic reaction to progestins. Also tell your health care professional if you are allergic to any other substances, such as foods, preservatives, or dyes.

Diet—Make certain your health care professional knows if you are on any special diet, such as a low-sodium or low-sugar diet.

Pregnancy—Use of progestin-only contraceptives during pregnancy is not recommended. Doctors should be told if pregnancy is suspected. When accidently used during pregnancy, progestins used for contraception have not caused problems.

Breast-feeding—Although progestins pass into the breast milk, the low doses of progestins used for contraception have not been shown to cause problems in nursing babies. Progestins used for contraception are recommended for nursing mothers when contraception is desired.

Teenagers—Progestins have been used by teenagers and have not been shown to cause different side effects or problems than they do in adults. You must take progestin-only oral contraceptives every day in order for them to work. Progestins do not protect against sexually transmitted diseases, a risk factor for teenagers. It is not known if *Depo-Provera Contraceptive Injection* causes problems with bone development and growth in teenagers and young women. It is important that your doctor check you regularly for growth problems, especially if you have been using this medicine for 2 years or longer.

Older adults—This medicine has been tested and has not been shown to cause different side effects or problems in older people than it does in younger adults.

Other medicines—Although certain medicines should not be used together at all, in other cases two different medicines may be used together even if an interaction might occur. In these cases, your doctor may want to change the dose, or other precautions may be necessary. When you are taking a progestin, it is especially important that your health care professional know if you are taking any of the following:

- Aminoglutethimide (e.g., Cytadren) or
- Carbamazepine (e.g., Tegretol) or
- Phenobarbital or
- Phenytoin (e.g., Dilantin) or
- Rifabutin (e.g., Mycobutin) or
- Rifampin (e.g., Rifadin, Rimactane)—These medicines may decrease the effects of progestins and increase your chance of pregnancy, so use of a second form of birth control is recommended

Other medical problems—The presence of other medical problems may affect the use of progestins. Make sure you tell your doctor if you have any other medical problems, especially:

- Asthma or
- Epilepsy (or history of) or
- Heart or circulation problems or
- Kidney disease (severe) or
- Migraine headaches—Progestins may cause fluid build-up and may cause these conditions to become worse
- Bleeding problems, undiagnosed, such as blood in urine or changes in vaginal bleeding—May make diagnosis of these problems more difficult
- Breast disease (such as breast lumps or cysts) (history of)—May make this condition worse in certain types of diseases that do not react in a positive way to progestins
- Central nervous system (CNS) disorders, such as mental depression (or history of) or
- High blood cholesterol—Effects of progestins may cause these conditions or may make these conditions worse
- Diabetes mellitus (sugar diabetes)—May cause a mild increase in your blood sugar and a need to change the amount of medicine you take for diabetes
- Liver disease—Effects of some progestins may be increased and may worsen this condition
- Other conditions that increase the chances for osteoporosis (brittle bones)—Since it is possible that certain doses of progestins may cause temporary thinning of the bones by changing your hormone balance, it is important that your doctor know if you have an increased risk of osteoporosis. Some things that can increase your risk for having osteoporosis include cigarette smoking, abusing alcohol, taking or drinking large amounts of caffeine, and having a family history of osteoporosis or easily broken bones. Some medicines, such as glucocorticoids (cortisone-like medicines) or anticonvulsants (seizure medicine), can also cause thinning of the bones. It is especially important that you tell your doctor about any of these risk factors if you are taking *Depo-Provera Contraceptive Injection* or *depo-subQ provera 104*. This contraceptive may cause loss of bone mineral density. Your doctor may replace this contraceptive with a different one. However, it is thought that progestins can help protect against osteoporosis in postmenopausal women.

Proper Use of This Medicine

To make the use of a progestin as safe and reliable as possible, you should understand how and when to take it and what effects may be expected. Progestins for contraception usually come with patient directions. Read them carefully before taking or using this medicine.

Progestins do not protect a woman from sexually transmitted diseases (STDs), including human immunodeficiency virus (HIV), or acquired immunodeficiency syndrome (AIDS). The use of latex (rubber) condoms or abstinence is recommended for protection from these diseases.

Take this medicine only as directed by your doctor. Do not take more of it and do not take it for a longer time than your doctor ordered. To do so may increase the chance of side effects. Try to take the medicine at the same time each day to reduce the possibility of side effects and to allow it to work better.

When using the levonorgestrel subdermal dosage form:

- For insertion:
  - Six implants are inserted under the skin of your upper arm by a health care professional. This usually takes about 15 minutes. No pain should be felt from the insertion process because you will receive a small injection from your doctor of a medicine that will numb your arm.
- For care of insertion site:
  - Keep the gauze wrap on for 24 hours after the insertion. Then, you should remove it. The sterile strips of tape should be left over the area for 3 days.

○ Be careful not to bump the site or get that area wet for at least 3 days after the procedure. Do not do any heavy lifting for 24 hours. Swelling and bruising are common for a few days.

- For contraceptive protection:
  ○ Full protection from pregnancy begins within 24 hours, if the insertion is done within 7 days of the beginning of your menstrual period. Otherwise, use another birth control method for the rest of your first cycle. Protection using implants lasts for 5 years or until removal, whichever comes first.

- For removal:
  ○ The implants need to be removed after 5 years. However, you may have them removed by a health care professional at any time before that.
  ○ If you want to continue using this form of birth control after 5 years, your health care professional may insert new implants in the same area where the old ones were or into the other arm.
  ○ After a local injection numbs the area on your arm, removal of the medication usually takes 20 minutes or longer. If the implants are hard to remove, your health care professional may want you to return another day to complete the removal process.
  ○ Keep a gauze wrap on for 24 hours after the removal. The sterile strips of tape underneath the gauze wrap should be left over the area for 3 days. Be careful not to bump the site or get that area wet until the area is healed.

When using levonorgestrel tablet dosage form for emergency contraception:

- The tablets may be taken at any time during the menstrual cycle.

When using medroxyprogesterone injection dosage form for contraception:

- Your injection is given by a health care professional *every* 3 months.

- To stop using medroxyprogesterone injection for contraception, simply do not have another injection.

- Full protection from pregnancy begins immediately if you receive the first injection within the first 5 days of your menstrual period or within 5 days after delivering a baby if you will not be breast-feeding. If you are going to breast-feed, you may have to wait for 6 weeks from your delivery date before receiving your first injection. If you follow this schedule, you do not need to use another form of birth control. Protection from that one injection ends at 3 months. You will need another injection every 3 months to have full protection from becoming pregnant. However, if the injection is given later than 5 days from the first day of your last menstrual period, you will need to use another method of birth control as directed by your doctor.

When using an oral progestin dosage form:

- Take a tablet every 24 hours each day of the year. Taking the medicine at the same time each day helps to reduce the possibility of side effects and makes it work as expected. Taking your tablet 3 hours late is the same as missing a dose and can cause the medicine to not work properly.

- Keep the tablets in the container in which you received them to help you to keep track of your dosage schedule.

- When switching from estrogen and progestin oral contraceptives, you should take the first dose of the progestin-only contraceptive the next day after the last active pill of the estrogen and progestin oral contraceptive has been taken. This means you will not take the last 7 days (placebo or nonactive pills) of a 28–day cycle of the estrogen and progestin oral contraceptive pack. You will begin a new pack of progestin-only birth control pills on the 22nd day.

- Also, when switching, full protection from pregnancy begins after 48 hours if the first dose of the progestin-only contraceptive is taken on the first day of the menstrual period. If the birth control is begun on other days, full protection may begin 3 weeks after you begin taking the medicine for the first time. You should *use a second method of birth control for at least the first 3 weeks to ensure full protection.* You are not fully protected if you miss pills. The chances of your getting pregnant are greater with each pill that is missed.

Dosing—*Follow your doctor's orders or the directions on the label.* Also, follow your health care professional's orders to schedule the proper time to remove the implants or receive an injection of progestins for contraception. You and your health care professional may choose to replace the implants sooner or begin a new method of birth control. The following information includes only the average doses of these medicines. *If your dose is different, do not change it* unless your doctor tells you to do so.

For levonorgestrel
- For *subdermal* dosage form (implants):
  ○ For preventing pregnancy:
    ▪ Adults and teenagers—Six implants (a total dose of 216 milligrams [mg]) inserted under the skin of the upper arm in a fan-like pattern. From this total dose, about 30 mcg is released every day for 5 years.
- For *oral* dosage form (tablet):
  ○ For emergency contraception for preventing pregnancy:
    ▪ Adults and teenagers—The first dose of 0.75 milligram (mg) should be taken as soon as possible within 72 hours of intercourse. The second dose must be taken 12 hours later.

For medroxyprogesterone
- For *muscular injection* dosage form:
  ○ For preventing pregnancy:
    ▪ Adults and teenagers—150 milligrams injected into a muscle in the upper arm or in the buttocks every three months (13 weeks).
- For *subcutaneous injection* dosage form:
  ○ For preventing pregnancy:
    ▪ Adults and teenagers—104 milligrams injected under the skin of the anterior thigh or abdomen every three months (12 to 14 weeks).

For norethindrone
- For *oral* dosage form (tablets):
  ○ For preventing pregnancy:
    ▪ Adults and teenagers—0.35 milligrams (mg) every 24 hours, beginning on the first day of your menstrual cycle whether menstrual bleeding begins or not. The first day of your menstrual cycle

can be figured out by counting 28 days from the first day of your last menstrual cycle.

For norgestrel
- For *oral* dosage form (tablets):
  - For preventing pregnancy:
    - Adults and teenagers—75 micrograms (mcg) every 24 hours, beginning on the first day of your menstrual cycle whether menstrual bleeding occurs or not. The first day of your menstrual cycle can be figured out by counting 28 days from the first day of your last menstrual cycle.

Missed dose—

- For *oral* dosage form (tablets): When you miss 1 day's dose of oral tablets or are 3 hours or more late in taking your dose, many doctors recommend that you take the missed dose immediately, continue your normal schedule, and use another method of contraception for 2 days. This is different from what is done after a person misses a dose of birth control tablets that contain more than one hormone.
- For *injection* dosage form: If you miss having your next injection and it has been longer than 13 weeks since your last injection, your doctor may want you to stop receiving the medicine. Use another method of birth control until your period begins or until your doctor determines that you are not pregnant.
- If your doctor has other directions, follow that advice. *Any time you miss a menstrual period within 45 days after a missed or delayed dose you will need to be tested for a possible pregnancy.*

Storage—To store this medicine:

- Keep out of the reach of children.
- Store away from heat. Light will fade some tablet colors but will not change the tablets' effect.
- Do not store in the bathroom, near the kitchen sink, or in other damp places. Heat or moisture may cause the medicine to break down.
- Keep the medicine from freezing. Do not refrigerate.
- Keep the injectable form of this medicine from freezing.
- Do not keep outdated medicine or medicine no longer needed. Be sure that any discarded medicine is out of the reach of children.

Precautions While Using This Medicine

It is very important that your health care professional check your progress at regular visits. This will allow your dosage to be adjusted to your changing needs, and will allow any unwanted effects to be detected. These visits are usually every 12 months when you are taking progestins by mouth for birth control.

- If you are receiving the medroxyprogesterone injection for contraception, a physical exam is needed only every 12 months, but you need an injection every 3 months. Your doctor will also want to check you for any bone development or growth problems, especially if you are a teenager or young adult.
- If you are using the levonorgestrel implants, your doctor will want to check the area where they were placed within 30 days after they are put into or removed from your arm.

After that, a visit every 12 months usually is all that is needed.

Progestins may cause some people to become dizzy. Make sure you know how you react to this medicine before you drive, use machines, or do anything else that could be dangerous if you are not alert.

Vaginal bleeding of various amounts may occur between your regular menstrual periods during the first 3 months of use. This is not unusual and does not mean you should stop the medicine. This is sometimes called spotting when the bleeding is slight, or breakthrough bleeding when it is heavier. If this occurs, continue on your regular dosing schedule. *Check with your doctor:*
- If vaginal bleeding continues for an unusually long time.
- If your menstrual period has not started within 45 days of your last period.

Missed menstrual periods may occur. *If you suspect a pregnancy, you should call your doctor immediately.*

If you are scheduled for any laboratory tests, tell your health care professional that you are taking a progestin. Progestins can change certain test results.

The following medicines might reduce the effectiveness of progestins for contraception:
- Aminoglutethimide (e.g., Cytadren)
- Carbamazepine (e.g., Tegretol)
- Phenobarbital
- Phenytoin (e.g., Dilantin)
- Rifabutin (e.g., Mycobutin)
- Rifampin (e.g., Rifadin)

Sometimes your doctor may use these medicines with progestins for contraception but will give you special directions to follow to make sure your progestin is working properly. *Use a second method of birth control* while using these medicines that reduce the effectiveness of progestins for contraception. If you are using medroxyprogesterone injection for contraception, continue using a back-up method of birth control until you have your next injection, even if those medicines that affect contraceptives are discontinued. If you are using the oral tablets or implants, continue using a back-up method of birth control for a full cycle (or 4 weeks), even if those medicines that affect contraceptives are discontinued.

If you vomit your oral progestin-only contraceptive for any reason within hours of taking it, do not take another dose. Return to your regular dosing schedule and use an additional back-up method of birth control for 48 hours.

If you are receiving levonorgestrel tablets for emergency contraception and vomiting occurs within 1 hour of taking either dose of the medicine, contact your physician to discuss whether the dose should be repeated.

Side Effects of This Medicine

Along with its needed effects, a medicine may cause some unwanted effects. Although not all of these side effects may occur, if they do occur they may need medical attention.

Check with your doctor as soon as possible if any of the following side effects occur:
More common
   Changes in uterine bleeding (increased amounts of menstrual bleeding occurring at regular monthly periods; lighter uterine bleeding between menstrual pe-

riods; heavier uterine bleeding between regular monthly periods; or stopping of menstrual periods

Less common

Mental depression; skin rash; unexpected or increased flow of breast milk

Incidence not known—for patients taking Depo-Provera Contraceptive Injection.

Cough; decrease in height; difficulty swallowing; fast heartbeat; hives, itching, puffiness, or swelling of the eyelids or around the eyes, face, lips or tongue; pain in back, ribs, arms, or legs; shortness of breath; pain or swelling in arms or legs without any injury; skin rash; tightness in chest; wheezing

Other side effects may occur that usually do not need medical attention. These side effects may go away during treatment as your body adjusts to the medicine. However, check with your doctor if any of the following side effects continue or are bothersome:

More common

Abdominal pain or cramping; diarrhea; dizziness; fatigue; mild headache; mood changes; nausea; nervousness; pain or irritation at place of injection or place where implants were inserted; swelling of face, ankles, or feet; unusual tiredness or weakness; vomiting; weight gain

Less common

Acne; breast pain or tenderness; brown spots on exposed skin, possibly long-lasting; hot flashes; loss or gain of body, facial, or scalp hair; loss of sexual desire; trouble in sleeping

Not all of the side effects listed above have been reported for each of these medicines, but they have been reported for at least one of them. All of the progestins are similar, so any of the above side effects may occur with any of these medicines.

After you stop using this medicine, your body may need time to adjust. The length of time this takes depends on the amount of medicine you were using and how long you used it. During this period of time check with your doctor if you notice any of the following side effects:

Delayed return to fertility; stopping of menstrual periods; unusual menstrual bleeding (continuing)

Other side effects not listed above may also occur in some patients. If you notice any other effects, check with your doctor.

PROGESTINS (Systemic)

Some commonly used brand names are:

In the U.S.—

Amen (3)	Hy/Gestrone (1)
Aygestin (5)	Hylutin (1)
Crinone (6)	Megace (4)
Curretab (3)	Prochieve (6)
Cycrin (3)	Prodrox (1)
Depo-Provera (3)	Prometrium (6)
depo-subQ provera 104 (3)	Pro-Span (1)
Gesterol 50 (6)	Provera (3)
Gesterol LA 250 (1)	

In Canada—

Alti-MPA (3)	Norlutate (5)
Apo-Megestrol (4)	Novo-Medrone (3)
Colprone (2)	PMS-Progesterone (6)
Depo-Provera (3)	Prometrium (6)
Gen-Medroxy (3)	Provera (3)
Megace (4)	Provera Pak (3)
Megace OS (4)	

This information applies to the following medicines

1. Hydroxyprogesterone (hye-drox-ee-proe-JES-te-rone)
2. Medrogestone (me-droe-JES-tone)
3. Medroxyprogesterone (me-DROX-ee-proe-JES-te-rone)
4. Megestrol (me-JES-trole)
5. Norethindrone (nor-eth-IN-drone)
6. Progesterone (proe-JES-ter-one)

Category

- **Antianorectic**—Megestrol
- **Anticachetic**—Megestrol
- **Antineoplastic**—Medroxyprogesterone; Megestrol
- **Diagnostic aid, estrogen production**—Hydroxyprogesterone; Medroxyprogesterone; Progesterone (parenteral)
- **Infertility therapy adjunct**—Progesterone (vaginal)
- **Ovarian hormone therapy agent adjunct**—Medroxyprogesterone (oral); Progesterone (oral)
- **Progestational agent**—Hydroxyprogesterone; Medrogestone; Medroxyprogesterone; Norethindrone; Progesterone

Description

Progestins (proe-JES-tins) are hormones. They are used by both men and women for different purposes.

Progestins are prescribed for several reasons:

- To properly regulate the menstrual cycle and treat unusual stopping of the menstrual periods (amenorrhea). Progestins work by causing changes in the uterus. After the amount of progestins in the blood drops, the lining of the uterus begins to come off and vaginal bleeding occurs (menstrual period). Progestins help other hormones start and stop the menstrual cycle.
- To help a pregnancy occur during egg donor or infertility procedures in women who do not produce enough progesterone. Also, progesterone is given to help maintain a pregnancy when not enough of it is made by the body.
- To prevent estrogen from thickening the lining of the uterus (endometrial hyperplasia) in women around menopause who are being treated with estrogen for ovarian hormone therapy (OHT). OHT is also called hormone replacement therapy (HRT) and estrogen replacement therapy (ERT).
- To treat pain that is related to endometriosis, a condition where the endometrial tissue which lines the uterus becomes displaced in other female organs.
- To treat a condition called endometriosis or unusual and heavy bleeding of the uterus (dysfunctional uterine bleeding) by starting or stopping the menstrual cycle.
- To help treat cancer of the breast, kidney, or uterus. Progestins help change the cancer cell's ability to react to

other hormones and proteins that cause tumor growth. In this way, progestins can stop the growth of a tumor.

- To test the body's production of certain hormones such as estrogen.
- To treat loss of appetite and severe weight or muscle loss in patients with acquired immunodeficiency syndrome (AIDS) or cancer by causing certain proteins to be produced that cause increased appetite and weight gain.

Progestins may also be used for other conditions as determined by your doctor.

Depending on how much and which progestin you use or take, a progestin can have different effects. For instance, high doses of progesterone are necessary for some women to continue a pregnancy while other progestins in low doses can prevent a pregnancy from occurring. Other effects include causing weight gain, increasing body temperature, developing the milk-producing glands for breast-feeding, and relaxing the uterus to maintain a pregnancy.

Progestins can help other hormones work properly. Progestins may help to prevent anemia (low iron in blood), too much menstrual blood loss, and cancer of the uterus.

Progestins are available only with your doctor's prescription, in the following dosage forms:

Oral
- Medrogestone
  - Tablets
- Medroxyprogesterone
  - Tablets
- Megestrol
  - Oral suspension
  - Tablets
- Norethindrone
  - Tablets
- Progesterone
  - Capsules

Parenteral
- Hydroxyprogesterone
  - Injection
- Medroxyprogesterone
  - Intramuscular injection
  - Subcutaneous injection
- Progesterone
  - Injection

Vaginal
- Progesterone
  - Gel
  - Suppositories

Before Using This Medicine

In deciding to use a medicine, the risks of taking the medicine must be weighed against the good it will do. This is a decision you and your health care professional will make. For progestins, the following should be considered:

Allergies—Tell your doctor if you have ever had any unusual reaction to progestins. If using progesterone capsules or injection, tell your doctor if you are allergic to peanuts. Also tell your health care professional if you are allergic to any other substances, such as foods, preservatives, or dyes.

Diet—Make certain your health care professional knows if you are on any special diet, such as a low-sodium or low-sugar diet.

Pregnancy—Progesterone, a natural hormone that the body makes during pregnancy, has not caused problems. In fact, it is sometimes used in women to treat a certain type of infertility and to aid in egg donor or infertility procedures.

Other progestins have not been studied in pregnant women. Be sure to tell your doctor if you become pregnant while using any of the progestins. It is best to use some kind of birth control method while you are receiving progestins in high doses. High doses of progestins are not recommended for use during pregnancy since there have been some reports that they may cause birth defects in the genitals (sex organs) of a male fetus. Also, some of these progestins may cause male-like changes in a female fetus and female-like changes in a male fetus, but these problems usually can be reversed. Low doses of progestins, such as those doses used for contraception, have not caused major problems when used accidentally during pregnancy.

Breast-feeding—Although progestins pass into the breast milk, they have not been shown to cause problems in nursing babies. However, progestins may change the quality or amount (increase or decrease) of the mother's breast milk. It may be necessary for you to take another medicine or to stop breast-feeding during treatment. Be sure you have discussed the risks and benefits of the medicine with your doctor.

Children—Although there is no specific information comparing use of progestins in children with use in other age groups, this medicine is not expected to cause different side effects or problems in children than it does in adults.

Teenagers—Although there is no specific information comparing use of progestins in teenagers with use in other age groups, this medicine is not expected to cause different side effects or problems in teenagers than it does in adults.

Older adults—This medicine has been tested and has not been shown to cause different side effects or problems in older people than it does in younger adults.

Other medicines—Although certain medicines should not be used together at all, in other cases two different medicines may be used together even if an interaction might occur. In these cases, your doctor may want to change the dose, or other precautions may be necessary. When you are taking a progestin, it is especially important that your health care professional know if you are taking any of the following:
- Aminoglutethimide (e.g., Cytadren) or
- Carbamazepine (e.g., Tegretol) or
- Phenobarbital or
- Phenytoin (e.g., Dilantin) or
- Rifabutin (e.g., Mycobutin) or
- Rifampin (e.g., Rifadin, Rimactane)—These medicines may decrease the effects of progestins

Other medical problems—The presence of other medical problems may affect the use of progestins. Make sure you tell your doctor if you have any other medical problems, especially:
- Asthma or
- Epilepsy (or history of) or
- Heart or circulation problems or
- Kidney disease (severe) or

- Migraine headaches—Progestins may cause fluid build-up and may cause these conditions to become worse
- Bleeding problems, undiagnosed, such as blood in urine or changes in vaginal bleeding—May make diagnosis of these problems more difficult
- Blood clots (or history of) or
- Stroke (or history of) or
- Varicose veins—May have greater chance of causing blood clots if these conditions are already present when high doses of progestins are taken
- Breast disease (such as breast lumps or cysts) (history of)—May make this condition worse in certain types of diseases that do not react in a positive way to progestins
- Central nervous system (CNS) disorders, such as mental depression (or history of) or
- High blood cholesterol—Effects of progestins may cause these conditions, or may make these conditions worse
- Diabetes mellitus (sugar diabetes)—May cause an increase in your blood sugar and a change in the amount of medicine you take for diabetes; progestins in high doses are more likely to cause this problem
- Liver disease—Effects of progestins may be increased and may make this condition worse
- Other conditions that increase the chances for osteoporosis (brittle bones)—Since it is possible that certain doses of progestins may cause temporary thinning of the bones by changing your hormone balance, it is important that your doctor know if you have an increased risk of osteoporosis. Some things that can increase your risk for having osteoporosis include cigarette smoking, abusing alcohol, taking or drinking large amounts of caffeine, and having a family history of osteoporosis or easily broken bones. Some medicines, such as glucocorticoids (cortisone-like medicines) or anticonvulsants (seizure medicine), can also cause thinning of the bones. However, it is thought that progestins can help protect against osteoporosis in postmenopausal women

Proper Use of This Medicine

To make the use of a progestin as safe and reliable as possible, you should understand how and when to take it and what effects may be expected. Progestins usually come with patient directions. Read them carefully before taking or using this medicine.

Take this medicine only as directed by your doctor. Do not take more of it and do not take it for a longer time than your doctor ordered. To do so may increase the chance of side effects. Try to take the medicine at the same time each day to reduce the possibility of side effects and to allow it to work better.

Progestins are often given together with certain medicines. If you are using a combination of medicines, make sure that you take each one at the proper time and do not mix them. Ask your health care professional to help you plan a way to remember to take your medicines at the right times.

Dosing—The dose of these medicines will be different for different patients. *Follow your doctor's orders or the directions on the label.* The following information includes only the average doses of these medicines. *If your dose is different, do not change it* unless your doctor tells you to do so.

The number of tablets, injections, or suppositories that you take, receive, or use depends on the strength of the medicine. Also, *the number of doses you take or use each day, the time allowed between doses, and the length of time you take or use the medicine depend on the medical problem for which you are taking progestins.*

For hydroxyprogesterone
- For *injection* dosage form:
  - For controlling unusual and heavy bleeding of the uterus (dysfunctional uterine bleeding) or treating unusual stopping of menstrual periods (amenorrhea):
    - Adults and teenagers—375 milligrams (mg) injected into a muscle as a single dose.
  - For preparing the uterus for the menstrual period:
    - Adults and teenagers—125 to 250 mg injected into a muscle as a single dose on Day 10 of the menstrual cycle (counting from the first day of the last menstrual cycle). May be repeated every seven days if needed.

For medrogestone
- For *oral* dosage form (tablets):
  - For preparing the uterus for the menstrual period, controlling unusual and heavy bleeding of the uterus (dysfunctional uterine bleeding), preventing estrogen from thickening the lining of the uterus (endometrial hyperplasia) when taking estrogen for ovarian hormone therapy in postmenopausal women, or treating unusual stopping of menstrual periods (amenorrhea):
    - Adults and teenagers—5 to 10 milligrams (mg) a day for ten to fourteen days each month as directed by your doctor.

For medroxyprogesterone
- For *oral* dosage form (tablets):
  - For controlling unusual and heavy bleeding of the uterus (dysfunctional uterine bleeding) or treating unusual stopping of menstrual periods (amenorrhea):
    - Adults and teenagers—5 to 10 milligrams (mg) a day for five to ten days as directed by your doctor.
  - For preparing the uterus for the menstrual period:
    - Adults and teenagers—10 mg daily for five or ten days as directed by your doctor.
  - For preventing estrogen from thickening the lining of the uterus (endometrial hyperplasia) when taking estrogen for ovarian hormone therapy in postmenopausal women:
    - Adults—When taking estrogen each day on Days 1 through 25: Oral, 5 to 10 mg of medroxyprogesterone daily for ten to fourteen or more days each month as directed by your doctor. Or, your doctor may want you to take 2.5 or 5 mg a day without stopping. Your doctor will help decide the number of tablets that is best for you and when to take them.
- For *intramuscular injection* dosage form:
  - For treating cancer of the kidneys or uterus:
    - Adults and teenagers—At first, 400 to 1000 milligrams (mg) injected into a muscle as a single dose once a week. Then, your doctor may lower your dose to 400 mg or more once a month.

- For *subcutaneous injection* dosage form:
  - For treating pain related to endometriosis:
    - Adults and teenagers—104 milligrams injected under the skin of the anterior thigh or abdomen every three months (12 to 14 weeks) for not more than 2 years.

For megestrol

- For *oral* dosage form (suspension):
  - For treating loss of appetite (anorexia), muscles (cachexia), or weight caused by acquired immunodeficiency syndrome (AIDS):
    - Adults and teenagers—800 milligrams (mg) a day for the first month. Then your doctor may want you to take 400 or 800 mg a day for three more months.
- For *oral* dosage form (tablets):
  - For treating cancer of the breast:
    - Adults and teenagers—160 mg a day as a single dose or in divided doses for two or more months.
  - For treating cancer of the uterus:
    - Adults and teenagers—40 to 320 mg a day for two or more months.
  - For treating loss of appetite (anorexia), muscles (cachexia), or weight caused by cancer:
    - Adults and teenagers—400 to 800 milligrams (mg) a day.

For norethindrone

- For *oral* dosage form (tablets):
  - For controlling unusual and heavy bleeding of the uterus (dysfunctional uterine bleeding) or treating unusual stopping of menstrual periods (amenorrhea):
    - Adults and teenagers—2.5 to 10 milligrams (mg) a day from Day 5 through Day 25 (counting from the first day of the last menstrual cycle). Or, your doctor may want you to take the medicine only for five to ten days as directed.
  - For treating endometriosis:
    - Adults and teenagers—At first, 5 mg a day for two weeks. Then, your doctor may increase your dose slowly up to 15 mg a day for six to nine months. Let your doctor know if your menstrual period starts. Your doctor may want you to take more of the medicine or may want you to stop taking the medicine for a short period of time.

For progesterone

- For *oral* dosage form (capsules):
  - For preventing estrogen from thickening the lining of the uterus (endometrial hyperplasia) when taking estrogen for ovarian hormone therapy in postmenopausal women:
    - Adults—200 mg a day at bedtime during the last fourteen days of estrogen treatment each month. Although other schedules are possible, usually treatment begins either on Day 8 through Day 21 of a twenty-eight–day cycle or on Day 12 through Day 25 of a thirty-day cycle. Your doctor may ask you not to take progestins or estrogens for the last five to seven days of each month. Sometimes your doctor may increase your dose to 100 mg in the morning to be taken 2 hours after breakfast and 200 mg to be taken at bedtime.

  - For treating unusual stopping of menstrual periods (amenorrhea):
    - Adults—400 mg a day in the evening for ten days.
- For *vaginal* dosage form (gel):
  - For treating unusual stopping of menstrual periods (amenorrhea):
    - Adults and teenagers—45 mg (one applicatorful of 4% gel) once every other day for up to six doses. Dose may be increased to 90 mg (one applicatorful of 8% gel) once every other day for up to six doses if needed.
  - For use with infertility procedures:
    - Adults and teenagers—90 mg (one applicatorful of 8% gel) one or two times a day. If pregnancy occurs, treatment can continue for up to ten to twelve weeks.
- For *injection* dosage form:
  - For controlling unusual and heavy bleeding of the uterus (dysfunctional uterine bleeding) or treating unusual stopping of menstrual periods (amenorrhea):
    - Adults and teenagers—5 to 10 milligrams (mg) a day injected into a muscle for six to ten days. Or, your doctor may want you to receive 100 or 150 mg injected into a muscle as a single dose. Sometimes your doctor may want you first to take another hormone called estrogen. If your menstrual period starts, your doctor will want you to stop taking the medicine.
- For *suppositories* dosage form (vaginal):
  - For maintaining a pregnancy (at ovulation and at the beginning of pregnancy):
    - Adults and teenagers—25 mg to 100 mg (one suppository) inserted into the vagina one or two times a day beginning near the time of ovulation. Your doctor may want you to receive the medicine for up to eleven weeks.

Missed dose—For all progestins, except for progesterone capsules for postmenopausal women: If you miss a dose of this medicine, take the missed dose as soon as possible. However, if it is almost time for your next dose, skip the missed dose and go back to your regular dosing schedule. Do not double doses.

For progesterone capsules for postmenopausal women: If you miss a dose of 200 mg of progesterone capsules at bedtime, take 100 mg in the morning then go back to your regular dosing schedule. If you take 300 mg of progesterone a day and you miss your morning and evening doses, you should not take the missed dose. Return to your regular dosing schedule.

Storage—To store this medicine:

- Keep out of the reach of children.
- Store away from heat.
- Do not store in the bathroom, near the kitchen sink, or in any other damp places. Heat or moisture may cause the medicine to break down.
- Keep the injectable form of this medicine from freezing.
- Do not keep outdated medicine or medicine no longer needed. Be sure that any discarded medicine is out of the reach of children.

Precautions While Using This Medicine

It is very important that your doctor check your progress at regular visits. This will allow your dosage to be adjusted to your changing needs, and will allow any unwanted effects to be detected. These visits will usually be every 6 to 12 months, but some doctors require them more often.

Progestins may cause some people to become dizzy. For oral or vaginal progesterone, dizziness or drowsiness may occur 1 to 4 hours after taking or using it. Make sure you know how you react to this medicine before you drive, use machines, or do anything else that could be dangerous if you are not alert.

Unusual or unexpected vaginal bleeding of various amounts may occur between your regular menstrual periods during the first 3 months of use. This is sometimes called spotting when slight, or breakthrough menstrual bleeding when heavier. If this should occur, continue on your regular dosing schedule. *Check with your doctor:*

- If unusual or unexpected vaginal bleeding continues for an unusually long time.
- If your menstrual period has not started within 45 days of your last period.

Missed menstrual periods may occur. *If you suspect a pregnancy, you should stop taking this medicine immediately and call your doctor.* Your doctor will let you know if you should continue taking the progestin.

If you are scheduled for any laboratory tests, tell your health care professional that you are taking a progestin. Progestins can change certain test results.

In some patients, tenderness, swelling, or bleeding of the gums may occur. Brushing and flossing your teeth carefully and regularly and massaging your gums may help prevent this. See your dentist regularly to have your teeth cleaned. Check with your medical doctor or dentist if you have any questions about how to take care of your teeth and gums, or if you notice any tenderness, swelling, or bleeding of your gums.

You will need to use a birth control method while taking progestins for noncontraceptive use if you are fertile and sexually active.

If you are using vaginal progesterone, avoid using other vaginal products for 6 hours before and for 6 hours after inserting the vaginal dose of progesterone.

Side Effects

Along with their needed effects, progestins used in high doses sometimes cause some unwanted effects such as blood clots, heart attacks, and strokes, or problems of the liver and eyes. Although these effects are rare, some of them can be very serious and cause death. It is not clear if these problems are due to the progestin. They may be caused by the disease or condition for which progestins are being used.

The following side effects may be caused by blood clots. Although not all of these side effects may occur, if they do occur they need immediate medical attention. *Get emergency help immediately* if any of the following side effects occur:

Rare
> Such as headache or migraine; loss of or change in speech, coordination, or vision; numbness of or pain in chest, arm, or leg; unexplained shortness of breath

Also, check with your doctor as soon as possible if any of the following side effects occur:

More common
> Changes in vaginal bleeding (increased amounts of menstrual bleeding occurring at regular monthly periods, lighter vaginal bleeding between menstrual periods, heavier vaginal bleeding between regular monthly periods, or stopping of menstrual periods); symptoms of blood sugar problems (dry mouth, frequent urination, loss of appetite, or unusual thirst)

Less common
> Mental depression; skin rash; unexpected or increased flow of breast milk

Rare
For megestrol—During chronic treatment
> Backache; dizziness; filling or rounding out of the face; irritability; mental depression; unusual decrease in sexual desire or ability in men; nausea or vomiting; unusual tiredness or weakness

Other side effects may occur that usually do not need medical attention. These side effects may go away during treatment as your body adjusts to the medicine. However, check with your doctor if any of the following side effects continue or are bothersome:

More common
> Abdominal pain or cramping; bloating or swelling of ankles or feet; blood pressure increase (mild); dizziness; drowsiness (progesterone only); headache (mild); mood changes; nervousness; pain or irritation at place of injection site; swelling of face, ankles, or feet; unusual or rapid weight gain

Less common
> Acne; breast pain or tenderness; brown spots on exposed skin, possibly long-lasting; hot flashes; loss or gain of body, facial, or scalp hair; loss of sexual desire; trouble in sleeping

Not all of the side effects listed above have been reported for each of these medicines, but they have been reported for at least one of them. All of the progestins are similar, so any of the above side effects may occur with any of these medicines.

After you stop using this medicine, your body may need time to adjust. The length of time this takes depends on the amount of medicine you were using and how long you used it. During this period of time check with your doctor if you notice the following side effect:

For megestrol
> Dizziness; nausea or vomiting; unusual tiredness or weakness

> Delayed return to fertility; stopping of menstrual periods; unusual menstrual bleeding (continuing)

Other side effects not listed above may also occur in some patients. If you notice any other effects, check with your doctor.

Additional Information

Once a medicine has been approved for marketing for a certain use, experience may show that it is also useful for other medical problems. Although these uses are not included in

product labeling, progestins are used in certain patients with the following medical conditions:

- Carcinoma of the prostate
- Corpus luteum insufficiency
- Endometrial hyperplasia
- Hot flashes
- Polycystic ovary syndrome
- Precocious puberty

Other than the above information, there is no additional information relating to proper use, precautions, or side effects for these uses.

PROPAFENONE (Oral route) - proe-pa-FEEN-one

Black Box Warning

In the National Heart, Lung and Blood Institute's Cardiac Arrhythmia Suppression Trial (CAST), a long-term, multi-center, randomized, double-blind study in patients with asymptomatic non-life-threatening ventricular arrhythmias who had a myocardial infarction more than six days but less than two years previously, an increased rate of death or reversed cardiac arrest rate (7.7%; 56/730) was seen in patients treated with encainide or flecainide (Class 1C antiarrhythmics) compared with that seen in patients assigned to placebo (3%; 22/725). The average duration of treatment with encainide or flecainide in this study was ten months.

The applicability of the CAST results to other populations (eg, those without recent myocardial infarction) or other antiarrhythmic drugs is uncertain, but at present, it is prudent to consider any 1C antiarrhythmic to have a significant risk in patients with structural heart disease. Given the lack of any evidence that these drugs improve survival, antiarrhythmic agents should generally be avoided in patients with non-life-threatening ventricular arrhythmias, even if the patients are experiencing unpleasant, but not life-threatening, symptoms or signs.

Commonly used brand name(s)

In the U.S.—
   Rythmol
   Rythmol SR

Available Dosage Forms:
- Tablet
- Capsule, Extended Release

Therapeutic Class: Antiarrhythmic, Group IC

Uses For This Medicine

Propafenone belongs to the group of medicines known as antiarrhythmics. It is used to treat abnormal heart rhythms.

Propafenone produces its helpful effects by slowing nerve impulses in the heart and making the heart tissue less sensitive.

There is a chance that propafenone may cause new heart rhythm problems or make worse those that already exist. Since similar medicines have been shown to cause severe problems in some patients, propafenone is only used to treat serious heart rhythm problems. Discuss this possible effect with your doctor.

This medicine is available only with your doctor's prescription.

Before Using This Medicine

In deciding to use a medicine, the risks of taking the medicine must be weighed against the good it will do. This is a decision you and your doctor will make. For this medicine, the following should be considered:

Allergies—Tell your doctor if you have ever had any unusual or allergic reaction to this medicine or any other medicines. Also tell your health care professional if you have any other types of allergies, such as to foods, dyes, preservatives, or animals. For non-prescription products, read the label or package ingredients carefully.

Pediatric—Propafenone can cause serious side effects in any patient. Therefore, it is especially important that you discuss with the child's doctor the good that this medicine may do as well as the risks of using it.

Geriatric—Many medicines have not been studied specifically in older people. Therefore, it may not be known whether they work exactly the same way they do in younger adults or if they cause different side effects or problems in older people. There is no specific information comparing use of propafenone in the elderly with use in other age groups.

Pregnancy—

	Pregnancy Category	Explanation
All Trimesters	C	Animal studies have shown an adverse effect and there are no adequate studies in pregnant women OR no animal studies have been conducted and there are no adequate studies in pregnant women.

Breast Feeding—There are no adequate studies in women for determining infant risk when using this medication during breastfeeding. Weigh the potential benefits against the potential risks before taking this medication while breastfeeding.

Other medicines—

Using this medicine with any of the following medicines is not recommended. Your doctor may decide not to treat you with this medication or change some of the other medicines you take.

Bepridil, Cisapride, Levomethadyl, Mesoridazine, Pimozide, Ritonavir, Saquinavir, Terfenadine, Thioridazine, Tipranavir, Ziprasidone

Interactions with Food/Tobacco/Alcohol—Certain medicines should not be used at or around the time of eating food or eating certain types of food since interactions may occur. Using alcohol or tobacco with certain medicines may also cause interactions to occur. Discuss with your healthcare professional the use of your medicine with food, alcohol, or tobacco.

Other medical problems—The presence of other medical problems may affect the use of this medicine. Make sure you tell your doctor if you have any other medical problems, especially:
- Asthma or
- Bronchitis or

- Emphysema—Propafenone can increase trouble in breathing
- Bradycardia (unusually slow heartbeat)—There is a risk of further decreased heart function
- Congestive heart failure or other heart disease or
- Myasthenia gravis or
- Severe low blood pressure—Propafenone may make these conditions worse
- Electrolyte (i.e., potassium) disorders—Propafenone may worsen heart rhythm problems
- Kidney disease or
- Liver disease—Effects of propafenone may be increased because of slower removal from the body
- If you have a pacemaker—Propafenone may interfere with the pacemaker and require more careful follow-up by the doctor

Proper Use of This Medicine

Take propafenone exactly as directed by your doctor. Do not take more or less of this medicine, and do not take it more often than your doctor ordered.

For patients taking the extended-release capsule form of this medicine

- Swallow capsules whole. Do not crush, break, or chew them.
- This medicine may be taken with or without food

Grapefruit and grapefruit juice may increase the effects of propafenone by increasing the amount of this medicine in the body. You should not eat grapefruit or drink grapefruit juice while you are taking this medicine.

This medicine works best when there is a constant amount in the blood. To help keep the amount constant, do not miss any doses. Also, it is best to take each dose at evenly spaced times day and night. For example, if you are to take 3 doses a day, doses should be spaced about 8 hours apart. If you need help in planning the best times to take your medicine, check with your health care professional.

Dosing—The dose of this medicine will be different for different patients. Follow your doctor's orders or the directions on the label. The following information includes only the average doses of this medicine. If your dose is different, do not change it unless your doctor tells you to do so.

The amount of medicine that you take depends on the strength of the medicine. Also, the number of doses you take each day, the time allowed between doses, and the length of time you take the medicine depend on the medical problem for which you are using the medicine.

- The number of extended-release capsule or tablets that you take depends on the strength of the medicine.
- For oral extended-release dosage form (capsules):
  - Adults—At first, 225 milligrams (mg) once every twelve hours. Your doctor may increase your dose as needed. However, the dose usually is not more than 450 mg every 12 hours
  - Children: Use and dose must be determined by your doctor
- For oral dosage forms (tablets):
  - Adults: 150 milligrams every eight hours. Your doctor may increase your dose if needed.
  - Children: Use and dose must be determined by your doctor.

Missed dose—If you miss a dose of this medicine, take it as soon as possible. However, if it is almost time for your next dose, skip the missed dose and go back to your regular dosing schedule. Do not double doses.

Storage—Store the medicine in a closed container at room temperature, away from heat, moisture, and direct light. Keep from freezing.

Keep out of the reach of children.

Do not keep outdated medicine or medicine no longer needed.

Precautions While Using This Medicine

It is important that your doctor check your progress at regular visits to make sure the medicine is working properly. This will allow changes to be made in the amount of medicine you are taking, if necessary.

Tell your doctor about all medications you are taking, prescription and over-the-counter (OTC)

Your doctor may want you to carry a medical identification card or bracelet stating that you are using this medicine.

Before having any kind of surgery (including dental surgery) or emergency treatment, tell the medical doctor or dentist in charge that you are taking this medicine.

Propafenone may cause some people to become dizzy or lightheaded. Make sure you know how you react to this medicine before you drive, use machines, or do anything else that could be dangerous if you are dizzy.

Side Effects of This Medicine

Along with its needed effects, a medicine may cause some unwanted effects. Although not all of these side effects may occur, if they do occur they may need medical attention.

Check with your doctor as soon as possible if any of the following side effects occur:

Less common
Chest pain; shortness of breath; fast, irregular, or slow heartbeat, dizziness, and/or fainting; swelling of feet or lower legs; weight gain

Rare
Chills, fever, and weakness; joint pain; trembling or shaking

Some side effects may occur that usually do not need medical attention. These side effects may go away during treatment as your body adjusts to the medicine. Also, your health care professional may be able to tell you about ways to prevent or reduce some of these side effects. Check with your health care professional if any of the following side effects continue or are bothersome or if you have any questions about them:

More common
Change in taste or bitter or metallic taste

Less common
Blurred vision; constipation or diarrhea; dryness of mouth; headache; nausea and/or vomiting; skin rash; unusual tiredness or weakness

Other side effects not listed may also occur in some patients. If you notice any other effects, check with your healthcare professional.

PSEUDOEPHEDRINE (Oral route) -
soo-doe-e-FED-rin

Commonly used brand name(s)

In the U.S.—

12 Hour Cold Maximum Strength	Efidac 24 Pseudoephedrine
Biofed	ElixSure Congestion
Cenafed	Children's
Chlor-Trimeton Nasal Decongestant	Genaphed
Contac 12–Hour	Pediacare Decongestant Infants
Dimetapp Decongestant	Simply Stuffy
	Sudafed

Available Dosage Forms:

- Tablet
- Tablet, Extended Release
- Tablet, Chewable
- Liquid
- Capsule, Extended Release
- Syrup
- Capsule
- Solution

Therapeutic Class: Decongestant
Pharmacologic Class: Sympathomimetic

Uses For This Medicine

Pseudoephedrine is used to relieve nasal or sinus congestion caused by the common cold, sinusitis, and hay fever and other respiratory allergies. It is also used to relieve ear congestion caused by ear inflammation or infection.

Some of these preparations are available only with your doctor's prescription.

Before Using This Medicine

In deciding to use a medicine, the risks of taking the medicine must be weighed against the good it will do. This is a decision you and your doctor will make. For this medicine, the following should be considered:

Allergies—Tell your doctor if you have ever had any unusual or allergic reaction to this medicine or any other medicines. Also tell your health care professional if you have any other types of allergies, such as to foods, dyes, preservatives, or animals. For non-prescription products, read the label or package ingredients carefully.

Pediatric—Pseudoephedrine may be more likely to cause side effects in infants, especially newborn and premature infants, than in older children and adults.

Geriatric—Many medicines have not been studied specifically in older people. Therefore, it may not be known whether they work exactly the same way they do in younger adults or if they cause different side effects or problems in older people. There is no specific information comparing use of pseudoephedrine in the elderly with use in other age groups.

Breast Feeding—There are no adequate studies in women for determining infant risk when using this medication during breastfeeding. Weigh the potential benefits against the potential risks before taking this medication while breastfeeding.

Other medicines—

Using this medicine with any of the following medicines is not recommended. Your doctor may decide not to treat you with this medication or change some of the other medicines you take.

Clorgyline, Dihydroergotamine, Furazolidone, Iproniazid, Isocarboxazid, Moclobemide, Nialamide, Pargyline, Phenelzine, Procarbazine, Rasagiline, Selegiline, Toloxatone, Tranylcypromine

Interactions with Food/Tobacco/Alcohol—Certain medicines should not be used at or around the time of eating food or eating certain types of food since interactions may occur. Using alcohol or tobacco with certain medicines may also cause interactions to occur. Discuss with your healthcare professional the use of your medicine with food, alcohol, or tobacco.

Other medical problems—The presence of other medical problems may affect the use of this medicine. Make sure you tell your doctor if you have any other medical problems, especially:

- Type 2 diabetes mellitus—Use of pseudoephedrine may cause an increase in blood glucose levels

- Enlarged prostate or

- Glaucoma, or a predisposition to glaucoma or

- Heart disease or blood vessel disease or

- High blood pressure—Pseudoephedrine may make the condition worse

- Overactive thyroid—Use of pseudoephedrine may make the condition worse

Proper Use of This Medicine

For patients taking pseudoephedrine extended-release capsules:

- Swallow the capsule whole. However, if the capsule is too large to swallow, you may mix the contents of the capsule with jam or jelly and swallow without chewing.
- Do not crush or chew before swallowing.

For patients taking pseudoephedrine extended-release tablets:

- Swallow the tablet whole.
- Do not break, crush, or chew before swallowing.

To help prevent trouble in sleeping, take the last dose of pseudoephedrine for each day a few hours before bedtime. If you have any questions about this, check with your doctor.

Take this medicine only as directed. Do not take more of it, do not take it more often, and do not take it for a longer period of time than recommended on the label (usually 7 days), unless otherwise directed by your doctor. To do so may increase the chance of side effects.

Dosing—The dose of this medicine will be different for different patients. Follow your doctor's orders or the directions on the label. The following information includes only the average doses of this medicine. If your dose is different, do not change it unless your doctor tells you to do so.

The amount of medicine that you take depends on the strength of the medicine. Also, the number of doses you take each day, the time allowed between doses, and the length of time you take the medicine depend on the medical problem for which you are using the medicine.

- For nasal or sinus congestion:
  - For regular (short-acting) oral dosage form (capsules, oral solution, syrup, or tablets):
    - Adults and children 12 years of age and older— 60 milligrams (mg) every four to six hours. Do not take more than 240 mg in twenty-four hours.
    - Children 6 to 12 years of age—30 mg every four to six hours. Do not take more than 120 mg in twenty-four hours.
    - Children 2 to 6 years of age—15 mg every four to six hours. Do not take more than 60 mg in twenty-four hours.
    - Children 4 months to 2 years of age—Dose must be determined by your doctor
    - Children up to 4 months of age—Use and dose must be determined by your doctor.
  - For long-acting oral dosage form (extended-release capsules or extended-release tablets):
    - Adults and children 12 years of age and older— 120 mg every 12 hours, or 240 mg every 24 hours. Do not take more than 240 mg in twenty-four hours.
    - Children up to 12 years of age—Use is not recommended.

Missed dose—If you miss a dose of this medicine, take it as soon as possible. However, if it is almost time for your next dose, skip the missed dose and go back to your regular dosing schedule. Do not double doses.

Storage—Store the medicine in a closed container at room temperature, away from heat, moisture, and direct light. Keep from freezing.

Keep out of the reach of children.

Do not keep outdated medicine or medicine no longer needed.

Precautions While Using This Medicine

If symptoms do not improve within 7 days or if you also have a high fever, check with your doctor since these signs may mean that you have other medical problems.

Side Effects of This Medicine

Along with its needed effects, a medicine may cause some unwanted effects. Although not all of these side effects may occur, if they do occur they may need medical attention.

Check with your doctor as soon as possible if any of the following side effects occur:

Rare—more common with high doses
Convulsions (seizures); hallucinations (seeing, hearing, or feeling things that are not there); irregular or slow heartbeat; shortness of breath or troubled breathing

Symptoms of overdose
Convulsions (seizures); fast breathing; hallucinations (seeing, hearing, or feeling things that are not there); increase in blood pressure; irregular heartbeat (continuing); shortness of breath or troubled breathing (severe or continuing); slow or fast heartbeat (severe or continuing); unusual nervousness, restlessness, or excitement

Some side effects may occur that usually do not need medical attention. These side effects may go away during treatment as your body adjusts to the medicine. Also, your health care professional may be able to tell you about ways to prevent or reduce some of these side effects. Check with your

health care professional if any of the following side effects continue or are bothersome or if you have any questions about them:

More common
Nervousness; restlessness; trouble in sleeping

Less common
Difficult or painful urination; dizziness or lightheadedness; fast or pounding heartbeat; headache; increased sweating; nausea or vomiting; trembling; unusual paleness; weakness

Other side effects not listed may also occur in some patients. If you notice any other effects, check with your healthcare professional.

PYRAZINAMIDE (Oral route) - peer-a-ZIN-a-mide

Uses For This Medicine

Pyrazinamide belongs to the family of medicines called anti-infectives. It is used, along with other medicines, to treat tuberculosis (TB).

To help clear up your tuberculosis (TB) infection completely, you must keep taking this medicine for the full time of treatment, even if you begin to feel better. This is very important. It is also important that you do not miss any doses.

Pyrazinamide is available only with your doctor's prescription.

Before Using This Medicine

In deciding to use a medicine, the risks of taking the medicine must be weighed against the good it will do. This is a decision you and your doctor will make. For this medicine, the following should be considered:

Allergies—Tell your doctor if you have ever had any unusual or allergic reaction to this medicine or any other medicines. Also tell your health care professional if you have any other types of allergies, such as to foods, dyes, preservatives, or animals. For non-prescription products, read the label or package ingredients carefully.

Pediatric—Pyrazinamide has been used in children and, in effective doses, has not been reported to cause different side effects or problems in children than it does in adults.

Geriatric—Many medicines have not been studied specifically in older people. Therefore, it may not be known whether they work exactly the same way they do in younger adults. Although there is no specific information comparing pyrazinamide in the elderly with use in other age groups, this medicine is not expected to cause different side effects or problems in older people than it does in younger adults.

Pregnancy—

	Pregnancy Category	Explanation
All Trimesters	C	Animal studies have shown an adverse effect and there are no adequate studies in pregnant women OR no animal studies have been conducted and there are no adequate studies in pregnant women.

Breast Feeding—There are no adequate studies in women for determining infant risk when using this medication during breastfeeding. Weigh the potential benefits against the potential risks before taking this medication while breastfeeding.

Other medicines—

Using this medicine with any of the following medicines is usually not recommended, but may be required in some cases. If both medicines are prescribed together, your doctor may change the dose or how often you use one or both of the medicines.

Cyclosporine, Ethionamide, Rifampin, Zidovudine

Interactions with Food/Tobacco/Alcohol—Certain medicines should not be used at or around the time of eating food or eating certain types of food since interactions may occur. Using alcohol or tobacco with certain medicines may also cause interactions to occur. Discuss with your healthcare professional the use of your medicine with food, alcohol, or tobacco.

Other medical problems—The presence of other medical problems may affect the use of this medicine. Make sure you tell your doctor if you have any other medical problems, especially:
- Gout (history of)—Pyrazinamide may worsen or cause a gout attack in patients with a history of gout
- Liver disease (severe)—Patients with severe liver disease who take pyrazinamide may have an increase in side effects

Proper Use of This Medicine

To help clear up your TB completely, it is important that you keep taking this medicine for the full time of treatment, even if you begin to feel better after a few weeks. It is important that you do not miss any doses.

Dosing—The dose of this medicine will be different for different patients. Follow your doctor's orders or the directions on the label. The following information includes only the average doses of this medicine. If your dose is different, do not change it unless your doctor tells you to do so.

The amount of medicine that you take depends on the strength of the medicine. Also, the number of doses you take each day, the time allowed between doses, and the length of time you take the medicine depend on the medical problem for which you are using the medicine.

- For oral dosage form (tablets):
  - For tuberculosis (TB):
    - Adults and children—Dose is based on body weight. The usual dose is 15 to 30 milligrams (mg) of pyrazinamide per kilogram (kg) (6.8 to 13.6 mg per pound) of body weight once a day; or 50 to 70 mg per kg (22.7 to 31.8 mg per pound) two times a week or three times a week, depending on the schedule your doctor chooses for you. This medicine must be taken along with other medicines used to treat TB.

Missed dose—If you miss a dose of this medicine, take it as soon as possible. However, if it is almost time for your next dose, skip the missed dose and go back to your regular dosing schedule. Do not double doses.

Storage—Store the medicine in a closed container at room temperature, away from heat, moisture, and direct light. Keep from freezing.

Keep out of the reach of children.

Do not keep outdated medicine or medicine no longer needed.

Precautions While Using This Medicine

It is very important that your doctor check your progress at regular visits.

If your symptoms do not improve within 2 to 3 weeks, or if they become worse, check with your doctor.

For diabetic patients:
- This medicine may cause false test results with urine ketone tests. Check with your doctor before changing your diet or the dosage of your diabetes medicine.

Side Effects of This Medicine

Along with its needed effects, a medicine may cause some unwanted effects. Although not all of these side effects may occur, if they do occur they may need medical attention.

Check with your doctor immediately if any of the following side effects occur:
> *More common*
>> Pain in large and small joints
> *Rare*
>> Loss of appetite; pain and swelling of joints, especially big toe, ankle, and knee; tense, hot skin over affected joints; unusual tiredness or weakness; yellow eyes or skin

Some side effects may occur that usually do not need medical attention. These side effects may go away during treatment as your body adjusts to the medicine. Also, your health care professional may be able to tell you about ways to prevent or reduce some of these side effects. Check with your health care professional if any of the following side effects continue or are bothersome or if you have any questions about them:
> *Rare*
>> Itching; skin rash

Other side effects not listed may also occur in some patients. If you notice any other effects, check with your healthcare professional.

PYRETHRUM EXTRACT AND PIPERONYL BUTOXIDE (Topical route) - pye-REE-thrum EX-trackt, PIP-er-oh-nil byoo-TOX-ide

Commonly used brand name(s)
In the U.S.—

A200 Maximum Strength	Pronto Maximum Strength
A200 Time-Tested Formula	Pyrinex
Lice-X	Pyrinyl
Licide	Rid
Medi-Lice Maximum Strength	Tisit

Available Dosage Forms:
- Shampoo
- Gel/Jelly
- Liquid
- Kit
- Foam

Therapeutic Class: Pediculicide

Uses For This Medicine

Medicine containing pyrethrins is used to treat head, body, and pubic lice infections. This medicine is absorbed by the lice and destroys them by acting on their nervous systems. It does not affect humans in this way. The piperonyl butoxide is included to make the pyrethrins more effective in killing the lice. This combination medicine is known as a pediculicide.

This medicine is available without a prescription.

Before Using This Medicine

In deciding to use a medicine, the risks of taking the medicine must be weighed against the good it will do. This is a decision you and your doctor will make. For this medicine, the following should be considered:

Allergies—Tell your doctor if you have ever had any unusual or allergic reaction to this medicine or any other medicines. Also tell your health care professional if you have any other types of allergies, such as to foods, dyes, preservatives, or animals. For non-prescription products, read the label or package ingredients carefully.

Pediatric—Although there is no specific information comparing use of pyrethrins and piperonyl butoxide combination in children with use in other age groups, this medicine is not expected to cause different side effects or problems in children than it does in adults.

Geriatric—Many medicines have not been studied specifically in older people. Therefore, it may not be known whether they work exactly the same way they do in younger adults. Although there is no specific information comparing use of pyrethrins and piperonyl butoxide combination medicine in the elderly with use in other age groups, this medicine is not expected to cause different side effects or problems in older people than it does in younger adults.

Pregnancy—

	Pregnancy Category	Explanation
All Trimesters	C	Animal studies have shown an adverse effect and there are no adequate studies in pregnant women OR no animal studies have been conducted and there are no adequate studies in pregnant women.

Breast Feeding—There are no adequate studies in women for determining infant risk when using this medication during breastfeeding. Weigh the potential benefits against the potential risks before taking this medication while breastfeeding.

Other medicines—Although certain medicines should not be used together at all, in other cases two different medicines may be used together even if an interaction might occur. In these cases, your doctor may want to change the dose, or other precautions may be necessary. Tell your healthcare professional if you are taking any other prescription or non-prescription (over-the-counter [OTC]) medicine.

Interactions with Food/Tobacco/Alcohol—Certain medicines should not be used at or around the time of eating food or eating certain types of food since interactions may occur. Using alcohol or tobacco with certain medicines may also cause interactions to occur. Discuss with your healthcare professional the use of your medicine with food, alcohol, or tobacco.

Other medical problems—The presence of other medical problems may affect the use of this medicine. Make sure you tell your doctor if you have any other medical problems, especially:
- Inflammation of the skin (severe)—Use of pyrethrins and piperonyl butoxide combination may make the condition worse

Proper Use of This Medicine

Pyrethrins and piperonyl butoxide combination medicine usually comes with patient directions. Read them carefully before using this medicine.

Use this medicine only as directed. Do not use more of it and do not use it more often than recommended on the label. To do so may increase the chance of absorption through the skin and the chance of side effects.

Keep pyrethrins and piperonyl butoxide combination medicine away from the mouth and do not inhale it. This medicine is harmful if swallowed or inhaled.

To lessen the chance of inhaling this medicine, apply it in a well-ventilated room (for example, one with free flowing air or with a fan turned on).

Keep this medicine away from the eyes and other mucous membranes, such as the inside of the nose, mouth, or vagina, because it may cause irritation. If you accidentally get some in your eyes, flush them thoroughly with water at once.

Do not apply this medicine to the eyelashes or eyebrows. If they become infected with lice, check with your doctor.

To use the gel or solution form of this medicine:
- Apply enough medicine to thoroughly wet the dry hair and scalp or skin. Allow the medicine to remain on the affected areas for exactly 10 minutes.
- Then, thoroughly wash the affected areas with warm water and soap or regular shampoo. Rinse thoroughly and dry with a clean towel.

To use the shampoo form of this medicine:
- Apply enough medicine to thoroughly wet the dry hair and scalp or skin. Allow the medicine to remain on the affected areas for exactly 10 minutes.
- Then use a small amount of water and work shampoo into the hair and scalp or skin until a lather forms. Rinse thoroughly and dry with a clean towel.

After rinsing and drying, use a nit removal comb (special fine-toothed comb, usually included with this medicine) to remove the dead lice and eggs (nits) from hair.

Immediately after using this medicine, wash your hands to remove any medicine that may be on them.

This medicine should be used again in 7 to 10 days after the first treatment in order to kill any newly hatched lice.

Lice can easily move from one person to another by close body contact. This can happen also by direct contact with such things as clothing, hats, scarves, bedding, towels, washcloths, hairbrushes and combs, or the hair of infected persons. Therefore, all members of your household should be examined for lice and receive treatment if they are found to be infected.

To use this medicine for pubic (crab) lice:

- Your sexual partner may also need to be treated, since the infection may spread to persons in close contact. If your partner is not being treated or if you have any questions about this, check with your doctor.

Dosing—The dose of this medicine will be different for different patients. Follow your doctor's orders or the directions on the label. The following information includes only the average doses of this medicine. If your dose is different, do not change it unless your doctor tells you to do so.

The amount of medicine that you take depends on the strength of the medicine. Also, the number of doses you take each day, the time allowed between doses, and the length of time you take the medicine depend on the medical problem for which you are using the medicine.

- For topical dosage forms (gel, solution shampoo, and topical solution):
  - For head, body, or pubic lice:
    - Adults and children—Use one time, then repeat one time in seven to ten days.

Storage—Store the medicine in a closed container at room temperature, away from heat, moisture, and direct light. Keep from freezing.

Keep out of the reach of children.

Do not keep outdated medicine or medicine no longer needed.

Precautions While Using This Medicine

To prevent reinfection or spreading of the infection to other people, good health habits are also required. These include the following:

- For head lice
  - Machine wash all clothing (including hats, scarves, and coats), bedding, towels, and washcloths in very hot water and dry them by using the hot cycle of a dryer for at least 20 minutes. Clothing or bedding that cannot be washed should be dry-cleaned or sealed in a plastic bag for 2 weeks.
  - Shampoo all wigs and hairpieces.
  - Wash all hairbrushes and combs in very hot soapy water (above 130 °F) for 5 to 10 minutes and do not share them with other people.
  - Clean the house or room by thoroughly vacuuming upholstered furniture, rugs, and floors.
- For body lice
  - Machine wash all clothing, bedding, towels, and washcloths in very hot water and dry them by using the hot cycle of a dryer for at least 20 minutes. Clothing or bedding that cannot be washed should be dry-cleaned or sealed in a plastic bag for 2 weeks.
  - Clean the house or room by thoroughly vacuuming upholstered furniture, rugs, and floors.
- For pubic lice
  - Machine wash all clothing (especially underwear), bedding, towels, and washcloths in very hot water and dry them by using the hot cycle of a dryer for at least 20 minutes. Clothing or bedding that cannot be washed should be dry-cleaned or sealed in a plastic bag for 2 weeks.
  - Scrub toilet seats frequently.

Side Effects of This Medicine

Along with its needed effects, a medicine may cause some unwanted effects. Although not all of these side effects may occur, if they do occur they may need medical attention.

Check with your doctor as soon as possible if any of the following side effects occur:

Less common or rare
  Skin irritation not present before use of this medicine; skin rash or infection; sneezing (sudden attacks of); stuffy or runny nose; wheezing or difficulty in breathing

Other side effects not listed may also occur in some patients. If you notice any other effects, check with your healthcare professional.

PYRIDOXINE   (Oral route, Injection route) - peer-i-DOX-een

Commonly used brand name(s)
In the U.S.—
  Aminoxin   Rodex
  Pyri-500   Vitabee 6

Available Dosage Forms:
- Tablet, Extended Release   • Capsule
- Solution   • Injectable
- Tablet   • Tablet, Enteric Coated

Therapeutic Class: Nutritive Agent
Pharmacologic Class: Vitamin B

Uses For This Dietary Supplement

Vitamins are compounds that you must have for growth and health. They are needed in small amounts only and are usually available in the foods that you eat. Pyridoxine (vitamin B_6) is necessary for normal breakdown of proteins, carbohydrates, and fats.

Some conditions may increase your need for pyridoxine. These include:
- Alcoholism
- Burns
- Diarrhea
- Dialysis
- Heart disease
- Intestinal problems
- Liver disease
- Overactive thyroid
- Stress, long-term illness, or serious injury
- Surgical removal of stomach

In addition, infants receiving unfortified formulas such as evaporated milk may need additional pyridoxine.

Increased need for pyridoxine should be determined by your health care professional.

Lack of pyridoxine may lead to anemia (weak blood), nerve damage, seizures, skin problems, and sores in the mouth. Your doctor may treat these problems by prescribing pyridoxine for you.

Claims that pyridoxine is effective for treatment of acne and other skin problems, alcohol intoxication, asthma, hemorrhoids, kidney stones, mental problems, migraine headaches, morning sickness, and menstrual problems, or to stimulate appetite or milk production have not been proven.

Injectable pyridoxine is given by or under the supervision of a health care professional. Other forms of pyridoxine are available without a prescription.

Importance of Diet—For good health, it is important that you eat a balanced and varied diet. Follow carefully any diet program your health care professional may recommend. For your specific dietary vitamin and/or mineral needs, ask your health care professional for a list of appropriate foods. If you think that you are not getting enough vitamins and/or minerals in your diet, you may choose to take a dietary supplement.

Pyridoxine is found in various foods, including meats, bananas, lima beans, egg yolks, peanuts, and whole-grain cereals. Pyridoxine is not lost from food during ordinary cooking, although some other forms of vitamin B_6 are.

Vitamins alone will not take the place of a good diet and will not provide energy. Your body also needs other substances found in food such as protein, minerals, carbohydrates, and fat. Vitamins themselves often cannot work without the presence of other foods.

The daily amount of pyridoxine needed is defined in several different ways.

For U.S.—
- Recommended Dietary Allowances (RDAs) are the amount of vitamins and minerals needed to provide for adequate nutrition in most healthy persons. RDAs for a given nutrient may vary depending on a person's age, sex, and physical condition (e.g., pregnancy).
- Daily Values (DVs) are used on food and dietary supplement labels to indicate the percent of the recommended daily amount of each nutrient that a serving provides. DV replaces the previous designation of United States Recommended Daily Allowances (USRDAs).

For Canada—
- Recommended Nutrient Intakes (RNIs) are used to determine the amounts of vitamins, minerals, and protein needed to provide adequate nutrition and lessen the risk of chronic disease.

Normal daily recommended intakes for pyridoxine are generally defined as follows:
- Infants and children—
  - Birth to 3 years of age: 0.3 to 1 milligram (mg).
  - 4 to 6 years of age: 1.1 mg.
  - 7 to 10 years of age: 1.4 mg.
- Adolescent and adult males—1.7 to 2 mg.
- Adolescent and adult females—1.4 to 1.6 mg.
- Pregnant females—2.2 mg.
- Breast-feeding females—2.1 mg.

Before Using This Dietary Supplement

If you are taking this dietary supplement without a prescription, carefully read and follow any precautions on the label. For this supplement, the following should be considered:

Allergies—Tell your doctor if you have ever had any unusual or allergic reaction to this medicine or any other medicines. Also tell your health care professional if you have any other types of allergies, such as to foods, dyes, preservatives,

or animals. For non-prescription products, read the label or package ingredients carefully.

Pediatric—Problems in children have not been reported with intake of normal daily recommended amounts.

Geriatric—Problems in older adults have not been reported with intake of normal daily recommended amounts.

Breast Feeding—There are no adequate studies in women for determining infant risk when using this medication during breastfeeding. Weigh the potential benefits against the potential risks before taking this medication while breastfeeding.

Other medicines—

Using this dietary supplement with any of the following medicines is usually not recommended, but may be required in some cases. If both medicines are prescribed together, your doctor may change the dose or how often you use one or both of the medicines.

Altretamine

Interactions with Food/Tobacco/Alcohol—Certain medicines should not be used at or around the time of eating food or eating certain types of food since interactions may occur. Using alcohol or tobacco with certain medicines may also cause interactions to occur. Discuss with your healthcare professional the use of your medicine with food, alcohol, or tobacco.

Proper Use of This Dietary Supplement

Dosing—The dose of this medicine will be different for different patients. Follow your doctor's orders or the directions on the label. The following information includes only the average doses of this medicine. If your dose is different, do not change it unless your doctor tells you to do so.

The amount of medicine that you take depends on the strength of the medicine. Also, the number of doses you take each day, the time allowed between doses, and the length of time you take the medicine depend on the medical problem for which you are using the medicine.

- For oral dosage forms (capsules, tablets, oral solution):
  - To prevent deficiency, the amount taken by mouth is based on normal daily recommended intakes:
    - Adult and teenage males—1.7 to 2 milligrams (mg) per day.
    - Adult and teenage females—1.4 to 1.6 mg per day.
    - Pregnant females—2.2 mg per day.
    - Breast-feeding females—2.1 mg per day.
    - Children 7 to 10 years of age—1.4 mg per day.
    - Children 4 to 6 years of age—1.1 mg per day.
    - Children birth to 3 years of age—0.3 to 1 mg per day.
  - To treat deficiency:
    - Adults, teenagers, and children—Treatment dose is determined by prescriber for each individual based on the severity of deficiency.

To use the extended-release capsule form of this dietary supplement:
- Swallow the capsule whole.
- Do not crush, break, or chew before swallowing.
- If the capsule is too large to swallow, you may mix the contents of the capsule with jam or jelly and swallow without chewing.

To use the extended-release tablet form of this dietary supplement:

- Swallow the tablet whole.
- Do not crush, break, or chew before swallowing.

Missed dose—If you miss a dose of this medicine, skip the missed dose and go back to your regular dosing schedule. Do not double doses.

Storage—Store the medicine in a closed container at room temperature, away from heat, moisture, and direct light. Keep from freezing.

Keep out of the reach of children.

Do not keep outdated medicine or medicine no longer needed.

Side Effects of This Dietary Supplement

Along with its needed effects, a medicine may cause some unwanted effects. Although not all of these side effects may occur, if they do occur they may need medical attention.

Check with your doctor as soon as possible if any of the following side effects occur:

With large doses
Clumsiness; numbness of hands or feet

Other side effects not listed may also occur in some patients. If you notice any other effects, check with your healthcare professional.

QUETIAPINE (Oral route) - kwe-TYE-a-peen

Black Box Warning

Elderly patients with dementia-related psychosis treated with atypical antipsychotic drugs are at an increased risk of death compared to placebo. Analyses of seventeen placebo-controlled trials (modal duration of 10 weeks) in these patients revealed a risk of death in the drug-treated patients of between 1.6 times to 1.7 times that seen in placebo-treated patients. Over the course of a typical 10 week controlled trial, the rate of death in drug-treated patients was about 4.5%, compared to a rate of about 2.6% in the placebo group. Although the causes of death were varied, most of the deaths appeared to be either cardiovascular (eg, heart failure, sudden death) or infectious (eg, pneumonia) in nature. Quetiapine fumarate is not approved for the treatment of patients with dementia-related psychosis.

Commonly used brand name(s)

In the U.S.—
Seroquel

Available Dosage Forms:
- Tablet

Therapeutic Class: Antipsychotic

Uses For This Medicine

Quetiapine is used to treat psychotic disorders, such as schizophrenia. This medicine has NOT been approved to treat behavioral problems in older adult patients who have dementia.

Quetiapine is available only with your doctor's prescription.

Before Using This Medicine

In deciding to use a medicine, the risks of taking the medicine must be weighed against the good it will do. This is a decision you and your doctor will make. For this medicine, the following should be considered:

Allergies—Tell your doctor if you have ever had any unusual or allergic reaction to this medicine or any other medicines. Also tell your health care professional if you have any other types of allergies, such as to foods, dyes, preservatives, or animals. For non-prescription products, read the label or package ingredients carefully.

Pediatric—Studies on this medicine have been done only in adult patients, and there is no specific information comparing use of quetiapine in children with use in other age groups.

Geriatric—This medicine has been tested in a limited number of patients 65 years of age or older and has not been shown to cause different side effects or problems in older people than it does in younger adults. However, quetiapine may be removed from the body more slowly in older adults, so an older adult may receive a lower dose than a younger adult. This medicine has NOT been approved to treat behavioral problems in older adults with dementia.

Pregnancy—

	Pregnancy Category	Explanation
All Trimesters	C	Animal studies have shown an adverse effect and there are no adequate studies in pregnant women OR no animal studies have been conducted and there are no adequate studies in pregnant women.

Breast Feeding—There are no adequate studies in women for determining infant risk when using this medication during breastfeeding. Weigh the potential benefits against the potential risks before taking this medication while breastfeeding.

Other medicines—

Using this medicine with any of the following medicines is not recommended. Your doctor may decide not to treat you with this medication or change some of the other medicines you take.

Bepridil, Cisapride, Mesoridazine, Terfenadine, Thioridazine

Interactions with Food/Tobacco/Alcohol—Certain medicines should not be used at or around the time of eating food or eating certain types of food since interactions may occur. Using alcohol or tobacco with certain medicines may also cause interactions to occur. The following interactions have been selected on the basis of their potential significance and are not necessarily all-inclusive.

Using this medicine with any of the following may cause an increased risk of certain side effects but may be unavoidable in some cases. If used together, your doctor may change the dose or how often you use this medicine, or give you special instructions about the use of food, alcohol, or tobacco.

Other medical problems—The presence of other medical problems may affect the use of this medicine. Make sure you tell your doctor if you have any other medical problems, especially:

- Alzheimer's disease—Quetiapine may cause problems with swallowing, which may increase the chance of pneumonia; also, the chance of seizures may be increased
- Breast cancer, or history of or
- Underactive thyroid—Quetiapine may make these conditions worse
- Dehydration—Decreased blood pressure caused by quetiapine may be more severe; chance of developing heatstroke may be increased
- Heart disease or
- Stroke, or history of—Decreased blood pressure caused by quetiapine may be more severe or may make these conditions worse
- Kidney disease (severe) or
- Liver disease—Higher blood levels of quetiapine may occur, increasing the chance of side effects; the dose may need to be changed
- Seizures, or history of—Chance of seizures may be increased

Proper Use of This Medicine

Take this medicine only as directed by your doctor to benefit your condition as much as possible. Do not take more or less of it and do not take it more or less often than your doctor ordered.

Quetiapine may be taken with or without food on a full or empty stomach. However, if your doctor tells you to take it a certain way, take it as directed.

Dosing—The dose of this medicine will be different for different patients. Follow your doctor's orders or the directions on the label. The following information includes only the average doses of this medicine. If your dose is different, do not change it unless your doctor tells you to do so.

The amount of medicine that you take depends on the strength of the medicine. Also, the number of doses you take each day, the time allowed between doses, and the length of time you take the medicine depend on the medical problem for which you are using the medicine.

- For oral dosage form (tablets):
  - For schizophrenia:
    - Adults—At first, 25 milligrams (mg) two times a day. The dose usually is increased to 300 to 400 mg a day, which is divided and given in two or three doses a day. Your doctor may increase your dose further, if needed. However, the dose usually is not more than 800 mg a day.
    - Children—Use and dose must be determined by the doctor.

Missed dose—If you miss a dose of this medicine, take it as soon as possible. However, if it is almost time for your next dose, skip the missed dose and go back to your regular dosing schedule. Do not double doses.

Storage—Store the medicine in a closed container at room temperature, away from heat, moisture, and direct light. Keep from freezing.

Keep out of the reach of children.

Do not keep outdated medicine or medicine no longer needed.

Precautions While Using This Medicine

Your doctor should check your progress at regular visits, especially during the first few months of treatment with this medicine. This will allow your dosage to be changed if necessary to meet your needs.

This medicine may add to the effects of alcohol and other CNS depressants (medicines that make you drowsy or less alert). Some examples of CNS depressants are antihistamines or medicine for hay fever, other allergies, or colds; sedatives, tranquilizers, or sleeping medicine; prescription pain medicine or narcotics; barbiturates; medicine for seizures; muscle relaxants; or anesthetics, including some dental anesthetics. Check with your doctor before taking any of the above while you are using quetiapine.

Quetiapine may cause drowsiness, especially during the first week of use. Make sure you know how you react to this medicine before you drive, use machines, or do anything else that could be dangerous if you are not alert.

Dizziness, lightheadedness, or fainting may occur, especially when you get up from a lying or sitting position. Getting up slowly may help. If the problem continues or gets worse, check with your doctor.

Quetiapine may make it more difficult for your body to cool down. Use extra care not to become overheated and to drink plenty of fluids during exercise or hot weather while you are taking this medicine. Overheating may result in heatstroke.

Side Effects of This Medicine

Along with its needed effects, quetiapine can sometimes cause serious side effects. Some side effects will have signs or symptoms that you can see or feel. Your doctor may watch for others, such as changes in the lenses of the eyes, by doing certain tests. Tardive dyskinesia (a movement disorder) may occur and may not go away after you stop using the medicine. Signs of tardive dyskinesia include fine, worm-like movements of the tongue, or other uncontrolled movements of the mouth, tongue, cheeks, jaw, or arms and legs. Another serious but rare side effect that may occur is the neuroleptic malignant syndrome (NMS). You and your doctor should discuss the good this medicine will do as well as the risks of taking it.

Stop taking this medicine and get emergency help immediately if any of the following effects occur:

Rare—Symptoms of NMS; two or more occur together; most of these effects do not require emergency medical attention if they occur alone

Convulsions (seizures); difficult or unusually fast breathing; fast heartbeat or irregular pulse; high fever; high or low (irregular) blood pressure; increased sweating; loss of bladder control; severe muscle stiffness; unusually pale skin; unusual tiredness or weakness

Check with your doctor as soon as possible if any of the following side effects occur:

Less common

Dizziness, lightheadedness, or fainting, especially when getting up from a lying or sitting position; fever, chills, muscle aches, or sore throat; loss of balance control; mask-like face; shuffling walk; skin rash; slowed movements; stiffness of arms or legs; swelling of feet or lower legs; trembling and shaking of hands and fingers; trouble in breathing, speaking, or swallowing

Rare

Fainting; fast, pounding, or irregular heartbeat; menstrual changes; unusual secretion of milk (in females)

Rare—Symptoms of underactive thyroid; usually two or more occur together; these effects do not require medical attention if they occur alone unless they continue or are bothersome

Dry, puffy skin; loss of appetite; tiredness; weight gain

Symptoms of overdose—May be similar to side effects seen at normal doses but may be more severe or two or more may occur together

Drowsiness; fast, slow, or irregular heartbeat; low blood pressure; weakness

Some side effects may occur that usually do not need medical attention. These side effects may go away during treatment as your body adjusts to the medicine. Also, your health care professional may be able to tell you about ways to prevent or reduce some of these side effects. Check with your health care professional if any of the following side effects continue or are bothersome or if you have any questions about them:

More common

Constipation; drowsiness; dry mouth; increased weight; indigestion

Less common

Abdominal pain; abnormal vision; decrease in appetite; decreased strength and energy; feeling of fast or irregular heartbeat; headache; increased muscle tone; increased sweating; stuffy or runny nose

Other side effects not listed may also occur in some patients. If you notice any other effects, check with your healthcare professional.

QUINIDINE (Oral route, Injection route, Intramuscular route) - KWIN-i-deen

Black Box Warning

In many trials of antiarrhythmic therapy for non-life threatening arrhythmias, active antiarrhythmic therapy has resulted in increased mortality; the risk of active therapy is probably greatest in patients with structural heart disease.

In the case of quinidine used to prevent or defer recurrence of atrial flutter/fibrillation, meta-analysis data has shown that in the patients studied in the trials there analyzed, the mortality associated with the use of quinidine was more than three times as great as the mortality associated with the use of placebo.

Another meta-analysis showed that in patients with various non-life-threatening ventricular arrhythmias, the mortality associated with the use of quinidine was consistently greater than that associated with the use of any of a variety of alternative antiarrhythmics.

Commonly used brand name(s)

In the U.S.—

Cardioquin Quinalan
Quinaglute Quinidex Extentabs

Available Dosage Forms:
- Tablet
- Tablet, Extended Release
- Solution
- Capsule

Therapeutic Class: Antiarrhythmic, Group IA

Uses For This Medicine

Quinidine is used to treat abnormal heart rhythms. It is also used to treat malaria.

Do not confuse this medicine with quinine, which, although related, has different medical uses.

Quinidine is available only with your doctor's prescription.

Before Using This Medicine

In deciding to use a medicine, the risks of taking the medicine must be weighed against the good it will do. This is a decision you and your doctor will make. For this medicine, the following should be considered:

Allergies—Tell your doctor if you have ever had any unusual or allergic reaction to this medicine or any other medicines. Also tell your health care professional if you have any other types of allergies, such as to foods, dyes, preservatives, or animals. For non-prescription products, read the label or package ingredients carefully.

Pediatric—Quinidine has not been widely studied in children; however, it is used in children to treat abnormal heart rhythms and to treat malaria. Children may be able to take higher doses than adults and may have fewer side effects (such as vomiting, loss of appetite, and diarrhea) than adults.

Geriatric—Many medicines have not been studied specifically in older people. Therefore, it may not be known whether they work exactly the same way they do in younger adults. Although there is no specific information comparing use of quinidine in the elderly with use in other age groups, this medicine is not expected to cause different side effects or problems in older people than it does in younger adults. However, quinidine may remain in the bodies of older adults longer than it does in younger adults, which may increase the risk of side effects and which may require lower doses.

Pregnancy—

	Pregnancy Category	Explanation
All Trimesters	C	Animal studies have shown an adverse effect and there are no adequate studies in pregnant women OR no animal studies have been conducted and there are no adequate studies in pregnant women.

Breast Feeding—There are no adequate studies in women for determining infant risk when using this medication during breastfeeding. Weigh the potential benefits against the potential risks before taking this medication while breastfeeding.

Other medicines—

Using this medicine with any of the following medicines is not recommended. Your doctor may decide not to treat you with this medication or change some of the other medicines you take.

Aurothioglucose, Bepridil, Cisapride, Grepafloxacin, Itraconazole, Levomethadyl, Mesoridazine, Nelfinavir, Pimozide, Ranolazine, Ritonavir, Saquinavir, Sparfloxacin, Terfenadine, Thioridazine, Tipranavir, Voriconazole, Ziprasidone

Interactions with Food/Tobacco/Alcohol—Certain medicines should not be used at or around the time of eating food or eating certain types of food since interactions may occur. Using alcohol or tobacco with certain medicines may also cause interactions to occur. The following interactions have been selected on the basis of their potential significance and are not necessarily all-inclusive.

Using this medicine with any of the following may cause an increased risk of certain side effects but may be unavoidable in some cases. If used together, your doctor may change the dose or how often you use this medicine, or give you special instructions about the use of food, alcohol, or tobacco.

Grapefruit Juice

Other medical problems—The presence of other medical problems may affect the use of this medicine. Make sure you tell your doctor if you have any other medical problems, especially:

- Electrolyte disorders—Quinidine may worsen heart rhythm problems
- Heart disease or
- Myasthenia gravis—Quinidine may make these conditions worse
- Kidney disease or
- Liver disease—Effects may be increased because of slower removal of quinidine from the body

Proper Use of This Medicine

Take this medicine exactly as directed. Do not take more of this medicine and do not take it more often than your doctor ordered. Do not miss any doses.

Taking quinidine with food may help lessen stomach upset.

For patients taking the extended-release tablet form of this medicine:

- Quinidex Extentabs or Biquin Durules—Swallow the tablets whole; do not break, crush, or chew before swallowing. Note that Biquin Durules may sometimes appear as a whole tablet in the stool; this tablet is just the empty shell that is left after the medicine has been absorbed into the body.
- Quinaglute Duratabs or Quin-Release—These tablets may be broken in half; however, they should not be crushed or chewed before swallowing.

Dosing—The dose of this medicine will be different for different patients. Follow your doctor's orders or the directions on the label. The following information includes only the average doses of this medicine. If your dose is different, do not change it unless your doctor tells you to do so.

The amount of medicine that you take depends on the strength of the medicine. Also, the number of doses you take each day, the time allowed between doses, and the length of time you take the medicine depend on the medical problem for which you are using the medicine.

- For regular (short-acting) oral dosage form (tablets):
  - For abnormal heart rhythm:
    - Adults—200 to 650 milligrams (mg) three or four times a day.
    - Children—30 to 40 mg per kilogram (kg) (13.6 to 18.2 mg per pound) of body weight per day. Your doctor may increase the dose if needed.
- For long-acting oral dosage form (tablets):
  - For abnormal heart rhythm:
    - Adults—300 to 660 mg every eight to twelve hours.
    - Children—30 to 40 mg per kilogram (kg) (13.6 to 18.2 mg per pound) of body weight per day. Your doctor may increase the dose if needed.
- For injection dosage form:
  - For abnormal heart rhythm:
    - Adults—190 to 380 mg injected into the muscle every two to four hours. Or, up to 0.25 mg per kg (0.11 mg per pound) of body weight per minute in a solution injected into a vein.
    - Children—Dose must be determined by your doctor.
  - For malaria:
    - Adults—10 mg per kg (4.54 mg per pound) of body weight in a solution injected slowly into a vein over one to two hours. Then, 0.02 mg per kg (0.009 mg per pound) of body weight per minute is given. Or, 24 mg per kg (10.91 mg per pound) of body weight in a solution injected slowly into a vein over a four-hour period. Then, eight hours after the first dose, 12 mg per kg (5.45 mg per pound) of body weight, injected slowly into a vein over a four-hour period, and repeated every eight hours.
    - Children—Dose must be determined by your doctor.

Missed dose—If you miss a dose of this medicine, take it as soon as possible. However, if it is almost time for your next dose, skip the missed dose and go back to your regular dosing schedule. Do not double doses.

Storage—Store the medicine in a closed container at room temperature, away from heat, moisture, and direct light. Keep from freezing.

Keep out of the reach of children.

Do not keep outdated medicine or medicine no longer needed.

Precautions While Using This Medicine

It is very important that your doctor check your progress at regular visits to make sure that the quinidine is working properly and does not cause unwanted effects.

Do not stop taking this medicine without first checking with your doctor, to avoid possible worsening of your condition.

Before having any kind of surgery (including dental surgery) or emergency treatment, tell the medical doctor or dentist in charge that you are taking this medicine.

Dizziness or lightheadedness may occur with this medicine, especially when you get up from a lying or sitting position. Getting up slowly may help.

Fainting may occur with this medicine. Do not drive or do anything else that could be dangerous if fainting occurs.

. Check with your doctor immediately if you faint or experience other side effects with this medicine.

Your doctor may want you to carry a medical identification card or bracelet stating that you are using this medicine.

Side Effects of This Medicine

Along with its needed effects, a medicine may cause some unwanted effects. Although not all of these side effects may occur, if they do occur they may need medical attention.

Check with your doctor immediately if any of the following side effects occur:

Less common

Abdominal pain and/or yellow eyes or skin; blurred and/or double vision, confusion, delirium, disturbed color perception, headache, noises or ringing in the ear, and/or visual intolerance of light; dizziness or lightheadedness; fainting; fever

Rare

Chest pain, fever, general discomfort, joint pain, joint swelling, muscle pain, and/or skin rash; nosebleeds or bleeding gums; unusual tiredness or weakness and/or pale skin

Some side effects may occur that usually do not need medical attention. These side effects may go away during treatment as your body adjusts to the medicine. Also, your health care professional may be able to tell you about ways to prevent or reduce some of these side effects. Check with your health care professional if any of the following side effects continue or are bothersome or if you have any questions about them:

More common

Diarrhea; loss of appetite; muscle weakness; nausea or vomiting

Other side effects not listed may also occur in some patients. If you notice any other effects, check with your healthcare professional.

QUININE   (Oral route) - KWYE-nine

Commonly used brand name(s)

In the U.S.—

Qualaquin
Quinamm
Quiphile

Available Dosage Forms:

- Capsule
- Tablet
- Tablet, Extended Release

Therapeutic Class: Musculoskeletal Agent

Uses For This Medicine

Quinine is used to treat malaria. This medicine usually is given with one or more other medicines for malaria.

Quinine may also be used for other problems as determined by your doctor. Do not confuse quinine with quinidine, a different medicine that is used for heart problems.

Quinine is available only with your doctor's prescription.

Once a medicine has been approved for marketing for a certain use, experience may show that it is also useful for other medical problems. Although these uses are not included in product labeling, quinine is used in certain patients with the following medical conditions:

- Babesiosis (infection caused by parasites)
- Nighttime leg cramps

Before Using This Medicine

In deciding to use a medicine, the risks of taking the medicine must be weighed against the good it will do. This is a decision you and your doctor will make. For this medicine, the following should be considered:

Allergies—Tell your doctor if you have ever had any unusual or allergic reaction to this medicine or any other medicines. Also tell your health care professional if you have any other types of allergies, such as to foods, dyes, preservatives, or animals. For non-prescription products, read the label or package ingredients carefully.

Pediatric—This medicine has been used to treat malaria in children and, in effective doses, has not been shown to cause different side effects or problems in children than it does in adults.

Geriatric—Many medicines have not been studied specifically in older people. Therefore, it may not be known whether they work exactly the same way they do in younger adults or if they cause different side effects or problems in older people. There is no specific information comparing use of quinine in the elderly with use in other age groups.

Pregnancy—

	Pregnancy Category	Explanation
All Trimesters	X	Studies in animals or pregnant women have demonstrated positive evidence of fetal abnormalities. This drug should not be used in women who are or may become pregnant because the risk clearly outweighs any possible benefit.

Breast Feeding—There are no adequate studies in women for determining infant risk when using this medication during breastfeeding. Weigh the potential benefits against the potential risks before taking this medication while breastfeeding.

Other medicines—

Using this medicine with any of the following medicines is not recommended. Your doctor may decide not to treat you with this medication or change some of the other medicines you take.

Astemizole, Aurothioglucose

Interactions   with   Food/Tobacco/Alcohol—Certain medicines should not be used at or around the time of eating food or eating certain types of food since interactions may occur. Using alcohol or tobacco with certain medicines may also cause interactions to occur. Discuss with your healthcare professional the use of your medicine with food, alcohol, or tobacco.

Other medical problems—The presence of other medical problems may affect the use of this medicine. Make sure you tell your doctor if you have any other medical problems, especially:

- Blackwater fever, history of, or
- Glucose-6–phosphate dehydrogenase (G6PD) deficiency or
- Purpura, or history of (purplish or brownish-red discoloration of skin)—Patients with a history of blackwater fever, G6PD deficiency, or purpura may have an increased risk of side effects affecting the blood
- Heart disease—Quinine can cause side effects affecting the heart, usually at higher doses
- Hypoglycemia—Quinine may cause low blood sugar
- Myasthenia gravis—Quinine may increase muscle weakness in patients with myasthenia gravis

Proper Use of This Medicine

Take this medicine only as directed. Do not take more of it, do not take it more often, and do not take it for a longer time than recommended on the label, unless otherwise directed by your doctor. To do so may increase the chance of side effects.

Take this medicine with or after meals to lessen possible stomach upset, unless otherwise directed by your doctor. If you are to take this medicine at bedtime, take it with a snack or with a glass of water, milk, or other beverage.

For patients taking quinine for malaria:

- To help clear up your infection completely, keep taking this medicine for the full time of treatment, even if you begin to feel better after a few days. If you stop taking this medicine too soon, your symptoms may return. Do not miss any doses.

Dosing—The dose of this medicine will be different for different patients. Follow your doctor's orders or the directions on the label. The following information includes only the average doses of this medicine. If your dose is different, do not change it unless your doctor tells you to do so.

The amount of medicine that you take depends on the strength of the medicine. Also, the number of doses you take each day, the time allowed between doses, and the length of time you take the medicine depend on the medical problem for which you are using the medicine.

- For treatment of malaria:
  - Adults and teenagers: 600 to 650 mg every eight hours for at least three days. This medicine must be taken with other medicine to treat malaria.
  - Children: Dose must be determined by the doctor.

Missed dose—If you miss a dose of this medicine, take it as soon as possible. However, if it is almost time for your next dose, skip the missed dose and go back to your regular dosing schedule. Do not double doses.

Storage—Store the medicine in a closed container at room temperature, away from heat, moisture, and direct light. Keep from freezing.

Keep out of the reach of children.

Do not keep outdated medicine or medicine no longer needed.

Precautions While Using This Medicine

Quinine may cause blurred vision or a change in color vision. Make sure you know how you react to this medicine before you drive, use machines, or do anything else that could be dangerous if you are not able to see well. If these reactions are especially bothersome, check with your doctor.

Side Effects of This Medicine

Along with its needed effects, a medicine may cause some unwanted effects. Although not all of these side effects may occur, if they do occur they may need medical attention.

Check with your doctor immediately if any of the following side effects occur:

More common
    Abdominal or stomach cramps or pain; diarrhea; nausea; vomiting

Less common
    Anxiety; behavior change, similar to drunkenness; black, tarry stools; blood in urine or stools; blurred vision; cold sweats; confusion; convulsions (seizures) or coma; cool pale skin; cough or hoarseness; difficulty in concentrating; drowsiness; excessive hunger; fast heartbeat; fever or chills; headache; lower back or side pain; nervousness; nightmares; painful or difficult urination; pinpoint red spots on skin; restless sleep; shakiness; slurred speech; sore throat; unusual bleeding or bruising; unusual tiredness or weakness

Rare
    Difficulty in breathing and/or swallowing; disturbed color perception; double vision; hives; increased sweating; muscle aches; night blindness; reddening of the skin, especially around ears; ringing or buzzing in ears; swelling of eyes, face, or inside of nose

Signs and symptoms of overdose
    Blindness; chest pain; dizziness; double vision; fainting; lightheadedness; rapid or irregular heartbeat; sleepiness

After you stop using this medicine, it may still produce some side effects that need attention. During this period of time, *check with your doctor immediately* if you notice the following side effects:
    Blurred vision or change in vision

Other side effects not listed may also occur in some patients. If you notice any other effects, check with your healthcare professional.

QUINUPRISTIN AND DALFOPRISTIN (Intravenous route) - kwi-NYOO-pris-tin, dal-FOE-pris-tin

Black Box Warning

One of dalfopristin/quinupristin's approved indications is for the treatment of patients with serious or life-threatening infections associated with vancomycin-resistant Enterococcus faecium (VREF) bacteremia. Dalfopristin/quinupristin has been approved for marketing in the United States for this indication under FDA's accelerated approval regulations that allow marketing of products for use in life-threatening conditions when other therapies are not available. Approval of drugs for marketing under these regulations is based upon a demonstrated effect on a surrogate endpoint that is likely to predict clinical benefit.

Approval of this indication is based upon dalfopristin/quinupristin's ability to clear VREF from the bloodstream, with clearance of bacteremia considered to be a surrogate endpoint. There are no results from well-controlled clinical studies that confirm the validity of this surrogate marker. However, a study to verify the clinical benefit of therapy with dalfopristin/quinupristin on traditional clinical endpoints (such as cure of the underlying infection) is presently underway.

Commonly used brand name(s)

In the U.S.—
   Synercid

Available Dosage Forms:
   • Powder for Solution

Therapeutic Class: Antibiotic

Uses For This Medicine

Quinupristin and dalfopristin belong to the family of medicine called antibiotics. Antibiotics are medicines used in the treatment of infections caused by bacteria. They work by killing bacteria or preventing their growth. Quinupristin and dalfopristin will not work for colds, flu, or other virus infections.

Quinupristin and dalfopristin injection is used to treat infection of the skin or the blood. It may also be used for other conditions as determined by your doctor. It is given by injection and is used mainly for serious infection for which other medicine may not work.

Quinupristin and dalfopristin injection is available only with your doctor's prescription.

Before Using This Medicine

In deciding to use a medicine, the risks of taking the medicine must be weighed against the good it will do. This is a decision you and your doctor will make. For this medicine, the following should be considered:

Allergies—Tell your doctor if you have ever had any unusual or allergic reaction to this medicine or any other medicines. Also tell your health care professional if you have any other types of allergies, such as to foods, dyes, preservatives, or animals. For non-prescription products, read the label or package ingredients carefully.

Pediatric—Studies on this medicine have been done only in adult patients, and there is no specific information comparing use of quinupristin and dalfopristin in children under 16 years old with use in other age groups.

Geriatric—In studies of patients 65 years or older, quinupristin and dalfopristin have not been shown to cause different side effects or problems than they do in younger adults.

Other medicines—

Using this medicine with any of the following medicines is not recommended. Your doctor may decide not to treat you with

this medication or change some of the other medicines you take.

Cisapride, Pimozide

Interactions with Food/Tobacco/Alcohol—Certain medicines should not be used at or around the time of eating food or eating certain types of food since interactions may occur. Using alcohol or tobacco with certain medicines may also cause interactions to occur. Discuss with your healthcare professional the use of your medicine with food, alcohol, or tobacco.

Other medical problems—The presence of other medical problems may affect the use of this medicine. Make sure you tell your doctor if you have any other medical problems, especially:
   • Liver disease—Liver disease may increase blood levels of this medicine, increasing the chance of side effects

Proper Use of This Medicine

Some medicine given by injection may sometimes be given at home to patients who do not need to be in the hospital. If you are using this medicine at home, make sure you clearly understand and carefully follow your doctor's instructions.

To help clear up your infection completely, this medicine must be given for the full time of treatment, even if you begin to feel better after a few days. Also, it works best when there is a constant amount in the blood. To help keep the amount constant, quinupristin and dalfopristin must be given on a regular schedule.

Dosing—The dose of this medicine will be different for different patients. Follow your doctor's orders or the directions on the label. The following information includes only the average doses of this medicine. If your dose is different, do not change it unless your doctor tells you to do so.

The amount of medicine that you take depends on the strength of the medicine. Also, the number of doses you take each day, the time allowed between doses, and the length of time you take the medicine depend on the medical problem for which you are using the medicine.

Side Effects of This Medicine

Along with its needed effects, a medicine may cause some unwanted effects. Although not all of these side effects may occur, if they do occur they may need medical attention.

Check with your doctor as soon as possible if any of the following side effects occur:
More common
   Swelling, redness, or pain at the injection area

Less common
   Joint pain; muscle pain; redness, burning sensation, or pain under the skin usually in the area of injection

Rare
   Chest pain; fast heartbeat; blood in urine; redness, burning sensation, or pain in vagina; severe bloody diarrhea; skin rash with red patches; hives

Other side effects not listed may also occur in some patients. If you notice any other effects, check with your healthcare professional.

RABEPRAZOLE (Oral route) - ra-BE-pray-zole

Commonly used brand name(s)

In the U.S.—
Aciphex

Available Dosage Forms:
- Tablet, Enteric Coated

Therapeutic Class: Antiulcer
Pharmacologic Class: Proton Pump Inhibitor

Uses For This Medicine

Rabeprazole is used to treat certain conditions in which there is too much acid in the stomach. It is used to treat duodenal ulcers and gastroesophageal reflux disease (GERD), a condition in which the acid in the stomach washes back up into the esophagus. Rabeprazole is also used to treat Zollinger-Ellison disease, a condition in which the stomach produces too much acid. Sometimes rabeprazole is used along with antibiotics to treat ulcers associated with infections caused by the *H. pylori* bacteria (germ).

Rabeprazole works by decreasing the amount of acid produced by the stomach.

This medicine is available only with your doctor's prescription.

Before Using This Medicine

In deciding to use a medicine, the risks of taking the medicine must be weighed against the good it will do. This is a decision you and your doctor will make. For this medicine, the following should be considered:

Allergies—Tell your doctor if you have ever had any unusual or allergic reaction to this medicine or any other medicines. Also tell your health care professional if you have any other types of allergies, such as to foods, dyes, preservatives, or animals. For non-prescription products, read the label or package ingredients carefully.

Pediatric—There is no specific information comparing the use of rabeprazole in children with use in other age groups.

Geriatric—In studies done to date that have included older adults, rabeprazole did not cause different side effects or problems than it did in younger adults.

Pregnancy—

	Pregnancy Category	Explanation
All Trimesters	B	Animal studies have revealed no evidence of harm to the fetus, however, there are no adequate studies in pregnant women OR animal studies have shown an adverse effect, but adequate studies in pregnant women have failed to demonstrate a risk to the fetus.

Breast Feeding—There are no adequate studies in women for determining infant risk when using this medication during breastfeeding. Weigh the potential benefits against the potential risks before taking this medication while breastfeeding.

Other medicines—
Using this medicine with any of the following medicines is usually not recommended, but may be required in some cases. If both medicines are prescribed together, your doctor may change the dose or how often you use one or both of the medicines.

Atazanavir

Interactions with Food/Tobacco/Alcohol—Certain medicines should not be used at or around the time of eating food or eating certain types of food since interactions may occur. Using alcohol or tobacco with certain medicines may also cause interactions to occur. Discuss with your healthcare professional the use of your medicine with food, alcohol, or tobacco.

Other medical problems—The presence of other medical problems may affect the use of this medicine. Make sure you tell your doctor if you have any other medical problems, especially:
- Liver disease—May increase chance of side effects
- Stomach infection—May make the condition worse

Proper Use of This Medicine

Swallow the tablet whole. Do not crush, chew, or split the tablet. Take this medicine for the full time of treatment, even if you begin to feel better. Also, keep your appointments with your doctor for check-ups so that your doctor will be better able to tell you when to stop taking this medicine.

Dosing—The dose of this medicine will be different for different patients. Follow your doctor's orders or the directions on the label. The following information includes only the average doses of this medicine. If your dose is different, do not change it unless your doctor tells you to do so.

The amount of medicine that you take depends on the strength of the medicine. Also, the number of doses you take each day, the time allowed between doses, and the length of time you take the medicine depend on the medical problem for which you are using the medicine.

- For oral dosage form (delayed-release tablet):
  - To treat gastroesophageal reflux disease (GERD):
    - Adults—20 mg once a day for 4 to 8 weeks.
    - Children up to 18 years of age—Use and dose must be determined by your doctor
  - To prevent gastroesophageal reflux disease (GERD):
    - Adults—20 mg once a day.
    - Children up to 18 years of age—Use and dose must be determined by your doctor
  - To treat duodenal ulcers:
    - Adults—20 mg once a day after the morning meal for up to 4 weeks.
    - Children up to 18 years of age—Use and dose must be determined by your doctor.
  - To treat duodenal ulcers related to infection with H. pylori:
    - Adults—20 mg twice a day, plus amoxicillin 1000 mg (1 gram) twice a day plus clarithromycin 500 mg twice a day, all taken together before the morning and evening meals for seven days.
    - Children up to 18 years of age—Use and dose must be determined by your doctor.

○ To treat conditions in which the stomach produces too much acid:
  ▪ Adults—At first, 60 mg once a day. Your doctor may increase your dose if needed.
  ▪ Children up to 18 years of age—Use and dose must be determined by your doctor.

Missed dose—If you miss a dose of this medicine, take it as soon as possible. However, if it is almost time for your next dose, skip the missed dose and go back to your regular dosing schedule. Do not double doses.

Storage—Store the medicine in a closed container at room temperature, away from heat, moisture, and direct light. Keep from freezing.

Keep out of the reach of children.

Do not keep outdated medicine or medicine no longer needed.

Ask your healthcare professional how you should dispose of any medicine you do not use.

Precautions While Using This Medicine

It is very important that your doctor check your progress at regular visits to make sure that this medicine is working properly and to check for unwanted effects. If your condition does not improve, or if it becomes worse, discuss this with your doctor.

Side Effects of This Medicine

Along with its needed effects, a medicine may cause some unwanted effects. Although not all of these side effects may occur, if they do occur they may need medical attention.

Check with your doctor as soon as possible if any of the following side effects occur:

Rare
Breathing interruptions; bloody urine; convulsions (seizures); chills, fever, or sore throat; continuing ulcers or sores in mouth; unusual bleeding or bruising; unusual tiredness or weakness; yellow eyes or skin

Incidence not known
Blistering, peeling, loosening of skin; change in consciousness; clay-colored stools; cloudy urine; confusion about identity, place, person, and time; continuing nausea or vomiting; cough; dark urine; difficult breathing; difficulty swallowing; fast heartbeat; greatly decreased frequency of urination or amount of urine; hallucinations; hives, itching, puffiness or swelling of the eyelids or around the eyes, face, lips or tongue; holding false beliefs that cannot be changed by fact; increase in frequency of seizures; itching; joint or muscle pain; large, hive-like swelling on face, eyelids, lips, tongue, throat, hands, legs, feet, sex organs; loss of appetite; loss of consciousness; muscle cramps or spasms; muscle pain or stiffness; no blood pressure; no breathing; no pulse; red, irritated eyes; red skin lesions, often with a purple center; shortness of breath; skin blisters; skin rash; sores, ulcers, or white spots in mouth or on lips; swelling of face; swelling of feet or lower legs; tightness in chest; tiredness and weakness; unusual excitement, nervousness or restlessness; wheezing

Some side effects may occur that usually do not need medical attention. These side effects may go away during treatment as your body adjusts to the medicine. Also, your health care professional may be able to tell you about ways to prevent or reduce some of these side effects. Check with your health care professional if any of the following side effects continue or are bothersome or if you have any questions about them:

More common
Headache

Less common or rare
Constipation; diarrhea; dizziness; feeling weak; gas; heartburn; itchy skin; nausea and vomiting; numbness, tingling, pain, or weakness in hands or feet; sleepiness; stomach pain

Other side effects not listed may also occur in some patients. If you notice any other effects, check with your healthcare professional.

RALOXIFENE (Oral route) - ral-OX-i-feen

Commonly used brand name(s)
In the U.S.—
  Evista

Available Dosage Forms:
  • Tablet

Therapeutic Class: Endocrine-Metabolic Agent
Pharmacologic Class: Selective Estrogen Receptor Modulator

Uses For This Medicine

Raloxifene is used to help prevent and treat thinning of the bones (osteoporosis) only in postmenopausal women.

It works like an estrogen to stop the bone loss that can develop in women after menopause, but it does not increase the bone density as much as daily 0.625 mg doses of conjugated estrogens. Raloxifene will not treat hot flashes of menopause and may cause hot flashes to occur. Also, raloxifene does not stimulate the breast or uterus as estrogen does.

Raloxifene lowers the blood concentrations of total and low-density lipoprotein (LDL) cholesterol, the bad cholesterols, but it does not increase concentrations of high-density lipoprotein (HDL) cholesterol, the good cholesterol, in your blood.

This medicine is available only with your doctor's prescription.

Before Using This Medicine

In deciding to use a medicine, the risks of taking the medicine must be weighed against the good it will do. This is a decision you and your doctor will make. For this medicine, the following should be considered:

Allergies—Tell your doctor if you have ever had any unusual or allergic reaction to this medicine or any other medicines. Also tell your health care professional if you have any other types of allergies, such as to foods, dyes, preservatives, or animals. For non-prescription products, read the label or package ingredients carefully.

Geriatric—This medicine has been tested only in women past menopause and has not been shown to cause different side effects or problems in elderly people than it does in adults who have just gone through menopause.

Pregnancy—

	Pregnancy Category	Explanation
All Trimesters	X	Studies in animals or pregnant women have demonstrated positive evidence of fetal abnormalities. This drug should not be used in women who are or may become pregnant because the risk clearly outweighs any possible benefit.

Breast Feeding—There are no adequate studies in women for determining infant risk when using this medication during breastfeeding. Weigh the potential benefits against the potential risks before taking this medication while breastfeeding.

Other medicines—Although certain medicines should not be used together at all, in other cases two different medicines may be used together even if an interaction might occur. In these cases, your doctor may want to change the dose, or other precautions may be necessary. Tell your healthcare professional if you are taking any other prescription or non-prescription (over-the-counter [OTC]) medicine.

Interactions with Food/Tobacco/Alcohol—Certain medicines should not be used at or around the time of eating food or eating certain types of food since interactions may occur. Using alcohol or tobacco with certain medicines may also cause interactions to occur. Discuss with your healthcare professional the use of your medicine with food, alcohol, or tobacco.

Other medical problems—The presence of other medical problems may affect the use of this medicine. Make sure you tell your doctor if you have any other medical problems, especially:
- Blood clot formation, active or history of, including deep vein thrombosis, pulmonary embolism, and retinal embolism—Raloxifene may slightly increase the chances of these conditions and, if they are already present, cause them to worsen
- Cancer or tumors or
- Congestive heart failure or
- Any other condition that increases the risk of blood clots—Taking raloxifene while having one of these conditions may worsen the chance that blood clots can form
- Liver disease—This condition may cause higher concentrations of raloxifene in the blood

---

Proper Use of This Medicine

A paper with information for the patient will be given to you with your filled prescription, and will provide many details concerning the use of raloxifene. Read this paper carefully and ask your health care professional if you need additional information or explanation.

Many patients trying to prevent or treat bone loss will not notice any signs of the problem. In fact, many may feel normal. It is very important that you take your medicine exactly as directed.

Dosing—The dose of this medicine will be different for different patients. Follow your doctor's orders or the directions on the label. The following information includes only the average doses of this medicine. If your dose is different, do not change it unless your doctor tells you to do so.

The amount of medicine that you take depends on the strength of the medicine. Also, the number of doses you take each day, the time allowed between doses, and the length of time you take the medicine depend on the medical problem for which you are using the medicine.
- For oral dosage form (tablets):
  - For preventing bone loss:
    - Adults—60 mg once a day, with or without meals.
  - For treating bone loss:
    - Adults—60 mg once a day, with or without meals.

Missed dose—If you miss a dose of this medicine, skip the missed dose and go back to your regular dosing schedule. Do not double doses.

Storage—Store the medicine in a closed container at room temperature, away from heat, moisture, and direct light. Keep from freezing.

Keep out of the reach of children.

Do not keep outdated medicine or medicine no longer needed.

Precautions While Using This Medicine

It is very important that you keep your appointments with your doctor even if you feel well.

Before you have any kind of surgery, tell the medical doctor in charge that you are using this medicine. Discuss discontinuing use of raloxifene 3 days before you think you will have a long period of inactivity, sitting, or bed rest, such as after having surgery or going on a long trip. The doctor may have you start the medicine again after you are back on your feet and fully mobile. If you are going on a trip and stay on raloxifene, you should walk regularly or move about when possible. Remaining still for long periods may cause blood clots for some people, and raloxifene may rarely worsen their condition.

If you are able to become pregnant, stop using the medicine immediately if you think you have become pregnant and check with your doctor. Raloxifene is recommended for women who are past menopause.

Raloxifene does not act like an estrogen to stimulate the uterus or breast. If you experience vaginal bleeding, breast pain or enlargement, or swelling of hands or feet while on raloxifene, you should report it to your doctor.

Other ways that may be used with raloxifene to help prevent or treat bone loss are taking calcium plus vitamin D supplements and getting weight-bearing exercise. You may want to discuss these options with your doctor.

Side Effects of This Medicine

Along with its needed effects, a medicine may cause some unwanted effects. Although not all of these side effects may occur, if they do occur they may need medical attention.

Stop taking this medicine and get emergency help immediately if any of the following effects occur:
Rare
> Coughing blood; headache or migraine headache; loss of or change in speech, coordination, or vision; pain or numbness in chest, arm, or leg; shortness of breath (unexplained)

Check with your doctor as soon as possible if any of the following side effects occur:

More common

Bloody or cloudy urine; chest pain; difficult, burning, or painful urination; fever; frequent urge to urinate; infection, including body aches or pain, congestion in throat, cough, dryness or soreness of throat, and loss of voice; runny nose; leg cramping; skin rash; swelling of hands, ankles, or feet; vaginal itching

Less common

Abdominal pain (severe); aching body pains; congestion in lungs; decreased vision or other changes in vision; diarrhea; difficulty in breathing; hoarseness; loss of appetite; nausea; trouble in swallowing; weakness

Some side effects may occur that usually do not need medical attention. These side effects may go away during treatment as your body adjusts to the medicine. Also, your health care professional may be able to tell you about ways to prevent or reduce some of these side effects. Check with your health care professional if any of the following side effects continue or are bothersome or if you have any questions about them:

More common

Hot flashes, including sudden sweating and feelings of warmth (especially common during the first 6 months of treatment); increased white vaginal discharge; joint or muscle pain; mental depression; problems of stomach or intestines, including passing of gas, upset stomach, or vomiting; swollen joints; trouble in sleeping; weight gain (unexplained)

Other side effects not listed may also occur in some patients. If you notice any other effects, check with your healthcare professional.

RALTITREXED   (Intravenous route) -
ral-ti-TREX-ed

Uses For This Medicine

Raltitrexed belongs to a group of medicines known as antimetabolites. It is used to treat cancer of the colon and rectum. It may also be used to treat other kinds of cancer, as determined by your doctor.

Raltitrexed blocks an enzyme needed by the cell to live. This interferes with the growth of cancer cells, which are eventually destroyed. Since the growth of normal body cells may also be affected by raltitrexed, other effects will also occur. Some of these may be serious and must be reported to your doctor. Other effects, like hair loss, may not be serious but may cause concern.

Before you begin treatment with raltitrexed, you and your doctor should talk about the good this medicine will do as well as the risks of using it.

Raltitrexed is to be administered only by or under the immediate supervision of your doctor.

Before Using This Medicine

In deciding to use a medicine, the risks of taking the medicine must be weighed against the good it will do. This is a decision you and your doctor will make. For this medicine, the following should be considered:

Allergies—Tell your doctor if you have ever had any unusual or allergic reaction to this medicine or any other medicines. Also tell your health care professional if you have any other types of allergies, such as to foods, dyes, preservatives, or animals. For non-prescription products, read the label or package ingredients carefully.

Pediatric—Studies on this medicine have been done only in adult patients, and there is no specific information comparing use of raltitrexed in children with use in other age groups.

Geriatric—Elderly people are especially sensitive to the effects of raltitrexed. Raltitrexed may be more likely to cause side effects such as cracked lips, diarrhea, difficulty in swallowing, sores, ulcers, or white spots on the lips, tongue, or inside the mouth in elderly patients.

Other medicines—

Using this medicine with any of the following medicines is not recommended. Your doctor may decide not to treat you with this medication or change some of the other medicines you take.

Rotavirus Vaccine, Live

Interactions with Food/Tobacco/Alcohol—Certain medicines should not be used at or around the time of eating food or eating certain types of food since interactions may occur. Using alcohol or tobacco with certain medicines may also cause interactions to occur. Discuss with your healthcare professional the use of your medicine with food, alcohol, or tobacco.

Other medical problems—The presence of other medical problems may affect the use of this medicine. Make sure you tell your doctor if you have any other medical problems, especially:

- Chickenpox (including recent exposure) or
- Herpes zoster (shingles)—Risk of severe disease affecting other parts of the body
- Infection—Raltitrexed can decrease your body's ability to fight infection
- Kidney disease or
- Liver disease—Effects of raltitrexed may be increased because of slower removal from the body; your doctor may need to change your dose

Proper Use of This Medicine

This medicine is sometimes given together with certain other medicines. If you are using a combination of medicines, it is important that you receive each one at the proper time. If you are taking some of these medicines by mouth, ask your health care professional to help you plan a way to take them at the right times.

This medicine usually causes nausea and vomiting that may be severe. However, it is very important that you continue to receive the medicine, even if you begin to feel ill. Ask your health care professional for ways to lessen these effects, especially if they are severe.

Dosing—The dose of this medicine will be different for different patients. Follow your doctor's orders or the directions on the label. The following information includes only the average doses of this medicine. If your dose is different, do not change it unless your doctor tells you to do so.

The amount of medicine that you take depends on the strength of the medicine. Also, the number of doses you take each day, the time allowed between doses, and the length of time you take the medicine depend on the medical problem for which you are using the medicine.

- For parenteral dosage form (injection):
  - For colorectal cancer
    - Adults—3 milligrams (mg) per square meter of body surface area given over a 15 minute period. The dose may be repeated every 3 weeks.
    - Children—Use and dose must be determined by your doctor.

Missed dose—Call your doctor or pharmacist for instructions.

Precautions While Using This Medicine

It is very important that your doctor check your progress at regular visits to make sure that this medicine is working properly and to check for unwanted effects.

This medicine may cause some people to feel unusually tired or ill. Make sure you know how you react to this medicine before you drive, use machines, or do anything else that could be dangerous if you are less alert.

While you are being treated with raltitrexed, and after you stop treatment with it, do not have any immunizations (vaccinations) without your doctor's approval. Raltitrexed may lower your body's resistance and there is a chance you might get the infection the immunization is meant to prevent. In addition, other persons living in your household should not take oral polio vaccine since there is a chance they could pass the polio virus on to you. Also, avoid persons who have taken oral polio vaccine within the last several months. Do not get close to them and do not stay in the same room with them for very long. If you cannot take these precautions, you should consider wearing a protective face mask that covers the nose and mouth.

Raltitrexed can temporarily lower the number of white blood cells in your blood, increasing the chance of getting an infection. It can also lower the number of platelets, which are necessary for proper blood clotting. If this occurs, there are certain precautions you can take, especially when your blood count is low, to reduce the risk of infection or bleeding:

- If you can, avoid people with infections. Check with your doctor immediately if you think you are getting an infection or if you get a fever or chills, cough or hoarseness, lower back or side pain, or painful or difficult urination.
- Check with your doctor immediately if you notice any unusual bleeding or bruising; black, tarry stools; blood in urine or stools; or pinpoint red spots on your skin.
- Be careful when using a regular toothbrush, dental floss, or toothpick. Your medical doctor, dentist, or nurse may recommend other ways to clean your teeth and gums. Check with your medical doctor before having any dental work done.
- Do not touch your eyes or the inside of your nose unless you have just washed your hands and have not touched anything else in the meantime.
- Be careful not to cut yourself when you are using sharp objects such as a safety razor or fingernail or toenail cutters.
- Avoid contact sports or other situations where bruising or injury could occur.

Side Effects of This Medicine

Along with its needed effects, a medicine may cause some unwanted effects. Although not all of these side effects may occur, if they do occur they may need medical attention.

Check with your doctor immediately if any of the following side effects occur:

More common
> Pale skin, troubled breathing, unusual bleeding or bruising, unusual tiredness or weakness; black, tarry stools, chest pain, chills, cough, fever, painful or difficult urination, shortness of breath, sore throat, sores, ulcers, or white spots on lips or in mouth, swollen glands; increase in bowel movements, loose stools, soft stools

Less common
> Dizziness, fainting, fast, slow, or irregular heartbeat, decreased urine output, dilated neck veins, extreme fatigue, irregular breathing, swelling of face, fingers, feet, or lower legs, tightness in chest, weight gain, wheezing

Some side effects may occur that usually do not need medical attention. These side effects may go away during treatment as your body adjusts to the medicine. Also, your health care professional may be able to tell you about ways to prevent or reduce some of these side effects. Check with your health care professional if any of the following side effects continue or are bothersome or if you have any questions about them:

More common
> Stomach or abdomen pain; loss of appetite, weight loss; constipation; nausea and vomiting; lack or loss of strength; general feeling of discomfort or illness, headache, joint pain, muscle aches and pains, runny nose, shivering, sweating, trouble sleeping; rash

Less common
> Bloating or swelling of face, arms, hands, lower legs, or feet, rapid weight gain, tingling of hands or feet

Some side effects may occur that usually do not need medical attention. These side effects may go away during treatment as your body adjusts to the medicine. Also, your health care professional may be able to tell you about ways to prevent or reduce some of these side effects. Check with your health care professional if any of the following side effects continue or are bothersome or if you have any questions about them:

More common
> Hair loss, thinning of hair

Less common
> Change in taste, bad unusual or unpleasant (after)taste

After you stop using this medicine, it may still produce some side effects that need attention. During this period of time, *check with your doctor immediately* if you notice the following side effects:

> Black, tarry stools, blood in urine or stools, cough or hoarseness, fever or chills, lower back or side pain, painful or difficult urination, pinpoint red spots on skin, unusual bleeding or bruising

Other side effects not listed may also occur in some patients. If you notice any other effects, check with your healthcare professional.

RAMELTEON   (Oral route) - ram-EL-tee-on

Commonly used brand name(s)

In the U.S.—
   Rozerem

Available Dosage Forms:
   • Tablet

Therapeutic Class: Nonbarbiturate Hypnotic
Pharmacologic Class: Melatonin Receptor Agonist

Uses For This Medicine

Ramelteon belongs to the group of medicines called central nervous system (CNS) depressants (medicines that slow down the nervous system). Ramelteon is used to treat insomnia (trouble in sleeping). Ramelteon helps you get to sleep faster and sleep through the night. In general, when sleep medicines are used every night for a long time, they may lose their effectiveness. In most cases, sleep medicines should be used only for short periods of time, such as 1 or 2 days, and generally for no longer than 1 or 2 weeks.

This medicine is available only with your doctor's prescription

Before Using This Medicine

In deciding to use a medicine, the risks of taking the medicine must be weighed against the good it will do. This is a decision you and your doctor will make. For this medicine, the following should be considered:

Allergies—Tell your doctor if you have ever had any unusual or allergic reaction to this medicine or any other medicines. Also tell your health care professional if you have any other types of allergies, such as to foods, dyes, preservatives, or animals. For non-prescription products, read the label or package ingredients carefully.

Pediatric—Studies on this medicine have been done only in adult patients, and there is no specific information comparing use of ramelteon in children with use in other age groups.

Geriatric—This medicine has been tested and has not been shown to cause different side effects or problems in older people than it does in younger adults.

Pregnancy—

	Pregnancy Category	Explanation
All Trimesters	C	Animal studies have shown an adverse effect and there are no adequate studies in pregnant women OR no animal studies have been conducted and there are no adequate studies in pregnant women.

Breast Feeding—There are no adequate studies in women for determining infant risk when using this medication during breastfeeding. Weigh the potential benefits against the potential risks before taking this medication while breastfeeding.

Other medicines—

Using this medicine with any of the following medicines is usually not recommended, but may be required in some cases. If both medicines are prescribed together, your doctor may change the dose or how often you use one or both of the medicines.

Fluvoxamine

Interactions with Food/Tobacco/Alcohol—Certain medicines should not be used at or around the time of eating food or eating certain types of food since interactions may occur. Using alcohol or tobacco with certain medicines may also cause interactions to occur. Discuss with your healthcare professional the use of your medicine with food, alcohol, or tobacco.

Other medical problems—The presence of other medical problems may affect the use of this medicine. Make sure you tell your doctor if you have any other medical problems, especially:

   • Emphysema, asthma, bronchitis, or other chronic lung disease or

   • Mental depression or

   • Sleep apnea (temporary stopping of breathing during sleep)—Ramelteon may make these conditions worse.

   • Liver disease—Higher blood levels of ramelteon may result, increasing the chance of side effects.

Proper Use of This Medicine

Take ramelteon just before going to bed, when you are ready to go to sleep. This medicine works very quickly to put you to sleep.

Take ramelteon on an empty stomach.

Dosing—The dose of this medicine will be different for different patients. Follow your doctor's orders or the directions on the label. The following information includes only the average doses of this medicine. If your dose is different, do not change it unless your doctor tells you to do so.

The amount of medicine that you take depends on the strength of the medicine. Also, the number of doses you take each day, the time allowed between doses, and the length of time you take the medicine depend on the medical problem for which you are using the medicine.

   • For oral dosage form (tablets):
     ○ For the treatment of insomnia (trouble in sleeping):
        ▪ Adults—8 milligrams (mg) at bedtime.
        ▪ Children—Use and dose must be determined by your doctor.

Missed dose—If you miss a dose of this medicine, skip the missed dose and go back to your regular dosing schedule. Do not double doses.

Storage—Keep out of the reach of children.

Store the medicine in a closed container at room temperature, away from heat, moisture, and direct light. Keep from freezing.

Do not keep outdated medicine or medicine no longer needed.

Precautions While Using This Medicine

Insomnia that lasts following a reasonable period of treatment may be a sign of another medical problem that should be evaluated. *Consult your doctor if new or worsening signs of insomnia occur.*

Avoid drinking alcohol while using this medicine. Ramelteon will add to the effects of alcohol.

If you develop any unusual and strange thoughts or behavior while you are taking ramelteon, be sure to discuss it with your doctor. Some changes that have occurred in people taking this medicine are like those seen in people who drink alcohol and then act in a manner that is not normal. Other changes may be more unusual and extreme, such as confusion, worsening of depression, hallucinations (seeing, hearing, or feeling things that are not there), suicidal thoughts, and unusual excitement, nervousness, or irritability.

This medicine may cause some people to become drowsy, dizzy, or less alert than they are normally. *Make sure you know how you react to this medicine before you drive, use machines, or do anything else that could be dangerous if you are dizzy or are not alert.*

If cessation of menstrual cycle (females), decreased libido, or problems with fertility occur, be sure to discuss it with your doctor.

Side Effects of This Medicine

Along with its needed effects, a medicine may cause some unwanted effects. Although not all of these side effects may occur, if they do occur they may need medical attention.

Some side effects may occur that usually do not need medical attention. These side effects may go away during treatment as your body adjusts to the medicine. Also, your health care professional may be able to tell you about ways to prevent or reduce some of these side effects. Check with your health care professional if any of the following side effects continue or are bothersome or if you have any questions about them:

More common
Dizziness; sleepiness or unusual drowsiness

Less common
Body aches or pain; change in taste; chills; cough; difficulty in breathing; difficulty in moving; discouragement; ear congestion; fatigue; feeling sad or empty; fever; general feeling of discomfort or illness; irritability; joint pain; loss of appetite; loss of interest or pleasure; loss of taste; loss of voice; muscle aching or cramping; muscle pain or stiffness; nasal congestion; nausea; pain in joints; runny nose; shivering; sleeplessness; sneezing; sore throat; sweating; swollen joints; trouble concentrating; trouble sleeping; unable to sleep; unusual tiredness or weakness; vomiting

Other side effects not listed may also occur in some patients. If you notice any other effects, check with your healthcare professional.

RASAGILINE (Oral route) - ra-SA-ji-leen

Commonly used brand name(s)

In the U.S.—
Azilect

Available Dosage Forms:
• Tablet

Therapeutic Class: Antiparkinsonian
Pharmacologic Class: Monoamine Oxidase Inhibitor, Type B

Uses For This Medicine

Rasagiline is used alone or with levodopa for the treatment of Parkinson's disease. Parkinson's disease is a condition of the brain that becomes worse over time and may cause movement problems, rigidity, tremors, and slowed physical movement.

This medicine is only available with your doctor's prescription.

Importance of Diet—If you take this medicine and consume tyramine-rich foods, beverages, or dietary supplements or amines (from over-the-counter medicines), you could experience a hypertensive crisis or "cheese reaction". A hypertensive crisis (increase in blood pressure) is very serious and requires immediate medical attention. It is very important that you restrict dietary tyramine by avoiding the following tyramine-rich foods and beverages:

• Aged cheese
• Air dried, aged and fermented meats, sausages and salamis (e.g., cacciatore, hard salami and mortadella)
• Animal livers that are spoiled or improperly stored
• Beers and tap beers, all varieties that have not been pasteurized so as to allow for ongoing fermentation
• Broad bean pods (e.g., fava bean pods)
• Meat, poultry, or fish that is spoiled or stored improperly (i.e., foods with changes in coloration, odor, or mold)
• OTC supplements containing tyramine
• Pickled herring
• Red wine
• Sauerkraut
• Soybean products including soy sauce and tofu
• Yeast extract, concentrated (e.g., Marmite)

Before Using This Medicine

In deciding to use a medicine, the risks of taking the medicine must be weighed against the good it will do. This is a decision you and your doctor will make. For this medicine, the following should be considered:

Allergies—Tell your doctor if you have ever had any unusual or allergic reaction to this medicine or any other medicines. Also tell your health care professional if you have any other types of allergies, such as to foods, dyes, preservatives, or animals. For non-prescription products, read the label or package ingredients carefully.

Pediatric—Appropriate studies have not been performed on the relationship of age to the effects of rasagiline in the pediatric population. Safety and efficacy have not been established.

Geriatric—Appropriate studies performed to date have not demonstrated geriatrics-specific problems that would limit the usefulness of rasagiline in the elderly.

Pregnancy—

	Pregnancy Category	Explanation
All Trimesters	C	Animal studies have shown an adverse effect and there are no adequate studies in pregnant women OR no animal studies have been conducted and there are no adequate studies in pregnant women.

Breast Feeding—Studies suggest that this medication may alter milk production or composition. If an alternative to this medication is not prescribed, you should monitor the infant for side effects and adequate milk intake.

Other medicines—

Using this medicine with any of the following medicines is not recommended. Your doctor may decide not to treat you with this medication or change some of the other medicines you take.

Amphetamine, Cyclobenzaprine, Dextromethorphan, Duloxetine, Ephedrine, Fluvoxamine, Meperidine, Methadone, Mirtazapine, Morphine, Morphine Sulfate Liposome, Phenelzine, Phenylephrine, Phenylpropanolamine, Propoxyphene, Pseudoephedrine, St John's Wort, Tramadol

Interactions with Food/Tobacco/Alcohol—Certain medicines should not be used at or around the time of eating food or eating certain types of food since interactions may occur. Using alcohol or tobacco with certain medicines may also cause interactions to occur. The following interactions have been selected on the basis of their potential significance and are not necessarily all-inclusive.

Using this medicine with any of the following is usually not recommended, but may be unavoidable in some cases. If used together, your doctor may change the dose or how often you use this medicine, or give you special instructions about the use of food, alcohol, or tobacco.

Tyramine Containing Food

Other medical problems—The presence of other medical problems may affect the use of this medicine. Make sure you tell your doctor if you have any other medical problems, especially:

- Mild liver problems—May cause an increased amount of rasagiline in your blood. Your doctor may lower your dose
- Moderate or severe liver problems—This medicine SHOULD NOT be used because it may cause an increased amount of rasagiline in your blood
- Pheochromocytoma (tumor on the adrenal gland)—This medicine SHOULD NOT be used.

Proper Use of This Medicine

The absorption of rasagiline is not affected by food, so this drug can be taken with or without food.

Dosing—The dose of this medicine will be different for different patients. Follow your doctor's orders or the directions on the label. The following information includes only the average doses of this medicine. If your dose is different, do not change it unless your doctor tells you to do so.

The amount of medicine that you take depends on the strength of the medicine. Also, the number of doses you take each day, the time allowed between doses, and the length of time you take the medicine depend on the medical problem for which you are using the medicine.

- For treatment of Parkinson's disease:
  - For oral dosage form (tablets):

  For rasagiline alone:
    - Adults—1 milligram (mg) once a day
    - Children—Use and dose must be determined by your doctor

  For rasagiline with levodopa:
    - Adults—At first, 0.5 mg once a day. Your doctor may increase your rasagiline dose to 1 mg once a day.
    - Children—Use and dose must be determined by your doctor.

Missed dose—If you miss a dose of this medicine, skip the missed dose and go back to your regular dosing schedule. Do not double doses.

Storage—Store the medicine in a closed container at room temperature, away from heat, moisture, and direct light. Keep from freezing.

Precautions While Using This Medicine

If you experience signs and symptoms of high blood pressure, you should seek immediate medical attention. Signs and symptoms include severe headache, blurred vision or visual disturbances, difficulty thinking, stupor or coma, seizures, chest pain, unexplained nausea or vomiting, or signs and symptoms of a stroke.

You should not use any of the following medicines while you are taking rasagiline, or for 2 weeks after stopping rasagiline:

- Analgesic agents (methadone [e.g., Methadose] propoxyphene [e.g., Darvon], tramadol [e.g., Ultram]) or
- Cold products containing ephedrine, phenylephrine, phenylpropanolamine, or pseudoephedrine or
- Cyclobenzaprine (e.g., Flexeril) or
- MAO inhibitors or
- Meperidine (e.g., Demerol) or
- Mirtazapine (e.g., Remeron)

You should tell your doctor before having any surgery that requires general anesthesia. Rasagiline should be discontinued at least 14 days before surgery.

Some studies have shown that patients with Parkinson's disease may have a higher risk of developing skin cancer. Therefore, it is very important that a dermatologist check you at regular visits for melanomas. You or your caregiver should also monitor for melanomas frequently and on a regular basis.

If you are taking this medicine with levodopa, you may experience increased dyskinesia (e.g., twitching, twisting, uncontrolled repetitive movements of tongue, lips, face, arms, or legs) and postural low blood pressure (e.g., chills, cold sweats, confusion, dizziness, faintness, or light-headedness when getting up from lying or sitting position).

Side Effects of This Medicine

Along with its needed effects, a medicine may cause some unwanted effects. Although not all of these side effects may occur, if they do occur they may need medical attention.

Check with your doctor immediately if any of the following side effects occur:

Less common
>Abdominal or stomach pain; arm, back, or jaw pain; black, tarry stools; chest pain or discomfort; chest tightness or heaviness; chills; cloudy urine; cough; diarrhea; difficulty swallowing; dizziness; fainting; fast or irregular heartbeat; fever; hives; itching; loss of appetite; nausea; painful or difficult urination; persistent, non-healing sore; pink growth on skin; puffiness or swelling of the eyelids or around the eyes; reddish patch or irritated area; redness, blistering, peeling, or loosening of the skin; seeing, hearing, or feeling things that are not there; shiny bump; shortness of breath; skin rash; sore throat; sores, ulcers, or white spots on lips or in mouth; sweating; swollen glands; tests that show problems with the liver; tightness in chest; unusual bleeding or bruising; unusual tiredness or weakness; weakness; wheezing; white, yellow or waxy scar-like area

Some side effects may occur that usually do not need medical attention. These side effects may go away during treatment as your body adjusts to the medicine. Also, your health care professional may be able to tell you about ways to prevent or reduce some of these side effects. Check with your health care professional if any of the following side effects continue or are bothersome or if you have any questions about them:

More common
>Acid or sour stomach; belching; difficulty in moving; headache; heartburn; indigestion; muscle pain or stiffness; pain in joints; stomach discomfort or upset

Less common
>Bruising; burning, crawling, itching, numbness, prickling, "pins and needles" or tingling feelings; burning, dry, or itching eyes; decreased interest in sexual intercourse; difficulty breathing; difficulty in moving; discouragement; excessive tearing; eye discharge; fall; feeling of constant movement of self or surroundings; feeling sad or empty; general feeling of discomfort or illness; hair loss; inability to have or keep an erection; irritability; joint pain; lack of appetite; large, flat, blue or purplish patches in the skin; light-headedness; loss in sexual ability, desire, drive, or performance; loss of interest or pleasure; muscle aches; neck pain; noisy breathing; redness, pain, swelling of eye, eyelid, or inner lining of eyelid; runny nose; sensation of spinning; shivering; sneezing; stuffy nose; swelling or redness in joints; thinning of hair; tiredness; trouble concentrating; trouble sleeping; vomiting; weight loss

Other side effects not listed may also occur in some patients. If you notice any other effects, check with your healthcare professional.

RASBURICASE (Intravenous route) -
ras-BYOOR-i-kayse

Black Box Warning

Rasburicase may cause severe hypersensitivity reactions including anaphylaxis. Rasburicase should be immediately and permanently discontinued in any patient developing clinical evidence of a serious hypersensitivity reaction.

Rasburicase administered to patients with glucose-6–phosphate dehydrogenase (G6PD) deficiency can cause severe hemolysis. Rasburicase administration should be immediately and permanently discontinued in any patient developing hemolysis. It is recommended that patients at higher risk for G6PD deficiency (eg, patients of African or Mediterranean ancestry) be screened prior to starting rasburicase therapy.

Rasburicase use has been associated with methemoglobinemia. Rasburicase administration should be immediately and permanently discontinued in any patient identified as having developed methemoglobinemia.

Rasburicase will cause enzymatic degradation of the uric acid within blood samples left at room temperature, resulting in spuriously low uric acid levels. To ensure accurate measurements, blood must be collected into pre-chilled tubes containing heparin anticoagulant and immediately immersed and maintained in an ice water bath; plasma samples must be assayed within 4 hours of sample collection.

Commonly used brand name(s)

In the U.S.—
>Elitek

Available Dosage Forms:
• Powder for Solution

Therapeutic Class: Endocrine-Metabolic Agent
Pharmacologic Class: Enzyme

Uses For This Medicine

Rasburicase helps your body remove the uric acid waste (hyperuricemia) from treatments for some types of cancer.

This medicine is available only with your doctor's prescription.

Before Using This Medicine

In deciding to use a medicine, the risks of taking the medicine must be weighed against the good it will do. This is a decision you and your doctor will make. For this medicine, the following should be considered:

Allergies—Tell your doctor if you have ever had any unusual or allergic reaction to this medicine or any other medicines. Also tell your health care professional if you have any other types of allergies, such as to foods, dyes, preservatives, or animals. For non-prescription products, read the label or package ingredients carefully.

Pediatric—This medicine has been tested in children (1 month to 17 years of age). Children less than 2 years of age may be at increased risk for adverse effects.

Geriatric—Many medicines have not been studied specifically in older people. Therefore, it may not be known whether they work the same way that they do in younger adults or if they cause different side effects or problems in older people. There is no specific information comparing the use of rasburicase in the elderly with use in other age groups.

Pregnancy—

	Pregnancy Category	Explanation
All Trimesters	C	Animal studies have shown an adverse effect and there are no adequate studies in pregnant women OR no animal studies have been conducted and there are no adequate studies in pregnant women.

Breast Feeding—There are no adequate studies in women for determining infant risk when using this medication during breastfeeding. Weigh the potential benefits against the potential risks before taking this medication while breastfeeding.

Other medicines—Although certain medicines should not be used together at all, in other cases two different medicines may be used together even if an interaction might occur. In these cases, your doctor may want to change the dose, or other precautions may be necessary. Tell your healthcare professional if you are taking any other prescription or nonprescription (over-the-counter [OTC]) medicine.

Interactions with Food/Tobacco/Alcohol—Certain medicines should not be used at or around the time of eating food or eating certain types of food since interactions may occur. Using alcohol or tobacco with certain medicines may also cause interactions to occur. Discuss with your healthcare professional the use of your medicine with food, alcohol, or tobacco.

Other medical problems—The presence of other medical problems may affect the use of this medicine. Make sure you tell your doctor if you have any other medical problems, especially:

- Anaphylaxis, hypersensitivity reaction, or a sudden, severe allergic reaction (or history of) or
- Glucose-6–phosphate dehydrogenase (G6PD) deficiency (a hereditary metabolic disorder affecting red blood cells) or
- Hemolytic reactions (or history of) or
- Methemoglobinemia reactions (or history of)—Rasburicase should not be used if you have or have had any of these medical problems
- Tumor lysis syndrome, risk of—Fluids may be injected into the vein.

Proper Use of This Medicine

You should take only one course of treatment (once a day for 5 days) of this medicine unless your doctor tells you differently. It is important that you follow your doctor's instructions to avoid a serious allergic reaction to rasburicase.

Dosing—The dose of this medicine will be different for different patients. Follow your doctor's orders or the directions on the label. The following information includes only the average doses of this medicine. If your dose is different, do not change it unless your doctor tells you to do so.

The amount of medicine that you take depends on the strength of the medicine. Also, the number of doses you take each day, the time allowed between doses, and the length of time you take the medicine depend on the medical problem for which you are using the medicine.

- For parenteral dosage form (injection):
  - For preventing or treating medical problems that may occur if certain treatments increase the amount of uric acid in the blood:
    - Adults—See the dose for children
    - Children—0.15 or 0.2 milligram (mg) per kilogram (kg) of body weight in a solution to be injected over 30 minutes into a vein as a single daily dose for five days. Chemotherapy should be initiated 4 to 24 hours after the first dose of rasburicase.

Storage—Store in the refrigerator. Do not freeze.

Keep out of the reach of children.

Do not keep outdated medicine or medicine no longer needed.

Ask your healthcare professional how you should dispose of any medicine you do not use.

Precautions While Using This Medicine

If your symptoms do not improve within a few days or if they become worse, check with your doctor. This is especially important for children under two years of age since they may have an increased level of side effects.

It is especially important to notify your healthcare professional immediately if you have any signs or symptoms of an allergic reaction, such as chest pain, dizziness, hives, skin rash, or trouble breathing.

Patients of African or Mediterranean ancestry are at higher risk of serious side effects and should be carefully evaluated by their healthcare professional before starting this medicine.

It is very important to use this medicine properly. The medicine must be given over time, and not administered all at once. There is a very specific 5 day treatment regimen that must be followed, and chemotherapy must be started 4 to 24 hours after the first dose of rasburicase.

Side Effects of This Medicine

Along with its needed effects, a medicine may cause some unwanted effects. Although not all of these side effects may occur, if they do occur they may need medical attention.

Check with your doctor immediately if any of the following side effects occur:

More common
    Cracked lips; diarrhea; difficulty in swallowing; sores, ulcers, or white spots on lips, tongue, or inside mouth

Less common
    Abdominal pain; agitation; black or red, tarry, stools; bleeding gums; bluish color of fingernails, lips, skin, palms, or nail beds; changes in skin color; changes in vision; coma; confusion; convulsions (seizures); chest pain or discomfort; chills; cough; coughing that sometimes produces a pink, frothy sputum; coughing up blood; decreased urination; depression; dilated neck veins; dizziness; dry mouth; fainting; fast, slow, or irregular heartbeat; fatigue; fever; headache; hostility; increased menstrual flow or vaginal bleeding; increased sweating; increased thirst; irritability; itching, pain, redness, swelling, tenderness or warmth on skin; light-

headedness; lower back or side pain; muscle twitching; nausea; no blood pressure or pulse; nosebleeds; pain or discomfort in arms, jaw, back or neck; pain, tenderness, swelling of foot or leg; painful or difficult urination; pains in chest, groin, or legs, especially calves of legs; pale skin; paralysis; prolonged bleeding from cuts; red or dark brown urine; severe constipation; severe headaches of sudden onset; shortness of breath; skin rash; sneezing; sore throat; stopping of heart; stupor; sudden onset of shortness of breath for no apparent reason; sudden loss of coordination; sudden onset of slurred speech; sunken eyes; sweating; swelling of face, fingers, feet, or lower legs; swollen glands; temporary blindness; thirst; tightness in chest; troubled breathing; unconsciousness; unexplained or unusual bleeding or bruising; unusual tiredness or weakness; vomiting; weight gain; wheezing; wrinkled skin

Rare
Back pain; hives; itching, puffiness or swelling of the eyelids or around the eyes, face, lips or tongue; yellow eyes or skin.

Some side effects may occur that usually do not need medical attention. These side effects may go away during treatment as your body adjusts to the medicine. Also, your health care professional may be able to tell you about ways to prevent or reduce some of these side effects. Check with your health care professional if any of the following side effects continue or are bothersome or if you have any questions about them:

More common
Difficulty having a bowel movement

Less common
Burning, crawling, itching, numbness, prickling, "pins and needles", or tingling feelings; feeling of warmth; feeling unusually cold; redness of the face, neck, arms and occasionally, upper chest; shivering

Other side effects not listed may also occur in some patients. If you notice any other effects, check with your healthcare professional.

REPAGLINIDE (Oral route) - re-pa-GLI-nide

Commonly used brand name(s)
In the U.S.—
Prandin

Available Dosage Forms:
• Tablet

Therapeutic Class: Hypoglycemic

Uses For This Medicine

Repaglinide is used to treat type 2 diabetes. When you have type 2 diabetes, insulin is still being produced by your pancreas. Sometimes the amount of insulin you produce may not be enough or your body may not be using it properly and you may still need more. Repaglinide works by causing your pancreas to release more insulin into the blood stream. Repag-

linide may be used alone or with another oral diabetes medicine called metformin.

This medicine is available only with your doctor's prescription.

Before Using This Medicine

In deciding to use a medicine, the risks of taking the medicine must be weighed against the good it will do. This is a decision you and your doctor will make. For this medicine, the following should be considered:

Allergies—Tell your doctor if you have ever had any unusual or allergic reaction to this medicine or any other medicines. Also tell your health care professional if you have any other types of allergies, such as to foods, dyes, preservatives, or animals. For non-prescription products, read the label or package ingredients carefully.

Pediatric—Studies on this medicine have been done only in adult patients, and there is no specific information comparing use of repaglinide in children with use in other age groups.

Geriatric—This medicine has been tested in a limited number of patients 65 years of age or older and has not been shown to cause different side effects or problems in older people than it does in younger adults. However, the first signs of low blood sugar are not easily seen or do not occur at all in older patients. This may increase the chance of low blood sugar developing during treatment.

Pregnancy—

	Pregnancy Category	Explanation
All Trimesters	C	Animal studies have shown an adverse effect and there are no adequate studies in pregnant women OR no animal studies have been conducted and there are no adequate studies in pregnant women.

Breast Feeding—There are no adequate studies in women for determining infant risk when using this medication during breastfeeding. Weigh the potential benefits against the potential risks before taking this medication while breastfeeding.

Other medicines—
Using this medicine with any of the following medicines is not recommended. Your doctor may decide not to treat you with this medication or change some of the other medicines you take.

Gemfibrozil

Interactions with Food/Tobacco/Alcohol—Certain medicines should not be used at or around the time of eating food or eating certain types of food since interactions may occur. Using alcohol or tobacco with certain medicines may also cause interactions to occur. Discuss with your healthcare professional the use of your medicine with food, alcohol, or tobacco.

Other medical problems—The presence of other medical problems may affect the use of this medicine. Make sure you tell your doctor if you have any other medical problems, especially:
• Infection or
• Ketones in the blood (diabetic ketoacidosis) or

- Surgery or
- Trauma or
- Type 1 (insulin-dependent) diabetes or
- Unusual stress—Insulin may be needed to control diabetes in patients with these conditions
- Kidney disease or
- Liver disease—Higher blood levels of repaglinide may occur; this may change the amount of medicine you need
- Underactive adrenal gland or
- Underactive pituitary gland or
- Undernourished condition or
- Weakened physical condition—Patients with these conditions may be more likely to develop low blood sugar while taking repaglinide

Proper Use of This Medicine

Follow carefully the special meal plan your doctor gave you. This is the most important part of controlling your condition, and is necessary if the medicine is to work properly. Also, exercise regularly and test for sugar in your blood or urine as directed.

This medicine usually is taken 15 minutes before a meal but may be taken up to 30 minutes before a meal.

Dosing—The dose of this medicine will be different for different patients. Follow your doctor's orders or the directions on the label. The following information includes only the average doses of this medicine. If your dose is different, do not change it unless your doctor tells you to do so.

The amount of medicine that you take depends on the strength of the medicine. Also, the number of doses you take each day, the time allowed between doses, and the length of time you take the medicine depend on the medical problem for which you are using the medicine.

- For oral dosage form (tablets):
  - For type 2 diabetes:
    - Adults:
      — For patients who have never taken medicine to lower their blood sugar or who have a glycosylated hemoglobin (hemoglobin A 1c) measurement that is less than 8%: At first the dose is 0.5 milligram (mg) fifteen to thirty minutes before each meal. The dose may then be adjusted by your doctor based on your fasting blood sugar level.
      — For patients who have taken medicine to lower their blood sugar and who have a hemoglobin A 1c measurement that is higher than 8%: At first the dose is 1 or 2 mg fifteen to thirty minutes before each meal. The dose may then be adjusted by your doctor based on your fasting blood sugar level.
    - Children: Use and dose must be determined by your doctor.

Missed dose—Call your doctor or pharmacist for instructions.

You should skip a dose of repaglinide if a meal is skipped and add a dose of repaglinide if you eat an extra meal.

Storage—Store the medicine in a closed container at room temperature, away from heat, moisture, and direct light. Keep from freezing.

Keep out of the reach of children.

Do not keep outdated medicine or medicine no longer needed.

Precautions While Using This Medicine

Your doctor will want to check your progress at regular visits, especially during the first few weeks you take this medicine.

It is very important to follow carefully any instructions from your health care team about:

- Alcohol—Drinking alcohol may cause severe low blood sugar. Discuss this with your health care team.
- Other medicines—Do not take other medicines during the time you are taking repaglinide unless they have been discussed with your doctor. This especially includes nonprescription medicines such as aspirin, and medicines for appetite control, asthma, colds, cough, hay fever, or sinus problems.
- Counseling—Other family members need to learn how to prevent side effects or help with side effects if they occur. Also, patients with diabetes may need special counseling about diabetes medicine dosing changes that might occur because of lifestyle changes, such as changes in exercise and diet. Furthermore, counseling on contraception and pregnancy may be needed because of the problems that can occur in patients with diabetes during pregnancy.
- Travel—Keep a recent prescription and your medical history with you. Be prepared for an emergency as you would normally. Make allowances for changing time zones and keep your meal times as close as possible to your usual meal times.

In case of emergency—There may be a time when you need emergency help for a problem caused by your diabetes. You need to be prepared for these emergencies. It is a good idea to wear a medical identification (ID) bracelet or neck chain at all times. Also, carry an ID card in your wallet or purse that says that you have diabetes and a list of all of your medicines.

Too much repaglinide can cause low blood sugar (hypoglycemia). Low blood sugar also can occur if you use repaglinide with another antidiabetic medicine, delay or miss a meal or snack, exercise more than usual, drink alcohol, or cannot eat because of nausea or vomiting. Symptoms of low blood sugar must be treated before they lead to unconsciousness (passing out). Different people may feel different symptoms of low blood sugar. It is important that you learn which symptoms of low blood sugar you usually have so that you can treat it quickly.

Symptoms of low blood sugar include anxiety; behavior change similar to being drunk; blurred vision; cold sweats; confusion; cool, pale skin; difficulty in thinking; drowsiness; excessive hunger; fast heartbeat; headache (continuing); nausea; nervousness; nightmares; restless sleep; shakiness; slurred speech; or unusual tiredness or weakness.

If symptoms of low blood sugar occur, eat glucose tablets or gel, corn syrup, honey, or sugar cubes; or drink fruit juice, nondiet soft drink, or sugar dissolved in water to relieve the symptoms. Also, check your blood for low blood sugar. Get to a doctor or a hospital right away if the symptoms do not improve. Someone should call for emergency help immediately if severe symptoms such as convulsions (seizures) or unconsciousness occur. Food or drink should not be forced because the patient could choke from not swallowing correctly.

Hyperglycemia (high blood sugar) may occur if you do not take enough or skip a dose of your antidiabetic medicine, overeat or do not follow your meal plan, have a fever or infection, or do not exercise as much as usual.

Symptoms of high blood sugar include blurred vision; drowsiness; dry mouth; flushed, dry skin; fruit-like breath odor; increased urination; ketones in urine; loss of appetite; stomachache, nausea, or vomiting; tiredness; troubled breathing (rapid and deep); unconsciousness; or unusual thirst.

If symptoms of high blood sugar occur, check your blood sugar level and then call your doctor for instructions.

Side Effects of This Medicine

Along with its needed effects, a medicine may cause some unwanted effects. Although not all of these side effects may occur, if they do occur they may need medical attention.

Check with your doctor immediately if any of the following side effects occur:

> *More common*
> Convulsions (seizures); unconsciousness

Check with your doctor as soon as possible if any of the following side effects occur:

> *More common*
> Cough; fever; low blood sugar, including anxious feeling, behavior change similar to being drunk, blurred vision, cold sweats, confusion, cool pale skin, difficulty in thinking, drowsiness, excessive hunger, fast heartbeat, headache, nausea, nervousness, nightmares, restless sleep, shakiness, slurred speech, or unusual tiredness or weakness; pain in the chest; runny or stuffy nose; shortness of breath; sinus congestion with pain; sneezing; sore throat

> *Less common*
> Bloody or cloudy urine; burning, painful, or difficult urination; chest pain; chills; frequent urge to urinate; problems with teeth; skin rash, itching, or hives; tearing of eyes; tightness in chest; trouble in breathing; vomiting; wheezing

> *Rare*
> Black, tarry stools; blood in stools; fast or irregular heartbeat; hoarseness; lower back or side pain; pinpoint red spots on skin; unusual bleeding or bruising

Some side effects may occur that usually do not need medical attention. These side effects may go away during treatment as your body adjusts to the medicine. Also, your health care professional may be able to tell you about ways to prevent or reduce some of these side effects. Check with your health care professional if any of the following side effects continue or are bothersome or if you have any questions about them:

> *More common*
> Back pain; diarrhea; joint pain

> *Less common*
> Constipation; feeling of burning, numbness, tightness, tingling, warmth, or heat; indigestion

Other side effects not listed may also occur in some patients. If you notice any other effects, check with your healthcare professional.

RESPIRATORY SYNCYTIAL VIRUS IMMUNE GLOBULIN, HUMAN
(Intravenous route) - RES-pi-ra-tor-ee sin-SISH-al VYE-rus im-MYOON GLOB-yoo-lin, HYOO-man

Commonly used brand name(s)
In the U.S.—
> Respigam

Available Dosage Forms:
- Solution

Therapeutic Class: Immune Serum

Uses For This Medicine

Respiratory syncytial virus immune globulin intravenous (RSV-IGIV) belongs to a group of medicines known as immunizing agents. RSV-IGIV is used to prevent infection caused by respiratory syncytial virus (RSV). RSV-IGIV works by giving your body the antibodies it needs to protect it against RSV infection.

RSV infection can cause serious problems, such as pneumonia and bronchitis, which affect the lungs; and in severe cases, even death. These problems are more likely to occur in infants and young children less than 6 months of age with chronic lung disease, those born with heart problems, and those with a history of premature birth.

Onset of RSV activity usually occurs in November and continues through April or early May, with peak activity occurring from late January through mid-February. A good way to help prevent RSV infection is to get RSV-IGIV before the start of the RSV season.

RSV-IGIV is used to prevent serious lower respiratory tract infection caused by the respiratory syncytial virus (RSV) in children less than 24 months of age with breathing problems or a history of premature birth.

RSV-IGIV is to be administered only by or under the supervision of your doctor or other health care professional.

Before Using This Medicine

In deciding to use a medicine, the risks of taking the medicine must be weighed against the good it will do. This is a decision you and your doctor will make. For this medicine, the following should be considered:

Allergies—Tell your doctor if you have ever had any unusual or allergic reaction to this medicine or any other medicines. Also tell your health care professional if you have any other types of allergies, such as to foods, dyes, preservatives, or animals. For non-prescription products, read the label or package ingredients carefully.

Pediatric—Children 24 months of age and older: Use is not recommended. Use is not recommended in children born with chronic heart disease. Also, too much fluid in the body is more likely to occur in infants and children with underlying lung disease.

Geriatric—RSV-IGIV has been tested only in infants and young children less than 24 months of age and there is no specific information about its use in older patients.

Pregnancy—

	Pregnancy Category	Explanation
All Trimesters	C	Animal studies have shown an adverse effect and there are no adequate studies in pregnant women OR no animal studies have been conducted and there are no adequate studies in pregnant women.

Breast Feeding—Studies in women suggest that this medication poses minimal risk to the infant when used during breastfeeding.

Other medicines—Although certain medicines should not be used together at all, in other cases two different medicines may be used together even if an interaction might occur. In these cases, your doctor may want to change the dose, or other precautions may be necessary. Tell your healthcare professional if you are taking any other prescription or non-prescription (over-the-counter [OTC]) medicine.

Interactions with Food/Tobacco/Alcohol—Certain medicines should not be used at or around the time of eating food or eating certain types of food since interactions may occur. Using alcohol or tobacco with certain medicines may also cause interactions to occur. Discuss with your healthcare professional the use of your medicine with food, alcohol, or tobacco.

Other medical problems—The presence of other medical problems may affect the use of this medicine. Make sure you tell your doctor if you have any other medical problems, especially:

- Allergic reaction to human immunoglobulins or
- Immunoglobulin A (IgA) deficiencies—RSV-IGIV may cause severe reactions

Proper Use of This Medicine

Make certain your health care professional knows if you are on any special diet, such as low-sodium or low-sugar diet.

Dosing—The dose of this medicine will be different for different patients. Follow your doctor's orders or the directions on the label. The following information includes only the average doses of this medicine. If your dose is different, do not change it unless your doctor tells you to do so.

The amount of medicine that you take depends on the strength of the medicine. Also, the number of doses you take each day, the time allowed between doses, and the length of time you take the medicine depend on the medical problem for which you are using the medicine.

- For injection dosage form:
  - For preventing respiratory syncytial virus (RSV) infection:
    - Adults and children 24 months of age and older— Use is not recommended.
    - Infants and children younger than 24 months of age—750 milligrams (mg) per kilogram (kg)

(340.9 mg per pound) of body weight injected into a vein once a month for five months.

Side Effects of This Medicine

Along with its needed effects, a medicine may cause some unwanted effects. Although not all of these side effects may occur, if they do occur they may need medical attention.

Check with your doctor immediately if any of the following side effects occur:

Rare

Difficulty in breathing and swallowing; hives; itching, especially of feet and hands; reddening of skin, especially around ears; swelling of eyes, face, or inside of nose; unusual tiredness or weakness, sudden and severe; fever of 39.2 °C (102.6 °F) or higher; increased heart rate; vomiting

Other side effects not listed may also occur in some patients. If you notice any other effects, check with your healthcare professional.

RIBAVIRIN (Inhalation, oral/ nebulization route, Oral route) - rye-ba-VYE-rin

Black Box Warning

- INHALATION
  - Use of aerosolized ribavirin in patients requiring mechanical ventilator assistance should be undertaken only by physicians and support staff familiar with the specific ventilator being used and this mode of administration of the drug. Strict attention must be paid to procedures that have been shown to minimize the accumulation of drug precipitate, which can result in mechanical ventilator dysfunction and associated increased pulmonary pressures.
  - Sudden deterioration of respiratory function has been associated with initiation of aerosolized ribavirin use in infants. Respiratory function should be carefully monitored during treatment. If initiation of aerosolized ribavirin treatment appears to produce sudden deterioration of respiratory function, treatment should be stopped and reinstituted only with extreme caution, continuous monitoring and consideration of concomitant administration of bronchodilators.
  - Ribavirin is not indicated for use in adults. Physicians and patients should be aware that ribavirin has been shown to produce testicular lesions in rodents and to be teratogenic in all animal species in which adequate studies have been conducted (rodents and rabbits).
- ORAL
  - Ribavirin monotherapy is not effective for the treatment of chronic hepatitis C virus infection and should not be used alone for this indication.
  - The primary clinical toxicity of ribavirin is hemolytic anemia. The anemia associated with ribavirin therapy may result in worsening of cardiac disease that led to fatal and nonfatal myocardial infarctions. Patients

with a history of significant or unstable cardiac disease should not be treated with ribavirin.

○ Significant teratogenic and/or embryocidal effects have been demonstrated in all animal species exposed to ribavirin. In addition, ribavirin has multiple-dose half-life of 12 days, and so it may persist in non-plasma compartments for as long as 6 months. Therefore, ribavirin therapy is contraindicated in women who are pregnant and in male partners of women who are pregnant. Extreme care must be taken to avoid pregnancy during therapy and for 6 months after completion of treatment in both female patients and in female partners of male patients who are taking ribavirin therapy. At least two reliable forms of effective contraception must be utilized during treatment and during the 6–month posttreatment follow-up period.

Commonly used brand name(s)

In the U.S.—

Copegus	Ribasphere
Rebetol	RibaTab
RibaPak	Virazole

Available Dosage Forms:

- Tablet
- Capsule
- Powder for Solution
- Solution

Therapeutic Class: Antiviral

Pharmacologic Class: Viral RNA Polymerase Inhibitor

Uses For This Medicine

Ribavirin is used to treat severe virus pneumonia in infants and young children. It is given by oral inhalation (breathing in the medicine as a fine mist through the mouth), using a special nebulizer (sprayer) attached to an oxygen hood or tent or face mask.

Ribavirin taken by mouth (oral) treats a viral liver infection known as hepatitis C. It can be used in patients who have hepatitis C and also have human immunodeficiency virus (HIV) infection. It is used in combination with injectable interferon alfa-2b or with injectable peginterferon alfa-2b. Ribavirin is used to treat virus infections. Interferons are substances naturally produced by cells in the body to help fight infections and tumors. Interferon alfa-2b and peginterferon alfa-2b are synthetic (man-made) versions of these substances. Interferon alfa-2b and peginterferon alfa-2b are used to treat a variety of tumors and viruses including the hepatitis C virus.

Once a medicine has been approved for marketing for a certain use, experience may show that it is also useful for other medical problems. Although these uses are not included in product labeling, ribavirin is used in certain patients with the following medical conditions:

- Influenza A and B (given by aerosol inhalation)
- Lassa fever (either given orally or by injection)

For patients taking this medicine by mouth or injection for Lassa fever:

- Check with your doctor immediately if any of the following side effects occur:

More common

○ Unusual tiredness and weakness

- Other side effects may occur that usually do not need medical attention. The following side effects may go away during treatment as your body adjusts to the medicine. However, check with your doctor if

any of the following side effects continue or are bothersome:

Less common

○ Headache; loss of appetite; nausea; trouble in sleeping; unusual tiredness or weakness

This medicine may also be used for other virus infections as determined by your doctor. However, it will not work for certain viruses, such as the common cold.

Before Using This Medicine

In deciding to use a medicine, the risks of taking the medicine must be weighed against the good it will do. This is a decision you and your doctor will make. For this medicine, the following should be considered:

Allergies—Tell your doctor if you have ever had any unusual or allergic reaction to this medicine or any other medicines. Also tell your health care professional if you have any other types of allergies, such as to foods, dyes, preservatives, or animals. For non-prescription products, read the label or package ingredients carefully.

Pediatric—Children may be sensitive to the effects of ribavirin. This may increase the chance of side effects or other problems during treatment. Be sure you have discussed the risks and benefits of this with your doctor.

Geriatric—Many medicines have not been studied specifically in older people. Therefore it may not be known if they work the same way that they do in younger adults or if they cause different side effects or problems in older people than they do in younger adults.

Pregnancy—

	Pregnancy Category	Explanation
All Trimesters	X	Studies in animals or pregnant women have demonstrated positive evidence of fetal abnormalities. This drug should not be used in women who are or may become pregnant because the risk clearly outweighs any possible benefit.

Breast Feeding—There are no adequate studies in women for determining infant risk when using this medication during breastfeeding. Weigh the potential benefits against the potential risks before taking this medication while breastfeeding.

Other medicines—

Using this medicine with any of the following medicines is usually not recommended, but may be required in some cases. If both medicines are prescribed together, your doctor may change the dose or how often you use one or both of the medicines.

Abacavir, Didanosine, Lamivudine, Stavudine, Zalcitabine, Zidovudine

Interactions with Food/Tobacco/Alcohol—Certain medicines should not be used at or around the time of eating food or eating certain types of food since interactions may occur. Using alcohol or tobacco with certain medicines may also cause interactions to occur. Discuss with your healthcare professional the use of your medicine with food, alcohol, or tobacco.

Other medical problems—The presence of other medical problems may affect the use of this medicine. Make sure you tell your doctor if you have any other medical problems, especially:

- Anemia (blood disorder) or
- Autoimmune hepatitis (liver inflammation)—Ribavirin could make these conditions worse and lead to very serious side effects.
- Heart disease—Patients with heart disease or a history of heart disease should not use ribavirin oral dosage forms because serious side effects can occur.
- Blood conditions such as
- Sickle cell anemia (red blood cell disorder) or
- Thalassemia major (genetic blood disorder)—Ribavirin should not be used in patients with these conditions.
- Hepatic decompensation—Ribavirin medicine should not be used in patients with this condition.
- Mental depression—Ribavirin should be used carefully in patients with this condition, especially adolescents as serious side effects can occur.
- Pancreatitis (inflammation of the pancreas)—Ribavirin should suspended in patients with symptoms of this condition and stopped in patients who have this condition.

Proper Use of This Medicine

To help clear up your infection completely, ribavirin must be given for the full time of treatment, even if you or your child begins to feel better after a few days. Also, ribavirin for inhalation works best when there is a constant amount in the lungs. To help keep the amount constant, ribavirin must be given on a regular or continuous schedule.

It is important that you read the patient information that comes with this medicine. Ask your doctor if you have any questions.

A negative pregnancy test is needed in women who are of childbearing age before starting treatment with oral ribavirin. Two forms of birth control must be used during oral ribavirin treatment and for six months after treatment ends.

Dosing—The dose of this medicine will be different for different patients. Follow your doctor's orders or the directions on the label. The following information includes only the average doses of this medicine. If your dose is different, do not change it unless your doctor tells you to do so.

The amount of medicine that you take depends on the strength of the medicine. Also, the number of doses you take each day, the time allowed between doses, and the length of time you take the medicine depend on the medical problem for which you are using the medicine.

- For the inhalation dosage form:
  - For treatment of respiratory syncytial virus (RSV) infection:
    - Adults and teenagers—Dose has not been determined since this medicine is not usually prescribed for teenagers or adults.
    - Infants and children—Dose must be determined by your doctor.
- For the oral dosage form:
  - For the treatment of hepatitis C virus infection:
  - For oral dosage forms (capsules):
    - Adults and children—Dose must be determined by your doctor

- For oral dosage form (oral solution):
  - Adults and teenagers—Dose must be determined by your doctor. The oral solution form of this medicine is not usually prescribed for teenagers or adults
  - Children—Dose must be determined by your doctor.
- For oral dosage form (tablets):
  - Adults—Dose must be determined by your doctor.
  - Children—Use and dose must be determined by your doctor. The tablet form of this medicine is not usually prescribed for children
  - For the treatment of hepatitis C virus infection with HIV infection:
    — Adults—Dose must be determined by your doctor.
    — Children—Use and dose must be determined by your doctor. The tablet form of this medicine is not usually prescribed for children.

Precautions While Using This Medicine

It is very important that your doctor check your progress at regular visits. This will allow your doctor to see if the medicine is working properly.

This medicine may cause some people to become dizzy, drowsy, or less alert than they are normally. Make sure you know how you react to this medicine before you drive, operate machinery or do anything else that could be dangerous if you are not alert.

It is very important that you stop this medicine and contact your doctor immediately if you think you might be pregnant.

Side Effects of This Medicine

Along with its needed effects, a medicine may cause some unwanted effects. Although not all of these side effects may occur, if they do occur they may need medical attention.

Check with your doctor as soon as possible if any of the following side effects occur:

More common

Black, tarry stools; bleeding gums; blood in urine or stools; chest pain; cough or hoarseness; difficult or labored breathing; fevers or chills; lower back or side pain; painful or difficult urination; pale skin; pinpoint red spots on skin; shortness of breath; sores, ulcers, or white spots in mouth; tightness in chest; troubled breathing with exertion; unusual bleeding or bruising; unusual tiredness or weakness; wheezing

Along with its needed effects, a medicine may cause some unwanted effects. Although not all of these side effects may occur, if they do occur they may need medical attention.

Some side effects may occur that usually do not need medical attention. These side effects may go away during treatment as your body adjusts to the medicine. Also, your health care professional may be able to tell you about ways to prevent or reduce some of these side effects. Check with your health care professional if any of the following side effects continue or are bothersome or if you have any questions about them:

More common

Acid or sour stomach; belching; discouragement; dizziness; feeling sad or empty; feeling unusually cold;

heartburn; indigestion; irritability; itching skin; lack of appetite; loss of interest or pleasure; lack or loss of strength; shivering; stomach discomfort, upset, or pain; tiredness; trouble concentrating; trouble sleeping

Less common

Change in taste; cough; crying; depersonalization; difficulty in moving; dysphoria; euphoria; fatigue; fever; gastrointestinal effects; headache; insomnia; joint pain; mental depression; muscle aching or cramping; muscle pains or stiffness; nervousness; pain or tenderness around eyes and cheekbones; paranoia; quick to react or overreact emotionally; rapidly changing moods; rash; shortness of breath; stuffy or runny nose; swollen joints; vomiting

Rare

Itching, redness, or swelling of eyes; skin rash or irritation

Other side effects not listed may also occur in some patients. If you notice any other effects, check with your healthcare professional.

RIBAVIRIN AND INTERFERON ALFA-2B (Oral route, Injection route) -
rye-ba-VYE-rin, in-ter-FEER-on AL-fa-2b

Commonly used brand name(s)

In the U.S.—
Rebetron

Available Dosage Forms:

- Solution
- Capsule
- Tablet

Uses For This Medicine

Ribavirin and interferon alfa-2b combination is used to treat a viral liver infection known as hepatitis C infection. Ribavirin is taken by mouth and interferon alfa-2b is administered beneath the skin (subcutaneously). Ribavirin is used to treat virus infections. Interferons are substances naturally produced by cells in the body to help fight infections and tumors. Interferon alfa-2b is a synthetic (man-made) version of these substances. Interferon alfa-2b is used to treat a variety of tumors and viruses including the hepatitis C virus.

Ribavirin is available for oral administration. Interferon alfa-2b is available only as an injectable form.

Before Using This Medicine

In deciding to use a medicine, the risks of taking the medicine must be weighed against the good it will do. This is a decision you and your doctor will make. For this medicine, the following should be considered:

Allergies—Tell your doctor if you have ever had any unusual or allergic reaction to this medicine or any other medicines. Also tell your health care professional if you have any other types of allergies, such as to foods, dyes, preservatives, or animals. For non-prescription products, read the label or package ingredients carefully.

Pediatric—Studies on this combination medicine have been done only in adult patients and there is no specific information comparing use of ribavirin and recombinant interferon alfa-2b combination in children younger than 18 years of age with use in other age group.

Geriatric—Many medicines have not been studied specifically in older people. Therefore, it may not be known whether they work exactly the same way they do in younger adults or if they cause different side effects or problems in older people. There is no specific information comparing use of ribavirin and interferon alfa-2b combination medicine in the elderly with use in other age group.

Other medicines—

Using this medicine with any of the following medicines is usually not recommended, but may be required in some cases. If both medicines are prescribed together, your doctor may change the dose or how often you use one or both of the medicines.

Abacavir, Didanosine, Lamivudine, Stavudine, Zalcitabine, Zidovudine

Interactions with Food/Tobacco/Alcohol—Certain medicines should not be used at or around the time of eating food or eating certain types of food since interactions may occur. Using alcohol or tobacco with certain medicines may also cause interactions to occur. Discuss with your healthcare professional the use of your medicine with food, alcohol, or tobacco.

Other medical problems—The presence of other medical problems may affect the use of this medicine. Make sure you tell your doctor if you have any other medical problems, especially:

- Anemia, severe or
- Autoimmune hepatitis or
- Bleeding disorders—May worsen with ribavirin and/or recombinant interferon alfa-2b
- Diabetes (increased sugar in blood)—May increase the risk of developing eye problems
- Heart disease—May worsen with ribavirin and/or recombinant interferon alfa-2b
- Hepatitis B or human immunodeficiency virus infection or
- Hepatitis C which has worsened or
- Hepatitis C which did not get better when treated with interferon alone—Safety and effectiveness in these conditions are unknown.
- High blood pressure—May increase the risk of developing eye problems
- Kidney problems—May worsen with ribavirin and/or recombinant interferon alfa-2b
- Liver or other organ transplant—Safety and effectiveness in these conditions are unknown.
- Lung problems—May worsen with ribavirin and/or recombinant interferon alfa-2b
- Mental problems (or history of)—May result in depression, aggressive, violent and suicidal behavior
- Problem with immune system or
- Psoriasis (inflammatory skin problem) or
- Thyroid problem—May worsen with ribavirin and/or recombinant interferon alfa-2b

- Virus infections, other—Use of ribavirin alone is not recommended.

Proper Use of This Medicine

If you are injecting interferon alfa-2b yourself, use it exactly as directed by your doctor. Do not use more or less of it, and do not use it more often than your doctor ordered. The exact amount of medicine you need has been carefully worked out. Using too much will increase the risk of side effects, while using too little may not improve your condition.

Interferon alfa-2b often cause unusual tiredness. This effect is less likely to cause problems if you inject this medicine at bedtime. Also, your doctor may want you to drink extra fluids, especially during the early phase of treatment.

Dosing—The dose of this medicine will be different for different patients. Follow your doctor's orders or the directions on the label. The following information includes only the average doses of this medicine. If your dose is different, do not change it unless your doctor tells you to do so.

The amount of medicine that you take depends on the strength of the medicine. Also, the number of doses you take each day, the time allowed between doses, and the length of time you take the medicine depend on the medical problem for which you are using the medicine.

Missed dose—Call your doctor or pharmacist for instructions.

Storage—Store in the refrigerator. Do not freeze.

Keep out of the reach of children.

Do not keep outdated medicine or medicine no longer needed.

Ask your healthcare professional how you should dispose of any medicine you do not use.

Precautions While Using This Medicine

It is very important that your doctor check your progress at regular visits to make sure that this medicine is working properly and to check for unwanted effects.

This medicine may cause some people to become unusually tired or dizzy, or less alert than they are normally. Make sure you know how you react to this medicine before you drive, use machines, or do anything else that could be dangerous if you are dizzy or if you are not alert.

This medicine may make you feel very sad, depressed or very angry. Call your doctor if you feel you cannot cope or you feel like you want to hurt yourself or someone else.

Interferon alfa-2b commonly causes a flu-like reaction, with aching muscles, fever and chills, and headache. To prevent problems from your temperature going too high, your doctor may ask you to take medicine for pain and fever such as acetaminophen (e.g., Anacin 3, Tylenol) before each dose of interferon alfa-2b. You may also need to take it after a dose to bring your temperature down. Follow your doctor's instructions carefully about taking your temperature, and how much and when to take the medicine such as acetaminophen.

Women of childbearing potential should use two reliable forms of effective contraception.

Alpha interferon can lower the number of white blood cells in your blood temporarily, increasing the chance of getting an infection. It can also lower the number of platelets, which are necessary for proper blood clotting. If this occurs, there are certain precautions you can take, especially when your blood count is low, to reduce the risk of infection or bleeding:

- If you can, avoid being close to people with infections. Check with your doctor immediately if you think you are getting an infection or if you get a fever or chills, cough or hoarseness, lower back or side pain, or have painful or difficult urination.
- Check with your doctor immediately if you notice any unusual bleeding or bruising; black, tarry stools; blood in urine or stools; or pinpoint red spots on your skin.
- Be careful when using a regular toothbrush, dental floss, or toothpick. Your medical doctor, dentist, or nurse may recommend other ways to clean your teeth and gums. Check with your medical doctor before having any dental work done
- Do not touch your eyes or the inside of your nose unless you have just washed your hands and have not touched anything else in the meantime.
- Be careful not to cut yourself when you are using sharp objects such as a safety razor or fingernail or toenail cutters.
- Avoid contact sports or other situations where bruising or injury could occur.

Side Effects of This Medicine

Along with its needed effects, a medicine may cause some unwanted effects. Although not all of these side effects may occur, if they do occur they may need medical attention.

Check with your doctor as soon as possible if any of the following side effects occur:

More common
> Chest pain; mood changes; trouble breathing; unusual tiredness or weakness

Rare
> Thoughts of suicide, attempts at suicide, changes in behavior

Some side effects may occur that usually do not need medical attention. These side effects may go away during treatment as your body adjusts to the medicine. Also, your health care professional may be able to tell you about ways to prevent or reduce some of these side effects. Check with your health care professional if any of the following side effects continue or are bothersome or if you have any questions about them:

More common
> Dizziness; fatigue; fever; headache; impaired concentration; impaired taste; influenza-like symptoms such as unusual tiredness or weakness; irritability; red itchy skin; large swing in moods; loss of appetite; muscle or joint pain; nausea, vomiting, or upset stomach; nervousness; redness and warm feeling at the site of injection; shaking; temporary thinning of hair; stuffy nose; trouble sleeping

Other side effects not listed may also occur in some patients. If you notice any other effects, check with your healthcare professional.

RIBOFLAVIN   (Oral route) - RYE-boe-flay-vin

Commonly used brand name(s)

In the U.S.—
  Ribo-100
  Ribo-2

Available Dosage Forms:

  • Tablet

  • Capsule

  • Tablet, Enteric Coated

Therapeutic Class: Nutritive Agent
Pharmacologic Class: Vitamin B

Uses For This Dietary Supplement

Vitamins are compounds that you must have for growth and health. They are needed in small amounts only and are usually available in the foods that you eat. Riboflavin (vitamin B_2) is needed to help break down carbohydrates, proteins, and fats. It also makes it possible for oxygen to be used by your body.

Lack of riboflavin may lead to itching and burning eyes, sensitivity of eyes to light, sore tongue, itching and peeling skin on the nose and scrotum, and sores in the mouth. Your doctor may treat this condition by prescribing riboflavin for you.

Some conditions may increase your need for riboflavin. These include:

  • Alcoholism

  • Burns

  • Cancer

  • Diarrhea (continuing)

  • Fever (continuing)

  • Illness (continuing)

  • Infection

  • Intestinal diseases

  • Liver disease

  • Overactive thyroid

  • Serious injury

  • Stress (continuing)

  • Surgical removal of stomach

In addition, riboflavin may be given to infants with high blood levels of bilirubin (hyperbilirubinemia).

Increased need for riboflavin should be determined by your health care professional.

Claims that riboflavin is effective for treatment of acne, some kinds of anemia (weak blood), migraine headaches, and muscle cramps have not been proven.

Oral forms of riboflavin are available without a prescription.

Importance of Diet—For good health, it is important that you eat a balanced and varied diet. Follow carefully any diet program your health care professional may recommend. For your specific dietary vitamin and/or mineral needs, ask your health care professional for a list of appropriate foods. If you think that you are not getting enough vitamins and/or minerals in your diet, you may choose to take a dietary supplement.

Riboflavin is found in various foods, including milk and dairy products, fish, meats, green leafy vegetables, and whole grain and enriched cereals and bread. It is best to eat fresh fruits and vegetables whenever possible since they contain the most vitamins. Food processing may destroy some of the vitamins, although little riboflavin is lost from foods during ordinary cooking.

Vitamins alone will not take the place of a good diet and will not provide energy. Your body also needs other substances found in food such as protein, minerals, carbohydrates, and fat. Vitamins themselves often cannot work without the presence of other foods.

The daily amount of riboflavin needed is defined in several different ways.

  For U.S.—
    • Recommended Dietary Allowances (RDAs) are the amount of vitamins and minerals needed to provide for adequate nutrition in most healthy persons. RDAs for a given nutrient may vary depending on a person's age, sex, and physical condition (e.g., pregnancy).

    • Daily Values (DVs) are used on food and dietary supplement labels to indicate the percent of the recommended daily amount of each nutrient that a serving provides. DV replaces the previous designation of United States Recommended Daily Allowances (USRDAs).

  For Canada—
    • Recommended Nutrient Intakes (RNIs) are used to determine the amounts of vitamins, minerals, and protein needed to provide adequate nutrition and lessen the risk of chronic disease.

Normal daily recommended intakes for riboflavin are generally defined as follows:

Persons	U.S. (mg)	Canada (mg)
Infants and children		
Birth to 3 years of age	0.4–0.8	0.3–0.7
4 to 6 years of age	1.1	0.9
7 to 10 years of age	1.2	1–1.3
Adolescent and adult males	1.4–1.8	1–1.6
Adolescent and adult females	1.2–1.3	1–1.1
Pregnant females	1.6	1.1–1.4
Breast-feeding females	1.7–1.8	1.4–1.5

Before Using This Dietary Supplement

If you are taking this dietary supplement without a prescription, carefully read and follow any precautions on the label. For this supplement, the following should be considered:

Allergies—Tell your doctor if you have ever had any unusual or allergic reaction to this medicine or any other medicines. Also tell your health care professional if you have any other types of allergies, such as to foods, dyes, preservatives, or animals. For non-prescription products, read the label or package ingredients carefully.

Pediatric—Problems in children have not been reported with intake of normal daily recommended amounts.

Geriatric—Problems in older adults have not been reported with intake of normal daily recommended amounts.

Breast Feeding—There are no adequate studies in women for determining infant risk when using this medication during

breastfeeding. Weigh the potential benefits against the potential risks before taking this medication while breastfeeding.

Other medicines—Although certain medicines should not be used together at all, in other cases two different medicines may be used together even if an interaction might occur. In these cases, your doctor may want to change the dose, or other precautions may be necessary. Tell your healthcare professional if you are taking any other prescription or non-prescription (over-the-counter [OTC]) medicine.

Interactions with Food/Tobacco/Alcohol—Certain medicines should not be used at or around the time of eating food or eating certain types of food since interactions may occur. Using alcohol or tobacco with certain medicines may also cause interactions to occur. Discuss with your healthcare professional the use of your medicine with food, alcohol, or tobacco.

Proper Use of This Dietary Supplement

Dosing—The dose of this medicine will be different for different patients. Follow your doctor's orders or the directions on the label. The following information includes only the average doses of this medicine. If your dose is different, do not change it unless your doctor tells you to do so.

The amount of medicine that you take depends on the strength of the medicine. Also, the number of doses you take each day, the time allowed between doses, and the length of time you take the medicine depend on the medical problem for which you are using the medicine.

- For oral dosage form (tablets):
  - To prevent deficiency, the amount taken by mouth is based on normal daily recommended intakes:

  For the U.S.
  - Adults and teenage males—1.4 to 1.8 milligrams (mg) per day.
  - Adults and teenage females—1.2 to 1.3 mg per day.
  - Pregnant females—1.6 mg per day.
  - Breast-feeding females—1.7 to 1.8 mg per day.
  - Children 7 to 10 years of age—1.2 mg per day.
  - Children 4 to 6 years of age—1.1 mg per day.
  - Children birth to 3 years of age—0.4 to 0.8 mg per day.

  For Canada
  - Adults and teenage males—1 to 1.6 mg per day.
  - Adults and teenage females—1 to 1.1 mg per day.
  - Pregnant females—1.1 to 1.4 mg per day.
  - Breast-feeding females—1.4 to 1.5 mg per day.
  - Children 7 to 10 years of age—1 to 1.3 mg per day.
  - Children 4 to 6 years of age—0.9 mg per day.
  - Children birth to 3 years of age—0.3 to 0.7 mg per day.

  - To treat deficiency:
    - Adults and teenagers—Treatment dose is determined by prescriber for each individual based on the severity of deficiency.

Missed dose—If you miss a dose of this medicine, skip the missed dose and go back to your regular dosing schedule. Do not double doses.

Storage—Store the dietary supplement in a closed container at room temperature, away from heat, moisture, and direct light. Keep from freezing.

Keep out of the reach of children.

Do not keep outdated medicine or medicine no longer needed.

Side Effects of This Dietary Supplement

Along with its needed effects, a dietary supplement may cause some unwanted effects. Riboflavin may cause urine to have a more yellow color than normal, especially if large doses are taken. This is to be expected and is no cause for alarm. Usually, however, riboflavin does not cause any side effects. Check with your health care professional if you notice any other unusual effects while you are using it.

RIFABUTIN (Oral route) - rif-a-BYOO-tin

Commonly used brand name(s)
In the U.S.—
  Mycobutin

Available Dosage Forms:
  - Capsule

Therapeutic Class: Antitubercular

Uses For This Medicine

Rifabutin is used to help prevent Mycobacterium avium complex (MAC) disease from causing disease throughout the body in patients with advanced human immunodeficiency virus (HIV) infection. MAC is an infection caused by two similar bacteria, Mycobacterium avium and Mycobacterium intracellulare. Mycobacterium avium is more common in patients with HIV infection. MAC also may occur in other patients whose immune system is not working properly. Symptoms of MAC in people with acquired immunodeficiency syndrome (AIDS) include fever, night sweats, chills, weight loss, and weakness. Rifabutin will not work for colds, flu, or most other infections.

Rifabutin is available only with your doctor's prescription.

Once a medicine has been approved for marketing for a certain use, experience may show that it is also useful for other medical problems. Although these uses are not included in product labeling, rifabutin is used in certain patients with the following medical condition:
  - Treatment of tuberculosis in patients with human immunodeficiency virus (HIV) infection

Before Using This Medicine

In deciding to use a medicine, the risks of taking the medicine must be weighed against the good it will do. This is a decision you and your doctor will make. For this medicine, the following should be considered:

Allergies—Tell your doctor if you have ever had any unusual or allergic reaction to this medicine or any other medicines. Also tell your health care professional if you have any other types of allergies, such as to foods, dyes, preservatives, or animals. For non-prescription products, read the label or package ingredients carefully.

Pediatric—Studies on this medicine have only been done in adult patients, and there is no specific information comparing use of rifabutin in children with use in other age groups. However, studies are being done to determine the best dose for children.

Geriatric—Many medicines have not been studied specifically in older people. Therefore, it may not be known whether they work exactly the same way they do in younger adults. Although there is no specific information comparing use of rifabutin in the elderly with use in other age groups, this medicine is not expected to cause different side effects or problems in older people than it does in younger adults.

Pregnancy—

	Pregnancy Category	Explanation
All Trimesters	B	Animal studies have revealed no evidence of harm to the fetus, however, there are no adequate studies in pregnant women OR animal studies have shown an adverse effect, but adequate studies in pregnant women have failed to demonstrate a risk to the fetus.

Breast Feeding—There are no adequate studies in women for determining infant risk when using this medication during breastfeeding. Weigh the potential benefits against the potential risks before taking this medication while breastfeeding.

Other medicines—Using this medicine with any of the following medicines is not recommended. Your doctor may decide not to treat you with this medication or change some of the other medicines you take.

Voriconazole

Interactions with Food/Tobacco/Alcohol—Certain medicines should not be used at or around the time of eating food or eating certain types of food since interactions may occur. Using alcohol or tobacco with certain medicines may also cause interactions to occur. Discuss with your healthcare professional the use of your medicine with food, alcohol, or tobacco.

Other medical problems—The presence of other medical problems may affect the use of this medicine. Make sure you tell your doctor if you have any other medical problems, especially:

- Kidney disease, mild to severe

Proper Use of This Medicine

Rifabutin may be taken on an empty stomach (either 1 hour before or 2 hours after a meal). However, if this medicine upsets your stomach, you may want to take it with food.

For patients unable to swallow capsules:

- The contents of the capsules may be mixed with applesauce. Be sure to take all the food to get the full dose of medicine.

To help prevent MAC disease, it is very important that you keep taking this medicine for the full time of treatment. You may have to take it every day for many months. It is important that you do not miss any doses.

Dosing—The dose of this medicine will be different for different patients. Follow your doctor's orders or the directions on the label. The following information includes only the average doses of this medicine. If your dose is different, do not change it unless your doctor tells you to do so.

The amount of medicine that you take depends on the strength of the medicine. Also, the number of doses you take each day, the time allowed between doses, and the length of time you take the medicine depend on the medical problem for which you are using the medicine.

- For oral dosage forms (capsules):
  - For the prevention of Mycobacterium avium complex (MAC):
    - Adults and teenagers—300 milligrams (mg) once a day, or 150 mg two times a day.
    - Children—Use and dose must be determined by your doctor.

Missed dose—If you miss a dose of this medicine, take it as soon as possible. However, if it is almost time for your next dose, skip the missed dose and go back to your regular dosing schedule. Do not double doses.

If this medicine is taken on an irregular schedule, side effects may occur more often and may be more serious than usual. If you have any questions about this, check with your health care professional.

Storage—Store the medicine in a closed container at room temperature, away from heat, moisture, and direct light. Keep from freezing.

Keep out of the reach of children.

Do not keep outdated medicine or medicine no longer needed.

Precautions While Using This Medicine

It is very important that your doctor check your progress at regular visits.

Rifabutin will cause your urine, stool, saliva, skin, sputum, sweat, and tears to turn reddish-orange to reddish-brown. This is to be expected while you are taking this medicine. This effect may cause soft contact lenses to become permanently discolored. Standard cleaning solutions may not take out all the discoloration. Therefore, it is best not to wear soft contact lenses while taking this medicine. Hard contact lenses are not discolored by rifabutin. If you have any questions about this, check with your doctor.

Be careful when using a regular toothbrush, dental floss, or toothpick. Your medical doctor, dentist, or nurse may recommend other ways to clean your teeth and gums. Check with your medical doctor before having any dental work done.

Side Effects of This Medicine

Along with its needed effects, a medicine may cause some unwanted effects. Although not all of these side effects may occur, if they do occur they may need medical attention.

Check with your doctor immediately if any of the following side effects occur:
More common
Diarrhea; fever; heartburn; indigestion; loss of appetite; nausea; skin itching and/or rash; sore throat; sour stomach; vomiting
Less common
Loss of strength or energy; muscle pain
Rare
Black, tarry, stools; bruising or purple spots on skin; change in taste; chills; cough; eye pain; joint pain; loss of vision; lower back or side pain; muscle inflammation

or pain; pale skin; painful or difficult urination; shortness of breath; ulcers, sores, or white spots in mouth; unusual bleeding or bruising; unusual tiredness or weakness; yellow skin

Some side effects may occur that usually do not need medical attention. These side effects may go away during treatment as your body adjusts to the medicine. Also, your health care professional may be able to tell you about ways to prevent or reduce some of these side effects. Check with your health care professional if any of the following side effects continue or are bothersome or if you have any questions about them:

More common

Abdominal pain; bad, unusual, or unpleasant (after) taste in mouth; belching; bloated, full feeling; change in taste; chest pain; excess air or gas in stomach or intestines; headache; passing gas; rash; trouble in sleeping

This medicine commonly causes reddish-orange to reddish-brown discoloration of urine, stools, saliva, skin, sputum, sweat, and tears. This side effect usually does not need medical attention. However, tears that have been discolored by this medicine may also discolor soft contact lenses (see Precautions While Using This Medicine).

Other side effects not listed may also occur in some patients. If you notice any other effects, check with your healthcare professional.

RIFAMPIN (Oral route, Intravenous route) - RIF-am-pin

Commonly used brand name(s)
In the U.S.—
  Rifadin
  Rifadin IV
  Rimactane

Available Dosage Forms:
  • Capsule
  • Tablet
  • Powder for Solution
  • Syrup

Therapeutic Class: Antitubercular

Uses For This Medicine

Rifampin is used to treat certain bacterial infections.

Rifampin is used with other medicines to treat tuberculosis (TB). Rifampin is also taken by itself by patients who may carry meningitis bacteria in their nose and throat (without feeling sick) and may spread these bacteria to others. This medicine may also be used for other problems as determined by your doctor. However, rifampin will not work for colds, flu, or other virus infections.

To help clear up your tuberculosis (TB) completely, you must keep taking this medicine for the full time of treatment, even if you begin to feel better. This is very important. It is also important that you do not miss any doses.

Rifampin is available only with your doctor's prescription.

Once a medicine has been approved for marketing for a certain use, experience may show that it is also useful for other medical problems. Although these uses are not included in product labeling, rifampin is used in certain patients with the following medical conditions:

  • Atypical mycobacterial infections, such as Mycobacterium avium complex (MAC)
  • Leprosy (Hansen's disease)
  • Prevention of Haemophilus influenzae infection
  • Treatment of serious staphylococcal (bacterial) infections

Before Using This Medicine

In deciding to use a medicine, the risks of taking the medicine must be weighed against the good it will do. This is a decision you and your doctor will make. For this medicine, the following should be considered:

Allergies—Tell your doctor if you have ever had any unusual or allergic reaction to this medicine or any other medicines. Also tell your health care professional if you have any other types of allergies, such as to foods, dyes, preservatives, or animals. For non-prescription products, read the label or package ingredients carefully.

Pediatric—This medicine has been tested in children and, in effective doses, has not been shown to cause different side effects or problems in children than it does in adults.

Geriatric—Many medicines have not been studied specifically in older people. Therefore, it may not be known whether they work exactly the same way they do in younger adults. Although there is no specific information comparing use of rifampin in the elderly with use in other age groups, this medicine is not expected to cause different side effects or problems in older people than it does in younger adults.

Pregnancy—

	Pregnancy Category	Explanation
All Trimesters	C	Animal studies have shown an adverse effect and there are no adequate studies in pregnant women OR no animal studies have been conducted and there are no adequate studies in pregnant women.

Breast Feeding—There are no adequate studies in women for determining infant risk when using this medication during breastfeeding. Weigh the potential benefits against the potential risks before taking this medication while breastfeeding.

Other medicines—

Using this medicine with any of the following medicines is not recommended. Your doctor may decide not to treat you with this medication or change some of the other medicines you take.

Saquinavir, Voriconazole

Interactions with Food/Tobacco/Alcohol—Certain medicines should not be used at or around the time of eating food or eating certain types of food since interactions may occur. Using alcohol or tobacco with certain medicines may also cause interactions to occur. Discuss with your healthcare professional the use of your medicine with food, alcohol, or tobacco.

Other medical problems—The presence of other medical problems may affect the use of this medicine. Make sure you tell your doctor if you have any other medical problems, especially:

- Alcohol abuse (or history of) or

- Liver disease—There may be an increased chance of side effects affecting the liver in patients with a history of alcohol abuse or liver disease

---

Proper Use of This Medicine

Rifampin is best taken with a full glass (8 ounces) of water on an empty stomach (either 1 hour before or 2 hours after a meal). However, if this medicine upsets your stomach, your doctor may want you to take it with food.

For patients unable to swallow capsules:

- Contents of the capsules may be mixed with applesauce or jelly. Be sure to take all the food to get the full dose of medicine.

- Your pharmacist can prepare an oral liquid form of this medicine if needed. The liquid form may be kept at room temperature or in the refrigerator. Follow the directions on the label. Shake the bottle well before using. Do not use after the expiration date on the label. The medicine may not work properly after that date. In addition, use a specially marked measuring spoon or other device to measure each dose accurately. The average household teaspoon may not hold the right amount of liquid.

To help clear up your tuberculosis (TB) infection completely, it is very important that you keep taking this medicine for the full time of treatment, even if you begin to feel better after a few weeks. You may have to take it every day for as long as 1 to 2 years or more. It is important that you do not miss any doses.

Dosing—The dose of this medicine will be different for different patients. Follow your doctor's orders or the directions on the label. The following information includes only the average doses of this medicine. If your dose is different, do not change it unless your doctor tells you to do so.

The amount of medicine that you take depends on the strength of the medicine. Also, the number of doses you take each day, the time allowed between doses, and the length of time you take the medicine depend on the medical problem for which you are using the medicine.

- For oral dosage form (capsules) and injection dosage form:
  - For the treatment of tuberculosis (TB):
    - Adults and older children—600 milligrams (mg) once a day. Your doctor may instruct you to take 600 mg two times a week or three times a week. Rifampin must be taken with other medicines to treat tuberculosis.
    - Infants and children—Dose is based on body weight and will be determined by your doctor. Rifampin is usually taken once a day. Your doctor may instruct you to take rifampin two times a week or three times a week. Rifampin must be taken with other medicines to treat tuberculosis.
  - For the treatment of patients in contact with the meningitis bacteria:
    - Adults and older children—600 mg once a day for four days.
    - Infants and children—Dose is based on body weight and will be determined by your doctor.

Missed dose—If you miss a dose of this medicine, take it as soon as possible. However, if it is almost time for your next dose, skip the missed dose and go back to your regular dosing schedule. Do not double doses.

If this medicine is taken on an irregular schedule, side effects may occur more often and may be more serious than usual. If you have any questions about this, check with your health care professional.

Storage—Store the medicine in a closed container at room temperature, away from heat, moisture, and direct light. Keep from freezing.

Keep out of the reach of children.

Do not keep outdated medicine or medicine no longer needed.

Precautions While Using This Medicine

It is very important that your doctor check your progress at regular visits.

If your symptoms do not improve within 2 to 3 weeks, or if they become worse, check with your doctor.

Oral contraceptives (birth control pills) containing estrogen may not work properly if you take them while you are taking rifampin. Unplanned pregnancies may occur. You should use a different means of birth control while you are taking rifampin. If you have any questions about this, check with your health care professional.

Liver problems may be more likely to occur if you drink alcoholic beverages regularly while you are taking this medicine. Also, the regular use of alcohol may keep this medicine from working properly. Therefore, you should not drink alcoholic beverages while you are taking this medicine.

If this medicine causes you to feel very tired or very weak or causes a loss of appetite, nausea, or vomiting, stop taking it and check with your doctor immediately. These may be early warning signs of more serious problems that could develop later.

Rifampin will cause the urine, stool, saliva, sputum, sweat, and tears to turn reddish-orange to reddish-brown. This is to be expected while you are taking this medicine. This effect may cause soft contact lenses to become permanently discolored. Standard cleaning solutions may not take out all the discoloration. Therefore, it is best not to wear soft contact lenses while taking this medicine. This condition will return to normal once you stop taking this medicine. Hard contact lenses are not discolored by rifampin. If you have any questions about this, check with your doctor.

Rifampin can lower the number of white blood cells in your blood temporarily, increasing the chance of getting an infection. It can also lower the number of platelets, which are necessary for proper blood clotting. These problems may result in a greater chance of getting certain infections, slow healing, and bleeding of the gums. Be careful when using a regular toothbrush, dental floss, or a toothpick. Dental work should be delayed until your blood counts have returned to normal. Check with your medical doctor or dentist if you have any questions about proper oral hygiene (mouth care) during treatment.

Before you have any medical tests, tell the doctor in charge that you are taking this medicine. The results of some tests may be affected by this medicine.

Side Effects of This Medicine

Along with its needed effects, a medicine may cause some unwanted effects. Although not all of these side effects may occur, if they do occur they may need medical attention.

Check with your doctor immediately if any of the following side effects occur:

Less common
Chills; difficult breathing; dizziness; fever; headache; itching; muscle and bone pain; shivering; skin rash and redness

Rare
Bloody or cloudy urine; greatly decreased frequency of urination or amount of urine; loss of appetite; nausea or vomiting; sore throat; unusual bleeding or bruising; unusual tiredness or weakness; yellow eyes or skin

Signs and symptoms of overdose
Itching over the whole body; mental changes; reddish-orange color of skin, mouth, and eyeballs; swelling around the eyes or the whole face

Some side effects may occur that usually do not need medical attention. These side effects may go away during treatment as your body adjusts to the medicine. Also, your health care professional may be able to tell you about ways to prevent or reduce some of these side effects. Check with your health care professional if any of the following side effects continue or are bothersome or if you have any questions about them:

More common
Diarrhea; stomach cramps

Less common
Sores on mouth or tongue

This medicine commonly causes reddish-orange to reddish-brown discoloration of urine, stool, saliva, sputum, sweat, and tears. This side effect does not usually need medical attention.

Other side effects not listed may also occur in some patients. If you notice any other effects, check with your healthcare professional.

RIFAMPIN AND ISONIAZID (Oral route) - RIF-am-pin, eye-soe-NYE-a-zid

Black Box Warning

Severe and sometimes fatal hepatitis associated with isoniazid therapy may occur and may develop even after many months of treatment. The risk of developing hepatitis is age related. Approximate case rates by age are: 0 per 1,000 for persons under 20 years of age, 3 per 1,000 for persons in the 20–34 year age group, 12 per 1,000 for persons in the 35–49 year age group, 23 per 1,000 for persons in the 50–64 year age group, and 8 per 1,000 for persons over 65 years of age. The risk of hepatitis is increased with daily consumption of alcohol. Precise data to provide a fatality rate for isoniazid-related hepatitis is not available; however, in a U.S. Public Health Service Surveillance Study of 13,838 persons taking isoniazid, there were 8 deaths among 174 cases of hepatitis.

Therefore, patients given isoniazid should be carefully monitored and interviewed at monthly intervals. Serum transaminase concentration becomes elevated in about 10–20 percent of patients, usually during the first few months of therapy, but it can occur at any time. Usually, enzyme levels return to normal despite continuance of drug, but in some cases progressive liver dysfunction occurs. Patients should be instructed to report immediately any of the prodromal symptoms of hepatitis, such as fatigue, weakness, malaise, anorexia, nausea, or vomiting. If these symptoms appear or if signs suggestive of hepatic damage are detected, isoniazid should be discontinued promptly, since continued use of the drug in these cases has been reported to cause a more severe form of liver damage.

Patients with tuberculosis should be given appropriate treatment with alternative drugs. If isoniazid must be reinstituted, it should be reinstituted only after symptoms and laboratory abnormalities have cleared. The drug should be restarted in very small and gradually increasing doses and should be withdrawn immediately if there is any indication of recurrent liver involvement. Treatment should be deferred in persons with acute hepatic diseases.

Commonly used brand name(s)

In the U.S.—
IsonaRif
Rifamate

Available Dosage Forms:

• Capsule

• Tablet

Therapeutic Class: Antitubercular Combination

Uses For This Medicine

Rifampin and isoniazid is a combination antibiotic and anti-infective medicine. This combination medication is used to treat tuberculosis (TB). It may be taken alone or with one or more other medicines for TB.

To help clear up your tuberculosis (TB) infection completely, you must keep taking this medicine for the full time of treatment, even if you begin to feel better. This is very important. It is also important that you do not miss any doses.

Rifampin and isoniazid combination is available only with your doctor's prescription.

Before Using This Medicine

In deciding to use a medicine, the risks of taking the medicine must be weighed against the good it will do. This is a decision you and your doctor will make. For this medicine, the following should be considered:

Allergies—Tell your doctor if you have ever had any unusual or allergic reaction to this medicine or any other medicines. Also tell your health care professional if you have any other types of allergies, such as to foods, dyes, preservatives, or animals. For non-prescription products, read the label or package ingredients carefully.

Pediatric—Rifampin and isoniazid combination is not recommended for use in children.

Geriatric—Liver problems are more likely to occur in patients over 50 years of age who are taking isoniazid-containing medicines.

Pregnancy—

	Pregnancy Category	Explanation
All Trimesters	C	Animal studies have shown an adverse effect and there are no adequate studies in pregnant women OR no animal studies have been conducted and there are no adequate studies in pregnant women.

Breast Feeding—There are no adequate studies in women for determining infant risk when using this medication during breastfeeding. Weigh the potential benefits against the potential risks before taking this medication while breastfeeding.

Other medicines—

Using this medicine with any of the following medicines is not recommended. Your doctor may decide not to treat you with this medication or change some of the other medicines you take.

Saquinavir, Voriconazole

Interactions with Food/Tobacco/Alcohol—Certain medicines should not be used at or around the time of eating food or eating certain types of food since interactions may occur. Using alcohol or tobacco with certain medicines may also cause interactions to occur. The following interactions have been selected on the basis of their potential significance and are not necessarily all-inclusive.

Using this medicine with any of the following is usually not recommended, but may be unavoidable in some cases. If used together, your doctor may change the dose or how often you use this medicine, or give you special instructions about the use of food, alcohol, or tobacco.

Ethanol

Using this medicine with any of the following may cause an increased risk of certain side effects but may be unavoidable in some cases. If used together, your doctor may change the dose or how often you use this medicine, or give you special instructions about the use of food, alcohol, or tobacco.

Tyramine Containing Food

Other medical problems—The presence of other medical problems may affect the use of this medicine. Make sure you tell your doctor if you have any other medical problems, especially:

- Alcohol abuse (or history of) or
- Liver disease—There may be an increased chance of getting hepatitis if you take this medicine and drink alcohol daily
- Convulsive disorders such as seizures or epilepsy—Rifampin and isoniazid combination may increase the frequency of seizures (convulsions) in some patients
- Kidney disease (severe)—There may be an increased chance of side effects in patients with severe kidney disease

Proper Use of This Medicine

If this medicine upsets your stomach, take it with food. Antacids may also help. However, do not take aluminum-containing antacids within 1 hour of the time you take rifampin and isoniazid combination. They may keep this medicine from working properly.

To help clear up your tuberculosis (TB) completely, it is very important that you keep taking this medicine for the full time of treatment, even if you begin to feel better after a few weeks. You may have to take it every day for as long as 1 to 2 years or more. It is important that you do not miss any doses.

Your doctor may also want you to take pyridoxine (e.g., Hexa-Betalin, vitamin B 6) every day to help prevent or lessen some of the side effects of isoniazid. If it is needed, it is very important to take pyridoxine every day along with this medicine. Do not miss any doses.

Dosing—The dose of this medicine will be different for different patients. Follow your doctor's orders or the directions on the label. The following information includes only the average doses of this medicine. If your dose is different, do not change it unless your doctor tells you to do so.

The amount of medicine that you take depends on the strength of the medicine. Also, the number of doses you take each day, the time allowed between doses, and the length of time you take the medicine depend on the medical problem for which you are using the medicine.

- For the oral dosage form (capsules):
  - For the treatment of tuberculosis:
    - Adults and older children—600 milligrams (mg) of rifampin and 300 mg of isoniazid once a day.
    - Children—This combination medicine is not recommended for use in children.

Missed dose—If you miss a dose of this medicine, take it as soon as possible. However, if it is almost time for your next dose, skip the missed dose and go back to your regular dosing schedule. Do not double doses.

Storage—Store the medicine in a closed container at room temperature, away from heat, moisture, and direct light. Keep from freezing.

Keep out of the reach of children.

Do not keep outdated medicine or medicine no longer needed.

Precautions While Using This Medicine

It is very important that your doctor check your progress at regular visits. In addition, you should check with your doctor immediately if blurred vision or loss of vision, with or without eye pain, occurs during treatment. He or she may want you to have your eyes checked by an ophthalmologist (eye doctor).

If your symptoms do not improve within 2 to 3 weeks, or if they become worse, check with your doctor.

Oral contraceptives (birth control pills) containing estrogen may not work properly if you take them while you are taking rifampin and isoniazid combination. Unplanned pregnancies may occur. You should use a different means of birth control while you are taking this medicine. If you have any questions about this, check with your health care professional.

Liver problems may be more likely to occur if you drink alcoholic beverages regularly while you are taking this medicine. Also, the regular use of alcohol may keep this medicine from working properly. Therefore, you should strictly limit the amount of alcoholic beverages you drink while you are taking this medicine.

Certain foods such as cheese (Swiss or Cheshire) or fish (tuna, skipjack, or Sardinella) may rarely cause reactions in some patients taking isoniazid-containing medicines. Check with your doctor if redness or itching of the skin, hot feeling, fast or pounding heartbeat, sweating, chills or clammy feeling, headache, or lightheadedness occurs after eating these foods while you are taking this medicine.

This medicine will cause the urine, stool, saliva, sputum, sweat, and tears to turn reddish-orange to reddish-brown. This is to be expected while you are taking this medicine. This effect may cause soft contact lenses to become permanently discolored. Standard cleaning solutions may not take out all the discoloration. Therefore, it is best not to wear soft contact lenses while taking this medicine. This condition will return to normal once you stop taking this medicine. Hard contact lenses are not discolored by this medicine. If you have any questions about this, check with your doctor.

If this medicine causes you to feel very tired or very weak; or causes clumsiness; unsteadiness; a loss of appetite; nausea; numbness, tingling, burning, or pain in the hands and feet; or vomiting, stop taking it and check with your doctor immediately. These may be early warning symptoms of more serious liver or nerve problems that could develop later.

Rifampin and isoniazid combination may cause blood problems. These problems may result in a greater chance of certain infections, slow healing, and bleeding of the gums. Therefore, you should be careful when using regular toothbrushes, dental floss, and toothpicks. Dental work should be delayed until your blood counts have returned to normal. Check with your medical doctor or dentist if you have any questions about proper oral hygiene (mouth care) during treatment.

Side Effects of This Medicine

Along with its needed effects, a medicine may cause some unwanted effects. Although not all of these side effects may occur, if they do occur they may need medical attention.

Check with your doctor immediately if any of the following side effects occur:

> *More common*
>> Clumsiness or unsteadiness; dark urine; loss of appetite; nausea and vomiting; numbness, tingling, burning, or pain in hands and feet; unusual tiredness or weakness; yellow eyes or skin

> *Less common*
>> Chills; difficult breathing; dizziness; fever; headache; itching; muscle and bone pain; shivering; skin rash and redness

> *Rare*
>> Bloody or cloudy urine; blurred vision or loss of vision, with or without eye pain; convulsions (seizures); depression; greatly decreased frequency of urination or amount of urine; mood or mental changes; sore throat; unusual bleeding or bruising

Some side effects may occur that usually do not need medical attention. These side effects may go away during treatment as your body adjusts to the medicine. Also, your health care professional may be able to tell you about ways to prevent or reduce some of these side effects. Check with your health care professional if any of the following side effects continue or are bothersome or if you have any questions about them:

> *More common*
>> Diarrhea; stomach pain or upset

> *Less common*
>> Sore mouth or tongue

This medicine commonly causes reddish-orange to reddish-brown discoloration of urine, stool, saliva, sputum, sweat, and tears. This side effect does not usually require medical attention.

Dark urine and yellowing of the eyes or skin (signs of liver problems) are more likely to occur in patients 50 years of age and older.

Other side effects not listed may also occur in some patients. If you notice any other effects, check with your healthcare professional.

RIFAMPIN, ISONIAZID, AND PYRAZINAMIDE (Oral route) - RIF-am-pin, eye-soe-NYE-a-zid, peer-a-ZIN-a-mide

Black Box Warning

Severe and sometimes fatal hepatitis associated with isoniazid therapy may occur and may develop even after many months of treatment. The risk of developing hepatitis is age related. Approximate case rates by age are: 0 per 1,000 for persons under 20 years of age, 3 per 1,000 for persons in the 20 to 34 year age group, 12 per 1,000 for persons in the 35 to 49 year age group, 23 per 1,000 for persons in the 50 to 64 year age group, and 8 per 1,000 for persons over 65 years of age. The risk of hepatitis is increased with daily consumption of alcohol. Precise data to provide a fatality rate for isoniazid-related hepatitis is not available; however, in a U.S. Public Health Service Surveillance Study of 13,838 persons taking isoniazid, there were 8 deaths among 174 cases of hepatitis.

Therefore, patients given isoniazid should be carefully monitored and interviewed at monthly intervals. Serum transaminase concentration becomes elevated in about 10% to 20% of patients, usually during the first few months of therapy, but it can occur at any time. Usually enzyme levels return to normal despite continuance of drug, but in some cases progressive liver dysfunction occurs. Patients should be instructed to report immediately any of the prodromal symptoms of hepatitis, such as fatigue, weakness, malaise, anorexia, nausea, or vomiting. If these symptoms appear or if signs suggestive of hepatic damage are detected, isoniazid should be discontinued promptly since continued use of the drug in these cases has been reported to cause a more severe form of liver damage.

Patients with tuberculosis should be given appropriate treatment with alternative drugs. If isoniazid must be reinstituted, it should be reinstituted only after symptoms and laboratory abnormalities have cleared. The drug should be restarted in very small and gradually increasing doses and should be withdrawn immediately if there is any indication of recurrent liver involvement. Treatment should be deferred in persons with acute hepatic diseases.

Commonly used brand name(s)

In the U.S.—
> Rifater

Available Dosage Forms:
  • Tablet

Therapeutic Class: Antitubercular Combination

Uses For This Medicine

Rifampin, isoniazid, and pyrazinamide is a combination anti-infective medicine. This combination medicine is used to treat tuberculosis (TB). It may be taken alone or with one or more of other medicines for TB.

To help clear up your tuberculosis (TB) infection completely, you must keep taking this medicine for the full time of treatment, even if you begin to feel better. This is very important. It is also important that you do not miss any doses.

Rifampin, isoniazid, and pyrazinamide combination is available only with your doctor's prescription.

Before Using This Medicine

In deciding to use a medicine, the risks of taking the medicine must be weighed against the good it will do. This is a decision you and your doctor will make. For this medicine, the following should be considered:

Allergies—Tell your doctor if you have ever had any unusual or allergic reaction to this medicine or any other medicines. Also tell your health care professional if you have any other types of allergies, such as to foods, dyes, preservatives, or animals. For non-prescription products, read the label or package ingredients carefully.

Pediatric—Rifampin, isoniazid, and pyrazinamide combination may not be appropriate for use in children and adolescents up to 15 years of age.

Geriatric—Liver problems are more likely to occur in patients over 50 years of age who are taking isoniazid-containing medicines.

Pregnancy—

	Pregnancy Category	Explanation
All Trimesters	C	Animal studies have shown an adverse effect and there are no adequate studies in pregnant women OR no animal studies have been conducted and there are no adequate studies in pregnant women.

Breast Feeding—There are no adequate studies in women for determining infant risk when using this medication during breastfeeding. Weigh the potential benefits against the potential risks before taking this medication while breastfeeding.

Other medicines—

Using this medicine with any of the following medicines is not recommended. Your doctor may decide not to treat you with this medication or change some of the other medicines you take.

Saquinavir, Voriconazole

Interactions with Food/Tobacco/Alcohol—Certain medicines should not be used at or around the time of eating food or eating certain types of food since interactions may occur. Using alcohol or tobacco with certain medicines may also cause interactions to occur. The following interactions

have been selected on the basis of their potential significance and are not necessarily all-inclusive.

Using this medicine with any of the following is usually not recommended, but may be unavoidable in some cases. If used together, your doctor may change the dose or how often you use this medicine, or give you special instructions about the use of food, alcohol, or tobacco.

Ethanol

Using this medicine with any of the following may cause an increased risk of certain side effects but may be unavoidable in some cases. If used together, your doctor may change the dose or how often you use this medicine, or give you special instructions about the use of food, alcohol, or tobacco.

Tyramine Containing Food

Other medical problems—The presence of other medical problems may affect the use of this medicine. Make sure you tell your doctor if you have any other medical problems, especially:

  • Alcohol abuse (or history of) or

  • Liver disease—There may be an increased chance of getting hepatitis if you take this medicine and drink alcohol daily

  • Convulsive disorders such as seizures or epilepsy—Rifampin, isoniazid, and pyrazinamide combination may increase the frequency of convulsions (seizures) in some patients

  • Gout (history of)—Rifampin, isoniazid, and pyrazinamide combination may worsen or cause a gout attack in patients with a history of gout

  • Kidney disease (severe)—There may be an increased chance of side effects in patients with severe kidney disease

Proper Use of This Medicine

If this medicine upsets your stomach, take it with food. Antacids may also help. However, do not take aluminum-containing antacids within 1 hour of the time you take rifampin, isoniazid, and pyrazinamide combination. They may keep this medicine from working properly.

To help clear up your tuberculosis (TB) completely, it is very important that you keep taking this medicine for the full time of treatment, even if you begin to feel better after a few weeks. It is important that you do not miss any doses.

Your doctor may also want you to take pyridoxine (e.g., Hexa-Betalin, vitamin B_6) every day to help prevent or lessen some of the side effects of isoniazid. If it is needed, it is very important to take pyridoxine every day along with this medicine. Do not miss any doses.

Dosing—The dose of this medicine will be different for different patients. Follow your doctor's orders or the directions on the label. The following information includes only the average doses of this medicine. If your dose is different, do not change it unless your doctor tells you to do so.

The amount of medicine that you take depends on the strength of the medicine. Also, the number of doses you take each day, the time allowed between doses, and the length of time you take the medicine depend on the medical problem for which you are using the medicine.

- For oral dosage form (tablets):
  - For the treatment of tuberculosis:
    - Adults and teenagers over 15 years of age weighing 44 kilograms (kg) (97 pounds) or less—4 tablets once a day.
    - Adults and teenagers over 15 years of age weighing between 45 and 54 kg (99 and 119 pounds)—5 tablets once a day.
    - Adults and teenagers over 15 years of age weighing 55 kg (121 pounds) or more—6 tablets once a day.
    - Children up to 15 years of age—This medicine is not recommended for this age group.

Missed dose—If you miss a dose of this medicine, take it as soon as possible. However, if it is almost time for your next dose, skip the missed dose and go back to your regular dosing schedule. Do not double doses.

If rifampin, isoniazid, and pyrazinamide combination is taken on an irregular schedule, side effects may occur more often and may be more serious than usual. If you have any questions about this, check with your health care professional.

Storage—Store the medicine in a closed container at room temperature, away from heat, moisture, and direct light. Keep from freezing.

Keep out of the reach of children.

Do not keep outdated medicine or medicine no longer needed.

Precautions While Using This Medicine

It is very important that your doctor check your progress at regular visits. In addition, you should check with your doctor immediately if blurred vision or loss of vision, with or without eye pain, occurs during treatment. He or she may want you to have your eyes checked by an ophthalmologist (eye doctor).

If your symptoms do not improve within 2 to 3 weeks, or if they become worse, check with your doctor.

Oral contraceptives (birth control pills) containing estrogen may not work properly if you take them while you are taking rifampin, isoniazid, and pyrazinamide combination. Unplanned pregnancies may occur. You should use a different method of birth control while you are taking this medicine. If you have any questions about this, check with your health care professional.

Liver problems may be more likely to occur if you drink alcoholic beverages regularly while you are taking this medicine. Also, the regular use of alcohol may keep this medicine from working properly. Therefore, you should strictly limit the amount of alcoholic beverages you drink while you are taking this medicine.

Certain foods such as cheese (Swiss or Cheshire) or fish (tuna, skipjack, or Sardinella) may rarely cause reactions in some patients taking isoniazid-containing medicines. Check with your doctor if redness or itching of the skin, hot feeling, fast or pounding heartbeat, sweating, chills or clammy feeling, headache, or lightheadedness occurs while you are taking this medicine.

This medicine will cause urine, stool, saliva, sputum, sweat, and tears to turn reddish-orange to reddish-brown. This is to be expected while you are taking this medicine. This effect may cause soft contact lenses to become permanently discolored. Standard cleaning solutions may not take out all the discoloration. Therefore, it is best not to wear soft contact lenses while taking this medicine. Hard contact lenses are not discolored by this medicine. This condition will return to normal once you stop taking this medicine. If you have any questions about this, check with your health care professional.

If this medicine causes you to feel very tired or very weak; or causes clumsiness; unsteadiness; a loss of appetite; nausea; numbness, tingling, burning, or pain in the hands and feet; or vomiting, stop taking it and check with your doctor immediately. These may be early warning symptoms of more serious liver or nerve problems that could develop later.

Rifampin, isoniazid, and pyrazinamide combination may cause blood problems. These problems may result in a greater chance of certain infections, slow healing, and bleeding of the gums. Therefore, you should be careful when using regular toothbrushes, dental floss, and toothpicks. Dental work should be delayed until your blood counts have returned to normal. Check with your medical doctor or dentist if you have any questions about proper oral hygiene (mouth care) during treatment.

For diabetic patients: This medicine may cause false test results with urine ketone tests. Check with your doctor before changing your diet or the dosage of your diabetes medicine.

Side Effects of This Medicine

Along with its needed effects, a medicine may cause some unwanted effects. Although not all of these side effects may occur, if they do occur they may need medical attention.

Check with your doctor immediately if any of the following side effects occur:
  More common
    Clumsiness or unsteadiness; dark urine; loss of appetite; nausea and vomiting; numbness, tingling, burning, or pain in hands and feet; pain in large and small joints; unusual tiredness or weakness; yellow eyes or skin
  Less common
    Chills; difficulty in breathing; dizziness; fever; headache; itching; muscle and bone pain; redness of skin; shivering; skin rash
  Rare
    Bloody or cloudy urine; blurred vision or loss of vision, with or without eye pain; convulsions (seizures); greatly decreased frequency of urination or amount of urine; mental depression; mood or mental changes; sore throat; unusual bleeding or bruising

Some side effects may occur that usually do not need medical attention. These side effects may go away during treatment as your body adjusts to the medicine. Also, your health care professional may be able to tell you about ways to prevent or reduce some of these side effects. Check with your health care professional if any of the following side effects continue or are bothersome or if you have any questions about them:
  More common
    Diarrhea; stomach pain
  Less common
    Sore mouth or tongue

This medicine commonly causes urine, stool, saliva, sputum, sweat, and tears to turn reddish-orange to reddish-brown. This side effect does not usually require medical attention.

Dark urine and yellowing of the eyes or skin (signs of liver problems) caused by isoniazid are more likely to occur in patients 50 years of age and older.

Other side effects not listed may also occur in some patients. If you notice any other effects, check with your healthcare professional.

RIFAPENTINE (Oral route) - RIF-a-pen-teen

Commonly used brand name(s)
In the U.S.—
   Priftin

Available Dosage Forms:
   • Tablet

Therapeutic Class: Antitubercular

Uses For This Medicine

Rifapentine is used with other medicines to treat tuberculosis.

To help clear up your tuberculosis completely, you must keep taking this medicine for the full time of treatment, even if you begin to feel better. This is very important. It is also important that you do not miss any doses.

Rifapentine is available only with your doctor's prescription.

Before Using This Medicine

In deciding to use a medicine, the risks of taking the medicine must be weighed against the good it will do. This is a decision you and your doctor will make. For this medicine, the following should be considered:

Allergies—Tell your doctor if you have ever had any unusual or allergic reaction to this medicine or any other medicines. Also tell your health care professional if you have any other types of allergies, such as to foods, dyes, preservatives, or animals. For non-prescription products, read the label or package ingredients carefully.

Pediatric—Safety and efficacy have not been established in infants and children younger than 12 years of age. For children 12 years of age and older, rifapentine is not expected to cause different side effects or problems than it does in adults.

Geriatric—Rifapentine is not expected to cause different side effects or problems in older people than it does in younger adults.

Pregnancy—

	Pregnancy Category	Explanation
All Trimesters	C	Animal studies have shown an adverse effect and there are no adequate studies in pregnant women OR no animal studies have been conducted and there are no adequate studies in pregnant women.

Breast Feeding—Studies suggest that this medication may alter milk production or composition. If an alternative to this medication is not prescribed, you should monitor the infant for side effects and adequate milk intake.

Other medicines—

Using this medicine with any of the following medicines is usually not recommended, but may be required in some cases. If both medicines are prescribed together, your doctor may change the dose or how often you use one or both of the medicines.

Amprenavir, Efavirenz, Erlotinib, Fosamprenavir, Indinavir, Nevirapine, Sunitinib

Interactions with Food/Tobacco/Alcohol—Certain medicines should not be used at or around the time of eating food or eating certain types of food since interactions may occur. Using alcohol or tobacco with certain medicines may also cause interactions to occur. Discuss with your healthcare professional the use of your medicine with food, alcohol, or tobacco.

Other medical problems—The presence of other medical problems may affect the use of this medicine. Make sure you tell your doctor if you have any other medical problems, especially:
   • Alcohol abuse (or history of) or
   • Liver disease—There may be an increased chance of side effects affecting the liver in patients with a history of alcohol abuse or liver disease

Proper Use of This Medicine

The treatment of tuberculosis may take months or years to complete. It is very important that you comply with the full course of therapy.

Dosing—The dose of this medicine will be different for different patients. Follow your doctor's orders or the directions on the label. The following information includes only the average doses of this medicine. If your dose is different, do not change it unless your doctor tells you to do so.

The amount of medicine that you take depends on the strength of the medicine. Also, the number of doses you take each day, the time allowed between doses, and the length of time you take the medicine depend on the medical problem for which you are using the medicine.

   • For oral dosage form (tablets):
      ○ For the treatment of tuberculosis (TB):
         ▪ Adults and children 12 years of age and older—600 milligrams (mg) twice a week with an interval of not less than three days (seventy-two hours) between doses. Rifapentine must be taken with other medicines to treat tuberculosis.
         ▪ Infants and children up to 12 years of age—Use and dose must be determined by your doctor.

Missed dose—If you miss a dose of this medicine, take it as soon as possible. However, if it is almost time for your next dose, skip the missed dose and go back to your regular dosing schedule. Do not double doses.

Storage—Store the medicine in a closed container at room temperature, away from heat, moisture, and direct light. Keep from freezing.

Keep out of the reach of children.

Do not keep outdated medicine or medicine no longer needed.

Precautions While Using This Medicine

It is very important that your doctor check your progress at regular visits.

If your symptoms do not improve within 2 to 3 weeks, or if they become worse, check with your doctor.

If this medicine causes you to feel very tired or very weak or causes a loss of appetite, nausea, or vomiting, stop taking it and check with your doctor immediately. These may be early warning signs of more serious problems that could develop later.

Oral contraceptives (birth control pills) may not work properly if you take them while you are taking rifapentine. Unplanned pregnancies may occur. You should use a different means of birth control while you are taking rifapentine. If you have any questions about this, check with your health care professional.

Liver problems may be more likely to occur if you drink alcoholic beverages regularly while you are taking this medicine. Also, the regular use of alcohol may keep this medicine from working properly. Therefore, you should not drink alcoholic beverages while you are taking this medicine.

Rifapentine will cause the urine, stools, saliva, sputum, sweat, and tears to turn reddish-orange to reddish-brown. This is to be expected while you are taking this medicine. This effect may cause soft contact lenses to become permanently discolored. Standard cleaning solutions may not take out all the discoloration. Therefore, it is best not to wear soft contact lenses while taking this medicine. Hard contact lenses are not discolored by rifapentine. If you have any question about this, check with your doctor.

Rifapentine can lower the number of white blood cells in your blood temporarily, increasing the chance of getting infection. It can also lower the number of platelets, which are necessary for proper blood clotting. These problems may result in a greater chance of getting certain infections, slow healing, and bleeding of the gums. Be careful when using a regular toothbrush, dental floss, or a toothpick. Dental work should be delayed until your blood counts have returned to normal. Check with your medical doctor or dentist if you have any questions about proper oral hygiene (mouth care) during treatment.

Before you have any medical tests, tell the doctor in charge that you are taking this medicine.

Side Effects of This Medicine

Along with its needed effects, a medicine may cause some unwanted effects. Although not all of these side effects may occur, if they do occur they may need medical attention.

Check with your doctor as soon as possible if any of the following side effects occur:

More common
> Blood in urine; joint pain; lower back or side pain; swelling of feet or lower legs

Less common
> Aggressive reaction; black, tarry stools; blood in stools; nausea; pinpoint red spots on skin; severe abdominal or stomach pain; sore throat and fever; unusual bleeding or bruising; unusual tiredness or weakness; yellow eyes or skin; vomiting

Rare
> Diarrhea; dizziness; severe or continuing headaches; increase in blood pressure

Some side effects may occur that usually do not need medical attention. These side effects may go away during treatment as your body adjusts to the medicine. Also, your health care professional may be able to tell you about ways to pre-

vent or reduce some of these side effects. Check with your health care professional if any of the following side effects continue or are bothersome or if you have any questions about them:

Less common
> Acne; constipation; loss of appetite

This medicine commonly causes reddish-orange to reddish-brown discoloration of urine, stools, saliva, sputum, sweat, and tears. This side effect does not usually need medical attention.

Other side effects not listed may also occur in some patients. If you notice any other effects, check with your healthcare professional.

RIFAXIMIN   (Oral route) - rif-AX-i-min

Commonly used brand name(s)

In the U.S.—
> Xifaxan

Available Dosage Forms:

- Tablet

Therapeutic Class: Antibiotic

Uses For This Medicine

Rifaximin is a medicine used to treat travelers' diarrhea caused by a bacteria called *E. coli*.

This medicine is available only with your doctor's prescription.

Before Using This Medicine

In deciding to use a medicine, the risks of taking the medicine must be weighed against the good it will do. This is a decision you and your doctor will make. For this medicine, the following should be considered:

Allergies—Tell your doctor if you have ever had any unusual or allergic reaction to this medicine or any other medicines. Also tell your health care professional if you have any other types of allergies, such as to foods, dyes, preservatives, or animals. For non-prescription products, read the label or package ingredients carefully.

Pediatric—Studies on this medicine have been done only in adult patients, and there is no specific information comparing the use of rifaximin in children under 12 years of age with use in other age groups.

Geriatric—Many medicines have not been studied specifically in older people. Therefore, it may not be known whether they work exactly the same way they do in younger adults or if they cause different side effects of problems in older people. There is no specific information comparing use of rifaximin in the elderly with use in other age groups.

Pregnancy—

	Pregnancy Category	Explanation
All Trimesters	C	Animal studies have shown an adverse effect and there are no adequate studies in pregnant women OR no animal studies have been conducted and there are no adequate studies in pregnant women.

Breast Feeding—There are no adequate studies in women for determining infant risk when using this medication during breastfeeding. Weigh the potential benefits against the potential risks before taking this medication while breastfeeding.

Other medicines—Although certain medicines should not be used together at all, in other cases two different medicines may be used together even if an interaction might occur. In these cases, your doctor may want to change the dose, or other precautions may be necessary. Tell your healthcare professional if you are taking any other prescription or non-prescription (over-the-counter [OTC]) medicine.

Interactions with Food/Tobacco/Alcohol—Certain medicines should not be used at or around the time of eating food or eating certain types of food since interactions may occur. Using alcohol or tobacco with certain medicines may also cause interactions to occur. Discuss with your healthcare professional the use of your medicine with food, alcohol, or tobacco.

Other medical problems—The presence of other medical problems may affect the use of this medicine. Make sure you tell your doctor if you have any other medical problems, especially:
- Pseudomembranous colitis—Rifaximin may also cause this serious side effect.

Proper Use of This Medicine

Do not use rifaximin to treat your diarrhea if you have a fever or if there is blood in your stools. Contact your doctor.

Importance of diet and fluid intake while treating diarrhea:

- In addition to using medicine for diarrhea, it is very important that you replace the fluid lost by the body and follow a proper diet. For the first 24 hours, you should eat gelatin, and drink plenty of caffeine-free clear liquids, such as ginger ale, decaffeinated cola, decaffeinated tea, and broth. During the next 24 hours you may eat bland foods, such as cooked cereals, bread, crackers, and applesauce. Fruits, vegetables, fried or spicy foods, bran, candy, caffeine, and alcoholic beverages may make the condition worse.
- If too much fluid has been lost by the body due to the diarrhea, a serious condition (dehydration) may develop. Check with your doctor as soon as possible if any of the following signs or symptoms of too much fluid loss occur:
  - Decreased urination
  - Dizziness and lightheadedness
  - Dryness of mouth
  - Increased thirst
  - Wrinkled skin

Dosing—The dose of this medicine will be different for different patients. Follow your doctor's orders or the directions on the label. The following information includes only the average doses of this medicine. If your dose is different, do not change it unless your doctor tells you to do so.

The amount of medicine that you take depends on the strength of the medicine. Also, the number of doses you take each day, the time allowed between doses, and the length of time you take the medicine depend on the medical problem for which you are using the medicine.

- For oral dosage form (tablets):
  - For diarrhea
    - Adults and children 12 years of age and older— 200 milligrams taken three times a day for 3 days.
    - Children under 12 years of age—Use and dose must be determined by your doctor.

Missed dose—If you miss a dose of this medicine, take it as soon as possible. However, if it is almost time for your next dose, skip the missed dose and go back to your regular dosing schedule. Do not double doses.

Storage—Store the medicine in a closed container at room temperature, away from heat, moisture, and direct light. Keep from freezing.

Keep out of the reach of children.

Do not keep outdated medicine or medicine no longer needed.

Ask your healthcare professional how you should dispose of any medicine you do not use.

Precautions While Using This Medicine

Check with your doctor if your diarrhea does not stop in 1 or 2 days or if you develop a fever or if you have blood in your stools.

Side Effects of This Medicine

Along with its needed effects, a medicine may cause some unwanted effects. Although not all of these side effects may occur, if they do occur they may need medical attention.

Check with your doctor immediately if any of the following side effects occur:
Incidence not determined
Hives or welts; itching skin; large, hive-like swelling on face, eyelids, lips, tongue, throat, hands, legs, feet, sex organs; rash; redness of skin

Some side effects may occur that usually do not need medical attention. These side effects may go away during treatment as your body adjusts to the medicine. Also, your health care professional may be able to tell you about ways to prevent or reduce some of these side effects. Check with your health care professional if any of the following side effects continue or are bothersome or if you have any questions about them:
More common
Headache

Less common
Difficulty having a bowel movement (stool); vomiting

Other side effects not listed may also occur in some patients. If you notice any other effects, check with your healthcare professional.

RILUZOLE   (Oral route) - RIL-yoo-zole

Commonly used brand name(s)
In the U.S.—
Rilutek

Available Dosage Forms:
• Tablet

Therapeutic Class: Central Nervous System Agent
Pharmacologic Class: Glutamate Antagonist

Uses For This Medicine

Riluzole is used to treat patients with amyotrophic lateral sclerosis (ALS), also known as Lou Gehrig's disease. Riluzole is not a cure for ALS, but it may extend survival in the early stages of the disease, and/or may extend the time until a tracheostomy may be needed.

Riluzole is available only with your doctor's prescription.

Before Using This Medicine

In deciding to use a medicine, the risks of taking the medicine must be weighed against the good it will do. This is a decision you and your doctor will make. For this medicine, the following should be considered:

Allergies—Tell your doctor if you have ever had any unusual or allergic reaction to this medicine or any other medicines. Also tell your health care professional if you have any other types of allergies, such as to foods, dyes, preservatives, or animals. For non-prescription products, read the label or package ingredients carefully.

Pediatric—Studies on this medicine have been done only in adult patients, and there is no specific information comparing use of riluzole in children with use in other age groups.

Geriatric—Many medicines have not been studied specifically in older people. Therefore, it may not be known whether they work exactly the same way they do in younger adults. Although there is no specific information comparing use of riluzole in the elderly with use in other age groups, this medicine has been used in elderly patients and is not expected to cause different side effects or problems in older people than it does in younger adults.

Pregnancy—

	Pregnancy Category	Explanation
All Trimesters	C	Animal studies have shown an adverse effect and there are no adequate studies in pregnant women OR no animal studies have been conducted and there are no adequate studies in pregnant women.

Breast Feeding—There are no adequate studies in women for determining infant risk when using this medication during breastfeeding. Weigh the potential benefits against the potential risks before taking this medication while breastfeeding.

Other medicines—

Using this medicine with any of the following medicines is usually not recommended, but may be required in some

cases. If both medicines are prescribed together, your doctor may change the dose or how often you use one or both of the medicines.

Sulfasalazine

Interactions with Food/Tobacco/Alcohol—Certain medicines should not be used at or around the time of eating food or eating certain types of food since interactions may occur. Using alcohol or tobacco with certain medicines may also cause interactions to occur. Discuss with your healthcare professional the use of your medicine with food, alcohol, or tobacco.

Other medical problems—The presence of other medical problems may affect the use of this medicine. Make sure you tell your doctor if you have any other medical problems, especially:
• Kidney disease or
• Liver disease—Higher blood levels of riluzole may occur, increasing the chance of side effects

Proper Use of This Medicine

Riluzole should be taken on a regular basis and at the same time of the day (for example, in the morning and the evening).

Riluzole should be taken on an empty stomach. Take this medicine at least one hour before meals or two hours after meals.

Dosing—The dose of this medicine will be different for different patients. Follow your doctor's orders or the directions on the label. The following information includes only the average doses of this medicine. If your dose is different, do not change it unless your doctor tells you to do so.

The amount of medicine that you take depends on the strength of the medicine. Also, the number of doses you take each day, the time allowed between doses, and the length of time you take the medicine depend on the medical problem for which you are using the medicine.

• For oral dosage form (tablets):
  ○ For ALS:
    ▪ Adults—Oral, 50 milligrams (mg) every twelve hours.
    ▪ Children up to 18 years of age—Use and dose must be determined by your doctor.

Missed dose—If you miss a dose of this medicine, skip the missed dose and go back to your regular dosing schedule. Do not double doses.

Storage—Store the medicine in a closed container at room temperature, away from heat, moisture, and direct light. Keep from freezing.

Keep out of the reach of children.

Do not keep outdated medicine or medicine no longer needed.

Precautions While Using This Medicine

If you become ill with a fever, report this to your doctor promptly. Fever may be a sign of infection.

This medicine may cause dizziness or drowsiness. Make sure you know how you react to this medicine before you drive, use machines, or do anything else that could be dangerous if you are dizzy or are not alert.

Avoid drinking alcoholic beverages. It is not known if drinking alcohol while taking riluzole may cause liver problems.

Side Effects of This Medicine

Along with its needed effects, a medicine may cause some unwanted effects. Although not all of these side effects may occur, if they do occur they may need medical attention.

Check with your doctor as soon as possible if any of the following side effects occur:

More common
Diarrhea; nausea; vomiting; worsening of some symptoms of ALS, including spasticity and tiredness or weakness

Less common
Difficulty in breathing; increased cough; pneumonia

Rare
Bloody or cloudy urine, frequent urge to urinate, or painful or difficult urination; convulsions (seizures); fast or pounding heartbeat; fever, chills, or continuing sores in mouth; hypertension (high blood pressure); increased thirst, irregular heartbeat, mood or mental changes, or muscle cramps, pain, or weakness; lack of coordination; lack of energy; mental depression; pain, tenderness, bluish color, or swelling of foot or leg; redness, scaling, or peeling of the skin; swelling of eyelids, mouth, lips, tongue, and/or throat; swelling of face; trouble in swallowing; yellow eyes or skin

Some side effects may occur that usually do not need medical attention. These side effects may go away during treatment as your body adjusts to the medicine. Also, your health care professional may be able to tell you about ways to prevent or reduce some of these side effects. Check with your health care professional if any of the following side effects continue or are bothersome or if you have any questions about them:

More common
Abdominal pain or gas; dizziness; drowsiness; loss of appetite; numbness or tingling around the mouth

Less common
Back or muscle pain or stiffness; constipation; general feeling of discomfort or illness; hair loss; headache; irritation or soreness of mouth; runny nose; skin rash or itching; trouble in sleeping

This medicine may also cause the following side effect that your doctor will watch for:

More common
Liver problems

Other side effects not listed may also occur in some patients. If you notice any other effects, check with your healthcare professional.

RIMANTADINE (Oral route) - ri-MAN-ta-deen

Commonly used brand name(s)
In the U.S.—
Flumadine

Available Dosage Forms:
• Syrup
• Tablet

Therapeutic Class: Antiviral

Uses For This Medicine

Rimantadine is an antiviral. It is used to prevent or treat certain influenza (flu) infections (type A). It may be given alone or along with flu shots. Rimantadine will not work for colds, other types of flu, or other virus infections.

Rimantadine is available only with your doctor's prescription.

Before Using This Medicine

In deciding to use a medicine, the risks of taking the medicine must be weighed against the good it will do. This is a decision you and your doctor will make. For this medicine, the following should be considered:

Allergies—Tell your doctor if you have ever had any unusual or allergic reaction to this medicine or any other medicines. Also tell your health care professional if you have any other types of allergies, such as to foods, dyes, preservatives, or animals. For non-prescription products, read the label or package ingredients carefully.

Pediatric—This medicine has been tested in children over one year of age and has not been shown to cause different side effects or problems in these children than it does in adults. There is no specific information comparing the use of rimantadine in children under one year of age with use in other age groups.

Geriatric—Elderly people are especially sensitive to the effects of rimantadine. Difficulty in sleeping, difficulty in concentrating, dizziness, headache, nervousness, and weakness may be especially likely to occur. Stomach pain, nausea, vomiting, and loss of appetite may also occur.

Pregnancy—

	Pregnancy Category	Explanation
All Trimesters	C	Animal studies have shown an adverse effect and there are no adequate studies in pregnant women OR no animal studies have been conducted and there are no adequate studies in pregnant women.

Breast Feeding—There are no adequate studies in women for determining infant risk when using this medication during breastfeeding. Weigh the potential benefits against the potential risks before taking this medication while breastfeeding.

Other medicines—Although certain medicines should not be used together at all, in other cases two different medicines may be used together even if an interaction might occur. In these cases, your doctor may want to change the dose, or other precautions may be necessary. Tell your healthcare professional if you are taking any other prescription or non-prescription (over-the-counter [OTC]) medicine.

Interactions with Food/Tobacco/Alcohol—Certain medicines should not be used at or around the time of eating food or eating certain types of food since interactions may

occur. Using alcohol or tobacco with certain medicines may also cause interactions to occur. Discuss with your healthcare professional the use of your medicine with food, alcohol, or tobacco.

Other medical problems—The presence of other medical problems may affect the use of this medicine. Make sure you tell your doctor if you have any other medical problems, especially:

- Epilepsy or other seizures (history of)—Rimantadine may increase the frequency of convulsions (seizures) in patients with a seizure disorder
- Kidney disease—Rimantadine is removed from the body by the kidneys; patients with severe kidney disease will need to receive a lower dose of rimantadine
- Liver disease—Patients with severe liver disease may need to receive a lower dose of rimantadine

Proper Use of This Medicine

Talk to your doctor about the possibility of getting a flu shot if you have not had one yet.

This medicine is best taken before exposure, or as soon as possible after exposure, to people who have the flu.

To help keep yourself from getting the flu, keep taking this medicine for the full time of treatment.

If you already have the flu, continue taking this medicine for the full time of treatment even if you begin to feel better after a few days. This will help to clear up your infection completely. If you stop taking this medicine too soon, your symptoms may return. This medicine should be taken for at least 5 to 7 days.

This medicine works best when there is a constant amount in the blood. To help keep the amount constant, do not miss any doses. Also, it is best to take the doses at evenly spaced times day and night.

If you are using the oral liquid form of rimantadine, use a specially marked measuring spoon or other device to measure each dose accurately. The average household teaspoon may not hold the right amount of liquid.

Dosing—The dose of this medicine will be different for different patients. Follow your doctor's orders or the directions on the label. The following information includes only the average doses of this medicine. If your dose is different, do not change it unless your doctor tells you to do so.

The amount of medicine that you take depends on the strength of the medicine. Also, the number of doses you take each day, the time allowed between doses, and the length of time you take the medicine depend on the medical problem for which you are using the medicine.

- For oral dosage forms (syrup, tablets):
  - For the prevention or treatment of flu:
    - Elderly adults—100 milligrams (mg) once a day.
    - Adults and children 10 years of age and older—100 mg two times a day.
    - Children up to 10 years of age—5 mg per kilogram (2.3 mg per pound) of body weight once a day. Children in this age group should not receive more than 150 mg a day.

Missed dose—If you miss a dose of this medicine, take it as soon as possible. However, if it is almost time for your next dose, skip the missed dose and go back to your regular dosing schedule. Do not double doses.

Storage—Store the medicine in a closed container at room temperature, away from heat, moisture, and direct light. Keep from freezing.

Keep out of the reach of children.

Do not keep outdated medicine or medicine no longer needed.

Precautions While Using This Medicine

This medicine may cause some people to become dizzy or confused, or to have trouble concentrating. Make sure you know how you react to this medicine before you drive, use machines, or do anything else that could be dangerous if you are dizzy or confused. If these reactions are especially bothersome, check with your doctor.

If your symptoms do not improve within a few days, or if they become worse, check with your doctor.

Side Effects of This Medicine

Along with its needed effects, a medicine may cause some unwanted effects. Although not all of these side effects may occur, if they do occur they may need medical attention.

Some side effects may occur that usually do not need medical attention. These side effects may go away during treatment as your body adjusts to the medicine. Also, your health care professional may be able to tell you about ways to prevent or reduce some of these side effects. Check with your health care professional if any of the following side effects continue or are bothersome or if you have any questions about them:

Less common
Difficulty in concentrating; dizziness; dryness of mouth; headache; loss of appetite; nausea; nervousness; stomach pain; trouble in sleeping; unusual tiredness; vomiting

Other side effects not listed may also occur in some patients. If you notice any other effects, check with your healthcare professional.

RIMEXOLONE   (Ophthalmic route) - ri-MEX-oh-lone

Commonly used brand name(s)

In the U.S.—
Vexol

Available Dosage Forms:
- Suspension

Therapeutic Class: Ophthalmologic Agent
Pharmacologic Class: Adrenal Glucocorticoid

Uses For This Medicine

Rimexolone belongs to the group of medicines known as corticosteroids (cortisone-like medicines). It is used to treat inflammation of the eye, which may occur following eye surgery or with certain eye problems.

This medicine is available only with your doctor's prescription.

Before Using This Medicine

In deciding to use a medicine, the risks of taking the medicine must be weighed against the good it will do. This is a decision you and your doctor will make. For this medicine, the following should be considered:

Allergies—Tell your doctor if you have ever had any unusual or allergic reaction to this medicine or any other medicines. Also tell your health care professional if you have any other types of allergies, such as to foods, dyes, preservatives, or animals. For non-prescription products, read the label or package ingredients carefully.

Pediatric—Studies on this medicine have been done only in adult patients, and there is no specific information comparing use of rimexolone in children with use in other age groups.

Geriatric—Many medicines have not been studied specifically in older people. Therefore, it may not be known whether they work exactly the same way they do in younger adults or if they cause different side effects or problems in older people. There is no specific information comparing use of rimexolone in the elderly with use in other age groups.

Other medicines—

Using this medicine with any of the following medicines is not recommended. Your doctor may decide not to treat you with this medication or change some of the other medicines you take.

Bupropion

Interactions with Food/Tobacco/Alcohol—Certain medicines should not be used at or around the time of eating food or eating certain types of food since interactions may occur. Using alcohol or tobacco with certain medicines may also cause interactions to occur. Discuss with your healthcare professional the use of your medicine with food, alcohol, or tobacco.

Other medical problems—The presence of other medical problems may affect the use of this medicine. Make sure you tell your doctor if you have any other medical problems, especially:

- Certain eye diseases that cause the cornea to get thin—Use of ophthalmic rimexolone could cause a hole to form (perforation)
- Fungus infection of the eye or
- Herpes infection of the eye or
- Virus infection of the eye or
- Yeast infection of the eye or
- Any other eye infection—Ophthalmic rimexolone may make existing infections worse or cause new infections

Proper Use of This Medicine

Shake the container very well before applying the eye drops.

To use:

- First, wash your hands. Tilt your head back and, pressing your finger gently on the skin just beneath the lower eyelid, pull the lower eyelid away from the eye to make a space. Drop the medicine into this space. Let go of the eyelid and gently close the eyes. Do not blink. Keep the eyes closed and apply pressure to the inner corner of the eye with your finger for 1 or 2 minutes to allow the medicine to be absorbed by the eye.
- If you think you did not get the drop of medicine into your eye properly, use another drop.
- To keep the medicine as germ-free as possible, do not touch the applicator tip to any surface (including the eye). Also, keep the container tightly closed.

Dosing—The dose of this medicine will be different for different patients. Follow your doctor's orders or the directions on the label. The following information includes only the average doses of this medicine. If your dose is different, do not change it unless your doctor tells you to do so.

The amount of medicine that you take depends on the strength of the medicine. Also, the number of doses you take each day, the time allowed between doses, and the length of time you take the medicine depend on the medical problem for which you are using the medicine.

- For ophthalmic dosage form (eye drops):
  - For inflammation after surgery:
    - Adults—Use one or two drops in the affected eye four times a day beginning twenty-four hours after surgery and continuing throughout the first two weeks after surgery.
    - Children—Use and dose must be determined by your doctor.
  - For anterior uveitis (inflammation in the iris of the eye):
    - Adults—Use one or two drops in the affected eye every hour, while awake, for the first week. Then use one drop in the affected eye every two hours, while awake, for the second week. Then gradually decrease the number of times the medicine is used each day according to your physician's instructions.
    - Children—Use and dose must be determined by your doctor.

Missed dose—If you miss a dose of this medicine, take it as soon as possible. However, if it is almost time for your next dose, skip the missed dose and go back to your regular dosing schedule. Do not double doses.

Storage—Store the medicine in a closed container at room temperature, away from heat, moisture, and direct light. Keep from freezing.

Keep out of the reach of children.

Do not keep outdated medicine or medicine no longer needed.

Precautions While Using This Medicine

An ophthalmologist (eye doctor) should examine your eyes at regular visits while you are using this medicine.

Side Effects of This Medicine

Along with its needed effects, a medicine may cause some unwanted effects. Although not all of these side effects may occur, if they do occur they may need medical attention.

Check with your doctor as soon as possible if any of the following side effects occur:

Less common or rare

Blurred vision or other change in vision; eye discharge, discomfort, dryness, or tearing; eye redness, irritation, or pain; feeling of something in the eye; itching; sore throat; stuffy or runny nose; swelling of the lining of the eyelids

Some side effects may occur that usually do not need medical attention. These side effects may go away during treatment as your body adjusts to the medicine. Also, your health care professional may be able to tell you about ways to prevent or reduce some of these side effects. Check with your health care professional if any of the following side effects continue or are bothersome or if you have any questions about them:

Less common or rare

Browache; change in taste; crusting in corner of eye; dizziness, lightheadedness, or faintness; headache; increased sensitivity of eyes to light; sticky sensation of eyelids; unusual tiredness or weakness

Other side effects not listed may also occur in some patients. If you notice any other effects, check with your healthcare professional.

RISEDRONATE (Oral route) - res-ED-roe-nate

Commonly used brand name(s)
In the U.S.—
Actonel

Available Dosage Forms:
- Tablet

Therapeutic Class: Calcium Regulator

Uses For This Medicine

Risedronate is used to prevent and treat osteoporosis (thinning of bone) in women after menopause. This medicine may also be used to increase bone mass in men who have osteoporosis, and It may be used in men and women to prevent and treat osteoporosis caused by long-term use of corticosteroids (cortisone-like medicine). Risedronate is also used to treat Paget's disease of the bone.

This medicine is available only with your doctor's prescription.

Before Using This Medicine

In deciding to use a medicine, the risks of taking the medicine must be weighed against the good it will do. This is a decision you and your doctor will make. For this medicine, the following should be considered:

Allergies—Tell your doctor if you have ever had any unusual or allergic reaction to this medicine or any other medicines. Also tell your health care professional if you have any other types of allergies, such as to foods, dyes, preservatives, or animals. For non-prescription products, read the label or package ingredients carefully.

Pediatric—There is no specific information comparing use of risedronate in children with use in other age groups.

Geriatric—Risedronate has been tested in elderly patients and has not been found to cause different side effects or problems in older people than it does in younger adults.

Pregnancy—

	Pregnancy Category	Explanation
All Trimesters	C	Animal studies have shown an adverse effect and there are no adequate studies in pregnant women OR no animal studies have been conducted and there are no adequate studies in pregnant women.

Breast Feeding—There are no adequate studies in women for determining infant risk when using this medication during breastfeeding. Weigh the potential benefits against the potential risks before taking this medication while breastfeeding.

Other medicines—Although certain medicines should not be used together at all, in other cases two different medicines may be used together even if an interaction might occur. In these cases, your doctor may want to change the dose, or other precautions may be necessary. Tell your healthcare professional if you are taking any other prescription or non-prescription (over-the-counter [OTC]) medicine.

Interactions with Food/Tobacco/Alcohol—Certain medicines should not be used at or around the time of eating food or eating certain types of food since interactions may occur. Using alcohol or tobacco with certain medicines may also cause interactions to occur. Discuss with your healthcare professional the use of your medicine with food, alcohol, or tobacco.

Other medical problems—The presence of other medical problems may affect the use of this medicine. Make sure you tell your doctor if you have any other medical problems, especially:

- Digestive system problems, including trouble swallowing, inflammation of the esophagus, or ulcer—Risedronate may make these conditions worse.

- Hypocalcemia (not enough calcium in the blood)—Hypocalcemia should be treated by your doctor before starting on risedronate.

- Inability to stand or sit upright for at least 30 minutes—This may effect the medicine getting to your stomach and it could cause your esophagus (digestive tract) to be irritated.

- Severe kidney problems—Effects of risedronate may be increased because of slower removal from the body.

Tell your doctor if you do weight-bearing exercises, smoke and/or drink excessively. Your doctor will need to take these into consideration in deciding your dose.

Proper Use of This Medicine

Take risedronate with a full glass (6 to 8 ounces) of plain water on an empty stomach. It should be taken in the morning at least 30 minutes before any food, beverage, or other medicines. Food and beverages will decrease the amount of risedronate absorbed by the body. Waiting longer than 30 minutes will allow more of the drug to be absorbed. Medicines such as antacids that contain calcium or calcium supplements also will decrease the absorption of risedronate.

Do not suck or chew on the tablet because it may cause throat irritation.

Do not lie down for 30 minutes after taking risedronate. This will help risedronate reach your stomach faster. It also will help prevent irritation to your esophagus.

It is important that you eat a well-balanced diet with adequate amounts of calcium and vitamin D (found in milk or other dairy products). However, do not take any foods, beverages, or calcium supplements within 30 minutes or longer after taking the risedronate. To do so may keep this medicine from working properly.

Follow your dosing instructions given to you by your doctor closely. It may affect the way this medicine works if you do not.

If you develop symptoms of esophageal problems such as difficulty or pain swallowing, pain behind your sternum, or severe heartburn that is continual and getting worse, tell your doctor before continuing to take this medicine.

Dosing—The dose of this medicine will be different for different patients. Follow your doctor's orders or the directions on the label. The following information includes only the average doses of this medicine. If your dose is different, do not change it unless your doctor tells you to do so.

The amount of medicine that you take depends on the strength of the medicine. Also, the number of doses you take each day, the time allowed between doses, and the length of time you take the medicine depend on the medical problem for which you are using the medicine.

- For oral dosage form (tablets):
  - For prevention and treatment of corticosteroid-induced osteoporosis:
    - Adults—5 milligrams (mg) daily at least 30 minutes before the first food or drink of the day other than water.
    - Children—Use and dose must be determined by your doctor.
  - For Paget's disease of the bone:
    - Adults—30 mg a day for two months. Your doctor may tell you to repeat this dose.
    - Children—Use and dose must be determined by your doctor.
  - For prevention and treatment of postmenopausal osteoporosis:
    - Adults—5 milligrams (mg) daily or 35 mg weekly at least 30 minutes before the first food or drink of the day other than water.
    - Children—Use and dose must be determined by your doctor.
  - For treatment of osteoporosis in men:
    - Adults—35 mg once a week at least 30 minutes before the first food or drink of the day other than water.
    - Children—Use and dose must be determined by your doctor.

Missed dose—If you miss a dose of this medicine, skip the missed dose and go back to your regular dosing schedule. Do not double doses.

If you are on a weekly schedule and miss a dose of this medicine, take it the next morning after you remember. Resume your usual schedule taking the medicine on your chosen day the next week.

Storage—Store the medicine in a closed container at room temperature, away from heat, moisture, and direct light. Keep from freezing.

Keep out of the reach of children.

Do not keep outdated medicine or medicine no longer needed.

Precautions While Using This Medicine

It is important that your doctor check your progress at regular visits to make sure this medicine is working properly and watch for unwanted effects.

It is important that you tell all of your health care providers that you are taking risedronate. If you are having dental procedures done while taking risedronate you may have an increased chance of getting a severe problem of your jaw.

Make sure you tell your doctor about any new medical problems, especially with your teeth or jaws. Tell your doctor if you have severe bone, joint, or muscle pain.

Side Effects of This Medicine

Along with its needed effects, a medicine may cause some unwanted effects. Although not all of these side effects may occur, if they do occur they may need medical attention.

Check with your doctor as soon as possible if any of the following side effects occur:
More common
    Abdominal or stomach pain; skin rash
Less common
    Abdominal or stomach pain (severe); belching; bone pain; cramping of stomach
Rare
    Red, sore eyes

Some side effects may occur that usually do not need medical attention. These side effects may go away during treatment as your body adjusts to the medicine. Also, your health care professional may be able to tell you about ways to prevent or reduce some of these side effects. Check with your health care professional if any of the following side effects continue or are bothersome or if you have any questions about them:
More common
    Back pain; cough or hoarseness; diarrhea; headache; fever or chills; joint pain; lower back or side pain; painful or difficult urination
Less common
    Acid or sour stomach; bladder pain; bloody or cloudy urine; blurred vision or change in vision; body aches or pains; chest pain; congestion; constipation; dizziness; difficult, burning, or painful urination; difficulty in moving; dry eyes; dryness or soreness of throat; frequent urge to urinate; general feeling of discomfort or illness; heartburn; indigestion; leg cramps; muscle pain or stiffness; nausea; nervousness; pain, swelling, or redness in joints; pounding in the ears; ringing in the ears; runny nose; slow or fast heartbeat; stomach discomfort, upset, or pain; swelling of feet or lower legs; tender swollen glands in neck; trouble swallowing; voice changes; weakness
Rare
    Abdominal discomfort; fainting; fear; itching skin; loss of appetite; pale skin; passing of gas; redness, swelling

or soreness of tongue; shortness of breath; sneezing; troubled breathing; sore throat; stomach fullness; tightness in chest; troubled breathing with exertion; unusual bleeding or bruising; unusual tiredness or weakness; vomiting; wheezing

Not known

Large, hive-like swelling on face, eyelids, lips, tongue, throat, hands, legs, feet, sex organs; muscle pain; rash; skin blisters

Other side effects not listed may also occur in some patients. If you notice any other effects, check with your healthcare professional.

RISPERIDONE (Oral route) - ris-PER-i-done

Black Box Warning

Elderly patients with dementia-related psychosis treated with atypical antipsychotic drugs are at an increased risk of death compared to placebo. Analyses of seventeen placebo controlled trials (modal duration of 10 weeks) in these patients revealed a risk of death in the drug-treated patients of between 1.6 times to 1.7 times that seen in placebo-treated patients. Over the course of a typical 10 week controlled trial, the rate of death in drug-treated patients was about 4.5%, compared to a rate of about 2.6% in the placebo group. Although the causes of death were varied, most of the deaths appeared to be either cardiovascular (eg, heart failure, sudden death) or infectious (eg, pneumonia) in nature. Risperidone is not approved for the treatment of patients with dementia-related psychosis.

Commonly used brand name(s)

In the U.S.—
Risperdal
Risperdal M-Tab

Available Dosage Forms:
- Tablet, Disintegrating
- Tablet
- Solution

Therapeutic Class: Antipsychotic

Uses For This Medicine

Risperidone is used to treat the symptoms of psychotic disorders, such as schizophrenia. This medicine should NOT be used to treat behavioral problems in older adult patients who have dementia.

Risperidone is available only with your doctor's prescription.

Before Using This Medicine

In deciding to use a medicine, the risks of taking the medicine must be weighed against the good it will do. This is a decision you and your doctor will make. For this medicine, the following should be considered:

Allergies—Tell your doctor if you have ever had any unusual or allergic reaction to this medicine or any other medi-

cines. Also tell your health care professional if you have any other types of allergies, such as to foods, dyes, preservatives, or animals. For non-prescription products, read the label or package ingredients carefully.

Pediatric—Studies on this medicine have been done only in adult patients, and there is no specific information comparing use of risperidone in children with use in other age groups.

Geriatric—Elderly people may be especially sensitive to the effects of risperidone. This may increase the chance of having side effects during treatment. This medicine should not be used for behavioral problems in older adults with dementia.

Pregnancy—

	Pregnancy Category	Explanation
All Trimesters	C	Animal studies have shown an adverse effect and there are no adequate studies in pregnant women OR no animal studies have been conducted and there are no adequate studies in pregnant women.

Breast Feeding—There are no adequate studies in women for determining infant risk when using this medication during breastfeeding. Weigh the potential benefits against the potential risks before taking this medication while breastfeeding.

Other medicines—

Using this medicine with any of the following medicines is not recommended. Your doctor may decide not to treat you with this medication or change some of the other medicines you take.

Bepridil, Cisapride, Levomethadyl, Mesoridazine, Pimozide, Terfenadine, Thioridazine, Ziprasidone

Interactions   with   Food/Tobacco/Alcohol—Certain medicines should not be used at or around the time of eating food or eating certain types of food since interactions may occur. Using alcohol or tobacco with certain medicines may also cause interactions to occur. Discuss with your healthcare professional the use of your medicine with food, alcohol, or tobacco.

Other medical problems—The presence of other medical problems may affect the use of this medicine. Make sure you tell your doctor if you have any other medical problems, especially:

- Aspiration pneumonia, risk or history of—May increase risk of adverse events

- Breast cancer or

- Heart or blood vessel problems, including stroke and unusual heartbeats or

- Parkinson's disease—Risperidone may make these conditions worse

- Dehydration or

- Blood circulation problems—These conditions may increase the chance of side effects from the medicine

- Dementia, such as decreasing mental ability or

- Difficulty swallowing—These conditions may increase the chance of side effects from the medicine

- Diabetes or family history of diabetes—May make condition worse and cause serious side effects
- Drug abuse problems in the past—These patients should be observed for any signs of abuse of this medicine.
- Epilepsy or other seizure disorders—Risperidone may increase the risk of having seizures
- Kidney disease or
- Liver disease—Higher blood levels of risperidone may occur, increasing the chance of side effects
- Other medical problems causing vomiting [e.g., brain tumor, bowel blockage, drug overdose, Reye's syndrome]—Risperidone may prevent vomiting and hide these medical problems from you and your doctor
- Phenylketonuria (PKU)—The oral disintegrating tablets may contain aspartame, which can make your condition worse.

Proper Use of This Medicine

Take this medicine only as directed by your doctor to benefit your condition as much as possible. Do not take more or less of it, do not take it more or less often, and do not take it for a longer or shorter time than your doctor ordered.

Dosing—The dose of this medicine will be different for different patients. Follow your doctor's orders or the directions on the label. The following information includes only the average doses of this medicine. If your dose is different, do not change it unless your doctor tells you to do so.

The amount of medicine that you take depends on the strength of the medicine. Also, the number of doses you take each day, the time allowed between doses, and the length of time you take the medicine depend on the medical problem for which you are using the medicine.

- For symptoms of psychotic disorder:
  - For oral solution dosage form—
    - Adults—At first, 1 milligram (mg) [1 milliliter (mL)] per day. The medicine can be given on a once a day or twice a day schedule. Your doctor may increase your dose as needed. However, the dose usually is not more than 16 mg (16 mL) a day.
    - Children younger than 18 years of age—Use and dose must be determined by the doctor.
    - Older adults—At first, 0.25 mg or 0.5 mg (0.5 mL) two times a day. The medicine can be given on a once a day schedule after your doctor has found the correct dose for you. Your doctor may increase your dose as needed. However, the dose usually is not more than 3 mg (3 mL) a day.
  - For oral tablet and orally disintegrating tablet dosage forms—
    - Adults—At first, 1 milligram (mg) per day. The medicine can be given on a once a day or twice a day schedule. Your doctor may increase your dose as needed. However, the dose usually is not more than 16 mg a day.
    - Children younger than 18 years of age—Use and dose must be determined by the doctor.
    - Older adults—At first, 0.25 mg or 0.5 mg two times a day. The medicine can be given on a once a day schedule after your doctor has found the correct dose for you. Your doctor may increase

your dose as needed. However, the dose usually is not more than 3 mg a day.

For patients taking the oral solution form of risperidone:

- Measure the dose with the measuring device provided with your medicine. Stir the dose into a small glass (3 to 4 ounces) of water, coffee, orange juice, or low-fat milk just before taking it. Do not mix this medicine with cola or tea.
- Rinse the empty measuring device with water and place it back in its storage case. Put the plastic cap back on the bottle of medicine.

For patients taking the orally disintegrating tablet form of risperidone:

- Do not open the package until you are ready to take your medicine. To remove one tablet, separate one of the four tablets by tearing apart on perforations. Bend the corner as shown on the package. Peel back the foil to get to the tablet, do not push the tablet through the foil because that could damage the tablet.
- Use dry hands and take the tablet out of the package and immediately place it on your tongue. The tablet needs to be used immediately because it can not be stored once it is taken out of the package. Once the tablet is on your tongue it will disintegrate in seconds. You can swallow it with or without liquid. It is important not to split or chew the tablet.

Missed dose—If you miss a dose of this medicine, take it as soon as possible. However, if it is almost time for your next dose, skip the missed dose and go back to your regular dosing schedule. Do not double doses.

Storage—Store the medicine in a closed container at room temperature, away from heat, moisture, and direct light. Keep from freezing.

Keep out of the reach of children.

Do not keep outdated medicine or medicine no longer needed.

Precautions While Using This Medicine

Your doctor should check your progress at regular visits, especially during the first few months of treatment with this medicine. This will allow the dosage to be changed if necessary to meet your needs.

Do not stop taking this medicine without first checking with your doctor. Your doctor may want you to reduce gradually the amount you are taking before stopping completely. This is to prevent side effects and to keep your condition from becoming worse.

This medicine may add to the effects of alcohol and other CNS depressants (medicine that makes you drowsy or less alert). Some examples of CNS depressants are antihistamines or medicine for hay fever, other allergies, or colds; sedatives, tranquilizers, or sleeping medicine; prescription pain medicine or narcotics; barbiturates; medicine for seizures; muscle relaxants; or anesthetics, including some dental anesthetics. Check with your doctor before taking any of the above while you are using this medicine.

Before having any kind of surgery, dental treatment, or emergency treatment, tell the medical doctor or dentist in charge that you are using this medicine. Taking risperidone together with medicines that are used during surgery, dental, or emergency treatments may increase the CNS depressant effects.

This medicine may cause blurred vision, dizziness, or drowsiness. Make sure you know how you react to this medicine before you drive, use machines, or do anything else that could be dangerous if you are not alert or able to see clearly.

Dizziness, lightheadedness, or fainting may occur, especially when you get up from a lying or sitting position. Getting up slowly may help. If the problem continues or gets worse, check with your doctor.

Risperidone may cause your skin to be more sensitive to sunlight than it is normally. Exposure to sunlight, even for brief periods of time, may cause a skin rash, itching, redness or other discoloration of the skin, or a severe sunburn. When you begin taking this medicine:

- Stay out of direct sunlight, especially between the hours of 10:00 a.m. and 3:00 p.m., if possible.
- Wear protective clothing, including a hat. Also, wear sunglasses.
- Apply a sun block product that has a skin protection factor (SPF) of at least 15. You may require a product with a higher SPF number, especially if you have a fair complexion. If you have any questions about this, check with your health care professional.
- Apply a sun block lipstick that has an SPF of at least 15 to protect your lips.
- Do not use a sunlamp or tanning bed or booth.

If you have a severe reaction from the sun, check with your doctor.

This medicine may make it more difficult for your body to keep a constant temperature. Use extra care not to become overheated during exercise or hot weather while you are taking this medicine, since overheating may result in heatstroke. Hot baths or saunas may make you feel dizzy or faint while you are taking this medicine. Also, use extra care not to become too cold while you are taking risperidone. If you become too cold, you may feel drowsy, confused, or clumsy.

Side Effects of This Medicine

Along with its needed effects, risperidone can sometimes cause serious side effects. Tardive dyskinesia (a movement disorder) may occur and may not go away after you stop using the medicine. Signs of tardive dyskinesia include fine, worm-like movements of the tongue, or other uncontrolled movements of the mouth, tongue, cheeks, jaw, or arms and legs. Other serious but rare side effects may also occur. These include neuroleptic malignant syndrome (NMS), which may cause severe muscle stiffness, fever, severe tiredness or weakness, fast heartbeat, difficult breathing, increased sweating, loss of bladder control, or seizures. You and your doctor should discuss the good this medicine will do as well as the risks of taking it.

Stop taking this medicine and get emergency help immediately if any of the following effects occur:

Rare

Convulsions (seizures); difficult or fast breathing; fast heartbeat or irregular pulse; fever (high); high or low blood pressure; increased sweating; loss of bladder control; muscle stiffness (severe); unusually pale skin; unusual tiredness or weakness (severe)

Check with your doctor immediately if any of the following side effects occur:

More common

Difficulty in speaking or swallowing; inability to move eyes; muscle spasms of face, neck, and back; twisting movements of body

Less common

speech or vision problems; sudden weakness or numbness in the face, arms or legs

Rare

High body temperature (dizziness; fast, shallow breathing; fast, weak heartbeat; headache; muscle cramps; pale, clammy skin; increased thirst); lip smacking or puckering; low body temperature (confusion, drowsiness, poor coordination, shivering); prolonged, painful, inappropriate erection of the penis; puffing of cheeks; rapid or worm-like movements of tongue; uncontrolled chewing movements; uncontrolled movements of arms and legs

Check with your doctor as soon as possible if any of the following side effects occur:

More common

Anxiety or nervousness; changes in vision, including blurred vision; decreased sexual desire or performance; loss of balance control; mask-like face; menstrual changes; mood or mental changes, including aggressive behavior, agitation, difficulty in concentration, and memory problems; problems in urination or increase in amount of urine; restlessness or need to keep moving (severe); shuffling walk; skin rash or itching; stiffness or weakness of arms or legs; tic-like or twitching movements; trembling and shaking of fingers and hands; trouble in sleeping

Less common

Back pain; chest pain; unusual secretion of milk

Rare

Extreme thirst; increased blinking or spasms of eyelid; loss of appetite; talking, feeling, and acting with excitement and activity that cannot be controlled; uncontrolled twisting movements of neck, trunk, arms, or legs; unusual bleeding or bruising; unusual facial expressions or body positions

Some side effects may occur that usually do not need medical attention. These side effects may go away during treatment as your body adjusts to the medicine. Also, your health care professional may be able to tell you about ways to prevent or reduce some of these side effects. Check with your health care professional if any of the following side effects continue or are bothersome or if you have any questions about them:

More common

Constipation; coughing; diarrhea; drowsiness; dryness of mouth; headache; heartburn; increased dream activity; increased length of sleep; nausea; sleepiness or unusual drowsiness; sore throat; stuffy or runny nose; unusual tiredness or weakness; weight gain

Less common

Back pain; body aches or pain; chills; dandruff; darkening of skin color; dry skin; ear congestion; fever; increase in body movements; increased sensitivity of the skin to sun; increased watering of mouth; joint pain; loss of voice; nasal congestion; oily skin; pain or tenderness around eyes and cheekbones; shortness of breath or troubled breathing; sneezing; stomach pain; toothache; tightness of chest or wheezing; vomiting; weight loss

Some side effects, such as uncontrolled movements of the mouth, tongue, and jaw, or uncontrolled movements of arms and legs, may occur after you have stopped taking this medicine. If you notice any of these effects, check with your doctor as soon as possible.

Other side effects not listed may also occur in some patients. If you notice any other effects, check with your healthcare professional.

RITODRINE   (Oral route, Intravenous route) - RI-toe-dreen

Uses For This Medicine

Ritodrine is used to stop premature labor. It is available only with your doctor's prescription.

Before Using This Medicine

In deciding to use a medicine, the risks of taking the medicine must be weighed against the good it will do. This is a decision you and your doctor will make. For this medicine, the following should be considered:

Allergies—Tell your doctor if you have ever had any unusual or allergic reaction to this medicine or any other medicines. Also tell your health care professional if you have any other types of allergies, such as to foods, dyes, preservatives, or animals. For non-prescription products, read the label or package ingredients carefully.

Pregnancy—

	Pregnancy Category	Explanation
All Trimesters	B	Animal studies have revealed no evidence of harm to the fetus, however, there are no adequate studies in pregnant women OR animal studies have shown an adverse effect, but adequate studies in pregnant women have failed to demonstrate a risk to the fetus.

Breast Feeding—There are no adequate studies in women for determining infant risk when using this medication during breastfeeding. Weigh the potential benefits against the potential risks before taking this medication while breastfeeding.

Other medicines—

Using this medicine with any of the following medicines is usually not recommended, but may be required in some cases. If both medicines are prescribed together, your doctor may change the dose or how often you use one or both of the medicines.

Clorgyline, Iproniazid, Isocarboxazid, Moclobemide, Nialamide, Pargyline, Phenelzine, Procarbazine, Selegiline, Toloxatone, Tranylcypromine

Interactions with Food/Tobacco/Alcohol—Certain medicines should not be used at or around the time of eating food or eating certain types of food since interactions may occur. Using alcohol or tobacco with certain medicines may also cause interactions to occur. Discuss with your healthcare professional the use of your medicine with food, alcohol, or tobacco.

Other medical problems—The presence of other medical problems may affect the use of this medicine. Make sure you tell your doctor if you have any other medical problems, especially:

- Type 2 diabetes mellitus—Ritodrine may make this condition worse
- Heart or blood vessel disease or
- Overactive thyroid, uncontrolled—Use of ritodrine may cause serious effects of the heart, including irregular heartbeat
- High blood pressure (hypertension), uncontrolled, or
- Migraine headaches (or history of)—Ritodrine may make these conditions worse. Rarely, use of ritodrine during a migraine headache may cause problems with blood circulation in the brain

---

Proper Use of This Medicine

Dosing—The dose of this medicine will be different for different patients. Follow your doctor's orders or the directions on the label. The following information includes only the average doses of this medicine. If your dose is different, do not change it unless your doctor tells you to do so.

The amount of medicine that you take depends on the strength of the medicine. Also, the number of doses you take each day, the time allowed between doses, and the length of time you take the medicine depend on the medical problem for which you are using the medicine.

- For oral dosage form (extended-release capsules):
  - Adults: In the first twenty-four hours after the doctor stops your intravenous ritodrine, your dose may be as high as 40 milligrams (mg) every eight hours. After that, the dose is usually 40 mg taken every eight to twelve hours. Your doctor may want you to take oral ritodrine up until it is time for you to deliver your baby or until your 37th week of pregnancy.
- For oral dosage form (tablets):
  - Adults: In the first twenty-four hours after the doctor stops your intravenous ritodrine, your dose may be as high as 10 mg every two hours. After that, the dose is usually 10 to 20 mg every four to six hours. Your doctor may want you to take oral ritodrine up until it is time for you to deliver your baby or until your 37th week of pregnancy.
- For injection dosage form:
  - Adults: 50 to 350 micrograms per minute, injected into a vein.

Missed dose—If you miss a dose of this medicine, take it as soon as possible. However, if it is almost time for your next dose, skip the missed dose and go back to your regular dosing schedule. Do not double doses.

Storage—Store the medicine in a closed container at room temperature, away from heat, moisture, and direct light. Keep from freezing.

Keep out of the reach of children.

Do not keep outdated medicine or medicine no longer needed.

Precautions While Using This Medicine

Check with your doctor right away if your contractions begin again or your water breaks.

Do not take other medicines unless they have been discussed with your doctor. This especially includes over-the-counter (nonprescription) medicines for appetite control, asthma, colds, cough, hay fever, or sinus problems since they may increase the unwanted effects of this medicine.

Side Effects of This Medicine

Along with its needed effects, a medicine may cause some unwanted effects. Although not all of these side effects may occur, if they do occur they may need medical attention.

Check with your doctor immediately if any of the following side effects occur:

  More common
    Chest pain or tightness; shortness of breath— rare with oral form

Check with your doctor as soon as possible if any of the following side effects occur:

  More common
    Blurred vision; dizziness or lightheadedness; drowsiness; dry mouth; flushed and dry skin; fast or irregular heartbeat—rare with oral form; fruit-like breath odor; increased urination; loss of appetite; nausea; severe pounding or racing heartbeat—rare with oral form; sleepiness; stomachache; tiredness; troubled breathing (rapid and deep); unusual thirst; vomiting

  Rare
    Sore throat or fever; yellow eyes or skin

  Symptoms of overdose
    Fast or irregular heartbeat (severe); nausea or vomiting (severe); nervousness or trembling (severe); shortness of breath (severe)

Some side effects may occur that usually do not need medical attention. These side effects may go away during treatment as your body adjusts to the medicine. Also, your health care professional may be able to tell you about ways to prevent or reduce some of these side effects. Check with your health care professional if any of the following side effects continue or are bothersome or if you have any questions about them:

  More common
    Headache; reddened skin; trembling

  Less common or rare
    Anxiety; emotional upset; jitteriness, nervousness, or restlessness; skin rash

After you stop using this medicine, it may still produce some side effects that need attention. During this period of time, *check with your doctor immediately* if you notice the following side effects:

    Shortness of breath

Other side effects not listed may also occur in some patients. If you notice any other effects, check with your healthcare professional.

RITONAVIR   (Oral route) - ri-TOE-na-veer

Black Box Warning

Co-administration of ritonavir with certain nonsedating antihistamines, sedative hypnotics, antiarrhythmics, or ergot alkaloid preparations may result in potentially serious and/or life-threatening adverse events due to possible effects of ritonavir on the hepatic metabolism of certain drugs.

Commonly used brand name(s)
In the U.S.—
    Norvir

Available Dosage Forms:
  • Capsule, Liquid Filled
  • Solution

Therapeutic Class: Antiretroviral Agent
Pharmacologic Class: Protease Inhibitor

Uses For This Medicine

Ritonavir is used, alone or in combination with other medicines, in the treatment of the infection caused by the human immunodeficiency virus (HIV). HIV is the virus that causes acquired immune deficiency syndrome (AIDS).

Ritonavir will not cure or prevent HIV infection or AIDS; however, it helps keep HIV from reproducing and appears to slow down the destruction of the immune system. This may help delay the development of problems usually related to AIDS or HIV disease. Ritonavir will not keep you from spreading HIV to other people. People who receive this medicine may continue to have other problems usually related to AIDS or HIV disease.

This medicine is available only with your doctor's prescription.

Before Using This Medicine

In deciding to use a medicine, the risks of taking the medicine must be weighed against the good it will do. This is a decision you and your doctor will make. For this medicine, the following should be considered:

Allergies—Tell your doctor if you have ever had any unusual or allergic reaction to this medicine or any other medicines. Also tell your health care professional if you have any other types of allergies, such as to foods, dyes, preservatives, or animals. For non-prescription products, read the label or package ingredients carefully.

Pediatric—This medicine has been tested in a limited number of childrenolder than 1 month of age. In effective doses, the medicine has not been shown to cause different side effects or problems than it does in adults.

Geriatric—Many medicines have not been studied specifically in older people. Therefore, it may not be known whether they work exactly the same way they do in younger adults.

There is no specific information comparing use of ritonavir in the elderly with use in other age groups.

Pregnancy—

	Pregnancy Category	Explanation
All Trimesters	B	Animal studies have revealed no evidence of harm to the fetus, however, there are no adequate studies in pregnant women OR animal studies have shown an adverse effect, but adequate studies in pregnant women have failed to demonstrate a risk to the fetus.

Breast Feeding—There are no adequate studies in women for determining infant risk when using this medication during breastfeeding. Weigh the potential benefits against the potential risks before taking this medication while breastfeeding.

Other medicines—

Using this medicine with any of the following medicines is not recommended. Your doctor may decide not to treat you with this medication or change some of the other medicines you take.

Alfuzosin, Amiodarone, Astemizole, Bepridil, Cisapride, Conivaptan, Dihydroergotamine, Encainide, Eplerenone, Ergoloid Mesylates, Ergonovine, Ergotamine, Flecainide, Methylergonovine, Methysergide, Midazolam, Pimozide, Propafenone, Quinidine, Ranolazine, St John's Wort, Terfenadine, Triazolam, Voriconazole

Interactions with Food/Tobacco/Alcohol—Certain medicines should not be used at or around the time of eating food or eating certain types of food since interactions may occur. Using alcohol or tobacco with certain medicines may also cause interactions to occur. Discuss with your healthcare professional the use of your medicine with food, alcohol, or tobacco.

Other medical problems—The presence of other medical problems may affect the use of this medicine. Make sure you tell your doctor if you have any other medical problems, especially:

- Diabetes mellitus (sugar diabetes)—Ritonavir may increase the amount of sugar in your blood.
- Hemophilia—Possible increased risk of bleeding
- Liver disease or other liver problems—Effects of ritonavir may be increased because of slower removal from the body

Proper Use of This Medicine

It is important that ritonavir be taken with food.

For patients taking the solution (liquid) form of this medicine:

- Shake the bottle well before using.
- Use a specially marked measuring syringe to measure each dose accurately. The average household teaspoon may not hold the right amount of liquid.

Take this medicine exactly as directed by your doctor. Do not take it more often, and do not take it for a longer time than your doctor ordered. Also, do not stop taking this medicine without checking with your doctor first.

Keep taking ritonavir for the full time of treatment, even if you begin to feel better.

This medicine works best when there is a constant amount in the blood. To help keep the amount constant, do not miss any doses. Also, it is best to take the doses at evenly spaced times, day and night. For example, if you are to take two doses a day, the doses should be spaced about 12 hours apart. If you need help in planning the best times to take your medicine, check with your health care professional.

Only take medicine that your doctor has prescribed specially for you. Do not share your medicine with others.

Dosing—The dose of this medicine will be different for different patients. Follow your doctor's orders or the directions on the label. The following information includes only the average doses of this medicine. If your dose is different, do not change it unless your doctor tells you to do so.

The amount of medicine that you take depends on the strength of the medicine. Also, the number of doses you take each day, the time allowed between doses, and the length of time you take the medicine depend on the medical problem for which you are using the medicine.

- For oral dosage form (capsules):
  - For treatment of HIV infection:
    - Adults—600 milligrams (mg) two times a day.
    - Children—This oral dosage form is usually not used for children. Please refer to oral solution dosage form.
- For oral dosage form (oral solution):
  - For treatment of HIV infection:
    - Adults—600 milligrams (mg) two times a day.
    - Infants and children older than 1 month of age—Dose is based on body size and must be determined by your doctor.
    - Infants 1 month of age or less—Use and dose must be determined by your doctor.

Note: Ritonavir can be used in combination with other medicines. Check with your doctor for more information on these doses.

Missed dose—If you miss a dose of this medicine, take it as soon as possible. However, if it is almost time for your next dose, skip the missed dose and go back to your regular dosing schedule. Do not double doses.

Storage—Keep out of the reach of children.

Do not keep outdated medicine or medicine no longer needed.

Store the capsule form of this medicine in the refrigerator. The oral solution form should not be refrigerated; it should be stored at room temperature.

Precautions While Using This Medicine

Do not take any other medicines without checking with your doctor first. To do so may increase the chance of side effects from ritonavir or the other medicines.

It is very important that your doctor check your progress at regular visits to make sure this medicine is working properly and check for unwanted effects, especially increases in blood sugar.

This medicine may decrease the effects of some oral contraceptives (birth control pills). To avoid unwanted pregnancy, it is a good idea to use some additional contraceptive measures while being treated with ritonavir.

Side Effects of This Medicine

Along with its needed effects, a medicine may cause some unwanted effects. Although not all of these side effects may occur, if they do occur they may need medical attention.

Check with your doctor as soon as possible if any of the following side effects occur:

Less common

Fainting; feeling faint, dizzy, or light-headedness; feeling of warmth or heat; flushing or redness of skin especially on face and neck; headache; sweating

Rare

Confusion; dehydration; dry or itchy skin; fatigue; fruity mouth odor; increased hunger; increased thirst; increased urination; nausea; vomiting; weight loss

Not known

Bloating; chills; constipation; convulsions; cough; darkened urine; decreased urination; difficulty breathing; dry mouth; fast heartbeat; fever; hives or welts; increase in heart rate; indigestion; itching; large, hive-like swelling on face, eyelids, lips, tongue, throat, hands, legs, feet, sex organs; loss of appetite; loss of bladder control; muscle spasm or jerking of all extremities; noisy breathing; pains in stomach, side, or abdomen, possibly radiating to the back; rapid breathing; redness of skin; shortness of breath; skin rash; sudden loss of consciousness; sunken eyes; thirst; tightness in chest; unusual tiredness or weakness; wheezing; wrinkled skin; yellow eyes or skin

Some side effects may occur that usually do not need medical attention. These side effects may go away during treatment as your body adjusts to the medicine. Also, your health care professional may be able to tell you about ways to prevent or reduce some of these side effects. Check with your health care professional if any of the following side effects continue or are bothersome or if you have any questions about them:

More common

Abdominal pain; acid or sour stomach; belching; burning, crawling, itching, numbness, prickling, pins and needles, or tingling feelings; Change in sense of taste; diarrhea; dizziness; heartburn; sleepiness or unusual drowsiness; sleeplessness; trouble sleeping; unable to sleep; weakness

Less common

Bloated, full feeling; body aches or pain; congestion; delusions; dementia; difficulty in moving; discouragement; dryness or soreness of throat; excess air or gas in stomach or intestines; fear; feeling sad or empty; general feeling of discomfort or illness; hoarseness; increased urge to urinate during the night; irritability; lack of appetite; loss of interest or pleasure; mood or mental changes; muscle pain or stiffness; nervousness; pain in joints or in unspecified location; passing gas; runny nose; tender, swollen glands in neck; throat irritation; tiredness; trouble concentrating; trouble in swallowing; voice changes; waking to urinate at night

Not known

Increased fat deposits on face, neck, and trunk

Other side effects not listed may also occur in some patients. If you notice any other effects, check with your healthcare professional.

RITUXIMAB　(Intravenous route) - ri-TUK-si-mab

Black Box Warning

Fatal Infusion Reactions: Deaths within 24 hours of rituximab infusion have been reported. These fatal reactions followed an infusion reaction complex which included hypoxia, pulmonary infiltrates, acute respiratory distress syndrome, myocardial infarction, ventricular fibrillation or cardiogenic shock. Approximately 80% of fatal infusion reactions occurred in association with the first infusion.

Patients who develop severe infusion reactions should have rituximab infusion discontinued and receive medical treatment.

Tumor Lysis Syndrome (TLS): Acute renal failure requiring dialysis with instances of fatal outcome has been reported in the setting of TLS following treatment with rituximab.

Severe mucocutaneous reactions, some with fatal outcome, have been reported in association with rituximab treatment.

Commonly used brand name(s)

In the U.S.—

Rituxan

Available Dosage Forms:

- Solution

Therapeutic Class: Antineoplastic Agent
Pharmacologic Class: Monoclonal Antibody

Uses For This Medicine

Rituximab is a monoclonal antibody. It is used to treat a type of cancer called non-Hodgkin's lymphoma. It can be used alone or with other cancer medicines or chemotherapy.

Rituximab is to be administered only by or under the immediate supervision of your doctor.

Once a medicine has been approved for marketing for a certain use, experience may show that it is also useful for other medical problems. Although these uses are not included in product labeling, rituximab is used in certain patients with the following medical conditions:

- Chronic lymphocytic leukemia (a type of cancer of the blood and lymph system)
- Waldenstrom's macroglobulinemia (a certain type of cancer of the blood)
- Immune or idiopathic thrombocytopenic purpura (ITP) (a blood disease)

Before Using This Medicine

In deciding to use a medicine, the risks of taking the medicine must be weighed against the good it will do. This is a decision

you and your doctor will make. For this medicine, the following should be considered:

Allergies—Tell your doctor if you have ever had any unusual or allergic reaction to this medicine or any other medicines. Also tell your health care professional if you have any other types of allergies, such as to foods, dyes, preservatives, or animals. For non-prescription products, read the label or package ingredients carefully.

Pediatric—Studies on this medicine have been done only in adult patients, and there is no specific information comparing use of rituximab in children with use in other age groups.

Geriatric—This medicine has been tested and has not been shown to cause different side effects or problems in older people than it does in younger adults.

Pregnancy—

	Pregnancy Category	Explanation
All Trimesters	C	Animal studies have shown an adverse effect and there are no adequate studies in pregnant women OR no animal studies have been conducted and there are no adequate studies in pregnant women.

Breast Feeding—There are no adequate studies in women for determining infant risk when using this medication during breastfeeding. Weigh the potential benefits against the potential risks before taking this medication while breastfeeding.

Other medicines—

Using this medicine with any of the following medicines is not recommended. Your doctor may decide not to treat you with this medication or change some of the other medicines you take.

Rotavirus Vaccine, Live

Interactions with Food/Tobacco/Alcohol—Certain medicines should not be used at or around the time of eating food or eating certain types of food since interactions may occur. Using alcohol or tobacco with certain medicines may also cause interactions to occur. Discuss with your healthcare professional the use of your medicine with food, alcohol, or tobacco.

Other medical problems—The presence of other medical problems may affect the use of this medicine. Make sure you tell your doctor if you have any other medical problems, especially:

The presence of other medical problems may affect the use of rituximab. Make sure you tell your doctor if you have any other medical problems, especially

- Heart problems (e.g., angina, arrhythmias) or
- Lung problems—Your doctor will want to check you periodically for heart and lung problems, especially if you have had serious problems in the past.
- Hepatitis B virus—Rituximab can cause the hepatitis B virus to worsen, resulting in serious liver problems.
- High number of cancerous cells in your body or
- Kidney problems—You may be at higher risk for very serious unwanted effects.

- Sensitivity or a previous severe allergic reaction to rituximab or to mouse proteins—Your doctor should not administer rituximab if you have experienced a previous allergic reaction.

Proper Use of This Medicine

Dosing—The dose of this medicine will be different for different patients. Follow your doctor's orders or the directions on the label. The following information includes only the average doses of this medicine. If your dose is different, do not change it unless your doctor tells you to do so.

The amount of medicine that you take depends on the strength of the medicine. Also, the number of doses you take each day, the time allowed between doses, and the length of time you take the medicine depend on the medical problem for which you are using the medicine.

Side Effects of This Medicine

Along with its needed effects, a medicine may cause some unwanted effects. Although not all of these side effects may occur, if they do occur they may need medical attention.

Check with your doctor as soon as possible if any of the following side effects occur:
More common
Black, tarry stools; bleeding gums; bloating or swelling of face, arms, hands, lower legs or feet; blood in urine or stools; blurred vision; cough or hoarseness; dizziness; dry mouth; fatigue; feeling of swelling of tongue or throat; fever and chills; flushed, dry skin; flushing of face; fruit-like breath odor; headache; increased hunger; increased thirst; increased urination; itching; lower back or side pain; nausea; nervousness; pain or tenderness around eyes and cheekbones; painful or difficult urination; pale skin; pinpoint red spots on skin; pounding in the ears; rapid weight gain; runny nose; shortness of breath; skin rash; slow or fast heartbeat; sore throat; sores, ulcers or white spots in mouth or on lips; stuffy or runny nose; sweating; swollen glands; tightness of chest; tingling of hands or feet; troubled breathing; troubled breathing with exertion; unexplained weight gain; unusual bleeding or bruising; unusual tiredness or weakness; unusual weight gain or loss; vomiting; wheezing

Less common
Blistering, peeling, loosening of the skin; blisters in the mouth; blisters on the trunk, scalp or other areas; burning, crawling, itching, numbness, prickling, "pins and needles", or tingling feeling; burning, tingling, numbness or pain in the hands, arms, feet, or legs,; confusion; decreased frequency and amount of urination; diarrhea; difficulty in moving; discouragement; feeling sad or empty; increased thirst; irregular heartbeat; irritability; joint or muscle pain; loss of appetite; loss of interest or pleasure; muscle pain or stiffness; muscle cramps; nervousness; numbness or tingling in hands, feet, or lips; pain at place of injection; pain, swelling, or redness in joints; red, itchy lining of eye; red skin lesions, often with a purple center; stabbing pain; trouble concentrating; trouble sleeping; swelling of face or fingers; swelling of feet or lower legs; weight gain

Rare

Chest pain

Incidence not known

Abdominal or stomach cramps or pain; blindness; blue-yellow color blindness; blurred vision or other change in vision; burning or stinging of skin; decreased vision; dry cough; eye pain, tearing; inflammation of joints; nosebleed; pain in many joints; painful cold sores or blisters on lips, nose, eyes, or genitals; redness of eye; redness, soreness or itching of skin; sensitivity of eye to light; severe abdominal pain; severe vomiting, sometimes with blood; sores, welting, or blisters; swelling, stiffness, redness, or warmth around many joints; swollen lymph glands; vision loss; weight loss

This medicine may also cause the following side effects that your doctor will watch for:

Less common

High blood pressure; low white blood cell count

Some side effects may occur that usually do not need medical attention. These side effects may go away during treatment as your body adjusts to the medicine. Also, your health care professional may be able to tell you about ways to prevent or reduce some of these side effects. Check with your health care professional if any of the following side effects continue or are bothersome or if you have any questions about them:

More common

Back pain; fear; increased cough; joint pain; lack or loss of strength; muscle aching or cramping; night sweats; pain; pain in joints; rash; swollen joints; throat irritation

Less common

Agitation or anxiety; change in taste; dry eyes; excessive muscle tone; feeling of constant movement of self or surroundings; feeling of weakness; general feeling of discomfort or illness; heartburn; increase in body movements; lightheadedness; muscle tension; pain at injection site; sensation of spinning; sleepiness or unusual drowsiness; swelling of stomach; trouble in sleeping

After you stop using this medicine, it may still produce some side effects that need attention. During this period of time, *check with your doctor immediately* if you notice the following side effects:

Black, tarry stools; blood in urine or stools; painful or difficult urination; pinpoint red spots on skin; unusual bleeding or bruising; unusual tiredness or weakness

Other side effects not listed may also occur in some patients. If you notice any other effects, check with your healthcare professional.

RIVASTIGMINE (Oral route) - ri-va-STIG-meen

Commonly used brand name(s)

In the U.S.—

Exelon

Available Dosage Forms:

- Solution
- Capsule

Therapeutic Class: Central Nervous System Agent

Pharmacologic Class: Cholinesterase Inhibitor, Centrally Acting

---

Uses For This Medicine

Rivastigmine is used to treat the symptoms of mild to moderate Alzheimer's disease. Rivastigmine will not cure Alzheimer's disease, and it will not stop the disease from getting worse. However, rivastigmine can improve thinking ability in some patients with Alzheimer's disease.

In Alzheimer's disease, many chemical changes take place in the brain. One of the earliest and biggest changes is that there is less of a chemical called acetylcholine (ACh). ACh helps the brain to work properly. Rivastigmine slows the breakdown of ACh, so it can build up and have a greater effect. However, as Alzheimer's disease gets worse, there will be less and less ACh, so rivastigmine may not work as well.

This medicine is available only with your doctor's prescription.

Before Using This Medicine

In deciding to use a medicine, the risks of taking the medicine must be weighed against the good it will do. This is a decision you and your doctor will make. For this medicine, the following should be considered:

Allergies—Tell your doctor if you have ever had any unusual or allergic reaction to this medicine or any other medicines. Also tell your health care professional if you have any other types of allergies, such as to foods, dyes, preservatives, or animals. For non-prescription products, read the label or package ingredients carefully.

Pediatric—Studies on this medicine have been done only in adult patients, and there is no specific information comparing use of rivastigmine in children with use in other age groups.

Geriatric—Studies on rivastigmine have been done only in middle-aged and older patients. Information on the effects of rivastigmine is based on these patients.

Pregnancy—

	Pregnancy Category	Explanation
All Trimesters	B	Animal studies have revealed no evidence of harm to the fetus, however, there are no adequate studies in pregnant women OR animal studies have shown an adverse effect, but adequate studies in pregnant women have failed to demonstrate a risk to the fetus.

Breast Feeding—There are no adequate studies in women for determining infant risk when using this medication during breastfeeding. Weigh the potential benefits against the potential risks before taking this medication while breastfeeding.

Other medicines—Although certain medicines should not be used together at all, in other cases two different medicines may be used together even if an interaction might occur. In these cases, your doctor may want to change the dose, or other precautions may be necessary. Tell your healthcare professional if you are taking any other prescription or non-prescription (over-the-counter [OTC]) medicine.

Interactions with Food/Tobacco/Alcohol—Certain medicines should not be used at or around the time of eating food or eating certain types of food since interactions may occur. Using alcohol or tobacco with certain medicines may also cause interactions to occur. Discuss with your healthcare professional the use of your medicine with food, alcohol, or tobacco.

Other medical problems—The presence of other medical problems may affect the use of this medicine. Make sure you tell your doctor if you have any other medical problems, especially:

- Asthma (or history of) or
- Blockage in the intestines or stomach, or
- Heart problems, including slow heartbeat or hypotension (low blood pressure), or
- Stomach ulcer (or history of) or
- Urinary tract blockage or difficult urination—Rivastigmine may make these conditions worse
- Epilepsy or history of seizures or
- Diabetes, hormone, or thyroid problems that are poorly controlled—Rivastigmine may cause seizures

Proper Use of This Medicine

Take this medicine only as directed by your doctor. Do not take more or less of it, and do not take it more or less often than your doctor ordered. Taking too much may increase the chance of side effects, while taking too little may not improve your condition.

Rivastigmine is best taken with food.

Rivastigmine seems to work best when it is taken at regularly spaced times, usually two times a day, in the morning and evening.

Dosing—The dose of this medicine will be different for different patients. Follow your doctor's orders or the directions on the label. The following information includes only the average doses of this medicine. If your dose is different, do not change it unless your doctor tells you to do so.

The amount of medicine that you take depends on the strength of the medicine. Also, the number of doses you take each day, the time allowed between doses, and the length of time you take the medicine depend on the medical problem for which you are using the medicine.

- For oral dosage form (capsules):
  - For treatment of Alzheimer's disease:
    - Adults—To start, 1.5 milligrams (mg) twice a day. Your doctor may increase your dose gradually if you are doing well on this medicine. However, the dose is usually not more than 6 mg twice a day.

Missed dose—If you miss a dose of this medicine, take it as soon as possible. However, if it is almost time for your next dose, skip the missed dose and go back to your regular dosing schedule. Do not double doses.

Storage—Store the medicine in a closed container at room temperature, away from heat, moisture, and direct light. Keep from freezing.

Keep out of the reach of children.

Do not keep outdated medicine or medicine no longer needed.

Ask your healthcare professional how you should dispose of any medicine you do not use.

Precautions While Using This Medicine

It is very important that your doctor check your progress at regular visits.

Tell your doctor if your symptoms get worse, or if you notice any new symptoms.

Before you have any kind of surgery, dental treatment, or emergency treatment, tell the doctor medical doctor or dentist in charge that you are taking this medicine. Taking rivastigmine together with medicines that are sometimes used during surgery or dental or emergency treatments may increase the effects of these medicines.

Rivastigmine may cause some people to become dizzy, clumsy, or unsteady. Make sure you know how you react to this medicine before you drive, use machines, or do anything else that could be dangerous if you are dizzy or are not alert.

Rivastigmine causes a large number of patients to have problems with their stomachs and intestines. Tell your doctor about any nausea, vomiting, stomach pain or loss of appetite.

Do not stop taking this medicine or decrease your dose without first checking with your doctor. Stopping this medicine suddenly or decreasing the dose by a large amount may cause mental or behavior changes.

If you think you or someone else may have taken an overdose of rivastigmine, get emergency help at once. Taking an overdose of rivastigmine may lead to convulsions (seizures) or shock. Some signs of shock are large pupils, irregular breathing, and fast weak pulse. Other signs of an overdose are severe nausea and vomiting, increasing muscle weakness, greatly increased sweating, and greatly increased watering of the mouth.

Side Effects of This Medicine

Along with its needed effects, a medicine may cause some unwanted effects. Although not all of these side effects may occur, if they do occur they may need medical attention.

Check with your doctor as soon as possible if any of the following side effects occur:

More common
   Diarrhea; indigestion; loss of appetite; loss of strength; nausea and vomiting; weight loss

Less common
   High blood pressure; fainting

Rare
   Aggression; convulsions (seizures); trembling and shaking of hands and fingers; trouble in urinating

Symptoms of overdose
   Seizures; fast weak pulse; greatly increased sweating; greatly increased watering of mouth; irregular breathing; increasing muscle weakness; large pupils; low blood pressure; nausea; slow heartbeat; vomiting (severe)

Some side effects may occur that usually do not need medical attention. These side effects may go away during treatment as your body adjusts to the medicine. Also, your health

care professional may be able to tell you about ways to prevent or reduce some of these side effects. Check with your health care professional if any of the following side effects continue or are bothersome or if you have any questions about them:

More common

Abdominal or stomach pain or cramping; bloated full feeling; confusion; constipation; mental depression; dizziness; fatigue; headache; seeing, hearing, or feeling things that are not there; trouble in sleeping

Less common

General feeling of discomfort or illness; increased sweating; runny nose

Other side effects not listed may also occur in some patients. If you notice any other effects, check with your healthcare professional.

RIZATRIPTAN   (Oral route) - rye-za-TRIP-tan

Commonly used brand name(s)

In the U.S.—
Maxalt
Maxalt-MLT

Available Dosage Forms:
• Tablet, Disintegrating
• Tablet

Therapeutic Class: Antimigraine
Pharmacologic Class: Serotonin Receptor Agonist, 5–HT1

Uses For This Medicine

Rizatriptan is used to treat severe migraine headaches. Many people find that their headaches go away completely after they take rizatriptan. Other people find that their headaches are much less painful, and that they are able to go back to their normal activities even though their headaches are not completely gone.

Rizatriptan is not an ordinary pain reliever. It should not be used to relieve any kind of pain other than migraine headaches.

Rizatriptan may cause serious side effects in some people, especially people who have heart or blood vessel disease. Be sure that you discuss with your doctor the risks of using this medicine as well as the good that it can do.

This medicine is available only with your doctor's prescription.

Before Using This Medicine

In deciding to use a medicine, the risks of taking the medicine must be weighed against the good it will do. This is a decision you and your doctor will make. For this medicine, the following should be considered:

Allergies—Tell your doctor if you have ever had any unusual or allergic reaction to this medicine or any other medicines. Also tell your health care professional if you have any other types of allergies, such as to foods, dyes, preservatives, or animals. For non-prescription products, read the label or package ingredients carefully.

Pediatric—There is no specific information comparing use of rizatriptan in children with use in other age groups.

Geriatric—Rizatriptan has been tested in elderly patients and has not been shown to cause different side effects or problems in older people than it does in younger adults.

Pregnancy—

	Pregnancy Category	Explanation
All Trimesters	C	Animal studies have shown an adverse effect and there are no adequate studies in pregnant women OR no animal studies have been conducted and there are no adequate studies in pregnant women.

Breast Feeding—There are no adequate studies in women for determining infant risk when using this medication during breastfeeding. Weigh the potential benefits against the potential risks before taking this medication while breastfeeding.

Other medicines—

Using this medicine with any of the following medicines is not recommended. Your doctor may decide not to treat you with this medication or change some of the other medicines you take.

Almotriptan, Clorgyline, Dihydroergotamine, Ergoloid Mesylates, Ergonovine, Ergotamine, Frovatriptan, Iproniazid, Isocarboxazid, Methylergonovine, Methysergide, Moclobemide, Naratriptan, Nialamide, Pargyline, Phenelzine, Procarbazine, Sumatriptan, Toloxatone, Tranylcypromine, Zolmitriptan

Interactions with Food/Tobacco/Alcohol—Certain medicines should not be used at or around the time of eating food or eating certain types of food since interactions may occur. Using alcohol or tobacco with certain medicines may also cause interactions to occur. Discuss with your healthcare professional the use of your medicine with food, alcohol, or tobacco.

Other medical problems—The presence of other medical problems may affect the use of this medicine. Make sure you tell your doctor if you have any other medical problems, especially:

• Angina (chest pain) or
• Heart or blood vessel disease or
• High blood pressure (uncontrolled) or
• Kidney disease or
• Liver disease—The chance of side effects may be increased. Heart or blood vessel disease and high blood pressure sometimes do not cause any symptoms, so some people do not know that they have these problems. Before deciding whether you should use rizatriptan, your doctor may need to do some tests to make sure that you do not have any of these conditions

Proper Use of This Medicine

Take this medicine exactly as directed by your doctor. It will work only if taken correctly.

Do not use rizatriptan for a headache that is different from your usual migraines. Instead, check with your doctor.

To relieve your migraine as soon as possible, use rizatriptan as soon as the headache pain begins. Even if you get warning signals of a coming migraine (an aura), you should wait until the headache pain starts before using rizatriptan.

Lying down in a quiet, dark room for a while after you use this medicine may help relieve your migraine.

Ask your doctor ahead of time about any other medicine you may take if rizatriptan does not work. After you take the other medicine, check with your doctor as soon as possible. Headaches that are not relieved by rizatriptan are sometimes caused by conditions that need other treatment.

If you feel much better after a dose of rizatriptan, but your headache comes back or gets worse after a while, you may use more rizatriptan. However, use this medicine only as directed by your doctor. Do not use more of it, and do not use it more often, than directed. Using too much rizatriptan may increase the chance of side effects.

Your doctor may direct you to take another medicine to help prevent headaches. It is important that you follow your doctor's directions, even if your headaches continue to occur. Headache-preventing medicines may take several weeks to start working. Even after they do start working, your headaches may not go away completely. However, your headaches should occur less often, and they should be less severe and easier to relieve. This can reduce the amount of rizatriptan or other pain medicines that you need. If you do not notice any improvement after several weeks of headache-preventing treatment, check with your doctor.

Dosing—The dose of this medicine will be different for different patients. Follow your doctor's orders or the directions on the label. The following information includes only the average doses of this medicine. If your dose is different, do not change it unless your doctor tells you to do so.

The amount of medicine that you take depends on the strength of the medicine. Also, the number of doses you take each day, the time allowed between doses, and the length of time you take the medicine depend on the medical problem for which you are using the medicine.

- For oral dosage form (tablets and orally disintegrating tablets):
  - For migraine headaches:
    - Adults—5 or 10 mg as a single dose. If the migraine comes back after being relieved, another dose may be taken two hours after the last dose.
- Children—Use and dose must be determined by your doctor.

Storage—Store the medicine in a closed container at room temperature, away from heat, moisture, and direct light. Keep from freezing.

Keep out of the reach of children.

Do not keep outdated medicine or medicine no longer needed.

Precautions While Using This Medicine

Drinking alcoholic beverages can make headaches worse or cause new headaches to occur. People who suffer from severe headaches should probably avoid alcoholic beverages, especially during a headache.

Some people feel drowsy or dizzy during or after a migraine, or after taking rizatriptan to relieve a migraine. As long as you are feeling drowsy or dizzy, do not drive, use machines, or do anything else that could be dangerous if you are dizzy or are not alert.

Side Effects of This Medicine

Along with its needed effects, a medicine may cause some unwanted effects. Although not all of these side effects may occur, if they do occur they may need medical attention.

Check with your doctor as soon as possible if any of the following side effects occur:

More common

Chest pain; heaviness, tightness, or pressure in chest and/or neck; pounding heartbeat; sensation of burning, warmth, heat, numbness, tightness, or tingling; shortness of breath

Less common

Increased heartbeat; irregular heartbeat; slow heartbeat

Symptoms of overdose

Dizziness; fainting; headache, severe or continuing; sleepiness; slow heartbeat; vomiting

Some side effects may occur that usually do not need medical attention. These side effects may go away during treatment as your body adjusts to the medicine. Also, your health care professional may be able to tell you about ways to prevent or reduce some of these side effects. Check with your health care professional if any of the following side effects continue or are bothersome or if you have any questions about them:

More common

Dizziness; dry mouth; hot flashes; nausea and/or vomiting; sleepiness; unusual tiredness or muscle weakness

Less common

Agitation; anxiety; blurred vision; chills; confusion; constipation; depression; diarrhea; difficulty swallowing; dry eyes; eye irritation; feeling of constant movement of self or surroundings; gas; headache; heartburn; heat sensitivity; inability to sleep; increased sweating; increased thirst; irritability; itching of the skin; muscle or joint stiffness, tightness, or rigidity; muscle pain or spasms; ringing or buzzing in ears; sudden large increase in frequency or quantity of urine; trembling of hands or feet; unusual feeling of well-being; warm and/or cold sensations

Other side effects not listed may also occur in some patients. If you notice any other effects, check with your healthcare professional.

ROPINIROLE (Oral route) - roe-PIN-i-role

Commonly used brand name(s)

In the U.S.—
Requip

Available Dosage Forms:
- Tablet

Therapeutic Class: Antiparkinsonian
Pharmacologic Class: Dopamine Agonist

Uses For This Medicine

Ropinirole is used alone or with other medicines to treat Parkinson's disease. It is also used to treat a condition called Restless Legs Syndrome (RLS). This condition is an overwhelming feeling of wanting to move your legs to make them comfortable from unpleasant sensations in the legs.

This medicine is available only with your doctor's prescription.

Before Using This Medicine

In deciding to use a medicine, the risks of taking the medicine must be weighed against the good it will do. This is a decision you and your doctor will make. For this medicine, the following should be considered:

Allergies—Tell your doctor if you have ever had any unusual or allergic reaction to this medicine or any other medicines. Also tell your health care professional if you have any other types of allergies, such as to foods, dyes, preservatives, or animals. For non-prescription products, read the label or package ingredients carefully.

Pediatric—Studies on this medicine have been done only in adult patients, and there is no specific information comparing use of ropinirole in children with use in other age groups.

Geriatric—Hallucinations (seeing, hearing, or feeling things that are not there) may be especially likely to occur in elderly patients, who are usually more sensitive than younger adults to the effects of ropinirole.

Pregnancy—

	Pregnancy Category	Explanation
All Trimesters	C	Animal studies have shown an adverse effect and there are no adequate studies in pregnant women OR no animal studies have been conducted and there are no adequate studies in pregnant women.

Breast Feeding—Studies suggest that this medication may alter milk production or composition. If an alternative to this medication is not prescribed, you should monitor the infant for side effects and adequate milk intake.

Other medicines—

Using this medicine with any of the following medicines may cause an increased risk of certain side effects, but using both drugs may be the best treatment for you. If both medicines are prescribed together, your doctor may change the dose or how often you use one or both of the medicines.

Ciprofloxacin, Kava

Interactions with Food/Tobacco/Alcohol—Certain medicines should not be used at or around the time of eating food or eating certain types of food since interactions may occur. Using alcohol or tobacco with certain medicines may also cause interactions to occur. The following interactions have been selected on the basis of their potential significance and are not necessarily all-inclusive.

Using this medicine with any of the following may cause an increased risk of certain side effects but may be unavoidable in some cases. If used together, your doctor may change the dose or how often you use this medicine, or give you special instructions about the use of food, alcohol, or tobacco.

Tobacco

Other medical problems—The presence of other medical problems may affect the use of this medicine. Make sure you tell your doctor if you have any other medical problems, especially:

- Eye problems, especially with the retina—Animal studies have shown that problems with the retina may occur; it is not certain if this may occur in humans
- Hallucinations (seeing, hearing, or feeling things that are not there) or
- Hypotension (low blood pressure) or
- Postural hypotension (dizziness, lightheadedness, or fainting when getting up from a lying or sitting position)—Ropinirole may make these conditions worse
- Kidney problems—May increase chance of side effects
- Liver problems—Higher blood levels of ropinirole may result, and cause an increase in side effects
- Lung problems resulting from treatment with some other Parkinson's disease medicines—Ropinirole may cause the condition to recur
- Sleep disorders or
- Sleepiness, history of in the past—May cause side effects to be worse

Proper Use of This Medicine

Take this medicine every day exactly as ordered by your doctor in order to improve your condition as much as possible. Do not take more of it or less of it, and do not take it more or less often than your doctor ordered.

Read the Patient Information leaflet before you take this medicine and each time you get your prescription refilled.

This medicine may be taken with or without food, or on an empty or full stomach. Taking this medicine with food may reduce nausea.

Dosing—The dose of this medicine will be different for different patients. Follow your doctor's orders or the directions on the label. The following information includes only the average doses of this medicine. If your dose is different, do not change it unless your doctor tells you to do so.

The amount of medicine that you take depends on the strength of the medicine. Also, the number of doses you take each day, the time allowed between doses, and the length of time you take the medicine depend on the medical problem for which you are using the medicine.

- For oral dosage form (tablets):
  - For Parkinson's disease:
    - Adults—At first, 0.25 milligrams (mg) three times a day. Your doctor will increase your dose as needed and tolerated. However, the dose is usually not more than 24 mg a day.
    - Children—Use and dose must be determined by the doctor.
  - For Restless Leg Syndrome:
    - Adults—At first, 0.25 milligram (mg) once a day, 1 to 3 hours before bedtime. Your doctor will increase your dose as needed and tolerated. However, the dose is usually not more than 4 mg a day.
    - Children—Use and dose must be determined by the doctor.

Missed dose—If you miss a dose of this medicine, take it as soon as possible. However, if it is almost time for your next dose, skip the missed dose and go back to your regular dosing schedule. Do not double doses.

Storage—Store the medicine in a closed container at room temperature, away from heat, moisture, and direct light. Keep from freezing.

Keep out of the reach of children.

Do not keep outdated medicine or medicine no longer needed.

Precautions While Using This Medicine

It is important that your doctor check your progress at regular visits. This is necessary to allow dose adjustments and to reduce any unwanted effects.

Do not stop taking this medicine without first checking with your doctor. Your doctor may want you to reduce gradually the amount you are taking before stopping completely.

This medicine may cause some people to become drowsy, dizzy or lightheaded, to be less alert than they are normally, or to have vision problems, weakness, or problems with co-ordination. Make sure you know how you react to this medicine before you drive, use machines, or do anything else that could be dangerous if you are not alert, well-coordinated, or able to think or see well. People taking this medicine have reported falling asleep without warning during activities of daily living, including driving which sometimes resulted in accidents. This may happen as late as one year after taking the medicine.

Alcohol or medicines that make you drowsy may add to the effects of this medicine. Be sure your doctor knows if you are taking alcohol or other medicines that may cause drowsiness.

Dizziness, lightheadedness, or fainting may occur, especially when you get up from a lying or sitting position. These symptoms are more likely to occur when you begin taking this medicine, or when the dose is increased. Getting up slowly may help. If you should have this problem, check with your doctor.

Hallucinations (seeing, hearing, or feeling things that are not there) may occur in some patients. This is more common with elderly patients.

It is important that your doctor check your skin for melanoma regularly if you have Parkinson's disease.

Side Effects of This Medicine

Along with its needed effects, a medicine may cause some unwanted effects. Although not all of these side effects may occur, if they do occur they may need medical attention.

Check with your doctor as soon as possible if any of the following side effects occur:

More common
> Confusion; dizziness; drowsiness; falling; lightheadedness or fainting, especially when standing up; nausea; seeing, hearing, or feeling things that are not there (hallucinations); swelling of legs; twisting, twitching, or other unusual body movements; unusual tiredness or weakness; worsening of parkinsonism

Less common
> Abdominal pain; blood in urine; burning, pain, or difficulty in urinating; chest pain; cough; double vision or other eye or vision problems; fast heartbeat; high or low blood pressure; irregular or pounding heartbeat; loss of memory; mental depression; pain; pain in arms or legs; shortness of breath; sore throat; tightness in chest; tingling, numbness, or prickly feelings; trouble in concentrating; troubled breathing; vomiting; wheezing

Rare
> Anxiety or nervousness; buzzing or ringing in ears; chills; cough; fever; headache; joint pain; loss of bladder control; muscle cramps, pain, or spasms; nasal congestion; runny nose; sneezing; trouble in swallowing

Symptoms of overdose
> Agitation; chest pain; confusion; dizziness or lightheadedness, especially when standing up; drowsiness; fainting; fatigue; grogginess; increase in unusual body movements, especially of the face or mouth; increased coughing; nausea; vomiting

Some side effects may occur that usually do not need medical attention. These side effects may go away during treatment as your body adjusts to the medicine. Also, your health care professional may be able to tell you about ways to prevent or reduce some of these side effects. Check with your health care professional if any of the following side effects continue or are bothersome or if you have any questions about them:

Less common
> Abnormal dreams; constipation; decrease in sexual desire or performance; diarrhea; dryness of mouth; flushing; general feeling of discomfort or illness; headache; heartburn or gas; hot flashes; increased sweating; loss of appetite; tremor; weight loss; yawning

Other side effects not listed may also occur in some patients. If you notice any other effects, check with your healthcare professional.

ROSIGLITAZONE (Oral route) - roh-si-GLI-ta-zone

Commonly used brand name(s)
In the U.S.—
> Avandia

Available Dosage Forms:
- Tablet

Therapeutic Class: Antidiabetic

Uses For This Medicine

Rosiglitazone is used to treat a certain type of diabetes mellitus (sugar diabetes) called type 2 diabetes. It may be used alone or with another type of diabetes medicine, such as metformin, insulin, a sulfonylurea, or sulfonylurea plus metformin.

This medicine is available only with your doctor's prescription.

Before Using This Medicine

In deciding to use a medicine, the risks of taking the medicine must be weighed against the good it will do. This is a decision

you and your doctor will make. For this medicine, the following should be considered:

Allergies—Tell your doctor if you have ever had any unusual or allergic reaction to this medicine or any other medicines. Also tell your health care professional if you have any other types of allergies, such as to foods, dyes, preservatives, or animals. For non-prescription products, read the label or package ingredients carefully.

Pediatric—Studies on this medicine have been done only in adult patients, and there is no specific information comparing use of rosiglitazone in children with use in other age groups.

Geriatric—This medicine has been tested in a limited number of patients 65 years of age or older and has not been shown to cause different side effects or problems in older people than it does in younger adults.

Pregnancy—

	Pregnancy Category	Explanation
All Trimesters	C	Animal studies have shown an adverse effect and there are no adequate studies in pregnant women OR no animal studies have been conducted and there are no adequate studies in pregnant women.

Breast Feeding—There are no adequate studies in women for determining infant risk when using this medication during breastfeeding. Weigh the potential benefits against the potential risks before taking this medication while breastfeeding.

Other medicines—

Using this medicine with any of the following medicines may cause an increased risk of certain side effects, but using both drugs may be the best treatment for you. If both medicines are prescribed together, your doctor may change the dose or how often you use one or both of the medicines.

Bitter Melon, Fenugreek, Gemfibrozil, Glucomannan, Guar Gum, Psyllium, Rifampin, St John's Wort, Trimethoprim

Interactions with Food/Tobacco/Alcohol—Certain medicines should not be used at or around the time of eating food or eating certain types of food since interactions may occur. Using alcohol or tobacco with certain medicines may also cause interactions to occur. Discuss with your healthcare professional the use of your medicine with food, alcohol, or tobacco.

Other medical problems—The presence of other medical problems may affect the use of this medicine. Make sure you tell your doctor if you have any other medical problems, especially:

- Diabetic ketoacidosis (ketones in the blood) or
- Lactic acidosis (lactic acid in the blood) or
- Metabolic acidosis (extra acids in the blood)—Patients with any of these conditions should not use this medicine.
- Diabetic macular edema (swelling of the retina)—May make this condition worse.
- Edema—May increase the side effects of rosiglitazone.
- Heart disease or
- Jaundice or

- Liver disease—Rosiglitazone may make these conditions worse.
- Type 1 diabetes—Insulin is needed to control these conditions.

Proper Use of This Medicine

Follow carefully the special meal plan your doctor gave you. This is the most important part of controlling your condition, and is necessary if the medicine is to work properly. Also, exercise regularly and test for sugar in your blood or urine as directed.

Rosiglitazone may be taken with or without food.

Dosing—The dose of this medicine will be different for different patients. Follow your doctor's orders or the directions on the label. The following information includes only the average doses of this medicine. If your dose is different, do not change it unless your doctor tells you to do so.

The amount of medicine that you take depends on the strength of the medicine. Also, the number of doses you take each day, the time allowed between doses, and the length of time you take the medicine depend on the medical problem for which you are using the medicine.

- For oral dosage form (tablets):
  - For type 2 diabetes:
    - Rosiglitazone alone:
      - Adults—At first, the dose is 4 milligrams (mg) once a day or 2 mg twice a day. After 8 to 12 weeks, the dose may be increased to 8 mg once a day or 4 mg twice a day.
      - Children—Use and dose must be determined by your doctor.
    - Rosiglitazone with insulin:
      - Adults—4 milligrams (mg) once a day. Your doctor may adjust your dose as needed.
      - Children—Use and dose must be determined by your doctor.
    - Rosiglitazone with metformin:
      - Adults—At first, the dose is 4 milligrams (mg) once a day or 2 mg twice a day. Any changes in dose will be determined by your doctor.
      - Children—Use and dose must be determined by your doctor.
    - Rosiglitazone with a sulfonylurea:
      - Adults—4 milligrams (mg) once a day or 2 mg twice a day. Any changes in the dose will be determined by your doctor.
      - Children—Use and dose must be determined by your doctor.
    - Rosiglitazone with sulfonylurea plus metformin:
      - Adults—4 milligrams (mg) once a day or 2 mg twice a day. Any changes in the dose will be determined by your doctor.
      - Children—Use and dose must be determined by your doctor.

Missed dose—If you miss a dose of this medicine, take it as soon as possible. However, if it is almost time for your next dose, skip the missed dose and go back to your regular dosing schedule. Do not double doses.

Storage—Store the medicine in a closed container at room temperature, away from heat, moisture, and direct light. Keep from freezing.

Keep out of the reach of children.

Do not keep outdated medicine or medicine no longer needed.

Precautions While Using This Medicine

If you experience abdominal or stomach pain, dark urine, loss of appetite, nausea or vomiting, unusual tiredness or weakness, or yellow eyes or skin, check with your doctor immediately. These may be symptoms of liver problems.

Check with your doctor immediately if blurred vision, difficulty in reading, or any other change in vision occurs during or after treatment. Your doctor will want you to have your eyes checked by an ophthalmologist (eye doctor).

If you are rapidly gaining weight, shortness of breath, or have excessive swelling of the hands, wrist, ankles, or feet. These may be symptoms of heart problems or your body keeping too much water.

Rosiglitazone may increase the chance of a premenopausal woman with type 2 diabetes getting pregnant. Reliable birth control is recommended. Talk to your health care professional about choices, risks, and benefits.

It is very important that your doctor check your progress at regular visits to make sure that this medicine is working properly and to check for unwanted effects.

It is very important to carefully follow any instructions from your health care team about:
- Alcohol—Drinking alcohol may cause severe low blood sugar. Discuss this with your health care team.
- Other medicines—Do not take other medicines during the time you are taking rosiglitazone unless they have been discussed with your doctor. This especially includes nonprescription medicines such as aspirin, and medicines for appetite control, asthma, colds, cough, hay fever, or sinus problems.
- Counseling—Other family members need to learn how to prevent side effects or help with side effects if they occur. Also, diabetic patients may need special counseling about diabetes medicine dosing changes that might occur because of lifestyle changes, such as changes in exercise and diet. Furthermore, counseling on contraception and pregnancy may be needed because of the problems that can occur in patients with diabetes during pregnancy.
- Travel—Keep a recent prescription and your medical history with you. Be prepared for an emergency as you would normally. Make allowances for changing time zones and keep your meal times as close as possible to your usual meal times.

In case of emergency—There may be a time when you need emergency help for a problem caused by your diabetes. You need to be prepared for these emergencies. It is a good idea to wear a medical identification (ID) bracelet or neck chain at all times. Also, carry an ID card in your wallet or purse that says that you have diabetes and a list of all of your medicines.

This medicine does not cause hypoglycemia (low blood sugar). However, low blood sugar can occur if you delay or miss a meal or snack, exercise more than usual, drink alcohol, cannot eat because of nausea or vomiting, take certain medicines, or take rosiglitazone with another type of diabetes medicine. Symptoms of low blood sugar must be treated before they lead to unconsciousness (passing out). Different people feel different symptoms of low blood sugar. It is im-portant that you learn which symptoms of low blood sugar you usually have so that you can treat it quickly.

Symptoms of low blood sugar include anxiety; behavior change similar to being drunk; blurred vision; cold sweats; confusion; cool, pale skin; difficulty in thinking; drowsiness; excessive hunger; fast heartbeat; headache (continuing); nausea; nervousness; nightmares; restless sleep; shakiness; slurred speech; or unusual tiredness or weakness.

If symptoms of low blood sugar occur, eat glucose tablets or gel, corn syrup, honey, or sugar cubes; or drink fruit juice, non-diet soft drink, or sugar dissolved in water to relieve the symptoms. Also, check your blood for low blood sugar. Glucagon is used in emergency situations when severe symptoms such as seizures (convulsions) or unconsciousness occur. Have a glucagon kit available, along with a syringe and needle, and know how to use it. Members of your family also should know how to use it.

Hyperglycemia (high blood sugar) may occur if you do not take enough or skip a dose of your antidiabetic medicine, overeat or do not follow your meal plan, have a fever or infection, or do not exercise as much as usual.

Symptoms of high blood sugar include blurred vision; drowsiness; dry mouth; flushed, dry skin; fruit-like breath odor; increased urination (frequency and amount); ketones in urine; loss of appetite; sleepiness; stomachache, nausea, or vomiting; tiredness; troubled breathing (rapid and deep); unconsciousness; or unusual thirst.

If symptoms of high blood sugar occur, check your blood sugar level and then call your doctor for instructions

Tell your healthcare provider right away if you have any of these symptoms: chest pain or discomfort, extreme tiredness or weakness, irregular breathing, irregular heartbeat, shortness of breath, swelling of your face, fingers, feet or lower legs, weight gain and wheezing.

It is important to tell your healthcare professional that you are taking this medicine if you are going to have any medical procedures or surgical procedures.

Side Effects of This Medicine

Along with its needed effects, a medicine may cause some unwanted effects. Although not all of these side effects may occur, if they do occur they may need medical attention.

Check with your doctor as soon as possible if any of the following side effects occur:

Less common
Abdominal or stomach pain; blurred vision; chest pain or discomfort; decrease in amount of urine; dry mouth; fatigue; flushed, dry skin; fruit-like breath odor; increased hunger; increased thirst; increased urination; irregular heartbeat; nausea; noisy, rattling breathing; pain in the shoulders, arms, jaw or neck; pale skin; shortness of breath; sweating; swelling of fingers, hands, feet, or lower legs; troubled breathing; unexplained weight loss; unusual bleeding or bruising; unusual tiredness or weakness; weight gain, rapid or unusual; vomiting

Rare
Anxiety; chills; cold sweats; coma; confusion; dark urine; depression; dizziness; fast heartbeat; headache; loss of appetite; nervousness; nightmares; seizures; shakiness; slurred speech

Frequency not known

Blue lips and fingernails; changes in vision; coughing that sometimes produces a pink frothy sputum; hive-like swelling on face, eyelids, lips, tongue, throat, hands, legs, feet, or sex organs; itching; light-colored stools; redness of skin; skin rash; wheezing; yellow eyes or skin

Some side effects may occur that usually do not need medical attention. These side effects may go away during treatment as your body adjusts to the medicine. Also, your health care professional may be able to tell you about ways to prevent or reduce some of these side effects. Check with your health care professional if any of the following side effects continue or are bothersome or if you have any questions about them:

More common

Ear congestion; fever; general feeling of discomfort or illness; hoarseness or other voice changes; injury; joint pain; muscle aches and pains; runny or stuffy nose; shivering; sneezing; sore throat; trouble sleeping

Less common

Back pain; cough; diarrhea; light-headedness; pain or tenderness around eyes and cheekbones

Other side effects not listed may also occur in some patients. If you notice any other effects, check with your healthcare professional.

ROSIGLITAZONE AND METFORMIN
(Oral route) - roh-si-GLI-ta-zone, met-FOR-min

Black Box Warning

- Metformin hydrochloride
  - Lactic Acidosis
    - Lactic acidosis is a rare, but serious, metabolic complication that can occur due to metformin accumulation during treatment with rosiglitazone maleate and metformin hydrochloride; when it occurs, it is fatal in approximately 50% of cases. Lactic acidosis may also occur in association with a number of pathophysiologic conditions, including diabetes mellitus, and whenever there is significant tissue hypoperfusion and hypoxemia. Lactic acidosis is characterized by elevated blood lactate levels (greater than 5 mmol/L), decreased blood pH, electrolyte disturbances with an increased anion gap, and an increased lactate/pyruvate ratio. When metformin is implicated as the cause of lactic acidosis, metformin plasma levels greater than 5 mcg/mL are generally found.
    - The reported incidence of lactic acidosis in patients receiving metformin hydrochloride is very low (approximately 0.03 cases/1,000 patient years of exposure, with approximately 0.015 fatal cases/1,000 patient years of exposure). Reported cases have occurred primarily in diabetic patients with significant renal insufficiency, including both intrinsic renal disease and renal hypoperfusion, often in the setting of multiple concomitant med-

ical/surgical problems and multiple concomitant medications. Patients with congestive heart failure requiring pharmacologic management, in particular those with unstable or acute congestive heart failure who are at risk of hypoperfusion and hypoxemia, are at increased risk of lactic acidosis. The risk of lactic acidosis increases with the degree of renal dysfunction and the patient's age. The risk of lactic acidosis may, therefore, be significantly decreased by regular monitoring of renal function in patients taking rosiglitazone maleate and metformin hydrochloride and by use of the minimum effective dose of rosiglitazone maleate and metformin hydrochloride. In particular, treatment of the elderly should be accompanied by careful monitoring of renal function. Treatment with rosiglitazone maleate and metformin hydrochloride should not be initiated in patients 80 years of age or older unless measurement of creatinine clearance demonstrates that renal function is not reduced, as these patients are more susceptible to developing lactic acidosis. In addition, rosiglitazone maleate and metformin hydrochloride should be promptly withheld in the presence of any condition associated with hypoxemia, dehydration, or sepsis. Because impaired hepatic function may significantly limit the ability to clear lactate, rosiglitazone maleate and metformin hydrochloride should generally be avoided in patients with clinical or laboratory evidence of hepatic disease. Patients should be cautioned against excessive alcohol intake, either acute or chronic, when taking rosiglitazone maleate and metformin hydrochloride, since alcohol potentiates the effects of metformin hydrochloride on lactate metabolism. In addition, rosiglitazone maleate and metformin hydrochloride should be temporarily discontinued prior to any intravascular radiocontrast study and for any surgical procedure.

- The onset of lactic acidosis often is subtle, and accompanied only by nonspecific symptoms such as malaise, myalgias, respiratory distress, increasing somnolence, and nonspecific abdominal distress. There may be associated hypothermia, hypotension, and resistant bradyarrhythmias with more marked acidosis. The patient and the patient's physician must be aware of the possible importance of such symptoms and the patient should be instructed to notify the physician immediately if they occur. Rosiglitazone maleate and metformin hydrochloride should be withdrawn until the situation is clarified. Serum electrolytes, ketones, blood glucose and, if indicated, blood pH, lactate levels, and even blood metformin levels may be useful. Once a patient is stabilized on any dose level of rosiglitazone maleate and metformin hydrochloride, gastrointestinal symptoms, which are common during initiation of therapy, are unlikely to be drug related. Later occurrence of gastrointestinal symptoms could be due to lactic acidosis or other serious disease.

- Levels of fasting venous plasma lactate above the upper limit of normal but less than 5 mmol/L in patients taking rosiglitazone maleate and metformin hydrochloride do not necessarily indicate impending lactic acidosis and may be explainable by other mechanisms, such as poorly controlled diabetes or obesity, vigorous physical activity or technical problems in sample handling.

- Lactic acidosis should be suspected in any diabetic patient with metabolic acidosis lacking evidence of ketoacidosis (ketonuria and ketonemia).
- Lactic acidosis is a medical emergency that must be treated in a hospital setting. In a patient with lactic acidosis who is taking rosiglitazone maleate and metformin hydrochloride, the drug should be discontinued immediately and general supportive measures promptly instituted. Because metformin hydrochloride is dialyzable (with a clearance of up to 170 mL/min under good hemodynamic conditions), prompt hemodialysis is recommended to correct the acidosis and remove the accumulated metformin. Such management often results in prompt reversal of symptoms and recovery.

Commonly used brand name(s)

In the U.S.—
Avandamet

Available Dosage Forms:
- Tablet

Therapeutic Class: Hypoglycemic

Uses For This Medicine

Rosiglitazone and metformin combination is used to treat high blood sugar levels that are caused by a type of diabetes mellitus or sugar diabetes called type 2 diabetes. In type 2 diabetes, your body does not work properly to store excess sugar and the sugar remains in your bloodstream. Chronic high blood sugar can lead to serious health problems in the future. Proper diet is the first step in managing type 2 diabetes, but often medicines are needed to help your body. Rosiglitazone helps your body use the insulin better and it reduces the amount of insulin in your body. Metformin reduces the absorption of sugar, reduces the release of stored sugar from the liver, and helps your body's cells use sugar better.

This medicine is available only with your doctor's prescription.

Before Using This Medicine

In deciding to use a medicine, the risks of taking the medicine must be weighed against the good it will do. This is a decision you and your doctor will make. For this medicine, the following should be considered:

Allergies—Tell your doctor if you have ever had any unusual or allergic reaction to this medicine or any other medicines. Also tell your health care professional if you have any other types of allergies, such as to foods, dyes, preservatives, or animals. For non-prescription products, read the label or package ingredients carefully.

Pediatric—Studies on this medicine have been done only in adult patients, and there is no specific information comparing use of rosiglitazone and metformin in children with use in other age groups.

Geriatric—Some older adults may be more sensitive than younger adults to the effects of these medicines. Older adults are more likely to have age-related problems such as kidney problems. Rosiglitazone and metformin should be used carefully as age increases and older adults may need a lower dose of this medicine.

Pregnancy—

	Pregnancy Category	Explanation
All Trimesters	C	Animal studies have shown an adverse effect and there are no adequate studies in pregnant women OR no animal studies have been conducted and there are no adequate studies in pregnant women.

Breast Feeding—There are no adequate studies in women for determining infant risk when using this medication during breastfeeding. Weigh the potential benefits against the potential risks before taking this medication while breastfeeding.

Other medicines—

Using this medicine with any of the following medicines is not recommended. Your doctor may decide not to treat you with this medication or change some of the other medicines you take.

Acetrizoic Acid, Diatrizoate, Ethiodized Oil, Iobenzamic Acid, Iobitridol, Iocarmic Acid, Iocetamic Acid, Iodamide, Iodipamide, Iodixanol, Iodohippuric Acid, Iodopyracet, Iodoxamic Acid, Ioglicic Acid, Ioglycamic Acid, Iohexol, Iomeprol, Iopamidol, Iopanoic Acid, Iopentol, Iophendylate, Iopromide, Iopronic Acid, Ioseric Acid, Iosimide, Iotasul, Iothalamate, Iotrolan, Iotroxic Acid, Ioversol, Ioxaglate, Ioxitalamic Acid, Ipodate, Metrizamide, Metrizoic Acid, Tyropanoate Sodium

Interactions with Food/Tobacco/Alcohol—Certain medicines should not be used at or around the time of eating food or eating certain types of food since interactions may occur. Using alcohol or tobacco with certain medicines may also cause interactions to occur. Discuss with your healthcare professional the use of your medicine with food, alcohol, or tobacco.

Other medical problems—The presence of other medical problems may affect the use of this medicine. Make sure you tell your doctor if you have any other medical problems, especially:

- Adrenal glands, not properly controlled or
- Alcohol intoxication or
- Caloric intake, deficient (not enough calories) or
- Elderly patients or
- Undernourished condition or
- Underactive pituitary gland, not properly controlled or
- Any other condition that causes low blood sugar—Patients with these conditions may be more likely to develop low blood sugar while taking a medication that contains rosiglitazone and metformin.
- Dehydration (not enough water in your body) or
- Heart attack or
- Sepsis (serious illness due to a bacterial infection) or
- Shock—These conditions can cause serious problems. If they happen, you should stop taking this medicine as soon as possible.
- Diabetic ketoacidosis (ketones in the blood) or
- Lactic acidosis (lactic acid in the blood) or

- Metabolic acidosis (extra acids in the blood)—Patients with any of these conditions should not use this medicine.
- Diabetic macular edema (swelling of the retina)—May make this condition worse.
- Edema—Patients with this condition should use this medicine with caution. Use of this medicine can increase the risk of serious side effects in these patients.
- Fever or
- Infection or
- Surgery or
- Trauma—These conditions may cause temporary problems with blood sugar control and your healthcare professional may want to treat you temporarily with insulin.
- Heart failure, congestive—Patients with this condition should not use this medicine.
- Jaundice—Patients with this condition should use this medicine with caution. Use of this medicine can increase the risk of serious side effects in these patients.
- Kidney disease—Patients with this condition should not use this medicine.
- Liver function, impaired—Patients with impaired liver conditions generally should not use this medicine.
- Radiologic procedures (e.g., x-rays, CT scans, and MRIs) that use intravenous contrast media—Use of this medicine should be discontinued before you have one of these procedures. The medicine should not be started again during the 48 hours after the procedure. You may begin taking your medicine again after the doctor checks your kidneys for normal function.
- Surgery—Use of this medicine should be stopped during surgical procedures (except for minor surgical procedures). You can take your medicine again after your healthcare professional makes sure your kidneys are normal.
- Type 1 diabetes—Patients with this condition should not use this medicine.

Proper Use of This Medicine

Follow carefully the special meal plan your doctor gave you. This is the most important part of controlling your condition, and is necessary if the medicine is to work properly. Also, exercise regularly and test for sugar in your blood or urine as directed.

Rosiglitazone and metformin combination should be taken with meals to help reduce the stomach and intestinal side effects that may occur while you are taking this medicine.

You may notice improvement in your blood glucose control in 1 to 2 weeks, but the full effect of blood glucose control may take up to 2 to 3 months. Ask your healthcare professional if you have any questions about this.

Dosing—The dose of this medicine will be different for different patients. Follow your doctor's orders or the directions on the label. The following information includes only the average doses of this medicine. If your dose is different, do not change it unless your doctor tells you to do so.

The amount of medicine that you take depends on the strength of the medicine. Also, the number of doses you take each day, the time allowed between doses, and the length of time you take the medicine depend on the medical problem for which you are using the medicine.

- For oral dosage form (tablets):
  - For type 2 diabetes:
    - For patients on metformin therapy:
      — Adults—4 milligrams (mg) rosiglitazone per day plus the dose of metformin already being taken, divided into two doses. Your doctor may gradually increase your dose until your blood sugar is controlled.
      — Children—Use and dose must be determined by your doctor.
    - For patients on rosiglitazone therapy:
      — Adults—1000 milligrams (mg) of metformin per day plus the dose of rosiglitazone already being taken, divided into two doses. Your doctor may gradually increase your dose until your blood sugar is controlled.
      — Children—Use and dose must be determined by your doctor.
    - For patients not on metformin or rosiglitazone therapy:
      — Adults—2 milligrams (mg) rosiglitazone and 500 mg metformin combination one or two times a day as directed by your doctor. Your doctor may gradually increase your dose as needed to control your blood sugar up to a maximum of 8 mg rosiglitazone and 2000 mg metformin per day, divided into two doses.
      — Children—Use and dose must be determined by your doctor.
    - For patients previously treated with rosiglitazone and metformin:
      — Adults—The dose is the same as the dose you are already taking. Your doctor may gradually increase your dose until your blood sugar is controlled.
      — Children—Use and dose must be determined by your doctor.

Missed dose—If you miss a dose of this medicine, take it as soon as possible. However, if it is almost time for your next dose, skip the missed dose and go back to your regular dosing schedule. Do not double doses.

Storage—Store the medicine in a closed container at room temperature, away from heat, moisture, and direct light. Keep from freezing.

Keep out of the reach of children.

Do not keep outdated medicine or medicine no longer needed.

Ask your healthcare professional how you should dispose of any medicine you do not use.

Precautions While Using This Medicine

It is very important that your doctor see you at regular visits to check your blood sugar control, and to check your kidneys and liver.

This medicine may cause women to ovulate, which could increase the chances of pregnancy. If you are a woman of child-bearing potential, you should discuss birth control options with your doctor.

It is very important to follow carefully any instructions from your health care team about:

- Alcohol—Drinking alcohol may cause severe low blood sugar. Discuss this with your health care team.
- Other medicines—Do not take other medicines unless they have been discussed with your doctor.

- Counseling—Other family members need to learn how to prevent side effects or help with side effects if they occur. Also, patients with diabetes may need special counseling about diabetes medicine dosing changes that might occur because of lifestyle changes, such as changes in exercise and diet. Furthermore, counseling on contraception and pregnancy may be needed because of the problems that can occur in patients with diabetes during pregnancy.
- Travel—Keep your recent prescription and your medical history with you. Be prepared for an emergency as you would normally. Make allowances for changing time zones and keep your meal times as close as possible to your usual meal times.

In case of emergency—There may be a time when you need emergency help for a problem caused by your diabetes. You need to be prepared for these emergencies. It is a good idea to wear a medical identification (ID) bracelet or neck chain at all times. Also, carry an ID card in your wallet or purse that says that you have diabetes and a list of all of your medicines.

Under certain conditions, too much rosiglitazone and metformin can cause lactic acidosis. Symptoms of lactic acidosis are severe and quick to appear and usually occur when other health problems not related to the medicine are present and are very severe, such as a heart attack or kidney failure. Symptoms of lactic acidosis include abdominal or stomach discomfort; decreased appetite; diarrhea; fast, shallow breathing; general feeling of discomfort; muscle pain or cramping; and unusual sleepiness, tiredness, or weakness.

If symptoms of lactic acidosis occur, you should check your blood sugar and get immediate emergency medical help.

Symptoms of hypoglycemia (low blood sugar) include anxiety; behavior change similar to being drunk; blurred vision; cold sweats; confusion; cool, pale skin; difficulty in thinking; drowsiness; excessive hunger; fast heartbeat; headache (continuing); nausea; nervousness; nightmares; restless sleep; shakiness; slurred speech; or unusual tiredness or weakness.

Rosiglitazone and metformin combination can cause low blood sugar. However, it also can occur if you delay or miss a meal or snack, drink alcohol, exercise more than usual, cannot eat because of nausea or vomiting, take certain medicines, or take rosiglitazone and metformin with another type of diabetes medicine. Symptoms of low blood sugar must be treated before they lead to unconsciousness (passing out). Different people feel different symptoms of low blood sugar. It is important that you learn which symptoms of low blood sugar you usually have so that you can treat it quickly.

If symptoms of low blood sugar occur, eat glucose tablets or gel, corn syrup, honey, or sugar cubes; or drink fruit juice, non-diet soft drink, or sugar dissolved in water. Also, check your blood for low blood sugar. Glucagon is used in emergency situations when severe symptoms such as seizures (convulsions) or unconsciousness occur. Have a glucagon kit available, along with a syringe or needle, and know how to use it. Members of your household also should know how to use it.

Symptoms of hyperglycemia (high blood sugar) include blurred vision; drowsiness; dry mouth; flushed, dry skin; fruit-like breath odor; increased urination (frequency and amount); ketones in urine; loss of appetite; sleepiness; stomachache, nausea, or vomiting; tiredness; troubled breathing (rapid and deep); unconsciousness; or unusual thirst.

High blood sugar may occur if you do not exercise as much as usual, have a fever or infection, do not take enough or skip a dose of your diabetes medicine, or overeat or do not follow your meal plan.

If symptoms of high blood sugar occur, check your blood sugar level and then call your health care professional for instructions.

Tell your healthcare provider right away if you have any of these symptoms: chest pain or discomfort, extreme tiredness or weakness, irregular breathing, irregular heartbeat, shortness of breath, swelling of your face, fingers, feet or lower legs, weight gain and wheezing.

It is important to tell your healthcare professional that you are taking this medicine if you are going to have any medical procedures or surgical procedures.

Check with your doctor immediately if blurred vision, difficulty in reading, or any other change in vision occurs during or after treatment. Your doctor will want you to have your eyes checked by an ophthalmologist (eye doctor).

Side Effects of This Medicine

Along with its needed effects, a medicine may cause some unwanted effects. Although not all of these side effects may occur, if they do occur they may need medical attention.

Check with your doctor immediately if any of the following side effects occur:

More common
Pale skin; troubled breathing with exertion; unusual bleeding or bruising; unusual tiredness or weakness

Less common
Anxiety; blurred vision; chest pain or discomfort; chills; cold sweats; coma; confusion; cool pale skin; depression; dilated neck veins; dizziness; extreme fatigue; fast heartbeat; headache; increased hunger; irregular breathing; irregular heartbeat; nausea; nervousness; nightmares; seizures; shakiness; shortness of breath; slurred speech; swelling of face, fingers, feet, or lower legs; weight gain; wheezing

Rare
Abdominal discomfort; decreased appetite; diarrhea; fast, shallow breathing; general feeling of discomfort; muscle pain or cramping; sleepiness

Incidence not known
Change in vision; dark urine; decreased urine output; hives or welts; itching; large, hive-like swelling on face, eyelids, lips, tongue, throat, hands, legs, feet, sex organs; redness of skin; skin rash; stomach pain

Some side effects may occur that usually do not need medical attention. These side effects may go away during treatment as your body adjusts to the medicine. Also, your health care professional may be able to tell you about ways to prevent or reduce some of these side effects. Check with your health care professional if any of the following side effects continue or are bothersome or if you have any questions about them:

More common
Body aches or pain; cough, fever, sneezing, or sore throat; difficulty in breathing; ear congestion; fever; loss of voice; nasal congestion; pain or tenderness around eyes and cheekbones; stuffy or runny nose; tightness of chest

Less common

Back pain; cold or flu-like symptoms; difficulty in moving; pain in joints

Other side effects not listed may also occur in some patients. If you notice any other effects, check with your healthcare professional.

ROSUVASTATIN (Oral route) - roe-SOO-va-sta-tin

Commonly used brand name(s)

In the U.S.—
Crestor

Available Dosage Forms:
• Tablet

Therapeutic Class: Antihyperlipidemic
Pharmacologic Class: HMG-COA Reductase Inhibitor

Uses For This Medicine

Rosuvastatin is used to lower cholesterol and triglyceride (fat-like substances) levels in the blood. Using this medicine may help prevent medical problems caused by such substances clogging the blood vessels.

Rosuvastatin belongs to the group of medicines called 3–hydroxy-3–methylglutaryl coenzyme A (HMG-CoA) reductase inhibitors. It works by blocking an enzyme that is needed by the body to make cholesterol, thereby reducing the amount of cholesterol in the blood.

Rosuvastatin is available only with your doctor's prescription.

Before Using This Medicine

In deciding to use a medicine, the risks of taking the medicine must be weighed against the good it will do. This is a decision you and your doctor will make. For this medicine, the following should be considered:

Allergies—Tell your doctor if you have ever had any unusual or allergic reaction to this medicine or any other medicines. Also tell your health care professional if you have any other types of allergies, such as to foods, dyes, preservatives, or animals. For non-prescription products, read the label or package ingredients carefully.

Pediatric—Studies on this medicine have been done only in adult patients and a small number of pediatric patients 8 years of age and older, and there is no specific information comparing use of rosuvastatin in children with use in other age groups.

Geriatric—This medicine has been tested in a limited number of patients 65 years of age or older and has not been shown to cause different problems in older people than it does in younger adults.

Pregnancy—

	Pregnancy Category	Explanation
All Trimesters	X	Studies in animals or pregnant women have demonstrated positive evidence of fetal abnormalities. This drug should not be used in women who are or may become pregnant because the risk clearly outweighs any possible benefit.

Breast Feeding—There are no adequate studies in women for determining infant risk when using this medication during breastfeeding. Weigh the potential benefits against the potential risks before taking this medication while breastfeeding.

Other medicines—

Using this medicine with any of the following medicines is usually not recommended, but may be required in some cases. If both medicines are prescribed together, your doctor may change the dose or how often you use one or both of the medicines.

Cyclosporine, Gemfibrozil, Niacin

Interactions with Food/Tobacco/Alcohol—Certain medicines should not be used at or around the time of eating food or eating certain types of food since interactions may occur. Using alcohol or tobacco with certain medicines may also cause interactions to occur. Discuss with your healthcare professional the use of your medicine with food, alcohol, or tobacco.

Other medical problems—The presence of other medical problems may affect the use of this medicine. Make sure you tell your doctor if you have any other medical problems, especially:

• Alcohol abuse (or history of) or

• Liver problems (or history of) or

• Liver enzymes, persistently high levels—Use of this medicine may make liver problems worse.

• Chinese or Japanese ancestry—May increase the amount of rosuvastatin in the body.

• Convulsions (seizures), not well-controlled, or

• Electrolyte or metabolic enzyme deficiencies or disorders or

• Infection, severe or

• Low blood pressure or

• Major surgery or trauma, recent—Patients with these conditions may be at risk of developing muscle problems (causing the release of muscle pigment into the urine) that may lead to kidney failure

• Kidney problems or

• Older adult or

• Underactive thyroid—May increase your chance of getting a serious side effect.

• Muscle problems—Use of this medicine may make muscle problems worse.

• Protein in the urine—Rosuvastatin may cause this problem. Your doctor may want to decrease the dose of rosuvastatin if you get this problem.

Proper Use of This Medicine

Use this medicine only as directed by your doctor. Do not use more or less of it, and do not use it more often or for a longer time than your doctor ordered. Also, this medicine works best if there is a constant amount in the blood. To help keep this amount constant, do not miss any doses and take the medicine at the same time each day.

Remember that this medicine will not cure your condition but it does help control it. Therefore, you must continue to take it as directed if you expect to keep your cholesterol levels down.

Before prescribing medicine for your condition, your doctor will probably try to control your condition by prescribing a personal diet for you. Such a diet may be low in fats, sugars, and/or cholesterol. Many people are able to control their condition by carefully following their doctor's orders for proper diet and exercise. Medicine is prescribed only when additional help is needed and is effective only when a schedule of diet and exercise is properly followed.

Follow carefully the special diet your doctor gave you. This is the most important part of controlling your condition and is necessary if the medicine is to work properly.

Dosing—The dose of this medicine will be different for different patients. Follow your doctor's orders or the directions on the label. The following information includes only the average doses of this medicine. If your dose is different, do not change it unless your doctor tells you to do so.

The amount of medicine that you take depends on the strength of the medicine. Also, the number of doses you take each day, the time allowed between doses, and the length of time you take the medicine depend on the medical problem for which you are using the medicine.

- For oral dosage form tablets:
  - Adult: Oral, 5 to 40 mg once daily
  - Children: Use and dose must be determined by your doctor

Missed dose—If you miss a dose of this medicine, take it as soon as possible. However, if it is almost time for your next dose, skip the missed dose and go back to your regular dosing schedule. Do not double doses.

Storage—Store the medicine in a closed container at room temperature, away from heat, moisture, and direct light. Keep from freezing.

Keep the medicine in the foil pouch until you are ready to use it. Store at room temperature, away from heat and direct light. Do not freeze.

Keep out of the reach of children.

Do not keep outdated medicine or medicine no longer needed.

Ask your healthcare professional how you should dispose of any medicine you do not use.

Precautions While Using This Medicine

It is very important that your doctor check your progress at regular visits. This will allow your doctor to see if the medicine is working properly to lower your cholesterol and triglyceride levels and to decide if you should continue to take it.

Check with your doctor immediately if you think that you may be pregnant. HMG-CoA reductase inhibitors may cause birth defects or other problems in the baby if taken during pregnancy.

Before having any kind of surgery (including dental surgery) or emergency treatment, tell the medical doctor or dentist in charge that you are taking this medicine.

Do not use excessive amounts of alcohol while taking rosuvastatin because it can worsen the adverse effects of this medicine on the liver.

Check with your doctor immediately if you experience unexplained muscle pain, tenderness, or weakness, especially if it is accompanied by unusual tiredness or fever, because the medicine's adverse effects on muscle can lead to serious kidney problems.

If your symptoms do not improve or if they become worse, check with your doctor.

Side Effects of This Medicine

Along with its needed effects, a medicine may cause some unwanted effects. Although not all of these side effects may occur, if they do occur they may need medical attention.

Check with your doctor immediately if any of the following side effects occur:

Rare
> Dark-colored urine; fever; muscular pain, tenderness, wasting or weakness; muscle cramps or spasms; muscle pain or stiffness; unusual tiredness or weakness

Incidence not known
> Abdominal or stomach pain; area rash; clay-colored stools; unpleasant breath odor; vomiting of blood; yellow eyes or skin

Some side effects may occur that usually do not need medical attention. These side effects may go away during treatment as your body adjusts to the medicine. Also, your health care professional may be able to tell you about ways to prevent or reduce some of these side effects. Check with your health care professional if any of the following side effects continue or are bothersome or if you have any questions about them:

More common
> Body aches or pain; congestion; cough; dryness or soreness of throat; headache; hoarseness; runny nose; tender, swollen glands in neck; trouble in swallowing; voice changes

Less common
> Accidental injury; accumulation of pus, swollen, red, tender area of infection near a tooth; acid or sour stomach; arm, back or jaw pain; arthritis; back pain; belching; bladder pain; bloated; bloody or cloudy urine; blurred vision; bruising; burning, crawling, itching, numbness, prickling, "pins and needles", or tingling feelings; burning feeling in chest or stomach; chest pain or discomfort; chest tightness or heaviness; chills; constipation; depression; diarrhea; difficult, burning, or painful urination; difficult or labored breathing; difficulty having a bowel movement (stool); difficulty in moving; discouragement; dizziness; dry mouth; excess air or gas in stomach or intestines; excessive muscle tone; fast, irregular, pounding, or racing heartbeat or pulse; fatigue; fear; feeling of constant movement of self or surroundings; feeling of warmth or heat; feeling faint; feeling sad or empty; flatulence; flushed, dry skin; flushing or redness of skin especially on face and neck; frequent urge to urinate; fruit-like breath odor; full

feeling; general feeling of discomfort or illness; heartburn; increased hunger; increased thirst; increased urination; indigestion; infection; irritability; itching skin; joint pain; lack of appetite; lack or loss of strength; large, flat, blue or purplish patches in the skin; lightheadedness; loss of appetite; loss of consciousness; loss of interest or pleasure; lower back or side pain; muscle tension or tightness; nausea; neck pain; nerve pain; nervousness; noisy breathing; pain; pain or swelling in arms or legs without any injury; pain, swelling, or redness in joints; pain or tenderness around eyes and cheekbones; painful or difficult urination; pale skin; passing gas; pounding in the ears; sensation of spinning; shivering; shortness of breath; sleeplessness; slow heartbeat; sneezing; sore throat; stomach pain, discomfort, tenderness, or upset; stuffy nose; sweating; swelling of hands, ankles, feet, or lower legs; tightness in chest; troubled breathing; trouble concentrating; trouble sleeping; unable to sleep; unexplained weight loss; unusual bleeding or bruising; vomiting; wheezing

Other side effects not listed may also occur in some patients. If you notice any other effects, check with your healthcare professional.

SALICYLATES (Systemic)

Some commonly used brand names are:

In the U.S.—

Acuprin 81 (1)	CMT (6)
Amigesic (8)	Cope (4)
Anacin Caplets (2)	Disalcid (8)
Anacin Maximum Strength (2)	Doan's Regular Strength Tablets (7)
Anacin Tablets (2)	Easprin (1)
Anaflex 750 (8)	Ecotrin Caplets (1)
Arthritis Pain Ascriptin (3)	Ecotrin Tablets (1)
Arthritis Pain Formula (3)	Empirin (1)
Arthritis Strength Bufferin (3)	Extended-release Bayer 8–Hour (1)
Arthropan (5)	
Aspergum (1)	Extra Strength Bayer Arthritis Pain Formula Caplets (1)
Aspirin Regimen Bayer Adult Low Dose (1)	Extra Strength Bayer Aspirin Caplets (1)
Aspirin Regimen Bayer Regular Strength Caplets (1)	Extra Strength Bayer Aspirin Tablets (1)
Aspir-Low (1)	Extra Strength Bayer Plus Caplets (3)
Aspirtab (1)	
Aspirtab-Max (1)	Gensan (2)
Backache Caplets (7)	Genuine Bayer Aspirin Caplets (1)
Bayer Children's Aspirin (1)	
Bayer Select Maximum Strength Backache Pain Relief Formula (7)	Genuine Bayer Aspirin Tablets (1)
	Halfprin (1)
Bufferin Caplets (3)	Healthprin Adult Low Strength (1)
Bufferin Tablets (3)	
Buffex (3)	Healthprin Full Strength (1)
Buffinol (3)	Healthprin Half-Dose (1)
Buffinol Extra (3)	Magan (7)
Cama Arthritis Pain Reliever (3)	Magnaprin (3)
	Marthritic (8)

Maximum Strength Arthritis Foundation Safety Coated Aspirin (1)	P-A-C Revised Formula (2)
	Regular Strength Ascriptin (3)
Maximum Strength Ascriptin (3)	Salflex (8)
	Salsitab (8)
Maximum Strength Doan's Analgesic Caplets (7)	Sloprin (1)
	St. Joseph Adult Chewable Aspirin (1)
Mobidin (7)	
Mono-Gesic (8)	Tricosal (6)
Norwich Aspirin (1)	Trilisate (6)
	ZORprin (1)

In Canada—

Anacin (2)	Doan's Backache Pills (7)
Anacin Extra Strength (2)	Dodd's Extra Strength (9)
Antidol (2)	Dodd's Pills (9)
Apo-Asa (1)	Dolomine (2)
Apo-ASEN (1)	Entrophen Caplets (1)
Arco Pain Tablet (2)	Entrophen Extra Strength (1)
Arthrisin (1)	Entrophen 15 Maximum Strength Tablets (1)
Artria S.R (1)	
Aspergum (1)	Entrophen 10 Super Strength Caplets (1)
Aspirin Caplets (1)	
Aspirin Children's Tablets (1)	Entrophen Tablets (1)
Aspirin, Coated (1)	Gin Pain Pills (9)
Aspirin Plus Stomach Guard Extra Strength (3)	Headache Tablet (1)
	Herbopyrine (2)
Aspirin Plus Stomach Guard Regular Strength (3)	Instantine (2)
	Kalmex (2)
Aspirin Tablets (1)	Nervine (2)
Astone (2)	Novasen (1)
Astrin (1)	Novasen Sp.C (1)
Bufferin Caplets (3)	Pain Aid (2)
Bufferin Extra Strength Caplets (3)	PMS-ASA (1)
	Sero-Gesic (7)
Calmine (2)	217 Strong (2)
C2 (2)	217 (2)
C2 Buffered (4)	Tri-Buffered ASA (3)
Coryphen (1)	Trilisate (6)
Disalcid (8)	

This information applies to the following medicines:

1. Aspirin (AS-pir-in)
2. Aspirin and Caffeine (AS-pir-in and KAF-een)
3. Buffered Aspirin
4. Buffered Aspirin and Caffeine
5. Choline Salicylate (KOE-leen sa-LI-si-late)
6. Choline and Magnesium Salicylates (KOE-leen and mag-NEE-zhum sa-LI-si-lates)
7. Magnesium Salicylate (mag-NEE-zhum sa-LI-si-late)
8. Salsalate (SAL-sa-late)
9. Sodium Salicylate (SOE-dee-um sa-LI-si-late)

Category

- **Analgesic**—Aspirin; Aspirin and Caffeine; Aspirin and Caffeine, Buffered; Aspirin, Buffered; Choline and Magnesium Salicylates; Choline Salicylate; Magnesium Salicylate; Salsalate; Sodium Salicylate

- **Anti-inflammatory, nonsteroidal**—Aspirin; Aspirin and Caffeine; Aspirin and Caffeine, Buffered; Aspirin, Buffered; Choline and Magnesium Salicylates; Choline Salicylate; Magnesium Salicylate; Salsalate; Sodium Salicylate

- **Antipyretic**—Aspirin; Aspirin and Caffeine; Aspirin and Caffeine, Buffered; Aspirin, Buffered; Choline and Magnesium Salicylates; Choline Salicylate; Magnesium Salicylate; Salsalate; Sodium Salicylate

- **Antirheumatic, nonsteroidal anti-inflammatory**—Aspirin; Aspirin and Caffeine; Aspirin and Caffeine, Buffered; Aspirin, Buffered; Choline and Magnesium Salicylates; Choline Salicylate; Magnesium Salicylate; Salsalate; Sodium Salicylate

- **Antithrombotic**—Aspirin; Aspirin and Caffeine; Aspirin and Caffeine, Buffered; Aspirin, Buffered
- **Myocardial infarction prophylactic**—Aspirin; Aspirin and Caffeine; Aspirin and Caffeine, Buffered; Aspirin, Buffered
- **Myocardial reinfarction prophylactic**—Aspirin; Aspirin and Caffeine; Aspirin and Caffeine, Buffered; Aspirin, Buffered
- **Platelet aggregation inhibitor**—Aspirin; Aspirin and Caffeine; Aspirin and Caffeine, Buffered; Aspirin, Buffered

---

Description

Salicylates are used to relieve pain and reduce fever. Most salicylates are also used to relieve some symptoms caused by arthritis (rheumatism), such as swelling, stiffness, and joint pain. However, they do not cure arthritis and will help you only as long as you continue to take them.

Aspirin may also be used to lessen the chance of heart attack, stroke, or other problems that may occur when a blood vessel is blocked by blood clots. Aspirin helps prevent dangerous blood clots from forming. However, this effect of aspirin may increase the chance of serious bleeding in some people. Therefore, aspirin should be used for this purpose only when your doctor decides, after studying your medical condition and history, that the danger of blood clots is greater than the risk of bleeding. *Do not take aspirin to prevent blood clots or a heart attack unless it has been ordered by your doctor.*

Salicylates may also be used for other conditions as determined by your doctor.

The caffeine present in some of these products may provide additional relief of headache pain or faster pain relief.

Some salicylates are available only with your medical doctor's or dentist's prescription. Others are available without a prescription; however, your medical doctor or dentist may have special instructions on the proper dose of these medicines for your medical condition.

These medicines are available in the following dosage forms:

Oral
- Aspirin
  - Tablets
  - Chewable tablets
  - Chewing gum tablets
  - Delayed-release (enteric-coated) tablets
  - Extended-release tablets
- Aspirin and Caffeine
  - Capsules
  - Tablets
- Buffered Aspirin
  - Tablets
- Buffered Aspirin and Caffeine
  - Tablets
- Choline Salicylate
  - Oral solution

- Choline and Magnesium Salicylates
  - Oral solution
  - Tablets
- Magnesium Salicylate
  - Tablets
- Salsalate
  - Capsules
  - Tablets
- Sodium Salicylate
  - Tablets
  - Delayed-release (enteric-coated) tablets

Rectal
- Aspirin
  - Suppositories

Before Using This Medicine

If you are taking this medicine without a prescription, carefully read and follow any precautions on the label. For salicylates, the following should be considered:

Allergies—Tell your doctor if you have ever had any unusual or allergic reaction to aspirin or other salicylates, including methyl salicylate (oil of wintergreen), or to any of the following medicines:

- Diclofenac (e.g., Voltaren)
- Diflunisal (e.g., Dolobid)
- Etodolac (e.g., Lodine)
- Fenoprofen (e.g., Nalfon)
- Floctafenine (e.g., Idarac)
- Flurbiprofen, oral (e.g., Ansaid)
- Ibuprofen (e.g., Motrin)
- Indomethacin (e.g., Indocin)
- Ketoprofen (e.g., Orudis)
- Ketorolac (e.g., Toradol)
- Meclofenamate (e.g., Meclomen)
- Mefenamic acid (e.g., Ponstel)
- Nabumetone (e.g., Relafen)
- Naproxen (e.g., Naprosyn)
- Oxaprozin (e.g., Daypro)
- Oxyphenbutazone (e.g., Tandearil)
- Phenylbutazone (e.g., Butazolidin)
- Piroxicam (e.g., Feldene)
- Sulindac (e.g., Clinoril)
- Suprofen (e.g., Suprol)
- Tenoxicam (e.g., Mobiflex)
- Tiaprofenic acid (e.g., Surgam)
- Tolmetin (e.g., Tolectin)
- Zomepirac (e.g., Zomax)

Also tell your health care professional if you are allergic to any other substances, such as foods, preservatives, or dyes.

Diet—Make certain your health care professional knows if you are on a low-sodium diet. Regular use of large amounts of sodium salicylate (as for arthritis) can add a large amount of sodium to your diet. Sodium salicylate contains 46 mg of sodium in each 325–mg tablet and 92 mg of sodium in each 650–mg tablet.

Pregnancy—Salicylates have not been shown to cause birth defects in humans. Studies on birth defects in humans have been done with aspirin but not with other salicylates. However, salicylates caused birth defects in animal studies.

Some reports have suggested that too much use of aspirin late in pregnancy may cause a decrease in the newborn's weight and possible death of the fetus or newborn infant. However, the mothers in these reports had been taking much larger amounts of aspirin than are usually recommended. Studies of mothers taking aspirin in the doses that are usually recommended did not show these unwanted effects. However, there is a chance that regular use of salicylates late in pregnancy may cause unwanted effects on the heart or blood flow in the fetus or in the newborn infant.

Use of salicylates, especially aspirin, during the last 2 weeks of pregnancy may cause bleeding problems in the fetus before or during delivery or in the newborn infant. Also, too much use of salicylates during the last 3 months of pregnancy may increase the length of pregnancy, prolong labor, cause other problems during delivery, or cause severe bleeding in the mother before, during, or after delivery. *Do not take aspirin during the last 3 months of pregnancy unless it has been ordered by your doctor.*

Studies in humans have not shown that caffeine (present in some aspirin products) causes birth defects. However, studies in animals have shown that caffeine causes birth defects when given in very large doses (amounts equal to those present in 12 to 24 cups of coffee a day).

Breast-feeding—Salicylates pass into the breast milk. Although salicylates have not been reported to cause problems in nursing babies, it is possible that problems may occur if large amounts are taken regularly, as for arthritis (rheumatism).

Caffeine passes into the breast milk in small amounts.

Children—*Do not give aspirin or other salicylates to a child or a teenager with a fever or other symptoms of a virus infection, especially flu or chickenpox, without first discussing its use with your child's doctor.* This is very important because salicylates may cause a serious illness called Reye's syndrome in children and teenagers with fever caused by a virus infection, especially flu or chickenpox.

Some children may need to take aspirin or another salicylate regularly (as for arthritis). However, your child's doctor may want to stop the medicine for a while if a fever or other symptoms of a virus infection occur. Discuss this with your child's doctor, so that you will know ahead of time what to do if your child gets sick.

Children who do not have a virus infection may also be more sensitive to the effects of salicylates, especially if they have a fever or have lost large amounts of body fluid because of vomiting, diarrhea, or sweating. This may increase the chance of side effects during treatment.

Older adults—Elderly people are especially sensitive to the effects of salicylates. This may increase the chance of side effects during treatment.

Other medicines—Although certain medicines should not be used together at all, in other cases two different medicines may be used together even if an interaction might occur. In these cases, your doctor may want to change the dose, or other precautions may be necessary. When you are taking a salicylate, it is especially important that your health care professional know if you are taking any of the following:

- Anticoagulants (blood thinners) or
- Carbenicillin by injection (e.g., Geopen) or
- Cefamandole (e.g., Mandol) or
- Cefoperazone (e.g., Cefobid) or
- Cefotetan (e.g., Cefotan) or
- Dipyridamole (e.g., Persantine) or
- Divalproex (e.g., Depakote) or
- Heparin or
- Inflammation or pain medicine, except narcotics, or
- Pentoxifylline (e.g., Trental) or
- Plicamycin (e.g., Mithracin) or
- Ticarcillin (e.g., Ticar) or
- Valproic acid (e.g., Depakene)—Taking these medicines together with a salicylate, especially aspirin, may increase the chance of bleeding
- Antidiabetics, oral (diabetes medicine you take by mouth)—Salicylates may increase the effects of the antidiabetic medicine; a change in dose may be needed if a salicylate is taken regularly
- Ciprofloxacin (e.g., Cipro) or
- Enoxacin (e.g., Penetrex) or
- Itraconazole (e.g., Sporanox) or
- Ketoconazole (e.g., Nizoral) or
- Lomefloxacin (e.g., Maxaquin) or
- Norfloxacin (e.g., Noroxin) or
- Ofloxacin (e.g., Floxin) or
- Tetracyclines (medicine for infection), taken by mouth—Buffered aspirin, choline and magnesium salicylates, and magnesium salicylate may keep these medicines from working properly if taken too close to them
- Methotrexate (e.g., Mexate) or
- Vancomycin (e.g., Vancocin)—The chance of serious side effects may be increased
- Probenecid (e.g., Benemid)—Salicylates can keep probenecid from working properly for treating gout
- Sulfinpyrazone (e.g., Anturane)—Salicylates can keep sulfinpyrazone from working properly for treating gout; also, taking a salicylate, especially aspirin, with sulfinpyrazone may increase the chance of bleeding
- Urinary alkalizers (medicine that makes the urine less acid, such as acetazolamide [e.g., Diamox], calcium-and/or magnesium-containing antacids, dichlorphenamide [e.g., Daranide], methazolamide [e.g., Neptazane], potassium or sodium citrate and/or citric acid, sodium bicarbonate [baking soda])—These medicines may make the salicylate less effective by causing it to be removed from the body more quickly

Other medical problems—The presence of other medical problems may affect the use of salicylates. Make sure you

tell your doctor if you have any other medical problems, especially:

- Anemia or
- Overactive thyroid or
- Stomach ulcer or other stomach problems—Salicylates may make your condition worse
- Asthma, allergies, and nasal polyps (history of) or
- Glucose-6–phosphate dehydrogenase (G6PD) deficiency or
- High blood pressure (hypertension) or
- Kidney disease or
- Liver disease—The chance of side effects may be increased.
- Gout—Salicylates can make this condition worse and can also lessen the effects of some medicines used to treat gout
- Heart disease—The chance of some side effects may be increased. Also, the caffeine present in some aspirin products can make some kinds of heart disease worse
- Hemophilia or other bleeding problems—The chance of bleeding may be increased, especially with aspirin

Proper Use of This Medicine

Take this medicine after meals or with food (except for enteric-coated capsules or tablets and aspirin suppositories) to lessen stomach irritation.

Take tablet or capsule forms of this medicine with a full glass (8 ounces) of water. Also, do not lie down for about 15 to 30 minutes after swallowing the medicine. This helps to prevent irritation that may lead to trouble in swallowing.

For patients taking *aspirin (including buffered aspirin and/or products containing caffeine)*:

- *Do not use any product that contains aspirin if it has a strong, vinegar-like odor.* This odor means the medicine is breaking down. If you have any questions about this, check with your health care professional.
- If you are to take any medicine that contains aspirin within 7 days after having your tonsils removed, a tooth pulled, or other dental or mouth surgery, be sure to swallow the aspirin whole. Do not chew aspirin during this time.
- Do not place any medicine that contains aspirin directly on a tooth or gum surface. This may cause a burn.
- There are several different forms of aspirin or buffered aspirin tablets. If you are using:
  - *chewable aspirin tablets*, they may be chewed, dissolved in liquid, crushed, or swallowed whole.
  - *delayed-release (enteric-coated) aspirin tablets*, they must be swallowed whole. Do not crush them or break them up before taking.
  - *extended-release (long-acting) aspirin tablets*, check with your pharmacist as to how they should be taken. Some may be broken up (but must not be crushed) before swallowing if you cannot swallow them whole. Others should not be broken up and must be swallowed whole.

To use *aspirin suppositories*:

- If the suppository is too soft to insert, chill it in the refrigerator for 30 minutes or run cold water over it before removing the foil wrapper.
- To insert the suppository: First remove the foil wrapper and moisten the suppository with cold water. Lie down on your side and use your finger to push the suppository well up into the rectum.

To take *choline and magnesium salicylates (e.g., Trilisate) oral solution*:

- The liquid may be mixed with fruit juice just before taking.
- Drink a full glass (8 ounces) of water after taking the medicine.

To take *enteric-coated sodium salicylate tablets*:

- The tablets must be swallowed whole. Do not crush them or break them up before taking.

Unless otherwise directed by your medical doctor or dentist:

- Do not take more of this medicine than recommended on the label, to lessen the chance of side effects.
- Children up to 12 years of age should not take this medicine more than 5 times a day.

When used for arthritis (rheumatism), this medicine must be taken regularly as ordered by your doctor in order for it to help you. Up to 2 to 3 weeks or longer may pass before you feel the full effects of this medicine.

Dosing—The dose of these medicines will be different for different patients. *Follow your doctor's orders or the directions on the label.* The following information includes only the average doses of these medicines. *If your dose is different, do not change it* unless your doctor tells you to do so.

The number of capsules or tablets or teaspoonfuls of solution that you take depends on the strength of the medicine. Also, *the number of doses you take each day, the time allowed between doses, and the length of time you take the medicine depend on whether you are taking a long-acting or a short-acting form of the medicine and the medical problem for which you are taking the salicylate.*

For aspirin

- For *short-acting tablet, chewable tablet, and delayed-release (enteric-coated) tablet oral* dosage forms:
  - For pain or fever:
    - Adults and teenagers—325 to 500 milligrams (mg) every three or four hours, 650 mg every four to six hours, or 1000 mg every six hours as needed.
    - Children up to 2 years of age—Dose must be determined by your doctor.
    - Children 2 to 4 years of age—160 mg every four hours as needed.
    - Children 4 to 6 years of age—240 mg every four hours as needed.
    - Children 6 to 9 years of age—320 to 325 mg every four hours as needed.
    - Children 9 to 11 years of age—320 to 400 mg every four hours as needed.
    - Children 11 to 12 years of age—320 to 480 mg every four hours as needed.
  - For arthritis:
    - Adults and teenagers—A total of 3600 to 5400 mg a day, divided into several smaller doses.
    - Children—A total of 80 to 100 mg per kilogram (kg) (32 to 40 mg per pound) of body weight a day, divided into several smaller doses.

- For preventing a heart attack, stroke, or other problems caused by blood clots:
  - Adults—Most people will take 81, 162.5, or 325 mg a day or 325 mg every other day. Some people taking aspirin to prevent a stroke may need as much as 1000 mg a day.
  - Children—Use and dose must be determined by your doctor.
- For *chewing gum tablet* dosage form:
  - For pain:
    - Adults and teenagers—2 tablets every four hours as needed.
    - Children up to 3 years of age—Dose must be determined by your doctor.
    - Children 3 to 6 years of age—1 tablet (227 mg) up to three times a day.
    - Children 6 to 12 years of age—1 or 2 tablets (227 mg each) up to four times a day.
- For *long-acting oral* dosage forms (extended-release tablets):
  - For pain:
    - Adults and teenagers—1 or 2 tablets twice a day.
    - Children—The long-acting aspirin tablets are too strong for use in children.
  - For arthritis:
    - Adults and teenagers—1 or 2 tablets twice a day, at first. Your doctor will then adjust your dose as needed.
    - Children—The long-acting aspirin tablets are too strong for use in children.
- For *rectal* dosage form (suppositories):
  - For pain or fever:
    - Adults and teenagers—325 to 650 mg every four hours as needed.
    - Children up to 2 years of age—Dose must be determined by your doctor.
    - Children 2 to 4 years of age—160 mg every four hours as needed.
    - Children 4 to 6 years of age—240 mg every four hours as needed.
    - Children 6 to 9 years of age—325 mg every four hours as needed.
    - Children 9 to 11 years of age—325 to 400 mg every four hours as needed.
    - Children 11 to 12 years of age—325 to 480 mg every four hours as needed.
  - For arthritis:
    - Adults and teenagers—A total of 3600 to 5400 mg a day, divided into several smaller doses.
    - Children—A total of 80 to 100 mg per kilogram (kg) (32 to 40 mg per pound) of body weight a day, divided into several smaller doses.

For aspirin and caffeine
- For *oral capsule* dosage form:
  - For pain or fever:
    - Adults and teenagers—325 to 500 milligrams (mg) of aspirin every three or four hours, 650 mg of aspirin every four to six hours, or 1000 mg of aspirin every six hours as needed.
    - Children up to 6 years of age—Aspirin and caffeine capsules are too strong for use in children up to 6 years of age.
    - Children 6 to 9 years of age—325 mg every four hours as needed.

- Children 9 to 12 years of age—325 to 400 mg every four hours as needed.
- For arthritis:
  - Adults and teenagers—A total of 3600 to 5400 mg of aspirin a day, divided into several smaller doses.
  - Children—A total of 80 to 100 mg per kilogram (kg) (32 to 40 mg per pound) of body weight a day, divided into several smaller doses.
- For preventing a heart attack, stroke, or other problems caused by blood clots:
  - Adults—325 mg a day or every other day. People who take smaller doses of aspirin will have to use a different product. Some people taking aspirin to prevent a stroke may need as much as 1000 mg a day.
  - Children—Use and dose must be determined by your doctor.
- For *oral tablet* dosage form:
  - For pain or fever:
    - Adults and teenagers—325 to 500 mg of aspirin every three or four hours, 650 mg of aspirin every four to six hours, or 1000 mg of aspirin every six hours as needed.
    - Children up to 9 years of age—Aspirin and caffeine tablets are too strong for use in children up to 9 years of age.
    - Children 9 to 12 years of age—325 to 400 mg every four hours as needed.
  - For arthritis:
    - Adults and teenagers—A total of 3600 to 5400 mg of aspirin a day, divided into several smaller doses.
    - Children—A total of 80 to 100 mg per kg (32 to 40 mg per pound) of body weight a day, divided into several smaller doses.
  - For preventing a heart attack, stroke, or other problems caused by blood clots:
    - Adults—325 mg a day or every other day. People who take smaller doses of aspirin will have to use a different product. Some people taking aspirin to prevent a stroke may need as much as 1000 mg a day.
    - Children—Use and dose must be determined by your doctor.

For buffered aspirin
- For *oral* dosage form (tablets):
  - For pain or fever:
    - Adults and teenagers—325 to 500 milligrams (mg) of aspirin every three or four hours, 650 mg of aspirin every four to six hours, or 1000 mg of aspirin every six hours as needed.
    - Children up to 2 years of age—Dose must be determined by your doctor.
    - Children 2 to 4 years of age—One-half of a 325–mg tablet every four hours as needed.
    - Children 4 to 6 years of age—Three-fourths of a 325–mg tablet every four hours as needed.
    - Children 6 to 9 years of age—One 325–mg tablet every four hours as needed.
    - Children 9 to 11 years of age—One or one and one-fourth 325–mg tablets every four hours as needed.

- Children 11 to 12 years of age—One or one and one-half 325–mg tablets every four hours as needed.
  - For arthritis:
    - Adults and teenagers—A total of 3600 to 5400 mg of aspirin a day, divided into several smaller doses.
    - Children—A total of 80 to 100 mg per kilogram (kg) (32 to 40 mg per pound) of body weight a day, divided into several smaller doses.
  - For preventing a heart attack, stroke, or other problems caused by blood clots:
    - Adults—325 mg a day or every other day. People who take smaller doses of aspirin will have to use a different product. Some people taking aspirin to prevent a stroke may need as much as 1000 mg a day.
    - Children—Use and dose must be determined by your doctor.

For buffered aspirin and caffeine
- For *oral* dosage form (tablets):
  - For pain or fever:
    - Adults and teenagers—325 or 421 milligrams (mg) of aspirin every three or four hours, 650 mg of aspirin every four to six hours, or 842 mg of aspirin every six hours as needed.
    - Children up to 2 years of age—Dose must be determined by your doctor.
    - Children 2 to 4 years of age—One-half of a 325–mg tablet every four hours as needed.
    - Children 4 to 6 years of age—Three-fourths of a 325–mg tablet every four hours as needed.
    - Children 6 to 9 years of age—One 325–mg or 421–mg tablet every four hours as needed.
    - Children 9 to 11 years of age—One or one and one-fourth 325–mg tablets every four hours as needed.
    - Children 11 to 12 years of age—One or one and one-half 325–mg tablets, or one 421–mg tablet, every four hours as needed.
  - For arthritis:
    - Adults and teenagers—A total of 3600 to 5400 mg of aspirin a day, divided into several smaller doses.
    - Children—A total of 80 to 100 mg per kilogram (kg) (32 to 40 mg per pound) of body weight a day, divided into several smaller doses.
  - For preventing a heart attack, stroke, or other problems caused by blood clots:
    - Adults—162.5 or 325 mg (one-half or one 325–mg tablet) a day or 325 mg every other day. People who need smaller doses of aspirin will have to use a different product. Some people taking aspirin to prevent a stroke may need as much as 1000 mg a day.
    - Children—Use and dose must be determined by your doctor.

For choline salicylate
- For *oral* dosage form (oral solution):
  - For pain or fever:
    - Adults and teenagers—One-half or three-fourths of a teaspoonful every three hours, one-half or one teaspoonful every four hours, or one or one and one-half teaspoonfuls every six hours as needed.
    - Children up to 2 years of age—Dose must be determined by your doctor.
    - Children 2 to 4 years of age—1.25 milliliters (mL) (one-fourth of a teaspoonful) every four hours as needed. This amount should be measured by a special dropper or measuring spoon.
    - Children 4 to 6 years of age—1.66 mL every four hours as needed. This amount should be measured by a special dropper or measuring spoon.
    - Children 6 to 11 years of age—2.5 mL (one-half of a teaspoonful) every four hours as needed. This amount should be measured by a special measuring spoon.
    - Children 11 to 12 years of age—2.5 to 3.75 mL (one-half to three-fourths of a teaspoonful) every four hours as needed. This amount should be measured by a special measuring spoon.
  - For arthritis:
    - Adults—A total of five and one-half to eight teaspoonfuls a day, divided into several smaller doses.
    - Children—A total of 0.6 to 0.7 mL per kilogram (kg) (0.25 to 0.28 mL per pound) of body weight a day, divided into several smaller doses.

For choline and magnesium salicylates
- For *oral* dosage forms (oral solution or tablets):
  - For pain or fever:
    - Adults and teenagers—A total of 2000 to 3000 milligrams (mg) a day, divided into two or three doses.
    - Children weighing up to 37 kilograms (kg) (about 89 pounds)—A total of 50 mg per kg (20 mg per pound) of body weight a day, divided into two doses.
    - Children weighing more than 37 kg (90 pounds or more)—2200 mg a day, divided into two doses.
  - For inflammation or arthritis:
    - Adults and teenagers—A total of 3000 mg a day, divided into two or three doses, to start. Your doctor will then adjust your dose as needed.
    - Children weighing up to 37 kg (about 89 pounds)—A total of 50 mg per kg (20 mg per pound) of body weight a day, divided into two doses.
    - Children weighing more than 37 kg (90 pounds or more)—2200 mg a day, divided into two doses.

For magnesium salicylate
- For *oral* dosage form (tablets):
  - For pain:
    - Adults and teenagers—2 regular-strength tablets every four hours, up to a maximum of 12 tablets a day, or 2 extra-strength tablets every eight hours, up to a maximum of 8 tablets a day.
    - Children—Dose must be determined by your doctor.

For salsalate
- For *oral* dosage forms (capsules or tablets):
  - For arthritis:
    - Adults and teenagers—500 to 1000 milligrams (mg) two or three times a day, to start. Your doctor will then adjust your dose as needed.
    - Children—Dose must be determined by your doctor.

For sodium salicylate
- For *oral* dosage forms (tablets or delayed-release [enteric-coated] tablets):
  - For pain or fever:
    - Adults and teenagers—325 or 650 milligrams (mg) every four hours as needed.
    - Children up to 6 years of age—This medicine is too strong for use in children younger than 6 years of age.
    - Children 6 years of age and older—325 mg every four hours as needed.
  - For arthritis:
    - Adults and teenagers—A total of 3600 to 5400 mg a day, divided into several smaller doses.
    - Children—A total of 80 to 100 mg per kilogram (kg) (32 to 40 mg per pound) of body weight a day, divided into several smaller doses.

Missed dose—If your medical doctor or dentist has ordered you to take this medicine according to a regular schedule and you miss a dose, take it as soon as you remember. However, if it is almost time for your next dose, skip the missed dose and go back to your regular dosing schedule. Do not double doses.

Storage—To store this medicine:
- Keep out of the reach of children. Overdose is very dangerous in young children.
- Store away from heat and direct light.
- Do not store tablets or capsules in the bathroom, near the kitchen sink, or in other damp places. Heat or moisture may cause the medicine to break down.
- Keep liquid forms of this medicine from freezing.
- Store aspirin suppositories in a cool place. It is usually best to keep them in the refrigerator, but keep them from freezing.
- Do not keep outdated medicine or medicine no longer needed. Be sure that any discarded medicine is out of the reach of children.

Precautions While Using This Medicine

Check the labels of all nonprescription (over-the-counter [OTC]) and prescription medicines you now take. If any contain aspirin or other salicylates (including bismuth subsalicylate [e.g., Pepto-Bismol] or any shampoo or skin medicine that contains salicylic acid or any other salicylate), check with your health care professional. Taking or using them together with this medicine may cause an overdose.

If you will be taking salicylates for a long time (more than 5 days in a row for children or 10 days in a row for adults) or in large amounts, *your doctor should check your progress at regular visits.*

Serious side effects can occur during treatment with this medicine. Sometimes serious side effects can occur without any warning. However, possible warning signs often occur, including swelling of the face, fingers, feet, and/or lower legs; severe stomach pain, black, tarry stools, and/or vomiting of blood or material that looks like coffee grounds; unusual weight gain; and/or skin rash. Also, signs of serious heart problems could occur such as chest pain, tightness in chest, fast or irregular heartbeat, or unusual flushing or warmth of skin. *Stop taking this medicine and check with your doctor immediately if you notice any of these warning signs.*

Check with your medical doctor or dentist:
- If you are taking this medicine to relieve pain and the pain lasts for more than 10 days (5 days for children) or if the pain gets worse, if new symptoms occur, or if redness or swelling is present. These could be signs of a serious condition that needs medical or dental treatment.
- If you are taking this medicine to bring down a fever, and the fever lasts for more than 3 days or returns, if the fever gets worse, if new symptoms occur, or if redness or swelling is present. These could be signs of a serious condition that needs treatment.
- If you are taking this medicine for a sore throat, and the sore throat is very painful, lasts for more than 2 days, or occurs together with or is followed by fever, headache, skin rash, nausea, or vomiting.
- If you are taking this medicine regularly, as for arthritis (rheumatism), and you notice a ringing or buzzing in your ears or severe or continuing headaches. These are often the first signs that too much salicylate is being taken. Your doctor may want to change the amount of medicine you are taking every day.

For patients taking *aspirin to lessen the chance of heart attack, stroke, or other problems caused by blood clots:*
- *Take only the amount of aspirin ordered by your doctor.* If you need a medicine to relieve pain, a fever, or arthritis, your doctor may not want you to take extra aspirin. It is a good idea to discuss this with your doctor, so that you will know ahead of time what medicine to take.
- *Do not stop taking this medicine for any reason without first checking with the doctor who directed you to take it.*

Taking certain other medicines together with a salicylate may increase the chance of unwanted effects. The risk will depend on how much of each medicine you take every day, and on how long you take the medicines together. If your doctor directs you to take these medicines together on a regular basis, follow his or her directions carefully. However, *do not take any of the following medicines together with a salicylate for more than a few days, unless your doctor has directed you to do so and is following your progress:*
- Acetaminophen (e.g., Tylenol)
- Diclofenac (e.g., Voltaren)
- Diflunisal (e.g., Dolobid)
- Etodolac (e.g., Lodine)
- Fenoprofen (e.g., Nalfon)
- Floctafenine (e.g., Idarac)
- Flurbiprofen, oral (e.g., Ansaid)
- Ibuprofen (e.g., Motrin)
- Indomethacin (e.g., Indocin)
- Ketoprofen (e.g., Orudis)
- Ketorolac (e.g., Toradol)
- Meclofenamate (e.g., Meclomen)
- Mefenamic acid (e.g., Ponstel)
- Nabumetone (e.g., Relafen)
- Naproxen (e.g., Naprosyn)
- Oxaprozin (e.g., Daypro)
- Phenylbutazone (e.g., Butazolidin)
- Piroxicam (e.g., Feldene)
- Sulindac (e.g., Clinoril)

- Tenoxicam (e.g., Mobiflex)
- Tiaprofenic acid (e.g., Surgam)
- Tolmetin (e.g., Tolectin)

For *diabetic patients:*
- False urine sugar test results may occur if you are regularly taking large amounts of salicylates, such as:
  - *Aspirin:* 8 or more 325–mg (5–grain), or 4 or more
500–mg or 650–mg (10–grain), or 3 or more 800–mg
(or higher strength), doses a day.
  - *Buffered aspirin or*
  - *Sodium salicylate:* 8 or more 325–mg (5–grain), or
4 or more 500–mg or 650–mg (10–grain), doses a
day.
  - *Choline salicylate:* 4 or more teaspoonfuls (each
teaspoonful containing 870 mg) a day.
  - *Choline and magnesium salicylates:* 5 or more
500–mg tablets or teaspoonfuls, 4 or more 750–mg
tablets, or 2 or more 1000–mg tablets, a day.
  - *Magnesium salicylate:* 7 or more regular-strength,
or 4 or more extra-strength, tablets a day.
  - *Salsalate:* 4 or more 500–mg doses, or 3 or more
750–mg doses, a day.
- Smaller doses or occasional use of salicylates usually
will not affect urine sugar tests. However, check with
your health care professional (especially if your diabetes
is not well-controlled) if:
  - you are not sure how much salicylate you are taking
every day.
  - you notice any change in your urine sugar test results.
  - you have any other questions about this possible
problem.

Do not take aspirin for 5 days before any surgery, including
dental surgery, unless otherwise directed by your medical
doctor or dentist. Taking aspirin during this time may cause
bleeding problems.

For patients taking *buffered aspirin, choline and magnesium salicylates (e.g., Trilisate), or magnesium salicylate
(e.g., Doan's):*
- Buffered aspirin, choline and magnesium salicylates, or
magnesium salicylate can keep many other medicines,
especially some medicines used to treat infections, from
working properly. This problem can be prevented by not
taking the 2 medicines too close together. Ask your
health care professional how long you should wait between taking a medicine for infection and taking buffered
aspirin, choline and magnesium salicylates, or magnesium salicylate.

If you are taking a laxative containing cellulose, take the salicylate at least 2 hours before or after you take the laxative.
Taking these medicines too close together may lessen the
effects of the salicylate.

For patients taking this medicine by mouth:
- Stomach problems may be more likely to occur if you
drink alcoholic beverages while being treated with this
medicine, especially if you are taking it in high doses or
for a long time. Check with your doctor if you have any
questions about this.

For patients using *aspirin suppositories:*
- Aspirin suppositories may cause irritation of the rectum.
Check with your doctor if this occurs.

Salicylates may interfere with the results of some medical
tests. Before you have any medical tests, tell the doctor in

charge if you have taken any of these medicines within the
past week. If possible, it is best to check with the doctor first,
to find out whether the medicine may be taken during the
week before the test.

For patients taking one of the products that contain *caffeine:*

- Caffeine may interfere with the result of a test that uses
adenosine (e.g., Adenocard) or dipyridamole (e.g., Persantine) to help find out how well your blood is flowing
through certain blood vessels. Therefore, you should not
have any caffeine for at least 8 to 12 hours before the
test.

*If you think that you or anyone else may have taken an
overdose, get emergency help at once.* Taking an overdose
of these medicines may cause unconsciousness or death.
Signs of overdose include convulsions (seizures), hearing
loss, confusion, ringing or buzzing in the ears, severe drowsiness or tiredness, severe excitement or nervousness, and
fast or deep breathing.

Side Effects of This Medicine

Along with its needed effects, a medicine may cause some
unwanted effects. When this medicine is used for short periods of time at low doses, side effects usually are rare. Although not all of the following side effects may occur, if they
do occur they may need medical attention.

Get emergency help immediately if any of the following side
effects occur:
> *Symptoms of overdose in children*
> Changes in behavior; drowsiness or tiredness (severe);
> fast or deep breathing

Any loss of hearing; bloody urine; confusion; convulsions
(seizures); diarrhea (severe or continuing); difficulty in
swallowing; dizziness, lightheadedness, or feeling faint
(severe); drowsiness (severe); excitement or nervousness
(severe); fast or deep breathing; flushing, redness, or
other change in skin color; hallucinations (seeing, hearing,
or feeling things that are not there); increased sweating;
increased thirst; nausea or vomiting (severe or continuing); shortness of breath, troubled breathing, tightness in
chest, or wheezing; stomach pain (severe or continuing);
swelling of eyelids, face, or lips; unexplained fever; uncontrollable flapping movements of the hands (especially in
elderly patients); vision problems

Also, check with your doctor as soon as possible if any of the
following side effects occur:
> *Less common or rare*
> Abdominal or stomach pain, cramping, or burning (se-
> vere); bloody or black, tarry stools; headache (severe
> or continuing); ringing or buzzing in ears (continuing);
> skin rash, hives, or itching; unusual tiredness or weak-
> ness; vomiting of blood or material that looks like coffee
> grounds

Other side effects may occur that usually do not need medical attention. These side effects may go away during treatment as your body adjusts to the medicine. However, check
with your health care professional if any of the following side
effects continue or are bothersome:
> *More common*
> Abdominal or stomach cramps, pain, or discomfort
> (mild to moderate); heartburn or indigestion; nausea or
> vomiting

Less common

    Trouble in sleeping, nervousness, or jitters (only for products containing caffeine)

Other side effects not listed above may also occur in some patients. If you notice any other effects, check with your doctor.

SAQUINAVIR (Oral route) - sa-KWIN-a-veer

Black Box Warning

Saquinavir mesylate (hard gelatin capsules and tablets) and saquinavir soft gelatin capsules are not bioequivalent and cannot be used interchangeably. Saquinavir mesylate may be used only if it is combined with ritonavir, which significantly inhibits saquinavir's metabolism to provide plasma saquinavir levels at least equal to those achieved with saquinavir soft gelatin capsules. When using saquinavir as the sole protease inhibitor in an antiviral regimen, saquinavir soft gelatin capsules is the recommended formulation.

Commonly used brand name(s)

In the U.S.—
    Fortovase
    Invirase

Available Dosage Forms:

- Capsule, Liquid Filled
- Tablet
- Capsule

Therapeutic Class: Antiretroviral Agent
Pharmacologic Class: Protease Inhibitor

Uses For This Medicine

Saquinavir is used, usually in combination with other HIV medicines including ritonavir (e.g., Norvir), in the treatment of the infection caused by the human immunodeficiency virus (HIV). HIV is the virus that causes acquired immune deficiency syndrome (AIDS).

Saquinavir will not cure or prevent HIV infection or AIDS; however, it helps keep HIV from reproducing and appears to slow down the destruction of the immune system. This may help delay the development of problems usually related to AIDS or HIV disease. Saquinavir will not keep you from spreading HIV to other people. People who receive this medicine may continue to have other problems usually related to AIDS or HIV disease.

This medicine is available only with your doctor's prescription.

Before Using This Medicine

In deciding to use a medicine, the risks of taking the medicine must be weighed against the good it will do. This is a decision you and your doctor will make. For this medicine, the following should be considered:

Allergies—Tell your doctor if you have ever had any unusual or allergic reaction to this medicine or any other medicines. Also tell your health care professional if you have any other types of allergies, such as to foods, dyes, preservatives, or animals. For non-prescription products, read the label or package ingredients carefully.

Pediatric—There is no specific information comparing use of saquinavir in children with use in other age groups.

Geriatric—Many medicines have not been studied specifically in older people. Therefore, it may not be known whether they work exactly the same way they do in younger adults. There is no specific information comparing use of saquinavir in the elderly with use in other age groups.

Pregnancy—

	Pregnancy Category	Explanation
All Trimesters	B	Animal studies have revealed no evidence of harm to the fetus, however, there are no adequate studies in pregnant women OR animal studies have shown an adverse effect, but adequate studies in pregnant women have failed to demonstrate a risk to the fetus.

Breast Feeding—There are no adequate studies in women for determining infant risk when using this medication during breastfeeding. Weigh the potential benefits against the potential risks before taking this medication while breastfeeding.

Other medicines—

Using this medicine with any of the following medicines is not recommended. Your doctor may decide not to treat you with this medication or change some of the other medicines you take.

Amiodarone, Astemizole, Bepridil, Cisapride, Dihydroergotamine, Ergoloid Mesylates, Ergonovine, Ergotamine, Flecainide, Methylergonovine, Midazolam, Pimozide, Propafenone, Quinidine, Ranolazine, Rifampin, St John's Wort, Terfenadine, Triazolam

Interactions with Food/Tobacco/Alcohol—Certain medicines should not be used at or around the time of eating food or eating certain types of food since interactions may occur. Using alcohol or tobacco with certain medicines may also cause interactions to occur. Discuss with your healthcare professional the use of your medicine with food, alcohol, or tobacco.

Other medical problems—The presence of other medical problems may affect the use of this medicine. Make sure you tell your doctor if you have any other medical problems, especially:

- Alcoholism or
- Cirrhosis of the liver or
- Hepatitis B or
- Hepatitis C—May cause liver problems to become worse
- Diabetes mellitus (sugar diabetes) or
- High blood sugar—May make these conditions worse.
- Hemophilia—Possible increased risk of bleeding
- Kidney disease, severe—Caution should be used
- Liver disease—Effects of saquinavir may be increased because of slower removal of the medicine from the body; also saquinavir has been reported to cause un-

wanted effects on the liver. If liver disease is severe, do not take saquinavir.

Proper Use of This Medicine

It is important that this medicine be taken with food in order to work properly. Take saquinavir within 2 hours after a meal.

Take this medicine exactly as directed by your doctor. Do not take it more often, and do not take it for a longer time than your doctor ordered. Also, do not stop taking this medicine without checking with your doctor first.

Keep taking saquinavir for the full time of treatment, even if you begin to feel better.

This medicine works best when there is a constant amount in the blood. To help keep the amount constant, do not miss any doses. Also, it is best to take the doses at evenly spaced times, day and night. For example, if you are to take three doses a day, the doses should be spaced about 8 hours apart. If you need help in planning the best times to take your medicine, check with your health care professional.

Take only the brand name of this medicine that the doctor has prescribed for you. Do not switch from one brand name to another unless your doctor tells you to. Different brands may not contain the same amount of medicine.

Only take medicine that your doctor has prescribed specially for you. Do not share your medicine with others.

Dosing—The dose of this medicine will be different for different patients. Follow your doctor's orders or the directions on the label. The following information includes only the average doses of this medicine. If your dose is different, do not change it unless your doctor tells you to do so.

The amount of medicine that you take depends on the strength of the medicine. Also, the number of doses you take each day, the time allowed between doses, and the length of time you take the medicine depend on the medical problem for which you are using the medicine.

- For oral dosage form (capsules and tablets [brand name Invirase]):
  - For treatment of HIV infection:
    - Adults—1000 milligrams (mg) two times a day, in combination with ritonavir (e.g., Norvir).
    - Children up to 16 years of age—Use and dose must be determined by your doctor.
  Note: Invirase must be used in combination with ritonavir (e.g., Norvir). Your doctor will tell you the dose of ritonavir that you should take.
- For oral dosage form (soft gelatin capsules [brand name Fortovase]):
  - For treatment of HIV infection:
    - Adults—1200 mg three times a day, alone or in combination with other medicines for HIV infection.
    - Children up to 16 years of age—Use and dose must be determined by your doctor.

Missed dose—If you miss a dose of this medicine, take it as soon as possible. However, if it is almost time for your next dose, skip the missed dose and go back to your regular dosing schedule. Do not double doses.

Storage—Keep out of the reach of children.

Do not keep outdated medicine or medicine no longer needed.

Store the soft gelatin capsule form (Fortovase) in the refrigerator. The Invirase capsules do not need to be refrigerated.

Precautions While Using This Medicine

Do not take any other medicines without checking with your doctor first. To do so may increase the chance of side effects from saquinavir or other medicines.

It is very important that your doctor check your progress at regular visits to make sure this medicine is working properly and to check for unwanted effects, especially increases in blood sugar.

This medicine may decrease the effects of some oral contraceptives (birth control pills). To avoid unwanted pregnancy, it is a good idea to use some additional contraceptive measures while being treated with saquinavir.

Saquinavir does not decrease the risk of transmitting the HIV infection to others through sexual contact or by contamination through blood. HIV may be acquired from or spread to others through infected body fluids, including blood, vaginal fluid, or semen. *If you are infected, it is best to avoid any sexual activity involving an exchange of body fluids with other people. If you do have sex, always wear (or have your partner wear) a condom ("rubber").* Only use condoms made of latex, and *use them every time you have vaginal, anal, or oral sex.* The use of a spermicide (such as nonoxynol-9) may also help prevent the spread of HIV if it is not irritating to the vagina, rectum, or mouth. Spermicides have been shown to kill HIV in lab tests. Do not use oil-based jelly, cold cream, baby oil, or shortening as a lubricant— these products can cause the condom to break. Lubricants without oil, such as *K-Y Jelly*, are recommended. Women may wish to carry their own condoms. Birth control pills and diaphragms will help protect against pregnancy, but they will not prevent someone from giving or getting the AIDS virus. *If you inject drugs,* get help to stop. *Do not share needles or equipment with anyone.* In some cities, more than half of the drug users are infected, and sharing even 1 needle or syringe can spread the virus. If you have any questions about this, check with your health care professional.

Side Effects of This Medicine

Along with its needed effects, a medicine may cause some unwanted effects. Although not all of these side effects may occur, if they do occur they may need medical attention.

Check with your doctor as soon as possible if any of the following side effects occur:

Less common
  Chest pain

Rare
  Burning or prickling sensation; confusion; dehydration; dry or itchy skin; fruity mouth odor; increased hunger; increased thirst; increased urination; nausea; skin rash; unusual tiredness; vomiting; weight loss

Some side effects may occur that usually do not need medical attention. These side effects may go away during treatment as your body adjusts to the medicine. Also, your health care professional may be able to tell you about ways to prevent or reduce some of these side effects. Check with your health care professional if any of the following side effects

continue or are bothersome or if you have any questions about them:

Less common or rare

Abdominal pain; acid or sour stomach; belching; bloated full feeling; change in taste; decreased interest in sexual intercourse; diarrhea; difficulty having a bowel movement (stool); discouragement; excess air or gas in stomach or intestines; fear; feeling sad or empty; headache; heartburn; inability to have or keep an erection; indigestion; irritability; lack of appetite; loss in sexual ability, desire, drive, or performance; loss of interest or pleasure; mouth ulcers; nervousness; passing gas; skin rash encrusted, scaly, and oozing; skin warts; sleeplessness; stomach upset, discomfort or pain; tiredness; trouble concentrating; trouble sleeping; unable to sleep; unusual tiredness or weakness; weakness

Other side effects not listed may also occur in some patients. If you notice any other effects, check with your healthcare professional.

SELEGILINE (Oral route) - se-LE-ji-leen

Commonly used brand name(s)

In the U.S.—
Eldepryl
Zelapar

Available Dosage Forms:

- Tablet
- Tablet, Disintegrating
- Capsule

Therapeutic Class: Antiparkinsonian
Pharmacologic Class: Monoamine Oxidase Inhibitor, Type B

Uses For This Medicine

Selegiline is used in combination with levodopa or levodopa and carbidopa combination to treat Parkinson's disease, sometimes called shaking palsy or paralysis agitans. This medicine works to increase and extend the effects of levodopa, and may help to slow the progress of Parkinson's disease.

Selegiline is available only with your doctor's prescription.

Before Using This Medicine

In deciding to use a medicine, the risks of taking the medicine must be weighed against the good it will do. This is a decision you and your doctor will make. For this medicine, the following should be considered:

Allergies—Tell your doctor if you have ever had any unusual or allergic reaction to this medicine or any other medicines. Also tell your health care professional if you have any other types of allergies, such as to foods, dyes, preservatives, or animals. For non-prescription products, read the label or package ingredients carefully.

Pediatric—Studies on this medicine have been done only in adult patients and there is no specific information about its use in children. Therefore, be sure to discuss with your doctor the use of this medicine in children.

Geriatric—In studies done to date that included elderly people, selegiline did not cause different side effects or problems in older people than it did in younger adults.

Pregnancy—

	Pregnancy Category	Explanation
All Trimesters	C	Animal studies have shown an adverse effect and there are no adequate studies in pregnant women OR no animal studies have been conducted and there are no adequate studies in pregnant women.

Breast Feeding—There are no adequate studies in women for determining infant risk when using this medication during breastfeeding. Weigh the potential benefits against the potential risks before taking this medication while breastfeeding.

Other medicines—

Using this medicine with any of the following medicines is not recommended. Your doctor may decide not to treat you with this medication or change some of the other medicines you take.

Amitriptyline, Amoxapine, Amphetamine, Apraclonidine, Atomoxetine, Benzphetamine, Brimonidine, Bupropion, Carbamazepine, Citalopram, Clomipramine, Cyclobenzaprine, Cyproheptadine, Desipramine, Dexfenfluramine, Dexmethylphenidate, Dextroamphetamine, Dextromethorphan, Diethylpropion, Duloxetine, Ephedrine, Escitalopram, Fenfluramine, Fluoxetine, Imipramine, Isometheptene, Levodopa, Levomethadyl, Maprotiline, Mazindol, Meperidine, Methadone, Methamphetamine, Methotrimeprazine, Methyldopa, Methylphenidate, Mirtazapine, Morphine, Morphine Sulfate Liposome, Nefopam, Nortriptyline, Opipramol, Paroxetine, Phendimetrazine, Phenelzine, Phenmetrazine, Phentermine, Phenylalanine, Phenylephrine, Phenylpropanolamine, Propoxyphene, Protriptyline, Pseudoephedrine, Reserpine, Sertraline, Sibutramine, St John's Wort, Tramadol, Trimipramine, Venlafaxine

Interactions with Food/Tobacco/Alcohol—Certain medicines should not be used at or around the time of eating food or eating certain types of food since interactions may occur. Using alcohol or tobacco with certain medicines may also cause interactions to occur. The following interactions have been selected on the basis of their potential significance and are not necessarily all-inclusive.

Using this medicine with any of the following is usually not recommended, but may be unavoidable in some cases. If used together, your doctor may change the dose or how often you use this medicine, or give you special instructions about the use of food, alcohol, or tobacco.

Tyramine Containing Food

Other medical problems—The presence of other medical problems may affect the use of this medicine. Make sure you tell your doctor if you have any other medical problems, especially:

- Stomach ulcer (history of)—Selegiline may make the condition worse

Proper Use of This Medicine

Take this medicine only as directed by your doctor. Do not take more of it, do not take it more often, and do not take it for a longer time than your doctor ordered.

Dosing—The dose of this medicine will be different for different patients. Follow your doctor's orders or the directions on the label. The following information includes only the average doses of this medicine. If your dose is different, do not change it unless your doctor tells you to do so.

The amount of medicine that you take depends on the strength of the medicine. Also, the number of doses you take each day, the time allowed between doses, and the length of time you take the medicine depend on the medical problem for which you are using the medicine.

For the treatment of Parkinson's disease, the usual dose of selegiline is 5 mg two times a day, taken with breakfast and lunch. Some patients may need less than this.

Missed dose—If you miss a dose of this medicine, take it as soon as possible. However, if it is almost time for your next dose, skip the missed dose and go back to your regular dosing schedule. Do not double doses.

Storage—Store the medicine in a closed container at room temperature, away from heat, moisture, and direct light. Keep from freezing.

Keep out of the reach of children.

Do not keep outdated medicine or medicine no longer needed.

Precautions While Using This Medicine

When selegiline is taken at doses of 10 mg or less per day for the treatment of Parkinson's disease, there are no restrictions on food or beverages you eat or drink. However, the chance exists that dangerous reactions, such as sudden high blood pressure, may occur if doses higher than those used for Parkinson's disease are taken with certain foods, beverages, or other medicines. These foods, beverages, and medicines include:

- Foods that have a high tyramine content (most common in foods that are aged or fermented to increase their flavor), such as cheeses; fava or broad bean pods; yeast or meat extracts; smoked or pickled meat, poultry, or fish; fermented sausage (bologna, pepperoni, salami, summer sausage) or other fermented meat; sauerkraut; or any overripe fruit. If a list of these foods and beverages is not given to you, ask your health care professional to provide one.
- Alcoholic beverages or alcohol-free or reduced-alcohol beer and wine.
- Large amounts of caffeine-containing food or beverages such as coffee, tea, cola, or chocolate.
- Any other medicine unless approved or prescribed by your doctor. This especially includes nonprescription (over-the-counter [OTC]) medicine, such as that for colds (including nose drops or sprays), cough, asthma, hay fever, and appetite control; "keep awake" products; or products that make you sleepy.

Also, for at least 2 weeks after you stop taking this medicine, these foods, beverages, and other medicines may continue to react with selegiline if it was taken in doses higher than those usually used for Parkinson's disease.

Check with your doctor or hospital emergency room immediately if severe headache, stiff neck, chest pains, fast heartbeat, or nausea and vomiting occur while you are taking this medicine. These may be symptoms of a serious side effect that should have a doctor's attention.

Dizziness, lightheadedness, or fainting may occur, especially when you get up from a lying or sitting position. Getting up

slowly may help. If the problem continues or gets worse, check with your doctor.

Selegiline may cause dryness of the mouth. For temporary relief, use sugarless candy or gum, melt bits of ice in your mouth, or use a saliva substitute. However, if your mouth continues to feel dry for more than 2 weeks, check with your medical doctor or dentist. Continuing dryness of the mouth may increase the chance of dental disease, including tooth decay, gum disease, and fungus infections.

Side Effects of This Medicine

When you start taking selegiline in addition to levodopa or carbidopa and levodopa combination, you may experience an increase in side effects. If this occurs, your doctor may gradually reduce the amount of levodopa or carbidopa and levodopa combination you take.

Along with its needed effects, a medicine may cause some unwanted effects. Although not all of these side effects may occur, if they do occur they may need medical attention.

Stop taking this medicine and get emergency help immediately if any of the following effects occur:
Symptoms of unusually high blood pressure (caused by reaction of higher than usual doses of selegiline with restricted foods or medicines)
   Chest pain (severe); enlarged pupils; fast or slow heartbeat; headache (severe); increased sensitivity of eyes to light; increased sweating (possibly with fever or cold, clammy skin); nausea and vomiting (severe); stiff or sore neck

Check with your doctor as soon as possible if any of the following side effects occur:
More common
   Increase in unusual movements of body; mood or other mental changes

Less common or rare
   Bloody or black, tarry stools; difficult or frequent urination; difficulty in breathing; difficulty in speaking; dizziness or lightheadedness, especially when getting up from a lying or sitting position; hallucinations (seeing, hearing, or feeling things that are not there); irregular heartbeat; lip smacking or puckering; loss of balance control; puffing of cheeks; rapid or worm-like movements of tongue; restlessness or desire to keep moving; severe stomach pain; swelling of feet or lower legs; tightness in chest; twisting movements of body; uncontrolled chewing movements; uncontrolled movements of face, neck, back, arms or legs; vomiting of blood or material that looks like coffee grounds; wheezing

Symptoms of overdose
   Agitation or irritability; chest pain; convulsions (seizures); difficulty opening mouth or lockjaw; dizziness (severe) or fainting; fast or irregular pulse (continuing); high fever; high or low blood pressure; increased sweating (possibly with fever or cold, clammy skin); severe spasm where the head and heels are bent backward and the body arched forward; troubled breathing

Some side effects may occur that usually do not need medical attention. These side effects may go away during treatment as your body adjusts to the medicine. Also, your health care professional may be able to tell you about ways to prevent or reduce some of these side effects. Check with your health care professional if any of the following side effects

continue or are bothersome or if you have any questions about them:

More common
   Abdominal or stomach pain; dizziness or feeling faint; dryness of mouth; nausea; trouble in sleeping; vomiting

Less common or rare
   Anxiety; back or leg pain; blurred or double vision; body ache; burning of lips, mouth, or throat; chills; constipation; diarrhea; drowsiness; headache; heartburn; high or low blood pressure; inability to move; frequent urge to urinate; increased sensitivity of skin to light; increased sweating; irritability (temporary); loss of appetite; memory problems; muscle cramps; nervousness; numbness of fingers or toes; pounding or fast heartbeat; red, raised, or itchy skin; restlessness; ringing or buzzing in ears; slow or difficult urination; slowed movements; taste changes; uncontrolled closing of eyelids; unusual feeling of well-being; unusual tiredness or weakness; unusual weight loss

With doses higher than 10 mg a day
   Clenching, gnashing, or grinding teeth; sudden jerky movements of body

Other side effects not listed may also occur in some patients. If you notice any other effects, check with your healthcare professional.

SERTACONAZOLE (Topical route) -
ser-ta-KON-a-zole

Commonly used brand name(s)
In the U.S.—
   Ertaczo

Available Dosage Forms:
• Cream

Therapeutic Class: Antifungal

Uses For This Medicine

Sertaconazole is used to treat infections caused by a fungus. It works by killing the fungus or yeast or preventing its growth. Sertaconazole is applied to your skin to treat athlete's foot (tinea pedis).

This medicine is available only with your doctor's prescription.

Before Using This Medicine

In deciding to use a medicine, the risks of taking the medicine must be weighed against the good it will do. This is a decision you and your doctor will make. For this medicine, the following should be considered:

Allergies—Tell your doctor if you have ever had any unusual or allergic reaction to this medicine or any other medicines. Also tell your health care professional if you have any other types of allergies, such as to foods, dyes, preservatives, or animals. For non-prescription products, read the label or package ingredients carefully.

Pediatric—This medicine has been tested in children and has not been shown to cause different side effects or prob-

lems than it does in adults. This medicine is to be used in children 12 years of age and older.

Geriatric—Many medicines have not been studied specifically in older people. Therefore, it may not be known whether they work exactly the same way they do in younger adults. Although there is no specific information comparing use of topical sertaconazole in the elderly with use in other age groups, this medicine is not expected to cause different side effects or problems in older people than it does in younger adults.

Pregnancy—

	Pregnancy Category	Explanation
All Trimesters	C	Animal studies have shown an adverse effect and there are no adequate studies in pregnant women OR no animal studies have been conducted and there are no adequate studies in pregnant women.

Breast Feeding—There are no adequate studies in women for determining infant risk when using this medication during breastfeeding. Weigh the potential benefits against the potential risks before taking this medication while breastfeeding.

Other medicines—Although certain medicines should not be used together at all, in other cases two different medicines may be used together even if an interaction might occur. In these cases, your doctor may want to change the dose, or other precautions may be necessary. Tell your healthcare professional if you are taking any other prescription or non-prescription (over-the-counter [OTC]) medicine.

Interactions with Food/Tobacco/Alcohol—Certain medicines should not be used at or around the time of eating food or eating certain types of food since interactions may occur. Using alcohol or tobacco with certain medicines may also cause interactions to occur. Discuss with your healthcare professional the use of your medicine with food, alcohol, or tobacco.

Proper Use of This Medicine

Use sertaconazole as directed by your doctor. Your hands should be washed after applying the medicine to the affected area(s) of your skin. Avoid contact with the eyes, nose, mouth and other mucus membranes. Sertaconazole is for external use only.

Dry the affected area(s) thoroughly before application, if you wish to use sertaconazole after bathing.

Use your medicine for the full treatment time recommended by your doctor, even though symptoms may have improved.

Avoid the use of bandages or gauze (occlusive dressings) unless otherwise directed by your doctor.

Dosing—The dose of this medicine will be different for different patients. Follow your doctor's orders or the directions on the label. The following information includes only the average doses of this medicine. If your dose is different, do not change it unless your doctor tells you to do so.

The amount of medicine that you take depends on the strength of the medicine. Also, the number of doses you take each day, the time allowed between doses, and the length of

time you take the medicine depend on the medical problem for which you are using the medicine.

- For topical dosage form (cream):
  - For athlete's foot:
    - Adults—Apply enough sertaconazole to cover the affected and surrounding skin areas and rub in gently
    - Children over the age of 12—Apply enough sertaconazole to cover the affected and surrounding skin areas and rub in gently

Missed dose—If you miss a dose of this medicine, take it as soon as possible. However, if it is almost time for your next dose, skip the missed dose and go back to your regular dosing schedule. Do not double doses.

Storage—Store the medicine in a closed container at room temperature, away from heat, moisture, and direct light. Keep from freezing.

Keep out of the reach of children.

Do not keep outdated medicine or medicine no longer needed.

Ask your healthcare professional how you should dispose of any medicine you do not use.

Precautions While Using This Medicine

Inform your doctor if the area of application shows signs of increased skin irritation, redness, itching, burning, blistering, swelling or oozing.

It is very important that you check with your doctor in 2 weeks if your symptoms are not improving or if your conditions become worse.

Side Effects of This Medicine

Some side effects may occur that usually do not need medical attention. These side effects may go away during treatment as your body adjusts to the medicine. Also, your health care professional may be able to tell you about ways to prevent or reduce some of these side effects. Check with your health care professional if any of the following side effects continue or are bothersome or if you have any questions about them:

Incidence unknown

Blistering, burning, crusting, dryness or flaking of skin; itching, redness, skin rash, swelling, or soreness at application site; darkening of skin; dry skin; flushing and redness of skin; scaling, severe redness, soreness or swelling of skin; peeling or loosening of skin; skin tenderness; unusually warm skin

Other side effects not listed may also occur in some patients. If you notice any other effects, check with your healthcare professional.

SERTRALINE (Oral route) - SER-tra-leen

Black Box Warning

Antidepressants increased the risk of suicidal thinking and behavior (suicidality) in short-term studies in children and adolescents with Major Depressive Disorder (MDD) and other psychiatric disorders. Anyone considering the use of sertraline hydrochloride or any other antidepressant in a child or adolescent must balance this risk with the clinical need. Patients who are started on therapy should be observed closely for clinical worsening, suicidality, or unusual changes in behavior. Families and caregivers should be advised of the need for close observation and communication with the prescriber. Sertraline hydrochloride is not approved for use in pediatric patients except for patients with obsessive compulsive disorder (OCD).

Pooled analyses of short-term (4 to 16 weeks) placebo-controlled trials of 9 antidepressant drugs (SSRIs and others) in children and adolescents with major depressive disorder (MDD), obsessive compulsive disorder (OCD), or other psychiatric disorders (a total of 24 trials involving over 4400 patients) have revealed a greater risk of adverse events representing suicidal thinking or behavior (suicidality) during the first few months of treatment in those receiving antidepressants. The average risk of such events in patients receiving antidepressants was 4%, twice the placebo risk of 2%. No suicides occurred in these trials.

Commonly used brand name(s)

In the U.S.—
  Zoloft

Available Dosage Forms:

- Capsule
- Tablet
- Solution

Therapeutic Class: Antidepressant
Pharmacologic Class: Serotonin Reuptake Inhibitor

Uses For This Medicine

Sertraline is used to treat mental depression, obsessive-compulsive disorder, panic disorder, premenstrual dysphoric disorder, posttraumatic stress disorder, and social anxiety disorder.

Sertraline belongs to a group of medicines known as selective serotonin reuptake inhibitors (SSRIs). These medicines are thought to work by increasing the activity of the chemical serotonin in the brain.

This medicine is available only with your doctor's prescription.

Once a medicine has been approved for marketing for a certain use, experience may show that it is also useful for other medical problems. Although these uses are not included in product labeling, sertraline is used in certain patients with the following medical conditions:

- Premature ejaculation

Before Using This Medicine

In deciding to use a medicine, the risks of taking the medicine must be weighed against the good it will do. This is a decision you and your doctor will make. For this medicine, the following should be considered:

Allergies—Tell your doctor if you have ever had any unusual or allergic reaction to this medicine or any other medicines. Also tell your health care professional if you have any other types of allergies, such as to foods, dyes, preservatives, or animals. For non-prescription products, read the label or package ingredients carefully.

Pediatric—Sertraline has been tested in children 6 to 17 years of age with obsessive-compulsive disorder. In effective doses, this medicine has not been shown to cause different side effects or problems than it does in adults. However, sertraline can cause a decrease in appetite and children who take this medicine for a long time should have their growth and body weight measured by the doctor at regular visits.

Sertraline must be used with caution in children with depression. Studies have shown occurrences of children thinking about suicide or attempting suicide in clinical trials for this medicine. More study is needed to be sure sertraline is safe and effective in children.

Geriatric—In studies done to date that have included elderly people, sertraline did not cause different side effects or problems in older people than it did in younger adults. However, this medicine may be removed from the body more slowly in older adults. An older adult may receive a lower dose of sertraline than a younger adult, especially when first starting treatment.

Pregnancy—

	Pregnancy Category	Explanation
All Trimesters	C	Animal studies have shown an adverse effect and there are no adequate studies in pregnant women OR no animal studies have been conducted and there are no adequate studies in pregnant women.

Breast Feeding—Studies in women suggest that this medication poses minimal risk to the infant when used during breastfeeding.

Other medicines—

Using this medicine with any of the following medicines is not recommended. Your doctor may decide not to treat you with this medication or change some of the other medicines you take.

Clorgyline, Furazolidone, Iproniazid, Isocarboxazid, Levomethadyl, Moclobemide, Nialamide, Pargyline, Phenelzine, Pimozide, Procarbazine, Selegiline, Toloxatone, Tranylcypromine

Interactions with Food/Tobacco/Alcohol—Certain medicines should not be used at or around the time of eating food or eating certain types of food since interactions may occur. Using alcohol or tobacco with certain medicines may also cause interactions to occur. The following interactions have been selected on the basis of their potential significance and are not necessarily all-inclusive.

Using this medicine with any of the following may cause an increased risk of certain side effects but may be unavoidable in some cases. If used together, your doctor may change the dose or how often you use this medicine, or give you special instructions about the use of food, alcohol, or tobacco.

Grapefruit Juice

Other medical problems—The presence of other medical problems may affect the use of this medicine. Make sure you tell your doctor if you have any other medical problems, especially:
- Bleeding problems, abnormal or

- Purpura, or history of (purplish or brownish-red discoloration of skin)—Sertraline may make these problems worse.
- Brain disease or damage or
- Mental retardation or
- Seizure disorders (history of)—The risk of seizures may be increased
- Dehydration or
- Hyponatremia (condition in which your body has too little sodium)—Sertraline may make these problems worse, especially in older adults.
- Heart attack, recent or
- Heart disease, unstable—The medicine has not been studied in patients with these medical problems.
- Kidney disease—It is not known whether the chance of side effects will be increased
- Liver disease—Higher blood levels of sertraline may occur, increasing the chance of side effects. Your doctor may want you to take a lower dose or to take your doses less often than a person without liver disease
- Mania (history of)—May be activated
- Weight loss—Sertraline may cause weight loss. This weight loss is usually small, but if a large weight loss occurs, it may be harmful in some patients

Proper Use of This Medicine

Take this medicine only as directed by your doctor, to benefit your condition as much as possible. Do not take more of it, do not take it more often, and do not take it for a longer time than your doctor ordered.

Sertraline may be taken with or without food on a full or empty stomach. This medicine should be taken once a day in the morning or at night. If your doctor tells you to take it a certain way, follow your doctor's instructions.

If you are taking the oral concentrate, mix it with 4 ounces of water, ginger ale, lemon-lime soda, lemonade or orange juice. Take it right away after mixing.

You may have to take sertraline for 4 weeks or longer before you begin to feel better. Your doctor should check your progress at regular visits during this time. Also, if you are taking this medicine for depression, you may need to keep taking it for 6 months or longer to help prevent the return of the depression.

Dosing—The dose of this medicine will be different for different patients. Follow your doctor's orders or the directions on the label. The following information includes only the average doses of this medicine. If your dose is different, do not change it unless your doctor tells you to do so.

The amount of medicine that you take depends on the strength of the medicine. Also, the number of doses you take each day, the time allowed between doses, and the length of time you take the medicine depend on the medical problem for which you are using the medicine.
- For oral dosage forms (capsules, oral solution or tablets):
  - Adults:
    - For mental depression or obsessive-compulsive disorder: To start, usually 50 milligrams (mg) once a day, taken either in the morning or evening. Your

doctor may increase your dose gradually if needed. However, the dose usually is not more than 200 mg a day.

- For panic disorder, posttraumatic stress disorder, or social anxiety disorder: To start, usually 25 mg once a day, taken either in the morning or evening. Your doctor may increase your dose gradually if needed. However, the dose usually is not more than 200 mg a day.
- For premenstrual dysphoric disorder: To start, 50 mg once a day throughout your menstrual cycle or just during the premenstrual time. Your doctor may increase your dose if needed. However, the dose usually is not more than 150 mg a day throughout your menstrual cycle or 100 mg a day if you are only taking it during your premenstrual time.
  ○ Children:
    - For mental depression, posttraumatic stress disorder, or panic disorder: Use and dose must be determined by the doctor.
    - For obsessive-compulsive disorder:
      — Children younger than 6 years old: Use and dose must be determined by the doctor.
      — Children 6 to 12 years old: To start, usually 25 mg once a day, taken either in the morning or evening. Your doctor may increase your dose gradually if needed. However, the dose usually is not more than 200 mg a day.
      — Children 13 to 17 years old: To start, usually 50 mg once a day, taken either in the morning or evening. Your doctor may increase your dose gradually if needed. However, the dose usually is not more than 200 mg a day.
  ○ Older adults:
    - For mental depression, obsessive-compulsive disorder, panic disorder, posttraumatic stress disorder, or social anxiety disorder (using capsules or tablets): To start, usually 12.5 to 25 mg once a day, taken either in the morning or evening. Your doctor may increase your dose gradually if needed.

Missed dose—Call your doctor or pharmacist for instructions.

Storage—Store the medicine in a closed container at room temperature, away from heat, moisture, and direct light. Keep from freezing.

Keep out of the reach of children.

Do not keep outdated medicine or medicine no longer needed.

Precautions While Using This Medicine

It is important that your doctor check your progress at regular visits, to allow for changes in your dose and to help reduce any side effects.

Do not take sertraline with or within 14 days of taking an MAO inhibitor (furazolidone, phenelzine, procarbazine, selegiline, tranylcypromine). Do not take an MAO inhibitor within 14 days of taking sertraline. If you do, you may develop extremely high blood pressure or convulsions (seizures).

Avoid drinking alcoholic beverages while taking sertraline.

This medicine may cause some people to become drowsy, to have trouble thinking, or to have problems with movement. Make sure you know how you react to sertraline before you drive, use machines, or do anything else that could be dangerous if you are not alert or well-coordinated.

Sertraline may cause some people to be agitated, irritable or display other abnormal behaviors. It may also cause some people to have suicidal thoughts and tendencies or to become more depressed. If you or your caregiver notice any of these adverse effects, tell your doctor right away.

Do not stop taking this medicine without first checking with your doctor. Your doctor may want you to reduce gradually the amount you are taking before stopping completely. This is to decrease the chance of having discontinuation symptoms such as agitation, anxiety, dizziness, feeling of constant movement of self or surroundings, headache, increased sweating, nausea, trembling or shaking, trouble in sleeping or walking, or unusual tiredness.

Side Effects of This Medicine

Along with its needed effects, a medicine may cause some unwanted effects. Although not all of these side effects may occur, if they do occur they may need medical attention. One rare, but very serious, effect that may occur is the serotonin syndrome. This syndrome (group of symptoms) is more likely to occur shortly after an increase in sertraline dose.

Check with your doctor as soon as possible if any of the following side effects occur:
  More common
    Decreased sexual desire or ability; failure to discharge semen (in men)

  Less common or rare
    Aggressive reaction; breast tenderness or enlargement; fast, pounding, irregular, or slow heartbeat; fast talking and excited feelings or actions that are out of control; fever; inability to sit still; increase in body movements; loss of bladder control; low blood sodium (confusion, convulsions [seizures], drowsiness, dryness of mouth, increased thirst, lack of energy); muscle spasm or jerking of all extremities; nose bleeds; red or purple spots on skin; restlessness; serotonin syndrome (diarrhea, fever, increased sweating, mood or behavior changes, overactive reflexes, racing heartbeat, restlessness, shivering or shaking); skin rash, hives, or itching; sudden loss of consciousness; unusual or sudden body or facial movements or postures; unusual secretion of milk (in females)

  Incidence not known
    Abdominal or stomach pain; bleeding gums; blindness; blistering, peeling, loosening of skin; bloating; bloody, black, tarry stools; blood in urine; blue-yellow color blindness; blurred vision; chest pain or discomfort; chills; clay-colored stools; coma; cough or hoarseness; darkened urine; decreased urine output; decreased vision; depressed mood; difficulty in breathing; difficulty in speaking; difficulty swallowing; drooling; dry skin and hair; eye pain; fainting; feeling cold; feeling of discomfort; feeling that others can hear your thoughts; feeling that others are watching you or controlling your behavior; feeling, seeing, or hearing things that are not there; fixed position of eye; general feeling of discom-

fort, illness, tiredness, or weakness; hair loss; high fever; high or low blood pressure; hoarseness or husky voice; hostility; increased coagulation times; indigestion; inflammation of joints; irritability; joint or muscle pain; large, hive-like swelling on face, eyelids, lips, tongue, throat, hands, legs, feet, and sex organs; lethargy; light-colored stools; lightheadedness; loss of appetite; loss of balance control; loss of bladder control; lower back or side pain; muscle aches; muscle cramps and stiffness; muscle trembling, jerking or stiffness; muscle twitching; painful or difficult urination; pains in stomach, side, or abdomen, possibly radiating to the back; pale skin; palpitations; puffiness or swelling of the eyelids or around the eyes, face, lips, or tongue; rapid weight gain; rash; red, irritated eyes; red skin lesions often with a purple center; redness, soreness or itching skin; right upper abdominal pain and fullness; seizures; severe mood or mental changes; severe muscle stiffness; shortness of breath; shuffling walk; sore throat; sores, ulcers, or white spots in mouth or on lips; sores, welting or blisters; stiffness of limbs; stupor; sweating; swelling of face, ankles, or hands; swollen lymph glands; swollen or painful glands; talking or acting with excitement you cannot control; tightness in chest; troubled breathing; twisting movements of body; twitching; uncontrolled movements, especially of face, neck, and back; unexplained bleeding or bruising; unpleasant breath odor; unusual behavior; unusual tiredness or weakness; upper right abdominal pain; vomiting of blood; weight gain; wheezing; yellow eyes and skin

Symptoms of overdose—may be more severe than side effects occurring at regular doses or several may occur together

Actions that are out of control; agitation; anxiety; bloating; blurred vision; change in consciousness; chest pain or discomfort; chills; coma; confusion; confusion as to time or place or person holding false beliefs that cannot be changed by fact; constipation; convulsions (seizures); darkened urine; decreased awareness or responsiveness; dizziness or fainting; drowsiness; fever; hallucinations; headache; indigestion; irritability; lightheadedness; loss of appetite; loss of consciousness; nausea; nervousness; pains in stomach, side, or abdomen, possibly radiating to the back; pounding in ears; seeing, hearing, or feeling things that are not there; serotonin syndrome (diarrhea, fever, increased sweating, mood or behavior changes, overactive reflexes, racing heartbeat, restlessness, shivering or shaking); severe sleepiness; shakiness in legs, arms, hands, feet; shortness of breath; slow or irregular heartbeat; sweating; trembling or shaking of hands or feet; unusual excitement, or restlessness; unusual tiredness or weakness; unusually fast heartbeat; unusually large pupils; vomiting; yellow eyes or skin

Some side effects may occur that usually do not need medical attention. These side effects may go away during treatment as your body adjusts to the medicine. Also, your health care professional may be able to tell you about ways to prevent or reduce some of these side effects. Check with your health care professional if any of the following side effects continue or are bothersome or if you have any questions about them:

More common

Acid or sour stomach; belching; decreased appetite or weight loss; diarrhea or loose stools; dizziness; drows-

iness; dryness of mouth; headache; heartburn; increased sweating; nausea; sleepiness or unusual drowsiness; stomach or abdominal cramps, gas, or pain; trembling or shaking; trouble in sleeping

Less common

Agitation, anxiety, or nervousness; bladder pain; burning, crawling, itching, numbness, prickling, "pins and needles", or tingling feelings; changes in vision, including blurred vision; cloudy urine; constipation; difficult, burning, or painful urination; flushing or redness of skin, with feeling of warmth or heat; frequent urge to urinate; increased appetite; pain or tenderness around eyes and cheekbones; stuffy or runny nose; vomiting

Incidence not known

flushed, dry skin; fruit-like breath odor; increased hunger; increased thirst; increased urination; redness or other discoloration of skin; severe sunburn; swelling of breasts (in women); unexplained weight loss; unusual secretion of milk (in women)

After you stop using this medicine, it may still produce some side effects that need attention. During this period of time, *check with your doctor immediately* if you notice the following side effects:

Abnormal dreams; agitation; anxiety; burning, crawling, itching, numbness, prickling, "pins and needles", or tingling feelings; dizziness; electric shock sensations; failure to discharge semen (in men); feeling of constant movement of self or surroundings; headache; increased sweating; nausea; sleepiness or unusual drowsiness; trembling or shaking; trouble in sleeping; trouble in walking; unusual tiredness

Other side effects not listed may also occur in some patients. If you notice any other effects, check with your healthcare professional.

SEVELAMER (Oral route) - se-VEL-a-mer

Commonly used brand name(s)

In the U.S.—
Renagel

Available Dosage Forms:
- Tablet
- Capsule

Therapeutic Class: Phosphate Binder

Uses For This Medicine

Sevelamer is used to treat hyperphosphatemia (too much phosphate in the blood) in patients with kidney disease who are on dialysis.

This medicine is available only with your doctor's prescription.

Before Using This Medicine

In deciding to use a medicine, the risks of taking the medicine must be weighed against the good it will do. This is a decision

you and your doctor will make. For this medicine, the following should be considered:

Allergies—Tell your doctor if you have ever had any unusual or allergic reaction to this medicine or any other medicines. Also tell your health care professional if you have any other types of allergies, such as to foods, dyes, preservatives, or animals. For non-prescription products, read the label or package ingredients carefully.

Pediatric—Studies on this medicine have been done only in adult patients, and there is no specific information comparing use of sevelamer in children with use in other age groups.

Geriatric—Many medicines have not been studied specifically in older people. Therefore, it may not be known whether they work exactly the same way they do in younger adults. Although there is no specific information comparing use of sevelamer in the elderly with use in other age groups, this medicine has been used in elderly patients and is not expected to cause different side effects or problems in older people than it does in younger adults.

Other medicines—Although certain medicines should not be used together at all, in other cases two different medicines may be used together even if an interaction might occur. In these cases, your doctor may want to change the dose, or other precautions may be necessary. Tell your healthcare professional if you are taking any other prescription or non-prescription (over-the-counter [OTC]) medicine.

Interactions with Food/Tobacco/Alcohol—Certain medicines should not be used at or around the time of eating food or eating certain types of food since interactions may occur. Using alcohol or tobacco with certain medicines may also cause interactions to occur. Discuss with your healthcare professional the use of your medicine with food, alcohol, or tobacco.

Other medical problems—The presence of other medical problems may affect the use of this medicine. Make sure you tell your doctor if you have any other medical problems, especially:

- Bowel obstruction (blockage) or other disorders affecting the gastrointestinal tract or
- Difficulty in swallowing or
- Major surgery on the gastrointestinal tract—Use of sevelamer may cause problems in these conditions
- Hypophosphatemia—Use of sevelamer may make this condition worse

Proper Use of This Medicine

Take this medicine with meals.

Take this medicine only as directed by your doctor. Do not take more or less of it, and do not take it more often than your doctor ordered.

Swallow the capsule whole. Do not break or chew the capsule before swallowing.

Do not open up the capsules before taking them. The medicine inside may swell if it comes in contact with water.

Follow carefully any diet program your doctor may recommend.

Dosing—The dose of this medicine will be different for different patients. Follow your doctor's orders or the directions on the label. The following information includes only the average doses of this medicine. If your dose is different, do not change it unless your doctor tells you to do so.

The amount of medicine that you take depends on the strength of the medicine. Also, the number of doses you take each day, the time allowed between doses, and the length of time you take the medicine depend on the medical problem for which you are using the medicine.

- For oral dosage form (capsules):
  - For high phosphorus levels in the blood:
    - Adults not taking a phosphate binder—The first dose is usually between 2 and 4 capsules three times a day, with each meal, depending on how high your blood phosphorus level is. After that, your doctor may change the dose, again depending on your blood phosphorus levels.
    - Adults switching from calcium acetate to sevelamer—The first dose of sevelamer is generally between 2 and 5 capsules three times a day, with each meal, depending on how many tablets of calcium acetate you are currently taking. After that the doctor may change the dose, depending on your blood phosphorus levels.
    - Children—Use and dose must be determined by your doctor.

- For oral dosage forms (tablets)
  - For high phosphorus levels in the blood:
    - Adults not taking a phosphate binder—The first dose is usually between 1 and 4 tablets three times a day, with each meal, depending on how high your blood phosphorus level is. After that, your doctor may change the dose, depending on your blood phosphorus levels.
    - Adults switching from calcium acetate to sevelamer—The first dose of sevelamer is generally between 1 and 5 tablets three times a day, with each meal, depending on how many tablets of calcium acetate you are currently taking. After that the doctor may change the dose, depending on your blood phosphorus levels.
    - Children—Use and dose must be determined by your doctor.

Missed dose—If you miss a dose of this medicine, take it as soon as possible. However, if it is almost time for your next dose, skip the missed dose and go back to your regular dosing schedule. Do not double doses.

Storage—Store the medicine in a closed container at room temperature, away from heat, moisture, and direct light. Keep from freezing.

Keep out of the reach of children.

Do not keep outdated medicine or medicine no longer needed.

Side Effects of This Medicine

Along with its needed effects, a medicine may cause some unwanted effects. Although not all of these side effects may occur, if they do occur they may need medical attention.

Some side effects may occur that usually do not need medical attention. These side effects may go away during treatment as your body adjusts to the medicine. Also, your health care professional may be able to tell you about ways to prevent or reduce some of these side effects. Check with your health

care professional if any of the following side effects continue or are bothersome or if you have any questions about them:

Less common

Bloating or gas; constipation; diarrhea; heartburn; nausea or vomiting

Other side effects not listed may also occur in some patients. If you notice any other effects, check with your healthcare professional.

SIBUTRAMINE (Oral route) - si-BYOO-tra-meen

Commonly used brand name(s)

In the U.S.—
Meridia

Available Dosage Forms:
- Capsule

Therapeutic Class: Appetite Suppressant, Centrally Acting
Pharmacologic Class: Serotonin/Norepinephrine Reuptake Inhibitor

---

Uses For This Medicine

Sibutramine is used together with a reduced-calorie diet to help you lose weight and to help keep the lost weight from returning. Sibutramine is thought to work by increasing the activity of certain chemicals, called norepinephrine and serotonin, in the brain. This medicine is approved for use only in people who are very overweight.

This medicine is available only with your doctor's prescription.

Before Using This Medicine

In deciding to use a medicine, the risks of taking the medicine must be weighed against the good it will do. This is a decision you and your doctor will make. For this medicine, the following should be considered:

Allergies—Tell your doctor if you have ever had any unusual or allergic reaction to this medicine or any other medicines. Also tell your health care professional if you have any other types of allergies, such as to foods, dyes, preservatives, or animals. For non-prescription products, read the label or package ingredients carefully.

Pediatric—Studies on this medicine have been done only in adult patients, and there is no specific information comparing use of sibutramine in children with use in other age groups.

Geriatric—Many medicines have not been studied specifically in older people. Therefore, it may not be known whether they work exactly the same way they do in younger adults. Although there is no specific information comparing use of sibutramine in the elderly with use in other age groups, this medicine is not expected to cause different side effects or problems in older people than it does in younger adults.

Pregnancy—

	Pregnancy Category	Explanation
All Trimesters	C	Animal studies have shown an adverse effect and there are no adequate studies in pregnant women OR no animal studies have been conducted and there are no adequate studies in pregnant women.

Breast Feeding—There are no adequate studies in women for determining infant risk when using this medication during breastfeeding. Weigh the potential benefits against the potential risks before taking this medication while breastfeeding.

Other medicines—

Using this medicine with any of the following medicines is not recommended. Your doctor may decide not to treat you with this medication or change some of the other medicines you take.

Amphetamine, Clorgyline, Dexfenfluramine, Dextroamphetamine, Diethylpropion, Fenfluramine, Iproniazid, Isocarboxazid, Mazindol, Moclobemide, Nialamide, Pargyline, Phendimetrazine, Phenelzine, Phenmetrazine, Phentermine, Phenylpropanolamine, Procarbazine, Selegiline, Toloxatone, Tranylcypromine

Interactions with Food/Tobacco/Alcohol—Certain medicines should not be used at or around the time of eating food or eating certain types of food since interactions may occur. Using alcohol or tobacco with certain medicines may also cause interactions to occur. Discuss with your healthcare professional the use of your medicine with food, alcohol, or tobacco.

Other medical problems—The presence of other medical problems may affect the use of this medicine. Make sure you tell your doctor if you have any other medical problems, especially:

- Anorexia nervosa (an eating disorder) or
- Glaucoma, narrow angle or
- High blood pressure (or history of)—Sibutramine may make these conditions worse
- Brain disease or damage, or mental retardation or
- Seizures (history of)—Sibutramine may increase the chance of having seizures
- Gallstones (or history of)—Weight loss may make this condition worse
- Heart disease (or history of) or
- Stroke (or history of)—Increased blood pressure or heart rate caused by sibutramine may make these conditions worse
- Kidney disease (severe) or
- Liver disease (severe)—Higher blood levels of sibutramine may occur, increasing the chance of having unwanted effects

---

Proper Use of This Medicine

Take this medicine only as directed. Do not take more of it, do not take it more often, and do not take it for a longer time than directed by your doctor. To do so may increase the chance of developing unwanted effects, such as high blood pressure.

Follow a reduced-calorie diet while taking sibutramine, as directed by your doctor.

Sibutramine may be taken with or without food, on a full or empty stomach. However, if your doctor tells you to take it in a certain way, take it as directed.

You must follow a reduced-calorie diet while taking sibutramine in order to lose weight and keep the lost weight from returning.

Dosing—The dose of this medicine will be different for different patients. Follow your doctor's orders or the directions on the label. The following information includes only the average doses of this medicine. If your dose is different, do not change it unless your doctor tells you to do so.

The amount of medicine that you take depends on the strength of the medicine. Also, the number of doses you take each day, the time allowed between doses, and the length of time you take the medicine depend on the medical problem for which you are using the medicine.

- For oral dosage form (capsules):
  - For weight loss:
    - Adults—At first, 10 milligrams (mg) one time a day, usually in the morning. Your doctor may increase or decrease your dose if needed. However, the dose is usually not more than 15 mg a day.
    - Children—Use and dose must be determined by the doctor.

Missed dose—If you miss a dose of this medicine, take it as soon as possible. However, if it is almost time for your next dose, skip the missed dose and go back to your regular dosing schedule. Do not double doses.

Storage—Store the medicine in a closed container at room temperature, away from heat, moisture, and direct light. Keep from freezing.

Keep out of the reach of children.

Do not keep outdated medicine or medicine no longer needed.

Precautions While Using This Medicine

It is important that your doctor check your progress at regular visits. Sibutramine may increase blood pressure or heart rate and your doctor will check for these effects. Your doctor may need to adjust your dose.

If sibutramine does not seem to be working well, do not increase your dosage. Check with your doctor.

Do not take sibutramine while you are taking or within 2 weeks of taking medicines with monoamine oxidase (MAO) inhibitor activity, such as isocarboxazid (e.g., Marplan), phenelzine (e.g., Nardil), procarbazine (e.g., Matulane), selegiline (e.g., Eldepryl), or tranylcypromine (e.g., Parnate). Do not take an MAO inhibitor within 2 weeks of taking sibutramine. To do so may cause severe seizures, extremely high blood pressure, or a life-threatening adverse effect called the serotonin syndrome.

Do not drink excess alcohol while taking sibutramine.

Notify your doctor as soon as possible if you develop a skin rash, hives, or other allergic symptoms.

Sibutramine may cause dizziness, drowsiness, or poor judgment. Be sure you know how you react to this medicine before you drive, operate machinery, or do other things that could be dangerous if you are not alert and able to think clearly.

Sibutramine may cause dryness of the mouth. For temporary relief, use sugarless candy or gum, melt bits of ice in your mouth, or use a saliva substitute. However, if your mouth continues to feel dry for more than 2 weeks, check with your medical doctor or dentist. Continuing dryness of the mouth may increase the chance of dental disease, including tooth decay, gum disease, and fungus infections.

Side Effects of This Medicine

Along with its needed effects, a medicine may cause some unwanted effects. Some of these effects, such as high blood pressure, may not have signs or symptoms that you can see or feel. While you are taking sibutramine, your doctor will check your blood pressure and heart rate at regular visits.

Although not all of these side effects may occur, if they do occur they may need medical attention.

Check with your doctor as soon as possible if any of the following side effects occur:

Less common
  Achiness; chills; fast or irregular heartbeat; increased blood pressure; mental depression; painful menstruation; swelling of body or of feet and ankles

Rare
  Bruising or red spots or patches on skin; convulsions (seizures); excessive bleeding following injury; headache (severe); rapidly changing moods; skin rash; weight gain (unusual)

Some side effects may occur that usually do not need medical attention. These side effects may go away during treatment as your body adjusts to the medicine. Also, your health care professional may be able to tell you about ways to prevent or reduce some of these side effects. Check with your health care professional if any of the following side effects continue or are bothersome or if you have any questions about them:

More common
  Anxiety; constipation; dizziness; dryness of mouth; headache; irritability or unusual impatience; nervousness; stuffy or runny nose; trouble in sleeping

Less common
  Abdominal pain; back pain; burning, itching, prickling, or tingling of skin; change in sense of taste; diarrhea; drowsiness; increase in appetite; increased sweating; increased thirst; indigestion; nausea; unusual warmth or flushing of skin

Other side effects not listed may also occur in some patients. If you notice any other effects, check with your healthcare professional.

SILDENAFIL (Oral route) - sil-DEN-a-fil

Commonly used brand name(s)

In the U.S.—
Revatio
Viagra

Available Dosage Forms:
- Tablet

Therapeutic Class: Antihypertensive, Peripheral Vasodilator
Pharmacologic Class: Phosphodiesterase Type 5 Inhibitor

Uses For This Medicine

Sildenafil belongs to a group of medicines that delay the enzymes called phosphodiesterases from working too quickly. The penis is one of the areas where these enzymes work. Sildenafil is used to treat men who have erectile dysfunction (also called sexual impotence).

By controlling the enzyme phosphodiesterase, sildenafil helps to maintain an erection that is produced when the penis is stroked. Without physical action to the penis, such as that occurring during sexual intercourse, sildenafil will not work to cause an erection.

Sildenafil is also used to treat the symptoms of pulmonary arterial hypertension. This is the high blood pressure that occurs in the main artery that carries blood from the right side of the heart (the ventricle) to the lungs. When the smaller blood vessels in the lungs become more resistant to blood flow, the right ventricle must work harder to pump enough blood through the lungs. Sildenafil helps by increasing the supply of blood to the lungs and reducing the workload of the heart.

This medicine is available only with your doctor's prescription.

Before Using This Medicine

In deciding to use a medicine, the risks of taking the medicine must be weighed against the good it will do. This is a decision you and your doctor will make. For this medicine, the following should be considered:

Allergies—Tell your doctor if you have ever had any unusual or allergic reaction to this medicine or any other medicines. Also tell your health care professional if you have any other types of allergies, such as to foods, dyes, preservatives, or animals. For non-prescription products, read the label or package ingredients carefully.

Geriatric—Elderly people are especially sensitive to the effects of sildenafil, which may increase their chance of having side effects. Patients 65 years of age and older who are taking this medicine for erectile dysfunction are started on a low dose, 25 mg, of sildenafil. Patients who are taking this medicine for pulmonary arterial hypertension may also need to be started at a lower dose. The dose may be increased by a doctor as needed and tolerated.

Pregnancy—

	Pregnancy Category	Explanation
All Trimesters	B	Animal studies have revealed no evidence of harm to the fetus, however, there are no adequate studies in pregnant women OR animal studies have shown an adverse effect, but adequate studies in pregnant women have failed to demonstrate a risk to the fetus.

Breast Feeding—There are no adequate studies in women for determining infant risk when using this medication during breastfeeding. Weigh the potential benefits against the potential risks before taking this medication while breastfeeding.

Other medicines—

Using this medicine with any of the following medicines is not recommended. Your doctor may decide not to treat you with this medication or change some of the other medicines you take.

Amyl Nitrite, Erythrityl Tetranitrate, Isosorbide Dinitrate, Isosorbide Mononitrate, Molsidomine, Nitroglycerin, Nitroprusside, Pentaerythritol Tetranitrate

Interactions with Food/Tobacco/Alcohol—Certain medicines should not be used at or around the time of eating food or eating certain types of food since interactions may occur. Using alcohol or tobacco with certain medicines may also cause interactions to occur. The following interactions have been selected on the basis of their potential significance and are not necessarily all-inclusive.

Using this medicine with any of the following may cause an increased risk of certain side effects but may be unavoidable in some cases. If used together, your doctor may change the dose or how often you use this medicine, or give you special instructions about the use of food, alcohol, or tobacco.

Grapefruit Juice

Other medical problems—The presence of other medical problems may affect the use of this medicine. Make sure you tell your doctor if you have any other medical problems, especially:
- Age greater than 50 years or
- Coronary artery disease or
- Diabetes or
- Hyperlipidemia (excess of lipids in the blood) or
- Hypertension (high blood pressure) or
- Low cup to disc ratio ('crowded disc') or
- Smoking—These conditions may increase risk for a serious eye problem called NAION.
- Arrhythmias (irregular heartbeat) or
- Coronary artery disease or
- Heart attack, history of (within the last 6 months) or
- High blood pressure or
- Low blood pressure or

- Stroke, history of (within the last 6 months)—Chance of problems occurring may be increased
- Abnormal penis, including curved penis and birth defects of the penis—Chance of problems occurring may be increased
- Bleeding problems or
- Retinitis pigmentosa—Chance of problems occurring may be increased. It is not known if the medicine is safe for use in these patients
- Conditions causing thickened blood or slower blood flow, including leukemia; multiple myeloma (tumors of the bone marrow); or polycythemia, sickle cell disease, and thrombocythemia (blood problems) or
- Priapism (history of)—Although sildenafil does not cause priapism (erection lasting longer than 6 hours), patients with these conditions have an increased risk of priapism and it could occur while using sildenafil
- Heart or blood disease—Sexual activity increases the heart rate and blood flow and can increase the chance of problems occurring for some patients who use any type of medicine, including sildenafil, that increases sexual ability
- Kidney problems (severe) or
- Liver problems (severe)—Chance of problems occurring may be increased. Lower starting doses may be used and doses increased as needed and as tolerated
- NAION (serious eye condition) in one or both eyes, previously—May increase your chance of getting NAION again
- Pulmonary veno-occlusive disease (high blood pressure in the blood vessels of the lungs)—May make heart problems worse in patients with this serious condition

Proper Use of This Medicine

Special patient directions come with sildenafil. Read the directions carefully before using the medicine.

This medicine usually begins to work within 30 minutes after taking it for erectile dysfunction. It continues to work for up to 4 hours, although its action is usually less after 2 hours.

Dosing—The dose of this medicine will be different for different patients. Follow your doctor's orders or the directions on the label. The following information includes only the average doses of this medicine. If your dose is different, do not change it unless your doctor tells you to do so.

The amount of medicine that you take depends on the strength of the medicine. Also, the number of doses you take each day, the time allowed between doses, and the length of time you take the medicine depend on the medical problem for which you are using the medicine.

- For oral dosage form (tablets):
  - For treatment of erectile dysfunction:
    - Adults up to 65 years of age—50 mg as a single dose no more than once a day, 1 hour before sexual intercourse. Alternatively, the medicine may be taken 30 minutes to 4 hours before sexual intercourse. If needed, your doctor may increase your daily dose to 100 mg or decrease your daily dose to 25 mg.
    - Adults 65 years of age and older—25 mg as a single dose no more than once a day, 1 hour before sexual intercourse. Alternatively, the medicine may be taken 30 minutes to 4 hours before sexual intercourse. If needed, your doctor may increase your daily dose.
    - If you are taking protease inhibitors, such as for the treatment of HIV, your doctor may recommend a 25 mg dose and may limit you to a maximum single dose of 25 mg of Viagra in a 48 hour period
  - For treatment of pulmonary arterial hypertension:
    - Adults—20 mg three times per day. Each dose should be taken about 4 to 6 hours apart and can be taken with or without food.
    - Children—Use and dose must be determined by your doctor.

Storage—Store the medicine in a closed container at room temperature, away from heat, moisture, and direct light. Keep from freezing.

Keep out of the reach of children.

Do not keep outdated medicine or medicine no longer needed.

Precautions While Using This Medicine

Sildenafil has not been studied with other medicines used for treatment of erectile dysfunction. Presently, using them together is not recommended.

It is important that you tell all of your healthcare providers that you take sildenafil. If you need emergency medical care for a heart problem, it is important that your healthcare provider knows when you last took sildenafil.

Use sildenafil exactly as directed by your doctor. Do not use more of it and do not use it more often than your doctor ordered. If too much is used, the chance of side effects is increased.

If you experience a prolonged or painful erection for 4 hours or more, contact your doctor immediately. This condition may require prompt medical treatment to prevent tissue damage of the penis and possible permanent impotence.

This medicine does not protect you against sexually transmitted diseases. Use protective measures and ask your doctor if you have any questions about this.

It is important to tell your doctor about any heart problems you may have now or may have had in the past. This medicine can cause serious side effects in patients with heart problems.

If you experience sudden loss of vision in one or both eyes, stop using sildenafil and contact your doctor immediately.

Side Effects of This Medicine

Along with its needed effects, a medicine may cause some unwanted effects. Although not all of these side effects may occur, if they do occur they may need medical attention.

Less common

Abnormal vision, including blurred vision, seeing shades of colors differently than before, or sensitivity to light; bladder pain; burning, crawling, itching, numbness, prickling, "pins and needles", or tingling feelings; burning feeling in chest or stomach; cloudy or bloody urine; dizziness; increased frequency of urination; indigestion; pain on urination; stomach upset; tenderness in stomach area

Rare

Bleeding of the eye; convulsions (seizures); decreased vision or other changes in vision; double vision; prolonged, painful, or inappropriate erection of penis; redness, burning, or swelling of the eye; vision loss, temporary

Note: The following rare side effects have not been completely established as being caused by sildenafil

Blood sugar problems (more likely with patients with diabetes mellitus), such as anxiety, behavior change similar to drunkenness, blurred vision, cold sweats, confusion, cool and pale skin, difficulty in concentrating, drowsiness, excessive hunger, fast heartbeat, headache, nausea, nervousness, nightmares, restless sleep, shakiness, slurred speech, and unusual tiredness or weakness; bone pain; breast enlargement; chest pain; chills; confusion; convulsions (seizures); deafness; decrease in amount of urine or in frequency of urination; dizziness or lightheadedness, especially when getting up from a lying or sitting position; dry eyes; dry mouth; dryness, redness, scaling, or peeling of the skin; eye pain; fainting or faintness; fast, irregular, or pounding heartbeat; feeling of something in the eye; groups of skin lesions with swelling; headache (severe or continuing); heart failure; hives; increase in size of pupil; increased sweating; increased thirst; itching of skin; low blood pressure; lower back or side pain; migraine headache; nausea (severe or continuing); nervousness; numbness of hands; painful, swollen joints; redness, itching, or tearing of eyes; shortness of breath or troubled breathing; skin paleness; skin rash; skin ulcers; sore throat and fever or chills; sudden weakness; swelling of face, hands, feet, or lower legs; twitching of muscles; unusual tiredness or weakness; unusual feeling of burning or stinging of skin

Incidence not known

Blindness

Some side effects may occur that usually do not need medical attention. These side effects may go away during treatment as your body adjusts to the medicine. Also, your health care professional may be able to tell you about ways to prevent or reduce some of these side effects. Check with your health care professional if any of the following side effects continue or are bothersome or if you have any questions about them:

More common

Aches or pains in muscles; bloody nose; diarrhea; difficult or labored breathing; flushing; headache; nasal congestion; pain or tenderness around eyes and cheekbones; redness of skin; sneezing; stomach discomfort following meals; stuffy or runny nose; trouble in sleeping; unusually warm skin

Rare

Anxiety

Note: The following rare side effects have not been completely established as being caused by sildenafil

Abdominal pain; abnormal dreams; clumsiness or unsteadiness; cough; diarrhea or stomach cramps (severe or continuing); difficulty in swallowing; ear pain; increased amount of saliva; increased skin sensitivity; lack of coordination; loss of bladder control; mental depression; nausea; numbness or tingling of hands, legs, or feet; rectal bleeding; redness or irritation of the tongue; redness, soreness, swelling, or bleeding of gums; ringing or buzzing in ears; sensation of motion,

usually whirling, either of one's self or of one's surroundings; sexual problems in men (continuing), including failure to experience a sexual orgasm; sleepiness; sores in mouth and on lips; tense muscles; tightness of chest or wheezing; trembling and shaking; vomiting; waking to urinate at night; worsening of asthma

Other side effects not listed may also occur in some patients. If you notice any other effects, check with your healthcare professional.

SILVER SULFADIAZINE (Topical route) - SIL-ver sul-fa-DYE-a-zeen

Commonly used brand name(s)

In the U.S.—

Silvadene   Thermazene
SSD AF

In Canada—

Flamazine
Ssd

Available Dosage Forms:

• Cream

Therapeutic Class: Antibacterial

Uses For This Medicine

Silver sulfadiazine, a sulfa medicine, is used to prevent and treat bacterial or fungus infections. It works by killing the fungus or bacteria.

Silver sulfadiazine cream is applied to the skin and/or burned area(s) to prevent and treat bacterial or fungus infections that may occur in burns. This medicine may also be used for other problems as determined by your doctor.

Other medicines are used along with this medicine for burns. Patients with severe burns or burns over a large area of the body must be treated in a hospital.

Silver sulfadiazine is available only with your doctor's prescription.

Before Using This Medicine

In deciding to use a medicine, the risks of taking the medicine must be weighed against the good it will do. This is a decision you and your doctor will make. For this medicine, the following should be considered:

Allergies—Tell your doctor if you have ever had any unusual or allergic reaction to this medicine or any other medicines. Also tell your health care professional if you have any other types of allergies, such as to foods, dyes, preservatives, or animals. For non-prescription products, read the label or package ingredients carefully.

Pediatric—Use is not recommended in premature or newborn infants up to 2 months of age. Sulfa medicines may cause liver problems in these infants. Although there is no specific information comparing use of silver sulfadiazine in older infants and children with use in other age groups, this medicine is not expected to cause different side effects or problems in older infants and children than it does in adults.

Geriatric—Many medicines have not been studied specifically in older people. Therefore, it may not be known whether they work exactly the same way they do in younger adults or if they cause different side effects or problems in older people. There is no specific information comparing use of silver sulfadiazine in the elderly with use in other age groups.

Pregnancy—

	Pregnancy Category	Explanation
All Trimesters	B	Animal studies have revealed no evidence of harm to the fetus, however, there are no adequate studies in pregnant women OR animal studies have shown an adverse effect, but adequate studies in pregnant women have failed to demonstrate a risk to the fetus.

Breast Feeding—There are no adequate studies in women for determining infant risk when using this medication during breastfeeding. Weigh the potential benefits against the potential risks before taking this medication while breastfeeding.

Other medicines—Although certain medicines should not be used together at all, in other cases two different medicines may be used together even if an interaction might occur. In these cases, your doctor may want to change the dose, or other precautions may be necessary. Tell your healthcare professional if you are taking any other prescription or non-prescription (over-the-counter [OTC]) medicine.

Interactions with Food/Tobacco/Alcohol—Certain medicines should not be used at or around the time of eating food or eating certain types of food since interactions may occur. Using alcohol or tobacco with certain medicines may also cause interactions to occur. Discuss with your healthcare professional the use of your medicine with food, alcohol, or tobacco.

Other medical problems—The presence of other medical problems may affect the use of this medicine. Make sure you tell your doctor if you have any other medical problems, especially:

- Blood problems or
- Glucose-6–phosphate dehydrogenase deficiency (lack of G6PD enzyme)—Use of this medicine may cause blood problems or make them worse
- Kidney disease or
- Liver disease—In persons with these conditions, use may result in higher blood levels of this medicine; a smaller dose may be needed
- Porphyria—Use of this medicine may result in a severe attack of porphyria

Proper Use of This Medicine

This medicine should not be used on premature or newborn infants up to 2 months of age, unless otherwise directed by your doctor. It may cause liver problems in these infants.

To use:

- Before applying this medicine, cleanse the affected area(s). Remove dead or burned skin and other debris.
- Wear a sterile glove to apply this medicine. Apply a thin layer (about 1/16 inch) of silver sulfadiazine to the af-

fected area(s). Keep the affected area(s) covered with the medicine at all times.

- If this medicine is rubbed off the affected area(s) by moving around or if it is washed off during bathing, showering, or the use of a whirlpool bath, reapply the medicine.
- After this medicine has been applied, the treated area(s) may be covered with a dressing or left uncovered as desired.

To help clear up your skin and/or burn infection completely, keep using silver sulfadiazine for the full time of treatment. You should keep using this medicine until the burned area has healed or is ready for skin grafting. Do not miss any doses.

Dosing—The dose of this medicine will be different for different patients. Follow your doctor's orders or the directions on the label. The following information includes only the average doses of this medicine. If your dose is different, do not change it unless your doctor tells you to do so.

The amount of medicine that you take depends on the strength of the medicine. Also, the number of doses you take each day, the time allowed between doses, and the length of time you take the medicine depend on the medical problem for which you are using the medicine.

- For topical dosage form (cream):
  - For burn wound infections:
    - Adults and children 2 months of age and older—Use one or two times a day.
    - Premature and newborn infants up to 2 months of age—Use and dose must be determined by the doctor.

Missed dose—If you miss a dose of this medicine, apply it as soon as possible. However, if it is almost time for your next dose, skip the missed dose and go back to your regular dosing schedule.

Storage—Store the medicine in a closed container at room temperature, away from heat, moisture, and direct light. Keep from freezing.

Keep out of the reach of children.

Do not keep outdated medicine or medicine no longer needed.

Precautions While Using This Medicine

It is important that your doctor check your progress at regular visits.

If your skin infection or burn does not improve within a few days or weeks (for more serious burns or burns over larger areas), or if it becomes worse, check with your doctor.

This medicine may rarely stain skin brownish gray.

Side Effects of This Medicine

Along with its needed effects, a medicine may cause some unwanted effects. Although not all of these side effects may occur, if they do occur they may need medical attention.

Check with your doctor as soon as possible if any of the following side effects occur:

Rare

Blistering, peeling or loosening of skin; bloody or cloudy urine; chills or fever; cough; decreased amount of urine or less frequent urination; increased sensitivity of skin to sunlight, especially in patients with burns on large areas; intense itching of burn wounds; pain at site of application; painful or difficult urination; red skin lesions, often with a purple center; shortness of breath; sore throat; sores, ulcers or white spots on lips or in mouth; swollen glands; unusual bleeding or bruising; unusual tiredness or weakness

Some side effects may occur that usually do not need medical attention. These side effects may go away during treatment as your body adjusts to the medicine. Also, your health care professional may be able to tell you about ways to prevent or reduce some of these side effects. Check with your health care professional if any of the following side effects continue or are bothersome or if you have any questions about them:

More common
    Burning feeling on treated area(s)
Less common or rare
    Brownish-gray skin discoloration; itching or skin rash

Other side effects not listed may also occur in some patients. If you notice any other effects, check with your healthcare professional.

SIMETHICONE (Oral route) - sye-METH-i-cone

Commonly used brand name(s)
In the U.S.—

Alka-Seltzer Anti-Gas	Genasyme
Anti-Gas Ultra Strength	Maalox Anti-Gas
Baby Gasz	Mylanta Gas
Equilizer Gas Relief	Mylicon
Gas Aid Maximum Strength	Mytab Gas
Gas-X	Phazyme

In Canada—
Ovol
Phazyme Liquid Gas Relief,
    Maximum Strength

Available Dosage Forms:

- Suspension
- Capsule, Liquid Filled
- Tablet, Chewable
- Liquid
- Capsule
- Solution
- Tablet
- Syrup

Therapeutic Class: Antiflatulent

Uses For This Medicine

Simethicone is used to relieve the painful symptoms of too much gas in the stomach and intestines.

Simethicone may also be used for other conditions as determined by your doctor.

Simethicone is available without a prescription.

Once a medicine has been approved for marketing for a certain use, experience may show that it is also useful for other medical problems. Although these uses are not included in product labeling, simethicone is used in certain patients before the following tests:

- Before a gastroscopy
- Before a radiography of the bowel

Before Using This Medicine

In deciding to use a medicine, the risks of taking the medicine must be weighed against the good it will do. This is a decision you and your doctor will make. For this medicine, the following should be considered:

Allergies—Tell your doctor if you have ever had any unusual or allergic reaction to this medicine or any other medicines. Also tell your health care professional if you have any other types of allergies, such as to foods, dyes, preservatives, or animals. For non-prescription products, read the label or package ingredients carefully.

Pediatric—This medicine has been tested in children and, in effective doses, has not been shown to cause different side effects or problems than it does in adults.

Geriatric—Many medicines have not been studied specifically in older people. Therefore, it may not be known whether they work exactly the same way they do in younger adults. There is no specific information comparing use of simethicone in the elderly with use in other age groups.

Other medicines—Although certain medicines should not be used together at all, in other cases two different medicines may be used together even if an interaction might occur. In these cases, your doctor may want to change the dose, or other precautions may be necessary. Tell your healthcare professional if you are taking any other prescription or non-prescription (over-the-counter [OTC]) medicine.

Interactions with Food/Tobacco/Alcohol—Certain medicines should not be used at or around the time of eating food or eating certain types of food since interactions may occur. Using alcohol or tobacco with certain medicines may also cause interactions to occur. Discuss with your healthcare professional the use of your medicine with food, alcohol, or tobacco.

Proper Use of This Medicine

For effective use of simethicone:

- Follow your doctor's instructions if this medicine was prescribed.
- Follow the manufacturer's package directions if you are treating yourself.

Take this medicine after meals and at bedtime for best results.

For patients taking the chewable tablet form of this medicine:

- It is important that you chew the tablets thoroughly before you swallow them. This is to allow the medicine to work faster and more completely.

For patients taking the oral liquid form of this medicine:

- This medicine is to be taken by mouth even if it comes in a dropper bottle. The amount you should take is to be measured with the specially marked dropper or measuring spoon.

Avoid foods that seem to increase gas. Chew food thoroughly and slowly. Reduce air swallowing by avoiding fizzy, carbonated drinks. Do not smoke before meals. Develop regular bowel habits and exercise regularly. Make certain your health care professional knows if you are on a low-sodium, low-sugar, or any other special diet. Most medicines contain more than their active ingredient.

Dosing—The dose of this medicine will be different for different patients. Follow your doctor's orders or the directions

on the label. The following information includes only the average doses of this medicine. If your dose is different, do not change it unless your doctor tells you to do so.

The amount of medicine that you take depends on the strength of the medicine. Also, the number of doses you take each day, the time allowed between doses, and the length of time you take the medicine depend on the medical problem for which you are using the medicine.

- For symptoms of too much gas:
  - For oral dosage forms (capsules or tablets):
    - Adults and teenagers—Usual dose is 60 to 125 milligrams (mg) four times a day, after meals and at bedtime. The dose should not be more than 500 mg in twenty-four hours.
    - Children—Dose must be determined by the doctor.
  - For oral dosage form (chewable tablets):
    - Adults and teenagers—Usual dose is 40 to 125 mg four times a day, after meals and at bedtime or the dose may be 150 mg three times a day, after meals. The dose should not be more than 500 mg in twenty-four hours.
    - Children—Dose must be determined by the doctor.
  - For oral dosage form (suspension):
    - Adults and teenagers—Usual dose is 40 to 95 mg four times a day, after meals and at bedtime. The dose should not be more than 500 mg in twenty-four hours.
    - Children—Dose must be determined by the doctor.

Missed dose—If you miss a dose of this medicine, take it as soon as possible. However, if it is almost time for your next dose, skip the missed dose and go back to your regular dosing schedule. Do not double doses.

Storage—Store the medicine in a closed container at room temperature, away from heat, moisture, and direct light. Keep from freezing.

Keep out of the reach of children.

Do not keep outdated medicine or medicine no longer needed.

Side Effects of This Medicine

There have not been any common or important side effects reported with this medicine. However, if you notice any side effects, check with your doctor.

SIROLIMUS (Oral route) - sir-OH-li-mus

Black Box Warning

Increased susceptibility to infection and the possible development of lymphoma may result from immunosuppression. Only physicians experienced in immunosuppressive therapy and management of renal transplant patients should use sirolimus. Patients receiving the drug should be managed in

facilities equipped and staffed with adequate laboratory and supportive medical resources. The physician responsible for maintenance therapy should have complete information requisite for the follow-up of the patient.

Commonly used brand name(s)

In the U.S.—
   Rapamune

Available Dosage Forms:
- Tablet
- Solution

Therapeutic Class: Immune Suppressant

Uses For This Medicine

Sirolimus belongs to a group of medicines known as immunosuppressive agents. It is used to lower the body's natural immunity in patients who receive kidney transplants.

When a patient receives an organ transplant, the body's white blood cells will try to get rid of (reject) the transplanted organ. Sirolimus works by preventing the white blood cells from getting rid of the transplanted organ.

Sirolimus is a very strong medicine. It can cause side effects that can be very serious, such as kidney problems. It may also reduce the body's ability to fight infections. You and your doctor should talk about the good this medicine will do as well as the risks of using it.

Sirolimus is available only with your doctor's prescription.

Before Using This Medicine

In deciding to use a medicine, the risks of taking the medicine must be weighed against the good it will do. This is a decision you and your doctor will make. For this medicine, the following should be considered:

Allergies—Tell your doctor if you have ever had any unusual or allergic reaction to this medicine or any other medicines. Also tell your health care professional if you have any other types of allergies, such as to foods, dyes, preservatives, or animals. For non-prescription products, read the label or package ingredients carefully.

Pregnancy—

	Pregnancy Category	Explanation
All Trimesters	C	Animal studies have shown an adverse effect and there are no adequate studies in pregnant women OR no animal studies have been conducted and there are no adequate studies in pregnant women.

Breast Feeding—There are no adequate studies in women for determining infant risk when using this medication during breastfeeding. Weigh the potential benefits against the potential risks before taking this medication while breastfeeding.

Other medicines—

Using this medicine with any of the following medicines is not recommended. Your doctor may decide not to treat you with this medication or change some of the other medicines you take.

Voriconazole

Interactions with Food/Tobacco/Alcohol—Certain medicines should not be used at or around the time of eating food or eating certain types of food since interactions may occur. Using alcohol or tobacco with certain medicines may also cause interactions to occur. The following interactions have been selected on the basis of their potential significance and are not necessarily all-inclusive.

Using this medicine with any of the following may cause an increased risk of certain side effects but may be unavoidable in some cases. If used together, your doctor may change the dose or how often you use this medicine, or give you special instructions about the use of food, alcohol, or tobacco.

Grapefruit Juice

Other medical problems—The presence of other medical problems may affect the use of this medicine. Make sure you tell your doctor if you have any other medical problems, especially:

- Cancer or
- Hyperlipidemia (high amount of cholesterol and fats in the blood)—Sirolimus can make these conditions worse
- Chickenpox (including recent exposure) or
- Herpes zoster (shingles)—Risk of severe disease affecting other parts of the body
- Infection—Sirolimus decreases the body's ability to fight infection
- Liver disease—A lower dose of sirolimus may be needed in patients with this condition
- Liver transplantation or
- Lung transplantation—Sirolimus is not recommended in liver or lung transplant patients

---

Proper Use of This Medicine

This medicine usually comes with patient information or directions. Read them carefully and make sure you understand them before taking this medicine. If you have any questions, ask your health care professional.

Take this medicine only as directed by your doctor. Do not use more or less of it, and do not use it more often than your doctor ordered. The exact amount of medicine you need has been carefully worked out. Using too much will increase the risk of side effects, while using too little may lead to rejection of your transplanted kidney.

To help you remember to take your medicine, try to get into the habit of taking it at the same time each day. This will help sirolimus work better by keeping a constant amount in the blood.

Absorption of this medicine may be changed if you change your diet. This medicine should be taken consistently with respect to meals. You should not change the type or amount of food you eat unless you discuss it with your health care professional.

Do not stop taking this medicine without first checking with your doctor. You may have to take this medicine for the rest of your life to prevent your body from rejecting the transplant.

Sirolimus usually is used along with a corticosteroid (cortisone-like medicine) and cyclosporine (another immunosuppressive agent). Sirolimus should be taken 4 hours after cyclosporine modified oral solution (Neoral) or cyclosporine modified capsules (Neoral). If you have any questions about this, ask your health care professional.

Mix sirolimus oral solution with at least 2 ounces (¼ cup, 60 milliliters [mL]) of water or orange juice in a glass or plastic container. Stir the mixture well and drink it immediately. Then, rinse the container with at least 4 ounces (½ cup, 120 mL) of additional water or orange juice, stir it well, and drink it to make sure that all of the medicine is taken.

Check with your doctor before you stop using cyclosporine when you have been taking sirolimus together with cyclosporine for 4 months after your transplant. Your doctor will tell you if you need to keep taking cyclosporine.

Dosing—The dose of this medicine will be different for different patients. Follow your doctor's orders or the directions on the label. The following information includes only the average doses of this medicine. If your dose is different, do not change it unless your doctor tells you to do so.

The amount of medicine that you take depends on the strength of the medicine. Also, the number of doses you take each day, the time allowed between doses, and the length of time you take the medicine depend on the medical problem for which you are using the medicine.

- For oral dosage form (oral solution or tablets):
  - Adults and children 13 years of age and older weighing 88 pounds (40 kilograms) or more: The usual dose is 2 milligrams (mg) a day after an initial one-time dose of 6 mg.
  - For children 13 years of age and older who weigh less than 88 pounds (40 kilograms): The dose is based on body size. It is usually 1 mg per square meter of body surface area once a day after an initial one-time dose of 3 mg per square meter of body surface area.
  - For children up to 13 years of age: Use and dose must be determined by your doctor.

Storage—Keep out of the reach of children.

Do not keep outdated medicine or medicine no longer needed.

Store tablets at room temperature. Store the oral liquid form in the refrigerator.

Precautions While Using This Medicine

It is very important that your doctor check your progress at regular visits to make sure that this medicine is working properly and to check for unwanted effects.

While you are taking sirolimus, it is important to maintain good dental hygiene and see a dentist regularly for teeth cleaning.

Raw oysters or other shellfish may contain bacteria that can cause serious illness and possibly death. This is more likely to be a problem if these foods are eaten by patients with certain medical conditions. Even eating oysters from "clean" water or good restaurants does not guarantee that the oysters do not contain the bacteria. Eating raw shellfish is not a problem for most healthy people; however, patients with the following conditions may be at greater risk: cancer, immune disorders, organ transplantation, long-term corticosteroid use (as for asthma, arthritis, or organ transplantation), liver disease (including viral hepatitis), excess alcohol intake (2 to 3 drinks or more per day), diabetes, stomach problems (including stomach surgery and low stomach acid), and hemochromatosis (an iron disorder). Do not eat raw oysters or other shellfish while you are taking sirolimus. Be sure oysters and shellfish are fully cooked.

While you are being treated with sirolimus, and after you stop treatment with it, it is important to see your doctor about the immunizations (vaccinations) you should receive. Do not get any immunizations without your doctor's approval. Sirolimus may lower your body's resistance and there is a chance you might get the infection the immunization is meant to prevent. In addition, other persons living in your household should not take or have recently taken oral polio vaccine since there is a chance they could pass the polio virus on to you. Also, avoid other persons who have taken the oral polio vaccine. Do not get close to them, and do not stay in the same room with them for very long. If you cannot take these precautions, you should consider wearing a protective face mask that covers the nose and mouth.

Treatment with sirolimus may also increase the chance of getting other infections. If you can, avoid people with colds or other infections. If you think you are getting a cold or other infection, check with your doctor.

Grapefruits and grapefruit juice may increase the effects of sirolimus by increasing the amount of this medicine in your body. You should not eat grapefruit or drink grapefruit juice while you taking this medicine.

Sirolimus may cause you to have a greater risk for getting skin cancer. When you begin taking this medicine:

- Stay out of direct sunlight, especially between the hours of 10:00 a.m. and 3:00 p.m., if possible.
- Wear protective clothing, including a hat. Also, wear sunglasses
- Apply a sun block product that has a skin protection factor (SPF) of at least 15. Some patients may require a product with a higher SPF number, especially if they have a fair complexion. If you have any questions about this, check with your health care professional.
- Apply a sun block lipstick that has an SPF of at least 15 to protect your lips
- Do not use a sunlamp or tanning bed or booth.

Check with your doctor right away if you notice a new mole; a change in size, shape or color of an existing mole; or a mole that leaks fluid or bleeds.

Side Effects of This Medicine

Along with its needed effects, a medicine may cause some unwanted effects. Although not all of these side effects may occur, if they do occur they may need medical attention.

Also, because of the way sirolimus acts on the body, there is a chance that it may cause effects that may not occur until years after the medicine is used. These delayed effects may include certain types of cancer, such as lymphoma.

Check with your doctor immediately if any of the following side effects occur:

More common
Black or red, tarry stools; chest pain; general feeling of discomfort or illness; shortness of breath; swollen glands; weight loss, unusual; yellow skin and eyes

Check with your doctor as soon as possible if any of the following side effects occur:

More common
Abdominal cramps or pain; accumulation of pus; anxiousness, unexplained; backache; bleeding from gums or nose; blindness; bloody or cloudy urine; blue lips and fingernails; blurred vision; body aches or pain; bone pain; bruising; burning while urinating; burning, dry, or itching eyes; burning or stinging of skin; burning, tingling, numbness, or pain in the hands, arms, feet, or legs; change in mental status; changes in skin color; chills; cold hands and feet; cold sweats; confusion; convulsions (seizures); cough; cough producing mucus; cough that sometimes produces a pink frothy sputum; coughing up blood; dark or bloody urine; deafness; decreased urge to urinate; decreased urine output; decreased vision; difficult, fast, noisy breathing sometimes with wheezing; difficulty in breathing or swallowing; difficulty speaking; dilated neck veins; discharge from eye; dizziness; drowsiness; dry mouth; ear congestion; earache; excessive tearing; extreme fatigue; eye pain; facial hair growth in females; fainting; faintness or lightheadedness when getting up from lying or sitting position; fast, slow, or irregular heartbeat; fatigue; feeling faint; feeling of warmth or heat; fever; flushed, dry skin; flushing or redness of skin, especially on face and neck; fractures; frequent urge to urinate; fruit-like breath odor; full or round face, neck, or trunk; increased menstrual flow or vaginal bleeding; increased hunger; increased sweating; increased thirst; increased urination; irregular breathing; irritability; itching, pain, redness, swelling, tenderness, warmth on skin; lab results that show problems with liver; large, flat, blue or purplish patches in the skin; lightheadedness; lack or loss of appetite; loss of consciousness; loss of sexual ability, desire, drive, or performance; loss of voice; lower back or side pain; lump in abdomen; menstrual irregularities; mood changes; muscle cramps in hands, arms, feet, legs, or face; muscle pain; muscle wasting; nasal congestion; nausea or vomiting; noisy breathing; numbness or tingling around lips, hands, or feet; pain in chest, groin, or legs, especially the calves; pain, tenderness, swelling of foot or leg; painful blisters on trunk of body; painful cold sores or blisters on lips, nose, eyes, or genitals; painful or difficult urination; pale skin; paralysis; pinpoint red spots on skin; pounding or racing heartbeat or pulse; prolonged bleeding from cuts; pus in urine; rapid heartbeat; rapid, shallow breathing; rash; red or dark brown urine; redness or swelling in ear; redness, pain, swelling of eye, eyelid, or inner lining of eyelid; ringing in the ears; runny nose; sensation of pins and needles; severe constipation; severe vomiting; severe, sudden headache; slurred speech; sneezing; sore mouth or tongue; sore throat; sores or white spots on lips or in mouth; stabbing pain; stomach pain or upset; stomachache; sudden decrease in amount of urine; sudden loss of coordination; sudden, severe weakness or numbness in arm or leg; sudden, unexplained shortness of breath; sweating; swelling of face, fingers, hands, ankles, feet, or lower legs; swollen glands; swollen, painful or tender lymph glands in neck, armpit, or groin; swollen, red, tender area of infection; tenderness, pain, swelling, warmth, skin discoloration, and prominent superficial veins over affected area; tightness in chest; tiredness; tremor; trouble breathing; ulcers on lips or in mouth; unusual bleeding or bruising; unusual tiredness or weakness; vision changes; weakness; weakness or heaviness of

legs; weight gain; wheezing; white patches in mouth and/or on tongue

Less common
Bloating; change is size, shape or color of existing mole; darkened urine; hoarseness; mole that leaks fluid or bleeds; new mole; pains in stomach, side or abdomen, possibly radiating to the back; skin ulcer or sores

Rare
Weight gain, unusual

Unknown frequency
Abnormal wound healing; hives; itching; large, hive-like swelling on face, eyelids, lips, tongue, throat, hands, legs, feet, or sex organs; nails loose or detached; puffiness or swelling of the eyelids or around the eyes, face, lips, or tongue; swelling of arms or legs; troubled breathing; yellow nails lacking a cuticle

Some side effects may occur that usually do not need medical attention. These side effects may go away during treatment as your body adjusts to the medicine. Also, your health care professional may be able to tell you about ways to prevent or reduce some of these side effects. Check with your health care professional if any of the following side effects continue or are bothersome or if you have any questions about them:

More common
Abdomen enlarged; abnormal vision; acne; belching; blistering, crusting, irritation, itching, or reddening of skin; bloated full feeling; burning feeling in chest or stomach; burning, crawling, itching, numbness, prickling, "pins and needles" or tingling feeling; constipation; continuing ring or buzzing or other unexplained noise in ears; cracked, dry, scaly skin; crying; decrease in frequency of urination; decrease in height; decreased interest in sexual intercourse; degenerative disease of the joint; depersonalization; diarrhea; difficulty in moving; difficulty in passing urine [dribbling]; discouragement; dysphoria; ear pain; euphoria; excess air or gas in stomach or intestines; excessive muscle tone, muscle tension or tightness; fear; feeling sad or empty; headache; hearing loss; heartburn; inability to have or keep an erection; increase in heart rate; increased hair growth, especially on the face; increased urge to urinate during the night; indigestion; irritation in mouth; itching skin; joint pain or swelling; kidney pain; leg cramps; loss of bladder control; loss of energy or weakness; loss of interest or pleasure; loss of strength; lower abdominal pain; mental depression; muscle aches, pain, stiffness, or weakness; nervousness; pain; pain in back, ribs, arms, or legs; pain or burning in throat; pain or tenderness around eyes and cheekbones; paranoia; passing gas; pelvic pain; quick to react or overreact emotionally; rapid breathing; rapidly changing moods; inflammation, redness, or swelling of gums or mouth; shaking or trembling; shivering; sleepiness; sunken eyes; swelling; swelling of the scrotum; tender, or enlarged gums; tenderness in stomach area; thickening of the skin; trouble concentrating; trouble in sleeping; waking to urinate at night; wrinkled skin

Other side effects not listed may also occur in some patients. If you notice any other effects, check with your healthcare professional.

SKELETAL MUSCLE RELAXANTS (Systemic)

Some commonly used brand names are:

In the U.S.—

EZE-DS (3)	Robaxin (5)
Maolate (2)	Robaxin-750 (5)
Paraflex (3)	Skelaxin (4)
Parafon Forte DSC (3)	Soma (1)
Relaxazone (3)	Strifon Forte DSC (3)
Remular (3)	Vanadom (1)
Remular-S (3)	

In Canada—
Robaxin (5)
Robaxin-750 (5)
Soma (1)

This information applies to the following medicines:
1. Carisoprodol (kar-eye-soe-PROE-dole)
2. Chlorphenesin (klor-FEN-e-sin)
3. Chlorzoxazone (klor-ZOX-a-zone)
4. Metaxalone (me-TAX-a-lone)
5. Methocarbamol (meth-oh-KAR-ba-mole)

Category

- **Skeletal muscle relaxant**—Carisoprodol; Chlorphenesin; Chlorzoxazone; Metaxalone; Methocarbamol

Description

Skeletal muscle relaxants are used to relax certain muscles in your body and relieve the stiffness, pain, and discomfort caused by strains, sprains, or other injury to your muscles. However, these medicines do not take the place of rest, exercise or physical therapy, or other treatment that your doctor may recommend for your medical problem. Methocarbamol also has been used to relieve some of the muscle problems caused by tetanus.

Skeletal muscle relaxants act in the central nervous system (CNS) to produce their muscle relaxant effects. Their actions in the CNS may also produce some of their side effects.

In the U.S., these medicines are available only with your doctor's prescription. In Canada, some of these medicines are available without a prescription.

These medicines are available in the following dosage forms:

Oral
- Carisoprodol
  - Tablets
- Chlorphenesin
  - Tablets
- Chlorzoxazone
  - Tablets
- Metaxalone
  - Tablets
- Methocarbamol
  - Tablets

Parenteral
- Methocarbamol
  - Injection

Before Using This Medicine

In deciding to use a medicine, the risks of taking the medicine must be weighed against the good it will do. This is a decision you and your doctor will make. For the skeletal muscle relaxants, the following should be considered:

Allergies—Tell your doctor if you have ever had any unusual or allergic reaction to any of the skeletal muscle relaxants or to carbromal, mebutamate, meprobamate (e.g., Equanil), or tybamate. Also tell your health care professional if you are allergic to any other substances, such as foods, preservatives, or dyes.

Pregnancy—Although skeletal muscle relaxants have not been shown to cause birth defects or other problems, studies on birth defects have not been done in pregnant women. Studies in animals with metaxalone have not shown that it causes birth defects.

Breast-feeding—Carisoprodol passes into the breast milk and may cause drowsiness or stomach upset in nursing babies. It is not known whether chlorphenesin, chlorzoxazone, metaxalone, or methocarbamol passes into the breast milk. However, these medicines have not been reported to cause problems in nursing babies.

Children—Studies with the skeletal muscle relaxants have been done only in adult patients, and there is no specific information comparing use of these medicines in children with use in other age groups. However, carisoprodol and chlorzoxazone have been used in children. They have not been reported to cause different side effects or problems in children than they do in adults.

Older adults—Many medicines have not been tested in older people. Therefore, it may not be known whether they work exactly the same way they do in younger adults or if they cause different side effects or problems in older people. There is no specific information about the use of skeletal muscle relaxants in the elderly.

Other medicines—Although certain medicines should not be used together at all, in other cases two different medicines may be used together even if an interaction might occur. In these cases, your doctor may want to change the dose, or other precautions may be necessary. When you are taking a skeletal muscle relaxant, it is especially important that your health care professional know if you are taking any of the following:

- Alcohol or
- Central nervous system (CNS) depressants or
- Tricyclic antidepressants (amitriptyline [e.g., Elavil], amoxapine [e.g., Asendin], clomipramine [e.g., Anafranil], desipramine [e.g., Pertofrane], doxepin [e.g., Sinequan], imipramine [e.g., Tofranil], nortriptyline [e.g., Aventyl], protriptyline [e.g., Vivactil], trimipramine [e.g., Surmontil])—The chance of side effects may be increased

Other medical problems—The presence of other medical problems may affect the use of a skeletal muscle relaxant. Make sure you tell your doctor if you have any other medical problems, especially:

- Allergies, history of, or
- Blood disease caused by an allergy or reaction to any other medicine, history of, or
- Drug abuse or dependence, or history of, or
- Kidney disease or
- Liver disease or

- Porphyria—Depending on which of the skeletal muscle relaxants you take, the chance of side effects may be increased; your doctor can choose a muscle relaxant that is less likely to cause problems
- Epilepsy—Convulsions may be more likely to occur if methocarbamol is given by injection

Proper Use of This Medicine

Chlorzoxazone, metaxalone, or methocarbamol tablets may be crushed and mixed with a little food or liquid if needed to make the tablets easier to swallow.

Dosing—The dose of these medicines will be different for different patients. *Follow your doctor's orders or the directions on the label.* The following information includes only the average doses of these medicines. *If your dose is different, do not change it* unless your doctor tells you to do so.

For carisoprodol
- For *oral* dosage form (tablets):
  - For relaxing stiff, sore muscles:
    - Adults and teenagers—350 milligrams (mg) four times a day.
    - Children up to 5 years of age—Dose must be determined by your doctor.
    - Children 5 to 12 years of age—6.25 mg per kilogram (2.5 mg per pound) of body weight four times a day.

For chlorphenesin
- For *oral* dosage form (tablets):
  - For relaxing stiff, sore muscles:
    - Adults and teenagers—800 milligrams (mg) three times a day, at first. Your doctor may decrease your dose after you begin to feel better.
    - Children—Use and dose must be determined by your doctor.

For chlorzoxazone
- For *oral* dosage form (tablets):
  - For relaxing stiff, sore muscles:
    - Adults and teenagers—500 milligrams (mg) three or four times a day.
    - Children—125 to 500 mg three or four times a day, depending on the child's size and weight.

For metaxalone
- For *oral* dosage form (tablets):
  - For relaxing stiff, sore muscles:
    - Adults and teenagers—800 milligrams (mg) three or four times a day.
    - Children—Use and dose must be determined by your doctor.

For methocarbamol
- For *oral* dosage form (tablets):
  - For relaxing stiff, sore muscles:
    - Adults and teenagers—1500 milligrams (mg) four times a day, at first. Your doctor may decrease your dose after you begin to feel better.
    - Children—Use and dose must be determined by your doctor.
- For *injection* dosage form:
  - For relaxing stiff, sore muscles:
    - Adults and teenagers—1 to 3 grams a day, injected into a muscle or a vein. This total daily dose may be divided into smaller amounts that are given

several times a day, especially when the medicine is injected into a muscle.

- Children—Use and dose must be determined by your doctor.

Missed dose—If you miss a dose of this medicine and remember within an hour or so of the missed dose, take it right away. But if you do not remember until later, skip the missed dose and go back to your regular dosing schedule. Do not double doses.

Storage—To store this medicine:

- Keep out of the reach of children.
- Store away from heat and direct light.
- Do not store this medicine in the bathroom, near the kitchen sink, or in other damp places. Heat or moisture may cause the medicine to break down.
- Do not keep outdated medicine or medicine no longer needed. Be sure that any discarded medicine is out of the reach of children.

Precautions While Using This Medicine

If you will be taking this medicine for a long time (for example, more than a few weeks), your doctor should check your progress at regular visits.

This medicine will add to the effects of alcohol and other CNS depressants (medicines that slow down the nervous system, possibly causing drowsiness). Some examples of CNS depressants are antihistamines or medicine for hay fever, other allergies, or colds; sedatives, tranquilizers, or sleeping medicine; prescription pain medicine or narcotics; barbiturates; medicine for seizures; other muscle relaxants; or anesthetics, including some dental anesthetics. *Do not drink alcoholic beverages, and check with your doctor before taking any of the medicines listed above, while you are using this medicine.*

Skeletal muscle relaxants may cause blurred vision or clumsiness or unsteadiness in some people. They may also cause some people to feel drowsy, dizzy, lightheaded, faint, or less alert than they are normally. *Make sure you know how you react to this medicine before you drive, use machines, or do anything else that could be dangerous if you are dizzy or are not alert, well-coordinated, and able to see well.*

For *diabetic patients:*

- Metaxalone (e.g., Skelaxin) may cause false test results with one type of test for sugar in your urine. If your urine sugar test shows an unusually large amount of sugar, or if you have any questions about this, check with your health care professional. This is especially important if your diabetes is not well controlled.

Side Effects of This Medicine

Along with its needed effects, a medicine may cause some unwanted effects. Although not all of these side effects may occur, if they do occur they may need medical attention.

Check with your doctor as soon as possible if any of the following side effects occur:

Less common

Fainting; fast heartbeat; fever; hive-like swellings (large) on face, eyelids, mouth, lips, and/or tongue; mental depression; shortness of breath, troubled breathing, tightness in chest, and/or wheezing; skin rash, hives, itching, or redness; slow heartbeat (meth-

ocarbamol injection only); stinging or burning of eyes; stuffy nose and red or bloodshot eyes

Rare

Blood in urine; bloody or black, tarry stools; convulsions (seizures) (methocarbamol injection only); cough or hoarseness; fast or irregular breathing; lower back or side pain; muscle cramps or pain (not present before treatment or more painful than before treatment); painful or difficult urination; pain, tenderness, heat, redness, or swelling over a blood vessel (vein) in arm or leg (methocarbamol injection only); pinpoint red spots on skin; puffiness or swelling of the eyelids or around the eyes; sores, ulcers, or white spots on lips or in mouth; sore throat and fever with or without chills; swollen and/or painful glands; unusual bruising or bleeding; unusual tiredness or weakness; vomiting of blood or material that looks like coffee grounds; yellow eyes or skin

Other side effects may occur that usually do not need medical attention. These side effects may go away during treatment as your body adjusts to the medicine. However, check with your doctor if any of the following side effects continue or are bothersome:

More common

Blurred or double vision or any change in vision; dizziness or lightheadedness; drowsiness

Less common or rare

Abdominal or stomach cramps or pain; clumsiness or unsteadiness; confusion; constipation; diarrhea; excitement, nervousness, restlessness, or irritability; flushing or redness of face; headache; heartburn; hiccups; muscle weakness; nausea or vomiting; pain or peeling of skin at place of injection (methocarbamol only); trembling; trouble in sleeping; uncontrolled movements of eyes (methocarbamol injection only)

Although not all of the side effects listed above have been reported for all of these medicines, they have been reported for at least one of them. However, since all of these skeletal muscle relaxants have similar effects, it is possible that any of the above side effects may occur with any of these medicines.

In addition to the other side effects listed above, chlorzoxazone may cause your urine to turn orange or reddish purple. Methocarbamol may cause your urine to turn black, brown, or green. This effect is harmless and will go away when you stop taking the medicine. However, if you have any questions about this, check with your doctor.

Other side effects not listed above may also occur in some patients. If you notice any other effects, check with your doctor.

SODIUM FLUORIDE (Oral route) -
soe-dee-um FLYOOR-ide

Commonly used brand name(s)

In the U.S.—

CaviRinse	Fluorigard
EtheDent	Fluorinse
Fluorabon	Flura-Drops
Fluor-A-Day	Flura-Loz

Luride
Neutragard
NeutraGard Plus
Pediaflor

Pharmaflur
Phos-Flur
Prevident

In Canada—
Fluorosol
Pdf
Pedi-Dent

Available Dosage Forms:

- Tablet
- Liquid
- Tablet, Chewable
- Solution
- Tablet, Enteric Coated

Therapeutic Class: Fluoride Supplement

Uses For This Medicine

Fluoride has been found to be helpful in reducing the number of cavities in the teeth. It is usually present naturally in drinking water. However, some areas of the country do not have a high enough level in the water to prevent cavities. To make up for this, extra fluorides may be added to the diet. Some children may require both dietary fluorides and topical fluoride treatments by the dentist. Use of a fluoride toothpaste or rinse may be helpful as well.

Taking fluorides does not replace good dental habits. These include eating a good diet, brushing and flossing teeth often, and having regular dental checkups.

Fluoride may also be used for other conditions as determined by your health care professional.

This medicine is available only with a prescription.

Importance of Diet—For good health, it is important that you eat a balanced and varied diet. Follow carefully any diet program your health care professional may recommend. For your specific dietary vitamin and/or mineral needs, ask your health care professional for a list of appropriate foods. If you think that you are not getting enough vitamins and/or minerals in your diet, you may choose to take a dietary supplement.

People get needed fluoride from fish, including the bones, tea, and drinking water that has fluoride added to it. Food that is cooked in water containing fluoride or in Teflon-coated pans also provides fluoride. However, foods cooked in aluminum pans provide less fluoride.

The daily amount of fluoride needed is defined in several different ways.

For U.S.—

- Recommended Dietary Allowances (RDAs) are the amount of vitamins and minerals needed to provide for adequate nutrition in most healthy persons. RDAs for a given nutrient may vary depending on a person's age, sex, and physical condition (e.g., pregnancy).
- Daily Values (DVs) are used on food and dietary supplement labels to indicate the percent of the recommended daily amount of each nutrient that a serving provides. DV replaces the previous designation of United States Recommended Daily Allowances (USRDAs).

For Canada—

- Recommended Nutrient Intakes (RNIs) are used to determine the amounts of vitamins, minerals, and protein needed to provide adequate nutrition and lessen the risk of chronic disease.

There is no RDA or RNI for fluoride. Daily recommended intakes for fluoride are generally defined as follows:

- Infants and children—
  - Birth to 3 years of age: 0.1 to 1.5 milligrams (mg).
  - 4 to 6 years of age: 1 to 2.5 mg.
  - 7 to 10 years of age: 1.5 to 2.5 mg.
- Adolescents and adults—1.5 to 4 mg.

Remember:

- The total amount of fluoride you get every day includes what you get from the foods and beverages that you eat and what you may take as a supplement.
- This total amount should not be greater than the above recommendations, unless ordered by your health care professional. Taking too much fluoride can cause serious problems to the teeth and bones.

Before Using This Medicine

In deciding to use a medicine, the risks of taking the medicine must be weighed against the good it will do. This is a decision you and your doctor will make. For this medicine, the following should be considered:

Allergies—Tell your doctor if you have ever had any unusual or allergic reaction to this medicine or any other medicines. Also tell your health care professional if you have any other types of allergies, such as to foods, dyes, preservatives, or animals. For non-prescription products, read the label or package ingredients carefully.

Pediatric—Problems in children have not been reported with intake of normal daily recommended amounts. Doses of sodium fluoride that are too large or are taken for a long time may cause bone problems and teeth discoloration in children.

Geriatric—Problems in older adults have not been reported with intake of normal daily recommended amounts. Older people are more likely to have joint pain, kidney problems, or stomach ulcers which may be made worse by taking large doses of sodium fluoride. You should check with your health care professional.

Breast Feeding—There are no adequate studies in women for determining infant risk when using this medication during breastfeeding. Weigh the potential benefits against the potential risks before taking this medication while breastfeeding.

Other medicines—Although certain medicines should not be used together at all, in other cases two different medicines may be used together even if an interaction might occur. In these cases, your doctor may want to change the dose, or other precautions may be necessary. Tell your healthcare professional if you are taking any other prescription or non-prescription (over-the-counter [OTC]) medicine.

Interactions with Food/Tobacco/Alcohol—Certain medicines should not be used at or around the time of eating food or eating certain types of food since interactions may occur. Using alcohol or tobacco with certain medicines may also cause interactions to occur. The following interactions have been selected on the basis of their potential significance and are not necessarily all-inclusive.

Using this medicine with any of the following may cause an increased risk of certain side effects but may be unavoidable in some cases. If used together, your doctor may change the dose or how often you use this medicine, or give you special instructions about the use of food, alcohol, or tobacco.

Dairy Food

Other medical problems—The presence of other medical problems may affect the use of this medicine. Make sure you tell your doctor if you have any other medical problems, especially:

- Brown, white, or black discoloration of teeth or
- Joint pain or
- Kidney problems (severe) or
- Stomach ulcer—Sodium fluoride may make these conditions worse

Proper Use of This Medicine

Take this medicine only as directed by your health care professional. Do not take more of it and do not take it more often than ordered. Taking too much fluoride over a period of time may cause unwanted effects.

For individuals taking the chewable tablet form of this medicine:

- Tablets should be chewed or crushed before they are swallowed.
- This medicine works best if it is taken at bedtime, after the teeth have been thoroughly brushed. Do not eat or drink for at least 15 minutes after taking sodium fluoride.

For individuals taking the oral liquid form of this medicine:

- This medicine is to be taken by mouth even though it comes in a dropper bottle. The amount to be taken is to be measured with the specially marked dropper.
- Always store this medicine in the original plastic container. Fluoride will affect glass and should not be stored in glass containers.
- This medicine may be dropped directly into the mouth or mixed with cereal, fruit juice, or other food. However, if this medicine is mixed with foods or beverages that contain calcium, the amount of sodium fluoride that is absorbed may be reduced.

Dosing—The dose of this medicine will be different for different patients. Follow your doctor's orders or the directions on the label. The following information includes only the average doses of this medicine. If your dose is different, do not change it unless your doctor tells you to do so.

The amount of medicine that you take depends on the strength of the medicine. Also, the number of doses you take each day, the time allowed between doses, and the length of time you take the medicine depend on the medical problem for which you are using the medicine.

- For oral dosage form (lozenges, solution, tablets, or chewable tablets):
  - To prevent cavities in the teeth (where there is not enough fluoride in the water):
    - Children—Dose is based on the amount of fluoride in drinking water in your area. Dose is also based on the child's age and must be determined by your health care professional.

Missed dose—If you miss a dose of this medicine, take it as soon as possible. However, if it is almost time for your next dose, skip the missed dose and go back to your regular dosing schedule. Do not double doses.

Storage—Store the medicine in a closed container at room temperature, away from heat, moisture, and direct light. Keep from freezing.

Keep out of the reach of children.

Do not keep outdated medicine or medicine no longer needed.

Precautions While Using This Medicine

The level of fluoride present in the water is different in different parts of the U.S. If you move to another area, check with a health care professional in the new area as soon as possible to see if this medicine is still needed or if the dose needs to be changed. Also, check with your health care professional if you change infant feeding habits (e.g., breast-feeding to infant formula), drinking water (e.g., city water to nonfluoridated bottled water), or filtration (e.g., tap water to filtered tap water).

Do not take calcium supplements or aluminum hydroxide–containing products and sodium fluoride at the same time. It is best to space doses of these two products 2 hours apart, to get the full benefit from each medicine.

Inform your health care professional as soon as possible if you notice white, brown, or black spots on the teeth. These are signs of too much fluoride in children when it is given during periods of tooth development.

Side Effects of This Medicine

Along with its needed effects, a medicine may cause some unwanted effects. Although not all of these side effects may occur, if they do occur they may need medical attention.

Check with your doctor as soon as possible if any of the following side effects occur:

Sores in mouth and on lips (rare)

Sodium fluoride in drinking water or taken as a supplement does not usually cause any side effects. However, taking an overdose of fluoride may cause serious problems.

Stop taking this medicine and get emergency help immediately if any of the following effects occur:

Black, tarry stools; bloody vomit; diarrhea; drowsiness; faintness; increased watering of mouth; nausea or vomiting; shallow breathing; stomach cramps or pain; tremors; unusual excitement; watery eyes; weakness

Check with your doctor as soon as possible if any of the following side effects occur:

Pain and aching of bones; stiffness; white, brown, or black discoloration of teeth— occur only during periods of tooth development in children

Other side effects not listed may also occur in some patients. If you notice any other effects, check with your healthcare professional.

SODIUM OXYBATE (Oral route) -
SOE-dee-um OX-i-bate

Black Box Warning

Central nervous system (CNS) depressant with abuse potential. Should not be used with alcohol or other CNS depressants.

Sodium oxybate is GHB, a known drug of abuse. Abuse has been associated with some important CNS adverse events (including death). Even at recommended doses, use has been associated with confusion, depression and other neuropsychiatric events. Reports of respiratory depression occurred in clinical trials. Almost all of the patients who received sodium oxybate during clinical trials were receiving CNS stimulants; whether this affected respiration during the night is unknown.

Important CNS adverse events associated with abuse GHB include seizure, respiratory depression and profound decreases in level of consciousness, with instances of coma and death. For events that occurred outside of clinical trials, in people taking GHB for recreational purposes, the circumstances surrounding the events are often unclear (eg, dose of GHB taken, the nature and amount of alcohol or any concomitant drugs).

Sodium oxybate is available through the Xyrem Success Program, using a centralized pharmacy 1–866–XYREM88 (1–866–997–3688). The Success Program provides educational materials to the prescriber and the patient explaining the risks and proper use of sodium oxybate, and the required prescription form. Once it is documented that the patient has read and/or understood the materials, the drug will be shipped to the patient. The Xyrem Success Program also recommends patient follow-up every 3 months. Physicians are expected to report all serious events to the manufacturer.

Commonly used brand name(s)

In the U.S.—
Xyrem

Available Dosage Forms:
• Solution

Therapeutic Class: Central Nervous System Agent

Uses For This Medicine

Sodium oxybate is used to reduce the number of cataplexy (weak or paralyzed muscles) attacks in people with narcolepsy. This medicine is available only with your healthcare professional's prescription, and you can only get it from one central pharmacy. Before you use sodium oxybate your healthcare professional should teach you about the safe and effective use of this medicine. You cannot get the medicine until you have read the information the pharmacy will send you about sodium oxybate.

Note: Sodium oxybate is a Schedule III, federally controlled substance. This means that if you sell, distribute, or give your medicine to anyone else, or if you use your sodium oxybate for purposes other than what it was prescribed for, you may be punished under federal and state law by jail and fines. Your sodium oxybate should be used only by you, as prescribed by your healthcare professional.

Before Using This Medicine

In deciding to use a medicine, the risks of taking the medicine must be weighed against the good it will do. This is a decision you and your doctor will make. For this medicine, the following should be considered:

Allergies—Tell your doctor if you have ever had any unusual or allergic reaction to this medicine or any other medicines. Also tell your health care professional if you have any other types of allergies, such as to foods, dyes, preservatives, or animals. For non-prescription products, read the label or package ingredients carefully.

Pediatric—Studies in this medicine have only been done in adult patients, and there is no specific information comparing the use of sodium oxybate in children with other age groups.

Geriatric—Elderly patients may be sensitive to the effects of sodium oxybate. This may increase the chance of side effects during treatment especially difficulty in movement or in thinking.

Pregnancy—

	Pregnancy Category	Explanation
All Trimesters	B	Animal studies have revealed no evidence of harm to the fetus, however, there are no adequate studies in pregnant women OR animal studies have shown an adverse effect, but adequate studies in pregnant women have failed to demonstrate a risk to the fetus.

Breast Feeding—There are no adequate studies in women for determining infant risk when using this medication during breastfeeding. Weigh the potential benefits against the potential risks before taking this medication while breastfeeding.

Other medicines—

Using this medicine with any of the following medicines is usually not recommended, but may be required in some cases. If both medicines are prescribed together, your doctor may change the dose or how often you use one or both of the medicines.

Adinazolam, Alfentanil, Alprazolam, Amobarbital, Anileridine, Aprobarbital, Bromazepam, Brotizolam, Butabarbital, Butalbital, Carisoprodol, Chlordiazepoxide, Chlorzoxazone, Clobazam, Clonazepam, Clorazepate, Codeine, Dantrolene, Diazepam, Estazolam, Fentanyl, Flunitrazepam, Flurazepam, Halazepam, Hydrocodone, Hydromorphone, Ketazolam, Levorphanol, Lorazepam, Lormetazepam, Medazepam, Meperidine, Mephenesin, Mephobarbital, Meprobamate, Metaxalone, Methocarbamol, Methohexital, Midazolam, Morphine, Morphine Sulfate Liposome, Nitrazepam, Nordazepam, Oxazepam, Oxycodone, Oxymorphone, Pentobarbital, Phenobarbital, Prazepam, Primidone, Propoxyphene, Quazepam, Remifentanil, Secobarbital, Sufentanil, Temazepam, Thiopental, Triazolam

Interactions with Food/Tobacco/Alcohol—Certain medicines should not be used at or around the time of eating food or eating certain types of food since interactions may occur. Using alcohol or tobacco with certain medicines may

also cause interactions to occur. Discuss with your healthcare professional the use of your medicine with food, alcohol, or tobacco.

Other medical problems—The presence of other medical problems may affect the use of this medicine. Make sure you tell your doctor if you have any other medical problems, especially:

- Breathing problems such as:
  - Hypopnea (abnormally slow, shallow breathing) or
  - Sleep apnea (stopping breathing during sleep)—Use of sodium oxybate may make these conditions worse
- Depression, history of, or
- Suicide, attempted—Use of sodium oxybate may worsen these conditions
- Drug abuse or dependence, history of—Dependence on sodium oxybate may be more likely to develop.
- Heart failure, history, or
- Hypertension (high blood pressure) or
- Kidney problems—The amount of sodium in this medicine may make these conditions worse.
- Liver problems—May increase the amount of sodium oxybate in the body and a smaller dose may be needed
- Succinic semialdehyde dehydrogenase deficiency (a rare, inborn metabolism deficiency)—Sodium oxybate should not be taken.

Proper Use of This Medicine

Dosing—The dose of this medicine will be different for different patients. Follow your doctor's orders or the directions on the label. The following information includes only the average doses of this medicine. If your dose is different, do not change it unless your doctor tells you to do so.

The amount of medicine that you take depends on the strength of the medicine. Also, the number of doses you take each day, the time allowed between doses, and the length of time you take the medicine depend on the medical problem for which you are using the medicine.

- For oral dosage form (oral solution):
  - For treatment of cataplexy
    - Adults—2.25 grams given at bedtime and repeated one time during the night. The first dose should be taken at bedtime and the second dose taken 2.5 to 4 hours later. The dose will be increased as needed by your healthcare professional up to a maximum of 9 grams. Food will decrease the amount of sodium oxybate that is absorbed by your body. It is best to take this medicine several hours after a meal.

Note: Sodium oxybate causes sleep very quickly. Take it only at bedtime and while in bed. Drink all of the first dose while sitting in bed, recap the cup, and then lie down right away. Right before going to sleep place your second dose (already prepared) in a secure location (locked if needed) near your bed. You may need to set an alarm to wake up to take the second dose. When you wake up to take the second dose, remove the cap from the second dosing cup. While sitting in bed, drink all of the second dose right before lying down to continue sleeping. Recap the second cup.

To take sodium oxybate, you must first mix it with water. Your healthcare professional and the medication guide that comes with your medicine will tell you how to prepare sodium oxybate. Prepare both doses before bedtime. Place the caps provided on the dosing cups and turn each cap so it locks in its child resistant position.

Missed dose—If you miss a dose of this medicine, take it as soon as possible. However, if it is almost time for your next dose, skip the missed dose and go back to your regular dosing schedule. Do not double doses.

Never take two doses of sodium oxybate at the same time. If you have any questions about this ask your healthcare professional.

Storage—Store the medicine in a closed container at room temperature, away from heat, moisture, and direct light. Keep from freezing.

Keep out of the reach of children.

Do not keep outdated medicine or medicine no longer needed.

Pour any unused sodium oxybate down the drain. Destroy the drug name on the label with a marker when you are finished with the medicine. Place the empty bottle in the trash so it is not used for illegal purposes.

Precautions While Using This Medicine

It is very important that your healthcare professional check your progress at regular visits to make sure the medicine is working properly and to check for any unwanted effects. This is especially important for elderly patients who may be more sensitive to the effects of this medicine.

Do not take other medicines unless they have been discussed with your healthcare professional. This medicine will add to the effects of CNS depressants (medicines that make you drowsy or less alert). Check with your healthcare professional or dentist before taking any of the above medicines while you are taking sodium oxybate.

While you are taking sodium oxybate, you should not drink alcohol. The effects of alcohol can increase the chance of dangerous side effects of sodium oxybate.

Other people living in your house should monitor you for the possibility of sleepwalking. If this happens, tell your healthcare professional.

Make sure you know how you react to this medicine before you drive, use machines, or do anything else that could be dangerous if you are dizzy or are not alert. Do not drive a car, operate heavy machinery, or perform any activity that is dangerous or requires mental alertness for at least 6 hours after taking sodium oxybate. When you first start taking sodium oxybate, until you know whether it makes you sleepy the next day, use extreme care while driving a car or doing anything else that could be dangerous or needs you to be fully mentally alert.

Side Effects of This Medicine

Along with its needed effects, a medicine may cause some unwanted effects. Although not all of these side effects may occur, if they do occur they may need medical attention.

Check with your doctor immediately if any of the following side effects occur:

More common

Blurred vision; burning, crawling, itching, numbness, prickling, "pins and needles" or tingling feeling; change in vision; confusion; discouragement; dizziness; feeling sad or empty; headache; impaired vision; irritability; lack of appetite; lack or loss of strength; loss of bladder control; loss of interest or pleasure; loss of memory; loss of strength or energy; muscle pain or weakness; nervousness; pounding in the ears; problems with memory; sleepwalking; slow or fast heartbeat; tiredness; trouble concentrating; trouble sleeping

Symptoms of overdose

Get emergency help immediately if any of the following symptoms of overdose occur:

Alternating periods of shallow and deep breathing; bluish lips or skin, not breathing; chest pain or discomfort; clumsiness; coma; confusion; confusional, agitated combative state; consciousness, depressed; convulsions; drowsiness; generalized slowing of mental and physical activity; headache; inability to hold bowel movement and/or urine; increased sweating; lightheadedness, dizziness or fainting; loss of strength or energy; low body temperature; muscle aches or weakness; muscle pain or weakness; shakiness and unsteady walk; shivering; shortness of breath; sleepiness; slow or irregular heartbeat; trembling, or other problems with muscle control or coordination; unusual tiredness; unusual weak feeling; vision, blurred; vomiting; weak or feeble pulse

Some side effects may occur that usually do not need medical attention. These side effects may go away during treatment as your body adjusts to the medicine. Also, your health care professional may be able to tell you about ways to prevent or reduce some of these side effects. Check with your health care professional if any of the following side effects continue or are bothersome or if you have any questions about them:

More common

Abdominal pain; abnormal thinking; acid or sour stomach; back pain; belching; body aches or pain; chills; congestion; cold; cough or hoarseness; cramps; diarrhea; dizziness; dreams, abnormal; dryness or soreness of throat; fear; fever; flu-like symptoms; general feeling of discomfort or illness; heartburn; heavy bleeding; hoarseness; indigestion; joint pain; lower back or side pain; nausea; pain; pain or tenderness around eyes and cheekbones; painful or difficult urination; runny nose; shivering; shortness of breath or troubled breathing; sleep disorder; sleepiness or unusual drowsiness; sneezing; sore throat; stomach discomfort, upset, or pain; stuffy nose; sweating; tender, swollen glands in neck; tightness of chest or wheezing; trouble in swallowing; unusual tiredness or weakness; voice changes; vomiting

Less common

Sleeplessness; unable to sleep

Other side effects not listed may also occur in some patients. If you notice any other effects, check with your healthcare professional.

SODIUM TETRADECYL SULFATE
(Injection route) - SOE-dee-um tet-ra-DEK-ul SUL-fate

Uses For This Medicine

Sodium tetradecyl sulfate is a type of medicine called a sclerosing agent. It is used for the treatment of small varicose veins of the lower extremities.

This medicine is available only with your doctor's prescription.

Before Receiving This Medicine

In deciding to use a medicine, the risks of taking the medicine must be weighed against the good it will do. This is a decision you and your doctor will make. For this medicine, the following should be considered:

Allergies—Tell your doctor if you have ever had any unusual or allergic reaction to this medicine or any other medicines. Also tell your health care professional if you have any other types of allergies, such as to foods, dyes, preservatives, or animals. For non-prescription products, read the label or package ingredients carefully.

Pediatric—Studies on this medicine have been done only in adult patients, and there is no specific information comparing use of sodium tetradecyl sulfate in children with use in other age groups.

Geriatric—Many medicines have not been studied specifically in older people. Therefore, it may not be known whether they work exactly the same way they do in younger adults or if they cause different side effects or problems in older people. There is no specific information comparing the use of sodium tetradecyl sulfate in the elderly with use in other age groups.

Pregnancy—

	Pregnancy Category	Explanation
All Trimesters	C	Animal studies have shown an adverse effect and there are no adequate studies in pregnant women OR no animal studies have been conducted and there are no adequate studies in pregnant women.

Breast Feeding—There are no adequate studies in women for determining infant risk when using this medication during breastfeeding. Weigh the potential benefits against the potential risks before taking this medication while breastfeeding.

Other medicines—Although certain medicines should not be used together at all, in other cases two different medicines may be used together even if an interaction might occur. In these cases, your doctor may want to change the dose, or other precautions may be necessary. Tell your healthcare professional if you are taking any other prescription or nonprescription (over-the-counter [OTC]) medicine.

Interactions with Food/Tobacco/Alcohol—Certain medicines should not be used at or around the time of eating food or eating certain types of food since interactions may occur. Using alcohol or tobacco with certain medicines may also cause interactions to occur. Discuss with your healthcare professional the use of your medicine with food, alcohol, or tobacco.

Other medical problems—The presence of other medical problems may affect the use of this medicine. Make sure you tell your doctor if you have any other medical problems, especially:

- Allergic conditions or
- Bedridden or
- Cellulitis or
- Deep vein incompetence or
- Huge superficial veins with connections to deeper veins or
- Infections or
- Phlebitis migrans or
- Respiratory diseases or
- Skin diseases or
- Thrombophlebitis or
- Valvular vein incompetence or
- Varicosities caused by abdominal and pelvic tumors (unless the tumor has been removed)—Sodium tetradecyl sulfate should not be administered.
- Asthma or
- Blood dyscrasias or
- Diabetes or
- Hyperthyroidism or
- Neoplasm or
- Sepsis or
- Tuberculosis—Sodium tetradecyl sulfate should not be administered.
- Peripheral arteriosclerosis or
- Thromboangiitis obliterans (Buerger's disease)—Extreme caution should be used; sodium tetradecyl sulfate may make these conditions worse.

Proper Use of This Medicine

It is important to have a preinjection evaluation.

It is important to give slow injections with a small amount (not over 2 milliliters) of sodium tetradecyl sulfate solution.

Dosing—The dose of this medicine will be different for different patients. Follow your doctor's orders or the directions on the label. The following information includes only the average doses of this medicine. If your dose is different, do not change it unless your doctor tells you to do so.

The amount of medicine that you take depends on the strength of the medicine. Also, the number of doses you take each day, the time allowed between doses, and the length of time you take the medicine depend on the medical problem for which you are using the medicine.

- For injection dosage form:
  - For varicose veins:
    - Adults—0.5 to 2 milliliters injected into the vein, depending on the size and degree of varicosity.
    - Children—Use and dose must be determined by your doctor.

Precautions After Receiving This Medicine

Embolism may occur up to 4 weeks following injection of sodium tetradecyl sulfate.

The possible development of deep vein thrombosis.

Side Effects of This Medicine

Along with its needed effects, a medicine may cause some unwanted effects. Although not all of these side effects may occur, if they do occur they may need medical attention.

Check with your doctor or nurse immediately if any of the following side effects occur:
Frequency not known
Anxiety; burning; chest pain; cough; difficulty breathing; difficulty swallowing; dizziness or light-headedness; fainting; fast heartbeat; hayfever; hives; itching; nausea; noisy breathing; pain, redness, or swelling in arm or leg; puffiness or swelling of the eyelids or around the eyes, face, lips or tongue; raised red swellings on the skin, lips, tongue, or in the throat; redness of skin; skin rash; sudden shortness of breath or troubled breathing; tightness in chest; unusual tiredness or weakness; vomiting; wheezing

Some side effects may occur that usually do not need medical attention. These side effects may go away during treatment as your body adjusts to the medicine. Also, your health care professional may be able to tell you about ways to prevent or reduce some of these side effects. Check with your health care professional if any of the following side effects continue or are bothersome or if you have any questions about them:
Frequency not known
Headache; pain, local; pain or redness at site of injection; pale skin at site of injection; peeling or sloughing of skin; ulceration at site of injection

Other side effects not listed may also occur in some patients. If you notice any other effects, check with your healthcare professional.

SOLIFENACIN (Oral route) - sol-i-FEN-a-cin

Commonly used brand name(s)
In the U.S.—
Vesicare

Available Dosage Forms:
  • Tablet

Therapeutic Class: Urinary Antispasmodic
Pharmacologic Class: Antimuscarinic

Uses For This Medicine

Solifenacin is used to treat bladder problems such as frequent need to urinate or loss of control of urinary function.

This medicine is available only with your doctor's prescription.

Before Using This Medicine

In deciding to use a medicine, the risks of taking the medicine must be weighed against the good it will do. This is a decision you and your doctor will make. For this medicine, the following should be considered:

Allergies—Tell your doctor if you have ever had any unusual or allergic reaction to this medicine or any other medicines. Also tell your health care professional if you have any other types of allergies, such as to foods, dyes, preservatives, or animals. For non-prescription products, read the label or package ingredients carefully.

Pediatric—Studies on this medicine have been done only in adult patients, and there is no specific information comparing use of solifenacin in children with use in other age groups.

Geriatric—This medicine has been tested and has not been shown to cause different side effects or problems in older people than is does in younger adults. However, elderly patients are more likely to be sensitive to anticholinergic agents and may require a lower dose.

Pregnancy—

	Pregnancy Category	Explanation
All Trimesters	C	Animal studies have shown an adverse effect and there are no adequate studies in pregnant women OR no animal studies have been conducted and there are no adequate studies in pregnant women.

Breast Feeding—There are no adequate studies in women for determining infant risk when using this medication during breastfeeding. Weigh the potential benefits against the potential risks before taking this medication while breastfeeding.

Other medicines—

Using this medicine with any of the following medicines may cause an increased risk of certain side effects, but using both drugs may be the best treatment for you. If both medicines are prescribed together, your doctor may change the dose or how often you use one or both of the medicines.

Ketoconazole

Interactions with Food/Tobacco/Alcohol—Certain medicines should not be used at or around the time of eating food or eating certain types of food since interactions may occur. Using alcohol or tobacco with certain medicines may also cause interactions to occur. Discuss with your healthcare professional the use of your medicine with food, alcohol, or tobacco.

Other medical problems—The presence of other medical problems may affect the use of this medicine. Make sure you tell your doctor if you have any other medical problems, especially:
  • Glaucoma or
  • Stomach problems or
  • Urinary retention—Solifenacin may make these conditions worse.
  • Kidney problems or
  • Liver problems—A lower dose of solifenacin may be necessary.
  • QT prolongation—Solifenacin may make this condition worse.

Proper Use of This Medicine

Dosing—The dose of this medicine will be different for different patients. Follow your doctor's orders or the directions on the label. The following information includes only the average doses of this medicine. If your dose is different, do not change it unless your doctor tells you to do so.

The amount of medicine that you take depends on the strength of the medicine. Also, the number of doses you take each day, the time allowed between doses, and the length of time you take the medicine depend on the medical problem for which you are using the medicine.
  • For oral dosage form (tablets):
    ○ To treat bladder problems:
      ▪ Adults—5 to 10 milligrams (mg) once a day.
      ▪ Children—Use and dose must be determined by your doctor.

Missed dose—If you miss a dose of this medicine, skip the missed dose and go back to your regular dosing schedule. Do not double doses.

Storage—Store the medicine in a closed container at room temperature, away from heat, moisture, and direct light. Keep from freezing.

Keep out of the reach of children.

Do not keep outdated medicine or medicine no longer needed.

Ask your healthcare professional how you should dispose of any medicine you do not use.

Precautions While Using This Medicine

This medicine may cause some people to have vision problems. Make sure your vision is clear before you drive or do anything else that could be dangerous if you are not able to see well.

Use caution during exercise or hot weather. Overheating may result in heat exhaustion.

This medicine may cause constipation, call your doctor if you get severe stomach pain or become constipated for 3 or more days.

This medicine may cause dryness of the mouth. For temporary relief of mouth dryness, use sugarless candy or gum, melt bits of ice in your mouth, or use a saliva substitute. However, if your mouth continues to feel dry for more than 2 weeks, check with your medical doctor or dentist.

Side Effects of This Medicine

Along with its needed effects, a medicine may cause some unwanted effects. Although not all of these side effects may occur, if they do occur they may need medical attention.

Check with your doctor immediately if any of the following side effects occur:

Symptoms of overdose

> *Get emergency help immediately if any of the following symptoms of overdose occur:*

> > Blurred vision; confusion; constipation; delirium or hallucinations; difficult urination; dizziness; drowsiness; dry eyes, mouth, nose, or throat; dry skin; eye pain; failure of heel-to-toe exam; fast heartbeat; fixed and dilated pupils; flushing or redness of face; nausea; tremors; troubled breathing; vomiting

Some side effects may occur that usually do not need medical attention. These side effects may go away during treatment as your body adjusts to the medicine. Also, your health care professional may be able to tell you about ways to prevent or reduce some of these side effects. Check with your health care professional if any of the following side effects continue or are bothersome or if you have any questions about them:

More common

> Difficulty having a bowel movement (stool); dry mouth

Less common

> Acid or sour stomach; belching; bladder pain; bloody or cloudy urine; blurred vision; body aches or pain; chills; congestion; cough; decrease in frequency of urination; decrease in urine volume; diarrhea; difficulty in passing urine; difficult, burning, or painful urination; discouragement; dizziness; [dribbling] painful urination; dry eyes; dryness or soreness of throat; feeling sad or empty; fever; frequent urge to urinate; general feeling of discomfort or illness; headache; heartburn; hoarseness; indigestion; irritability; joint pain; lack of appetite; loss of interest or pleasure; lower back or side pain; muscle aches and pains; nausea; nervousness; pounding in the ears; runny nose; shivering; slow or fast heartbeat; sore throat; stomach discomfort upset or pain; sweating; swelling of the legs; tender, swollen glands in neck; tiredness; trouble concentrating; trouble sleeping; trouble in swallowing; unusual tiredness or weakness; upper stomach pain; voice changes; vomiting

Other side effects not listed may also occur in some patients. If you notice any other effects, check with your healthcare professional.

SORAFENIB   (Oral route)

Commonly used brand name(s)

In the U.S.—
   Nexavar

Available Dosage Forms:
   • Tablet

Therapeutic Class: Antineoplastic Agent

Uses For This Medicine

Sorafenib is an anticancer medicine used to treat adults with kidney cancer called advanced renal carcinoma.

This medicine is available only with your doctor's prescription.

Before Using This Medicine

In deciding to use a medicine, the risks of taking the medicine must be weighed against the good it will do. This is a decision you and your doctor will make. For this medicine, the following should be considered:

Allergies—Tell your doctor if you have ever had any unusual or allergic reaction to this medicine or any other medicines. Also tell your health care professional if you have any other types of allergies, such as to foods, dyes, preservatives, or animals. For non-prescription products, read the label or package ingredients carefully.

Pediatric—Studies on this medicine have been done only in adult patients, and there is no specific information comparing use of sorafenib in children with use in other age groups.

Geriatric—This medicine has been tested and has not been shown to cause different side effects or problems in older people than it does in younger adults. However, elderly patients are more likely to be sensitive and may require a lower dose.

Pregnancy—

	Pregnancy Category	Explanation
All Trimesters	D	Studies in pregnant women have demonstrated a risk to the fetus. However, the benefits of therapy in a life threatening situation or a serious disease, may outweigh the potential risk.

Breast Feeding—There are no adequate studies in women for determining infant risk when using this medication during breastfeeding. Weigh the potential benefits against the potential risks before taking this medication while breastfeeding.

Other medicines—

Using this medicine with any of the following medicines may cause an increased risk of certain side effects, but using both drugs may be the best treatment for you. If both medicines are prescribed together, your doctor may change the dose or how often you use one or both of the medicines.

Doxorubicin, Irinotecan

Interactions   with   Food/Tobacco/Alcohol—Certain medicines should not be used at or around the time of eating food or eating certain types of food since interactions may occur. Using alcohol or tobacco with certain medicines may also cause interactions to occur. Discuss with your healthcare professional the use of your medicine with food, alcohol, or tobacco.

Proper Use of This Medicine

Read the patient information leaflet before taking sorafenib and each time the prescription is refilled.

Take this medicine exactly as prescribed.

Swallow the tablet whole with water.

Take on an empty stomach (at least 1 hour before or 2 hours after a meal).

Use of effective birth control during sorafenib treatment and for at least 2 weeks after stopping treatment for both male and female patients.

Dosing—The dose of this medicine will be different for different patients. Follow your doctor's orders or the directions on the label. The following information includes only the average doses of this medicine. If your dose is different, do not change it unless your doctor tells you to do so.

The amount of medicine that you take depends on the strength of the medicine. Also, the number of doses you take each day, the time allowed between doses, and the length of time you take the medicine depend on the medical problem for which you are using the medicine.

- For oral dosage form (tablets):
  - Kidney cancer
    - Adults—400 milligrams (2 x 200 milligram tablets) taken twice daily, without food (at least 1 hour before or 2 hours after a meal).
    - Children—Use and dose must be determined by your doctor.

Missed dose—If you miss a dose of this medicine, take it as soon as possible. However, if it is almost time for your next dose, skip the missed dose and go back to your regular dosing schedule. Do not double doses.

Storage—Keep out of the reach of children.

Store the medicine in a closed container at room temperature, away from heat, moisture, and direct light. Keep from freezing.

Do not keep outdated medicine or medicine no longer needed.

Precautions While Using This Medicine

Regular visits: If you will be taking this medicine for a long time, *it is very important that your doctor check you at regular visits* for high blood pressure that may be caused by this medicine.

Check with your doctor if any redness, pain, swelling or blisters on the palms of your hands or soles of your feet occur.

Check with your doctor if you have any chest pain.

Report any bleeding.

Side Effects of This Medicine

Along with its needed effects, a medicine may cause some unwanted effects. Although not all of these side effects may occur, if they do occur they may need medical attention.

Check with your doctor immediately if any of the following side effects occur:
More common
Bleeding gums; blurred vision; coughing up blood; difficulty in breathing or swallowing; dizziness; headache;

increased menstrual flow or vaginal bleeding; nervousness; nosebleeds; paralysis; pounding in the ears; prolonged bleeding from cuts; red or black, tarry stools; red or dark brown urine; shortness of breath; slow or fast heartbeat
Reported during clinical trials
Area rash; bloating; blood in urine or stools; bone pain; chest pain or discomfort; chills; clammy skin; clay-colored stools; coma; confusion; continuing ringing or buzzing or other unexplained noise in ears; constipation; convulsions; cough; dark urine; decreased urine output; depressed mood; difficulty in moving; dry skin and hair; feeling cold; enlarged pupils; fever; hair loss; hearing loss; hives; hoarseness or husky voice; increased sensitivity of eyes to light; increased sweating, possibly with fever or cold; increased thirst; indigestion; itching; joint pain; loss of appetite; lower back or side pain; muscle cramps and stiffness; muscle pain or cramps; nausea or vomiting; pains in stomach, side, or abdomen, possibly radiating to the back; pain or discomfort in arms, jaw, back or neck; painful or difficult urination; pale skin; pinpoint red spots on skin; reddening of the skin, especially around ears; severe chest pain; severe headache; stiff or sore neck; sore throat; sores, ulcers, or white spots on lips or in mouth; stomach discomfort, upset, or pain; sweating; swelling of eyes, face, or inside of nose; swelling of face, ankles, or hands; swollen glands; swollen joints; troubled breathing with exertion; unpleasant breath odor; unusual bleeding or bruising; unusual tiredness or weakness; vomiting of blood; weight gain; yellow eyes or skin

Get emergency help immediately if any of the following symptoms of overdose occur:

Diarrhea; flushing; impaired wound healing; increased sweating; suppressed reaction to skin tests; thin, fragile skin

Some side effects may occur that usually do not need medical attention. These side effects may go away during treatment as your body adjusts to the medicine. Also, your health care professional may be able to tell you about ways to prevent or reduce some of these side effects. Check with your health care professional if any of the following side effects continue or are bothersome or if you have any questions about them:
More common
Blistering, peeling, redness, and/or swelling of palms of hands or bottoms of feet; burning, tingling, numbness or pain in the hands, arms, feet, or legs; diarrhea; difficulty having a bowel movement (stool); numbness, pain, tingling, or unusual sensations in palms of hands or bottoms of feet; sensation of pins and needles; stabbing pain; thinning of hair; tightness in chest; weight loss; wheezing
Reported during clinical trials
Acid or sour stomach; acne; belching; blistering, peeling, loosening of skin; burning feeling in chest or stomach; burning, itching, and pain in hairy areas; cracked lips; cracks in the skin; decreased appetite; decreased interest in sexual intercourse; discouragement; dry mouth; fainting; feeling of warmth, redness of the face, neck, arms and occasionally, upper chest; feeling sad or empty; flushing, redness of skin; gas; general feeling of discomfort or illness; heartburn; in-

ability to have or keep an erection; increase in heart rate; irritability; lack or loss of strength; light-headedness; loss in sexual ability, desire, drive, or performance; loss of ability to use or understand speech or language; loss of heat from the body; loss of interest or pleasure; mouth pain; pus at root of hair; rapid breathing; red irritated eyes; red, swollen skin, scaly skin; rough, scratchy sound to voice; runny nose; shivering; skin rash encrusted, scaly, and oozing; sunken eyes; swelling of the breasts or breast soreness in both females and males; swelling or inflammation of the mouth; tenderness in stomach area; thirst; trouble concentrating; trouble sleeping; unusually warm skin; wrinkled skin

Other side effects not listed may also occur in some patients. If you notice any other effects, check with your healthcare professional.

SPERMICIDES   (Vaginal)

Some commonly used brand names are:

In the U.S.—

Advantage 24 (2)	Koromex Cream (3)
Because (2)	Koromex Crystal Clear Gel (2)
Conceptrol Contraceptive	Koromex Foam (2)
Inserts (2)	Koromex Jelly (2)
Conceptrol Gel (2)	K-Y Plus (2)
Delfen (2)	Ortho-Creme (2)
Emko (2)	Ortho-Gynol (3)
Emko Pre-Fil (2)	Ramses Crystal Clear Gel (2)
Encare (2)	Semicid (2)
Gynol II Extra Strength	Shur-Seal (2)
Contraceptive Jelly (2)	VCF (2)
Gynol II Original Formula	
Contraceptive Jelly (2)	

In Canada—

Advantage 24 (2)	Ortho-Gynol (3)
Delfen (2)	Pharmatex (1)
Emko (2)	Ramses Contraceptive Foam
Encare (2)	(2)

This information applies to the following medicines

1. Benzalkonium Chloride (benz-al-KOE-nee-um KLOR-ide)
2. Nonoxynol 9 (no-NOX-i-nole nine)
3. Octoxynol 9 (awk-TOX-i-nole nine)

Category

• **Contraceptive, vaginal**—Benzalkonium Chloride; Nonoxynol 9; Octoxynol 9

Description

Vaginal spermicides are a type of contraceptive (birth control). These products are inserted into the vagina *before* any genital contact occurs or sexual intercourse begins. They work by damaging and killing sperm in the vagina. Therefore, the sperm are not able to travel from the vagina into the uterus and fallopian tubes, where fertilization usually takes place.

Vaginal spermicides when used alone are much less effective in preventing pregnancy than birth control pills or the IUD or spermicides used with another form of birth control, such as cervical caps, condoms, or diaphragms. *Studies have shown that when spermicides are used alone, pregnancy usually occurs in 21 of each 100 women during the first year of spermicide use.* The number of pregnancies is reduced when spermicides are used with another method, especially the condom. Discuss with a doctor what your options are for birth control and the risks and benefits of each method.

Laboratory studies have shown that nonoxynol 9 kills or stops the growth of the AIDS virus (HIV) and herpes simplex I and II viruses. It was also shown to be effective against other types of organisms that cause gonorrhea, chlamydia, syphilis, trichomoniasis, and other sexually transmitted diseases (venereal disease, VD, STDs). Benzalkonium chloride also killed the AIDS virus in laboratory studies. Although this has *not* been proven in *human* studies, some scientists *believe* that if spermicides are put into the vagina or on the inside and outside of a latex (rubber) condom, they *may* kill these germs before they are able to come in contact with the vagina or rectum (lower bowel).

The most effective way to protect yourself against STDs (such as AIDS) is by abstinence (not having sexual intercourse) or by having one partner who you can be sure is not already infected or is not going to get an STD. However, if either of these methods is not likely or possible, using latex (rubber) condoms with a spermicide is the best way of protecting yourself.

The use of a spermicide is recommended even when you are using nonbarrier methods of birth control such as birth control pills (the Pill) or intrauterine devices (IUDs), since these do not offer any protection from STDs.

The safety of using spermicides in the rectum (lower bowel), anus, or rectal area is not known. However, no side effects or problems have been reported that are different from those reported for use in the vagina.

Vaginal spermicides are available without a prescription, in the following dosage forms:

Vaginal
- Benzalkonium chloride
  - Suppositories
- Nonoxynol 9
  - Cream
  - Film
  - Foam
  - Gel
  - Jelly
  - Suppositories
- Octoxynol 9
  - Cream
  - Jelly

Before Using This Medicine

In deciding to use vaginal spermicides, the risks of using them must be weighed against the good they will do. This is a decision you and possibly your doctor will make. The following information may help you in making your decision:

Allergies—If you have ever had any unusual or allergic reaction to benzalkonium chloride, nonoxynol 9, or octoxynol 9, it is best to check with your doctor before using vaginal spermicides.

Pregnancy—Many studies have shown that the use of vaginal spermicides does not increase the risk of birth defects or miscarriage.

Breast-feeding—It is not known if vaginal spermicides pass into breast milk in humans. However, their use has not been reported to cause problems in nursing babies.

Children—These products have been used by teenagers and have not been shown to cause different side effects or problems than they do in adults. However, some younger users may need extra counseling and information on the importance of using spermicides exactly as they are supposed to be used so they will work properly.

Other medicines—If you are using this medicine without a prescription, carefully read and follow any precautions on the label. For spermicides, the following should be considered:

- Salicylates used on the skin (e.g., some types of ointments for muscle aches) or
- Sulfonamides (sulfa medicine) for use in the vagina or
- Chemicals or substances such as aluminum, citrate, cotton dressings, hydrogen peroxide, iodides, lanolin, nitrates, permanganates, some forms of silver, soaps, detergents, or tartrates—Benzalkonium chloride may not work if it comes in direct contact with these as well as many other chemicals
- Vaginal douches and rectal or vaginal cleansing products—For spermicides to work properly to prevent pregnancy, they must stay in contact with the sperm in the vagina for at least 6 or 8 hours (depending upon which brand of spermicide you use) after sexual intercourse. *Vaginal douching is not necessary after use of these medicines.* Douching too soon (even with just water) may stop the spermicide from working. Also, washing or rinsing the vaginal or rectal area may also make the spermicide ineffective in helping to prevent sexually transmitted diseases

Other medical problems—The presence of certain medical problems may affect the use of vaginal spermicides. Since in some cases spermicides should not be used, check with your doctor if you have any of the following:

- Allergies, irritations, or infections of the genitals—Using vaginal spermicides may cause moderate to severe irritation in these conditions. Also, benzalkonium suppositories may be less effective in women with vaginal infections
- Conditions or medical problems where it is important that pregnancy does not occur—Vaginal spermicides when used alone are much less effective than birth control pills or the IUD or spermicides used with another form of birth control such as cervical caps, condoms, or diaphragms. Discuss with your doctor what your options are for birth control and the risks and benefits of each method
- Recent childbirth or abortion or
- Toxic shock syndrome (history of)—Cervical caps or diaphragms should not be used in these cases because there is an increased chance of developing toxic shock syndrome
- Sores on the genitals (sex organs) or
- Irritation of the vagina—It is not known whether spermicides can cause breaks in the skin that could increase the chances of getting a sexually transmitted disease, especially AIDS. Discuss this with a doctor if you have any questions

If you develop any medical problem or begin using any new medicine (prescription or nonprescription) while you are using this medicine, you may want to check with your doctor.

Proper Use of This Medicine

Make sure you carefully read and follow the directions that come with each spermicide product. Each product may have different directions for using the product. The directions tell you how much to use, how long you must wait before having intercourse, and how long you must leave it in the vagina after intercourse.

Vaginal douching is not needed or advised after using these medicines. When using a spermicide, douching within 6 to 8 hours after the last sexual intercourse (even with just water) may stop the spermicide from working properly. Also, washing or rinsing the vaginal or rectal area may wash the spermicide away before it has had time to work properly.

Cervical caps and diaphragms are not recommended for use during your menstrual period because of an increased chance of developing toxic shock syndrome. Your doctor may advise you to use condoms with a spermicide instead during your menstrual periods when protection is needed.

For proper use of spermicide when used alone:

- Follow directions carefully to make sure the spermicide is properly placed in the vagina. The spermicide should be inserted deep into the vagina, directly on the cervix (opening to the uterus).
- Use the correct amount, according to the product directions.
- Use another dose for *each* act of intercourse.
- After you have applied or inserted the spermicide, wait the correct amount of time before having intercourse so that the spermicide can begin to work.
- If you do not have intercourse within half an hour, read the product directions to see if you need to apply more spermicide.

For proper use of spermicide with cervical caps, condoms, or diaphragms:

- *Make sure the directions for the spermicide you choose state that it is safe for use with latex cervical caps, condoms, or diaphragms.* If the directions do not say the spermicide is safe to use with latex products, the spermicide may cause cervical caps, condoms, or diaphragms to weaken and leak or cause condoms to break during intercourse.
- If there is a leak or break during intercourse, it may be a good idea for the female partner to immediately place more spermicide in the vagina.
- *If you need an extra lubricant, make sure it is a water-based product safe for use with cervical caps, condoms, or diaphragms.* Spermicides, especially gels and jellies, provide some lubrication during sexual intercourse.
- Oil-based products such as hand, face, or body cream; petroleum jelly; cooking oils or shortenings; or baby oil should *not* be used because they weaken the latex rubber. (Even some products that easily rinse away with water are oil-based and should not be used.) Use of oil-based products increases the chances of the condom breaking during sexual intercourse. These products can also cause the rubber in cervical caps or diaphragms to break down faster and wear out sooner.

For patients using spermicides with a cervical cap:

- *To be most effective at preventing pregnancy, the cervical cap must always be used with a spermicide.* Both must be used every time you have sexual intercourse.

- Before inserting the cervical cap, inspect it for holes, tears, or cracks. If there are holes or defects, the cervical cap will not work effectively, even with a spermicide. It must be replaced.

- Before you put the cervical cap over the cervix (opening to the uterus), a spermicide cream, foam, gel, or jelly should be put into the cup of the cervical cap. Follow the manufacturer's directions on how long before sexual intercourse you may apply the spermicide. Fill the cervical cap one-third full with spermicide.

- To insert the cervical cap, squeeze the rim between your thumb and forefinger so that it is narrow enough to fit into the vagina. While in a comfortable position, push the cervical cap as deeply into the vagina as it will go. Release the rim and press it into place around the cervix with your finger. The rim should be round again and be directly on the cervix. The cervical cap is held onto the cervix by suction.

- Some doctors may recommend that you put more spermicide into the vagina each time you repeat sexual intercourse using a cervical cap. You should also check to make sure the cervical cap is in the proper position on the cervix before and after each time you have intercourse. You may wear the cervical cap for up to 48 hours (2 days).

- *Do not remove the cervical cap if it has been less than 8 hours since the last time you had sexual intercourse.* For the cervical cap to be most effective at preventing pregnancy, it must remain in the vagina for at least 8 hours after sexual intercourse.

- To remove the cervical cap, use 1 or 2 fingers to push the rim away from the cervix. This will break the suction seal with the cervix. Then gently pull the cervical cap out of the vagina. *Call your doctor if you have trouble removing the cervical cap.*

For patients using spermicides with condoms:

- Condoms do not have to be used with spermicides, but the spermicide may provide a back-up birth control method in case the condom breaks or leaks.

- Spread some spermicide on the outside of the condom, after it is unrolled over the penis. It is even more important that the female partner also use a spermicide inside the vagina.

- Each time you repeat intercourse, a new condom must be used. *Condoms should never be reused.* Spermicide should also be applied to the outside of the new condom. The female partner must also put more spermicide in the vagina each time she has intercourse.

For patients using spermicides with a diaphragm:

- *To be most effective at preventing pregnancy, diaphragms must always be used with a spermicide.* Some women may choose to insert a diaphragm every night, to avoid the chance of unprotected sexual intercourse and unplanned pregnancy happening.

- Inspect the diaphragm for holes by holding it up to a light. If there are holes or defects, the diaphragm will not work effectively, even with a spermicide. It must be replaced.

- Before you put the diaphragm over the cervix (opening to the uterus), a spermicide cream, foam, gel, or jelly should be put into the cup of the diaphragm. Follow the manufacturer's directions on how much spermicide to use and how long before sexual intercourse you may apply the spermicide. Also, spread some spermicide all around the rim of the diaphragm that will be touching the cervix. Some doctors also advise spreading more spermicide on the outside of the cup of the diaphragm.

- To insert the diaphragm, squeeze the rim between your thumb and forefinger so that it is narrow enough to fit into the vagina. While in a comfortable position, push the diaphragm as deeply into the vagina as it will go. (Some women use a special applicator that makes it easier to insert the diaphragm.) Release the rim. The diaphragm rim should be round again and be directly on the cervix.

- Each time you repeat sexual intercourse, you should put more spermicide into the vagina. *Do not remove the diaphragm if it has been less than 6 or 8 hours (depending upon which brand of spermicide you use) since the last sexual intercourse.* For the diaphragm to be most effective at preventing pregnancy, it must remain in the vagina for at least 6 or 8 hours (depending upon which brand of spermicide you use) after sexual intercourse. Be careful not to move the diaphragm out of place while you are applying more spermicide.

- Do not wear the diaphragm for more than 24 hours, since doing so increases the risk of getting toxic shock syndrome or a urinary tract (bladder) infection.

- To remove the diaphragm, hook one finger over the rim nearest the front. Pull the diaphragm downward and out of the vagina. *Call your doctor if you have trouble removing the diaphragm.*

Dosing—*Follow your doctor's orders or the directions on the label.* The following information includes the usual way that spermicides are used.

For benzalkonium chloride
- For preventing pregnancy:
  - For *vaginal suppositories* dosage form:
    - Adults and teenagers:
      - For use alone: One suppository inserted into the vagina at least ten minutes but not longer than four hours before each time you have sexual intercourse.
      - For use with a diaphragm: After the diaphragm with spermicide has been placed into the vagina, insert one suppository at least ten minutes, but not longer than four hours, before each time you have sexual intercourse. Also, insert another suppository before sexual intercourse if six hours have passed since you inserted the diaphragm.

For nonoxynol 9
- For preventing pregnancy:
  - For *vaginal cream* dosage form:
    - Adults and teenagers:
      - For use alone: One applicatorful of a 5% cream inserted into the vagina just before each time you have sexual intercourse.
      - For use with a diaphragm: One applicatorful of a 2 or 5% cream inserted into the cup of the diaphragm. Spread more spermicide along the rim of the diaphragm. Insert the diaphragm into the vagina just before, but not

longer than six hours before, sexual intercourse. Also, insert one applicatorful just before each time you have intercourse or if six hours have passed since you inserted the diaphragm.

○ For *vaginal film* dosage form:
  ▪ Adults and teenagers—One film inserted into the vagina from five to fifteen minutes (but not longer than one and one-half hours) before each time you have sexual intercourse.

○ For *vaginal foam* dosage form:
  ▪ Adults and teenagers:
    — For use alone: One applicatorful inserted into the vagina just before, but not longer than one hour before, each time you have sexual intercourse.
    — For use with a diaphragm: One applicatorful inserted into either the vagina or into the cup of the diaphragm, depending on the product. Spread more spermicide along the rim of the diaphragm. Insert the diaphragm into the vagina just before, but not longer than one hour before, sexual intercourse. Also, insert another applicatorful into the vagina just before, but not longer than one hour before, each time you have sexual intercourse.

○ For *vaginal gel* dosage form:
  ▪ Adults and teenagers:
    — For use alone: One applicatorful of a 3.5, 4, or 5% gel inserted into the vagina before each time you have sexual intercourse. The 3.5% gel may be used up to twenty-four hours before each act of intercourse. The 4% gel may be used up to one hour before each act of intercourse. The 5% gel must used just before intercourse.
    — For use with a diaphragm: One or two teaspoonfuls (depending on the product) or the contents of one packet of gel is placed into the cup of the diaphragm. Spread more spermicide along the rim of the diaphragm. Insert the diaphragm into the vagina just before, or up to six hours before, sexual intercourse. Also, insert another applicatorful or the contents of one packet into the vagina before each time you have sexual intercourse or if six hours have passed since you inserted the diaphragm.

○ For *vaginal jelly* dosage form:
  ▪ Adults and teenagers:
    — For use alone: One applicatorful of 2.2 or 3% jelly inserted into the vagina just before each time you have sexual intercourse. The contraceptive effect of the 2.2 or 3% jelly will last one hour.
    — For use with a diaphragm: One applicatorful or two teaspoonfuls of jelly (depending on the product) placed into the cup of the diaphragm. Spread more spermicide along the rim of the diaphragm. Insert the diaphragm into the vagina just before, but not longer than six hours before, sexual intercourse. Also, insert another applicatorful before each time you have sexual intercourse or if six hours have passed since you inserted the diaphragm.

○ For *vaginal suppositories* dosage form:
  ▪ Adults and teenagers:
    — For use alone: One suppository inserted into the vagina from ten to fifteen minutes (depending on the product) before, but not longer than one hour before, each time you have sexual intercourse.
  ▪ Adults and teenagers:
    — For use with a diaphragm: After the diaphragm with spermicide has been placed into the vagina, insert one suppository into the vagina from ten to fifteen minutes (depending on the product) before, but not longer than one hour before, sexual intercourse. Also, insert another suppository before each time you have sexual intercourse or if six hours have passed since you have inserted the diaphragm.

For octoxynol 9
• For preventing pregnancy:
  ○ For *vaginal cream* dosage form:
    ▪ Adults and teenagers:
      — For use with a diaphragm: Two teaspoonfuls placed into the cup of the diaphragm. Spread more spermicide along the rim of the diaphragm. Insert the diaphragm into the vagina just before, but not longer than six hours before, sexual intercourse. Also, insert one applicatorful of the vaginal cream just before each time you have sexual intercourse or if six hours have passed since you inserted the diaphragm.
  ○ For *vaginal jelly* dosage form:
    ▪ Adults and teenagers:
      — For use with a diaphragm: One applicatorful placed into the cup of the diaphragm. Spread more spermicide along the rim of the diaphragm. Insert the diaphragm into the vagina just before, but not longer than six hours before, sexual intercourse. Also, insert another applicatorful just before each time you have sexual intercourse or if six hours have passed since you inserted the diaphragm.

Storage—To store this medicine:
• Keep out of the reach of children.
• Store away from heat and direct light.
• Do not store in the bathroom, near the kitchen sink, or in other damp places. Heat or moisture may cause the medicine to break down.
• Do not refrigerate.
• Do not keep outdated products or products no longer needed. Be sure that any discarded products are out of the reach of children.

Precautions While Using This Medicine

During use of spermicides, either partner may feel burning, stinging, warmth, itching, or other irritation of the skin, sex organs, anus, or rectum. Using a weaker strength of vaginal spermicide or one with different ingredients may be necessary. If you are using benzalkonium chloride suppositories, it may help to wet them before they are inserted into the vagina. If any of these effects continue after you have changed products, you may have an allergy to these products or an infection, and should contact a doctor as soon as possible.

Side Effects

Along with its needed effects, a medicine may cause some unwanted effects. Although not all of these side effects may occur, if they do occur they may need medical attention.

Check with a doctor *immediately* if any of the following side effects occur:

Rare
Signs of toxic shock syndrome— for cervical caps or diaphragms
Chills; confusion; dizziness; fever; lightheadedness; muscle aches; sunburn-like skin rash that is followed by peeling of the skin; unusual redness of the inside of the nose, mouth, throat, vagina, or insides of the eyelids

Also, check with a doctor as soon as possible if any of the following side effects occur:

Rare
For females and males
Skin rash, redness, irritation, or itching that does not subside or go away within a short period of time
For females only
Cloudy or bloody urine; increased frequency of urination; pain in the bladder or lower abdomen; pain on urination; thick, white, or curd-like vaginal discharge— with use of cervical caps or diaphragms only; vaginal irritation, redness, rash, dryness, or whitish discharge

Other side effects may occur that usually do not need medical attention. However, check with a doctor if any of the following side effects continue or are bothersome:

Less common
Vaginal discharge (temporary)— for creams, foams, and suppositories; vaginal dryness or odor

Other side effects not listed above may also occur in some people. If you notice any other effects, check with your doctor.

STAVUDINE (Oral route) - STAV-yoo-deen

Black Box Warning

Lactic acidosis and severe hepatomegaly with steatosis including fatal cases, have been reported with the use of nucleoside analogues alone or in combination, including stavudine and other antiretrovirals. Fatal lactic acidosis has been reported in pregnant women who received the combination of stavudine and didanosine with other antiretroviral agents. The combination of stavudine and didanosine should be used with caution during pregnancy and is recommended only if the potential benefit clearly outweighs the potential risk.

Fatal and nonfatal pancreatitis have occurred during therapy when stavudine was part of a combination regimen that included didanosine, with or without hydroxyurea, in both treatment-naive and treatment-experienced patients, regardless of degree of immunosuppression.

Commonly used brand name(s)

In the U.S.—
Zerit

In Canada—
Zerit Pediatrics

Available Dosage Forms:
- Capsule
- Powder for Suspension

Therapeutic Class: Antiretroviral Agent
Pharmacologic Class: Nucleoside Reverse Transcriptase Inhibitor

Uses For This Medicine

Stavudine (also known as d4T) is used in the treatment of the infection caused by the human immunodeficiency virus (HIV). HIV is the virus responsible for acquired immune deficiency syndrome (AIDS).

Stavudine (d4T) will not cure or prevent HIV infection or AIDS; however, it helps to keep HIV from reproducing and appears to slow down the destruction of the immune system. This may help delay the development of problems usually related to AIDS or HIV disease. Stavudine will not keep you from spreading HIV to other people. People who receive this medicine may continue to have the problems usually related to AIDS or HIV disease.

Stavudine may cause some serious side effects, including peripheral neuropathy. Symptoms of peripheral neuropathy include tingling, burning, numbness, and pain in the hands or feet. Check with your doctor if any new health problems or symptoms occur while you are taking stavudine.

Stavudine is available only with your doctor's prescription.

Before Using This Medicine

In deciding to use a medicine, the risks of taking the medicine must be weighed against the good it will do. This is a decision you and your doctor will make. For this medicine, the following should be considered:

Allergies—Tell your doctor if you have ever had any unusual or allergic reaction to this medicine or any other medicines. Also tell your health care professional if you have any other types of allergies, such as to foods, dyes, preservatives, or animals. For non-prescription products, read the label or package ingredients carefully.

Pediatric—This medicine has been tested in children from birth through adolescence and, in effective doses, has not been shown to cause different side effects or problems than it does in adults. Studies on the extended-release capsule form of this medicine have been done only in adult patients, and there is no specific information comparing use of extended-release stavudine capsules in children with use in other age groups.

Geriatric—Stavudine has not been studied specifically in older people. Therefore, it is not known whether it causes different side effects or problems in the elderly than it does in younger adults. Elderly patients should be closely monitored for signs and symptoms of peripheral neuropathy.

Pregnancy—

	Pregnancy Category	Explanation
All Trimesters	C	Animal studies have shown an adverse effect and there are no adequate studies in pregnant women OR no animal studies have been conducted and there are no adequate studies in pregnant women.

Breast Feeding—There are no adequate studies in women for determining infant risk when using this medication during breastfeeding. Weigh the potential benefits against the potential risks before taking this medication while breastfeeding.

Other medicines—

Using this medicine with any of the following medicines is usually not recommended, but may be required in some cases. If both medicines are prescribed together, your doctor may change the dose or how often you use one or both of the medicines.

Didanosine, Doxorubicin Hydrochloride, Hydroxyurea, Ribavirin, Zidovudine

Interactions with Food/Tobacco/Alcohol—Certain medicines should not be used at or around the time of eating food or eating certain types of food since interactions may occur. Using alcohol or tobacco with certain medicines may also cause interactions to occur. Discuss with your healthcare professional the use of your medicine with food, alcohol, or tobacco.

Other medical problems—The presence of other medical problems may affect the use of this medicine. Make sure you tell your doctor if you have any other medical problems, especially:

- Alcohol abuse, active or a history of, or
- Liver disease or
- Obesity (being overweight) or
- Use of other HIV medicines over a long period of time— Stavudine may make liver disease worse in patients with liver disease, active alcohol abuse, history of alcohol abuse, obesity and other HIV medicine use.
- Kidney disease—Patients with kidney disease may have an increased chance of side effects
- Peripheral neuropathy—Stavudine may make this condition worse

Proper Use of This Medicine

Take this medicine exactly as directed by your doctor. Do not take more of it, do not take it more often, and do not take it for a longer time than your doctor ordered. Also, do not stop taking this medicine without checking with your doctor first.

Keep taking stavudine for the full time of treatment, even if you begin to feel better.

This medicine works best when there is a constant amount in the blood. To help keep the amount constant, do not miss any doses. If you need help in planning the best times to take your medicine, check with your health care professional.

Only take medicine that your doctor has prescribed specifically for you. Do not share your medicine with others.

Dosing—The dose of this medicine will be different for different patients. Follow your doctor's orders or the directions on the label. The following information includes only the average doses of this medicine. If your dose is different, do not change it unless your doctor tells you to do so.

The amount of medicine that you take depends on the strength of the medicine. Also, the number of doses you take each day, the time allowed between doses, and the length of time you take the medicine depend on the medical problem for which you are using the medicine.

- For short-acting oral dosage forms (capsules, oral solution):
  - For treatment of HIV infection:
    - Adults and teenagers weighing 60 kilograms (kg) (132 pounds) or more—40 milligrams (mg) every twelve hours.
    - Adults and teenagers weighing up to 60 kg (132 pounds)—30 mg every twelve hours.
    - Children weighing 30 kg (66 pounds) or more— 30 mg every twelve hours.
    - Infants and children at least 14 days old and weighing less than 30 kg (66 pounds)—1 mg per kg (0.45 mg per pound) of body weight, every twelve hours.
    - Infants from birth to 13 days old—0.5 mg per kg of body weight, every twelve hours
- For long-acting oral dosage form (extended-release capsules):
  - For treatment of HIV infection:
    - Adults and teenagers weighing 60 kilograms (kg) (132 pounds) or more—100 milligrams (mg) one time per day.
    - Adults and teenagers weighing up to 60 kg (132 pounds)—75 mg one time per day.
    - Children—Long-acting capsules have not been studied in children. Your doctor will determine which short-acting dosage form is right for your child.

Note: These capsules should be swallowed whole. Do not chew, crush or dissolve. If you have trouble swallowing a capsule whole, the capsule can be opened and all of the beads inside sprinkled over 2 tablespoons of yogurt or applesauce. You should not chew or crush the beads while swallowing.

Missed dose—If you miss a dose of this medicine, take it as soon as possible. However, if it is almost time for your next dose, skip the missed dose and go back to your regular dosing schedule. Do not double doses.

Storage—Store the medicine in a closed container at room temperature, away from heat, moisture, and direct light. Keep from freezing.

Keep out of the reach of children.

Do not keep outdated medicine or medicine no longer needed.

Store the oral solution form in the refrigerator.

Precautions While Using This Medicine

It is very important that your doctor check your progress at regular visits.

Do not take any other medicines without checking with your doctor first. To do so may increase the chance of side effects from stavudine.

HIV may be acquired from or spread to other people through infected body fluids, including blood, vaginal fluid, or semen. If you are infected, it is best to avoid any sexual activity involving an exchange of body fluids with other people. If you do have sex, always wear (or have your partner wear) a condom ("rubber"). Only use condoms made of latex, and use them every time you have vaginal, anal, or oral sex. The use of a spermicide (such as nonoxynol-9) may also help prevent transmission of HIV if it is not irritating to the vagina, rectum, or mouth. Spermicides have been shown to kill HIV in lab tests. Do not use oil-based jelly, cold cream, baby oil, or short-ening as a lubricant— these products can cause the condom to break. Lubricants without oil, such as K-Y Jelly, are rec-ommended. Women may wish to carry their own condoms. Birth control pills and diaphragms will help protect against pregnancy, but they will not prevent someone from giving or getting the AIDS virus. If you inject drugs, get help to stop. Do not share needles or equipment with anyone. In some cities, more than half of the drug users are infected, and sharing even 1 needle or syringe can spread the virus. If you have any questions about this, check with your health care professional.

Side Effects of This Medicine

Along with its needed effects, a medicine may cause some unwanted effects. Although not all of these side effects may occur, if they do occur they may need medical attention.

Check with your doctor immediately if any of the following side effects occur:

More common
Tingling, burning, numbness, or pain in the hands or feet

Less common
Cough; difficulty swallowing; dizziness; fast heartbeat; hives; itching; joint pain; muscle pain; puffiness or swelling of the eyelids or around the eyes, face, lips or tongue; shortness of breath; skin rash; tightness in chest; unusual tiredness or weakness; wheezing

Rare
Nausea and vomiting; stomach pain (severe)

Some side effects may occur that usually do not need med-ical attention. These side effects may go away during treat-ment as your body adjusts to the medicine. Also, your health care professional may be able to tell you about ways to pre-vent or reduce some of these side effects. Check with your health care professional if any of the following side effects continue or are bothersome or if you have any questions about them:

More common
Chills with fever; loss of appetite; weight loss

Less common
Diarrhea; difficulty in sleeping; headache; lack of strength or energy; stomach pain (mild)

Other side effects not listed may also occur in some patients. If you notice any other effects, check with your healthcare professional.

SUCRALFATE   (Oral route) - soo-KRAL-fate

Commonly used brand name(s)

In the U.S.—
Carafate

In Canada—
Sulcrate Suspension Plus

Available Dosage Forms:
- Suspension
- Tablet

Therapeutic Class: Antiulcer, Protectant

Uses For This Medicine

Sucralfate is used to treat and prevent duodenal ulcers. This medicine may also be used for other conditions as deter-mined by your doctor.

Sucralfate works by forming a "barrier" or "coating" over the ulcer. This protects the ulcer from the acid of the stomach, allowing it to heal. Sucralfate contains an aluminum salt.

This medicine is available only with your doctor's prescription.

Once a medicine has been approved for marketing for a cer-tain use, experience may show that it is also useful for other medical problems. Although these uses are not included in product labeling, sucralfate is used in certain patients with the following medical conditions:
- Gastric ulcers
- Gastroesophageal reflux disease (a condition in which stomach acid washes back into the esophagus)
- Stomach or intestinal ulcers resulting from stress or trauma damage or from damage caused by medication used to treat rheumatoid arthritis

Before Using This Medicine

In deciding to use a medicine, the risks of taking the medicine must be weighed against the good it will do. This is a decision you and your doctor will make. For this medicine, the following should be considered:

Allergies—Tell your doctor if you have ever had any un-usual or allergic reaction to this medicine or any other medi-cines. Also tell your health care professional if you have any other types of allergies, such as to foods, dyes, preservatives, or animals. For non-prescription products, read the label or package ingredients carefully.

Pediatric—This medicine has been tested in a limited number of children. In effective doses, the medicine has not been shown to cause different side effects or problems than it does in adults.

Geriatric—Many medicines have not been studied specifi-cally in older people. Therefore, it may not be known whether they work exactly the same way they do in younger adults. Although there is no specific information comparing the use of sucralfate in the elderly with use in other age groups, this medicine is not expected to cause different side effects or problems in older people than it does in younger adults.

Pregnancy—

	Pregnancy Category	Explanation
All Trimesters	B	Animal studies have revealed no evidence of harm to the fetus, however, there are no adequate studies in pregnant women OR animal studies have shown an adverse effect, but adequate studies in pregnant women have failed to demonstrate a risk to the fetus.

Breast Feeding—There are no adequate studies in women for determining infant risk when using this medication during breastfeeding. Weigh the potential benefits against the potential risks before taking this medication while breastfeeding.

Other medicines—

Using this medicine with any of the following medicines is usually not recommended, but may be required in some cases. If both medicines are prescribed together, your doctor may change the dose or how often you use one or both of the medicines.

Ciprofloxacin

Interactions with Food/Tobacco/Alcohol—Certain medicines should not be used at or around the time of eating food or eating certain types of food since interactions may occur. Using alcohol or tobacco with certain medicines may also cause interactions to occur. Discuss with your healthcare professional the use of your medicine with food, alcohol, or tobacco.

Other medical problems—The presence of other medical problems may affect the use of this medicine. Make sure you tell your doctor if you have any other medical problems, especially:

- Gastrointestinal tract obstruction disease—Sucralfate may bind with other foods and drugs and cause obstruction of the gastrointestinal tract

- Kidney failure—Use may lead to a toxic increase of aluminum blood levels

Proper Use of This Medicine

Sucralfate is best taken with water on an empty stomach 1 hour before meals and at bedtime, unless otherwise directed by your doctor.

Take this medicine for the full time of treatment, even if you begin to feel better. Also, it is important that you keep your doctor's appointments for check-ups so that your doctor will be better able to tell you when to stop taking this medicine.

Dosing—The dose of this medicine will be different for different patients. Follow your doctor's orders or the directions on the label. The following information includes only the average doses of this medicine. If your dose is different, do not change it unless your doctor tells you to do so.

The amount of medicine that you take depends on the strength of the medicine. Also, the number of doses you take each day, the time allowed between doses, and the length of time you take the medicine depend on the medical problem for which you are using the medicine.

- For oral dosage form (suspension):
  - To treat duodenal ulcers:
    - Adults and teenagers—One gram four times a day, one hour before each meal and at bedtime. Some people may take two grams two times a day, when they wake up and at bedtime on an empty stomach.
    - Children—Dose must be determined by your doctor.
- For oral dosage form (tablets):
  - To treat duodenal ulcers:
    - Adults and teenagers—One gram four times a day, one hour before each meal and at bedtime.
    - Children—Dose must be determined by your doctor.
  - To prevent duodenal ulcers:
    - Adults and teenagers—One gram two times a day on an empty stomach.
    - Children—Dose must be determined by your doctor.

Missed dose—If you miss a dose of this medicine, take it as soon as possible. However, if it is almost time for your next dose, skip the missed dose and go back to your regular dosing schedule. Do not double doses.

Storage—Store the medicine in a closed container at room temperature, away from heat, moisture, and direct light. Keep from freezing.

Keep out of the reach of children.

Do not keep outdated medicine or medicine no longer needed.

Precautions While Using This Medicine

Antacids may be taken with sucralfate to help relieve any stomach pain, unless your doctor has told you not to use them. However, antacids should not be taken within 30 minutes before or after sucralfate. Taking these medicines too close together may keep sucralfate from working properly.

Side Effects of This Medicine

Along with its needed effects, a medicine may cause some unwanted effects. Although not all of these side effects may occur, if they do occur they may need medical attention.

Check with your doctor immediately if any of the following side effects occur:

Signs of aluminum toxicity
   Drowsiness; convulsions (seizures)

Some side effects may occur that usually do not need medical attention. These side effects may go away during treatment as your body adjusts to the medicine. Also, your health care professional may be able to tell you about ways to prevent or reduce some of these side effects. Check with your health care professional if any of the following side effects continue or are bothersome or if you have any questions about them:

More common
   Constipation

Less common or rare
   Backache; diarrhea; dizziness or lightheadedness; dryness of mouth; indigestion; nausea; skin rash, hives, or itching; stomach cramps or pain

Other side effects not listed may also occur in some patients. If you notice any other effects, check with your healthcare professional.

SULCONAZOLE   (Topical route) - sul-KON-a-zole

Commonly used brand name(s)

In the U.S.—
    Exelderm

In Canada—
    Sulcosyn

Available Dosage Forms:
- Cream
- Solution

Therapeutic Class: Antifungal

Uses For This Medicine

Sulconazole is used to treat infections caused by a fungus. It works by killing the fungus or preventing its growth.

Sulconazole is applied to the skin to treat the following:
- ringworm of the body (tinea corporis);
- ringworm of the foot (tinea pedis; athlete's foot);
- ringworm of the groin (tinea cruris; jock itch);
- "sun fungus" (tinea versicolor; pityriasis versicolor).

Sulconazole may also be used for other conditions as determined by your doctor.

Topical sulconazole is available only with your doctor's prescription.

Once a medicine has been approved for marketing for a certain use, experience may show that it is also useful for other medical problems. Although this use is not included in product labeling, sulconazole is used in certain patients with the following medical condition:
- Cutaneous candidiasis

Before Using This Medicine

In deciding to use a medicine, the risks of taking the medicine must be weighed against the good it will do. This is a decision you and your doctor will make. For this medicine, the following should be considered:

Allergies—Tell your doctor if you have ever had any unusual or allergic reaction to this medicine or any other medicines. Also tell your health care professional if you have any other types of allergies, such as to foods, dyes, preservatives, or animals. For non-prescription products, read the label or package ingredients carefully.

Pediatric—Studies on this medicine have been done only in adult patients, and there is no specific information comparing use of sulconazole in children with use in other age groups.

Geriatric—Many medicines have not been studied specifically in older people. Therefore, it may not be known whether they work exactly the same way they do in younger adults. Although there is no specific information comparing use of topical sulconazole in the elderly with use in other age groups, this medicine is not expected to cause different side effects or problems in older people than it does in younger adults.

Pregnancy—

	Pregnancy Category	Explanation
All Trimesters	C	Animal studies have shown an adverse effect and there are no adequate studies in pregnant women OR no animal studies have been conducted and there are no adequate studies in pregnant women.

Breast Feeding—There are no adequate studies in women for determining infant risk when using this medication during breastfeeding. Weigh the potential benefits against the potential risks before taking this medication while breastfeeding.

Other medicines—Although certain medicines should not be used together at all, in other cases two different medicines may be used together even if an interaction might occur. In these cases, your doctor may want to change the dose, or other precautions may be necessary. Tell your healthcare professional if you are taking any other prescription or non-prescription (over-the-counter [OTC]) medicine.

Interactions with Food/Tobacco/Alcohol—Certain medicines should not be used at or around the time of eating food or eating certain types of food since interactions may occur. Using alcohol or tobacco with certain medicines may also cause interactions to occur. Discuss with your healthcare professional the use of your medicine with food, alcohol, or tobacco.

Proper Use of This Medicine

Apply enough sulconazole to cover the affected and surrounding skin areas, and rub in gently.

Keep this medicine away from the eyes.

When sulconazole is used to treat certain types of fungus infections of the skin, occlusive dressing (airtight covering, such as kitchen plastic wrap) should not be applied over the medicine. To do so may irritate the skin. Do not apply an airtight covering over this medicine unless you have been directed to do so by your doctor.

To help clear up your infection completely, it is very important that you keep using sulconazole for the full time of treatment, even if your symptoms begin to clear up after a few days. Since fungus infections may be very slow to clear up, you may have to continue using this medicine every day for several weeks or more. If you stop using this medicine too soon, your symptoms may return.

Do not miss any doses.

Dosing—The dose of this medicine will be different for different patients. Follow your doctor's orders or the directions on the label. The following information includes only the average doses of this medicine. If your dose is different, do not change it unless your doctor tells you to do so.

The amount of medicine that you take depends on the strength of the medicine. Also, the number of doses you take each day, the time allowed between doses, and the length of time you take the medicine depend on the medical problem for which you are using the medicine.
- For topical cream dosage form:
  - For ringworm of the body or ringworm of the groin or "sun fungus":

- Adults—Use one or two times a day for at least three weeks.
- Children—Use and dose must be determined by your doctor.
  - For athlete's foot:
    - Adults—Use two times a day for at least four weeks.
    - Children—Use and dose must be determined by your doctor.
- For topical solution dosage form:
  - For ringworm of the body or ringworm of the groin or "sun fungus":
    - Adults—Use one or two times a day for at least three weeks.
    - Children—Use and dose must be determined by your doctor.

Missed dose—If you miss a dose of this medicine, apply it as soon as possible. However, if it is almost time for your next dose, skip the missed dose and go back to your regular dosing schedule.

Storage—Store the medicine in a closed container at room temperature, away from heat, moisture, and direct light. Keep from freezing.

Keep out of the reach of children.

Do not keep outdated medicine or medicine no longer needed.

Precautions While Using This Medicine

If your skin problem does not improve within 4 to 6 weeks or if it becomes worse, check with your doctor.

To help clear up your infection completely and to help make sure it does not return, good health habits are also required. The following measures will help reduce chaffing and irritation and will also help keep the area cool and dry:

- For patients using sulconazole for ringworm of the groin (tinea cruris; jock itch):
  - Avoid wearing underwear that is tight-fitting or made from synthetic materials (for example, rayon or nylon). Instead, wear loose-fitting, cotton underwear.
- For patients using sulconazole for ringworm of the foot (tinea pedis; athlete's foot):
  - Carefully dry the feet, especially between the toes, after bathing.
  - Avoid wearing socks made from wool or synthetic materials (for example, rayon or nylon). Instead wear clean, cotton socks and change them daily or more often if the feet sweat a lot.
  - Wear sandals or other well-ventilated shoes.
- For patients using sulconazole for ringworm of the body (tinea corporis):
  - Carefully dry yourself after bathing.
  - Avoid too much heat and humidity if possible.
  - Wear well-ventilated, loose-fitting clothing.

If you have any questions about these measures, check with your health care professional.

Side Effects of This Medicine

Along with its needed effects, a medicine may cause some unwanted effects. Although not all of these side effects may occur, if they do occur they may need medical attention.

Check with your doctor as soon as possible if any of the following side effects occur:

Less common

Burning or stinging, itching, redness of the skin, or other signs of irritation not present before use of this medicine

Other side effects not listed may also occur in some patients. If you notice any other effects, check with your healthcare professional.

SULFASALAZINE (Oral route, Rectal route) - sul-fa-SAL-a-zeen

Commonly used brand name(s)

In the U.S.—
Azulfidine
Azulfidine Entabs
Sulfazine

Sulfazine EC

In Canada—
Alti-Sulfasalazine
Salazopyrin

Available Dosage Forms:

- Tablet
- Enema
- Suppository
- Tablet, Enteric Coated

Therapeutic Class: Gastrointestinal Agent

Uses For This Medicine

Sulfasalazine, a sulfa medicine, is used to prevent and treat inflammatory bowel disease, such as ulcerative colitis. It works inside the bowel by helping to reduce the inflammation and other symptoms of the disease. Sulfasalazine is sometimes given with other medicines to treat inflammatory bowel disease.

Sulfasalazine is also used to treat rheumatoid arthritis in patients who have not been helped by or who cannot tolerate other medicines for rheumatoid arthritis.

Sulfasalazine is available only with your doctor's prescription.

Once a medicine has been approved for marketing for a certain use, experience may show that it is also useful for other medical problems. Although these uses are not included in product labeling, sulfasalazine is used in certain patients with the following medical conditions:

- Ankylosing spondylitis

Before Using This Medicine

In deciding to use a medicine, the risks of taking the medicine must be weighed against the good it will do. This is a decision you and your doctor will make. For this medicine, the following should be considered:

Allergies—Tell your doctor if you have ever had any unusual or allergic reaction to this medicine or any other medi-

cines. Also tell your health care professional if you have any other types of allergies, such as to foods, dyes, preservatives, or animals. For non-prescription products, read the label or package ingredients carefully.

Pediatric—Sulfasalazine should not be used in children up to 2 years of age because it may cause brain problems. However, sulfasalazine has not been shown to cause different side effects or problems in children over the age of 2 years than it does in adults.

Geriatric—This medicine has been tested and has not been shown to cause different side effects or problems in older people than it does in younger adults.

Pregnancy—

	Pregnancy Category	Explanation
All Trimesters	B	Animal studies have revealed no evidence of harm to the fetus, however, there are no adequate studies in pregnant women OR animal studies have shown an adverse effect, but adequate studies in pregnant women have failed to demonstrate a risk to the fetus.

Breast Feeding—There are no adequate studies in women for determining infant risk when using this medication during breastfeeding. Weigh the potential benefits against the potential risks before taking this medication while breastfeeding.

Other medicines—

Using this medicine with any of the following medicines is usually not recommended, but may be required in some cases. If both medicines are prescribed together, your doctor may change the dose or how often you use one or both of the medicines.

Riluzole

Interactions with Food/Tobacco/Alcohol—Certain medicines should not be used at or around the time of eating food or eating certain types of food since interactions may occur. Using alcohol or tobacco with certain medicines may also cause interactions to occur. Discuss with your healthcare professional the use of your medicine with food, alcohol, or tobacco.

Other medical problems—The presence of other medical problems may affect the use of this medicine. Make sure you tell your doctor if you have any other medical problems, especially:

- Allergies, severe or
- Asthma, bronchial—The risk of an allergic reaction to sulfasalazine may be increased
- Blood problems or
- Glucose-6–phosphate dehydrogenase deficiency (lack of G6PD enzyme)—Patients with these problems may have an increase in side effects affecting the blood
- Intestinal blockage—Sulfasalazine will not reach the site of action in the bowel
- Kidney disease or

- Liver disease—Patients with kidney disease or liver disease may have an increased chance of side effects
- Porphyria—Use of sulfasalazine may cause an attack of porphyria
- Urinary blockage—Sulfasalazine may not be eliminated properly, causing an increased risk of side effects

Proper Use of This Medicine

Do not give sulfasalazine to infants and children up to 2 years of age, unless otherwise directed by your doctor. It may cause brain problems.

Sulfasalazine is best taken right after meals or with food to lessen stomach upset. If stomach upset continues or is bothersome, check with your doctor.

Each dose of sulfasalazine should also be taken with a full glass (8 ounces) of water. Several additional glasses of water should be taken every day, unless otherwise directed by your doctor. Drinking extra water will help to prevent some unwanted effects of the sulfa medicine.

For patients taking the enteric-coated tablet form of this medicine:

- Swallow tablets whole. Do not break or crush.

Keep taking this medicine for the full time of treatment, even if you begin to feel better after a few days. Do not miss any doses.

Dosing—The dose of this medicine will be different for different patients. Follow your doctor's orders or the directions on the label. The following information includes only the average doses of this medicine. If your dose is different, do not change it unless your doctor tells you to do so.

The amount of medicine that you take depends on the strength of the medicine. Also, the number of doses you take each day, the time allowed between doses, and the length of time you take the medicine depend on the medical problem for which you are using the medicine.

- For prevention or treatment of inflammatory bowel disease:
  - For oral dosage forms (tablets, enteric-coated tablets):
    - Adults and teenagers—To start, 500 milligrams (mg) to 1000 mg (1 gram) every six to eight hours. Your doctor may then decrease the dose to 500 mg every six hours. Later, your doctor may change your dose as needed.
    - Children 2 years of age and over—Dose is based on body weight and must be determined by your doctor.
      — To start, the dose is usually:
        - 6.7 to 10 mg per kilogram (kg) (3.05 to 4.55 mg per pound) of body weight every four hours or
        - 10 to 15 mg per kg (4.55 to 6.82 mg per pound) of body weight every six hours or
        - 13.3 to 20 mg per kg (6.05 to 9.09 mg per pound) of body weight every eight hours.
      — Then, the dose is usually 7.5 mg per kg (3.41 mg per pound) of body weight every six hours.

- Infants and children up to 2 years of age—Use is not recommended.
  - For rectal dosage form (enema):
    - Adults and teenagers—3 grams (1 unit), used rectally as directed, every night.
    - Children 2 years of age and over—Dose must be determined by your doctor.
    - Infants and children up to 2 years of age—Use is not recommended.
- For treatment of rheumatoid arthritis:
  - For oral dosage forms (tablets, enteric-coated tablets):
    - Adults and teenagers—To start, 500 mg to 1000 mg (1 gram) daily. Your doctor may increase your dose as needed, but the dose is generally not more than 3000 mg (3 grams) a day.
    - For children ages 6 and over—30 to 50 mg per kg of body weight daily, divided into two doses. The medicine is usually started at a lower amount and gradually increased to the actual amount over a month. Typically the amount that is needed does not exceed 2 grams per day. The dose must be determined by your doctor.
    - Infants and children up to 2 years of age—Use is not recommended.

Missed dose—If you miss a dose of this medicine, take it as soon as possible. However, if it is almost time for your next dose, skip the missed dose and go back to your regular dosing schedule. Do not double doses.

Storage—Store the medicine in a closed container at room temperature, away from heat, moisture, and direct light. Keep from freezing.

Keep out of the reach of children.

Do not keep outdated medicine or medicine no longer needed.

Precautions While Using This Medicine

It is very important that your doctor check your progress at regular visits. This medicine may cause blood problems, especially if it is taken for a long time.

If your symptoms (including diarrhea) do not improve within 1 or 2 months, or if they become worse, check with your doctor.

Sulfasalazine may cause blood problems. These problems may result in a greater chance of certain infections, slow healing, and bleeding of the gums. Therefore, you should be careful when using regular toothbrushes, dental floss, and toothpicks. Dental work should be delayed until your blood counts have returned to normal. Check with your medical doctor or dentist if you have any questions about proper oral hygiene (mouth care) during treatment.

Sulfasalazine may cause your skin to be more sensitive to sunlight than it is normally. Exposure to sunlight, even for brief periods of time, may cause a skin rash, itching, redness or other discoloration of the skin, or a severe sunburn. When you begin taking this medicine:

- Stay out of direct sunlight, especially between the hours of 10:00 a.m. and 3:00 p.m., if possible.
- Wear protective clothing, including a hat. Also, wear sunglasses.
- Apply a sun block product that has a skin protection factor (SPF) of at least 15. Some patients may require a product with a higher SPF number, especially if they have a fair complexion. If you have any questions about this, check with your health care professional.
- Apply a sun block lipstick that has an SPF of at least 15 to protect your lips.
- Do not use a sunlamp or tanning bed or booth.

If you have a severe reaction from the sun, check with your doctor.

This medicine may also cause some people to become dizzy. Make sure you know how you react to this medicine before you drive, use machines, or do anything else that could be dangerous if you are dizzy. If this reaction is especially bothersome, check with your doctor.

Before you have any medical tests, tell the doctor in charge that you are taking this medicine. The results of the bentiromide (e.g., Chymex) test for pancreas function are affected by this medicine.

Side Effects of This Medicine

Along with its needed effects, a medicine may cause some unwanted effects. Although not all of these side effects may occur, if they do occur they may need medical attention.

Check with your doctor immediately if any of the following side effects occur:
  More common
    Aching of joints; fever; headache (continuing); itching; skin rash; vomiting
  Less common or rare
    Aching of joints and muscles; back, leg, or stomach pains; bloody diarrhea; bluish fingernails, lips, or skin; chest pain; cough; difficult breathing; difficulty in swallowing; chills, or sore throat; general feeling of discomfort or illness; loss of appetite; pale skin; redness, blistering, peeling, or loosening of skin; unusual bleeding or bruising; unusual tiredness or weakness; yellow eyes or skin

Check with your doctor as soon as possible if any of the following side effects occur:
  More common
    Increased sensitivity of skin to sunlight

Some side effects may occur that usually do not need medical attention. These side effects may go away during treatment as your body adjusts to the medicine. Also, your health care professional may be able to tell you about ways to prevent or reduce some of these side effects. Check with your health care professional if any of the following side effects continue or are bothersome or if you have any questions about them:
  More common
    Abdominal or stomach pain or upset; diarrhea; loss of appetite; nausea

In some patients this medicine may also cause the urine or skin to become orange-yellow. This side effect does not need medical attention.

Other side effects not listed may also occur in some patients. If you notice any other effects, check with your healthcare professional.

SULFONAMIDES (Systemic)

Some commonly used brand names are:

In the U.S.—

Gantanol (3)	Thiosulfil Forte (2)
Gantrisin (4)	Urobak (3)

In Canada—

Apo-Sulfamethoxazole (3)	Novo-Soxazole (4)
Apo-Sulfisoxazole (4)	Sulfizole (4)

This information applies to the following medicines:

1. Sulfadiazine (sul-fa-DYE-a-zeen)
2. Sulfamethizole (sul-fa-METH-a-zole)
3. Sulfamethoxazole (sul-fa-meth-OX-a-zole)
4. Sulfisoxazole (sul-fi-SOX-a-zole)

Category

- **Antibacterial, systemic**—Sulfadiazine; Sulfamethoxazole; Sulfisoxazole
- **Antibacterial, urinary**—Sulfamethizole
- **Antiprotozoal**—Sulfamethoxazole; Sulfisoxazole

Description

Sulfonamides (sul-FON-a-mides) or sulfa medicines are used to treat infections. They will not work for colds, flu, or other virus infections.

Sulfonamides are available only with your doctor's prescription, in the following dosage forms:

Oral
- Sulfadiazine
  - Tablets
- Sulfamethizole
  - Tablets
- Sulfamethoxazole
  - Tablets
- Sulfisoxazole
  - Oral suspension
  - Syrup
  - Tablets

Before Using This Medicine

In deciding to use a medicine, the risks of taking the medicine must be weighed against the good it will do. This is a decision you and your doctor will make. For sulfonamides, the following should be considered:

Allergies—Tell your doctor if you have ever had any unusual or allergic reaction to sulfa medicines, furosemide (e.g., Lasix) or thiazide diuretics (water pills), oral antidiabetics (diabetes medicine you take by mouth), glaucoma medicine you take by mouth (for example, acetazolamide [e.g., Diamox], dichlorphenamide [e.g., Daranide], or methazolamide [e.g., Neptazane]). Also tell your health care professional if you are allergic to any other substances, such as foods, preservatives, or dyes.

Pregnancy—Studies have not been done in pregnant women. However, studies in mice, rats, and rabbits have shown that some sulfonamides cause birth defects, including cleft palate and bone problems. Sulfonamides are not recommended for use at the time of labor and delivery. These medicines may cause unwanted effects in the baby.

Breast-feeding—Sulfonamides pass into the breast milk. This medicine is not recommended for use during breast-feeding. It may cause liver problems, anemia, and other unwanted effects in nursing babies, especially those with glucose-6–phosphate dehydrogenase (G6PD) deficiency.

Children—Sulfonamides should not be given to infants under 2 months of age unless directed by the child's doctor, because they may cause unwanted effects.

Older adults—Elderly people are especially sensitive to the effects of sulfonamides. Severe skin problems and blood problems may be more likely to occur in the elderly. These problems may also be more likely to occur in patients who are taking diuretics (water pills) along with this medicine.

Other medicines—Although certain medicines should not be used together at all, in other cases two different medicines may be used together even if an interaction might occur. In these cases, your doctor may want to change the dose, or other precautions may be necessary. When you are taking sulfonamides, it is especially important that your health care professional knows if you are taking any of the following:

- Acetaminophen (e.g., Tylenol) (with long-term, high-dose use) or
- Amiodarone (e.g., Cordarone) or
- Anabolic steroids (nandrolone [e.g., Anabolin], oxandrolone [e.g., Anavar], oxymetholone [e.g., Anadrol], stanozolol [e.g., Winstrol]) or
- Androgens (male hormones) or
- Antithyroid agents (medicine for overactive thyroid) or
- Carbamazepine (e.g., Tegretol) or
- Carmustine (e.g., BiCNU) or
- Chloroquine (e.g., Aralen) or
- Dantrolene (e.g., Dantrium) or
- Daunorubicin (e.g., Cerubidine) or
- Disulfiram (e.g., Antabuse) or
- Divalproex (e.g., Depakote) or
- Estrogens (female hormones) or
- Etretinate (e.g., Tegison) or
- Gold salts (medicine for arthritis) or
- Hydroxychloroquine (e.g., Plaquenil) or
- Mercaptopurine (e.g., Purinethol) or
- Naltrexone (e.g., Trexan) (with long-term, high-dose use) or
- Oral contraceptives (birth control pills) containing estrogens or
- Other anti-infectives by mouth or by injection (medicine for infection) or
- Phenothiazines (acetophenazine [e.g., Tindal], chlorpromazine [e.g., Thorazine], fluphenazine [e.g., Prolixin], mesoridazine [e.g., Serentil], perphenazine [e.g., Trilafon], prochlorperazine [e.g., Compazine], promazine [e.g., Sparine], promethazine [e.g., Phenergan], thioridazine [e.g., Mellaril], trifluoperazine [e.g., Stelazine], triflupromazine [e.g., Vesprin], trimeprazine [e.g., Temaril]) or
- Plicamycin (e.g., Mithracin) or

- Valproic acid (e.g., Depakene)—Use of sulfonamides with these medicines may increase the chance of side effects affecting the liver
- Acetohydroxamic acid (e.g., Lithostat) or
- Dapsone or
- Furazolidone (e.g., Furoxone) or
- Nitrofurantoin (e.g., Furadantin) or
- Primaquine or
- Procainamide (e.g., Pronestyl) or
- Quinidine (e.g., Quinidex) or
- Quinine (e.g., Quinamm) or
- Sulfoxone (e.g., Diasone) or
- Vitamin K (e.g., AquaMEPHYTON, Synkayvite)—Use of sulfonamides with these medicines may increase the chance of side effects affecting the blood
- Anticoagulants (blood thinners) or
- Ethotoin (e.g., Peganone) or
- Mephenytoin (e.g., Mesantoin)—Use of sulfonamides with these medicines may increase the chance of side effects of these medicines
- Antidiabetics, oral (diabetes medicine you take by mouth)—Use of oral antidiabetics with sulfonamides may increase the chance of side effects affecting the blood and/or the side effects of oral antidiabetics
- Methenamine (e.g., Mandelamine)—Use of this medicine with sulfonamides may increase the chance of side effects of sulfonamides
- Methotrexate (e.g., Mexate) or
- Phenytoin (e.g., Dilantin)—Use of these medicines with sulfonamides may increase the chance of side effects affecting the liver and/or the side effects of these medicines
- Methyldopa (e.g., Aldomet)—Use of methyldopa with sulfonamides may increase the chance of side effects affecting the liver and/or the blood

Other medical problems—The presence of other medical problems may affect the use of sulfonamides. Make sure you tell your doctor if you have any other medical problems, especially:

- Anemia or other blood problems or
- Glucose-6-phosphate dehydrogenase (G6PD) deficiency—Patients with these problems may have an increase in side effects affecting the blood
- Kidney disease or
- Liver disease—Patients with kidney and/or liver disease may have an increased chance of side effects
- Porphyria—This medicine may bring on an attack of porphyria

Proper Use of This Medicine

Sulfonamides should not be given to infants less than 2 months of age unless directed by the patient's doctor because sulfonamides may cause serious unwanted effects.

Sulfonamides are best taken with a full glass (8 ounces) of water. Several additional glasses of water should be taken every day, unless otherwise directed by your doctor.

Drinking extra water will help to prevent some unwanted effects of sulfonamides.

For patients taking the *oral liquid form* of this medicine:

- Use a specially marked measuring spoon or other device to measure each dose accurately. The average household teaspoon may not hold the right amount of liquid.

To help clear up your infection completely, *keep taking this medicine for the full time of treatment,* even if you begin to feel better after a few days. If you stop taking this medicine too soon, your symptoms may return.

This medicine works best when there is a constant amount in the blood or urine. *To help keep the amount constant, do not miss any doses. Also, it is best to take the doses at evenly spaced times day and night.* If you need help in planning the best times to take your medicine, check with your health care professional.

Dosing—The dose of these medicines will be different for different patients. *Follow your doctor's orders or the directions on the label.* The following information includes only the average doses of these medicines. *If your dose is different, do not change it* unless your doctor tells you to do so.

For sulfadiazine
- For *tablet* dosage form:
  - For bacterial or protozoal infections:
    - Adults and teenagers—2 to 4 grams for the first dose, then 1 gram every four to six hours.
    - Children up to 2 months of age—Use is not recommended.
    - Children 2 months of age and older—Dose is based on body weight. The usual dose is 75 milligrams (mg) per kilogram (kg) (34 mg per pound) of body weight for the first dose, then 37.5 mg per kg (17 mg per pound) of body weight every six hours, or 25 mg per kg (11.4 mg per pound) of body weight every four hours.

For sulfamethizole
- For *tablet* dosage form:
  - For bacterial infections:
    - Adults and teenagers—500 milligrams (mg) to 1 gram every six to eight hours.
    - Children up to 2 months of age—Use is not recommended.
    - Children 2 months of age and older—Dose is based on body weight. The usual dose is 7.5 to 11.25 mg per kilogram (kg) (3.4 to 5.1 mg per pound) of body weight every six hours.

For sulfamethoxazole
- For *tablet* dosage form:
  - For bacterial or protozoal infections:
    - Adults and teenagers—2 to 4 grams for the first dose, then 1 to 2 grams every eight to twelve hours.
    - Children up to 2 months of age—Use and dose must be determined by your doctor.
    - Children 2 months of age and older—Dose is based on body weight. The usual dose is 50 to 60 milligrams (mg) per kilogram (kg) (22.7 to 27.3 mg per pound) of body weight for the first dose, then 25 to 30 mg per kg (11.4 to 13.6 mg per pound) of body weight every twelve hours.

For sulfisoxazole
- For *suspension, syrup, or tablet* dosage forms:
  - For bacterial or protozoal infections:
    - Adults and teenagers—2 to 4 grams for the first dose, then 750 milligrams (mg) to 1.5 grams every four hours; or 1 to 2 grams every six hours.
    - Children up to 2 months of age—Use and dose must be determined by your doctor.
    - Children 2 months of age and older—Dose is based on body weight. The usual dose is 75 mg per kilogram (kg) (34 mg per pound) of body weight for the first dose, then 25 mg per kg (11.4 mg per pound) of body weight every four hours, or 37.5 mg per kg (17 mg per pound) of body weight every six hours.

Missed dose—If you miss a dose of this medicine, take it as soon as possible. This will help to keep a constant amount of medicine in the blood or urine. However, if it is almost time for your next dose, skip the missed dose and go back to your regular dosing schedule. Do not double doses.

Storage—To store this medicine:
- Keep out of the reach of children.
- Store away from heat and direct light.
- Do not store the tablet form of this medicine in the bathroom, near the kitchen sink, or in other damp places. Heat or moisture may cause the medicine to break down.
- Keep the oral liquid forms of this medicine from freezing.
- Do not keep outdated medicine or medicine no longer needed. Be sure that any discarded medicine is out of the reach of children.

Precautions While Using This Medicine

It is very important that your doctor check your progress at regular visits. This medicine may cause blood problems, especially if it is taken for a long time.

If your symptoms do not improve within a few days, or if they become worse, check with your doctor.

Sulfonamides may cause blood problems. These problems may result in a greater chance of certain infections, slow healing, and bleeding of the gums. Therefore, you should be careful when using regular toothbrushes, dental floss, and toothpicks. Dental work should be delayed until your blood counts have returned to normal. Check with your medical doctor or dentist if you have any questions about proper oral hygiene (mouth care) during treatment.

Sulfonamides may cause your skin to be more sensitive to sunlight than it is normally. Exposure to sunlight, even for brief periods of time, may cause a skin rash, itching, redness or other discoloration of the skin, or a severe sunburn. When you begin taking this medicine:
- Stay out of direct sunlight, especially between the hours of 10:00 a.m. and 3:00 p.m., if possible.
- Wear protective clothing, including a hat. Also, wear sunglasses.
- Apply a sun block product that has a skin protection factor (SPF) of at least 15. Some patients may require a product with a higher SPF number, especially if they have a fair complexion. If you have any questions about this, check with your health care professional.
- Apply a sun block lipstick that has an SPF of at least 15 to protect your lips.
- Do not use a sunlamp or tanning bed or booth.

If you have a severe reaction from the sun, check with your doctor.

This medicine may also cause some people to become dizzy. *Make sure you know how you react to this medicine before you drive, use machines, or do anything else that could be dangerous if you are dizzy or are not alert.* If this reaction is especially bothersome, check with your doctor.

Side Effects

Along with its needed effects, a medicine may cause some unwanted effects. Although not all of these side effects may occur, if they do occur they may need medical attention.

Check with your doctor immediately if any of the following side effects occur:

More common
   Itching; skin rash

Less common
   Aching of joints and muscles; difficulty in swallowing; pale skin; redness, blistering, peeling, or loosening of skin; sore throat and fever; unusual bleeding or bruising; unusual tiredness or weakness; yellow eyes or skin

Rare
   Abdominal or stomach cramps and pain (severe); abdominal tenderness; blood in urine; diarrhea (watery and severe), which may also be bloody; greatly increased or decreased frequency of urination or amount of urine; increased thirst; lower back pain; mood or mental changes; pain or burning while urinating; swelling of front part of neck

Also, check with your doctor as soon as possible if the following side effect occurs:

More common
   Increased sensitivity of skin to sunlight

Other side effects may occur that usually do not need medical attention. These side effects may go away during treatment as your body adjusts to the medicine. However, check with your doctor if any of the following side effects continue or are bothersome:

More common
   Diarrhea; dizziness; headache; loss of appetite; nausea or vomiting; tiredness

Other side effects not listed above may also occur in some patients. If you notice any other effects, check with your doctor.

SULFONAMIDES   (Vaginal)

Some commonly used brand names are:

In the U.S.—
AVC (1)	Trysul (2)
Sultrin (2)	

In Canada—
AVC (1)
Sultrin (2)

This information applies to the following medicines
1. Sulfanilamide (sul-fa-NILL-a-mide)
2. Triple Sulfa (TRI-pel SUL-fa)

Category

- **Anti-infective, vaginal—**

Description

Sulfonamides (sul-FON-a-mides), or sulfa medicines, are used to treat bacterial infections. They work by killing bacteria or preventing their growth.

Vaginal sulfonamides are used to treat bacterial infections. These medicines may also be used for other problems as determined by your doctor.

Vaginal sulfonamides are available only with your doctor's prescription, in the following dosage forms:

Vaginal
- Sulfanilamide
  ○ Cream
  ○ Suppositories
- Triple Sulfa
  ○ Cream
  ○ Tablets

Before Using This Medicine

In deciding to use a medicine, the risks of using the medicine must be weighed against the good it will do. This is a decision you and your doctor will make. For vaginal sulfonamides, the following should be considered:

Allergies—Tell your doctor if you have ever had any unusual or allergic reaction to any of the sulfa medicines, furosemide (e.g., Lasix) or thiazide diuretics (water pills), oral antidiabetics (diabetes medicine you take by mouth), or glaucoma medicine you take by mouth (for example, acetazolamide [e.g., Diamox], dichlorphenamide [e.g., Daranide], or methazolamide [e.g., Neptazane]). Also tell your health care professional if you are allergic to any other substances, such as foods, preservatives, or dyes, including to parabens, lanolin, or peanut oil.

Pregnancy—Studies have not been done in humans. However, vaginal sulfonamides are absorbed through the vagina into the bloodstream and appear in the bloodstream of the fetus. Studies in rats and mice given high doses by mouth have shown that certain sulfonamides cause birth defects.

Breast-feeding—Vaginal sulfonamides are absorbed through the vagina into the bloodstream and pass into the breast milk. Use is not recommended in nursing mothers. Vaginal sulfonamides may cause liver problems in nursing babies. These medicines may also cause anemia in nursing babies with glucose-6–phosphate dehydrogenase (G6PD) deficiency.

Children—Studies on this medicine have been done only in adult patients and there is no specific information comparing the use of vaginal sulfonamides in children with use in other age groups.

Older adults—Many medicines have not been studied specifically in older people. Therefore, it may not be known whether they work exactly the same way they do in younger adults or if they cause different side effects or problems in older people. There is no specific information comparing the use of vaginal sulfonamides in the elderly with use in other age groups.

Other medicines—Although certain medicines should not be used together at all, in other cases two different medicines may be used together even if an interaction might occur. In these cases, your doctor may want to change the dose, or other precautions may be necessary. Tell your health care professional if you are taking or using any other prescription or nonprescription (over-the-counter [OTC]) medicine.

Other medical problems—The presence of other medical problems may affect the use of vaginal sulfonamides. Make sure you tell your doctor if you have any other medical problems, especially:
- Glucose-6–phosphate dehydrogenase (G6PD) deficiency—Anemia (a blood problem) can occur if sulfonamides are used
- Kidney disease
- Porphyria—Sulfonamides can cause porphyria attacks

Proper Use of This Medicine

Vaginal sulfonamides usually come with patient directions. Read them carefully before using this medicine.

This medicine is usually inserted into the vagina with an applicator. However, if you are pregnant, check with your doctor before using the applicator.

To help clear up your infection completely, *it is very important that you keep using this medicine for the full time of treatment*, even if your symptoms begin to clear up after a few days. If you stop using this medicine too soon, your symptoms may return. *Do not miss any doses.* Also, *do not stop using this medicine if your menstrual period starts during the time of treatment.*

Dosing—The dose of these medicines will be different for different patients. *Follow your doctor's orders or the directions on the label.* The following information includes only the average doses of these medicines. *If your dose is different, do not change it* unless your doctor tells you to do so.

For sulfanilamide
- For *vaginal cream* dosage form:
  ○ For bacterial infections:
    ▪ Adults and teenagers—One applicatorful (approximately 6 grams) inserted into the vagina one or two times a day for thirty days.
    ▪ Children—Use and dose must be determined by your doctor.
- For *vaginal suppositories* dosage form:
  ○ For bacterial infections:
    ▪ Adults and teenagers—One suppository inserted into the vagina one or two times a day for thirty days.
    ▪ Children—Use and dose must be determined by your doctor.

For triple sulfa
- For *vaginal cream* dosage form:
  ○ For bacterial infections:
    ▪ Adults and teenagers—At first, one applicatorful (approximately 4 to 5 grams) inserted into the vagina two times a day for four to six days. Then, your doctor may lower your dose to one-half to one-quarter applicatorful two times a day. Use when you wake up and just before you go to bed.

- Children—Use and dose must be determined by your doctor.
- For *vaginal tablets* dosage form:
  - For bacterial infections:
    - Adults and teenagers—One tablet inserted into the vagina two times a day for ten days.
    - Children—Use and dose must be determined by your doctor.

Missed dose—If you miss a dose of this medicine, insert it as soon as possible. However, if it is almost time for your next dose, skip the missed dose and go back to your regular dosing schedule.

Storage—To store this medicine:

- Keep out of the reach of children.
- Store away from heat and direct light.
- Do not store the vaginal tablet or vaginal suppository form of this medicine in the bathroom, near the kitchen sink, or in other damp places. Heat or moisture may cause the medicine to break down.
- Keep the vaginal cream and vaginal suppository forms of this medicine from freezing.
- Do not keep outdated medicine or medicine no longer needed. Be sure that any discarded medicine is out of the reach of children.

Precautions While Using This Medicine

If your symptoms do not improve within a few days, or if they become worse, check with your doctor.

Vaginal medicines usually will slowly work their way out of the vagina during treatment. To keep the medicine from soiling or staining your clothing, a sanitary napkin may be worn. Minipads, clean paper tissues, or paper diapers may also be used. However, the use of tampons is not recommended since they may soak up too much of the medicine. In addition, tampons may be more likely to slip out of the vagina if you use them during treatment with this medicine.

To help clear up your infection completely and to help make sure it does not return, good health habits are also required.

- Wear cotton panties (or panties or pantyhose with cotton crotches) instead of synthetic (for example, nylon or rayon) underclothes.
- Wear only freshly washed underclothes.

If you have any questions about this, check with your health care professional.

Many vaginal infections are spread by sexual intercourse. The male sexual partner may carry the fungus or other organism in his reproductive tract. Therefore, it may be desirable that your partner wear a condom (prophylactic) during intercourse to keep the infection from returning. Also, it may be necessary for your partner to be treated at the same time you are being treated to avoid passing the infection back and forth. In addition, *do not stop using this medicine if you have intercourse during treatment.*

Some patients who use vaginal medicines may prefer to use a douche for cleansing purposes before inserting the next dose of medicine. Some doctors recommend a vinegar and water or other douche. However, others do not recommend douching at all. If you do use a douche, *do not overfill the vagina with douche solution.* To do so may force the solution up into the uterus (womb) and may cause inflammation

or infection. Also, *do not douche if you are pregnant since this may harm the fetus.* If you have any questions about this or which douche products are best for you, check with your health care professional.

Side Effects

Studies in rats have shown that long-term use of sulfonamides may cause cancer of the thyroid gland. In addition, studies in rats have shown that sulfonamides may increase the chance of goiters (noncancerous tumors of the thyroid gland).

Along with its needed effects, a medicine may cause some unwanted effects. Although not all of these side effects may occur, if they do occur they may need medical attention.

Check with your doctor immediately if any of the following side effects occur:
  Less common
    Itching, burning, skin rash, redness, swelling, or other sign of irritation not present before use of this medicine
  Rare
    Burning at site of application

Other side effects may occur that usually do not need medical attention. These side effects may go away during treatment as your body adjusts to the medicine. However, check with your doctor if either of the following side effects continues or is bothersome:
  Less common or rare
    Rash or irritation of penis of sexual partner

Other side effects not listed above may also occur in some patients. If you notice any other effects, check with your doctor.

SULFONAMIDES AND TRIMETHOPRIM (Systemic)

Some commonly used brand names are:

In the U.S.—

Bactrim (2)	Septra DS (2)
Bactrim DS (2)	Septra I.V. (2)
Bactrim I.V. (2)	Septra Suspension (2)
Bactrim Pediatric (2)	Septra Grape Suspension (2)
Cofatrim Forte (2)	Sulfatrim (2)
Cotrim (2)	Sulfatrim-DS (2)
Cotrim DS (2)	Sulfatrim Pediatric (2)
Cotrim Pediatric (2)	Sulfatrim S/S (2)
Septra (2)	Sulfatrim Suspension (2)

In Canada—

Apo-Sulfatrim (2)	Novo-Trimel D.S. (2)
Apo-Sulfatrim DS (2)	Nu-Cotrimox (2)
Bactrim (2)	Nu-Cotrimox DS (2)
Bactrim DS (2)	Roubac (2)
Coptin (1)	Septra (2)
Coptin 1 (1)	Septra DS (2)
Novo-Trimel (2)	

This information applies to the following medicines:

1. Sulfadiazine and Trimethoprim (sul-fa-DYE-a-zeen and trye-METH-oh-prim)

2. Sulfamethoxazole and Trimethoprim (sul-fa-meth-OX-a-zole and trye-METH-oh-prim)

Category

- **Antibacterial, systemic**—Sulfadiazine and Trimethoprim; Sulfamethoxazole and Trimethoprim
- **Antiprotozoal**—Sulfamethoxazole and Trimethoprim

Description

Sulfonamide (sul-FON-ah-mide) and trimethoprim combinations are used to prevent and treat infections. Sulfadiazine and trimethoprim combination is used to treat urinary tract infections. Sulfamethoxazole and trimethoprim combination is used to treat infections, such as bronchitis, middle ear infection, urinary tract infection, and traveler's diarrhea. It is also used for the prevention and treatment of Pneumocystis carinii pneumonia (PCP). These medicines will not work for colds, flu, or other virus infections. They may also be used for other conditions as determined by your doctor.

Sulfonamide and trimethoprim combinations are available only with your doctor's prescription, in the following dosage forms:

Oral
- Sulfadiazine and Trimethoprim
  - Oral suspension
  - Tablets
- Sulfamethoxazole and Trimethoprim
  - Oral suspension
  - Tablets

Parenteral
- Sulfamethoxazole and Trimethoprim
  - Injection

Before Using This Medicine

In deciding to use a medicine, the risks of taking the medicine must be weighed against the good it will do. This is a decision you and your doctor will make. For sulfonamide and trimethoprim combinations, the following should be considered:

Allergies—Tell your doctor if you have ever had any unusual or allergic reaction to sulfa medicines, furosemide (e.g., Lasix) or thiazide diuretics (water pills), oral antidiabetics (diabetes medicine you take by mouth), glaucoma medicine you take by mouth (for example, acetazolamide [e.g., Diamox], dichlorphenamide [e.g., Daranide], methazolamide [e.g., Neptazane]), or trimethoprim (e.g., Trimpex). Also tell your health care professional if you are allergic to any other substances, such as foods, preservatives (e.g., sulfites), or dyes.

Pregnancy—Sulfamethoxazole and trimethoprim combination has not been reported to cause birth defects or other problems in humans. However, studies in mice, rats, and rabbits have shown that some sulfonamides cause birth defects, including cleft palate and bone problems. Studies in rabbits have also shown that trimethoprim causes birth defects, as well as a decrease in the number of successful pregnancies. Sulfonamides are not recommended for use at the time of labor and delivery because these medicines may cause unwanted effects in the baby.

Breast-feeding—Sulfonamides and trimethoprim pass into the breast milk. These medicines are not recommended for use during breast-feeding. They may cause liver problems, anemia, and other unwanted effects in nursing babies, especially those with glucose-6–phosphate dehydrogenase (G6PD) deficiency.

Children—Sulfadiazine and trimethoprim combination should not be given to infants less than 3 months of age. Sulfamethoxazole and trimethoprim combination should not be given to infants less than 2 months of age unless directed by the child's doctor. These combinations may cause unwanted effects. In special situations, sulfamethoxazole and trimethoprim combination may be given to infants less than 2 months of age.

Older adults—Elderly people are especially sensitive to the effects of sulfonamide and trimethoprim combinations. Severe skin problems and blood problems may be more likely to occur in the elderly. These problems may also be more likely to occur in patients who are taking diuretics (water pills) along with this medicine.

Other medicines—Although certain medicines should not be used together at all, in other cases two different medicines may be used together even if an interaction might occur. In these cases, your doctor may want to change the dose, or other precautions may be necessary. When you are taking sulfonamide and trimethoprim combinations, it is especially important that your health care professional know if you are taking any of the following:

- Acetaminophen (e.g., Tylenol) (with long-term, high-dose use) or
- Amiodarone (e.g., Cordarone) or
- Anabolic steroids (nandrolone [e.g., Anabolin], oxandrolone [e.g., Anavar], oxymetholone [e.g., Anadrol], stanozolol [e.g., Winstrol]) or
- Androgens (male hormones) or
- Antithyroid agents (medicine for overactive thyroid) or
- Carbamazepine (e.g., Tegretol) or
- Carmustine (e.g., BiCNU) or
- Chloroquine (e.g., Aralen) or
- Dantrolene (e.g., Dantrium) or
- Daunorubicin (e.g., Cerubidine) or
- Disulfiram (e.g., Antabuse) or
- Divalproex (e.g., Depakote) or
- Estrogens (female hormones) or
- Etretinate (e.g., Tegison) or
- Gold salts (medicine for arthritis) or
- Mercaptopurine (e.g., Purinethol) or
- Naltrexone (e.g., Trexan) (with long-term, high-dose use) or
- Oral contraceptives (birth control pills) containing estrogens or
- Other anti-infectives by mouth or by injection (medicine for infection) or
- Phenothiazines (acetophenazine [e.g., Tindal], chlorpromazine [e.g., Thorazine], fluphenazine [e.g., Prolixin], mesoridazine [e.g., Serentil], perphenazine [e.g., Trilafon], prochlorperazine [e.g., Compazine], promazine [e.g., Sparine], promethazine [e.g., Phenergan], thioridazine [e.g., Mellaril], trifluoperazine [e.g., Stelazine], triflupromazine [e.g., Vesprin], trimeprazine [e.g., Temaril]) or
- Plicamycin (e.g., Mithracin) or

- Valproic acid (e.g., Depakene)—Use of sulfonamide and trimethoprim combinations with these medicines may increase the chance of side effects affecting the liver
- Acetohydroxamic acid (e.g., Lithostat) or
- Furazolidone (e.g., Furoxone) or
- Nitrofurantoin (e.g., Furadantin) or
- Primaquine or
- Procainamide (e.g., Pronestyl) or
- Quinidine (e.g., Quinidex) or
- Quinine (e.g., Quinamm) or
- Sulfoxone (e.g., Diasone)—Use of sulfonamide and trimethoprim combinations with these medicines may increase the chance of side effects affecting the blood
- Anticoagulants (blood thinners) or
- Digoxin (e.g., Lanoxin) or
- Ethotoin (e.g., Peganone) or
- Mephenytoin (e.g., Mesantoin) or
- Methotrexate (e.g., Mexate) or
- Phenytoin (e.g., Dilantin)—Use of sulfonamide and trimethoprim combinations with these medicines may increase the chance of side effects of these medicines
- Antidiabetics, oral (diabetes medicine you take by mouth)—Use of oral antidiabetics with sulfonamide and trimethoprim combinations may increase the chance of side effects affecting the blood and/or the side effects of the oral antidiabetics
- Methenamine (e.g., Mandelamine)—Use of methenamine with sulfonamide and trimethoprim combinations may increase the chance of side effects of the sulfonamide
- Methyldopa (e.g., Aldomet)—Use of methyldopa with sulfonamide and trimethoprim combinations may increase the chance of side effects affecting the liver and/or the blood

Other medical problems—The presence of other medical problems may affect the use of sulfonamide and trimethoprim combinations. Make sure you tell your doctor if you have any other medical problems, especially:

- Anemia or other blood problems or
- Glucose-6–phosphate dehydrogenase (G6PD) deficiency—Patients with these problems may have an increase in side effects affecting the blood
- Kidney disease or
- Liver disease—Patients with kidney and/or liver disease may have an increased chance of side effects
- Porphyria—This medicine may bring on an attack of porphyria

---

Proper Use of This Medicine

Sulfadiazine and trimethoprim combination should not be given to infants less than 3 months of age, and sulfamethoxazole and trimethoprim combination should not be given to infants less than 2 months of age unless directed by the child's doctor. These medicines may cause unwanted effects in the baby. In special situations, sulfamethoxazole and trimethoprim combination may be given to infants less than 2 months of age.

Sulfonamide and trimethoprim combinations are best taken with a full glass (8 ounces) of water. Several additional glasses of water should be taken every day, unless otherwise directed by your doctor. Drinking extra water will help to prevent some unwanted effects of sulfonamides.

For patients taking the *oral liquid form* of this medicine:

- Use a specially marked measuring spoon or other device to measure each dose accurately. The average household teaspoon may not hold the right amount of liquid.

To help clear up your infection completely, *keep taking this medicine for the full time of treatment*, even if you begin to feel better after a few days. If you stop taking this medicine too soon, your symptoms may return.

This medicine works best when there is a constant amount in the blood or urine. *To help keep the amount constant, do not miss any doses. Also, it is best to take the doses at evenly spaced times day and night.* If you need help in planning the best times to take your medicine, check with your health care professional.

Dosing—The dose of these medicines will be different for different patients. *Follow your doctor's orders or the directions on the label.* The following information includes only the average doses of these medicines. *If your dose is different, do not change it* unless your doctor tells you to do so.

The number of tablets or teaspoonfuls of suspension that you take depends on the strength of the medicine. Also, *the number of doses you take each day, the time allowed between doses, and the length of time you take the medicine depend on the medical problem for which you are taking sulfonamide and trimethoprim combinations.*

For sulfadiazine and trimethoprim combination
- For *oral* dosage forms (suspension, tablets):
  - For bacterial infections:
    - Adults and teenagers—820 milligrams (mg) of sulfadiazine and 180 mg of trimethoprim once a day.
    - Infants less than 3 months of age—Use is not recommended.
    - Infants 3 months of age and older and children up to 12 years of age—Dose is based on body weight. The usual dose is 7 mg of sulfadiazine and 1.5 mg of trimethoprim per kilogram (kg) (3.2 mg of sulfadiazine and 0.7 mg of trimethoprim per pound) of body weight every twelve hours.

For sulfamethoxazole and trimethoprim combination
- For *oral* dosage forms (suspension, tablets):
  - For bacterial infections:
    - Adults and children 40 kilograms (kg) of body weight (88 pounds) and over—800 milligrams (mg) of sulfamethoxazole and 160 mg of trimethoprim every twelve hours.
    - Infants less than 2 months of age—Use is not recommended.
    - Infants 2 months of age and older and children up to 40 kg of weight (88 pounds)—Dose is based on body weight. The usual dose is 20 to 30 mg of sulfamethoxazole and 4 to 6 mg of trimethoprim per kg (9.1 to 13.6 mg of sulfamethoxazole and 1.8 to 2.7 mg of trimethoprim per pound) of body weight every twelve hours.

○ For the treatment of Pneumocystis carinii pneumonia (PCP):

- Adults and children older than 2 months—Dose is based on body weight. The usual dose is 18.75 to 25 mg of sulfamethoxazole and 3.75 to 5 mg of trimethoprim per kg (8.5 to 11.4 mg of sulfamethoxazole and 1.7 to 2.3 mg of trimethoprim per pound) of body weight every six hours.

○ For the prevention of Pneumocystis carinii pneumonia (PCP):

- Adults and teenagers—800 mg of sulfamethoxazole and 160 mg of trimethoprim once a day.
- Infants and children 4 weeks of age and older—Dose is based on body size and must be determined by your doctor. There are several dosing regimens available that your doctor may choose from. One dosing regimen is 375 mg of sulfamethoxazole and 75 mg of trimethoprim per square meter of body surface two times a day, three times a week on consecutive days (e.g., Monday, Tuesday, Wednesday).

- For *injection* dosage form:

○ For bacterial infections:

- Adults and children older than 2 months—The usual total daily dose is 40 to 50 mg of sulfamethoxazole and 8 to 10 mg of trimethoprim per kg (18.2 to 22.7 mg of sulfamethoxazole and 3.6 to 4.5 mg of trimethoprim per pound) of body weight. This total daily dose may be divided up and injected into a vein every six, eight, or twelve hours.
- Infants less than 2 months of age—Use is not recommended.

○ For the treatment of Pneumocystis carinii pneumonia (PCP):

- Adults and children older than 2 months—The usual dose is 18.75 to 25 mg of sulfamethoxazole and 3.75 to 5 mg of trimethoprim per kg (8.5 to 11.4 mg of sulfamethoxazole and 1.7 to 2.3 mg of trimethoprim per pound) of body weight. This is injected into a vein every six hours.
- Infants less than 2 months of age—Use is not recommended.

Missed dose—If you miss a dose of this medicine, take it as soon as possible. This will help to keep a constant amount of medicine in the blood or urine. However, if it is almost time for your next dose, skip the missed dose and go back to your regular dosing schedule. Do not double doses.

Storage—To store this medicine:

- Keep out of the reach of children.
- Store away from heat and direct light.
- Do not store the tablet form of this medicine in the bathroom, near the kitchen sink, or in other damp places. Heat or moisture may cause the medicine to break down.
- Keep the oral liquid form of this medicine from freezing.
- Do not keep outdated medicine or medicine no longer needed. Be sure that any discarded medicine is out of the reach of children.

Precautions While Using This Medicine

It is very important that your doctor check your progress at regular visits. This medicine may cause blood problems, especially if it is taken for a long time.

If your symptoms do not improve within a few days, or if they become worse, check with your doctor.

Sulfonamide and trimethoprim combinations may cause blood problems. These problems may result in a greater chance of certain infections, slow healing, and bleeding of the gums. Therefore, you should be careful when using regular toothbrushes, dental floss, and toothpicks. Dental work should be delayed until your blood counts have returned to normal. Check with your medical doctor or dentist if you have any questions about proper oral hygiene (mouth care) during treatment.

Sulfonamide and trimethoprim combinations may cause your skin to be more sensitive to sunlight than it is normally. Exposure to sunlight, even for brief periods of time, may cause a skin rash, itching, redness or other discoloration of the skin, or a severe sunburn. When you begin taking this medicine:

- Stay out of direct sunlight, especially between the hours of 10:00 a.m. and 3:00 p.m., if possible.
- Wear protective clothing, including a hat and sunglasses.
- Apply a sun block product that has a skin protection factor (SPF) of at least 15. Some patients may require a product with a higher SPF number, especially if they have a fair complexion. If you have any questions about this, check with your health care professional.
- Apply a sun block lipstick that has an SPF of at least 15 to protect your lips.
- Do not use a sunlamp or tanning bed or booth.

If you have a severe reaction from the sun, check with your doctor.

This medicine may also cause some people to become dizzy. *Make sure you know how you react to this medicine before you drive, use machines, or do anything else that could be dangerous if you are dizzy or are not alert.* If this reaction is especially bothersome, check with your doctor.

Side Effects

Along with its needed effects, a medicine may cause some unwanted effects. Although not all of these side effects may occur, if they do occur they may need medical attention.

Check with your doctor immediately if any of the following side effects occur:

More common
Itching; skin rash

Less common
Aching of joints and muscles; difficulty in swallowing; pale skin; redness, blistering, peeling, or loosening of skin; sore throat and fever; unusual bleeding or bruising; unusual tiredness or weakness; yellow eyes or skin

Rare
Abdominal or stomach cramps and pain (severe); abdominal or stomach tenderness; anxiety; blood in urine; bluish fingernails, lips, or skin; confusion; diarrhea (watery and severe), which may also be bloody; difficult breathing; drowsiness; fever; general feeling of illness; greatly increased or decreased frequency of urination or amount of urine; hallucinations; headache, severe; increased thirst; lower back pain; mental depression; muscle pain or weakness; nausea; nervousness; pain at site of injection; pain or burning while urinating; sei-

zures (convulsions); stiff neck and/or back; swelling of front part of neck

Also, check with your doctor as soon as possible if the following side effect occurs:

More common

Increased sensitivity of skin to sunlight

Other side effects may occur that usually do not need medical attention. These side effects may go away during treatment as your body adjusts to the medicine. However, check with your doctor if any of the following side effects continue or are bothersome:

More common

Diarrhea; dizziness; headache; loss of appetite; mouth sores or swelling of the tongue; nausea or vomiting; tiredness

Other side effects not listed above may also occur in some patients. If you notice any other effects, check with your doctor.

Additional Information

Once a medicine has been approved for marketing for a certain use, experience may show that it is also useful for other medical problems. Although these uses are not included in product labeling, sulfamethoxazole and trimethoprim combination is used in certain patients for the following medical conditions:

- Bile infections
- Bone and joint infections
- HIV-related infections in Africa
- Sexually transmitted diseases, such as gonorrhea
- Sinus infections
- Toxoplasmosis (prevention of)
- Urinary tract infections (prevention of)
- Whipple's disease

Other than the above information, there is no additional information relating to proper use, precautions, or side effects for these uses.

SULFONYLUREA (Oral route, Intravenous route)

Commonly used brand name(s)

In the U.S.—

Amaryl	Glycron
Diabeta	Glynase Pres-Tab
Diabinese	Micronase
Glucotrol	Tolinase
Glucotrol XL	Tol-Tab

Available Dosage Forms:

- Tablet
- Tablet, Extended Release
- Powder for Solution

Uses For This Medicine

Sulfonylurea antidiabetic agents (also known as sulfonylureas) are used to treat a certain type of diabetes mellitus (sugar diabetes) called type 2 diabetes. When you have type 2 diabetes, insulin is still being produced by your pancreas. Sometimes the amount of insulin you produce may not be enough or your body may not be using it properly and you may still need more. Sulfonylureas work by causing your pancreas to release more insulin into the blood stream. All of the cells in your body need insulin to help turn the food you eat into energy. This is done by using sugar (or glucose) in the blood as quick energy. Or the sugar may be stored in the form of fats, sugars, and proteins for use later, such as for energy between meals.

Sometimes insulin that is being produced by the body is not able to help sugar get inside the body's cells. Sulfonylureas help insulin get into the cells where it can work properly to lower blood sugar. In this way, sulfonylureas will help lower blood sugar and help restore the way you use food to make energy.

Chlorpropamide may also be used for other conditions as determined by your doctor.

Once a medicine has been approved for marketing for a certain use, experience may show that it is also useful for other medical problems. Although this use is not included in product labeling, chlorpropamide is used in certain patients with the following medical condition:

- Diabetes insipidus (water diabetes)

If you are taking this medicine for water diabetes, the advice listed above that relates to diet for patients with *sugar* diabetes *does not apply to you*. However, the advice about hypoglycemia (low blood sugar) *does* apply to you. Call your doctor right away if you feel any of the symptoms described.

Before Using This Medicine

Allergies—Tell your doctor if you have ever had any unusual or allergic reaction to medicines in this group or any other medicines. Also tell your health care professional if you have any other types of allergies, such as to foods dyes, preservatives, or animals. For non-prescription products, read the label or package ingredients carefully.

Pediatric—There is little information about the use of sulfonylureas in children. Type 2 diabetes is unusual in this age group. Type 2 diabetes is unusual in this age group.

Geriatric—Some elderly patients may be more sensitive than younger adults to the effects of sulfonylureas, especially when more than one antidiabetic medicine is being taken or if other medicines that affect blood sugar are also being taken. This may increase the chance of developing low blood sugar during treatment. Furthermore, the first signs of low or high blood sugar are not easily seen or do not occur at all in older patients. This may increase the chance of low blood sugar developing during treatment.

Also, elderly patients who take chlorpropamide are more likely to hold too much body water.

Pregnancy—Sulfonylureas are rarely used during pregnancy. The amount of insulin needed changes during and after pregnancy. For this reason, it is easier to control blood sugar using injections of insulin, rather than with the use of sulfonylureas. Close control of blood sugar can reduce the chance of having high blood sugar during the pregnancy and of the baby gaining too much weight, or having birth defects. Be sure to tell your doctor if you plan to become pregnant or if you think you are pregnant. If insulin is not available or cannot be used and sulfonylureas are used during pregnancy, they should be stopped at least 2 weeks before the delivery date (one month before for chlorpropamide and glipizide). Glimepiride should not be used at all during pregnancy. Lowering of blood sugar can occur as a rebound effect at delivery and for several days following birth and will be watched closely by your health care professionals.

Breast Feeding—Chlorpropamide and tolbutamide pass into human breast milk and glimepiride passes into the milk of rats. Chlorpropamide is not recommended in nursing mothers but, in some cases, tolbutamide has been used. Nursing mothers should not take glimepiride. It is not known if other sulfonylureas pass into breast milk. Check with your doctor if you are thinking about breast-feeding.

Other medicines—

Using medicines in this class with any of the following medicines is not recommended. Your doctor may decide not to treat you with a medication in this class or change some of the other medicines you take.

Bosentan

Using medicines in this class with any of the following medicines is usually not recommended, but may be required in some cases. If both medicines are prescribed together, your doctor may change the dose or how often you use one or both of the medicines.

Acarbose, Alatrofloxacin, Balofloxacin, Ciprofloxacin, Clinafloxacin, Enoxacin, Fleroxacin, Flumequine, Gatifloxacin, Gemifloxacin, Grepafloxacin, Levofloxacin, Lomefloxacin, Moxifloxacin, Norfloxacin, Ofloxacin, Pefloxacin, Prulifloxacin, Rufloxacin, Sparfloxacin, Temafloxacin, Tosufloxacin, Trovafloxacin Mesylate

Using this medicine with any of the following may cause an increased risk of certain side effects but using both medicines may be the best treatment for you. If both medicines are prescribed together, your doctor may change the dose or how often you use one or both of the medicines.

Acebutolol, Aceclofenac, Acemetacin, Alclofenac, Alprenolol, Apazone, Aprepitant, Aspirin, Atenolol, Benoxaprofen, Betaxolol, Bevantolol, Bisoprolol, Bitter Melon, Bromfenac, Bucindolol, Bufexamac, Carprofen, Carteolol, Carvedilol, Celiprolol, Chloramphenicol, Chlorthalidone, Cimetidine, Clofibrate, Clometacin, Clonixin, Clorgyline, Cyclosporine, Dexketoprofen, Diazoxide, Diclofenac, Dicumarol, Diflunisal, Dilevalol, Dipyrone, Droxicam, Esmolol, Etodolac, Etofenamate, Felbinac, Fenbufen, Fenoprofen, Fentiazac, Fenugreek, Floctafenine, Fluconazole, Flufenamic Acid, Flurbiprofen, Fosphenytoin, Gemfibrozil, Glucomannan, Guar Gum, Hydrochlorothiazide, Ibuprofen, Indomethacin, Indoprofen, Iproniazid, Isocarboxazid, Isoxicam, Ketoconazole, Ketoprofen, Ketorolac, Labetalol, Levobunolol, Lornoxicam, Meclofenamate, Mefenamic Acid, Meloxicam, Mepindolol, Metipranolol, Metoprolol, Moclobemide, Nabumetone, Nadolol, Naproxen, Nebivolol, Nialamide, Niflumic Acid, Nimesulide, Oxaprozin, Oxprenolol, Oxyphenbutazone, Pargyline, Penbutolol, Phenelzine, Phenylbutazone, Phenytoin, Pindolol, Pirazolac, Piroxicam, Pirprofen, Procarbazine, Propranolol, Propyphenazone, Proquazone, Psyllium, Ranitidine, Rifampin, Rifapentine, Selegiline, Sotalol, St John's Wort, Sulfadiazine, Sulfamethoxazole, Sulfaphenazole, Sulfisoxazole, Sulindac, Suprofen, Talinolol, Tenidap, Tenoxicam, Tertatolol, Tiaprofenic Acid, Timolol, Tolmetin, Toloxatone, Tranylcypromine, Trimethoprim, Voriconazole, Warfarin, Zomepirac

Interactions with Food/Tobacco/Alcohol—Certain medicines should not be used at or around the time of eating food or eating certain types of food since interactions may occur. Using alcohol or tobacco with certain medicines may also cause interactions to occur. The following interactions have been selected on the basis of their potential significance and are not necessarily all-inclusive.

Using medicines in this class with any of the following is usually not recommended, but may be unavoidable in some cases. If used together, your doctor may change the dose or how often you use your medicine, or give you special instructions about the use of food, alcohol, or tobacco.

Ethanol

Other medical problems—The presence of other medical problems may affect the use of medicines in this class. Make sure you tell your doctor if you have any other medical problems, especially:

- Acid in the blood (acidosis) or
- Burns (severe) or
- Diabetic coma or
- Fever, high or
- Injury, severe or
- Ketones in the blood (diabetic ketoacidosis) or
- Surgery, major or
- Any other condition in which insulin needs change rapidly—Insulin may be needed temporarily to control diabetes in patients with these conditions because changes in blood sugar may occur rapidly and without much warning. Also, your blood sugar may need to be tested more often.
- Diarrhea, continuing or
- Female hormone changes for some women (e.g., during puberty, pregnancy, or menstruation) or
- Infection, severe or
- Mental stress, severe or
- Overactive adrenal gland, not properly controlled or
- Problems with intestines, severe or
- Slow stomach emptying or
- Vomiting, continuing or
- Any other condition that causes severe blood sugar changes—Insulin may be needed temporarily to control diabetes mellitus in patients with these conditions because changes in blood sugar may occur rapidly and without much warning. Also, your blood sugar may need to be tested more often
- Heart disease—Chlorpropamide or tolbutamide causes some patients to retain (keep) more body water than usual. Heart disease may be worsened by this extra body water.
- Kidney disease or
- Liver disease—Your blood sugar may be increased or decreased, partly because of slower removal of sulfonylurea from the body. This may change the amount of sulfonylurea you need.
- Underactive adrenal gland, not properly controlled or
- Underactive pituitary gland, not properly controlled or
- Undernourished condition or
- Weakened physical condition or

- Any other condition that causes low blood sugar—Patients with these conditions may be more likely to develop low blood sugar while taking sulfonylureas.

Proper Use of This Medicine

Use this medicine only as directed even if you feel well and do not notice any signs of high blood sugar. Do not take more of this medicine and do not take it more often than your doctor ordered. To do so may increase the chance of serious side effects. Remember that this medicine will not cure your diabetes but it does help control it. Therefore, you must continue to take it as directed if you expect to lower your blood sugar and keep it low. You may have to take an antidiabetic medicine for the rest of your life. If high blood sugar is not treated, it can cause serious problems, such as heart failure, blood vessel disease, eye disease, or kidney disease.

Your doctor will give you instructions about diet, exercise, how to test your blood sugar levels, and how to adjust your dose when you are sick.

- Diet—The daily number of calories in the meal plan should be adjusted by your doctor or a registered dietitian to help you reach and maintain a healthy body weight. In addition, regular meals and snacks are arranged to meet the energy needs of your body at different times of the day. It is very important that you follow your meal plan carefully.

- Exercise—Ask your doctor what kind of exercise to do, the best time to do it, and how much you should do each day.

- Blood tests—This is the best way to tell whether your diabetes is being controlled properly. Blood sugar testing helps you and your health care team adjust the dose of your medicine, meal plan, or exercise schedule.

- On sick days—When you become sick with a cold, fever, or the flu, you need to take your usual dose of sulfonylurea, even if you feel too ill to eat. This is especially true if you have nausea, vomiting, or diarrhea. Infection usually increases your need to produce more insulin. Sometimes you may need to be switched from your sulfonylurea to insulin for a short period of time while you are sick to properly control blood sugar. Call your doctor for specific instructions. Continue taking your sulfonylurea and try to stay on your regular meal plan. If you have trouble eating solid food, drink fruit juices, nondiet soft drinks, or clear soups, or eat small amounts of bland foods. A dietitian or your health care professional can give you a list of foods and the amounts to use for sick days. Test your blood sugar level at least every 4 hours while you are awake and check your urine for ketones. If ketones are present, call your doctor at once. If you have severe or prolonged vomiting, check with your doctor. Even when you start feeling better, let your doctor know how you are doing.

For patients taking glipizide extended-release tablets:

- Swallow the tablet whole, without breaking, crushing, or chewing it.

- You may sometimes notice what looks like a tablet in your stool. Do not worry. After you swallow the tablet, the medicine in the tablet is absorbed inside your body. Then the tablet passes into your stool without changing its shape. The medicine has entered your body and will work properly.

Dosing—The dose medicines in this class will be different for different patients. Follow your doctor's orders or the directions on the label. The following information includes only the average doses of these medicines. If your dose is different, do not change it unless your doctor tells you to do so.

The amount of medicine that you take depends on the strength of the medicine. Also, the number of doses you take each day, the time allowed between doses, and the length of time you take the medicine depend on the medical problem for which you are using the medicine.

- For acetohexamide:
  - For treating type 2 diabetes:
    - For oral dosage form (tablets):
      - Adults—At first, 250 milligrams (mg) once a day. Some elderly people may need a lower dose at first. Then, your doctor may change your dose a little at a time if needed. The dose is usually not more than 1.5 grams a day. If your dose is 1 gram or more, the dose is usually divided into two doses. These doses are taken before the morning and evening meals.
      - Children—The type of diabetes treated with this medicine is rare in children. However, if a child needs this medicine, the dose would have to be determined by the doctor.

- For chlorpropamide:
  - For treating type 2 diabetes:
    - For oral dosage form (tablets):
      - Adults—At first, 250 milligrams (mg) once a day. Some elderly people may need a lower dose of 100 to 125 mg a day at first. Then, your doctor may change your dose a little at a time if needed. The dose is usually not more than 750 mg a day.
      - Children—The type of diabetes treated with this medicine is rare in children. However, if a child needs this medicine, the dose would have to be determined by the doctor.

- For gliclazide:
  - For treating type 2 diabetes:
    - For oral dosage form (tablets):
      - Adults—80 milligrams (mg) a day with a meal as a single dose or 160 to 320 mg divided into two doses taken with the morning and evening meals.
      - Children—The type of diabetes treated with this medicine is rare in children. However, if a child needs this medicine, the dose would have to be determined by the doctor.

- For glimepiride:
  - For treating type 2 diabetes:
    - For oral dosage form (tablets):
      - Adults—Glimepiride alone: At first, 1 to 2 milligrams (mg) once a day with breakfast or the first main meal. The dose then may be increased by your doctor based on your blood sugar level.
      - Adults—Glimepiride with metformin: The usual dose is 8 mg once a day with breakfast or the first main meal.
      - Adults—Glimepiride with insulin: The usual dose is 8 mg once a day with breakfast or the first main meal.

— Children—The type of diabetes treated with this medicine is rare in children. However, if a child needs this medicine, the dose would have to be determined by the doctor.

- For glipizide:
  - For treating type 2 diabetes:
    - For oral dosage form (tablets):
      — Adults—At first, 5 milligrams (mg) once a day. Some elderly people may need a lower dose of 2.5 mg a day at first. Then, your doctor may change your dose a little at a time if needed. The dose is usually not more than 40 mg a day. If your dose is 15 mg or more, the dose is usually divided into two doses. These doses are taken thirty minutes before the morning and evening meals.
      — Children—The type of diabetes treated with this medicine is rare in children. However, if a child needs this medicine, the dose would have to be determined by the doctor.
    - For oral dosage form (extended-release tablets):
      - Adults—At first, 5 mg once a day with breakfast. Then, your doctor may change your dose a little at a time if needed. The dose is usually not more than 20 mg a day.
      - Children—The type of diabetes treated with this medicine is rare in children. However, if a child needs this medicine, the dose would have to be determined by the doctor.

- For glyburide:
  - For treating type 2 diabetes:
    - For oral dosage form (nonmicronized tablets):
      — Adults—At first, 2.5 to 5 milligrams (mg) once a day. Some elderly people may need a lower dose of 1.25 to 2.5 mg a day at first. Then, your doctor may change your dose a little at a time if needed. The dose is usually not more than 20 mg a day. If your dose is 10 mg or more, the dose usually is divided into two doses. These doses are taken with the morning and evening meals.
      — Children—The type of diabetes treated with this medicine is rare in children. However, if a child needs this medicine, the dose would have to be determined by the doctor.
    - For oral dosage form (micronized tablets):
      - Adults—At first, 1.5 to 3 mg a day. Some elderly people may need a low dose of 0.75 to 3 mg a day at first. Then, your doctor may change your dose a little at a time if needed. The dose is usually not more than 12 mg a day. If your dose is 6 mg or more, the dose is usually divided into two doses. These doses are taken with the morning and evening meals. A single dose is taken with breakfast or with the first meal.
      - Children—The type of diabetes treated with this medicine is rare in children. However, if a child needs this medicine,

the dose would have to be determined by the doctor.

- For tolazamide:
  - For treating type 2 diabetes:
    - For oral dosage form (tablets):
      — Adults—At first, 100 to 250 milligrams (mg) once a day in the morning. Then, your doctor may change your dose a little at a time if needed. The dose is usually not more than 1 gram a day. If your dose is 500 mg or more, the dose is usually divided into two doses. These doses are taken with the morning and evening meals.
      — Children—The type of diabetes treated with this medicine is rare in children. However, if a child needs this medicine, the dose would have to be determined by the doctor.

- For tolbutamide:
  - For treating type 2 diabetes:
    - For oral dosage form (tablets):
      — Adults—At first, 1000 to 2000 milligrams (mg) a day. Some elderly people may need lower doses to start. The dose is usually divided into two doses. These doses are taken before the morning and evening meals. Your doctor may change your dose a little at a time if needed. The dose is usually not more than 3000 mg a day.
      — Children—The type of diabetes treated with this medicine is rare in children. However, if a child needs this medicine, the dose would have to be determined by the doctor.

Missed dose—If you miss a dose of this medicine, take it as soon as possible. However, if it is almost time for your next dose, skip the missed dose and go back to your regular dosing schedule. Do not double doses.

Storage—Store the medicine in a closed container at room temperature, away from heat, moisture, and direct light. Keep from freezing.

Keep out of the reach of children.

Do not keep outdated medicine or medicine no longer needed.

Precautions While Using This Medicine

Your doctor will want to check your progress at regular visits, especially during the first few weeks that you take this medicine.

It is very important to follow carefully any instructions from your health care team about:

- Alcohol—Drinking alcohol may cause severe low blood sugar. Discuss this with your health care team.
- Tobacco—If you have been smoking for a long time and suddenly stop, your dosage of sulfonylurea may need to be reduced. If you decide to quit, tell your doctor first.
- Other medicines—Do not take other medicines unless they have been discussed with your doctor. This especially includes nonprescription medicines, such as aspirin, and medicines for appetite control, asthma, colds, cough, hay fever, or sinus problems.
- Counseling—Other family members need to learn how to prevent side effects or help with side effects in the patient if they occur. Also, patients with diabetes, espe-

cially teenagers, may need special counseling about sulfonylurea or insulin dosing changes that might occur because of lifestyle changes, such as changes in exercise and diet. Furthermore, counseling on contraception and pregnancy may be needed because of the problems that can occur in women with diabetes who become pregnant.

- Travel—Carry a recent prescription and your medical history. Be prepared for an emergency as you would normally. Make allowances for changing time zones, and keep your meal times as close as possible to your usual meal times.

- Protecting skin from sunlight—Sulfonylureas can make you more sensitive to the sun. Use of sunblock products that have a skin protection factor (SPF) of at least 15 on your skin and lips can help to prevent sunburn. Do not use a sunlamp or tanning bed or booth.

In case of emergency—There may be a time when you need emergency help for a problem caused by your diabetes. You need to be prepared for these emergencies. It is a good idea to:

- Wear a medical identification (I.D.) bracelet or neck chain at all times. Also, carry an I.D. card in your wallet or purse that says that you have diabetes and a list of all of your medicines.

- Keep some kind of quick-acting sugar handy to treat low blood sugar.

- Have a glucagon kit and a syringe and needle available in case severe low blood sugar occurs. Check and replace any expired kits regularly.

- Too much of a sulfonylurea can cause low blood sugar (also called hypoglycemia). Symptoms of low blood sugar must be treated before they lead to unconsciousness (passing out). Different people may feel different symptoms of low blood sugar. It is important that you learn which symptoms of low blood sugar you usually have so that you can treat it quickly.

- Symptoms of low blood sugar can include: anxious feeling, behavior change similar to being drunk, blurred vision, cold sweats, confusion, cool pale skin, difficulty in concentrating, drowsiness, excessive hunger, fast heartbeat, headache, nausea, nervousness, nightmares, restless sleep, shakiness, slurred speech, and unusual tiredness or weakness.

- The symptoms of low blood sugar may develop quickly and may result from:
  - delaying or missing a scheduled meal or snack.
  - exercising more than usual.
  - drinking a significant amount of alcohol.
  - taking certain medicines.
  - taking too high a dose of sulfonylurea.
  - if using insulin, using too much insulin.

- Know what to do if symptoms of low blood sugar occur. Eating some form of quick-acting sugar when symptoms of low blood sugar first appear will usually prevent them from getting worse. Good sources of sugar include:
  - Glucose tablets or gel, fruit juice or nondiet soft drink (4 to 6 ounces [one-half cup]), corn syrup or honey (1 tablespoon), sugar cubes (6 one-half-inch sized), or table sugar (dissolved in water).

- Do not use chocolate because its fat slows down the sugar entering the bloodstream.
- If a snack is not scheduled for an hour or more you should also eat a light snack, such as crackers or a half sandwich, or drink an 8-ounce glass of milk.
- Glucagon is used in emergency situations such as unconsciousness. Have a glucagon kit available, along with a syringe and needle, and know how to prepare and use it. Members of your household also should know how and when to use it.

High blood sugar (hyperglycemia) is another problem related to uncontrolled diabetes. If you have any symptoms of high blood sugar, contact your health care team right away. If high blood sugar is not treated, severe hyperglycemia can occur, leading to ketoacidosis (diabetic coma) and death.

- Symptoms of high blood sugar appear more slowly than those of low blood sugar. Symptoms can include: blurred vision; drowsiness; dry mouth; flushed and dry skin; fruit-like breath odor; increased urination; loss of appetite; stomachache, nausea, or vomiting; tiredness; troubled breathing (rapid and deep); and unusual thirst.

- Symptoms of severe high blood sugar (called ketoacidosis or diabetic coma) that need immediate hospitalization include: flushed dry skin, fruit-like breath odor, ketones in urine, passing out, troubled breathing (rapid and deep).

- High blood sugar symptoms may occur if you:
  - have a fever, diarrhea, or an infection.
  - if using insulin, do not take enough insulin or skip a dose of insulin.
  - do not exercise as much as usual.
  - overeat or do not follow your meal plan.
  - Know what to do if high blood sugar occurs. Your doctor may recommend changes in your sulfonylurea dose or meal plan to avoid high blood sugar. Symptoms of high blood sugar must be corrected before they progress to more serious conditions. Check with your doctor often to make sure you are controlling your blood sugar, but do not change the dose of your medicine without checking with your doctor. Your doctor might discuss the following with you:
    - Decreasing your dose for a short time for special needs, such as when you cannot exercise as you normally do.
    - Increasing your dose when you plan to eat an unusually large dinner, such as on holidays. This type of increase is called an anticipatory dose.
    - Delaying a meal if your blood sugar is over 200 mg/dL to allow time for your blood sugar to go down. An extra dose or an injection of insulin may be needed if your blood sugar does not come down shortly.
    - Not exercising if your blood sugar is over 240 mg/dL and reporting this to your doctor immediately.
    - Being hospitalized if ketoacidosis or diabetic coma occurs with a possible change of treatment.

Side Effects of This Medicine

The use of sulfonylurea antidiabetic agents has been reported, but not proven in all studies, to increase the risk of death from heart and blood vessel disease. Patients with diabetes are already more likely to have these problems if they do not control their blood sugar. Some sulfonylureas, such as glyburide and gliclazide, can have a positive effect on heart and blood vessel disease. It is important to know that problems can occur, but it is also not known if other sulfonylureas, particularly tolbutamide, help to cause these problems. It is known that if blood sugar is not controlled, such problems can occur.

Along with its needed effects, a medicine may cause some unwanted effects. Although not all of these side effects may occur, if they do occur they may need medical attention.

Check with your doctor immediately if any of the following side effects occur:
> *Less common*
>> Convulsions (seizures); unconsciousness

Check with your doctor as soon as possible if any of the following side effects occur:
> *More common*
>> Low blood sugar; unusual weight gain; including anxious feeling; behavior change similar to being drunk; blurred vision; cold sweats; confusion; cool pale skin; difficulty in concentrating; drowsiness; excessive hunger; fast heartbeat; headache; nausea; nervousness; nightmares; restless sleep; shakiness; slurred speech; unusual tiredness or weakness
> *Less common*
>> Peeling of skin; skin redness, itching, or rash
> *Rare*
>> Chest pain; chills; coughing up blood; dark urine; fever; fluid-filled skin blisters; general feeling of illness; increased amounts of sputum (phlegm); increased sweating; light-colored stools; pale skin; sensitivity to the sun; shortness of breath; sore throat; thinning of the skin; unusual bleeding or bruising; unusual tiredness or weakness; yellow eyes or skin
> *Rarely, for patients taking chlorpropamide or tolbutamide*
>> Depression; retain (keep) more body water than usual, even less often with tolbutamide; swelling or puffiness of face, ankles, or hands

Some side effects may occur that usually do not need medical attention. These side effects may go away during treatment as your body adjusts to the medicine. Also, your health care professional may be able to tell you about ways to prevent or reduce some of these side effects. Check with your health care professional if any of the following side effects continue or are bothersome or if you have any questions about them:
> *More common*
>> Changes in sense of taste; constipation; diarrhea; dizziness; heartburn; increased amount of urine or more frequent urination; increased or decreased appetite; passing of gas; stomach pain, fullness, or discomfort; vomiting
> *Less common or rare*
>> Difficulty in focusing the eyes; increased sensitivity of skin to sun

Other side effects not listed may also occur in some patients. If you notice any other effects, check with your healthcare professional.

SUMATRIPTAN (Nasal route, Oral route, Subcutaneous route) - soo-ma-TRIP-tan

Commonly used brand name(s)

In the U.S.—
Imitrex

Available Dosage Forms:
- Spray
- Tablet
- Kit
- Solution

Therapeutic Class: Antimigraine
Pharmacologic Class: Serotonin Receptor Agonist, 5–HT1

Uses For This Medicine

Sumatriptan is used to treat severe migraine headaches. Many people find that their headaches go away completely after they take sumatriptan. Other people find that their headaches are much less painful, and that they are able to go back to their normal activities even though their headaches are not completely gone. Sumatriptan often relieves other symptoms that occur together with a migraine headache, such as nausea, vomiting, sensitivity to light, and sensitivity to sound.

Sumatriptan is not an ordinary pain reliever. It will not relieve any kind of pain other than migraine headaches. This medicine is usually used for people whose headaches are not relieved by acetaminophen, aspirin, or other pain relievers.

Sumatriptan injection is also used to treat cluster headaches.

Sumatriptan has caused serious side effects in some people, especially people who have heart or blood vessel disease. Be sure that you discuss with your doctor the risks of using this medicine as well as the good that it can do.

Sumatriptan is available only with your doctor's prescription.

Before Using This Medicine

In deciding to use a medicine, the risks of taking the medicine must be weighed against the good it will do. This is a decision you and your doctor will make. For this medicine, the following should be considered:

Allergies—Tell your doctor if you have ever had any unusual or allergic reaction to this medicine or any other medicines. Also tell your health care professional if you have any other types of allergies, such as to foods, dyes, preservatives, or animals. For non-prescription products, read the label or package ingredients carefully.

Pediatric—This medicine has been tested in a limited number of children aged 12 to 17 years, however use is not recommend in children younger than 18 years of age.

Geriatric—Use of sumatriptan in elderly patients is not recommended.

Pregnancy—

	Pregnancy Category	Explanation
All Trimesters	C	Animal studies have shown an adverse effect and there are no adequate studies in pregnant women OR no animal studies have been conducted and there are no adequate studies in pregnant women.

Breast Feeding—There are no adequate studies in women for determining infant risk when using this medication during breastfeeding. Weigh the potential benefits against the potential risks before taking this medication while breastfeeding.

Other medicines—

Using this medicine with any of the following medicines is not recommended. Your doctor may decide not to treat you with this medication or change some of the other medicines you take.

Almotriptan, Clorgyline, Dihydroergotamine, Ergoloid Mesylates, Ergonovine, Ergotamine, Frovatriptan, Iproniazid, Isocarboxazid, Methylergonovine, Methysergide, Moclobemide, Naratriptan, Nialamide, Pargyline, Phenelzine, Procarbazine, Rizatriptan, Toloxatone, Tranylcypromine, Zolmitriptan

Interactions with Food/Tobacco/Alcohol—Certain medicines should not be used at or around the time of eating food or eating certain types of food since interactions may occur. Using alcohol or tobacco with certain medicines may also cause interactions to occur. Discuss with your healthcare professional the use of your medicine with food, alcohol, or tobacco.

Other medical problems—The presence of other medical problems may affect the use of this medicine. Make sure you tell your doctor if you have any other medical problems, especially:

- Angina (chest pain) or
- Fast or irregular heartbeat or
- Heart or blood vessel disease or
- High blood pressure or
- Kidney disease or
- Liver disease or
- Stroke (history of)—The chance of side effects may be increased. Heart or blood vessel disease and high blood pressure sometimes do not cause any symptoms, so some people do not know that they have these problems. Before deciding whether you should use sumatriptan, your doctor may need to do some tests to make sure that you do not have any of these conditions.

Proper Use of This Medicine

Do not use sumatriptan for a headache that is different from your usual migraines. Instead, check with your doctor.

To relieve your migraine as soon as possible, use sumatriptan as soon as the headache pain begins. Even if you get warning signals of a coming migraine (an aura), you should wait until the headache pain starts before using sumatriptan. Using sumatriptan during the aura probably will not prevent the headache from occurring. However, even if you do not use sumatriptan until your migraine has been present for several hours, the medicine will still work.

Lying down in a quiet, dark room for a while after you use this medicine may help relieve your migraine.

If you are not much better in 1 or 2 hours after an injection of sumatriptan or after sumatriptan nasal solution, or in 2 to 4 hours after a tablet is taken, do not use any more of this medicine for the same migraine. A migraine that is not relieved by the first dose of sumatriptan probably will not be relieved by a second dose, either. Ask your doctor ahead of time about other medicine to be taken if sumatriptan does not work. After taking the other medicine, check with your doctor as soon as possible. Headaches that are not relieved by sumatriptan are sometimes caused by conditions that need other treatment. However, even if sumatriptan does not relieve one migraine, it may still relieve the next one.

If you feel much better after a dose of sumatriptan, but your headache comes back or gets worse after a while, you may use more sumatriptan. However, use this medicine only as directed by your doctor. Do not use more of it, and do not use it more often, than directed. Using too much sumatriptan may increase the chance of side effects.

Your doctor may direct you to take another medicine to help prevent headaches. It is important that you follow your doctor's directions, even if your headaches continue to occur. Headache-preventing medicines may take several weeks to start working. Even after they do start working, your headaches may not go away completely. However, your headaches should occur less often, and they should be less severe and easier to relieve. This can reduce the amount of sumatriptan or pain relievers that you need. If you do not notice any improvement after several weeks of headache-preventing treatment, check with your doctor.

For patients taking sumatriptan tablets:

- Sumatriptan tablets are to be swallowed whole with a full glass of water. Do not break, crush, or chew the tablets before swallowing them.

For patients using sumatriptan injection:

- This medicine comes with patient directions. Read them carefully before using the medicine, and check with your health care professional if you have any questions.
- Your health care professional will teach you how to inject yourself with the medicine. Be sure to follow the directions carefully. Check with your health care professional if you have any problems using the medicine.
- After you have finished injecting the medicine, be sure to follow the precautions in the patient directions about safely discarding the empty cartridge and the needle. Always return the empty cartridge and needle to their container before discarding them. Do not throw away the autoinjector unit, because refills are available.

For patients using sumatriptan nasal solution:

- This medicine comes with patient directions. Read them carefully before using the medicine, and check with your health care professional if you have any questions.

Dosing—The dose of this medicine will be different for different patients. Follow your doctor's orders or the directions

on the label. The following information includes only the average doses of this medicine. If your dose is different, do not change it unless your doctor tells you to do so.

The amount of medicine that you take depends on the strength of the medicine. Also, the number of doses you take each day, the time allowed between doses, and the length of time you take the medicine depend on the medical problem for which you are using the medicine.

- For nasal dosage form (nasal solution):
  ○ For migraine headaches:
    ▪ Adults—5 milligrams (mg) (1 spray into one nostril) or 10 mg (2 sprays in one nostril or 1 spray in each nostril) or 20 mg (1 spray into one nostril). If pain is not relieved, another spray (5 mg, 10 mg, or 20 mg) should not be used for the same migraine attack. Another spray (5 mg, 10 mg, or 20 mg) may be used for a migraine that occurs at a later time as long as it has been at least two hours since the last spray. Do not use more than 40 mg in a twenty-four-hour period (one day).
    ▪ Children—Use and dose must be determined by your doctor.
- For oral dosage form (tablets):
  ○ For migraine headaches:
    ▪ Adults—25, 50 or 100 mg as a single dose. If you get some relief, or if the migraine comes back after being relieved, another dose may be taken two hours after the last dose. Do not take more than 200 mg in any twenty-four-hour period. If you are taking the tablets after using an injection, you may take single doses up to 100 mg a day with two hours between doses. Do not take more than 200 mg in a twenty-four-hour period.
    ▪ Children—Use and dose must be determined by your doctor.
- For parenteral dosage form (injection):
  ○ For migraine or cluster headaches:
    ▪ Adults—One 6–mg injection. One more 6–mg dose may be injected, if necessary, if the migraine comes back after being relieved. However, the second injection should not be given any sooner than one hour after the first one. Do not use more than two 6–mg injections in a twenty-four-hour period (one day). However, some people may be directed to use no more than two 6–mg doses in a forty-eight-hour period (two days).
    ▪ Children—Use and dose must be determined by your doctor.

Storage—Store the medicine in a closed container at room temperature, away from heat, moisture, and direct light. Keep from freezing.

Keep out of the reach of children.

Do not keep outdated medicine or medicine no longer needed.

Precautions While Using This Medicine

Check with your doctor if you have used sumatriptan for three headaches, and have not had good relief. Also, check with your doctor if your migraine headaches are worse, or if they are occurring more often, than before you started using sumatriptan.

Drinking alcoholic beverages can make headaches worse or cause new headaches to occur. People who suffer from severe headaches should probably avoid alcoholic beverages, especially during a headache.

Some people feel drowsy or dizzy during or after a migraine, or after taking sumatriptan to relieve a migraine. As long as you are feeling drowsy or dizzy, do not drive, use machines, or do anything else that could be dangerous if you are dizzy or are not alert.

Side Effects of This Medicine

Along with its needed effects, a medicine may cause some unwanted effects. Most side effects of sumatriptan are milder and occur less often with the tablets than with the injection. Although not all of these side effects may occur, if they do occur they may need medical attention.

Stop taking this medicine and get emergency help immediately if any of the following effects occur:
Rare
Chest pain (severe); changes in skin color on face; convulsions (seizures); fast or irregular breathing; puffiness or swelling of eyelids, area around the eyes, face, or lips; shortness of breath, troubled breathing, or wheezing

Check with your doctor immediately if any of the following side effects occur:
Less common
Chest pain (mild); heaviness, tightness, or pressure in chest and/or neck

Check with your doctor as soon as possible if any of the following side effects occur:
Less common
Difficulty in swallowing; pounding heartbeat; skin rash, hives, itching, or bumps on skin

Other side effects may occur that usually do not need medical attention. Some of the following effects, such as nausea, vomiting, drowsiness, dizziness, and general feeling of illness or tiredness, often occur during or after a migraine, even when sumatriptan has not been used. Most of the side effects caused by sumatriptan go away within a short time (less than 1 hour after an injection or 2 hours after a tablet). However, check with your doctor if any of the following side effects continue or are bothersome:
More common
Burning, discharge, pain, and/or soreness in the nose; burning, pain, or redness at place of injection; change in sense of taste; discomfort in jaw, mouth, tongue, throat, nose, or sinuses; dizziness; drowsiness; feeling of burning, warmth, heat, numbness, tightness, or tingling; feeling cold, "strange," or weak; flushing; lightheadedness; muscle aches, cramps, or stiffness; nausea or vomiting

Less common or rare
Anxiety; general feeling of illness or tiredness; vision changes

Other side effects not listed may also occur in some patients. If you notice any other effects, check with your healthcare professional.

TACRINE (Oral route) - TAK-reen

Commonly used brand name(s)
In the U.S.—
  Cognex

Available Dosage Forms:
  • Capsule

Therapeutic Class: Central Nervous System Agent
Pharmacologic Class: Cholinesterase Inhibitor, Centrally Acting

Uses For This Medicine

Tacrine is used to treat the symptoms of mild to moderate Alzheimer's disease. Tacrine will not cure Alzheimer's disease, and it will not stop the disease from getting worse. However, tacrine can improve thinking ability in some patients with Alzheimer's disease.

In Alzheimer's disease, many chemical changes take place in the brain. One of the earliest and biggest changes is that there is less of a chemical messenger called acetylcholine (ACh). ACh helps the brain to work properly. Tacrine slows the breakdown of ACh, so it can build up and have a greater effect. However, as Alzheimer's disease gets worse, there will be less and less ACh, so tacrine may not work as well.

Tacrine may cause liver problems. While taking this medicine, you must have blood tests regularly to see if the medicine is affecting your liver.

This medicine is available only with your doctor's prescription.

Before Using This Medicine

In deciding to use a medicine, the risks of taking the medicine must be weighed against the good it will do. This is a decision you and your doctor will make. For this medicine, the following should be considered:

Allergies—Tell your doctor if you have ever had any unusual or allergic reaction to this medicine or any other medicines. Also tell your health care professional if you have any other types of allergies, such as to foods, dyes, preservatives, or animals. For non-prescription products, read the label or package ingredients carefully.

Pediatric—Studies on this medicine have been done only in adult patients, and there is no specific information comparing use of tacrine in children with use in other age groups.

Geriatric—Studies on tacrine have been done only in middle-aged and older patients. Information on the effects of tacrine is based on these patients.

Pregnancy—

	Pregnancy Category	Explanation
All Trimesters	C	Animal studies have shown an adverse effect and there are no adequate studies in pregnant women OR no animal studies have been conducted and there are no adequate studies in pregnant women.

Breast Feeding—There are no adequate studies in women for determining infant risk when using this medication during breastfeeding. Weigh the potential benefits against the potential risks before taking this medication while breastfeeding.

Other medicines—
Using this medicine with any of the following medicines may cause an increased risk of certain side effects, but using both drugs may be the best treatment for you. If both medicines are prescribed together, your doctor may change the dose or how often you use one or both of the medicines.

Estradiol, Fluvoxamine, Haloperidol, Ibuprofen, Levonorgestrel, Riluzole, Theophylline

Interactions with Food/Tobacco/Alcohol—Certain medicines should not be used at or around the time of eating food or eating certain types of food since interactions may occur. Using alcohol or tobacco with certain medicines may also cause interactions to occur. Discuss with your healthcare professional the use of your medicine with food, alcohol, or tobacco.

Other medical problems—The presence of other medical problems may affect the use of this medicine. Make sure you tell your doctor if you have any other medical problems, especially:
  • Asthma (or history of) or
  • Heart problems, including slow heartbeat or hypotension (low blood pressure), or
  • Intestinal blockage or
  • Liver disease (or history of) or
  • Parkinson's disease or
  • Stomach ulcer (or history of) or
  • Urinary tract blockage or difficult urination—Tacrine may make these conditions worse
  • Brain disease, other, or
  • Epilepsy or history of seizures or
  • Head injury with loss of consciousness—Tacrine may cause seizures

Proper Use of This Medicine

Take this medicine only as directed by your doctor. Do not take more or less of it, and do not take it more or less often than your doctor ordered. Taking too much may increase the chance of side effects, while taking too little may not improve your condition.

Tacrine is best taken on an empty stomach (1 hour before or 2 hours after meals). However, if this medicine upsets your stomach, your doctor may want you to take it with food.

Tacrine seems to work best when it is taken at regularly spaced times, usually four times a day.

Dosing—The dose of this medicine will be different for different patients. Follow your doctor's orders or the directions on the label. The following information includes only the average doses of this medicine. If your dose is different, do not change it unless your doctor tells you to do so.

The amount of medicine that you take depends on the strength of the medicine. Also, the number of doses you take each day, the time allowed between doses, and the length of time you take the medicine depend on the medical problem for which you are using the medicine.

  • For oral dosage form (capsules):
    ◦ For treatment of Alzheimer's disease:
      ▪ Adults—To start, 10 milligrams (mg) four times a day. Your doctor may increase your dose gradually if you are doing well on this medicine and your liver tests are normal. However, the dose is usually not more than 40 mg four times a day.

Missed dose—If you miss a dose of this medicine, take it as soon as possible. However, if it is almost time for your next dose, skip the missed dose and go back to your regular dosing schedule. Do not double doses.

Storage—Store the medicine in a closed container at room temperature, away from heat, moisture, and direct light. Keep from freezing.

Keep out of the reach of children.

Do not keep outdated medicine or medicine no longer needed.

Precautions While Using This Medicine

It is important that your doctor check your progress at regular visits. Also, you must have your blood tested every other week for at least the first 4 to 16 weeks when you start using tacrine to see if this medicine is affecting your liver. If all of the blood tests are normal, you will still need regular testing, but then your doctor may decide to do the tests less often.

Tell your doctor if your symptoms get worse, or if you notice any new symptoms.

Before you have any kind of surgery, dental treatment, or emergency treatment, tell the medical doctor or dentist in charge that you are taking this medicine. Taking tacrine together with medicines that are sometimes used during surgery or dental or emergency treatments may increase the effects of these medicines.

Tacrine may cause some people to become dizzy, clumsy, or unsteady. Make sure you know how you react to this medicine before you do anything that could be dangerous if you are dizzy, clumsy, or unsteady.

Do not stop taking this medicine or decrease your dose without first checking with your doctor. Stopping this medicine suddenly or decreasing the dose by a large amount may cause mental or behavior changes.

If you think you or someone else may have taken an overdose of tacrine, get emergency help at once. Taking an overdose of tacrine may lead to seizures or shock. Some signs of shock are large pupils, irregular breathing, and fast weak pulse. Other signs of an overdose are severe nausea and vomiting, increasing muscle weakness, greatly increased sweating, and greatly increased watering of the mouth.

Side Effects of This Medicine

Along with its needed effects, a medicine may cause some unwanted effects. Some side effects will have signs or symptoms that you can see or feel. Your doctor may watch for others by doing certain tests

Tacrine may cause some serious side effects, including liver problems. You and your doctor should discuss the good this medicine will do as well as the risks of receiving it.

Check with your doctor as soon as possible if any of the following side effects occur:

More common
Clumsiness or unsteadiness; diarrhea; loss of appetite; nausea; vomiting

Less common
Fainting; fast or pounding heartbeat; fever; high or low blood pressure; skin rash; slow heartbeat

Rare
Aggression, irritability, or nervousness; change in stool color; convulsions (seizures); cough, tightness in chest, troubled breathing, or wheezing; stiffness of arms or legs, slow movement, or trembling and shaking of hands and fingers; trouble in urinating; yellow eyes or skin

Symptoms of overdose
Convulsions (seizures); greatly increased sweating; greatly increased watering of mouth; increasing muscle weakness; low blood pressure; nausea (severe); shock (fast weak pulse, irregular breathing, large pupils); slow heartbeat; vomiting (severe)

This medicine may also cause the following side effect that your doctor will watch for:

More common
Liver problems

Some side effects may occur that usually do not need medical attention. These side effects may go away during treatment as your body adjusts to the medicine. Also, your health care professional may be able to tell you about ways to prevent or reduce some of these side effects. Check with your health care professional if any of the following side effects continue or are bothersome or if you have any questions about them:

More common
Abdominal or stomach pain or cramping; dizziness; headache; indigestion; muscle aches or pain

Less common
Belching; fast breathing; flushing of skin; general feeling of discomfort or illness; increased sweating; increased urination; increased watering of eyes; increased watering of mouth; runny nose; swelling of feet or lower legs; trouble in sleeping

Other side effects not listed may also occur in some patients. If you notice any other effects, check with your healthcare professional.

TACROLIMUS (Oral route, Intravenous route) - ta-KROE-li-mus

Black Box Warning

• INTRAVENOUS/ORAL

Increased susceptibility to infection and the possible development of lymphoma may result from immunosuppression. Only physicians experienced in immunosuppressive therapy and management of organ transplant patients should prescribe tacrolimus. Patients receiving the drug should be managed in facilities equipped and staffed with adequate laboratory and supportive medical resources. The physician responsible for maintenance therapy should have complete information requisite for the follow-up of the patient.

• TOPICAL

Long-term safety of topical calcineurin inhibitors has not been established. Although a causal relationship has not been established, rare cases of malignancy (eg, skin and lymphoma) have been reported in patients treated with topical calcineurin inhibitors, including tacrolimus ointment. Therefore:

Continuous long-term use of topical calcineurin inhibitors, including tacrolimus ointment, in any age group should be avoided, and application limited to areas of involvement with atopic dermatitis. Tacrolimus ointment is not indicated for use in children less than 2 years of age. Only 0.03% tacrolimus ointment is indicated for use in children 2–15 years of age

Commonly used brand name(s)

In the U.S.—
    Prograf

Available Dosage Forms:
- Solution
- Capsule

Therapeutic Class: Immune Suppressant

Uses For This Medicine

Tacrolimus belongs to a group of medicines known as immunosuppressive agents. It is used to lower the body's natural immunity in patients who receive organ (for example, kidney, liver, pancreas, lung, and heart) transplants.

When a patient receives an organ transplant, the body's white blood cells will try to get rid of (reject) the transplanted organ. Tacrolimus works by preventing the white blood cells from getting rid of the transplanted organ.

Tacrolimus may also be used for other indications, as determined by your doctor.

Tacrolimus is a very strong medicine. It can cause side effects that can be very serious, such as kidney problems. It may also reduce the body's ability to fight infections. You and your doctor should talk about the good this medicine will do as well as the risks of using it.

Tacrolimus is available only with your doctor's prescription.

Once a medicine has been approved for marketing for a certain use, experience may show that it is also useful for other medical problems. Although not specifically included in the product labeling, tacrolimus is used in certain patients with the following medical conditions:
- Bone marrow transplantation
- Uveitis, severe, refractory (an eye condition)

For patients receiving bone marrow transplantation, tacrolimus may work by preventing the cells from the transplanted bone marrow from attacking the cells of the patient. The dose of tacrolimus for patients receiving bone marrow transplantation is based on body weight. The usual dose is 0.12 to 0.3 mg per kg (0.05 to 0.14 mg per pound) of body weight a day for patients taking tacrolimus by mouth, and 0.04 to 0.1 mg per kg (0.018 to 0.045 mg per pound) of body weight a day for patients receiving tacrolimus by injection.

The dose of tacrolimus for patients with severe, refractory uveitis is based on body weight. For severe, refractory uveitis, the usual dose is 0.1 to 0.15 mg per kg (0.045 to 0.068 mg per pound) of body weight a day.

Before Using This Medicine

In deciding to use a medicine, the risks of taking the medicine must be weighed against the good it will do. This is a decision you and your doctor will make. For this medicine, the following should be considered:

Allergies—Tell your doctor if you have ever had any unusual or allergic reaction to this medicine or any other medicines. Also tell your health care professional if you have any other types of allergies, such as to foods, dyes, preservatives, or animals. For non-prescription products, read the label or package ingredients carefully.

Pediatric—This medicine does not cause different types of side effects or problems in children than it does in adults, although some side effects may occur more or less often than they do in adult patients.

Geriatric—There is no specific information comparing the use of tacrolimus in the elderly with the use in other age groups. Tacrolimus is not expected to cause different side effects or problems in older people than it does in younger adults. However, older patients may need lower doses of tacrolimus.

Pregnancy—

	Pregnancy Category	Explanation
All Trimesters	C	Animal studies have shown an adverse effect and there are no adequate studies in pregnant women OR no animal studies have been conducted and there are no adequate studies in pregnant women.

Breast Feeding—There are no adequate studies in women for determining infant risk when using this medication during breastfeeding. Weigh the potential benefits against the potential risks before taking this medication while breastfeeding.

Other medicines—

Using this medicine with any of the following medicines is not recommended. Your doctor may decide not to treat you with this medication or change some of the other medicines you take.

Ziprasidone

Interactions with Food/Tobacco/Alcohol—Certain medicines should not be used at or around the time of eating food or eating certain types of food since interactions may occur. Using alcohol or tobacco with certain medicines may also cause interactions to occur. The following interactions have been selected on the basis of their potential significance and are not necessarily all-inclusive.

Using this medicine with any of the following may cause an increased risk of certain side effects but may be unavoidable in some cases. If used together, your doctor may change the dose or how often you use this medicine, or give you special instructions about the use of food, alcohol, or tobacco.

Grapefruit Juice

Other medical problems—The presence of other medical problems may affect the use of this medicine. Make sure you tell your doctor if you have any other medical problems, especially:
- Cancer—Tacrolimus can make this condition worse.
- Chickenpox (including recent exposure) or
- Herpes zoster (shingles)—The risk of severe disease affecting other parts of the body may be increased.
- Diabetes mellitus (sugar diabetes)—Tacrolimus can increase the amount of sugar in the blood.
- Hepatitis or
- Kidney disease or
- Liver disease—Tacrolimus can have harmful effects on the kidney in patients with these conditions; a lower dose

of tacrolimus may be needed in patients with these conditions.

- Hyperkalemia (high amount of potassium in the blood) or
- Nervous system problems—Tacrolimus can make these conditions worse.
- Infection—Tacrolimus decreases the body's ability to fight infection.

Proper Use of This Medicine

Take this medicine only as directed by your doctor. Do not take more or less of it and do not take it more often than your doctor ordered. The exact amount of medicine you need has been carefully worked out. Taking too much may increase the chance of side effects, while taking too little may lead to rejection of your transplanted organ.

To help you remember to take your medicine, try to get into the habit of taking it at the same time each day. This will also help tacrolimus work better by keeping a constant amount in the blood.

Absorption of this medicine may be changed if you change your diet. This medicine should be taken consistently with respect to meals. You should not change the type or amount of food you eat unless you discuss it with your health care professional.

Grapefruit and grapefruit juice may increase the effects of tacrolimus by increasing the amount of this medicine in the body. *You should not eat grapefruit or drink grapefruit juice while you are taking this medicine.*

Do not stop taking this medicine without first checking with your doctor. You may have to take medicine for the rest of your life to prevent your body from rejecting the transplant.

Dosing—The dose of this medicine will be different for different patients. Follow your doctor's orders or the directions on the label. The following information includes only the average doses of this medicine. If your dose is different, do not change it unless your doctor tells you to do so.

The amount of medicine that you take depends on the strength of the medicine. Also, the number of doses you take each day, the time allowed between doses, and the length of time you take the medicine depend on the medical problem for which you are using the medicine.

- For oral dosage form (capsules):
  - Adults, teenagers, or children—Dose is based on body weight and will be determined by your doctor.
- For injection dosage form:
  - Adults, teenagers, or children—Dose is based on body weight and will be determined by your doctor.

Storage—Store the medicine in a closed container at room temperature, away from heat, moisture, and direct light. Keep from freezing.

Keep out of the reach of children.

Do not keep outdated medicine or medicine no longer needed.

Precautions While Using This Medicine

The effects of tacrolimus may cause increased infections and delayed healing. Dental work, whenever possible, should be completed prior to beginning this medicine.

It is very important that your doctor check your progress at regular visits. Your doctor will want to do laboratory tests to make sure that tacrolimus is working properly and to check for unwanted effects.

Tacrolimus may *increase your risk for getting skin cancer* when exposed to sunlight.

- Stay out of direct sunlight, especially between the hours of 10:00 AM and 3:00 PM if possible.
- Wear protective clothing, including a hat. Also, wear sunglasses
- Apply a sun block product that has a skin protection factor (SPF) of 15 or higher. If you have questions about this, check with your health care professional.
- Apply a sun block lipstick that has an SPF of at least 15 to protect your lips.
- Do not use a sun lamp or a tanning bed.
- If you notice any unusual changes to your skin, check with your doctor.

While you are taking tacrolimus, it is important to maintain good dental hygiene and see a dentist regularly for teeth cleaning.

Raw oysters or other shellfish may contain bacteria that can cause serious illness, and possibly death. This is more likely to be a problem if these foods are eaten by patients with certain medical conditions. Even eating oysters from "clean" water or good restaurants does not guarantee that the oysters do not contain the bacteria. Symptoms of this infection include sudden chills, fever, nausea, vomiting, blood poisoning, and sometimes death. Eating raw shellfish is not a problem for most healthy people; however, patients with the following conditions may be at greater risk: cancer, immune disorders, organ transplantation, long-term corticosteroid use (as for asthma, arthritis, or organ transplantation), liver disease (including viral hepatitis), excess alcohol intake (2 to 3 drinks or more per day), diabetes, stomach problems (including previous stomach surgery and low stomach acid), and hemochromatosis (an iron disorder). *Do not eat raw oysters or other shellfish while you are taking tacrolimus. Be sure oysters and shellfish are fully cooked.*

While you are being treated with tacrolimus, and after you stop treatment with it, *it is important to see your doctor about the immunizations (vaccinations) you should receive. Do not get any immunizations without your doctor's approval.* Tacrolimus lowers your body's resistance. For some immunizations, there is a chance you might get the infection the immunization is meant to prevent. For other immunizations, it may be especially important to receive the immunization to prevent a disease. In addition, other persons living in your house should not take oral poliovirus vaccine since there is a chance they could pass the poliovirus on to you. Also, avoid persons who have recently taken oral poliovirus vaccine. Do not get close to them, and do not stay in the same room with them for very long. If you cannot take these precautions, you should consider wearing a protective face mask that covers the nose and mouth.

Treatment with tacrolimus may also increase the chance of getting other infections. If you can, avoid people with colds or other infections. If you think you are getting a cold or other infection, check with your doctor.

Tacrolimus is not available in all countries. *If you are traveling to another country, be sure you will have an adequate supply of your medicine.*

Side Effects of This Medicine

Along with its needed effects, a medicine may cause some unwanted effects. Some side effects will have signs or symptoms that you can see or feel. Your doctor will watch for others by doing certain tests.

Also, because of the way tacrolimus acts on the body, there is a chance that it may cause effects that may not occur until years after the medicine is used. These delayed effects may include certain types of cancer, such as lymphomas or skin cancers.

Check with your doctor immediately if any of the following side effects occur:

More common
Abdominal pain; abnormal dreams; agitation; anxiety; chills; confusion; convulsions (seizures); diarrhea; dizziness; fever and sore throat; flu-like symptoms; frequent urination; hallucinations (seeing or hearing things that are not there); headache; infection; itching; loss of appetite; loss of energy or weakness; mental depression; muscle trembling or twitching; nausea; nervousness; pale skin; shortness of breath; skin rash; swelling of feet or lower legs; tingling; trembling and shaking of hands; trouble in sleeping; unusual bleeding or bruising; unusual tiredness or weakness; vomiting

Less common
Blurred vision; chest pain; increased sensitivity to pain; muscle cramps; numbness or pain in legs; ringing in ears; sweating

Rare
Enlarged heart; flushing of face or neck; general feeling of discomfort or illness; weight loss; wheezing

Incidence not determined—Observed during clinical practice with tacrolimus; estimates of frequency cannot be determined.
Black, tarry stools; blistering, peeling, loosening of skin; bloating; blood in urine; blurred vision; constipation; convulsions (seizures); cough; cramping or burning; drowsiness; fainting; fast, slow, or irregular heartbeat; heartburn; increased blood pressure; increased thirst; indigestion; irregular heartbeat; itching; joint or muscle pain; lightheadedness; loss of appetite; lower back or side pain; nausea; pinpoint red spots on skin; pounding or rapid pulse; recurrent fainting; red, irritated eyes; red skin lesions, often with a purple center; shortness of breath; sores; stomach pain; sugar in the urine; troubled breathing; ulcers or white spots in mouth or on lips; weakness; weight gain; yellow eyes or skin

This medicine may also cause the following side effects that your doctor will watch for:

More common
Hyperkalemia (too much potassium in the blood); hypomagnesemia (not enough magnesium in the blood); kidney problems

Less common
Hyperlipidemia (high cholesterol); hypertension (high blood pressure)

Other side effects not listed may also occur in some patients. If you notice any other effects, check with your healthcare professional.

TACROLIMUS (Topical route) - ta-KROE-li-mus

Black Box Warning

• INTRAVENOUS/ORAL

Increased susceptibility to infection and the possible development of lymphoma may result from immunosuppression. Only physicians experienced in immunosuppressive therapy and management of organ transplant patients should prescribe tacrolimus. Patients receiving the drug should be managed in facilities equipped and staffed with adequate laboratory and supportive medical resources. The physician responsible for maintenance therapy should have complete information requisite for the follow-up of the patient.

• TOPICAL

Long-term safety of topical calcineurin inhibitors has not been established. Although a causal relationship has not been established, rare cases of malignancy (eg, skin and lymphoma) have been reported in patients treated with topical calcineurin inhibitors, including tacrolimus ointment. Therefore:

Continuous long-term use of topical calcineurin inhibitors, including tacrolimus ointment, in any age group should be avoided, and application limited to areas of involvement with atopic dermatitis. Tacrolimus ointment is not indicated for use in children less than 2 years of age. Only 0.03% tacrolimus ointment is indicated for use in children 2–15 years of age

Commonly used brand name(s)

In the U.S.—
Protopic

Available Dosage Forms:
• Ointment

Therapeutic Class: Antipsoriatic

Uses For This Medicine

Tacrolimus ointment is used for moderate to severe atopic dermatitis. This is a skin condition where there is itching, redness and inflammation, much like an allergic reaction. Tacrolimus helps to suppress these symptoms which are a reaction caused by the body's immune system. It can be used for short-term or long-term intermittent treatment. It is often used when other types of treatment are not working or not tolerated by the patient.

Tacrolimus is available only with your doctor's prescription.

Before Using This Medicine

In deciding to use a medicine, the risks of taking the medicine must be weighed against the good it will do. This is a decision you and your doctor will make. For this medicine, the following should be considered:

Allergies—Tell your doctor if you have ever had any unusual or allergic reaction to this medicine or any other medicines. Also tell your health care professional if you have any other types of allergies, such as to foods, dyes, preservatives, or animals. For non-prescription products, read the label or package ingredients carefully.

Pediatric—Some side effects may occur more or less often in children than they do in adult patients. This medicine has not been tested and should not be used in children under 2 years of age. Only the lower concentration of 0.03% tacrolimus ointment should be used in children 2 to 15 years of age.

Geriatric—Tacrolimus ointment has been tested and has not been shown to cause different side effects or problems in older people than it does in younger adults.

Pregnancy—

	Pregnancy Category	Explanation
All Trimesters	C	Animal studies have shown an adverse effect and there are no adequate studies in pregnant women OR no animal studies have been conducted and there are no adequate studies in pregnant women.

Breast Feeding—There are no adequate studies in women for determining infant risk when using this medication during breastfeeding. Weigh the potential benefits against the potential risks before taking this medication while breastfeeding.

Other medicines—

Using this medicine with any of the following medicines is not recommended. Your doctor may decide not to treat you with this medication or change some of the other medicines you take.

Ziprasidone

Interactions with Food/Tobacco/Alcohol—Certain medicines should not be used at or around the time of eating food or eating certain types of food since interactions may occur. Using alcohol or tobacco with certain medicines may also cause interactions to occur. Discuss with your healthcare professional the use of your medicine with food, alcohol, or tobacco.

Other medical problems—The presence of other medical problems may affect the use of this medicine. Make sure you tell your doctor if you have any other medical problems, especially:

- Chickenpox, existing or recent (including recent exposure) or
- Herpes simplex virus infections (skin blisters) or
- Varicella zoster virus infection (shingles)—Increased risk may be associated with these conditions.
- Immunocompromised patients (weakened immune system)—May cause serious problems; this medicine should not be used by these patients
- Kidney problems or
- Tendency to develop kidney problems—You should use this medicine with caution. It may cause your kidney problems to become worse.
- Precancerous condition of the skin or
- Skin cancer—You should not use this medicine.
- Skin infections, other—Safety is unknown
- Cancer of the lymph system—May increase risk in transplant patients receiving oral or injected immunosuppressant therapy and topical tacrolimus
- Netherton's syndrome—May cause too much of the tacrolimus to be absorbed into the body

Proper Use of This Medicine

Infections in the affected areas should be treated before starting treatment with tacrolimus ointment.

Dry skin completely before applying tacrolimus ointment.

Apply a thin layer of tacrolimus ointment and rub it in well to cover the affected areas

Do not swallow this medicine.

Wash hand thoroughly after applying tacrolimus ointment, if hands are not any area for treatment.

Use of this medicine may cause reactions at the site of application such as a mild to moderate feeling of warmth and/or sensation of burning. You should contact your doctor if this reaction is severe or persists for more than 1 week.

While using tacrolimus, if symptoms of your skin condition go away, consult your doctor.

Do not use any occlusive dressings (a dressing that seals the are that is being treated such as a plastic exercise suit or plastic wraps used to store foods).

Do not bathe, shower or swim right after applying this medicine. This could wash off the ointment.

Dosing—The dose of this medicine will be different for different patients. Follow your doctor's orders or the directions on the label. The following information includes only the average doses of this medicine. If your dose is different, do not change it unless your doctor tells you to do so.

The amount of medicine that you take depends on the strength of the medicine. Also, the number of doses you take each day, the time allowed between doses, and the length of time you take the medicine depend on the medical problem for which you are using the medicine.

- For ointment dosage form
  - For atopic dermatitis:
    - Adults—Gently apply 0.03% or 0.1% ointment to skin that is clean and dry two times a day. Do not cover the area with a bandage that sticks to the skin. Stop using when the signs and symptoms of eczema, such as itching, rash, and redness go away, as directed by your doctor.
    - Children 2 to 15 years old—Gently apply 0.03% ointment to skin that is clean and dry two times a day. Do not cover the area with a bandage that sticks to the skin. Stop using when the signs and symptoms of eczema, such as itching, rash, and redness go away, as directed by your doctor.
    - Children under 2 years of age—Use and dose must be determined by your doctor.

Storage—Store the medicine in a closed container at room temperature, away from heat, moisture, and direct light. Keep from freezing.

Keep out of the reach of children.

Do not keep outdated medicine or medicine no longer needed.

Ask your healthcare professional how you should dispose of any medicine you do not use.

Precautions While Using This Medicine

It is very important that your doctor check your progress at regular visits. Your doctor will want to make sure the tacrolimus ointment is working properly and to check for unwanted effects. If your condition has not improved after 6 weeks, your doctor will want to reexamine you.

Report any adverse reactions or side effects to your doctor.

Use this medicine only for the condition for which it was prescribed by your doctor.

You should not use this medicine beyond a year.

Tacrolimus ointment may increase the risk of skin tumors, when patients are also exposed to sunlight. The association between topical tacrolimus and the incidence of skin tumors has not been proven. When you begin taking this medicine:

- Stay out of direct sunlight, especially between the hours of 10:00 a.m. and 3:00 p.m., if possible.
- Wear protective clothing, including a hat. Also, wear sunglasses.
- Apply a sun block product that has a skin protection factor (SPF) of at least 15. Some patients may require a product with a higher SPF number, especially if they have a fair complexion. If you have any questions about this, check with your health care professional.
- Apply a sun block lipstick that has an SPF of at least 15 to protect your lips.
- Do not use a sunlamp or tanning bed or booth.

If you have a severe reaction from the sun, check with your doctor.

Side Effects of This Medicine

Along with its needed effects, a medicine may cause some unwanted effects. Although not all of these side effects may occur, if they do occur they may need medical attention.

Check with your doctor as soon as possible if any of the following side effects occur:

Incidence not known
> Agitation; black, tarry stools; bloody urine; burning or stinging sensation of face; change in size, shape, or color of existing mole; coma; confusion; convulsions; decreased frequency/amount of urine; depression; fever; general feeling of illness; growth or bump on skin; hostility; increase in bone pain; increased blood pressure; increased thirst; irritability; lethargy; looks very ill; loss of appetite; loss of bladder control; lower back/side pain; mole that leaks fluid or bleeds; muscle spasm or jerking of all extremities; muscle twitching; nausea; new mole; rapid weight gain; red rash with watery, yellow-colored, or pus filled blisters; redness of face; seizures; small, red skin lesion, growth, or bump usually on face, ears, neck, hands, or arms; sore that will not heal; spider-like blood vessels on the face; stupor; sudden loss of consciousness; swelling of face, ankles, lower legs, hands, or fingers; swollen glands; thick yellow to honey-colored crusts; unusual tiredness or weakness; vomiting; weight gain; weight loss; yellow skin and eyes

Some side effects may occur that usually do not need medical attention. These side effects may go away during treatment as your body adjusts to the medicine. Also, your health care professional may be able to tell you about ways to prevent or reduce some of these side effects. Check with your health care professional if any of the following side effects continue or are bothersome or if you have any questions about them:

More common
> Cough; fever; general aches and pains; headache; itching skin– in children; loss of appetite; skin burning; skin flushing in areas of ointment application when drinking alcohol; sneezing; weakness

Less common
> Acid or sour stomach; acne; back pain; belching; burning, itching, or pain in hairy areas; chills; cyst; flushing; heartburn; increased sensitivity to sunlight; increased skin sensitivity; indigestion; itching eyes; joint pain; muscle aches or pain; pain in eye; pain or tenderness around eyes and cheekbones; pus at root of hair; rash; redness in eye; runny nose; severe skin rash or hives; skin blisters—in children; skin tingling; stomach discomfort, upset, or pain; stuffy nose; swelling of eye, eyelid, or inner lining of eyelid; swollen glands; tightness of chest; troubled breathing or wheezing; watery eyes

Other side effects not listed may also occur in some patients. If you notice any other effects, check with your healthcare professional.

TADALAFIL   (Oral route) - tah-DA-la-fil

Commonly used brand name(s)

In the U.S.—
  Cialis

Available Dosage Forms:

- Tablet

Therapeutic Class: Erectile Dysfunction Agent
Pharmacologic Class: Phosphodiesterase Type 5 Inhibitor

Uses For This Medicine

Tadalafil is a medicine used to treat erectile dysfunction in men. Erectile dysfunction is a condition where the penis does not harden and expand when a man is sexually excited, or when he cannot keep an erection. When a man is sexually stimulated, his body's normal response is to increase blood flow to his penis. This results in an erection. Tadalafil helps increase blood flow to the penis and may help men with erectile dysfunction get and keep an erection satisfactory for sexual activity. Once a man has completed sexual activity, blood flow to his penis decreases, and his erection goes away.

This medicine is available only with your doctor's prescription.

Before Using This Medicine

In deciding to use a medicine, the risks of taking the medicine must be weighed against the good it will do. This is a decision you and your doctor will make. For this medicine, the following should be considered:

Allergies—Tell your doctor if you have ever had any unusual or allergic reaction to this medicine or any other medicines. Also tell your health care professional if you have any other types of allergies, such as to foods, dyes, preservatives, or animals. For non-prescription products, read the label or package ingredients carefully.

Pediatric—Tadalafil is not for use in children.

Geriatric—This medicine has been tested in a limited number of patients 65 years of age or older and has not been shown to cause different side effects or problems in older people than it does in younger adults.

Pregnancy—

	Pregnancy Category	Explanation
All Trimesters	B	Animal studies have revealed no evidence of harm to the fetus, however, there are no adequate studies in pregnant women OR animal studies have shown an adverse effect, but adequate studies in pregnant women have failed to demonstrate a risk to the fetus.

Breast Feeding—There are no adequate studies in women for determining infant risk when using this medication during breastfeeding. Weigh the potential benefits against the potential risks before taking this medication while breastfeeding.

Other medicines—

Using this medicine with any of the following medicines is not recommended. Your doctor may decide not to treat you with this medication or change some of the other medicines you take.

Erythrityl Tetranitrate, Isosorbide Dinitrate, Isosorbide Mononitrate, Nitroglycerin, Pentaerythritol Tetranitrate

Interactions with Food/Tobacco/Alcohol—Certain medicines should not be used at or around the time of eating food or eating certain types of food since interactions may occur. Using alcohol or tobacco with certain medicines may also cause interactions to occur. The following interactions have been selected on the basis of their potential significance and are not necessarily all-inclusive.

Using this medicine with any of the following may cause an increased risk of certain side effects but may be unavoidable in some cases. If used together, your doctor may change the dose or how often you use this medicine, or give you special instructions about the use of food, alcohol, or tobacco.

Ethanol

Other medical problems—The presence of other medical problems may affect the use of this medicine. Make sure you tell your doctor if you have any other medical problems, especially:

- Age greater than 50 years or
- Coronary artery disease or
- Diabetes or
- Hyperlipidemia (excess of lipids in the blood) or
- Hypertension (high blood pressure) or
- Low cup to disc ratio (' crowded disc') or
- Smoking—These conditions may increase risk for a serious eye problem called NAION.
- Angina (reoccurring chest pain) or
- Arrhythmia (irregular heartbeat) or
- Hypotension (low blood pressure) or
- Hypertension (high blood pressure) or
- Stroke (recent history of) or
- Heart attack (within the last 3 months) or

- Heart failure (within the last 6 months) or
- Retinal disorders (rare hereditary eye problem)—Tadalafil has not been studied in patients with these medical conditions and should not be used.
- Kidney disease (severe)—Tadalafil should be used with caution in these patients and a lower dose may be needed.
- Liver disease—Tadalafil should not be used in patients with serious liver disease; in patients with less serious liver disease, tadalafil should be used with caution and a lower dose may be needed.
- Abnormal penis, including curved penis and birth defects of the penis—Chance of problems occurring may be increased and this medicine should be used with caution in these patients
- Bleeding disorders or
- Stomach ulcers—Chance of problems occurring may be increased; it is not known if the medicine is safe for use in these patients.
- Heart disease, underlying—Chance of low blood pressure occurring is greater; tadalafil should be used carefully in these patients.
- Heart blood flow problems—These conditions may cause you to be more sensitive to tadalafil.
- Sickle-cell anemia (blood disorder) or
- Bone marrow cancer or
- Leukemia (blood related cancer)—Tadalafil should be used with caution in these patients as problems with prolonged erection of the penis may occur.
- NAION (serious eye condition) in one or both eyes, previously—May increase your chance of getting NAION again

Proper Use of This Medicine

Special patient directions come with tadalafil. Read the directions carefully before you start using tadalafil and each time you get a refill of your medicine.

Use tadalafil exactly as directed by your doctor. Do not use more of it and do not use it more often than your doctor ordered. If too much is used, the chance of side effects or other problems is increased.

Dosing—The dose of this medicine will be different for different patients. Follow your doctor's orders or the directions on the label. The following information includes only the average doses of this medicine. If your dose is different, do not change it unless your doctor tells you to do so.

The amount of medicine that you take depends on the strength of the medicine. Also, the number of doses you take each day, the time allowed between doses, and the length of time you take the medicine depend on the medical problem for which you are using the medicine.

- For oral dosage form (tablets):
  - For treatment of erectile dysfunction:
    - Adults—10 mg as a single dose no more than once a day, taken before you think sexual activity may occur. The ability to have sexual activity may be improved up to 36 hours after taking tadalafil when compared to placebo (sugar pill). If needed, your doctor may change your dose.

Storage—Store the medicine in a closed container at room temperature, away from heat, moisture, and direct light. Keep from freezing.

Keep out of the reach of children.

Do not keep outdated medicine or medicine no longer needed.

Ask your healthcare professional how you should dispose of any medicine you do not use.

Precautions While Using This Medicine

Tadalafil has not been studied with other medicines used for treatment of erectile dysfunction. Using them together is not recommended.

It is important that you tell all of your healthcare providers that you take tadalafil. If you need emergency medical care for a heart problem, it is important that your healthcare provider knows when you last took tadalafil.

If you experience a prolonged or painful erection for 4 hours or more, contact your doctor immediately. This condition may require prompt medical treatment to prevent serious and permanent damage to your penis.

This medicine does not protect you against sexually transmitted diseases. Use protective measures and ask your doctor if you have any questions about this.

It is important to tell your doctor about any heart problems you may have now or may have had in the past. This medicine can cause serious side effects in patients with heart problems.

Do not drink alcohol to excess (for example, 5 glasses of wine or 5 shots of whiskey) when taking tadalafil. When taken in excess alcohol can increase your chances of getting a headache or getting dizzy, increasing your heart rate, or lowering your blood pressure.

If you experience sudden loss of vision in one or both eyes, stop using tadalafil and contact your doctor immediately.

Side Effects of This Medicine

Along with its needed effects, a medicine may cause some unwanted effects. Although not all of these side effects may occur, if they do occur they may need medical attention.

Check with your doctor immediately if any of the following side effects occur:

Less common
Arm, back or jaw pain; blurred vision; chest pain or discomfort; chest tightness or heaviness; chills; cold sweats; confusion; dizziness; fainting; faintness, or lightheadedness when getting up from a lying or sitting position suddenly; fast or irregular heartbeat; headache; nausea; nervousness; pain or discomfort in arms, jaw, back or neck; pounding in the ears; shortness of breath; slow or fast heartbeat; sweating; unusual tiredness or weakness; vomiting

Rare
Painful or prolonged erection of the penis

Incidence not known
Abdominal or stomach pain; blistering, peeling, loosening of skin; cracks in the skin; decrease or change in vision; difficulty in speaking; double vision; hives or welts; inability to move arms, legs, or facial muscles; inability to speak; loss of heat from the body; numbness or tingling of face, hands or feet; red irritated eyes; red skin lesions, often with a purple center; red, swollen skin; redness or soreness of eyes; redness of skin;

scaly skin; slow speech; sore throat; sores in mouth; swelling of feet or lower legs

Some side effects may occur that usually do not need medical attention. These side effects may go away during treatment as your body adjusts to the medicine. Also, your health care professional may be able to tell you about ways to prevent or reduce some of these side effects. Check with your health care professional if any of the following side effects continue or are bothersome or if you have any questions about them:

More common
Acid or sour stomach; belching; heartburn; indigestion; stomach discomfort, upset, or pain

Less common
Bloody nose; burning, crawling, itching, numbness, prickling, "pins and needles", or tingling feelings; burning feeling in chest or stomach; burning, dry or itching eyes; body aches or pain; congestion; cough; diarrhea; difficulty in moving; difficulty swallowing; dry mouth; dryness or soreness of throat; eye pain; excessive eye discharge; fever; feeling of constant movement of self or surroundings; feeling of warmth redness of the face, neck, arms and occasionally, upper chest; hoarseness; increased erection; itching skin; joint pain; lack or loss of strength; loose stools; muscle aching or cramping; muscle pains or stiffness; nasal congestion; neck pain; pain; pain in arms and/or legs; pain or burning in throat; rash; redness, pain, swelling of eye, eyelid, or inner lining of eyelid; reduced sensitivity to touch; runny nose; sensation of spinning; sleepiness or unusual drowsiness; sleeplessness; sores, ulcers, or white spots on lips or tongue or inside the mouth; spontaneous penile erection; stomach upset; swelling of eyelids; swelling or puffiness of eye or face; swollen joints; tearing; tender, swollen glands in neck; tenderness in stomach area; trouble sleeping; unable to sleep; upper abdominal pain; voice changes; watering of eyes

Other side effects not listed may also occur in some patients. If you notice any other effects, check with your healthcare professional.

Rare
Changes in color vision

TAMOXIFEN   (Oral route) - ta-MOX-i-fen

Black Box Warning

For Women with Ductal Carcinoma in Situ (DCIS) and Women at High Risk for Breast Cancer: Serious and life-threatening events associated with tamoxifen citrate in the risk reduction setting (women at high risk for cancer and women with DCIS) include uterine malignancies, stroke and pulmonary embolism. Incidence rates for these events were estimated from the National Surgical Adjuvant Breast and Bowel Project's P-1 (NSABP P-1) trial. Uterine malignancies consist of both endometrial adenocarcinoma (incidence rate per 1,000 women-years of 2.20 for tamoxifen citrate versus 0.71 for placebo) and uterine sarcoma (incidence rate per 1,000 women-years of 0.17 for tamoxifen citrate versus 0.4 for placebo). For stroke, the incidence rate per 1,000 women-years was 1.43 for tamoxifen citrate versus

1 for placebo. For pulmonary embolism, the incidence rate per 1,000 women-years was 0.75 for tamoxifen citrate versus 0.25 for placebo.

Some of the strokes, pulmonary emboli, and uterine malignancies were fatal.

Health care providers should discuss the potential benefits versus the potential risks of these serious events with women at high risk of breast cancer and women with DCIS considering tamoxifen citrate to reduce their risk of developing breast cancer.

The benefits of tamoxifen citrate outweigh its risks in women already diagnosed with breast cancer.

Commonly used brand name(s)

In the U.S.—
Nolvadex
Soltamox

Available Dosage Forms:
- Solution
- Tablet

Therapeutic Class: Antiestrogen

Uses For This Medicine

Tamoxifen is a medicine that blocks the effects of the estrogen hormone in the body. It is used to treat breast cancer in women or men. It may also be used to treat other kinds of cancer, as determined by your doctor.

Tamoxifen also may be used to reduce the risk of developing breast cancer in women who have a high risk of developing breast cancer. Women at high risk for developing breast cancer are at least 35 years of age and have a combination of risk factors that make their chance of developing breast cancer 1.67% or more over the next 5 years. Your doctor will help to determine your risk of developing breast cancer.

   The following are risk factors that may increase your chance of developing breast cancer:
   - If you have close family members (mother, sister, or daughter) with breast cancer
   - If you have ever had a breast biopsy or if high-risk changes in your breast(s) have been found from a breast biopsy
   - If you have never been pregnant or if your first pregnancy occurred at a late age
   - If your first menstrual period occurred at an early age

The exact way that tamoxifen works against cancer is not known, but it may be related to the way it blocks the effects of estrogen on the body.

Before you begin treatment with tamoxifen, you and your doctor should talk about the good this medicine will do as well as the risks of using it.

Tamoxifen is available only with your doctor's prescription.

Once a medicine has been approved for marketing for a certain use, experience may show that it is also useful for other medical problems. Although these uses are not included in product labeling, tamoxifen is used in certain patients with the following medical conditions:
   - Malignant melanoma (a certain type of skin cancer)
   - Cancer of the endometrium (lining of the uterus)

Before Using This Medicine

In deciding to use a medicine, the risks of taking the medicine must be weighed against the good it will do. This is a decision you and your doctor will make. For this medicine, the following should be considered:

Allergies—Tell your doctor if you have ever had any unusual or allergic reaction to this medicine or any other medicines. Also tell your health care professional if you have any other types of allergies, such as to foods, dyes, preservatives, or animals. For non-prescription products, read the label or package ingredients carefully.

Geriatric—Many medicines have not been studied specifically in older people. Therefore, it may not be known whether they work exactly the same way they do in younger adults. Although there is no specific information comparing use of tamoxifen in the elderly with use in other age groups, this medicine is not expected to cause different side effects or problems in older people than it does in younger adults.

Pregnancy—

	Pregnancy Category	Explanation
All Trimesters	D	Studies in pregnant women have demonstrated a risk to the fetus. However, the benefits of therapy in a life threatening situation or a serious disease, may outweigh the potential risk.

Breast Feeding—There are no adequate studies in women for determining infant risk when using this medication during breastfeeding. Weigh the potential benefits against the potential risks before taking this medication while breastfeeding.

Other medicines—

Using this medicine with any of the following medicines is usually not recommended, but may be required in some cases. If both medicines are prescribed together, your doctor may change the dose or how often you use one or both of the medicines.

Acenocoumarol, Cyclophosphamide, Dicumarol, Fluorouracil, Genistein, Ipriflavone, Methotrexate, Mitomycin, Phenprocoumon, Red Clover, St John's Wort, Warfarin

Interactions with Food/Tobacco/Alcohol—Certain medicines should not be used at or around the time of eating food or eating certain types of food since interactions may occur. Using alcohol or tobacco with certain medicines may also cause interactions to occur. Discuss with your healthcare professional the use of your medicine with food, alcohol, or tobacco.

Other medical problems—The presence of other medical problems may affect the use of this medicine. Make sure you tell your doctor if you have any other medical problems, especially:
   For all patients
   - Blood problems or
   - Cataracts or other eye problems—Tamoxifen may also cause these problems
   - High cholesterol levels in the blood—Tamoxifen can increase cholesterol levels
   When used for reducing the risk for developing breast cancer in high-risk women or in women with Ductal Carcinoma in Situ (DCIS)

- Blood clots (or history of) or
- Pulmonary embolism (or history of) or
- Stroke or
- Uterine (womb) cancer—May increase risk of serious side effects from tamoxifen.

Proper Use of This Medicine

Use this medicine only as directed by your doctor. Do not use more or less of it, and do not use it more often than your doctor ordered. The exact amount of medicine you need has been carefully worked out. Taking too much may increase the chance of side effects, while taking too little may not improve your condition.

Tamoxifen sometimes causes mild nausea and vomiting. However, it may have to be taken for several weeks or months to be effective. Even if you begin to feel ill, do not stop using this medicine without first checking with your doctor. Ask your health care professional for ways to lessen these effects.

Swallow the tablets whole with a drink of water. You can take the tablets with or without food.

If you vomit shortly after taking a dose of tamoxifen, check with your doctor. You will be told whether to take the dose again or to wait until the next scheduled dose.

Dosing—The dose of this medicine will be different for different patients. Follow your doctor's orders or the directions on the label. The following information includes only the average doses of this medicine. If your dose is different, do not change it unless your doctor tells you to do so.

The amount of medicine that you take depends on the strength of the medicine. Also, the number of doses you take each day, the time allowed between doses, and the length of time you take the medicine depend on the medical problem for which you are using the medicine.

- For oral dosage form (tablets)
  - For breast cancer in women or men:
    - Adults—20 to 40 milligrams (mg) daily.
  - For reducing the risk of developing breast cancer in high-risk women:
    - Adults—20 milligrams (mg) a day, for five years
  - For reducing the risk of developing invasive breast cancer in women with ductal carcinoma in situ:
    - Adults—20 milligrams (mg) a day, for five years

Missed dose—If you miss a dose of this medicine, skip the missed dose and go back to your regular dosing schedule. Do not double doses.

Call your doctor or pharmacist for instructions.

Storage—Store the medicine in a closed container at room temperature, away from heat, moisture, and direct light. Keep from freezing.

Keep out of the reach of children.

Do not keep outdated medicine or medicine no longer needed.

Precautions While Using This Medicine

It is very important that your doctor check your progress at regular visits to make sure that this medicine is working properly and to check for unwanted effects.

A woman should contact her healthcare profession right away if she develops:

- Changes in vaginal discharge or
- Changes in vision or
- Coughing up blood or
- Leg swelling or tenderness or
- Menstrual irregularities or
- New breast lumps or
- Pelvic pain or pressure or
- Sudden chest pain or
- Unexplained shortness of breath or
- Vaginal bleeding

If you seek medical attention for any reason, be sure to tell your healthcare professional that you take tamoxifen or have taken tamoxifen.

For women: Tamoxifen may make you more fertile. It is best to use some type of birth control while you are taking it. However, do not use oral contraceptives ("the Pill") since they may change the effects of tamoxifen. Tell your doctor right away if you think you have become pregnant while taking this medicine.

Side Effects of This Medicine

Along with its needed effects, a medicine may cause some unwanted effects. Some side effects will have signs or symptoms that you can see or feel. Your doctor will watch for others by doing certain tests.

Also, because of the way this medicine acts on the body, there is a chance that it might cause other unwanted effects that may not occur until months or years after the medicine is used. Tamoxifen increases the chance of cancer of the uterus (womb) in some women taking it. Tamoxifen may cause blockages to form in a vein, lung, or brain. In women, tamoxifen may cause cancer or other problems of the uterus (womb). It also causes liver cancer in rats. In addition, tamoxifen has been reported to cause cataracts and other eye problems. Discuss these possible effects with your doctor.

Check with your doctor as soon as possible if any of the following side effects occur:

For both females and males
  Less common or rare
    Anxiety; blistering, peeling, or loosening of skin and mucous membranes; blurred vision; chest pain; confusion; cough; dizziness; fainting; fast heartbeat; lightheadedness; pain or swelling in legs; shortness of breath or trouble breathing; weakness or sleepiness; yellow eyes or skin

For females only
  Less common or rare
    Change in vaginal discharge; chills; fever; hoarseness; lower back or side pain; pain or feeling of pressure in pelvis; pain, redness, or swelling in your arm or leg; painful or difficult urination; rapid shallow breathing; skin rash or itching over the entire body; sweating; vaginal bleeding; wheezing

For females and males
  Frequency not determined
    Bloating; constipation; darkened urine; diarrhea; difficult breathing; indigestion; itching; joint or muscle pain; large, hard skin blisters; large hive-like swelling on face, eyelids, lips, tongue, throat, hands, legs, feet, and sex organs; loss of appetite; nausea; pain in stomach or side, possibly radiating to the back; red, irritated eyes; red skin lesions, often with a

purple center; sore throat; sores, ulcers or white spots in mouth or on lips; unusual tiredness or weakness; vomiting

This medicine may also cause the following side effect that your doctor will watch for:

For both females and males
Less common or rare
Cataracts in the eyes or other eye problems; liver problems

Some side effects may occur that usually do not need medical attention. These side effects may go away during treatment as your body adjusts to the medicine. Also, your health care professional may be able to tell you about ways to prevent or reduce some of these side effects. Check with your health care professional if any of the following side effects continue or are bothersome or if you have any questions about them:

For both females and males
Less common
Bone pain; headache; nausea and/or vomiting (mild); skin rash or dryness

For females only
More common
Absent, missed, or irregular periods; confusion; decrease in amount of urine; feeling of warmth redness of the face, neck, arms and occasionally, upper chest; lower back or side pain; menstrual changes; nausea; noisy, rattling breathing; painful or difficult urination; rapid, shallow breathing; skin changes; stopping of menstrual bleeding; swelling of fingers, hands, feet, or lower legs; troubled breathing at rest; vaginal bleeding; weight gain; weight loss; white or brownish vaginal discharge

Less common or rare
Abdominal cramps; black, tarry stools; bleeding gums; blood in urine or stools; Bluish color changes in skin color; discouragement; feeling sad or empty; irritability; itching in genital area; lack of appetite; loss of interest or pleasure; pain; pinpoint red spots on skin; stomach or pelvic discomfort, aching or heaviness; swelling; trouble concentrating; trouble sleeping; unusual bleeding or bruising

For males only
Less common
Decreased interest in sexual intercourse; inability to have or keep an erection; loss in sexual ability, desire, drive, or performance

This medicine may infrequently cause hair thinning or partial loss of hair.

Other side effects not listed may also occur in some patients. If you notice any other effects, check with your healthcare professional.

TAMSULOSIN (Oral route) - tam-SOO-loe-sin

Commonly used brand name(s)
In the U.S.—
Flomax

Available Dosage Forms:
• Capsule

Therapeutic Class: Benign Prostatic Hypertrophy Agent
Pharmacologic Class: Alpha-1 Adrenergic Blocker

Uses For This Medicine

Tamsulosin is used to treat the signs and symptoms of benign enlargement of the prostate (benign prostatic hyperplasia or BPH). Benign enlargement of the prostate is a problem that can occur in men as they get older. The prostate gland is located below the bladder. As the prostate gland enlarges, certain muscles in the gland may become tight and get in the way of the tube that drains urine from the bladder. This can cause problems in urinating, such as a need to urinate often, a weak stream when urinating, or a feeling of not being able to empty the bladder completely.

Tamsulosin helps relax the muscles in the prostate and the opening of the bladder. This may help increase the flow of urine and/or decrease the symptoms. However, tamsulosin will not shrink the prostate. The prostate may continue to get larger. This may cause the symptoms to become worse over time. Therefore, even though tamsulosin may lessen the problems caused by enlarged prostate now, surgery still may be needed in the future.

This medicine is available only with your doctor's prescription.

Before Using This Medicine

In deciding to use a medicine, the risks of taking the medicine must be weighed against the good it will do. This is a decision you and your doctor will make. For this medicine, the following should be considered:

Allergies—Tell your doctor if you have ever had any unusual or allergic reaction to this medicine or any other medicines. Also tell your health care professional if you have any other types of allergies, such as to foods, dyes, preservatives, or animals. For non-prescription products, read the label or package ingredients carefully.

Geriatric—This medicine has been tested and has not been shown to cause different side effects or problems in older people than it does in younger adults. However, older people may be more sensitive to the effects of this medicine.

Pregnancy—

	Pregnancy Category	Explanation
All Trimesters	B	Animal studies have revealed no evidence of harm to the fetus, however, there are no adequate studies in pregnant women OR animal studies have shown an adverse effect, but adequate studies in pregnant women have failed to demonstrate a risk to the fetus.

Breast Feeding—There are no adequate studies in women for determining infant risk when using this medication during breastfeeding. Weigh the potential benefits against the potential risks before taking this medication while breastfeeding.

Other medicines—

Using this medicine with any of the following medicines is usually not recommended, but may be required in some cases. If both medicines are prescribed together, your doctor

may change the dose or how often you use one or both of the medicines.

Vardenafil

Interactions with Food/Tobacco/Alcohol—Certain medicines should not be used at or around the time of eating food or eating certain types of food since interactions may occur. Using alcohol or tobacco with certain medicines may also cause interactions to occur. Discuss with your healthcare professional the use of your medicine with food, alcohol, or tobacco.

Other medical problems—The presence of other medical problems may affect the use of this medicine. Make sure you tell your doctor if you have any other medical problems, especially:

- Cataract surgery—An eye problem called Intraoperative Floppy Iris Syndrome (IFIS) has occurred in patients who are taking or who have recently taken this medicine when they are having cataract surgery. You should tell your eye doctor before your surgery if you are taking or have taken tamsulosin in the past 9 months.
- Sulfa drug (antibiotics such as sulfamethoxazole/trimethoprim [e.g., Bactrim, Septra]) allergy—An allergic reaction to tamsulosin has been rarely reported in patients with sulfa allergy. If you have ever had a serious or life-threatening sulfa allergy, you should tell your doctor before taking tamsulosin.

Proper Use of This Medicine

To help you remember to take your medicine, try to get into the habit of taking it at the same time each day. Take it approximately 30 minutes after the same meal each day.

Swallow the capsules whole. Do not crush, chew, or open them, unless otherwise directed by your doctor.

Dosing—The dose of this medicine will be different for different patients. Follow your doctor's orders or the directions on the label. The following information includes only the average doses of this medicine. If your dose is different, do not change it unless your doctor tells you to do so.

The amount of medicine that you take depends on the strength of the medicine. Also, the number of doses you take each day, the time allowed between doses, and the length of time you take the medicine depend on the medical problem for which you are using the medicine.

- For oral dosage form (capsules):
  - For benign enlargement of the prostate:
    - Adults—At first, 0.4 milligram (mg) once a day, about thirty minutes after the same meal each day. Your doctor may increase the dose if necessary.

Missed dose—If you miss a dose of this medicine, skip the missed dose and go back to your regular dosing schedule. Do not double doses.

Storage—Store the medicine in a closed container at room temperature, away from heat, moisture, and direct light. Keep from freezing.

Keep out of the reach of children.

Do not keep outdated medicine or medicine no longer needed.

Precautions While Using This Medicine

It is important that your doctor check your progress at regular visits to make sure that this medicine is working properly.

Dizziness, lightheadedness, or fainting may occur after you take this medicine, especially when you get up from a lying or sitting position. Getting up slowly may help lessen this problem. *If you feel dizzy, lie down so you do not faint.* Then sit for a few moments before standing to prevent the dizziness from returning.

Because tamsulosin may cause some people to become dizzy, *make sure you know how you react to this medicine before you drive, use machines, or do anything else that could be dangerous if you are dizzy.*

You should seek medical attention right away, if you experience a prolonged erection. This is an extremely rare side effect, but if it goes untreated, can result in permanent erectile dysfunction (impotence).

Side Effects of This Medicine

Along with its needed effects, a medicine may cause some unwanted effects. Although not all of these side effects may occur, if they do occur they may need medical attention.

Some side effects may occur that usually do not need medical attention. These side effects may go away during treatment as your body adjusts to the medicine. Also, your health care professional may be able to tell you about ways to prevent or reduce some of these side effects. Check with your health care professional if any of the following side effects continue or are bothersome or if you have any questions about them:

More common

Abnormal ejaculation; back pain; diarrhea; dizziness; headache; stuffy or runny nose; unusual weakness

Less common

Chest pain; decreased sexual drive or performance; difficulty in sleeping; drowsiness; fainting or lightheadedness, especially when getting up from a lying or sitting position; nausea

Other side effects not listed may also occur in some patients. If you notice any other effects, check with your healthcare professional.

TAZAROTENE (Topical route) - taz-AR-oh-teen

Commonly used brand name(s)

In the U.S.—
Avage
Tazorac

Available Dosage Forms:
- Gel/Jelly
- Cream

Therapeutic Class: Dermatological Agent

Uses For This Medicine

Tazarotene is used to treat acne on the face and and to treat psoriasis.

It works to help clear acne on the face partly by keeping skin pores clear. It works in the treatment of psoriasis by making the skin less red and reducing the number and size of lesions of the skin.

This medicine is available only with your doctor's prescription.

Before Using This Medicine

In deciding to use a medicine, the risks of taking the medicine must be weighed against the good it will do. This is a decision you and your doctor will make. For this medicine, the following should be considered:

Allergies—Tell your doctor if you have ever had any unusual or allergic reaction to this medicine or any other medicines. Also tell your health care professional if you have any other types of allergies, such as to foods, dyes, preservatives, or animals. For non-prescription products, read the label or package ingredients carefully.

Pediatric—Studies of this medicine have been done only in adult patients, and there is no specific information comparing use of tazarotene in children up to 12 years of age (gel) and up to 18 years of age (cream) with use in other age groups.

Geriatric—Many medicines have not been studied specifically in older people. Therefore, it may not be known whether or not they work in exactly the same way they do in younger adults or if they cause different side effects or problems in older people. There is no specific information comparing the use of tazarotene in the elderly with use in other age groups.

Pregnancy—

	Pregnancy Category	Explanation
All Trimesters	X	Studies in animals or pregnant women have demonstrated positive evidence of fetal abnormalities. This drug should not be used in women who are or may become pregnant because the risk clearly outweighs any possible benefit.

Breast Feeding—There are no adequate studies in women for determining infant risk when using this medication during breastfeeding. Weigh the potential benefits against the potential risks before taking this medication while breastfeeding.

Other medicines—Although certain medicines should not be used together at all, in other cases two different medicines may be used together even if an interaction might occur. In these cases, your doctor may want to change the dose, or other precautions may be necessary. Tell your healthcare professional if you are taking any other prescription or non-prescription (over-the-counter [OTC]) medicine.

Interactions with Food/Tobacco/Alcohol—Certain medicines should not be used at or around the time of eating food or eating certain types of food since interactions may occur. Using alcohol or tobacco with certain medicines may also cause interactions to occur. Discuss with your healthcare professional the use of your medicine with food, alcohol, or tobacco.

Other medical problems—The presence of other medical problems may affect the use of this medicine. Make sure you tell your doctor if you have any other medical problems, especially:
- Eczema—Tazarotene may cause skin irritation and may worsen this condition

Proper Use of This Medicine

It is very important that you use this medicine only as directed. Do not use more of it, do not use it more often, and do not use it for a longer time than your doctor ordered. To do so may cause irritation of the skin.

Read the patient information that will come with your medicine.

For acne—Before applying tazarotene to acne areas of the skin, wash the skin with a mild soap or cleanser and warm water, then gently pat dry. Wait at least 20 to 30 minutes before applying this medicine.

For acne or psoriasis—*Do not use this medicine in or around the eyes or lips, or inside of the nose*. Spread the medicine away form these areas when applying

Do not apply this medicine to windburned or sunburned skin or on open wounds.

When using tazarotene, apply medicine to dry skin. If skin has just been washed and dried, *wait at least 20 to 30 minutes before applying this medicine*. Applying to wet or damp skin may cause skin irritation.

Apply a thin layer of this medicine only to lesions of psoriasis on the body or areas on face prone to developing acne. Rub medicine in gently and well. Wash medicine off skin areas not intended to be treated.

After applying the medicine, wash your hands to remove any medicine that might remain on them.

Dosing—The dose of this medicine will be different for different patients. Follow your doctor's orders or the directions on the label. The following information includes only the average doses of this medicine. If your dose is different, do not change it unless your doctor tells you to do so.

The amount of medicine that you take depends on the strength of the medicine. Also, the number of doses you take each day, the time allowed between doses, and the length of time you take the medicine depend on the medical problem for which you are using the medicine.

- For topical dosage form (gel):
  - For acne:
    - Adults and children 12 years of age and older—Apply 0.1% tazarotene to clean, dry affected areas of the face once a day, usually in the evening or at bedtime.
    - Children up to 12 years of age—Use and dose must be determined by the doctor.
  - For psoriasis:
    - Adults and children 12 years of age and older—Apply 0.05% or 0.1% tazarotene to dry affected areas of the body once a day, usually in the evening or at bedtime. Do not treat a larger area of the skin than your doctor tells you to treat.
    - Children up to 12 years of age—Use and dose must be determined by the doctor.
- For topical dosage form (cream):
  - For psoriasis:
    - Adults and children 18 years of age and older—Apply 0.05% or 0.1% tazarotene to dry affected areas of the body once a day, usually in the evening or at bedtime. Do not treat a larger area of the skin than your doctor tells you to treat.
    - Children up to 18 years of age—Use and dose must be determined by the doctor.

Missed dose—If you miss a dose of this medicine, skip the missed dose and go back to your regular dosing schedule. Do not double doses.

Storage—Store the medicine in a closed container at room temperature, away from heat, moisture, and direct light. Keep from freezing.

Keep out of the reach of children.

Do not keep outdated medicine or medicine no longer needed.

Precautions While Using This Medicine

If you think that you may be pregnant, stop using the medicine immediately and check with your doctor.

If you are using this medicine to treat acne of the face, your condition may seem to worsen at first before it begins to improve in about 4 weeks. Check with your doctor if your condition does not improve within 8 to 12 weeks.

If your are using this medicine to treat psoriasis, scaly patches on skin may begin to improve in about 1 to 4 weeks but redness may take longer to improve. Check with your doctor if your condition becomes worse.

Do not cover the treated area with a bandage.

When using tazarotene, do not use skin products such as abrasive soaps or cleansers; alcohol-containing products; cosmetics or soaps that dry the skin; hair products that are irritating, such as permanents or hair removal products; skin products containing spices, limes, or other ingredients that may make the skin more sensitive to the sun; or other topical medicine for the skin on the same area as tazarotene, unless otherwise directed. To do so may cause severe irritation of the skin.

Ask your doctor before taking vitamin A supplements by mouth while using this medicine.

During treatment with this medicine, avoid exposing the treated areas to sunlight when possible, since the skin may be more likely to become sunburned. Do not use a sunlamp.

Some people who use this medicine may become more sensitive to wind or cold weather, as well as to sunlight. Avoiding exposure to these conditions by using sunscreen products with a sun protection factor (SPF) of 15 or more and wearing protective clothing will help protect your skin against becoming too dry, irritated, or sunburned.

Side Effects of This Medicine

It is likely that your skin may become irritated with normal use of this medicine. You should not stop using tazarotene unless your skin becomes too red, dry, puffy, or otherwise irritated. If severe irritation occurs, contact your doctor.

Along with its needed effects, a medicine may cause some unwanted effects. Although not all of these side effects may occur, if they do occur they may need medical attention.

Check with your doctor as soon as possible if any of the following side effects occur:
> *More common*
>> Burning or stinging of the skin (severe); changes in color of treated skin; deep grooves or lines in skin; dryness, itching, peeling, or redness of the skin (severe); pain or swelling of treated skin; skin rash (in patients with psoriasis only)

Some side effects may occur that usually do not need medical attention. These side effects may go away during treatment as your body adjusts to the medicine. Also, your health care professional may be able to tell you about ways to pre-

vent or reduce some of these side effects. Check with your health care professional if any of the following side effects continue or are bothersome or if you have any questions about them:
> *More common*
>> Burning or stinging after application; dryness, itching, peeling, or redness of the skin (mild)

Other side effects not listed may also occur in some patients. If you notice any other effects, check with your healthcare professional.

TEGASEROD (Oral route) - teg-a-SER-od

Commonly used brand name(s)
In the U.S.—
 Zelnorm

Available Dosage Forms:
 • Tablet

Therapeutic Class: Gastrointestinal Agent
Pharmacologic Class: Serotonin Receptor Agonist, 5–HT4

Uses For This Medicine

Tegaserod is a medicine for short term treatment of women who have irritable bowel syndrome (IBS) with constipation (not enough or hard bowel movements) as their main bowel problem. Tegaserod is also used to treat women younger than 65 years of age who have chronic constipation with an unknown cause. Tegaserod increases the movement of stools (bowel movement) through the bowels. Tegaserod does not cure irritable bowel syndrome. Tegaserod decreases pain and discomfort in the abdominal area, bloating, and constipation. If you stop taking tegaserod your irritable bowel syndrome symptoms may return in one to two weeks.

This medicine is available only with your healthcare professional's prescription.

Before Using This Medicine

In deciding to use a medicine, the risks of taking the medicine must be weighed against the good it will do. This is a decision you and your doctor will make. For this medicine, the following should be considered:

Allergies—Tell your doctor if you have ever had any unusual or allergic reaction to this medicine or any other medicines. Also tell your health care professional if you have any other types of allergies, such as to foods, dyes, preservatives, or animals. For non-prescription products, read the label or package ingredients carefully.

Pediatric—Studies on this medicine have been done only in adult patients and there is no specific information comparing the use of tegaserod in children and adolescents under the age of 18 with use in other age groups.

Geriatric—Many medicines have not been specifically studied in older people. Therefore it may not be known whether they work the same way they do in younger adults or if they cause different side effects or problems in older people. There is no specific information comparing the use of tegaserod in older patients with use in other age groups for treatment of irritable bowel syndrome

This medicine is not approved for patients 65 years of age or older for treatment of chronic constipation.

Pregnancy—

	Pregnancy Category	Explanation
All Trimesters	B	Animal studies have revealed no evidence of harm to the fetus, however, there are no adequate studies in pregnant women OR animal studies have shown an adverse effect, but adequate studies in pregnant women have failed to demonstrate a risk to the fetus.

Breast Feeding—There are no adequate studies in women for determining infant risk when using this medication during breastfeeding. Weigh the potential benefits against the potential risks before taking this medication while breastfeeding.

Other medicines—Although certain medicines should not be used together at all, in other cases two different medicines may be used together even if an interaction might occur. In these cases, your doctor may want to change the dose, or other precautions may be necessary. Tell your healthcare professional if you are taking any other prescription or nonprescription (over-the-counter [OTC]) medicine.

Interactions with Food/Tobacco/Alcohol—Certain medicines should not be used at or around the time of eating food or eating certain types of food since interactions may occur. Using alcohol or tobacco with certain medicines may also cause interactions to occur. Discuss with your healthcare professional the use of your medicine with food, alcohol, or tobacco.

Other medical problems—The presence of other medical problems may affect the use of this medicine. Make sure you tell your doctor if you have any other medical problems, especially:

- Abdominal adhesions or
- Bowel obstructions or intestinal blockage (or history of) or
- Gallbladder disease or gallstones (or history of) or
- Liver disease or
- Kidney disease or
- Sphincter of Oddi dysfunction (severe stomach pain with nausea and vomiting)—Tegaserod should not be used if you have any of these conditions
- Abdominal pain, new or sudden worsening of—Tegaserod should be stopped immediately
- Diarrhea—Serious side effects such as dizziness, lightheadedness, and dehydration can occur when using tegaserod. If you have any of these symptoms, notify your doctor immediately and stop taking this medicine. Tegaserod should not be used if you are currently experiencing or frequently experience diarrhea.

Proper Use of This Medicine

Dosing—The dose of this medicine will be different for different patients. Follow your doctor's orders or the directions on the label. The following information includes only the average doses of this medicine. If your dose is different, do not change it unless your doctor tells you to do so.

The amount of medicine that you take depends on the strength of the medicine. Also, the number of doses you take each day, the time allowed between doses, and the length of time you take the medicine depend on the medical problem for which you are using the medicine.

- For oral dosage form (tablets):
  - For chronic constipation:
    - Adults—Oral, 6 milligrams (mg) twice daily on an empty stomach shortly before you eat a meal. Your doctor will decide how long you should continue to take this medicine.
  - For irritable bowel syndrome:
    - Adults—Oral, 6 milligrams (mg) twice daily on an empty stomach shortly before you eat a meal. You will take tegaserod for 4 to 6 weeks. If you feel better your healthcare professional might want to continue the medicine for an additional 4 to 6 weeks.

Missed dose—If you miss a dose of this medicine, skip the missed dose and go back to your regular dosing schedule. Do not double doses.

Storage—Store the medicine in a closed container at room temperature, away from heat, moisture, and direct light. Keep from freezing.

Keep out of the reach of children.

Do not keep outdated medicine or medicine no longer needed.

Ask your healthcare professional how you should dispose of any medicine you do not use.

Precautions While Using This Medicine

Your healthcare professional will want to check your progress at regular visits, especially during the first few weeks that you take this medicine.

It is important to check with your healthcare professional or pharmacist if you are taking or plan to take any prescription or over-the-counter medicines while taking tegaserod

It is very important to tell your healthcare professional immediately if you become pregnant

You should consult your healthcare professional if you experience severe diarrhea, or if the diarrhea is accompanied by severe cramping, abdominal pain, or dizziness. You should also consult your healthcare professional if you experience new or worsening abdominal pain.

Do not take this medication if you have diarrhea now or have diarrhea often.

This medicine may cause some people to become dizzy. Make sure you know how you react to this medicine before you drive, use machines, or do anything else that could be dangerous if you are dizzy.

Side Effects of This Medicine

Along with its needed effects, a medicine may cause some unwanted effects. Although not all of these side effects may occur, if they do occur they may need medical attention.

Check with your doctor immediately if any of the following side effects occur:

More common

Diarrhea; stomach pain

Less common

Dizziness; feeling of warmth; itching skin; redness of the face, neck, arms and occasionally, upper chest; swelling or puffiness of face

Frequency not determined

Black, tarry stools; bloody diarrhea; bloody stools; constipation; fainting; indigestion; nausea; new or worsening abdominal pain; rectal bleeding; severe stomach pain with nausea and vomiting; vomiting

Symptoms of overdose

Get emergency help immediately if any of the following symptoms of overdose occur:

Bloated, full feeling; chills; cold sweats; confusion; diarrhea; dizziness, faintness, or lightheadedness when getting up from lying or sitting position; excess air or gas in stomach or intestines; headache; nausea; passing gas; stomach pain; vomiting

Some side effects may occur that usually do not need medical attention. These side effects may go away during treatment as your body adjusts to the medicine. Also, your health care professional may be able to tell you about ways to prevent or reduce some of these side effects. Check with your health care professional if any of the following side effects continue or are bothersome or if you have any questions about them:

More common

Bloated, full feeling; excess air or gas in stomach or intestines; headache; nausea; passing gas

Less common or rare

Back pain; disease or abnormality of the joint; headache, severe and throbbing; leg pain

Other side effects not listed may also occur in some patients. If you notice any other effects, check with your healthcare professional.

TELITHROMYCIN (Oral route) - tel-ith-roe-MYE-sin

Commonly used brand name(s)

In the U.S.—

Ketek

Ketek Pak

Available Dosage Forms:

• Tablet

Therapeutic Class: Antibiotic

Uses For This Medicine

Telithromycin belongs to the family of medicines called antibiotics. Antibiotics are medicines used in the treatment of infections caused by bacteria. They work by killing bacteria or preventing their growth. However, this medicine will not work for colds, flu, or other virus infections.

This medicine is available only with your doctor's prescription.

Before Using This Medicine

In deciding to use a medicine, the risks of taking the medicine must be weighed against the good it will do. This is a decision you and your doctor will make. For this medicine, the following should be considered:

Allergies—Tell your doctor if you have ever had any unusual or allergic reaction to this medicine or any other medicines. Also tell your health care professional if you have any other types of allergies, such as to foods, dyes, preservatives, or animals. For non-prescription products, read the label or package ingredients carefully.

Pediatric—Studies on this medicine have been done only in adult patients, and there is no specific information comparing the use of telithromycin in children with use in other age groups.

Geriatric—This medicine has been tested in a limited number of elderly patients and has not been shown to cause different side effects or problems in older people than it does in younger adults.

Pregnancy—

	Pregnancy Category	Explanation
All Trimesters	C	Animal studies have shown an adverse effect and there are no adequate studies in pregnant women OR no animal studies have been conducted and there are no adequate studies in pregnant women.

Breast Feeding—There are no adequate studies in women for determining infant risk when using this medication during breastfeeding. Weigh the potential benefits against the potential risks before taking this medication while breastfeeding.

Other medicines—

Using this medicine with any of the following medicines is not recommended. Your doctor may decide not to treat you with this medication or change some of the other medicines you take.

Bepridil, Cisapride, Mesoridazine, Pimozide, Terfenadine, Thioridazine, Ziprasidone

Interactions with Food/Tobacco/Alcohol—Certain medicines should not be used at or around the time of eating food or eating certain types of food since interactions may occur. Using alcohol or tobacco with certain medicines may also cause interactions to occur. Discuss with your healthcare professional the use of your medicine with food, alcohol, or tobacco.

Other medical problems—The presence of other medical problems may affect the use of this medicine. Make sure you tell your doctor if you have any other medical problems, especially:

• Bradycardia (slow heartbeat) or

• Heart rhythm problems or

• Hypokalemia (not enough potassium in your blood) or

• Hypomagnesemia (not enough magnesium in your blood) or

- QTc prolongation (rare heart rhythm problem)—Telithromycin may cause these conditions to become worse.
- Hepatitis or
- Jaundice or
- Other liver problems—This medicine should not be used in patients who have had hepatitis or jaundice related to telithromycin use or any other macrolide antibiotic use in the past.
- Kidney disease—Patients with severe kidney disease may have an increased chance of side effects.
- Myasthenia gravis—Telithromycin may make this condition worse.

Proper Use of This Medicine

Telithromycin may be taken with or without food.

To help clear up your infection completely, keep taking telithromycin for the full time of treatment, even if you begin to feel better after a few days. If you stop taking this medicine too soon, your symptoms may return.

Dosing—The dose of this medicine will be different for different patients. Follow your doctor's orders or the directions on the label. The following information includes only the average doses of this medicine. If your dose is different, do not change it unless your doctor tells you to do so.

The amount of medicine that you take depends on the strength of the medicine. Also, the number of doses you take each day, the time allowed between doses, and the length of time you take the medicine depend on the medical problem for which you are using the medicine.

- For oral dosage form (tablets):
  - For acute bacterial infections in patients with chronic bronchitis or sinusitis:
    - Adults—800 milligrams (mg) once daily for 5 days
    - Children—Use and dose must be determined by your doctor.
  - For community-acquired pneumonia:
    - Adults—800 milligrams (mg) once daily for 7 to 10 days
    - Children—Use and dose must be determined by your doctor.

Missed dose—If you miss a dose of this medicine, take it as soon as possible. However, if it is almost time for your next dose, skip the missed dose and go back to your regular dosing schedule. Do not double doses.

Storage—Store the medicine in a closed container at room temperature, away from heat, moisture, and direct light. Keep from freezing.

Keep out of the reach of children.

Do not keep outdated medicine or medicine no longer needed.

Ask your healthcare professional how you should dispose of any medicine you do not use.

Precautions While Using This Medicine

Telithromycin should not be taken with cisapride or pimozide. Doing so may increase the risk of serious side effects.

If your symptoms do not improve within a few days, or if they become worse, check with your doctor.

Stop taking telithromycin and contact your doctor immediately if you experience symptoms of liver disease. These symptoms include tiredness, body aches, loss of appetite, nausea, yellow skin and eyes, dark urine, light-colored stools, itchy skin, or stomach pains. Severe liver problems and liver failure have been reported, and in some cases, liver injury developed very quickly after only a few doses of telithromycin.

This medicine may cause changes in your vision. Make sure you know how you react to this medicine before you drive, use machines, or do anything else that could be dangerous if you are having vision problems.

Side Effects of This Medicine

Along with its needed effects, a medicine may cause some unwanted effects. Although not all of these side effects may occur, if they do occur they may need medical attention.

Check with your doctor immediately if any of the following side effects occur:

Rare

Abdominal pain; blistering, peeling, loosening of skin; blood bilirubin, elevated; blurred vision; chest pain or discomfort; chills; confusion; convulsions; cough; dark urine; decreased urine; difficulty in breathing, chewing, swallowing, or talking; dizziness; double vision; drooping eyelids; dry mouth; fainting; faintness, or lightheadedness when getting up from a lying or sitting position suddenly; fast, slow, or irregular heartbeat; fever with or without chills; increased blood alkaline phosphatase; increased eosinophil count; increased thirst; itching; joint pain; large, hive-like swelling on face, eyelids, lips, tongue, throat, hands, legs, feet, sex organs; light-colored stools; loss of appetite; mood changes; muscle pain or cramps; muscle weakness; nausea; nervousness; numbness or tingling in hands, feet, or lips; red irritated eyes; shortness of breath; skin rash; sores, ulcers, or white spots in mouth or on lips or tongue; stomach cramps, tenderness, or pain; sweating; tightness in chest; unusual tiredness or weakness; upper right abdominal pain; vomiting; watery or bloody diarrhea; weakness or heaviness of legs; wheezing; yellow eyes and skin

Frequency not known

Black, tarry stools; clay-colored stools; continuous vomiting; dark-colored urine; decreased appetite; general feeling of tiredness or weakness; swelling of feet or lower legs; unpleasant breath odor; vomiting of blood

Some side effects may occur that usually do not need medical attention. These side effects may go away during treatment as your body adjusts to the medicine. Also, your health care professional may be able to tell you about ways to prevent or reduce some of these side effects. Check with your health care professional if any of the following side effects continue or are bothersome or if you have any questions about them:

More common

Diarrhea

Less common or rare

Abnormal dream; acid or sour stomach; belching; bloated or full feeling or pressure in the stomach; burning, crawling, itching, numbness, prickling, "pins and needles", or tingling feelings; burning feeling in chest or stomach; change in color, amount or odor of vaginal discharge; change in sense of smell; change in taste; difficulty focusing eyes; difficulty having a bowel movement (stool); disturbed attention; dry lips; dry skin; excess air or gas in stomach or intestines; fear; feeling of constant movement of self or surroundings; feeling of warmth, redness of the face, neck, arms and occasionally, upper chest; frequent urination; headache; heartburn; increased platelet count; increased volume of pale, dilute urine; indigestion; itching of the vagina or outside genitals; lack or loss of strength; light-headedness; loose stools; loss of appetite; loss of sense of taste; pain during sexual intercourse; pain or tenderness around eyes and cheekbones; passing gas; redness of skin; redness, swelling, or soreness of tongue; reflux; sensation of spinning; shakiness in legs, arms, hands, or feet; skin rash encrusted, scaly and oozing; sleeplessness; sore mouth or tongue; sore throat; stomach upset or pain; stuffy or runny nose; swelling or puffiness of face; tenderness in stomach area; thick, white curd-like vaginal discharge without odor or with mild odor; tooth discoloration; trouble sleeping; unable to sleep; weight loss; white patches in mouth and/or on tongue

Other side effects not listed may also occur in some patients. If you notice any other effects, check with your healthcare professional.

TELMISARTAN (Oral route) - tel-mi-SAR-tan

Black Box Warning

When used in pregnancy during the second and third trimesters, drugs that act directly on the renin-angiotensin system can cause injury and even death to the developing fetus. When pregnancy is detected, telmisartan tablets should be discontinued as soon as possible.

Commonly used brand name(s)

In the U.S.—
Micardis

Available Dosage Forms:
- Tablet

Therapeutic Class: Cardiovascular Agent
Pharmacologic Class: Angiotensin II Receptor Antagonist

Uses For This Medicine

Telmisartan belongs to the class of medicines called angiotensin II receptor blockers (ARB). It is used to treat high blood pressure (hypertension).

High blood pressure adds to the workload of the heart and arteries. If it continues for a long time, the heart and arteries may not function properly. This can damage the blood vessels of the brain, heart, and kidneys, resulting in a stroke, heart failure, or kidney failure. High blood pressure may also increase the risk of heart attacks. These problems may be less likely to occur if blood pressure is controlled.

Telmisartan works by blocking the action of a substance in the body that causes blood vessels to tighten. As a result, telmisartan relaxes blood vessels. This lowers blood pressure.

This medicine is available only with your doctor's prescription.

Before Using This Medicine

In deciding to use a medicine, the risks of taking the medicine must be weighed against the good it will do. This is a decision you and your doctor will make. For this medicine, the following should be considered:

Allergies—Tell your doctor if you have ever had any unusual or allergic reaction to this medicine or any other medicines. Also tell your health care professional if you have any other types of allergies, such as to foods, dyes, preservatives, or animals. For non-prescription products, read the label or package ingredients carefully.

Pediatric—Studies on this medicine have been done only in adult patients, and there is no specific information comparing use of telmisartan in children with use in other age groups.

Geriatric—This medicine has been tested in patients 65 years of age or older and has not been shown to cause different side effects or problems in older people than it does in younger adults.

Pregnancy—

	Pregnancy Category	Explanation
1st Trimester	C	Animal studies have shown an adverse effect and there are no adequate studies in pregnant women OR no animal studies have been conducted and there are no adequate studies in pregnant women.
2nd Trimester	D	Studies in pregnant women have demonstrated a risk to the fetus. However, the benefits of therapy in a life threatening situation or a serious disease, may outweigh the potential risk.
3rd Trimester	D	Studies in pregnant women have demonstrated a risk to the fetus. However, the benefits of therapy in a life threatening situation or a serious disease, may outweigh the potential risk.

Breast Feeding—There are no adequate studies in women for determining infant risk when using this medication during breastfeeding. Weigh the potential benefits against the potential risks before taking this medication while breastfeeding.

Other medicines—

Using this medicine with any of the following medicines may cause an increased risk of certain side effects, but using both drugs may be the best treatment for you. If both medicines are prescribed together, your doctor may change the dose or how often you use one or both of the medicines.

Digoxin

Interactions with Food/Tobacco/Alcohol—Certain medicines should not be used at or around the time of eating food or eating certain types of food since interactions may occur. Using alcohol or tobacco with certain medicines may also cause interactions to occur. Discuss with your healthcare professional the use of your medicine with food, alcohol, or tobacco.

Other medical problems—The presence of other medical problems may affect the use of this medicine. Make sure you tell your doctor if you have any other medical problems, especially:

- Aortic valve damage—Risk of decreased blood flow through the heart
- Congestive heart failure (severe)—Lowering of blood pressure by telmisartan may make this condition worse
- Dehydration (fluid and electrolyte loss due to excessive perspiration, vomiting, diarrhea, prolonged diuretic therapy, dialysis, or dietary salt restriction)—Blood pressure-lowering effects of telmisartan may be increased
- Kidney disease—Effects of telmisartan may make this condition worse
- Liver disease, severe—Blood levels of telmisartan may be higher in patients with this condition

Proper Use of This Medicine

Take this medicine only as directed by your doctor. Do not take more of it and do not take it more often than your doctor ordered. This medicine also works best when there is a constant amount in the blood. *To help keep the amount constant, do not miss any doses. Also, it is best to take the doses at the same time each day.*

Protect the tablets from moisture and do not remove from the blister pack until you are ready to use them.

Dosing—The dose of this medicine will be different for different patients. Follow your doctor's orders or the directions on the label. The following information includes only the average doses of this medicine. If your dose is different, do not change it unless your doctor tells you to do so.

The amount of medicine that you take depends on the strength of the medicine. Also, the number of doses you take each day, the time allowed between doses, and the length of time you take the medicine depend on the medical problem for which you are using the medicine.

- For oral dosage form (tablets):
  - For high blood pressure:
    - Adults—40 milligrams (mg) once a day. Your doctor may increase your dose if needed.
    - Children—Use and dose must be determined by your doctor.

Missed dose—If you miss a dose of this medicine, take it as soon as possible. However, if it is almost time for your next dose, skip the missed dose and go back to your regular dosing schedule. Do not double doses.

Storage—Store the medicine in a closed container at room temperature, away from heat, moisture, and direct light. Keep from freezing.

Keep out of the reach of children.

Do not keep outdated medicine or medicine no longer needed.

Precautions While Using This Medicine

It is important that your doctor check your progress at regular visits to make sure that this medicine is working properly and to check for unwanted effects.

Check with your doctor immediately if you think that you may be pregnant. Telmisartan may cause birth defects or other problems in the baby if taken during pregnancy.

Do not take other medicines unless they have been discussed with your doctor. This especially includes over-the-counter (nonprescription) medicines for appetite control, asthma, colds, cough, hay fever, or sinus problems, since they may increase your blood pressure.

Dizziness or lightheadedness may occur, especially if you have been taking a diuretic (water pill). Make sure you know how you react to this medicine before you drive, use machines, or do anything else that could be dangerous if you experience these effects.

Check with your doctor right away if you become sick while taking this medicine, especially with severe or continuing nausea and vomiting or diarrhea. These conditions may cause you to lose too much water and lead to low blood pressure.

Dizziness, lightheadedness, or fainting also may occur if you exercise or if the weather is hot. Heavy sweating can cause loss of too much water and result in low blood pressure. Use extra care during exercise or hot weather.

Black patients may have a smaller response to the blood pressure-lowering effects of telmisartan.

Side Effects of This Medicine

Along with its needed effects, a medicine may cause some unwanted effects. Although not all of these side effects may occur, if they do occur they may need medical attention.

Check with your doctor as soon as possible if any of the following side effects occur:

Rare

Changes in vision; dizziness, lightheadedness, or fainting; fast heartbeat; large hives

Incidence not known

Blurred vision; chest pain or discomfort; confusion; dark-colored urine; decreased urine output; difficult breathing; dilated neck veins; extreme fatigue; fast or irregular heartbeat; flushing; hives or welts; hoarseness; irregular breathing; irritation; itching; joint pain, stiffness or swelling; large, hive-like swelling on face, eyelids, lips, tongue, throat, hands, legs, feet, sex organs; muscle cramps or stiffness; numbness or tingling in hands, feet, or lips; pain or discomfort in arms, jaw, back or neck; pounding in the ears; rash; redness of skin; shortness of breath; slow or fast heartbeat; sweating; swelling of eyelids, face, or lips; tightness in chest; troubled breathing or swallowing; trouble speaking or walking; trouble thinking; unusual tiredness or weakness; unusually warm skin; weakness or heaviness of legs; weakness, numbness or tingling in arms or legs; weight gain; wheezing

Some side effects may occur that usually do not need medical attention. These side effects may go away during treatment as your body adjusts to the medicine. Also, your health

care professional may be able to tell you about ways to prevent or reduce some of these side effects. Check with your health care professional if any of the following side effects continue or are bothersome or if you have any questions about them:

Less common

Abdominal pain; back pain; bloating or gas; changes in appetite; coughing, ear congestion or pain, fever, head congestion, nasal congestion, runny nose, sneezing, and/or sore throat; diarrhea; dry mouth; general tiredness or weakness; headache; heartburn; increased sweating; muscle pain or spasm; nausea; nervousness; painful urination or changes in urinary frequency; skin rash; swelling in hands, lower legs, and feet

Incidence not known

Acid or sour stomach; belching; coughing; decreased interest in sexual intercourse; difficulty in moving; inability to have or keep an erection; indigestion; joint pain; lack or loss of strength; leg cramps; loss in sexual ability, desire, drive, or performance; muscle aching; stomach discomfort, upset or pain; swelling; swelling or puffiness of face; weakness

Other side effects not listed may also occur in some patients. If you notice any other effects, check with your healthcare professional.

TEMOZOLOMIDE (Oral route) - te-moe-ZOE-loe-mide

Commonly used brand name(s)
In the U.S.—
   Temodar

Available Dosage Forms:
- Capsule

Therapeutic Class: Antineoplastic Agent
Pharmacologic Class: Alkylating Agent

Uses For This Medicine

Temozolomide belongs to the general group of medicines known as antineoplastics. It is used to treat specific types of cancer of the brain in adults whose tumors have returned and whose tumors have just been diagnosed.

Temozolomide seems to interfere with the growth of cancer cells, which are then eventually destroyed by the body. Since the growth of normal body cells may also be affected by temozolomide, other effects will also occur. Some of these may be serious and must be reported to your doctor.

Before you begin treatment with temozolomide, you and your doctor should talk about the good this medicine will do as well as the risks of using it.

Temozolomide is to be administered only by or under the immediate supervision of your doctor.

Once a medicine has been approved for marketing for a certain use, experience may show that it is also useful for other medical problems. Although this use is not included in product labeling, temozolomide is used in certain patients with the following medical condition:

- Metastatic melanoma (a certain type of skin cancer that has spread to other areas of the body, including the brain)

Before Using This Medicine

In deciding to use a medicine, the risks of taking the medicine must be weighed against the good it will do. This is a decision you and your doctor will make. For this medicine, the following should be considered:

Allergies—Tell your doctor if you have ever had any unusual or allergic reaction to this medicine or any other medicines. Also tell your health care professional if you have any other types of allergies, such as to foods, dyes, preservatives, or animals. For non-prescription products, read the label or package ingredients carefully.

Pediatric—Studies on this medicine have been done only in adult patients, and there is no specific information comparing the use of temozolomide in children with use in other age groups.

Geriatric—Elderly patients may be more sensitive to the effects of temozolomide. Blood problems such as low platelet (the cell that helps blood to clot) counts and low white blood cell (the cell that helps fight off infections) counts may be especially likely to occur in patients 70 years of age or older.

Pregnancy—

	Pregnancy Category	Explanation
All Trimesters	D	Studies in pregnant women have demonstrated a risk to the fetus. However, the benefits of therapy in a life threatening situation or a serious disease, may outweigh the potential risk.

Breast Feeding—There are no adequate studies in women for determining infant risk when using this medication during breastfeeding. Weigh the potential benefits against the potential risks before taking this medication while breastfeeding.

Other medicines—Although certain medicines should not be used together at all, in other cases two different medicines may be used together even if an interaction might occur. In these cases, your doctor may want to change the dose, or other precautions may be necessary. Tell your healthcare professional if you are taking any other prescription or non-prescription (over-the-counter [OTC]) medicine.

Interactions with Food/Tobacco/Alcohol—Certain medicines should not be used at or around the time of eating food or eating certain types of food since interactions may occur. Using alcohol or tobacco with certain medicines may also cause interactions to occur. Discuss with your healthcare professional the use of your medicine with food, alcohol, or tobacco.

Other medical problems—The presence of other medical problems may affect the use of this medicine. Make sure you tell your doctor if you have any other medical problems, especially:

- Bone marrow depression, existing or

- Infection—There may be an increased risk of infections or worsening infections because of the body's reduced ability to fight them

- Chickenpox (including recent exposure) or
- Herpes zoster (shingles)—Risk of severe disease affecting other parts of the body
- Kidney disease or
- Liver disease—Temozolomide should be used with caution

Proper Use of This Medicine

Take this medicine only as directed. Do not take more or less of it and do not take it for a longer time than directed. To do so may increase the chance of unwanted side effects. This is especially important for elderly patients, who may be more sensitive to the effects of this medicine.

Temozolomide often causes nausea and vomiting. However, it is very important that you continue to take the medicine, even if you begin to feel ill. Taking the medicine on an empty stomach or at bedtime may help to lessen the nausea. Ask your health care professional for other ways to help lessen these effects.

Temozolomide should be taken at the same time each day in relation to meals.

Temozolomide capsules should be swallowed whole with a full glass of water. The capsules should not be chewed, crushed or broken open. If the capsules are opened accidentally, do not allow the powder to come into contact with your skin or into your mouth or nose. Be careful not to inhale the contents of the capsule.

Dosing—The dose of this medicine will be different for different patients. Follow your doctor's orders or the directions on the label. The following information includes only the average doses of this medicine. If your dose is different, do not change it unless your doctor tells you to do so.

The amount of medicine that you take depends on the strength of the medicine. Also, the number of doses you take each day, the time allowed between doses, and the length of time you take the medicine depend on the medical problem for which you are using the medicine.

Missed dose—Call your doctor or pharmacist for instructions.

If you miss a dose of this medicine, do not double the next one.

Storage—Store the medicine in a closed container at room temperature, away from heat, moisture, and direct light. Keep from freezing.

Keep out of the reach of children.

Do not keep outdated medicine or medicine no longer needed.

Ask your healthcare professional how you should dispose of any medicine you do not use.

Precautions While Using This Medicine

It is very important that your doctor check your progress at regular visits to make sure that this medicine is working properly and to check for unwanted effects.

While you are being treated with temozolomide, and after you stop treatment with it, do not have any immunizations (vaccinations) without your doctor's approval. Temozolomide may lower your body's resistance, and there is a chance you might get the infection that the immunization is meant to prevent. In addition, other persons living in your household should not take oral polio vaccine, since there is a chance they could pass the polio virus on to you. Also, avoid persons who have taken oral polio vaccine within the last several months. Do not get close to them, and do not stay in the room with them for very long. If you cannot take these precautions, you should consider wearing a protective face mask that covers the nose and mouth.

Temozolomide can temporarily lower the number of white blood cells in your blood, increasing the chance of getting an infection. It can also lower the number of platelets, which are necessary for proper blood clotting. If this occurs, there are certain precautions you can take, especially when your blood count is low, to reduce the risk of infection or bleeding:

- If you can, avoid people with infections. Check with your doctor immediately if you think you are getting an infection or if you get a fever or chills, cough or hoarseness, lower back or side pain, or painful or difficult urination.
- Check with your doctor immediately if you notice any unusual bleeding or bruising; black, tarry stools; blood in urine or stools; or pinpoint red spots on your skin.
- Be careful when using a regular toothbrush, dental floss, or toothpick. Your medical doctor, dentist, or nurse may recommend other ways to clean your teeth and gums. Check with your medical doctor before having any dental work done.
- Do not touch your eyes or the inside of your nose unless you have just washed your hands and have not touched anything else in the meantime.
- Be careful not to cut yourself when you are using sharp objects such as a safety razor or fingernail or toenail cutters.
- Avoid contact sports or other situations where bruising or injury could occur.

Side Effects of This Medicine

Along with its needed effects, a medicine may cause some unwanted effects. Although not all of these side effects may occur, if they do occur they may need medical attention.

Also, because of the way these medicines act on the body, there is a chance that they might cause other unwanted effects that may not occur until months or years after the medicine is used. These may include certain types of cancer, such as leukemia. Discuss these possible effects with your doctor.

Check with your doctor immediately if any of the following side effects occur:

Less common or rare

Amnesia; black, tarry stools; blood in urine or stools; convulsions (seizures); cough or hoarseness; fever or chills; infection; lower back or side pain; muscle weakness or paralysis on one or both sides of the body; painful or difficult urination; pinpoint red spots on skin; swelling of feet or lower legs; unusual bleeding or bruising

Incidence not determined—Observed during clinical practice; estimates of frequency cannot be determined

Blistering, peeling, loosening of skin; chest pain; cough; difficulty swallowing; dizziness; fast heartbeat; fever or chills; hives; itching; joint or muscle pain; puffiness or swelling of the eyelids or around the eyes, face, lips or tongue; sneezing; shortness of breath; skin rash; sore throat; troubled breathing; tightness in chest; unusual tiredness or weakness; wheezing

Some side effects may occur that usually do not need medical attention. These side effects may go away during treatment as your body adjusts to the medicine. Also, your health care professional may be able to tell you about ways to prevent or reduce some of these side effects. Check with your health care professional if any of the following side effects continue or are bothersome or if you have any questions about them:

More common

Constipation; headache; nausea and vomiting; unusual tiredness or weakness

Less common or rare

Abdominal or stomach pain; anxiety; blurred or double vision; breast pain (in females); burning or prickling feeling on the skin; confusion; diarrhea; difficulty in speaking; dizziness; drowsiness; loss of appetite; loss of muscle coordination; mental depression; muscle pain; runny or stuffy nose; skin rash or itching; sore throat; trouble in sleeping; unusual weight gain; urinary incontinence or increased urge to urinate

Other side effects not listed may also occur in some patients. If you notice any other effects, check with your healthcare professional.

TENIPOSIDE (Intravenous route) - ten-i-POE-side

Black Box Warning

Teniposide injection is a cytotoxic drug, which should be administered under the supervision of a qualified physician experienced in the use of cancer chemotherapeutic agents. Appropriate management of therapy and complications is possible only when adequate treatment facilities are readily available.

Severe myelosuppression with resulting infection or bleeding may occur. Hypersensitivity reactions, including anaphylaxis-like symptoms, may occur with initial dosing or at repeated exposure to teniposide. Epinephrine, with or without corticosteroids and antihistamines, has been employed to alleviate hypersensitivity reaction symptoms.

Commonly used brand name(s)

In the U.S.—
   Vumon

Available Dosage Forms:
   • Solution

Therapeutic Class: Antineoplastic Agent
Pharmacologic Class: Mitotic Inhibitor

Uses For This Medicine

Teniposide belongs to the group of medicines called antineoplastics. Teniposide injection is used along with other medicines to treat acute lymphoblastic leukemia (ALL), non-Hodgkin's lymphoma (NHL), and neuroblastoma.

Teniposide interferes with the growth of cancer cells, which are eventually destroyed. Since the growth of normal body cells may also be affected by teniposide, other effects will also occur. Some of these may be serious and must be reported to your doctor. Other effects may not be serious but may cause concern.

Teniposide is to be administered only by or under the immediate supervision of your doctor.

Before Using This Medicine

In deciding to use a medicine, the risks of taking the medicine must be weighed against the good it will do. This is a decision you and your doctor will make. For this medicine, the following should be considered:

Allergies—Tell your doctor if you have ever had any unusual or allergic reaction to this medicine or any other medicines. Also tell your health care professional if you have any other types of allergies, such as to foods, dyes, preservatives, or animals. For non-prescription products, read the label or package ingredients carefully.

Pediatric—Children with Down syndrome may be more sensitive to the effects of this medicine compared to other children. Your doctor may decide to start treatment with this medicine at a lower dose.

Geriatric—Many medicines have not been studied specifically in older people. Therefore, it may not be known whether they work exactly the same way they do in younger adults or if they cause different side effects or problems in older people. There is no specific information comparing use of teniposide in the elderly with use in other age groups.

Pregnancy—

	Pregnancy Category	Explanation
All Trimesters	D	Studies in pregnant women have demonstrated a risk to the fetus. However, the benefits of therapy in a life threatening situation or a serious disease, may outweigh the potential risk.

Breast Feeding—There are no adequate studies in women for determining infant risk when using this medication during breastfeeding. Weigh the potential benefits against the potential risks before taking this medication while breastfeeding.

Other medicines—

Using this medicine with any of the following medicines is not recommended. Your doctor may decide not to treat you with this medication or change some of the other medicines you take.

Rotavirus Vaccine, Live

Interactions with Food/Tobacco/Alcohol—Certain medicines should not be used at or around the time of eating food or eating certain types of food since interactions may occur. Using alcohol or tobacco with certain medicines may also cause interactions to occur. Discuss with your healthcare professional the use of your medicine with food, alcohol, or tobacco.

Other medical problems—The presence of other medical problems may affect the use of this medicine. Make sure you tell your doctor if you have any other medical problems, especially:

- Blood disorders due to bone marrow depression or
- Infection—There may be an increased risk of infections or worsening infections because of the body's reduced ability to fight them
- Chickenpox (including recent exposure) or
- Herpes zoster (shingles)—Risk of severe disease affecting other parts of the body
- Down syndrome—Patients who have this condition may be more sensitive to this medicine
- Hypoalbuminemia or
- Kidney disease or
- Liver disease—These conditions may cause the level of teniposide in the body to be higher than usual, which may increase the chance of unwanted effects

Proper Use of This Medicine

Teniposide often causes nausea and vomiting, which usually are not severe. However, it is very important that you continue to receive the medicine, even if you begin to feel ill. Ask your doctor, nurse, or pharmacist for ways to lessen these effects.

Dosing—The dose of this medicine will be different for different patients. Follow your doctor's orders or the directions on the label. The following information includes only the average doses of this medicine. If your dose is different, do not change it unless your doctor tells you to do so.

The amount of medicine that you take depends on the strength of the medicine. Also, the number of doses you take each day, the time allowed between doses, and the length of time you take the medicine depend on the medical problem for which you are using the medicine.

Precautions While Using This Medicine

It is very important that your doctor check your progress at regular visits to make sure that teniposide is working properly and to check for unwanted effects.

It is important to tell your doctor or nurse right away if redness, pain, swelling, or a lump under the skin occurs in the area where the injection is given.

While you are being treated with teniposide, and after you stop treatment, do not have any immunizations (vaccinations) without your doctor's approval. Teniposide may lower your body's resistance, and there is a chance you might get the infection the immunization is meant to prevent. In addition, other persons living in your household should not take oral polio vaccine, since there is a chance they could pass the polio virus on to you. Also, avoid persons who have taken oral polio vaccine within the last several months. Do not get close to them, and do not stay in the same room with them for very long. If you cannot take these precautions, you should consider wearing a protective face mask that covers the nose and mouth.

Teniposide can temporarily lower the number of white blood cells in your blood, increasing the chance of getting an infection. It can also lower the number of platelets, which are necessary for proper blood clotting. If this occurs, there are certain precautions you can take, especially when your blood count is low, to reduce the risk of infection or bleeding:

- If you can, avoid people with infections. Check with your doctor immediately if you think you are getting an infec-

tion or if you get a fever or chills, cough or hoarseness, lower back or side pain, or painful or difficult urination.

- Check with your doctor immediately if you notice any unusual bleeding or bruising; black, tarry stools; blood in urine or stools; or pinpoint red spots on your skin.
- Be careful when using a regular toothbrush, dental floss, or toothpick. Your medical doctor, dentist, or nurse may recommend other ways to clean your teeth and gums. Check with your medical doctor before having any dental work done.
- Do not touch your eyes or the inside of your nose unless you have just washed your hands and have not touched anything else in the meantime.
- Be careful not to cut yourself when you are using sharp objects such as a safety razor or fingernail or toenail cutters.
- Avoid contact sports or other situations where bruising or injury could occur.

Side Effects of This Medicine

Along with its needed effects, a medicine may cause some unwanted effects. Although not all of these side effects may occur, if they do occur they may need medical attention.

Check with your doctor immediately if any of the following side effects occur:
More common
   Black, tarry stools; blood in urine or stools; chills; cough or hoarseness; fever; hives; lower back or side pain; painful or difficult urination; pinpoint red spots on skin; shortness of breath; tightness in chest, or wheezing; troubled breathing; unusual bleeding or bruising

Check with your doctor as soon as possible if any of the following side effects occur:
More common
   Flushing of face; sores in mouth or on lips; unusually fast heartbeat; unusual tiredness

Less common
   Skin rash

Rare
   Decreased urination; swelling of face, fingers, feet, or lower legs; yellow eyes or skin

Some side effects may occur that usually do not need medical attention. These side effects may go away during treatment as your body adjusts to the medicine. Also, your health care professional may be able to tell you about ways to prevent or reduce some of these side effects. Check with your health care professional if any of the following side effects continue or are bothersome or if you have any questions about them:
More common
   Diarrhea; nausea and vomiting

This medicine often causes a temporary loss of hair. After treatment with teniposide has ended, normal hair growth should return.

Other side effects not listed may also occur in some patients. If you notice any other effects, check with your healthcare professional.

TENOFOVIR DISOPROXIL FUMARATE (Oral route) - te-NOE-fo-veer dye-soe-PROX-il FOO-ma-rate

Black Box Warning

Lactic acidosis and severe hepatomegaly with steatosis, including fatal cases, have been reported with the use of nucleoside analogs alone or in combination with other antiretrovirals.

Tenofovir disoproxil fumarate is not indicated for the treatment of chronic hepatitis B virus (HBV) infection and the safety and efficacy of tenofovir disoproxil fumarate have not been established in patients coinfected with HBV and HIV. Severe acute exacerbations of hepatitis B have been reported in patients who are coinfected with HBV and HIV and have discontinued tenofovir disoproxil fumarate. Hepatic function should be monitored closely with both clinical and laboratory follow-up for at least several months in patients who discontinue tenofovir disoproxil fumarate and are coinfected with HIV and HBV. If appropriate, initiation of anti-hepatitis B therapy may be warranted.

Commonly used brand name(s)

In the U.S.—
  Viread

Available Dosage Forms:
  • Tablet

Therapeutic Class: Antiretroviral Agent
Pharmacologic Class: Nucleotide Reverse Transcriptase Inhibitor

Uses For This Medicine

Tenofovir is used, in combination with other medicines, in the treatment of the infection caused by the human immunodeficiency virus (HIV). HIV is the virus that causes acquired immunodeficiency syndrome (AIDS).

Tenofovir will not cure or prevent HIV infection or AIDS; however, it may help keep HIV from reproducing which may slow down the destruction of the immune system. This may help delay the development of problems usually related to AIDS or HIV disease. Tenofovir will not keep you from spreading HIV to other people. People who receive this medicine may continue to have other problems usually related to AIDS or HIV disease.

This medicine is available only with your doctor's prescription.

Once a medicine has been approved for marketing for a certain use, experience may show that it is also useful for other medical problems. Although this use is not included in product labeling, tenofovir is used in certain patients with the following medical condition:

  • Human immunodeficiency virus (HIV) infection in combination with hepatitis B virus (HBV) infection

Before Using This Medicine

In deciding to use a medicine, the risks of taking the medicine must be weighed against the good it will do. This is a decision you and your doctor will make. For this medicine, the following should be considered:

Allergies—Tell your doctor if you have ever had any unusual or allergic reaction to this medicine or any other medi-cines. Also tell your health care professional if you have any other types of allergies, such as to foods, dyes, preservatives, or animals. For non-prescription products, read the label or package ingredients carefully.

Pediatric—Studies on this medicine have been done only in adult patients, and there is no specific information comparing use of tenofovir in children with use in other age groups.

Geriatric—Many medicines have not been studied specifically in older people. Therefore, it may not be known whether they work exactly the same way they do in younger adults. Although there is no specific information comparing use of tenofovir in the elderly with use in other age groups, this medicine is not expected to cause different side effects or problems in older people than it does in younger adults.

Pregnancy—

	Pregnancy Category	Explanation
All Trimesters	B	Animal studies have revealed no evidence of harm to the fetus, however, there are no adequate studies in pregnant women OR animal studies have shown an adverse effect, but adequate studies in pregnant women have failed to demonstrate a risk to the fetus.

Breast Feeding—There are no adequate studies in women for determining infant risk when using this medication during breastfeeding. Weigh the potential benefits against the potential risks before taking this medication while breastfeeding.

Other medicines—

Using this medicine with any of the following medicines is usually not recommended, but may be required in some cases. If both medicines are prescribed together, your doctor may change the dose or how often you use one or both of the medicines.

Atazanavir, Didanosine

Interactions with Food/Tobacco/Alcohol—Certain medicines should not be used at or around the time of eating food or eating certain types of food since interactions may occur. Using alcohol or tobacco with certain medicines may also cause interactions to occur. Discuss with your healthcare professional the use of your medicine with food, alcohol, or tobacco.

Other medical problems—The presence of other medical problems may affect the use of this medicine. Make sure you tell your doctor if you have any other medical problems, especially:

  • Hepatitis B virus infection—May be worsened if tenofovir is discontinued.

  • Kidney disease or

  • Liver disease—May be worsened by tenofovir.

Proper Use of This Medicine

Take this medicine exactly as directed by your doctor. Do not take it more often, and do not take it for a longer time than your doctor ordered. Also, do not stop taking this medicine without checking with your doctor first.

This medicine may be taken with or without food.

This medicine works best when there is a constant amount in the blood. To help keep the amount constant, do not miss any doses.

Dosing—The dose of this medicine will be different for different patients. Follow your doctor's orders or the directions on the label. The following information includes only the average doses of this medicine. If your dose is different, do not change it unless your doctor tells you to do so.

The amount of medicine that you take depends on the strength of the medicine. Also, the number of doses you take each day, the time allowed between doses, and the length of time you take the medicine depend on the medical problem for which you are using the medicine.

- For oral dosage form (tablets):
  - For HIV infection:
    - Adults—300 milligrams (mg) once a day with a meal. You may take this medicine less often if you have kidney problems.
    - Children—Use and dose must be determined by your doctor.

Missed dose—If you miss a dose of this medicine, take it as soon as possible. However, if it is almost time for your next dose, skip the missed dose and go back to your regular dosing schedule. Do not double doses.

Storage—Store the medicine in a closed container at room temperature, away from heat, moisture, and direct light. Keep from freezing.

Keep out of the reach of children.

Do not keep outdated medicine or medicine no longer needed.

Precautions While Using This Medicine

It is very important that your doctor check you at regular visits to make sure this medicine is working properly and to check for unwanted effects.

This medicine may cause serious problems with your liver or cause too much acid in your blood. If untreated, it can lead to severe low blood pressure and even death. Check with your doctor immediately if you notice abdominal discomfort; decreased appetite; diarrhea; fast, shallow breathing; general feeling of discomfort; muscle pain or cramping; nausea; shortness of breath; sleepiness; or unusual tiredness or weakness.

Side Effects of This Medicine

Along with its needed effects, a medicine may cause some unwanted effects. Although not all of these side effects may occur, if they do occur they may need medical attention.

Check with your doctor immediately if any of the following side effects occur:
  Rare
    Abdominal discomfort; decreased appetite; diarrhea; fast, shallow breathing; general feeling of discomfort; muscle pain or cramping; nausea; shortness of breath; sleepiness; unusual tiredness or weakness
  Incidence not known
    Agitation; bloating; bloody or cloudy urine; bone pain; chills; coma; confusion; constipation; convulsions or seizures; darkened urine; decreased frequency or amount of urine; depression; difficult or painful urination; dizziness; fast heartbeat; fever; headache; hostility; increased blood pressure; increased thirst; indi-

gestion; irritability; lethargy; loss of appetite; muscle twitching; pains in stomach, side, or abdomen, possibly radiating to the back; stupor; swelling of face, fingers, lower legs; trouble breathing; vomiting; weight gain; yellow eyes or skin

Some side effects may occur that usually do not need medical attention. These side effects may go away during treatment as your body adjusts to the medicine. Also, your health care professional may be able to tell you about ways to prevent or reduce some of these side effects. Check with your health care professional if any of the following side effects continue or are bothersome or if you have any questions about them:
  More common
    Lack or loss of strength
  Less common
    Passing of gas; weight loss

Other side effects not listed may also occur in some patients. If you notice any other effects, check with your healthcare professional.

TERAZOSIN (Oral route) - ter-AY-zoe-sin

Commonly used brand name(s)
In the U.S.—
  Hytrin

Available Dosage Forms:
- Tablet
- Capsule, Liquid Filled
- Capsule

Therapeutic Class: Cardiovascular Agent
Pharmacologic Class: Alpha-1 Adrenergic Blocker

Uses For This Medicine

Terazosin is used to treat high blood pressure (hypertension).

High blood pressure adds to the work load of the heart and arteries. If it continues for a long time, the heart and arteries may not function properly. This can damage the blood vessels of the brain, heart, and kidneys, resulting in a stroke, heart failure, or kidney failure. High blood pressure may also increase the risk of heart attacks. These problems may be less likely to occur if blood pressure is controlled.

Terazosin helps to lower blood pressure by relaxing blood vessels so that blood passes through them more easily.

Terazosin is also used to treat benign enlargement of the prostate (benign prostatic hyperplasia [BPH]). Benign enlargement of the prostate is a problem that can occur in men as they get older. The prostate gland is located below the bladder. As the prostate gland enlarges, certain muscles in the gland may become tight and get in the way of the tube that drains urine from the bladder. This can cause problems in urinating, such as a need to urinate often, a weak stream when urinating, or a feeling of not being able to empty the bladder completely.

Terazosin helps relax the muscles in the prostate and the opening of the bladder. This may help increase the flow of urine and/or decrease the symptoms. However, terazosin will not help shrink the prostate. The prostate may continue to grow. This may cause the symptoms to become worse over time. Therefore, even though terazosin may lessen the problems caused by enlarged prostate now, surgery still may be needed in the future.

Terazosin is available only with your doctor's prescription.

Before Using This Medicine

In deciding to use a medicine, the risks of taking the medicine must be weighed against the good it will do. This is a decision you and your doctor will make. For this medicine, the following should be considered:

Allergies—Tell your doctor if you have ever had any unusual or allergic reaction to this medicine or any other medicines. Also tell your health care professional if you have any other types of allergies, such as to foods, dyes, preservatives, or animals. For non-prescription products, read the label or package ingredients carefully.

Pediatric—Studies on this medicine have been done only in adult patients, and there is no specific information comparing use of terazosin in children with use in other age groups.

Geriatric—Dizziness, lightheadedness, or fainting (especially when getting up from a lying or sitting position) may be more likely to occur in the elderly, who are more sensitive to the effects of terazosin.

Pregnancy—

	Pregnancy Category	Explanation
All Trimesters	C	Animal studies have shown an adverse effect and there are no adequate studies in pregnant women OR no animal studies have been conducted and there are no adequate studies in pregnant women.

Breast Feeding—There are no adequate studies in women for determining infant risk when using this medication during breastfeeding. Weigh the potential benefits against the potential risks before taking this medication while breastfeeding.

Other medicines—

Using this medicine with any of the following medicines is usually not recommended, but may be required in some cases. If both medicines are prescribed together, your doctor may change the dose or how often you use one or both of the medicines.

Tadalafil, Vardenafil

Interactions with Food/Tobacco/Alcohol—Certain medicines should not be used at or around the time of eating food or eating certain types of food since interactions may occur. Using alcohol or tobacco with certain medicines may also cause interactions to occur. Discuss with your healthcare professional the use of your medicine with food, alcohol, or tobacco.

Other medical problems—The presence of other medical problems may affect the use of this medicine. Make sure you tell your doctor if you have any other medical problems, especially:

- Angina (chest pain)—Terazosin may make this condition worse

- Heart disease (severe)—Terazosin may make this condition worse

- Kidney disease—Possible increased sensitivity to the effects of terazosin

Proper Use of This Medicine

For patients taking this medicine for high blood pressure:

- In addition to the use of the medicine your doctor has prescribed, treatment for your high blood pressure may include weight control and care in the types of foods you eat, especially foods high in sodium. Your doctor will tell you which of these are most important for you. You should check with your doctor before changing your diet.

- Many patients who have high blood pressure will not notice any signs of the problem. In fact, many may feel normal. It is very important that you take your medicine exactly as directed and that you keep your appointments with your doctor even if you feel well.

- Remember that terazosin will not cure your high blood pressure but it does help control it. Therefore, you must continue to take it as directed if you expect to lower your blood pressure and keep it down. You may have to take high blood pressure medicine for the rest of your life. If high blood pressure is not treated, it can cause serious problems such as heart failure, blood vessel disease, stroke, or kidney disease.

For patients taking this medicine for benign enlargement of the prostate:

- Remember that terazosin will not shrink the size of your prostate but it does help to relieve the symptoms.

- It may take up to 6 weeks before your symptoms get better.

To help you remember to take your medicine, try to get into the habit of taking it at the same time each day.

Dosing—The dose of this medicine will be different for different patients. Follow your doctor's orders or the directions on the label. The following information includes only the average doses of this medicine. If your dose is different, do not change it unless your doctor tells you to do so.

The amount of medicine that you take depends on the strength of the medicine. Also, the number of doses you take each day, the time allowed between doses, and the length of time you take the medicine depend on the medical problem for which you are using the medicine.

- For oral dosage form (tablets):
  - For benign enlargement of the prostate:
    - Adults—At first, 1 milligram (mg) taken at bedtime. Then, 5 to 10 mg once a day.
  - For high blood pressure:
    - Adults—At first, 1 mg taken at bedtime. Then, 1 to 5 mg once a day.
    - Children—Use and dose must be determined by your doctor.

Missed dose—If you miss a dose of this medicine, take it as soon as possible. However, if it is almost time for your next dose, skip the missed dose and go back to your regular dosing schedule. Do not double doses.

Storage—Store the medicine in a closed container at room temperature, away from heat, moisture, and direct light. Keep from freezing.

Keep out of the reach of children.

Do not keep outdated medicine or medicine no longer needed.

Precautions While Using This Medicine

It is important that your doctor check your progress at regular visits to make sure that this medicine is working properly.

For patients taking this medicine for high blood pressure:

- Do not take other medicines unless they have been discussed with your doctor. This especially includes over-the-counter (nonprescription) medicines for appetite control, asthma, colds, cough, hay fever, or sinus problems, since they may tend to increase your blood pressure.

Dizziness, lightheadedness, or sudden fainting may occur after you take this medicine, especially when you get up from a lying or sitting position. These effects are more likely to occur when you take the first dose of this medicine. Taking the first dose at bedtime may prevent problems. However, be especially careful if you need to get up during the night. These effects may also occur with any doses you take after the first dose. Getting up slowly may help lessen this problem. If you feel dizzy, lie down so that you do not faint. Then sit for a few moments before standing to prevent the dizziness from returning.

The dizziness, lightheadedness, or fainting is more likely to occur if you drink alcohol, stand for long periods of time, exercise, or if the weather is hot. While you are taking this medicine, be careful to limit the amount of alcohol you drink. Also, use extra care during exercise or hot weather or if you must stand for long periods of time.

Terazosin may cause some people to become drowsy or less alert than they are normally. Make sure you know how you react to this medicine before you drive, use machines, or do anything else that could be dangerous if you are dizzy, drowsy, or are not alert. After you have taken several doses of this medicine, these effects should lessen.

Side Effects of This Medicine

Along with its needed effects, a medicine may cause some unwanted effects. Although not all of these side effects may occur, if they do occur they may need medical attention.

Check with your doctor as soon as possible if any of the following side effects occur:

More common
  Dizziness

Less common
  Chest pain; dizziness or lightheadedness when getting up from a lying or sitting position; fainting (sudden); fast or irregular heartbeat; pounding heartbeat; shortness of breath; swelling of feet or lower legs

Rare
  Weight gain

Some side effects may occur that usually do not need medical attention. These side effects may go away during treatment as your body adjusts to the medicine. Also, your health care professional may be able to tell you about ways to prevent or reduce some of these side effects. Check with your health care professional if any of the following side effects continue or are bothersome or if you have any questions about them:

More common
  Headache; unusual tiredness or weakness

Less common
  Back or joint pain; blurred vision; drowsiness; nausea and vomiting; stuffy nose

Other side effects not listed may also occur in some patients. If you notice any other effects, check with your healthcare professional.

TERBINAFINE (Oral route) - TER-bin-a-feen

Commonly used brand name(s)
In the U.S.—
  Lamisil

Available Dosage Forms:
- Tablet

Therapeutic Class: Antifungal

Uses For This Medicine

Terbinafine belongs to the group of medicines called antifungals. It is used to treat fungus infections of the scalp, body, groin (jock itch), feet (athlete's foot), fingernails, and toenails.

Terbinafine is available only with your doctor's prescription.

Before Using This Medicine

In deciding to use a medicine, the risks of taking the medicine must be weighed against the good it will do. This is a decision you and your doctor will make. For this medicine, the following should be considered:

Allergies—Tell your doctor if you have ever had any unusual or allergic reaction to this medicine or any other medicines. Also tell your health care professional if you have any other types of allergies, such as to foods, dyes, preservatives, or animals. For non-prescription products, read the label or package ingredients carefully.

Pediatric—Studies on this medicine have been done only in adult patients, and there is no specific information comparing use of terbinafine in children with use in other age groups.

Geriatric—Many medicines have not been studied specifically in older people. Therefore, it may not be known whether they work exactly the same way they do in younger adults or if they cause different side effects or problems in older people. There is no specific information comparing use of terbinafine in the elderly with use in other age groups.

Pregnancy—

	Pregnancy Category	Explanation
All Trimesters	B	Animal studies have revealed no evidence of harm to the fetus, however, there are no adequate studies in pregnant women OR animal studies have shown an adverse effect, but adequate studies in pregnant women have failed to demonstrate a risk to the fetus.

Breast Feeding—There are no adequate studies in women for determining infant risk when using this medication during breastfeeding. Weigh the potential benefits against the potential risks before taking this medication while breastfeeding.

Other medicines—

Using this medicine with any of the following medicines may cause an increased risk of certain side effects, but using both drugs may be the best treatment for you. If both medicines are prescribed together, your doctor may change the dose or how often you use one or both of the medicines.

Cyclosporine, Nortriptyline, Warfarin

Interactions with Food/Tobacco/Alcohol—Certain medicines should not be used at or around the time of eating food or eating certain types of food since interactions may occur. Using alcohol or tobacco with certain medicines may also cause interactions to occur. Discuss with your healthcare professional the use of your medicine with food, alcohol, or tobacco.

Other medical problems—The presence of other medical problems may affect the use of this medicine. Make sure you tell your doctor if you have any other medical problems, especially:

- Alcohol abuse (or history of)—Problems with alcohol may increase the chance of side effects caused by terbinafine
- Kidney disease or
- Liver disease, active or chronic—Terbinafine is not recommended for patients with liver or kidney problems

Proper Use of This Medicine

Terbinafine may be taken with food or on an empty stomach.

To help clear up your infection completely, it is very important that you keep taking this medicine for the full time of treatment, even if your symptoms begin to clear up or you begin to feel better after a few days. Since fungus infections may be very slow to clear up, you may need to take this medicine for several weeks or months. If you stop taking this medicine too soon, your symptoms may return.

This medicine works best when there is a constant amount in the blood. To help keep the amount constant, do not miss any doses. Also, it is best to take the doses at the same times every day. If you need help in planning the best time to take your medicine, check with your health care professional.

Dosing—The dose of this medicine will be different for different patients. Follow your doctor's orders or the directions on the label. The following information includes only the average doses of this medicine. If your dose is different, do not change it unless your doctor tells you to do so.

The amount of medicine that you take depends on the strength of the medicine. Also, the number of doses you take each day, the time allowed between doses, and the length of time you take the medicine depend on the medical problem for which you are using the medicine.

- For oral dosage form (tablets):
  - For onychomycosis (fungus infections of the fingernails or toenails):
    - Adults and teenagers—250 milligrams (mg) once a day for six to twelve weeks.
    - Children—Use and dose must be determined by the doctor.
  - For tinea corporis (ringworm of the body):
    - Adults and teenagers—250 mg once a day for two to four weeks.
    - Children—Use and dose must be determined by the doctor.
  - For tinea cruris (ringworm of the groin; jock itch):
    - Adults and teenagers—250 mg once a day for two to four weeks.
    - Children—Use and dose must be determined by the doctor.
  - For tinea pedis (ringworm of the foot; athlete's foot):
    - Adults and teenagers—250 mg once a day for two to six weeks.
    - Children—Use and dose must be determined by the doctor.

Missed dose—If you miss a dose of this medicine, take it as soon as possible. However, if it is almost time for your next dose, skip the missed dose and go back to your regular dosing schedule. Do not double doses.

Storage—Store the medicine in a closed container at room temperature, away from heat, moisture, and direct light. Keep from freezing.

Keep out of the reach of children.

Do not keep outdated medicine or medicine no longer needed.

Precautions While Using This Medicine

It is important that your doctor check your progress at regular visits. This will allow your doctor to check for any unwanted effects.

If your symptoms do not improve within a few weeks (or months for onychomycosis), or if they become worse, check with your doctor.

Liver problems may be more likely to occur if you drink alcoholic beverages while you are taking this medicine. Therefore, you should not drink alcoholic beverages while you are taking this medicine.

It is important that you check with your doctor immediately if you persistently experience any discomforts of liver disease (e.g., nausea or vomiting, lack or loss of appetite, general feeling of tiredness or weakness, stomach pain, yellow eyes or skin, dark urine, or pale stools).

Side Effects of This Medicine

Along with its needed effects, a medicine may cause some unwanted effects. Although not all of these side effects may occur, if they do occur they may need medical attention.

Check with your doctor immediately if any of the following side effects occur:

Less common
    Skin rash or itching

Rare
    Aching joints and muscles; dark urine; difficulty in swallowing; fever, chills, or sore throat; loss of appetite; pale skin; pale stools; redness, blistering, peeling, or loosening of skin; unusual bleeding or bruising; unusual tiredness or weakness; yellow skin or eyes; continuing headache; stomach pain or vomiting; general feeling of tiredness or weakness

Some side effects may occur that usually do not need medical attention. These side effects may go away during treat-

ment as your body adjusts to the medicine. Also, your health care professional may be able to tell you about ways to prevent or reduce some of these side effects. Check with your health care professional if any of the following side effects continue or are bothersome or if you have any questions about them:

    More common

        Diarrhea; nausea and vomiting; stomach pain (mild)

    Less common

        Change of taste or loss of taste

Other side effects not listed may also occur in some patients. If you notice any other effects, check with your healthcare professional.

TERBINAFINE (Topical route) - TER-bin-a-feen

Commonly used brand name(s)

In the U.S.—
  Lamisil
  Lamisil AT Athlete's Foot
  Lamisil AT Jock Itch

In Canada—
  Lamisil Dermgel

Available Dosage Forms:
- Gel/Jelly
- Cream
- Spray
- Solution

Therapeutic Class: Antifungal

Uses For This Medicine

Terbinafine is used to treat infections caused by a fungus. It works by killing the fungus or preventing its growth.

Terbinafine is applied to the skin to treat:
- ringworm of the body (tinea corporis);
- ringworm of the foot (interdigital and plantar tinea pedis; athlete's foot);
- ringworm of the groin (tinea cruris; jock itch);
- tinea versicolor (sometimes called "sun fungus"); and
- yeast infection of the skin (cutaneous candidiasis).

Terbinafine is available only with your doctor's prescription.

Before Using This Medicine

In deciding to use a medicine, the risks of taking the medicine must be weighed against the good it will do. This is a decision you and your doctor will make. For this medicine, the following should be considered:

Allergies—Tell your doctor if you have ever had any unusual or allergic reaction to this medicine or any other medicines. Also tell your health care professional if you have any other types of allergies, such as to foods, dyes, preservatives, or animals. For non-prescription products, read the label or package ingredients carefully.

Pediatric—Studies on this medicine have been done only in adult patients, and there is no specific information com-

paring use of terbinafine in children under the age of 12 with use in other age groups.

Geriatric—Many medicines have not been studied specifically in older people. Therefore, it may not be known whether they work exactly the same way they do in younger adults. Although there is no specific information comparing use of terbinafine in the elderly with use in other age groups, this medicine is not expected to cause different side effects or problems in older people than it does in younger adults.

Pregnancy—

	Pregnancy Category	Explanation
All Trimesters	B	Animal studies have revealed no evidence of harm to the fetus, however, there are no adequate studies in pregnant women OR animal studies have shown an adverse effect, but adequate studies in pregnant women have failed to demonstrate a risk to the fetus.

Breast Feeding—There are no adequate studies in women for determining infant risk when using this medication during breastfeeding. Weigh the potential benefits against the potential risks before taking this medication while breastfeeding.

Other medicines—

Using this medicine with any of the following medicines may cause an increased risk of certain side effects, but using both drugs may be the best treatment for you. If both medicines are prescribed together, your doctor may change the dose or how often you use one or both of the medicines.

Cyclosporine, Nortriptyline, Warfarin

Interactions with Food/Tobacco/Alcohol—Certain medicines should not be used at or around the time of eating food or eating certain types of food since interactions may occur. Using alcohol or tobacco with certain medicines may also cause interactions to occur. Discuss with your healthcare professional the use of your medicine with food, alcohol, or tobacco.

Other medical problems—The presence of other medical problems may affect the use of this medicine. Make sure you tell your doctor if you have any other medical problems, especially:
- Fungus infection of the nails—Condition may decrease the effect of terbinafine when this medicine is used to treat a type of ringworm of the foot (plantar tinea pedis)

Proper Use of This Medicine

Apply enough terbinafine cream to cover the affected and surrounding skin areas and rub in gently.

Apply enough terbinafine solution to wet and cover the affected and surrounding skin areas. Allow it to dry.

Keep this medicine away from the eyes, nose, mouth, and other mucous membranes. The solution may be especially irritating to the eyes.

Terbinafine spray solution contains alcohol and should not be applied to the face.

Do not apply an occlusive dressing (airtight covering, such as a tight bandage or plastic kitchen wrap) over this medicine unless you have been directed to do so by your doctor.

Dosing—The dose of this medicine will be different for different patients. Follow your doctor's orders or the directions on the label. The following information includes only the average doses of this medicine. If your dose is different, do not change it unless your doctor tells you to do so.

The amount of medicine that you take depends on the strength of the medicine. Also, the number of doses you take each day, the time allowed between doses, and the length of time you take the medicine depend on the medical problem for which you are using the medicine.

- For topical dosage form (cream):
  - For cutaneous candidiasis:
    - Adults—Use one or two times a day for seven to fourteen days.
    - Children—Use and dose must be determined by your doctor.
  - For tinea corporis or tinea cruris:
    - Adults and children 12 years of age and older—Use one or two times a day for seven to twenty-eight days.
    - Infants and children younger than 12 years of age—Use and dose must be determined by your doctor.
  - For tinea pedis (interdigital):
    - Adults and children 12 years of age and older—Use two times a day for seven to twenty-eight days.
    - Infants and children younger than 12 years of age—Use and dose must be determined by your doctor.
  - For tinea pedis (plantar):
    - Adults and children 12 years of age and older—Use two times a day for fourteen days.
    - Infants and children younger than 12 years of age—Use and dose must be determined by your doctor.
  - For tinea versicolor:
    - Adults—Use one or two times a day for fourteen days.
    - Children—Use and dose must be determined by your doctor.
- For topical dosage form (spray solution):
  - For tinea corporis or tinea cruris:
    - Adults—Use once a day for seven days.
    - Children—Use and dose must be determined by your doctor.
  - For tinea pedis or tinea versicolor:
    - Adults—Use two times a day for seven days.
    - Children—Use and dose must be determined by your doctor.

To help clear up your infection completely, it is very important that you keep using terbinafine for the full time of treatment, even if your symptoms begin to clear up after a few days. Since fungus infections may be very slow to clear up, you may have to continue using this medicine every day for several weeks or more. If you stop using this medicine too soon, your symptoms may return. Do not miss any doses.

Missed dose—If you miss a dose of this medicine, apply it as soon as possible. However, if it is almost time for your next dose, skip the missed dose and go back to your regular dosing schedule.

Storage—Store the medicine in a closed container at room temperature, away from heat, moisture, and direct light. Keep from freezing.

Keep out of the reach of children.

Do not keep outdated medicine or medicine no longer needed.

Precautions While Using This Medicine

Discontinue using this medicine and check with your doctor if increased irritation or possible sensitization (redness, itching, burning, blistering, swelling, or oozing) occurs while using the medication.

If your skin problem does not improve within 4 to 7 weeks, or if it becomes worse, check with your doctor.

To help clear up your infection completely and to help make sure it does not return, good health habits are also needed. The following measures will help reduce chafing and irritation and will also help keep the area cool and dry.

- For patients using terbinafine for ringworm of the body:
  - Carefully dry yourself after bathing.
  - Avoid too much heat and humidity if possible. Try to keep moisture from building up on affected areas of the body.
  - Wear well-ventilated, loose-fitting clothing.
  - Use a bland, absorbent powder (for example, talcum powder) once or twice a day. Be sure to use the powder after terbinafine cream or solution has been applied and has disappeared into the skin.
- For patients using terbinafine for ringworm of the groin:
  - Avoid wearing underwear that is tight-fitting or made from synthetic (man-made) materials (for example, rayon or nylon). Instead, wear loose-fitting, cotton underwear.
  - Use a bland, absorbent powder (for example, talcum powder) on the skin. It is best to use the powder between the times you use terbinafine.
- For patients using terbinafine for ringworm of the foot:
  - Carefully dry the feet, especially between the toes, after bathing.
  - Avoid wearing socks made from wool or synthetic materials (for example, rayon or nylon). Instead, wear clean, cotton socks and change them daily or more often if the feet sweat a lot.
  - Wear sandals or well-ventilated shoes (for example, shoes with holes).
  - Use a bland, absorbent powder (for example, talcum powder) between the toes, on the feet, and in socks and shoes once or twice a day. It is best to use the powder between the times you use terbinafine.

If you have any questions about these measures, check with your health care professional.

Side Effects of This Medicine

Along with its needed effects, a medicine may cause some unwanted effects. Although not all of these side effects may occur, if they do occur they may need medical attention.

Check with your doctor as soon as possible if any of the following side effects occur:
  Rare
    Dryness; redness; itching; burning; peeling; rash; stinging; tingling; or other signs of skin irritation not present before use of this medicine

Other side effects not listed may also occur in some patients. If you notice any other effects, check with your healthcare professional.

TETANUS IMMUNE GLOBULIN
(Intramuscular route) - TET-n-us im-MYOON GLOB-yoo-lin

Commonly used brand name(s)

In the U.S.—
Baytet

Available Dosage Forms:
- Solution

Therapeutic Class: Immune Serum

Uses For This Medicine

Tetanus immune globulin is used to prevent tetanus infection (also known as lockjaw). Tetanus is a serious illness that causes convulsions (seizures) and severe muscle spasms that can be strong enough to cause bone fractures of the spine. Tetanus causes death in 30 to 40 percent of cases.

In recent years, two thirds of all tetanus cases have been in persons 50 years of age and older. A tetanus infection in the past does not make you immune to tetanus in the future.

Tetanus immune globulin works by giving your body the antibodies it needs to protect it against tetanus infection. This is called passive protection. This passive protection lasts long enough to protect your body until your body can produce its own antibodies against tetanus.

Tetanus immune globulin is to be administered only by or under the supervision of your doctor or other health care professional.

Before Using This Medicine

In deciding to use a medicine, the risks of taking the medicine must be weighed against the good it will do. This is a decision you and your doctor will make. For this medicine, the following should be considered:

Allergies—Tell your doctor if you have ever had any unusual or allergic reaction to this medicine or any other medicines. Also tell your health care professional if you have any other types of allergies, such as to foods, dyes, preservatives, or animals. For non-prescription products, read the label or package ingredients carefully.

Pediatric—Although there is no specific information comparing use of tetanus immune globulin in children with use in other age groups, this medicine is not expected to cause different side effects or problems in children than it does in adults.

Geriatric—Many medicines have not been studied specifically in older people. Therefore, it may not be known whether they work exactly the same way they do in younger adults or if they cause different side effects or problems in older people. There is no specific information comparing use of tetanus immune globulin in the elderly with use in other age groups. However, there is no evidence that the effects of tetanus immune globulin in older adults differ from those in younger persons.

Pregnancy—

	Pregnancy Category	Explanation
All Trimesters	C	Animal studies have shown an adverse effect and there are no adequate studies in pregnant women OR no animal studies have been conducted and there are no adequate studies in pregnant women.

Breast Feeding—There are no adequate studies in women for determining infant risk when using this medication during breastfeeding. Weigh the potential benefits against the potential risks before taking this medication while breastfeeding.

Other medicines—Although certain medicines should not be used together at all, in other cases two different medicines may be used together even if an interaction might occur. In these cases, your doctor may want to change the dose, or other precautions may be necessary. Tell your healthcare professional if you are taking any other prescription or nonprescription (over-the-counter [OTC]) medicine.

Interactions with Food/Tobacco/Alcohol—Certain medicines should not be used at or around the time of eating food or eating certain types of food since interactions may occur. Using alcohol or tobacco with certain medicines may also cause interactions to occur. Discuss with your healthcare professional the use of your medicine with food, alcohol, or tobacco.

Other medical problems—The presence of other medical problems may affect the use of tetanus immune globulin. Make sure you tell your doctor if you have any other medical problems.

Proper Use of This Medicine

Dosing—The dose of this medicine will be different for different patients. Follow your doctor's orders or the directions on the label. The following information includes only the average doses of this medicine. If your dose is different, do not change it unless your doctor tells you to do so.

The amount of medicine that you take depends on the strength of the medicine. Also, the number of doses you take each day, the time allowed between doses, and the length of time you take the medicine depend on the medical problem for which you are using the medicine.

- For injection dosage form:
  - For preventing tetanus infection:
    - Adults and children—250 units injected into a muscle.

Side Effects of This Medicine

Along with its needed effects, a medicine may cause some unwanted effects. Although not all of these side effects may occur, if they do occur they may need medical attention.

Check with your doctor immediately if any of the following side effects occur:
Rare
Difficulty in breathing or swallowing; hives; itching, especially of soles or palms; reddening of skin, especially around ears; swelling of eyes, face, or inside of nose; unusual tiredness or weakness, sudden and severe

Other side effects not listed may also occur in some patients. If you notice any other effects, check with your healthcare professional.

TETANUS TOXOID (Intramuscular route, Injection route) - TET-n-us TOX-oyd

Commonly used brand name(s)

In the U.S.—
TE Anatoxal Berna

In Canada—
Tetanus Toxoid Adsorbed

Available Dosage Forms:
- Suspension
- Solution

Therapeutic Class: Toxoid

Uses For This Medicine

Tetanus toxoid is used to prevent tetanus (also known as lockjaw). Tetanus is a serious illness that causes convulsions (seizures) and severe muscle spasms that can be strong enough to cause bone fractures of the spine. Tetanus causes death in 30 to 40 percent of cases.

Immunization against tetanus is recommended for all infants 6 to 8 weeks of age and older, all children, and all adults. Immunization against tetanus consists first of a series of either 3 or 4 injections, depending on which type of tetanus toxoid you receive. In addition, it is very important that you get a booster injection every 10 years for the rest of your life. Also, if you get a wound that is unclean or hard to clean, you may need an emergency booster injection if it has been more than 5 years since your last booster. In recent years, two-thirds of all tetanus cases have been in persons 50 years of age and older. A tetanus infection in the past does not make you immune to tetanus in the future.

This vaccine is to be administered only by or under the supervision of your doctor or other health care professional.

Before Using This Medicine

In deciding to use a medicine, the risks of taking the medicine must be weighed against the good it will do. This is a decision you and your doctor will make. For this medicine, the following should be considered:

In deciding to receive this vaccine, the risks of receiving the vaccine must be weighed against the good it will do. This is a decision you and your doctor will make. For tetanus toxoid, the following should be considered:

Allergies—Tell your doctor if you have ever had any unusual or allergic reaction to this medicine or any other medicines. Also tell your health care professional if you have any other types of allergies, such as to foods, dyes, preservatives, or animals. For non-prescription products, read the label or package ingredients carefully.

Pediatric—Use is not recommended for infants up to 6 weeks of age. For infants and children 6 weeks of age and older, tetanus toxoid is not expected to cause different side effects or problems than it does in adults.

Geriatric—This vaccine is not expected to cause different side effects or problems in older people than it does in younger adults. However, the vaccine may be slightly less effective in older persons than in younger adults.

Pregnancy—

	Pregnancy Category	Explanation
All Trimesters	C	Animal studies have shown an adverse effect and there are no adequate studies in pregnant women OR no animal studies have been conducted and there are no adequate studies in pregnant women.

Breast Feeding—There are no adequate studies in women for determining infant risk when using this medication during breastfeeding. Weigh the potential benefits against the potential risks before taking this medication while breastfeeding.

Other medicines—

Using this medicine with any of the following medicines may cause an increased risk of certain side effects, but using both drugs may be the best treatment for you. If both medicines are prescribed together, your doctor may change the dose or how often you use one or both of the medicines.

Chloramphenicol

Interactions with Food/Tobacco/Alcohol—Certain medicines should not be used at or around the time of eating food or eating certain types of food since interactions may occur. Using alcohol or tobacco with certain medicines may also cause interactions to occur. Discuss with your healthcare professional the use of your medicine with food, alcohol, or tobacco.

Other medical problems—The presence of other medical problems may affect the use of this medicine. Make sure you tell your doctor if you have any other medical problems, especially:

- A severe reaction or a fever greater than 103 °F (39.4 °C) following a previous dose of tetanus toxoid—May increase the chance of side effects with future doses of tetanus toxoid; be sure your doctor knows about this before you receive the next dose of tetanus toxoid
- Bronchitis, pneumonia, or other illness involving lungs or bronchial tubes, or
- Severe illness with fever—Possible side effects from tetanus toxoid may be confused with the symptoms of the condition

---

Proper Use of This Medicine

Dosing—The dose of this medicine will be different for different patients. Follow your doctor's orders or the directions on the label. The following information includes only the average doses of this medicine. If your dose is different, do not change it unless your doctor tells you to do so.

The amount of medicine that you take depends on the

The amount of medicine that you take depends on the strength of the medicine. Also, the number of doses you take each day, the time allowed between doses, and the length of time you take the medicine depend on the medical problem for which you are using the medicine.

- For injection dosage forms:
  - For prevention of tetanus (lockjaw):
    - Adults, children, and infants 6 weeks of age and older—One dose is given at your first visit, then a second dose is given four to eight weeks later. Depending on the product given, you may receive a third dose four to eight weeks after the second dose, and a fourth dose six to twelve months after that; or you may receive a third dose six to twelve months after the second dose. Everyone should receive a booster dose every ten years. The doses are injected under the skin or into a muscle. In addition, if you get a wound that is unclean or hard to clean, you may need an emergency booster injection if it has been more than 5 years since your last booster dose.

Side Effects of This Medicine

Along with its needed effects, a medicine may cause some unwanted effects. Although not all of these side effects may occur, if they do occur they may need medical attention.

Check with your doctor immediately if any of the following side effects occur:

Symptoms of allergic reaction
Difficulty in breathing or swallowing; hives; itching, especially of feet or hands; reddening of skin, especially around ears; swelling of eyes, face, or inside of nose; unusual tiredness or weakness (sudden and severe)

Check with your doctor as soon as possible if any of the following side effects occur:

Rare
Confusion; convulsions (seizures); fever over 103 °F (39.4 °C); headache (severe or continuing); sleepiness (excessive); swelling, blistering, or pain at place of injection (severe or continuing); swelling of glands in armpit; unusual irritability; vomiting (severe or continuing)

Some side effects may occur that usually do not need medical attention. These side effects may go away during treatment as your body adjusts to the medicine. Also, your health care professional may be able to tell you about ways to prevent or reduce some of these side effects. Check with your health care professional if any of the following side effects continue or are bothersome or if you have any questions about them:

More common
Redness or hard lump at place of injection

Less common
Chills, fever, irritability, or unusual tiredness; pain, tenderness, itching, or swelling at place of injection; skin rash

Other side effects not listed may also occur in some patients. If you notice any other effects, check with your healthcare professional.

TETRACYCLINES (Systemic)

Some commonly used brand names are:

In the U.S.—

Achromycin V (5)
Declomycin (1)
Doryx (2)
Dynacin (3)
Minocin (3)

Monodox (2)
Terramycin (4)
Vibramycin (2)
Vibra-Tabs (2)

In Canada—

Alti-Doxycycline (2)
Alti-Minocycline (3)
Apo-Doxy (2)
Apo-Doxy-Tabs (2)
Apo-Minocycline (3)
Apo-Tetra (5)
Declomycin (1)
Doxycin (2)
Doxytec (2)
Gen-Minocycline (3)

Minocin (3)
Novo-Doxylin (2)
Novo-Minocycline (3)
Novo-Tetra (5)
Nu-Doxycycline (2)
Nu-Tetra (5)
Vibramycin (2)
Vibra-Tabs (2)
Vibra-Tabs C-Pak (2)

This information applies to the following medicines:

1. Demeclocycline (dem-e-kloe-SYE-kleen)
2. Doxycycline (dox-i-SYE-kleen)
3. Minocycline (mi-noe-SYE-kleen)
4. Oxytetracycline (ox-i-tet-ra-SYE-kleen)
5. Tetracycline (tet-ra-SYE-kleen)

Category

- **Antiacne agent, systemic**—Minocycline; tetracycline
- **Antibacterial, systemic**—Demeclocycline; doxycycline; minocycline; oxytetracycline; tetracycline
- **Antiprotozoal**—Demeclocycline; doxycycline; minocycline; oxytetracycline; tetracycline
- **Antirheumatic**—Minocycline
- **Diuretic, syndrome of inappropriate antidiuretic hormone**—Demeclocycline
- **Intrapleural sclerosing agent**—Doxycycline; tetracycline

Description

Tetracyclines are used to treat infections and to help control acne. Demeclocycline, doxycycline, and minocycline also may be used for other problems as determined by your doctor. Tetracyclines will not work for colds, flu, or other virus infections.

Tetracyclines are available only with your doctor's prescription, in the following dosage forms:

Oral
- Demeclocycline
  - Tablets
- Doxycycline
  - Capsules
  - Delayed-release capsules (U.S.)
  - Oral suspension
  - Tablets
- Minocycline
  - Capsules
  - Oral suspension

- Oxytetracycline
  - Capsules
- Tetracycline
  - Capsules
  - Oral suspension

Parenteral
- Doxycycline
  - Injection
- Minocycline
  - Injection
- Oxytetracycline
  - Injection

Before Using This Medicine

In deciding to use a medicine, the risks of taking the medicine must be weighed against the good it will do. This is a decision you and your doctor will make. For tetracyclines, the following should be considered:

Allergies—Tell your doctor if you have ever had any unusual or allergic reaction to any of the tetracyclines or combination medicines containing a tetracycline. Also tell your health care professional if you are allergic to any other substances, such as foods, preservatives, or dyes. In addition, if you are going to be given oxytetracycline by injection, tell your doctor if you have ever had an unusual or allergic reaction to "caine-type" anesthetics (e.g., lidocaine).

Pregnancy—Use is not recommended during the last half of pregnancy. If tetracyclines are taken during that time, they may cause the unborn infant's teeth to become discolored and may slow down the growth of the infant's teeth and bones. In addition, liver problems may occur in pregnant women, especially those receiving high doses by injection into a vein.

Breast-feeding—Use is not recommended since tetracyclines pass into breast milk. They may cause the nursing baby's teeth to become discolored and may slow down the growth of the baby's teeth and bones. They may also increase the sensitivity of nursing babies' skin to sunlight and cause fungus infections of the mouth and vagina. In addition, minocycline may cause dizziness, light-headedness, or unsteadiness in nursing babies.

Children—Tetracyclines may cause permanent discoloration of teeth and slow down the growth of bones. These medicines should not be given to children 8 years of age and younger unless directed by the child's doctor.

Older adults—Many medicines have not been studied specifically in older people. Therefore, it may not be known whether they work exactly the same way they do in younger adults or if they cause different side effects or problems in older people. There is no specific information comparing use of tetracyclines in the elderly with use in other age groups.

Other medicines—Although certain medicines should not be used together at all, in other cases two different medicines may be used together even if an interaction might occur. In these cases, your doctor may want to change the dose, or other precautions may be necessary. When you are taking tetracyclines, it is especially important that your health care professional know if you are taking any of the following:
- Antacids or
- Calcium supplements such as calcium carbonate or
- Cholestyramine (e.g., Questran) or

- Choline and magnesium salicylates (e.g., Trilisate) or
- Colestipol (e.g., Colestid) or
- Iron-containing medicine or
- Laxatives (magnesium-containing) or
- Magnesium salicylate (e.g., Magan)—Use of these medicines with tetracyclines may decrease the effect of tetracyclines
- Oral contraceptives (birth control pills) containing estrogen—Use of birth control pills with tetracyclines may decrease the effect of the birth control pills and increase the chance of unwanted pregnancy
- Penicillins—Use of tetracyclines with penicillins may decrease the effect of penicillins

Other medical problems—The presence of other medical problems may affect the use of tetracyclines. Make sure you tell your doctor if you have any other medical problems, especially:
- Diabetes insipidus (water diabetes)—Demeclocycline may make the condition worse
- Kidney disease (does not apply to doxycycline or minocycline)—Patients with kidney disease may have an increased chance of side effects
- Liver disease—Patients with liver disease may have an increased chance of side effects if they use doxycycline or minocycline

Proper Use of This Medicine

Do not give tetracyclines to infants or children 8 years of age and younger unless directed by your doctor. Tetracyclines may cause permanently discolored teeth and other problems in patients in these age groups.

Tetracyclines should be taken with a full glass (8 ounces) of water to prevent irritation of the esophagus (tube between the throat and stomach) or stomach. In addition, most tetracyclines (except doxycycline and minocycline) are best taken on an empty stomach (either 1 hour before or 2 hours after meals). However, if this medicine upsets your stomach, your doctor may want you to take it with food.

Do not take milk, milk formulas, or other dairy products within 1 to 2 hours of the time you take tetracyclines (except doxycycline and minocycline) by mouth. They may keep this medicine from working properly.

If this medicine has changed color or tastes or looks different, has become outdated (old), or has been stored incorrectly (too warm or too damp area or place), do not use it. To do so may cause *serious side effects.* Throw away the medicine. If you have any questions about this, check with your health care professional.

For patients taking the *oral liquid form* of this medicine:
- Use a specially marked measuring spoon or other device to measure each dose accurately. The average household teaspoon may not hold the right amount of liquid.
- Do not use after the expiration date on the label since the medicine may not work properly after that date. Check with your pharmacist if you have any questions about this.

For patients taking *doxycycline* or *minocycline:*
- These medicines may be taken with food or milk if they upset your stomach.

- Swallow the capsule (with enteric-coated pellets) form of doxycycline whole. Do not break or crush it.

To help clear up your infection completely, *keep taking this medicine for the full time of treatment*, even if you begin to feel better after a few days. If you stop taking this medicine too soon, your symptoms may return.

This medicine works best when there is a constant amount in the blood or urine. *To help keep the amount constant, do not miss any doses. Also, it is best to take the doses at evenly spaced times day and night.* For example, if you are to take four doses a day, the doses should be spaced about 6 hours apart. If this interferes with your sleep or other daily activities, or if you need help in planning the best times to take your medicine, check with your health care professional.

Dosing—The dose of these medicines will be different for different patients. *Follow your doctor's orders or the directions on the label.* The following information includes only the average doses of these medicines. *If your dose is different, do not change it* unless your doctor tells you to do so.

The number of capsules, tablets, or teaspoonfuls of suspension that you take depends on the strength of the medicine. Also, *the number of doses you take each day, the time allowed between doses, and the length of time you take the medicine depend on the medical problem for which you are taking a tetracycline.*

For demeclocycline
- For *oral* dosage form (tablets):
  - For bacterial or protozoal infections:
    - Adults and teenagers—150 milligrams (mg) every six hours; or 300 mg every twelve hours. Gonorrhea is treated with 600 mg on the first day, then 300 mg every twelve hours for four days.
    - Children older than 8 years of age—Dose is based on body weight. The usual dose is 1.65 to 3.3 mg per kilogram (kg) (0.8 to 1.5 mg per pound) of body weight every six hours; or 3.3 to 6.6 mg per kg (1.5 to 3 mg per pound) of body weight every twelve hours.
    - Infants and children 8 years of age and younger— Tetracyclines usually are not used in young children because tetracyclines can permanently stain teeth.

For doxycycline
- For *oral* dosage forms (capsules, suspension, and tablets):
  - For bacterial or protozoal infections:
    - Adults and children older than 8 years of age who weigh more than 45 kilograms (kg) (99 pounds)— 100 milligrams (mg) every twelve hours the first day, then 100 mg once a day or 50 to 100 mg every twelve hours.
    - Children older than 8 years of age who weigh 45 kg (99 pounds) or less—Dose is based on body weight. The usual dose is 2.2 mg per kg (1 mg per pound) of body weight two times a day on the first day, then 2.2 to 4.4 mg per kg (1 to 2 mg per pound) of body weight once a day or 1.1 to 2.2 mg per kg (0.5 to 1 mg per pound) of body weight twice a day.
    - Infants and children 8 years of age and younger— Tetracyclines are usually not used in young chil-

dren because tetracyclines can permanently stain teeth.
  - For the prevention of malaria:
    - Adults and teenagers—100 mg once a day. You should take the first dose one or two days before travel to an area where malaria may occur, and continue taking the medicine every day throughout travel and for four weeks after you leave the malarious area.
    - Children older than 8 years of age—Dose is based on body weight. The usual dose is 2 mg per kg (0.9 mg per pound) of body weight once a day. You should take the first dose one or two days before travel to an area where malaria may occur, and continue taking the medicine every day throughout travel and for four weeks after you leave the malarious area.
    - Infants and children 8 years of age and younger— Tetracyclines are usually not used in young children because tetracyclines can permanently stain teeth.
- For *injection* dosage form:
  - For bacterial or protozoal infections:
    - Adults and children older than 8 years of age who weigh more than 45 kg of body weight (99 pounds)—200 mg injected slowly into a vein once a day; or 100 mg injected slowly into a vein every twelve hours the first day, then 100 to 200 mg injected slowly into a vein once a day or 50 to 100 mg injected slowly into a vein every twelve hours.
    - Children older than 8 years of age who weigh 45 kg of body weight (99 pounds) or less—Dose is based on body weight. The usual dose is 4.4 mg per kg (2 mg per pound) of body weight injected slowly into a vein once a day; or 2.2 mg per kg (1 mg per pound) of body weight injected slowly into a vein every twelve hours the first day, then 2.2 to 4.4 mg per kg (1 to 2 mg per pound) of body weight once a day, or 1.1 to 2.2 per kg (0.5 to 1 mg per pound) of body weight every twelve hours.
    - Infants and children 8 years of age and younger— Tetracyclines are usually not used in young children because tetracyclines can permanently stain teeth.

For minocycline
- For *oral* dosage forms (capsules and suspension):
  - For bacterial or protozoal infections:
    - Adults and teenagers—200 milligrams (mg) at first, then 100 mg every twelve hours; or 100 to 200 mg at first, then 50 mg every six hours.
    - Children older than 8 years of age—Dose is based on body weight. The usual dose is 4 mg per kilogram (kg) (1.8 mg per pound) of body weight at first, then 2 mg per kg (0.9 mg per pound) of body weight every twelve hours.
    - Infants and children 8 years of age and younger— Tetracyclines are usually not used in young children because tetracyclines can permanently stain teeth.
- For *injection* dosage form:
  - For bacterial or protozoal infections:
    - Adults and teenagers—200 mg at first, then 100 mg every twelve hours, injected slowly into a vein.

- Children older than 8 years of age—Dose is based on body weight. The usual dose is 4 mg per kg (1.8 mg per pound) of body weight at first, then 2 mg per kg (0.9 mg per pound) of body weight every twelve hours, injected slowly into a vein.
- Infants and children 8 years of age and younger—Tetracyclines are usually not used in young children because tetracyclines can permanently stain teeth.

For oxytetracycline
- For *oral* dosage form (capsules):
  - For bacterial or protozoal infections:
    - Adults and teenagers—250 to 500 milligrams (mg) every six hours.
    - Children older than 8 years of age—Dose is based on body weight. The usual dose is 6.25 to 12.5 mg per kilogram (kg) (2.8 to 5.7 mg per pound) of body weight every six hours.
    - Infants and children 8 years of age and younger—Tetracyclines are usually not used in young children because tetracyclines can permanently stain teeth.

- For *injection* dosage form (muscle injection):
  - For bacterial or protozoal infections:
    - Adults and teenagers—100 mg every eight hours; or 150 mg every twelve hours; or 250 mg once a day, injected into a muscle.
    - Children older than 8 years of age—Dose is based on body weight. The usual dose is 5 to 8.3 mg per kg (2.3 to 3.8 mg per pound) of body weight every eight hours; or 7.5 to 12.5 mg per kg (3.4 to 5.7 mg per pound) of body weight every twelve hours, injected into a muscle.
    - Infants and children 8 years of age and younger—Tetracyclines are usually not used in young children because tetracyclines can permanently stain teeth.

For tetracycline
- For *oral* dosage forms (capsules and suspension):
  - For bacterial or protozoal infections:
    - Adults and teenagers—250 to 500 milligrams (mg) every six hours; or 500 mg to 1 gram every twelve hours. Gonorrhea is treated with 1.5 grams as the first dose, then 500 mg every six hours for four days.
    - Children older than 8 years of age—Dose is based on body weight. The usual dose is 6.25 to 12.5 mg per kilogram (kg) (2.8 to 5.7 mg per pound) of body weight every six hours; or 12.5 to 25 mg per kg (5.7 to 11.4 mg per pound) of body weight every twelve hours.
    - Infants and children 8 years of age and younger—Tetracyclines are usually not used in young children because tetracyclines can permanently stain teeth.

Missed dose—If you miss a dose of this medicine, take it as soon as possible. This will help to keep a constant amount of medicine in the blood or urine. However, if it is almost time for your next dose, skip the missed dose and go back to your regular dosing schedule. Do not double doses.

Storage—To store this medicine:
- Keep out of the reach of children.
- Store away from heat and direct light.

- Do not store the capsule or tablet form of this medicine in the bathroom, near the kitchen sink, or in other damp places. Heat or moisture may cause the medicine to break down.
- Keep the oral liquid forms of this medicine from freezing.
- Do not keep outdated medicine or medicine no longer needed. Be sure that any discarded medicine is out of the reach of children.

Precautions While Using This Medicine

If your symptoms do not improve within a few days (or a few weeks or months for acne patients), or if they become worse, check with your doctor.

Oral contraceptives (birth control pills) containing estrogen may not work properly if you take them while you are taking tetracyclines. Unplanned pregnancies may occur. You should use a different or additional means of birth control while you are taking tetracyclines. If you have any questions about this, check with your health care professional.

Before having surgery (including dental surgery) with a general anesthetic, tell the medical doctor or dentist in charge that you are taking a tetracycline. This does not apply to doxycycline, however.

Tetracyclines may cause your skin to be more sensitive to sunlight than it is normally. Exposure to sunlight, even for brief periods of time, may cause a skin rash, itching, redness or other discoloration of the skin, or a severe sunburn. When you begin taking this medicine:
- Stay out of direct sunlight, especially between the hours of 10:00 a.m. and 3:00 p.m., if possible.
- Wear protective clothing, including a hat. Also, wear sunglasses.
- Apply a sun block product that has a skin protection factor (SPF) of at least 15. Some patients may require a product with a higher SPF number, especially if they have a fair complexion. If you have any questions about this, check with your health care professional.
- Apply a sun block lipstick that has an SPF of at least 15 to protect your lips.
- Do not use a sunlamp or tanning bed or booth.

You may still be more sensitive to sunlight or sunlamps for 2 weeks to several months or more after stopping this medicine. *If you have a severe reaction, check with your doctor.*

For patients taking *minocycline:*
- Minocycline may also cause some people to become dizzy, lightheaded, or unsteady. *Make sure you know how you react to this medicine before you drive, use machines, or do anything else that could be dangerous if you are dizzy or are not alert.* If these reactions are especially bothersome, check with your doctor.

Side Effects of This Medicine

Along with its needed effects, a medicine may cause some unwanted effects. In some infants and children, tetracyclines may cause the teeth to become discolored. Even though this may not happen right away, check with your doctor as soon as possible if you notice this effect or if you have any questions about it.

For all tetracyclines
More common
Increased sensitivity of skin to sunlight (rare with minocycline)
Rare
Abdominal pain; bulging fontanel (soft spot on head) of infants; headache; loss of appetite; nausea and vomiting; visual changes; yellowing skin

For demeclocycline only
Less common
Greatly increased frequency of urination or amount of urine; increased thirst; unusual tiredness or weakness

For minocycline only
Less common
Pigmentation (darker color or discoloration) of skin and mucous membranes

Other side effects may occur that usually do not need medical attention. These side effects may go away during treatment as your body adjusts to the medicine. However, check with your doctor if any of the following side effects continue or are bothersome:

For all tetracyclines
More common
Cramps or burning of the stomach; diarrhea
Less common
Itching of the rectal or genital (sex organ) areas; sore mouth or tongue

For minocycline only
More common
Dizziness, light-headedness, or unsteadiness

In some patients tetracyclines may cause the tongue to become darkened or discolored. This effect is only temporary and will go away when you stop taking this medicine.

Other side effects not listed above may also occur in some patients. If you notice any other effects, check with your doctor.

Additional Information

Once a medicine has been approved for marketing for a certain use, experience may show that it is also useful for other medical problems. Although these uses are not included in product labeling, tetracyclines are used in certain patients with the following medical conditions:

- Gonococcal arthritis
- Leprosy (for minocycline)
- Lyme disease (for doxycycline and tetracycline)
- Malaria treatment (for doxycycline and tetracycline)
- Nocardiosis (a type of bacterial infection) (for doxycycline and minocycline)
- Ocular rosacea (a type of eye infection) (for doxycycline and tetracycline)
- Pneumothorax (a pocket of air in the space surrounding the lungs) (for doxycycline and tetracycline)
- Rheumatoid arthritis (for minocycline)
- Shigellosis (a type of intestinal infection) (for doxycycline and tetracycline)
- Syndrome of inappropriate antidiuretic hormone (SIADH) (for demeclocycline)

For patients taking this medicine for *SIADH:*

- Some doctors may prescribe demeclocycline for certain patients who retain (keep) more body water than usual. Although demeclocycline works like a diuretic (water pill) in these patients, it will not work that way in other patients who may need a diuretic.

Other than the above information, there is no additional information relating to proper use, precautions, or side effects for these uses.

THALIDOMIDE (Oral route) - tha-LI-doe-mide

Black Box Warning

- WARNING: SEVERE, LIFE-THREATENING HUMAN BIRTH DEFECTS
  - If thalidomide is taken during pregnancy, it can cause severe birth defects or death to an unborn baby. Thalidomide should never be used by women who are pregnant or who could become pregnant while taking the drug. Even a single dose [1 capsule (50 mg, 100 mg or 200 mg)] taken by a pregnant woman during her pregnancy can cause severe birth defects.
  - Because of this toxicity and in an effort to make the chance of fetal exposure to thalidomide as negligible as possible, thalidomide is approved for marketing only under a special restricted distribution program approved by the Food and Drug Administration. This program is called the "System for Thalidomide Education and Prescribing Safety (S.T.E.P.S.(R))."
  - Under this restricted distribution program, only prescribers and pharmacists registered with the program are allowed to prescribe and dispense the product. In addition, patients must be advised of, agree to, and comply with the requirements of the S.T.E.P.S.(R) program in order to receive product.
  - Please see the following containing special information for prescribers, female patients, and male patients about this restricted distribution program.

- PRESCRIBERS
  - Thalidomide may be prescribed only by licensed prescribers who are registered in the S.T.E.P.S.(R) program and understand the risk of teratogenicity if thalidomide is used during pregnancy. Major human fetal abnormalities related to thalidomide administration during pregnancy have been documented: amelia (absence of limbs), phocomelia (short limbs), hypoplasticity of the bones, absence of bones, external ear abnormalities (including anotia, micro pinna, small or absent external auditory canals), facial palsy, eye abnormalities (anophthalmos, microphthalmos), and congenital heart defects. Alimentary tract, urinary tract, and genital malformations have also been documented. Mortality at or shortly after birth has been reported at about 40%.
  - Effective contraception must be used for at least 4 weeks before beginning thalidomide therapy, during thalidomide therapy, and for 4 weeks following discontinuation of thalidomide therapy. Reliable contraception is indicated even where there has been a

history of infertility, unless due to hysterectomy or because the patient has been postmenopausal for at least 24 months. Two reliable forms of contraception must be used simultaneously unless continuous abstinence from heterosexual sexual contact is the chosen method. Women of childbearing potential should be referred to a qualified provider of contraceptive methods, if needed. Sexually mature women who have not undergone a hysterectomy or who have not been postmenopausal for at least 24 consecutive months (i.e., who have had menses at some time in the preceding 24 consecutive months) are considered to be women of childbearing potential.

- Before starting treatment, women of childbearing potential should have a pregnancy test (sensitivity of at least 50 mIU/mL). The test should be performed within the 24 hours prior to beginning thalidomide therapy. A prescription for thalidomide for a woman of childbearing potential must not be issued by the prescriber until a written report of a negative pregnancy test has been obtained by the prescriber.
- Male Patients: Because thalidomide is present in the semen of patients receiving the drug, males receiving thalidomide must always use a latex condom during any sexual contact with women of childbearing potential even if he has undergone a successful vasectomy.
- Once treatment has started, pregnancy testing should occur weekly during the first 4 weeks of use, then pregnancy testing should be repeated at 4 weeks in women with regular menstrual cycles. If menstrual cycles are irregular, the pregnancy testing should occur every 2 weeks. Pregnancy testing and counseling should be performed if a patient misses her period or if there is any abnormality in menstrual bleeding.
- If pregnancy does occur during thalidomide treatment, thalidomide must be discontinued immediately. Any suspected fetal exposure to thalidomide must be reported immediately to the FDA via the MedWatch number at 1–800–FDA-1088 and also to Celgene Corporation. The patient should be referred to an obstetrician/gynecologist experienced in reproductive toxicity for further evaluation and counseling.

- FEMALE PATIENTS
  - Thalidomide is contraindicated in women of childbearing potential unless alternative therapies are considered inappropriate and the patient meets all of the following conditions (i.e., she is essentially unable to become pregnant while on thalidomide therapy): 1) she understands and can reliably carry out instructions, 2) she is capable of complying with the mandatory contraceptive measures, pregnancy testing, patient registration, and patient survey as described in the System for Thalidomide Education and Prescribing Safety (S.T.E.P.S.(R)) program, 3) she has received both oral and written warnings of the hazards of taking thalidomide during pregnancy and of exposing a fetus to the drug, 4) she has received both oral and written warnings of the risk of possible contraception failure and of the need to use two reliable forms of contraception simultaneously, unless continuous abstinence from heterosexual sexual contact is the chosen method. Sexually mature women who have not undergone a hysterectomy or who have not

been postmenopausal for at least 24 consecutive months (i.e., who have had menses at some time in the preceding 24 consecutive months) are considered to be women of childbearing potential, 5) she acknowledges, in writing, her understanding of these warnings and of the need for using two reliable methods of contraception for 4 weeks prior to beginning thalidomide therapy, during thalidomide therapy, and for 4 weeks after discontinuation of thalidomide therapy, 6) she has had a negative pregnancy test with a sensitivity of at least 50 mIU/mL, within the 24 hours prior to beginning therapy, and 7) if the patient is between 12 and 18 years of age, her parent or legal guardian must have read this material and agreed to ensure compliance with the above.

- MALE PATIENTS
  - Thalidomide is contraindicated in sexually mature males unless the patient meets all of the following conditions: 1) he understands and can reliably carry out instructions, 2) he is capable of complying with the mandatory contraceptive measures that are appropriate for men, patient registration, and patient survey as described in the S.T.E.P.S.(R) program, 3) he has received both oral and written warnings of the hazards of taking thalidomide and exposing a fetus to the drug, 4) he has received both oral and written warnings of the risk of possible contraception failure and of the presence of thalidomide in semen. He has been instructed that he must always use a latex condom during any sexual contact with women of childbearing potential, even if he has undergone a successful vasectomy, 5) he acknowledges, in writing, his understanding of these warnings and of the need to use a latex condom during any sexual contact with women of childbearing potential, even if he has undergone a successful vasectomy. Sexually mature women who have not undergone a hysterectomy or who have not been postmenopausal for at least 24 consecutive months (i.e., who have had menses at any time in the preceding 24 consecutive months) are considered to be women of childbearing potential, and 6) if the patient is between 12 and 18 years of age, his parent or legal guardian must have read this material and agreed to ensure compliance with the above.

- VENOUS THROMBOEMBOLIC EVENTS
  - The use of thalidomide in multiple myeloma results in an increased risk of venous thromboembolic events, such as deep venous thrombosis and pulmonary embolus. The risk increases significantly when thalidomide is used in combination with standard chemotherapeutic agents including dexamethasone. In one controlled trial, the rate of venous thromboembolic events was 22.5% in patients receiving thalidomide in combination with dexamethasone compared to 4.9% in patients receiving dexamethasone alone (p=0.002). Patients and physicians are advised to be observant for the signs and symptoms of thromboembolism. Patients should be instructed to seek medical care if they develop symptoms such as shortness of breath, chest pain, or arm or leg swelling. Preliminary data suggest that patients who are appropriate candidates may benefit from concurrent prophylactic anticoagulation or aspirin treatment.

Commonly used brand name(s)

In the U.S.—
   Thalomid

Available Dosage Forms:
- Capsule

Therapeutic Class: Leprostatic

Uses For This Medicine

Thalidomide is used to treat and prevent erythema nodosum leprosum (ENL), a painful skin disease associated with leprosy. It is also used together with dexamethasone (e.g., Decadron®) to treat patients who have just been diagnosed with multiple myeloma (a certain type of cancer of the blood). This medicine may also be used for other diseases as determined by your doctor.

Thalidomide is available only from your doctor. It has not been widely available since the early 1960s because it was found to cause birth defects. However, under special conditions, your doctor may decide that this medicine will be useful for your treatment.

This medicine is available only with your doctor's prescription.

Once a medicine has been approved for marketing for a certain use, experience may show that it is also useful for other medical problems. Although these uses are not included in product labeling, thalidomide is used in certain patients with the following medical condition:
- Esophagus ulcers in patients with human immunodeficiency virus (HIV) infection

Before Using This Medicine

In deciding to use a medicine, the risks of taking the medicine must be weighed against the good it will do. This is a decision you and your doctor will make. For this medicine, the following should be considered:

Allergies—Tell your doctor if you have ever had any unusual or allergic reaction to this medicine or any other medicines. Also tell your health care professional if you have any other types of allergies, such as to foods, dyes, preservatives, or animals. For non-prescription products, read the label or package ingredients carefully.

Pediatric—Appropriate studies have not been performed on the relationship of age to the effects of thalidomide in children up to 12 years of age. Safety and efficacy have not been established.

Geriatric—This medicine has been tested in a limited number of patients up to 90 years of age and has not been shown to cause different side effects or problems in older people than it does in younger adults.

Pregnancy—

	Pregnancy Category	Explanation
All Trimesters	X	Studies in animals or pregnant women have demonstrated positive evidence of fetal abnormalities. This drug should not be used in women who are or may become pregnant because the risk clearly outweighs any possible benefit.

Breast Feeding—There are no adequate studies in women for determining infant risk when using this medication during breastfeeding. Weigh the potential benefits against the potential risks before taking this medication while breastfeeding.

Other medicines—

Using this medicine with any of the following medicines is usually not recommended, but may be required in some cases. If both medicines are prescribed together, your doctor may change the dose or how often you use one or both of the medicines.

Darbepoetin Alfa, Dexamethasone, Docetaxel

Interactions with Food/Tobacco/Alcohol—Certain medicines should not be used at or around the time of eating food or eating certain types of food since interactions may occur. Using alcohol or tobacco with certain medicines may also cause interactions to occur. Discuss with your healthcare professional the use of your medicine with food, alcohol, or tobacco.

Other medical problems—The presence of other medical problems may affect the use of this medicine. Make sure you tell your doctor if you have any other medical problems, especially:
- Decreased white blood cell counts or
- Epilepsy or risk of seizures or
- Peripheral neuropathy—Thalidomide may make these conditions worse.

Proper Use of This Medicine

You should take this medicine with water, preferably at bedtime and at least 1 hour after the evening meal.

Take this medicine exactly as directed by your doctor. Do not take more of it, do not take it more often, and do not take it for a longer time than your doctor ordered. Also, do not stop taking this medicine without checking with your doctor first.

Only take medicine that your doctor has prescribed specifically for you. Do not share your medicine with others.

Dosing—The dose of this medicine will be different for different patients. Follow your doctor's orders or the directions on the label. The following information includes only the average doses of this medicine. If your dose is different, do not change it unless your doctor tells you to do so.

The amount of medicine that you take depends on the strength of the medicine. Also, the number of doses you take each day, the time allowed between doses, and the length of time you take the medicine depend on the medical problem for which you are using the medicine.

- For oral dosage form (capsules):
  - For erythema nodosum leprosum (ENL):
    - Adults and teenagers—100 to 400 milligrams (mg) once a day until the condition improves. Then, the dose may be decreased as determined by your doctor.
    - Children—Use and dose must be determined by your doctor.
  - For multiple myeloma:
    - Adults and teenagers—200 mg once a day in combination with dexamethasone in 28–day treatment cycles as instructed by your doctor. The dose of dexamethasone that you need to take will be determined by your doctor.

- Children—Use and dose must be determined by your doctor.

Missed dose—If you miss a dose of this medicine, take it as soon as possible. However, if it is almost time for your next dose, skip the missed dose and go back to your regular dosing schedule. Do not double doses.

Storage—Store the medicine in a closed container at room temperature, away from heat, moisture, and direct light. Keep from freezing.

Keep out of the reach of children.

Do not keep outdated medicine or medicine no longer needed.

Precautions While Using This Medicine

This medicine will add to the effects of alcohol and other CNS depressants (medicines that may make you drowsy or less alert). Some examples of CNS depressants are antihistamines or medicines for hay fever, other allergies, or colds; sedatives, tranquilizers, or sleeping medicine; prescription pain medicine or narcotics; barbiturates; medicine for seizures; muscle relaxants; or anesthetics, including some dental anesthetics. *Check with your doctor before taking any of these while you are using thalidomide.*

Your doctor will inform you of a safety program called S.T.E.P.S.® that you must agree to and comply with in order to receive your thalidomide prescription. Be sure to ask your doctor or pharmacist if you have any questions about this program.

For women of childbearing age: *If you are able to bear children, you must have a pregnancy test within 24 hours before starting thalidomide treatment, once a week during the first month of treatment, and every 2 to 4 weeks after that. Also, you must not have heterosexual sexual contact unless you use two effective birth control methods at the same time for at least 1 month before starting thalidomide treatment, during treatment, and for at least 1 month after you stop taking thalidomide.*

For men taking thalidomide: *If you have heterosexual sexual contact with women of childbearing potential, you must always use a condom during sexual contact while taking thalidomide and for 4 weeks after you stop taking it, even if you have had a vasectomy.*

Your doctor may prescribe an anticoagulant (prevents the clotting of blood) or aspirin treatment while you are taking thalidomide to prevent blood clots. You should take this medicine as instructed by your doctor.

You should contact your doctor right away if you develop shortness of breath, chest pain, or arm or leg swelling. These could be symptoms of blood clots that require immediate attention.

It is very important that your doctor check you at regular visits for any nerve problems that may be caused by this medicine. If you notice any symptoms of peripheral neuropathy (tingling, burning, numbness, or pain in the hands or feet), stop taking this medicine and call your doctor right away.

Side Effects of This Medicine

Along with its needed effects, a medicine may cause some unwanted effects. Although not all of these side effects may occur, if they do occur they may need medical attention.

Check with your doctor immediately if any of the following side effects occur:

More common

Anxiety; chest pain; cough; dizziness or lightheadedness; fainting; fast heartbeat; muscle weakness; pain, redness, or swelling in arm or leg; sudden shortness of breath or troubled breathing; tingling, burning, numbness, or pain in the hands, arms, feet, or legs

Rare

Blood in urine; decreased urination; fever, alone or with chills and sore throat; irregular heartbeat; low blood pressure; skin rash

Incidence not known

Blistering of skin; convulsions; itching skin; muscle jerking of arms and legs; peeling and loosening of skin; red, irritated eyes; red skin lesions, often with a purple center; sores, ulcers, or white spots in mouth or on lips; sudden loss of consciousness

Some side effects may occur that usually do not need medical attention. These side effects may go away during treatment as your body adjusts to the medicine. Also, your health care professional may be able to tell you about ways to prevent or reduce some of these side effects. Check with your health care professional if any of the following side effects continue or are bothersome or if you have any questions about them:

More common

Constipation; diarrhea; drowsiness; nausea; stomach pain

Less common

Dry skin; dryness of mouth; headache; increased appetite; mood changes

Other side effects not listed may also occur in some patients. If you notice any other effects, check with your healthcare professional.

THIAMINE   (Oral route, Injection route)
- THYE-a-min

Commonly used brand name(s)

In the U.S.—
Thiamilate

Available Dosage Forms:

- Capsule
- Tablet
- Tablet, Enteric Coated
- Solution

Therapeutic Class: Nutritive Agent
Pharmacologic Class: Vitamin B

Uses For This Dietary Supplement

Vitamins are compounds that you must have for growth and health. They are needed in small amounts only and are usually available in the foods that you eat. Thiamine (vitamin B 1) is needed for the breakdown of carbohydrates.

Some conditions may increase your need for thiamine. These include:

- Alcoholism
- Burns

- Diarrhea (continuing)
- Fever (continuing)
- Illness (continuing)
- Intestinal disease
- Liver disease
- Overactive thyroid
- Stress (continuing)
- Surgical removal of stomach

Also, the following groups of people may have a deficiency of thiamine:

- Patients using an artificial kidney (on hemodialysis)
- Individuals who do heavy manual labor on a daily basis

Increased need for thiamine should be determined by your health care professional.

Lack of thiamine may lead to a condition called beriberi. Signs of beriberi include loss of appetite, constipation, muscle weakness, pain or tingling in arms or legs, and possible swelling of feet or lower legs. In addition, if severe, lack of thiamine may cause mental depression, memory problems, weakness, shortness of breath, and fast heartbeat. Your health care professional may treat this by prescribing thiamine for you.

Thiamine may also be used for other conditions as determined by your health care professional.

Claims that thiamine is effective for treatment of skin problems, chronic diarrhea, tiredness, mental problems, multiple sclerosis, nerve problems, and ulcerative colitis (a disease of the intestines), or as an insect repellant or to stimulate appetite have not been proven.

Injectable thiamine is administered only by or under the supervision of your health care professional. Other forms of thiamine are available without a prescription.

Once a medicine or dietary supplement has been approved for marketing for a certain use, experience may show that it is also useful for other medical problems. Although this use is not included in product labeling, thiamine is used in certain patients with the following medical conditions:

- Enzyme deficiency diseases such as encephalomyelopathy, maple syrup urine disease, pyruvate carboxylase, and hyperalaninemia

Importance of Diet—For good health, it is important that you eat a balanced and varied diet. Follow carefully any diet program your health care professional may recommend. For your specific dietary vitamin and/or mineral needs, ask your health care professional for a list of appropriate foods. If you think that you are not getting enough vitamins and/or minerals in your diet, you may choose to take a dietary supplement.

Thiamine is found in various foods, including cereals (whole-grain and enriched), peas, beans, nuts, and meats (especially pork and beef). Some thiamine in foods is lost with cooking.

Vitamins alone will not take the place of a good diet and will not provide energy. Your body also needs other substances found in food such as protein, minerals, carbohydrates, and fat. Vitamins themselves often cannot work without the presence of other foods.

The daily amount of thiamine needed is defined in several different ways.

For U.S.—
- Recommended Dietary Allowances (RDAs) are the amount of vitamins and minerals needed to provide for adequate nutrition in most healthy persons. RDAs for a given nutrient may vary depending on a person's age, sex, and physical condition (e.g., pregnancy).
- Daily Values (DVs) are used on food and dietary supplement labels to indicate the percent of the recommended daily amount of each nutrient that a serving provides. DV replaces the previous designation of United States Recommended Daily Allowances (USRDAs).

For Canada—
- Recommended Nutrient Intakes (RNIs) are used to determine the amounts of vitamins, minerals, and protein needed to provide adequate nutrition and lessen the risk of chronic disease.

Normal daily recommended intakes in milligrams (mg) for thiamine are generally defined as follows:

Persons	U.S. (mg)	Canada (mg)
Infants and children		
Birth to 3 years of age	0.3–0.7	0.3–0.6
4 to 6 years of age	0.9	0.7
7 to 10 years of age	1	0.8–1
Adolescent and adult males	1.2–1.5	0.8–1.3
Adolescent and adult females	1–1.1	0.8–0.9
Pregnant females	1.5	0.9–1
Breast-feeding females	1.6	1–1.2

Before Using This Dietary Supplement

If you are taking this dietary supplement without a prescription, carefully read and follow any precautions on the label. For this supplement, the following should be considered:

Allergies—Tell your doctor if you have ever had any unusual or allergic reaction to this medicine or any other medicines. Also tell your health care professional if you have any other types of allergies, such as to foods, dyes, preservatives, or animals. For non-prescription products, read the label or package ingredients carefully.

Pediatric—Problems in children have not been reported with intake of normal daily recommended amounts.

Geriatric—Problems in older adults have not been reported with intake of normal daily recommended amounts. Studies have shown that older adults may have lower blood levels of thiamine than younger adults. Your health care professional may recommend that you take a vitamin supplement that contains thiamine.

Breast Feeding—Studies in women suggest that this medication poses minimal risk to the infant when used during breastfeeding.

Other medicines—Although certain medicines should not be used together at all, in other cases two different medicines may be used together even if an interaction might occur. In these cases, your doctor may want to change the dose, or other precautions may be necessary. Tell your healthcare professional if you are taking any other prescription or non-prescription (over-the-counter [OTC]) medicine.

Interactions with Food/Tobacco/Alcohol—Certain medicines should not be used at or around the time of eating food or eating certain types of food since interactions may occur. Using alcohol or tobacco with certain medicines may also cause interactions to occur. Discuss with your healthcare professional the use of your medicine with food, alcohol, or tobacco.

Proper Use of This Dietary Supplement

Dosing—The dose of this medicine will be different for different patients. Follow your doctor's orders or the directions on the label. The following information includes only the average doses of this medicine. If your dose is different, do not change it unless your doctor tells you to do so.

The amount of medicine that you take depends on the strength of the medicine. Also, the number of doses you take each day, the time allowed between doses, and the length of time you take the medicine depend on the medical problem for which you are using the medicine.

- For oral dosage forms (tablets, oral solution):
  - To prevent deficiency, the amount taken by mouth is based on normal daily recommended intakes:

  For the U.S.
  - Adult and teenage males—1.2 to 1.5 milligrams (mg) per day.
  - Adult and teenage females—1 to 1.1 mg per day.
  - Pregnant females—1.5 mg per day.
  - Breast-feeding females—1.6 mg per day.
  - Children 7 to 10 years of age—1 mg per day.
  - Children 4 to 6 years of age—0.9 mg per day.
  - Children birth to 3 years of age—0.3 to 0.7 mg per day.

  For Canada
  - Adult and teenage males—0.8 to 1.3 mg per day.
  - Adult and teenage females—0.8 to 0.9 mg per day.
  - Pregnant females—0.9 to 1 mg per day.
  - Breast-feeding females—1 to 1.2 mg per day.
  - Children 7 to 10 years of age—0.8 to 1 mg per day.
  - Children 4 to 6 years of age—0.7 mg per day.
  - Children birth to 3 years of age—0.3 to 0.6 mg per day.

  - To treat deficiency:
    - Adults and teenagers—Treatment dose is determined by prescriber for each individual based on the severity of deficiency. The following dosage has been established: Beriberi—Oral, 5 to 10 mg three times a day.
    - Children—Treatment dose is determined by prescriber for each individual based on the severity of deficiency. The following dosage has been established: Beriberi—Oral, 10 a day.

Missed dose—If you miss a dose of this medicine, take it as soon as possible. However, if it is almost time for your next dose, skip the missed dose and go back to your regular dosing schedule. Do not double doses.

If you miss taking a vitamin for 1 or more days there is no cause for concern, since it takes some time for your body to become seriously low in vitamins. However, if your health care professional has recommended that you take this vitamin, try to remember to take it as directed every day.

Storage—Store the dietary supplement in a closed container at room temperature, away from heat, moisture, and direct light. Keep from freezing.

Keep out of the reach of children.

Do not keep outdated medicine or medicine no longer needed.

Side Effects of This Dietary Supplement

Along with its needed effects, a medicine may cause some unwanted effects. Although not all of these side effects may occur, if they do occur they may need medical attention.

Check with your doctor immediately if any of the following side effects occur:
> *Rare*—Soon after receiving injection only
>> Coughing; difficulty in swallowing; hives; itching of skin; swelling of face, lips, or eyelids; wheezing or difficulty in breathing

Other side effects not listed may also occur in some patients. If you notice any other effects, check with your healthcare professional.

THROMBOLYTIC AGENTS
(Systemic)

Some commonly used brand names are:

In the U.S.—

Abbokinase (5)	Eminase (2)
Abbokinase Open-Cath (5)	Retavase (3)
Activase (1)	Streptase (4)

In Canada—

Abbokinase (5)	Eminase (2)
Abbokinase Open-Cath (5)	Streptase (4)
Activase rt-PA (1)	

This information applies to the following medicines:

1. Alteplase, Recombinant (AL-te-plase)
2. Anistreplase (a-NISS-tre-place)
3. Reteplase, Recombinant (RE-te-plays)
4. Streptokinase (strep-toe-KIN-ace)
5. Urokinase (yoor-oh-KIN-ace)

Category

- **Thrombolytic**—Alteplase, Recombinant; Anistreplase; Reteplase, Recombinant; Streptokinase; Urokinase

Description

Thrombolytic agents are used to dissolve blood clots that have formed in certain blood vessels. These medicines are usually used when a blood clot seriously lessens the flow of blood to certain parts of the body.

Thrombolytic agents are also used to dissolve blood clots that form in tubes that are placed into the body. The tubes allow treatments (such as dialysis or injections into a vein) to be given over a long period of time.

These medicines are to be given only by or under the direct supervision of a doctor.

These medicines are available in the following dosage forms:

Parenteral
- Alteplase, Recombinant
  - Injection
- Anistreplase
  - Injection

- Reteplase, Recombinant
  - Injection
- Streptokinase
  - Injection
- Urokinase
  - Injection

Before Receiving This Medicine

In deciding to use a medicine, the risks of using the medicine must be weighed against the good it will do. This is a decision you and your doctor will make. For thrombolytic agents, the following should be considered:

Allergies—Tell your doctor if you have ever had any unusual or allergic reaction to alteplase, anistreplase, streptokinase, or urokinase. Also tell your health care professional if you are allergic to any other substances, such as foods, preservatives, or dyes.

Pregnancy—Tell your doctor if you are pregnant or if you have recently had a baby.

There is a slight chance that use of a thrombolytic agent during the first five months of pregnancy may cause a miscarriage. However, both streptokinase and urokinase have been used in pregnant women and have not been reported to cause this problem. Also, studies in pregnant women (for streptokinase) and studies in animals (for urokinase) have not shown that these medicines cause either miscarriage or harm to the fetus (including birth defects). Studies on birth defects with alteplase and anistreplase have not been done in either pregnant women or animals.

Breast-feeding—It is not known whether thrombolytic agents pass into the breast milk. Although most medicines pass into breast milk in small amounts, many of them may be used safely while breast-feeding. Mothers who are taking any of these medicines and who wish to breast-feed should discuss this with their doctor.

Children—Studies on these medicines have been done only in adult patients, and there is no specific information comparing the use of thrombolytic agents in children with use in other age groups. However, streptokinase has occasionally been used in children to dissolve blood clots in certain blood vessels. Bleeding may be more likely to occur in children, who are usually more sensitive than adults to the effects of streptokinase.

Older adults—The need for treatment with a thrombolytic agent (instead of other kinds of treatment) may be increased in elderly patients with blood clots. However, the chance of bleeding may also be increased. It is especially important that you discuss the use of this medicine with your doctor.

Other medicines—Although certain medicines should not be used together at all, in other cases two different medicines may be used together even if an interaction might occur. In these cases, your doctor may want to change the dose, or other precautions may be necessary. Before you receive a thrombolytic agent, it is especially important that your doctor know if you are taking any of the following:

- Anticoagulants (blood thinners) or
- Aspirin or
- Cefamandole (e.g., Mandol) or
- Cefoperazone (e.g., Cefobid) or

- Cefotetan (e.g., Cefotan) or
- Dipyridamole (e.g., Persantine)
- Divalproex (e.g., Depakote) or
- Enoxaparin (e.g., Lovenox) or
- Heparin or
- Indomethacin (e.g., Indocin) or
- Inflammation or pain medicine (except narcotics) or
- Phenylbutazone (e.g., Butazolidin) or
- Plicamycin (e.g., Mithracin) or
- Sulfinpyrazone (e.g., Anturane) or
- Thrombolytic agents, other or
- Ticlopidine (e.g., Ticlid) or
- Valproic acid (e.g., Depakene)—The chance of bleeding may be increased

Also, tell your doctor if you have had an injection of anistreplase or streptokinase within the past year. If you have, these medicines may not work properly if they are given to you again. Your doctor may decide to use alteplase or urokinase instead.

Other medical problems—The presence of other medical problems or recent delivery of a child may affect the use of thrombolytic agents. Make sure you tell your doctor if you have any other medical problems, especially:

- Allergic reaction to streptokinase, anistreplase, or urokinase (or history of)—Increased risk of an allergic reaction
- Blood disease, bleeding problems, or a history of bleeding in any part of the body or
- Brain disease or tumor or
- Heart or blood vessel disease, including irregular heartbeat or
- High blood pressure or
- Liver disease (severe) or
- Stroke, especially with seizure (or history of)—The chance of serious bleeding may be increased
- Streptococcal ("strep") infection (recent)
- Surgery within the last two months—Anistreplase or streptokinase may not work properly after a streptococcal infection; your doctor may decide to use a different thrombolytic agent

Also, tell your doctor if you have recently had any of the following conditions:

- Falls or blows to the body or head or any other injury or
- Injections into a blood vessel or
- Placement of any tube into the body or
- Surgery, including dental surgery—The chance of serious bleeding may be increased

If you have recently had a baby, use of these medicines may cause serious bleeding.

Proper Use of This Medicine

Dosing—The dose of these medicines will be different for different patients. The dose you receive will depend on the medicine you receive and will be based on the condition for which you are receiving the medicine. In some cases, the dose will also depend on your body weight.

Precautions While Using This Medicine

Thrombolytic agents can cause bleeding that usually is not serious. However, serious bleeding may occur in some people. *To help prevent serious bleeding, carefully follow any instructions given by your health care professional. Also, move around as little as possible, and do not get out of bed on your own, unless your health care professional tells you it is all right to do so.*

Side Effects

Along with its needed effects, a medicine may cause some unwanted effects. Although not all of these side effects may occur, if they do occur they may need medical attention.

Tell your health care professional immediately if any of the following side effects occur:
More common
Bleeding or oozing from cuts, gums, wounds, or around the place of injection; fever; low blood pressure
Less common or rare
Agitation; bloating; blue or purple toes; blurred vision; bruising; changes in facial skin color; chest pain or discomfort; chills; coma; confusion; darkened urine; decreased urine output; depression; dizziness; double vision; fast or irregular breathing; flushing or redness of skin; gangrenous fingers or toes; headache (mild or severe); hostility; indigestion; irritability; lethargy; loss of appetite; muscle cramps or spasms; muscle pain or stiffness; muscle twitching; nausea; nervousness; numbness or tingling in face, arms, legs; pain in side or abdomen, possibly radiating to the back; pain in toes; pain or discomfort in arms, jaw, back or neck; pounding in the ears; purplish red, net-like, blotchy spots on skin; rapid weight gain; seizures; shortness of breath, troubled breathing, tightness in chest, and/or wheezing; skin rash, hives, or itching; slow or fast heartbeat; stupor; sweating; swelling of eyes, face, lips, or tongue; swelling of hands or ankles; trouble in speaking or walking; unusual tiredness or weakness; vomiting; weakness in arms or legs; yellow eyes or skin
Frequency not determined
Bluish color of fingernails, lips, skin, palms, or nail beds; cough; difficulty breathing; drowsiness; faintness or lightheadedness when getting up from a lying or sitting position suddenly; fatigue; noisy breathing; welts
Symptoms of bleeding inside the body
Abdominal or stomach pain or swelling; back pain or backaches; blood in urine; bloody or black, tarry stools; constipation; coughing up blood; dizziness; headaches (sudden, severe, or continuing); joint pain, stiffness, or swelling; muscle pain or stiffness (severe or continuing); nosebleeds; unexpected or unusually heavy bleeding from vagina; vomiting of blood or material that looks like coffee grounds

Other side effects not listed above may also occur in some patients. If you notice any other effects, check with your doctor.

Additional Information

Once a medicine has been approved for marketing for a certain use, experience may show that it is also useful for other medical problems. Although this use is not included in product labeling, alteplase may be used in certain patients with the following condition:

 • Peripheral arterial occlusive disease

Other than the above information, there is no additional information relating to proper use, precautions, or side effects for this use.

THYROID HORMONES   (Systemic)

Some commonly used brand names are:
In the U.S.—

Armour Thyroid (5)	Thyrar (5)
Cytomel (2)	Thyroid Strong (5)
Levo-T (1)	Thyrolar (3)
Levothroid (1)	Triostat (2)
Levoxyl (1)	Westhroid (5)
Synthroid (1)	

In Canada—

Cytomel (2)	PMS-Levothyroxine Sodium (1)
Eltroxin (1)	Synthroid (1)

This information applies to the following medicines:
1. Levothyroxine (lee-voe-thye-ROX-een)
2. Liothyronine (lye-oh-THYE-roe-neen)
3. Liotrix (LYE-oh-trix)
4. Thyroglobulin (thye-roe-GLOB-yoo-lin)
5. Thyroid (THYE-roid)

Category

 • **Antineoplastic—**Levothyroxine; Liothyronine; Liotrix; Thyroglobulin; Thyroid
 • **Diagnostic aid, thyroid function—**Levothyroxine; Liothyronine
 • **Thyroid hormone—**Levothyroxine; Liothyronine; Liotrix; Thyroglobulin; Thyroid

Description

Thyroid medicines belong to the general group of medicines called hormones. They are used when the thyroid gland does not produce enough hormone. They are also used to help decrease the size of enlarged thyroid glands (known as goiter) and to treat thyroid cancer.

These medicines are available only with your doctor's prescription, in the following dosage forms:
Oral
 • Levothyroxine
   ○ Tablets
 • Liothyronine
   ○ Tablets
 • Liotrix
   ○ Tablets
 • Thyroglobulin
   ○ Tablets
 • Thyroid
   ○ Tablets

Parenteral
- Levothyroxine
  - Injection
- Liothyronine
  - Injection

Before Using This Medicine

In deciding to use a medicine, the risks of taking the medicine must be weighed against the good it will do. This is a decision you and your doctor will make. For thyroid hormones, the following should be considered:

Allergies—Tell your doctor if you have ever had any unusual or allergic reaction to thyroid hormones. Also tell your health care professional if you are allergic to any other substances, such as foods, preservatives, or dyes.

Pregnancy—Use of proper amounts of thyroid hormone during pregnancy has not been shown to cause birth defects or other problems. However, your doctor may want you to change your dose while you are pregnant. This will make regular visits to your doctor important.

Breast-feeding—Use of proper amounts of thyroid hormones by mothers has not been shown to cause problems in nursing babies.

Children—Thyroid hormones have been tested in children and have not been shown to cause different side effects or problems in children than they do in adults.

Older adults—This medicine has been tested and has not been shown to cause different side effects or problems in older people than it does in younger adults. However, a different dose may be needed in the elderly. Therefore, it is important to take the medicine only as directed by the doctor.

Other medicines—Although certain medicines should not be used together at all, in other cases two different medicines may be used together even if an interaction might occur. In these cases, your doctor may want to change the dose, or other precautions may be necessary. When you are taking thyroid hormones, it is especially important that your health care professional know if you are taking any of the following:

- Amphetamines
- Anticoagulants (blood thinners)
- Appetite suppressants (diet pills)
- Cholestyramine (e.g., Questran)
- Colestipol (e.g., Colestid)
- Medicine for asthma or other breathing problems
- Medicine for colds, sinus problems, or hay fever or other allergies (including nose drops or sprays)

Other medical problems—The presence of other medical problems may affect the use of thyroid hormones. Make sure you tell your doctor if you have any other medical problems especially:
- Diabetes mellitus (sugar diabetes)
- Hardening of the arteries
- Heart disease
- High blood pressure
- Overactive thyroid (history of)
- Underactive adrenal gland
- Underactive pituitary gland

Proper Use of This Medicine

Use this medicine only as directed by your doctor. Do not use more or less of it, and do not use it more often than your doctor ordered. Your doctor has prescribed the exact amount your body needs and if you take different amounts, you may experience symptoms of an overactive or underactive thyroid. Take it at the same time each day to make sure it always has the same effect.

If your condition is due to a lack of thyroid hormone, you may have to take this medicine for the rest of your life. It is very important that you *do not stop taking this medicine without first checking with your doctor.*

Dosing—The dose of these medicines will be different for different patients. *Follow your doctor's orders or the directions on the label.* The following information includes only the average doses of these medicines. *If your dose is different, do not change it* unless your doctor tells you to do so.

The number of tablets that you take depends on the strength of the medicine. The amount of thyroid hormone that you need to take every day depends on the results of your thyroid tests. However, treatment is usually started with lower doses that are increased a little at a time until you are taking the full amount. This helps prevent side effects.

For levothyroxine
- For *oral* dosage form (tablets):
  - For replacing the thyroid hormone:
    - Adults and teenagers—At first, 0.0125 to 0.05 milligrams (mg) once a day. Then, your doctor may increase your dose a little at a time to 0.075 to 0.125 mg a day. The dose is usually no higher than 0.15 mg once a day.
    - Children less than 6 months of age—The dose is based on body weight and must be determined by your doctor. The usual dose is 0.025 to 0.05 mg once a day.
    - Children 6 months to 12 months of age—The dose is based on body weight and must be determined by your doctor. The usual dose is 0.05 to 0.075 mg once a day.
    - Children 1 to 5 years of age—The dose is based on body weight and must be determined by your doctor. The usual dose is 0.075 to 0.1 mg once a day.
    - Children 6 to 10 years of age—The dose is based on body weight and must be determined by your doctor. The usual dose is 0.1 to 0.15 mg once a day.
    - Children over 10 years of age—The dose is based on body weight and must be determined by your doctor. The usual dose is 0.15 to 0.2 mg once a day.
- For *injection* dosage form:
  - For replacing the thyroid hormone:
    - Adults and teenagers—50 to 100 micrograms (mcg) injected into a muscle or into a vein once a day. People with very serious conditions caused by too little thyroid hormone may need higher doses.
    - Children less than 6 months of age—The dose is based on body weight and must be determined by your doctor. The usual dose is 0.019 to 0.038 mg once a day.

- Children 6 months to 12 months of age—The dose is based on body weight and must be determined by your doctor. The usual dose is 0.038 to 0.056 mg once a day.
- Children 1 to 5 years of age—The dose is based on body weight and must be determined by your doctor. The usual dose is 0.056 to 0.075 mg once a day.
- Children 6 to 10 years of age—The dose is based on body weight and must be determined by your doctor. The usual dose is 0.075 to 0.113 mg once a day.
- Children over 10 years of age—The dose is based on body weight and must be determined by your doctor. The usual dose is 0.113 to 0.15 mg once a day.

For liothyronine sodium
- For *oral* dosage form (tablets):
  - For replacing the thyroid hormone:
    - Adults and teenagers—At first, 25 micrograms (mcg) a day. Some patients with very serious conditions caused by too little thyroid hormone may need to take only 2.5 to 5 mcg a day at first. Also, some patients with heart disease or the elderly may need lower doses at first. Then, your doctor may increase your dose a little at a time to up to 50 mcg a day if needed. Your doctor may want you to divide your dose into smaller amounts that are taken two or more times a day.
  - For treating a large thyroid gland (goiter):
    - Adults—At first, 5 mcg a day. Some patients with heart disease or the elderly may need lower doses at first. Then, your doctor may increase your dose a little at a time to 50 to 100 mcg a day.
- For *injection* dosage form:
  - For replacing the thyroid hormone in very serious conditions (myxedema coma):
    - Adults—At first, 10 to 50 mcg injected into a vein every four to twelve hours. Then, your doctor may want to adjust your dose depending on your condition.
    - Children—Use and dose must be determined by your doctor.

For liotrix (levothyroxine and liothyronine combination)
- For *oral* dosage form (tablets):
  - For replacing the thyroid hormone:
    - Adults, teenagers, and children—At first, 50 micrograms (mcg) of levothyroxine and 12.5 mcg of liothyronine once a day. Some people with very serious conditions caused by too little thyroid hormone may need only 12.5 mcg of levothyroxine and 3.1 mcg of liothyronine once a day. Also, some elderly patients may need lower doses at first. Then, your doctor may want to increase your dose a little at a time to up to 100 mcg of levothyroxine and 25 mcg of liothyronine.

For thyroglobulin
- For *oral* dosage form (tablets):
  - For replacing the thyroid hormone:
    - Adults, teenagers, and children—At first, 32 milligrams (mg) a day. Some people with very serious conditions caused by too little thyroid hormone may need to take only 16 to 32 mg a day at first.

Then, the doctor may want you to increase your dose a little at a time to 65 to 160 mg a day.

For thyroid
- For *oral* dosage form (tablets):
  - For replacing thyroid hormone:
    - Adults, teenagers, and children—60 milligrams (mg) a day. Some people with very serious conditions caused by too little thyroid hormone may need to take only 15 mg a day at first. Also, some elderly patients may need lower doses at first. Then, your doctor may want you to increase your dose a little at a time to 60 to 120 mg a day.

Missed dose—If you miss a dose of this medicine, take it as soon as possible. However, if it is almost time for your next dose, skip the missed dose and go back to your regular dosing schedule. Do not double doses. If you miss 2 or more doses in a row or if you have any questions about this, check with your doctor.

Storage—To store this medicine:
- Keep out of the reach of children.
- Store away from heat and direct light.
- Do not store in the bathroom, near the kitchen sink, or in other damp places. Heat or moisture may cause the medicine to break down.
- Do not keep outdated medicine or medicine no longer needed. Be sure that any discarded medicine is out of the reach of children.

Precautions While Using This Medicine

It is very important that your doctor check your progress at regular visits, to make sure that this medicine is working properly.

If you have certain kinds of heart disease, this medicine may cause chest pain or shortness of breath when you exert yourself. If these occur, do not overdo exercise or physical work. If you have any questions about this, check with your doctor.

Before having any kind of surgery (including dental surgery) or emergency treatment, *tell the medical doctor or dentist in charge that you are taking this medicine.*

Do not take any other medicine unless prescribed by your doctor. Some medicines may increase or decrease the effects of thyroid on your body and cause problems in controlling your condition. Also, thyroid hormones may change the effects of other medicines.

Side Effects

Along with its needed effects, a medicine may cause some unwanted effects. Although not all of these side effects may occur, if they do occur they may need medical attention.

Check with your doctor as soon as possible if any of the following side effects occur since they may indicate an overdose or an allergic reaction:

Less common or rare
   Headache (severe) in children; skin rash or hives

Signs and symptoms of overdose
   Chest pain; confusion; fast or irregular heartbeat; mood swings; muscle weakness; psychosis; restlessness (extreme); yellow eyes or skin; shortness of breath

For patients taking this medicine for underactive thyroid:
- This medicine usually takes several weeks to have a noticeable effect on your condition. Until it begins to work, you may experience no change in your symptoms. Check with your doctor if the following symptoms continue:

Clumsiness; coldness; constipation; dry, puffy skin; listlessness; muscle aches; sleepiness; tiredness; weakness; weight gain

Other effects may occur if the dose of the medicine is not exactly right. These side effects will go away when the dose is corrected. Check with your doctor if any of the following symptoms occur:

Changes in appetite; changes in menstrual periods; diarrhea; fever; hand tremors; headache; increased sensitivity to heat; irritability; leg cramps; nervousness; sweating; trouble in sleeping; vomiting; weight loss

Other side effects not listed above may also occur in some patients. If you notice any other effects, check with your doctor.

TIAGABINE (Oral route) - tye-AG-a-been

Commonly used brand name(s)

In the U.S.—
Gabitril

Available Dosage Forms:
- Capsule
- Tablet

Therapeutic Class: Anticonvulsant
Pharmacologic Class: Gamma Aminobutyric Acid Uptake Inhibitor

Uses For This Medicine

Tiagabine is used to help control some types of seizures in the treatment of epilepsy. This medicine cannot cure epilepsy and will only work to control seizures for as long as you continue to take it.

Tiagabine is available only with your doctor's prescription.

Before Using This Medicine

In deciding to use a medicine, the risks of taking the medicine must be weighed against the good it will do. This is a decision you and your doctor will make. For this medicine, the following should be considered:

Allergies—Tell your doctor if you have ever had any unusual or allergic reaction to this medicine or any other medicines. Also tell your health care professional if you have any other types of allergies, such as to foods, dyes, preservatives, or animals. For non-prescription products, read the label or package ingredients carefully.

Pediatric—Although there is no specific information comparing use of tiagabine in children younger than 12 years of age with use in other age groups, this medicine is not expected to cause different side effects or problems in children than it does in adults.

Geriatric—Many medicines have not been studied specifically in older people. Therefore, it may not be known whether they work exactly the same way they do in younger adults. Although there is no specific information comparing use of tiagabine in the elderly with use in other age groups, this medicine is not expected to cause different side effects or problems in older people than it does in younger adults.

Pregnancy—

	Pregnancy Category	Explanation
All Trimesters	C	Animal studies have shown an adverse effect and there are no adequate studies in pregnant women OR no animal studies have been conducted and there are no adequate studies in pregnant women.

Breast Feeding—There are no adequate studies in women for determining infant risk when using this medication during breastfeeding. Weigh the potential benefits against the potential risks before taking this medication while breastfeeding.

Other medicines—

Using this medicine with any of the following medicines may cause an increased risk of certain side effects, but using both drugs may be the best treatment for you. If both medicines are prescribed together, your doctor may change the dose or how often you use one or both of the medicines.

Carbamazepine, Fosphenytoin, Ginkgo, Phenobarbital, Phenytoin, Primidone

Interactions with Food/Tobacco/Alcohol—Certain medicines should not be used at or around the time of eating food or eating certain types of food since interactions may occur. Using alcohol or tobacco with certain medicines may also cause interactions to occur. Discuss with your healthcare professional the use of your medicine with food, alcohol, or tobacco.

Other medical problems—The presence of other medical problems may affect the use of this medicine. Make sure you tell your doctor if you have any other medical problems, especially:
- Liver problems—Higher blood levels of tiagabine may result, leading to an increase in the chance of side effects
- Status epilepticus—Tiagabine may cause the condition to recur

Proper Use of This Medicine

Take this medicine only as directed by your doctor, to help your condition as much as possible. Do not take more or less of it, and do not take it more or less often than your doctor ordered.

Tiagabine should be taken with food or on a full stomach.

Dosing—The dose of this medicine will be different for different patients. Follow your doctor's orders or the directions on the label. The following information includes only the average doses of this medicine. If your dose is different, do not change it unless your doctor tells you to do so.

The amount of medicine that you take depends on the strength of the medicine. Also, the number of doses you take each day, the time allowed between doses, and the length of

time you take the medicine depend on the medical problem for which you are using the medicine.

- For oral dosage form (tablets):
  - For epilepsy:
    - Adults and teenagers 12 years of age and older— At first, 4 milligrams (mg) once a day. Your doctor may increase your dose slowly as needed and tolerated. However, the dose usually is not greater than 56 mg a day.
    - Children up to 12 years of age—Use and dose must be determined by the doctor.

Missed dose—If you miss a dose of this medicine, take it as soon as possible. However, if it is almost time for your next dose, skip the missed dose and go back to your regular dosing schedule. Do not double doses.

Storage—Store the medicine in a closed container at room temperature, away from heat, moisture, and direct light. Keep from freezing.

Keep out of the reach of children.

Do not keep outdated medicine or medicine no longer needed.

Precautions While Using This Medicine

Tiagabine may cause dizziness, drowsiness, trouble in thinking, trouble with motor skills, or vision problems. Make sure you know how you react to this medicine before you drive, use machines, or do anything else that could be dangerous if you are not alert, well-coordinated, or able to think or see well.

This medicine will add to the effects of alcohol and other CNS depressants (medicines that make you drowsy or less alert). Some examples of CNS depressants are antihistamines or medicine for hay fever, other allergies, or colds; sedatives, tranquilizers, or sleeping medicine; prescription pain medicine or narcotics; barbiturates; other medicines for seizures; muscle relaxants; or anesthetics, including some dental anesthetics. Check with your medical doctor or dentist before taking any of the above while you are taking tiagabine.

Do not stop taking tiagabine without first checking with your doctor. Stopping the medicine suddenly may cause your seizures to return or to occur more often. Your doctor may want you to gradually reduce the amount you are taking before stopping completely.

Side Effects of This Medicine

Along with its needed effects, a medicine may cause some unwanted effects. Although not all of these side effects may occur, if they do occur they may need medical attention.

Check with your doctor as soon as possible if any of the following side effects occur:

More common
> Blue or purple spots on skin; difficulty in concentrating or paying attention

Less common
> Burning, numbness, or tingling sensations; clumsiness or unsteadiness; confusion; itching; mental depression; speech or language problems

Rare
> Agitation; bloody or cloudy urine; burning, pain, or difficulty in urinating; frequent urge to urinate; generalized weakness; hostility; memory problems; quick to react or overreact emotionally; rash; uncontrolled back-and-

forth and/or rolling eye movements; walking in unusual manner

Symptoms of overdose
> Agitation (severe); clumsiness or unsteadiness (severe); coma; confusion (severe); drowsiness (severe); increase in seizures; mental depression; severe muscle twitching or jerking; sluggishness; speech problems (severe); weakness

Some side effects may occur that usually do not need medical attention. These side effects may go away during treatment as your body adjusts to the medicine. Also, your health care professional may be able to tell you about ways to prevent or reduce some of these side effects. Check with your health care professional if any of the following side effects continue or are bothersome or if you have any questions about them:

More common
> Chills; diarrhea; dizziness; drowsiness; fever; headache; muscle aches or pain; nervousness; sore throat; tremor; unusual tiredness or weakness; vomiting

Less common
> Abdominal pain; flushing; impaired vision; increased appetite; increased cough; mouth ulcers; muscle weakness; nausea; pain; trouble in sleeping

Other side effects not listed may also occur in some patients. If you notice any other effects, check with your healthcare professional.

TICLOPIDINE   (Oral route) - tye-KLOE-pi-deen

Black Box Warning

Ticlopidine hydrochloride can cause life-threatening hematological adverse reactions, including neutropenia/agranulocytosis, thrombotic thrombocytopenic purpura (TTP) and aplastic anemia.

Among 2,048 patients in clinical trials, there were 50 cases (2.4%) of neutropenia (less than 1,200 neutrophils/mm(3)), and the neutrophil count was below 450/mm(3) in 17 of these patients (0.8% of the total population).

One case of thrombotic thrombocytopenic purpura (TTP) was reported during clinical trials. Based on postmarketing data, US physicians reported about 100 cases between 1992 and 1997. Based on an estimated patient exposure of 2 million to 4 million, and assuming an event reporting rate of 10% (the true rate is not known), the incidence of ticlopidine-associated TTP may be as high as one case in every 2,000 to 4,000 patients exposed.

Aplastic anemia was not seen during clinical trials, but US physicians reported about 50 cases between 1992 and 1998. Based on an estimated patient exposure of 2 million to 4 million, and assuming an event reporting rate of 10% (the true rate is not known), the incidence of ticlopidine-associated aplastic anemia may be as high as one case in every 4,000 to 8,000 patients exposed.

Severe hematological adverse reactions may occur within a few days of the start of therapy. The incidence of TTP peaks after about 3 to 4 weeks of therapy and neutropenia peaks at approximately 4 to 6 weeks. The incidence of aplastic anemia peaks after about 4 to 8 weeks of therapy. The incidence of the hematologic adverse reactions declines thereafter. Only a few cases of neutropenia, TTP, or aplastic anemia have arisen after more than 3 months of therapy.

Hematological adverse reactions cannot be reliably predicted by any identified demographic or clinical characteristics. During the first 3 months of treatment, patients receiving ticlopidine hydrochloride must, therefore, be hematologically and clinically monitored for evidence of neutropenia or TTP. If any such evidence is seen, ticlopidine hydrochloride should be immediately discontinued.

Commonly used brand name(s)
In the U.S.—
   Ticlid

Available Dosage Forms:
   • Tablet

Therapeutic Class: Platelet Aggregation Inhibitor
Pharmacologic Class: ADP-Induced Aggregation Inhibitor

Uses For This Medicine

Ticlopidine is used to lessen the chance of having a stroke. It is given to people who have already had a stroke and to people with certain medical problems that may lead to a stroke. Because ticlopidine can cause serious side effects, especially during the first 3 months of treatment, it is used mostly for people who cannot take aspirin to prevent strokes.

A stroke may occur when blood flow to the brain is interrupted by a blood clot. Ticlopidine reduces the chance that a harmful blood clot will form, by preventing certain cells in the blood from clumping together. This effect of ticlopidine may also increase the chance of serious bleeding in some people.

This medicine is available only with a doctor's prescription.

Before Using This Medicine

In deciding to use a medicine, the risks of taking the medicine must be weighed against the good it will do. This is a decision you and your doctor will make. For this medicine, the following should be considered:

Allergies—Tell your doctor if you have ever had any unusual or allergic reaction to this medicine or any other medicines. Also tell your health care professional if you have any other types of allergies, such as to foods, dyes, preservatives, or animals. For non-prescription products, read the label or package ingredients carefully.

Pediatric—There is no specific information comparing use of ticlopidine in children with use in other age groups.

Geriatric—This medicine has been tested and has not been shown to cause different side effects or problems in older people than it does in younger adults.

Pregnancy—

	Pregnancy Category	Explanation
All Trimesters	B	Animal studies have revealed no evidence of harm to the fetus, however, there are no adequate studies in pregnant women OR animal studies have shown an adverse effect, but adequate studies in pregnant women have failed to demonstrate a risk to the fetus.

Breast Feeding—There are no adequate studies in women for determining infant risk when using this medication during breastfeeding. Weigh the potential benefits against the potential risks before taking this medication while breastfeeding.

Other medicines—

Using this medicine with any of the following medicines is usually not recommended, but may be required in some cases. If both medicines are prescribed together, your doctor may change the dose or how often you use one or both of the medicines.

Abciximab, Aspirin, Ginkgo, Tinzaparin, Tizanidine

Interactions with Food/Tobacco/Alcohol—Certain medicines should not be used at or around the time of eating food or eating certain types of food since interactions may occur. Using alcohol or tobacco with certain medicines may also cause interactions to occur. Discuss with your healthcare professional the use of your medicine with food, alcohol, or tobacco.

Other medical problems—The presence of other medical problems may affect the use of this medicine. Make sure you tell your doctor if you have any other medical problems, especially:
- Blood clotting problems, such as hemophilia and von Willebrand's disease, or
- Liver disease (severe) or
- Stomach ulcers—The chance of serious bleeding may be increased
- Blood disease—The chance of serious side effects may be increased
- Kidney disease (severe)—Ticlopidine is removed from the body more slowly when the kidneys are not working properly. This may increase the chance of side effects

Also, tell your doctor if you have ever had a problem called thrombotic thrombocytopenic purpura (TTP). This problem could reoccur if you take ticlopidine.

Proper Use of This Medicine

Ticlopidine should be taken with food. This increases the amount of medicine that is absorbed into the body. It may also lessen the chance of stomach upset.

Take this medicine only as directed by your doctor. Ticlopidine will not work properly if you take less of it than directed. Taking more ticlopidine than directed may increase the chance of serious side effects without increasing the helpful effects.

Dosing—The dose of this medicine will be different for different patients. Follow your doctor's orders or the directions on the label. The following information includes only the average doses of this medicine. If your dose is different, do not change it unless your doctor tells you to do so.

The amount of medicine that you take depends on the strength of the medicine. Also, the number of doses you take each day, the time allowed between doses, and the length of time you take the medicine depend on the medical problem for which you are using the medicine.
- For oral dosage form (tablets):
  - For prevention of strokes:
    - Adults—1 tablet (250 mg) two times a day, with food.
    - Children—It is not likely that ticlopidine would be used to help prevent strokes in children. If a child

needs this medicine, however, the dose would have to be determined by the doctor.

- ○ For prevention of strokes or heart attack following heart stent procedure:
  - ▪ Adults—1 tablet (250 mg) two times a day, with food together with your doctor's recommended dose of aspirin for up to 30 days following the procedure
  - ▪ Children—It is not likely that ticlopidine would be used to help prevent strokes or heart attack in children. If a child needs this medicine, however, the dose would have to be determined by the doctor

Missed dose—If you miss a dose of this medicine, take it as soon as possible. However, if it is almost time for your next dose, skip the missed dose and go back to your regular dosing schedule. Do not double doses.

Storage—Store the medicine in a closed container at room temperature, away from heat, moisture, and direct light. Keep from freezing.

Keep out of the reach of children.

Do not keep outdated medicine or medicine no longer needed.

Precautions While Using This Medicine

It is very important that blood tests be done before treatment is started with ticlopidine, and repeated every 2 weeks for the first 3 months of treatment with ticlopidine. The tests are needed to find out whether certain side effects are occurring. Finding these side effects early helps to prevent them from becoming serious. Your doctor will arrange for the blood tests to be done. Be sure that you do not miss any appointments for these tests. You will probably not need to have your blood tested so often after the first 3 months of treatment, because the side effects are less likely to occur after that time.

Tell all medical doctors, dentists, nurses, and pharmacists you go to that you are taking this medicine. Ticlopidine may increase the risk of serious bleeding during an operation or some kinds of dental work. Therefore, treatment may have to be stopped about 10 days to 2 weeks before the operation or dental work is done.

Ticlopidine may cause serious bleeding, especially after an injury. Sometimes, bleeding inside the body can occur without your knowing about it. Ask your doctor whether there are certain activities you should avoid while taking this medicine (for example, sports that can cause injuries). Also, check with your doctor immediately if you are injured while being treated with this medicine.

Check with your doctor immediately if you notice any of the following side effects:

- Bruising or bleeding, especially bleeding that is hard to stop. Bleeding inside the body sometimes appears as bloody or black, tarry stools, or faintness. Also, bleeding may occur from the gums when brushing or flossing teeth.
- Any sign of infection, such as fever, chills, or sore throat.
- Sores, ulcers, or white spots in the mouth.
- Dark or bloody urine, difficulty in speaking, fever, pale color of skin, pinpoint red spots on skin, convulsions (seizures), weakness, or yellow eyes or skin.

After you stop taking ticlopidine, the chance of bleeding may continue for 1 or 2 weeks. During this period of time, continue to follow the same precautions that you followed while you were taking the medicine.

Side Effects of This Medicine

Along with its needed effects, a medicine may cause some unwanted effects. Although not all of these side effects may occur, if they do occur they may need medical attention.

Check with your doctor immediately if any of the following side effects occur:

Less common or rare

Abdominal or stomach pain (severe) or swelling; back pain; blistering, peeling, or loosening of the skin or lips or mucous membranes (moist lining of many body cavities, including the mouth, lips, inside of nose, anus, and vagina); blood in eyes; bloody or black tarry stools; bruising or purple areas on skin; change in mental status; convulsions (seizures); coughing up blood; dark or bloody urine; decreased alertness; dizziness; fever, chills, or sore throat; headache (severe or continuing); joint pain or swelling; nosebleeds; pale color of skin; paralysis or problems with coordination; pinpoint red spots on skin; red lesions on the skin, often with a purple center; red, thickened, or scaly skin; sores, ulcers, or white spots in mouth; stammering or other difficulty in speaking; unusually heavy bleeding or oozing from cuts or wounds; unusual tiredness; unusually heavy or unexpected menstrual bleeding; vomiting of blood or material that looks like coffee grounds; weakness; yellow eyes or skin

Check with your doctor as soon as possible if any of the following side effects occur:

More common

Skin rash

Less common or rare

General feeling of discomfort or illness; hives or itching of skin; ringing or buzzing in ears

Some side effects may occur that usually do not need medical attention. These side effects may go away during treatment as your body adjusts to the medicine. Also, your health care professional may be able to tell you about ways to prevent or reduce some of these side effects. Check with your health care professional if any of the following side effects continue or are bothersome or if you have any questions about them:

More common

Abdominal or stomach pain (mild); diarrhea; indigestion; nausea

Less common

Bloating or gas; dizziness; vomiting

Other side effects not listed may also occur in some patients. If you notice any other effects, check with your healthcare professional.

TILUDRONATE (Oral route) - tye-LOO-droe-nate

Commonly used brand name(s)

In the U.S.—

Skelid

Available Dosage Forms:

- Tablet

Therapeutic Class: Calcium Regulator

Uses For This Medicine

Tiludronate is used to treat Paget's disease of the bone.

This medicine is available only with your doctor's prescription.

Before Using This Medicine

In deciding to use a medicine, the risks of taking the medicine must be weighed against the good it will do. This is a decision you and your doctor will make. For this medicine, the following should be considered:

Allergies—Tell your doctor if you have ever had any unusual or allergic reaction to this medicine or any other medicines. Also tell your health care professional if you have any other types of allergies, such as to foods, dyes, preservatives, or animals. For non-prescription products, read the label or package ingredients carefully.

Pediatric—Studies on this medicine have been done only in adult patients, and there is no specific information comparing use of tiludronate in children with use in other age groups.

Geriatric—Tiludronate has been tested in elderly patients and has not been found to cause different side effects or problems in older people than it does in younger adults.

Pregnancy—

	Pregnancy Category	Explanation
All Trimesters	C	Animal studies have shown an adverse effect and there are no adequate studies in pregnant women OR no animal studies have been conducted and there are no adequate studies in pregnant women.

Breast Feeding—There are no adequate studies in women for determining infant risk when using this medication during breastfeeding. Weigh the potential benefits against the potential risks before taking this medication while breastfeeding.

Other medicines—Although certain medicines should not be used together at all, in other cases two different medicines may be used together even if an interaction might occur. In these cases, your doctor may want to change the dose, or other precautions may be necessary. Tell your healthcare professional if you are taking any other prescription or non-prescription (over-the-counter [OTC]) medicine.

Interactions with Food/Tobacco/Alcohol—Certain medicines should not be used at or around the time of eating food or eating certain types of food since interactions may occur. Using alcohol or tobacco with certain medicines may also cause interactions to occur. Discuss with your healthcare professional the use of your medicine with food, alcohol, or tobacco.

Other medical problems—The presence of other medical problems may affect the use of this medicine. Make sure you tell your doctor if you have any other medical problems, especially:

- Hypocalcemia (low calcium levels in the blood)
- Overactive parathyroid gland or
- Vitamin D deficiency—Tiludronate may make these conditions worse

- Kidney disease—Effects may be increased because of slower removal of tiludronate from the body
- Stomach or intestine problems, including trouble swallowing, inflammation of the esophagus, or ulcer—Tiludronate may make these conditions worse

Proper Use of This Medicine

Take tiludronate with a full glass (6 to 8 ounces) of plain water on an empty stomach.

It is important that you eat a well-balanced diet with an adequate amount of calcium and vitamin D (found in milk or other dairy products). However, do not take any beverages (including mineral water), dietary supplements, food, or other medicines at least 2 hours before or after taking the tiludronate. To do so may keep this medicine from working properly.

Dosing—The dose of this medicine will be different for different patients. Follow your doctor's orders or the directions on the label. The following information includes only the average doses of this medicine. If your dose is different, do not change it unless your doctor tells you to do so.

The amount of medicine that you take depends on the strength of the medicine. Also, the number of doses you take each day, the time allowed between doses, and the length of time you take the medicine depend on the medical problem for which you are using the medicine.

- For oral dosage form (tablets):
  - For treating Paget's disease of the bone:
    - Adults and teenagers—400 milligrams (mg) a day for at least three months.
    - Children—Use and dose must be determined by your doctor.

Missed dose—If you miss a dose of this medicine, take it as soon as possible. However, if it is almost time for your next dose, skip the missed dose and go back to your regular dosing schedule. Do not double doses.

Storage—Store the medicine in a closed container at room temperature, away from heat, moisture, and direct light. Keep from freezing.

Keep out of the reach of children.

Do not keep outdated medicine or medicine no longer needed.

Side Effects of This Medicine

Along with its needed effects, a medicine may cause some unwanted effects. Although not all of these side effects may occur, if they do occur they may need medical attention.

Check with your doctor as soon as possible if any of the following side effects occur:

More common
Cough; fever; head congestion; hoarseness or other voice changes; nasal congestion; runny nose; sneezing; sore throat

Less common
Blurred or decreased vision; chest pain; eye pain; headache; swelling of face, feet, or lower legs; unusual weight gain

Some side effects may occur that usually do not need medical attention. These side effects may go away during treatment as your body adjusts to the medicine. Also, your health care professional may be able to tell you about ways to prevent or reduce some of these side effects. Check with your health care professional if any of the following side effects continue or are bothersome or if you have any questions about them:

More common
  Back pain; body pain (general); diarrhea; nausea; upset stomach

Less common
  Dizziness; joint pain; muscle pain; pain in throat; red or irritated eyes; skin rash; stomach gas; vomiting

Other side effects not listed may also occur in some patients. If you notice any other effects, check with your healthcare professional.

TINIDAZOLE (Oral route) - tye-NI-da-zole

Black Box Warning

Carcinogenicity has been seen in mice and rats treated chronically with another agent in the nitroimidazole class (metronidazole). Although such data have not been reported for tinidazole, unnecessary use of tinidazole should be avoided.

Commonly used brand name(s)

In the U.S.—
  Tindamax

Available Dosage Forms:
  • Tablet

Therapeutic Class: Antibiotic

Uses For This Medicine

Tinidazole is used to treat infections caused by protozoa (tiny, one-celled animals). It works by killing the protozoa.

Tinidazole is available only with your doctor's prescription.

Before Using This Medicine

In deciding to use a medicine, the risks of taking the medicine must be weighed against the good it will do. This is a decision you and your doctor will make. For this medicine, the following should be considered:

Allergies—Tell your doctor if you have ever had any unusual or allergic reaction to this medicine or any other medicines. Also tell your health care professional if you have any other types of allergies, such as to foods, dyes, preservatives, or animals. For non-prescription products, read the label or package ingredients carefully.

Pediatric—Tinidazole has been used in children three years of age and older for the treatment of giardiasis.

Geriatric—Many medicines have not been studied specifically in older people. Therefore, it may not be known whether they work exactly the same way they do in younger adults or if they cause different side effects or problems in older people. There is no specific information comparing use of tinidazole in the elderly with use in other age groups.

Pregnancy—

	Pregnancy Category	Explanation
All Trimesters	C	Animal studies have shown an adverse effect and there are no adequate studies in pregnant women OR no animal studies have been conducted and there are no adequate studies in pregnant women.

Breast Feeding—There are no adequate studies in women for determining infant risk when using this medication during breastfeeding. Weigh the potential benefits against the potential risks before taking this medication while breastfeeding.

Other medicines—Although certain medicines should not be used together at all, in other cases two different medicines may be used together even if an interaction might occur. In these cases, your doctor may want to change the dose, or other precautions may be necessary. Tell your healthcare professional if you are taking any other prescription or non-prescription (over-the-counter [OTC]) medicine.

Interactions with Food/Tobacco/Alcohol—Certain medicines should not be used at or around the time of eating food or eating certain types of food since interactions may occur. Using alcohol or tobacco with certain medicines may also cause interactions to occur. Discuss with your healthcare professional the use of your medicine with food, alcohol, or tobacco.

Other medical problems—The presence of other medical problems may affect the use of this medicine. Make sure you tell your doctor if you have any other medical problems, especially:

  • Blood disease or a history of blood disease—Tinidazole may make this condition worse.

  • Central nervous system (CNS) disease, including epilepsy—Tinidazole may increase the chance of seizures (convulsions) or other CNS side effects.

  • Liver disease, severe—Patients with severe liver disease may have an increase in side effects.

  • Oral thrush or vaginal yeast infection—Tinidazole may make yeast infections worse.

Proper Use of This Medicine

If this medicine upsets your stomach, it may be taken with meals or a snack. If stomach upset (nausea, vomiting, stomach pain, or diarrhea) continues, check with your doctor.

To help clear up your infection completely, keep taking this medicine for the full time of treatment, even if you begin to feel better after a few days. If you stop taking this medicine too soon, your symptoms may return.

In some kinds of infections, this medicine works best when there is a constant amount in the blood. To help keep the amount constant, do not miss any doses. Also, it is best to take the doses at evenly spaced times, day and night. For example, if you are to take one dose a day, the doses should be spaced about 24 hours apart. If this interferes with your sleep or other daily activities, or if you need help in planning the best times to take your medicine, check with your health care professional.

Some types of infections are treated with one dose of tinidazole.

Dosing—The dose of this medicine will be different for different patients. Follow your doctor's orders or the directions on the label. The following information includes only the average doses of this medicine. If your dose is different, do not change it unless your doctor tells you to do so.

The amount of medicine that you take depends on the strength of the medicine. Also, the number of doses you take each day, the time allowed between doses, and the length of time you take the medicine depend on the medical problem for which you are using the medicine.

- For oral dosage form (tablets):
  - For amebiasis, intestinal infections:
    - Adults—2 grams per day for three days.
    - Children—50 milligrams per kilogram of body weight per day (up to to 2 grams per day) for three days.
  - For amebiasis, liver access:
    - Adults—2 grams per day for 3 to 5 days.
    - Children—50 milligrams per kilogram of body weight per day (up to to 2 grams per day) for 3 to 5 days.
  - For giardiasis infections:
    - Adults—2 grams per day for just one day.
    - Children—50 milligrams per kilogram of body weight per day (up to to 2 grams per day) for just one day.
  - For trichomoniasis infections:
    - Adults—2 grams given once as a single dose.
    - Children—Use and dose must be determined by your doctor.

Missed dose—If you miss a dose of this medicine, take it as soon as possible. However, if it is almost time for your next dose, skip the missed dose and go back to your regular dosing schedule. Do not double doses.

Storage—Store the medicine in a closed container at room temperature, away from heat, moisture, and direct light. Keep from freezing.

Keep out of the reach of children.

Do not keep outdated medicine or medicine no longer needed.

Precautions While Using This Medicine

If your symptoms do not improve within a few days, or if they become worse, check with your doctor.

Drinking alcoholic beverages while taking this medicine may cause stomach pain, nausea, vomiting, headache, or flushing or redness of the face. Other alcohol-containing preparations (for example, elixirs, cough syrups, tonics) may also cause problems. These problems may last for at least 3 days after you stop taking tinidazole. Also, this medicine may cause alcoholic beverages to taste different. Therefore, you should not drink alcoholic beverages or take other alcohol-containing preparations while you are taking this medicine and for at least 3 days after stopping it.

If you are taking this medicine for trichomoniasis (an infection of the sex organs in males and females), your doctor may want to treat your sexual partner at the same time you are being treated, even if he or she has no symptoms. Also, it may be desirable to use a condom (prophylactic) during intercourse. These measures will help keep you from getting the infection back again from your partner. If you have any questions about this, check with your doctor.

Side Effects of This Medicine

Along with its needed effects, a medicine may cause some unwanted effects. Although not all of these side effects may occur, if they do occur they may need medical attention.

Check with your doctor immediately if any of the following side effects occur:

Rare

Change in consciousness; cough; difficulty breathing; loss of consciousness; noisy breathing; shortness of breath; tightness in chest; wheezing

Incidence unknown

Black, tarry stools; bleeding gums; blood in urine or stools; burning, numbness, tingling, or painful sensations; chest pain; chills; difficulty swallowing; fast, irregular, pounding, or racing heartbeat or pulse; fever; hives; increased transaminase levels; large, hive-like swelling on face, eyelids, lips, tongue, throat, hands, legs, feet, sex organs; lower back or side pain; nausea; painful or difficult urination; pale skin; pinpoint red spots on skin; reddening of the skin, especially around ears; seizures; sore throat; sores, ulcers, or white spots on lips or in mouth; swelling of eyes, face, or inside of nose; swollen glands; ulcers; unsteadiness or awkwardness; unusual bleeding or bruising; unusual tiredness or weakness; weakness in arms, hands, legs, or feet

Some side effects may occur that usually do not need medical attention. These side effects may go away during treatment as your body adjusts to the medicine. Also, your health care professional may be able to tell you about ways to prevent or reduce some of these side effects. Check with your health care professional if any of the following side effects continue or are bothersome or if you have any questions about them:

More common

Bitter taste; metallic taste

Less common

Acid or sour stomach; belching; cramps; difficulty having a bowel movement (stool); dizziness; general feeling of discomfort or illness; headache; heartburn; indigestion; loss of appetite; pain or discomfort in chest, upper stomach, or throat; vomiting; weight loss

Rare

Body aches or pain; coating on tongue; congestion; depression; dryness or soreness of throat; hoarseness; mood or mental changes; runny nose; tender, swollen glands in neck; voice changes

Incidence unknown

Abnormal liver; darkened urine; diarrhea; difficulty in moving; feeling of constant movement of self or surroundings; giddiness; lightheadedness; muscle pain or stiffness; pain; swelling, or redness in joints; shakiness and unsteady walk; sleepiness; trembling, or other problems with muscle control or coordination; sensation of spinning; sleeplessness; swelling or inflammation of the mouth; tongue discoloration; trouble sleeping; unable to sleep; white or brownish vaginal discharge; white patches in the mouth or throat or on the tongue

Other side effects not listed may also occur in some patients. If you notice any other effects, check with your healthcare professional.

TINZAPARIN (Subcutaneous route) -
tin-ZA-pa-rin

Black Box Warning

When neuraxial anesthesia (epidural/spinal anesthesia) or spinal puncture is employed, patients anticoagulated or scheduled to be anticoagulated with low molecular weight heparins or heparinoids for prevention of thromboembolic complications are at risk of developing an epidural or spinal hematoma which can result in long-term or permanent paralysis.

The risk of these events is increased by the use of indwelling epidural catheters for administration of analgesia or by the concomitant use of drugs affecting hemostasis such as non-steroidal anti-inflammatory drugs (NSAIDs), platelet inhibitors, or other anticoagulants. The risk also appears to be increased by traumatic or repeated epidural or spinal puncture.

Patients should be frequently monitored for signs and symptoms of neurological impairment. If neurological compromise is noted, urgent treatment is necessary.

The physician should consider the potential benefit versus risk before neuraxial intervention in patients anticoagulated or to be anticoagulated for thromboprophylaxis.

Commonly used brand name(s)

In the U.S.—
Innohep

Available Dosage Forms:
• Solution

Therapeutic Class: Anticoagulant
Pharmacologic Class: Low Molecular Weight Heparin

Uses For This Medicine

Tinzaparin is used for the prevention and/or treatment of deep venous thrombosis, a condition in which harmful blood clots form in the blood vessels of the legs. These blood clots can travel to the lungs and can become lodged in the blood vessels of the lungs, causing a condition called pulmonary embolism. Tinzaparin is used for several days after surgery, while you are unable to walk. It is during this time that blood clots are most likely to form. Tinzaparin also may be used for other conditions as determined by your doctor.

This medicine is available only with your doctor's prescription.

Before Using This Medicine

In deciding to use a medicine, the risks of taking the medicine must be weighed against the good it will do. This is a decision you and your doctor will make. For this medicine, the following should be considered:

Allergies—Tell your doctor if you have ever had any unusual or allergic reaction to this medicine or any other medicines. Also tell your health care professional if you have any other types of allergies, such as to foods, dyes, preservatives, or animals. For non-prescription products, read the label or package ingredients carefully.

Pediatric—Studies on this medicine have been done only in adult patients, and there is no specific information comparing use of tinzaparin in children with use in other age groups.

Geriatric—This medicine has been tested and has not been shown to cause different side effects or problems in older people than it does in younger adults.

Pregnancy—

	Pregnancy Category	Explanation
All Trimesters	B	Animal studies have revealed no evidence of harm to the fetus, however, there are no adequate studies in pregnant women OR animal studies have shown an adverse effect, but adequate studies in pregnant women have failed to demonstrate a risk to the fetus.

Breast Feeding—There are no adequate studies in women for determining infant risk when using this medication during breastfeeding. Weigh the potential benefits against the potential risks before taking this medication while breastfeeding.

Other medicines—

Using this medicine with any of the following medicines is usually not recommended, but may be required in some cases. If both medicines are prescribed together, your doctor may change the dose or how often you use one or both of the medicines.

Abciximab, Aceclofenac, Acemetacin, Acenocoumarol, Alclofenac, Alteplase, Recombinant, Ancrod, Anisindione, Anistreplase, Antithrombin III Human, Apazone, Ardeparin, Argatroban, Benoxaprofen, Bivalirudin, Bromfenac, Bufexamac, Carprofen, Certoparin, Clometacin, Clonixin, Clopidogrel, Dalteparin, Danaparoid, Defibrotide, Dermatan Sulfate, Desirudin, Dexketoprofen, Dextran, Diclofenac, Dicumarol, Diflunisal, Dipyrone, Droxicam, Enoxaparin, Eptifibatide, Etodolac, Etofenamate, Felbinac, Fenbufen, Fenoprofen, Fentiazac, Floctafenine, Flufenamic Acid, Flurbiprofen, Fondaparinux, Heparin, Ibuprofen, Indomethacin, Indoprofen, Isoxicam, Ketoprofen, Ketorolac, Lamifiban, Lornoxicam, Meclofenamate, Mefenamic Acid, Meloxicam, Nabumetone, Nadroparin, Naproxen, Niflumic Acid, Nimesulide, Oxaprozin, Oxyphenbutazone, Parnaparin, Pentosan Polysulfate Sodium, Phenindione, Phenprocoumon, Phenylbutazone, Pirazolac, Piroxicam, Pirprofen, Propyphenazone, Proquazone, Reteplase, Recombinant, Reviparin, Sibrafiban, Streptokinase, Sulindac, Suprofen, Tenecteplase, Tenidap, Tenoxicam, Tiaprofenic Acid, Ticlopidine, Tinzaparin, Tirofiban, Tolmetin, Urokinase, Warfarin, Xemilofiban, Zomepirac

Interactions with Food/Tobacco/Alcohol—Certain medicines should not be used at or around the time of eating food or eating certain types of food since interactions may occur. Using alcohol or tobacco with certain medicines may also cause interactions to occur. Discuss with your healthcare professional the use of your medicine with food, alcohol, or tobacco.

Other medical problems—The presence of other medical problems may affect the use of this medicine. Make sure you tell your doctor if you have any other medical problems, especially:
  • Prosthetic heart valve—Tinzaparin may not protect these patients from developing a blood clot
  • Blood disease or bleeding problems or
  • Eye problems caused by diabetes or high blood pressure or

- Heart infection or
- High blood pressure (hypertension) or
- Kidney disease or
- Liver disease or
- Stomach or intestinal ulcer (active) or
- Stroke—The risk of bleeding may be increased
- Also, tell your doctor if you have received tinzaparin or heparin before and had a reaction to either of them called thrombocytopenia (a low platelet count in the blood), or if new blood clots formed while you were receiving the medicine.
- In addition, tell your doctor if you have recently had surgery. This may increase the risk of serious bleeding when you are taking tinzaparin.

Proper Use of This Medicine

If you are using tinzaparin at home, your health care professional will teach you how to inject yourself with the medicine. Be sure to follow the directions carefully. Check with your health care professional if you have any problems using the medicine.

Put used syringes in a puncture-resistant, disposable container, or dispose of them as directed by your health care professional.

Dosing—The dose of this medicine will be different for different patients. Follow your doctor's orders or the directions on the label. The following information includes only the average doses of this medicine. If your dose is different, do not change it unless your doctor tells you to do so.

The amount of medicine that you take depends on the strength of the medicine. Also, the number of doses you take each day, the time allowed between doses, and the length of time you take the medicine depend on the medical problem for which you are using the medicine.

- For injection dosage form:
  - For prevention of deep venous thrombosis (leg clots) due to surgery:

  Adults
  - General surgery—3500 International Units (IU) 2 hours before surgery then 3500 IU once daily for seven to ten days.
  - Hip surgery—50 International Units (IU) per kilogram (kg) of body weight 2 hours before surgery then 50 IU per kg of body weight once daily for seven to ten days, or 75 IU per kg of body weight given after surgery once daily for seven to ten days.
  - Knee surgery—75 International Units (IU) per kilogram (kg) of body weight given after surgery once daily for seven to ten days.

  - Children—Use and dose must be determined by your doctor.
  - For treatment of deep venous thrombosis (leg clots) with or without pulmonary embolism (lung clots):
    - Adults—175 International Units (IU) per kilogram (kg) of body weight once daily for six to seven days.
    - Children—Use and dose must be determined by your doctor.

Missed dose—Call your doctor or pharmacist for instructions.

Storage—Store the medicine in a closed container at room temperature, away from heat, moisture, and direct light. Keep from freezing.

Keep out of the reach of children.

Do not keep outdated medicine or medicine no longer needed.

Precautions While Using This Medicine

Tell all your medical doctors, dentists, and other health care professionals that you are using this medicine.

This medicine may cause severe side effects in babies.

Check with your doctor immediately if you notice any of the following side effects:
- Bruising or bleeding, especially bleeding that is hard to stop. (Bleeding inside the body sometimes appears as bloody or black, tarry stools or causes faintness.)
- Back pain; burning, pricking, tickling, or tingling sensation; leg weakness; numbness; paralysis; or problems with bowel or bladder function.

Side Effects of This Medicine

Along with its needed effects, a medicine may cause some unwanted effects. Although not all of these side effects may occur, if they do occur they may need medical attention.

Check with your doctor immediately if any of the following side effects occur:

More common
Deep, dark purple bruise, pain, or swelling at place of injection

Less common
Bladder pain; bleeding gums; blood in urine; bloody or cloudy urine; blurred vision; chest pain; chest tightness; chills; confusion; cough; coughing up blood; difficulty in breathing or swallowing; dizziness; faintness, or lightheadedness when getting up from a lying or sitting position suddenly; fast, slow, or irregular heartbeat; fever; frequent urge to urinate; headache; increased menstrual flow or vaginal bleeding; lower back pain or side pain; nosebleeds; pain or burning while urinating; painful or difficult urination; pale skin; palpitations; paralysis; pounding in the ears; prolonged bleeding from cuts; red or dark brown urine; red or black, tarry stools; severe or continuing dull nervousness; shortness of breath; skin rash; sore throat; sores, ulcers, or white spots on lips or in mouth; sweating; swollen glands; troubled breathing, exertional; unexplained pain, swelling, or discomfort, especially in the chest, abdomen, joints, or muscles; unusual bleeding or bruising; unusual tiredness or weakness; vomiting of blood or coffee ground-like material

Rare
Blue-green to black skin discoloration; bowel/bladder dysfunction; hives; itching; leg weakness; numbness; pain, redness, or sloughing of skin at place of injection; paresthesia; puffiness or swelling of the eyelids or around the eyes, face, lips, or tongue; wheezing

Incidence not known
Abdominal or stomach pain; accumulation of pus; bloody or black, tarry stools; break in the skin, espe-

cially associated with blue-black discoloration, swelling, or drainage of fluid; change in vision; clay-colored stools; collection of blood under the skin; dark urine; diarrhea; excessive thirst; fatigue; hoarseness; large, flat, blue or purplish patches in the skin; large, hive-like swelling on face, eyelids, lips, tongue, throat, hands, legs, feet, sex organs; loss of appetite; malaise; muscle cramps; numbness and tingling of face, fingers, or toes; pain in arms, legs, or lower back, especially pain in calves and/or heels upon exertion; pain, redness or swelling; painful knees and ankles; pale, bluish-colored, or cold hands or feet; problems with vision or hearing; raised, red swellings on the skin, the buttocks, legs or ankles; redness, tenderness, burning, blistering or peeling of skin (usually on the backs of arms and the fronts of legs, mouth, eyes or hands and feet; red or irritated eyes; seeing floating spots before the eyes; swollen, red, tender area of infection; unpleasant breath odor; weak or absent pulses in legs; yellow eyes or skin

Some side effects may occur that usually do not need medical attention. These side effects may go away during treatment as your body adjusts to the medicine. Also, your health care professional may be able to tell you about ways to prevent or reduce some of these side effects. Check with your health care professional if any of the following side effects continue or are bothersome or if you have any questions about them:

Less common or rare
    Constipation; nausea and vomiting; prolonged, painful, inappropriate erection of the penis; trouble in sleeping

Incidence not known
    Hives or welts; redness of skin

Other side effects not listed may also occur in some patients. If you notice any other effects, check with your healthcare professional.

TIOCONAZOLE   (Topical route) - tye-oh-KONE-a-zole

Commonly used brand name(s)
In Canada—
   Gyne Cure   Trosyd J
   Trosyd Af

Available Dosage Forms:
• Cream

Uses For This Medicine

Tioconazole belongs to the family of medicines called antifungals, which are used to treat infections caused by a fungus or yeast. They work by killing the fungus or yeast or preventing its growth.

Tioconazole cream is applied to the skin to treat:
• ringworm of the body (tinea corporis);
• ringworm of the foot (tinea pedis; athlete's foot);
• ringworm of the groin (tinea cruris; jock itch);
• tinea versicolor (sometimes called "sun fungus"); and
• yeast infection of the skin (cutaneous candidiasis).

Tioconazole is available in the following dosage forms:
   Topical
     • Cream (Canada)

Before Using This Medicine

In deciding to use a medicine, the risks of taking the medicine must be weighed against the good it will do. This is a decision you and your doctor will make. For this medicine, the following should be considered:

Allergies—Tell your doctor if you have ever had any unusual or allergic reaction to this medicine or any other medicines. Also tell your health care professional if you have any other types of allergies, such as to foods, dyes, preservatives, or animals. For non-prescription products, read the label or package ingredients carefully.

Pediatric—Although there is no specific information comparing use of this medicine in children with use in other age groups, this medicine is not expected to cause different side effects or problems in children than it does in adults.

Geriatric—Many medicines have not been studied specifically in older people. Therefore, it may not be known whether they work exactly the same way they do in younger adults. Although there is no specific information comparing use of tioconazole in the elderly with use in other age groups, this medicine is not expected to cause different side effects or problems in older people than it does in younger adults.

Other medicines—Although certain medicines should not be used together at all, in other cases two different medicines may be used together even if an interaction might occur. In these cases, your doctor may want to change the dose, or other precautions may be necessary. Tell your healthcare professional if you are taking any other prescription or non-prescription (over-the-counter [OTC]) medicine.

Interactions with Food/Tobacco/Alcohol—Certain medicines should not be used at or around the time of eating food or eating certain types of food since interactions may occur. Using alcohol or tobacco with certain medicines may also cause interactions to occur. Discuss with your healthcare professional the use of your medicine with food, alcohol, or tobacco.

Proper Use of This Medicine

Apply enough tioconazole to cover the affected and surrounding skin areas, and rub in gently.

Keep this medicine away from the eyes.

Do not apply an occlusive dressing (airtight covering, such as kitchen plastic wrap) over this medicine unless you have been directed to do so by your doctor. To do so may cause irritation of the skin.

To help clear up your infection completely, it is very important that you keep using tioconazole for the full time of treatment, even if your symptoms begin to clear up after a few days. Since fungus infections may be very slow to clear up, you may have to continue using this medicine every day for several weeks or more. If you stop using this medicine too soon, your symptoms may return. Do not miss any doses.

Dosing—The dose of this medicine will be different for different patients. Follow your doctor's orders or the directions on the label. The following information includes only the average doses of this medicine. If your dose is different, do not change it unless your doctor tells you to do so.

The amount of medicine that you take depends on the strength of the medicine. Also, the number of doses you take each day, the time allowed between doses, and the length of time you take the medicine depend on the medical problem for which you are using the medicine.

- For topical cream dosage form:
  - For ringworm of the body or yeast infection of the skin:
    - Adults—Use two times a day for 2 to 4 weeks.
    - Children—Dose must be determined by your doctor.
  - For ringworm of the foot:
    - Adults—Use two times a day for up to 6 weeks.
    - Children—Dose must be determined by your doctor.
  - For ringworm of the groin:
    - Adults—Use two times a day for up to 2 weeks.
    - Children—Dose must be determined by your doctor.
  - For tinea versicolor ("sun fungus"):
    - Adults—Use two times a day for 1 to 4 weeks.
    - Children—Dose must be determined by your doctor.

Missed dose—If you miss a dose of this medicine, apply it as soon as possible. However, if it is almost time for your next dose, skip the missed dose and go back to your regular dosing schedule.

Storage—Store the medicine in a closed container at room temperature, away from heat, moisture, and direct light. Keep from freezing.

Keep out of the reach of children.

Do not keep outdated medicine or medicine no longer needed.

Ask your healthcare professional how you should dispose of any medicine you do not use.

Precautions While Using This Medicine

If your skin problem does not improve within:

- 2 weeks for ringworm of the body or yeast infection of the skin, tinea versicolor, or ringworm of the groin;
- 4 to 6 weeks for ringworm of the foot;

or if it becomes worse, check with your doctor.

To help clear up your infection completely and to help make sure it does not return, good health habits are also required. The following measures will help reduce chaffing and irritation and will also help keep the area cool and dry:

- For patients using tioconazole for ringworm of the groin (tinea cruris; jock itch):
  - Avoid wearing underwear that is tight-fitting or made from synthetic materials (for example, rayon or nylon). Instead, wear loose-fitting, cotton underwear.
- For patients using tioconazole for ringworm of the foot (tinea pedis; athlete's foot):
  - Carefully dry the feet, especially between the toes, after bathing.
  - Avoid wearing socks made from wool or synthetic materials (for example, rayon or nylon). Instead wear clean, cotton socks and change them daily or more often if the feet sweat a lot.
  - Wear sandals or other well-ventilated shoes.
- For patients using tioconazole for ringworm of the body (tinea corporis):
  - Carefully dry yourself after bathing.
  - Avoid too much heat and humidity if possible.
  - Wear well-ventilated, loose-fitting clothing.

If you have any questions about these measures, check with your health care professional.

Side Effects of This Medicine

Along with its needed effects, a medicine may cause some unwanted effects. Although not all of these side effects may occur, if they do occur they may need medical attention.

Check with your doctor as soon as possible if any of the following side effects occur:

Less common
Burning; itching; redness; skin rash; swelling; or other signs of skin irritation not present before use of this medicine

Other side effects not listed may also occur in some patients. If you notice any other effects, check with your healthcare professional.

TIOTROPIUM (Inhalation, oral/nebulization route) - tye-oh-TROE-pee-um

Commonly used brand name(s)

In the U.S.—
Spiriva

Available Dosage Forms:
- Capsule

Therapeutic Class: Bronchodilator
Pharmacologic Class: Antimuscarinic

Uses For This Medicine

Tiotropium is a medicine used to treat bronchospasm (wheezing or difficulty in breathing) that is associated with Chronic obstructive pulmonary disease. Chronic obstructive pulmonary disease is a long-term lung disease. It is also called COPD. COPD also includes breathing problems like chronic bronchitis (swelling of the airways or tubes leading to the lungs) and emphysema (damage to the air sacs in the lungs).

Tiotropium is a bronchodilator. A bronchodilator is a medicine that opens up narrowed breathing passages. It is taken by inhalation (an inhaler) to help decrease coughing, wheezing, shortness of breath, and troubled breathing by increasing the flow of air into the lungs

This medicine is available only with your doctor's prescription.

Before Using This Medicine

In deciding to use a medicine, the risks of taking the medicine must be weighed against the good it will do. This is a decision you and your doctor will make. For this medicine, the following should be considered:

Allergies—Tell your doctor if you have ever had any unusual or allergic reaction to this medicine or any other medi-

cines. Also tell your health care professional if you have any other types of allergies, such as to foods, dyes, preservatives, or animals. For non-prescription products, read the label or package ingredients carefully.

Pediatric—Studies on this medicine have only been done in adult patients, and there is no specific information comparing the use of tiotropium in children with use in other age groups. The disease that this medicine treats does not normally occur in children.

Geriatric—This medicine has been tested and has not been shown to cause different side effects or problems in older people than it does in younger adults.

Pregnancy—

	Pregnancy Category	Explanation
All Trimesters	C	Animal studies have shown an adverse effect and there are no adequate studies in pregnant women OR no animal studies have been conducted and there are no adequate studies in pregnant women.

Breast Feeding—There are no adequate studies in women for determining infant risk when using this medication during breastfeeding. Weigh the potential benefits against the potential risks before taking this medication while breastfeeding.

Other medicines—Although certain medicines should not be used together at all, in other cases two different medicines may be used together even if an interaction might occur. In these cases, your doctor may want to change the dose, or other precautions may be necessary. Tell your healthcare professional if you are taking any other prescription or non-prescription (over-the-counter [OTC]) medicine.

Interactions with Food/Tobacco/Alcohol—Certain medicines should not be used at or around the time of eating food or eating certain types of food since interactions may occur. Using alcohol or tobacco with certain medicines may also cause interactions to occur. Discuss with your healthcare professional the use of your medicine with food, alcohol, or tobacco.

Other medical problems—The presence of other medical problems may affect the use of this medicine. Make sure you tell your doctor if you have any other medical problems, especially:

- Difficulty urinating (bladder problems) or
- Narrow angle glaucoma (eye condition) or
- Enlarged prostate—This medicine can make these conditions worse

Proper Use of This Medicine

Inhaled tiotropium is used with a special inhaler (HandiHaler) and usually comes with patient directions. Read the directions carefully before using this medicine. If you do not understand the directions or you are not sure how to use the inhaler, ask your health care professional to show you what to do. There are four main steps to take your medicine. Open the blister and the HandiHaler device, insert the tiotropium capsule, press the HandiHaler button and inhale your medication. Ask your health care professional to check regularly how you use the inhaler to make sure you are using it properly.

The HandiHaler is an inhalation device (inhaler) that has been specially designed for use with tiotropium capsules for inhalation. The HandiHaler must not be used to take other medicines.

Capsules should always be stored in sealed blisters and only removed immediately before use. The blister strip should be carefully opened to expose only one capsule at a time. Open the blister foil as far as the STOP line to remove only one capsule at a time. The medicine should be used immediately after the packaging over an individual capsule is opened, or else it may not be as effective as it should be. After using the first capsule, the 2 remaining capsules should be used over the next 2 consecutive days. Capsules should always be stored in the blister and only removed immediately before use. Capsules that are accidently exposed to air and that are not intended for immediate use should be discarded.

Inhaled tiotropium is a once daily maintenance medicine that opens narrowed airways and keeps them open for 24 hours. This medicine should not be used for immediate relief of breathing problems, such as a rescue medication.

Tiotropium capsules are to be used for oral inhalation only. The capsules should not be swallowed.

Dosing—The dose of this medicine will be different for different patients. Follow your doctor's orders or the directions on the label. The following information includes only the average doses of this medicine. If your dose is different, do not change it unless your doctor tells you to do so.

The amount of medicine that you take depends on the strength of the medicine. Also, the number of doses you take each day, the time allowed between doses, and the length of time you take the medicine depend on the medical problem for which you are using the medicine.

- For inhalation dosage form (capsules):
  - For bronchospasm associated with Chronic Obstructive Pulmonary Disease (COPD)
    - Adults—1 capsule (18 micrograms [mcg]) inhaled once daily; capsules should only be used with the HandiHaler inhalation device (inhaler).
    - Children—Use and dose must be determined by your doctor.

Missed dose—If you miss a dose of this medicine, take it as soon as possible. However, if it is almost time for your next dose, skip the missed dose and go back to your regular dosing schedule. Do not double doses.

Storage—Store the medicine in a closed container at room temperature, away from heat, moisture, and direct light. Keep from freezing.

Keep out of the reach of children.

Do not keep outdated medicine or medicine no longer needed.

Ask your healthcare professional how you should dispose of any medicine you do not use.

Precautions While Using This Medicine

Care must be taken not to allow powder from the capsules to get into your eyes. If the powder does get into your eye it can cause blurring of vision and pupil dilation (decreasing pupil size).

If symptoms of eye pain, eye discomfort, blurred vision, visual halos, or colored images in association with red eyes occur, contact a physician immediately.

It is very important that your doctor check you at regular visits.

Side Effects of This Medicine

Along with its needed effects, a medicine may cause some unwanted effects. Although not all of these side effects may occur, if they do occur they may need medical attention.

Check with your doctor immediately if any of the following side effects occur:

More common
Arm, back or jaw pain; chest pain or discomfort; chest tightness or heaviness; fast or irregular heartbeat; nausea; shortness of breath; sweating

Less common
Cough; difficulty swallowing; dizziness; hives; itching; painful blisters on trunk of body; puffiness or swelling of the eyelids or around the eyes, face, lips or tongue; skin rash; tightness in chest; unusual tiredness or weakness; wheezing

Rare
Fainting; large, hive-like swelling on face, eyelids, lips, tongue, throat, hands, legs, feet, sex organs; palpitations; pounding, or irregular heartbeat or pulse

Some side effects may occur that usually do not need medical attention. These side effects may go away during treatment as your body adjusts to the medicine. Also, your health care professional may be able to tell you about ways to prevent or reduce some of these side effects. Check with your health care professional if any of the following side effects continue or are bothersome or if you have any questions about them:

More common
Acid or sour stomach; belching; bladder pain; bloody or cloudy urine; body aches or pain; chest pain; chills; congestion; cough; difficult, burning, or painful urination; difficulty in breathing; dry mouth; dryness of throat; ear congestion; fever; frequent urge to urinate; headache; heartburn; hoarseness; indigestion; loss of voice; lower back or side pain; nasal congestion; pain or tenderness around eyes and cheekbones; runny nose; sneezing; sore throat; stomach discomfort, upset or pain; stuffy nose; tender, swollen glands in neck; trouble in swallowing; troubled breathing; unusual tiredness or weakness; voice changes

Less common
Abdominal pain; bloody nose; blurred vision; burning, crawling, itching, numbness, prickling, "pins and needles", or tingling feelings; canker sores; difficulty having a bowel movement (stool); discouragement; fatigue; feeling sad or empty; flushed, dry skin; fruit-like breath odor; increased hunger; increased thirst; increased urination; irritability; lack of appetite; large amount of cholesterol in the blood; leg pain; loss of interest or pleasure; muscle pain; nausea; painful or difficult urination; skeletal pain; sore mouth or tongue; sores, ulcers, or white spots on lips or tongue or inside the mouth; sweating; swelling; swelling or inflammation of the mouth; tiredness; troubled breathing; trouble concentrating; trouble sleeping; unexplained weight loss; vomiting; white patches in mouth and/or on tongue

Incidence rare
Painful or difficult urination

Incidence unknown
Hives or welts; irregular heartbeat; itching; itching skin; redness of skin; skin rash

Other side effects not listed may also occur in some patients. If you notice any other effects, check with your healthcare professional.

TIZANIDINE   (Oral route) - tye-ZAN-i-deen

Commonly used brand name(s)

In the U.S.—
Zanaflex

Available Dosage Forms:

- Capsule
- Tablet

Therapeutic Class: Skeletal Muscle Relaxant, Centrally Acting

Uses For This Medicine

Tizanidine is used to help relax certain muscles in your body. It relieves the spasms, cramping, and tightness of muscles caused by medical problems such as multiple sclerosis or certain injuries to the spine. Tizanidine does not cure these problems, but it may allow other treatment, such as physical therapy, to be more helpful in improving your condition.

Tizanidine acts on the central nervous system (CNS) to produce its muscle relaxant effects. Its actions on the CNS may also cause some of the medicine's side effects.

This medicine is available only with your doctor's prescription.

Before Using This Medicine

In deciding to use a medicine, the risks of taking the medicine must be weighed against the good it will do. This is a decision you and your doctor will make. For this medicine, the following should be considered:

Allergies—Tell your doctor if you have ever had any unusual or allergic reaction to this medicine or any other medicines. Also tell your health care professional if you have any other types of allergies, such as to foods, dyes, preservatives, or animals. For non-prescription products, read the label or package ingredients carefully.

Pediatric—Studies on this medicine have been done only in adult patients, and there is no specific information comparing use of tizanidine in children with use in other age groups.

Geriatric—Studies in older adults show that tizanidine stays in the body a little longer than it does in younger adults. Your doctor will consider this when deciding on your dose.

Pregnancy—

	Pregnancy Category	Explanation
All Trimesters	C	Animal studies have shown an adverse effect and there are no adequate studies in pregnant women OR no animal studies have been conducted and there are no adequate studies in pregnant women.

Breast Feeding—There are no adequate studies in women for determining infant risk when using this medication during breastfeeding. Weigh the potential benefits against the potential risks before taking this medication while breastfeeding.

Other medicines—

Using this medicine with any of the following medicines is not recommended. Your doctor may decide not to treat you with this medication or change some of the other medicines you take.

Ciprofloxacin, Fluvoxamine

Interactions with Food/Tobacco/Alcohol—Certain medicines should not be used at or around the time of eating food or eating certain types of food since interactions may occur. Using alcohol or tobacco with certain medicines may also cause interactions to occur. Discuss with your healthcare professional the use of your medicine with food, alcohol, or tobacco.

Other medical problems—The presence of other medical problems may affect the use of this medicine. Make sure you tell your doctor if you have any other medical problems, especially:

- Kidney disease or
- Liver disease—The chance of side effects may be increased; higher blood levels of tizanidine may result and a smaller dose may be needed

Proper Use of This Medicine

When you take the different dosage forms (tablets, capsules, capsule contents sprinkled over applesauce) of tizanidine with food, it effects the amount of the medicine absorbed into your blood differently. Follow your doctor's instructions for when to take this medicine and whether or not you should take it with food.

Take this medicine only as directed. Do not take more of it and do not take it more often than recommended on the label, unless otherwise directed by your doctor. To do so may increase the chance of side effects.

Dosing—The dose of this medicine will be different for different patients. Follow your doctor's orders or the directions on the label. The following information includes only the average doses of this medicine. If your dose is different, do not change it unless your doctor tells you to do so.

The amount of medicine that you take depends on the strength of the medicine. Also, the number of doses you take each day, the time allowed between doses, and the length of time you take the medicine depend on the medical problem for which you are using the medicine.

- For oral dosage form (capsules and tablets):
  - For muscle relaxation:
    - Adults—The dose is 8 milligrams (mg) every six to eight hours as needed. No more than 36 mg should be taken within a twenty-four-hour period.
    - Children—Use and dose must be determined by your doctor.

Missed dose—If you miss a dose of this medicine, take it as soon as possible. However, if it is almost time for your next dose, skip the missed dose and go back to your regular dosing schedule. Do not double doses.

Storage—Store the medicine in a closed container at room temperature, away from heat, moisture, and direct light. Keep from freezing.

Keep out of the reach of children.

Do not keep outdated medicine or medicine no longer needed.

Precautions While Using This Medicine

Your doctor should check your progress at regular visits, especially during the first few weeks of treatment with this medicine. During this time the amount of medicine you are taking may have to be changed often to meet your individual needs.

Do not suddenly stop taking this medicine. Unwanted effects may occur if the medicine is stopped suddenly. Check with your doctor for the best way to reduce gradually the amount you are taking before stopping completely.

This medicine will add to the effects of alcohol and other CNS depressants (medicines that make you drowsy or less alert). Some examples of CNS depressants are antihistamines or medicine for hay fever, other allergies, or colds; sedatives, tranquilizers, or sleeping medicine; prescription pain medicine or narcotics; barbiturates; medicine for seizures; other muscle relaxants; or anesthetics, including some dental anesthetics. Check with your doctor before taking any of the above while you are using tizanidine.

This medicine may cause dizziness, drowsiness, lightheadedness, clumsiness or unsteadiness, or vision problems in some people. Make sure you know how you react to this medicine before you drive, use machines, or do anything else that could be dangerous if you are not alert, well-coordinated, and able to see well.

Tizanidine may cause dryness of the mouth. For temporary relief, use sugarless candy or gum, melt bits of ice in your mouth, or use a saliva substitute. However, if dry mouth continues for more than 2 weeks, check with your medical doctor or dentist. Continuing dryness of the mouth may increase the chance of dental disease, including tooth decay, gum disease, and fungus infections.

Dizziness, lightheadedness, or fainting may occur when you get up suddenly from a lying or sitting position. Getting up slowly may help lessen this problem.

Side Effects of This Medicine

Along with its needed effects, a medicine may cause some unwanted effects. Although not all of these side effects may occur, if they do occur they may need medical attention.

Check with your doctor as soon as possible if any of the following side effects occur:

More common

Chest pain or discomfort; fever; loss of appetite; lower back or side pain; nausea and/or vomiting; nervousness; pain or burning while urinating; painful or difficult urination; sores on the skin; tingling, burning, or prickling sensations; unusual tiredness; yellow eyes or skin

Less common

Black, tarry stools; bloody vomit; blurred vision; chills or sore throat; coldness; convulsions (seizures); cough or hoarseness; dark urine; dry, puffy skin; eye pain; fainting; influenza (flu)-like symptoms; irregular heartbeat; kidney stones; persistent anorexia; pruritus; right upper quadrant tenderness; seeing things that are not there; shortness of breath; slow or irregular heartbeat; unusual tiredness or weakness; weight gain

Incidence not known

Continuing vomiting; general feeling of tiredness or weakness; headache; light-colored stools

Get emergency help immediately if any of the following symptoms of overdose occur:

Symptoms of overdose

Blurred vision; change in consciousness; chest pain or discomfort; confusion; decreased awareness or responsiveness; difficult or troubled breathing; dizziness, faintness or lightheadedness when getting up from a lying position; irregular, fast or slow, or shallow breathing; lightheadedness, dizziness or fainting; loss of consciousness; pale or blue lips, fingernails, or skin; severe sleepiness; shortness of breath; sleepiness or unusual drowsiness; slow or irregular heartbeat; sweating; unusual tiredness or weakness

Some side effects may occur that usually do not need medical attention. These side effects may go away during treatment as your body adjusts to the medicine. Also, your health care professional may be able to tell you about ways to prevent or reduce some of these side effects. Check with your health care professional if any of the following side effects continue or are bothersome or if you have any questions about them:

More common

Anxiety; back pain; constipation; depression; diarrhea; difficulty in speaking; dizziness or lightheadedness, especially when getting up from a lying or sitting position; drowsiness; dry mouth; heartburn; increased sweating; increased muscle spasms or tone; muscle weakness; pain or burning in throat; runny nose; skin rash; sleepiness; stomach pain; uncontrolled movements of the body

Less common

Difficulty swallowing; dry skin; general feeling of discomfort or illness; increased need to urinate; joint or muscle pain or stiffness; loss of hair; migraine headache; mood changes; neck pain; passing urine more often; shivering; swelling of feet or lower legs; swollen area that feels warm and tender; trembling or shaking; trouble sleeping; unusual feeling of well-being; unusual tiredness or weakness; weight loss

Other side effects not listed may also occur in some patients. If you notice any other effects, check with your healthcare professional.

TOBRAMYCIN (Ophthalmic route) -
toe-bra-MYE-sin

Commonly used brand name(s)

In the U.S.—
AKTob
Tobrasol
Tobrex

In Canada—
Apo-Tobramycin   Tomycine
Sab-Tobramycin

Available Dosage Forms:
- Solution
- Ointment

Therapeutic Class: Antibiotic

Uses For This Medicine

Ophthalmic tobramycin is used in the eye to treat bacterial infections of the eye. Tobramycin works by killing bacteria.

Ophthalmic tobramycin may be used alone or with other medicines for eye infections. Either the drops or the ointment form of this medicine may be used alone during the day. In addition, both forms may be used together, with the drops being used during the day and the ointment at night.

Tobramycin ophthalmic preparations are available only with your doctor's prescription.

Before Using This Medicine

In deciding to use a medicine, the risks of taking the medicine must be weighed against the good it will do. This is a decision you and your doctor will make. For this medicine, the following should be considered:

Allergies—Tell your doctor if you have ever had any unusual or allergic reaction to this medicine or any other medicines. Also tell your health care professional if you have any other types of allergies, such as to foods, dyes, preservatives, or animals. For non-prescription products, read the label or package ingredients carefully.

Pediatric—This medicine has been tested in children and, in effective doses, has not been shown to cause different side effects or problems than it does in adults.

Geriatric—Many medicines have not been studied specifically in older people. Therefore, it may not be known whether they work exactly the same way they do in younger adults or if they cause different side effects or problems in older people. There is no specific information comparing use of ophthalmic tobramycin in the elderly with use in other age groups.

Pregnancy—

	Pregnancy Category	Explanation
All Trimesters	D	Studies in pregnant women have demonstrated a risk to the fetus. However, the benefits of therapy in a life threatening situation or a serious disease, may outweigh the potential risk.

Breast Feeding—There are no adequate studies in women for determining infant risk when using this medication during breastfeeding. Weigh the potential benefits against the potential risks before taking this medication while breastfeeding.

Other medicines—

Using this medicine with any of the following medicines is usually not recommended, but may be required in some cases. If both medicines are prescribed together, your doctor may change the dose or how often you use one or both of the medicines.

Alcuronium, Atracurium, Cidofovir, Cisatracurium, Decamethonium, Doxacurium, Fazadinium, Gallamine, Hexafluorenium, Lysine, Metocurine, Mivacurium, Pancuronium, Pipecuronium, Rapacuronium, Rocuronium, Succinylcholine, Tacrolimus, Tubocurarine, Vecuronium

Interactions with Food/Tobacco/Alcohol—Certain medicines should not be used at or around the time of eating food or eating certain types of food since interactions may occur. Using alcohol or tobacco with certain medicines may also cause interactions to occur. Discuss with your healthcare professional the use of your medicine with food, alcohol, or tobacco.

Proper Use of This Medicine

For patients using tobramycin ophthalmic solution (eye drops):

- The bottle is only partially full to provide proper drop control.
- To use:
  - First, wash your hands. Tilt the head back and with the index finger of one hand, press gently on the skin just beneath the lower eyelid and pull the lower eyelid away from the eye to make a space. Drop the medicine into this space. Let go of the eyelid and gently close the eyes. Do not blink. Keep the eyes closed for 1 or 2 minutes, to allow the medicine to come into contact with the infection.
  - If you think you did not get the drop of medicine into your eye properly, use another drop.
  - To keep the medicine as germ-free as possible, do not touch the applicator tip to any surface (including the eye). Also, keep the container tightly closed.
- If your doctor ordered two different ophthalmic solutions to be used together, wait at least 5 minutes between the times you apply the medicines. This will help to keep the second medicine from "washing out" the first one.

For patients using tobramycin ophthalmic ointment (eye ointment):

- To use:
  - First, wash your hands. Tilt the head back and with the index finger of one hand, press gently on the skin just beneath the lower eyelid and pull the lower eyelid away from the eye to make a space. Squeeze a thin strip of ointment into this space. A 1.25-cm (approximately ½-inch) strip of ointment usually is enough, unless you have been told by your doctor to use a different amount. Let go of the eyelid and gently close the eyes and keep them closed for 1 or 2 minutes, to allow the medicine to come into contact with the infection.
  - To keep the medicine as germ-free as possible, do not touch the applicator tip to any surface (including the eye). After using tobramycin eye ointment, wipe the tip of the ointment tube with a clean tissue and keep the tube tightly closed.

To help clear up your eye infection completely, keep using tobramycin for the full time of treatment, even if your symptoms have disappeared. Do not miss any doses.

Dosing—The dose of this medicine will be different for different patients. Follow your doctor's orders or the directions on the label. The following information includes only the average doses of this medicine. If your dose is different, do not change it unless your doctor tells you to do so.

The amount of medicine that you take depends on the strength of the medicine. Also, the number of doses you take each day, the time allowed between doses, and the length of time you take the medicine depend on the medical problem for which you are using the medicine.

- For ophthalmic ointment dosage forms:
  - For mild to moderate infections:
    - Adults and children—Use every eight to twelve hours.
  - For severe infections:
    - Adults and children—Use every three to four hours until improvement occurs.
- For ophthalmic solution (eye drops) dosage forms:
  - For mild to moderate infections:
    - Adults and children—One drop every four hours.
  - For severe infections:
    - Adults and children—One drop every hour until improvement occurs.

Missed dose—If you miss a dose of this medicine, take it as soon as possible. However, if it is almost time for your next dose, skip the missed dose and go back to your regular dosing schedule. Do not double doses.

Storage—Store the medicine in a closed container at room temperature, away from heat, moisture, and direct light. Keep from freezing.

Keep out of the reach of children.

Do not keep outdated medicine or medicine no longer needed.

Precautions While Using This Medicine

If your eye infection does not improve within a few days, or if it becomes worse, check with your doctor.

Side Effects of This Medicine

Along with its needed effects, a medicine may cause some unwanted effects. Although not all of these side effects may occur, if they do occur they may need medical attention.

Check with your doctor immediately if any of the following side effects occur:

Less common
Itching, redness, swelling, or other sign of eye or eyelid irritation not present before use of this medicine

Symptoms of overdose
Increased watering of the eyes; itching, redness, or swelling of the eyes or eyelids; painful irritation of the clear front part of the eye

Some side effects may occur that usually do not need medical attention. These side effects may go away during treatment as your body adjusts to the medicine. Also, your health care professional may be able to tell you about ways to prevent or reduce some of these side effects. Check with your health care professional if any of the following side effects continue or are bothersome or if you have any questions about them:

> *Less common*
>> Burning or stinging of the eyes

Eye ointments usually cause your vision to blur for a few minutes after application.

Other side effects not listed may also occur in some patients. If you notice any other effects, check with your healthcare professional.

TOLCAPONE (Oral route) - TOLE-ka-pone

Black Box Warning

Because of the risk of potentially fatal, acute fulminant liver failure, tolcapone should ordinarily be used in patients with Parkinson's disease on levodopa/carbidopa who are experiencing symptom fluctuations and are not responding satisfactorily to or are not appropriate candidates for other adjunctive therapies.

Because of the risk of liver injury and because tolcapone, when it is effective, provides an observable symptomatic benefit, the patient who fails to show substantial clinical benefit within 3 weeks of initiation of treatment, should be withdrawn from tolcapone.

Tolcapone therapy should not be initiated if the patient exhibits clinical evidence of liver disease or two SGPT/ALT or SGOT/AST values greater than the upper limit of normal. Patients with severe dyskinesia or dystonia should be treated with caution.

Patients who develop evidence of hepatocellular injury while on tolcapone and are withdrawn from the drug for any reason may be at increased risk for liver injury if tolcapone is reintroduced. Accordingly, such patients should not ordinarily be considered for retreatment.

Cases of severe hepatocellular injury, including fulminant liver failure resulting in death, have been reported in post-marketing use. As of May 2005, 3 cases of fatal fulminant hepatic failure have been reported from more than 40,000 patient years of worldwide use. This incidence may be 10–fold to 100–fold higher than the background incidence in the general population. Underreporting of cases may lead to significant underestimation of the increased risk associated with the use of tolcapone. All 3 cases were reported within the first six months of initiation of treatment with tolcapone. Analysis of the laboratory monitoring data in over 3,400 tolcapone-treated patients participating in clinical trials indicated that increases in SGPT/ALT or SGOT/AST, when present, generally occurred within the first 6 months of treatment with tolcapone.

A prescriber who elects to use tolcapone in face of the increased risk of liver injury is strongly advised to monitor patients for evidence of emergent liver injury. Patients should be advised of the need for self-monitoring for both the classical signs of liver disease (eg, clay colored stools, jaundice) and the nonspecific ones (eg, fatigue, loss of appetite, lethargy).

Although a program of periodic laboratory monitoring for evidence of hepatocellular injury is recommended, it is not clear that periodic monitoring of liver enzymes will prevent the occurrence of fulminant liver failure. However, it is generally believed that early detection of drug-induced hepatic injury along with immediate withdrawal of the suspect drug enhances the likelihood for recovery. Accordingly, the following liver monitoring program is recommended.

Before starting treatment with tolcapone, the physician should conduct appropriate tests to exclude the presence of liver disease. In patients determined to be appropriate candidates for treatment with tolcapone, serum glutamic-pyruvic transaminase (SGPT/ALT) and serum glutamic-oxaloacetic transaminase (SGOT/AST) levels should be determined at baseline and periodically (i.e. every 2 to 4 weeks) for the first 6 months of therapy. After the first six months, periodic monitoring is recommended at intervals deemed clinically relevant. Although more frequent monitoring increases the chances of early detection, the precise schedule for monitoring is a matter of clinical judgement. If the dose is increased to 200 mg three times a day, liver enzyme monitoring should take place before increasing the dose then be conducted every 2 to 4 weeks for the following 6 months of therapy. After six months, periodic monitoring is recommended at intervals deemed clinically relevant.

Tolcapone should be discontinued if SGPT/ALT or SGOT/AST exceeds 2 times the upper limit of normal or if clinical signs and symptoms suggest the onset of hepatic dysfunction (persistent nausea, fatigue, lethargy, anorexia, jaundice, dark urine, pruritus, and right upper quadrant tenderness).

Commonly used brand name(s)

In the U.S.—
> Tasmar

Available Dosage Forms:
- Tablet

Therapeutic Class: Antiparkinsonian

Pharmacologic Class: Catechol-O-Methyltransferase Inhibitor

Uses For This Medicine

Tolcapone is used in combination with levodopa and carbidopa for the treatment of the symptoms of Parkinson's disease.

This medicine is available only with your doctor's prescription.

Before Using This Medicine

In deciding to use a medicine, the risks of taking the medicine must be weighed against the good it will do. This is a decision you and your doctor will make. For this medicine, the following should be considered:

Allergies—Tell your doctor if you have ever had any unusual or allergic reaction to this medicine or any other medicines. Also tell your health care professional if you have any other types of allergies, such as to foods, dyes, preservatives, or animals. For non-prescription products, read the label or package ingredients carefully.

Pediatric—Studies on this medicine have been done only in adult patients. There is no identified potential use of tolcapone in children.

Geriatric—The risk of hallucinations (seeing, hearing, or feeling things that are not there) may be increased in patients older than 75 years of age.

Pregnancy—

	Pregnancy Category	Explanation
All Trimesters	C	Animal studies have shown an adverse effect and there are no adequate studies in pregnant women OR no animal studies have been conducted and there are no adequate studies in pregnant women.

Breast Feeding—There are no adequate studies in women for determining infant risk when using this medication during breastfeeding. Weigh the potential benefits against the potential risks before taking this medication while breastfeeding.

Other medicines—

Using this medicine with any of the following medicines is usually not recommended, but may be required in some cases. If both medicines are prescribed together, your doctor may change the dose or how often you use one or both of the medicines.

Iproniazid, Isocarboxazid, Nialamide, Pargyline, Phenelzine, Procarbazine, Tranylcypromine

Interactions with Food/Tobacco/Alcohol—Certain medicines should not be used at or around the time of eating food or eating certain types of food since interactions may occur. Using alcohol or tobacco with certain medicines may also cause interactions to occur. Discuss with your healthcare professional the use of your medicine with food, alcohol, or tobacco.

Other medical problems—The presence of other medical problems may affect the use of this medicine. Make sure you tell your doctor if you have any other medical problems, especially:

- Hallucinations (seeing, hearing, or feeling things that are not there)—Condition may become worse.
- High fever and confusion or
- Muscle injury, aches, cramps—You should not take tolcapone.
- Kidney problems, severe—Elimination of tolcapone may be decreased, which increases the risk of unwanted effects.
- Liver problems or
- Liver tests higher than normal—This medicine can increase chances of serious liver problems. You should not start taking this medicine if you have these problems.
- Low blood pressure or
- Orthostatic or postural low blood pressure (dizziness or lightheadedness when getting up suddenly from a sitting or lying position)—Condition may become worse.

Proper Use of This Medicine

Take this medicine only as directed by your doctor, to help your condition as much as possible. Do not take more or less of it, and do not take it more or less often than your doctor ordered.

It is important that you and your doctor discuss the risks of this medicine and that you read and sign a written informed consent before you begin taking this medicine.

Dosing—The dose of this medicine will be different for different patients. Follow your doctor's orders or the directions on the label. The following information includes only the average doses of this medicine. If your dose is different, do not change it unless your doctor tells you to do so.

The amount of medicine that you take depends on the strength of the medicine. Also, the number of doses you take each day, the time allowed between doses, and the length of time you take the medicine depend on the medical problem for which you are using the medicine.

- For oral dosage form (tablets):
  - For Parkinson's disease:
    - Adults—100 milligrams (mg) three times a day, taken in addition to levodopa and carbidopa.
    - Children—Use and dose must be determined by your doctor.

Missed dose—If you miss a dose of this medicine, take it as soon as possible. However, if it is almost time for your next dose, skip the missed dose and go back to your regular dosing schedule. Do not double doses.

Storage—Store the medicine in a closed container at room temperature, away from heat, moisture, and direct light. Keep from freezing.

Keep out of the reach of children.

Do not keep outdated medicine or medicine no longer needed.

Precautions While Using This Medicine

It is important that your doctor check your progress at regular visits. Tolcapone may have serious effects on your liver. You must have regular blood tests done to make sure this medicine is not affecting your liver.

Because tolcapone may have serious effects on your liver, you should watch for any signs of these effects. Signs include dark urine; itching; light-colored stools; loss of appetite; nausea (continuing); tenderness in upper right part of abdomen; unusual drowsiness, dullness, or feeling sluggish; unusual tiredness or weakness; or yellow eyes or skin. *If you notice any of these signs, contact your doctor.*

Do not stop taking tolcapone without first checking with your doctor. Your doctor may want you to gradually reduce the amount you are taking before stopping completely.

Tolcapone may cause dizziness or lightheadedness, drowsiness, weakness, or trouble in thinking or concentrating. *Make sure you know how you react to this medicine before you drive, use machines, or do anything else that could be dangerous if you are not alert, well-coordinated, or able to think clearly.*

Dizziness, lightheadedness, or fainting may occur, especially when you get up from a lying or sitting position. Getting up slowly may help. If you should have this problem, check with your doctor.

Hallucinations (seeing, hearing, or feeling things that are not there) may occur in some patients. This is more common in elderly patients.

You may experience nausea, especially when you first begin taking this medicine.

Tolcapone causes the urine to turn bright yellow. This is to be expected while you are taking it. This effect is harmless and will go away after you stop taking the medicine.

Side Effects of This Medicine

Along with its needed effects, a medicine may cause some unwanted effects. Although not all of these side effects may occur, if they do occur they may need medical attention.

Check with your doctor immediately if any of the following side effects occur:

Incidence not known
Dark urine; itching; light-colored stools; loss of appetite; nausea (continuing); tenderness in upper right part of abdomen; unusual drowsiness, dullness, or feeling sluggish; unusual tiredness or weakness; yellow eyes or skin

Check with your doctor as soon as possible if any of the following side effects occur:

More common
Abdominal pain; cough; diarrhea; dizziness; dizziness or lightheadedness when getting up from a lying or sitting position; drowsiness; fainting; fever; hallucinations (seeing, hearing, or feeling things that are not there); headache; nasal congestion (stuffy nose); nausea; runny nose; sneezing; sore throat; trouble in sleeping; twitching, twisting, or other unusual body movements; vomiting

Less common
Absence of or decrease in body movement; blood in urine; chest pain; chills; confusion; falling; general feeling of discomfort or illness; hyperactivity; loss of balance control; muscle pain; troubled breathing

Rare
Agitation; bloody or cloudy urine; burning of feet; burning, prickling, or tingling sensations; chest discomfort; difficult or painful urination; difficulty in thinking or concentrating; frequent urge to urinate; irritability; joint pain, redness, or swelling; low blood pressure; muscle cramps; neck pain; stiffness

Some side effects may occur that usually do not need medical attention. These side effects may go away during treatment as your body adjusts to the medicine. Also, your health care professional may be able to tell you about ways to prevent or reduce some of these side effects. Check with your health care professional if any of the following side effects continue or are bothersome or if you have any questions about them:

More common
Constipation; dryness of mouth; excessive dreaming; increased sweating

Less common
Bleeding; difficulty in sleeping; excessive muscle tone; fever; heartburn; gas; muscle stiffness; muscle tension or tightness; trouble in holding or releasing urine

After you stop using this medicine, it may still produce some side effects that need attention. During this period of time, *check with your doctor immediately* if you notice the following side effects:
Confusion; fever; muscle rigidity

Other side effects not listed may also occur in some patients. If you notice any other effects, check with your healthcare professional.

TOLTERODINE   (Oral route) - tohl-TER-oh-deen

Commonly used brand name(s)

In the U.S.—
Detrol
Detrol LA

Available Dosage Forms:
• Capsule, Extended Release
• Tablet

Therapeutic Class: Urinary Antispasmodic
Pharmacologic Class: Antimuscarinic

Uses For This Medicine

Tolterodine (TOLE-tear-oh-deen) is used to treat bladder problems such as frequent need to urinate or loss of control of urinary function.

This medicine is available only with your doctor's prescription.

Before Using This Medicine

In deciding to use a medicine, the risks of taking the medicine must be weighed against the good it will do. This is a decision you and your doctor will make. For this medicine, the following should be considered:

Allergies—Tell your doctor if you have ever had any unusual or allergic reaction to this medicine or any other medicines. Also tell your health care professional if you have any other types of allergies, such as to foods, dyes, preservatives, or animals. For non-prescription products, read the label or package ingredients carefully.

Pediatric—Appropriate studies performed to date have not demonstrated that tolterodine is useful in children.

Geriatric—This medicine has been tested and has not been shown to cause different side effects or problems in older people than is does in younger adults.

Pregnancy—

	Pregnancy Category	Explanation
All Trimesters	C	Animal studies have shown an adverse effect and there are no adequate studies in pregnant women OR no animal studies have been conducted and there are no adequate studies in pregnant women.

Breast Feeding—There are no adequate studies in women for determining infant risk when using this medication during breastfeeding. Weigh the potential benefits against the potential risks before taking this medication while breastfeeding.

Other medicines—

Using this medicine with any of the following medicines may cause an increased risk of certain side effects, but using both drugs may be the best treatment for you. If both medicines are prescribed together, your doctor may change the dose or how often you use one or both of the medicines.

Clarithromycin, Cyclosporine, Erythromycin, Itraconazole, Ketoconazole, Miconazole, Vinblastine, Warfarin

Interactions with Food/Tobacco/Alcohol—Certain medicines should not be used at or around the time of eating food or eating certain types of food since interactions may occur. Using alcohol or tobacco with certain medicines may also cause interactions to occur. Discuss with your healthcare professional the use of your medicine with food, alcohol, or tobacco.

Other medical problems—The presence of other medical problems may affect the use of this medicine. Make sure you tell your doctor if you have any other medical problems, especially:

- Glaucoma or
- Intestinal blockage or
- Intestinal problems or
- Stomach problems or
- Urinary retention—Tolterodine may make these conditions worse.
- Liver problems—A lower dose of tolterodine may be necessary.
- Kidney problems—A lower dose of tolterodine may be necessary.

Proper Use of This Medicine

Take this medicine only as directed. Do not take more of it, do not take it more often, and do not take it for a longer time than your doctor ordered. To do so may increase the chance of side effects. The extended release capsules should be taken with liquids and swallowed whole.

Dosing—The dose of this medicine will be different for different patients. Follow your doctor's orders or the directions on the label. The following information includes only the average doses of this medicine. If your dose is different, do not change it unless your doctor tells you to do so.

The amount of medicine that you take depends on the strength of the medicine. Also, the number of doses you take each day, the time allowed between doses, and the length of time you take the medicine depend on the medical problem for which you are using the medicine.

- For oral dosage form (tablets):
  - To treat bladder problems:
    - Adults—1 to 2 milligrams (mg) two times a day. Your doctor may change your dose.
    - Children—Use and dose must be determined by your doctor.
- For oral dosage form (extended release capsules):
  - To treat bladder problems:
    - Adults—4 milligrams (mg) once a day. Your doctor may change your dose.
    - Children—Use and dose must be determined by your doctor.

Missed dose—If you miss a dose of this medicine, take it as soon as possible. However, if it is almost time for your next dose, skip the missed dose and go back to your regular dosing schedule. Do not double doses.

Storage—Store the medicine in a closed container at room temperature, away from heat, moisture, and direct light. Keep from freezing.

Keep out of the reach of children.

Do not keep outdated medicine or medicine no longer needed.

Precautions While Using This Medicine

This medicine may cause some people to have vision problems. Make sure your vision is clear before you drive or do anything else that could be dangerous if you are not able to see well.

This medicine, especially in high doses, may cause some people to become dizzy or drowsy. Make sure you know how you react to this medicine before you drive, use machines, or do anything else that could be dangerous if you are dizzy or are not alert.

This medicine may cause dryness of the mouth, nose, and throat. For temporary relief of mouth dryness, use sugarless candy or gum, melt bits of ice in your mouth, or use a saliva substitute. However, if your mouth continues to feel dry for more than 2 weeks, check with your medical doctor or dentist. Continuing dryness of the mouth may increase the chance of dental disease, including tooth decay, gum disease, and fungus infections.

Side Effects of This Medicine

Along with its needed effects, a medicine may cause some unwanted effects. Although not all of these side effects may occur, if they do occur they may need medical attention.

Check with your doctor as soon as possible if any of the following side effects occur:

More common

Abnormal vision, including difficulty adjusting to distances; bloody or cloudy urine; difficult, burning, or painful urination; frequent urge to urinate

Some side effects may occur that usually do not need medical attention. These side effects may go away during treatment as your body adjusts to the medicine. Also, your health care professional may be able to tell you about ways to prevent or reduce some of these side effects. Check with your health care professional if any of the following side effects continue or are bothersome or if you have any questions about them:

More common

Abdominal pain; chest pain; constipation; diarrhea; dizziness; drowsiness; dry eyes; dry mouth; fatigue; headache; joint pain; nausea; upset stomach

Less common

Blurred vision; difficult urination

Other side effects not listed may also occur in some patients. If you notice any other effects, check with your healthcare professional.

TOPIRAMATE (Oral route) - toe-PYRE-a-mate

Commonly used brand name(s)

In the U.S.—
Topamax

Available Dosage Forms:
- Tablet
- Capsule

Therapeutic Class: Anticonvulsant

Uses For This Medicine

Topiramate is used to help control some types of seizures in the treatment of epilepsy. This medicine cannot cure epilepsy and will only work to help control seizures for as long as you continue to take it. Topiramate is also used to help prevent migraine headaches in adults.

This medicine is available only with your doctor's prescription.

Before Using This Medicine

In deciding to use a medicine, the risks of taking the medicine must be weighed against the good it will do. This is a decision you and your doctor will make. For this medicine, the following should be considered:

Allergies—Tell your doctor if you have ever had any unusual or allergic reaction to this medicine or any other medicines. Also tell your health care professional if you have any other types of allergies, such as to foods, dyes, preservatives, or animals. For non-prescription products, read the label or package ingredients carefully.

Pediatric—Although there is no specific information comparing the use of topiramate in children with use in other age groups, this medicine is not expected to cause different side effects or problems in children than it does in adults. This medicine is not approved for use to help prevent migraine headaches in children.

Note: Studies in children have shown that some children are at higher risk for oligohidrosis (decreased sweating) and hyperthermia (unusually high body temperature), especially in warm or hot weather. This can sometimes result in heat stroke and hospitalization.

Geriatric—In studies done to date that have included adults older than 60 years of age, topiramate has not been shown to cause different side effects or problems in older people than it does in younger adults.

Pregnancy—

	Pregnancy Category	Explanation
All Trimesters	C	Animal studies have shown an adverse effect and there are no adequate studies in pregnant women OR no animal studies have been conducted and there are no adequate studies in pregnant women.

Breast Feeding—There are no adequate studies in women for determining infant risk when using this medication during breastfeeding. Weigh the potential benefits against the potential risks before taking this medication while breastfeeding.

Other medicines—
Using this medicine with any of the following medicines may cause an increased risk of certain side effects, but using both drugs may be the best treatment for you. If both medicines are prescribed together, your doctor may change the dose or how often you use one or both of the medicines.

Carbamazepine, Desogestrel, Ethinyl Estradiol, Ethynodiol, Etonogestrel, Fosphenytoin, Ginkgo, Hydrochlorothiazide, Levonorgestrel, Mestranol, Metformin, Norelgestromin, Norethindrone, Norgestimate, Norgestrel, Phenobarbital, Phenytoin, Pioglitazone, Risperidone, Valproic Acid

Interactions with Food/Tobacco/Alcohol—Certain medicines should not be used at or around the time of eating food or eating certain types of food since interactions may occur. Using alcohol or tobacco with certain medicines may also cause interactions to occur. Discuss with your healthcare professional the use of your medicine with food, alcohol, or tobacco.

Other medical problems—The presence of other medical problems may affect the use of this medicine. Make sure you tell your doctor if you have any other medical problems, especially:
- Diarrhea or
- Fatty diet or
- Kidney disease or
- Lung problems, severe or
- Status epilepticus (e.g., a state of epilepsy where you have many seizures in a row and do not gain consciousness) or
- Surgery—These problems may make a condition called metabolic acidosis (e.g., abnormal amounts of acid in your blood) occur or make it worse.
- History of kidney stones—Risk of having kidney stones again may be increased
- Kidney problems or
- Liver problems—Higher blood levels of topiramate may result and increase the chance of side effects

Proper Use of This Medicine

Take this medicine every day exactly as ordered by your doctor in order to improve your condition as much as possible. Do not take more or less of it, and do not take it more or less often than your doctor ordered.

Topiramate may be taken with or without food, on a full or an empty stomach. Swallow the tablets whole, without breaking, crushing, or chewing them. The bitter taste may be more noticeable if the tablets are held in the mouth or chewed. The capsules may be swallowed whole, or the contents of the capsule may be opened and the contents sprinkled on a small amount (teaspoonful) of soft food (such as applesauce, custard, ice cream, oatmeal, pudding, or yogurt) and swallowed immediately without chewing

Dosing—The dose of this medicine will be different for different patients. Follow your doctor's orders or the directions on the label. The following information includes only the average doses of this medicine. If your dose is different, do not change it unless your doctor tells you to do so.

The amount of medicine that you take depends on the strength of the medicine. Also, the number of doses you take each day, the time allowed between doses, and the length of time you take the medicine depend on the medical problem for which you are using the medicine.

- For oral dosage form (tablets or capsules):
  - To help prevent seizures (taken with other medicines):
    - Adults—At first, 25 or 50 milligrams (mg) a day for the first week. Your doctor may increase your dose gradually every week if needed and tolerated, but the usual dose is not greater than 400 mg a day.
    - Children (age 2 to 16 years)—At first, 25 milligrams (mg) nightly for the first week. Your doctor may increase your dose gradually every 1 or 2 weeks to be taken in two divided doses.
  - To help prevent seizures:
    - Adults and Children (age 10 years or older)—At first, 50 milligrams (mg) a day in 2 divided doses for the first week. Your doctor may increase your dose gradually every week if needed and tolerated, but the usual dose is not greater than 400 mg a day taken in 2 divided doses.
  - To help prevent migraine headaches:
    - Adults—At first, 25 milligrams (mg) a day for the first week. Your doctor may increase your dose gradually every week if needed and tolerated, but the usual dose is not greater than 100 mg a day.
    - Children—Use and dose must be determined by your doctor.

Missed dose—If you miss a dose of this medicine, take it as soon as possible. However, if it is almost time for your next dose, skip the missed dose and go back to your regular dosing schedule. Do not double doses.

Storage—Store the medicine in a closed container at room temperature, away from heat, moisture, and direct light. Keep from freezing.

Keep out of the reach of children.

Do not keep outdated medicine or medicine no longer needed.

Precautions While Using This Medicine

It is very important that your doctor check your progress at regular visits. This will allow your doctor to see if the medicine is working properly, and to check for unwanted effects.

This medicine may cause some people to have blurred vision, double vision, clumsiness or unsteadiness, or to become dizzy, drowsy, or have trouble in thinking. Make sure you know how you react to this medicine before you drive, use machines, or do anything else that could be dangerous if you are not alert, well-coordinated, or able to think or see well.

This medicine will add to the effects of alcohol and other CNS depressants (medicines that make you drowsy or less alert). Some examples of CNS depressants are antihistamines or medicine for hay fever, other allergies, or colds; prescription pain medicines, or sleep medicines. Do not take other medicines unless they have been discussed with your doctor. This especially includes nonprescription medicines for appetite control, asthma, colds, cough, hay fever, or sinus problems.

Check with your doctor immediately if you experience a decrease in vision, blurred vision, double vision or pain around the eyes.

Check with your doctor right away if you experience fatigue, loss of appetite, abnormal heart rate, decreased awareness, or severe sleepiness.

Oral contraceptives (birth control pills) containing estrogen may not work properly if you take them while you are taking topiramate. Unplanned pregnancies may occur. You should use a different or additional means of birth control while you are using topiramate. If you have any questions about this, check with your doctor or pharmacist.

These medicines may make you sweat less, causing your body temperature to increase. Use extra care not to become overheated during exercise or hot weather while you are taking this medicine, since overheating may result in heat stroke. Also, hot baths or saunas may make you dizzy or faint while you are taking this medicine.

Do not stop taking topiramate without first checking with your doctor. Stopping the medicine suddenly may cause your seizures to return or to occur more often. Your doctor may want you to gradually reduce the amount you are taking before stopping completely.

It is important that you drink plenty of fluids every day during therapy with topiramate to help prevent kidney stones from forming.

Side Effects of This Medicine

Along with its needed effects, a medicine may cause some unwanted effects. Although not all of these side effects may occur, if they do occur they may need medical attention.

Check with your doctor as soon as possible if any of the following side effects occur:

More common
Any vision problems, especially blurred vision, double vision, eye pain or rapidly decreasing vision; burning, prickling, or tingling sensations; clumsiness or unsteadiness; confusion; continuous, uncontrolled back-and-forth or rolling eye movements; dizziness; drowsiness; eye redness; generalized slowing of mental and physical activity; increased eye pressure; memory problems; menstrual changes; menstrual pain; nervousness; speech or language problems; trouble in concentrating or paying attention; unusual tiredness or weakness

Less common
Abdominal pain; fever, chills, or sore throat; lessening of sensations or perception; loss of appetite; mood or mental changes, including aggression, agitation, apathy, irritability, and mental depression; red, irritated, or bleeding gums; weight loss

Rare
Blood in urine; decrease in sexual performance or desire; difficult or painful urination; eye pain; frequent urination; hearing loss; itching; loss of bladder control; lower back or side pain; nosebleeds; pale skin; red or irritated eyes; ringing or buzzing in ears; skin rash; swelling; troubled breathing

Incidence not determined
Abdominal or stomach pain; Blistering, peeling, loosening of skin; blisters in the mouth; blisters on the trunk, scalp, or other areas; bloating; clay-colored stools; confusion; constipation; cough; diarrhea; fatigue; fever; increased rate of breathing; itching; joint or muscle pain; loss of appetite; pain or tenderness in upper abdomen;

red, irritated eyes; red skin lesions, often with a purple center; sores, ulcers, or white spots in mouth or on lips; unusual tiredness or weakness; yellow eyes or skin

Some side effects may occur that usually do not need medical attention. These side effects may go away during treatment as your body adjusts to the medicine. Also, your health care professional may be able to tell you about ways to prevent or reduce some of these side effects. Check with your health care professional if any of the following side effects continue or are bothersome or if you have any questions about them:

More common
   Breast pain in women; nausea; tremors
Less common
   Back pain; chest pain; constipation; heartburn; hot flushes; increased sweating; leg pain

Topiramate may cause a change in your sense of taste.

Other side effects not listed may also occur in some patients. If you notice any other effects, check with your healthcare professional.

TOPOTECAN   (Intravenous route) - toe-poe-TEE-kan

Black Box Warning

Topotecan hydrochloride for injection should be administered under the supervision of a physician experienced in the use of cancer chemotherapeutic agents. Appropriate management of complications is possible only when adequate diagnostic and treatment facilities are readily available.

Therapy with topotecan hydrochloride should not be given to patients with baseline neutrophil counts of less than 1,500 cells/mm(3). In order to monitor the occurrence of bone marrow suppression, primarily neutropenia, which may be severe and result in infection and death, frequent peripheral blood cell counts should be performed on all patients receiving topotecan hydrochloride.

Commonly used brand name(s)

In the U.S.—
   Hycamtin

Available Dosage Forms:
   • Powder for Solution

Therapeutic Class: Antineoplastic Agent
Pharmacologic Class: Topoisomerase I Inhibitor

Uses For This Medicine

Topotecan belongs to the group of medicines known as antineoplastics. It is used to treat cancer of the ovaries and certain types of lung cancer.

Topotecan interferes with the growth of cancer cells, which are eventually destroyed. Since the growth of normal cells may also be affected by the medicine, other effects may also occur. Some of these may be serious and must be reported to your doctor. Other effects, like hair loss, may not be serious but may cause concern. Some effects may occur after treatment with topotecan has been stopped.

This medicine is available only with your doctor's prescription.

Once a medicine has been approved for marketing for a certain use, experience may show that it is also useful for other medical problems. Although these uses are not included in product labeling, topotecan is used in certain patients with the following medical conditions:
   • Chronic myelomonocytic leukemia (CMML)
   • Myelodysplastic syndrome (MDS)

Before Using This Medicine

In deciding to use a medicine, the risks of taking the medicine must be weighed against the good it will do. This is a decision you and your doctor will make. For this medicine, the following should be considered:

Allergies—Tell your doctor if you have ever had any unusual or allergic reaction to this medicine or any other medicines. Also tell your health care professional if you have any other types of allergies, such as to foods, dyes, preservatives, or animals. For non-prescription products, read the label or package ingredients carefully.

Pediatric—Topotecan has been studied in a limited number of children. One study showed that seriously low blood counts may be more likely to occur in children than in adults.

Geriatric—This medicine has been tested in elderly patients and has not been shown to cause different side effects or problems in older people than it does in younger adults.

Pregnancy—

	Pregnancy Category	Explanation
All Trimesters	D	Studies in pregnant women have demonstrated a risk to the fetus. However, the benefits of therapy in a life threatening situation or a serious disease, may outweigh the potential risk.

Breast Feeding—There are no adequate studies in women for determining infant risk when using this medication during breastfeeding. Weigh the potential benefits against the potential risks before taking this medication while breastfeeding.

Other medicines—

Using this medicine with any of the following medicines is not recommended. Your doctor may decide not to treat you with this medication or change some of the other medicines you take.

Rotavirus Vaccine, Live

Interactions with Food/Tobacco/Alcohol—Certain medicines should not be used at or around the time of eating food or eating certain types of food since interactions may occur. Using alcohol or tobacco with certain medicines may also cause interactions to occur. Discuss with your healthcare professional the use of your medicine with food, alcohol, or tobacco.

Other medical problems—The presence of other medical problems may affect the use of this medicine. Make sure you tell your doctor if you have any other medical problems, especially:
   • Chickenpox (including recent exposure) or

- Herpes zoster (shingles)—Topotecan may cause these conditions to get worse and spread to other parts of your body
- Infection—Topotecan may decrease your body's ability to fight an infection
- Kidney disease—Higher blood levels of topotecan can occur, which increases the risk of serious side effects

Proper Use of This Medicine

Topotecan often causes nausea and vomiting. It is very important that you continue to receive the medicine even if it makes you feel ill. Ask your health care professional for ways to lessen these effects.

Dosing—The dose of this medicine will be different for different patients. Follow your doctor's orders or the directions on the label. The following information includes only the average doses of this medicine. If your dose is different, do not change it unless your doctor tells you to do so.

The amount of medicine that you take depends on the strength of the medicine. Also, the number of doses you take each day, the time allowed between doses, and the length of time you take the medicine depend on the medical problem for which you are using the medicine.

Precautions While Using This Medicine

It is very important that your doctor check your progress at regular visits to make sure that this medicine is working properly and to check for unwanted effects. Some of the side effects of this medicine do not have any symptoms and must be found with a blood test.

While you are being treated with topotecan, and after you stop treatment with it, do not have any immunizations (vaccinations) without your doctor's approval. Topotecan may lower your body's resistance, and there is a chance you might get the infection the immunization is meant to prevent. In addition, other persons living in your household should not take oral polio vaccine, since there is a chance they could pass the polio virus on to you. Also, avoid persons who have taken oral polio vaccine within the past several months. Do not get close to them and do not stay in the same room with them for very long. If you cannot take these precautions, you should consider wearing a protective face mask that covers the nose and mouth.

Topotecan can temporarily lower the number of white blood cells in your blood, increasing the chance of getting an infection. It can also lower the number of platelets, which are needed for proper blood clotting. If this occurs, there are certain precautions you can take, especially when your blood count is low, to reduce the risk of infection or bleeding:

- If you can, avoid people with infections. Check with your doctor immediately if you think you are getting an infection or if you get a fever or chills, cough or hoarseness, lower back or side pain, or painful or difficult urination.
- Check with your doctor immediately if you notice any unusual bleeding or bruising; black, tarry stools; blood in urine or stools; or pinpoint red spots on your skin.
- Be careful when using a regular toothbrush, dental floss, or toothpick. Your medical doctor, dentist, or nurse may recommend other ways to clean your teeth and gums. Also, check with your medical doctor before having any dental work done.

- Do not touch your eyes or the inside of your nose unless you have just washed your hands and have not touched anything else in the meantime.
- Be careful not to cut yourself when you are using sharp objects such as a safety razor or fingernail or toenail cutters.
- Avoid contact sports or other situations where bruising or injury could occur.

Side Effects of This Medicine

Along with its needed effects, a medicine may cause some unwanted effects. Although not all of these side effects may occur, if they do occur they may need medical attention.

Check with your doctor immediately if any of the following side effects occur:
  More common
    Black, tarry stools; blood in urine or stools; cough or hoarseness (accompanied by fever or chills); fever or chills; lower back or side pain (accompanied by fever or chills); painful or difficult urination (accompanied by fever or chills); pinpoint red spots on skin; shortness of breath or troubled breathing; unusual bleeding or bruising

  Rare
    Fast or irregular breathing; large, hive-like swellings on the face, eyelids, mouth, lips, and/or tongue; puffiness or swelling of the eyelids or around the eyes; tightness in chest or wheezing

Check with your doctor as soon as possible if any of the following side effects occur:
  More common
    Unusual tiredness or weakness
  Rare
    Changes in the skin color of the face; skin rash, hives, and/or itching

Some of the above side effects may occur, or continue to occur, after treatment with topotecan has ended. Check with your doctor if you notice any of them after you stop receiving the medicine.

Some side effects may occur that usually do not need medical attention. These side effects may go away during treatment as your body adjusts to the medicine. Also, your health care professional may be able to tell you about ways to prevent or reduce some of these side effects. Check with your health care professional if any of the following side effects continue or are bothersome or if you have any questions about them:
  More common
    Abdominal or stomach pain; burning or tingling in hands or feet; constipation; diarrhea; fatigue; headache; loss of appetite; muscle weakness; nausea or vomiting; sores, ulcers, or white spots on lips or tongue or inside the mouth

Topotecan sometimes causes bruising or redness at the place of injection. Check with your doctor or nurse if these effects are especially bothersome.

Topotecan may also cause a temporary loss of hair in some people. After treatment with topotecan has ended, normal hair growth should return.

Other side effects not listed may also occur in some patients. If you notice any other effects, check with your healthcare professional.

TOREMIFENE (Oral route) - TORE-em-i-feen

Commonly used brand name(s)
In the U.S.—
Fareston

Available Dosage Forms:
• Tablet

Therapeutic Class: Antiestrogen

Uses For This Medicine

Toremifene is a medicine that blocks the effects of the estrogen hormone in the body. It is used to treat breast cancer in women.

The exact way that toremifene works against cancer is not known but it may be related to the way it blocks the effects of estrogen in the body.

Before you begin treatment with toremifene, you and your doctor should talk about the good this medicine will do as well as the risks of using it.

Toremifene is available only with your doctor's prescription.

Before Using This Medicine

In deciding to use a medicine, the risks of taking the medicine must be weighed against the good it will do. This is a decision you and your doctor will make. For this medicine, the following should be considered:

Allergies—Tell your doctor if you have ever had any unusual or allergic reaction to this medicine or any other medicines. Also tell your health care professional if you have any other types of allergies, such as to foods, dyes, preservatives, or animals. For non-prescription products, read the label or package ingredients carefully.

Pregnancy—

	Pregnancy Category	Explanation
All Trimesters	D	Studies in pregnant women have demonstrated a risk to the fetus. However, the benefits of therapy in a life threatening situation or a serious disease, may outweigh the potential risk.

Breast Feeding—There are no adequate studies in women for determining infant risk when using this medication during breastfeeding. Weigh the potential benefits against the potential risks before taking this medication while breastfeeding.

Other medicines—Although certain medicines should not be used together at all, in other cases two different medicines may be used together even if an interaction might occur. In these cases, your doctor may want to change the dose, or other precautions may be necessary. Tell your healthcare professional if you are taking any other prescription or non-prescription (over-the-counter [OTC]) medicine.

Interactions with Food/Tobacco/Alcohol—Certain medicines should not be used at or around the time of eating food or eating certain types of food since interactions may occur. Using alcohol or tobacco with certain medicines may also cause interactions to occur. Discuss with your healthcare professional the use of your medicine with food, alcohol, or tobacco.

Other medical problems—The presence of other medical problems may affect the use of this medicine. Make sure you tell your doctor if you have any other medical problems, especially:
• Blood clots (history of)—Use of toremifene is usually not recommended
• Unusual growth of the lining of the uterus (womb)—Long-term use of toremifene is usually not recommended

Proper Use of This Medicine

Dosing—The dose of this medicine will be different for different patients. Follow your doctor's orders or the directions on the label. The following information includes only the average doses of this medicine. If your dose is different, do not change it unless your doctor tells you to do so.

The amount of medicine that you take depends on the strength of the medicine. Also, the number of doses you take each day, the time allowed between doses, and the length of time you take the medicine depend on the medical problem for which you are using the medicine.
• For oral dosage form (tablets):
  ○ For breast cancer:
    ▪ Adults—60 milligrams (mg) once a day.

Storage—Store the medicine in a closed container at room temperature, away from heat, moisture, and direct light. Keep from freezing.

Keep out of the reach of children.

Do not keep outdated medicine or medicine no longer needed.

Side Effects of This Medicine

Along with its needed effects, a medicine may cause some unwanted effects. Some side effects will have signs or symptoms that you can see or feel. Your doctor will watch for others by doing certain tests.

Also, because of the way this medicine acts on the body, there is a chance that it might cause other unwanted effects that may not occur until months or years after the medicine is used. Some patients who have used toremifene have developed cancer of the uterus (womb), although it is not known for sure if it was caused by the medicine. Discuss this possible effect with your doctor.

Check with your doctor as soon as possible if any of the following side effects occur:
Less common
Blurred vision; change in vaginal discharge; changes in vision; confusion; increased urination; loss of appe-

tite; pain or feeling of pressure in pelvis; unusual tiredness; vaginal bleeding
  Rare
    Chest pain; pain or swelling of feet or legs; shortness
    of breath

This medicine may also cause the following side effect(s) that
your doctor will watch for:
  Less common
    Liver problems

Some side effects may occur that usually do not need medical attention. These side effects may go away during treatment as your body adjusts to the medicine. Also, your health
care professional may be able to tell you about ways to prevent or reduce some of these side effects. Check with your
health care professional if any of the following side effects
continue or are bothersome or if you have any questions
about them:
  More common
    Nausea; sudden sweating and feelings of warmth
  Less common
    Bone pain; dizziness; dry eyes; vomiting

Other side effects not listed may also occur in some patients.
If you notice any other effects, check with your healthcare
professional.

TORSEMIDE (Oral route, Intravenous route) - TORE-se-mide

Commonly used brand name(s)
In the U.S.—
  Demadex

Available Dosage Forms:
  • Tablet
  • Solution

Therapeutic Class: Cardiovascular Agent
Pharmacologic Class: Diuretic, Loop

Uses For This Medicine

Torsemide belongs to the group of medicines called loop diuretics. Torsemide is given to help reduce the amount of
water in the body in certain conditions, such as congestive
heart failure, severe liver disease (cirrhosis), or kidney disease. It works by acting on the kidneys to increase the flow
of urine.

Torsemide is also used to treat high blood pressure (hypertension). High blood pressure adds to the work load of the
heart and arteries. If it continues for a long time, the heart
and arteries may not function properly. This can damage the
blood vessels of the brain, heart, and kidneys, resulting in a
stroke, heart failure, or kidney failure. High blood pressure
may also increase the risk of heart attacks. These problems
may be less likely to occur if blood pressure is controlled.

Torsemide is available only with your doctor's prescription.

Before Using This Medicine

In deciding to use a medicine, the risks of taking the medicine
must be weighed against the good it will do. This is a decision

you and your doctor will make. For this medicine, the following
should be considered:

Allergies—Tell your doctor if you have ever had any unusual or allergic reaction to this medicine or any other medicines. Also tell your health care professional if you have any
other types of allergies, such as to foods, dyes, preservatives,
or animals. For non-prescription products, read the label or
package ingredients carefully.

Pediatric—Studies on this medicine have been done only
in adult patients, and there is no specific information comparing use of torsemide in children with use in other age
groups.

Geriatric—Many medicines have not been studied specifically in older people. Therefore, it may not be known whether
they work exactly the same way they do in younger adults.
Although there is no specific information comparing use of
torsemide in the elderly with use in other age groups, this
medicine is not expected to cause different side effects or
problems in older people than it does in younger adults.

Pregnancy—

	Pregnancy Category	Explanation
All Trimesters	B	Animal studies have revealed no evidence of harm to the fetus, however, there are no adequate studies in pregnant women OR animal studies have shown an adverse effect, but adequate studies in preg-nant women have failed to demonstrate a risk to the fetus.

Breast Feeding—There are no adequate studies in women
for determining infant risk when using this medication during
breastfeeding. Weigh the potential benefits against the potential risks before taking this medication while breastfeeding.

Other medicines—

Using this medicine with any of the following medicines is
usually not recommended, but may be required in some
cases. If both medicines are prescribed together, your doctor
may change the dose or how often you use one or both of
the medicines.

Arsenic Trioxide, Digitoxin, Dofetilide, Droperidol, Ketanserin,
Levomethadyl, Lithium, Sotalol

Interactions with Food/Tobacco/Alcohol—Certain
medicines should not be used at or around the time of eating
food or eating certain types of food since interactions may
occur. Using alcohol or tobacco with certain medicines may
also cause interactions to occur. Discuss with your healthcare
professional the use of your medicine with food, alcohol, or
tobacco.

Other medical problems—The presence of other medical
problems may affect the use of this medicine. Make sure you
tell your doctor if you have any other medical problems, especially:
  • Type 2 diabetes mellitus—Torsemide may increase the
    amount of sugar in the blood
  • Gout or
  • Hearing problems—Torsemide may make these condi-
    tions worse

- Heart attack (recent)—Use of torsemide after a recent heart attack may make this condition worse

- Kidney disease (severe) or

- Liver disease—Higher blood levels of torsemide may occur, which may increase the chance of side effects

Proper Use of This Medicine

This medicine may cause you to have an unusual feeling of tiredness when you begin to take it. You may also notice an increase in the amount of urine or in your frequency of urination. After you have taken the medicine for a while, these effects should lessen.

It is best to plan your dose or doses according to a schedule that will least affect your personal activities and sleep. Ask your health care professional to help you plan the best time to take this medicine.

To help you remember to take your medicine, try to get into the habit of taking it at the same time each day.

For patients taking this medicine for high blood pressure:

- In addition to the use of the medicine your doctor has prescribed, treatment for your high blood pressure may include weight control and care in the types of foods you eat, especially foods high in sodium. Your doctor will tell you which of these are most important for you. You should check with your doctor before changing your diet.

- Many patients who have high blood pressure will not notice any signs of the problem. In fact, many may feel normal. It is very important that you take your medicine exactly as directed and that you keep your appointments with your doctor even if you feel well.

- Remember that this medicine will not cure your high blood pressure but it does help control it. Therefore, you must continue to take it as directed if you expect to lower your blood pressure and keep it down. You may have to take high blood pressure medicine for the rest of your life. If high blood pressure is not treated, it can cause serious problems, such as heart failure, blood vessel disease, stroke, or kidney disease.

Dosing—The dose of this medicine will be different for different patients. Follow your doctor's orders or the directions on the label. The following information includes only the average doses of this medicine. If your dose is different, do not change it unless your doctor tells you to do so.

The amount of medicine that you take depends on the strength of the medicine. Also, the number of doses you take each day, the time allowed between doses, and the length of time you take the medicine depend on the medical problem for which you are using the medicine.

- For oral dosage form (tablets):
  - For lowering the amount of water in the body:
    - Adults—Dose is usually 5 to 20 milligrams (mg) once a day. However, your doctor may increase your dose as needed.
    - Children—Use and dose must be determined by your doctor.
  - For high blood pressure:
    - Adults—5 to 10 mg once a day.
    - Children—Use and dose must be determined by your doctor.

- For injection dosage form:
  - For lowering the amount of water in the body:
    - Adults—Dose is usually 5 to 20 mg injected into a vein once a day. However, your doctor may increase your dose as needed.
    - Children—Use and dose must be determined by your doctor.

Missed dose—If you miss a dose of this medicine, take it as soon as possible. However, if it is almost time for your next dose, skip the missed dose and go back to your regular dosing schedule. Do not double doses.

Storage—Store the medicine in a closed container at room temperature, away from heat, moisture, and direct light. Keep from freezing.

Keep out of the reach of children.

Do not keep outdated medicine or medicine no longer needed.

Precautions While Using This Medicine

It is important that your doctor check your progress at regular visits to make sure that this medicine is working properly.

This medicine may cause a loss of potassium from your body:

- To help prevent this, your doctor may want you to:
  - eat or drink foods that have a high potassium content (for example, orange or other citrus fruit juices), or
  - take a potassium supplement, or
  - take another medicine to help prevent the loss of the potassium in the first place.

- It is very important to follow these directions. Also, it is important not to change your diet on your own. This is more important if you are already on a special diet (as for diabetes) or if you are taking a potassium supplement or a medicine to reduce potassium loss. Extra potassium may not be necessary and, in some cases, too much potassium could be harmful.

To prevent the loss of too much water and potassium, tell your doctor if you become sick, especially with severe or continuing nausea and vomiting or diarrhea.

Before having any kind of surgery (including dental surgery) or emergency treatment, make sure the medical doctor or dentist in charge knows that you are taking this medicine.

Dizziness, lightheadedness, or fainting may occur, especially when you get up from a lying or sitting position. This is more likely to occur in the morning. Getting up slowly may help. When you get up from lying down, sit on the edge of the bed with your feet dangling for 1 or 2 minutes. Then stand up slowly. If the problem continues or gets worse, check with your doctor.

The dizziness, lightheadedness, or fainting is also more likely to occur if you drink alcohol, stand for long periods of time, or exercise, or if the weather is hot. While you are taking this medicine, be careful to limit the amount of alcohol you drink. Also, use extra care during exercise or hot weather or if you must stand for long periods of time.

For diabetic patients:

- This medicine may affect blood sugar levels. While you are using this medicine, be especially careful in testing for sugar in your blood or urine.

For patients taking this medicine for high blood pressure:

• Do not take other medicines unless they have been discussed with your doctor. This especially includes over-the-counter (nonprescription) medicines for appetite control, asthma, colds, cough, hay fever, or sinus problems, since they may tend to increase your blood pressure.

Side Effects of This Medicine

Along with its needed effects, a medicine may cause some unwanted effects. Although not all of these side effects may occur, if they do occur they may need medical attention.

Check with your doctor as soon as possible if any of the following side effects occur:

Less common
Dryness of mouth; fast or irregular heartbeat; increased thirst; mood or mental changes; muscle pain or cramps; nausea or vomiting; unusual tiredness or weakness

Rare
Black, tarry stools; dizziness when getting up from a sitting or lying position; ringing or buzzing in the ears or any hearing loss; skin rash

Some side effects may occur that usually do not need medical attention. These side effects may go away during treatment as your body adjusts to the medicine. Also, your health care professional may be able to tell you about ways to prevent or reduce some of these side effects. Check with your health care professional if any of the following side effects continue or are bothersome or if you have any questions about them:

More common
Constipation; dizziness; headache; stomach upset

TOSITUMOMAB (Intravenous route) -
tos-IT-too-moe-mab

Commonly used brand name(s)
In the U.S.—
Bexxar

Available Dosage Forms:
• Solution

Therapeutic Class: Antineoplastic Agent
Pharmacologic Class: Monoclonal Antibody

Uses For This Medicine

Tositumomab and iodine I 131 tositumomab is a protein called a monoclonal antibody. It is used to treat a type of cancer called non-Hodgkin's lymphoma.

Tositumomab and iodine I 131 tositumomab is to be administered only by or under the immediate supervision of your doctor.

Before Using This Medicine

In deciding to use a medicine, the risks of taking the medicine must be weighed against the good it will do. This is a decision you and your doctor will make. For this medicine, the following should be considered:

Allergies—Tell your doctor if you have ever had any unusual or allergic reaction to this medicine or any other medicines. Also tell your health care professional if you have any other types of allergies, such as to foods, dyes, preservatives, or animals. For non-prescription products, read the label or package ingredients carefully.

Pediatric—Studies on this medicine have been done only in adult patients, and there is no specific information comparing use of tositumomab and iodine I 131 tositumomab in children with use in other age groups.

Geriatric—Many medicines have not been studied specifically in older people. Therefore, it may not be known whether they work exactly the same way they do in younger adults. Although there is no specific information comparing use of tositumomab and iodine I 131 tositumomab in the elderly with use in other age groups, this medicine is not expected to cause different side effects or problems in older people than it does in younger adults.

Pregnancy—

	Pregnancy Category	Explanation
All Trimesters	X	Studies in animals or pregnant women have demonstrated positive evidence of fetal abnormalities. This drug should not be used in women who are or may become pregnant because the risk clearly outweighs any possible benefit.

Breast Feeding—Studies in women breastfeeding have demonstrated harmful infant effects. An alternative to this medication should be prescribed or you should stop breastfeeding while using this medicine.

Other medicines—Although certain medicines should not be used together at all, in other cases two different medicines may be used together even if an interaction might occur. In these cases, your doctor may want to change the dose, or other precautions may be necessary. Tell your healthcare professional if you are taking any other prescription or non-prescription (over-the-counter [OTC]) medicine.

Interactions with Food/Tobacco/Alcohol—Certain medicines should not be used at or around the time of eating food or eating certain types of food since interactions may occur. Using alcohol or tobacco with certain medicines may also cause interactions to occur. Discuss with your healthcare professional the use of your medicine with food, alcohol, or tobacco.

Other medical problems—The presence of other medical problems may affect the use of tositumomab and iodine I 131 tositumomab. Make sure you tell your doctor if you have any other medical problems, or bone marrow problems.

Proper Use of This Medicine

Dosing—The dose of this medicine will be different for different patients. Follow your doctor's orders or the directions on the label. The following information includes only the average doses of this medicine. If your dose is different, do not change it unless your doctor tells you to do so.

The amount of medicine that you take depends on the strength of the medicine. Also, the number of doses you take each day, the time allowed between doses, and the length of time you take the medicine depend on the medical problem for which you are using the medicine.

Precautions While Using This Medicine

It is very important that your doctor check your progress at regular visits to make sure that this medicine is working properly and to check for unwanted effects.

While you are being treated with tositumomab and iodine I 131 tositumomab, and after you stop treatment with it, do not have any immunizations (vaccinations) without your doctor's approval. Tositumomab and iodine I 131 tositumomab may lower your body's resistance and there is a chance you might get the infection the immunization is meant to prevent.

Patients should be informed of the risks of hypothyroidism and be advised to take thyroid blocking agents during treatment.

Tositumomab and iodine I 131 tositumomab can temporarily lower the number of white blood cells in your blood, increasing the chance of getting an infection. It can also lower the number of platelets, which are necessary for proper blood clotting. If this occurs, there are certain precautions you can take, especially when your blood count is low, to reduce the risk of infection or bleeding:

- Avoid people with infections. Check with your doctor immediately if you think you are getting an infection or if you get a fever or chills, cough or hoarseness, lower back or side pain, or painful or difficult urination.
- Check with your doctor immediately if you notice any unusual bleeding or bruising; black, tarry stools; blood in urine or stools; or pinpoint red spots on your skin.
- Be careful when using a regular toothbrush, dental floss, or toothpick. Your medical doctor, dentist, or nurse may recommend other ways to clean your teeth and gums. Check with your medical doctor before having any dental work done.
- Do not touch your eyes or the inside of your nose unless you have just washed your hands and have not touched anything else in the meantime.
- Be careful not to cut yourself when you are using sharp objects such as a safety razor or fingernail or toenail cutters.
- Avoid sports or other situations where bruising or injury could occur.

Side Effects of This Medicine

Along with its needed effects, a medicine may cause some unwanted effects. Although not all of these side effects may occur, if they do occur they may need medical attention.

Check with your doctor immediately if any of the following side effects occur:
More common
Bleeding gums; bone pain; chills; constipation; cough; coughing up blood; depressed mood; difficulty breathing; difficulty swallowing; dizziness; dry skin and hair; fast heartbeat; feeling cold; fever or chills; hair loss; headache; hives; hoarseness or husky voice; increased menstrual flow or vaginal bleeding; itching;

large, hive-like swelling on face, eyelids, lips, tongue, throat, hands, legs, feet, sex organs; lower back or side pain; muscle cramps and stiffness; noisy breathing; nosebleeds; painful or difficult urination; pale skin; paralysis; pinpoint red spots on skin; prolonged bleeding from cuts; puffiness or swelling of the eyelids or around the eyes, face, lips or tongue; red or dark brown urine; red or black, tarry stools; shortness of breath; skin rash; slowed heartbeat; sore throat; sores, ulcers, or white spots on lips or in mouth; swollen glands; tightness in chest; troubled breathing with exertion; unusual bleeding or bruising; unusual tiredness or weakness; weight gain; or wheezing

Some side effects may occur that usually do not need medical attention. These side effects may go away during treatment as your body adjusts to the medicine. Also, your health care professional may be able to tell you about ways to prevent or reduce some of these side effects. Check with your health care professional if any of the following side effects continue or are bothersome or if you have any questions about them:
More common
Abdominal pain or stomach pain; acid or sour stomach; belching; blurred vision; body aches or pain; confusion; congestion; diarrhea or increased bowel movements; difficult or labored breathing; difficulty having a bowel movement (stool); difficulty in moving; dryness or soreness of throat; faintness or lightheadedness when getting up from a lying or sitting position; feeling of warmth or heat; flushing or redness of skin, especially on face and neck; headache; heartburn; indigestion; itching skin; joint pain; swollen joints; muscle aching or cramping; muscle pains or stiffness; difficulty in moving; lack or loss of strength; loose or liquid stools; muscle pain or stiffness; nausea or feeling of upset stomach or feeling like you may vomit; pain in joints; runny nose; stomach discomfort, upset or pain; sudden sweating; swelling of hands, ankles, feet, or lower legs; swollen joints; tender, swollen glands in neck; trouble in swallowing; voice changes; vomiting

TRAMADOL (Oral route) - TRA-ma-dole

Commonly used brand name(s)

In the U.S.—
Ultram
Ultram ER

Available Dosage Forms:
- Tablet, Extended Release
- Tablet

Therapeutic Class: Analgesic

Uses For This Medicine

Tramadol is used to relieve pain, including pain after surgery. The long-acting tablets are used for chronic ongoing pain.. The effects of tramadol are similar to those of narcotic analgesics. Although tramadol is not classified as a narcotic, it may become habit-forming, causing mental or physical dependence.

Tramadol is available only with your doctor's prescription.

Before Using This Medicine

In deciding to use a medicine, the risks of taking the medicine must be weighed against the good it will do. This is a decision you and your doctor will make. For this medicine, the following should be considered:

Allergies—Tell your doctor if you have ever had any unusual or allergic reaction to this medicine or any other medicines. Also tell your health care professional if you have any other types of allergies, such as to foods, dyes, preservatives, or animals. For non-prescription products, read the label or package ingredients carefully.

Pediatric—There is no specific information on the relationship of age to the effects of tramadol tablets in patients less than 16 years of age, and tramadol extended-release tablets in patients less than 18 years of age.

Geriatric—Studies in older adults show that tramadol stays in the body a little longer than it does in younger adults. Your doctor will consider this when deciding on your doses.

Pregnancy—

	Pregnancy Category	Explanation
All Trimesters	C	Animal studies have shown an adverse effect and there are no adequate studies in pregnant women OR no animal studies have been conducted and there are no adequate studies in pregnant women.

Breast Feeding—There are no adequate studies in women for determining infant risk when using this medication during breastfeeding. Weigh the potential benefits against the potential risks before taking this medication while breastfeeding.

Other medicines—

Using this medicine with any of the following medicines is not recommended. Your doctor may decide not to treat you with this medication or change some of the other medicines you take.

Rasagiline, Selegiline

Interactions with Food/Tobacco/Alcohol—Certain medicines should not be used at or around the time of eating food or eating certain types of food since interactions may occur. Using alcohol or tobacco with certain medicines may also cause interactions to occur. The following interactions have been selected on the basis of their potential significance and are not necessarily all-inclusive.

Using this medicine with any of the following is usually not recommended, but may be unavoidable in some cases. If used together, your doctor may change the dose or how often you use this medicine, or give you special instructions about the use of food, alcohol, or tobacco.

Ethanol

Other medical problems—The presence of other medical problems may affect the use of this medicine. Make sure you

tell your doctor if you have any other medical problems, especially:

- Abdominal or stomach conditions (severe)—Tramadol may hide signs of other medical conditions.
- Addiction problems or
- Suicidal—Tramadol should not be used.
- Alcohol or drug abuse, or history of—May increase the serious side effects of tramadol.
- Epilepsy or
- History of seizures or
- Increased risk for seizures caused by alcohol and drug withdrawal, brain or spinal cord infections, or head trauma—Risk of seizures may be increased.
- Head injury—Tramadol can hide signs of other medical conditions.
- Kidney disease or
- Liver disease—The chance of side effects may be increased. Your doctor will consider this when deciding on your doses.

Proper Use of This Medicine

If you think that this medicine is not working as well after you have been taking it for a few weeks, do not increase the dose. Instead, check with your medical doctor or dentist.

Dosing—The dose of this medicine will be different for different patients. Follow your doctor's orders or the directions on the label. The following information includes only the average doses of this medicine. If your dose is different, do not change it unless your doctor tells you to do so.

The amount of medicine that you take depends on the strength of the medicine. Also, the number of doses you take each day, the time allowed between doses, and the length of time you take the medicine depend on the medical problem for which you are using the medicine.

- For chronic pain:
  - For oral dosage form (long-acting tablets):
    - Adults—100 mg once a day. Your doctor may increase your dose as needed. You should not take more than 300 mg per day.
    - Children up to 18 years of age—Use and dose must be determined by your doctor.

- For pain:
  - For oral dosage form (tablets):
    - Adults—One-half to two 50–milligram (mg) tablets every four to six hours as needed, no more than 8 tablets in a day Your healthcare professional may want you to break the tablets in half for the first dose and increase your dose by half-tablets, up to a maximum of 2 full tablets per dose. By starting at a lower dose and slowly increasing the amount of medicine you take, this will help you get used to the medicine gradually. Your healthcare professional may want you to take 2 tablets for the first dose if you are having severe pain. This helps the medicine start working a little faster.
    - Children up to 16 years of age—Use and dose must be determined by your doctor.

Missed dose—If you miss a dose of this medicine, take it as soon as possible. However, if it is almost time for your next dose, skip the missed dose and go back to your regular dosing schedule. Do not double doses.

Storage—Store the medicine in a closed container at room temperature, away from heat, moisture, and direct light. Keep from freezing.

Keep out of the reach of children.

Do not keep outdated medicine or medicine no longer needed.

Precautions While Using This Medicine

This medicine will add to the effects of alcohol and other CNS depressants (medicine that causes drowsiness). Some examples of CNS depressants are antihistamines or medicine for hay fever, other allergies, or colds; sedatives, tranquilizers, or sleeping medicine; prescription pain medicine or narcotics; barbiturates; medicine for seizures; muscle relaxants; or anesthetics, including some dental anesthetics. Do not drink alcoholic beverages, and check with your medical doctor or dentist before taking any of the medicines listed above while you are using this medicine.

This medicine may cause some people to become drowsy, dizzy, or lightheaded. Make sure you know how you react to this medicine before you drive, use machines, or do anything else that could be dangerous if you are dizzy or are not alert.

Dizziness, lightheadedness, or fainting may occur, especially when you get up suddenly from a lying or sitting position. Getting up slowly may help lessen this problem.

Nausea or vomiting may occur, especially after the first couple of doses. This effect may go away if you lie down for awhile. However, if nausea or vomiting continues, check with your medical doctor or dentist. Lying down for a while may also help relieve some other side effects, such as dizziness or lightheadedness, that may occur.

Before having any kind of surgery (including dental surgery) or emergency treatment, tell the medical doctor or dentist in charge that you are taking this medicine. Taking tramadol together with medicines that are used during surgery or dental or emergency treatments may cause increased side effects.

If you think you or someone else may have taken an overdose of tramadol, get emergency help at once. Signs of an overdose include convulsions (seizures) and pinpoint pupils of the eyes.

Side Effects of This Medicine

Along with its needed effects, a medicine may cause some unwanted effects. Although not all of these side effects may occur, if they do occur they may need medical attention.

Get emergency help immediately if any of the following symptoms of overdose occur:

Change in consciousness; chest pain or discomfort; convulsions (seizures); decreased awareness or responsiveness; difficulty in breathing; dizziness or fainting; lack of muscle tone; lightheadedness; loss of consciousness; pinpointed pupils of the eyes; severe sleepiness; shortness of breath; slow or irregular heartbeat; unusual tiredness

Check with your doctor as soon as possible if any of the following side effects occur:

Less common or rare
Abdominal fullness; abnormal or decreased touch sensation; blisters under the skin; bloating; blood in urine; blood pressure increased; blurred vision; change in walking and balance; chest pain or discomfort; chills; convulsions (seizures); darkened urine; difficult urination; dizziness or lightheadedness when getting up from a lying or sitting position; fainting; fast heartbeat; frequent urge to urinate; gaseous abdominal pain; heart rate increased; indigestion; irregular heartbeat; loss of memory; numbness and tingling of face, fingers, or toes; numbness, tingling, pain, or weakness in hands or feet; pain in arms, legs, or lower back, especially pain in calves and/or heels upon exertion; pain or discomfort in arms, jaw, back or neck; pains in stomach, side, or abdomen, possibly radiating to the back; pale bluish-colored or cold hands or feet; recurrent fever; seeing, hearing, or feeling things that are not there; severe cramping; severe nausea; severe redness, swelling, and itching of the skin; shortness of breath; sweats; trembling and shaking of hands or feet; trouble performing routine tasks; weak or absent pulses in legs; yellow eyes or skin

Some side effects may occur that usually do not need medical attention. These side effects may go away during treatment as your body adjusts to the medicine. Also, your health care professional may be able to tell you about ways to prevent or reduce some of these side effects. Check with your health care professional if any of the following side effects continue or are bothersome or if you have any questions about them:

More common
Abdominal or stomach pain; agitation; anxiety; constipation; cough; diarrhea; discouragement; dizziness; drowsiness; dry mouth; feeling of warmth; feeling sad or empty; feeling unusually cold; fever; general feeling of discomfort or illness; headache; heartburn; irritability; itching of the skin; joint pain; loss of appetite; loss of interest or pleasure; loss of strength or weakness; muscle aches and pains; nausea; nervousness; redness of the face, neck, arms and occasionally, upper chest; restlessness; runny nose; shivering; skin rash; sleepiness or unusual drowsiness; sore throat; stuffy nose; sweating; tiredness; trouble concentrating; unusual feeling of excitement; unusual tiredness or weakness; vomiting; weakness

Less common or rare
Abnormal dreams; appetite decreased; back pain; bladder pain; blistering, crusting, irritation, itching, or reddening of skin; bloody or cloudy urine; body aches or pain; change in hearing; clamminess; cold flu-like symptoms; confusion; cough producing mucus; cracked, dry, scaly skin; decreased interest in sexual intercourse; difficult, burning, or painful urination; difficulty breathing; difficulty in moving; disturbance in attention; ear congestion; ear drainage; earache or pain in ear; excessive gas; fall; false or unusual sense of well-being; feeling hot; feeling jittery; flushing or redness of the skin; general feeling of bodily discomfort; goosebumps; headache, severe and throbbing; hoarseness; hot flashes; inability to have or keep an erection; itching, pain, redness, swelling, tenderness, warmth on skin; joint sprain; joint stiffness; joint swelling; loss in sexual ability, desire, drive, or performance; loss of voice; lower back or side pain; muscle aching or cramping; muscle injury; muscle pain or stiffness; muscle spasms or twitching; nasal congestion; neck pain; night sweats; pain; pain in limb; pain or tenderness around eyes and cheekbones; pain, swelling, or redness in joints; skin discoloration; swelling;

swelling of hands, ankles, feet, or lower legs; tightness of chest; trouble in holding or releasing urine; trouble in sleeping; troubled breathing; weight increased or decreased

After you stop using this medicine, it may still produce some side effects that need attention. During this period of time, *check with your doctor immediately* if you notice the following side effects:

Anxiety; body aches; diarrhea; fast heartbeat; fever, runny nose, or sneezing; gooseflesh; high blood pressure; increased sweating; increased yawning; loss of appetite; nausea or vomiting; nervousness, restlessness or irritability; shivering or trembling; stomach cramps; trouble in sleeping; unusually large pupils; weakness

Other side effects not listed may also occur in some patients. If you notice any other effects, check with your healthcare professional.

TRAMADOL AND ACETAMINOPHEN (Oral route) - TRA-ma-dole, a-seet-a-MIN-oh-fen

Commonly used brand name(s)
In the U.S.—
Ultracet

Available Dosage Forms:
• Tablet

Therapeutic Class: Opioid/Acetaminophen Combination

Uses For This Medicine

Combination medicines containing narcotic analgesics such as tramadol and acetaminophen are used to relieve pain. An opioid analgesic and acetaminophen used together may provide better pain relief than either medicine used alone. In some cases, you may get relief with lower doses of each medicine.

Opioid analgesics act in the central nervous system (CNS) to relieve pain. Many of their side effects are also caused by actions in the CNS. When opioids are used for a long time, your body may get used to them so that larger amounts are needed to relieve pain. This is called tolerance to the medicine. Also, when opioids are used for a long time or in large doses, they may become habit-forming (causing mental or physical dependence). Physical dependence may lead to withdrawal symptoms when you stop taking the medicine.

Acetaminophen does not become habit-forming when taken for a long time but it may cause other unwanted effects, when taken in large doses including liver damage, if too much is taken.

This medicine is available only with your doctor's prescription.

Before Using This Medicine

In deciding to use a medicine, the risks of taking the medicine must be weighed against the good it will do. This is a decision you and your doctor will make. For this medicine, the following should be considered:

Allergies—Tell your doctor if you have ever had any unusual or allergic reaction to this medicine or any other medicines. Also tell your health care professional if you have any other types of allergies, such as to foods, dyes, preservatives, or animals. For non-prescription products, read the label or package ingredients carefully.

Pediatric—Studies on this medicine have been done only in adult patients, and there is no specific information comparing use of tramadol and acetaminophen in children up to 16 years of age with use in other age groups.

Geriatric—This medicine has been tested and has not been shown to cause different side effects or problems in older people than it does in younger adults.

Other medicines—

Using this medicine with any of the following medicines is not recommended. Your doctor may decide not to treat you with this medication or change some of the other medicines you take.

Rasagiline, Selegiline

Interactions with Food/Tobacco/Alcohol—Certain medicines should not be used at or around the time of eating food or eating certain types of food since interactions may occur. Using alcohol or tobacco with certain medicines may also cause interactions to occur. The following interactions have been selected on the basis of their potential significance and are not necessarily all-inclusive.

Using this medicine with any of the following is usually not recommended, but may be unavoidable in some cases. If used together, your doctor may change the dose or how often you use this medicine, or give you special instructions about the use of food, alcohol, or tobacco.

Ethanol

Using this medicine with any of the following may cause an increased risk of certain side effects but may be unavoidable in some cases. If used together, your doctor may change the dose or how often you use this medicine, or give you special instructions about the use of food, alcohol, or tobacco.

Cabbage

Other medical problems—The presence of other medical problems may affect the use of this medicine. Make sure you tell your doctor if you have any other medical problems, especially:

• Alcohol and/or other drug abuse, or history of, or

• Convulsions (seizures), history of, or

• Head injury, or

• Hormonal problems or

• Infections of the central nervous system or

• Kidney disease or

• Liver disease, or

• Respiratory difficulty or troubled breathing, or

• Severe abdominal problems—The chance of serious side effects may be increased

Proper Use of This Medicine

Take this medicine only as directed by your medical doctor or dentist. Do not take more of it, do not take it more often, and do not take it for a longer time than your medical doctor or dentist ordered. This is especially important for young children and elderly patients, who may be more sensitive than other people to the effects of analgesics. If too much of a analgesic is taken, it may become habit-forming (causing mental or physical dependence) or lead to medical problems because of an overdose. Taking too much acetaminophen may cause liver damage.

Dosing—The dose of this medicine will be different for different patients. Follow your doctor's orders or the directions on the label. The following information includes only the average doses of this medicine. If your dose is different, do not change it unless your doctor tells you to do so.

The amount of medicine that you take depends on the strength of the medicine. Also, the number of doses you take each day, the time allowed between doses, and the length of time you take the medicine depend on the medical problem for which you are using the medicine.

- For oral dosage form (tablets):
  - For pain:
    - Adults and adolescents 16 years and older—Take 2 tablets every 4–6 hours as needed for up to 5 days.
    - Children under 16 years of age– use and dose must be determined by your doctor.

Storage—Store the medicine in a closed container at room temperature, away from heat, moisture, and direct light. Keep from freezing.

Keep out of the reach of children.

Do not keep outdated medicine or medicine no longer needed.

Ask your healthcare professional how you should dispose of any medicine you do not use.

Precautions While Using This Medicine

The analgesic in this medicine will add to the effects of alcohol and other CNS depressants (medicines that slow down the nervous system, possibly causing drowsiness). Some examples of CNS depressants are antihistamines or medicine for hay fever, other allergies, or colds; sedatives, tranquilizers, or sleeping medicine; other prescription pain medicine or narcotics; opioids; barbiturates; medicine for seizures; muscle relaxants; or anesthetics, including some dental anesthetics. Also, there may be a greater risk of liver damage if you drink three or more alcoholic beverages while you are taking acetaminophen. Do not drink alcoholic beverages, and check with your medical doctor or dentist before taking any of the medicines listed above, while you are using this medicine.

This medicine may cause some people to become drowsy, dizzy, or less alert than they are normally. Make sure you know how you react to this medicine before you drive, use machines, or do anything else that could be dangerous if you are dizzy or are not alert.

Dizziness, lightheadedness, or fainting may occur, especially when you get up suddenly from a lying or sitting position. Getting up slowly may help lessen this problem.

Nausea or vomiting may occur, especially after the first couple of doses. This effect may go away if you lie down for a while. However, if nausea or vomiting continues, check with your medical doctor or dentist. Lying down for a while may also help relieve some other side effects, such as dizziness or lightheadedness, that may occur.

Before having any kind of surgery (including dental surgery) or emergency treatment, tell the medical doctor or dentist in charge that you are taking this medicine.

Analgesics may cause dryness of the mouth. For temporary relief, use sugarless candy or gum, melt bits of ice in your mouth, or use a saliva substitute. However, if dry mouth continues for more than 2 weeks, check with your dentist. Continuing dryness of the mouth may increase the chance of dental disease, including tooth decay, gum disease, and fungus infections.

If you have been taking this medicine regularly, do not suddenly stop taking it without first checking with your doctor. Your doctor may want you to reduce gradually the amount you are taking before stopping completely, to lessen the chance of withdrawal side effects. This will depend on which of these medicines you have been taking, and the amount you have been taking every day.

Side Effects of This Medicine

Along with its needed effects, a medicine may cause some unwanted effects. Although not all of these side effects may occur, if they do occur they may need medical attention.

Check with your doctor immediately if any of the following side effects occur:
  Rare
    Burning, itching, and redness of skin; vomiting; chest pain; cough; difficulty swallowing; dizziness; fast heartbeat; hives; itching; puffiness or swelling of the eyelids or around the eyes, face, lips or tongue; shortness of breath; skin rash; tightness in chest; unusual tiredness or weakness; wheezing; seizures

Symptoms of overdose

  Get emergency help immediately if any of the following symptoms of overdose occur:

    Chest pain or discomfort; convulsions; difficulty breathing

Some side effects may occur that usually do not need medical attention. These side effects may go away during treatment as your body adjusts to the medicine. Also, your health care professional may be able to tell you about ways to prevent or reduce some of these side effects. Check with your health care professional if any of the following side effects continue or are bothersome or if you have any questions about them:
  Less common
    Abdominal pain; aches, pains or weakness of muscles; numbness or tingling of hands, legs, and feet; acid or

sour stomach; belching; heartburn; indigestion; stomach discomfort; anxiety; bloated full feeling; excess air or gas in stomach or intestines; confusion; constipation; dizziness; dry mouth; false or unusual sense of well-being; feeling of warmth; redness of the face, neck, arms, and occasionally the upper chest; headache; increased sweating; increase in bowel movements; loose stools; soft stools; itching skin; loss of appetite; weight loss; loss of strength or energy; muscle pain or weakness; mood or mental changes; nausea; nervousness; painful or difficult urination; rash; sleepiness or unusual drowsiness; sleeplessness; trouble sleeping; unable to sleep; unusual tiredness or weakness; vomiting

Rare

Abnormal thinking; bloody or black, tarry stools; vomiting of blood or material that looks like coffee grounds; sever stomach pain; constipation; blurred vision; dizziness; severe or continuing, dull headache; pounding in the ears; slow or fast heartbeat; change in vision; chills; cold sweats; confusion; dizziness; faintness, or light-headedness when getting up from lying or sitting position; continuing ringing or buzzing or other unexplained noise in ears; crying; depersonalization; dysphoria; euphoria; mental depression; paranoia; quick to react or overreact emotionally; rapidly changing moods; decreased awareness or responsiveness; decrease in amount of urine; decrease in urine volume; decrease in frequency of urination; difficulty in passing urine [dribbling]; painful urination; depression; difficulty swallowing; dizziness or lightheadedness; feeling of constant movement of self or surroundings; sensation of spinning; drug abuse and dependence; fainting; fast, pounding, or irregular heartbeat or pulse; palpitations; feeling unusually cold; shivering; high or low blood pressure; dizziness; lightheadedness; increased muscle tone; involuntary muscle contractions; loss in sexual ability, desire, drive, or performance; decreased interest in sexual intercourse; inability to have or keep an erection; loss of memory; problems with memory; loss of sense of reality; morbid dreaming; migraine headache; seeing, hearing, or feeling things that are not there; shakiness and unsteady walk; clumsiness, unsteadiness, trembling, or other problems with muscle control or coordination; shortness of breath; difficult or labored breathing; tightness in chest; wheezing; swelling of tongue; trouble in holding or releasing urine; painful urination; unusual tiredness or weakness; weight loss; yellow eyes or skinAfter you stop using this medicine, it may still produce some side effects that need attention. During this period of time, *check with your doctor immediately* if you notice the following side effects:

Anxiety; diarrhea; fever, runny nose, or sneezing; gooseflesh; increased sweating; nausea or vomiting; nervousness, restlessness, or irritability; pain; seeing, hearing, or feeling things that are not there; shivering or trembling; trouble in sleeping

Other side effects not listed may also occur in some patients. If you notice any other effects, check with your healthcare professional.

TRANDOLAPRIL AND VERAPAMIL
(Oral route) - tran-DOE-la-pril, ver-AP-a-mil

Black Box Warning

When used in pregnancy during the second and third trimesters, ACE inhibitors can cause injury and even death to the developing fetus. When pregnancy is detected, trandolapril/verapamil hydrochloride should be discontinued as soon as possible.

Commonly used brand name(s)

In the U.S.—
  Tarka

Available Dosage Forms:

  • Tablet, Extended Release

Therapeutic Class: ACE Inhibitor/Calcium Channel Blocker Combination
Pharmacologic Class: ACE Inhibitor

Uses For This Medicine

Trandolapril and verapamil combination belongs to the class of medicines called high blood pressure medicines (antihypertensives). It is used to treat high blood pressure (hypertension).

High blood pressure adds to the workload of the heart and arteries. If it continues for a long time, the heart and arteries may not function properly. This can damage the blood vessels of the brain, heart, and kidneys, resulting in a stroke, heart failure, or kidney failure. High blood pressure may also increase the risk of heart attacks. These problems may be less likely to occur if blood pressure is controlled.

The exact way in which this medicine works is not known. Trandolapril is a type of medicine known as an angiotensin-converting enzyme (ACE) inhibitor. It blocks an enzyme in the body that is necessary in producing a substance that causes blood vessels to tighten. Verapamil is a type of medicine known as a calcium channel blocker. Calcium channel blocking agents affect the movement of calcium into the cells of the heart and blood vessels. The actions of both medicines relax blood vessels, lower blood pressure, and increase the supply of blood and oxygen to the heart.

This medicine is available only with your doctor's prescription.

Before Using This Medicine

In deciding to use a medicine, the risks of taking the medicine must be weighed against the good it will do. This is a decision you and your doctor will make. For this medicine, the following should be considered:

Allergies—Tell your doctor if you have ever had any unusual or allergic reaction to this medicine or any other medicines. Also tell your health care professional if you have any other types of allergies, such as to foods, dyes, preservatives, or animals. For non-prescription products, read the label or package ingredients carefully.

Pediatric—Studies on this medicine have been done only in adult patients, and there is no specific information com-

paring use of trandolapril and verapamil in children with use in other age groups.

Geriatric—Although this medicine has not been shown to cause different side effects or problems in older people than it does in younger adults, blood levels of trandolapril and verapamil may be increased in the elderly. Elderly people also may be more sensitive to the effects of this medicine.

Other medicines—

Using this medicine with any of the following medicines is not recommended. Your doctor may decide not to treat you with this medication or change some of the other medicines you take.

Dofetilide, Ranolazine

Interactions with Food/Tobacco/Alcohol—Certain medicines should not be used at or around the time of eating food or eating certain types of food since interactions may occur. Using alcohol or tobacco with certain medicines may also cause interactions to occur. The following interactions have been selected on the basis of their potential significance and are not necessarily all-inclusive.

Using this medicine with any of the following may cause an increased risk of certain side effects but may be unavoidable in some cases. If used together, your doctor may change the dose or how often you use this medicine, or give you special instructions about the use of food, alcohol, or tobacco.

Grapefruit Juice

Other medical problems—The presence of other medical problems may affect the use of this medicine. Make sure you tell your doctor if you have any other medical problems, especially:

* Bee-sting allergy treatments or
* Dialysis treatments—Increased risk of serious allergic reaction occurring
* Dehydration—Lowering effects on blood pressure may be increased
* Type 2 diabetes mellitus—Increased risk of potassium levels in the body becoming too high
* Duchenne's muscular dystrophy—Verapamil may make this condition worse
* Heart disease or
* Hypotension (low blood pressure)—Further lowering of blood pressure may make problems resulting from these conditions worse
* Kidney disease or
* Liver disease—Effects may be increased because of slower removal of the medicine from the body
* Scleroderma or
* Systemic lupus erythematosus (SLE) (or history of)—Increased risk of blood problems with ACE inhibitors
* Previous reaction to any ACE inhibitor involving hoarseness; swelling of face, mouth, hands, or feet; or sudden trouble in breathing—Reaction is more likely to occur again with ACE inhibitors

Proper Use of This Medicine

Take this medicine exactly as directed by your doctor, at the same time each day. Do not take more of it and do not take it more often than directed.

Swallow the tablets whole, without breaking, crushing, or chewing them.

Take this medicine with food or milk.

Dosing—The dose of this medicine will be different for different patients. Follow your doctor's orders or the directions on the label. The following information includes only the average doses of this medicine. If your dose is different, do not change it unless your doctor tells you to do so.

The amount of medicine that you take depends on the strength of the medicine. Also, the number of doses you take each day, the time allowed between doses, and the length of time you take the medicine depend on the medical problem for which you are using the medicine.

* For oral dosage form (extended-release tablets):
  * For high blood pressure:
    * Adults—1 or 2 tablets a day.
    * Children—Use and dose must be determined by your doctor.

Missed dose—If you miss a dose of this medicine, take it as soon as possible. However, if it is almost time for your next dose, skip the missed dose and go back to your regular dosing schedule. Do not double doses.

Storage—Store the medicine in a closed container at room temperature, away from heat, moisture, and direct light. Keep from freezing.

Keep out of the reach of children.

Do not keep outdated medicine or medicine no longer needed.

Precautions While Using This Medicine

It is very important that your doctor check your progress at regular visits. This will allow your doctor to make sure the medicine is working properly, to check for unwanted effects, and to change the dosage if needed.

If you think that you may have become pregnant, check with your doctor immediately. Use of this medicine, especially during the second and third trimesters (after the first 3 months) of pregnancy, may cause serious injury or even death to the unborn child.

Do not take any other medicines, especially potassium supplements, or salt substitutes that contain potassium unless approved or prescribed by your doctor.

Dizziness, lightheadedness, or fainting may occur after the first dose, especially if you have been taking a diuretic (water pill). Make sure you know how you react to the medicine before you drive, use machines, or do other things that could be dangerous if you experience these effects.

Check with your doctor if you notice any signs of fever, sore throat, or chills. These could be symptoms of an infection resulting from low white blood cell counts.

Check with your doctor immediately if you notice difficult breathing or swelling of the face, arms, or legs. These could be symptoms of a serious allergic reaction.

Check with your doctor if you become sick while taking this medicine, especially with severe or continuing vomiting or diarrhea. These conditions may cause you to lose too much water, possibly resulting in low blood pressure.

Dizziness, lightheadedness, or fainting may also occur if you exercise or if the weather is hot. Heavy sweating can cause loss of too much water which can result in low blood pressure. Use extra care during exercise or hot weather.

Before having any kind of surgery (including dental surgery) or emergency treatment, tell the medical doctor or dentist in charge that you are taking this medicine.

Side Effects of This Medicine

Along with its needed effects, a medicine may cause some unwanted effects. Although not all of these side effects may occur, if they do occur they may need medical attention.

Check with your doctor immediately if any of the following side effects occur:

Rare

Swelling of face, mouth, hands, or feet; trouble in swallowing or breathing (sudden) accompanied by hoarseness

Check with your doctor as soon as possible if any of the following side effects occur:

Rare

Chest pain; cough (with mucus); dark urine, yellow eyes or skin, or pain in right side; lightheadedness or fainting; fever, chills, or sore throat; general feeling of discomfort or illness; shortness of breath; slow heartbeat; wheezing

Signs and symptoms of too much potassium in the body

Confusion; irregular heartbeat; nervousness; numbness or tingling in hands, feet, or lips; weakness or heaviness of legs

Some side effects may occur that usually do not need medical attention. These side effects may go away during treatment as your body adjusts to the medicine. Also, your health care professional may be able to tell you about ways to prevent or reduce some of these side effects. Check with your health care professional if any of the following side effects continue or are bothersome or if you have any questions about them:

Less common or rare

Constipation; cough (dry, continuing); diarrhea; dizziness; itching; joint pain or pain in arms or legs; nausea; unusual tiredness

Other side effects not listed may also occur in some patients. If you notice any other effects, check with your healthcare professional.

TRAZODONE   (Oral route) - TRAZ-oh-done

Black Box Warning

Antidepressants increased the risk of suicidal thinking and behavior (suicidality) in short-term studies in children and adolescents with Major Depressive Disorder (MDD) and other psychiatric disorders. Anyone considering the use of trazodone hydrochloride or any other antidepressant in a child or adolescent must balance this risk with the clinical need. Patients who are started on therapy should be observed closely for clinical worsening, suicidality, or unusual changes in behavior. Families and caregivers should be advised of the need for close observation and communication with the pre-

scriber. Trazodone hydrochloride is not approved for use in pediatric patients.

Pooled analyses of short-term (4 weeks to 16 weeks) placebo-controlled trials of 9 antidepressant drugs (SSRIs and others) in children and adolescents with major depressive disorder (MDD), obsessive compulsive disorder (OCD), or other psychiatric disorders (a total of 24 trials involving over 4,400 patients) have revealed a greater risk of adverse events representing suicidal thinking or behavior (suicidality) during the first few months of treatment in those receiving antidepressants. The average risk of such events in patients receiving antidepressants was 4%, twice the placebo risk of 2%. No suicides occurred in these trials.

Commonly used brand name(s)

In the U.S.—
    Desyrel
    Desyrel Dividose

Available Dosage Forms:
    • Tablet

Therapeutic Class: Antidepressant

Uses For This Medicine

Trazodone belongs to the group of medicines known as antidepressants or "mood elevators." It is used to relieve mental depression and depression that sometimes occurs with anxiety.

Trazodone is available only with your doctor's prescription.

Before Using This Medicine

In deciding to use a medicine, the risks of taking the medicine must be weighed against the good it will do. This is a decision you and your doctor will make. For this medicine, the following should be considered:

Allergies—Tell your doctor if you have ever had any unusual or allergic reaction to this medicine or any other medicines. Also tell your health care professional if you have any other types of allergies, such as to foods, dyes, preservatives, or animals. For non-prescription products, read the label or package ingredients carefully.

Pediatric—Trazodone must be used with caution in children with depression. Studies have shown occurrences of children thinking about suicide or attempting suicide in clinical trials for this medicine. More study is needed to be sure trazodone is safe and effective in children

Geriatric—Drowsiness, dizziness, confusion, vision problems, dryness of mouth, and constipation may be more likely to occur in the elderly, who are usually more sensitive to the effects of trazodone.

Pregnancy—

	Pregnancy Category	Explanation
All Trimesters	C	Animal studies have shown an adverse effect and there are no adequate studies in pregnant women OR no animal studies have been conducted and there are no adequate studies in pregnant women.

Breast Feeding—There are no adequate studies in women for determining infant risk when using this medication during

breastfeeding. Weigh the potential benefits against the potential risks before taking this medication while breastfeeding.

Other medicines—

Using this medicine with any of the following medicines is usually not recommended, but may be required in some cases. If both medicines are prescribed together, your doctor may change the dose or how often you use one or both of the medicines.

Droperidol, Fluoxetine, Ginkgo, Linezolid, Paroxetine, St John's Wort

Interactions with Food/Tobacco/Alcohol—Certain medicines should not be used at or around the time of eating food or eating certain types of food since interactions may occur. Using alcohol or tobacco with certain medicines may also cause interactions to occur. Discuss with your healthcare professional the use of your medicine with food, alcohol, or tobacco.

Other medical problems—The presence of other medical problems may affect the use of this medicine. Make sure you tell your doctor if you have any other medical problems, especially:

- Alcohol abuse (or history of)—Drinking alcohol with trazodone will increase the central nervous system (CNS) depressant effects
- Heart disease—Trazodone may make the condition worse
- Kidney disease or
- Liver disease—Higher blood levels of trazodone may occur, increasing the chance of side effects

Proper Use of This Medicine

To lessen stomach upset and to reduce dizziness and lightheadedness, take this medicine with or shortly after a meal or light snack, even for a daily bedtime dose, unless your doctor has told you to take it on an empty stomach.

Take trazodone only as directed by your doctor, to benefit your condition as much as possible.

Sometimes trazodone must be taken for up to 4 weeks before you begin to feel better, although most people notice improvement within 2 weeks.

Dosing—The dose of this medicine will be different for different patients. Follow your doctor's orders or the directions on the label. The following information includes only the average doses of this medicine. If your dose is different, do not change it unless your doctor tells you to do so.

The amount of medicine that you take depends on the strength of the medicine. Also, the number of doses you take each day, the time allowed between doses, and the length of time you take the medicine depend on the medical problem for which you are using the medicine.

- Adults—Oral, to start, 50 milligrams per dose taken three times a day, or 75 milligrams per dose taken two times a day. Your doctor may increase your dose if needed.
- Children 6 to 18 years of age—Your doctor will tell you what dose to take based on your body weight.
- Children up to 6 years of age—Dose must be determined by the doctor.
- Elderly patients—Oral, to start, 25 milligrams per dose taken three times a day. Your doctor may increase your dose if needed.

Missed dose—If you miss a dose of this medicine, take it as soon as possible. However, if it is almost time for your next dose, skip the missed dose and go back to your regular dosing schedule. Do not double doses.

Storage—Store the medicine in a closed container at room temperature, away from heat, moisture, and direct light. Keep from freezing.

Keep out of the reach of children.

Do not keep outdated medicine or medicine no longer needed.

Precautions While Using This Medicine

It is very important that your doctor check your progress at regular visits. This will allow your doctor to check the medicine's effects and to change the dose if needed.

Do not stop taking this medicine without first checking with your doctor. To prevent a possible return of your medical problem, your doctor may want you to reduce gradually the amount of medicine you are using before you stop completely.

Before having any kind of surgery, dental treatment, or emergency treatment, tell the medical doctor or dentist in charge that you are using this medicine. Taking trazodone together with medicines that are used during surgery or dental or emergency treatments may increase the CNS depressant effects.

Trazodone may cause some people to be agitated, irritable or display other abnormal behaviors. It may also cause some people to have suicidal thoughts and tendencies or to become more depressed. If you or your caregiver notice any of these adverse effects, tell your doctor right away.

This medicine will add to the effects of alcohol and other CNS depressants (medicines that slow down the nervous system, possibly causing drowsiness). Some examples of CNS depressants are antihistamines or medicine for hay fever, other allergies, or colds; sedatives, tranquilizers, or sleeping medicine; prescription pain medicine or narcotics; barbiturates; medicine for seizures; muscle relaxants; or anesthetics, including some dental anesthetics. Check with your doctor before taking any of the above while you are using this medicine.

This medicine may cause some people to become drowsy or less alert than they are normally. Make sure you know how you react to this medicine before you drive, use machines, or do anything else that could be dangerous if you are not alert.

Dizziness, lightheadedness, or fainting may occur, especially when you get up from a lying or sitting position. Getting up slowly may help. If this problem continues or gets worse, check with your doctor.

Trazodone may cause dryness of the mouth. For temporary relief, use sugarless gum or candy, melt bits of ice in your mouth, or use a saliva substitute. However, if your mouth continues to feel dry for more than 2 weeks, check with your medical doctor or dentist. Continuing dryness of the mouth may increase the chance of dental disease, including tooth decay, gum disease, and fungus infections.

Side Effects of This Medicine

Along with its needed effects, a medicine may cause some unwanted effects. Although not all of these side effects may occur, if they do occur they may need medical attention.

Stop taking this medicine and get emergency help immediately if any of the following effects occur:

Rare
   Painful, inappropriate erection of the penis, continuing

Check with your doctor as soon as possible if any of the following side effects occur:

Less common
   Confusion; fainting; muscle tremors

Rare
   Fast or slow heartbeat; skin rash; unusual excitement

Symptoms of overdose
   Drowsiness; loss of muscle coordination; nausea and vomiting

Some side effects may occur that usually do not need medical attention. These side effects may go away during treatment as your body adjusts to the medicine. Also, your health care professional may be able to tell you about ways to prevent or reduce some of these side effects. Check with your health care professional if any of the following side effects continue or are bothersome or if you have any questions about them:

More common
   Dizziness or lightheadedness; drowsiness; dryness of mouth (usually mild); headache; nausea and vomiting; unpleasant taste

Less common
   Blurred vision; constipation; diarrhea; muscle aches or pains; unusual tiredness or weakness

Other side effects not listed may also occur in some patients. If you notice any other effects, check with your healthcare professional.

TREPROSTINIL (Subcutaneous route)
- tre-PROS-ti-nil

Commonly used brand name(s)

In the U.S.—
   Remodulin

Available Dosage Forms:
   • Solution

Therapeutic Class: Antihypertensive
Pharmacologic Class: Prostaglandin

Uses For This Medicine

Treprostinil belongs to a group of agents called prostaglandins. Prostaglandins occur naturally in the body and are involved in many biological functions. Treprostinil is used to treat the symptoms of primary pulmonary hypertension, or the high blood pressure that occurs in the main artery that carries blood from the right side of the heart (the ventricle) to the lungs. When the smaller blood vessels in the lungs become more resistant to blood flow, the right ventricle must work harder to pump enough blood through the lungs. Treprostinil works by relaxing blood vessels and increasing the supply of blood to the lungs, reducing the workload of the heart.

This medicine is available only with your doctor's prescription.

Before Using This Medicine

In deciding to use a medicine, the risks of taking the medicine must be weighed against the good it will do. This is a decision you and your doctor will make. For this medicine, the following should be considered:

Allergies—Tell your doctor if you have ever had any unusual or allergic reaction to this medicine or any other medicines. Also tell your health care professional if you have any other types of allergies, such as to foods, dyes, preservatives, or animals. For non-prescription products, read the label or package ingredients carefully.

Pediatric—Studies on this medicine have been done only in adult patients, and there is no specific information comparing use of treprostinil in children with other age groups.

Geriatric—Many medicines have not been studied specifically in older people. Therefore, it may not be known whether they work exactly the same way they do in younger adults or if they cause different side effects or problems in older people. There is no specific information comparing use of treprostinil in the elderly with use in other age groups.

Pregnancy—

	Pregnancy Category	Explanation
All Trimesters	B	Animal studies have revealed no evidence of harm to the fetus, however, there are no adequate studies in pregnant women OR animal studies have shown an adverse effect, but adequate studies in pregnant women have failed to demonstrate a risk to the fetus.

Breast Feeding—There are no adequate studies in women for determining infant risk when using this medication during breastfeeding. Weigh the potential benefits against the potential risks before taking this medication while breastfeeding.

Other medicines—

Using this medicine with any of the following medicines is usually not recommended, but may be required in some cases. If both medicines are prescribed together, your doctor may change the dose or how often you use one or both of the medicines.

Ginkgo

Interactions with Food/Tobacco/Alcohol—Certain medicines should not be used at or around the time of eating food or eating certain types of food since interactions may occur. Using alcohol or tobacco with certain medicines may also cause interactions to occur. Discuss with your healthcare professional the use of your medicine with food, alcohol, or tobacco.

Other medical problems—The presence of other medical problems may affect the use of this medicine. Make sure you tell your doctor if you have any other medical problems, especially:
   • Kidney disease or
   • Liver disease—Treprostinil effects may increase because of slower removal of medicine from the body

Proper Use of This Medicine

Your doctor or nurse will teach you how to prepare the medicine and use the pump for administering the medicine. Treprostinil must be administered continuously by a portable pump that is operated by a small computer. The medicine will be delivered directly under your skin or into a vein through a catheter.

The instructions for the use of the pump may vary depending on the particular make and model of the pump. Your doctor or nurse will give you detailed instructions on how to use and care for the particular pump and accessories that you will use for administering your medicine.

Dosing—The dose of this medicine will be different for different patients. Follow your doctor's orders or the directions on the label. The following information includes only the average doses of this medicine. If your dose is different, do not change it unless your doctor tells you to do so.

The amount of medicine that you take depends on the strength of the medicine. Also, the number of doses you take each day, the time allowed between doses, and the length of time you take the medicine depend on the medical problem for which you are using the medicine.

The amount of medicine that you take depends on the concentration of the medicine and the rate at which the infusion pump delivers the medicine.

- For injection dosage form:
  - For pulmonary arterial hypertension:
    - Adults—Initially, 1.25 nanograms per kilogram (kg) (0.6 nanogram per pound) of body weight per minute. Your doctor may increase or decrease your dose as necessary. Your doctor may also need to use another similar medicine called epoprostenol (e.g., Flolan) to help treat your pulmonary arterial hypertension.
    - Children—Use and dose must be determined by your doctor.

Missed dose—Call your doctor or pharmacist for instructions.

Storage—Store the medicine in a closed container at room temperature, away from heat, moisture, and direct light. Keep from freezing.

Keep out of the reach of children.

Do not keep outdated medicine or medicine no longer needed.

If the medicine has particles in it or is discolored, it should be discarded.

Precautions While Using This Medicine

Treprostinil has to be administered by a continuous subcutaneous (under the skin) or intravenous (into a vein) infusion and it must never be stopped suddenly.

It is important that your doctor check your progress at regular visits. This will allow your doctor to make sure the medicine is working properly and to change the dosage if needed.

Be sure to report any signs of infection or reaction at the catheter site to your doctor. Also, if you develop a sudden fever, contact your doctor as soon as possible.

Avoid the use of saunas, hot baths, or sunbathing, or other situations that may cause blood vessels to dilate, resulting in low blood pressure and increasing the possibility of dizziness, light-headedness, or fainting.

Do not suddenly stop using this medicine. Stopping suddenly may bring on symptoms of your condition and can be dangerous. Check with your doctor before stopping completely.

Your doctor may want you to carry a medical identification card stating that you are using this medicine.

Do not reuse syringes and needles. Put used syringes and needles in a puncture-resistant disposable container, or dispose of them as directed by your health care professional.

Side Effects of This Medicine

Along with its needed effects, a medicine may cause some unwanted effects. Although not all of these side effects may occur, if they do occur they may need medical attention.

Check with your doctor immediately if any of the following side effects occur:
  More common
    Edema, such as, swelling; infusion site reaction, such as, accumulation of blood at site of injection; dry, red, hot, or irritated skin; hardening of site of injection; vasodilation, such as, feeling of warmth or heat, flushing or redness of skin, especially on face and neck, feeling faint, dizzy, or light-headed

  Less common
    Hypotension, such as, blurred vision, confusion, dizziness, faintness, lightheadedness when getting up from a lying or sitting position, sudden sweating, unusual tiredness or weakness

  Symptoms of overdose

    Get emergency help immediately if any of the following symptoms of overdose occur:

      Diarrhea; flushing, such as, feeling of warmth and redness of the face, neck, arms, and occasionally, upper chest; headache; hypotension, such as, blurred vision, confusion, dizziness, faintness, lightheadedness when getting up from a lying or sitting position, sudden sweating, unusual tiredness or weakness; nausea and vomiting

Some side effects may occur that usually do not need medical attention. These side effects may go away during treatment as your body adjusts to the medicine. Also, your health care professional may be able to tell you about ways to prevent or reduce some of these side effects. Check with your health care professional if any of the following side effects continue or are bothersome or if you have any questions about them:
  More common
    Diarrhea; dizziness; headache; infusion site pain; jaw pain; nausea; pruritus, such as itching skin; rash

Other side effects not listed may also occur in some patients. If you notice any other effects, check with your healthcare professional.

TRETINOIN (Oral route) - TRET-i noyn

Black Box Warning

- Experienced Physician and Institution
  - Patients with acute promyelocytic leukemia (APL) are at high risk in general and can have severe adverse reactions to tretinoin. tretinoin should therefore be administered only to patients with APL under the strict supervision of a physician who is experienced in the management of patients with acute leukemia and ni a facility with laboratory and supportive services sufficient to monitor drug tolerance and protect and maintain a patient compromised by drug toxicity, including respiratory compromise. Use of tretinoin requires that the physician concludes that the possible benefit to the patient outweighs the following known adverse effects of the therapy.

- Retinoic Acid-APL Syndrome
  - About 25% of patients with APL treated with tretinoin have experienced a syndrome called the retinoic acid-APL (RA-APL) syndrome characterized by fever, dyspnea, acute respiratory distress, weight gain, radiographic pulmonary infiltrates, pleural and pericardial effusions, edema, and hepatic, renal and multi-organ failure. This syndrome has occasionally been accompanied by impaired myocardial contractility and episodic hypotension. It has been observed with or without concomitant leukocytosis. Endotracheal intubation and mechanical ventilation have been required in some cases due to progressive hypoxemia, and several patients have expires with multi-organ failure. The syndrome generally occurs during the first month of treatment, with some cases reported following the first dose of tretinoin.
  - The management of the syndrome has not been defined rigorously, but high-dose steroids given at the first suspicion of the RA-APL syndrome appear to reduce morbidity and mortality. At the first signs suggestive of the syndrome (unexplained fever, dyspnea and/or weight gain, abnormal chest auscultatory findings or radiographic abnormalties), high-dose steroids (dexamethasone 10 mg intravenously administered every 12 hours for 3 days or until the resolution of symptoms) should be immediately initiated, irrespective of the leukocyte count. The majority of patients do not require termination of tretinoin therapy during treatment of the RA-APL syndrome. However, in cases of moderate and severe RA-APL syndrome, temporary interruption of tretinoin therapy should be considered.

- Leukocytosis at Presentation and Rapidly Evolving Leukocytosis During Tretinoin Treatment
  - During tretinoin treatment about 40% of patients will develop rapidly evolving leukocytosis. Patients who present with high WBC at diagnosis (greater than 5x10(9)/L) have an increased risk of a further rapid increase in WBC counts. Rapidly evolving leukocytosis is associated with a higher risk of life-threatening complications.
  - If signs and symptoms of the RA-APL syndrome are present together with leukocytosis, treatment with high-dose steroids should be initiated immediately. Some investigators routinely add chemotherapy to tretinoin treatment in the case of patients presenting with a WBC count of greater than 5x10(9)/L or in the case of a rapid increase in WBC count for patients leukopenic at start of treatment, and have reported a lower incidence of the RA-APL syndrome. Consideration could be given to adding full-dose chemotherapy (including an anthracycline if not contraindicated) to the tretinoin therapy on day 1 or 2 for patients presenting with a WBC count of greater than 5x10(9)/L, or immediately, for patients presenting with a WBC count of <5x10(9)/L, if the WBC count reaches greater than or equal to 6x10(9)/L by day 5, or greater than or equal to 10x10(9)/L by day 10, or greater than or equal to 15x10(9)/L by day 28.

- Teratogenic Effects. Pregnancy Category D
  - There is a high risk that a severely deformed infant will result if tretinoin is administered during pregnancy. If, nonetheless, it is determined that tretinoin represents the best available treatment for a pregnant woman or a woman of childbearing potential, it must be assured that the patient has received full information and warnings of the risk to the fetus if she were to be pregnant and of the risk of possible contraception failure and has been instructed in the need to use two reliable forms of contraception simultaneously during therapy and for 1 month following discontinuation of therapy, and has acknowledged her understanding of the need for using dual contraception, unless abstinence in the chosen method.
  - Within 1 week prior to the institution of tretinoin therapy, the patient should have blood or urine collected for a serum or urine pregnancy test with a sensitivity of at least 50 mIU/mL. When possible, tretinoin therapy should be delayed until a negative result from this test is obtained. When a delay is not possible, the patient should be placed on two reliable forms of contraception. Pregnancy testing and contraception counseling should be repeated monthly throughout the period of tretinoin treatment.

Commonly used brand name(s)

In the U.S.—
  Vesanoid

Available Dosage Forms:
- Capsule, Liquid Filled

Therapeutic Class: Antineoplastic Agent

Uses For This Medicine

Tretinoin belongs to the group of medicines known as retinoids (RET-i-noyds). It is used to treat a form of leukemia (acute promyelocytic leukemia [APL]).

Tretinoin has side effects that can be very serious. Be sure that you discuss with your doctor the good that this medicine can do as well as the risks of taking it.

This medicine is available only with your doctor's prescription.

Before Using This Medicine

In deciding to use a medicine, the risks of taking the medicine must be weighed against the good it will do. This is a decision

you and your doctor will make. For this medicine, the following should be considered:

Allergies—Tell your doctor if you have ever had any unusual or allergic reaction to this medicine or any other medicines. Also tell your health care professional if you have any other types of allergies, such as to foods, dyes, preservatives, or animals. For non-prescription products, read the label or package ingredients carefully.

Pediatric—Studies in a limited number of children between 1 and 16 years of age have shown that children may be especially sensitive to the effects of this medicine, and may be more likely than adults to experience severe headaches and some other side effects during treatment.

Geriatric—Many medicines have not been studied specifically in older people. Therefore, it may not be known whether they work exactly the same way they do in younger adults or if they cause different side effects or problems in older people. There is no specific information comparing use of tretinoin in the elderly with use in other age groups.

Pregnancy—

	Pregnancy Category	Explanation
All Trimesters	D	Studies in pregnant women have demonstrated a risk to the fetus. However, the benefits of therapy in a life threatening situation or a serious disease, may outweigh the potential risk.

Breast Feeding—There are no adequate studies in women for determining infant risk when using this medication during breastfeeding. Weigh the potential benefits against the potential risks before taking this medication while breastfeeding.

Other medicines—

Using this medicine with any of the following medicines is usually not recommended, but may be required in some cases. If both medicines are prescribed together, your doctor may change the dose or how often you use one or both of the medicines.

Aminocaproic Acid, Aprotinin, Paclitaxel, Paclitaxel Protein-Bound, Tetracycline, Tranexamic Acid

Interactions with Food/Tobacco/Alcohol—Certain medicines should not be used at or around the time of eating food or eating certain types of food since interactions may occur. Using alcohol or tobacco with certain medicines may also cause interactions to occur. Discuss with your healthcare professional the use of your medicine with food, alcohol, or tobacco.

Proper Use of This Medicine

It is very important that you take tretinoin only as directed by your doctor. Do not take more of it, do not take it more often, and do not take it for a longer time than your doctor ordered. To do so may increase the chance of side effects.

Dosing—The dose of this medicine will be different for different patients. Follow your doctor's orders or the directions on the label. The following information includes only the average doses of this medicine. If your dose is different, do not change it unless your doctor tells you to do so.

The amount of medicine that you take depends on the strength of the medicine. Also, the number of doses you take each day, the time allowed between doses, and the length of time you take the medicine depend on the medical problem for which you are using the medicine.

- For oral dosage form (capsules):
  - For acute promyelocytic leukemia (APL):
    - Adults—Dose is based on body size and must be determined by your doctor. The usual dose is 45 milligrams (mg) for each square meter of body surface area a day, given in two equally divided doses.
    - Children—The dose will be determined by your doctor.

Missed dose—If you miss a dose of this medicine, take it as soon as possible. However, if it is almost time for your next dose, skip the missed dose and go back to your regular dosing schedule. Do not double doses.

If it is almost time for your next dose, check with your health care professional to find out how much medicine to take for the next dose.

Storage—Store the medicine in a closed container at room temperature, away from heat, moisture, and direct light. Keep from freezing.

Keep out of the reach of children.

Do not keep outdated medicine or medicine no longer needed.

Precautions While Using This Medicine

Your doctor should check your progress at regular visits to make sure that the medicine is working properly and to check for unwanted effects.

Tretinoin causes fever, headache, tiredness, and weakness in most people who take it. It is very important that you continue taking the medicine even if it makes you feel ill. Your health care professional may be able to suggest ways to relieve some of these effects. However, if you develop a very severe headache or a headache that occurs together with nausea, vomiting, or vision problems, check with your doctor right away.

Tretinoin sometimes causes a severe reaction that affects the lungs at first, but can later spread to other parts of the body. Signs of this reaction include breathing problems, bone pain, chest pain, and fever. Check with your doctor right away if any of these effects occur during treatment.

Side Effects of This Medicine

Along with its needed effects, a medicine may cause some unwanted effects. Although not all of these side effects may occur, if they do occur they may need medical attention.

Check with your doctor immediately if any of the following side effects occur:
More common
　　Black, tarry stools; bleeding; blistering; bloody stools; bone pain; burning; coldness; difficulty in moving; discomfort or pain in chest; enlarged heart; feeling of pressure; fever; hives; infection; inflammation; joint pain; lumps; numbness; paleness of skin; rash; redness; scaring; seizures; shortness of breath, troubled breathing, tightness in chest, or wheezing; soreness; stinging; sweating increased; swelling; swollen joints;

tenderness; tingling; ulceration; unusual tiredness or weakness; vomiting of blood or material that looks like coffee grounds; warmness at site; weight gain (occurring together with any of the other symptoms listed before)

Less common

Blue lips and fingernails; convulsions (seizures); difficulty in speaking, slow speech, or inability to speak; faintness; feeling of heaviness in chest; headache (severe); inability to move arms, legs, or muscles of the face; nausea and vomiting (occurring together with a headache); no blood pressure or pulse; pain in back or left arm; painful, red lumps under the skin, mostly on the legs; prominent superficial veins over affected area; stopping of heart; unconsciousness; vision problems (occurring together with a headache); warmth

Check with your doctor as soon as possible if any of the following side effects occur:

More common

Any change in vision (not occurring with a headache); coughing, sneezing, sore throat, and stuffy or runny nose; cracked lips; crusting, redness, pain, or sores in mouth or nose; decreased urination; earache or feeling of fullness in the ear; increase or decrease in blood pressure; irregular heartbeat; mental depression; pain in stomach, side, abdomen or back; pain and swelling in leg or foot; skin rash; swelling of abdomen (stomach area); swelling of face, fingers, hands, feet, or lower legs

Less common

Bone swelling; cramping or pain in stomach (severe); difficult or painful urination; drowsiness (very severe and continuing); hallucinations (seeing, hearing, or feeling things that are not there); hearing loss; heartburn, indigestion, or nausea (severe and continuing); mood, mental, or personality changes; pain in lower back or side; swollen area that feels sore and tender; yellow eyes or skin

Some side effects may occur that usually do not need medical attention. These side effects may go away during treatment as your body adjusts to the medicine. Also, your health care professional may be able to tell you about ways to prevent or reduce some of these side effects. Check with your health care professional if any of the following side effects continue or are bothersome or if you have any questions about them:

More common

Acid or sour stomach; agitation; anxiety; belching; blurred vision; bloating; burning, crawling, or tingling feeling in the skin; chills; confusion; constipation; darkened urine; diarrhea; dizziness; dryness of skin, mouth, or nose; fast heartbeat; flushing; general feeling of discomfort or illness; hair loss; headache (mild and not occurring together with other side effects); indigestion; irritability; itching of skin; loss of appetite; mood or mental changes; muscle pain; nausea and vomiting (not occurring together with a headache); shivering; trouble sleeping; weakness; weight loss

Less common

Anxiety and restlessness (occurring together); clumsiness or unsteadiness when walking; difficulty sleeping; disorientation; forgetfulness; frequent urination; lethargy; lightheadedness; low body temperature; redness, soreness or itching skin; sores, welting or blisters; sores on genitals; swelling of feet or lower legs; thirst;

trembling, sometimes with a flapping movement; weak or feeble pulse; weakness in legs

Other side effects not listed may also occur in some patients. If you notice any other effects, check with your healthcare professional.

TRETINOIN   (Topical route) - TRET-i noyn

Commonly used brand name(s)

In the U.S.—

Avita	Retin-A Micro
Renova	Tretin-X
Retin-A	

In Canada—

Rejuva-A	Stieva-A Gel
Stieva-A Cream	Stieva-A Solution
Stieva-A Cream Forte	Vitamin A Acid

Available Dosage Forms:

- Cream
- Gel/Jelly
- Solution
- Liquid

Therapeutic Class: Dermatological Agent

Uses For This Medicine

Tretinoin is used to treat acne. It works partly by keeping skin pores clear.

One of the tretinoin creams is used to treat fine wrinkles, dark spots, or rough skin on the face caused by damaging rays of the sun. It works by lightening the skin, replacing older skin with newer skin, and by slowing down the way the body removes skin cells that may have been harmed by the sun. Tretinoin works best when used within a skin care program that includes protecting the treated skin from the sun. However, it does not completely or permanently erase these skin problems or greatly improve more obvious changes in the skin, such as deep wrinkles caused by sun or the natural aging process.

Tretinoin may also be used to treat other skin diseases as determined by your doctor.

Tretinoin is available only with your doctor's prescription.

Once a medicine has been approved for marketing for a certain use, experience may show that it is also useful for other medical problems. Although this use is not included in product labeling, tretinoin is used in certain patients with the following medical conditions:

- Keratosis follicularis (skin disorder of small, red bumps)
- Verruca plana (flat warts)

Before Using This Medicine

In deciding to use a medicine, the risks of taking the medicine must be weighed against the good it will do. This is a decision you and your doctor will make. For this medicine, the following should be considered:

Allergies—Tell your doctor if you have ever had any unusual or allergic reaction to this medicine or any other medicines. Also tell your health care professional if you have any other types of allergies, such as to foods, dyes, preservatives,

or animals. For non-prescription products, read the label or package ingredients carefully.

Pediatric—Studies on this medicine have been done only in adult patients, and there is no specific information comparing use of this medicine in children with use in other age groups. Children are unlikely to have skin problems due to the sun. In older children treated for acne, tretinoin is not expected to cause different side effects or problems than it does in other age groups.

Geriatric—Many medicines have not been studied specifically in older people. Therefore, it may not be known whether they work exactly the same way they do in younger adults or if they cause different side effects or problems in older people. There is no specific information comparing use of tretinoin in patients 50 years of age and older with use in other age groups.

Pregnancy—

	Pregnancy Category	Explanation
All Trimesters	D	Studies in pregnant women have demonstrated a risk to the fetus. However, the benefits of therapy in a life threatening situation or a serious disease, may outweigh the potential risk.

Breast Feeding—There are no adequate studies in women for determining infant risk when using this medication during breastfeeding. Weigh the potential benefits against the potential risks before taking this medication while breastfeeding.

Other medicines—

Using this medicine with any of the following medicines is usually not recommended, but may be required in some cases. If both medicines are prescribed together, your doctor may change the dose or how often you use one or both of the medicines.

Aminocaproic Acid, Aprotinin, Tetracycline, Tranexamic Acid

Interactions with Food/Tobacco/Alcohol—Certain medicines should not be used at or around the time of eating food or eating certain types of food since interactions may occur. Using alcohol or tobacco with certain medicines may also cause interactions to occur. Discuss with your healthcare professional the use of your medicine with food, alcohol, or tobacco.

Other medical problems—The presence of other medical problems may affect the use of this medicine. Make sure you tell your doctor if you have any other medical problems, especially:

- Dermatitis, seborrheic or
- Eczema or
- Sunburn—Use of this medicine may cause or increase the irritation associated with these problems

Proper Use of This Medicine

It is very important that you use this medicine only as directed. Do not use more of it, do not use it more often, and do not use it for a longer time than your doctor ordered. To do so may cause irritation of the skin.

Do not apply this medicine to windburned or sunburned skin or on open wounds.

Do not use this medicine in or around the eyes or lips, or inside of the nose. Spread the medicine away from these areas when applying. If the medicine accidentally gets on these areas, wash with water at once.

This medicine usually comes with patient directions. Read them carefully before using the medicine.

Before applying tretinoin, wash the skin with a mild soap or cleanser and warm water by using the tips of your fingers. Then gently pat dry. Do not scrub your face with a sponge or washcloth. Wait 20 to 30 minutes before applying this medicine to make sure the skin is completely dry. Applying tretinoin to wet skin can irritate the skin.

To use the cream or gel form of this medicine:

- Apply just enough medicine to very lightly cover the affected areas, and rub in gently but well. A pea-sized amount is enough to cover the whole face.

To use the solution form of this medicine:

- Using your fingertips, a gauze pad, or a cotton swab, apply enough tretinoin solution to cover the affected areas. If you use a gauze pad or a cotton swab for applying the medicine, avoid getting it too wet. This will help prevent the medicine from running into areas not intended for treatment.

After applying the medicine, wash your hands to remove any medicine that might remain on them.

Dosing—The dose of this medicine will be different for different patients. Follow your doctor's orders or the directions on the label. The following information includes only the average doses of this medicine. If your dose is different, do not change it unless your doctor tells you to do so.

The amount of medicine that you take depends on the strength of the medicine. Also, the number of doses you take each day, the time allowed between doses, and the length of time you take the medicine depend on the medical problem for which you are using the medicine.

- For topical dosage forms (cream, gel, or solution):
  - For acne:
    - Adults and teenagers—Apply to the affected area(s) of the skin once a day, at bedtime.
- For cream dosage form (brand name Renova only):
  - For fine wrinkles, dark spots, or rough skin caused by the sun:
    - Adults up to 50 years of age—Apply to the affected area(s) of the skin once a day, at bedtime.
    - Adults 50 years of age and older—Use and dose must be determined by your doctor.

Missed dose—If you miss a dose of this medicine, skip the missed dose and go back to your regular dosing schedule. Do not double doses.

Storage—Store the medicine in a closed container at room temperature, away from heat, moisture, and direct light. Keep from freezing.

Keep out of the reach of children.

Do not keep outdated medicine or medicine no longer needed.

The gel product is flammable and should be kept away from fire or excessive heat.

Precautions While Using This Medicine

During the first 3 weeks you are using tretinoin, your skin may become irritated. Also, your acne may seem to get worse before it gets better. It may take longer than 12 weeks before you notice full improvement of your acne, even if you use the medicine every day. Check with your health care professional at any time skin irritation becomes severe or if your acne does not improve within 8 to 12 weeks.

You should avoid washing the skin treated with tretinoin for at least 1 hour after applying it.

Avoid using any topical medicine on the same area within 1 hour before or after using tretinoin. Otherwise, tretinoin may not work properly or skin irritation might occur.

Unless your doctor tells you otherwise, it is especially important to avoid using the following skin products on the same area as tretinoin:

- Any other topical acne product or skin product containing a peeling agent (such as benzoyl peroxide, resorcinol, salicylic acid, or sulfur)
- Hair products that are irritating, such as permanents or hair removal products
- Skin products that cause sensitivity to the sun, such as those containing spices or limes
- Skin products containing a large amount of alcohol, such as astringents, shaving creams, or after-shave lotions
- Skin products that are too drying or abrasive, such as some cosmetics, soaps, or skin cleansers

Using these products along with tretinoin may cause mild to severe irritation of the skin. Although skin irritation can occur, some doctors sometimes allow benzoyl peroxide to be used with tretinoin to treat acne. Usually tretinoin is applied at night so that it does not cause a problem with any other topical products that you might use during the day. Check with your doctor before using topical medicines with tretinoin.

During the first 6 months of use, avoid overexposing the treated areas to sunlight, wind, or cold weather. The skin will be more prone to sunburn, dryness, or irritation, especially during the first 2 or 3 weeks. However, you should not stop using this medicine unless the skin irritation becomes too severe. Do not use a sunlamp.

To help tretinoin work properly, regularly use sunscreen or sunblocking lotions with a sun protection factor (SPF) of at least 15. Also, wear protective clothing and hats, and apply creams, lotions, or moisturizers often.

Check with your doctor at any time your skin becomes too dry and irritated. Your health care professional can help you choose the right skin products for you to reduce skin dryness and irritation and may include the following:

- For patients using tretinoin for the treatment of acne:
  - Regular use of water-based creams or lotions helps to reduce skin irritation or dryness that may be caused by the use of tretinoin.
- For patients using tretinoin for the treatment of fine wrinkling, dark spots, and rough skin caused by the sun:
  - This medicine should be used as part of an ongoing program to avoid further damage to your skin from the sun. This program includes staying out of the sun when possible or wearing proper clothing or hats to protect your skin from sunlight.
  - Regular use of oil-based creams or lotions helps to reduce skin irritation or dryness caused by the use of tretinoin.

Side Effects of This Medicine

In some animal studies, tretinoin has been shown to cause skin tumors to develop faster when the treated area is exposed to ultraviolet light (sunlight or artificial sunlight from a sunlamp). Other studies have not shown the same result and more studies need to be done. It is not known if tretinoin causes skin tumors to develop faster in humans.

Along with its needed effects, a medicine may cause some unwanted effects. Although not all of these side effects may occur, if they do occur they may need medical attention.

Check with your doctor as soon as possible if any of the following side effects occur:

More common
 Burning feeling or stinging skin (severe); lightening of skin of treated area, unexpected; peeling of skin (severe); redness of skin (severe); unusual dryness of skin (severe)

Rare
 Darkening of treated skin

Some side effects may occur that usually do not need medical attention. These side effects may go away during treatment as your body adjusts to the medicine. Also, your health care professional may be able to tell you about ways to prevent or reduce some of these side effects. Check with your health care professional if any of the following side effects continue or are bothersome or if you have any questions about them:

More common
 Burning feeling, stinging, or tingling of skin (mild)—lasting for a short time after first applying the medicine; chapping or slight peeling of skin (mild); redness of skin (mild); unusual dryness of skin (mild); unusually warm skin (mild)

The side effects will go away after you stop using tretinoin. On the rare chance that your skin color changes, this effect may last for several months before your skin color returns to normal.

Other side effects not listed may also occur in some patients. If you notice any other effects, check with your healthcare professional.

TRIFLURIDINE   (Ophthalmic route) -
trye-FLURE-i-deen

Commonly used brand name(s)

In the U.S.—
 Viroptic

Available Dosage Forms:
- Solution

Therapeutic Class: Antiviral
Pharmacologic Class: Viral DNA Thymidylate Synthetase Inhibitor

Uses For This Medicine

Trifluridine ophthalmic preparations are used to treat virus infections of the eye.

Trifluridine is available only with your doctor's prescription.

Before Using This Medicine

In deciding to use a medicine, the risks of taking the medicine must be weighed against the good it will do. This is a decision

you and your doctor will make. For this medicine, the following should be considered:

Allergies—Tell your doctor if you have ever had any unusual or allergic reaction to this medicine or any other medicines. Also tell your health care professional if you have any other types of allergies, such as to foods, dyes, preservatives, or animals. For non-prescription products, read the label or package ingredients carefully.

Pediatric—Although there is no specific information comparing the use of trifluridine in children with use in other age groups, it is not expected to cause different side effects or problems in children than it does in adults.

Geriatric—Many medicines have not been studied specifically in older people. Therefore, it may not be known whether they work exactly the same way they do in younger adults or if they cause different side effects or problems in older people. There is no specific information comparing the use of trifluridine in the elderly with use in other age groups.

Other medicines—Although certain medicines should not be used together at all, in other cases two different medicines may be used together even if an interaction might occur. In these cases, your doctor may want to change the dose, or other precautions may be necessary. Tell your healthcare professional if you are taking any other prescription or non-prescription (over-the-counter [OTC]) medicine.

Interactions with Food/Tobacco/Alcohol—Certain medicines should not be used at or around the time of eating food or eating certain types of food since interactions may occur. Using alcohol or tobacco with certain medicines may also cause interactions to occur. Discuss with your healthcare professional the use of your medicine with food, alcohol, or tobacco.

Proper Use of This Medicine

The bottle is only partially full to provide proper drop control.

To use:

- First, wash your hands. Then tilt the head back and pull the lower eyelid away from the eye to form a pouch. Drop the medicine into the pouch and gently close the eyes. Do not blink. Keep the eyes closed for 1 or 2 minutes to allow the medicine to come into contact with the infection.
- If you think you did not get the drop of medicine into your eye properly, use another drop.
- To keep the medicine as germ-free as possible, do not touch the applicator tip to any surface (including the eye). Also, keep the container tightly closed.

Do not use this medicine more often or for a longer time than your doctor ordered. To do so may cause problems in the eyes. If you have any questions about this, check with your doctor.

To help clear up your infection completely, keep using this medicine for the full time of treatment, even if your symptoms have disappeared. Do not miss any doses.

Dosing—The dose of this medicine will be different for different patients. Follow your doctor's orders or the directions on the label. The following information includes only the average doses of this medicine. If your dose is different, do not change it unless your doctor tells you to do so.

The amount of medicine that you take depends on the strength of the medicine. Also, the number of doses you take each day, the time allowed between doses, and the length of

time you take the medicine depend on the medical problem for which you are using the medicine.

- For ophthalmic solution dosage forms:
  - For viral eye infection:
    - Adults and children 6 years of age and older— One drop every two hours while you are awake. After healing has occurred, the dose may be reduced for seven more days to one drop every four hours (at least 5 doses a day) while you are awake.
    - Children up to 6 years of age—Use and dose must be determined by your doctor.

Missed dose—If you miss a dose of this medicine, apply it as soon as possible. However, if it is almost time for your next dose, skip the missed dose and go back to your regular dosing schedule.

Storage—Store in the refrigerator. Do not freeze.

Keep out of the reach of children.

Do not keep outdated medicine or medicine no longer needed.

Precautions While Using This Medicine

It is very important that you keep your appointment with your doctor. If your symptoms become worse, check with your doctor sooner.

Side Effects of This Medicine

Along with its needed effects, a medicine may cause some unwanted effects. Although not all of these side effects may occur, if they do occur they may need medical attention.

Check with your doctor as soon as possible if any of the following side effects occur:
    Rare
        Blurred vision or other change in vision; dryness of eye; irritation of eye; itching, redness, swelling, or other sign of irritation not present before use of this medicine

Some side effects may occur that usually do not need medical attention. These side effects may go away during treatment as your body adjusts to the medicine. Also, your health care professional may be able to tell you about ways to prevent or reduce some of these side effects. Check with your health care professional if any of the following side effects continue or are bothersome or if you have any questions about them:
    More common
        Burning or stinging

Other side effects not listed may also occur in some patients. If you notice any other effects, check with your healthcare professional.

TRIMETHOPRIM (Oral route) - trye-METH-oh-prim

Commonly used brand name(s)

In the U.S.—
    Primsol
    Proloprim
    Trimpex

Available Dosage Forms:
- Tablet
- Solution

Therapeutic Class: Antibiotic
Pharmacologic Class: Folic Acid Antagonist

Uses For This Medicine

Trimethoprim is used to treat infections of the urinary tract. It may also be used for other problems as determined by your doctor. It will not work for colds, flu, or other virus infections.

Trimethoprim is available only with your doctor's prescription.

Once a medicine has been approved for marketing for a certain use, experience may show that it is also useful for other medical problems. Although these uses are not included in product labeling, trimethoprim is used in certain patients for the following medical conditions:
- Prevention of urinary tract infections
- Treatment of Pneumocystis carinii pneumonia (PCP)

For patients taking this medicine for prevention of urinary tract infections:
- Your doctor may have prescribed this medicine to prevent infections of the urinary tract. It is usually given once a day and may be given for a long time for this purpose. If you have any questions about this, check with your doctor.

Before Using This Medicine

In deciding to use a medicine, the risks of taking the medicine must be weighed against the good it will do. This is a decision you and your doctor will make. For this medicine, the following should be considered:

Allergies—Tell your doctor if you have ever had any unusual or allergic reaction to this medicine or any other medicines. Also tell your health care professional if you have any other types of allergies, such as to foods, dyes, preservatives, or animals. For non-prescription products, read the label or package ingredients carefully.

Pediatric—This medicine has been used in a limited number of children 2 months of age or older, and tested in children 12 years of age or older. In effective doses, the medicine has not been shown to cause different side effects or problems in children than it does in adults.

Geriatric—Elderly people may be more sensitive to the effects of trimethoprim. Blood problems may be more likely to occur in elderly patients who are taking diuretics (water pills) along with this medicine.

Pregnancy—

	Pregnancy Category	Explanation
All Trimesters	C	Animal studies have shown an adverse effect and there are no adequate studies in pregnant women OR no animal studies have been conducted and there are no adequate studies in pregnant women.

Breast Feeding—Studies in women suggest that this medication poses minimal risk to the infant when used during breastfeeding.

Other medicines—
Using this medicine with any of the following medicines is not recommended. Your doctor may decide not to treat you with this medication or change some of the other medicines you take.

Bepridil, Cisapride, Dofetilide, Levomethadyl, Mesoridazine, Pimozide, Terfenadine, Thioridazine, Ziprasidone

Interactions with Food/Tobacco/Alcohol—Certain medicines should not be used at or around the time of eating food or eating certain types of food since interactions may occur. Using alcohol or tobacco with certain medicines may also cause interactions to occur. The following interactions have been selected on the basis of their potential significance and are not necessarily all-inclusive.

Using this medicine with any of the following is usually not recommended, but may be unavoidable in some cases. If used together, your doctor may change the dose or how often you use this medicine, or give you special instructions about the use of food, alcohol, or tobacco.

Ethanol

Other medical problems—The presence of other medical problems may affect the use of this medicine. Make sure you tell your doctor if you have any other medical problems, especially:
- Anemia—Patients with anemia may have an increased chance of side effects affecting the blood
- Kidney disease—Patients with kidney disease may have an increased chance of side effects
- Liver disease—Patients with liver disease may have an increased chance of side effects

---

Proper Use of This Medicine

Do not give this medicine to infants or children under 12 years of age unless otherwise directed by your doctor.

Trimethoprim may be taken on an empty stomach or, if it upsets your stomach, it may be taken with food.

To help clear up your infection completely, keep taking this medicine for the full time of treatment even if you begin to feel better after a few days. If you stop taking this medicine too soon, your symptoms may return.

This medicine works best when there is a constant amount in the body. To help keep the amount constant, do not miss any doses. Also, it is best to take the doses at evenly spaced times day and night. For example, if you are to take 2 doses a day, the doses should be spaced about 12 hours apart. If this interferes with your sleep or other daily activities, or if you need help in planning the best times to take your medicine, check with your health care professional.

Dosing—The dose of this medicine will be different for different patients. Follow your doctor's orders or the directions on the label. The following information includes only the average doses of this medicine. If your dose is different, do not change it unless your doctor tells you to do so.

The amount of medicine that you take depends on the strength of the medicine. Also, the number of doses you take each day, the time allowed between doses, and the length of time you take the medicine depend on the medical problem for which you are using the medicine.
- For the treatment of urinary tract infections:
  - Adults and children 12 years of age and older: 100 milligrams every twelve hours for ten days, or 200 milligrams once a day for ten days.

- Children up to 12 years of age: Dose must be determined by the doctor.

Missed dose—If you miss a dose of this medicine, take it as soon as possible. However, if it is almost time for your next dose, skip the missed dose and go back to your regular dosing schedule. Do not double doses.

Storage—Store the medicine in a closed container at room temperature, away from heat, moisture, and direct light. Keep from freezing.

Keep out of the reach of children.

Do not keep outdated medicine or medicine no longer needed.

Precautions While Using This Medicine

It is important that your doctor check your progress at regular visits if you will be taking this medicine for a long time. This will allow your doctor to check for any unwanted effects that may be caused by this medicine.

If your symptoms do not improve within a few days, or if they become worse, check with your doctor.

If this medicine causes anemia, your doctor may want you to take folic acid (a vitamin) every day to help clear up the anemia. If so, it is important to take folic acid every day along with this medicine; do not miss any doses.

Trimethoprim may cause blood problems. These problems may result in a greater chance of certain infections, slow healing, and bleeding of the gums. Therefore, you should be careful when using regular toothbrushes, dental floss, and toothpicks. Dental work should be delayed until your blood counts have returned to normal. Check with your medical doctor or dentist if you have any questions about proper oral hygiene (mouth care) during treatment.

Some people who take trimethoprim may become more sensitive to sunlight than they are normally. Exposure to sunlight, even for brief periods of time, may cause severe sunburn or skin rash, redness, itching, or discoloration. When you begin taking this medicine:

- Stay out of direct sunlight, especially between the hours of 10:00 a.m. and 3:00 p.m., if possible.
- Apply a sun block product that has a skin protection factor (SPF) of at least 15. Some patients may require a product with a higher SPF number, especially if they have a fair complexion. If you have any questions about this, check with your health care professional.
- Do not use a sunlamp or tanning bed or booth.

If you have a severe reaction from the sun, check with your doctor.

Side Effects of This Medicine

Along with its needed effects, a medicine may cause some unwanted effects. Although not all of these side effects may occur, if they do occur they may need medical attention.

Check with your doctor immediately if any of the following side effects occur:

Less common
 Skin rash or itching

Rare
 Black, tarry stools; blood in urine or stools; bluish fingernails, lips, or skin; changes in facial skin color; chills; difficult breathing or shortness of breath; fever with or without chills; general feeling of discomfort or illness;

headache; joint or muscle pain; nausea; neck stiffness; pale skin; pinpoint red spots on skin; redness, blistering, burning, tenderness, peeling, or loosening of skin or mucous membranes; redness, swelling, or soreness of tongue; red skin lesions, often with a purple center; sore throat; swelling; thickened or scaly skin; unusual bleeding or bruising; unusual tiredness or weakness

Some side effects may occur that usually do not need medical attention. These side effects may go away during treatment as your body adjusts to the medicine. Also, your health care professional may be able to tell you about ways to prevent or reduce some of these side effects. Check with your health care professional if any of the following side effects continue or are bothersome or if you have any questions about them:

Less common
 Diarrhea; loss of appetite; nausea or vomiting; stomach cramps or pain

Other side effects not listed may also occur in some patients. If you notice any other effects, check with your healthcare professional.

TRIMETREXATE (Intravenous route) - tri-me-TREX-ate

Black Box Warning

Trimetrexate glucuronate for injection must be used with concurrent leucovorin (leucovorin protection) to avoid potentially serious or life-threatening toxicities.

Commonly used brand name(s)

In the U.S.—
 NeuTrexin

Available Dosage Forms:
- Powder for Solution

Therapeutic Class: Antibiotic
Pharmacologic Class: Antimetabolite

Uses For This Medicine

Trimetrexate is used, together with leucovorin, to treat Pneumocystis carinii pneumonia (PCP), a very serious kind of pneumonia. This kind of pneumonia occurs commonly in patients whose immune system is not working normally, such as cancer patients, transplant patients, and patients with acquired immune deficiency syndrome (AIDS).

Trimetrexate may cause some serious, even life-threatening, side effects. To prevent these effects, you must take another medicine, leucovorin, together with trimetrexate and for 3 days after you stop receiving trimetrexate. Before you begin treatment with trimetrexate, you and your doctor should talk about the good this medicine will do as well as the risks of using it.

Trimetrexate is to be administered only by or under the immediate supervision of your doctor.

Once a medicine has been approved for marketing for a certain use, experience may show that it is also useful for other medical problems. Although this use is not included in product labeling, trimetrexate is used in certain patients with the following medical condition:

- Cancer of the colon

Before Receiving This Medicine

In deciding to use a medicine, the risks of taking the medicine must be weighed against the good it will do. This is a decision you and your doctor will make. For this medicine, the following should be considered:

Allergies—Tell your doctor if you have ever had any unusual or allergic reaction to this medicine or any other medicines. Also tell your health care professional if you have any other types of allergies, such as to foods, dyes, preservatives, or animals. For non-prescription products, read the label or package ingredients carefully.

Pediatric—This medicine has been tested in a limited number of children younger than 18 years of age. Trimetrexate can cause serious side effects in any patient. However, in effective doses, this medicine did not cause different side effects or problems in the few children who received it than it does in adults.

Geriatric—Many medicines have not been studied specifically in older people. Therefore, it may not be known whether they work exactly the same way they do in younger adults or if they cause different side effects or problems in older people. There is no specific information comparing use of trimetrexate in the elderly with use in other age groups.

Pregnancy—

	Pregnancy Category	Explanation
All Trimesters	D	Studies in pregnant women have demonstrated a risk to the fetus. However, the benefits of therapy in a life threatening situation or a serious disease, may outweigh the potential risk.

Breast Feeding—There are no adequate studies in women for determining infant risk when using this medication during breastfeeding. Weigh the potential benefits against the potential risks before taking this medication while breastfeeding.

Other medicines—

Using this medicine with any of the following medicines is not recommended. Your doctor may decide not to treat you with this medication or change some of the other medicines you take.

Rotavirus Vaccine, Live

Interactions with Food/Tobacco/Alcohol—Certain medicines should not be used at or around the time of eating food or eating certain types of food since interactions may occur. Using alcohol or tobacco with certain medicines may also cause interactions to occur. Discuss with your healthcare professional the use of your medicine with food, alcohol, or tobacco.

Other medical problems—The presence of other medical problems may affect the use of this medicine. Make sure you tell your doctor if you have any other medical problems, especially:

- Anemia or
- Blood problems or
- Low platelet count or
- Low white blood cell count—Trimetrexate may make any blood diseases that you have worse
- Mouth ulcers or other mouth sores or
- Stomach ulcer or other stomach or intestinal problems—Trimetrexate may make these conditions that you have worse
- Kidney disease or
- Liver disease—Kidney or liver disease may increase the chance of side effects from trimetrexate

Proper Use of This Medicine

When you take leucovorin:

- Leucovorin must be taken with trimetrexate to help prevent very serious, possibly life-threatening, unwanted side effects. Leucovorin should be taken during trimetrexate treatment and for 3 days after trimetrexate is stopped. It is very important to take this medicine exactly as your doctor told you. Failure to do this can result in very serious side effects.
- Take oral leucovorin exactly as directed by your doctor. Do not take more of it, do not take it more often, and do not take it for a longer time than your doctor ordered. Also, do not stop taking this medicine without checking with your doctor first.
- Oral leucovorin works best when there is a constant amount in the blood. To help keep the amount constant, do not miss any doses. If you need help in planning the best times to take your medicine, check with your health care professional.
- If you vomit shortly after taking an oral dose of leucovorin, check with your doctor. You will be told whether to take the dose again or to wait until the next scheduled dose.

Dosing—The dose of this medicine will be different for different patients. Follow your doctor's orders or the directions on the label. The following information includes only the average doses of this medicine. If your dose is different, do not change it unless your doctor tells you to do so.

The amount of medicine that you take depends on the strength of the medicine. Also, the number of doses you take each day, the time allowed between doses, and the length of time you take the medicine depend on the medical problem for which you are using the medicine.

For trimetrexate
- For the treatment of Pneumocystis carinii pneumonia:
  - For injection dosage form:
    - Adults—45 milligrams per square meter of body surface area (mg/m2) injected into a vein once a day for twenty-one days. Your doctor will check your blood counts and may change your dose based on these counts. Your doctor may want to give you a dose you based on how much you weigh. Your dose will be determined by your doctor.
    - Children and teenagers—Use and dose must be determined by your doctor.

For leucovorin
- For the prevention of serious side effects of trimetrexate in the treatment of Pneumocystis carinii pneumonia:
  - For the oral or injection dosage forms:
    - Adults—20 milligrams per square meter of body surface area (mg/m 2) taken by mouth or injected

into a vein every six hours for twenty-four days. Your doctor will check your blood counts and may change your dose based on these counts. Your doctor may want to give you a dose you based on how much you weigh. Your dose will be determined by your doctor.

- Children and teenagers—Use and dose must be determined by your doctor.

Missed dose—If you miss a dose of this medicine, take it as soon as possible. However, if it is almost time for your next dose, skip the missed dose and go back to your regular dosing schedule. Do not double doses.

Storage—Store the medicine in a closed container at room temperature, away from heat, moisture, and direct light. Keep from freezing.

Keep out of the reach of children.

Do not keep outdated medicine or medicine no longer needed.

Precautions After Receiving This Medicine

If your symptoms do not improve within a few days, or if they become worse, check with your doctor.

It is very important that your doctor check your progress at regular visits to make sure that this medicine is working properly and to check for unwanted effects.

Trimetrexate can lower the number of white blood cells in your blood temporarily, increasing your chance of getting an infection. It can also lower the number of platelets, which are necessary for proper blood clotting. If this occurs, there are certain precautions you can take, especially when your blood count is low, to reduce the risk of infection or bleeding:

- If you can, avoid people with infections. Check with your doctor immediately if you think you are getting an infection or if you get a fever or chills, cough or hoarseness, lower back or side pain, or painful or difficult urination.
- Check with your doctor immediately if you notice any unusual bleeding or bruising; black, tarry stools; blood in urine or stools; or pinpoint red spots on your skin.
- Be careful when using a regular toothbrush, dental floss, or toothpick. Your medical doctor, dentist, or nurse may recommend other ways to clean your teeth and gums. Check with your medical doctor before having any dental work done.
- Be careful not to cut yourself when you are using sharp objects such as a safety razor or fingernail or toenail cutters.

Check with your doctor right away if you experience symptoms of an allergic reaction such as cough, difficulty swallowing, dizziness, fainting or loss of consciousness, fast heartbeat, fast or irregular breathing, hives, itching, puffiness or swelling of the eyelids or around the eyes, face, lips or tongue, shortness of breath, skin rash, swelling of eyes or eyelids, tightness in chest, trouble in breathing, unusual tiredness or weakness, and/or wheezing.

Side Effects of This Medicine

Along with its needed effects, a medicine may cause some unwanted effects. Although not all of these side effects may occur, if they do occur they may need medical attention.

Check with your doctor immediately if any of the following side effects occur:
More common
  Abdominal pain or tenderness; black, tarry stools; blood in urine or stools; clay colored stools; dark urine; decreased appetite; fever and sore throat; headache; itching; loss of appetite; nausea and vomiting; pinpoint red spots on skin; skin rash; swelling of feet or lower legs; unusual bleeding or bruising; unusual tiredness or weakness; yellow eyes or skin
Less common
  Abdominal cramps; coma; confusion; convulsions; decreased urine output; difficulty in breathing; dizziness; fast or irregular heartbeat; hypocalcemia; increased thirst; mood or mental changes; muscle cramps in hands, arms, feet, legs, or face; muscle pain; mouth sores or ulcers; numbness and tingling around the mouth, fingertips, or feet; skin rash and itching; shortness of breath; tremor
Rare
  Cough; difficulty swallowing; fainting or loss of consciousness; fast or irregular breathing; hives; puffiness or swelling of the eyelids or around the eyes, face, lips or tongue; swelling of eyes or eyelids; tightness in chest; trouble in breathing; wheezing

Some side effects may occur that usually do not need medical attention. These side effects may go away during treatment as your body adjusts to the medicine. Also, your health care professional may be able to tell you about ways to prevent or reduce some of these side effects. Check with your health care professional if any of the following side effects continue or are bothersome or if you have any questions about them:
Less common
  Fatigue; stomach pain

Other side effects not listed may also occur in some patients. If you notice any other effects, check with your healthcare professional.

TRIPTORELIN (Intramuscular route, Injection route) - trip-toe-REL-in

Commonly used brand name(s)
In the U.S.—
  Trelstar Depot
  Trelstar LA

Available Dosage Forms:
  - Injectable
  - Powder for Suspension

Therapeutic Class: Antineoplastic Agent
Pharmacologic Class: Luteinizing Hormone Releasing Hormone Agonist

Uses For This Medicine

Triptorelin is similar to a hormone normally released from the hypothalamus gland.

When given regularly to men, triptorelin decreases testosterone levels. Reducing the amount of testosterone in the body is one way of treating cancer of the prostate.

Triptorelin is to be given only under the supervision of your doctor. It is to be injected into a muscle.

Before Using This Medicine

In deciding to use a medicine, the risks of taking the medicine must be weighed against the good it will do. This is a decision you and your doctor will make. For this medicine, the following should be considered:

Allergies—Tell your doctor if you have ever had any unusual or allergic reaction to this medicine or any other medicines. Also tell your health care professional if you have any other types of allergies, such as to foods, dyes, preservatives, or animals. For non-prescription products, read the label or package ingredients carefully.

Pediatric—Studies on this medicine have been done only in adult patients, and there is no specific information comparing use of triptorelin in children with use in other age groups.

Geriatric—Many medicines have not been tested in older people. Therefore, it may not be known whether they work exactly the same way they do in younger adults. Although there is no specific information comparing use of triptorelin in the elderly with use in other age groups, it has been used mostly in elderly patients and is not expected to cause different side effects or problems in older people than it does in younger adults.

Pregnancy—

	Pregnancy Category	Explanation
All Trimesters	X	Studies in animals or pregnant women have demonstrated positive evidence of fetal abnormalities. This drug should not be used in women who are or may become pregnant because the risk clearly outweighs any possible benefit.

Breast Feeding—There are no adequate studies in women for determining infant risk when using this medication during breastfeeding. Weigh the potential benefits against the potential risks before taking this medication while breastfeeding.

Other medicines—Although certain medicines should not be used together at all, in other cases two different medicines may be used together even if an interaction might occur. In these cases, your doctor may want to change the dose, or other precautions may be necessary. Tell your healthcare professional if you are taking any other prescription or nonprescription (over-the-counter [OTC]) medicine.

Interactions with Food/Tobacco/Alcohol—Certain medicines should not be used at or around the time of eating food or eating certain types of food since interactions may occur. Using alcohol or tobacco with certain medicines may also cause interactions to occur. Discuss with your healthcare professional the use of your medicine with food, alcohol, or tobacco.

Other medical problems—The presence of other medical problems may affect the use of this medicine. Make sure you tell your doctor if you have any other medical problems, especially:
- Cancer that has spread to the backbone or

- Problems in passing urine—Conditions may get worse for a short time after treatment with triptorelin is started

Proper Use of This Medicine

Triptorelin sometimes causes unwanted effects such as hot flashes or decreased sexual ability. It may also cause a temporary increase in pain or difficulty in urinating. However, it is very important that you continue to use the medicine. Do not stop using this medicine without first checking with your doctor.

Dosing—The dose of this medicine will be different for different patients. Follow your doctor's orders or the directions on the label. The following information includes only the average doses of this medicine. If your dose is different, do not change it unless your doctor tells you to do so.

The amount of medicine that you take depends on the strength of the medicine. Also, the number of doses you take each day, the time allowed between doses, and the length of time you take the medicine depend on the medical problem for which you are using the medicine.
- For long-acting (1–month) injection dosage forms:
  - For cancer of the prostate:
    - Adults—3.75 milligrams (mg) injected into a muscle once a month.

Missed dose—If you miss a dose of this medicine, take it as soon as possible. However, if it is almost time for your next dose, skip the missed dose and go back to your regular dosing schedule. Do not double doses.

Storage—Store the medicine in a closed container at room temperature, away from heat, moisture, and direct light. Keep from freezing.

Keep out of the reach of children.

Do not keep outdated medicine or medicine no longer needed.

Dispose of used syringes properly in the container provided.

Precautions While Using This Medicine

It is very important that your doctor check your progress at regular visits to make sure that this medicine is working properly and to check for unwanted effects.

Side Effects of This Medicine

Along with its needed effects, a medicine may cause some unwanted effects. Although not all of these side effects may occur, if they do occur they may need medical attention.

Check with your doctor as soon as possible if any of the following side effects occur:
Less common
Bladder pain; bloody or cloudy urine; decrease in urine volume or frequency of urination; difficulty in passing urine; frequent urge to urinate; high blood pressure; lower back or side pain; painful urination; pale skin; troubled breathing; unusual bleeding or bruising; unusual tiredness or weakness

Some side effects may occur that usually do not need medical attention. These side effects may go away during treatment as your body adjusts to the medicine. Also, your health care professional may be able to tell you about ways to prevent or reduce some of these side effects. Check with your health care professional if any of the following side effects

continue or are bothersome or if you have any questions about them:

More common

Decreased interest in sexual intercourse; feeling of warmth or redness of the face, neck, arms and occasionally, upper chest; headache; inability to have or keep an erection; loss in sexual ability, desire, drive, or performance; sudden sweating

Less common

Crying; diarrhea; dizziness; injection site pain; itching; leg pain; mental depression; paranoia; rapidly changing moods; trouble sleeping or getting to sleep; vomiting

Other side effects not listed may also occur in some patients. If you notice any other effects, check with your healthcare professional.

TROSPIUM (Oral route) - TROSE-pee-um

Commonly used brand name(s)

In the U.S.—

Sanctura

Available Dosage Forms:

• Tablet

Therapeutic Class: Urinary Antispasmodic
Pharmacologic Class: Antimuscarinic

Uses For This Medicine

Trospium is used to treat bladder problems such as frequent need to urinate or loss of control of urinary function.

This medicine is available only with your doctor's prescription.

Before Using This Medicine

In deciding to use a medicine, the risks of taking the medicine must be weighed against the good it will do. This is a decision you and your doctor will make. For this medicine, the following should be considered:

Allergies—Tell your doctor if you have ever had any unusual or allergic reaction to this medicine or any other medicines. Also tell your health care professional if you have any other types of allergies, such as to foods, dyes, preservatives, or animals. For non-prescription products, read the label or package ingredients carefully.

Pediatric—Studies on this medicine have been done only in adult patients, and there is no specific information comparing use of trospium in children with use in other age groups.

Geriatric—This medicine has been tested and has not been shown to cause different side effects or problems in older people than is does in younger adults. However, elderly patients are more likely to be sensitive to anticholinergic agents and may require a lower dose.

Pregnancy—

	Pregnancy Category	Explanation
All Trimesters	C	Animal studies have shown an adverse effect and there are no adequate studies in pregnant women OR no animal studies have been conducted and there are no adequate studies in pregnant women.

Breast Feeding—There are no adequate studies in women for determining infant risk when using this medication during breastfeeding. Weigh the potential benefits against the potential risks before taking this medication while breastfeeding.

Other medicines—Although certain medicines should not be used together at all, in other cases two different medicines may be used together even if an interaction might occur. In these cases, your doctor may want to change the dose, or other precautions may be necessary. Tell your healthcare professional if you are taking any other prescription or non-prescription (over-the-counter [OTC]) medicine.

Interactions with Food/Tobacco/Alcohol—Certain medicines should not be used at or around the time of eating food or eating certain types of food since interactions may occur. Using alcohol or tobacco with certain medicines may also cause interactions to occur. Discuss with your healthcare professional the use of your medicine with food, alcohol, or tobacco.

Other medical problems—The presence of other medical problems may affect the use of this medicine. Make sure you tell your doctor if you have any other medical problems, especially:

• Glaucoma or

• Stomach problems or

• Urinary retention—Trospium may make these conditions worse.

• Kidney problems or

• Liver problems—A lower dose of trospium may be necessary.

Proper Use of This Medicine

Dosing—The dose of this medicine will be different for different patients. Follow your doctor's orders or the directions on the label. The following information includes only the average doses of this medicine. If your dose is different, do not change it unless your doctor tells you to do so.

The amount of medicine that you take depends on the strength of the medicine. Also, the number of doses you take each day, the time allowed between doses, and the length of time you take the medicine depend on the medical problem for which you are using the medicine.

• For oral dosage form (tablets):
  ○ To treat bladder problems:
    ▪ Adults—20 milligrams (mg) one or two times a day 1 hour before meal.
    ▪ Children—Use and dose must be determined by your doctor.

Missed dose—If you miss a dose of this medicine, take it as soon as possible. However, if it is almost time for your next

dose, skip the missed dose and go back to your regular dosing schedule. Do not double doses.

Storage—Store the medicine in a closed container at room temperature, away from heat, moisture, and direct light. Keep from freezing.

Keep out of the reach of children.

Do not keep outdated medicine or medicine no longer needed.

Precautions While Using This Medicine

This medicine may cause some people to have vision problems. Make sure your vision is clear before you drive or do anything else that could be dangerous if you are not able to see well.

This medicine, especially in high doses, may cause some people to become dizzy or drowsy. Make sure you know how you react to this medicine before you drive, use machines, or do anything else that could be dangerous if you are dizzy or are not alert.

Avoid use of alcohol. Alcohol may increase your risk of drowsiness.

Use caution during exercise or hot weather. Overheating may result in heat stroke.

This medicine may cause dryness of the mouth, nose, and throat. For temporary relief of mouth dryness, use sugarless candy or gum, melt bits of ice in your mouth, or use a saliva substitute. However, if your mouth continues to feel dry for more than 2 weeks, check with your medical doctor or dentist.

Side Effects of This Medicine

Along with its needed effects, a medicine may cause some unwanted effects. Although not all of these side effects may occur, if they do occur they may need medical attention.

Check with your doctor immediately if any of the following side effects occur:

Frequency not determined—Observed during clinical practice

Blistering, peeling, loosening of skin; changes in vision; chills; clammy skin; confusion as to time, place, or person; cough; dark-colored urine; diarrhea; difficulty swallowing; dizziness; enlarged pupils; fast or slow heartbeat; fever; hallucinations; hives; holding false beliefs that cannot be changed by fact; increased sensitivity of eyes to light; increased sweating, possibly with fever or cold; itching; joint or muscle pain; muscle cramps or spasms; muscle pain or stiffness; puffiness or swelling of the eyelids or around the eyes, face, lips or tongue; red irritated eyes; red skin lesions, often with a purple center; seeing, hearing, or feeling things that are not there; severe chest pain; severe headache; shortness of breath; skin rash; sore throat; sores, ulcers, or white spots in mouth or on lips; stiff or sore neck; tightness in chest; unusual excitement, nervousness, or restlessness; unusual tiredness or weakness; wheezing

Symptoms of overdose

Get emergency help immediately if any of the following symptoms of overdose occur:

Bigger, dilated, or enlarged pupils [black part of eye] blurred vision; confusion; constipation; delirium; difficult urination; dizziness; drowsiness;

dry eyes, mouth, nose, or throat; eye pain; fast, pounding, or irregular heartbeat or pulse; flushing or redness of face; hallucinations; increased sensitivity of eyes to light; nausea; troubled breathing; vomiting

Some side effects may occur that usually do not need medical attention. These side effects may go away during treatment as your body adjusts to the medicine. Also, your health care professional may be able to tell you about ways to prevent or reduce some of these side effects. Check with your health care professional if any of the following side effects continue or are bothersome or if you have any questions about them:

More common

Difficulty having a bowel movement (stool); dry mouth

Less common

Acid or sour stomach; belching; bloated full feeling; dry eyes; excess air or gas in stomach or intestines; headache; heartburn; indigestion; passing gas; stomach discomfort upset or pain; trouble in urinating; unable to have a bowel movement; upper stomach pain

Incidence unknown

Change in taste; dry skin; dry throat; loss of taste; swelling of abdominal or stomach area; vision blurred; vomiting

Frequency not determined—Observed during clinical practice

Burning feeling in chest or stomach; fainting; indigestion; tenderness in stomach area

Other side effects not listed may also occur in some patients. If you notice any other effects, check with your healthcare professional.

TRYPTOPHAN   (Oral route) - TRIP-toe-fan

Commonly used brand name(s)

In the U.S.—
Aminomine

Available Dosage Forms:
- Tablet
- Capsule

Therapeutic Class: Nutriceutical

Uses For This Medicine

L-tryptophan is used along with other medications to treat mental depression. Also, L-tryptophan is used along with lithium to treat bipolar disorder.

Before Using This Medicine

In deciding to use a medicine, the risks of taking the medicine must be weighed against the good it will do. This is a decision you and your doctor will make. For this medicine, the following should be considered:

Allergies—Tell your doctor if you have ever had any unusual or allergic reaction to this medicine or any other medicines. Also tell your health care professional if you have any other types of allergies, such as to foods, dyes, preservatives,

or animals. For non-prescription products, read the label or package ingredients carefully.

Pediatric—Studies on this medicine have been done only in adult patients, and there is no specific information comparing use of L-tryptophan in children with use in other age groups.

Geriatric—Many medicines have not been studied specifically in older people. Therefore, it may not be known whether they work exactly the same way they do in younger adults or if they cause different side effects or problems in older people. There is no specific information comparing use of L-tryptophan in the elderly with use in other age groups.

Other medicines—

Using this medicine with any of the following medicines is not recommended. Your doctor may decide not to treat you with this medication or change some of the other medicines you take.

Isocarboxazid, Phenelzine, Tranylcypromine

Interactions with Food/Tobacco/Alcohol—Certain medicines should not be used at or around the time of eating food or eating certain types of food since interactions may occur. Using alcohol or tobacco with certain medicines may also cause interactions to occur. Discuss with your healthcare professional the use of your medicine with food, alcohol, or tobacco.

Other medical problems—The presence of other medical problems may affect the use of this medicine. Make sure you tell your doctor if you have any other medical problems, especially:

- Achlohydria or malabsorption (digestion problems)—L-tryptophan may cause breathing problems in patients with certain types of digestion problems
- Bladder cancer—L-tryptophan may increase the risk of bladder cancer
- Cataracts—L-tryptophan may cause cataracts
- Diabetes mellitus (sugar diabetes)—L-tryptophan may cause diabetes in patients with a family history of diabetes

Proper Use of This Medicine

Take with a low-protein, carbohydrate-rich meal or snack to prevent an upset stomach.

Dosing—The dose of this medicine will be different for different patients. Follow your doctor's orders or the directions on the label. The following information includes only the average doses of this medicine. If your dose is different, do not change it unless your doctor tells you to do so.

The amount of medicine that you take depends on the strength of the medicine. Also, the number of doses you take each day, the time allowed between doses, and the length of time you take the medicine depend on the medical problem for which you are using the medicine.

- For oral dosage forms (capsules or tablets):
  - For mental depression:
    - Adults—8 to 12 grams per day, given in 3 to 4 equally divided doses.
    - Children—Use and dose must be determined by your doctor.

Missed dose—If you miss a dose of this medicine, skip the missed dose and go back to your regular dosing schedule. Do not double doses.

Storage—Store the medicine in a closed container at room temperature, away from heat, moisture, and direct light. Keep from freezing.

Keep out of the reach of children.

Do not keep outdated medicine or medicine no longer needed.

Precautions While Using This Medicine

It is important that your doctor check your progress at regular visits, to allow dosage adjustments and help reduce any side effects.

This medicine may cause some people to become drowsy, dizzy, or less alert than they are normally. Make sure you know how you react to this medicine before you drive, use machines, or do anything else that could be dangerous if you are dizzy or are not alert.

This medicine may cause dryness of the mouth. Using sugarless candy or gum, ice, or a saliva substitute may be helpful. Check with your physician or dentist if dry mouth continues for more than 2 weeks.

Avoid excessive exposure to ultraviolet light to reduce the chance of cataract formation.

Side Effects of This Medicine

Along with its needed effects, a medicine may cause some unwanted effects. Although not all of these side effects may occur, if they do occur they may need medical attention.

Symptoms of overdose

Get emergency help immediately if any of the following symptoms of overdose occur:

Agitation; confusion; diarrhea; fever; overactive reflexes; poor coordination; restlessness; shivering; sweating; talking or acting with excitement you cannot control; trembling or shaking; twitching; vomiting

Some side effects may occur that usually do not need medical attention. These side effects may go away during treatment as your body adjusts to the medicine. Also, your health care professional may be able to tell you about ways to prevent or reduce some of these side effects. Check with your health care professional if any of the following side effects continue or are bothersome or if you have any questions about them:

Dizziness; drowsiness; dry mouth; headache; loss of appetite; nausea

Other side effects not listed may also occur in some patients. If you notice any other effects, check with your healthcare professional.

TUBERCULIN (Intradermal route) - too-BER-kyoo-lin

Commonly used brand name(s)

In the U.S.—
Aplisol
Tubersol

Available Dosage Forms:

• Solution

Therapeutic Class: Diagnostic Agent, Tuberculin

Uses For This Medicine

Tuberculin, purified protein derivative (PPD) is used as a test to help diagnose tuberculous infection.

How the test is done: Tuberculin PPD is injected into the surface layers of the skin. If the test is positive, a reaction will be seen at and around the place of injection or puncture. If the test is given using an injection, this reaction is usually a hard, raised area with clear margins. If the test is given using the puncture devices, the reaction is usually a swollen area at the puncture site. Forty-eight to 72 hours after administration of the injection the size of the reaction is measured and recorded and the results of the test are studied.

Tuberculin PPD is to be used only by or under the supervision of a doctor.

Before Using This Medicine

In deciding to use a medicine, the risks of taking the medicine must be weighed against the good it will do. This is a decision you and your doctor will make. For this medicine, the following should be considered:

In deciding to use a diagnostic test, the risks of the test must be weighed against the good it will do. This is a decision you and your doctor will make. For tuberculin PPD, the following should be considered:

Allergies—Tell your doctor if you have ever had any unusual or allergic reaction to this medicine or any other medicines. Also tell your health care professional if you have any other types of allergies, such as to foods, dyes, preservatives, or animals. For non-prescription products, read the label or package ingredients carefully.

Pediatric—Although there is no specific information comparing use of tuberculin PPD in children with use in other age groups, this diagnostic test is not expected to cause different side effects or problems in children than it does in adults.

Geriatric—Reactions to tuberculin PPD in older patients may be more likely to develop slowly and may not reach the peak effect until after 72 hours.

Pregnancy—

	Pregnancy Category	Explanation
All Trimesters	C	Animal studies have shown an adverse effect and there are no adequate studies in pregnant women OR no animal studies have been conducted and there are no adequate studies in pregnant women.

Breast Feeding—There are no adequate studies in women for determining infant risk when using this medica-

tion during breastfeeding. Weigh the potential benefits against the potential risks before taking this medication while breastfeeding.

Other medicines—Although certain medicines should not be used together at all, in other cases two different medicines may be used together even if an interaction might occur. In these cases, your doctor may want to change the dose, or other precautions may be necessary. Tell your healthcare professional if you are taking any other prescription or non-prescription (over-the-counter [OTC]) medicine.

Interactions with Food/Tobacco/Alcohol—Certain medicines should not be used at or around the time of eating food or eating certain types of food since interactions may occur. Using alcohol or tobacco with certain medicines may also cause interactions to occur. Discuss with your healthcare professional the use of your medicine with food, alcohol, or tobacco.

Other medical problems—The presence of other medical problems may affect the use of this medicine. Make sure you tell your doctor if you have any other medical problems, especially:

• Positive tuberculin reaction (previous)—The reaction to tuberculin PPD may be severe, possibly causing sores on the skin where the test is given

Proper Use of This Medicine

Dosing—The dose of this medicine will be different for different patients. Follow your doctor's orders or the directions on the label. The following information includes only the average doses of this medicine. If your dose is different, do not change it unless your doctor tells you to do so.

The amount of medicine that you take depends on the strength of the medicine. Also, the number of doses you take each day, the time allowed between doses, and the length of time you take the medicine depend on the medical problem for which you are using the medicine.

Side Effects of This Medicine

Along with its needed effects, a medicine may cause some unwanted effects. Although not all of these side effects may occur, if they do occur they may need medical attention.
   Rare
      Skin rash or itching; redness, blistering, peeling, or loosening of the skin

Some side effects may occur that usually do not need medical attention. These side effects may go away during treatment as your body adjusts to the medicine. Also, your health care professional may be able to tell you about ways to prevent or reduce some of these side effects. Check with your health care professional if any of the following side effects continue or are bothersome or if you have any questions about them:
   Less common
      Pain; redness at the site of injection; sores at and around the place of injection

Other side effects not listed may also occur in some patients. If you notice any other effects, check with your healthcare professional.

VACCINIA IMMUNE GLOBULIN, HUMAN   (Intravenous route)

Black Box Warning

- VIGIV FROM DYNPORT
  - Immune globulin intravenous (Human) (IGIV) products have been reported to be associated with renal dysfunction, acute renal failure, osmotic nephrosis, proximal tubular nephropathy, and death. Although these reports of renal dysfunction and acute renal failure have been associated with the use of many licensed IGIV products, those that contained sucrose as a stabilizer and were administered at daily doses of 400 mg/kg or greater have accounted for a disproportionate share of the total number. VIGIV contains sucrose (5%) as a stabilizer, and the recommended dose is 100 mg/kg. Patients predisposed to acute renal failure include the following: patients with any degree of pre-existing renal insufficiency, diabetes mellitus, volume depletion, sepsis, or paraproteinemia, patients who are at least 65 years of age, or patients who are receiving known nephrotoxic drugs. Especially in such patients, VIGIV should be administered at the minimum concentration available and at the minimum rate of infusion practical.

Commonly used brand name(s)

In the U.S.—
  Vaccinia IVIG

Available Dosage Forms:
- Solution

Therapeutic Class: Immune Serum

Uses For This Medicine

Vaccinia immune globulin is used to treat infections caused by the vaccinia virus.

Before Using This Medicine

In deciding to use a medicine, the risks of taking the medicine must be weighed against the good it will do. This is a decision you and your doctor will make. For this medicine, the following should be considered:

Allergies—Tell your doctor if you have ever had any unusual or allergic reaction to this medicine or any other medicines. Also tell your health care professional if you have any other types of allergies, such as to foods, dyes, preservatives, or animals. For non-prescription products, read the label or package ingredients carefully.

Pediatric—Studies on this medicine have been done only in adult patients, and there is no known specific information comparing use of vaccinia immune globulin in children with use in other age groups.

Geriatric—Many medicines have not been studied specifically in older people. Therefore, it may not be known whether they work exactly the same way they do in younger adults or if they cause different side effects or problems in older people. There is no specific information comparing use of vaccinia immune globulin in the elderly with use in other age groups.

Pregnancy—

	Pregnancy Category	Explanation
All Trimesters	C	Animal studies have shown an adverse effect and there are no adequate studies in pregnant women OR no animal studies have been conducted and there are no adequate studies in pregnant women.

Breast Feeding—There are no adequate studies in women for determining infant risk when using this medication during breastfeeding. Weigh the potential benefits against the potential risks before taking this medication while breastfeeding.

Other medicines—Although certain medicines should not be used together at all, in other cases two different medicines may be used together even if an interaction might occur. In these cases, your doctor may want to change the dose, or other precautions may be necessary. Tell your healthcare professional if you are taking any other prescription or non-prescription (over-the-counter [OTC]) medicine.

Interactions with Food/Tobacco/Alcohol—Certain medicines should not be used at or around the time of eating food or eating certain types of food since interactions may occur. Using alcohol or tobacco with certain medicines may also cause interactions to occur. Discuss with your healthcare professional the use of your medicine with food, alcohol, or tobacco.

Other medical problems—The presence of other medical problems may affect the use of this medicine. Make sure you tell your doctor if you have any other medical problems, especially:

- Vaccinia keratitis—Use is not recommended.
- Hyperviscosity, known or suspected—May increase chance for serious side effects.
- Immunoglobulin A (IgA) deficiency—Increased risk for allergic reaction.

Proper Use of This Medicine

Make sure you discuss the risks and benefits of this medicine with your doctor.

Report all infections thought to have been possibly transmitted by this product by having your doctor call Cangene Corporation at 1–877–CANGENE.

Dosing—The dose of this medicine will be different for different patients. Follow your doctor's orders or the directions on the label. The following information includes only the average doses of this medicine. If your dose is different, do not change it unless your doctor tells you to do so.

The amount of medicine that you take depends on the strength of the medicine. Also, the number of doses you take each day, the time allowed between doses, and the length of time you take the medicine depend on the medical problem for which you are using the medicine.

- For injectable dosage form:
  - For treatment and/or medical problems due to vaccinia virus

- Adults—Dose is based on weight and will be determined by your doctor.
- Children—Use and dose must be determined by your doctor.

Precautions While Using This Medicine

Tell your healthcare provider if you have ever had a reaction to a vaccination.

Side Effects of This Medicine

Along with its needed effects, a medicine may cause some unwanted effects. Although not all of these side effects may occur, if they do occur they may need medical attention.

Check with your doctor immediately if any of the following side effects occur:

Incidence unknown
Fever; headache; nausea; stiff neck or back

Observed postmarketing
Back, leg or stomach pain; black, tarry stools; bleeding gums; blistering, peeling, loosening of skin; bluish color of fingernails, lips, skin, palms, or nail beds; blurred vision; change in consciousness; chest pain; chills; cold, clammy, pale skin; confusion; convulsions; cough; coughing that produces a pink frothy sputum; dark urine; decreased urination; diarrhea; difficulty or labored breathing; dizziness, faintness, or lightheadedness when getting up from a lying or sitting position; fatigue; general body swelling; itching; irregular heartbeats; joint or muscle pain; light-colored stools; loss of appetite; loss of bladder control; loss of consciousness; muscle spasms or jerking of all extremities; nausea or vomiting; no blood pressure or pulse; noisy breathing; nosebleeds; not breathing; pain in chest, groin, or legs, especially the calves; painful or difficult urination; red irritated eyes; red skin lesions, often with a purple center; severe, sudden headache; severe weakness or numbness in arm or leg; shortness of breath; slow heart rate; slurred speech; sore throat; sores, ulcers, or white spots in mouth or on lips; stopping of heart; sudden loss of coordination; suddenly sweating; swelling in legs and ankles; swollen glands; tightness in chest; troubled breathing; unconsciousness; unusual bleeding or bruising; unusual tiredness or weakness; vision changes; wheezing; yellowing of the eyes or skin

Some side effects may occur that usually do not need medical attention. These side effects may go away during treatment as your body adjusts to the medicine. Also, your health care professional may be able to tell you about ways to prevent or reduce some of these side effects. Check with your health care professional if any of the following side effects continue or are bothersome or if you have any questions about them:

More common
Burning, crawling, itching, numbness, prickling, "pins and needles", or tingling feelings; eye disorder; energy increased; feeling unusually cold; feeling hot; lack or loss of strength; lip dry; muscle pain; shakiness in legs, arms, hands, feet; shivering; trembling or shaking of hands or feet

Other side effects not listed may also occur in some patients. If you notice any other effects, check with your healthcare professional.

VALACYCLOVIR (Oral route) - val-ay-SYE-kloe-veer

Commonly used brand name(s)
In the U.S.—
  Valtrex

Available Dosage Forms:
- Tablet

Therapeutic Class: Antiviral
Pharmacologic Class: Viral DNA Polymerase Inhibitor

Uses For This Medicine

Valacyclovir is used to treat the symptoms of herpes zoster (also known as shingles), a herpes virus infection of the skin; it is also used to treat and prevent genital herpes infections. In your body, valacyclovir becomes the anti-herpes medicine, acyclovir. Although valacyclovir will not cure shingles or genital herpes, it does help relieve the pain and discomfort and helps the sores heal faster.

Valacyclovir is available only with your doctor's prescription.

Before Using This Medicine

In deciding to use a medicine, the risks of taking the medicine must be weighed against the good it will do. This is a decision you and your doctor will make. For this medicine, the following should be considered:

Allergies—Tell your doctor if you have ever had any unusual or allergic reaction to this medicine or any other medicines. Also tell your health care professional if you have any other types of allergies, such as to foods, dyes, preservatives, or animals. For non-prescription products, read the label or package ingredients carefully.

Pediatric—Studies on this medicine have been done only in adult patients. There is no specific information comparing use of valacyclovir in children with use in other age groups.

Geriatric—Valacyclovir has been used in elderly patients and has not been shown to cause different side effects or problems in older people than it does in younger adults. Elderly patients are at a high risk for dehydration and should drink plenty of fluids.

Pregnancy—

	Pregnancy Category	Explanation
All Trimesters	B	Animal studies have revealed no evidence of harm to the fetus, however, there are no adequate studies in pregnant women OR animal studies have shown an adverse effect, but adequate studies in pregnant women have failed to demonstrate a risk to the fetus.

Breast Feeding—Studies in women suggest that this medication poses minimal risk to the infant when used during breastfeeding.

Other medicines—

Using this medicine with any of the following medicines may cause an increased risk of certain side effects, but using both drugs may be the best treatment for you. If both medicines are prescribed together, your doctor may change the dose or how often you use one or both of the medicines.

Mycophenolate Mofetil, Mycophenolic Acid

Interactions with Food/Tobacco/Alcohol—Certain medicines should not be used at or around the time of eating food or eating certain types of food since interactions may occur. Using alcohol or tobacco with certain medicines may also cause interactions to occur. Discuss with your healthcare professional the use of your medicine with food, alcohol, or tobacco.

Other medical problems—The presence of other medical problems may affect the use of this medicine. Make sure you tell your doctor if you have any other medical problems, especially:

- Advanced human immunodeficiency virus (HIV) infection or
- Bone marrow transplantation or
- Kidney transplantation—Patients with these medical problems may have an increased risk of severe side effects
- Kidney disease—Kidney disease may increase blood levels of this medicine, increasing the chance of side effects

Proper Use of This Medicine

Valacyclovir works best if it is used within 48 hours after the first symptoms of shingles or genital herpes (for example, pain, burning, or blisters) begin to appear. For recurrent outbreaks of genital herpes, valacyclovir works best if it is used within 24 hours after the symptoms begin to appear.

Valacyclovir may be taken with meals.

Keep taking valacyclovir for the full time of treatment, even if your symptoms begin to clear up after a few days. Do not miss any doses. However, do not use this medicine more often or for a longer time than your doctor ordered.

Dosing—The dose of this medicine will be different for different patients. Follow your doctor's orders or the directions on the label. The following information includes only the average doses of this medicine. If your dose is different, do not change it unless your doctor tells you to do so.

The amount of medicine that you take depends on the strength of the medicine. Also, the number of doses you take each day, the time allowed between doses, and the length of time you take the medicine depend on the medical problem for which you are using the medicine.

- For oral dosage form (tablets):
  - For treatment of genital herpes, first outbreak:
    - Adults—1 gram two times a day for ten days.
    - Children—Use and dose must be determined by your doctor.
  - For treatment of genital herpes, recurrent outbreaks:
    - Adults—500 milligrams (mg) two times a day for three days.
    - Children—Use and dose must be determined by your doctor.
  - To prevent recurrent outbreaks of genital herpes:
    - Adults—500 mg or 1 gram once a day.
    - Children—Use and dose must be determined by your doctor.

  - For treatment of shingles:
    - Adults—1 gram three times a day for seven days.
    - Children—Use and dose must be determined by your doctor.

Missed dose—If you miss a dose of this medicine, take it as soon as possible. However, if it is almost time for your next dose, skip the missed dose and go back to your regular dosing schedule. Do not double doses.

Storage—Store the medicine in a closed container at room temperature, away from heat, moisture, and direct light. Keep from freezing.

Keep out of the reach of children.

Do not keep outdated medicine or medicine no longer needed.

Precautions While Using This Medicine

If your symptoms do not improve within a few days, or if they become worse, check with your doctor.

The areas affected by genital herpes or shingles should be kept as clean and dry as possible. Also, wear loose-fitting clothing to avoid irritating the sores (blisters).

Side Effects of This Medicine

Along with its needed effects, a medicine may cause some unwanted effects. Although not all of these side effects may occur, if they do occur they may need medical attention.

Check with your doctor as soon as possible if any of the following side effects occur:

Less common
　Painful menstruation, including abdominal cramps, diarrhea, or nausea

Rare
　Black, tarry stools; chest pain; chills; cough; decreased frequency/output of urine; fever; flu-like symptoms; headache; lower back/side pain; reduced mental alertness; shortness of breath; unusual tiredness; yellow eyes or skin

Frequency not determined
　Back, leg or stomach pains; changes in behavior, especially in interactions with other people; difficulty breathing or swallowing; fast, pounding, or irregular heartbeat; high blood pressure; itching; lightheadedness when getting up from a lying or sitting position; redness of skin; seeing, hearing, or feeling things that are not there; skin rash; swelling or puffiness of face, hands, legs, or feet; wheezing

Symptoms of overdose with intravenous acyclovir
　Anxiety; convulsions (seizures); decrease in urine output; decreased frequency of urination; dry mouth; hallucinations (seeing, hearing, or feeling things that are not there); irritability; loss of consciousness; lower back/side pain; nervousness; restlessness

Note: Because the information on valacyclovir overdose is limited, information on intravenous acyclovir overdose is provided. In the body, valacyclovir is converted into acyclovir.

Some side effects may occur that usually do not need medical attention. These side effects may go away during treatment as your body adjusts to the medicine. Also, your health care professional may be able to tell you about ways to prevent or reduce some of these side effects. Check with your health care professional if any of the following side effects

continue or are bothersome or if you have any questions about them:

More common
> Headache; nausea

Less common
> Constipation; diarrhea; dizziness; joint pain; loss of appetite; stomach pain; unusual tiredness or weakness; vomiting

Frequency not determined
> Anxiety; dry mouth; irritability; mood or mental changes; nervousness; restlessness

Other side effects not listed may also occur in some patients. If you notice any other effects, check with your healthcare professional.

VALGANCICLOVIR (Oral route) - val-gan-SYE-kloe-veer

Black Box Warning

The clinical toxicity of valganciclovir hydrochloride, which is metabolized to ganciclovir, includes granulocytopenia, anemia and thrombocytopenia. In animal studies ganciclovir was carcinogenic, teratogenic and caused aspermatogenesis.

Commonly used brand name(s)

In the U.S.—
> Valcyte

Available Dosage Forms:
- Tablet

Therapeutic Class: Antiviral
Pharmacologic Class: Viral DNA Polymerase Inhibitor

Uses For This Medicine

Valganciclovir is an antiviral. It is used to treat infections caused by viruses.

Valganciclovir is used to treat the symptoms of cytomegalovirus (CMV) retinitis, an infection in the eyes of people with acquired immunodeficiency syndrome (AIDS). Valganciclovir will not cure this eye infection, but it may help to keep the symptoms from becoming worse.

This medicine may cause some serious side effects, including anemia and other blood problems. Before you begin treatment with valganciclovir, you and your doctor should talk about the good this medicine will do as well as the risks of using it.

This medicine is available only with your doctor's prescription.

Before Using This Medicine

In deciding to use a medicine, the risks of taking the medicine must be weighed against the good it will do. This is a decision you and your doctor will make. For this medicine, the following should be considered:

Allergies—Tell your doctor if you have ever had any unusual or allergic reaction to this medicine or any other medicines. Also tell your health care professional if you have any other types of allergies, such as to foods, dyes, preservatives, or animals. For non-prescription products, read the label or package ingredients carefully.

Pediatric—Studies on this medicine have been done only in adult patients, and there is no specific information comparing use of valganciclovir in children with use in other age groups.

Geriatric—Many medicines have not been studied specifically in older people. Therefore, it may not be known whether they work exactly the same way they do in younger adults or if they cause different side effects or problems in older people. There is no specific information comparing use of valganciclovir in the elderly with use in other age groups.

Pregnancy—

	Pregnancy Category	Explanation
All Trimesters	C	Animal studies have shown an adverse effect and there are no adequate studies in pregnant women OR no animal studies have been conducted and there are no adequate studies in pregnant women.

Breast Feeding—There are no adequate studies in women for determining infant risk when using this medication during breastfeeding. Weigh the potential benefits against the potential risks before taking this medication while breastfeeding.

Other medicines—Although certain medicines should not be used together at all, in other cases two different medicines may be used together even if an interaction might occur. In these cases, your doctor may want to change the dose, or other precautions may be necessary. Tell your healthcare professional if you are taking any other prescription or non-prescription (over-the-counter [OTC]) medicine.

Interactions with Food/Tobacco/Alcohol—Certain medicines should not be used at or around the time of eating food or eating certain types of food since interactions may occur. Using alcohol or tobacco with certain medicines may also cause interactions to occur. The following interactions have been selected on the basis of their potential significance and are not necessarily all-inclusive.

Using this medicine with any of the following may cause an increased risk of certain side effects but may be unavoidable in some cases. If used together, your doctor may change the dose or how often you use this medicine, or give you special instructions about the use of food, alcohol, or tobacco.

High Fat Food

Other medical problems—The presence of other medical problems may affect the use of this medicine. Make sure you tell your doctor if you have any other medical problems, especially:
- Kidney disease—Valganciclovir may build up in the blood in patients with kidney disease, increasing the chance of side effects
- Low platelet count or
- Low red blood cell count or
- Low white blood cell count—Valganciclovir may make these blood diseases worse

Proper Use of This Medicine

It is important that you take valganciclovir tablets with food. This is to make sure the medicine is fully absorbed into the body and will work properly.

To get the best results, valganciclovir must be given for the full time of treatment. Also, this medicine works best when there is a constant amount in the blood. To help keep the amount constant, valganciclovir must be taken on a regular schedule.

Dosing—The dose of this medicine will be different for different patients. Follow your doctor's orders or the directions on the label. The following information includes only the average doses of this medicine. If your dose is different, do not change it unless your doctor tells you to do so.

The amount of medicine that you take depends on the strength of the medicine. Also, the number of doses you take each day, the time allowed between doses, and the length of time you take the medicine depend on the medical problem for which you are using the medicine.

- For oral dosage form (tablets):
  - For treatment of CMV in the eyes:
    - Adults—To start, 900 milligrams (mg) two times a day with food. As you improve the dose may be changed to 900 mg once a day with food.
    - Children—Use and dose must be determined by your doctor.

Storage—Store the medicine in a closed container at room temperature, away from heat, moisture, and direct light. Keep from freezing.

Keep out of the reach of children.

Do not keep outdated medicine or medicine no longer needed.

Ask your healthcare professional how you should dispose of any medicine you do not use.

Precautions While Using This Medicine

It is very important that your doctor check you at regular visits for any blood problems that may be caused by this medicine.

It is also very important that your ophthalmologist (eye doctor) check your eyes every 4 to 6 weeks since it is still possible that you may have some loss of eyesight during valganciclovir treatment.

Valganciclovir can lower the number of white blood cells in your blood, increasing the chance of getting an infection. It can also lower the number of platelets, which are necessary for proper blood clotting. If this occurs, there are certain precautions you can take to reduce the risk of infection or bleeding:

- If you can, avoid people with infections. Check with your doctor immediately if you think you are getting an infection or if you get a fever or chills, cough or hoarseness, lower back or side pain, or painful or difficult urination.
- Check with your doctor immediately if you notice any unusual bleeding or bruising; black, tarry stools; blood in urine or stools; or pinpoint red spots on your skin.
- Be careful when using a regular toothbrush, dental floss, or toothpick. Your medical doctor, dentist, or nurse may recommend other ways to clean your teeth and gums.

Check with your medical doctor before having any dental work done.

- Be careful not to cut yourself when you are using sharp objects such as a safety razor or fingernail or toenail cutters.

Be careful not to handle crushed or broken tablets. If you have contact with broken or crushed tablets, wash your skin with soap and clear water. If the medicine gets into your eyes, rinse them with clear water.

Side Effects of This Medicine

Along with its needed effects, a medicine may cause some unwanted effects. Although not all of these side effects may occur, if they do occur they may need medical attention.

Check with your doctor immediately if any of the following side effects occur:

More common
   Black, tarry stools; blood in urine or stools; chills; cough; fever; hoarseness; lower back or side pain; painful or difficult urination; pale skin; pinpoint red spots on skin; sore throat; seeing flashes or sparks of light; seeing floating spots before the eyes; troubled breathing; ulcers, sores, or white spots in the mouth; unusual bleeding or bruising; unusual tiredness or weakness; veil or curtain appearing across part of vision

Less common
   Changes in facial skin color; fast or irregular breathing; hives, itching, and skin rash; large, hive-like swellings on eyelids, face, lips, mouth, and/or tongue; puffiness or swelling of the eyelids or around the eyes; runny or stuffy nose; shortness of breath; tightness in chest and/or wheezing

Check with your doctor as soon as possible if any of the following side effects occur:

Less common
   Confusion; false beliefs; feeling, hearing, or seeing things that are not there; illogical thinking; seizures

Some side effects may occur that usually do not need medical attention. These side effects may go away during treatment as your body adjusts to the medicine. Also, your health care professional may be able to tell you about ways to prevent or reduce some of these side effects. Check with your health care professional if any of the following side effects continue or are bothersome or if you have any questions about them:

More common
   Abdominal pain; diarrhea; headache; nausea and vomiting; numbness, tingling, pain, or weakness of hands or feet; sleeplessness; tingling, burning, or prickly sensations; trouble sleeping

Less common
   Agitation

Other side effects not listed may also occur in some patients. If you notice any other effects, check with your healthcare professional.

VALPROIC ACID   (Systemic)

Some commonly used brand names are:

In the U.S.—

Depacon (2)	Depakote (1)
Depakene (3)	Depakote Sprinkle (1)

In Canada—

Alti-Valproic (3)	Novo-Valproic (3)
Depakene (3)	Nu-Valproic (3)
Deproic (3)	Penta-Valproic (3)
Dom-Valproic (3)	pms-Valproic Acid (3)
Epival (1)	pms-Valproic Acid E.C. (3)
Med Valproic (3)	

This information applies to the following medicines:

1. Divalproex (dye-VAL-pro-ex)
2. Valproate Sodium (val-PRO-ate SO-dee-um)
3. Valproic Acid (val-PRO-ic acid)

Category

- **Anticonvulsant**—Divalproex; Valproate Sodium; Valproic Acid
- **Antimanic**—Divalproex
- **Migraine headache prophylactic**—Divalproex

Description

Valproic acid, valproate sodium, and divalproex belong to the group of medicines called anticonvulsants. They are used to control certain types of seizures in the treatment of epilepsy. Valproic acid, valproate sodium, and divalproex may be used alone or with other seizure medicine. Divalproex is also used to treat the manic phase of bipolar disorder (manic-depressive illness), and to help prevent migraine headaches.

Divalproex and valproate sodium form valproic acid in the body. Therefore, the following information applies to all of these medicines.

These medicines are available only with your doctor's prescription, in the following dosage forms:

Oral
- Divalproex
  - Delayed-release capsules
  - Delayed-release tablets
- Valproic Acid
  - Capsules
  - Syrup

Parenteral
- Valproate Sodium
  - Injection

Before Using This Medicine

In deciding to use a medicine, the risks of taking the medicine must be weighed against the good it will do. This is a decision you and your doctor will make. For valproic acid, valproate sodium, and divalproex, the following should be considered:

Allergies—Tell your doctor if you have ever had any unusual or allergic reaction to valproic acid, valproate sodium, or divalproex. Also tell your health care professional if you are allergic to any other substances, such as foods, preservatives, or dyes.

Pregnancy—Valproic acid, valproate sodium, and divalproex have been reported to cause birth defects when taken by the mother during the first 3 months of pregnancy. Also, animal studies have shown that valproic acid, valproate sodium, and divalproex cause birth defects when taken in doses several times greater than doses used in humans. However, these medicines may be necessary to control seizures in some pregnant patients. Be sure you have discussed this with your doctor.

Breast-feeding—Valproic acid, valproate sodium, and divalproex pass into the breast milk, but their effect on the nursing baby is not known. It may be necessary for you to take another medicine or to stop breast-feeding during treatment with valproic acid, valproate sodium, or divalproex. Be sure you have discussed the risks and benefits of this medicine with your doctor.

Children—Abdominal or stomach cramps, nausea or vomiting, tiredness or weakness, and yellow eyes or skin may be especially likely to occur in children, who are usually more sensitive to the effects of these medicines. Children up to 2 years of age, those taking more than one medicine for seizure control, and children with certain other medical problems may be more likely to develop serious side effects.

Older adults—Elderly people are especially sensitive to the effects of these medicines. This may increase the chance of side effects during treatment. The dose of this medicine may be lower for older adults.

Other medicines—Although certain medicines should not be used together at all, in other cases two different medicines may be used together even if an interaction might occur. In these cases, your doctor may want to change the dose, or other precautions may be necessary. When you are taking valproic acid, valproate sodium, or divalproex, it is especially important that your health care professional knows if you are taking any of the following:

- Acetaminophen (e.g., Tylenol) (with long-term, high-dose use) or
- Amiodarone (e.g., Cordarone) or
- Amitriptyline and nortriptyline or
- Anabolic steroids (nandrolone [e.g., Anabolin], oxandrolone [e.g., Anavar], oxymetholone [e.g., Anadrol], stanozolol [e.g., Winstrol]) or
- Androgens (male hormones) or
- Anticoagulants or
- Aspirin or
- Barbiturates or
- Carbamazepine (e.g., Tegretol) or
- Carmustine (e.g., BiCNU) or
- Dantrolene (e.g., Dantrium) or
- Daunorubicin (e.g., Cerubidine) or
- Disulfiram (e.g., Antabuse) or
- Estrogens (female hormones) or
- Ethosuximide or
- Etretinate (e.g., Tegison) or
- Gold salts (medicine for arthritis) or
- Mercaptopurine (e.g., Purinethol) or
- Methotrexate (e.g., Mexate) or

- Methyldopa (e.g., Aldomet) or
- Naltrexone (e.g., Trexan) (with long-term, high-dose use) or
- Phenothiazines (acetophenazine [e.g., Tindal], chlorpromazine [e.g., Thorazine], fluphenazine [e.g., Prolixin], mesoridazine [e.g., Serentil], perphenazine [e.g., Trilafon], prochlorperazine [e.g., Compazine], promazine [e.g., Sparine], promethazine [e.g., Phenergan], thioridazine [e.g., Mellaril], trifluoperazine [e.g., Stelazine], triflupromazine [e.g., Vesprin], trimeprazine [e.g., Temaril]) or
- Plicamycin (e.g., Mithracin)—There is an increased risk of serious side effects to the liver
- Central nervous system (CNS) depressants (medicines that cause drowsiness) or
- Tricyclic antidepressants (medicine for depression)—There may be an increase in CNS depressant effects
- Carbenicillin by injection (e.g., Geopen) or
- Dipyridamole (e.g., Persantine) or
- Inflammation or pain medicine, except narcotics, or
- Pentoxifylline (e.g., Trental) or
- Sulfinpyrazone (e.g., Anturane) or
- Ticarcillin (e.g., Ticar)—Valproic acid, valproate sodium, or divalproex may increase the chance of bleeding because of decreased blood clotting ability; the potential of aspirin, medicine for inflammation or pain, or sulfinpyrazone to cause stomach ulcer and bleeding may also increase the chance of bleeding in patients taking valproic acid, valproate sodium, or divalproex
- Heparin—There is an increased risk of side effects that may cause bleeding
- Mefloquine—The amount of valproic acid, valproate sodium, or divalproex that you need to take may change
- Other anticonvulsants (medicine for seizures)—There is an increased risk of seizures or other unwanted effects

Other medical problems—The presence of other medical problems may affect the use of these medicines. Make sure you tell your doctor if you have any other medical problems, especially:
- Blood disease or
- Brain disease or
- Kidney disease—There is an increased risk of serious side effects
- Liver disease—Valproic acid, valproate sodium, or divalproex may make the condition worse
- Pancreatitis— may be life threatening, stop using valproate if you have this condition
- Urea cycle disorders— my lead to serious side effects or death

Proper Use of This Medicine

For patients taking the *capsule form* of valproic acid:
- Swallow the capsule whole without chewing, crushing, or breaking. This is to prevent irritation of the mouth or throat.

For patients taking the *delayed-release capsule form* of divalproex:
- Swallow the capsule whole, or sprinkle the contents on a small amount of soft food, such as applesauce or pudding, and swallow without chewing.

For patients taking the *delayed-release tablet form* of divalproex:
- Swallow the tablet whole without chewing, breaking, or crushing. This is to prevent damage to the special coating that helps lessen irritation of the stomach.

For patients taking the *syrup form* of valproic acid:
- The syrup may be mixed with any liquid or added to food for a better taste.

For patients taking the oral dosage forms of valproic acid and divalproex:
- These medicines may be taken with meals or snacks to reduce stomach upset.

This medicine must be taken exactly as directed by your doctor to prevent seizures and lessen the possibility of side effects.

Dosing—The dose of valproic acid, valproate sodium, or divalproex will be different for different patients. *Follow your doctor's orders or the directions on the label.* The following information includes only the average doses of valproic acid, valproate sodium, or divalproex. *If your dose is different, do not change it* unless your doctor tells you to do so.

The number of capsules or tablets or teaspoonfuls of syrup that you take or the number of injections you receive depends on the strength of the medicine. Also, *the number of doses you take each day, the time allowed between doses, and the length of time you take the medicine depend on the medical problem for which you are using valproic acid, valproate sodium, or divalproex.*

- If valproic acid or divalproex is the only medicine you are taking for seizures:
  - Adults and adolescents: Dose is based on body weight. The usual dose is 5 to 15 milligrams (mg) per kilogram (kg) (2.3 to 6.9 mg per pound) of body weight to start. Your doctor may increase your dose gradually every week by 5 to 10 mg per kg of body weight if needed. However, the dose is usually not more than 60 mg per kg of body weight a day. If the total dose a day is greater than 250 mg, it is usually divided into smaller doses and taken two or more times during the day.
  - Children 1 to 12 years of age: Dose is based on body weight. The usual dose is 15 to 45 mg per kg (6.9 to 20.7 mg per pound) of body weight to start. The doctor may increase the dose gradually every week by 5 to 10 mg per kg of body weight if needed.
- If you are taking more than one medicine for seizures:
  - Adults and adolescents: Dose is based on body weight. The usual dose is 10 to 30 mg per kg (4.6 to 13.8 mg per pound) of body weight to start. Your doctor may increase your dose gradually every week by 5 to 10 mg per kg of body weight if needed. If the total dose a day is greater than 250 mg, it is usually divided into smaller doses and taken two or more times during the day.
  - Children 1 to 12 years of age: Dose is based on body weight. The usual dose is 30 to 100 mg per kg (13.8 to 45.5 mg per pound) of body weight.

- If you are using valproate sodium for seizures because you temporarily cannot take oral medication:
  - Adults, adolescents, and children: Dose is based on body weight, and will be determined by your doctor. The dose is injected into a vein.
- If you are taking divalproex for treatment of mania:
  - Adults: At first, 750 mg a day, usually divided into smaller doses and taken two or more times during the day. Your doctor may increase your dose if needed.
  - Children: Use and dose must be determined by your doctor.
- If you are taking divalproex for prevention of migraine headaches:
  - Adults: At first, 250 mg two times a day. Your doctor may increase your dose if needed. However, the dose is usually not more than 1000 mg a day.
  - Children: Use and dose must be determined by your doctor.

Missed dose—If you miss a dose of this medicine, and your dosing schedule is:

- One dose a day—Take the missed dose as soon as possible. However, if you do not remember until the next day, skip the missed dose and go back to your regular dosing schedule. Do not double doses.
- Two or more doses a day—If you remember within 6 hours of the missed dose, take it right away. Then take the rest of the doses for that day at equally spaced times. Do not double doses.

If you have any questions about this, check with your doctor.

Storage—To store this medicine:

- Keep out of the reach of children.
- Store away from heat and direct light.
- Do not store the capsule or tablet form of this medicine in the bathroom, near the kitchen sink, or in other damp places. Heat or moisture may cause the medicine to break down.
- Keep the syrup form of this medicine from freezing.
- Do not keep outdated medicine or medicine no longer needed. Be sure that any discarded medicine is out of the reach of children.

Precautions While Using This Medicine

Your doctor should check your progress at regular visits, especially for the first few months that you take this medicine. This is necessary to allow dose adjustments and to reduce any unwanted effects.

Do not stop taking this medicine without first checking with your doctor. Your doctor may want you to gradually reduce the amount you are taking before stopping completely.

Before you have any medical tests, tell the doctor in charge that you are taking this medicine. The results of the metyrapone and thyroid function tests may be affected by this medicine.

Before having any kind of surgery, dental treatment, or emergency treatment, tell the medical doctor or dentist in charge that you are taking this medicine. Valproic acid, valproate sodium, or divalproex may change the time it takes your blood to clot, which may increase the chance of

bleeding. Also, taking valproic acid, valproate sodium, or divalproex together with medicines that are used during surgery or dental or emergency treatments may increase the CNS depressant effects.

Valproic acid, valproate sodium, and divalproex will add to the effects of alcohol and other CNS depressants (medicines that make you drowsy or less alert). Some examples of CNS depressants are antihistamines or medicine for hay fever, other allergies, or colds; sedatives, tranquilizers, or sleeping medicine; prescription pain medicine or narcotics; barbiturates; medicine for seizures; muscle relaxants; or anesthetics, including some dental anesthetics. *Check with your doctor before taking any of the above while you are using this medicine.*

For diabetic patients:

- This medicine may interfere with urine tests for ketones and give false-positive results.

Your doctor may want you to carry a medical identification card or bracelet stating that you are taking this medicine.

This medicine may cause some people to become drowsy or less alert than they are normally. *Make sure you know how you react to this medicine before you drive, use machines, or do anything else that could be dangerous if you are drowsy or not alert.*

Side Effects of This Medicine

Along with its needed effects, a medicine may cause some unwanted effects. Although not all of these side effects may occur, if they do occur they may need medical attention.

Check with your doctor as soon as possible if any of the following side effects occur:
More common
 body aches or pain; congestion; cough; dryness or soreness of throat; fever; hoarseness runny nose; tender, swollen glands in neck; trouble in swallowing; voice changes
Less common
 Abdominal or stomach cramps (severe); behavioral, mood, or mental changes; blurred vision;; confusion;; continuous, uncontrolled back-and-forth and/or rolling eye movements; earache, redness or swelling in ear; dizziness,; double vision; faintness, or light-headedness when getting up from a lying or sitting position suddenly; sweating; unusual tiredness or weakness; fast, irregular, pounding, or racing heartbeat or pulse; heavy, nonmenstrual vaginal bleeding; increase in seizures; loss of appetite; nausea or vomiting (continuing); rapid weight gain; spots before eyes; swelling of face, arms, hands, lower legs, or feet; tingling of hands or feet; tiredness and weakness; unusual bleeding or bruising; unusual weight gain or loss; vomiting of blood or material that looks like coffee grounds; yellow eyes or skin

Other side effects may occur that usually do not need medical attention. These side effects may go away during treatment as your body adjusts to the medicine. However, check with your doctor if any of the following side effects continue or are bothersome:
More common
 Abdominal or stomach cramps (mild); acid or sour stomach; belching; heartburn; indigestion; stomach discomfort, upset or pain; change in menstrual periods;

crying paranoia; quick to react or overreact emotionally; rapidly changing moods; depersonalization; dysphoria; diarrhea; euphoria; hair loss; indigestion; lack or loss of strength; loss of appetite; loss of bowel control; mental depression; nausea and vomiting; paranoia; quick to react or overreact emotionally; rapidly changing moods; sleepiness or unusual drowsiness; trembling of hands and arms; unusual weight loss or gain

Less common or rare

Absence of or decrease in body movement; absent, missed, or irregular menstrual periods; stopping of menstrual bleeding; anxiety; nervousness; restlessness; bloated full feeling; bloody or cloudy urine; bloody nose; bruising; burning, crawling, itching, numbness, prickling, "pins and needles", or tingling feelings; burning, dry or itching eyes; change in taste; chills; clumsiness or unsteadiness; coin-shaped lesions on skin; cold sweats; confusion; constipation; cramps; decreased awareness or responsiveness; degenerative disease of the joint; difficult, burning, or painful urination; difficulty in moving; discharge; excessive tearing of eye; discouragement; dizziness; drowsiness; dry mouth; excess air or gas in stomach or intestines; excessive muscle tone; muscle tension or tightness; muscle stiffness; feeling of constant movement of self or surroundings; feeling sad or empty; feeling of warmth or heat;; flushing or redness of skin, especially on face and neck; frequent urge to urinate; headache; heavy bleeding; irregular heartbeats; irritability; joint pain; swollen joints; lack of appetite; lip smacking; uncontrolled chewing movements; loss of hair; loss of interest or pleasure; loss of memory; problems with memory; mimicry of speech or movements; muscle aching or cramping; muscle pains or stiffness; mutism; negativism; normal menstrual bleeding occurring earlier, possibly lasting longer than expected; pain; passing gas; peculiar postures or movements, mannerisms or grimacing; puffing of cheeks; rapid or worm-like movements of tongue; redness, swelling, or soreness of tongue; severe sleepiness; shortness of breath; difficult or labored breathing; small red or purple spots on skin; stuffy nose; runny nose; sneezing; redness, pain, swelling of eye, eyelid, or inner lining of eyelid; seeing, hearing, or feeling things that are not there; sensation of spinning; shaking; shortness of breath; hyperventilation; skin rash; sweating; tightness in chest; tiredness; trouble concentrating; trouble in speaking; slurred speech; trouble sleeping; uncontrolled chewing movements; uncontrolled movements of arms and legs; unusual excitement, restlessness, or irritability; wheezing

Other side effects not listed above may also occur in some patients. If you notice any other effects, check with your doctor.

VALSARTAN (Oral route) - val-SAR-tan

Black Box Warning

When used in pregnancy during the second and third trimesters, drugs that act directly on the renin-angiotensin system can cause injury and even death to the developing fetus. When pregnancy is detected, valsartan should be discontinued as soon as possible.

Commonly used brand name(s)

In the U.S.—
Diovan

Available Dosage Forms:
- Tablet
- Capsule

Therapeutic Class: Cardiovascular Agent
Pharmacologic Class: Angiotensin II Receptor Antagonist

Uses For This Medicine

Valsartan belongs to the class of medicines called angiotensin II inhibitors. It is used to treat high blood pressure (hypertension). It is also used to treat heart failure and it can lower the need for hospitalization that happens from heart failure. Valsartan can also treat left ventricular dysfunction after a heart attack. Left ventricular dysfunction occurs when the left ventricle (the main pumping chamber of the heart) stiffens and enlarges and can cause the lungs to fill with blood.

High blood pressure adds to the workload of the heart and arteries. If it continues for a long time, the heart and arteries may not function properly. This can damage the blood vessels of the brain, heart, and kidneys, resulting in a stroke, heart failure, or kidney failure. High blood pressure may also increase the risk of heart attacks. These problems may be less likely to occur if blood pressure is controlled.

Valsartan works by blocking the action of a substance in the body that causes blood vessels to tighten. As a result, valsartan relaxes blood vessels. This lowers blood pressure.

This medicine is available only with your doctor's prescription.

Before Using This Medicine

In deciding to use a medicine, the risks of taking the medicine must be weighed against the good it will do. This is a decision you and your doctor will make. For this medicine, the following should be considered:

Allergies—Tell your doctor if you have ever had any unusual or allergic reaction to this medicine or any other medicines. Also tell your health care professional if you have any other types of allergies, such as to foods, dyes, preservatives, or animals. For non-prescription products, read the label or package ingredients carefully.

Pediatric—Studies on this medicine have been done only in adult patients, and there is no specific information comparing use of valsartan in children with use in other age groups.

Geriatric—This medicine has been tested in patients 65 years of age or older and has not been shown to cause different side effects or problems in older people than it does in younger adults. However, blood levels of valsartan and the time it takes for it to be eliminated from the body are increased in the elderly. Additionally, elderly patients may be more sensitive to its effects.

Pregnancy—

	Pregnancy Category	Explanation
1st Trimester	C	Animal studies have shown an adverse effect and there are no adequate studies in pregnant women OR no animal studies have been conducted and there are no adequate studies in pregnant women.
2nd Trimester	D	Studies in pregnant women have demonstrated a risk to the fetus. However, the benefits of therapy in a life threatening situation or a serious disease, may outweigh the potential risk.
3rd Trimester	D	Studies in pregnant women have demonstrated a risk to the fetus. However, the benefits of therapy in a life threatening situation or a serious disease, may outweigh the potential risk.

Breast Feeding—There are no adequate studies in women for determining infant risk when using this medication during breastfeeding. Weigh the potential benefits against the potential risks before taking this medication while breastfeeding.

Other medicines—

Using this medicine with any of the following medicines is usually not recommended, but may be required in some cases. If both medicines are prescribed together, your doctor may change the dose or how often you use one or both of the medicines.

Lithium

Interactions with Food/Tobacco/Alcohol—Certain medicines should not be used at or around the time of eating food or eating certain types of food since interactions may occur. Using alcohol or tobacco with certain medicines may also cause interactions to occur. Discuss with your healthcare professional the use of your medicine with food, alcohol, or tobacco.

Other medical problems—The presence of other medical problems may affect the use of this medicine. Make sure you tell your doctor if you have any other medical problems, especially:

- Dehydration—Blood pressure-lowering effects of valsartan may be increased.
- Heart failure or problems—May cause a decrease in blood pressure
- Kidney disease—Effects of valsartan may make this condition worse.
- Liver disease—Effects of valsartan may be increased because of slower removal of medicine from the body.

Proper Use of This Medicine

Take this medicine only as directed by your doctor. Do not take more of it and do not take it more often than your doctor ordered. This medicine also works best when there is a constant amount in the blood. To help keep the amount constant, do not miss any doses. Also, it is best to take the doses at the same time each day.

Valsartan may be taken with or without food.

Dosing—The dose of this medicine will be different for different patients. Follow your doctor's orders or the directions on the label. The following information includes only the average doses of this medicine. If your dose is different, do not change it unless your doctor tells you to do so.

The amount of medicine that you take depends on the strength of the medicine. Also, the number of doses you take each day, the time allowed between doses, and the length of time you take the medicine depend on the medical problem for which you are using the medicine.

- For oral dosage form (tablets):
  - For high blood pressure:
    - Adults—80 milligrams (mg) or 160 mg once a day. Your doctor may increase your dose as needed.
    - Children—Use and dose must be determined by your doctor.
  - For heart failure:
    - Adults—40 mg twice a day. Your doctor may increase your dose as needed.
    - Children—Use and dose must be determined by your doctor.
  - For left ventricular dysfunction after a heart attack:
    - Adults—20 mg twice a day as early as 12 hours after a heart attack. Your doctor may increase your dose as needed.
    - Children—Use and dose must be determined by your doctor.

Missed dose—If you miss a dose of this medicine, take it as soon as possible. However, if it is almost time for your next dose, skip the missed dose and go back to your regular dosing schedule. Do not double doses.

Storage—Store the medicine in a closed container at room temperature, away from heat, moisture, and direct light. Keep from freezing.

Keep out of the reach of children.

Do not keep outdated medicine or medicine no longer needed.

Precautions While Using This Medicine

It is important that your doctor check your progress at regular visits to make sure that this medicine is working properly and to check for unwanted effects.

Check with your doctor immediately if you think that you may be pregnant. Valsartan may cause birth defects or other problems in the baby if taken during pregnancy.

Do not take other medicines unless they have been discussed with your doctor. This especially includes over-the-counter (nonprescription) medicines for appetite control, asthma, colds, cough, hay fever, or sinus problems, since they may tend to increase your blood pressure.

Dizziness or lightheadedness may occur, especially if you have been taking a diuretic (water pill). Make sure you know how you react to this medicine before you drive, use machines, or do anything else that could be dangerous if you experience these effects.

Check with your doctor right away if you become sick while taking this medicine, especially with severe or continuing nausea and vomiting or diarrhea. These conditions may cause you to lose too much water and lead to low blood pressure.

Dizziness, lightheadedness, or fainting may also occur if you exercise or if the weather is hot. Heavy sweating can cause loss of too much water and result in low blood pressure. Use extra care during exercise or hot weather.

Side Effects of This Medicine

Along with its needed effects, a medicine may cause some unwanted effects. Although not all of these side effects may occur, if they do occur they may need medical attention.

Check with your doctor immediately if any of the following side effects occur:

Less common
  Bloody urine; cold sweats; confusion; decreased frequency/amount of urine; difficult breathing; dizziness, faintness, or lightheadedness when getting up from lying position; fainting; increased blood pressure; increased thirst; irregular heartbeat; loss of appetite; lower back/side pain; nausea; nervousness; numbness or tingling in hands, feet or lips; shortness of breath; swelling of face, fingers, lower legs; troubled breathing; unusual tiredness or weakness; vomiting; weakness or heaviness of legs; weight gain

Rare
  Chills, fever, or sore throat; swelling of face, mouth, hands, or feet; trouble in swallowing or breathing (sudden)

Incidence not known
  Dark urine; general tiredness and weakness; light-colored stools; upper right abdominal pain; yellow eyes and skin

Check with your doctor as soon as possible if any of the following side effects occur:

Rare
  Dizziness, lightheadedness, or fainting; hoarseness

Some side effects may occur that usually do not need medical attention. These side effects may go away during treatment as your body adjusts to the medicine. Also, your health care professional may be able to tell you about ways to prevent or reduce some of these side effects. Check with your health care professional if any of the following side effects continue or are bothersome or if you have any questions about them:

Less common
  Abdominal pain; blurred vision; back pain; cold or flu-like symptoms; coughing; diarrhea; difficulty in moving; headache; muscle pain or stiffness; pain, swelling, or redness in joints; unusual tiredness

Incidence not known
  Hair loss; thinning of hair

Other side effects not listed may also occur in some patients. If you notice any other effects, check with your healthcare professional.

VARDENAFIL (Oral route) - var-DEN-a-fil

Commonly used brand name(s)
In the U.S.—
  Levitra

Available Dosage Forms:
  • Tablet

Therapeutic Class: Erectile Dysfunction Agent
Pharmacologic Class: Phosphodiesterase Type 5 Inhibitor

Uses For This Medicine

Vardenafil belongs to a group of medicines that delay the enzymes (proteins in your body) called phosphodiesterases from working too quickly. The penis is one of the areas where these enzymes work. Vardenafil is used to treat men who have erectile dysfunction (also called sexual impotence). Erectile dysfunction is a condition where the penis does not harden and expand when a man is sexually excited, or when he cannot keep an erection. Vardenafil may help a man get and keep an erection when he is sexually excited. Vardenafil helps to increase the blood flow to the penis and may help men with erectile dysfunction get and keep an erection satisfactory for sexual activity. Once a man has completed sexual activity, blood flow to his penis decreases, and his erection goes away. Vardenafil does not help to cure erectile dysfunction.

This medicine is available only with your doctor's prescription.

Before Using This Medicine

In deciding to use a medicine, the risks of taking the medicine must be weighed against the good it will do. This is a decision you and your doctor will make. For this medicine, the following should be considered:

Allergies—Tell your doctor if you have ever had any unusual or allergic reaction to this medicine or any other medicines. Also tell your health care professional if you have any other types of allergies, such as to foods, dyes, preservatives, or animals. For non-prescription products, read the label or package ingredients carefully.

Geriatric—Elderly people are especially sensitive to the effects of vardenafil, which may increase their chance of having side effects. Patients 65 years of age and older are started on a lower dose than younger adults. The dose may be increased by a doctor as needed and tolerated.

Pregnancy—

	Pregnancy Category	Explanation
All Trimesters	B	Animal studies have revealed no evidence of harm to the fetus, however, there are no adequate studies in pregnant women OR animal studies have shown an adverse effect, but adequate studies in pregnant women have failed to demonstrate a risk to the fetus.

Breast Feeding—There are no adequate studies in women for determining infant risk when using this medication during breastfeeding. Weigh the potential benefits against the potential risks before taking this medication while breastfeeding.

Other medicines—

Using this medicine with any of the following medicines is not recommended. Your doctor may decide not to treat you with this medication or change some of the other medicines you take.

Erythrityl Tetranitrate, Isosorbide Dinitrate, Isosorbide Mononitrate, Nitroglycerin, Pentaerythritol Tetranitrate

Interactions with Food/Tobacco/Alcohol—Certain medicines should not be used at or around the time of eating food or eating certain types of food since interactions may occur. Using alcohol or tobacco with certain medicines may also cause interactions to occur. Discuss with your healthcare professional the use of your medicine with food, alcohol, or tobacco.

Other medical problems—The presence of other medical problems may affect the use of this medicine. Make sure you tell your doctor if you have any other medical problems, especially:

- Age greater than 50 years or
- Coronary artery disease or
- Diabetes or
- Hyperlipidemia (excess of lipids in the blood) or
- Hypertension (high blood pressure) or
- Low cup to disc ratio (' crowded disc') or
- Smoking—These conditions may increase risk for a serious eye problem called NAION.
- Angina (reoccurring chest pain) or
- Arrhythmia (irregular heartbeat) or
- Heart attack (within the last 6 months) or
- Heart failure or
- Hypertension (high blood pressure) or
- Hypotension (low blood pressure) or
- Liver disease (severe) or
- Kidney disease (severe) or
- Retinal disorders (rare hereditary eye problem) or
- Stroke (recent history of)—Vardenafil has not been studied in patients with these medical conditions and should not be used.
- Abnormal penis, including curved penis and birth defects of the penis—Chance of problems occurring may be increased and should be used with caution in these patients.
- Bleeding disorders or
- Stomach ulcers—Chance of problems occurring may be increased; it is not known if the medicine is safe for use in these patients.
- Bone marrow cancer or
- Leukemia or
- Sickle-cell anemia—Vardenafil may cause this condition to become worse.
- Heart disease, underlying—Chance of low blood pressure occurring is greater; vardenafil should be used carefully in these patients.
- Liver disease, moderate—This condition may cause there to be more vardenafil in your body; your doctor may want to start these patients on a lower dose.
- Heart blood flow problems—These conditions may cause you to be more sensitive to vardenafil.
- NAION (serious eye condition) in one or both eyes, previously—May increase your chance of getting NAION again

- QT prolongation (rare heart condition)—Vardenafil may cause this condition to become worse.

Proper Use of This Medicine

Special patient directions come with vardenafil. Read the directions carefully before you start using vardenafil and each time you get a refill of your medicine.

This medicine usually begins to work within 60 minutes after taking it. It continues to work for up to 4 hours. Stimulation is required for an erection. If you have any questions about the use and benefits of vardenafil ask your health care professional.

Dosing—The dose of this medicine will be different for different patients. Follow your doctor's orders or the directions on the label. The following information includes only the average doses of this medicine. If your dose is different, do not change it unless your doctor tells you to do so.

The amount of medicine that you take depends on the strength of the medicine. Also, the number of doses you take each day, the time allowed between doses, and the length of time you take the medicine depend on the medical problem for which you are using the medicine.

- For oral dosage form (tablets):
  - For treatment of erectile dysfunction:
    - Adults up to 65 years of age—10 mg as a single dose no more than once a day, 1 hour before sexual activity. If needed, your doctor may change your dose.
    - Adults 65 years of age and older—5 mg as a single dose no more than once a day, 1 hour before sexual intercourse. If needed, your doctor may change your dose.

Storage—Store the medicine in a closed container at room temperature, away from heat, moisture, and direct light. Keep from freezing.

Keep out of the reach of children.

Do not keep outdated medicine or medicine no longer needed.

Ask your healthcare professional how you should dispose of any medicine you do not use.

Precautions While Using This Medicine

Vardenafil has not been studied with other medicines used for treatment of erectile dysfunction. Using them together is not recommended.

Use vardenafil exactly as directed by your doctor. Do not use more of it and do not use it more often than your doctor ordered. If too much is used, the chance of side effects is increased.

It is important that you tell all of your healthcare providers that you take vardenafil. If you need emergency medical care for a heart problem, it is important that your healthcare provider knows when you last took vardenafil.

If you experience a prolonged or painful erection for 4 hours or more, contact your doctor immediately. This condition may require prompt medical treatment to prevent serious and permanent damage to your penis.

This medicine does not protect you against sexually transmitted diseases. Use protective measures and ask your doctor if you have any questions about this.

It is important to tell your doctor about any heart problems you may have now or may have had in the past. This medicine can cause serious side effects in patients with heart problems.

If you experience sudden loss of vision in one or both eyes, stop using vardenafil and contact your doctor immediately.

Side Effects of This Medicine

Along with its needed effects, a medicine may cause some unwanted effects. Although not all of these side effects may occur, if they do occur they may need medical attention.

Check with your doctor immediately if any of the following side effects occur:

Less common

Arm, back or jaw pain; blindness; blurred vision; chest pain or discomfort; chest tightness or heaviness; chills; cold sweats; confusion; decreased vision; difficult or labored breathing; difficulty swallowing; dizziness; dizziness, faintness, or lightheadedness when getting up from lying or sitting position; eye pain; fainting; fast, irregular, pounding, or racing heartbeat or pulse; headache; hives; itching; nausea; nervousness; pain or discomfort in arms, jaw, back or neck; pounding in the ears; puffiness or swelling of the eyelids or around the eyes, face, lips or tongue; shortness of breath; skin rash; slow or fast heartbeat; sweating; tearing; tightness in chest; unusual tiredness or weakness; vomiting; wheezing

Some side effects may occur that usually do not need medical attention. These side effects may go away during treatment as your body adjusts to the medicine. Also, your health care professional may be able to tell you about ways to prevent or reduce some of these side effects. Check with your health care professional if any of the following side effects continue or are bothersome or if you have any questions about them:

More common

Feeling of warmth and redness of the face, neck, arms and occasionally, upper chest; sneezing; stuffy nose

Less common

Abnormal ejaculation; abnormal vision; abdominal pain; acid or sour stomach; back pain; belching; bloody nose; body aches or pain; burning, crawling, itching, numbness, prickling, "pins and needles", or tingling feelings; burning feeling in chest or stomach; changes in color vision; changes in vision; congestion; cough; diarrhea; difficulty in moving; difficulty seeing at night; difficulty swallowing; dim vision; dry mouth; dryness or soreness of throat; eye pain; excessive muscle tone; face swelling; fast heartbeat; feeling of constant movement of self or surroundings; fever; general feeling of discomfort or illness; heartburn; hoarseness; increased redness of the eye; increased sensitivity of eyes to sunlight; indigestion; itching skin; joint pain; lack or loss of strength; loss of appetite; muscle aches and pains; muscle cramping; muscle stiffness; muscle tension or tightness; neck pain; pain; pain or burning in throat; runny nose; sensation of spinning; shivering; sleepiness or unusual drowsiness; sleeplessness; sore throat; sores, ulcers, or white spots on lips or tongue or inside the mouth; stomach discomfort, upset, or pain; swollen joints; tenderness in stomach area; tender,

swollen glands in neck; trouble in swallowing; trouble sleeping; unable to sleep; voice changes; watery eyes

Other side effects not listed may also occur in some patients. If you notice any other effects, check with your healthcare professional.

VARENICLINE (Oral route) - var-EN-i-kleen

Commonly used brand name(s)

In the U.S.—
Chantix

Available Dosage Forms:
- Tablet

Therapeutic Class: Smoking Cessation Agent

Uses For This Medicine

Varenicline is used as part of a support program to help you stop smoking. Educational materials and necessary counseling should also be provided as part of the support program.

This medicine is available only with your doctor's prescription.

Before Using This Medicine

In deciding to use a medicine, the risks of taking the medicine must be weighed against the good it will do. This is a decision you and your doctor will make. For this medicine, the following should be considered:

Allergies—Tell your doctor if you have ever had any unusual or allergic reaction to this medicine or any other medicines. Also tell your health care professional if you have any other types of allergies, such as to foods, dyes, preservatives, or animals. For non-prescription products, read the label or package ingredients carefully.

Pediatric—Appropriate studies have not been performed on the relationship of age to the effects of varenicline in in children up to 18 years of age. Safety and efficacy have not been established and use is not recommended.

Geriatric—Appropriate studies performed to date have not demonstrated geriatrics-specific problems that would limit the usefulness of varenicline in the elderly. However, elderly patients are more likely to have age-related kidney problems, which may require care in dosing and monitoring in patients receiving varenicline.

Pregnancy—

	Pregnancy Category	Explanation
All Trimesters	C	Animal studies have shown an adverse effect and there are no adequate studies in pregnant women OR no animal studies have been conducted and there are no adequate studies in pregnant women.

Breast Feeding—There are no adequate studies in women for determining infant risk when using this medication during

breastfeeding. Weigh the potential benefits against the potential risks before taking this medication while breastfeeding.

Other medicines—Although certain medicines should not be used together at all, in other cases two different medicines may be used together even if an interaction might occur. In these cases, your doctor may want to change the dose, or other precautions may be necessary. Tell your healthcare professional if you are taking any other prescription or nonprescription (over-the-counter [OTC]) medicine.

Interactions with Food/Tobacco/Alcohol—Certain medicines should not be used at or around the time of eating food or eating certain types of food since interactions may occur. Using alcohol or tobacco with certain medicines may also cause interactions to occur. Discuss with your healthcare professional the use of your medicine with food, alcohol, or tobacco.

Other medical problems—The presence of other medical problems may affect the use of this medicine. Make sure you tell your doctor if you have any other medical problems, especially:

- Kidney problems—Caution should be used. For severe kidney problems, your doctor will start you on a lower dose.

Proper Use of This Medicine

You should set a date to stop smoking. You should start taking varenicline *one week before* this date.

You should take this medicine with a full glass of water after eating.

Dosing—The dose of this medicine will be different for different patients. Follow your doctor's orders or the directions on the label. The following information includes only the average doses of this medicine. If your dose is different, do not change it unless your doctor tells you to do so.

The amount of medicine that you take depends on the strength of the medicine. Also, the number of doses you take each day, the time allowed between doses, and the length of time you take the medicine depend on the medical problem for which you are using the medicine.

- For an aid to stop smoking:
  - For oral dosage form (tablet):
    - Adults:
      - Days 1 to 3: 0.5 mg one time a day
      - Days 4 to 7: 0.5 mg two times a day
      - Days 8 to End of treatment: 1 mg twice a day
    - Children: Use and dose will be determined by your doctor.

If you have successfully stopped smoking at the end of 12 weeks, your doctor may prescribe another 12 weeks of this medicine to increase your long-term abstinence.

If you do not succeed in stopping smoking during the first 12 weeks or if you relapse during treatment, you should make another attempt after you have addressed concerns with your doctor.

Storage—Store the medicine in a closed container at room temperature, away from heat, moisture, and direct light. Keep from freezing.

Precautions While Using This Medicine

If your symptoms, especially nausea and insomnia, do not improve or if they persist, check with your doctor.

You should inform your doctor of any medicines that you are taking. After you quit smoking, your doctor may need to adjust doses on some of your medicines.

Side Effects of This Medicine

Along with its needed effects, a medicine may cause some unwanted effects. Although not all of these side effects may occur, if they do occur they may need medical attention.

Check with your doctor immediately if any of the following side effects occur:

Less common
> Difficult or labored breathing; shortness of breath; tightness in chest; wheezing

Some side effects may occur that usually do not need medical attention. These side effects may go away during treatment as your body adjusts to the medicine. Also, your health care professional may be able to tell you about ways to prevent or reduce some of these side effects. Check with your health care professional if any of the following side effects continue or are bothersome or if you have any questions about them:

More common
> Abnormal dreams; bloated, full feeling; difficulty having a bowel movement (stool); dry mouth; excess air or gas in stomach or intestines; general feeling of discomfort or illness; headache; lack or loss of strength; nausea; passing gas; sleeplessness; stomach pain; trouble sleeping; unable to sleep; unusual tiredness or weakness

Less common
> Acid or sour stomach; belching; body aches or pain; change in taste; chills; cough; decreased appetite; ear congestion; fever; heartburn; increased appetite; indigestion; itching skin; loss of appetite; loss of taste; loss of voice; nasal congestion; nightmare; rash; runny nose; sleepiness or unusual drowsiness; sneezing or sore throat; stomach discomfort or upset; unusual drowsiness, dullness, or feeling of sluggishness; vomiting

Other side effects not listed may also occur in some patients. If you notice any other effects, check with your healthcare professional.

VENLAFAXINE (Oral route) - VEN-la-fax-een

Black Box Warning

Antidepressants increased the risk of suicidal thinking and behavior (suicidality) in short-term studies in children and adolescents with Major Depressive Disorder (MDD) and other psychiatric disorders. Anyone considering the use of venlafaxine hydrochloride or any other antidepressant in a child or adolescent must balance this risk with the clinical need. Patients who are started on therapy should be observed closely for clinical worsening, suicidality, or unusual changes in behavior. Families and caregivers should be advised of the need for close observation and communication with the prescriber. Venlafaxine hydrochloride is not approved for use in pediatric patients.

Pooled analyses of short-term (4 to 6 weeks) placebo-controlled trials of 9 anti depressant drugs (SSRIs and others) in children and adolescents with MDD, obsessive compulsive disorder (OCD), or other psychiatric disorders (a total of 24 trials involving over 4400 patients) have revealed a greater risk of adverse events representing suicidal thinking or behavior (suicidality) during the first few months of treatment in those receiving antidepressants. The average risk of such events in patients receiving antidepressants was 4%, twice the placebo risk of 2%. No suicides occurred in these trials.

Commonly used brand name(s)

In the U.S.—
   Effexor
   Effexor-XR

Available Dosage Forms:
- Capsule, Extended Release
- Tablet

Therapeutic Class: Antidepressant
Pharmacologic Class: Antidepressant, Bicyclic

Uses For This Medicine

Venlafaxine is used to treat mental depression. It is also used to treat certain anxiety disorders or to relieve the symptoms of anxiety. However, it usually is not used for anxiety or tension caused by the stress of everyday life. Venlafaxine is also used to treat panic disorders.

This medicine is available only with your doctor's prescription.

Once a medicine has been approved for marketing for a certain use, experience may show that it is also useful for other medical problems. Although this use is not included in product labeling, venlafaxine is used in certain patients with the following medical condition:
- Hot flashes

Before Using This Medicine

In deciding to use a medicine, the risks of taking the medicine must be weighed against the good it will do. This is a decision you and your doctor will make. For this medicine, the following should be considered:

Allergies—Tell your doctor if you have ever had any unusual or allergic reaction to this medicine or any other medicines. Also tell your health care professional if you have any other types of allergies, such as to foods, dyes, preservatives, or animals. For non-prescription products, read the label or package ingredients carefully.

Pediatric—Venlafaxine must be used with caution in children with depression. Studies have shown occurrences of children thinking about suicide or attempting suicide in clinical trials for this medicine. More study is needed to be sure venlafaxine is safe and effective in children.

Geriatric—In studies done to date that have included elderly people, venlafaxine did not cause different side effects or problems in older people than it did in younger adults.

Pregnancy—

	Pregnancy Category	Explanation
All Trimesters	C	Animal studies have shown an adverse effect and there are no adequate studies in pregnant women OR no animal studies have been conducted and there are no adequate studies in pregnant women.

Breast Feeding—Studies in women suggest that this medication poses minimal risk to the infant when used during breastfeeding.

Other medicines—

Using this medicine with any of the following medicines is not recommended. Your doctor may decide not to treat you with this medication or change some of the other medicines you take.

Bepridil, Cisapride, Clorgyline, Furazolidone, Iproniazid, Isocarboxazid, Levomethadyl, Mesoridazine, Moclobemide, Nialamide, Pargyline, Phenelzine, Pimozide, Procarbazine, Selegiline, Terfenadine, Thioridazine, Toloxatone, Tranylcypromine, Trifluoperazine

Interactions with Food/Tobacco/Alcohol—Certain medicines should not be used at or around the time of eating food or eating certain types of food since interactions may occur. Using alcohol or tobacco with certain medicines may also cause interactions to occur. Discuss with your healthcare professional the use of your medicine with food, alcohol, or tobacco.

Other medical problems—The presence of other medical problems may affect the use of this medicine. Make sure you tell your doctor if you have any other medical problems, especially:
- Bipolar disorder (mood disorder with alternating episodes of mania and depression) or risk of—May make condition worse. Your doctor will check you for this condition.
- Brain disease or damage, or mental retardation or
- Seizures (history of)—The risk of seizures may be increased
- Dehydration—Venlafaxine may cause serious problems in patients who are dehydrated.
- Glaucoma or
- Pressure within the eye—Venlafaxine may cause abnormal dilation of the pupil or other eye problems in these patients.
- Heart attack or
- Heart failure or
- Hyperthyroidism (overactive thyroid)—Venlafaxine may cause an increase in heart rate and should be used with caution in these patients.
- Heart disease or
- High or low blood pressure—Venlafaxine may make these conditions worse
- Kidney disease or
- Liver disease or

- Cirrhosis of the liver—Higher blood levels of venlafaxine may occur, increasing the chance of side effects; your doctor may need to adjust your venlafaxine dose.
- Mania (history of)—The risk of developing mania may be increased
- Weight loss—Venlafaxine may cause weight loss; this weight loss is usually small, but if a large weight loss occurs, it may be harmful in some patients

Proper Use of This Medicine

Take this medicine only as directed by your doctor to benefit your condition as much as possible. Do not take more of it, do not take it more often, and do not take it for a longer time than your doctor ordered.

You may have to take venlafaxine for 4 weeks or longer before you begin to feel better. Also, you will probably need to keep taking this medicine for at least 6 months, even if you feel better, to help prevent your depression from returning. Your doctor should check your progress at regular visits during this time.

Venlafaxine should be taken with food or on a full stomach to lessen the chance of stomach upset. However, if your doctor tells you to take the medicine a certain way, take it exactly as directed.

If you are taking the extended-release capsule dosage form, swallow the capsule whole with fluid; do not break, crush, chew, or place the capsule in liquid.

Dosing—The dose of this medicine will be different for different patients. Follow your doctor's orders or the directions on the label. The following information includes only the average doses of this medicine. If your dose is different, do not change it unless your doctor tells you to do so.

The amount of medicine that you take depends on the strength of the medicine. Also, the number of doses you take each day, the time allowed between doses, and the length of time you take the medicine depend on the medical problem for which you are using the medicine.

- For mental depression:
  - For oral extended-release capsule dosage form:
    - Adults—At first, 75 milligrams (mg) a day, taken in one dose in the morning or evening. Your doctor may increase your dose if needed. However, the dose is usually not more than 225 mg a day.
    - Children—Use and dose must be determined by your doctor.
  - For oral tablet dosage form:
    - Adults—At first, a total of 75 mg a day, taken in smaller doses two or three times during the day. Your doctor may increase your dose if needed. However, the dose is usually not more than 375 mg a day.
    - Children up to 18 years of age—Use and dose must be determined by your doctor.
- For anxiety:
  - For oral extended-release capsule dosage form:
    - Adults—At first, 75 mg a day, taken in one dose in the morning or evening. Your doctor may increase your dose if needed. However, the dose is usually not more than 225 mg per day.
    - Children—Use and dose must be determined by your doctor.

- For panic disorder:
  - For oral extended-release capsule dosage form:
    - Adults—At first, 37.5 mg a day, taken in one dose in the morning or evening for 7 days. Your doctor may increase your dose if needed. However, the dose is usually not more than 225 mg per day.
    - Children—Use and dose must be determined by your doctor.

Missed dose—If you miss a dose of this medicine, take it as soon as possible. However, if it is almost time for your next dose, skip the missed dose and go back to your regular dosing schedule. Do not double doses.

Storage—Store the medicine in a closed container at room temperature, away from heat, moisture, and direct light. Keep from freezing.

Keep out of the reach of children.

Do not keep outdated medicine or medicine no longer needed.

Precautions While Using This Medicine

It is important that your doctor check your progress at regular visits, to allow for changes in your dose and to help reduce any side effects.

Tell your doctor right away if you develop any allergic reactions, such as skin rash or hives, while taking venlafaxine.

Venlafaxine may cause some people to be agitated, irritable or display other abnormal behaviors. It may also cause some people to have suicidal thoughts and tendencies or to become more depressed. If you or your caregiver notice any of these adverse effects, tell your doctor right away.

Do not stop taking this medicine without first checking with your doctor. Your doctor may want you to reduce gradually the amount you are taking before stopping completely. This is to decrease the chance of side effects.

It is not known how venlafaxine will interact with alcohol and other central nervous system (CNS) depressants (medicines that may make you drowsy or less alert). Some examples of CNS depressants are antihistamines or medicine for hay fever, other allergies, or colds; sedatives, tranquilizers, or sleeping medicine; prescription pain medicine or narcotics; barbiturates; medicine for seizures; muscle relaxants; or anesthetics, including some dental anesthetics. Check with your doctor before taking any of the above while you are using this medicine.

Venlafaxine may cause some people to become drowsy or have blurred vision. Make sure you know how you react to this medicine before you drive, use machines, or do anything else that could be dangerous if you are not alert or able to see clearly.

Dizziness, lightheadedness, or fainting may occur, especially when you get up from a lying or sitting position. Getting up slowly may help. If this problem continues or gets worse, check with your doctor.

Side Effects of This Medicine

Along with its needed effects, a medicine may cause some unwanted effects. Although not all of these side effects may occur, if they do occur they may need medical attention.

Check with your doctor as soon as possible if any of the following side effects occur:

More common

Changes in vision, such as blurred vision; headache

Less common

Chest pain; fast or irregular heartbeat; mood or mental changes; ringing or buzzing in ears

Rare

Convulsions (seizures); itching or skin rash; lightheadedness or fainting, especially when getting up suddenly from a sitting or lying position; lockjaw; menstrual changes; problems in urinating or in holding urine; swelling; talking, feeling, and acting with excitement and activity you cannot control; trouble in breathing

Incidence not known

Abdominal or stomach pain; agitation; black, tarry stools; bleeding gums; blistering, peeling, loosening of skin; bloating of abdomen; blood in eye; bloody urine; bloody, black, or tarry stools; blue-green to black skin; chest pain or discomfort; coma; confusion; confusion as to time, place, or person; cough or hoarseness; coughing up blood; dark urine; decreased awareness or responsiveness; decreased frequency/amount of urine; depression; difficulty in breathing or swallowing; discoloration, pain, redness, or sloughing of skin at place of injection; dry cough; extra heartbeats; eye pain; fast, pounding, or irregular heartbeat or pulse; fast, slow, or irregular heartbeat; fever with or without chills; general feeling of tiredness or weakness; hallucinations; hearing loss; high fever; hives; holding false beliefs that can not be changed by fact; hostility; increased menstrual flow or vaginal bleeding; increased thirst; indigestion; involuntary movements; irregular heartbeats; irritability; joint or muscle pain; lethargy; light-colored stools; lip smacking or puckering; low blood pressure; lower back or side pain; mimicry of speech or movements; muscle cramps or spasms; muscle pain or stiffness; muscle twitching; mutism; negativism; nosebleeds; overactive reflexes; pain, redness or swelling in arm or leg; painful or difficult urination; pains in stomach, side, or abdomen, possibly radiating to the back; palpitations; panic; paralysis; peculiar postures or movements, mannerisms, or grimacing; poor coordination; pounding or rapid pulse; prolonged bleeding from cuts; puffiness or swelling of the eyelids or around the eyes, face, lips, or tongue; puffing of cheeks; rapid breathing; rapid or worm-like movements of tongue; rapid weight gain; rash; recurrent fainting; red or dark brown urine; red skin lesions, often with a purple center; red, irritated eyes; redness in whites of eyes; restlessness; seizures; severe muscle stiffness; severe sleepiness; shivering; shock-like electrical sensations; sore throat; sores, ulcers, or white spots in mouth or on lips; stupor; sweating; swelling of face, lower legs, ankles, hands, or fingers; swollen or painful glands; talking or acting with excitement you cannot control; tightness in chest; tiredness; twitching; twitching, twisting, uncontrolled repetitive movements of tongue, lips, face, arms, or legs; uncontrolled chewing movements; uncontrolled movements of arms and legs; unexplained bleeding or bruising; unpleasant breath odor; unusual excitement, nervousness or restlessness; unusually pale skin; vomiting of blood or material that looks like coffee grounds; weight gain; wheezing; yellow eyes or skin

Symptoms of overdose

Agitation; convulsions (seizures); drowsiness; extreme tiredness or weakness; fast heartbeat; tingling, burning, or prickling sensations; trembling or shaking

This medicine may also cause the following side effect that your doctor will watch for:

More common

High blood pressure

Some side effects may occur that usually do not need medical attention. These side effects may go away during treatment as your body adjusts to the medicine. Also, your health care professional may be able to tell you about ways to prevent or reduce some of these side effects. Check with your health care professional if any of the following side effects continue or are bothersome or if you have any questions about them:

More common

Abnormal dreams; anxiety or nervousness; chills; constipation; decrease in sexual desire or ability; diarrhea; dizziness; drowsiness; dryness of mouth; heartburn; increased sweating; loss of appetite; nausea; stuffy or runny nose; stomach pain or gas; tingling, burning, or prickly sensations; trembling or shaking; trouble in sleeping; unusual tiredness or weakness; vomiting; weight loss

Less common

Change in sense of taste; muscle tension; yawning

Incidence not known

Night sweats

After you stop using this medicine, it may still produce some side effects that need attention. During this period of time, *check with your doctor immediately* if you notice the following side effects:

Actions that are out of control; anxiety; changes in dreaming; continuing ringing or buzzing or other unexplained noise in ears; convulsions; crying; depersonalization; diarrhea; difficulty with coordination; dizziness; dryness of mouth; dysphoria; euphoria; fear; feeling of constant movement of self or surroundings; feeling unwell or unhappy; headache; hearing loss; hyperventilation; increased sweating; irregular heartbeats; irritability; lightheadedness; loss of appetite; loss of bladder control; mental depression; mood or mental changes; muscle spasm or jerking of all extremities; nausea; nervousness; nightmares; paranoia; quick to react or overreact emotionally; rapidly changing moods; restlessness; sensation of spinning; sensory disturbances (including shock-like electrical sensations; shakiness in legs, arms, hands, feet; shaking; shaking of hands or feet; shortness of breath; sleeping or unusual drowsiness; sudden loss of consciousness; talking, feeling, and acting with excitement; trembling or shaking of hands or feet; trouble in sleeping; twitches of the muscle visible under the skin; unusual drowsiness, dullness or feeling of sluggishness; unusual tiredness or weakness; vomiting; weight loss

Other side effects not listed may also occur in some patients. If you notice any other effects, check with your healthcare professional.

VERTEPORFIN (Intravenous route, Injection route) - ver-te-POR-fin

Commonly used brand name(s)

In the U.S.—

Visudyne

Available Dosage Forms:
* Powder for Solution

Therapeutic Class: Photosensitizing Agent

Uses For This Medicine

Verteporfin is used together with a special laser light, to treat abnormal blood vessel formation in a part of the eye which, if left untreated, can lead to a loss of eyesight.

Verteporfin may also be used for the following problems:
* Pathologic myopia (changes in the eyeball causing vision problems);
* Ocular histoplasmosis (damage to the eye from a fungus found in the soil)

This medicine is to be administered only by or under the immediate supervision of your doctor.

Before Using This Medicine

In deciding to use a medicine, the risks of taking the medicine must be weighed against the good it will do. This is a decision you and your doctor will make. For this medicine, the following should be considered:

Allergies—Tell your doctor if you have ever had any unusual or allergic reaction to this medicine or any other medicines. Also tell your health care professional if you have any other types of allergies, such as to foods, dyes, preservatives, or animals. For non-prescription products, read the label or package ingredients carefully.

Pediatric—Studies on this medicine have been done only in adult patients, and there is no specific information comparing use of verteporfin in children with use in other age groups.

Geriatric—Studies show that the effects of verteporfin are less in patients 75 years of age or older.

Pregnancy—

	Pregnancy Category	Explanation
All Trimesters	C	Animal studies have shown an adverse effect and there are no adequate studies in pregnant women OR no animal studies have been conducted and there are no adequate studies in pregnant women.

Breast Feeding—There are no adequate studies in women for determining infant risk when using this medication during breastfeeding. Weigh the potential benefits against the potential risks before taking this medication while breastfeeding.

Other medicines—Although certain medicines should not be used together at all, in other cases two different medicines may be used together even if an interaction might occur. In these cases, your doctor may want to change the dose, or other precautions may be necessary. Tell your healthcare professional if you are taking any other prescription or nonprescription (over-the-counter [OTC]) medicine.

Interactions with Food/Tobacco/Alcohol—Certain medicines should not be used at or around the time of eating food or eating certain types of food since interactions may occur. Using alcohol or tobacco with certain medicines may also cause interactions to occur. Discuss with your healthcare professional the use of your medicine with food, alcohol, or tobacco.

Other medical problems—The presence of other medical problems may affect the use of this medicine. Make sure you tell your doctor if you have any other medical problems, especially:
* Liver function impairment
* Porphyria—Sensitivity to light may be increased
* Previous reaction to verteporfin—Reaction is more likely to occur again

Proper Use of This Medicine

Treatment with verteporfin and laser light occurs in two steps. First, the verteporfin is injected into your body. Second, 15 minutes later, a laser light is directed at the affected eye.

Dosing—The dose of this medicine will be different for different patients. Follow your doctor's orders or the directions on the label. The following information includes only the average doses of this medicine. If your dose is different, do not change it unless your doctor tells you to do so.

The amount of medicine that you take depends on the strength of the medicine. Also, the number of doses you take each day, the time allowed between doses, and the length of time you take the medicine depend on the medical problem for which you are using the medicine.

Precautions While Using This Medicine

For 5 days after you receive an injection of verteporfin, your eyes will be extra sensitive to light, including sunlight and bright indoor lights. Certain types of sunglasses can help protect your eyes during this time. Check with your doctor about which sunglasses to use.

For 5 days after you receive an injection of verteporfin, your skin will be extra sensitive to sunlight and to very bright indoor lights, such as tanning lamps, bright halogen lighting and lights in dental offices or operating rooms. Do not expose your skin to direct sunlight or to bright indoor lights during this time. Sunscreens will not protect your skin from a severe reaction to light (blistering, burning, and swelling of the skin). However, exposure to normal amounts of indoor light (for example, daylight or light from lamps with shades) will help clear up the verteporfin remaining in your skin. Therefore, do not protect your skin from normal amounts of indoor light. If you have any questions about whether the light in your home is too bright, check with your doctor or nurse. If you do have a severe reaction to light, call your doctor immediately.

Side Effects of This Medicine

Along with its needed effects, a medicine may cause some unwanted effects. Although not all of these side effects may occur, if they do occur they may need medical attention.

Check with your doctor immediately if any of the following side effects occur:
> *More common*
> Blurred vision or other change in vision
>
> *Less common*
> Decrease in vision, may be severe; dizziness; dull nervousness; eye pain; fainting; fast, slow, or irregular heartbeat; itching, redness, or other irritation of eye; pale skin; pounding in the ears; troubled breathing on

exertion; unusual bleeding or bruising; unusual tiredness or weakness

Some side effects may occur that usually do not need medical attention. These side effects may go away during treatment as your body adjusts to the medicine. Also, your health care professional may be able to tell you about ways to prevent or reduce some of these side effects. Check with your health care professional if any of the following side effects continue or are bothersome or if you have any questions about them:

More common
Bleeding, blistering, burning, coldness, discoloration of skin, feeling of pressure, infection, itching, numbness, pain, rash, redness, scarring, stinging, swelling, tenderness, tingling, ulceration, and/or warmth at the injection site; headache

Less common
Back pain (during infusion of verteporfin); chills; cloudy urine; constipation; cough; decreased hearing; decreased sensitivity to touch; diarrhea; difficult or painful urination; difficulty in moving; double vision; dry eyes; feeling of constant movement of self or surroundings; fever; general feeling of discomfort or illness; hoarseness; increased sensitivity of skin to sunlight; joint pain; light headedness; loss of appetite; loss of strength or energy; muscle pain or stiffness; nausea; pain, swelling, or redness in joints; pelvic discomfort; redness or other discoloration of skin; runny nose; severe sunburn; shivering; skin rash; sore throat; sweating; tearing; tender, swollen glands in neck; throat congestion; trouble in sleeping; trouble in swallowing; trouble sleeping; varicose veins; voice changes; vomiting

Other side effects not listed may also occur in some patients. If you notice any other effects, check with your healthcare professional.

VIGABATRIN (Oral route) - vye-GA-ba-trin

Commonly used brand name(s)

In Canada—
Sabril

Available Dosage Forms:
- Powder
- Tablet

Therapeutic Class: Anticonvulsant
Pharmacologic Class: Gamma Aminobutyric Acid Transaminase Inhibitor

Uses For This Medicine

Vigabatrin increases the amount of the brain chemical GABA. It is thought that epileptic seizures are the result of low levels of GABA. By increasing the amount of GABA, vigabatrin reduces the likelihood of an epileptic seizure.

This medicine is available only with your doctor's prescription.

Before Using This Medicine

In deciding to use a medicine, the risks of taking the medicine must be weighed against the good it will do. This is a decision you and your doctor will make. For this medicine, the following should be considered:

Allergies—Tell your doctor if you have ever had any unusual or allergic reaction to this medicine or any other medicines. Also tell your health care professional if you have any other types of allergies, such as to foods, dyes, preservatives, or animals. For non-prescription products, read the label or package ingredients carefully.

Pediatric—This medicine has been tested in children and, in effective doses, has not been shown to cause different problems than it does in adults.

Geriatric—Many medicines have not been studied specifically in older people. Therefore, it may not be known whether they work exactly the same way they do in younger adults or if they cause different side effects or problems in older people. There is no specific information comparing use of vigabatrin in the elderly with use in other age groups.

Breast Feeding—There are no adequate studies in women for determining infant risk when using this medication during breastfeeding. Weigh the potential benefits against the potential risks before taking this medication while breastfeeding.

Other medicines—

Using this medicine with any of the following medicines is usually not recommended, but may be required in some cases. If both medicines are prescribed together, your doctor may change the dose or how often you use one or both of the medicines.

Carbamazepine

Interactions with Food/Tobacco/Alcohol—Certain medicines should not be used at or around the time of eating food or eating certain types of food since interactions may occur. Using alcohol or tobacco with certain medicines may also cause interactions to occur. Discuss with your healthcare professional the use of your medicine with food, alcohol, or tobacco.

Other medical problems—The presence of other medical problems may affect the use of this medicine. Make sure you tell your doctor if you have any other medical problems, especially:
- Mental illness—Patients with a history of emotional or behavioral disturbances may be more likely to have an episode following vigabatrin therapy.
- Kidney disease—Vigabatrin is removed from the body by the kidney; slower removal from the body may increase the chance of side effects

Proper Use of This Medicine

Dosing—The dose of this medicine will be different for different patients. Follow your doctor's orders or the directions on the label. The following information includes only the average doses of this medicine. If your dose is different, do not change it unless your doctor tells you to do so.

The amount of medicine that you take depends on the strength of the medicine. Also, the number of doses you take each day, the time allowed between doses, and the length of time you take the medicine depend on the medical problem for which you are using the medicine.

- For oral dosage form (powder):
  - For epilepsy
    - Adults—To start, 1000 milligrams (mg) a day. The doctor may need to adjust the dose depending on your response to the medicine. However, the dose is usually not more than 4000 mg a day.
    - Children—The dose is based on body weight and will be determined by your doctor. To start, 40 milligrams (mg) per kilogram (kg) (18.2 mg per pound) of body weight per day. Your doctor may increase your dose as needed. However, the dose is usually not more than 100 mg per kg (45.5 mg per pound) of body weight a day, taken in two smaller doses.
  - For infantile spasms
    - Children—The dose is based on body weight and will be determined by your doctor. The usual dose is 50 to 100 mg per kg (22.7 to 45.5 mg per pound) of body weight per day, given in smaller doses twice a day. The doctor may need to adjust the dose based on your response to the medicine.
- For oral dosage form (tablets):
  - For epilepsy
    - Adults—To start, 1000 milligrams (mg) a day. The doctor may need to adjust the dose depending on your response to the medicine. However, the dose is usually not more than 4000 mg a day.
    - Children—The dose is based on body weight and will be determined by your doctor. To start, 40 mg per kg (18.2 mg per pound) of body weight a day. Your doctor may increase your dose as needed. However, the dose is usually not more than 100 mg per kg (45.5 mg per pound) of body weight a day, taken in two smaller doses.

Missed dose—If you miss a dose of this medicine, take it as soon as possible. However, if it is almost time for your next dose, skip the missed dose and go back to your regular dosing schedule. Do not double doses.

Storage—Store the medicine in a closed container at room temperature, away from heat, moisture, and direct light. Keep from freezing.

Keep out of the reach of children.

Do not keep outdated medicine or medicine no longer needed.

Ask your healthcare professional how you should dispose of any medicine you do not use.

Precautions While Using This Medicine

It is important that you visit your physician.

If you will be taking this medicine for a long time, it is very important that your eye doctor check you approximately every 3 months for any visual problems.

If your symptoms do not improve or if they become worse, check with your doctor.

Do not take other medicines unless they have been discussed with your doctor.

This medicine may cause some people to become drowsy, dizzy, or less alert than they are normally. Make sure you know how you react to this medicine before you drive, use machines, or do anything else that could be dangerous if you are dizzy, drowsy, or not alert,.

Do not suddenly stop taking this medicine without first checking with your doctor. Your doctor may want to reduce your dose gradually. Stopping this medicine suddenly may cause seizures.

Side Effects of This Medicine

Along with its needed effects, a medicine may cause some unwanted effects. Although not all of these side effects may occur, if they do occur they may need medical attention.

Check with your doctor immediately if any of the following side effects occur:
  More common
    Amnesia; blurred vision; blue-yellow color blindness; decreased vision or other vision changes; eye pain; increase in seizures

  Less common or rare
    Uncontrolled rolling eye movements

  Symptoms of overdose

  Get emergency help immediately if any of the following symptoms of overdose occur:
    Mood or mental changes

Some side effects may occur that usually do not need medical attention. These side effects may go away during treatment as your body adjusts to the medicine. Also, your health care professional may be able to tell you about ways to prevent or reduce some of these side effects. Check with your health care professional if any of the following side effects continue or are bothersome or if you have any questions about them:
  More common
    Abdominal pain; abnormal coordination; agitation; anxiety; clumsiness; confusion; constipation; mental depression; diarrhea; dizziness; drowsiness; double vision or seeing double; fatigue; hyperactivity; increased movement; joint pain; burning, tingling, or prickly sensations; shakiness; sleepiness or unusual drowsiness; trembling; tremor; unsteadiness

  Less common
    Aggression; concentration impaired; headache; increased saliva; insomnia; muscle weakness; nausea; speech disorder; thinking abnormal; vomiting; weight gain

Other side effects not listed may also occur in some patients. If you notice any other effects, check with your healthcare professional.

VINBLASTINE   (Intravenous route) -
vin-BLAS-teen

Black Box Warning

Caution - This preparation should be administered by individuals experienced in the administration of vinblastine sulfate. It is extremely important that the needle be properly positioned in the vein before this product is injected. If leakage into surrounding tissue should occur during intravenous administration of vinblastine sulfate, it may cause considerable irritation. The injection should be discontinued immediately, and any remaining portion of the dose should then be introduced into another vein. Local injection of hyaluronidase and the application of moderate heat to the area of leakage help disperse the drug and are thought to minimize discomfort and the possibility of cellulitis.

Fatal if given intrathecally. For intravenous use only.

Commonly used brand name(s)

In the U.S.—
 Velban

Available Dosage Forms:

- Solution
- Powder for Solution

Therapeutic Class: Antineoplastic Agent
Pharmacologic Class: Mitotic Inhibitor

Uses For This Medicine

Vinblastine belongs to the group of medicines known as antineoplastic agents. It is used to treat certain kinds of cancer, including lymphoma and cancer of the breast or testicles, as well as some noncancerous conditions.

Vinblastine interferes with the growth of cancer cells, which are eventually destroyed. Since the growth of normal body cells may also be affected by vinblastine, other effects will also occur. Some of these may be serious and must be reported to your doctor. Other effects, such as hair loss, may not be serious but may cause concern. Some effects do not occur until months or years after the medicine is used.

Before you begin treatment with vinblastine, you and your doctor should talk about the good this medicine will do as well as the risks of using it.

Vinblastine is to be administered only by or under the immediate supervision of your doctor.

Once a medicine has been approved for marketing for a certain use, experience may show that it is also useful for other medical problems. Although these uses are not included in product labeling, vinblastine is used in certain patients with the following medical conditions:

- Cancer of the bladder
- Cancer of the kidneys
- Cancer of the lungs
- Cancer of the prostate
- Germ cell ovarian tumors (a certain type of cancer of the ovaries)
- Malignant melanoma

Before Using This Medicine

In deciding to use a medicine, the risks of taking the medicine must be weighed against the good it will do. This is a decision you and your doctor will make. For this medicine, the following should be considered:

Allergies—Tell your doctor if you have ever had any unusual or allergic reaction to this medicine or any other medicines. Also tell your health care professional if you have any other types of allergies, such as to foods, dyes, preservatives, or animals. For non-prescription products, read the label or package ingredients carefully.

Pediatric—This medicine has been tested in children and has not been shown to cause different side effects or problems than it does in adults.

Geriatric—Many medicines have not been tested in older people. Therefore, it may not be known whether they work exactly the same way they do in younger adults or if they cause different side effects or problems in older people. There is no specific information about the use of vinblastine in the elderly.

Pregnancy—

	Pregnancy Category	Explanation
All Trimesters	D	Studies in pregnant women have demonstrated a risk to the fetus. However, the benefits of therapy in a life threatening situation or a serious disease, may outweigh the potential risk.

Breast Feeding—There are no adequate studies in women for determining infant risk when using this medication during breastfeeding. Weigh the potential benefits against the potential risks before taking this medication while breastfeeding.

Other medicines—

Using this medicine with any of the following medicines is not recommended. Your doctor may decide not to treat you with this medication or change some of the other medicines you take.

Rotavirus Vaccine, Live

Interactions with Food/Tobacco/Alcohol—Certain medicines should not be used at or around the time of eating food or eating certain types of food since interactions may occur. Using alcohol or tobacco with certain medicines may also cause interactions to occur. Discuss with your healthcare professional the use of your medicine with food, alcohol, or tobacco.

Other medical problems—The presence of other medical problems may affect the use of this medicine. Make sure you tell your doctor if you have any other medical problems, especially:

- Chickenpox (including recent exposure) or
- Herpes zoster (shingles)—Risk of severe disease affecting other parts of the body
- Gout (history of) or
- Kidney stones (history of)—Vinblastine may increase levels of uric acid in the body, which can cause gout or kidney stones
- Infection—Vinblastine may decrease your body's ability to fight infection
- Liver disease—Effects may be increased because of slower removal of vinblastine from the body

Proper Use of This Medicine

Vinblastine is sometimes given together with certain other medicines. If you are using a combination of medicines, it is important that you receive each one at the proper time. If you are taking some of these medicines by mouth, ask your health care professional to help you plan a way to take them at the right times.

While you are using this medicine, your doctor may want you to drink extra fluids so that you will pass more urine. This will help prevent kidney problems and keep your kidneys working well.

Vinblastine sometimes causes nausea and vomiting. However, it is very important that you continue to receive the medicine, even if you begin to feel ill. Ask your health care professional for ways to lessen these effects.

Dosing—The dose of this medicine will be different for different patients. Follow your doctor's orders or the directions on the label. The following information includes only the average doses of this medicine. If your dose is different, do not change it unless your doctor tells you to do so.

The amount of medicine that you take depends on the strength of the medicine. Also, the number of doses you take each day, the time allowed between doses, and the length of time you take the medicine depend on the medical problem for which you are using the medicine.

Precautions While Using This Medicine

It is very important that your doctor check your progress at regular visits to make sure that this medicine is working properly and to check for unwanted effects.

While you are being treated with vinblastine, and after you stop treatment with it, do not have any immunizations (vaccinations) without your doctor's approval. Vinblastine may lower your body's resistance and there is a chance you might get the infection the immunization is meant to prevent. Other people living in your household should not take oral polio vaccine since there is a chance they could pass the polio virus on to you. Also, avoid persons who have taken oral polio vaccine within the past several months. Do not get close to them, and do not stay in the same room with them for very long. If you cannot take these precautions, you should consider wearing a protective face mask that covers the nose and mouth.

Vinblastine can temporarily lower the number of white blood cells in your blood, increasing the chance of getting an infection. It can also lower the number of platelets, which are necessary for proper blood clotting. If this occurs, there are certain precautions you can take, especially when your blood count is low, to reduce the risk of infection or bleeding:

- If you can, avoid people with infections. Check with your doctor immediately if you think you are getting an infection or if you get a fever or chills, cough or hoarseness, lower back or side pain, or painful or difficult urination.

- Check with your doctor immediately if you notice any unusual bleeding or bruising; black, tarry stools; blood in urine or stools; or pinpoint red spots on your skin.

- Be careful when using a regular toothbrush, dental floss, or toothpick. Your medical doctor, dentist, or nurse may recommend other ways to clean your teeth and gums. Check with your medical doctor before having any dental work done.

- Do not touch your eyes or the inside of your nose unless you have just washed your hands and have not touched anything else in the meantime.

- Be careful not to cut yourself when you are using sharp objects such as a safety razor or fingernail or toenail cutters.

- Avoid contact sports or other situations where bruising or injury could occur.

If vinblastine accidentally seeps out of the vein into which it is injected, it may damage the skin and cause some scarring. Tell the doctor or nurse right away if you notice redness, pain, or swelling at the place of injection.

Side Effects of This Medicine

Along with their needed effects, medicines like vinblastine can sometimes cause unwanted effects such as blood problems, loss of hair, and other side effects. These and other effects are described below. Also, because of the way these medicines act on the body, there is a chance that they might cause other unwanted effects that may not occur until months or years after the medicine is used. These delayed effects may include certain types of cancer, such as leukemia. Discuss these possible effects with your doctor.

Although not all of these side effects may occur, if they do occur they may need medical attention.

Check with your doctor immediately if any of the following side effects occur:
> *More frequent*
>> Cough or hoarseness accompanied by fever or chills; fever or chills; lower back or side pain accompanied by fever or chills; painful or difficult urination accompanied by fever or chills
>
> *Less common*
>> Blood in urine or stools; pain or redness at place of injection; pinpoint red spots on skin; unusual bleeding or bruising
>
> *Rare*
>> Black, tarry stools

Check with your doctor as soon as possible if any of the following side effects occur:
> *Less common*
>> Joint pain; sores in mouth and on lips; swelling of feet or lower legs
>
> *Rare*
>> Difficulty in walking; dizziness; double vision; drooping eyelids; headache; jaw pain; mental depression; numbness or tingling in fingers and toes; pain in fingers and toes; pain in testicles; weakness

Some side effects may occur that usually do not need medical attention. These side effects may go away during treatment as your body adjusts to the medicine. Also, your health care professional may be able to tell you about ways to prevent or reduce some of these side effects. Check with your health care professional if any of the following side effects continue or are bothersome or if you have any questions about them:
> *Less common*
>> Bone or muscle pain; nausea and vomiting

This medicine often causes a temporary loss of hair. After treatment with vinblastine has ended, or sometimes even during treatment, normal hair growth should return.

Other side effects not listed may also occur in some patients. If you notice any other effects, check with your healthcare professional.

VINCRISTINE   (Intravenous route) - vin-KRIS-teen

Black Box Warning

Vincristine sulfate injection should be administered by individuals experienced in the administration of vincristine sulfate.

Caution- It is extremely important that the intravenous needle or catheter be properly positioned before any vincristine is injected. Leakage into surrounding tissue during intravenous administration of vincristine sulfate may cause considerable irritation. If extravasation occurs, the injection should be discontinued immediately, and any remaining portion of the dose should then be introduced into another vein. Local injection of hyaluronidase and the application of moderate heat to the area of leakage help disperse the drug and are thought to minimize discomfort and the possibility of cellulitis.

Fatal if given intrathecally. For intravenous use only.

Commonly used brand name(s)

In the U.S.—
    Oncovin
    Vincasar PFS

Available Dosage Forms:
  • Powder for Solution
  • Solution

Therapeutic Class: Antineoplastic Agent
Pharmacologic Class: Mitotic Inhibitor

Uses For This Medicine

Vincristine belongs to the group of medicines known as antineoplastic agents. It is used to treat some kinds of cancer as well as some noncancerous conditions.

Vincristine interferes with the growth of cancer cells, which are eventually destroyed. Since the growth of normal body cells may also be affected by vincristine, other effects will also occur. Some of these may be serious and must be reported to your doctor. Other effects, such as hair loss, may not be serious but may cause concern. Some effects may not occur for months or years after the medicine is used.

Before you begin treatment with vincristine, you and your doctor should talk about the good this medicine will do as well as the risks of using it.

Vincristine is to be administered only by or under the immediate supervision of your doctor.

Before Using This Medicine

In deciding to use a medicine, the risks of taking the medicine must be weighed against the good it will do. This is a decision you and your doctor will make. For this medicine, the following should be considered:

Allergies—Tell your doctor if you have ever had any unusual or allergic reaction to this medicine or any other medicines. Also tell your health care professional if you have any other types of allergies, such as to foods, dyes, preservatives, or animals. For non-prescription products, read the label or package ingredients carefully.

Pediatric—This medicine has been tested in children and has not been shown to cause different side effects or problems than it does in adults.

Geriatric—Nervous system effects may be more likely to occur in the elderly, who are usually more sensitive to the effects of vincristine.

Pregnancy—

	Pregnancy Category	Explanation
All Trimesters	D	Studies in pregnant women have demonstrated a risk to the fetus. However, the benefits of therapy in a life threatening situation or a serious disease, may outweigh the potential risk.

Breast Feeding—There are no adequate studies in women for determining infant risk when using this medication during breastfeeding. Weigh the potential benefits against the potential risks before taking this medication while breastfeeding.

Other medicines—

Using this medicine with any of the following medicines is not recommended. Your doctor may decide not to treat you with this medication or change some of the other medicines you take.

Rotavirus Vaccine, Live

Interactions with Food/Tobacco/Alcohol—Certain medicines should not be used at or around the time of eating food or eating certain types of food since interactions may occur. Using alcohol or tobacco with certain medicines may also cause interactions to occur. Discuss with your healthcare professional the use of your medicine with food, alcohol, or tobacco.

Other medical problems—The presence of other medical problems may affect the use of this medicine. Make sure you tell your doctor if you have any other medical problems, especially:
  • Chickenpox (including recent exposure) or
  • Herpes zoster (shingles)—Risk of severe disease affecting other parts of the body
  • Gout (history of) or
  • Kidney stones (history of)—Vincristine may increase levels of uric acid in the body, which can cause gout or kidney stones
  • Infection—Vincristine can reduce immunity to infection
  • Liver disease—Effects may be increased because of slower removal of vincristine from the body
  • Nerve or muscle disease—May be worsened

Proper Use of This Medicine

Vincristine is often given together with certain other medicines. If you are using a combination of medicines, it is important that you receive each one at the proper time. If you are taking some of these medicines by mouth, ask your health care professional to help you plan a way to take them at the right times.

While you are using this medicine, it may be necessary to drink extra fluids so that you will pass more urine. This will help prevent kidney problems and keep your kidneys working well. Ask your doctor if this is necessary for you.

This medicine sometimes causes nausea and vomiting. However, it is very important that you continue to receive the medicine, even if you begin to feel ill. Ask your health care professional for ways to lessen these effects.

Vincristine frequently causes constipation and stomach cramps. Your doctor may want you to take a laxative. However, do not decide to take these medicines on your own without first checking with your doctor.

Dosing—The dose of this medicine will be different for different patients. Follow your doctor's orders or the directions on the label. The following information includes only the average doses of this medicine. If your dose is different, do not change it unless your doctor tells you to do so.

The amount of medicine that you take depends on the strength of the medicine. Also, the number of doses you take each day, the time allowed between doses, and the length of time you take the medicine depend on the medical problem for which you are using the medicine.

Precautions While Using This Medicine

It is very important that your doctor check your progress at regular visits to make sure that vincristine is working properly and to check for unwanted effects.

While you are being treated with vincristine, and after you stop treatment with it, do not have any immunizations (vaccinations) without your doctor's approval. Vincristine may lower your body's resistance and there is a chance you might get the infection the immunization is meant to prevent. Other people living in your household should not take or should not have recently taken oral polio vaccine since there is a chance they could pass the polio virus on to you. Also, avoid other persons who have taken oral polio vaccine. Do not get close to them, and do not stay in the same room with them for very long. If you cannot take these precautions, you should consider wearing a protective face mask that covers the nose and mouth.

If vincristine accidentally seeps out of the vein into which it is injected, it may damage some tissues and cause scarring. Tell the doctor or nurse right away if you notice redness, pain, or swelling at the place of injection.

Side Effects of This Medicine

Along with their needed effects, medicines like vincristine can sometimes cause unwanted effects such as blood problems, nervous system problems, loss of hair, and other side effects. These and others are described below. Also, because of the way these medicines act on the body, there is a chance that they might cause other unwanted effects that may not occur until months or years after the medicine is used. Discuss these possible effects with your doctor.

Check with your doctor immediately if any of the following side effects occur:
Less common
Pain or redness at place of injection
Rare
Black, tarry stools; blood in urine or stools; cough or hoarseness; fever or chills; pinpoint red spots on skin; unusual bleeding or bruising

Check with your doctor as soon as possible if any of the following side effects occur:
More common
Blurred or double vision; constipation; difficulty in walking; drooping eyelids; headache; jaw pain; joint pain; lower back or side pain; numbness or tingling in fingers and toes; pain in fingers and toes; pain in testicles; stomach cramps; swelling of feet or lower legs; weakness
Less common
Agitation; bed-wetting; confusion; convulsions (seizures); decrease or increase in urination; dizziness or lightheadedness when getting up from a lying or sitting position; hallucinations (seeing, hearing, or feeling things that are not there); lack of sweating; loss of appetite; mental depression; painful or difficult urination; trouble in sleeping; unconsciousness
Rare
Sores in mouth and on lips

Some side effects may occur that usually do not need medical attention. These side effects may go away during treatment as your body adjusts to the medicine. Also, your health care professional may be able to tell you about ways to prevent or reduce some of these side effects. Check with your health care professional if any of the following side effects continue or are bothersome or if you have any questions about them:
Less common
Bloating; diarrhea; loss of weight; nausea and vomiting; skin rash

Other side effects may occur that usually do not need medical attention. This medicine often causes a temporary loss of hair. After treatment with vincristine has ended, or sometimes even during treatment, normal hair growth should return.

Other side effects not listed may also occur in some patients. If you notice any other effects, check with your healthcare professional.

VINORELBINE   (Intravenous route) - vi-NOR-el-been

Commonly used brand name(s)
In the U.S.—
Navelbine

Available Dosage Forms:
• Solution

Therapeutic Class: Antineoplastic Agent
Pharmacologic Class: Mitotic Inhibitor

Uses For This Medicine

Vinorelbine belongs to the general group of medicines known as antineoplastics. It is used to treat some kinds of lung cancer. It may also be used to treat other kinds of cancer, as determined by your doctor.

Vinorelbine interferes with the growth of cancer cells, which are eventually destroyed. Since the growth of normal cells also may be affected by vinorelbine, other effects will occur. Some of these may be serious and must be reported to your doctor. Other effects, such as hair loss, may not be serious but may cause concern. Some effects may not occur until months or years after the medicine is used.

Before you begin treatment with vinorelbine, you and your doctor should talk about the good this medicine will do as well as the risks of using it.

Vinorelbine is to be administered only by or under the immediate supervision of your doctor.

Once a medicine has been approved for marketing for a certain use, experience may show that it is also useful for other medical problems. Although this use is not included in product labeling, vinorelbine is used in certain patients with the following medical condition:

- Breast cancer
- Cervical cancer
- Ovarian cancer (epithelial)

Before Receiving This Medicine

In deciding to use a medicine, the risks of taking the medicine must be weighed against the good it will do. This is a decision you and your doctor will make. For this medicine, the following should be considered:

Allergies—Tell your doctor if you have ever had any unusual or allergic reaction to this medicine or any other medicines. Also tell your health care professional if you have any other types of allergies, such as to foods, dyes, preservatives, or animals. For non-prescription products, read the label or package ingredients carefully.

Pediatric—There is no specific information comparing use of vinorelbine in children with use in other age groups. Safety and efficacy of vinorelbine in children have not been established.

Geriatric—Vinorelbine has been studied in the elderly. Although patients older than 65 years of age have shown a slight increase in side effects compared with patients younger than 65 years of age, the overall safety and efficacy of vinorelbine are not different for older people.

Pregnancy—

	Pregnancy Category	Explanation
All Trimesters	D	Studies in pregnant women have demonstrated a risk to the fetus. However, the benefits of therapy in a life threatening situation or a serious disease, may outweigh the potential risk.

Breast Feeding—There are no adequate studies in women for determining infant risk when using this medication during breastfeeding. Weigh the potential benefits against the potential risks before taking this medication while breastfeeding.

Other medicines—

Using this medicine with any of the following medicines is not recommended. Your doctor may decide not to treat you with this medication or change some of the other medicines you take.

Rotavirus Vaccine, Live

Interactions with Food/Tobacco/Alcohol—Certain medicines should not be used at or around the time of eating food or eating certain types of food since interactions may occur. Using alcohol or tobacco with certain medicines may also cause interactions to occur. Discuss with your healthcare professional the use of your medicine with food, alcohol, or tobacco.

Other medical problems—The presence of other medical problems may affect the use of this medicine. Make sure you tell your doctor if you have any other medical problems, especially:

- Chickenpox (including recent exposure) or
- Herpes zoster (shingles)—Risk of severe disease affecting other parts of the body
- Infection—Vinorelbine may decrease your body's ability to fight infections

Proper Use of This Medicine

Vinorelbine is sometimes given together with certain other medicines. If you are using a combination of medicines, it is important that you receive each one at the proper time. If you are taking some of these medicines by mouth, ask your health care professional to help you plan a way to take them at the right times.

While you are receiving vinorelbine, your doctor may want you to drink extra fluids so that you will pass more urine. This will help prevent kidney problems and keep your kidneys working well.

This medicine often causes nausea and vomiting. However, it is very important that you continue to receive it, even if you begin to feel ill. Ask your health care professional for ways to lessen these effects.

Dosing—The dose of this medicine will be different for different patients. Follow your doctor's orders or the directions on the label. The following information includes only the average doses of this medicine. If your dose is different, do not change it unless your doctor tells you to do so.

The amount of medicine that you take depends on the strength of the medicine. Also, the number of doses you take each day, the time allowed between doses, and the length of time you take the medicine depend on the medical problem for which you are using the medicine.

Precautions After Receiving This Medicine

It is very important that your doctor check your progress at regular visits to make sure that this medicine is working properly and to check for unwanted effects.

While you are being treated with vinorelbine, and after you stop treatment with it, do not have any immunizations (vaccinations) without your doctor's approval. Vinorelbine may lower your body's resistance and there is a chance you might get the infection the immunization is meant to prevent. In addition, other persons living in your household should not take oral poliovirus vaccine, since there is a chance they could pass the poliovirus on to you. Also, avoid persons who have taken oral poliovirus vaccine within the last several months. Do not get close to them, and do not stay in the same room with them for very long. If you cannot take these precautions, you should consider wearing a protective face mask that covers the nose and the mouth.

Vinorelbine can temporarily lower the number of white blood cells in your blood, increasing the chance of getting an infection. It can also lower the number of platelets, which are necessary for proper blood clotting. If this occurs, there are certain precautions you can take, especially when your blood count is low, to reduce the risk of infection or bleeding:

- If you can, avoid people with infection. Check with your doctor immediately if you think you are getting an infection or if you get a fever or chills, cough or hoarseness, lower back or side pain, or have painful or difficult urination.

- Check with your doctor immediately if you notice any unusual bleeding or bruising; black, tarry stools; blood in urine or stools; or pinpoint red spots on your skin.

- Do not touch your eyes or the inside of your nose, unless you have just washed your hands and have not touched anything else in the meantime.

- Be careful not to cut yourself when you are using sharp objects, such as a safety razor or fingernail or toenail cutters.

- Avoid contact sports or other situations where bruising or injury can occur.

If vinorelbine accidentally seeps out of the vein into which it is injected, it may damage some tissue and cause scarring. Tell the doctor or nurse right away if you notice redness, pain, or swelling at the place of injection.

Be careful when using a regular toothbrush, dental floss, or toothpick. Your medical doctor, dentist, or nurse may recommend other ways to clean your teeth and gums. Check with your medical doctor before having any dental work done.

Side Effects of This Medicine

Along with its needed effects, a medicine may cause some unwanted effects. Although not all of these side effects may occur, if they do occur they may need medical attention.

Check with your doctor immediately if any of the following side effects occur:
More common
    Cough or hoarseness, accompanied by fever or chills; fever or chills; lower back or side pain, accompanied by fever or chills; painful or difficult urination, accompanied by fever or chills; redness, increased warmth, pain, or discoloration of vein at place of injection; sore throat, accompanied by fever or chills

Less common
    Chest pain; shortness of breath; sores in mouth and on lips

Rare
    Black, tarry stools; bloating; blood in urine or stools; chills; darkened urine; fast heartbeat; fever; indigestion; loss of appetite; nausea; painful urination; pains in stomach; pinpoint red spots on skin; skin rash; unusual bleeding or bruising; vomiting; yellow eyes or skin

Check with your doctor as soon as possible if any of the following side effects occur:
More common
    Loss of strength and energy; unusual tiredness or weakness

Less common
    Numbness or tingling in fingers and toes
Symptoms of overdose
    Chest pain; cough or hoarseness, accompanied by fever or chills; fever or chills; heartburn; lower back or side pain, accompanied by fever or chills; mild abdominal pain and constipation; numbness or tingling in fingers and toes; painful or difficult urination, accompanied by fever or chills; sore throat, accompanied by fever or chills; unusual bleeding or bruising; unusual tiredness or weakness; vomiting

Some side effects may occur that usually do not need medical attention. These side effects may go away during treatment as your body adjusts to the medicine. Also, your health care professional may be able to tell you about ways to prevent or reduce some of these side effects. Check with your health care professional if any of the following side effects continue or are bothersome or if you have any questions about them:
More common
    Constipation; loss of appetite; nausea and vomiting
Less common
    Diarrhea; jaw pain; joint or muscle pain

Other side effects not listed may also occur in some patients. If you notice any other effects, check with your healthcare professional.

VITAMIN A (Oral route, Intramuscular route) - VYE-ta-min A

Commonly used brand name(s)
In the U.S.—
    Aquasol A
    Palmitate-A

Available Dosage Forms:

- Tablet
- Capsule
- Capsule, Liquid Filled
- Liquid
- Tablet, Chewable
- Solution

Therapeutic Class: Nutritive Agent
Pharmacologic Class: Vitamin A (class)

Uses For This Dietary Supplement

Vitamins are compounds that you must have for growth and health. They are needed in small amounts only and are usually available in the foods that you eat. Vitamin A is needed for night vision and for growth of skin, bones, and male and female reproductive organs. In pregnant women vitamin A is necessary for the growth of a healthy fetus.

Lack of vitamin A may lead to a rare condition called night blindness (problems seeing in the dark), as well as dry eyes, eye infections, skin problems, and slowed growth. Your health care professional may treat these problems by prescribing vitamin A for you.

Some conditions may increase your need for vitamin A. These include:

- Diarrhea
- Eye diseases

- Intestine diseases
- Infections (continuing or chronic)
- Measles
- Pancreas disease
- Stomach removal
- Stress (continuing)

In addition, infants receiving unfortified formula may need vitamin A supplements.

Vitamin A absorption will be decreased in any condition in which fat is poorly absorbed.

Increased need for vitamin A should be determined by your health care professional.

Claims that vitamin A is effective for treatment of conditions such as acne or lung diseases, or for treatment of eye problems, wounds, or dry or wrinkled skin not caused by lack of vitamin A have not been proven. Although vitamin A is being used to prevent certain types of cancer, some experts feel there is not enough information to show that this is effective, particularly in well-nourished individuals.

Injectable vitamin A is given by or under the supervision of a health care professional. Other forms of vitamin A are available without a prescription.

Importance of Diet—For good health, it is important that you eat a balanced and varied diet. Follow carefully any diet program your health care professional may recommend. For your specific dietary vitamin and/or mineral needs, ask your health care professional for a list of appropriate foods. If you think that you are not getting enough vitamins and/or minerals in your diet, you may choose to take a dietary supplement.

Vitamin A is found in various foods including yellow-orange fruits and vegetables; dark green, leafy vegetables; vitamin A-fortified milk; liver; and margarine. Vitamin A comes in two different forms, retinols and beta-carotene. Retinols are found in foods that come from animals (meat, milk, eggs). The form of vitamin A found in plants is called beta-carotene (which is converted to vitamin A in the body). Food processing may destroy some of the vitamins. For example, freezing may reduce the amount of vitamin A in foods.

Vitamins alone will not take the place of a good diet and will not provide energy. Your body needs other substances found in food, such as protein, minerals, carbohydrates, and fat. Vitamins themselves often cannot work without the presence of other foods. For example, small amounts of fat are needed so that vitamin A can be absorbed into the body.

The daily amount of vitamin A needed is defined in several different ways.

For U.S.—
- Recommended Dietary Allowances (RDAs) are the amount of vitamins and minerals needed to provide for adequate nutrition in most healthy persons. RDAs for a given nutrient may vary depending on a person's age, sex, and physical condition (e.g., pregnancy).
- Daily Values (DVs) are used on food and dietary supplement labels to indicate the percent of the recommended daily amount of each nutrient that a serving provides. DV replaces the previous designation of United States Recommended Daily Allowances (USRDAs).
- Normal daily recommended intakes in the United States for vitamin A are generally defined according

to age or condition and to the form of vitamin A as follows:

Age or Condition	Form of Vitamin A		
	RE or mcg of Retinol	Amount in Units as Retinol	Amount in Units as a Combination of Retinol and Beta-carotene
Infants and children			
Birth to 3 years	375–400	1250–1330	1875–2000
4 to 6 years	500	1665	2500
7 to 10 years	700	2330	3500
Teenage and adult males	1000	3330	5000
Teenage and adult females	800	2665	4000
Pregnant females	800	2665	4000
Breast-feeding females	1200–1300	4000–4330	6000–6500

Note: Based on 1980 U.S. Recommended Dietary Allowances (RDAs) for vitamin A in the diet that is a combination of retinol and beta-carotene.

For Canada—
- Recommended Nutrient Intakes (RNIs) are used to determine the amounts of vitamins, minerals, and protein needed to provide adequate nutrition and lessen the risk of chronic disease.
- Normal daily recommended intakes in Canada for vitamin A are generally defined according to age or condition and to the form of vitamin A as follows:

Age or Condition	Form of Vitamin A		
	RE or mcg of Retinol	Amount in Units as Retinol	Amount in Units as a Combination of Retinol and Beta-carotene
Infants and children			
Birth to 3 years	400	1330	2000
4 to 6 years	500	1665	2330
7 to 10 years	700–800	2330–2665	3500
Teenage and adult males	1000	3330	5000
Teenage and adult females	800	2665	4000
Pregnant females	900	2665–3000	4000–4500
Breast-feeding females	1200	4000	6000

Note: Based on 1980 U.S. Recommended Dietary Allowances (RDAs) for vitamin A in the diet that is a combination of retinol and beta-carotene.

In the past, the RDA and RNI for vitamin A have been expressed in Units. This term Units has been replaced by retinol equivalents (RE) or micrograms (mcg) of retinol, with 1 RE equal to 1 mcg of retinol. This was done to better describe the two forms of vitamin A, retinol and beta-carotene. One RE of vitamin A is equal to 3.33 Units of retinol and 10 Units of beta-carotene. Some products available have not changed their labels and continue to be labeled in Units.

Before Using This Dietary Supplement

If you are taking this dietary supplement without a prescription, carefully read and follow any precautions on the label. For this supplement, the following should be considered:

Allergies—Tell your doctor if you have ever had any unusual or allergic reaction to this medicine or any other medicines. Also tell your health care professional if you have any other types of allergies, such as to foods, dyes, preservatives, or animals. For non-prescription products, read the label or package ingredients carefully.

Pediatric—Problems in children have not been reported with intake of normal daily recommended amounts. However, side effects from high doses and/or prolonged use of vitamin A are more likely to occur in young children than adults.

Geriatric—Problems in older adults have not been reported with intake of normal daily recommended amounts. However, some studies have shown that the elderly may be at risk of high blood levels of vitamin A with long-term use.

Pregnancy—

	Pregnancy Category	Explanation
All Trimesters	X	Studies in animals or pregnant women have demonstrated positive evidence of fetal abnormalities. This drug should not be used in women who are or may become pregnant because the risk clearly outweighs any possible benefit.

Breast Feeding—There are no adequate studies in women for determining infant risk when using this medication during breastfeeding. Weigh the potential benefits against the potential risks before taking this medication while breastfeeding.

Other medicines—

Using this dietary supplement with any of the following medicines may cause an increased risk of certain side effects, but using both drugs may be the best treatment for you. If both medicines are prescribed together, your doctor may change the dose or how often you use one or both of the medicines.

Abciximab, Acenocoumarol, Ancrod, Anisindione, Antithrombin III Human, Argatroban, Bexarotene, Bivalirudin, Clopidogrel, Danaparoid, Defibrotide, Dermatan Sulfate, Desirudin, Dicumarol, Eptifibatide, Fondaparinux, Heparin, Lamifiban, Minocycline, Pentosan Polysulfate Sodium, Phenindione, Phenprocoumon, Sibrafiban, Tirofiban, Warfarin, Xemilofiban

Interactions with Food/Tobacco/Alcohol—Certain medicines should not be used at or around the time of eating food or eating certain types of food since interactions may occur. Using alcohol or tobacco with certain medicines may also cause interactions to occur. Discuss with your healthcare professional the use of your medicine with food, alcohol, or tobacco.

Other medical problems—The presence of other medical problems may affect the use of this dietary supplement. Make sure you tell your doctor if you have any other medical problems, especially:

- Alcohol abuse (or history of) or
- Liver disease—Vitamin A use may make liver problems worse

- Kidney disease—May cause high blood levels of vitamin A, which may increase the chance of side effects

Proper Use of This Dietary Supplement

If you miss taking a vitamin for one or more days there is no cause for concern, since it takes some time for your body to become seriously low in vitamins. However, if your health care professional has recommended that you take this vitamin, try to remember to take it as directed every day.

Dosing—The dose of this medicine will be different for different patients. Follow your doctor's orders or the directions on the label. The following information includes only the average doses of this medicine. If your dose is different, do not change it unless your doctor tells you to do so.

The amount of medicine that you take depends on the strength of the medicine. Also, the number of doses you take each day, the time allowed between doses, and the length of time you take the medicine depend on the medical problem for which you are using the medicine.

- For oral dosage form (capsules, tablets, oral solution):
  - To prevent deficiency, the amount taken by mouth is based on normal daily recommended intakes:

  For the U.S.
  - Adult and teenage males—1000 retinol equivalents (RE) (3330 Units of retinol or 5000 Units as a combination of retinol and beta-carotene) per day.
  - Adult and teenage females—800 RE (2665 Units of retinol or 4000 Units as a combination of retinol and beta-carotene) per day.
  - Pregnant females—800 RE (2665 Units of retinol or 4000 Units as a combination of retinol and beta-carotene) per day.
  - Breast-feeding females—1200 to 1300 RE (4000 to 4330 Units of retinol or 6000 to 6500 Units as a combination of retinol and beta-carotene) per day.
  - Children 7 to 10 years of age—700 RE (2330 Units of retinol or 3500 Units as a combination of retinol and beta-carotene) per day.
  - Children 4 to 6 years of age—500 RE (1665 Units of retinol or 2500 Units as a combination of retinol and beta-carotene) per day.
  - Children birth to 3 years of age—375 to 400 RE (1250 to 1330 Units of retinol or 1875 to 2000 Units as a combination of retinol and beta-carotene) per day.

  For Canada
  - Adult and teenage males—1000 RE (3330 Units of retinol or 5000 Units as a combination of retinol and beta-carotene) per day.
  - Adult and teenage females—800 RE (2665 Units of retinol or 4000 Units as a combination of retinol and beta-carotene) per day.
  - Pregnant females—900 RE (2665 to 3000 Units of retinol or 4000 to 4500 Units as a combination of retinol and beta-carotene) per day.
  - Breast-feeding females—1200 RE (4000 Units of retinol or 6000 Units as a combination of retinol and beta-carotene) per day.
  - Children 7 to 10 years of age—700 to 800 RE (2330 to 2665 Units of retinol or 3500 Units as a combination of retinol and beta-carotene) per day.

- Children 4 to 6 years of age—500 RE (1665 Units of retinol or 2500 Units as a combination of retinol and beta-carotene) per day.
- Children birth to 3 years of age—400 RE (1330 Units or 2000 Units as a combination of retinol and beta-carotene) per day.
  - ○ To treat deficiency:
    - Adults and teenagers—Treatment dose is determined by prescriber for each individual based on severity of deficiency. The following dose has been determined for xerophthalmia (eye disease): Oral, 7500 to 15,000 RE (25,000 to 50,000 Units) a day.
    - Children—Treatment dose is determined by prescriber for each individual based of severity of deficiency. The following doses have been determined:
      - — For measles—
        - Children 6 months to 1 year of age: Oral, 30,000 RE (100,000 Units) as a single dose.
        - For children 1 year of age and older: Oral, 60,000 RE (200,000 Units) as a single dose.
      - — Xerophthalmia (eye disease)—
        - Children 6 months to 1 year of age: Oral, 30,000 RE (100,000 Units) as a single dose, the same dose being repeated the next day and again at 4 weeks.
        - Children 1 year of age and older: Oral, 60,000 RE (200,000 Units) as a single dose, the same dose being repeated the next day and again at 4 weeks.

      Note: Vitamin A is used in measles and xerophthalmia only when vitamin A deficiency is a problem as determined by your health care professional. Vitamin A deficiency occurs in malnutrition or in certain disease states.

For individuals taking the oral liquid form of vitamin A:

- This preparation is to be taken by mouth even though it comes in a dropper bottle.
- This dietary supplement may be dropped directly into the mouth or mixed with cereal, fruit juice, or other food.

Missed dose—If you miss a dose of this medicine, skip the missed dose and go back to your regular dosing schedule. Do not double doses.

Storage—Store the medicine in a closed container at room temperature, away from heat, moisture, and direct light. Keep from freezing.

Keep out of the reach of children.

Do not keep outdated medicine or medicine no longer needed.

Precautions While Using This Dietary Supplement

Vitamin A is stored in the body; therefore, when you take more than the body needs, it will build up in the body. This may lead to poisoning and even death. Problems are more likely to occur in:

- Adults taking 7500 RE (25,000 Units) a day for 8 months in a row, or 450,000 RE (1,500,000 Units) all at once; or
- Children taking 5400 RE (18,000 Units) to 15,000 RE (50,000 Units) a day for several months in a row, or

- 22,500 RE (75,000 Units) to 105,100 RE (350,000 Units) all at once.
- Pregnant women taking more than 1800 RE (6000 Units) a day.

Remember that the total amount of vitamin A you get every day includes what you get from foods that you eat and what you take as a supplement.

High doses and/or prolonged use of vitamin A may cause bleeding from the gums; dry or sore mouth; or drying, cracking, or peeling of the lips.

Side Effects of This Dietary Supplement

Along with its needed effects, a medicine may cause some unwanted effects. Although not all of these side effects may occur, if they do occur they may need medical attention.

Check with your doctor immediately if any of the following side effects occur:

Bleeding from gums or sore mouth; bulging soft spot on head (in babies); confusion or unusual excitement; diarrhea; dizziness or drowsiness; double vision; headache (severe); irritability (severe); peeling of skin, especially on lips and palms; vomiting (severe)

Check with your doctor as soon as possible if any of the following side effects occur:

Bone or joint pain; convulsions (seizures); drying or cracking of skin or lips; dry mouth; fever; general feeling of discomfort or illness or weakness; headache; increased sensitivity of skin to sunlight; increase in frequency of urination, especially at night, or in amount of urine; irritability; loss of appetite; loss of hair; stomach pain; unusual tiredness; vomiting; yellow-orange patches on soles of feet, palms of hands, or skin around nose and lips

Other side effects not listed may also occur in some patients. If you notice any other effects, check with your healthcare professional.

VITAMIN D AND RELATED COMPOUNDS (Systemic)

Some commonly used brand names are:

In the U.S.—

Calciferol (6)	Drisdol (6)
Calciferol Drops (6)	Drisdol Drops (6)
Calcijex (3)	Hectorol (5)
Calderol (2)	Hytakerol (4)
DHT (4)	Rocaltrol (3)
DHT Intensol (4)	Zemplar (7)

In Canada—

Calciferol (6)	One-Alpha (1)
Calcijex (3)	Ostoforte (6)
Drisdol (6)	Radiostol Forte (6)
Hytakerol (4)	Rocaltrol (3)

This information applies to the following:

1. Alfacalcidol (al-fa-KAL-si-dol)
2. Calcifediol (kal-si-fe-DYE-ole)
3. Calcitriol (kal-si-TRYE-ole)
4. Dihydrotachysterol (dye-hye-droh-tak-ISS-ter-ole)
5. Doxercalciferol (docks-er-kal-SIF-e-role)
6. Ergocalciferol (er-goe-kal-SIF-e-role)
7. Paricalcitol (par-i-KAL-si-trole)

Category

• **Antihypocalcemic—**
• **Antihypoparathyroid—**
• **Nutritional supplement, vitamin—**

Description

Vitamins (VYE-ta-mins) are compounds that you *must* have for growth and health. They are needed in small amounts only and are available in the foods that you eat. Vitamin D is necessary for strong bones and teeth.

Lack of vitamin D may lead to a condition called rickets, especially in children, in which bones and teeth are weak. In adults it may cause a condition called osteomalacia, in which calcium is lost from bones so that they become weak. Your doctor may treat these problems by prescribing vitamin D for you. Vitamin D is also sometimes used to treat other diseases in which calcium is not used properly by the body.

Ergocalciferol is the form of vitamin D used in vitamin supplements.

Some conditions may increase your need for vitamin D. These include:

• Alcoholism
• Intestine diseases
• Kidney disease
• Liver disease
• Overactivity of the parathyroid glands with kidney failure
• Pancreas disease
• Surgical removal of stomach

In addition, individuals and breast-fed infants who lack exposure to sunlight, as well as dark-skinned individuals, may be more likely to have a vitamin D deficiency. Increased need for vitamin D should be determined by your health care professional.

Alfacalcidol, calcifediol, calcitriol, and dihydrotachysterol are forms of vitamin D used to treat hypocalcemia (not enough calcium in the blood). Alfacalcidol, calcifediol, and calcitriol are also used to treat certain types of bone disease that may occur with kidney disease in patients who are undergoing kidney dialysis.

Claims that vitamin D is effective for treatment of arthritis and prevention of nearsightedness or nerve problems have not been proven. Some psoriasis patients may benefit from vitamin D supplements; however, controlled studies have not been performed.

Injectable vitamin D is given by or under the supervision of a health care professional. Some strengths of ergocalciferol and all strengths of alfacalcidol, calcifediol, calcitriol, and dihydrotachysterol are available only with your doctor's prescription. Other strengths of ergocalciferol are available without a prescription. However, it may be a good idea to check with your health care professional before taking vitamin D on your own. *Taking large amounts over long periods may cause serious unwanted effects.*

Vitamin D and related compounds are available in the following dosage forms:

Oral
• Alfacalcidol
  ◦ Capsules
  ◦ Oral solution
  ◦ Oral drops
• Calcifediol
  ◦ Capsules
• Calcitriol
  ◦ Capsules
  ◦ Oral solution
• Dihydrotachysterol
  ◦ Capsules
  ◦ Oral solution
  ◦ Tablets
• Doxercalciferol
  ◦ Capsules
• Ergocalciferol
  ◦ Capsules
  ◦ Oral solution
  ◦ Tablets
• Paricalcitol
  ◦ Capsules

Parenteral
• Alfacalcidol
  ◦ Injection
• Calcitriol
  ◦ Injection
• Ergocalciferol
  ◦ Injection
• Paricalcitol
  ◦ Injection

Importance of Diet

For good health, it is important that you eat a balanced and varied diet. Follow carefully any diet program your health care professional may recommend. For your specific dietary vitamin and/or mineral needs, ask your health care professional for a list of appropriate foods. If you think that you are not getting enough vitamins and/or minerals in your diet, you may choose to take a dietary supplement.

Vitamin D is found naturally only in fish and fish-liver oils. However, it is also found in milk (vitamin D– fortified). Cooking does not affect the vitamin D in foods. Vitamin D is sometimes called the "sunshine vitamin" since it is made in your skin when you are exposed to sunlight. If you eat a balanced diet and get outside in the sunshine at least 1.5 to 2 hours a week, you should be getting all the vitamin D you need.

Vitamins alone will not take the place of a good diet and will not provide energy. Your body also needs other substances found in food such as protein, minerals, carbohydrates, and fat. Vitamins themselves often cannot work without the presence of other foods. For example, fat is needed so that vitamin D can be absorbed into the body.

The daily amount of vitamin D needed is defined in several different ways.

For U.S.—
• Recommended Dietary Allowances (RDAs) are the amount of vitamins and minerals needed to provide for adequate nutrition in most healthy persons. RDAs for a given nutrient may vary depending on a person's age, sex, and physical condition (e.g., pregnancy).

• Daily Values (DVs) are used on food and dietary supplement labels to indicate the percent of the recommended daily amount of each nutrient that a serving provides. DV replaces the previous designation of United States Recommended Daily Allowances (USRDAs).

For Canada—

- Recommended Nutrient Intakes (RNIs) are used to determine the amounts of vitamins, minerals, and protein needed to provide adequate nutrition and lessen the risk of chronic disease.

In the past, the RDA and RNI for vitamin D have been expressed in Units (U). This term has been replaced by micrograms (mcg) of vitamin D.

Normal daily recommended intakes in mcg and Units are generally defined as follows:

Persons	U.S. (mcg)	U.S. Units	Canada (mcg)	Canada Units
Infants and children				
Birth to 3 years of age	7.5–10	300–400	5–10	200–400
4 to 6 years of age	10	400	5	200
7 to 10 years of age	10	400	2.5–5	100–200
Adolescents and adults	5–10	200–400	2.5–5	100–200
Pregnant and breast-feeding females	10	400	5–7.5	200–300

Remember:

- The total amount of each vitamin that you get every day includes what you get from the foods that you eat *and* what you may take as a supplement.

- Your total amount should not be greater than the RDA or RNI, unless ordered by your doctor. *Taking too much vitamin D over a period of time may cause harmful effects.*

Before Using This Dietary Supplement

If you are taking this dietary supplement without a prescription, carefully read and follow any precautions on the label. For vitamin D and related compounds, the following should be considered:

Allergies—Tell your health care professional if you have ever had any unusual or allergic reaction to alfacalcidol, calcifediol, calcitriol, dihydrotachysterol, doxercalciferol, ergocalciferol, or paricalcitol. Also, tell your health care professional if you are allergic to any other substances, such as foods, preservatives, or dyes.

Pregnancy—It is especially important that you are receiving enough vitamin D when you become pregnant and that you continue to receive the right amounts of vitamins throughout your pregnancy. The healthy growth and development of the fetus depend on a steady supply of nutrients from the mother.

You may need vitamin D supplements if you are a strict vegetarian (vegan-vegetarian) and/or have little exposure to sunlight and do not drink vitamin D-fortified milk.

Taking too much alfacalcidol, calcifediol, calcitriol, dihydrotachysterol, or ergocalciferol can also be harmful to the fetus. Taking more than your health care professional has recommended can cause your baby to be more sensitive than usual to its effects, can cause problems with a gland called the parathyroid, and can cause a defect in the baby's heart.

Doxercalciferol or paricalcitol have not been studied in pregnant women. However, studies in animals have shown that paricalcitol causes problems in newborns. Before taking this medicine, make sure your doctor knows if you are pregnant or if you may become pregnant.

Breast-feeding—It is especially important that you receive the right amounts of vitamins so that your baby will also get the vitamins needed to grow properly. Infants who are totally breast-fed and have little exposure to the sun may require vitamin D supplementation. However, taking large amounts of a dietary supplement while breast-feeding may be harmful to the mother and/or baby and should be avoided.

Only small amounts of alfacalcidol, calcifediol, calcitriol, or dihydrotachysterol pass into breast milk and these amounts have not been reported to cause problems in nursing babies.

It is not known whether doxercalciferol or paricalcitol passes into breast milk. Be sure you have discussed the risks and benefits of the supplement with your doctor.

Children—Problems in children have not been reported with intake of normal daily recommended amounts. Some studies have shown that infants who are totally breast-fed, especially with dark-skinned mothers, and have little exposure to sunlight may be at risk of vitamin D deficiency. Your health care professional may prescribe a vitamin/mineral supplement that contains vitamin D. Some infants may be sensitive to even small amounts of alfacalcidol, calcifediol, calcitriol, dihydrotachysterol, or ergocalciferol. Also, children may show slowed growth when receiving large doses of alfacalcidol, calcifediol, calcitriol, dihydrotachysterol, or ergocalciferol for a long time.

Studies on doxercalciferol or paricalcitol have been done only in adult patients, and there is no specific information comparing the use of doxercalciferol or paricalcitol in children with use in other age groups.

Older adults—Problems in older adults have not been reported with intake of normal daily recommended amounts. Studies have shown that older adults may have lower blood levels of vitamin D than younger adults, especially those who have little exposure to sunlight. Your health care professional may recommend that you take a vitamin supplement that contains vitamin D.

Medicines or other dietary supplements—Although certain medicines or dietary supplements should not be used together at all, in other cases they may be used together even if an interaction might occur. In these cases, your health care professional may want to change the dose, or other precautions may be necessary. When you are taking vitamin D and related compounds, it is especially important that your health care professional know if you are taking any of the following:

- Antacids containing magnesium—Use of these products with any vitamin D– related compound may result in high blood levels of magnesium, especially in patients with kidney disease

- Calcium-containing preparations or

- Thiazide diuretics (water pills)—Use of these preparations with vitamin D may cause high blood levels of calcium and increase the chance of side effects

- Vitamin D and related compounds, other—Use of vitamin D with a related compound may cause high blood levels of vitamin D and increase the chance of side effects.

Other medical problems—The presence of other medical problems may affect the use of vitamin D and related compounds. Make sure you tell your health care professional if you have any other medical problems, especially:

- Heart or blood vessel disease—Alfacalcidol, calcifediol, calcitriol, or dihydrotachysterol may cause hypercalcemia (high blood levels of calcium), which may make these conditions worse

- Kidney disease—High blood levels of alfacalcidol, calcifediol, calcitriol, dihydrotachysterol, or ergocalciferol may result, which may increase the chance of side effects
- Sarcoidosis—May increase sensitivity to alfacalcidol, calcifediol, calcitriol, dihydrotachysterol, or ergocalciferol and increase the chance of side effects

Proper Use of This Dietary Supplement

For use as a dietary supplement:

- *Do not take more than the recommended daily amount.* Vitamin D is stored in the body, and taking too much over a period of time can cause poisoning and even death.

If you have any questions about this, check with your health care professional.

For individuals taking the *oral liquid form* of this dietary supplement:

- This preparation should be taken by mouth even though it comes in a dropper bottle.
- This dietary supplement may be dropped directly into the mouth or mixed with cereal, fruit juice, or other food.

While you are taking alfacalcidol, calcifediol, calcitriol, dihydrotachysterol, doxercalciferol or paricalcitol, your health care professional may want you to follow a special diet or take a calcium supplement. Be sure to follow instructions carefully. If you are already taking a calcium supplement or any medicine containing calcium, make sure your health care professional knows.

Dosing—The dose of these vitamin D and related compounds will be different for different patients. *Follow your doctor's orders or the directions on the label.* The following information includes only the average doses of these medicines. *If your dose is different, do not change it* unless your health care professional tells you to do so.

The number of milliliters (mL) of solution that you take, or the number of capsules or tablets you take, depends on the strength of the medicine. Also, *the number of doses you take each day, the time allowed between doses, and the length of time you take the medicine depend on the medical problem for which you are taking the combination medicine.*

For alfacalcidol
- To treat bone disease in kidney patients undergoing kidney dialysis:
  - For *oral* dosage form (capsules):
    - Adults and teenagers—At first, 1 microgram (mcg) a day. Your doctor may change your dose if needed. However, most people will take not more than 3 mcg a day.
  - For *oral* dosage form (drops):
    - Adults and teenagers—At first, 1 microgram (mcg) a day. Your doctor may change your dose if needed. However, most people will take not more than 3 mcg a day.
  - For *oral* dosage form (solution):
    - Adults and teenagers—At first, 1 mcg a day. Your doctor may change your dose if needed. However, most people will take not more than 3 mcg a day.

  - For *parenteral* dosage form (injection):
    - Adults and teenagers—At first, 1 mcg a day. Your doctor may change your dose if needed. However, most people will take not more than 12 mcg a week.
- To treat diseases in which calcium is not used properly by the body
  - For *oral* dosage form (capsules):
    - Adults and teenagers—At first, 0.25 microgram (mcg) a day. Your doctor may change your dose if needed. However, most people will take not more than 1 mcg a day.
  - For *oral* dosage form (drops):
    - Adults and teenagers—At first, 0.25 microgram (mcg) a day. Your doctor may change your dose if needed. However, most people will take not more than 1 mcg a day.
  - For *oral* dosage form (solution):
    - Adults and teenagers—At first, 0.25 mcg a day. Your doctor may change your dose if needed. However, most people will take not more than 1 mcg a day.

For calcifediol
- To treat diseases in which calcium is not used properly by the body or to treat bone disease in kidney patients undergoing kidney dialysis:
  - For *oral* dosage form (capsules):
    - Adults, teenagers, and children over 10 years of age—At first, 300 to 350 micrograms (mcg) a week, taken in divided doses either once a day or every other day. Your doctor may change your dose if needed.
    - Children up to 2 years of age—20 to 50 mcg a day.
    - Children 2 to 10 years of age—50 mcg a day.

For calcitriol
- To treat diseases in which calcium is not used properly by the body or to treat bone disease in kidney patients undergoing kidney dialysis:
  - For *oral* dosage form (capsules and solution):
    - Adults, teenagers, and children—At first, 0.25 micrograms (mcg) a day. Your doctor may change your dose if needed.
  - For *injection* dosage form:
    - Adults and teenagers—At first, 0.5 mcg injected into a vein three times a week. Your doctor may change your dose if needed.
    - Children—Use and dose must be determined by your doctor.

For dihydrotachysterol
- To treat diseases in which calcium is not used properly by the body:
  - For *oral* dosage forms (capsules, solution, or tablets):
    - Adults and teenagers—At first, 100 micrograms (mcg) to 2.5 milligrams (mg) a day. Your doctor may change your dose if needed.
    - Children—At first, 1 to 5 mg a day. Your doctor may change your dose if needed.

For doxercalciferol
- To treat an overactive parathyroid gland in patients with kidney failure:
  - For *oral* dosage form (capsules):

- Adults: 10 micrograms (mcg) three times weekly at dialysis. The doctor may change your dose if needed.
- Children: Use and dose must be determined by your doctor.

For ergocalciferol

- For *oral* dosage forms (capsules, tablets, oral solution):
  - The amount of vitamin D to meet normal daily recommended intakes will be different for different individuals. The following information includes only the average amounts of vitamin D.
  - To prevent deficiency, the amount taken by mouth is based on normal daily recommended intakes:

  For the U.S.
  - Adults and teenagers: 5 to 10 micrograms (mcg) (200 to 400 Units) per day.
  - Pregnant and breast-feeding females: 10 mcg (400 Units) per day.
  - Children 4 to 10 years of age: 10 mcg (400 Units) per day.
  - Children birth to 3 years of age: 7.5 to 10 mcg (300 to 400 Units) per day.

  For Canada
  - Adults and teenagers: 2.5 to 5 mcg (100 to 200 Units) per day.
  - Pregnant and breast-feeding females: 5 to 7.5 mcg (200 to 300 Units) per day.
  - Children 7 to 10 years of age: 2.5 to 5 mcg (100 to 200 Units) per day.
  - Children 4 to 6 years of age: 5 mcg (200 Units) per day.
  - Children birth to 3 years of age: 5 to 10 mcg (200 to 400 Units) per day.
  - To treat deficiency:
    - Adults, teenagers, and children: Treatment dose is determined by prescriber for each individual based on severity of deficiency.
  - To treat diseases in which calcium and phosphate are not used properly by the body:
    - Adults and teenagers: At first, 1000 to 500,000 Units a day. The doctor may change your dose if needed.
    - Children: At first, 1000 to 200,000 Units a day. The doctor may change your dose if needed.

For paricalcitol

- To treat an overactive parathyroid gland in patients with kidney failure:
  - For *oral* dosage form (capsules):
    - Adults: 1 to 2 micrograms (mcg) one time per day or 2 to 4 mcg three times a week (not more often than every other day). The doctor may change your dose if needed.
    - Children: Use and dose must be determined by your doctor.
  - For *injection* dosage form:
    - Adults: 0.04 to 0.1 micrograms (mcg) per kg no more than every other day during dialysis. The doctor may change your dose if needed.
    - Children: Use and dose must be determined by your doctor.

Missed dose—If you have any questions about this, check with your health care professional.

- *For use as a dietary supplement:* If you miss taking a dietary supplement for one or more days there is no cause for concern, since it takes some time for your body to become seriously low in vitamins. However, if your health care professional has recommended that you take this dietary supplement, try to remember to take it as directed every day.
- If you are taking this medicine for a reason other than as a dietary supplement and you miss a dose and your dosing schedule is:
  - One dose every other day: Take the missed dose as soon as possible if you remember it on the day it should be taken. However, if you do not remember the missed dose until the next day, take it at that time. Then skip a day and start your dosing schedule again. Do not double doses.
  - One dose a day: Take the missed dose as soon as possible. Then go back to your regular dosing schedule. However, if you do not remember the missed dose until the next day, skip the missed dose and go back to your regular dosing schedule. Do not double doses.
  - More than one dose a day: Take the missed dose as soon as possible. Then go back to your regular dosing schedule. However, if it is almost time for your next dose, skip the missed dose and go back to your regular dosing schedule. Do not double doses.

If you have any questions about this, check with your health care professional.

Storage—To store this dietary supplement:

- Keep out of the reach of children.
- Store away from heat and direct light.
- Do not store in the bathroom, near the kitchen sink, or in other damp places. Heat or moisture may cause the dietary supplement to break down.
- Keep the oral liquid form of the dietary supplement from freezing.
- Do not keep outdated dietary supplements or those no longer needed. Be sure that any discarded dietary supplement is out of the reach of children.

Precautions While Using This Dietary Supplement

For individuals taking vitamin D *without a prescription:*

- Vitamin D is stored in the body; therefore, when you take more than the body needs, it will build up in the body. This may lead to poisoning. Problems are more likely to occur in:
  - Adults taking 20,000 to 80,000 Units a day and more for several weeks or months.
  - Children taking 2,000 to 4,000 Units a day for several months.
- Remember that the total amount of vitamin D you get every day includes what you get from foods that you eat and what you take as a supplement.

If you are taking this medicine for a reason other than as a dietary supplement, *your doctor should check your progress at regular visits* to make sure that it does not cause unwanted effects.

Do not take any nonprescription (over-the-counter [OTC]) medicine or dietary supplement that contains calcium, phosphorus, or vitamin D while you are taking any of these dietary supplements unless you have been told to do so by your health care professional. The extra calcium, phosphorus, or vitamin D may increase the chance of side effects.

Do not take antacids or other medicines containing magnesium while you are taking any of these medicines. Taking these medicines together may cause unwanted effects.

Side Effects of This Dietary Supplement

Along with its needed effects, a dietary supplement may cause some unwanted effects. Alfacalcidol, calcifediol, calcitriol, dihydrotachysterol, and ergocalciferol do not usually cause any side effects when taken as directed. However, *taking large amounts over a period of time may cause some unwanted effects that can be serious.*

Check with your doctor immediately if any of the following effects occur:

Late symptoms of severe overdose
High blood pressure; high fever; irregular heartbeat; stomach pain (severe)

Check with your health care professional as soon as possible if any of the following effects occur:

Early symptoms of overdose
Bone pain; constipation (especially in children or adolescents); diarrhea; drowsiness; dryness of mouth; headache (continuing); increased thirst; increase in frequency of urination, especially at night, or in amount of urine; irregular heartbeat; itching skin; loss of appetite; metallic taste; muscle pain; nausea or vomiting (especially in children or adolescents); unusual tiredness or weakness

Late symptoms of overdose
Bone pain; calcium deposits (hard lumps) in tissues outside of the bone; cloudy urine; drowsiness; increased sensitivity of eyes to light or irritation of eyes; itching of skin; loss of appetite; loss of sex drive; mood or mental changes; muscle pain; nausea or vomiting; protein in the urine; redness or discharge of the eye, eyelid, or lining of the eyelid; runny nose; weight loss

Other side effects not listed above may also occur in some individuals. If you notice any other effects, check with your health care professional.

VITAMIN E (Oral route) - VYE-ta-min E

Commonly used brand name(s)

In the U.S.—

Alpha-E	Formula E 400
Aqua Gem-E	Gamma E-Gems
Aquasol E	Gamma E Plus
D-Alpha Gems	Key-E
E-400	Natural Vitamin Blend E-
E-600	400IU
E-Gems	Nutr-E-Sol

Available Dosage Forms:
- Capsule, Liquid Filled
- Tablet
- Solution
- Liquid
- Tablet, Chewable
- Powder for Solution
- Capsule

Therapeutic Class: Nutritive Agent
Pharmacologic Class: Vitamin E (class)

Uses For This Dietary Supplement

Vitamins are compounds that you must have for growth and health. They are needed in only small amounts and are available in the foods that you eat. Vitamin E prevents a chemical reaction called oxidation, which can sometimes result in harmful effects in your body. It is also important for the proper function of nerves and muscles.

Some conditions may increase your need for vitamin E. These include:
- Intestine disease
- Liver disease
- Pancreas disease
- Surgical removal of stomach

Increased need for vitamin E should be determined by your health care professional.

Infants who are receiving a formula that is not fortified with vitamin E may be likely to have a vitamin E deficiency. Also, diets high in polyunsaturated fatty acids may increase your need for vitamin E.

Claims that vitamin E is effective for treatment of cancer and for prevention or treatment of acne, aging, loss of hair, bee stings, liver spots on the hands, bursitis, diaper rash, frostbite, stomach ulcer, heart attacks, labor pains, certain blood diseases, miscarriage, muscular dystrophy, poor posture, sexual impotence, sterility, infertility, menopause, sunburn, and lung damage from air pollution have not been proven. Although vitamin E is being used to prevent certain types of cancer, there is not enough information to show that this is effective.

Lack of vitamin E is extremely rare, except in people who have a disease in which it is not absorbed into the body.

Vitamin E is available without a prescription.

Importance of Diet—For good health, it is important that you eat a balanced and varied diet. Follow carefully any diet program your health care professional may recommend. For your specific dietary vitamin and/or mineral needs, ask your health care professional for a list of appropriate foods. If you think that you are not getting enough vitamins and/or minerals in your diet, you may choose to take a dietary supplement.

Vitamin E is found in various foods including vegetable oils (corn, cottonseed, soybean, safflower), wheat germ, wholegrain cereals, and green leafy vegetables. Cooking and storage may destroy some of the vitamin E in foods.

Vitamin supplements alone will not take the place of a good diet and will not provide energy. Your body also needs other substances found in food such as protein, minerals, carbohydrates, and fat. Vitamins themselves often cannot work without the presence of other foods. For example, small amounts of fat are needed so that vitamin E can be absorbed into the body.

The daily amount of vitamin E needed is defined in several different ways.

For U.S.—
- Recommended Dietary Allowances (RDAs) are the amount of vitamins and minerals needed to provide for adequate nutrition in most healthy persons. RDAs for a given nutrient may vary depending on a person's age, sex, and physical condition (e.g., pregnancy).
- Daily Values (DVs) are used on food and dietary supplement labels to indicate the percent of the recommended daily amount of each nutrient that a serving provides. DV replaces the previous designation of United States Recommended Daily Allowances (USRDAs).

For Canada—
- Recommended Nutrient Intakes (RNIs) are used to determine the amounts of vitamins, minerals, and protein needed to provide adequate nutrition and lessen the risk of chronic disease.

Vitamin E is available in various forms, including d- or dl-alpha tocopheryl acetate, d- or dl-alpha tocopherol, and d- or dl-alpha tocopheryl acid succinate. In the past, the RDA for vitamin E have been expressed in Units. This term has been replaced by alpha tocopherol equivalents (alpha-TE) or milligrams (mg) of d-alpha tocopherol. One Unit is equivalent to 1 mg of dl-alpha tocopherol acetate or 0.6 mg d-alpha tocopherol. Most products available in stores continue to be labeled in Units.

Normal daily recommended intakes in milligrams (mg) of alpha tocopherol equivalents (mg alpha-TE) and Units for vitamin E are generally defined as follows:

Persons	U.S.		Canada	
	mg alpha-TE	Units	mg alpha-TE	Units
Infants and children				
Birth to 3 years of age	3–6	5–10	3–4	5–6.7
4 to 6 years of age	7	11.7	5	8.3
7 to 10 years of age	7	11.7	6–8	10–13
Adolescent and adult males	10	16.7	6–10	10–16.7
Adolescent and adult females	8	13	5–7	8.3–11.7
Pregnant females	10	16.7	8–9	13–15
Breast-feeding females	11–12	18–20	9–10	15–16.7

Before Using This Dietary Supplement

If you are taking this dietary supplement without a prescription, carefully read and follow any precautions on the label. For this supplement, the following should be considered:

Allergies—Tell your doctor if you have ever had any unusual or allergic reaction to this medicine or any other medicines. Also tell your health care professional if you have any other types of allergies, such as to foods, dyes, preservatives, or animals. For non-prescription products, read the label or package ingredients carefully.

Pediatric—Problems in children have not been reported with intake of normal daily recommended amounts. You should check with your health care professional if you are giving your baby an unfortified formula. In that case, the baby must get the vitamins needed some other way. Some studies have shown that premature infants may have low levels of vitamin E. Your health care professional may recommend a vitamin E supplement.

Geriatric—Problems in older adults have not been reported with intake of normal daily recommended amounts.

Breast Feeding—There are no adequate studies in women for determining infant risk when using this medication during breastfeeding. Weigh the potential benefits against the potential risks before taking this medication while breastfeeding.

Other medicines—

Using this dietary supplement with any of the following medicines is usually not recommended, but may be required in some cases. If both medicines are prescribed together, your doctor may change the dose or how often you use one or both of the medicines.

Dicumarol

Interactions with Food/Tobacco/Alcohol—Certain medicines should not be used at or around the time of eating food or eating certain types of food since interactions may occur. Using alcohol or tobacco with certain medicines may also cause interactions to occur. Discuss with your healthcare professional the use of your medicine with food, alcohol, or tobacco.

Other medical problems—The presence of other medical problems may affect the use of this dietary supplement. Make sure you tell your doctor if you have any other medical problems, especially:
- Bleeding problems—Vitamin E, when taken in doses greater than 800 Units a day for long periods of time, may make this condition worse

Proper Use of This Dietary Supplement

Dosing—The dose of this medicine will be different for different patients. Follow your doctor's orders or the directions on the label. The following information includes only the average doses of this medicine. If your dose is different, do not change it unless your doctor tells you to do so.

The amount of medicine that you take depends on the strength of the medicine. Also, the number of doses you take each day, the time allowed between doses, and the length of time you take the medicine depend on the medical problem for which you are using the medicine.

- For oral solution dosage form:
  - To prevent the following deficiencies in infants:
    - Infants receiving a formula high in polyunsaturated fatty acids—15 to 25 Units per day or 7 Units per 32 ounces of formula.
    - Infants with certain colon problems—15 to 25 Units per kilogram (kg) (6.8 to 11 Units per pound) of body weight per day. The water-soluble form of vitamin E must be used.
    - Infants of normal birthweight—5 Units per 32 ounces of formula.
- For oral dosage forms (capsules, tablets, oral solution):
  - To prevent deficiency for individuals (other than infants), the amount taken by mouth is based on normal daily recommended intakes:

For the U.S.
  - Adult and teenage males—10 milligrams (mg) of alpha tocopherol equivalents (mg alpha-TE) or 16.7 Units per day.
  - Adult and teenage females—8 mg alpha-TE or 13 Units per day.
  - Pregnant females—10 mg alpha-TE or 16.7 Units per day.
  - Breast-feeding females—11 to 12 mg alpha-TE or 18 to 20 Units per day.
  - Children 4 to 10 years of age—7 mg alpha-TE or 11.7 Units per day.
  - Children birth to 3 years of age—3 to 6 mg alpha-TE or 5 to 10 Units per day.

For Canada
  - Adult and teenage males—6 to 10 mg alpha-TE or 10 to 16.7 Units per day.
  - Adult and teenage females—5 to 7 mg alpha-TE or 8.3 to 11.7 Units per day.
  - Pregnant females—8 to 9 mg alpha-TE or 13 to 15 Units per day.
  - Breast-feeding females—9 to 10 mg alpha-TE or 15 to 16.7 Units per day.
  - Children 7 to 10 years of age—6 to 8 mg alpha-TE or 10 to 13 Units per day.
  - Children 4 to 6 years of age—5 mg alpha-TE or 8.3 Units per day.
  - Children birth to 3 years of age—3 to 4 mg alpha-TE or 5 to 6.7 Units per day.
  ○ To treat deficiency:
    - Adults, teenagers, and children—Treatment dose is determined by prescriber for each individual based on the severity of deficiency.

For individuals taking the oral liquid form of this dietary supplement:

  - This preparation should be taken by mouth even though it comes in a dropper bottle.
  - This dietary supplement may be dropped directly into the mouth or mixed with cereal, fruit juice, or other food.

Missed dose—If you miss a dose of this medicine, skip the missed dose and go back to your regular dosing schedule. Do not double doses.

Storage—Store the dietary supplement in a closed container at room temperature, away from heat, moisture, and direct light. Keep from freezing.

Keep out of the reach of children.

Do not keep outdated medicine or medicine no longer needed.

Side Effects of This Dietary Supplement

Along with its needed effects, a medicine may cause some unwanted effects. Although not all of these side effects may occur, if they do occur they may need medical attention.

Check with your doctor as soon as possible if any of the following side effects occur:

  With doses greater than 400 Units a day and long-term use
    Blurred vision; diarrhea; dizziness; headache; nausea or stomach cramps; unusual tiredness or weakness

Other side effects not listed may also occur in some patients. If you notice any other effects, check with your healthcare professional.

VITAMIN K   (Systemic)

Some commonly used brand names are:

In the U.S.—
   AquaMEPHYTON (2)
   Mephyton (2)

This information applies to the following medicines:

1. Menadiol (men-a-DYE-ole)
2. Phytonadione (fye-toe-na-DYE-one)

Category

  - **Antidote, to drug-induced hypoprothrombinemia—** Menadiol; Phytonadione
  - **Antihemorrhagic—**Phytonadione
  - **Nutritional supplement, vitamin, prothrombogenic—** Menadiol; Phytonadione

Description

Vitamins (VYE-ta-mins) are compounds that you *must* have for growth and health. They are needed in only small amounts and usually are available in the foods that you eat. Vitamin K is necessary for normal clotting of the blood.

Vitamin K is found in various foods including green leafy vegetables, meat, and dairy products. If you eat a balanced diet containing these foods, you should be getting all the vitamin K you need. Little vitamin K is lost from foods with ordinary cooking.

If you are taking anticoagulant medicine (blood thinners), the amount of vitamin K in your diet may affect how well these medicines work. Your doctor or health care professional may recommend changes in your diet to help these medicines work better.

Lack of vitamin K is rare but may lead to problems with blood clotting and increased bleeding. Your doctor may treat this by prescribing vitamin K for you.

Vitamin K is routinely given to newborn infants to prevent bleeding problems.

This medicine is available only with your doctor's prescription, in the following dosage forms:

  Oral
  - Phytonadione
    ○ Tablets
  Parenteral
  - Phytonadione
    ○ Injection (U.S.)

Before Using This Medicine

In deciding to use a medicine, the risks of taking the medicine must be weighed against the good it will do. This is a decision you and your doctor will make. For vitamin K, the following should be considered:

Allergies—Tell your doctor if you have ever had any unusual or allergic reaction to vitamin K. Also tell your health care professional if you are allergic to any other substances, such as foods, preservatives, or dyes.

Pregnancy—Vitamin K has not been reported to cause birth defects or other problems in humans. However, the use of vitamin K supplements during pregnancy is not recommended because it has been reported to cause jaundice and other problems in the baby.

Breast-feeding—Vitamin K taken by the mother has not been reported to cause problems in nursing babies. You should check with your doctor if you are giving your baby an unfortified formula. In that case, the baby must get the vitamins needed some other way.

Children—Children may be especially sensitive to the effects of vitamin K, especially menadiol or high doses of phytonadione. This may increase the chance of side effects during treatment. Newborns, especially premature babies, may be more sensitive to these effects than older children.

Older adults—Many medicines have not been tested in older people. Therefore, it may not be known whether they work exactly the same way they do in younger adults or if they cause different side effects or problems in older people. There is no specific information about the use of vitamin K in the elderly.

Other medicines—Although certain medicines should not be used together at all, in other cases two different medicines may be used together even if an interaction might occur. In these cases, your doctor may want to change the dose, or other precautions may be necessary. When you are taking vitamin K, it is especially important that your health care professional know if you are taking any of the following:
- Acetohydroxamic acid (e.g., Lithostat) or
- Antidiabetics, oral (diabetes medicine you take by mouth) or
- Dapsone or
- Furazolidone (e.g., Furoxone) or
- Methyldopa (e.g., Aldomet) or
- Nitrofurantoin (e.g., Furadantin) or
- Primaquine or
- Procainamide (e.g., Pronestyl) or
- Quinidine (e.g., Quinidex) or
- Quinine (e.g., Quinamm) or
- Sulfonamides (sulfa medicine) or
- Sulfoxone (e.g., Diasone)—The chance of a serious side effect may be increased, especially with menadiol
- Anticoagulants (blood thinners)—Vitamin K decreases the effects of these medicines and is sometimes used to treat bleeding caused by anticoagulants; however, patients receiving an anticoagulant should not take any supplement that contains vitamin K (alone or in combination with other vitamins or nutrients) unless it has been ordered by their doctor

Other medical problems—The presence of other medical problems may affect the use of vitamin K. Make sure you tell your doctor if you have any other medical problems, especially:
- Cystic fibrosis or other diseases affecting the pancreas or
- Diarrhea (prolonged) or
- Gallbladder disease or
- Intestinal problems—These conditions may interfere with absorption of vitamin K into the body when it is taken by mouth; higher doses may be needed, or the medicine may have to be injected

- Glucose-6–phosphate dehydrogenase (G6PD) deficiency—The chance of side effects may be increased, especially with menadiol
- Liver disease—The chance of unwanted effects may be increased

Proper Use of This Medicine

Take this medicine only as directed by your doctor. Do not take more or less of it, do not take it more often, and do not take it for a longer time than your doctor ordered. To do so may cause serious unwanted effects, such as blood clotting problems.

Dosing—The dose of these medicines will be different for different patients. *Follow your doctor's orders or the directions on the label.* The following information includes only the average doses of these medicines. *If your dose is different, do not change it* unless your doctor tells you to do so.

The number of tablets or injections that you take depends on the strength of the medicine. Also, *the number of doses you take each day, the time allowed between doses, and the length of time you take the medicine depend on the medical problem for which you are taking the medicine.*

For menadiol
- For *oral* dosage form (tablets):
  - For problems with blood clotting or increased bleeding, or for dietary supplementation:
    - Adults and children—The usual dose is 5 to 10 milligrams (mg) a day.
- For *injection* dosage form:
  - For problems with blood clotting or increased bleeding, or for dietary supplementation:
    - Adults and teenagers—The usual dose is 5 to 15 mg, injected into a muscle or under the skin, one or two times a day.
    - Children—The usual dose is 5 to 10 mg, injected into a muscle or under the skin, one or two times a day.

For phytonadione
- For *oral* dosage form (tablets):
  - For problems with blood clotting or increased bleeding:
    - Adults and teenagers—The usual dose is 2.5 to 25 milligrams (mg), rarely up to 50 mg. The dose may be repeated, if needed.
    - Children—Use is not recommended.
- For *injection* dosage form:
  - For problems with blood clotting or increased bleeding:
    - Adults and teenagers—The usual dose is 2.5 to 25 mg, rarely up to 50 mg, injected under the skin. The dose may be repeated, if needed.
  - For prevention of bleeding in newborns:
    - The usual dose is 0.5 to 1 mg, injected into a muscle or under the skin, right after delivery. The dose may be repeated after six to eight hours, if needed.

Missed dose—If you miss a dose of this medicine, take it as soon as possible. However, if it is almost time for your next dose, skip the missed dose and go back to your regular dosing schedule. Do not double doses. *Tell your doctor about any doses you miss.*

Storage—To store this medicine:

- Keep out of the reach of children.
- Store away from heat and direct light.
- Do not store in the bathroom, near the kitchen sink, or in other damp places. Heat or moisture may cause the medicine to break down.
- Do not keep outdated medicine or medicine no longer needed. Be sure that any discarded medicine is out of the reach of children.

Precautions While Using This Medicine

Tell all medical doctors and dentists you go to that you are taking this medicine.

Always check with your health care professional before you start or stop taking any other medicine. This includes any nonprescription (over-the-counter [OTC]) medicine, even aspirin. Other medicines may change the way this medicine affects your body.

Your doctor should check your progress at regular visits. A blood test must be taken regularly to see how fast your blood is clotting. This will help your doctor decide how much medicine you need.

Side Effects of This Medicine

Along with its needed effects, a medicine may cause some unwanted effects. Although not all of these side effects may occur, if they do occur they may need medical attention.

Check with your doctor as soon as possible if any of the following side effects occur:

Less common—With menadiol or high doses of phytonadione in newborns

Decreased appetite; decreased movement or activity; difficulty in breathing; enlarged liver; general body swelling; irritability; muscle stiffness; paleness; yellow eyes or skin

Rare—With injection only

Difficulty in swallowing; fast or irregular breathing; light-headedness or fainting; shortness of breath; skin rash, hives and/or itching; swelling of eyelids, face, or lips; tightness in chest; troubled breathing and/or wheezing

Rare

Blue color or flushing or redness of skin; dizziness; fast and/or weak heartbeat; increased sweating; low blood pressure (temporary)

Other side effects may occur that usually do not need medical attention. These side effects may go away during treatment as your body adjusts to the medicine. However, check with your doctor if any of the following side effects continue or are bothersome:

Less common

Flushing of face; redness, pain, or swelling at place of injection; skin lesions at place of injection (rare); unusual taste

Other side effects not listed above may also occur in some patients. If you notice any other effects, check with your doctor.

VITAMINS AND FLUORIDE
(Systemic)

Some commonly used brand names are:

In the U.S.—

Adeflor (1)	Poly-Vi-Flor (1)
Cari-Tab (2)	Tri-Vi-Flor (2)
Mulvidren-F (1)	Vi-Daylin/F (1)

In Canada—

Adeflor (1)
Poly-Vi-Flor (1)
Tri-Vi-Flor (2)

This information applies to the following medicines:

1. Multiple Vitamins and Fluoride
2. Vitamins A, D, and C and Fluoride

Category

- **Vitamin replenisher– dental caries prophylactic—** Vitamins and Fluoride

Description

This medicine is a combination of vitamins and fluoride. Vitamins are used when the daily diet does not include enough of the vitamins needed for good health.

Fluoride has been found to be helpful in reducing the number of cavities in the teeth. It is usually present naturally in drinking water. However, some areas of the country do not have a high enough level of fluoride in the water. To make up for this, extra fluorides may be added to the diet. Some children may require both dietary fluorides and fluoride treatments by the dentist. Use of a fluoride toothpaste or rinse may be helpful, as well.

Taking fluorides does not replace good dental habits. These include eating a good diet, brushing and flossing teeth frequently, and having regular dental checkups.

This medicine is available only with your medical doctor's or dentist's prescription, in the following dosage forms:

Oral

- Oral solution
- Chewable Tablets

Before Using This Dietary Supplement

In deciding to use a dietary supplement, the risks of taking the dietary supplement must be weighed against the good it will do. This is a decision you and your medical doctor or dentist will make. For multiple vitamins and fluoride, the following should be considered:

Allergies—Tell your medical doctor or dentist if you have ever had any unusual or allergic reactions to fluoride. Also, tell your medical doctor, dentist, and pharmacist if you are allergic to any other substances, such as foods, preservatives, or dyes.

Pregnancy—Fluoride occurs naturally in water and has not been shown to cause problems in infants of mothers who drank fluoridated water or took recommended doses of supplements.

Breast-feeding—Small amounts of fluoride pass into breast milk; however, problems have not been documented with normal intake.

Children—Doses of fluoride that are too large or are taken for a long time may cause bone problems and teeth discoloration in children.

Older adults—This dietary supplement has not been shown to cause different side effects or problems in older people than it does in younger adults.

Medicines or other dietary supplements—Although certain medicines or dietary supplements should not be used together at all, in other cases they may be used together even if an interaction might occur. In these cases, your medical doctor or dentist may want to change the dose, or other precautions may be necessary. When you are taking multiple vitamins and fluoride it is especially important that your medical doctor or dentist, and pharmacist know if you are taking any of the following:

- Anticoagulants, coumarin- or indandione-derivative (blood thinners)—Use with vitamin K (in the multiple vitamins and fluoride preparations) may prevent the anticoagulant from working properly
- Iron supplements—Use with vitamin E (in the multiple vitamins and fluoride preparation) may prevent the iron supplement from working properly
- Vitamin D and related compounds—Use with vitamin D (in the multiple vitamins and fluoride preparations) may cause high blood levels of vitamin D, which may increase the chance of side effects

Other medical problems—The presence of other medical problems may affect the use of multiple vitamins and fluoride. Make sure you tell your medical doctor or dentist if you have any other medical problems, especially:

- Dental fluorosis (teeth discoloration)—Fluorides may make this condition worse

Proper Use of This Dietary Supplement

Take this dietary supplement only as directed by your medical doctor or dentist. Do not take more of it and do not take it more often than ordered. Taking too much fluoride and some vitamins (especially vitamins A and D) over a period of time may cause unwanted effects.

Do not take multiple vitamins and fluoride products at the same time as taking foods that contain calcium. It is best to space them 1 to 2 hours apart, to get the full benefit from the medicine.

For patients taking the *chewable tablet form* of this dietary supplement:

- Tablets should be chewed or crushed before they are swallowed.
- This dietary supplement works best if it is taken at bedtime, after the teeth have been thoroughly brushed.

For patients taking the *oral liquid form of* this dietary supplement:

- This dietary supplement is to be taken by mouth even though it comes in a dropper bottle. The amount to be taken is to be measured with the specially marked dropper.
- *Always store this dietary supplement in the original plastic container.* It has been designed to give you the correct dose. Also, fluoride will interact with glass and should not be stored in glass containers.

- This dietary supplement may be dropped directly into the mouth or mixed with cereal, fruit juice, or other food.

Missed dose—If you miss a dose of this dietary supplement, take it as soon as you remember. However, if it is almost time for the next dose, skip the missed dose and go back to your regular dosing schedule. Do not double doses.

Storage—To store this dietary supplement:

- Keep this dietary supplement out of the reach of children, since overdose is especially dangerous in children.
- Store away from heat and direct light.
- Do not store in the bathroom, near the kitchen sink, or in other damp places. Heat or moisture may cause the dietary supplement to break down.
- Protect the oral solution from freezing.
- Do not keep outdated dietary supplements or those no longer needed. Be sure that any discarded dietary supplement is out of the reach of children.

Precautions While Using This Dietary Supplement

The level of fluoride present in the water is different in different parts of the country. If you move to another area, check with a medical doctor or dentist in the new area as soon as possible to see if this medicine is still needed or if the dose needs to be changed. Also, check with your medical doctor or dentist if you change infant feeding habits (e.g., breastfeeding to infant formula), drinking water (e.g., city water to nonfluoridated bottled water), or filtering systems (e.g., tap water to filtered tap water).

Inform your medical doctor or dentist as soon as possible if you notice white, brown, or black spots on the teeth. These are signs of too much fluoride.

Side Effects of This Dietary Supplement

Along with its needed effects, a dietary supplement may cause some unwanted effects. Although not all of these side effects may occur, if they do occur they may need medical attention.

When the correct amount of this dietary supplement is used, side effects usually are rare. However, *taking an overdose of fluoride may cause serious problems.*

Stop taking this dietary supplement and check with your medical doctor immediately if any of the following side effects occur, as they may be signs of severe fluoride overdose:

Black, tarry stools; bloody vomit; diarrhea; drowsiness; faintness; increased watering of mouth; nausea or vomiting; shallow breathing; stomach cramps or pain; tremors; unusual excitement; watery eyes; weakness

Check with your medical doctor or dentist as soon as possible if the following side effects occur, as some may be early signs of possible chronic fluoride overdose:

Pain and aching of bones; skin rash; sores in the mouth and on the lips; stiffness; white, brown, or black discoloration of teeth

Other side effects not listed above may also occur in some patients. If you notice any other effects, check with your medical doctor or dentist.

VORICONAZOLE (Oral route, Intravenous route) - vor-i-KON-a-zole

Commonly used brand name(s)

In the U.S.—
  Vfend
  Vfend I.V.

Available Dosage Forms:

- Tablet
- Powder for Suspension
- Powder for Solution

Therapeutic Class: Antifungal

Uses For This Medicine

Voriconazole is used to treat different kinds of serious fungal infections. It may also be used to treat patients with serious fungal infections who cannot tolerate other types of treatment or do not respond to other types of treatment.

This medicine is available only with your doctor's prescription.

Before Using This Medicine

In deciding to use a medicine, the risks of taking the medicine must be weighed against the good it will do. This is a decision you and your doctor will make. For this medicine, the following should be considered:

Allergies—Tell your doctor if you have ever had any unusual or allergic reaction to this medicine or any other medicines. Also tell your health care professional if you have any other types of allergies, such as to foods, dyes, preservatives, or animals. For non-prescription products, read the label or package ingredients carefully.

Pediatric—Studies on this medicine have been done only in patients 12 and older, and there is no specific information comparing the use of voriconazole in children with use in other age groups.

Geriatric—Many medicines have not been studied specifically in older people. Therefore, it may not be known whether they work exactly the same way they do in younger adults or if they cause different side effects or problems in older people. Voriconazole is not expected to cause different side effects or problems in older people than it does in younger adults.

Pregnancy—

	Pregnancy Category	Explanation
All Trimesters	D	Studies in pregnant women have demonstrated a risk to the fetus. However, the benefits of therapy in a life threatening situation or a serious disease, may outweigh the potential risk.

Breast Feeding—There are no adequate studies in women for determining infant risk when using this medication during breastfeeding. Weigh the potential benefits against the potential risks before taking this medication while breastfeeding.

Other medicines—

Using this medicine with any of the following medicines is not recommended. Your doctor may decide not to treat you with this medication or change some of the other medicines you take.

Amobarbital, Aprobarbital, Astemizole, Butabarbital, Carbamazepine, Cisapride, Dihydroergotamine, Efavirenz, Ergoloid Mesylates, Ergonovine, Ergotamine, Eterobarb, Heptabarbital, Hexobarbital, Mephobarbital, Methylergonovine, Methysergide, Pentobarbital, Phenobarbital, Pimozide, Quinidine, Rifabutin, Rifampin, Ritonavir, Secobarbital, Sirolimus, Terfenadine

Interactions with Food/Tobacco/Alcohol—Certain medicines should not be used at or around the time of eating food or eating certain types of food since interactions may occur. Using alcohol or tobacco with certain medicines may also cause interactions to occur. Discuss with your healthcare professional the use of your medicine with food, alcohol, or tobacco.

Other medical problems—The presence of other medical problems may affect the use of this medicine. Make sure you tell your doctor if you have any other medical problems, especially:

- Hypersensitivity to voriconazole, other azole antifungal agents, or any of the ingredients in voriconazole.

Proper Use of This Medicine

Dosing—The dose of this medicine will be different for different patients. Follow your doctor's orders or the directions on the label. The following information includes only the average doses of this medicine. If your dose is different, do not change it unless your doctor tells you to do so.

The amount of medicine that you take depends on the strength of the medicine. Also, the number of doses you take each day, the time allowed between doses, and the length of time you take the medicine depend on the medical problem for which you are using the medicine.

For the oral suspension, shake well before measuring the dose. Use the oral dispenser supplied with your medicine to measure the dose.

- For oral dosage forms (oral suspension or tablets):
  - For serious fungal infections:
    - Adults—Your dose will be determined based on your weight and other medicines you are taking. Check with your doctor for more dosage information. Oral suspension or tablets should be taken 1 hour before or after a meal.
    - Children—Safety and effectiveness have not been established in children less than 12 years of age. For children over 12 years of age, use and dose will be determined by your doctor.
- For injection dosage form:
  - For serious fungal infections:
    - Adults—Your dose will be determined based on your weight and other medicines you are taking. The dose should be infused over 1 to 2 hours.

Check with your doctor for more dosage information.

- Children—Safety and effectiveness have not been established in children less than 12 years of age. For children over 12 years of age, use and dose will be determined by your doctor.

Missed dose—If you miss a dose of this medicine, take it as soon as possible. However, if it is almost time for your next dose, skip the missed dose and go back to your regular dosing schedule. Do not double doses.

Storage—Store the medicine in a closed container at room temperature, away from heat, moisture, and direct light. Keep from freezing.

Keep out of the reach of children.

Do not keep outdated medicine or medicine no longer needed.

Ask your healthcare professional how you should dispose of any medicine you do not use.

Throw away any unused oral suspension after the date listed on the label.

Precautions While Using This Medicine

It is very important that your doctor check you at regular visits to see if the medicine is working properly and decide if you should continue to take it.

If your symptoms do not improve within a few days or if they become worse, check with your doctor.

Do not take other medicines unless they have been discussed with your doctor. Your doctor will discuss with you any changes in your medicine. Ask your doctor if you have any questions.

This medicine may cause some people to have changes in vision, such as blurred vision and seeing bright spots or wavy lines. Make sure you know how you react to this medicine before you drive, use machines, or do anything else that could be dangerous if you have vision changes.

It is important that contraception (birth control) be used in women during treatment with this medicine.

Side Effects of This Medicine

Along with its needed effects, a medicine may cause some unwanted effects. Although not all of these side effects may occur, if they do occur they may need medical attention.

Check with your doctor immediately if any of the following side effects occur:

More common
Rash

Less common
Abdominal or stomach pain; bloating or swelling of face, arms, hands, lower legs, or feet; blurred vision; chills; clay-colored stools; confusion; convulsions; dark urine; decreased urine; dizziness; dry mouth; faintness or light-headedness when getting up from a lying or sitting position; fever; headache; increased thirst; irregular or pounding heartbeat; itching; loss of appetite; mood or mental changes; muscle pain or cramps; muscle spasms or twitching; nausea; nervousness; numbness or tingling in hands, feet, or lips; pounding in the ears; rapid weight gain; rash with flat lesions or

small raised lesions on the skin; shortness of breath; slow or fast heartbeat; suddenly sweating; trembling; unpleasant breath odor; unusual tiredness or weakness; vomiting of blood; vasodilation (flushing); yellow eyes or skin

Rare
Abnormal kidney function; black, bloody, or tarry stools; bleeding gums; blood in eye; blood in urine or stools; chest pain; eye pain; painful or difficult urination; pale skin; pinpoint red spots on skin; redness in whites of eyes; sores, ulcers, or white spots on lips or in mouth; sore throat; sudden kidney failure; swollen glands; trouble breathing with activity; unusual bleeding or bruising

Some side effects may occur that usually do not need medical attention. These side effects may go away during treatment as your body adjusts to the medicine. Also, your health care professional may be able to tell you about ways to prevent or reduce some of these side effects. Check with your health care professional if any of the following side effects continue or are bothersome or if you have any questions about them:

More common
Changes in vision; seeing things that are not there

Less common
Diarrhea; difficulty seeing at night; disturbance in vision; dry mouth; feeling unusually cold; increased sensitivity of eyes to sunlight; shivering; vomiting

Other side effects not listed may also occur in some patients. If you notice any other effects, check with your healthcare professional.

YOHIMBINE (Oral route) - yo-HIM-been

Uses For This Medicine

Yohimbine is used to increase peripheral blood flow. It is also used to dilate the pupil of the eye.

Yohimbine is available only with your doctor's prescription.

Once a medicine has been approved for marketing for a certain use, experience may show that it is also useful for other medical problems. Yohimbine is used to treat men with the following medical condition:

- Impotence (not able to have erections)

The way yohimbine works is not known for sure. It is thought, however, to work by increasing the body's production of certain chemicals that help produce erections. It does not work in all men who are impotent.

This medicine usually begins to work about 2 to 3 weeks after you begin to take it.

The dose of yohimbine will be different for different patients. Follow your doctor's orders or the directions on the label. The following information includes only the average doses of yohimbine. If your dose is different, do not change it unless your doctor tells you to do so.

The number of tablets that you take depends on the strength of the medicine.

- For oral dosage form (tablets):
  - For treating impotence:
    - Adults—5.4 to 6 milligrams (mg) three times a day.

Before Using This Medicine

In deciding to use a medicine, the risks of taking the medicine must be weighed against the good it will do. This is a decision you and your doctor will make. For this medicine, the following should be considered:

Allergies—Tell your doctor if you have ever had any unusual or allergic reaction to this medicine or any other medicines. Also tell your health care professional if you have any other types of allergies, such as to foods, dyes, preservatives, or animals. For non-prescription products, read the label or package ingredients carefully.

Geriatric—Many medicines have not been studied specifically in older people. Therefore, it may not be known whether they work exactly the same way they do in younger adults. Although there is no specific information comparing use of yohimbine in the elderly with use in other age groups, this medicine has been used in some elderly patients and has not been shown to cause different side effects or problems in older people than it does in younger adults.

Other medicines—

Using this medicine with any of the following medicines may cause an increased risk of certain side effects, but using both drugs may be the best treatment for you. If both medicines are prescribed together, your doctor may change the dose or how often you use one or both of the medicines.

Clomipramine, Clonidine, Guanabenz, Guanadrel, Guanethidine, Guanfacine, Lithium, Morphine, Morphine Sulfate Liposome, Naloxone, Naltrexone, Reserpine

Interactions with Food/Tobacco/Alcohol—Certain medicines should not be used at or around the time of eating food or eating certain types of food since interactions may occur. Using alcohol or tobacco with certain medicines may also cause interactions to occur. The following interactions have been selected on the basis of their potential significance and are not necessarily all-inclusive.

Using this medicine with any of the following may cause an increased risk of certain side effects but may be unavoidable in some cases. If used together, your doctor may change the dose or how often you use this medicine, or give you special instructions about the use of food, alcohol, or tobacco.

Ethanol

Other medical problems—The presence of other medical problems may affect the use of this medicine. Make sure you tell your doctor if you have any other medical problems, especially:

- Angina pectoris or
- Depression or
- Other psychiatric illness or
- Heart disease or
- High blood pressure or
- Kidney disease—Yohimbine may make these conditions worse
- Liver disease—Effects of yohimbine may be increased because of slower removal from the body

Proper Use of This Medicine

Take this medicine only as directed by your doctor to help your condition as much as possible. Do not take more or less of it, and do not take it more or less often than your doctor ordered.

Dosing—The dose of this medicine will be different for different patients. Follow your doctor's orders or the directions on the label. The following information includes only the average doses of this medicine. If your dose is different, do not change it unless your doctor tells you to do so.

The amount of medicine that you take depends on the strength of the medicine. Also, the number of doses you take each day, the time allowed between doses, and the length of time you take the medicine depend on the medical problem for which you are using the medicine.

Missed dose—If you miss a dose of this medicine, take it as soon as possible. However, if it is almost time for your next dose, skip the missed dose and go back to your regular dosing schedule. Do not double doses.

Storage—Store the medicine in a closed container at room temperature, away from heat, moisture, and direct light. Keep from freezing.

Keep out of the reach of children.

Do not keep outdated medicine or medicine no longer needed.

Precautions While Using This Medicine

It is important that your doctor check your progress at regular visits to make sure that this medicine is working properly.

Use yohimbine exactly as directed by your doctor. Do not use more of it and do not use it more often than ordered. If too much is used, the risk of side effects such as fast heartbeat and high blood pressure is increased.

Side Effects of This Medicine

Along with its needed effects, a medicine may cause some unwanted effects. Although not all of these side effects may occur, if they do occur they may need medical attention.

Check with your doctor as soon as possible if any of the following side effects occur:
Less common
   Fast heartbeat; increased blood pressure

Some side effects may occur that usually do not need medical attention. These side effects may go away during treatment as your body adjusts to the medicine. Also, your health care professional may be able to tell you about ways to prevent or reduce some of these side effects. Check with your health care professional if any of the following side effects continue or are bothersome or if you have any questions about them:
Less common
   Dizziness; headache; irritability; nervousness or restlessness
Rare
   Nausea and vomiting; skin flushing; sweating; tremor

Other side effects not listed may also occur in some patients. If you notice any other effects, check with your healthcare professional.

ZAFIRLUKAST (Oral route) - za-FIR-loo-kast

Commonly used brand name(s)

In the U.S.—
   Accolate

Available Dosage Forms:
   • Tablet

Therapeutic Class: Anti-Inflammatory
Pharmacologic Class: Leukotriene Pathway Inhibitor

Uses For This Medicine

Zafirlukast is used by patients with mild-to-moderate asthma to decrease the symptoms of asthma and the number of acute asthma attacks. However, this medicine should not be used to relieve an asthma attack that has already started.

This medicine is available only with your doctor's prescription.

Before Using This Medicine

In deciding to use a medicine, the risks of taking the medicine must be weighed against the good it will do. This is a decision you and your doctor will make. For this medicine, the following should be considered:

Allergies—Tell your doctor if you have ever had any unusual or allergic reaction to this medicine or any other medicines. Also tell your health care professional if you have any other types of allergies, such as to foods, dyes, preservatives, or animals. For non-prescription products, read the label or package ingredients carefully.

Pediatric—Studies on this medicine have been done only in adult patients and there is no specific information comparing use of zafirlukast in children up to 7 years of age with use in other age groups.

Geriatric—In studies, mild to moderate respiratory tract infections were more likely to occur in patients 55 years of age or older taking zafirlukast. It is not known whether these infections were caused by taking zafirlukast or by other factors.

Pregnancy—

	Pregnancy Category	Explanation
All Trimesters	B	Animal studies have revealed no evidence of harm to the fetus, however, there are no adequate studies in pregnant women OR animal studies have shown an adverse effect, but adequate studies in pregnant women have failed to demonstrate a risk to the fetus.

Breast Feeding—There are no adequate studies in women for determining infant risk when using this medication during breastfeeding. Weigh the potential benefits against the potential risks before taking this medication while breastfeeding.

Other medicines—
Using this medicine with any of the following medicines may cause an increased risk of certain side effects, but using both drugs may be the best treatment for you. If both medicines

are prescribed together, your doctor may change the dose or how often you use one or both of the medicines.

Erythromycin, Terfenadine, Theophylline, Warfarin

Interactions with Food/Tobacco/Alcohol—Certain medicines should not be used at or around the time of eating food or eating certain types of food since interactions may occur. Using alcohol or tobacco with certain medicines may also cause interactions to occur. Discuss with your healthcare professional the use of your medicine with food, alcohol, or tobacco.

Proper Use of This Medicine

Zafirlukast is used to prevent asthma attacks. It is not used to relieve an attack that has already started. For relief of an asthma attack that has already started, you should use another medicine. If you do not have another medicine to use for an attack or if you have any questions about this, check with your health care professional.

Food may change the amount of zafirlukast that is absorbed. For this reason, it should be taken on an empty stomach, 1 hour before or 2 hours after a meal.

Dosing—The dose of this medicine will be different for different patients. Follow your doctor's orders or the directions on the label. The following information includes only the average doses of this medicine. If your dose is different, do not change it unless your doctor tells you to do so.

The amount of medicine that you take depends on the strength of the medicine. Also, the number of doses you take each day, the time allowed between doses, and the length of time you take the medicine depend on the medical problem for which you are using the medicine.

   • For oral dosage form (tablets):
      ○ For asthma:
         ▪ Adults and children 12 years of age and older—20 milligrams (mg) two times a day, on an empty stomach, at least 1 hour before or 2 hours after meals.
         ▪ Children between 7 and 11 years of age—10 milligrams two times a day, on an empty stomach, at least 1 hour before or 2 hours after meals.
         ▪ Children up to 7 years of age—Use and dose must be determined by your doctor.

Missed dose—If you miss a dose of this medicine, take it as soon as possible. However, if it is almost time for your next dose, skip the missed dose and go back to your regular dosing schedule. Do not double doses.

Storage—Store the medicine in a closed container at room temperature, away from heat, moisture, and direct light. Keep from freezing.

Keep out of the reach of children.

Do not keep outdated medicine or medicine no longer needed.

Precautions While Using This Medicine

To work properly, zafirlukast must be taken every day at regularly spaced times, even if your asthma seems better.

You may be taking other medicines for asthma along with zafirlukast. Do not stop taking or reduce the dose of the other medicines, even if your asthma seems better, unless you are told to do so by your doctor.

Side Effects of This Medicine

Along with its needed effects, a medicine may cause some unwanted effects. Although not all of these side effects may occur, if they do occur they may need medical attention.

Some side effects may occur that usually do not need medical attention. These side effects may go away during treatment as your body adjusts to the medicine. Also, your health care professional may be able to tell you about ways to prevent or reduce some of these side effects. Check with your health care professional if any of the following side effects continue or are bothersome or if you have any questions about them:

Less common
Headache; nausea

ZALCITABINE (Oral route) - zal-SITE-a-been

Black Box Warning

The use of zalcitabine has been associated with significant clinical adverse reactions, some of which are potentially fatal. Zalcitabine can cause severe peripheral neuropathy and because of this should be used with extreme caution in patients with preexisting neuropathy. Zalcitabine may also rarely cause pancreatitis and patients who develop any symptoms suggestive of pancreatitis while using zalcitabine should have therapy suspended immediately until this diagnosis is excluded.

Lactic acidosis and severe hepatomegaly with steatosis, including fatal cases, have been reported with the use of antiretroviral nucleoside analogues alone or in combination, including zalcitabine.

In addition, rare cases of hepatic failure and death considered possibly related to underlying hepatitis B and zalcitabine have been reported.

Commonly used brand name(s)

In the U.S.—
Hivid

Available Dosage Forms:
• Tablet

Therapeutic Class: Antiretroviral Agent
Pharmacologic Class: Nucleoside Reverse Transcriptase Inhibitor

Uses For This Medicine

Zalcitabine (also known as ddC) is used in the treatment of the infection caused by the human immunodeficiency virus (HIV). HIV is the virus that causes acquired immune deficiency syndrome (AIDS).

Zalcitabine (ddC) will not cure or prevent HIV infection or AIDS; however, it helps keep HIV from reproducing and appears to slow down the destruction of the immune system. This may help delay the development of problems usually related to AIDS or HIV disease. Zalcitabine will not keep you from spreading HIV to other people. People who receive this medicine may continue to have other problems usually related to AIDS or HIV disease.

Zalcitabine may cause some serious side effects, including peripheral neuropathy (a problem involving the nerves). Symptoms of peripheral neuropathy include tingling, burning, numbness, or pain in the hands or feet. Zalcitabine may also cause pancreatitis (inflammation of the pancreas). Symptoms of pancreatitis include stomach pain, and nausea and vomiting. Check with your doctor if any new health problems or symptoms occur while you are taking zalcitabine.

Zalcitabine is available only with your doctor's prescription.

Before Using This Medicine

In deciding to use a medicine, the risks of taking the medicine must be weighed against the good it will do. This is a decision you and your doctor will make. For this medicine, the following should be considered:

Allergies—Tell your doctor if you have ever had any unusual or allergic reaction to this medicine or any other medicines. Also tell your health care professional if you have any other types of allergies, such as to foods, dyes, preservatives, or animals. For non-prescription products, read the label or package ingredients carefully.

Pediatric—Zalcitabine can cause serious side effects in any patient. Therefore, it is especially important that you discuss with your child's doctor the good that this medicine may do as well as the risks of using it. Your child must be seen frequently and your child's progress carefully followed by the doctor while the child is taking zalcitabine.

Geriatric—Zalcitabine has not been studied specifically in older people. Therefore, it is not known whether it causes different side effects or problems in the elderly than it does in younger adults.

Pregnancy—

	Pregnancy Category	Explanation
All Trimesters	C	Animal studies have shown an adverse effect and there are no adequate studies in pregnant women OR no animal studies have been conducted and there are no adequate studies in pregnant women.

Breast Feeding—There are no adequate studies in women for determining infant risk when using this medication during breastfeeding. Weigh the potential benefits against the potential risks before taking this medication while breastfeeding.

Other medicines—

Using this medicine with any of the following medicines is usually not recommended, but may be required in some cases. If both medicines are prescribed together, your doctor may change the dose or how often you use one or both of the medicines.

Cimetidine, Didanosine, Lamivudine, Probenecid, Ribavirin

Interactions with Food/Tobacco/Alcohol—Certain medicines should not be used at or around the time of eating food or eating certain types of food since interactions may occur. Using alcohol or tobacco with certain medicines may

also cause interactions to occur. Discuss with your healthcare professional the use of your medicine with food, alcohol, or tobacco.

Other medical problems—The presence of other medical problems may affect the use of this medicine. Make sure you tell your doctor if you have any other medical problems, especially:

- Alcohol abuse or
- Increased amylase (or a history of) or
- Increased blood triglycerides (or a history of) or
- Pancreatitis (or a history of, or at risk for) or
- Receiving nutrition in your veins—Patients with these medical problems may be at increased risk of pancreatitis (inflammation of the pancreas)
- Abnormal liver function, or
- Alcohol abuse, history of, or
- At risk for liver disease, or
- Hepatitis, or
- Liver disease, or
- Obesity, or
- Taking medicines called nucleosides for a long time—Zalcitabine may make liver disease worse in patients with liver disease or a history of alcohol abuse
- Allergy to zalcitabine, or
- Allergy to any part of the medicine—Serious allergic reactions can occur
- Bone marrow disease—Patients with this condition may develop severe blood problems when taking zalcitabine
- Heart problems, or
- Congestive heart failure—Zalcitabine may make these conditions worse.
- Kidney disease—Patients with kidney disease may have an increased chance of side effects
- Low CD4 cell count—Zalcitabine may cause serious side effects in patients with very low CD4 cell counts.
- Peripheral neuropathy or at risk of developing peripheral neuropathy, or
- Diabetes, or
- Low CD4 cell count, or
- Weight loss—Zalcitabine may increase your chance of developing neuropathy or worsening neuropathy.

Proper Use of This Medicine

Take this medicine exactly as directed by your doctor. Do not take more of it, do not take it more often, and do not take it for a longer time than your doctor ordered. Also, do not stop taking this medicine without checking with your doctor first.

Keep taking zalcitabine for the full time of treatment, even if you begin to feel better.

This medicine works best when there is a constant amount in the blood. To help keep the amount constant, do not miss any doses. If you need help in planning the best times to take your medicine, check with your health care professional.

Only take medicine that your doctor has prescribed specifically for you. Do not share your medicine with others.

Dosing—The dose of this medicine will be different for different patients. Follow your doctor's orders or the directions

on the label. The following information includes only the average doses of this medicine. If your dose is different, do not change it unless your doctor tells you to do so.

The amount of medicine that you take depends on the strength of the medicine. Also, the number of doses you take each day, the time allowed between doses, and the length of time you take the medicine depend on the medical problem for which you are using the medicine.

- For oral dosage form (tablets):
  - For treatment of HIV infection:
    - Adults and children 12 years of age and older—0.75 milligrams (mg)
    - Children up to 12 years of age—Use and dose must be determined by your doctor.

Missed dose—If you miss a dose of this medicine, take it as soon as possible. However, if it is almost time for your next dose, skip the missed dose and go back to your regular dosing schedule. Do not double doses.

Storage—Store the medicine in a closed container at room temperature, away from heat, moisture, and direct light. Keep from freezing.

Keep out of the reach of children.

Do not keep outdated medicine or medicine no longer needed.

Precautions While Using This Medicine

It is very important that your doctor check your progress at regular visits.

Do not take any other medicines without checking with your doctor first. To do so may increase the chance of side effects from zalcitabine.

HIV may be acquired from or spread to other people through infected body fluids, including blood, vaginal fluid, or semen. If you are infected, it is best to avoid any sexual activity involving an exchange of body fluids with other people. If you do have sex, always wear (or have your partner wear) a condom ("rubber"). Only use condoms made of latex, and use them every time you have vaginal, anal, or oral sex. The use of a spermicide (such as nonoxynol-9) may also help prevent transmission of HIV if it is not irritating to the vagina, rectum, or mouth. Spermicides have been shown to kill HIV in lab tests. Do not use oil-based jelly, cold cream, baby oil, or shortening as a lubricant— these products can cause the condom to break. Lubricants without oil, such as K-Y Jelly, are recommended. Women may wish to carry their own condoms. Birth control pills and diaphragms will help protect against pregnancy, but they will not prevent someone from giving or getting the AIDS virus. If you inject drugs, get help to stop. Do not share needles or equipment with anyone. In some cities, more than half of the drug users are infected, and sharing even 1 needle or syringe can spread the virus. If you have any questions about this, check with your health care professional.

Side Effects of This Medicine

Along with its needed effects, a medicine may cause some unwanted effects. Although not all of these side effects may occur, if they do occur they may need medical attention.

Check with your doctor immediately if any of the following side effects occur:

More common
Lab results that show problems with liver; tingling, burning, numbness, or pain in the hands, arms, feet, or legs

Less common
Fever; joint pain; muscle pain; nausea and vomiting; seizures; skin rash; stomach pain (severe); ulcers in the mouth and throat

Rare
Discouragement, feeling sad or empty, irritability, lack of appetite, loss of interest or pleasure, tiredness, trouble concentrating, trouble sleeping; fever and sore throat; yellow eyes or skin

Some side effects may occur that usually do not need medical attention. These side effects may go away during treatment as your body adjusts to the medicine. Also, your health care professional may be able to tell you about ways to prevent or reduce some of these side effects. Check with your health care professional if any of the following side effects continue or are bothersome or if you have any questions about them:

Less common
Constipation; diarrhea; headache; hives or welts; itching skin; swelling or inflammation of the mouth

Other side effects not listed may also occur in some patients. If you notice any other effects, check with your healthcare professional.

ZALEPLON (Oral route) - ZAL-e-plon

Commonly used brand name(s)
In the U.S.—
Sonata

Available Dosage Forms:
• Capsule

Therapeutic Class: Nonbarbiturate Hypnotic

Uses For This Medicine

Zaleplon belongs to the group of medicines called central nervous system (CNS) depressants (medicines that make you drowsy or less alert). Zaleplon is used to treat insomnia (trouble sleeping). In general, when sleep medicines are used every night for a long time, they may lose their effectiveness. In most cases, sleep medicines should be used only for short periods of time, such as 1 or 2 days, and generally for no longer than 1 or 2 weeks.

This medicine is available only with your doctor's prescription.

Before Using This Medicine

In deciding to use a medicine, the risks of taking the medicine must be weighed against the good it will do. This is a decision you and your doctor will make. For this medicine, the following should be considered:

Sleep medicines may cause a special type of memory loss or "amnesia". When this occurs, a person does not remember what has happened during the several hours between use of the medicine and the time when its effects wear off. This is usually not a problem since most people fall asleep after taking the medicine. In most instances, memory problems can be avoided by taking zaleplon only when you are able to get at least 4 hours of sleep before you need to be active again. Be sure to talk to your doctor if you think you are having memory problems.

Allergies—Tell your doctor if you have ever had any unusual or allergic reaction to this medicine or any other medicines. Also tell your health care professional if you have any other types of allergies, such as to foods, dyes, preservatives, or animals. For non-prescription products, read the label or package ingredients carefully.

Pediatric—Studies on this medicine have been done only in adult patients, and there is no specific information comparing use of zaleplon in children younger than 18 years with adults.

Geriatric—Elderly patients are usually more sensitive than younger adults to the effects of zaleplon.

Pregnancy—

	Pregnancy Category	Explanation
All Trimesters	C	Animal studies have shown an adverse effect and there are no adequate studies in pregnant women OR no animal studies have been conducted and there are no adequate studies in pregnant women.

Breast Feeding—Studies in women suggest that this medication poses minimal risk to the infant when used during breastfeeding.

Other medicines—

Using this medicine with any of the following medicines may cause an increased risk of certain side effects, but using both drugs may be the best treatment for you. If both medicines are prescribed together, your doctor may change the dose or how often you use one or both of the medicines.

Cimetidine, Rifampin

Interactions with Food/Tobacco/Alcohol—Certain medicines should not be used at or around the time of eating food or eating certain types of food since interactions may occur. Using alcohol or tobacco with certain medicines may also cause interactions to occur. The following interactions have been selected on the basis of their potential significance and are not necessarily all-inclusive.

Using this medicine with any of the following may cause an increased risk of certain side effects but may be unavoidable in some cases. If used together, your doctor may change the dose or how often you use this medicine, or give you special instructions about the use of food, alcohol, or tobacco.

Ethanol

Other medical problems—The presence of other medical problems may affect the use of this medicine. Make sure you tell your doctor if you have any other medical problems, especially:
• Alcohol abuse (or history of) or
• Drug abuse or dependence (or history of)—Dependence on zaleplon may develop
• Breathing problems or

- Mental depression—Zaleplon may make the condition worse
- Liver disease—Higher blood levels of zaleplon may result, increasing the chance of side effects.

Proper Use of This Medicine

Take this medicine only as directed by your doctor. Do not take more of it, do not take it more often, and do not take it for a longer time than your doctor ordered. If too much is taken, it may become habit-forming (causing mental or physical dependence).

Take zaleplon just before going to bed, when you are ready to go to sleep. This medicine works very quickly to put you to sleep.

Do not take this medicine when your schedule does not permit you to get at least 4 hours of sleep. If you must wake up before this, you may continue to feel drowsy and may experience memory problems, because the effects of the medicine have not had time to wear off.

Zaleplon may be taken with or without food or on a full or empty stomach. However, taking this medicine with or immediately after a heavy or a high fat meal may make zaleplon not work as fast.

Dosing—The dose of this medicine will be different for different patients. Follow your doctor's orders or the directions on the label. The following information includes only the average doses of this medicine. If your dose is different, do not change it unless your doctor tells you to do so.

The amount of medicine that you take depends on the strength of the medicine. Also, the number of doses you take each day, the time allowed between doses, and the length of time you take the medicine depend on the medical problem for which you are using the medicine.

- For oral dosage form (capsules):
  - For the treatment of insomnia (trouble in sleeping):
    - Adults—10 milligrams (mg) at bedtime.
    - Older adults—5 mg at bedtime.
    - Children up to 18 years of age—Use and dose must be determined by doctor.

Missed dose—If you miss a dose of this medicine, skip the missed dose and go back to your regular dosing schedule. Do not double doses.

Storage—Store the medicine in a closed container at room temperature, away from heat, moisture, and direct light. Keep from freezing.

Keep out of the reach of children.

Do not keep outdated medicine or medicine no longer needed.

Precautions While Using This Medicine

If you think you need to take zaleplon for more than 7 to 10 days, be sure to discuss it with your doctor. Insomnia that lasts longer than this may be a sign of another medical problem.

This medicine will add to the effects of alcohol and other central nervous system (CNS) depressants (medicines that cause drowsiness). Some examples of CNS depressants are antihistamines or medicine for hay fever, other allergies or colds; sedatives, tranquilizers, or sleeping medicines; prescription pain medicine or narcotics; barbiturates; medicine for seizures; muscle relaxants; or anesthetics, including some

dental anesthetics. Check with your doctor before taking any of the above while you are using this medicine.

This medicine may cause some people, especially older persons, to become drowsy, dizzy, lightheaded, clumsy or unsteady, or less alert than they are normally. Even though zaleplon is taken at bedtime, it may cause some people to feel drowsy or less alert on arising. Make sure you know how you react to zaleplon before you drive, use machines, or do anything else that could be dangerous if you are dizzy, unsteady, or are not alert or able to see well.

If you develop any unusual and strange thoughts or behavior while taking zaleplon, be sure to discuss it with your doctor. Some changes that have occurred in people taking this medicine are like those seen in people who drink alcohol and then act in a manner that is not normal. Other changes may be more unusual and extreme, such as confusion, hallucinations (seeing, hearing, smelling, or feeling things that are not there), and unusual excitement, nervousness, or irritability.

If you will be taking zaleplon for a long time, do not stop taking it without first checking with your doctor. Your doctor may want you to reduce gradually the amount you are taking before stopping completely. Stopping this medicine suddenly may cause withdrawal side effects.

After taking zaleplon for insomnia, you may have difficulty sleeping (rebound insomnia) for the first few nights after you stop taking it.

If you think you or someone else may have taken an overdose of this medicine, get emergency help at once. Taking an overdose of zaleplon or taking alcohol or other CNS depressants with zaleplon may lead to breathing problems and unconsciousness. Some signs of an overdose are clumsiness or unsteadiness, confusion, severe drowsiness, low blood pressure, unusual dullness or feeling sluggish, and troubled breathing.

Side Effects of This Medicine

Along with its needed effects, a medicine may cause some unwanted effects. Although not all of these side effects may occur, if they do occur they may need medical attention.

Check with your doctor as soon as possible if any of the following side effects occur:

Less common
Anxiety; blurred or double vision; not feeling like oneself

Rare
Nosebleed; seeing, hearing, smelling, or feeling things that are not there

Symptoms of overdose
Confusion; clumsiness or unsteadiness, severe; dizziness or fainting; drowsiness, severe; weak muscle tone; troubled breathing; unusual dullness or feeling sluggish

Some side effects may occur that usually do not need medical attention. These side effects may go away during treatment as your body adjusts to the medicine. Also, your health care professional may be able to tell you about ways to prevent or reduce some of these side effects. Check with your health care professional if any of the following side effects continue or are bothersome or if you have any questions about them:

More common
Dizziness; headache; muscle pain; nausea

Less common

Abdominal pain; burning, prickling, or tingling sensation; constipation; cough; difficulty concentrating; drowsiness; dryness of mouth; excess muscle tone; eye pain; fever; heartburn, indigestion, or acid stomach; itching; itching or burning eyes; joint stiffness and/or pain; memory loss; menstrual pain; mental depression; nervousness; sensitive hearing; severe headache; shortness of breath; skin rash; tightness in chest; trembling or shaking; troubled breathing; unusual weakness or tiredness; wheezing

After you stop using this medicine, it may still produce some side effects that need attention. During this period of time, *check with your doctor immediately* if you notice the following side effects:

Abdominal and muscle cramps; convulsions (seizures); increased sweating; sadness; trembling or shaking; vomiting

ZANAMIVIR (Inhalation, oral/ nebulization route) - za-NA-mi-veer

Commonly used brand name(s)

In the U.S.—
Relenza

Available Dosage Forms:
• Disk

Therapeutic Class: Antiviral
Pharmacologic Class: Neuraminidase Inhibitor, Influenza A&B Virus

Uses For This Medicine

Zanamivir is used in the treatment of the infection caused by the flu virus (influenza A and influenza B). Zanamivir may reduce flu symptoms (weakness, headache, fever, cough, and sore throat) by 1 to 1.5 days. Zanamivir does not prevent influenza infection.

This medicine must be started within 2 days of having flu symptoms (weakness, headache, fever, cough, and sore throat). Zanamivir will not keep you from spreading the flu virus to other people. Zanamivir may not work for everybody. Zanamivir may not be for you if you are severely sick or have a breathing problem (like asthma or chronic obstructive pulmonary disease). If you receive the flu vaccine every year, continue to do so.

Once a medicine has been approved for marketing for a certain use, experience may show that it is also useful for other medical problems. Although this use is not included in product labeling, zanamivir is used in certain patients:

• To prevent the infection caused by the flu virus (influenza A or influenza B).

Before Using This Medicine

In deciding to use a medicine, the risks of taking the medicine must be weighed against the good it will do. This is a decision you and your doctor will make. For this medicine, the following should be considered:

Allergies—Tell your doctor if you have ever had any unusual or allergic reaction to this medicine or any other medi-

cines. Also tell your health care professional if you have any other types of allergies, such as to foods, dyes, preservatives, or animals. For non-prescription products, read the label or package ingredients carefully.

Pediatric—This medicine is not recommended for use in children younger than 7 years of age. This medicine has been tested in children 12 years and older and has not been shown to cause different side effects or problems in these children than it does in adults.

Note: This medicine is available in Canada. It is not recommended in children younger than 12 years of age.

Geriatric—This medicine has been tested in older adults and has not been shown to cause different side effects or problems in older adults than it does in younger adults.

Pregnancy—

	Pregnancy Category	Explanation
All Trimesters	C	Animal studies have shown an adverse effect and there are no adequate studies in pregnant women OR no animal studies have been conducted and there are no adequate studies in pregnant women.

Breast Feeding—There are no adequate studies in women for determining infant risk when using this medication during breastfeeding. Weigh the potential benefits against the potential risks before taking this medication while breastfeeding.

Other medicines—Although certain medicines should not be used together at all, in other cases two different medicines may be used together even if an interaction might occur. In these cases, your doctor may want to change the dose, or other precautions may be necessary. Tell your healthcare professional if you are taking any other prescription or non-prescription (over-the-counter [OTC]) medicine.

Interactions with Food/Tobacco/Alcohol—Certain medicines should not be used at or around the time of eating food or eating certain types of food since interactions may occur. Using alcohol or tobacco with certain medicines may also cause interactions to occur. Discuss with your healthcare professional the use of your medicine with food, alcohol, or tobacco.

Other medical problems—The presence of other medical problems may affect the use of this medicine. Make sure you tell your doctor if you have any other medical problems, especially:

• Lung disease—Patients with lung disease (chronic obstructive pulmonary disease or asthma) may experience trouble breathing with the use of zanamivir. Zanamivir may not work in patients with chronic lung disease.

• Heart disease—Zanamivir may not work in patients with heart disease.

Proper Use of This Medicine

Talk to your doctor about the possibility of getting a flu shot if you have not had one yet. This medicine works best if taken as soon as possible after exposure to people who have the flu. If you already have the flu, continue taking this medicine for the full time of treatment even if you begin to feel better after a few days. This will help to clear up your infection completely. If you stop taking this medicine too soon, your symptoms may return. This medicine should be taken for 5 days.

Inhaled zanamivir is used with a special inhaler and usually comes with patient directions. Read the directions carefully before using this medicine. If you do not understand the directions or you are not sure how to use the inhaler, ask your health care professional to show you what to do.

To load the inhaler:

- Pull off the blue cover. Make sure the mouthpiece is clean and free of foreign objects.
- Pull the white mouthpiece until the tray is extended.
- Hold the corners of the white tray and pull out gently until you can see all the raised ridges on the sides of the tray.
- Put your finger and thumb on the ridges, squeeze inward, and gently pull the tray out of the body of the inhaler.
- Place a disk on the wheel and then slide the tray back into the inhaler
- To replace the empty disk with a full disk, follow the same steps you used to load the inhaler.

To use the inhaler:

- Hold the inhaler flat in your hand.
- A plastic needle will break the blister containing one inhalation of medicine. When the flap is raised as far as it will go, the blister will be pierced. Do not lift the flap if the cartridge is not in the inhaler. Doing this will break the needle and you will need a new inhaler.
- After the blister is broken open, close the lid. Keeping the inhaler flat and well away from your mouth, breathe out to the end of a normal breath.
- Raise the inhaler to your mouth, and place the mouthpiece in your mouth.
- Close your lips around the mouthpiece and tilt your head slightly back. Do not bite down on the mouthpiece. Do not block the mouthpiece with your teeth or tongue. Do not cover the air holes on the side of the mouthpiece.
- Breathe in through your mouth as steadily and as deeply as you can until you have taken a full deep breath.
- Hold your breath and remove the mouthpiece from your mouth. Continue holding your breath as long as you can up to 10 seconds before breathing out. This gives the medicine time to settle in your airways and lungs.
- Hold the inhaler well away from your mouth and breathe out to the end of a normal breath.
- Prepare the cartridge for your next inhalation. Pull the mouthpiece to extend the tray then push it in until it clicks. The disk will turn to the next dose. Do not pierce the blister until just before the inhalation.
- Take the second puff following exactly the same steps you used for the first puff.
- When you are finished, wipe off the mouthpiece and replace the cover to keep the mouthpiece clean and free of foreign objects.

Dosing—The dose of this medicine will be different for different patients. Follow your doctor's orders or the directions on the label. The following information includes only the average doses of this medicine. If your dose is different, do not change it unless your doctor tells you to do so.

The amount of medicine that you take depends on the strength of the medicine. Also, the number of doses you take each day, the time allowed between doses, and the length of time you take the medicine depend on the medical problem for which you are using the medicine.

- For treatment of flu (Influenza A and Influenza B)
  - Adults and children 7 years and older—Two puffs twice daily (approximately 12 hours apart in the morning and evening) for 5 days. Two doses should be taken on the first day of treatment whenever possible provided there are at least 2 hours between doses. Zanamivir must be started within 48 hours after the onset of signs and symptoms of the flu.
- Canada: For treatment of flu (Influenza A and Influenza B)
  - Adults and children 12 years and older—Two puffs twice daily (approximately 12 hours apart in the morning and evening) for 5 days. Two doses should be taken on the first day of treatment whenever possible provided there are at least 2 hours between doses. Zanamivir must be started within 48 hours after the onset of signs and symptoms of the flu.

Missed dose—If you miss a dose of this medicine, take it as soon as possible. However, if it is almost time for your next dose, skip the missed dose and go back to your regular dosing schedule. Do not double doses.

Storage—Store the medicine in a closed container at room temperature, away from heat, moisture, and direct light. Keep from freezing.

Keep out of the reach of children.

Do not keep outdated medicine or medicine no longer needed.

Precautions While Using This Medicine

Zanamivir will not keep you from spreading the flu virus to other people. This medicine may cause people with lung disease (chronic obstructive lung disease or asthma) to experience trouble breathing. If this should happen contact your doctor immediately. Zanamivir may not work in patients with lung disease, heart disease, or serious medical conditions.

Bronchospasm (wheezing) is a risk for patients with asthma or chronic respiratory disease. Always have a fast-acting inhaled bronchodilator available for your use.

Side Effects of This Medicine

Along with its needed effects, a medicine may cause some unwanted effects. Although not all of these side effects may occur, if they do occur they may need medical attention.

Stop taking this medicine and get emergency help immediately if any of the following effects occur:

Rare
  Convulsions; dizziness and fainting; heartbeat, fast, slow, or irregular; increased sensitivity to sunlight; itching, pain, redness, swelling or watering of eye or eyelid; flushing or reddening of skin; joint pain; severe skin rash or hives; shortness of breath or troubled breathing; swelling or puffiness of face; swollen glands or tightness in throat; tightness in chest or wheezing

Some side effects may occur that usually do not need medical attention. These side effects may go away during treatment as your body adjusts to the medicine. Also, your health care professional may be able to tell you about ways to prevent or reduce some of these side effects. Check with your health care professional if any of the following side effects

continue or are bothersome or if you have any questions about them:

Less common

Change in hearing; cough; cough producing mucus; diarrhea; dizziness; earache; ear drainage; ear, nose and throat infections; headache; nasal signs and symptoms; nausea; pain and pressure over cheeks; pain in ear; shortness of breath; tightness in chest; vomiting; wheezing

Other side effects not listed may also occur in some patients. If you notice any other effects, check with your healthcare professional.

ZIDOVUDINE (Oral route, Intravenous route) - zye-DOE-vyoo-deen

Black Box Warning

Zidovudine has been associated with hematologic toxicity, including neutropenia and severe anemia, particularly in patients with advanced HIV disease. Prolonged use of zidovudine has been associated with symptomatic myopathy.

Lactic acidosis and severe hepatomegaly with steatosis, including fatal cases, have been reported with the use of nucleoside analogues alone or in combination, including zidovudine and other antiretrovirals.

Commonly used brand name(s)

In the U.S.—
Retrovir

Available Dosage Forms:
- Capsule
- Syrup
- Tablet
- Solution

Therapeutic Class: Antiretroviral Agent
Pharmacologic Class: Nucleoside Reverse Transcriptase Inhibitor

Uses For This Medicine

Zidovudine (also known as AZT) is used in combination with other anti-virus medicines in the treatment of the infection caused by the human immunodeficiency virus (HIV). HIV is the virus responsible for acquired immune deficiency syndrome (AIDS). Zidovudine is used to slow the progression of disease in patients infected with HIV who have advanced symptoms, early symptoms, or no symptoms at all. This medicine also is used to help prevent pregnant women who have HIV from passing the virus to their babies during pregnancy and at birth.

Zidovudine will not cure or prevent HIV infection or AIDS; however, it helps keep HIV from reproducing and appears to slow down the destruction of the immune system. This may help delay the development of problems usually related to AIDS or HIV disease. Zidovudine will not keep you from spreading HIV to other people. People who receive this medicine may continue to have the problems usually related to AIDS or HIV disease.

Zidovudine may cause some serious side effects, including bone marrow problems. Symptoms of bone marrow problems include fever, chills, or sore throat; pale skin; and unusual tiredness or weakness. These problems may require blood transfusions or temporarily stopping treatment with zidovudine. Check with your doctor if any new health problems or symptoms occur while you are taking zidovudine.

Zidovudine is available only with your doctor's prescription.

Once a medicine has been approved for marketing for a certain use, experience may show that it is also useful for other medical problems. Although this use is not included in product labeling, zidovudine is used in certain patients with the following medical condition:
- Human immunodeficiency virus (HIV) infection due to occupational exposure (possible prevention of)

Before Using This Medicine

In deciding to use a medicine, the risks of taking the medicine must be weighed against the good it will do. This is a decision you and your doctor will make. For this medicine, the following should be considered:

Allergies—Tell your doctor if you have ever had any unusual or allergic reaction to this medicine or any other medicines. Also tell your health care professional if you have any other types of allergies, such as to foods, dyes, preservatives, or animals. For non-prescription products, read the label or package ingredients carefully.

Pediatric—Zidovudine can cause serious side effects in any patient. Therefore, it is especially important that you discuss with your child's doctor the good that this medicine may do as well as the risks of using it. Your child must be carefully followed, and frequently seen, by the doctor while he or she is taking zidovudine.

Geriatric—Zidovudine has not been studied specifically in older people. Therefore, it is not known whether it causes different side effects or problems in the elderly than it does in younger adults.

Pregnancy—

	Pregnancy Category	Explanation
All Trimesters	C	Animal studies have shown an adverse effect and there are no adequate studies in pregnant women OR no animal studies have been conducted and there are no adequate studies in pregnant women.

Breast Feeding—There are no adequate studies in women for determining infant risk when using this medication during breastfeeding. Weigh the potential benefits against the potential risks before taking this medication while breastfeeding.

Other medicines—

Using this medicine with any of the following medicines is usually not recommended, but may be required in some cases. If both medicines are prescribed together, your doctor may change the dose or how often you use one or both of the medicines.

Dapsone, Doxorubicin Hydrochloride, Flucytosine, Ganciclovir, Interferon Alfa, Pyrazinamide, Pyrimethamine, Ribavirin, Stavudine, Vinblastine, Vincristine, Vincristine Liposome

Interactions with Food/Tobacco/Alcohol—Certain medicines should not be used at or around the time of eating food or eating certain types of food since interactions may occur. Using alcohol or tobacco with certain medicines may also cause interactions to occur. Discuss with your healthcare

professional the use of your medicine with food, alcohol, or tobacco.

Other medical problems—The presence of other medical problems may affect the use of this medicine. Make sure you tell your doctor if you have any other medical problems, especially:

- Anemia or other blood problems—Zidovudine may make these conditions worse

- Liver disease—Patients with liver disease may have an increase in side effects from zidovudine

- Low amounts of folic acid or vitamin B12 in the blood— Zidovudine may worsen anemia caused by a decrease of folic acid or vitamin B12

- At risk for liver disease, or

- Obesity, or

- Taking medicines called nucleosides for a long time— Zidovudine may increase the chance for liver disease

Proper Use of This Medicine

Patient information sheets about zidovudine are available. Read this information carefully.

Take this medicine exactly as directed by your doctor. Do not take more of it, do not take it more often, and do not take it for a longer time than your doctor ordered. Also, do not stop taking this medicine without checking with your doctor first.

Keep taking zidovudine for the full time of treatment, even if you begin to feel better.

For patients using zidovudine oral solution:

- Use a specially marked measuring spoon or other device to measure each dose accurately. The average household teaspoon may not hold the right amount of liquid.

This medicine works best when there is a constant amount in the blood. To help keep the amount constant, do not miss any doses. If you need help in planning the best times to take your medicine, check with your health care professional.

Dosing—The dose of this medicine will be different for different patients. Follow your doctor's orders or the directions on the label. The following information includes only the average doses of this medicine. If your dose is different, do not change it unless your doctor tells you to do so.

The amount of medicine that you take depends on the strength of the medicine. Also, the number of doses you take each day, the time allowed between doses, and the length of time you take the medicine depend on the medical problem for which you are using the medicine.

- For the treatment of HIV infection:
  - For oral dosage forms (capsules, oral solution, and tablets):
    - Adults and children 12 years of age and older— 600 milligrams (mg) a day in divided doses in combination with other anti-virus medicine.
    - Children up to 12 years of age—Dose is based on body weight or body size and must be determined by your doctor. Zidovudine is given in combination with other anti-virus medicine.
  - For injection dosage form:
    - Adults and teenagers—Dose is based on body weight and must be determined by your doctor. The usual dose is 1 to 2 mg per kilogram (kg) (0.45 to 0.9 mg per pound) of body weight, injected slowly into a vein every four hours five to six times

a day. The injection dosage form is given until you can take zidovudine by mouth.
    - Children up to 12 years of age—Dose is based on body weight or body size and must be determined by your doctor.

- To help prevent pregnant women from passing HIV to their babies during pregnancy and at birth:
  - For capsule dosage form:
    - Pregnant women (after 14 weeks of pregnancy, up to the start of labor)—100 milligrams (mg) five times a day, 200 mg every eight hours, or 300 mg every twelve hours until the start of labor.
  - For oral solution dosage form:
    - Pregnant women (after 14 weeks of pregnancy, up to the start of labor)—100 milligrams (mg) five times a day, 200 mg every eight hours, or 300 mg every twelve hours until the start of labor.
    - Newborn infants—Dose is based on body weight and must be determined by your doctor. The usual dose of oral solution is 2 mg per kilogram (kg) (0.9 mg per pound) of body weight every six hours starting within eight to twelve hours of birth and continuing through six weeks of age.
  - For injection dosage form:
    - Pregnant women (during labor and delivery)— Dose is based on body weight and must be determined by your doctor. The usual dose is 2 milligrams (mg) per kilogram (kg) (0.9 mg per pound) of body weight infused into a vein over the first hour, followed by 1 mg per kg (0.45 mg per pound) of body weight infused into a vein each hour until the umbilical cord is clamped.
    - Newborn infants—If the infant is unable to receive zidovudine oral solution, the injection form may be used instead. Dose is based on body weight and must be determined by your doctor. The usual dose is 1.5 mg per kilogram (kg) (0.7 mg per pound) of body weight every six hours.

Missed dose—If you miss a dose of this medicine, take it as soon as possible. However, if it is almost time for your next dose, skip the missed dose and go back to your regular dosing schedule. Do not double doses.

Storage—Store the medicine in a closed container at room temperature, away from heat, moisture, and direct light. Keep from freezing.

Keep out of the reach of children.

Do not keep outdated medicine or medicine no longer needed.

Precautions While Using This Medicine

It is very important that your doctor check your progress at regular visits. This medicine may cause blood problems.

Do not take any other medicines without checking with your doctor first. To do so may increase the chance of side effects from zidovudine.

Zidovudine may cause blood problems. These problems may result in a greater chance of certain infections and slow healing. Therefore, you should be careful when using regular toothbrushes, dental floss, and toothpicks not to damage your gums. Check with your medical doctor or dentist if you have any questions about proper oral hygiene (mouth care) during treatment.

HIV may be acquired from or spread to other people through infected body fluids, including blood, vaginal fluid, or semen.

If you are infected, it is best to avoid any sexual activity involving an exchange of body fluids with other people. If you do have sex, always wear (or have your partner wear) a condom ("rubber"). Only use condoms made of latex, and use them every time you have vaginal, anal, or oral sex. The use of a spermicide (such as nonoxynol-9) may also help prevent the spread of HIV if it is not irritating to the vagina, rectum, or mouth. Spermicides have been shown to kill HIV in lab tests. Do not use oil-based jelly, cold cream, baby oil, or shortening as a lubricant—these products can cause the condom to break. Lubricants without oil, such as K-Y Jelly, are recommended. Women may wish to carry their own condoms. Birth control pills and diaphragms will help protect against pregnancy, but they will not prevent someone from giving or getting the AIDS virus. If you inject drugs, get help to stop. Do not share needles with anyone. In some cities, more than half of the drug users are infected, and sharing even one needle can spread the virus. If you have any questions about this, check with your health care professional.

Side Effects of This Medicine

Along with its needed effects, a medicine may cause some unwanted effects. Although not all of these side effects may occur, if they do occur they may need medical attention.

Check with your doctor immediately if any of the following side effects occur:

More common
 Fever, chills, or sore throat; pale skin; unusual tiredness or weakness

Rare
 Abdominal discomfort; confusion; convulsions (seizures); diarrhea; fast, shallow breathing; general feeling of discomfort; loss of appetite; mood or mental changes; muscle pain, tenderness, weakness, or cramping; nausea; shortness of breath; sleepiness

Note: Some of the above side effects may also occur up to weeks or months after you stop taking this medicine.

Some side effects may occur that usually do not need medical attention. These side effects may go away during treatment as your body adjusts to the medicine. Also, your health care professional may be able to tell you about ways to prevent or reduce some of these side effects. Check with your health care professional if any of the following side effects continue or are bothersome or if you have any questions about them:

More common
 Difficulty having a bowel movement (stool); general feeling of discomfort or illness; headache (severe); lack or loss of strength; muscle soreness; nausea; trouble in sleeping; vomiting; weight loss

Less common
 Bluish-brown colored bands on nails; changes in skin color

Other side effects not listed may also occur in some patients. If you notice any other effects, check with your healthcare professional.

Incidence unknown
 acid or sour stomach; belching; burning, tingling, numbness or pain in the hands, arms, feet, or legs; sensation of pins and needles, stabbing pain; heartburn; muscle or bone pain; indigestion; stomach cramps; stomach pain; yellow eyes or skin

ZILEUTON (Oral route) - zye-LOO-ton

Commonly used brand name(s)
In the U.S.—
 Zyflo Filmtab

Available Dosage Forms:
 • Tablet

Therapeutic Class: Anti-Inflammatory
Pharmacologic Class: Leukotriene Pathway Inhibitor

Uses For This Medicine

Zileuton is used by patients with mild to moderate chronic asthma to decrease the symptoms of asthma and the number of acute asthma attacks. However, this medicine should not be taken to relieve an asthma attack that has already started.

This medicine is available only with your doctor's prescription.

Before Using This Medicine

In deciding to use a medicine, the risks of taking the medicine must be weighed against the good it will do. This is a decision you and your doctor will make. For this medicine, the following should be considered:

Allergies—Tell your doctor if you have ever had any unusual or allergic reaction to this medicine or any other medicines. Also tell your health care professional if you have any other types of allergies, such as to foods, dyes, preservatives, or animals. For non-prescription products, read the label or package ingredients carefully.

Pediatric—Studies on this medicine have been done only in adult patients and there is no specific information comparing use of zileuton in children up to 12 years of age with use in other age groups.

Geriatric—This medicine has been tested and has not been shown to cause different side effects or problems in older people than it does in younger adults.

Pregnancy—

	Pregnancy Category	Explanation
All Trimesters	C	Animal studies have shown an adverse effect and there are no adequate studies in pregnant women OR no animal studies have been conducted and there are no adequate studies in pregnant women.

Breast Feeding—There are no adequate studies in women for determining infant risk when using this medication during breastfeeding. Weigh the potential benefits against the potential risks before taking this medication while breastfeeding.

Other medicines—

Using this medicine with any of the following medicines is not recommended. Your doctor may decide not to treat you with this medication or change some of the other medicines you take.

Dihydroergotamine, Ergoloid Mesylates, Ergonovine, Ergotamine, Methylergonovine

Interactions with Food/Tobacco/Alcohol—Certain medicines should not be used at or around the time of eating

food or eating certain types of food since interactions may occur. Using alcohol or tobacco with certain medicines may also cause interactions to occur. Discuss with your healthcare professional the use of your medicine with food, alcohol, or tobacco.

Other medical problems—The presence of other medical problems may affect the use of this medicine. Make sure you tell your doctor if you have any other medical problems, especially:

- Active alcoholism or
- Liver disease—The chance of serious side effects may be increased

Proper Use of This Medicine

Zileuton is used to prevent asthma attacks. It is not used to relieve an attack that has already started. For relief of an asthma attack that has already started, you should use another medicine. If you do not have another medicine to use for an attack or if you have any question about this, check with your health care professional.

Dosing—The dose of this medicine will be different for different patients. Follow your doctor's orders or the directions on the label. The following information includes only the average doses of this medicine. If your dose is different, do not change it unless your doctor tells you to do so.

The amount of medicine that you take depends on the strength of the medicine. Also, the number of doses you take each day, the time allowed between doses, and the length of time you take the medicine depend on the medical problem for which you are using the medicine.

- For oral dosage form (tablets):
  - For asthma:
    - Adults and children 12 years of age and older— 600 milligrams (mg) four times a day.
    - Children up to 12 years of age—Use and dose must be determined by your doctor.

Missed dose—If you miss a dose of this medicine, take it as soon as possible. However, if it is almost time for your next dose, skip the missed dose and go back to your regular dosing schedule. Do not double doses.

Storage—Store the medicine in a closed container at room temperature, away from heat, moisture, and direct light. Keep from freezing.

Keep out of the reach of children.

Do not keep outdated medicine or medicine no longer needed.

Precautions While Using This Medicine

To work properly, zileuton must be taken every day at regularly spaced times, even if your asthma seems better.

It is very important that your doctor check your progress at regular visits. Your doctor will want to have certain tests done regularly to see if side effects may be occurring in your liver without your knowing it.

Check with your health care professional if more inhalations (puffs) than usual of an inhaled, short-acting bronchodilator are needed to relieve an acute attack or if more than the maximum number of puffs of the bronchodilator prescribed for a 24–hour period are needed.

You may be taking other medicines for asthma along with zileuton. Do not stop taking or reduce the dose of the other medicines, even if your asthma seems better, unless you are told to do so by your health care professional.

Side Effects of This Medicine

Along with its needed effects, a medicine may cause some unwanted effects. Although not all of these side effects may occur, if they do occur they may need medical attention.

Check with your doctor as soon as possible if any of the following side effects occur:

Rare
Flu-like symptoms; itching; right upper abdominal pain; unusual tiredness or weakness; yellow eyes or skin

Some side effects may occur that usually do not need medical attention. These side effects may go away during treatment as your body adjusts to the medicine. Also, your health care professional may be able to tell you about ways to prevent or reduce some of these side effects. Check with your health care professional if any of the following side effects continue or are bothersome or if you have any questions about them:

More common
Nausea; upset stomach

Less common
Abdominal pain; weakness

Other side effects not listed may also occur in some patients. If you notice any other effects, check with your healthcare professional.

ZIPRASIDONE (Oral route, Intramuscular route) - zi-PRAY-si-done

Black Box Warning

Elderly patients with dementia-related psychosis treated with atypical antipsychotic drugs are at an increased risk of death compared to placebo. Analyses of seventeen placebo controlled trials (modal duration of 10 weeks) in these patients revealed a risk of death in the drug-treated patients of between 1.6 times to 1.7 times that seen in placebo-treated patients. Over the course of a typical 10 week controlled trial, the rate of death in drug-treated patients was about 4.5%, compared to a rate of about 2.6% in the placebo group. Although the causes of death were varied, most of the deaths appeared to be either cardiovascular (eg, heart failure, sudden death) or infectious (eg, pneumonia) in nature. Ziprasidone hydrochloride is not approved for the treatment of patients with dementia-related psychosis.

Commonly used brand name(s)

In the U.S.—
Geodon

Available Dosage Forms:
- Powder for Solution
- Capsule

Therapeutic Class: Antipsychotic

Uses For This Medicine

Ziprasidone is used to treat schizophrenia and bipolar disorder which are mental disorders. This medicine should NOT be used to treat behavioral problems in older adult patients who have dementia.

This medicine is available only with your doctor's prescription.

Before Using This Medicine

In deciding to use a medicine, the risks of taking the medicine must be weighed against the good it will do. This is a decision you and your doctor will make. For this medicine, the following should be considered:

Allergies—Tell your doctor if you have ever had any unusual or allergic reaction to this medicine or any other medicines. Also tell your health care professional if you have any other types of allergies, such as to foods, dyes, preservatives, or animals. For non-prescription products, read the label or package ingredients carefully.

Pediatric—Studies on this medicine have been done only in adult patients, and there is no specific information comparing use of ziprasidone in children with use in other age groups.

Geriatric—Many medicines have not been studied specifically in older people. Therefore, it may not be known whether they work exactly the same way they do in younger adults or if they cause different side effects or problems in older people. There is no specific information comparing use of ziprasidone in the elderly with use in other age groups. This medicine should not be used for behavioral problems in older adults with dementia.

Pregnancy—

	Pregnancy Category	Explanation
All Trimesters	C	Animal studies have shown an adverse effect and there are no adequate studies in pregnant women OR no animal studies have been conducted and there are no adequate studies in pregnant women.

Breast Feeding—There are no adequate studies in women for determining infant risk when using this medication during breastfeeding. Weigh the potential benefits against the potential risks before taking this medication while breastfeeding.

Other medicines—

Using this medicine with any of the following medicines is not recommended. Your doctor may decide not to treat you with this medication or change some of the other medicines you take.

Acecainide, Ajmaline, Amiodarone, Amisulpride, Amitriptyline, Amoxapine, Aprindine, Arsenic Trioxide, Astemizole, Azimilide, Bepridil, Bretylium, Chloral Hydrate, Chloroquine, Chlorpromazine, Cisapride, Clarithromycin, Desipramine, Dibenzepin, Disopyramide, Dofetilide, Dolasetron, Doxepin, Droperidol, Enflurane, Erythromycin, Flecainide, Fluconazole, Foscarnet, Gatifloxacin, Gemifloxacin, Halofantrine, Haloperidol, Halothane, Hydroquinidine, Ibutilide, Imipramine, Isoflurane, Isradipine, Levomethadyl, Lidoflazine, Lor-

cainide, Mefloquine, Mesoridazine, Moxifloxacin, Nortriptyline, Octreotide, Pentamidine, Pimozide, Pirmenol, Prajmaline, Probucol, Procainamide, Prochlorperazine, Propafenone, Protriptyline, Quinidine, Ranolazine, Risperidone, Sematilide, Sertindole, Sotalol, Sparfloxacin, Spiramycin, Sulfamethoxazole, Sultopride, Tacrolimus, Tedisamil, Telithromycin, Terfenadine, Thioridazine, Trifluoperazine, Trimethoprim, Trimipramine, Vasopressin, Zolmitriptan, Zotepine

Interactions with Food/Tobacco/Alcohol—Certain medicines should not be used at or around the time of eating food or eating certain types of food since interactions may occur. Using alcohol or tobacco with certain medicines may also cause interactions to occur. Discuss with your healthcare professional the use of your medicine with food, alcohol, or tobacco.

Other medical problems—The presence of other medical problems may affect the use of this medicine. Make sure you tell your doctor if you have any other medical problems, especially:

- Heart attack (recent) or
- Heart disease or
- Irregular heartbeat or
- Heart failure—Ziprasidone may make these conditions worse
- High level of sugar in the blood or
- Diabetes mellitus (sugar diabetes)—Ziprasidone may make these conditions worse
- Low level of magnesium in your blood or
- Low level of potassium in your blood—This increases chance for heart problems
- Neuroleptic malignant syndrome (NMS) or
- Tardive dyskinesia—May appear or worsen with ziprasidone therapy
- Seizures or
- Alzheimer's disease—Increased risk of seizures and aspiration pneumonia

Proper Use of This Medicine

Do not chew the capsules, swallow whole.

Dosing—The dose of this medicine will be different for different patients. Follow your doctor's orders or the directions on the label. The following information includes only the average doses of this medicine. If your dose is different, do not change it unless your doctor tells you to do so.

The amount of medicine that you take depends on the strength of the medicine. Also, the number of doses you take each day, the time allowed between doses, and the length of time you take the medicine depend on the medical problem for which you are using the medicine.

- For oral dosage form (capsules):
  - For treating bipolar disorder
    - Adults—To start, 40 milligrams (mg) twice a day with food. The dose will be increased to either 60 or 80 mg on the second day. Your doctor may increase your dose if needed. However, the dose is usually not more than 80 mg twice a day.
  - For treating schizophrenia:
    - Adults—To start, 20 mg twice a day with food. Your doctor may increase your dose if needed.

However, the dose is usually not more than 80 mg twice a day.

- Children—Use and dose must be determined by your doctor.
- For parenteral dosage form (for injection):
  - For treating acute agitation in schizophrenic patients
    - Adults—To start, 10 to 20 mg per day. Your doctor may increase your dose if needed. However, the dose is usually not more than 40 mg a day.

Missed dose—If you miss a dose of this medicine, take it as soon as possible. However, if it is almost time for your next dose, skip the missed dose and go back to your regular dosing schedule. Do not double doses.

Storage—Store the medicine in a closed container at room temperature, away from heat, moisture, and direct light. Keep from freezing.

Keep out of the reach of children.

Do not keep outdated medicine or medicine no longer needed.

Ask your healthcare professional how you should dispose of any medicine you do not use.

Precautions While Using This Medicine

It is very important that your doctor check you at regular visits to make sure your medicine is working for you. Your doctor will check your blood to make sure your potassium is normal.

Check with doctor if fainting, dizziness, fast, racing, pounding, or irregular heartbeat, or other unusual symptoms occur

Symptoms of hyperglycemia (high blood sugar) include blurred vision; drowsiness; dry mouth; flushed, dry skin; fruit like breath odor; increased urination; ketones in urine; loss of appetite; stomach ache; nausea or vomiting; tiredness; trouble breathing; unconsciousness; or unusual thirst.

This medicine may cause some people to become drowsy, dizzy, or less alert than they are normally. Make sure you know how you react to this medicine before you drive, use machines, or do anything else that could be dangerous if you are dizzy or are not alert. Avoid use of alcohol.

Avoid activities involving high temperature or humidity. This medicine may reduce your body's ability to adjust to the heat.

Side Effects of This Medicine

Along with its needed effects, a medicine may cause some unwanted effects. Although not all of these side effects may occur, if they do occur they may need medical attention.

Less common

Chest pain; fast, pounding, or irregular heartbeat or pulse; palpitations

Rare

Dizziness; fainting or feeling faint; persistent, painful erection; seizures

Symptoms of overdose

Get emergency help immediately if any of the following symptoms of overdose occur:

Drowsiness; sleepiness; slurred speech

Some side effects may occur that usually do not need medical attention. These side effects may go away during treatment as your body adjusts to the medicine. Also, your health care professional may be able to tell you about ways to prevent or reduce some of these side effects. Check with your health care professional if any of the following side effects continue or are bothersome or if you have any questions about them:

More common

Acid or sour stomach; belching; constipation; diarrhea; difficulty speaking; dizziness; drooling; heartburn; indigestion; lack or loss of strength; loss of balance control; muscle trembling, jerking or stiffness; nausea; rash; restlessness; shuffling walk; stiffness of limbs; stomach discomfort, upset or pain; twisting movements of body; uncontrollable movements of body parts; weakness; weight gain

Less common

Change in vision; cough increased; depression; dry mouth; feeling faint upon standing; inability to move eyes; increasing blinking or spasms of eyelid; itching or reddening of skin; loss of appetite; muscle ache; muscle tightness; runny nose; sneezing; sore throat; sticking out of tongue; stuffy nose; swelling; trouble in breathing, speaking or swallowing; uncontrolled twisting movements of neck, trunk, arms, or legs; unusual facial expressions; vomiting; weakness of arms and legs; weight loss

Other side effects not listed may also occur in some patients. If you notice any other effects, check with your healthcare professional.

ZOLEDRONIC ACID (Intravenous route) - ZOE-le-dron-ik AS-id

Commonly used brand name(s)

In the U.S.—
  Zometa

Available Dosage Forms:

- Solution
- Powder for Solution

Therapeutic Class: Calcium Regulator

Uses For This Medicine

Zoledronic acid is used to treat hypercalcemia (high levels of blood calcium) that may occur in patients with some types of cancer. It is also used to treat cancer called multiple myeloma (tumors formed by the cells of the bone marrow) or certain types of bone metastases (the spread of cancer).

This medicine may also be used for other conditions as determined by your doctor.

This medicine is to be administered only by or under the supervision of your doctor.

Once a medicine has been approved for marketing for a certain use, experience may show that it is also useful for other medical problems. Although these uses are not included in product labeling, zoledronic acid is used in certain patients with the following medical conditions:

- Bone loss, in men, from taking certain medicines for prostate cancer.

Before Using This Medicine

In deciding to use a medicine, the risks of taking the medicine must be weighed against the good it will do. This is a decision you and your doctor will make. For this medicine, the following should be considered:

Allergies—Tell your doctor if you have ever had any unusual or allergic reaction to this medicine or any other medicines. Also tell your health care professional if you have any other types of allergies, such as to foods, dyes, preservatives, or animals. For non-prescription products, read the label or package ingredients carefully.

Pediatric—Studies on this medicine have been done only in adult patients, and there is no specific information comparing use of zoledronic acid in children with use in adults. Because of bone problems, this medicine should only be used in children if the benefit outweighs the risk.

Geriatric—Many medicines have not been studied specifically in older people. Therefore, it may not be known whether they work exactly the same way they do in younger adults or if they cause different side effects or problems in older people. However, because kidney problems occur more often in older adults, kidney function will need to be monitored.

Pregnancy—

	Pregnancy Category	Explanation
All Trimesters	D	Studies in pregnant women have demonstrated a risk to the fetus. However, the benefits of therapy in a life threatening situation or a serious disease, may outweigh the potential risk.

Breast Feeding—There are no adequate studies in women for determining infant risk when using this medication during breastfeeding. Weigh the potential benefits against the potential risks before taking this medication while breastfeeding.

Other medicines—Although certain medicines should not be used together at all, in other cases two different medicines may be used together even if an interaction might occur. In these cases, your doctor may want to change the dose, or other precautions may be necessary. Tell your healthcare professional if you are taking any other prescription or non-prescription (over-the-counter [OTC]) medicine.

Interactions with Food/Tobacco/Alcohol—Certain medicines should not be used at or around the time of eating food or eating certain types of food since interactions may occur. Using alcohol or tobacco with certain medicines may also cause interactions to occur. Discuss with your healthcare professional the use of your medicine with food, alcohol, or tobacco.

Other medical problems—The presence of other medical problems may affect the use of this medicine. Make sure you tell your doctor if you have any other medical problems, especially:

- Previous allergic reaction to zoledronic acid or other drugs—May cause severe reaction
- Asthma—Certain types of asthma may be worsened by zoledronic acid
- Heart disease—May be worsened by zoledronic acid
- Kidney disease—May be worsened by zoledronic acid
- Cancer or
- Cancer treatment or
- Dental procedures or surgery or
- Poor dental hygiene—May put you at risk for a serious jaw problem
- Dehydration (not enough water or fluids in your body)—May increase risk of severe kidney problems
- Liver problems—Safety of this medicine not known in patients with liver problems.

Proper Use of This Medicine

Note: Your health care professional my also give you vitamins containing Vitamin D and calcium

Your doctor may adjust your dose for kidney problems. Take the dose that your doctor instructs you to take.

Dosing—The dose of this medicine will be different for different patients. Follow your doctor's orders or the directions on the label. The following information includes only the average doses of this medicine. If your dose is different, do not change it unless your doctor tells you to do so.

The amount of medicine that you take depends on the strength of the medicine. Also, the number of doses you take each day, the time allowed between doses, and the length of time you take the medicine depend on the medical problem for which you are using the medicine.

- For intravenous dosage form
  - For treating multiple myeloma and bone metastases and,
  - For treating hypercalcemia (too much calcium in the blood):
    - Adults—4 milligrams (mg) in a solution to be injected into a vein in not less than 15 minutes.
    - Children—Use and dose must be determined by your doctor.

Precautions While Using This Medicine

It is important that your doctor check your progress at regular visits after you have received zoledronic acid. If your condition has improved, your progress must still be checked. The results of laboratory tests or the occurrence of certain symptoms will tell your doctor if your condition is coming back and if a second treatment is needed.

Tell your doctor right away if you experience symptoms of agitation, blood in urine, coma, confusion, decreased urine output, depression, dizziness, headache, irritability, lethargy, muscle twitching, nausea, rapid weight gain, seizures, stupor, swelling of face, ankles, or hands, or unusual tiredness or weakness. These could be a sign of serious kidney problems.

It is important that you check with your doctor before having any dental procedures or surgeries done while you are receiving zoledronic acid. Tell your doctor right away if you experience jaw tightness, swelling, numbing, or pain or a loose tooth. It could be the sign of a serious jaw disease.

Side Effects of This Medicine

Along with its needed effects, a medicine may cause some unwanted effects. Although not all of these side effects may occur, if they do occur they may need medical attention.

Check with your doctor immediately if any of the following side effects occur:

More common

Agitation; black, tarry stools; blurred vision; chest pain; chills; coma; confusion; convulsions; cough; depression; dizziness, faintness, or lightheadedness when getting up from a lying or sitting position; dizziness; fever; irregular heartbeat; irritability; lack or loss of strength; lethargy; lower back or side pain; mood or mental changes, confusion; muscle pain or cramps; muscle trembling or twitching, shaking of hands, arms, feet, legs, or face; nausea or vomiting; numbness and tingling around mouth, fingertips, or feet; painful or difficult urination; pale skin; rapid weight gain; seizures; shortness of breath, difficult or labored breathing; skin rash, cracks in skin at the corners of mouth, soreness or redness around fingernails and toenails; sore throat; sores, ulcers, or white spots on lips or mouth; stupor; sudden sweating; swollen glands; tightness in chest; trouble breathing with exercise; unusual bleeding or bruising; unusual tiredness or weakness; wheezing

Incidence not known—occurred during clinical practice

Decreased frequency/amount of urine; heavy jaw feeling; increased blood pressure; increased thirst; loosening of a tooth; pain, swelling, or numbness in the mouth or jaw; swelling of face, hands, fingers, lower legs, ankles; troubled breathing; weight gain

Some side effects may occur that usually do not need medical attention. These side effects may go away during treatment as your body adjusts to the medicine. Also, your health care professional may be able to tell you about ways to prevent or reduce some of these side effects. Check with your health care professional if any of the following side effects continue or are bothersome or if you have any questions about them:

More common

Abdominal pain; anxiety, nervousness, restlessness or irritability; bad, unusual or unpleasant (after) taste; back pain; bladder pain, bloody or cloudy urine; blistering, crusting, irritation, itching, or reddening of skin; bone pain; burning, crawling, itching, numbness, prickling, "pins and needles", or tingling feelings; change in taste; cracked, dry scaly skin; cracked lips; constipation; dehydration; diarrhea; difficulty swallowing; discouragement; dry mouth; ear congestion; fear or nervousness; feeling sad, or empty; frequent urge to urinate; hair loss, or thinning hair; headache; hyperventilation; irregular heartbeats; joint pain, or swollen joints; loss of appetite; loss of interest, or pleasure; loss of voice; muscle pain, stiffness or difficulty in moving; pain, swelling, or redness in joints; partial loss of feeling; nasal congestion, or runny nose; seeing, hearing, or feeling things that are not there; sleepiness or unusual drowsiness; sleeplessness, trouble sleeping, unable to sleep; swelling; swelling of leg; swelling or inflammation of the mouth; thirst; trouble concentrating; unusually cold, shivering; vomiting; weight loss; white spots on lips, tongue, or inside mouth

Other side effects not listed may also occur in some patients. If you notice any other effects, check with your healthcare professional.

ZOLMITRIPTAN (Oral route) - zohl-mi-TRIP-tan

Commonly used brand name(s)

In the U.S.—

Zomig

Zomig-ZMT

Available Dosage Forms:

- Tablet
- Tablet, Disintegrating

Therapeutic Class: Antimigraine

Pharmacologic Class: Serotonin Receptor Agonist, 5–HT1

Uses For This Medicine

Zolmitriptan is used to treat severe migraine headaches. Many people find that their headaches go away completely after they take zolmitriptan. Other people find that their headaches are much less painful, and that they are able to go back to their normal activities even though their headaches are not completely gone. Zolmitriptan often relieves symptoms that occur together with a migraine headache, such as nausea, vomiting, sensitivity to light, and sensitivity to sound.

Zolmitriptan is not an ordinary pain reliever. It should not be used to relieve any kind of pain other than migraine headaches.

Zolmitriptan may cause serious side effects in some people, especially people who have heart or blood vessel disease. Be sure that you discuss with your doctor the risks of using this medicine as well as the good that it can do.

Zolmitriptan is available only with your doctor's prescription.

Before Using This Medicine

In deciding to use a medicine, the risks of taking the medicine must be weighed against the good it will do. This is a decision you and your doctor will make. For this medicine, the following should be considered:

Allergies—Tell your doctor if you have ever had any unusual or allergic reaction to this medicine or any other medicines. Also tell your health care professional if you have any other types of allergies, such as to foods, dyes, preservatives, or animals. For non-prescription products, read the label or package ingredients carefully.

Pediatric—There is no specific information comparing use of zolmitriptan in children or teenagers with use in other age groups.

Geriatric—There is no specific information comparing use of zolmitriptan in patients older than 65 years of age with use in younger adults.

Pregnancy—

	Pregnancy Category	Explanation
All Trimesters	C	Animal studies have shown an adverse effect and there are no adequate studies in pregnant women OR no animal studies have been conducted and there are no adequate studies in pregnant women.

Breast Feeding—There are no adequate studies in women for determining infant risk when using this medication during breastfeeding. Weigh the potential benefits against the potential risks before taking this medication while breastfeeding.

Other medicines—

Using this medicine with any of the following medicines is not recommended. Your doctor may decide not to treat you with this medication or change some of the other medicines you take.

Almotriptan, Cisapride, Clorgyline, Dihydroergotamine, Ergoloid Mesylates, Ergonovine, Ergotamine, Frovatriptan, Iproniazid, Isocarboxazid, Levomethadyl, Mesoridazine, Methylergonovine, Methysergide, Moclobemide, Naratriptan, Nialamide, Pargyline, Phenelzine, Pimozide, Procarbazine, Rizatriptan, Sumatriptan, Terfenadine, Thioridazine, Toloxatone, Tranylcypromine, Ziprasidone

Interactions with Food/Tobacco/Alcohol—Certain medicines should not be used at or around the time of eating food or eating certain types of food since interactions may occur. Using alcohol or tobacco with certain medicines may also cause interactions to occur. Discuss with your healthcare professional the use of your medicine with food, alcohol, or tobacco.

Other medical problems—The presence of other medical problems may affect the use of this medicine. Make sure you tell your doctor if you have any other medical problems, especially:

- Angina (chest pain) or
- Fast or irregular heartbeat or
- Heart or blood vessel disease or
- High blood pressure or
- Kidney disease or
- Liver disease or
- Stroke (history of)—The chance of side effects may be increased. Heart or blood vessel disease and high blood pressure sometimes do not cause any symptoms, so some people do not know that they have these problems. Before deciding whether you should use zolmitriptan, your doctor may need to do some tests to make sure that you do not have any of these conditions.
- Phenylketonuria (PKU)—The oral disintegrating tablets may contain aspartame, which can make your condition worse

Proper Use of This Medicine

Do not use zolmitriptan for a headache that is different from your usual migraines. Instead, check with your doctor.

To relieve your migraine as soon as possible, use zolmitriptan as soon as the headache pain begins. Even if you get warning signals of a coming migraine (an aura), you should wait until the headache pain starts before using zolmitriptan.

Lying down in a quiet, dark room for a while after you use this medicine may help relieve your migraine.

Ask your doctor ahead of time about other medicine you might take if zolmitriptan does not work. After you take the other medicine, check with your doctor as soon as possible. Headaches that are not relieved by zolmitriptan are sometimes caused by conditions that need other treatment.

If you feel much better after a dose of zolmitriptan, but your headache comes back or gets worse after a while, you may

use more zolmitriptan. However, use this medicine only as directed by your doctor. Do not use more of it, and do not use it more often, than directed. Using too much zolmitriptan may increase the chance of side effects.

Your doctor may direct you to take another medicine to help prevent headaches. It is important that you follow your doctor's directions, even if your headaches continue to occur. Headache-preventing medicines may take several weeks to start working. Even after they do start working, your headaches may not go away completely. However, your headaches should occur less often, and they should be less severe and easier to relieve. This can reduce the amount of zolmitriptan or other pain medicines that you need. If you do not notice any improvement after several weeks of headache-preventing treatment, check with your doctor.

For patients using the oral disintegrating tablet form of this medicine:

- Make sure your hands are dry.
- Remove tablet from package, and immediately place the tablet on top of your tongue.
- The tablet will dissolve in seconds, and you may swallow it with your saliva. You do not need to drink water or other liquid to swallow the tablet.

Dosing—The dose of this medicine will be different for different patients. Follow your doctor's orders or the directions on the label. The following information includes only the average doses of this medicine. If your dose is different, do not change it unless your doctor tells you to do so.

The amount of medicine that you take depends on the strength of the medicine. Also, the number of doses you take each day, the time allowed between doses, and the length of time you take the medicine depend on the medical problem for which you are using the medicine.

- For oral dosage form (tablets):
  - For migraine headaches:
    - Adults—2.5 mg or lower (tablet may be broken in half) as a single dose. If the migraine comes back after being relieved, another dose may be taken two hours after the last dose. Do not take more than 10 mg in any twenty-four-hour period (one day).
    - Children—Use and dose must be determined by your doctor.
- For oral dosage form (oral disintegrating tablets):
  - For migraine headaches:
    - Adults—2.5 mg placed on top of your tongue. If the migraine comes back after being relieved, another dose may be taken two hours after the last dose. Do not take more than 10 mg in any twenty-four-hour period (one day).
    - Children—Use and dose must be determined by your doctor.

Storage—Store the medicine in a closed container at room temperature, away from heat, moisture, and direct light. Keep from freezing.

Keep out of the reach of children.

Do not keep outdated medicine or medicine no longer needed.

Precautions While Using This Medicine

Drinking alcoholic beverages can make headaches worse or cause new headaches to occur. People who suffer from severe headaches should probably avoid alcoholic beverages, especially during a headache.

Some people feel drowsy or dizzy during or after a migraine, or after taking zolmitriptan to relieve a migraine. As long as you are feeling drowsy or dizzy, do not drive, use machines, or do anything else that could be dangerous if you are dizzy or are not alert.

Side Effects of This Medicine

Along with its needed effects, a medicine may cause some unwanted effects. Although not all of these side effects may occur, if they do occur they may need medical attention.

Stop taking this medicine and get emergency help immediately if any of the following effects occur:

More common
Chest pain (severe); heaviness, tightness, or pressure in chest and/or neck; sensation of burning, warmth, heat, numbness, tightness, or tingling

Less common or rare
Abdominal pain (severe); changes in facial skin color; cough or hoarseness; diarrhea; fast or irregular heartbeat; fever or chills; loss of appetite; lower back or side pain; nausea; painful or difficult urination; puffiness or swelling of the eyelids or around the eyes, face, or lips; shortness of breath, troubled breathing, tightness in chest, and/or wheezing; skin rash, hives, and/or itching; weakness

Other side effects may occur that usually do not need medical attention. Some of the following effects, such as nausea, vomiting, drowsiness, dizziness, and general feeling of illness or tiredness, often occur during or after a migraine, even when zolmitriptan has not been used. However, check with your doctor if any of the following side effects continue or are bothersome:

More common
Dizziness; nausea; sleepiness; unusual tiredness or muscle weakness

Less common
Agitation; anxiety; depression; discomfort in jaw, mouth, or throat; difficulty in swallowing; dry mouth; fainting; heartburn; itching of the skin; large nonelevated blue or purplish patches in the skin; muscle aches; pounding heartbeat; sudden large increase in frequency and quantity of urine; sweating; swelling of face, fingers, feet and/or lower legs

Other side effects not listed may also occur in some patients. If you notice any other effects, check with your healthcare professional.

ZOLPIDEM (Oral route) - zole-PI-dem

Commonly used brand name(s)
In the U.S.—
Ambien
Ambien CR

Available Dosage Forms:
• Tablet, Extended Release
• Tablet

Therapeutic Class: Nonbarbiturate Hypnotic

Uses For This Medicine

Zolpidem belongs to the group of medicines called central nervous system (CNS) depressants (medicines that slow down the nervous system). Zolpidem is used to treat insomnia (trouble in sleeping). Zolpidem helps you get to sleep faster and sleep through the night. In general, when sleep medicines are used every night for a long time, they may lose their effectiveness. In most cases, sleep medicines should be used only for short periods of time, such as 1 or 2 days, and generally for no longer than 1 or 2 weeks.

This medicine is available only with your doctor's prescription.

Before Using This Medicine

In deciding to use a medicine, the risks of taking the medicine must be weighed against the good it will do. This is a decision you and your doctor will make. For this medicine, the following should be considered:

Sleep medicines may cause a special type of memory loss or "amnesia". When this occurs, a person does not remember what has happened during the several hours between use of the medicine and the time when its effects wear off. This is usually not a problem since most people fall asleep after taking the medicine. In most instances, memory problems can be avoided by taking zolpidem only when you are able to get a full night's sleep (7 to 8 hours) before you need to be active again. Be sure to talk to your doctor if you think you are having memory problems.

Allergies—Tell your doctor if you have ever had any unusual or allergic reaction to this medicine or any other medicines. Also tell your health care professional if you have any other types of allergies, such as to foods, dyes, preservatives, or animals. For non-prescription products, read the label or package ingredients carefully.

Pediatric—Studies on this medicine have been done only in adult patients, and there is no specific information comparing use of zolpidem in children with use in other age groups.

Geriatric—Confusion and falling are more likely to occur in the elderly, who are usually more sensitive than younger adults to the effects of zolpidem.

Pregnancy—

	Pregnancy Category	Explanation
All Trimesters	C	Animal studies have shown an adverse effect and there are no adequate studies in pregnant women OR no animal studies have been conducted and there are no adequate studies in pregnant women.

Breast Feeding—There are no adequate studies in women for determining infant risk when using this medication during breastfeeding. Weigh the potential benefits against the potential risks before taking this medication while breastfeeding.

Other medicines—

Using this medicine with any of the following medicines may cause an increased risk of certain side effects, but using both drugs may be the best treatment for you. If both medicines are prescribed together, your doctor may change the dose or how often you use one or both of the medicines.

Bupropion, Desipramine, Ketoconazole, Rifampin, Sertraline, Venlafaxine

Interactions with Food/Tobacco/Alcohol—Certain medicines should not be used at or around the time of eating food or eating certain types of food since interactions may occur. Using alcohol or tobacco with certain medicines may also cause interactions to occur. The following interactions have been selected on the basis of their potential significance and are not necessarily all-inclusive.

Using this medicine with any of the following may cause an increased risk of certain side effects but may be unavoidable in some cases. If used together, your doctor may change the dose or how often you use this medicine, or give you special instructions about the use of food, alcohol, or tobacco.

Ethanol

Other medical problems—The presence of other medical problems may affect the use of this medicine. Make sure you tell your doctor if you have any other medical problems, especially:

- Alcohol abuse (or history of) or
- Drug abuse or dependence (or history of)—Dependence on zolpidem may develop
- Emphysema, asthma, bronchitis, or other chronic lung disease or
- Mental depression or
- Sleep apnea (temporary stopping of breathing during sleep)—Zolpidem may make these conditions worse
- Kidney disease or
- Liver disease—Higher blood levels of zolpidem may result, increasing the chance of side effects

Proper Use of This Medicine

Take this medicine only as directed by your doctor. Do not take more of it, do not take it more often, and do not take it for a longer time than your doctor ordered. If too much is taken, it may become habit-forming (causing mental or physical dependence).

Take zolpidem just before going to bed, when you are ready to go to sleep. This medicine works very quickly to put you to sleep.

You should swallow the extended-release tablets whole. Do not crush or chew them.

Do not take this medicine when your schedule does not permit you to get a full night's sleep (7 to 8 hours). If you must wake up before this, you may continue to feel drowsy and may experience memory problems, because the effects of the medicine have not had time to wear off.

Zolpidem should be taken without food on an empty stomach. It will work faster if you take it on an empty stomach. However, if your doctor tells you to take the medicine a certain way, take it exactly as directed.

Dosing—The dose of this medicine will be different for different patients. Follow your doctor's orders or the directions on the label. The following information includes only the average doses of this medicine. If your dose is different, do not change it unless your doctor tells you to do so.

The amount of medicine that you take depends on the strength of the medicine. Also, the number of doses you take each day, the time allowed between doses, and the length of time you take the medicine depend on the medical problem for which you are using the medicine.

- For oral dosage form (tablets):
  - For the treatment of insomnia (trouble in sleeping):
    - Adults—10 milligrams (mg) at bedtime.
    - Older adults—5 mg at bedtime.
    - Children up to 18 years of age—Use and dose must be determined by the doctor.
- For oral dosage form (extended-release [long-acting] tablets):
  - For the treatment of insomnia (trouble in sleeping):
    - Adults—12.5 milligrams (mg) at bedtime.
    - Older adults—6.25 mg at bedtime.
    - Children up to 18 years of age—Use and dose must be determined by the doctor.

Missed dose—If you miss a dose of this medicine, skip the missed dose and go back to your regular dosing schedule. Do not double doses.

Storage—Store the medicine in a closed container at room temperature, away from heat, moisture, and direct light. Keep from freezing.

Keep out of the reach of children.

Do not keep outdated medicine or medicine no longer needed.

Precautions While Using This Medicine

If you think you need to take zolpidem for more than 7 to 10 days, be sure to discuss it with your doctor. Insomnia that lasts longer than this may be a sign of another medical problem.

This medicine will add to the effects of alcohol and other CNS depressants (medicines that slow down the nervous system, possibly causing drowsiness). Some examples of CNS depressants are antihistamines or medicine for hay fever, other allergies, or colds; sedatives, tranquilizers, or sleeping medicine; prescription pain medicine or narcotics; barbiturates; medicine for seizures; muscle relaxants; or anesthetics, including some dental anesthetics. Check with your doctor before taking any of the above while you are using this medicine.

This medicine may cause some people, especially older persons, to become drowsy, dizzy, lightheaded, clumsy or unsteady, or less alert than they are normally. Even though zolpidem is taken at bedtime, it may cause some people to feel drowsy or less alert on arising. Also, this medicine may cause double vision or other vision problems. Make sure you know how you react to zolpidem before you drive, use machines, or do anything else that could be dangerous if you are dizzy, or are not alert or able to see well.

If you develop any unusual and strange thoughts or behavior while you are taking zolpidem, be sure to discuss it with your doctor. Some changes that have occurred in people taking this medicine are like those seen in people who drink alcohol and then act in a manner that is not normal. Other changes may be more unusual and extreme, such as confusion, worsening of depression hallucinations (seeing, hearing, or feeling things that are not there), suicidal thoughts, and unusual excitement, nervousness, or irritability.

If you will be taking zolpidem for a long time, do not stop taking it without first checking with your doctor. Your doctor may want you to reduce gradually the amount you are taking before stopping completely. Stopping this medicine suddenly may cause withdrawal side effects.

After taking zolpidem for insomnia, you may have difficulty sleeping (rebound insomnia) for the first few nights after you stop taking it.

If you think you or someone else may have taken an overdose of this medicine, get emergency help at once. Taking an overdose of zolpidem or taking alcohol or other CNS depressants with zolpidem may lead to breathing problems and unconsciousness. Some signs of an overdose are severe drowsiness, severe nausea or vomiting, staggering, and troubled breathing.

Side Effects of This Medicine

Along with its needed effects, a medicine may cause some unwanted effects. Although not all of these side effects may occur, if they do occur they may need medical attention.

Check with your doctor as soon as possible if any of the following side effects occur:

Less common
Clumsiness or unsteadiness; confusion—more common in older adults; mental depression

Rare
Dizziness, lightheadedness, or fainting; falling—more common in older adults; fast heartbeat; hallucinations (seeing, hearing, or feeling things that are not there); skin rash; swelling of face; trouble in sleeping; unusual excitement, nervousness, or irritability; wheezing or difficulty in breathing

Symptoms of overdose
Clumsiness or unsteadiness (severe); dizziness (severe); double vision or other vision problems; drowsiness (severe); nausea (severe); slow heartbeat; troubled breathing; vomiting (severe)

Some side effects may occur that usually do not need medical attention. These side effects may go away during treatment as your body adjusts to the medicine. Also, your health care professional may be able to tell you about ways to prevent or reduce some of these side effects. Check with your health care professional if any of the following side effects continue or are bothersome or if you have any questions about them:

More common
Sleepiness or unusual drowsiness

Less common
Abdominal or stomach pain; abnormal or decreased touch sensation; abnormal sensation of movement; appetite disorder; balance disorder; binge eating; bladder pain; bloody or cloudy urine; burning, crawling, itching, numbness, prickling, "pins and needles", or tingling feelings; change in hearing; chest discomfort; chills; confusion about identity, place, and time; constipation; continuing ringing or buzzing or other unexplained noise in ears; daytime drowsiness; diarrhea; difficult, burning, or painful urination; difficulty in moving; difficulty swallowing; discouragement; double vision or other vision problems; drugged feelings; dryness of mouth; ear drainage; earache; eye redness; false or unusual sense of well-being; fear; feeling of unreality; feeling sad or empty; fever; flatulence; frequent bowel movements; frequent urge to urinate; general feeling of discomfort or illness; generalized slowing of mental and physical activity; headache; hearing loss; heartburn; hives or welts; itching ears; joint pain; lack of appetite; lack of feeling or emotion; lack or loss of self-control;

lack or loss of strength; longer or heavier menstrual periods; loss of balance; loss of interest or pleasure; memory problems; mood swings; muscle aches, cramping, pain or stiffness; nausea; nervousness; nightmares or unusual dreams; pain in joints; redness of skin; redness or soreness of throat; sense of detachment from self or body; shortness of breath or troubled breathing; skin rash; skin wrinkling; sneezing; sore throat; stress symptoms; stuffy or runny nose; swollen joints; tiredness; trouble concentrating; trouble sleeping; vision blurred; visual depth perception altered; vomiting

After you stop using this medicine, it may still produce some side effects that need attention. During this period of time, *check with your doctor immediately* if you notice the following side effects:

Abdominal or stomach cramps or discomfort; agitation, nervousness, or feelings of panic; convulsions (seizures); flushing; lightheadedness; muscle cramps; nausea; sweating; tremors; uncontrolled crying; unusual tiredness or weakness; vomiting; worsening of mental or emotional problems

Other side effects not listed may also occur in some patients. If you notice any other effects, check with your healthcare professional.

ZONISAMIDE (Oral route) - zoe-NIS-a-mide

Commonly used brand name(s)

In the U.S.—
Zonegran

Available Dosage Forms:
- Capsule
- Tablet

Therapeutic Class: Anticonvulsant

Uses For This Medicine

Zonisamide is used to control some kinds of seizures in the treatment of epilepsy.

This medicine is available only with your doctor's prescription.

Before Using This Medicine

In deciding to use a medicine, the risks of taking the medicine must be weighed against the good it will do. This is a decision you and your doctor will make. For this medicine, the following should be considered:

Allergies—Tell your doctor if you have ever had any unusual or allergic reaction to this medicine or any other medicines. Also tell your health care professional if you have any other types of allergies, such as to foods, dyes, preservatives, or animals. For non-prescription products, read the label or package ingredients carefully.

Pediatric—Safety and efficacy have not been established in children who are under 16 years of age and is not approved for use.

Note: Studies in children have shown that some children are at higher risk for oligohidrosis (decreased sweating) and hyperthermia (unusually high body temperature), especially in warm or hot weather. This can sometimes result in heat stroke and hospitalization.

Geriatric—Many medicines have not been studied specifically in older people. Therefore, it may not be known whether they work exactly the same way they do in younger adults. Although there is no specific information comparing use of zonisamide in the elderly with use in other age groups, this medicine is not expected to cause different side effects or problems in older people than it does in younger adults.

Pregnancy—

	Pregnancy Category	Explanation
All Trimesters	C	Animal studies have shown an adverse effect and there are no adequate studies in pregnant women OR no animal studies have been conducted and there are no adequate studies in pregnant women.

Breast Feeding—There are no adequate studies in women for determining infant risk when using this medication during breastfeeding. Weigh the potential benefits against the potential risks before taking this medication while breastfeeding.

Other medicines—

Using this medicine with any of the following medicines may cause an increased risk of certain side effects, but using both drugs may be the best treatment for you. If both medicines are prescribed together, your doctor may change the dose or how often you use one or both of the medicines.

Ginkgo

Interactions with Food/Tobacco/Alcohol—Certain medicines should not be used at or around the time of eating food or eating certain types of food since interactions may occur. Using alcohol or tobacco with certain medicines may also cause interactions to occur. Discuss with your healthcare professional the use of your medicine with food, alcohol, or tobacco.

Other medical problems—The presence of other medical problems may affect the use of this medicine. Make sure you tell your doctor if you have any other medical problems, especially:

- Kidney disease or
- Liver disease

Proper Use of This Medicine

Take this medicine only as directed by your doctor to help your condition as much as possible. Do not take more or less of it, and do not take it more or less often than your doctor ordered.

Zonisamide may be taken with or without food, on a full or empty stomach. Swallow capsule whole. Do not break or crush.

Dosing—The dose of this medicine will be different for different patients. Follow your doctor's orders or the directions on the label. The following information includes only the average doses of this medicine. If your dose is different, do not change it unless your doctor tells you to do so.

The amount of medicine that you take depends on the strength of the medicine. Also, the number of doses you take each day, the time allowed between doses, and the length of time you take the medicine depend on the medical problem for which you are using the medicine.

- For oral dosage form (capsules):
  - For partial seizures (epilepsy)
    - Adults and teenagers 16 years of age and older— At first, 100 milligrams (mg) a day for two weeks. The dose may then be increased by 100 mg a day once every two weeks, as decided by your doctor. However, the dose is usually not more than 400 mg a day, taken one or two times a day.
    - Children up to 16 years of age—Use and dose must be determined by the doctor.

Missed dose—If you miss a dose of this medicine, take it as soon as possible. However, if it is almost time for your next dose, skip the missed dose and go back to your regular dosing schedule. Do not double doses.

Storage—Store the medicine in a closed container at room temperature, away from heat, moisture, and direct light. Keep from freezing.

Keep out of the reach of children.

Do not keep outdated medicine or medicine no longer needed.

Ask your healthcare professional how you should dispose of any medicine you do not use.

Precautions While Using This Medicine

It is very important that your doctor check your progress at regular visits. This will allow your doctor to see if the medicine is working properly, and to check for unwanted effects.

If your condition does not improve within a few weeks or if it becomes worse, check with your doctor.

This medicine may cause some people to become drowsy, dizzy, or less alert than they are normally. Make sure you know how you react to this medicine before you drive, use machines, or do anything else that could be dangerous if you are dizzy or are not alert.

This medicine will add to the effects of alcohol and other CNS depressants (medicines that make you drowsy or less alert). Some examples of CNS depressants are antihistamines or medicine for hay fever, other allergies, or colds; prescription pain medicines, or sleep medicines. Do not take other medicines unless they have been discussed with your doctor. This especially includes nonprescription medicines for appetite control, asthma, colds, cough, hay fever, or sinus problems.

Contact your doctor immediately if you develop skin rash, experience fever, sore throat, oral ulcers, easy bruising, or worsening of seizures.

These medicines may make you sweat less, causing your body temperature to increase. Use extra care not to become overheated during exercise or hot weather while you are taking this medicine, since overheating may result in heat stroke. Also, hot baths or saunas may make you dizzy or faint while you are taking this medicine.

Use effective birth control methods to prevent pregnancy if you are sexually active and able to become pregnant.

Do not stop taking zonisamide without first checking with your doctor. Stopping the medicine suddenly may cause your seizures to return or to occur more often. Your doctor may want you to gradually reduce the amount you are taking before stopping completely.

It is important that you drink plenty of fluids every day during therapy with zonisamide to help prevent kidney stones from forming.

Side Effects of This Medicine

Along with its needed effects, a medicine may cause some unwanted effects. Although not all of these side effects may occur, if they do occur they may need medical attention.

Symptoms of overdose

Get emergency help immediately if any of the following symptoms of overdose occur:

Confusion; difficult or labored breathing; faintness; loss of consciousness; slow or irregular heartbeat

Check with your doctor immediately if any of the following side effects occur:

More common

Discouragement; feeling sad or empty; irritability; lack of appetite; loss of interest or pleasure; mood or mental changes; shakiness or unsteady walking; tiredness; trouble concentrating; trouble sleeping

Less common

Agitation; bruising; delusions; hallucinations; large, flat blue or purplish patches on the skin; rash

---

Some side effects may occur that usually do not need medical attention. These side effects may go away during treatment as your body adjusts to the medicine. Also, your health care professional may be able to tell you about ways to prevent or reduce some of these side effects. Check with your health care professional if any of the following side effects continue or are bothersome or if you have any questions about them:

More common

Abdominal pain; anxiety; difficulty with memory; dizziness; double vision; headache; loss of appetite; nausea; restlessness; sleepiness; sleeplessness; unusual drowsiness; unusual tiredness or weakness

Less common

Aching muscles or joints; acid or sour stomach; bad, unusual, or unpleasant taste in mouth; belching; change in taste; chills; constipation; diarrhea; difficulty in speaking; difficulty in thinking; dry mouth; fever; general ill feeling; headache; heartburn; indigestion; mental slowness; nervousness; runny or stuffy nose; sneezing; tingling, burning, or prickly feelings on skin; uncontrolled, back and forth, or rolling eye movements; weight loss

Other side effects not listed may also occur in some patients. If you notice any other effects, check with your healthcare professional.

you to gradually reduce the amount you are taking before stopping completely.

It's important that you drink plenty of fluids every day during therapy with zonisamide to help prevent kidney stones from forming.

Side Effects of This Medicine

Along with its needed effects, a medicine may cause some unwanted effects. Although not all of these side effects may occur, if they do occur they may need medical attention.

Check with your doctor immediately if any of the following side effects occur:

More common

Discouragement, feeling sad or empty, irritability, loss of interest or pleasure, need or mental sharpness, tiredness or unusual weariness or tiredness, trouble concentrating, trouble sleeping

Less common

Agitation, delusions, hallucinations, tremor, blue-black or purplish patches on the skin, rash

Some side effects may occur that usually do not need medical attention. These side effects may go away during treatment as your body adjusts to the medicine. Also, your health care professional may be able to tell you about ways to prevent or reduce some of these side effects. Check with your health care professional if any of the following side effects continue or are bothersome or if you have any questions about them:

More common

Abdominal pain, anxiety, difficulty with memory, dizziness or lightheadedness, headache, loss of appetite, nausea, nervousness, sleepiness, sleeplessness, unusual drowsiness, unusual tiredness or weakness

Less common

Acid or sour stomach, aching muscles or joints, bad, unusual, or unpleasant taste in mouth, belching, diarrhea, difficulty in speaking, difficulty in breathing, dry mouth, fever, general feeling of discomfort or illness, heartburn, indigestion, mental slowness, nervousness, runny or stuffy nose, sneezing, tingling, numbness, or prickly feelings on skin, uncontrolled back and forth or rolling eye movements, weight loss

Other side effects not listed may also occur in some patients. If you notice any other effects, check with your healthcare professional.

Glossary

Abdomen—The body area between the chest and pelvis; the belly. It contains the stomach and intestines.

Abnormal—Not normal or usual.

Abortifacient—Agent that causes abortion.

Abrade—Scrape or rub away the outer cover or layer of a part.

Abrasion—Minor wound or injury caused by scraping, rubbing, or wearing.

Absorption—Passing of substances into or across tissues of the body, for example, digested food into the blood from the small intestine, or poisons through the skin.

Achlorhydria—Absence of acid that normally would be found in the stomach.

Acidic—1. Refers to sharp, sour taste. 2. Referring to an acid (a chemical characterized by the way it combines with certain other substances). Opposite of alkaline.

Acidifier, urinary—Medicine that makes the urine more acidic.

Acidosis—A condition in which certain body fluids and tissues become too acidic.

Acne—Condition caused by inflammation of certain glands and hair follicles of the face, neck, and upper back, marked by red raised areas, pimples, and cysts.

Acromegaly—Enlargement of the face, body, hands, and feet because of too much growth hormone.

Acute—Describes a condition that begins suddenly, often has severe symptoms, and usually lasts a short time.

Added fiber—In food labeling, at least 2.5 grams or more fiber per serving than reference food.

Addison's disease—Disease caused by not enough corticosteroid hormones being produced by the adrenal glands; causes brownish discoloration of the skin, weakness, salt loss, and low blood pressure.

ADHD (attention-deficit hyperactivity disorder)—Syndrome marked by short attention span, disruptive behavior, learning difficulties, and an excessive level of activity.

Adhesion—The joining together, by fibrous tissue, of body parts and tissues that are normally separate.

Adjunct—An additional or secondary treatment that is helpful but may not be necessary for treatment of a particular condition; not effective for that condition if used alone.

Adjuvant—1. A substance added to or used with another substance to assist its action. 2. Something that assists or enhances the effectiveness of medical treatment.

Adrenal cortex—Outer layer of tissue of the adrenal gland, which produces corticosteroid (cortisone-like) hormones.

Adrenal glands—Two organs located next to the kidneys. They produce the hormones epinephrine (adrenaline) and norepinephrine and corticosteroid (cortisone-like) hormones.

Adrenaline—*See* Epinephrine.

Adrenal medulla—Inner part of the adrenal gland, which produces epinephrine (adrenaline) and norepinephrine.

Adrenocorticoids—*See* Corticosteroids.

Adverse effect—Any unwanted effect produced by a drug or therapy that is harmful to the patient.

Aerosol—Suspension of very small liquid or solid particles in compressed gas. Drugs in aerosol form are dispensed in the form of a mist by releasing the gas.

African sleeping sickness—*See* Trypanosomiasis, African.

Agent—A force or substance able to cause a change.

Agoraphobia—Abnormal fear and avoidance of public places or open spaces.

Agranulocytosis—Disease marked by a severe decrease in the number of granulocytes (one type of white blood cell) normally present in the blood. Also called *granulocytopenia*.

AIDS (acquired immunodeficiency syndrome)—Disease caused by human immunodeficiency virus (HIV). The disease results in a breakdown of the body's immune system, which makes a person more likely to get some other infections and some forms of cancer.

Alcohol-abuse deterrent—Medicine used to help alcoholics avoid the use of alcohol.

Alkaline—Referring to an alkali (a chemical characterized by the way it combines with certain other substances). Opposite of acidic.

Alkalizer, urinary—Medicine that makes the urine more alkaline.

Alkalosis—A condition in which certain body fluids and tissues become too alkaline.

Allergen—Any substance that induces an allergic reaction.

Allergy—Abnormal, high sensitivity to particular substances that are ordinarily harmless; common reactions include hives, itching, sneezing, stuffy nose, and swelling of mucous membranes, such as the tissues lining the nose, mouth, and throat.

Alopecia—Loss or absence of hair from areas where it normally is present.

Altitude sickness agent—Medicine used to prevent or lessen some of the effects of high altitude on the body.

Alzheimer's disease—Disease of the brain, usually beginning in late middle age, that is marked by gradual and worsening loss of mental performance, changes in personality and/or behavior, and inability to perform daily tasks.

Amenorrhea—Abnormal absence of menstrual periods.

Amino acid—One of a large group of compounds that contain carbon and nitrogen. Amino acids are the building blocks of protein and also the end product of protein digestion.

Aminoglycosides—A class of chemically related antibiotics used to treat some serious types of bacterial infections.

Ampul—Small sealed glass or plastic container holding a sterile solution, usually for injection. Also, *ampule*.

Anabolic steroid—Any of a group of compounds resembling testosterone that aid in the building of body tissues.

Analgesic—Medicine that relieves pain.

Anaphylaxis—Sudden, life-threatening allergic reaction.

Androgen—Hormone, such as testosterone, that promotes male characteristics, such as a deep voice and beard growth.

Anemia—Reduction, to below normal, of hemoglobin (the oxygen-carrying substance found in red blood cells) in the blood.

Anesthesiologist—A physician who is qualified to give an anesthetic and other medicines to a patient before and during surgery.

Anesthetic—Medicine that causes a loss of feeling or sensation, especially of pain, sometimes through loss of consciousness.

Aneurysm—A balloon-like swelling that forms at a weak place in the wall of an artery, vein, or the heart.

Angina—Pain, tightness, or feeling of heaviness in the chest, due to a lack of oxygen supply for the heart muscle. The pain may be felt in the left shoulder, jaw, or arm instead of or in addition to the chest. Symptoms often occur during physical activity.

Angioedema—Condition marked by hives and continuing swelling of areas of the skin, usually in the head and neck area. Swelling of the tongue or the tissues lining the mouth and throat may also occur, causing breathing problems.

Anorexia—Loss of appetite for food.

Anoxia—Absence of oxygen. (The term is sometimes incorrectly used for hypoxia.)

Antacid—Medicine used to neutralize excess acid in the stomach.

Antagonist—Drug or other substance that blocks or works against the action of another.

Anthelmintic—Medicine used to destroy or expel intestinal worms.

Antiacne agent—Medicine used to treat acne.

Antianemic—Agent that prevents or corrects anemia.

Antianginal—Medicine used to prevent or treat angina attacks.

Antianxiety agent—Medicine used to treat excessive nervousness, tension, or anxiety.

Antiarrhythmic—Medicine used to prevent or correct irregular heartbeats.

Antiasthmatic—Medicine used to treat asthma.

Antibacterial—Agent that kills or slows the growth of bacteria.

Antibiotic—Medicine used to treat certain types of infections.

Antibody—Protein produced by the immune system that acts against a specific antigen. Antibodies help the body fight infection and are involved in allergic reactions. Also called *immunoglobulin*.

Antibulimic—Medicine used to treat bulimia.

Anticholelithic—Medicine used to dissolve gallstones.

Anticoagulant—Medicine used to decrease or slow the clotting of blood.

Anticonvulsant—Medicine used to prevent or treat convulsions (seizures).

Antidepressant—Medicine used to treat mental depression.

Antidiabetic agent—Medicine used to control blood sugar levels in patients with diabetes mellitus (sugar diabetes).

Antidiarrheal—Medicine used to treat diarrhea.

Antidiuretic—Medicine used to decrease urine output (for example, in patients with diabetes insipidus).

Antidiuretic hormone—*See* Vasopressin.

Antidote—Medicine used to prevent or treat harmful effects of another medicine or a poison.

Antidyskinetic—Medicine used to help treat the loss of muscle control caused by certain diseases or by some other medicines.

Antidysmenorrheal—Medicine used to treat menstrual cramps.

Antiemetic—Medicine used to prevent or relieve nausea and vomiting.

Antiendometriotic—Medicine used to treat endometriosis.

Antienuretic—Medicine used to help prevent bedwetting.

Antifibrotic—Medicine used to treat fibrosis.

Antiflatulent—Medicine used to help relieve excess gas in the stomach or intestines.

Antifungal—Medicine used to treat infections caused by a fungus.

Antigen—Any substance that causes an immune reaction.

Antiglaucoma agent—Medicine used to treat glaucoma.

Antigout agent—Medicine used to prevent or relieve gout attacks.

Antihemorrhagic—Medicine used to prevent or help stop serious bleeding.

Antihistamine—Medicine used to prevent or relieve the symptoms of allergic reactions, such as itching, rash, swelling, runny nose, and sneezing.

Antihypercalcemic—Medicine used to help lower the amount of calcium in the blood.

Antihyperlipidemic—Medicine used to help lower high levels of lipids (fatty substances) in the blood.

Antihyperphosphatemic—Medicine used to help lower the amount of phosphate in the blood.

Antihypertensive—Medicine used to help lower high blood pressure.

Antihyperuricemic—Medicine used to prevent or treat gout or other medical problems caused by too much uric acid in the blood.

Antihypocalcemic—Medicine used to increase calcium blood levels in patients with too little calcium.

Antihypoglycemic—Medicine used to increase blood sugar levels in patients with low blood sugar.

Antihypokalemic—Medicine used to increase potassium blood levels in patients with too little potassium.

Anti-infective—Medicine used to treat infection.

Anti-inflammatory—Medicine used to relieve pain, swelling, and other symptoms of inflammation.

Anti-inflammatory, nonsteroidal—An anti-inflammatory medicine that is not a cortisone-like medicine. Also called *NSAID*.

Anti-inflammatory, steroidal—A cortisone-like anti-inflammatory medicine.

Antimetabolite—Substance that interferes with the normal processes within cells, preventing their growth.

Antimuscarinic—Medicine used to block the effects of a certain chemical in the body; often used to reduce smooth muscle spasms, especially abdominal or stomach cramps or spasms.

Antimyasthenic—Medicine used to treat myasthenia gravis.

Antimyotonic—Medicine used to prevent or relieve night-time leg cramps or muscle spasms.

Antineoplastic—Medicine used to treat cancer.

Antineuralgic—Medicine used to treat nerve pain (neuralgia).

Antioxidant—Substance that protects tissues of the body against oxygen damage. Examples of antioxidants are vitamins A, C, and E, and beta-carotene.

Antiprotozoal—Medicine used to treat infections caused by protozoa.

Antipruritic—Medicine used to prevent or relieve itching.

Antipsoriatic—Medicine used to treat psoriasis.

Antipsychotic—Medicine used to treat certain mental and emotional conditions, including psychosis.

Antipyretic—Medicine used to reduce fever.

Antirheumatic—Medicine used to treat arthritis (rheumatism).

Antirosacea—Medicine used to treat rosacea (a form of acne).

Antiseborrheic—Medicine used to treat dandruff and seborrhea.

Antiseptic—Medicine that stops the growth of germs. Antiseptics are used on the skin or mucous membranes to prevent or treat infections.

Antispasmodic—Medicine used to reduce smooth muscle spasms (for example, stomach, intestinal, or urinary tract spasms).

Antispastic—Medicine used to treat muscle spasms.

Antithyroid agent—Medicine used to treat an overactive thyroid gland.

Antitremor agent—Medicine used to treat tremors (trembling or shaking).

Antitubercular—Medicine used to treat tuberculosis (TB).

Antitussive—Medicine used to relieve cough.

Antiulcer agent—Medicine used to treat stomach and duodenal ulcers.

Antivertigo agent—Medicine used to prevent dizziness (vertigo).

Antiviral—Medicine used to treat infections caused by a virus.

Anus—The opening at the end of the digestive tract through which waste matter (feces) passes out of the body.

Anxiety—An emotional state with apprehension, worry, or tension in reaction to real or imagined danger or dread; accompanied by sweating, increased pulse, trembling, weakness, and fatigue.

Apnea—Temporary absence of breathing.

Apoplexy—*See* Stroke.

Appendicitis—Inflammation of the appendix.

Appetite—A desire for food.

Appetite stimulant—Medicine used to help increase the desire for food.

Appetite suppressant—Medicine used in weight control programs to help decrease the desire to eat.

Arrhythmia—Abnormal heart rhythm.

Arteritis, temporal—Inflammation of arteries in the area around the eyes; occurs in older people.

Artery—Blood vessel that carries blood away from the heart.

Arthralgia—Pain in a joint.

Arthritis, rheumatoid—Chronic disease, mainly of the joints, marked by inflammation (pain, redness, and swelling).

Ascites—Accumulation of fluid in the abdominal cavity.

Asthma—Disease marked by inflammation with constriction (narrowing) of the bronchial tubes (air passages). The constricted airways result in wheezing and difficult breathing. Attacks may be brought on by allergens, virus infection, cold air, or exercise.

Atherosclerosis—Common disease of the arteries in which artery walls thicken and harden.

Athlete's foot—Fungus infection or ringworm of the feet. Also called *tinea pedis*.

Atrophy—A wasting away or reduction in size and function of a cell, tissue, or part.

Avoid—To keep away from deliberately.

Backbone—*See* Spinal column.

Bacteremia—Presence of bacteria in the blood.

Bacteria—Any of a group of one-celled microorganisms found widely in nature. Many diseases and infections are caused by bacteria.

Bancroft's filariasis—Disease transmitted by mosquitoes in which an infection with the filarial worm occurs; affects the lymph system, producing inflammation.

Basophil—One type of white blood cell; plays a role in allergic reactions.

Beriberi—Disorder caused by too little vitamin B_1 (thiamine), marked by an accumulation of fluid in the body, extreme weight loss, inflammation of nerves, or paralysis.

Bile—Thick fluid produced by the liver and stored in the gallbladder; helps in the digestion of fats.

Bile duct—Tube which carries bile from the liver to the gallbladder, or from the gallbladder to the intestine.

Bilharziasis—*See* Schistosomiasis.

Biliary—Relating to bile, the bile duct, or the gallbladder.

Bilirubin—The bile pigment that is orange-colored or yellow; an excess in the blood may cause jaundice.

Biofeedback—Process that aims to help the patient gain some control over blood pressure, skin temperature, or other involuntary function.

Bipolar disorder—Severe mental illness marked by repeated episodes of depression and mania. Also called *manic-depressive illness.*

Bisexual—One who is sexually attracted to both sexes.

Black fever—*See* Leishmaniasis, visceral.

Blood cell—Any of the cells that are present in the blood. Major types are red blood cells (erythrocytes, which carry oxygen to the tissues), white blood cells (leukocytes, which help protect against infection), and platelets (thrombocytes, which are necessary for blood clotting).

Blood plasma—The liquid in which blood cells and other substances are carried through the arteries and veins.

Blood pressure—Pressure of the blood upon the walls of the arteries; usually measured by both the highest (systolic) and lowest (diastolic) pressures.

Bone marrow—Soft material filling the cavities of bones. Bone marrow is the main place in the body where blood cells and platelets are formed.

Bone marrow depression—Condition in which the production of red blood cells, white blood cells, or platelets by the bone marrow is decreased.

Bone resorption inhibitor—Medicine used to prevent or treat certain types of bone disorders; helps prevent bone loss.

Bowel—Intestine.

Bowel disease, inflammatory, suppressant—Medicine used to treat certain intestinal disorders, such as colitis and Crohn's disease.

Bradycardia—Slow heart rate, usually less than 60 beats per minute in adults.

Bronchitis—Inflammation of the bronchial tubes (air passages) of the lungs.

Bronchodilator—Medicine used to open up the bronchial tubes (air passages) of the lungs to increase the flow of air through them.

Bruise—Discoloration of the skin caused by an injury to the tissue beneath without a break in the skin. Most bruises slowly change in color from reddish purple to bluish to greenish yellow.

Buccal—Relating to the cheek. A buccal medicine is taken by placing it between the cheek and the gum and letting it slowly dissolve.

Bulimia—Eating disorder, mostly of females, marked by bouts of excessive eating followed by self-induced vomiting, hard exercise, or fasting.

Bulk—In nutrition, fiber that absorbs water while in the intestine; helps formation and movement of the stool. Also called *roughage.*

Bursa—Small fluid-filled sac that helps reduce friction; located between body parts that move over one another (such as in a joint).

Bursitis—Inflammation of a bursa.

Calorie—Unit of heat that measures the energy value of food.

Calorie free—In food labeling, fewer than 5 calories per serving.

Candidiasis of the mouth—Overgrowth of the yeast *Candida* in the mouth; marked by white patches on the tongue or in side the mouth. Also called *thrush* or *white mouth.*

Candidiasis of the vagina—Yeast infection of the vagina caused by the yeast *Candida;* associated with itching, burning, and a curd-like white discharge.

Canker sore—Acute, painful ulcer inside the mouth.

Carbohydrate—Any one of a large group of compounds from plants, including sugars and starches, that contain only carbon, hydrogen, and oxygen. Carbohydrates are a source of energy and fiber for animals and humans.

Carbon dioxide—A colorless, odorless gas. In the body, it is a final product in the breakdown of foods and is breathed out of the body through the lungs.

Cardiac—Relating to the heart.

Cardiac arrhythmia—*See* Arrhythmia.

Cardiac load–reducing agent—Medicine used to ease the workload of the heart by allowing the blood to flow through the blood vessels more easily.

Cardiotonic—Medicine used to improve the strength and efficiency of the heart.

Cardiovascular—Relating to the heart and blood vessels.

Caries, dental—Tooth decay, sometimes causing pain, leading to tooth damage. Also called *cavities.*

Cartilage—Type of connective tissue; it is elastic and softer than bone and makes up a part of the skeleton.

Cataract—A cloudiness in the lens of the eye that impairs vision or causes blindness.

Catheter—Tube inserted into various openings or blood vessels in the body so that fluids can be put in or taken out.

Caustic—1. Burning or corrosive. 2. Substance that is irritating and destructive to living tissue.

Cavity—1. Hollow space within the body. 2. Hole in a tooth caused by dental caries.

Cell—Basic unit that makes up the tissues of all living animals and plants. A cell usually consists of a nucleus, which contains the cell's genetic material, and various other structures outside of the nucleus that are enclosed within a cell membrane.

Central nervous system—The brain and spinal cord.

Cerebral—Relating to the brain.

Cerebral palsy—Permanent disorder of motor weakness and loss of coordination due to damage to the brain.

Cervix—Lower end or necklike opening of the uterus into the vagina.

Characterized by—Term used to describe properties that identify a particular condition (for example, measles is a disease characterized by a high fever, cough, and a blotchy rash).

Chemotherapy—Treatment of illness or disease by chemical agents. The term most commonly refers to the use of drugs to treat cancer.

Chickenpox—*See* Varicella.

Chlamydia—A family of microorganisms that cause a variety of diseases in humans. One form is commonly transmitted by sexual contact. Infection can be transmitted to a baby during the birth process.

Cholesterol—Fatlike substance made by the liver but also absorbed from the diet; found only in animal tissues. Too much blood cholesterol is associated with several potential health risks, especially atherosclerosis (hardening of the arteries) and heart disease.

Cholesterol free—In food labeling, less than 2 milligrams of cholesterol and 2 grams or less of saturated fat per serving.

Chromosome—The structure in the cell nucleus that contains the DNA and carries the genes. Most human cells normally contain 46 chromosomes.

Chronic—Describes a condition of long duration, which is often of gradual onset and may involve very slow changes.

Cirrhosis—Chronic liver disease marked by destruction of its cells and abnormal tissue growth, resulting in abnormal function.

Clitoris—Small, erectile organ that is part of the female external sex organs.

Clotting factor—Any of a group of substances in blood plasma that are involved in the process of blood clotting.

CNS—*See* Central nervous system.

Coagulation, blood (blood clotting)—Process that changes blood from a liquid to a solid, forming a clot.

Cold sores—*See* Herpes simplex.

Colic—Waves of sudden, severe abdominal pain, which are usually separated by relatively pain-free intervals. Often occurs in infants, causing crying and irritability.

Colitis—Inflammation of the colon (large bowel).

Collagen—A tough, strong protein found mostly in bone, skin, tendons, and ligaments.

Colon—Large intestine (bowel), from the end of the ileum to the rectum.

Colony stimulating factor—Protein that stimulates the production of one or more kinds of cells made in the bone marrow.

Colostomy—Operation in which part of the colon (large bowel) is brought through the abdominal wall to create an artificial opening (stoma). The contents of the intestine are passed out of the body through the opening.

Coma—Sleeplike state from which a person cannot be aroused.

Coma, hepatic—Disturbances in alertness and mental function caused by severe liver disease.

Compliance—The extent to which a patient follows medical advice.

Component—Any ingredient that helps make up a substance.

Compound—Substance made up of two or more units, elements, ingredients, or parts.

Condom, male—Thin sheath or cover, made of latex (rubber) or animal intestine, that is worn over the penis during sexual intercourse to prevent pregnancy. Condoms made of latex (rubber) are also used to prevent infection.

Congestion—Abnormal accumulation of fluid, especially of blood, within an organ or part of the body.

Congestive heart failure—Condition of inadequate blood flow caused by the inability of the heart to pump strongly enough; characterized by breathlessness and edema.

Conjugated estrogens—A mixture of naturally occurring estrogens (female hormones) that have been processed and made into a medicine.

Conjunctiva—Delicate mucous membrane covering the front of the eye and the inside of the eyelid.

Conjunctivitis—Inflammation of the conjunctiva.

Connective tissue—Material of the body that joins and supports other tissue and body parts; includes skin, bone, and tendons.

Constipation—A condition in which hard bowel movements are passed infrequently and/or with difficulty.

Constriction—Squeezing together and becoming narrower or smaller, such as constriction of blood vessels or eye pupils.

Contagious disease—Most often refers to disease that can be transmitted from one person to another. May also refer to disease that can be transmitted from an animal to a person.

Contamination—The introduction of germs or unclean material into or on normally sterile substances or objects.

Contraceptive—Medicine or device used to prevent pregnancy.

Contraction—A shortening or tightening, as in the normal function of muscles.

Convulsion—*See* Seizure.

Corrosive—Causing slow wearing away by a destructive agent.

Corticosteroids—Group of cortisone-like hormones that are secreted by the adrenal cortex and are critical to the body. The two major groups of corticosteroids are glucocorticoids, which affect fat and body metabolism, and mineralocorticoids, which regulate salt/water balance. Also called *adrenocorticoids*.

Cortisol—Natural cortisone-like hormone produced by the adrenal cortex, important for carbohydrate, protein, and fat metabolism and for the normal response to stress; synthetic cortisol (hydrocortisone) is used to treat inflammations, allergies, collagen diseases, rheumatic disorders, and adrenal failure.

Cot death—*See* Sudden infant death syndrome (SIDS).

Cowpox—*See* Vaccinia.

Creutzfeldt-Jakob disease—Rare disease, probably caused by a slow-acting virus that affects the brain and nervous system.

Crib death—*See* Sudden infant death syndrome (SIDS).

Criteria—Standards on which a judgment or decision is based.

Crohn's disease—A chronic inflammatory disease of the digestive tract, usually the lower portion of the small intestine (the ileum) or the large intestine.

Croup—Inflammation and blockage of the larynx (voice box) and air passages in young children. Symptoms of croup include harsh, difficult breathing and a barking cough.

Crystalluria—Crystals in the urine.

Cushing's syndrome—Condition caused by too much cortisone-like hormone, leading to weight gain, round face, osteoporosis (thinning of bones), diabetes mellitus (sugar diabetes), and high blood pressure.

Cycloplegia—Paralysis of certain eye muscles; can be caused by medication for certain eye tests.

Cycloplegic—Medicine used to induce cycloplegia.

Cyst—Abnormal sac or closed cavity filled with liquid or semisolid matter.

Cystic—Marked by cysts.

Cystic fibrosis—Hereditary disease of children and young adults which mainly affects the lungs. Exocrine glands do not function normally, and excess mucus is produced.

Cystine—An amino acid found in most proteins; it is released by the breakdown of the protein.

Cystitis, interstitial—Inflammation of the bladder that occurs mainly in women and is associated with pain, frequent urge to urinate, and burning urination.

Cytomegalovirus—One of a group of viruses. One form may be transmitted sexually or by infected blood and can cause death in patients with weakened immune systems.

Cytoplasm—The contents of a cell outside the nucleus.

Cytotoxic agent—Chemical that kills cells or stops cell division; used to treat cancer.

Daily Value (DV)—Value used on food and dietary supplement labels to indicate the percent of the recommended daily amount of each nutrient that a serving provides. DV takes the place of USRDA (United States Recommended Daily Allowance).

Dandruff—Scalp condition marked by the shedding of thin, dry flakes of dead skin.

Decongestant, nasal—Medicine used to help relieve nasal congestion (stuffy nose).

Decongestant, ophthalmic—Medicine used in the eye to relieve redness, burning, itching, or other eye irritation.

Decubitus ulcer—Bedsore; damage to the skin and underlying tissues caused by constant pressure.

Dehydration—Condition that results from an excessive loss or a deficiency of body water. Vomiting, diarrhea, sweating, or inadequate water intake may lead to dehydration.

Dental—Related to the teeth and gums.

Depression, mental—Condition marked by deep sadness; associated with lack of any pleasurable interest in life. Other symptoms include disturbances in sleep, appetite, and concentration, and difficulty in performing day-to-day tasks.

Dermatitis herpetiformis—Skin disease marked by sores that develop suddenly and by intense itching.

Dermatitis, seborrheic—Type of eczema found on the scalp and face.

Dermatomyositis—Inflammatory disorder, mainly of the skin and muscle fibers.

Deterioration—Process of growing worse in quality, ability, or state.

Diabetes insipidus—Disorder in which the patient produces large amounts of dilute urine and is constantly thirsty. This condition is caused by a lack of the hormone vasopressin, and is different from diabetes mellitus (sugar diabetes). Also called *water diabetes*.

Diabetes mellitus—Disorder in which the body does not produce enough insulin or else the body tissues are unable to use the insulin present. This leads to hyperglycemia (high blood sugar). Also called *sugar diabetes*.

Diagnose—Find out the cause or nature of a disorder. This often includes physical examination, laboratory tests, or other tests.

Diagnostic procedure—A process carried out to determine the cause or nature of a condition, disease, or disorder.

Dialysis, renal—Process using mechanical or other means to remove waste materials or poisons from the blood when the kidneys are not working well.

Diarrhea—Frequent passing of abnormally soft or liquid stools.

Dietary fiber—The part of food that cannot be broken down and digested; recommended as part of a balanced diet. Also called *bulk* or *roughage*.

Dietary supplement—Nutrient eaten or taken into the body in addition to the usual food.

Digestant—Agent that helps digestion.

Dilatation—Condition of being stretched or expanded beyond normal dimensions.

Diplopia—Awareness of two images of a single object at one time; double vision.

Discharge—1. Material that is released and flows away from an organ or body part. 2. Release of electrical energy by a nerve cell.

Disintegration—The process of breaking down into small pieces. In relation to medicines, a measure of how fast a tablet or capsule breaks into small pieces in stomach fluids.

Disorder—Abnormal physical or mental state.

Dissolution—1. The breaking down of a substance into its separate parts. 2. The act of being dissolved (completely merged with a liquid). In relation to medicines, a measure of how fast the contents of a tablet or capsule dissolve in body fluids.

Diuretic—Medicine used to increase the amount of urine produced by helping the kidneys get rid of water and salt.

Diverticulitis—Inflammation of a diverticulum (sac or pouch) in the intestinal tract.

Diverticulum—Sac or pouch formed at a weak place in the mucous membrane lining the wall of a canal or cavity, such as the intestine or bladder.

DNA—Deoxyribonucleic acid; the genetic material that controls heredity. DNA is found chiefly in the cell nucleus.

Down syndrome—Disorder associated with the presence of an extra chromosome 21. People with Down syndrome are mentally retarded and are marked physically by a round head, flat nose, slightly slanted eyes, and short stature. Formerly called *mongolism*.

Drug interaction—The action of one drug upon another when taken close together; depending on the drugs and the patient's medical condition, may be harmful to the patient.

Duct—Tube or channel, especially one that serves to carry secretions from a gland.

Dumdum fever—*See* Leishmaniasis, visceral.

Duodenal ulcer—Open sore in that part of the small intestine closest to the stomach.

Duodenum—First of the three parts of the small intestine.

Dyskinesia—Refers to abnormal, involuntary movement or having difficulty in performing voluntary movement.

Dysmenorrhea—Painful menstruation.

Dyspnea—Shortness of breath; difficult breathing.

Eczema—Inflammation of the skin, marked by itching, a red rash, and oozing sores that become crusted and scaly.

Edema—Swelling of body tissue due to accumulation of excess fluids.

Eighth-cranial-nerve disease—Disease of the eighth cranial nerve, which serves the inner ear; results in dizziness, loss of balance, impaired hearing, nausea, or vomiting.

Electrolyte—In medical use, chemicals (ions), such as bicarbonate, chloride, sodium, and potassium, in body fluids and tissues. Healthy functioning of the body depends on correct amounts and balances of electrolytes.

Element—In chemistry, a simple substance that cannot be broken down into simpler substances by chemical means; made up of atoms of only one kind.

Elimination—The act of expelling waste products (urine, feces) and other substances from the body.

Embolism—Sudden blocking of a blood vessel by a blood clot or other substances carried by the blood.

Embryo—In humans, a developing fertilized egg within the uterus (womb) from about two to eight weeks after fertilization.

Emergency—Extremely serious unexpected or sudden happening or situation that calls for immediate action.

Emetic—Substance that causes vomiting; used in some cases of drug overdose and poisonings.

Emollient—Substance that soothes and softens, such as an emollient lotion.

Emphysema—Lung condition in which the air spaces are enlarged and damaged, causing poor exchange of oxygen and carbon dioxide during the process of breathing in and out.

Encephalitis—Inflammation of the brain.

Encephalopathy—Any degenerative disease of the brain; caused by many different medical conditions.

Endemic—Refers to a disease that is normally present in a specific human community or geographic location.

Endocarditis—Inflammation of the lining of the heart; may lead to fever, heart murmurs, and heart failure.

Endocrine gland—A gland that has no duct, but releases its secretion directly into the blood or lymph.

Endometriosis—Condition in which material similar to the lining of the uterus (womb) appears at other sites, usually within the pelvic cavity, causing pain or bleeding.

Endoscope—An instrument inserted through an opening into the body, such as the mouth or anus, so that the doctor can see the inside of a body structure, such as the esophagus, stomach, or intestine.

Enema—Solution introduced into the rectum and colon to help empty the bowel, give nutrients or medicine, or help x-ray the lower intestines.

Enteric coating—Special coating on tablets or on the contents of capsules that allows them to pass through the stomach unchanged. The tablets or capsule contents are broken up in the intestine and absorbed.

Enteritis—Inflammation of the small intestine, usually causing diarrhea.

Enuresis—Urinating while asleep (bedwetting).

Enzyme—One type of protein produced by cells. Enzymes usually bring about or speed up normal chemical body reactions.

Eosinophil—One type of white blood cell; plays a role in allergic reactions and in fighting parasite infections.

Eosinophilia—Condition in which the number of eosinophils in the blood is abnormally high.

Epidemic—Refers to a disease that is present in a community only occasionally, but affects a large number of people when it is present.

Epidural space—Area in the spinal column into which medicines (usually for pain or local anesthesia) can be administered.

Epilepsy—Any of a group of brain disorders marked by sudden seizures or other symptoms that are brought on by abnormal electrical brain activity.

Epinephrine—Hormone produced by the adrenal gland. It stimulates the heart, constricts blood vessels, and relaxes some smooth muscles. Also called *adrenaline*.

EPO—*See* Erythropoietin.

Ergot alkaloids—A class of medicines that cause narrowing of blood vessels; some are used to treat migraine headaches, and others are used to reduce bleeding in childbirth.

Erythrocyte—Red blood cell. Erythrocytes contain hemoglobin and transport oxygen.

Erythropoietin—Hormone, secreted by the kidney, that controls the production of red blood cells by the bone marrow; also available as a synthetic drug (EPO). It is used to treat anemia in some patients with cancer, HIV, or kidney disease.

Esophagus—The part of the digestive tract that connects the pharynx (throat) to the stomach.

Estrogen—Principal female sex hormone necessary for the normal sexual development of the female. During the menstrual cycle, its actions help prepare for possible pregnancy.

Excessive—Describes an amount or degree that is more than what is proper, usual, or normal.

Excrete—To throw off or eliminate waste material from the body, blood, or organs.

Exocrine gland—Any gland that discharges its secretion through a duct directly onto or into a body part, but not into the blood.

Exophthalmic goiter—*See* Graves' disease.

Exophthalmos—Thrusting forward of the eyeballs in their sockets giving the appearance of the eyes sticking out too far; commonly associated with hyperthyroidism.

Expectorant—Medicine used to help the patient cough up and expel mucus from the air passages.

Expel—To force out.

Extrapyramidal symptoms—Movement disorders occurring with certain diseases or with use of certain drugs, including trembling and shaking of hands and fingers, twisting movements of the body, shuffling walk, and stiffness of arms or legs.

Facial—Relating to the face.

Factor—Substance that is necessary to produce a result in a specific process of the body.

Familial Mediterranean fever—Inherited condition involving inflammation of the lining of the chest, abdomen, and joints. Also called *recurrent polyserositis.*

Fasciculation—Small, repeated contraction of a few muscle fibers, which is visible through the skin; muscular twitching.

Fat—An energy-rich organic compound that occurs naturally in animals and plants. Fats are an essential nutrient for humans.

Fat free—In food labeling, less than 0.5 grams of fat per serving.

Fatty acid—One of the basic organic compounds that make up lipids.

Favism—Inherited condition resulting from sensitivity to broad (fava) beans; marked by fever, vomiting, diarrhea, and acute destruction of red blood cells.

Feces—Waste material remaining after food has been digested, which is passed out of the intestine through the anus. Also called *stool.*

Fertility—Ability to bring about the start of pregnancy or produce offspring.

Fertilization—Union of an ovum with a sperm.

Fetal—Relating to the fetus.

Fetus—In humans, a developing baby within the uterus (womb) from about the beginning of the third month of pregnancy.

Fewer calories—In food labeling, at least 25 percent fewer calories per serving than the reference food.

Fiber—1. In nutrition, the carbohydrate material of food that cannot be digested. Fiber adds bulk to the diet. 2. In medicine, a thin, threadlike structure that combines with others to form certain tissues, for example, muscles and nerves.

Fibrocystic—Describes a benign (noncancerous) tumor that consists of a cyst surrounded by fibrous tissue.

Fibroid tumor—A noncancerous tumor of the uterus formed of fibrous or fully developed connective tissue.

Fibrosis—Scarring and thickening of connective tissue causing it to tighten and become less flexible.

Fibrous—Made up of fibers or containing fibers.

Fistula—Abnormal tubelike passage connecting two internal organs or one that leads from an abscess or internal organ to the body surface.

Flatulence—Excessive amount of gas in the stomach or intestine.

Flu—*See* Influenza.

Flushing—Temporary redness of the face and/or neck.

Folic acid—A vitamin of the B complex. Lack of folic acid may lead to anemia.

Follicle—A sac or pouchlike cavity. For example, a hair follicle is a small cavity from which a hair grows.

Food Guide Pyramid—An eating plan developed by Health and Human Services and the Department of Agriculture that describes the basic food groups. It serves as a guide for having a proper diet.

Fungus—Any of a group of simple organisms, including molds and yeasts.

Fungus infection—Infection caused by a fungus. Some common fungus infections are tinea pedis (athlete's foot), tinea capitis (ringworm of the scalp), tinea cruris (ringworm of the groin or jock itch), and mouth or vaginal candidiasis (yeast infections).

Gait—Manner of walk.

Gallbladder—An organ that stores bile. It is attached to the liver.

Gamma globulin—A group of proteins in the blood that act as antibodies in fighting infection.

Gastric—Relating to the stomach.

Gastric acid secretion inhibitor—Medicine used to decrease the amount of acid produced by the stomach.

Gastritis—Inflammation of the stomach, especially of the stomach lining.

Gastroenteritis—Inflammation of the stomach and intestine.

Gastroesophageal reflux—Backward flow of stomach contents into the esophagus. The condition is often characterized by "heartburn."

Gene—A part of a DNA molecule that acts as a basic unit of genetic information, located on a chromosome. Genes transmit the traits that a parent passes on to its offspring.

Generic—General in nature; relating to an entire group or class. In relation to medicines, generic refers to a medicine's chemical name, which is not protected by a trademark and can therefore be used by all manufacturers or providers of the medicine.

Genetics—The study of genes and their passing on of a quality or trait from parent to offspring.

Genital—1. Relating to the organs concerned with reproduction; the sexual organs. 2. Relating to reproduction.

Genital warts—Small growths found on the genitals or around the anus; caused by a virus. The disease may be transmitted by sexual contact.

Geriatric—Relating to the care of elderly people and the treatment of disorders that commonly affect them.

Gilles de la Tourette syndrome—See Tourette's disorder.

Gingiva—Tissue that surrounds the teeth, or the gums.

Gingival hyperplasia—Excessive growth of the gums.

Gingivitis—Inflammation of the gums.

Gland—Group of cells or an organ specialized to produce one or more secretions.

Glandular fever—See Mononucleosis.

Glaucoma—Condition of abnormally high pressure in the eye; may lead to loss of vision if not treated.

Glomeruli—Clusters of capillaries (tiny blood vessels) in the kidney that act as filters of the blood.

Glomerulonephritis—Inflammation of the glomeruli of the kidney; not directly caused by infection.

Glucose—A simple sugar. In living organisms, it is formed by the breakdown of carbohydrates and is the chief source of energy.

Glucose-6-phosphate dehydrogenase (G6PD) deficiency—Lack of or reduced amounts of an enzyme (glucose-6-phosphate dehydrogenase) that helps the breakdown of certain sugar compounds in the body. People with this condition may be more likely to develop a form of anemia.

Gluten—Type of protein found primarily in wheat and rye.

Goiter—Enlargement of the thyroid gland that causes the neck to swell; usually results from a lack of iodine in the diet or overactivity of the thyroid gland.

Gonadotropin—Any hormone that stimulates the activities of the ovaries or testes.

Gonorrhea—An infectious disease, usually transmitted by sexual contact. It causes infection in the genital organs in both men and women, and may result in disease in other parts of the body.

Good source of fiber—In food labeling, 2.5 grams to 4.9 grams of fiber per serving.

Gout—Disorder caused by uric acid in the joints and kidneys, leading to painful inflammation of the joints and kidney stones.

Granulation—Small, fleshy outgrowths on the healing surface of a wound or ulcer; a normal stage in healing.

Granulocyte—One type of white blood cell.

Granulocytopenia—See Agranulocytosis.

Granuloma—A granular growth or mass produced in response to chronic infection, inflammation, a foreign body, or to unknown causes.

Graves' disease—Enlargement of the thyroid gland (goiter) and overproduction of thyroid hormones, causing fast heart beat, bulging eyes, tremor, sweating, and weight loss. Also called *exophthalmic goiter*.

Groin—The area where the abdomen meets the thigh.

Growth factor—Substance, usually a vitamin, hormone, or mineral, that promotes the process of growing.

Guillain-Barré syndrome—Nerve disease marked by sudden numbness and weakness in the limbs that may progress to paralysis; recovery usually follows.

Gynecomastia—Excessive development of the breast tissue in the male.

Haemophilus—Closely related group of bacteria. Some varieties are found normally in the upper respiratory tract (the nose and throat) but may sometimes cause infections, including infections of the respiratory tract, eyes, and the tissues covering the brain and spinal cord. Also *Hemophilus*.

Hair follicle—Sheath of tissue surrounding a hair root.

Hansen's disease—*See* Leprosy.

Hartnup disease—Hereditary defect in protein metabolism that leads to mental retardation, rough skin, and poor control of muscle movement.

Healthy—1. Food labeling term that may be used if the food is low in fat and saturated fat and a serving does not contain more than 480 milligrams of sodium or more than 95 milligrams of cholesterol. The food must also contain at least 10% of the daily value (DV) per serving of vitamin A, vitamin C, calcium, iron, protein, and fiber. 2. Being in a state of physical, mental, and social wellness.

Heart attack—*See* Myocardial infarction.

Heartburn—Warmth or burning felt behind the breastbone. Heartburn is usually caused by stomach contents rising toward the mouth.

Helicobacter pylori—Organism that has been associated with gastritis and certain ulcers.

Hematologic—Relating to the blood.

Hematuria—Presence of blood or red blood cells in the urine.

Heme—A blood pigment containing iron; a component of hemoglobin.

Hemoglobin—Iron-containing substance found in red blood cells that transports oxygen from the lungs to the tissues of the body.

Hemolytic anemia—Type of anemia resulting from breakdown of red blood cells.

Hemophilia—Hereditary disease marked by delayed blood clotting, leading to uncontrolled bleeding even after minor injuries. Generally, only males have the disease.

Hemorrhoids—Enlarged veins in the walls of the anus. Also called *piles*.

Hepatic—Relating to the liver.

Hepatitis—Inflammation of the liver; may be caused by virus infection.

Hereditary—Genetically passed on from parent to offspring.

Hernia, hiatal—Condition in which the stomach passes partly into the chest cavity through the opening for the esophagus in the diaphragm.

Herpes simplex—The virus that causes genital herpes infections and "cold sores," both of which are marked by the appearance of painful blisters that can be transmitted from one person to another. In genital herpes, the blisters appear on the genitals (sex organs) and are often transmitted by sexual contact. "Cold sores" may appear on the lips, in or around the mouth, or around the nose.

Herpes zoster—The virus that causes chickenpox and shingles. Shingles is an infectious disease usually marked by pain and blisters along one nerve, often on the face, chest, stomach, or back.

Heterosexual—One who is sexually attracted to persons of the opposite sex.

High blood pressure—*See* Hypertension.

High fiber—In food labeling, 5 grams or more of fiber per serving. (Foods making high-fiber claims must meet the definition for low fat, or the level of total fat must appear next to the high-fiber claim.)

Hirsutism—Excessive hair growth or the growth of hair in unusual places, especially in women.

Histamine—Chemical, found in all body tissues, that dilates capillaries (small blood vessels), contracts smooth muscle, and stimulates gastric (stomach) secretions. Histamine is released during allergic reactions, producing swelling and inflammation.

HIV (human immunodeficiency virus)—Virus that causes AIDS.

Hives—*See* Urticaria.

Hoarseness—Gruff, husky, quality of the voice.

Hodgkin's disease—Malignant condition marked by swelling of the lymph nodes, with weight loss and fever.

Homosexual—One who is sexually attracted to persons of the same sex.

Hormone—A chemical substance, produced in the body, that controls or regulates the activity of specific organs or cells. The term hormone may also refer to manufactured substances that act like a hormone.

Hot flashes—Sensations of heat of the face, neck, and upper body, often accompanied by sweating and flushing; commonly associated with menopause.

Hydrocortisone—*See* Cortisol.

Hyperactivity—Abnormally increased activity and shortened attention span.

Hypercalcemia—Abnormally high amount of calcium in the blood.

Hypercalciuria—Abnormally high amount of calcium in the urine.

Hypercholesterolemia—Excessive amount of cholesterol in the blood.

Hyperglycemia—Abnormally high amount of glucose in the blood.

Hyperkalemia—Abnormally high amount of potassium in the blood.

Hyperkeratosis—Overgrowth or thickening of the outer layer of the skin.

Hyperlipidemia—General term for an abnormally high level of lipids (fats or fatlike substances) in the blood.

Hyperphosphatemia—Abnormally high amount of phosphate in the blood.

Hypersensitivity—An excessive response by the body to a foreign substance.

Hypertension—Blood pressure in the arteries (blood vessels) that is higher than normal for the patient's age group. Hypertension may lead to a number of serious health problems. Also called *high blood pressure*.

Hyperthermia—Abnormally high body temperature; fever.

Hyperthyroidism—Condition in which there is too much thyroid hormone in the body, leading to fast heart beat, trembling, sweating, bulging of the eyes, and weight loss.

Hypertrophy—Increase in bulk or size of a body part, brought about by excessive development rather than an increase in the number of cells.

Hypocalcemia—Abnormally low amount of calcium in the blood.

Hypoglycemia—Abnormally low amount of glucose in the blood.

Hypokalemia—Abnormally low amount of potassium in the blood.

Hypotension, orthostatic—Excessive fall in blood pressure that occurs when standing or upon standing up.

Hypothalamus—Area of the brain that controls many body functions, including body temperature, certain metabolic and endocrine processes, and some activities of the nervous system.

Hypothermia—Abnormally low body temperature.

Hypothyroidism—Condition caused by thyroid hormone deficiency, which results in a decrease in metabolism.

Hypoxia—Broad term meaning that not enough oxygen is being supplied to, or used by, body tissues.

Ileostomy—Operation in which the ileum is brought through the abdominal wall to create an artificial opening (stoma). The contents of the intestine are discharged through the opening.

Ileum—Last of the three portions of the small intestine, farthest from the mouth.

Immune—Having protection against infectious disease.

Immune deficiency condition—Lack of immune response to protect against infectious disease.

Immune system—Complex network of the body that defends against foreign substances or organisms that may harm the body.

Immunity—The body's ability to resist infection.

Immunizing agent, active—Agent that causes the body to pro duce its own antibodies for protection against certain infections or substances.

Immunocompromised—Decreased natural immunity caused by certain medicines, diseases, genetic disorders, or use of immunosuppressants.

Immunoglobulin—*See* Antibody.

Immunosuppressant—Medicine that reduces the body's natural immunity.

Impair—To decrease, weaken, or damage ability or function, usually because of injury or disease.

Impairment—Decrease in strength or ability, often because of illness or injury (for example, hearing impairment).

Impetigo—Contagious bacterial skin infection most common in babies and children. The infection starts as a red patch, which develops into blisters that break and form a thick crust.

Implant—1. Special form of medicine, often a small pellet or rod, that is inserted into the body or beneath the skin so that the medicine will be released continuously over a period of time. 2. To insert or graft material or an object into a body site. 3. Material or an object inserted into a body site, such as a lens implant or a breast implant. 4. Action of a fertilized ovum becoming attached or embedded in the uterus.

Impotence—Difficulty or inability of a male to have or maintain an erection of the penis.

Incontinence—Inability to control natural passage of urine or of bowel movements.

Induce—To cause or bring about.

Infection—Invasion and multiplication of a disease-causing microorganism in body tissue.

Infertility—Refers to the inability of a woman to become pregnant or of a man to cause pregnancy.

Inflammation—Pain, redness, swelling, and heat in a part of the body, usually in response to injury or illness.

Inflammatory bowel disease—Irritation of the intestinal tract; usually refers to a chronic condition, such as Crohn's disease or ulcerative colitis.

Influenza—Highly contagious respiratory virus infection, marked by coughing, headache, chills, fever, muscle pain, and general weakness. Also called *flu.*

Ingredient—One of the parts or substances that make up a mixture or compound.

Inhalation—1. Act of drawing in the breath or drawing air into the lungs. 2. Medicine that is breathed (inhaled) into the lungs. Some inhalations work locally in the lungs, while others produce their effects elsewhere in the body. Also called *inhalant.*

Inhalator—Device used to help the patient breathe in air, anesthetics, or other gases, or medicinal mists or vapors. Also called *inhaler.*

Inhibitor—Substance that prevents or slows a process or reaction.

Inner ear—The liquid-filled system of cavities and ducts deep inside the ear that make up the organs of hearing and balance.

Inorganic—Being made up of matter that is not living and has never lived.

Insomnia—Inability to sleep or remain asleep.

Insulin—Hormone that controls the way the body uses and stores sugar (glucose). Injections of insulin are used to treat diabetes mellitus (sugar diabetes) that cannot be controlled by diet, exercise, or other medicines.

Interferon—Substance produced by cells that stops the growth and the spread of viruses; may also have effects on cells fighting cancer.

Intestine—The part of the digestive tract that extends from the stomach to the anus.

Intra-amniotic—Within the sac that contains the fetus and amniotic fluid (fluid surrounding the fetus).

Intra-arterial—Within an artery.

Intracavernosal—Into the corpus cavernosa (cavities in the penis that, when filled with blood, produce an erection).

Intracavitary—Into a body cavity (for example, the chest cavity or bladder).

Intramuscular—Into a muscle.

Intrauterine device (IUD)—Small plastic or metal device placed in the uterus (womb) to prevent pregnancy.

Intravenous—Into a vein.

Involuntary—Not under conscious control (for example, digestion of food is an involuntary action).

Ion—Atom or group of atoms carrying an electric charge.

Irrigation—Washing of a body cavity or wound with a stream of sterile water or a solution of a medicine.

Ischemia—Condition caused by inadequate blood flow to a part of the body; usually caused by constriction or blocking of blood vessels that supply the part of the body affected.

Jaundice—Yellowing of the eyes and skin due to the presence of bilirubin, a substance that may be released into the blood and tissues of patients with certain medical problems, such as hepatitis (inflammation of the liver, often caused by a virus infection).

Jock itch—Ringworm of the groin or the area around the scrotum.

Kala-azar—*See* Leishmaniasis, visceral.

Kaposi's sarcoma—Malignant (cancerous) tumor that usually first appears as purple or brown patches on the skin of the feet. The tumors slowly grow in number and size, spreading toward the upper part of the body. One severe form occurs in immunocompromised patients, including transplant recipients and AIDS patients.

Keratin—Tough protein substance found in hair, nails, and the outer layer of the skin.

Keratolytic—Medicine used to soften thickened or hardened areas of the skin, such as warts.

Ketoacidosis—A condition in which acidosis and large amounts of ketones are present in the body tissues and fluids. This condition occurs when the body burns fat, instead of carbohydrates, for energy. It is especially likely to occur in patients with poorly controlled diabetes mellitus (sugar diabetes).

Kidney—Organ that removes waste products from the blood and excretes them in the form of urine. Also, controls the amounts of several ions, such as hydrogen, sodium, potassium, and phosphate, in body fluids.

Lactation—Secretion of breast milk.

Lactose—A sugar found in milk.

Larva—The immature form of life of some insects and other animal groups that hatch from eggs.

Larynx—Organ that serves as a passage for air from the pharynx (throat) to the lungs; it contains the vocal cords.

Laxative—Natural or synthetic substances used to stimulate passage of bowel movements.

Laxative, bulk-forming—Laxative that acts by absorbing liquid and swelling to form a soft, bulky stool. The bowel is then stimulated normally by the presence of the bulky mass.

Laxative, hyperosmotic—Laxative that acts by drawing water into the bowel from surrounding body tissues. This provides a soft stool mass and increased bowel action.

Laxative, lubricant—Laxative that acts by coating the bowel and the stool mass with a waterproof film. This keeps moisture in the stool. The stool remains soft and its passage is made easier.

Laxative, stimulant—Laxative that acts directly on the intestinal wall. The direct stimulation increases the muscle contractions that move the stool mass along. Also called *contact laxative.*

Laxative, stool softener—Laxative that acts by helping liquids mix into the stool and prevent dry, hard stool masses. The stool remains soft and its passage is made easier. Also called *emollient laxative.*

Lean—Food labeling term for seafood or game meat, meals, and main dishes. May be used if a serving contains less than 10 grams of total fat, 4.5 grams or less of saturated fat, and less than 95 milligrams of cholesterol. Seafood and game meat must meet these criteria per 100 grams of food. Meals and main dishes must meet these criteria per 100 grams of food and per labeled serving.

Legionnaires' disease—A severe bacterial infection in the lungs, which causes a high fever and pneumonia. It sometimes also affects other parts of the body.

Leishmaniasis, visceral—Tropical disease, transmitted by sandfly bites, which causes liver and spleen enlargement, anemia, weight loss, and fever. Also called *black fever, Dumdum fever,* or *kala-azar.*

Lennox-Gastaut syndrome—Type of childhood epilepsy.

Leprosy—Chronic infectious disease marked by skin lesions. It is slowly progressive and leads to loss of feeling, tissue destruction, and deformity. Also called *Hansen's disease.*

Lesion—A defined area of diseased or injured tissue.

Less cholesterol—In food labeling, at least 25 percent less cholesterol and 2 grams or less of saturated fat per serving than the reference food.

Less fat—In food labeling, at least 25 percent less fat per serving than the reference food.

Less saturated fat—In food labeling, at least 25 percent less saturated fat per serving than the reference food.

Less sodium—In food labeling, at least 25 percent less sodium per serving than the reference food.

Less sugar—In food labeling, at least 25 percent less sugar per serving than the reference food.

Leukemia—Malignant disease of the blood and bone marrow in which too many white blood cells are produced; results in anemia, bleeding, and low resistance to infections.

Leukocyte—White blood cell. Leukocytes help protect the body against foreign substances and are active in antibody production.

Leukoderma—*See* Vitiligo.

Leukopenia—Abnormally low number of leukocytes in the blood.

Ligament—Tough, fibrous tissue that connects one bone to an other or supports organs.

Lipid—Term applied generally to fat or fatlike substances not soluble in water.

Local effect—Affecting a limited area at or near the place to which the medicine is applied, rather than the whole body (for example, local anesthetics causing numbness only around the place of injection).

Long-acting—Refers to a medicine that is made up in a special way so that it is slowly released in the body; the medicine's effect lasts longer than usual.

Low calorie—In food labeling, 40 calories or less per serving. However, for small servings (30 grams or less or 2 tablespoons or less), low calorie is 40 calories or less per 50 grams of the food.

Low cholesterol—In food labeling, 20 milligrams or less of cholesterol and 2 grams or less of saturated fat per serving. However, for small servings (30 grams or less or 2 tablespoons or less), low cholesterol is 20 milligrams or less of cholesterol per 50 grams of the food and 2 grams or less of saturated fat per serving.

Low fat—In food labeling, 3 grams or less of fat per serving. However, for small servings (30 grams or less or 2 tablespoons or less), low fat is 3 grams or less of fat per 50 grams of the food.

Low saturated fat—One gram or less of fat per serving and not more than 15 percent of calories from saturated fatty acids.

Low sodium—In food labeling, 140 milligrams or less of sodium per serving. However, for small servings (30 grams or less or 2 tablespoons or less), low sodium is 140 milligrams or less of sodium per 50 grams of the food.

Lozenge—A dry, medicated tablet or disk to be placed in the mouth and allowed to dissolve slowly. Also called *troche*.

Lugol's solution—Deep brown liquid containing iodine and potassium iodide.

Lupus—*See* Lupus erythematosus, systemic.

Lupus erythematosus, systemic—Chronic inflammatory disease most often affecting the skin, joints, and various internal organs. Also called *lupus* or *SLE* (systemic lupus erythematosus).

Lyme disease—Acute disease transmitted by the bite of certain ticks. The disease is marked by a slowly spreading rash, and fever, headache, and flu-like symptoms. Left untreated, the disease may later cause heart or nerve disorders, arthritis, or joint pain.

Lymph—Fluid that bathes the tissues. It is formed in tissue spaces in all parts of the body and circulated by the lymphatic system.

Lymphatic system—Network of vessels that conveys lymph from the spaces between the cells of the body back to the bloodstream.

Lymph node—A small rounded body found at intervals along the lymphatic system. The nodes act as filters for the lymph by keeping bacteria and other foreign particles from entering the bloodstream. They also produce lymphocytes.

Lymphocyte—A type of white blood cell found in the blood, lymph, and lymphatic tissues. They are involved in immunity.

Lymphoma—Malignant tumors that arise in lymph nodes or the tissue where lymphocytes are formed.

Lyse—To cause breakdown. In cells, damage or rupture of the membrane results in destruction of the cell.

Macrobiotic—Vegetarian diet consisting mostly of whole grains.

Malaise—General feeling of discomfort, uneasiness, and being unwell.

Malaria—Tropical blood infection caused by protozoa (tiny, one-celled animals); symptoms include chills, fever, sweats, headaches, and anemia. Malaria is spread to humans by the bite of an infected mosquito.

Malignant—Refers to a condition, usually a cancer, that can become life-threatening if untreated.

Malnutrition—Condition caused by a diet that is not balanced or one that does not provide the right amount of food for maintaining good health.

Mammogram—X-ray picture of the breast.

Mania—Mental state in which fast talking and excited feelings or actions are out of control.

Mast cells—Cells that release histamine and other chemicals that cause inflammation and signs of allergic reactions.

Mastocytosis—Accumulation of too many mast cells in tissues.

Mediate—To bring about or accomplish.

Medicinal—Refers to a substance that has the ability to cure, heal, or relieve.

Megavitamin therapy—Taking very large doses of vitamins to prevent or treat certain medical problems.

Melanoma—Highly malignant (cancerous) tumor, usually occurring on the skin.

Meniere's disease—Disease affecting the inner ear that is characterized by ringing in the ears, nausea, dizziness, and progessive hearing loss.

Meningitis—Inflammation of the tissues that cover the brain and spinal cord; often caused by an infection.

Menopause—The time in a woman's life when the ovaries no longer produce an egg cell at regular times and menstruation stops.

Menstruation—Monthly flow of blood and small pieces of tissue from the uterus through the vagina. Normally, menstruation occurs from puberty to menopause, except during pregnancy.

Metabolism—Sum of all physical and chemical processes that occur in cells to maintain growth and function, including building-up processes, breaking-down processes, and energy changes.

Methemoglobin—Substance formed when hemoglobin has been chemically changed; in this form, hemoglobin cannot act as an oxygen carrier.

Methemoglobinemia—Presence of excessive amounts of methemoglobin in the blood.

Microorganism—Any organism too small to be seen by the naked eye.

Middle ear—Chamber of the ear lying behind the eardrum; contains the three bones that transmit sound waves.

Migraine—Throbbing headache, usually affecting one side of the head; often accompanied by nausea, vomiting, and sensitivity to light.

Mineral—One of many elements needed in small amounts for many body functions, including blood clotting, muscle movement, and fluid balance.

Miotic—Medicine used in the eye that causes the pupil to constrict (become smaller).

Mongolism—*See* Down syndrome.

Mono—*See* Mononucleosis.

Monoclonal—Derived from a single cell; related to production of certain drugs by genetic engineering, such as monoclonal antibodies.

Mononucleosis—Infectious viral disease occurring mostly in adolescents and young adults, marked by fever, sore throat, swelling of the lymph nodes in the neck and armpits, and by severe fatigue. Also called *mono* or *glandular fever*.

More fiber—*See* Added fiber.

Motility—Ability to move without outside aid, force, or cause.

Motor—Relating to structures that bring about movement, such as nerves and muscles.

MRI (magnetic resonance imaging)—Technique that produces an image of internal body tissue by computer. The technique uses radio waves and a strong magnetic field, but no x-rays.

Mucolytic—Medicine that breaks down or dissolves mucus.

Mucosal—Relating to mucous membrane.

Mucous membrane—Moist layer of tissue surrounding or lining many body structures and cavities, including the mouth, lips, inside of nose, throat, digestive tract (esophagus, stomach, intestines, and anus), and vagina.

Mucus—Thick fluid produced by the mucous membranes and glands.

Multiple sclerosis (MS)—Chronic, inflammatory nerve disease marked by weakness, unsteadiness, shakiness, and speech and vision problems.

Muscular dystrophy—Hereditary disease characterized by gradual wasting of muscles and increasing disability.

Myalgia—Tenderness or pain in a muscle or muscles.

Myasthenia gravis—Chronic disease marked by abnormal weakness, and sometimes paralysis, of certain muscles.

Mydriatic—Medicine used in the eye that causes the pupil to dilate (become larger).

Myelogram—X-ray picture of the spinal cord.

Myeloma, multiple—Cancerous bone marrow disease.

Myocardial infarction—Interruption of blood supply to the heart, leading to symptoms such as tightness or feeling of heaviness in the chest and/or pain in the chest, left shoulder, jaw, or arm, and damage to the heart muscle. Also called *heart attack*.

Myocardial reinfarction prophylactic—Medicine used to help prevent additional heart attacks in patients who have already had one attack.

Myotonia congenita—Hereditary muscle disorder marked by difficulty in relaxing a muscle or releasing a grip after any strong effort.

Narcolepsy—Condition in which the patient is unable to prevent himself or herself from repeatedly falling asleep, often at inappropriate times and places.

Nasal—Relating to the nose.

Nasogastric (NG) tube—Tube that is inserted through the nose, down the throat, and into the stomach. It may be used to remove fluid or gas from the stomach or to give medicine, fluid, or nutrients to the patient.

Nausea—Uncomfortable sensation in the stomach along with an urge to vomit.

Nebulizer—Instrument that changes a liquid into a fine spray.

Necrosis—Death of tissue, cells, or a part of a structure or organ, surrounded by healthy parts.

Neonate—A newborn baby less than four weeks old.

Neoplasm—New and abnormal growth of tissue in or on a part of the body, in which the multiplication of cells is uncontrolled and progressive. Also called *tumor*.

Nephron—Unit of the kidney that contributes to formation of urine by filtering the blood, adding substances to the fluid formed, and removing substances from it.

Nerve—Bundle of fibers that carries messages, in the form of electrical impulses, between the brain or spinal cord and other parts of the body.

Neuralgia—Severe stabbing or throbbing pain along the course of one or more nerves.

Neuralgia, trigeminal—Severe burning or stabbing pain along certain nerves in the face. Also called *tic douloureux*.

Neural tube—Hollow tube in the embryo that gives rise to the brain and spinal cord.

Neural tube defects—Severe, abnormal conditions resulting when the nerve tract in the fetus fails to close fully. *See* Spina bifida.

Neuritis, optic—Disease of the nerves in the eye.

Neuritis, peripheral—Inflammation of nerves or nerve endings located at or near the surface of the body, usually associated with pain, abnormal sensations (such as a burning or prickling feeling), muscle wasting, and loss of reflexes.

Neutropenia—Abnormally small number of neutrophils (a type of white blood cell) in the blood.

Neutrophil—The most common type of granulocyte (a type of white blood cell); important in the body's protection against infection.

Nit—Egg of a louse.

No added sugar—In food labeling, no sugars added to food during processing or packing. This includes ingredients that contain sugars, for example, fruit juices, applesauce, or dried fruit.

No sugar added—*See* No added sugar.

Nodule—Small, rounded mass, lump, or swelling.

Nonsuppurative—Not discharging pus.

NSAID (nonsteroidal anti-inflammatory drug)—*See* Anti-inflammatory, nonsteroidal.

Nucleus—The part of the cell that contains the chromosomes.

Nutrient—Food substance that provides a source of energy or aids in growth and repair. Nutrients include carbohydrates, fats, proteins, minerals, and vitamins.

Nutrition—1. Study of food and drink relating to the building of sound bodies and promoting health. 2. All the body processes that are part of taking in food and using it.

Nutrition Labeling and Education Act (NLEA) of 1990—The law that required the Food and Drug Administration to develop new labeling requirements for foods and dietary supplements.

Nystagmus—Rapid, rhythmic, involuntary movements of the eyeball; may be from side to side, up and down, or around.

Obesity—Excess accumulation of fat in the body along with an increase in body weight that exceeds the healthy range for the body's frame.

Obstetrics—Field of medicine concerned with the care of women during pregnancy and childbirth.

Obstruction—Something that blocks or closes up a passage or structure.

Occlusive dressing—Dressing (such as plastic kitchen wrap) that cuts off air to the skin.

Occult—In medicine, refers to an abnormality that cannot be seen by the human eye (for example, occult blood in the stools or feces can be detected only by microscope or chemical testing).

Offspring—Children or descendants of parents.

Ooze—To slowly give out or pass off moist material.

Ophthalmic—Relating to the eye.

Opioid—1. Any synthetic narcotic with opium-like actions; not derived from opium. 2. Natural chemicals that act at the same cell sites where opium exerts its actions.

Oral—Relating to the mouth.

Orchitis—Inflammation of the testis.

Organ—A body part that performs a particular function or functions.

Organic—1. In nutrition, a term used to describe plants that have been treated with animal or vegetable fertilizers instead of chemicals. 2. Refers to matter that is part of or produced by living organisms, including animals and plants.

Organism—Any individual living thing; may consist of a single cell or may be made up of many cells.

Osteitis deformans—*See* Paget's disease of bone.

Osteomalacia—Softening of the bones due to lack of vitamin D.

Osteoporosis—A condition in which thinning of bone tissue occurs, producing bones that are easily fractured (broken). Often occurs in elderly people because of a loss of calcium from bone tissue.

OTC (over the counter)—Refers to medicine or devices available without a prescription.

Otic—Relating to the ear.

Otitis media—Inflammation of the middle ear.

Ototoxicity—Having a harmful effect on the organs or nerves of the ear concerned with hearing and balance.

Ovary—Female sex organ that produces egg cells and sex hormones.

Overactive thyroid—*See* Hyperthyroidism.

Ovulation—Process by which an ovum (egg cell) is released from the ovary. In human menstruating females, this usually occurs once a month.

Ovum—Mature female sex cell or egg cell. If fertilization of an ovum occurs, a new individual begins to develop.

Oxidize—To lose electrons or to combine with oxygen.

Paget's disease of bone—A chronic, painful bone disease in which the bones gradually become thickened, deformed (abnormal in shape), and weak. Also called *osteitis deformans*.

Palpitation—Rapid, forceful, or throbbing heart beat.

Pancreas—Large gland that secretes digestive enzymes into the intestine and hormones, including insulin, into the bloodstream.

Pancreatitis—Inflammation of the pancreas.

Pancytopenia—Reduction in the number of red cells, all types of white cells, and platelets in the blood.

Pap test—Test that helps detect cancerous or precancerous conditions or certain infections of the female genital tract (vagina, cervix, and uterus). The test, in which cells from this area are examined under a microscope, can also help determine whether the cells are working normally. Also called *Papanicolaou test*.

Paralysis agitans—*See* Parkinson's disease.

Parathyroid glands—Four small bodies situated beside the thyroid gland; secrete parathyroid hormone that regulates calcium and phosphorus metabolism.

Parenteral—Most often refers to injecting a medicine directly into a body part (for example, into a vein or a muscle).

Parkinsonism—*See* Parkinson's disease.

Parkinson's disease—Brain disease marked by tremor (shaking), stiffness, and difficulty in moving. In addition to brain disease, symptoms similar to those of Parkinson's disease may be caused by certain medications, head injury, or other causes. Also called *Parkinsonism, paralysis agitans,* or *shaking palsy.*

Patent ductus arteriosus (PDA)—Condition in babies in which an important fetal blood vessel fails to close as it should, resulting in faulty circulation and serious health problems.

Pathogen—Any microorganism that causes a disease.

Pediculicide—Medicine that kills lice.

Pediculosis—Infestation of the body, most often of the pubis (genital region) or scalp, with lice.

Pellagra—Disease caused by too little niacin, which results in scaly skin, diarrhea, and mental depression.

Pelvis—Bony structure of the skeleton that includes the hip bones and the bottom part of the backbone. It is located at the lowest part of the trunk, just above the legs.

Pemphigus—Skin disease marked by successive outbreaks of blisters.

Peptic ulcer—Open sore in the esophagus, stomach, or duodenum.

Peritoneum—Membrane lining the abdominal wall and covering the liver, stomach, spleen, gallbladder, and intestines.

Peritonitis—Inflammation of the peritoneum.

Peyronie's disease—Dense, fiber-like growth in the penis, which can be felt as an irregular hard lump, and which usually causes bending and pain when the penis is erect.

Pharynx—Space just behind the mouth that serves as a passageway for food from the mouth to the esophagus and for air from the nose and mouth to the larynx; the throat.

Phenol—Substance used as a preservative for some injectable medicines. It is also used as an antiseptic and pain reliever in some mouth and throat products (mouthwashes, throat lozenges, etc.)

Pheochromocytoma—Tumor of the adrenal medulla.

Phlebitis—Inflammation of a vein; often caused by a blood clot.

Phlegm—Thick mucus produced in the respiratory passages.

Piles—*See* Hemorrhoids.

Pituitary gland—Pea-sized body located at the base of the brain. It produces a number of hormones that are essential to normal body growth and functioning.

Placebo—Medicine that, unknown to the patient, has no active medicinal substance; its use may relieve or improve a condition because the patient believes it will. In some studies it may be used as a "control" against which the medicine being studied can be compared. Also called *sugar pill*.

Plaque, dental—Mixture of saliva, bacteria, and carbohydrates that forms on the teeth, leading to caries (cavities) and gum disease.

Platelet—Small, disk-shaped body found in the blood. Platelets play an important role in blood clotting.

Platelet aggregation inhibitor—Medicine used to help prevent the platelets in the blood from clumping together. This effect reduces the chance of heart attack or stroke in certain patients.

Pledget—Small mass of gauze or cotton used to apply or absorb fluids, cover a wound, or act as a plug to keep out air.

Pleura—Membrane covering the lungs and lining the chest cavity.

PMS—*See* Premenstrual syndrome.

Pneumococcal—Relating to certain bacteria that cause pneumonia and certain other infections.

Pneumocystis carinii—Organism that causes pneumocystis carinii pneumonia.

Pneumocystis carinii pneumonia—A lung infection of infants and weakened persons, including those with AIDS or those receiving drugs that weaken the immune system.

Polymorphous light eruption—A skin problem in certain people, which results from exposure to sunlight.

Polymyalgia rheumatica—A rheumatic disease, most common in elderly patients, which causes aching and stiffness in the shoulders and hips.

Polyp—Tumor or mass of tissue attached with a stalk or broad base; found in cavities such as the nose, uterus, or rectum.

Porphyria—A group of uncommon, usually inherited diseases of defective porphyrin metabolism.

Porphyrin—One of a number of chemicals that can combine with certain metal ions. Porphyrins occur in living organisms throughout nature (for example, as constituents in heme, chlorophyll, vitamin B_{12} and certain enzymes).

Potency—The strength of a medicine, chemical, or vitamin that will bring about a certain effect.

Pregnancy—Condition during which a woman is carrying a developing embryo or fetus in the uterus.

Pregnant—Containing one or more developing young within the body.

Premenstrual syndrome—Condition of physical or mental changes, including anxiety, headache, depression, bloating, and fatigue, that occurs in some women during the two-week period before menstruation.

Prenatal—Refers to the stage or period before birth.

Preservative—Substance added to a product to destroy or prevent the growth of microorganisms.

Prevent—To stop or to keep from happening.

Priapism—Prolonged abnormal, painful erection of the penis.

Prickling—Stinging or tingling sensation.

Proctitis—Inflammation of the rectum.

Progesterone—Natural steroid hormone responsible for preparing the uterus for pregnancy. If fertilization occurs, progesterone's actions carry on or maintain the pregnancy.

Progestin—A natural or synthetic hormone that has progesterone-like actions.

Progressive—In medicine, refers to an illness or condition that continues to worsen or become more severe with time.

Prolactin—Hormone secreted by the pituitary gland that stimulates and maintains milk flow in women following childbirth.

Prolactinoma—A pituitary tumor; results in secretion of excess prolactin.

Prophylactic—1. Agent or medicine used to prevent the occurrence of a specific condition. 2. Condom.

Prostate—Gland surrounding the neck of the male urethra just below the base of the bladder. It secretes a fluid that helps make up semen.

Prostatitis—Inflammation of the prostate gland.

Prosthesis—Any artificial substitute for a missing body part.

Protein—One of a group of compounds that make up the greatest part of plant and animal tissues. Enzymes, immunoglobulins, and several body structures, including muscles, are proteins. They are responsible for or involved in many body functions and are an essential nutrient in the diet.

Protozoa—Tiny, one-celled animals; some cause diseases in humans.

Psoralen—Chemical found in plants and used in certain perfumes and medicines. Exposure to a psoralen and then to sunlight may increase the risk of severe burning.

Psoriasis—Chronic skin disease marked by itchy, scaly, red patches.

Psychosis—Severe mental illness marked by loss of contact with reality, often involving delusions, hallucinations, and disordered thinking.

Puberty—Period in life during which sexual organs mature, making reproduction possible.

Pulmonary—Relating to the lungs.

Puncture—Wound or opening made by piercing with a pointed object or instrument.

Purity—Describes a measure of freedom from contamination.

Purpura—Tiny, purple-colored spots that appear at areas where bleeding into the skin occurs; similar to, but much smaller than, a bruise. May be caused by defects in the capillaries or a decreased number of platelets.

Pus—Yellowish liquid matter formed in certain infections, made up of leukocytes, bacteria, and dead tissue.

PUVA (psoralen plus ultraviolet light A)—Treatment for psoriasis and other conditions by use of a psoralen, such as methoxsalen or trioxsalen, and long-wave ultraviolet light.

Rachischisis—*See* Spina bifida.

Radiation—General term for any form of energy moving in all directions from a common center, including radioactive elements and x-ray tubes.

Radiopaque agent—Substance that makes it easier to see an area of the body with x-rays. Radiopaque agents are used to help diagnose a variety of medical problems.

Radiopharmaceutical—Radioactive agent used to diagnose certain medical problems or treat certain diseases.

Raynaud's syndrome—Condition caused by poor blood circulation in the hands; marked by numbness, tingling, and color change (white, blue, then red) in the fingers when they are exposed to cold.

Receptor—Structure within the cell or on the cell surface that binds with a specific substance to bring about a response.

Recommended Dietary Allowances (RDAs)—In the U.S., the amount of vitamins and minerals needed to provide for adequate nutrition in most healthy persons. RDAs for a given nutrient may vary depending on a person's age, sex, and physical condition (for example, pregnancy).

Recommended Nutrient Intakes (RNIs)—In Canada, values used to determine the amounts of vitamins, minerals, and protein needed to provide adequate nutrition and lessen the risk of chronic disease.

Rectal—Relating to the rectum.

Reduced calories—*See* Fewer calories.

Reduced cholesterol—*See* Less cholesterol.

Reduced fat—*See* Less fat.

Reduced saturated fat—*See* Less saturated fat.

Reduced sodium—*See* Less sodium.

Reduced sugar—*See* Less sugar.

Reference food—A basic food item. In food labeling, reference food is compared against the same food that has had something added to it or taken away from it.

Relapse—To fall back into illness after recovery has begun or after a remission.

Remission—State of an illness or disease during which symptoms lessen or disappear.

Renal—Relating to the kidneys.

Reproduction—Process in animals and plants that gives rise to new individuals or offspring.

Respiratory tract—The structures that are associated with breathing, including the nose, larynx, trachea, bronchial tree, and lungs.

Reye's syndrome—Serious disease affecting the liver and brain that sometimes occurs after a virus infection, such as influenza or chickenpox. It occurs most often in young children and teenagers, especially those who have been treated with aspirin during the illness. The first sign of Reye's syndrome is usually severe, prolonged vomiting.

Rheumatic heart disease—Heart disease marked by scarring and chronic inflammation of the heart and its valves, occurring after rheumatic fever.

Rhinitis—Inflammation of the mucous membrane inside the nose; often caused by an infection (such as a cold) or an allergy. Symptoms include runny or stuffy nose and sneezing.

Rickets—Bone disease usually caused by too little vitamin D, resulting in soft and malformed bones.

Rigidity—Lacking the ability to bend or be bent; stiffness.

Ringworm—*See* Tinea.

Risk—The possibility of injury or of suffering harm.

River blindness—Tropical disease produced by infection with worms of the Onchocerca type. The condition usually causes severe itching and may cause blindness.

Rosacea—Skin disease of the face, usually in middle-aged and older persons. Also called *adult acne*.

Saliva—Liquid secreted into the mouth by salivary glands; breaks down starch and moistens food for easy swallowing.

Sarcoidosis—Chronic disorder marked by enlarged lymph nodes in many parts of the body and inflammation, often in the muscles, eye, lungs, liver, and spleen.

Saturated fat—In chemistry, a fat that has all of the possible hydrogen atoms present on the carbon atoms and no double or triple bonds between the carbon atoms.

Saturated fat free—In food labeling, less than 0.5 grams of fat and less than 0.5 grams trans fatty acid per serving.

Scabicide—Medicine used to treat scabies (itch mite) infection.

Scabies—Contagious dermatitis caused by a mite burrowing into the skin; marked by tiny skin eruptions and severe itching.

Schistosomiasis—Tropical infection in which worms enter the skin from infested water and settle in the bladder or intestines, causing inflammation and scarring. Also called *bilharziasis*.

Schizophrenia—Severe mental disorder. The patient loses contact with reality, expresses disturbed thinking and behavior, and may become agitated (anxious and restless) or withdrawn.

Scintigram—Image obtained by photographing emissions made by a radiopharmaceutical introduced into the body.

Scleroderma—Chronic disease first seen as hardening, thickening, and shrinking of the skin; later, certain organs also are affected.

Scotoma—Area of decreased vision or total loss of vision in a part of the visual field; a blind spot.

Scrotum—Sac that holds the testes (male sex glands).

Scurvy—Disease caused by a deficiency of vitamin C (ascorbic acid), marked by bleeding gums, bleeding beneath the skin, and body weakness.

Sebaceous gland—Skin gland that secretes sebum.

Seborrhea—Skin condition caused by the excess release of sebum from the sebaceous glands, accompanied by dandruff and oily skin.

Sebum—Fatty secretion produced by sebaceous (oil) glands of the skin.

Secretion—1. Process in which a gland in the body or on the surface of the body releases a substance for use. 2. The substance released by the gland.

Sedative-hypnotic—Medicine used to treat excessive nervousness, restlessness, or insomnia.

Sedation—A profoundly relaxed or calmed state.

Seizure—A sudden attack, usually referring to contractions of muscles as seen in some forms of epilepsy or other disorders.

Semen—Fluid released from the penis at sexual climax. It is made up of sperm suspended in secretions from the reproductive tract.

Sensory—Relating to the senses (smell, taste, hearing, sight, and touch).

Severe—Of a great degree (for example, severe pain or distress).

Sexually transmitted disease (STD)—Any disease that is spread by sexual contact. Formerly called *venereal disease*.

Shaking palsy—*See* Parkinson's disease.

Shingles—*See* Herpes zoster.

Shock—A condition in which blood supply to the tissues is dangerously low, often caused by severe bleeding, overwhelming infection, or heart problems. Signs of shock include very low blood pressure, fast heartbeat, and mental confusion.

Short-acting—Refers to a medicine that is effective for a short amount of time.

Shunt—A passage that transfers or channels blood or other fluid from one part of the body to another. Shunts may occur naturally or they may be created for a specific purpose by a surgical procedure.

SIADH (secretion of inappropriate antidiuretic hormone) syndrome—Disease caused by excess production of antidiuretic hormone; the body retains (keeps) more fluid than normal. A syndrome similar to SIADH may also be a side effect of some medicines.

Sickle cell anemia—Hereditary disorder of chronic anemia caused by abnormal hemoglobin. The name of the disorder comes from the sickle-shaped red blood cells that are formed in the blood of patients. The disorder mainly affects people of African or Arabian ancestry.

Sign—Possible evidence of a disease or other change in condition that can be seen or measured by someone other than the person experiencing it (for example, a skin rash or high blood pressure). *See also* Symptom.

Sinusitis—Inflammation of a sinus.

Sjögren's syndrome—Condition usually occurring in older women, marked by dry eyes, dry mouth, inflamed salivary glands, and other problems such as rheumatoid arthritis, systemic lupus erythematosus (SLE), or scleroderma.

Skeletal muscle relaxant—Medicine used to relax certain muscles and help relieve the pain and discomfort caused by strains, sprains, or other injury to the muscles.

Skeleton—The bony framework of the body that supports the soft tissues and organs.

SLE—*See* Lupus erythematosus, systemic.

Sloughing of skin—Peeling away of dead skin tissue (for example, after a sunburn).

Sodium fluoride—A chemical that makes teeth stronger and helps prevent cavities; in many communities, small amounts are added to the drinking water.

Sodium free—In food labeling, less than 5 milligrams of sodium per serving.

Soluble—Able to be dissolved in a fluid.

Soothe—To relieve or make less painful.

Spasticity—Increase in normal muscular tone, causing stiff, awkward movements.

Spastic paralysis—Paralysis marked by muscle rigidity or spasticity in the part of the body that is paralyzed.

Sperm—Mature male reproductive or sex cell. When a sperm fertilizes an ovum, a new organism begins developing.

Spermicide—Substance that kills sperm.

Spina bifida—Birth defect caused by failure of the neural tube of the fetus, a structure that develops into the backbone, to close normally. In many cases, part of the infant's spinal cord and its coverings are not completely surrounded by the spinal column (backbone). Also called *rachischisis*.

Spinal column—The column made up of vertebrae that extends from the base of the skull to the end of the trunk. Also called *spine* or *backbone*. It helps to support the body and protects the spinal cord, which passes through it.

Spine—*See* Spinal column.

STD—*See* Sexually transmitted disease.

Stenosis—Abnormal narrowing of a canal or duct of the body.

Sterility—1. Inability to produce offspring. 2. The state of being free of living microorganisms.

Stimulant, respiratory—Medicine used to stimulate breathing.

Stimulate—To promote greater activity of a body part or function.

Stomatitis—Inflammation of the mucous membrane of the mouth; causes ulcers or sores that may be painful.

Stool—*See* Feces.

Strength—1. In relation to medicines, a measure of the amount of active ingredient present. 2. In nutrition, the measure of a vitamin's health value.

Streptokinase—Enzyme that dissolves blood clots.

Stroke—Very serious event in which blood flow to the brain is stopped; an artery to the brain may become clogged by a blood clot or it may burst and cause hemorrhage. Stroke can affect speech, memory, and behavior, and may result in paralysis. Also called *apoplexy*.

Stye—Infection of one or more sebaceous glands of the eyelid, marked by swelling.

Subcutaneous—Under the skin.

Sublingual—Under the tongue. A sublingual medicine is taken by placing it under the tongue and letting it slowly dissolve.

Sudden infant death syndrome (SIDS)—Sudden death of an apparently well infant from an unknown cause; death usually occurs during sleep. Also called *crib death* or *cot death*.

Sugar diabetes—*See* Diabetes mellitus.

Sugar free—In food labeling, less than 0.5 grams of sugar per serving.

Sugar pill—*See* Placebo.

Sulfite—Type of preservative; causes allergic reactions, such as asthma, in sensitive people.

Sunscreen—Substance that blocks ultraviolet light and helps prevent sunburn when applied to the skin.

Suppository—Mass of medicated material shaped for insertion into a body cavity, such as the rectum or vagina. A suppository is solid at room temperature but melts at body temperature or dissolves in body fluids.

Suppressant—Medicine that slows or stops an action or condition.

Suspension—A form of medicine in which the drug particles are mixed with a liquid but not dissolved in it. When left standing, some suspensions may separate, with the particles settling at the bottom of the container and the liquid rising to the top. Most suspensions must be shaken before use.

Symptom—Possible evidence of a disease or other change in condition that is apparent only to the person experiencing it (for example, a headache). *See also* Sign.

Syncope—Sudden loss of consciousness due to inadequate blood flow to the brain; fainting.

Syndrome—Group of signs and symptoms that occur together and characterize a particular disorder.

Synthetic—A substance that is manufactured rather than occurring naturally.

Syphilis—An infectious disease, usually transmitted by sexual contact. The three stages of the disease may be separated by months or years.

Syringe—Medical device used to inject liquids into the body or remove material from a part of the body. Some types are used to help wash out a body cavity.

Systemic—Having general effects throughout the body; applies to most medicines when taken by mouth or given by injection into a blood vessel or a muscle.

Tachycardia—Abnormal rapid beating of the heart, usually at a rate over 100 beats per minute in adults.

Tardive dyskinesia—Slow, involuntary movements, often of the tongue, lips, or arms, usually brought on by certain drugs.

TB—*See* Tuberculosis.

Temporomandibular joint (TMJ)—Hinge that connects the lower jaw to the skull.

Tendinitis—Inflammation of a tendon.

Tendon—Band of tough tissue that attaches a muscle to bone.

Teratogenic—Causing abnormal development in an embryo or fetus, resulting in birth defects.

Testicle—Male sex organ that produces sperm and testosterone.

Testosterone—Principal male sex hormone.

Tetany—Condition marked by spasm and twitching of the muscles, particularly those of the hands, feet, and face; caused by a decrease in the calcium ion concentration in the blood.

Therapeutic—Relating to the treatment of a specific condition.

Thimerosal—Chemical used as a preservative in some medicines, and as an antiseptic and disinfectant; contains mercury.

Thorax—The part of the body between the neck and abdomen; the chest.

Thrombolytic agent—Substance that dissolves blood clots.

Thrombophlebitis—Inflammation of a vein accompanied by the formation of a blood clot.

Thrombus—Blood clot that obstructs a cavity of the heart or a blood vessel.

Thrush—*See* Candidiasis of the mouth.

Thyroid gland—Gland in the lower front of the neck. It releases thyroid hormones, which control body metabolism.

Thyrotoxicosis—Condition resulting from excessive amounts of thyroid hormones in the blood, causing increased metabolism, fast heartbeat, tremors, nervousness, bulging eyes, and increased sweating.

Tic—Repeated involuntary movement or spasm of a muscle.

Tic douloureux—*See* Neuralgia, trigeminal.

Tinea—Fungus infection of the surface of the skin, particularly the scalp, feet, and nails. Also called *ringworm.*

Tinnitus—Ringing in the ears.

Tone—In medicine, the normal amount of tension or resistance to stretching of a tissue, such as a muscle or the skin.

Topical—In medicine, refers to a medicine being applied to a particular surface area, usually the skin.

Tourette's disorder—Rare condition beginning in childhood, marked by tics and other unnecessary movements and barks, sniffs, or grunts (may be swearing). Also called *Gilles de la Tourette syndrome.*

Toxemia—Blood poisoning caused by bacterial production of toxins.

Toxemia of pregnancy—Condition occurring in pregnant women marked by hypertension, edema, excess protein in the urine, convulsions, and possibly coma.

Toxic—Poisonous; related to or caused by a toxin or poison.

Toxin—A substance that may cause damage to body tissues or disturb body functions, causing illness or even death; a poison.

Toxoplasmosis—Disease caused by a protozoa in the blood, usually transmitted to humans from cats or by eating raw meat; generally the symptoms are mild and self-limited.

Tracheostomy—A surgical opening through the throat into the trachea (windpipe) to bypass an obstruction to breathing.

Trait—In genetics, any characteristic that is inherited.

Tranquilizer—Medicine that produces a calming effect. It is used to relieve mental anxiety and tension.

Transdermal—A method of applying a medicine to the skin that produces a prolonged systemic effect rather than a local effect. The medicine is contained in a special patch, disk, or ointment, from which it slowly passes through the skin and is absorbed into the bloodstream, which carries it through the body.

Transmit—In medicine, to pass or spread infection or disease from one person to another.

Tremble—Shake or shiver.

Trichomoniasis—Infection of the vagina and the male genital tract resulting in inflammation of genital tissues; symptoms may include itching, burning (in men, burning while urinating), and discharge. The infection can be passed between sex partners.

Triglyceride—A molecular form in which fats are present in food and the body; triglycerides are stored in the body as fat.

Troche—*See* Lozenge.

Trypanosome fever—*See* Trypanosomiasis, African.

Trypanosomiasis, African—Tropical disease, transmitted by tsetse fly bites, which causes fever, headache, and chills, followed by enlarged lymph nodes and anemia. Months or even years later, the disease affects the central nervous system, causing drowsiness and lethargy, coma, and death. Also called *African sleeping sickness.*

Tuberculosis (TB)—Infectious disease that most commonly affects the lungs, producing symptoms that include cough, fever, night sweats, weight loss, and spitting up blood.

Tumor—Abnormal growth or enlargement in or on a part of the body.

Tyramine—Chemical present in many foods and beverages. Its structure and action in the body are similar to epinephrine.

Ulcer—Open sore or break in the skin or mucous membrane; often fails to heal and is accompanied by inflammation.

Ulcerative colitis—Chronic, recurrent inflammation and ulceration of the colon.

Ulceration—1. Formation or development of an ulcer. 2. Condition of an area marked with ulcers loosely associated with one another.

Ultraviolet rays—Invisible radiation having a wavelength shorter than that of visible light but longer than that of x-rays. These rays are responsible for sunburns, tanning, damage to skin cells, and skin cancers.

Underactive thyroid—*See* Hypothyroidism.

Ureter—Tube through which urine passes from the kidney to the bladder.

Urethra—Tube through which urine passes from the bladder to the outside of the body.

Uric acid—Product of protein metabolism, excreted in the urine. High levels of uric acid in the body can lead to gout and kidney stones.

Urination—Act of passing urine from the bladder.

Urine—Fluid containing waste products that is formed and excreted by the kidneys. It is then stored in the urinary bladder until the individual urinates.

Urticaria—An eruption of itching wheals on the skin. Also called *hives.*

USRDA—Labeling term formerly used to indicate how much of a nutrient a serving provided. This term is now stated as Daily Value (DV).

Uterus—Hollow organ in the female in which the fetus develops until birth.

Vaccine—Preparation, usually made from specially treated microorganisms or parts of microorganisms, that is given to stimulate production of antibodies that protect against the disease that the microorganisms cause.

Vaccinia—The skin and sometimes body reactions associated with smallpox vaccine. Also called *cowpox.*

Vagina—Passage in the female leading from the cervix of the uterus to the outside of the body.

Vaginal—Relating to the vagina.

Varicella—Very infectious virus disease marked by fever and itchy rash that develops into blisters and then scabs. Also called *chickenpox.*

Vasoconstrictor—Medicine or enzyme that causes smooth muscles of blood vessels to contract, raising blood pressure.

Vascular—Relating to the blood vessels.

Vasodilator—Medicine that dilates the blood vessels, permitting increased blood flow. Sometimes used to lower blood pressure.

Vasopressin—A hormone that prevents excessive water loss by its action on the kidney and raises blood pressure by constricting small blood vessels. Also called *antidiuretic hormone, ADH.*

Vein—Blood vessel that carries blood from various parts of the body toward the heart.

Venous—Relating to veins.

Ventricular fibrillation—Life-threatening condition of fine, quivering, irregular movements of many muscle fibers of certain heart muscle; replaces the normal heart beat and interrupts pumping function.

Ventricle—A small cavity, such as one of the two lower chambers of the heart or one of the several cavities of the brain.

Vertebra—Any of the thirty-three bones that make up the spinal column.

Vertigo—Sensation of motion, usually whirling, or dizziness, either of oneself or of one's surroundings.

Very low sodium—In food labeling, 35 milligrams or less of sodium per serving. However, for small servings (30 grams or less or 2 tablespoons or less), very low sodium is 35 milligrams or less of sodium per 50 grams of the food.

Veterinary—Relating to animals and their diseases and treatment.

Virus—Any of a group of simple microbes too small to be seen by a light microscope. They grow and reproduce only in living cells. Viruses cause many diseases in humans, including the common cold.

Visual—Relating to vision or sight.

Vitamin—Any of a group of substances, needed in small amounts only, for growth and health. Vitamins are usually found naturally in food, but may also be man-made.

Vitamin, natural—A vitamin that comes from natural sources such as plants.

Vitamin, synthetic—A vitamin that does not come from natural sources, but instead is man-made.

Vitamins, fat-soluble—Vitamins that can be dissolved in fat (vitamins A, D, E, K). They are stored in fat tissue.

Vitamins, water-soluble—Vitamins that can be dissolved in water (vitamin C and the B-complex vitamins). They are stored in small amounts by the body.

Vitiligo—Condition in which some areas of skin lose pigment and turn white. Also called *leukoderma.*

von Willebrand's disease—Hereditary blood disorder characterized by delayed blood clotting, which leads to excessive bleeding even after minor injuries.

Wart—Small, usually hard, benign growth on the skin, caused by a virus.

Wasting—Gradual loss of weight and strength.

Water diabetes—*See* Diabetes insipidus.

Water pill—*See* Diuretic.

Wheal—Temporary, small, raised area of the skin, usually accompanied by itching or burning; welt.

Wheezing—A whistling sound made when there is difficulty in breathing.

White mouth—*See* Candidiasis of the mouth.

Wilson's disease—Inborn defect in the body's ability to process copper. Too much copper may accumulate and lead to jaundice, cirrhosis, mental retardation, or symptoms like those of Parkinson's disease.

Without added sugar—*See* No added sugar.

Zollinger-Ellison syndrome—Disorder in which a tumor of the pancreas causes overproduction of stomach acid, leading to diarrhea and ulcers.

Appendix I

ADDITIONAL LIST OF DRUG INFORMATION NOW AVAILABLE ONLINE

The following monographs are not included in the published version of the book but are available online. Refer to the inside front cover for access information.

Abciximab (Intravenous Route)
ACE Inhibitor (Oral Route, Injection Route)
Acetaminophen, Sodium Bicarbonate, And Citric Acid (Oral Route)
Acetone, Isopropyl Alcohol, And Polysorbate (Topical Route)
Agalsidase Beta (Intravenous Route)
Alemtuzumab (Intravenous Route)
Alglucerase (Intravenous Route)
Allopurinol (Intravenous Route)
Almotriptan (Oral Route)
Alpha-1 Proteinase Inhibitor Human (Intravenous Route)
Aminobenzoate Potassium (Oral Route)
Aminoglutethimide (Oral Route)
Aminosalicylate Sodium (Oral Route)
Amiodarone (Intravenous Route)
Amlexanox (Mucous Membrane, Oral Route)
Ammoniated Mercury (Topical Route)
Ammonium Molybdate (Intravenous Route, Injection Route)
Amphotericin B (Intravenous Route, Injection Route)
Amphotericin B (Topical Route)
Amphotericin B Cholesteryl Sulfate Complex (Intravenous Route)
Amphotericin B Lipid Complex (Intravenous Route, Injection Route)
Amphotericin B Liposome (Intravenous Route)
Amprenavir (Oral Route)
Amsacrine (Intravenous Route)
Amyl Nitrite (Inhalation, Oral/Nebulization Route)
Anesthetic, Local (Ophthalmic Route)
Anesthetics (Dental)
Anesthetics (Parenteral-Local)
Anesthetics, General (Systemic)
Angiotensin-Converting Enzyme (ACE) Inhibitors And Hydrochlorothiazide (Systemic)
Anticonvulsants, Dione (Systemic)
Antihemophilic Factor (Intravenous Route, Injection Route)
Anti-Inflammatory Drugs, Nonsteroidal (Ophthalmic)
Antithymocyte Globulin Rabbit (Intravenous Route)
Antivenin (Crotalidae) Polyvalent (Injection Route)
Antivenin (Crotalidae) Polyvalent Immune Fab (Intravenous Route)
Antivenin (Latrodectus Mactans) (Injection Route)
Antivenin (Micrurus Fulvius) (Intravenous Route)
Ardeparin (Subcutaneous Route)
Aromatic Ammonia Spirit (Inhalation, Oral/Nebulization Route)
Arsenic Trioxide (Intravenous Route)
Atovaquone (Oral Route)
Atovaquone And Chloroguanide (Oral Route)
Atropine, Hyoscyamine, Methenamine, Methylene Blue, Phenyl Salicylate, And Benzoic Acid (Oral Route)
Atropine/Homatropine/Scopolamine (Ophthalmic)
Attapulgite (Oral Route)
Bacillus Of Calmette And Guerin Vaccine, Live (Intradermal Route)
Bacillus Of Calmette And Guerin Vaccine, Live (Intravesical Route)
Basiliximab (Intravenous Route)
Belladonna Alkaloids And Barbiturates (Systemic)
Bentiromide (Oral Route)
Beta-Adrenergic Blocking Agents (Ophthalmic)
Beta-Adrenergic Blocking Agents And Thiazide Diuretics (Systemic)
Betaine (Oral Route)
Bimatoprost (Ophthalmic Route)
Biotin (Oral Route)
Bismuth Subsalicylate (Oral Route)
Botulinum Toxin Type B (Intramuscular Route)
Brimonidine (Ophthalmic Route)
Brinzolamide (Ophthalmic Route)
Bromfenac (Ophthalmic Route)

Budesonide/Formoterol (Inhalation Route)
Calamine (Topical Route)
Calcipotriene (Topical Route)
Calcitonin (Salmon) (Nasal Route)
Calcium Acetate (Oral Route)
Candesartan And Hydrochlorothiazide (Oral Route)
Carbetocin (Intravenous Route)
Carbol-Fuchsin Solution (Topical Route)
Carboprost (Intramuscular Route)
Carmustine (Implantation Route)
Chlophedianol (Oral Route)
Chloral Hydrate (Oral Route, Rectal Route)
Chlorhexidine (Oral Route)
Chlorhexidine (Subgingival Route)
Cholecystographic Agents, Oral (Diagnostic)
Cholecystokinin (Injection Route)
Cholera Vaccine (Injection Route)
Chondrocytes, Autologous Cultured (Implantation Route)
Chromic Phosphate P 32 (Injection Route)
Chromium Supplements (Systemic)
Chymopapain (Injection Route)
Cinoxacin (Oral Route)
Cisapride (Oral Route)
Clioquinol (Topical Route)
Clioquinol And Hydrocortisone (Topical Route)
Clodronic Acid (Oral Route, Injection Route)
Cocaine (Topical Route)
Colistin Sulfate, Neomycin Sulfate, Hydrocortisone Acetate, And Thonzonium Bromide (Otic Route)
Copper Supplements (Systemic)
Corticosteroids (Dental)
Corticosteroids (Ophthalmic)
Corticosteroids (Otic)
Corticosteroids (Rectal)
Cyclandelate (Oral Route)
Cyproterone (Oral Route, Intramuscular Route)
Cysteamine (Oral Route)
Dapsone (Oral Route)
Daunorubicin Citrate Liposome (Intravenous Route)
Desflurane (Inhalation, Oral/Nebulization Route)
Diethylcarbamazine (Oral Route)
Diethyltoluamide (Topical Route)
Difenoxin And Atropine (Oral Route)
Dinoprost (Injection Route)
Diphenidol (Oral Route)
Diphtheria Antitoxin (Injection Route)
Dirithromycin (Oral Route)
Domperidone (Oral Route)
Doxycycline (Oral Route)
Doxycycline (Subgingival Route)
Drospirenone And Ethinyl Estradiol (Oral Route)
Dyphylline (Oral Route, Intramuscular Route)
Efavirenz/Emtricitabine/Tenofovir (Oral Route)
Eflornithine (Injection Route)
Epinephrine (Ophthalmic)
Epoprostenol (Intravenous Route)
Eptacog Alfa (Intravenous Route)
Ethchlorvynol (Oral Route)
Factor IX Complex (Intravenous Route, Injection Route)
Fat Emulsion (Intravenous Route, Injection Route)
Fluticasone (Nasal Route)
Fomivirsen (Intraocular Route)
Framycetin (Ophthalmic Route)
Fructose, Dextrose, And Phosphoric Acid (Oral Route)
Furazolidone (Oral Route)
Fusidic Acid (Oral Route, Injection Route)
Gallium Nitrate (Intravenous Route)
Gentamicin (Topical Route)
Gentian Violet (Topical Route)
Gentian Violet (Vaginal Route)
Glatiramer Acetate (Subcutaneous Route)
Glycerin (Oral Route)
Gold Compounds (Systemic)
Guanabenz (Oral Route)

Guanadrel (Oral Route)
Guanethidine (Oral Route)
Guanfacine (Oral Route)
Halofantrine (Oral Route)
Heparin (Intravenous Route, Injection Route)
Histamine (Injection Route)
Histrelin (Implantation Route)
Hyaluronate Sodium (Injection Route)
Hyaluronidase (Subcutaneous Route, Injection Route)
Hydralazine And Hydrochlorothiazide (Oral Route)
Hydroxyamphetamine And Tropicamide (Ophthalmic Route)
Hylan Polymers A And B (Injection Route)
Hypromellose (Intraocular Route)
Ibritumomab Tiuxetan (Intravenous Route)
Idursulfase (Intravenous Route)
Imiglucerase (Intravenous Route)
Inulin (Intravenous Route)
Iobenguane I 131 (Intravenous Route)
Iodine (Topical Route)
Iodine And Potassium Iodide (Strong Iodine) (Oral Route)
Iodoquinol (Oral Route)
Isoxsuprine (Oral Route, Injection Route)
Ivermectin (Oral Route)
Japanese Encephalitis Virus Vaccine (Subcutaneous Route)
Kanamycin (Oral Route)
Kaolin And Pectin (Oral Route)
Levamisole (Oral Route)
Levocabastine (Ophthalmic Route)
Levocarnitine (Oral Route, Intravenous Route)
Levomethadyl (Oral Route)
Lidocaine (Topical Route)
Lidocaine And Prilocaine (Topical Route)
Lincomycin (Oral Route, Injection Route)
Lodoxamide (Ophthalmic Route)
Lomustine (Oral Route)
Losartan And Hydrochlorothiazide (Oral Route)
Lyme Disease Vaccine (Recombinant OspA) (Intramuscular Route)
Magnesium Supplements (Systemic)
Magnetic Resonance Imaging Contrast Agents (Diagnostic)
Magnetic Resonance Imaging Contrast Agents, Iron-Containing (Diagnostic)
Malathion (Topical Route)
Mangafodipir (Intravenous Route)
Manganese Supplements(Systemic)
Measles And Rubella Virus Vaccine Live (Intramuscular Route, Injection Route)
Mecamylamine (Oral Route)
Mechlorethamine (Topical Route)
Meglumine Antimoniate (Intravenous Route, Injection Route)
Meprobamate (Oral Route)
Meropenem (Intravenous Route)
Mesalamine (Rectal Route)
Mesna (Intravenous Route)
Methenamine (Oral Route)
Methionine (Oral Route)
Methyldopa And Thiazide Diuretics (Systemic)
Methylene Blue (Oral Route, Intravenous Route)
Methysergide (Oral Route)
Metyrapone (Oral Route)
Micafungin (Intravenous Route)
Midazolam (Injection Route)
Moclobemide (Oral Route)
Mometasone (Nasal Route)
Monoctanoin (Injection Route)
Moricizine (Oral Route)
Mumps Virus Vaccine, Live (Subcutaneous Route)
Mupirocin (Nasal Route)
Muromonab-CD3 (Intravenous Route)
Nabilone (Oral Route)
Naftifine (Topical Route)

Nalidixic Acid (Oral Route)
Naltrexone (Oral Route)
Natamycin (Ophthalmic Route)
Neomycin (Ophthalmic Route)
Niclosamide (Oral Route)
Nitrofurazone (Topical Route)
Nylidrin (Oral Route)
Nystatin And Triamcinolone (Topical Route)
Opium Preparations (Systemic)
Oprelvekin (Subcutaneous Route)
Oxiconazole (Topical Route)
Oxtriphylline And Guaifenesin (Oral Route)
Pantothenic Acid (Oral Route)
Papaverine (Injection Route)
Papaverine (Oral Route, Injection Route)
Paraldehyde (Oral Route, Injection Route, Rectal
     Route)
Pegademase Bovine (Intramuscular Route)
Pemoline (Oral Route)
Penicillamine (Oral Route)
Pentamidine (Injection Route)
Pentetate Zinc Trisodium (Intravenous Route,
     Inhalation, Oral/Nebulization Route)
Pentostatin (Intravenous Route)
Perflubron (Oral Route)
Perphenazine And Amitriptyline (Oral Route)
Phenolsulfonphthalein (Injection Route)
Phentolamine (Injection Route)
Phenylephrine (Ophthalmic Route)
Physostigmine (Ophthalmic Route)
Pilocarpine (Oral Route)
Pioglitazone And Glimepiride (Oral Route)
Piperazine (Oral Route)
Podophyllum (Topical Route)
Poliovirus Vaccine (Systemic)
Poliovirus Vaccine, Live (Oral Route)
Polyethylene Glycol, Sodium Sulfate, Sodium
     Chloride, Potassium Chloride, Sodium Ascorbate,
     And Ascorbic Acid (Oral Route)
Porfimer (Intravenous Route)
Potassium Iodide (Oral Route)
Pralidoxime (Injection Route)
Praziquantel (Oral Route)
Prazosin And Polythiazide (Oral Route)
Primaquine (Oral Route)
Proguanil (Oral Route)
Protirelin (Intravenous Route)
Prussian Blue (Oral Route)
Pyrantel (Oral Route)
Pyrimethamine (Oral Route)
Pyrimethamine And Sulfadoxine (Oral Route)
Pyrithione (Topical Route)
Pyrvinium (Oral Route)
Rabies Immune Globulin (Intramuscular Route)
Rabies Vaccine (Systemic)
Radiopaque Agents (Diagnostic)
Radiopaque Agents (Local)

Radiopharmaceuticals (Diagnostic)
Rauwolfia Alkaloids (Systemic)
Rauwolfia Alkaloids And Thiazide Diuretics
     (Systemic)
Reserpine, Hydralazine, And Hydrochlorothiazide
     (Oral Route)
Resorcinol (Topical Route)
Resorcinol And Sulfur (Topical Route)
Rho (D) Immune Globulin (Intravenous Route,
     Intramuscular Route, Injection Route)
Rofecoxib (Oral Route)
Ropivacaine (Injection Route)
Rubella And Mumps Virus Vaccine Live
     (Intramuscular Route)
Rubella Virus Vaccine, Live (Subcutaneous Route)
Sacrosidase (Oral Route)
Salicylic Acid (Topical Route)
Salicylic Acid And Sulfur (Topical Route)
Salicylic Acid, Sulfur, And Coal Tar (Topical Route)
Samarium Sm 153 Lexidronam (Intravenous Route)
Selenium Sulfide (Topical Route)
Selenium Supplement (Oral Route)
Sermorelin (Injection Route)
Sevoflurane (Inhalation, Oral/Nebulization Route)
Sincalide (Intravenous Route)
Sodium Benzoate And Sodium Phenylacetate (Oral
     Route)
Sodium Bicarbonate (Oral Route, Intravenous Route,
     Subcutaneous Route)
Sodium Cellulose Phosphate (Oral Route)
Sodium Chloride (Injection Route)
Sodium Chloride (Ophthalmic Route)
Sodium Iodide (Oral Route, Injection Route,
     Intravenous Route)
Sodium Iodide I 131 (Oral Route)
Sodium Phenylbutyrate (Oral Route)
Sodium Phosphate P 32 (Intravenous Route)
Sodium Thiosulfate (Intramuscular Route)
Sparfloxacin (Oral Route)
Spectinomycin (Intramuscular Route)
Spiramycin (Oral Route, Injection Route, Rectal
     Route)
Streptozocin (Intravenous Route)
Strontium Chloride Sr 89 (Intravenous Route,
     Injection Route)
Succimer (Oral Route)
Sulfapyridine (Oral Route)
Sulfinpyrazone (Oral Route)
Sulfonamides (Ophthalmic)
Sulfonamides And Phenazopyridine (Systemic)
Sulfur (Topical Route)
Suramin (Injection Route)
Talc (Intrapleural Route)
Telmisartan And Hydrochlorothiazide (Oral Route)
Tenecteplase (Intravenous Route)
Teriparatide (Subcutaneous Route)
Testolactone (Oral Route)

Testosterone (Buccal Route)
Testosterone (Transdermal Route)
Tetracycline (Mucous Membrane, Oral Route)
Tetracyclines (Ophthalmic)
Tetracyclines (Topical)
Theophylline And Guaifenesin (Oral Route)
Theophylline, Ephedrine, And Phenobarbital (Oral
     Route)
Thiabendazole (Oral Route)
Thiabendazole (Topical Route)
Thiethylperazine (Oral Route, Intramuscular Route,
     Rectal Route)
Thioguanine (Oral Route)
Thiotepa (Injection Route)
Thioxanthenes (Systemic)
Thyrotropin (Injection Route)
Tiopronin (Oral Route)
Tobramycin And Dexamethasone (Ophthalmic Route)
Tocainide (Oral Route)
Tolnaftate (Topical Route)
Trastuzumab (Intravenous Route)
Travoprost (Ophthalmic Route)
Trientine (Oral Route)
Trimethobenzamide (Oral Route, Intramuscular Route,
     Rectal Route)
Trioxsalen (Oral Route)
Tropicamide (Ophthalmic Route)
Trovafloxacin (Oral Route)
Typhoid Vaccine, Inactivated (Subcutaneous Route,
     Injection Route)
Typhoid Vaccine, Live (Oral Route)
Typhoid Vi Polysaccharide Vaccine (Intramuscular
     Route)
Undecylenic Acid (Topical Route)
Unoprostone (Ophthalmic Route)
Urea (Injection Route)
14c Urea (Oral Route)
Urofollitropin (Intramuscular Route, Subcutaneous
     Route, Injection Route)
Ursodiol (Oral Route)
Valdecoxib (Oral Route)
Valrubicin (Intravesical Route)
Valsartan And Hydrochlorothiazide (Oral Route)
Vancomycin (Intravenous Route, Injection Route)
Vancomycin (Oral Route)
Varicella Virus Vaccine (Subcutaneous Route)
Vasopressin (Injection Route)
Vidarabine (Ophthalmic Route)
Vindesine (Injection Route)
Vitamin B12 (Systemic)
Xylometazoline (Nasal Route)
Yellow Fever Vaccine (Subcutaneous Route, Injection
     Route)
Ziconotide (Intrathecal Route)
Zinc Supplements (Systemic)
Zopiclone (Oral Route)

Appendix II

POISON CONTROL CENTER LISTING

The following is a list of emergency telephone numbers for United States and Canadian poison control centers.

UNITED STATES
American Association of Poison Control Centers
U.S. Poison Control Center Members
Updated May 2003

ALABAMA
Alabama Poison Center
2503 Phoenix Drive
Tuscaloosa, AL 35405
Emergency Phone: (800) 222-1222

Regional Poison Control Center
Children's Hospital
1600 7th Avenue South
Birmingham, AL 35233
Emergency Phone: (800) 222-1222

ALASKA
Oregon Poison Center
Oregon Health and Science University
3181 SW Sam Jackson Park Road
CB550
Portland, OR 97201
Emergency Phone: (800) 222-1222
(Voice and TTY/TDD)

ARIZONA
Arizona Poison & Drug Info Center
Arizona Health Sciences Center
Room 1156
1501 North Campbell Avenue
Tucson, AZ 85724
Emergency Phone: (800) 222-1222

Banner Poison Control Center
901 Willetta St.
Room 2701
Phoenix, AZ 85006
Emergency Phone: (800) 222-1222

ARKANSAS
Arkansas Poison & Drug Information Center
College of Pharmacy
University of Arkansas for Medical Sciences
4301 W. Markham
Mail Slot 522-2
Little Rock, AR 72205
Emergency Phone: (800) 222-1222
TDD/TTY: (800) 641-3805

CALIFORNIA
California Poison Control System - Fresno/Madera Division
Children's Hospital Central California
9300 Valley Children's Place, MB 15
Madera, CA 93638-8762
Emergency Phone: (800) 222-1222
TDD/TTY: (800) 972-3323

California Poison Control System - Sacramento Division
UC Davis Medical Center
2315 Stockton Boulevard
Sacramento, CA 95817
Emergency Phone: (800) 222-1222
TDD/TTY: (800) 972-3323

California Poison Control System - San Diego Division
University of California, San Diego, Medical Center
200 West Arbor Drive
San Diego, CA 92103-8925
Emergency Phone: (800) 222-1222
TDD/TTY: (800) 972-3323

California Poison Control System - San Francisco Division
UCSF Box 1369
San Francisco, CA 94143-1369
Emergency Phone: (800) 222-1222
TDD/TTY: (800) 972-3323

COLORADO
Rocky Mountain Poison & Drug Ctr
777 Bannock Street
Mail Code 0180
Denver, CO 80204-4507
Emergency Phone: (800) 222-1222
TDD/TTY: (303) 739-1127
Emergency Phone: (800) 332-3073
(CO only/outside metro area)

CONNECTICUT
Connecticut Poison Control Center
University of Connecticut Health Center
263 Farmington Avenue
Farmington, CT 06030-5365
Emergency Phone: (800) 222-1222
TTY/TDD: (866) 218-5372

DELAWARE
The Poison Control Center
Children's Hospital of Philadelphia
3400 Civic Center Blvd
Philadelphia, PA 19104-4303
Emergency Phone: (800) 222-1222
TDD/TTY: (215) 590-8789

DISTRICT OF COLUMBIA
National Capital Poison Center
3201 New Mexico Avenue, NW
Suite 310
Washington, DC 20016
Emergency Phone: (800) 222-1222
(Voice and TTY)

FLORIDA
Florida Poison Information Center - Jacksonville
655 West Eighth Street
Jacksonville, FL 32209
Emergency Phone: (800) 222-1222
(Voice and TTY/TDD)

Florida Poison Information Center - Miami
University of Miami, Department of Pediatrics
P.O. Box 110626 (R-131)
Miami, FL 33101
Emergency Phone: (800) 222-1222

Florida Poison Information Center - Tampa
Tampa General Hospital
P.O. Box 1289
Tampa, FL 33601
Emergency Phone: (800) 222-1222

GEORGIA
Georgia Poison Center
Hughes Spalding Children's Hospital
Grady Health System
80 Butler Street, SE
P.O. Box 26066
Atlanta, GA 30335-3801
Emergency Phone: (800) 222-1222
TDD/TTY: (404) 616-9287

HAWAII
Rocky Mountain Poison & Drug Ctr
777 Bannock Street
Mail Code 0180
Denver, CO 80204-4507
Emergency Phone: (800) 222-1222
TDD/TYY: (303) 739-1127

IDAHO
Rocky Mountain Poison & Drug Center
777 Bannock Street
Mail Code 0180
Denver, CO 80204-4507
Emergency Phone: (800) 222-1222
(800) 860-0620 (ID only)

ILLINOIS
Illinois Poison Center
222 S. Riverside Plaza, Suite 1900
Chicago, IL 60606
Emergency Phone: (800) 222-1222
TDD/TTY: (312) 906-6185

INDIANA
Indiana Poison Center
Methodist Hospital
Clarian Health Partners
I-65 at 21st Street
Indianapolis, IN 46206-1367
Emergency Phone: (800) 222-1222
TDD/TTY: (317) 962-2336 (TTY)

IOWA
Iowa Statewide Poison Control Center
St. Luke's Regional Medical Center
2720 Stone Park Boulevard
Sioux City, IA 51104
Emergency Phone: (800) 222-1222

KANSAS
Mid-America Poison Control Center
University of Kansas Medical Center
3901 Rainbow Blvd., Room B-400
Kansas City, KS 66160-7231
Emergency Phone: (800) 222-1222
TDD/TTY: (913) 588-6639 (TDD)

KENTUCKY
Kentucky Regional Poison Center
Medical Towers South, Suite 572
234 East Gray Street
Louisville, KY 40202
Emergency Phone: (800) 222-1222

LOUISIANA
**Louisiana Drug and Poison Information
   Center**
University of Louisiana at Monroe
College of Pharmacy
Sugar Hall
Monroe, LA 71209-6430
Emergency Phone: (800) 222-1222

MAINE
Northern New England Poison
22 Bramhall Street
Portland, ME 04102
Emergency Phone: (800) 222-1222
TDD/TTY: (877) 299-4447 (ME only)
        (207) 871-2879

MARYLAND
Maryland Poison Center
University of MD at Baltimore
School of Pharmacy
20 North Pine Street, PH 772
Baltimore, MD 21201
Emergency Phone: (800) 222-1222
TDD/TTY: (410) 706-1858 (TDD)

National Capital Poison Center
Montgomery and Prince Georges Counties
   only
3201 New Mexico Avenue, NW
Suite 310
Washington, DC 20016
Emergency Phone & TDD/TTY: (800) 222-1222

MASSACHUSETTS
**Regional Center for Poison Control and
   Prevention Serving Massachusetts &
   Rhode Island**
300 Longwood Avenue
Boston, MA 02115
Emergency Phone: (800) 222-1222
TDD/TTY: (888) 244-5313

MICHIGAN
Children's Hospital of Michigan
Regional Poison Control Center
4160 John R Harper Professional Office
   Building
Suite 616
Detroit, MI 48201
Emergency Phone: (800) 222-1222
TDD/TTY: (800) 356-3232 (TDD)

**DeVos Children's Hospital Regional
   Poison Center**
1300 Michigan, NE
Suite 203
Grand Rapids, MI 49506-2968
Emergency Phone: (800) 222-1222
(Voice and TTY)

MINNESOTA
Hennepin Regional Poison Center
Hennepin County Medical Center
701 Park Avenue
Minneapolis, MN 55415
Emergency Phone: (800) 222-1222
TDD/TTY: (800) 222-1222 (Voice and TTY)

MISSISSIPPI
Mississippi Regional Poison Control Center
University of Mississippi Medical Center
2500 N. State Street
Jackson, MS 39216
Emergency Phone: (800) 222-1222

MISSOURI
Missouri Regional Poison Center
7980 Clayton Rd
Suite 200
St. Louis, MO 63117
Emergency Phone: (800) 222-1222
TDD/TTY: (314) 612-5705

MONTANA
Rocky Mountain Poison & Drug Ctr
777 Bannock Street
Mail Code 0180
Denver, CO 80204-4028
Emergency Phone: (800) 222-1222
(800) 525-5042 (MT only)
TDD/TTY: (303) 739-1127

NEBRASKA
Nebraska Regional Poison Center
8401 W. Dodge Rd, Ste 115
Omaha, NE 68114
Emergency Phone: (800) 222-1222

NEVADA
**Northern Nevada
Oregon Poison Center**
Oregon Health Sciences University
3181 SW Sam Jackson Park Road
CB550
Portland, OR 97201
Emergency Phone: (800) 222-1222
(Voice and TTY/TDD)

**Southern Nevada
Rocky Mountain Poison & Drug Ctr**
777 Bannock Street
Mail Code 0180
Denver, CO 80204-4028
Emergency Phone: (800) 222-1222
(800) 446-6179 (NV only)
TDD/TTY: (303) 739-1127

NEW HAMPSHIRE
New Hampshire Poison Information Center
Dartmouth-Hitchcock Medical Center
One Medical Center Drive
Lebanon, NH 03756
Emergency Phone: (800) 222-1222
TTY/TDD (877) 299-4447 (ME only)
   (207) 871-2879

NEW JERSEY
**New Jersey Poison Information and
   Education System**
located at Univ of Medicine and Dentistry of
   New Jersey
65 Bergen Street
Newark, NJ 07107-3001
Emergency Phone: (800) 222-1222
TDD/TTY: (973) 926-8008

NEW MEXICO
**New Mexico Poison & Drug Information
   Center**
MSC09 5080
University of New Mexico
Albuquerque, NM 87131-0001
Emergency Phone: (800) 222-1222

NEW YORK
Central New York Poison Center
750 East Adams Street
Syracuse, NY 13210
Emergency Phone: (800) 222-1222

**Finger Lakes Regional Poison & Drug Info
   Center**
University of Rochester Medical Center
601 Elmwood Avenue
Box 321
Rochester, NY 14642
Emergency Phone: (800) 222-1222
TDD/TTY: (585) 273-3854

**Long Island Regional Poison and Drug
   Information Center**
Winthrop University Hospital
259 First Street
Mineola, NY 11501
Emergency Phone: (800) 222-1222
TDD/TTY: (516) 924-8811 (TDD Suffolk)
        (516) 747-3323 (TDD Nassau)

New York City Poison Control Center
NYC Bureau of Labs
455 First Avenue
Room 123, Box 81
New York, NY 10016
Emergency Phone: (800) 222-1222
TDD/TTY: (212) 689-9014

**Western New York Regional Poison
   Control Center**
Children's Hospital of Buffalo
219 Bryant Street
Buffalo, NY 14222
Emergency Phone: (800) 222-1222

NORTH CAROLINA
Carolinas Poison Center
Carolinas Medical Center
5000 Airport Center Parkway, Suite B
Charlotte, NC 28208
Emergency Phone: (800) 222-1222

NORTH DAKOTA
Hennepin Regional Poison Center
Hennepin County Medical Center
701 Park Avenue
Minneapolis, MN 55415
Emergency Phone: (800) 222-1222
TDD/TTY: (800) 222-1222
        (612) 904-4691 (TTY)

OHIO
Central Ohio Poison Center
700 Children's Drive, Room L032
Columbus, OH 43205
Emergency Phone: (800) 222-1222
TDD/TTY: (614) 228-2272 (TTY)

**Cincinnati Drug & Poison Information
   Center**
Regional Poison Control System
3333 Burnet Avenue
Vernon Place - 3rd Floor
Cincinnati, OH 45229
Emergency Phone: (800) 222-1222
TDD/TTY: (800) 253-7955

Greater Cleveland Poison Control Center
11100 Euclid Avenue
Cleveland, OH 44106-6010
Emergency Phone: (800) 222-1222

OKLAHOMA
Oklahoma Poison Control Center
Children's Hospital at OU Medical Center
940 N.E. 13th Street
Room 3510
Oklahoma City, OK 73104
Emergency Phone: (800) 222-1222
(Voice and TDD/TTY)

OREGON
Oregon Poison Center
Oregon Health Sciences University
3181 SW Sam Jackson Park Road
CB550
Portland, OR 97201
Emergency Phone: (800) 222-1222
(Voice and TTY/TDD)

PENNSYLVANIA
Pittsburgh Poison Center
Children's Hospital of Pittsburgh
3705 Fifth Avenue
Pittsburgh, PA 15213
Emergency Phone: (800) 222-1222

The Poison Control Center
Children's Hospital of Philadelphia
3400 Civic Center Blvd
Philadelphia, PA 19104-4303
Emergency Phone: (800) 222-1222
TDD/TTY: (215) 590-8789

PUERTO RICO
Puerto Rico Poison Center
Calle San Jorge #252
Santurce, Puerto Rico 00912
Emergency Phone: (800) 222-1222

RHODE ISLAND
Regional Center for Poison Control and Prevention
Serving Massachusetts and Rhode Island
300 Longwood Avenue
Boston, MA 02115
Emergency Phone: (800) 222-1222
TDD/TTY: (888) 244-5313

SOUTH CAROLINA
Palmetto Poison Center
College of Pharmacy
University of South Carolina
Columbia, SC 29208
Emergency Phone: (800) 222-1222

SOUTH DAKOTA
Hennepin Regional Poison Center
Hennepin County Medical Center
701 Park Avenue
Minneapolis, MN 55415
Emergency Phone: (800) 222-1222
(Voice and TDD/TTY)

TENNESSEE
Middle Tennessee Poison Center
501 Oxford House
1161 21st Avenue South
Nashville, TN 37232-4632
Emergency Phone: (800) 222-1222
TDD/TTY: (615) 936-2047

TEXAS
Central Texas Poison Center
Scott and White Memorial Hospital
2401 South 31st Street
Temple, TX 76508
Emergency Phone: (800) 222-1222

North Texas Poison Center
Parkland Memorial Hospital
5201 Harry Hines Blvd.
Dallas, TX 75235
Emergency Phone: (800) 222-1222

South Texas Poison Center
The Univ of Texas Health Science Ctr - San Antonio
Department of Surgery
Mail Code 7849
7703 Floyd Curl Drive
San Antonio, TX 78229-3900
Emergency Phone: (800) 222-1222
(Voice and TTY/TDD)

Southeast Texas Poison Center
The University of Texas Medical Branch
3.112 Trauma Building
Galveston, TX 77555-1175
Emergency Phone: (800) 222-1222

Texas Panhandle Poison Center
1501 S. Coulter
Amarillo, TX 79106
Emergency Phone: (800) 222-1222

West Texas Regional Poison Center
Thomason Hospital
4815 Alameda Avenue
El Paso, TX 79905
Emergency Phone: (800) 222-1222

UTAH
Utah Poison Control Center
585 Komas Drive, Suite 200
Salt Lake City, UT 84108
Emergency Phone: (800) 222-1222

VERMONT
Northern New England Poison Center
22 Bramhall Street
Portland, ME 04102
Emergency Phone: (800) 222-1222
TDD/TTY: (877) 299-4474 (ME only)
(207) 871-2879

VIRGINIA
Blue Ridge Poison Center
Jefferson Park Place
1222 Jefferson Park Avenue
Charlottesville, VA 22903
Emergency Phone: (800) 222-1222

National Capital Poison Center
3201 New Mexico Avenue, NW
Suite 310
Washington, DC 20016
Emergency Phone: (800) 222-1222
(Voice and TTY/TDD)

Virginia Poison Center
Medical College of Virginia Hospitals
Virginia Commonwealth University
P.O. Box 980522
Richmond, VA 23298-0522
Emergency Phone: (800) 222-1222

WASHINGTON
Washington Poison Center
155 NE 100th Street, Suite 400
Seattle, WA 98125-8012
Emergency Phone: (800) 222-1222
TDD/TTY: (206) 517-2394 (TDD)
(800) 572-0638 (TDD WA only)

WEST VIRGINIA
West Virginia Poison Center
3110 MacCorkle Ave, S.E.
Charleston, WV 25304
Emergency Phone: (800) 222-1222

WISCONSIN
Children's Hospital of Wisconsin Poison Center
PO Box 1997, Mail Station 677A
Milwaukee, WI 53201-1997
Emergency Phone: (800) 222-1222
TDD/TTY: (414) 266-2542

WYOMING
Nebraska Regional Poison Center
Children's Hospital
8200 Dodge Street
Omaha, NE 68114
Emergency Phone: (800) 222-1222

ANIMAL POISON CONTROL

ASPCA Animal Poison Control Center
Animal Poison Control Center
1717 South Philo Road, Suite 36
Urbana, IL 61802
Emergency Phone: (888) 426-4435

CANADA
Source: Canadian Poison Control Centres.

ALBERTA
Foothills Medical Center
1403 29th Street N.W.
Calgary, AB T2N 2T9
1-800-332-1414 toll-free
(403) 944-1414 local
(403) 944-1472 fax

BRITISH COLUMBIA
**British Columbia Drug and Poison
 Information Centre**
St. Paul's Hospital
1081 Burrard Street
Vancouver, B.C. V6Z 1Y6
1-800-567-8911 toll-free
(604) 682-5050 Greater Vancouver & lower
 mainland
(604) 631-5262 fax

MANITOBA
Provincial Poison Information Centre
Children's Hospital Health Science Centre
840 Sherbrook Street
Winnipeg. MB R3A 1S1
(204) 787-2591 local
(204) 787-1775 fax

NEW BRUNSWICK
Poison Information Centre
Clinidata
774 Main St. 6th floor
Moncton, NB E1C 9Y3
(506) 857-5555
(506) 867-3259 fax

NEWFOUNDLAND
Poison Control Centre
The Janeway Child Health Centre
710 Janeway Place
St. John's, NF A1A 1R8
(709) 722-1110
(709) 726-0830 fax

NOVA SCOTIA / PEI
Poison Control Centre
**The IWK/Grace Health Care
 Centre**
P.O. Box 3070
Halifax, NS B3J 3G9
1-800-565-8161
(902) 470-8161
(902) 470-7213 fax

ONTARIO
**Ontario Regional Poison Information
 Centre**
Children's Hospital of Eastern Ontario
401 Smyth Road
Ottawa, ON K1V 8L1
1-800-267-1373 toll-free
(613) 737-1100 local
(613) 738-4862 fax

**Ontario Regional Poison Information
 Centre**
The Hospital for Sick Children
555 University Avenue
Toronto, ON M5G 1X8
1-800-268-9017 toll-free
(416) 598-5900 local
(416) 813-7489 fax

QUEBEC
Centre Anti-Poison du Québec
1050 Chemin Ste-Foy, 1er étage
Quebec, QC G1S 4L8
1-800-463-5060 Toll-free
(418) 656-8090 local
(418) 654-2747 fax

SASKATCHEWAN
Saskatchewan Poison Centre
(866) 454-1212

Appendix III

PREGNANCY PRECAUTION LISTING

The following medicines, selected from those included in this publication, have specific precautions in regard to use during pregnancy. For specific information, consult the individual drug entry; look in the index for the page number.

The use of any medicine during pregnancy must be carefully considered. The physician and the patient must balance the expected benefits against the possible risks.

Absence of a drug from the list is not meant to imply that it is safe for use in pregnant patients. For many drugs, it is not known whether a problem exists; experimentation on pregnant women is generally not done. Knowledge is usually gained only from the accumulated experience over many years in giving a drug to pregnant women who needed its benefits. Also, well-planned studies in pregnant animals may reveal problems, although the relation of such findings to pregnant humans and their babies may not be known. Problems suggested by animal studies are often included in the warnings in this book.

Readers are reminded that the information in this text is selected and not considered to be complete.

A

Abarelix (Intramuscular Route)
Abciximab (Intravenous Route)
Acamprosate (Oral Route)
Acarbose (Oral Route)
Acenocoumarol (Systemic)
Acetaminophen and Codeine (Systemic)
Acetaminophen, Aspirin, and Caffeine (Systemic)
Acetaminophen, Aspirin, and Caffeine, Buffered (Systemic)
Acetaminophen, Aspirin, Salicylamide, and Caffeine (Systemic)
Acetaminophen, Codeine, and Caffeine (Systemic)
Acetaminophen, Salicylamide, and Caffeine (Systemic)
Acetazolamide (Systemic)
Acetylcysteine (Inhalation, Oral/Nebulization Route)
Acitretin (Oral Route)
Acrivastine and Pseudoephedrine (Systemic)
Acyclovir (Oral Route, Intravenous Route)
Acyclovir (Topical Route)
Adalimumab (Subcutaneous Route)
Adapalene (Topical Route)
Adefovir Dipivoxil (Oral Route)
Agalsidase Beta (Intravenous Route)
Albendazole (Oral Route)
Albuterol (Inhalation)
Albuterol (Oral/Injection)
Alclometasone (Topical)
Aldesleukin (Intravenous Route)
Alefacept (Intravenous Route, Intramuscular Route)
Alemtuzumab (Intravenous Route)
Alendronate (Oral Route)
Alfacalcidol (Systemic)
Alfentanil (Systemic)
Alfuzosin (Oral Route)
Alglucerase (Intravenous Route)
Allopurinol (Intravenous Route)
Almotriptan (Oral Route)
Alosetron (Oral Route)
Alpha-1 Proteinase Inhibitor Human (Intravenous Route)
Alprazolam (Systemic)

Alprostadil (Intraurethral Route, Intravenous Route, Intracavernosal Route)
Alteplase, Recombinant (Systemic)
Altretamine (Oral Route)
Alumina and Magnesia (Oral)
Alumina and Magnesium Carbonate (Oral)
Alumina and Magnesium Trisilicate (Oral)
Alumina, Magnesia, and Magnesium Carbonate (Oral)
Alumina, Magnesia, and Simethicone (Oral)
Alumina, Magnesia, Calcium Carbonate, and Simethicone (Oral)
Alumina, Magnesium Alginate, and Magnesium Carbonate (Oral)
Alumina, Magnesium Carbonate, and Simethicone (Oral)
Alumina, Magnesium Trisilicate, and Sodium Bicarbonate (Oral)
Aluminum Carbonate, Basic (Oral)
Aluminum Hydroxide (Oral)
Amantadine (Oral Route)
Ambenonium (Systemic)
Amcinonide (Topical)
Amifostine (Intravenous Route)
Amikacin (Systemic)
Amiloride (Systemic)
Amiloride and Hydrochlorothiazide (Systemic)
Aminoglutethimide (Oral Route)
Aminolevulinic Acid (Topical Route)
Aminophylline (Systemic)
Aminosalicylate Sodium (Oral Route)
Amiodarone (Intravenous Route)
Amitriptyline (Systemic)
Amlexanox (Mucous Membrane, Oral Route)
Amlodipine (Oral Route)
Amobarbital (Systemic)
Amoxapine (Systemic)
Amphetamine (Systemic)
Amphotericin B (Intravenous Route, Injection Route)
Amphotericin B Cholesteryl Sulfate Complex (Intravenous Route)
Amphotericin B Lipid Complex (Intravenous Route, Injection Route)
Amphotericin B Liposome (Intravenous Route)

Amprenavir (Oral Route)
Anagrelide (Oral Route)
Anakinra (Subcutaneous Route)
Anastrozole (Oral Route)
Anidulafungin (Intravenous Route)
Anisindione (Systemic)
Anistreplase (Systemic)
Anthralin (Topical Route)
Antihemophilic Factor (Intravenous Route, Injection Route)
Antithymocyte Globulin Rabbit (Intravenous Route)
Antivenin (Crotalidae) Polyvalent Immune Fab (Intravenous Route)
Apomorphine (Injection Route)
Apraclonidine (Ophthalmic Route)
Aprepitant (Oral Route)
Aprobarbital (Systemic)
Ardeparin (Subcutaneous Route)
Aripiprazole (Oral Route)
Articaine (Parenteral-Local)
Ascorbic Acid (Oral Route)
Asparaginase (Injection Route)
Aspirin (Systemic)
Aspirin and Caffeine (Systemic)
Aspirin and Caffeine, Buffered (Systemic)
Aspirin and Codeine (Systemic)
Aspirin, Buffered (Systemic)
Aspirin, Caffeine, and Dihydrocodeine (Systemic)
Aspirin, Codeine, and Caffeine (Systemic)
Aspirin, Codeine, and Caffeine, Buffered (Systemic)
Aspirin, Sodium Bicarbonate, And Citric Acid (Oral Route)
Atazanavir Sulfate (Oral Route)
Atenolol and Chlorthalidone (Systemic)
Atomoxetine (Oral Route)
Atorvastatin (Oral Route)
Atovaquone (Oral Route)
Atropine (Systemic)
Atropine and Phenobarbital (Systemic)
Atropine, Hyoscyamine, Methenamine, Methylene Blue, Phenyl Salicylate, And Benzoic Acid (Oral Route)
Atropine, Hyoscyamine, Scopolamine, and Phenobarbital (Systemic)
Auranofin (Systemic)
Aurothioglucose (Systemic)

Azacitidine (Subcutaneous Route)
Azatadine and Pseudoephedrine (Systemic)
Azathioprine (Oral Route, Intravenous Route)
Azelaic Acid (Topical Route)
Azelastine (Nasal Route)
Azelastine (Ophthalmic Route)
Azithromycin (Intravenous Route)
Aztreonam (Intravenous Route, Injection Route)

B

Bacillus Of Calmette And Guerin Vaccine, Live (Intradermal Route)
Bacillus Of Calmette And Guerin Vaccine, Live (Intravesical Route)
Baclofen (Intrathecal Route)
Baclofen (Oral Route)
Balsalazide (Oral Route)
Basiliximab (Intravenous Route)
Beclomethasone (Inhalation)
Beclomethasone (Topical)
Belladonna and Butabarbital (Systemic)
Belladonna and Phenobarbital (Systemic)
Benazepril and Hydrochlorothiazide (Systemic)
Bendroflumethiazide (Systemic)
Benzonatate (Oral Route)
Benzphetamine (Systemic)
Benzthiazide (Systemic)
Bepridil (Systemic)
Betaine (Oral Route)
Betamethasone (Ophthalmic)
Betamethasone (Otic)
Betamethasone (Rectal)
Betamethasone (Systemic)
Betamethasone (Topical)
Betaxolol (Ophthalmic)
Bethanechol (Oral Route, Subcutaneous Route)
Bevacizumab (Intravenous Route)
Bexarotene (Oral Route)
Bexarotene (Topical Route)
Bicalutamide (Systemic)
Bimatoprost (Ophthalmic Route)
Bisprolol and Hydrochlorothiazide (Systemic)
Bitolterol (Inhalation)
Bleomycin (Injection Route)
Bortezomib (Intravenous Route)
Bosentan (Oral Route)
Botulinum Toxin Type A (Intramuscular Route)
Botulinum Toxin Type B (Intramuscular Route)
Brimonidine (Ophthalmic Route)
Brinzolamide (Ophthalmic Route)
Bromazepam (Systemic)
Bromfenac (Ophthalmic Route)
Bromocriptine (Oral Route)
Bromodipheniramine (Systemic)
Brompheniramine (Systemic)
Brompheniramine and Phenylephrine (Systemic)
Brompheniramine and Pseudoephedrine (Systemic)

Brompheniramine, Pseudoephedrine, and Acetaminophen
Brompheniramine, Pseudoephedrine, and Dextromethorphan (Systemic)
Budesonide (Inhalation)
Budesonide (Rectal)
Budesonide (Systemic)
Budesonide/Formoterol (Inhalation Route)
Bupivacaine (Parenteral-Local)
Buprenorphine (Systemic)
Bupropion (Oral Route)
Buspirone (Oral Route)
Busulfan (Intravenous Route)
Butabarbital (Systemic)
Butalbital and Acetaminophen (Systemic)
Butalbital and Aspirin (Systemic)
Butalbital, Acetaminophen, and Caffeine (Systemic)
Butalbital, Acetaminophen, Caffeine, And Codeine (Oral Route)
Butalbital, Aspirin, and Caffeine (Systemic)
Butenafine (Topical Route)
Butoconazole (Vaginal)
Butorphanol (Nasal Route)
Butorphanol (Systemic)
Butorphenol (Systemic)

C

Cabergoline (Oral Route)
Caffeine (Systemic)
Caffeine and Sodium Benzoate (Systemic)
Caffeine, Citrated (Systemic)
Calcifediol (Systemic)
Calcipotriene (Topical Route)
Calcitonin (Salmon) (Nasal Route)
Calcitriol (Systemic)
Calcium Acetate (Oral Route)
Calcium and Magnesium Carbonates (Oral)
Calcium and Magnesium Carbonates and Sodium Bicarbonate (Oral)
Calcium Carbonate (Oral)
Calcium Carbonate and Magnesia (Oral)
Calcium Carbonate and Simethicone (Oral)
Calcium Carbonate, Magnesia, and Simethicone (Oral)
Candesartan Cilexetil (Oral Route)
Candesartan Cilexetil and Hydrochlorothiazide (Oral Route)
Capecitabine (Oral Route)
Capreomycin (Injection Route)
Captopril and Hydrochlorothiazide (Systemic)
Carbachol (Ophthalmic Route)
Carbamazepine (Oral Route)
Carbinoxamine and Pseudoephedrine (Systemic)
Carbinoxamine, Pseudoephedrine, and Dextromethorphan (Systemic)
Carboplatin (Intravenous Route)
Carboprost (Intramuscular Route)
Carmustine (Implantation Route)
Carmustine (Intravenous Route)

Carteolol (Ophthalmic)
Carvedilol (Oral Route)
Caspofungin (Intravenous Route)
Castor Oil (Oral)
Cefditoren Pivoxil (Oral Route)
Cefuroxime (Injection Route, Intravenous Route)
Celecoxib (Oral Route)
Cetirizine (Systemic)
Cetrorelix (Subcutaneous Route)
Cetuximab (Intravenous Route)
Cevimeline (Oral Route)
Chlorambucil (Oral Route)
Chlordiazepoxide (Systemic)
Chlorhexidine (Oral Route)
Chlorhexidine (Subgingival Route)
Chloroprocaine (Parenteral-Local)
Chloroquine (Oral Route, Intramuscular Route)
Chlorothiazide (Systemic)
Chloroxine (Topical Route)
Chlorpheniramine and Codeine (Systemic)
Chlorpheniramine and Dextromethorphan (Systemic)
Chlorpheniramine and Hydrocodone (Systemic)
Chlorpheniramine and Phenylephrine (Systemic)
Chlorpheniramine and Pseudoephedrine (Systemic)
Chlorpheniramine, Ephedrine, and Guaifenesin (Systemic)
Chlorpheniramine, Ephedrine, Phenylephrine, and Carbetapentane (Systemic)
Chlorpheniramine, Ephedrine, Phenylephrine, Dextromethorphan, Ammonium Chloride, and Ipecac (Systemic)
Chlorpheniramine, Pheniramine, Pyrilamine, Phenylephrine, Hydrocodone, Salicylamide, Caffeine, and Ascorbic Acid (Systemic)
Chlorpheniramine, Phenylephrine, and Acetaminophen (Systemic)
Chlorpheniramine, Phenylephrine, and Dextromethorphan (Systemic)
Chlorpheniramine, Phenylephrine, and Hydrocodone (Systemic)
Chlorpheniramine, Phenylephrine, and Methscopolamine (Systemic)
Chlorpheniramine, Phenylephrine, Codeine, and Ammonium Chloride (Systemic)
Chlorpheniramine, Phenylephrine, Codeine, and Potassium Iodide (Systemic)
Chlorpheniramine, Phenylephrine, Dextromethorphan, and Guaifenesin (Systemic)
Chlorpheniramine, Phenylephrine, Dextromethorphan, Guaifenesin, and Ammonium Chloride (Systemic)
Chlorpheniramine, Phenylephrine, Hydrocodone, Acetaminophen, and Caffeine (Systemic)
Chlorpheniramine, Phenyltoloxamine, and Phenylephrine (Systemic)

Chlorpheniramine, Phenyltoloxamine, Ephedrine, Codeine, and Guaiacol Carbonate (Systemic)

Chlorpheniramine, Pseudoephedrine, and Acetaminophen (Systemic)

Chlorpheniramine, Pseudoephedrine, and Codeine (Systemic)

Chlorpheniramine, Pseudoephedrine, and Dextromethorphan (Systemic)

Chlorpheniramine, Pseudoephedrine, and Hydrocodone (Systemic)

Chlorpheniramine, Pseudoephedrine, and Methscopolamine (Systemic)

Chlorpheniramine, Pseudoephedrine, Codeine, and Acetaminophen (Systemic)

Chlorpheniramine, Pseudoephedrine, Dextromethorphan, and Acetaminophen (Systemic)

Chlorpheniramine, Pseudoephedrine, Dextromethorphan, and Guaifenesin (Systemic)

Chlorpheniramine, Pyrilamine, and Phenylephrine (Systemic)

Chlorpheniramine, Pyrilamine, Phenylephrine, and Acetaminophen (Systemic)

Chlorpromazine (Systemic)

Chlorprothixene (Systemic)

Chlorthalidone (Systemic)

Cholera Vaccine (Injection Route)

Cholestyramine (Oral Route)

Choline and Magnesium Salicylates (Systemic)

Choline Salicylate (Systemic)

Chorionic Gonadotropin (Subcutaneous Route, Intramuscular Route, Injection Route)

Chromic Phosphate P 32 (Therapeutic)

Cidofovir (Intravenous Route)

Cilostazol (Oral Route)

Cinacalcet (Oral Route)

Cinoxacin (Oral Route)

Ciprofloxacin (Ophthalmic Route)

Cisapride (Oral Route)

Cisplatin (Intravenous Route)

Citalopram (Oral Route)

Cladribine (Intravenous Route)

Clarithromycin (Oral Route)

Clemastine (Systemic)

Clindamycin (Oral Route, Injection Route, Intravenous Route)

Clindamycin (Topical Route)

Clindamycin (Vaginal Route)

Clobazam (Systemic)

Clobetasol (Topical)

Clobetasone (Topical)

Clocortolone (Topical)

Clofarabine (Intravenous Route)

Clofazimine (Oral Route)

Clofibrate (Oral Route)

Clomiphene (Oral Route)

Clomipramine (Systemic)

Clonazepam (Systemic)

Clonidine (Epidural Route)

Clonidine (Oral Route, Transdermal Route)

Clopidogrel (Oral Route)

Clorazepate (Systemic)

Clotrimazole (Mucous Membrane, Oral Route)

Clotrimazole (Topical Route)

Clotrimazole (Vaginal)

Clozapine (Oral Route)

Cocaine (Topical Route)

Codeine (Systemic)

Codeine and Guaifenesin (Systemic)

Codeine, Ammonium Chloride, and Guaifenesin (Systemic)

Colchicine (Oral Route, Intravenous Route)

Colesevelam (Oral Route)

Colistin Sulfate, Neomycin Sulfate, Hydrocortisone Acetate, And Thonzonium Bromide (Otic Route)

Conjugated Estrogens and Medroxyprogesterone (Systemic)

Conjugated Estrogens, and Conjugated Estrogens and Medroxyprogesterone (Systemic)

Cortisone (Systemic)

Cromolyn (Inhalation, Oral/Nebulization Route)

Cromolyn (Nasal Route)

Cromolyn (Oral Route)

Crotamiton (Topical Route)

Cyanocobalamin Co 57 (Diagnostic)

Cyclobenzaprine (Oral Route)

Cyclopentolate (Ophthalmic Route)

Cyclophosphamide (Oral Route, Intravenous Route)

Cycloserine (Oral Route)

Cyclosporine (Oral Route, Intravenous Route)

Cyclothiazide (Systemic)

Cyproheptadine (Systemic)

Cysteamine (Oral Route)

Cytarabine (Oral Route)

Cytarabine Liposome (Intrathecal Route)

D

Dacarbazine (Intravenous Route, Injection Route)

Daclizumab (Intravenous Route)

Dactinomycin (Intravenous Route)

Dalteparin (Subcutaneous Route, Injection Route)

Danaparoid (Subcutaneous Route)

Danazol (Oral Route)

Dantrolene (Oral Route, Intravenous Route)

Dapiprazole (Ophthalmic Route)

Dapsone (Oral Route)

Dapsone (Topical Route)

Daptomycin (Intravenous Route)

Darbepoetin Alfa (Injection Route)

Darifenacin (Oral Route)

Daunorubicin (Intravenous Route)

Daunorubicin Citrate Liposome (Intravenous Route)

Deferoxamine (Injection Route)

Delavirdine (Oral Route)

Demecarium (Ophthalmic)

Demeclocycline (Systemic)

Denileukin Diftitox (Intravenous Route)

Deserpidine (Systemic)

Deserpidine and Hydrochlorothiazide (Systemic)

Deserpidine and Methyclothiazide (Systemic)

Desflurane (Inhalation, Oral/Nebulization Route)

Desipramine (Systemic)

Desloratadine (Oral Route)

Desloratadine And Pseudoephedrine (Oral Route)

Desmopressin (Nasal Route, Oral Route, Injection Route)

Desogestrel and Ethinyl Estradiol (Systemic)

Desonide (Topical)

Desoximetasone (Topical)

Dexamethasone (Inhalation)

Dexamethasone (Nasal)

Dexamethasone (Ophthalmic)

Dexamethasone (Otic)

Dexamethasone (Topical)

Dexbrompheniramine and Pseudoephedrine (Systemic)

Dexbrompheniramine, Pseudoephedrine, and Acetaminophen (Systemic)

Dexchlorpheniramine (Systemic)

Dexmethylphenidate (Oral Route)

Dexrazoxane (Intravenous Route)

Dextroamphetamine (Systemic)

Dextromethorphan and Acetaminophen (Systemic)

Dextromethorphan and Guaifenesin (Systemic)

Diatrizoate and Iodipamide (Diagnostic, Local)

Diatrizoates (Diagnostic)

Diatrizoates Meglumine (Local)

Diatrizoates Sodium (Local)

Diazepam (Systemic)

Diazoxide (Oral Route)

Dichlorphenamide (Systemic)

Diclofenac (Ophthalmic)

Diclofenac (Systemic)

Diclofenac (Topical Route)

Diclofenac And Misoprostol (Oral Route)

Dicumarol (Systemic)

Dicyclomine (Systemic)

Didanosine (Oral Route)

Dienestrol (Vaginal)

Diethylpropion (Systemic)

Diethylstilbestrol (Systemic)

Diethylstilbestrol and Methyltestosterone (Systemic)

Difenoxin And Atropine (Oral Route)

Diflorasone (Topical)

Diflucortolone (Topical)

Diflunisal (Systemic)

Digitoxin (Systemic)

Digoxin (Systemic)

Dihydrocodeine, Acetaminophen, and Caffeine (Systemic)

Dihydroergotamine (Systemic)

Dihydrotachysterol (Systemic)

Diltiazem (Systemic)
Dimenhydrinate (Systemic)
Dimethyl Sulfoxide (Intravesical Route)
Dinoprostone (Vaginal Route)
Diphenhydramine (Systemic)
Diphenhydramine and Pseudoephedrine (Systemic)
Diphenhydramine, Codeine, and Ammonium Chloride (Systemic)
Diphenhydramine, Dextromethorphan, and Ammonium Chloride (Systemic)
Diphenhydramine, Pseudoephedrine, and Acetaminophen (Systemic)
Diphenoxylate And Atropine (Oral Route)
Diphtheria and Tetanus Toxoids and Pertussis Vaccine Adsorbed and Haemophilus B Conjugate Vaccine (Systemic)
Diphtheria and Tetanus Toxoids for Adult Use (Systemic)
Diphtheria and Tetanus Toxoids for Pediatric Use (Systemic)
Diphtheria Toxoid, Tetanus Toxoid, And Acellular Pertussis Vaccine (Intramuscular Route)
Dipivefrin (Ophthalmic Route)
Dipyridamole (Oral Route, Intravenous Route)
Dirithromycin (Oral Route)
Disopyramide (Oral Route)
Divalproex (Systemic)
Docetaxel (Intravenous Route)
Dofetilide (Oral Route)
Dolasetron (Oral Route, Intravenous Route)
Donepezil (Oral Route)
Dorzolamide (Ophthalmic Route)
Doxazosin (Oral Route)
Doxepin (Systemic)
Doxepin (Topical Route)
Doxorubicin (Intravenous Route)
Doxycycline (Oral Route)
Doxycycline (Subgingival Route)
Doxylamine, Codeine, and Acetaminophen (Systemic)
Doxylamine, Etafedrine, and Hydrocone (Systemic)
Doxylamine, Pseudoephedrine, Dextromethorphan, and Acetaminophen (Systemic)
Dronabinol (Oral Route)
Droperidol (Injection Route)
Drospirenone And Estradiol (Oral Route)
Drospirenone And Ethinyl Estradiol (Oral Route)
Drotrecogin Alfa (Intravenous Route)
Duloxetine (Oral Route)
Dutasteride (Oral Route)
Dyphylline (Oral Route, Intramuscular Route)

E

Echothiophate (Ophthalmic)
Econazole (Vaginal)
Efalizumab (Subcutaneous Route)

Efavirenz (Oral Route)
Efavirenz/Emtricitabine/Tenofovir (Oral Route)
Eflornithine (Injection Route)
Eletriptan (Oral Route)
Emedastine (Ophthalmic Route)
Emtricitabine (Oral Route)
Enalapril and Hydrochlorothiazide (Systemic)
Enflurane (Systemic)
Enfuvirtide (Subcutaneous Route)
Enoxaparin (Subcutaneous Route)
Entacapone (Oral Route)
Entecavir (Oral Route)
Ephedrine and Guaifenesin (Systemic)
Epinastine (Ophthalmic Route)
Epinephrine (Inhalation)
Epinephrine (Oral/Injection)
Epirubicin (Intravenous Route, Injection Route)
Eplerenone (Oral Route)
Epoprostenol (Intravenous Route)
Eprosartan (Oral Route)
Eptacog Alfa (Intravenous Route)
Ergocalciferol (Systemic)
Ergonovine (Systemic)
Ergotamine (Systemic)
Ergotamine and Caffeine (Systemic)
Ergotamine, Caffeine, and Belladonna Alkaloids (Systemic)
Ergotamine, Caffeine, and Cyclizine (Systemic)
Ergotamine, Caffeine, and Dimenhydrinate (Systemic)
Ergotamine, Caffeine, and Diphenhydramine (Systemic)
Ergotamine, Caffeine, Belladonna Alkaloids, and Pentobarbital (Systemic)
Erlotinib (Oral Route)
Ertapenem (Injection Route)
Erythromycin And Sulfisoxazole (Oral Route)
Erythromycin Estolate (Systemic)
Erythropoietin (Injection Route)
Escitalopram (Oral Route)
Esomeprazole (Oral Route)
Estazolam (Systemic)
Estradiol (Systemic)
Estradiol (Vaginal)
Estrogens, Conjugated (Systemic)
Estrogens, Conjugated (Vaginal)
Estrogens, Conjugated, and Methyltestosterone (Systemic)
Estrogens, Esterified (Systemic)
Estrogens, Esterified, and Methyltestosterone (Systemic)
Estrone (Systemic)
Estrone (Vaginal)
Estropipate (Systemic)
Estropipate (Vaginal)
Eszopiclone (Oral Route)
Etanercept (Subcutaneous Route)
Ethambutol (Oral Route)
Ethchlorvynol (Oral Route)
Ethinyl Estradiol (Systemic)

Ethinyl Estradiol And Norelgestromin (Transdermal Route)
Ethionamide (Oral Route)
Ethosuximide (Systemic)
Ethotoin (Systemic)
Ethynodiol Diacetate and Ethinyl Estradiol (Systemic)
Etidocaine (Parenteral-Local)
Etidronate (Oral Route, Intravenous Route)
Etodolac (Systemic)
Etomidate (Systemic)
Etoposide (Oral Route, Intravenous Route)
Exemestane (Oral Route)
Exenatide (Subcutaneous Route)
Ezetimibe (Oral Route)

F

Factor IX Complex (Intravenous Route, Injection Route)
Famciclovir (Oral Route)
Fat Emulsion (Intravenous Route, Injection Route)
Felbamate (Oral Route)
Felodipine (Systemic)
Fenofibrate (Oral Route)
Fenoprofen (Systemic)
Fentanyl (Buccal Route)
Fentanyl (Transdermal Route)
Ferrous Citrate Fe 59 (Diagnostic)
Ferumoxides (Diagnostic)
Fexofenadine (Oral Route)
Finasteride (Oral Route)
Flavoxate (Oral Route)
Flecainide (Oral Route)
Floctafenine (Systemic)
Floxuridine (Injection Route)
Fluconazole (Systemic)
Flucytosine (Oral Route)
Fludarabine (Oral Route)
Fludrocortisone (Oral Route)
Flumethasone (Topical)
Flunarizine (Systemic)
Flunisolide (Inhalation)
Fluocinolone (Topical)
Fluocinonide (Topical)
Fluorometholone (Ophthalmic)
Fluorouracil (Intravenous Route, Injection Route)
Fluorouracil (Topical Route)
Fluoxetine (Oral Route)
Fluoxymesterone (Systemic)
Fluoxymesterone and Ethinyl Estradiol (Systemic)
Flupenthixol (Systemic)
Fluphenazine (Systemic)
Flurandrenolide (Topical)
Flurazepam (Systemic)
Flurbiprofen (Ophthalmic)
Flurbiprofen (Systemic)
Flutamide (Systemic)
Fluticasone (Inhalation, Oral/Nebulization Route)
Fluticasone (Nasal Route)

Fluticasone (Topical)
Fluvoxamine (Oral Route)
Follitropin Alfa (Subcutaneous Route)
Follitropin Beta (Subcutaneous Route)
Fomivirsen (Intraocular Route)
Fondaparinux (Subcutaneous Route)
Formoterol (Inhalation, Oral/Nebulization Route)
Fosamprenavir (Oral Route)
Foscarnet (Intravenous Route)
Fosfomycin (Oral Route)
Fosphenytoin (Systemic)
Frovatriptan (Oral Route)
Fructose, Dextrose, And Phosphoric Acid (Oral Route)
Fulvestrant (Intramuscular Route)
Furazolidone (Oral Route)

G

Gabapentin (Oral Route)
Gadodiamide (Diagnostic)
Gadopentetate (Diagnostic)
Gadoteridol (Diagnostic)
Gadoversetamide (Diagnostic)
Galantamine (Oral Route)
Gallium Citrate Ga 67 (Diagnostic)
Gallium Nitrate (Intravenous Route)
Ganciclovir (Oral Route, Intravenous Route)
Ganirelix (Subcutaneous Route)
Gatifloxacin (Ophthalmic Route)
Gefitinib (Oral Route)
Gemcitabine (Intravenous Route)
Gemfibrozil (Oral Route)
Gemifloxacin (Oral Route)
Gemtuzumab Ozogamicin (Intravenous Route)
Gentamicin (Ophthalmic Route)
Gentamicin (Systemic)
Glatiramer Acetate (Subcutaneous Route)
Glipizide And Metformin (Oral Route)
Glucagon (Injection Route)
Glutamine (Oral Route)
Glyburide And Metformin (Oral Route)
Glycerin (Oral Route)
Glycopyrrolate (Systemic)
Gold Sodium Thiomalate (Systemic)
Gonadorelin (Intravenous Route, Injection Route)
Goserelin (Subcutaneous Route)
Granisetron (Oral Route, Intravenous Route)
Guaifenesin (Oral Route)
Guanabenz (Oral Route)
Guanadrel (Oral Route)
Guanethidine (Oral Route)
Guanfacine (Oral Route)

H

Haemophilus B Polysaccharide Vaccine (Intramuscular Route, Injection Route)
Halazepam (Systemic)
Halcinonide (Topical)
Halobetasol (Topical)

Halofantrine (Oral Route)
Haloperidol (Oral Route, Intramuscular Route, Injection Route)
Halothane (Systemic)
Heparin (Intravenous Route, Injection Route)
Hepatitis A Vaccine Inactivated And Hepatitis B Vaccine Recombinant (Intramuscular Route)
Hepatitis A Vaccine, Inactivated (Intramuscular Route)
Hepatitis B Immune Globulin (Intramuscular Route)
Hepatitis B Vaccine Recombinant (Intramuscular Route)
Histrelin (Implantation Route)
Hyaluronidase (Subcutaneous Route, Injection Route)
Hydralazine (Oral Route, Injection Route, Intravenous Route)
Hydralazine And Hydrochlorothiazide (Oral Route)
Hydrochlorothiazide (Systemic)
Hydrocodone (Systemic)
Hydrocodone and Acetaminophen (Systemic)
Hydrocodone and Aspirin (Systemic)
Hydrocodone and Guaifenesin (Systemic)
Hydrocodone and Homatropine (Systemic)
Hydrocodone and Potassium Guaiacolsulfonate (Systemic)
Hydrocortisone (Dental)
Hydrocortisone (Ophthalmic)
Hydrocortisone (Rectal)
Hydrocortisone (Systemic)
Hydrocortisone (Topical)
Hydrocortisone Acetate (Topical)
Hydrocortisone And Acetic Acid (Otic Route)
Hydrocortisone Butyrate (Topical)
Hydrocortisone Valerate (Topical)
Hydroflumethiazide (Systemic)
Hydromorphone (Systemic)
Hydroxyprogesterone (Systemic)
Hydroxyurea (Oral Route)
Hydroxyzine (Systemic)
Hyoscyamine (Systemic)
Hyoscyamine and Phenobarbital (Systemic)

I

Ibandronate (Oral Route, Injection Route)
Ibritumomab Tiuxetan (Intravenous Route)
Ibuprofen (Systemic)
Idarubicin (Intravenous Route)
Idursulfase (Intravenous Route)
Ifosfamide (Intravenous Route)
Iloprost (Inhalation, Oral/Nebulization Route)
Imatinib (Oral Route)
Imiglucerase (Intravenous Route)
Imipenem And Cilastatin (Intravenous Route, Intramuscular Route)
Imipramine (Systemic)

Imiquimod (Topical Route)
Immune Globulin (Intramuscular Route, Intravenous Route, Injection Route)
Inamrinone (Intravenous Route)
Indapamide (Oral Route)
Indinavir (Oral Route)
Indium In 111 Oxyquinoline (Diagnostic)
Indium In 111 Pentetate (Diagnostic)
Indium In 111 Pentetreotide (Diagnostic)
Indium In 111 Satumomab Pendetide (Diagnostic)
Indomethacin (Ophthalmic)
Indomethacin (Systemic)
Infliximab (Injection Route, Intravenous Route)
Influenza Virus Vaccine (Intramuscular Route, Nasal Route)
Insulin (Systemic)
Insulin Aspart, Recombinant (Subcutaneous Route)
Insulin Detemir (Injection Route)
Insulin Glargine, Recombinant (Subcutaneous Route)
Insulin Glulisine (Subcutaneous Route)
Insulin Human (Systemic)
Insulin Human, Buffered (Systemic)
Insulin Lispro, Recombinant (Subcutaneous Route)
Insulin Zinc (Systemic)
Insulin Zinc, Extended (Systemic)
Insulin Zinc, Extended, Human (Systemic)
Insulin Zinc, Human (Systemic)
Insulin Zinc, Prompt (Systemic)
Insulin, Isophane (Systemic)
Insulin, Isophane, Human (Systemic)
Insulin, Isophane, Human, and Insulin Human (Systemic)
Interferon Alfacon-1 (Subcutaneous Route)
Interferon Beta-1a (Intramuscular Route, Subcutaneous Route, Injection Route)
Interferon Beta-1b (Subcutaneous Route)
Interferon Gamma (Subcutaneous Route, Injection Route)
Iobenguane, Radioiodinated (Diagnostic)
Iocetamic Acid (Diagnostic)
Iodipamide (Diagnostic)
Iodohippurate Sodium I 123 (Diagnostic)
Iodohippurate Sodium I 131 (Diagnostic)
Iofetamine I 123 (Diagnostic)
Iohexol (Diagnostic)
Iohexol (Diagnostic, Local)
Iopamidol (Diagnostic)
Iopanoic Acid (Diagnostic)
Iothalamate (Diagnostic)
Iothalamate (Diagnostic, Local)
Iothalamate Sodium I 125 (Diagnostic)
Ioversol (Diagnostic)
Ioxaglate (Diagnostic)
Ioxaglate (Diagnostic, Local)

Ipodate (Diagnostic)
Ipratropium (Inhalation, Oral/Nebulization Route)
Ipratropium (Nasal Route)
Irbesartan (Oral Route)
Irbesartan (Oral Route)
Irbesartan (Oral Route)
Irinotecan (Intravenous Route)
Iron Dextran (Systemic)
Iron Sorbitol (Systemic)
Isoflurane (Systemic)
Isoflurophate (Ophthalmic)
Isoproterenol (Oral/Injection)
Isosorbide Dinitrate—Oral (Systemic)
Isosorbide Dinitrate—Sublingual, Chewable, or Buccal (Systemic)
Isosorbide Mononitrate—Oral (Systemic)
Isotretinoin (Oral Route)
Isradipine (Systemic)
Itraconazole (Systemic)
Ivermectin (Oral Route)

J

Japanese Encephalitis Virus Vaccine (Subcutaneous Route)

K

Kanamycin (Oral Route)
Ketamine (Systemic)
Ketazolam (Systemic)
Ketoconazole (Systemic)
Ketoprofen (Systemic)
Ketorolac (Oral Route, Intravenous Route, Injection Route, Intramuscular Route)
Ketotifen (Ophthalmic Route)
Krypton Kr 81m (Diagnostic)

L

Lamivudine (Oral Route)
Lamotrigine (Oral Route)
Lansoprazole (Oral Route)
Lanthanum Carbonate (Oral Route)
Laronidase (Intravenous Route)
Leflunomide (Oral Route)
Lenalidomide (Oral Route)
Letrozole (Oral Route)
Leucovorin (Oral Route, Intravenous Route, Injection Route)
Leuprolide (Intramuscular Route, Subcutaneous Route, Intradermal Route, Injection Route)
Levalbuterol (Inhalation, Oral/Nebulization Route)
Levamisole (Oral Route)
Levetiracetam (Oral Route)
Levobunolol (Ophthalmic)
Levocabastine (Ophthalmic Route)
Levocarnitine (Oral Route, Intravenous Route)
Levodopa (Oral Route)
Levofloxacin (Ophthalmic Route)
Levofloxacin (Oral Route, Intravenous Route)

Levomethadyl (Oral Route)
Levonorgestrel (Systemic)
Levonorgestrel and Ethinyl Estradiol (Systemic)
Levorphanol (Systemic)
Levothyroxine (Systemic)
Lidocaine (Parenteral-Local)
Lidocaine (Topical Route)
Lincomycin (Oral Route, Injection Route)
Lindane (Topical Route)
Linezolid (Intravenous Route, Oral Route)
Liothyronine (Systemic)
Liotrix (Systemic)
Lisinopril and Hydrochlorothiazide (Systemic)
Lithium (Oral Route)
Lomustine (Oral Route)
Loperamide (Oral Route)
Loracarbef (Oral Route)
Loratadine (Systemic)
Loratadine and Pseudoephedrine (Systemic)
Lorazepam (Systemic)
Losartan (Oral Route)
Losartan and Hydrochlorothiazide (Oral Route)
Loxapine (Oral Route, Intramuscular Route)
Lutropin Alfa (Subcutaneous Route)
Lyme Disease Vaccine (Recombinant Ospa) (Intramuscular Route)

M

Mafenide (Topical Route)
Magaldrate (Oral)
Magaldrate and Simethicone (Oral)
Magnesium Carbonate and Sodium Bicarbonate (Oral)
Magnesium Citrate (Oral)
Magnesium Hydroxide (Oral)
Magnesium Hydroxide and Cascara Sagrada (Oral)
Magnesium Hydroxide and Mineral Oil (Oral)
Magnesium Oxide (Oral)
Magnesium Salicylate (Systemic)
Magnesium Sulfate (Oral)
Malathion (Topical Route)
Mangafodipir (Intravenous Route)
Maprotiline (Oral Route)
Mazindol (Systemic)
Measles And Rubella Virus Vaccine Live (Intramuscular Route, Injection Route)
Measles Virus Vaccine, Live (Subcutaneous Route)
Measles, Mumps, And Rubella Virus Vaccine Live (Subcutaneous Route, Intramuscular Route)
Mebendazole (Oral Route)
Mecamylamine (Oral Route)
Mecasermin (Subcutaneous Route)
Mechlorethamine (Intravenous Route)
Mechlorethamine (Topical Route)
Meclocycline (Topical)
Meclofenamate (Systemic)

Medrogestone (Systemic)
Medroxyprogesterone (Systemic)
Medrysone (Ophthalmic)
Mefenamic Acid (Systemic)
Mefloquine (Oral Route)
Megestrol (Systemic)
Meloxicam (Oral Route)
Melphalan (Oral Route, Intravenous Route)
Memantine (Oral Route)
Menadiol (Systemic)
Meningococcal Polysaccharide Vaccine (Subcutaneous Route)
Meningococcal Vaccine, Diphtheria Conjugate (Intramuscular Route)
Meperidine (Systemic)
Mephenytoin (Systemic)
Mephobarbital (Systemic)
Mepivacaine (Parenteral-Local)
Meprobamate (Oral Route)
Meprobamate And Aspirin (Oral Route)
Mercaptopurine (Oral Route)
Meropenem (Intravenous Route)
Mesalamine (Oral Route)
Mesalamine (Rectal Route)
Mesna (Intravenous Route)
Mesoridazine (Systemic)
Metaproterenol (Inhalation)
Metaproterenol (Oral/Injection)
Metformin (Oral Route)
Metformin And Pioglitazone (Oral Route)
Methadone (Systemic)
Methamphetamine (Systemic)
Metharbital (Systemic)
Methazolamide (Systemic)
Methdilazine (Systemic)
Methenamine (Oral Route)
Methimazole (Systemic)
Methocarbamol (Systemic)
Methohexital (Systemic)
Methotrexate (Oral Route, Injection Route)
Methotrimeprazine (Systemic)
Methoxsalen (Injection Route)
Methoxsalen (Oral Route)
Methoxsalen (Topical Route)
Methoxyflurane (Systemic)
Methsuximide (Systemic)
Methyclothiazide (Systemic)
Methyldopa (Oral Route, Intravenous Route)
Methyldopa and Chlorothiazide (Systemic)
Methyldopa and Hydrochlorothiazide (Systemic)
Methylene Blue (Oral Route, Intravenous Route)
Methylergonovine (Systemic)
Methylphenidate (Oral Route)
Methylprednisolone (Systemic)
Methyltestosterone (Systemic)
Methysergide (Oral Route)
Metipranolol (Ophthalmic)
Metoclopramide (Oral Route, Intravenous Route)
Metolazone (Systemic)

Metoprolol and Hydrochlorothiazide (Systemic)
Metrizamide (Diagnostic)
Metronidazole (Oral Route, Intravenous Route)
Metronidazole (Vaginal Route)
Metyrosine (Oral Route)
Mexiletine (Oral Route)
Micafungin (Intravenous Route)
Miconazole (Vaginal)
Midazolam (Injection Route)
Midodrine (Oral Route)
Mifepristone (Oral Route)
Miglitol (Oral Route)
Miglustat (Oral Route)
Mineral Oil (Oral)
Mineral Oil and Cascara Sagrada (Oral)
Mineral Oil and Glycerin (Oral)
Mineral Oil and Phenolphthalein (Oral)
Mineral Oil, Glycerin, and Phenolphthalein (Oral)
Minocycline (Subgingival Route)
Minocycline (Systemic)
Minoxidil (Oral Route)
Minoxidil (Topical Route)
Mirtazapine (Oral Route)
Misoprostol (Oral Route)
Mitotane (Oral Route)
Mitoxantrone (Intravenous Route, Injection Route)
Modafinil (Oral Route)
Moexipril and Hydrochlorothiazide (Systemic)
Molindone (Oral Route)
Mometasone (Inhalation, Oral/Nebulization Route)
Mometasone (Nasal Route)
Mometasone (Topical)
Montelukast (Oral Route)
Moricizine (Oral Route)
Morphine (Systemic)
Moxifloxacin (Ophthalmic Route)
Mumps Virus Vaccine, Live (Subcutaneous Route)
Mupirocin (Topical Route)
Muromonab-Cd3 (Intravenous Route)
Mycophenolate Mofetil (Oral Route, Intravenous Route)

N

Nabilone (Oral Route)
Nabumetone (Systemic)
Nadolol and Bendroflumethiazide (Systemic)
Nafarelin (Nasal Route)
Naftifine (Topical Route)
Nalbuphine (Systemic)
Nalidixic Acid (Oral Route)
Naltrexone (Oral Route)
Nandrolone (Systemic)
Naphazoline (Ophthalmic Route)
Naproxen (Systemic)
Naratriptan (Oral Route)
Natalizumab (Intravenous Route)
Natamycin (Ophthalmic Route)
Nateglinide (Oral Route)

Nedocromil (Inhalation, Oral/Nebulization Route)
Nedocromil (Ophthalmic Route)
Nefazodone (Oral Route)
Nelfinavir (Oral Route)
Neomycin (Oral Route)
Neomycin (Topical Route)
Neomycin And Polymyxin B (Topical Route)
Neomycin, Polymyxin B, And Bacitracin (Topical Route)
Neostigmine (Systemic)
Nepafenac (Ophthalmic Route)
Nesiritide (Intravenous Route)
Netilmicin (Systemic)
Nevirapine (Oral Route)
Niacin (Oral Route)
Nicardipine (Systemic)
Niclosamide (Oral Route)
Nicotine (Inhalation, Oral/Nebulization Route)
Nicotine (Nasal Route)
Nicotine (Oral Route, Transdermal Route)
Nifedipine (Systemic)
Nilutamide (Systemic)
Nimodipine (Systemic)
Nisoldipine (Oral Route)
Nitazoxanide (Oral Route)
Nitisinone (Oral Route)
Nitrazepam (Systemic)
Nitrofurantoin (Oral Route)
Nitroglycerine—Oral (Systemic)
Nitroglycerin—Sublingual, Chewable, or Buccal (Systemic)
Nitrous Oxide (Systemic)
Norethindrone (Systemic)
Norethindrone Acetate and Ethyl Estradiol (Systemic)
Norethindrone and Ethinyl Estradiol (Systemic)
Norethindrone and Mestranol (Systemic)
Norgestimate and Ethinyl Estradiol (Systemic)
Norgestrel (Systemic)
Norgestrel and Ethinyl Estradiol (Systemic)
Nortriptyline (Systemic)

O

Octreotide (Injection Route, Intramuscular Route)
Ofloxacin (Ophthalmic Route)
Ofloxacin (Otic Route)
Olanzapine (Intramuscular Route)
Olmesartan Medoxomil (Oral Route)
Olmesartan Medoxomil and Hydrochlorothiazide (Oral Route)
Olopatadine (Ophthalmic Route)
Olsalazine (Oral Route)
Omalizumab (Subcutaneous Route)
Omega-3-Acid Ethyl Esters (Oral Route)
Omeprazole (Oral Route)
Ondansetron (Oral Route, Injection Route, Intravenous Route)

Opium Injection (Systemic)
Opium Tincture (Systemic)
Oprelvekin (Subcutaneous Route)
Orlistat (Oral Route)
Orphenadrine (Oral Route, Injection Route)
Orphenadrine, Aspirin, And Caffeine (Oral Route)
Oseltamivir (Oral Route)
Oxaliplatin (Intravenous Route)
Oxandrolone (Systemic)
Oxaprozin (Systemic)
Oxazepam (Systemic)
Oxcarbazepine (Oral Route)
Oxiconazole (Topical Route)
Oxtriphylline (Systemic)
Oxtriphylline And Guaifenesin (Oral Route)
Oxybutynin (Oral Route)
Oxycodone (Systemic)
Oxycodone and Acetaminophen (Systemic)
Oxycodone and Aspirin (Systemic)
Oxycodone And Ibuprofen (Oral Route)
Oxymetholone (Systemic)
Oxymorphone (Systemic)
Oxytetracycline (Systemic)

P

Paclitaxel (Intravenous Route)
Paclitaxel Protein-Bound (Injection Route)
Palifermin (Intravenous Route)
Palivizumab (Intramuscular Route)
Palonosetron (Intravenous Route)
Pamidronate (Intravenous Route)
Pancrelipase (Oral Route)
Pantoprazole (Intravenous Route)
Papaverine (Injection Route)
Papaverine (Oral Route)
Paramethadione (Systemic)
Paregoric (Systemic)
Paroxetine (Oral Route)
Pegademase Bovine (Intramuscular Route)
Pegaspargase (Intramuscular Route, Intravenous Route)
Pegfilgrastim (Subcutaneous Route)
Peginterferon Alfa-2a (Subcutaneous Route)
Peginterferon Alfa-2b (Subcutaneous Route)
Pegvisomant (Subcutaneous Route)
Pemetrexed (Intravenous Route)
Pemirolast (Ophthalmic Route)
Pemoline (Oral Route)
Penciclovir (Topical Route)
Penicillamine (Oral Route)
Pentamidine (Inhalation, Oral/Nebulization Route)
Pentamidine (Injection Route)
Pentazocine (Systemic)
Pentazocine and Acetaminophen (Systemic)
Pentazocine and Aspirin (Systemic)
Pentermine (Systemic)

Pentetate Calcium Trisodium (Intravenous Route, Inhalation, Oral/Nebulization Route)

601091

Pentetate Zinc Trisodium (Intravenous Route, Inhalation, Oral/Nebulization Route)

Pentobarbital (Systemic)

Pentosan Polysulfate Sodium (Oral Route)

Pentostatin (Intravenous Route)

Pentoxifylline (Oral Route)

Perflutren Protein Type A Microsphere (Intravenous Route)

Pergolide (Oral Route)

Pericyazine (Systemic)

Permethrin (Topical Route)

Perphenazine (Systemic)

Phenazopyridine (Oral Route)

Phendimetrazine (Systemic)

Phenelzine (Systemic)

Phenindamine (Systemic)

Pheniramine and Phenylephrine

Pheniramine, Codeine, and Guaifenesin (Systemic)

Pheniramine, Phenylephrine, and Acetaminophen (Systemic)

Pheniramine, Phenylephrine, and Dextromethorphan (Systemic)

Pheniramine, Phenylephrine, Codeine, Sodium Citrate, Sodium Salicylate, and Caffeine (Systemic)

Pheniramine, Phenylephrine, Sodium Salicylate, and Caffeine (Systemic)

Pheniramine, Pyrilamine, Hydrocodone, Potassium Citrate, and Ascorbic Acid (Systemic)

Phenobarbital (Systemic)

Phenobarbital, Aspirin, and Codeine (Systemic)

Phenoxybenzamine (Oral Route)

Phentolamine (Injection Route)

Phenylbutazone (Systemic)

Phenylephrine (Nasal Route)

Phenylephrine (Ophthalmic Route)

Phenylephrine and Acetaminophen (Systemic)

Phenylephrine and Guaifenesin (Systemic)

Phenylephrine and Hydrocodone (Systemic)

Phenylephrine, Guaifenesin, Acetaminophen, Salicylamide, and Caffeine (Systemic)

Phenylephrine, Hydrocodone, and Guaifenesin (Systemic)

Phenyltoloxamine and Hydrocodone (Systemic)

Phenytoin (Systemic)

Physostigmine (Ophthalmic Route)

Phytonadione (Systemic)

Pilocarpine (Ophthalmic Route)

Pilocarpine (Oral Route)

Pimecrolimus (Topical Route)

Pimozide (Oral Route)

Pindolol and Hydrochlorothiazide (Systemic)

Pioglitazone (Oral Route)

Pioglitazone And Glimepiride (Oral Route)

Pipotiazine (Systemic)

Pirbuterol (Inhalation)

Piroxicam (Systemic)

Plicamycin (Intravenous Route)

Pneumococcal Vaccine, Diphtheria Conjugate (Intramuscular Route)

Podofilox (Topical Route)

Poliovirus Vaccine Inactivated (Systemic)

Poliovirus Vaccine Inactivated Enhanced Potency (Systemic)

Poliovirus Vaccine, Live (Oral Route)

Polyethylene Glycol, Potassium Chloride, Sodium Bicarbonate, Sodium Chloride, And Sodium Sulfate (Oral Route)

Polyethylene Glycol, Sodium Sulfate, Sodium Chloride, Potassium Chloride, Sodium Ascorbate, , And Ascorbic Acid (Oral Route)

Polythiazide (Systemic)

Porfimer (Intravenous Route)

Pralidoxime (Injection Route)

Pramipexole (Oral Route)

Pramlintide (Subcutaneous Route)

Prazepam (Systemic)

Praziquantel (Oral Route)

Prazosin (Oral Route)

Prednisolone (Ophthalmic)

Prednisolone (Systemic)

Prednisone (Systemic)

Pregabalin (Oral Route)

Prilocaine (Parenteral-Local)

Primidone (Oral Route)

Probenecid (Oral Route)

Probenecid And Colchicine (Oral Route)

Probucol (Oral Route)

Procainamide (Oral Route, Intravenous Route)

Procaine (Parenteral-Local)

Procarbazine (Oral Route)

Prochlorperazine (Systemic)

Progesterone (Systemic)

Promazine (Systemic)

Promethazine (Systemic)

Promethazine and Codeine (Systemic)

Promethazine and Dextromethorphan (Systemic)

Promethazine and Phenylephrine (Systemic)

Promethazine and Potassium Guaiacolsulfonate (Systemic)

Promethazine, Codeine, and Potassium Guaiacolsulfonate (Systemic)

Promethazine, Phenylephrine, and Codeine (Systemic)

Promethazine, Phenylephrine, and Potassium Guaiacolsulfonate (Systemic)

Propafenone (Oral Route)

Propofol (Systemic)

Propoxyphene (Systemic)

Propoxyphene and Acetaminophen (Systemic)

Propoxyphene and Aspirin (Systemic)

Propoxyphene, Aspirin, and Caffeine (Systemic)

Propranolol and Hydrochlorothiazide (Systemic)

Propylthiouracil (Systemic)

Protirelin (Intravenous Route)

Protriptyline (Systemic)

Pseudoephedrine and Dextromethorphan (Systemic)

Pseudoephedrine and Guaifenesin (Systemic)

Pseudoephedrine and Ibuprofen (Systemic)

Pseudoephedrine, Codeine, and Guaifenesin (Systemic)

Pseudoephedrine, Dextromethorphan, and Acetaminophen (Systemic)

Pseudoephedrine, Dextromethorphan, and Guaifenesin (Systemic)

Pseudoephedrine, Dextromethorphan, Guaifenesin, and Acetaminophen (Systemic)

Pseudoephedrine, Hydrocodone, and Guaifenesin (Systemic)

Pseudoephedrine, Hydrocodone, and Potassium Guaiacolsulfonate (Systemic)

Pyrantel (Oral Route)

Pyrazinamide (Oral Route)

Pyrethrum Extract And Piperonyl Butoxide (Topical Route)

Pyridostigmine (Systemic)

Pyrilamine and Codeine (Systemic)

Pyrilamine, Phenylephrine, Hydrocodone, and Ammonium Chloride (Systemic)

Pyrilamine, Pseudoephedrine, Dextromethorphan, and Acetaminophen (Systemic)

Pyrimethamine (Oral Route)

Q

Quazepam (Systemic)

Quetiapine (Oral Route)

Quinapril and Hydrochlorothiazide (Systemic)

Quinethazone (Systemic)

Quinidine (Oral Route, Injection Route, Intramuscular Route)

Quinine (Oral Route)

R

Rabeprazole (Oral Route)

Rabies Immune Globulin (Intramuscular Route)

Radioiodinated Albumin (Diagnostic)

Raloxifene (Oral Route)

Ramelteon (Oral Route)

Rasagiline (Oral Route)

Rasburicase (Intravenous Route)

Rauwolfia Serpentina (Systemic)

Rauwolfia Serpentina and Bendroflumethiazide (Systemic)

Remifentanil (Systemic)

Repaglinide (Oral Route)

Reserpine (Systemic)

Reserpine and Chlorothiazide (Systemic)
Reserpine and Chlorthalidone (Systemic)
Reserpine and Hydrochlorothiazide (Systemic)
Reserpine and Hydroflumethiazide (Systemic)
Reserpine and Methyclothiazide (Systemic)
Reserpine and Trichlormethiazide (Systemic)
Reserpine, Hydralazine, And Hydrochlorothiazide (Oral Route)
Respiratory Syncytial Virus Immune Globulin, Human (Intravenous Route)
Rho(D) Immune Globulin (Intravenous Route, Intramuscular Route, Injection Route)
Ribavirin (Inhalation, Oral/Nebulization Route, Oral Route)
Rifabutin (Oral Route)
Rifampin (Oral Route, Intravenous Route)
Rifampin And Isoniazid (Oral Route)
Rifampin, Isoniazid, And Pyrazinamide (Oral Route)
Rifapentine (Oral Route)
Rifaximin (Oral Route)
Riluzole (Oral Route)
Rimantadine (Oral Route)
Risedronate (Oral Route)
Risperidone (Oral Route)
Ritodrine (Oral Route, Intravenous Route)
Ritonavir (Oral Route)
Rituximab (Intravenous Route)
Rivastigmine (Oral Route)
Rizatriptan (Oral Route)
Rofecoxib (Oral Route)
Ropinirole (Oral Route)
Ropivacaine (Injection Route)
Rosiglitazone (Oral Route)
Rosiglitazone And Metformin (Oral Route)
Rosuvastatin (Oral Route)
Rubella And Mumps Virus Vaccine Live (Intramuscular Route)
Rubella Virus Vaccine, Live (Subcutaneous Route)
Rubidium Rb 82 (Diagnostic)

S

Sacrosidase (Oral Route)
Salsalate (Systemic)
Saquinavir (Oral Route)
Secobarbital (Systemic)
Secobarbital and Amobarbital (Systemic)
Selegiline (Oral Route)
Sermorelin (Injection Route)
Sertaconazole (Topical Route)
Sertraline (Oral Route)
Sevoflurane (Inhalation, Oral/Nebulization Route)
Sibutramine (Oral Route)
Sildenafil (Oral Route)

Silver Sulfadiazine (Topical Route)
Sincalide (Intravenous Route)
Sirolimus (Oral Route)
Sodium Bicarbonate (Oral Route, Intravenous Route, Subcutaneous Route)
Sodium Chloride (Injection Route)
Sodium Chromate Cr 51 (Diagnostic)
Sodium Iodide I 123 (Diagnostic)
Sodium Iodide I 131 (Diagnostic)
Sodium Oxybate (Oral Route)
Sodium Pertechnetate Tc 99m (Diagnostic)
Sodium Phosphate (Oral)
Sodium Salicylate (Systemic)
Sodium Tetradecyl Sulfate (Injection Route)
Solifenacin (Oral Route)
Sorafenib (Oral Route)
Sparfloxacin (Oral Route)
Spectinomycin (Intramuscular Route)
Spironolactone (Systemic)
Spironolactone and Hydrochlorothiazide (Systemic)
Stanozolol (Systemic)
Stavudine (Oral Route)
Streptokinase (Systemic)
Streptomycin (Systemic)
Streptozocin (Intravenous Route)
Strontium Chloride Sr 89 (Intravenous Route, Injection Route)
Succimer (Oral Route)
Sucralfate (Oral Route)
Sufentanil (Systemic)
Sulconazole (Topical Route)
Sulfadiazine (Systemic)
Sulfadiazine and Trimethoprim (Systemic)
Sulfamethizole (Systemic)
Sulfamethoxazole (Systemic)
Sulfamethoxazole and Phenazopyridine (Systemic)
Sulfamethoxazole and Trimethoprim (Systemic)
Sulfasalazine (Oral Route, Rectal Route)
Sulfisoxazole (Systemic)
Sulfisoxazole and Phenazopyridine (Systemic)
Sulindac (Systemic)
Sumatriptan (Nasal Route, Oral Route, Subcutaneous Route)
Suprofen (Ophthalmic)

T

Tacrine (Oral Route)
Tacrolimus (Oral Route, Intravenous Route)
Tacrolimus (Topical Route)
Tadalafil (Oral Route)
Talc (Intrapleural Route)
Tamoxifen (Oral Route)
Tamsulosin (Oral Route)
Tazarotene (Topical Route)
Technetium Tc 99m (Pyro- and trimeta-) Phosphates (Diagnostic)

Technetium Tc 99m Albumin (Diagnostic)
Technetium Tc 99m Albumin Aggregated (Diagnostic)
Technetium Tc 99m Albumin Colloid (Diagnostic)
Technetium Tc 99m Apcitide (Diagnostic)
Technetium Tc 99m Arcitumomab (Diagnostic)
Technetium Tc 99m Bicisate (Diagnostic)
Technetium Tc 99m Disofenin (Diagnostic)
Technetium Tc 99m Exametazime (Diagnostic)
Technetium Tc 99m Fanolesomab (Systemic)
Technetium Tc 99m Gluceptate (Diagnostic)
Technetium Tc 99m Lidofenin (Diagnostic)
Technetium Tc 99m Mebrofenin (Diagnostic)
Technetium Tc 99m Medronate (Diagnostic)
Technetium Tc 99m Mertiatide (Diagnostic)
Technetium Tc 99m Nofetumomab Merpentan (Diagnostic)
Technetium Tc 99m Oxidronate (Diagnostic)
Technetium Tc 99m Pentetate (Diagnostic)
Technetium Tc 99m Pyrophosphate (Diagnostic)
Technetium Tc 99m Sestamibi (Diagnostic)
Technetium Tc 99m Succimer (Diagnostic)
Technetium Tc 99m Sulfur Colloid (Diagnostic)
Technetium Tc 99m Teboroxime (Diagnostic)
Technetium Tc 99m Tetrofosmin (Diagnostic)
Tegaserod (Oral Route)
Telithromycin (Oral Route)
Telmisartan (Oral Route)
Telmisartan and Hydrochlorothiazide (Oral Route)
Temazepam (Systemic)
Temozolomide (Oral Route)
Tenecteplase (Intravenous Route)
Teniposide (Intravenous Route)
Tenofovir Disoproxil Fumarate (Oral Route)
Tenoxicam (Systemic)
Terazosin (Oral Route)
Terbinafine (Oral Route)
Terbinafine (Topical Route)
Terbutaline (Inhalation)
Terbutaline (Oral/Injection)
Terconazole (Vaginal)
Terfenadine (Systemic)
Terfenadineand Pseudoephedrine (Systemic)
Teriparatide (Subcutaneous Route)

Teriparatide (Systemic)
Testolactone (Oral Route)
Testosterone (Buccal Route)
Testosterone (Transdermal Route)
Testosterone and Estradiol (Systemic)
Tetanus Immune Globulin (Intramuscular Route)
Tetanus Toxoid (Intramuscular Route, Injection Route)
Tetracaine (Parenteral-Local)
Tetracycline (Systemic)
Thalidomide (Oral Route)
Thallous Chloride Tl 201 (Diagnostic)
Theophylline (Systemic)
Theophylline And Guaifenesin (Oral Route)
Theophylline, Ephedrine, And Phenobarbital (Oral Route)
Thiabendazole (Oral Route)
Thiabendazole (Topical Route)
Thioguanine (Oral Route)
Thiopental (Systemic)
Thioproperazine (Systemic)
Thioridazine (Systemic)
Thiotepa (Injection Route)
Thiothixene (Systemic)
Thyroglobulin (Systemic)
Thyroid (Systemic)
Thyrotropin (Injection Route)
Tiagabine (Oral Route)
Tiaprofenic Acid (Systemic)
Ticlopidine (Oral Route)
Tiludronate (Oral Route)
Timolol (Ophthalmic)
Timolol and Hydrochlorothiazide (Systemic)
Tinidazole (Oral Route)
Tinzaparin (Subcutaneous Route)
Tioconazole (Vaginal)
Tiopronin (Oral Route)
Tiotropium (Inhalation, Oral/Nebulization Route)
Tixocortol (Rectal)
Tizanidine (Oral Route)
Tobramycin (Ophthalmic Route)
Tobramycin (Systemic)
Tobramycin And Dexamethasone (Ophthalmic Route)
Tocainide (Oral Route)
Tolcapone (Oral Route)
Tolmetin (Systemic)
Tolterodine (Oral Route)
Topiramate (Oral Route)
Topotecan (Intravenous Route)
Toremifene (Oral Route)
Torsemide (Oral Route, Intravenous Route)
Tositumomab (Intravenous Route)
Tramadol (Oral Route)

Tranylcypromine (Systemic)
Trastuzumab (Intravenous Route)
Travoprost (Ophthalmic Route)
Trazodone (Oral Route)
Treprostinil (Subcutaneous Route)
Tretinoin (Oral Route)
Tretinoin (Topical Route)
Triamcinolone (Dental)
Triamcinolone (Inhalation)
Triamcinolone (Topical)
Triamterene (Systemic)
Triamterene and Hydrochlorothiazide (Systemic)
Triazolam (Systemic)
Trichlormethiazide (Systemic)
Trientine (Oral Route)
Trifluoperazine (Systemic)
Triflupromazine (Systemic)
Trimeprazine (Systemic)
Trimethadione (Systemic)
Trimethoprim (Oral Route)
Trimetrexate (Intravenous Route)
Trimipramine (Systemic)
Triplennamine (Systemic)
Triprolidine and Pseudoephedrine (Systemic)
Triprolidine, Pseudoephedrine, and Acetaminophen (Systemic)
Triprolidine, Pseudoephedrine, and Codeine (Systemic)
Triprolidine, Pseudoephedrine, Codeine, and Guaifenesin (Systemic)
Triptorelin (Intramuscular Route, Injection Route)
Tropicamide (Ophthalmic Route)
Trospium (Oral Route)
Trovafloxacin (Oral Route)
Tuberculin (Intradermal Route)
Typhoid Vaccine, Inactivated (Subcutaneous Route, Injection Route)
Typhoid Vaccine, Live (Oral Route)
Typhoid Vi Polysaccharide Vaccine (Intramuscular Route)
Tyropanoate (Diagnostic)

U

Urofollitropin (Intramuscular Route, Subcutaneous Route, Injection Route)
Urokinase (Systemic)
Ursodiol (Oral Route)

V

Vaccinia Immune Globulin, Human (Intravenous Route)
Valacyclovir (Oral Route)
Valdecoxib (Oral Route)

Valganciclovir (Oral Route)
Valproate Sodium (Systemic)
Valproic Acid (Systemic)
Valrubicin (Intravesical Route)
Valsartan (Oral Route)
Valsartan and Hydrochlorothiazide (Oral Route)
Vancomycin (Intravenous Route, Injection Route)
Vancomycin (Oral Route)
Vardenafil (Oral Route)
Varenicline (Oral Route)
Varicella Virus Vaccine (Subcutaneous Route)
Vasopressin (Injection Route)
Venlafaxine (Oral Route)
Verapamil (Systemic)
Verteporfin (Intravenous Route, Injection Route)
Vinblastine (Intravenous Route)
Vincristine (Intravenous Route)
Vinorelbine (Intravenous Route)
Vitamin A (Oral Route, Intramuscular Route)
Voriconazole (Oral Route, Intravenous Route)

W

Warfarin (Systemic)

X

Xenon Xe 127 (Diagnostic)
Xenon Xe 133 (Diagnostic)

Y

Yellow Fever Vaccine (Subcutaneous Route, Injection Route)

Z

Zafirlukast (Oral Route)
Zalcitabine (Oral Route)
Zaleplon (Oral Route)
Zanamivir (Inhalation, Oral/Nebulization Route)
Ziconotide (Intrathecal Route)
Zidovudine (Oral Route, Intravenous Route)
Zileuton (Oral Route)
Ziprasidone (Oral Route, Intramuscular Route)
Zoledronic Acid (Intravenous Route)
Zolmitriptan (Oral Route)
Zolpidem (Oral Route)
Zonisamide (Oral Route)

Appendix IV

BREAST-FEEDING PRECAUTION LISTING

The following medicines, selected from those included in this publication, have specific precautions in regard to use while breast-feeding. For specific information, consult the individual drug entry; look in the index for the page number.

The use of any medicine while breast-feeding must be carefully considered. The physician and the patient must balance the expected benefits against the possible risks.

Absence of a drug from the list is not meant to imply that it is safe for use while breast-feeding. For many drugs, it is not known whether a problem exists; experimentation on women who are breast-feeding is generally not done. Knowledge is usually gained only from the accumulated experience over many years in giving a drug to breast-feeding women who needed its benefits. Also, well-planned studies in breast-feeding animals may reveal problems, although the relation of such findings to humans may not be known. Problems suggested by animal studies are often included in the warnings in this book.

Readers are reminded that the information in this text is selected and not considered to be complete.

A

Abarelix (Intramuscular Route)
Abciximab (Intravenous Route)
Acamprosate (Oral Route)
Acarbose (Oral Route)
Acenocoumarol (Systemic)
Acetaminophen (Oral Route, Rectal Route)
Acetazolamide (Systemic)
Acetylcysteine (Inhalation, Oral/Nebulization Route)
Acitretin (Oral Route)
Acrivastine and Pseudoephedrine (Systemic)
Acyclovir (Oral Route, Intravenous Route)
Acyclovir (Topical Route)
Adalimumab (Subcutaneous Route)
Adapalene (Topical Route)
Adefovir Dipivoxil (Oral Route)
Agalsidase Beta (Intravenous Route)
Albendazole (Oral Route)
Albuterol (Inhalation)
Alclometasone (Topical)
Aldesleukin (Intravenous Route)
Alefacept (Intravenous Route, Intramuscular Route)
Alemtuzumab (Intravenous Route)
Alendronate (Oral Route)
Alfuzosin (Oral Route)
Alglucerase (Intravenous Route)
Allopurinol (Intravenous Route)
Almotriptan (Oral Route)
Alosetron (Oral Route)
Alpha-1 Proteinase Inhibitor Human (Intravenous Route)
Alprazolam (Systemic)
Alprostadil (Intraurethral Route, Intravenous Route, Intracavernosal Route)
Altretamine (Oral Route)
Amantadine (Oral Route)
Amcinonide (Topical)
Amifostine (Intravenous Route)
Amiloride and Hydrochlorothiazide (Systemic)
Aminoglutethimide (Oral Route)
Aminolevulinic Acid (Topical Route)
Aminophylline (Systemic)
Aminosalicylate Sodium (Oral Route)
Amiodarone (Intravenous Route)
Amlexanox (Mucous Membrane, Oral Route)
Amlodipine (Oral Route)
Amobarbital (Systemic)
Amoxicillin and Clavulanate (Systemic)

Amphetamine (Systemic)
Amphotericin B (Intravenous Route, Injection Route)
Amphotericin B Cholesteryl Sulfate Complex (Intravenous Route)
Amphotericin B Lipid Complex (Intravenous Route, Injection Route)
Amphotericin B Liposome (Intravenous Route)
Ampicillin and Sulbactam (Systemic)
Amprenavir (Oral Route)
Amsacrine (Intravenous Route)
Amyl Nitrite (Inhalation, Oral/Nebulization Route)
Anagrelide (Oral Route)
Anakinra (Subcutaneous Route)
Anastrozole (Oral Route)
Anidulafungin (Intravenous Route)
Anisotropine (Systemic)
Anthralin (Topical Route)
Antihemophilic Factor (Intravenous Route, Injection Route)
Antithymocyte Globulin Rabbit (Intravenous Route)
Antivenin (Crotalidae) Polyvalent (Injection Route)
Antivenin (Crotalidae) Polyvalent Immune Fab (Intravenous Route)
Apomorphine (Injection Route)
Apraclonidine (Ophthalmic Route)
Aprepitant (Oral Route)
Aprobarbital (Systemic)
Ardeparin (Subcutaneous Route)
Aripiprazole (Oral Route)
Ascorbic Acid (Oral Route)
Asparaginase (Injection Route)
Aspirin (Systemic)
Aspirin and Caffeine (Systemic)
Aspirin and Caffeine, Buffered (Systemic)
Aspirin and Codeine (Systemic)
Aspirin, Buffered (Systemic)
Aspirin, Caffeine, and Dihydrocodeine (Systemic)
Aspirin, Codeine, and Caffeine (Systemic)
Aspirin, Codeine, and Caffeine, Buffered (Systemic)
Aspirin, Sodium Bicarbonate, And Citric Acid (Oral Route)
Atazanavir Sulfate (Oral Route)
Atenolol and Chlorthalidone (Systemic)
Atomoxetine (Oral Route)
Atorvastatin (Oral Route)
Atovaquone (Oral Route)

Atropine (Ophthalmic)
Atropine (Systemic)
Atropine and Phenobarbital (Systemic)
Atropine, Hyoscyamine, Methenamine, Methylene Blue, Phenyl Salicylate, And Benzoic Acid (Oral Route)
Atropine, Hyoscyamine, Scopolamine, and Phenobarbital (Systemic)
Auranofin (Systemic)
Aurothioglucose (Systemic)
Azacitidine (Subcutaneous Route)
Azatadine and Pseudoephedrine (Systemic)
Azathioprine (Oral Route, Intravenous Route)
Azelaic Acid (Topical Route)
Azelastine (Nasal Route)
Azelastine (Ophthalmic Route)
Azithromycin (Intravenous Route)
Aztreonam (Intravenous Route, Injection Route)

B

Bacillus Of Calmette And Guerin Vaccine, Live (Intradermal Route)
Bacillus Of Calmette And Guerin Vaccine, Live (Intravesical Route)
Baclofen (Intrathecal Route)
Baclofen (Oral Route)
Balsalazide (Oral Route)
Basiliximab (Intravenous Route)
Beclomethasone (Topical)
Belladonna (Systemic)
Belladonna and Butabarbital (Systemic)
Belladonna and Phenobarbital (Systemic)
Bendroflumethiazide (Systemic)
Bentiromide (Oral Route)
Benzonatate (Oral Route)
Benztropine (Systemic)
Beta Carotene (Oral Route)
Betaine (Oral Route)
Betamethasone (Otic)
Betamethasone (Rectal)
Betamethasone (Systemic)
Betamethasone (Topical)
Bethanechol (Oral Route, Subcutaneous Route)
Bevacizumab (Intravenous Route)
Bexarotene (Oral Route)
Bexarotene (Topical Route)
Bimatoprost (Ophthalmic Route)
Biperiden (Systemic)
Bismuth Subsalicylate (Oral Route)

Bisprolol and Hydrochlorothiazide (Systemic)
Bleomycin (Injection Route)
Bortezomib (Intravenous Route)
Bosentan (Oral Route)
Botulinum Toxin Type A (Intramuscular Route)
Botulinum Toxin Type B (Intramuscular Route)
Brimonidine (Ophthalmic Route)
Brinzolamide (Ophthalmic Route)
Bromazepam (Systemic)
Bromfenac (Ophthalmic Route)
Bromocriptine (Oral Route)
Brompheniramine (Systemic)
Brompheniramine and Phenylephrine (Systemic)
Brompheniramine and Pseudoephedrine (Systemic)
Brompheniramine, Pseudoephedrine, and Acetaminophen
Brompheniramine, Pseudoephedrine, and Dextromethorphan (Systemic)
Budesonide (Rectal)
Budesonide (Systemic)
Budesonide/Formoterol (Inhalation Route)
Buprenorphine (Systemic)
Buprenorphine (Systemic)
Bupropion (Oral Route)
Bupropion (Systemic)
Buspirone (Oral Route)
Busulfan (Intravenous Route)
Butabarbital (Systemic)
Butalbital and Acetaminophen (Systemic)
Butalbital and Aspirin (Systemic)
Butalbital, Acetaminophen, and Caffeine (Systemic)
Butalbital, Acetaminophen, Caffeine, And Codeine (Oral Route)
Butalbital, Aspirin, and Caffeine (Systemic)
Butalbital, Aspirin, Caffeine, and Codeine (Systemic)
Butenafine (Topical Route)
Butorphanol (Nasal Route)

C

Cabergoline (Oral Route)
Caffeine (Systemic)
Caffeine and Sodium Benzoate (Systemic)
Caffeine, Citrated (Systemic)
Calcipotriene (Topical Route)
Calcitonin (Salmon) (Nasal Route)
Calcium Acetate (Oral Route)
Candesartan Cilexetil (Oral Route)
Capecitabine (Oral Route)
Capreomycin (Injection Route)
Carbachol (Ophthalmic Route)
Carbamazepine (Oral Route)
Carbetocin (Intravenous Route)
Carbinoxamine and Pseudoephedrine (Systemic)
Carbinoxamine, Pseudoephedrine, and Dextromethorphan (Systemic)
Carboplatin (Intravenous Route)
Carboprost (Intramuscular Route)
Carisoprodol (Systemic)
Carmustine (Implantation Route)
Carmustine (Intravenous Route)
Carvedilol (Oral Route)
Cascara Sagrada (Oral)
Cascara Sagrada and Aloe (Oral)
Cascara Sagrada and Phenolphthalein (Oral)

Caspofungin (Intravenous Route)
Cefditoren Pivoxil (Oral Route)
Cefuroxime (Injection Route, Intravenous Route)
Celecoxib (Oral Route)
Cetirizine (Systemic)
Cetrorelix (Subcutaneous Route)
Cetuximab (Intravenous Route)
Cevimeline (Oral Route)
Chloral Hydrate (Oral Route, Rectal Route)
Chlorambucil (Oral Route)
Chloramphenicol (Ophthalmic Route)
Chloramphenicol (Oral Route, Intravenous Route, Injection Route)
Chloramphenicol (Otic Route)
Chlordiazepoxide (Systemic)
Chlordiazepoxide And Amitriptyline (Oral Route)
Chlorhexidine (Oral Route)
Chlorhexidine (Subgingival Route)
Chloroquine (Oral Route, Intramuscular Route)
Chlorothiazide (Systemic)
Chloroxine (Topical Route)
Chlorpheniramine (Systemic)
Chlorpheniramine and Codeine (Systemic)
Chlorpheniramine and Dextromethorphan (Systemic)
Chlorpheniramine and Hydrocodone (Systemic)
Chlorpheniramine and Phenylephrine (Systemic)
Chlorpheniramine and Pseudoephedrine (Systemic)
Chlorpheniramine, Ephedrine, and Guaifenesin (Systemic)
Chlorpheniramine, Ephedrine, Phenylephrine, and Carbetapentane (Systemic)
Chlorpheniramine, Ephedrine, Phenylephrine, Dextromethorphan, Ammonium Chloride, and Ipecac (Systemic)
Chlorpheniramine, Pheniramine, Pyrilamine, Phenylephrine, Hydrocodone, Salicylamide, Caffeine, and Ascorbic Acid (Systemic)
Chlorpheniramine, Phenylephrine, and Acetaminophen (Systemic)
Chlorpheniramine, Phenylephrine, and Dextromethorphan (Systemic)
Chlorpheniramine, Phenylephrine, and Hydrocodone (Systemic)
Chlorpheniramine, Phenylephrine, and Methscopolamine (Systemic)
Chlorpheniramine, Phenylephrine, Codeine, and Ammonium Chloride (Systemic)
Chlorpheniramine, Phenylephrine, Codeine, and Potassium Iodide (Systemic)
Chlorpheniramine, Phenylephrine, Dextromethorphan, and Guaifenesin (Systemic)
Chlorpheniramine, Phenylephrine, Dextromethorphan, Guaifenesin, and Ammonium Chloride (Systemic)
Chlorpheniramine, Phenylephrine, Hydrocodone, Acetaminophen, and Caffeine (Systemic)
Chlorpheniramine, Phenyltoloxamine, and Phenylephrine (Systemic)
Chlorpheniramine, Pseudoephedrine, and Acetaminophen (Systemic)
Chlorpheniramine, Pseudoephedrine, and Codeine (Systemic)
Chlorpheniramine, Pseudoephedrine, and Dextromethorphan (Systemic)

Chlorpheniramine, Pseudoephedrine, and Hydrocodone (Systemic)
Chlorpheniramine, Pseudoephedrine, and Methscopolamine (Systemic)
Chlorpheniramine, Pseudoephedrine, Codeine, and Acetaminophen (Systemic)
Chlorpheniramine, Pseudoephedrine, Dextromethorphan, and Acetaminophen (Systemic)
Chlorpheniramine, Pseudoephedrine, Dextromethorphan, and Guaifenesin (Systemic)
Chlorpheniramine, Pyrilamine, and Phenylephrine (Systemic)
Chlorpheniramine, Pyrilamine, Phenylephrine, and Acetaminophen (Systemic)
Chlorpromazine (Systemic)
Chlorprothixene (Systemic)
Chlorthalidone (Systemic)
Cholera Vaccine (Injection Route)
Cholestyramine (Oral Route)
Choline and Magnesium Salicylates (Systemic)
Choline Salicylate (Systemic)
Chorionic Gonadotropin (Subcutaneous Route, Intramuscular Route, Injection Route)
Chymopapain (Injection Route)
Cidofovir (Intravenous Route)
Cilostazol (Oral Route)
Cinacalcet (Oral Route)
Cinoxacin (Oral Route)
Ciprofloxacin (Ophthalmic Route)
Cisapride (Oral Route)
Cisplatin (Intravenous Route)
Citalopram (Oral Route)
Cladribine (Intravenous Route)
Clarithromycin (Oral Route)
Clemastine (Systemic)
Clidinium (Systemic)
Clindamycin (Oral Route, Injection Route, Intravenous Route)
Clindamycin (Topical Route)
Clindamycin (Vaginal Route)
Clioquinol (Topical Route)
Clioquinol And Hydrocortisone (Topical Route)
Clobazan (Systemic)
Clobetasol (Topical)
Clobetasone (Topical)
Clocortolone (Topical)
Clofarabine (Intravenous Route)
Clofazimine (Oral Route)
Clofibrate (Oral Route)
Clomiphene (Oral Route)
Clonazepam (Systemic)
Clonidine (Epidural Route)
Clonidine (Oral Route, Transdermal Route)
Clopidogrel (Oral Route)
Clorazepate (Systemic)
Clotrimazole (Mucous Membrane, Oral Route)
Clotrimazole (Topical Route)
Clozapine (Oral Route)
Coal Tar (Topical Route)
Cocaine (Topical Route)
Codeine and Guaifenesin (Systemic)
Codeine, Ammonium Chloride, and Guaifenesin (Systemic)
Colchicine (Oral Route, Intravenous Route)
Colesevelam (Oral Route)
Colestipol (Oral Route)
Colistin Sulfate, Neomycin Sulfate, Hydrocortisone Acetate, And Thonzonium Bromide (Otic Route)

Conjugated Estrogens and Medroxyprogesterone (Systemic)
Conjugated Estrogens, and Conjugated Estrogens and Medroxyprogesterone (Systemic)
Cortisone (Systemic)
Cromolyn (Inhalation, Oral/Nebulization Route)
Cromolyn (Nasal Route)
Cromolyn (Oral Route)
Crotamiton (Topical Route)
Cyanocobalamin Co 57 (Diagnostic)
Cyclandelate (Oral Route)
Cyclobenzaprine (Oral Route)
Cyclopentolate (Ophthalmic Route)
Cyclophosphamide (Oral Route, Intravenous Route)
Cycloserine (Oral Route)
Cyclosporine (Oral Route, Intravenous Route)
Cyproheptadine (Systemic)
Cyproterone (Oral Route, Intramuscular Route)
Cysteamine (Oral Route)
Cytarabine (Oral Route)
Cytarabine Liposome (Intrathecal Route)

D

Dacarbazine (Intravenous Route, Injection Route)
Daclizumab (Intravenous Route)
Dactinomycin (Intravenous Route)
Dalteparin (Subcutaneous Route, Injection Route)
Danaparoid (Subcutaneous Route)
Danazol (Oral Route)
Danthron and Docusate (Oral)
Dantrolene (Oral Route, Intravenous Route)
Dapiprazole (Ophthalmic Route)
Dapsone (Oral Route)
Dapsone (Topical Route)
Daptomycin (Intravenous Route)
Darbepoetin Alfa (Injection Route)
Darifenacin (Oral Route)
Daunorubicin (Intravenous Route)
Daunorubicin Citrate Liposome (Intravenous Route)
Deferoxamine (Injection Route)
Delavirdine (Oral Route)
Demecarium (Ophthalmic)
Demeclocycline (Systemic)
Denileukin Diftitox (Intravenous Route)
Deserpidine (Systemic)
Deserpidine and Hydrochlorothiazide (Systemic)
Deserpidine and Methyclothiazide (Systemic)
Desflurane (Inhalation, Oral/Nebulization Route)
Desloratadine (Oral Route)
Desloratadine And Pseudoephedrine (Oral Route)
Desmopressin (Nasal Route, Oral Route, Injection Route)
Desogestrel and Ethinyl Estradiol (Systemic)
Desonide (Topical)
Desoximetasone (Topical)
Dexamethasone (Nasal)
Dexamethasone (Otic)
Dexamethasone (Systemic)
Dexamethasone (Topical)
Dexbrompheniramine and Pseudoephedrine (Systemic)

Dexbrompheniramine, Pseudoephedrine, and Acetaminophen (Systemic)
Dexchlorpheniramine (Systemic)
Dexmethylphenidate (Oral Route)
Dexrazoxane (Intravenous Route)
Dextromethorphan (Oral Route)
Dextromethorphan and Acetaminophen (Systemic)
Dextromethorphan and Guaifenesin (Systemic)
Dextromethorphan and Iodinated Glycerol (Systemic)
Diatrizoate and Iodipamide (Diagnostic, Local)
Diatrizoate Meglumine (Local)
Diatrizoate Sodium (Local)
Diatrizoates (Diagnostic)
Diazepam (Systemic)
Diazoxide (Oral Route)
Dichlorphenamide (Systemic)
Diclofenac (Topical Route)
Diclofenac And Misoprostol (Oral Route)
Dicyclomine (Systemic)
Didanosine (Oral Route)
Dienestrol (Vaginal)
Diethylpropion (Systemic)
Diethylstilbestrol (Systemic)
Diethylstilbestrol and Methyltestosterone (Systemic)
Difenoxin And Atropine (Oral Route)
Diflorasone (Topical)
Diflucortolone (Topical)
Digitoxin (Systemic)
Digoxin (Systemic)
Dihydroergotamine (Nasal Route)
Dihydroergotamine (Systemic)
Dimenhydrinate (Systemic)
Dimethyl Sulfoxide (Intravesical Route)
Dinoprost (Injection Route)
Dinoprostone (Vaginal Route)
Diphenhydramine (Systemic)
Diphenhydramine and Pseudoephedrine (Systemic)
Diphenhydramine, Codeine, and Ammonium Chloride (Systemic)
Diphenhydramine, Dextromethorphan, and Ammonium Chloride (Systemic)
Diphenhydramine, Pseudoephedrine, and Acetaminophen (Systemic)
Diphenidol (Oral Route)
Diphenoxylate And Atropine (Oral Route)
Diphtheria and Tetanus Toxoids for Adult Use (Systemic)
Diphtheria and Tetanus Toxoids for Pediatric Use (Systemic)
Diphtheria Antitoxin (Injection Route)
Diphtheria Toxoid, Tetanus Toxoid, And Acellular Pertussis Vaccine (Intramuscular Route)
Dipivefrin (Ophthalmic Route)
Dipyridamole (Oral Route, Intravenous Route)
Dirithromycin (Oral Route)
Disopyramide (Oral Route)
Disulfiram (Oral Route)
Divalproex (Systemic)
Docetaxel (Intravenous Route)
Dofetilide (Oral Route)
Dolasetron (Oral Route, Intravenous Route)
Domperidone (Oral Route)
Donepezil (Oral Route)
Dorzolamide (Ophthalmic Route)
Doxazosin (Oral Route)

Doxepin (Systemic)
Doxepin (Topical Route)
Doxorubicin (Intravenous Route)
Doxycycline (Oral Route)
Doxycycline (Subgingival Route)
Doxylamine (Systemic)
Doxylamine, Codeine, and Acetaminophen (Systemic)
Doxylamine, Etafedrine, and Hydrocone (Systemic)
Doxylamine, Pseudoephedrine, Dextromethorphan, and Acetaminophen (Systemic)
Dronabinol (Oral Route)
Droperidol (Injection Route)
Drospirenone And Estradiol (Oral Route)
Drospirenone And Ethinyl Estradiol (Oral Route)
Drotrecogin Alfa (Intravenous Route)
Duloxetine (Oral Route)
Dutasteride (Oral Route)
Dyphylline (Oral Route, Intramuscular Route)

E

Echothiophate (Ophthalmic)
Efalizumab (Subcutaneous Route)
Efavirenz (Oral Route)
Efavirenz/Emtricitabine/Tenofovir (Oral Route)
Eflornithine (Injection Route)
Eletriptan (Oral Route)
Emedastine (Ophthalmic Route)
Emtricitabine (Oral Route)
Enfuvirtide (Subcutaneous Route)
Enoxaparin (Subcutaneous Route)
Entacapone (Oral Route)
Entecavir (Oral Route)
Ephedrine (Oral/Injection)
Ephedrine and Guaifenesin (Systemic)
Epinastine (Ophthalmic Route)
Epinephrine (Inhalation)
Epirubicin (Intravenous Route, Injection Route)
Eplerenone (Oral Route)
Epoprostenol (Intravenous Route)
Eprosartan (Oral Route)
Eptacog Alfa (Intravenous Route)
Ergoloid Mesylates (Oral Route, Sublingual Route)
Ergonovine (Systemic)
Ergotamine (Systemic)
Ergotamine and Caffeine (Systemic)
Ergotamine, Caffeine, and Belladonna Alkaloids (Systemic)
Ergotamine, Caffeine, and Cyclizine (Systemic)
Ergotamine, Caffeine, and Dimenhydrinate (Systemic)
Ergotamine, Caffeine, and Diphenhydramine (Systemic)
Ergotamine, Caffeine, Belladonna Alkaloids, and Pentobarbital (Systemic)
Erlotinib (Oral Route)
Ertapenem (Injection Route)
Erythromycin And Sulfisoxazole (Oral Route)
Erythropoietin (Injection Route)
Escitalopram (Oral Route)
Esomeprazole (Oral Route)
Estazolam (Systemic)
Estradiol (Systemic)
Estradiol (Vaginal)

Estramustine (Oral Route)
Estrogens, Conjugated (Systemic)
Estrogens, Conjugated (Vaginal)
Estrogens, Conjugated, and Methyltestosterone (Systemic)
Estrogens, Esterified (Systemic)
Estrogens, Esterified, and Methyltestosterone (Systemic)
Estrone (Systemic)
Estrone (Vaginal)
Estropipate (Systemic)
Estropipate (Vaginal)
Eszopiclone (Oral Route)
Etanercept (Subcutaneous Route)
Ethambutol (Oral Route)
Ethchlorvynol (Oral Route)
Ethinyl Estradiol (Systemic)
Ethinyl Estradiol And Norelgestromin (Transdermal Route)
Ethinyl Estradiol And Norelgestromin (Transdermal Route)
Ethionamide (Oral Route)
Ethopropazine (Systemic)
Ethotoin (Systemic)
Ethynodiol Diacetate and Ethinyl Estradiol (Systemic)
Etidronate (Oral Route, Intravenous Route)
Etoposide (Oral Route, Intravenous Route)
Exemestane (Oral Route)
Exenatide (Subcutaneous Route)
Ezetimibe (Oral Route)

F

Factor IX Complex (Intravenous Route, Injection Route)
Famciclovir (Oral Route)
Fat Emulsion (Intravenous Route, Injection Route)
Felbamate (Oral Route)
Fenofibrate (Oral Route)
Fentanyl (Buccal Route)
Fentanyl (Transdermal Route)
Ferrous Citrate Fe 59 (Diagnostic)
Fexofenadine (Oral Route)
Finasteride (Oral Route)
Flavocoxid (Oral Route)
Flavoxate (Oral Route)
Flecainide (Oral Route)
Floxuridine (Injection Route)
Flucytosine (Oral Route)
Fludarabine (Oral Route)
Fludrocortisone (Oral Route)
Flumethasone (Topical)
Fluocinolone (Topical)
Fluocinonide (Topical)
Fluorouracil (Intravenous Route, Injection Route)
Fluorouracil (Topical Route)
Fluoxetine (Oral Route)
Fluoxymesterone (Systemic)
Fluoxymesterone and Ethinyl Estradiol (Systemic)
Flupenthixol (Systemic)
Fluphenazine (Systemic)
Flurandrenolide (Topical)
Flurandrenolide (Topical)
Flurazepam (Systemic)
Fluticasone (Inhalation, Oral/Nebulization Route)
Fluticasone (Nasal Route)
Fluticasone (Topical)
Fluvoxamine (Oral Route)

Folic Acid (Oral Route, Injection Route)
Follitropin Alfa (Subcutaneous Route)
Follitropin Beta (Subcutaneous Route)
Fomivirsen (Intraocular Route)
Fondaparinux (Subcutaneous Route)
Formoterol (Inhalation, Oral/Nebulization Route)
Fosamprenavir (Oral Route)
Foscarnet (Intravenous Route)
Fosfomycin (Oral Route)
Fosphenytoin (Systemic)
Frovatriptan (Oral Route)
Fructose, Dextrose, And Phosphoric Acid (Oral Route)
Fulvestrant (Intramuscular Route)
Furazolidone (Oral Route)
Fusidic Acid (Oral Route, Injection Route)

G

Gabapentin (Oral Route)
Gadopentetate (Diagnostic)
Gadoversetamide (Systemic)
Galantamine (Oral Route)
Gallium Citrate Ga 67 (Diagnostic)
Gallium Nitrate (Intravenous Route)
Ganciclovir (Oral Route, Intravenous Route)
Ganirelix (Subcutaneous Route)
Gatifloxacin (Ophthalmic Route)
Gefitinib (Oral Route)
Gemcitabine (Intravenous Route)
Gemfibrozil (Oral Route)
Gemifloxacin (Oral Route)
Gemtuzumab Ozogamicin (Intravenous Route)
Gentamicin (Ophthalmic Route)
Glatiramer Acetate (Subcutaneous Route)
Glipizide And Metformin (Oral Route)
Glucagon (Injection Route)
Glutamine (Oral Route)
Glyburide And Metformin (Oral Route)
Glycerin (Oral Route)
Glycopyrrolate (Systemic)
Gold Sodium Thiomalate (Systemic)
Gonadorelin (Intravenous Route, Injection Route)
Goserelin (Subcutaneous Route)
Granisetron (Oral Route, Intravenous Route)
Griseofulvin (Oral Route)
Guaifenesin (Oral Route)
Guanabenz (Oral Route)
Guanadrel (Oral Route)
Guanethidine (Oral Route)
Guanfacine (Oral Route)

H

Haemophilus B Polysaccharide Vaccine (Intramuscular Route, Injection Route)
Halazepam (Systemic)
Halcinonide (Topical)
Halobetasol (Topical)
Halofantrine (Oral Route)
Haloperidol (Oral Route, Intramuscular Route, Injection Route)
Heparin (Intravenous Route, Injection Route)
Hepatitis A Vaccine Inactivated And Hepatitis B Vaccine Recombinant (Intramuscular Route)
Hepatitis A Vaccine, Inactivated (Intramuscular Route)

Hepatitis B Immune Globulin (Intramuscular Route)
Hepatitis B Vaccine Recombinant (Intramuscular Route)
Histamine (Injection Route)
Histrelin (Implantation Route)
Homatropine (Systemic)
Hyaluronate Sodium (Injection Route)
Hyaluronidase (Subcutaneous Route, Injection Route)
Hydralazine (Oral Route, Injection Route, Intravenous Route)
Hydralazine And Hydrochlorothiazide (Oral Route)
Hydralazine And Hydrochlorothiazide (Oral Route)
Hydrochlorothiazide (Systemic)
Hydrocodone and Aspirin (Systemic)
Hydrocodone and Guaifenesin (Systemic)
Hydrocodone and Homatropine (Systemic)
Hydrocodone and Potassium Guaiacolsulfonate (Systemic)
Hydrocortisone (Dental)
Hydrocortisone (Rectal)
Hydrocortisone (Systemic)
Hydrocortisone (Topical)
Hydrocortisone Acetate (Topical)
Hydrocortisone And Acetic Acid (Otic Route)
Hydrocortisone Butyrate (Topical)
Hydrocortisone Valerate (Topical)
Hydroflumethiazide (Systemic)
Hydroxychloroquine (Oral Route)
Hydroxyprogesterone (Systemic)
Hydroxyurea (Oral Route)
Hydroxyzine (Systemic)
Hyoscyamine (Systemic)
Hyoscyamine and Phenobarbital (Systemic)

I

Ibandronate (Oral Route, Injection Route)
Ibritumomab Tiuxetan (Intravenous Route)
Idarubicin (Intravenous Route)
Idursulfase (Intravenous Route)
Ifosfamide (Intravenous Route)
Iloprost (Inhalation, Oral/Nebulization Route)
Imatinib (Oral Route)
Imiglucerase (Intravenous Route)
Imipenem And Cilastatin (Intravenous Route, Intramuscular Route)
Imiquimod (Topical Route)
Immune Globulin (Intramuscular Route, Intravenous Route, Injection Route)
Inamrinone (Intravenous Route)
Indapamide (Oral Route)
Indinavir (Oral Route)
Indium In 111 Oxyquinoline (Diagnostic)
Indium In 111 Pentetate (Diagnostic)
Indium In 111 Pentetreotide (Diagnostic)
Indium In 111 Satumomab Pendetide (Diagnostic)
Indomethacin (Systemic)
Infliximab (Injection Route, Intravenous Route)
Influenza Virus Vaccine (Intramuscular Route, Nasal Route)
Insulin (Systemic)
Insulin Aspart, Recombinant (Subcutaneous Route)
Insulin Detemir (Injection Route)
Insulin Glulisine (Subcutaneous Route)

Insulin Human (Systemic)
Insulin Human, Buffered (Systemic)
Insulin Lispro, Recombinant (Subcutaneous Route)
Insulin Zinc (Systemic)
Insulin Zinc, Extended (Systemic)
Insulin Zinc, Extended, Human (Systemic)
Insulin Zinc, Human (Systemic)
Insulin Zinc, Prompt (Systemic)
Insulin, Isophane (Systemic)
Insulin, Isophane, Human (Systemic)
Insulin, Isophane, Human, and Insulin Human (Systemic)
Interferon Alfacon-1 (Subcutaneous Route)
Interferon Beta-1a (Intramuscular Route, Subcutaneous Route, Injection Route)
Interferon Beta-1b (Subcutaneous Route)
Interferon Gamma (Subcutaneous Route, Injection Route)
Iobenguane, Radioiodinated (Diagnostic)
Iocetamic Acid (Diagnostic)
Iodine And Potassium Iodide (Strong Iodine) (Oral Route)
Iodine And Potassium Iodide (Strong Iodine) (Oral Route)
Iodipamide (Diagnostic)
Iodohippurate Sodium I 123 (Diagnostic)
Iodohippurate Sodium I 131 (Diagnostic)
Iodoquinol (Oral Route)
Iofetamine I 123 (Diagnostic)
Iohexol (Diagnostic)
Iohexol (Diagnostic, Local)
Iopamidol (Diagnostic)
Iopanoic Acid (Diagnostic)
Iothalamate (Diagnostic)
Iothalamate (Diagnostic, Local)
Iothalamate Sodium I 125 (Diagnostic)
Ioversol (Diagnostic)
Ioxaglate (Diagnostic)
Ioxaglate (Diagnostic, Local)
Ipecac (Oral Route)
Ipodate (Diagnostic)
Ipratropium (Inhalation, Oral/Nebulization Route)
Ipratropium (Nasal Route)
Irbesartan (Oral Route)
Irinotecan (Intravenous Route)
Isoflurophate (Ophthalmic)
Isoniazid (Oral Route, Intramuscular Route)
Isotretinoin (Oral Route)
Isoxsuprine (Oral Route, Injection Route)
Ivermectin (Oral Route)
Japanese Encephalitis Virus Vaccine (Subcutaneous Route)

K

Kanamycin (Oral Route)
Ketazolam (Systemic)
Ketorolac (Oral Route, Intravenous Route, Injection Route, Intramuscular Route)
Ketotifen (Ophthalmic Route)
Krypton Kr 81m (Diagnostic)

L

Lamivudine (Oral Route)
Lamotrigine (Oral Route)
Lansoprazole (Oral Route)
Lanthanum Carbonate (Oral Route)
Laronidase (Intravenous Route)
Leflunomide (Oral Route)
Lenalidomide (Oral Route)

Letrozole (Oral Route)
Leucovorin (Oral Route, Intravenous Route, Injection Route)
Leuprolide (Intramuscular Route, Subcutaneous Route, Intradermal Route, Injection Route)
Levalbuterol (Inhalation, Oral/Nebulization Route)
Levamisole (Oral Route)
Levetiracetam (Oral Route)
Levocabastine (Ophthalmic Route)
Levocarnitine (Oral Route, Intravenous Route)
Levodopa (Oral Route)
Levofloxacin (Ophthalmic Route)
Levofloxacin (Oral Route, Intravenous Route)
Levomethadyl (Oral Route)
Levonorgestrel and Ethinyl Estradiol (Systemic)
Lidocaine (Topical Route)
Lincomycin (Oral Route, Injection Route)
Lindane (Topical Route)
Linezolid (Intravenous Route, Oral Route)
Lithium (Oral Route)
Lomustine (Oral Route)
Loperamide (Oral Route)
Loracarbef (Oral Route)
Loratadine (Systemic)
Loratadine and Pseudoephedrine (Systemic)
Lorazepam (Systemic)
Losartan (Oral Route)
Loxapine (Oral Route, Intramuscular Route)
Lutropin Alfa (Subcutaneous Route)
Lyme Disease Vaccine (Recombinant Ospa) (Intramuscular Route)

M

Mafenide (Topical Route)
Magnesium Hydroxide and Cascara Sagrada (Oral)
Magnesium Salicylate (Systemic)
Malathion (Topical Route)
Mangafodipir (Intravenous Route)
Maprotiline (Oral Route)
Mazindol (Systemic)
Measles And Rubella Virus Vaccine Live (Intramuscular Route, Injection Route)
Measles Virus Vaccine, Live (Subcutaneous Route)
Measles, Mumps, And Rubella Virus Vaccine Live (Subcutaneous Route, Intramuscular Route)
Mebendazole (Oral Route)
Mecamylamine (Oral Route)
Mecasermin (Subcutaneous Route)
Mechlorethamine (Intravenous Route)
Mechlorethamine (Topical Route)
Meclofenamate (Systemic)
Medrogestone (Systemic)
Medroxyprogesterone (Systemic)
Mefloquine (Oral Route)
Megestrol (Systemic)
Meloxicam (Oral Route)
Melphalan (Oral Route, Intravenous Route)
Memantine (Oral Route)
Menadiol (Systemic)
Meningococcal Polysaccharide Vaccine (Subcutaneous Route)
Meningococcal Vaccine, Diphtheria Conjugate (Intramuscular Route)

Mepenzolate (Systemic)
Mephobarbital (Systemic)
Meprobamate (Oral Route)
Meprobamate And Aspirin (Oral Route)
Mercaptopurine (Oral Route)
Meropenem (Intravenous Route)
Mesalamine (Oral Route)
Mesalamine (Rectal Route)
Mesna (Intravenous Route)
Mesoridazine (Systemic)
Metformin (Oral Route)
Metformin And Pioglitazone (Oral Route)
Methadone (Oral Route)
Methantheline (Systemic)
Metharbital (Systemic)
Methazolamide (Systemic)
Methdilazine (Systemic)
Methenamine (Oral Route)
Methimazole (Systemic)
Methotrexate (Oral Route, Injection Route)
Methotrimeprazine (Systemic)
Methoxsalen (Injection Route)
Methoxsalen (Oral Route)
Methoxsalen (Topical Route)
Methscopolamine (Systemic)
Methyclothiazide (Systemic)
Methyldopa (Oral Route, Intravenous Route)
Methyldopa and Chlorothiazide (Systemic)
Methyldopa and Hydrochlorothiazide (Systemic)
Methylene Blue (Oral Route, Intravenous Route)
Methylergonovine (Systemic)
Methylphenidate (Oral Route)
Methylprednisolone (Systemic)
Methyltestosterone (Systemic)
Methysergide (Oral Route)
Metoclopramide (Oral Route, Intravenous Route)
Metolazone (Systemic)
Metoprolol and Hydrochlorothiazide (Systemic)
Metrizamide (Diagnostic)
Metronidazole (Oral Route, Intravenous Route)
Metronidazole (Vaginal Route)
Metyrosine (Oral Route)
Mexiletine (Oral Route)
Micafungin (Intravenous Route)
Midazolam (Injection Route)
Midodrine (Oral Route)
Mifepristone (Oral Route)
Miglitol (Oral Route)
Miglustat (Oral Route)
Minocycline (Subgingival Route)
Minoxidil (Oral Route)
Minoxidil (Topical Route)
Mirtazapine (Oral Route)
Misoprostol (Oral Route)
Mitomycin (Intravenous Route)
Mitotane (Oral Route)
Mitoxantrone (Intravenous Route, Injection Route)
Modafinil (Oral Route)
Molindone (Oral Route)
Mometasone (Inhalation, Oral/Nebulization Route)
Mometasone (Nasal Route)
Mometasone (Topical)
Monoctanoin (Injection Route)
Montelukast (Oral Route)
Moricizine (Oral Route)

Moxifloxacin (Ophthalmic Route)
Mumps Virus Vaccine, Live (Subcutaneous Route)
Mupirocin (Topical Route)
Muromonab-CD3 (Intravenous Route)
Mycophenolate Mofetil (Oral Route, Intravenous Route)

N

Nabilone (Oral Route)
Nadolol and Bendroflumethiazide (Systemic)
Nafarelin (Nasal Route)
Naftifine (Topical Route)
Nalidixic Acid (Oral Route)
Naltrexone (Oral Route)
Naphazoline (Ophthalmic Route)
Naratriptan (Oral Route)
Natalizumab (Intravenous Route)
Natamycin (Ophthalmic Route)
Nateglinide (Oral Route)
Nedocromil (Inhalation, Oral/Nebulization Route)
Nedocromil (Ophthalmic Route)
Nefazodone (Oral Route)
Nelfinavir (Oral Route)
Neomycin (Oral Route)
Neomycin (Topical Route)
Neomycin And Polymyxin B (Topical Route)
Neomycin, Polymyxin B, And Bacitracin (Ophthalmic Route)
Neomycin, Polymyxin B, And Bacitracin (Topical Route)
Neomycin, Polymyxin B, And Gramicidin (Ophthalmic Route)
Nepafenac (Ophthalmic Route)
Nesiritide (Intravenous Route)
Nevirapine (Oral Route)
Niacin (Oral Route)
Niclosamide (Oral Route)
Nicotine (Inhalation, Oral/Nebulization Route)
Nicotine (Nasal Route)
Nicotine (Oral Route, Transdermal Route)
Nisoldipine (Oral Route)
Nitazoxanide (Oral Route)
Nitisinone (Oral Route)
Nitrazepam (Systemic)
Nitrofurantoin (Oral Route)
Norethindrone (Systemic)
Norethindrone Acetate and Ethinyl Estradiol (Systemic)
Norethindrone Acetate and Ethinyl Estradiol (Systemic)
Norethindrone and Ethinyl Estradiol (Systemic)
Norethindrone and Mestranol (Systemic)
Norgestimate and 17 Beta-Estradiol (Systemic)
Norgestimate and Ethinyl Estradiol (Systemic)
Norgestrel and Ethinyl Estradiol (Systemic)
Nylidrin (Oral Route)

O

Octreotide (Injection Route, Intramuscular Route)
Ofloxacin (Ophthalmic Route)
Ofloxacin (Otic Route)
Olanzapine (Intramuscular Route)
Olmesartan Medoxomil (Oral Route)
Olopatadine (Ophthalmic Route)

Olsalazine (Oral Route)
Omalizumab (Subcutaneous Route)
Omega-3-Acid Ethyl Esters (Oral Route)
Omeprazole (Oral Route)
Ondansetron (Oral Route, Injection Route, Intravenous Route)
Oprelvekin (Subcutaneous Route)
Orlistat (Oral Route)
Orphenadrine (Oral Route, Injection Route)
Orphenadrine, Aspirin, And Caffeine (Oral Route)
Oseltamivir (Oral Route)
Oxaliplatin (Intravenous Route)
Oxazepam (Systemic)
Oxcarbazepine (Oral Route)
Oxiconazole (Topical Route)
Oxtriphylline (Systemic)
Oxtriphylline And Guaifenesin (Oral Route)
Oxybutynin (Oral Route)
Oxycodone and Aspirin (Systemic)
Oxycodone And Ibuprofen (Oral Route)
Oxymetazoline (Nasal Route)
Oxymetazoline (Ophthalmic Route)
Oxytetracycline (Systemic)
Oxytocin (Nasal Route, Intravenous Route, Injection Route)

P

Paclitaxel (Intravenous Route)
Paclitaxel Protein-Bound (Injection Route)
Palifermin (Intravenous Route)
Palivizumab (Intramuscular Route)
Palonosetron (Intravenous Route)
Pamidronate (Intravenous Route)
Pancrelipase (Oral Route)
Pantoprazole (Intravenous Route)
Papaverine (Oral Route, Injection Route)
Paraldehyde (Oral Route, Injection Route, Rectal Route)
Paregoric (Systemic)
Paroxetine (Oral Route)
Pegademase Bovine (Intramuscular Route)
Pegaspargase (Intramuscular Route, Intravenous Route)
Pegfilgrastim (Subcutaneous Route)
Peginterferon Alfa-2a (Subcutaneous Route)
Peginterferon Alfa-2b (Subcutaneous Route)
Pegvisomant (Subcutaneous Route)
Pemetrexed (Intravenous Route)
Pemirolast (Ophthalmic Route)
Pemoline (Oral Route)
Penciclovir (Topical Route)
Penicillamine (Oral Route)
Pentamidine (Inhalation, Oral/Nebulization Route)
Pentamidine (Injection Route)
Pentazocine and Aspirin (Systemic)
Pentetate Calcium Trisodium (Intravenous Route, Inhalation, Oral/Nebulization Route)
601091
Pentetate Zinc Trisodium (Intravenous Route, Inhalation, Oral/Nebulization Route)
Pentobarbital (Systemic)
Pentosan Polysulfate Sodium (Oral Route)
Pentostatin (Intravenous Route)
Pentoxifylline (Oral Route)
Perflutren Protein Type A Microsphere (Intravenous Route)

Pergolide (Oral Route)
Pericyazine (Systemic)
Permethrin (Topical Route)
Perphenazine (Systemic)
Phenazopyridine (Oral Route)
Phendimetrazine (Systemic)
Phenindamine (Systemic)
Pheniramine and Phenylephrine (Systemic)
Pheniramine, Codeine, and Guaifenesin (Systemic)
Pheniramine, Phenylephrine, and Acetaminophen (Systemic)
Pheniramine, Phenylephrine, and Dextromethorphan (Systemic)
Pheniramine, Phenylephrine, Codeine, Sodium Citrate, Sodium Salicylate, and Caffeine (Systemic)
Pheniramine, Phenylephrine, Sodium Salicylate, and Caffeine (Systemic)
Pheniramine, Pyrilamine, Hydrocodone, Potassium Citrate, and Ascorbic Acid (Systemic)
Phenobarbital (Systemic)
Phenobarbital, Aspirin, and Codeine (Systemic)
Phenoxybenzamine (Oral Route)
Phentermine (Systemic)
Phentolamine (Injection Route)
Phenylbutazone (Systemic)
Phenylephrine (Nasal Route)
Phenylephrine (Ophthalmic Route)
Phenylephrine and Guaifenesin (Systemic)
Phenylephrine and Hydrocodone (Systemic)
Phenylephrine, Dextromethorphan, and Guaifenesin (Systemic)
Phenylephrine, Hydrocodone, and Guaifenesin (Systemic)
Phenyltoloxamine and Hydrocodone (Systemic)
Phenytoin (Systemic)
Physostigmine (Ophthalmic Route)
Phytonadione (Systemic)
Pilocarpine (Ophthalmic Route)
Pilocarpine (Oral Route)
Pimecrolimus (Topical Route)
Pimozide (Oral Route)
Pindolol and Hydrochlorothiazide (Systemic)
Pioglitazone (Oral Route)
Pioglitazone And Glimepiride (Oral Route)
Piperacillin and Tazobactam (Systemic)
Pipotiazine (Systemic)
Pirenzepine (Systemic)
Piroxicam (Systemic)
Plicamycin (Intravenous Route)
Pneumococcal Vaccine, Diphtheria Conjugate (Intramuscular Route)
Podofilox (Topical Route)
Poliovirus Vaccine, Live (Oral Route)
Polyethylene Glycol, Potassium Chloride, Sodium Bicarbonate, Sodium Chloride, And Sodium Sulfate (Oral Route)
Polythiazide (Systemic)
Porfimer (Intravenous Route)
Potassium Iodide (Oral Route)
Pralidoxime (Injection Route)
Pramipexole (Oral Route)
Pramlintide (Subcutaneous Route)
Prazepam (Systemic)
Praziquantel (Oral Route)
Prazosin (Oral Route)
Prednisolone (Systemic)
Prednisone (Systemic)

Pregabalin (Oral Route)
Primaquine (Oral Route)
Primidone (Oral Route)
Probenecid (Oral Route)
Probenecid And Colchicine (Oral Route)
Probucol (Oral Route)
Procainamide (Oral Route, Intravenous Route)
Procarbazine (Oral Route)
Prochlorperazine (Systemic)
Procyclidine (Systemic)
Progesterone (Systemic)
Proguanil (Oral Route)
Promazine (Systemic)
Promethazine (Systemic)
Promethazine and Codeine (Systemic)
Promethazine and Dextromethorphan (Systemic)
Promethazine and Phenylephrine (Systemic)
Promethazine and Potassium Guaiacolsulfonate (Systemic)
Promethazine, Codeine, and Potassium Guaiacolsulfonate (Systemic)
Promethazine, Phenylephrine, and Codeine (Systemic)
Promethazine, Phenylephrine, and Potassium Guaiacolsulfonate (Systemic)
Propafenone (Oral Route)
Propantheline (Systemic)
Propoxyphene and Aspirin (Systemic)
Propoxyphene, Aspirin, and Caffeine (Systemic)
Propranolol and Hydrochlorothiazide (Systemic)
Propylthiouracil (Systemic)
Protirelin (Intravenous Route)
Pseudoephedrine (Oral Route)
Pseudoephedrine and Dextromethorphan (Systemic)
Pseudoephedrine and Guaifenesin (Systemic)
Pseudoephedrine, Codeine, and Guaifenesin (Systemic)
Pseudoephedrine, Dextromethorphan, and Acetaminophen (Systemic)
Pseudoephedrine, Dextromethorphan, and Guaifenesin (Systemic)
Pseudoephedrine, Dextromethorphan, Guaifenesin, and Acetaminophen (Systemic)
Pseudoephedrine, Hydrocodone, and Guaifenesin (Systemic)
Pseudoephedrine, Hydrocodone, and Potassium Guaiacolsulfonate (Systemic)
Pyrantel (Oral Route)
Pyrazinamide (Oral Route)
Pyrethrum Extract And Piperonyl Butoxide (Topical Route)
Pyridoxine (Oral Route, Injection Route)
Pyrilamine and Codeine (Systemic)
Pyrilamine, Phenylephrine, Hydrocodone, and Ammonium Chloride (Systemic)
Pyrilamine, Pseudoephedrine, Dextromethorphan, and Acetaminophen (Systemic)
Pyrimethamine (Oral Route)
Pyrvinium (Oral Route)

Q

Quazepam (Systemic)
Quetiapine (Oral Route)
Quinethazone (Systemic)

Quinidine (Oral Route, Injection Route, Intramuscular Route)
Quinine (Oral Route)

R

Rabeprazole (Oral Route)
Rabies Immune Globulin (Intramuscular Route)
Radioiodinated Albumin (Diagnostic)
Raloxifene (Oral Route)
Ramelteon (Oral Route)
Rasagiline (Oral Route)
Rasburicase (Intravenous Route)
Rauwolfia Serpentina (Systemic)
Rauwolfia Serpentina and Bendroflumethiazide (Systemic)
Repaglinide (Oral Route)
Reserpine (Systemic)
Reserpine and Chlorothiazide (Systemic)
Reserpine and Chlorthalidone (Systemic)
Reserpine and Hydrochlorothiazide (Systemic)
Reserpine and Hydroflumethiazide (Systemic)
Reserpine and Methyclothiazide (Systemic)
Reserpine and Trichlormethiazide (Systemic)
Reserpine, Hydralazine, And Hydrochlorothiazide (Oral Route)
Resorcinol And Sulfur (Topical Route)
Respiratory Syncytial Virus Immune Globulin, Human (Intravenous Route)
Rho(D) Immune Globulin (Intravenous Route, Intramuscular Route, Injection Route)
Ribavirin (Inhalation, Oral/Nebulization Route, Oral Route)
Riboflavin (Oral Route)
Rifabutin (Oral Route)
Rifampin (Oral Route, Intravenous Route)
Rifampin And Isoniazid (Oral Route)
Rifampin, Isoniazid, And Pyrazinamide (Oral Route)
Rifapentine (Oral Route)
Rifaximin (Oral Route)
Riluzole (Oral Route)
Rimantadine (Oral Route)
Risedronate (Oral Route)
Risperidone (Oral Route)
Ritodrine (Oral Route, Intravenous Route)
Ritonavir (Oral Route)
Rituximab (Intravenous Route)
Rivastigmine (Oral Route)
Rizatriptan (Oral Route)
Rofecoxib (Oral Route)
Ropinirole (Oral Route)
Ropivacaine (Injection Route)
Rosiglitazone (Oral Route)
Rosiglitazone And Metformin (Oral Route)
Rosuvastatin (Oral Route)
Rubella And Mumps Virus Vaccine Live (Intramuscular Route)
Rubella Virus Vaccine, Live (Subcutaneous Route)
Rubidium Rb 82 (Diagnostic)

S

Sacrosidase (Oral Route)
Salicylic Acid (Topical Route)
Salicylic Acid And Sulfur (Topical Route)
Salicylic Acid, Sulfur, And Coal Tar (Topical Route)

Salsalate (Systemic)
Saquinavir (Oral Route)
Scopolamine (Systemic)
Secobarbital (Systemic)
Secobarbital and Amobarbital (Systemic)
Selegiline (Oral Route)
Sermorelin (Injection Route)
Sertaconazole (Topical Route)
Sertraline (Oral Route)
Sevoflurane (Inhalation, Oral/Nebulization Route)
Sibutramine (Oral Route)
Sildenafil (Oral Route)
Silver Sulfadiazine (Topical Route)
Sincalide (Intravenous Route)
Sirolimus (Oral Route)
Sodium Bicarbonate (Oral Route, Intravenous Route, Subcutaneous Route)
Sodium Chloride (Injection Route)
Sodium Chromate Cr 51 (Diagnostic)
Sodium Fluoride (Oral Route)
Sodium Iodide (Oral Route, Injection Route, Intravenous Route)
Sodium Iodide I 123 (Diagnostic)
Sodium Iodide I 131 (Diagnostic)
Sodium Oxybate (Oral Route)
Sodium Pertechnetate Tc 99m (Diagnostic)
Sodium Phenylbutyrate (Oral Route)
Sodium Salicylate (Systemic)
Sodium Tetradecyl Sulfate (Injection Route)
Sodium Thiosulfate (Intramuscular Route)
Solifenacin (Oral Route)
Sorafenib (Oral Route)
Sparfloxacin (Oral Route)
Spectinomycin (Intramuscular Route)
Spironolactone and Hydrochlorothiazide (Systemic)
Stavudine (Oral Route)
Streptozocin (Intravenous Route)
Strontium Chloride Sr 89 (Intravenous Route, Injection Route)
Succimer (Oral Route)
Sucralfate (Oral Route)
Sulconazole (Topical Route)
Sulfadiazine (Systemic)
Sulfadiazine and Trimethoprim (Systemic)
Sulfamethizole (Systemic)
Sulfamethoxazole (Systemic)
Sulfamethoxazole and Phenazopyridine (Systemic)
Sulfamethoxazole and Trimethoprim (Systemic)
Sulfapyridine (Oral Route)
Sulfasalazine (Oral Route, Rectal Route)
Sulfinpyrazone (Oral Route)
Sulfisoxazole (Systemic)
Sulfisoxazole and Phenazopyridine (Systemic)
Sulfur (Topical Route)
Sumatriptan (Nasal Route, Oral Route, Subcutaneous Route)
Suramin (Injection Route)

T

Tacrine (Oral Route)
Tacrolimus (Oral Route, Intravenous Route)
Tacrolimus (Topical Route)
Tadalafil (Oral Route)
Talc (Intrapleural Route)
Tamoxifen (Oral Route)
Tamsulosin (Oral Route)
Tazarotene (Topical Route)

Technetium Tc 99m (Pyro- and trimeta-) Phosphates (Diagnostic)
Technetium Tc 99m Albumin (Diagnostic)
Technetium Tc 99m Albumin Aggregated (Diagnostic)
Technetium Tc 99m Albumin Colloid (Diagnostic)
Technetium Tc 99m Apcitide (Diagnostic)
Technetium Tc 99m Arcitumomab (Diagnostic)
Technetium Tc 99m Bicisate (Diagnostic)
Technetium Tc 99m Disofenin (Diagnostic)
Technetium Tc 99m Exametazime (Diagnostic)
Technetium Tc 99m Gluceptate (Diagnostic)
Technetium Tc 99m Lidofenin (Diagnostic)
Technetium Tc 99m Mebrofenin (Diagnostic)
Technetium Tc 99m Medronate (Diagnostic)
Technetium Tc 99m Mertiatide (Diagnostic)
Technetium Tc 99m Nofetumomab Merpentan (Diagnostic)
Technetium Tc 99m Oxidronate (Diagnostic)
Technetium Tc 99m Pentetate (Diagnostic)
Technetium Tc 99m Pyrophosphate (Diagnostic)
Technetium Tc 99m Sestamibi (Diagnostic)
Technetium Tc 99m Succimer (Diagnostic)
Technetium Tc 99m Sulfur Colloid (Diagnostic)
Technetium Tc 99m Teboroxime (Diagnostic)
Technetium Tc 99m Tetrofosmin (Diagnostic)
Tegaserod (Oral Route)
Telithromycin (Oral Route)
Telmisartan (Oral Route)
Temazepam (Systemic)
Temozolomide (Oral Route)
Tenecteplase (Intravenous Route)
Teniposide (Intravenous Route)
Tenofovir Disoproxil Fumarate (Oral Route)
Terazosin (Oral Route)
Terbinafine (Oral Route)
Terbinafine (Topical Route)
Terbutaline (Inhalation)
Terbutaline (Oral/Injection)
Terfenadine (Systemic)
Teriparatide (Subcutaneous Route)
Testolactone (Oral Route)
Testosterone (Buccal Route)
Testosterone (Transdermal Route)
Testosterone and Estradiol (Systemic)
Tetanus Immune Globulin (Intramuscular Route)
Tetanus Toxoid (Intramuscular Route, Injection Route)
Tetracycline (Systemic)
Thalidomide (Oral Route)
Thallous Chloride Tl 201 (Diagnostic)
Theophylline (Systemic)
Theophylline And Guaifenesin (Oral Route)
Theophylline, Ephedrine, And Phenobarbital (Oral Route)
Thiabendazole (Oral Route)
Thiabendazole (Topical Route)
Thiamine (Oral Route, Injection Route)
Thiethylperazine (Oral Route, Intramuscular Route, Rectal Route)
Thioguanine (Oral Route)
Thioproperazine (Systemic)

Thioridazine (Systemic)
Thiotepa (Injection Route)
Thiothixene (Systemic)
Thyrotropin (Injection Route)
Tiagabine (Oral Route)
Ticarcillin and Clavulanate (Systemic)
Ticlopidine (Oral Route)
Tiludronate (Oral Route)
Timolol and Hydrochlorothiazide (Systemic)
Tinidazole (Oral Route)
Tinzaparin (Subcutaneous Route)
Tiopronin (Oral Route)
Tiotropium (Inhalation, Oral/Nebulization Route)
Tixocortol (Rectal)
Tizanidine (Oral Route)
Tobramycin (Ophthalmic Route)
Tobramycin And Dexamethasone (Ophthalmic Route)
Tocainide (Oral Route)
Tolcapone (Oral Route)
Tolterodine (Oral Route)
Topiramate (Oral Route)
Topotecan (Intravenous Route)
Toremifene (Oral Route)
Torsemide (Oral Route, Intravenous Route)
Tositumomab (Intravenous Route)
Tramadol (Oral Route)
Trastuzumab (Intravenous Route)
Travoprost (Ophthalmic Route)
Trazodone (Oral Route)
Treprostinil (Subcutaneous Route)
Tretinoin (Oral Route)
Tretinoin (Topical Route)
Triamcinolone (Dental)
Triamcinolone (Systemic)
Triamcinolone (Topical)
Triamterene and Hydrochlorothiazide (Systemic)
Triazolam (Systemic)
Trichlormethiazide (Systemic)
Trientine (Oral Route)
Trifluoperazine (Systemic)
Triflupromazine (Systemic)
Trihexyphenidyl (Systemic)
Trimeprazine (Systemic)
Trimethobenzamide (Oral Route, Intramuscular Route, Rectal Route)
Trimethoprim (Oral Route)
Trimetrexate (Intravenous Route)
Trioxsalen (Oral Route)
Triprolidine and Pseudoephedrine (Systemic)
Triprolidine, Pseudoephedrine, and Acetaminophen (Systemic)
Triprolidine, Pseudoephedrine, and Codeine (Systemic)
Triprolidine, Pseudoephedrine, and Dextromethorphan (Systemic)
Triprolidine, Pseudoephedrine, Codeine, and Guaifenesin (Systemic)
Triptorelin (Intramuscular Route, Injection Route)
Tropicamide (Ophthalmic Route)
Trospium (Oral Route)
Trovafloxacin (Oral Route)
Tuberculin (Intradermal Route)
Typhoid Vaccine, Inactivated (Subcutaneous Route, Injection Route)
Typhoid Vaccine, Live (Oral Route)
Typhoid Vi Polysaccharide Vaccine (Intramuscular Route)
Tyropanoate (Diagnostic)

U

Urea (Injection Route)
Urofollitropin (Intramuscular Route, Subcutaneous Route, Injection Route)
Ursodiol (Oral Route)

V

Vaccinia Immune Globulin, Human (Intravenous Route)
Valacyclovir (Oral Route)
Valdecoxib (Oral Route)
Valganciclovir (Oral Route)
Valproate Sodium (Systemic)
Valproic Acid (Systemic)
Valrubicin (Intravesical Route)
Valsartan (Oral Route)
Vancomycin (Intravenous Route, Injection Route)
Vancomycin (Oral Route)
Vardenafil (Oral Route)
Varenicline (Oral Route)
Varicella Virus Vaccine (Subcutaneous Route)
Vasopressin (Injection Route)
Venlafaxine (Oral Route)
Verteporfin (Intravenous Route, Injection Route)
Vigabatrin (Oral Route)
Vinblastine (Intravenous Route)
Vincristine (Intravenous Route)
Vindesine (Injection Route)
Vinorelbine (Intravenous Route)
Vitamin A (Oral Route, Intramuscular Route)
Vitamin E (Oral Route)
Voriconazole (Oral Route, Intravenous Route)

W

Warfarin (Systemic)

X

Xenon Xe 127 (Diagnostic)
Xenon Xe 133 (Diagnostic)
Xylometazoline (Nasal Route)

Y

Yellow Fever Vaccine (Subcutaneous Route, Injection Route)

Z

Zafirlukast (Oral Route)
Zalcitabine (Oral Route)
Zaleplon (Oral Route)
Zanamivir (Inhalation, Oral/Nebulization Route)
Ziconotide (Intrathecal Route)
Zidovudine (Oral Route, Intravenous Route)
Zileuton (Oral Route)
Ziprasidone (Oral Route, Intramuscular Route)
Zoledronic Acid (Intravenous Route)
Zolmitriptan (Oral Route)
Zolpidem (Oral Route)
Zonisamide (Oral Route)
Zopiclone (Oral Route)

DRUG INFORMATION CENTERS

ALABAMA

BIRMINGHAM

Drug Information Service
University of Alabama
UAB Hospital Pharmacy
Drug Information-JT1720
619 S. 19th St.
Birmingham, AL 35249-6860
Mon.-Fri. 8 AM-5 PM
  205-934-2162
www.health.uab.edu/pharmacy

Global Drug
Information Service
Samford University
McWhorter School
of Pharmacy
800 Lakeshore Dr.
Birmingham, AL 35229-7027
Mon.-Wed. 8 AM-9 PM
Thurs.-Fri. 8 AM-4:30 PM
  205-726-2519 or 2891
www.samford.edu/schools/
pharmacy/dic/index.html

HUNTSVILLE

Huntsville Hospital Drug
Information Center
101 Sivley Rd.
Huntsville, AL 35801
Mon.-Fri. 7 AM-3:30 PM
  256-265-8284

ARIZONA

TUCSON

Arizona Poison and Drug
Information Center
Arizona Health
Sciences Center
University Medical Center
1501 N. Campbell Ave.
Room 1156
Tucson, AZ 85724
7 days/week, 24 hours
  520-626-6016
  800-222-1222 (**Emergency**)
www.pharmacy.arizona.edu

ARKANSAS

LITTLE ROCK

Arkansas Drug Information Center
4301 W. Markham St.
Slot 522-2
Little Rock, AR 72205
Mon.-Fri. 8:30 AM-5 PM
  501-686-5072
  (Little Rock area only -
  for healthcare
  professionals only)
  800-228-1233
  (AR only - **for healthcare**
  professionals only)

CALIFORNIA

LOS ANGELES

Los Angeles Regional
Drug Information Center
LAC & USC Medical Center
1200 N. State St.
Trailer 25
Los Angeles, CA 90033
Mon.-Fri. 8 AM-4 PM
Closed 12 PM to 1 PM
  323-226-7741

SAN DIEGO

Drug Information Service
University of California
San Diego Medical Center
200 West Arbor Dr.
MC 8925
San Diego, CA 92103-8925
Mon.-Fri. 9 AM-5 PM
  619-543-6971
  (**for healthcare**
  professionals only)

SAN FRANCISCO

Drug Information Analysis Service
University of California,
San Francisco
533 Parnassus Ave.
Room U12
San Francisco, CA 94143-0622
Mon.-Fri. 8:30 AM-4:30 PM
  415-502-9540
  (**for healthcare**
  professionals only)

STANFORD

Drug Information Center
University of California
Stanford Hospital and Clinics
300 Pasteur Dr.
Room H-0301
Stanford, CA 94305
Mon.-Fri. 8 AM-4 PM
  650-723-6422

COLORADO

DENVER

Rocky Mountain Poison
and Drug Center
990 Bannock St.
(Physical address)
777 Bannock St.
(Mailing address)
Denver, CO 80264
  303-739-1123
  800-222-1222 (**Emergency**)
www.rmpdc.org

CONNECTICUT

FARMINGTON

Drug Information Service
University of Connecticut Health
Center
263 Farmington Ave.
Farmington, CT 06030
Mon.-Fri. 7:30 AM-4 PM
  860-679-2783

HARTFORD

Drug Information Center
Hartford Hospital
P.O. Box 5037
80 Seymour St.
Hartford, CT 06102
Mon.-Fri. 8:30 AM-5 PM
  860-545-2221
  860-545-2961(After 5 PM)
www.hartfordhospital.org

NEW HAVEN

Drug Information Center
Yale-New Haven Hospital
20 York St.
New Haven, CT 06540-3202
Mon.-Fri. 8:30 AM-5 PM
  203-688-2248
www.ynhh.org

DISTRICT OF COLUMBIA

Drug Information Service
Howard University Hospital
Room BB06
2041 Georgia Ave. NW
Washington, DC 20060
Mon.-Fri. 8:30 AM-4 PM
  202-865-1325
  800-222-1222 (**Emergency**)
www.huhosp.org/patientpublic/
pharmacy.htm

FLORIDA

FT. LAUDERDALE

Nova Southeastern University
College of Pharmacy
Drug Information Center
3200 S. University Dr.
Ft. Lauderdale, FL 33328
Mon.-Fri. 9 AM-5 PM
  954-262-3103
http://pharmacy.nova.edu

GAINESVILLE

Drug Information &
Pharmacy Resource Center
Shands Hospital at
University of Florida
P.O. Box 100316
Gainesville, FL 32610-0316
Mon.-Fri. 9 AM-5 PM
  352-265-0408
  (**for healthcare**
  professionals only)
http://shands.org/professional/drugs

JACKSONVILLE

Drug Information Service
Shands Jacksonville
655 W. 8th St.
Jacksonville, FL 32209
Mon.-Fri. 8:30 AM-5 PM
  904-244-4185
  (**for healthcare**
  professionals only)
  904-244-4700
  (**for consumers,**
  Mon.-Fri. 9:30 AM-4 PM)

ORLANDO

Orlando Regional Drug
Information Service
Orlando Regional
Healthcare System
1414 Kuhl Ave., MP 192
Orlando, FL 32806
Mon.-Fri. 8 AM-4 PM
  321-841-8717

TALLAHASSEE

Drug Information
Education Center
Florida Agricultural and
Mechanical University
College of Pharmacy and
Pharmaceutical Sciences
Tallahassee, FL 32307
Mon.-Fri. 9 AM-5 PM
  850-488-5239

WEST PALM BEACH

Drug Information Center
Nova Southeastern University,
West Palm Beach
3970 RCA Blvd., Suite 7006A
Palm Beach Gardens, FL 33410
Mon.-Fri. 9 AM-5 PM
  561-622-0658
  (**for healthcare**
  professionals only)

GEORGIA

ATLANTA

Emory University Hospital
Dept. of Pharmaceutical Services-
Drug Information
1364 Clifton Rd. NE
Atlanta, GA 30322
Mon.-Fri. 8 AM-1 PM
    404-712-4644
    (for healthcare
    professionals only)

Drug Information Service
Northside Hospital
1000 Johnson Ferry Rd. NE
Atlanta, GA 30342
Mon.-Fri. 9 AM-5 PM
    404-851-8676 (GA only)

AUGUSTA

Drug Information Center
Medical College of Georgia
Hospital and Clinic
BI2101
1120 15th St.
Augusta, GA 30912
Mon.-Fri. 8:30 AM-5 PM
    706-721-2887

COLUMBUS

Columbus Regional Drug
Information Center
710 Center St.
Columbus, GA 31902
Mon.-Fri. 8 AM-5 PM
    706-571-1934
    (for healthcare
    professionals only)

IDAHO

POCATELLO

Drug Information Center
Idaho State University
School of Pharmacy
970 S. 5th St.
Campus Box 8092
Pocatello, ID 83209
Mon.-Thur. 8:30 AM-5 PM
Fri. 8:30 AM-3 PM
    208-282-4689
    800-334-7139 (ID only)
http://pharmacy.isu.edu

ILLINOIS

CHICAGO

Drug Information Center
Northwestern Memorial Hospital
Feinberg Pavilion, LC 700
251 E. Huron St.
Chicago, IL 60611
Mon.-Fri. 8:30 AM-5 PM
    312-926-7573

Drug Information Services
University of Chicago Hospitals
5841 S. Maryland Ave.
MC 0010
Chicago, IL 60637-1470
Mon.-Fri. 9 AM-5 PM
    773-702-1388

Drug Information Center
University of Illinois at Chicago
833 S. Wood St.
MC 886
Chicago, IL 60612-7231
Mon.-Fri. 8 AM-4 PM
    312-996-5332
    (for healthcare
    professionals only)
    312-996-3682
    (for consumers,
    Mon.-Fri. 9 AM-12 PM)
www.uic.edu/pharmacy/
services/di/index.html

HARVEY

Drug Information Center
Ingalls Memorial Hospital
1 Ingalls Dr.
Harvey, IL 60426
Mon.-Fri. 8 AM-4:30 PM
    708-333-2300

HINES

Drug Information Service
Hines Veterans Administration
Hospital
2100 S. 5th Ave.
Pharmacy Services
MC119
P.O. Box 5000
Hines, IL 60141-5000
Mon.-Fri. 8 AM-4:30 PM
    708-202-8387,
    ext. 23780

PARK RIDGE

Drug Information Center
Advocate Lutheran General
Hospital
1775 Dempster St.
Park Ridge, IL 60068
Mon.-Fri. 7:30 AM-4 PM
    847-723-8128
    (for healthcare
    professionals only)

INDIANA

INDIANAPOLIS

Drug Information Center
St. Vincent Hospital
and Health Services
2001 W. 86th St.
Indianapolis, IN 46260
Mon.-Fri. 8 AM-4 PM
    317-338-3200
    (for healthcare
    professionals only)

Drug Information Service
Clarian Health Partners
Pharmacy Department I-65
at 21st St.
Room CG04
Indianapolis, IN 46202
Mon.-Fri. 8 AM-4:30 PM
    317-962-1750

MUNCIE

Drug Information Center
Ball Memorial Hospital
2401 University Ave.
Muncie, IN 47303
Mon.-Fri. 8 AM-4:30 PM
    765-747-3035

IOWA

DES MOINES

Regional Drug
Information Center
Mercy Medical Center-
Des Moines
1111 Sixth Ave.
Des Moines, IA 50314
Mon.-Fri. 8 AM-4:30 PM
    (regional service; in-house
    service answered 7 days/
    week, 24 hours)
    515-247-3286

IOWA CITY

Drug Information Center
University of Iowa
Hospitals and Clinics
200 Hawkins Dr.
Iowa City, IA 52242
Mon.-Fri. 8 AM-4:30 PM
    319-356-2600

KANSAS

KANSAS CITY

Drug Information Center
University of Kansas
Medical Center
3901 Rainbow Blvd.
Kansas City, KS 66160
Mon.-Fri. 8:30 AM-4:30 PM
    913-588-2328
    (for healthcare
    professionals only)

KENTUCKY

LEXINGTON

University of Kentucky
Central Pharmacy
Chandler Medical Center
800 Rose St., C-114
Lexington, KY 40536-0293
7 days/week, 24 hours
    859-323-5642

LOUISIANA

MONROE

Louisiana Drug and Poison
Information Center
University of Louisiana at Monroe
College of Pharmacy
Sugar Hall
Monroe, LA 71209-6430
Mon.-Fri. 8 AM-4:30 PM
    318-342-1710

NEW ORLEANS

Xavier University Drug
Information Center
Tulane University
Hospital and Clinic
1440 Canal St.
Suite 808
New Orleans, LA 70112
Mon.-Fri. 9 AM-5 PM
    504-588-5670

MARYLAND

ANDREWS AFB

Drug Information Services
79 MDSS/SGQP
1050 W. Perimeter Rd.
Suite D1-119
Andrews AFB, MD 20762-6660
Mon.-Fri. 7:30 AM-5 PM
    240-857-4565

BALTIMORE

Drug Information Service
Johns Hopkins Hospital
600 N. Wolfe St.
Carnegie 180
Baltimore, MD 21287-6180
Mon.-Fri. 8:30 AM-5 PM
    410-955-6348

Drug Information Service
University of Maryland
School of Pharmacy
Pharmacy Hall Room 760
20 North Pine St.
Baltimore, MD 21201
Mon.-Fri. 8:30 AM-5 PM
    410-706-7568
    (consumers only)
    410-706-0898
    (for healthcare
    professionals only)
www.pharmacy.umaryland.edu/umdi

EASTON

Drug Information
Pharmacy Dept.
Memorial Hospital
219 S. Washington St.
Easton, MD 21601
7 days/week, 7 AM-5:30 PM
    410-822-1000, ext. 5645

MASSACHUSETTS

BOSTON

Drug Information Services
Brigham and Women's Hospital
75 Francis St.
Boston, MA 02115
Mon.-Fri. 7 AM-3 PM
    617-732-7166

WORCESTER

Drug Information Pharmacy
UMass Memorial
Medical Center
Healthcare Hospital
55 Lake Ave. North
Worcester, MA 01655
Mon.-Fri. 8:30 AM-5 PM
    508-856-3456
    508-856-2775 (24-hour)

MICHIGAN

ANN ARBOR

Drug Information Service
Dept. of Pharmacy Services
University of Michigan
Health System
1500 East Medical
Center Dr.
UH B2D301
Box 0008
Ann Arbor, MI 48109-0008
Mon.-Fri. 8 AM-5 PM
    734-936-8200

DETROIT

Drug Information Center
Department of Pharmacy Services
Detroit Receiving Hospital and
University Health Center
4201 St. Antoine Blvd.
Detroit, MI 48201
Mon.-Fri. 9 AM-5 PM
    313-745-4556
www.dmcpharmacy.org

LANSING

Drug Information Services
Sparrow Hospital
1215 East Michigan Ave.
Lansing, MI 48912
7 days/week, 24 hours
    517-364-2444

PONTIAC

Drug Information Center
St. Joseph Mercy Oakland
44405 Woodward Ave.
Pontiac, MI 48341
Mon.-Fri. 8 AM-4:30 PM
    248-858-3055

ROYAL OAK

Drug Information Services
William Beaumont Hospital
3601 West 13 Mile Rd.
Royal Oak, MI 48073-6769
Mon.-Fri. 8 AM-4:30 PM
    248-898-4077

SOUTHFIELD

Drug Information Service
Providence Hospital
16001 West 9 Mile Rd.
Southfield, MI 48075
Mon.-Fri. 8 AM-4 PM
    248-849-3125

MISSISSIPPI

JACKSON

Drug Information Center
University of Mississippi
Medical Center
2500 N. State St.
Jackson, MS 39216
Mon.-Fri. 8 AM-4:30 PM
    601-984-2060

MISSOURI

KANSAS CITY

University of
Missouri-Kansas City
Drug Information Center
2411 Holmes St., MG-200
Kansas City, MO 64108
Mon.-Fri. 9 AM-4 PM
    816-235-5490
http://druginfo.umkc.edu/

SPRINGFIELD

Drug Information Center
St. John's Hospital
1235 E. Cherokee St.
Springfield, MO 65804
Mon.-Fri. 8 AM-4:30 PM
    417-820-3488

ST. JOSEPH

Regional Medical Center
Pharmacy
5325 Faraon St.
St. Joseph, MO 64506
7 days/week, 24 hours
    816-271-6141

MONTANA

MISSOULA

Drug Information Service
University of Montana School of
Pharmacy and Allied Health
Sciences
32 Campus Dr.
1522 Skaggs Bldg.
Missoula, MT 59812-1522
Mon.-Fri. 8 AM-5 PM
    406-243-5254
    800-501-5491
www.umt.edu/druginfo

NEBRASKA

OMAHA

Drug Informatics Service
School of Pharmacy
Creighton University
2500 California Plaza
Health Science Library
Room 204
Omaha, NE 68178
Mon.-Fri. 8:30 AM-4:30 PM
    402-280-5101
http://druginfo.creighton.edu

NEW JERSEY

NEWARK

New Jersey Poison Information
and Education System
65 Bergen St.
Newark, NJ 07107
Mon.-Fri. 8 AM- 5 PM
    973-972-9280
    800-222-1222 (Emergency)
www.njpies.org

NEW BRUNSWICK

Drug Information Service
Robert Wood Johnson
University Hospital
Pharmacy Department
1 Robert Wood Johnson Pl.
New Brunswick, NJ 08901
Mon.-Fri. 8:30 AM-4:30 PM
    732-937-8842

NEW MEXICO

ALBUQUERQUE

New Mexico Poison Center
University of New Mexico
Health Sciences Center
MSC09 5080
1 University of New Mexico
Albuquerque, NM 87131
7 days/week, 24 hours
    505-272-4261
    800-222-1222 (**Emergency**)
http://hsc.unm.edu/pharmacy/poison

NEW YORK

BROOKLYN

International Drug
Information Center
Long Island University
Arnold & Marie Schwartz College
of Pharmacy & Health Sciences
75 DeKalb Ave.
RM-HS509
Brooklyn, NY 11201
Mon.-Fri. 9 AM-5 PM
    718-488-1064
www.liu.edu

NEW HYDE PARK

Drug Information Center
St. John's University at Long
Island Jewish Medical Center
270-05 76th Ave.
New Hyde Park, NY 11040
Mon.-Fri. 8 AM-3 PM
    718-470-DRUG (3784)

NEW YORK CITY

Drug Information Center
Memorial Sloan-Kettering
Cancer Center
1275 York Ave.
RM S-702
New York, NY 10021
Mon.-Fri. 9 AM-5 PM
    212-639-7552

Drug Information Center
Mount Sinai Medical Center
1 Gustave Levy Pl.
New York, NY 10029
Mon.-Fri. 9 AM-5 PM
    212-241-6619
(for in-house healthcare
professionals only)

Drug Information Service
New York Presbyterian Hospital
Room K04
525 E. 68th St.
New York, NY 10021
Mon.-Fri. 9 AM-5 PM
    212-746-0741

ROCHESTER

Finger Lakes
Poison and Drug
Information Center
University of Rochester
601 Elmwood Ave.
Rochester, NY 14642
Mon.-Fri. 8 AM-5 PM
    585-275-3718

ROCKVILLE CENTER

Drug Information Center
Mercy Medical Center
1000 North Village Ave.
Rockville Center, NY 11571-9024
Mon.-Fri. 8 AM-4 PM
    516-705-1053

NORTH CAROLINA

BUIES CREEK

Drug Information Center
School of Pharmacy
Campbell University
P.O. Box 1090
Buies Creek, NC 27506
Mon.-Fri. 8:30 AM-4:30 PM
   910-893-1200
    x2701
   800-760-9697 (Toll free)
    x2701
   800-327-5467 (NC only)

CHAPEL HILL

University of North
Carolina Hospitals
Drug Information Center
Dept. of Pharmacy
101 Manning Dr.
Chapel Hill, NC 27514
Mon.-Fri. 8 AM-4:30 PM
   919-966-2373

DURHAM

Drug Information Center
Duke University Health
Systems
DUMC Box 3089
Durham, NC 27710
Mon.-Fri. 8 AM-5 PM
   919-684-5125

GREENVILLE

Eastern Carolina Drug
Information Center
Pitt County
Memorial Hospital
Dept. of Pharmacy Service
P.O. Box 6028
2100 Stantonsburg Rd.
Greenville, NC 27835
Mon.-Fri. 8 AM-5 PM
   252-847-4257

WINSTON-SALEM

Drug Information
Service Center
Wake-Forest University
Baptist Medical Center
Medical Center Blvd.
Winston-Salem, NC 27157
Mon.-Fri. 8 AM-5 PM
   336-716-2037
   (for healthcare
   professionals only)

OHIO

ADA

Drug Information Center
Raabe College of Pharmacy
Ohio Northern University
Ada, OH 45810
Mon.-Thurs. 8:30 AM-5 PM,
    7-10 PM
Fri. 8:30 AM- 4 PM;
Sun. 2 PM-10 PM
   419-772-2307
www.onu.edu/pharmacy/druginfo

CINCINNATI

Drug and Poison
Information Center
Children's Hospital
Medical Center
3333 Burnet Ave. VP-3
Cincinnati, OH 45229
Mon.-Fri. 9 AM-5 PM
   513-636-5054 (Administration)
   513-636-5111
   (7 days/week, 24 hours)

CLEVELAND

Drug Information Service
Cleveland Clinic Foundation
9500 Euclid Ave.
Cleveland, OH 44195
Mon.-Fri. 8:30 AM-4:30 PM
   216-444-6456
   (for healthcare
   professionals only)

COLUMBUS

Drug Information Center
Ohio State University Hospital
Dept. of Pharmacy
Doan Hall 368
410 W. 10th Ave.
Columbus, OH 43210-1228
7 days/week, 24 hours
   614-293-8679
   (for in-house healthcare
   professionals only)

Drug Information Center
Riverside Methodist Hospital
3535 Olentangy River Road
Columbus, OH 43214
7 days/week, 24 hours
   614-566-5425

TOLEDO

Drug Information Services
St. Vincent Mercy Medical Center
2213 Cherry St.
Toledo, Ohio 43608-2691
Mon.-Fri. 7 AM-5 PM
   419-251-4227
www.rx.medctr.ohio-state.edu

OKLAHOMA

OKLAHOMA CITY

Drug Information Service
Integris Health
3300 Northwest Expressway
Oklahoma City, OK 73112
Mon.-Fri. 8 AM-4:30 PM
   405-949-3660

Drug Information Center
OU Medical Center
Presbyterian Tower
700 NE 13th St.
Oklahoma City, OK 73104
Mon.-Fri. 8 AM-4:30 PM
   405-271-6226
   Fax: 405-271-6281

TULSA

Drug Information Center
Saint Francis Hospital
6161 S. Yale Ave.
Tulsa, OK 74136
Mon.-Fri. 8 AM-4:30 PM
   918-494-6339
   (for healthcare
   professionals only)

PENNSYLVANIA

PHILADELPHIA

Drug Information Center
Temple University Hospital
Dept. of Pharmacy
3401 N. Broad St.
Philadelphia, PA 19140
Mon.-Fri. 8 AM-4:30 PM
   215-707-4644

Drug Information Service
Tenet Health System
Hahnemann University Hospital
Department of Pharmacy
MS 451
Broad and Vine Streets
Philadelphia, PA 19102
Mon.-Fri. 8 AM-4 PM
   215-762-DRUG (3784)
   (for healthcare
   professionals only)

Drug Information Service
Dept. of Pharmacy
Thomas Jefferson
University Hospital
111 S. 11th St.
Philadelphia, PA 19107-5089
Mon.-Fri. 8 AM-5 PM
   215-955-8877

University of Pennsylvania
Health System Drug Information
Service
Hospital of the University of
Pennsylvania
Department of Pharmacy
3400 Spruce St.
Philadelphia, PA 19104
Mon.-Fri. 8:30 AM-4 PM
   215-662-2903

PITTSBURGH

Pharmaceutical
Information Center
Mylan School of Pharmacy
Duquesne University
431 Mellon Hall
Pittsburgh, PA 15282
Mon.-Fri. 8 AM-4 PM
   412-396-4600

Drug Information Center
University of Pittsburgh
302 Scaife Hall
200 Lothrop St.
Pittsburgh, PA 15213
Mon.-Fri. 8:30 AM-4:30 PM
   412-647-3784
   (for healthcare
   professionals only)

UPLAND

Drug Information Center
Crozer-Chester Medical Center
Dept. of Pharmacy
1 Medical Center Blvd.
Upland, PA 19013
Mon.-Fri. 8 AM-4:30 PM
   610-447-2851
   (for in-house healthcare
   professionals only)

PUERTO RICO

PONCE

Centro Informacion
Medicamentos
Escuela de Medicina de Ponce
P.O. Box 7004
Ponce, PR 00732-7004
Mon.-Fri. 8 AM-4:30 PM
   787-840-2575

SAN JUAN

Centro de Informacion de
Medicamentos-CIM
Escuela de Farmacia-RCM
P.O. Box 365067
San Juan, PR 00936-5067
Mon.-Fri. 8 AM-5:30 PM
   787-758-2525, ext. 1516

SOUTH CAROLINA

CHARLESTON

Drug Information Service
Medical University of
South Carolina
150 Ashley Ave.
Rutledge Tower Annex
Room 604
P.O. Box 250584
Charleston, SC 29425-0810
Mon.-Fri. 9 AM-5:30 PM
   843-792-3896
   800-922-5250

COLUMBIA

Drug Information Service
University of South Carolina
College of Pharmacy
Columbia, SC 29208
Mon.-Fri. 8 AM-5 PM
803-777-7804
www.pharm.sc.edu

SPARTANBURG

Drug Information Center
Spartanburg Regional
Healthcare System
101 E. Wood St.
Spartanburg, SC 29303
Mon.-Fri. 8 AM-4:30 PM
864-560-6910

TENNESSEE

KNOXVILLE

Drug Information Center
University of Tennessee
Medical Center at Knoxville
1924 Alcoa Highway
Knoxville, TN 37920-6999
Mon.-Fri. 8 AM-4:30 PM
865-544-9124

MEMPHIS

South East Regional Drug
Information Center
VA Medical Center
1030 Jefferson Ave.
Memphis, TN 38104
Mon.-Fri. 6:30 AM-4 PM
901-523-8990, ext. 6720

Drug Information Center
University of Tennessee
875 Monroe Ave.
Suite 116
Memphis, TN 38163
Mon.-Fri. 8 AM-5 PM
901-448-5556

TEXAS

AMARILLO

Drug Information Center
Texas Tech Health
Sciences Center
School of Pharmacy
1300 Coulter Rd.
Amarillo, TX 79106
Mon.-Fri. 8 AM-5 PM
806-356-4008

GALVESTON

Drug Information Center
University of Texas
Medical Branch
301 University Blvd.
Galveston, TX 77555-0701
Mon.-Fri. 8 AM-5 PM
409-772-2734

HOUSTON

Drug Information Center
Ben Taub General Hospital
Texas Southern University/HCHD
1504 Taub Loop
Houston, TX 77030
Mon.-Fri. 8:30 AM-5 PM
713-873-3710

LACKLAND A.F.B.

Drug Information Center
Dept. of Pharmacy
Wilford Hall Medical Center
2200 Bergquist Dr.
Suite 1
Lackland A.F.B., TX 78236
7 days/week, 24 hours
210-292-5414

LUBBOCK

Drug Information and
Consultation Service
Covenant Medical Center
3615 19th St.
Lubbock, TX 79410
Mon.-Fri. 8 AM-5 PM
806-725-0408

SAN ANTONIO

Drug Information Service
University of Texas
Health Science Center
at San Antonio
Department of Pharmacology
7703 Floyd Curl Drive
San Antonio, TX 78229-3900
Mon.-Fri. 8 AM-4 PM
210-567-4280

TEMPLE

Drug Information Center
Scott and White
Memorial Hospital
2401 S. 31st St.
Temple, TX 76508
Mon.-Fri. 8 AM-5 PM
254-724-4636

UTAH

SALT LAKE CITY

Drug Information Service
University of Utah Hospital
421 Wakara Way
Suite 204
Salt Lake City, UT 84108
Mon.-Fri. 7 AM-5 PM
801-581-2073

VIRGINIA

HAMPTON

Drug Information Center
Hampton University School
of Pharmacy
Hampton Harbors Annex
Hampton, VA 23668
Mon.-Fri. 9 AM-4 PM
757-728-6693

WEST VIRGINIA

MORGANTOWN

West Virginia Center for
Drug and Health Information
West Virginia University
Robert C. Byrd
Health Sciences Center
1124 HSN, P.O. Box 9520
Morgantown, WV 26506
Mon.-Fri. 8:30 AM-5 PM
304-293-6640
800-352-2501 (WV)
www.hsc.wvu.edu/SOP

WYOMING

LARAMIE

Drug Information Center
University of Wyoming
P.O. Box 3375
Laramie, WY 82071
Mon.-Fri. 8:30 AM-4:30 PM
307-766-6988

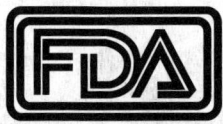

U.S. FOOD AND DRUG ADMINISTRATION

Medical Product Reporting Programs

MedWatch (24-hour service) **800-332-1088**
Reporting of problems with drugs, devices, biologics (except vaccines), medical foods, and dietary supplements.

Vaccine Adverse Event Reporting System (24-hour service) **800-822-7967**
Reporting of vaccine-related problems.

Mandatory Medical Device Reporting **240-276-3000**
Reporting required from user facilities regarding device-related deaths and serious injuries.

Veterinary Adverse Drug Reaction Program **888-332-8387**
Reporting of adverse drug events in animals.

Division of Drug Marketing, Advertising, and Communication (DDMAC) **301-796-1200**
Inquiries from health professionals regarding product promotion.

USP Medication Errors **800-233-7767**
Reporting of medication errors or near-errors to help avoid future problems through improvement in product names and packaging.

Information for Health Professionals

Center for Drug Evaluation and Research Drug Information Hotline **301-827-4573**
Information on human drugs including hormones.

Center for Biologics Office of Communications **301-827-2000**
Information on biological products including vaccines and blood.

Center for Devices and Radiological Health **800-638-2041**
Automated request for information on medical devices and radiation-emitting products.

Emergency Operations **301-443-1240**
Emergencies involving FDA-regulated products, tampering reports, and emergency Investigational New Drug requests.

Office of Orphan Products Development **301-827-3666**
Information on products for rare diseases.

General Information

General Consumer Inquiries **888-463-6332**
Consumer information on regulated products/issues.

Freedom of Information **301-827-6500**
Requests for publicly available FDA documents.

Office of Public Affairs **301-827-6250**
Interviews/press inquiries on FDA activities.

Center for Food Safety and Applied Nutrition **888-723-3366**
Information on food safety, seafood, dietary supplements, women's nutrition, and cosmetics.

Consumer Information Service, Center for Devices and Radiological Health **800-638-2041**
Information on medical devices, mammography facilities, and radiation-emitting products.

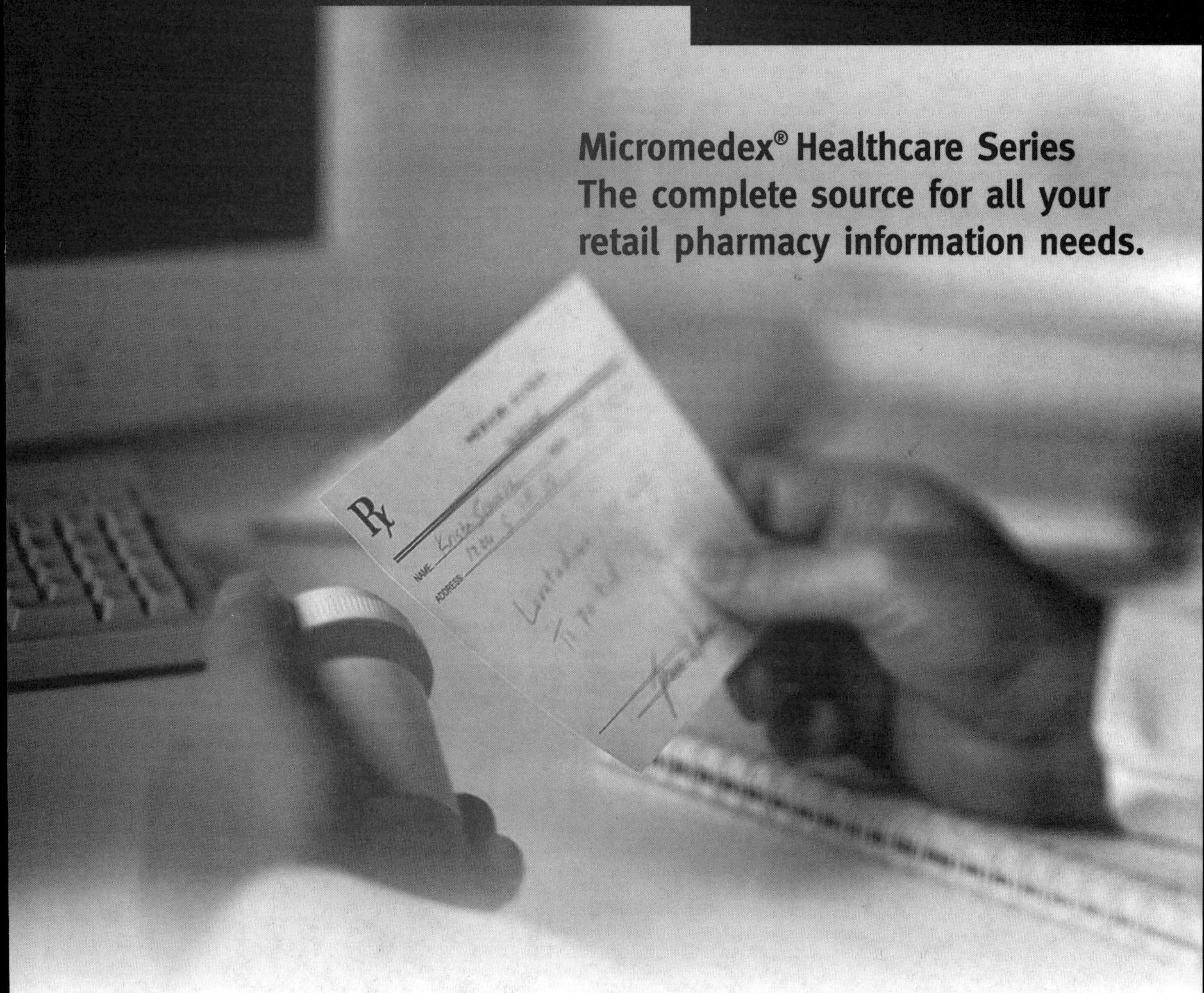

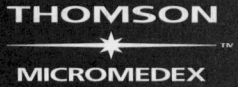

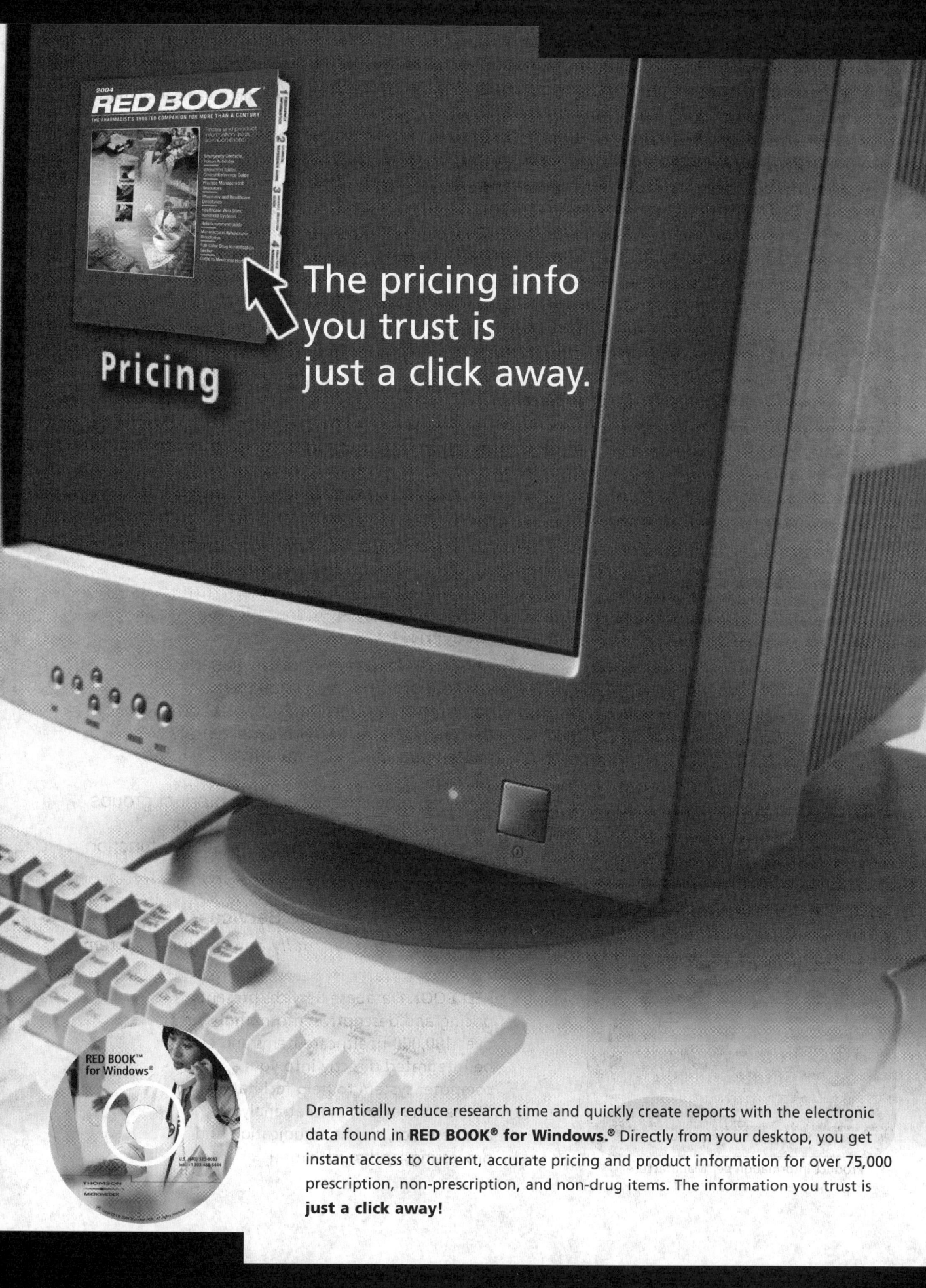

The pricing info you trust is just a click away.

Pricing

Dramatically reduce research time and quickly create reports with the electronic data found in **RED BOOK® for Windows.®** Directly from your desktop, you get instant access to current, accurate pricing and product information for over 75,000 prescription, non-prescription, and non-drug items. The information you trust is **just a click away!**

FREE Shipping! Details on back...

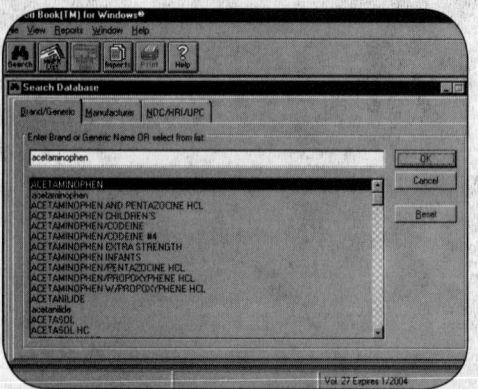

Search by Brand or Generic Name

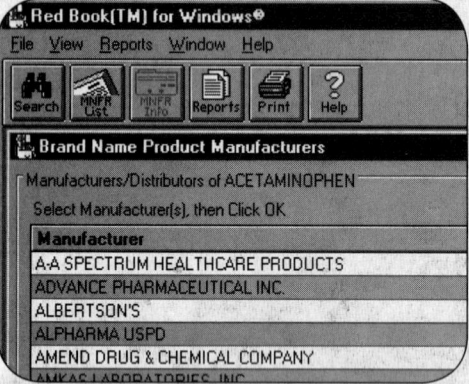

Specific Drug Manufacturer Listings

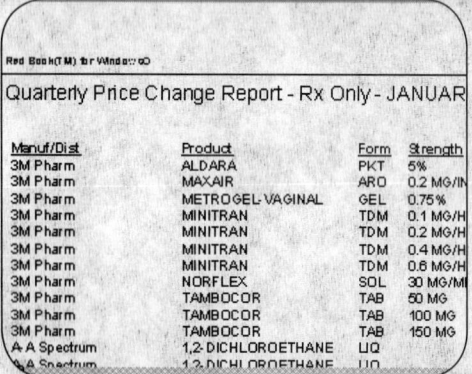

Report View

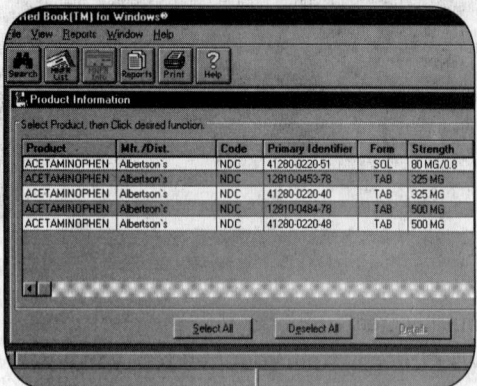

Product Information per Manufacturer

RED BOOK for Windows®...

- Instantly searches by brand or generic name, manufacturer, or NDC number
- Conveniently lists manufacturer names, address, phone, etc...
- Reports on the latest price changes, new products, and deactivated products
- Easily enables the export of data into spreadsheets for further analysis and manipulation
- Also includes non-drug items such as medical devices and supplies

Don't miss this special offer for 2007...

FREE shipping on all first-time orders.

RED BOOK for Windows is available as an annual or quarterly subscription.

Call **(800) 737-2577** for more information or to place an order.

Also available...

ReadyPrice®

This easy-to-use, Windows-based application provides the same comprehensive product information as RED BOOK for Windows, but also gives you access to advanced features such as:

- User-created custom product groups
- Historical pricing information
- Therapeutic category search function

RED BOOK Database Services

Compatible with virtually any computer system!

RED BOOK Database Services presents pricing and descriptive information for over 180,000 healthcare items and can be integrated directly into your computer system to help facilitate utilization review, market analysis and research, claims adjudication and processing, and much more!

(800) 525-9083
www.micromedex.com

HC-3753 10/06

Ordering Information

Mail Order:	Thomson Micromedex USP DI Customer Service	**Phone Order**: (800) 877-6209
	P.O. Box 187	**Fax Order:** (201) 722-2680
	Montvale, NJ 07645-0187 USA	
International Phone Order:	For international orders, please call +1 201 358-2233 for a distributor near you.	
Order On-line:	www.pdrbookstore.com	

Payment Required in advance in U.S. dollars drawn on a U.S. bank. Any bank fees, customs duties, tariffs, and taxes are the customer's responsibility. Errors in fax transmissions are the responsibility of the sender. Prices subject to change without notice.

Sales Tax: Add appropriate sales tax to product costs for orders according to the sales tax schedule below the order form.

Drug Information Publications

2007 USP DI® Volume I
Drug Information for the Health Care Professional

Organized in a concise, outline format, *Drug Information for the Health Care Professional* contains medically accepted uses—labeled and off-label—of more than 11,000 generic and brand-name drug products throughout the United States and Canada.

Item Number: U20061   **ISBN**: 1-56363-574-7   **Price**: $174.00 plus S&H ($9.95)

2007 USP DI® Volume II
Advice for the Patient® Drug Information in Lay Language

Written in patient-friendly terms, *Advice for the Patient* is specifically designed to make important drug information easy to grasp. Simplified monographs provide detailed information on proper drug use, available dosage forms, precautions, side effects, and special consideration.

Item Number: U20062   **ISBN**: 1-56363-575-5   **Price**: $93.00 plus S&H ($9.95)

2007 USP DI® Volume III
Approved Drug Products and Legal Requirements

Contains important therapeutic equivalence information and selected federal requirements that affect the prescribing and dispensing of prescription drugs and controlled substances.

Item Number: U20063   **ISBN**: 1-56363-576-3   **Price**: $145.00 plus S&H ($9.95)

FREE USP DI On-Line

With your purchase of any USP DI print book, you have FREE access to the USP DI On-line site, containing over 400 additional monographs.

To visit USP DI On-line, log on to the Micromedex Web site at http://uspdi.micromedex.com. Then enter the USER NAME and PASSWORD listed below.

USERNAME: **usp2007**   PASSWORD: **moredrugs**

If you have questions regarding USP DI On-line, please contact Thomson Micromedex at (800) 877-6209, (303) 486-6400, or http://www.micromedex.com/support/request

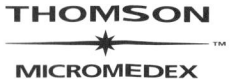
THOMSON
MICROMEDEX

Change of Address Notification
If your address has changed, please send your new address with your latest mailing label to:
Thomson Micromedex USP DI   P.O. Box 187   Montvale, NJ 07645-0187

To order, remove this form, fill out completely, and mail to Thomson Micromedex Customer Service Department with payment or credit card information. For faster service, order by phone or fax.

Mail Order
Thomson Micromedex USP DI Customer Service Department
P.O. Box 187
Montvale, NJ 07645-0187

Phone Order (800) 877-6209
Fax Order (201) 722-2680
International Phone Order For international orders, please call +1 201 358-2233 for a distributor near you.

Ordered By:

Name _____

Title _____

Company _____

E-mail _____

Street Address _____

City _____ State _____ ZIP _____ Country _____

Phone (_____) _____ Fax (_____) _____

Ship To (Only complete if different):

Name _____

Title _____

Company _____

Street Address _____

City _____ State _____ ZIP _____ Country _____

Phone (_____) _____ Fax (_____) _____

Payment is required in advance in U.S. dollars drawn on a U.S. bank. Any bank fees, customs duties, tariffs, and taxes are the customer's responsibility. Errors in fax transmissions are the responsibility of the sender. Prices subject to change without notice. Please allow 2-4 weeks for normal delivery. Inquire for faster delivery (additional charge).

Valid for 2007 editions only; prices and shipping and handling higher outside U.S.

Payment Method

❑ Enclosed is my check payable to Thomson Micromedex.

❑ VISA ❑ MasterCard ❑ AmFex ❑ Discover

Card No. _____ Exp. Date_____

Signature _____

Item #	Description	Price	Quantity	Total Price	Domestic Shipping	Shipping Quantity	Total Shipping
160101	2007 USP DI® Volume I, *Drug Information for the Health Care Professional* ISBN 1-56363-574-7	$174.00			$9.95		
160119	2007 USP DI® Volume II, Advice for the Patient® *Drug Information in Lay Language* ISBN 1-56363-575-5	$ 93.00			$9.95		
160127	2007 USP DI® Volume III, *Approved Drug Products and Legal Requirements* ISBN 1-56363-576-3	$145.00			$9.95		

Total Price

Add Sales Tax in FL, IA, NJ

Subtotal

Shipping

← Shipping Total

GRAND TOTAL

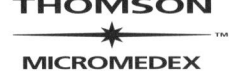

THOMSON
MICROMEDEX

341M00A